Mercer's Textbook of Orthopaedics and Trauma

Mercer's Textbook of Orthopaedics and Trauma

Tenth edition

Sureshan Sivananthan MD FRCS (Tr&Orth)
Consultant Orthopaedic Surgeon and Visiting Assistant Professor, Department of Orthopaedic Surgery, Stanford University School of Medicine, Palo Alto, California, USA

Eugene Sherry MBChB MPH MD FRACS FAOrthA
Senior Orthopaedic Consultant, Sydney Private Hospital, Ashfield, New South Wales, Australia

Patrick Warnke Dr Med DrMed Dent PhD Habil
Professor of Surgery, Faculty of Health Sciences and Medicine, Bond University, Queensland, Australia

Mark D Miller MD
Professor of Orthopaedic Surgery, Head of the Division of Sports Medicine, University of Virginia, Charlottesville, USA

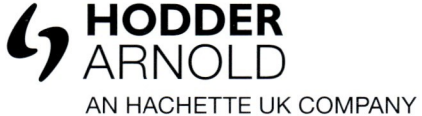

AN HACHETTE UK COMPANY

First published in Great Britain in 1932 as Orthopaedic Surgery by Edward Arnold & Co.
Second edition 1937, Third edition 1945
Fourth edition 1950, Fifth edition 1959
Sixth edition 1964, Seventh edition 1973
Eighth edition 1983, Ninth edition 1996

This 10th edition published in 2012 by Hodder Arnold, an imprint of Hodder Education, an Hachette UK Company, 338 Euston Road, London NW1 3BH

http://www.hodderarnold.com

© 2012 Edward Arnold (Publishers) Ltd

All rights reserved. Apart from any use permitted under UK copyright law, this publication may only be reproduced, stored or transmitted, in any form, or by any means with prior permission in writing of the publishers or in the case of reprographic production in accordance with the terms of licences issued by the Copyright Licensing Agency. In the United Kingdom such licences are issued by the Copyright Licensing Agency: Saffron House, 6-10 Kirby Street, London EC1N 8TS

Whilst the advice and information in this book are believed to be true and accurate at the date of going to press, neither the author1s nor the publisher can accept any legal responsibility or liability for any errors or omissions that may be made. In particular (but without limiting the generality of the preceding disclaimer) every effort has been made to check drug dosages; however it is still possible that errors have been missed. Furthermore, dosage schedules are constantly being revised and new side-effects recognized. For these reasons the reader is strongly urged to consult the drug companies' printed instructions before administering any of the drugs recommended in this book.

British Library Cataloguing in Publication Data
A catalogue record for this book is available from the British Library

Library of Congress Cataloging-in-Publication Data
A catalog record for this book is available from the Library of Congress

978 0 340 942 031 (main edition)
978 1 444 172 317 (Indian hardback edition)
978 1 444 172 300 (Indian paperback edition)

1 2 3 4 5 6 7 8 9 10

Commissioning Editor:	Gavin Jamieson
Project Editors:	Francesca Naish and Joanna Silman
Production Controller:	Joanna Walker
Cover Designer:	Helen Townson

Cover image © Science Photo Library

Typeset in 10/12pt Minion by MPS Limited, A Macmillan Company, Chennai, India and Phoenix Photosetting, Chatham, Kent, UK
Printed and bound in India

> What do you think about this book? Or any other Hodder Arnold title?
> Please visit our website: www.hodderarnold.com

To my father Dato KS Sivananthan, mentor and surgeon extraordinaire, for all his invaluable guidance, knowledge and wisdom and for buying me my first copy of Mercers, while exhorting me to "read it cover to cover" and to my mother, Chella, for her constant encouragement.
SS

Dedicated to my judicious wife, Raquel, and my intrepid sons, Declan and Conor. Cogito et seco
ES

Dedicated to my wonderful wife, Frauke, and to my audacious daughters, Ginger and Vivien. Let their generation judge if we have done our best and by doing so, inspire them to do even better.
PHW

To all orthopaedic surgeons throughout the world in hopes that you will never lose your quest for knowledge and pursuit of life long learning. And to my wife, Ann, the CEO of Mark Miller Enterprises!
MDM

Contents

Contributors	xiii
Foreword by Sam Weisel, Department of Orthopaedics, Georgetown University Hospital, Washington DC, USA	xix
Foreword by David Stanley, Chairman of the Intercollegiate Examination Board in Trauma and Orthopaedics, UK	xix
Preface to the tenth edition	xx

PART ONE: INTRODUCTION   EUGENE SHERRY AND SURESHAN SIVANANTHAN

1	History of orthopaedic surgery *Behrooz Mostofi*	3
2	History and examination techniques *Henry Colaco, Sureshan Sivananthan, Laurence James*	8
3	Orthopaedic research: research methods, epidemiology and statistics *Jenna Godfrey, Eric McCarty*	36

PART TWO: MUSCULOSKELETAL STRUCTURE, FUNCTION AND HEALING   NICOLA MAFFULLI

4	Surgical anatomy and embryology of the musculoskeletal system *Franklin D Shuler*	51
5	The structure and development of bone tissue *Bodo Kurz*	82
6	Metabolic bone diseases *Eugene Sherry*	92
7	Soft tissue physiology and healing *Pankaj Sharma, Nicola Maffulli*	100
8	The physiology of ageing *Marco V Narici, Filippo Spiezia, Nicola Maffulli*	120
9	Principles of orthopaedic pharmacology *Chezhiyan Shanmugam, Umile Giuseppe Longo, Nicola Maffulli*	126

PART THREEE: BASIC SCIENCE   NICOLA MAFFULLI

10	Molecular and cell biology, immunology and genetics *Chezhiyan Shanmugam, Umile Giuseppe Longo, Nicola Maffulli*	139
11	Musculoskeletal imaging *Mark W Anderson*	155
12	Biomechanics and biomaterials *Duncan ET Shepherd, David WL Hukins*	173
13	Clinical principles of kinesiology *Jim Richards, James Selfe*	202
14	Infections of the musculoskeletal system *Sureshan Sivananthan, Eugene Sherry*	219

PART FOUR: TRAUMA   SURESHAN SIVANANTHAN

Section 1: General considerations

15	Advanced trauma life support and polytrauma *Peter V Giannoudis, George M Kontakis*	231
16	Mass casualty management *James P Stannard, Michael P Rusnak*	244
17	Open injuries of limbs *Shanmuganathan Rajasekaran, P Rishi Mugesh Kanna, Jayaramaraju Dheenadhayalan*	247
18	Closed treatment of common fractures *Peter V Giannoudis, Fareed Kagda*	258
19	Principles of operative fracture fixation *Peter V Giannoudis, Costas Papacostidis*	269
20	Clinical aspects in acute limb compartment syndrome *Rajiv Malhotra, Nikolaos Giotakis*	278

Section 2: Upper Extremity Fractures & Dislocations

SHOULDER GIRDLE INJURIES

21	Acromioclavicular joint injuries *Shanmuganathan Rajasekaran, Rishi Mugesh Kanna, Jayaramaraju Dheenadhayalan*	285
22	Clavicular fractures *Shanmuganathan Rajasekaran, Rishi Mugesh Kanna, Jayaramaraju Dheenadhayalan*	288
23	Sternoclavicular joint injuries *Shanmuganathan Rajasekaran, Rishi Mugesh Kanna, Jayaramaraju Dheenadhayalan*	291
24	Scapular fractures *Shanmuganathan Rajasekaran, Rishi Mugesh Kanna, Jayaramaraju Dheenadhayalan*	294
25	Dislocations of the glenohumeral joint *Shanmuganathan Rajasekaran, Rishi Mugesh Kanna, Jayaramaraju Dheenadhayalan*	297

HUMERAL FRACTURES

26	Fractures of the proximal humerus *Shanmuganathan Rajasekaran, Rishi Mugesh Kanna, Jayaramaraju Dheenadhayalan*	303
27	Humeral shaft fractures *Shanmuganathan Rajasekaran, Rishi Mugesh Kanna, Jayaramaraju Dheenadhayalan*	307
28	Fractures of the distal humerus *Shanmuganathan Rajasekaran, Rishi Mugesh Kanna, Jayaramaraju Dheenadhayalan*	311

ELBOW AND FOREARM

29	Fractures and dislocations of the elbow *Shanmuganathan Rajasekaran, Rishi Mugesh Kanna, Jayaramaraju Dheenadhayalan*	316
30	Fractures of the shaft of the radius and ulna *Shanmuganathan Rajasekaran, Rishi Mugesh Kanna, Jayaramaraju Dheenadhayalan*	322
31	Fractures of the distal radius *Shanmuganathan Rajasekaran, Rishi Mugesh Kanna, Jayaramaraju Dheenadhayalan*	327

Section 3: Lower Extremity Fractures & Dislocations

32	Dislocations and fracture dislocations of the hip *Shanmuganathan Rajasekaran, Vijay Kamath, Jayaramaraju Dheenadhayalan*	335

PROXIMAL FEMORAL INJURIES

33	Femoral neck fractures *Shanmuganathan Rajasekaran, Vijay Kamath, Jayaramaraju Dheenadhayalan*	340
34	Intertrochanteric fractures *Shanmuganathan Rajasekaran, Vijay Kamath, Jayaramaraju Dheenadhayalan*	346
35	Subtrochanteric fractures *Shanmuganathan Rajasekaran, Vijay Kamath, Jayaramaraju Dheenadhayalan*	350

36	Femoral shaft fractures	353
	Shanmuganathan Rajasekaran, Vijay Kamath, Jayaramaraju Dheenadhayalan	
37	Distal femoral fractures	358
	Shanmuganathan Rajasekaran, Vijay Kamath, Jayaramaraju Dheenadhayalan	

KNEE INJURIES

38	Patellar dislocation	363
	Shanmuganathan Rajasekaran, Rishi Mugesh Kanna, Jayaramaraju Dheenadhayalan	
39	Knee dislocations	365
	Shanmuganathan Rajasekaran, Rishi Mugesh Kanna, Jayaramaraju Dheenadhayalan	
40	Patellar fractures and extension mechanism injuries	368
	Shanmuganathan Rajasekaran, Rishi Mugesh Kanna, Jayaramaraju Dheenadhayalan	

LOWER LEG, FOOT AND ANKLE FRACTURES

41	Tibial plateau fractures	372
	Shanmuganathan Rajasekaran, Vijay Kamath, Jayaramaraju Dheenadhayalan	
42	Fractures of the tibial and fibular shaft	377
	Shanmuganathan Rajasekaran, Rishi Mugesh Kanna, Jayaramaraju Dheenadhayalan	
43	Tibial plafond fractures	382
	Shanmuganathan Rajasekaran, Vijay Kamath, Jayaramaraju Dheenadhayalan	
44	Injuries of the ankle joint	386
	Shanmuganathan Rajasekaran, Rishi Mugesh Kanna, Jayaramaraju Dheenadhayalan	
45	Talar fractures and dislocation	394
	Sureshan Sivananthan, Shanmuganathan Rajasekaran	
46	Calcaneum fractures	398
	Sureshan Sivananthan, Shanmuganathan Rajasekaran	
47	Fractures of the midfoot	403
	Shanmuganathan Rajasekaran, Vijay Kamath, Jayaramaraju Dheenadhayalan	
48	Injuries of the tarsometatarsal (Lisfranc) joint	407
	Shanmuganathan Rajasekaran, Rishi Mugesh Kanna, Jayaramaraju Dheenadhayalan	
49	Fractures of the forefoot	411
	Shanmuganathan Rajasekaran, Rishi Mugesh Kanna, Jayaramaraju Dheenadhayalan	
50	Metatarsophalangeal joint, phalangeal and interphalangeal joint injuries	414
	Shanmuganathan Rajasekaran, Rishi Mugesh Kanna, Jayaramaraju Dheenadhayalan	
51	Acetabular fractures	419
	Anish Potty, Sureshan Sivananthan	
52	Pelvic fractures	425
	Anish Potty	
53	Spinal fractures	439
	Shanmuganathan Rajasekaran, Rishi Mugesh Kanna, Ajoy Prasad Shetty	
54	Head and face trauma	466
	Patrick H Warnke	
55	Paediatric fractures and dislocations	481
	Dorien Schneidmueller, Christoph Nau, Ingo Marzi	
56	Compartment syndrome	503
	Ashish K Sharma, Edward T Mah	
57	Management of fracture complications	515
	Robert B Simons, Andrew M Richards, David S Elliott	

PART FIVE: PAEDIATRIC ORTHOPAEDIC SURGERY BENJAMIN JOSEPH

58	Clinical assessment of the paediatric patient	535
	Michael P Horan, Forest Walker, Todd A Milbrandt	
59	Developmental disorders of human skeleton	541
	Chezhiyan Shanmugam, Umile Giuseppe Longo, Nicola Maffulli	

60	Normal and pathological gait in children *Richard Beauchamp*	563
61	Developmental diseases of the skeleton *Sunil Bajaj, Sanjeev S Madan*	570
62	Bone and joint infections in children *Vrisha Madhuri, Hamish Crawford, James Huntley*	578
63	Juvenile idiopathic arthritis *Tracy V Ting, Brent Graham*	589
64	Neuromuscular disorders *Kishore Mulpuri, Sanjeev Madan, Uni Narayanan, Nick Nicolaou, Shahryar Noordin, Renjit A Varghese, Janet Walker*	598
65	Spinal disorders in children *Stephen Tredwell, Christopher Reilly*	626
66	Hip disorders in children *Hamish Crawford, James A Fernandes, James HP Hui, Arjandas Mahadev, Kishore Mulpuri, Kiran AN Saldanha, Jean-Claude Theis, Simon P Kelley*	642
67	Knee disorders in children *Kevin Lim, James HP Hui, Andrew Lim, Azura Mansor, Ismail Munajat, Kishore Mulpuri, Simon P Kelley*	664
68	Disorders of the leg in children *Stanley Jones, Sunil Bajaj, Nicolas Nicolaou, James A Fernandes, Kiran AN Saldanha*	673
69	Disorders of the foot in children *Haemish A Crawford, James S Huntley, Benjamin Joseph*	688

PART SIX: SPORTS MEDICINE   MARK D MILLER

70	Exercise physiology, epidemiology and special considerations *Chealon D Miller, Joseph M Hart*	697
71	Essential arthroscopic skills *Kimberly A Turman, Mark D Miller*	712
72	Head and spine injuries in sport *James Brezina, Dino Samartzis, Francis H Shen*	720
73	The evaluation and treatment of glenohumeral instability, superior labrum anterior to posterior tears and rotator cuff tears *Matthew T Provencher, Allison McNickle, Janeth Kim, Brian J Cole, Neil Ghodadra*	729
74	Athletic injuries of the elbow, wrist and hand *A Bobby Chhabra, Jesse Seamon*	750
75	Pelvis, hip and thigh *Benjamin G Domb, JW Thomas Byrd*	772
76	Diagnosis and treatment of non-ligamentous knee injuries *Samir G Tejwani, Jessica E Ellerman, Freddie H Fu*	782
77	Diagnosis and management of ligamentous injuries of the knee *Randy Mascarenhas, Eric J Kropf, Christopher D Harner*	805
78	Leg, ankle and foot injuries *John E Femino, Ned Amendola*	821

PART SEVEN: MUSCULOSKELETAL ONCOLOGY   PAUL COOL

79	Clinical evaluation, principles of biopsy and staging *Theodore W Parsons III, Scot E Campbell4*	863
80	Principles of chemotherapy and radiotherapy *Hamid Sheikh, Michael Leahy, James Wylie*	874
81	Bone tumours *David C Mangham and Paul Cool*	882
82	Soft-tissue sarcomas *Gillian L Cribb*	912
83	Skeletal metastases and pathological fractures *Jonathan James Gregory, Paul Cool*	925
84	Limb reconstruction for musculoskeletal tumours *Emma K Reay and Craig H Gerrand*	940

85	Amputations, prosthetics and orthotics *Frank Gottschalk, Ruth M O'Sullivan, Daniel Porter*	954

PART EIGHT: THE SPINE   ALEX VACCARO AND STEPHAN BECKER

86	Pathophysiology of low back pain *Joseph M Hart, Noelle M Selkow, Nicole Cosby, Matthew C Bessette*	975
87	Spinal infections *Shanmuganathan Rajasekaran, P Rishi Mugesh Kanna, T Ajoy Prasad Shetty*	982
88	Degenerative disc disease *Mun Keong Kwan*	993
89	Adult spinal deformity *William C Lauerman, Ryan J Caufield*	1007
90	Surgical options in the osteoporotic spine *Stephan Becker*	1024
91	Spondylolysis and spondylolisthesis *István Hovorka*	1048
92	Tumours of the spine *Stephan Becker, Jason Beng Teck Lim, Volker Schirrmacher, Himanshu Sharma*	1058

PART NINE: ADULT RECONSTRUCTION SURGERY   EUGENE SHERRY AND SURESHAN SIVANANTHAN

Section 1: General considerations

93	Arthritis *Sureshan Sivananthan, Ram Shah*	1077

Section 2: The Hip

94	History of the development of total hip arthroplasty *Mukesh Hemmady*	1097
95	Biomechanics of the hip and total hip arthroplasty *Asim Rajpura, Timothy N Board*	1105
96	Materials in hip arthroplasty *Samuel S Rajaratnam, William L Walter*	1114
97	Perioperative considerations *Daniel Kendoff, Thomas P Sculco, Friedrich Boettner*	1123
98	Primary total hip arthroplasty *Ramankutty Sreekumar, Peter R Kay*	1135
99	Minimal incision surgery/mini-invasive total hip replacement *Eugene Sherry, Declan O Sherry*	1147
100	Revision total hip arthroplasty *Ardeshir Bonshahi, Timothy N Board, Martyn L Porter*	1153

Section 3: The Knee

101	Development of knee arthroplasty *Shi-Lu Chia, Ser Kiat Tan*	1171
102	Total knee arthroplasty *Shi-Lu Chia, Boon Keng Tay*	1176
103	Unicompartmental knee arthroplasty *Seo-Kiat Goh, Seng Jin Yeo, Boon Keng Tay*	1186
104	Patellofemoral arthroplasty of the knee *Erica D Taylor, Mark D Miller*	1193
105	Revision knee arthroplasty *Shi-Lu Chia, Ngai-Nung Lo*	1198

Section 4: The Shoulder

106	Shoulder arthroplasty *Gerald Williams*	1207

Section 5: The ankle

107	Ankle arthroplasty	1241
	Norman Espinosa, Gerardo Juan Maquieira	

Section 6: Arthritis in the younger adult

108	Special considerations in young patients	1253
	Minoo Patel	
109	Osteotomies around the knee	1260
	Andy Williams, Ali Narvani	
110	Joint arthrodesis	1268
	Nikolaos Giotakis, Rajiv Malhotra, Muhammed Arshad Nazar	

PART TEN: HAND AND UPPER LIMB — TED MAH

111	Finger injuries	1277
	A Bobby Chhabra, Jesse Seamon	
112	Tendon injuries	1292
	S Raja Sabapathy, Praveen Bhardwaj	
113	Nerve injuries	1302
	Rolfe Birch	
114	Hand infections	1309
	Tunku Kamarul Zaman	
115	Replantation and microsurgery	1315
	Tunku Kamarul Zaman	
116	Dupuytren's contracture	1324
	William YC Loh, Wee-Leon Lam	
117	Arthritis of the hand	1333
	Ashish Sharma, Edward T Mah	
118	Carpal instability	1351
	Ng Eng Seng, Edward T Mah	
119	The distal radial ulnar joint	1365
	Edward T Mah, Ng Eng Seng	
120	Hand tumours	1373
	Graham Cheung, Gillian L Cribb	
121	The elbow	1382
	Ashish K Sharma, Kamarul Khalid, Edward T Mah	

PART ELEVEN: FOOT AND ANKLE — ANISH KADAKIA

122	Tendon pathologies	1421
	Clifford L Jeng	
123	Hallux valgus	1434
	Shamal Das De, Krishna Lingaraj	
124	Disorders of the hallucal sesamoids and related great toe pathologies	1442
	Andrew Moore, Anish Raj Kadakia	
125	Lesser toe deformities	1449
	Andrew P Molloy, Moez S Ballal	
126	Pes cavus and pes planus	1460
	Anthony Perera, Mark S Myerson	
127	The diabetic foot	1466
	Aziz Nather, Fu Cai Han	
128	Neurological disorders	1472
	Norman Espinosa	
129	Inflammatory and osteoarthritis of the foot and ankle	1484
	Andrew P Molloy, Edward V Wood	

130	Nerve compression syndromes of the foot and ankle *Giselle Tan, Norman Espinosa, Anish Raj Kadakia*	1500

PART TWELVE: NEW TECHNOLOGIES AND BEST CLINICAL PRACTICE   PATRICK WARNKE AND SURESHAN SIVANANTHAN

131	Computer-assisted navigation in orthopaedic surgery *Kamal Deep*	1511
132	Orthopaedic tissue engineering *Patrick H Warnke*	1524
133	Medical ethics *Rachel G Geddes, Suresh Sivananthan*	1531
134	Outcomes, databanks (joint registries), medical coding *Eugene Sherry, Sureshan Sivananthan, Raquel Gehr*	1536
135	Informed consent *Eugene Sherry, Raquel Gehr*	1539
136	Work-related injuries and assessment for compensation *Eugene Sherry, Raquel Gehr*	1542
137	Evidence-based medicine and orthopaedic surgeons *Patrick H Warnke, Eugene Sherry, Conor sherry*	1545
138	Risk management through burnout prevention in orthopaedic surgeons *Sue Besomo*	1549

Subject Index	1555

Contributors

T Ajoy Prasad Shetty
Ganga Hospital, Coimbatore, Tamilnadu, India

Ned Amendola MD
Professor and Director, University of Iowa Sports Medicine Center, Iowa City, USA

Mark W Anderson MD
Professor of Radiology and Orthopaedic Surgery Chief, Division of Musculoskeletal Radiology, University of Virginia School of Medicine, Charlottesville, VA, USA

Sunil Bajaj
Sheffield Children's NHS Foundation Trust, Sheffield, UK

Moez S Ballal MBBS, MRCSEd,
Department of Paediatric Orthopaedics, Royal Liverpool Children's NHS Trust, Liverpool, UK

Richard Beauchamp
Department of Orthopaedic Surgery, Children's & Women's Health Centre of British Columbia, Vanocuver, Canada

Stephan Becker
Institute for Musculoskeletal Analysis, Research and Therapy IMSART, Medimpuls Zentrum für Therapie, Diagnostik und Training, Vienna, Austria

Sue Besomo
Assistant Professor Personal and Professional Development, School of Medicine, Bond University, Queensland, Australia

Matthew C Bessette
University of Virginia, Charlottesville, Virginia, USA

Praveen Bhardwaj MBBS, MS (Ortho), DNB (Ortho)
National Board Fellow in Hand & Reconstructive Microsurgery at Ganga Hospital, Coimbatore, India

Rolfe Birch
Orthopaedic Surgeon, Peripheral Nerve Injury Unit, Royal National Orthopaedic Hospital, Stanmore, Middlesex, UK

Timothy N Board
Consultant Orthopaedic Surgeon, Wrightington Hospital, Wigan; and Lecturer in Orthopaedics, University of Manchester, UK

Friedrich Boettner MD
Assistant Attending Orthopaedic Surgeon, Hospital for Special Surgery, Assistant Professor of Orthopaedic Surgery, Weill Cornell Medical College, New York, USA

Ardeshir Bonshahi
Wrightington Hospital, Wigan, Lancashire, UK

James Brezina MD
Spine Fellow, Department of Orthopaedic Surgery, University of Virginia, Charlottesville, VA, USA

JW Thomas Byrd M.D.
Nashville Sports Medicine & Orthopaedic Center, Nashville, TN, USA

Scot E Campbell
Department of Radiology, Wilford Hall Medical Center, TX, USA

Ryan J Caufield MD
Orthopedic Surgery Specialist, Washington DC, USA

Graham Cheung SpR
Robert Jones and Agnes Hunt Orthopaedic and District Hospital, Oswestry, Shropshire, UK

A Bobby Chhabra
Associate Professor, Division Head, Hand & Upper Extremity Surgery, Co-Director, University of Virginia Hand Center, Residency Program Director, Orthopaedic Surgery, University of Virginia Department of Orthopaedics, USA

Shi-Lu Chia
Orthopaedic Surgeon Singapore General Hospital, Singapore

Henry Colaco
Clinical Research Fellow, University College Hospital, London, UK

Brian J Cole MD
Professor of the Departments of Orthopaedics Anatomy and Cell Biology, Rush University Medical Centre, Chicago, IL, USA

Paul Cool MD MMedSc(Res) FRCS(Ed) FRCS(Orth),
Consultant Orthopaedic & Oncological Surgeon, Orthopaedic Hospital, Shropshire, UK

Nicole Cosby MA ATC
University of Virginia, Curry School of Education, VA, USA

Haemish A Crawford MBChB, FRACS
Orthopaedic Surgery Auckland Hip & Knee Specialist, Starship Children's Hospital, Auckland, New Zealand

Gillian L Cribb MBChB, MRCS, FRCS (Trauma and Orthopaedics)
Queensland Orthopaedic Oncology Fellow, Wesley and Princess Alexander Hospitals, Brisbane, Australia

Shamal Das De MChOrth Liv., MBBS Calc., FRCS (Ed), FRCS (Orth) Ed, FRCS, AM Sing., MD NUS
Professor, Department of Orthopaedic Surgery, Yong Loo Lin School of Medicine, National University of Singapore, Singapore

Kamal Deep
Consultant Orthopaedic Suregon, Golden Jubilee National Hospital NHS Trust, Glasgow, UK

Jayaramaraju Dheenadhayalan MBBS, MS
Department of Orthopedics, Traumatology, and Spine Surgery, Ganga Hospital, Coimbatore, Tamil Nadu, India

Benjamin G Domb MD
Staff Physician, Sports Medicine & Arthroscopic Surgery, Hinsdale Orthopaedics, Ilinois, USA

Jessica E Ellerman
Faculty of Medicine, University of Pittsburgh, Pittsburgh, Pennsylvania, USA

David S Elliot FRCS(Orth)
Rowley Bristow Orthopaedic Unit Ashford & St Peters Hospital, Chertsey, Surrey, UK

Norman Espinosa MD
Director of Foot and Ankle Service, University of Zurich, Zurich, Switzerland

John E Femino MD
Clinical Assistant Professor, Department of Orthopaedics and Rehabilitation, University of Iowa, Iowa, USA

James A Fernandes MD
Consultant Paediatric Orthopaedic Surgeon, Sheffield Children's Foundation NHS Trust, Sheffield, UK

Freddie H Fu
Professor and Chairman, Department of Orthopaedic Surgery, University of Pittsburgh, Pittsburgh, Pennsylvania, USA

Raquel Gehr
Sydney, Australia

Craig H Gerrand MB ChB, FRCSEd (Trauma and Orthopaedics), MD, MBA
Consultant Orthopaedic Surgeon, Freeman Hospital, Newcastle Upon Tyne, UK

Neil Ghodadra
Newcastle Upon Tyne, United Kingdom

Peter V Giannoudis
Professor of Trauma and Orthopaedic Surgery at St James' University Hospital, Leeds, UK.

Nikolaos Giotakis
Royal Liverpool University hospital, Liverpool

Jenna Godfrey
University of Colorado School of Medicine Department of Orthopaedics Denver, Colorado USA

Seo-Kiat Goh MA MBBChir(Cambridge) MMed(Orth Surg) MRCSEd FRCSEd (Orth)
Consultant, Department of Orthopaedic Surgery, Singapore General Hopsital, Singapor

Frank Gottschalk MD
Professor in the Department of Orthopaedic Surgery at U.T. Southwestern Medical Center, Dallas, USA

Brent Graham
Monroe Carell Jr. Children's Hospital at Vanderbilt, Division of Pediatric Rheumatology, Nashville, TN, USA

Jonathan James Gregory
Specialist Registrar Trauma and Orthopaedics, Robert Jones and Agnes Hunt Orthopaedic & District General Hospital, Shropshire, UK

Fu Cai Han
Resident, Department of Orthopaedic Surgery, National University of Singapore and National University Hospital, Singapore

Christopher D Harner
Blue Cross of Western Pennsylvania Professor of Orthopaedic Surgery, University of Pittsburgh School of Medicine, Medical Director, UPMC Center for Sports Medicine, USA

Joseph M Hart PhD ATC
Assistant Professor of Orthopaedic Research, Department of Orthopaedic Surgery, University of Virginia, USA

Mukesh Hemmady
Consultant Orthopaedic Surgeon, The Centre for Hip Surgery Wrightington Hospital, Wigan, UK

Michael P Horan
Department of Orthopaedics Surgery and Sports Medicine, Shriners Hospital, Lexington, Kentucky, USA

István Hovorka MD
Department of Orthopaedics and Sports Traumatology, University of Nice; and Monaco Institute of Sports Medicine and Surgery, Monaco

James HP Hui MBBS, FRCS, FAMS
Assistant Professor, Senior Consultant, Department of Orthopaedic Surgery, National University Hospital, Singapore

David WL Hukins PhD, DSc, FRSE
Professor of Bio-medical Engineering, School of Mechanical Engineering, University of Birmingham, Birmingham, UK

James S Huntley
Orthopaedic Department, Royal Hospital for Sick Children, Glasgow, UK

Laurence James
Consultant Orthopaedic and Trauma Surgeon, Honorary Lecturer at The Institute of Orthopaedics, University College London, London, UK

Clifford L Jeng MD
Attending Orthopedic Surgeon, The Institute for Foot and Ankle Reconstruction, Mercy, Baltimore, USA

Stanley Jones
Consultant Orthopaedic Surgeon, Dept of Orthopaedics, Sheffield Children's Hospital, Sheffield, UK

Benjamin Joseph D'Ortho, MS Ortho
Professor of Orthopaedics, Kasturba Medical College and Hospital, Manipal, India.

Anish Raj Kadakia MD
University of Michigan, Department of Orthopedic Surgery, Division of Foot and Ankle Surgery, USA

Fareed Kagda MBBS (Sing), FRCS (Glas), FRCSEd(Orth)
Visiting Consultant, University Orthopaedics, Hand and Reconstructive Microsurgery Cluster, Singapore

Vijay Kamath MS (Orth) FNBE (Spine)
Senior Spine Registrar, Department of Orthopaedics and Spine Surgery, Ganga Hospital, Coimbatore, India

P. Rishi Mugesh Kanna
Department of Orthopaedics, Traumatology and Spine Surgery, Ganga Hospita, Coimbatore, India

Peter R Kay FRCS
Consultant Orthopaedic Surgeon at Wrightington Hospital (WWL NHS Foundation Trust), Honorary Clinical Professor University of Central Lancashire and Reader in Orthopaedics, University of Manchester, Manchester, UK

Simon P Kelley MBChB, FRCS (Tr and Orth)
Assistant Professor . The Hospital for Sick Children, Limb Reconstruction and Hip Surgery, Division of Orthopaedic Surgery, University of Toronto, Toronto, Canada

Daniel Kendoff MD, PhD
Computer Assisted Surgery Center at Hospital for Special Surgery, New York, USA

Kamarul Khalid
Department of Orthopaedics and Trauma, Queen Elizabeth Hospital, Adelaide, Australia

Janeth Kim LCDR Janeth Kim, MD, MC, USN
Naval Medical Center, San Diego, USA

George M Kontakis
Department of Trauma & Orthopaedic Surgery, School of Medicine, University of Crete, Crete, Greece

Eric J Kropf MD
Chief Resident, Department of Orthopaedic Surgery, University of Pittsburgh Medical Center, USA

Bodo Kurz
Associate Professor of Anatomy & Histology, Faculty of Health Sciences & Medicine, Bond University, Gold Coast, Queensland, Australia

Mun Keong Kwan
Department of Orthopaedic Surgery Faculty of Medicine University of Malaya Lembah Pantai, Kuala Lumpur, Malaysia

Wee-Leon Lam
Specialist Registrar in Plastic Surgery North Western Deanery, Leeds, UK

William C Lauerman MD
Georgetown University, Washington, DC, USA

Michael Leahy MD
Department of Haematology, Fremantle Hospital, Fremantle, Australia

Andrew Lim MD
South Bay Orthopaedic Specialists Medical Centre, Torrance, CA, USA

Kevin Lim
Senior Consultant, Dy Chairman, Division of Surgery, KK Women's and Children's Hospital, Singapore

Jason Teng Beck Lim
University of Glasgow, Glasgow, UK

Krishna Lingaraj MBBS (Singapore), M.Med (Orth), MRCSEd, FRCSEd (Orth)
Consultant, Assistant Professor, Associate Program Director and Core Faculty for Hip & Knee Division, NUHS Orthopaedics Residency Program, Singapore

Ngai-Nung Lo
Department of Orthopaedic Surgery, Adult Reconstruction Service, Singapore General Hospital, Singapore

William Yc Loh
Department of Orthopaedic Surgery, Southport and Ormskirk Hospital NHS Trust, Ormskirk and District General Hospital, Lancashire, UK

Umile Giuseppe Longo MD
Department of Orthopaedic and Trauma Surgery, Campus Biomedico University, Rome, Italy

Sanjeev S Madan
Consultant Orthopaedic Surgeon, Sheffield Children's NHS Foundation Trust, Sheffield, UK

Vrisha Madhuri
Department of Orthopaedics, Christian Medical College, Vellore, India

Nicola Maffulli MS, PhD, FRCS(Orth)
Centre Lead and Professor of Sports and Exercise Medicine Consultant Trauma and Orthopaedic Surgeon Centre for Sports and Exercise Medicine Barts and The London School of Medicine and Dentistry Mile End Hospital, London, UK

Edward T Mah
Calvary Orthopaedic & Hand Care Centre, North Adelaide, Australia

Arjandas Mahadev MBBS, FAMS, FRCS (Edin)
Head & Senior Consultant, Department of Orthopaedic Surgery, KK Women's and Children's Hospital, Singapore

Rajiv Malhotra
Department of Orthopaedics, Royal Liverpool University Hospital, Liverpool, UK

David C. Mangham
The Royal Orthopaedic Hospital Oncology Service, The Royal Orthopaedic Hospital NHS Trust, Bristol Road South, Northfield, Birmingham, UK

Azura Mansor
University of Malaya Medical School, Malaya

Gerardo Juan Maquieira
Department of Orthopedics, University Hospital Balgrist, University of Zurich, Zurich, Switzerland.

Ingo Marzi
Department of Trauma, Hand and Reconstructive Surgery, Hospital of the J.W. Goethe-University of Frankfurt, Frankfurt am Main, Germany

Randy Mascarenhas MD
Orthopaedic Clinical Research Fellow, Department of Orthopaedic Surgery, University of Pittsburgh School of Medicine, USA

Eric McCarty MD
Orthopaedic Sports Medicine, Department of Orthopaedics, University of Colorado, Boulder, USA

Allison McNickle BA
Research Assistant, Division of Sports Medicine, Rush University Medical Center, Department of Orthopaedic Surgery, Chicago, IL, USA

Todd A Milbrandt
University of Kentucky School of Medicine, USA

Mark D Miller MD
Professor of Orthopaedic Surgery, University of Virginia, James Madison University, Charlottesville, VA, USA

Chealon D Miller MD
Department Orthopaedic Surgery, University of Virginia, Charlottesville, VA, USA.

Andrew P Molloy FRCS(Tr&Orth), MR
Department of Trauma and Orthopaedics, Uni Hospital Aintree, Liverpool, UK

Andrew Moore
Department of Orthopaedic Surgery, University of Michigan, Michigan, USA

Behrooz Mostofi
Trauma and Othopaedics, William Harvey Hospital, Kent, UK

Kishore Mulpuri MBBS; MS(Ortho); MHSc(Epi)
Paediatric Orthopaedic Surgeon, BC Childrens Hospital, Vancouver, BC, Canada

Ismail Munajat
Department of Orthopaedics, School of Medical Sciences, Kelantan, Malaysia

Mark S Myerson MD
Mercy Medical Centre, Baltimore, Maryland, USA

Uni Narayanan MB BS
The Hospital for Sick Children and University of Toronto, Toronto, Canada

Marco V Narici
Centre for Biophysical and Clinical Research into Human Movement, Manchester Metropolitan University, UK

Ali Narvani
University of Leeds School of Medicine, Academic Department of Trauma and Orthopaedics, Leeds General Infirmary, Leeds, UK

Aziz Nather
Associate Professor & Senior Consultant, Department of Orthopaedic Surgery, National University of Singapore and National University Hospital, Singapore

Christoph Nau
Hospital of the J.W. Goethe-University of Frankfurt, Frankfurt am Main, Germany

Muhammed Arshad Nazar
Royal Liverpool University hospital, Liverpool, UK

Nick Nicolaou
Conquest Hospital, East Sussex Hospital Trust Hastings, UK

Shahryar Noordin MBBS, FCPS,
Department of Orthopaedics, University of British Columbia, Vancouver, British Columbia, Canada

Costas Papacostidis
Department of Trauma and Orthopaedics, Leeds General Infirmary University Hospital, Leeds, UK

Theodore W Parsons MD, FACS
Theodore William Parsons III, Breech Chair and Chief, Department of Orthopaedic Surgery, Detroit, USA

Minoo Patel
The Epworth Centre, Epworth Hospital, Richmond, Australia

Anthony Perera MBChB MRCS MFSEM (RCP & SI) FRCS (Orth)
Consultant Orthopaedic Surgeon, Cardiff & Vale NHS, Wales

Daniel Porter
Consultant Orthopaedic and Trauma Surgeon, Senior Lecturer, Department of Orthopaedics Edinburgh University, The Royal Infirmary of Edinburgh at Little France, Scotland

Martyn L Porter FRCS
Wrightington Hospital in Lancashire, UK

Anish Potty
Department of Trauma and Orthopaedics, University College Hospital, London, UK

Matthew T Provencher LCDR, MD, MC, USN
Division of Shoulder and Sports Surgery, Dept of Orthopaedic Surgery, Naval Medical Center San Diego, San Diego, CA, USA

Samuel S Rajaratnam FRCS (Tr & Orth), BSc (Hons),
Senior Hip & Knee Fellow, Peninsula Orthopaedic Research Institute, Sydney, Australia

Shanmuganathan Rajasekaran Ph.D.,
Director & Head, Dept of Orthopaedic & Spine Surgery, Ganga Hospital, Coimbatore, India

Asim Rajpura MRCS
Department of Orthopedics, Hope Hospital, Salford, UK

Emma K Reay MBBS
Freeman Hospital, Newcastle-upon-Tyne, UK

Christopher Reilly MD, FRCSC
Department of Orthopaedics, University of British Columbia, Canada

Jim Richards
Professor of Biomechanics, Department of Allied Health Professions, Faculty of Health, University of Central Lancashire, Preston, UK

Andrew M Richards
Limb Reconstruction Unit, Rowley Bristow Unit, St. Peter's Hospitals NHS Trust, Surrey, UK

Michael P Rusnak
Orthopaedic & Spine Center of the Rockies, Fort Collins, Colorado, USA

S Raja Sabapathy
Director & Head Department of Plastic Surgery, Hand Surgery, Reconstructive Microsurgery and Burns, Ganga Hospital, Coimbatore, India

Kiran AN Saldanha
Sheffield Children's Foundation NHS Trust, Sheffield, UK

Dino Samartzis DSc, MSc, Dip EBHC
Research Fellow, Department of Epidemiology, Radiation Effects Research Foundation, Hiroshima, Japan

Volker Schirrmacher
Division of Cellular Immunology, German Cancer Research Center, Heidelberg, Germany

Dorien Schneidmueller
Department of Trauma, Hand and Reconstructive Surgery, Hospital of the J.W. Goethe-University of Frankfurt, Frankfurt am Main, Germany

Thomas P Sculco
Department of Orthopaedic Surgery, Hospital for Special Surgery, New York, NY, USA

Jesse Seamon
University of Virginia School of Medicine, VA, USA

James Selfe
Professor of Physiotherapy, School of Sport, Tourism and The Outdoors, University of Central Lancashire, Preston, UK

Noelle M Selkow MEd ATC
University of Virginia, Charlottesville, Virginia, USA

Ng Eng Seng MBBS (MAL) MS ORTH (MAL)
Consultant Hand and Microsurgeon, Sime Darby Medical Centre, Subanj Jaya, Malaysia

Ram Shah
Department of Orthopaedics Nepal Medical College, Kathmandu, Nepal

Chezhiyan Shanmugam
Registrar in Orthopaedics, Weston General Hospital, Weston-Super-Mare, UK

Himanshu Sharma
Spinal Surgeon, Orthopaedic Consultant, Western Infirmary, Glasgow, UK

Ashish K Sharma
Calvary Orthopaedic & Hand Care Centre, North Adelaide, South Australia, Australia

Pankaj Sharma
Specialist Registrar in Trauma and Orthopaedic Surgery, Southampton University Hospital, Southampton, UK

Hamid Sheikh
Dept of Clinical Oncology, The Christie NHS Foundation Trust, Manchester, UK

Francis H Shen
Assistant Professor, Division of Spine Surgery, Co-Director Spine Fellowship, Department of Orthpaedic Surgery, University of Virginia, Charlottesville, Virginia, USA

Duncan ET Shepherd Du PhD, CEng, FIMechE
Reader in Bio-medical Engineering, School of Mechanical Engineering, University of Birmingham, Birmingham, UK

Eugene Sherry
Faculty of Health Sciences and Medicine, Bond University, Gold Coast, Queensland, Australia

Declan O Sherry
Department of Civil Engineering, University of Melbourne, Victoria, Australia

Ajoy Prasad Shetty
Department of Orthopaedics, Traumatology and Spine Surgery, Ganga Hospital, Coimbatore, India

Franklin D Shuler M.D., Ph.D
Department of Orthopaedic Surgery Division of Orthopaedic Trauma Robert C Byrd HSC Morgantown, USA

Robert B Simonis
Consultant Orthopaedic Surgeon, London

Sureshan Sivananthan MD FRCS (Tr&Orth)
Consultant Orthopaedic Surgeon and Visiting Assistant Professor, Department of Orthopaedic Surgery, Stanford University School of Medicine, Palo Alto, California, USA

Filippo Spiezia MD
Fourth Year resident in Trauma and Orthopaedic Surgery, Universita' Campus Biomedico, Rome, Italy

Ramankutty Sreekumar
Wrightington Hospital, Wigan, UK

James P Stannard MD
Chairman and Professor of Orthopaedic Surgery, Department of Orthopaedic Surgery, Columbia, MO, USA

Ser Kiat Tan MBBS, FRCS (Glasg), FAMS, Clinical Professor
GCEO SingHealth, Emeritus Consultant, Singapore General Health, Singapore

Giselle Tan MD
Orthopaedic Surgery, Michigan, USA

Boon Keng Tay MBBS, FRCS (Edin), FRCS (Edin)(Ortho), FAMS, FACS, Clinical Professor
Emeritus Consultant, Department of Orthopaedic Singapore General Hospital, Singapore

Erica D Taylor MD
Clinical Research Training Program Fellow, National Institute of Child Health and Human Development Resident, Orthopedic Surgery, University of Virginia, USA

Samir G Tejwani MD
Associate Department of Orthopaedic Surgery, Kaiser Permanente, Fontana, California, USA

Jean-Claude Theis
Head of Section, Surgical Sciences - Orthopaedic Surgery, University of Otago, New Zealand

Tracy V Ting MD
Assistant Professor, UC Department of Pediatrics, USA

Stephen Tredwell
Department of Orthopaedics, University of British Columbia, Canada

Kimberly A Turman MD
Department of Orthopaedic Surgery, University of Virginia, Virginia, USA

Renjit A Varghese
Orthopedic Surgeon, Massachusetts General Hospital, Boston, MA, USA

Janet Walker
University of Kentucky Department of Orthopaedic Surgery and Shriners Hospital for Children, Lexington, KY, USA

Forest Walker
University of Kentucky Department of Orthopaedics, KY, USA

William L Walter MBBS (Syd), FRACS (Orth), FAOrthA, PhD (surgery)
Orthopaedic Surgeon, Mater Sydney, Australia

Patrick H Warnke Dr Med DrMed Dent PhD Habil
Professor of Surgery, Faculty of Health Sciences and Medicine, Bond University, Australia

Gerald Williams
The Rothman Institute, Philadelphia, Pennsylvania, USA

Andy Williams MBBS, FRCS, FRCS (Ortho)
Consultant, The Wellington Hospital, London UK

Edward V Wood MB ChB FRCS(Tr&Orth)
Consultant orthopaedic surgeon, Countess of Chester Hospital, UK

James Wylie MBBS, MRCP (UK), FRCR
Consultant Clinical Oncologist, The Alexandra Hospital, UK

Seng Jin Yeo MBBS, FRCS (Edin), FAMS
Senior Consultant & Director, Adult Reconstruction Service, Department of Orthopaedic Surgery, Singapore General Hospital, Singapore

Tunkuk Kamarul Zaman
Upper Limb and Microsurgery Unit, Department of Orthopaedic Surgery, Faculty of Medicine, University of Malaya, Kuala Lumpur, Malaysia

Foreword by Sam Wiesel MD

The tenth edition of *Mercer's Textbook of Orthopaedics and Trauma* continues its tradition of excellence for the education of medical students, residents and registrars who are in training to become orthopaedic surgeons. The editors have created a comprehensive, readable resource for orthopaedic students and residents during the early years of their training. Mercer himself described it in the Preface to the first edition as "a volume of modest size containing the essentials of the old, and a summary of the new". Orthopaedics is changing rapidly with a large infusion of new knowledge and techniques over the past decade. Therefore, Mercers' will be most useful to the student for the personal expertise and experience of the authors.

The content of the first three parts cover the significant points of basic science and physiology of the musculoskeletal system. The next section provides a succinct review of trauma and the final set of chapters cover information on all of the orthopaedic sub-specialties.

The contributors have synthesized and prioritized the importance of their considered knowledge. The editors in turn have maintained this balance of information, and included all aspects of elective orthopaedics and trauma in both children and adults within a single volume. National board standards and key learning points are given for most topics to emphasize significant facts for retention and recall.

I feel this is an essential resource for any orthopaedic resident or registrar preparing for their board examinations. The book will also be useful for trauma and general orthopaedics. We should be grateful to the current set of authors for providing orthopaedic trainees with a highly informative, eminently readable, and well organized textbook.

Sam Wiesel, MD
Professor and Chair, Department of Orthopaedics
Georgetown University Hospital
Washington DC, USA

Foreword by David Stanley FRCS

This tenth edition of *Mercer's Textbook of Orthopaedics and Trauma* is a valuable addition to the medical literature. It covers topics that the young surgeon in training must be familiar with both on a day-to-day basis and when studying for postgraduate examinations. The chapters are comprehensive and of an appropriate length to allow the key information to be conveyed in an easily readable form. In addition, for those who wish to delve deeper into the subject, there are key references at the end of each chapter.

The illustrations are clear and of good quality so that they complement the text making it easier for the reader to more fully understand the points that are being made.

The editors have done an excellent job updating this classic textbook and I believe it will be particularly valuable for orthopaedic trainees preparing for the FRCS Intercollegiate examination in trauma and orthopaedics.

David Stanley FRCS
Chairman of the Intercollegiate Examination Board
in Trauma and Orthopaedics
Edinburgh, UK

Preface to the tenth edition

With the advent of the Internet and web 2.0, all the information contained in any textbook is available online. So why buy this book? The most important reason is that the words contained in these pages represent expert opinion and best current practice which is not easily accessible online. We have brought together the finest minds in modern orthopaedic and related surgery. Secondly, it serves as a guide to residents and trainees the world over who have started their journey in Orthopaedics. Ideally the first year resident should start reading this book on day one and read a few pages every day thus allowing the book to be covered a few times over by the time they come up to the final exit examinations. Certainly in the 4th year most trainees would opt to arm themselves with a review book, with "Miller" being the most popular. However we hope that this book will serve as an underlying base on which one can build a solid foundation of orthopaedic knowledge.

For the practicing orthopaedist what you know is what your patient gets. Therefore it is always a good idea to have an up-to-date textbook which has condensed the most current and evidence based orthopaedic and trauma practice into a single volume complete with high quality images, illustrations and references. Most important is that the information contained in these pages has been filtered and checked by world renowned orthopaedic specialists and rigorously edited by the editorial team to ensure, as far as possible, an accurate picture of current orthopaedic best practice.

Mercer's has been around for over 80 years and this tenth edition has been completely revamped and updated by the new editorial team, with a totally new arrangement of chapters and topics. Although the readership is worldwide, we have introduced "Board Standards" for most chapters which are points that summarize important concepts that may be tested in examinations. Where pertinent, key learning points have also been included. All the images are new and the figures have been drawn in a two colour format for clarity and added precision. Bearing in mind the worldwide readership we have sought to maintain a balance of topics and included all aspects of trauma surgery and elective orthopaedics in both children and adults within a single volume. We have retained and updated the material on diseases and disorders prevalent in rural and developing areas. In addition we have added topics such as medical ethics and burnout prevention in order to engender good medical practice. With regard to the new chapter authors, we have sought out key opinion leaders from around the world and asked them to contribute.

As mentioned in previous editions, good patient selection is paramount in ensuring a good outcome. This requires an excellent knowledge of the basic sciences in orthopaedics and also the natural history of a disorder or disease. We have therefore ordered the chapters in such a way that the reader is rapidly able to find the relevant information. We hope that we have retained Mercer's original concept which was to produce, in a single volume, "the essentials of the old and a summary of the new". If you the reader find any mistakes, omissions or typos please do not hesitate to email us at mercers.textbook@gmail.com.

SS, ES, PHW, MDM

PART 1

INTRODUCTION

EUGENE SHERRY AND SURESHAN SIVANATHAN

1 **History of orthopaedic surgery** 3
  Behrooz Mostofi
2 **History and examination techniques** 8
  Henry Colaco, Sureshan Sivananthan, Laurence James
3 **Orthopaedic research: research methods, epidemiology and statistics** 36
  Jenna Godfrey, Eric McCarty

1

History of orthopaedic surgery

BEHROOZ MOSTOFI

Introduction	3	Technique development	5
Early pioneers and founding fathers	3	Creative orthopaedics for the twenty-first century	6
Anaesthesia and antisepsis	4	Conclusion	6
Orthopaedic evolution	4	References	7

INTRODUCTION

From an ancient history and tradition of bone setting, and a millennia-spanning reliance on the wisdom of Hippocrates, the seeds of orthopaedic surgery were sowed. It took many years, as well as an impressive array of physicians, inventors and scientists, to develop the art and practice of musculoskeletal surgery as we know it today.

EARLY PIONEERS AND FOUNDING FATHERS

The ancient Greeks were prone to injuries resulting from an agrarian society and athletic pursuits. Hippocrates (c. 460–370 BC), born on the Greek island of Cos, routinely faced the problem of shoulder dislocation in his burgeoning medical practice. Among his many advances in establishing medicine as a discipline, Hippocrates dealt with acute dislocation, faced the problems of delayed reduction and saw cases of pathological dislocations attributable to supperative conditions such as tuberculosis. With this, he established a form of orthopaedic best practices that lasted for nearly 2000 years.

Nicholas Andry (1658–1742), Professor of Medicine at the University of Paris and Dean of the Faculty of Physick, was the first figure after Hippocrates to signal a change in orthopaedic medicine. In 1741, at the age of 81, he published the first book on orthopaedic surgery, called *L'Orthopédie*. Of the title, Andry said:

> ... I have formed it of two Greek Words, Orthos, which signifies streight, free from Deformity, and Pais, a Child. Out of these two Words I have compounded that of Orthopaedia, to express in one Term the Design I propose, which is to teach the different Methods of preventing and correcting the Deformities of Children.

Thus began orthopaedic medicine, and with it orthopaedic surgery. Today we still see the influence of Andry – the 'Orthos Pais', or great seal of the American Orthopaedic Association, and the emblem of the crooked tree straightened by a splint, used by the British Orthopaedic Association, are tributes to Nicolas Andry.

After Andry, more medical explorers stepped into the new specialty. In the case of two physicians, personal injury pointed the way. Percivall Pott (1714–88) of London, UK, is perhaps the best known English surgeon of the pre-antiseptic era, and is known to orthopaedic surgeons for his clear descriptions of bone injuries and diseases. In 1756, Pott was thrown from his horse, suffering a compound fracture of the leg. At a consultation of surgeons, the case was thought so desperate as to require immediate amputation. But a late arriving surgeon, Mr Nourse, believed it to be in his power to preserve the leg, and succeeded. Pott's fracture, Pott's disease and Pott's puffy tumour are some of Pott's contributions to the knowledge of surgery.

In 1767, John Hunter (1728–93) ruptured his tendo-Achillis while dancing. Following his injury, he studied the means and methods of joining divided tendons in animals. He studied the structure of innumerable living organisms, and observed the effects of disease and injury upon it.

Dissected specimens were preserved carefully, and, from this collection, Hunter formed an anatomical and pathological museum that became the bedrock of the scientific study of surgery in England.

Not long after, Jacques-Malthieu Delpech's (1777–1832) work marked the beginning of the modern era of orthopaedics. In 1816, Delpech performed a subcutaneous tenotomy for the first time. In 1828, he published *De l'Orthomorphie*, a comprehensive work consisting of two small volumes and plentiful illustrations concerning deformities and diseases of bones and joints.

ANAESTHESIA AND ANTISEPSIS

Before orthopaedic surgery could advance further, the process of surgery needed improvement. It was the development of anaesthesia and antisepsis that revolutionized the practice of surgery and led to phenomenal advance in all fields.

At the beginning of the nineteenth century, anaesthesia was introduced into surgical practice. Sir Humphry Davy routinely worked with nitrous oxide in his laboratory and, after experiencing the narcotic effect of the vapour upon himself, he declared in 1800 that the gas might have its uses in surgery. In 1824, Henry Hickman proved its efficacy in operations upon small animals. Horace Wells in the USA used the gas successfully in his private practice as a dental surgeon. Upon attempting to demonstrate its use in general surgery, however, he failed and garnered unceasing ridicule. Finally, in 1846, W.T.G. Morton, a former student of Wells, succeeded in inducing anaesthesia at the Massachusetts General Hospital during surgery for removal of a tumour.

After anaesthesia became a functioning reality, scientists and physicians turned to further improvements of the surgical environment. Surgery had always been crippled by infections, complications and the other side-effects of an unsterile setting. Joseph Lister (1827–1912) became acquainted with the writings of Pasteur in 1865. After many investigations he adopted carbolic acid as a permanent feature of his technique. Acceptance of the antiseptic principle soon followed, laying the groundwork for millions of saved lives. Sir William Macewen (1848–1924) was Lister's dresser for 4 years. He watched the dawn of antisepsis, grasped its implications and eagerly played a leading part in the expansion of surgery. Macewen went on to become the earliest innovator of neurosurgery and thoracic surgery. In 1878, he performed a linear osteotomy for the first time for correction of genu valgum. He also designed an all-metal osteotome, led research on the growth of bone and, in 1879, successfully transplanted bone in a human. Robert Hamilton Russell (1860–1933) worked for Joseph Lister as a house officer. His description of a method of skin traction for the treatment of fractures of the femur made his name well known to surgeons throughout the world.

William Arbuthnot Lane (1856–1943) perfected aseptic surgery by introducing the no-touch technique. He conducted early research on skeletal function that led him to study restoration of function in skeletal injury and disease. When Lane operated upon a man with oblique fractures of the tibia and fibula in 1894, inserting screws, he soon realized that, if the operative treatment of fractures was to be safe, a rigorous aseptic technique was essential. His technique allowed further development of the sterile surgical environment.

ORTHOPAEDIC EVOLUTION

William John Little (1810–94) was afflicted with a clubfoot as a result of infantile paralysis at the age of 4 years and wore a leg appliance. From the time he began to study medicine, Little sought a means of curing, or at least minimizing, the disability. He turned to Louis Stromeyer of Hanover, Germany, who had studied Delpech's work, proposed important modifications of his plans and treated two patients successfully. Stromeyer divided Little's tendo-Achillis and gradually corrected the deformity of his foot. Encouraged and motivated, Little returned home and carried out the first subcutaneous tenotomy in London in 1837. Three years later, Little opened the Orthopaedic Infirmary in Bloomsbury Square, London, the first hospital in the UK to be devoted solely to the study and treatment of disabilities of the limbs and spine.

Hugh Owen Thomas (1834–91), descended from a well-known family of bone-setters, acquired an extensive practice in the treatment of fractures and bone and joint diseases in Liverpool, UK. Rest and alignment were his watchwords; to ensure this, he used splints. He introduced many devices, such as the cock-up splint, the wrench, and the cuff and collar sling, as well as the practice of percussing for non-united fractures and the clinical test for flexion deformity of the hip. In 1875, in his first book, *Diseases of the Hip, Knee, and Ankle Joints*, he described for the first time his hip and knee splints. The splint was adapted for treatment of femoral fractures during the First World War, and drastically reduced the mortality rate of open fractures from 60% to 25%. In 1864, he married, but he and his wife had no children; in 1873, they offered their young nephew, Robert Jones, a home in Liverpool in order that he might study medicine.

Robert Jones (1857–1933), general surgeon to the Liverpool hospitals, published the first report of the clinical use of a radiograph to locate a bullet in a wrist in 1896. He founded several associations and orthopaedic hospitals and wrote books, including *Injuries of Joints* (1915) and *Notes on Military Orthopaedics* (1917). His textbook *Orthopaedic Surgery* is said to be the first to have dealt systematically with the diagnosis and treatment of fresh fractures. During the First World War, Jones headed the orthopaedic section of the British forces. After the war, he realized that industrial, domestic and road accidents would increasingly call upon the services of orthopaedic surgeons, creating the basis for 'fracture clinics'.

Gathorne Robert Girdlestone (1881–1950) was prevented from serving overseas in the First World War by the effects of a serious chest injury, the result of a motorcycle accident. However, he was placed in charge of the orthopaedic division of a military hospital in Oxford, UK, and came into contact with Robert Jones. Immediately after the war, the two surgeons launched their campaign for the establishment of regional orthopaedic services. His operations for Pott's paraplegia, hallux valgus, osteoarthritis of the hip and claw toes were particularly valuable contributions.

TECHNIQUE DEVELOPMENT

With groundwork for an exciting and essential medical specialty, physicians the world over drove the momentum forward. With new tools and techniques developed in the late nineteenth century and throughout the twentieth century, orthopaedic surgery expanded and improved.

Edward Bradford (1848–1926) was the third President of the American Orthopaedic Association. Some of his great technical contributions were treatment of tuberculosis coxitis and of congenital hip disease, and a complete study of clubfeet.

Alessandro Codivilla (1861–1912) developed the world famous Instituto Ortopeclico Rizzoli, where he made original and important contributions to the surgery of fractures and the methods of tendon transplantation, and to the development and standing of the specialty. After his death in 1912, Codivilla was succeeded by Vittorio Putti (1880–1940). Putti's contributions included advances in the treatment of congenital dislocation of the hip, arthritis, arthroplasty, adult clubfeet, the open treatment of fractures and the use of skeletal traction and metal fixation, bone lengthening, spinal anomalies, and the surgical treatment of the residual effects of poliomyelitis.

In Vienna, Austria, Lorenz Böhler (1885–1973) formed the Unfallkrankenhaus (Accident Hospital) in 1925, serving as the director until his retirement in 1963. Böhler became the greatest authority on the treatment of fractures in the first half of the twentieth century.

Albin Lambotte (1866–1955) of Antwerp, Belgium, designed and forged devices for fixation and the instruments for manipulating them. Fritz Steinmann (1872–1932) of Bern, Switzerland, described a new method for the reduction and the treatment of fractures using a specially designed pin to be inserted through a distal fragment and controlled by direct skeletal traction.

Fred Houdlette Albee (1876–1945) conducted his bone-graft operation for fusion of a tuberculur spine. Albee also designed a special fracture table, developed an electric saw, and worked on original arthroplasty of the knee and the elbow.

In the UK, Sir Reginald Watson-Jones (1902–72) published *Fractures and Joint Injuries* in January 1940. In the early part of the Second World War, Watson-Jones was appointed civilian consultant in orthopaedic surgery to the Royal Air Force. He inspired and trained the young surgeons who were later to become leading orthopaedic consultants in civilian practice.

Gerhard Küntscher (1900–72), from the University of Kiel in Germany, is known throughout the medical community for developing intramedullary nailing. Kiel, in the northernmost part of Germany, on the Baltic sea, was the main port for German U-boats during the war. During the Second World War, Küntscher served as a surgeon on the Eastern Front and performed the operation on war victims and Luftwaffe pilots, allowing them a quicker return to action. Later, Küntscher developed the distractor that made it possible to carry out closed nailing of malaligned pseudarthroses and old fractures. The internal medullary osteotome was the final culmination of his work in the field of closed bone surgery. Robin Denham introduced Küntscher's techniques to the UK at the end of the war.

In 1950, Frederick Roeck Thompson (1907–83) developed the hip prosthesis that bears his name. This design became a prototype for many later prostheses, including the femoral component for the total hip replacement in use today.

Austin Talley Moore (1899–1963) was also a pioneer in the use of the femoral prosthesis; his work on this made available the techniques and materials that have restored function to thousands of elderly patients. Robert Judet (1909–80), the son of an orthopaedic surgeon, is best known for his work in joint replacement. With his brother, Jean, he was one of the first to use an acrylic prosthesis to replace the femoral head, in 1946. He worked for years to improve the acrylic material, developing a cementless total hip arthroplasty in 1971.

John Charnley (1911–82) published *Closed Treatment of Common Fractures* in 1950. In the late 1940s, arthrodesis was regarded as an acceptable treatment for a stiff and painful joint, but no entirely reliable procedures were available. After extensive experimentation with Teflon shells, Charnley conceived 'low frictional torque arthroplasty'. While Teflon eventually failed, high-density polyethylene enabled his efforts to be directed towards a more perfect mechanical solution for total hip replacement. His report 'Low friction arthroplasty of the hip: theory and practice' was published in 1979. Kenneth McKee, John Watson Farrar and Peter Ring were other early pioneers in the field of total hip arthroplasty, whereas John Insall and Mike Freeman were pioneers in the field of total knee arthroplasty, introducing such key concepts as flexion extension gaps and balancing techniques.

Gavriil Abramovich Ilizarov (1921–92) was based in Kurgan, a town in the middle of Siberia, and applied the concept of distraction osteogenesis to orthopaedics, successfully treating the Russian Olympic high jumper Valery Brumel. After a motorcycle accident, Brumel had chronically infected non-united fractures of both legs, even after 14 operations by the best surgeons in Moscow. With Ilizarov's treatment, Brumel's fractures healed and he went on to jump again in competition. By 1986, North American orthopaedic surgeons had learned the Ilizarov techniques from the Italians, who had worked directly with him and were performing Ilizarov limb-saving operations.

Robert Danis (1880–1962) was a Belgian professor of clinical surgery with very broad interests. He invented a clamp to be used for portocaval shunts, studied the use of vein grafts to reconstruct defects in arteries and bile ducts, and further developed the operative treatment of fractures, demonstrating that primary union of fractures could occur without callus formation. The results of his clinical and laboratory experience were published in his book *Theorie et Pratique de l'Osteosynthese*. Impressed by his book, Maurice E. Müller visited Robert Danis in March 1950. Müller later gathered about him a small group of Swiss surgeons who shared his interests, including Robert Schneider, Hans Willenegger and Martin Allgöwer. They formed a study group in 1958, called the Arbeitsgemeinschaft für Osteosynthesefragen, or AO, to conduct research into bone healing and the influence of the mechanical environment on fracture healing. They also established a Laboratory for Experimental Surgery, created the Documentation Centre and worked closely with Robert Mathys for development of implants and instruments. Many of today's recent inventions are from the AO group.

Ronald L. Huckstep (1926–) developed simple surgical techniques, orthotics and wheelchairs for the treatment of patients with poliomyelitis in Africa (the same-styled wheelchairs are now used by paralympians). He later produced a standard and popular textbook of trauma, championed the surgical care of patients with cancer and contributed to modern arthroplasty and trauma (Huckstep hip and nail).

CREATIVE ORTHOPAEDICS FOR THE TWENTY-FIRST CENTURY

The major elements of this century are the emergence of China and India as a dominant influence; globalization and rebuilding the environment; and the Internet, which is now central to our modern lives. Social and professional interactions have been rebranded as social networking on Twitter and Facebook.

The central theme for modern orthopaedics will be the biological production of new joints, replacement bone and novel ways in which to glue fractured bones together. Also, the demand for surgery with minimal disturbance of tissues or minimally invasive surgery will grow in popularity as patients and administrators realize that less invasive surgery means shorter hospital stays and faster rehabilitation.

As the 'baby boomers' age, demand for orthopaedic services, especially joint replacement, is set to increase dramatically. A patient aged 60 years in a developed country is as physically active and productive as a 30 year old from previous generations. These patients want modern and high-technology medicine. There is a saying among surgeons that '70 is the new 40'. It is all too easy to equate modern medicine with expensive medicine; it does not need to be if we think and innovate. But we should never forget that orthopaedics is a large part of healthcare, especially in the area of trauma and worn-out joints. It's 'easy' to have highly technical operations with complex navigation systems for trauma fixation or knee replacement in Berlin, Germany, or Manhattan, USA, but it takes real genius to reproduce the same great care in rural environments or developing countries.

It can, however, be done. For example, Küntscher proposed battle-front nailing of femurs in the 1930s; Rush developed a brilliant, cheap system for fracture fixation in the 1950s; Huckstep did it with poliomyelitis in the 1960s in Uganda; even Virginia Apgar in the 1950s provided encouragement ('you know it, now do it'). We need creative orthopaedics, not just a slavish observance of current thinking and practice, in the same way that Fred Hollows, a famous eye surgeon in Australia, brought high-technology cataract surgery to the outback communities of Australia and the poor of Vietnam.

Let us arm these doctors with good and accessible technology (forget cumbersome government-based telemedicine, just use Google or an iPhone). YouTube and Wikipedia, built by individuals (not institutions or governments), have provided more education since their beginnings in 2005/07 than all the great universities over the last 500 years (YouTube with 3 billion views in January 2008 alone, and Wikipedia with 10 million articles from volunteers – a tribute to global civic duty).

Along with these, MacDonald's (with 31 000 restaurants) has been able to teach more young people good manners and a work ethic than any schooling system.

The future is being masterminded by entrepreneurial individuals. We hope that reading this book will enable you to become a thinking orthopaedic surgeon.

CONCLUSION

The history of orthopaedic surgery is one of a quest – one that has ranged from ancient times to today. Passionate physicians, scientists and innovators dedicated to creating solutions to devastating problems have made orthopaedic surgery the environment of excellence it is today. As we are entering the bionic age, the quest will continue in the future with its new pioneers.

KEY LEARNING POINTS

- It took many years, as well as an impressive array of physicians, inventors and scientists, to develop the art and practice of musculoskeletal surgery as we know it today.
- The future will be driven by the bionic biological age, the Internet and innovation.

REFERENCES

Butler FH. John Hunter. In: *Encyclopaedia Britannica*. London, UK: Encyclopaedia Britannica, 1910.

Delpech JM. *Precis Elementaire des Maladies Reputees Chirurgicales*. Paris, France: Méquignon-Marvis, 1816.

Delpech JM. *Chirurgie Clinique de Montpellier*, vol. 1. Paris, France: Gabon, 1823–8.

Delpech JM. *De l'Orthomorphie*. Paris, France: Gabon, 1828.

Horder TJ. Life and works of Percivall Pott. *St Bartholomew's Hospital Reports* 1894;**30**:163.

Jones AR. The evolution of orthopaedic surgery in Great Britain. *Proceedings of the Royal Society of Medicine (Section of Orthopaedics)* 1937;**31**:19–26.

Keith A. *Menders of the Maimed*. London, UK: Henry Frowde and Holder & Stoughton, 1919.

Little WJ. *A Treatise on the Nature of Club Foot and Analogous Distortions*. London, UK: W. Jeffs, 1839.

Little WJ. On the influence of abnormal parturition, difficult labour, premature birth and asphyxia neonatorum, on the mental and physical condition of the child, especially in relation to deformities. *Transactions of the Obstetrical Society of London* 1862;**3**:293.

Lloyd GM. Life and works of Percivall Pott. *St Bartholomew's Hospital Reports* 1933;**66**:291.

Palmer JF. *The Works of John Hunter, F.R.S., with Notes*. London, UK: Longmans, 1835.

Paget S. *John Hunter*. London, UK: T. Fisher Unwin, 1897.

Pott P. *The Chirurgical Works of Percivall Pott, F.R.S., to which are added 'a short Account of the Life of the Author, by James Earle, Esq.*, vols. 1–3. London, UK: J. Johnson, 1790.

Power D'A. Percivall Pott: his own fracture. *British Journal of Surgery* 1923;**10**:313.

Power D'A. The works of Percivall Pott. *British Journal of Surgery* 1929;**17**:1.

Rochard J. *Histoire de la Chirurgie Franpaise au XIX Siecle*. Paris, France: B. Bailliere et Fils, 1875.

Valentin B. *Geschichte der Orthopaedie*. Stuttgart, Germany: Georg Thieme Verlag, 1961.

History and examination techniques

HENRY COLACO, SURESHAN SIVANANTHAN, LAURENCE JAMES

The clinical examination of an orthopaedic case	8	CLINICAL EXAMINATION OF THE LOWER LIMB	17
CLINICAL EXAMINATION OF THE UPPER LIMB	9	The hip	17
The shoulder	9	The knee	22
The elbow	11	Gait foot and ankle	26
The wrist	13	The spine	31
The hand	15	References	35

THE CLINICAL EXAMINATION OF AN ORTHOPAEDIC CASE

No part of orthopaedic training is more important than developing a systematized method of examination. It cannot be too strongly emphasized that a true knowledge of disease, which forms the basis of successful diagnosis and treatment, can be found only on the careful and accurate study of individual cases. Scientific and orderly investigation is essential in orthopaedic conditions.

The history

At the first consultation it is necessary to elicit a complete and accurate history of the patient's complaint, the mode of its onset and the order in which the symptoms were first observed.

THE COMPLAINT

The chief complaint may suggest to some extent the nature of the affection, while it always focuses attention on some definite part of the body.

MANNER OF ONSET

The illness may begin suddenly, or it may be gradual and insidious in its development. Apart from trauma, the most likely cause of sudden derangement is acute infection. When the onset is insidious, it may be due to a low-grade inflammation, granuloma or tumour, a slow degenerative process or a postural anomaly.

TYPICAL SYMPTOMS

The typical symptoms to be inquired for in any injury, disease or deformity (congenital or acquired) of the musculoskeletal system and its associated structures are:

1. pain and its features
2. disturbed sensation (e.g. paraesthesia)
3. deformity: its onset and progress
4. weakness or paralysis of muscle power
5. limitation of movement of a joint
6. instability of a joint
7. crepitus.

THE QUESTION OF PRECEDING INJURY

There is a distinct tendency to ascribe all orthopaedic symptoms and errors to some injury, often sustained at a date considerably remote. An attempt should always be made to ascertain the extact details of any alleged trauma, and to establish its exact relation to the actual lesion as this may have important medicolegal aspects. Such an inquiry should be directed towards discovering whether the symptoms arose at the time of the injury, existed previously, or only appeared subsequently.

CLINICAL EXAMINATION OF THE UPPER LIMB

THE SHOULDER

Introduction

The shoulder is a complex joint and is by design inherently unstable because of its large range of movement. It mainly relies on soft-tissue structures around it for stability. Examination of the shoulder follows the standard 'look, feel, move' order of proceedings but there are a plethora of special tests that must be borne in mind when taking the history and examining the patient. Depending on the history and initial 'look, feel, move' examination, the examiner should then home in on the area of concern and bring out the 'special test' that is going to prove or disprove that probable or differential diagnosis. For example, if a patient complains of pain in the shoulder and this is localized to the acromioclavicular joint (AC) joint, then the Scarf test is performed as the first 'special test'. The five commonest pathologies encountered in the shoulder examination are instability, rotator cuff tear, arthritis, AC joint pathology and impingement. Cervical spine problems should also be ruled out as a cause of pain. A complete upper limb examination should include assessment of neurology (Table 2.1 and Table 2.2).

History

As with other parts of the musculoskeletal system, age, occupation and dominant hand should be ascertained. Age alone will give plenty of clues as to the nature of the problem. Instability is usually seen in the second and third decades, frozen shoulder in diabetics and in the fourth decade, inflammatory joint diseases in the fifth decade and degenerative joint diseases and rotator cuff tears in the sixth and seventh decades. In the history, specific questions regarding pain, weakness, stiffness, clicking and instability should be asked. The duration and onset of symptoms should be ascertained.

Table 2.1 Upper limb myotomes

Root value	Action	Muscles
C5	Shoulder abduction	Deltoid, supraspinatus
C5, C6	Elbow flexion	Biceps brachii, brachialis
C6, C7	Wrist extension	ECRL, ECRB, ECU
C6, C7, C8	Elbow extension	Triceps brachii
C7, C8	Finger extension	Extensor digitorum communis/pollicis/indicis
C8	Finger flexion	FDS, FDP, FPL, FPB
C8, T1	Finger adduction	Palmar interossei
C8, T1	Finger abduction	Dorsal interossei

ECRL, extensor carpi radialis longus; ECRB, extensor carpi radialis brevis; ECU, extensor carpi ulnaris; FDS, flexor digitorum superficialis; FDP, flexor digitorum profundus; FPL, flexor pollicis longus; FPB, flexor pollicis brevis.

Table 2.2 Deep DTRs

Root value	Reflex	Action	Muscles
C5, C6	Biceps jerk	Elbow flexion	Biceps brachii
C5, C6	Supinator jerk	Forearm supination	Brachioradialis
C6, C7	Triceps jerk	Elbow extension	Triceps
L3, L4	Knee jerk	Knee extension	Quadriceps femoris
S1, S2	Ankle jerk	Ankle plantarflexion	Gastrocnemius

Examination

INSPECTION

Inspection should follow a systematic approach. The patient should be standing and undressed to the waist. Female patients should have a strapless garment or a drape to cover the breasts. Note the difficulty with which the patient gets undressed as this will correlate with the severity of the symptoms. Document any scars, sinuses or redness around the shoulder area. Starting from the anterior aspect, check for prominent sternoclavicular joint (subluxation), deformity of the clavicle (old fracture), prominent AC joint (subluxation or osteoarthritis (OA)) or deltoid wasting. From the lateral aspect check for any swelling which may suggest infection or inflammatory reaction. From the posterior aspect check for normal-shaped and situated scapulae and also if any winging is present. From the superior aspect (from above) check for swelling, deformity, and asymmetry of the supraclavicular fossae.

PALPATION

Palpation should also be systematic, as with inspection. It is a good idea to stand behind the patient with the patient facing a mirror so you can see their facial expression while palpating the shoulder. Remember to palpate with one hand only and press only on one point at a time. Start with the sternoclavicular joint medially and move along the clavicle, examining the bony prominences from anterior to posterior. Note any point tenderness in the AC joint and the long head of biceps. However, diffuse tenderness is more suggestive of infection or supraspinatus tendinitis. Palpate the coracoid and the area around it. Tenderness lateral to the coracoid is suggestive of inflammatory arthropathy or frozen shoulder. Continue the palpation distally. The intertubercular sulcus is palpated approximately 7 cm distal to the acromion, and tenderness here may reflect a bicipital tendinitis. However, tenderness in a particular area is rather non-specific for any particular diagnosis, although it does offer pointers towards the correct diagnosis when taken with the history and other clinical examination findings.

MOVEMENT

First assess active movement followed by passive movement. It is more efficient to ask the patient to perform an active movement first and then passively assess if the range can be extended. Then one can record active and passive movements in one go. (For example 'active abduction to 120° and further passive abduction to 170°'.) Check the scapulohumeral rhythm. If restricted then repeat with the scapula fixed to check the amount of glenohumeral movement passively. It is also prudent to examine the cervical spine quickly to ensure that the symptoms present in the shoulder area are not referred from the cervical spine.

SPECIAL TESTS

There are many special tests for the shoulder and the general orthopaedist is not expected to know them all. However, the authors recommend the excellent monograph by TD Tennant which outlines the key tests.[1,2]

Key special tests are as follows:

1. Subacromial impingement
    a. Hawkin test. Shoulder flexed 90°, elbow flexed 90°, internal rotation will cause pain.[3]
    b. Neer's sign. Pain at mid-arc of passive abduction in the scapula plane.[4]
2. AC joint pathology
    a. Scarf test. Forced cross body adduction in 90° flexion, pain at the extreme of motion *over the AC joint* is indicative of AC joint pathology.
3. Rotator cuff tears
    Rotator cuff tests can be divided into resistance tests and lag tests.
    a. Supraspinatus. Jobe's test (also known as 'empty can' test): arm abducted to 20°, in the plane of the scapula, thumb pointing down and ask the patient to resist abduction.[5] A positive test signifies supraspinatus tear.
    b. Posterior cuff (infraspinatus and teres minor)
        i. External rotation lag test: the patient is asked to flex the elbow at 90° and the arm is fully externally rotated by the side and released. If the forearm drops forward this signifies a massive infraspinatus tear. This is known as a lag test for infraspinatus.[6]
        ii. Patte's test: shoulder is flexed 90°, flexed elbow and resisted external rotation. This is a resistance test for infraspinatus and teres minor. The Zasloff test is similar.[1,2]
        iii. The Hornblower's sign is an inability to externally rotate and abduct the hand from in front of the mouth against gravity. This is therefore a *lag test for infraspinatus and teres minor*.[5]
    c. Subscapularis (anteroinferior cuff)
        i. Gerber's lift-off test involves the patient's hand behind their back pushing the examiner's hand away from the 'hand behind the back position'. This eliminates pectoralis major and is a resistance test for subscapularis.[7] This test is often performed incorrectly so ensure that the patient has a full range of passive internal rotation and that active internal rotation is not limited by pain. Also the hand should be at the level of the mid-lumbar spine and not the buttock (Fig. 2.1).
        ii. Napoleon/LaFosse belly-press test (Fig. 2.2). The patient is asked to push their hand on their belly. If the patient cannot fully internally rotate and push on their belly, an elbow will drop backwards signifying a positive test. Scheibel described a modification where the examiner tries to pull the hand away from the abdomen.

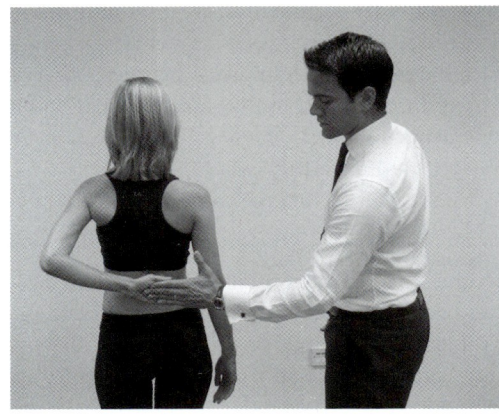

Figure 2.1 Gerber's lift-off test.

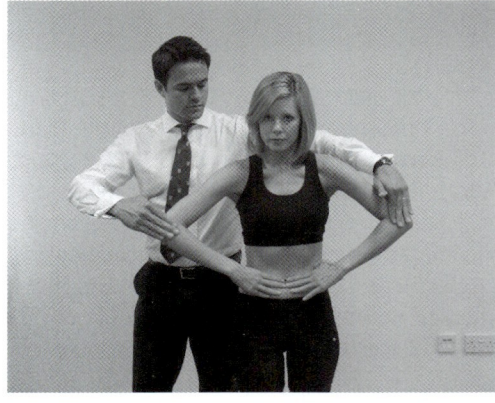

Figure 2.2 Belly presses.

4. Biceps
   a. Looking at the biceps one may see a Popeye sign signifying a long head of biceps rupture.
   b. Speed's test involves a supinated arm flexed against resistance. Pain felt in the bicipital groove indicates biceps tendon pathology.
   c. Yergason's test involves feeling for subluxation of the biceps tendon out of the bicipital groove when the arm is gently internally and externally rotated in extension and adduction.
5. Instability
   a. Laxity tests examine the amount of translation allowed by the shoulder starting from positions where the ligaments are normally loose. Many normally stable shoulders, such as those of gymnasts, will demonstrate substantial translation on these laxity tests even though they are asymptomatic. Use the contralateral shoulder as an example of what is 'normal' for the patient. The standard tests are the anterior and posterior drawer tests and the inferior drawer test. The inferior drawer test is performed by gentle axial traction on the upper arm in a downward direction. Formation of a 'sulcus' as the humeral head slides inferiorly is indicative of a lax capsule.[7]
   b. Apprehension tests examine the stability of the shoulder. The patient can lie supine or sit with the back towards the examiner. The arm is held in 90° of abduction and external rotation. The examiner pulls back on the patient's wrist with one hand while stabilizing the back of the shoulder with the other. The patient with anterior instability usually will become apprehensive with this manoeuvre. The relocation test of Jobe is then performed immediately after a positive result for the anterior apprehension test. The examiner applies posterior force on the proximal humerus while externally rotating the patient's arm. A decrease in pain or apprehension suggests anterior glenohumeral instability.[8] This can be performed standing, sitting or supine. The original description is with the patient supine.

THE ELBOW

As with the other joints a full history is obtained, bearing in mind that certain conditions are more prevalent in certain age groups; for example, locking of the elbow in a young patient is likely to be due to osteochondritis dissecans whereas the same symptoms in an older patient would be due to loose bodies. It is important to note if there are any other associated symptoms and if there is any instability to document the position at which the elbow feels most unstable. Also, as with all upper limb disorders it is vital to specifically ask the patient about neck symptoms as cervical spine pathology can cause referred pain to the elbow.

Inspection

Note the position in which the elbow is held. A painful elbow is usually pronated with the forearm being supported by the contralateral hand. Also look closely at the skin for previous scars due to either trauma or surgery and also assess the condition of the skin. Finally look for the presence of swelling in the joint or for rheumatoid nodules on the extensor aspect of the elbow.

Palpation

As much of the elbow is a subcutaneous joint systematic palpation will reveal the site of maximal tenderness and the cause of the patient's symptoms. Ask the patient to abduct the shoulder 45° and stand at the side or behind the patient. This position allows the examiner to easily palpate the anterior, posterior, medial and lateral aspects of the elbow (Fig. 2.1).

LATERAL

Start at the supracondylar ridge and palpate down the ridge to the lateral epicondyle, common extensor origin and lateral collateral ligament (LCL). At this point the extensor carpi radialis brevis (ECRB) and extensor carpi radialis longus (ECRL) muscles can be assessed by resisted wrist extension in neutral and radial deviation. Point tenderness over the ECRB indicates tennis elbow (lateral epicondylitis). Continue by palpating the radiocapitellar joint line, where tenderness may indicate articular injury or osteochondritis dissecans. Look for the infracondylar sulcus between the lateral condyle and the radial head. Palpation in this area will reveal boggy swelling if there is synovial hypertrophy due to rheumatoid arthritis or fluctuation if there is fluid in the joint. Following this, palpate the radial head and check for congruency with the capitellum. Ask the patient to pronate and supinate to check that the radial head is well oriented to the capitellum and that there is no dislocation. Also check for pain or crepitus, as this will signify a recent injury, radial head fracture or degenerative change in that joint.

ANTERIOR

The anterior structures from lateral to medial are the biceps tendon (together with the lacertus fibrosus), the brachial artery and median nerve (mnemonic: TAN). Look for biceps tendon insertion rupture (proximal bulge) or long head of biceps rupture (distal bulge), which is more common. Occasionally, anterior myositis ossificans may be palpated after elbow dislocation.

MEDIAL

Feel for tenderness over the medial epicondyle and common flexor origin which indicates medial epicondylitis (golfer's elbow) whereas tenderness over the pronator teres indicates pronator syndrome. In pronator syndrome percussion of the median nerve at the elbow results in tingling distally.[1] Provocation tests for this syndrome include resisted middle finger flexion at the proximal interphalangeal joint, pain on resisted pronation and resisted elbow flexion.

The ulnar nerve should also be palpated and is easily felt behind the medial epicondyle (Fig. 2.3). Check the position of the ulnar nerve during flexion and extension movements of the elbow to ascertain if there is subluxation of the nerve, as up to 10% of patients have an anterior subluxing ulnar nerve, which is a recognized cause of medial elbow pain.

Be sure to know the common sites of compression of the ulnar nerve in this area. They are from proximal to distal (see Chapter 121).

POSTERIOR

Palpate the bony prominences of the triad which includes the tip of the olecranon process and the medial and lateral epicondyles, which should form a straight line with the elbow extended. With the elbow flexed to 90°, these landmarks should form an isosceles triangle. Any disruption of this arrangement signifies previous bony injury.

Movement

Elbow flexion (140°) and extension (0°) can most easily be demonstrated in the coronal plane at 90° of shoulder abduction (Figs 2.4 and 2.5), comparing both sides.

Provocation tests for elbow pathology

There are a number of provocation tests that can be used to elicit various conditions as detailed below.

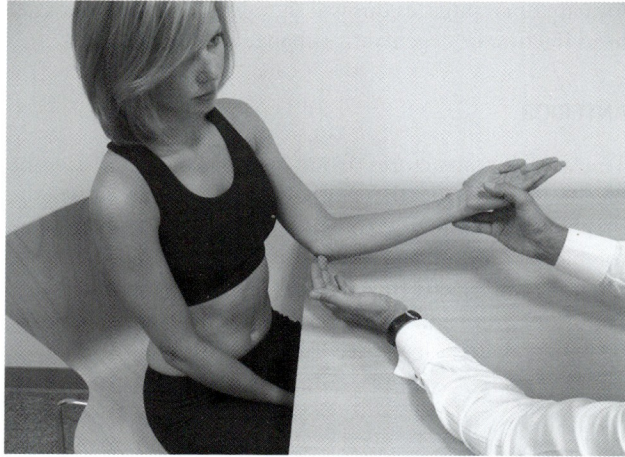

Figure 2.3 Tinel's test (ulnar nerve in cubital tunnel).

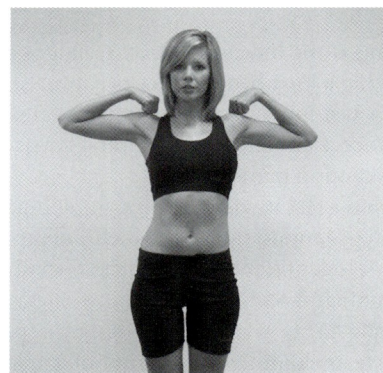

Figure 2.4 Elbow flexion.

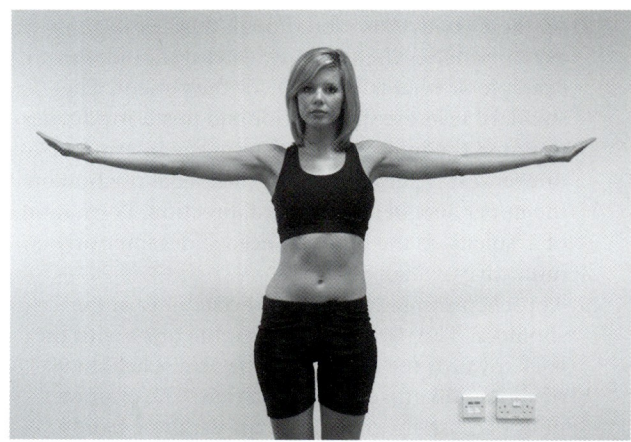

Figure 2.5 Elbow extension.

1. Lateral epicondylitis ('tennis elbow'). With the wrist in neutral, resisted wrist dorsiflexion results in localized pain over the lateral epicondyle. Pain may also occur if the test is done with the wrist in extension and radial deviation and on resisted extension of the middle finger. Another provocative test includes pain at the lateral epicondyle on passive volar flexion of the wrist with elbow extension and pronation. Pinch grip is also found to be weak and painful. Resolution of the pain with an injection of local anaesthetic at the attachment of ECRB will confirm the diagnosis by eliminating symptoms.

    Lateral epicondylitis should not be confused with PIN syndrome, which is compression of the posterior interosseous nerve at one of the following sites:
    a. arcade of Frohse (most common location)
    b. fibrous bands anterior to radial head (least common location)
    c. radial recurrent vessels (leash of Henry)
    d. tendinous origin of ECRB.
2. Medial epicondylitis ('golfer's elbow'). This is characterized by tenderness at the common flexor origin. There is pain on resisted palmar flexion of the wrist.

Medial epicondylitis should not be confused with pronator syndrome, which is a compressive neuropathy of the median nerve at one of the following sites:
a. between the two heads of the pronator teres muscle (commonest cause)
b. compression of the nerve from the fibrous arch of the flexor digitorum superficialis
c. compression at the thickening of the bicipital aponeurosis.

SPECIAL TESTS

Instability

Both valgus and varus testing are performed with the elbow in full extension and several degrees of flexion to about 30° to unlock the olecranon from the olecranon fossa.

Valgus testing is then performed with the elbow fully pronated so that posterolateral rotatory instability is not mistaken for valgus instability, which occurs because the ulna and radius as a unit rotate away from the humerus in response to valgus stress when the LCL is disrupted. Forced pronation prevents this from happening by using the intact medial soft tissues as a hinge or fulcrum, just as the periosteum is used for this purpose during the reduction of a supracondylar fracture in a child.

Varus testing is easiest to perform with the shoulder fully internally rotated.

Lateral pivot-shift test for posterolateral instability

Posterolateral rotatory instability is diagnosed by the lateral pivot-shift test of the elbow. With the patient in the supine position and the affected extremity overhead, the elbow is supinated with a mild force at the wrist and a valgus movement is applied to the elbow during flexion. This action results in a typical apprehension response with reproduction of the patient's symptoms and a sense that the elbow is about to dislocate. Reproducing the actual subluxation and the clunk that occurs with reduction can usually only be accomplished with the patient under general anaesthetic, or after injecting local anaesthetic into the elbow joint.

THE WRIST

Examination of the wrist follows the familiar 'look, feel, move' sequence followed by special tests. The hand, wrist and forearm should be exposed.

Inspection

Look for deformity, swellings, scars or muscle wasting. As the wrist is subcutaneous any deformity due to previous fracture or swellings should be easily visible.

Palpation

After asking the patient if there is a tender spot, start at the radial side of the wrist and move in a circle around the wrist, palpating the tender area last and with care.

Movement

Start with active followed by passive movements.

- Normal dorsiflexion is 75° test with palms together and lifting up the elbows (Fig. 2.6).
- Normal palmar flexion is 75°. Dorsum of hands should be in contact, and drop the elbows (Fig. 2.7).
- Normal radial deviation is 20° and ulnar deviation 35° in the neutral position.
- Test pronation–supination with elbows tucked in by the side. Ask the patient to hold a pen, and measure the angle between vertical and pen.
- Normal pronation is 75° and supination is normally 80° (Figs 2.8 and 2.9).

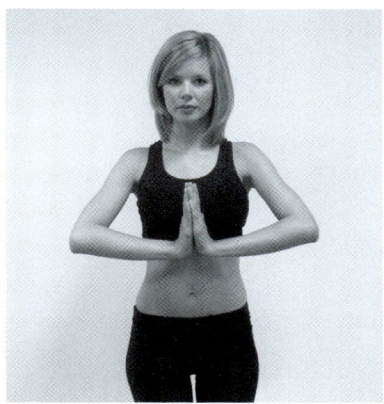

Figure 2.6 Wrist dorsiflexion (extension).

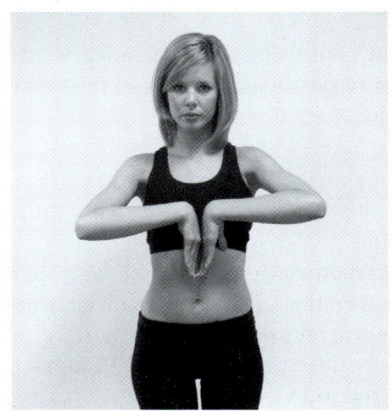

Figure 2.7 Wrist (palmar) flexion.

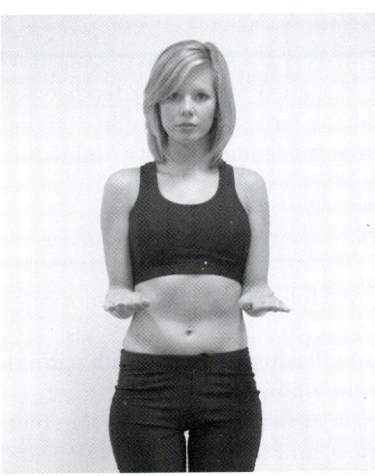

Figure 2.8 Forearm pronation.

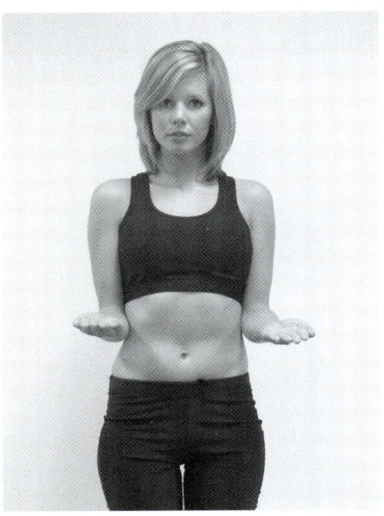

Figure 2.9 Forearm supination.

SPECIAL TESTS

If the patient complains of radial-sided wrist pain, there are a number of possible diagnoses so the following special tests should be done first.

- Finkelstein's test to rule out De Quervain's tenosynovitis – ulnar deviation with thumb in palm causes pain[9]
- Thumb carpometacarpal (CMC) joint arthritis test – pressing over the CMC joint and circumducting the thumb with axial pressure causes pain
- Scaphotrapeziotrapezoidal (STT) joint arthritis – resisted pronation causes pain.
- Wartenburg's test is done to check for intersection syndrome or superficial radial nerve irritation[10].

Distal radioulnar joint

The *piano key sign* is a test for distal radioulnar joint (DRUJ) instability. There is a prominence of ulna, and ballottement of the ulnar head is possible

In *the squeeze and turn test* the examiner stabilizes the patient's forearm with one hand while, with the other hand, he/she grasps the patient's hand as if for a handshake. When the patient resists forced passive rotation, or when there is active rotation against resistance, pain usually is elicited.

Triangular fibrocartilage complex

The *ulna impingement test* aims to elucidate triangular fibrocartilage complex (TFCC) problems. The examiner shakes hands with the patient, and ulnar deviates the wrist while rotating the forearm. Pain signifies a positive test.

Scapholunate instability

1. *Scapholunate ballottement* involves using both index fingers and both thumbs to stabilize the lunate between the thumb and index finger of one hand and the scaphoid between the thumb and index finger of the other; the scaphoid is then pushed in a volar to dorsal direction; discomfort in this area suggest the possibility of injury to the scapholunate ligament (SLL).
2. *Kirk Watson's scaphoid shift test* involves the examiner's thumb on the scaphoid tubercle and an index finger on the scapholunate ligament. The SLL initiates scaphoid flexion on radial deviation of the wrist. In the normal scenario one can feel the scaphoid flexing on radial deviation. With SLL injury, pressure of the examiner's thumb prevents initiation of flexion of the scaphoid as there is no SLL to pull the scaphoid into flexion. Therefore, palpation of a clunk on radial deviation of the wrist occurs due to sudden pressure from the surrounding bones.

Also the patient may withdraw the hand with pain. However, it is essential to compare with the contralateral wrist as up to 20% of 'normal' people have a positive test.[11] Watson's original description is reproduced below.

The patient is approached by the examiner as if to engage in arm wrestling, face to face across a table with diagonally opposed hands raised (right to right or left to left) and elbows resting on the surface in between. With the patient's forearm slightly pronated, the examiner grasps the wrist from the radial side, placing his thumb on the scaphoid tuberosity (as if pushing a button to open a car door) and wrapping his fingers around the distal radius. The examiner's other hand grasps at the metacarpal level, controlling the wrist position. Starting in ulnar deviation and slight extension, the wrist is moved radially and slightly flexed with constant thumb pressure on the scaphoid. This radial deviation causes the scaphoid to flex. The examiner's thumb pressure opposes this normal rotation, causing the scaphoid to shift in relation to the other bones of the carpus. This scaphoid shift may be subtle or dramatic. A truly positive test requires both pain on the back of the wrist (not just where you are pressing on the scaphoid tuberosity), and comparison with the opposite wrist is essential.

Lunotriquetral instability

1. *Lunotriquetral ballottement test (Reagan test)* – stabilize the lunate between the thumb and index finger of one hand and the triquetrum between the thumb and index finger of the other; the pisiform and triquetrum are pushed in a volar to dorsal direction; discomfort in this area suggests the possibility of injury to the lunotriquetral interosseous ligament.[9]
2. *Kleinman shear test (shuck test)* – the examiner sits opposite the patient, the contralateral thumb over the dorsum of the lunate, index finger over the pisiform. Pushing the pisiform dorsally arouses pain in the lunotriquetral joint.

Carpal tunnel syndrome

There are numerous tests described for carpal tunnel syndrome (Chapter 118).

- In Phalen's test, the elbows are placed on the table allowing the wrists to passively flex. If symptoms are provoked within 60 seconds then the test is positive.[13]
- This test has 61% sensitivity and 83% specificity.
- The carpal compression test is similar to Phalen's test, but with direct pressure from the examiner's fingers over the carpal tunnel, which makes the test more sensitive.
- Finally Tinel's test is done, which involves tapping lightly over the median nerve which reproduces symptoms in the nerve's sensory distribution – radial three fingers (Fig. 2.9)
- Always assess from distal to proximal.
- 74% sensitivity, 91% specifically.

Table 2.3 presents the differential diagnosis for wrist pain.

THE HAND

Examination of the hand is covered in more detail in Chapters 92 to 99 as it is always disease specific. This means that, in other words, the site and nature of the pain or deformity will determine your approach to the examination.

The broad topics in examination of the hand are deformities, neurological conditions and painful conditions. The principles of look, feel, move followed by special tests still apply.

Table 2.3 Wrist pain - differential diagnosis

Location	Cause
Radial	1. De Quervain's tenosynovitis
	2. 1st CMCJ OA
	3. STT OA
	4. Scaphoid non-union
	5. Ganglion
Dorsal/central	1. Ganglion
	2. Kienbock's disease
	3. Scapholunate dissociation
	4. Intra-osseous ganglion
	5. SLAC
Ulnar	1. Distorted DRUJ after distal radius fracture
	2. DRUJ OA
	3. TFCC tear with ulnar impaction
	4. Unstable DRUH
	5. Piso-triquetral OA
	6. Hamate hook fracture non-union

CMCJ, carpometacarpal joint; DRUJ, distal radio-ulnar joint; OA, osteoarthritis; SLAC, scapholunate advanced collapse; TFCC, triangular fibrocartilage complex.

Inspection

Expose the whole forearm and hand. Look at the dorsum and the palm and check for muscle wasting of the thenar, hypothenar and first dorsal interosseus. Ask the patient to open and close the hand quickly to assess mass movement of the hand.

Palpation

Ask for and feel the tender area if there is one. Pay particular attention to any swellings and nodules that may be present.

Movement

Ask the patient to make a fist (active mass motion) and then extend all fingers. Then examine the thumb, asking for opposition to all fingers in turn followed by adduction, abduction and flexion. The extensor pollicis longus (EPL) is then tested by asking the patient to lift the thumb off the table while the hand is held palm down on table.

The extensor digitorum communis is then tested by asking the patient to extend the fingers at the metacarpophalangeal (MCP) joints. The interossei are tested by asking the patient to abduct and adduct fingers. Remember that dorsal interossei abduct (DAB) and palmar interossei adduct (PAD).

Be sure to check the flexor digitorum superficialis (FDS) individually by holding other fingers in hyperextension, followed by the flexor digitorum profundus (FDP), which is tested by fixing the proximal interphalangeal (PIP) joint and thus isolating the distal interphalangeal (DIP) joint.

A *quadriga* is an ancient Greek four-horse chariot; thus the quadriga phenomenon describes the situation when testing for FDS where the FDP is defunctioned because the FDP tendons are combined while the FDS muscles are separate in the forearm.

Therefore, following repair or reconstruction of an FDP tendon, the tension must be identical to the other FDPs, since the excursion of the combined tendons is equal to the shortest tendon.

Special tests

SENSATION

In the hand sensation is vital. Therefore, sensory testing should be performed at the autogenous zones to ensure that the three major nerves are intact. The autogenous zones are: for the median nerve, the volar aspect of the index finger; for the ulnar nerve, the volar aspect of the little finger; and for the radial nerve, over the first dorsal interosseous muscle (dorsum of the first web space).

In addition, the superficial branch of median nerve sensation is over the thenar eminence. This helps discriminate between high and low median nerve lesions.

Dermatomes: C6, thumb and index finger; C7, middle finger; C8, ring and little fingers.

MOTOR

1. The median nerve is tested by testing the power of abductor pollicis brevis (APB) with the examiner's hand over the thenar muscles.
2. The ulnar nerve is tested by testing the power of
   a. The abductor digiti minimi (ADM) and first dorsal interosseous muscle together, by abducting fingers against resistance.
   b. *Wartenburg's sign* is where the little finger lies abducted due to the unopposed action of the extensor digiti minimi (EDM) and signifies a high ulnar nerve lesion.
   c. *Froment's test* is done by asking the patient to hold a piece of paper between the thumb and index finger and trying to pull the paper away. The key point is to ensure that the thumb is performing an adducting manoeuvre. In an ulnar nerve lesion the thumb will flex at the IP (median nerve) joint to prevent the paper from being pulled away. Froment describes this after watching a train commuter reading the newspaper with one thumb flexed and the other straight (Fig. 2.10).

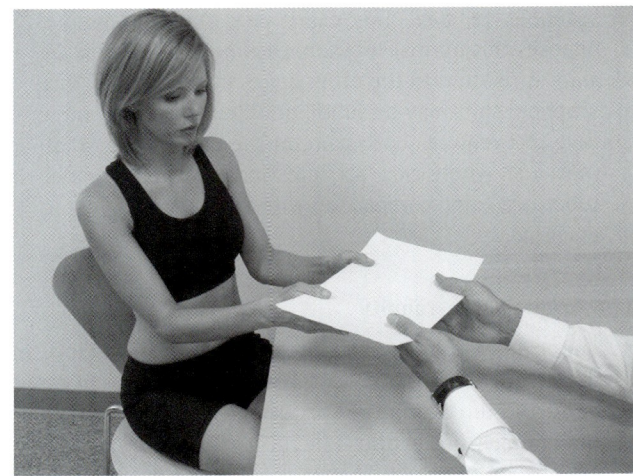

Figure 2.10   Frament's test.

   d. The *ulnar paradox* describes less clawing of the fingers than in a high ulnar nerve lesion than a low lesion, because the FDP is involved in high lesions, thus relaxing the IP joints.
3. The anterior interosseous nerve is tested by loss of precise pinch (unable to make 'OK' sign) due to loss of flexor pollicis longus (FPL) and FDP to the index finger (Fig. 2.11).[14]
4. The posterior interosseous nerve is tested when wrist dorsiflexion results in radial deviation (Fig. 2.7) (since the extensor carpi ulnaris (ECU) is supplied by the PIN, but the brachioradialis and ECRL are supplied by the radial nerve).
5. Superficial branch of radial nerve compression at the insertion of brachioradialis results in Wartenburg's neuritis.
6. The radial nerve is tested by asking the patient to extend the fingers and wrist against resistance.

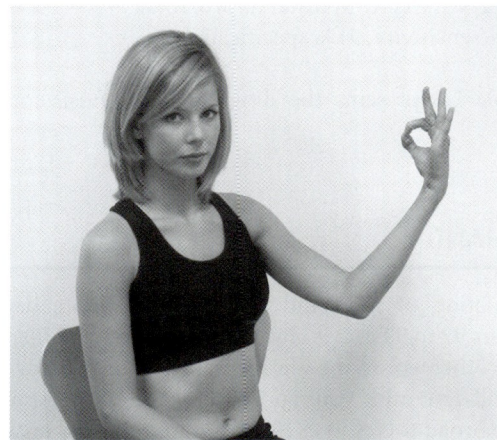

Figure 2.11   The OK sign for anterior interosseous nerve function.

Functional tests include power grip and precision pinch (AIN). Key grip pinch and strength is tested using a dynamometer.

Intrinsic tests are carried out in patients with hand deformity in order to differentiate intrinsic from extrinsic weakness or contracture.

To differentiate intrinsic contracture from forearm flexor contracture

Flexing the wrist relaxes the patient's FDS and FDP (long flexor) tendons; if the patient can then flex the IP joints with the wrist flexed there is intrinsic tightness; if they cannot it is a Volkmann's contracture (long flexors).

The *Bunnel–Littler test* is carried out for intrinsic tightness.

1. With the MCP joint in extension the intrinsics are put on a stretch. Try to flex the PIP joint with the MCP joint in extension. If it does not flex then there is joint capsule contracture or tight intrinsics.
2. With the MCP joint in flexion the intrinsics are relaxed. Thus, if the patient is unable to flex the PIP joint then the capsule is tight. Note that prior to the test check that passive motion of the PIP joint is possible (i.e. normal PIP joint). Tight intrinsics occur in 'intrinsic plus' hands due to ischaemia or fibrosis of intrinsics or rheumatoid arthritis.

Bouvier's test is carried out to determine if the PIP joint capsule and extensor mechanism are working normally.

If the PIP joint capsule and extensor mechanism are functionally normal, then blocking MCP joint hyperextension allows IP joint extension.

A positive test occurs as a result of attenuation of central slip, adherent central slip at the PIP joint or volar subluxation of the lateral bands.

Tests for traumatic boutonniere deformity

There are a number of tests for traumatic boutonnière deformity which are important to master. They are as follows:

1. *Elson's test.* Put the finger over edge of the table, with the PIP joint flexed to 90° and ask the patient to extend against resistance. Weakness of resisted extension of the PIP joint and hyperextension of the DIP joint occurs if the central slip is ruptured.
2. *Passive test.* Flex wrist and the MCP joints. Poor passive resistance to pushing over the middle phalanx indicates weak extensor mechanism.
3. *Boye's test* (1970). If the PIP joint is held passively extended, it is then possible for the normal individual to flex the terminal IP joint in isolation. However, if the central slip has been ruptured, there is increasing difficulty in performing this action. This test only becomes positive when the proximal part of the rupture's central slip has retracted and has become adherent to the surrounding tissues.

CLINICAL EXAMINATION OF THE LOWER LIMB

THE HIP

History

Hip conditions can present with a range of symptoms: stiffness, limping, instability, clicking, snapping, clunking, recurrent falls and pain. The cardinal symptom is often pain, and an accurate history of the timing, onset and exact nature can be a useful tool to aid diagnosis. The location of pain may be vague and non-specific, and patients can present with groin, outer thigh and pain referred to the back, buttock or knee. The timing of pain may also be relevant: early-morning pain that improves with activity throughout the day is suggestive of an inflammatory process, whereas pain which worsens with activity is suggestive of OA. Night pain which occurs in certain positions may be due to bursitis or tendinopathy. Constant night pain must raise the suspicion of joint pathology, including OA, infection or malignancy. Enquire about associated systemic symptoms of weight loss, fever and night sweats.

The nature of the pain can also give clues to the diagnosis; if the pain is sharp and acute with associated symptoms of 'locking' or giving way, consider labral pathology. Pain associated with specific movements can be related to a single musculotendinous unit, tendinitis or bursitis.

If the patient complains of stiffness, ask them what it most restricts them doing, and any exacerbating or relieving factors. The pattern of capsular restriction in the hip joint is internal rotation > flexion > abduction = extension > other movements. Exclude other anatomical sites as a source of 'hip' pain. In the lumbar spine, consider lumbar disc prolapse, OA, ankylosing spondylitis and malignancy. Enquire about peripheral neurological symptoms and consider peripheral nerve entrapment syndromes. Inguinal herniae, previous surgery in the inguinal region, psoas pathology, abdominal wall or intra-abdominal pathology can all present with hip pain and you should enquire about genitourinary or abdominal symptoms.

It is important to ask the patient about relevant past medical history: primary or secondary spine, hip, knee or ankle OA or any previous hip surgery. Ask if they had any hip problems or surgery in childhood, specifically developmental dysplasia of the hip (DDH), Perthes' disease, transient synovitis, slipped capital femoral epiphysis (SCFE) and hip dysplasia. Past history of rheumatoid arthritis, Reiter's syndrome, tuberculosis, or any other cause of septic arthritis in the hip joint is also relevant.

There are several validated scoring systems that assess different functional parameters, including pain, gait, activities of daily living, and some incorporate radiological findings. The modified Harris score is measured by an examiner and scored out of 100. Other widely used scores include the Oxford hip score, which is a questionnaire

Table 2.4 Lower limb myotomes

	Action	Muscles
L1, L2	Hip flexion	Iliopsoas
L2/L3	Hip adduction	Adductor longus/magnus
L3, L4	Knee extension	Quadriceps femoris
L4	Ankle dorsiflexion	Tibialis anterior
L5	Toe extension	Extensor digitorum longus/hallucis longus
L4/L5	Hip abduction	Gluteus medius/minimis
L5, S1	Hip extension	Gluteus maximus
S1	Knee flexion	Hamstrings
S1, S2	Ankle plantarflexion	Gastrocnemius, soleus
S1, S2	Toe flexion	Flexor digitorum/hallucis longus

completed by the patient, and the WOMAC Osteoarthritis Index, which is not specific for the hip.

Examination

Examination of the hip should be performed with a systematic, ordered approach, but using positive or negative findings to direct the examination and which special tests should be performed or other anatomical regions examined in detail. Follow the general principle of 'look, feel, move' and include assessment of the knee, lumbar spine and pelvis. Hip examination can be quicker and smoother if you perform all the relevant inspection, palpation, movements and special tests with the patient first standing, then supine, and finally in the lateral position and prone rather than asking the patient to constantly change positions.

LOOK

Begin with the patient standing, exposed to their underwear from the waist down. Inspect the hips for any obvious deformity or asymmetry, muscle wasting (particularly gluteal and quadriceps), skin changes, sinuses, previous surgical scars, bony prominences and leg length. Expose the spine and look for scoliosis, excessive lumbar lordosis, other deformity or scars from previous surgery.

Gait

Ask the patient to walk several paces away and then back towards you while watching the gait and posture. In particular, look for a Trendelenburg, antalgic or extensor lurch gait (see 'Gait' section, p.31).

Trendelenburg test

This important test was initially described by Trendelenburg in 1895 in children with developmental dysplasia of the hip. It is performed with the patient facing the examiner with outstretched palms facing the floor, resting on the examiner's hands. Alternatively, the examiner can rest the patient's palms on their forearms as they feel for the anterior superior iliac spine (ASIS) bilaterally. As the patient stands on each leg in turn, the pelvis should remain level, and if the pelvis drops to the unsupported side, or the patient uses the contralateral upper limb for support on the examiner, the test is positive in the standing limb. This identifies abductor weakness, which can be due to pain, atrophy, polio or a mechanical disadvantage due to longstanding DDH or coxa vara.

Leg length

Leg length inequality can be assessed in several ways. Initially with the patient standing, look for obvious limb shortening and compensatory posture; the patient may stand with a tilted pelvis, or have developed a lumbar scoliosis. Alternatively, the longer limb can be held with the knee flexed or the shorter limb with the ankle in plantarflexion with the heel off the ground. With the patient standing, wooden blocks can be placed under the short leg to correct the limb length inequality while assessing the lumbar spine and pelvis.

With the patient supine, feel for the ASIS bilaterally and ensure the pelvis is square on the couch. To assess the apparent leg length, measure from a fixed midline point (e.g. xiphisternum) to the medial malleolus bilaterally. Apparent leg length shortening can be due to a fixed adduction deformity. To assess 'true' leg length, measure from the ASIS to the medial malleolus on each side and compare, placing the unaffected limb in the same position as the affected side if there is a fixed flexion or adduction deformity (Fig. 2.12).

Shortening can be 'true', where there is shortening of the femur or tibia, or apparent. Apparent shortening can be due to a fixed adduction deformity in OA. True shortening of the femur can originate from above or below the greater

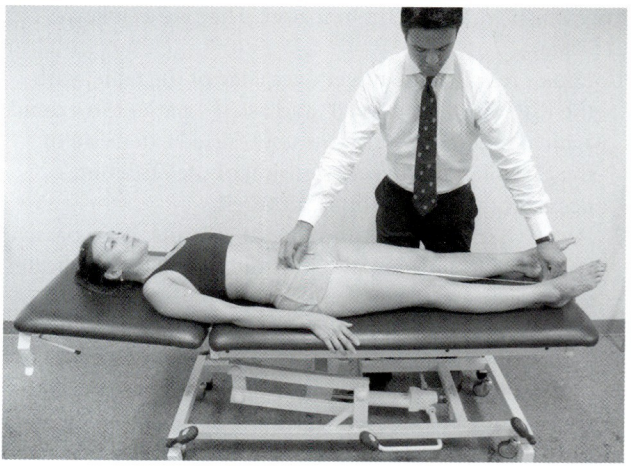

Figure 2.12 Measurement of leg length from ASIS to medial malleolus ('true' leg length).

trochanter, which can be assessed clinically. The simplest test is to place the thumbs under the ASIS bilaterally and the index fingers over the greater trochanters, and compare the distance between the two sides. This forms one line of Bryant's triangle, which is completed by a vertical line from the ASIS to the couch, and a horizontal connecting line. A difference in length of this horizontal line between the sides suggests unilateral shortening above the trochanter. The tip of the greater trochanter should not be palpable above Nelaton's line, between the ASIS and the ischial tuberosity, a finding which would again suggest shortening above the trochanter.

Perform Galleazzi's test with the knees flexed to 90°, the heels placed together on the couch and look from the side; if the femur is shortened, the knee will lie more proximal; if the tibia is shortened, it will lie more distal to the opposite knee. With the patient in the prone position tibial shortening can be clearly demonstrated with the knees flexed to 90° and the heels together; any difference in length should be apparent and easily measureable. Femoral anteversion can also be assessed by palpating the greater trochanter while internally and externally rotating the femur with the knee flexed to 90°.

Feel

The hip is the deepest joint in the body and cannot be palpated directly; however, there are several important bony and tendinous landmarks that can be palpated around the hip joint. The ASIS is an important structure; it is used to determine alignment of the pelvis and marks the origin of sartorius and the tensor fascia latae. The pubic tubercle is palpable lateral to the pubic symphysis at the medial end of the inguinal ligament. The origins of rectus abdominus and adductor longus tendons lie distally, and in the normal hip the pubic tubercle lies at the same level as the greater trochanter. This is more easily palpable along the posterior border, where there is less muscle coverage, and provides attachments for the abductors (gluteus medius, gluteus minimus) and short external rotators of the hip. From behind, the posterior superior iliac spine can be palpated in the area of the sacral dimples, in addition to the ischial tuberosity, which provides attachments for the hamstrings and adductor magnus.

The origin of adductor longus can be palpated distal to the pubic tubercle with the patient supine, knee flexed and hip abducted, which can be tender following an acute adductor strain and contracted in longstanding OA. The insertion of iliopsoas can be palpated at the lesser trochanter with the patient supine while externally rotating the hip in neutral.

Move

Movements of the hip can be active, passive or resisted. Active movements of the hip can give an indication of the range of movement and integrity of musculotendinous structures. Passive movements are performed by the examiner to elucidate the maximal range of each movement, and the end-feel can be assessed: hard (bone), capsular, ligamentous or soft (soft-tissue approximation), elastic (e.g. hip flexion with knee in extension) or have an abrupt end due to protective muscle spasm. Resisted movements test the integrity and power of individual or groups of musculotendinous units. This examination can elicit pain and weakness, which can be present alone or in combination. Weakness can be due to muscle/tendon rupture, tendinopathy, atrophy or pain. Muscle atrophy can be due to a central or peripheral neurological condition or result from disuse (e.g. as a result of hip pain from OA).

FLEXION (MAXIMUM 100–140°)

With the patient relaxed in the supine position, the examiner flexes the knee with one hand stabilizing with gentle pressure over the patella, and moves it towards the patient's chest. In the normal hip, maximal flexion is often limited by soft-tissue apposition between the abdomen and thigh. To assess the power of the iliopsoas, the principal hip flexor, the patient is seated on the edge of the couch with legs hanging freely. The patient then lifts the thigh off the couch against resistance from the examiner.

EXTENSION (MAXIMUM 10–30°)

With the patient in the prone position, the pelvis is stabilized by exerting downward pressure with one hand and the thigh is lifted off the couch until the pelvis starts to rotate anteriorly. To assess the power of the gluteus maximus, the principal hip extensor, ask the patient to lift the leg off the couch with the knee flexed to 90° while still in the prone position. Extension can also be assessed in the lateral position with the contralateral limb on the couch.

ABDUCTION (MAXIMUM 30–60°)

With the patient the supine position, the pelvis is stabilized by placing a hand on the contralateral ASIS and exerting gentle pressure, with the forearm resting on the ipsilateral ASIS. The hip is abducted with the knee in extension. To assess the power of the abductors in the lateral position, flex the knee to relax the iliotibial band and ask the patient to abduct the lower limb against resistance.

ADDUCTION (MAXIMUM 20–45°)

With the patient in the supine position, the pelvis is again stabilized by placing a hand on the contralateral ASIS. Ideally, adduction is assessed with the contralateral lower limb out of the plane of movement by either abduction of the limb or flexion of the hip by an assistant. Otherwise, lift the affected lower limb into minimal flexion to clear the opposite limb during adduction. Adductor power can be assessed on both sides simultaneously in the supine position by adducting against resistance.

INTERNAL ROTATION (IR) IN 90° FLEXION (MAXIMUM 20–45°) IN EXTENSION (MAXIMUM 20–35°)

With the patient in the supine position, rotate the lower limb with the knee in extension, then flex the knee and hip to 90° and stabilize by holding the knee. Pull the foot laterally, which rotates the hip internally. In the prone position with the knees flexed to 90°, the two sides can be internally rotated and compared. This is a sensitive test and is useful for detecting minor restrictions of movement in early OA. Power can be assessed bilaterally in the same position by asking the patient to swing their feet outwards against resistance.

EXTERNAL ROTATION (ER) IN 90° FLEXION (MAXIMUM 40–60°) IN EXTENSION (MAXIMUM 40–50°)

With the patient in the supine position, rotate the lower limb with the knee in extension, then flex the knee and hip to 90° and stabilize by holding the knee. Bring the foot medially, which rotates the hip externally. In the prone position with the knees flexed, the two sides can be externally rotated and compared by crossing the legs. Power can again be assessed bilaterally in the same position by asking the patient to swing their feet together against resistance. External rotation is limited by significant femoral neck anteversion.

Special tests

MODIFIED THOMAS' TEST

The modified Thomas test is used to assess fixed flexion deformity due to either hip joint pathology or iliopsoas or rectus femoris contracture. The hips may initially appear to be in 0° of flexion if the patient is compensating with an exaggerated lumbar lordosis. There are a number of variants of this test, and we describe one below. With the patient supine, the examiner first places a hand under the lumbar spine to assess for any lumbar lordosis at rest. Fully flex both hips and knees, which should obliterate the lumbar lordosis, and ask the patient to hold the knee on the unaffected side against their body. The patient is then asked to attempt to fully extend the affected hip. In a positive test, the hip remains flexed and the angle between the shaft of the femur and the couch demonstrates the degree of fixed flexion deformity. The affected hip should then be flexed up and the opposite side lowered to assess for contralateral fixed flexion (Fig. 2.13).

DUNCAN ELY TEST (RECTUS FEMORIS)

Ely's test is performed with the patient in a prone position to assess rectus femoris contracture. The ipsilateral thigh

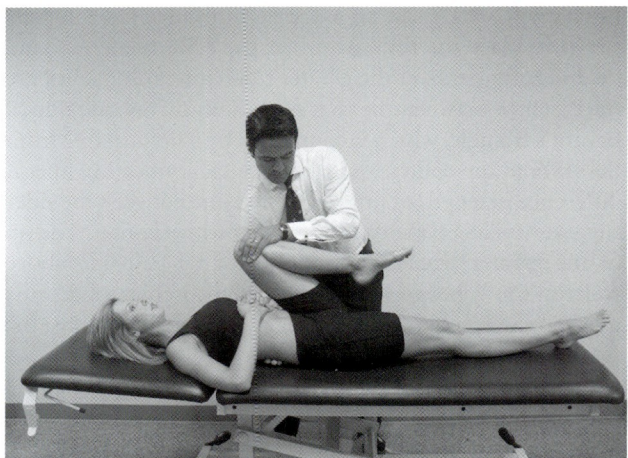

Figure 2.13 Thomas' test.

should remain horizontal, but a test is positive if the ipsilateral thigh and buttock rise off the couch. Recent research has suggested that intra- and interobserver reliability is only moderate.

OBER'S TEST

The Ober test is performed with the patient in a lateral position resting on the unaffected hip. The affected hip is placed in abduction and extension, and left unsupported. If it maintains the same position, the test is positive, indicating a tight illiotibial band.

FABER/PATRICK TEST

The FABER (flexion abduction external rotation) test (Patrick test) is performed with the patient supine by flexion, abduction, and external rotation of the affected hip by flexing the hips and knees bilaterally. To assess the right hip, the right foot is placed over the left knee in the 'figure-of-four' position and gentle downward pressure is exerted on the right knee, increasing the degree of external rotation. This manoeuvre can elicit pain in an osteoarthritic hip, and is often the first demonstrable sign, although it can also be positive with sacroiliac (SI) joint or psoas pathology.

CRAIG'S TEST (FEMORAL NECK ANTEVERSION)

Femoral neck anteversion is assessed with the patient in the prone position, the hip in neutral and the knee flexed to 90°. Anteversion ranges from 30° to 40° at birth and on average measures 8° in men and 14° in women; greater than this is abnormal. The affected hip is externally and internally rotated until the prominence of the greater tuberosity is felt laterally with the other hand. Anteversion is estimated as the angle between the leg and the vertical, and accuracy can be improved with the use of a gravity goniometer.

ANTERIOR/POSTERIOR IMPINGEMENT TESTS

The acetabular labrum is assessed by two separate tests for anterior and posterior labral tears with the patient in the supine position. The anterior impingement test or apprehension test is performed by passive flexion, internal rotation and adduction of the hip. A positive test is indicated by reproduction of symptoms of pain with or without a clicking sensation. The posterior impingement test is performed with the supine patient's hips at the end of the couch and the contralateral hip and knee held flexed by the patient. A positive test is indicated by pain as the affected hip is moved into extension and external rotation (Fig. 2.14).

FLEXION–ADDUCTION TEST

The flexion–adduction test is a provocative test for early hip pathology, which compresses groin structures and stretches posterior structures. With the patient in the supine position and hip flexed, the examiner exerts pressure on the flexed knee towards the contralateral iliac crest while stabilizing the pelvis. The end-feel, range of movement and discomfort can be compared with the unaffected side.

TELESCOPING OF THE HIP

Telescoping or pistoning of the hip can occur with previous DDH or following a total hip replacement with laxity of the soft-tissue structures.

SACROILIAC PROVOCATION

There are several different tests for SI joint pathology, which involve either direct stress across the SI joints or passively moving the hips. A simple screening test for SI joint pathology can be performed by pushing the ASIS apart with the patient supine and compressing the pelvis with the patient in a lateral position; this will identify anterior or posterior SI joint instability.

STRAIGHT LEG RAISE

Straight leg raise (SLR) can be used to assess hamstring length and sciatica. SLR is initially performed with the patient in the supine position with the knee in extension. The patient lifts their leg off the couch as high as possible and the examiner attempts gentle further flexion, noting the angle reached before any discomfort. With the leg at the maximal comfortable angle, the ankle is dorsiflexed by the examiner, and reproduction of radicular symptoms is a positive Lasègue's sign. SLR can then be repeated with the hip and knee starting at 90° flexion, and the patient is asked to extend the knee. The angle of knee flexion reached is noted and compared with the other side.

NOBLE COMPRESSION TEST

The Noble compression test assesses iliotibial band syndrome at the knee. With the patient supine, the hip partly flexed and the knee in 90° flexion, the examiner applies pressure 1–2 cm above the lateral femoral condyle while the patient actively extends the knee. A positive test is indicated by pain when the patient reaches 30° knee flexion.

PIRIFORMIS TEST

The piriformis test is performed with the patient in the lateral position lying on the unaffected side. With the knee flexed and the hip flexed to 60° on the affected side, downward pressure over the knee will elicit pain in the area of the piriformis in a positive test.

THE KNEE

History

Knee symptoms at presentation are not always pathognomonic, and delay from the time of injury to presentation can alter the pattern of symptoms. The patient's age, occupation, level of sporting activity and mechanism of injury are important clues to aid diagnosis. Enquire about any relevant past medical history (e.g. rheumatoid arthritis) or previous hip, ankle or foot injuries in addition to pre-existing knee conditions. Ask if the patient has had any previous treatment for the condition, or uses any walking aids or orthotics. Prevalence of conditions vary with age, and there is a range of patients seen in orthopaedic practice with knee problems,

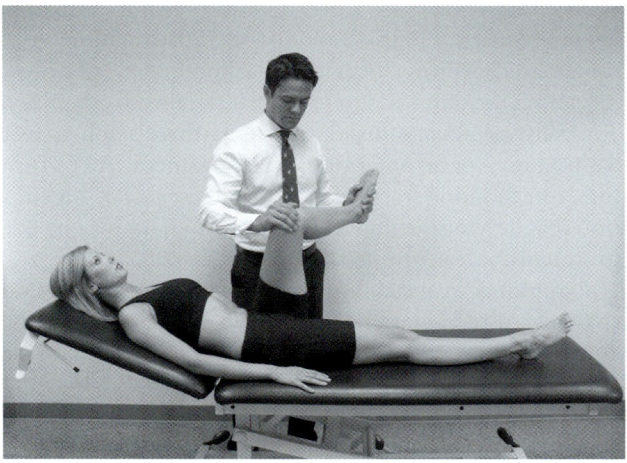

Figure 2.14 Internal rotation.

> ### Sample examination schedule: hip
>
> Now Mr Smith I would like you to take off your trousers, shoes and socks and sit here. Please start with your shoes. You may keep your shirt and underwear on.
>
> **Shoes: inspection**
>
> 1. These are off-the-shelf shoes.
> 2. There is no abnormal wear pattern.
> 3. There is no external or internal raise.
> 4. There is no arch support or orthotic.
> 5. No abnormal wear in the toe box.
> 6. There are no walking aids or wheelchair in the room.
>
> Now I am going to examine you standing, walking and lying down.
>
> - Check the gait – antalgic, extensor lurch, etc.
> - Perform the Trendelenburg test.
> - Look standing – from the front, side and back.
> - Inspection – swelling, wasting:
>   – Scars, sinus – e.g. Smith Petersen anterior scar.
>   – Deformity – e.g. hip flex, knee flex, foot equines, lumbar lodrosis present?
>   – From the back – shoulders same level? Scoliosis or kyphosis?
>   – Now place the patient supine and complete inspection of the groin.
>   – Feel – temperature – just lateral to femoral pulse is the femoral head.
> - Tenderness
>   1. ASIS.
>   2. Trochanteric bursa (bursitis).
>   3. Femoral head, capsule.
>   4. Adductor longus.
>   5. Hernia – cough.
>   6. ITB? Fascial defect.
> - Move
>   – Perform Thomas' test. For example, if right-sided pathology then
>   i. Place hand in lumbar lordosis to rule out exaggerated lumbar lordosis.
>   ii. Ask patient to actively flex the normal hip (left) and hold it – LL is obliterated.
>   iii. Look for flexion deformity on right side – check it is fixed. Check active and passive movement; for example – actively can extend 10 short of full extension, passively 5° so the FFD is 5°!
>   iv. With right hip flexed then bring (left) hip down – should be full.
>   v. Bring the right hip down.
> - Now flexion/extension is checked.
> - Next check rotation – no active – passive only
>   – Rotation in extension IR 0–30/40 ER 0–40.
>   – Rotation in flexion IR 0–30/40 ER 0–40/50.
>   – If there is differential rotation then this is a sign of early OA – the anterolateral (superior) part of head is affected and is painful during IR in flexion.
>   – Next check adduction and abduction. Now must square the pelvis.
>   – (Unmask fixed adduction or abduction deformity.)
>   – Make the ASIS Level. (ASIS lower = abduction deformity; ASIS higher = adduction deformity.)
> - Then measure leg lengths in that same position, with the squared pelvis.
> - Special tests as appropriate, e.g.
>   – Rectus femoris (Elys).
>   – ITB contracture (Ober).
>   – Apprehension (labrum), etc.

including anterior knee pain in adolescents, acute and chronic sports injuries, trauma, and inflammatory and degenerative conditions.

Pain is the commonest presenting symptom; ask the patient to describe the nature, severity, onset, location and any exacerbating or relieving factors. Anterior knee pain is a common complaint with a wide range of underlying aetiologies, e.g. patellofemoral pain syndrome, Osgood Schlatter's disease, etc. Patellar tendinopathy presents with pain and tenderness over the tendon, aggravated by jumping, squatting and lunging, which may become constant. Joint line pain can indicate meniscal pathology. Popliteal cysts can present with posterior knee swelling with or without pain. Synovial plica syndrome can cause intermittent anteromedial knee pain, and iliotibial band syndrome often presents with intermittent lateral knee pain triggered by running, and worse on descending stairs.

Swelling may be due to fluid (joint effusion, haemarthrosis, bursitis) or tissue inflammation (e.g. rheumatoid arthritis, pigmented villonodular synovitis). Ask about the onset and in particular the time from injury. Typically, an acute effusion or haemarthrosis will appear within hours of an anterior cruciate ligament (ACL) rupture, ostechondral fracture or large meniscal tear. An effusion that develops within 24 hours of an injury may be due to a meniscal tear or osteochondral injury.

Symptoms of instability or 'giving way', especially on changing direction rapidly, twisting movements of the knee or walking on uneven ground, are reported following an ACL rupture. If there is additional damage to other structures, e.g. medial or lateral meniscal and medial collateral ligament (MCL) injury, the knee can become very unstable and give way during normal daily activities. Instability is covered later in this section.

Patients with chronic meniscal tears will give a history of pain on turning, with recurrent episodes of localized pain and a small joint effusion. Acutely, they may present with restricted rotation, particularly external rotation and a loss of full extension with a springy block, which indicates locking. Locking is a commonly reported symptom, but true locking due to a displaced flap from a meniscal tear impinging on knee joint movement is less common. The locked joint may be held in one position, have a restricted range of movement, or lock intermittently as the flap moves in and out of the tibiofemoral articulation. Spontaneous unlocking may be accompanied by a 'clunk' with sudden reduction of pain and increased range of movement. Joint movement may be voluntarily or reflexively restricted if movement is painful, and lack of extension is the key symptom in true locking.

The mechanism of injury can give important clues to the damage sustained, prognosis and management. A high-energy road traffic accident, fall from height or other direct impact which suggests a significant force across the knee is likely to have caused significant injury. ACL rupture is typically a non-contact injury where the femur and upper body rotate with the foot planted. In a sporting context, the inability to continue sporting activity, inability to weight bear, or a 'popping' or 'snapping' sensation at the moment of injury are all significant.

Medial compartment knee OA presents with pain, stiffness and varus deformity, whereas lateral compartment knee OA more commonly presents with pain on climbing or descending stairs and episodes of 'giving way'. Patellofemoral OA can present with intermittent anterior knee pain, with or without crepitus, exacerbated by climbing stairs or standing from a seated position.

Examination

The patient's lower limbs should be adequately exposed, ideally wearing shorts or appropriate underwear. A complete examination of the knee should also include the hip and spine, which must be excluded as sources of referred pain. Clinical gait assessment is essential; the patient should walk several steps away from the examiner and return. Femoral anteversion (see 'Hip' section) and tibial torsion (see 'Foot and ankle' section) should also be assessed.

LOOK

With the patient standing, inspect the knee for varus or valgus deformity, swellings, erythema, scars, muscle atrophy or asymmetry, and any deformity of the ankles. Compare the two sides, check for any posterior swellings, and note the size, position and symmetry of the patellae. Ask the patient to walk the length of the room and return; look for any gait abnormality, including a fixed flexion deformity, locked knee or antalgic gait, noting any walking aids or orthotics (see 'Gait' section). With the patient supine, look for any fixed flexion deformity and compare quadriceps bulk with the contralateral side. Measure 'true' and apparent leg length, and determine if a true shortening is above or below the knee (see 'Hip' section).

FEEL

With the patient lying relaxed, supine on a couch, several important anatomical structures in the knee can be palpated as much of the joint is subcutaneous. Test for an effusion with the knee in extension (covered below). With the knee relaxed, resting in a few degrees of flexion, apply medial and lateral stress to the patella to assess the lateral and medial patellofemoral ligaments. With the knee flexed to 90° and the foot resting on the couch, palpate the menisci along the medial and lateral joint lines, which can elicit point tenderness over an area of meniscal pathology. Palpate the MCLs and LCLs for tenderness. The LCL is best felt with the leg in the 'figure-of-four' position with the leg crossed and the ankle resting on the opposite leg. This stresses the ligament, and helps to differentiate it from meniscal tenderness. Finally, palpate behind the knee in the popliteal fossa for any tenderness or swellings.

MOVE

The normal range of knee movement is 0–140° flexion, although a few degrees of hyperflexion is normal. Ask the patient to flex their knee, bringing their heel towards their backside testing active flexion, and then gently flex the knee further with the hip in flexion to test passive range of movement. During flexion and extension, the palm of one hand is rested on the patella, to feel for patellofemoral crepitus. With the patient sitting on the edge of the couch, patellar tracking can be assessed by asking the patient to actively flex and extend the knee and watching or feeling the patella. Compare extension and flexion of the affected knee with the contralateral limb.

Effusion

Gently ballot the patella in the fully extended knee. A positive *patellar tap* as the patella engages with the trochlea and femoral condyles denotes a large effusion. A small or moderate effusion can be detected by the *'bulge' test* (Fig. 2.15). After emptying the suprapatellar bursa into the joint and sweeping fluid from the medial compartment, a brisk sweep down the lateral compartment will cause a sudden, visible 'bulge' of fluid on the medial side.

Instability

Knee instability can occur as a result of trauma, overuse or a degenerative condition, and clinical examination can

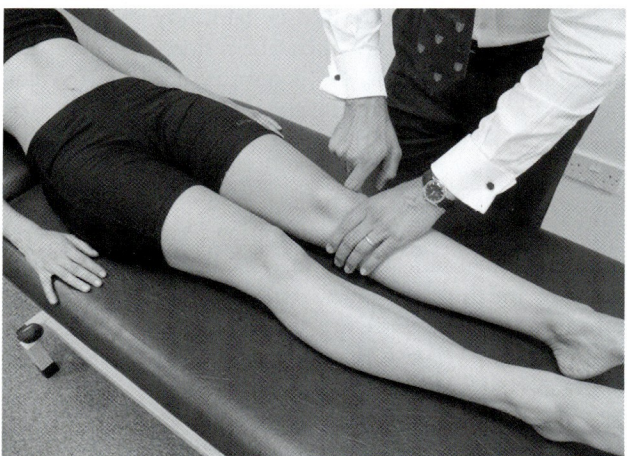

Figure 2.15 Patellar 'bulge' test for knee effusion.

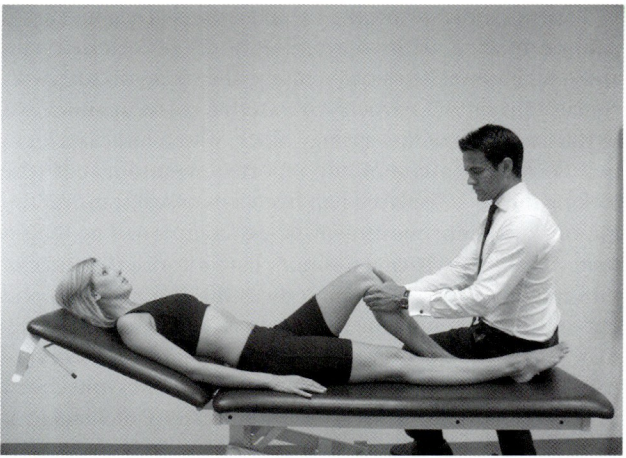

Figure 2.16 Anterior drawer test.

elicit the direction of instability, which can be defined as one plane, rotatory or combined. Combined instability can be anterolateral/anteromedial, anterolateral/posterolateral, or anteromedial/posteromedial, which can occur as a result of multiple ligament injuries and dislocations of the knee.

One-plane instability can occur in isolation or in combination and can be defined as medial, lateral, anterior, or posterior. Medial (or valgus) instability results from damage to the medial structures: joint capsule, MCL, posterior oblique ligament, semimembranosus tendon. Lateral (or varus) instability results from damage to the lateral structures: joint capsule, patellar retinaculum and expansions from the quadriceps tendon, iliotibial band, LCL and arcuate ligament. Posterior instability occurs as a result of damage to the posterior cruciate ligament (PCL) and posterior structures: the arcuate ligament posterolaterally, and the oblique popliteal ligament medially. The popliteus muscle adds stability, particularly in the flexed knee. Anterior instability results from rupture of the ACL.

Rotatory instability can be classified as anteromedial, anterolateral (flexion, extension), posteromedial and posterolateral. Anteromedial instability is due to MCL damage, augmented by ACL damage. Excessive external rotation of the tibia can be tested by repeating the anterior drawer test in external rotation (Fig. 2.16).

Anterolateral instability is due to ACL rupture, augmented by damage to lateral joint structures. Excessive internal rotation of the tibia with anterior subluxation of the lateral tibial condyle can be elicited by the pivot shift test and by repeating the anterior drawer test in internal rotation. Posteromedial instability is most pronounced with a combined PCL and MCL injury, and can be demonstrated as posterior sag with internal rotation.

Posterolateral rotatory instability (PLRI) indicates insufficiency of the posterolateral corner structures, particularly the arcuate and popliteofibular ligaments. Abnormal lateral rotation and posterior subluxation of the

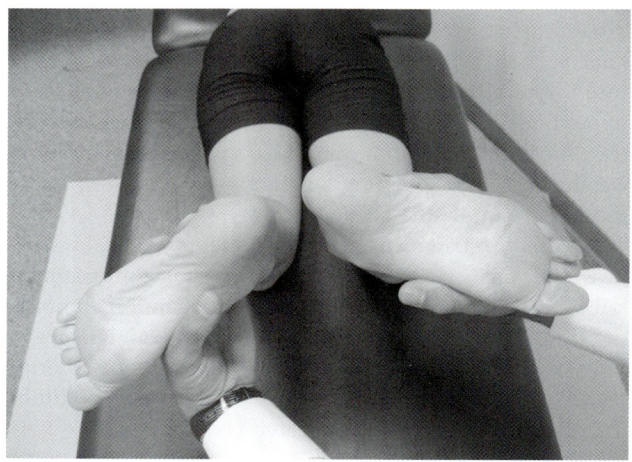

Figure 2.17 Dial test.

lateral tibial condyle can be demonstrated by the *external rotation/recurvatum test*. In a positive test, when the relaxed lower limb is lifted off the couch by the toes, the knee joint falls into slight varus, hyperextension with external rotation. With the patient prone, a positive '*dial*' *test* can be demonstrated by increased passive external rotation with the knee in 30° flexion. In a combined PCL and posterolateral corner injury the dial test is also positive at 90° of knee flexion (Fig. 2.17).

Medial collateral ligament and lateral collateral ligament

Apply gentle valgus stress to the knee with the joint in full extension and repeat in 30° of flexion, which tests the superficial fibres of the MCL. Feel for the degree of laxity and a firm endpoint. Apply varus stress in extension and 30° flexion to test the LCL. Palpate for the point of maximal tenderness following an MCL injury to localize the damage to the femoral attachment, mid-substance or tibial attachment. Opening of the joint by 5–8 mm more than the contralateral knee may indicate complete ligament disruption.

Grade I injury is a sprain of the superficial MCL with no demonstrable laxity. There is minimal or no effusion, with tenderness at the site of injury (usually femoral attachment) and pain on valgus stress in 30° of flexion but no instability, and the patient is able to weight bear. *Grade II* injury is a partial tear of the superficial MCL with laxity and intact deep MCL. Application of a valgus stress will demonstrate 10–15° laxity with a firm painful endpoint in 30° flexion. There will be swelling and tenderness localized to the site of injury (again, usually femoral attachment). *Grade III* injury is a complete tear of the superficial and deep layers of the MCL. On examination, over 15° laxity may be present and the endpoint has a 'mushy' feel in 30° of knee flexion.

Anterior cruciate ligament

The *anterior drawer test* is performed with the knee in 90° of flexion. Relax the hamstrings with the index fingers of both hands and, with thumbs adjacent to the patellar tendon, pull the tibia forwards. The degree of movement can be graded, but is subject to interobserver variation, although more than 6 mm is considered positive. The presence or absence of an endpoint is a useful finding.

Lachman's test (Fig. 2.18) works on the same principle but at 30° of flexion, and the distal femur is held in one hand while the proximal tibia is held with the other hand and brought forwards.[16] The feel of the endpoint can be assessed, and the displacement graded: grade I (5 mm), grade II (5–10 mm), grade III (>10 mm). In larger patients, it is sometimes easier to fix the femur between

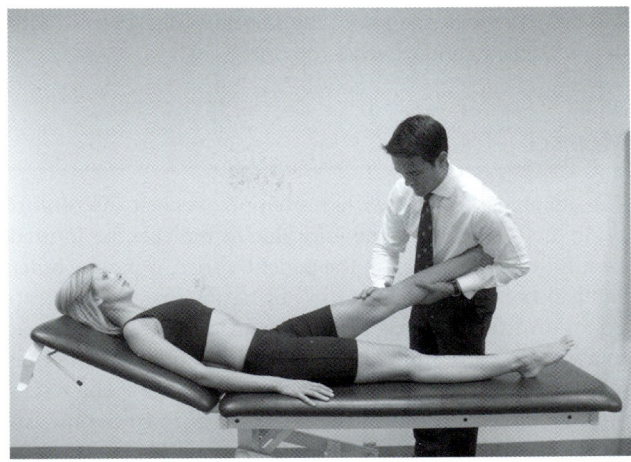

Figure 2.19 Pivot shift test.

the examiner's hand and flexed knee resting on the couch.

The *pivot shift test* (Fig. 2.19) recreates anterolateral subluxation of the tibia. The knee is held in full extension with the tibia in internal rotation between the examiner's upper arm and torso, and a valgus stress is applied with one hand. The knee is gently flexed, and, if the test is positive, the knee will suddenly reduce at around 20° flexion. The *jerk test* is undertaken the other way round – from flexion to extension, recreating the subluxation.

Posterior cruciate ligament

The action of gravity will cause a *posterior sag* of the tibia with the knees flexed at 90°; compare the two sides, as this can also help to exclude a false-positive anterior drawer sign in PCL rupture. The *step-off sign* is performed by the examiner sliding a thumb up the anterior tibia; normally there is a step-off posteriorly to the anterior surface of the medial femoral condyle. Following a PCL rupture, the tibia can sit flush or posterior to the medial femoral condyle, when a posterolateral corner injury should be suspected. The *posterior drawer test* is carried out at the same time as anterior drawer, and the degree of laxity and endpoint can be assessed: grade 1, lax but the tibia remains anterior to the femoral condyles; grade 2, anterior tibia lies flush with the femoral condyles; grade 3, the tibia lies behind the femoral condyles (with or without a palpable endpoint).

The *reverse pivot-shift test* describes the sudden reduction of the posteriorly subluxed lateral tibial plateau at 30° as the knee is held in external rotation and slowly brought from 90° flexion into extension. The *external rotation/recurvatum test* can also be performed to detect posterolateral instability. In a positive test, when the relaxed lower limb is lifted off the

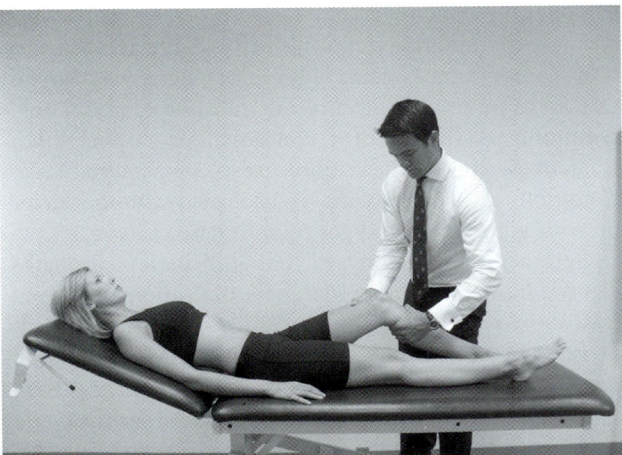

Figure 2.18 Lachman's test.

couch by the toes, the knee joint falls into slight varus, with hyperextension and external rotation.

Menisci

The adapted *McMurray's test* attempts to elicit discomfort along the medial or lateral joint line to indicate the injured area. Resting one hand on the patient's knee, using the other hand to hold the patient's foot, bring the knee slowly into extension from a flexed position with the knee in internal rotation, palpating the lateral joint line, and then external rotation, while palpating the medial joint line.[17] The test is most specific for a tear of the posterior horn of the medial meniscus. The *Childress duck waddle test*, where the patient waddles in a deep squatting position, may be useful in diagnosing a posterior horn medial meniscal tear in younger patients, and is positive when it provokes localized pain and clicking during early extension from the fully flexed position.

Coronary ligament sprain. The patient with medial coronary ligament sprain will have discomfort on full extension with localized tenderness and associated thickening along the joint line.

Plicae

The *'stutter' test* is performed with the patient sitting on the edge of the couch with legs hanging freely. Rest a hand over the patella and ask the patient to extend their knee; a 'stuttering' movement of the patella between 40° and 60° flexion indicates a positive test for a medial plica. Other tests for medial plicae include the *mediopatellar plica test* and *Hughston's plica test*.

Patellofemoral

The pull of the quadriceps on the patella is in line with the femur, whereas the patellar tendon, which inserts into the tibia, is almost vertical. This discrepancy between these two directions is known as the Q angle, which is made by a line drawn from the anterior superior iliac spine to the centre of the patella and a line drawn from the centre of the patella through the tibial tubercle. Average Q-angle values are 14° in men and 17° in women.

Look for vastus medialis obliquus (VMO) bulk, *patella alta* or *baja*, and lateral patellar tilt on sitting and standing, in addition to scars from previous surgery. Lateral deviation of the patella as the knee nears full extension is known as the *'J' sign*, which may be due to VMO dysfunction, tight lateral structures, trochlear dysplasia or a lateral tibial tubercle. Palpate the retinacular structures surrounding the patella, noting the location of any tenderness, in particular the medial patellofemoral ligament.

The *glide test* assesses patellar mobility: <25% indicates tight lateral structures, and >50% indicates hypermobility if present bilaterally, which is a common finding in adolescent females. The *patellar tilt test* is performed in 20° flexion, with the patella held between the examiner's thumb and index finger. If the patella cannot be tilted upwards laterally above neutral, this suggests tightness of the lateral structures.

The *patellar apprehension test* is performed by subluxing the patella laterally and flexing the knee; a positive test of pain, reflex muscular contraction and apprehension indicates previous dislocation. The *patellar compression test* is positive if flexion and extension cause pain while the patella is displaced inferiorly into the trochlear groove by the examiner. *Clarke's sign* indicates patellofemoral pathology, and is performed by asking the patient to contract their quads with the knee in extension while the examiner places a hand on the superior border of the patella and displaces the patella distally; pain and reproduction of symptoms is a positive sign.

FOOT AND ANKLE

History

Pain is the commonest presenting feature of a foot or ankle condition, and the exact location, nature and timing of the pain is important. Other presenting symptoms include stiffness, swelling, deformity, instability, weakness, numbness, burning and limping. Enquire about any symptoms or underlying conditions of lower back, hips or knees, as an abnormality in the lower limb can lead to compensatory alterations in foot and ankle biomechanics. Establish if the patient had any foot disorders during childhood, e.g. tarsal coalition, tibial torsion, etc. It is also important to gain an understanding of how the symptoms impact on the patient's daily life, work and sporting activities. Ask if the patient uses any orthotics or walking aids. If the patient presents following trauma, a detailed description of the mechanism of injury should be obtained.

Foot and ankle pathology can also present as part of a systemic condition, so a clear history and directed examination is important. Cardiac failure, peripheral vascular disease and venous insufficiency can all cause foot and ankle symptoms. A history of a congenital (e.g. spina bifida, Charcot–Marie–Tooth, cerebral palsy) or acquired spinal condition (e.g. poliomyelitis) is associated with foot deformities, e.g. pes cavus and pes equinovalgus.

Peripheral neuropathy, including diabetic neuropathy, can result in an insensate foot, with ulceration and degenerative (Charcot) joints. Rheumatoid arthritis may initially present with foot or ankle symptoms, as the forefoot, midtarsal joint and hindfoot can all be affected. These patients can develop metatarsalgia, claw toes, hammer toes, talonavicular arthritis, tibialis posterior tenosynovitis leading to rupture and pes planus, and a progressive hindfoot valgus deformity.

Patients may describe a sensation of walking on marbles or pebbles with metatarsalgia in rheumatoid arthritis or intractable plantar keratosis. Plantar fasciitis typically causes burning pain near the calcaneal origin of the plantar fascia, which is worse on the first few steps after getting out of bed in the morning, whereas the pain from foot or ankle OA tends to worsen with activity. The patient may describe a 'snapping' sensation over the lateral malleolus in peroneal tendon subluxation

Examination

The anatomy of the foot and ankle is complex, and there are several bones, joints, tendons and supportive structures to be considered. Range of movement should be assessed individually in the ankle joint, subtalar (talocalcaneal) joint and midtarsal (talonavicular and calcaneocuboid) joint. The relative alignment of the hindfoot, midfoot and forefoot, and the arches of the foot (medial longitudinal, lateral longitudinal, transverse and anterior) should be assessed in weight-bearing and non-weight-bearing positions. Ankle stability is assessed by examining the lateral ligament complex (anterior and posterior talofibular and calcaneofibular ligaments) and medial deltoid ligament complex (see 'Special tests' section).

The ankle supports up to 1.5 times bodyweight during walking, and up to five times body weight when running. To aid weight distribution and balance, the bony structure of the foot comprises several arches: the medial longitudinal arch is formed by the calcaneus, talus, navicular, cuneiforms and first three metatarsals. Support is provided by the spring ligament, plantar fascia, abductor hallucis, flexor hallucis longus and tibialis anterior and posterior. Disruption of any or all of these structures can contribute to pes cavus and pes planus deformities. The shallower lateral longitudinal arch is formed by the calcaneus, cuboid, and fourth and fifth metatarsals, supported by the plantar fascia, plantar ligaments and the peronei. The transverse and anterior arches are of less clinical significance.

The ankle and subtalar joints work in combination during gait, and any reduction in joint mobility can alter the load-bearing distribution and result in an abnormal gait. This can lead to pain and degenerative change in adjacent joints as the biomechanics are altered. When describing a deformity, one should comment on whether it is fixed or flexible, as this has implications for prognosis and management. Complete examination of the foot and ankle should include neurovascular assessment of the lower limbs and clinical gait analysis.

LOOK

With the patient adequately exposed, inspect the anterior, posterior, medial and lateral aspects of the feet and ankles as well as the soles. Inspect footwear for abnormal or asymmetrical wear patterns, orthoses or insoles, and look for any walking aids. Ask the patient to remove any orthotic insoles from their footwear, place on the floor and stand on them; assess if the deformity is corrected. Perform a general inspection of the foot and ankle, looking for skin changes including those of peripheral arterial disease or venous insufficiency, old surgical or traumatic scars, erythema and fungal infection. Look for ankle oedema – is it localized or diffuse, unilateral or bilateral, pitting or non-pitting?

From in front, look for any asymmetry, splay foot, hallux valgus, abnormal swellings or exostoses, lesser toe deformities, bunions, bunionettes, nail changes or ingrowing toenails, and inspect between the toes. Inspect the sole, looking for distribution of callus, discrete keratoses, plantar warts, thickening of Dupuytren's disease. From behind look for swellings associated with the Achilles tendon, including a prominent posterosuperior calcaneal tuberosity. Look for movement of any swelling relative to the tendon to distinguish inflammation of the tendon from inflammation of the tendon sheath. If the posture of the hindfeet is asymmetrical, examine the spine, knees and hips with particular attention to leg length measurement.

Look at the general posture of the ankle and foot, including the medial arch, and any asymmetry or abnormalities in the hallux and the lesser toes. There are three common foot types in the general population; the hallux is the longest digit in the Egyptian foot (69%), the second digit in the Greek foot (22%), and the hallux and second toes are equal length in the squared foot (9%). Abnormalities to look for include pes planus, pes cavus, splaying of the forefoot, hallux valgus, metatarsus primus varus and lesser toe deformities (e.g. under-riding/over-riding toes, claw toe, hammer toe, mallet toe).

In the normal foot, there is a narrow lateral weight-bearing area, and moderate callus under the heel and first metatarsal head. In pes planus, the lateral weight-bearing area is widened, and there is increased callus under the metatarsal heads. With the patient standing, attempt to insert two fingers under the medial arch and repeat with the great toes dorsiflexed. The examiner should be able to insert two fingers at least 2 cm easily; any less indicates pes planus, and more indicates pes cavus.

The heel is normally in 5° of valgus when weight bearing, and can be measured at the intersection of a line along the long axis of the tibia and the calcaneum. The fourth and fifth digits should be visible from behind, but in pes planus the second and third digits may also be seen – the 'too many toes' sign. In metatarsus adductus, the hallux and second toe may be seen medially. As the patient stands on tip-toes, the heel should move into varus; failure to do so may be due to a fixed subtalar joint (OA, tarsal coalition) or tibialis posterior insufficiency. The *Windlass mechanism* describes the action of the plantar fascia, which tightens and supports the medial longtitudinal arch as the great toe is dorsiflexed. It can be examined passively with the patient seated, or observed from behind as the patient stands on

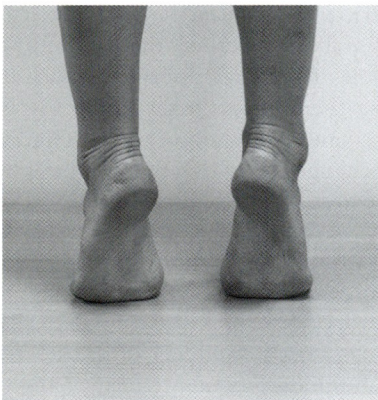

Figure 2.20 Heel raise stance.

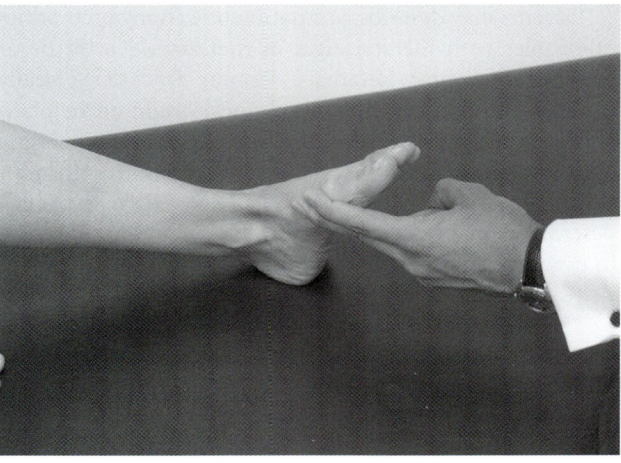

Figure 2.21 Tibialis anterior.

tip toes (Fig. 2.20). The effectiveness of this mechanism is reduced by lateral subluxation of the first metatarsophalangeal (MTP) joint in hallux valgus. Comment on whether a pes planus or planovalgus deformity is fixed (rigid) or flexible (correctable).

FEEL

Palpation of bony landmarks and important soft-tissue structures should be performed in a systematic manner, considering the hindfoot, midfoot and forefoot sequentially. A complete examination should always include assessment of peripheral pulses.

From medial to lateral across the dorsum of the ankle, medial malleolus, tibialis anterior (TA), extensor hallucis longus, extensor digitorum longus, peroneus tertius, and lateral malleolus can be palpated. Peroneus brevis and peroneus longus can be palpated in the peroneal sulcus behind the lateral malleolus, and tibialis posterior behind the medial malleolus. The medial and lateral malleoli are prominent and easily palpable subcutaneous structures and the tendons are most easily visualized and palpated by contraction against resistance (see 'Move' section). Tenderness along the course of a tendon may signify tendinitis or tenosynovitis. To distinguish between the two conditions, move the tendon passively with a finger over the point of tenderness; if the mass moves or the pain diminishes, this indicates tendinitis, if not it indicates tenosynovitis.

From behind, the calcaneum (os calcis) can be palpated; medial–lateral compression can cause tenderness in the presence of a stress fracture. Palpate the insertion of the TA, and the tendon itself, noting the location of any tenderness or swelling (Fig. 2.21).

The sinus tarsi, a bony tunnel between the talus and the calcaneum covered by the extensor retinaculum, can be palpated distal to the lateral malleolus. The tarsal tunnel lies distal to the medial malleolus covered by the flexor retinaculum, and contains several structures including the posterior tibial nerve. In a patient with tarsal tunnel syndrome causing nerve compression, percussion over the posterior tibial nerve can elicit pain and paraesthesia (positive Tinel's sign) over the area of the sole supplied by the medial and lateral plantar nerves. This sensation can also be replicated by stretching the nerve by passive toe dorsiflexion.

Laterally, the anterior talofibular ligament (ATFL) can be felt in front of the lateral malleolus with the ankle passively plantarflexed and inverted, and the calcaneofibular ligament (CFL) can be felt at the posteroinferior aspect of the lateral malleolus with the ankle inverted. The posterior talofibular ligament (PTFL) can also be felt by pressing firmly behind the lateral malleolus with the ankle dorsiflexed. Medially, the components of the deltoid ligament and spring ligament can be palpated, although less easily, in addition to the sustentaculum tali. More distally, the talar head and navicular tuberosity, first tarsometatarsal (TMT) joint, and first MTP joint can be palpated medially, and the calcaneocuboid joint, base of the fifth metatarsal and fifth TMT joint laterally.

The plantar fascia and its origin at the anteromedial tuberosity of the calcaneum should be palpated, noting tenderness and fibromatoses. Tenderness under the metatarsal heads on the plantar surface caused by synovitis may be due to rheumatoid arthritis. A positive *squeeze test*, pain elicited by mediolateral compression of the forefoot, is found in these patients. A discrete, tender callus under a lesser metatarsal head is typical of intractable plantar keratosis, and the patient will commonly have a long second metatarsal. Tenderness and swelling over the dorsum and pain on passive movement of the lesser MTP joints, particularly the second and third MTP joint, is indicative of Freiberg's disease. Morton's neuroma, most common between the third and fourth metatarsal heads, can cause pain and paraesthesia radiating to the adjacent toes. You may find a well-localized area of tenderness, a positive squeeze test, and a positive Mulder's sign (see 'Special tests' section).

In addition to the deformity of the great toe in hallux valgus, there may be tenderness and abnormal callus under the second metatarsal head from transfer metatarsalgia. Tender dorsal/medial osteophytes may be found in a stiff first metatarsophalangeal joint in hallux rigidus.

MOVE

Active movements

Ask the patient to perform plantarflexion, dorsiflexion, inversion and eversion at the ankle in addition to flexion, extension, abduction and adduction of the toes.

Passive movements

Most movements are easily assessed with the patient in a seated position on an examination couch with legs hanging freely. Pain, crepitus and reduced range of movement are found in OA.

Combined movements: supination (35°) and pronation (20°)

The ankle, subtalar and midtarsal joints are involved in complex combined movements. Supination of the foot is achieved by a combination of inversion at the subtalar joint, adduction at the midtarsal joint and plantarflexion. Pronation is achieved by a combination of eversion at the subtalar joint, abduction at the midtarsal joint and dorsiflexion.

Ankle: plantarflexion (40–55°) and dorsiflexion (10–20°)

This is best assessed by grasping the calcaneum firmly in one hand, resting the foot on the examiner's forearm, while holding the distal lower leg above the ankle. In this position, the ankle can be plantarflexed up to 50°, and dorsiflexed up to 20°. The *Silfverskiold test* can be used to distinguish a tight gastrocnemius from other causes of reduced dorsiflexion (Fig. 2.22). Ankle dorsiflexion should be reassessed in maximal inversion.

Subtalar: inversion (20–30°) and eversion (5–10°)

By applying varus and valgus stress to the calcaneus with the ankle in neutral and the talar neck stabilized, the contribution of inversion and eversion of the subtalar joint to supination and pronation can also be assessed.

Midtarsal (Chopart) joint

By grasping the midfoot in one hand and stabilizing the hindfoot, the movement at the midtarsal joint can be assessed. Movement at this composite joint contributes to overall inversion, eversion, abduction, adduction, dorsiflexion and plantarflexion.

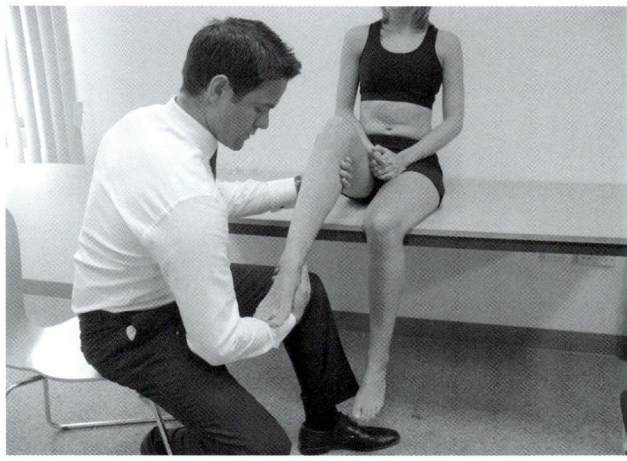

Figure 2.22 Ankle range of movement.

Tarsometatarsal (Lisfranc) joints

With the midfoot stabilized, the forefoot can be moved superiorly and inferiorly in the sagittal plane. The first, second and third tarsometatarsal (TMT) joints (medial longtitudinal arch) are much less mobile than the fourth and fifth TMT joints (lateral longtitudinal arch), which articulate with the cuboid, and the first ray should be assessed for hypermobility.

Metatarsophalangeal joints

The great toe (hallux) can be plantarflexed (70–90°) and dorsiflexed (60–90°) with the forefoot stabilized. A hallux valgus deformity may be rigid, but an attempt should be made to correct the deformity before performing these movements if it is flexible. Any pain, stiffness, impingement or crepitus should be noted, and the test should be repeated in the lesser toes, again noting any stiffness or deformity (e.g. hammer toe) and whether it is fixed or flexible.

Resisted movements

Resisted movements can be used to assess the strength of individual muscles or groups of muscles according to the Medical Research Council (MRC) grading system. They are also useful to identify individual tendons, and palpate for tenderness and localized swelling seen in tendinitis or tenosynovitis. *Peroneus brevis* (Fig. 2.23) can be easily identified behind the lateral malleolus during resisted eversion, and the adjacent *peroneus longus* by resisted plantarflexion of the first metatarsal ray with a finger held under the first metatarsal head. Peroneal subluxation can be demonstrated as the peroneal tendons snap forwards over the lateral malleolus during resisted eversion with dorsiflexion. The *tibialis anterior* has a large tendon that can be easily palpated over the medial side of the dorsum of the ankle during resisted inversion in dorsiflexion, while the *tibialis posterior* can be palpated behind the medial malleolus during resisted inversion in plantarflexion

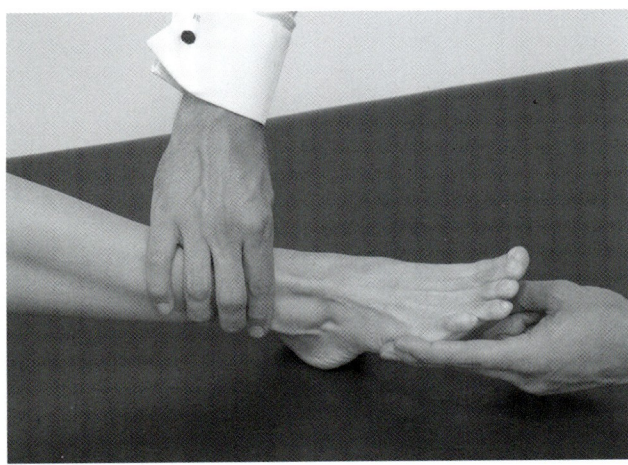

Figure 2.23 Peroneus brevis.

Special tests

ANTERIOR DRAWER TEST

The anterior drawer test assesses the integrity of the anterior talofibular ligament. With the patient sitting on the edge of the couch, the distal leg is stabilized and an anterior force is applied to the heel with the ankle in slight plantarflexion and medial rotation. A positive sign is defined as >8 mm of anterior translation, which can be confirmed on stress radiographs, and a 'suction sign' may be demonstrated anterolaterally.

TALAR TILT TEST

Talar tilt of >15° inversion when applying a varus stress implies anterior talofibular and calcaneofibular ligament rupture.

KLEIGER'S TEST

Kleiger's test assesses the integrity of the medial deltoid ligament and the distal tibiofibular syndesmosis. The examiner externally rotates the foot with the patient seated on the edge of the couch and ankle in neutral; increased rotation compared with the other side, which may be painful, implies deltoid ligament rupture. A syndesmotic injury can be more subtle, particularly in athletes, and its integrity can be tested by the examiner rotating the patient's body to mimic external rotation with the patient standing on the affected limb.

TIBIAL TORSION AND METATARSUS ADDUCTUS

Tibial torsion can be assessed with the patient prone with the knees together, flexed to 90°. The angle made by the medial border of the foot and the midline is normally 13–18°. Internal tibial torsion is associated in some cases with metatarsus adductus and can result in an in-toeing gait.

Femoral anteversion should also be assessed with the patient in the same position. Tibial torsion can also be measured with the patient prone, noting the angle between the transmalleolar axis and the bicondylar axis of the knee.

In children with an in-toeing gait, a number of clinical measurements can be made. The *foot progression angle* can be determined by a line in the direction of walking and a line down the long axis of the foot; a negative angle represents in-toeing. The *heel bisector* is a line drawn down the centre of the long axis of the hindfoot; this should bisect the forefoot between the second and third toes. If this bisects the third, fourth or fifth toes, this indicates metatarsus adductus. The *foot–thigh angle* is measured prone at the intersection of a line down the centre of the thigh and the heel bisector and is normally 0–10°, and represents the amount of tibial torsion.

FEISS LINE

The Feiss line is drawn between the apex of the medial malleolus and the plantar aspect of the first MTP joint. With the patient standing, the navicular tuberosity should be palpable at a point on the line. The degree of pes planus can be graded according to the distance it falls below this line: one-third of the distance to the floor equates to a first-degree pes planus, two-thirds below is found in second-degree pes planus, and, if it rests on the floor, this represents third-degree pes planus.

COLEMAN BLOCK TEST

The Coleman block test is used to differentiate between fixed and mobile hindfoot varus. The patient is observed from behind standing with one foot squarely on a 2 cm high wooden block. The foot is then moved medially so that the first metatarsal is unsupported, and the heel will adopt a more valgus position if the deformity is mobile.

TINEL'S SIGN

Percussion over the posterior tibial nerve behind the medial malleolus in tarsal tunnel syndrome can elicit paraesthesia over the area of the sole supplied by the medial and lateral plantar nerves.

MULDER'S SIGN

In a patient with Morton's neuroma, reproduction of symptoms and an audible 'click' produced by applying pressure over the plantar aspect of the affected interdigital space, while applying medial–lateral compression across the metatarsal heads, is a positive Mulder's sign.[19]

THOMPSON'S TEST/SIMMOND'S TEST

With the patient in a prone position or kneeling, compression of the calf muscles should result in plantarflexion of the ankle if the Achilles tendon is intact. Failure of the ankle to move due to a complete rupture of the Achilles tendon is a positive Thompson test.[20]

SILFVERSKIÖLD'S TEST

In a positive test, a patient with an isolated tight gastrocnemius will have significantly greater passive ankle dorsiflexion with the knee flexed than fully extended. If passive dorsiflexion is reduced with the knee extended, and does not significantly increase with the knee flexed, this indicates a tight gastrosoleus complex or an osseous equinus deformity.[21]

Gait

Ask the patient to walk several paces away and then back towards you across the room, while watching the gait and posture. Note also if the patient has any walking aids or orthotics, and comment on the wear pattern of the patient's footwear. The gait is divided into two main phases: stance (support) and swing (unsupported). The stance phase (60% of normal gait cycle) consists of the heel strike, mid-stance period and toe-off. The swing phase (40%) consists of acceleration and deceleration of the unsupported limb. The stance phases of the left and right lower limbs overlap, as a double support phase. Observe the alignment of the lower limbs in the sagittal, coronal and transverse planes and note where malalignment occurs, whether it is at the hip, knee, etc. Gage described five prerequisites which are essential to achieve a normal, efficient gait which should be considered (acronym: PACES):

1. Appropriate *P*repositioning of the foot during the swing phase.
2. *A*dequate step length.
3. Sufficient foot *C*learance during swing phase.
4. *E*nergy conservation.
5. *S*tance phase stability.

Comment on the pattern of any gait abnormality, e.g. antalgic, Trendelenburg, circumducting, steppage, etc. Neurological gaits can result from congenital or degenerative conditions, or trauma. The gait in cervical myelopathy is typically *broad-based* and *ataxic*. Hip flexors and extensors both work phasically in the initiation of gait, and eccentrically as the flexors slow and control extension and vice versa. The hip abductors are integral in maintaining the single stance phase (see 'Trendelenburg test'). A few commoner gait abnormalities are described below.

ANTALGIC GAIT

An antalgic gait arises from an attempt to minimize the load through the affected limb, resulting in a limp with a shorter single stance phase on the affected side, a shortened stride length on the contralateral side, and a longer double support phase. If the condition is bilateral (e.g. OA), this may be more difficult to detect, but the gait will be slow and deliberate.

TRENDELENBURG GAIT

A Trendelenburg gait can be caused by abductor, femoral neck or joint pathology resulting in the pelvis dropping towards the opposite side during the stance phase on the affected side. To compensate, the patient bends their trunk towards the affected side during the stance phase to reduce the moment of force acting on the affected hip by moving their centre of gravity closer. The *Trendelenburg test* is used to identify hip abductor weakness (see 'Hip' section).

EXTENSOR LURCH (GLUTEUS MAXIMUS GAIT)

The gluteus maximus muscle is the principal hip extensor, and is activated at the point of heel strike, slowing flexion and initiating extension to propel the body forwards. Reduced power in the gluteus maximus will result in an 'extensor lurch' at the point of heel strike, and forward motion is temporarily halted.

SCIATIC LIST

A patient with unilateral lumbar nerve root compression can walk with a sciatic list as they lean away from the side of the affected nerve root in an attempt to reduce the compression on the affected nerve root. This should be differentiated from a Trendelenburg gait, as the pathologies underlying the gait abnormalities are different.

LEG LENGTH DISCREPANCY

Patients with a true or apparent leg length discrepancy can demonstrate several different gait abnormalities in an attempt to compensate. This can be achieved by functionally shortening the longer limb: a *steppage* or *high-stepping gait* where hip flexion is exaggerated is used to compensate for a foot drop, and can be employed in combination with a *circumducting gait*, where the longer limb is abducted during swing phase. Alternatively, the shorter limb can be functionally lengthened, such as in a *vaulting gait*, where the ankle of the shorter limb is plantar flexed into a 'tiptoe' pattern during stance.

THE SPINE

Examination of the spine requires inspection, palpation, movements and special tests for the cervical, thoracic and lumbar region, although, in the clinical setting, a single region should rarely be examined in isolation.

History

Patients may present with a congenital deformity, degenerate condition or following trauma to the spine, and different conditions are obviously more prevalent in different age groups. If a patient presents with neck or back pain, enquire about the nature, exact location, timing of onset, and any radiation or referred pain. Other neurological symptoms include paraesthesia, loss of sensation, weakness, loss of coordination, gait disturbance and bladder or bowel dysfunction.

Ask how the symptoms impact on the patient's daily activities, work and exercise, and establish if there is any potential for secondary gain, e.g. from ongoing legal proceedings. There are several validated disability scoring systems, e.g. Oswestry Disability Index. Enquire about any relevant past medical history or previous surgery, as many conditions can present with symptoms of spinal origin, e.g. rheumatoid arthritis, ankylosing spondylitis, tuberculosis, primary and secondary tumours, OA and degenerative neurological conditions. Ask what treatment they have had in the past, e.g. medication, physiotherapy, acupuncture, etc.

Patients with cervical spondylotic myelopathy can present with neck pain and stiffness with brachialgia, numb, clumsy hands or weakness, which is worse in the upper than in the lower limbs. The pattern of dysfunction is of a lower motor neurone deficit at the level of the compression with upper motor neurone signs below due to compression of the dorsal column of the spinal cord. Cervical radiculopathy will present with pain, numbness and weakness in a specific dermatome or myotome in the upper limb. Thoracic cord compression is rare, as is thoracic nerve root impingement, which presents with rib or interscapular pain.

Thoracic outlet syndrome (TOS) can present with symptoms of arterial, venous or nerve compression. Vascular TOS can present with a gradual worsening of upper limb pain and fatigue, particularly on overhead activity. Neurogenic symptoms include painless atrophy of the intrinsic muscles of the hand, paraesthesia and reduced sensation in a C8/T1 dermatomal distribution, and less commonly pain.

Mechanical lower back pain is common, and may be postural or caused by discogenic pain of a degenerate lumbar spine. Nerve root impingement is commoner at the L4/5 and L5/S1 levels than in the upper lumbar region, and commonly presents with pain, paraesthesia, reduced sensation, and even weakness in a sciatic nerve distribution (L4/L5/S1), although patients can present with femoral nerve (L1/L2/L3) symptoms. Bladder or bowel dysfunction and loss of perineal sensation are signals of cauda equina syndrome and warrant urgent further investigation and treatment. Patients with lumbar canal stenosis (spinal claudication) often present with pain radiating down both legs not associated with a single nerve root. The pain is exacerbated by walking or standing for prolonged periods and is relieved by sitting or leaning forwards. Patients with spondylolisthesis at L4/5 or L5/S1 often present with lower back pain with or without sciatic symptoms.

Lower back pain is extremely common, but there are a number of features in the history which may indicate a sinister cause for the pain, including age under 20 or over 55 years, significant trauma, bilateral sciatica, systemic features of sepsis or neoplasia, and pain that is progressive, continuous and unrelated to activity. Any of these or a number of other 'red flag' symptoms warrants further investigation.

Examination

Depending on the presentation and the location of symptoms, examination of the spine should be accompanied by examination of other areas; cranial nerves, chest, abdomen, rectal examination, peripheral neurovascular examination and screening of relevant joints, e.g. shoulder, hip, knee, foot and ankle. Gait should always be assessed as part of the examination, and may reveal a characteristic abnormality, e.g. a patient with cervical myelopathy typically has a broad-based, ataxic gait (see 'Gait' section).

Cervical spine

LOOK

With the patient adequately exposed, look for any surgical scars, swellings, skin changes, asymmetry or differences between the upper limbs. Look at the posture of the neck. Is it held flexed? Is it hyperextended to compensate for a thoracic kyphosis? Does the patient have torticollis? In congenital torticollis, the sternomastoid muscle is larger on the side the head is tilted towards, whereas the opposite sternomastoid is larger in torticollis because of atlanto-axial subluxation.

FEEL

Standing behind the patient, palpate the spinous processes along the midline, working downwards from the occiput to include the prominent spinous process of C7 and the upper few thoracic vertebrae. Palpate the erector spinae muscles over the lateral aspects of the vertebrae, noting any tenderness and crepitus on flexion and extension. Palpate the anterior and posterior triangles of the neck, and for a cervical rib in the supraclavicular fossa. Finally, palpate the sternomastoid muscles, noting tension, swelling and asymmetry.

MOVE

Ask the patient to touch their chin onto their chest (forward flexion 75°), look up at the ceiling (extension 50°), touch their ear to their right and left shoulders in turn (lateral flexion 45°), and turn their head to the right and left (rotation 80°). Flexion and extension occurs mainly from C3–C7, with approximately 50° of rotation occurring at the atlanto-axial (C1/C2) joint.

Special tests

TESTS FOR CERVICAL RADICULOPATHY

Spurling's compression test (Fig. 2.24) is used to assess cervical radiculopathy by narrowing the vertebral foramina and compressing the affected nerve roots. The examiner applies gentle downward pressure on the patient's head with the neck laterally flexed towards the affected side. If the test is still negative, it can be repeated with additional lateral rotation and hyperextension of the neck.

The *shoulder abduction (relief) test* can immediately provide relief from symptoms of radiculopathy (especially C4, C5) by passively abducting the ipsilateral shoulder of a patient who is symptomatic at rest, or from the laterally flexed position in a patient who has a positive *Spurling's test*.

TESTS FOR CERVICAL MYELOPATHY

Lhermitte's sign is positive if hip and neck flexion in a seated position with the patient's legs on the couch elicit sharp shooting pain and paraesthesia down the spine radiating into the upper or lower limbs. *Romberg's sign* is positive if the patient is unable to stand still with feet together and eyes closed for 30 seconds without losing balance, and indicates an upper motor neurone lesion. *Hoffman's sign* is performed by rapidly flicking the patient's middle fingertip. Reflex contraction of thumb or index finger flexors is a positive test. The reflex can be reinforced by neck flexion or extension.

The 'finger escape sign' is positive if the little and possibly ring fingers drift into abduction or flexion when the patient attempts to hold the fingers extended and adducted. The 'finger fatigue test' is positive if the patient fatigues and is unable to rapidly flex and extend the fingers for 20 seconds. Other myelopathic signs include an inverted supinator reflex, a positive Babinski reflex (upgoing plantar response), and more than three beats of ankle clonus.

TESTS FOR THORACIC OUTLET SYNDROME

Adson's test is performed by passively abducting, extending and externally rotating the upper limb while palpating the radial pulse. The patient then rotates their head towards the affected side and holds a deep breath. A positive test will result in a reduced or absent radial pulse.

Roos' test is performed by the patient clenching and unclenching the fists repeatedly with the shoulder abducted and externally rotated to 90° with the elbows flexed to 90°. The test is positive if vascular or neurogenic symptoms return, or the radial pulse is absent.

T-spine

LOOK

From the side, look for a kyphosis (increased thoracic spine convexity) or an acute angled gibbus, both of which may be congenital or acquired. Ankylosing spondylitis leads to a loss of the normal thoracic spine curvature and a reduced range of movement and lung expansion. From behind, look for swellings, café-au-lait spots, and any scars from previous spinal or lung surgery, in addition to scoliosis (abnormal lateral curvature of the spine). Scoliosis which corrects on sitting, bending forwards in a seated position with or without lateral flexion is considered mobile (postural), and can develop secondary to leg length asymmetry. If these manoeuvres do not correct the deformity, or a rib hump becomes visible, the scoliosis is considered fixed (structural). A plumb line can be used to demonstrate the degree of scoliosis, and the curves can be described as primary and secondary.

FEEL

Palpate the thoracic spine in a similar manner to the cervical spine, and gently percuss the vertebrae with the lateral border of a closed fist, noting any significant tenderness with the patient in a flexed forward position.

MOVE

The principal movement of the thoracic spine is rotation (40°); ask the patient to rotate from side to side with their arms folded across their chest while the examiner stabilizes the pelvis. Lateral flexion is approximately 15°, extension 5–10°, and flexion is limited by the orientation of the thoracic facet joints and the ribs. The thoracic and lumbar spines work as a unit, and movements are the result of these actions are achieved by movement in both sections of spine.

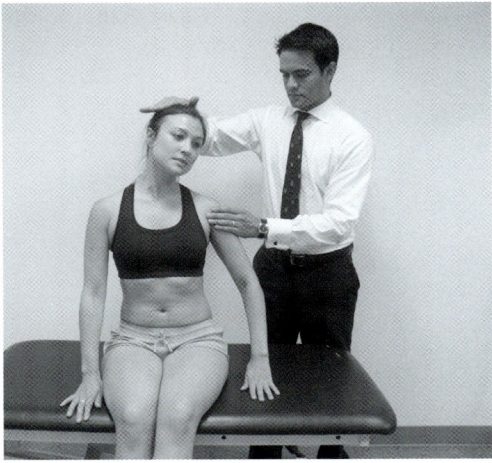

Figure 2.24 Spurling's test.

SPECIAL TESTS

The *slump test (dural stretch test)* is used to assess thoracic and lumbar nerve root impingement, by increasing dural tension incrementally. To begin, the patient sits on the edge of the couch in an erect posture, then flexes the thoracic and lumbar spine by slumping forwards while the examiner keeps the cervical spine extended by supporting the chin. The patient then flexes the neck forwards and the examiner gently applies pressure over the occiput to increase the degree of flexion. Lastly, the examiner extends the patient's knee and dorsiflexes the foot. Note the stage at which symptoms are reproduced and do not progress further with the test. Additionally, the dural tension can be increased on the thoracic nerve roots by rotation in the slumped position.

Lumbar spine

LOOK

Look for scars of previous surgery and a hairy patch over the lumbar spine, indicative of spina bifida occulta. Look for scoliosis, which may be a secondary protective adaptation to sciatic nerve root impingement (sciatic list) or thoracic scoliosis. Measure leg length with the patient standing, noting any pelvic obliquity, and supine on the examination couch. Loss of the lumbar lordosis occurs commonly with OA and ankylosing spondylitis, and also with a prolapsed intervertebral disc. An exaggerated lumbar lordosis may be normal, especially in women, or found in conjunction with an abrupt step in spondylolisthesis.

FEEL

With the patient standing, palpate and percuss the lumbar spine along with the thoracic spine. The sacrum can also be palpated, along with the coccyx *per rectum* if indicated. The sacroiliac joints should be assessed with the patient on the couch (see 'Hip' section). An abrupt step may be felt at the L4/L5 level, or at the lumbosacral junction due to spondylolisthesis.

MOVE

The lumbar spine has a good range of forward flexion (60°), extension (35°) and lateral flexion (30°). Only a few degrees of rotation is possible, and most rotation occurs in the thoracic spine. Ask the patient to bend forward and touch their toes, recording the distance from fingertip to floor, and perform a modified Schober's test. Ask the patient to lean back as far as possible without losing balance, and slide their right hand down the side of their right leg and repeat on the left, comparing the two sides.

SPECIAL TESTS

Modified Schober's test

The modified Schober's test can be used to evaluate the contribution of the lumbar spine to total flexion. Draw a horizontal line between the posterior superior iliac spines, which lie beneath the skin dimples, and a vertical line in the midline (Fig. 2.25a) which extends 10 cm above and 5 cm below this level. When the patient bends forwards, the midline marking should increase in length by 5–7 cm (Fig. 2.25b).

Tests for Lumbar nerve root compression

The *straight leg raise (SLR) test* (Fig. 2.26) is used to assess a prolapsed intervertebral disc as a possible cause of lumbar back pain. In the supine position, hold the patient's leg just proximal to the ankle and slowly lift the leg up off the couch with the knee in full extension. Note the angle at

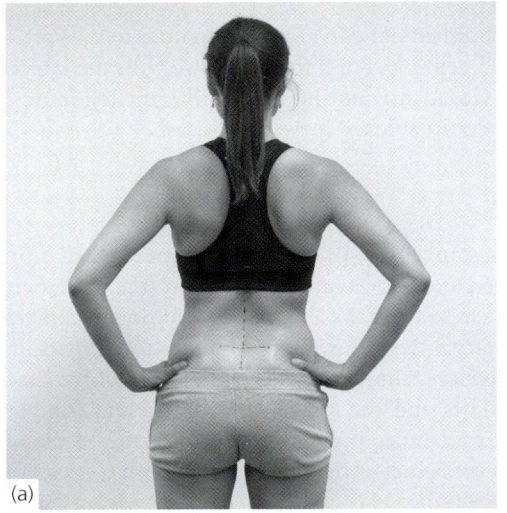
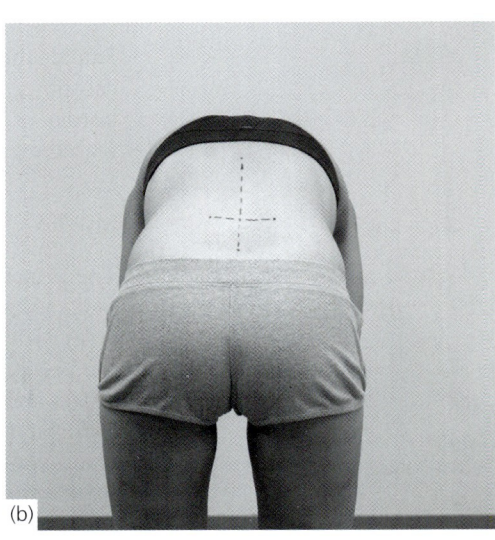

(a) (b)

Figure 2.25 Schober's test.

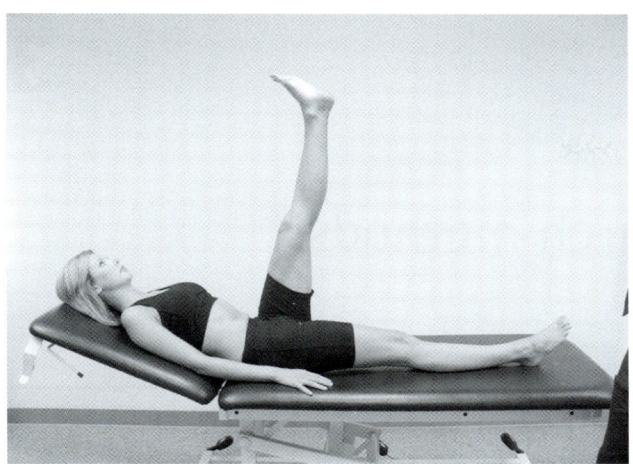

Figure 2.26 Straight leg raise.

which the patient's sciatic (L4, L5, S1) symptoms are reproduced. The *Lasègue sign (sciatic stretch test)* is elicited by lowering the limb slightly from this position and dorsiflexing the ankle; reproduction of the symptoms indicates sciatic nerve involvement. From this position, return the ankle to neutral and slightly flex the knee. Reproduction of sciatic symptoms by applying pressure over the popliteal nerve in the popliteal fossa is a positive *'bowstring test'*. The *'crossover sign'* is positive when the patient's symptoms are reproduced by straight leg raise of the contralateral limb, which suggests a large disc protrusion medial to the affected nerve root.

To confirm the validity of a positive finding, attempt to get the patient to perform the equivalent of a 90° SLR while distracted. Ask the patient to sit up with their legs still on the couch; the ability to do so without flexing the knees or falling backwards suggests that the problem may not be entirely organic in origin. A variation of this test is performed by asking the patient to extend their knee in a seated position on the edge of the couch.

Consider *Waddell's five signs of inorganic behaviour*: tenderness (superficial, diffuse, non-anatomical), simulation (e.g. on axial loading), distraction (described above for SLR), regional disturbances (non-dermatomal/myotomoal), over-reaction (subjective, susceptible to observer bias). Finding three or more of these signs suggests a non-organic origin of symptoms, but does not exclude an organic cause, and should therefore be interpreted with caution.

The *reverse Lasègue test (femoral stretch test)* is performed with the patient prone and the knee flexed to 90°. Lift the affected limb off the couch while stabilizing the pelvis, and note any reproduction of symptoms in an L2, L3, L4 distribution. L4/5 and L5/S1 intervertebral disc prolapses are more common than the higher lumbar disc prolapses, and femoral nerve symptoms are therefore much less common than sciatic nerve symptoms.

ACKNOWLEDGEMENTS

The authors would like to thank the following people for their input into sections of this chapters: Professor T Kamaruizaman (upper limb) Mr Jonathan Bird (hip and knee), and Mr Stephen James (spine).

REFERENCES

- ● = Key primary paper
- ◆ = Major review article

1. Tennent TD, Beach WR, Meyers JF. A review of the special tests associated with shoulder examination. Part I: the rotator cuff tests. *Am J Sports Med* 2003;**31**(1):154–60. Review.
2. Tennent TD, Beach WR, Meyers JF. A review of the special tests associated with shoulder examination. Part II: laxity, instability, and superior labral anterior and posterior (SLAP) lesions. *Am J Sports Med* 2003;**31**(2):301–7. Review.
3. Hawkins RJ, Abrams JS. Impingement syndrome in the absence of rotator cuff tear. *Orthop Clin North Am* 1987;**18**:373–82.
4. Neer CS. Impingement lesions. *Clin Orthop* 1983;**173**: 70–7.
5. Jobe FW, Moynes DR Delineation of diagnostic criteria and a rehabilitation program for rotator cuff injuries. *Am J Sports Med* 1982;**10**(6):336–9.
6. Hertel R, Ballmer FT, Lombert SM, Gerber C. Lag signs in the diagnosis of rotator cuff rupture. *J Shoulder Elbow Surg* 1996;**5**(4):307–13.
7. Gerber C, Krushell RJ. Isolated rupture of the tendon of the subscapularis muscle. Clinical features in 16 cases. *J Bone Joint Surg Br* 1991;**73**(3):389–94.
8. Hamner DL, Pink MM, Jobe FW. A modification of the relocation test: arthroscopic findings associated with a positive test. *J Shoulder Elbow Surg* 2000;**9**(4):263–7.
9. Finkelstein H. Stenosing tendovaginitis at the radial styloid process. *J Bone Joint Surg Am* 1930;**12**:509–540
10. Wartenberg R. Cheiralgia Paraesthetica. Neuritis des ramus superficialis nervi radialis. *Z Neurol Pschiatr* 1932;**141**: 145–155.
11. Watson HK, Ashmead D 4th, Makhlouf MV. Examination of the scaphoid. J Hand Surg Am 1988;**13**(5):657–60.
12. Reagan DS, Linscheid RL, Dobyns JH. Lunotriquetral sprains. *J Hand Surg Am* 1984;**9**(4):502–14.
13. Phalen GS. Spontaneous compression of the median nerve at the wrist. *JAMA* 1951;**145**:1128–1131.
14. Kiloh LG, Nevin S. Isolated neuritis of the anterior interosseous nerve. *Br Med J* 1952;**19**;1(4763):850–1.
15. Trendelenburg F. Trendelenburg's test: 1895. *Clin Orthop Relat Res* 1998;**355**:3–7.
16. Gurtler RA, Stine R, Torg JS. Lachman test evaluated. Quantification of a clinical observation. *Clin Orthop Relat Res* 1987;**216**:141–50.

3

Orthopaedic research: research methods, epidemiology and statistics

JENNA GODFREY, ERIC McCARTY

Introduction	36	Statistical analyses	44
Terminology	37	Evidence-based medicine	46
Hypothesis testing	39	Conclusion	47
Experimental study designs	40	References	47
Statistics	43		

NATIONAL BOARD STANDARDS

- Understand commonly used terms and statistical tests and when to use them. For example, P-value, positive predictive value, Student's t-test
- Interpret results of research investigations
- Be able to interpret data in peer-reviewed papers
- Be familiar with the setting up of clinical trials
- Be familiar with survivorship analysis of hip and knee implants
- Understand regression analysis

INTRODUCTION

Epidemiology is an important part of orthopaedic research. Thus, one must begin by asking what is epidemiology and why is it important to the practising clinician? There are several definitions of epidemiology:

> Epidemiology is the study of the distribution and determinants of health-related states or events in specified populations and the application of this study to the control of health problems.[1]

> Epidemiology represents the recognition that the patterns of occurrence of disease and disability in communities are determined by forces that can be identified and measured, and these forces include, but are not limited to, medical concepts of etiology, and that modification of these forces is the most effective way to prevent disease.[2]

The definition posited by Stallones[2] argues for the relevance of epidemiology to the practising clinician. Epidemiology is the identification of patterns of disease, with the purpose of modifying forces affecting disease patterns and the goal of preventing disease. Is this the fundamental force behind the daily practice of medicine, with the goal of preventing the occurrence or progression of disease in our patients? Of note, the word 'disease' can easily be replaced with 'injury'.

In the past, clinicians relied on experience, prevailing practice, professional training and peer opinion as guides for day-to-day decisions about patient care. The majority of techniques and treatments taught had not been subjected to scientifically rigorous investigation. In the 1970s, clinicians and researchers at McMaster's University began to address this clinical information overload by developing tools to help clinicians discern the clinically valid, important and applicable details, and thus evidence-based medicine (EBM) was born. EBM is an approach to healthcare that promotes the collection, interpretation and integration of valid, important and applicable patient-reported, clinician-observed and research-derived evidence. The EBM movement asserts that potential advances in healthcare must be tested and proven to do more good than harm before they are incorporated into medical practice.[3]

In this chapter, we will discuss several fundamental epidemiological concepts, how to conduct clinical research from hypothesis formulation to statistical analysis, and the relevance of EBM to your clinical practice. Topics will include terminology, types of studies, designing a research study, statistical analysis and a discussion on EBM.

TERMINOLOGY

Incidence *vs* prevalence

Epidemiology is the study of disease occurrence at a population level. The occurrence of disease can be measured using *rates* and *proportions*.[4] Rates indicate how fast a disease is occurring in a population, and proportions tell us what fraction of individuals in a population are disease positive. Two terms are commonly used to quantify the burden of disease in populations: *incidence* and *prevalence*. An incidence rate is the 'number of new cases of a disease that occur during a specified *period* of time in a population at risk for developing disease'.[4] The numerator consists of *new* cases developing over a specific time interval. The denominator is composed of individuals at risk for developing the disease during the same specified time interval.

Consider the following hypothetical example. An orthopaedic surgeon practising in a ski resort is in charge of caring for the 250-member ski patrol and the 250 ski instructors at the resort. During the course of the skiing season, which spans November to April, 50 employees sustain a new anterior cruciate ligament (ACL) tear while skiing at work, effectively ending their ski season and limiting their work duties.

The cumulative incidence (or risk) of having an ACL tear would be calculated in the following way:

$$\text{Cumulative incidence} = \frac{[50 \text{ new ACL tears during the ski season sustained by resort employees (over 6 months)}]}{[500 \text{ resort employees at risk for sustaining a skiing-related injury at work (at risk over 6 months)}]}$$

Incidence is expressed as per 1000 (or 100 000) per time period. In this example, the cumulative incidence is 100 ACL tears per 1000 individuals per ski season, or a 10% chance of developing an ACL tear.

The incidence rate (per unit time) estimates the number of new ACL tears that occurred per day, week, month, etc.

$$\text{Incidence rate} = \frac{[50 \text{ new tears (over the 6 month period)}]}{[500 \text{ resort employees at risk each month} \times 6 \text{ months} \ (= 3000 \text{ person-months at risk})]}$$

$$= \frac{0.0167}{\text{month}}$$

= 1.67 per 100 person-months of skiing (or 16.7 per 1000 person-months – the units can be scaled as needed)

Thus, these two measures tell you that there is a 10% risk of developing an ACL tear during the skiing season, and that about 1–2% of employees per month will develop a tear and arrive for care.

Prevalence, on the other hand, is the 'number of affected persons present in the population at a *specific time* divided by the number of persons in the population at that time'.[4] For example, you are interested in determining the number of individuals with osteoarthritis in your practice. You have electronic medical records, so you perform a search of the database for all those individuals who are currently diagnosed with osteoarthritis. This number is the numerator, and the number of individuals in your database is the denominator:

$$\text{Prevalence of osteoarthritis in patients seen at your clinic} = \frac{[75 \text{ patients diagnosed with osteoarthritis}]}{[1500 \text{ patients seen in your clinic}]}$$

= 0.05 or 50 per 1000

This is an example of point prevalence. Point prevalence is the prevalence of disease at one point in time.[4]

One commonly confused difference between incidence and prevalence is that incidence is an estimate of risk, but prevalence is not. Prevalence does not estimate risk because it does not address when the individuals in the numerator developed the disease. Individuals in the numerator may have been diagnosed with the disease the previous day or may have been diagnosed with the disease 10 years ago. Therefore, when we survey a population to estimate the prevalence of disease, we do not take into account the duration of the disease.[4] Incidence, on the other hand, starts with a group of disease-free individuals and watches them for a period of time for the development of disease. Because incidence looks only at *new* cases of disease, it is an estimate of risk.

However, there is a relationship between incidence and prevalence:

$$\text{Prevalence} = \text{incidence} \times \text{duration}$$

If the duration of a disease is very short (say hours for a child with a displaced wrist fracture), the prevalence of disease would be low, whereas the incidence could be high. Therefore, you may set 30 wrist fractures in 1 month (incidence), but the prevalence of displaced wrist fractures on any given day in that month may be 1 or even 0 because a fracture is displaced only for hours (we hope). On the other hand, if the duration of the disease is long (seen in incurable diseases such as osteoarthritis), the prevalence of individuals may be large, but the incidence of new disease in a given period of time is low. Therefore, you may only diagnose five people in a year with osteoarthritis, but you have accumulated 75 individuals with a diagnosis of osteoarthritis over the past 15 years of practising.

Populations and sampling

A *population* of patients have a common characteristic of clinical or scientific interest.[5] For example, all patients with shoulder osteoarthritis, or every individual with an Achilles tendon rupture. In the majority of cases, a population is prohibitively large.[5] Consider, for example, the number of individuals who have suffered a femur fracture in the USA in the past year. Because testing an entire population is financially and logistically impossible in nearly every situation, a *sample* of the population is tested and the results are generalized to the population. Random sampling provides the entire population with an equal chance of being selected for the sample.[5]

Screening and diagnostic tests

In order to accurately assess the burden of disease in a community, it is necessary to distinguish individuals with disease from those who are disease free.[4] Screening and diagnostic tests are used to identify individuals with disease in a population. The difference between a screening test and a diagnostic test is that screening tests are performed on individuals with no clinical indications of disease, whereas diagnostic tests are used to confirm disease in individuals with a high index of suspicion for disease.

Specificity and sensitivity

While the timing and use of these two types of tests are different, the methods used to evaluate the quality of screening and diagnostic tests are the same. In order to convey the utility of a test, e.g. how good the test is at separating disease-positive individuals from disease-negative individuals, sensitivity, specificity, positive predictive value (PPV) and negative predictive value (NPV) are calculated.

The simplest way to conceptualize these parameters is to draw a 2 × 2 table (Table 3.1).

A 2 × 2 table compares two different tests: the screening or diagnostic test in question and a 'gold standard'

Table 3.1 A 2 × 2 table

	Gold standard disease +	Gold standard disease −	
Test +	A True positives	B False positives	A + B
Test −	C False negatives	D True negatives	C + D
	A + C	B + D	Total

diagnostic test. A 'gold standard' diagnostic test is any test that has been previously validated and definitively identifies disease in an individual. Before calculating specificity and sensitivity, let us first consider what each cell in Table 3.1 represents. True positives (cell A) are individuals with a positive screening test who are disease positive according to the gold standard. False positives (cell B) are individuals with a positive screening test who are actually disease negative according to the gold standard. True negatives (cell D) are individuals with a negative screening test who are disease negative according to the gold standard. False negatives (cell C) are individuals with negative test results who are actually disease positive according to the gold standard. Ideally, the results of a screening or diagnostic test would maximize the number of correctly identified individuals with disease while avoiding falsely alarming patients and missing diagnoses.

Sensitivity is the proportion of individuals with disease who were correctly identified as positive by the screening test.[4] Specificity is the proportion of individuals without disease who were correctly identified as disease free by the screening test.[4]

Using the 2 × 2 table:

$$\text{Sensitivity} = \frac{A}{(A + C)}$$

$$\text{Specificity} = \frac{D}{(B + D)}$$

In a recent study, the sensitivity and specificity of an MRI for diagnosis of an ACL tear were found to be 99% and 95%, respectively.[6] In this study, 300 patients with traumatic knee injuries warranting a surgical intervention underwent both MRI testing and arthroscopic evaluation of the structures in the knee. The exact number of individuals in each group was not reported, so for simplicity we will assume that 100 patients actually had a torn ACL based on arthroscopy (disease +) and 200 patients did not (disease −). Using these hypothetical data, let us look at how these numbers were calculated (Table 3.2):

$$\text{Sensitivity} = \frac{99}{100} = 99\%$$

$$\text{Specificity} = \frac{190}{200} = 95\%$$

Positive and negative predictive values

Sensitivity and specificity are not easy to apply in a clinical setting because the clinician does not know whether the patient has a disease during the screening and diagnostic process. Instead, clinicians are given test results to interpret to determine a diagnosis. From this standpoint, PPVs and NPVs can be more practically applicable.

PPVs and NPVs use test results to estimate the probability of actually having the disease given the test result. The PPV is the proportion of individuals with a positive test who actually have the disease. The NPV is the proportion of individuals with a negative test who are disease negative.[4,7]

Using the 2 × 2 table:

$$PPV = \frac{A}{(A + B)}$$

$$NPV = \frac{D}{(D + C)}$$

In our example:

$$PPV = \frac{99}{109} = 91\%$$

$$NPV = \frac{190}{191} = 99\%$$

Therefore, 91% of patients with a positive MRI will have a torn ACL, whereas 99% of patients with a negative MRI will not have a torn ACL (Table 3.3).

Validity, reliability and responsiveness

Outcomes assessment has become a hot topic in medicine because of the desire of physicians to quantify the effectiveness of their interventions. Outcomes measures include generic measures (such as the Short Form 36 for quality of life assessment), condition-specific measures (the American Shoulder and Elbow Surgeons (ASES) shoulder scale) and measures of patient satisfaction.[7] A new trend towards psychometric assessment of outcomes instruments includes assessing each instrument for its reliability, validity and responsiveness to change.[7] *Reliability* refers to the reproducibility of the measure. *Interobserver reliability* is the ability of the instrument to perform the same regardless of the person administering the instrument. *Test–retest reliability* is a measure of intraobserver reliability, e.g. if a subject is given a test and then retested within a given time frame, during which the outcome is unchanged, does the score change? *Validity*, simply stated, is the instrument's ability to test what it was designed to test. *Content validity*, or face validity, looks directly at the instrument's ability to accurately reflect the outcome of interest, as determined by a panel of experts in the field. *Construct validity* looks at whether or not the instrument follows an expected non-controversial hypothesis. *Criterion validity* compares the instrument with the 'gold standard' in measuring that outcome. *Responsiveness* is the instrument's ability to detect change in an outcome owing to time or intervention, e.g. if the patient is given the instrument before beginning rehabilitation and again after several weeks of rehabilitation, the instrument should reflect improvements in the outcome.

External validity, or generalizability, is the extent to which the study results (from a sample group) are representative of all patients with a disease (the population).[4] Bias threatens the validity of a study. Bias can corrupt a study during patient selection (selection bias), study performance (performance or information bias), patient follow-up (non-responder or transfer bias) and outcome determination (detection, recall, acceptability and interviewer bias).[5]

HYPOTHESIS TESTING

In medicine, clinical studies share one common goal: improving patient outcomes. Improvement in outcomes can come from a variety of places, such as improved screening and diagnostic techniques, better treatments, less invasive procedural techniques, or greater symptom control resulting in improved quality of life. Any idea for improving outcomes needs to be rigorously tested before it can be applied to patients, and thus clinical studies are conducted. Designing and conducting a clinical study require the following steps: identifying a specific question, performing a literature search, choosing an appropriate study design, picking measurement tools, collecting data, statistical analysis and, finally, writing up the results.

Independent and dependent variables

Clinical studies are designed to look for associations between variables. *Variables* are entities that can be manipulated or changed during the course of the study.

Table 3.2 Calculating sensitivity and specificity

	Disease +	Disease −	
Test +	99	10	109
Test −	1	190	191
	100	200	300

Table 3.3 Calculating predictive values

	Gold standard disease +	Gold standard disease −	
Test +	A True positives	B False positives	A + B
Test −	C False negatives	D True negatives	C + D
	A + C	B + D	Total

The exposure of interest and the outcome are both such variables, as are other factors that may influence the outcome. An *independent variable* may be manipulated by the researcher and contributes to the outcome of interest.[7] A *dependent variable* is the outcome of interest and is affected by the independent variable.[7] An association is the relationship between the independent and dependent variable such that manipulating the independent variable has a measurable affect on the dependent variable.

Hypothesis generation: null hypothesis *vs* alternative hypothesis

Clinical studies start with a well-formulated clinical question. Clinical questions involve a simple relationship between the patient, an exposure (to a treatment, a screening test, a new procedural technique, etc.) and one or more outcomes of interest.[8] Consider the following clinical question: does intra-articular morphine (exposure) improve postoperative pain (outcome) in patients after ACL reconstruction?[9]

A well-formed clinical question is used to generate two hypotheses: the null hypothesis and the alternative hypothesis. The null hypothesis is that there is no relationship between exposure and outcome. In our case, the null hypothesis is that intra-articular morphine injections will not change patients' pain following an ACL reconstruction. The alternative hypothesis for every clinical question is that an association between exposure and outcome exists. In our example, the alternative hypothesis is that an intra-articular morphine injection will influence patients' postoperative pain level following an ACL reconstruction. Since the alternative and null hypotheses are two sides of the same question, it is not uncommon to refer to the alternative hypothesis as 'the hypothesis' for the study, and then infer the null hypothesis. From now on, when we refer to the study hypothesis, we will be referring to the alternative hypothesis

Study design

After a hypothesis is formed and the exposure and outcome variables have been defined, the next step is to choose an appropriate study design. There are two major categories of study design: experimental and observational.[4,7] The primary and fundamental difference between experimental study designs and observational study designs is that an experimental design involves researcher intervention, whereas an observational study design does not involve researcher intervention. Study designs can also be categorized temporally: studies which start with the enrolment of the first participant and follow participants forward are prospective studies; studies which use pre-existing data on outcomes and look back for exposures of interest are retrospective studies. Experimental study designs include randomized control trials (RCTs) and controlled laboratory experiments, whereas observational study designs include cohort studies, case–control studies, cross-sectional surveys and case series.[7] Finally, a meta-analysis may be used to aggregate multiple similar studies to look for similar (or different) effects across studies.

EXPERIMENTAL STUDY DESIGNS

Randomized control trials

The RCT is the gold standard in study design. In RCTs, participants are randomly assigned to an experimental group or a control group. The experimental group is exposed to the variable in question (intervention), while the control group is followed without exposure to the variable. Why is randomization so important? Outcomes are influenced by multiple factors, including underlying severity of the illness, comorbid conditions and other prognostic factors (known or unknown).[10] Completely random assignment of participants into experimental and control groups should evenly allocate these 'other' factors between the two groups. Randomization also minimizes selection bias. Selection bias occurs when patients are specifically selected for certain study groups, which would result in an uneven distribution of comorbid factors (or other factors) between groups and would invalidate the study.

Let us return to our example of postoperative pain control using intra-articular morphine injections. Patients were randomly assigned to receive either an injection of morphine (exposure) or a bolus of saline (control) prior to surgery and postoperative pain was measured using a visual analogue pain scale (outcome). The results of the study indicated that intra-articular morphine injections did not significantly change patients' pain following ACL reconstruction.[9]

Evaluation of outcomes in RCTs can be subjective, so it is common to blind both the researchers and study participants (if possible) to group assignments. Blinding, or masking, is an element of the study design which hides study group assignments from individuals participating in the study, either study participants themselves or clinical investigators involved in evaluating study outcomes, or both (double blinding).[7] Blinding is done because predetermined expectations concerning the effects of the exposure on the outcome could alter the participants' or evaluators' subjective evaluation of the outcome. Consider pain scales. If participants are aware that postoperative morphine was withheld because they are in the control group, their subjective pain reporting could be biased. In order to keep the participants from guessing their group assignment, sham procedures and placebo pills or other interventions are commonly used.

RCTs are the gold standard study, but it is not uncommon that implementing them is unethical. Withholding a beneficial treatment or administering a potentially harmful intervention is not reasonable. Thorough evaluation of all purposed research studies is performed by institutional review boards, whose primary focus is to determine whether the intervention proposed in the study could cause unreasonable harm to research participants.

Observational study designs

In cases in which assigning exposure to a variable of interest is unreasonable, impractical or unethical, other study designs are available for hypothesis testing. The most commonly used observational study designs are cohort (or prospective) studies, case–control (or retrospective) studies, cross-sectional surveys or case series.

Prospective trials begin with a group of patients and follow them over time looking for the outcome of interest. Retrospective trials begin with individuals who already have the outcome of interest (cases) and look backwards for exposures influencing the outcome.

COHORT STUDY

In a cohort study, the investigator 'selects a group of exposed individuals and a group of nonexposed individuals and follows up both groups to compare the incidence of disease'.[4] Let us consider an example. Multiligament knee injuries are significant and often involve not only the damaged ligaments but the meniscus and chondral surface as well. A recent study indicated a higher incidence of lateral meniscus injuries in patients with multiligament knee injuries compared with a single ligament knee injury.[11] The authors of this study chose to address this topic using a prospective cohort design. Patients were enrolled in the study upon diagnosis of a ligamentous injury to the knee. Patients with a multiligament injury were assigned to one cohort (exposure group) and patients with injury to the ACL only were assigned to the other cohort (non-exposed group). All patients had no prior history of traumatic knee injury, meniscal injuries or known chondral injuries. During surgery to repair the ligament tear, meniscal injury and chondral injury were documented. The incidence of meniscal injuries (lateral or medial) and the incidence of chondral injuries were compared between the two groups.

Cohort studies are either prospective or retrospective. In a prospective cohort study, participants are assigned to a cohort based on a known exposure and followed forward, often for years, to monitor for the outcome of interest. In a retrospective cohort study, previously obtained patient data are used to determine exposure and to assess for the outcome of interest, which must be captured in the record over the preceding interval of time. The obvious benefit of a retrospective cohort study is time, because the data already exist. However, the investigator may be limited in the amount of information available on each participant. In a prospective cohort study, investigators have the ability to continuously re-evaluate the progress of the study, collect more data as needed and modify the study if necessary. The most important and limiting aspects of a prospective cohort study are time and money, because it may take years for an outcome to develop.

An observational cohort study design is useful when assigning exposure to an individual is unethical. This design is also useful for rare exposures. In this instance, the investigator can seek out study participants with a rare exposure from multiple clinical centres and follow them forward for the outcome of interest.

CASE–CONTROL STUDY

Another observational study design is a case–control (or retrospective) study. In a case–control study, individuals with a disease of interest (cases) are compared with a group of similar non-diseased individuals (controls), and the proportion of cases who were exposed is compared with the proportion of exposed controls.[4] Let us consider another example from the literature. Shoulder osteoarthritis is a problem for many older patients. There are many proposed risk factors for developing shoulder osteoarthritis, including a history of shoulder dislocations. A recent study indicated that there is, in fact, a higher risk of developing osteoarthritis in patients with a history of shoulder dislocations.[12] The authors of the study chose to use a case–control design to address this clinical question. Patients identified as having osteoarthritis of the shoulder during shoulder arthroplasty (cases) were compared with individuals with osteoarthritis of the knee identified during a knee arthroplasty (controls). To assess exposure, both groups were given a questionnaire asking about a history of shoulder dislocations (exposure). A higher proportion of cases had a positive history of shoulder dislocations (11 out of 91) than controls (two out of 282), which would suggest an increased risk of shoulder osteoarthritis in individuals with a history of shoulder dislocations (odds ratio 19.3).

Choosing a control group is often the most difficult challenge in a case–control study. Again, the central tenet of clinical research is that groups should be as similar as possible. The control group should be as similar as possible to the cases in all dimensions, other than exposure. If the cases are all young, fit soccer players, controls should also be young fit soccer players. The diversity of cases will dictate the generalizability of the results (e.g. young fit soccer players).

A common misconception is that case–control studies and cohort studies differ only in time; cohort studies look forward and case–control studies look back. In fact, as discussed, cohort studies can be retrospective. The important difference between cohort and case–control studies is group assignment. In cohort studies, individuals are selected based on exposure status. In case–control studies, individuals are selected based on disease status.[4] Since cohort studies start from exposure and watch for outcomes, it is possible to calculate an incidence rate. Statistical analysis of cohort studies involves comparison of incidence rates using relative risks. Case–control studies start with the outcome and look for exposure; the results are conveyed as the proportion of patients in each group with an exposure. Statistical analysis of case–control studies involves comparing the proportion of individuals exposed using an odds ratio.

OTHER OBSERVATIONAL STUDY DESIGNS

Cross-sectional surveys and case series are observational study designs. Cross-sectional surveys involve surveying a group of individuals on a topic of interest, and can be done in person, via mail or email, or on the phone. A case series is a retrospective descriptive account of individuals with an interesting aspect of disease, a common exposure or who have undergone a similar intervention.[7] These two designs are not generally considered to be as scientifically rigorous as the study designs previously discussed. Their utility lies in providing information relating to a clinical question, which may aid in the development of a more rigorous trial.

Systematic review and meta-analyses

It is not uncommon to find conflicting results on the same topic in the literature. A systematic review is the systematic process of amassing studies on a topic of interest and evaluating them with the purpose of integrating the results. After an exhaustive literature search is completed, the studies are usually weighted based on sample size. Studies are then evaluated for quality and are often rated or graded. Studies that are determined to be similar enough in their methods and analysis can then be combined. For example, a recent systematic analysis published in the *Archives of Internal Medicine* reviewed all RCTs looking at interventions for preventing sports-related injuries.[13] The analysis revealed sufficient evidence for three methods of sports injury prevention: shoe inserts, external joint support and specific training programmes. A meta-analysis is a systematic review using advanced statistical techniques to combine the study results into one analysis, giving a pooled size of the effect of the exposure on the outcome.[4] Systematic reviews and meta-analyses are becoming much more common given the breadth of medical literature available now and because of the utility of synthesizing it into one article.

Error

Clinical studies are used to *estimate* the true association between exposure and outcome variables. The true relationship between variables can never be known because testing an entire population is not possible, but this true relationship exists. Either the experimental results accurately reflect this truth or they misrepresent this truth. When experimental results and absolute truth are the same, the study has been a success. A 2 × 2 table can be helpful to understand the concepts of experimental results and truth (Table 3.4).

Table 3.4 Experimental results and truth

Experimental results	Truth – no association	Truth – association
No association	Correct	Type II error
Association	Type I error	Correct

Type I or alpha errors occur when a statistically significant association is found in an experimental setting, but in truth no association exists.[7] In other words, alpha is the probability that your claim of an association is incorrect. The *P*-value is a statistical value calculated using the data that represents the strength of evidence provided in favour of the null hypothesis. If the *P*-value is less than the alpha level, the strength of evidence in favour of the null hypothesis is not strong enough to accept it and it is rejected. A type II error or beta error occurs when no association is found in an experimental setting, but in truth an association does exist. In other words, beta is the probability that you will find an association that truly exists.

Power

Power is the probability of finding no association when an association truly exists, and is defined as 1 − the probability of a type II error.[7] Power is often set at 80% or 90%. A power level of 80% can be interpreted to mean that there is less than a 20% chance that the experimental results missed a true association. A primary reason why a study may fail to find an association when one truly exists is that the sample size was insufficient (often called an 'underpowered' study).

Sample size

Calculating the appropriate sample size prior to initiation of a study is necessary in avoiding a type II error. The following decisions need to be made in order to calculate sample size: effect size (i.e. how big a difference the treatment or exposure make in the outcome), variance (or noise in an exposure), alpha, beta, and one-sided *vs* two-sided test analysis. Effect size requires the clinician to define changes in the outcome that are clinically significant.[7] This process typically involves both a subjective approach and a literature search, and in some instances may also involve a pilot study. Although it may seem wasteful to run a 'mini' version of the study to aid in determining effect size, the alternative is far worse, because selecting too few patients may result in a type II error, thereby missing a real effect and wasting resources. Variance describes the spread of the data by looking at how far each datum point is from the mean. Two-sided analyses are most commonly used as they are more conservative and improve the power of the study.

STATISTICS

In their classic statistics textbook, Mendenhall and Beaver[14] define statistics as 'an area of science concerned with extraction of information from numerical data and its use in making inferences about a population from which data are obtained'. The practice of statistical analysis can be daunting owing to the numerous complicated equations. For the busy clinician, a knowledge of the principles of statistical analysis is necessary for practising evidence-based medicine. The goal of the educated clinician should be to have a rudimentary understanding of data collection and statistical analysis. Memorizing equations is not necessary.

Types of data

Data can take many different forms. Data can fall into three categories: categorical, ordinal or continuous.[7] Categorical data are data in categories with no inherent order, such as type of athlete (rugby, soccer or basketball player). Dichotomous is a special case of categorical, in which all individuals fit into either one category or the other (e.g. male or female, smoker or non-smoker). Categorical data can also be ordinal, which indicates that there is an inherent order to the categories, such as cancer stages and injury grades. Categorical data are often reported as percentages or proportions (e.g. 51% female) and presented in tables or bar graphs. Continuous data are observations measured on a continuum, so that the interval between them does hold meaning, such as test scores, blood pressure values, age and weight. Continuous data are often reported using means and standard deviation (the mean weight was 75 kg with a standard deviation of 10 kg) and presented in tables or line graphs. Different statistical tests are appropriate for each data type.

Descriptive *vs* inferential statistics

There are two different categories of statistics: *descriptive statistics* and *inferential statistics*. Descriptive statistics describe the basic features of the study data. Commonly mentioned descriptive statistics include mean, median, mode and standard deviation. *Inferential statistics* determine whether the differences seen in the study are real or the result of chance, and are used to generalize sample data to the entire population.[15]

Descriptive statistics look at the distribution of the data collected. Mean, median and mode are measures of the central tendency of the data and standard deviation is a measurement of the spread of the data.[7] Data can be plotted to look for either a normal distribution (Gaussian (bell shaped)) or a skewed distribution of data (Fig. 3.1). A skew in the data indicates that the mean and median are not equal, usually indicating a large spread of data with a congregation of a large percentage of the data around a point that is either greater than (left skew) or less than (right skew) the mean.

Standard deviation estimates the variation among individual observations and indicates the spread of the data (Fig. 3.2). Looking at the curve, 95% of patients fall within two standard deviations of the mean.

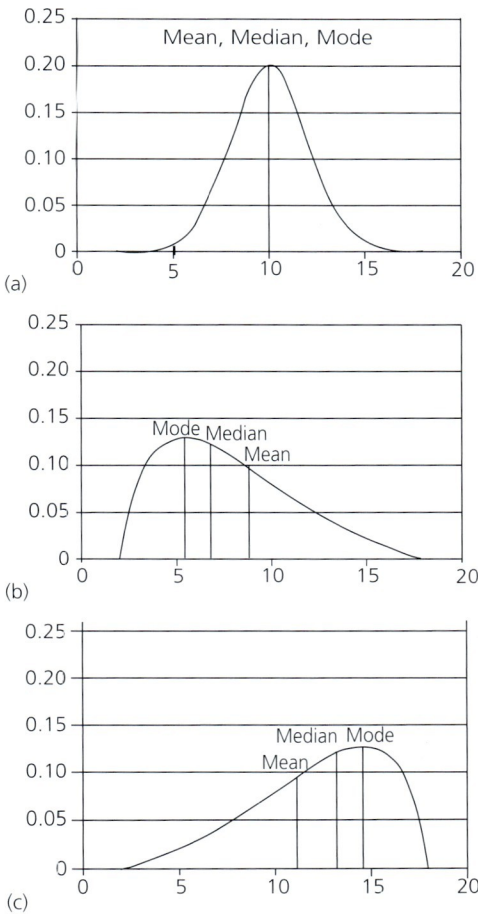

Figure 3.1 Normal compared with skewed graphs. (a) Normal curve; (b) positive skew; (c) negative skew.

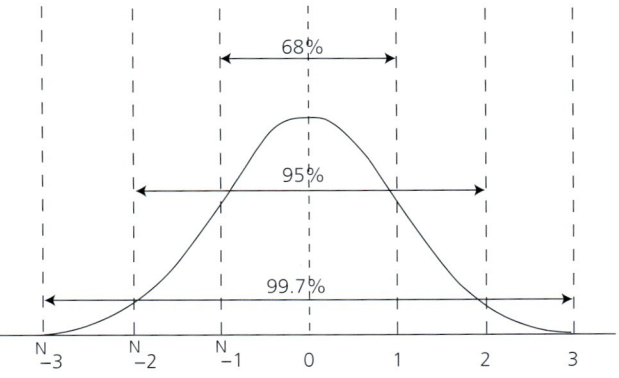

Figure 3.2 Standard deviation.

Inferential statistics are commonly used in hypothesis-driven experimental research, and are used to evaluate the relationship between variables. The goal of inferential statistics is to estimate parameters with the intent of generalizing the results from the sample group to the population.[15] *Parametric statistics* are based on the following assumptions: observations between groups are independent, the data are *distributed normally* and the variance is similar between groups. Violation of these assumptions results in unreliable parametric tests. *Non-parametric statistics* are not based on these assumptions and are applied when the data are not normally distributed.

STATISTICAL ANALYSES

t-tests and analysis of variance

After determining the type and distribution of the data collected, the next step is to choose the appropriate statistical test. First, determine what you are looking to do: quantify the difference between variables or look at the relationship between variables.

Tests to compare continuous data are *t*-tests and analysis of variance (ANOVA). Tests to compare discrete data are the chi-squared test and Fisher's exact test. Tests addressing the relationship between variables include correlations and regression analysis (Table 3.5).[16,17]

There are two tests commonly used to compare two groups of continuous data: *paired* t-*test* and *Student's* t-*test*. *Paired* t-*tests* are used when repeated measures of the same subject are being tested (e.g. before and after surgery). The corresponding non-parametric test is the Wilcoxon signed rank. *Student's* t-*test* compares independent continuous measures from two different groups (e.g. patients enrolled in rehabilitation programme A compared with patients enrolled in rehabilitation programme B). The corresponding non-parametric test is the Wilcoxon rank-sum test or the Mann–Whitney *U*-test. ANOVA is used to look for differences among three or more groups. After the ANOVA test, specific differences between groups are identified using several different methods.[16]

Correlations

Correlation and regression are measures of association between variables. These analyses calculate an '*r*', which represents the strength and directions of a relationship between two variables. The '*r*' value is usually categorized as a weak, moderate, or strong correlation (Fig. 3.3).

A Pearson correlation test is used for normally distributed data, and a Spearman rank order is used for non-parametric data.[18] Remember that correlation does not equal causation. Therefore, a correlation between variables A and B does not indicate that A caused B, only that as A changes, B changes. A positive correlation would indicate that the variables are directly related; a negative correlation would indicate that the variables are indirectly related. The strength of the relationship, as indicated by the score which falls between 0 and 1, indicates how close the data fall to a linear relationship. A score of 0 indicates that the data are completely scattered and a linear relationship between the two variables does not exist. A score of 1 would indicate that all data points fall into a straight line, indicating a direct relationship between the two variables.

One common pitfall is to assume that, because a correlation is statistically significant, it must be clinically significant, e.g. a correlation may have a *P*-value of 0.001, but the actual correlation is only 0.12. Be careful to look at both the *P*-value and the correlation coefficient before determining whether the statistically significant correlation is clinically significant.

Regression analyses

Multivariate analysis looks at the relationship between multiple independent variables and the outcome of interest. Regression is a method for obtaining a mathematical relationship between independent variables and the outcome.[7] Linear regression is calculated using an r^2. Simple linear regression looks for one predictor variable, whereas multiple regression looks at several predictor variables. The r^2 describes to what extent you can predict an outcome variable given the score of the predictor variable. For example, an r^2 of 0.81 means that the predictor variable explains 81% of the variance in the outcome variable.[19]

Table 3.5 Parametric and non-parametric tests

	Normally distributed data: parametric test	Not normally distributed data: non-parametric test
Descriptive statistics	Mean, median, standard deviation	Median, ranks
Compare 2 unpaired groups	Independent samples *t*-test	Wilcoxon rank-sum test (Mann–Whitney *U*-test)
Compare 2 paired groups	Paired *t*-test	Wilcoxon signed-rank
Compare 3 or more groups	Analysis of variance (ANOVA)	Kruskal–Wallis test
Describe the relationship between two variables	Pearson correlation coefficient	Spearman rank-correlation coefficient
Predict value from other value(s)	Linear regression, multiple-regression analysis	Non-parametric regression analysis

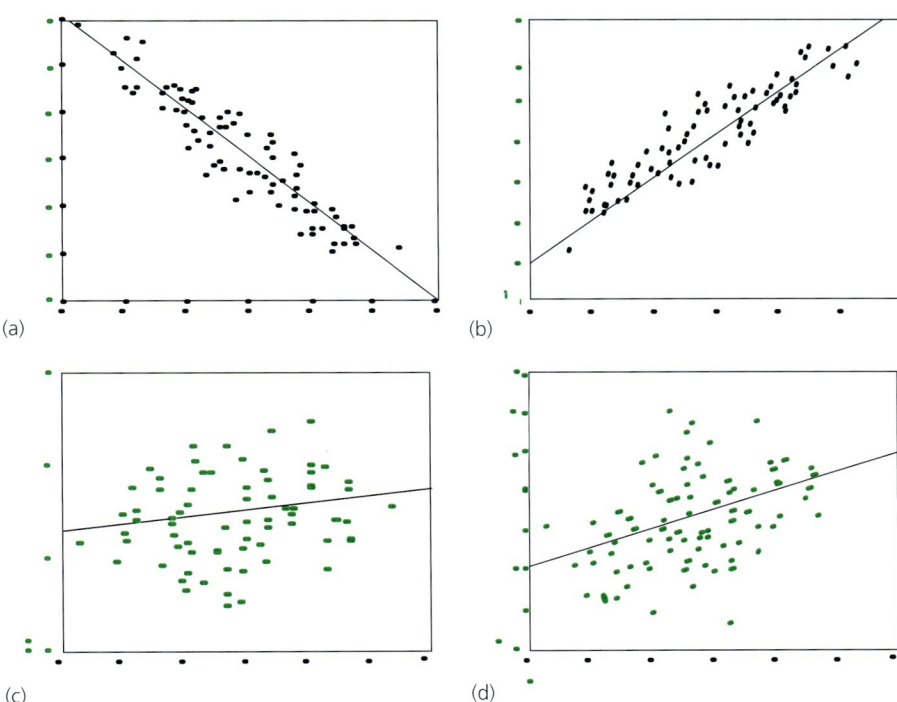

Figure 3.3 Correlations. (a) $r = -0.94$: strong negative correlation. (b) $r = 0.85$: strong positive correlation. (c) $r = 0.17$: weak positive correlation. (d) $r = 0.42$: moderate positive correlation.

Relative risks *vs* odds ratios

Cohort study and case–control study results are analysed using two specific methods: relative risks and odds ratios, respectively. A relative risk is the ratio of the incidence of disease in exposed compared with the incidence of disease in the non-exposed:[4]

$$\text{Relative risk} = \frac{\text{incidence in exposed}}{\text{incidence in non-exposed}}$$

Using a 2×2 table, relative risk is calculated in the following manner (Table 3.6):

$$\text{Incidence in exposed} = \frac{A}{(A + B)}$$

$$\text{Incidence in non-exposed} = \frac{C}{(C + D)}$$

$$\text{Relative risk} = \frac{\left[\frac{A}{(A + B)}\right]}{\left[\frac{C}{(C + D)}\right]}$$

Let us try an example problem using data from the study on multiligamentous knee injuries (exposure) and the occurrence of meniscal injury (outcome) (Table 3.7):[11]

$$\text{Relative risk} = \frac{\left[\frac{126}{184}\right]}{\left[\frac{1009}{1986}\right]} = 1.33$$

The risk of a lateral meniscus tear is 1.3 in those with a multiligament injury (ACL/medial collateral ligament) compared with those with an ACL injury only. What does this mean? It means that people with the exposure are 30% more likely to get the disease than people without the exposure. A relative risk of 1.0 would indicate that the incidence in exposed is the same as the incidence in non-exposed. A relative risk greater than 1 would indicate that the incidence in the numerator (exposed) is greater than that in the denominator (non-exposed). A relative risk less than 1 would indicate that the incidence in the denominator (non-exposed) is greater than the incidence in the numerator (exposed). Relative risks are interpreted as 'given exposure to X, the likelihood of disease is (RR)'.

In case–control studies, it is not possible to calculate an incidence rate; therefore, a relative risk calculation cannot be made. Instead, the proportion of exposed cases is compared with the proportion of exposed controls using an odds ratio (Table 3.8):[4]

Table 3.6 Relative risk

	Disease +	Disease −
Exposed	A	B
Non-exposed	C	D

Table 3.7 Example calculation of relative risk

	Lateral meniscus tear	No lateral meniscus tear	Total
ACL/MCL	126	58	184
ACL only	1009	977	1986

ACL, anterior cruciate ligament; MCL, medial collateral ligament.

$$\text{Odds that a case was exposed} = \frac{A}{C}$$

$$\text{Odds that a control was exposed} = \frac{B}{D}$$

$$\text{Odds ratio} = \frac{\left[\frac{A}{C}\right]}{\left[\frac{B}{D}\right]} = \frac{AD}{BC}$$

Let us try an example using data from our example case–control study looking at the patients with documented shoulder osteoarthritis and their exposure to shoulder dislocation (Table 3.9):[12]

$$\text{Odds ratio} = \frac{(11 \times 280)}{(80 \times 2)} = 19.3$$

The odds ratio is interpreted similarly to the relative risk. An odds ratio of 1.0 indicates that the odds of being exposed in cases are the same as the odds of being exposed in the controls. An odds ratio greater than 1.0 would indicate that the odds of exposure in the cases is higher than that in controls, and an odds ratio less than 1.0 would indicate that the odds of exposure in the controls is higher than that in cases. The odds ratio is interpreted as 'given disease X, the likelihood of exposure is (odds ratio)'. In this case, patients with shoulder osteoarthritis are 19.3 times more likely to have a history of dislocation.

Confidence intervals

Finally, there is an increasing trend of reporting confidence intervals with statistical results. Confidence intervals quantify the precision of the measurement and are usually reported as the 95% confidence interval.[7] A 95% confidence interval contains 95% of the possible values for the given statistical result, such that the true value lies somewhere within this interval. For example, if the mean is 40.0 and the confidence interval is (37.33, 42.67), and the distribution of patients was normal, the graph would look like that shown in Fig. 3.4.

In other words, we are 95% confident that the mean will fall between 37.33 and 42.67.

Confidence intervals are important for relative risks and odds ratios. If the confidence interval of a relative risk or odds ratio contains 1.0 then there is the possibility that no true difference in incidence or odds exists between groups and the findings are not statistically significant. Confidence intervals are also useful to evaluate the precision of the study. A wide confidence interval would tend to indicate a low number of subjects and uncertainty surrounding the results. A narrow confidence interval is usually seen in studies with a sufficiently large number of participants and

Table 3.8 The odds ratio

	Cases	Controls
Exposed	A	B
Non-exposed	C	D

Table 3.9 Calculation of the odds ratio

	Cases: osteoarthritis	Controls: no shoulder osteoarthritis
History of shoulder dislocation	11	2
No shoulder dislocation	80	280

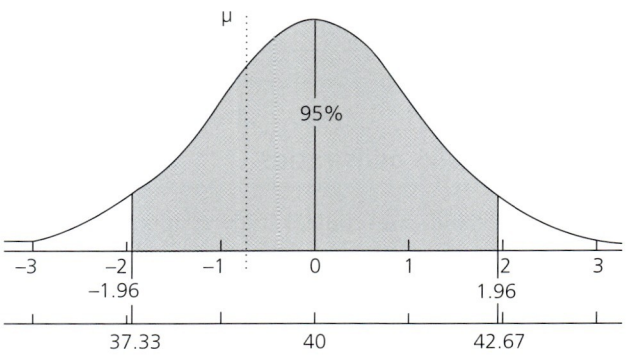

Figure 3.4 Confidence interval.

a more precise estimate of the relationship between the exposure and outcome.

EVIDENCE-BASED MEDICINE

According to the Centre of Evidence Based Medicine, 'evidence-based medicine is the conscientious, explicit and judicious use of current best evidence in making decisions about the care of individual patients. The practice of evidence-based medicine means integrating individual clinical expertise with the best available external clinical evidence from systematic research'.[20]

It is difficult to keep up with all of the latest clinical research in the field of orthopaedics. However, it is not uncommon for an interesting study to cross your desk, to hear about a new technique from colleagues, or to seek out the latest information for treating a complicated case. How can prudent clinicians evaluate the latest research and practise EBM in their clinic?

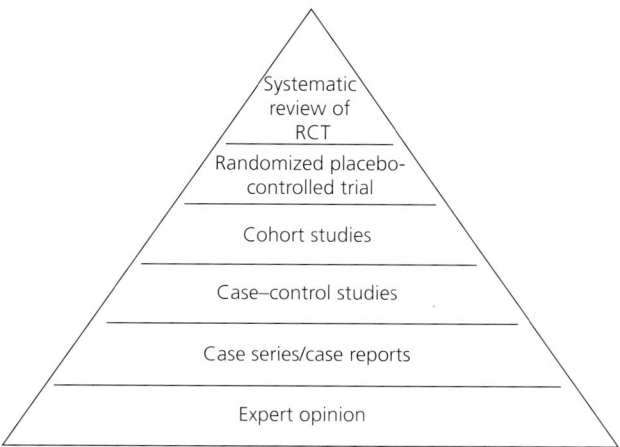

Figure 3.5 Evidence pyramid. RCT, randomized control trial.

Level of evidence

Systems for ranking the level of evidence of a study have been developed, such as the evidence pyramid (Fig. 3.5).

While the presentation may differ, the sequential increase in level of evidence from low-evidence studies, such as case reports, to high-evidence studies, such as RCTs and systematic reviews, is the same. Also notice that, as the level of evidence increases, the amount of bias decreases, again indicating improvement in the level of evidence from the bottom of the pyramid to the top. When possible, the highest level of evidence should be sought to answer a clinical query.

Reviewing articles for applicability to your practice

A systematic approach to evaluating clinical research is suggested to ensure that a thorough evaluation of the article has been completed before deciding on the applicability of the study to your practice. Suggestions regarding this approach have been made, ranging from developing a detailed outline of the article starting with the hypothesis and ending with the statistical analysis used, to an approach that looks at the biological, social, economic and epidemiological influences on the participants in the study in order to assess the study's applicability to a real clinical setting.[21] However you choose to approach this, it is important to keep one key question in mind: are the results of the article valid?[8]

Some questions that might help guide your reading include the following:[8,21]

- Was the assignment of patients to treatments randomized? If no, why not?
- Were all of the patients who entered the trial accounted for?
- What were the treatment groups? Were they similar? (Hint: look for a Table 1 containing data on patient demographics.)
- How were the exposure and outcomes measured?
- Were the appropriate statistical tests used?
- Were the power and sample size calculated prior to the study? (Note: this is often omitted from the publication.)
- Do the results seem reasonable?
- Who are the patients in this study and are they similar to patients seen in your clinic?
- Is there a compelling reason why this study would not be applicable to your practice?
- Do other studies support this finding? Is there a consensus in the literature that this finding is valid?

CONCLUSION

Epidemiology is the study of disease at a population level. Instead of focusing on each individual patient, it forces the perceptive clinician to look for trends across patients. The EBM movement has further encouraged us to con-

> **KEY LEARNING POINTS**
>
> - Understand basic epidemiological concepts and terminology, including incidence, prevalence, population, sample, bias, sensitivity, specificity, positive predictive value, negative predictive value, validity, reliability and responsiveness.
> - Know the fundamental steps involved in planning and executing a clinical trial, beginning with hypothesis generation and finishing with the final statistical analysis.
> - Understand basic statistical analysis techniques and when they are used.
> - Be able to create a 2 × 2 table and use it to determine sensitivity and specificity and to calculate odds ratios and relative risks.
> - Understand how to practically apply evidence-based medicine techniques to your everyday practice.

tinue to evaluate and re-evaluate current clinical practices using rigorous analysis techniques. A basic understanding of the concepts employed in epidemiology, the process of creating and running a clinical trial, statistical analysis and EBM will help you to create and maintain a progressive practice in order to provide your patients with the best care possible.

REFERENCES

1. Last JM. *A Dictionary of Epidemiology*, 2nd edn. New York, NY: Oxford University Press, 1988.
2. Stallones RA. To advance epidemiology. *Annual Review of Public Health* 1980;**1**:69–82.
3. Evidence-Based Medicine Working Group. Evidence-based medicine: a new approach to teaching the practice of medicine. *Journal of the American Medical Association* 1992;**268**:2420–5.
4. Gordis L. *Epidemiology*, 2nd edn. Baltimore, MD: W.B. Saunders, 2000:308.
5. Greenfield ML, Kuhn JE, Wojtys EM. A statistics primer. *American Journal of Sports Medicine* 1996;**24**:393–5.
6. Vaz CE, Camargo OP, Santana PJ, Valezi AC. Accuracy of magnetic resonance in identifying traumatic intraarticular knee lesions. *Clinics* 2005;**60**:445–50.
7. Kocher MS, Zurakowski D. Clinical epidemiology and biostatistics: a primer for orthopaedic surgeons. *Journal of Bone and Joint Surgery (American)* 2004;**86A**:607–20.
8. Oxman AD, Sackett DL, Guyatt GH. Users' guides to the medical literature. I. How to get started. Evidence-Based Medicine Working Group. *Journal of the American Medical Association* 1993;**270**:2093–5.
9. McCarty EC, Spindler KP, Tingstad E, *et al.* Does intraarticular morphine improve pain control with femoral nerve block after anterior cruciate ligament reconstruction? *American Journal of Sports Medicine* 2001;**29**:327–32.
10. Guyatt GH, Sackett DL, Cook DJ. Users' guides to the medical literature. II. How to use an article about therapy or prevention. A. Are the results of the study valid? Evidence-Based Medicine Working Group. *Journal of the American Medical Association* 1993;**270**:2598–601.
11. Kaeding CC, Pedroza AD, Parker RD, *et al.* Intra-articular findings in the reconstructed multiligament-injured knee. *Arthroscopy* 2005;**21**:424–30.
12. Marx RG, McCarty EC, Montemurno TD, *et al.* Development of arthrosis following dislocation of the shoulder: a case-control study. *Journal of Shoulder and Elbow Surgery* 2002;**11**:1–5.
13. Aaltonen S, Karjalainen H, Heinonen A, *et al.* Prevention of sports injuries: systematic review of randomized controlled trials. *Archives of Internal Medicine* 2007;**167**:1585–92.
14. Mendenhall W, Beaver R. *Introduction to Probability and Statistics*. Boston, MA: PWS-Kent Publishing Company, 1991.
15. Motulsky H. *Intuitive Biostatistics*. New York, NY: Oxford University Press, Inc., 1995.
16. Greenfield ML, Wojtys EM, Kuhn JE. A statistics primer. Tests for continuous data. *American Journal of Sports Medicine* 1997;**25**:882–4.
17. Kuhn JE, Greenfield ML, Wojtys EM. A statistics primer. Statistical tests for discrete data. *American Journal of Sports Medicine* 1997;**25**:585–6.
18. Lane D. *HyperStat*, 2nd edn. Mason, OH: Atomic Dog Publishing, 2007:244.
19. Greenfield ML, Kuhn JE, Wojtys EM. A statistics primer. Correlation and regression analysis. *American Journal of Sports Medicine* 1998;**26**:338–43.
20. Sackett DL, Rosenberg WM, Gray JA, *et al.* Evidence based medicine: what it is and what it isn't. *British Medical Journal* 1996;**312**:71–2.
21. Dans AL, Dans LF, Guyatt GH, Richardson S. Users' guides to the medical literature. XIV. How to decide on the applicability of clinical trial results to your patient. Evidence-Based Medicine Working Group. *Journal of the American Medical Association* 1998;**279**:545–9.

PART 2

MUSCULOSKELETAL STRUCTURE, FUNCTION AND HEALING

NICOLA MAFFULLI AND PATRICK WARNKE

4	Surgical anatomy and embryology of the musculoskeletal system *Franklin D Shuler*	51
5	The structure and development of bone tissue *Bodo Kurz*	82
6	Metabolic bone diseases *Eugene Sherry*	92
7	Soft tissue physiology and healing *Pankaj Sharma, Nicola Maffulli*	100
8	The physiology of ageing *Marco V. Narici, Filippo Spiezia, Nicola Maffulli*	120
9	Principles of orthopaedic pharmacology *Chezhiyan Shanmugam, Umile Giuseppe Longo, Nicola Maffulli*	126

4

Surgical anatomy and embryology of the musculoskeletal system

FRANKLIN D SHULER

Introduction	51	Spine	64
Surgical anatomy	52	Pelvis and hip	69
Shoulder	52	Thigh	73
Arm	56	Knee and leg	75
Forearm	61	Ankle and foot	77
Wrist and hand	64	Further reading	80

NATIONAL BOARD STANDARDS

- How does bone grow? Be able to draw the primary and secondary centres
- Be able to draw the growth plate (physis) and explain it
- Have a thorough knowledge of all extensile approaches
- Know the different stabilizers of the shoulder and innervation of the rotator cuff
- Be able to draw cross-sections of mid-tibia, femur, etc., showing the various structures, compartments and neurovascular bundles
- Know the anatomy of vertebrae and the exiting and traversing nerve roots
- Know the consequences of injury to nerves at various levels: what to look for clinically
- Know the course of all major nerves
- Know the structure and function of ligaments and tendons, especially the anterior cruciate ligament and the posterior cruciate ligament
- Be able to draw and explain the brachial plexus in under 1 minute

INTRODUCTION

Embryology

During the third week of human embryonic development, three basic germ layers are formed (ectoderm, mesoderm and endoderm). During the period of organogenesis (the fourth to eighth week of embryonic development) these three germ layers give rise to very specific tissues and organ systems, with the musculoskeletal system being derived from mesoderm. Ectoderm derivatives include the central and peripheral nervous system, epidermis (including hair, nails), glands (pituitary, sweat and mammary), tooth enamel and sensory epithelium of the eye, ears and nose. Mesoderm derivatives include cartilage, bone, muscle (smooth and striated), connective tissue, vascular structures and cells (arteries, veins, lymph system, heart and blood cells), and the urogenital system except the bladder, spleen and suprarenal glands. Endoderm derivatives include the epithelial linings (respiratory tract, gastrointestinal tract, tympanic cavity, Eustachian tube and urinary bladder), and parenchyma of the tonsils, thyroid, parathyroid, thymus, liver and pancreas. Alterations in musculoskeletal development can occur and are often traced to congenital (e.g. autosomal dominant point mutation in chromosome 4 producing achrondroplasia dwarfism) or environmental (e.g. radiation, drugs (thalidomide producing limb abnormalities)) factors interfering with the process of organogenesis.

Osteology (mesoderm origin)

The human skeleton has 206 bones: 80 bones in the axial skeleton and 126 bones in the appendicular skeleton. Ossification, the formation of bone, can be intramembranous (without a cartilage model; as in the skull) or enchondral (with a cartilage model; most bones). Enchondral growth begins in the diaphyses of long bones at a primary ossification centre, most of which are present at birth. Secondary ossification centres usually develop in the periphery of bones and are important for growth and the treatment of childhood fractures. The first bone to ossify at 5 weeks of fetal development is the medial and lateral primary ossification centre of the clavicle. Of interest, the clavicle's medial ossification centre is the last skeletal bone to fuse at 21–25 years old.

SURGICAL ANATOMY

Surgically important anatomy is reviewed in this chapter. Readers should refer to excellent resources such as the third edition of *Surgical Exposures in Orthopaedics: The Anatomic Approach* by Hoppenfield and deBoer for a more in-depth illustrative coverage of this material.

SHOULDER

Osteology

SCAPULA

The scapula is triangular shaped and spans the second to seventh ribs posteriorly and serves as an attachment for 17 muscles and four ligaments. Key anatomical processes are the scapular spine, coracoid and acromion. The scapular spine separates the supraspinatus and infraspinatus fossae and terminates laterally as the acromion. The scapular glenoid is retroverted approximately 5°. Attachments to the anterior coracoid process include the coracoacromial ligament, coracoclavicular ligaments (conoid and trapezoid (lateral)), conjoined tendon (coracobrachialis and short head of biceps) and pectoralis minor. There are three intrinsic ligaments of the scapula (superior transverse scapular ligament, inferior transverse scapular ligament and the coracoacromial ligament). The suprascapular notch has the superior transverse scapular ligament separating the suprascapular artery (superior) from the suprascapular nerve (inferior). The spinoglenoid notch has both the artery and nerve inferior to the inferior transverse scapular ligament. Long-term nerve compression at the spinoglenoid notch results in infraspinatus muscle atrophy. The coracoacromial ligament is important in superior–anterior restraint in rotator cuff deficiencies and should be preserved when debriding painful massive rotator cuff tears that cannot be surgically repaired. The acromial branch of the thoracoacromial artery runs on the medial aspect of the coracoacromial ligament.

CLAVICLE

The clavicle is the most frequently fractured bone, and a fractured clavicle is the most common musculoskeletal birth injury. The clavicle has a double curvature (sternal–ventral, acromial–dorsal) and serves as a fulcrum for lateral movement of the arm.

Arthrology

GLENOHUMERAL JOINT

The shoulder area has one major (glenohumeral) and several minor (sternoclavicular, acromioclavicular, scapulothoracic) articulations. The spheroidal (ball and socket) glenohumeral joint has the greatest range of motion of any joint, but motion is at the expense of stability that is kept in check by static and dynamic restraints. Static restraints include articular anatomy, glenoid labrum, negative pressure, capsule and ligaments (Table 4.1). Dynamic restraints include the rotator cuff, biceps tendon and scapulothoracic motion.

STERNOCLAVICULAR JOINT

A double gliding joint with an articular disc. Its ligaments include the capsule, anterior and posterior sternoclavicular ligaments, an interclavicular ligament and a costoclavicular ligament. The sternoclavicular joint rotates 30° with shoulder motion.

Table 4.1 Glenohumeral stabilizers

Structure	Function
Coracohumeral ligament	Primary restraint to inferior translation of the adducted arm and to ER
Glenoid labrum	Increases surface area, static stabilizer
SGHL	Primary restraint to ER in adducted or slightly abducted arm
	Primary restraint to inferior translation in the adducted arm
MGHL (absent in up to 30%)	Primary stabilizer to anterior translation with the arm abducted to 45°
IGHLC	Primary stabilizer for anterior and inferior instability in abduction

ER, external rotation; IGHLC, inferior glenohumeral ligament complex; MGHL, middle glenohumeral ligament; SGHL, superior glenohumeral ligament.

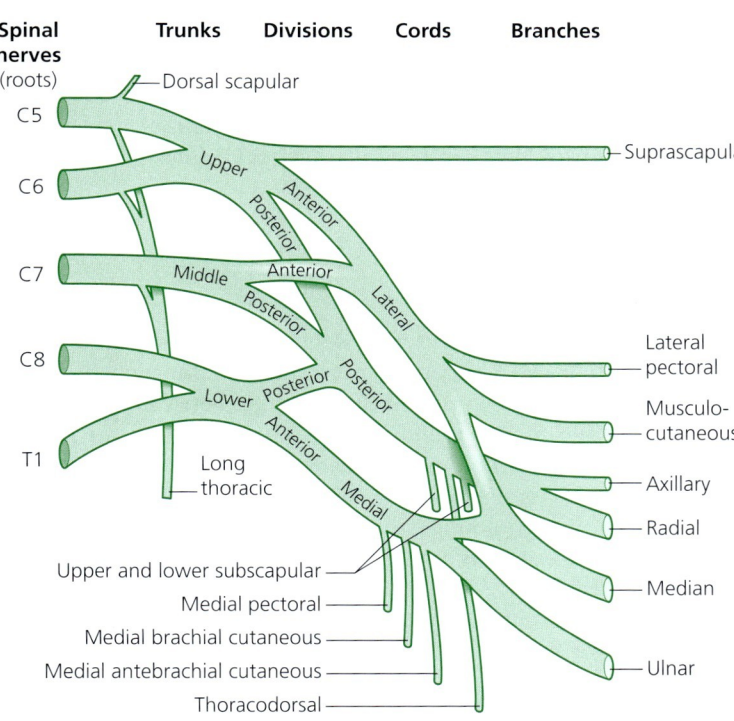

Figure 4.1 Brachial plexus: ventral primary rami C5–T1. There are four preclavicular/supraclavicular branches: long thoracic nerve (serratus anterior muscle), dorsal scapular nerve (rhomboid muscle), suprascapular nerve (supraspinatus and infraspinatus muscle) and the nerve to the subclavius (not shown). Redrawn with permission from DB Jenkins *Hollinshead's Functional Anatomy of the Limbs and Back*, 6th edn. Philadelphia, PA: WB Saunders, 1991.

ACROMIOCLAVICULAR JOINT

A plane/gliding joint that also possesses a fibrocartilaginous disc. Its ligaments include the capsule, acromioclavicular ligament and coracoclavicular ligament (with trapezoid (anterolateral) and conoid (posteromedial and stronger) component ligaments). The acromioclavicular ligaments prevent anteroposterior displacement of the distal clavicle. The coracoclavicular ligament prevents superior displacement of the distal clavicle. When the arm is maximally elevated, about 5–8° of rotation occurs at the acromioclavicluar joint, although the clavicle rotates approximately 40–50°.

SCAPULOTHORACIC JOINT

Although not a true joint, this attachment allows scapular movement against the posterior rib cage. It is fixed primarily by the scapular muscular attachments. Glenohumeral motion, as compared with scapulothoracic motion, is in approximately a 2:1 ratio.

Neuromuscular anatomy

MUSCLES OF THE SHOULDER

Five muscles help to connect the upper limb to the vertebral column (trapezius, latissimus, both rhomboids and the levator scapulae). Four muscles connect the upper limb to the thoracic wall (both pectoralis muscles, subclavius and serratus anterior). Finally, six muscles act on the shoulder joint itself (deltoid, teres major and the four rotator cuff muscles (supraspinatus, infraspinatus, teres minor, subscapularis)). The rotator cuff muscles serve to depress and stabilize the humeral head against the glenoid. The greater tuberosity of the humerus serves as an attachment for three rotator cuff muscles: supraspinatus, infraspinatus and the teres minor. The lesser tuberosity of the humerus serves as the attachment site for the subscapularis muscle (shoulder internal rotator). The shoulder internal rotators (pectoralis major, lattisimus dorsi and subscapularis) are stronger than the external rotators (teres minor and infraspinatus), which is why posterior shoulder dislocations happen more commonly with electrical shock and seizures.

Table 4.2 Rotator cuff muscle innervation: all C5, C6

Muscle	Innervation
External rotators	
Supraspinatus	Suprascapular nerve (C5, C6)
Infraspinatus	Suprascapular nerve (C5, C6)
Teres minor	Axillary nerve (C5, C6)
Internal rotators	
Subscapularis	Upper (C5) and lower subscapular nerve (C5, C6)

NERVES OF THE SHOULDER

The brachial plexus (Fig. 4.1) is formed from the ventral primary rami of C5–T1 and lies under the clavicle between the scalenus anterior and scalenus medius. Innervation of all rotator cuff muscles is derived from C5, C6 of the brachial plexus (Table 4.2).

There are four preclavicular nerve branches (from roots and upper trunk): dorsal scapular nerve, long thoracic nerve, suprascapular nerve and nerve to subclavius. Preganglionic (proximal to the dorsal root ganglion) brachial plexus lesions would be expected to produce scapular winging (owing to paralysis of the preclavicular long thoracic nerve) and Horner syndrome (injury to brachial plexus at C8–T1 involving the inferior/stellate ganglion). Patients with post-ganglionic brachial plexus injuries should therefore not have Horner syndrome, winged scapula, diaphragmatic paralysis or rhomboid paralysis. Additional review of obstetrical brachial plexus palsies is shown in Table 4.3.

Injury to the spinal accessory nerve causes scapular–trapezius winging, resulting in shoulder depression with scapular translation laterally and the inferior angle rotated laterally because of the unopposed pull of the serratus anterior. Injury to the long thoracic nerve causes serratus anterior scapular winging, resulting in superior elevation with scapular translation medially and the inferior angle rotated medially. Cutaneous innervation of the shoulder is from the supraclavicular nerve (C3,C4) and the axillary nerve.

Vessels

The subclavian artery arises either directly from the aorta (left subclavian) or from the brachiocephalic trunk (right subclavian). It then emerges between the scalenus anterior and medius muscles and becomes the axillary artery at the outer border of the first rib. The axillary artery is divided into three portions based on its relationship to the pectoralis minor (the first is medial to it, the second is under it, and the third is lateral to it) (Table 4.4). Each part of the artery has as many branches as the number of that portion (e.g. the second part has two branches). The third part of the axillary artery at the origin of the anterior and posterior humeral circumflex arteries is most vulnerable to traumatic vascular injury. See Fig. 4.2.

Surgical approaches to the shoulder

These include the anterior approach (reconstruction and arthroplasty), lateral and anterolateral approach (acromioplasty and rotator cuff repair) and posterior

Table 4.3 Brachial plexus palsy summary

Palsy	Roots	Deficit	Prognosis
Erb–Duchenne	C5, C6	Deltoid, rotator cuff, elbow flexors, wrist and hand extensors, 'waiter's tip'	Best
Klumpke	C8, T1	Wrist flexors, intrinsics, Horner syndrome	Poor
Total plexus	C5–T1	Flaccid arm	Worst

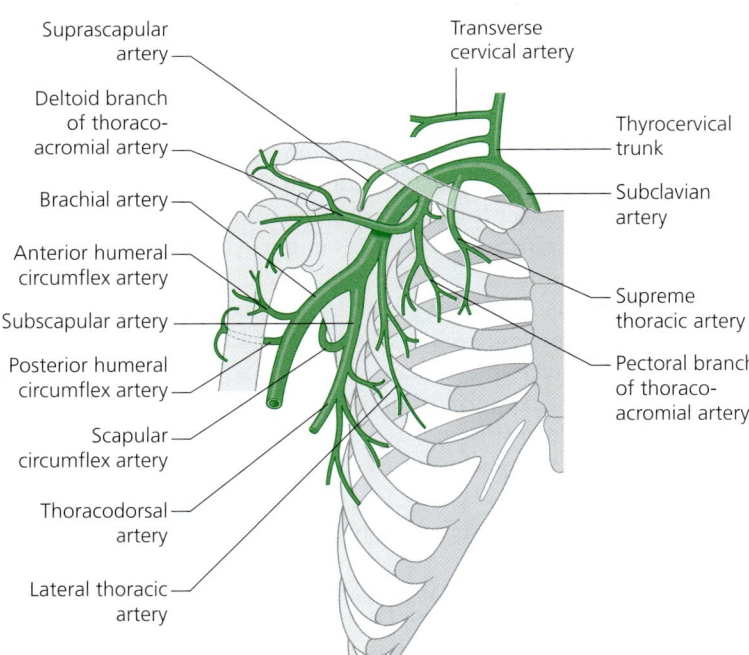

Figure 4.2 Branches of the axillary artery. When the subclavian artery passes beneath the clavicle, it becomes the axillary artery. The axillary artery is divided into three sections based on the relationship to the pectoralis minor muscle (not shown but attaches to coracoid). The first part of the axillary artery is medial to the pectoralis minor and supplies the supreme thoracic artery. The second part is beneath the muscle and supplies the thoracoacromial artery and the lateral thoracic artery. The third part is lateral to the pectoralis minor and supplies the subscapular artery and the posterior and anterior humeral circumflex arteries. The third part of the axillary artery, at the origin of the anterior and posterior humeral circumflex arteries, is the most vulnerable to injury. Redrawn with permission from DB Jenkins *Hollinshead's Functional Anatomy of the Limbs and Back*, 6th edn. Philadelphia, PA: WB Saunders, 1991.

Table 4.4 Axillary artery branches

Part	Branch	Course
1	Supreme thoracic	Medial to serratus anterior and pectoralis minor
2	Thoracoacromial	Four branches (deltoid, acromial, pectoralis, clavicular)
	Lateral thoracic	Descends to serratus anterior
3	Subscapular	Two branches (thoracodorsal and circumflex scapular (triangular space))
	Anterior humeral circumflex	Blood supply to humeral head: arcuate artery lateral to bicipital groove
	Posterior humeral circumflex	Branch in the quadrangular space accompanying the axillary nerve

Table 4.5 Shoulder surgical approaches

Approach	Interval	Risks
Anterior (Henry)	Deltoid (axillary nerve) and pectoralis major (medial and lateral pectoral nerve)	Axillary nerve limits inferior exposure (place arm in adduction and ER)
		Musculocutaneous nerve: avoid vigorous retraction and medial dissection to the conjoined tendon/coracobrachialis
Lateral	Deltoid splitting (axillary nerve)	Avoid deltoid split >5 cm below the acromion to avoid damaging the axillary nerve. Division of the acromial branch of the coracoacromial artery
Posterior	Infraspinatus (suprascapular nerve) and teres minor (axillary nerve)	Dissection inferior to the teres minor risks quadrangular space structures: axillary nerve and posterior humeral circumflex artery
		Avoid excessive medial retraction on infraspinatus, which can injure suprascapular nerve

ER, external rotation.

approach (posterior reconstruction). A summary chart is shown in Table 4.5.

ANTERIOR APPROACH (HENRY) (FIG. 4.3)

This explores the interval between the deltoid (axillary nerve) and the pectoralis major (medial and lateral pectoral nerve). The cephalic vein is identified in the deltopectoral groove and retracted either laterally with the deltoid or medially with the pectoralis major. If preferred, the surgeon can improve deep exposure by performing a coracoid osteotomy with arm adduction, releasing the conjoined tendon (short head of biceps and coracobrachialis). Protect the musculocutaneous nerve by avoiding vigorous retraction of the conjoined tendon and by avoiding dissection medial to the coracobrachialis. The subscapularis transversely oriented muscle fibres are noted deep, with the muscle inferior border marked with a leash of three vessels (one artery and the superior and inferior venae comitantes). With the arm held in external rotation to move the planned incision away from the axillary nerve (inferior to the shoulder capsule), the subscapularis tendon is incised with a longitudinal incision, with some surgeons preserving the inferior fibres of the supscapularis to add a measure of safety in axillary nerve protection. Retraction of the subscapularis with tag sutures reveals the anterior shoulder joint capsule. With capsular incision, the humeral head and glenoid are exposed, completing the anterior approach to the shoulder.

LATERAL AND ANTEROLATERAL APPROACH

There is no internervous plane with these approaches. Following incision, the deltoid muscle is visualized and is either vertically split or subperiosteally elevated from the acromion. The deltoid should not be split more than 5 cm below the acromion to avoid injury to the axillary nerve. If dissection extends >5 cm inferior, denervation of the deltoid can occur in a location anterior to the muscle split owing to the posterior innervation of the muscle. If the anterolateral approach is used for rotator cuff repair, the coracoacromial ligament is noted and detached from the acromion (bleeding noted from the acromial branch of the thoracoacromial artery). Preservation of this ligament is important for superior

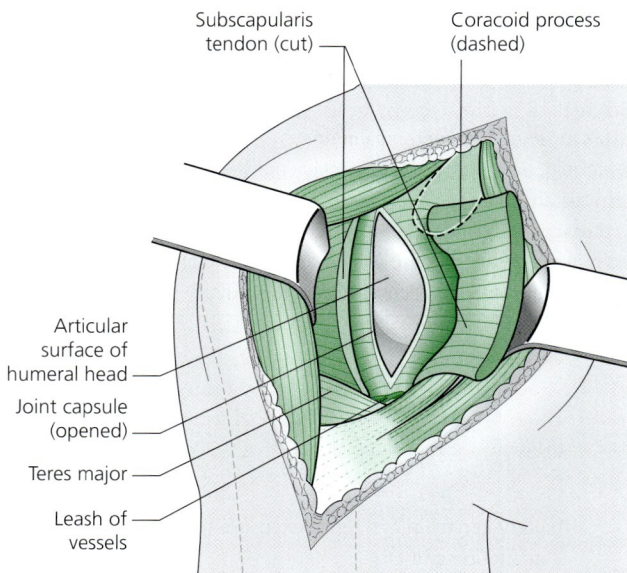

Figure 4.3 Anterior (Henry) approach to the shoulder. The interval between the deltoid (axillary nerve) and the pectoralis major (medial and lateral pectoral nerve) is explored. Avoid excessive medial retraction on the coracobrachialis or dissection medial to this muscle to prevent injury to the musculocutaneous nerve. Avoid the axillary nerve, which is inferior to the shoulder capsule. Positioning the arm in adduction and external rotation helps displace the axillary nerve from the surgical field. The deep exposure is assisted following coracoid osteotomy (shown with predrilling). The tag sutures in the subscapularis tendon aid with retraction with a longitudinal incision in the anterior shoulder capsule exposing the glenohumeral articulation.

humeral head restraint when debriding painful massive rotator cuff tears. Deep exposure of the supraspinatus is achieved with humeral rotation bringing other rotator cuff insertions into view.

POSTERIOR APPROACH

This approach (Fig. 4.4) explores the internervous plane between the infraspinatus (suprascapular nerve) and teres minor (axillary nerve). This plane can be approached by detaching the deltoid from the scapular spine or by splitting the deltoid (Rockwood's). Following retraction of the infraspinatus superiorly (avoid excessive medial retraction and possible suprascapular nerve injury) and the teres minor inferiorly, the posterior shoulder capsule is visualized. Following capsule incision, the glenohumeral joint is exposed, completing the approach. The axillary nerve and the posterior circumflex humeral artery both run in the quadrangular space below the teres minor, so it is important that dissections stay above this muscle.

ARM

Osteology

HUMERUS

The humerus is the largest and longest bone of the upper extremity. The hemispherical head, directed superiorly, medially and slightly dorsally, articulates with the much smaller scapular glenoid cavity. Unlike the femoral head, there is no fossa for ligamentous attachments on the

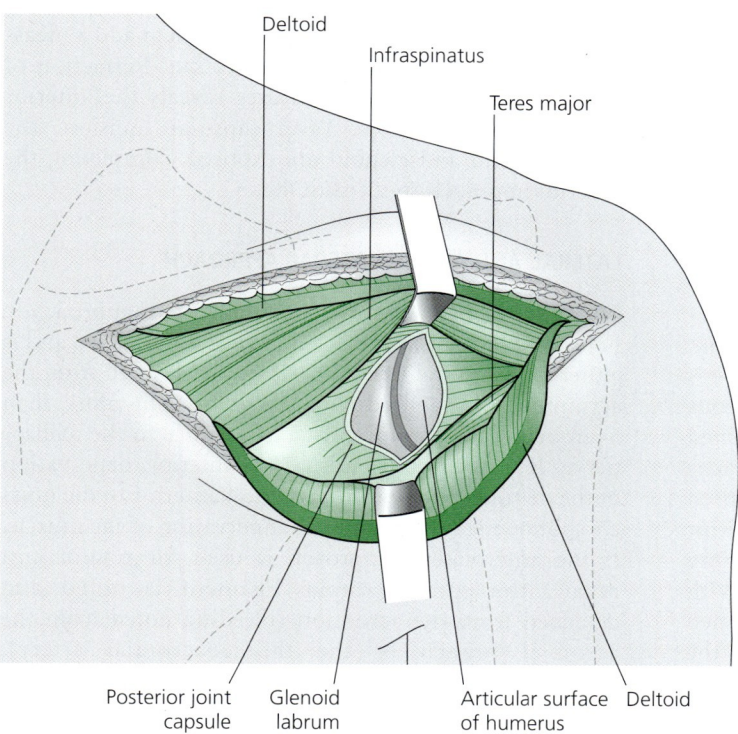

Figure 4.4 Posterior approach to the shoulder. The interval between the infraspinatus (suprascapular nerve) and teres minor (axillary nerve) is explored. Do not dissect below the teres minor. Dissections below the teres minor risk injury to the structures in the quadrangular space: posterior humeral circumflex artery and the axillary nerve. The axillary nerve divides into the deep (deltoid) and superficial branches (teres minor and cutaneous branch (Hilton's law)) within the quadrangular space. Also avoid excessive retraction of the infraspinatus to avoid suprascapular nerve palsy.

humeral head. Like the glenoid, the humeral head is retroverted approximately 30° (widely variable) with respect to the transepicondylar axis. The anatomical neck, directly below the head, serves as an attachment for the shoulder capsule. The surgical neck is lower and is more often involved in fractures. The greater tuberosity, lateral to the head, serves as the attachment for the supraspinatus, infraspinatus and teres minor muscles (anterior to posterior, respectively). The lesser tuberosity, located anteriorly, has only one muscular insertion: the subscapularis. The bicipital or intertubercular groove (for the tendon of the long head of the biceps) is situated between these two tuberosities. The blood supply to the humeral head (arcuate artery: anterolateral ascending branch of the anterior humeral circumflex artery) is located in the lateral portion of the bicipital groove. The posterior humeral shaft has a spiral groove for the radial nerve located approximately 13 cm above the articular surface of the trochlea. Distally, the humerus flares into medial and lateral epicondyles. Medially, the spool-shaped trochlea articulates with the olecranon of the ulna. Laterally, the globular capitellum articulates with the radial head. The normal articular alignment of the distal humerus has a 7° valgus tilt (carrying angle).

Arthrology

GLENOHUMERAL AND ELBOW JOINTS

The humerus articulates with the scapula on its upper end, forming the glenohumeral joint (discussed earlier), and, with the radius and ulna on its lower end, forming the elbow joint. The elbow is composed of a compound ginglymus (hinge) joint (the humeroulnar articulation) and a trochoid (pivot) joint (the humeroradial articulation). The axis of rotation for the elbow is centred through the trochlea and capitellum and passes through a point anteroinferior on the medial epicondyle. The elbow capsule allows maximal distension at approximately 70–80° of flexion, which is why patients with effusions hold their arms in this most comfortable position. Also, the anterior capsule attaches at a point approximately 6 mm distal to the tip of the coronoid. Because of this, the coronoid tip is an intra-articular structure that is visualized during elbow arthroscopy. Other coronoid attachments include the anterior bundle of the medial collateral ligament (18 mm distal to the medial coronoid tip) and brachialis (11 mm distal to the coronoid tip). Chapter 74 addresses the clinically important elbow capsuloligamentous structures with a quick review provided in Table 4.6. The medial collateral ligament (anterior bundle, posterior bundle and transverse bundle) arises from the anteroinferior portion of the medial humeral epicondyle and provides stability to valgus stress. The anterior bundle is most important in helping resist valgus forces. Remember that valgus stability with the arm in pronation suggests an intact band of the medial collateral ligament. The lateral collateral ligament or radial collateral ligament (annular, radial and ulnar parts) originates on the lateral humeral epicondyle near the axis of elbow rotation. The lateral ulnar collateral ligament (LUCL) is an essential elbow stabilizer and runs from the lateral epicondyle to the ulna crista supinatoris (supinator crest). Deficiency of the LUCL manifests as posterolateral rotatory instability of the elbow.

Neuromuscular anatomy

MUSCLES OF THE ARM

The four muscles of the arm are the coracobrachialis, biceps, brachialis and triceps. From posterior, the long head of the triceps serves as an important landmark in defining the quadrangular space, the triangular space and the triangular interval (Table 4.7).

NERVES OF THE ARM

Two nerves give rise to arm muscle innervation. The musculocutaneous nerve innervates the coracobrachialis, biceps and the brachialis (dual innervation with radial nerve). The radial nerve innervates the triceps. A summary of the four major nerves in the arm is provided below.

Table 4.6 Elbow ligaments

Ligament	Components	Comments
MCL	Anterior bundle MCL (ulnar collateral) Posterior bundle Transverse bundle (Cooper's ligament)	Anterior bundle (strongest of all elbow ligaments): anterior band taut from 60° flexion to full extension, posterior band taut from 60° to 120° flexion
Lateral collateral	LUCL Annular ligament Quadrate (annular ligament to radial neck) and oblique cord	Deficiency of LUCL results in posterolateral rotatory instability

LUCL, lateral ulnar collateral; MCL, medial collateral.

Table 4.7 Shoulder spaces and intervals

Space	Borders	Nerve	Vessel
Quadrangular (quadrilateral) space	Superior: lower border teres minor Lateral: surgical neck of humerus Medial: long head of triceps Inferior: upper border of teres major	Axillary nerve	Posterior humeral circumflex artery
Triangular space	Superior: lower border of teres minor Lateral: long head of triceps Medial: teres major		Circumflex scapular artery
Triangular interval	Superior: lower border teres major Lateral: shaft of humerus Medial: long head of triceps	Radial nerve	Profunda brachii artery

Table 4.8 Arm surgical approaches

Approach	Interval	Risks
Anterior	Proximal: deltoid (axillary nerve) and pectoralis major (medial and lateral pectoral nerve) Distal: brachialis (radial and musculocutaneous nerve)	Radial nerve Axillary nerve Anterior humeral circumflex artery
Posterior	Triceps (radial nerve): lateral and long heads with split of the deep head	Radial nerve Deep brachial artery
Anterolateral–distal	Brachialis (musculocutaneous and radial nerve) and brachioradialis (radial nerve)	Radial nerve

Musculocutaneous nerve (lateral cord brachial plexus)

Pierces the coracobrachialis 5–8 cm distal to the coracoid and then branches to supply this muscle, the biceps and the brachialis. It also gives off a branch to the elbow joint before it becomes the lateral antebrachial cutaneous nerve of the forearm, which is located lateral to the cephalic vein.

Radial nerve (posterior cord brachial plexus)

Spirals around the humerus (medial to lateral) in the posterior spiral groove at a distance of approximately 13 cm from the trochlea. It emerges on the lateral side of the arm after piercing the lateral intermuscular septum approximately 7.5 cm above the trochlea between the brachialis and brachioradialis anterior to the lateral epicondyle (where it supplies the anconeus muscle).

Median nerve (medial and lateral cords brachial plexus)

Accompanies the brachial artery along the arm, crossing it during its course (lateral to medial). It supplies some branches to the elbow joint.

Ulnar nerve (medial cord brachial plexus)

Medial to the brachial artery in the arm and then runs behind the medial epicondyle of the humerus, where it is quite superficial. It also supplies some branches to the elbow joint.

Cutaneous nerves

Most of the cutaneous innervation of the arm arises directly from the brachial plexus.

Vessels

The brachial artery originates at the lower border of the tendon of the teres major and continues to the elbow, where it bifurcates into the radial and ulnar arteries. Lying medial in the arm, the brachial artery curves laterally to enter the cubital fossa (formed by the distal humerus proximally, the brachioradialis laterally and the pronator teres medially). Its principal branches include the profunda or deep brachial artery that accompanies the radial nerve posteriorly in the triangular interval, the superior and inferior ulnar collaterals, and the nutrient and muscular branches.

Surgical approaches to the arm

These include the anterior and posterior approaches to the arm and distal humerus. A summary is shown in Table 4.8.

ANTERIOR APPROACH TO THE HUMERUS

There are two internervous planes: proximal and distal. The proximal plane is between the deltoid (axillary nerve)

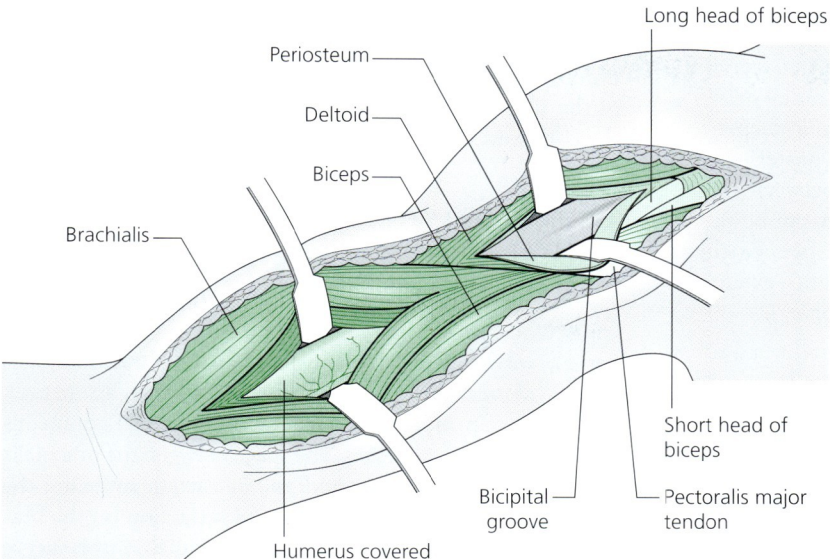

Figure 4.5 Anterior approach to the humerus. The two internervous planes are illustrated. The proximal plane is between the deltoid (axillary nerve) and the pectoralis major (medial and lateral pectoral nerves) and the distal plane is between the medial and lateral fibres of the brachialis (musculocutaneous nerve and radial nerve, respectively).

and the pectoralis major (medial and lateral pectoral nerves) with the distal plane between the medial and lateral fibres of the brachialis (musculocutaneous nerve and radial nerve, respectively). See Fig. 4.5. The proximal humeral shaft is approached after locating the cephalic vein and retracting the deltoid and pectoralis major. The insertions of the deltoid (deltoid tuberosity) and the pectoralis major (lateral bicipital groove) are exposed with the anterior humeral circumflex artery crossing the surgical field. Subperiosteal dissection with anterior humeral circumflex artery ligation completes the approach to the proximal humeral shaft. Careful lateral deltoid retraction is used to decrease the chance of axillary nerve injury. Radial nerve injury is minimized by meticulous attention to avoid deep posterior humeral cortical penetration with drills, taps, screws and depth gauges, especially in the region 13 cm proximal to the trochlea (humeral spiral radial groove). The distal humeral shaft is approached following retraction of the biceps medially exposing the underlying brachialis. A midline longitudinal split of the brachialis fibres exposes the distal humeral shaft. Lateral brachialis retraction places an additional compressive force against the radial nerve that has pierced the lateral intramuscular septum and lies between the brachialis and brachioradialis. A midline brachialis split leaves enough muscle to help cushion against compressive injury to the radial nerve during lateral brachialis retraction.

POSTERIOR APPROACH TO THE HUMERUS

This is illustrated in Fig. 4.6. There is no internervous plane with the interval between the lateral and long heads of the triceps split superficially and a muscle-splitting approach used on the deep medial triceps. The radial nerve limits proximal extension of this approach and the radial nerve and groove separates the origins of the lateral head and the

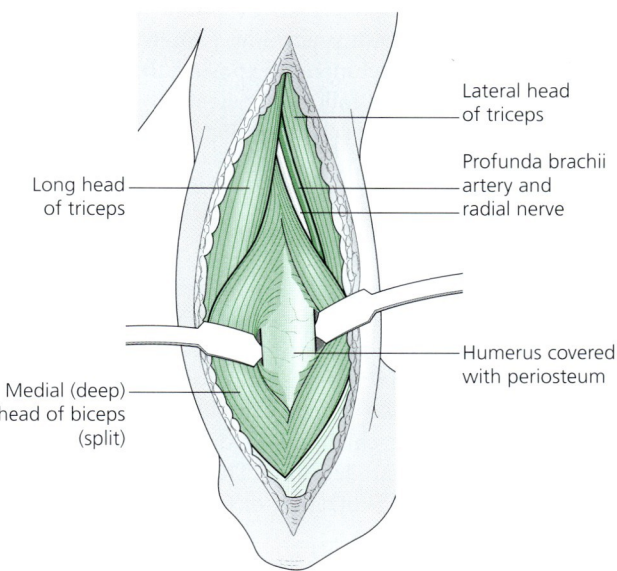

Figure 4.6 Posterior approach to the humerus. The medial or deep head of the triceps is split in this approach. As illustrated, the radial nerve and profunda brachii artery limit the proximal extent of this approach.

medial head of the triceps. Following separation of the lateral and long triceps heads, midline incision of the triceps tendon distally exposes the deep medial triceps. In the superior deep surgical field, the radial nerve and deep or profunda brachial artery are seen at the superior extent/origin of the medial triceps and protected. Midline medial triceps split exposes the humeral shaft. Subperiosteal dissection completes the surgical approach and also helps protect the ulnar nerve as it passes anterior to posterior at the lateral intermuscular septum.

LATERAL APPROACH TO THE DISTAL HUMERUS

There is no internervous plane with dissection between the brachioradialis (radial nerve) and the triceps (radial nerve). The lateral incision at the supracondylar ridge is deepened to expose the anterior brachioradialis and the posterior triceps. Exposure to bone is done by cutting between these muscles and with retraction. Distal extension can be used to visualize the radiocapitellar articulation (see Kocher elbow approach: anconeus (radial nerve) and extensor carpi radialis ulnaris (posterior interosseus nerve)).

Surgical approaches to the elbow

Surgical approaches include the anterior, posterior and anterolateral approaches. A summary is given in Table 4.9.

POSTERIOR APPROACH TO THE ELBOW

There is no internervous plane. The arm extensor mechanism is detached following an olecranon osteotomy (a chevron osteotomy with predrilling is preferred to facilitate anatomical reattachment). Exposure to the posterior elbow joint is achieved following osteotomy, which completes the surgical approach. The ulnar nerve is protected throughout this approach.

MEDIAL APPROACH TO THE ELBOW

The internervous plane is between the brachialis (musculocutaneous nerve) and the triceps (radial nerve) proximally and the brachialis and pronator teres (median nerve) distally. Following skin incision, the ulnar nerve is palpated in the medial epicondylar groove. The interval between the pronator teres and brachialis is seen directly anterior to the medial intermuscular septum. The pronator teres is retracted gently with protection of the median nerve that enters this muscle. A medial epicondyle osteotomy provides access to the elbow joint and visualization of the ulnohumeral articulation, including the coronoid process of the ulna with the brachialis attaching 11 mm distal to the coronoid tip.

ANTEROLATERAL APPROACH TO THE ELBOW (HENRY'S)

The internervous plane proximally is between the brachialis (musculocutaneous nerve) and the brachioradialis (radial nerve), with the distal plane between the brachioradialis (radial nerve) and the pronator teres (median nerve). Following skin incision, the lateral antebrachial cutaneous nerve is seen and protected. The space between the brachialis and brachioradialis is entered and retracted, revealing the radial nerve and its branches. Careful retraction on the brachioradialis helps prevent injury to the radial sensory nerve branch. Ligation of the recurrent radial artery facilitates retraction of the brachioradialis laterally and retraction of the pronator teres and radial artery medially. The anterior radiocapitellar articulation is exposed following incision into the anterior joint capsule between the radial nerve and the brachialis. With the arm in supination, the supinator muscle is subperiosteally elevated to expose the proximal radial shaft, completing the surgical approach. See Fig. 4.7.

POSTEROLATERAL (KOCHER'S) APPROACH TO THE ELBOW

The internervous plane is between the anconeus (radial nerve) and the extensor carpi ulnaris (ECU) (posterior interosseous nerve; PIN). Following skin incision, the interval between the anconeus and the ECU is noted distally (proximally, the two muscles share the same aponeurosis). The anconeus and ECU are separated, exposing the deep supinator. With the forearm in pronation, the supinator is

Table 4.9 Elbow surgical approaches

Approach	Interval	Risks
Posterior	Detach triceps or olecranon osteotomy	Ulnar nerve
		Olecranon non-union
Medial	Proximally: brachialis (musculocutaneous nerve) and triceps (radial nerve)	Ulnar nerve
		Medial antebrachial cutaneous nerve
	Distally: brachialis and pronator teres (median nerve)	Median nerve with pronator teres retraction
Anterolateral (Henry's)	Proximally: brachialis (musculocutaneous nerve) and brachioradialis (radial nerve)	Lateral antebrachial cutaneous nerve
		Radial nerve and its branches
	Distally: pronator teres (median nerve) and brachioradialis (radial nerve)	Ligation of radial recurrent artery
		Supinate forearm during supinator subperiosteal elevation
Posterolateral (Kocher's)	Anconeus (radial nerve) and ECU (PIN of radial nerve)	PIN (pronation moves PIN anteriorly and radially)
		Pronate forearm

ECU, extensor carpi ulnaris; PIN, posterior interosseous nerve.

Forearm

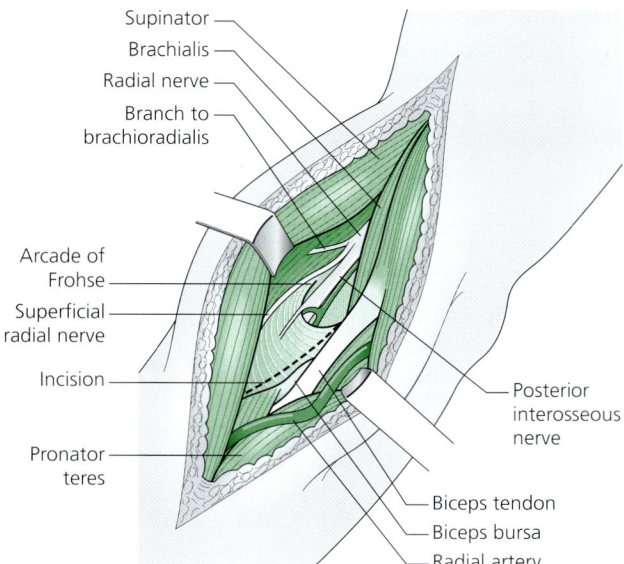

Figure 4.7 Anterolateral approach to the elbow (Henry's). The internervous plane proximally is between the brachialis (musculocutaneous nerve) and the brachioradialis (radial nerve), with the distal plane between the brachioradialis (radial nerve) and the pronator teres (median nerve). As illustrated, with the arm in supination, the supinator muscle is subperiosteally elevated (dotted line) to expose the proximal radial shaft. The radial nerve three terminal branches are noted: posterior interosseous nerve, sensory radial nerve, and a motor branch to the extensor carpi radialis brevis.

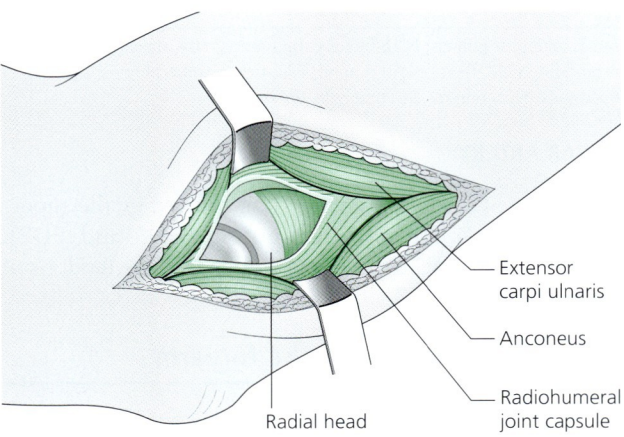

Figure 4.8 Posterolateral (Kocher's) approach to the elbow. The internervous plane is between the anconeus (radial nerve) and the extensor carpi ulnaris (posterior interosseous nerve). With the forearm in pronation, the supinator is incised, exposing the radial head and radiocapitellar articulation.

incised exposing the radial head and radiocapitellar articulation, completing the approach. Pronation of the forearm moves the PIN anteriorly and radially away from the planned supinator incision. The surgical approach is not extended distally past the annular ligament to avoid increasing the risk of damage to the PIN. See Fig. 4.8.

FOREARM

Osteology

ULNA

Proximally, the ulna is composed of two curved processes, the olecranon and the coronoid, with an intervening trochlear notch. Distally, the ulna tapers and ends in a lateral head and a medial styloid process.

RADIUS

The proximal radius is composed of a head with a central fovea, a neck and a proximal medial radial tuberosity (for insertion of the biceps tendon). The radius has a gradual bend (convex laterally) and gradually increases in size distally. Restoration of the radial bow is important in fixation of radial shaft fractures. The distal extremity of the radius is composed of the carpal articular surface, an ulnar notch, a dorsal tubercle (Lister's tubercle, which is at the level of the scapholunate joint) and a lateral styloid process.

Arthrology

The ulnohumeral and radiocapitellar articulations were discussed earlier. The wrist has a radiocarpal joint, a distal radioulnar articulation that is most stable in supination, and a triangular fibrocartilage complex.

RADIOCARPAL JOINT

An ellipsoid joint involving the distal radius and the scaphoid, lunate and triquetrum. This joint is usually located at the level of the proximal wrist flexion crease. Covered by a loose capsule, the wrist relies heavily on ligaments, especially volar ligaments, for stability. They include the volar and dorsal radiocarpal ligaments and the ulnar and radial collateral ligaments.

TRIANGULAR FIBROCARTILAGE COMPLEX

This originates from the most ulnar portion of the radius and extends into the caput ulna and the ulnar wrist to the base of the fifth metacarpal. Clinically relevant anatomy of the triangular fibrocartilage complex is covered in Chapter 74.

Neuromuscular anatomy

MUSCLES OF THE FOREARM

The forearm muscles include the superficial flexors (pronator teres, flexor carpi radialis, palmaris longus, flexor carpi ulnaris and flexor digitorum superficialis), the deep flexors (flexor digitorum profundus, flexor pollicis longus and pronator quadratus), the superficial extensors (brachioradialis, extensor carpi radialis longus and brevis, extensor digitorum, extensor digiti minimi, extensor carpi ulnaris and the anconeus) and the deep extensors (supinator, abductor pollicis longus, extensor pollicis brevis, extensor pollicis longus and extensor indicis proprius).

NERVES OF THE FOREARM

Clinically relevant anatomy is highlighted in Chapter 45 with a discussion of compression neuropathies of the radial, median and ulnar nerves.

Radial nerve

Lying anterior to the lateral epicondyle, the radial nerve runs between the brachialis and brachioradialis when entering the forearm. A summary of the radial nerve innervation is given in Table 4.10.

Median nerve

This lies medial to the brachial artery at the elbow, and superficial to the brachialis muscle. In the forearm the median nerve splits the two heads of the pronator teres. The median nerve runs between the flexor digitorum superficialis (FDS) and flexor digitorum profundus (FDP), becoming more superficial at the flexor retinaculum, where it continues into the hand. A summary of the median nerve innervation is given in Table 4.11.

Ulnar nerve

The ulnar nerve enters the forearm between the two heads of the flexor carpi ulnaris (FCU), which it supplies. The ulnar nerve runs between the FCU and FDP (and innervates the ulnar half of this muscle). It lies more superficial at the wrist and enters the hand through Guyon's canal. A summary of the ulnar nerve innervation is given in Table 4.12.

Cutaneous nerves

The forearm has the lateral antebrachial cutaneous nerve (the continuation of the musculocutaneous nerve that passes lateral to the cephalic vein after emerging laterally from between the biceps and brachialis at the elbow), the medial antebrachial cutaneous nerve (a branch from the medial cord of the brachial plexus) and the posterior antebrachial cutaneous nerve (a branch of the radial nerve given off in the arm).

Vessels

At the elbow the brachial artery enters the cubital fossa (bordered by the two epicondyles, the brachioradialis, the pronator teres and overlying the brachialis and supinator). It then divides at the level of the radial neck into the radial and ulnar arteries.

RADIAL ARTERY

This runs initially on the pronator teres, deep to the brachioradialis, and continues to the wrist between this muscle and the flexor carpi radialis (FCR).

Table 4.10 Radial nerve innervation

Nerve	Innervation
Radial nerve (post cord)	Triceps, brachioradialis, ECRL, ECRB
PIN	Supinator, ECU, ED, EDM, AbdPL, EPL, EPB, EI

AbdPL, abductor pollicis longus; ECRL, extensor carpi radialis longus; ECRB, extensor carpi radialis brevis; ECU, extensor carpi ulnaris; ED, extensor digitorum; EDM, extensor digiti minimi; EI, extensor indicis proprius; EPB, extensor pollicis brevis; EPL, extensor pollicis longus; PIN, posterior interosseous nerve.

Table 4.11 Median nerve innervation

Nerve	Innervation
Median nerve (med and lat cord)	PT, FCR, PL, FDS, AbdPB, FPB superficial head, OP, 1st and 2nd lumbrical
AIN	FDP (I and II), FPL, PQ

AbdPB, abductor pollicis brevis; AIN, anterior interosseous nerve; FCR, flexor carpi radialis; FDP, flexor digitorum profundus; FDS, flexor digitorum superficialis; FPB, flexor pollicis brevis; FPL, flexor pollicis longus; OP, opponens pollicis; PL, palmaris longus; PQ, pronator quadratus; PT, pronator teres.

Table 4.12 Ulnar nerve innervation

Nerve	Innervation
Ulnar nerve (medial cord)	FCU, FDP (III and IV), PB, AbdDM, ODM, FDM, 3rd and 4th lumbrical, interossei, AddP, deep head FPB

AddP, adductor pollicis; FCU, flexor carpi ulnaris; FDP, flexor digitorum profundus; FDM, flexor digiti minimi; FPB, flexor pollicis brevis; ODM, opponens digiti minimi; PB, peroneus brevis.

ULNAR ARTERY

The larger of the two branches; it is covered by the superficial flexors proximally (between the FDS and FDP). Distally, the artery lies on the FDP, between the tendons of the FCU and FDS.

Surgical approaches to the forearm

See Table 4.13 for a summary of approaches.

ANTERIOR APPROACH TO THE RADIUS (HENRY'S)

The internervous plane is between the brachioradialis (radial nerve) and the pronator teres proximally and the FCR distally (median nerve). See Fig. 4.9. Following incision, the brachioradialis and the FCR are identified distally. This interval is opened with gentle retraction on the brachio-radialis to protect the superficial radial nerve with the recurrent radial vessels ligated to assist with tissue retraction. Deep dissection in the proximal forearm is located lateral to the bicipital tendon to avoid the medial and more superficial radial artery. With the forearm in

Table 4.13 Forearm surgical approaches

Approach	Interval	Risks
Anterior (Henry's)	Brachioradialis (radial nerve) and pronator teres proximally and FCR distally (median nerve)	Radial artery – stay lateral to bicipital tendon Superficial branch radial nerve and PIN (remove supinator with forearm supination)
Dorsal posterior (Thompson's)	ECRB (radial nerve) and EDC, proximally (PIN) EPL, distally (PIN)	PIN. Avoid excessive retraction of supinator and identify and protect the PIN
Ulna	ECU (PIN) and FCU (ulnar nerve)	

ECRB, extensor carpi radialis brevis; EDC, extensor digitorum communis; ECU, extensor carpi ulnaris; EPL, extensor pollicis longus; FCR, flexor carpi radialis; FCU, flexor carpi ulnaris; PIN, posterior interosseous nerve.

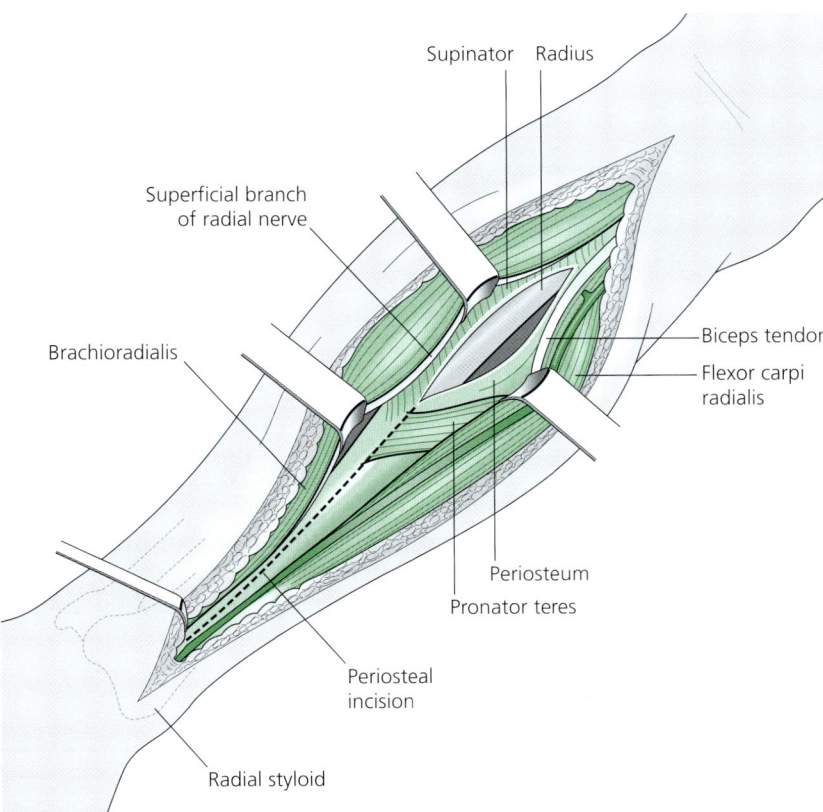

Figure 4.9 Anterior approach to the radius (Henry's). The internervous plane is between the brachioradialis (radial nerve) and the pronator teres proximally and the flexor carpi radialis distally (median nerve). The dotted line illustrates the planned incision to remove the insertion of the pronator teres (arm in pronation) to expose the midshaft of the radius. Proximally, dissection is carried out lateral to the bicipital tendon.

supination to protect the PIN, the supinator is incised and elevated subperiosteally, exposing the proximal radial shaft. Deep dissection in the middle forearm requires forearm pronation to identify the insertion of the pronator teres. The insertion of the pronator teres is incised, exposing the radial shaft. Deep dissection in the distal forearm continues lateral to the pronator quadratus and flexor pollicis longus. Following elevation, the distal radial shaft is exposed.

POSTERIOR APPROACH TO THE RADIUS (THOMPSON)

The internervous plane is between the extensor carpi radialis brevis (ECRB; radial nerve) and the extensor digitorum communis (EDC), proximally, or extensor pollicis longus, distally (PIN). See Fig. 4.10. Following skin incision, the ECRB and the EDC are identified with the first extensor compartment muscles assisting with defining this interval distally. Retraction and dissection of the ECRB and EDC reveal the supinator proximally. The PIN must be identified and protected when using this surgical approach, with dissection of the supinator exposing the proximal third of the radial shaft. Exposure of the mid-radial shaft is accomplished by elevation of the abductor pollicis longus and the extensor pollicis brevis. Distal radial shaft exposure is through separation of the ECRB and extensor pollicis longus.

EXPOSURE OF THE ULNA

The internervous plane is between the extensor carpi ulnaris (PIN) and the FCU (ulnar nerve). Following skin

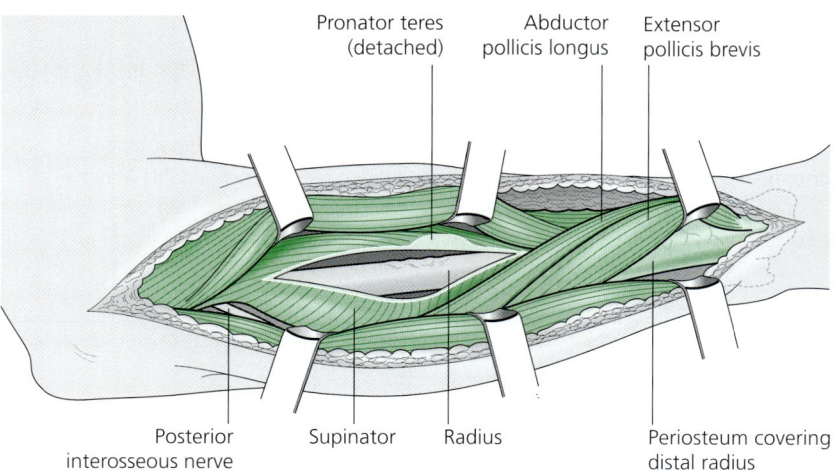

Figure 4.10 Posterior approach to the radius (Thompson). The internervous plane is between the extensor carpi radialis brevis (radial nerve) and the extensor digitorum communis, proximally, or extensor pollicis longus, distally (posterior interosseous nerve (PIN)). The PIN must be identified and protected when using this surgical approach with dissection of the supinator exposing the proximal third of the radial shaft.

incision, the ulnar shaft is easily palpated and can be approached by subperiosteal elevation on either the flexor or extensor surface.

WRIST AND HAND

Osteology

CARPAL BONES

Each carpal bone has six surfaces, with proximal, distal, medial and lateral surfaces for articulation and palmar and dorsal surfaces for ligamentous insertion. Ossification begins at the capitate (usually present at 1 year old) and proceeds in a counterclockwise direction. Therefore, the hamate is the second carpus to ossify (1–2 years), followed by the triquetrum (3 years), lunate (4–5 years), scaphoid (5 years), trapezium (6 years) and trapezoid (7 years). The pisiform, which is a large sesamoid bone, is the last to ossify (9 years).

METACARPALS

These have two ossification centres: one for the body (primary centre of ossification), which ossifies at 8 weeks of fetal life (like most long bones), and one at the neck, which usually appears before age 3. The first metacarpal is a primordial phalanx and has its secondary ossification centre located at the base (like the phalanges).

PHALANGES

The 14 phalanges (three for each finger and two for the thumb) are similar. They all have secondary ossification centres at their bases that appear at ages 3 (proximal), 4 (middle) and 5 (distal). The bases of the proximal phalanges are oval and concave, with smaller heads ending in two condyles. The middle phalanges have two concave facets at their bases and pulley-shaped heads. The distal phalanges are smaller and have palmar ungual tuberosities distally.

Table 4.14 Key topographical spinal anatomical landmarks

Topographical landmark	Spinal level
Mandible	C2/3
Hyoid cartilage	C3
Thyroid cartilage	C4/5
Cricoid cartilage	C6
Vertebra prominens	C7
Scapular spine	T3
Distal tip of scapula	T7
Iliac crest	L4/5

Arthrology and neuromuscular anatomy

Clinically relevant anatomy of the hand and wrist is covered in Chapters 74 and 106.

SPINE

Osteology

The spine contains 33 vertebrae: seven cervical, 12 thoracic, five lumbar, five fused sacral and four fused coccygeal vertebrae. The vertebral bodies generally increase in width craniocaudally with the exception of T1–T3. Normal spinal curves include cervical lordosis, thoracic kyphosis, lumbar lordosis and sacral kyphosis. Key topographical spinal anatomical landmarks are shown in Table 4.14.

CERVICAL SPINE

The atlas (C1) has no vertebral body and no spinous process. C1 has two concave superior facets that articulate with the occipital condyles. The highest percentage of neck flexion and extension occur at the occiput–C1 articulation (50% of total). The axis (C2) develops from five ossification centres with an initial cartilaginous junction between the dens and the vertebral body (subdental synchondrosis) that fuses at 7 years old. The base of the dens narrows because of the transverse ligament. The atlantoaxial articulation is responsible for the majority of neck rotation, with 50% of total rotation occurring at the C1–C2 articulation. The atlantoaxial joint is a diarthrodial joint, which explains why pannus in rheumatoid arthritis can affect this articulation, resulting in instability. This also explains why patients with rheumatoid arthritis require cervical radiographs prior to elective orthopaedic procedures to rule out cervical instability. Vertebrae C2–C7 have foramina in each transverse process and bifid spinous processes (except for the C7 non-bifid posterior spinous process – vertebral prominens). The vertebral artery travels in the transverse foramina of C6–C1. The carotid (Chassaingnac's) tubercle is found at C6. The cervical spine canal diameter is normally 17 mm and the cervical cord becomes compromised when the diameter is reduced to less than 13 mm.

THORACIC SPINE

Unique features include costal facets (present on all 12 vertebral bodies and the transverse processes of T1–T9) and a rounded vertebral foramen. The thoracic vertebrae articulation with the rib cage makes this the most rigid region of the axial skeleton.

LUMBAR SPINE

These vertebrae are the largest and are higher anteriorly than posteriorly, contributing to the lumbar lordosis. Lumbar lordosis ranges from 55° to 60° with the apex at L3, and with most of the lordosis due to the intervertebral disc spaces. The majority of lumbar lordosis (66%) occurs from L4 to the sacrum. Lumbar vertebrae contain short laminae and pedicles. They also have mammillary processes (separate ossification centres) that project posteriorly from the superior articular facet. Do not forget that spondylolysis is a defect in the pars interarticularis and the most common cause of back pain in children and adolescents.

SACRUM

Fusion of five spinal elements. The sacral promontory is the anterosuperior portion that projects into the pelvis. There are usually four pairs of pelvic sacral foramina located both anteriorly and posteriorly that transmit, respectively, the ventral and dorsal branches of the upper four sacral nerves. There is also a sacral canal, which opens caudally into the sacral hiatus.

COCCYX

Fusion of the lowest four spinal elements; it attaches dorsally to the gluteus maximus, the external anal sphincter and the coccygeal muscles.

SPINAL LIGAMENTS

These include the anterior and posterior longitudinal ligaments, ligamentum flavum and the supraspinous, interspinous and intertransverse ligaments.

General arrangement

The vertebral bodies are bound together by the strong anterior longitudinal ligament (ALL) and the weaker posterior longitudinal ligament (PLL). The ALL is usually thickest at the centre of the vertebral body and thins at the periphery. Separate fibres extend from one to five levels. The ALL resists hyperextension. The PLL extends from the occiput (tectoral membrane) to the posterior sacrum. It is separated from the centre of the vertebral body by a space that allows passage of the dorsal branches of the spinal artery and veins. The PLL is hourglass shaped, with the wider (yet thinner) sections located over the discs. Ruptured discs tend to occur lateral to these expansions. Ligamentous capsules overlying the zygapophyseal joints and the intertransverse ligaments contribute little to interspinous stability. The ligamentum flavum is a strong, yellow, elastic ligament connecting the laminae. It runs from the anterior surface of the superior lamina to the posterior surface of the inferior lamina and is constantly in tension. Hypertrophy of the ligamentum flavum is said to contribute to nerve root compression. The supraspinous and interspinous ligaments lie dorsal to and between the spinous processes, respectively. The supraspinous ligament begins at C7 and is in continuity with the ligamentum nuchae (which runs from C7 to the occiput).

Spine stability (Denis)

The three-column system is summarized in Table 4.15.

Specialized ligaments

Atlanto-occipital joint

Consists of two articular capsules (anterior and posterior) and the tectoral membrane (a cephalad extension of the PLL). It is further stabilized by the ligamentous attachments to the dens.

Atlantoaxial joint

The transverse ligament is the major stabilizer of the median atlantoaxial joint. This articulation is further stabilized

Table 4.15 Denis spine columns

Column	Composition
Anterior	ALL, anterior two-thirds of annulus and vertebral body
Middle	Posterior one-third of body and annulus, PLL
Posterior	Pedicles, facets and facet capsules, spinous processes, posterior ligaments including interspinous and supraspinous ligaments, ligamentum flavum

ALL, anterior longitudinal ligament; PLL, posterior longitudinal ligament.

by the apical ligament (longitudinal), which together with the transverse ligament composes the cruciate ligament. Additionally, a pair of alar, or 'check', ligaments run obliquely from the tip of the dens to the occiput. Do not forget that an atlantodens interval of >7–10 mm or a posterior space of <13 mm is a relative contraindication to elective orthopaedic surgery and the spine should be stabilized first.

Iliolumbar ligament

This stout ligament connects the transverse process of L5 with the ilium. Tension on this ligament in patients with unstable vertical shear pelvic fractures can lead to avulsion fractures of the transverse process.

Facet (apophyseal) joints

The orientation of the facets of the spine dictates the plane of motion at each relative level. The facet orientation varies with spinal level and is summarized in Table 4.16.

In the cervical spine the superior articular facet is anterior and inferior to the inferior articular process of the vertebra above. Nerve roots exit near the superior articulating process. In the lumbar spine the superior articular facet is anterior and lateral to the inferior articular facet.

Intervertebral discs

The intervertebral discs are fibrocartilaginous, with an obliquely oriented annulus fibrosus composed of type I collagen and a softer central nucleus pulposus made of type II collagen. The nucleus pulposus has a high polysaccharide content and is approximately 88% water. Ageing results in the loss of water and conversion to fibrocartilage. The discs account for 25% of the total spinal columnar height. They are attached to the vertebral bodies by hyaline cartilage, which is responsible for the vertical growth of the column. Intradiscal pressure is position dependent: pressure is lowest when lying supine, and highest when sitting and flexed forward with weights in hands.

Neuromuscular anatomy

NECK

The neck is divided, for functional purposes, into the anterior and posterior regions.

Table 4.16 Orientation of spine facets

Spine region	Sagittal facet orientation	Coronal facet orientation
Cervical	35° at C2 increasing to 55° at C7	Neutral 0°
Thoracic	60° at T1 increasing to 70° at T12	20° posterior
Lumbar	137° at L1 decreasing to 118° at L5	45° anterior

Anterior

The anterior neck muscles include the superficial platysma muscle (CN VII innervated), stylohyoid and digastric muscles (CN XII) above the hyoid, and 'strap' muscles below the hyoid. Important strap muscles include the sternohyoid and omohyoid in the superficial layer and the thyrohyoid and sternothyroid in the deep layer; all are innervated by the ansa cervicalis (C1–C3). Laterally, the sternocleidomastoid (CN XI and ansa) runs obliquely across the neck, rotating the head to the contralateral side. The anterior triangle (borders: sternocleidomastoid, midline of the neck and the lower border of the mandible) is the largest area. Three smaller triangles include the submandibular, carotid (bordered by the posterior aspect of the digastric and the omohyoid, and used for the anterior approach to C5) and posterior (bordered by the trapezius, sternocleidomastoid and clavicle).

Posterior

The posterior neck muscles form the borders of the suboccipital triangle. The superior and inferior heads of the obliquus capitis muscle and the rectus capitis posterior major muscle forms this triangle. The vertebral artery and the first cervical nerve are within this triangle, and the greater occipital nerve (C2) is superficial.

BACK

The back is blanketed by the trapezius (superiorly) and the latissimus dorsi (inferiorly). The rhomboids and levator scapulae are deep to this layer. The deep muscles of the back are arranged into two groups: erector spinae and transversospinalis group. The erector spinae run from the transverse and spinous processes of the inferior vertebrae to the spinous processes of the superior vertebrae. They stabilize and extend the back. All of the deep back musculature is innervated by dorsal primary rami of spinal nerves.

NERVES

Spinal cord

The cord extends from the brainstem to the inferior border of L1, where it terminates as the conus medullaris. It is enclosed within the bony spinal canal with variable amounts of space (greatest in the upper cervical spine). The cord also varies in diameter (widest at the origin of plexi). In cross-section, the cord has both geographic and functional boundaries (Fig. 4.11). It is divided in the midline anteriorly by a fissure and posteriorly by the sulcus. Functions of the ascending (sensory) and descending (motor) tracts are summarized in Table 4.17.

The posterior funiculi (dorsal columns) are located dorsally and receive ascending fibres, which deliver deep touch, proprioception and vibratory sensation. The lateral spinothalamic tract transmits pain and temperature (it is the site for chordotomy for intractable pain). Descending in the lateral corticospinal tract are fibres that transmit instructions for voluntary muscle contraction. Sacral structures are most peripheral in the lateral corticospinal tracts with cervical structures more medial. (This is why central cord syndrome affects the upper extremities more than the lower extremities; see Table 4.18.) The ventral (anterior) spinothalamic tract transmits light touch sensation, and the ventral (anterior) corticospinal tract delivers cortical messages of voluntary contraction. Deficits associated with incomplete spinal cord injury patterns are predicted by the anatomy of the ascending and descending tracts. Do not forget that prognosis with incomplete spinal cord injury is unaffected by the bulbocavernosis reflex. A summary is provided in Table 4.18.

The spinal cord tapers at L1 (conus medullaris), and a small filum terminale continues with surrounding nerve roots contained within a common dural sac (cauda equina) to its termination in the coccyx. Spinal cord injury at this level may permanently interrupt the bulbocavernosis reflex.

Nerve roots

There are thirty-one pairs of spinal nerves: eight cervical, 12 thoracic, five lumbar, five sacral and one coccygeal. Within the subarachnoid space the dorsal root (and ganglia) and ventral roots converge to form the spinal nerve (Fig. 4.12). The nerve becomes 'extradural' as it approaches the intervertebral foramen (dura becomes epineurium) at all levels above L1. Below this level, the nerves are contained within the cauda equina. After exiting the foramen the spinal nerve delivers dorsal primary rami, which supply the muscles and skin of the neck and back regions. Innervation of structures within the spinal canal, including periosteum, meninges, vascular structures and articular connective tissue, is due to the sinuvertebral nerve. The ventral rami supply the anteromedial trunk and the limbs. With the exception of the thoracic nerves, ventral rami are grouped in plexuses before delivering sensorimotor functions to a general region. In the cervical spine the numbered nerve exits at a level *above* the pedicle of the corresponding vertebral level (e.g. C2 exits at C1–C2). In the lumbar spine the nerve root traverses the respective disc space above the named vertebral body and exits the respective foramen under the pedicle. Herniated discs usually impinge on the traversing nerve root and the facet joint. For example, a disc herniation at L4–L5 would cause compression of the traversing L5 nerve root, resulting in a positive tension sign (straight leg raise) and diminished strength in the hip abductors, extensor hallucis longus (EHL) and pain and numbness in the lateral leg to the dorsum of the foot. A far lateral L4–L5 disc herniation would compress the exiting L4 nerve root, resulting in a positive tension sign (femoral

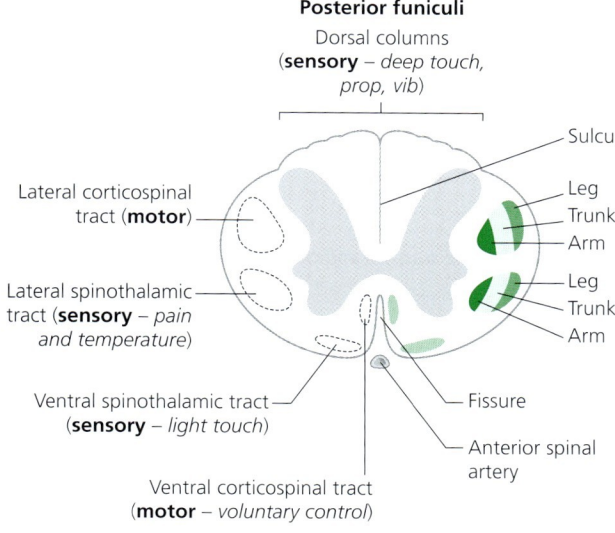

Figure 4.11 Cross-section of the spinal cord illustrating the functions of the ascending and descending tracts. Ascending tracts (sensory): dorsal columns, lateral spinothalamic, ventral or anterior spinothalamic. Descending (motor) tracts: lateral corticospinal and ventral or anterior corticospinal.

Table 4.17 Spinal cord tracts

	Tracts	Function
Ascending (sensory)	Dorsal columns	Deep touch, proprioception, vibratory
	Lateral spinothalamic	Pain and temperature
	Anterior spinothalamic	Light touch
Descending (motor)	Lateral corticospinal	Voluntary motor
	Anterior corticospinal	Voluntary motor

Table 4.18 Incomplete spinal cord injury patterns

Injury pattern	Functional deficit	Recovery
Central (most common)	UE>LE, usually quadriplegic with sacral sparing. Flaccid paralysis of UE and spastic paralysis of LE	75%
Anterior	Complete motor deficit	10% (worst prognosis)
Posterior	Loss of deep pressure, deep pain and proprioception	
Brown–Séquard syndrome	Unilateral cord injury with ipsilateral motor deficit and contralateral pain and temperature deficit (two levels below injury)	>90% recovery

LE, lower extremity; UE, upper extremity.

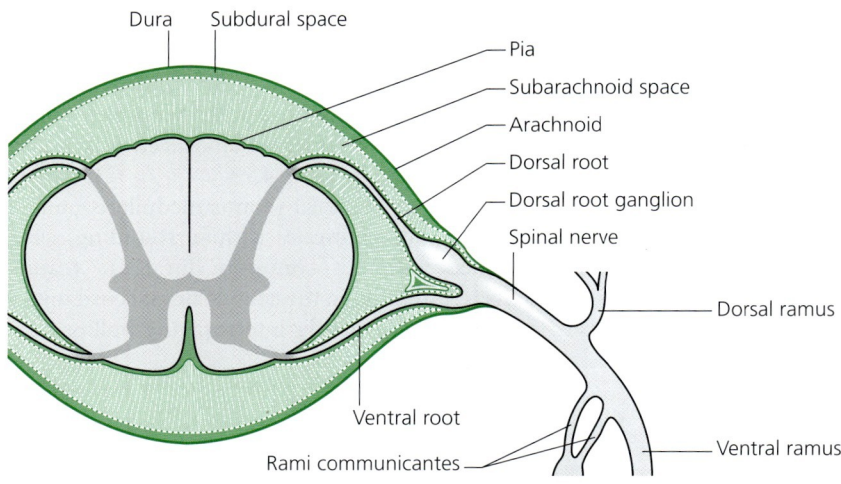

Figure 4.12 Spinal nerves. The subarachnoid space houses the dorsal root ganglion and the ventral root, forming the more lateral spinal nerve. The spinal nerve becomes extradural at all levels above L1, with the remaining distal branches part of the cauda equina. Structures within the spinal canal are innervated by the sinuvertebral nerve. Ventral rami supply the anteromedial trunk and the limbs. Facet joints are innervated by the medial branch of the dorsal primary ramus and sinuvertebral nerve. Redrawn from Jenkins 1991, with permission.

Table 4.19 Cervical sympathetic ganglia

Ganglia	Location	Other
Superior	C2–C3	Largest
Middle	C6	Variable
Inferior	C7–T1	Stellate

Table 4.20 Spine surgical approaches

Approach	Interval	Risks
Anterior cervical	Carotid sheath and the trachea	Recurrent laryngeal nerve Sympathetic ganglion
Posterior cervical	Midline approach between paracervical muscles	Vertebral artery
Anterior lumbar (transperitoneal)	Between segmentally innervated rectus abdominis	Presacral plexus of parasympathetic nerve

nerve stretch test) and L4 compromise. Do not forget that the L5 nerve root is relatively fixed to the anterior sacral ala and can be damaged by sacral fractures and errant anteriorly placed iliosacral screws.

Sympathetic chain

The cervical sympathetic chain lies posterior and medial to the carotid sheath. It is anterior to the longus capitus muscle. The cervical sympathetic chain has three ganglia (Table 4.19): superior, middle and inferior. Disruption of the inferior ganglia can lead to Horner syndrome. There are three ganglia in the cervical region, 11 in the thoracic region, four in the lumbar region and four in the sacral region.

Vascular supply to the spine

Spinal blood supply is usually derived from the segmental arteries located at vertebral midbodies via the aorta (which lies on the left side of the vertebral column with the inferior vena cava and azygos vein on the right). The primary supply to the dura and posterior elements is from the dorsal branches. The ventral branches supply the vertebral bodies via ascending and descending branches, which are delivered underneath the PLL in four separate ostia. The vertebral artery (a branch of the subclavian) ascends through the transverse foramina of C1–C6 (anterior to and not through C7), posterior to the longus colli muscle, then posterior to the lateral masses, along the cephalad surface of the posterior arch of C1 (atlas), passes ventromedially around the spinal cord and through the foramen magnum before uniting at the midline basilar artery. The distance from the spinous process of C1 laterally to the vertebral artery is 2 cm (the safe distance for dissections would, therefore, be less than 2 cm). The artery of Adamkiewicz (great anterior medullary artery) enters through the left intervertebral foramen in the lower thoracic spine from T8 to T12. It supplies the interior two-thirds of the anterior cord. Arterial supply to the spinal cord is from the anterior and posterior spinal arteries and segmental branches of the vertebral artery and dorsal arteries, which travel via the dorsal and ventral rootlets to the respective dorsal and anterolateral portions of the cord. The venous drainage of the vertebral bodies is primarily via the central sinusoid located on the dorsum of each vertebral body.

Surgical approaches to the spine

These are summarised in Table 4.20.

ANTERIOR APPROACH TO THE CERVICAL SPINE

A transverse incision is based on the desired level. Following skin incision, the platysma is incised and split in line with the vertically oriented fibres. With the sternocleidomastoid muscle retracted laterally, the pretracheal fascia medial to the carotid sheath is exposed. The pretracheal fascia is incised between the interval of the carotid sheath (contains the internal and common carotid arteries, the internal jugular vein and the vagus nerve (CN X)) and the trachea. Carotid sheath lateral retraction reveals the prevertebral fascia over the ALL. The prevertebral fascia is sharply incised and the longus colli muscle gently retracted (protecting the recurrent laryngeal nerve (a branch of the vagus nerve that lies outside the sheath)) to expose the vertebral body. Increased risk of injury to the recurrent laryngeal nerve occurs with right-sided approaches (paralysis is identified by a hoarse, scratchy voice due to unilateral vocal cord paralysis, which can be visualized with direct laryngoscopy). The recurrent laryngeal nerve arises from the vagus at the level of the subclavian artery on the right with the left arising at the level of the aortic arch. Lower left-sided anterior cervical approaches risk injury to the thoracic duct that is posterior to the carotid sheath. By dissecting the longus muscles subperiosteally, one also protects the stellate ganglion (avoiding possible Horner syndrome). The anterior surface of the vertebral body is exposed, completing the approach.

POSTERIOR APPROACH TO THE CERVICAL SPINE

Following identification of the appropriate level, a midline posterior skin incision is made. After a midline approach through the ligamentum nuchae, the superficial layer (trapezius) and intermediate layer (splenius, semispinalis, longissimus capitis) are subperiosteally reflected laterally, and the vertebrae are exposed. The vertebral artery is especially vulnerable as it leaves the foramen transversarium and travels above and medially to pierce the atlanto-occipital membrane at its lateral angle. The greater occipital nerve (C2) and the third occipital nerve (C3) should be protected in the suboccipital region. Access to the spinal canal is via laminectomy or facetectomy, completing the approach.

THORACIC SPINE

For approaches to the thoracic spine, please refer to more detailed anatomical exposure texts (see Further Reading list, p. 80.).

POSTERIOR APPROACH TO THE LUMBAR SPINE

At the appropriate level, a posterior longitudinal incision is made over the spinous processes. Subperiosteal dissection is used to detach the paraspinal muscles, exposing the lamina and the facet joints. Exposure of the spinal canal is achieved following ligamentum flavum removal beginning at the superior edge of the inferior lamina.

ANTERIOR APPROACH TO THE LUMBAR SPINE (TRANSPERITONEAL)

Following the longitudinal skin incision from the umbilicus to just above the pubic symphysis, skin and fat retraction reveals rectus abdominis fascia. Vertically separate the rectus abdominis muscles and incise the peritoneum. Protect and retract the bladder distally and bowel cephalad and incise the posterior peritoneum longitudinally over the sacral promontory. The aorta bifurcation is revealed and the middle sacral artery is ligated. Expose the L5–S1 disc space. Injury to the lumbar plexus, particularly the superior hypogastric plexus of the sympathetic plexus that lies over the L5 vertebral body, can cause sexual dysfunction and retrograde ejaculation. Do not forget that ejaculation is a predominantly sympathetic nervous system function and erection is a predominantly parasympathetic nervous system function. Exposure of the L4–L5 interval using this approach requires great vessel and ureter mobilization.

ANTEROLATERAL APPROACH TO THE LUMBAR SPINE (RETROPERITONEAL)

This approach provides access from L1 to the sacrum. An oblique incision is centred over the twelfth rib to the lateral border of the rectus abdominis muscle. The external oblique, internal oblique and transversus abdominis muscles are incised in line with the skin incision. Elevate the retroperitoneal fat, revealing the psoas major muscle and genitofemoral nerve. Ligate the segmental lumbar vessels and mobilize the aorta and vena cava to expose the desired vertebral level. Protect the sympathetic chain (medial to the psoas and lateral to the vertebral body) and ureters (between peritoneum and psoas fascia).

PELVIS AND HIP

Osteology

The pelvic girdle is composed of two innominate (coxal) bones that articulate with the sacrum. Each innominate bone is composed of three united bones: the ilium, ischium and pubis. The ilium has two important anterior prominences: the anterior superior and anterior inferior iliac spines. The anterior superior iliac spine is palpable at the lateral edge of the inguinal ligament. It is the origin for the sartorius muscle and the transverse and internal abdominal muscles. The anterior inferior iliac spine is less prominent and provides the origin of the direct head of the rectus femoris and the iliofemoral ligament (Y ligament of Bigelow). The iliopectineal eminence is a raised region anteriorly that represents the union of the ilium and pubis. The iliopsoas muscle traverses a groove between this eminence and the anteroinferior iliac spine. The ilium also has a posterior superior iliac spine that is usually located 4–5 cm lateral to the S2 spinous process. The greater sciatic notch is located posterior and superior to the acetabulum. The acetabulum is anteverted (15°) and obliquely oriented (45° caudally). The posterosuperior articular surface is thickened to accommodate weight bearing. The inferior surface is deficient and contains the acetabular, or cotyloid, notch bound by the transverse acetabular ligament. The proximal femur is composed of the femoral head, neck, and greater and lesser trochanters. The femoral neck is anteverted approximately 14° in relation to the femoral condyles. The femoral neck shaft angle averages 127°.

Arthrology

HIP

The hip joint is a spheroidal, or ball and socket, type of diarthrodial joint. Its stability is based primarily on the bony architecture. The acetabulum is deepened by the fibrocartilaginous labrum. The joint capsule extends anteriorly across the femoral neck to the trochanteric crest; however, posteriorly it extends only partially across the femoral neck, leaving the basicervical and intertrochanteric crest regions extracapsular. A series of three ligaments compose the capsule anteriorly. The iliofemoral, or Y ligament of Bigelow, is the strongest ligament in the body and attaches the anterior inferior iliac spine to the intertrochanteric line in an inverted Y fashion. The remaining anterior ligaments, the ischiofemoral and pubofemoral ligaments, are weaker but lend additional stability. Inside the joint, the ligament of teres arises from the apex of the cotyloid notch and attaches to the fovea of the femoral head. It transmits an arterial branch of the posterior division of the obturator artery to the femoral head. Blood supply to the femoral head changes with age and key points are highlighted in Table 4.21. This table helps to explain why the standard antegrade femoral nailing start point is undesirable for paediatric femur fractures. Using the piriformis start point would damage the posterosuperior retinacular vessels, risking avascular necrosis of the femoral head. Additionally, in adults, one avoids completely transecting the quadratus femoris muscle in the posterior acetabular and hip approaches to avoid damage to the main blood supply to the femoral head – the medial femoral circumflex artery.

Table 4.21 Age-dependent changes to femoral head blood supply

Age	Blood supply
Birth to 4 years	Primary medial and lateral circumflex arteries (from deep femoral artery)
	Ligamentum teres with obturator artery posterior division
4 years to adult	Negligible lateral circumflex artery
	Minimal ligamentum teres
	Posterosuperior and posteroinferior retinacular from medial femoral circumflex artery
Adult	Medial femoral circumflex to lateral epiphyseal artery

SACROILIAC JOINT

A true diarthrodial-gliding joint supported by three groups of ligaments: posterior sacroiliac ligaments, anterior sacroiliac ligaments and interosseous ligaments.

SYMPHYSIS PUBIS

Connects the two hemipelvi anteriorly and is united with a fibrocartilaginous disc and supported by the superior pubic ligament and the arcuate pubic ligament.

OTHER LIGAMENTS

Other ligaments include the sacrospinous and sacrotuberous ligaments, which outline the boundaries for the greater and lesser sciatic foramina. The sacrospinous ligament (anterior sacrum ischial spine) is the inferior border of the greater sciatic foramen and the superior border of the lesser sciatic foramen. The lesser sciatic foramen is bordered inferiorly by the sacrotuberous ligament (anterior sacrum ischial tuberosity). The piriformis, sciatic nerve and other important structures exit the greater sciatic foramen. The short external rotators of the hip exit the lesser sciatic foramen.

Neuromuscular anatomy

Principal hip flexor muscles are the iliopsoas, rectus femoris and sartorius. Hip extensor muscles are the gluteus maximus and hamstrings (semitendinosus, semimembranosus and long head of biceps femoris). Hip abduction is primarily due to the actions of the gluteus medius and minimus. The tensor fascia lata also helps with abduction in a flexed hip. Hip adduction is due primarily to the actions of the adductor brevis, longus and magnus, pectineus and gracilis. Hip external rotation is due to the action of the obturator internus, obturator externus, superior and inferior gemellus, quadratus femoris and the piriformis. Hip internal rotation is provided by secondary actions of the anterior fibres of the gluteus medius and minimus, tensor fascia lata, semimembranosus, semitendinosus, pectineus and posterior part of the adductor magnus.

NERVES

Lumbosacral plexus

The lumbosacral plexus is composed of ventral rami from T12 to S3 and lies posterior to the psoas muscle. The sciatic nerve (L4–S3) has an anterior preaxial tibial nerve division and a postaxial peroneal nerve division. The spatial orientation of the sciatic nerve also places the peroneal division more lateral than the tibial division. This orientation makes it more vulnerable to injury at the time of surgery.

Anatomical spatial relationships

The lumbar plexus is found on the anterior surface of the quadratus lumborum under (and within) the substance of the psoas major muscle. The genitofemoral nerve pierces the psoas and then lies on the anteromedial surface of the psoas. The femoral nerve lies between the iliacus and the psoas. The lateral femoral cutaneous nerve lies on the surface of the iliacus muscle and exits the pelvis under the lateral attachment of the inguinal ligament. Virtually all important nerves about the hip leave the pelvis by way of the sciatic foramen. The major reference point for the greater sciatic nerve and related structures in the hip is the piriformis muscle ('key' to the sciatic foramen). The superior gluteal nerve and artery lie above the piriformis, and virtually everything else leaves below the muscle (remember POP'S IQ (lateral to medial nerves): *p*udendal, *o*bturator internus, *p*osterior femoral cutaneous, *s*ciatic, *i*nferior gluteal, *q*uadratus femoris). Two nerves leave the greater sciatic foramen and re-enter the pelvis via the lesser foramen (pudendal and nerve to obturator internus). Anteriorly, the great nerves and vessels enter the thigh (and into the femoral triangle) under the inguinal ligament. The borders of this triangle include the sartorius laterally, the pectineus medially, and the inguinal ligament superiorly. Within the triangle, from lateral to medial, are the femoral *n*erve, *a*rtery, and *v*ein *a*nd the *l*ymphatic vessels (remember NAVAL). The floor of the femoral triangle (again, lateral to medial) is made up of the iliacus, psoas, pectineus and the adductor longus. The femoral nerve descends between the iliacus and psoas and delivers numerous branches to muscle, overlying skin and the hip joint (in accordance with Hilton's law). A spontaneous iliacus haematoma may irritate the femoral nerve owing to its proximity. At the apex of the triangle the saphenous nerve branches off and travels under the sartorius muscle. The obturator nerve exits the pelvis via the obturator canal. It splits into anterior and posterior divisions within the canal. The anterior division proceeds anteriorly to the obturator externus and posteriorly to the pectineus, supplying the adductor longus and brevis and the gracilis; it then delivers cutaneous branches to the medial thigh. The posterior division supplies the obturator externus, adductor brevis and the upper part of the adductor magnus, and it delivers other branches to the knee joint. Referred pain from the hip to the knee can be from the continuation of the obturator nerve anterior that can provide sensation to the medial side of the knee. A summary of the neurological levels responsible for lower extremity motion is given in Table 4.22.

Vessels

The aorta branches into the common iliac arteries anterior to the L4 vertebral body. The common iliac vessels, in turn, divide into the internal (or hypogastric; medial) and external (lateral) iliacs at the S1 level. Important internal iliac artery branches include the obturator (the posterior branch supplies the transverse acetabular ligament), superior gluteal (can be injured in the sciatic notch), inferior gluteal (supplies the gluteus maximus and the short external rotators) and internal pudendal (re-enters the pelvis through

Table 4.22 Summary of important lower extremity neurology

Joint	Function	Neurological level
Hip	Flexion	T12, L1–L3
	Extension	S1
	Adduction	L2–L4
	Abduction	L5
Knee	Flexion	L5, S1
	Extension	L2–L4
Ankle	Dorsiflexion	L4, L5
	Plantarflexion	S1, S2
	Inversion	L4
	Eversion	S1

Table 4.23 Acetabular screw placement zones

Acetabular zone	Structures at risk
Posterior superior	Safe zone
Posterior inferior	Safe zone
Anterior superior	External iliac artery and vein
Anterior inferior	Anterior inferior obturator nerve, obturator artery and vein

the lesser sciatic notch). Anteroinferior screws and acetabular retractors jeopardize the obturator artery and vein. The external iliac artery continues under the inguinal ligament to become the femoral artery. It can be injured by anterosuperior quadrant acetabular screw placement during total hip arthroplasty. A summary of key issues for acetabular screw placement is shown in Table 4.23.

The femoral artery enters the femoral triangle and delivers the profunda femoris, which supplies the anteromedial portion of the thigh and the perforators, which pierce the lateral intermuscular septum to supply the vastus lateralis muscle. The profunda has two other important branches: the medial and lateral femoral circumflex arteries. The lateral femoral circumflex travels obliquely and deep to the sartorius and rectus femoris. It delivers an ascending branch (at risk during anterolateral approaches) that proceeds to the greater trochanteric region and a descending branch that travels laterally under the rectus femoris. The medial femoral circumflex, which supplies most of the blood to the femoral head, runs between the pectineus and the iliopsoas and then in the interval between the obturator externus and adductor brevis muscles and in the interval between the adductor magnus and brevis. It proceeds distally anterior to the quadratus femoris on its cranial edge just distal to the obturator externus. The cruciate anastomosis is the confluence of the ascending branch of the first perforating artery, the descending branch of the inferior gluteal artery and the transverse branches of the medial and lateral femoral circumflex arteries. It lies at the inferior margin of the quadratus femoris muscle. The superficial femoral artery continues on the medial side of the thigh

Table 4.24 Hip surgical approaches

Approach	Interval	Risks
Anterior (Smith–Peterson)	Sartorius/rectus femoris (femoral nerve) and tensor fascia lata/gluteus medius (superior gluteal nerve)	Lateral femoral cutaneous nerve (6–8 cm below **anterior** superior iliac spine anterior or medial to sartorius) Ligation of ascending branch of lateral femoral circumflex artery (lies superficial to rectus femoris muscle)
Anterolateral (Watson–Jones)	Between tensor fascia lata (superior gluteal nerve) and gluteus medius (superior gluteal nerve)	Femoral nerve due to excessive medial retraction Injury to descending branch of lateral femoral circumflex artery
Lateral (Hardinge)	Gluteus medius (superior gluteal nerve) and vastus lateralis (femoral nerve)	Femoral nerve, artery, vein Superior gluteal nerve if dissection carried 3 cm above the tip of the greater trochanter
Posterior (Moore–Southern)	Gluteus maximus (inferior gluteal nerve) gluteus medius/tensor fascia lata (superior gluteal nerve)	Sciatic nerve and inferior gluteal artery during the gluteus maximus muscle split. If quadratis femoris transected, ligation of medial femoral circumflex artery

(between the vastus medialis and adductor longus) toward the adductor (Hunter's) canal. In the posteromedial thigh it becomes the popliteal artery in the popliteal fossa.

Surgical approaches to the pelvis and hip

See Table 4.24 for a summary.

ANTERIOR (SMITH–PETERSON) APPROACH TO THE HIP

This approach (Fig. 4.13) explores the internervous plane between the sartorius (femoral nerve) and the tensor fascia lata (superior gluteal nerve) and the deeper plane between the rectus femoris (femoral nerve) and the gluteus medius (superior gluteal nerve). Following skin incision, the lateral femoral cutaneous nerve is identified and protected. The fascia between the tensor fascia lata and sartorius is incised. Muscle retraction reveals the ascending branch of the lateral femoral circumflex artery (superficial to the rectus), which is ligated. For deeper dissection, approach the interval between the gluteus medius and rectus femoris. Detach the origin of both heads of the rectus femoris. Reflection of the conjoined rectus tendon too distally can risk injury to the descending branch of the lateral femoral circumflex artery. Retract the rectus medially and the gluteus medius laterally. Dissect any attachments of the iliopsoas to the inferior capsule and perform a capsulotomy that completes this approach.

ANTEROLATERAL (WATSON–JONES) APPROACH TO THE HIP (FIG. 4.14)

There is no true internervous plane, but this approach utilizes the intermuscular plane between the tensor fascia lata and gluteus medius. After the incision and superficial dissection, the fascia lata is split to expose the gluteus medius and vastus lateralis. Retraction of the gluteus medius and gluteus minimus posteriorly helps to expose the anterior

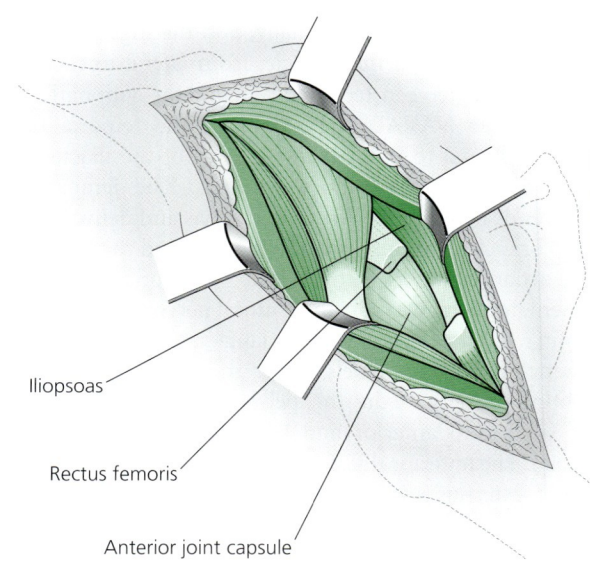

Figure 4.13 Anterior (Smith–Peterson) approach to the hip. The deeper internervous plane is shown between rectus femoris (femoral nerve) and the gluteus medius (superior gluteal nerve). The ascending branch of the lateral femoral circumflex artery has been ligated with the rectus femoris origin release shown. Dissect any attachments of the iliopsoas to the inferior capsule. A capsulotomy completes this approach.

joint capsule. Reflection of the vastus lateralis origin assists with exposure. Dissect the reflected head of the rectus femoris (and capsular attachment of the iliopsoas if necessary) and retract medially. Performing a capsulotomy completes this approach.

LATERAL (HARDINGE) APPROACH TO THE HIP

This approach (Fig. 4.15) utilizes an incision that splits both the gluteus medius and the vastus lateralis in tandem; therefore, there is no true internervous plane. Incise the

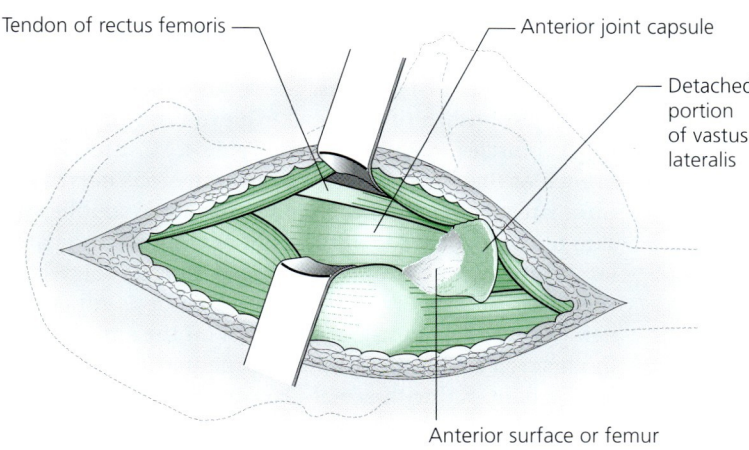

Figure 4.14 Anterolateral (Watson–Jones) approach to the hip. There is no true internervous plane, but this approach utilizes the intermuscular plane between the tensor fascia lata and gluteus medius. The vastus lateralis origin is reflected inferiorly, assisting with exposure of the hip capsule. A capsulotomy completes this approach.

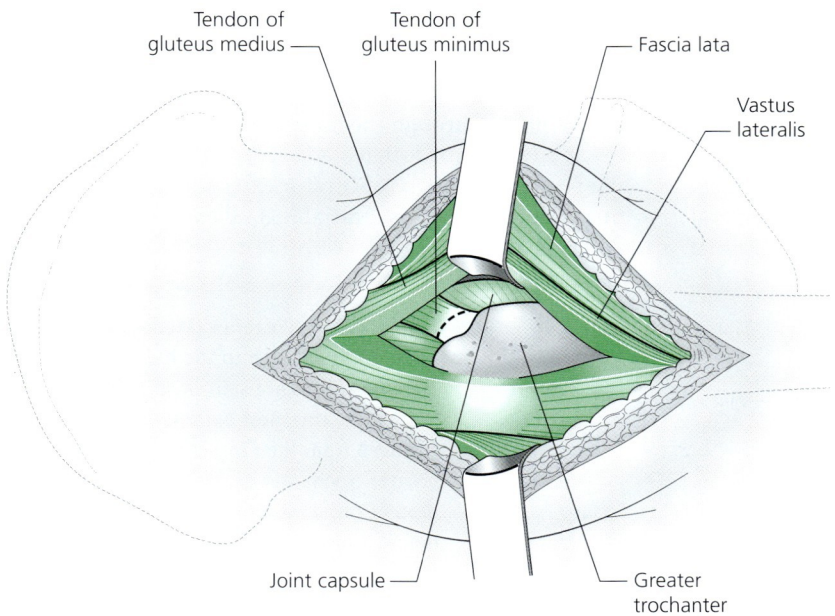

Figure 4.15 Lateral (Hardinge) approach to the hip. The gluteus medius and the vastus lateralis is split in tandem; therefore, there is no true internervous plane. Development of an anterior cuff of tissue exposes the joint capsule and the gluteus minimus tendon (dotted line), which will be released. Capsulotomy completes this approach.

skin and the fascia lata to expose the gluteus medius and the vastus. Over the tip of the greater trochanter, the gluteus medius fibres are split with incision carried proximally for about 2 cm and distally into the vastus lateralis for 2 cm. The anterior cuff of tissue is elevated to expose the anterior femoral neck and joint capsule. Capsulotomy completes this approach.

POSTERIOR (MOORE OR SOUTHERN) APPROACH TO THE HIP

Following a curved posterior incision, the fascia lata is incised over the greater trochanter. See Fig. 4.16. The fibres of the gluteus maximus are split and retracted. The short external rotators are exposed close to their insertion into the greater trochanter. Reflect them laterally to protect the sciatic nerve and expose the posterior hip capsule. A portion of the quadratus femoris may be taken down with the short external rotators, but one must be aware of the significant bleeding that can come from the inferior portion of this muscle (ascending branches of medial femoral circumflex artery). Capsulotomy completes this approach.

ACETABULAR APPROACHES

Acetabular surgical approaches are beyond the scope of this text; please refer to more detailed anatomical exposure texts (e.g. Hoppenfield 2003, see Further Reading list).

THIGH

Osteology

The femur is the largest bone of the body. Important areas of femoral ossification include the head and the distal femur. The femoral head is usually not present at birth but appears as one large physis that includes both trochanters at about 11 months and fuses at 18 years. The distal femoral physis appears at birth and fuses at 19 years, making a knee stress examination important for detecting physeal fractures. The neck–shaft angle is 141° in the fetus, with the adult angle averaging 127°. The femoral neck anteversion varies from 1° to 40° but averages 14°. The anterior bow of the femur is accounted for with improved radius of curvatures of intramedullary implants.

Neuromuscular anatomy

A useful way to summarize thigh neuromuscular components is shown in Table 4.25.

The sciatic nerve (L4–S3) emerges from its foramen anterior to the piriformis muscle (through the piriformis in 2% of people) and lies posterior to the other short external rotators. It descends below the gluteus maximus and proceeds posteriorly to the adductor magnus and between the long head of the biceps and the semimembranosus. Before it emerges from the popliteal fossa, it divides into the common peroneal nerve and the tibial nerve. The peroneal division has one innervation in the thigh – short head of biceps femoris. The common peroneal nerve diverges laterally and traverses the lateral knee region under cover of the biceps femoris. The tibial nerve emerges into the popliteal fossa laterally, proceeds posteriorly to the vessel, and then descends between the heads of the gastrocnemius. The femoral nerve (L2–4) is the largest branch of the lumbar plexus and supplies the thigh muscles highlighted in Table 4.25. The largest branch of the femoral nerve is the saphenous nerve. The infrapatellar branch of the saphenous nerve supplies the skin of the medial side of the front of the knee and patellar ligament, and can be damaged during total knee replacement surgery. The lateral femoral cutaneous nerve (L2,3) supplies skin and fascia on the anterolateral thigh surface from the greater trochanter to the knee. It can be damaged with acetabular approaches that dissect around its course underneath the lateral end of the inguinal ligament. The obturator nerve (L2–4) can be damaged during various hip and acetabular approaches (screw placement in anteroinferior quadrant), resulting in sensation decrease in the medial thigh and loss of hip adductor function. The obturator nerve has two branches after it passes through the obturator foramen: the anterior branch (adductor longus, adductor brevis, gracilis) and the posterior branch (obturator externus, adductor magnus, adductor brevis (variable)). Please note that the anterior branch of the obturator nerve can provide

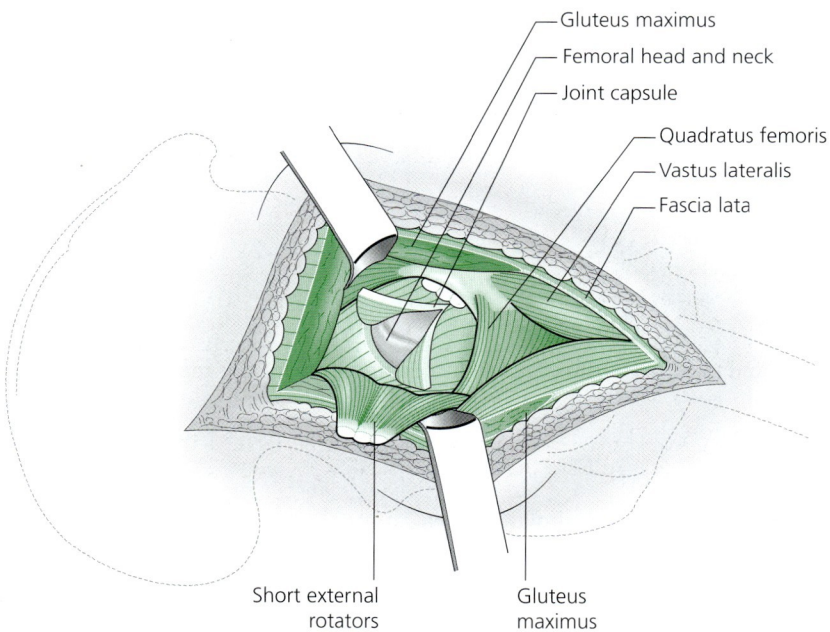

Figure 4.16 Posterior (Moore or Southern) approach to the hip. The gluteus maximus fibres are split in this approach. As illustrated, the short external rotators are removed from their insertion onto the greater trochanter and reflected posterior to protect the sciatic nerve and to expose the hip capsule. A portion of the quadratus femoris may be taken down with the short external rotators, but one must be aware of the significant bleeding that can come from the inferior portion of this muscle (ascending branches of the medial femoral circumflex artery). Ligation of this artery will devascularize the femoral head, but this is not an issue if this approach is used for prosthetic replacement. A T-capsulotomy is shown exposing the femoral head and neck.

Table 4.25 Thigh muscle innervation

Nerve in thigh	Components	Innervation
Femoral	L2–4	Iliacus, psoas major (lower part), sartorius, pectineus, quadriceps, articularis genus muscle
Obturator	L2–4	Obturator externus, hip adductors (brevis, longus, magnus), gracilis
Sciatic	L4–S3	Peroneal division: short head biceps femoris
		Tibial division: hamstrings (semitendinosus, semimembranosus), part of adductor magnus, long head biceps femoris

sensation to the medial side of the knee and can be a source of referred pain from hip pathology. Always evaluate clinically and radiographically a joint above and below the patient's complaint.

The arterial branches in the thigh are worth discussing. The external iliac artery becomes the femoral artery after traversing the inguinal ligament arriving into the femoral triangle. The femoral artery branches to become the deep femoral artery and the superficial femoral artery. The deep femoral artery gives rise to the medial and lateral femoral circumflex arteries. The medial femoral circumflex artery is the major blood supply to the femoral head in the adult and lies anterior to the quadratus femoris muscle. After supplying the profundus (described earlier), the superficial femoral artery descends under cover of the sartorius muscle and proceeds between the adductor group and the vastus medialis into the adductor canal. At the level above the medial femoral condyle, the artery supplies a descending geniculate branch, then passes through a defect in the adductor magnus (adductor hiatus) and emerges in the popliteal fossa. The vein is usually posterior to the artery. The obturator artery is a branch of the internal iliac artery and its posterior branch supplies the ligamentum teres acetabular artery. This arterial supply is an important blood supply to the femoral head from birth to 4 years. The internal iliac artery also supplies the superior and inferior gluteal arteries.

Surgical approaches to the thigh

See Table 4.26 for a summary of approaches.

LATERAL APPROACH TO THE THIGH

There is no true internervous plane. Following a lateral incision, the fascia lata is split in line with the femoral shaft. Then bluntly dissect the vastus lateralis in line with its fibres or dissect the fibres of the intermuscular septum. Identify and coagulate the various perforators from the profunda femoris. The lateral surface of the femur is exposed, completing this approach.

POSTEROLATERAL APPROACH TO THE THIGH

The internervous plane is between the vastus lateralis (femoral nerve) and the hamstrings (sciatic nerve). Following a lateral incision, the deep fascia is incised, exposing the vastus lateralis. The vastus is elevated and the lateral intermuscular septum is visualized. The perforating vessels from the profundus are ligated. The lateral femur is visualized following periosteal incision at the linea aspera, completing this approach.

ANTEROMEDIAL APPROACH TO THE DISTAL FEMUR

The interval between the rectus femoris and vastus medialis (femoral nerve) is explored. Following incision, the vastus medialis and rectus femoris are retracted, exposing the vastus intermedius. It may be necessary to open the knee joint. If so, incise the medial patellar retinaculum and split a portion of the quadriceps tendon just lateral to the medial border. After identifying the vastus intermedius, split it along its fibres to expose the femur, completing this approach.

KNEE AND LEG

Osteology

PATELLA

The patella is the largest sesamoid bone. It serves three functions: it is a fulcrum for the quadriceps; it protects the knee joint; and it enhances lubrication and nutrition of the knee. An accessory or 'bipartite' patella may represent failure of fusion of the superolateral corner of the patella and is commonly confused with patellar fractures.

TIBIA

The tibia articulates with the distal femur with proximal medial (oval and concave) and lateral (circular and convex) facets. Gerdy's tubercle lies on the lateral side of the proximal tibia and is the insertion of the iliotibial tract. The tibial shaft is triangular in cross-section and tapers to its thinnest point at the junction of the middle and distal thirds and then again widens to form the tibial plafond. Distally, the tibia forms an inferior quadrilateral surface for articulation with the talus and the pyramid-shaped medial malleolus. Laterally, the fibular notch forms an articulation with the fibula.

Table 4.26 Thigh surgical approaches

Approach	Interval	Risks
Lateral	Vastus lateralis (femoral nerve)	Perforators from the profunda femoris artery
Posterolateral	Vastus lateralis (femoral nerve) and hamstrings (sciatic nerve)	Perforators from the profunda femoris artery Distal exposure: lateral superior geniculate artery
Anteromedial (distal)	Rectus femoris (femoral nerve) and vastus medialis (femoral nerve)	Medial superior geniculate artery Infrapatellar branch of saphenous nerve

Table 4.27 Compartment releases of leg

Compartment	Muscles	Neurovascular structures released
Anterior	TA, EHL, EDL, PT	Deep peroneal nerve and anterior tibial artery
Lateral	PL, PB	Superficial peroneal nerve
Superficial posterior	GSC, plantaris	Sural nerve
Deep posterior	Popliteus, FHL, FDL, TP	Posterior tibial artery and vein; tibial nerve; peroneal artery and vein

EDL, extensor digitorum longus; EHL, extensor hallucis longus; FDL, flexor digitorum longus; FHL, flexor hallucis longus; GSC, gastrocsoleus; PB, peroneus brevis; PL, peroneus longus; PT, peroneus tertius; TA, tibiais anterior; TP, tibialis posterior.

FIBULA

The styloid process of the head serves as the attachment for the fibular collateral ligament and the biceps tendon. Lying just below the head, the neck of the fibula is grooved by the common peroneal nerve. The expanded distal fibula is known as the lateral malleolus and extends beyond the distal margin of the medial malleolus. Together with the inferior distal surface of the tibia, these structures make up the ankle mortise.

Arthrology

KNEE

Clinically relevant knee anatomy is covered in Chapter 47.

Neuromuscular anatomy

Leg muscles are commonly divided into groups based on four compartments (anterior, lateral, superficial posterior and deep posterior). The posterior compartments are supplied by the tibial nerve and contain pre-axial muscles. The anterior and lateral compartments are supplied by the common peroneal nerve (anterior – deep, lateral – superficial) and contain post-axial muscles. Four-compartment fascial release of the leg is summarized in Table 4.27.

NERVES

Tibial nerve (L4–S3)

Continues in the thigh deep to the long head of the biceps and enters the popliteal fossa. It then crosses over the popliteus muscle and splits the two heads of the gastrocnemius, passing deep to the soleus on its course to the posterior aspect of the medial malleolus. It terminates as the medial and lateral plantar nerves. Muscular branches supply the posterior leg along its course (superficial and deep posterior compartments). See Table 4.28.

Common peroneal nerve (L4–S2)

The smaller terminal division of the sciatic, this nerve runs laterally in the popliteal fossa in the interval between the medial border of the biceps and the lateral head of the gastrocnemius. Then it winds around the neck of the fibula deep to the peroneus longus, where it divides into superficial and deep branches. This nerve can be injured with traction and with lateral meniscal repair.

Superficial peroneal nerve

Runs along the border between the lateral and anterior compartments in the leg, supplying muscular branches to the peroneus longus and brevis (lateral compartment). It terminates in two cutaneous branches (medial dorsal and intermediate dorsal cutaneous nerve) supplying the dorsal foot. Please note that the superficial peroneal nerve supplies dorsal medial sensation to the great toe. See Table 4.29.

Deep peroneal nerve

Sometimes known as the anterior tibial nerve, this nerve runs along the anterior surface of the interosseous membrane, supplying the musculature of the anterior compartment (TA, EHL, extensor digitorum longus (EDL), PT). The first web space sensation is provided by the deep peroneal nerve. See Table 4.30.

Table 4.28 Tibial nerve innervation

Nerve	Innervation distal to knee
Tibial nerve	Gastrocnemius, soleus, tibialis posterior, FDL, FHL, medial and lateral plantar nerve

FDL, flexor digitorum longus; FHL, flexor hallucis longus.

Table 4.29 Superficial peroneal nerve innervation

Nerve	Innervation
Superficial peroneal nerve	Peroneus longus and brevis

Table 4.30 Deep peroneal nerve innervation

Nerve	Innervation
Deep peroneal nerve	Tibialis anterior, EDL, EHL, PT, EDB

EDB, extensor digitorum brevis; EDL, extensor digitorum longus; EHL, extensor hallucis longus; PT, peroneus tertius.

Cutaneous nerves

Important cutaneous nerves include the saphenous nerve (L3,4) and the sural nerve (S1,2). The saphenous nerve is the continuation of the femoral nerve of the thigh, and it becomes subcutaneous on the medial aspect of the knee between the sartorius and gracilis (where it is sometimes injured during procedures about the knee, e.g. meniscal repair). The saphenous nerve supplies sensation to the medial aspect of the leg and foot. The sural nerve, which is often used for nerve grafting and which can cause painful neuromas when inadvertently cut, is formed by cutaneous branches of both the tibial (medial sural cutaneous) and common peroneal (lateral sural cutaneous) nerves. It lies on the lateral aspect of the leg and foot.

Vessels

Branches of the popliteal artery, the continuation of the femoral artery, supply the leg. The artery enters the popliteal fossa between the biceps and semimembranosus and descends underneath the tibial nerve and terminates between the medial and lateral heads of the gastrocnemius, dividing into the anterior and posterior tibial arteries. Several genicular branches are given off in the popliteal fossa, including the medial and lateral geniculates (which supply the menisci) and the middle geniculate artery (which supplies the cruciate ligaments). The superior lateral geniculate can be injured during lateral release procedures. The descending geniculate artery (a branch of the femoral artery proximal to Hunter's canal) supplies the vastus medialis at the anterior border of the intermuscular septum. The inferior geniculate artery passes between the popliteal tendon and fibular collateral ligament in the posterolateral corner of the knee.

Anterior tibial artery

The first branch of the popliteal artery, this vessel passes between the two heads of the tibialis posterior and the interosseous membrane to lie on the anterior surface of that membrane between the tibialis anterior and EHL until it terminates as the dorsalis pedis artery.

Posterior tibial artery

Continues in the deep posterior compartment of the leg, coursing obliquely to pass behind the medial malleolus, where it terminates by dividing into medial and lateral plantar arteries. Its main branch, the peroneal artery, is given off 2.5 cm distal to the popliteal fossa and continues in the deep posterior compartment, lateral to its parent artery, between the tibialis posterior and flexor hallucis longus (FHL), eventually terminating in calcaneal branches.

Surgical approaches to the knee and leg

Surgically relevant knee and leg approaches are covered in Chapters 76 and 77.

ANKLE AND FOOT

Osteology

The 26 bones of the foot include: seven tarsal bones, five metatarsals and 14 phalanges. The foot is divided into the hindfoot (talus and calcaneus), midfoot (navicular, cuboid, and three cuneiforms) and forefoot (metatarsals and phalanges).

TARSUS

This includes the talus, calcaneus, cuboid, navicular and three cuneiforms.

Talus

Articulates with the tibia and fibula in the ankle mortise and with the calcaneus and navicular distally. It is made up of a body that is wider anteriorly with three articular surfaces (the trochlea (including surfaces for the malleoli articulations), and the posterior and middle calcaneal facets) and a posterior process (for the posterior talofibular ligament). The neck of the talus connects with the head, which in turn articulates with the navicular distally and the calcaneus inferiorly. The talus has no muscular attachments but has a groove posteriorly for the tendon of the FHL. Additionally, two-thirds of the talus is covered with cartilage. The primary blood supply to the talar body is from the artery of the tarsal canal (posterior tibial artery). The other blood supplies include the superior neck vessels (anterior tibial artery) and the artery of the tarsal sinus (dorsalis pedis).

Calcaneus

The largest and strongest bone in the foot. It has three surfaces that articulate with the talus: a large posterior facet, an anterior facet and a middle facet. Distally, there is an articular surface that receives the cuboid bone. The sustentaculum tali is an overhanging horizontal eminence on the anteromedial surface of the calcaneus. The sustentaculum tali supports the middle articular surface above it and has an inferior groove for the FHL tendon.

Cuboid

This lies on the lateral aspect of the foot, is grooved on the plantar surface by the peroneus longus and has four facets for articulation with the calcaneus, the lateral cuneiform, and the fourth and fifth metatarsals.

Navicular

The most medial tarsal bone; it lies between the talus and the cuneiforms. Proximally, the surface is oval and concave for its articulation with the head of the talus. Distally, the navicular has three articular surfaces, one for each of the cuneiforms. The medial plantar projection serves as the insertion for the posterior tibial tendon.

Cuneiforms

Medial, intermediate and lateral, these three bones articulate with the navicular and posterior cuboid (lateral cuneiform) and the first three metatarsals. The intermediate cuneiform does not extend as far distally as the medial cuneiform, allowing the second metatarsal to 'key' into place.

METATARSALS

Five bones, numbered from medial to lateral, span the distance between the tarsals and the phalanges. In general, their shape and function are similar to those of the metacarpals of the hand. The first metatarsal has a plantar crista that articulates with the fibular and tibial sesamoids contained within the flexor hallucis brevis tendon.

PHALANGES

Also similar to the hand. The great toe has two phalanges, and the remaining digits have three.

OSSIFICATION

Each tarsus has a single ossification centre, except the calcaneus, which has a second centre posteriorly. The calcaneus, talus and usually the cuboid are present at birth. The lateral cuneiform appears during the first year, the medial cuneiform during the second year, and the intermediate cuneiform and navicular during the third year. The posterior centre for the calcaneus usually appears in the eighth year. The second to fifth metatarsals have two ossification centres: a primary centre in the shaft and a secondary centre for the head that appears at age 5–8. The phalanges and first metatarsal have secondary centres at their bases that appear during the third or fourth year proximally and the sixth to seventh year distally.

Arthrology

INFERIOR TIBIOFIBULAR JOINT

Formed by the medial distal fibula and the notched lateral distal tibia, this joint is supported by four ligaments: anterior and posterior inferior tibiofibular ligaments, transverse tibiofibular ligament and an interosseous ligament. The anteroinferior tibiofibular ligament is an oblique band that connects the bones anteriorly. Avulsion of this ligament may result in a Tillaux fracture.

ANKLE JOINT

The ankle is a ginglymus, or hinge, joint formed by the malleoli and the talus. The medial collateral (deltoid) ligament comprises two layers: (1) superficial – tibionavicular and tibiocalcaneal; (2) deep – anterior and posterior tibiotalar. The lateral fibular ligaments are the anterior talofibular (ATFL), calcaneofibular (CFL) and posterior talofibular (PTFL). The ATFL is the weakest and is intracapsular (intracapsular thickening). The position of the ankle is critical when testing the lateral ligament complex: plantarflexion tightens the ATFL and inversion with neutral flexion tightens the CFL.

SUBTALAR JOINT

Talar plantar facets articulate with the calcaneus. Stability is derived from four ligaments: the medial, lateral and interosseous talocalcaneal and cervical ligaments.

OTHER JOINTS

Tarsometatarsal joints are gliding joints supported by dorsal, plantar and interosseous ligaments. The base of the first metatarsal is not ligamentously connected to the second metatarsal. The Lisfranc ligament connects the medial (shortest) cuneiform to the second (longest) metatarsal. In about 20% of patients, it exists as a plantar and dorsal structure. The deep transverse metatarsal ligaments interconnect the metatarsal heads. The digital nerve courses plantar under the transverse metatarsal ligament and is the spot where interdigital neuritis (Morton's neuroma – usually the second or third interdigital space) occurs. Additionally, the transverse metatarsal ligament attaches the second metatarsal head to the fibular sesamoid. This ligament holds the hallucal sesamoids in place and gives the appearance of sesamoid subluxation when the first metatarsal moves medially in hallux valgus. Plantar and collateral ligaments support the metatarsophalangeal joints. The primary stabilizing structure of the metatarsophalangeal joint is the plantar plate. Interphalangeal joints are supported mainly by their capsules.

Neuromuscular anatomy

A total of 13 tendons cross the ankle joint: posterior, Achilles; lateral, peroneals with longus (superficial) and brevis (deep); anterior (from lateral to medial), peroneus tertius, EDL, EHL, TA; and medial ('Tom, Dick and Harry'), tibialis posterior, flexor digitorum longus, FHL. Please note that the Achilles tendon maximum normal anteroposterior dimension on MRI is 8 mm. There is one dorsal intrinsic muscle of the foot – extensor digitorum brevis (EDB) (lateral terminal branch of the deep peroneal nerve). Plantar heel spurs originate in the flexor digitorum brevis (medial plantar nerve innervation).

NERVES

Nerves of the ankle and foot are summarized above. A functional summary of ankle motion is provided in Table 4.31.

Please note that the posterior tibial tendon is the initiator of hindfoot inversion during gait. This explains why a person cannot single stance toe rise with posterior tibial tendon deficiency and a normal Achilles.

Tibial nerve

The tibial nerve supplies all intrinsic foot muscles except the EDB (deep peroneal nerve). The tibial nerve splits into two branches under the flexor retinaculum: medial and lateral plantar nerves (Table 4.32). Both of these nerves run in the second layer of the foot. The medial plantar nerve runs deep to the abductor hallucis, and the lateral plantar nerve runs obliquely under the cover of the quadratus plantae. The most proximal branch of the lateral plantar nerve is the nerve to the abductor digiti quinti (Baxter's nerve). The distribution of the sensory and motor branches of the plantar nerves is similar to that in the hand. The medial plantar nerve (like the median nerve of the hand) supplies plantar sensation to the medial 3½ digits and motor to only a few plantar muscles (flexor hallucis brevis, abductor hallucis, flexor digitorum brevis and first lumbrical). The lateral plantar nerve (like the ulnar nerve in the hand) supplies plantar sensation to the lateral 1½ digits and the remaining intrinsic muscles of the foot. The third web space digital nerve consists of branches from both the medial and lateral plantar nerves.

Common peroneal nerve

Splits into superficial and deep branches in the leg and has terminal branches in the foot as well. The lateral terminal branch of the deep peroneal nerve ends in the proximal dorsal foot by supplying the EDB muscle. The medial terminal branch of the deep peroneal nerve supplies sensation to the first web space. The medial and intermediate dorsal cutaneous nerves of the superficial peroneal nerve supply the bulk of the remaining sensation to the dorsal foot. The dorsal intermediate branch is at risk during placement of the anterolateral ankle arthroscopic portal discussed below. All sensation of the foot is supplied by the sciatic nerve except the medial ankle and foot (saphenous nerve (termination of femoral nerve)). Please note that the dorsal medial cutaneous nerve (branch of the superficial peroneal nerve) crosses the EHL from lateral to medial and supplies sensation to the dorsomedial aspect of the great toe.

A summary of lower extremity innervation is shown in Table 4.33.

Vessels

Like the nerves that run with them, there are two main arteries that supply the ankle and foot.

DORSALIS PEDIS ARTERY

Continuation of the anterior tibial artery of the leg, it provides the blood supply to the dorsum of the foot via

Table 4.31 Ankle neuromuscular interactions

Foot function	Muscle	Innervation
Inversion	Tibialis anterior	Deep peroneal nerve (L4)
	Tibialis posterior	Tibial nerve (S1)
Dorsiflexion	Tibialis anterior, EDL, EHL	Deep peroneal nerve: TA (L4), EDL and EHL (L5)
Eversion	Peroneus longus and brevis	Superficial peroneal nerve (S1)
Plantarflexion	Gastrocsoleus, FDL, FHL, tibialis posterior (also hindfoot inverter)	Tibial nerve (S1)

EDL, extensor digitorum longus; EHL, extensor hallucis longus; FDL, flexor digitorum longus; FHL, flexor hallucis longus; TA, tibialis anterior.

Table 4.32 Medial and lateral plantar nerve innervation

Nerve	Innervation
Medial plantar nerve	FHB, abductor hallucis, FDB, first lumbrical
Lateral plantar nerve	QP, ADM, FDM, AdHal, interossei, 2–4th lumbricals

ADM, abductor digiti minimi; FDB, flexor digitorum brevis; FDM, flexor digiti minimi; FHB, flexor hallucis brevis; QP, quadratus plantae..

Table 4.33 Summary of lower extremity innervation

Nerve	Innervation
Femoral nerve	Iliacus, psoas, quadriceps femoris (rectus femoris and the vastus lateralis, intermedius and medialis)
Obturator nerve	Adductor brevis, longus and magnus (along with tibial nerve), gracilis
Superior gluteal nerve	Gluteus medius, gluteus minimus, tensor fascia lata
Inferior gluteal nerve	Gluteus maximus
Sciatic nerve	Semitendinosus, semimembranosus, biceps femoris (long head (tibial division) and short head (peroneal division)), adductor magnus (with obturator nerve)
Tibial nerve	Gastrocnemius, soleus, tibialis posterior, FDL, FHL, medial and lateral plantar nerve
Deep peroneal nerve	Tibialis anterior, EDL, EHL, PT, EDB
Superficial peroneal nerve	Peroneus longus and brevis

EDB, extensor digitorum brevis; EDL, extensor digitorum longus; EHL, extensor hallucis longus; FDL, flexor digitorum longus; FHL, flexor hallucis longus; PT, peroneus tertius.

Table 4.34 Foot and ankle surgical approaches

Approach	Interval	Risks
Anterior ankle	EHL (deep peroneal nerve) EDL (deep peroneal nerve)	Superficial and deep peroneal nerve, anterior tibial artery
Anterior medial malleolus ankle		Saphenous nerve and vein
Distal fibula		Sural nerve (posterolateral) and superficial peroneal nerve (anterior with variable position)

EDL, extensor digitorum longus; EHL, extensor hallucis longus.

its lateral tarsal, medial tarsal, arcuate and first dorsal metatarsal branches. Its largest branch, the deep plantar artery, runs between the first and second metatarsals and contributes to the plantar arch.

POSTERIOR TIBIAL ARTERY

This divides into medial and lateral plantar branches under the abductor hallucis muscle. The larger lateral branch receives the deep plantar artery and forms the plantar arch in the fourth layer of the plantar foot.

Surgical approaches to the foot and ankle (Table 4.34)

The approaches are summarised in Table 4.34.

ANTERIOR APPROACH TO THE ANKLE

This approach utilizes the interval between the EHL and EDL (both deep peroneal nerve). Before incising the extensor retinaculum, care must be taken to protect the superficial peroneal nerve. The deep peroneal nerve and anterior tibial artery, which lie directly in this interval, must be retracted medially with the EHL.

APPROACH TO THE MEDIAL MALLEOLUS

The medial malleolus is superficial and can be approached anteriorly or posteriorly. The anterior approach jeopardizes the saphenous nerve and the long saphenous vein; the posterior approach places the structures running behind the medial malleolus (posterior tibial artery; flexor digitorum longus; posterior tibial artery, vein and nerve; and FHL) at risk. A posteromedial approach, behind the medial malleolus, can be made through the tendon sheath of the posterior tibialis.

LATERAL APPROACH TO THE FIBULA

This approach is subcutaneous. The sural nerve (posterolateral) and the superficial peroneal nerve (anterior) must be avoided.

FURTHER READING

Arnoczky SP, Warren RF. Microvasculature of the human meniscus. *American Journal of Sports Medicine* 1982;**10**:90–5.

Bohlman HH. The neck. In: D'Ambrosia R (ed.) *Musculoskeletal Disorders*. Philadelphia, PA: J.B. Lippincott, 1977.

Bora FW. *The Pediatric Upper Extremity*. Philadelphia, PA: W.B. Saunders, 1986.

Browner BD, Jupiter JB, Levine AM, *et al*. *Skeletal Trauma*. Philadelphia, PA: W.B. Saunders, 1992.

Callaghan JJ (ed.). *Anatomy Self-Assessment Examination*. Park Ridge, IL: American Academy of Orthopaedic Surgeons, 1991.

Callaghan JJ (ed.). *Anatomy Self-Assessment Examination*. Park Ridge, IL, American Academy of Orthopaedic Surgeons, 1996.

Cervical Spine Research Education Committee. *The Cervical Spine*, 2nd edn. Philadelphia, PA: J.B. Lippincott, 1989.

Chapman MW (ed.). *Operative Orthopaedics*. Philadelphia, PA: J.B. Lippincott, 1988.

Chapman MW (ed.). *Gray's Anatomy*, 30th edn. Philadelphia, PA: Lea & Febiger, 1985.

Cohen MS, Bruno RJ. The collateral ligaments of the elbow. *Clinical Orthopaedics and Related Research* 2001;**383**:123–30.

Cooper DE, O'Brien SJ, Warren RF. Supporting layers of the glenohumeral joint. *Clinical Orthopaedics and Related Research* 1993;**289**:144–55.

Corley FG (ed.). *Shoulder and Elbow Self-Assessment Examination*. Park Ridge, IL: American Academy of Orthopaedic Surgeons, 1996.

Corley FG (ed.). *Shoulder and Elbow Self-Assessment Examination*. Park Ridge, IL: American Academy of Orthopaedic Surgeons, 1999.

Crock HV. An atlas of the arterial supply of the head and neck of the femur in man. *Clinical Orthopaedics and Related Research* 1980;**152**:17.

DeCoster TA (ed.). *Anatomy Self-Assessment Examination*. Park Ridge, IL: American Academy of Orthopaedic Surgeons, 1999.

DeCoster TA (ed.). *Anatomy Self-Assessment Examination*. Park Ridge, IL: American Academy of Orthopaedic Surgeons, 2002.

DeLee JC, Drez D Jr. *Orthopaedic Sports Medicine: Principles and Practice*. Philadelphia, PA: W.B. Saunders, 1994.

Doyle JR. Anatomy of the finger flexor tendon sheath and pulley system. *Journal of Hand Surgery (American)* 1988;**13**:473–84.

Girgis FG, Marshall JL, Monajem ARS. The cruciate ligaments of the knee joint: anatomical, functional, and experimental analysis. *Clinical Orthopaedics and Related Research* 1975;**106**:216–31.

Green DP, Hotchkiss RN, Pederson WC. *Green's Operative Hand Surgery*, 4th edn. New York, NY: Churchill Livingstone, 1999.

Harding K. The direct lateral approach to the hip. *Journal of Bone and Joint Surgery (British)* 1982;**64**:17–19.

Henry AK. *Extensive Exposure*, 2nd edn. New York, NY: Churchill Livingstone, 1973.

Hollinshead WH. *Anatomy for Surgeons*, vol. 3, 2nd edn. New York, NY: Harper & Row, 1969.

Hoppenfield S, DeBoer P. *Surgical Exposures in Orthopaedics: The Anatomic Approach*. Philadelphia, PA: J.B. Lippincott, 2003.

Hoppenfeld S. *Orthopaedic Neurology: A Diagnostic Guide to Neurological Levels*. Philadelphia, PA: Lippincott-Raven, 1997.

Jahss MH. *Disorders of the Foot*. Philadelphia, PA: W.B. Saunders, 1987.

Jenkins DB. *Hollinshead's Functional Anatomy of the Limbs and Back*, 6th edn. Philadelphia, PA: W.B. Saunders, 1991.

Kaplan EB. *Surgical Approaches to the Neck, Cervical Spine, and Upper Extremity*. Philadelphia, PA: W.B. Saunders, 1966.

Ludloff K. The open reduction of the congenital hip dislocation by an anterior incision. *American Journal of Orthopedic Surgery* 1913;**10**:438.

Magee DJ. *Orthopaedic Physical Assessment*. Philadelphia, PA: W.B. Saunders, 1987.

Mooney JF, Siegel DB, Koman LA. Ligamentous injuries of the wrist in athletes. *Clinics in Sports Medicine* 1992;**11**:129–39.

Morrey BF, An KN. Articular and ligamentous contributions to the stability of the elbow joint. *Journal of Sports Medicine* 1983;**11**:315–19.

Morrey BF, An KN. Functional anatomy of the ligaments of the elbow. *Clinical Orthopaedics and Related Research* 1985;**210**:84–90.

Myerson MS (ed.). *Foot and Ankle Self-Assessment Examination*. Park Ridge, IL: American Academy of Orthopaedic Surgeons, 1997.

Myerson MS (ed.). *Foot and Ankle Self-Assessment Examination*. Park Ridge, IL: American Academy of Orthopaedic Surgeons, 2000.

Netter FH. *The CIBA Collection of Medical Illustrations*. Vol. 8. *Musculoskeletal System, Part I*. Summit, NJ: Ciba-Geigy, 1987.

Orthopaedic Knowledge Update. *Home Study Syllabus I*. Chicago, IL: American Academy of Orthopaedic Surgeons, 1984.

Orthopaedic Knowledge Update. *Home Study Syllabus II*. Chicago, IL: American Academy of Orthopaedic Surgeons, 1987.

Orthopaedic Knowledge Update. *Home Study Syllabus III*. Chicago, IL: American Academy of Orthopaedic Surgeons, 1990.

Place HM (ed.). *Adult Spine Self-Assessment Examination*. Park Ridge, IL: American Academy of Orthopaedic Surgeons, 1997.

Place HM (ed.). *Adult Spine Self-Assessment Examination*. Park Ridge, IL: American Academy of Orthopaedic Surgeons, 2000.

Rockwood CA Jr, Green DP (eds). *Fractures in Adults*, 3rd edn. Philadelphia, PA: J.B. Lippincott, 1991.

Rothman RH, Simeon FA. *The Spine*, 2nd edn. Philadelphia, PA: W.B. Saunders, 1982.

Ruge D, Wiltse LL (eds). *Spinal Disorders: Diagnosis and Treatment*. Philadelphia, PA: Lea & Febiger, 1977.

Sadler TW. *Langman's Medical Embryology*, 5th edn. Baltimore, MD: Williams & Wilkins, 1985.

Sarrafian SK. *Anatomy of the Foot and Ankle*. Philadelphia, PA: J.B. Lippincott, 1983.

Seebacher JR, Inglis AE, Marshall JL, *et al*. The structure of the posterolateral aspect of the knee. *Journal of Bone and Joint Surgery (American)* 1982;**64**:536–41.

Steinberg ME. *The Hip and Its Disorders*. Philadelphia, PA: W.B. Saunders, 1991.

Tubiana R. *The Hand*. Philadelphia, PA: W.B. Saunders, 1985.

Turkel SJ, Panio MW, Marshall JL, Girgis FG. Stabilizing mechanisms preventing anterior dislocation of the glenohumeral joint. *Journal of Bone and Joint Surgery (American)* 1981;**63**:1208–17.

Verbiest HA. Lateral approach to the cervical spine: technique and indications. *Journal of Neurosurgery* 1968;**28**:191–203.

Warren IF, Marshall JL. The supporting structures and layers on the medial side of the knee. *Journal of Bone and Joint Surgery (American)* 1979;**61**:56–62.

Watkins RG. *Surgical Approaches to the Spine*. New York, NY: Springer-Verlag, 1983.

Weissman BN, Sledge CB. *Orthopedic Radiology*. Philadelphia, PA: W.B. Saunders, 1986.

Wilson FC, Dirschl DR. *Orthopaedics: PreTest® and Self-Assessment and Review*. New York, NY: McGraw-Hill, 1996.

Woodburne RT, Burkel WE. *Essentials of Human Anatomy*, 9th edn. New York, NY: Oxford University Press, 1994.

5

The structure and development of bone tissue

BODO KURZ

Components of bone tissue and biomechanical properties	82	Periosteum and endosteum	87
Types of bone tissue	83	Bone remodelling	88
Structure and function of bone cells	86	Bone development and growth	88
		References	91

NATIONAL BOARD STANDARDS

- Know the different bone cells and their function during bone formation, resorption or maintenance of bone tissue.
- Learn about the extracellular matrix (ECM) produced and remodelled by these cells, and how the organic and inorganic components of the ECM contribute to the tensile strength, the compressive strength and the bending strength of bone tissue.
- Be able to differentiate the kinds of bone tissue, such as woven (immature) and lamellar (mature; arranged as either compact or cancellous bone) bone.
- Understand the function and structure of the periosteum and endosteum – specialized tissue layers that cover all surfaces of bone tissue.
- Know about the two major kinds of bone development and growth: intramembranous and chondral/endochondral ossification (including the growth plate).

COMPONENTS OF BONE TISSUE AND BIOMECHANICAL PROPERTIES

Bone tissue consists of different cell types, a mineralized extracellular matrix (ECM) and a highly organized neurovascular supply. Chemically, it contains about 45% inorganic minerals (predominantly calcium phosphate in the form of hydroxyapatite), 30% organic material (mostly type I collagen) and 25% water. The inorganic components are deposited by a process called mineralization, which is initiated by osteoblasts (see below). Because of its mineralization, bone is able to carry high compressive loads (compressive strengths of the tissue). The organic matrix and, especially, the collagen fibres and their distribution are able to withstand tensile forces (tensile strength of the tissue). Together, the inorganic and organic components enable bone tissue to carry bending and shearing stresses (bending strength). The compressive strength is higher than the tensile and, especially, the bending strength, which appears to be the weakest. Since all components are arranged in specific axes, bone tissue is an anisotropic material; therefore, the mechanical properties are different in different directions. The water content of bone tissue has also been shown to be important, since bone is to some extent a viscoelastic tissue that shows stiffening with increasing loading rates, a behaviour which is usually related to increasing friction during interstitial fluid flow. Drying of the tissue, therefore, increases the moduli of elasticity, hardness and even the tensile strengths. It is suggested that bone tissue-related biomechanics studies should always be carried out under normal moisture content conditions.

Even though type I collagen makes up more than 90% of the organic matrix, the other components of this ECM

Table 5.1 Extracellular matrix proteins

Protein	Bone-related function	Human disease
Collagen-related proteins		
Type I	Most abundant bone matrix protein	Osteogenesis imperfecta
Type X	Found in hypertrophic cartilage	None
Type III	Trace amounts in bone; may regulate collagen fibril diameter	Ehlers–Danlos syndrome
Type V	Trace amounts in bone; may regulate collagen fibril diameter	
Serum proteins in bone matrix		
Albumin	Decreases hydroxyapatite crystal growth	None
α_2-HS glycoprotein	Bovine analogue is fetuin	None
Glycoaminoglycan-containing proteins and leucine-rich repeat proteins		
Aggrecan	Matrix organization, retention of calcium/phosphorus	None
Versican	Defines space destined to become bone	None
Decorin	Regulates collagen fibril diameter; binds TGF-β	Progeroid form of Ehlers–Danlos syndrome with decorin/biglycan double knockout
Biglycan	Binds collagen; binds TGF-β; genetic determinant of peak bone mass	
Hyaluronan	May work with versican to define space destined to become bone	None
Glycoproteins		
Alkaline phosphatase	Hydrolyses mineral deposition inhibitors	Hypophosphatasia
Osteonectin	Regulates collagen fibril diameter	None
SIBLING proteins		
Osteopontin	Inhibits mineralization and remodelling	None
Bone sialoprotein	Initiates mineralization	None
MEPE	Regulator of phosphate metabolism	Tumour-induced osteomalacia
RGD-containing glycoproteins		
Thrombospondins	Cell attachment	None
Fibronectin	Binds to cells	None
Vitronectin	Cell attachment	None
Fibrillin 1 and 2	Regulates elastic fibre formation	Fibrillin 1: Marfan syndrome
γ-Carboxy glutamic acid-containing proteins		
Matrix Gla protein	Inhibits mineralization	None
Osteocalcin	Regulates osteoclasts; inhibits mineralization	None
Protein S	Liver product, may be made by osteoblasts	Osteopenia

Gla, gamma-carboxyglutamic acid; MEPE, matrix extracellular phosphoglycoprotein; RGD, tripeptide arginine–glycine–aspartic acid; SIBLING, small integrin-binding ligand, *N*-glycosylated; TGF, transforming growth factor.
Adapted from Clarke.[1]

appear to add important contributions to the organization, maintenance and stability of bone tissue. Table 5.1 lists some of the organic components together with their major functions and, if known, their involvement in certain human diseases.

TYPES OF BONE TISSUE

There are different types of bone tissue in the human body that primarily differ in the way the cells a) are distributed, b) the type I collagen fibres have been arranged and c) the blood supply is structured. The two major types of bone tissue are (1) woven bone (also described as immature bone) and (2) lamellar bone (which is further divided into compact bone and cancellous bone).

Woven bone

In woven bone the collagen fibres run in various directions and appear to be less organized than in lamellar bone (Fig. 5.1). This type of bone is usually found in early phases of bone development, bone remodelling or fracture healing, especially when bone formation is needed more rapidly. Woven bone is mineralized, but has less biomechanical strength than lamellar bone and is therefore replaced by the latter after some time. This replacement can take many years, but in an adult most parts of the bones consist of lamellar bone tissue.

Lamellar bone

In lamellar bone the collagen fibres are oriented in layers (lamellae). Within each layer all collagen fibres are parallel to each other, but the direction of fibres differs from layer to layer, which provides a tensile strength in more than one direction. The somas of osteocytes are located at the borders between these lamellae, but the cells have long processes that bridge the extracellular layers in order to stay in contact with neighbour cells (Figs 5.1 and 5.2). Depending on where the lamellar bone tissue is located, the shape of the layers can be different. It can be structured either in osteons, which are found in cortical compact bone, or in trabeculae, which are found in cancellous (spongy) bone.

COMPACT BONE

Compact or cortical bone forms a shell-like structure at the surface of all bones. It gives a bone its shape and

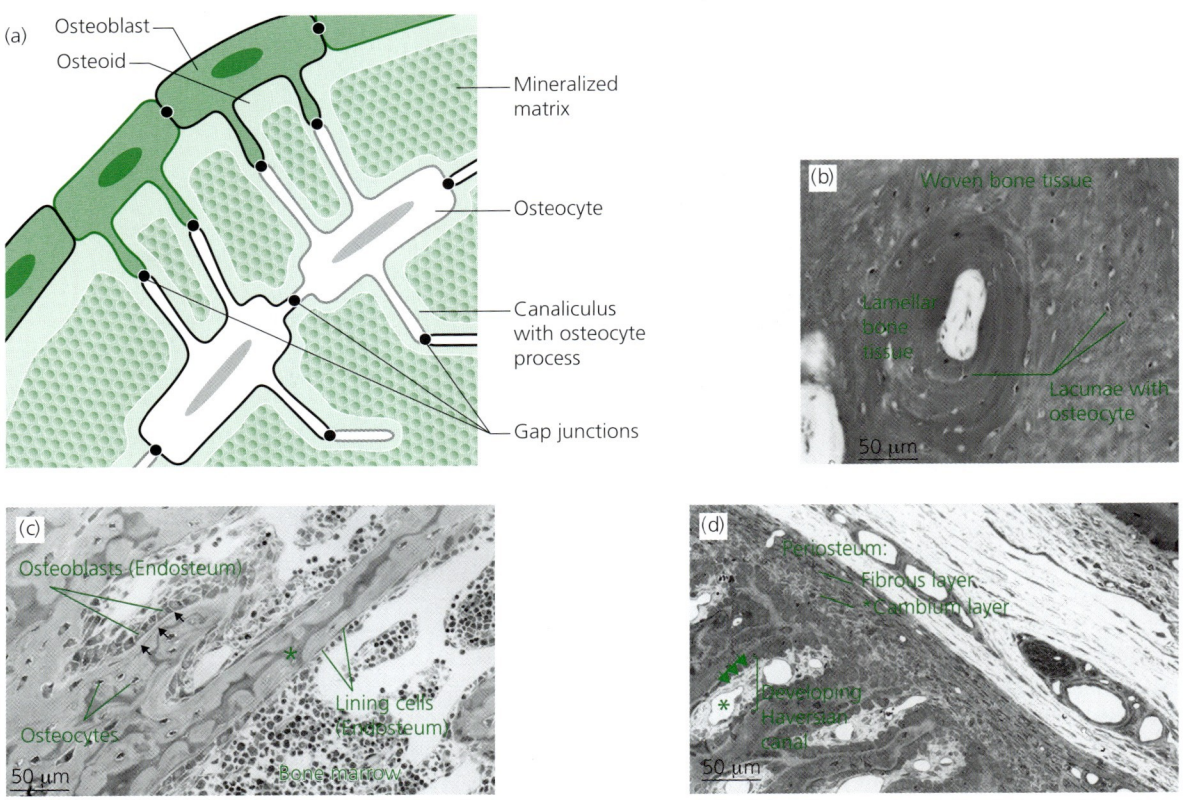

Figure 5.1 (a) Osteoblasts form bone tissue by secretion of extracellular matrix (osteoid) and subsequent induction of mineralization. The osteoblasts have cellular processes that are surrounded by the matrix and connected to other cells via gap junctions. Osteoblasts can be walled in by the next generation of osteoblasts, which turns them into osteocytes. (b) Woven bone tissue and lamellar bone tissue in the alveolar bone (pig; Goldner's trichrome). (c) Cancellous bone in the tibia. The trabeculae are covered by endosteum; lining cells are squamous, whereas active osteoblasts are cuboidal. Arrows indicate the deposition of fresh osteoid (thin grey line); asterisk marks the cartilage core in the trabeculae (primary trabeculae) (mouse; toluidine blue). (d) Periosteum covers the developing tibial bone of a mouse; the fibrous layer is like a dense connective tissue; the cambium layer contains osteoprogenitor cells. The bone tissue shows developing Haversian systems with endosteum lining the canal (arrows) and vessels (asterisk) (mouse; toluidine blue). All histological slides were provided by the Department of Anatomy, University of Kiel, Germany.

contributes significantly to its biomechanical strength. In the shaft region (diaphysis) of long bones, compact bone can be extremely thick (up to 1 cm in the femur), but other bones, such as the vertebral bodies, have a very thin shell of compact bone. In compact bone the density of bone tissue is very high, which demands a specialized architecture. This is provided by osteons (Haversian systems), which are cylinder-like structures that are mainly oriented parallel to the long axis of the bone (each is several millimetres in length and 300–400 ∝m in diameter). Osteons contain concentric layers of lamellae and have centrally a canal (Haversian canal) that is lined by endosteum (Figs 5.1 and 5.2) and filled with a neurovascular bundle and connective tissue. Osteocytes within this lamellar bone tissue obtain their nutritional supply from the vessels within the Haversian canal. Osteons can branch and produce tree-like systems of osteons, but they can also end blindly. Some bigger vessels penetrate the compact bone at a 90° angle to the long axis. They are the origin of the smaller vessels in the Haversian systems. These main vessels may be surrounded by a few layers of lamellar bone tissue, and are called Volkmann's vessels, located in Volkmann's canals (Fig. 5.2a). Within the compact bone, completely intact osteons lie directly adjacent to incomplete osteons; this is the result of an ongoing remodelling process and turnover of the bone tissue, which is described below in further detail. At the outer surface and sometimes also at the inner surface of the compact bone a few layers of lamellae cover or line the complete circumference of the bone, like rings in a cross-section of a tree; these are called circumferential bone lamellae. Their nutritional supply is provided by vessels close to the bone surface or within the bone marrow.

Except for articular surfaces or at apophyses the surfaces of compact bone are covered by periosteum, and the inner surface of compact bone (including Haversian and Volkmann's canals) is lined by endosteum, which is important for further bone formation, remodelling or repair (see below).

CANCELLOUS BONE

Cancellous bone is porous or spongy, and the layers of this lamellar bone form trabeculae (wall-like structures) that are usually oriented parallel to the axes of the highest compression and tension forces. The cavities between the trabeculae are filled with bone marrow and blood vessels (Fig. 5.1). Cancellous bone is found inside the shell of compact cortical bone, and is more frequently present in the epiphysis or metaphysis than in the diaphysis of long bones, where it can be missing. Both sides of the trabeculae are covered by endosteum, which is important for

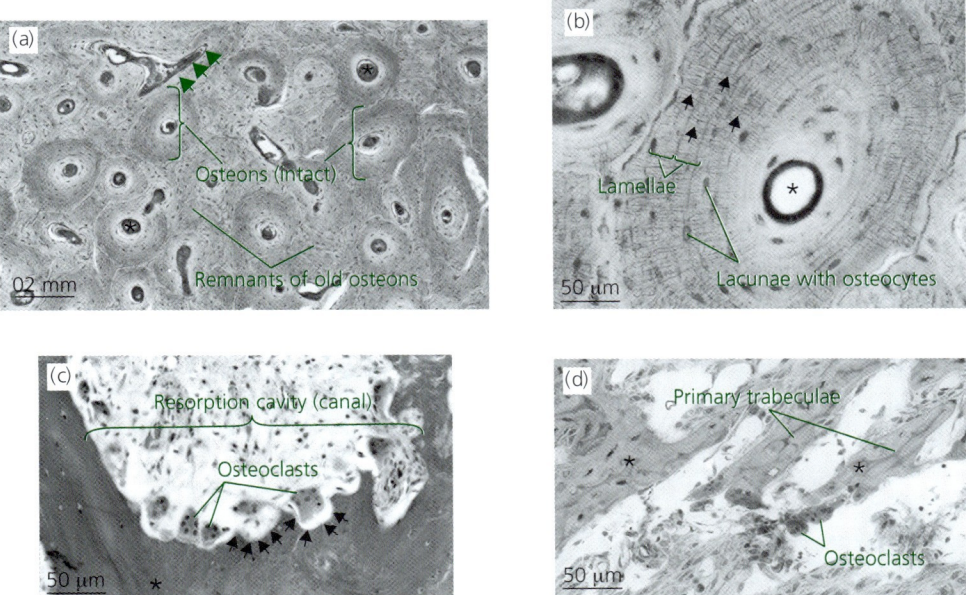

Figure 5.2 (a) Cross-section through compact bone, showing intact osteons with Haversian canals (asterisks) and remnants of older and partially removed osteons. Arrows indicate a Volkmann's canal (human; Schmorl staining). (b) Cross-section through an osteon. In the centre is the Haversian canal (asterisk) surrounded by certain layers of lamellae. Lacunae with osteocytes inside are located at the borders between the lamellae. Arrows indicate canaliculi in the matrix (human; Schmorl staining). (c) Resorption cavity (or canal) in the alveolar bone. Osteoclasts resorb mineralized matrix (arrows) and produce a canal that can be filled with a new osteon (pig; Goldner's trichrome; asterisk indicates the surrounding bone tissue). (d) Osteoclasts resorb parts of a primary trabecula (asterisk indicates cartilage matrix in the core of the trabeculae), so that the latter can be replaced by new lamellar bone (mouse; toluidine blue). All histological slides were provided by the Department of Anatomy, University of Kiel, Germany.

further trabecular formation or remodelling (see below). Nutritional supply comes from the blood vessels within the bone marrow tissue. Since nutrients need to be transported along a chain of osteocytes within the bone tissue (a process with limited capacity), the maximum thickness of trabeculae is about 300–400 µm.

STRUCTURE AND FUNCTION OF BONE CELLS

Bone tissue contains four types of cells (osteoprogenitor cells, osteoblasts, osteocytes and osteoclasts), which are involved in all processes of bone formation, maintenance, remodelling or repair (Table 5.2).

Osteoprogenitor cells

Osteoprogenitor cells derive from mesenchymal stem cells and are the precursor cells for osteoblasts. They can be found in endosteum and the cambium layer of periosteum – tissue layers which cover the external surface or line all the cavities inside bones, respectively (see below) – or they differentiate from mesenchymal stem cells during intramembranous ossification.

Osteoblasts (bone formation and mineralization)

Osteoblasts play a central role in bone formation and turnover since they are the only cells that actually produce the organic components and induce formation of the anorganic components of the ECM; they also control the formation and activity of osteoclasts (see Osteoblast – osteoclast interaction). Osteoblasts differentiate from mesenchymal stem or osteoprogenitor cells. They have a cuboidal shape and usually start their activity as a single layer of cells attached to an appropriate surface (Fig. 5.1), such as bone tissue or mineralized cartilage tissue (only in intramembranous ossification do the cells produce bone matrix without a pre-existing surface; see below). For bone tissue formation osteoblasts first secrete and deposit the organic components of the ECM at the site of attachment.

This freshly deposited and still unmineralized ECM is called *osteoid*. The cells thereby control the three-dimensional arrangement of the collagen fibres in an unknown manner, a function which is important for the tensile strength of the tissue. In order to begin the mineralization process,[2] osteoblasts release matrix vesicles that are rich in calcium-binding proteins (annexin, phosphatidyl serine) and phosphatases (alkaline phosphatase, pyrophosphatase) concentrated in the vesicles or the vesicles' membranes. Calcium and phosphate ions are then concentrated within the vesicles and, together with the activity of the different proteins, crystal formation is initiated. The latter starts with precipitation of $CaPO_4$, which then transforms into insoluble hydroxyapatite crystals. At some point, the vesicles rupture and further growth of the crystals occurs extracellularly under the guidance of the organic ECM. Extracellular inorganic pyrophosphate inhibits hydroxyapatite formation, whereas the tissue non-specific alkaline phosphatase (TNAP) hydrolyses pyrophosphate, which provides inorganic phosphate and promotes mineralization.

When osteoblasts secrete osteoid, they also form cellular processes that are walled in by the newly formed matrix (Fig. 5.1). These processes are important for the interaction of the cells, since each process is connected to the process of another osteoblast or osteocyte via gap junctions. In addition to the nutritional supply, these cell contacts are probably important for signal transmission, but little is known about the kind of information that is transported from cell to cell in response to changes in the microenvironment. Once a cell and its processes are completely surrounded by ECM, it differentiates into an osteocyte. There is always a narrow unmineralized gap between the cellular membrane and the mineralized ECM. The gap surrounding the osteocyte soma is called the *lacuna*; the gaps surrounding the processes are called *canaliculi*. When the osteoblasts are inactive they become bone-lining cells.

Osteocytes

Osteocytes are distributed throughout the bone tissue and are important for tissue maintenance. Even though the cells lie individually surrounded by mineralized ECM

Table 5.2 Bone cells and their major functions

Cell	Function
Osteoprogenitor cells	Mesenchymal precursor cells that self-duplicate or differentiate into bone-forming cells (osteoblasts/osteocytes)
Osteoblasts	Bone-forming cells, produce osteoid (unmineralized organic extracellular matrix) and induce mineralization; mediate control of osteoclast formation and activity
Osteocytes	Derive from osteoblasts during bone formation, measure the microenvironment in the tissue (probably induce or prevent bone remodelling)
Osteoclasts	Bone tissue-resorbing cells (differentiate from monocytes); important cells in calcium metabolism

they still have contact with neighbouring cells via their processes (Figs 5.1 and 5.2). Recent studies indicate that osteocytes function (1) as sensors for mechanical changes and other events in the microenvironment and (2) induce bone remodelling by sending out signals (this can involve osteocyte cell death, i.e. apoptosis). The cell processes of osteocytes form a network that is thought to be important for signal transmission and nutritional supply. The effectiveness of nutrient transport along a chain of cells is limited; therefore, the distance between an osteocyte and its corresponding blood vessel is limited to about 150–200 μm (see above).

Osteoclasts

Osteoclasts are the only cells that are able to degrade and resorb mineralized bone tissue. They are therefore vital for all remodelling processes in bone and are central cells in calcium metabolism. Osteoclasts form by fusion of their progenitor cells, the monocytes, and are therefore multinucleated bone marrow-derived cells (size 50–100 μm). This process is initialized by an interaction of monocytes with osteoblasts, which suggests that osteoclastogenesis is primarily controlled by osteoblasts. This is supported by the fact that osteoblasts are actually the target cells for most of the hormones that influence bone resorption (see Osteoblast – osteoclast interaction). Osteoclasts are recruited by an unknown mechanism to those sites where bone tissue needs to be resorbed. The osteoclasts attach to the surface of the mineralized bone matrix and form a tight annular seal (a ring-like zone stabilized by bundles of actin; integrins connect the cell to the ECM). This creates a sealed cavity (resorption cavity) in between the osteoclast cell and the matrix (Fig. 5.2). The plasma membrane facing the resorption cavity is increased in size and folded many times ('ruffled' membrane) in order to allow extensive transport mechanisms. The cells secrete HCl and release lysosomal matrix-degrading enzymes (such as cathepsin K) into the resorption cavity: HCl lowers the pH (pH 4–5) and dissolves the hydroxyapatite crystals, which uncovers the organic parts of the ECM. The latter is then cleaved and degraded by the specialized enzymes. The osteoclasts transfer the fragments of the cleaved matrix from the resorption cavity into the interstitial space by transcytosis. HCl formation in osteoclasts is comparable to that of parietal cells in the stomach mucosa – osteoclasts have a carbonic anhydrase that catalyses the production of carbonic acid from CO_2 and water. Carbonic acid dissociates into H^+ and HCO_3^-, and H^+ is then actively transported into the resorption cavity by a proton pump (H^+-ATPase) located in the ruffled membrane. HCO_3^- is released into the interstitial space by a HCO_3^-/Cl^- exchange mechanism, which promotes accumulation of Cl^- in the cell. Cl^- is finally released into the resorption cavity through a Cl^- channel in the ruffled membrane.

Osteoblast – osteoclast interaction

Osteoclast formation and activity is mediated by osteoblasts, which have receptors for the most relevant hormones in bone remodelling (such as parathyroid hormone (PTH) and calcitriol (vitamin D)). The production and activity of osteoclasts is controlled by two substances that are produced by the osteoblasts: monocyte colony-stimulating factor (M-CSF) and receptor activator of nuclear factor kappa B ligand (RANKL). M-CSF stimulates proliferation and osteoclastogenesis (fusion of monocytes and differentiation). With RANKL osteoblasts bind to the cell surface receptor RANK, which is found on osteoclast progenitor cells and mature osteoclasts and which stimulates further differentiation and activity of these cells. Osteoblasts also secrete osteoprotegerin (OPG), a molecule which masks the RANKL–RANK interaction and therefore inhibits osteoclast formation and activity. It is suggested that oestradiol stimulates OPG production, and that this is one of the mechanisms in oestradiol-dependent bone protection.

Calcitonin, which is produced by the parafollicular cells of the thyroid gland, is the only known hormone that directly interacts with osteoclasts. It induces the detachment of osteoclasts and therefore inhibits their activity. However, under normal circumstances calcitonin is suggested to have a minor role in bone turnover and calcium metabolism. This is mostly controlled by PTH and vitamin D, which stimulate osteoblasts in bone formation as well as osteoclast activation.

PERIOSTEUM AND ENDOSTEUM

Most surfaces of bones are covered by specialized tissue layers called periosteum and endosteum. These are activated during bone growth, tissue turnover, injury or certain diseases. *Periosteum* covers the outer surface of a bone (except for articular surfaces and apophyses). It consists of two layers: an external fibrous layer (which is a dense connective tissue and which might protect the second inner layer against tension or bending forces) and an internal osteogenic layer (cambium layer), containing osteoprogenitor cells, osteoblasts and osteoclasts (Fig. 5.1d). The periosteum is attached to the bone and is fixed by bundles of collagen fibres that are anchored deep within the bone tissue (Sharpey's fibres). Activation of the cambium layer is an important part in the growth of bone width (appositional growth). *Endosteum* lines the inner surfaces/cavities in a bone (including Haversian canals; Fig. 5.1c,d). This single layer of cells (mesenchymal stem cells, osteoprogenitor cells, osteoblasts, osteoclasts) is connected to a thin network of collagen fibres. Inactive endost cells are squamous and called *bone-lining cells*; they change to a more cuboidal cell layer after activation.

BONE REMODELLING

Bone tissue is a vital tissue that has a regular turnover and remodelling during its lifetime. Adaptation of the tissue to changes in the mechanical environment has been described and the load-dependent response of the bone has been termed *Wolff's law*. Changes in the mechanical axis or loading of bone results in changes in the orientation and density of trabeculae in the cancellous bone. It is hypothesized that some of the bone cells sense alterations in the biomechanical microenvironment. However, these mechanisms remain mostly unknown. In an adult healthy person, the turnover rate is expected to be balanced, with bone formation and degradation being the same. The rate of turnover is higher in cancellous bone than in compact bone (28% compared with 4%, respectively), which is obvious in diseases such as osteoporosis in which cancellous bone mass drops significantly, while compact bone appears to be more stable. About 25% of the bone in the human body is cancellous and 75% is compact bone, so that all bone tissue is thought to be replaced by new tissue every 10 years. These very broad calculations vary dramatically depending on the individual's activity, age or sex, and especially in the case of certain diseases.

Bone remodelling is a complex mechanism that involves all cells of bone tissue and even other associated tissues, such as vessels. Measurement of the microenvironment in the tissue, recruitment of monocytes for osteoclastogenesis, activation of osteoblasts and angiogenesis are just some of the major events that are involved. Some of the signal pathways and interactions of the different cells have recently been reviewed.[3] In general, osteoclasts and osteoblasts form team-like groups of cells, called bone multicellular units (BMUs), that coordinate the remodelling process. These remodelling processes can last for months, so the BMUs need to be replaced regularly. Bone remodelling occurs differently, depending on the type of bone tissue. In cancellous bone, osteoclasts remove parts of the surface of trabeculae, which results in the formation of excavations (Howship's lacunae; Fig. 5.2d). Osteoblasts then fill the lacunae with new lamellae or add new bone tissue somewhere else instead. Remodelling in compact bone is more complex: troops of osteoclasts drill tunnels (resorption cavities; Fig. 5.2c) into the solid compact bone tissue. These tunnels are like moulds for the formation of new osteons. It is not known how osteoclasts determine the direction of drilling; however, this direction does not seem to depend on pre-existing osteons because the latter are partially or completely removed by this drilling. This is the reason why compact bone always contains remnants of older osteons distributed in between the newer, intact osteons (Fig. 5.2a). Each tunnel is then filled with a new osteon either by a neurovascular bundle growing into the tunnel or by osteoprogenitor cells growing into the tunnel and lining it completely. The osteoprogenitor cells differentiate into active osteoblasts, which first produce a layer of cement that forms the outer edge of the osteon. Then, the first layer of the ECM is deposited, forming the outermost lamella of the osteon, and then the next layer is deposited, until the tunnel is filled with multiple lamellae. Finally, the osteoblasts become inactive and transform into lining cells of the endosteum, which remains attached to the inner surface of the last lamella. Inside this endosteum, connective tissue is deposited, and, together with the neurovascular bundle, these structures form the new Haversian canal as the core of the new osteon. The region with active osteoclasts at the tip of the canal is called the cutting cone. The region where osteoblasts fill the canal with new lamellae is called the closing cone. The region in between the cutting and the closing cones is called the reversal zone.

BONE DEVELOPMENT AND GROWTH

All bone tissue formation (ossification) in the human body starts with condensation of mesenchymal cells, which differentiate either directly into osteoblasts (*intramembranous ossification*) or into cartilage tissue, which forms a primordial cartilage model of the bone and is replaced by bone tissue afterwards (*chondral ossification*). Areas showing the first occurrence of bone tissue in a developing bone are called *primary centres of ossification*. Some parts of bones, such as the epiphyses, demonstrate later onsets of ossification; these regions are called *secondary centres of ossification*. The starting point of ossification varies for all different bones in the human skeleton but shows a common pattern for all individuals, which can be used for ageing a skeleton. Especially the secondary centres of ossification occur at late stages of development, sometimes even years after birth.

Intramembranous ossification

Intramembranous ossification is the kind of bone tissue formation found in the clavicle, skull bones and some of the facial bones. Osteoblasts usually deposit new ECM on suitable pre-existing surfaces (such as bone matrix or calcified cartilage tissue) only. However, in intramembranous ossification, osteoprogenitor cells in the areas of condensed mesenchymal stem cells differentiate directly into osteoblasts, which have cell processes connected via gap junctions to those of neighbouring cells. A system of capillaries functions as a mechanical stabilizer in the beginning, since osteoblasts need an environment free of mechanical deformation. The osteoblasts deposit osteoid in the surrounding interstitial space, which is subsequently mineralized. Cells completely surrounded by mineralized ECM differentiate into osteocytes. The ECM of neighbouring cells fuses with time and creates bigger pieces of woven bone tissue, which further increases mechanical stability. The surface of the pieces is then covered with more osteoblasts, which deposit bone matrix (appositional growth). These primarily needle-like pieces of bone tissue are called spicules, which finally unite with each other in order to form the first trabeculae (primary spongiosa). However, the primary spongiosa will be replaced later by lamellar bone tissue during a process of maturation and remodelling. The outer parts are replaced by osteon-like lamellar bone tissue and turn into the compact, cortical bone; the inner parts turn into spongy, trabecular (cancellous) bone.

Chondral ossification

The majority of bones in the body are generated by a process called chondral ossification. This is a complex mechanism, which can differ depending on where in the developing bone the ossification takes place. In the beginning, mesenchymal cells form a condensed area with high cell density that further develops into a small but enlarging cartilage model of the future bone (cartilage model or primordial skeleton; Fig. 5.3). The cartilage is covered by a perichondrium, and in the diaphysis (shaft) region of the future bone progenitor cells within this perichondrium differentiate directly into osteoblasts and produce bone tissue in a comparable way to that of intramembranous ossification (see above). This finally results in the production of a cuff or frill-like cortical bone structure in the shaft region (Fig. 5.3). The rest of the cartilage model is replaced by bone in a process called *endochondral ossification*. This endochondral ossification involves cartilage mineralization and subsequent replacement by bone tissue, and is similar for the diaphysis (shaft) and epiphyseal regions, but further specialized in the growth plate (see below).

ENDOCHONDRAL OSSIFICATION IN THE DIAPHYSIS AND EPIPHYSIS

Endochondral ossification starts in the diaphysis, when the cuff-like cortical bone tissue formation from the perichondrium has already started (see above). Unknown mechanisms result in the hyaline cartilage cells inside the cortical bone cuff of the diaphysis differentiating into hypertrophic chondrocytes, and starting to mineralize the surrounding cartilage matrix (Fig. 5.3). Additionally, the cells secrete vascular endothelial growth factor (VEGF), which induces ingrowth of blood vessels. First, osteoclasts and chondroclasts penetrate the cortical bone shell and the mineralized cartilage and create cavities in the cartilage (primary bone marrow cavities). The blood vessels grow into these cavities and pave the way for osteoprogenitor cells and cells of bone marrow tissue. The osteoprogenitor cells differentiate into osteoblasts and cover the walls of the cavities and begin the deposition and subsequent mineralization of osteoid, which results in the formation of primary trabeculae (primary spongiosa). The process continues, until all mineralized cartilage has been replaced by bone tissue, bone marrow or blood vessels. When the primary and immature trabeculae are replaced by lamellar mature bone tissue, they are called secondary trabeculae (secondary spongiosa) and are surrounded by a secondary bone marrow cavity. The ossification in the epiphysis generally uses the same mechanism; however, this process starts much later during bone development, and proceeds from the centre of the epiphyseal cartilage to the outside (centrifugal). These secondary centres of ossification can be visualized on radiographs, and appear as isolated islets in the centres of the epiphyses.

ENDOCHONDRAL OSSIFICATION IN THE GROWTH PLATE

The growth plate is a specialized part of the cartilage model located in between the future epiphysis and the metaphysis (Fig. 5.3a). As in the rest of the cartilage model, it consists of hyaline cartilage, but here the chondrocytes form columns that are oriented parallel to the long axis of the future bone; proliferation activity in the growth plate elongates the cartilage model (longitudinal growth).

The growth plate consists of different horizontal zones, which have different functions and histological appearances (Fig. 5.3c). Textbooks of histology will use as many versions of nomenclature as there are textbooks; for that reason, in this chapter, only the main zones are discussed.

The first zone close to the epiphysis is the *resting or reserve zone*. This is a thin zone with a few layers of flat chondroprogenitor cells that divide in order to add new generations of chondrocytes. The next zone is the *proliferative zone*, where chondrocytes proliferate quickly, resulting in column-like chondrons that are largely elongated. The ECM produced by the cells can be divided into *longitudinal septa*, which are oriented parallel to the longitudinal axis and which separate columns of cells that are lying next to each other, and *transverse septa*, which lie in between individual cells within one column. At a given moment, chondrocytes stop proliferation and start to differentiate into hypertrophic chondrocytes, which is the beginning of the *hypertrophic zone*. The cells increase in size dramatically, and start to mineralize the ECM in the longitudinal septa; the transverse septa remain unmineralized. The hypertrophic chondrocytes secrete zone-specific molecules, such as type X collagen and VEGF. Finally, at the lower end of the hypertrophic zone, the chondrocytes die by apoptosis. The next zone connects the growth plate to

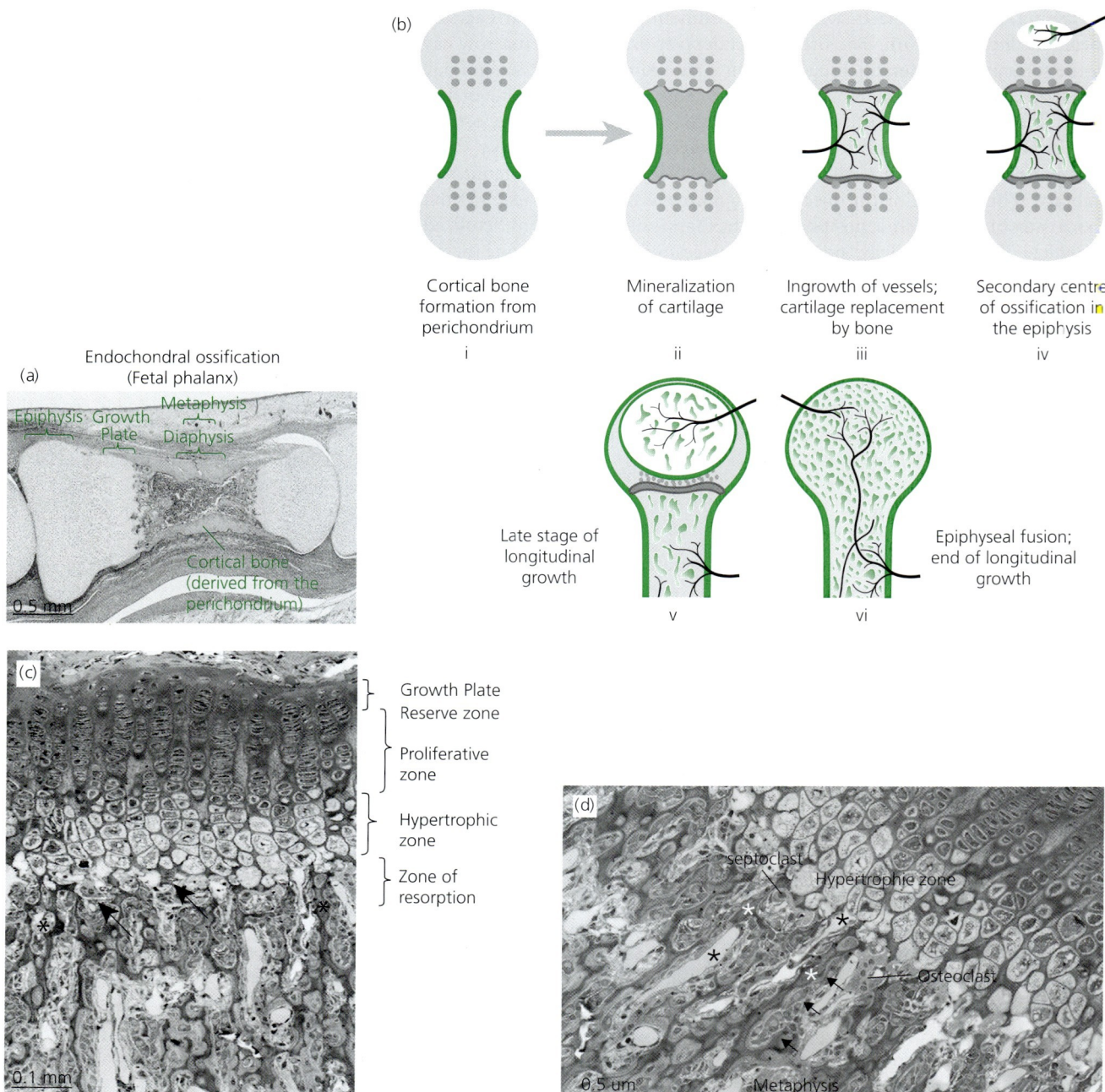

Figure 5.3 (a) Fetal bone of the finger, middle phalanx. The proximal and distal ends (epiphyses and growth plates) still represent the hyaline cartilage model, whereas the diaphysis is covered by a cortical bone shell, which is derived from the perichondrium. Inside the diaphysis, most of the mineralized cartilage has been removed and a primary bone marrow cavity and trabecular bone are visible instead (human; haematoxylin and eosin). (b) Different stages of endochondral ossification (adapted from Lüllmann-Rauch[4]). (i–iv) The upper row shows the formation of cortical bone from the perichondrium (green cuff surrounding the diaphysis) and the development and growth of the growth plates (grey areas). Then, in the diaphysis, the cartilage is mineralized, and vessels penetrate the diaphysis. The cartilage is replaced by primary bone trabeculae, vessels and bone marrow. In the epiphysis the same mechanisms result in the formation of secondary centres of ossification. (v, vi) With time, all cartilage tissue (except for the articular cartilage) is replaced by bone tissue and finally the growth plates fuse, which ends the longitudinal growth. (c) Growth plate showing the different zones. Asterisks indicate longitudinal septae of mineralized cartilage matrix; arrows indicate osteoclasts (mouse; toluidine blue). (d) Zone of resorption showing the lower end of the hypertrophic zone, where septoclasts remove transverse septae in order to open the lacunae of apoptotic chondrocytes. Vessels (black asterisks) grow into the lacuna, and osteoblasts (arrows) cover the remaining longitudinal septae of the cartilage (white asterisks). Osteoclasts remove some of the longitudinal septae (mouse; toluidine blue). All histological slides were provided by the Department of Anatomy, University of Kiel, Germany.

the metaphysis (metaphysis/growth plate junction) and is called the *zone of resorption or degeneration* (Fig. 5.3d). Attracted by VEGF, macrophage-like cells (sometimes called septoclasts) resorb the matrix of the transverse septa and open the lacunae with the apoptotic chondrocytes. After removal of the dead cells the opened lacunae are entered by blood vessels and bone marrow cells, which are attracted by the VEGF from the hypertrophic zone cells. The vessels pave the way for osteoprogenitor cells. The mineralized longitudinal septa remain and are now occupied and covered by these osteoprogenitor cells, which differentiate into active osteoblasts. The osteoblasts deposit osteoid and initiate mineralization on both sides of the longitudinal septa, so that the septa display a sandwich-like structure, with bone matrix at the surfaces surrounding a core of mineralized cartilage matrix. The septa are now called *primary trabeculae* and form the *primary spongiosa*. About two out of three of the longitudinal septa are removed by chondroclasts immediately, in order to allow the other septa to grow thicker. The primary trabeculae will be removed by osteoclasts after some time and replaced by secondary, mature trabeculae (secondary spongiosa). When the bone has reached its final length, the chondrocytes in the growth plate stop the proliferation. The remaining chondrocytes go through the process of differentiation described above until the last chondrocyte has died and been removed; this final replacement of cartilage is called the closure of the growth plate or epiphyseal fusion. No further longitudinal growth of the bone is possible after this event. The mechanisms that initiate the epiphyseal fusion are complex and poorly understood. They might include senescence of the progenitor cells in the resting zone and endocrine changes in the maturing individual (such as alterations in the production of growth hormone or sex hormones).

There is a range of hormones that influence the activity of the growth plate.[5,6] Growth hormone (GH) and insulin-like growth factors (IGFs) are potent stimulators of longitudinal bone growth, and it is suggested that the effect of GH on growth is mediated by liver-derived IGF-I, but GH might also stimulate local IGF-I production. Premature oestrogen exposure, as in precocious puberty, accelerates skeletal maturation, thus causing premature epiphyseal fusion and decreased final height. Conversely, lack of oestrogen, as in hypogonadism, results in delayed fusion and tall stature. Long-term, high-dose glucocorticoid treatment often leads to growth failure; glucocorticoids decrease the rate of chondrocyte proliferation and may stimulate apoptosis of growth plate chondrocytes. Other factors that seem to be important in the growth plate include Indian hedgehog, PTH-related peptide, fibroblast growth factors, bone morphogenic proteins and VEGF (see above). A feedback loop of the Indian hedgehog/PTH-related peptide pathway, for example, seems to influence the width of the proliferative zone, since it delays the hypertrophic differentiation in the lower proliferating zone. However, little is currently known about these complex pathways.

KEY LEARNING POINTS

- Bone tissue consists of bone cells and extracellular matrix (ECM).
- Bone cells include osteoprogenitor cells, osteoblasts, osteocytes and osteoclasts, all of which are involved differently in the production and maintenance of bone tissue.
- Organic (such as type I collagen) and inorganic components of the ECM (such as hydroxyapatite) contribute differently to the tensile strength, the compressive strength and the bending strength of bone tissue.
- There are different types of bone tissue, such as woven (immature) and lamellar (mature; arranged as either compact bone with osteons or cancellous bone with trabecular) bone tissue.
- All surfaces of bone tissue are covered by either periosteum (outside) or endosteum (inside), tissue layers which are important during bone development, remodelling and repair.
- Bone development and growth occur by two major kinds of ossification: intramembranous and chondral/endochondral ossification (including the growth plate).
- Bone development and growth involves the activity of hormones, growth factors and angiogenesis factors, such as growth hormone, insulin-like growth factor or vascular endothelial growth factor.

ACKNOWLEDGEMENT

B.K. thanks the Department of Anatomy, Christian-Albrechts-University, Kiel, Germany, for support and provision of histological slides. These were produced by Mrs Bettina Facompre and Prof. Dr. Renate Lüllmann-Rauch.

REFERENCES

1. Clarke B. Normal bone anatomy and physiology. *Clinical Journal of the American Society of Nephrology* 2008;**3**:S131–9.
2. Orimo H. The mechanism of mineralization and the role of alkaline phosphatase in health and disease. *Journal of the Nippon Medical School* 2010;**77**:4–12.
3. Nakahama K. Cellular communications in bone homeostasis and repair. *Cellular and Molecular Life Sciences* 2010;**67**:4001–9.
4. Lüllmann-Rauch R. *Taschenlehrbuch Histologie*, 3rd edn. Stuttgart, Germany: Thieme Verlag, 2009
5. Burdan F, Szumi J, Korobowicz A, *et al*. Morphology and physiology of the epiphyseal growth plate. *Folia Histochemica et Cytobiologica* 2009;**47**:5–16.
6. Nilsson O, Marino R, De Luca F, *et al*. Endocrine regulation of the growth plate. *Hormone Research* 2005;**64**:157–65.

Metabolic bone diseases

EUGENE SHERRY

Background	92	Normal bone metabolism	92
Connective tissue syndromes	92	References	99

NATIONAL BOARD STANDARDS

- To know about bone mineralization
- To understand the causes of bone metabolic diseases

BACKGROUND

The body has been described as a set of mechanical levers, packed with offal (viscera), controlled by a lump of fat on top (the brain) with the soul as its indentity card. Orthopaedic surgeons deal with mechanical failure of this machine from wear (age-related) or trauma. Therefore, it is highly relevant that surgeons know about disorders of the substrate that they are working with, i.e. metabolic bone diseases.

In essence, these disorders are related to disorders of bone mineralization (calcium and phosphate metabolism) and bone density (decreased, osteopenia and osteopetrosis; increased, Paget disease and osteopetrosis) (Table 6.1).[1-3]

CONNECTIVE TISSUE SYNDROMES

Marfan syndrome

- Is an autosomal dominant disorder of the a1 unit of collagen synthesis.
- Features are: arachnodactyly, pectus deformities, scoliosis, spondylolisthesis, heart valve abnormalities, superior lens dislocation, joint laxity, protrusio acetabuli.
- Treatment is to monitor joint laxity; scoliosis and spondylolisthesis may need surgery. Consider for protrusio acetabuli triradiate cartilage fusion.

Ehlers–Danlos syndrome

- An autosomal dominant disorder with skin laxity, joint hypermobility and vascular fragility. There are 11 types. Types 2 and 3 are the most common and least disabling.
- Treatment is orthotics, physiotherapy and soft-tissue surgery.

Homocystinuria

- An autosomal recessive inborn error of methionine metabolism, in which there is accumulation of homocysteine. Clinical features are osteoporosis, marfanoid habitus, but with stiffening and inferior lens dislocation. Also central nervous system effects.
- Associated with increased homocysteine in urine (use the cyanide nitroprusside test).
- Beware of thrombosis after minor procedures.
- Treatment is vitamin B6 and reduced methionine diet.

NORMAL BONE METABOLISM

- This is regulated by parathyroid hormone, vitamin calcitonin, oestrogens, corticosteroids, thyroid hormones, growth hormone and growth factors (Table 6.2 and Figs 6.1 and 6.2).[4,5]

Table 6.1 Metabolic bone diseases

Metabolic bone disease	Aetiology	Clinical features/treatment	Radiographic findings	Blood chemistry
Hypercalcaemia	Malignancy - do not forget			
Primary hyperparathyroidism	PTH overproduction: adenoma - hyperplasia	Often asymptomatic Age 40-65; F/M, 2:1 10% have kidney stone, hyper-reflexia (bones, moans, stones, abdominal groans); polyuria Treatment: parathyroidectomy (beware of hungry bone syndrome postoperatively due to hypocalcaemia from brisk formation of new bone)	Osteopenia, osteitis fibrosa cystica (brown tumours), destructive metaphyseal lesions	↑Calcium ↑PTH ↓Phosphate ↑/N, alkaline phosphatase
Familial syndromes	PTH overproduction: adenoma - MEN/renal	Endocrine/renal abnormalities	Osteopenia	
Secondary hypoparathyroidism	Response to chronic hypocalcaemia (rickets, osteomalacia)			
Other causes of hypercalcaemia	Hyperthyroidism, Addison disease, steroids, peptic ulcers, kidney disease, sarcoidosis			
Hypocalcaemia				
Primary hypoparathyroidism	PTH underproduction: adenoma – idiopathic	Neuromuscular irritability, tetany, seizures, Chvostek's sign, cataracts, fungal infections, prolonged QT on ECG	Calcified basal ganglia	↓Calcium ↑Phosphate
Pseudohypoparathyroidism/Albright syndrome	Rare; X-linked dominant; PTH receptor abnormality (lack of effect)	Short MC/MT, obesity, low IQ	Brachydactylic, exostosis. Short 1st, 4th, 5th metacarpals and metatarsals	↑/N, PTH ↓Calcium ↑Phosphate
Renal osteodystrophy	CRF leads to ↓phosphate excretion	Renal abnormalities Long-term dialysis	Rugger jersey spine, soft-tissue calcification	↓/N, calcium ↑Alkaline phosphatase
Rickets (osteomalacia in adults)[3]; a failure of mineralization; changes in physis (zone of provisional calcification)	A defect in mineralization, with a large amount of mineralized osteoid (qualitative defect) Chronic alcoholism Types are: nutritional, GI	Rickets: tetany, failure to thrive, listless, muscular flaccidity, craniotabes, thickening of wrists from epiphyseal overgrowth, bowed legs, stunted growth, rachitic rosary, spinal curves, coxa vara, fractures of long bones	Rickets: thickening and widening of physes, cupping of metaphysis, bowing of diaphysis, wide metaphysis Osteomalacia: Looser's zones, incomplete stress fractures, codfish vertebrae, trefoil pelvis, radiographic changes of	↓Calcium ↓Phosphate ↑Alkaline phosphatase, urinary excretion of calcium Ca × phosphate is <2.4 (N is 3)

(continued)

Table 6.1 (Continued)

Metabolic bone disease	Aetiology	Clinical features/treatment	Radiographic findings	Blood chemistry
	absorption defects (post-gastrectomy, biliary disease, enteric absorption defects), renal tubular defects (renal phosphate leak), renal osteodystrophy (miscellaneous, soft-tissue tumours such as fibrous dysplasia, anticonvulsant therapy, heavy metal intoxication)	Osteomalacia: aches and pains, muscle weakness; short, stress fractures	Secondary hyperparathyroidism	
Vitamin D/Ca/phosphate: nutritional deficiency rickets; rare	Decreased vitamin D in diet; malabsorption (post-gastrectomy, biliary disease, small bowel disease)	Bone deformities, hypotonia Histology: Swiss cheese trabeculae, widened osteoid seams, gross distortion at the maturation zone of the physis, poorly defined zone of calcification Treatment: vitamin D (5000 g day^{-1}) and calcium (3 mg day^{-1})	Rachitic rosary, wide growth planes, fractures	
Vitamin D-dependent (types I and II) rickets; hereditary		Total baldness	Poor mineralization	
Vitamin D-resistant (hypophosphataemic) rickets; familial; the most common type, X-linked dominant	Decreased renal tubular phosphate resorption	Bone deformities, hypotonia Treatment: phosphate and vitamin D replacement	Poor mineralization	↓25-HCC
Hypophosphatasia Autosomal recessive	Decreased alkaline phosphatase Autosomal recessive	Bone deformities, hypotonia Diagnosis from ↑urinary phosphoethanolamine Treatment: phosphate therapy	Poor mineralization	
(Decreased) bone density Osteopenia[4] Osteoporosis, defined by the WHO as lumbar (L2-4) density 25 SDs less than the peak bone mass at 25 years old, is a qualitative not quantitative defect in bone. Mineralization remains normal	Decreased oestrogen leads to decreased bone mass. Seen in sedentary, thin Caucasian women of North European descent, smokers, drinkers, on phenytoin, diets low in calcium and vitamin D, who breastfed. Two	Kyphosis, vertebral fractures	Compression vertebral fractures (codfish) Hip fractures	

Metabolic bone disease	Aetiology	Clinical features/ treatment	Radiographic findings	Blood chemistry
Two types: type I, post-menopausal – trabecular bone, vertebrae and wrist fractures; type II, >75 years old, poor calcium absorption. Hip and pelvic fractures. Radiographs not helpful until bone loss >30%. DEXA is most accurate measure. Oestrogen therapy in type I needs to be started within 6 years of menopause Idiopathic transient osteoporosis: uncommon, self-limiting, seen in pregnancy Bone loss from spinal cord injury (for first 16 months) Osteopenia of rickets (see above)	vertebral fractures predicts another vertebral fracture in post-menopausal women. Also positive family history and premature menopause. Affects cancellous bone			
Scurvy	Vitamin C deficiency: decreased chondroitin sulphate synthesis, which leads to defective collagen growth and repair	Fatigue, bleeding, effusions	Thin cortices, corner sign. Affects the metaphysis	
Myeloma, leukaemia Osteogenesis imperfecta	Abnormal collagen synthesis. Mutation of genes for synthesis of type I collagen	Deformities, fractures, short stature, blue sclerae, scoliosis, tooth defects, hearing defects, lax ligaments, autosomal dominant and recessive types. Sillence classification (four types) is useful.[6] Treatment is with telescoping intramedullary rods, bisphosphonates and corrective scoliosis surgery	Radiographs show thin cortices and widespread osteopenia	
Idiopathic juvenile osteoporosis	Rare, self-limited disorder, big reduction in bone mass, onset 8–14 years old but resolves within 2 years	Back pain, leg pain, osteopenia, fractures, kyphosis		

(continued)

Table 6.1 (Continued)

Metabolic bone disease	Aetiology	Clinical features/ treatment	Radiographic findings	Blood chemistry
(Increased) bone density				
Osteopetrosis (marble bone disease) (Fig. 6.2). One type is Albers-Schonberg disease: autosomal dominant tarda variant	Decreased osteoclast and chondroblast function from defect in thymus. Mild form is autosomal dominant, malignant form is autosomal recessive	Hepatosplenomegaly, anaemia. Brittle bones. Necrotic calcified cartilage. May need bone marrow transplant in childhood. Also calcitriol and steroids	Bone within bone. Rugger jersey spine, marble bone, 'Erlenmeyer flask' proximal humerus/distal humerus	
Osteopoikilosis (spotted bone disease)	Island of cortical bone in cancellous bone (long bones and hands/feet)	Asymptomatic		
Infantile cortical hyperostosis (Caffey syndrome)	Age 0-9 months, soft-tissue swelling and bony cortical thickening after febrile illness	Exclude child abuse, hypervitaminosis A, infection and scurvy Prognosis is benign and self-limiting	Periosteal reactions of ulna and jaw	
Paget disease (Fig. 6.1)	Osteoclastic abnormality: increased bone turnover. Increased serum alkaline phosphatase and urinary hydroxyproline. Virus-like inclusion bodies seen in osteoclasts	Deformities, pain, CHF, fractures. Has active (lytic, mixed, sclerotic phases) and inactive phases	Coarse trabeculation, picture frame vertebra	
Conditions of bone viability				
Osteonecrosis; blood supply loss (Fig. 6.3)	Idiopathic osteonecrosis of femoral head and Perthes disease when there are coagulation abnormalities. Steroid use, alcohol use, radiation, Gaucher disease. Related to enlargement of marrow fat cells. Phases I (mechanical), II (chemical) and III (thrombotic) Histology: autolysis, inflammation, new woven bone on the dead bone, resorption/remodelling. Creeping substitution		MRI shows earliest sign. Femoral head pressure >30 mmHg. Core decompression controversial. Crescent sign on radiograph	
Osteochondroses	Same path as osteonecrosis. Traction apophysis, children. Trauma, inflammation, vascular insult, thrombosis			

25-HCC, 25-hydroxycholecalciferol; CHF, congestive heart failure; CRF, chronic renal failure; DEXA, dual-emission X-ray absorptiometry; F, female; GI, gastrointestinal; M, male; MC, ; MEN, multiple endocrine neoplasia; MT, ; N, normal; PTH, parathyroid hormone; WHO, World Health Organization.

Modified with permission from Miller MD. *Review of Orthopaedics*, 5th edn. Philadelphia, PA: Saunders, Elsevier, 2008:21.

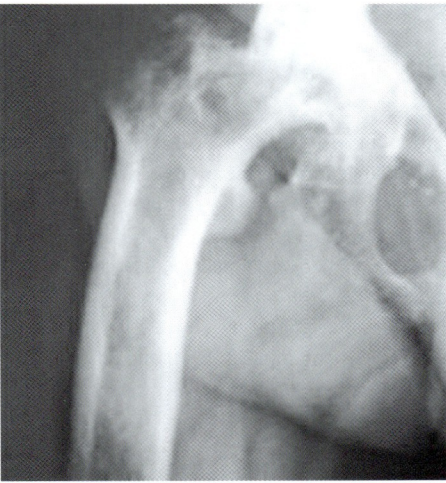

Figure 6.1 Paget disease of the femur with deformity and osteoarthritis.

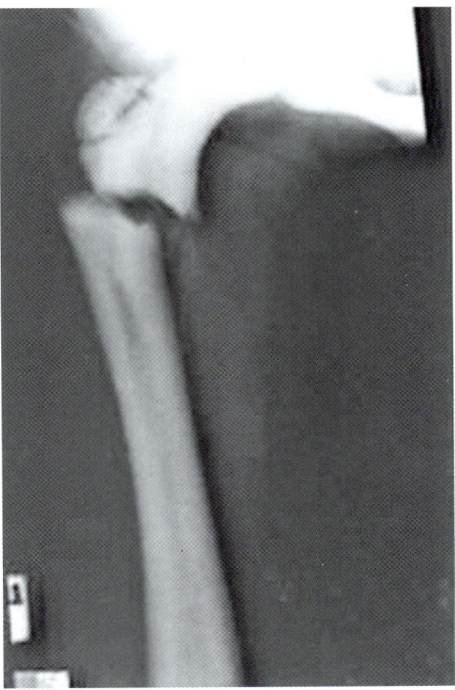

Figure 6.2 Subtrochanteric fracture of osteopetrotic bone.

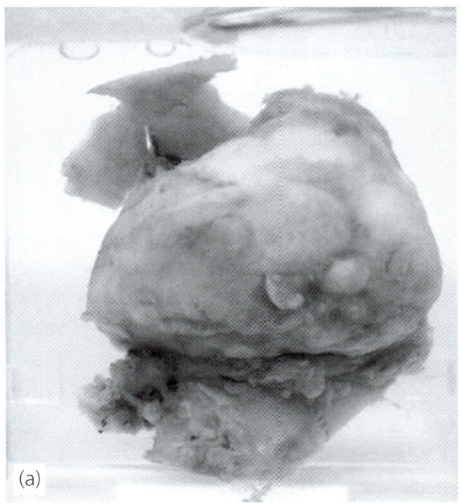

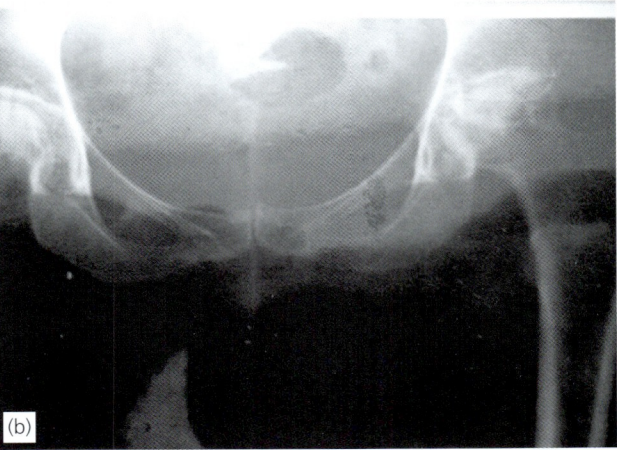

Figure 6.3 Osteochondral flap of femoral head avascular necrosis from steroids.

- Calcium is mainly found in bone (99%). Its main actions are muscle and nerve function and clotting. Plasma calcium is 50% free; the other 50% is bound to albumin.
- Dietary needs are: children (600 mg day^{-1}), adolescents (1300 mg day^{-1}), adults (750 mg day^{-1}), pregnancy (1500 mg day^{-1}) and when breastfeeding (2 g day^{-1}).
- It is absorbed in the duodenum (active transport) and in the jejunum (by diffusion); 98% is reabsorbed in the kidney proximal tubule and it may be excreted in stool.
- Calcium balance is positive for the first three decades of life and then becomes negative.
- Phosphate: 85% is in bone. Its functions are metabolite and as a buffer in enzyme systems. Plasma phosphate is mainly unbound. The daily requirement is 1–1.5 g day^{-1}.
- The regulation of calcium and phosphate metabolism[5] is summarized in Table 6.3 and vitamin D metabolism is summarized in Fig. 6.4.
- In all conditions except osteoporosis there is coupling of calcium metabolism.

Table 6.2 Regulation of bone metabolism

Chemical	Feature
Calcium	Bone is reservoir for 99%. For muscle and nerve function, clotting and other functions. Plasma calcium (<1% of body store) is free and bound (to albumin). Ca absorbed in the duodenum (active transport via ATP, calcium-binding protein, regulated by 1,25-(OH)$_2$ vitamin D3 and passive diffusion. Kidney reabsorbs 98%. Serum Ca is regulated by PTH and 1,25-(OH)$_2$ vitamin D3. Post-menopausal women and patients with healing fracture require 1500 mg day^{-1} (normal, 1300 mg day^{-1}). Most people have negative Ca balance after age 40
Phosphate	Bone minerals (85%), enzyme systems, molecular interactions
PTH	84 amino acid peptide. Activates osteoblasts and controls renal phosphate filtration
Vitamin D	Steroid activated by sunlight, or from the diet. Hydroxylated to 25-(OH) vitamin D3 (liver) and again hydroxylated (kidney). 1,25-(OH)$_2$ vitamin D3 is active form; 24,25-(OH)$_2$ is inactive
Calcitonin	32 amino acid peptide inhibits osteoclastic bone resorption and decreases serum calcium
Oestrogens	Decrease bone formations
Corticosteroids	Increase bone loss (decrease gut absorption of Ca, inhibit collagen synthesis and osteoblast formation). No affect on mineralization
Thyroid hormones	Affect bone resorption > bone formation, so leads to osteoporosis. Regulate growth by affects at physis on chondrocyte growth
Growth hormone	Increases gut absorption of Ca
Growth factors, TGF-β, PDGF	Affect bone and cartilage repair
Peak bone mass	Between 16 and 25 years old; greater in men and African Americans
Bone loss	After peak bone mass, loss at 0.3–0.5% per year (2.3% per year, untreated women and 6–10 years post-menopausal). In menopause, increased bone formation and loss (net loss)

ATP, adenosine triphosphate; PDGF, platelet-derived growth factor; PTH, parathyroid hormone; TGF-β, transforming growth factor β.

Table 6.3

	Origin	Factors →↑	Factors →↓	Effects on intestine	Effects on kidney	Effects on bone	Effects on [calcium]	Effects on [phosphate]
PTH peptide	Chief cells parathyroid gland	↓[Ca^{2+}]	↑[Ca^{2+}] ↑1,25(OH)D	No direct affect ↑Absorption of Ca indirectly via ↑1,25(OH)D	↑Production of 1,25(OH)D ↑Reabsorption of calcium ↑Excretion of phosphate	Stimulates osteoclasts to absorb bone Stimulates recruitment of preosteoclasts	↑	↓
1,25(OH)$_2$D steroid	Proximal 1 tubule of kidney	↓[Ca^{2+}] ↓[phosphate] ↑PTH	↑[Ca^{2+}] 9↑[phosphate] ↓PTH	↑↑Absorption of Ca ↑↑Absorption of phosphate		Stimulates reabsorption of bone (osteoclastic)	↑	↑
Calcitonin	Parafollicular cells of thyroid	↑[Ca^{2+}]	↓[Ca^{2+}]			Inhibits osteoclastic reabsorption of bone	Transient ↓	

PTH, parathyroid hormone.

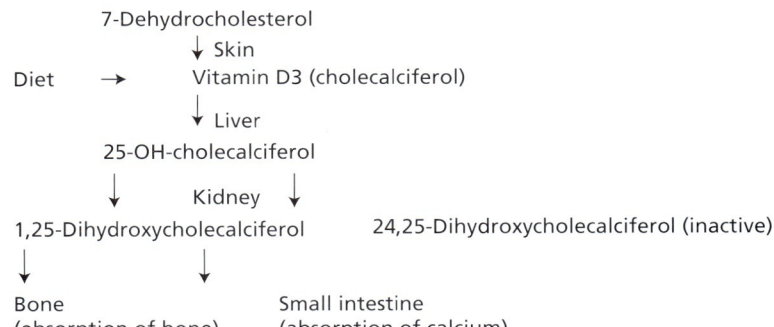

Figure 6.4 Vitamin D metabolism.

KEY LEARNING POINTS

- Metabolic bone diseases are related to hypercalcaemia, hypocalcaemia, hypophosphatasia, decreased bone density (osteopenia, osteoporosis), osteopoikilosis, increased bone density (Paget disease, osteopetrosis), myeloma, leukaemia, osteoporosis imperfecta and conditions of bone viability.
- Malignancy is a common cause of hypercalcaemia.
- Rickets (osteomalacia in adults) is failure of bony mineralization.
- Osteoporosis, defined by the World Health Organization as lumbar (L2–4) density 25 SDs less than the peak bone mass at 25 years old, is a quantitative not qualitative defect in bone. But mineralization remains normal.
- Osteogenesis imperfecta is caused by abnormal collagen synthesis.
- Paget disease is an osteoclastic abnormality with increased bone turnover, caused by a virus.
- Osteopetrosis (marble bone disease) is from decreased osteoclastic and chondroblast function.
- Conditions of bone viability include: osteonecrosis of the femoral head and Perthes disease, in which there is blood supply loss and abnormality of coagulation.
- Normal bone metabolism is mainly regulated by parathyroid hormone, vitamin D and calcitonin, and is affected by oestrogens, corticosteroids, thyroid hormones, growth hormone and growth factors.

REFERENCES

- ● = Key primary paper
- ◆ = Major review article

◆1. Miller MD. *Review of Orthopaedics*, 5th edn. Philadelphia, PA: Saunders Elsevier, 2008:18–36.
◆2. Mankin HJ. Rickets, osteomalacia and renal osteodystrophy. An update. *Orthopaedic Clinics of North America* 1990;**21**:80–96.
◆3. Frymoyer JW. Bone metabolism and metabolic bone disease. In: Frymoyer JW (ed.) *Orthopaedic Knowledge Update 4: Home Study Syllabus.* Rosemont, IL: AAOS, 1993:77.
●4. Lane JM, Vigorita VJ. Osteoporosis. *Journal of Bone and Joint Surgery American* 1983;**65**:274–8.
◆5. Orthoteers. Available from www.orthoteers.org.
●6. Sillence DO, Senn A, Danks DM. Genetic heterogeneity in osteogenesis imperfect. *Journal of Medical Genetics* 1979;**16**:101–16.

Soft tissue physiology and healing

PANKAJ SHARMA, NICOLA MAFFULLI

Introduction	100	Intervertebral disc	105
Collagen	100	Skeletal muscle	107
Articular cartilage	101	Ligament and tendon	110
Meniscus	103	References	114

NATIONAL BOARD STANDARDS

- Understand the structure and function of meniscus and cartilage and be able to draw a representation and explain the layers and arrangement of collagen fibres therein.
- Know the structure of collagen and the composition of the extracellular matrix.
- Understand the degenerative processes that affect musculoskeletal soft tissues.
- Know the healing responses in musculoskeletal soft tissues.
- Know about autologous chondrocyte implantation and various repair techniques for cartilage.
- Know about the various repair techniques for meniscus, including graft options.

INTRODUCTION

Soft tissues form a major component of the musculoskeletal system, and play vital roles in normal skeletal function. Unlike bone, intrinsic soft-tissue healing has a limited potential. Consequently, healed soft tissues have significantly reduced mechanical properties. This often causes problems for patients, when, after severe injuries, bony union takes place but function remains impaired secondary to soft-tissue compromise. In recent times, advances in gene therapy and tissue engineering hold promise for improved soft-tissue healing and regeneration.

In the human body, soft tissues are composed of a cellular component and an extracellular matrix (ECM) component. The ECM is primarily composed of water, usually between 60% and 80% of weight depending on tissue type. The primary constituent of the ECM is collagen; collagen structure and configuration are responsible for the unique mechanical properties of soft tissue.

COLLAGEN

Collagen is the most abundant protein in the animal kingdom. At least 16 subtypes of collagen have been identified, although 80–90% of the body's collagen is composed of types I, II and III.[1] Type I collagen was the first to be identified and structurally characterized. It is composed of three polypeptide chains containing precisely 1050 amino acids. Type I collagen consists of two identical α_1 and one distinct α_2 polypeptide chains.[2] These three polypeptide chains wind round each other and produce the characteristic right-handed triple helix structure of collagen.[1] Collagen synthesis occurs in several stages, with both intracellular and extracellular steps. Messenger ribonucleic acid (mRNA) translation initiates synthesis of polypeptide chains in the rough endoplasmic reticulum. Subsequently, the signal peptide is cleaved and lysine and proline amino acids are hydroxylated, and hydroxylysine residues are glycosylated. The resultant pro-collagen is packaged into secretory vesicles in the Golgi apparatus.

Table 7.1 Types of collagen found in the human musculoskeletal system

Collagen subtype	Representative tissue
Type I	Tendon, bone, ligament, meniscus, annulus fibrosus
Type II	Articular cartilage, nucleus pulposus
Type III	Muscle
Type IV	Basement membrane
Type IX	Articular cartilage: cross-links collagen type II
Type X	Articular cartilage: present in calcified cartilage zone and hypertrophic zone of growth plate
Type XI	Regulates type II fibril diameter

On release into the ECM, the ends of the pro-collagen are cleaved to form tropocollagen fibrils. Subsequent cross-linkage between lysine and hydroxylysine residues results in the formation of collagen fibres.

Table 7.1 shows the types of collagen that are relevant to the musculoskeletal system.

ARTICULAR CARTILAGE

Structure and function

Articular cartilage, also known as hyaline cartilage, is a visco-elastic, composite material consisting of water, chondrocytes and the ECM. Articular cartilage lacks a blood supply, and has no nerve supply or lymphatic drainage. Articular cartilage is inert and is incapable of inciting an immunological response. Nutrition is derived via diffusion from synovial fluid. Articular cartilage has an extremely low coefficient of friction, which aids in joint lubrication. An additional function of articular cartilage is shock absorption, which is accomplished by distributing joint loads and thereby reducing contact stress.

Composition

The primary cell present in articular cartilage is the chondrocyte, which accounts for approximately 5% of its wet weight. Water accounts for 65–80% of the ECM and is held in place by negatively charged proteoglycans. Collagen, which is predominantly type II, accounts for 10–20% of wet weight. The nascent type II collagen fibril is a heteropolymer, with collagen IX molecules covalently linked to the surface and collagen XI forming the filamentous template of the fibril as a whole.[3] Immunolocalization studies and analyses of cross-linked peptides have shown that the collagen XI pool is intimately copolymerized with type II collagen.[4,5] It has been postulated that this relationship allows collagen type XI to prevent further growth of collagen type II, and thus regulate fibril diameter.[6] The calcified zone of cartilage that interfaces with bone and the hypertrophic zone of the growth plate also include small amounts of type X collagen.[7] Type X collagen is associated with cartilage calcification; hence, it is also seen during endochondral ossification, in fracture callus and in heterotopic ossification.

Proteoglycans

In addition, the ECM contains a large variety of non-collagenous proteins. One such group of proteins are the proteoglycans, which are large hydrophilic molecules containing chains of glycosaminoglycans (keratan sulphate and chondroitin sulphate). The predominant proteoglycan in articular cartilage is aggrecan.[8] Aggrecan endows articular cartilage with a turgid nature and is responsible for its compressive strength. Aggrecan consists of a core protein, linked to multiple glycosaminoglycan side chains via sugar bonds. The bound glycosaminoglycans are highly negatively charged, owing to attached carboxyl and sulphate groups, and are responsible for the hydrophilic nature of aggrecan. Aggrecan is synthesized by chondrocytes and is then secreted into the ECM, where it forms large proteoglycan aggregates by attaching to hyaluronic acid via link proteins (Fig. 7.1).

In addition, several less well-studied proteoglycans are also present. These include biglycan, decorin, fibromodulin, lumican and superficial zone protein. These proteoglycans play vital roles in a variety of tissue and extracellular matrices, comprising binding and regulation of collagen fibrils as well as modulation of cellular responses.[9] The superficial zone protein is synthesized by the superficial chondrocytes of articular cartilage and by synoviocytes, and is responsible for the lubrication and extremely low friction motion of the cartilage surface.[10]

Glycoproteins

The ECM also contains glycoproteins. The best studied of these glycoproteins is the cartilage oligomeric matrix protein (COMP). COMP can bind chondrocytes, and serves

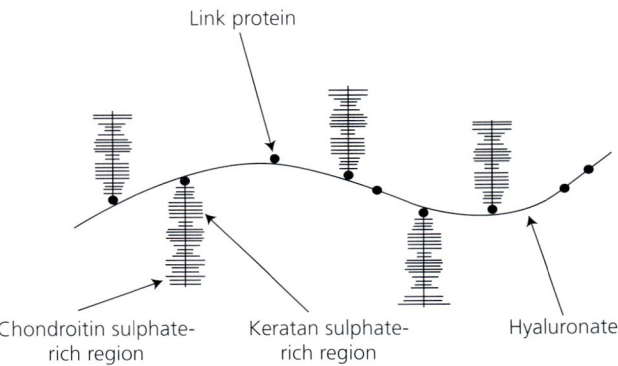

Figure 7.1 A proteoglycan aggregate.

Table 7.2 Layers of articular cartilage

Zone	Collagen fibre arrangement	Features	Mechanical resistance
Superficial tangential	Parallel to surface	Thinnest layer Greatest tensile stiffness Highest water and collagen content Lowest proteoglycan synthesis	Shear
Intermediate transitional	Oblique	Increased metabolic activity	Compression
Deep radial	Perpendicular	Largest layer Increased size of collagen fibres	Compression
Tidemark		Undulating boundary between calcified and uncalcified cartilage	Shear
Calcified cartilage		Hydroxyapatite crystals anchor cartilage to subchondral bone	Anchor

as an adhesive factor for these cells.[11] COMP can coordinate with bone morphogenetic protein 2 to promote the early stages of chondrogenic differentiation of mesenchymal stem cells.[12] COMP is present in all types of cartilage, but it is most abundant in the growth plate during development. The importance of COMP for cartilage development is illustrated by individuals with mutations of the *COMP* gene, who develop pseudochondroplasia or multiple epiphyseal dysplasia.[13]

Extracellular matrix enzymes

Matrix metalloproteinases (MMPs) are a large group of degradative enzymes present in the ECM. MMPs are calcium- and zinc-dependent endopeptidases with the capacity to cleave most of the ECM components.[14] They are responsible for maintaining the composition of the ECM, and degrade collagen and proteoglycan aggregates as part of this normal turnover of matrix constituents. Tissue inhibitors of metalloproteinases (TIMPs) are acidic polypeptides that counteract the action of MMPs. The expression of TIMP is tightly regulated during development and tissue remodelling, helping to maintain the composition of the ECM.[15,16]

Mechanical properties and microstructure

The unique structural arrangement of cartilage is ideally adapted for the functions of shock absorption and load dissipation. Cartilage is viscoelastic, and the properties of creep and stress relaxation account for its ability to dissipate load. Cartilage is freely permeable to water, and water redistribution under compressive loading helps in its ability to bear high loads. Cartilage is anisotropic; therefore, it has different mechanical properties depending on the direction of loading. This property is secondary to the characteristic arrangement of collagen fibres. Articular cartilage can be divided into distinct zones on the basis of collagen fibre arrangement (Table 7.2). The tidemark can be seen on histological staining, and represents the boundary between calcified and uncalcified cartilage.

Changes with ageing and osteoarthritis

Articular cartilage undergoes characteristic changes in response to ageing. Typical changes are also seen with osteoarthritis, but these changes are distinct from those seen in ageing.[17] Although osteoarthritis is more common in elderly individuals, it is not a direct consequence of ageing. Age-related changes in joint tissues do not directly cause osteoarthritis, but rather increase the susceptibility of older adults to developing osteoarthritis when other factors, such as joint incongruity or instability, are present.[18,19] In osteoarthritis, collagen disruption occurs secondary to direct trauma or from an increase in MMP concentration. Once the collagen meshwork is disrupted, proteoglycans attract more water, resulting in reduced stiffness and a decreased ability to bear load. Chondrocytes proliferate and hypertrophy in an attempt to counteract these changes, thus increasing the rate of collagen and proteoglycan synthesis. Expression of collagen type X, alkaline phosphatase and matrix vesicles is increased, along with increased matrix calcification. Eventually, chondrocytes are unable to maintain this compensation, and proteoglycan chains become shorter and proteoglycan levels decrease. However, the ratio of chondroitin sulphate to keratan sulphate increases. Increased levels of interleukin 1 and MMPs are noted, which has a further catabolic effect on cartilage. Table 7.3 compares the changes seen in ageing and osteoarthritis.

Injury and healing

Articular cartilage damage is common: in one study, it was associated with 16% (21 of 132) injuries of the knee that were sufficient to cause intra-articular bleeding.[20] In particular, knee injuries are associated with bone

Table 7.3 Changes observed in articular cartilage with ageing and osteoarthritis

Property	Ageing	Osteoarthritis
Water content	Decreased	Increased
Synthetic activity	Decreased	Increased
Collagen	Unchanged	Decreased
Proteoglycan content	Decreased	Decreased
Proteoglycan synthesis	Decreased	Increased
Proteoglycan degradation	Decreased	Increased significantly
Chondroitin sulphate	Decreased	Increased
Keratan sulphate	Increased	Decreased
Chondrocyte size	Increased	
Chondrocyte number	Decreased	
Stiffness	Increased	Decreased
Matrix metalloproteinase activity		Increased

bruising. Approximately 80% of patients are noted to have bone bruising in the presence of an anterior or posterior cruciate ligament injury.[21–23] Bone bruising may represent a supraphysiological injury, and lead to progressive chondral damage.[24]

Given its avascular nature, articular cartilage has a very limited healing potential. Articular cartilage injuries can be divided into three types. Type I and type II injuries are superficial. In type I injuries, microscopic damage to chondrocytes and the ECM occurs, whereas in type II injuries macroscopic damage occurs resulting in chondral fracture or fissuring. Type III injuries are deeper, and result in penetration of the subchondral bone. The tidemark is not breached in superficial injuries; therefore, healing potential is extremely limited. Superficial injury to articular cartilage stimulates only a slight reaction in adjacent chondrocytes, producing a transient increase in cell replication and matrix turnover.[25] In general, this response is largely ineffective in producing healing of articular cartilage defects.

In deeper type III injuries, penetration of the subchondral bone leads to a more pronounced inflammatory healing response. A fibrin clot is formed, and undifferentiated mesenchymal stem cells are recruited from marrow elements. The stem cells produce a reparative tissue; this is not hyaline cartilage, but fibrocartilage. Fibrocartilage predominantly consists of type I collagen. Consequently, it has a reduced ability to withstand cyclical loading and is prone to early degenerative change.

MENISCUS

Composition and ultrastructure

The menisci are crescentic, viscoelastic, fibrocartilaginous structures located between the tibial and femoral condyles of the knee joint. The meniscus is more elastic and less

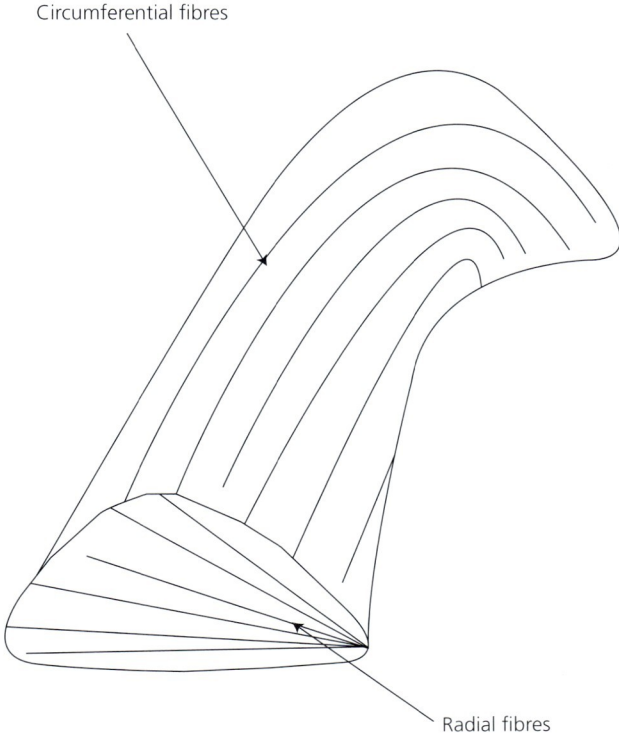

Figure 7.2 The collagen fibre ultrastructure of meniscus.

permeable than articular cartilage. The primary cell of menisci is the fibrochondrocyte, which is responsible for synthesis and maintenance of the ECM. The ECM is composed of 70% water, along with interlacing collagen fibres, elastin, proteoglycans and glycoproteins.[26] Ninety per cent of collagen present in the meniscus is type I, with smaller amounts of types II, III, V and VI present. Between 8% and 13% of dry weight is made up of non-collagenous proteins.[27–29] Elastin constitutes less than 0.06% of meniscal tissue. However, it plays a vital role, and aids in the recovery of shape after load deformation.[30]

Ultrastructural analysis demonstrates three collagen fibre layers, which are specifically arranged to convert compressive loads into circumferential or 'hoop' stresses. In the superficial layer, fibres are arranged randomly, similar to articular cartilage. The function of this layer is to facilitate smooth gliding of the femoral condyles. In the next layer, collagen fibres are arranged circumferentially to resist hoop stresses during weight bearing. Interspersed among this layer are radial fibres, which serve as 'ties' that resist shearing or splitting (Fig. 7.2).[31]

Anatomy and blood supply

In the knee, each meniscus covers approximately two-thirds of the corresponding tibial plateau. The peripheral border of the menisci is attached to the joint capsule and is thickened and convex in shape; it tapers to a thin free edge towards its inner border. Meniscal blood supply is a major determinant in healing of meniscal tears. The menisci derive their blood supply from a circumferential perimeniscal plexus, which is present in the synovial and capsular tissues of the knee. This plexus receives branches from the medial, lateral and middle geniculate arteries, which in turn are branches of the popliteal artery.[32,33] However, only 10–30% of the peripheral medial meniscus and 10–25% of the peripheral lateral meniscus receive a direct blood supply from this plexus.[32,33] The remaining, inner, portion of each meniscus (65–75%) receives nutrition by diffusion from the synovial fluid.[34] The peripheral zone is known as the 'red zone' and has a good healing potential given its good blood supply. The inner zone is known as the 'white zone' and has a poor healing potential secondary to its avascular nature. The area in between these two zones is referred to as the 'red–white zone', and its healing potential is variable (Fig. 7.3).

Nerve supply

The posterior articular branch of the posterior tibial nerve and branches of the obturator and femoral nerves innervate the knee joint. Small nerve fibres from these branches penetrate the joint capsule, along with the vascular supply, and supply the substance of the menisci.[35,36] Several different types of receptors, such as Ruffini, Pacinian and Golgi tendon mechanoreceptors, have been identified in the knee joint capsule and in the peripheral menisci.[37] The meniscal horns contain the highest concentration of mechanoreceptors, in particular Pacinian mechanoreceptors.

Functions of the meniscus

The important role played by the meniscus was initially elucidated by observing severe degenerative changes in knees that had undergone total meniscectomy.[38,39] Virtually all meniscectomized knees will develop degenerative changes over time, and the severity of these changes is directly proportional to the amount of meniscus resected.[40,41] The meniscus plays a vital role in load transmission and stress distribution across the knee joint. The menisci achieve this by compensating for tibial and femoral articular incongruity, and their presence leads to improved articular conformity. In the standing position, menisci transmit 30–55% of compressive load through the knee joint, and transmit up to 85% when the knee is flexed to 90°.[42] After total meniscectomy, joint contact stress doubles in conjunction with a 50–70% reduction in contact area.[43] A 10% reduction in meniscal contact area following partial meniscectomy produces a 65% increase in peak joint-contact stresses, which in turn leads to the development of early osteoarthritis.[43,44]

Articular conformity is maintained by motion of the menisci as the knee progresses through its arc of flexion.[45,46] As the knee flexes, the femoral condyles glide posteriorly on the tibial plateau and the tibia rotates internally relative to the femur. The menisci translate posteriorly during this motion, preventing the femur from contacting the posterior margin of the tibia. The lateral meniscus undergoes twice the anteroposterior translation of the medial meniscus during knee flexion.[47] The lateral meniscus can better accommodate this mobility by translating with the femoral condyles and is thereby less susceptible to injury than the medial meniscus.[48] The medial meniscus also enhances the anteroposterior stability of the knee, as demonstrated by the significantly increased laxity observed in anterior cruciate ligament-deficient knees that also lack a medial meniscus.

The meniscus also plays an important role in shock absorption and joint lubrication.[26,49] Meniscal shock absorption is time dependent because of the exudation of water out of the ECM. As water leaves the proteoglycans of the ECM, it enters the joint space, where it helps to enhance joint lubrication. In addition, as water leaves, the meniscus becomes stiffer, thus allowing it to bear greater compressive loads. As an adaptation to this function, the highest concentrations of glycosaminoglycans are found in the meniscal horns and the inner half of the menisci, coinciding with the primary weight-bearing areas.[50] Box 7.1 shows a summary of the functions of the meniscus.

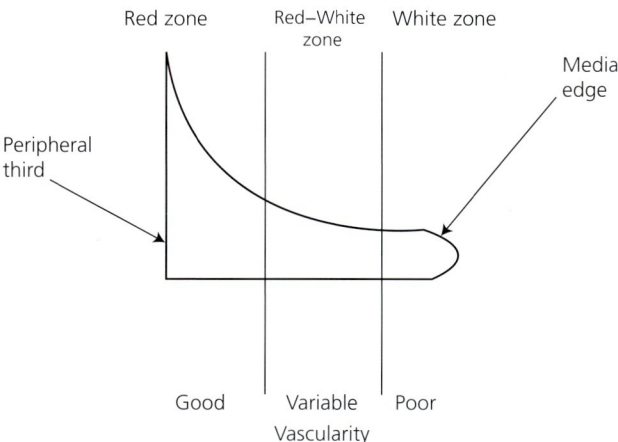

Figure 7.3 Coronal cross-section through meniscus showing the zones of vascularity.

> **BOX 7.1: Important functions of the meniscus**
>
> - Tibiofemoral load transmission
> - Shock absorption
> - Lubrication
> - Prevent synovial impingement
> - Distribute synovial fluid
> - Contribute to joint stability
> - Assist in gliding motion
> - Prevent hyperextension

Meniscal healing

As with all biological tissues, the key determinant of healing in meniscal injuries is its blood supply. Soft-tissue healing follows the sequence of haematoma formation, regeneration via cellular proliferation and remodelling. A reliable blood supply allows delivery of cells and inflammatory mediators to the site of injury. The resultant haematoma functions as a scaffold for matrix formation and is a chemotactic stimulus for the cellular elements involved in healing.[27] Vessels from the perimeniscal capillary plexus proliferate and enter this fibrin scaffold. Undifferentiated mesenchymal cells also arrive and proliferate to effect healing. Eventually, a cellular, fibrovascular scar tissue forms within the defect, causing the wound edges to come together and appear continuous with normal adjacent meniscal fibrocartilage.[51] By 10 weeks, meniscal defects in the vascular zone are filled by a fibrovascular scar tissue. However, remodelling of this scar tissue to a more normal-appearing fibrocartilage takes several months.[52]

Only the peripheral portion of meniscus is vascularized. The aforementioned healing process takes place in this vascularized region with the production of a cellular fibrovascular scar tissue. *In vitro* experiments have demonstrated that meniscal cells can proliferate and synthesize an ECM when exposed to factors normally present in wound haematoma.[53] However, as the central 65–75% of the meniscus does not have a viable blood supply, no haematoma forms in response to injury; therefore, the healing potential in this zone is very limited.

The healing potential of meniscal tears varies according to location, vascular supply, age of the patient, nature of the tear and chronicity of the tear. As the many important functions of the meniscus are now more clearly understood, substantial efforts have been directed towards enhancing meniscal healing. The division of meniscus into zones allows the healing potential to be predicted. The peripheral red–red zone is fully vascular and therefore has an excellent healing prognosis. The intermediate red–white zone is at the border of the vascular supply and has a less predictable, albeit good, healing prognosis. The white–white zone is avascular and has a poor prognosis for healing.[51,54,55] The ability of peripheral tears to heal forms the rationale for surgical repair of these tears, which is accomplished via open or arthroscopic techniques. Indications for surgical repair are traumatic tears within the vascular zone of the meniscus that have caused minimum damage to the meniscal body fragment.[56] Vertical–longitudinal tears, which are 1 cm or greater in length and are located within 3 mm of the vascular periphery, are ideal tears to repair.[57,58] In addition, an improved outcome has been noted when repair is performed within 8 weeks of initial injury.[59] Early intervention is also advocated because the chance of developing osteoarthritis increases when the time from injury to repair increases.[60] Variable long-term results have been reported for meniscal repair, with success rates between 67% and 92%.[61–64] Factors associated with a favourable outcome include time from injury to surgery of less than 8 weeks, peripheral location of the tear, patient age less than 30 years, tear length less than 2.5 cm and a tear in the lateral meniscus.[63] The chondroprotective effect of successful meniscal repair is preserved at an average follow-up of 10.9 years; 85% of compartments were normal on plane radiographs and 15% had only grade 1 degenerative changes.[62]

Given the poor healing potential of meniscal tears in the white–white zone, considerable energy has been invested in techniques to improve healing for these tears. One of the described options consists of injection of a fibrin clot into the meniscal lesion to promote healing by delivery of haematoma chemotactic factors.[27] Vascular access channels can be produced by trephination of the meniscus from vascular portions in the red zone to a more central avascular area within the white zone. Good to excellent results in 90% of patients have been reported for incomplete meniscal tears managed by creation of vascular access channels.[65] Synovial abrasion is commonly used when performing surgery for meniscal tears. Such abrasion should promote the formation of a vascular pannus that will migrate into the meniscal tear and support a reparative response.[56] A recent interesting development is meniscal allograft transplantation. Early animal studies confirmed that meniscal allografts healed to the peripheral tissues of the recipient knee.[66,67] More recent studies have demonstrated that, over time, the allograft becomes repopulated with host cells that are capable of synthesizing ECM components, and revascularization of the graft also occurs.[68–70] Favourable short- to medium-term results have been reported following meniscal transplantation. However, longer term results from higher quality trials are still awaited. As with any new evolving technique, guidelines for the exact indications for meniscal transplantation also remain to be developed.

INTERVERTEBRAL DISC

Structure

The intervertebral disc is a heterogeneous, avascular, aneural, cartilaginous structure that contributes to flexibility and load bearing in the spine. In the spine, a motion segment is composed of two adjacent vertebral bodies and the intervening intervertebral disc. The intervertebral disc forms the primary articulation between the vertebral bodies. The intervertebral disc is separated from the vertebral bodies by hyaline cartilage end plates, and serves as a major constraint to motion between vertebral bodies. In older adults, these cartilaginous end plates often become calcified. In general, intervertebral disc size increases with caudal progression, with the largest disc found at the L4/5 level. The intervertebral disc is composed of three anatomical zones: the outer annulus fibrosus, the central nucleus pulposus and the transitional intermediate zone.

The collagen content of discs increases from the centre of the nucleus pulposus to the outer annulus. Collagen fibres primarily function to provide a tough, three-dimensional scaffold, which supports cells and provides a framework to confine the proteoglycans, which in turn trap water.

Annulus fibrosus

The outer annulus fibrosus is attached to the anterior and posterior longitudinal ligaments, and to both superior and inferior vertebrae. The outer annulus fibrosus is composed predominantly of type I collagen, which is arranged in a dense lamellar formation, imparting high tensile strength to this region. The direction of collagen fibres alternates in neighbouring lamellae and they are arranged at approximately 30° to the horizontal axis, enabling them to resist both distractive and shear forces. The predominant cell type in this zone is the fibroblast. The inner segment of the annulus fibrosus forms an intermediate transitional zone. The predominant cell type in this region is the chondrocyte, and mainly collagen type II is found. Proteoglycan concentration and the proportion of type II collagen gradually increase, moving centrally from the outer region of the annulus fibrosus into the nucleus pulposus.[71] Given the dense collagen network in the outer annulus, permeability is lower than in the inner annulus.[72] Nerve fibres supply the outer portion of the annulus fibrosus; dorsally these arise from the sinuvertebral nerve, and ventrally from the sympathetic chain. The outer annulus is supplied by capillaries, which also feed the surrounding ligaments and soft tissue in this area. The other areas of the disc depend on diffusion of nutrients from blood vessels in the vertebral bodies through the end plate to reach the cells present in the disc centre.

Nucleus pulposus

The nucleus pulposus lies most centrally within the intervertebral disc. At birth, cells derived from the notochord are present, but are gradually replaced so that in adults only chondrocytes are present. The ECM of the nucleus pulposus is a gelatinous, isotropic tissue that consists of a proteoglycan–water gel enmeshed in a randomly oriented network of type II collagen fibres and non-collagenous proteins. In young adults, approximately 90% of the nucleus pulposus is water.

Extracellular matrix

The ECM of the intervertebral disc is synthesized and maintained by the cellular components – fibroblasts and chondrocytes. However, the intervertebral disc has a low cell density, and only about 1% of disc volume is composed of cells.[73] The ECM has three major components: collagen fibres, proteoglycans and glycoproteins.[74] The bulk of the disc matrix is composed of collagen types I and II, although other collagen types such as collagen types V, VI, IX, XI, XII and XIV are also found in lesser amounts.[75] The ECM consists of proteoglycan aggregates, which are large, hydrophilic, negatively charged molecules that hold water in the ECM. This interaction confers to the intervertebral disc the properties of viscoelasticity, stiffness and resistance to compression.

Function

The intervertebral disc functions to maintain flexibility and motion within an otherwise rigid spine. With the facet joints, discs are responsible for carrying all the compressive loads to which the trunk is subjected. Intervertebral discs are subjected to a varied pattern of loading and stresses, which includes dynamic or static loading, and tensile, torsional, shear or compressive stresses. These forces may act on the disc alone or in combination. The specific parts of the intervertebral disc are uniquely adapted to be able to withstand such forces. The alternating lamellar organization of collagen fibres in the annulus fibrosus allows it to resist tensile, torsional and shear stresses. The nucleus pulposus is ideally suited to withstand high compressive stresses, given its high proteoglycan and water content. The nucleus pulposus exhibits viscoelastic creep, secondary to hydrostatic pressure in the interstitial fluid, and Donnan osmotic pressure from fixed negative charges on proteoglycan molecules. The high osmotic pressure exerted by the proteoglycans allows intervertebral discs to withstand a mechanical pressure of several atmospheres without significant loss of hydration.[76] This property allows the intervertebral disc to deform in response to loading, thus producing intradiscal fluid flow and allowing dissipation of energy. The intervertebral disc behaves in a biphasic manner, whereby compression of the nucleus pulposus results in the generation of hoop stresses in the outer layers of the annulus, and the deformed inner layers of the disc act as shock absorbers.

Ageing and disc degeneration

Degenerative changes occur within the intervertebral disc as part of the natural ageing process. However, environmental and genetic factors also play a part in the process of disc degeneration.[77–79] Extrinsic environmental factors such as heavy lifting, use of vibrating machinery, immobilization and trauma can accelerate the degenerative process, as can intrinsic factors such as smoking, diabetes, infection and vascular disease. The process of degeneration initially begins in the nucleus pulposus during the third decade, when loss of chondrocytes and ECM changes are seen. Changes are observed in the pericellular matrix of chondrocytes and collagen, and elastin networks become more disorganized and weaken.[80–82] Progression of degeneration causes the outer annulus fibrosus to lose its normal lamellar arrangement, which compromises the mechanical strength of the disc.[83] The annulus becomes fibrotic, and macroscopically appears firm and white. The most significant biochemical change to occur in disc degeneration is loss of proteoglycans. This loss results in a fall in osmotic pressure and a loss of hydration, with a major impact on the disc's load-bearing behaviour. The degenerate disc no longer behaves hydrostatically under loading and inappropriate stress peaks may occur, resulting in cleft and tear formation.[84] These degenerative changes alter spinal biomechanics, and can lead to secondary adverse effects such as facet joint arthrosis. These age-related degenerative changes are usually complete by the sixth or seventh decade of life, when almost the entire disc, except the fibrotic outer annulus, becomes stiff fibrocartilage.

Injury and healing

Intervertebral disc injury occurs secondary to a defect in the annulus fibrosus, which allows herniation of the contents of the nucleus pulposus. Pain is thought to arise from irritation of the outer innervated layer of the annulus fibrosus. When the outer layer of the annulus fibrosus remains intact, a disc bulge or prolapse occurs. However, if this outer layer is breached, then a disc extrusion occurs. If the herniated contents break free into the spinal canal, a disc sequestration occurs. Any form of intervertebral disc herniation can cause neurological symptoms, secondary to spinal cord or nerve root compression. Intervertebral disc herniation most commonly occurs in the more mobile cervical and lumbar spine regions.

As the intervertebral disc is largely avascular, it has very little intrinsic healing potential. However, despite this, 90% of patients with lumbar disc herniations experience sufficient pain relief within 6 weeks not to warrant surgery.[85] Furthermore, sequential magnetic resonance images demonstrate that the herniated portion of the disc tends to regress over time, with partial to complete resolution after 6 months in two-thirds of patients.[86] Even massive disc herniations resolve over time, although on average this takes 24 months.[87]

Rates for recurrent intervertebral disc herniation after surgical discectomy range from 29% to 41%.[88,89] Animal models have been used to evaluate the effect of surgical repair of the annulus fibrosus following discectomy. However, such a repair does not significantly alter the healing strength of the intervertebral disc after lumbar discectomy.[90] This study supports the notion that intervertebral discs have poor healing ability. Efforts to prevent recurrent disc herniation have therefore focused on techniques that do not rely on intervertebral disc healing. Implantation of non-cell-based material, such as gelfoam, has shown promise in preventing recurrent disc herniation in a porcine model.[91] Intervertebral disc allograft transplantation and tissue engineering interventions have been reported.[92,93] However, both these technologies are in the preliminary stages of development, and further research is required prior to clinically applicable treatment options being available.

SKELETAL MUSCLE

Structure

Skeletal muscle is a vital component of the musculoskeletal system. Coordinated muscle contraction facilitates many important functions, including joint movement and locomotion. Skeletal muscle represents the largest tissue mass in the human body, accounting for 40–45% of total body weight. Skeletal muscle is a composite structure that consists of myocytes, an organized network of nerves and blood vessels, and ECM.[94] The basic structural unit of skeletal muscle is the myofibre, which is composed of multiple myofibrils. Myofibre cytoplasm, known as sarcoplasm, contains organelles vital to cell metabolism such as Golgi apparatus, mitochondria and the sarcoplasmic reticulum. Lipid droplets, glycogen and myoglobin are present in the sarcoplasm, and provide the energy necessary for cell function. The skeletal muscle fibre is a differentiated multinucleated syncytium, which is formed by the fusion of multiple immature mononucleated myoblasts. Muscle fibre size and length varies according to genetic and physiological influences.[95] Fibres in muscles controlling fine, precise movements, such as the small muscles of the hand, tend to be smaller than muscle fibres in large powerful muscles, such as the quadriceps.

Myofibres are surrounded by a connective tissue sheath, known as endomysium. Several myofibres group together to form a fascicle, which in turn is enclosed within the perimysium. Multiple muscle fascicles group together to form the body of the muscle, which is covered by epimysium. Muscle fibre arrangement is an important determinant of the contractile properties of skeletal muscle, and can be parallel or oblique to the long axis of the muscle.

Muscle cells are characterized by a high concentration of contractile proteins in their sarcoplasm. Almost 80% of cell volume is taken up by contractile proteins arranged in a highly organized fashion. The cell nuclei are marginalized as a result of this architectural arrangement. By convention, muscle fibres are termed mature when nuclear marginalization is noted within myocytes. Particularly high concentrations of cell nuclei are observed in the vicinity of the neuromuscular junction.

The plasma membrane that surrounds each myofibre unit is known as the sarcolemma. In addition to myofibres, separate cells called satellite cells are located between the basal lamina and plasma membrane, and play a key role in the muscle regeneration process.[96,97] The multiple small myofibrils, which coalesce to compose muscle fibres, are surrounded by a membranous sac, the sarcoplasmic reticulum. The sarcoplasmic reticulum serves as a reservoir for calcium, which is released during muscle contraction. T-tubules (transverse tubules) are invaginations of the sarcolemma that run perpendicular to the long axis of myofibres. The T-tubule carries the depolarization wave from the surface of the sarcolemma to the interior of the muscle fibre. Multiple interconnections exist between T-tubules and the sarcoplasmic reticulum. As the T-tubules become depolarized, calcium release is initiated from the sarcoplasmic reticulum.

Ultrastructure and contractile proteins

Actin and myosin are the major contractile proteins present in skeletal muscle. The grouped functional unit of these filaments is referred to as a myofibril. In skeletal muscle, myofibrils are arranged into functional, contractile units known as sarcomeres. A sarcomere is approximately 2 μm long and 1 μm in diameter. A muscle cell from the biceps muscle may contain up to 100 000 sarcomeres. Sarcomeres are responsible for the striated appearance of skeletal muscle, and a number of bands can be identified on either light or electron microscopy (Table 7.4 and Fig. 7.4).

Table 7.4 Bands present in the muscle sarcomere

Band	Description
A band	Interdigitating actin and myosin filaments
H band	Lies within A band, contains myosin filaments only
I band	Actin filaments only
M line	Anchors myosin filaments
Z line	Anchors actin filaments

Actin is the main component of thin filaments, although tropomyosin and troponin are also present. The thick filaments are composed of myosin. Myosin molecules are composed of two heavy and four light chains and the heavy chains articulate with actin during muscle contraction. The articulating head component of the myosin heavy chain is termed the S1 segment, and the neck portion, which moves to allow articulation of the head, is termed the S2 segment.

Blood supply

In human muscle, a main artery enters the muscle and branches rapidly into a series of arcades. Arterioles arise from these arcades and penetrate the perimysium, which encloses the muscle fascicles. Upon entering the muscle fascicle, arterioles run parallel to muscle fibres. Terminal capillaries are associated with muscle fibre nuclei.

Neuromuscular junction

The point at which a nerve enters a skeletal muscle is known as the motor point. Multiple axonal branches arise from each motor neurone, and each myofibre is innervated by a single axonal branch. The synapse formed between a nerve axon and a myofibre is known as the neuromuscular junction (Fig. 7.5). No clear architectural arrangement exists in the axonal supply of myofibres; therefore, adjacent myofibres are rarely supplied by the same parent motor neurone. A single motor neurone and all the muscle fibres supplied by its branches are termed a motor unit. Figure 7.5 illustrates the

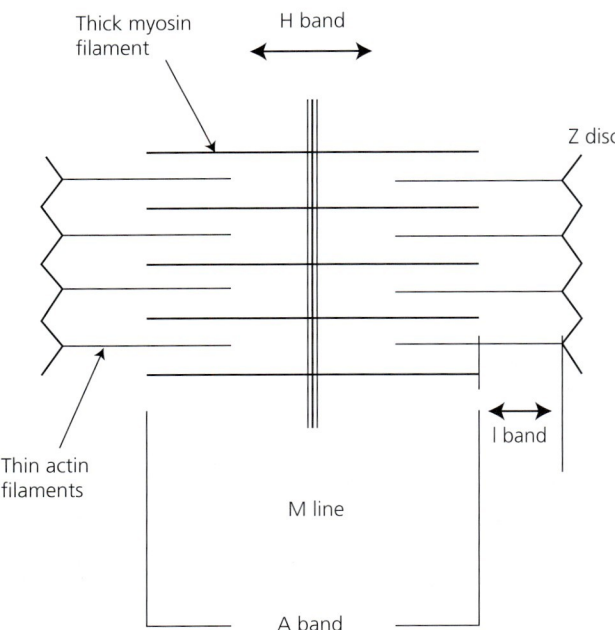

Figure 7.4 The muscle ultrastructural arrangement.

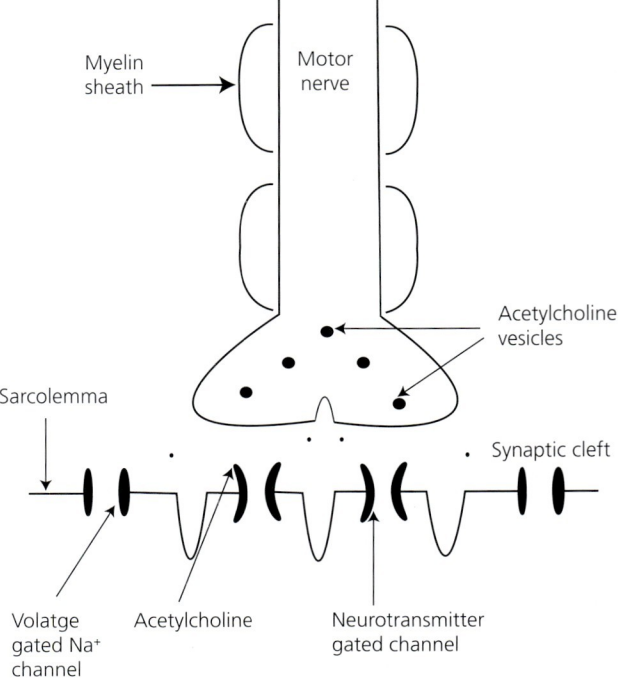

Figure 7.5 The neuromuscular junction.

three major structural components of the neuromuscular junction: the presynaptic axon, the synaptic cleft and the post-synaptic area on the myofibres. Skeletal muscle composition varies, in terms of the number of myofibres per motor unit and the number of motor units present, according to the function performed by the muscle. Muscles responsible for fine motor control and highly coordinated motion contain very few myofibres within each motor unit. Large powerful muscles, such as the gastrocnemius, may contain up to 1000 myofibres per single motor unit.

Action potential propagation along a motor neurone results in depolarization of the presynaptic motor axon membrane.[98] This depolarization allows an influx of calcium ions through voltage-sensitive ion channels. Calcium influx results in preformed acetylcholine vesicles fusing with the presynaptic motor axon membrane, leading to acetylcholine release into the synaptic cleft. The released acetylcholine binds to specific acetylcholine receptors, which are present in the post-junctional folds of the myofibres in the post-synaptic area, and leads to depolarization of the myofibre. Depolarization triggers an action potential that passes along the entire length of the myofibre. Following depolarization of the neuromuscular junction, the action potential travels along the transverse tubules to reach the interior of the muscle. This initiates a transient release of calcium from the sarcoplasmic reticulum.[94]

In response to myofibre depolarization and calcium release from the sarcoplasmic reticulum, the actin and myosin contractile filaments move relative to each other to produce muscle contraction.[99] The process by which movement of contractile filaments takes place is known as the sliding filament theory. Calcium released from the sarcoplasmic reticulum binds to troponin, a component of the thin filament. Troponin is actually composed of three subunits, known as troponin C, troponin I and troponin T.[100] These subunits play an important role in facilitating sliding of the contractile filaments. Initially, calcium binds to the troponin C subunit; this allows troponin C to displace the inhibitory troponin I subunit from the actin–myosin complex. Troponin T interacts with tropomyosin, resulting in a conformational change that allows the head of a myosin molecule to bind to actin. The myosin heads flex and pull the actin strand, which results in muscle contraction. After contraction, adenosine triphosphate (ATP) binds to myosin. Binding of ATP causes disengagement of the actin–myosin cross-bridge and hydrolysis of ATP. The energy released from ATP hydrolysis is stored in the myosin molecule to power the next contractile sequence.[101] At the end of muscle contraction, acetylcholine is degraded by the enzyme acetylcholinesterase, leading to muscle relaxation. Intracellular calcium is taken up by the sarcoplasmic reticulum and the troponin unit returns to its original formation to once again inhibit muscle contraction. The main events that occur during skeletal muscle contraction are summarized in Box 7.2.

> **BOX 7.2: Sequence of events in skeletal muscle contraction**
>
> - Motor nerve action potential
> - Acetylcholine release
> - Muscle depolarization
> - Calcium released from sarcoplasmic reticulum
> - Calcium binds to troponin C
> - Troponin I displaced
> - Troponin T–tropomyosin conformational change
> - Actin–myosin cross-bridge formation
> - Muscle contraction

Muscle kinesiology

To produce movement of a joint, the muscles around the joint must function in a controlled and coordinated fashion. The group of muscles initiating a movement are known as agonists. Muscles that provide resistance, generally on the opposite side of a joint, are called antagonists.[100] Muscle can contract in a variety of ways, depending on the specific requirements. In concentric contraction, tension within the muscle is proportional to the externally applied load. The force produced by the muscle is larger than the resisting load and the muscle shortens in response to loading. In eccentric contraction, the resisting load is larger than the force produced by the muscle; consequently, the muscle lengthens in response to loading. Eccentric contraction of tibialis anterior and gastrocsoleus is seen during the highly coordinated movements of the normal gait cycle. Eccentric contraction is the most efficient way to strengthen a muscle, but it also carries the greatest risk of injury. In isometric contraction, the force generated by the muscle is equal to the resisting load and, therefore, the length of the muscle does not change. In isotonic contraction, a constant tension is maintained in the muscle throughout the range of motion, although muscle length changes through the range of motion. An isotonic contraction can be concentric or eccentric. An isoinertial contraction is a muscle contraction against the same weight; again, an isoinertial contraction can be concentric or eccentric. In isokinetic motion, the muscle contracts maximally at a constant velocity through the full range of motion. An isokinetic contraction can be concentric or eccentric. Special computer-equipped exercise machines are required to perform isokinetic exercises.

The force that a muscle is able to produce at any given length is proportional to its cross-sectional area. More sarcomeres, acting in parallel, can be recruited in thicker muscles; therefore, they are able to generate more force. The longer the muscle, the greater is the change in length per unit time, upon contraction. Hence, contraction velocity is greater for longer muscles. Power generated by a muscle is the product of force and velocity.

Three main types of myofibre are present in human skeletal muscle: type 1, which are slow myofibres highly resistant to fatigue; type 2A, fast myofibres with intermediate resistance to fatigue; and type 2B, fast, but easily fatigable myofibres.[94] A mixture of these fibre types is usually present in most human skeletal muscles. Activity pattern and exercise regime are the most important determinants of fibre type expression.[102] Muscle biopsies performed on elite sprinters are more likely to show a larger number of type 2 myofibres, whereas distance runners are more likely to have a large proportion of type 1 myofibres.[102] Table 7.5 summarizes the salient properties of the different muscle fibre types.

Muscle injury and healing

Injury to muscle can occur through a variety of direct or indirect mechanisms (Box 7.3).[103–105] The mechanism of injury does not influence the sequence of events seen in muscle healing, although functional recovery may be altered depending on the type of injury sustained. Following injury, an interrelated and temporal sequence of events occurs. For descriptive purposes, the healing response can be divided into the following phases: degeneration, inflammation, regeneration and fibrosis.

Muscle injury resulting from direct trauma mechanically damages the myofibre sarcolemma and basal lamina, which causes an influx of calcium ions.[106,107] The influx of calcium triggers the activation of degradative enzymes, such as proteases and phospholipases. This results in autodigestion of the myofibres and leads to muscle necrosis.[108,109] Muscle damage occurs secondary to free radical production.[110] Local swelling and haematoma formation occur, leading to further muscle degeneration.[111,112] The degenerative phase typically occurs in the first few days after injury. The necrotic area is invaded by newly formed, small blood vessels. This initiates the inflammatory phase, which is also seen within the first few days following injury. An inflammatory infiltrate, consisting of monocytes, macrophages and T lymphocytes, is seen at the site of injury. The inflammatory cells secrete cytokines, which are chemotactic and further perpetuate the inflammatory response. Adhesion molecules, interleukins and tumour necrosis factor α are among the inflammatory mediators found at the site of injury.[113–117] Many growth factors are also released at the site of injury; these consist of insulin-like growth factor 1, hepatocyte growth factor, epidermal growth factor, transforming growth factors α and β and platelet-derived growth factors AA and BB. Growth factors regulate myoblast proliferation and differentiation, thus promoting muscle regeneration and repair. During this phase, satellite cells become activated. After focal muscle injury, disruption of the sarcolemma and basal lamina leads to satellite cell activation.[96,118] In response to the various growth factors present, satellite cells become activated, proliferate and differentiate into multinucleated myotubes and eventually into regenerated myofibres.[119–121] This process of myofibre regeneration following injury is equivalent to muscle histogenesis in the embryo. The regenerative phase usually commences 7–10 days after injury. The regenerative process usually peaks 2 weeks after injury and then gradually declines by about 3–4 weeks after injury. The final phase of healing is fibrosis. During this period, scar tissue is formed at the site of injury. This phase typically begins between the second and third weeks after injury, with the scar tissue increasing in size over time. The appearance of scar tissue is the final stage of the muscle repair process. Consequently, complete regeneration of injured muscle does not take place, and the healed, fibrotic muscle has inferior mechanical properties. Prevention of fibrosis during the muscle-healing process may improve the potential for muscle regeneration after injury. Various techniques have been investigated to achieve this, but no definitive method has emerged.[99]

Table 7.5 Types of muscle fibre

Fibre type	Properties
Type 1	Slow contraction
	Red: high myoglobin content
	Oxidative: high aerobic capacity
	Fatigue resistant
	(mnemonic: slow red ox)
Type 2A	Fast contraction
	White fibres
	Intermediate fatigue resistance
	Anaerobic and aerobic metabolism
Type 2B	Fast contraction
	White fibres
	Fatigable
	Anaerobic metabolism

BOX 7.3: Modes of muscle injury

- Muscle belly tear
- Muscle laceration
- Muscle contusion
- Musculotendinous junction injury
- Denervation
- Crush injury and rhabdomyolysis
- Malignant hyperthermia
- Delayed-onset muscle soreness (typically presents 24–72 hours after intense activity)

LIGAMENT AND TENDON

Ligaments and tendons are unique constituents of the musculoskeletal system, and have many important features in common. Consequently, they will be discussed together. Despite the similarities that they share, some important differences do exist, and these will be highlighted. Ligaments connect bone to bone and function to augment the static and dynamic stability of joints. In addition, they may also play an important role in proprioceptive feedback. Tendons attach muscle to bone, and allow muscles to generate motion. Tendons transmit load from muscles to bones, and also act as a buffer by storing energy, thus preventing damage to muscles.[122]

Structure

Healthy ligaments and tendons are white and have a fibroelastic texture. Tendons can be rounded cords, strap-like bands or flattened ribbons.[123] Fibroblasts lie within the ECM network and constitute 90–95% of the cellular elements.[124] The remaining 5–10% consists of chondrocytes at the bone attachment and insertion sites, synovial cells of the tendon sheath and vascular cells, including capillary endothelial cells and smooth muscle cells of arterioles. Fibroblasts are active in energy generation and synthesize collagen and all components of the ECM.[125]

The dry mass of human tendons is approximately 30% of the total tendon mass. Collagen type I accounts for 65–80% and elastin accounts for approximately 2% of the dry mass of tendons.[125–128] Typically, tendons contain more collagen than ligaments, and ligaments contain more elastin. Fibroblasts lie between the collagen fibres along the long axis of the tendon.[129]

Soluble tropocollagen molecules form cross-links to produce insoluble collagen molecules that aggregate to form collagen fibrils. Collagen is arranged in hierarchical levels of increasing complexity, beginning with tropocollagen, a triple-helix polypeptide chain that merges into fibrils; fibres (primary bundles); fascicles (secondary bundles); tertiary bundles; and the tendon itself (Fig. 7.6).[130,131] A collagen fibre is the smallest tendon unit that can be mechanically tested and is visible on light microscopy. Although collagen fibres are mainly orientated longitudinally, fibres also run transversely and horizontally, forming spirals and plaits.[132–134] The ground substance of the ECM, which surrounds the collagen and the tenocytes, is composed of proteoglycans, glycosaminoglycans, glycoproteins and several other small molecules.[124] Proteoglycans are strongly hydrophilic, enabling rapid diffusion of water-soluble molecules and migration of cells. Adhesive glycoproteins, such as fibronectin and thrombospondin, participate in repair and regeneration processes in tendon.[135,136] The epitenon is a fine, loose connective-tissue sheath containing the vascular, lymphatic and nerve supply to the tendon. It covers the whole tendon, and extends deep within it between the tertiary bundles as the endotenon. The endotenon is a thin reticular network of connective tissue investing each tendon fibre.[137,138] Similar loose connective tissue surrounds ligaments, although this has no specific name. Superficially, the epitenon is surrounded by paratenon, a loose areolar connective tissue consisting of type I and III collagen fibrils, some elastic fibrils and an inner lining of synovial cells.[139] Synovial tendon sheaths are present in areas subjected to increased mechanical stress, such as tendons of the hands and feet, where very efficient lubrication is required. Synovial sheaths consist of an outer fibrotic sheath and an inner synovial sheath, which consists of thin visceral and parietal sheets.[130]

Attachment to bone

At the myotendinous junction (MTJ), tendinous collagen fibrils are inserted into deep recesses formed by myocyte processes, allowing the tension produced by intracellular contractile proteins of muscle fibres to be transmitted to the collagen fibrils.[140–144] This complex architecture reduces the tensile stress exerted on the tendon during muscle contraction. However, the MTJ still remains the weakest point of the muscle–tendon unit.[144–147] The osteotendinous junction (OTJ) is composed of four zones: a zone of dense collagen fibres, fibrocartilage, mineralized fibrocartilage and bone.[148] The specialized structure of the OTJ prevents collagen fibre bending, fraying, shearing and failure.[149,150] Ligaments display two types of insertion into bone: direct and indirect. Direct tendon insertion is seen in the attachment of the native anterior cruciate ligament, and is the same as the four zones seen at the osteotendinous junction. In indirect insertion, seen at the tibial attachment of the medial collateral ligament, the superficial layer connects directly to periosteum, and the deep layer anchors to bone via Sharpey's fibres.

Blood supply

In ligaments, the blood supply mainly originates at the insertion sites. Blood vessels tend to run longitudinally, and the blood supply is fairly uniform throughout the body of the ligaments. Tendons receive their blood supply from three

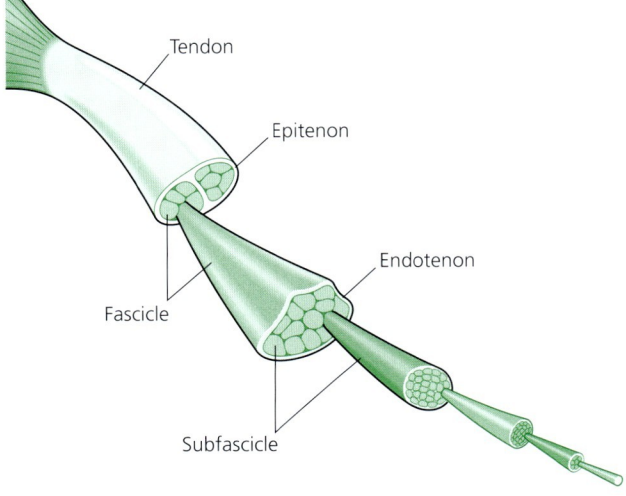

Figure 7.6 The ultrastructure of tendon.

main sources: the intrinsic systems at the MTJ and OTJ, and the extrinsic system via the paratenon or the synovial sheath. At the MTJ, perimyseal vessels from the muscle continue between the fasciculi of the tendon, and supply approximately the proximal third of the tendon.[151] The blood supply from the OTJ is sparse and limited to the insertion zone of the tendon, although vessels from the extrinsic system communicate with periosteal vessels at the OTJ. In tendons with sheaths, branches from major vessels pass through the vincula (mesotenon) to reach the visceral sheet of the synovial sheath, where they form a plexus. This plexus supplies the superficial part of the tendon, while some vessels from the vinculae penetrate the epitenon. These vessels run in the endotenon septae, and form a connection between the peri- and intratendinous vascular networks. In the absence of a synovial sheath, the paratenon provides the extrinsic component of the vasculature. Vessels entering the paratenon run transversely and branch repeatedly to form a complex vascular network. Arterial branches from the paratenon penetrate the epitenon to run in the endotenon septae, where an intratendinous vascular network with abundant anastomoses is formed. Tendon vascularity is compromised at junctional zones and sites of torsion, friction or compression. In the Achilles tendon, classical angiographic injection techniques have demonstrated a zone of hypovascularity 2–7 cm proximal to the tendon insertion,[152] although the real presence of an area of hypovascularity has been disputed by some authors. A similar zone of hypovascularity is present on the dorsal surface of the flexor digitorum profundus tendon subjacent to the volar plate, within 1 cm of the tendon insertion.[153] In general, tendon blood flow declines with increasing age and mechanical loading.

Nerve supply

Tendon innervation originates from cutaneous, muscular and peritendinous nerve trunks. At the myotendinous junction, nerve fibres cross and enter the endotenon septa. Nerve fibres form rich plexuses in the paratenon, and branches penetrate the epitenon. Most nerve fibres do not actually enter the main body of the tendon but terminate as nerve endings on its surface. Nerve endings of myelinated fibres function as specialized mechanoreceptors to detect changes in pressure or tension. These mechanoreceptors, the Golgi tendon organs, are most numerous at the insertion of tendons into the muscle. Golgi tendon organs consist of a thin, delicate capsule of connective tissue that encloses a group of branches of large myelinated nerve fibres. These fibres terminate with a spray of fibre endings between bundles of collagen fibres of the tendon.[154,155] Golgi tendon organs play an important protective and proprioceptive role. They are activated during rapid loading and help to prevent the development of excessive tension within tendons or ligaments. Unmyelinated nerve endings act as nociceptors, and they sense and transmit pain. Both sympathetic and parasympathetic fibres are present in tendon.

Biomechanics

Ligaments and tendons exhibit high mechanical strength, good flexibility and an optimal level of elasticity to perform their unique role.[156,157] Ligaments and tendons are viscoelastic tissues which display stress relaxation, creep and hysteresis. A stress–strain curve helps to demonstrate the behaviour of tendon (Fig. 7.7). At rest, collagen fibres and fibrils display a crimped configuration. If the strain remains below 4%, a tendon behaves in an elastic fashion and returns to its original length when unloaded.[158] Microscopic failure occurs when the strain exceeds 4%, and beyond 8–10% strain macroscopic failure occurs because of intrafibril damage by molecular slippage.[159,160] After this, complete failure occurs rapidly, and the fibres recoil into a tangled bud at the ruptured end.

Ligament and tendon injury

Injuries can be acute or chronic, and are caused by intrinsic or extrinsic factors, either alone or in combination. In acute trauma, extrinsic factors predominate. Overuse injuries generally have a multifactorial origin. In chronic tendon disorders, interaction between intrinsic and extrinsic factors is common. Excessive loading of tendons during vigorous physical training is regarded as the main pathological stimulus for degeneration.[161] Tendons respond to repetitive overload beyond the physiological threshold by inflammation of their sheath, degeneration of their body or a combination of both.[162] It remains unclear whether different stresses induce different responses. Active repair of fatigue damage must occur, or tendons would weaken and eventually rupture.[163] The repair mechanism is probably mediated by resident tenocytes that continually monitor the ECM. Failure to adapt to recurrent excessive loads

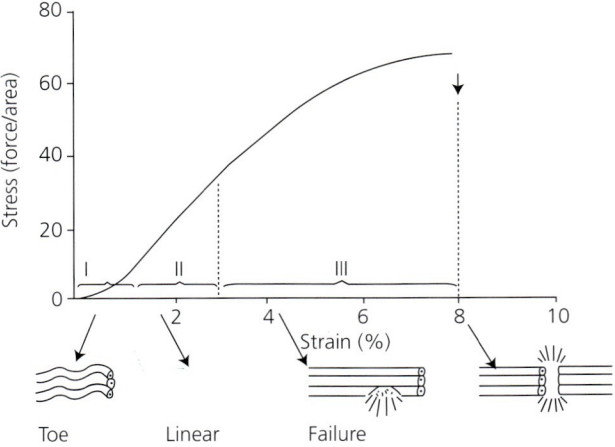

Figure 7.7 A stress–strain curve for tendon.

results in the release of cytokines, leading to further modulation of cell activity.[164] Tendon damage may even occur from stresses within physiological limits, as frequent cumulative microtrauma may not allow enough time for repair.[161] Microtrauma can also result from non-uniform stress within tendons, producing abnormal load concentrations and frictional forces between the fibrils, resulting in localized fibre damage.[165] The aetiology of tendinopathy remains unclear, and many factors, such as ischaemia, free radical damage, hyperthermia, impaired apoptosis, inflammatory mediators and an imbalance in MMP levels, have all been implicated.[166] Histologically, tendinopathy is characterized by an absence of inflammatory cells and a poor healing response, with non-inflammatory intratendinous collagen degeneration, fibre disorientation and thinning, hypercellularity, scattered vascular ingrowth and increased interfibrillar glycosaminoglycans.

Acute rupture occurs when a force greater than the ultimate tensile strength is applied. Specific mechanisms are more likely to cause such injuries; for example, a valgus force to the knee results in disruption of the medial collateral ligament, and eccentric loading is usually associated with Achilles tendon rupture. An advanced failed healing response is the most common histological finding in spontaneous tendon ruptures.[167] In ligaments, at low loading rates, the weakest zone is at the insertion sites. At higher loading rates, the ligament itself is more likely to fail. In tendon, the musculotendinous junction is the weakest area, and thus most likely to fail. In the presence of a significant failure of the normal healing response within the body of the tendon, tensile strength is reduced, leading to a predisposition to rupture. Indeed, ruptured Achilles tendons are more degenerate than tendinopathic tendons.

Healing

Tendons and ligaments are relatively avascular structures, and have 7.5 times lower oxygen consumption than skeletal muscles.[168] Their low metabolic rate and well-developed anaerobic energy-generating capacity are essential to carry loads and maintain tension for long periods, reducing the risk of ischaemia and subsequent necrosis. However, a low metabolic rate results in slow healing after injury. Tendon-healing studies have predominantly been performed on transected animal tendons or ruptured human tendons, and their relevance to degenerate human tendons remains unclear. Tendon healing occurs in three overlapping phases: the inflammatory phase, the regenerative phase and the remodelling phase. However, for the purposes of description, these phases will be considered separately.

- *Inflammatory phase.* Following injury, erythrocytes and inflammatory cells, particularly neutrophils, enter the site of damage. In the first 24 hours monocytes and macrophages predominate and phagocytosis of necrotic materials occurs. Vasoactive and chemotactic factors are released, leading to increased vascular permeability, initiation of angiogenesis, stimulation of fibroblast proliferation and recruitment of more inflammatory cells.[169,170] Fibroblasts gradually migrate to the wound, and type III collagen synthesis is initiated.
- *Regenerative phase.* Commences a few days after injury. Synthesis of type III collagen peaks during this stage, and lasts for a few weeks. Water content and glycosaminoglycan concentrations remain high during this stage.[171]
- *Remodelling phase.* After approximately 6 weeks, the remodelling stage commences, with decreased cellularity and decreased collagen and glycosaminoglycan synthesis. The remodelling phase can be divided into a consolidation and a maturation stage.[172] The consolidation stage commences at about 6 weeks and continues up to 10 weeks. In this period, the repair tissue changes from cellular to fibrous. Fibroblast metabolism remains high during this period, and fibroblasts and collagen fibres become aligned in the direction of stress.[173] A higher proportion of type I collagen is synthesized during this stage.[174] After 10 weeks, the maturation stage occurs, with a gradual change of fibrous tissue to scar-like tendon tissue.[173,175] The maturation stage continues for up to a year. However, during the latter half of this stage, fibroblast metabolism and tendon vascularity decline.[176]

Tendon healing consists of intrinsic and extrinsic components. Extrinsic healing is mediated by fibroblasts that migrate from the tendon sheath or surrounding tissues. In the process, adhesions are formed that limit tendon excursion. Intrinsic healing is mediated by internal fibroblasts, and results in improved biomechanics and fewer complications. Both processes are likely to occur during healing, although their relative contributions may vary depending on factors such as the type of trauma sustained, anatomical position, presence of a synovial sheath, and the amount of post-repair motion stress.[177]

MMPs are important regulators of ECM remodelling, and their levels are altered during tendon healing, suggesting that they play an important role.[178–180] Growth factors act as regulators of the phases of tendon healing.[181–186] Wounding and inflammation provoke release of growth factors from platelets, polymorphonuclear leucocytes and macrophages.[182,183,186] These growth factors induce neovascularization and chemotaxis for fibroblasts and for stimulating fibroblast proliferation and synthesis of collagen.[187,188]

The healing response in ligaments differs depending on whether the injured ligament is intra-articular or extra-articular. The medial collateral ligament heals more readily than the anterior cruciate ligament, because a fibrin clot forms at the site of injury and functions as a scaffold, which is invaded by fibroblasts and gradually replaced by collagen fibres.[189,190] Anterior cruciate ligament healing is impaired because formation of a fibrin clot is prevented by fibrinolytic enzymes which are present in the intra-articular milieu.[191,192]

Factors affecting healing

Controlled mobilization has a beneficial effect on healing. Animal studies demonstrate that immobilization leads to reduced tensile strength and stiffness of ligaments and tendons, along with a reduction in water and proteoglycan content.[193] Controlled motion increases collagen and proteoglycan synthesis, improves collagen fibre orientation and increases tensile strength.

The roles of growth factor therapy, gene therapy and tissue engineering are being intensively researched to enhance tendon healing, although such methods are currently not in routine clinical use.[194]

> **KEY LEARNING POINTS**
>
> - Collagen is the basic building block for soft tissue, and several types of collagen exist.
> - Proteoglycans are hydrophilic, non-collagenous proteins, which serve to trap water in soft tissue.
> - Proteoglycan levels decline in ageing and osteoarthritis.
> - Soft tissue integrity is vital for normal musculoskeletal function.
> - Unlike bone, soft tissues have a limited repair capacity. Healing generally leads to a reduction in tensile strength.
> - Therefore it is vital to minimize soft tissue trauma during surgery.

REFERENCES

1. Lodish H, Berk A, Zipursky LS, *et al.* (eds). *Molecular Cell Biology.* New York, NY: W.H. Freeman, 2000.
2. Van der Rest M, Garrone R. Collagen family of proteins. *FASEB Journal* 2001;**5**:2814–23.
3. Eyre DR, Weis MA, Wu JJ. Articular cartilage collagen: an irreplaceable framework? *European Cells and Materials* 2006;**12**:57–63.
4. Mendler M, Eich-Bender SG, Vaughan L, *et al.* Cartilage contains mixed fibrils of collagen types II, IX, and XI. *Journal of Cell Biology* 1989;**108**:191–7.
5. Wu JJ, Eyre DR. Structural analysis of cross-linking domains in cartilage type XI collagen: insights on polymeric assembly. *Journal of Biological Chemistry* 1995;**270**:18865–70.
6. Gregory KE, Oxford JT, Chen Y, *et al.* Structural organization of distinct domains within the non-collagenous N-terminal region of collagen type XI. *Journal of Biological Chemistry* 2000;**275**:11498–506.
7. Gannon JM, Walker G, Fischer M, *et al.* Localization of type X collagen in canine growth plate and adult canine articular cartilage. *Journal of Orthopaedic Research* 1991;**9**:485–94.
8. Watanabe H, Yamada Y, Kimata K. Roles of aggrecan, a large chondroitin sulfate proteoglycan, in cartilage structure and function. *Journal of Biochemistry* 1998;**124**:687–93.
9. Iozzo RV. The biology of the small leucine-rich proteoglycans. *Journal of Biological Chemistry* 1999;**274**:18843–6.
10. Flannery CR, Hughes CE, Schumacher BL, *et al.* Articular cartilage superficial zone protein (SZP) is homologous to megakaryocyte stimulating factor precursor and is a multifunctional proteoglycan with potential growth-promoting, cytoprotective, and lubricating properties in cartilage metabolism. *Biochemical and Biophysical Research Communications* 1999;**254**:535–41.
11. Chen FH, Thomas AO, Hecht JT, *et al.* Cartilage oligomeric matrix protein/thrombospondin 5 supports chondrocyte attachment through interaction with integrins. *Journal of Biological Chemistry* 2005;**280**:32655–61.
12. Kipnes J, Carlberg AL, Loredo GA, *et al.* Effect of cartilage oligomeric matrix protein on mesenchymal chondrogenesis in vitro. *Osteoarthritis and Cartilage* 2003;**11**:442–54.
13. Briggs MD, Hoffman SM, King LM, *et al.* Pseudoachondroplasia and multiple epiphyseal dysplasia due to mutations in the cartilage oligomeric matrix protein gene. *Nature Genetics* 1995;**10**:330–6.
14. Mannello F, Luchetti F, Falcieri E, *et al.* Multiple roles of matrix metalloproteinases during apoptosis. *Apoptosis* 2005;**10**:19–24.
15. Mannello F, Gazzanelli G. Tissue inhibitors of metalloproteinases and programmed cell death: conundrums, controversies and potential implications. *Apoptosis* 2001;**6**:479–82.
16. Visse R, Nagase H. Matrix metalloproteinases and tissue inhibitors of metalloproteinases. *Circulation Research* 2003;**92**:827–39.
17. Loeser Jr RF. Aging cartilage and osteoarthritis: what's the link? *Science of Aging Knowledge Environment* 2004;**29**:31.
18. Felson DT, Zhang Y. An update on the epidemiology of knee and hip osteoarthritis with a view to prevention. *Arthritis and Rheumatism* 1998;**41**:1343–1355.
19. Sharma L, Song J, Felson DT, *et al.* The role of knee alignment in disease progression and functional decline in knee osteoarthritis. *Journal of the American Medical Association* 2001;**286**:188–95.
20. Hardaker Jr WT, Garrett Jr WE, Barrett 3rd FH. Evaluation of acute traumatic hemarthrosis of the knee joint. *Southern Medical Journal* 1990;**83**:640–4.
21. Graf BK, Cook DA, De Smet AA, Keene JS. 'Bone bruises' on magnetic resonance imaging evaluation of anterior cruciate ligament injuries. *American Journal of Sports Medicine* 1993;**21**:220–3.
22. Nakamae A, Engebretsen L, Bahr R, *et al.* Natural history of bone bruises after acute knee injury: clinical outcome and histopathological findings. *Knee Surgery, Sports Traumatology, Arthroscopy* 2006;**14**:1252–8.
23. Mair SD, Schlegel TF, Gill TJ, *et al.* Incidence and location of bone bruises after acute posterior cruciate ligament injury. *American Journal of Sports Medicine* 2004;**32**:1681–7.

24. Mankin HJ. The response of articular cartilage to mechanical injury. *Journal of Bone and Joint Surgery (American)* 1982;**64A**:462–6.
25. O'Driscoll SW. Current concepts review: the healing and regeneration of articular cartilage. *Journal of Bone and Joint Surgery* 1998;**80**:1795–812.
26. Fithian DC, Kelly MA, Mow VC. Material properties and structure-function relationships in the menisci. *Clinical Orthopaedics and Related Research* 1990;**252**:19–31.
27. Arnoczky SP, Warren RF, Spivak JM. Meniscal repair using exogenous fibrin clot: an experimental study in dogs. *Journal of Bone and Joint Surgery (American)* 1988;**70**:1209–17.
28. Ingman A, Ghosh P, Taylor T. Variations of collagenous and non-collagenous proteins of human knee joint menisci with age and degeneration. *Gerontology* 1974;**20**:212–33.
29. Peters TJ, Smillie IS. Studies on the chemical composition of the menisci of the knee joint with special reference to the horizontal cleavage lesion. *Clinical Orthopaedics and Related Research* 1972;**86**:245–52.
30. Adams M, Hukins D. The extracellular matrix of the meniscus. In: Mow VC, Arnoczky S, Jackson D (eds) *Knee Meniscus: Basic and Clinical Foundations*. New York, NY: Raven Press, 1992:15–28.
31. Mcdermott I, Masouros S, Amis A. Biomechanics of the menisci of the knee. *Current Orthopaedics* 2008;**22**:193–201.
32. Arnoczky SP, Warren RF. Microvasculature of the human meniscus. *American Journal of Sports Medicine* 1982;**10**:90–5.
33. Danzig L, Resnik D, Gonsalves M, et al. Blood supply to the normal and abnormal meniscus of the human knee. *Clinical Orthopaedics and Related Research* 1983;**172**:271–6.
34. Mow V, Fithian D, Kelly M. Fundamentals of articular cartilage and meniscus biomechanics. In: Ewing JW (ed.) *Articular Cartilage and Knee Joint Function: Basic Science and Arthroscopy*. New York, NY: Raven Press, 1989:1–18.
35. Assimakopoulos AP, Katonis PG, Agapitos MV, et al. The innervation of the human meniscus. *Clinical Orthopaedics and Related Research* 1992;**275**:232–6.
36. O'Donoghue D, Kennedy JC, Alexander IJ, Hayes KC. Nerve supply of the human and its functional importance. *American Journal of Sports Medicine* 1982;**10**:329–35.
37. Zimny ML. Mechanoreceptors in articular tissues. *American Journal of Anatomy* 1988;**182**:16–32.
38. Noble J, Turner PG. The function, pathology, and surgery of the meniscus. *Clinical Orthopaedics and Related Research* 1986;**210**:62–8.
39. Jorgensen U, Sonne-Holm S, Lauridsen F, et al. Long-term follow-up of meniscectomy in athletes a prospective longitudinal study. *Journal of Bone and Joint Surgery (British)* 1987;**69**:80–3.
40. Hede A, Svalastoga E, Reimann I. Articular cartilage changes following meniscal lesions. Repair and meniscectomy studied in the rabbit knee. *Acta Orthopaedica Scandinavica* 1991;**62**:319–22.
41. Henning CE, Lynch MA. Current concepts of meniscal function and pathology. *Clinics in Sports Medicine* 1985;**4**:259–65.
42. Krause WR, Pope MH, Johnson RJ, et al. Mechanical changes in the knee after meniscectomy. *Journal of Bone and Joint Surgery (American)* 1976;**58**:599–604.
43. Baratz ME, Fu FH, Mengato R. Meniscal tears: the effect of meniscectomy and of repair on intraarticular contact areas and stress in the human knee. A preliminary report. *American Journal of Sports Medicine* 1986;**14**:270–5.
44. Jones RE, Smith EC, Reisch JS. Effects of medial meniscectomy in patients older than forty years. *Journal of Bone and Joint Surgery (American)* 1978;**60**:783–6.
45. Arnoczky S. Gross and vascular anatomy of the meniscus and its role in meniscal healing. In: Mow VC, Arnoczky S, Jackson D (eds) *Knee Meniscus: Basic and Clinical Foundations*. New York, NY: Raven Press, 1992:1–14.
46. Mow VC. Structure and function relationships of the meniscus in the knee. In: Mow VC, Arnoczky S, Jackson D (eds) *Knee Meniscus: Basic and Clinical Foundations*. New York, NY: Raven Press, 1992:37–58.
47. Thompson WD, Thaete FL, Fu FH, et al. Tibial meniscal dynamics using three-dimensional reconstruction of magnetic resonance images. *American Journal of Sports Medicine* 1991;**19**:210–15.
48. Shapeero LB, Dye SF, Lipton MJ, et al. Functional dynamics of the knee joint by ultrafast, cine CT. *Investigative Radiology* 1988;**23**:118–23.
49. Voloshin AS, Wosk J. Shock absorption of meniscectomized and painful knees: a comparative in vivo study. *Journal of Biomedical Engineering* 1983;**5**:157–61.
50. Herwig J, Egner E, Buddecke E. Chemical changes of the human knee joint menisci in various stages of degeneration. *Annals of the Rheumatic Diseases* 1984;**43**:635–40.
51. Arnoczky SP, Warren RF. The microvasculature of the meniscus and its response to injury. An experimental study in the dog. *American Journal of Sports Medicine* 1983;**11**:131–41.
52. Cabaud HE, Rodkey WG, Fitzwater JE. Medical meniscus repairs. An experimental and morphologic study. *American Journal of Sports Medicine* 1981;**9**:129–34.
53. Webber RJ, Harris MG, Hough Jr AJ. Cell culture of rabbit meniscal fibrochondrocytes: proliferative and synthetic response to growth factors and ascorbate. *Journal of Orthopaedic Research* 1985;**3**:36–42.
54. Cannon WD, Vittori J. Meniscal repair. In: Aichroth P, Cannon WD (eds) *Knee Surgery: Current Practice*. New York, NY: Raven Press, 1992:71–84.
55. Weiss CB, Lundeberg M, Hamberg P, et al. Non-operative treatment of meniscal tears. *Journal of Bone and Joint Surgery (American)* 1989;**71**:811–21.
56. Dehaven KE, Arnoczky SP. Meniscal repair. Part I. Basic science, indications for repair, and open repair. *Journal of Bone and Joint Surgery (American)* 1994;**76**:140–52.
57. Turman KA, Diduch DR. Meniscal repair: indications and techniques. *Journal of Knee Surgery* 2008;**21**:154–62.

58. DeHaven KE, Stone R. Meniscal repair. In: Shahriaree H (ed.) *O'Connor's Textbook of Arthroscopic Surgery*. Philadelphia, PA: Lippincott, 1983:327–38.
59. Henning CE. Current status of meniscal salvage. *Clinics in Sports Medicine* 1990;**9**:567–76.
60. Barber F. Accelerated rehabilitation for meniscus repairs. *Arthroscopy* 1994;**10**:206–10.
61. Barber F, Click SD. Meniscus repair rehabilitation with concurrent anterior cruciate reconstruction. *Arthroscopy* 1997;**13**:433–7.
62. DeHaven KE, Lohrer WA, Lovelock JE. Long-term results of open meniscal repair. *American Journal of Sports Medicine* 1995;**23**:524–30.
63. Eggli S, Wegmueller H, Kosina J, *et al*. Long-term results of arthroscopic meniscal repair. An analysis of isolated tears. *American Journal of Sports Medicine* 1995;**23**:715–20.
64. Chang HC, The KL, Leong KL, *et al*. Clinical evaluation of arthroscopic-assisted allograft meniscal transplantation. *Annals of the Academy of Medicine Singapore* 2008;**37**:266–72.
65. Fox JM, Rintz KG, Ferkel RD. Trephination of incomplete meniscal tears. *Arthroscopy* 1993;**9**:451–5.
66. Canham W, Stanish W. A study of the biological behavior of the meniscus as a transplant in the medial compartment of a dog's knee. *American Journal of Sports Medicine* 1986;**14**:376–9.
67. Milachowski KA, Weismeier K, Wirth CJ. Homologous meniscus transplantation. Experimental and clinical results. *International Orthopaedics* 1989;**13**:1–11.
68. Goble EM, Kohn D, Verdonk R, *et al*. Meniscal substitutes: human experience. *Scandinavian Journal of Medicine and Science in Sports* 1999;**9**:146–57.
69. Wada Y, Amiel M, Harwood F, *et al*. Architectural remodeling in deep frozen meniscal allografts after total meniscectomy. *Arthroscopy* 1998;**14**:250–7.
70. Jackson DW, McDevitt CA, Simon TM, *et al*. Meniscal transplantation using fresh and cryopreserved allografts. An experimental study in goats. *American Journal of Sports Medicine* 1992;**20**:644–56.
71. Stoeckelhuber M, Brueckner S, Spohr G, *et al*. Proteoglycans and collagen in the intervertebral disc of the rhesus monkey (*Macaca mulatta*). *Annals of Anatomy* 2005;**187**:35–42.
72. Houben GB, Drost MR, Huyghe JM, *et al*. Nonhomogeneous permeability of canine annulus fibrosus. *Spine* 2007;**22**:7–16.
73. Bibby SR, Jones DA, Lee RB, *et al*. The pathophysiology of the intervertebral disc. *Joint, Bone, Spine* 2001;**68**:537–42.
74. Culav EM, Clark CH, Merrilees MJ. Connective tissues: matrix composition and its relevance to physical therapy. *Physical Therapy* 1999;**79**:308–19.
75. Eyre DR, Matsui Y, Wu JJ. Collagen polymorphisms of the intervertebral disc. *Biochemical Society Transactions* 2002;**30**:844–8.
76. Urban JP, Maroudas A, Bayliss MT, *et al*. Swelling pressures of proteoglycans at the concentrations found in cartilaginous tissues. *Biorheology* 1979;**16**:447–64.
77. Prescher A. Anatomy and pathology of the aging spine. *European Journal of Radiology* 1998;**27**:181–95.
78. Skaggs DL, Weidenbaum M, Iatridis JC. Regional variation in tensile properties and biochemical composition of the human lumbar annulus fibrosus. *Spine* 1994;**19**:1310–19.
79. Urban JP, Smith S, Fairbank J. Nutrition of the intervertebral disc. *Spine* 2004;**29**:2700–9.
80. Nerlich GA, Schleicher E, Boos N. Immunohistologic markers for age-related changes of human lumbar intervertebral discs. *Spine* 1997;**22**:2781–95.
81. Roughley PJ. Biology of intervertebral disc aging and degeneration: involvement of the extracellular matrix. *Spine* 2004;**29**:2691–9.
82. Urban JP, Roberts SR. Degeneration of the intervertebral disc. *Arthritis Research & Therapy* 2003;**5**(63):120–30.
83. Berlemann U, Gries NC, Moore RJ. The relationship between height, shape and histological changes in early degeneration of the lower lumbar discs. *European Spine Journal* 1998;**7**:212–17.
84. Wognum S, Huyghe JM, Baaijens FP. Influence of osmotic pressure changes on the opening of existing cracks in 2 intervertebral disc models. *Spine* 2006;**31**:1783–8.
85. Jordon J, Konstantinou K, Shawver Morgan T, *et al*. Herniated lumbar disk. *Clinical Evidence Concise* 2005;**14**:366–8.
86. Deyo RA, Weinstein JN. Low back pain. *New England Journal of Medicine* 2001;**344**:365–70.
87. Cribb GL, Jaffray DC, Cassar-Pullicino VN. Observations on the natural history of massive lumbar disc herniation. *Journal of Bone and Joint Surgery (British)* 2007;**89**:782–4.
88. Jonsson B, Stromqvist B. Repeat decompression of lumbar nerve roots. A prospective two-year evaluation. *Journal of Bone and Joint Surgery (British)* 1993;**75**:894–7.
89. Erbayraktar S, Acar F, Tekinsoy B, *et al*. Outcome analysis of reoperations after lumbar discectomies: a report of 22 patients. *Kobe Journal of Medical Sciences* 2002;**48**(1–2):33–41.
90. Ahlgren BD, Lui W, Herkowitz HN, *et al*. Effect of annular repair on the healing strength of the intervertebral disc: a sheep model. *Spine* 2000;**25**:2165–70.
91. Wang YH, Kuo TF, Wang JL. The implantation of non-cell-based materials to prevent the recurrent disc herniation: an in vivo porcine model using quantitative discomanometry examination. *European Spine Journal* 2007;**16**:1021–7.
92. Ruan D, He Q, Ding Y, *et al*. Intervertebral disc transplantation in the treatment of degenerative spine disease: a preliminary study. *Lancet* 2007;**369**:993–9.
93. Abbushi A, Endres M, Cabraja M, *et al*. Regeneration of intervertebral disc tissue by resorbable cell-free polyglycolic acid-based implants in a rabbit model of disc degeneration. *Spine* 2008;**33**:1527–32.
94. Garrett Jr WE, Best TM. Anatomy, physiology, and mechanics of skeletal muscle. In: Simon SR (ed.) *Orthopaedic Basic Science*. Rosemont, IL: American Academy of Orthopaedic Surgeons, 1994:89–125.
95. Stewart CE, Rittweger J. Adaptive processes in skeletal muscle: molecular regulators and genetic influences. *Journal of Musculoskeletal and Neuronal Interactions* 2006;**6**:73–86.

96. Bischoff R. The satellite cell and muscle regeneration. In: Engel AG, Franzini-Armstrong C (eds) *Myology. Basic and Clinical*. New York, NY: McGraw-Hill, 1994:97–118.
97. Hurme T, Kalimo H. Activation of myogenic precursor cells after muscle injury. *Medicine and Science in Sports and Exercise* 1992;**24**:197–205.
98. Katz B, Miledi R. The timing of calcium action during neuromuscular transmission. *Journal of Physiology* 1967;**189**:535–44.
99. Huard J, Li Y, Fu FH. Muscle injuries and repair: current trends in research. *Journal of Bone and Joint Surgery (American)* 2002;**84A**:822–32.
100. Greaser ML, Gergely J. Reconstitution of troponin activity from three protein components. *Journal of Biological Chemistry* 1971;**246**:4226–33.
101. Gordon AM, Homsher E, Regnier M. Regulation of contraction in striated muscle. *Physiological Reviews* 2000;**80**:853–924.
102. Andersen JL, Schjerling P, Saltin B. Muscle, genes and athletic performance. *Scientific American* 2000;**283**:48–55.
103. Menetrey J, Kasemkijwattana C, Day CS, et al. Growth factors improve muscle healing in vivo. *Journal of Bone and Joint Surgery (British)* 2000;**82**:131–7.
104. Nikolaou PK, Macdonald BL, Glisson RR, et al. Biomechanical and histological evaluation of muscle after controlled strain injury. *American Journal of Sports Medicine* 1987;**15**:9–14.
105. Jarvinen TA, Kaariainen M, Jarvinen M, et al. Muscle strain injuries. *Current Opinion in Rheumatology* 2000;**12**:155–61.
106. Kasemkijwattana C, Menetrey J, Day CS, et al. Biologic intervention in muscle healing and regeneration. *Sports Medicine and Arthroscopy Review* 1998;**6**:95–102.
107. Best TM, Fiebig R, Corr DT, et al. Free radical activity, antioxidant enzyme, and glutathione changes with muscle stretch injury in rabbits. *Journal of Applied Physiology* 1999;**87**:74–82.
108. Lille ST, Lefler SR, Mowlavi A, et al. Inhibition of the initial wave of NF-kappaB activity in rat muscle reduces ischemia/reperfusion injury. *Muscle and Nerve* 2001;**24**:534–41.
109. St Pierre BA, Tidball JG. Differential response of macrophage subpopulations to soleus muscle reloading after rat hindlimb suspension. *Journal of Applied Physiology* 1994;**77**:290–7.
110. Supinski GS, Callahan LA. Free radical-mediated skeletal muscle dysfunction in inflammatory conditions. *Journal of Applied Physiology* 2007;**102**:2056–63.
111. Hurme T, Kalimo H, Lehto H, et al. Healing of skeletal muscle injury: an ultrastructural and immunohistochemical study. *Medicine and Science in Sports and Exercise* 1991;**23**:801–10.
112. Honda H, Kimura H, Rostami A. Demonstration and phenotypic characterization of resident macrophages in rat skeletal muscle. *Immunology* 1990;**70**:272–7.
113. Aronson D, Wojtaszewski JF, Thorell A. Extracellular-regulated protein kinase cascades are activated in response to injury in human skeletal muscle. *American Journal of Physiology* 1998;**275**(2 Pt 1):555–61.
114. Pimorady-Esfahani A, Grounds MD, McMenamin PG. Macrophages and dendritic cells in normal and regenerating murine skeletal muscle. *Muscle and Nerve* 1997;**20**:158–66.
115. Tidball JG. Inflammatory cell response to acute muscle injury. *Medicine and Science in Sports and Exercise* 1995;**27**:1022–32.
116. Cannon JG, St Pierre BA. Cytokines in exertion-induced skeletal muscle injury. *Molecular and Cellular Biochemistry* 1998;**179**:159–67.
117. Altstaedt J, Kirchner H, Rink L. Cytokine production of neutrophils is limited to interleukin-8. *Immunology* 1996;**89**:563–8.
118. Hurme T, Kalimo H. Activation of myogenic precursor cells after muscle injury. *Medicine and Science in Sports and Exercise* 1992;**24**:197–205.
119. Best TM, Hunter KD. Muscle injury and repair. *Physical Medicine and Rehabilitation Clinics of North America* 2000;**11**:251–66.
120. Li Y, Cummins J, Huard J. Muscle injury and repair. *Current Opinion in Orthopaedics* 2001;**12**:409–15.
121. Russell B, Dix DJ, Haller DL, et al. Repair of injured skeletal muscle: a molecular approach. *Medicine and Science in Sports and Exercise* 1992;**24**:189–96.
122. Best TM, Garrett WE. Basic science of soft tissue: muscle and tendon. In: DeLee JC, Drez D (eds) *Orthopaedic Sports Medicine*. Philadelphia, PA: W.B. Saunders, 1994:1–45.
123. Benjamin M, Ralphs J. Functional and developmental anatomy of tendons and ligaments. In: Gordon SL, Blair SJ, Fine LJ (eds) *Repetitive Motion Disorders of the Upper Extremity*. Rosemont, IL: American Academy of Orthopaedic Surgeons, 1995:185–203.
124. Kannus P, Jozsa L, Jarvinnen M. Basic science of tendons. In: Garrett WJ, Speer K, Kirkendall DT (eds) *Principles and Practice of Orthopaedic Sports Medicine*. Philadelphia, PA: Lippincott Williams and Wilkins, 2000:21–37.
125. O'Brien M. Structure and metabolism of tendons. *Scandinavian Journal of Medicine and Science in Sports* 1997;**7**:55–61.
126. Hess GP, Cappiello WL, Poole RM, Hunter SC. Prevention and treatment of overuse tendon injuries. *Sports Medicine* 1989;**8**:371–84.
127. Jozsa L, Lehto M, Kannus P, et al. Fibronectin and laminin in Achilles tendon. *Acta Orthopaedica Scandinavica* 1989;**60**:469–71.
128. Tipton CM, Matthes RD, Maynard JA, et al. The influence of physical activity on ligaments and tendons. *Medicine and Science in Sports* 1975;**7**:165–75.
129. Kirkendall DT, Garrett WE. Function and biomechanics of tendons. *Scandinavian Journal of Medicine and Science in Sports* 1997;**7**:62–6.

130. Jozsa L, Kannus P. *Human Tendons: Anatomy, Physiology and Pathology.* Champaign, IL: Human Kinetics, 1997.
131. Movin T, Kristoffersen-Wiberg M, Shalabi A, et al. Intratendinous alterations as imaged by ultrasound and contrast medium-enhanced magnetic resonance in chronic achillodynia. *Foot and Ankle International* 1998;**19**:311–17.
132. Jozsa L, Kannus P, Balint JB, et al. Three-dimensional ultrastructure of human tendons. *Acta Anatomica* 1991;**142**:306–12.
133. Balint BJ, Jozsa L. [Investigation on the construction and spatial structure of human tendons.] *Magyar Traumatológia Orthopaedia és Helyreállító Sebészet* 1978;**21**:293–9.
134. Hueston JT, Wilson WF. The aetiology of trigger finger explained on the basis of intratendinous architecture. *Hand* 1972;**4**:257–60.
135. Lawler J. The structural and functional properties of thrombospondin. *Blood* 1986;**67**:1197–209.
136. Miller RR, McDevitt CA. Thrombospondin in ligament, meniscus and intervertebral disc. *Biochimica et Biophysica Acta* 1991;**1115**:85–8.
137. Elliott D. Structure and function of mammalian tendon. *Biological Reviews of the Cambridge Philosophical Society* 1965;**40**:392.
138. Kastelic J, Galeski A, Baer E. The multicomposite structure of tendon. *Connective Tissue Research* 1978;**6**:11–23.
139. Kvist M, Jozsa L, Jarvinen M, et al. Fine structural alterations in chronic Achilles paratendonitis in athletes. *Pathology, Research and Practice* 1985;**180**:416–23.
140. Kvist M, Jozsa L, Kannus P, et al. Morphology and histochemistry of the myotendineal junction of the rat calf muscles. Histochemical, immunohistochemical and electron-microscopic study. *Acta Anatomica (Basel)* 1991;**141**:199–205.
141. Michna H. A peculiar myofibrillar pattern in the murine muscle-tendon junction. *Cell and Tissue Research* 1983;**233**:227–31.
142. Trotter JA, Baca JM. A stereological comparison of the muscle-tendon junctions of fast and slow fibers in the chicken. *Anatomical Record (Hoboken, NJ)* 1987;**218**:256–66.
143. Tidball JG. Myotendinous junction of tonic muscle cells: structure and loading. *Cell and Tissue Research* 1986;**245**:315.
144. Tidball JG. Myotendinous junction injury in relation to junction structure and molecular composition. *Exercise and Sports Sciences Reviews* 1991;**19**:419–45.
145. Nikolaou PK, Macdonald BL, Glisson RR, et al. Biomechanical and histological evaluation of muscle after controlled strain injury. *American Journal of Sports Medicine* 1987;**15**:9–14.
146. Garrett WE. Muscle strain injuries: clinical and basic aspects. *Medicine and Science in Sports and Exercise* 1990;**22**:436–43.
147. Jarvinen M, Kannus P, Kvist M, et al. Macromolecular composition of the myotendinous junction. *Experimental and Molecular Pathology* 1991;**55**:230–7.
148. Benjamin M, Ralphs JR. Fibrocartilage in tendons and ligaments – an adaptation to compressive load. *Journal of Anatomy* 1998;**193**:481–94.
149. Benjamin M, Qin S, Ralphs JR. Fibrocartilage associated with human tendons and their pulleys. *Journal of Anatomy* 1995;**187**:625–33.
150. Evans EJ, Benjamin M, Pemberton DJ. Fibrocartilage in the attachment zones of the quadriceps tendon and patellar ligament of man. *Journal of Anatomy* 1990;**171**:155–62.
151. Carr AJ, Norris SH. The blood supply of the calcaneal tendon. *Journal of Bone and Joint Surgery (British)* 1989;**71**:100–1.
152. Niculescu V, Matusz P. The clinical importance of the calcaneal tendon vasculature (tendo calcaneus). *Morphologie et Embryologie* 1988;**34**:5–8.
153. Leversedge FJ, Ditsios K, Goldfarb CA, et al. Vascular anatomy of the human flexor digitorum profundus tendon insertion. *Journal of Hand Surgery* 2002;**27**:806–12.
154. Brodal A (ed.). *Neurological Anatomy in Relation to Clinical Medicine.* New York, NY: Oxford University Press, 1981.
155. Barr ML, Kiernan JA (eds). *The Human Nervous System: an Anatomical Viewpoint.* Philadelphia, PA: Lippincott, 1988.
156. O'Brien M. Functional anatomy and physiology of tendons. *Clinics in Sports Medicine* 1992;**11**:505.
157. Oxlund H. Relationships between the biomechanical properties, composition and molecular structure of connective tissues. *Connective Tissue Research* 1986;**15**(1–2):65–72.
158. Curwin SL, Stanish WD (eds). *Tendinitis: its Etiology and Treatment.* Lexington, KT: Collamore Press, 1984.
159. Butler DL, Grood ES, Noyes FR, Zernicke RF. Biomechanics of ligaments and tendons. *Exercise and Sport Sciences Reviews* 1978;**6**:125–81.
160. Kastelic J, Baer E. Deformation in tendon collagen. *Symposia of the Society for Experimental Biology* 1980;**34**:397–435.
161. Selvanetti A, Cipolla M, Puddu G. Overuse tendon injuries: basic science and classification. *Operative Techniques in Sports Medicine* 1997;**5**:110–17.
162. Benazzo F, Maffulli N. An operative approach to Achilles tendinopathy. *Sports Medicine and Arthroscopy Review* 2000;**8**:96–101.
163. Ker RF. The implications of the adaptable fatigue quality of tendons for their construction, repair and function. *Comparative Biochemistry and Physiology. Part A. Molecular and Integrative Physiology* 2002;**133**:987–1000.
164. Leadbetter WB. Cell-matrix response in tendon injury. *Clinics in Sports Medicine* 1992;**11**:533–78.
165. Arndt AN, Komi PV, Bruggemann GP, et al. Individual muscle contributions to the in vivo Achilles tendon force. *Clinical Biomechanics* 1998;**13**:532–41.
166. Sharma P, Maffulli N. Tendon injury and tendinopathy: healing and repair. *Journal of Bone and Joint Surgery (American)* 2005;**87**:187–202.
167. Kannus P, Jozsa L. Histopathological changes preceding spontaneous rupture of a tendon. A controlled study of 891 patients. *Journal of Bone and Joint Surgery (American)* 1991;**73**:1507–25.

168. Vailas AC, Tipton CM, Laughlin HL, et al. Physical activity and hypophysectomy on the aerobic capacity of ligaments and tendons. *Journal of Applied Physiology* 1978;**44**:542–46.
169. Murphy PG, Loitz CB, Frank CB, et al. Influence of exogenous growth factors on the synthesis and secretion of collagen types I and III by explants of normal and healing rabbit ligaments. *Biochemistry and Cell Biology* 1994;**72**:403–9.
170. Pierce GF, Mustoe TA, Lingelbach J, et al. Platelet derived growth factor and transforming growth factor-β enhance tissue repair activities by unique mechanisms. *Journal of Cell Biology* 1989;**109**:429–40.
171. Oakes BW. Tissue healing and repair: tendons and ligaments. In: Frontera WR (ed.) *Rehabilitation of Sports Injuries: Scientific Basis*. Oxford, UK: Blackwell Science, 2003:56–98.
172. Tillman LJ, Chasan NP. Properties of dense connective tissue and wound healing. In: Hertling D, Kessler RM (eds) *Management of Common Musculoskeletal Disorders*. Philadelphia, PA: Lippincott Williams and Wilkins, 1996:8–21.
173. Hooley CJ, Cohen RE. A model for the creep behaviour of tendon. *International Journal of Biological Macromolecules* 1979;**1**:123–32.
174. Abrahamsson SO. Matrix metabolism and healing in the flexor tendon. Experimental studies on rabbit tendon. *Scandinavian Journal of Plastic and Reconstructive Surgery and Hand Surgery* 1991;**23**(Suppl.):1–51.
175. Farkas LG, McCain WG, Sweeney P, et al. An experimental study of changes following silastic rod preparation of new tendon sheath and subsequent tendon grafting. *Journal of Bone and Joint Surgery (American)* 1973;**55**:149–58.
176. Amiel D, Akeson W, Harwood FL, et al. Stress deprivation effect on metabolic turnover of medial collateral ligament collagen. *Clinical Orthopaedics and Related Research* 1987;**172**:25–7.
177. Koob TJ. Biomimetic approaches to tendon repair. *Comparative Biochemistry and Physiology. Part A. Molecular and Integrative Physiology* 2002;**133**:1171–92.
178. Vu TH, Werb Z. Matrix metalloproteinases: effectors of development and normal physiology. *Genes and Development* 2000;**14**:2123–33.
179. Birkedal-Hansen H. Proteolytic remodeling of extracellular matrix. *Current Opinion in Cell Biology* 1995;**7**:728–35.
180. Ireland D, Harrall R, Curry V, et al. Multiple changes in gene expression in chronic human Achilles tendinopathy. *Matrix Biology* 2001;**20**:159–69.
181. Evans CH. Cytokines and the role they play in the healing of ligaments and tendons. *Sports Medicine* 1999;**28**:71–6.
182. Sciore P, Boykiw R, Hart DA. Semiquantitative reverse transcription-polymerase chain reaction analysis of mRNA for growth factors and growth factor receptors from normal and healing rabbit medial collateral ligament tissue. *Journal of Orthopaedic Research* 1998;**16**:429–37.
183. Chang J, Most D, Stelnicki E, et al. Gene expression of transforming growth factor beta-1 in rabbit zone II flexor tendon wound healing: evidence for dual mechanisms of repair. *Plastic and Reconstructive Surgery* 1997;**100**:937–44.
184. Chang J, Most D, Thunder R, et al. Molecular studies in flexor tendon wound healing: the role of basic fibroblast growth factor gene expression. *Journal of Hand Surgery* 1998;**23A**:1052–8.
185. Woo SL, Hildebrand K, Watanabe N, et al. Tissue engineering of ligaments and tendon healing. *Clinical Orthopaedics and Related Research* 1999;**367**:S312–23.
186. Natsuume T, Nakamura N, Shino K, et al. Temporal and spatial expression of transforming growth factor-beta in the healing patellar ligament of the rat. *Journal of Orthopaedic Research* 1997;**15**:837.
187. Marui T, Niyibizi C, Georgescu HI, et al. Effect of growth factors on matrix synthesis by ligament fibroblasts. *Journal of Orthopaedic Research* 1997;**15**:18–23.
188. Abrahamsson SO, Lohmander S. Differential effects of insulin-like growth factor-I on matrix and DNA synthesis in various regions and types of rabbit tendons. *Journal of Orthopaedic Research* 1996;**14**:370–6.
189. Murray MM, Martin SD, Martin TL, et al. Histological changes in the human anterior cruciate ligament after rupture. *Journal of Bone and Joint Surgery (American)* 2000;**82**:1387–97.
190. Frank C, Amiel D, Akeson WH. Healing of the medial collateral ligament of the knee. A morphological and biochemical assessment in rabbits. *Acta Orthopaedica Scandinavica* 1983;**54**:917–23.
191. Andersen RB, Gormsen J. Fibrin dissolution in synovial fluid. *Acta Rheumatologica Scandinavica* 1970;**16**:319–33.
192. Harrold AJ. The defect of blood coagulation in joints. *Journal of Clinical Pathology* 1961;**14**:305–8.
193. Kvist M, Hurme T, Kannus P, et al. Vascular density at the myotendinous junction of the rat gastrocnemius muscle after immobilization and remobilization. *American Journal of Sports Medicine* 1995;**23**:359–64.
194. Sharma P, Maffulli N. Tendinopathy and tendon injury: The future. *Disability and Rehabilitation* 2008;**9**:1–13.

8

The physiology of ageing

MARCO V. NARICI, FILIPPO SPIEZIA, NICOLA MAFFULLI

Introduction	120	References	123
The physiology of ageing	120		

NATIONAL BOARD STANDARDS

- Understand that older patients will form a significant part of your workload in the years to come
- Understand the pathophysiology of tendon and ligament disorders in the older patient group
- Know the pathophysiology of osteoporosis and its management guidelines
- Know about DXA scan, Z-score, T-score

INTRODUCTION

As we go into the second decade of the twenty-first century human beings are living longer and healthier lives. Many of the patients you see in your daily practice will be from the 'baby boomer' generation, which is only now contemplating retirement. Most of these individuals will tell you that '70 is the new 50!' Which is why this textbook devotes an entire chapter to ageing and the science and art of treating this group of patients.

The process of ageing is intrinsic to human beings, and should be considered not pathological, but innate to our genetic design.[1] The rate of ageing is highly individual and depends on many factors, including genetics, lifestyle and former disease processes.[2] Tendons, bones and muscles are involved in the ageing process. In this century, the proportion of elderly citizens will overcome that of young people, hence a full understanding of the muscle, tendon and bone changes associated with old age is essential to combat physical frailty in old age and maintain an active role in life. This chapter discusses some of the processes associated with ageing.

THE PHYSIOLOGY OF AGEING

The degenerative changes associated with ageing may be present at the third decade in musculoskeletal and cardiovascular systems.[3,4] Tendons are also subjected to early degenerative changes. The collagen and non-collagenous matrix components of tendons show qualitative and quantitative changes, and many cellular and vascular changes may happen in the ageing tendon. Hence, aged tendon is weaker than its younger counterpart.[5] Given these degenerative changes, an aged tendon is more prone to injury.[5] Changes at the cellular level consist in tenoblasts, which may become tenocytes, and the volume density of these cells may be decreased. The number of tendon cells per unit of surface area is also decreased. Qualitative changes of the tendon cells have been shown as they become longer, more slender, and more uniform in shape.[6,7] The nucleus-to-cytoplasm ratio increases. The metabolic activity of tenoblasts is impaired in ageing, and the healing process is likely to be less effective. The metabolic pathway shifts from aerobic to more anaerobic.[8] Extracellular changes are also detected in ageing tendons. The extracellular matrix is composed of collagen and non-collagenous components. These may show qualitative and quantitative changes. The proteoglycan and glycoprotein content decreases, even though the collagen content remains unchanged. The extracellular water content of a tendon is also decreased.[8] The ageing process also involves collagen. Collagen turnover and synthesis diminish.[9] Changes in the collagen cross-linking profile impair mechanical properties and are considered biomarkers of ageing. The increase in the number of cross-links may be responsible for an increased resistance to degradative enzymes, reduced solubility of collagen, increased stability to thermal denaturation, and increased mechanical stiffness.[10,2,11] Elastic fibres show quantitative and qualitative changes in ageing tendons.[9] Synthesis of fibrillar glycoproteins is increased and has been associated with partial degeneration of elastin by tissue elastases.[12] The extracellular water content and mucopolysaccharide content is decreased.[6,2] Vascular supply and hence nutrition to tendons are decreased.[13]

In ageing tendons, tensile strength is decreased and also other parameters of mechanical properties of the tendon may be impaired, such as the ultimate strain, ultimate load, modulus of elasticity, and tensile strength, and there may be an increase in mechanical stiffness.[14]

Accumulations of lipids, ground substance (glycosaminoglycans) and calcium deposits have been shown in aged tendons.[9]

The term 'sarcopenia' was proposed for the first time by Rosenberg in 1989. It indicates the loss of muscle mass associated with ageing. A common definition of sarcopenia[15] is based on a skeletal muscle mass index obtained by dividing the appendicular skeletal muscle mass (ASM), evaluated by dual-emission X-ray absorptiometry (DXA), by height squared (ASM/h^2). According to this definition, individuals presenting an ASM/h^2 ratio of sarcopenia between −1 and −2 standard deviations (SD) of the gender-specific mean value of young control subjects are categorized as having class I sarcopenia, and those with an ASM/h^2 ratio below −2 SD are categorized as having class II sarcopenia.

The total lean body mass declines by about 15% in men and by 18% in women from the second to the eighth decade of life. Women have a considerably smaller muscle mass than men at all ages. However, the decline in lean body mass becomes detectable after the age of 45 years because the total body mass increases from 18 to 40 years whereas skeletal muscle mass remains constant.

Both men and women lose about 24–27% of muscle mass (or volume since muscle has a density of 1.056 g cm^{-3}) between the second and seventh decade.[16] Some conditions may accelerate the process of sarcopenia, such as disuse, disease or anorexia. If the muscle mass decreases too much, women more than men risk losing independence and spending the last years of life under institutional care. 'Myosteatosis' indicates infiltration of fat and connective tissue in the muscles and can be associated with sarcopenia, as has been shown by imaging studies.[17–24] Hence, muscle mass is smaller than that measured by a simple muscle cross-sectional area (CSA).[23]

The amount of intramuscular fat and connective tissue seems to be inversely related to the level of physical activity.[23] When sarcopenia is combined with obesity in older people it is called sarcopenic obesity (SO). This can be defined as a ASM/h^2 ratio less than 2 SD below the sex-specific mean of a younger reference group and as a percentage of body fat greater than 27% in men and 38% in women. Studies imply chronic inflammation as a mechanism for stimulating insulin resistance and all the abnormalities also known as 'metabolic syndrome'. Loss of muscle mass associated with sarcopenia promotes insulin resistance and this may start a vicious circle, resulting in further loss of muscle mass and mobility, insulin resistance and risk of metabolic syndrome development.[25]

The sarcopenic shows changes in muscle fibre size (atrophy), number (hypoplasia) and composition. In contrast, disuse atrophy involves a decrease in fibre size but not the number. Type II fibres are more vulnerable to atrophy than type I fibres in the ageing process.[26–28] Studies showed that in old people the areas occupied by type I and type II fibres were smaller than those found in young subjects,[29,27,30] but in all cases type II fibre was more damaged than type I fibre.[31,15,32]

Morphological and electrophysiological studies have shown changes in fibre number associated with ageing.[33,30] Motor unit (MU) number remained fairly constant up to the sixth decade but from 60 to 80 years of age it declined by 50%.[34,28] With ageing loss of muscle fibres occurs, but this loss has a different pattern for each muscle fibre type and is greater for type II fibres up to the late 70s and past 80 years. Type I fibres are also lost and a new 'balance' between the two types of fibres is reached, as suggested by the finding of a similar type I/II fibre ratio in individuals aged 85–97 years.[31]

Sarcopenia is characterized by the reduction in muscle cross-sectional area and volume, and remodelling of the muscle architecture. The muscle architecture determines the mechanical characteristics of muscle, namely the length–force (L–F) and the force–velocity (F–V) relationships.[35] The maximum shortening velocity depends on the number of sarcomeres placed in series and on fibre length. Ultrasound imaging shows that both the length of muscle fibre fascicles and their angle of insertion into the tendon aponeurosis (angle of pennation) decrease with ageing.[36,37] The decrease in fascicle length is related to the loss of sarcomeres in series and causes loss of muscle-shortening velocity. A decrease in the pennation angle reflects a loss of sarcomeres in parallel, hence in muscle CSA and thus in muscle force-generating potential.[38]

Sarcopenia is caused by different alterations in the central and peripheral nervous systems, and in hormonal, nutritional, immunological and physical activity changes. Neuropathic processes are responsible for α-motor neurone degeneration and muscle fibre denervation, resulting in a loss of motor units.[39] Denervated type II muscle fibres are reinnervated through axonal sprouting from type I fibres.[40–43] This may produce a motor unit with a very large action potential. This could probably be a mechanism of compensation against the loss of force because it increases the innervation ratio of the affected motor units, even though fine control of force during motor unit recruitment is decreased. The degenerative changes of the nervous system damage the neuromuscular junction. Degenerative changes of the neuromuscular system may also damage the muscle cell itself, because apoptosis of skeletal myocytes seems to contribute to sarcopenia.[44] Mitochondrial dysfunction and sarcoplasmic reticulum stress could induce apoptosis of skeletal muscle cells and reactive oxygen species (ROS), which may trigger these events.[45,46]

Age-related muscle atrophy is characterized by reduction in fibre size, probably due to a decrease in satellite cell proliferation. Levels of growth factors such as insulin-like growth factor 6, as well as a reduction in mechanical stimuli due to decreased physical activity may be related to muscle atrophy. Recent studies have shown that older people (70–79 years) are about 20% less active than individuals aged 20–29 years.[47] Nutritional, hormonal and immunological factors have been associated with sarcopenia. Malnutrition is common in older people due to appetite loss and reduction in food intake. Lower levels of vitamin D are associated with high parathyroid hormone levels and have been related to increase the risk of muscle wasting in old age.[48] No significant difference has been shown in protein breakdown and synthesis between younger and older individuals,[49–53] only in protein synthesis in response to feeding and exercise. Older people show a lower increase in muscle protein synthesis in response to amino acid feeding under insulin clamping conditions,[50] and also in response to acute exercise activity. Sarcopenia seems also to be related to a reduced sensitivity to the inhibitory effect of insulin on protein breakdown.[54]

What are the functional consequences of sarcopenia? The decline in muscle power with increasing age[55] is 3–4% per year. Isometric force decline is 1–2% per year.[56]

A difference of 40% in isometric force and a difference of 60% in peak power have been reported between older people and young controls.[38] The loss of muscle strength and power exceeds that of muscle size and volume (force depends on muscle cross-sectional area, whereas power depends on muscle volume). Consequently, a decline in force per unit of muscle cross-sectional area and in peak power per unit volume have be reported by some authors.[18,26,57,47,58,59] This may be caused by deterioration in muscle quality, which comprehends neuromuscular and tendinous changes. Reduction in single fibre force per cross-sectional area (specific tension) is associated with the decline in intrinsic muscle force. Recently the association between reduction in single fibre force per cross-sectional area and decrease in the number of actomyosin cross-bridges has been shown.[60] Loss in shortening velocity in old age depends on selective loss of fast twitch fibres (whose power is about 10 times higher than that of slow fibres)[61] and on the reduction in the intrinsic speed of shortening of the myosin molecule.[62]

Reduction in neural drive to the agonist muscles and an increase in neural drive to the antagonist muscles have been reported in older people.[17,63–65] Motor unit recruitment and firing frequency have been also found to be reduced in older adults.[44,105] An increased co-activation of antagonist muscles has also been suggested as a possible mechanism for the loss of force with ageing.[66,67]

Osteoporosis is a systemic skeletal disorder characterized by low bone mass and microarchitectural deterioration of bone tissue, with a consequent increase in bone fragility and susceptibility to fracture.[2] Osteoporosis is common in older men and women,[68,69] and is often under-recognized and undertreated. It is common for an older osteoporotic person to fall[70] resulting in a fracture, which then has a high risk of mortality.[71] Those who survive after fractures may be disabled for the rest of their life.[72] The risk of osteoporotic fractures increases with ageing.[73] Fractures in elderly individuals are due in the most part to reduced bone mass. Risk factors for developing osteoporosis are insufficient bone mass at the time of skeletal maturity and rapid loss of bone after the menopause in women, but also low body weight, recent weight loss, history of fractures, family history of fractures and smoking.[74]

Bone remodelling allows replacing of old bone and constant renewing of the tissue. It is responsible for the stochastic removal of trabeculae.[75] Bone loss consequent to high bone turnover can cause trabecular perforation and consequently thinning of trabeculae, which reduces bone strength.[76] Osteoclasts target the narrowest region of a trabecula.[77] The aged bone is characterized by an increase in the outside dimensions due to periosteal apposition.[78] Bone loss is not uniform along the skeleton and may be worse in specific regions; this is called regional bone loss. For example, the superior region of the neck has a higher rate of bone resorption than the inferior region.[79] Ageing impairs the capacity of bone marrow stem cells to differentiate into bone cells.[80,81] Also the stem cells of the periosteum lose the ability to differentiate into chondrocytes.[82] This could explain the less efficient healing process in older people.[83] Changes in the osteocyte network may be responsible for the decreased capacity of the bone to respond to mechanical loads that produce new bone.[84]

Quantitative changes also affect the aged bone. The number of osteocytes decreases with age, but the pathological implications of this phenomenon are still unclear.[85]

Osteoblasts have receptors for oestrogens. These hormones affect mineral metabolism by increasing calcium absorption across the gut and by preserving renal calcium.

Women's oestrogen levels decline with age, even though it is the menopause which causes a true deficiency. Women after the menopause lose skeletal bone at a rate of about 2% per year. Administration of oestrogen to perimenopausal women can decrease the loss in all bones, particularly those rich in trabecular bone; however, there is an increased risk of breast cancer. However, a 10-year follow-up study has shown that the total mortality among women who use post-menopausal hormones is lower than in non-users, probably because of the beneficial effects of oestrogens on cardiovascular diseases.[86–89]

REFERENCES

1. Tuite DJ, Renstrom PA, O'Brien M. The aging tendon. *Scandinavian Journal of Medicine & Science in Sports* 1997;**7**:72–7.
2. Menard D, Stanish WD. The aging athlete. *American Journal of Sports Medicine* 1989;**17**:187–96.
3. Bosco C, Komi PV. Influence of aging on the mechanical behavior of leg extensor muscles. *European Journal of Applied Physiology and Occupational Physiology* 1980;**45**:209–19.
4. Kannus P, Niittymaki S, Jarvinen M, Lehto M. Sports injuries in elderly athletes: a three-year prospective, controlled study. *Age Ageing* 1989;**18**:263–70.
5. O'Brien M. Functional anatomy and physiology of tendons. *Clinical Sports Medicine* 1992;**11**:505–20.
6. Ippolito E, Natali PG, Postacchini F, et al. Morphological, immunochemical, and biochemical study of rabbit Achilles tendon at various ages. *Journal of Bone and Joint Surgery (American)* 1980;**62**:583–98.
7. Nakagawa Y, Majima T, Nagashima K. Effect of ageing on ultrastructure of slow and fast skeletal muscle tendon in rabbit Achilles tendons. *Acta Physiologica Scandinavica* 1994;**152**:307–13.
8. Hess GP, Cappiello WL, Poole RM, Hunter SC. Prevention and treatment of overuse tendon injuries. *Sports Medicine* 1989;**8**:371–84.
9. Kannus P, Jozsa L. Histopathological changes preceding spontaneous rupture of a tendon. A controlled study of 891 patients. *Journal of Bone and Joint Surgery (American)* 1991;**73**:1507–25.
10. Carlstedt CA. Mechanical and chemical factors in tendon healing. Effects of indomethacin and surgery in the rabbit. *Acta Orthopaedica Scandinavica Supplementum* 1987;**224**:1–75.
11. Shadwick RE. Elastic energy storage in tendons: mechanical differences related to function and age. *Journal of Applied Physiology* 1990;**68**:1033–40.
12. Robert L, Moczar M, Robert M. Biogenesis, maturation and aging of elastic tissue. *Experientia* 1974;**30**:211–12.
13. Jozsa L, Kvist M, Balint BJ, et al. The role of recreational sport activity in Achilles tendon rupture. A clinical, pathoanatomical, and sociological study of 292 cases. *American Journal of Sports Medicine* 1989;**17**:338–43.
14. Vogel HG. Influence of maturation and age on mechanical and biochemical parameters of connective tissue of various organs in the rat. *Connective Tissue Research* 1978;**6**:161–6.
15. Baumgartner RN, Waters DL, Gallagher D, Morley JE, Garry PJ. Predictors of skeletal muscle mass in elderly men and women. *Mechanisms of Ageing and Development* 1999;**107**:123–36.
16. Janssen I, Heymsfield SB, Wang ZM, Ross R. Skeletal muscle mass and distribution in 468 men and women aged 18–88 yr. *Journal of Applied Physiology* 2000;**89**:81–8.
17. Harridge SD, Kryger A, Stensgaard A. Knee extensor strength, activation, and size in very elderly people following strength training. *Muscle and Nerve* 1999;**22**:831–9.
18. Jubrias SA, Odderson IR, Esselman PC, Conley KE. Decline in isokinetic force with age: muscle cross-sectional area and specific force. *Pflugers Archives* 1997;**434**:246–53.
19. Kent-Braun JA, Ng AV, Young K. Skeletal muscle contractile and noncontractile components in young and older women and men. *Journal of Applied Physiology* 2000;**88**:662–8.
20. Lang T, Streeper T, Cawthon P, et al. Sarcopenia: etiology, clinical consequences, intervention, and assessment. *Osteoporosis International* 2010;**21**:543–59.
21. Rice CL, Cunningham DA, Paterson DH, Lefcoe MS. Arm and leg composition determined by computed tomography in young and elderly men. *Clinical Physiology* 1989;**9**:207–20.
22. Taaffe DR, Henwood TR, Nalls MA, et al. Alterations in muscle attenuation following detraining and retraining in resistance-trained older adults. *Gerontology* 2009;**55**:217–23.
23. Brack AS, Bildsoe H, Hughes SM. Evidence that satellite cell decrement contributes to preferential decline in nuclear number from large fibres during murine age-related muscle atrophy. *Journal of Cell Science* 2005;**118**(Pt 20):4813–21.
24. Sipila S, Suominen H. Knee extension strength and walking speed in relation to quadriceps muscle composition and training in elderly women. *Clinical Physiology* 1994;**14**:433–42.
25. Roubenoff R. Sarcopenic obesity: the confluence of two epidemics. *Obesity Research* 2004;**12**:887–8.
26. Klitgaard H, Mantoni M, Schiaffino S, et al. Function, morphology and protein expression of ageing skeletal muscle: a cross-sectional study of elderly men with different training backgrounds. *Acta Physiologica Scandinavica* 1990;**140**:41–54.
27. Larsson L. Morphological and functional characteristics of the ageing skeletal muscle in man. A cross-sectional study. *Acta Physiologica Scandinavica Supplementum* 1978;**457**:1–36.
28. Lexell J, Henriksson-Larsen K, Winblad B, Sjostrom M. Distribution of different fiber types in human skeletal muscles: effects of aging studied in whole muscle cross sections. *Muscle and Nerve* 1983;**6**:588–95.
29. Coggan AR, Spina RJ, King DS, et al. Histochemical and enzymatic comparison of the gastrocnemius muscle of young and elderly men and women. *Journal of Gerontology* 1992;**47**:B71–6.
30. Lexell J, Taylor CC, Sjostrom M. What is the cause of the ageing atrophy? Total number, size and proportion of different fiber types studied in whole vastus lateralis muscle from 15- to 83-year-old men. *Journal of Neurological Sciences* 1988;**84**:275–94.

31. Andersen JL. Muscle fibre type adaptation in the elderly human muscle. *Scandinavian Journal of Medicine & Science in Sports* 2003;**13**:40–7.
32. Klitgaard H, Zhou M, Schiaffino S, et al. Ageing alters the myosin heavy chain composition of single fibres from human skeletal muscle. *Acta Physiologica Scandinavica* 1990;**140**:55–62.
33. Lexell J, Henriksson-Larsen K, Sjostrom M. Distribution of different fibre types in human skeletal muscles. 2. A study of cross-sections of whole m. vastus lateralis. *Acta Physiologica Scandinavica* 1983;**117**:115–22.
34. Campbell MJ, McComas AJ, Petito F. Physiological changes in ageing muscles. *Journal of Neurology, Neurosurgery, and Psychiatry* 1973;**36**:174–82.
35. Lieber RL, Friden J. Functional and clinical significance of skeletal muscle architecture. *Muscle and Nerve* 2000;**23**:1647–66.
36. Kubo K, Kanehisa H, Azuma K, et al. Muscle architectural characteristics in young and elderly men and women. *International Journal of Sports Medicine* 2003;**24**:125–30.
37. Narici MV, Maganaris CN, Reeves ND, Capodaglio P. Effect of aging on human muscle architecture. *Journal of Applied Physiology* 2003;**95**:2229–34.
38. Thom JM, Morse CI, Birch KM, Narici MV. Influence of muscle architecture on the torque and power-velocity characteristics of young and elderly men. *European Journal of Applied Physiology* 2007;**100**:613–19.
39. Brown WF. A method for estimating the number of motor units in thenar muscles and the changes in motor unit count with ageing. *Journal of Neurology, Neurosurgery, and Psychiatry* 1972;**35**:845–52.
40. Frey D, Schneider C, Xu L, et al. Early and selective loss of neuromuscular synapse subtypes with low sprouting competence in motoneuron diseases. *Journal of Neuroscience* 2000;**20**:2534–42.
41. Gardiner P, Michel R, Olha A, Pettigrew F. Force and fatiguability of sprouting motor units in partially denervated rat plantaris. *Experimental Brain Research* 1987;**66**:597–606.
42. Larsson L, Ansved T. Effects of ageing on the motor unit. *Progress in Neurobiology* 1995;**45**:397–458.
43. Lexell J. Human aging, muscle mass, and fiber type composition. *Journals of Gerontology. Series A, Biological Sciences and Medical Sciences* 1995;**50**:11–16.
44. Dirks AJ, Leeuwenburgh C. The role of apoptosis in age-related skeletal muscle atrophy. *Sports Medicine* 2005;**35**:473–83.
45. Drew B, Phaneuf S, Dirks A, et al. Effects of aging and caloric restriction on mitochondrial energy production in gastrocnemius muscle and heart. *American Journal of Physiology. Regulatory, Integrative and Comparative Physiology* 2003;**284**:R474–80.
46. Short KR, Bigelow ML, Kahl J, et al. Decline in skeletal muscle mitochondrial function with aging in humans. *Proceedings of the National Academy of Sciences USA* 2005;**102**:5618–23.
47. Morse CI, Thom JM, Davis MG, et al. Reduced plantarflexor specific torque in the elderly is associated with a lower activation capacity. *European Journal of Applied Physiology* 2004;**92**:219–26.
48. Visser M, Deeg DJ, Lips P. Low vitamin D and high parathyroid hormone levels as determinants of loss of muscle strength and muscle mass (sarcopenia): the Longitudinal Aging Study Amsterdam. *Journal of Clinical Endocrinology and Metabolism* 2003;**88**:5766–72.
49. Balagopal P, Rooyackers OE, Adey DB, Ades PA, Nair KS. Effects of aging on in vivo synthesis of skeletal muscle myosin heavy-chain and sarcoplasmic protein in humans. *American Journal of Physiology* 1997;**273**(4 Pt 1):E790–800.
50. Cuthbertson D, Smith K, Babraj J, et al. Anabolic signaling deficits underlie amino acid resistance of wasting, aging muscle. *FASEB Journal* 2005;**19**:422–4.
51. Volpi E, Rasmussen BB. Nutrition and muscle protein metabolism in the elderly. *Diabetes, Nutrition & Metabolism* 2000;**13**:99–107.
52. Volpi E, Sheffield-Moore M, Rasmussen BB, Wolfe RR. Basal muscle amino acid kinetics and protein synthesis in healthy young and older men. *Journal of the American Medical Association* 2001;**286**:1206–12.
53. Welle S, Thornton C, Statt M. Myofibrillar protein synthesis in young and old human subjects after three months of resistance training. *American Journal of Physiology* 1995;**268**(3 Pt 1):E422–7.
54. Wilkes EA, Selby AL, Atherton PJ, et al. Blunting of insulin inhibition of proteolysis in legs of older subjects may contribute to age-related sarcopenia. *American Journal of Clinical Nutrition* 2009;**5**:1343–50.
55. Macaluso A, De Vito G. Muscle strength, power and adaptations to resistance training in older people. *European Journal of Applied Physiology* 2004;**91**:450–72.
56. Skelton DA, Greig CA, Davies JM, Young A. Strength, power and related functional ability of healthy people aged 65–89 years. *Age Ageing* 1994;**23**:371–7.
57. Macaluso A, Nimmo MA, Foster JE, et al. Contractile muscle volume and agonist-antagonist coactivation account for differences in torque between young and older women. *Muscle and Nerve* 2002;**25**:858–63.
58. Phillips SK, Rook KM, Siddle NC, et al. Muscle weakness in women occurs at an earlier age than in men, but strength is preserved by hormone replacement therapy. *Clinical Science (London)* 1993;**84**:95–8.
59. Young A, Stokes M, Crowe M. The size and strength of the quadriceps muscles of old and young men. *Clinical Physiology* 1985;**5**:145–54.
60. D'Antona G, Pellegrino MA, Adami R, et al. The effect of ageing and immobilization on structure and function of human skeletal muscle fibres. *Journal of Physiology* 2003;**552**:499–511.
61. Bottinelli R, Reggiani C. Human skeletal muscle fibres: molecular and functional diversity. *Progress in Biophysics and Molecular Biology* 2000;**73**:195–262.

62. Hook P, Sriramoju V, Larsson L. Effects of aging on actin sliding speed on myosin from single skeletal muscle cells of mice, rats, and humans. *American Journal of Cell Physiology* 2001;**280**:C782–8.
63. Scaglioni G, Ferri A, Minetti AE, et al. Plantar flexor activation capacity and H reflex in older adults: adaptations to strength training. *Journal of Applied Physiology* 2002;**92**:2292–302.
64. Winegard KJ, Hicks AL, Sale DG, Vandervoort AA. A 12-year follow-up study of ankle muscle function in older adults. *Journals of Gerontology. Series A, Biological Sciences and Medical Sciences* 1996;**51**:B202–7.
65. Yue GH, Ranganathan VK, Siemionow V, et al. Older adults exhibit a reduced ability to fully activate their biceps brachii muscle. *Journals of Gerontology. Series A, Biological Sciences and Medical Sciences* 1999;**54**:M249–53.
66. de Boer MD, Morse CI, Thom JM, et al. Changes in antagonist muscles' coactivation in response to strength training in older women. *The Journals of Gerontology. Series A, Biological Sciences and Medical Sciences* 2007;**62**:1022–7.
67. Klein CS, Rice CL, Marsh GD. Normalized force, activation, and coactivation in the arm muscles of young and old men. *Journal of Applied Physiology* 2001;**91**:1341–9.
68. Assessment of fracture risk and its application to screening for postmenopausal osteoporosis. Report of a WHO Study Group. *World Health Organization Technical Report Series* 1994;**843**:1–129.
69. Jones G, Nguyen T, Sambrook PN, et al. Symptomatic fracture incidence in elderly men and women: the Dubbo Osteoporosis Epidemiology Study (DOES). *Osteoporosis International* 1994;**4**:277–82.
70. Winner SJ, Morgan CA, Evans JG. Perimenopausal risk of falling and incidence of distal forearm fracture. *British Medical Journal* 1989;**298**:1486–8.
71. Center JR, Nguyen TV, Schneider D, Sambrook PN, Eisman JA. Mortality after all major types of osteoporotic fracture in men and women: an observational study. *Lancet* 1999;**353**:878–82.
72. Magaziner J, Fredman L, Hawkes W, et al. Changes in functional status attributable to hip fracture: a comparison of hip fracture patients to community-dwelling aged. *American Journal of Epidemiology* 2003;**157**:1023–31.
73. Lane JM, Nydick M. Osteoporosis: current modes of prevention and treatment. *Journal of American Academy of Orthopedic Surgeons* 1999;**7**:19–31.
74. Cummings SR, Nevitt MC, Browner WS, et al. Risk factors for hip fracture in white women. Study of Osteoporotic Fractures Research Group. *New England Journal of Medicine* 1995;**332**:767–73.
75. Khosla S, Riggs BL, Atkinson EJ, et al. Effects of sex and age on bone microstructure at the ultradistal radius: a population-based noninvasive in vivo assessment. *Journal of Bone and Mineral Research* 2006;**21**:124–31.
76. Guo XE, Kim CH. Mechanical consequence of trabecular bone loss and its treatment: a three-dimensional model simulation. *Bone* 2002;**30**:404–11.
77. McNamara LM, Van der Linden JC, Weinans H, Prendergast PJ. Stress-concentrating effect of resorption lacunae in trabecular bone. *Journal of Biomechanics* 2006;**39**:734–41.
78. Seeman E. Periosteal bone formation—a neglected determinant of bone strength. *New England Journal of Medicine* 2003;**349**:320–3.
79. Yoshikawa T, Turner CH, Peacock M, et al. Geometric structure of the femoral neck measured using dual-energy x-ray absorptiometry. *Journal of Bone and Mineral Research* 1994;**9**:1053–64.
80. Bonab MM, Alimoghaddam K, Talebian F, et al. Aging of mesenchymal stem cell in vitro. *BMC Cell Biology* 2006;**7**:14.
81. Tyan ML. Femur mass: modulation by marrow cells from young and old donors. *Proceedings of the Society for Experimental Biology and Medicine* 1980;**164**:89–92.
82. Bak B, Andreassen TT. The effect of aging on fracture healing in the rat. *Calcified Tissue International* 1989;**45**:292–7.
83. O'Driscoll SW, Saris DB, Ito Y, Fitzimmons JS. The chondrogenic potential of periosteum decreases with age. *Journal of Orthopaedic Research* 2001;**19**:95–103.
84. Turner CH TY, Owan I. Aging changes mechanical loading thresholds for bone formation in rats. *Journal of Bone and Mineral Research* 1995;**10**:1544–9.
85. Vashishth D, Verborgt O, Divine G, et al. Decline in osteocyte lacunar density in human cortical bone is associated with accumulation of microcracks with age. *Bone* 2000;**26**:375–80.
86. Grady D, Rubin SM, Petitti DB, et al. Hormone therapy to prevent disease and prolong life in postmenopausal women. *Annals of Internal Medicine* 1992;**117**:1016–37.
87. Grodstein F, Stampfer MJ, Colditz GA, et al. Postmenopausal hormone therapy and mortality. *New England Journal of Medicine* 1997;**336**:1769–75.
88. Lane JM, Riley EH, Wirganowicz PZ. Osteoporosis: diagnosis and treatment. *Instructional Course Lectures* 1997;**46**:445–58.
89. Lindsay R, Bush TL, Grady D, et al. Therapeutic controversy: Estrogen replacement in menopause. *Journal of Clinical Endocrinology and Metabolism* 1996;**81**:3829–38.

9

Principles of orthopaedic pharmacology

CHEZHIYAN SHANMUGAM, UMILE GIUSEPPE LONGO, NICOLA MAFFULLI

Introduction	126	Thrombolytics	132
Analgesics and anti-inflammatory drugs	126	Anti-osteoporotic drugs	132
Glucocorticoids	129	References	134
Anticoagulants	130		

NATIONAL BOARD STANDARDS

- Know the mode of action of various antibiotics
- Understand the mechanism of development of antibiotic resistance
- Understand and define surgical prophylaxis
- Know treatment regimes for tuberculosis
- Understand empirical antibacterial therapy for osteomyelitis and septic arthritis

- Know current agents used as deep vein thrombosis prophylaxis
- Know the mode of action of various classes of drugs used in management of osteoporosis
- Understand the analgesic ladder and various options for analgesia

INTRODUCTION

Practising orthopaedic surgeons need to maintain basic pharmacological knowledge for a comprehensive care of orthopaedic patients. Orthopaedic pharmacology deals with common classes of drugs that are used in the management of pre-operative, intra-operative and postoperative orthopaedic conditions. This chapter covers analgesics and anti-inflammatory drugs, glucocorticoids, anticoagulants, thrombolytics, anti-osteoporotic drugs and nutraceuticals. Antibiotics and anti-neoplastic drugs are described elsewhere in this textbook.

ANALGESICS AND ANTI-INFLAMMATORY DRUGS

Four classes of drugs are used to alleviate pain in orthopaedic patients:

1. opioid analgesics
2. non-steroidal anti-inflammatory drugs
3. non-opioid analgesic drugs
4. local anaesthetics.

Opioid analgesics

Opiates are derived from the juice of the opium poppy (*Papaver somniferum*), from which morphine, codeine, thebaine and many other semisynthetic opioids are derived.

MECHANISM OF ACTION

Opioids exert their therapeutic effects by mimicking the action of endogenous opioid peptides, the enkephalins, endorphins and dynorphins, at opioid receptors, namely μ, δ, and κ. They are present in areas of the central nervous system (CNS) related to the perception of pain, e.g. laminae I and II of the spinal cord, the spinal trigeminal nucleus and the peri-aqueductal grey matter. The receptors in endogenous neuronal settings are coupled via pertussis toxin-sensitive GTP-binding protein inhibition of adenyl cyclase activity (Herz, receptor-operated K^+ currents, and suppression of voltage-gated Ca^{2+} currents.[1] The hyperpolarization of the membrane potential by K^+ current activation and limitation of Ca^{2+} entry by suppression of Ca^{2+} currents modulates the pain transmission in varying neuronal pathways.

CLASSIFICATION OF OPIOIDS

- High efficacy for severe pain: Morphine, diamorphine (heroin), tramadol, pethidine (Meperidine), alfenatil and phenoperidine, fentanyl, and buprenorphine. Tramadol, phenoperidine and fentanyl are highly effective opioids used for anaesthetic purpose.
- Low efficacy for mild to moderate pain: codeine, dihydrocodeine, dextropropoxyphene.

MORPHINE

Morphine is rapidly absorbed when given subcutaneously or intramuscularly, is metabolized by both liver and kidney, and is largely excreted by the kidneys.

CLINICAL USE

Sir William Osler described morphine as 'god's own medicine'. It is used to produce analgesia, sedation, production of euphoria as well as pain relief in the dying, and brief relief of anxiety in serious and frightening disease accompanied by pain, e.g. trauma.

ROUTES OF ADMINISTRATION

Oral morphine is subjected to extensive presystemic or first-pass metabolism, and only 20% of a given dose enters the systemic circulation.

PATIENT CONTROLLED ANALGESIA

Patient controlled analgesia (PCA) can be used for intravenous or epidural infusion. This technique avoids any delays in administration and allows greater dosing flexibility, giving patients a greater sense of control. PCA is suitable for both adults and children, and it is preferred over intramuscular injections for postoperative pain control.[2] Currently, there is no evidence that self-administration of opioids for analgesic purposes increases risk of addiction.

COMPUTER-ASSISTED CONTINUOUS INFUSION

Computer-assisted continuous infusion enables the clinicians to titrate intravenous agents in a fashion similar to that used in delivering volatile agents.[3,4]

PERIPHERAL ANALGESIA

Although it was thought that 1 mg of intra-articular morphine would significantly reduce pain following knee surgery,[5] this was proven not to be the case.[6]

RECTAL ADMINISTRATION

In the United States, morphine, hydromorphine and oxymorphone are available in rectal suppository formulations.

INHALATION

Inhalation is a cost-effective, convenient method of analgesic delivery for chronic pain.

ORAL TRANSMUCOSAL

Buprenorphine is an effective analgesic when given sublingually.

TRANSDERMAL OR IONTOPHORETIC ADMINISTRATION

Fentanyl patches can be given transdermally for chronic pain. It may take up to 12 hours to develop analgesia, and up to 16 hours to observe the full clinical effect. The plasma half-life after patch removal is about 17 hours.

Iontophoresis is the transport of soluble ions through the skin by using a mild electric current. Iontophoresed morphine appeared to be a promising agent for postoperative pain relief in total knee or hip arthroplasty,[7] but no recent studies on this modality of administration have been published.

SIDE-EFFECTS

The side-effects are respiratory depression, nausea and vomiting, constipation, tolerance and dependence, postural hypotension due to depression of the vasomotor centre and release of histamine, biliary spasm, pruritus and bronchoconstriction.

TREATMENT OF OPIOID OVERDOSAGE

Naloxone hydrochloride is used to antagonize the respiratory-depressant actions without eliciting a full withdrawal syndrome.

MORPHINE ANALOGUES

- *Diamorphine (heroin)*: This semi-synthetic drug was first made from morphine at St Mary's Hospital, London, in 1874. It was introduced in 1898 as a remedy for cough and for morphine addiction. It 'cured' morphine addiction by substituting itself as the addicting agent.
- *Codeine (methylmorphine)* ($t_{1/2}$ 3 hours): This is a low-efficacy opioid that binds to μ-receptors; 10% is converted to morphine. It is used for mild and moderate musculoskeletal pain (co-codamol) and as codeine linctus for cough.
- *Tramadol* ($t_{1/2}$ 6 h): This inhibits the neuronal noradrenaline (norepinephrine) uptake and serotonin release. Tramadol is approximately as effective as pethidine for postoperative pain and as morphine for moderate chronic pain. Tramadol is claimed to be less likely to constipate, depress respiration and addict.
- *Dextropropoxyphene*: This interacts with warfarin by enhancing its anticoagulant effect, so co-proxamol should be avoided when the patient is anticoagulated with warfarin.

PAIN IN OPIOID ADDICTS

Nefopam (Acupan), being neither an opioid nor a non-steroidal anti-inflammatory drug (NSAID), is effective against moderate pain. Its mode of action is not fully understood.

Non-steroidal anti-inflammatory drugs

NSAIDS are analgesics, anti-inflammatory and antipyretics. NSAIDs exert this anti-inflammatory action by inhibiting cyclo-oxygenase (COX), resulting in inhibition of prostaglandin synthesis (Fig. 9.1). COX-1 is present in many tissues, including platelets, stomach and kidney; and COX-2 is induced by cytokines and endotoxins at sites of inflammation, e.g. joints. NSAIDs exert their anti-inflammatory actions via inhibition of COX-2. The inhibition of COX-1 by NSAIDs results in loss of the gastroprotective effects of prostaglandins E2 (PGE_2) and I2 (PGI_2). COX-2 inhibitors are more selective in their action. All NSAIDs are reversible non-selective competitive inhibitors of prostaglandin G/H synthase (cyclooxygenase) except aspirin.

CLASSIFICATION OF NSAIDs

- Para-aminophenol group: paracetamol
- Propionic acids: ibuprofen, flurbiprofen, ketoprofen
- Fenamic acids: mefenamic acid
- Salicylic acids: acetylsalicylic acid (aspirin)
- Acetic acids: diclofenac, indomethacin
- Enolic acids: piroxicam, tenoxicam, phenylbutazone
- Non-acidic drug: nabumetone.

The vast majority of NSAIDs are weakly acidic drugs and act preferentially on the synovial tissue of inflamed joints.

ADVERSE EFFECTS

Bleeding, dyspepsia, nausea and gastritis, analgesic nephropathy, and Samter's syndrome (the triad of aspirin sensitivity, asthma and nasal polyposis).

ACETYLSALICYLIC ACID (ASPIRIN)

Aspirin is the most commonly used antiplatelet agent. It irreversibly acetylates cyclooxygenase, the enzyme responsible for the first step in the formation of prostaglandin H2 (Fig. 9.1). Aspirin can prevent formation of both thromboxane A_2 and prostacyclin for its lifetime (8–10 days).

Pre-operative consideration

Aspirin should be discontinued 10 days prior to any elective surgery to allow replenishment with new platelets to avoid the risk of intra-operative bleeding.

ACETAMINOPHEN (PARACETAMOL)

Acetaminophen is a 'coal tar analgesic', is available over the counter, and is an antipyretic. It acts via the production of reactive metabolites by peroxidase function of COX-2, which could deplete glutathione, a cofactor of enzymes such as prostaglandin E synthase. Acetaminophen acts on COX-3, an isoenzyme of COX-1 found in the central nervous system. The central action of acetaminophen may also be due to activation of descending serotonergic pathways.

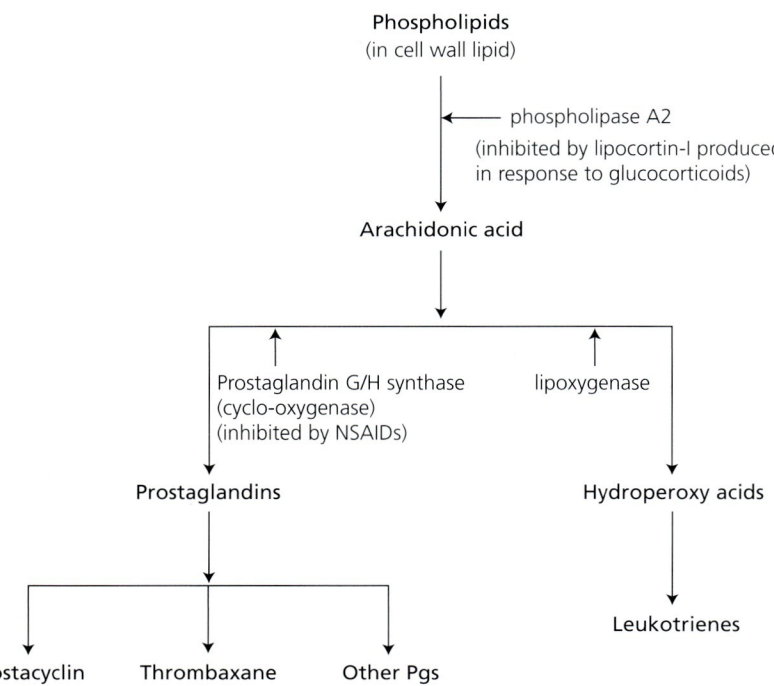

Figure 9.1 Biosynthetic pathway of eicosanoids. NSAIDs, non-steroidal anti-inflammatory drugs; Pg, prostaglandin.

Side-effects

- Analgesic-associated nephropathy.
- Fatal liver damage can occur by saturation of the normal conjugating enzymes causing acetaminophen to be converted by cytochrome p450s to N-acetyl-para-benzoquinonimine, which is electrophilic. The principal antidote treatment is administration of N-acetylcysteine (Mucomyst), which acts by replenishing hepatic stores of glutathione.

IBUPROFEN

Ibuprofen and its analogues have similar properties and are most useful in painful musculoskeletal disorders. Patients often prefer one to another. Naproxen and fenbufen are suitable for twice-daily dosing because of their long duration of action. The main advantage over aspirin is a lower incidence of adverse effects, particularly in the gastrointestinal tract. However, epigastric discomfort, activation of peptic ulcer and bleeding may occur. Side-effects include headaches, dizziness, fever and rashes.

Local anaesthetics

A typical local anaesthetic has hydrophilic and hydrophobic moieties that are separated by an ester or amide linkage (Fig. 9.2). Local anaesthetics block action potential initiation and propagation in neurones by reducing the passage through sodium voltage-activated Na^+ ion channels. They raise the threshold of excitability and thereby block conduction. The smallest fibres (autonomic and sensory) are affected first, and then the larger (motor) fibres. Paradoxically, they stimulate the central nervous system.

CLASSIFICATION OF LOCAL ANAESTHETICS

- Ester compounds: cocaine, procaine, amethocaine, benzocaine.
- Amide compounds: lignocaine, bupivacaine, prilocaine ropivacaine.

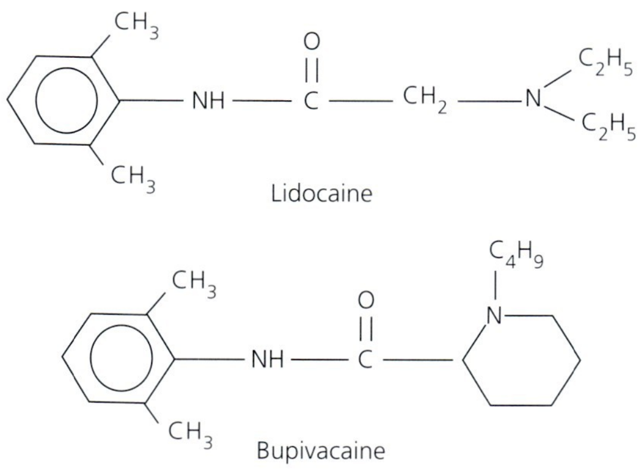

Figure 9.2 Lidocaine and bupivacaine.

PHARMACOKINETICS

Most local anaesthetics are acid salts, which dissociate in the tissues to liberate the free base, which is biologically active. This dissociation is delayed in an acidic environment, e.g. inflamed tissues (abscess). Given the risk of spreading infection, their use should be limited in infected areas. The duration of action of local anaesthetics can be enhanced by adding epinephrine or norepinephrine (1 : 200 000). This combination should be avoided in the extremities (fingers, toes, nose and penis), as the whole blood supply may be cut off by the intense vasoconstriction. A synthetic vasopressin, felypressin, can be used in patients with cardiovascular disease.

CLINICAL USE

- Surface anaesthesia
- Infiltration anaesthesia

This is the most often used method of local anaesthetic, e.g. haematoma block, skin laceration repair, carpal tunnel decompression, percutaneous tendo-Achilles repair, and immediate pre-, per- and postoperative pain relief.

- Regional anaesthesia
- Spinal anaesthesia.

Side-effects

Agitation, confusion, tremors progressing to convulsions, respiratory depression, myocardial depression, and vasodilatation leading to a drop in blood pressure.

GLUCOCORTICOIDS

Steroids are lipophilic. The glucocorticoid receptor is normally bound to heat shock protein HSP90. Once the steroid is bound to the receptor, HSP90 dissociates from the occupied receptor and translocates to the nucleus. Steroids have multiple actions due to the presence of glucocorticoid response elements (GREs) in the promoter region of several genes. Steroids induce transcription of a protein, IkB, which traps activated NF-kB in inactive cytoplasmic complexes. Steroids inhibit the pathways of synthesis of eicosanoids (anti-inflammatory), and also directly depress monocyte/lymphocyte/macrophage functions, and decrease circulating T-cell levels and antibody production.

Classification of steroids based on their potency

- Mildly potent: hydrocortisone
- Moderately potent: triamcinolone
- Potent: methylprednisolone
- Very potent: betamethasone dipropionate, dexamethasone.

Pharmacokinetics

Glucocorticoids are given by oral, topical, intravenous and intramuscular routes. They are absorbed systemically from the sites of local administration, such as synovial spaces. In the circulation, they are bound to corticosteroid-binding globulin (CBG or transcortin) and albumin, both secreted by the liver. All biologically active steroids have a double bond in the 4, 5 position and a ketone group at C3. Reduction of the double bond, and subsequent reduction of 3-ketone substituent to the 3-hydroxyl group, forming tetrahydrocortisol, occurs in the liver. The resultant sulphate esters and glucuronides are water soluble and are excreted by the kidneys.

Clinical use

1. Organ transplantation.
2. Acute spinal cord injury.

A double-blind, randomized controlled trial of 499 patients diagnosed in National Acute Spinal Cord Injury Study (NASCIS) centres within 8 hours of injury showed that patients who received methylprednisolone for 24 hours within 3 hours of injury and for 48 hours between 3 and 8 hours after injury showed improvement to one full neurological grade ($p = 0.03$) at 6 months.
The following are the two treatment regimens.

1. *24 hour regimen*: within 3 hours of injury, methylprednisolone prescribed as a bolus intravenous infusion of 30 mg per kilogram of body weight over 15 minutes, and then 45 minutes later, by an infusion of 5.4mg per kilogram of body weight per hour for 23 hours.
2. *48 hour regimen*: between 3 and 8 hours of injury, dosage is same as above. This regimen is associated with high risk of complications such as sepsis and severe pneumonia relative to 24 hours regimen.[8]

Nevertheless, several researchers believe that NASCIS data are insufficient to support the use of high-dose methylprednisolone as a treatment standard or as a guideline for treatment following an acute closed spinal cord injury.[9–12]

3. Methylprednisolone + bupivacaine combinations are used in various musculotendinous problems such as rotator cuff injury, frozen shoulders, patellar and Achilles tendinopathy, golfers and tennis elbow, writers cramp and trigger finger.

Side-effects

- Iatrogenic Cushing syndrome
- Infection
- Proximal myopathy (due to protein loss)
- Adrenal insufficiency
- Hyperglycaemia, and diabetes
- Hypotension
- Osteoporosis (propably due to inhibition of vitamin D_3-mediated induction of the osteocalcin gene in osteoblasts)
- Peptic ulcer
- Pancreatitis
- Central obesity (lemon on toothpick appearance), easy bruising and hirsutism
- Avascular necrosis of the femoral head
- Glaucoma, cataracts
- Psychological disturbances.

ANTICOAGULANTS

The haemostatic system is complex. Coagulation is formation of fibrin, which stabilizes the platelet plug. Fibrinolysis is the degradation of fibrin. The extrinsic system is monitored by the prothrombin time, which is expressed as the international normalized ratio (INR). The intrinsic system is monitored by activated partial thromboplastin time (APTT). The blood coagulation pathways are illustrated in Fig. 9.3. Anticoagulants are drugs that can interfere with the coagulation pathways.

Classification of anticoagulants

There are two types of anticoagulant.

INDIRECT-ACTING

- Coumarine: warfarin, nicoumalone
- Indandione: phenindione.

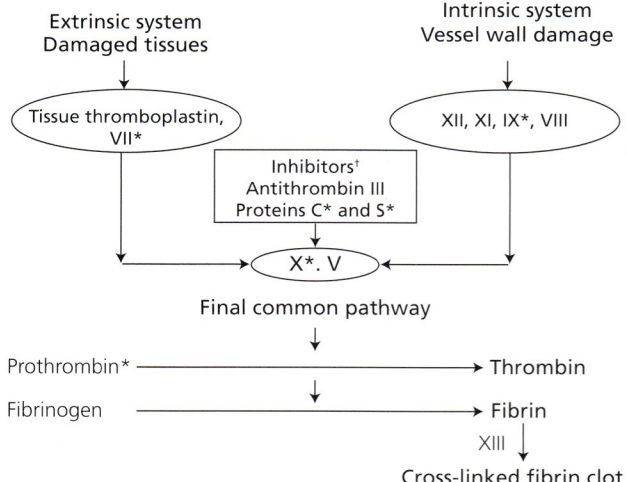

Warfarin acts on *vitamin K-dependent factors.
Heparin acts on †antithrombin III, inhibits IX, X, XI, XII and thrombin.
Proteins C and S inhibit V and VIII.
Rivaroxaban acts as activated factor Xa, by direct competitive reversible inhibition.

Figure 9.3 Blood coagulation pathways.

DIRECT-ACTING

- Heparin
- Low-molecular-weight heparins (LMWHs): delteparin, enoxaparin and tinzaparin.
- Direct inhibitors of thrombin (Dabigatran) and factor Xa (Rivaroxaban) are also now available.

Warfarin

Warfarin blocks γ-carboxylation of vitamin K (coagulant)-dependent factors II, VII, IX and X, and the proteins C and S in the liver. Active vitamin K (coagulant) is oxidized to an epoxide, and must be reduced by the enzyme vitamin K epoxide reductase to become active again. Warfarin is structurally similar to vitamin K, and competitively inhibits epoxide reductase, so limiting availability of the active form of the vitamin to form coagulant proteins.

It takes 72 hours to anticoagulate completely until the clotting factors already present in the circulation have been completely exhausted. A similar time lag is observed when the warfarin dose is altered or discontinued, as the $t_{1/2}$ of the malfunctioning proteins is approximately that of functioning proteins. Warfarin therapy is optimized by measuring the INR.

Clinical use

An initial dose of 10 mg is started daily for 2 days, and then the maintenance dose is adjusted according to the INR.[13] The level of anticoagulation should match the perceived level of danger of thrombosis by following the guidelines.[14,15] Warfarin is considered when there is a requirement for longstanding anticoagulation in patients who are already on heparin.

INR 2.0–2.5	Prophylaxis of deep vein thrombosis (DVT) in hip surgery and fractured femur operations.
INR 2.0–3.0	Treatment of DVT, pulmonary embolism, systemic embolism, prevention of venous thromboembolism in myocardial infarction, mitral stenosis with embolism, transient ischaemic attacks and atrial fibrillation.
INR 3.0–4.5	Recurrent DVT and pulmonary embolism, arterial disease including myocardial infarction and mechanical prosthetic heart valves.

Side-effects

Bleeding is the commonest. Kounis et al. reported haemorrhage in gastrocnemius muscles.[16] Acute compartmental syndromes resulting from anticoagulant treatment have also been reported.[17]

Management of bleeding

LIFE- OR MAJOR ORGAN-THREATENING HAEMORRHAGE

In addition to blood replacement, prothrombin complex concentrate or fresh frozen plasma should be given. If full reversal of anticoagulation is deemed necessary, phytomenadione 5 mg is then given by slow i.v. injection and repeated if necessary.

LESSER BLEEDING

Warfarin should be withheld and phytomenadione 0.5–2 mg may be given by slow i.v. injection.

Pre-operative consideration

ELECTIVE SURGERY

Warfarin should be withdrawn 5 days before the operation, and resumed after 3 days of surgery. LMWH may be used in the intervening period.

In patients with mechanical prosthetic valves, heparin is substituted at full dosage 4 days before surgery, and restarted 12–24 hours after the operation. Warfarin is restarted when the patient resumes oral intake. Once the target INR is achieved, then heparin should be withdrawn.

EMERGENCY SURGERY

Proceed as per bleeding. Adopt the principles of management of bleeding as detailed previously.

Drug Interactions

Drugs that can induce hepatic microsomal enzymes will decrease the anticoagualant effect, e.g. co-proxamol, rifampicin, phenytoin.

Drugs that can inhibit hepatic microsomal enzymes potentiate the effect of warfarin, e.g. trimethoprim, amoxycillin, serotonin re-uptake inhibitors, omeprazole and simvastatin.

HEPARIN

Heparin complexes with antithrombin III, and it inhibits activated factor Xa, which is needed to covert prothrombin to thrombin. It also inhibits thrombin directly preventing the formation of fibrin threads. Heparin also inhibits platelet aggregation and certain aspects of the inflammatory response; this is evident in the rapid resolution of inflammation that accompanies DVT when LMWH is given. Heparin therapy is controlled by the APTT.

LMWHs (delteparin, enoxaparin, tinzaparin) are safe and effective in patients with thrombosis of popliteal or more proximal veins.[18] This simplified therapy may allow patients with uncomplicated DVT to be treated without admission to hospital and even prevent death from fatal pulmonary embolism following lower limb arthroplasty.[19]

Cinical use

- *Prophylaxis of venous thromboembolism.* Enoxaparin 30 mg s.c. or tinzaparin 4500 units s.c. once a day appears promising.
- *Treatment of venous thromboembolism.* The site and extent of thrombosis should be established by venous ultrasound or venography.
- *Small distal thrombi.* Require only elevation of the limb and no anticoagulant.
- *Thrombus less than 10 cm.* Tinzaparin 175 units kg^{-1} is sufficient until the patient is fully mobile.
- *Thrombus 10 cm and above.* Uncomplicated by pulmonary embolus, 3 months of anticoagulant therapy appears adequate. Where there is evidence of pulmonary embolus it is a safe practice to continue therapy for 6 months.

Side-effects

The side-effects are bleeding, osteoporosis, hypersensitivity reactions, skin necrosis, and transient alopecia.

HEPARIN ANTAGONISM

Heparin effects wear off so rapidly that an antagonist is seldom required. Protamine sulphate is an antidote given by slow i.v. injection, and 1 mg neutralizes about 100 units of heparin.

THROMBOLYTICS

These drugs act on the blood fibrinolytic system.

Streptokinase ($t_{1/2}$ 80 minutes) is a protein derived from β-haemolytic streptococci.

Alteplase ($t_{1/2}$ 30 minutes) is produced by recombinant DNA technology.

Clinical use

- *Pulmonary embolism.* Thrombolysis is superior to LMWH at relieving radiologically visualized obstructed veins. Alteplase 100 mg may be infused over 2 hours, followed by an i.v. infusion of heparin.
- *DVT.* Thrombolysis may be justified where the affected vessels are proximal and the risk of pulmonary embolism is high.
- *Systemic or local thrombolysis.* This may be considered for arterial occlusions distal to the popliteal artery. Fogarty catheter embolectomy is the usual therapeutic approach for occlusion of <24 hours' duration proximal to the popliteal artery.[20,21]

NEWER AGENTS IN PROPHYLAXIS OF VENOUS THROMBOEMBOLISM

In recent years, National Institute for Clinical Excellence (NICE), UK had issued guidelines on newer oral anticoagulants in the prevention of venous thromboembolism following hip and knee arthroplasty in adults. The duration of treatment of oral anticoagulant depends on the individual risk of the patient for VTE that is determined by the type of orthopaedic surgery.

In major joint replacement surgeries:

Dabigatran etexilate, 110 mg, once a day should be started within 1–4 hours of surgery. Thereafter, a standard dose of 220 mg once daily should be given for 10 days after knee replacement and for 28–35 days after hip replacement.[22]

Rivaroxaban, 10 mg, once a day should be taken 6–10 hours after surgery, provided that haemostasis has been established. And it is continued for 2 weeks in knee replacement and for 5 weeks in hip replacement.[23]

Recent studies showed oral dabigatran 220 mg once-daily was as effective as subcutaneous enoxaparin 40 mg once-daily in reducing the risk of VTE after total hip arthroplasty, and superior to enoxaparin for reducing the risk of major VTE.[24] The risk of bleeding and safety profiles were similar.[24,25] Enoxaparin was less effective than rivaroxaban but had a lower risk of bleeding.[25]

In view of concerns among the orthopaedic surgeons with subspecialty interest in hips and knees replacement surgeries with regard to the risk of bleeding and increased chances of infection at operative site, they may prefer to use LMWH, Clexane 40 mg started on the evening a day before surgery and continued till the patients become ambulant. Thereafter, either low dose warfarin or newer agents such as dabigatran or rivaroxaban should be given for an extended thromboembolic prophylaxis. The regimen for Warfarin is 1 mg in patients aged >60 years and 2 mg in patients <60 years old, once a day for 6 weeks. INR check once a week is sufficient.

ANTI-OSTEOPOROTIC DRUGS

The bone physiology, repair and pathophysiology of osteoporosis are described in Parts 2, 7 and 8 of this textbook. Those who are at risk of osteoporosis should maintain adequate intake of calcium and vitamin D, and any deficiency should be corrected by increasing dietary intake or taking supplements.

Classification of anti-osteoporotic drugs

- Bisphosphonates: alendronic acid, tiludronic acid, zoledronic acid
- Selective oestrogen receptor modulator: raloxifene

- Calcitonin
- Vitamin D derivatives: ergocalciferol (calciferol, vitamin D_2), colecalciferol (vitamin D_3), dihydrotachysterol, alfacalcidol (1α-hydroxycholecalciferol) and calcitriol (1, 25-dihydroxycholecalciferol)
- Parathyroid hormone (PTH): teriparatide
- Strontium ranelate
- Miscellaneous: monoclonal antibodies, nitrates, beta-blockers and cathepsin K inhibitors are being researched.

BISPHOSPHONATES

Bisphosphonates are adsorbed onto hydroxyapatite crystals in bone, slowing both their rate of growth and their dissolution, and thereby reducing the rate of bone turnover. They are used in the prophylaxis and management of osteoporosis and steroid-induced osteoporosis. They may be given orally or intravenously, and are eliminated unchanged by the kidney.

Side-effects

- *Common*: oesophageal irritation; to avoid this, a 70 mg tablet once a week is taken on an empty stomach 1 hour before breakfast in an erect posture. The patient should stand or sit upright for at least 30 minutes after taking the tablet.
- *Rarely*: urticaria, angioedema, and transient drop in serum calcium and phosphate.
- *Very rarely*: Steven Johnson syndrome, osteonecrosis of jaw.
- *Selective oestrogen receptor modulator*: raloxifene is given as an alternative to biphosphonates.

CALCITONIN

Calcitonin is involved with PTH in the regulation of bone turnover, and thereby controlling calcium homeostasis. Calcitonin is available for clinical use in natural (porcine calcitonin) and synthetic (recombinant salmon calcitonin – salcatonin) forms. Its calcium-lowering effect is utilized to treat hypercalcaemia of malignant disease. Calcitonin is commonly used to treat bony pain in Paget's disease of bone. It can also be used in the prevention and management of post-menopausal osteoporosis. It may be administered subcutaneously, intramuscularly, or via the intranasal route.

VITAMIN D DERIVATIVES

The term vitamin D is used for a range of compounds that prevent or cure rickets. It can be administered by oral or intravenous routes.

Clinical use

- *Prevention of osteoporosis*: oral supplement of 10 μg (400 units) of calciferol, once a day, is given. Calcitriol is used in the management of post-menopausal osteoporosis.
- *Intestinal malabsorbtion or chronic liver disease*: 1 mg of calciferol (40 000 units) is given.
- *Hypocalcaemia of hypoparathyroidism*: 2.5 mg of calciferol (100 000 units) is given.
- *Severe renal failure*: calcitriol is given.

Side-effects

Nausea, vomiting, thirst, weight loss, polyuria and raised concentrations of calcium and phosphate in plasma and urine.

PARATHYROID HORMONE

Teriparatide (recombinant human PTH (1-34)), represents a new class of anabolic therapy for the treatment of severe osteoporosis, having the potential to improve skeletal microarchitecture. PTH induces substantial gains in bone mass density.[26,27] Significant reductions in both vertebral and appendicular fracture rates have been demonstrated in the phase III trial of teriparatide, involving elderly women with at least one prevalent vertebral fracture before the onset of therapy. However, currently there is no evidence that the antifracture efficacy of PTH is superior to that of bisphosphonates.[28] Teriparatide is significantly more expensive than bisphosphonates.

STRONTIUM (PROTELOS)

Strontium is an alkaline, dazzling, silvery earth metal with a molecular mass of 513.491 g mol^{-1} and an atomic number of 38 (Fig. 9.4). It is formed on its own in minerals such as celestial and strontianite, and is much softer than calcium.

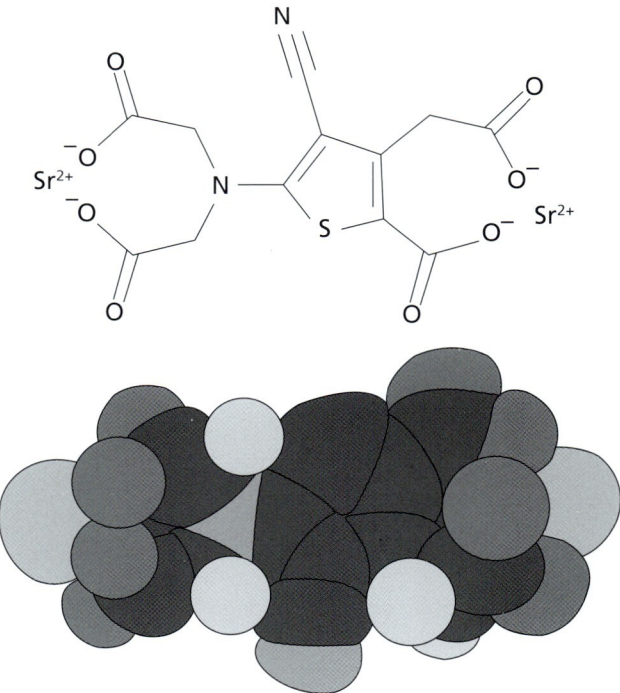

Figure 9.4 The structure of strontium ranelate.

Strontium ranelate is a dual-action bone agent (DABA), which simultaneously inhibits bone resorption and stimulates bone formation, resulting in a rebalance of bone turnover in favour of new bone formation. A dose of 2 g of strontium ranelate, taken daily at bedtime diluted in a glass of water, is effective in post-menopausal osteoporosis, and reduces the risk of vertebral and hip fractures.[29,30] Strontium ranelate is contraindicated in severe renal failure and in patients at high risk of DVT. Strontium should be taken 2 hours before the intake of chelators such as milk, dairy products and antacids. Treatment should be suspended when taking tetracycline and quinolone antibiotics.

NEUTRACEUTICALS

Neutraceuticals are over-the-counter nutritional supplements.

Glucosamine hydrochloride and chondroitin sulphate

Glucosamine salts (glucosamine hydrochloride (GH)) and chondroitin sulphate (CS) preparations are the most commonly used neutraceuticals in the conservative management of osteoarthritis (OA). The combination of GH and CS may be effective in the subgroup of patients with moderate to severe knee pain.[31] An *in vitro* study demonstrated downregulation of mRNA expression for inflammatory mediators and matrix-degrading enzymes while increasing TIMP-3 transcripts.[32] With respect to the structure-modifying effect, there is compelling evidence that GS and CS may interfere with progression of OA.[31] Contrary to this, a double-blind, placebo-controlled, randomized trial[33] showed that the GH/CS group was not superior to the placebo group in function, pain or mobility after both phases of the intervention (phase 1, pill only and phase 2, pill plus exercise). Their long-term efficacy and safety are still to be established.[34]

KEY LEARNING POINTS

- Opioids exert their therapeutic effects by mimicking the action of endogenous opioid peptides, the enkephalins, endorphins and dynorphins, at opioid receptors.
- Patient controlled analgesia (PCA) can be used for intravenous or epidural infusion. This technique avoids any delays in administration and allows greater dosing flexibility.
- Non-steroidal anti-inflammatory drugs are analgesics, anti-inflammatory and antipyretics. NSAIDs exert this anti-inflammatory action by inhibiting cyclo-oxygenase (COX), resulting in inhibition of prostaglandin synthesis.
- Aspirin is the most commonly used antiplatelet agent. It irreversibly acetylates cyclooxygenase, the enzyme responsible for the first step in the formation of prostaglandins H2.
- Local anaesthetics block action potential initiation and propagation in neurons by reducing the passage of sodium voltage-activated Na+ ion channels.
- Steroids have multiple actions due to the presence of glucocorticoids response elements (GREs) in the promoter region of several genes. Steroids induce transcription of a protein, IkB, which traps activated NF-kB in inactive cytoplasmic complexes.
- Heparin complexes with antithrombin III, and it inhibits activated factor Xa, which is needed to covert prothrombin to thrombin.

REFERENCES

- ● = Key primary paper
- ◆ = Major review article

●1. Duggan AW, North RA. Electrophysiology of opioids. *Pharmacological Reviews* 1983;**35**:219–81.
●2. Rodgers BM, Webb CJ, Stergios D, Newman BM. Patient-controlled analgesia in pediatric surgery. *Journal of Pediatric Surgery* 1988;**23**:259–62.
●3. Bressan N, Castro A, Braga C, Lages J, Silva NR, Portela P, et al. Automation in anesthesia: computer controlled propofol infusion and data acquisition. Conference proceedings: *Annual International Conference of the IEEE Engineering in Medicine and Biology Society IEEE Engineering in Medicine and Biology Society Conference.* 2008;**2008**:5543–7.
●4. Fivel PA. Computer-controlled drug doses for IV drug self-administration. *Experimental and Clinical Psychopharmacology* 2011;**19**:131–3.
●5. Stein C, Comisel K, Haimerl E, et al. Analgesic effect of intraarticular morphine after arthroscopic knee surgery. *New England Journal of Medicine* 1991;**325**:1123–6.
◆6. Hege-Scheuing G, Michaelsen K, Buhler A, et al. [Analgesia with intra-articular morphine following knee joint arthroscopy? A double-blind, randomized study with patient-controlled analgesia]. *Anaesthesist* 1995;**44**:351–8.
●7. Ashburn MA, Stephen RL, Ackerman E, et al. Iontophoretic delivery of morphine for postoperative analgesia. *Journal of Pain Symptom Management* 1992;**7**:27–33.
◆8. Bracken MB, Shepard MJ, Holford TR, et al. Administration of methylprednisolone for 24 or 48 hours or tirilazad mesylate for 48 hours in the treatment of acute spinal cord injury. Results of the Third National Acute Spinal Cord Injury Randomized Controlled Trial. National Acute Spinal Cord Injury Study. *Journal of the American Medical Association* 1997;**277**:1597–604.
●9. Sorensen, P. [High-dose methylprednisolone in acute spinal injury]. *Ugeskrift for Laeger* 2008;**170**:315–17.
●10. Hugenholtz H, Cass DE, Dvorak MF, et al. High-dose methylprednisolone for acute closed spinal cord

injury – only a treatment option. *Canadian Journal of Neurological Sciences* 2002;**29**:227–35.

●11. Kronvall E, Sayer FT, Nilsson OG. [Methylprednisolone in the treatment of acute spinal cord injury has become more and more questioned]. *Lakartidningen* 2005;**102**:1887–90.

●12. Hurlbert RJ. Methylprednisolone for acute spinal cord injury: an inappropriate standard of care. *Journal of Neurosurgery* 2000;**193**:1–7.

●13. Fennerty A Campbell IA and Routledge PA. Anticoagulants in venous thromboembolism. *British Medical Journal* 1988;**297**:1285–8.

●14. Svensson P, Sodermark A, Schulman S. Experiences of a low-intensity anticoagulation regimen for extended secondary prevention of venous thromboembolism. *Hematology Journal* 2002;**3**:311–14.

15. Guidelines on oral anticoagulation. British Society for Haematology, second edition. British Committee for Standards in Haematology. Haemostasis and Thrombosis Task Force. *Journal of Clinical Pathology* 1990;**43**:177–83.

●16. Kounis NG, Alexandridis T, Gogos CA. Calf haematoma masquerading as veno-occlusive disease during anticoagulation. *The British Journal of Clinical Practice* 1986;**40**:541–2.

●17. Hay SM, Allen MJ, Barnes MR. Acute compartment syndromes resulting from anticoagulant treatment. *British Medical Journal* 1992;**305**:1474–5.

●18. Hull RD, Raskob GE, Pineo GF, *et al*. Subcutaneous low-molecular-weight heparin compared with continuous intravenous heparin in the treatment of proximal-vein thrombosis. *New England Journal of Medicine* 1992; **326**:975–82.

19. Frostick SP. Death after joint replacement. *Haemostasis* 2000;**30**(Suppl 2):84–7; Discussion 82–3.

●20. Wolosker N, Kuzniec S, Gaudencio A, *et al*. Arterial embolectomy in lower limbs. *Sao Paulo Medical Journal* 1996;**114**:1226–30.

21. Borioni R, Garofalo M, Albano P, *et al*. [Thromboembolectomy with a Fogarty catheter. Our clinical experience]. *Minerva Cardioangiology* 2000;**48**:111–16.

●22. NICE. UK2011 [updated 17 June 2011]; Available from: http://www.nice.org.uk/TA157.

●23. NICE. 2010 [updated 01 December 2010]; Available from: http://www.nice.org.uk/guidance/TA170.

◆24. Eriksson BI, Dahl OE, Huo MH, Kurth AA, Hantel S, Hermansson K, *et al*. Oral dabigatran versus enoxaparin for thromboprophylaxis after primary total hip arthroplasty (RE-NOVATE II*). A randomised, double-blind, non-inferiority trial. *Thrombosis and Haemostasis.* 2011;**105**:721–9.

◆25. Huisman MV, Quinlan DJ, Dahl OE, Schulman S. Enoxaparin versus dabigatran or rivaroxaban for thromboprophylaxis after hip or knee arthroplasty: Results of separate pooled analyses of phase III multicenter randomized trials. *Circulation Cardiovascular Quality and Outcomes* 2010;**3**:652–60.

●26. Lane NE, Sanchez S, Modin GW, *et al*. Parathyroid hormone treatment can reverse corticosteroid-induced osteoporosis. Results of a randomized controlled clinical trial. *Journal of Clinical Investigation* 1998;**102**:1627–33.

●27. Orwoll ES, Scheele WH, Paul S, *et al*. The effect of teriparatide [human parathyroid hormone (1–34)] therapy on bone density in men with osteoporosis. *Journal of Bone and Mineral Research* 2003;**18**:9–17.

◆28. Hodsman AB, Bauer DC, Dempster DW, *et al*. (2005) Parathyroid hormone and teriparatide for the treatment of osteoporosis: a review of the evidence and suggested guidelines for its use. *Endocrine Reviews* **26**:688–703.

◆29. Blake GM, Fogelman I. Strontium ranelate: a novel treatment for postmenopausal osteoporosis: a review of safety and efficacy. *Clinical Interventions in Aging* 2006;**1**:367–75.

●30. Burlet N, Reginster JY. Strontium ranelate: the first dual acting treatment for postmenopausal osteoporosis. *Clinical Orthopaedics and Related Research* 2006;**443**:55–60.

●31. Bruyere O, Reginster JY. Glucosamine and chondroitin sulfate as therapeutic agents for knee and hip osteoarthritis. *Drugs Aging* 2007;**24**:573–80.

●32. Chan PS, Caron JP, Orth MW. Effects of glucosamine and chondroitin sulfate on bovine cartilage explants under long-term culture conditions. *American Journal of Veterinary Research* 2007;**68**:709–15.

33. Messier SP, Mihalko S, Loeser RF, *et al*. Glucosamine/chondroitin combined with exercise for the treatment of knee osteoarthritis: a preliminary study. *Osteoarthritis Cartilage* 2007;**15**:1256–66.

34. Lozada, CJ. Glucosamine in osteoarthritis: questions remain. *Cleveland Clinic Journal of Medicine* 2007;**74**:65–71.

PART 3

BASIC SCIENCE

NICOLA MAFFULLI AND PATRICK WARNKE

10	**Molecular and cell biology, immunology and genetics** *Chezhiyan Shanmugam, Umile Giuseppe Longo, Nicola Maffulli*	139
11	**Musculoskeletal imaging** *Mark W Anderson*	155
12	**Biomechanics and biomaterials** *Duncan ET Shepherd, David WL Hukins*	173
13	**Clinical principles of kinesiology** *Jim Richards, James Selfe*	202
14	**Infections of the musculoskeletal system** *Sureshan Sivananthan, Eugene Sherry*	219

10

Molecular and cell biology, immunology and genetics

CHEZHIYAN SHANMUGAM, UMILE GIUSEPPE LONGO, NICOLA MAFFULLI

Introduction	139	Genetics	150
Molecular and cell biology	139	References	153
Immunology	145		

NATIONAL BOARD STANDARDS

- Understand the structure and function of DNA and RNA
- Understand the process of protein synthesis and gene expression
- Know about the various growth factors
- Understand the function of cytokines
- Understand cell matrix interactions
- Know how the immune system works
- Understand the genetic basis of common orthopaedic conditions

INTRODUCTION

Molecular and cell biology, immunology and genetics are three rapidly evolving basic science fields that are currently being explored to provide a better understanding of the basic defects underlying musculoskeletal diseases. There is much research and development pertaining to orthopaedics, and the knowledge accumulated in these fields over the last few years is enormous. One chapter could never cover the entirety of these three major fields. Therefore, this chapter addresses only those major topics of each of these disciplines that are relevant to the understanding of musculoskeletal conditions.

MOLECULAR AND CELL BIOLOGY

DNA (deoxyribonucleic acid)

DNA is composed of two nucleotide chains (forming a double helix), each consisting of a deoxyribose sugar–phosphate (phosphodiester bonds) backbone with bases bonded with complementary bases on the opposite chain (Fig. 10.1a). There are only two types of complementary base pairs possible in nature: adenosine–thymine (A–T) and guanine–cytosine (G–C). The A–T base pair has a double-ring structure called a purine, and the G–C base pair has a single-ring structure called a pyrimidine. Most DNA is located in the cell nucleus and is known as nuclear DNA; the small amount found in the mitochondria is called mitochondrial DNA. Each type of DNA has the following three inherent cellular functions.

1. *Replication.* The two DNA strands separate, and each serves as a template for building a new complementary strand. For example, if one strand has the base sequence of TGACCAGT (in the 3′-to-5′ direction), then its complementary strand ACTGGTCA (5′-to-3′ direction) is formed (Fig. 10.1c). DNA polymerase builds new DNA strands during the process of duplication. (Note that DNA polymerase III is the main enzyme involved in DNA replication; DNA polymerase II is a minor enzyme involved in DNA repair; and DNA polymerase I is the main polymerase involved in DNA repair and plays a specialized role in DNA replication, using its 5′-to-3′ exonuclease activity.)

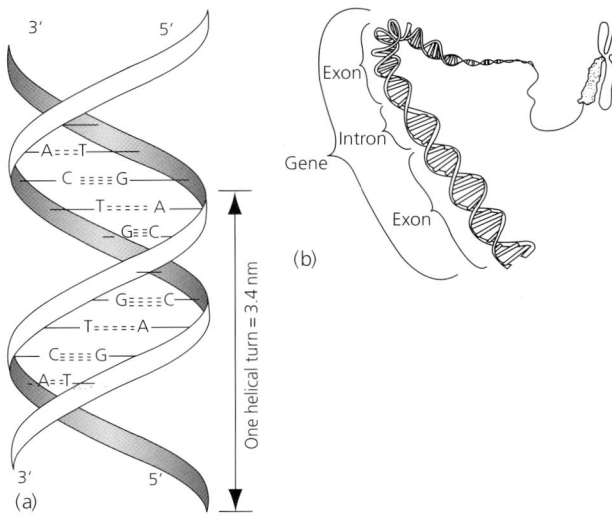

2. *Hereditary information.* The specific base pair/nucleotide sequence represents the hereditary information necessary for building and maintaining an organism.
3. *Regulation of cell division.* This occurs through expression of messenger ribonucleic acid (mRNA).

Nucleotides

Nucleotides are the structural units of RNA, DNA and several cofactors, such as coenzyme A, flavin adenine dinucleotide, flavin mononucleotide, adenosine triphosphate (ATP) and nicotinamide adenine dinucleotide phosphate. The current genome sequence (Build 35, which is based on 2004 data) contains 2.85 billion nucleotides interrupted by only 341 gaps. It covers 99% of the euchromatic genome and is accurate to an error rate of one event per 100 000 bases.[1] Nucleotides consist of three portions: a nitrogenous base, a sugar and one or more phosphate groups. They have important roles in metabolism and signalling in the cell. Three nucleotides constitute a codon, which encodes for an amino acid. The codon specifies one of the possible 20 amino acids that are the building blocks of all proteins.

Chromosomes

The 46 human chromosomes are located in the nucleus of every cell. We have 44 autosomes and two allosomes. The genes that determine somatic characteristics are in the autosomes, or somatic chromosomes, and do not exert any influence on determining the sex of the organism. The allosomes are the sex chromosomes – they carry the genes responsible for sexual characteristics. Chromosomes contain both DNA and RNA. Each chromosome contains >150 000 genes. A chromosomal DNA molecule contains three specific nucleotide sequences that are required for replication. They are DNA replication origin, a centromere to attach the DNA to the mitotic spindle, and a telomere located at each end of the linear chromosome. DNA occupies a relatively large space in the cell despite the fact that it is highly condensed. Nucleosomes pack these DNA molecules into smaller units to compact the intracellular space.

Genes (alleles) (Fig. 10.1b)

In its simplest form, a gene is a sequence of DNA codifying for a protein. A gene is a union of genomic sequences encoding a coherent set of potentially overlapping functional products.[2] The base pair information of a gene is copied into the mRNA (transcription). Then, the mRNA travels out of the nucleus into the cytoplasm to ribosomes. There, the mRNA assembles the amino acids to form specific proteins (translation). The Human Genome Project, started in 1990, produced a working draft of the genome in 2000, and a complete sequence in 2003, with

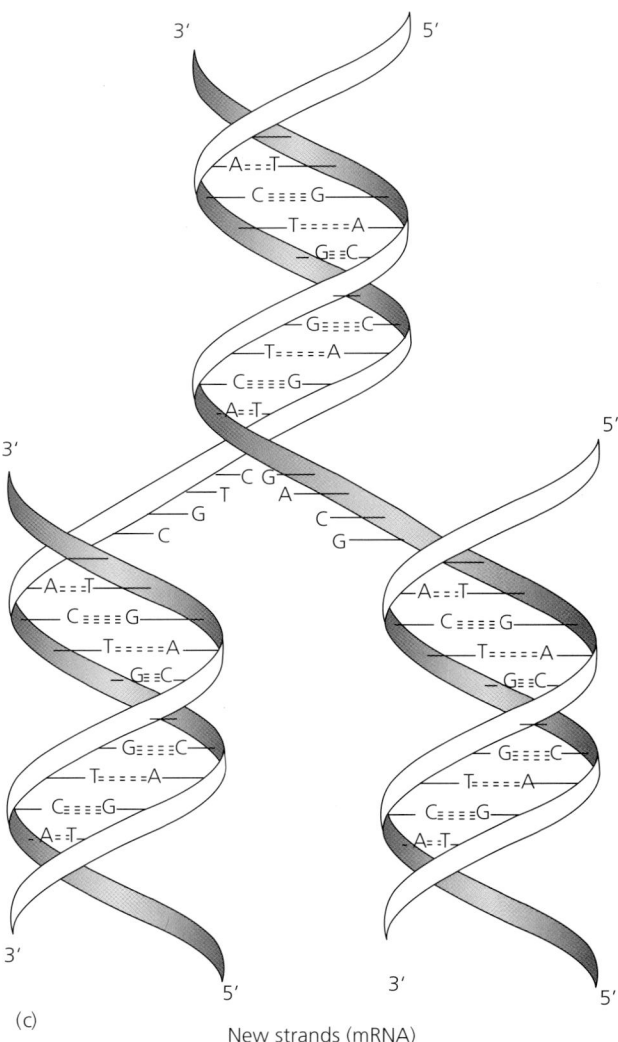

Figure 10.1 (a) The structure of DNA. (b) The structure of a gene. (c) A simple rule of faithful duplication.

further analysis still being published. The genes are regulated so that a relatively small number of genes are expressed for any given cell. Regulation of gene expression determines the unique biological qualities of each cell. The Human Genome Project has found only 20 000–25 000 protein-coding genes, contrary to the expectation of as high as 2 000 000 before the start of the project.[1]

TECHNIQUES USED TO STUDY GENETIC DISORDERS

Restriction enzymes

Restriction endonucleases are used to cut double-stranded DNA at nucleotide sequences specific for each restriction endonuclease. Such sequences are known as restriction sites, and the action of the restriction endonuclease produces restriction fragments. Restriction enzymes enable a DNA sequence to be 'cut' from the rest of the DNA, and further manipulation will allow such a sequence to be spliced into a plasmid. This technology has opened the way to cloning of genes. This technique is commonly used to estimate the probability of a genetic trait or disease associated with various polymorphisms identified in the restriction fragments.

Oligonucleotide ligation assay[3]

Oligonucleotides are used as primers in polymerase chain reactions (PCRs) to match their target sequence, which will then generate a product. This approach is also known as the amplification refractory mutation system (ARMS), and is often used to detect common cystic fibrosis mutations and certain mutations involved in familial breast cancer.

Single-stranded conformation polymorphism analysis

The principle of single-stranded conformation polymorphism (SSCP) analysis is based on the fact that the secondary structure of single-stranded DNA is dependent on its base composition. Any change to the base composition introduced by a mutation or polymorphism will cause a modification to the secondary structure of the DNA strand. This altered conformation affects its migration through a non-denaturing polyacrylamide gel electrophoresis.

Heteroduplex analysis

Heteroduplexes are double-stranded DNA molecules that are formed from two complementary strands that are imperfectly matched. If a mutation is present in one copy of a gene being amplified using PCR, heteroduplexes will be formed from the hybridization of the normal and the mutant PCR product. In practice, SSCP and heteroduplex analysis can be carried out simultaneously on the same polyacrylamide gel to increase the sensitivity of the analysis.

Protein truncation test

This analysis is based on the protein product generated from the DNA sequence, and it detects the premature protein truncation caused by nonsense mutations. Samples with nonsense mutations generate smaller protein products than their normal counterparts, which are then separated by polyacrylamide gel electrophoresis.

DNA ligation

DNA ligation involves producing a phosphodiester bond between the 3′ hydroxyl of one nucleotide and the 5′ phosphate of another to produce a useful DNA molecule. A ligation reaction requires three ingredients in addition to water: (1) fragments of DNA with either blunt or cohesive (sticky) ends; (2) a buffer which contains ATP; and (3) T4 DNA ligase. T4 ligase, which originates from the T4 bacteriophage, is used for ligation. This enzyme will ligate DNA fragments, repairing the defects in duplex DNA.

A typical reaction for inserting a fragment into a plasmid vector (subcloning) would utilize about 0.01 (sticky ends) to 1 (blunt ends) units of ligase. The optimal incubation temperature for T4 DNA ligase is 16°C.

Almost all DNA fragments produced by digestion of a plasmid with two restriction enzymes when incubated with ligase for 5 minutes will ligate to one another, and shift to a higher molecular weight.

Genomic screening

This tool identifies the unique patterns of genes that are 'turned on' or 'turned off' by specific environmental stressors.[4] This will enable better understanding of the pathways from exposure to outcome that can be achieved for building computational toxicology. This technology will ultimately reduce the uncertainty in assessing risk of stressors in the environment.

Polymerase chain reaction

DNA polymerase is used to amplify a piece of DNA by *in vitro* enzymatic replication. As PCR progresses, the DNA thus generated is itself used as the template for replication. This chain reaction exponentially amplifies the DNA template. PCR is used for genetic fingerprinting, a forensic technique used to identify a person or organism by comparing DNA molecules through different PCR-based methods. PCR amplification has also been used for the prenatal diagnosis of sickle cell disease and screening DNA for gene mutations, e.g. methicillin-resistant *Staphylococcus aureus*.[5] This analysis is feasible even if there are very small amounts of starting material.

Agarose gel electrophoresis

This technique is used to separate DNA or RNA molecules by size. By subjecting the sample to an electrical field, negatively charged nucleic acid molecules move through an agarose matrix. The gel acts as a sieve. Shorter molecules move faster and migrate further than longer ones. Clinically, agarose gel electrophoresis is commonly used after or in conjunction with restriction enzymes to estimate the size of DNA molecules, e.g. in restriction mapping of cloned DNA. If the sample is homozygous for the common allele, there will be two bands of DNA, because the cut will have occurred at the restriction site by restriction enzymes. If the sample is homozygous for the rarer allele, the sample will show only one band, because the cut will not have occurred. If the sample is heterozygous at that single nucleotide polymorphism, there will be three bands of DNA.

Denaturing high-performance liquid chromatography

Denaturing high-performance liquid chromatography (DHPLC) uses a high-pressure system to force the products through a column under partially denaturing conditions. The DNA molecules that are progressively eluted from the column are monitored by an ultraviolet detector, with data being collected by computer.

Southern blotting

This method is used to detect large deletions in the DNA, well out of the range of PCR. The DNA is transferred by capillary blotting onto a nylon membrane before radio-labelled probes are used to investigate the region of interest by pulsed-field gel electrophoresis (PFGE). PFGE uses specialized restriction enzymes and electrophoresis conditions to fractionate the genomic DNA to a high resolution. The mnemonic 'SNOW DROP' can be used: Southern for DNA, Northern for RNA and Western for Proteins.

Plasmid vectors

These are used to produce large quantities of a gene in a bacterium. The gene is ligated into a plasmid (which is then known as a recombinant plasmid), and inserted into a bacterium (the vector) using a process called transformation. The recombinant plasmid replicates inside the bacterium at 30°C, and thus increases the recombinant DNA and the gene. This plasmid is finally eliminated from the cells by increasing the temperature of the culture to 44°C.[6]

Transgenic animals

A transgenic animal (Fig. 10.2) is produced by inserting a foreign gene (transgene) into a single-cell embryo, which then replicates and carries the transgene to every cell in the body.[7] In addition to a structural gene, the DNA contains other sequences to be incorporated into the DNA of the host, and to be expressed correctly by the cells of the host. For example, transgenic sheep and goats have been produced that express foreign proteins in their milk, and transgenic chickens are now able to synthesize human proteins by as much as 0.1 g in each egg that they lay. Using sperm-mediated gene transfer, we may be able to produce transgenic pigs that can serve as a source of transplanted organs for humans.[8]

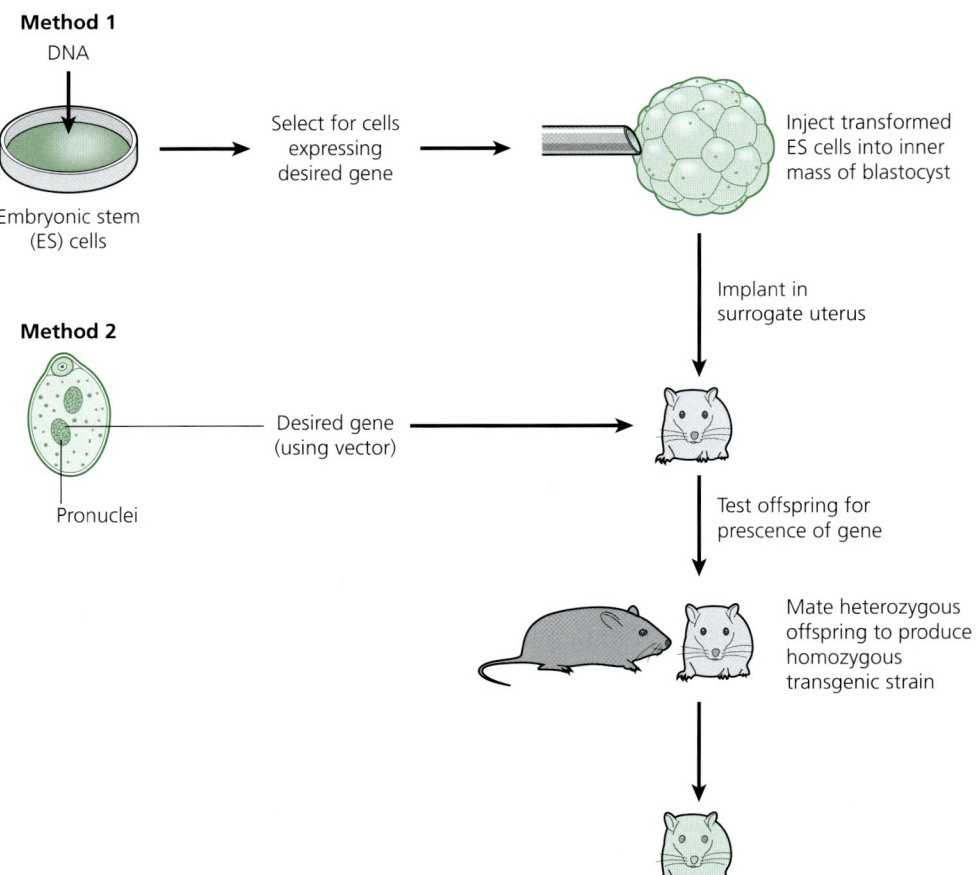

Figure 10.2 Transgenic animals, e.g. mouse. Method 1, knock-out mice lacking specific genes of interest are produced by homologous recombination in embryonic stem (ES) cells followed by injection into blastocysts to create chimeric mice. Method 2, microinjection of DNA into the pronuclei of fertilized eggs performed out to produce a heterozygous transgenic mouse which expresses the desired gene. By mating with another heterozygous offspring, a homozygous strain is produced.

Gene chip technology

Thousands of short DNA probe molecules are first attached to silica-based support materials. The DNA under investigation is then fluorescently labelled and hybridized to the probe matrix. The large number of probes used enables the pattern of hybridization to be translated into sequence information. The high cost of this approach limits its use to the analysis of rare disease genes in a diagnostic setting.

HUMAN CLONING

Human cloning is an *in vitro* process of producing a genetically identical copy of a human cell, human tissue or human being. Genes influence behaviour and cognition. Cloned humans, even though they are genetically identical, they may not necessarily be identical altogether. Identical twins are natural human clones. Even though they have identical DNA, they are separate people with different experiences and personalities.[9]

In the UK, the government, after an amendment to the Human Fertilization and Embryology Act 1990, introduced legislation to allow licensed therapeutic cloning in January 2001, but prohibited reproductive cloning, The first license was granted in August 2004 to researchers at the University of Newcastle to allow them to investigate treatments for diabetes, Parkinson's disease and Alzheimer's disease.[10,11]

Somatic cell nuclear transfer allows therapeutic and reproductive cloning. The nucleus of a donor somatic cell (46 chromosomes – a diploid set) to be cloned is removed, and the rest of the cell is discarded. At the same time, the surrogate egg is enucleated using a micropipette. Thereafter, the nucleus of the somatic cell is injected into the enucleated egg cell, and it is stimulated with an electric shock. The somatic cell nucleus starts to divide, and, after many mitotic divisions in culture, forms a blastocyst with an almost identical DNA to the original somatic cell.

There are three types of cloning, as follows.

Therapeutic cloning

Somatic cell nuclear transfer is adopted initially as detailed above. From the embryo, the stem cells are removed, and cultured using appropriate growth factors. The remaining embryo dies. This process guides the stem cell to differentiate into a desired lineage of cells, tissues or an organ. Then, the cloned cells, tissues or organ are transplanted back to the patient, thereby avoiding organ rejection and the complications due to concurrent use of life-long immunosuppressant.

Reproductive cloning

The somatic cell nuclear transfer is adopted initially as explained above. When the clone reaches the embryo stage, it is implanted into a surrogate uterus and allowed to develop. Currently, reproductive cloning is banned worldwide. The first hybrid human clone was created in November 1998 by American Cell Technologies.[12] A man's leg cell nucleus was used in an enucleated cow's egg. However, it was destroyed after 12 days, as a normal embryo implants at 14 days.

Embryo cloning

The first human embryo was cloned by *in vitro* fertilization of an egg cell with sperm (Fig. 10.3).[13] The zygote was allowed to develop into a blastula. At the 100 cell stage, acidic Tyrode's solution was added to remove the zona pellucida covering. This provided nutrients to the cells to promote cell division. The blastula was then divided into individual cells, which were deposited on individual dishes (Fig. 10.3a). They were either covered with an artificial zona pellucida to develop into an independent embryo or left uncovered to yield stem cells. The stem cells were then coaxed to grow a variety of cells, such as nerve cells, haemopoietic cells, pancreatic cells and cardiac cells (Fig. 10.3b,c).[13] For ethical reasons, the researchers selected human embryos that had no possibility of ever maturing into newborn babies.[14] Currently, embryo cloning is used to safeguard endangered animal species.[10,11]

GENE THERAPY

Gene therapy has been a promising strategy for various orthopaedic applications over the last two decades.[3] Correcting or compensating for a mutation is the goal of gene therapy. The identification of alterations in the signalling peptides underlying many diseases led to speculation that genetic disorders could be treated by gene therapy. An increasing amount of evidence has indicated that gene transfer can aid the repair of articular cartilage, menisci, intervertebral discs, ligaments and tendons. In orthopaedic oncology, gene therapy may induce tumour necrosis and increased tumour sensitivity to chemotherapy.[15] Polypeptide growth factors have shown promising results in enhancing the structural quality of the repair tissue by stimulating chondrocyte proliferation, maturation and matrix synthesis via direct or cell transplantation-mediated approaches.[3] Kaul *et al.*[16] demonstrated chondrogenesis in cartilage defects *in vivo* by transplanting genetically modified articular chondrocytes with human fibroblast growth factor 2 (FGF-2). The localized overexpression of FGF-2 enhanced the repair of cartilage defects via stimulation of chondrogenesis, without adverse effects on the synovial membrane.

Efforts have focused on somatic gene therapy, in which the function of mutated genes is corrected in specific cells or organs rather than in egg or sperm cells or early embryos (germline therapy). Two approaches have been used: *ex vivo* and *in vivo* gene delivery. In *ex vivo* delivery, cells are taken from a patient, the new gene is inserted and the cells are then placed back into the patient. The *in vivo* delivery involves delivering the gene directly to the patient's tissues, usually by infecting the patient with a virus that contains the new gene.

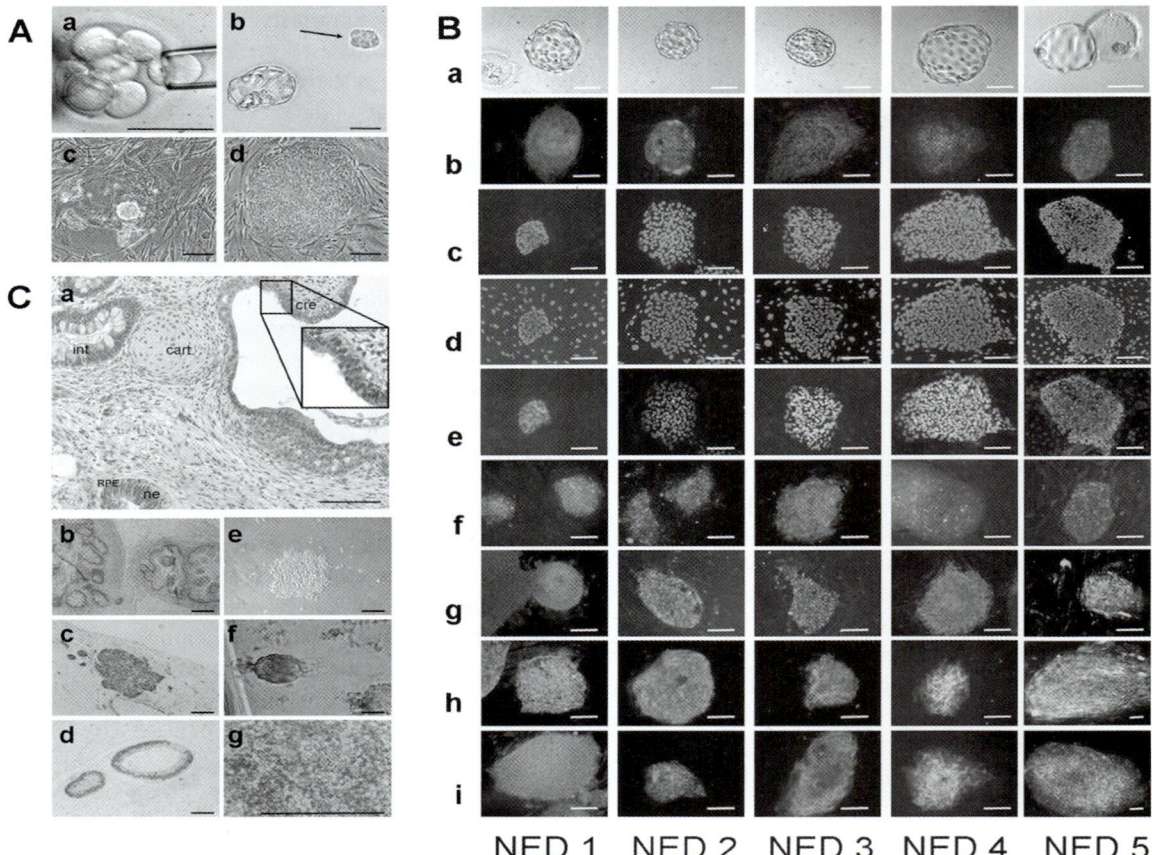

Figure 10.3 Derivation and characterization of human embryonic stem cell (HESC) lines from single blastomeres without embryo destruction. (A) Stages of derivation of HESCs from a single blastomere. (a) Blastomere biopsy; (b) biopsied blastomere (arrow) and parent embryo are developing next to each other; (c) initial outgrowth of single blastomere on mouse embryonic fibroblasts (MEFs), 6 days; and (d) colony of single blastomere-derived HESCs. (B) Blastocysts formed by the biopsied parental embryos (a) and markers of pluripotency in single blastomere-derived HESC lines (b–i). (b) Alkaline phosphatase; (c) Oct-4; (d) DAPI corresponding to Oct-4 and (e) Nanog; (f) SSEA-3; (g) SSEA-4; (h) TRA-1-60; and (i) TRA-1-81. (C) Differentiation of single blastomere-derived HESCs into three germ layers *in vivo* (a–d) and *in vitro* (e–g). (a) Teratoma showing derivatives of all three germ layers. Ciliated respiratory epithelium (cre); intestinal epithelium (int); cartilage (cart); and columnar neuroepithelium (ne) with associated retinal pigmented epithelium (RPE). (b) Bronchiolar nests. (c) Muscle stained for smooth muscle actin. (d) Intestinal epithelium stained for cdx2. (e) Haemangioblast colony with both haematopoietic and endothelial potential. (f) An embryoid body with beating heart cells. (g) Retinal pigment epithelium. DAPI = Diamidino-2-phenylindole dihydrocloride DNA dye; SSEA- SSEA-3 and -4 are cell surface globoseries glycosphingolipid epitopes that are commonly used as markers for human embryonic stem cells; TRA = embryonic stem cell marker; NED = no embryo destruction. Oct-4 and nanog are transcription factors required to maintain the pluripotency and self-renewal of embryonic stem (ES) cells. Reproduced with permission from Chung *et al.*[12]

Prerequisites of gene therapy

- The gene must have been cloned and sequenced so that it is fully characterized and readily available in its correct form.
- The gene should be safely introducible into appropriate target cells.
- The gene should express in its new site.

Classification of gene vectors

- Viral delivery systems
  - RNA viruses: retroviral vectors
  - adenoviruses
  - herpes simplex virus type 1
  - adeno-associated viruses
  - lentivirus.
- Non-viral delivery systems
  - naked DNA
  - plasmid DNA.

The most common approach has been to incorporate the gene into a virus, which is then used to infect the target cells. Modified viruses can incorporate nucleic acid into cells and induce new gene expression, often without cytotoxicity. They are thus ideally suited to achieve a high efficiency of gene transfer and expression.

The potential risks of viral vectors include:

- viral vectors that integrate into the genome may cause DNA mutations (insertional mutagenesis)
- recombination of the disabled viral vector with wild-type virus may lead to infectious complications
- the virus can induce an inflammatory and immune response.

Gene therapy is still in the research realm. The challenge remains in integrating therapeutic DNA into the genome to increase its duration of expressivity. Currently, researchers face the potential toxicity of viral vectors. The death of a patient from systemic administration of an adenoviral vector and recent reports of leukaemia in two patients in a clinical gene therapy trial have produced serious setbacks in the safety of gene therapy. In the near future, tissue repair may become one of the earliest clinical successes (phase III) for gene therapy as a whole.[15]

IMMUNOLOGY

Immunology is the study of the human defence system. As we move around in our environment, we are invariably exposed to attack by a variety of micro-organisms and other factors of one kind or another. To defend against these, we have a robust immune system. The immune system can be divided into the innate and adaptive immune systems. These systems rely on a complex network of organs, cells and circulating proteins. The principal organs of the immune system are the bone marrow, the thymus, the spleen, the lymph nodes and the lymphoid tissues associated with the epithelia that line the gut and airways (known as mucosa-associated lymphoid tissue). Collectively, they are known as the lymphoid organs. The cells of the immune system include the leucocytes (or white blood cells), mast cells and various accessory cells that are scattered throughout the body. The accessory cells include phagocytic cells that are found in many organs, including the bone, lungs, liver, spleen and kidneys. Most of these cells also function as antigen-presenting cells. The antibodies and complement form the proteins of the immune system.

Innate immune system

The natural immune system consists of defence mechanisms that do not change very much either with age or following infections. It consists of four kinds of cells and three different classes of proteins. The cells of the natural immune system are:

- phagocytes
- natural killer cells
- mast cells
- eosinophils.

The classes of proteins are:

- complement
- interferons
- acute phase proteins.

The phagocytes include macrophages and neutrophils, which engulf small invading organisms (e.g. bacteria) and kill them using highly reactive oxygen and nitrogen intermediates. They then digest the remains and release the contents for use by the host. Cells that become infected with a virus are destroyed by natural killer cells before the virus can replicate. Natural killer cells are large granular lymphocytes that are believed to recognize virus-infected cells via modified cell surface markers. They release granules by exocytosis on the target cells, which responds by undergoing preprogrammed cell death. This ensures that viruses lack the ability to use the genetic machinery of host cells to make copies of themselves. Mast cells release histamine, which causes local vasodilatation and increases the chances of leucocytes being exposed to the inflammatory site. Eosinophils play an important role in helminth infections. Eosinophils are particularly attracted to parasites whose outer membranes have been coated with antibody of the immunoglobulin E (IgE) class. Major basic proteins, perforins, peroxidase and phospholipase D attack the outer membrane of the parasites to inactivate or kill them.

THE COMPLEMENT SYSTEM

The complement system (Fig. 10.4) plays an important role in the innate immune system in eradicating infections, particularly those caused by bacteria and fungi. The complement system may also be recruited by the adaptive immune system in case of overwhelming inflammation. The complement proteins can be sequentially activated by either microbial cell surfaces or antibody secreted by the lymphocytes. There are three pathways that activate the complement system: classical, alternative and lectin pathways. The major component of the complement system is the C3, which can be activated in a variety of ways (Fig. 10.4). Once activated, C3 produces a fraction, C3b, which binds to the surface of microbes and so facilitates their uptake by phagocytes. The C3b fragment cleaves C5 into C5a and C5b. C5a is an important chemotactic protein, and helps in recruiting inflammatory cells. Both C3a and C5a have anaphylatoxin activity, directly triggering degranulation of mast cells and increasing vascular permeability and smooth muscle contraction. C5b combines with C6, C7, C8 and polymeric C9, forming the membrane attack complex (MAC). The MAC is the cytolytic end product of the complement cascade that forms a transmembrane channel leading to osmotic lysis of the target cell.

ACUTE PHASE PROTEINS

The acute phase proteins are a group of plasma proteins synthesized by the liver that show a huge increase in

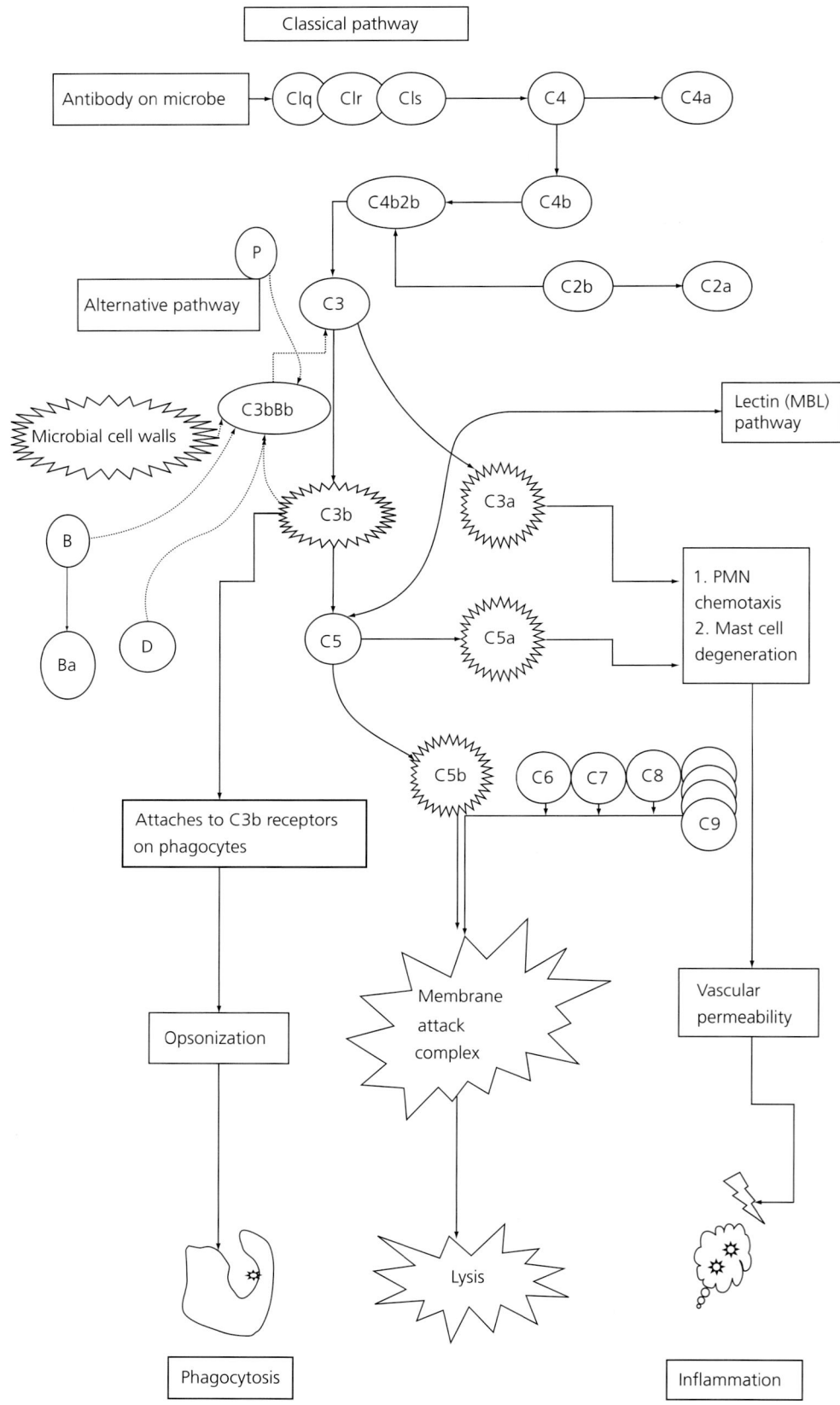

Figure 10.4 Activation and regulation of complement system. MBL, mannose-binding lectin; PMN, polymorphonuclear.

concentration during an infection. They include C-reactive protein and mannose-binding protein, both of which bind to the surface of invading organisms. This surface coating is known as opsonization. The complement and antibodies can also opsonize foreign organisms. As the phagocytes have receptors for the coating proteins, they are able to recognize opsonized particles and engulf them.

INTERFERONS

Interferons belong to the large class of glycoproteins known as cytokines. The virus-infected cells release interferons. The interferons then bind to receptors on neighbouring cells, which respond by reducing the rate of mRNA translation. This results in the infected cell being surrounded by a layer of cells that cannot replicate the virus, so that a barrier is formed preventing the spread of the infection. Thereafter, the natural killer cells identify and destroy any infected cells. The interferon family is summarized in Table 10.1.

THE ACUTE INFLAMMATORY RESPONSE

When the body becomes injured, e.g. following trauma, fracture, soft-tissue injury, surgery or infection, the four cardinal signs of inflammation identified by Celsus are observed: (1) redness, as vasoactive peptides (histamine) are released by mast cells; (2) heat, as capillary permeability increases, allowing exudation of serum proteins (antibody, complement, kinikogens, etc.) required to control the inflammation; (3) swelling, as exudation of fluids and cellular migration (diapedesis of leucocytes) occurs – the type of cells recruited depends on the nature of the antigenic challenge and on the site where the reactions occur; (4) pain, which results from activation of nerve endings. The trigger for the inflammatory response is mast cell degranulation. Various components of complement (Fig. 10.4) and factor XII (Hageman factor) are the two plasma mediators that come into play in inflammation. Polymorphonuclear and mononuclear phagocytes migrate into the damaged tissues, where they engulf and digest bacteria and necrotic cells.

The tissue heals by formation of granulation tissue, which is a combination of proliferation of capillaries and fibroblasts, and by scarring. In bone fracture, cartilage is formed either from primitive mesenchymal cells or from demodulation of other cells when subjected to physiological strain at the fracture site. Connective tissue and the cartilage tissue are together described as callus. Dormant osteogenic cells of the periosteum become osteoblasts. These osteoblasts and the osteogenic buds from fracture fragments invade and replace the fibrocartilaginous callus with bony callus. Then, after fracture healing, remodelling of the bone takes place over months to years.

The acute inflammatory reaction may either subside or persist to become chronic. If the offending material persists, it is sealed off by a layer of macrophages, lymphocytes and other cells to form a granuloma. Chronic inflammation occurs as a result of many types of bacterial infection, such as tuberculosis, syphilis and fungal infection. It is also characteristically seen in autoimmune diseases, such as rheumatoid arthritis and systemic lupus erythematosus, and in response to the introduction of foreign bodies, e.g. suture material or particulate debris generated by total joint replacement procedures.

The adaptive immune system

This can be divided into cell-mediated immunity and humoral antibody-mediated immunity (Fig. 10.5).

CELL-MEDIATED IMMUNITY

Cell-mediated immunity (Fig. 10.5a) is mediated by T lymphocytes, which are present throughout the body. T cells are activated when they encounter antigens on tumour cells or viruses. They enlarge, divide and release lymphokines, substances of high molecular weight that participate in the attack on the foreign protein. Effector T lymphocytes are specialized in recognizing histocompatibility antigens (human leucocyte antigens) that identify self from non-self. Once activated, the cytotoxic or killer T lymphocytes enlarge, divide and produce complement-independent lysis of the foreign cells.

HUMORAL ANTIBODY-MEDIATED IMMUNITY

Humoral antibody-mediated immunity (Fig. 10.5b) is dependent on B lymphocytes. When stimulated by an antigen, a B lymphocyte becomes a plasma cell that secretes antibodies. The antibodies have B-cell receptor-specific affinity. A particular antigen will stimulate only those B

Table 10.1 The interferon family; comparison of type I and II interferons

Interferon type	Source	Antiviral activity	Effects on	Increased HLA expression
Type I (IFN-α/β)	Virus-infected cells	+++	NK cells	Class I
Type II (IFN-γ)	Activated NK and T cells	+	Macrophages	Class I and II

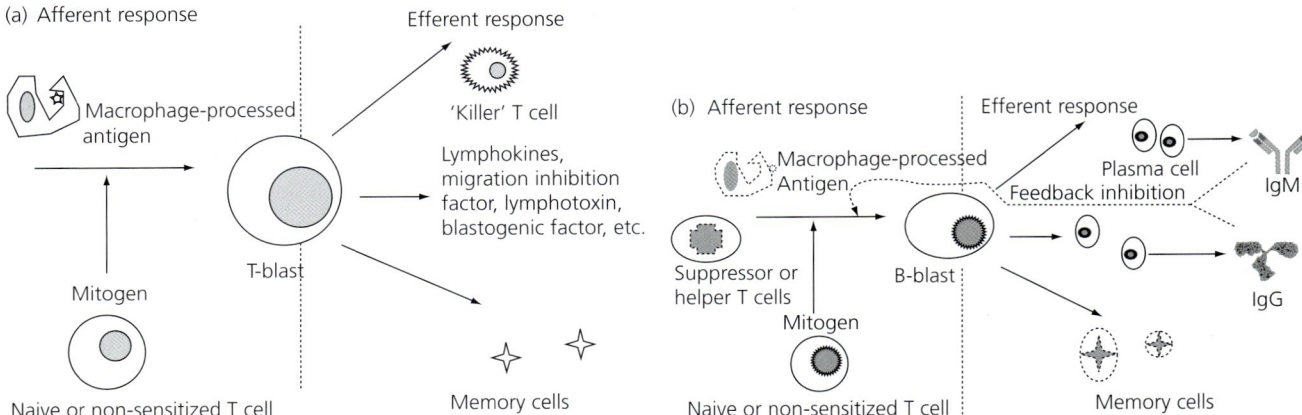

Figure 10.5 Basic structure of the human immune system. (a) Structure of cell-mediated immune response. (b) Structure of the humoral antibody-mediated immune response. Adapted from Friedlander GE. Immunology. In: Albright JA, Brand RA (eds) *The Scientific Basis of Orthopaedics*, 2nd edn. Norwalk, CT: Appleton & Lange, 1987: 492.

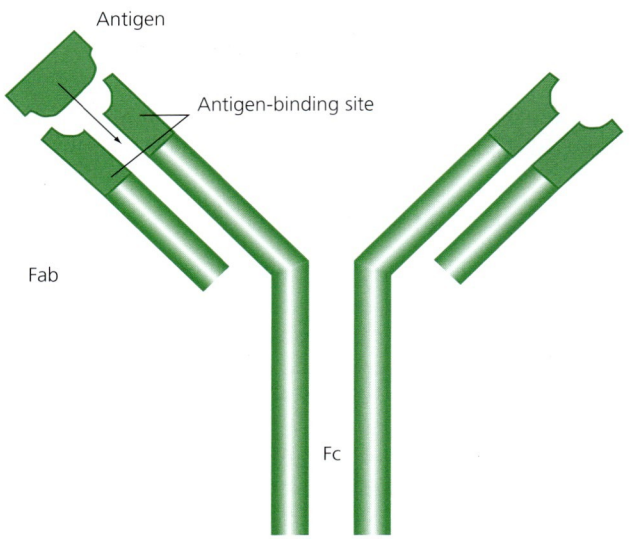

Figure 10.6 Structure of immunoglobulin.

cells that will respond by secreting an appropriate antibody, e.g. IgM or IgG. In this way, the secretion of a particular antibody is specific to the nature of the infection. The antibodies (immunoglobulins) have the same basic structure, consisting of two identical light chains and two identical heavy chains linked to give a Y-shaped molecule (Fig. 10.6). The antigen-binding domains (Fab) are highly variable in structure. This variable region permits an antibody to distinguish one antigen from another. The antibody will recognize and bind to a particular part of an antigen. Antibodies do not bind to the whole molecule, but only to specific structural motifs. The stem of an immunoglobulin molecule is known as the Fc region, and this is used by the cells of the immune system to recognize particles that have been coated with antibody, e.g. viruses or bacteria.

There are five classes of antibody, namely IgA, IgD, IgE, IgG and IgM:

- IgA is the most common immunoglobulin found in secretions such as saliva, bile and colostrum
- IgD acts as a surface receptor on B cells together with IgM
- IgE binds to Fc receptors on mast cells to facilitate an inflammatory response to antigens
- IgG is the most abundant immunoglobulin in plasma; in addition, this protein can cross the placental membrane and protect the fetus *in utero* and for some months after birth
- IgM is the first antibody to be produced during development and during the primary immune response; it also activates the complement system.

Antibodies bind with an antigen, and elicit a response that results in the removal of the antigen from the body. The antibody acts together with the complement to stimulate the phagocytes, with the result that the organism carrying the antigen is killed and digested. The combination of antibody, complement and phagocyte is very effective to mount an effective immune response.

Allograft bone transplantation

Allografting is a technique used to transplant tissues or organs between individuals of the same species. Xenografting is transplantation of tissues between genetically non-identical species, e.g. porcine valves in humans. Transplanted tissue or organ may function well during the initial 2 weeks. Thereafter, between 2 and 3 weeks, organ rejection is encountered from attack by the host's adaptive immune system. The T-lymphocyte system is responsible for the rejection of transplanted organs.

Kawabe and Yoshinao[17] confirmed this phenomenon by performing cartilage transplants in rabbits, which showed excellent healing during the first 2 weeks. After 2 weeks, the host lymphocytes had accumulated around the allografts. Most of the implanted cartilage had died and was replaced by fibrous tissue. A ^{51}Cr release assay on these specimens indicated that the implanted cartilage began to degenerate 2–3 weeks after implantation, partially because of a humoral immune response but more importantly because of cell-mediated cytotoxicity.

In a similar rabbit experiment, Siliski et al.,[18] who performed vascularized whole knee allograft transplantation on 21 rabbits, showed rejection at 2–3 weeks in four of six rabbits in the group that had not received immunosuppressants. Arteriography showed occluded popliteal vessels in these four rabbits. In the eight rabbits that were immunosuppressed with cyclosporine at 15 mg kg^{-1} day^{-1}, one allograft failed at 10 days owing to femoral fracture; none of the remaining seven was rejected acutely, and three of them had patent vessels by arteriography and live bone and cartilage by light microscopy when harvested 100 days after transplantation.

However, with the advent of new techniques in processing the allograft, specialized antigen-presenting cells in the grafts are destroyed during the processing.[19] A number of treatments have been developed to overcome the rejection of transplanted organs in humans. The goal of treatment is to stop rejection without leaving the patient vulnerable to massive infections. One approach is to kill T lymphocytes with drugs such as azathioprine, a purine antimetabolite, glucocorticoids, cyclosporine and antilymphocyte globulin. Long-term immunosuppressive medication is not required in bone transplantation, unlike other organ transplantation. Freezing markedly reduces the immunogenicity, and freeze drying reduces it even further.[20]

Oncology

Approximately one person in five in industrialized countries will die of cancer.[21] Most of the cancers are probably initiated by a change in the cell's DNA sequence. Only for teratocarcinoma does the evidence favour an epigenetic origin. Three classes of agents are clearly implicated for mutagenesis and carcinogenesis: chemical carcinogens, which cause a change in the nucleotide sequence of DNA; ionizing radiation, which causes chromosome breaks and translocations; and viruses, which introduce foreign DNA into the cell.[22] A single genetic change is rarely sufficient for the development of a malignant tumour. The current evidence points to a multistep process of sequential alterations in oncogenes, tumour suppressor genes or micro-RNA genes in cancer cells.[23]

ONCOGENES

Oncogenes encode proteins that control cell proliferation, apoptosis or both. They can be activated by structural alterations resulting from mutation or gene fusion,[24] by juxtaposition to enhancer elements[25] and by amplification. Translocations and mutations can occur as initiating events[26] or during tumour progression, whereas amplification usually occurs during progression. Oncogene-induced DNA damage may explain two key features of cancer: genomic instability and the high frequency of p53 mutations.[27]

Proto-oncogenes

These code for proteins that transduce signals from membrane-bound receptors, via multiple downstream effector pathways. Thereby, they affect fundamental cellular processes, including proliferation, apoptosis and differentiation. Mutations in proto-oncogenes may play a key role in neoplastic progression.[28]

TUMOUR SUPPRESSOR GENES

RB1 and p53 are well-known tumour suppressor genes in humans. In the cell, p53 protein binds to DNA and, by interacting with another gene, produces a protein called p21. When p21 locks with cdk2 (cell division-stimulating protein), the cell stops progressing to the next stage of cell division. Li–Fraumeni syndrome is caused by mutations in p53 that result in the development of several independent tumours in a variety of tissues in early adult life.

MICRO-RNA GENES

Micro-RNA genes have been implicated more recently in carcinogenesis. They do not encode proteins, unlike other genes involved in cancer. Instead, they regulate gene expression. A micro-RNA molecule can anneal to a messenger RNA (mRNA) containing a nucleotide sequence that is complementary to the sequence of the micro-RNA. In this way, the micro-RNA blocks protein translation or causes degradation of the mRNA, thereby causing neoplasms; for example, miR-15a and miR-16-1, which are deleted or downregulated in most indolent cases of chronic lymphocytic leukaemia.[30] As a result, dormant oncogenes can be switched on and can permit cells to become invasive and to metastasize. These capabilities are possessed by embryonic cells and cancer cells, but not by differentiated adult cells.

Hypersensitivity

The adaptive immune system is very powerful and capable of responding to a wide variety of antigens. In normal people, the response is appropriate and correctly targeted against the invading organism. Sometimes, the activity of the immune system leads to pathological changes in the host tissues. Such reactions are called hypersensitivity reactions.

Hypersensitivity reactions can be grouped under one of the six types:

1. Type I is an acute allergic and anaphylactic type that is mediated by IgE antibodies and mast cells, e.g. hay fever and asthma. The immunopathological steps are:
   a. the generation of an IgE specific for a particular allergen (e.g. pollen)
   b. IgE binds to mast cells and basophils
   c. further contact with allergen cross-links to the bound IgE results in degranulation of the mast cells and the secretion of vasoactive materials that cause vascular permeability, mucus secretion and bronchial constriction. This may provoke an anaphylactic shock, if the allergen reaches the circulation, and is a potentially fatal condition; it can be tested for by an immediate skin test.
2. Type II is an antibody-dependent cytotoxic hypersensitivity, e.g. autoimmune haemolytic anaemia. The following are the immunopathological reactions:
   a. opsonization, and complement and Fc receptor-mediated phagocytosis
   b. complement and Fc receptor-mediated inflammation
   c. IgG antibody-mediated cellular dysfunction. This unwanted reaction may follow a transfusion of incompatible blood. It may also follow skin or organ transplants, leading to the rejection of the graft or transplant.
3. Type III is an immune complex-mediated hypersensitivity, e.g. serum sickness. At times, the complex of antigen and antibody, instead of being removed by phagocytic cells, remains in the tissues or in the circulation. These complexes are attacked by complement and neutrophils, damaging the endothelium and compromising the function of the affected organ (e.g. glomerulonephritis), which results from the deposition of immune complexes in the glomerular capillaries and is a cause of renal failure. Other classic examples are serum sickness, following repeated intravenous injections of animal serum, and the arthus reaction, which is necrosis following subcutaneous injection.
4. Type IV is a cell-mediated delayed hypersensitivity, and is also described as 'tuberculin type', e.g. tuberculosis granuloma. The activation of macrophages as a result of prolonged T-cell responses often accompanies parasitic infections, e.g. bacteria and fungi resulting in granuloma formation in solid organs. It may cause contact dermatitis from sensitization to a chemical agent, or from the rejection of a tissue graft or transplant. It is mediated principally by the T cells. It can be tested for by delayed skin test, e.g. the Mantoux test.
5. Type V is a stimulator, e.g. Graves disease. This disease is also considered to be a type II hypersensitivity reaction. Antibodies recognize and bind to the cell surface receptors instead of binding to cell surface components. They either prevent the intended ligand binding with the receptor or mimic the effects of the ligand, thus impairing cell signalling, e.g. Graves disease and myasthenia gravis.[31]
6. Type VI is natural killer cell-mediated hypersensitivity, which is newly described. Natural killer cells lyse the cells that have been coated in antibody. This type is implicated in some autoimmune diseases, tumour rejection and parasite rejection.

GENETICS

Genes encode the cell's RNA molecules and proteins, which constitute the structural components and signalling molecules of an organism or act as enzymes to direct the formation of these components. Finding mutations and determining how they affect health and disease are key goals of current biomedical research.

Gregor Mendel, an Austrian monk, described the basic laws of inheritance based on seven traits of garden peas by observing how they were passed down through several generations. He concluded that each trait is independent of the others and is transmitted by two particles, one inherited from each parent. They are called alleles.

Mechanisms of inheritance

Mendelian law is based on two phenomena:

1. segregation: the two alleles for each gene segregate into different germ cells (sperm or eggs)
2. independence: genes controlling different traits assort independently.

Mendelian inheritance

Four different patterns of inheritance depend on whether the nuclear gene is dominant or recessive and whether it is carried on the X chromosome or an autosome. Y-linked diseases are nearly unknown in humans. Typical Mendelian patterns of inheritance can be demonstrated in families in which a trait can be tracked through several generations (Fig. 10.7). The most clinically relevant traits are caused by changes in genes that predispose to certain diseases, often through disruptions in a metabolic or signalling pathway.

AUTOSOMAL DOMINANT

These mutations affect people of either sex. The mutation is either inherited from one parent or arises *de novo*. Heterozygous alleles can influence the phenotype. Each child

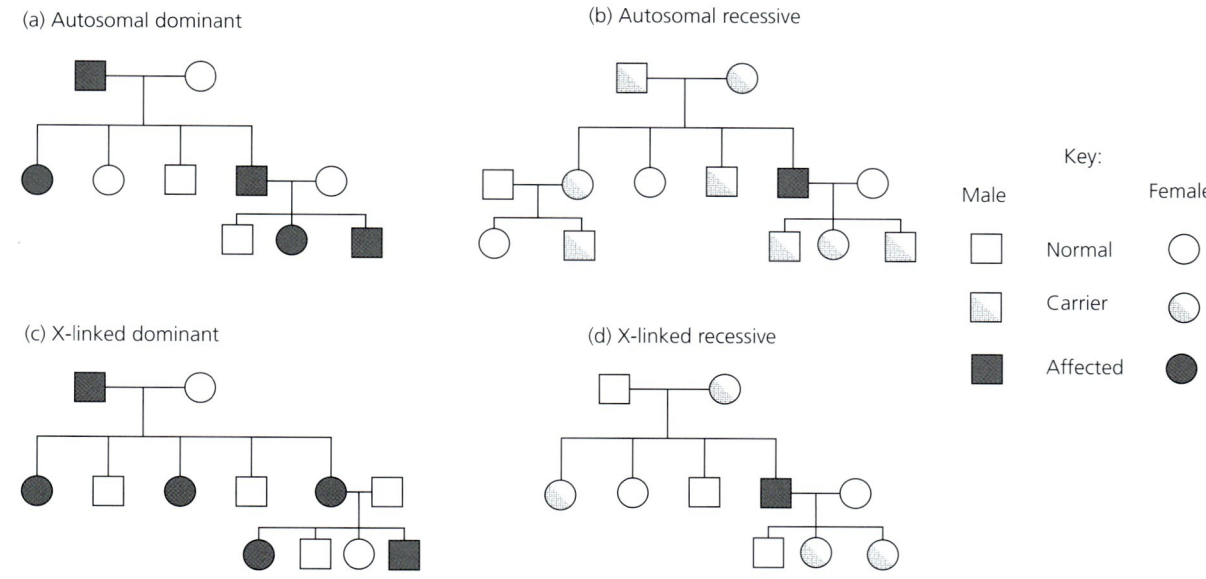

Figure 10.7 Pedigree charts demonstrate representative patterns of Mendelian gene inheritance. For recessive alleles, homozygotes are affected and heterozygotes are asymptomatic carriers. For dominant alleles, there are no carriers because heterozygotes are affected.

of an affected parent has a 50% chance of being affected (Fig. 10.7a).

AUTOSOMAL RECESSIVE

This type of inheritance affects people of either sex born to parents who are asymptomatic carriers. The risk of having an affected child is increased if the parents are related because the two inherited alleles are more likely to be identical. Each child has a 25% chance of being affected, a 50% chance of being a carrier and a 25% chance of being normal (Fig. 10.7b).

X-LINKED DOMINANT

X-linked dominant mutations affect sons more severely than daughters, because the daughters receive their second X chromosome from the unaffected parent. Some X-linked dominant alleles are lethal in males because their sole X chromosome is the disease-carrying chromosome. In the next generation, sons of an affected father are unaffected because their X chromosome is from their mother. Daughters of an affected father are always affected because one of their X chromosomes is inherited from their father. Each child of an affected mother has a 50% chance of being affected (Fig. 10.7c).

X-LINKED RECESSIVE

Males are almost always affected. Each son of a carrier mother has a 50% chance of being affected whereas each daughter of a female carrier has a 50% chance of being a carrier, like her mother. There is no father to son transmission. In females, those with homozygous X chromosomes will express the phenotype. Heterozygous daughters may show some mild disease characteristics because of non-random inactivation of the X chromosome (Fig. 10.7d).

Trinucleotide repeat disorder

The hallmark of trinucleotide repeat disorders is genetic anticipation, which is a pattern of disease worsening over generations. The increased severity and earlier onset of symptoms may well correlate with the increasing numbers of repeated trinucleotide. As explained earlier in molecular biology, three nucleotides constitute a codon, which encodes an amino acid. Several of these diseases are characterized by aberrant proteins with repeated amino acids, e.g. spinocerebellar ataxia type 12 is also caused by CAG repeats.

Non-Mendelian inheritance

IMPRINTING

We inherit two copies of all genes, except those that reside on the sex chromosomes. There is a subset of these genes that are functional only if the paternal or maternal copy is inherited. This phenomenon of monoallelic, parent-of-origin expression of genes is termed genomic imprinting.[32] Imprinted genes are normally involved in embryonic growth and behavioural development, but occasionally they also function inappropriately as oncogenes and tumour suppressor genes.

Table 10.2 Overview of musculoskeletal-related disorders and their inheritance patterns. Autosomal dominant conditions are usually structural whereas autosomal recessive conditions are enzyme linked

Autosomal dominant	Autosomal recessive	X-linked dominant	X-linked recessive
Achondroplasia	Metaphyseal chondrodysplasia (McKusick type)	Hypophosphataemic rickets	Spondyloepiphyseal dysplasia (tarda form)
Spondyloepiphyseal dysplasia (congenital form)	Diastrophic dysplasia		Haemophilia
Multiple epiphyseal dysplasia	Laron's dysplasia		Hunter syndrome
Metaphyseal chondrodysplasia (Schmid and Jansen types)	Sickle cell anaemia		Duchenne muscular dystrophy
Kniest's dysplasia	Hurler syndrome		
Malignant hyperthermia	Osteogenesis imperfecta (types II and III)		
Marfan syndrome	Hypophosphatasia		
Ehlers–Danlos syndrome	Hereditary vitamin D-dependent rickets		
Osteogenesis imperfecta (types I and IV)	Homocystinuria		
Osteochondromatosis			
Polydactyly			

ANEUPLOIDY

Aneuploidy is an aberrant chromosome number from the normal ($n = 23$). Aneuploidy usually results from a failure of homologous chromosomes to separate during mitosis or meiosis (non-disjunction). The most common changes are one more ($2n + 1$; trisomy) or less ($2n - 1$; monosomy) chromosome. The other aberrations are nullisomy ($2n - 2$) and disomy ($n + 1$).

TRISOMY

The most common viable human aneuploidy is trisomy 21, causing Down syndrome. The frequency of trisomy 21 increases with maternal age. The long delay between the first meiotic division, which occurs before birth, and the second meiotic division, which begins in some eggs at the onset of each menstrual cycle, may be the reason.

UNIPARENTAL DISOMY

The most frequent cause of uniparental disomy is an unequal recombination between the chromosomes. Translocation and non-disjunction during the first meiotic division can also cause chromosome imbalance. The incidence is unknown because it is not always detected. Uniparental disomy may cause several syndromes. For example, uniparental chromosome disomy 1 can cause concurrent Charcot–Marie–Tooth and Gaucher disease type 3.[33]

Orthopaedic disorders with underlying genetic aberration

An overview of musculoskeletal-related conditions and their inheritance patterns is given in Table 10.2.

KEY LEARNING POINTS

Molecular and cell biology

- DNA is double helix nucleotide chains, each consisting of deoxyribose sugar–phosphate with bases bonded with complementary bases on the opposite chain.
- The A–T base pair are purines, and the G–C base pair are pyrimidines. They are the only two types of complementary base pairs possible in nature.
- A gene (allele) is a sequence of DNA coded to produce a specific protein.
- Each human cell has 46 chromosomes in its nucleus. Out of 46, 44 are autosomes that determine somatic characteristics, and two are allosomes that influences sexual characteristics.
- Gene therapy is transfecting the target cell with therapeutic DNA to effect a new gene expression.

Immunology

- There are two types of immune systems: innate and adaptive.
- The innate immune system consists of four kinds of cells (phagocytes, natural killer cells, mast cells, eosinophils), and three different classes of proteins (complement, interferons, acute phase proteins).
- An adaptive immune system comprises of cell-mediated and humoral antibody-mediated immunity.
- Bone allograft transplantation may elicit type IV cell-mediated delayed hypersensitivity reaction if they are not properly processed.

- Freeze-drying is a technique in processing the allograft that markedly reduces the immunogenicity to avoid rejection and massive infections.

Oncology

- Oncogenes encode proteins that control cell proliferation, apoptosis or both.
- Proto-oncogenes affect fundamental cellular processes and mutations in proto-oncogenes may play a key role in neoplastic progression.
- *RB1* and *p53* are tumour suppressor genes in humans. *p53* and *RB1* gene mutations are implicated in osteosarcoma tumorigenicity.
- *P53* gene mutations result in the development of several independent tumours in a variety of tissues in early adult life and is described as Li–Fraumeni syndrome.

REFERENCES

1. International Human Genome Sequencing Consortium. Finishing the euchromatic sequence of the human genome. *Nature* 2004;**431**:931–45.
2. Pearson H. Genetics: what is a gene? *Nature* 2006;**441**:398–401.
3. Lattanzi W, Pola E, Pecorini G, et al. Gene therapy for in vivo bone formation: recent advances. *European Review for Medical and Pharmacological Sciences* 2005;**9**:167–74.
4. Gallegos Ruiz MI, Floor K, et al. Integration of gene dosage and gene expression in non-small cell lung cancer, identification of HSP90 as potential target. *PLoS One* 2008;**3**:e0001722.
5. Renwick L, Hardie A, Girvan EK, et al. Detection of meticillin-resistant Staphylococcus aureus and Panton-Valentine leukocidin directly from clinical samples and the development of a multiplex assay using real-time polymerase chain reaction. *European Journal of Clinical Microbiology and Infectious Diseases*, 2008;**27**:791–6.
6. Le Borgne S, Bolivar F, Gosset G. Plasmid vectors for marker-free chromosomal insertion of genetic material in Escherichia coli. *Methods in Molecular Biology* 2004;**267**:135–43.
7. Spadafora C. Sperm-mediated gene transfer: mechanisms and implications. *Society of Reproduction and Fertility Supplement* 2007;**65**:459–67.
8. Lavitrano M, Busnelli M, Cerrito MG, et al. Sperm-mediated gene transfer. *Reproduction, Fertility, and Development* 2006;**18**:19–23.
9. Baker MR. Cloning humans. *Nature* 1997;**387**:19.
10. Wikipedia. *Cloning*, 2008. Available from: http://en.wikipedia.org/w/index.php?title=Cloning&oldid=200343210.
11. Wikipedia. *Human Cloning*, 2008. Available from: http://en.wikipedia.org/w/index.php?title=Human_cloning&oldid=197992657.
12. Chung Y, Klimanskaya I, Becker S, et al. Human embryonic stem cell lines generated without embryo destruction. *Cell Stem Cell* 2008;**2**:113–17.
13. Jose BC, Robert PL, West MD. The first human cloned embryo. *Sci Am* 2001; November 24.
14. Robinson BA. *Embryo Cloning of Humans: (a.k.a. Artificial Twinning)*. Ontario, Canada: Ontario Consultants on Religious Tolerance, 1997. Available from: http://64.233.183.104/search?q=cache:fGxVkPFSP5cJ:www.religioustolerance.org/clo_intr.htm+For+ethical+reasons,+in+human+embryo%E2%80%99s,+the+researchers+selected+embryos+which+had+no+possibility+of+ever+maturing+into+newborn+babies.&hl=en&ct=clnk&cd=1.
15. Giannoudis PV, Tzioupis CC, Tsiridis E. Gene therapy in orthopaedics. *Injury* 2006;**37**(Suppl. 1):S30–40.
16. Kaul G, Cucchiarini M, Arntzen D, et al. Local stimulation of articular cartilage repair by transplantation of encapsulated chondrocytes overexpressing human fibroblast growth factor 2 (FGF-2) in vivo. *Journal of Gene Medicine* 2006;**8**:100–11.
17. Kawabe N, Yoshinao M. The repair of full-thickness articular cartilage defects. Immune responses to reparative tissue formed by allogeneic growth plate chondrocyte implants. *Clinical Orthopaedics and Related Research* 1991;**268**:279–93.
18. Siliski JM, Simpkin S, Green CJ. Vascularized whole knee joint allografts in rabbits immunosuppressed with cyclosporin A. *Archives of Orthopaedic and Traumatic Surgery* 1984;**103**:26–35.
19. Elves MW. Humoral immune response to allografts of bone. *International Archives of Allergy and Applied Immunology* 1974;**47**:708–15.
20. Leong JCY. Bone and cartilage transplant. *Journal of the Hong Kong Medical Association* 1993;**45**:130–5.
21. Alberts B, Bray D, Lewis J, et al. Cancer. In: Alberts B, Bray D, Lewis J, et al. (eds) *Molecular Biology of the Cell*, 3rd edn. New York, NY: Garland Publishing, 1994:1269–90.
22. Ames BN, Durston WE, Yamasaki E, Lee FD. Carcinogens are mutagens: a simple test system combining liver homogenates for activation and bacteria for detection. *Proceedings of the National Academy of Sciences of the USA* 1973;**70**:2281–5.
23. Croce CM. Oncogenes and cancer. *New England Journal of Medicine* 2008;**358**:502–11.
24. Konopka JB, Watanabe SM, Singer JW, et al. Cell lines and clinical isolates derived from Ph1-positive chronic myelogenous leukemia patients express c-abl proteins with a common structural alteration. *Proceedings of the National Academy of Sciences of the USA* 1985;**82**:1810–14.
25. Tsujimoto Y, Gorham J, Crossman J, et al. The t(14;18) chromosome translocations involved in B-cell neoplasms result from mistakes in VDJ joining. *Science* 1985;**229**:1390–3.

26. Finger LR, Harvey RC, Moore RC, *et al.* A common mechanism of chromosomal translocation in T- and B-cell neoplasia. *Science* 1986;**234**:982–5.
27. Halazonetis TD, Gorgoulis VG, Bartek J. An oncogene-induced DNA damage model for cancer development. *Science* 2008;**319**:1352–5.
28. James RM, Arends MJ, Plowman SJ, *et al.* K-ras proto-oncogene exhibits tumor suppressor activity as its absence promotes tumorigenesis in murine teratomas. *Molecular Cancer Research* 2003;**1**:820–5.
29. Isfort RJ, Cody DB, Lovell GJ, *et al.* Analysis of oncogene, tumor suppressor gene, and chromosomal alterations in HeLa x osteosarcoma somatic cell hybrids. *Molecular Carcinogenesis* 1999;**25**:30–41.
30. Calin GA, Dumitru CD, Shimizu M, *et al.* Frequent deletions and down-regulation of micro-RNA genes miR15 and miR16 at 13q14 in chronic lymphocytic leukemia. *Proceedings of the National Academy of Sciences of the USA* 2002;**99**:15524–9.
31. Rajan TV. The Gell-Coombs classification of hypersensitivity reactions: a re-interpretation. *Trends in Immunology* 2003;**24**:376–9.
32. Jirtle RL. Genomic imprinting and cancer. *Experimental Cell Research* 1999;**248**:18–24.
33. Benko WS, Hruska KS, Nagan N, *et al.* Uniparental disomy of chromosome 1 causing concurrent Charcot-Marie-Tooth and Gaucher disease type 3. *Neurology* 2008;**70**:976–8.

11

Musculoskeletal imaging

MARK W ANDERSON

| Introduction | 155 | Imaging modalities | 156 |
| History | 155 | References | 172 |

NATIONAL BOARD STANDARDS

- Know how radiographs, MRI and CT work; basic principles
- Know how to differentiate between infection and neoplasm on radiographs
- Understand how the image-intensifier works
- Understand the difference between T_1, T_2, short tau inversion–recovery and fat suppression and when to use each modality
- Understand how bone densitometry works

INTRODUCTION

From the discovery of the X-ray in 1895 to the present day, the role of diagnostic imaging has continued to expand within the world of medicine. From trauma to tumours, the ability to provide exquisite anatomical and physiological information has revolutionized the way that we do business as physicians. The goal of this chapter is to provide basic information about the numerous imaging modalities available to the orthopaedic surgeon today, as well as the strengths and weaknesses of each, with a primary emphasis on MRI.

HISTORY

On 22 December 1895, using the 'X-rays' he had been investigating, Wilhelm Conrad Röntgen produced the first human image, a radiograph of his wife Bertha's hand. As such, the discipline of radiology and subspecialty of musculoskeletal imaging were created simultaneously.[1]

Technological advances began immediately, and, by 1896, Charles Thurstan Holland, a physician who was encouraged to experiment with these new rays by Robert Jones, an eminent orthopaedic surgeon, exposed numerous photographic plates that were used to diagnose fractures, congenital deformities and foreign bodies. When addressing the Roentgen Society in 1897, Sylvanus Thompson stated, 'Excepting only the introduction into surgery by Lord Lister of antiseptics, and the discovery of anesthetics, no discovery in the present century has done so much for the operative surgery as this of the roentgen rays. The first great application has been the use of the rays by the surgeon for the diagnosis of fractures and dislocations, the study of bone disease and the detection of foreign bodies in various parts of the human frame.' Amazingly, the first medical malpractice case in which a radiograph was introduced as evidence occurred in late 1896, in which the failure to diagnose a femoral fracture was alleged.[1]

By the 1920s, the concept of the tomogram was introduced with the idea that images could be focused at various levels within the body, with blurring of overlying structures. This became commercially available in the late 1930s, and provided the only 'tomographic' imaging capability until the advent of CT in the 1970s, which produced tomographic slices in the axial plane. The advent of spiral/helical CT in the 1990s provided another quantum leap forward in diagnostic imaging by making possible the rapid acquisition of extremely thin slices, thereby allowing for the production of detailed reformatted images in virtually any plane, as well as exquisite three-dimensional reconstructions.

Also in the 1970s, radionuclide imaging provided a relatively efficient method for assessing both anatomical and physiological abnormalities of the entire skeleton. By attaching a radionuclide to compounds taken up in areas of bone turnover, the level of 'activity' of a skeletal lesion could be assessed. Positron emission tomography (PET) imaging is the latest development in radionuclide imaging, and its role in the diagnosis of musculoskeletal disorders is still evolving.

Finally, MRI became commercially available in the early 1980s, and, although its application in the musculoskeletal system initially lagged behind its use in other parts of the body, it has become the imaging modality of choice in many musculoskeletal disorders and has greatly facilitated the diagnosis of most types of orthopaedic pathology.

IMAGING MODALITIES

Radiography

Radiography (Table 11.1) is still the most commonly used diagnostic imaging modality, and remains the screening method of choice for most musculoskeletal disorders. It is a relatively cost-effective option for evaluating skeletal and, to a much lesser degree, soft-tissue abnormalities, and is readily available throughout the world. The development of digital radiography has also resulted in the ability to instantaneously transmit images anywhere in the world for an initial interpretation or second opinion from an expert. As in its early days, radiography is still widely used in the evaluation of skeletal trauma (Fig. 11.1), and its ability to provide information regarding the nature and aggressiveness of an osseous neoplasm is unsurpassed. Similarly, the radiographic appearances of most arthritides are quite characteristic (Fig. 11.1).

Unfortunately, radiographs are insensitive for detecting bone contusions and subtle fractures (hence the term 'radiographically occult fracture') as well as neoplastic infiltration of the medullary cavity. Radiography is also very limited in its ability to assess soft tissues given its relatively poor contrast resolution.

Table 11.1 Radiography

Strengths	Weaknesses
Trauma screening	Medullary pathology
Primary bone lesion	Occult fracture
Arthritis	Tumour
Osteomyelitis	Soft tissues
Metabolic bone disease	

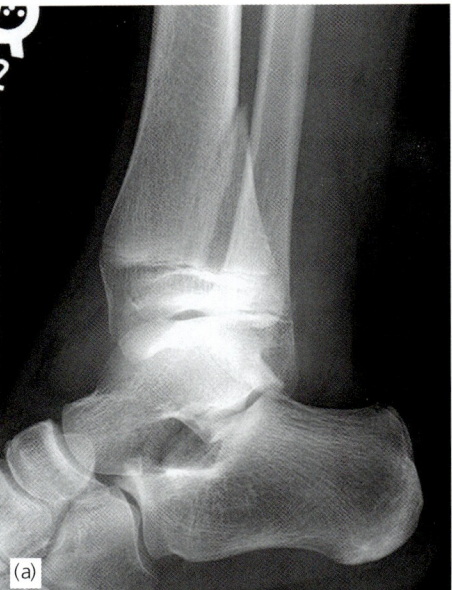

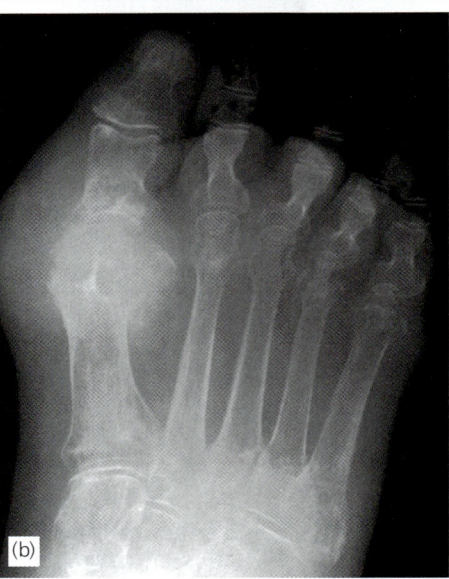

Figure 11.1 Radiography. (a) Lateral radiograph of the ankle reveals an oblique metaphyseal fracture of the distal tibia, part of a triplane fracture. (b) Classic radiographic findings of gout are present at the first metatarsophalangeal joint on this frontal radiograph of the foot.

Bone scan

With the advent of radionuclide scanning techniques, the ability to efficiently scan (Table 11.2) the entire skeleton became possible. Technetium-99m diphosphonate, a bone-seeking radioactive material, is a phosphorus analogue that is taken up in areas of increased bone turnover such as tumour, infection or fracture. Imaging is performed with a gamma scintillation camera.

Typically, the patient is scanned 4–6 hours after the radiopharmaceutical has been injected intravenously, and

Table 11.2 Radionuclide bone scan

Strengths	Weaknesses
Whole body evaluation	Low specificity
Osseous metastases	Multiple myeloma
Physiological information	Radiographs more sensitive
Areas of increased bone turnover	Soft tissues
Tumour	False-negative examinations
Fracture	Initial 24–72 hours, especially in elderly patients
Osteomyelitis	
Sensitive	

produce tomographic images in the axial, sagittal and coronal planes.

Given its whole body capability and sensitivity for detecting areas of active bone turnover, a radionuclide bone scan is the imaging study of choice when assessing a patient for skeletal metastases. Similarly, a bone scan is useful for determining the degree of activity of a focal bone lesion discovered with radiography, and this technique is often useful for assessing for loosening or infection of a prosthetic joint (Fig. 11.3).[2] Osseous stress injuries and osteomyelitis can be assessed with radionuclide scanning, and, in the case of suspected osteomyelitis, other radionuclides, such as indium-111 (typically tagged to white blood cells) and gallium, provide increased specificity. However, today, these types of pathology are more often evaluated with MRI, as will be discussed below.

Weaknesses of radionuclide bone scanning include poor spatial resolution, limited soft-tissue evaluation and poor specificity. For example, a focus of increased activity in the proximal femur of an elderly patient presenting with hip pain could be due to an insufficiency fracture or tumour. In these cases, cross-sectional imaging (typically MRI) is needed for better characterization. Bone scans have been shown to be especially insensitive for detecting malignant myeloma, with radiographs actually being more sensitive in this regard. Additionally, false-negative radionuclide examinations may be encountered within the first 24–72 hours after trauma, especially in elderly patients.[3]

PET scanning uses a metabolically active tracer, typically ^{18}F-fluorodeoxyglucose (^{18}F-FDG), a glucose analogue that is taken up in tissues proportional to glucose utilization. Pathological processes typically show increased metabolic

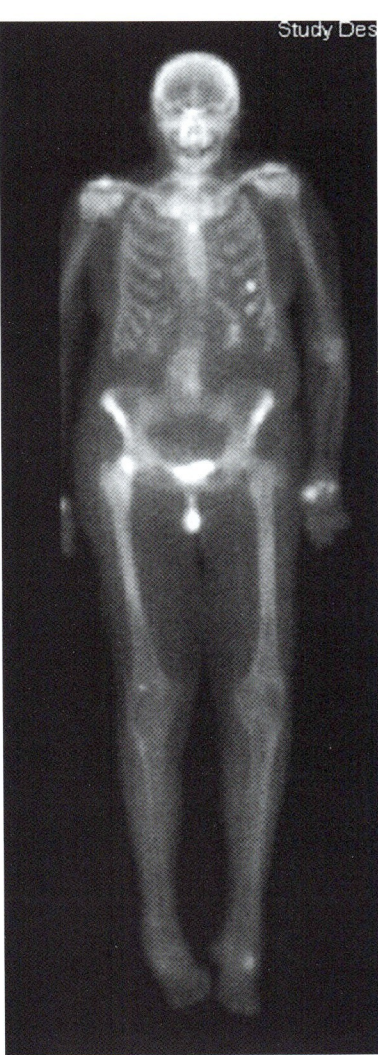

Figure 11.2 Bone scan. Anterior view from a whole body radionuclide scan reveals a focus of abnormal activity at the site of an insufficiency fracture of the right femoral neck.

whole body images are obtained (Fig. 11.2). More localized, 'spot' images focused on a smaller anatomical region may also be acquired in areas of specific clinical concern, and the use of single-photon emission CT (SPECT) technology can

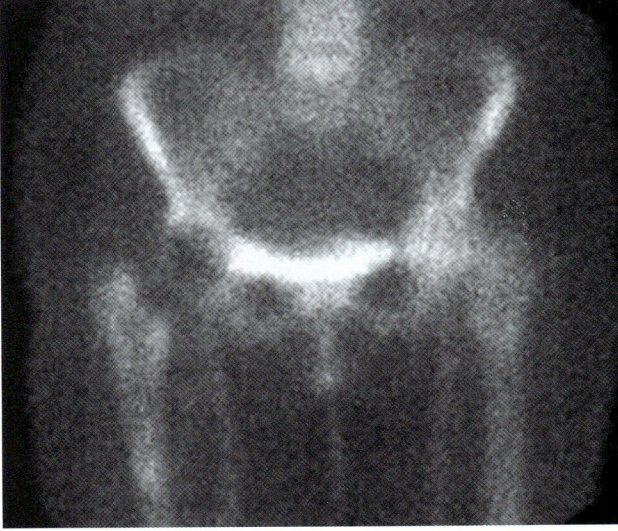

Figure 11.3 Bone scan: prosthesis. Anterior spot view of the pelvis from a radionuclide bone scan reveals abnormal activity compatible with loosening or infection along the proximal and distal portions of the femoral component of a right total hip prosthesis. Note also the area of decreased activity in the right hip relative to the left secondary to the prosthetic femoral head and neck.

activity and increased ^{18}F-FDG uptake. Its ability to detect tumours in bone and soft tissues has led to an increasing role for this technique in the staging work-up for many primary tumours arising in the lung, colon, and head and neck as well as lymphoma. This modality also has theoretical value for the evaluation of a variety of neoplastic, infectious and inflammatory conditions of the musculoskeletal system; although promising results have been reported for its use in the evaluation of infections of the spine and joint prostheses, the detection and staging of multiple myeloma and lymphomatous involvement of the marrow, the response of tumours to therapy and the work-up of rheumatoid arthritis, the number of studies has been limited to date, and further investigation is needed.[4]

Computed tomography

CT scans (Table 11.3) are obtained when an X-ray source is rotated around the patient so that the tissues are scanned through a complete 360° cycle. Tomographic slices are then created from the acquired data, typically in the axial plane. With the advent of multidetector helical CT scanners, scan times have been markedly reduced with an increase in spatial resolution, such that isotropic imaging voxels (the same dimension in all three planes) can be obtained, thereby allowing for the creation of seamless high-resolution reconstructions in the sagittal, coronal or any plane desired. This capability has revolutionized the use of CT throughout the body, including the musculoskeletal system.[5,6]

With regard to musculoskeletal imaging, CT is most often used in trauma patients, and is especially useful for evaluating the spine. Given its ability to scan through the entire spine in a matter of seconds and produce detailed two-dimensional or three-dimensional reconstructions, it has essentially replaced the use of plain films in patients with a high probability of spinal injury (e.g. high-speed motor vehicle accident with ejection from the vehicle, complex facial injuries, etc.). Its ability to detect fractures in this setting is unsurpassed. In several studies, helical CT revealed 50–70% of fractures not identified on radiographs, with many of the injuries considered to be significant (Fig. 11.4).[7] Similarly, complex pelvic fractures are readily

Table 11.3 Computed tomography

Strengths	Weaknesses
Rapid acquisition	Soft-tissue contrast
Two-dimensional and three-dimensional reconstructions	Relative to MRI
	Fracture detection
Any plane	With significant osteopenia
Trauma	Uses ionizing radiation
Spine	
Pelvic/acetabular fractures	
Complex extremity fractures	
Postoperative imaging	
Fracture union	
Degree of fusion	

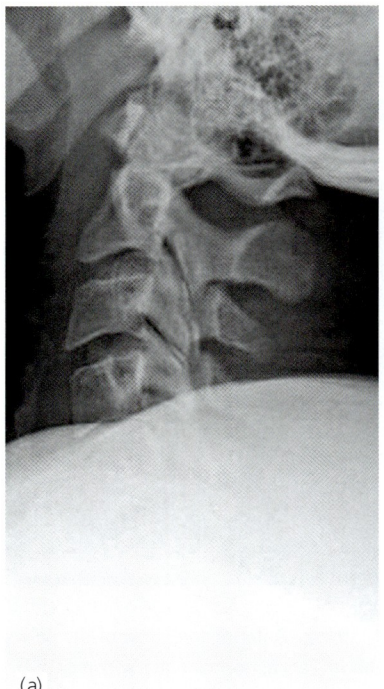
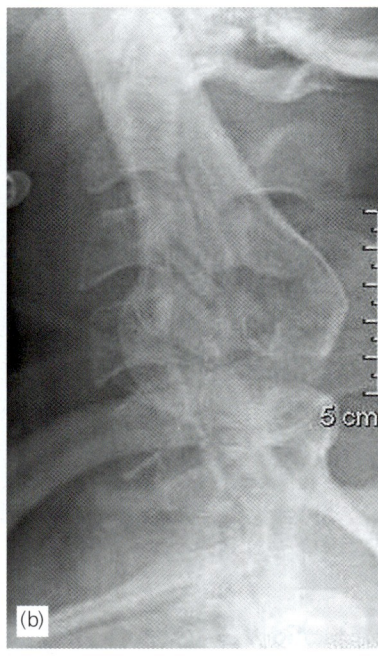
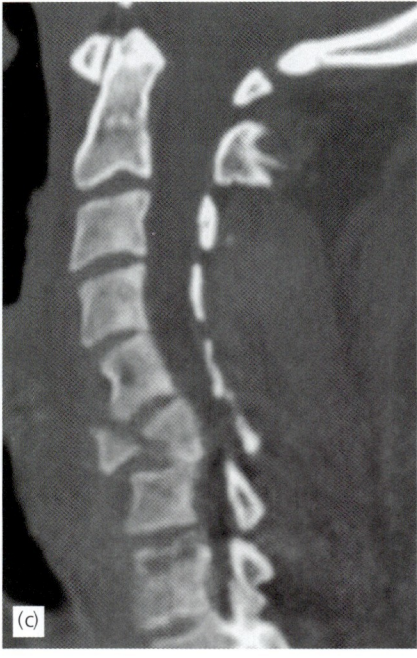

Figure 11.4 CT: spine trauma. (a) Lateral and (b) 'swimmer's' views of the cervical spine result in limited visualization of the lower cervical vertebrae and the cervicothoracic junction. (c) Sagittal reformatted image from a cervical CT scan reveals a burst fracture of C6.

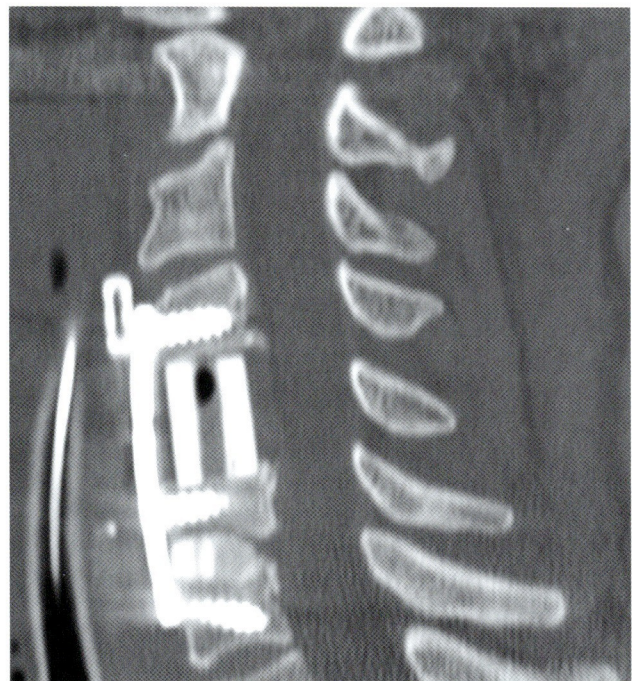

Figure 11.5 CT: metal artefact. Sagittal reformatted image from a helical CT scan of the cervical spine demonstrates minimal scanning artefact arising from the surgical hardware in this postoperative patient.

displayed from virtually any angle, and the same holds true for comminuted tibial plateau or hindfoot fractures.

CT has also become the study of choice for assessing fracture union, especially in the presence of metallic hardware. With the multidetector technique, metal-related artefact is markedly reduced such that it is usually possible to 'see around' hardware to evaluate the adjacent bone, something not possible with older scanners (Fig. 11.5).[8]

Despite these strengths, one of the weaknesses of CT is poorer soft-tissue contrast than MRI. It is also much less sensitive than MRI or bone scan for detecting trabecular/marrow injury (e.g. bone contusion), and has limited sensitivity for fracture detection in patients with significant osteopenia. One other concern has to do with the possibility of increased radiation dose when multidetector scanning is performed. Although the newer scanners have built-in dose reduction components, this concern is heightened for paediatric patients undergoing examinations of the cervical spine and neck (thyroid dose) or studies of the brain and skull base (dose to the lens of the eye).[9]

Ultrasound

Diagnostic ultrasound (Table 11.4) has become the imaging modality of choice for evaluating certain musculoskeletal disorders. It is especially useful for assessing tendons and soft-tissue masses as well as developmental dysplasia of the hip. It is also effective for demonstrating foreign bodies in the soft tissues, and can provide real-time guidance for percutaneous interventional procedures.[10,11]

With regard to tendon assessment, ultrasound has long been used to evaluate the integrity of the rotator cuff and other accessible tendons (Fig. 11.6). Additionally, its ability to demonstrate not only intrinsic tendon structure but also dynamic tendon motion during real-time observation sets ultrasound apart from other static imaging modalities such as MRI and CT. Partial or complete tendon tears can be identified along with abnormal tendon motion, which can be seen with stenosing tenosynovitis (e.g. 'trigger'

Table 11.4 Ultrasound

Strengths	Weaknesses
Real-time, dynamic assessment	Assessment of deeper tissues/bone
Tendons	
Soft-tissue masses	
Developmental dysplasia of the hip	
Foreign body detection	
Real-time interventional guidance	

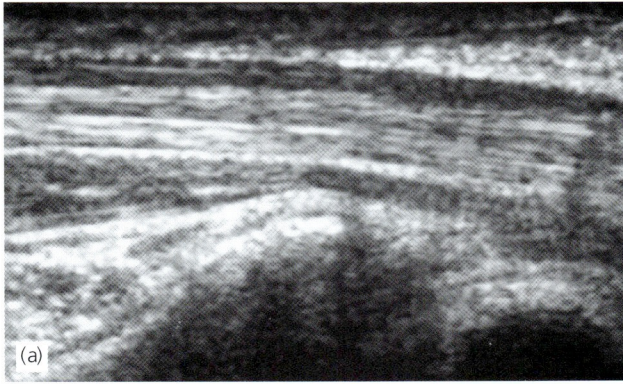

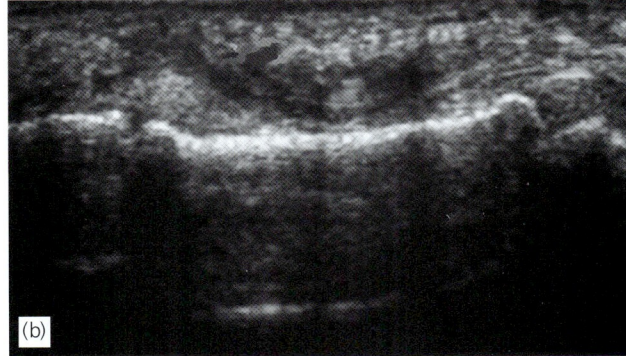

Figure 11.6 Ultrasound: tendons. (a) Longitudinal scan of the normal flexor tendons of the finger. (b) Longitudinal scan of the finger in a different patient reveals complete disruption of the flexor digitorum profundus tendon with retraction of the tendon to the level of the proximal interphalangeal joint.

finger) or tendon subluxation (e.g. peroneal tendons). Sonographic evaluation of tendon pathology in a potential surgical candidate may help determine the most appropriate therapy, such as in the assessment of the margins of a torn Achilles tendon to determine whether they can be approximated with plantarflexion of the foot.

In the case of a soft-tissue mass, ultrasound is useful for determining whether a mass is cystic or solid, assessing its degree of vascularity and/or necrosis and for providing valuable real-time guidance during a percutaneous biopsy.

Foreign bodies are often extremely difficult, if not impossible, to detect with radiography or even CT, but ultrasound provides a method for their rapid detection and localization, thereby aiding in their removal (Fig. 11.7).

Magnetic resonance imaging

More than any other modality, MRI has revolutionized the evaluation of the musculoskeletal system on several fronts. Its ability to display intra-articular anatomy and pathology is unsurpassed, and for some indications its performance is enhanced when it is combined with the intra-articular injection of gadolinium (Gd) contrast material (magnetic resonance (MR) arthrography). Radiographically occult osseous injuries (contusion, fractures) are readily displayed with MRI. Similarly, MRI has been shown to be more sensitive than radionuclide bone scanning for detecting neoplastic infiltration of the marrow. More than with other modalities, a basic understanding of the technical factors involved in acquiring MR images is important to ensure accurate image interpretation.

HARDWARE

The process of MRI depends primarily on a large magnet and a source of radiofrequency waves. The hardware involved can range from a top of the range 3 tesla (T) machine (tesla is the measure of the strength of the magnetic field) capable of scanning any part of the body with maximal scanning options to low field strength (0.2 T) 'niche' machines in which a only a portion of an extremity can be imaged (e.g. knee, wrist, etc.).

Potential drawbacks of the larger 'high field strength' units (>1 T) include higher price, a need for significant magnetic and radiofrequency (RF) shielding of the scanning room and higher maintenance costs. However, the image quality obtained with these units is unquestionably superior to lower field strength units. Although the lower strength units have the advantage of lower costs, they typically require longer scan times and often do not have some of the basic functions necessary to produce high-quality images.

In summary, there is no question that the higher field strength machines produce superior images, but, ultimately, the essential question is whether or not the images obtained are of *diagnostic* quality (i.e. 'they may not be pretty, but do they get the job done?'). While this question is ultimately determined in the clinical arena, there is a quality threshold below which the imaging study is likely to be non-diagnostic, and will not add any value to the patient's work-up.

In addition to the scanner itself, another type of hardware that is essential for obtaining optimal images is the surface coil. Surface coils come in a variety of shapes and sizes, but they all provide better images, especially in the extremities, since they can be placed closer to the body part of interest. In so doing, the amount of signal detected from the tissues is markedly increased, leading to much better image quality. In general, the smallest coil should be used that still provides the field of view needed to cover the area of interest.

IMAGING PLANES

One of the major advantages of MRI is its ability to provide images in virtually any plane desired. While the standard orthogonal sagittal, coronal and axial planes are typically used for most applications, certain anatomical regions are best viewed in an oblique orientation. This is most notable in the shoulder, in which oblique coronal and oblique sagittal imaging is performed along the axis of the supraspinatus tendon, allowing for optimal demonstration of the rotator cuff and adjacent structures.

Within a joint, certain structures will be best evaluated in certain planes. For example, the intrinsic ligaments of the wrist (scapholunate and lunotriquetral) as well as the triangular fibrocartilage are best evaluated in the coronal plane, whereas the tendons of the wrist, as well as the median and ulnar nerves, are optimally assessed on axial images.

BASIC PRINCIPLES OF MAGNETIC RESONANCE

MRI exploits the fact that hydrogen atoms act like small bar magnets in the presence of a magnetic field since they contain an unpaired electron, and therefore an ionic charge. As a result, when a patient is placed into the bore of the magnet, a certain percentage of the hydrogen atoms will align themselves with the magnetic field, and, when

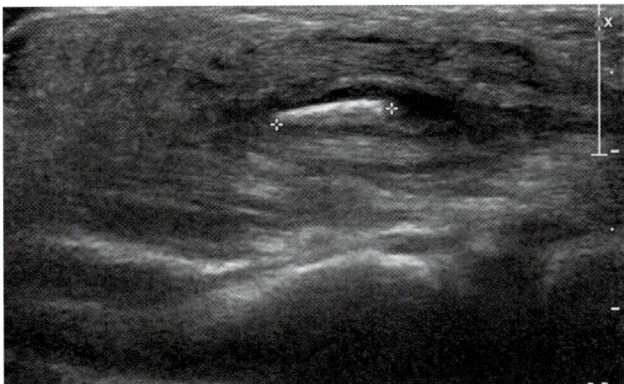

Figure 11.7 Ultrasound: foreign body. Ultrasound of the volar soft tissues of the wrist reveals a linear, hyperechoic focus with surrounding hypoechoic tissue compatible with a foreign body (wood splinter) and surrounding soft-tissue reaction.

energy is added to the tissues in the form of RF waves, some of these protons absorb the energy and 'flip' into a higher energy state. After the RF pulse is turned off, the higher energy protons will relax back to their baseline state, while simultaneously releasing the absorbed energy, again in the form of RF waves. These are then detected by the machine and form the basis of the image that is ultimately produced. This process is known as 'resonance' and is repeated multiple times during the scan to capture enough information to produce an image.

T_1 AND T_2

The manner in which a proton relaxes during this process is dependent upon inherent properties of the tissue in which it resides (e.g. fat, water, muscle, tendon, etc.). These properties are designated as T_1 and T_2 relaxation times and form the basis for the MRI appearances of different tissues.

PULSE SEQUENCES

The combination of scanning parameters that are chosen at the scanner console results in a specific 'pulse sequence'. If parameters are chosen to emphasize T_1 relaxation properties it is considered a 'T_1-weighted' (T_1W) sequence, whereas a pulse sequence that emphasizes T_2 relaxation properties is designated a 'T_2-weighted' (T_2W) sequence. By noting the appearance of a tissue on T_1W and T_2W images, some information can be inferred as to the nature of the tissue and whether or not it is normal. The MRI appearances of common musculoskeletal tissues will be discussed below, and are summarized in Table 11.5 (Figs 11.8 and 11.9).

There are a few other sequences that are commonly used in MRI. When scanning parameters are selected that emphasize a balance of T_1 and T_2 properties, a 'proton density' sequence is obtained. Images will look somewhat like they are T_1W (bright fat, etc.), but fluid is light grey rather than dark.

Table 11.5 Tissue characterization on MR images

Tissue	T_1	T_2	Fat-saturated T_2
Fluid	− −	+ +	+ + +
Fat	+ +	+	− −
Tendon	− −	− −	− −
Ligament	− −	− −	− −
Fibrocartilage	− −	− − −	− − −
Hyaline cartilage	+	− −	− −
Cortical bone	− − −	− − −	− − −
Red marrow	+	=	+ +
Yellow marrow	+ +	+ +	− −
Fibrous tissue/scar	− −	− −	− −
Air	− − −	− − −	− − −

Signal intensity of tissue (relative to muscle): =, equal; −, lower; +, brighter.

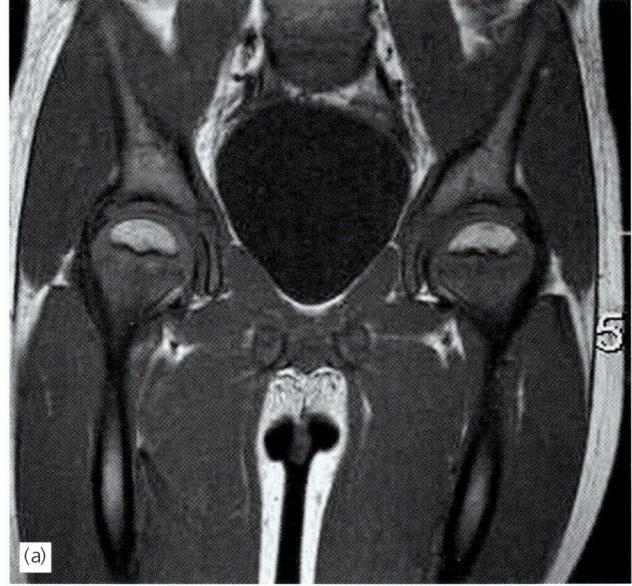

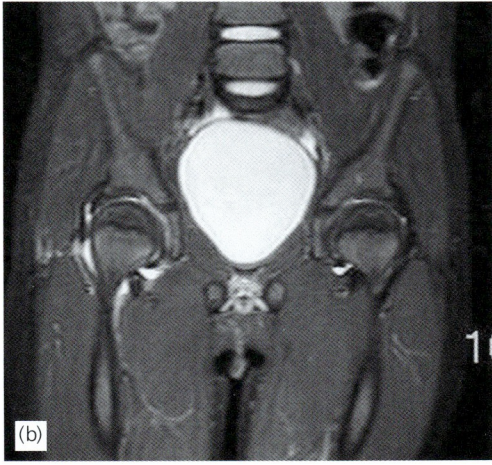

Figure 11.8 MRI: fluid. (a) Coronal T_1-weighted image of the pelvis demonstrates low signal intensity fluid within the bladder. (b) Coronal T_2-weighted image reveals increased signal fluid within the bladder and hip joints, as well as high signal within the normally hydrated nucleus pulposus of the L4–5 and L5–S1 intervertebral discs.

A gradient echo (GRE) sequence uses a different scanning technique from that used to produce conventional T_1W, T_2W and proton density-weighted images. As a result, the tissue contrast appears different on GRE images, which vary widely depending on the exact type of GRE sequence used (e.g. it may be relatively 'T_1' or 'T_2' weighted). One of the most important features of the GRE technique is what is known as 'susceptibility' artefact, which occurs when there are adjacent tissues or materials within the body that vary widely in their magnetic properties, such as metal or air. An artefactual dropout of signal (also known as a 'blooming' artefact) is seen in these regions, such that this type of sequence should not be used in a patient with known hardware

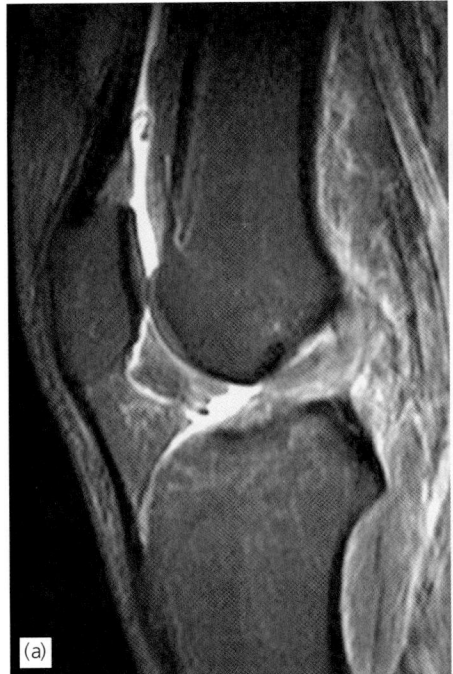
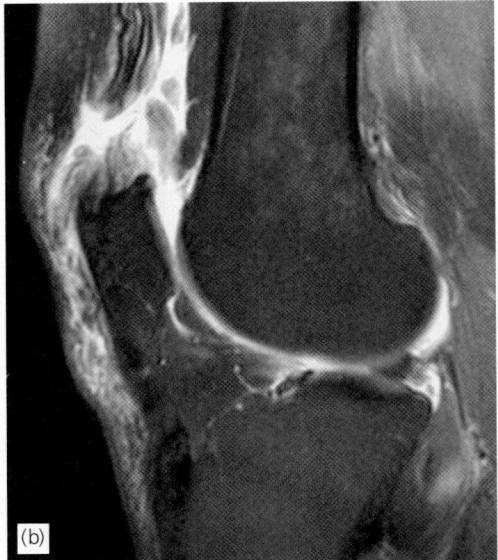

Figure 11.9 MRI: tendon. (a) Sagittal short tau inversion–recovery (STIR) image reveals normal quadriceps and patellar tendons. (b) Sagittal STIR image in a different patient demonstrates complete disruption of the quadriceps tendon with extensive adjacent high-signal oedema/haemorrhage.

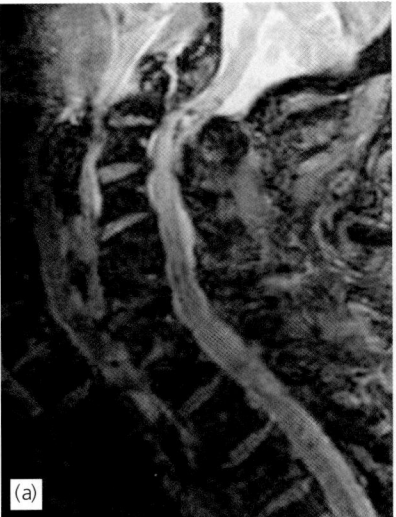
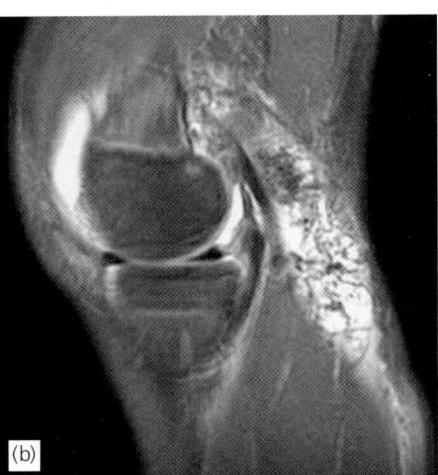
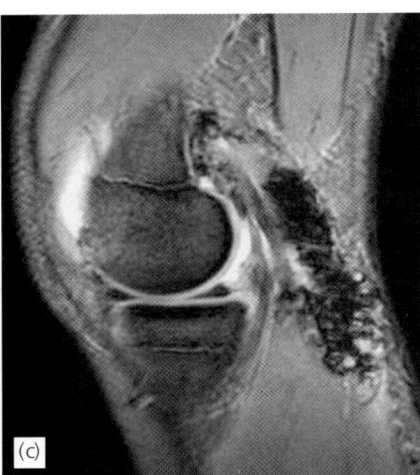

Figure 11.10 MRI: susceptibility artefact (gradient echo (GRE) sequence). (a) Sagittal GRE image of the cervical spine shows low-signal foci within the upper cervical cord compatible with intraparenchymal haemorrhage at the level of the oblique dens fracture. (b) Sagittal T_2-weighted image of the knee reveals a mildly heterogeneous Baker's cyst. (c) Sagittal GRE image demonstrates a profound 'blooming' artefact within the cyst related to haemosiderin deposition within foci of pigmented villonodular synovitis.

because of the resulting image degradation. However, this artefact can be advantageous when looking for haemorrhage within the spinal cord since the iron within the blood products will produce this type of dark, 'blooming' artefact, making the haemorrhagic foci much more conspicuous. Similarly, mass-like tissue within a joint that demonstrates this type of artefact on a GRE sequence is nearly pathgnomonic of pigmented villonodular synovitis, and is related to the haemosiderin deposited within the affected tissues (Fig. 11.10).

FAT SATURATION

When imaging musculoskeletal tissues the addition of 'fat saturation' (a technique in which the fat is turned dark) to a T_1W or T_2W sequence can be very advantageous. A fat-saturated T_2W image is extremely sensitive for detecting most types of bone marrow pathology such as traumatic contusion, osteomyelitis or tumour. Because of the increased fluid content in these areas, they will usually be bright on T_2W images. However, on a routine T_2W image,

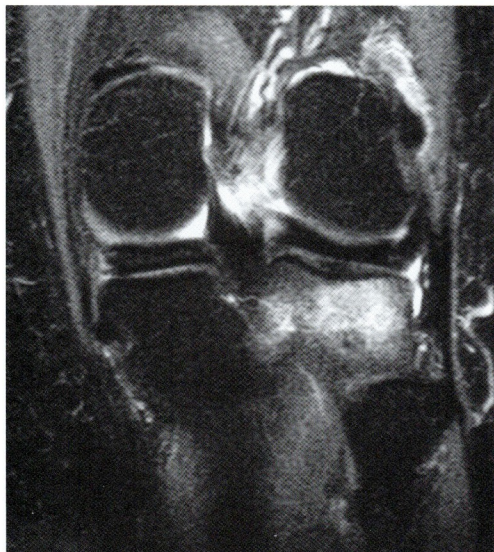

Figure 11.11 MRI: bone contusion. Coronal short tau inversion–recovery image demonstrates an ill-defined area of increased signal within the marrow of the posterolateral aspect of the tibial plateau compatible with a bone contusion.

the adjacent fat within the marrow will also be relatively bright, making the areas of pathology less conspicuous because of their similar signal intensities. When the fat is 'saturated' (turned dark), the areas of marrow pathology become much more noticeable because of the heightened contrast between the pathological areas of increased signal intensity and background of darkened, normal fat (Fig. 11.11).[12]

Similarly, fat saturation can be advantageous when applied to a T_1W sequence in some situations, especially when Gd contrast is used. Gd is a paramagnetic contrast agent that can be administered intravenously or in a dilute form directly into a joint (an MR arthrogram). In either case the Gd produces increased signal intensity on T_1W images, either in vascular tissues after its intravenous injection or within the joint in the case of an MR arthrogram. The addition of fat saturation to a T_1W sequence will increase the conspicuity of subtle areas of vascular enhancement against the background of dark fat, or better delineate intra-articular structures in the case of an MR arthrogram.

THE USE OF GADOLINIUM CONTRAST AGENTS

Whether administered intravenously or directly into a joint, Gd contrast media should be used only for certain indications, especially in light of recent reports of an apparent link between Gd agents and a rare, but potentially devastating, condition, nephrogenic systemic fibrosis. This is most commonly seen in patients with poor renal function; further information about this topic is given in Broom *et al.*[13]

Intravenous gadolinium

Evaluation of a soft-tissue mass

Some solid neoplasms may appear quite cystic on routine MR images. A true cyst will demonstrate only thin, peripheral enhancement around its central non-enhancing fluid on a post-contrast T_1W image (Fig. 11.12), whereas a cystic-appearing solid mass will demonstrate diffuse, often heterogeneous, enhancement (Fig. 11.13). Similarly, intravenous Gd may assist in directing a percutaneous biopsy by differentiating enhancing viable tissue from non-enhancing areas of tumour necrosis.

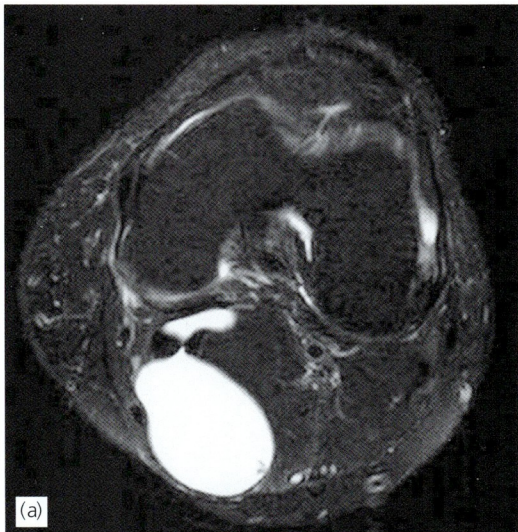
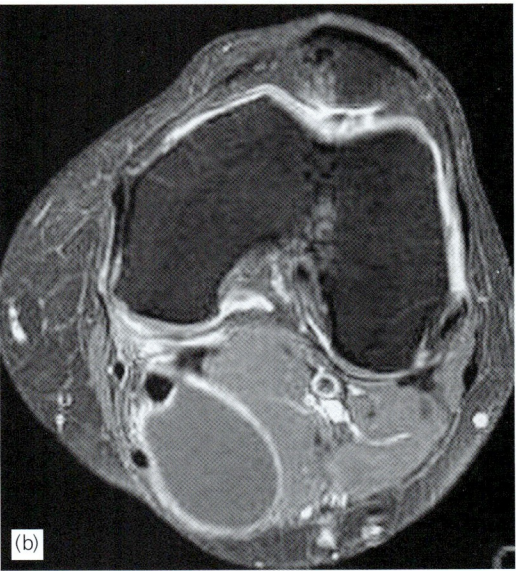

Figure 11.12 Gadolinium contrast: cyst. (a) Large Baker's cyst demonstrating homogeneous internal high signal intensity on this T_2-weighted image. (b) T_1-weighted fat-saturated image obtained after the intravenous administration of gadolinium contrast confirms the cystic nature of the mass with non-enhancing fluid centrally and smooth peripheral enhancement of the cyst wall.

Follow-up after tumour resection

Although postoperative granulation tissue will enhance on a baseline scan obtained after tumour resection, the degree of enhancement of the postoperative changes should gradually decrease over time on subsequent scans. The appearance of a nodular focus of enhancing tissue on a follow-up scan is highly suspicious for tumour recurrence, which can then be biopsied, typically under CT or ultrasound guidance.

Soft-tissue infection

In the case of known or suspected soft-tissue infection, intravenous Gd can increase the conspicuity of a soft-tissue abscess (thick, enhancing wall surrounding a central area of non-enhancement) or sinus tract (enhancing walls along a non-enhancing central fluid-filled tract) (Fig. 11.14). When assessing for osteomyelitis, intravenous Gd is less useful since both infected bone and areas of hyperaemic non-infected/reactive bone marrow may also enhance.

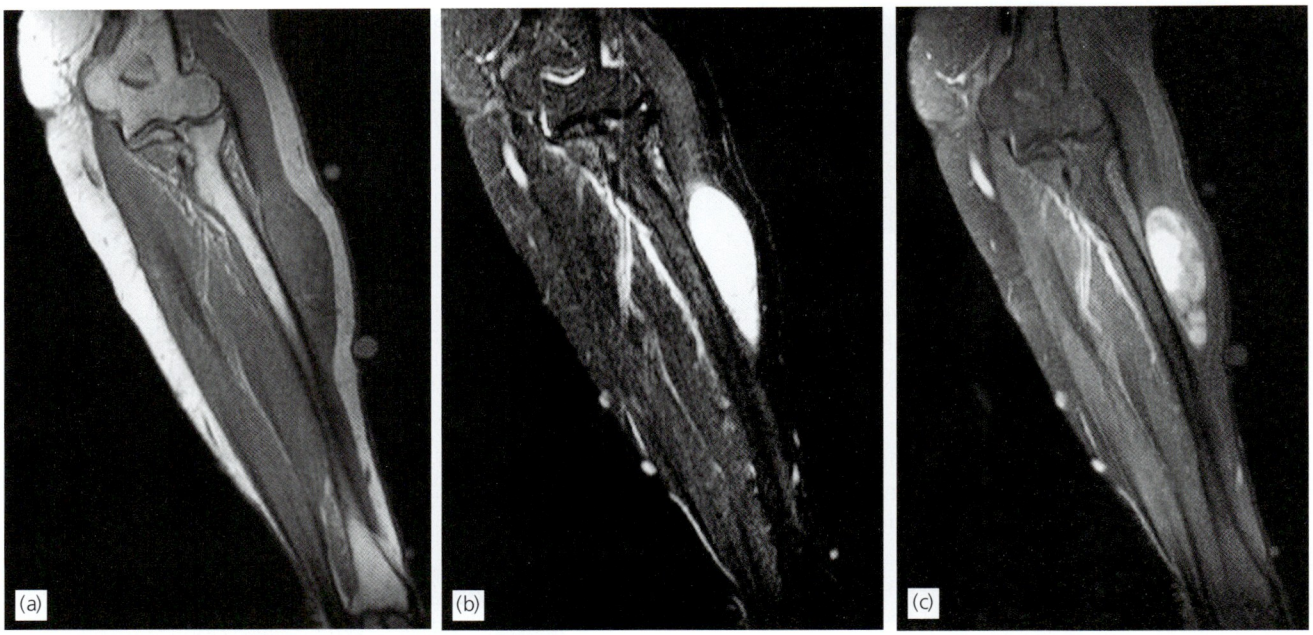

Figure 11.13 Gadolinium contrast: solid mass. (a) Sagittal T_1-weighted (T_1W) and (b) short tau inversion–recovery images of the forearm reveal an elongated cystic-appearing mass. (c) Sagittal fat-saturated post-gadolinium T_1W image shows heterogeneous enhancement throughout this solid neurofibroma.

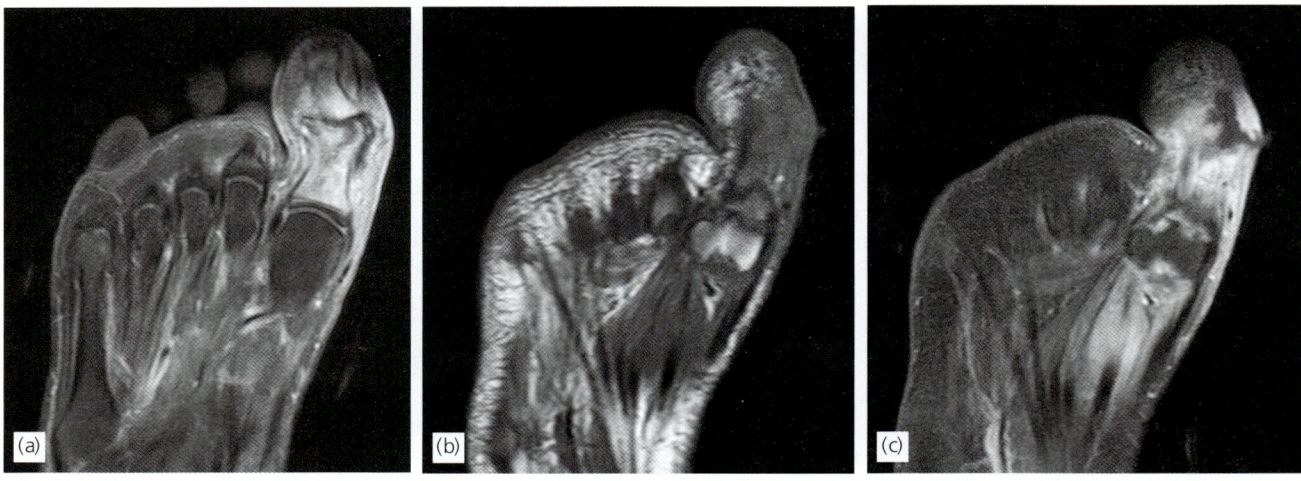

Figure 11.14 Gadolinium contrast: infection. (a) Long-axis T_2-weighted image of the forefoot reveals diffusely abnormal increased signal intensity throughout the proximal and distal phalanges of the great toe and adjacent soft tissues, compatible with osteomyelitis. (b) T_1-weighted (T_1W) pre- and (c) T_1W fat-saturated post-gadolinium images demonstrate a small non-enhancing abscess within the plantar soft tissues of the toe as well as a small sinus tract communicating with the overlying skin.

Spine

In the postoperative lumbar spine, intravenous Gd helps to differentiate residual or recurrent disc from postoperative scar tissue since granulation tissue will enhance whereas disc material will not (Fig. 11.15). It is also helpful for assessing cord pathology (tumour, demyelinating disease) as well as intradural/extramedullary lesions (metastases, nerve sheath tumours).

Inflammatory arthritis

The use of Gd-enhanced MRI is rapidly increasing in patients with suspected inflammatory arthropathies, especially those in which there is a high degree of clinical suspicion for rheumatoid arthritis but normal radiographs. The enhancing synovial pannus present in active disease is very conspicuous on fat-saturated T_1W images (Fig. 11.16).[14]

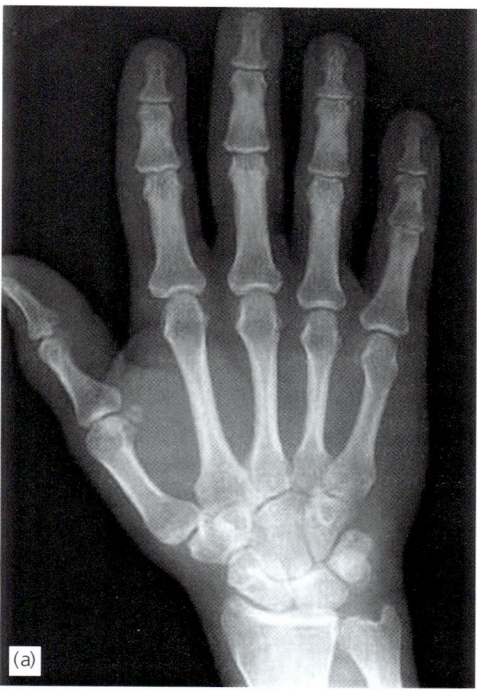

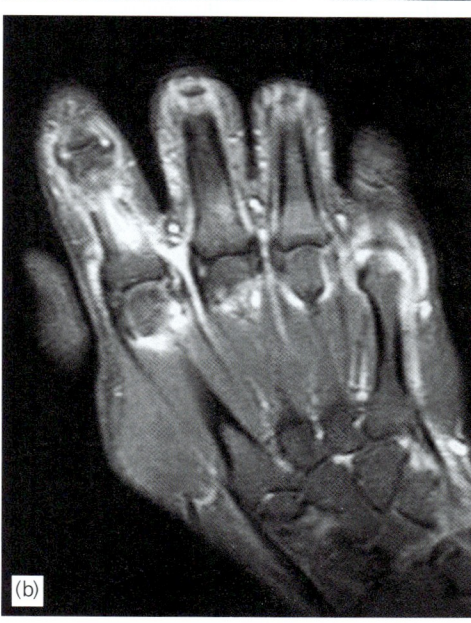

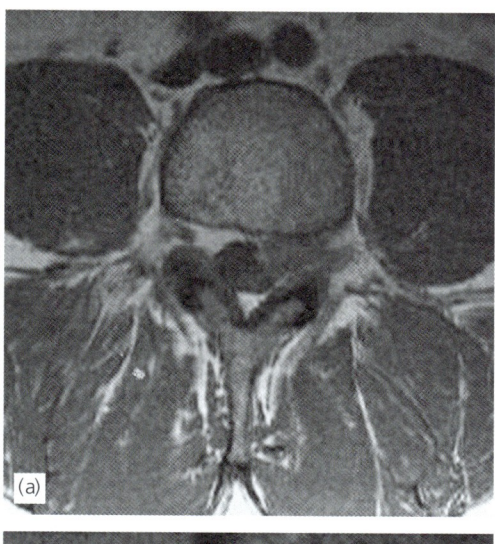

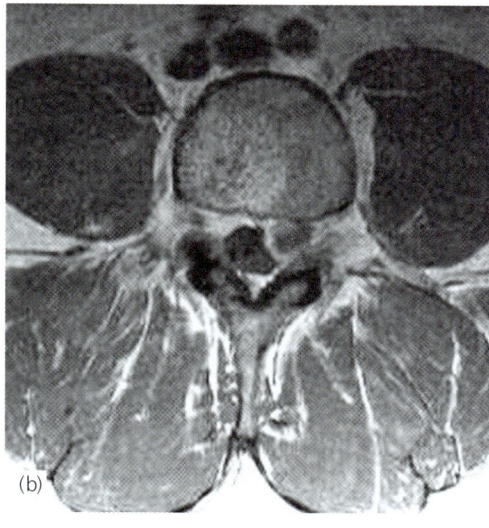

Figure 11.15 Gadolinium contrast: scar versus disc. (a) Axial T_1-weighted (T_1W) image of the lumbar spine reveals intermediate signal intensity tissue in the left ventral epidural space, deforming the thecal sac in this postoperative patient. Note also the low signal 'flow voids' within the distal aorta and proximal common iliac veins. (b) Axial T_1W post-gadolinium image at the same level allows for differentiation between the higher signal enhancing granulation tissue that surrounds a low-intensity disc fragment.

Figure 11.16 Gadolinium: inflammatory arthritis. (a) Normal posteroanterior radiograph of the hand in a 33 year old man with suspected rheumatoid arthritis. (b) Coronal T_1-weighted fat-saturated image obtained after the intravenous injection of gadolinium contrast demonstrates intensely enhancing, hypertrophied synovium in the second and fifth metacarpophalangeal joints as well as in the intercarpal joints compatible with an inflammatory arthritis.

MR arthrography

The direct injection of a dilute solution of Gd into a joint is an 'off-label' use, but can be advantageous in certain situations. The contrast must be diluted since pure, concentrated Gd will actually cause a paradoxical decrease in signal intensity when injected into a joint. For example, for shoulder arthrography, 0.1 mL of Gd contrast is typically mixed with 15 mL of diluent (usually a combination of saline and radiographic contrast).

Labral pathology

Labral abnormalities in the shoulder or hip are much better evaluated after distending the joint with contrast.

Osteochondral lesion

Intra-articular Gd can be used to help assess the stability of an osteochondral fragment. If the contrast is seen to extend between the fragment and native bone, the fragment is considered unstable. Similarly, intra-articular Gd can highlight subtle abnormalities of articular cartilage, although it is not typically administered solely for this purpose.

Postoperative knee

In the case of a prior meniscal repair, distension of the knee with a dilute Gd solution can be helpful to separate a healed tear from a residual or recurrent tear. In the case of a healed tear, the granulation tissue within it will continue to display intermediate signal that mimics an acute tear on conventional imaging, whereas with an MR arthrogram Gd will not extend into that portion of the meniscus (Fig. 11.17).

IMAGE ANALYSIS

When analysing tissues on an MRI study, the first task is to determine what type of sequence is being viewed. This can be accomplished by 'learning the numbers' (the numerals and text included on the images) or by finding a fluid-filled structure (e.g. cerebrospinal fluid in the spine, the bladder in the pelvis or a joint effusion in an extremity) and then observing whether the fluid is bright or dark. Fluid is very bright on T_2W images, and some people find it helpful to think of H_2O as being bright on a T_2W image. As a result, most types of pathology are relatively bright on a T_2W image because of the higher fluid content in areas of injury, inflammation or neoplasm. Alternatively, fluid is relatively dark on a T_1W image.

APPEARANCE OF MUSCULOSKELETAL TISSUES ON MR IMAGES

Next, the tissue signal intensity of structures (Table 11.5) should be compared on T_1W and T_2W images to determine whether there is any pathology present; therefore, it is critically important to become familiar with the normal MR appearances of tissues on these pulse sequences.

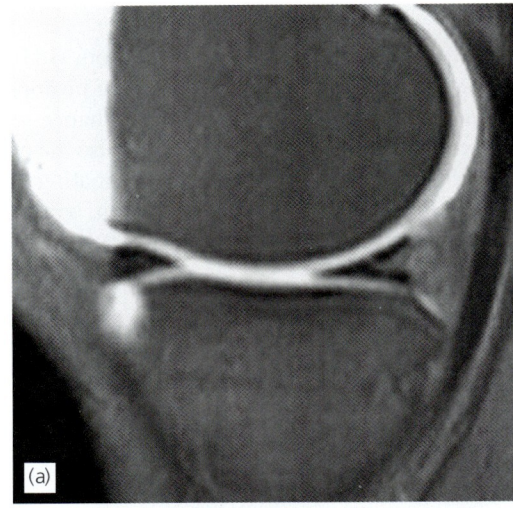

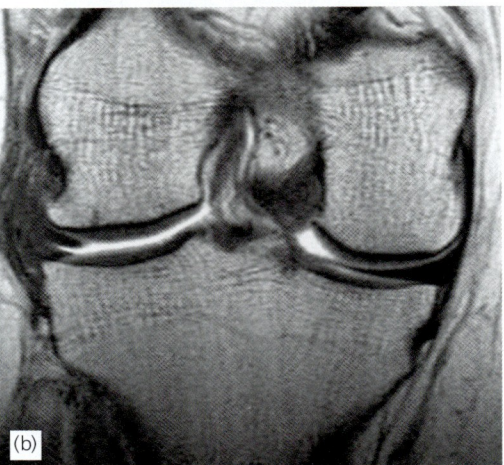

Figure 11.17 MRI arthrography: knee. (a) Sagittal T_1-weighted (T_1W) fat-suppressed image after the injection of a dilute solution of gadolinium contrast into the knee joint reveals abnormal signal within the posterior horn of the medial meniscus. The absence of gadolinium with this portion of the meniscus indicates that this is a healed tear. (b) Coronal T_1W image from a gadolinium arthrogram demonstrates extension of gadolinium into a tear in the body of the lateral meniscus.

Fat

Fat/adipose tissue is easily recognized on MRI because of its unique T_1 and T_2 properties. It is very bright (typically the brightest tissue) on a T_1W image. Very few tissues other than fat demonstrate increased signal intensity on T_1W images. These include subacute haemorrhage, proteinaceous fluid (as found in an abscess or proteinaceous cyst) and occasionally melanin. Adipose tissue maintains relatively bright signal intensity on non-fat-suppressed T_2W images, and displays moderately low signal intensity when fat saturation is applied to either a T_1W or T_2W sequence, thereby helping to confirm its fatty nature (Fig. 11.18).

Fluid

Simple fluid is dark (isointense to, or darker than, skeletal muscle) on T_1W images and becomes homogeneously bright on T_2W images.

Cortical bone

The protons within cortical bone are unable to participate in the resonance phenomenon because they are locked in a matrix; as a result, normal cortical bone displays an absence of signal (it is *black*) on all pulse sequences. Other materials that appear dark black on all pulse sequences include air, areas of soft-tissue calcification and haemosiderin (e.g. within a chronic haematoma or pigmented villonodular synovitis). On many pulse sequences, flowing blood in a vessel produces a dark 'flow void' within its lumen because the protons that were excited by the initial RF pulse have flowed out of the plane of the section by the time the tissue is sampled for returning signal at that level (Fig. 11.15a).

Trabecular/medullary bone

The MR appearance of the medullary cavity of a bone depends on the amount and type of marrow present. Yellow, non-haematopoietic marrow contains a preponderance of fat and is therefore bright on T_1W images and very dark grey on fat-saturated T_2W images. Red, haematopoietic marrow also contains fat (about 40% of its content) but also contains about 60% cellular elements. As a result, red marrow appears light grey (slightly hypointense relative to fat) on T_1W images and somewhat brighter than yellow marrow and subcutaneous fat on fat-saturated T_2W images (Fig. 11.19).

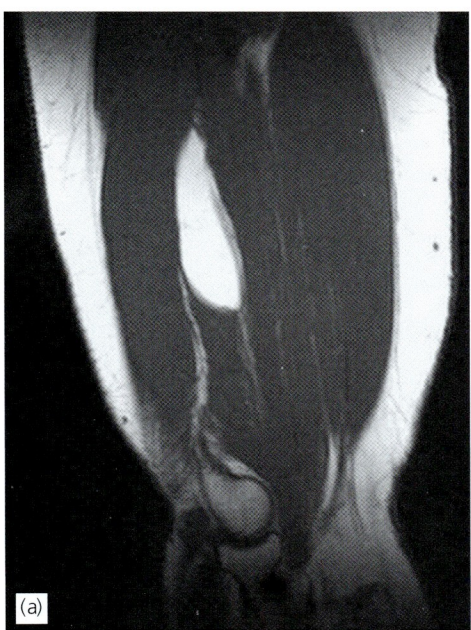
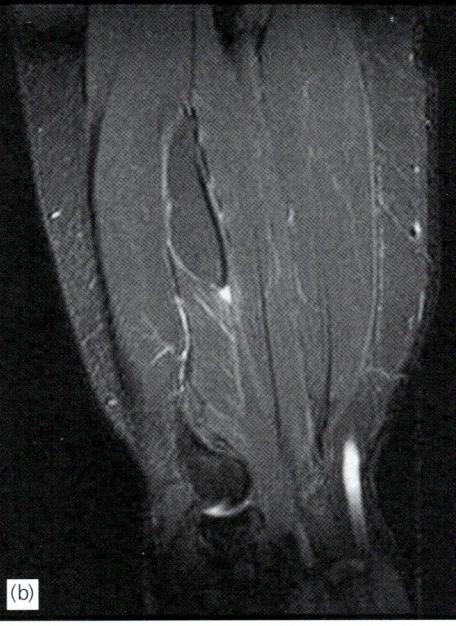

Figure 11.18 MRI signal characteristics: fat. (a) Sagittal T_1-weighted image reveals a smoothly marginated high signal intensity mass within the musculature of the upper arm compatible with a benign lipoma. (b) Sagittal short tau inversion–recovery image demonstrates complete suppression of the fat within the lesion.

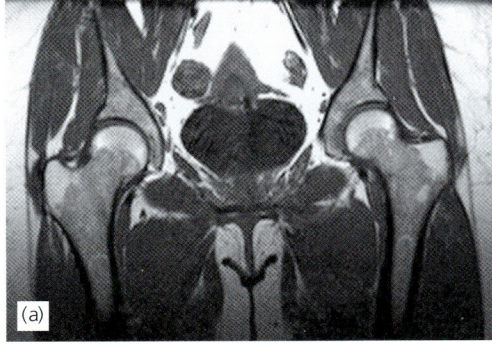
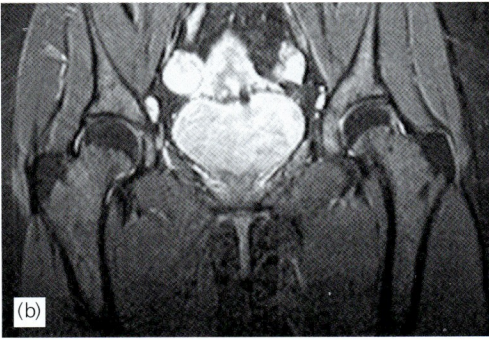

Figure 11.19 MRI signal characteristics: normal marrow. (a) Coronal T_1-weighted image of the pelvis shows geographic areas of haematopoietic marrow, with signal intensity slightly higher than that of skeletal muscle and lower than that of adjacent fatty marrow within the femoral heads and greater trochanters. (b) Coronal short tau inversion–recovery image demonstrates relatively increased signal within the areas of haematopoietic marrow relative to the suppressed fatty marrow.

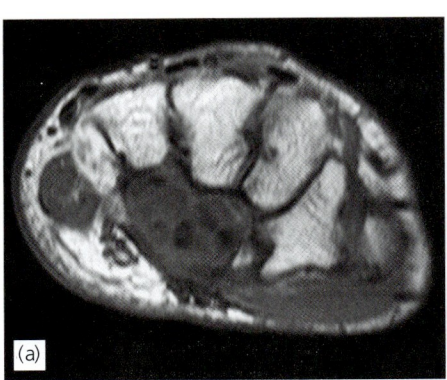 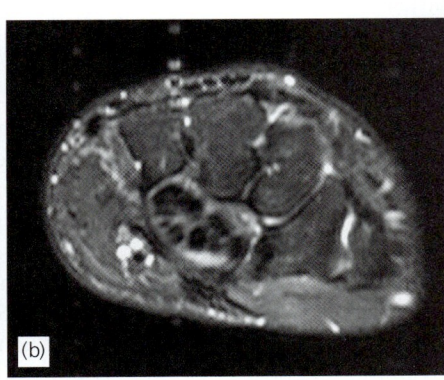 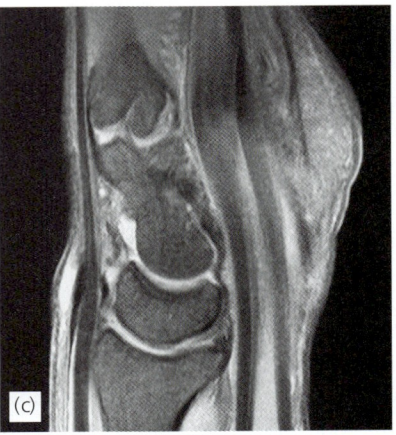

Figure 11.20 MRI signal characteristics: magic angle artefact. (a) Axial T_1-weighted image of the wrist shows diffuse, abnormal intermediate signal throughout the flexor tendons in the carpal tunnel. (b) Axial fat-saturated T_2-weighted image at the same level demonstrates normal signal intensity within the tendons confirming the magic angle artefact. (c) Sagittal proton density fat-saturated image displays the angled course of the tendons at this level, resulting in the artefactually increased signal.

Tendons/ligaments

Owing to their collagen-based structure, with few exceptions normal tendons and ligaments are of moderately low signal intensity on all pulse sequences. Two exceptions include the anterior cruciate ligament and the quadriceps tendon, both of which display intermediate signal intensity striations within their substance on T_1W and T_2W images. Another source of increased signal intensity within a normal tendon or ligament is the 'magic angle' artefact. This occurs in a highly ordered collagen-based structure that is positioned at an oblique angle within the magnetic field (typically 55° to the main magnetic field that runs longitudinally down the bore of the magnet). On T_1, proton density and most GRE pulse sequences, artefactual intermediate signal intensity is present within the tendon or ligament, and, in some cases, the structure may appear to be completely disrupted. The key to its recognition is that the abnormal signal intensity 'magically' disappears on T_2W images and the tendon or ligament appears normal (Fig. 11.20).[15]

Fibrocartilage

Normal fibrocartilaginous structures such as the menisci of the knee, triangular fibrocartilage of the wrist and labral tissue in the shoulder and hip also display very low signal intensity on T_1W and T_2W images.

Articular cartilage

Hyaline articular cartilage demonstrates variable signal intensity depending on the sequence used. It is grey on T_1W images; since it is virtually indistinguishable from joint fluid, this sequence is not typically used for its evaluation. A fat-saturated T_2W technique is more useful for evaluating articular cartilage owing to the excellent contrast between the high-signal joint fluid and dark-grey cartilage (Fig. 11.21). Similarly, a relatively

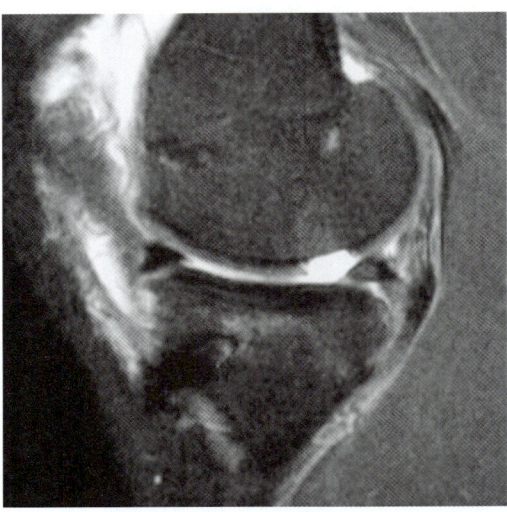

Figure 11.21 MRI: articular cartilage injury. Sagittal short tau inversion–recovery image demonstrates a focal defect within the posterior weight-bearing cartilage of the medial femoral condyle filled with high signal intensity fluid.

T_1W GRE technique may be used since the opposite tissue contrast is produced (low-signal joint fluid and high-signal cartilage).

Muscle

Normal skeletal muscle demonstrates a very characteristic MR appearance on T_1W images, in which it appears predominantly low in signal but with thin, high-signal striations coursing through it that represent normal intramuscular fat ('fatty marbling') (Fig. 11.22). Normal muscle remains of relatively low signal intensity (dark grey) on T_2W images, and the fatty striations are less apparent, especially if fat saturation is applied.

Imaging modalities 169

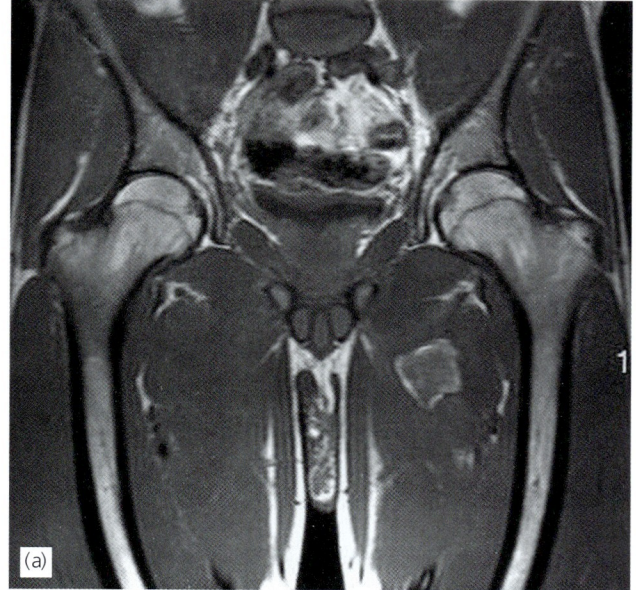
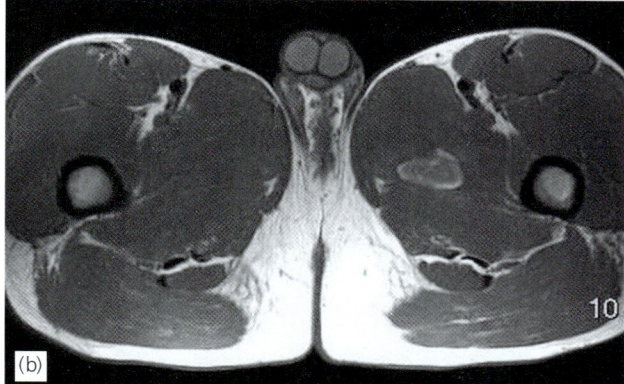
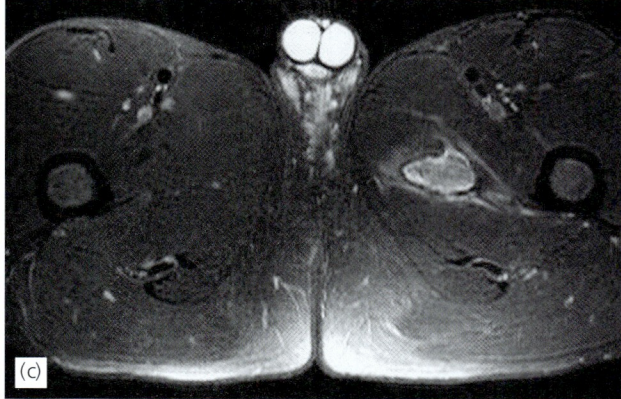

Figure 11.22 MRI: muscle injury. (a) Coronal T_1-weighted (T_1W), (b) axial T_1W and (c) axial T_2-weighted images reveal a mass-like area of mixed signal intensity in the left adductor musculature in a soccer player after injury. MRI signal characteristics are compatible with a partial tear and intramuscular haematoma. Note the normal fatty 'marbling' within the uninvolved muscles on the T_1W images.

Synovium

Normal synovium is not readily visible with routine MRI sequences. However, it may be detected if it is hypertrophied, and even normal synovium will demonstrate avid enhancement on fat-saturated, post-Gd T_1W images.

MUSCULOSKELETAL APPLICATIONS

The potential applications of MRI in the musculoskeletal system are myriad, and only a brief general discussion of its major applications will be included in this chapter. More extensive discussion of specific uses and indications will be addressed throughout the text in the appropriate chapters.

Osseous trauma

Acute traumatic injuries to bone occur along a spectrum of severity from a bone contusion to a frank fracture. Most osseous injuries are radiographically occult, but are readily evident on MR images because of the associated marrow oedema and haemorrhage that is present from the time of injury. These types of injury are most conspicuous on fat-saturated T_2W images, in which they appear as ill-defined areas of increased signal. In the case of a radiographically occult fracture, a linear signal abnormality will be observed within the oedema and is often more conspicuous on a T_1W image (Fig. 11.23).

Chronic stress injury to bone may lead to a fatigue injury when abnormal stresses are applied to normal bone, or an insufficiency fracture when normal stresses are applied to abnormal bone. In both cases, repetitive submaximal forces result in the accumulation of osseous microdamage, and these stress injuries range from an asymptomatic 'stress reaction' to a true stress fracture. MRI findings depend on the stage of injury at the time of the scan and are again most conspicuous on fat-saturated T_2W images. A mild stress reaction may manifest as only high-signal fluid/oedema along the periosteal surface of the bone on fat-saturated T_2W images, or, in the case of a more severe stress reaction, with prominent high-signal 'oedema' in the medullary cavity. A stress fracture is diagnosed if a linear component is detected (Fig. 11.24).

Sports injuries

MRI has revolutionized the practice of sports medicine. In addition to detecting the radiographically occult osseous injuries described above, MR is able to exquisitely define both intra-articular and extra-articular soft-tissue structures.

Ligament and tendon injuries are most apparent on fat-saturated T_2W images, in which the normally low signal intensity structure will demonstrate abnormal increased intrasubstance signal intensity. In the case of sprains or partial tears, intact fibres will be seen along with areas of abnormally increased intrasubstance signal intensity. In the case of a complete tear, the structure will appear completely disrupted (Fig. 11.25).

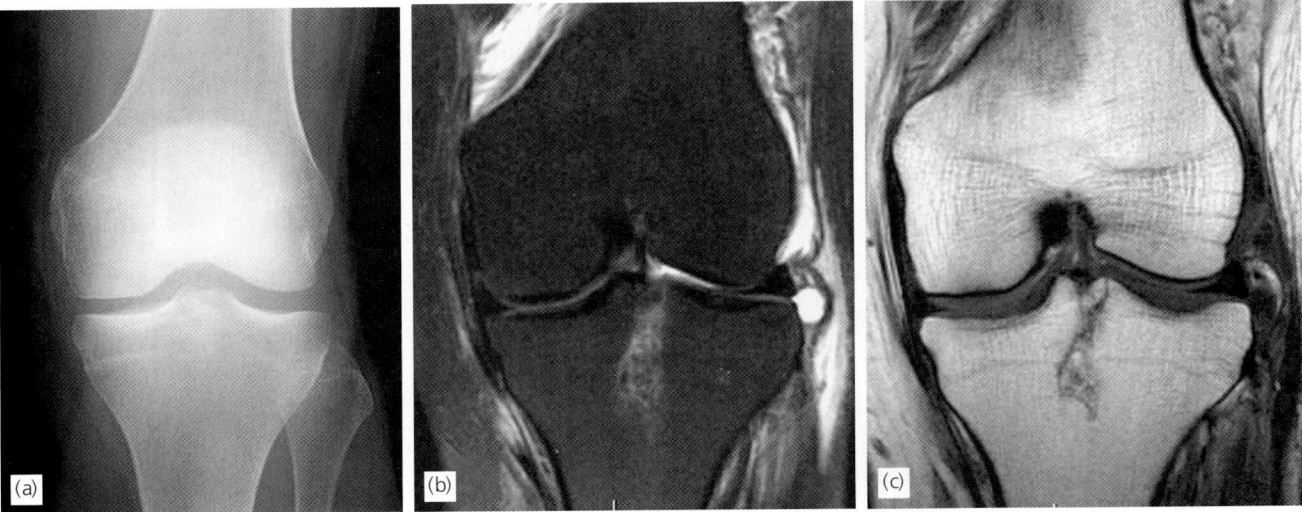

Figure 11.23 MRI: radiographically occult fracture. (a) Anteroposterior radiograph in a patient with knee pain shows no evidence of fracture. (b) Coronal short tau inversion–recovery demonstrates oedema-like signal in the mid-tibial plateau. (c) T_1-weighted coronal image shows the vertically oriented fracture line to better advantage.

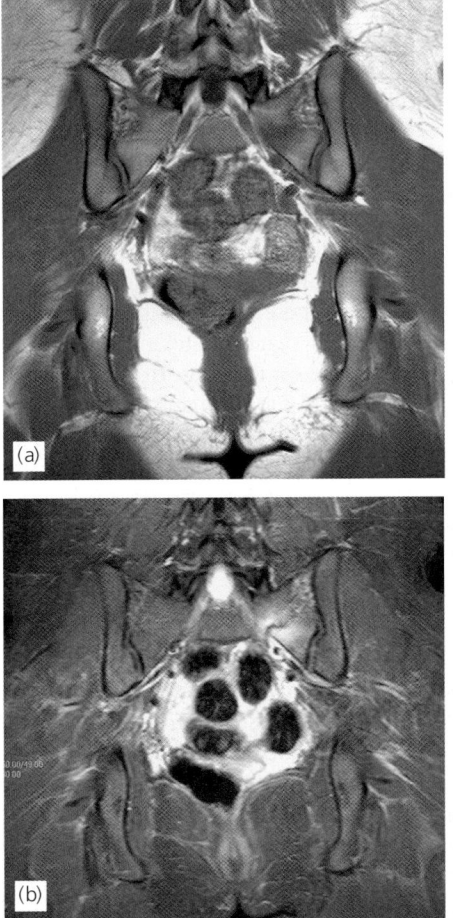

Figure 11.24 MRI: stress fracture. (a) Coronal T_1-weighted and (b) coronal short tau inversion–recovery images reveal abnormal, oedema-like signal intensity in the left sacral ala with an incomplete fracture line.

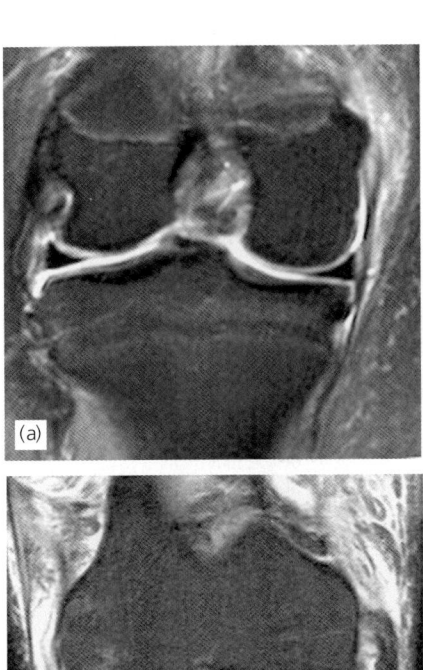

Figure 11.25 MRI: ligament injury. (a) Coronal short tau inversion–recovery (STIR) image shows a partial tear of the proximal medial collateral ligament. (b) Coronal STIR image in a different patient reveals a complete tear of the medial collateral ligament with a thickened, retracted ligament.

Muscle injuries most typically occur at the musculotendinous junction and are again best detected on fat-saturated T_2W images. These can be similarly classified based on their MR appearance as a strain (feathery, increased, oedema-like signal infiltrating otherwise intact muscle fibres), partial tear (increased signal with focal disruption of some muscle fibres) or complete rupture (Fig. 11.22). Chronic injury resulting in fatty atrophy of a muscle will be most conspicuous on T_1W images owing to the increased intensity of the infiltrating fat, which is best displayed on that sequence.

A tear of a fibrocartilaginous structure (meniscus, labrum) will manifest as abnormal signal that extends to involve one or both of its articular surfaces. Often, these injuries are best seen on T_1, proton density or GRE images, and are actually less apparent on more heavily T_2W images.

The ability to detect articular cartilage injury is dependent upon the use of an appropriate pulse sequence that produces a high degree of contrast between the cartilage and joint fluid. As mentioned, these are typically either a fat-saturated T_2W sequence (bright fluid/dark cartilage) or a relatively T_1W GRE sequence (bright cartilage/dark fluid) (Fig. 11.21).

Tumour

With a primary bone tumour, radiographs still provide the most accurate assessment of the aggressiveness of the lesion, and the most specific information regarding its nature. MRI, however, plays an integral role in the local staging of a primary bone neoplasm, providing a comprehensive depiction of its local and regional extent.

In the case of osseous metastases and myeloma, MRI is more sensitive for detecting these lesions than radiographs, CT or bone scan because of its ability to directly demonstrate the abnormal intramedullary tissue, not just its effects on adjacent bone (Fig. 11.26). Both T_1W and fat-saturated T_2W sequences are quite sensitive in this regard.

When investigating a soft-tissue mass, MRI is able to provide a tissue-specific diagnosis in approximately 25–30% of cases based solely on the MRI characteristics of the mass (Figs 11.10, 11.12 and 11.16).[16] Identifiable lesions include lipoma, simple cyst, haemangioma/vascular malformation, pigmented villonodular synovitis/giant cell tumour of the tendon sheath and haematoma. Care must be taken when haematoma is observed since it may be the result of an underlying tumour that bled; therefore, it must be followed to resolution either clinically or with imaging.

As with an osseous lesion, MRI is able to provide essential information regarding the local stage of a soft-tissue lesion as well.

Infection

The accurate diagnosis of osteomyelitis is important since its detection will determine the need for long-term antibiotic therapy. Radiographs are quite insensitive in this regard. Historically, radionuclide bone scanning – in particular ^{111}In-labelled white cell scanning – has been the gold standard; however, in recent years, MRI has become the modality of choice given its ability to detect not only abnormal marrow signal at the site of infection but also adjacent soft-tissue abnormalities (abscess, sinus tract) that may require surgical intervention.

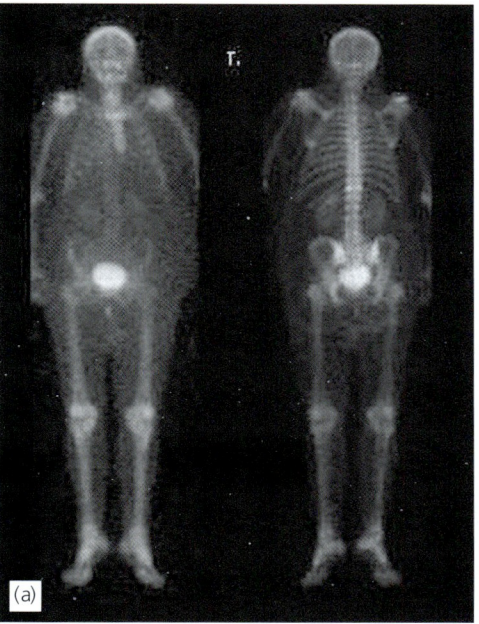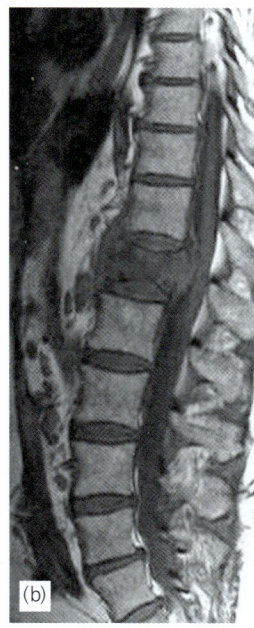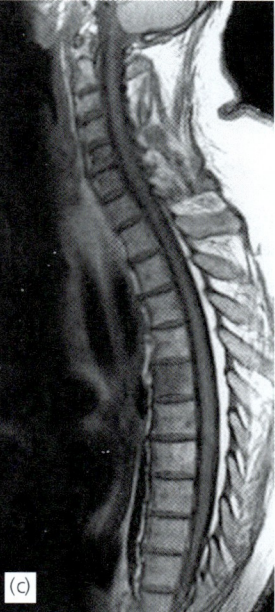

Figure 11.26 MRI occult bone tumour. (a) Bone scan reveals abnormal activity within the T12 vertebral body, corresponding to a pathological burst fracture secondary to metastatic tumour involvement that is well demonstrated on a T_1-weighted (T_1W) sagittal image of that region (b). No other tumour focus is evident elsewhere in the spine on the bone scan. (c) Sagittal T_1W image of the cervicothoracic spine reveals additional areas of low-signal tumour involvement in the lower cervical and mid-thoracic spine.

REFERENCES

1. Murphy WA. Radiologic history exhibit: introduction to the history of musculoskeletal imaging. *Radiographics* 1990;**10**:915–43.
2. Love C, Din AS, Tomas MB, et al. Radionuclide bone imaging: an illustrative review. *Radiographics* 2003;**23**:341–58.
3. Rizzo PF, Gould ES, Lyden JP, Asnis SE. Diagnosis of occult fractures about the hip: magnetic resonance imaging compared with bone scanning. *Journal of Bone and Joint Surgery (American)* 1993;**75**:395–401.
4. Duet M, Pouchot J, Liote F, Faraggi M. Role for positron emission tomography in skeletal diseases. *Joint, Bone, Spine* 2007;**74**:14–23.
5. Imhof H, Mang T. Advances in musculoskeletal radiology: multidetector computed tomography. *Orthopedic Clinics of North America* 2006;**37**:287–98.
6. Geijer M, El-Khoury GY. MDCT in the evaluation of skeletal trauma: principles, protocols, and clinical applications. *Emergency Radiology* 2006;**13**:7–18.
7. Holmes JF, Mirvis SE, Panacek EA, et al. Variability in computed tomography and magnetic resonance imaging in patients with cervical spine injuries. *Journal of Trauma* 2002;**53**:524–30.
8. Vande Berg B, Malghem J, Maldague B, Lecouvet F. Multi-detector CT imaging in the postoperative orthopedic patient with metal hardware. *European Journal of Radiology* 2006;**60**:470–9.
9. National Cancer Institute. *Radiation Risks and Pediatric Computed Tomography (CT); a Guide for Health Care Providers.* Available from: www.cancer.gov.cancertopics/causes/radiation-risks-pediatric-CT.
10. Khoury V, Cardinal E, Bureau NJ. Musculoskeletal sonography: a dynamic tool for usual and unusual disorders. *AJR American Journal of Roentgenology* 2007;**188**:W63–W73.
11. Roberts CS, Beck DJ, Heinsen J, Seligson D. Diagnostic ultrasonography: applications in orthopaedic surgery. *Clinical Orthopaedics and Related Research* 2002;**401**:248–64.
12. Kapelov SR, Teresi LM, Bradley WG, et al. Bone contusions of the knee: increased lesion detection with fast spin-echo MR imaging with spectroscopic fat saturation. *Radiology* 1993;**189**:901–4.
13. Broome DR, Girquis MS, Baron PW, et al. Gadodiamide-associated nephrogenic systemic sclerosis: why radiologists should be concerned. *AJR American Journal of Roentgenology* 2007;**188**:586–92.
14. Farrant JM, O'Connor PJ, Grainger AJ. Advanced imaging in rheumatoid arthritis. Part 1. Synovitis. *Skeletal Radiology* 2007;**36**:269–79.
15. Hayes CW, Parellada JA. The magic angle effect in musculoskeletal MR imaging. *Topics in Magnetic Resonance Imaging* 1996;**8**:51–6.
16. Gielen JL, De Schepper AM, Vanhoenacker F, et al. Accuracy of MRI in characterization of soft tissue tumors and tumor like lesions. A prospective study in 548 patients. *European Radiology* 2004;**14**:2320–30.

12

Biomechanics and biomaterials

DUNCAN ET SHEPHERD, DAVID WL HUKINS

Introduction	173	Joint replacement of synovial joints	189
Mechanical principles	173	Fracture fixation devices	195
Mechanical properties of materials	178	Spinal implants	196
Dynamics and control	184	Preclinical testing	197
Biomechanics of joints	186	References	199
Biomaterials	188		

NATIONAL BOARD STANDARDS

- Know how to draw the stress–strain curve and understand the concept of modulus of elasticity
- Be able to draw joint reaction forces around major joints
- Understand viscoelasticity and the hysteresis loop
- Understand the different types of failure of materials
- Know about wear in different types of hip replacements
- Understand the basic principles of mechanical testing of implants

INTRODUCTION

This chapter gives an overview of biomechanics and biomaterials. The first part of the chapter will detail basic mechanical principles, the mechanical properties of materials, and dynamics and control. Further reading on these sections can be found in many standard textbooks and review papers.[1-5] The biomechanics of joints will then be presented. The second part of the chapter will discuss biomaterials. In the first section, the mechanical properties of natural tissues associated with orthopaedics will be discussed, followed by an overview of synthetic biomaterials used in the manufacture of orthopaedic devices. Examples of orthopaedic devices (synovial joint replacement implants, fracture fixation devices and spinal implants) will be given and the reasons why specific materials are used explained. Finally, a section on preclinical testing will be given, describing ways of modelling implants and the importance of subjecting them to mechanical testing before they are implanted into patients.

MECHANICAL PRINCIPLES

Vectors

Biomechanics is not the same as functional anatomy because it uses a branch of physics (mechanics) to explain how our bodies work and so, inevitably, some mathematical concepts are involved. This section covers the first important mathematical concept – vectors.

A *vector* is a number that has a direction associated with it. Because it has a direction, it is not the same as an ordinary number or *scalar*. Consider what happens when we flex the elbow with the wrist rigid. The distance, x, between the hand and the elbow does not change; x is a scalar. However, the position of the hand, with respect to the elbow, does change. We can denote the position of the hand by a vector **x** that can be represented by an arrow, as shown in Fig. 12.1. The length of this vector is the constant distance between the elbow and the hand but its direction changes as the elbow flexes. The vector is sometimes called

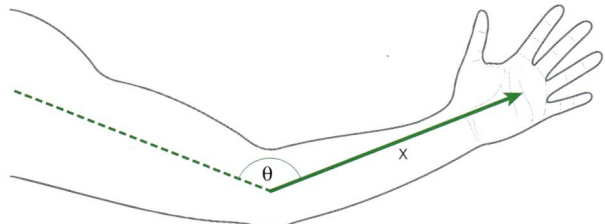

Figure 12.1 Description of flexion at the elbow. The vector **x** denotes the position of the hand with respect to the elbow. When the elbow flexes, the direction, but not the length, of **x** changes. The position of the hand can also be denoted by the angle θ, measured from the upper arm. When the elbow flexes, θ increases. Sometimes this angle is denoted by the vector $\boldsymbol{\theta}$, whose direction defines the axis about which positive rotation occurs (through the elbow towards you because anticlockwise rotations are positive).

the *displacement* of the hand, with respect to the elbow, or the *position vector* of the hand. Notice that it is conventional to represent a vector, like **x**, in bold type but not the number associated with it (sometimes called its modulus). We measure the displacement vector **x** in metres, in exactly the same way as we measure the distance x. Other vectors (such as force) are measured in different units.

In general, movement can involve changes in the displacement x as well as of the vector **x**. During subsidence, the femoral component of a total hip prosthesis sinks down into the medulla of the femur. In this case, the distance changes, but there is very little change in direction during subsidence; the motion occurs more or less along a straight line. We can then represent the motion reasonably well by a change in x, and can represent it graphically by a graph of x against time, t. In the unlikely event that the prosthesis moved upwards, out of the femur, we could express this mathematically by simply defining movement in this direction to be negative.

Rates of change

The rate at which x changes with time is called *speed*, and the rate at which **x** changes with time is called *velocity*. Notice that speed is the modulus of velocity. If **x** changes to $\mathbf{x} + \Delta\mathbf{x}$ in a time interval Δt, the *average velocity* is $\Delta\mathbf{x}/\Delta t$ and the *average speed* is $\Delta x/\Delta t$. The symbol Δ just represents an increment of something; if x becomes bigger, the value of Δx is positive, but if it becomes smaller the value is negative.

Unfortunately, average speeds and velocities are not much use to us, which is why calculus was invented. Although we will not be using calculus in this chapter, it will be useful to understand why it is needed. If we calculate the average speed over the time interval Δt, shown in Fig. 12.2, we obtain a single number. However, we can see from the graph that, initially, x is changing very slowly but it gradually speeds up. We really need to know the speed at

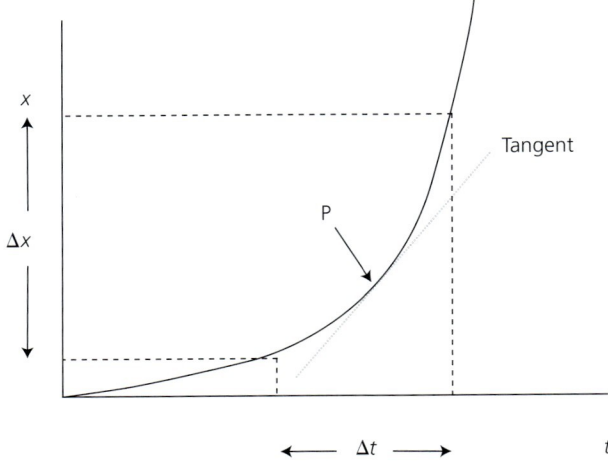

Figure 12.2 A graph showing the distance, x, moved by an object plotted against time, t. Then Δx is the distance the object moves during a time interval Δt so that its average speed is $\Delta x/\Delta t$. The smaller the value of Δt, the more closely the slope $\Delta x/\Delta t$ resembles a straight line. When Δt becomes zero, the slope collapses to the point P, at which the slope of the curve is given by the tangent shown on the graph. The value of $\Delta x/\Delta t$ at a point is denoted by dx/dt and gives the slope of the tangent that defines the instantaneous speed.

an instant in time. Figure 12.2 explains how the slope at an instant in time, written dx/dt, can be calculated. Then the speed at an instant in time, as the one denoted by the point P in Fig. 12.2, is defined by

$$v = \frac{dx}{dt}, \qquad (12.1)$$

and the velocity is defined by

$$\mathbf{v} = \frac{d\mathbf{x}}{dt}. \qquad (12.2)$$

Angular motion

Alternatively, we may describe the motion of a joint by a change in angle; flexion of the elbow can be described as a decrease in the angle θ shown in Fig. 12.1. Angles can be measured in degrees, but, when describing motion, they are usually measured in *radians*. In the same way as a circle is arbitrarily divided up into 360°, it can also be divided into 2π radians so that 1 radian is equal to $360/2\pi = 180/\pi$ degrees, which is approximately equal to 57.3°. The *angular speed* is defined by

$$\omega = \frac{d\theta}{dt}. \qquad (12.3)$$

Sometimes an *angular displacement*, which is a vector, is used to describe position, as described in the caption to Fig. 12.1. Then the angular displacement can be represented by the vector, **θ**, and the angular velocity is defined by

$$\boldsymbol{\omega} = \frac{d\boldsymbol{\theta}}{dt}. \qquad (12.4)$$

However, all the time that angular motion is confined to a plane, like flexion of the elbow, angular speed and angular velocity are the same.

Kinematics

Kinematics is simply the description of the motion of an object. We first have to define the initial position vector of the object with respect to some arbitrarily defined point called the *origin*. Its position, as time, t, changes, is then given by the parameters listed in Table 12.1, in which *acceleration*, the rate of change of velocity, is defined by

$$\mathbf{a} = \frac{d\mathbf{v}}{dt}. \qquad (12.5)$$

Table 12.1 also lists the units used to measure the values of these parameters. These are derived from the units of length and time, the metre (m) and second (s), respectively. Note that there are standard abbreviations that should always be used for these units and that they should never be made plural, e.g. 5 m represents five metres but 5 ms represents five milliseconds or 0.005 s. Table 12.2 lists the parameters of angular motion that may be used as an alternative for measuring the motion of a joint, in which displacements are measured in radians (rad). The prefixes that are sometimes used for large (such as the kilometre) and small (such as the millisecond) units are listed in Table 12.3. However, these large and small units must always be converted into the basic units before they are substituted into a formula to make any calculations.

Table 12.1 Kinematic parameters for translational motion

Name	Abbreviation	Units
Displacement	x	m
Time	t	s
Velocity	v	m s^{-1}
Acceleration	a	m s^{-2}

Table 12.2 Kinematic parameters for angular motion

Name	Abbreviation	Units
Angular displacement	θ	rad
Time	t	s
Angular velocity	ω	rad s^{-1}
Angular acceleration	α	rad s^{-2}

Table 12.3 Prefixes used for large and small units

Prefix	Abbreviation	Number	Power
Tera	T	1 000 000 000 000	10^{12}
Giga	G	1 000 000 000	10^{9}
Mega	M	1 000 000	10^{6}
Kilo	k	1000	10^{3}
Milli	m	0.001	10^{-3}
Micro	μ	0.000 001	10^{-6}
Nano	n	0.000 000 001	10^{-9}
Pico	p	0.000 000 000 001	10^{-12}

Note that, although abbreviations for units are standard, the symbols that represent parameters such as velocity and acceleration are not. In this chapter, we have used symbols that are commonly used but they are not really standard. It is, therefore, very important to define the meaning of any symbol that is used in a scientific article on biomechanics.

Kinematics is usually measured by video-recording the body after markers have been attached to identify specific anatomical points; further details are given in Ferrari *et al.*[6] The main problem with this technique is that, when a joint moves, the skin tends to move over its surface. The marker then moves with the skin to which it is attached, instead of remaining at a defined anatomical point. This problem has been overcome by inserting pins into bone to measure movement.[7] Radiographic techniques are less invasive, and video-fluoroscopy is commonly used to measure the kinematics of, for example, the knee joint.[8] Open bore MRI enables some kinematic measurements to be made without exposure to ionizing radiation.[9]

It is sometimes adequate to measure kinematics in a plane (two dimensions), e.g. to determine the range of motion of a joint in flexion. However, in other cases, it is necessary to measure three-dimensional motion; for example to determine whether rotation accompanies flexion of a joint. It is then necessary to reconstruct three-dimensional measurements from two or more images, as in RSA (called either *roentgen stereophotometric analysis* or *radiostereometric analysis*) or a tomographic technique such as MRI.

Force

A force changes the size, shape or motion of an object. A *tensile force* pulls an object, and can make it longer. A *compressive force* pushes an object and can make it shorter. A *shear force* changes the shape of an object without changing its dimensions, as shown in Fig. 12.3.

When we are concerned solely with the motion of an object, we can sometimes ignore the effect of the force on its size and shape, since they are usually relatively small. We are then making the assumption that the object is perfectly rigid. The object then resists the tendency of the force to change its motion because it has *mass*. Confusingly, the

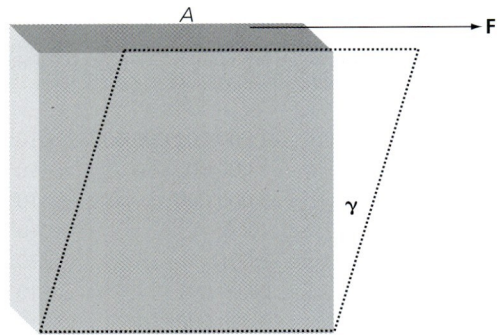

Figure 12.3 The force **F** acts on the upper face of the cube. In pure shear, the dimensions of the cube do not change. **F** is then a shear force and the angle γ is called the *shear strain*. (Strictly speaking, this diagram does not represent pure shear but has been simplified to make the explanation easier.) If the upper face of the cube has an area A, F/A is called the *shear stress*. Both stress and strain are vectors. However, shear strain is only a vector because it represents an angular displacement, so it is often represented as a scalar.

standard unit of mass is the kilogram (not the gram), and so masses must be converted to kilograms if they are to be used in a formula to make any calculations.

If the mass of the object does not change, which is invariably the case in biomechanics, the force is defined by

$$\mathbf{F} = m\mathbf{a}, \tag{12.6}$$

where the acceleration, **a**, is a measure of the change in the motion of the object, and the mass, *m*, is a measure of the ability of the object to resist this change. The ability to resist change in motion is called *inertia*. Force is measured in newtons (N), and is a vector. It is ultimately measured in terms of mass, distance and time, because acceleration is defined solely by distance and time (equations (12.2)–(12.5)). This dependence on mass, distance and time is true for all the mechanical parameters listed in Table 12.4. Most of the parameters listed in Table 12.4 will be explained in subsequent sections. They are all involved in explaining the motion of an object. This branch of mechanics is called *dynamics* and includes kinematics, which simply describes the motion.

Objects have *weight* because gravity pulls them towards the centre of the Earth. Their acceleration, often denoted by **g**, is approximately 9.81 m s^{-2}. According to equation (12.6), the Earth exerts a gravitation force *m***g** on an object of mass *m*. So weight is a force, and is measured in newtons not in kilograms, which are a measure of mass.

A *component of a force* is a measure of its effect in a given direction. The component of a force *F* in a direction that makes an angle θ with respect to its line of action is given by $F \cos θ$; the component at right angles to this direction is $F \sin θ$. Note that the components of forces are not vectors; they are scalars.

Table 12.4 Dynamic parameters for translational motion, in addition to those of Table 12.1

Name	Abbreviation	Definition	Units
Mass	*m*	Measure of inertia	kilograms (kg)
Momentum	**p**	*m***v**	kg m s^{-1}
Force	**F**	*m***a***	newtons (N)
Work	W	FΔx†	joules (J)
Energy	E	Ability to do work	J
Potential energy	U	Stored energy†	J
Kinetic energy	K	$mv^2/2$†	J
Power	P	dE/dt	watts (W)

*Strictly speaking, **F** is defined by d**p**/d*t* but, if the mass of the object stays constant, this is the same as *m***a**.

†The general definition of work requires mathematics that is beyond the scope of this chapter. However, when a constant force, **F**, gives an object a displacement Δ**x**, the work done is given by **F**Δ**x**cosθ, where θ is the angle between the vectors **F** and Δ**x**. Since the movement is usually in the direction of the force, W = FΔx provides a simple definition. Notice that the definition depends only on the moduli of **F** and Δ**x**, and not on their directions, so W is a scalar.

‡Potential and kinetic energy are simply different forms of energy, U. Note that the definition of kinetic energy uses the modulus of **v**, and is independent of its direction, because energy is the ability to do work and is, therefore, a scalar.

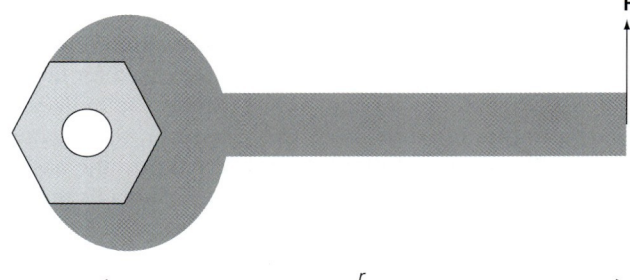

Figure 12.4 A spanner of length *r* being used to loosen a nut on a bolt (with a right-hand thread). A force, **F**, is exerted, perpendicular to the shaft of the spanner, to turn the nut in an anticlockwise direction. The task is made easier by increasing *r* and/or the magnitude of **F**. Therefore, the torque is defined to be F*r*. Note that the point of application of **F** defines a circle of radius *r*.

Torque

Torque changes the angular motion of an object, such as putting a screw-cap on a bottle or tightening a nut on a bolt; Fig. 12.4 shows that the effectiveness of these actions depends on the force, *F*, exerted and the perpendicular distance, *r*, from the line of action of the force to the axis around which the object is turning. The torque is then defined by

$$T = rF. \tag{12.7}$$

Table 12.5 Examples of rotational inertia for some simple shapes

Example	Rotational inertia	Possible biomechanical application*
Rotation of a cylinder of length L, radius r and mass m about an axis through the end of the cylinder and perpendicular to its axis	$I = \dfrac{mr^2}{4} + \dfrac{mL^2}{3}$	Raising the arm
Rotation of a rectangular plate of length L, width w, height h and mass m about an axis along one of its shortest sides	$I = \dfrac{mh^2}{12} + \dfrac{mL^2}{3}$	Flexion of the hand at the wrist
Rotation of a rectangular plate of length L, width w, height h and mass m about an axis perpendicular to one of its shortest sides	$I = \dfrac{mw^2}{12} + \dfrac{mL^2}{3}$	Lateral bending of the hand at the wrist

*These examples are simple models for movement of limbs since the arm is not a cylinder and the hand is not rectangular. However, simple models of this kind can often provide useful mechanical insights.

Table 12.6 Dynamic parameters for angular motion, in addition to those of Table 12.2

Name	Abbreviation	Definition	Units
Rotational inertia	I_r	Measure of inertia	kg m²
Angular momentum		$I_r \theta$	kg m² rad s⁻¹
Torque	T	$I_r \alpha$*	N m
Kinetic energy	K	$I_r \omega^2/2$	J

*Either equation (12.7) or the table entry could be considered as a definition of torque; one then follows from the other. Equation (12.7) leads directly to the units in the table; the alternative definition has equivalent units.

Torque, like the other angular motion parameters in Table 12.2, is defined to be a vector, but the mathematics involved is beyond the scope of this chapter. Fortunately, we can often treat it as a scalar that acts in either a clockwise or an anticlockwise direction.

Torque has to overcome the *rotational inertia* of an object. Rotational inertia, sometimes called *moment of inertia*, depends on the dimensions, shape and mass of an object. The definition of rotational inertia depends on mathematics that is beyond the scope of the chapter. Table 12.5 gives formulae for calculating the rotational inertia for different shapes. Table 12.6 lists some of the other parameters used to describe angular motion which sometimes appear in the biomechanics literature.

Equilibrium

An object is in equilibrium when all the forces acting on it cancel each other out, and all the torques acting on it cancel each other out. To calculate the conditions of equilibrium, it is useful to construct a *free body diagram* that shows all the forces acting. This diagram can indicate anatomical structures or be highly schematic, as in Fig. 12.5.

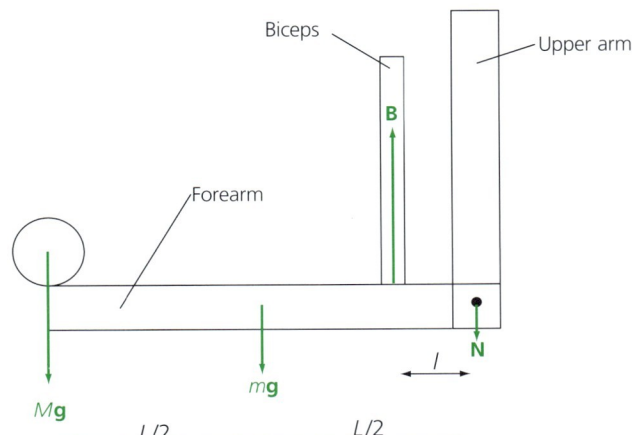

Figure 12.5 Free body diagram of a horizontal forearm, of length L, supporting an object of mass M in the hand. The upper arm is vertical. **B** is the force exerted by the biceps, whose point of attachment is a distance l from the elbow joint. The weight, m**g**, of the arm can be considered to act at a point called its centre of gravity. For a uniform object, the centre of gravity is at its geometric centre so, for this calculation, we will assume that the arm is uniform. Calculation of the position of the centre of gravity for non-uniform objects is beyond the scope of this chapter. The force **N** is generated at the elbow by the weight of the object being held and of the arm itself.

Since all the forces must cancel each other out, we can write

$$M\mathbf{g} + m\mathbf{g} + \mathbf{N} - \mathbf{B} = 0. \quad (12.8)$$

All the symbols used in this paragraph are defined in the caption to Fig. 12.5. Now, we consider the torques tending to turn the arm about the elbow. Since the arm is stationary, it is in equilibrium, so all the torques must cancel each other out, i.e.

$$Bl - mgL/2 - MgL = 0, \quad (12.9)$$

where anticlockwise torques are positive. From equation (12.9), we can work out that the force that the biceps needs to exert to hold the forearm horizontal is

$$\mathbf{B} = \frac{L(m+2M)}{2l}\mathbf{g}. \qquad (12.10)$$

Substituting the expression for **B** from equation (12.10) into equation (12.8), we can calculate the force, **N**, generated at the elbow.

The body is not always in equilibrium. For example, when we are running, we lean so that we are tending to fall forwards. We are only in equilibrium when we are stationary; the branch of mechanics that deals with equilibrium is called *statics*. Dynamic stability is a more difficult problem (see the section on Movement).

Work, energy and power

When a force moves an object, or changes its dimensions or shape, it performs *work*. The concept of work, measured in joules (J), is described in greater detail in Table 12.4. When work is done on an object, this is said to be given *mechanical energy*, *E*. This energy can be stored, as *potential energy* (Table 12.4), or dissipated, often as heat. When the force is removed, any potential energy is used to return the object towards its initial state.

A moving object can affect a second object in the same way, i.e. by moving it or changing its dimensions or shape. A moving hammer and a moving bullet provide examples of this phenomenon. The energy that the moving object possesses, and that it can transfer to a second object, is called *kinetic energy* (Table 12.4).

This behaviour of a force can be illustrated by two extreme examples. The first is lifting an object in which all the work done is stored as potential energy. When the force is removed, the object uses its potential energy to drop to the floor, at which point all its potential energy has been converted to kinetic energy.

In complete contrast, when an object is pushed or pulled across a horizontal surface, the force exerted simply has to overcome friction (see the section on Friction). Then all the energy given to the object is dissipated (as heat). So, when the force is removed, the object has no potential energy and remains in its final position.

The rate at which energy is transferred is called *power*, and is measured in watts (W); further details are given in Table 12.4.

MECHANICAL PROPERTIES OF MATERIALS

Elasticity

As well as being able to change the motion of an object, a force can change its size or shape. For example, the long, thin object in Fig. 12.6 is extended by the action of the

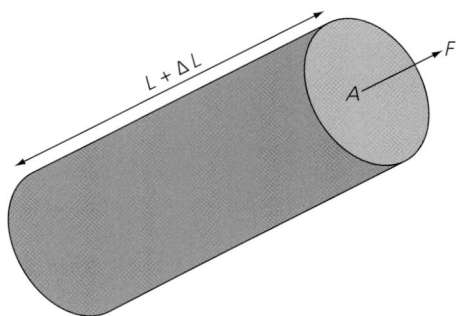

Figure 12.6 A tensile force of magnitude *F* acting along the axis of an object of initial length *L* and cross-sectional area *A* so as to increase its length by ΔL.

tensile force, of magnitude *F*, acting along the direction of its axis but compressed by a compressive force, acting along the same axis in an opposite direction. If the object has an initial length *L*, and the action of the force is to extend it by an increment ΔL, we define its tensile *stiffness* to be

$$k = \frac{F}{\Delta L}. \qquad (12.11)$$

We can calculate compressive stiffness in exactly the same way.

We can use equation (12.11) to describe the stiffness of an object, but we often need to describe the stiffness of a material; the two are not the same. For example, a very thick cylinder of silicone rubber could be stiffer than a very thin steel wire. But when objects of similar dimensions are compared, silicone is less stiff than steel.

To compare stiffnesses of materials we define *stress* by

$$\sigma = \frac{F}{A}, \qquad (12.12)$$

where *A* is the cross-sectional area of the object (perpendicular to the direction in which the force acts), and the strain by

$$\varepsilon = \frac{\Delta L}{L}. \qquad (12.13)$$

Since an object becomes thinner as it stretches, *A*, in equation (12.12), is not really a constant when an object extends. However, we usually neglect this effect when calculating stress; the resulting approximate definition is sometimes called *engineering stress*. A similar problem occurs in the definition of strain; because the initial extension of some materials is easier than further extension; the definition of ε, in equation (12.13), can then be affected by the size of ΔL. However, we often ignore this effect, and call the strain defined by equation (12.13) *engineering strain*. If we take these effects into account, the stress and strain are usually called *true stress* and *true strain*.

Stress is a force divided by an area, and so is measured in newtons per square metre (N m^{-2}); however, this unit is encountered so often that is has a special name – the pascal (abbreviated to Pa). Note that pressure is also measured in Pa, but is not the same as stress; stress has a direction associated with it, but pressure acts equally in all directions. Strain is a dimensionless number because it is calculated by dividing a length by a length.

It is conventional to define ΔL as positive when an object becomes longer. If a force makes the object longer, it is then defined to act along the axis in a positive direction. As a result, tensile stresses and strains are positive, but compressive stresses and strains are negative.

We can represent the effect of stretching or compressing a material by plotting a graph of σ against ε. The result is called a *stress–strain curve*. For some materials, especially metals such as those used in orthopaedic devices, the graph will be a straight line. For others, like most body tissues, it will be some form of curve, as shown in Fig. 12.7.

When the stress–strain curve is a straight line, its slope is a measure of the stiffness of the material: the slope is called *Young's modulus* of the material and is given by

$$E = \frac{\sigma}{\varepsilon}. \qquad (12.14)$$

A material with a linear stress–strain curve is said to obey *Hooke's law*. However, Young's modulus of a ligament (in Fig. 12.7) is not constant; initially, the ligament is easy to stretch, but it then becomes much stiffer. Many authors try to describe these curves by linear regions, in order to calculate Young's modulus. Mathematically, such a curve has a changing slope that can be calculated exactly at a chosen value of ε, like ε' in Fig. 12.7. Geometrically, this slope can be determined by drawing a tangent to the curve at this point. However, it can be calculated if the definition of E, in equation (12.14), is generalized to

$$E = \frac{d\sigma}{d\varepsilon}. \qquad (12.15)$$

A method for using equation (12.15) to calculate E at any value of ε' has been described.[10] Whatever method is chosen, Young's modulus of most biological tissues, and many synthetic materials such as gels and elastomers, has to be calculated at more than a single strain value.

In this chapter, we have E to represent both energy (Table 12.4) and Young's modulus. It is unfortunate that E is commonly used to denote these two very different variables. Fortunately, in this chapter, it should not cause confusion because it should be clear, from the context, which one we mean. If there had been any risk of confusion, we could have used different symbols or simply distinguished them with different subscripts.

Qualitatively, a material or structure that is easily deformed (stretched or compressed) is said to be *compliant*. Unfortunately, the term *elastic* is often used as a synonym for compliant in the orthopaedics literature. This is incorrect, as elasticity has a very different meaning from compliance – as we shall see in the next paragraph.

When the stress is removed from a metal, it rapidly returns to its original dimensions; this process is called *recoil*. Recoil occurs because all the work done in deforming the object is stored as potential energy; this energy is used to return the object to its original dimensions. Materials that behave in this way are said to be *elastic*; the metals used in orthopaedic devices tend to be elastic. However, most biological tissues are more complicated because they are *viscoelastic*; viscoelasticity is described in a later section.

If we stretch an elastic material from zero strain to strain ε (Fig. 12.8), the area under the stress–strain curve is the work done (i.e. energy used) to stretch a unit volume of the material. If the material is elastic, this energy is stored as potential energy, and, if the stress–strain curve is linear, the area is simply the area of the shaded triangle so that

$$U = \frac{1}{2}\sigma\varepsilon = \frac{1}{2E}\sigma^2 = \frac{1}{2}E\varepsilon^2. \qquad (12.16)$$

The various forms of equation (12.16) arise from applying equation (12.14) to the original area calculation. Since

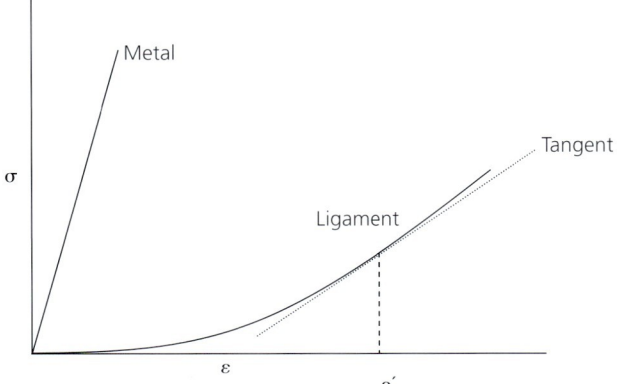

Figure 12.7 Stress–strain curves for a material (such as a metal) that obeys Hooke's law compared with another (such as a ligament) that does not. The non-Hookean curve is not a straight line and so does not have a unique value of Young's modulus, E. However, E can be calculated at any given strain, like ε', from the slope of the tangent to the curve.

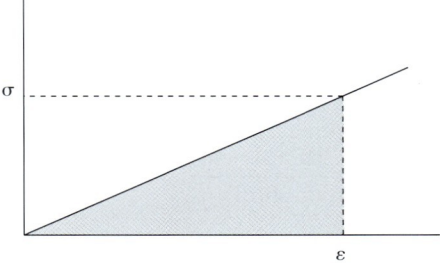

Figure 12.8 The shaded area under the stress–strain curve represents the work done to increase the strain from zero to ε. In this example, the material obeys Hooke's law so the stress–strain curve is a straight line and the shaded area is simply the area of a right-angled triangle whose perpendicular sides are ε and σ, where σ is the stress required to induce the strain ε.

an elastic material stores all this energy and dissipates it in recoil, an elastic material deforms and recoils along the same path on the stress–strain graph.

When an object is stretched, it usually becomes thinner. If we consider a cylindrical object, it then experiences a negative radial strain, σ_r, as well as a positive axial strain, σ, as the result of the application of an axial tensile stress. The relative value of these strains depends on the properties of the material, and is quantified by a quantity called *Poisson's ratio* defined by

$$\nu = -\frac{\sigma_r}{\sigma}. \qquad (12.17)$$

Most metals have ν values of about 0.3; rubber-like materials (e.g. silicones), which show very small volume changes during extension and compression, have values of about 0.5. Many elementary textbooks state that Poisson's ratio cannot be less than zero; this is not necessarily true for materials with complicated internal structures (like many biological tissues).

The *rigidity* or *shear modulus*, G, describes the ability of a material to resist change in shape rather than change in dimensions. G is calculated by dividing shear stress by shear strain (both defined in Fig. 12.3). For isotropic materials (whose properties do not depend on direction) at small strains, G is related to E by

$$G = \frac{E}{2(1+\nu)}. \qquad (12.18)$$

Equation (12.18) is a good approximation for metals and polymers that are not in fibre or sheet form (e.g. the polyethylene in the acetabular cups of total hip prostheses), but is not likely to be a good approximation for materials such as ligaments, whose preferred orientations of collagen fibres make than anisotropic.

Bending and twisting

An object that provides support in bending is called a *beam*. The most common type of beam encountered in orthopaedics is one that is fixed at both ends; examples are a plate and an intramedullary nail used to stabilize a fracture. If a force F is applied at a distance a from one end of a beam of length L, the beam deflects a distance

$$y_1 = \frac{Fa^2(3L-4a)}{48EI}. \qquad (12.19)$$

In equation (12.19), E is Young's modulus of the material of the beam and I depends on its cross-sectional shape. Table 12.7 explains how to calculate I for some common cross-sectional shapes. If the beam is loaded at its centre, equation (12.19) simplifies to

$$y_2 = \frac{FL^3}{192EI}. \qquad (12.20)$$

Table 12.7 Formulae for I, the second moment of area, for use in beam deflection calculations. Note that, if dimensions are measured in m, I is measured in m⁴

Shape	I
Plate of width w and thickness t	$wt^3/12$
Cylindrical rod of radius r	$\pi r^4/4$
Hollow cylindrical rod, internal radius r_i, external radius r_o	$\frac{\pi}{4}(r_o^4 - r_i^4)$

If the beam is subjected to a uniformly distributed force along its length, its maximum deflection is at the centre and is given by

$$y_3 = \frac{FL^3}{384EI}. \qquad (12.21)$$

An object which provides support in torsion or which transmits torque is called a *shaft*. An intramedullary nail (with its associated screws) can be considered as a shaft (as well as a beam) because it prevents bone ends being twisted about its axis. When a torque is applied to a shaft, it is twisted through an angle, θ (as shown in Fig. 12.9), given by

$$\theta = \frac{2}{\pi(r_o^4 - r_i^4)} \cdot \frac{TL}{G}, \qquad (12.22)$$

where T is the applied torque, L is the length of the shaft and G is the rigidity modulus of the material of the shaft; r_o and r_i are the outer and inner radii of a hollow shaft. To perform the calculation for a solid shaft, r_i is set equal to zero.

Flow

When a shear stress is applied to a fluid (either a liquid or a gas), it flows because, unlike an elastic solid, it does not store any of the energy used to deform it. However, fluids can resist flow; this resistance is called *viscosity*. For example, blood is more viscous than water because it flows less easily, i.e. blood has a higher viscosity (about 3.1×10^{-3} Pa s) than water (8.9×10^{-4} Pa s).

The viscosity, η, dictates, for example, the rate at which fluid will flow through a long, thin tube of radius r and length L. If a volume ΔV flows in a time interval Δt, this flow rate is given by

$$\frac{\Delta V}{\Delta t} = \frac{\pi r^4}{8\eta} \cdot \frac{\Delta P}{L}, \qquad (12.23)$$

where ΔP is the pressure difference between the ends. Equation (12.23) is sometimes applied to the flow of blood in vessels. However, it is, at best, an approximation, because blood vessels are compliant (so r is not constant) and because biological fluids tend to exhibit non-Newtonian viscosity, as explained in the next paragraph.

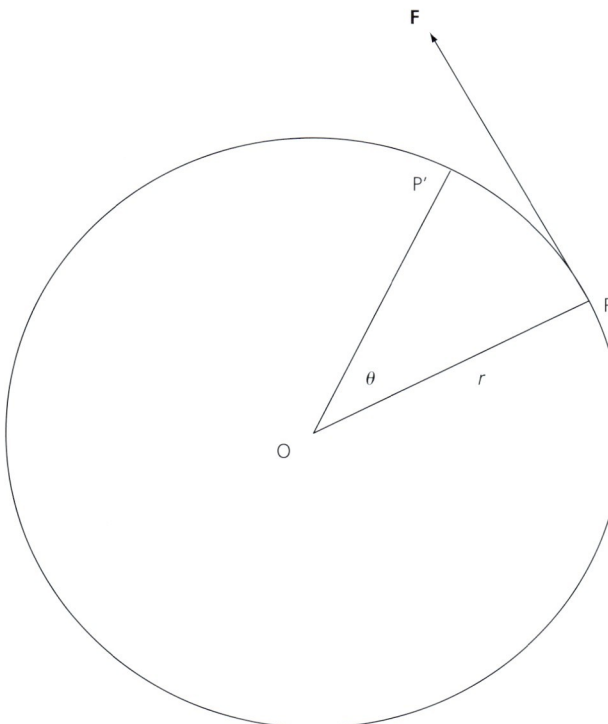

Figure 12.9 Torsion of a circular shaft viewed perpendicular to an end. The tangential force **F**, acts at a point P and so twists it to P'. (The extent of this twist is very much exaggerated in the diagram.) If O is the centre of the end, the lengths OP and OP' are equal to the radius, r, of the shaft. The twisting motion (torsion) is produced by a torque of magnitude rF and can be represented by a torsion angle, θ, between the lines OP and OP'.

For biological fluids and most gels, the value of η depends on the shear stress applied. This behaviour contrasts with that of simple fluids (like water) that are said to be *Newtonian fluids*; more complicated fluids are *non-Newtonian*. The most common non-Newtonian behaviour is *shear thinning* (sometimes called *thixotropy*), in which η decreases with increasing shear stress (this is why you can easily spread non-drip paint with a brush); *shear thickening* is the opposite behaviour.

Viscoelasticity

Most biological tissues are viscoelastic. A *viscoelastic* material is intermediate in properties between an elastic solid (that stores all the energy used to deform it) and a viscous liquid (that dissipates all the energy used to deform it by flow). As a result, viscoelastic materials exhibit the properties of creep, stress relaxation and mechanical hysteresis that will be explained in the following paragraphs.

A viscoelastic material continues to deform when a constant stress is applied to it; this continuing deformation is called *creep*. The creep rate decreases with time, as shown in Fig. 12.10a. It then follows that, if a viscoelastic material is

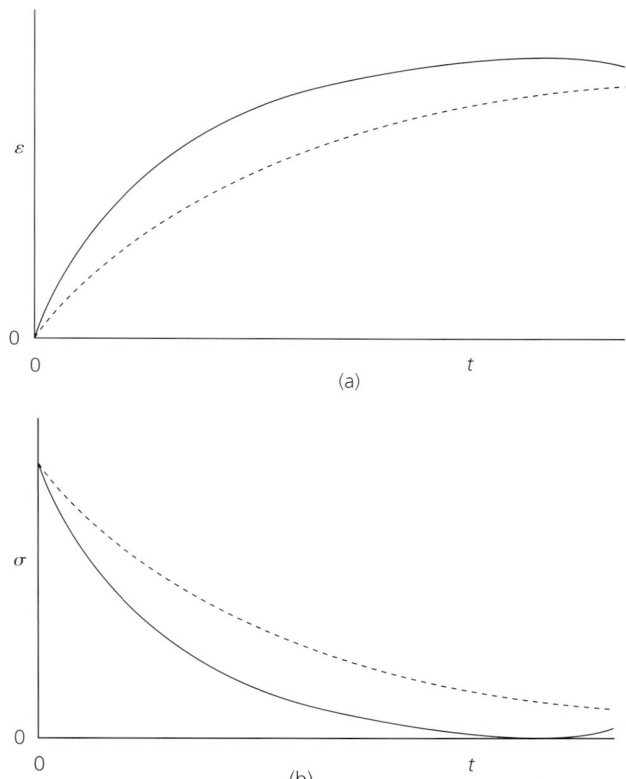

Figure 12.10 Stress, σ, or strain, ε, plotted against time, t, for a viscoelastic material for (a) creep (σ is constant and ε varies) and (b) stress relaxation (ε is constant and σ varies). For single energy dissipation processes, these curves are represented by (a) $\varepsilon = \varepsilon_0 (1 - e^{-t/\tau})$, where ε_0 is the value of ε at infinite time, and (b) $\sigma = \sigma_0 e^{-t/\tau}$, where σ_0 is the value of ε at infinite time; in both equations τ is a relaxation time whose value is η/E'; here, η is the viscosity that appears in equation (12.23) and E' is the storage modulus. In the figure, continuous curves show results for short relaxation times and dashed curves for longer relaxation times. Further details on equations of this kind and their application are given by Holmes and Hukins.[11]

held at a constant strain, the stress will decrease with time; this is called *stress relaxation*. Once again, the stress relaxation rate decreases with time, as shown in Fig. 12.10b. Finally, a viscoelastic material does not follow the same path on a stress–strain graph when it recoils as it did when it was initially loaded, as shown in Fig. 12.11; this effect is called mechanical *hysteresis*. It occurs because the area under the initial loading phase represents the energy (per unit volume) used to deform the material. Some of this energy is dissipated, so not all of it is available for recoil. The energy (per unit volume) used for recoil is the area under the unloading curve, and is less than the energy used to deform the material. Consequently, the area between the two curves is the energy dissipated per unit volume of material.

The behaviour of a viscoelastic material in tension and compression can be represented by two moduli: the storage modulus, E', that represents its elastic response and

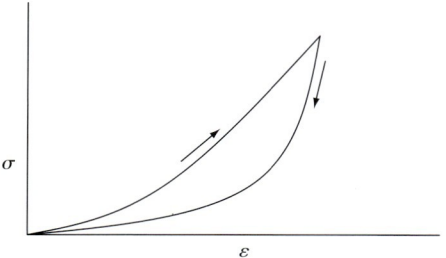

Figure 12.11 Hysteresis in the stress–strain curve of a viscoelastic material showing that it follows a different path during extension (upper curve) and recoil (lower curve). The area enclosed between the two curves represents the energy dissipated per unit volume of material.

the loss modulus, E'', that represents its viscous response; E'' is related to, but is not the same as, viscosity. Similar storage and loss moduli, G' and G'', represent the response to shear. We can still use equation (12.14) to relate stress and strain provided we replace E by E^* where

$$E^* = \sqrt{E'^2 + E''^2}. \qquad (12.24)$$

However, E^* may depend on the loading rate. This rate dependence is often represented by a dependence on loading frequency, f, measured in hertz (abbreviated to Hz) that is simply a reciprocal second or on $\omega = 2\pi f$ (measured in rad s^{-1}).

A further consequence of viscoelasticity is that when a material is deformed cyclically, as shown in Fig. 12.12, the peak stress and peak strain will not occur at the same time. If the time period of a loading cycle is T and Δt represents the time difference between the stress and strain peaks, the *phase difference* is defined by

$$\delta = 2\pi \frac{\Delta t}{T}. \qquad (12.25)$$

The phase difference is related to the storage and loss moduli by

$$\tan \delta = E''/E'. \qquad (12.26)$$

One reason why biological tissues may be viscoelastic is because they contain fluids. Application of a stress to the tissue may induce fluid flow. Since fluids are viscous, this flow dissipates some of the mechanical energy supplied to the tissue. This mechanism for energy dissipation is sometimes called *poroelasticity*. However, it is not usually necessary to distinguish poroelasticity from other viscoelastic mechanisms because the overall effects are the same.

Fracture

If the stress applied to a material is sufficiently high, it will cause damage. The first sign of damage is that the slope of the stress–strain curve decreases; this occurs at a point called the *yield point*, as shown in Fig. 12.13. The exact behaviour after the yield point depends on the nature of the material. Typically the stress–strain curve becomes less steep, and may become parallel, as less stress is required to increase the strain. The strain induced in the material is then irreversible and is described as *plastic deformation*. In fibre-reinforced composite materials, like tendons and ligaments that are reinforced by collagen, this stage may involve fibre debonding from the surrounding material, fibre breakage and fibre pull-out.[12] Ultimately, the material will fracture and so be unable to support applied stress. This occurs when the *ultimate tensile strength* is attained, as shown in Fig. 12.13, i.e. the ultimate tensile strength is the stress at which the material has fractured.

A brittle material fails suddenly, soon after the yield point. The resulting *brittle fracture* is characterized by a clearly defined fracture surface generated across the material (Fig. 12.14a). If there is considerable deformation, after the yield point, before the material fractures, the resulting

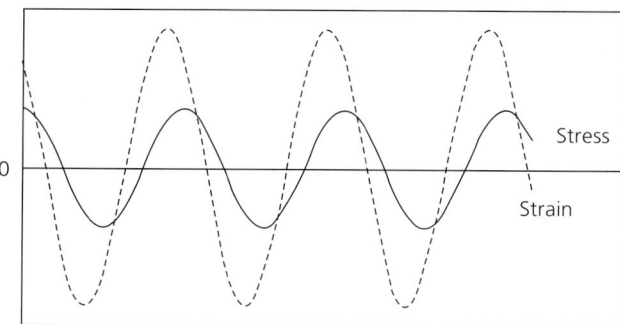

Figure 12.12 When a repetitive stress is applied to a viscoelastic material, there is a time difference between the peak stress and the peak strain. This time difference can be converted into a phase difference (equation (12.25)) that is related to the values of the storage and loss moduli (equation (12.26)).

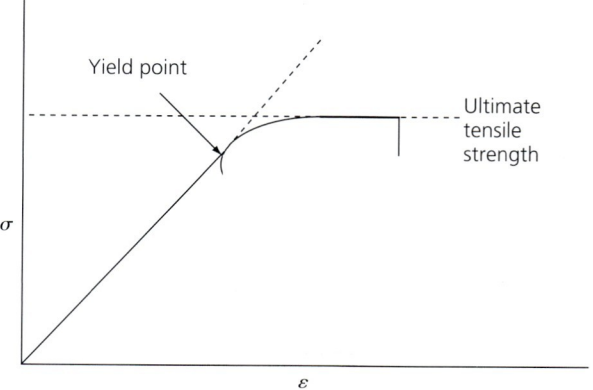

Figure 12.13 Schematic stress–strain curve for a material showing the yield point (where the stiffness of the curve starts to decrease) and the ultimate tensile strength (the stress at which the material fails).

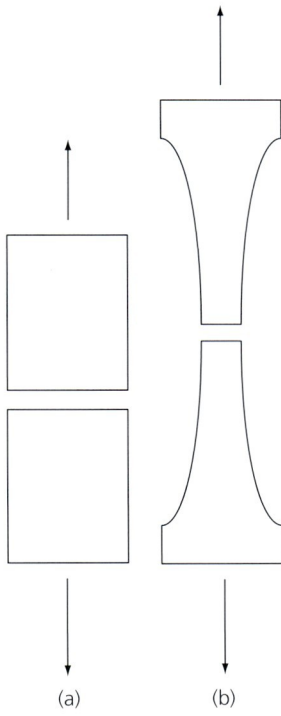

Figure 12.14 Appearance of (a) a brittle fracture and (b) a ductile fracture.

ductile fracture has a characteristic 'drawn-out' appearance (Fig. 12.14b). In some viscoelastic materials, rapid loading can lead to brittle fracture, whereas slower loading leads to ductile fracture. In orthopaedics, the term 'fracture' is usually reserved for fracture of bone; failure of soft tissues, such as ligaments or tendons, is usually referred to as 'rupture' or 'tear'. However, in mechanics, 'fracture' can refer to any material and so these concepts also apply to ligaments and other soft tissues.[13]

It is incorrect to describe osteoporotic bone as more brittle than normal bone. In osteoporosis, bone tissue is lost. As a result, a bone (a structure) contains less bone tissue (a material). As a result, the area of bone tissue within the structure decreases so that the stress produced when a force acts upon the bone increases. When the quantity of bone is so small that the stress produced by everyday forces reaches the ultimate tensile strength of bone, the material will fracture. This has nothing to do with brittle behaviour as described in the previous paragraph.

A *strong material* has a high ultimate tensile strength; a *tough material* does not fail until considerable energy has been supplied to it. Strength alone may not be desirable because the material may be brittle and fracture suddenly. The early steel femoral components of total hip prostheses were made of strong steel that was prone to fracture; replacing it with high-ductile steel provided a tougher material that deformed plastically, bending the prosthesis, if subjected to excessive load, and so avoided fracture. Ideally, tough materials have a high ultimate tensile strength and can continue to withstand applied stress long after the yield point, i.e. they can be supplied with energy after the yield point and before failure. Fibre reinforcing enables a material to withstand stress after the yield point, for the reasons described previously. Viscoelastic materials can be tough because they dissipate some of the energy supplied to them. Thus biological tissues tend to be tough because they are viscoelastic fibre-reinforced materials.

In practice, materials may fail under a variety of loading conditions that can be much more complicated than pulling them apart in simple tension. The *von Mises stress* then enables us to determine whether the material is likely to fail. Details on von Mises stress are beyond the scope of this chapter, but further details can be found in engineering books.[4]

In complicated structures, further damage mechanisms may occur. The failure of fibre-reinforced composite materials has already been described in the first paragraph of this section. Failure of laminated structures may involve separation of their lamellae – *delamination*. Delamination failure of the annulus fibrosus of the intervertebral disc has been observed in post-mortem specimens and attributed to excessive shear stress generated by twisting of the spine.[14]

Biological tissues differ from the synthetic materials used in implants in that they can repair themselves. Toughening mechanisms, which enable the tissue to remain intact after the yield point, are then especially important because they allow integrity of the damaged tissue, and so enable natural repair.

Fatigue

A material can fracture at stress levels much lower than the ultimate tensile strength, if it is subjected to repeated loading. This phenomenon is known as fatigue. Generally, the greater the number of cycles of loading applied to a material, the lower the fracture stress will be. Fatigue is particularly important to consider in synthetic biomaterials used for the manufacture of orthopaedic devices. For example, with a total hip replacement, the device may be subjected to 1 million loading cycles per year.

Friction

Consider a stationary box in contact with a surface (Fig. 12.15). If we then try and move the box from right to left, there will be a resistance to motion owing to the contact between the box and the surface This resistance is known as the friction force, whose magnitude is defined as

$$F = \mu W, \tag{12.27}$$

where μ is the coefficient of friction and W is the resultant force acting perpendicular to the direction of motion,[15] i.e. in Fig. 12.15 it is the weight of the object. Note that in this section, and the next, W denotes the magnitude of a force and not work as in Table 12.4.

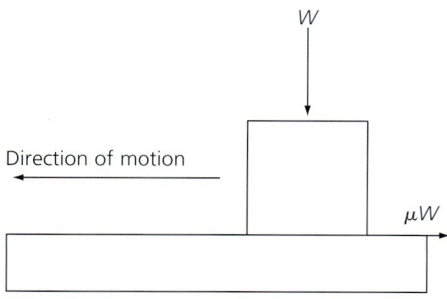

Figure 12.15 Friction of a box in contact with a surface.

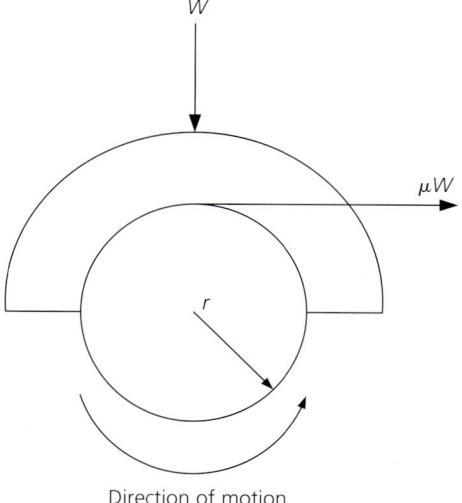

Figure 12.16 Friction of a ball in contact with a socket.

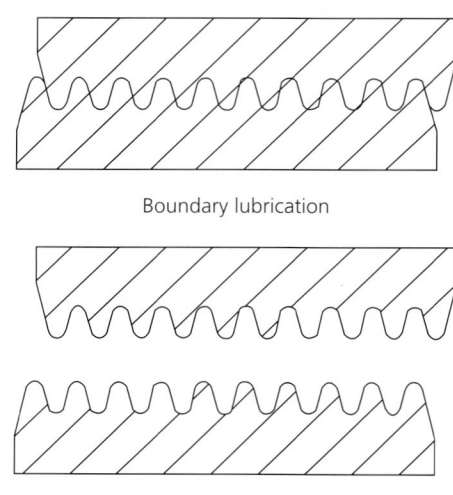

Figure 12.17 Boundary and fluid-film lubrication. On a microscale, a surface is not smooth, but consists of a series of peaks and troughs.

The coefficient of friction varies between different pairs of materials. For example, the coefficient of friction of ice against ice is 0.1, whereas steel against steel is 0.8. The laws of friction state that the friction force is independent of the contact area and also speed.

Let us now consider the situation with a ball-and-socket configuration (Fig. 12.16), in which the ball moves relative to the socket, as in a total hip replacement. The friction force has a magnitude of μW. A frictional torque can be defined as

$$T = \mu W r, \tag{12.28}$$

where r is the radius of the ball.

Wear

Wear is defined as progressive loss of material from a surface (or surfaces) due to the relative motion between them.[15] The volume of wear generated can be defined as

$$V = \frac{k_1 W x}{H}, \tag{12.29}$$

where W is the magnitude of the applied force, x is the sliding distance, H is the hardness of the softer material and k_1 is a dimensionless wear coefficient. Hardness of a material is defined as the resistance to indentation. Many investigators include H within the wear coefficient to create a wear factor, k, with the dimensions of $mm^3\ N\ m^{-1}$. Therefore, the volume of wear generated can be defined as

$$V = kWx. \tag{12.30}$$

Lubrication

The use of a lubricant between two surfaces moving relative to each other is used to reduce friction and wear.[15] Examples of lubricants include oil in a gearbox and synovial fluid in a joint. Fluid-film and boundary are the two main types of lubrication (Fig. 12.17), with the transition zone between them known as mixed lubrication. With fluid-film lubrication there is complete separation of the two surfaces by a thin film of fluid. With boundary lubrication there is contact between the surfaces, and therefore wear will occur. In reality, different lubrication regimes will act at different times. Typically, when something is starting or stopping there will be boundary lubrication until a sufficient velocity has been achieved to generate a film of fluid.

DYNAMICS AND CONTROL

Dynamics

Most accounts of biomechanics cover only statics (the mechanics of objects in equilibrium) and ignore dynamics (the mechanics of objects in motion). This can lead to the mistaken impression that, when we move, we pass through a series of equilibrium states. There are many examples which show that this is not true. When we bend forward quickly, we would fall if we did not stop ourselves. The need to stop ourselves means that dynamics is inseparable from the control of motion.

We initiate movement by contracting our muscles to apply a force to a joint or series of joints. This force can do three things:[16]

1. it can deform the tissues of the body (described by equation (12.11))
2. it can do work that leads simply to energy dissipation (e.g. by fluid flow)
3. it can accelerate part or all of the body (see Table 12.4).

This list gives rise to the three terms on the right-hand side of equation (12.31):

$$\mathbf{F} = k\mathbf{x} + \Omega\mathbf{v} + m\mathbf{a}. \quad (12.31)$$

In this equation, the object moves a distance $\mathbf{x}$ at speed $\mathbf{v}$ with an acceleration $\mathbf{a}$; k is the stiffness of the joint, or joints, being moved (defined in equation (12.11)) and Ω is the measure of the resistance to viscous flow (it bears the same resemblance to η, of equation (12.25), as stiffness bears to Young's modulus). Because we vary $\mathbf{F}$ with time, by constantly changing the muscles we relax and contract, and because $\mathbf{v}$ and $\mathbf{a}$ both depend on time, the solution of equation (12.31) requires mathematics well beyond the scope of this chapter; this is probably why it so widely ignored in biomechanics. Therefore, in this chapter we will simply describe two consequences of equation (12.31).

Because energy dissipation takes time (e.g. fluid flow through the tissues of the body takes a finite time), the response of an object, like the human body, can depend on the rate at which a force is applied. This means that, for some systems, the value of x (the displacement that is the response of the system) depends on the rate at which $\mathbf{F}$ is applied.

A system that does not move when a force is applied to it for a very short duration is called a *shock absorber*. Many authors in biomechanics appear to confuse the ability to act as a shock absorber with the ability to withstand a compressive load.

Neither the intervertebral disc[17] nor the articular cartilage[18] appear to be shock absorbers despite many statements, invariably unsupported by evidence, that they are. Both tissues need to withstand high compressive loads, but there is no evidence that either of them dissipates the energy supplied by short duration application of force.

Control

Once an object is in motion, a force has to be applied to stop it. We are familiar with the need to apply brakes, to generate the force to stop a car, but, in most everyday experiences, the force that stops a moving object is friction, and so we are not always aware that a force is being applied.

A system described by equation (12.32) will eventually come to rest because the second term on its right-hand side means that energy dissipation leads to damping of the motion. This is the reason that bathroom scales settle to a final position after their initial oscillations. Figure 12.18 then shows that there are three possible outcomes when we apply a force to move a system from one position to another:

1. it moves smoothly (critical damping)
2. it never quite manages to reach its intended position (overdamped)
3. it oscillates about its final position before gradually settling (underdamped).

The type of damping that occurs depends on k, Ω and m, as described in the caption to Fig. 12.18. Ideally, we expect to move our bodies smoothly to adopt new postures (case 1), but the other two types of motion are characteristic of some musculoskeletal and neurological disorders.[16]

The motion of the body is more complicated because it can be controlled by antagonistic muscles. This *active damping* leads to more rapid control than the *passive damping* that relies on processes such as fluid flow. The time-scale for nerve conduction that leads to muscle contraction is measured in milliseconds, but the shortest relaxation time (see legend to Fig. 12.10) associated with viscoelasticity of the intervertebral disc is about 16 minutes.[11] The effect of using antagonistic muscles is to rapidly increase the value of Ω in equation (12.31), under the control of the nervous system.

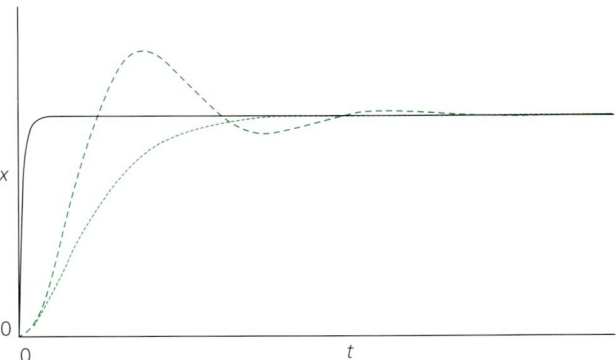

Figure 12.18 Displacement, x, of a system, plotted against time, t, when changing its position when critically (solid line), over (dotted line) and under (dashed line) damped. The type of damping depends on the value of a damping factor $f = \sqrt{\Omega^2/(4km)}$, where the symbols on the right-hand side of the equation are the coefficients of equation (12.31). When $f = 1$ the system is critically damped; when f is greater than 1 the system is overdamped; and when f is less than 1 the system is underdamped.

BIOMECHANICS OF JOINTS

Hip

The hip joint is the articulation between the femoral head and the acetabulum. The hip joint provides a large range of motion with typical values of 120° flexion, 20° extension and 45° of abduction and adduction.[19] Forces acting on the hip joint are large during walking. Figure 12.19 shows a free body diagram of the hip joint when a person is standing on one leg. During walking, you stand on one leg for a short period of time. The forces acting are body weight minus the weight of one leg, **F**, the force exerted by the abductor muscles, **f**, and a joint reaction force between the femoral head and the acetabulum, **R**. To have equilibrium, all the forces and moments must balance. In this example, we will consider the forces in scalar form.

If we take moments (force multiplied by a distance) about O we have

$$FD - fd = 0, \quad (12.32)$$

$$\therefore f = \frac{FD}{d}. \quad (12.33)$$

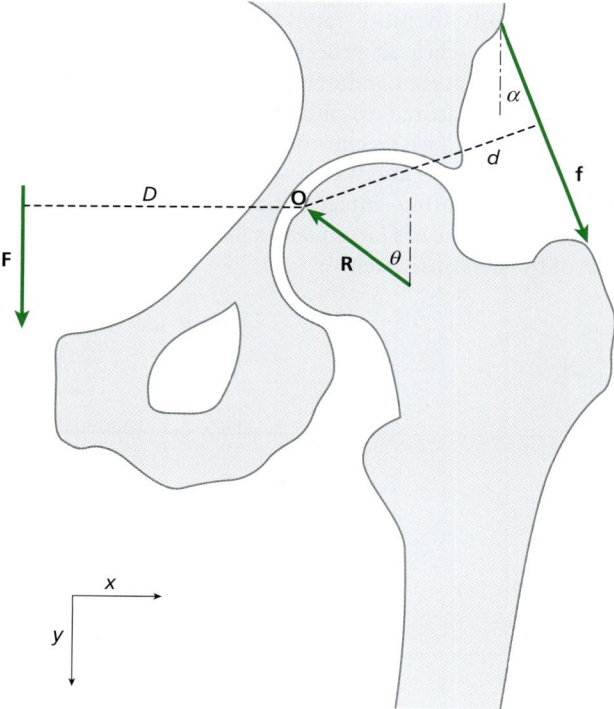

Figure 12.19 Free body diagram of the hip joint. **F** is the body weight minus the weight of one leg, **f** is the force exerted by the abductor muscles, **R** is the force acting on the hip joint, **D** is the distance from the origin O to **F**, **d** is the distance from O to **f**, and θ and α are angles of **R** and **f** from the vertical. Note that in this example it is necessary to resolve the **R** and **f** into their vertical ($R\cos\theta$ and $f\cos\alpha$) and horizontal ($R\cos\theta$ and $f\cos\alpha$) components.

The resultant force in the y-direction must be zero so we have

$$F - R\cos\theta + f\cos\alpha = 0, \quad (12.34)$$

$$\therefore R\cos\theta = F + f\cos\alpha. \quad (12.35)$$

The resultant force in the x-direction must be zero so we have

$$R\sin\theta - f\sin\alpha = 0, \quad (12.36)$$

$$\therefore R\sin\theta = f\sin\alpha. \quad (12.37)$$

Now $\tan\theta = \dfrac{\sin\theta}{\cos\theta}$, so dividing equation (12.37) by equation (12.35) we obtain

$$\tan\theta = \frac{f\sin\alpha}{F + f\cos\alpha}. \quad (12.38)$$

Some of the values are known based on anatomical measurements, so we can assume that $D = 0.09$ m, $d = 0.05$ m and $\alpha = 15°$. Let us calculate the magnitude of the hip joint force, R, for a person with $F = 600$ N (we will assume they have a body weight of 750 N and that one leg is 20% of body weight).

Putting the values into equation (12.33), we obtain $f = 1080$ N. From equation (12.38) we obtain $\theta = 10°$. Now from equation (12.37) we obtain $R = 1610$ N. So you can see that during walking the force acting on the hip joint is over two times body weight. This simple example has been confirmed where the actual force *in vivo* has been measured using an instrumented total hip implant.[20]

Ankle

The ankle joint is the articulation between the distal ends of the tibia and fibula and the talus. The ankle is capable of dorsiflexion, plantarflexion, eversion and inversion. During the walking cycle, the range of motion of the ankle is typically 12° dorsiflexion and 15° plantarflexion.[21] The resultant force acting on the ankle joint during walking has been found to be three to five times body weight. For a person of mass 70 kg, the maximum force in the ankle would be in the range 2060–3434 N.[21]

Knee

The knee joint comprises the distal femur, proximal tibia and patellar. The articulations of the knee joint are tibiofemoral and patellofemoral. To move, the human body requires large flexions of the knee. For walking, 70° of flexion is required, while flexions of up to 120° may be required when rising from a chair.[19]

There is some confusion in the literature concerning the kinematics of the tibiofemoral joint.[22] The joint surfaces, together with the cruciate ligaments, are sometimes considered as a rigid 'four-bar linkage'. However, this is incorrect because the ligaments are stiff only in tension. Flexion of the tibiofemoral joint involves translation ('femoral roll-back') as well as flexion. Attempts have been made to quantify this translation by calculating how the instantaneous centre of rotation of the knee shifts during flexion. These attempts have not provided quantifiable results because the calculation is mathematically inherently unreliable.

Tibiofemoral forces are around three times body weight for walking, but can be up to four times body weight when walking down stairs. The patellofemoral forces are lower than the tibiofemoral forces, with walking around 0.6 times body weight and walking down stairs three times body weight.[19]

Shoulder

The shoulder joint is considered to be the articulation between the glenoid and humerus, although other joints in the shoulder (scapulothoracic, acromioclavicular and sternoclavicular) help with the global motion of the shoulder. The main motions in the shoulder joint are 180° of flexion and abduction and 45° of extension.[23] An instrumented shoulder implant has been used to measure the contact forces between the glenoid and humerus, with force of up to 1.5 times body weight measured.[24]

Fingers

The metacarpophalangeal (MCP) joint is the most common finger joint replaced with a joint replacement implant, and the biomechanics of this joint will be discussed here.

The MCP joint consists of the articulation between the metacarpal head and the proximal phalanx. The primary motion of the joint is flexion extension, with a healthy joint capable of 90° of flexion and 20–30° of extension.[25] The MCP joint is also capable of abduction and adduction as well as a small amount of rotation about its longitudinal axis. During most activities of daily living, the full range of motion of the MCP joint is not used. The resultant force acting on the MCP joint has been estimated in many studies, with typical values for a static pinch grip being 490 N for males and 350 N for females.[25]

Wrist

The main movements of the wrist are flexion/extension, radial/ulnar deviation, although small degrees of rotation take place between the carpal bones and the radius. Typical values of movement for a healthy wrist joint are 76° for flexion, 75° for extension, 22° for radial deviation, 36° for ulnar deviation and 2–12° of rotation.[26] The resultant force acting through the wrist joint is typically in the range 118–143 N.[26]

Spine

The structure of the spine allows a large range of motion, but the motion at adjacent vertebral bodies is relatively small. For example, in the lumbar spine typical values of motion between two adjacent vertebrae would be flexion 8°, extension 6°, lateral bending 6° and torsion 3°.[27] The compressive forces in the spine arise from the posterior muscles producing a counterbalance moment to the weight of the body above the level of the spine being considered. Figure 12.20 shows a simple free body diagram of the spine. The forces acting are the weight of the body above the level of the spine being considered, **F**, the posterior

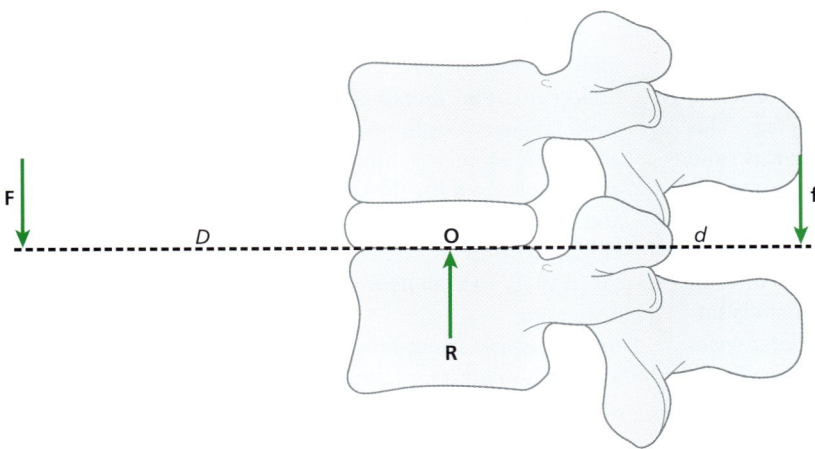

Figure 12.20 Free body diagram of the spine. **F** is the weight of the body above the section of spine being considered, **f** is the force exerted by posterior muscles, **R** is the force acting between two vertebrae, *D* is the distance from the origin O to **F** and *d* is the distance from O to **f**.

muscle force, **f**, and a compressive force acting through the vertebral bodies, **R**. To have equilibrium all the forces and moments must balance. Scalar form will be used in this example.

If we take moments (force multiplied by a distance) about O we have

$$FD - fd = 0, \quad (12.39)$$

$$\therefore f = \frac{FD}{d}. \quad (12.40)$$

The resultant force in the vertical direction must be zero so we have

$$F - R + f = 0, \quad (12.41)$$

$$\therefore R = F + f. \quad (12.42)$$

Some of the values are known based on anatomical measurements, so we can assume that $D = 0.08$ m and $d = 0.05$ m. Let us calculate the magnitude of the force through the vertebral bodies, R, for a person with $F = 450$ N (we will assume they have a body weight of 750 N and that upper body is 60% of body weight). Putting the values into equation (12.40), we obtain $f = 720$ N. Now from equation (12.42) we obtain $R = 1170$ N. So you can see that, during walking, the force acting between vertebral bodies is over 1.5 times body weight. The compressive force acting during walking can fluctuate between 1.5 and three times body weight. Higher forces can be generated during activities such as lifting an object with the arms outstretched as the distance D will increase resulting in a larger moment to be resisted.[28]

In reality, simple calculations such as these do not yield reliable numbers because the spine is a flexible structure.[29] However, they do enable us to understand, qualitatively, why compressive forces are generated in the spine.

BIOMATERIALS

Natural tissues

It is extremely important to have a good understanding of the mechanical properties of natural tissues in order to understand how they function and why they fail. This information enables the design of medical devices, and their fixation, to be improved and synthetic biomaterials that closely match the mechanical properties of natural tissues to be developed. Natural tissues consist of an extracellular matrix, cells and a large volume of water. As a result their behaviour is viscoelastic. However, if movement is sufficiently slow that it can be considered to consist of a series of equilibrium positions (so-called 'quasistatic' behaviour), their properties can be considered as being elastic, enabling them to be described by single values for the

Table 12.8 Values of Young's modulus for various natural tissues

Tissue	Young's modulus	Reference
Cortical bone	6–24.5 GPa	Jutley et al.[30]
Cancellous bone	0.04–2.2 GPa	Jutley et al.[30]
Articular cartilage	4.5–18.6 MPa	Shepherd and Seedhom[31]
Annulus fibrosus	0.1–1000 MPa	Meakin and Hukins[32]
Nucleus pulposus	1 MPa	Johannessen and Elliott[33]
	1098–2114 MPa (bulk modulus)	Yang and Kish[34]

parameters listed in Table 12.8. It is important to note that the mechanical properties of natural tissues are then wide ranging. These differences arise from differences in experimental technique, such as the rate of loading and the size and geometry of specimens. However, differences in mechanical properties of natural tissues also arise between individuals and different joints or different areas within the same individual. For example, with articular cartilage it has been observed that there are topographical variations in Young's modulus over the surfaces of human joints as well as differences between joints.[31,35,36]

Synthetic biomaterials

All materials for use in the human body share a number of characteristics in that they are required to be biocompatible,[37] i.e. the materials must not cause an adverse effect on the body (e.g. non-toxic) and the body should not cause an adverse effect on the material (e.g. no corrosion or degradation by body fluids). The choice of materials for use in the manufacture of orthopaedic medical devices is wide ranging, including metals, polymers, ceramics and elastomers. Table 12.9 shows these materials and their typical mechanical properties. The choice of materials for a device depends on the requirements and performance that the device must meet.

Metals have high strength to prevent fracture and a high enough Young's modulus to prevent appreciable deflection. The metals chosen for implants should have good fatigue strength to be able to survive the cyclic loading encountered in the human body. Metals are, therefore, commonly used for the stems of implants and fracture fixation devices. Stainless steel (commonly Ortron 90 or 316L), cobalt–chrome–molybdenum alloy and titanium alloy (Ti–6Al–4V) are all used in the manufacture of orthopaedic devices.[41]

Metals are also commonly used as one of the bearing materials in joint replacement implants, with stainless steel and cobalt–chrome–molybdenum alloys being commonly used. A titanium alloy with aluminium and vanadium

Table 12.9 Typical mechanical properties of synthetic materials used for orthopaedic devices

Material	Young's modulus (GPa)	Ultimate tensile strength (MPa)
Metals		
Stainless steel	193	1100
Cobalt–chrome–molybdenum alloy	200	655
Titanium alloy	114	860
Aluminium*	70	310
Polymers		
Ultra-high-molecular-weight polyethylene	0.5	30
Polyetheretherketone	3.6	93
Bone cement	3	75
Hydrogels[†]	1×10^{-3}	0.3
Polyglycolide[‡]	8.4	890
Ceramics		
Alumina	380	400
Zirconia	180	600
Elastomers		
Silicone	0.03	7

All values from Brown[38] unless otherwise indicated.
*Gere and Timoshenko.[3]
[†]Jones et al.[39]
[‡]Chu.[40]

(Ti–6Al–4V) has poor wear characteristics on its own as a bearing material. However, if nitrogen is incorporated in the surface of the alloy, it will become a highly wear-resistant bearing surface.[41]

The ceramics alumina and zirconia have been used as bearing surfaces in hip joint replacement implants, as they have excellent wear resistance. However, ceramics have a much lower fracture toughness than metals, and this did lead to some brittle fractures in the bearing surfaces in the early days of their use. Improved manufacturing processes for ceramics have generally prevented this problem, leading to an increase in their use.[41]

The polymer ultra-high-molecular-weight polyethylene (UHMWPE) is most commonly used as one of the bearing surfaces in joint replacement implants.[42] It has low friction when articulated against a metal or ceramic. A newer variation of the material is highly cross-linked polyethylene, where radiation is used to increase the cross-links in the polymer. This material has lower wear rates in joint replacement implants than UHMWPE, although there has been some concern about reduced mechanical properties.[43]

The replacement of joints of the hand and wrist has typically involved the use of implants manufactured from elastomers, normally silicone.[44] Silicone (sometimes known under trade names such as Silastic or Flexspan) has excellent fatigue properties over a wide range of strains. However, silicone has been shown to have poor crack growth resistance once a crack has been initiated in the material. At present, the use of such implants has been criticized, and it is not as common as it was only a decade ago.

JOINT REPLACEMENT OF SYNOVIAL JOINTS

Introduction

Joint replacement is a common method for treating diseased synovial joints with the intention of relieving pain and restoring function. Large joints, such as the hip and knee, are replaced by an implant that has articulating bearing surfaces. The main design and material requirements are low friction between the bearing surfaces, low wear of the materials, low contact stresses and good fixation with the host bone. Joint replacement of the finger joints and the wrist is different from the large weight-bearing joints as the forces are smaller. This section will discuss the materials used in the manufacture of various joint replacement implants for synovial joints.

Hip

The conventional design of a hip joint replacement consists of a femoral component, with a stem and femoral head, and an acetabular component. Some designs are modular, and so different femoral heads can be fitted to a stem. Other designs consist of a one-piece combined stem and head (Fig. 12.21). The stems of hip implants are generally made from implantable grade stainless steel, cobalt–chrome–molybdenum alloy or a titanium alloy. The materials used for the manufacture of various stems are shown in Table 12.10.

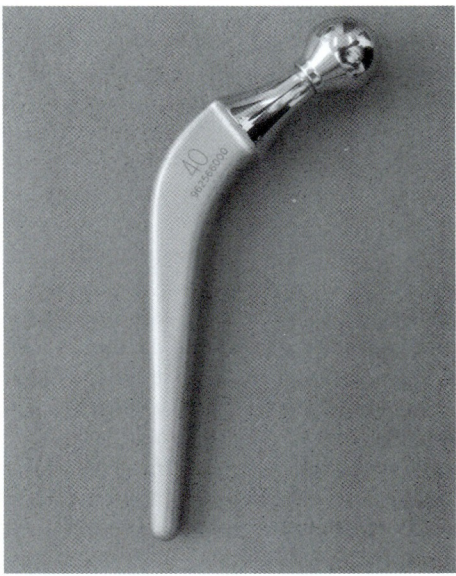

Figure 12.21 Charnley modular hip (DePuy, Leeds, UK).

Table 12.10 Materials used for various stems

Implant	Company	Femoral Stem material
Lubinus SP II	Waldemar Link (Hamburg, Germany)	Cobalt–chrome–molybdenum alloy
Spectron EF	Smith & Nephew (Memphis, TN, USA)	Cobalt–chrome–molybdenum alloy
Charnley	DePuy (Leeds, UK)	Stainless steel (Ortron 90)
Exeter	Stryker (NJ, USA)	Stainless steel (Orthinox)
Bi-Metric	Biomet (Swindon, UK)	Titanium alloy

Table 12.11 Materials used for various heads

Implant	Company	Femoral head bearing material
Lubinus SP II	Waldemar Link (Hamburg, Germany)	Cobalt–chrome–molybdenum alloy
Femoral heads	Smith & Nephew (Memphis, TN, USA)	Alumina, cobalt–chrome–molybdenum alloy, Oxinium, zirconia
Charnley	DePuy (Leeds, UK)	Stainless steel (Ortron 90)
Exeter	Stryker (Mahwah, NJ, USA)	Stainless steel (Orthinox)

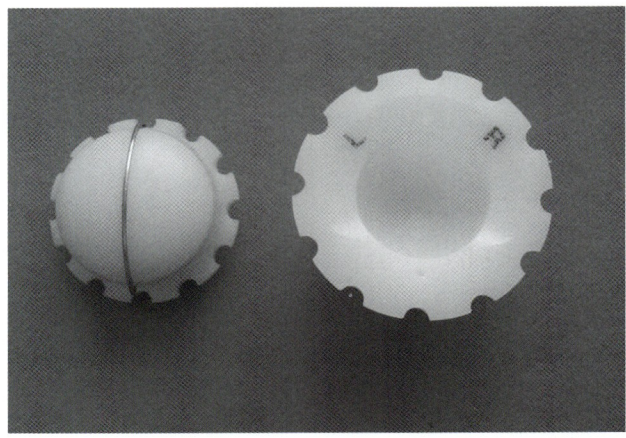

Figure 12.22 Ultra-high-molecular-weight polyethylene acetabular cups.

Table 12.12 Materials used for various acetabular cups

Implant	Company	Acetabular cup bearing material
Lubinus	Waldemar Link (Hamburg, Germany)	Ultra-high-molecular-weight polyethylene
Lineage	Wright Medical Technology (Arlington, TN, USA)	Alumina, cobalt–chrome–molybdenum alloy or ultra-high-molecular-weight polyethylene
Charnley	DePuy (Leeds, UK)	Ultra-high-molecular-weight polyethylene
Ceracup	Biomet (Swindon, UK)	Alumina

For the femoral head, metals are also conventionally used, with the head made from either implantable grade stainless steel or cobalt–chrome–molybdenum alloy. An alternative material to the use of metals for the femoral head is to use ceramics, such as alumina or zirconia. Smith and Nephew have produced a material known as Oxinium, a metal with a ceramic surface, that should have extremely high wear resistance.[45] The materials for various femoral heads are shown in Table 12.11. Depending on the design the diameter of the femoral head is typically between 22 mm (Charnley hip, DePuy, Leeds, UK) and 32 mm (Muller hip, Biomet, Dordrecht, The Netherlands). There is a design trade-off for the dimensions of the femoral head. From equation (12.12) it can been seen that a larger radius will lead to a larger contact area and therefore a lower stress. However, from equation (12.28) it can be seen that an increase in the radius of the femoral head will lead to higher friction torque.

The acetabular component of a hip replacement can be either a one- or two-piece design. The one-piece designs attach directly to the acetabular bone and are generally manufactured from UHMWPE, as shown in Fig. 12.22. With this type of design a metal wire is attached to the polymer to enable it to be seen on plain radiographs. Other one-piece designs of the acetabular component are made from cobalt–chrome–molybdenum alloy. Two-piece designs of the acetabular component consist of a metal shell that attaches to the acetabular bone, and an insert that fixes into the shell and acts as the bearing surface. The inserts are manufactured from UHMWPE or a ceramic. Table 12.12 shows some of the materials used for various acetabular cups. Another form of polyethylene that is now being used is highly cross-linked polyethylene; early clinical results show that the wear rates are far reduced compared with UHMWPE.[43]

The range of bearing material combinations available for traditional hip replacement implants are: metal against polymer, metal against metal, ceramic against polymer and ceramic against ceramic. An alternative to the traditional design of hip replacement implants is hip resurfacing (Fig. 12.23), which is for use in young or active patients. This implant design has a large radius femoral head, and the traditional femoral stem has been replaced with a short peg. Hip-resurfacing implants involve a cobalt–chrome–molybdenum alloy against cobalt–chrome–molybdenum

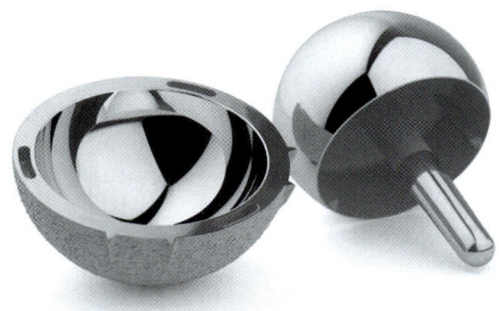

Figure 12.23 Cormet hip resurfacing. Reproduced with kind permission from Corin, Cirencester, UK. © Corin.

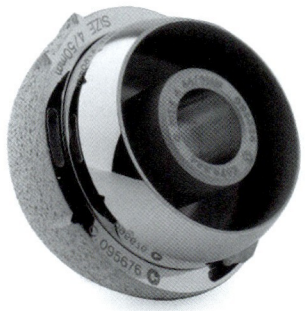

Figure 12.24 Optimom large diameter metal-on-metal Total Hip Replacement System. Reproduced with kind permission from Corin, Cirencester, UK. © Corin.

Table 12.13 Hip resurfacing implants

Implant	Company
Adept	Finsbury Orthopaedics (Leatherhead, UK)
ASR	DePuy (Leeds, UK)
Birmingham hip	Smith & Nephew (Memphis, TN, USA)
Conserve	Wright Medical Technology, (Arlington, TN, USA)
Cormet	Corin (Cirencester, UK)
Durom	Zimmer (Warsaw, IN, USA)
ReCap	Biomet (Swindon, UK)

alloy articulation. Normally, a bearing surface consisting of two identical metals leads to high friction. However, this alloy can be polished to give a very smooth surface that leads to low friction. Table 12.13 shows various hip-resurfacing implants available. Large diameter femoral heads are also available for attachment to conventional femoral stems when a patient might not be suitable for a peg (Fig. 12.24).

Knee

The material combinations of the bearing surfaces of total knee replacement devices are not as wide as those used for hip implants. The design of total knee replacement devices consists of femoral and tibial components; and in some designs a patellar component may also be included. Designs vary depending on whether the cruciate ligaments are preserved or sacrificed. The femoral component is a one-piece design, and is generally made from cobalt–chrome–molybdenum alloy. Alternative materials for the femoral component include Oxinium or a titanium alloy whose surface has been treated with nitrogen. The tibial component is generally a two-piece design comprising a tibial tray and an insert. The insert is made from UHMWPE (although one-piece tibial components, made from UHMWPE, are available for some designs). With fixed bearing designs (Fig. 12.25) of knee replacement implants,

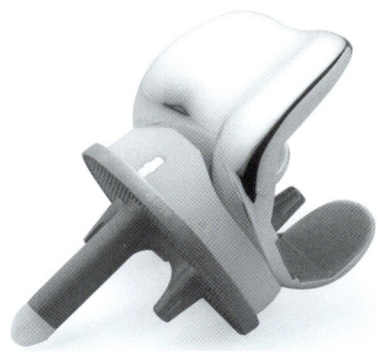

Figure 12.25 Rotaglide+ fixed bearing Total Knee System. Reproduced with kind permission from Corin, Cirencester, UK. © Corin.

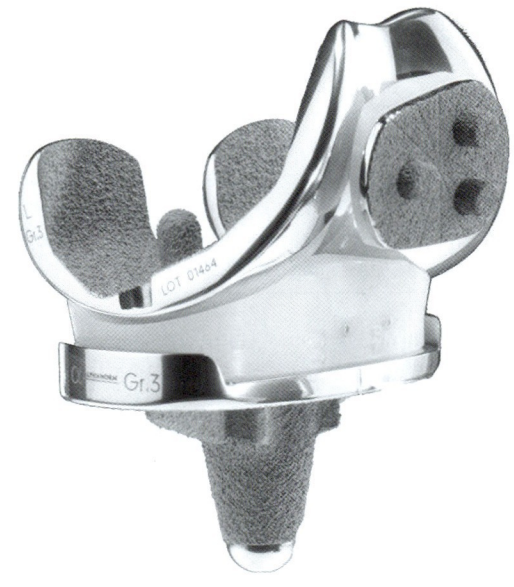

Figure 12.26 AMC Mobile Knee System. Reproduced with kind permission from Corin, Cirencester, UK. © Corin.

the insert is attached to the tray. With mobile bearing designs (Fig. 12.26) the insert is free to move relative to the tray. The trays for the fixed bearing designs are generally made from titanium alloy, whereas the mobile bearings trays are made from cobalt–chrome–molybdenum alloy since there is movement between the tray and the insert, and titanium alloy has been shown to have poor wear characteristics. Patellar components have an UHMWPE bearing surface. Table 12.14 shows some commonly available knee replacement implants.

In the knee joint where the damage to the joint surface is confined to either the medial or lateral side, a unicondylar (or unicompartmental) implant can be used as an alternative to the use of a total knee replacement implant. The material combinations used are the same as for the total knee system, with fixed and mobile bearings designs available.[46]

Other large synovial joint replacement implants

Materials used in the manufacture of joint replacement implants for the ankle, elbow and shoulder are generally based on the experience gained from hip and knee arthroplasty devices. All implants involve either a cobalt–chrome–molybdenum alloy or stainless steel bearing articulating against UHMWPE. Some commonly used implants for the ankle, elbow and shoulder are shown in Table 12.15.

Ankle joint replacement implants (Fig. 12.27) generally consist of three parts: a metal tibial part, a metal talar part and a polymer insert. Early designs had a fixed bearing design where the polymer insert was rigidly attached to the tibial part. Newer designs now have mobile bearings, where the polymer part is free to articulate against the metal parts attached to the tibia and talus.[21,47,48] Elbow implants have had three main designs: hinged, semiconstrained and unconstrained.[49] Shoulder joint replacement (Fig. 12.28) has generally comprised a metal humeral component articulating against an UHMWPE glenoid component.[50]

Joint replacement of the joints of the hand and wrist

For the finger joints the most common joint replacement implant is a single-piece silicone joint,[51] shown in Fig. 12.29. The Swanson finger implant (Wright Medical Technology, Arlington, TN, USA) has been in use since the 1960s, and consists of two stems joined to a central barrel. The Swanson implants suffer from fractures

Table 12.14 Materials used for various knee replacement implants

Implant	Company	Tibial tray bearing material	Tibial insert	Femoral bearing material
PFC Sigma	DePuy (Leeds, UK)	Titanium alloy	Ultra-high-molecular-weight polyethylene	Cobalt–chrome–molybdenum alloy
PFC Sigma RP	DePuy (Leeds, UK)	Cobalt–chrome–molybdenum alloy	Ultra-high-molecular-weight polyethylene	Cobalt–chrome–molybdenum alloy
AGC	Biomet (Swindon, UK)	Titanium alloy	Ultra-high-molecular-weight polyethylene	Cobalt–chrome–molybdenum alloy
Rotaglide+ Mobile/Fixed	Corin (Cirencester, UK)	Cobalt–chrome–molybdenum alloy	Ultra-high-molecular-weight polyethylene	Cobalt–chrome–molybdenum alloy
AMC mobile	Corin (Cirencester, UK)	Titanium nitride	Ultra-high-molecular-weight polyethylene	Titanium nitride
Genesis 2	Smith & Nephew (Memphis, TN, USA)	Titanium alloy	Ultra-high-molecular-weight polyethylene	Cobalt–chrome–molybdenum alloy or Oxinium

Table 12.15 Examples of ankle, elbow and shoulder joint replacement implants

Implant type	Implant name	Company
Ankle	Box	Finsbury Orthopaedics, (Leatherhead, Surrey, UK)
Ankle	Agility	DePuy (Leeds, UK)
Ankle	Hintegra	Newdeal (Lyon, France)
Elbow	Coonrad/Morrey	Zimmer (Warsaw, IN, USA)
Elbow	Souter/Strathclyde	Stryker (NJ, USA)
Elbow	Kudo	Biomet (Swindon, UK)
Shoulder	Cofield 2	Smith & Nephew (Memphis, TN, USA)
Shoulder	Oxford	Corin (Cirencester, UK)
Shoulder	Global Advantage	DePuy (Leeds, UK)

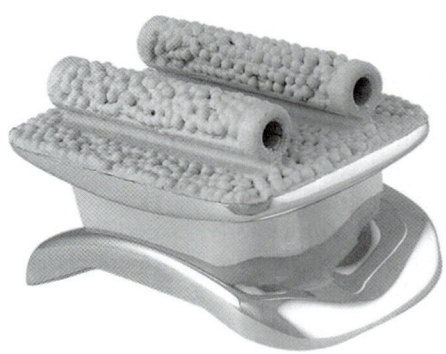

Figure 12.27 Box Total Ankle Replacement. Reproduced with kind permission from Finsbury Orthopaedics, Leatherhead, Surrey, UK. © Finsbury Orthopaedics.

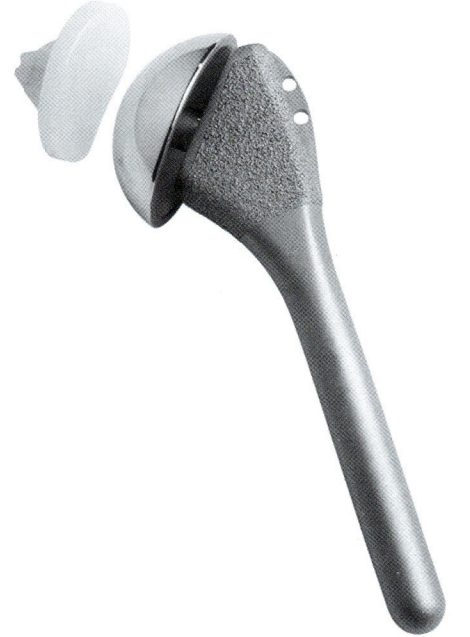

Figure 12.28 Oxford shoulder replacement. Reproduced with kind permission from Corin, Cirencester, UK. © Corin.

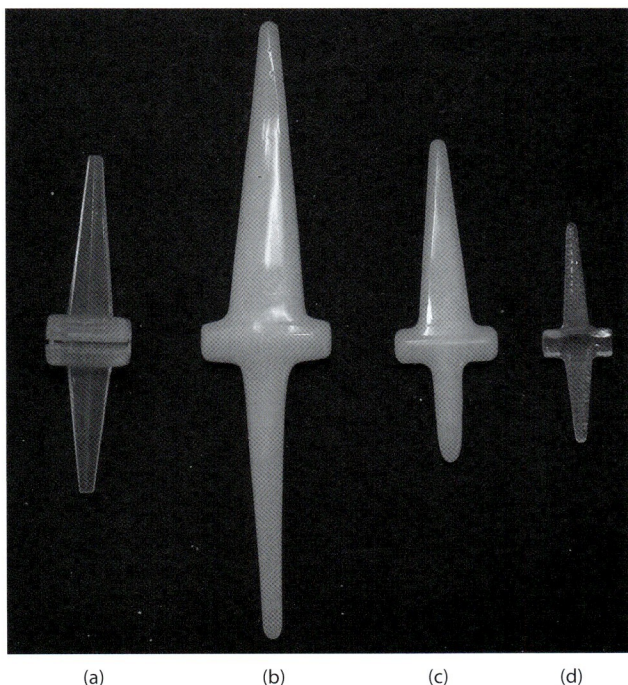

Figure 12.29 Various single-piece finger and wrist implants. (a) Avanta finger; (b) Swanson wrist (large); (c) Swanson wrist (small); (d) Swanson finger.

not fixed in position, but pistons in and out of the bone during finger movement. Titanium grommets were introduced for use with the Swanson implant to shield the implant from the bones edges; however, fractures have still been observed. The Sutter implant, now known as the Avanta Soft Skeletal Implant (Avanta Orthopaedics, San Diego, California, USA), is a similar design to the Swanson, but the problems of fracture have also been seen clinically.

Newer designs of single-piece silicone implants that have been designed for the finger joint have the neutral position of the implant with one stem at an angle of 30° to the other.[51] The idea with this type of design is that the natural resting position of the hand has the MCP joint at about 30°. If the implant is straight, as with the Swanson, the neutral position of the hand at 30° will induce a higher strain in the material These newer designs include the Preflex (Avanta Orthopaedics) and Neuflex (DePuy).

As an alternative to the use of single-piece silicone finger implants, some manufacturers have designs that have articulating bearing surfaces. For the MCP joint, these designs comprise metacarpal and phalangeal parts that form a ball-and-socket joint. Examples of articulating bearing surface implants include the Total Metacarpophalangeal Replacement (TMPR; Finsbury Orthopaedics, Leatherhead, Surrey, UK), which has a cobalt–chrome–molybdenum alloy against UHMWPE articulation, and the SR (Small Bone Innovations, Morrisville, PA, USA). The TMPR design (Fig. 12.30) has a mechanical fixation with a series of UHMWPE fins that wedge against the inside of the bone. Other designs of articulating finger joint replacements include the Pyrocarbon Total Joint (Ascension Orthopaedics, Austin, TX, USA) which has an articulation of pyrocarbon against itself.

Joint replacement of the wrist is not common because of the high failure rates of wrist implants. A single-piece

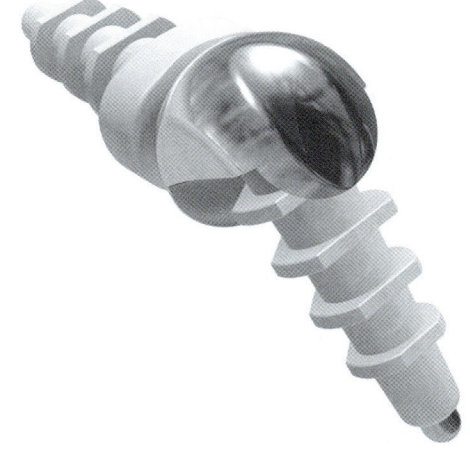

Figure 12.30 Total Metacarpophalangeal Replacement, TMPR. Reproduced with kind permission from Finsbury Orthopaedics, Leatherhead, Surrey, UK. © Finsbury Orthopaedics.

occurring at the junction between the distal stem and the barrel. It is believed that a crack is initiated from contact with the sharp bone edges or from abrasion against the bone during finger movement. The Swanson implant is silicone Swanson implant is available for the wrist (Fig. 12.29), with the design along similar lines to the Swanson finger implant, with stems joined to a central barrel. Titanium grommets are also available to shield the silicone from the edges of the bone. The Swanson wrist implant also suffers from the same problems as the Swanson finger implant, with fractures occurring at the junction between the barrel and the distal stem. Fracture rates of up to 65% have been reported at follow-up studies of 6 years.[26,52]

Articulating surface implants are also available for wrist replacement implants (Fig. 12.31). Designs generally involve a cobalt–chrome–molybdenum alloy against UHMWPE bearing surfaces. Articulating surface designs include the Biaxial (DePuy), Universal 2 (Integra, Plainsboro, NJ, USA) and Re-motion (Small Bone Innovations).[26]

Fixation

The secure fixation of joint replacement implants within the host bone is essential. The methods of fixation are: bone cement, bone in-growth and mechanical. Polymethylmethacrylate (PMMA) has been successfully used as bone cement for the fixation of implant stems within the host bone for over 40 years. The cement is made by mixing together PMMA powder, liquid methylmethacrylate, benzoyl peroxide (which acts as an accelerator) and barium sulphate (radiopaque additive so the cement can be seen on plain radiographs). Mixing these components together causes an exothermic reaction. The cement can then be manually applied or, preferably, injected into the bone cavity.[53] It is important that pressure is applied to the cement so that it can be forced into the interstices of the bone: this will increase the strength at the cement/bone interface. In some cases, such as the acetabular component of a hip replacement, holes may be drilled into the bone so that cement can enter deeper. Implant stems are generally tapered, so that, as the stem is pushed into the bone cement, it will cause pressurization of the cement. After the implant is in place, the cement will harden in around 10 minutes. The cement is not an adhesive, but acts as a filler between the bone and the implant stem, and therefore relies on mechanical interlock. The main advantage of using bone cement is that, after it has hardened, there is immediate fixation of the implant within the bone. Disadvantages can include bone necrosis from the exothermic reaction, blood contamination of the cement, and fatigue failure of the cement.[54]

Fixation can also be achieved through bone in-growth with the use of a roughened or porous surface on the implant, into which bone will grow. Bone in-growth techniques do require good bone stock to be present, and the ultimate fixation is not immediate, as time is required for the bone to grow into the porous coating. There are a variety of techniques for producing a porous surface such as sintered titanium alloy beads or the use of hydroxyapatite.[55,56]

Mechanical fixation includes the use of an interference fit and screws. An interference, or press, fit involves a component being pushed into the bone, where the size of the implant is slightly larger than the hole in the bone. This can be used for hip and knee joint replacement implants, but generally there is a roughened or porous surface for bone in-growth as well. Some implants rely completely on mechanical fixation. The TMPR (Finsbury Orthopaedics) has a series of UHMWPE fins that wedge against the inside of the bone. Screw fixation has been used in the Hintegra total ankle prosthesis (Newdeal, Lyon, France) to augment the porous coat fixation.

Tribology of joint replacement implants

Tribology is the study of friction, lubrication and wear. The tribological performance of joint replacement implants with articulating bearing surfaces is essential to their long-term survival. Joint replacement implants with metal against polymer articulating bearing surfaces operate with a boundary or mixed lubrication regime.[57] This means that there will be contact between the bearing surfaces leading to the generation of wear debris. The UHMWPE wear debris can cause loosening of the implants as a result of osteolysis. This is a reaction of the cells to the wear debris that causes bone resorption. It is not the overall volume of wear that causes the adverse cellular reaction, but the size range of the wear particles, typically in the range 0.2–0.8 μm.[58]

Bearing material combinations of metal-on-metal and ceramic-on-ceramic generally operate with a mixed lubrication regime, implying that they produce some wear debris. However, there is evidence of fluid-film lubrication during some loading conditions, which would mean separation of the bearing surfaces. The improved lubrication regimes of metal-on-metal and ceramic-on-ceramic bearing combinations is shown by the production of lower volumes of wear debris than UHMWPE. However, the long-term effects of metal and ceramic wear debris in the body are not fully known.[59–61]

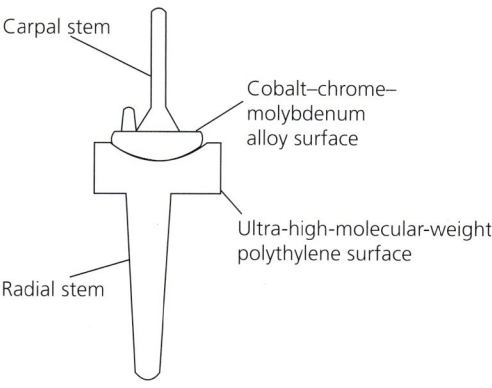

Figure 12.31 Biaxial wrist implant.

FRACTURE FIXATION DEVICES

Introduction

The aim of a fracture fixation device is to stabilize the bone while the fracture heals. Fracture fixation devices will become a redundant structure in the body once the fracture has healed. Therefore, the loading conditions that need to be considered in the design of these devices is not as severe as those for joint replacement implants. In this section screws, plates, intramedullary nails and external fixators will be discussed.

Screws

Screws can be used on their own or in combination with other devices such as plates and intramedullary nails. The aim of the screw is to either hold bone fragments together or to fix a plate or nail in position. The screw thread will vary depending on the type of bone it is to be used in. Cortical screws have a small thread depth, whereas cancellous screws have a large thread depth to increase the contact area with the bone, as cancellous bone has a lower shear strength than cortical bone. Figure 12.32 shows cortical and cancellous screw threads. Screw types can be further divided into self-tapping and self-drilling. Self-tapping screws cut their own thread into a drilled hole, while self-drilling screws will also drill the hole. If a screw is not self-tapping it will generally be necessary to use a tap to cut a thread into the bone before insertion of the screw. The pull-out strength of a screw increases with increasing screw length, outside diameter and thread depth, as well as bone strength.[54,62] The pull-out strength of a screw (the magnitude of the force required to dislodge it) is given by

$$F = S \times (L \times \pi \times D) \times T, \quad (12.43)$$

where S is the shear strength of the bone, L is the length of the screw thread, D is the outside thread diameter and T is the *thread shape factor* given by

$$T = 0.5 \times \frac{0.58t}{p}, \quad (12.44)$$

where t is the thread depth and p is the thread pitch. Note that the symbol T is not being used the same way here as in equation (12.7).

Let us consider a screw of outside diameter 6.4 mm, thread depth 0.8 mm, pitch 1 mm and length 45 mm being pulled from a bone of shear strength 1.6 MPa. Putting the numbers into equation (12.43) we obtain the pull-out strength, $F = 1396$ N. In diseased bone, such as osteoporotic or rheumatoid, the shear strength of the bone will be reduced, and therefore the pull-out strength will be lower than that of a screw inserted in normal bone.

Screws are generally manufactured from stainless steel or titanium alloy. However, screws made from bioabsorbable materials that gradually decompose and are replaced by bone have been used for treating a variety of fractures. These devices are made from polymers such as polyglycolide, polylactide and polydioxanone.[63]

Plates

The design of plates is wide ranging to cover a variety of fractures in different bones. Plates are fixed to the outside of bones and are subjected to large bending moments so they require high stiffness in bending to avoid excessive deflections. This can only be controlled through the geometry of the plate and Young's modulus of the material used. Therefore, stainless steel and titanium alloy are used as they have a high enough Young's modulus to resist bending. If two plates have identical geometry and are subjected to bending, a titanium alloy plate will deflect more than a stainless steel plate as it has a lower Young's modulus.[54] Conventional plates have holes for the screws to pass through. Fixation of the plate is achieved from the compression of the screw against the plate causing friction at the plate/bone interface. Newer designs of plates have a threaded hole so that the screw head can be locked with the plate. It is believed that locking the screws with the plate will provide improved stability in torsion.[64]

Intramedullary nails

Intramedullary nails are commonly used to treat long-bone fractures.[65] These tube-like implants are inserted down the medullary canal of a bone and fixed in position with screws (Fig. 12.33). The requirements of the implants are to have sufficient strength to avoid fracture and a high enough Young's modulus to avoid deflection. For these reasons metals, either stainless steel or titanium alloy, are used to manufacture the intramedullary nails.

Let us consider an intramedullary nail made from stainless steel with a Young's modulus of 193 GPa and a shear modulus of 80 GPa. The nail is 345 mm long and has an outside radius of 5.5 mm and an inside radius of 4 mm.

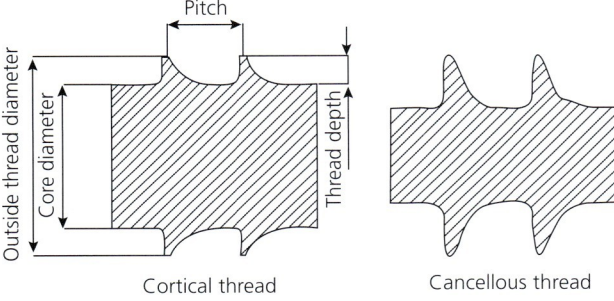

Figure 12.32 Cortical and cancellous screw threads.

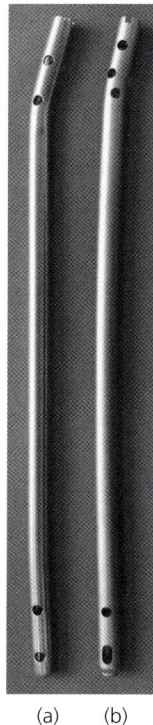

(a) (b)

Figure 12.33 Russell Taylor (a) and Trigen (b) intramedullary nails (Smith & Nephew, Memphis, TN, USA).

If the nail is considered to be a beam fixed at both ends and subjected to a central force of 200 N, we can use equation (12.20) to calculate the deflection

$$y_2 = \frac{200 \times 0.345^3}{192 \times 193 \times 10^9}\left(\frac{4}{\pi\left(0.0055^4 - 0.004^4\right)}\right) = 0.4 \text{ mm}.$$

Let us now consider the same nail, fixed at one end and subjected to torsion at the other end with the application of a torque of 6 N m. From equation (12.22) we can calculate the angle of twist

$$\theta = \frac{2}{\pi\left(0.0055^4 - 0.004^4\right)}\left(\frac{6 \times 0.345}{80 \times 10^9}\right)$$

$$= 0.025 \text{ radians} = 1.4°.$$

External ring fixators

External ring fixators (Fig. 12.34) are used for fracture fixation and the correction of limb deformities. The fixator assembly consists of the number of parts (rings, wires and longitudinal elements) that are assembled around a bone in various configurations. The rings distribute the loads from the wires to the longitudinal elements. Materials used for the manufacture of the rings include aluminium, stainless

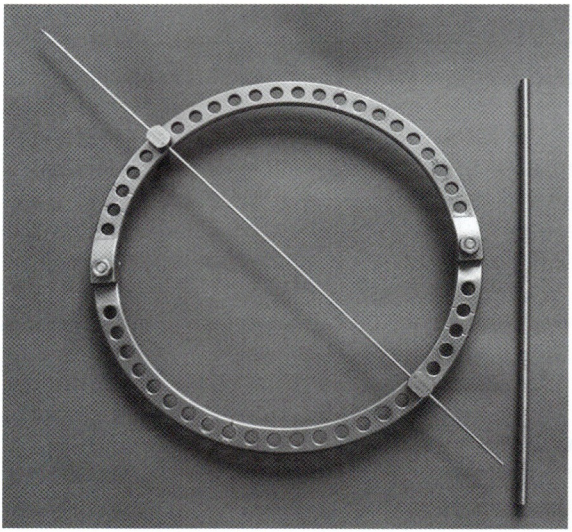

Figure 12.34 Parts of an Ilizarov external fixation device.

steel and carbon composite. The wires, made from stainless steel, suspend the bone to the rings. A wire is clamped to one side of the ring, and tension is applied with a tensioning device. The other end of the wire is then clamped to the ring. The longitudinal elements connect between the rings and are generally made from stainless steel. The chosen configuration and the tension applied to the wires control the overall stiffness of the fixator assembly.[66]

SPINAL IMPLANTS

Introduction

The traditional surgical method of treating back pain is spinal fusion, where two vertebrae are encouraged to grow together with the use of bone graft material. While fusion eliminates back pain, it also removes motion at that vertebral level, and this can change the mechanics of the adjacent vertebral levels. Recently, a range of devices have been developed that partially or totally replace the intervertebral disc, with the major advantage over spinal fusion of preserving spinal motion. This section will describe the materials used for fusion devices and devices for partially or totally replacing the intervertebral disc.

Fusion devices

Traditionally, the spine has been stabilized, while fusion is taking place, by a combination of rods, plates, hooks and screws. Fusion is now generally achieved with the use of an interbody fusion cage.[67] Fusion cages are designed to contain bone graft material and maintain the height between the two vertebral bodies to allow fusion to occur. They can be divided into three main types: horizontal

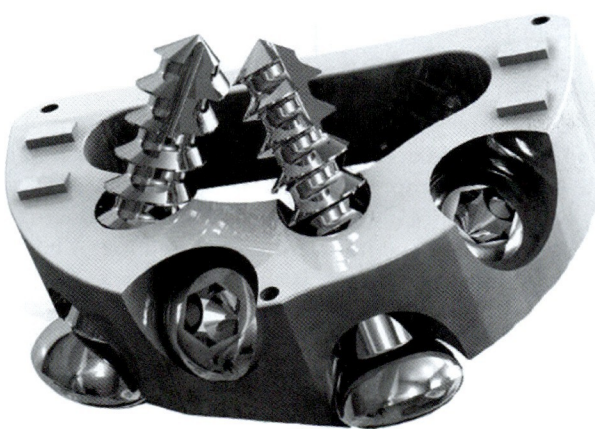

Figure 12.35 STALIF TT. Reproduced with kind permission from Surgicraft Ltd, Redditch, UK. © Surgicraft Ltd.

threaded cylinders, vertical rings and open boxes.[68] The horizontal threaded fusion cages were originally made from titanium alloy, with current examples including the BAK/L (Zimmer, Warsaw, IN, USA). However, there has been concern that the titanium alloy obscures the view when medical imaging is used, and it is not possible to determine whether fusion has occurred. For this reason, poly(etheretherketone) (PEEK) is now commonly used to manufacture fusion cages. The BAK Vista (Zimmer) is a threaded horizontal cage made from carbon-reinforced PEEK. Other PEEK cages include the Stalif (Surgicraft Ltd, Redditch, UK) which uses screws for fixation (Fig. 12.35).

Nucleus replacement devices

The natural nucleus in the human body has a low Young's modulus of about 1 MPa. Therefore, devices for replacing the nucleus have tended to involve synthetic materials of low modulus, such as hydrogels and elastomers. The Raymedica (Minneapolis, MN, USA) prosthetic disc nucleus (PDN) consists of a woven polyethylene jacket wrapped around a hydrogel core. When hydrated, the device expands to fill the space of the removed nucleus and restores disc height.[69] Other designs proposed and currently under clinical investigation include the Aquarelle (Stryker Spine, Allendale, NJ, USA), which is made from a polyvinyl alcohol hydrogel, and the Dascor Disc Arthroplasty System (Disc Dynamics, Inc., Eden Prairie, MN, USA), which involves injecting a curable polyurethane elastomer into a balloon.[70]

Total disc replacement devices

The successful combination of materials used in hip and knee arthroplasty has led to a range of total disc replacement devices that have articulating bearing surfaces. The Charité (DePuy Spine, Raynham, MA, USA) was the first

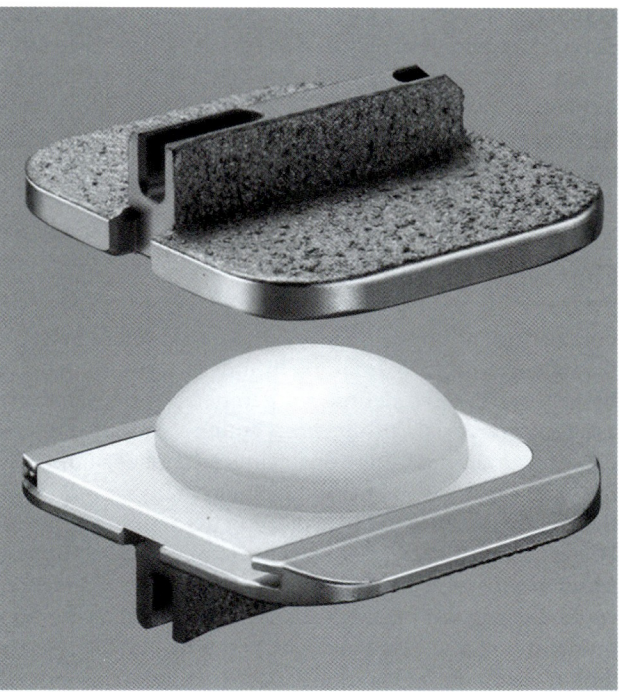

Figure 12.36 ProDisc C. Reproduced with kind permission from Synthes, Solothurn, Switzerland. © Synthes.

artificial disc, and is designed for use in the lumbar spine.[71] It was given US Food and Drug Administration (FDA) approval in October 2004. While only gaining approval for use in the USA recently, the disc has been used in Europe for over 15 years. The Charité consists of an UHMWPE spacer sandwiched between two metal endplates made from cobalt–chrome–molybdenum alloy. The ProDisc (Synthes, Solothurn, Switzerland) also has an UHMWPE against cobalt–chrome–molybdenum alloy articulation (Fig. 12.36). Other disc devices, such as the Maverick (Medtronic, Minneapolis, MN, USA) and Flexicore (Stryker, Allendale, NJ, USA) have utilized a metal-against-metal articulation (cobalt–chrome–molybdenum alloy against cobalt–chrome–molybdenum alloy). Fixation methods for these devices avoid the use of bone cement. The Charité and Flexicore have teeth or spikes that will grip into the vertebral body. The ProDisc and Maverick use a keel, whereby a section of bone is cut out from the vertebral body and the keel of the implant is placed within the cut bone. A textured surface may also be used to enhance fixation.

PRECLINICAL TESTING

Introduction

The ultimate test of any orthopaedic device or biomaterial is once it has been implanted into the human body. However, the regulations of the FDA (for devices in the

USA) and the Medical Device Directive (for devices in Europe) require medical device companies to verify and validate that the design of a device will perform once implanted in the human body. Within the design process for medical devices, finite-element modelling and mechanical testing are used.

Finite-element modelling

Finite-element modelling is a computational method that gives an approximate solution to a problem. The basic steps involve defining a geometry for the model, assigning materials properties (Young's modulus, etc.), creating a mesh, adding constraints and loads, and solving. The results from a finite-element analysis will show the stresses, strains and displacements within a model. When calculating stresses, it is usual to calculate the *von Mises stress*; this is simply a measure of the stress that could damage the material of the implant. Finite-element modelling is a widely used technique in medical device design, and can be used to verify whether a design will have sufficient strength to withstand the loading conditions in the human body.[72] For example, finite-element modelling has been used to investigate the effect of introducing holes into the femoral component of a total hip replacement implant to engage with a stem introducer instrument,[73] the stiffness of different configurations of the Ilizarov external fixation device[74] and stresses in fusion cages.[75] Finite-element modelling can also be used to simulate wear in total joint replacement implants.[76] One important aspect of finite-element modelling is that its results depend on the assumptions made in building the model and the values assigned to its parameters. Therefore, these results need to be validated either by independent calculations or by the results of mechanical testing.

Mechanical testing

Mechanical testing allows the mechanical conditions in the human body to be simulated in the laboratory and to validate a design. Mechanical testing typically addresses questions such as how strong is the device, how long will it last and at what rate will it wear? Mechanical testing will typically use a materials testing machine or a joint simulator. These machines can apply forces and motions to attempt to simulate the conditions encountered in the human body. However, mechanical testing is unlikely to exactly replicate the mechanical loading conditions in the body, and cannot allow for any biological response within the body. To enable comparison between different designs of orthopaedic devices, a range of national and international standards have been adopted. For example, with a total hip replacement it would be necessary to undertake testing to measure the wear of the bearing surfaces using a hip simulator to International Organization for Standardization (ISO) 14242-1,[77] and to determine the fatigue strength of the femoral stem to ISO 7206-4.[78]

To perform wear testing, it is necessary to mount a femoral head and acetabular cup into a simulator that is able to apply a compressive force of up to 3000 N and to be able to apply motions of abduction/adduction, flexion/extension and inward/outward rotation. A lubricant of diluted calf serum is maintained at 37°C. The forces and motions are applied to the hip implant at a frequency of 1 Hz. The machine is stopped after 0.5 million cycles have been completed and the wear determined, typically by measuring the mass of the femoral head and acetabular cup. The simulator is then restarted, and wear measurements made at 1 million cycles and then every 1 million cycles, up to maximum of 5 million. To test the fatigue strength of the femoral stem, the stem is potted into a container (Fig. 12.37). The hip stem is placed into a container of fluid, and a testing machine is used to apply a cyclic force to the femoral head to produce bending and torsion of the stem (Fig. 12.38). Testing continues until failure of the stem occurs or 5 million cycles are reached.[73]

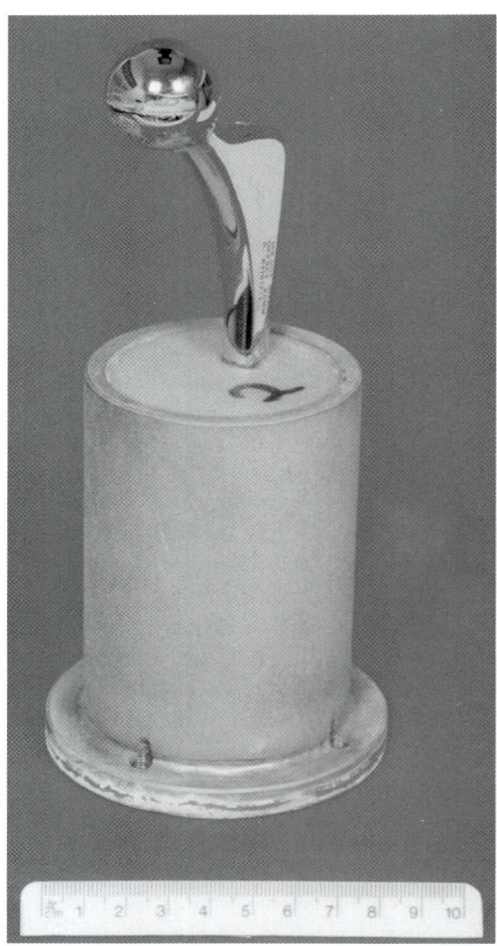

Figure 12.37 Femoral part prepared for mechanical testing.

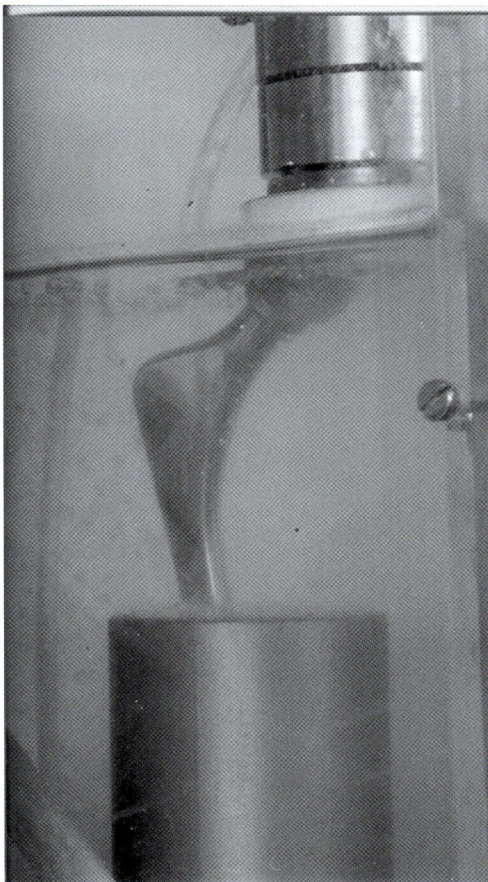

Figure 12.38 Femoral part subjected to mechanical testing.

KEY LEARNING POINTS

- It is important to understand mechanical terms such as stress, strain, force, stiffness, Young's modulus, elasticity and viscoelasticity and to use them correctly, as they have specific meanings.
- Mechanics can be used to understand the forces acting through human joints. The magnitudes of typical forces can be multiples of body weight; for example, the magnitude of the resultant force acting thorough the tibiofemoral joint of the knee can be three times body weight during walking.
- Synthetic biomaterials used in the manufacture of orthopaedic devices include metals, polymers, ceramics and elastomers. The choice of materials will depend on the requirements of the implant.
- Preclinical testing is essential to verify how a device will perform in the human body from a mechanical point of view; testing can include wear testing and assessment of fatigue performance.

REFERENCES

1. Cordey J. Introduction: basic concepts and definitions in mechanics. *Injury* 2000;**31**(Suppl. 2):1–13.
2. Dowson D. Basic mechanics. In: Dowson D, Wright V (eds) *Introduction to the Biomechanics of Joints and Joint Replacement*. London, UK: Mechanical Engineering Publications, 1981:11–20.
3. Gere JM, Timoshenko SP (eds) *Mechanics of Materials*. Cheltenham, UK: Stanley Thornes, 1999.
4. Stephens JH (ed.) *Kempe's Engineers Year-book*. Tonbridge, UK: Miller Freeman, 1998.
5. Wilcox RK. An introduction to basic mechanics. *Current Orthopaedics* 2006;**20**:1–8.
6. Ferrari A, Benedetti MG, Pavan E, et al. Quantitative comparison of five current protocols in gait analysis. *Gait & Posture* 2008;**28**:207–16.
7. Benoit DL, Ramsey DK, Lamontagne M, et al. Effect of skin movement artifact on knee kinematics during gait and cutting motions measured in vivo. *Gait & Posture* 2006;**24**:152–64.
8. Isaac DL, Beard DJ, Price AJ, et al. In-vivo sagittal plane knee kinematics: ACL intact, deficient and reconstructed knees. *Knee* 2005;**12**:25–31.
9. Harvey SB, Smith FW, Hukins DWL. Measurement of lumbar spine flexion-extension using a low-field open-magnet magnetic resonance scanner. *Investigative Radiology* 1998;**33**:439–43.
10. Wands I, Shepherd DET, Hukins DWL. Viscoelastic properties of composites of calcium alginate and hydroxyapatite. *Journal of Materials Science: Materials in Medicine* 2008;**19**:2417–21.
11. Holmes AD, Hukins DWL. Analysis of load-relaxation in compressed segments of lumbar spine. *Medical Engineering and Physics* 1996;**18**:99–104.
12. Hukins DWL, Kirby MC, Sikoryn TA, et al. Comparison of structure, mechanical properties and functions of lumbar spinal ligaments. *Spine* 1990;**15**:787–95.
13. Azangwe G, Mathias KJ, Marshall D. Preliminary comparison of the rupture of human and rabbit anterior cruciate ligaments. *Clinical Biomechanics* 2001;**16**:913–17.
14. Farfan HF, Cossette JW, Robertson GH, et al. The effects of torsion on the lumbar intervertebral joints: the role of torsion in the production of disc degeneration. *Journal of Bone & Joint Surgery* 1970;**52A**:468–97.
15. Jin ZM, Stone M, Ingham E, Fisher J. Biotribology. *Current Orthopaedics* 2006;**20**:32–40.
16. Hukins DWL. What is lumbar instability? In: Aspden RM, Porter RW (eds) *Lumbar Spine Disorders: Current Concepts*. London, UK: World Scientific, 1995:26–37.
17. Smeathers JE. Shocking news about discs. *Current Orthopaedics* 1994;**8**:45–8.
18. Radin EL, Paul IL. Does cartilage compliance reduce skeletal impact loads: relative force-attenuating properties of articular cartilage, synovial fluid, periarticular soft tissues and bone. *Arthritis and Rheumatism* 1970;**13**:139–44.

19. Dowson D, Seedhom BB, Johnson GR. Biomechanics of the lower limb. In: Dowson D, Wright V (eds) *Introduction to the Biomechanics of Joints and Joint Replacement.* London, UK: Mechanical Engineering Publications, 1981:78–84.
20. Bergmann G, Deuretzbacher G, Heller M, et al. Hip contact forces and gait patterns from routine activities. *Journal of Biomechanics* 2001;**34**:859–71.
21. Vickerstaff JA, Miles AW, Cunningham JL. A brief history of total ankle replacement and a review of the current status. *Medical Engineering & Physics* 2007;**29**:1056–64.
22. Long AJ, Monsell FP, Porter ML, et al. A method for the kinematic evaluation of the knee following anterior cruciate ligament injury and reconstruction. *Journal of Engineering in Medicine* 1993;**207**:73–7.
23. Jobbins B, Amis AA, Unsworth A. Biomechanics of the upper limb. In: Dowson D, Wright V (eds) *Introduction to the Biomechanics of Joints and Joint Replacement.* London, UK: Mechanical Engineering Publications, 1981:85–102.
24. Bergmann G, Graichen F, Bender A, et al. In vivo glenohumeral contact forces: measurements in the first patient 7 months postoperatively. *Journal of Biomechanics* 2007;**40**:2139–49.
25. Pylios T, Shepherd DET. Biomechanics of the normal and diseased metacarpophalangeal joint: implications on the design of joint replacement implants. *Journal of Mechanics in Medicine and Biology* 2007;**7**:163–74.
26. Shepherd DET, Johnstone AJ. Design considerations for a wrist implant. *Medical Engineering & Physics* 2002;**24**:641–50.
27. Cripton PA, Kroeker SG, Saari A. Musculature actuation and biomechanics of the spine. In: Kurtz SM, Edidin AA (eds) *Spine Technology Handbook.* London, UK: Elsevier, 2006:99–143.
28. Stewart TD, Hall RM. Basic biomechanics of human joints: hips, knees and the spine. *Current Orthopaedics* 2006;**20**:23–31.
29. Aspden RM. The spine as an arch. *Spine* 1989;**14**:266–74.
30. Jutley RS, Watson MA, Shepherd DET, Hukins DWL. Finite element analysis of stress around a sternum screw used to prevent sternal dehiscence after heart surgery. *Journal of Engineering in Medicine* 2002;**216**:315–21.
31. Shepherd DET, Seedhom BB. The 'instantaneous' compressive modulus of human articular cartilage in joints of the lower limb. *Rheumatology* 1999;**38**:124–32.
32. Meakin JR, Hukins DWL. Replacing the nucleus pulposus of the intervertebral disk: prediction of suitable properties of a replacement material using finite element analysis. *Journal of Materials Science: Materials in Medicine* 2001;**12**:207–13.
33. Johannessen W, Elliott DM. Effects of degeneration on the biphasic material properties of human nucleus pulposus in confined compression. *Spine* 2005;**30**:E724–9.
34. Yang KH, Kish VL. Compressibility measurement of human intervertebral nucleus pulposus. *Journal of Biomechanics* 1988;**21**:865.
35. Kempson GE, Spivey CJ, Swanson SAV, Freeman MAR. Patterns of cartilage stiffness on normal and degenerate human femoral heads. *Journal of Biomechanics* 1971;**4**:597–609.
36. Swann AC, Seedhom BB. The stiffness of normal articular cartilage and the predominant acting stress levels: implications for the aetiology of osteoarthrosis. *British Journal of Rheumatology* 1993;**32**:16–25.
37. Williams DF. On the mechanisms of biocompatibility. *Biomaterials* 2008;**29**:2941–53.
38. Brown SA. Synthetic biomaterials for spinal applications. In: Kurtz SM, Edidin AA (eds) *Spine Technology Handbook.* London, UK: Elsevier, 2006:11–33.
39. Jones DS, McLaughlin DWJ, McCoy CP, Gorman SP. Physicochemical characterisation and biological evaluation of hydrogel-poly(e-caprolactone) interpenetrating polymer networks as novel urinary biomaterials. *Biomaterials* 2005;**26**:1761–70.
40. Chu C-C. Biodegradable polymeric biomaterials: an updated overview. In: Bronzino JD (ed.) *The Biomedical Engineering Handbook.* Boca Raton, FL: CRC Press, 2000:1–22.
41. Dearnley PA. A review of metallic, ceramic and surface-treated metals used for bearing surfaces in human joint replacements. *Journal of Engineering in Medicine* 1999;**213**:107–35.
42. Li S, Burstein AH. Ultra-high-molecular-weight polyethylene: the material and its use in total joint implants. *Journal of Bone and Joint Surgery (American)* 1994;**76A**:1080–90.
43. Glyn-Jones S, Saac S, Hauptfleisch J, et al. Does highly cross-linked polyethylene wear less than conventional polyethylene in total hip arthroplasty? *Journal of Arthroplasty* 2008;**23**:337–43.
44. Yoda R. Elastomers for biomedical applications. *Journal of Biomaterials Science: Polymer Edition* 1998;**9**:561–626.
45. Good V, Widding K, Hunter G, Heuer D. Oxidized zirconium: a potentially longer lasting hip implant. *Materials & Design* 2005;**26**:618–22.
46. Tanavalee A, Choi YJ, Tria AJ. Unicondylar knee arthroplasty: past and present. *Orthopedics* 2005;**28**:1423–33.
47. Lewis G. Biomechanics of and research challenges in uncemented total ankle replacement. *Clinical Orthopaedics and Related Research* 2004;**424**:89–97.
48. Guyer AJ, Richardson EG. Current concepts review: total ankle arthroplasty. *Foot & Ankle International* 2008;**29**:256–64.
49. Gregory JJ, Ennis O, Hay SM. Total elbow arthroplasty. *Current Orthopaedics* 2008;**22**:80–9.
50. Gregory T, Hansen U, Emery RJ, et al. Developments in shoulder arthroplasty. *Journal of Engineering in Medicine* 2007;**221**:87–96.
51. Joyce TJ. Currently available metacarpophalangeal prostheses: their designs and prospective considerations. *Expert Review of Medical Devices* 2004;**1**:193–204.

52. Costi J, Krishnan J, Pearcy M. Total wrist arthroplasty: a quantitative review of the last 30 years. *Journal of Rheumatology* 1998;**25**:451–8.
53. Kapoor B, Datir SP, Davies B, *et al*. Femoral cement pressurisation in hip arthroplasty: a laboratory comparison of three techniques. *Acta Orthopaedica Scandinavica* 2004;**75**:708–12.
54. Park SH, Llinás A, Goel VK, Keller JC. Hard tissue replacements. In: Bronzino JD (ed.) *The Biomedical Engineering Handbook*. Boca Raton, FL: CRC Press, 2000:1–35.
55. Kienapfel H, Sprey C, Wilke A, Griss P. Implant fixation by bone ingrowth. *Journal of Arthroplasty* 1999;**14**:355–68.
56. Sun LM, Berndt CC, Gross KA, Kucuk A. Material fundamentals and clinical performance of plasma-sprayed hydroxyapatite coatings: a review. *Journal of Biomedical Materials Research* 2001;**58**:570–92.
57. Fisher J, Dowson D. Tribology of total artificial joints. *Journal of Engineering in Medicine* 1991;**205**:73–9.
58. Ingham E, Fisher J. Biological reactions to wear debris in total joint replacement. *Journal of Engineering in Medicine* 2000;**214**:21–37.
59. Dowson D. New joints for the millennium: wear control in total replacement hip joints. *Journal of Engineering in Medicine* 2001;**215**:335–58.
60. Dowson D, Jin ZM. Metal-on-metal hip joint tribology. *Journal of Engineering in Medicine* 2006;**220**:107–18.
61. Scholes SC, Unsworth A. Comparison of friction and lubrication of different hip prostheses. *Journal of Engineering in Medicine* 2000;**214**:49–57.
62. Chapman JR, Harrington RM, Lee KM, *et al*. Factors affecting the pullout strength of cancellous bone screws. *Journal of Biomechanical Engineering* 1996;**118**:391–8.
63. Rokkanen PU, Bostman O, Hirvensalo E, *et al*. Bioabsorbable fixation in orthopaedic surgery and traumatology. *Biomaterials* 2000;**21**:2607–13.
64. Miller DL, Goswmi T. A review of locking compression plate biomechanics and their advantages as internal fixators in fracture healing. *Clinical Biomechanics* 2007;**22**:1049–62.
65. Eveleigh RJ. A review of biomechanical studies of intramedullary nails. *Medical Engineering & Physics* 1995;**17**:323–31.
66. Watson MA, Mathias KJ, Maffulli N. External ring fixators: an overview. *Journal of Engineering in Medicine* 2000;**214**:459–70.
67. Villarraga ML. Historical review of spinal instrumentation for fusion: rods, plates, screws and cages. In: Kurtz SM, Edidin AA (eds) *Spine Technology Handbook*. London, UK: Elsevier, 2006:183–207.
68. Weiner BK, Fraser RD. Lumbar interbody cages. *Spine* 1998;**23**:634–40.
69. Ray CD. The PDN® prosthetic disc-nucleus device. *European Spine Journal* 2002;**11**:S137–42.
70. Di Martino A, Vaccaro AR, Lee JY, *et al*. Nucleus pulposus replacement: basic science and indications for clinical use. *Spine* 2005;**30**(Suppl.):S16–22.
71. Anderson PA, Rouleau JP. Intervertebral disc arthroplasty. *Spine* 2004;**29**:2779–86.
72. Contro R, Vena P. Computational models for biological tissues and biomedical implants. *Engineering Computations* 2003;**20**:513–23.
73. Mathias KJ, Leahy JC, Heaton A, *et al*. Hip joint prosthesis design: effect of stem introducers. *Medical Engineering & Physics* 1998;**20**:620–4.
74. Watson MA, Mathias KJ, Maffulli N, *et al*. Finite element modelling of the Ilizarov external fixation system. *Journal of Engineering in Medicine* 2007;**221**:863–71.
75. Fantigrossi A, Galbusera F, Raimondi MT, *et al*. Biomechanical analysis of cages for posterior lumbar interbody fusion. *Medical Engineering & Physics* 2007;**29**:101–9.
76. Fialho JC, Fernandes PR, Eca L, Folgado J. Computational hip joint simulator for wear and heat generation. *Journal of Biomechanics* 2007;**40**:2358–66.
77. ISO 14242-1:2002. *Implants for Surgery. Wear of Total Hip Joint Prostheses. Loading and Displacement Parameters for Wear-testing Machines and Corresponding Environmental Conditions for Test*. London, UK: British Standards Institution.
78. ISO 7206-4:2002. *Implants for Surgery. Partial and Total Hip Joint Prostheses. Determination of Endurance Properties of Stemmed Femoral Components*. London, UK: British Standards Institution.

13

Clinical principles of kinesiology

JIM RICHARDS, JAMES SELFE

The International Classification of Functioning, Disability and Health and its relevance to kinesiology	202	Muscle strength testing	211
		Muscle action	213
The six fundamental principles of joint assessment	202	Proprioception	214
Open and closed kinetic chains	203	Summary	215
Joint movement	204	Further Reading	216
Joint control and stability	207	References	216

NATIONAL BOARD STANDARDS

- Understand the International Classification of Functioning, Disability and Health
- Understand the gait cycle
- Understand the joint reaction forces at major joints
- Understand knee and hip kinematics
- Understand the methods of joint assessment

THE INTERNATIONAL CLASSIFICATION OF FUNCTIONING, DISABILITY AND HEALTH AND ITS RELEVANCE TO KINESIOLOGY

The International Classification of Functioning, Disability and Health (ICF)[1] was endorsed by the World Health Organization (WHO) in 2001; it presents a holistic biopsychosocial paradigm in which to view a person's health status. The ICF stresses health and function rather than disability, with a focus on impact rather than cause. The medical model of health views disability as a problem of the individual, caused by injury or disease, whereas the social model of health defines disability as a lack of integration of individuals into society.[2] The ICF framework is divided into two parts, each with two components, which can be expressed in either positive or negative terms (Fig. 13.1).

From a clinical perspective patients will tend to seek medical help when they experience negative changes in their *functioning* leading to *disability*. These changes are often a consequence of alterations in *body structure* or function due to pathological processes, which have led to restrictions in *activities and participation*.

THE SIX FUNDAMENTAL PRINCIPLES OF JOINT ASSESSMENT

The ICF presents a holistic biopsychosocial paradigm in which to view a person's health status. To determine the health status, we often need to assess the specific function of individual joints. There are many important factors to take into consideration when performing an assessment of joint function; these include: the control of the joint movement in open and closed kinetic chain (CKC) situations, the type of muscle contraction, whether the muscles surrounding the joint act across more than one joint, the rotational and translational stability of the joint and the joint proprioception (Fig. 13.2).

Each of these factors will not only affect the overall joint function but may also affect the interactions between all the factors simultaneously. This presents a

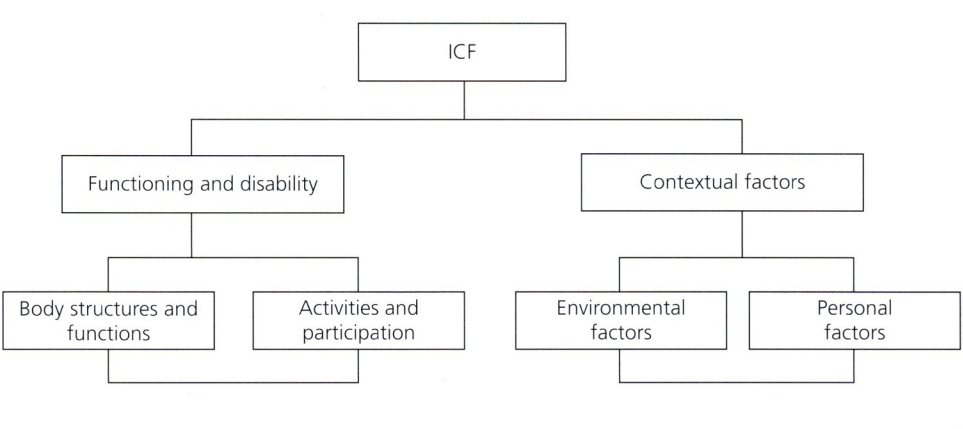

Figure 13.1 Structure of the International Classification of Functioning, Disability and Health (ICF) (adapted from Greenhalgh and Selfe 2009).[3]

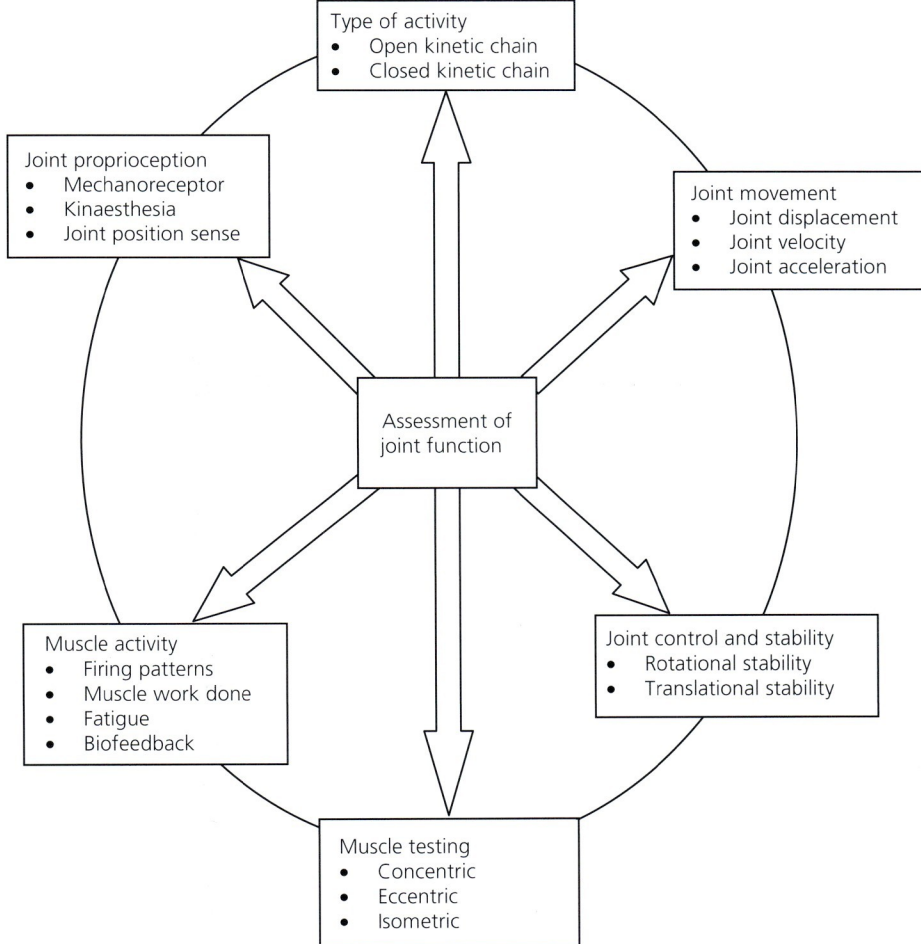

Figure 13.2 The six fundamental principles of joint assessment.

difficult set of problems when assessing a joint for a specific functional deficit. For example, an individual may have pain at the knee due to rotational or translational instability. To compensate for this the knee flexion/extension angle and angular velocity control is likely to be affected, which in turn will affect the moments about the knee, the muscle firing patterns and the concentric/eccentric control from specific muscles around the knee. Therefore, the challenge in joint assessment is to measure or record the factors which are directly clinically relevant rather than secondary effects, which may give misleading information.

OPEN AND CLOSED KINETIC CHAINS

Differences between open and closed chain

Steindler is credited with introducing the concept of open and CKCs to the study of human movement.[4]

Steindler's *Kinesiology of the Human Body*[5] introduced useful terminology adapted from mechanical engineering. In mechanical engineering, the link concept considers rigid overlapping bars that are connected in series by pin joints. The system is considered closed if both ends are connected to an immovable framework, thus preventing translation of either the distal or proximal joint centre. This creates a system where movement at one joint produces movement at all other joints in a predictable manner.[6] When applied to human movement it is apparent that there can never be a situation where there is a truly CKC and certainly the movement of the knee joint for example is more complex than that occurring around a pin joint. In the lower limb an open kinetic chain (OKC) is said to occur when the foot is free to move in space with little or no resistance. A CKC occurs in the lower limb when the foot meets considerable resistance, e.g. the ground.[6] However, Ellenbecker and Davies[4] point out that there is some controversy over the definition of considerable resistance, particularly when it comes to classifying activities such as cycling as either open or closed chain.

Functionality of open and closed kinetic chain exercises

CKC exercises such as standing squats and step ascent and descent are assumed to be more functional than OKC exercises such as seated leg extensions or straight leg raises (SLRs).[7,8]

The combined simultaneous segmental motion and movement in multiple planes around multiple axes increases the demand for dynamic stabilization and joint control, which increases muscle co-contraction activity.[4] This is particularly important at the knee when the hamstrings provide an active dynamic restraint to prevent excessive anterior shearing at the tibiofemoral joint during strong quadriceps contractions. Without the hamstring co-contraction, the anterior cruciate ligament is potentially exposed to dangerously high forces. Another important difference in motor control between OKC and CKC is the contraction of the bi-articular muscles. During CKC exercise, simultaneous hip and knee extension occurs when rising from the flexed position, causing the rectus femoris to simultaneously eccentrically lengthen across the hip, but concentrically shorten across the knee. Conversely, the hamstrings lengthen across the hip but shorten at the knee. This form of pseudoisometric muscle contraction has been referred to as 'concurrent shift'.[6]

JOINT MOVEMENT

Joint control may be considered in terms of linear and angular movement. Linear movement relates to the movement of the body or a body segment in the vertical, anterior/posterior or medial/lateral directions or a combination of all three. Angular movement relates to flexion/extension, abduction/adduction and transverse plane motion of a joint. For both linear and angular movements, joint displacement, velocity and acceleration may be measured and assessed.

The methods described in this section include the calculation and interpretation of linear and angular joint displacement, velocity and acceleration. These can be applied to any joints of the body; however, to demonstrate this we will consider the movement of the hand during an upper limb reaching task and the movement of the knee during walking.

Linear displacement, velocity and acceleration

LINEAR DISPLACEMENT

Linear displacement, which is given the symbol (s), refers to the movement of an object over a particular distance in a particular direction. Displacement may also be calculated by the average velocity multiplied by time (t). The average velocity may be calculated by adding the initial (u) and final (v) velocities and dividing by two:

$$\text{Average velocity} = 1/2\,(u + v)$$
$$\text{Displacement} = 1/2\,(u + v)t$$

LINEAR VELOCITY

Linear velocity is the rate of change of displacement; that is, the distance covered in a particular time. This is the speed of movement in any particular direction or anatomical plane:

$$\text{Velocity} = \text{change in displacement time}$$

This is sometimes written as ds/dt.

LINEAR ACCELERATION

Acceleration is the rate of change of velocity; that is, the change in velocity over a given time. Acceleration tells us about the rate of change of velocity. This is an important aspect of all movement which relates to the muscles overcoming inertial forces to either start or stop movement. This relates directly to Newton's Second Law of Motion, $F = m \times a$, which states that the rate of change of velocity (acceleration) is directly proportional to the forces applied on the body, which, in the case of human movement, come from the action of muscles. Therefore, muscle forces can cause either an acceleration or deceleration of a body segment.

$$\text{Acceleration} = \text{change in velocity time}$$

This is sometimes written as dv/dt.

Kinematics of a reaching task

The above equations can be used to examine the quality of movement of different tasks. We will consider linear control by evaluating what information may be gained from the study of the movement of the hand forwards during a reaching task, such as reaching to pick up a cup, in a subject who is pain and pathology free and a patient who has a painful unstable shoulder. The motion of the upper limb during reaching can be examined by studying the displacement, velocity and acceleration graphs. All of these are derived from the same displacement data; however, they all yield significantly different information that may be used to help us to describe functional aspects of the task.

LINEAR DISPLACEMENT OF THE HAND DURING REACHING WITH AND WITHOUT SHOULDER DYSFUNCTION

The graphs in Fig. 13.3a,b show the hand starting at a position zero and moving forwards in a reaching motion. The gradient of the curve indicates the velocity at which the hand is moving throughout the task. Figure 13.3a shows an individual who is pain and pathology free, and Fig. 13.3b shows an individual with a painful unstable shoulder. Both graphs show a similar pattern, both indicating a similar amount of hand movement. The individual with the painful unstable shoulder appears to have a less smooth pattern of movement; however, we cannot measure this directly from the linear displacement graph.

LINEAR VELOCITY OF THE HAND DURING REACHING WITH AND WITHOUT SHOULDER DYSFUNCTION

The velocity graph is found by measuring the change in the linear displacement over successive time intervals. The linear velocity graph for the hand of the individual who is pain and pathology free shows a bell-shaped curve (Fig. 13.4a). Initially the velocity of the hand is zero; the hand then accelerates to its maximum velocity at approximately the mid-point of the reaching movement. The hand then decelerates; this takes slightly longer than the acceleration phase to ensure accuracy of hand positioning. The individual with a painful unstable shoulder (Fig. 13.4b) shows a marked difference with a continuously varying velocity which is followed by a decrease then an increase in velocity, indicating either an unstable or painful part of the movement. The peak velocity may be measured from this graph, indicating the level of performance of the task. The unsmooth nature of the pattern gives us a further insight to the control of the task; however, we cannot measure this directly from the linear velocity graph.

LINEAR ACCELERATION OF THE HAND DURING REACHING WITH AND WITHOUT SHOULDER DYSFUNCTION

Acceleration is calculated by measuring the change in the linear velocity over successive time intervals. The pain- and pathology-free individual (Fig. 13.5a) shows an initial acceleration peak early in the movement. The acceleration then decreases to zero as the hand reaches its maximum velocity. The hand then goes into a deceleration phase as the hand reaches its target. The peak deceleration is lower than the acceleration phase, but it lasts longer as shown by the velocity curve; this is to ensure accuracy of positioning the hand at the target. The individual with a painful unstable shoulder (Fig. 13.5b) shows a marked difference when considering the linear acceleration graph; this shows a rapidly changing graph, indicating a lack of smooth controlled movement with no clear acceleration and deceleration period. This lack of smoothness gives us important

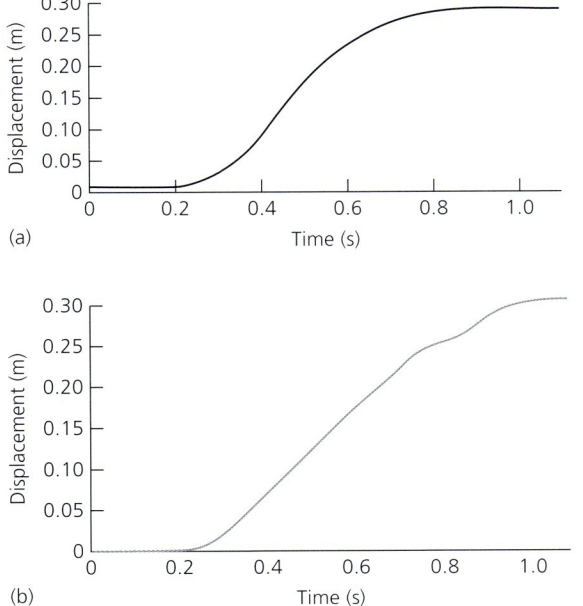

Figure 13.3 Displacement versus time of a reaching task. (a) Pain and pathology free, and (b) with shoulder dysfunction.

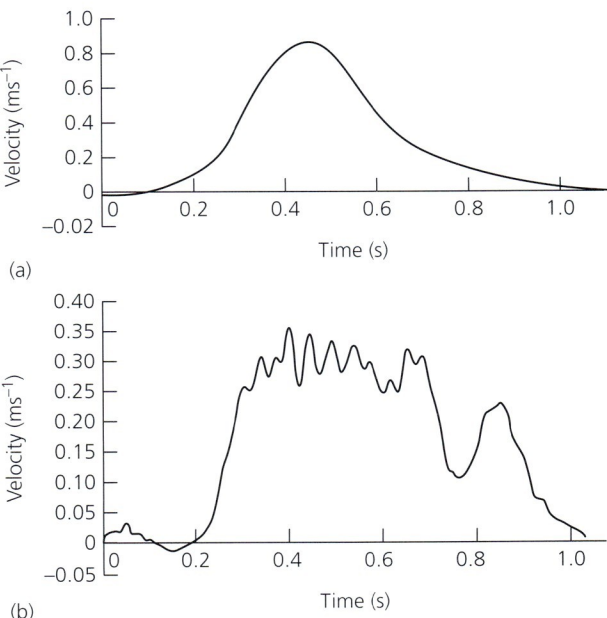

Figure 13.4 Velocity versus time of a reaching task. (a) Pain and pathology free, and (b) with shoulder dysfunction.

information about a lack of control, which could arise from poor control at the shoulder. One way of considering this lack of stability is to measure the frequency of oscillation or the number of zero crossings of the acceleration graph. If we consider the number of zero crossings, we can see that the pain- and pathology-free individual has only one zero crossing, dividing the graph into an acceleration and a deceleration phase. However, the individual with a painful unstable shoulder has more than 10 zero crossings, giving a clear objective measurement of poor control.

Angular displacement, velocity and acceleration

ANGULAR DISPLACEMENT

Angular displacement is given the symbol Θ and refers to the movement of an object through an angle. Angular displacement can be measured in two ways, either in degrees or in radians.

ANGULAR VELOCITY

Angular velocity is the rate of change of angular displacement, or the rate at which an angle is covered in a particular time. This is referred to as the angular velocity and is given the symbol ω. Angular velocity can be expressed in degrees/s or radians/s.

ANGULAR ACCELERATION

Angular acceleration is the rate of change of angular velocity and is given the symbol $\pm$. As with linear acceleration this relates to the muscles overcoming inertial forces to either start or stop movement, although this is not commonly used as an outcome measure on its own. Angular acceleration can be written in degree/s^2 or radians/s^2.

Kinematics of the knee during walking

As with the linear movement of the hand during reaching tasks, we can use the above angular motion equations to examine the quality of movement of joints during different tasks.

KNEE ANGULAR DISPLACEMENT OF NORMAL KNEE FUNCTION AND MILD CEREBRAL PALSY DURING WALKING

During normal walking the motion of the knee joint in the sagittal plane varies between 0° and 70° (Fig. 13.6a), although there is some variation in the exact amount of peak flexion occurring. At heel strike, or initial contact, the knee is flexed. After the initial contact there is a controlled increase in knee flexion to about 20° when the knee is flexed under maximum weight-bearing load. During this time the knee extensors are acting eccentrically. After this first peak of knee flexion the knee joint extends; this relates to a smooth eccentrically controlled movement of the

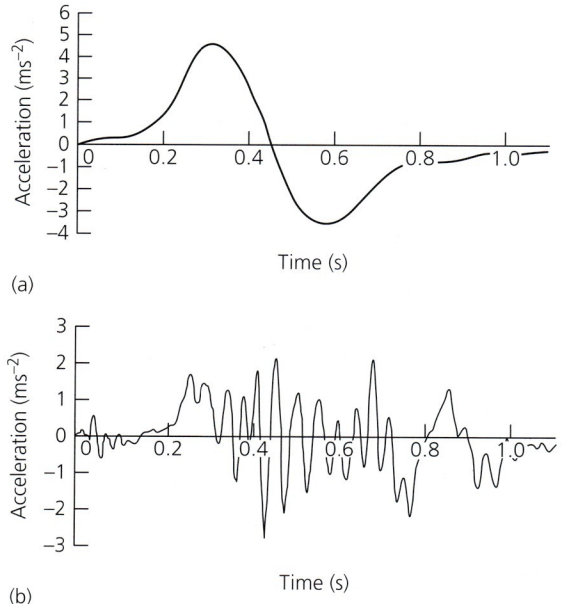

Figure 13.5 Acceleration versus time of a reaching task. (a) Pain and pathology free, and (b) with shoulder dysfunction.

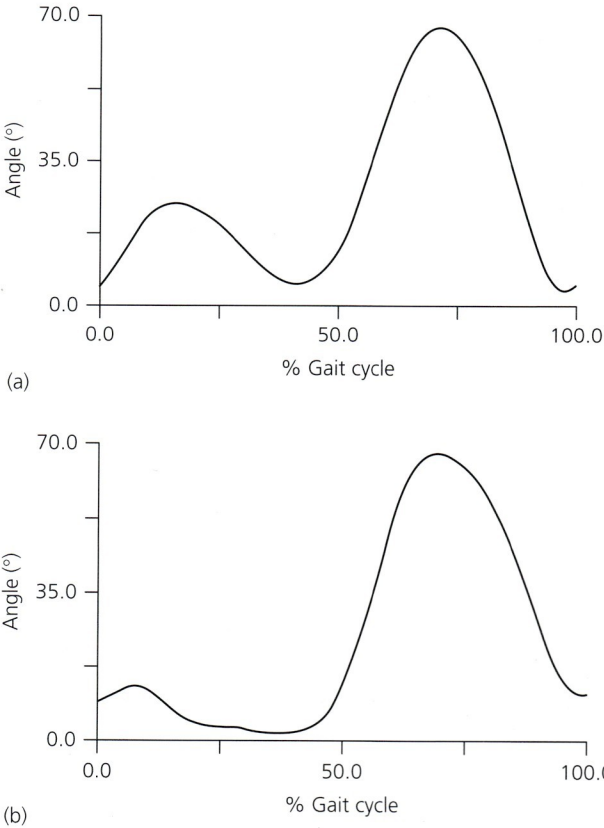

Figure 13.6 Knee angular displacement during walking. (a) An adult who is pain and pathology free, and (b) an adult with mild cerebral palsy.

body over the stance limb. The knee undergoes a rapid flexion in preparation for swing phase. Toe-off marks the start of swing phase, which allows the toe to clear the ground. During initial to mid-swing the knee continues to flex to a maximum of 65–70°. During late swing, the knee undergoes a rapid extension to prepare for the second heel strike.

In the patient with mild cerebral palsy (Fig. 13.6b) the knee starts with slightly greater knee flexion; however, the amount of knee flexion attained is significantly lower than that of normal, indicating that the eccentric control may be affected. The knee then does re-extend; however, the pattern of movement is not consistent with that of normal, again indicating that control may be affected. Swing phase appears to follow a normal pattern of movement but with slightly elevated knee flexion at mid-swing.

The comparison of the angle against time graphs allows us to identify the positions of the joint at different stages during walking, although we cannot take any direct measures of performance and control of movement from these graphs.

KNEE ANGULAR VELOCITY OF NORMAL KNEE FUNCTION AND MILD CEREBRAL PALSY DURING WALKING

Velocity is found by plotting the change in the angular displacement over successive time intervals. This allows us to show the speed of movement into flexion or extension during walking.

During normal walking (Fig. 13.7a) the knee flexes to approximately 200°/s during loading; this gives a measure of the eccentric control of the knee during loading. The knee then extends at a rate of approximately 100°/s, which shows a smooth controlled movement over the stance limb as the body moves forwards. During swing phase the knee flexes and extends with an angular velocity of approximately 400°/s.

In the patient with mild cerebral palsy (Fig. 13.7b) the knee flexes with a reduced angular velocity; therefore, the eccentric speeds and the control of the knee during loading are substantially reduced. The knee extension then occurs earlier than normal and lasts for a shorter length of time, which again shows a substantial deficit in the control of the movement over the stance limb. Interestingly, during the OKC, i.e. swing phase, the control of the knee flexion extension appears close to that of normal but with a slightly elevated knee flexion velocity during early swing.

The comparison of the angular velocity allows us to take measurements that relate to the eccentric and concentric control of the joint. Therefore, we are not just looking at what joint angle is attained at different points during walking but how the joint is controlled between these points.

Clinical importance of assessment of control

Linear and angular control of joints is clearly important for the 'quality of movement' during activities of daily

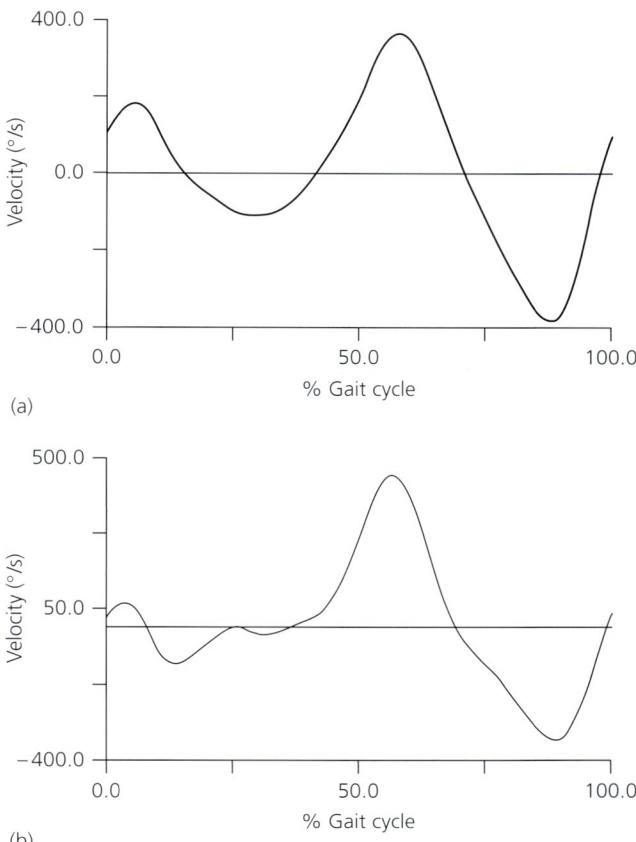

Figure 13.7 Knee angular velocity during walking. (a) An adult who is pain and pathology free, and (b) an adult with mild cerebral palsy.

living. This has been demonstrated both in neurological conditions[9] and in patients recovering from knee arthroplasty (Jevsevar et al., 1993).

JOINT CONTROL AND STABILITY

The latest techniques in biomechanics model each body segment in 'six degrees of freedom'. This allows the movement of the body segments to be measured in rotation and translation independently, although there is still a debate regarding the accuracy of translational movements due to skin and soft-tissue artefacts (Fig. 13.8).

For some joints, the use of six degrees of freedom may not be strictly necessary to gain clinically useful information; therefore, simple anatomical models are extremely useful for determining function changes due to surgical and conservative management. However, simple anatomical models do not give a full picture of the functioning and stability of different joints. Consider the measurement of knee valgus. With a simple model what may appear as a valgus knee may, in fact, be nothing of the sort. If an individual were to stand, for instance, with their knee flexed and their hip internally rotated then this would

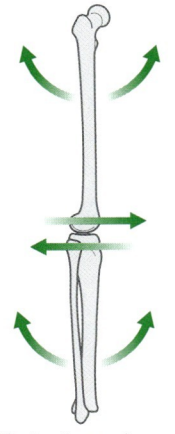
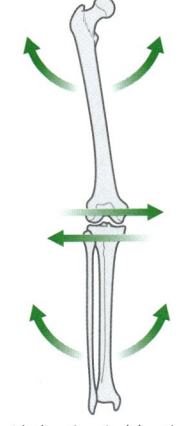
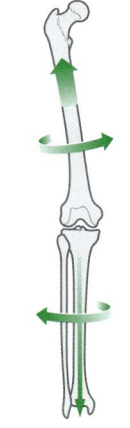

Flexion/extension
Anterior/posterior translation

Abduction/adduction
Medial/lateral translation

Internal/external rotation
Distraction/compression

Figure 13.8 Six degrees of freedom modelling of the knee.

appear as an extremely valgus knee, far beyond what the anatomy would in fact be capable of (Fig. 13.9). In this case the measurements could give misleading information about the position and stability of the knee joint in the coronal plane (Fig. 13.9).

Rotational stability in the sagittal plane

CONTROL OF SAGITTAL PLANE MOMENTS DURING WALKING

During quiet upright stance the knee is in the close pack position where there is maximum joint congruence and hence maximum joint stability. This position is achieved through the screw home mechanism which occurs mainly because of the articular geometry of the femur and tibia and the ligamentous orientation of the cruciate and collateral ligaments. Importantly, once this position has been attained the quadriceps become minimally active as the line of gravity passes anterior to the axis of the knee joint. The moment about the knee in the close pack position is one of extension, which helps to keep the knee in the locked position without requiring any muscle force. This energy-saving system is one of the key features that allows humans to stand in upright postures.

The locking mechanism is less important during gait. However, during non-pathological human gait, at heel strike it is important that the knee is in a position of nearly full extension and that this should continue as the weight is accepted onto the standing leg. Because the knee of the standing leg is near to extension, the flexion turning moment, which would cause the leg to collapse, is minimized, therefore reducing the eccentric effort required from the quadriceps to maintain an upright position. The importance of this effect is illustrated clearly when comparing the gait of the great apes such as gorillas with humans or in pathological conditions such as cerebral palsy, where a crouch gait is adopted that increases the knee flexion moment.

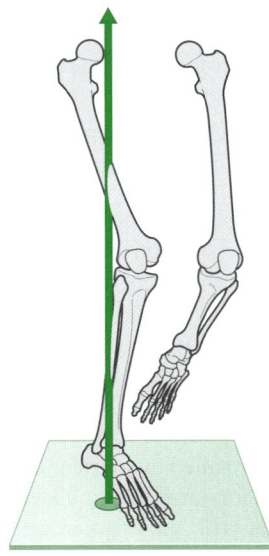

Figure 13.9 Errors in valgus knee measurements due to internal rotation.

Rotational stability in the coronal plane

CORONAL PLANE KNEE STABILITY DURING WALKING IN KNEE OSTEOARTHRITIS

The importance of the coronal plane of movement of the knee was highlighted by Kowalk et al.,[10] who reported that, although the knee abduction–adduction moment is not in the primary plane of motion, it should not be ignored when assessing the stability and function of the knee.

One example of this is knee osteoarthritis, which affects the medial compartment far more than the lateral compartment of the knee joint with an estimated 10:1 ratio between the occurrence of medial compartment to lateral compartment knee osteoarthritis. This has been attributed to the mechanics of the knee in the coronal plane, with particular areas of concern being the greater loading on the medial compartment during gait,[11–13] with between 60% and 80% of total load at the knee passing through the medial compartment.[14]

The load distribution between the medial and lateral compartments is to be expected since medial compartment knee osteoarthritis is closely associated with a knee varus deformity which will give rise to an external adduction moment at the knee throughout stance (Fig. 13.10).

The knee adduction moment is the product of the ground reaction force passing medial to the knee joint centre of rotation in the coronal plane. The knee adduction moment has therefore been used in many biomechanical studies of knee osteoarthritis as an indirect measure of medial joint loading.[15,16] In a comparison of normal and medial compartment knee osteoarthritis adduction moments Kim et al.[17] found a significant difference in the adduction moment between the osteoarthritis group and an age- and gender-matched normal group, with the medial compartment knee osteoarthritis group having on average a 50% increase in their adduction moments (Fig. 13.11).

Whether the knee starts in a varus position that leads to the adduction moment, which will then exacerbate the varus deformity, or whether the presence of an adduction moment causes the varus deformity is unclear. However, the importance of the varus deformity and knee adduction moment on the mechanics of medial compartment knee osteoarthritis is clear.[11–19]

ALIGNMENT CORRECTION DUE TO SURGICAL MANAGEMENT

There are several surgical approaches to the management of medial compartment knee osteoarthritis. These include total knee arthroplasty (TKA), unicompartment knee replacement and high tibial osteotomy (HTO). The aim of all these procedures is to reduce excessive loading on the medial compartment of the knee by correcting varus deformity, thereby reducing pain and improving function. In all surgical procedures, the focus is on obtaining the best possible anatomical realignment of the pathological joint (Fig. 13.10), which in turn aims to reduce the knee adduction moments to that of a pain- and pathology-free knee (Fig. 13.11).

Mandeville et al.[20] investigated the effect of total knee replacement on the knee varus angle and adduction moments during walking pre- and postoperatively and compared with healthy control subjects. During level walking the knee varus angle of the patient group was significantly greater than controls at pre-surgery. However, post surgery the coronal plane knee angle was restored to similar values to the healthy control, with a mean reduction after surgery of approximately 4°. The mean knee adduction moment of the patient group also showed a significant reduction between pre- and post surgery of 25%, which also restored the surgical group to similar values to the healthy controls. Mandeville et al.[20] also found a significant correlation between the change in the coronal knee angle and adduction moments during level walking and described the critical effect of knee alignment on the knee adduction moments in subjects undergoing total knee replacement.

Briem et al.[21] studied the effects of the amount of valgus correction using HTO for medial compartment knee osteoarthritis. Physical function improved significantly overall. However, those subjects whose knee alignment was further away from the group's postoperative mean tended to improve less than those closer to the mean and have higher adduction moments 1 year after surgery. This illustrates the importance of correct alignment during

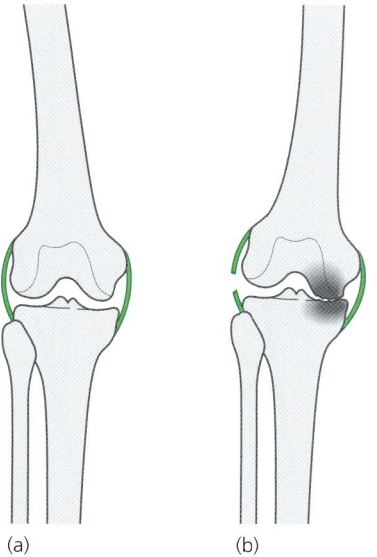

Figure 13.10 Loading on the ligamentous structures and condyles (a) in a pain- and pathology-free knee and (b) in a knee with medial compartment osteoarthritis.

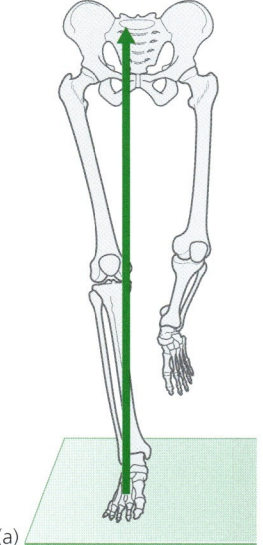 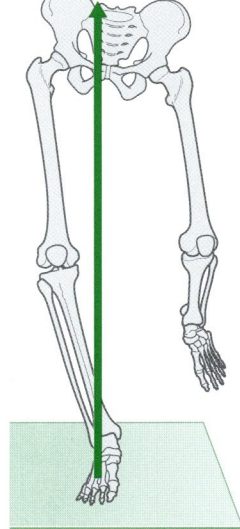

Figure 13.11 Knee adduction moments in (a) a pain- and pathology-free individual and (b) an individual with medial compartment knee osteoarthritis.

surgery and its relevance to adduction moments, joint loading and clinical outcome scores.

DIRECT AND INDIRECT ORTHOTIC MANAGEMENT

Knee braces (direct orthotic management) and wedged insoles (indirect orthotic management) are becoming popular orthotic approaches to managing medial compartment osteoarthritis.

Valgus bracing in knee osteoarthritis

The use of valgus bracing in the management of knee osteoarthritis has been a point of debate for some time. To determine the effect of osteoarthritis bracing we will consider the immediate effect of an individual walking with and without a valgus brace[20,22–28] (Fig. 13.12).

The aims of knee valgus braces are to unload the painful compartment, through bending moments applied proximally and distally to the knee joint, and reducing the varus deformity.[23] Several studies have been conducted into the use of valgus knee braces for medial compartment osteoarthritis, and have reported that patients experience significant pain relief and an improvement in physical function[24–28] and also a reduction in medial compartment load.[22,29]

Lateral wedging of the foot in knee osteoarthritis

Another conservative treatment that has been suggested is the use of lateral wedging of the foot. A lateral wedged insole has a thicker lateral border and applies a valgus moment to the heel, attempting to move it into an everted position. It has been theorized that by changing the position of the ankle and subtalar joints during weight bearing the lateral wedges may apply a valgus moment across the knee as well as the rear foot. In essence, this is achieved by moving the centre of pressure laterally on the foot and therefore reducing the moment arm of the ground reaction force at the knee (Fig. 13.13).

Lateral wedging has been shown to significantly decrease the knee adduction moment in subjects with medial compartment osteoarthritis using laterally wedged insoles.[30–33] However, Kakihana et al.[34] found some inconsistency in knee varus moment reduction. With such indirect management of the knee, many biomechanical factors come into play, including the position of the centre of pressure, the medial ground reaction force, the loading of the ligaments around the ankle, the foot type and foot contact area.

Transverse plane knee stability

The tibiofemoral and patellofemoral joints are often considered in terms of flexion/extension control and stability, as they are part of the knee extensor mechanism. However, the knee is clearly not a simple hinge mechanism and its stability should be considered in all three anatomical planes, sagittal (flexion/extension), coronal (abduction/adduction) and transverse (internal/external rotation).

The nature of much surgical and conservative management of joints focuses on the transverse or torsional stability. One example is the conservative management of the patellofemoral pain, which often uses taping or bracing. Most bracing and taping techniques aim to control the patella in the coronal and transverse planes. Selfe et al.[8,35]

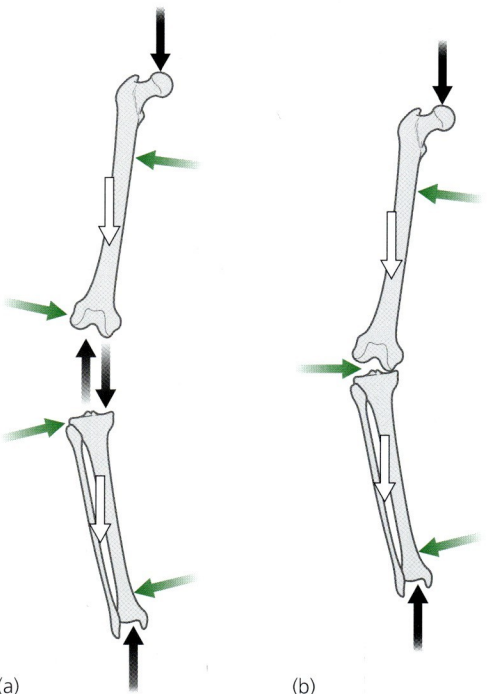

Figure 13.12 Osteoarthritis bracing force system for the lower limb. (a) Combined segments and (b) three-point force system.

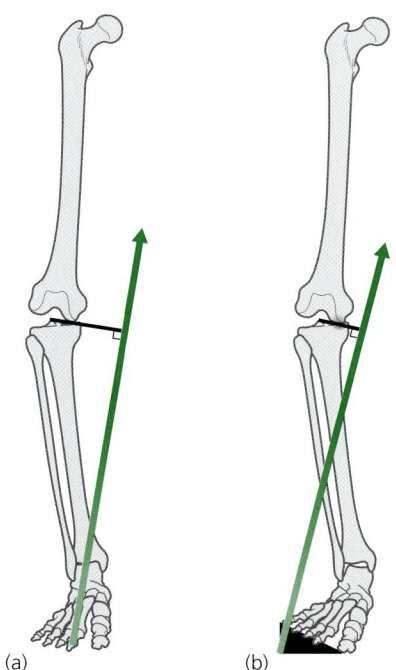

Figure 13.13 (a and b) Mechanics of lateral wedging for medial compartment osteoarthritis.

between 60% and 80% of total load at the knee passing through the medial compartment.[14]

The load distribution between the medial and lateral compartments is to be expected since medial compartment knee osteoarthritis is closely associated with a knee varus deformity which will give rise to an external adduction moment at the knee throughout stance (Fig. 13.10).

The knee adduction moment is the product of the ground reaction force passing medial to the knee joint centre of rotation in the coronal plane. The knee adduction moment has therefore been used in many biomechanical studies of knee osteoarthritis as an indirect measure of medial joint loading.[15,16] In a comparison of normal and medial compartment knee osteoarthritis adduction moments Kim et al.[17] found a significant difference in the adduction moment between the osteoarthritis group and an age- and gender-matched normal group, with the medial compartment knee osteoarthritis group having on average a 50% increase in their adduction moments (Fig. 13.11).

Whether the knee starts in a varus position that leads to the adduction moment, which will then exacerbate the varus deformity, or whether the presence of an adduction moment causes the varus deformity is unclear. However, the importance of the varus deformity and knee adduction moment on the mechanics of medial compartment knee osteoarthritis is clear.[11–19]

ALIGNMENT CORRECTION DUE TO SURGICAL MANAGEMENT

There are several surgical approaches to the management of medial compartment knee osteoarthritis. These include total knee arthroplasty (TKA), unicompartment knee replacement and high tibial osteotomy (HTO). The aim of all these procedures is to reduce excessive loading on the medial compartment of the knee by correcting varus deformity, thereby reducing pain and improving function. In all surgical procedures, the focus is on obtaining the best possible anatomical realignment of the pathological joint (Fig. 13.10), which in turn aims to reduce the knee adduction moments to that of a pain- and pathology-free knee (Fig. 13.11).

Mandeville et al.[20] investigated the effect of total knee replacement on the knee varus angle and adduction moments during walking pre- and postoperatively and compared with healthy control subjects. During level walking the knee varus angle of the patient group was significantly greater than controls at pre-surgery. However, post surgery the coronal plane knee angle was restored to similar values to the healthy control, with a mean reduction after surgery of approximately 4°. The mean knee adduction moment of the patient group also showed a significant reduction between pre- and post surgery of 25%, which also restored the surgical group to similar values to the healthy controls. Mandeville et al.[20] also found a significant correlation between the change in the coronal knee angle and adduction moments during level walking and described the critical effect of knee alignment on the knee adduction moments in subjects undergoing total knee replacement.

Briem et al.[21] studied the effects of the amount of valgus correction using HTO for medial compartment knee osteoarthritis. Physical function improved significantly overall. However, those subjects whose knee alignment was further away from the group's postoperative mean tended to improve less than those closer to the mean and have higher adduction moments 1 year after surgery. This illustrates the importance of correct alignment during

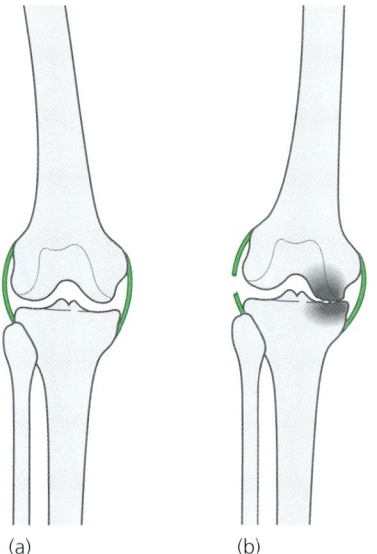

Figure 13.10 Loading on the ligamentous structures and condyles (a) in a pain- and pathology-free knee and (b) in a knee with medial compartment osteoarthritis.

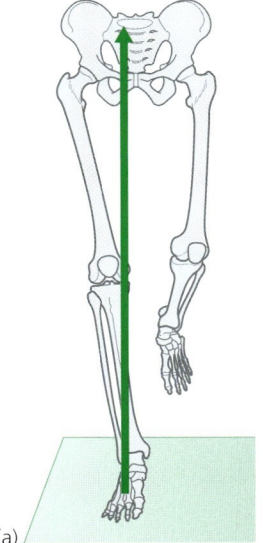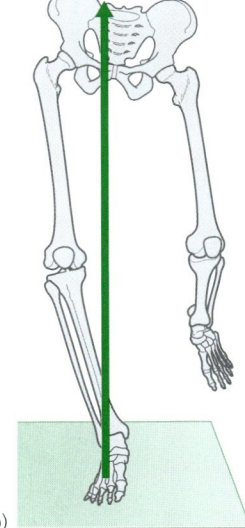

Figure 13.11 Knee adduction moments in (a) a pain- and pathology-free individual and (b) an individual with medial compartment knee osteoarthritis.

surgery and its relevance to adduction moments, joint loading and clinical outcome scores.

DIRECT AND INDIRECT ORTHOTIC MANAGEMENT

Knee braces (direct orthotic management) and wedged insoles (indirect orthotic management) are becoming popular orthotic approaches to managing medial compartment osteoarthritis.

Valgus bracing in knee osteoarthritis

The use of valgus bracing in the management of knee osteoarthritis has been a point of debate for some time. To determine the effect of osteoarthritis bracing we will consider the immediate effect of an individual walking with and without a valgus brace[20,22–28] (Fig. 13.12).

The aims of knee valgus braces are to unload the painful compartment, through bending moments applied proximally and distally to the knee joint, and reducing the varus deformity.[23] Several studies have been conducted into the use of valgus knee braces for medial compartment osteoarthritis, and have reported that patients experience significant pain relief and an improvement in physical function[24–28] and also a reduction in medial compartment load.[22,29]

Lateral wedging of the foot in knee osteoarthritis

Another conservative treatment that has been suggested is the use of lateral wedging of the foot. A lateral wedged insole has a thicker lateral border and applies a valgus moment to the heel, attempting to move it into an everted position. It has been theorized that by changing the position of the ankle and subtalar joints during weight bearing the lateral wedges may apply a valgus moment across the knee as well as the rear foot. In essence, this is achieved by moving the centre of pressure laterally on the foot and therefore reducing the moment arm of the ground reaction force at the knee (Fig. 13.13).

Lateral wedging has been shown to significantly decrease the knee adduction moment in subjects with medial compartment osteoarthritis using laterally wedged insoles.[30–33] However, Kakihana et al.[34] found some inconsistency in knee varus moment reduction. With such indirect management of the knee, many biomechanical factors come into play, including the position of the centre of pressure, the medial ground reaction force, the loading of the ligaments around the ankle, the foot type and foot contact area.

Transverse plane knee stability

The tibiofemoral and patellofemoral joints are often considered in terms of flexion/extension control and stability, as they are part of the knee extensor mechanism. However, the knee is clearly not a simple hinge mechanism and its stability should be considered in all three anatomical planes, sagittal (flexion/extension), coronal (abduction/adduction) and transverse (internal/external rotation).

The nature of much surgical and conservative management of joints focuses on the transverse or torsional stability. One example is the conservative management of the patellofemoral pain, which often uses taping or bracing. Most bracing and taping techniques aim to control the patella in the coronal and transverse planes. Selfe et al.[8,35]

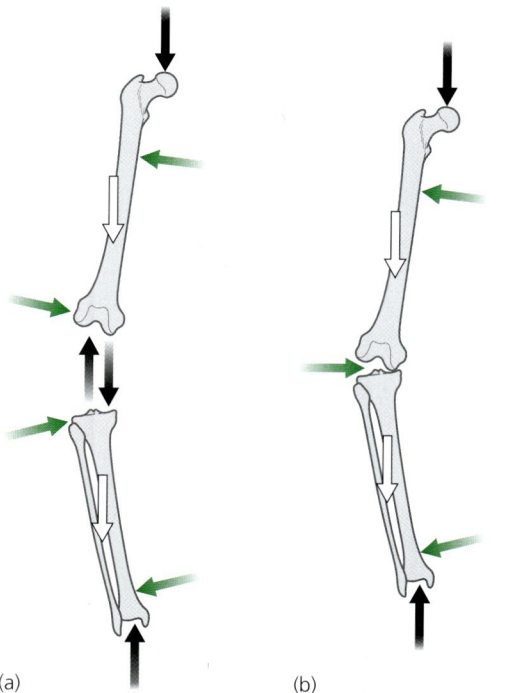

Figure 13.12 Osteoarthritis bracing force system for the lower limb. (a) Combined segments and (b) three-point force system.

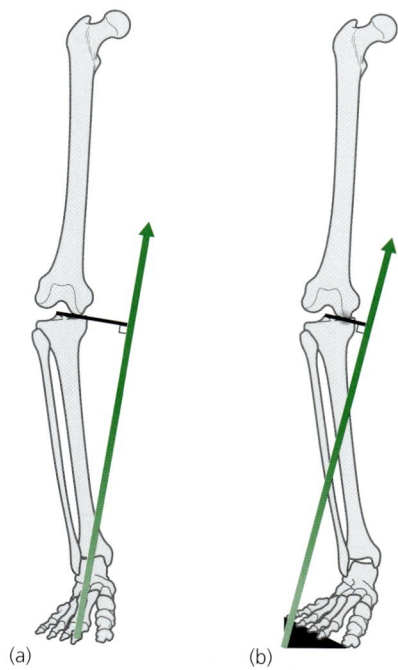

Figure 13.13 (a and b) Mechanics of lateral wedging for medial compartment osteoarthritis.

showed that patellofemoral bracing and taping have a significant effect on the coronal and torsional mechanics of the knee, which had not been previously identified. This led to an eccentric step descent with considerably more control with bracing showing more torsional and coronal plane control than taping.

Translational stability

The balance of the recruitment between the quadriceps and the hamstring muscles is crucial to functional knee stability. However, quadriceps activity may in fact contribute to anterior cruciate ligament injury as quadriceps contraction has been shown to increase anterior cruciate ligament strain between 10° and 30° of knee flexion.[37] One mechanism for the increase in anterior cruciate ligament strain is the balance of the muscle power between the hamstrings relative to the quadriceps. If the quadriceps produce a larger anterior force relative to the posterior force from the hamstrings then this would produce an anterior shear and pull the tibia forwards as the quadriceps overpower the hamstrings. Such an anterior draw would lead to the pre-stressing of the anterior cruciate ligament; the hamstrings are often referred to as 'stress shielders'. According to mechanical calculations, an eccentric quadriceps muscle contraction can in fact produce forces beyond those required for anterior cruciate ligament tensile failure.[38] It is also well established that open-chain quadriceps extension exercises should be avoided during the early postoperative period to prevent harmful stress to the anterior cruciate ligament graft.[39] This again suggests that any imbalance between quadriceps and hamstrings can lead to anterior/posterior instability.

ANTERIOR/POSTERIOR DRAW TESTING

Much has been written on the use of anterior drawer testing to diagnose a tear of the anterior cruciate ligament. This test looks for translational movement between the tibia and femur (Fig. 13.14b).

Figure 13.14c demonstrates the nature of the anterior drawer test and how it relates to anterior cruciate ligament translational dysfunction.

MANAGEMENT OF THE ANTERIOR CRUCIATE LIGAMENT-DEFICIENT KNEE

Surgical reconstruction of the anterior cruciate ligament aims to replace the ligament with either an artificial ligament or, more commonly, with a graft harvested from the central third of the patellar tendon or a hamstrings tendon. This rebalances the internal forces in the knee and gives translational stability back to the knee (Fig. 13.14).

Another treatment which aims to regain translational stability is anterior cruciate ligament bracing. Anterior cruciate ligament bracing has a similar end functional goal to surgical management; however, this is achieved by applying an external system of forces, which aims to replace the forces from the anterior cruciate ligament and to return translational stability to the knee (Fig. 13.15).

MUSCLE STRENGTH TESTING

Considerations for muscle testing

One way in which we often talk about muscle and joint performance is strength, or the capacity to resist force. However, a better way of thinking about muscle strength is the amount of force a particular muscle or muscle group can produce. When evaluating muscle strength, the measures taken are not directly measuring the actual strength of the muscle or muscle group, and what is usually recorded is the effective moment being produced by the muscle. Therefore, most measures taken in the clinical setting do not go as far as to estimate actual muscle forces. However, there are a number of methods of indirect evaluation. Indirect evaluation of the force produced by a muscle can be influenced, however, by a number of factors; each method has its own advantages and disadvantages (Table 13.1).

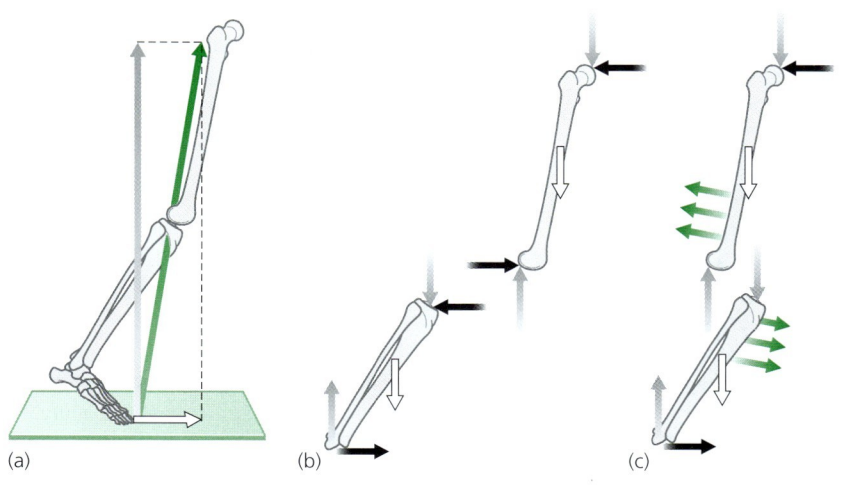

Figure 13.14 (a) Ground reaction forces and (b) internal ligament forces. (c) Force system with an anterior cruciate ligament-deficient knee.

(a) (b) (c)

Methods of objective assessment

CLINICAL METHODS OF MUSCLE TESTING

The Oxford scale is a common clinical assessment method for muscle strength. The Oxford scale classifies muscle strength using the following criteria:

0 = No contraction
1 = Flicker of a contraction
2 = Active movement with gravity eliminated
3 = Active movement against gravity
4 = Active movement against light resistance
5 = Full functional strength (full range of motion against strong resistance).

The aim of the Oxford scale is to assess the functional ability of an individual. Scores 0–3 give a very useful functional progression by assessing if the individual can

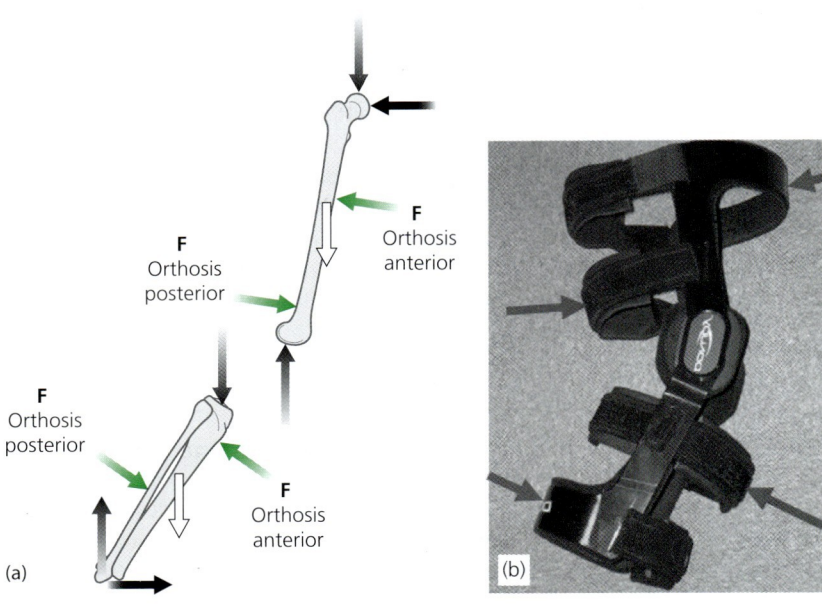

Figure 13.15 (a) Four-point force system to achieve translational stability. (b) 4Titude Ligament Knee Brace, DJO Inc.

Table 13.1 Advantages and disadvantages of the clinical methods of measuring muscle performance

	Advantages	Disadvantages
Oxford scale	No cost or equipment required Minimal training required Ease and speed of testing	Subjectivity of tester No data storage Insensitive to small changes
Free weights and springs	Relatively inexpensive Relatively portable Ease of testing Minimal training required Able to test through a range of motion	The initial weight has to be determined by trial and error No data storage
Hand-held dynamometers	Relatively inexpensive Minimal training required Objective data Highly portable Ease and speed of testing Intratester and intertester reliability moderate to high (Bohannon 1990)	Limited or no data storage Results dependent on strength of tester Static testing only
Isokinetic dynamometers	Objective data Intratester and intertester reliability high Data storage and processing functions Multiple variables assessed Able to test through a range of motion	High cost Intensive training required Not portable Time required for setting up Testing at low speeds (30°/s or less) has the potential to cause overload and injury

support the weight of a limb against gravity; however, care must be taken that the body segments are constantly placed to ensure a consistent and 'correct' effect due to the weight of the body segment, and associated muscle action. Scores 3–5, however, are open to considerable variability as the exact definition of light resistance and strong resistance will vary from clinician to clinician. The position of the applied load on the body segments will be variable and will depend on the length of the body segment and the position the clinician chooses to offer the resistance, and also the velocity with which the joint moves. This leads to difficulties in the comparison of assessments using the Oxford scale between different clinicians and the individuals tested.

FREE WEIGHTS AND SPRINGS

DeLorme is credited with introducing the concept of repetition maximum (RM) in 1945.[40] RM is defined as the weight that can be moved a given number of times and no more; therefore a 1 RM is the maximum amount of weight that can be lifted once whereas a 10 RM is the maximum weight that can be lifted 10 times.

The use of spring balances to measure muscle strength is also clinically popular and is incorporated into a number of standardized functional assessment protocols; one of the best known examples of these is the Constant Score for the shoulder.[41]

HAND-HELD DYNAMOMETERS

A wide variety of these relatively inexpensive and portable instruments are available. They comprise a variety of force-detecting systems including hydraulics, springs, load cells and strain gauges. Similar to testing when using the Oxford scale, care is required in the positioning of the force sensors on the body segments to ensure repeatable and useful measurements. Bohannon (1990) stated that, when using hand-held dynamometers, it is particularly important that the dynamometer should be placed perpendicular to the tested limb. It is also very important that the tester stabilizes the tested limb appropriately during the test in order to prevent unwanted substitution movements. Clear explanation of test procedures is also required and an opportunity to practise is also crucial and should be standardized. Clinicians should however be aware of the potential for greater patient discomfort during break tests than make tests and should use appropriate clinical reasoning to inform their decision as to which type of test is appropriate to conduct for individual patients.

ISOKINETIC AND ISOMETRIC TESTING

The use of isokinetics allows for a standardized assessment by controlling, or presetting, the angular velocity and measuring the resistance that can be produced by an individual. In controlling the angular velocity and measuring the resistance, muscle power produced becomes easy to calculate. Isokinetics machines also allow concentric, eccentric and isometric moments (commonly referred to as torque in isokinetics) and concentric and eccentric power to be measured separately.

MUSCLE BALANCE/IMBALANCE

It is often important to assess the balance between antagonist muscle groups. To assess this balance, the peak torque or peak power of the two muscle groups can be found and a ratio calculated. A common ratio to see quoted is the concentric/concentric hamstring/quadriceps ratio or HQ ratio. It is well documented that the HQ ratio is approximately 0.67:1, the hamstrings being two-thirds of the strength of the quadriceps in normal subjects. However, in many sporting activities one muscle group may be disproportionately trained and this may lead to an imbalance between the antagonist muscles. The HQ ratio gives a measure of this muscle imbalance. This may be found for any antagonistic pair of muscles. A low HQ ratio indicates a reduced capacity of the hamstrings relative to the quadriceps and would mean that there is more likelihood of anterior shear of the tibia forwards as the quadriceps overpowers hamstrings. Such an anterior draw would lead to the pre-stressing of the anterior cruciate ligament. It is interesting to note that professional soccer players have very well-developed quadriceps, but also often have relatively poor defined hamstrings, leading to a very low HQ ratio. Therefore, this imbalance between quadriceps and hamstrings, should be considered as one of the possible risk factors for both anterior cruciate ligament injury and hamstring tears.

MUSCLE ACTION

What is EMG?

Nerve impulses cause twitch responses in muscle fibres, and these combined cause the bulk contractions of a muscle. The electromyogram (EMG) signal itself is the electrical signal associated with the contraction of a muscle. The signal is produced by the depolarizing of motor units, often referred to as motor unit action potential. This electrical signal is usually proportional to the level of the muscle activity, or motor unit activity, although this does not obey the same relationship for the different types of contraction. An EMG is sometimes also referred to as a myogram. EMGs can be used to detect abnormal muscle electrical activity in many diseases and conditions. An EMG is a record of the electrical activity of muscles. The threshold of the signal is often used to give information as to whether the muscle is firing or not. The threshold is often determined by measuring the noise amplitude and finding the value of 2 or 3 standard deviations of the noise; this will include 95% or 99.7% of the noise amplitude

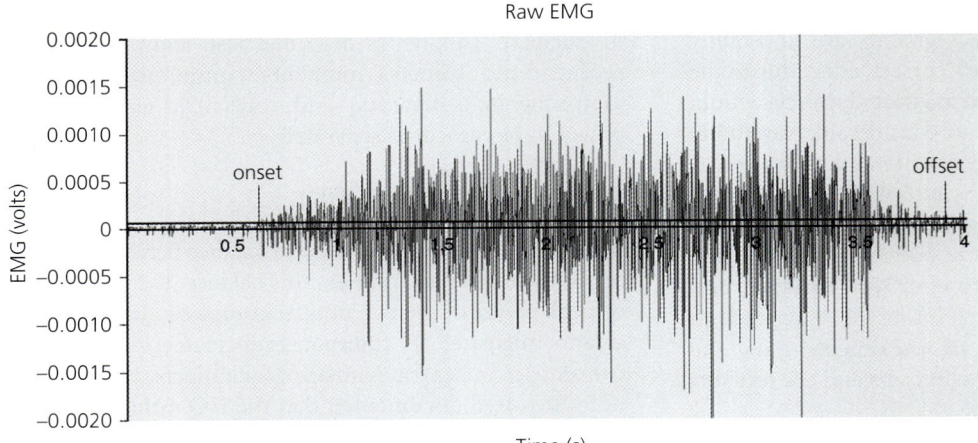

Figure 13.16 Onset and offset using raw electromyogram.

respectively. This gives an on/off measurement of whether the muscle is active or not, or muscle activity onset and offset. This is by far the most common clinical use of EMG (Fig. 13.16).

Clinical EMG and biofeedback

The term biofeedback was first coined in 1969 by a group of workers who went on to found the Biofeedback Society of America. They defined biofeedback as 'the use of appropriate instrumentation to bring covert physiological processes to the conscious awareness of one or more individuals'.[41]

Biofeedback provides instant feedback as to whether an exercise is performed correctly. This is particularly useful when the exercises are not easy to perform. With the use of biofeedback the patient can be taught much more quickly what a particular muscle contraction feels like. This is particularly important as it enables them to take that sensation away with them out of the clinic, so when they perform the exercise at home they know exactly what it feels like. This instant feedback is especially useful in the early stages of rehabilitation.

During neurological or stress rehabilitation programmes, we often require the patient to relax more. In this case the threshold of the EMG signal is reduced, therefore increasing the sensitivity; this is called negative shaping. More commonly used in musculoskeletal work is positive shaping, whereby the threshold of the EMG signal is increased as the patient progresses. This elicits a stronger contraction in order to reach the required level of feedback, therefore making the patient work harder using this process.

PROPRIOCEPTION

What is proprioception?

Proprioception is a broad term describing a range of complex sensorimotor or neuromuscular control parameters.

> **BOX 13.1: Components of proprioception**
>
> - Detection of movement from joints (joint position sense)
> - Sensation of force and contraction
> - Sensation of body segment orientation
> - Sensation of whole body orientation
> - Kinaesthesia is a constituent of proprioception; it is a combined sense of movement from a variety of anatomical structures
>
> Based on Williams and Krishnan[49] and Lephart et al.[43]

It is not a description of any individual sensory modalities (Box 13.1).

Lephart and Fu[44] define proprioception as 'the acquisition of stimuli from conscious and unconscious processes in the sensorimotor system'. Proprioception can be appreciated and measured consciously by a complex system involving a variety of neural receptors known as mechanoreceptors; these are thought to mediate the sensations of kinaesthesia and joint position sense (JPS) (Table 13.2).

It is interesting to consider Table 13.2 as traditionally cutaneous receptors have not been thought to play a significant role in joint stability. However, the table shows that five out of the eight receptors thought to be involved in proprioception are found distributed in the skin. Sensory feedback through the skin may therefore have a greater importance than previously assumed. A number of studies, particularly of the knee, have provided evidence which supports this case. Prymka et al.[45] found significant differences between 43 patellofemoral pain syndrome (PFPS) patients and 30 healthy control subjects in isolated JPS testing of the knee. The poor proprioceptive performance associated with PFPS was improved after applying a simple elastic bandage. A proposed mechanism for this finding was that the bandage stimulated rapidly adapting superficial receptors in the skin during joint motion and increased pressure on the underlying muscles and joint capsule. Proprioceptive deficits have been found in

Table 13.2 Mechanoreceptors involved in proprioception

Receptor type	Location	Stimulus
Ruffini ending	Capsule, ligament, menisci, skin	Stretch, strain
Pacinian corpuscle	Capsule, ligament, menisci, fat pads, skin	Compression
Golgi tendon organ-like	Capsule, ligament, menisci	Strain
Free nerve ending	Capsule, ligament, menisci, skin	Nociceptive
Muscle spindle	Throughout whole muscle	Stretch
Golgi tendon organ	Musculotendinous junction	Strain
Meissner's corpuscles	Skin	Deformation caused by light touch
Merkel's discs	Skin	Continuous pressure

Based on Williams and Krishnan.[42]

- anterior cruciate-deficient knees[46]
- osteoarthritic knees[47,48]
- knees with chronic effusion[49]
- patellofemoral dislocation[50]
- patellofemoral pain syndrome.[51]

Functional relevance of proprioception

Proprioception is thought to play a more significant role than pain in preventing injury in the aetiology of chronic injury and in degenerative joint disease (Box 13.2).[52]

Assessment of deficit in proprioception

There are many methods for testing proprioceptive acuity; one of the most common is to use isokinetic dynamometers (Box 13.3). Using this type of equipment is beneficial as isokinetic dynamometers are often available in clinical environments. Performing joint position sense testing usually involves isolating individual joints, which although providing a high degree of control during testing and accuracy of results is sometimes criticized due to its non-functional nature. Common proprioceptive tests are listed in Box 13.3.

BOX 13.2: Factors leading to decreased proprioceptive acuity

- Inherited predisposition
- Joint effusion
- Joint pain
- Muscle atrophy
- Decreased cutaneous sensitivity
- Older age

Based on Williams and Krishnan[42] and Callaghan and Selfe et al. 2002.

BOX 13.3: Common proprioceptive tests

- Passive angle reproduction
- Active angle reproduction
- Threshold to detect passive motion

SUMMARY

The principles of kinesiology give a series of techniques to investigate the severity of pathological joint function and provide a framework for joint assessment. From these techniques we are able to determine

- objective measures that are relevant to the ICF
- quality and performance of individual joint movement patterns during functional tasks
- joint control and stability and relate this to functional deficits
- muscle function by considering the action of muscle groups through strength testing and individual muscle function using EMG
- functional deficits due to lack of proprioception.

This arsenal of methods can provide useful information in the assessment of the efficacy and effectiveness of surgical and conservative management. However, much care needs to be taken to determine which of these methods and associated measures are appropriate to measure or record factors which are directly clinically relevant. So the questions that we should ask before any tests are conducted are 'What do we need to know?', 'What does this method actually tell us?' and 'How does this inform clinical practice?'. With this in mind kinesiology may be used to investigate important clinical questions and provide a significant contribution to clinical assessment and research.

KEY LEARNING POINTS

- Kinesiology provides important objective measures which are relevant to the International Classification of Function, Disability and Health.
- The principles of kinesiology provide methods of assessment of joint control and stability during functional tasks.
- Muscle strength and power can be assessed using indirect methods and individual muscle function may be assessed directly using an electromyogram.
- Proprioception is a complex system involving mechanoreceptors and cutaneous receptors; these play a significant role in preventing injury and should be assessed.

FURTHER READING

Callaghan MJ, Selfe J, Bagley PJ, and Oldham JA. The effects of Patellar taping on knee joint proprioception. *Journal of Athletic Training* 2002; **37(1)**:19-24.

Jeysevar DS, Riley PO, Hodge WA, Krebs DE. Knee kinematics and kinetics during locomotoractivities of daily living in subjects with knee arthroplasty and in healthy control subjects. *Physical Therapy* 1993;**73**:229-242.

Bohannon RW. Hand-held compared with isokinetic dynamometry for measurement of static knee extension torque (parallel reliability of dynamometers). *Clinical Physics and Physiological Measurement* 1990;**11(3)**: 217-222.

Selfe J, Thewlis D, Hill S, Whitaker J, Sutton C, Richards J. A clinical study of the biomechanics of step descent using different treatment modalities for patellofemoral pain. *Gait and Posture* 2011;**34(1)**:92-6.

REFERENCES

1. World Health Organization. *International Classification of Functioning, Disability and Health*. Geneva, Switzerland: World Health Organization, 2001.
2. Mittrach R, Grill E, Walchner-Bonjean M, et al. Goals of physiotherapy interventions can be described using the International Classification of Functioning, Disability and Health. *Physiotherapy* 2008;**94**:150-7.
3. Greenhalgh S, Selfe J. *Red Flags 2: Clinical cases of serious spinal pathology*. Edinburgh, UK: Churchill and Livingstone, 2009.
4. Ellenbecker S, Davies GJ. *Closed Kinetic Chain Exercise*. Champaign, IL: Human Kinetics, 2001.
5. Steindler A. *Kinesiology of the Human Body*. Springfield, IL: Charles Thomas, 1955.
6. Palmitier RA, An KN, Scott SG, Chao EY. Kinetic chain exercise in knee rehabilitation. *Sports Medicine* 1991;**11**:402-13.
7. Doucette SA, Child DD. The effect of open and closed chain exercise and knee joint position on patellar tracking in lateral patellar compression syndrome. *Journal of Orthopaedic and Sports Physical Therapy* 1996;**23**: 104-10.
8. Selfe J, Richards J, Thewlis D, Kilmurray S. The biomechanics of step descent under different treatment modalities used in patellofemoral pain. *Gait and Posture* 2008;**27**:258-63.
9. Richards JD, Pramanik A, Sykes L, Pomeroy VM. A comparison of knee kinematic characteristics of stroke patients and age-matched healthy volunteers. *Clinical Rehabilitation* 2003;**17**:565-71.
10. Kowalk D, Duncan J, Vaughan C. Abduction–adduction moments at the knee during stair ascent and descent. *Journal of Biomechanics* 1996;**29**:383-8.
11. Andriacchi TP. Dynamics of knee malalignment. *Orthopaedic Clinics of North America* 1994;**25**:395-403.
12. Baliunas AJ, Hurwitz DE, Ryals AB, et al. Increased knee joint loads during walking are present in subjects with knee osteoarthritis. *Osteoarthritis and Cartilage* 2002;**10**:573-9.
13. Hurwitz DE, Ryals AB, Case JP, et al. The knee adduction moment during gait in subjects with knee osteoarthritis is more closely correlated with static alignment than radiographic disease severity, toe out angle and pain. *Journal of Orthopaedic Research* 2002;**20**:101-7.
14. Schipplein OD, Andriacchi TP. Interaction between active and passive knee stabilizers during level walking. *Journal of Orthopaedic Research* 1991;**9**:113-19.
15. Prodromos CC, Andriacchi TP, Galante JO. A relationship between gait and clinical changes following high tibial osteotomy. *Journal of Bone and Joint Surgery (American)* 1985;**67**:1188-94.
16. Goh JC, Bose K, Khoo BC. Gait analysis study on patients with varus osteoarthrosis of the knee. *Clinical Orthopaedics and Related Research* 1993;**294**:223-31.
17. Kim WY, Richards J, Jones RK, Hegab A. A new biomechanical model for the functional assessment of knee osteoarthritis. *The Knee* 2004;**11**:225-231.
18. Crenshaw SJ, Pollo FE, Calton EF. Effect of lateral-wedged insoles on kinetics of the knee. *Clinical Orthopaedics and Related Research* 2000;**375**:185-92.
19. Hurwitz DE, Sumner DR, Andriacchi TP, Sugar DA. Dynamic knee loads during gait predict proximal tibial bone distribution. *Journal of Biomechanics* 1998;**31**: 423-30.
20. Mandeville D, Osternig LR, Lantz BA, et al. The effect of total knee replacement on the knee varus angle and moment during walking and stair ascent. *Clinical Biomechanics (Bristol, Avon)* 2008;**23**:1053-8.
21. Briem K, Ramsey DK, Newcomb W, et al. Effects of the amount of valgus correction for medial compartment knee osteoarthritis on clinical outcome, knee kinetics and muscle co-contraction after opening wedge high tibial osteotomy. *Orthopaedic Research* 2007;**25**: 311-18.

22. Jones RK, Nester CJ, Kim WY, et al. Direct and Indirect Orthotic Management of Medial Compartment Osteoarthritis of the Knee. ESMAC & GCMAS meeting, Amsterdam, 25–30 September, 2006.
23. Pollo FE. Bracing and heel wedging for unicompartmental osteoarthritis of the knee. American Journal of Knee Surgery 1998;**11**:47–50.
24. Hewett TE, Noyes FR, Barber-Westin SD, Heckmann TP. Decrease in knee joint pain and increase in function in patients with medial compartment arthrosis: a prospective analysis of valgus bracing. Ortopedica 1998;**21**:131–8.
25. Kirkley A, Webster-Bogaert S, Litchfield R, et al. The effect of bracing on varus gonarthrosis. Journal of Bone and Joint Surgery (American) 1999;**81A**:539–48.
26. Lindenfeld TN, Hewett TE, Andriacchi TP. Joint loading with valgus bracing in patients with varus gonarthrosis. Clinical Orthopaedics and Related Research 1997;**344**:290–7.
27. Matsumo H, Kadowaki K, Tsuji H. Generation II knee bracing for severe medial compartment osteoarthritis of the knee. Archives of Physical Medicine and Rehabilitation 1997;**78**:745–9.
28. Richards JD, Sanchez-Ballester J, Jones RK, et al. A comparison of knee braces during walking for the treatment of osteoarthritis of the medial compartment of the knee. Journal of Bone and Joint Surgery (British) 2005;**87**:937–9.
29. Pollo FE, Otis JC, Backus SL, et al. Reduction of medial compartment loads with valgus bracing of the osteoarthritic knee. American Journal of Sports Medicine 2002;**23**:496–502.
30. Keating EM, Faris PM, Ritter MA, Kane J. Use of lateral heel and sole wedges in the treatment of medial osteoarthritis of the knee. Orthopaedic Review 1993;**19**:921–4.
31. Toda Y, Segal N, Kato A, et al. Effect of a novel insole on the subtalar joint of patients with medial compartment osteoarthritis of the knee. Journal of Rheumatology 2001;**28**:2705–10.
32. Shimada S, Kobayashi S, Wada M, et al. Effect of disease severity on response to lateral wedged shoe insole for medial compartment knee osteoarthritis. Archives of Physical Medicine and Rehabilitation 2006;**87**:1436–51.
33. Butler RJ, Marchesi S, Royer T, Davis JS. The effect of a subject-specific amount of lateral wedge on knee mechanics in patients with medial knee osteoarthritis. Journal of Orthopaedic Research 2007;**25**:1121–7.
34. Kakihana W, Akai M, Nakazawa K, et al. Inconsistent knee varus moment reduction caused by a lateral wedge in knee osteoarthritis. American Journal of Physical Medicine and Rehabilitation 2007;**86**:446–54.
35. Selfe J, Thewlis D, Hill S, et al. A clinical study of the biomechanics of step descent using different treatment modalities for patellofemoral pain. Gait and Posture 2011;**348(17)**:92–6.
36. Boden BP, Dean GS, Feagin JA Jr, Garrett WE Jr. Mechanisms of ACL injury. Orthopedics 2000;**23**:573–8
37. Woo SL, Hollis JM, Adams DJ, et al. Tensile properties of the human femur-anterior cruciate ligament-tibia complex: the effects of specimen age and orientation. American Journal of Sports Medicine 1991;**19**:217–25.
38. Wilk KE, Escamilla RF, Fleisig GS, et al. A comparison of tibiofemoral joint forces and electromyographic activity during open and closed kinetic chain exercises. American Journal of Sports Medicine 1996;**24**:518–27.
39. Wilk K. Dynamic muscle strength testing. In: Amundsen LT (ed.) Muscle Strength Testing Instrumented and Non-Instrumented Systems. New York, NY: Churchill Livingstone: Chapter 5.
40. Consant CR, Murley AHG. A clinical method of functional assessment of the shoulder. Clinical Orthopaedics and Related Research 1987;**214**:160–4.
41. Wolff SL. Essential considerations in the use of EMG biofeedback. Physical Therapy 1978;**58**:25.
42. Williams GN, Krishnan C. Articular neurophysiology and sensorimotor control. In: Magee DJ, Zachewski JE, Quillen WS (eds) Scientific Foundations and Principles of Practice in Musculoskeletal Rehabilitation. St Louis, MO: Saunders, 2007: Chapter 9.
43. Lephart SM, Perrin DH, Fu FH, et al. Relationship between selected physical characteristics and functional capacity in the anterior cruciate ligament-insufficient athlete. Journal of Orthopaedic and Sports Physical Therapy 1992;**16**:174–81.
44. Lephart SM, Fu FH. Proprioception and Neuromuscular Control in Joint Stability. Champaign, IL: Human Kinetics, 2000.
45. Prymka M, Schmidt K, Jerosch J. Proprioception in patients suffering from chondropathia patellae. International Journal of Sports Medicine 1998;**19**:S60.
46. Beynnon BD, Ryder SH, Konradsen L, et al. The effect of anterior cruciate ligament trauma and bracing on knee proprioception. American Journal of Sports Medicine 1999;**27**:150–5.
47. Sharma L, Pai YC, Holtkamp K, Rymer WZ. Is knee joint proprioception worse in the arthritic knee versus the unaffected knee in unilateral knee osteoarthritis? Arthritis and Rheumatism 1997;**40**:1518–25.
48. Hewitt BA, Refshauge KM, Kilbreath SL. Kinesthesia at the knee: the effect of osteoarthritis and bandage application. Arthritis and Rheumatism 2002;**47**:479–83.
49. Guido J Jr, Voight ML, Blackburn TA, et al. The effects of chronic effusion on knee joint proprioception: a case study. Journal of Orthopaedic and Sports Physical Therapy 1997;**25**:208–12.
50. Jerosch J, Prymka M. Knee joint proprioception in patients with posttraumatic recurrent patella dislocation. Knee Surgery, Sports Traumatology, Arthroscopy 1996;**4**:14–18.

51. Baker V, Bennell K, Stillman B, et al. Abnormal knee joint position sense in individuals with patellofemoral pain syndrome. *Journal of Orthopaedic Research* 2002;**20**:208–14.

52. Lephart SM, Henry TJ. Functional rehabilitation for the upper and lower extremity. *Orthopaedic Clinics of North America* 1995;**26**:579–92.

14

Infections of the musculoskeletal system

SURESHAN SIVANANTHAN, EUGENE SHERRY

Introduction	219	Septic arthritis	225
Soft-tissue infections	219	References	227
Osteomyelitis	221		

NATIONAL BOARD STANDARDS

- Understand the pathogenesis and pathological anatomy of osteomyelitis and septic arthritis
- Know the presentation, salient features, investigations, differential diagnosis, treatment, complications and sequelae

INTRODUCTION

Infections in the bones, joints and muscles are acute, chronic or granulomatous. Granulomatous infection is a 'catch all' term used to describe evidence of prior or inactive infection that results in the formation of granulomas which wall off the substances that the immune system perceives as foreign but is unable to eliminate. In histological terms, an important feature of granulomas is whether or not they contain necrosis (mass of dead cells without nuclei). The presence of necrosis indicates that the granuloma has an infective cause. Two types of necrosis have been identified – caseous, which describes the appearance as being 'cheese-like', and non-caseous. In the musculoskeletal system, caseous necrosis usually indicates the presence of tuberculosis (TB). Other infections characterized by granulomas include histoplasmosis, cryptococcosis, coccidiomycosis, blastomycosis, leprosy and cat scratch disease. Non-infectious causes of granulomas include sarcoidosis, Crohn disease, Wegener disease, Churg–Strauss syndrome and pulmonary rheumatoid nodules.

Musculoskeletal infections encountered by orthopaedic surgeons include soft-tissue infections, osteomyelitis and joint infections (septic arthritis). These infections have specific pathophysiologies, particular characteristics and specific organisms that are associated with each infection.

One must be aware of the most likely organism found in particular types of infection so that therapy can be guided (Table 14.1).

SOFT-TISSUE INFECTIONS

The usual soft-tissue infections are cellulitis and wound infection. The resulting acute inflammation usually presents with the five cardinal signs described over 2000 years ago by Celsus and later by Galen, who added the fifth sign. These are pain, heat, redness, swelling and loss of function of the affected part. Acute inflammation is initiated and sustained by neutrophils, macrophages, lymphocytes, plasma cells, eosinophils and the substances that they release. Other important soft-tissue infections are summarized in Table 14.1.

The most common organisms found in cellulitis are *Staphylococcus aureus*, *Staphylococcus epidermidis* and *Streptococcus pyogenes*. Wound infections following surgery can develop from a wide variety of pathogens, most commonly *S. aureus* and *S. epidermidis*. Meticillin-resistant *S. aureus* and *Pseudomonas aeruginosa* are also increasingly common nosocomial infections. Wound infections also occur with open fractures, with the incidence of infection related to the grade of injury.

Table 14.1 Types of infection and antibiotics used to treat them (may differ according to local antibiotic policy)

Soft-tissue Problem	Tissues involved	Clinical features	Microbes	Treatment
Cellulitis	Subcutaneous	Erythema, tenderness, warm, glands swollen	Group A *Streptococcus* and *Staphylococcus aureus*	PRSPs (nafcillin, oxacillin)
Erysipelas	Superficial, demarcated	As above	Diabetics, above plus Enterobacteriaceae and clostridia	
Necrotizing fasciitis (**life threatening**)	Muscle fascia	Aggressive, associated with vascular disease such as diabetes. Occurs after trauma, surgery and streptococcal skin infections	Group A, C and G *Streptococcus*, *Clostridium*, polymicrobial infections (aerobic and anaerobic), MRSA	Urgent, extensive debridement and intravenous antibiotics. Penicillin G (for *Streptococcus* and clostridia), imipenem, cilastatin, meropenem (for polymicrobial). Vancomycin for MRSA
Gas gangrene	Muscle, where gross contamination, especially if closed too early	Severe pain, swelling, foul-smelling, discharge. Toxaemia, crepitus. Radiographs show widespread gas	*Clostridium perfringens*, *Clostridium specticum* and other *Clostridium* spp. produce toxic exotoxins	Debridement, fasciotomies, hyperbaric oxygen, clindamycin and penicillin G (or ceftriaxone and erythromycin)
Toxic shock syndrome	Toxaemia from colonization of wounds	Septic shock, erythematous macular rash	Toxins from *S. aureus* or group A, B, C, G *Streptococcus*, *Streptococcus pyogenes*	Irrigate, debride, PRSPs (or cephalosporins) For *Streptococcus* clindamycin, penicillin G and intravenous immune globulin
Surgical wound infection	Varies		Usually *S. aureus*, groups A, B, C, G *Streptococcus*, Enterobacteriaceae MRSA increasing VMRSA has also been reported	Vancomycin. For VMRSA, consider using quinupristin, linezolid, daptomycin
Marine injuries		History of fishing or other marine activity. Positive cultures may be difficult	Indolent infections. *Vibrio vulnificus* or atypical mycobacterium (e.g. *Mycobacterium marinarum*)	Use ceftazidime for *V. vulnificus* (doxycycline for penicillin allergy or in addition to ceftazidime). Alternatives include cefotaxime or ciprofloxacin *M. marinarum* is best treated with the standard drugs, which are rifampicin + ethambutol

MRSA, meticillin-resistant *Staphylococcus aureus*; PRSP, penicillinase-resistant synthetic penicillin; VMRSA, vancomycin-meticillin-resistant *Staphylococcus aureus*.
Adapted from Miller MD (ed.). *Miller's Review of Orthopaedics*, 5th edn. Philadelphia, PA: Elsevier Saunders, 2008:Table 1–40, p. 84.

Table 14.2 Mechanism of action of common antibiotics

Antibiotic class	Mechanism of action
β-Lactam antibiotics (e.g. penicillin, cephalosporin)	Inhibition of cell wall synthesis (via binding to the penicillin-binding proteins on the surface of the bacterial cell membrane)
Aminoglycosides (e.g. gentamicin)	Inhibition of protein synthesis (by binding to cytoplasmic rRNA)
Macrolides (e.g. erythromycin, clarithromycin)	Binds 50s ribosomal subunit and prevents transfer of RNA during translocation
Rifampicin	Inhibits DNA-dependent RNA polymerase, thus inhibiting RNA synthesis in bacteria
Tetracyclines	Inhibit protein synthesis on 70s and 80s ribosomes
Glycopeptides (e.g. vancomycin, teicoplanin)	Prevent insertion of glycan subunits into cell wall
Quinolones (ciprofloxacin, levofloxacin)	Inhibit DNA gyrase
Oxazolidinones (e.g. linezolid)	Inhibit protein synthesis by blocking formation of the 70s ribosomal translation complex
Polyenes (amphotericin, nystatin)	Interact with ergosterol in cell membranes, forming a transmembrane channel that leads to ion leakage causing fungal cell death
Metronidazole	Selectively absorbed by anaerobic bacteria where it causes DNA strand breakage and degradation

Management

Patients are usually admitted for intravenous antibiotics, which can be converted to oral antibiotics once the infection shows signs of resolution. The classes of commonly used antibiotics are listed in Table 14.2. Deep infection requires surgical debridement of all non-viable tissue and may require the application of a vacuum dressing (or packing of the wound) to allow healing by secondary intention. Bleeding is the key characteristic of viable tissue. Bone infection is discussed in more detail in the section Osteomyelitis, and deep infection following total joint arthroplasty is discussed in more detail in Part 9.

OSTEOMYELITIS

Definitions

- *Osteomyelitis* is defined as infection of bone or bone marrow. The infection can be a direct inoculation (e.g. open fracture) or blood borne (haematogenous). Note that deep cultures are usually required to diagnose the causative organism for chronic osteomyelitis.
- *Sequestrum* is a term used almost exclusively in osteomyelitis and is a fragment of necrotic (usually cortical) bone found at the nidus of the infection within bone. These fragments usually begin as part of the cortex and are surrounded by pus and infected granulation tissue.
- *Involucrum* (from *volvere*, to wrap) is when reactive bone is newly formed at the interface between diseased bone and healthy tissue. Radiographically, it appears as newly formed radiodense bone around the radiolucent sequestrum.
- *Glycocalyx* is a mucopolysaccharide biofilm synthesized by bacteria and is produced freely once it has assisted bacterial adhesion to a solid substrate such as necrotic bone, surgical implants or a foreign body.[1,2] This biofilm provides a mechanical barrier to antibodies, antibiotics and phagocytosis while allowing the bacteria to thrive.[1,3]

Classification

The classification is based upon the timing of the onset and method of spread.

ACUTE HAEMATOGENOUS OSTEOMYELITIS

This is caused by blood-borne organisms and is most common in children (boys more often than girls) and is covered in detail in Chapter 35. In adults aged over 21, *S. aureus* is the commonest cause of acute haematogenous osteomyelitis. In patients with sickle cell anaemia, *Salmonella* is the usual cause of acute haematogenous osteomyelitis and the causative organisms in patients who are intravenous drug abusers are usually *S. epidermidis* and *P. aeruginosa* (Table 14.1).

ACUTE OSTEOMYELITIS

Acute osteomyelitis occurs after direct inoculation, usually following an open fracture (Chapter 17) or open reduction with internal fixation. Clinical findings include a rapid presentation of pain, temperature, redness and a non-healing soft-tissue envelope and, occasionally, the classic draining sinus tract with abscess formation. Inflammatory markers will be raised and, as with acute haematogenous osteomyelitis, C-reactive protein (CRP) is the most sensitive marker of the course of infection as it has a short half-life and decreases about a week after effective treatment. Deep infection in the presence of a fracture fixation implant requires surgical debridement of all non-viable tissue as inadequate debridement is the commonest cause of failure of infection control.[4] Bleeding is the key characteristic of viable tissue. Viable bone is characterized by punctuate bleeding ('paprika sign'). Inadequate debridement results in recurrence of infection despite antibiotic therapy because non-viable or infected tissue is secluded from the microcirculation, which results in biofilm formation, thus protecting pathogens from antibiotics and host defence mechanisms.[3] Specimens of purulent fluid, soft tissue and bone from the affected area are sent for aerobic and anaerobic cultures. Skeletal stabilization of ununited fractures is necessary for the control of infection, but the presence of internal fixation implants encourages the formation of biofilm, which protects the infective organisms. Thus, the decision to retain or remove infected implants is individualized and depends on several factors, including the location of the fracture, the status of bone healing and whether or not the implant is providing stability (Fig. 14.1). If the fracture is unstable in the early postoperative period, retention of internal fixation is useful to maintain fracture reduction and stability. Management in this case includes irrigation and debridement as usual but also brushing of the implant to mechanically remove biofilm, and the administration of specific antibiotics. Loose hardware not providing stability should be removed and the fracture stabilized by other means, for example with an external fixator, which can be used until the infection has resolved and definitive stabilization can be performed. Alternatively, if the fracture was fixed with an intramedullary rod, exchange nailing with reaming of the medullary canal should be performed. An open wound may require plastic surgical input and local or free muscle flaps to achieve soft-tissue coverage.

CHRONIC OSTEOMYELITIS

The commonest causes of chronic osteomyelitis are poorly treated acute osteomyelitis, trauma or soft-tissue spread, especially in the immunosuppressed host (Cierny type C).

Cierny's anatomical classification of adult chronic osteomyelitis is shown in Fig. 14.2. Published in 1985, the Cierny–Mader classification of adult osteomyelitis is the first system to articulate treatment with the natural history of the disease. In this system, the biofilm nidus is characterized by one of four anatomical types whose complexity and associated risk for treatment failure escalate numerically (Fig. 14.2). In type I, medullary osteomyelitis, the nidus is endosteal, whereas in type II, superficial osteomyelitis, it is confined to an outer surface of bone that remains exposed, usually unprotected by a refractory, soft-tissue deficit. Localized osteomyelitis, type III, is a well-marginated sequestration of an attached or floating fragment of bone, often combining the features of both types I and II osteomyelitis. In localized osteomyelitis, the entire nidus can be excised with a wide margin without causing the osseous segment to become unstable. In type IV lesions, diffuse osteomyelitis, the process is permeative and involves a segment of bone

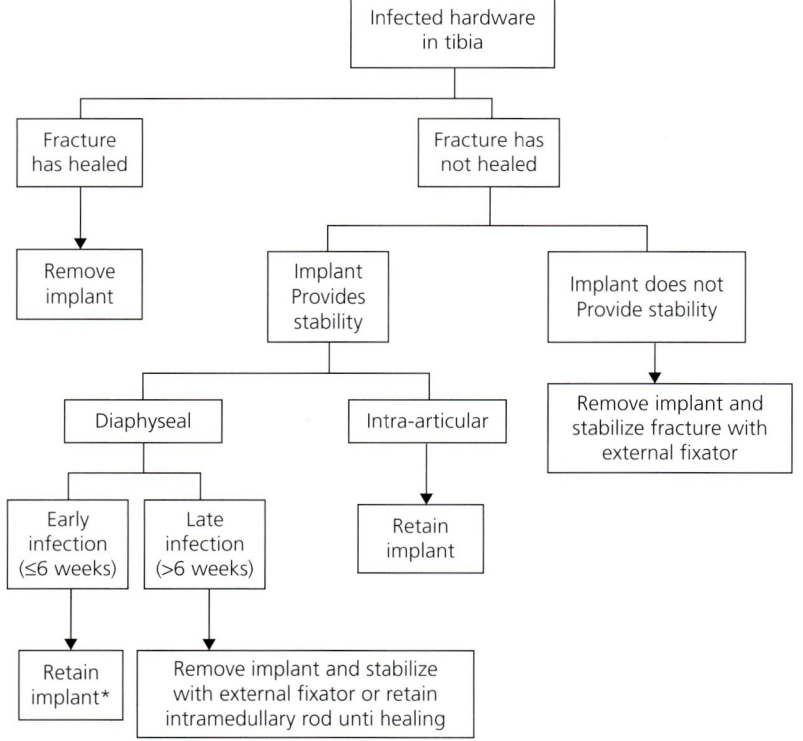

Figure 14.1 Algorithm for removing or retaining infected hardware in patients with chronic osteomyelitis of the tibia. Asterisk, intramedullary abscess formation and discharge may require removal of an intramedullary rod.

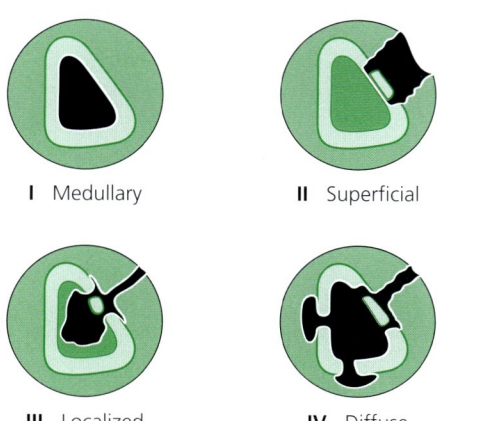

Figure 14.2 Cierny's anatomical classification of adult chronic osteomyelitis. There are four anatomical types of osteomyelitis, matched with their respective treatment formats and components of their reconstruction. Adapted from Cierny G III. Chronic osteomyelitis: results of treatment. *Instructional Course Lectures* 1990;**39**:495–508.

Table 14.3 Cierny's infected host types

Type	Description	Risk
A	Normal immune response, non-smoker	Minimal
B	Local or mild systemic deficiency, smoker	Moderate
C	Major nutritional or systemic disorder	High

and/or an entire joint and it often exhibits characteristics of types I, II and III. Type IV lesions are mechanically unstable either before and/or after a complete and thorough debridement. Examples for each anatomical type include the following: type I, haematogenous osteomyelitis, or an infected fracture union following medullary stabilization; type II, full-thickness wounds resulting from pressure or venous stasis ulcers; type III, infected fracture union with butterfly fragment sequestration or previous plate fixation; and type IV, periprosthetic infections, chronic septic arthritis or infected non-unions. In this same system, the patient host is stratified with regard to his or her physiological capacity to detour infection, withstand treatment and/or benefit from cure.

Cierny's infected host types are shown in Table 14.3.

Skin and soft tissues are often involved and squamous cell carcinoma may develop in sinus tracts. Quiescence may be followed by exacerbations.

Diagnosing chronic osteomyelitis requires a careful history and examination followed by special tests, including radiographs, CT scans, which help delineate the extent of bony involvement, and scintigraphy, which can be used as a diagnostic tool as well as a gauge of response to treatment. The gold standard for diagnosing infection remains isolation of pathogens in culture.[3] Gram stains of specimens may also be helpful, but prior administration of antibiotics or improper handling of specimens may preclude the growth of the correct pathogens. Multiple deep intra-operative samples are required to diagnose the pathological organism. These samples should include sinus tract material, purulent fluid, soft tissue, curetted bone and the bed of the involved bone. Common organisms include *S. aureus*, Enterobacteriaceae and *P. aeruginosa*.

The tibia is the commonest site of infected non-union and chronic post-traumatic osteomyelitis.[5] Approximately 10% of open tibial fractures result in chronic osteomyelitis.[6] In contrast, the infection rate following intramedullary nailing of closed tibial fractures is approximately 1%.[7]

Management is long and difficult and involves culture-specific intravenous antibiotics, adequate debridement and removal of hardware (Fig. 14.1). As discussed above, biofilm formation is the key in the development and persistence of infection in chronic osteomyelitis[8] as the biofilm shields the infecting micro-organisms from antibiotics and the immune system. Local antibiotic delivery in carriers such as polymethylmethacrylate cement or calcium sulphate pellets has also shown good results in a number of studies. Adequacy of debridement remains the most important clinical predictor of success;[4] therefore, adopting an oncological approach to complete excision is important. Once infection is resolved, reconstruction can then be performed using a variety of methods (distraction osteogenesis or vascularized bone graft, etc.). It is also important to evaluate the soft-tissue envelope and the neurovascular and functional status of the extremity along with patient factors (smoking, immune compromise, etc.) during the pre-operative evaluation. Therefore, proper patient selection and staging are vital in ensuring a successful outcome. The ideal dosing regimens for intravenous antibiotics vary and it is important to follow local hospital guidelines. Again, local or free muscle flaps may be necessary to achieve soft-tissue coverage.

UNUSUAL EXPRESSIONS OF OSTEOMYELITIS

Subacute osteomyelitis

This may arise as a result of poorly treated acute osteomyelitis and, rarely, can develop in a fracture haematoma. It may present as an incidental finding on radiographs where a Brodie's abscess is seen as a localized radiolucency in the metaphyses of long bones. The differential diagnosis in children would include Ewing's sarcoma. The white cell count (WCC) and blood cultures are frequently normal. However, the erythrocyte sedimentation rate (ESR) may be raised and deep bone cultures may give a positive result. Subacute osteomyelitis may cross the physis. Epiphyseal osteomyelitis is caused almost exclusively by *S. aureus* and requires surgical drainage if pus is present. The treatment of subacute osteomyelitis includes surgical drainage and intravenous antibiotics followed by 6 weeks of oral antibiotics once the levels of inflammatory markers have decreased.

Chronic sclerosing osteomyelitis

First described by Garre in 1891, chronic sclerosing osteomyelitis involves the diaphysis of long bones of adolescents, symmetrical thickening of the cortex and narrowing of the medulla. Radiographs show a dense progressive sclerosis. It has an insidious onset and malignancy must be ruled out. Where pain is persistent, either drilling multiple holes or guttering the bone may result in resolution of symptoms.

Chronic multifocal osteomyelitis

Chronic multifocal osteomyelitis is described in children, has no systemic symptoms and, except for a raised ESR, other markers are normal. Radiographs show multiple metaphyseal lytic lesions (medial clavicle, distal tibia, distal femur) and the condition resolves spontaneously.

Osteomyelitis with unusual organisms

It is important to know the characteristics of infections with syphilis and TB.

Syphilis

Syphilitic infections of bone can be congenital or acquired, and, in the latter, are more serious in the tertiary stage. Syphilis differs from bone TB in that the shaft is more frequently involved whereas the joints escape. In TB, it is the other way round – there is destruction on both sides of a joint. Radiographs in syphilitic infection show metaphyseal lucency. The inflammation is a result of infection with *Treponema pallidum*, which may be demonstrated in biopsies 36 hours after infection and prior to the appearance of clinical evidence of disease. The tibia, femur, humerus and the cranial bones are the most common sites of syphilitic osseous disease (Fig. 14.3). The bone pain in syphilis usually occurs at night and is not relieved by salicylates. Blood serological tests will confirm the diagnosis and appropriate antibiotics are rapidly effective. Diffuse osteoperiostitis is a chronic inflammation affecting the whole bone inside its periosteal envelope. Radiographs show a double outline that is very characteristic of syphilis. This is usually a bilaterally symmetrical polyostotic lesion affecting tubular bones (Fig. 14.3). Syphilitic dactylitis most commonly affects the proximal phalanx of the index finger or thumb. More than one finger may be affected and results in marked shortening and deformity. Open sores may form as the lesion consists of a gummatous osteomyelitis. The patient usually presents with other signs of congenital syphilis, and complete recovery is possible with appropriate antibiotic treatment.

Tuberculosis

There has been a steady decline in the incidence of bone and joint TB in developed countries over the years, but TB is still a major cause of death and disability in developing countries. Two-thirds of the world's population live in countries defined as 'developing' by World Health Organization standards.[9] With the resurgence of immunosuppression owing to HIV infection, TB infection rates have increased in many parts of the world. Bacille Calmette–Guérin (BCG) vaccination carried out in school children aged 10–14 years has gone a long way towards decreasing the incidence of TB. Infection of a bone or joint with *Mycobacterium tuberculosis* is nearly always secondary to an infection from some other area, usually the lymphatic glands at the root of the lung, or the mesentery. Spread to the bone is usually haematogenous, but occasionally can be from a neighbouring joint or from infected soft tissues. Spinal TB (>50% of skeletal TB) is covered in Chapter 63.

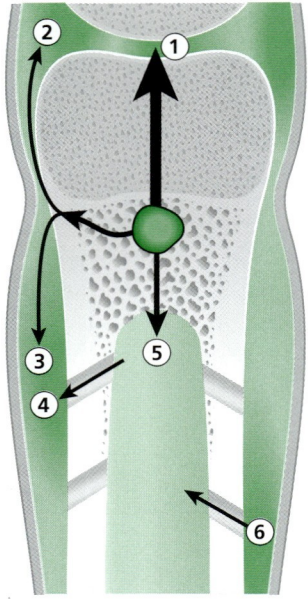

Figure 14.3 Methods of spread of osteomyelitis.

- *Natural history.* The disease progresses slowly and caseation usually occurs. Ultimately, the pus extends peripherally and a subperiosteal abscess forms. If the disease is not controlled, the periosteum bursts open and tuberculous debris is extruded into the soft tissues or joints. The skin overlying the abscess then reddens but is not warm to the touch; hence, the term 'cold abscess'. The skin then becomes progressively thinner and finally yields, forming a tuberculous sinus. If this sinus is then superinfected with pyogenic organisims, the prognosis is grave.
- *Diagnosis.* Ziehl–Neelsen staining is used to identify acid-fast bacilli in the aspirate or excised tissues. A positive Mantoux test is of significance only up to the age of 3 or 4 years, after which time 50% of the population give a positive reaction. On the other hand, a negative Mantoux reaction does not preclude active bone or joint TB. Traditionally, Lowenstein–Jensen medium has been used to culture *M. tuberculosis*, but newer automated systems (e.g. Bactec MGIT 960) give faster and more accurate results. Polymerase chain reaction is very sensitive and can distinguish *M. tuberculosis* from other mycobacteria.
- *Radiographic appearance.* The earliest sign may be a decalcification or localized area of diminished density. This is followed by an increased joint space and irregularity of the joint outline. The later films show a gross destructive lesion of the joint with absorption of bone, loss of continuity of the joint and subluxation or dislocation. With healing, there is gradual replacement and condensation of bone but any gross deformity persists. CT scans and MRI are particularly useful in determining the size and extent of the bony lesion and its soft-tissue component.
- *Treatment.* Treatment strategies are divided into local treatment of the lesion and systemic chemotherapy. The traditional triple chemotherapy regime is still used as it discourages the emergence of resistant strains. The Medical Research Council has funded a succession of controlled clinical trials in Masan and Pusan, South Korea; Hong Kong; Bulawayo, Zimbabwe; and Madras, India, where guidelines were laid down for the management of spinal TB (more details are given in Chapter 63):
    - The standard drugs were potent for florid spinal TB in children and bed rest was not necessary (Masan, Korea).
    - Streptomycin is not necessary and a plaster of Paris jacket offers no benefit (Pusan, Korea; MRC 1973b).
    - Debridement is not a good operation. Clinical diagnosis assisted with radiographs was sufficient to start the treatment, as was later confirmed by histopathology and/or bacteriology in 83% of patients (Bulawayo, Zimbabwe).
    - Radical anterior excision is a better operation with positive HP and/or bacteriology in 85% of patients (Hong Kong).

Local treatment includes non-operative and operative interventions. The majority of cases can be treated non-operatively. The indications for operative intervention include tuberculous abscess or sinus formation or joint destruction. Non-operative treatment involves reduction of the deformity, and fixation of the joint in the desired position with plaster of Paris. Reduction of a deformed joint is usually achieved by gradual traction.

SEPTIC ARTHRITIS

The incidence of pyogenic septic arthritis peaks in the first few years of life, and more than 50% of cases occur in young children. Also, more than 50% of cases are caused by *S. aureus*. This condition in children is discussed in more detail in Chapter 35.

Septic arthritis is a surgical emergency that requires prompt surgical wash-out of the joint. Delayed treatment can result in permanent joint damage and long-term disability. Most cases of septic arthritis arise from either direct inoculation as a result of trauma or surgery or contiguous spread from adjacent osteomyelitis. Once the infection starts, release of proteolytic enzymes and inflammatory mediators can result in cartilage damage within 8 hours. In the hip, increased fluid pressure may cause avascular necrosis.

Diagnosis

The patient often appears toxic and the *sine qua non* of this condition is the inability or refusal to move the joint or bear weight, as septic joints have an associated tense effusion, and warmth and any motion causes excruciating pain. The extremity rests in the position that maximizes the volume of the joint involved; in the case of the hip, this results in flexion, abduction and external rotation (the 'FABER' position). Laboratory findings include a raised WCC with a left shift in up to 60% of individuals, elevated ESR and CRP. Blood cultures are often positive as well. Plain radiographs may show an increased joint space and ultrasound of the hip will confirm the presence of an effusion which can be aspirated. Joint aspiration will yield pus-coloured fluid, which should be sent for cell count with differential, Gram stain and culture. The following signs are important diagnostic predictors of septic arthritis (in decreasing order of significance): (1) fever >38.5°C, (2) elevated CRP and ESR, (3) refusal to bear weight and (4) elevated WCC.

Differential diagnosis

The differential diagnosis includes reactive arthritis, arthritis associated with gonorrhoea, inflammatory bowel disease, gastroenteritis or Reiter syndrome, TB, Lyme disease, viral arthritis, syphilis, brucellosis and haemophilia.

Tuberculous arthritis presents in a more insidious fashion and has no associated leucocytosis. The patient may present with complete limitation of joint movement. Radiographs, however, are characteristic and help to differentiate this condition from pyogenic septic arthritis. The other tests for TB will also be positive.

The incidence of gonococcal arthritis in modern times is rare, but worth knowing about. It usually develops in sexually active adults aged between 20 and 30 and manifests during the third week of the infection. It is five times more common in men than in women and occasionally may occur in newborn babies from the first week onwards. The joint manifestations have a tendency to relapse and recur. The main aetiological factor is untreated gonorrhoea. The organism is carried through the bloodstream to the affected joint. The disease is monoarticular in 40% of cases but frequently can involve multiple joints. The knee is the most frequently affected joint.

Syphilitic infection of the joints can occur in all stages of the disease and a negative blood serological test for syphilis does not rule out syphilis as the cause of the arthritis. Syphilitic arthritis can occur in congenital syphilis or acquired syphilis later in life. In the early stages, there is joint arthralgia and increased joint effusion. In the later stages, there may be gummatous arthritis, which may further progress to a Charcot joint (also known as tabetic arthropathy).

Treatment

Once joint aspiration has been performed, empirical antibiotics are started (Table 14.1). An arthrotomy is then performed to remove all purulent fluid and irrigate the joint. For the hip the anterolateral approach is preferred to minimize the risk of avascular necrosis. Other joints such as the knee or shoulder may be amenable to arthroscopic drainage and wash-out if suitable equipment and support is available.

> ### KEY LEARNING POINTS
>
> **Osteomyelitis**
>
> - Osteomyelitis is defined as inflammation or infection of bone or bone marrow.
> - Osteomyelitis is most often acute haematogenous, but can also be acute, chronic, subacute, chronic sclerosing, chronic multifocal and from unusual organisms.
> - The infection begins in the sinusoids of the metaphysis and spreads with increased intra-osseous pressure. Periosteal elevation, sequestrum and involucrum may occur.
> - Physical signs include: localized area of tenderness/warmth/erythema at the metaphysis.
> - Investigations include white cell count, blood cultures (positive in 50% of cases), erythrocyte sedimentation rate (ESR) and C-reactive protein (CRP).
> - Radiographic changes include soft-tissue swelling (early), bone demineralization (10–14 days) and, much later, sequestrum (dead bone) and involucrum (periosteal new bone).
> - A firm diagnosis is possible when two of the following four are present:
>   - pus aspirated from the bone
>   - positive bone or blood culture
>   - symptoms of pain/swelling/warmth/decreased range of motion
>   - raised inflammatory markers.
> - Treatment consists of identifying the organism, selecting the right antibiotic and getting the antibiotics to the site, surgical treatment if indicated, and limiting tissue destruction.
> - In chronic osteomyelitis, multiple deep samples are required to diagnose the pathological organism.
> - In acute osteomyelitis, removal of metalwork may be required.
> - For soft-tissue injuries the most serious infections are gas gangrene and necrotizing fasciitis. Both require extensive debridement, fasciotomies and the right antibiotics.
> - Other types include: subacute osteomyelitis (e.g. Brodie's abscess), chronic sclerosing osteomyelitis, chronic multifocal osteomyelitis and from unusual organisms.
>
> **Septic arthritis**
>
> - Septic arthritis is a pyogenic bacterial infection of a joint.
> - It may result from haematogenous infection of the synovium, spontaneous decompression of a contiguous osteomyelitis, direct inoculation from trauma (in the neonate metaphyseal blood vessels extend into the epiphysis across the physis, facilitating spread of infection to the joint by this route).
> - It presents with acute pain, high fever and swelling of the affected joint plus irritability, malaise, anorexia, body ache, limp and pseudoparalysis.
> - There is fever, local warmth, erythema and oedema, tender swelling of the joint and typical positioning of the joint; associated septicaemia may result in generalized constitutional features.
> - Do white blood cell count, ESR and CRP tests.
> - An ultrasound examination is useful and can give 100% sensitivity in diagnosing effusion.
> - Culture of synovial fluid is key to establishing a diagnosis (positive in less than two-thirds of cases).

- *Staphylococcus aureus* is the most common pathogen, then streptococci; *Haemophilus influenzae* type b is declining as a result of vaccination. Neonates are prone to Gram-negative bacilli and group B *Streptococcus*. Patients with sickle cell anaemia are prone to *Salmonella* infection.
- Needs to be differentiated from rheumatoid arthritis and seronegative spondyloarthropathy, toxic synovitis, irritable hip and post-infectious arthritis.
- Osteomyelitis can usually be ruled out by ultrasound examination.
- Septic arthritis is a surgical emergency – treat with arthrotomy and drainage.
- Empirical antibiotic therapy is started after aspiration for culture and then rest the joint.
- Complications are due to delay in treatment or inadequate surgical drainage.

REFERENCES

- ● = Key primary paper
- ◆ = Major review article

●1. Gristina AG, Costerton JW. Bacterial adhesion and the glycocalyx and their role in musculoskeletal infection. *Orthopedic Clinics of North America* 1984;**15**:517.

2. Gristina AG, Costerton JW, Hobgood CD, Webb LX. Bacterial adhesion, biomaterials, the foreign body effect and infection from natural ecosystems to infection in man: a brief overview. *Contemporary Orthopaedics* 1987;**14**:27.

●3. Patzakis MJ, Zalavras CG. Chronic posttraumatic osteomyelitis and infected nonunion of the tibia: current management concepts. *Journal of the American Academy of Orthopaedic Surgeons* 2005;**13**:417–27.

4. Forsberg JA, Potter BK, Cierny G, Webb L. Diagnosis and management of chronic infection. *Journal of the American Academy of Orthopaedic Surgeons* 2011;**19**:S8–S19.

5. Patzakis MJ, Abdollahi K, Sherman R, *et al*. Treatment of chronic osteomyelitis with muscle flaps. *Orthopedic Clinics of North America* 1993;**24**:505–9.

6. Gustilo RB, Anderson JT. Prevention of infection in the treatment of one thousand and twenty five open fractures of long bones: retrospective and prospective analyses. *Journal of Bone and Joint Surgery (American)* 1976;**58**:453–8.

7. Blachut PA, O'Brien PJ, Meek RN, Broekhuyse HM. Interlocking intramedullary nailing with and without reaming for the treatment of closed fractures of the tibial shaft: a prospective randomized study. *Journal of Bone and Joint Surgery (American)* 1997;**79**:640–6.

8. Gristina AG, Costerton JW. Bacterial adherence to biomaterials and tissue: the significance of its role in clinical sepsis. *Journal of Bone and Joint Surgery (American)* 1985;**67**:264–73.

9. Dormans JP, Fisher RC, Pill SG. Orthopaedics in the developing world: present and future concerns. *Journal of the American Academy of Orthopaedic Surgeons* 2001;**9**:289–96.

PART 4

TRAUMA

SURESHAN SIVANANTHAN

15	**Advanced trauma life support and polytrauma**	233
	Peter V Giannoudis, George M Kontakis	
16	**Mass casualty management**	244
	James P Stannard, Michael P Rusnak	
17	**Open injuries of limbs**	247
	Shanmuganathan Rajasekaran, P. Rishi Mugesh Kanna, Jayaramaraju Dheenadhayalan	
18	**Closed treatment of common fractures**	258
	Peter V Giannoudis, Fareed Kagda	
19	**Principles of operative fracture fixation**	269
	Peter V Giannoudis, Costas Papacostidis	
20	**Clinical aspects in acute limb compartment syndrome**	278
	Rajiv Malhotra, Nikolaos Giotakis	

SECTION 1

General considerations

15	**Advanced trauma life support and polytrauma** *Peter V Giannoudis, George M Kontakis*	233
16	**Mass casualty management** *James P Stannard, Michael P Rusnak*	244
17	**Open injuries of limbs** *Shanmuganathan Rajasekaran, P. Rishi Mugesh Kanna, J Dheenadhayalan*	247
18	**Closed treatment of common fractures** *Peter V Giannoudis, Fareed Kagda*	258
19	**Principles of operative fracture fixation** *Peter V Giannoudis, Costas Papacostidis*	269
20	**Clinical aspects in acute limb compartment syndrome** *Rajiv Malhotra, Nikolaos Giotakis*	278

15

Advanced trauma life support and polytrauma

PETER V GIANNOUDIS, GEORGE M KONTAKIS

Introduction	233	Secondary survey	238
Pre-hospital care	234	Specific orthopaedic trauma situations in ATLS	238
Initial assessment – trauma room	235	Operating room – surgical strategy	239
Primary survey	235	References	241
Definition of the patient's condition	237		

NATIONAL BOARD STANDARDS

- Understand the advance trauma life support principles
- Know about multiple organ dysfunction syndrome and systemic inflammatory response syndrome
- Know the different classes of haemorrhage and management thereof
- Know about damage control orthopaedics
- Understand the classification and principles of management of open fractures

INTRODUCTION

Trauma is the leading cause of death particularly in younger people (<45 years old). In the United Kingdom approximately 14 500 deaths per year are attributed to contemporary trauma causes.[1] Polytrauma is a generic term describing the condition of a person who has been subjected to traumatic injuries to more than one body region (head, neck and cervical spine; face, chest and thoracic spine; abdomen and lumbar spine; limbs and bony pelvis; and external (skin).[2] Polytrauma represents 15–20% of the overall trauma population.[3] It constitutes a huge burden on society due to the associated long-term disability and loss of earnings.[4] It is defined as an injury severity score (ISS) ≥16.[5] The ISS is an anatomical scoring system (virtually the only anatomical scoring system in use) that provides an overall score for patients with multiple injuries.[6] It correlates with mortality, morbidity and hospital stay after trauma. Its base is the abbreviated injury scale (AIS).[6] According to the AIS, injuries are ranked on a scale of 1 to 6, with 1 being minor, 2 moderate, 3 serious, 4 severe, 5 critical and 6 an unsurvivable injury. One of these scores is allocated to each of six body regions (head, face, chest, abdomen, extremities (including pelvis), external). Only the highest AIS score in each body region is used. The three most severely injured body regions have their score squared and added together to produce the ISS. The ISS takes values from 0 to 75. If an injury is assigned an AIS score of 6 (unsurvivable injury), the ISS is automatically assigned to 75. Its weaknesses are that any error in AIS scoring increases the ISS error, many different injury patterns can yield the same ISS and injuries to different body regions are not weighted (for example bilateral femoral fractures). Also, as a full description of patient injuries is not known prior to full investigation and operation, the ISS (along with other anatomical scoring systems) is not useful as a triage tool.[5]

Over the years, it has been shown that deaths after severe injury have a trimodal distribution. Approximately 50% of deaths occur immediately at the scene of trauma because of severe neurotrauma or massive haemorrhage. These deaths are reduced by improvements in safety and accident prevention. The second peak (approximately 30% of deaths) occurs during the initial post-injury hours. Within this time frame, deaths can be reduced by the use of a standardized protocol ATLS (advance trauma life support) for the initial assessment and management of polytraumatized patients. The third peak – due to sepsis and multiple organ failure – occurs within 1–2 weeks in the intensive care environment. Advances in critical care have reduced these 'late' deaths.[7]

The pathway of clinical interventions of patients with multiple injuries is unique and requires the involvement of a variety of medical specialties such as paramedics, emergency physicians, radiologists, anaesthetists, intensivists, orthopaedic and trauma surgeons, neurosurgeons, urologists, and cardiothoracic and plastic surgeons.

This pathway of active medical treatment is initiated at the scene of the accident by the paramedics or by a physician, depending on the service provided by the regional and nationally developed trauma systems. Subsequently and following safe transportation of the patient to the nearest medical facility, treatment is continued in the resuscitation room. The different steps of the pathway can be divided as follows: scene of the accident and transport to a medical facility, resuscitation room, diagnostics (radiological investigations), operating theatre, intensive care unit, ward care, in-hospital rehabilitation and discharge home.

In general terms the management of a polytrauma patient can be divided grossly into the pre-hospital phase and the in-hospital one. The chance of survival and the extent of recovery are highly dependent on the medical care that follows the injury. The speed with which lethal processes are identified and halted makes the difference between life and death, recovery and disability. Time is an independent and cynical challenger of any physician managing multiply injured patients. Thus the adopted approach to this peculiar clinical setting should be based on getting most things right and very few things wrong. Owing to the inherent imperfections of the human nature of the medical personnel, this approach should be based on simple and practical principles, well organized and standardized.

Starting from the pre-hospital phases of extrication and transfer to the hospital, the initial evaluation and management, despite its inherent limitations due to lack of time and means, has been proven decisive for the severely injured patient. The effect on survival of early extrication,[8] initial management from trained emergency personnel (physicians or paramedics)[9–11] and, equally importantly, fast transfer to the designated trauma centre[12,13] has been evaluated and highlighted in numerous studies. The introduction and the universal acceptance, primarily, of the ATLS[14] and, to a lesser degree, of the PHTLS[15,16] (pre-hospital trauma life support) protocols have contributed immensely towards an improved and standardized initial evaluation and management of the trauma patient.

Following the principles and the structured initial diagnostic evaluation of the traumatized patient, the priorities of airway, breathing, circulation and disability (neurological deficit) have been proven to be the gold standard. Together with direct triage towards the appropriate health centre, protection of the spine, early aggressive pre-hospital resuscitation, the implications of telemedicine and informatics, advances in the means of transport and the rationalization of the location of trauma centres has resulted in minimizing pre-hospital mortality and achieving mortality rates lower than those predicted by mathematical models.[17,18]

The ATLS protocol of the American College of Surgeons' Committee on Trauma has been developed in the last 30 years and has become globally established, aiming at assessing and managing the patient during the 'early hours' after injury to increase survival.[14] Today, ATLS is the internationally recognized standard for the initial assessment and management of the severely injured patient. It aims to guide the resuscitation and evaluation of trauma patients. The objective is to reduce the mortality rate during the 'golden hour' after injury. It is based on the fact that trauma kills reproducibly in a particular way. Airway damage kills people earlier than loss of breathing, which causes death earlier than circulated blood volume loss, which in turn kills earlier than an expanding intracranial mass. The easily recalled mnemonic 'ABCDE' determines the sequence of priorities that will be followed during the evaluation and management of all patients.

A	Airway maintenance and cervical spine protection
B	Breathing evaluation and maintenance of the respiratory function
C	Circulation evaluation and maintenance, haemorrhage control
D	Disability assessment – neurological examination
E	Exposure removing the patient's clothes and environment control (protection from hypothermia).

PRE-HOSPITAL CARE

The traumatized patient's resuscitation and assessment begins at the site of injury. Usually, the first people at the scene of an accident are not familiar with medicine. Paramedics usually follow. There are certain rules applied in the initial evaluation and management of these patients. In any case, the goal is to get the right patient to the right hospital at the right time.[19] The application of ATLS principles depends on several factors such as the expertise of the field personnel, the patient's condition and the time needed for the transportation of the patient to hospital.[20]

Active airway management as guided by the ATLS requires skilled and experienced paramedics or physicians. This presumes a properly designed trauma care system providing such pre-hospital medical skills.[21] Controversy exists on whether fluid administration in the field is beneficial in such systems. There is a balance between prolonged cellular shock in cases of no intervention, and haemodilution and coagulation disturbances produced by administered intravenous fluids.[22–24] However, things seem different in cases of accidental entrapment, where the time needed for extrication and transportation to hospital is unknown. In such cases, ATLS procedures could be valuable.[5] Protection of the cervical spine as early as possible at the scene of the accident is of paramount importance to minimize the risk of secondary spinal trauma. Immobilization of the rest of the spine can be safely performed by using a long backboard.

INITIAL ASSESSMENT – TRAUMA ROOM

The established trauma team at the receiving hospital is usually notified by the paramedics about the physiological state of the injured patient and the anticipated time of arrival. The trauma team is constantly in a state of alertness and all the necessary preparations in the resuscitation room of the hospital are in place. The initial assessment of the injured patient must have a stepwise approach with planned diagnostic, clinical assessment and operative strategies to avoid mistakes that could have a negative impact on the patient's prognosis. It is well recognized that the clinical course of the patient may change rapidly, and treatment plans must be adapted accordingly.

The ATLS course has had a great impact on providing a common language for all clinical staff who initially manage the injured patient. It has helped to develop an organized and systematic approach for the evaluation and treatment of patients. The primary goal of initial management is to rapidly diagnose and treat immediately life-threatening conditions. These include

- airway obstruction or injury and asphyxia (e.g. laryngeal trauma)
- tension pneumothorax or haemothorax
- open thoracic injury and flail chest
- cardiac tamponade
- massive internal or external haemorrhage.

PRIMARY SURVEY

Airway maintenance and C-spine immobilization

All trauma patients receive 100% oxygen and have the cervical spine protected by a collar. Conditions that may lead to airway obstruction are mandibular or midfacial fractures, direct damage to the larynx or trachea, aspiration of blood or vomit, and foreign bodies. Any accessible obstacle in the airway must be removed and in some cases emergency cricothyroidotomy or tracheostomy may be indicated, although the common practice is endotracheal intubation, which is feasible in the majority of cases where active airway intervention is needed.[25]

Breathing: maintenance of respiration

Disorders of the respiratory system can be diagnosed clinically from symptoms and signs including dyspnoea, cyanosis, stridor, depressed conscious level, abnormal chest expansion and the presence of major thoracic injuries (lung contusion, tension pneumothorax and haemothorax). The management of pneumothorax and haemothorax should include the insertion of a chest drain to decompress the chest. Severe head injury or brain injury secondary to cerebral hypoxia due to severe hypovolaemia can result in respiratory impairment too. Direct cardiac trauma as well as secondary myocardial infarction may lead to pulmonary oedema, which also occurs after thoracic compression. In the patient with severe polytrauma, immediate intubation and ventilation with a tidal volume of $8–10$ mL kg^{-1} body weight, positive end-expiratory pressure of 5 mL and 50% O_2 saturation are prerequisites of adequate ventilation.[25]

Circulation evaluation and maintenance, haemorrhage control

Once the airway and breathing are secured, the next step is to optimize O_2 delivery in the tissues via maximization of the cardiovascular function. Three distinguishable types of shock may be present: cardiogenic, neurogenic and hypovolaemic (the most likely).[14]

CARDIOGENIC SHOCK

Heart dysfunction may be caused by cardiac tamponade, tension pneumothorax, haemothorax or, rarely, intra-abdominal bleeding. Ischaemia or cardiac failure *per se* may cause myocardial infarction. This may be difficult to distinguish from cardiac contusion following blunt anterior thoracic wall trauma. Both conditions in this setting require management of cardiac arrhythmias, so the exact diagnosis does not influence the initial treatment. Hypovolaemia should be restored. Cardiac tamponade needs pericardiocentesis, and tension pneumothorax necessitates urgent placement of a chest drain. In some cases an emergency thoracotomy may be indicated to address the cause of dysfunction.[14]

NEUROGENIC SHOCK

When a spinal cord injury occurs, loss of the sympathetic tone in the distal vessels leads to blood pooling in the periphery and relative hypovolaemia, which is the cause of neurogenic shock. Neurogenic shock does not preclude true hypovolaemia. Classically, neurogenic shock appears with hypotension but without tachycardia or vasoconstriction in the extremities. Failure to reverse shock with intravenous fluid administration means neurogenic shock or ongoing haemorrhage.[14]

HYPOVOLAEMIC SHOCK

This is the most common type of shock in traumatized patients and it is due to the acute loss of blood. Every patient with hypotension must be considered to be in shock, although patients in shock may be normotensive. Hypotension is considered a late manifestation of hypovolaemia in a patient with adequate compensatory mechanisms. Assessment of the nail beds and conjunctiva will reveal diminished peripheral capillary flow, which may be considered as the most sensitive indicator of intravascular volume. Urine output normally should exceed 1 mL kg^{-1} h^{-1}, and is reduced in cases of blood volume loss. It is also a sensitive indicator of shock and can be used to monitor the response of the patient in resuscitation. Other manifestations of haemorrhagic shock are tachycardia, decreased pulse pressure, anxiety, cold and wet extremities.[14]

Hypovolaemic shock can be divided into four stages. In stage 1, there is up to 15% blood volume loss (750 mL). The blood pressure is maintained. Pallor of the skin exists. The respiratory rate is normal, as is mental status and capillary refill. Compensation is achieved by constriction of the vascular bed. In stage 2, there is 15–30% blood volume loss (750–1500 mL). Cardiac output cannot be maintained by arterial constriction. There is increased tachycardia >100 bpm, increased respiratory rate, delayed capillary refill, sweating from sympathetic stimulation and narrow pulse pressure. Stage 3 is characterized by 30–40% blood volume loss (1500–2000 mL). Alteration of mental status is present, and there is sweating with cool, pale skin, delayed capillary refill, marked tachycardia >120 bpm and tachypnoea >30 breaths per minute. The systolic blood pressure falls to 100 mmHg or less and there is also a decrease in urinary output. Finally in stage 4 there is blood volume loss of greater than 40% (>2000 mL). Pronounced tachypnoea and tachycardia are present. The systolic blood pressure is 70 mmHg or less. Moreover, capillary refill is absent, and there is negligible urine output, lethargy or even coma.

The management of hypovolaemic shock includes rapid and adequate restoration of the circulated volume by the use of fluid and blood administered intravenously. Any external or internal source of bleeding must be identified and addressed properly. Thoracic and pelvic anteroposterior (AP) radiographs as well as abdominal ultrasonography should provide helpful information to reveal the source of bleeding.

Disability assessment

When circulation problems have been addressed, a quick neurological evaluation of the patient is performed. In conscious patients, the Glasgow Coma Scale (GCS) provides a rapid evaluation of the neurological status and can be used to detect any subsequent deterioration.[26] Motor deficits signify spinal cord or peripheral nerve injury. In the patient with a severe open fracture or a mangled extremity, the degree of nerve damage may determine the decision for an amputation. It is very important to have in mind that in every case before intubation and sedation the neurological status of the patient should be recorded. A GCS score of 8 or less necessitates tracheal intubation and continuous intracranial pressure monitoring.[27] The size and the reaction of the pupils, the light reflex, and the oculocephalic and corneal reflexes should show the presence of any central impairment. If a cranial CT scan is indicated (deteriorated GCS or GCS <10), it should be done later during the secondary survey.[3,14]

Exposure and environment control

The clothes of the patient are removed (by the use of scissors) and the whole body is examined. Hypothermia, a common manifestation of severely traumatized patients (due to a variety of intrinsic or iatrogenic causes), should be prevented. After exposure, the patients are covered with warming blankets. Administration of cold fluids or blood will lower the core temperature, so fluid warmers are recommended.[3]

Overall, if lines in the peripheral veins are not feasible, venous cutdown can be conducted by using the long saphenous vein around the ankle. Ideally, fully cross-matched blood should be used, but in an emergency universal donor O-negative blood can be used immediately. A sample should be drawn for cross-match prior to administration, as the transfusion of O-negative blood can interfere with subsequent analysis. The blood bank should be able to deliver type-specific blood within 15–20 minutes of the patient's arrival in the emergency room. Coagulopathy should be anticipated in the victims of severe trauma as a result of haemodilution, hypothermia, consumption and disseminated intravascular coagulation. Correction and avoidance of hypothermia and the administration of warmed fluids is of utmost importance. The administration of platelets, fresh-frozen plasma and other blood products should be guided by laboratory results alongside clinical judgement. Response to volume replacement therapy is usually monitored initially using the clinical response of the patient and simple measurements including pulse, blood pressure, capillary refill and urine output. Urinary catheterization is mandatory.

In the severely injured or complex patient, invasive techniques including invasive arterial monitoring and central venous or pulmonary artery pressure recording should be considered at an early stage. Although controversy still exists in specific situations, current goals include normalization of vital signs and maintenance of central venous pressure between 8 and 15 mmHg. Serial recording of acid–base parameters, the base excess and serum lactate in particular, has been shown to be particularly useful in assessing response to therapy and detecting the presence of occult hypoperfusion in apparently stable patients. Ongoing requirement for blood transfusion should be monitored by regular measurement of the haemoglobin concentration; this can be rapidly estimated where necessary using the majority of bedside arterial blood gas analysers. Ongoing excessive fluid or blood requirement should always prompt a repeated search for sources of haemorrhage. Shock treatment is a dynamic process and, in cases where there is ongoing bleeding, surgical intervention is often indicated.

The issue of 'resuscitation' in polytraumatized patients has been a point of lively discussion among clinicians over the years. Although early administration of volume substitutes in trauma victims seems biologically rational and clinically sensible, it has not been proven through randomized studies.[28] The so-called 'damage control resuscitation'[29] brings about the idea of early administration of increased amounts of plasma and red blood cells in order to prevent coagulopathy, and implementation of measures to restore normal temperature and acid–base balance. This concept of resuscitation emphasizes the importance of simultaneous fluid replacement in the form of fresh whole blood and the implementation of damage control surgical techniques.

'Permissive hypotension' or 'low-volume resuscitation' is gaining considerable attention and nowadays it applies not only to the pre-hospital setting.[30] Through this approach, the major side-effects of high-volume resuscitation (i.e. cooling the patient), diluting the coagulation factors and increasing the blood pressure at the wound site are avoided; however, at the same time, tissue perfusion is maintained.[31,32] Low-volume resuscitation is contraindicated in brain and spinal cord injuries. 'Closed loop' fluid control is an experimental innovative approach that utilizes 'smart' resuscitation systems that link sensors of physiological variables with intravenous infusion pumps with microreceptors programmed with treatment algorithms in order to titrate fluid delivery in hypovolaemic victims.[33]

Regarding the type of fluids that should be given, the age-old controversy between crystalloids (normal saline, Ringer's lactate) and colloids (albumin, starch) has not yet been resolved. No superiority of colloids over crystalloids in terms of a reduction in the number of deaths of trauma victims is evident from published studies.[34] Consequently, an evidence-based approach does not call for the use of colloids as the primary means of volume replacement in a trauma setting. In addition, although it is yet unclear which type of fluid should be administered in traumatized patients, crystalloids are considered the initial treatment in bleeding patients.[32] Hypertonic–hyperoncotic saline solutions are promising volume replacements, especially in traumatic brain injury patients,[35] although no difference in neurological status 6 months post injury compared with patients treated with other fluids has been shown.[36] Red blood cell transfusion optimizes oxygen delivery to the tissues and is mainly indicated to maintain the haemoglobin level between 7 and 9 g dL^{-1}.[32] Antifibrinolytic agents such as tranexamic acid, ε-aminocaproic acid and aprotinin should be considered in bleeding management and discontinued when haemorrhage is controlled.[32]

DEFINITION OF THE PATIENT'S CONDITION

Following the initial ATLS assessment and primary interventions, the physiological condition of the patient must be assessed as being in one of four categories to direct the subsequent treatment protocol. This assessment is performed on the basis of overall injury severity, the presence of specific injuries and haemodynamic status. The four categories are stable, borderline, unstable and *in extremis*.[37,38] In order for the physician to be able to categorize the patient appropriately, he/she must be in a position to assess whether the patient has been adequately resuscitated. Endpoints of resuscitation include the evaluation of the following parameters: stable blood pressure and pulse rate, stable oxygen saturation, lactate level <2 mmol L^{-1}, no coagulation disturbances, normal temperature, urinary output >1 mL kg^{-1} h^{-1} and no requirement for inotropic support. Achieving the endpoints of resuscitation is of paramount importance for the stratification of the patient into the appropriate category.

Stable

These patients respond to initial therapy and are haemodynamically stable. They have no immediately life-threatening injuries and there are no signs of physiological disturbance such as coagulopathy or respiratory distress, or ongoing occult hypoperfusion, manifesting as abnormalities of the acid–base status. The endpoints of resuscitation are shown in Table 15.1.

Table 15.1 Endpoints of resuscitation (serially measured parameters employed to assess the adequacy of oxygen delivery to tissues)

Clinical signs	Haemodynamic and oxygen transport measures	Laboratory markers of
Heart rate	Central venous pressure	Gastric muscle ischaemia
Blood pressure	Arterial haemoglobin	and subcutaneous ischaemia
Urine output	Oxygen saturation	
Prolonged capillary refill	Cardiac output	
Mental status	Arterial haemoglobin concentration	
Pulse pressure	Base deficit	
	Lactate levels	

Borderline

Borderline patients have stabilized in response to initial resuscitative attempts but have clinical features or combinations of injury that have been associated with poor outcome and put them at risk of rapid deterioration. The criteria defining a borderline polytrauma patient are shown in Box 15.1.

> **BOX 15.1: Parameters to identify the borderline patient**
>
> - Multiple injuries in association with severe abdominal or pelvic injury and haemorrhagic shock at presentation (systolic blood pressure <90 mmHg)
> - Patients with bilateral femoral fractures
> - Radiographic evidence of pulmonary contusion
> - Hypothermia below 35°C
> - Patients with additional moderate or severe head injuries (AIS ≥3)
> - Patients with moderate or severe head injuries (AIS >3) ISS >40
> - Multiple injuries (ISS >20) in association with thoracic trauma (AIS >2)
> - Initial mean pulmonary arterial pressure >24 mmHg or a >6 mmHg rise in pulmonary artery pressure during intramedullary nailing or other operative intervention

Unstable

Despite initial intervention, patients remain haemodynamically unstable and are at greatly increased risk of rapid deterioration, subsequent multiple organ failure and death. Treatment in these cases includes rapid life-saving surgery only if absolutely necessary and timely transfer to the intensive care unit for further stabilization and monitoring. Temporary stabilization of fractures using external fixation, haemorrhage control and exteriorization of gastrointestinal injuries where possible is advocated.

In extremis

These patients frequently have ongoing uncontrolled blood loss. They are very close to death having suffered severe injuries. They remain physiologically unstable despite ongoing resuscitative efforts. They are usually suffering the effects of a 'deadly triad' of hypothermia, acidosis and coagulopathy. A damage control approach is certainly advocated, although only absolutely life-saving procedures are attempted so as not to drive this process further. The patients should then be transferred directly to intensive care for invasive monitoring and advanced haematological, pulmonary and cardiovascular support. Orthopaedic injuries can be stabilized rapidly in the emergency department or intensive care unit using external fixation and this should not delay other therapy. Any reconstructive surgery is again delayed and can be performed if the patient survives.

SECONDARY SURVEY

When physiological stability has been achieved, a secondary survey can be performed. The secondary survey includes a thorough clinical examination of the whole body, gathering the patient's information (history) and a complete diagnostic imaging evaluation. During this, any deterioration of the patient's condition necessitates return to the primary survey, starting with the assessment of the airway.[6] During all aspects of the secondary survey, the spine is protected, avoiding dangerous manipulation.

The secondary survey is carried out after airway, breathing, circulation and disability concerns have been addressed and the vital signs have been stabilized. It includes a thorough evaluation of the patient from head to toe, and collection of information regarding the patient's history. If the patient is unable to give information, family members, transporting paramedics or possibly other persons who know about the patient should be asked. The mnemonic to guide the initial history is 'AMPLE' (allergies, medications, past illness, last meal, events of accident). A detailed neurological examination must be performed. Additional radiographs are taken of the anatomical sites of suspected injuries (extremities, etc.), as well as other radiological investigations such as CT scans and MRI. The patient must be re-evaluated continuously. The secondary survey will reveal all other concomitant injuries with less immediate impact on the patient's survival.

SPECIFIC ORTHOPAEDIC TRAUMA SITUATIONS IN ATLS

Spinal fractures: spinal cord injuries

In all severely injured patients the spine should be protected during the primary and secondary surveys to avoid secondary nervous tissue damage as a result of any underlying existing spinal instability. Spinal injury should be considered to exist in every case until proven otherwise. The majority of cervical spine injuries in live adult patients admitted to emergency departments involve the C5–C7 levels.[39] Contemporarily with airway preservation, the cervical spine is protected with a collar; during intubation – if necessary – care should be taken not to jeopardize the spinal cord with forced manipulation. In the initial trauma series radiographs, a lateral view of the cervical spine should be obtained from occiput to the first thoracic vertebrae. If there is suspicion of fracture, AP and transoral radiographs for the odontoid peg will give further diagnostic information. A CT scan of the cervical spine should be taken during the secondary survey. The documented incidence of spinal fractures at multiple levels has been reported to range between 7% and 12%.[40] In unconscious patients, whole spine radiological examination is recommended.

Pelvic injuries

Pelvic fractures from a high-energy trauma are usually associated with injuries in other organ systems. The mortality rates from pelvic fracture have been reported to be as high as 30%.[41,42] The major concern in these fractures is haemorrhage, which may be profound. Open pelvic fractures bleed more because of loss of the internal tamponade effect of clotting in a closed space. Other sources of bleeding (open wounds, thoracic, intra-abdominal, etc.) may aggravate the clinical condition of the patient and lead to more severe shock. The life-threatening nature of pelvic fractures demands increased awareness, a standardized approach and aggressive resuscitation.[43]

In general, the ABCDE sequence of the primary survey should be followed in each case. Because haemorrhage is the major concern (estimated blood loss 1.5–4.5 L) in pelvic injuries, rapid fluid administration and blood transfusion is required. Rapid infusion of 1–2 L of isotonic Ringer's lactate solution or normal saline is carried out until cross-matched blood is available. When necessary, O-positive blood is transfused. Sterile and compressive dressings should cover any wound. Abdominal and thoracic sources of bleeding must be excluded and pelvic stability must be assessed at once. A circumferential pelvic sheet can be applied to compress the pelvis and control haemorrhage.[43,44] During the secondary survey, injuries to long bones and the spine should be evaluated and splinted temporarily. Retrograde urethrocystogram may be performed when there is suspicion of urethral injury. If the patient is haemodynamically stable, further radiographic evaluation is carried out (Judet, inlet/outlet views) as well as a CT scan of the abdomen and pelvis. Haemodynamically unstable or in extremis patients should be rapidly transferred to the operating room, where an external fixator (C clamp) should be applied.[44,45] If the patient's condition remains unstable, laparotomy may be indicated and/or pelvic packing may be necessary.[46–48] In patients with bowel rupture a diverting colostomy is performed. In some cases hemipelvectomy should be attempted in order to save the patient's life.

Long bone fractures

Long bone fractures should be addressed for the first time during the C component of the primary survey as potential bleeding sites. Grossly, certain closed fractures should lead to an estimated blood loss. As a rule, a closed fracture of the hip or femur has a blood loss 1.0–2.5 L. Humeral, tibial or knee fractures may lead to blood loss of 1.0–1.5 L, whereas elbow, forearm and ankle fractures separately may result in loss of 0.5–1 L.[40] Multiple fractures have an additional impact on blood loss and must be considered more severe injuries. Also, long bone fractures may be associated with injuries in other organ systems, a fact that has additional impact for the injured patient.

In the emergency department, long bone fractures that may be considered as potential sources of great blood loss (for example a femoral fracture) should be realigned and stabilized by closed means. In this way, the muscles surrounding the fracture should be stretched, bony fragments should be opposed to each other and bleeding may be reduced.[47]

Obviously an open fracture may be associated with more bleeding. A large quantity of blood may be lost at the scene of the accident or during the pre-hospital phase of care. All open fractures are inspected immediately after airway and breathing concerns are addressed. If they have been covered by dressings during pre-hospital care, they are exposed and evaluated. Superficial vessels that are bleeding are ligated. Deep bleeding is controlled initially by digital pressure or by sterile packing. A deep vessel is ligated only if it is easily accessible without putting a neighbouring nerve in jeopardy. Blind ligation of deep vessels is not recommended.[47] A large open fracture that is unexpectedly 'silent' during inspection may be indicative of severe exsanguination, because hypotension and reduced intravascular volume temporarily help to stop bleeding that recurs as the blood pressure is elevated to normal.[48] Fracture realignment and temporary stabilization are performed as in closed fractures and also have a positive impact on haemorrhage control. Fractures of lower severity are stabilized during the secondary survey. A neurovascular evaluation is followed by realignment and splinting of fractured bones. Radiographs are taken when the patient's condition is stable and may be of secondary priority after completion of screening, with a CT scan of the head and/or thorax and/or abdomen. Sometimes radiographic evaluation of simple fractures is carried out in the operating theatre after an intervention (such as thoracotomy, laparotomy, etc.) for a life-threatening condition.

OPERATING ROOM: SURGICAL STRATEGY

Two surgical strategies that have evolved over the years are the early total care (ETC) approach and the damage control orthopaedic (DCO) concept (Fig. 15.1). The ETC approach implies that all the patient's injuries will be stabilized early, within 24 hours of injury and during the same operative setting. However, it has become clear that not all patients benefit from this kind of approach. In the early 1990s a variety of unexpected complications related to early stabilization of long bone fractures was reported.[49–51]

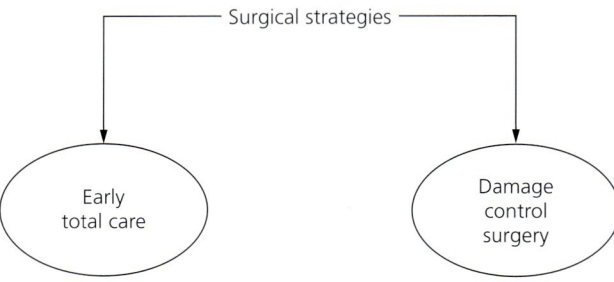

Figure 15.1 Strategies of fracture fixation.

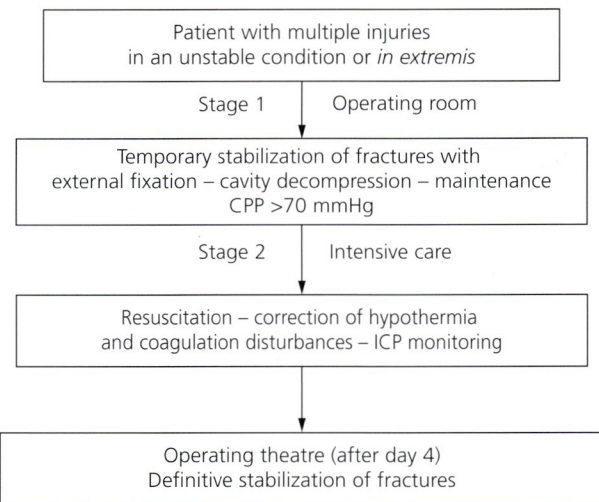

Figure 15.2 Stages of treatment of patients managed with the damage control surgery concept. CPP, cerebral perfusion pressure; ICP, intracranial pressure.

It was then realized that ETC was not appropriate for all multiply injured patients, as an increased incidence of adult respiratory distress syndrome (ARDS) and multiple organ dysfunction syndrome (MODS) was observed. The increased understanding of the pathophysiological mechanisms governing trauma and more specifically the knowledge acquired from the immuno-inflammatory response to injury provided the explanation for why these unexpected complications were taking place.

The initial traumatic insult stimulates, to variable degrees of activation, the immune system leading to a state of systematic inflammation. Several mediators have been implicated in this process, such as cytokines (interleukin (IL)-6), IL-8, IL-13, tumour necrosis factor α, etc.) as well as cellular elements (polymorphonuclear leucocytes, monocytes, dendritic cells, etc.).[52] The magnitude of this physiological process (systemic inflammatory response syndrome) correlates with the degree of injury sustained. This response is also known as the 'first hit phenomenon'; if it becomes overactive or exaggerated it can cause remote organ injury and the patient can progress rapidly to ARDS and MODS.[16,53] In addition it soon becomes clear that the type of surgery performed early or late on the patient, 'the second hit phenomenon', produces a varying burden on the biological reserve of the patient, which has already been compromised by the magnitude of the 'first hit'. In this context if the magnitude of the 'second hit' (type of surgery) exceeds the regulatory mechanisms of homeostasis, the patient enters a malignant inflammatory state and again rapidly progresses to ARDS or MODS and is at an increased risk of mortality.[54]

Besides the impact of the 'first and second hit phenomena' on the physiological state, it is now accepted that the individual biological response regulated by the genetic make-up of the patient could predispose to an adverse outcome. Clearly, only the second hit phenomenon can be modulated by medical treatment and thus inappropriate clinical decisions may have a detrimental effect on the well-being of the patient.

In the past, our capacity to characterize and to quantify the impact of surgical procedures on the inflammatory system was limited and thus it was difficult to appreciate the effect of our actions on the physiological state of the patient until several hours later when complications had been established and mortality was an expected outcome. Nowadays, with the advances made in molecular medicine and molecular biology, we have the capacity to measure all the important molecules known to participate in pathophysiological mechanisms. Several studies have been published illustrating that surgical procedures cause a variety of subclinical changes in the inflammatory system which become clinically relevant, with a cumulative effect if there are several impacts. Based on these observations, the concept of damage control orthopaedics for the management of patients with multiple injuries was developed. This concept of management is based on the principle of damage limitation and attempts to minimize the magnitude of the 'second hit or the inflammatory reaction' induced by the operative procedure.

Damage control orthopaedics provides a stepwise approach to the management of patients with polytrauma and is designed to take into account the difficulties encountered in patients who are haemodynamically unstable, or in an *in extremis* clinical condition. The manoeuvres used focus on the rapid resuscitation of the patient by providing temporary stabilization and minimizing the biological load of surgery, allowing the biological reserve of the patient to compensate better when in a physiological crisis struggling for survival. Damage control orthopaedics is the outcome of enhanced utilization of the increased knowledge acquired of the inflammatory response to trauma and its application in the operating theatre. The clinical course of the patient being treated by the damage control principle is shown in Fig. 15.2.

In general terms, the severity of the injuries sustained and the clinical condition of the patient are the major factors governing which line of treatment should be implemented in patients with polytrauma. For the stable patient the ETC approach is still valid and advisable. Definitive fracture

Table 15.2 Parameters for evaluation of the physiological state of the patient and selection of the appropriate treatment strategy

	Parameter	Stable	Borderline	Unstable	In extremis
Shock	Blood pressure (mmHg)	100 or more	80–100	60–90	<50–60
	Blood units (2 hours)	0–2	2–8	5–15	>15
	Lactate levels	Normal range	Around 2.5	>2.5	Severe acidosis
	Base deficit (mmol L^{-1})	Normal range	No data	No data	>6–8
	ATLS classification	I	II–III	III–IV	IV
Coagulation	Platelet count (μg mL^{-1})	>110 000	90 000–110 000	<70 000–90 000	<70 000
	Factors II and V (%)	90–100	70–80	50–70	<50
	Fibrinogen (g dL^{-1})	>1	Around 1	<1	DIC
	D-Dimer	Normal range	Abnormal	Abnormal	DIC
Temperature		>34°C	33–35°C	30–32°C	30°C or less
Soft-tissue injuries	Lung function; Pao_2/Fio_2	350–400	300–350	200–300	<200
	Chest trauma scores; AIS	AIS I or II	AIS 2 or more	AIS 2 or more	AIS 3 or more
	Chest trauma score; TTS	0	I–II	II–III	IV
	Abdominal trauma (Moore)	≤II	≤II	III	III or >III
	Pelvic trauma (AO class.)	A type (AO)	B or C	C	C (crush, rollover abd.)
		AIS I–II	AIS II–III	AIS III–IV	Crush, rollover extrem.
Surgical strategy	DCO or definitive surgery (ETC)	DCO	DCO if uncertain; ETC if stable	DCO	DCO

AIS, abbreviated injury scale; DCO, damage control orthopaedic; DIC, disseminated intravascular coagulation; ETC, early total care; TTS, thoracic trauma severity score.

stabilization can be performed safely within 24 hours of injury when resuscitation has been accomplished. For the borderline patient, ETC may still be used with caution and the surgeon will have to be alert, observing potential physiological changes occurring during surgery. There should not be any hesitation in converting to the damage control concept at any time throughout the procedure if the clinical condition of the patient deteriorates. For the patient who is unstable or in an *in extremis* situation, the damage control approach is recommended (Table 15.2).[37] Any surgical intervention here must be considered as life saving and should be quick and well performed. In the presence of severe head injuries the damage control approach is also advocated. The treatment and protection of the central nervous system must be the priorities in patients with considerable intracranial trauma since secondary brain injury may lead to further morbidity and disability.

KEY LEARNING POINTS

- Understand the management of the polytraumatized patient using advanced trauma life support principles.
- Know the different classes of haemorrhage.
- Classify early the physiological state of the patient.
- Appropriate selection of patients for the early total care or the damage control orthopaedic treatment strategies.

REFERENCES

● = Key primary paper
◆ = Major review article

◆1. The Trauma Audit and Research Network. TARN 2007. Available from: https://www.tarn.ac.uk.
2. *Dorland's Medical Dictionary for Health Consumers.* Available from: http://medical-dictionary.thefreedictionary.com/polytrauma.
◆3. ACS/COT. *National Trauma Data Bank Annual Report 2005*, dataset version 5.0. American College of Surgeons Committee on Trauma, 2005.
●4. Sikand M, Williams K, White C, Moran CG. The financial cost of treating polytrauma: implications for tertiary referral centres in the United Kingdom. *Injury* 2005;**36**:733–7.
◆5. Pape H-C, Giannoudis PV. Management of the multiply injured patient. In: Browner BD, Jupiter J, Levine A, Trafton P (eds) *Fracture in Adults*, 6th edn. Philadelphia, PA: Lippincott, Williams & Wilkins, 2004:59–92.
●6. Baker SP, O'Neill B, Haddon W Jr, Long WB. The Injury Severity Score: a method for describing patients with multiple injuries and evaluating emergency care. *Journal of Trauma* 1974;**14**:187–96.
◆7. American College of Surgeons: Committee on Trauma. *Advanced Trauma Life Support for Doctors*, 7th edn. Chicago, IL: ACS, 2004.
●8. Wilmink AB, Samra GS, Watson LM, *et al.* Vehicle entrapment rescue and pre-hospital trauma care. *Injury* 1996;**27**:21–5.
●9. Jones JH, Murphy MP, Dickson RL, *et al.* Emergency physician-verified out-of-hospital intubation: miss rates by paramedics. *Academic Emergency Medicine* 2004;**11**:707–9.

◆10. Sethi D, Kwan I, Kelly AM, et al. Advanced trauma life support training for ambulance crews. *Cochrane Database of Systematic Reviews* 2001;**2**:CD003109.

◆11. Timmermann A, Russo SG, Hollmann MW. Paramedic versus emergency physician emergency medical service: role of the anaesthesiologist and the European versus the Anglo-American concept. *Current Opinions in Anaesthesiology* 2008;**21**:222-7.

◆12. Thomas SH. Helicopter emergency medical services transport outcomes literature: annotated review of articles published 2000-2003. *Prehospital Emergency Care* 2004;**8**:322-33.

●13. Ringburg AN, Spanjersberg WR, Frankema SP, et al. Helicopter emergency medical services (HEMS): impact on on-scene times. *Journal of Trauma* 2007;**63**:258-62.

◆14. American College of Surgeons. *ATLS, Advanced Trauma Life Support, Student's manual*. Chicago, IL: ACS, 1997.

●15. Ali J, Adam RU, Gana TJ, et al. Trauma patient outcome after the Prehospital Trauma Life Support program. *Journal of Trauma* 1997;**42**:1018-21.

16. Wolfl CG, Bouillon B, Lackner CK, et al. [Prehospital Trauma Life Support(R) (PHTLS(R)): An interdisciplinary training in preclinical trauma care.] *Unfallchirurgie* 2008;**111**:688-94.

◆17. Sanson G, Di Bartolomeo S, Nardi G, et al. Road traffic accidents with vehicular entrapment: incidence of major injuries and need for advanced life support. *European Journal of Emergency Medicine* 1999;**6**:285-91.

●18. Osterwalder JJ. Can the 'golden hour of shock' safely be extended in blunt polytrauma patients? Prospective cohort study at a level I hospital in eastern Switzerland. *Prehospital Disaster Medicine* 2002;**17**:75-80.

●19. Trunkey DD. What's wrong with trauma care? *Bulletin of the American College of Surgeons* 1990;**75**:10-15.

◆20. Stahel PF, Heyde CE, Wyrwich W, Ertel W. Current concepts of polytrauma management: from ATLS to 'damage control'. *Orthopade* 2005;**34**:823-36.

●21. Copass MK, Oreskovich MR, Bladergroen MR, Carrico CJ. Prehospital cardiopulmonary resuscitation of the critically injured patient. *American Journal of Surgery* 1984;**148**:20-6.

●22. Bickell WH, Wall MJ Jr, Pepe PE, et al. Immediate versus delayed fluid resuscitation for hypotensive patients with penetrating torso injuries. *New England Journal of Medicine* 1994;**331**:1105-9.

●23. Soucy DM, Rudé M, Hsia WC, et al. The effects of varying fluid volume and rate of resuscitation during uncontrolled hemorrhage. *Journal of Trauma* 1999;**46**:209-15.

●24. Burris D, Rhee P, Kaufmann C, et al. Controlled resuscitation for uncontrolled hemorrhagic shock. *Journal of Trauma* 1999;**46**:216-23.

◆25. Moore FA, Moore EE. Trauma resuscitation. In: Souba WW (ed.) *ACS Surgery: Principles and Practice*. New York, NY; WebMD Inc., 2005.

●26. Teasdale G, Jennett B. Assessment of coma and impaired consciousness. A practical scale. *Lancet* 1974,**2**:81-84.

●27. Chesnut RM, Marshall LF, Klauber MR, et al. The role of secondary brain injury in determining outcome from severe head injury. *Journal of Trauma* 1993;**34**:216-22.

●28. Bagshaw SM, Bellomo R. The influence of volume management on outcome. *Current Opinion in Critical Care* 2007;**13**:541-8.

●29. Beekley AC. Damage control resuscitation: a sensible approach to the exsanguinating surgical patient. *Critical Care Medicine* 2008;**36**(7 Suppl):S267-74.

◆30. Boldt J. Fluid choice for resuscitation of the trauma patient: a review of the physiological, pharmacological, and clinical evidence. *Canadian Journal of Anaesthesia* 2004;**51**:500-13.

●31. Stern SA. Low-volume fluid resuscitation for presumed hemorrhagic shock: helpful or harmful? *Current Opinion in Critical Care* 2001;**7**:422-30.

◆32. Spahn DR, Cerny V, Prough DS, et al. Management of bleeding following major trauma: a European guideline. *Critical Care* 2007;**11**:R17.

●33. Kramer GC, Kinsky, MP, Prough DS, et al. Closed-loop control of fluid therapy for treatment of hypovolemia. *Journal of Trauma* 2008;**64**(4 Suppl):S333-41.

●34. Perel P, Roberts I. Colloids versus crystalloids for fluid resuscitation in critically ill patients. *Cochrane Database of Systematic Reviews* 2007:CD000567.

◆35. Chiara O, Bucci L, Sara A, et al. Quality and quantity of volume replacement in trauma patients. *Minerva Anestesiologica* 2008;**74**:303-6.

●36. Cooper DJ, Myles PS, McDermott FT, et al. Prehospital hypertonic saline resuscitation of patients with hypotension and severe traumatic brain injury: a randomized controlled trial. *Journal of the American Medical Association* 2004;**291**:1350-7.

●37. Pape HC, Giannoudis PV, Krettek C, Trentz O. Timing of fixation of major fractures in blunt polytrauma: role of conventional indicators in clinical decision making. *Journal of Orthopaedic Trauma* 2005;**19**:551-62.

●38. Pape HC, Giannoudis PV, Krettek C. The timing of fracture treatment in polytrauma patients: relevance of damage control orthopaedic surgery. *American Journal of Surgery* 2002;**183**:622-29.

●39. Ducker TB, Russo GL, Bellegarrique R, Lucas JT. Complete sensorimotor paralysis after cord injury: mortality, recovery, and therapeutic implications. *Journal of Trauma* 1979;**19**:837-40.

◆40. Cole PA. The diagnosis and management of musculoskeletal trauma. In: Swiontkowski MF, Stovits SD (eds) *Manual of Orthopaedics*, 6th edn. Philadelphia, PA: Lippincott, Williams & Wilkins, 2006.

◆41. Brenneman FD, Katyal D, Boulanger BR, et al. Long-term outcomes in open pelvic fractures. *Journal of Trauma* 1997;**42**:773-7.

●42. Ertel W, Keel M, Eid K, et al. Control of severe hemorrhage using C-clamp and pelvic packing in multiply injured patients with pelvic ring disruption. *Journal of Orthopaedic Trauma* 2001;**15**:468-74.

◆43. Rommens PM, Hessmann MH. Staged reconstruction of pelvic ring disruption: differences in morbidity, mortality, radiologic results, and functional outcomes between B1, B2/B3, and C-type lesions. *Journal of Orthopaedic Trauma* 2002;**16**:92-8.

- ●44. Katsoulis E, Giannoudis PV. Shock-room management of pelvic ring injuries. *European Journal of Trauma* 2005;**31**:22–30.
- ●45. Tile M. Pelvic ring fractures: should they be fixed? *Journal of Bone and Joint Surgery (British)* 1988;**70**:1–12.
- ●46. Grimm MR, Vrahas MS, Thomas KA. Pressure-volume characteristics of the intact and disrupted pelvic retroperitoneum. *Journal of Trauma* 1998;**44**:454–9.
- ●47. Pryor JP, Reilly PM. Initial care of the patient with blunt polytrauma. *Clinical Orthopaedics and Related Research* 2004;**422**:30–6.
- ◆48. Pedowitz RA, Shackford SR. Non-cavitary hemorrhage producing shock in trauma patients: incidence and severity. *Journal of Trauma* 1989;**29**:219–22.
- ●49. Giannoudis PV, Smith RM, Banks RA, *et al.* Stimulation of inflammatory markers after blunt trauma. *British Journal of Surgery* 1998;**85**:986–90.
- ●50. Giannoudis PV, Smith RM, Windsor AJ, *et al.* Monocyte HLA-DR expression correlates with intrapulmonary shunting after major trauma. *American Journal of Surgery* 1999;**177**:454–9.
- ●51. Giannoudis PV, Abbott C, Stone M, *et al.* Fatal systemic inflammatory response syndrome following early bilateral femoral nailing. *Intensive Care Medicine* 1998;**24**:641–2.
- ◆52. Giannoudis PV. Current concepts of the inflammatory response after major trauma: an update. *Injury* 2003;**34**:397–404.
- ●53. Giannoudis PV, Smith RM, Bellamy MC, *et al.* Stimulation of the inflammatory system by reamed and unreamed nailing of femoral fractures; an analysis of the second hit. *Journal Bone Joint Surgery (British)* 1999;**81**:356–61.
- ◆54. Giannoudis PV, Pape HC. Damage control orthopaedics in unstable pelvic ring injuries. *Injury* 2004;**35**:671–7.

16

Mass casualty management

JAMES P STANNARD, MICHAEL P RUSNAK

Introduction 244
References 246

NATIONAL BOARD STANDARDS

- Understand mass casualty management
- Know the importance of the chain of command

INTRODUCTION

The definition of a mass casualty accident is a large-scale occurrence with destruction requiring personnel and resources not normally available.[1] The damages exceed the ability of the local community to cope with the event. A major part of this unique demand on the community involves medical care of the victims. The orthopaedic surgeon is an integral member of the response team in a mass casualty accident. He or she is intimately involved with multiple disciplines, particularly with severe extremity injuries often requiring life-saving stabilization.

Successful stabilization must follow some general principles. One of the difficulties in mass casualty preparation is establishing a system to handle an unknown problem. An 'all hazards approach' is necessary to apply management principles universally whether war, nature or man-made disasters occur.[1] Much has been learned from the military in war time and has started to make its way into the civilian realm. Preparation must be focused on the population as a whole, rather than the individual.[2] The first and most important step in establishing an efficient system is through education. This chapter attempts to highlight the most important concepts in mass casualty management.

One of the great challenges of mass casualty management is overseeing the rapid and coordinated response of the multiple individuals and agencies. A system is needed to evaluate, communicate and coordinate the victim's care from the initial search and rescue to the definitive medical evacuation. This type of sophisticated trauma care system has its roots in the military. The US military has established five levels of care for wounded soldiers.[3] These five levels include (1) immediate care, or 'first aid'; (2) surgical resuscitation within mobile field units; (3) highest level medical, surgical and trauma care still within the combat zone (similar to a civilian trauma centre); (4) the first step in definitive care outside the combat zone; and (5) definitive stabilization and management of wounds, including reconstructive and limb salvage decisions.[4] Each level of care is progressively more sophisticated and further removed from the epicentre of the mass casualty incident. The civilian equivalent in the USA is the ICS, or Incident Command System. This organizational tool was implemented by the US government to oversee and implement its four major management activities, of which medical care is only one part. These are (1) command operations; (2) planning; (3) logistics; and (4) finance or administration. The entire operation is overseen by an incident commander. Each management activity is assigned a chief officer and his/her own general staff creating a top-down hierarchal structure.[1] The system must be flexible and able to adapt to the many possibilities of a disaster.

Medical personnel are involved in the command operations in addition to fire and police personnel. The importance of the medical unit in executing a successful mission is reflected in the establishment of a separate system called the Hospital Incident Command System (HICS).

This was established in the USA in 1991 to coordinate the transition from first responders at the scene to the hospital scene.[5]

Just like the ABCs of trauma care, mass casualty management's backbone of care follows a stepwise checklist. This includes four elements: search and rescue; triage and initial stabilization; medical evacuation; and definitive medical care. The efficiency of the triage system is likely to have the greatest impact on whether a mass casualty management operation will be successful. Typically 5–25% of surviving casualties are critically injured and will be hidden among the larger crowd with less severe injuries.[2] The objective of the medical personnel is to identify these patients and allocate resources appropriately.

Triage personnel are faced with four categories of patients: immediate, delayed, expectant and dead.[1] The greatest impact on potentially exhausting resources occurs within the expectant group. These patients are defined as those with extensive injuries requiring significant time and resources for definitive care. These are casualties whose survival would be questionable if they were the only patients injured. Expending a large proportion of a medical facility's resources on such patients leads to poor results during mass casualty situations. 'Overtriage' should be avoided in this group so as to prevent overextending limited resources better suited for salvageable casualties. This is counter-intuitive in today's emergency room, where the most severe injuries take precedence for immediate care and overtriage is considered appropriate with the abundant resources available. A direct correlation has been shown between overtriage and the critical mortality rate in major bombing disasters.[2] The critical mortality rate has been defined as the death rate among survivors with critical injuries.

In addition to triage, another method of reducing the critical mortality rate and avoiding overtriage is medical evacuation. This will decompress the scene and allow for better utilization of resources at the scene of the disaster. This involves transferring stable victims, or victims who will exhaust resources, to offsite facilities or hospitals. This will improve care for the critical and provide specialized care for the expectant and delayed group of victims.

Errors and mistakes are common in mass casualty situations. The key to success is limiting those mistakes by learning from prior experiences. Triage errors are common and can be devastating. Examples of avoiding these are by decompressing the site as much as possible, as already mentioned. A common impediment to the flow of victims can occur from bottlenecks in which numerous victims with varying injuries come to one checkpoint. This can be limited by increasing the number of checkpoints at each consecutive stage of triage, a simple step implemented in training prior to any disaster. Increasing the capacity and instituting these guidelines comes from a well-organized facility with an appropriate chain of command. A recent disaster in the USA, Hurricane Katrina, compounded the difficulty of evacuation secondary to the mass destruction of roads and transportation. Although this is difficult to plan for, you must assume that normal transportation routes may be compromised during a disaster. We should learn from Hurricane Katrina and recognize that evacuation is a key to success, and a flexible system must include alternative medical evacuation options.

The chain of command in decision-making is critical, and must be established prior to the occurrence of a disaster. A conflict in the ultimate authority to determine which patients went to the operating theatre was one of the lessons learned from Bellevue Hospital in New York City during the World Trade Center disaster on 11 September 2001.[6] Another common problem also encountered during 9/11 was dealing with communication barriers. This can occur when there is damage to power lines and mobile masts. Alternatives must be investigated and available, including walkie-talkies, internal communication systems or satellite-based systems.

Mass casualty incidents are rare events, making preparation and planning critical. Exercises must be conducted, resources maintained and personnel trained on a regular basis in order to be successful. This takes very dedicated individuals and often requires local and national organizations to be involved in providing the resources and money to run such an operation.

A committed foundation for coping with disasters must be in place, with regular training, education and a prepared system. This system must be structured and systematic with the ability to adapt to changing circumstances. All the people involved should be aware of and familiar with the available resources and other personnel who will be able to provide assistance. With time, experience and training, there is potential for a more efficient and successful response to mass casualty disasters.

KEY LEARNING POINTS

- A mass casualty is a large-scale occurrence with destruction requiring personnel and resources not normally available.
- An 'all hazards approach' is necessary to apply management principles universally whether war, nature or man-made disasters occur.
- The US military has established five levels of care for wounded soldiers: (1) immediate care, or 'first aid'; (2) surgical resuscitation within mobile field units; (3) highest level medical, surgical and trauma care still within the combat zone (similar to a civilian trauma centre); (4) the first step in definitive care outside the combat zone; and (5) definitive stabilization and management of wounds, including reconstructive and limb salvage decisions.

- The importance of the medical unit in executing a successful mission is reflected in the establishment of a separate system called the Hospital Incident Command System (HICS).
- Mass casualty management's backbone of care follows a stepwise checklist: search and rescue; triage and initial stabilization; medical evacuation; and definitive medical care.
- Triage personnel are faced with four categories of patients: immediate, delayed, expectant and dead.
- Errors and mistakes are common in mass casualty situations.
- The chain of command in decision-making is critical.
- A committed foundation for coping with disasters must be in place.

REFERENCES

- ● = Key primary paper
- ◆ = Major review article

◆1. Born CT, Briggs SM. Disasters and mass casualties. I. General principles of response and management. *Journal of the American Academy of Orthopaedic Surgeons* 2007;**15**:388–96.

◆2. Frykberg ER. Medical management of disasters and mass casualties from terrorist bombings: How can we cope? *Journal of Trauma* 2002;**53**:201–12.

◆3. Szul AC, Davis LB, *et al.* (eds) *Emergency War Surgery: Third United States Revision.* Washington, DC: Department of the Army, 2004:4.1–4.9.

●4. Bagg M, Covey D, Powell E. Levels of medical care in the global war on terrorism. *Journal of the American Academy of Orthopaedic Surgeons* 2006;**14**:S7–S9.

◆5. San Mateo County Department of Health Services Emergency Medical Services Agency. *The Hospital Emergency Incident Command System,* 3rd edn. San Mateo, CA: San Mateo County Department of Health Services Emergency Medical Services Agency, 1998.

●6. Wolinsky PR, Tejwani NC, Testa N, Zuckerman J. Lessons learned from the activation of a disaster plan: 9/11. *Journal of Bone and Joint Surgery (American)* 2003;**85A**:1844–6.

Open injuries of limbs

SHANMUGANATHAN RAJASEKARAN, P RISHI MUGESH KANNA, J DHEENADHAYALAN

Introduction	247	Classification systems	249
Pathophysiology	247	Treatment	253
Initial evaluation and management	248	References	257

NATIONAL BOARD STANDARDS

- Know the pathophysiology of open fractures
- Be able to classify injuries
- Be able to do the initial evaluation and know emergency room management
- Understand the principles of debridement and stabilization of bone

INTRODUCTION

An open fracture is defined as an injury in which the fracture and the fracture haematoma communicate with the external environment owing to a break in the overlying skin and surrounding soft tissue (Fig. 17.1). The term 'compound fracture' was previously used to describe this injury but is obsolete now as it is considered archaic. These are usually high-energy injuries with severe bone and soft-tissue involvement and are often associated with decreased vascular supply, contamination, degloving of the skin and a variable degree of soft-tissue damage (Table 17.1). Many of them occur as a part of major polytrauma, and a team approach is essential to save the life and restore the function of the limb. Improvements in intensive care management, the availability of powerful antibiotics and development of surgical principles of radical debridement, immediate bone stabilization and early soft-tissue cover have largely improved the outcome. However, these injuries continue to remain a major challenge to the trauma surgeon as there is still a high incidence of amputation, infection and poor outcome at the end of treatment.

PATHOPHYSIOLOGY

The amount of injury dissipated to a limb during an impact is determined by the equation, $KE = mv^2/2$ where KE is the kinetic energy, m is the mass and v represents the speed. During impact, the energy is absorbed by the soft and hard tissues until the strength of the respective tissues is exceeded. High-energy injuries typically thus result in serious comminution of bone with extensive periosteal stripping and soft-tissue damage. The comminuted bone pieces may acquire significant velocities which propel them into surrounding soft tissues, resulting in additional local damage and even neurovascular injuries. The skin can be torn apart creating a momentary vacuum that sucks in adjacent foreign material, which may be deposited in the depths of the wound, reaching the intramedullary areas of the bone and the intermuscular spaces.

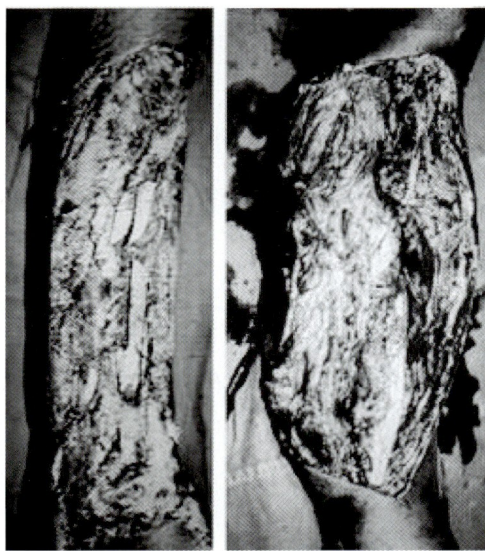

Figure 17.1 Extensive open injury of the leg with a large soft-tissue loss and free fragments of tibia lying free with minimal soft-tissue attachments.

Table 17.1 Energy transmitted by injury mechanism

Fall from curb	100
Skiing injury	300–500
High-velocity gunshot wound (single missile)	2000
20 mph bumper injury (assumes bumper strikes fixed target)	100 000

Data from Chapman MW. Role of bone stability in open fractures. *Instructional Course Lectures* 1982;**31**:75–87.

One must be aware that often the external wound may not clearly indicate the extent of damage to the deeper structures. The open wound may also not lie directly over the fracture and can be situated either proximally or distally communicating with the fracture through the degloved skin. Hence any fracture with a wound in the same limb segment must be suspected to be an open fracture and carefully evaluated. Although the injury may expose one compartment of the limb, the ensuing swelling may result in severe compartment syndrome of the other intact compartments of the same limb. The incidence of compartment syndrome is in fact more frequent in open injuries than in closed fractures.

An open injury is thus not a simple combination of a fracture and a wound. Contamination of the fracture by exposure to the external environment and devitalization of the soft tissues cause an increased susceptibility to infection. Management of the fracture and its healing potential could be affected. Also, such high-velocity injuries can result in damage and loss of function to the muscle, tendon, ligament, nerves and vascular structures. This in turn affects the initial treatment plan as well as the final outcome of the patient.

INITIAL EVALUATION AND MANAGEMENT

Up to 30% of patients with an open injury have other associated injuries, which can be potentially life threatening. The initial assessment should be on the established principles of advanced trauma life support (ATLS) with thorough evaluation of the airway, breathing and circulation. The primary survey must exclude injuries to the chest, abdomen and pelvis, which demand urgent intervention on the principles of damage control surgery. Loss of blood volume must be quickly evaluated and resuscitative measures for shock immediately instituted, as shock has been demonstrated to increase mortality and morbidities such as pulmonary complications, infections, wound-healing problems and non-unions.

A quick evaluation of the wound must be performed and the neurovascular status must be evaluated and documented. The wound must be quickly given a sterile dressing as there is hardly any benefit for elaborate examination of the wound in the emergency room. This may in fact result in unnecessary bleeding and increases the chances of secondary contamination and nosocomial infections. Bleeding from the wound must be controlled by elevation of the limb and application of compression bandages. No attempt must be made to blindly clamp a bleeding vein or artery, as it may lead to permanent damage of the neurovascular structures by inadvertent clamping of neighbouring nerve or artery.

Examination and documentation of the vascular status is important (Box 17.1). If pulses are absent, the limb must be re-examined after the limbs are anatomically aligned and splinted, as the vessels could have undergone kinking due to deformity and shortening of the limb. If pulses are still absent, additional investigations by an arterial Doppler or a CT angiogram must be performed. CT angiograms are of special benefit as they indicate the exact location and type of the block and also the status of the collateral flow. However, they are not easily available in

> **BOX 17.1: Signs of vascular injury**
>
> *Hard signs*
> - Absent pulses
> - Severe haemorrhage
> - Expanding and pulsatile haematoma
> - Bruit or thrill
>
> *Associated signs*
> - Associated numbness and neurological deficit
> - Difference in skin temperature distal to injury
> - Absence of pulse oximeter reading, no capillary blanching

all centres and are time-consuming. This can prolong the ischaemia time and delay the start of definitive treatment. Once the primary and secondary survey has been completed, radiographs of the injured extremity are obtained. Wherever necessary, a full regular trauma survey that includes lateral cervical spine film and anteroposterior views of the chest, abdomen and pelvis must be performed.

CLASSIFICATION SYSTEMS

Open injuries considerably vary from each other in the extent of severity of the injury to the different structures of the limb, and a thorough evaluation is usually possible only at the end of debridement. Clinical photographs of the wound in the emergency room, at the end of debridement and at different stages of management greatly help in accurate documentation.

Gustilo–Anderson classification

Until 1960, fractures were classified merely as open or closed. Although many classifications have been proposed thereafter, Gustilo and Anderson's classification (1976)[1] is the most commonly followed classification system worldwide (Table 17.2). In 1984, type III open fractures were subdivided into three types depending upon the size of the wound, degree of contamination, amount of periosteal stripping and the presence of arterial injury, which requires vascular repair for viability.[2] It should be understood that, apart from the size of the wound, factors such as the extent of degloving of skin, degree of contamination, extent of periosteal damage, crushing and devitalization of soft tissues and delay in debridement are also important factors in determining the Gustilo grade of injury as well as the outcome.

While Gustilo's classification has shown some prognostic value for predicting the rate of infection, incidence of non-union and requirement of soft-tissue reconstruction, it has many inherent limitations. It does not clearly address the question of salvage in IIIB injuries where the vascularity may be intact but the degree of injury to the soft tissues is so extensive that a useful salvage is not possible. The system also relies on subjective terms such as 'extensive soft-tissue damage' or 'significant periosteal stripping', which leads to wide variation of interpretation between surgeons. The interobserver agreement of Gustilo's classification has been found to be only moderate to poor, highly case dependent and varying with the experience of the surgeon. In practice, type IIIB injuries include a wide spectrum of injuries, ranging from the easily manageable to the almost unsalvageable[3] (Fig. 17.2). The management and prognosis of these injuries are highly variable, making this classification generalized, non-specific and not of much use in prognostication. The above disadvantages of the Gustilo system have led to the formation of other scores that are more successful in predicting salvage and also limb salvage pathways.

Ganga Hospital Open Injury Severity Score

The Ganga Hospital Open Injury Severity Score was proposed to fill in the need for a single scoring system that has a high sensitivity and specificity for salvage in type IIIB injuries and which can predict clinical outcome.[4] One to five points are allocated according to the severity of injury to each of the three components of the limb, i.e. the covering

Table 17.2 Gustilo and Anderson's classification of open fractures

Type	Wound	Level of contamination	Soft-tissue injury	Bone injury
I	<1 cm long	Clean	Minimal	Simple, minimal comminution
II	>1 cm long	Moderate	Moderate, some muscle damage	Moderate comminution
IIIA	Usually <10 cm long	High	Severe with crushing	Usually comminuted; soft-tissue coverage of bone possible
IIIB	Usually >10 cm long	High	Very severe loss of coverage; usually requires soft-tissue reconstructive surgery	Moderate to severe comminution
IIIC	Usually >10 cm long	High	Very severe loss of skin coverage plus vascular injury requiring repair; may require soft-tissue reconstructive surgery	Bone coverage poor; variable, may be moderate to severe comminution

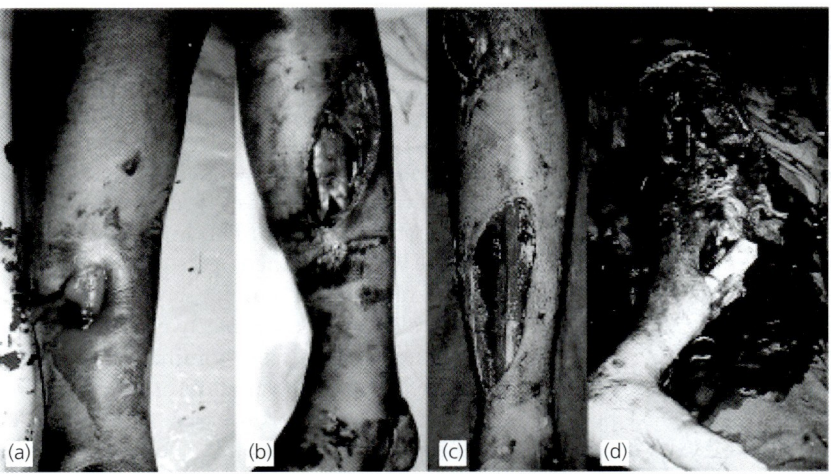

Figure 17.2 One of the main criticisms regarding Gustilo's classification is that the IIIB classification includes injuries of a wide spectrum of severity of injury. (a–d) All four of the injuries shown are by definition type IIIB injuries as they involve soft-tissue loss, exposure of the fracture site and moderate to severe damage to the soft tissues. However, it is clearly seen that the injuries vary from the easily manageable to the barely salvageable. The treatment requirements and prognosis vary widely between these injuries. It is difficult to prognosticate the outcome and also to compare the results of IIIB injuries from different institutions.

tissues (skin and fascia), the skeleton (bones and joints) and the functional tissues (muscles, tendons and nerve units). Systemic factors, which may influence treatment and outcome, are given 2 points each and the final score is arrived at by adding the individual scores together (Table 17.3).

COVERING TISSUES (SKIN AND FASCIA)

Wounds without skin loss which have an adequate soft-tissue bed and can be approximated without tension after debridement are given a score of 1 if they do not overlie the fracture and 2 if they expose it. Wounds with primary skin loss or which require extensive debridement of the skin because of friction burns or degloving have a score of 3 if they are not over the fracture site and 4 if they expose it. Wounds with skin loss over the entire circumference of the limb have a score of 5 (Fig. 17.3).

SKELETAL STRUCTURES (BONE AND JOINTS)

Transverse and oblique fractures with butterfly fragments involving less than 50% of the circumference have a score of 1. The presence of a large butterfly fragment involving more than 50% of the circumference indicates a score of 2, and extensive comminution or segmental fractures without loss of bone have a score of 3. Loss of bone of less than 4 cm has a score of 4 and of more than 4 cm a score of 5 (Fig. 17.4).

FUNCTIONAL TISSUES (MUSCLES, TENDONS AND NERVE UNITS)

Exposure of musculotendinous units of any size with only partial direct damage of muscle units has a score of 1, a complete but repairable injury with no resultant loss of function a score of 2, and irreparable injury resulting in partial loss of a compartment or a complete injury to the posterior tibial nerve has a score of 3. Extensive damage of one entire compartment has a score of 4 and loss of more than one compartment a score of 5 (Fig. 17.5).

Table 17.3 Ganga Hospital Injury Severity Score

Covering structures: skin and fascia	
Wounds without skin loss	
Not over the fracture	1
Exposing the fracture	2
Wounds with skin loss	
Not over the fracture	3
Over the fracture	4
Circumferential wound with skin loss	5
Skeletal structures: bone and joints	
Transverse/oblique fracture/butterfly fragment <50% circumference	1
Large butterfly fragment >50% circumference	2
Comminution/segmental fractures without bone loss	3
Bone loss <4 cm	4
Bone loss >4 cm	5
Functional tissues: musculotendinous (MT) and nerve units	
Partial injury to MT unit	1
Complete but repairable injury to MT units	2
Irreparable injury to MT units/partial loss of a compartment/complete injury to posterior tibial nerve	3
Loss of one compartment of MT units	4
Loss of two or more compartments/subtotal amputation	5
Comorbid conditions: add 2 points for each condition present	
Injury–debridement interval >12 hours	
Sewage or organic contamination/farmyard injuries	
Age >65 years	
Drug-dependent diabetes mellitus/cardiorespiratory diseases leading to increased anaesthetic risk	
Polytrauma involving chest or abdomen with injury severity	
Score >25/fat embolism	
Hypotension with systolic blood pressure <90 mmHg at presentation	
Another major injury to the same limb/compartment syndrome	

Classification systems

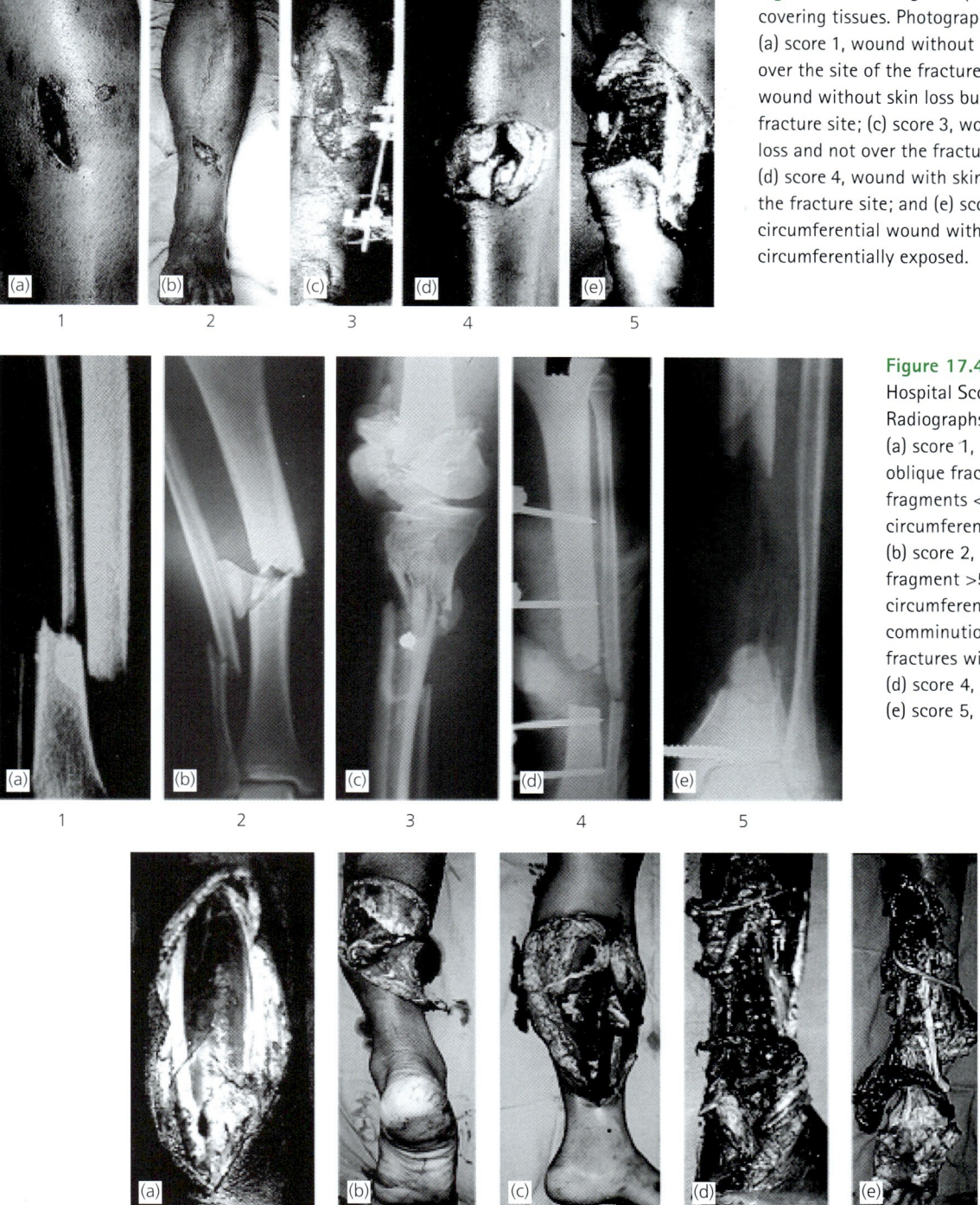

Figure 17.3 Ganga Hospital Score for covering tissues. Photographs showing (a) score 1, wound without skin loss and not over the site of the fracture; (b) score 2, wound without skin loss but exposing the fracture site; (c) score 3, wound with skin loss and not over the fracture site; (d) score 4, wound with skin loss and over the fracture site; and (e) score 5, circumferential wound with bone circumferentially exposed.

Figure 17.4 Ganga Hospital Score for bones. Radiographs showing (a) score 1, transverse/oblique fractures/butterfly fragments <50% circumference; (b) score 2, large butterfly fragment >50% circumference; (c) score 3, comminution/segmental fractures without bone loss; (d) score 4, bone loss <4 cm; (e) score 5, bone loss >4 cm.

Figure 17.5 Ganga Hospital score for functional tissues. Photographs showing (a) score 1, partial injury to musculotendinous units; (b) score 2, complete but repairable injury to musculotendinous units; (c) score 3, irreparable injury to musculotendinous units involving one or more muscles in a compartment or complete injury to the posterior tibial nerve; (d) score 4, loss of one entire compartment; and (e) score 5, loss of two or more compartments or subtotal amputation.

The scoring is assessed after debridement when the severity of injury to all components of the limb has been established accurately. By adding the individual scores, a total score is obtained. In a study by Rajasekaran et al.,[4] the total score was used to assess the possibilities of salvage in type III injuries. The outcome was measured by dividing the injuries into four groups according to their total scores: group 1 scored less than 5; group II 6–10; group III

Table 17.4 Mangled Extremity Severity Score (MESS)

Type	Definition	Points
A	Skeletal/soft-tissue injury	
	Low energy (stab; simple fracture; 'civilian' gun shot wounds (GSWs))	1
	Medium energy (open or multiple fractures; dislocation)	2
	High energy (close-range shotgun or 'military' GSW; crush injury)	3
	Very high energy (above and gross contamination; soft-tissue avulsion)	4
B	Limb ischaemia	1*
	Pulse reduced or absent but perfusion normal; pulseless; paraesthesias; diminished capillary refill	2*
	Cool; paralysed; insensate; numb	3*
C	Shock	
	Systolic BP always >90 mmHg	0
	Hypotensive transiently	1
	Persistent hypotension	2
D	Age (years)	
	<30	0
	30–50	1
	>50	2

*Score doubled for ischaemia >6 hours.

11–15; and group IV 16 or more. All limbs in group IV and one in group III underwent amputation. A threshold score of 14 was found to have a high sensitivity and specificity to predict amputation. The score was found to have better predictive rates than the Mangled Extremity Severity Score (MESS) for predicting amputation, especially in patients who had a very severe crush injury of the limb with intact vascularity. MESS has been designed to predict the likelihood of amputation based on four criteria[5] (Table 17.4). A score of >7 has been reported to predict amputation accurately in both retrospective and prospective studies.[6] In comparison, a Ganga Hospital Open Injury Severity Score of more than 14 was observed to be a better predictor of amputation with >90% positive predictive value. Of the salvaged limbs, it was observed that there was a significant difference in the three groups for the requirement of a flap for wound cover, the time to union, the number of surgical procedures required, the total days as an inpatient and the incidence of deep infection.[4]

Limb salvage vs amputation

The decision-making logistics in Gustilo grade III injuries whether to salvage or amputate the limb are controversial. The question of salvage must be addressed by the surgeon not only when there is an obvious vascular insult but also when there is a severely mangled viable limb. It is important that the question of salvage is addressed collectively by an experienced team along with the patient and relatives. Amputation when necessary should be discussed in depth and decided on the day of injury or as soon as possible, as postponement of the decision prolongs the agony of the patient.

> **BOX 17.2: Indications for primary amputation**
>
> - Warm ischemia time over 8 hours and the limb is completely non-viable
> - Vascular injury which is non-repairable with no collateral flow seen in arteriograms
> - Limb is severely crushed with minimal viable tissue
> - Presence of severe and debilitating systemic diseases where lengthy surgical procedures to preserve the limb will endanger life
> - Presence of severe multisystem injuries with an injury severity score of 25 or more where salvage may lead to MODS and death
> - Damage is so severe that ultimate function will be less satisfactory than prosthesis

Immediate or primary amputation may be indicated in certain instances (Box 17.2). However, many patients may fall into a grey zone of indeterminate prognosis where the decision of an experienced team is invaluable. The surgeon must not fall into the trap of 'victory of surgical enthusiasm over practical wisdom' and must not embark on a risky multistaged reconstruction procedure that may endanger the life of the patient or lead to a salvaged but non-functional or painful limb. The local factors commanding attention are the mechanism of injury, fracture patterns, extent of vascular injury, presence of neurological injury, associated ipsilateral extremity injury and the degree of contamination. Apart from the severity of the injury to the limb, patient-related factors such as age, severity of shock, the presence of comorbid factors such as uncontrolled diabetes mellitus, pre-existing vascular diseases, smoking behaviour and any systemic disease which can make a lengthy operation unduly risky must be considered.

Based on the above discussed variables, many predictive scoring systems have been proposed, all of which may assist the surgeon but cannot completely substitute experience. Of these, the most extensively used is MESS.[7] A score greater than or equal to 7 has a high predictive value for amputation. In the authors' experience, this score is very reliable in patients who have had a vascular injury. However, in situations where the limb is mangled but without a vascular injury, MESS often gives a very low score leading to failed salvages and secondary amputations.

On the contrary, the Ganga Hospital Open Injury Severity Score has been found to be more reliable in such injuries where a score of 14 and below supports salvage, and those above 17 indicate amputation; those in between can be decided by an experienced team depending upon the nature of injury and the expectations of the patient. The important influencing factors in managing grey zone injuries is the expertise of the treating team, the social and cultural background of the patient, the cost provider and the personality of the patient.

TREATMENT

The aim of treatment in open injury is to achieve early healing of the soft tissues with good bone union and avoiding the complications of infection, non-union and stiffness of joints.[8] Infection is the major problem that leads to delayed and non-unions, failures of soft-tissue reconstructions and in rare cases even to amputation. While the typical infection rates in type I fractures range from 0% to 2% and in type II fractures from 2% to 7%, the rates are very high ranging from 10% to 25% in type IIIB injuries. The commonly isolated organisms from established infections of open fractures are *Staphylococcus aureus*, *Pseudomonas*, *Proteus* and *Escherichia coli*. These organisms have not been isolated from the environment where accidents occur. Hence there is no role for wound cultures either in the pre-debridement stage or in the post-debridement phase. The factors leading to increased risk of infection are listed in Box 17.3 and must be carefully looked into.

Antibiotic therapy

All patients with open injuries must have intravenous antibiotics at the earliest possible opportunity. The fractures can be contaminated from different sources (Fig. 17.6) and it is now considered that antibiotic therapy is compulsory and therapeutic and not prophylactic. Typically for types I, II and III fractures without organic contamination, first- or second-generation cepholosporins are instituted intravenously, usually in the emergency room itself. An aminoglycoside is also prescribed for type III injuries. Penicillin with or without metronidazole is added for patients with gross organic contamination. Tetanus prophylaxis should also be given in the emergency room. In patients with extensive muscle crushing, anti-gas gangrene therapy also needs to be administered (Table 17.5).

> **BOX 17.3: Factors increasing risk for infection**
>
> *Local factors*
> - Organic, farmyard or sewage contamination
> - Poor debridement with retention of foreign debris and non-viable tissues
> - Inadequate skeletal stabilization
> - Presence of dead space
> - Debridement later than 12 hours
>
> *Systemic factors*
> - Presence of shock and acute respiratory distress syndrome
> - Presence of comorbid factors such as age above 65 years, metabolic disorders such as diabetes mellitus
> - Compartment syndrome
> - Prolonged hospital stay and exposure to resistant organisms
> - Poor nutrition

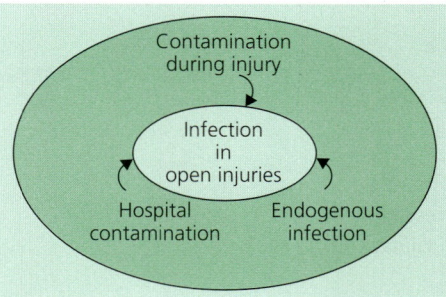

Figure 17.6 The organism for wound infection in open injuries is from three main sources. Although the majority of grade IIIB injuries are contaminated, their significance in subsequent infections is debated. Endogenous infections are common in patients with severe shock where the mucosal barrier of the gut is lost and there is bacteraemia of coliform organisms. Hospital contamination with resistant strains is however the most common cause for infection.

Principles of debridement

Debridement is the single most important factor that determines the outcome in open injuries. It must be done as soon as possible, by experienced and senior members of the team, in a systematic manner with an aim of excising all contaminated and non-viable tissues (Table 17.6). Debridement is best performed with a tourniquet, as a bloodless field during debridement helps to identify contamination, protect the vital structures, carefully explore the various compartments and muscle planes, explore the joint cavities and also save unnecessary blood loss in a patient who may already be in shock. At the end of the debridement, the tourniquet is released and the viability of all tissues ascertained comfortably. Vascular tissues appear pale while under tourniquet and blush immediately on release, whereas avascular muscles appear dark red even while under tourniquet with no change after release of the tourniquet. Wounds must be adequately enlarged in an extensile fashion so as to preserve skin viability and allow for suitable skeletal stabilization. Skin must be carefully debrided up to the bleeding margins and all necrotic fascia and muscles carefully excised. The viability of muscles is evaluated on the basis of the four 'Cs': contractality, colour, consistency and capacity to bleed. One should not hesitate to excise even entire muscle bellies, as whole compartments can become avascular in severe crush injuries.

Fractured bone fragments must be carefully evaluated for periosteal and muscular attachments which determine blood supply. Whenever in doubt, they must be considered as potential sequestrum and removed. Large metaphyseal fragments and osteochondral fragments that are important for joint alignment and reconstruction can be retained if not severely contaminated. The ends of the bone may contain deep impregnation of paint, mud and other organic material and it is important to nibble away the edges till adequate clearance is achieved.

During the process of debridement and after completion, the wound is frequently washed thoroughly by copious lavage (Box 17.4). It is frequently mentioned that the

Table 17.5 Intravenous antibiotic therapy for open fractures

Antibiotic	Type I	Type II	Type III	Organic contamination
Cefazolin, 1 g every 8 hours	*	*	*	*
Aminoglycoside, 3–5 mg/kg/day			*	*
Penicillin, 2 000 000 units every 4 hours (or metronidazole, 500 mg every 6 hours)				*

Data from Bucholz RW, Heckman JD, Court-Brown C, *et al*. (eds). *Rockwood and Green's Fractures in Adults*, 6th edn. Philadelphia, PA: Lippincott Williams & Wilkins, 2006.

BOX 17.4: Wound lavage in open injuries

- Adequate quantity of fluid must be used for lavage. For example, 9 litres of fluid are used for type IIIB fractures
- Lavage clears blood clot, non-viable tissues and debris from tissue planes and dead spaces
- Lavage reduces bacterial population
- No advantage in adding antiseptic solutions to lavage fluid
- Use of hydrogen peroxide, alcohol solution, povidone iodine and other chemical agents may impair osteoblast function, inhibit wound healing and cause cartilage damage
- Advantage of addition of antibiotics in the lavage solution has not been documented
- High-pressure pulsatile lavage can reduce bacterial load by 100-fold but has the disadvantages of microscopic damage to the bone, considerable soft-tissue damage and may push the bacteria contamination to a deeper tissue plane
- Low-pressure pulsatile lavage (14 psi @ 550 pulsations) is equally effective as high-pressure pulsatile lavage (70 psi @ 1050 pulsation per minute) and has fewer disadvantages

---

Table 17.6 Principles of debridement

Debridement - principles	Must be performed by an experienced team and as early as possible
	Involvement of orthopaedic and plastic surgeon at this stage is essential
Steps	A pre-debridement photograph is taken
	A tourniquet must be inflated without exsanguination
Skin and fascia	Wounds must be longitudinally extended to provide adequate visualization of deeper structures
	Margins must be trimmed up to bleeding dermis to create a clean wound edge
	Gentle handling of the skin and prevention of degloving is a must
	All avascular fascia must be excised
Muscle	All muscles in the compartment must be evaluated for viability and debrided
Bone	Bone ends and medullary cavity must be carefully examined for impregnated paint, mud and organic material
	All fragments without soft-tissue attachment must be excised
Lavage	Adequate quantity of fluid with low-pressure pulsatile lavage is preferable
Completion	Deflate tourniquet and evaluate viability of all retained structures
	Assess loss of tissues and document with photograph for future reference and planning
	Decide on method and timing of wound closure or coverage and bone stabilization
	Document sequence of reconstruction

solution for pollution is dilution and at least 15–20 L of fluid is necessary during the debridement of a type IIIB wound. Once debridement and lavage are complete, it is good practice to completely drape the limb again and proceed to bone fixation with a clean set of instruments.

Bone stabilization

Restoring the alignment and length of the limb and stabilizing the bone is important, as it removes the kink in the neurovascular structures, improves venous return, reduces oedema, decreases inflammatory response, decreases pain and permits wound care and better mobilization of the patient. Stable fixation also reduces dead space that predisposes to haematoma and infection.

Three main choices of skeletal stabilization are available – the external fixator, the interlocking nails and the plate–screw fixation systems. Although external fixation was considered the work horse in open injuries, advances in techniques for early coverage of wounds, availability of powerful antibiotics and a new generation of intramedullary and plate fixation systems have allowed definitive fixation of fractures in many cases. The choice of stabilization must be made carefully depending on the nature and size of the wound, the pattern of fracture, the degree of contamination, the presence of comorbid factors and the provision for immediate soft-tissue cover.

External fixators are the most commonly used in type IIIB fractures (Fig. 17.7). They are cost-effective and can be used in a modular fashion, allowing the surgeon to provide a versatile and stable fixation without additional stripping or damage to soft tissues (Box 17.5). They are usually used for temporary stabilization, with the definitive internal fixation performed either before or after the final soft-tissue reconstruction. When conversion to intramedullary devices is performed within the first week, the infection rates are low.

Although there was an initial phobia for the use of intramedullary nails, their usage has become widespread

> **BOX 17.5: External fixators in open injuries**
>
> *Advantages*
> - Provides easy and versatile mechanism for fixation
> - Can be modular to suit any anatomical region and fracture pattern
> - No additional exposure or periosteal stripping required
> - Less time consuming and allows early vascular repair
> - Cost-effective
>
> *Disadvantages*
> - Usually a temporary mechanism and needs revision procedures
> - Transfixes the soft tissues and can produce stiffness
> - Pin tract infections are common and can interfere with secondary internal fixations
> - Pins can interfere with plastic surgical procedures

not only in grades I and II but even in grade III injuries[9] (Fig. 17.8). Unreamed nails were initially preferred as they are quicker, considered to be more biological, cause less cortical devascularization and also have a low incidence of fat embolism and thermal necrosis. However, their usage was associated with increased implant failure, with a higher rate of non-union and malunion. The current trend is to use reamed nails as they allow larger and stronger nails with the advantages of early weight bearing and less implant failure.[10] Over-reaming, which can lead to weakening of the bone and thermal necrosis, must be avoided.

Fractures involving metaphysis and intra-articular fractures frequently require the use of plate–screw systems to achieve exact anatomical restoration and stable fixation (Fig. 17.9). Plate osteosynthesis is also the primary choice for all open fractures of the upper limb, especially in the forearm.[11] Locking plates have further improved the possibility of achieving excellent stability even in the

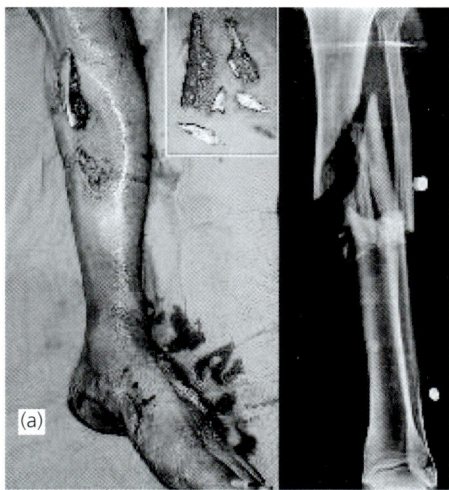
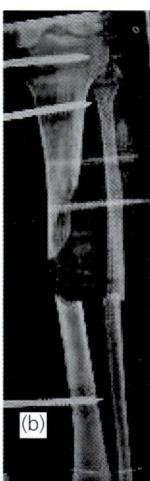
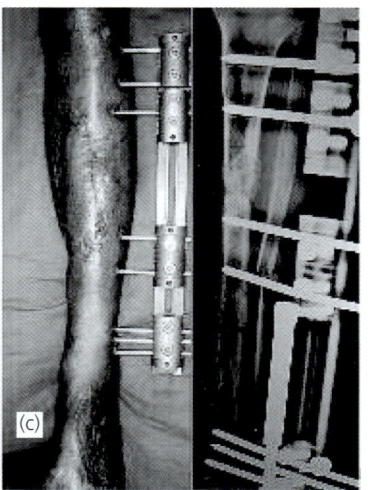

Figure 17.7 (a–c) Grade IIIB injury of tibia with extensive comminution, free fragments with minimal soft tissue attachment and doubtful viability. Removal of the fragments led to a bone gap which was reconstructed successfully by bone transport. Modern techniques of bone transport allow even large gaps in bone to be bridged successfully provided there is no infection.

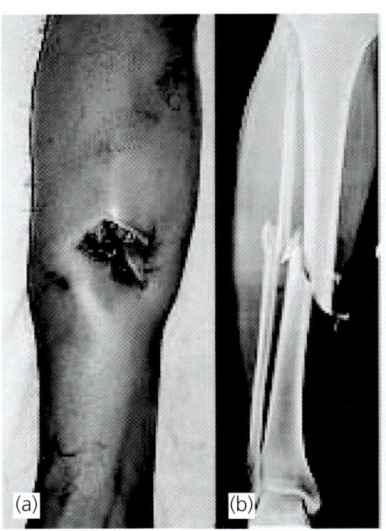
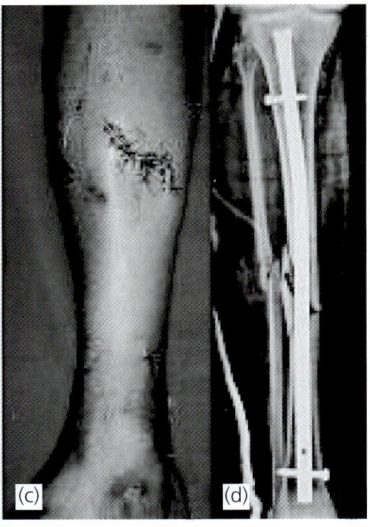

Figure 17.8 (a–d) Open injury of the tibia treated by debridement followed by stabilization with a locking nail and primary closure. There is ample evidence that locking nails do not lead to additional complications provided debridement is adequate.

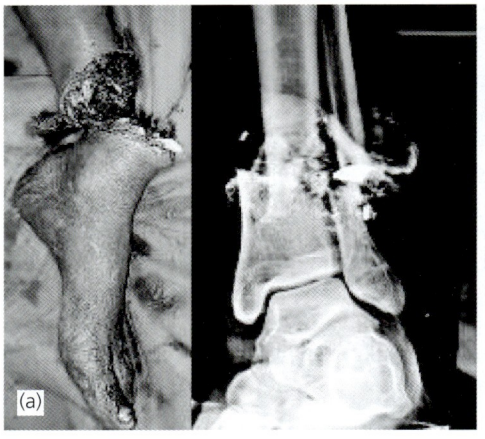
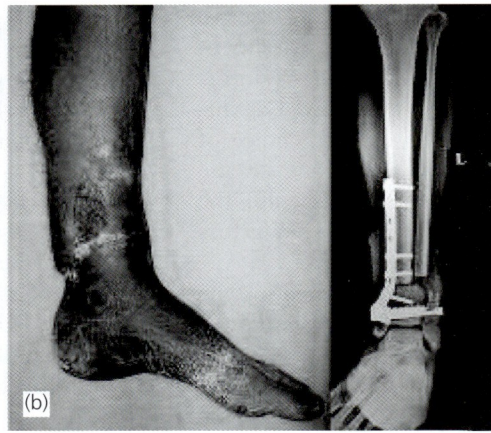

Figure 17.9 (a and b) A type IIIC fracture of the lower end of the tibia which required immediate fixation and vascular repair. After debridement, the bone was stabilized by a buttress plate which afforded good stability for vascular reconstruction and soft-tissue cover.

presence of comminution without further disruption of soft tissues.

Soft-tissue reconstruction

Along with good debridement, the other most important factor that ensures success in open injury management is to quickly convert an open injury to a closed injury by providing adequate soft-tissue cover. Leaving a wound open has numerous disadvantages. It leads to desiccation of tissues, causing secondary loss of tissues and contamination by multidrug-resistant organisms leading to a poor result. The importance of involving a plastic surgeon even from the stages of initial evaluation, debridement and reconstruction cannot be overemphasized. Best results are achieved in institutions where there is adequate team work and established protocols for both the orthopaedic and plastic surgeons to work together through all stages of reconstruction of these injuries.

Primary closure of wounds should rarely be performed in open injuries for fear of infection and wound-healing problems. After adequate debridement, it may be possible to close the wound primarily in small, clean wounds. This should not be done in cases with gross contamination or when there is a need for a second-look debridement. The second rung in the reconstructive ladder is delayed primary closure. If at the time of second or third debridement, the wound is clean and healthy, a delayed primary closure is carried out. The next level of reconstruction is the use of a split thickness skin graft. Wounds even with minimal skin loss are better treated by a skin graft when there is adequate soft-tissue cover over the fracture. In wounds where the bone, tendon or the neurovascular structures remain exposed at the end of debridement, there is a need for a flap.

A flap refers to a tissue transferred from one anatomic site to another. The vascularity of the flap is derived from nutrient vessels within the pedicle of the flap. The pedicle may either remain attached at its origin or be divided during the transfer and anastomosed to recipient vessels using microsurgical techniques. Microsurgical transfer of tissue is known as a free flap. Flaps are useful to close defects too large for primary closure and where skin

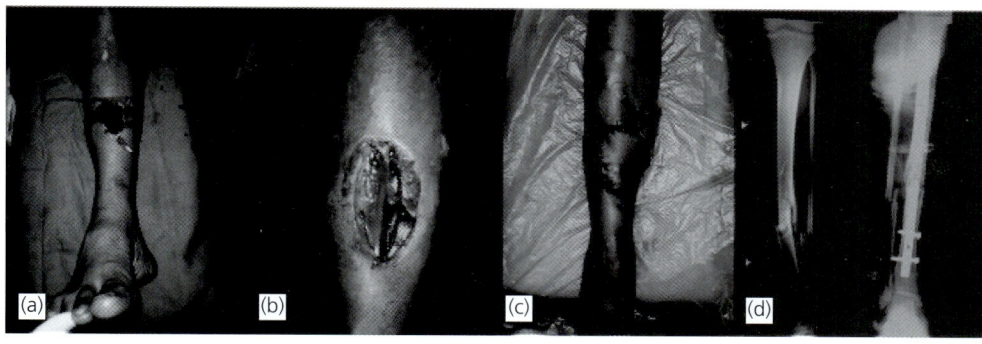

Figure 17.10 (a–d) Open fracture of the tibia which after debridement required a flap. A local transposition flap has been performed. In these situations, if the wound looks clean and healthy, the fracture can be stabilized by internal fixation in the same sitting along with the soft-tissue reconstruction.

grafts are inadequate. Flaps can contain more than one type of tissue and are named based on the tissues they contain. A typical example would be fasciocutaneous flaps, which contain skin and underlying fascia. Rotation flaps, such as muscle, skin and fascia or a combination, from adjacent regions are used to obliterate dead space, and help to close the wound without tension (Fig. 17.10). When such options are limited, free flaps must be considered, which are complex reconstruction procedures requiring expertise.

KEY LEARNING POINTS

- An open fracture is defined as an injury where the fracture communicates with the external environment because of a break in the overlying skin and surrounding soft tissue.
- The magnitude of force applied, the injury environment, the type of bone involved, the fracture pattern, coexisting injuries and medical illnesses affect the management and prognosis.
- The injuries are classified traditionally based on the Gusti–Anderson classification system.
- Ambiguity in classifying and managing type IIIB injuries has led to the proposal of newer classification systems, such as the Ganga Hospital Open Injury Severity Score, which also help in formulating limb reconstruction pathways and in predicting salvage.
- Appropriate antibiotic therapy, early and adequate surgical debridement, stabilization of bone and early soft-tissue cover are the key issues in the management of open fractures.
- The prognosis in open fractures is determined primarily by the amount of devitalized soft tissue and the level and type of bacterial contamination.
- The ultimate functional results depend on viable soft-tissue coverage, neurovascular integrity, prevention of infection and healing of the fracture.

REFERENCES

● = Key primary paper
◆ = Major review article

●1. Gustilo RB, Anderson JT. Prevention of infection in the treatment of one thousand and twenty-five open fractures of long bones: retrospective and prospective analyses. *Journal of Bone and Joint Surgery (American)* 1976;**58A**:453.
◆2. Gustilo RB, Mendoza RM, Williams DN. Problems in the management of type III (severe) open fractures: a new classification of type III open fractures. *Journal of Trauma* 1984;**24**:742.
●3. Horn BD, Rettig ME. Interobserver reliability in the Gustilo and Anderson classification of open fractures. *Journal of Orthopaedic Trauma* 1993;**7**:357–60.
●4. Rajasekaran S, Naresh Babu J, Dheenadhayalan J, *et al.* A score for predicting salvage and outcome in Gustilo type-IIIA and type IIIB open tibial fractures. *Journal of Bone and Joint Surgery (British)* 2006;**88B**:1351.
◆5. Helfet DL, Howery T, Sanders R, *et al.* Limb salvage versus amputation: preliminary results of the mangled extremity severity score. *Clinical Orthopaedics and Related Research* 1990;**256**:80.
◆6. Johansen K, Daines M, Howey T, *et al.* Objective criteria accurately predict amputation following lower extremity trauma. *Journal of Trauma* 1990;**30**:568–72.
◆7. Bosse MJ, MacKenzie EJ, Kellam JF, *et al.* A prospective evaluation of the clinical utility of the lower-extremity injury-severity scores. *Journal of Bone and Joint Surgery (American)* 2001;**83A**:3.
●8. Rajasekaran S, Sabapathy SR. A philosophy of care of open injuries based on the Ganga hospital score. *Injury* 2007;**38**:137–46.
9. Anderson JT, Gustilo RB. Immediate internal fixation in open fractures. *Orthopaedic Clinics of North America* 1980;**11**:569.
●10. Fischer MD, Gustilo RB, Varecka TF. The timing of flap coverage, bone-grafting, and intramedullary nailing in patients who have a fracture of the tibial shaft with extensive soft tissue injury. *Journal of Bone and Joint Surgery (American)* 1991;**73A**:1316.
◆11. Okike K, Bhattacharyya T. Current concepts review: trends in the management of open fractures: a critical analysis. *Journal of Bone and Joint Surgery (American)* 2006; **88A**:2739.

18

Closed treatment of common fractures

PETER V GIANNOUDIS, FAREED KAGDA

Introduction	258	Complications	260
Principles of closed reduction	259	Common fractures treated non-operatively	261
Cast and splinting techniques	260	References	267

NATIONAL BOARD STANDARDS

- Understand the concept of three-point fixation
- Know the different types of cast and the formula for plaster of Paris
- Understand the different types of traction and be able to draw them
- Know when to treat any particular fracture non-operatively

INTRODUCTION

Until the early 1950s non-operative treatment of fractures was very common and was associated with either the application of traction and bed rest or immobilization of the limb with plaster of Paris. It was not long, however, before it was realized that this approach of fracture care led to increased local complications such as bed pressure sores, muscle atrophy, joint stiffness and malunion with a variable degree of morbidity. Systemic complications were also a common finding including pneumonia, the fat embolism syndrome, deep vein thrombosis and pulmonary embolism.[1]

Subsequently, the positive effect of skeletal stabilization became apparent with the implementation of standardized techniques of fracture fixation by the AO (Arbeitsgemeinschaft für Osteosynthesefragen) group in Switzerland.[2] The initial effectiveness of compression plate fixation techniques and subsequently the spreading of intramedullary nailing for stabilization of long bone fractures set the scene for operative treatment of fractures.

Lately, the concepts of biological fixation and minimal invasive plate osteosynthesis (MIPO) have been popularized, emphasizing the change in the mind-set of the surgical community towards preservation of vascularity and of the local biological substrate in general.[3] This approach is the outcome of the knowledge acquired relevant to the physiological mechanisms governing the fracture-healing processes. During the past 30 years, therefore, the relative ease of treatment of fractures with surgical intervention and the overall efficacy of this strategy set the foundation for the advances made in fracture fixation and the modern osteosynthesis techniques that are currently practised.

Despite all of the advances made in terms of the operative treatment of fractures, surgical intervention is not free of complications and this practice is also frequently associated with another surgical procedure (reoperation) required for implant removal. Therefore, non-operative management of fractures, despite being considered out of date by a number of surgeons, can still be used in an effective way, especially in cases where there are contraindications for surgical treatment of the index fracture. Not all fractures however can be considered for non-operative treatment. It is widely accepted that intra-articular fractures as well as many metaphyseal fractures demand open reduction internal fixation (ORIF) as the only procedure through which fracture pain is abolished and early resumption of movement can be achieved.[4] Non-operative treatment in these cases therefore is not recommended. Certain fractures that could be treated non-operatively include the distal radius, proximal humerus, forearm and tibia, especially in children. Consequently, Charnley's classic manuscript on closed treatment of common fractures remains unsurprisingly up to date given that adhering to the proposed guidelines would lead to the successful treatment of most fractures including diaphyseal ones.[5]

In the era when the human genome project was completed and the universal acceptance of the existence of biological variation, it is reasonable for the surgeon to approach every patient and every fracture as a special entity. In other words, operative and/or non-operative treatment of a fracture in a specific patient must be considered on an individual basis. Not every fracture is amenable to surgical treatment and vice versa to non-operative treatment. Schatzker,[4] being one of the first who wanted to give emphasis to this principle, used the term 'fracture personality', which in a sense represented a number of important factors that the clinician had to take into account prior to his decision-making process. These factors included the age of the patient, the mechanism of the accident, the extent of the damage to the soft tissues (open/closed), other associated injuries above or below the site of injury, the degree of fracture fragmentation and the presence of comorbidities in the host, such as diabetes, osteoporosis, peripheral vascular disease and systemic inflammatory disease processes (i.e. rheumatoid arthritis).

Before a surgeon decides whether a common fracture such as that of a midshaft clavicle should be treated non-operatively, an analysis of the parameters composing the fracture personality should be carried out. In cases where there is pressure on the soft tissues by one of the fracture edges to the extent that there is an increased risk of skin breakdown, then operative treatment of this fracture should be carried out rather than non-operative, and has been proven to be successful over the years. For any fracture where a non-operative treatment approach is considered, the concept of the term 'fracture personality' must be applied.

Theoretically the vast majority of fractures could be treated non-operatively. Nowadays, common fractures in adults that can be considered for non-operative treatment include those of the clavicle, proximal and midshaft of the humerus, distal radius, metacarpi, tibia shaft, ankle and metatarsi.

PRINCIPLES OF CLOSED REDUCTION

Achieving satisfactory closed reduction of a fracture is of vital significance for successful bone healing. Closed reduction of fractures should be considered a work. Cooperation among the whole team involved in this process, the surgeon, the assistant, the anaesthetist, the radiographer and the patient, is a prerequisite. Adequate analgesia and muscle relaxation is of paramount importance, especially when dealing with children. The anaesthetist can facilitate the process by utilizing different methods of analgesia including blocks (local, regional and intravenous), sedation (conscious and deep) and dissociative anaesthesia (ketamine sedation). The assistant can provide support and countertraction of the affected limb while the radiologist with the appropriate positioning of the C-arm can provide good-quality imaging to reduce the period of both screening and the overall procedure. As with any technique, proper monitoring and adherence to safety guidelines is essential.[6]

The value of traction in the reduction of many fractures is well known. The concept of using axial traction and reversal of the mechanism of injury should be undertaken, although the aim is to correct and maintain optimal length, rotation and angulation.

In general terms, traction can be achieved by manipulation or with the help of pulleys or weights.[5] The latter could be used for the purpose of generating continuous traction and producing a relative fixation of the fragments with the help of tension in the surrounding soft tissues. If tension can be maintained while muscles relax and swelling subsides, length can be restored.[7] It is recommended that, during this process, muscle compartments should be monitored, for the purpose of avoiding a compartment syndrome, since lengthening of a limb segment will be followed by a decrease in the volume of muscle compartments, which tends to increase compartment pressure.[7]

Continuous traction can be applied through bones or skin and has the drawback of lengthy immobilization, with all the inevitable unpleasant consequences for the patient's general health. When skin traction is in use, it must be taken into account that there is a limitation to the force that can be applied, which cannot exceed 10 lb (4.5 kg). Special attention is warranted in elderly patients and in the presence of rheumatoid arthritis.[8] On the other hand, skeletal traction is more powerful, and up to 20% of body weight for the lower extremity can be applied.[8] It has to be emphasized that traction devices work only when the fragments are still connected to some soft tissue. Skeletal traction entails the insertion of either a Kirschner (K) wire or Steinman pin through the bone.[9] Regarding the upper extremity, olecranon skeletal traction is rarely used nowadays for humeral fractures. Traction pins for the lower extremity are placed in the supracondylar femur, proximal tibia and calcaneus, and are associated with possible complications such as quadriceps injury, neurovascular injury and infection. Calcaneal traction should be avoided because of the high infection rate.

Traction is the method of choice of temporizing long bone, pelvic and acetabular fractures until operative treatment can be performed.[8] When the use of long-term skeletal pins is required, local injection of antibiotic at the site of insertion to prevent infection and early loosening of the pin is recommended by some authors.[10]

CAST AND SPLINTING TECHNIQUES

Following manipulation of a fracture, immobilization of the injured limb and control of position is maintained with the help of casts or splints.

Casts

Cast immobilization includes two basic types: a holding cast or a moulded cast. A holding cast does not require extensive moulding. It is used for stable or non-displaced fractures, whereas a moulded cast has specific external moulding contours and aims to maintain a closed reduction of the fracture.[7]

A cast made of plaster of Paris is the most widely used method of immobilizing a fracture, despite a few disadvantages accompanying this practice. A plaster bandage and splints are made by impregnating crinoline with plaster of Paris $((CaSO_4)_2H_2O)$. When this material is dipped into water, the powdery plaster of Paris is transformed into a solid crystalline form of gypsum, and heat is given off:

$$(CaSO_4)_2H_2O + 3H_2O \leftrightarrow (CaSO_4 \cdot 2H_2O) + heat$$

Anhydrous calcium sulphate (plaster of Paris) ↔ Hydrated calcium sulphate (gypsum)

The three-point rule as proposed by Charnley should be applied to maintain closed reduction.[5] According to this rule the 'three-point' plaster exerts pressure at certain precisely determined points on the skeleton and no pressure at the others. Two of the three points are those where the surgeon moulds the cast firmly while setting against the proximal and distal portions of the extremity. In order to neutralize the turning couple of these two points and to prevent the plaster from rotating away from the limb, the third point is located directly opposite the apex of the cast.[11] Whether one or two joints should be immobilized with the cast (application of a forearm cast or an above-elbow cast) depends purely on the fracture personality.

Nowadays, synthetic casting materials are increasingly used as alternatives for plaster of Paris. They are characterized by certain advantages such as being stronger, lighter, relatively radiolucent, more water resistant and allowing weight bearing sooner after application than their plaster counterparts.[12,13] For these reasons they may be considered more convenient from the patient's point of view. It has been reported that the mean duration of usage before failure for synthetic forearm, scaphoid and below-knee casts was found to be approximately twice that of plaster casts.[14] Besides the aforementioned advantages, these commonly used synthetic materials also provide the benefit that when in use they do not create temperatures high enough to cause burns.[15] On the other hand, they are more expensive, leave less room for swelling and are more difficult to mould than plaster of Paris.[16] Concerns that synthetic materials generate higher pressures on and within the extremity and accommodate less swelling have led some investigators to discourage the use of casts made of such materials in the acute period after an injury or an operation.[17]

Splints

Splints are composed of a relatively rigid material that does not encompass the entire limb.[18] Coaptation splints and hanging casts have been widely used by many surgeons, implicitly indicating acceptance that immobilization of joints above and below the fracture and rigid fixation of fragments were not essential for uneventful healing.[19] Common splitting techniques generally in use include the coaptation or U-shaped slab for humeral fractures, the ulnar gutter splint, the volar/dorsal hand splint and the thumb spica splint. Their placement follows the same principles as those of a cast. In general, several other different splints are in use according to the fracture site.

Functional braces

Functional bracing was introduced in the 1960s as an alternative, conservative method for the treatment of selected fractures of long bones. After the initial treatment of diaphyseal tibial fractures, the technique was soon extended to fractures of the femoral shaft, the humerus, both bones of the forearm, the isolated ulnar shaft, and the distal radius.[20–22] This technique gained approval for the care of low-energy injuries, on the premise that motion at the fracture site encourages osteogenesis. Functional bracing is predicated on the belief that immobilization of the fragments and the joints above and below the fracture is not necessary for fracture healing. It also proposes that the soft tissues of the injured extremity play a major role in providing the stability necessary to allow uninterrupted osteogenesis.[23] In an animal study, Sarmiento and Latta,[22] compared the biomechanical properties of rigid compression plating and functional braces for closed non-displaced fractures and concluded that fractures treated with functional braces and followed by early activity demonstrated a cytologically more active endosteal callus and increased biomechanical strength characteristics at the fracture site.

According to Latta et al.,[23] during ambulation the brace encapsulates the water-rich soft tissues of the extremity and this hydraulic environment contributes to the prevention of limb shortening. In addition, the fact that functional bracing does not immobilize the joints adjacent to the fracture makes early restoration of motion possible.

COMPLICATIONS

Most of the complications associated with the application of a cast or splint are a result of improper application of the device or poor management of the patient. Drawbacks recorded after closed fracture treatment include pressure and rub sores, leg swelling, compartment syndrome, dermatitis, joint laxity or stiffness, cast or splint breakage, malunion or non-union and refracture.[24,25]

Middle-aged patients treated non-operatively with above-knee casts who are non-weight bearing are at special risk for deep vein thrombosis and pulmonary embolism.[26] Careful consideration should therefore be given to the necessity of non-weight bearing in a patient with a lower limb injury, and also prophylaxis against thrombosis should be instituted among high-risk individuals who must undergo case immobilization for injuries to the lower extremity.[27] As the incidence of deep vein thrombosis after isolated ankle fractures is low, routine thromboprophylaxis is not recommended for this kind of fracture treated non-operatively with a plaster.

Regarding plaster cast immobilization during aircraft transportation, a recent study supported that patients can be transported with a plaster cast split to the skin with no strict elevation needed.[28]

COMMON FRACTURES TREATED NON-OPERATIVELY

Distal radius

Colles fractures or extra-articular distal radial fractures can often be treated non-operatively. The distal radius has an 11° volar tilt, and a radial inclination of 22° with an average radial height of 11 mm.[29] These parameters are important, as restoration of such enable a better outcome. The deformity in a Colles-type fracture is a typical 'dinner fork' deformity, with shortening, radial deviation and dorsal displacement as well as dorsal comminution of the fracture (Fig. 18.1). A prominence of the ulna and dorsal part of the distal radius occurs.

Common indications for non-operative treatment of distal radius fractures are an extra-articular fracture in a low-demand patient and of a stable configuration. This 'stability' is inferred from there being less than 20° of dorsal angulation, less than 5 mm of shortening and minimal dorsal comminution.[30] Unfortunately, low-demand patients with extra-articular fractures are usually of the osteoporotic type.

Plain radiographs will define the anatomy and help delineate the indications for non-operative treatment. Analgesia given for the reduction of the fracture is either general or intralesional block (a haematoma block with local anaesthetic) or a Biers block, taking great care in monitoring the cardiac function in an elderly patient on release of the tourniquet.

Reduction is carried out with countertraction on the distal humerus by an assistant. The wrist is supinated, the deformity exaggerated dorsally and then traction and reduction in flexion to achieve cortical contact and volar inclination in pronation. Ulnar deviation is maintained to achieve the radial tilt and restore radial height.[31]

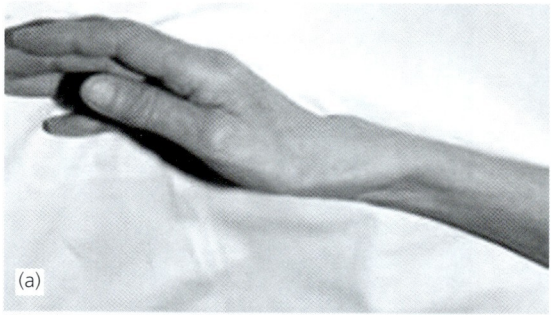
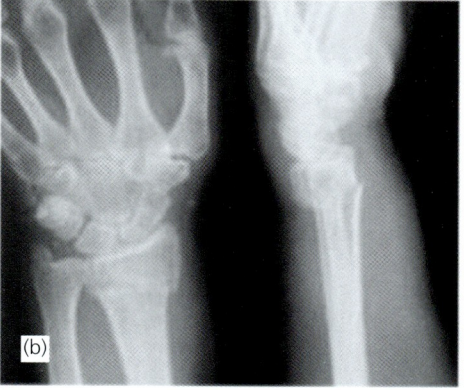

Figure 18.1 (a) Dinner fork-type deformity of the wrist secondary to a distal radius (Colles) fracture. (b) Anteroposterior and lateral radiographs of the wrist illustrating the fracture.

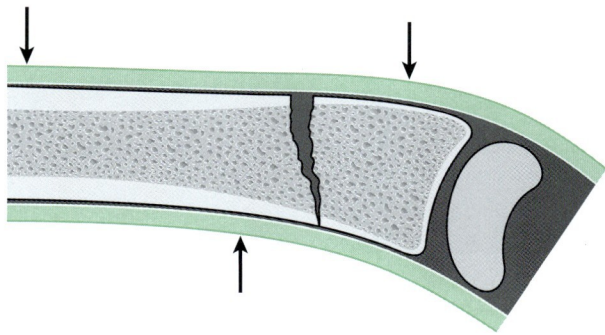

Figure 18.2 The plaster should be moulded adequately to provide the three-point fixation principle.

A below-elbow full cast with a 4 inch (10.2 cm) plaster may be applied and moulded to the wrist after the prominences are padded. The three-point fixation principle is applied to prevent a recurrent dorsal angular deformity (Fig. 18.2). The metacarpophalangeal joints must be left free to allow for finger movements and the elbow and shoulder joints mobilized early. Another alternative is a sugar tong splint as described for the forearm. This allows swelling to reduce and application of a full cast in the same position of reduction when the swelling is reduced. The arm is placed in an arm sling for a week or two but no more to facilitate elbow and shoulder mobilization. Elevation is necessary for reduction of swelling.

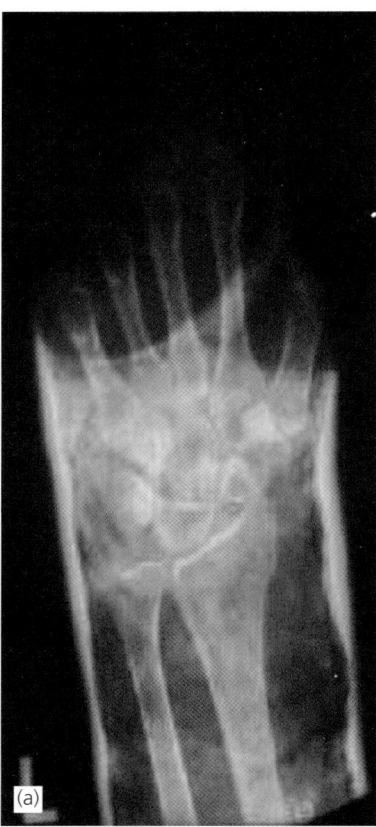

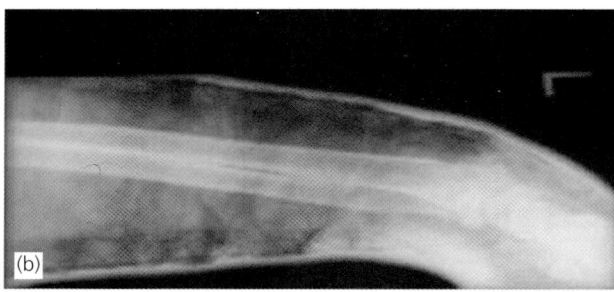

Figure 18.3 (a and b) Anteroposterior and lateral radiographs of the left wrist 2 weeks after the injury demonstrating good alignment with no loss of original reduction achieved.

Radiographs are done at weekly intervals for 2 weeks and then at 4 weeks (Fig. 18.3). The cast may be removed at 6 weeks and active mobilization of the wrist commenced.

Median nerve neuropathy may occur as a result of the flexed position of the wrist, and this should be carefully assessed during the first 2 weeks. Possible complications include loss of reduction (often because of dorsal comminution) and malunion, stiffness of the wrist and complex regional pain syndrome.

As long as good radiocarpal alignment is restored, the vast majority of patients gain 90% of motion after 1 year, although the arm and hand may be weaker than before.

Forearm fractures

Radius and ulna fractures in adults are rarely treated non-operatively. This is because the radius and ulna are considered part of one large rectangular joint. Accurate reduction of radius and ulna shaft fractures is required for optimal function at the proximal and distal radioulnar joints. This is to ensure that supination and pronation of the forearm are restored. The ulna is the flagpole of the forearm with the radius rotating around it. The radial bow should be restored. Single-bone fractures often are associated with injury or dislocations of the radioulnar joints. Accurate reduction will facilitate reduction of the proximal and distal joints.

Paediatric radius and ulna shaft fractures, however, are often treated non-operatively. The paucity of cast immobilization sequelae, the potential for remodelling, the relatively faster union time, the need for implant removal and cosmetic problems with the scars all add to the popularity of non-operative treatment. However, with the increasing expectations of parents and increasing cost of frequent follow-up and of plaster casts, there is a significant trend towards treating these fractures with closed reduction and percutaneous flexible intramedullary nailing.

Common indications currently for adults treated non-operatively for forearm fractures include (1) undisplaced fracture where the mechanism suggests minimal initial displacement and intact soft tissues, (2) less than 10% angulation and (3) less than 50% displacement and no shortening or joint dislocation. Nightstick fractures – i.e. isolated fractures of the ulna with less than 50% displacement and less than 10° of angulation – are ideal for non-operative management.

When treating the forearm bones, the restoration of length, the radial bow and reduction of rotational deformity are of paramount importance. Shortening is not acceptable and a minimum of 50% cortical contact is required.

Radiology is very important in identifying specific features relevant to achieving reduction. The level of the radial shaft fracture is important. If the fracture is in the proximal third, the proximal fragment is maintained in supination by the supinators, and any reduction of the distal fragment of the radius must be finally positioned in supination to avoid malrotation. Midshaft and distal shaft fractures will have the proximal radius in neutral rotation as both the supinator and pronator actions will be present; this will require the placement of the forearm in the mid-prone or neutral position after reduction.

The radial bow is an important consideration as this will affect the length of the radius and its ability to rotate around the flagpole of the ulna. The radial bow can be restored by thumb pressure on the interosseous membrane after achieving cortical contact of the fracture ends. This separates the shafts of the ulna and radius, helping to restore the radial bow as well as preventing synostosis (Fig. 18.4).

Finally, it is important to check that the proximal and distal radioulnar joints are in a good position after

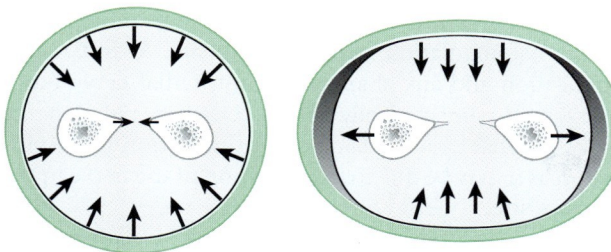

Figure 18.4 The cross-section of forearm casts should be made oval in order to avoid possible cross-union of the fracture.

manipulation. A line drawn through the centre of the neck and head of the radius must pass through the capitellum in all views and the ulnar level with respect to the distal radius, and the position on the lateral view must be restored.

Analgesia for reduction can be a Biers block or general anaesthesia. Usually at least three people are required for the procedure. Countertraction is given by someone holding on to the distal radius and someone pulling on the hand with radial deviation. Traction, exaggeration of the deformity and then reduction are performed to achieve cortical contact first. Oblique fractures may be difficult to reduce at the more acute angle of the end, and often the distal fragment can be rotated around the proximal shaft to the other end where the less acute angle of the fracture is present and the above-mentioned manoeuvre performed again. Once cortical contact of both bones is achieved, the ulnar reduction is fine-tuned using the subcutaneous border as a guide. Thumb pressure is then applied to the interosseous membrane to restore the radial bow. The wrist is then placed in supination or mid-prone depending on the considerations mentioned above.

An alternative method is to suspend the arm from a stable post using a clove hitch-type 2 inch (5.1 cm) bandage attached to the thumb separately and the index and middle finger. One assistant is required to provide downward countertraction and the forearm is vertically suspended. Manipulation is carried out as above and reduction manoeuvres are similar. The advantage of this method is that more consistent traction is applied (the post does not tire out) and less dependent angulation occurs on placing the splint.

Once reduced, the fracture can be placed in a full above-elbow cast (which can be split to prevent the complication of compartment syndrome). Reduction is maintained during cast application by consistent traction. A good but quick and easy alternative is to apply a sugar tong splint and reinforce it later, once the swelling is reduced. The sugar tong splint controls rotation and envelops most of the forearm, yet it allows for swelling of the soft tissues. The elbow is usually maintained at 90° of flexion. A 4 inch (10.2 cm) plaster is usually used and immobilization is from above the elbow to the metacarpal–phalangeal joint, allowing free finger movements. The wrist should be in neutral flexion and minimal ulnar deviation.

An arm sling is used to suspend the arm and elevation is advised. Compartment syndrome advice should be given to the patient. A neurovascular examination must be carried out after the manipulation. Radiographs are repeated after the splint is applied and at weekly intervals for 2 weeks. Following this radiographs will be taken in a cast at 4 weeks and 6 weeks and consideration then given for removal of the cast.

Finger and shoulder movement must be encouraged immediately and continued throughout the treatment period. Malrotation is possible and stiffness of the elbow joint, including limitation of supination and pronation, may occur. Synostosis is rare.

Proximal humerus fractures

Proximal humeus fractures that are undisplaced, impacted or minimally angulated or stable under image intensifier manipulation may be treated non-operatively. By Neer's criteria, fractures with less than 1 cm of displacement and less than 45° of angulation are considered relatively stable.[32] Other factors for non-operative treatment may include the patient's wishes and medical comorbidities.

Treatment is with a collar and cuff. The elbow is left unsupported. This allows gravity traction of the fracture. Early pendulum motion may be initiated. Hand, wrist and elbow motion should also be encouraged as soon as pain allows. However, early active abduction may cause a greater tuberosity fragment to displace and cause impingement. Thus, active abduction is avoided initially. Two weeks after injury, passive abduction may be initiated followed by active assisted and active range of motion exercises after 6 weeks. Early, staged rehabilitation will minimize secondary complications of stiffness or posttraumatic frozen shoulder.

Radiographs can be done 2 weeks after initial radiographs and at 6 weeks and finally 3 months after the injury.

Humeral shaft fractures

Closed humeral shaft fractures have shown good results when treated non-operatively.[33] The very large range of motion afforded by the glenohumeral joint can compensate for a certain degree of malunion and malrotation. Shortening is not much of a problem in the single-bone upper arm. Several factors should be considered in the choice of treatment modality, such as the fracture pattern. A spiral or oblique pattern would be more successfully treated non-operatively than a transverse or segmental fracture. A Holstein–Lewis pattern with a distal lateral spike may also caution against closed treatment. This is due to the larger surface area for healing provided in the spiral patterns. Body habitus may also play a part, as those generously endowed in the upper chest may cause unacceptable amounts of angulation at the fracture site.

Deforming forces acting on the humerus would be the rotator cuff, which would abduct and externally rotate attached fragments. The pectoralis major muscle adducts the proximal fragment and the deltoid causes abduction of the proximal fragment. Fractures just distal to the deltoid insertion may have exaggerated abduction and can, in patients with a small soft-tissue envelope, pierce through the skin in a U-slab, but this is an exception.

Radial nerve palsy is not a contraindication to closed non-operative treatment. Closed fractures with radial nerve palsy are considered to have a neuropraxia. Expectant treatment has been shown to have good recovery rates and recovery is only expected to begin after 3–4 months. An advancing Tinel's sign and nerve conduction studies done at 6 week intervals may be used to monitor progress of nerve recovery.

Acceptable displacement and angulation is less than 3 cm of shortening, less than 20° of shortening in the sagittal plane and less than 30° of angulation in the coronal plane (varus–valgus).

Once suitable radiological investigations are performed and a decision is made for non-operative treatment, a U-slab or sugar tong plaster splint is applied together with a collar and cuff (Fig. 18.5a–c). A hanging cast may be used in place of a U-slab, if excessive shortening is present or further reduction is required. The U-slab or hanging cast is made from a 4 inch (10.2 cm) plaster. Active finger, wrist and elbow range of motion exercises are encouraged from the beginning. While using a U-slab/hanging cast, it is advisable for the patient to be upright most of the time and to sleep propped up so as to allow gravity traction to the arm. An arm sling should not be used. The splint and arm weight will act as gravity traction to aid/maintain reduction of the fracture.

It is important that the medial proximal edge of the U-slab or proximal extent of the hanging cast does not end at the fracture site, as this may cause hinging and additional angulation at the fracture site. At initial slab application and any change of splint, radial nerve function should be clinically tested. Delayed radial nerve palsy is considered by some as an indication for exploration as it may be due to interposition of the nerve in the fracture site.

After 3–4 weeks the slab or cast may be changed to a removable humeral brace (Fig. 18.6a,b). This follows Sarmiento functional bracing principles. This is continued for 8–10 weeks. During the time the functional brace is on (it should be strapped on as tight as possible), active and active assisted rehabilitative activities may be commenced. Tight bracing muscle movement will help maintain reduction and provide stimuli for early bone healing with callus. The brace may be removed for hygiene maintenance purposes but otherwise should be worn most of the time.

Clinical healing usually precedes radiological callus formation, and rehabilitative exercises are initiated and progressed according to clinical tolerance. Good outcomes have been reported in the literature and indeed a large number of humeral fractures are treated non-operatively.[34,35]

Tibial shaft fractures

The tibia is the most commonly fractured long bone. The mechanism can be low energy or high energy. Low-energy fractures occur with minimal displacement and have simple fracture patterns such as spiral or oblique and transverse. Non-operative treatment is reserved for patients whose soft tissues are good, have minimal displacement and have a simple fracture pattern (Fig. 18.7).

The presence of an intact fibula bone may make non-operative treatment a little more difficult and predispose

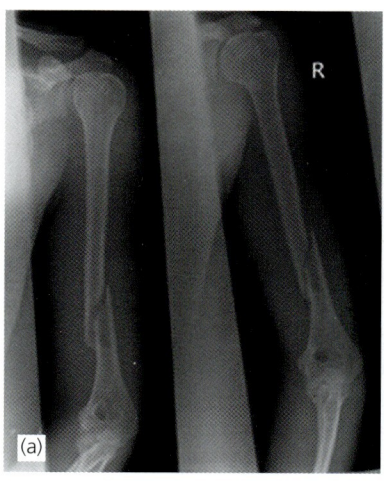
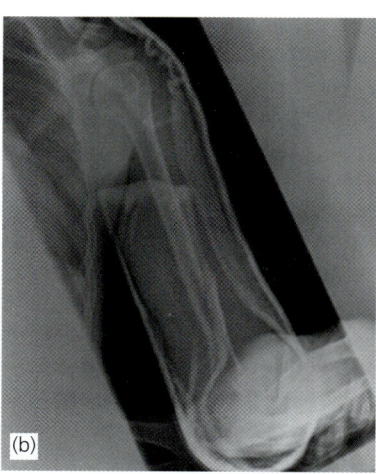
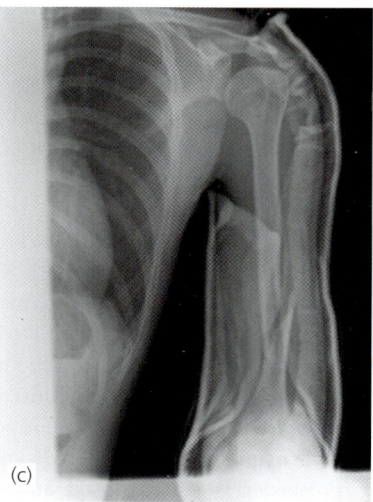

Figure 18.5 (a) Anteroposterior and lateral radiographs of a fracture at the middle to distal third junction of the humerus. (b and c) Anteroposterior and lateral radiographs of a humeral fracture treated with a U-slab.

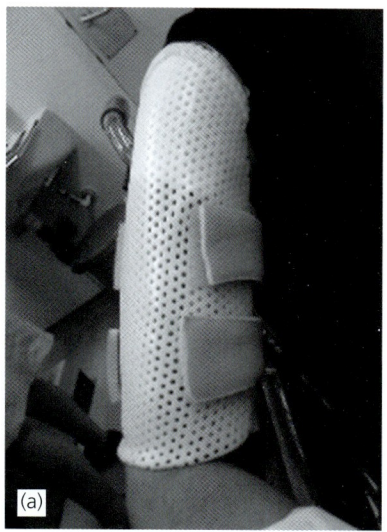 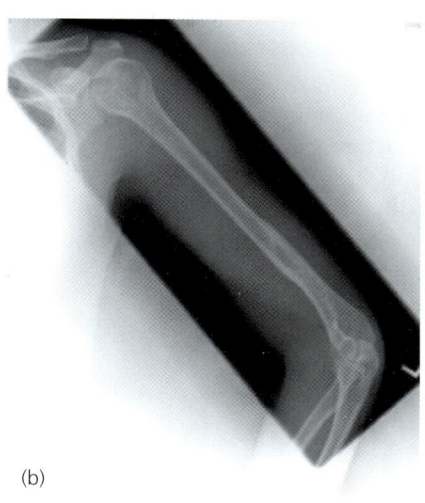

Figure 18.6 (a) Fracture stabilized with a humeral brace. (b) Lateral radiograph showing union of the fracture 12 weeks after injury.

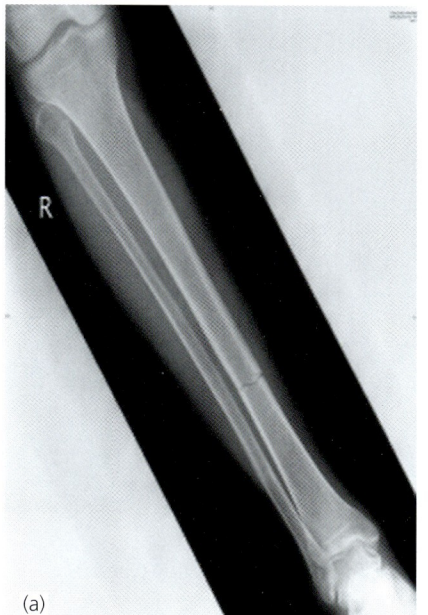 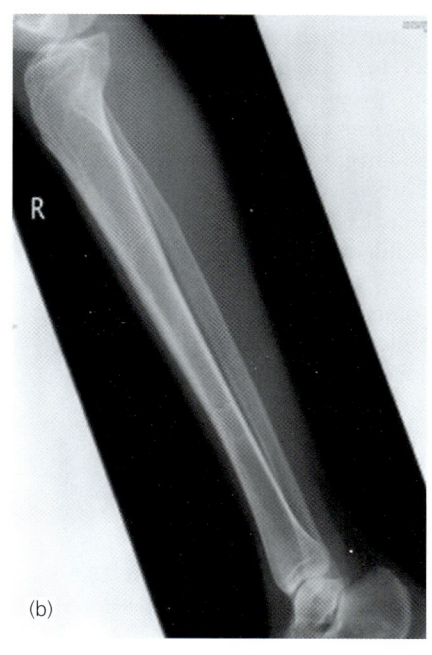

Figure 18.7 (a and b) Anteroposterior and lateral radiographs of a transverse tibial shaft fracture undisplaced.

the patient to varus malunion. Acceptable alignment of shaft fractures amenable to conservative treatment would be less than 10° of recurvatum/antecurvatum, 5° or less of varus/valgus angulation, less than 10° of malrotation and up to 1 cm of shortening.

Manipulation and reduction of the fracture is usually carried out under general anaesthesia.

The leg is hung down over the side of the operating table and traction applied to the ankle by means of an ankle strap and direct traction. The subcutaneous border of the tibia is used as a guide to reduction, and rotation can be estimated from the flexed knee and by using the second toe as a point of reference (15° external rotation of the ankle). This can be compared with the external rotation of the ankle of the contralateral side.

A full cast can be applied and then bivalved to allow for swelling. A 6 inch (15.2 cm) plaster is used for the tibia. The bony prominences – malleoli and the back of the heel – and the fibular head are padded with felt. After a stocking net and a thin layer of padding is applied, plaster is then first applied to the shaft of the tibia in single layers and the cast moulded to maintain the fracture reduction. While this is hardening the cast can be continued to cover the ankle, with the ankle in a plantigrade position if possible. Control of rotation of the distal fracture site must be maintained so as to not have a malrotation deformity.

The plaster is then completed proximally above the knee and the knee kept in 20–30° of flexion. It is good to mark the fracture site on the cast, in case wedging of the cast is required in future.

Postoperative radiographs are obtained. If the alignment needs to be corrected, wedging of the cast may be performed over the next few days and within 2 weeks. Wedging is done by estimating the apex of the angular deformity from the radiographs. The cast is circumferentially cut at the level of the fracture for three-quarters of the circumference for plaster of Paris the full circumference for fibreglass. Padding is not cut. A wooden spacer of the required size is inserted between the cut ends at 180° opposite the apex of the fracture to correct the angulation. Another layer of plaster is applied over this and a repeat radiograph is done to assess the alignment.

The cast is maintained for 4–6 weeks and radiographed weekly for the first 2 weeks to ensure alignment is maintained. This is followed by radiographs 2 weekly for 4 weeks. Non-weight-bearing ambulation is commenced with crutches. After 6 weeks, the cast is converted to a weight-bearing Sarmiento cast brace for another 6–8 weeks and the patient is allowed to progressively weight bear. The Sarmiento-type brace (patellar tendon-bearing cast) is a well-moulded below-knee weight-bearing cast moulded to the tibia and tibial condyles allowing flexion of the knee at the same time. Knee mobilization is commenced and 3 weekly radiographs performed to assess healing (Fig. 18.8a–d).

Complications of compartment syndrome, malunion, non-union and stiffness of the knee and ankle can occur. Carefully chosen low-energy isolated injuries treated by this method can have good results with up to 98% union and shortening of less than 5 mm. Union takes approximately 14–18 weeks as described by Sarmiento and Latta.[22]

Ankle fractures

Certain ankle fractures can be treated non-operatively. A very important consideration is the potential for talar shift in the mortise. If the deltoid ligament is ruptured or the medial malleolus is fractured then the potential for talar shift is high with an associated fibula fracture. Isolated medial malleolus fractures tend to non-union if treated non-operatively when a gap is present.

If there is no talar shift and an undisplaced or minimally displaced fibular fracture is present, this would be ideal for non-operative treatment. Examination for tenderness or bruising on the medial side raises suspicion of deltoid rupture and the potential for talar shift.

Adequate radiographic views of the fracture include anteroposterior, lateral and mortise views. Radiographs should be repeated routinely for the first 2 weeks after the injury for assessment of loss of position.

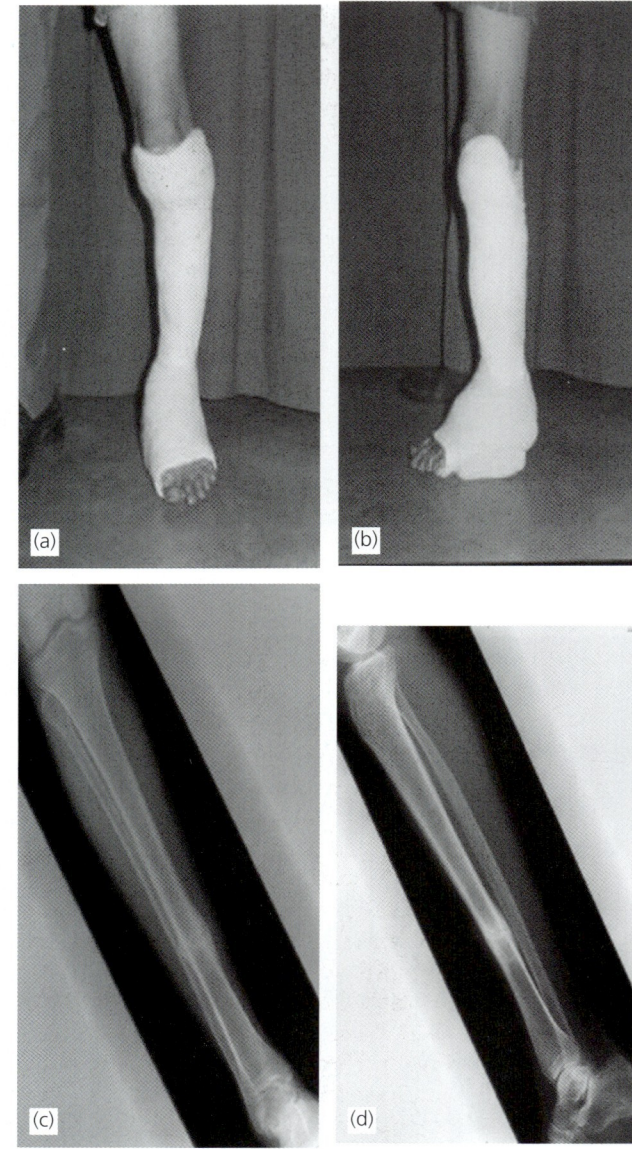

Figure 18.8 (a and b) Illustration of a Sarmiento-type brace (patellar tendon-bearing cast) for the midshaft tibial shaft fracture previously shown in Fig. 18.7. (c and d) Anteroposterior and lateral radiographs showing union of the fracture after 11 weeks.

Ankle fractures treated in a cast can initially be placed in a posterior splint or backslab and converted to a full cast within 3–7 days after the swelling subsides. It is important to pad the malleoli and the posterior heel to prevent pressure effects of the cast. With such fractures partial weight bearing may be commenced after 2 weeks and an aircast walker or weight-bearing cast applied. The cast can be removed after 4–6 weeks and progressive weight bearing commenced. Complications include stiffness of the ankle and the possibility of talar shift, which must be looked out for in all radiographs performed.

KEY LEARNING POINTS

- The benefits of skeletal stabilization became apparent with the Arbeitsgemeinschaft für Osteosynthesefragen (AO) techniques.
- The concepts of biological fixation and minimal invasive plate osteosynthesis have been popularized.
- Surgical intervention is not free of complications.
- Non-operative management of fractures can still be used in an effective way, especially in cases where there are contraindications for surgical treatment of the index fracture.
- Intra-articular fractures as well as many metaphyseal fractures demand open reduction and internal fixation.
- Fractures that could be treated non-operatively include the distal radius, proximal humerus, forearm and tibia, especially in children.
- The value of traction in the reduction of many fractures is well known.
- A cast made of plaster of Paris is the most widely used method of immobilizing a fracture.
- The three-point rule as proposed by charnley should be applied to maintain closed reduction.
- Splints are composed of a relatively rigid material that does not encompass the entire limb.
- Functional bracing is predicated on the belief that immobilization of the fragments and the joints above and below the fracture is not necessary for fracture healing.
- Most of the complications associated with the application of a cast or splint are a result of improper application of the device or poor management of the patient.
- Certain ankle fractures can be treated non-operatively. A very important consideration is the potential for talar shift in the mortise.

REFERENCES

- ● = Key primary paper
- ◆ = Major review article

● 1. Pape HC, Giannoudis PV, Krettek C. The timing of fracture treatment in polytrauma patients: relevance of damage control orthopaedic surgery. *American Journal of Surgery* 2002;**183**:622–9.

● 2. Giannoudis PV. Surgical priorities in damage control in polytrauma. *Joint of Bone and Joint Surgery (British)* 2003;**85**:478–84.

● 3. Papakostidis C, Grotz MRW, Papadokostakis G, et al. Femoral biological plate fixation. *Clinical Orthopaedics and Related Research* 2006;**450**:193–202.

◆ 4. Schatzker J. Intra-articular fractures. In: Schatzker J, Tile M (eds) *The Rationale of Operative Fracture Care*, 3rd edn. Berlin, Germany: Springer, 2005.

● 5. Charnley J. *The Closed Treatment of Common Fractures*, 4th edn. Cambridge, UK: The John Charnley Trust, 1999.

6. Migita RT, Klein EJ, Garrison MM. Sedation and analgesia for pediatric fracture reduction in the emergency department: a systematic review. *Archives of Pediatrics & Adolescent Medicine* 2006;**160**:46–51.

◆ 7. Latta LL, Sarmiento A, Zych G. Principles of nonoperative fracture treatment. In: Browner BD, Levine A, Jupiter J, Trafton P (eds) *Skeletal Trauma*. Philadelphia, PA: Saunders, 2003:159–78.

◆ 8. Koval KJ, Zuckerman JD. Closed reduction, casting, and traction. In: Koval KJ, Zuckerman JD (eds) *Handbook of Fractures*, 3rd edn. Philadelphia, PA: Philadelphia, PA: Lippincott Williams & Wilkins, 2006.

◆ 9. Taljanovic MS, Jones MD, Ruth JT, et al. Fracture fixation. *Radiographics* 2003;**23**:1569–90.

● 10. Nigam V, Jaiswal A, Dhaon BK. Local antibiotics: panacea for long term skeletal traction. *Injury* 2005;**36**:199–202.

◆ 11. Swiontkowski M, Stovitz S. Cast and bandaging techniques. In: Swiontkowski M, Stovitz S (eds) *Manual of Orthopaedics*, 6th edn. Philadelphia, PA: Lippincott Williams & Wilkins, 2001.

12. Kowalski KL, Pitcher JD Jr, Bickley B. Evaluation of fiberglass versus plaster of Paris for immobilization of fractures of the arm and leg. *Military Medicine* 2002;**167**:657–61.

◆ 13. Berman AT, Parks BG. A comparison of the mechanical properties of fiberglass cast materials and their clinical relevance. *Journal of Orthopaedic Trauma* 1990;**4**:85–92.

14. Marshall PD, Dibble AK, Walters TH, Lewis D. When should a synthetic casting material be used in preference to plaster-of-Paris? A cost analysis and guidance for casting departments. *Injury* 1992;**23**:542–4.

15. Pope MH, Callahan G, Lavalette R. Setting temperatures of synthetic casts. *Journal of Bone and Joint Surgery (American)* 1985;**67**:262–4.

16. Smith GD, Hart RG, Tsai TM. Fiberglass cast application. *American Journal of Emergency Medicine* 2005;**23**:347–50.

● 17. Davids JR, Frick SL, Skewes E, Blackhurst DW. Skin surface pressure beneath an above-the-knee cast: plaster casts compared with fiberglass casts. *Journal of Bone and Joint Surgery (American)* 1997;**79**:565–9.

● 18. Weinstein J, Ralphs SC. External coaptation. *Clinical Techniques in Small Animal Practice* 2004;**19**:98–104.

◆ 19. Sarmiento A, Latta LL. Functional fracture bracing. *Journal of the American Academy of Orthopaedic Surgeons* 1999;**7**:66–75.

◆ 20. Zagorski JB, Zych GA, Latta LL, McCollough NC 3rd. Modern concepts in functional fracture bracing: the upper limb. *Instructional Course Lectures* 1987;**36**:377–401.

◆ 21. Handoll HH, Pearce PK. Interventions for isolated diaphyseal fractures of the ulna in adults. *Cochrane Database of Systematic Reviews* 2004; CD000523.

◆ 22. Sarmiento A, Latta L. The evolution of functional bracing of fractures. *Journal of Bone and Joint Surgery (British)* 2006;**88**:141–8.

- ◆23. Latta LL, Sarmiento A, Tarr RR. The rationale of functional bracing of fractures. *Clinical Orthopaedics and Related Research* 1980;**Jan–Feb**:28–36.
- ◆24. Coles CP, Gross M. Closed tibial shaft fractures: management and treatment complications. A review of the prospective literature. *Canadian Journal of Surgery* 2000;**43**:256–62.
- ●25. Davids JR, Frick SL, Skewes E, Blackhurst DW. Skin surface pressure beneath an above-the-knee cast: plaster casts compared with fiberglass casts. *Journal of Bone and Joint Surgery (American)* 1997;**79**:565–9.
- ●26. Patil S, Gandhi J, Curzon I, Hui AC. Incidence of deep-vein thrombosis in patients with fractures of the ankle treated in a plaster cast. *Journal of Bone and Joint Surgery (British)* 2007;**89**:1340–3.
- ●27. Lassen MR, Borris LC, Nakov RL. Use of the low-molecular-weight heparin reviparin to prevent deep-vein thrombosis after leg injury requiring immobilization. *New England Journal of Medicine* 2002;**347**:726–30.
- 28. Senbaga N, Davies EM, Miller R, *et al*. Plaster cast immobilisation during air travel: analysis of current practice and aircraft-simulated experimental study. *Injury* 2006;**37**:138–44.
- ◆29. Simic PM, Weiland AJ. Fractures of the distal aspect of the radius: changes in treatment over the past two decades. *Instructional Course Lectures* 2003;**52**:185–95.
- ◆30. Handoll HH, Madhok R. Conservative interventions for treating distal radial fractures in adults. *Cochrane Database of Systematic Reviews* 2003;CD000314.
- ●31. Chen NC, Jupiter JB. Management of distal radial fractures. *Journal of Bone and Joint Surgery (American)* 2007;**89**:2051–62.
- ●32. Neer CS II. Displaced proximal humeral fractures. Part I. Classification and evaluation. *Journal of Bone and Joint Surgery (American)* 1970;**52**:1077–89.
- ●33. Sarmiento AMJ. Functional bracing for the treatment of fractures of the humeral diaphysis. *Journal of Bone and Joint Surgery (American)* 2000;**82**:478–86.
- ●34. Jawa A, McCarty P, Doornberg J, *et al*. Extra-articular distal-third diaphyseal fractures of the humerus. A comparison of functional bracing and plate fixation. *Journal of Bone and Joint Surgery (American)* 2006;**88**:2343–7.
- ●35. Rutgers M, Ring D. Treatment of diaphyseal fractures of the humerus using a functional brace. *Journal of Orthopaedic Trauma* 2006;**20**:597–601.

19

Principles of operative fracture fixation

PETER V GIANNOUDIS, COSTAS PAPACOSTIDIS

Introduction	269	Methods of achieving absolute stability	271
The concept of stable fixation	269	Methods of achieving relative stability	272
Biomechanics of fracture healing	270	References	276

NATIONAL BOARD STANDARDS

- Understand the biomechanical basis of fracture healing
- Know the different types of internal fixation system
- Understand techniques for internal fixation of osteoporotic bone
- Understand the mechanism of healing following intramedullary nailing
- Understand the biomechanics and mechanism of healing following locked plating

INTRODUCTION

A fracture can be described as an abrupt disruption of the continuity of a living bone with concomitant injury of various degrees to the adjacent soft-tissue envelope. The basic goals of fracture treatment are restoration of the disrupted osseous anatomy and sufficient stabilization of the fractured bone that will facilitate soft-tissue healing and permit early painless motion, resulting ultimately in an optimal functional recovery of the injured extremity.

Although the above principles were introduced almost 50 years ago by the AO (Arbeitsgemeinschaft für Osteosynthesefragen) group and have remained virtually unaltered since then, the operative techniques designed to serve these principles have been evolving up to the present time.

The scope of this chapter is to review these techniques and their evolution, with special emphasis on the current 'state of the art' operative fracture treatment.

THE CONCEPT OF STABLE FIXATION

The basic element of the AO philosophy regarding fracture treatment was the concept of 'early functional rehabilitation'.[1] This concept could only be applied in fractures that had been anatomically reduced and stably fixed. Stable fixation eliminates fracture pain and allows for early and full mobilization of the injured extremity. A stable fixation is the one that eliminates motion at the fracture site. Stability, in terms of fracture fixation, is either absolute, when even micro-motions are abolished at the fracture site under functional loading, or relative, when gross motion is prevented, although micro-motions still exist at the fracture zone.

Absolute stability

Absolute stability is synonymous with compression. Therefore, an absolutely stable fixation is the one that restores structural continuity of the fracture zone through

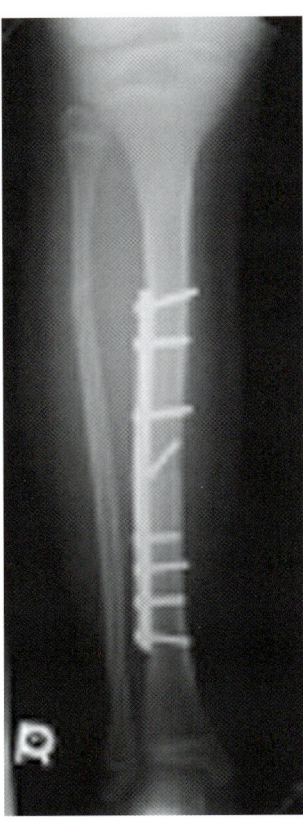

Figure 19.1 Anteroposterior radiograph of a healed tibia shaft fracture stabilized with a lag screw and plate. Absolute stability (no callus formation).

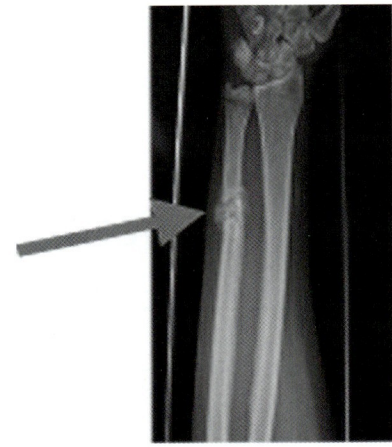

Figure 19.2 Anteroposterior radiograph of a distal ulna fracture stabilized with plaster of Paris (relative stability – healed by callus formation).

anatomical reduction and stabilizes the fractured fragments by means of interfragmentary compression.[2] With absolute stability, any micro-motion is abolished at the fracture zone. The initial bone resorption is eliminated and fracture healing progresses without external callus formation through the process of direct (primary) bone healing[3] (Fig. 19.1).

Relative stability

With relative stability, some degree of interfragmentary motion is allowed under functional loading. Under these mechanical conditions fracture healing progresses through the indirect healing process with abundant callus formation[3] (Fig. 19.2).

BIOMECHANICS OF FRACTURE HEALING

Modern principles of fracture fixation aim at securing a fine balance between optimal mechanical and biological conditions at the fracture zone. Operative intervention on a fracture should minimize any potential damage to the vascularity (biological environment) of the fracture fragments, while, at the same time, achieving the optimal degree of fracture stability (mechanical environment), so that the healing process progresses uneventfully.

Mechanical environment and fracture healing

Fracture fixation obviously aims to create the optimal mechanical stability that will permit both early functional rehabilitation of the injured limb and timely fracture healing. The interfragmentary strain theory provides a better insight to the optimal mechanical environment of fractures.[4] In the setting of fractures, strain (ε) is expressed as the ratio of the displacement (Δl) of the fracture fragments to the fracture gap (L), i.e. $\varepsilon = \Delta l / L$. Strain is proportional to the degree of displacement of fracture fragments and inversely proportional to the initial fracture gap. According to this theory, the pluripotent cells of the granulation tissue at the fracture gap respond according to the deformation of the fracture gap (strain) and are gradually differentiated into cartilage-forming and eventually bone-forming cells. The various repair tissues, on the other hand, present at the fracture gap at different stages of fracture healing have different strain tolerances (critical strain) before they yield and fail under conditions of mechanical instability. Although the critical strain of granulation tissue is 100%, cartilage can tolerate a much lesser degree of strain (10%) and bone can tolerate only 2%. The evolution of the fracture-healing process, according to the strain theory, is possible only if the strain at the fracture gap does not exceed the critical value of the next, in order of differentiation, repair tissue. Consequently, under conditions of gross mechanical instability and fracture gap strain exceeding the critical limit of strain of the next repair tissue to be developed, the differentiation process comes to a halt. According to

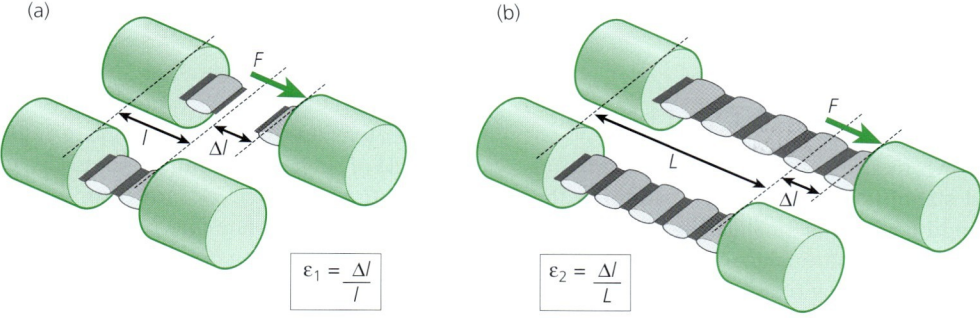

Figure 19.3 Illustration of the influence of the fracture pattern on strain. Simple fracture pattern with a small fracture gap (a) cannot tolerate conditions of mechanical instability (displacement Δl), as the resultant strain (ε_1) is well above the critical value. In this case the 'chain of reparative tissues' within the fracture gap ruptures and the healing process stops. In the multifragmentary fracture pattern (b) the same degree of displacement (Δl) will keep the overall strain (ε_2) to low levels, well below the critical value, due to the larger fracture gap (L). The healing process, therefore, progresses uneventfully.

strain definition, different fracture patterns can tolerate different degrees of instability in order to keep strain at optimal levels for propagation of the healing process. In a simple fracture pattern with a small fracture gap (L) of 1 mm, the degree of instability (Δl) that can be tolerated so that the cartilaginous tissue at the fracture site can be differentiated to bone (optimal strain levels, $\varepsilon < 2\%$) is less than 0.02 mm. In contrast, a comminuted fracture pattern with a large gap between the main fragments can tolerate a larger degree of instability while keeping strain at low levels. It is thus clear that simple fracture patterns, having been reduced with close apposition of the fracture fragments, cannot tolerate unstable conditions and need an absolutely stable fixation, whereas comminuted fractures can tolerate conditions of relative instability without compromising the progression of the healing process (Fig. 19.3).

Biological environment and fracture healing

Adequate blood supply of the fracture area is of paramount importance for the evolution of the healing process. When a fracture occurs, the absorbed energy causes interruption of endosteal circulation and various degrees of periosteum and soft-tissue stripping.[5] While in an intact tubular bone, blood circulation is centrifugal (from the endosteal towards periosteal network); in cases of a fracture with rupture of the blood vessels of the medullary canal, the periosteal circulation takes precedence and the blood flow is directed centripetally from the periosteal plexus through the cortex towards the medullary canal.[6] The surgical approach potentially results in additional damage to the soft-tissue envelope of fractures, whereas the bone–implant interface could contribute to further disturbance of cortical vascularity.[7] Based on the above observations, it is clear that meticulous soft-tissue and bone fragment handling during surgical exposure of a fracture will minimize additional disturbance of the biological environment of the fracture and secure the evolution of the bone-healing process.

METHODS OF ACHIEVING ABSOLUTE STABILITY

Lag screw fixation

The simplest and most effective way of exerting interfragmentary compression is by means of a lag screw.[8] A lag screw is optimally inserted perpendicular to the fracture plane and takes purchase only in the far fracture fragment while it glides through the near fragment. When a lag screw is being tightened, the two fracture fragments are compressed (lagged) together. A partially threaded screw (shaft screw) can be readily used as a lag screw. A fully threaded cortical screw can function as a lag screw if overdrilling of the near cortex to the outer diameter of the screw thread is performed (thus creating a gliding hole that does not permit any purchase with the screw threads), with concomitant drilling of a pilot hole (thread hole) in the far cortex. Lag screws are predominantly used in intra-articular fractures, where anatomical reduction and absolute stability are mandatory for preservation of the cartilage and recovery of the joint function. In long oblique or spiral fractures of the diaphysis, however, where at least two or even three such screws are necessary for stable fixation, the merits of their application should be weighed against biological considerations of extensive soft-tissue and periosteal stripping that their use could entail.

Plating

Plates can be used as a means of achieving absolute stability of fractures under different principles. Such plates are referred to as neutralization, buttress, compression or tension band plates, according to the principle of their application and function.[9,10]

NEUTRALIZATION AND BUTTRESS PLATES

Although lag screw fixation achieves interfragmental compression and stability of a fracture, it cannot withstand alone all bending, torsional or shearing forces exerted on the fracture during functional loading. The simplest method of protecting lag screw fixation is by means of a plate that takes most of the forces across the fracture zone. In the diaphyseal region, a plate used to neutralize forces across the fracture surface and, consequently, to protect the compressive osteosynthesis achieved by lag screws is referred to as a *neutralization* or *protection plate*. Such a plate does not exert axial compression at the fracture level but bypasses most of the load from one main fragment of the fracture to the other, thus protecting the lag screw fixation from overloading and potential failure. The metaphyseal area, on the other hand, consisting mainly of cancellous bone with a thin cortical shell, is subjected to compressive and shearing forces during functional loading. Lag screw fixation in this area also needs protection in order to prevent fracture displacement with subsequent malalignment or articular incongruity. A plate used to support the underlying cortex in the metaphyseal area is called a buttress plate.

COMPRESSION AND TENSION BAND PLATES

Although a major shift in the philosophy of osteosynthesis of long bone fractures towards more flexible forms of fixation has taken place over the last few decades, techniques of absolute stability are still practised. A simple fracture pattern that needs anatomical reduction (in order to obtain complete functional recovery of the injured limb) is not compatible with high strain conditions and it requires a rigid, absolutely stable fixation. Short oblique or transverse fractures are not amenable to lag screw fixation. In these cases plates can be utilized to achieve stable fixation by exerting compression at the fracture plane (compression plates). A compression plate generates compression along the long axis of the bone, either by means of the tension device or by taking advantage of the specific hole design of the self-compression plates, which allows for axial compression by eccentric screw insertion. Whenever possible, self-compression plates can be combined with lag screws to achieve the maximal effect of interfragmental compression. Axial compression of a simple fracture by means of a self-compression plate creates a gap in the opposite cortex, which could jeopardize the stability of fixation. Compression of the opposite cortex and subsequent enhancement of the stability of fixation can be achieved by means of pre-bending of the plate before its final application onto the fractured bone. Appropriate insertion of the screws (in compression mode) through the holes of the plate will press the pre-bent plate against the underlying cortex. The plate, acting like a spring, will exert compression across the opposite cortex, closing the gap. In eccentrically loaded bones (such as the femur), one cortex is being loaded under compression whereas the opposite one is under tension. A compression plate applied on the tension side of such a bone will be put under tension and will convert the tensile forces into compressive forces on the opposite cortex. A plate that functions in the above way is referred to as a *tension band plate*. A basic prerequisite for application of the principle of tension band plating is the integrity of the cortex opposite the plate, so as to withstand the compressive forces generated by the conversion of the tensile force by the plate. Otherwise the plate will be subject to cyclic bending and, eventually, fatigue failure.

METHODS OF ACHIEVING RELATIVE STABILITY

They fall into three categories:

1. biological plate fixation
2. external fixation
3. intramedullary nail fixation.

The common denominator of all three methods of elastic fixation is the absence of interfragmentary compression. According to the strain theory these methods should be applied in comminuted fracture patterns that can tolerate relatively unstable conditions while keeping strain to low, permissive levels for bone healing. The indications of elastic fixation, however, can be extended even to simple fracture patterns, provided that the reduction is not accurate, leaving larger gap widths that maintain strain within 'permissive limits'.[11]

Biological plate fixation

The importance of periosteal blood supply for fracture healing is well established. In the presence of a fracture and interruption of the endosteal circulation, the periosteal circulation takes precedence and it is responsible for the blood supply to the fracture zone.[5,12] The 'mechanistic' concept of fixation, already described, requires wide exposure of the fracture zone and an accurate reduction. This approach increases operative trauma to the soft-tissue envelope (muscles, periosteum) of the fracture area, which is superimposed on the damage inflicted by the initial trauma, often leading to unfavourable results (non-union, implant failure). On the other hand, the excellent results of closed intramedullary nailing of fractures of long bones have prompted a shift in the philosophy of internal fixation with plates and screws towards more atraumatic techniques, particularly regarding the soft-tissue envelope. A new concept of biological plate fixation has thus been created based on the following principles of indirect reduction and bridge plating.[11,13–18]

INDIRECT REDUCTION

The principle of indirect reduction is applied only on diaphyseal long bone fractures aiming at restoring proper length as well as, axial and torsional alignment of the fractured bone by means of traction. Anatomical reduction by means of direct handling of all the bone fragments in the zone of comminution is avoided in an effort to preserve their vascularity. These bone fragments, provided that their soft-tissue attachments remain intact, will act as vascularized bone grafts that, along with the elasticity of fixation, will promote fracture healing with abundant callus formation. Traction can be applied either by using the specific fracture table in an identical manner to that in the intramedullary nailing procedure, or by means of a traction device.

BRIDGE PLATES

The term 'bridge plate' refers to a long plate applied epiperiosteally, adequately spanning the fracture zone and fixed onto the two main fragments with the least possible number of screws (Fig. 19.4). Such a plate acts as an extramedullary splint, securing the two main fragments of the long bone fracture to proper length and axial and rotational alignment without compression. Any plate can be used as a bridge plate, provided that the basic principles of biological plate fixation are met. However, conventional plates (such as the dynamic compression plate (DCP)) provide a wide contact area with the underlying cortex and were found to induce partial cortical necrosis. This fact could compromise both the healing capacity and local resistance to infection.[7,19] In an effort to reduce the contact area between the plate and the underlying cortical bone, plate design has evolved, introducing first the limited contact (LC)-DCP[20] and culminating recently in the introduction of the locking compression plate (LCP).[21-24] This plate incorporates the dynamic compression principle of the DCP along with the principle of locking between screws and plate. The locking principle is due to the presence of an extra thread in the head of the screws which allows them to be locked rigidly on the plate. The LCP plate functioning as a fixed-angle device offers certain biological advantages compared with conventional plates. First, tight contact with the underlying bone is eliminated, preserving the cortical blood supply. Second, it provides increased stability and so it can be used as a single implant in highly unstable fractures (e.g. comminuted bicondylar fractures of tibia) for which conventional double plate fixation would be required. Subsequently, extensive soft-tissue dissection is spared, local vascularity is preserved and bone healing potential is enhanced.[11,25] The biological aspect of the use of LCPs

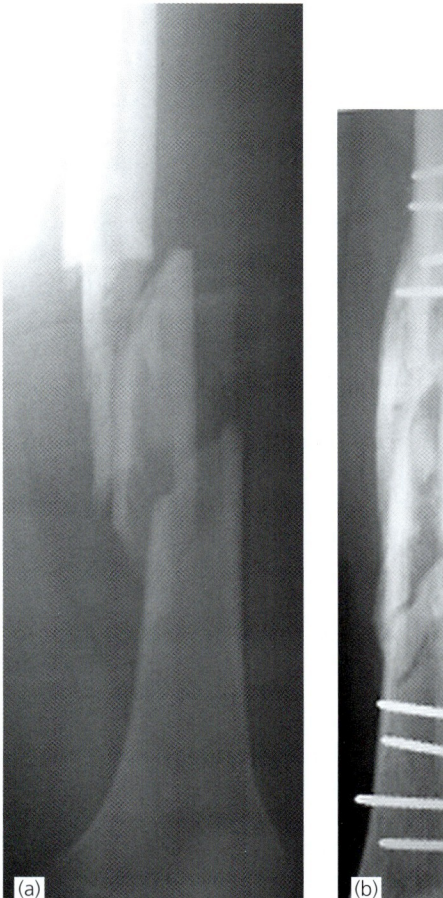
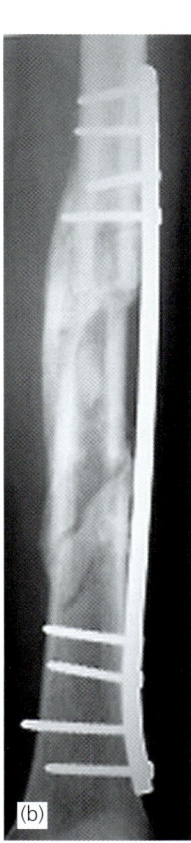
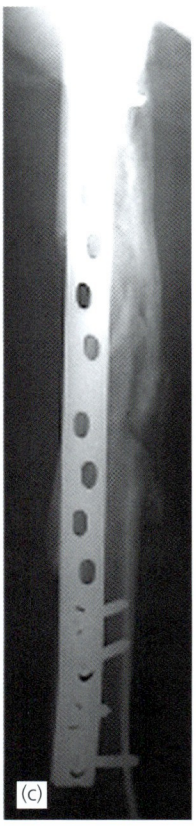

Figure 19.4 (a) Anteroposterior (AP) radiograph of a femoral shaft fracture with the zone of fragmentation. (b, c) AP and lateral radiographs showing fracture healing after 5 months with the technique of bridge plating.

has been further emphasized by the development of percutaneous surgical techniques allowing their placement through small incisions, remote to the fracture zone, and blind insertion of the locking screws with the use of specifically designed aiming devices. The MIPPO (minimally invasive percutaneous plate osteosynthesis) epitomizes recent advances in the biological approach of plate osteosynthesis.[26–28]

External fixation

This method utilizes pins or wires inserted in the main bone fragments proximal and distal to the fracture site and connected outside the skin to one or more longitudinal bars or rods (Fig. 19.5). The basic characteristic of external fixation is penetration of the soft-tissue envelope of bones by the pins of the external fixator, which in turn is associated with certain disadvantages, such as pin track infection and joint stiffness due to restriction of the normal gliding mechanism of the soft-tissue envelope by pins inserted through fascia and muscles. The above disadvantages along with the cumbersome nature of bulky frames make routine use of external fixation a less attractive option. Nevertheless, there are certain indications for its use either as a temporary or even as a definitive means of fracture fixation.[29] These include

1. open fractures
2. closed fractures with precarious skin conditions
3. polytrauma patients (damage control orthopaedics)
4. children's fractures
5. specific intra-articular fractures (e.g. distal radius fractures) as a joint-spanning device
6. distraction osteogenesis and bone transport techniques.

A basic concern of the use of external fixation as a temporary fixation device is the risk of deep infection after conversion to internal fixation, particularly intramedullary nail fixation.[29,30] Direct conversion to intramedullary nail fixation is recommended within the first 2 weeks of external fixation, provided that there are no local signs of pin track infection. At a later time, it is advisable that the procedure is performed in two stages, consisting of removal of the external frame, pin track toilette and application of a cast for temporary immobilization of the injured limb, followed by a definitive nailing procedure when pin tracks are completely healed without signs of infection. When plating is contemplated, the conversion follows the above principles, but direct, one-stage conversion can be attained within 3–4 weeks in the absence of infection.[29] In order to overcome the problem of potential infection, a specific device, the pinless fixator, has been devised. This fixator consists of forceps-like pins that are attached firmly to the cortical surface without violating the intramedullary canal.

There are several parameters influencing the rigidity of the construct and thus the stability of a fracture managed with external fixation, such as the diameter and spread of the pins, the distance between bone and longitudinal rod and the type of frame (bilateral, delta or triangular frame). As a general rule the rigidity of the frame should be individualized according to the type of fracture.[31]

Intramedullary nailing

Intramedullary nails are placed within the medullary canal acting as intramedullary splints (Fig. 19.6). The classical Küntscher nail represents the early efforts of fixing diaphyseal fractures of long bones by means of intramedullary splints. The stability of the Küntscher nail relied on the tight fit of the elastic slotted nail with the endosteal surface of the cortical bone of the diaphysis as well as the interdigitation of the bone fragments at the fracture level. In an effort to

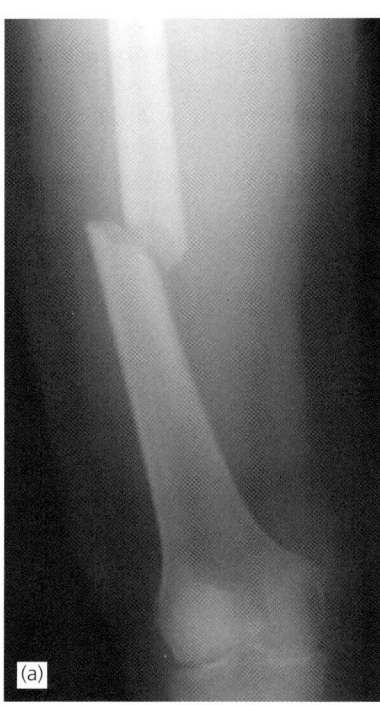

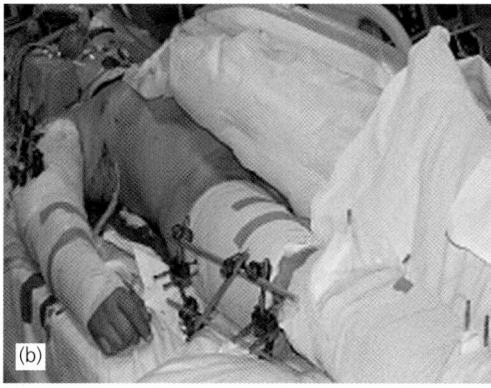

Figure 19.5 (a) Anteroposterior radiograph of a femoral shaft fracture. (b) The patient had sustained multiple injuries. The femoral fracture was stabilized with an external fixator as shown.

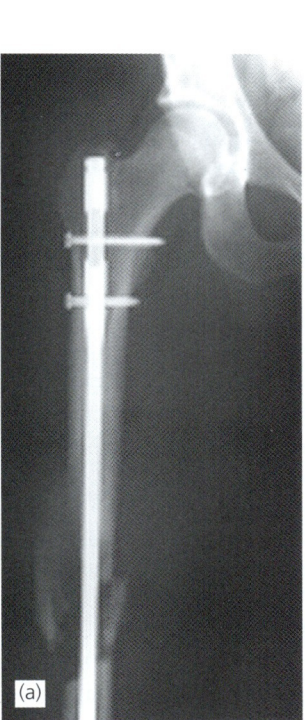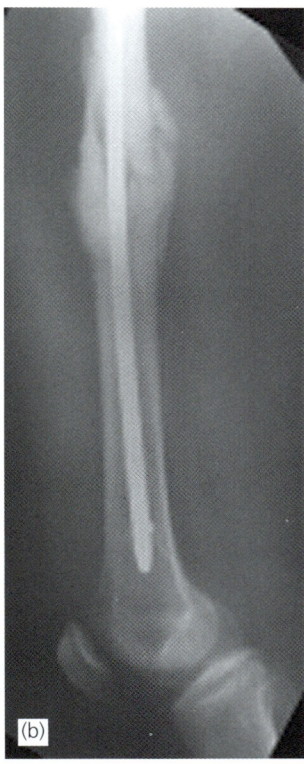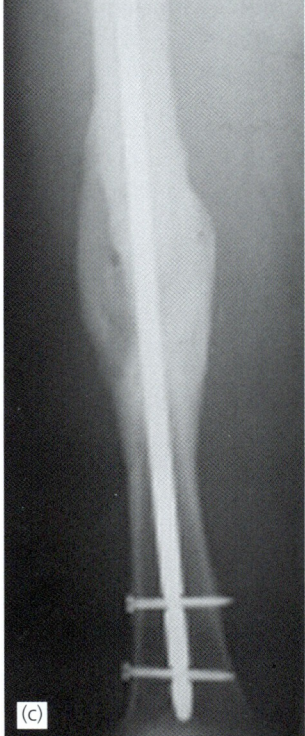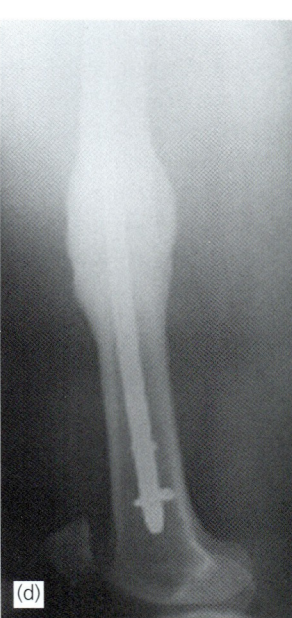

Figure 19.6 Femoral fracture. (a, b) Anteroposterior and lateral radiographs stabilized with an intramedullary nail. (c, d) Healing of the fracture 5 months later by callus formation.

increase the contact area between endosteal bone and nail and thus enhance the stability of the fracture, Küntscher introduced reaming of the medullary canal. Nevertheless, the indications for this nail were limited to transverse midshaft fractures. The addition of interlocking screws by Grosse and Kempf expanded the indications of nailing for any fracture type in any location of the diaphysis of long bones.[32] These first-generation interlocking nails, however, were not suitable for certain fracture types such as subtrochanteric fractures of femur or femur fractures with intertrochanteric extension. This fact prompted the development of second-generation intramedullary nails, such as the reconstruction nail or short and long cephalomedullary nails. Moreover, retrograde nails made management of fractures of the distal femoral metaphysis feasible. Currently, closed intra-medullary nailing is considered to be the standard method of treatment of long bone shaft fractures.[33] A still controversial topic regarding modern intramedullary nailing techniques is reaming of the medullary canal. Proponents of reaming maintain that this technique allows for the insertion of nails of larger diameter with improved mechanical features. From the biological aspect, the reaming process is considered to produce an intramedullary bone grafting effect at the fracture site, potentiating the healing process.[33] However, the osteoinductive effects of the reaming material have been questioned.[33] Opponents of reaming emphasize both local and general adverse effects of the reaming process. With respect to local effects, the reaming process has been associated with cortical bone necrosis and predisposition to infection.[34] Therefore, reamed nails are not considered as first choice implants in open fractures. As for the systematic manifestations, reaming appears to stimulate the inflammatory system causing pulmonary embolic phenomena and disturbances of the coagulation system.[35,36] These effects are particularly potentiated in the context of polytrauma and, consequently, intramedullary nailing, particularly with reaming, should be deferred until the condition of the polytrauma victim is stabilized (damage control orthopaedics).[37,38]

KEY LEARNING POINTS

- A fracture can be described as an abrupt disruption of the continuity of a living bone with concomitant injury of various degrees to the adjacent soft-tissue envelope.
- The basic goals of fracture treatment are restoration of the disrupted osseous anatomy and sufficient stabilization of the fractured bone that will facilitate soft-tissue healing and permit early painless motion, resulting ultimately in an optimal functional recovery of the injured extremity.
- A stable fixation is the one that eliminates motion at the fracture site (relative or absolute).

- Absolute stability is synonymous with compression; in relative stability, some degree of interfragmentary motion is allowed under functional loading.
- Operative intervention on a fracture should minimize any potential damage to the vascularity (biological environment) and achieve the optimal degree of fracture stability (mechanical environment), so that the healing process progresses uneventfully.
- Adequate blood supply of the fracture area is of paramount importance for the evolution of the healing process.
- To achieve absolute stability, the simplest and most effective way of exerting interfragmentary compression is by means of a lag screw; and so can plates (neutralization and buttress plates, compression and tension band plates) be used as a means of achieving absolute stability of fractures under different principles.
- To achieve relative stability there is: biological plate fixation (indirect reduction, bridge plates); external fixation; and intramedullary nail fixation. In all there is the absence of interfragmentary compression.

REFERENCES

- ● = Key primary paper
- ◆ = Major review article

◆1. Muller ME, Allgower M, Schneider R, Willeneger H. *Manual of Internal Fixation*, 2nd edn. Heidelberg, Germany: Springer-Verlag, 1979.

◆2. Muller ME, Allgower M, Schneider R, Willeneger H. *Manual of Internal Fixation*, 3rd edn. Heidelberg, Germany: Springer-Verlag, 1991.

◆3. Perren SM. Physical and biological aspects of fracture healing with special reference to internal fixation. *Clinical Orthopaedics and Related Research* 1979;**138**:175–96.

◆4. Perren SM, Cordey J. The concept of interfragmentary strain. In: Uhthoff HK, Stahl E (eds) *Current Concepts of Internal Fixation of Fractures*. Berlin, Germany: Springer, 1980:63–77.

◆5. Trueta J. Blood supply and the rate of healing of tibial fractures. *Clinical Orthopaedics and Related Research* 1974;**105**:11–26.

●6. Rhinelander FW. The normal microcirculation of diaphyseal cortex and its response to fracture. *Journal of Bone and Joint Surgery (American)* 1968;**50A**:784–800.

◆7. Gautier E, Cordey J, Mathys R, *et al*. *Porosity and Remodeling of Plated Bone after Internal Fixation: Result of Stress Shielding or Vascular Damage?* Amsterdam, The Netherlands: Elsevier Science Publishers, 1984:195–200.

◆8. Perren SM, Frigg R, Hehli M, *et al*. Lag screw. In: Ruedi TP, Murphy WM (eds) *AO Principles of Fracture Management*. Stuttgart, Germany: Thieme, 2000:157–67.

◆9. Wittner B, Holz U. Plates. In: Ruedi TP, Murphy WM (eds) *AO Principles of Fracture Management*. Stuttgart, Germany: Thieme, 2000:169–85.

◆10. Schatzker J. Principles of internal fixation. In: *The Rationale of Operative Fracture Care*. Berlin, Germany: Springer, 2005:3–33.

◆11. Perren SM. Evolution of the internal fixation of long bone fractures. The scientific basis of biological internal fixation: choosing a new balance between stability and biology. *Journal of Bone and Joint Surgery (British)* 2002;**84**:1093–110.

●12. Strachan RK, McCarthy I, Fleming R, Hughes SP. The role of the tibial nutrient artery. Microsphere estimation of blood flow in the osteotomised canine tibia. *Journal of Bone and Joint Surgery (British)* 1990;**72**:391–4.

13. Heitemeyer U, Hierholzer G. Die Uberbruckende Osteosynthese bei geschlossenen Stuckfrakturen des femurschaftes. *Aktuelle Traumatologie* 1985;**15**:205–9.

●14. Mast J, Ganz R, Jakob RP. *Preoperative Planning and Reduction Techniques*. Heidelberg, Germany: Springer-Verlag, 1988.

●15. Gerber C, Mast JW, Ganz R. Biological internal fixation of fractures. *Archives of Orthopaedic and Trauma Surgery* 1990;**109**:295–303.

16. Baumgaertel F, Perren SM, Rahn B. Animal experiment studies of 'biological' plate osteosynthesis of multifragment fractures of the femur. *Unfallchirurgie* 1994;**97**:19–27.

◆17. Rozbruch SR, Muller U, Gautier E, Ganz R. The evolution of femoral shaft plating technique. *Clinical Orthopaedics and Related Research* 1998;**354**:195–208.

◆18. Baumgaertel F. Bridge plating. In: Ruedi TP, Murphy WM (eds) *AO Principles of Fracture Management*. Stuttgart, Germany: Thieme, 2000:221–31.

19. Gautier E, Perren SM. Die Limited Contact Dynamic Compression Plate (LC-DCP): Biomechanische Forschung als Grundlage des neuen Plattendesigns. *Orthopaede* 1992;**21**:11–23.

◆20. Perren SM. The concept of biological plating using the limited contact-dynamic compression plate (LC-DCP). Scientific background, design and application. *Injury* 1991;**22**(Suppl. 1):5.

◆21. Fernandez A, Regazzoni P. Internal fixation: a new technology. In: *AO Principles of Fracture Management*. Stuttgart, Germany: Thieme, 2000:249–53.

◆22. Gautier E, Sommer CH. Guidelines for the clinical application of the LCP. *Injury* 2003;**34**:S-B63–S-B76.

23. Egol KA, Kubiak EN, Fulkerson E, *et al*. Biomechanics of locked plates and screws. *Journal of Orthopaedic Trauma* 2004;**18**:488–93.

24. Kubiak EN, Fulkerson E, Strauss E, *et al*. The evolution of locked plates. *Journal of Bone and Joint Surgery (American)* 2006;**88A**:189–200.

25. Wagner M. General principles for the clinical use of the LCP. *Injury* 2003;**34**(Suppl. 2):B31–42.
●26. Krettek C, Schandelmaier P, Miclau T, *et al*. Minimally invasive percutaneous plate osteosynthesis (MIPPO) using the DCS in proximal and distal femoral fractures. *Injury* 1997;**28**:A20–A30.
●27. Krettek C. Concepts of minimally invasive plate osteosynthesis. *Injury* 1997;**28**(Suppl. 1):1–6.
●28. Farouk O, Krettek C, Miclau T, *et al*. Minimally invasive plate osteosynthesis and vascularity: preliminary results of a cadaver injection study. *Injury* 1997;**28**(Suppl. 1):7–12.
29. Fernandez A. External fixation. In: Ruedi TP, Murphy WM (eds) *AO Principles of Fracture Management*. Stuttgart, Germany: Thieme, 2000:233–47.
●30. Nowotarski PJ, Turen CH, Brumback RJ. Conversion of external fixation to intramedullary nailing for fractures of the shaft of the femur in multiply injured patients. *Journal of Bone and Joint Surgery (American)* 2000;**82A**:781–8.
◆31. Behrens F, Searls K. External fixation of the tibia. Basic concepts and prospective evaluation. *Journal of Bone and Joint Surgery (British)* 1986;**68B**:246–54.
●32. Kempf I, Grosse A, Beck G. Closed locked intramedullary nailing. Its application to comminuted fractures of the femur. *Journal of Bone and Joint Surgery (American)* 1985;**67A**:709–20.
◆33. Krettek C. Intramedullary nailing. In: *AO Principles of Fracture Management*. Stuttgart, Germany: Thieme, 2000:195–219.
●34. Schemitsch EH, Kowalski MJ, Swiontkowski MF, *et al*. Cortical bone blood flow in reamed and unreamed locked intramedullary nailing: a fractured tibia model in sheep. *Journal of Orthopaedic Trauma* 1994;**8**:373–82.
●35. Bosse MJ, Mackenzie EZ, Riemer BL, *et al*. Adult respiratory distress syndrome, pneumonia, and mortality following thoracic injury and a femoral fracture treated either with intramedullary nailing with reaming or with a plate. A comparative study. *Journal of Bone and Joint Surgery (American)* 1997;**79A**:799–809.
●36. Grosse A, Christie J, Taglang G, *et al*. Open adult femoral shaft fractures treated by early IM nailing. *Journal of Bone and Joint Surgery (British)* 1993;**75B**:562–5.
◆37. Giannoudis PV. Aspects of current management. Surgical priorities in damage control in polytrauma. *Journal of Bone and Joint Surgery (British)* 2003;**85**:478–83.
◆38. Pape HC, Hildebrand F, Pertschy S, *et al*. Changes in the management of femoral shaft fractures in polytrauma patients: from early total care to damage control orthopaedic surgery. *Journal of Trauma* 2002;**53**:452–61.

20

Clinical aspects in acute limb compartment syndrome

RAJIV MALHOTRA, NIKOLAOS GIOTAKIS

Introduction	278	Clinical features	280
Definition	278	Investigations	280
Pathophysiology	278	Management	280
Causes of acute compartment syndrome	278	Summary	281
Common causes of compartment syndrome	279	References	281

INTRODUCTION

There are few true orthopaedic emergencies that a junior doctor will come across and acute compartment syndrome of the limb is one of them. It is a condition that can be easily missed and has serious consequences if left untreated. The most important determinant of poor outcome from acute compartment syndrome is delay in the diagnosis.[1]

DEFINITION

Acute compartment syndrome is a condition in which high pressure within a closed fascial space reduces capillary blood perfusion below a level necessary for tissue viability.[2]

PATHOPHYSIOLOGY

Compartment syndromes develop in muscles enclosed by non-compliant fascia. Any build-up of pressure within the compartment is therefore not easily dissipated and can affect vascular supply to muscles and nerves. If this raised intracompartmental pressure (ICP) continues for 6 hours,[3] myoneural necrosis will result.[3] The sequelae of untreated compartment syndrome include loss of function of the affected limb and the development of contractures. (Fig. 20.1). With muscle infarction there is the risk of developing systemic complications (crush syndrome), which include myoglobinuria, renal failure, shock, cardiac arrhythmias and death.

The commonest sites of compartment syndrome are in the leg and the forearm.[2] The leg consists of four compartments: the anterior compartment, the lateral compartment, and the superficial and deep posterior compartments. The most commonly involved compartment is the *anterior* compartment, which contains the anterior tibial artery and deep peroneal nerve.

The forearm consists of two compartments: the ventral compartment, which contains the median and ulnar nerves and arteries, and the dorsal compartment, which is more rarely affected.

CAUSES OF ACUTE COMPARTMENT SYNDROME[2]

The cause of an increased intracompartmental pressure (ICP) can be due to either an increase in compartmental content or a decrease in compartment size.[4] Increased content can be divided into

1. oedema – prolonged limb compression, post trauma
2. haemorrhage – vessel laceration
3. combination of both – fractures.

A decrease in compartment size can occur with constrictive casts, circular dressings and extensive burns.

COMMON CAUSES OF COMPARTMENT SYNDROME

- Fractures.
- Soft-tissue injuries.
- Arterial injury.
- Prolonged limb compression.
- Burns.

Fractures

Fractures account for 69% of acute compartment syndromes, with the most common being tibial fractures and distal radial and ulnar fractures. The incidence of ischaemic contracture after tibial fractures ranges from 3% to 10% (Fig. 20.2).

Comminuted fractures (more than two fragments), involving both the tibia and fibula at the same height and particularly of the proximal tibia, carry a higher risk of compartment syndrome owing to the high energy needed to cause such fractures and the limited expansibility of the fascial envelope.

Orthopaedic treatment strategies such as traction, application of casts and manipulation can all increase the ICP and the risk of developing compartment syndrome.

Despite the two most common sites for compartment syndrome being the leg and the forearm, compartment syndrome can develop in a number of other sites, including the thigh and the foot.

Soft-tissue injuries

Acute compartment syndrome can occur from a severe soft-tissue injury without a fracture being present but as a result of massive oedema. Patients with bleeding diatheses are particularly at risk.

Arterial injuries

Repair of arterial injuries can result in a post-revascularization compartment syndrome. This occurs because of tissue swelling mediated by such factors as free radicals. The necessity for fasciotomy as a complementary procedure to arterial repair varies from 6% to 33%; indeed many surgeons perform this pre-emptively.

Prolonged limb compression

Compression of a forearm or elbow by a patient's body or head can result in ICPs of over 50 mmHg, which if left untreated can result in muscle and nerve necrosis.

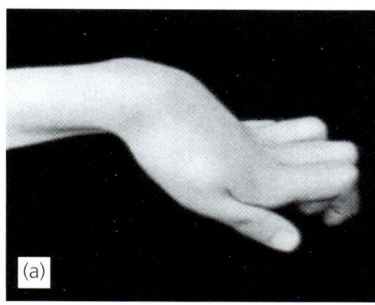
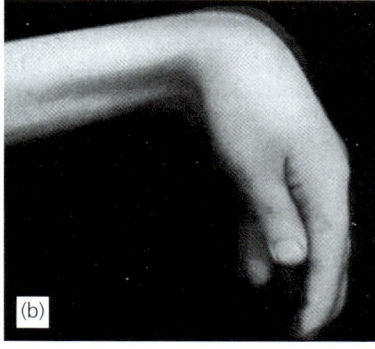

Figure 20.1 Volkmann's ischaemic contractures.

Figure 20.2 Tibial and fibular fracture.

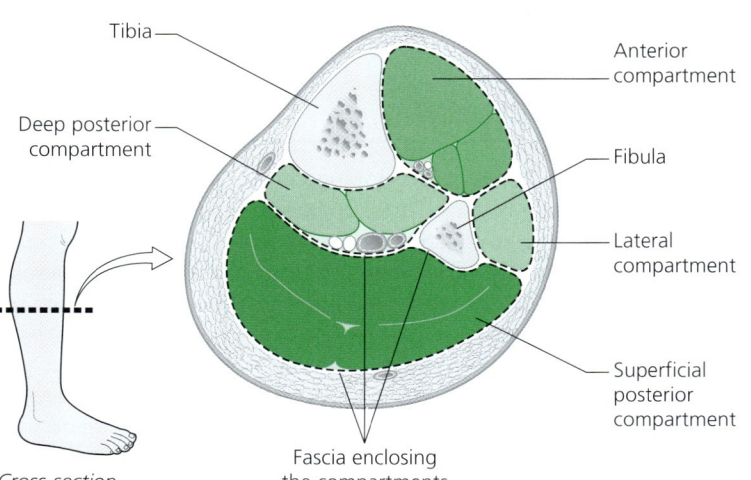

Therefore, measurement of ICP may be needed in patients who have been unconscious in the same position for some hours (e.g. drug overdose).

CLINICAL FEATURES

As a junior doctor, the most common presentation of a compartment syndrome will probably be the patient complaining of increasing pain in the affected part. The difficulty comes in distinguishing the pain associated with a tibial fracture itself, for example, and the pain associated with an impending compartment syndrome. In acute compartment syndrome, the pain experienced is much greater than that expected from the primary problem. Pain on passive stretching of the muscles involved is a common feature, as ischaemic muscle is highly sensitive to stretch. This sign, in combination with a tense and swollen limb, is the most reliable early finding of an acute compartment syndrome.[4]

A less reliable physical finding is a sensory deficit, such as paraesthesia or loss of two-point discrimination. Pallor and pulselessness imply a vascular injury, but the presence of peripheral pulses does NOT exclude a compartment syndrome. Paresis and paralysis are difficult to interpret as these signs can arise secondary to nerve involvement.

Signs and symptoms of compartment syndrome

- Pain (on passive stretching).
- Swollen, tense compartment.
- Paraesthesia.
- Pallor.
- Pulselessness (not reliable).
- Paralysis (late sign).

INVESTIGATIONS

The majority of compartment syndromes can be diagnosed from the clinical assessment of the patient. However, there are methods of measuring the ICP, which are often carried out to confirm the diagnosis. It is of particular value in three groups of patients:[5]

1. uncooperative or unreliable patients (e.g. children, intoxicated adults)
2. unresponsive patients (e.g. unconscious)
3. patients with a nerve deficit owing to another cause.

To measure the ICP, a catheter is placed into the compartment at a level close to that of the fracture (approximately 1.5 cm). One must ideally measure the ICP in all compartments of the limb, not just those that are most affected.

This often is not practical, particularly in the leg, so in a conscious patient measurement needs to be performed in the compartment that appears more swollen.

In case of fractures the measurement is best done at a distance of about 2 cm from the fracture site.

There are several different methods of measuring the ICP, such as a wick catheter or simple needle manometry, so become familiar with the one available in your hospital. Most departments have dedicated compartmental monitoring devices that can give continuous readings. If there is not one, use an arterial line set-up.

There has been much debate over the level of ICP that necessitates a fasciotomy. The normal resting ICP is 0–8 mmHg, with pain and paraesthesia appearing at pressures between 20 and 30 mmHg.[5] Some authors use an ICP of more than 30 mmHg as the cut-off point for doing a fasciotomy.[6] A prospective study by McQueen and Court-Brown[7] used a differential pressure (difference between the diastolic blood pressure and the ICP) of less than 30 mmHg as an indication for fasciotomy in compartment syndrome; this led to no compartment syndromes being missed and appears to be a more reliable method than the use of an absolute value of ICP alone. Indeed, if an ICP of more than 30 mmHg was used as the critical ICP, 50 patients (43%) would have had unnecessary fasciotomies.

Much of the variability in reported pressure thresholds may be due to differences in the perfusion state of the limbs. It is thought that a patient with a diastolic pressure of 80 mmHg is likely to tolerate a tissue pressure of 30 mmHg without ischaemia, but a hypotensive patient with a diastolic pressure similar to the tissue pressure will not.

The ideal pressure threshold for performing fasciotomy is still unknown and the literature recommends treating each patient on the basis of their clinical presentation and the progression of their signs and symptoms. In recent times, a differential pressure of 30 mmHg or less is seen as the limit to consider an urgent fasciotomy. It is important to note that, in the presence of clinical suspicion of compartment syndrome, a negative ICP measurement should not exclude the diagnosis, but close observation of symptom progression and serial measurements should be performed. It is important to note whether the trend of ICP variation and clinical symptoms evolves towards improvement or deterioration.

MANAGEMENT

If you suspect a developing compartment syndrome in a patient you must first recognize this as an emergency that needs prompt action. A fasciotomy is the definitive treatment but it must be done before any myoneural necrosis has occurred to be of maximal benefit. Irreversible damage begins after 6 hours.

As with any patient who has a serious condition, you must follow the ABCDE (airway, breathing, circulation, disability, exposure) approach; indeed the patient may have systemic complications (e.g. crush syndrome) and need urgent initial resuscitation.

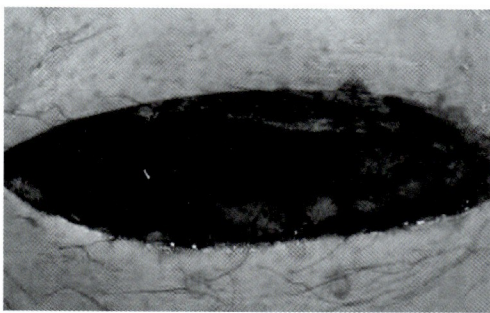

Figure 20.3 Necrotic muscle after compartment syndrome.

There are certain measures that junior doctors can perform to lower the ICP. The main one involves urgently removing any casts or constrictive bandages on the affected area; splitting the cast will not decompress the compartment effectively. Do not be tempted to raise the leg to help reduce the oedema; it has been shown that this decreases the end-capillary pressure and so worsens the myoneural ischaemia, so nurse the affected area flat.

An urgent assessment by the on-call orthopaedic resident is needed, who will normally measure the ICP if the diagnosis is not certain, but it is a useful skill for you to have too.

A decision will be made either to take the patient to theatre immediately or to monitor the condition. If the patient is not going to theatre immediately then the clinical signs, symptoms and ICP should be reassessed every 15–30 minutes to look for any progression.

The ultimate management is to perform a fasciotomy to relieve the raised ICP and to allow normal myoneural vascular supply. In the lower limb all four compartments must be decompressed and this is normally achieved via two long longitudinal incisions.[8] Superficial debridement may be needed if there is necrotic tissue (Fig. 20.3), and then the wound can be packed. The patient can be taken back to theatre 3 or 4 days later, at which time re-examination, further debridement and partial skin closure can occur. It is important to remember that skin closure can increase ICP and to remain vigilant for this.

SUMMARY

Acute compartment syndrome is an orthopaedic emergency that requires prompt fasciotomy to prevent long-term damage. The frequency and severity of complications are inversely related to the promptness of decompression.

Junior doctors must recognize the clinical features of this condition and have them in mind when assessing orthopaedic patients who are complaining of increasing pain. Clinical findings are the key when making a diagnosis, with ICP measurements proving useful in certain circumstances. With this knowledge, limbs and lives can be saved.

> ### KEY LEARNING POINTS
>
> - Acute compartment syndrome is an orthopaedic emergency that can result in loss of limb or even death if left untreated.
> - Common causes include fractures of the tibia and the forearm bones.
> - Clinical features include pain beyond what would normally be expected, a bulky compartment and sensory loss, which is a late sign.
> - Measurement of the intracompartmental pressure can be of use in some patients.
> - The definitive management is a fasciotomy.

REFERENCES

1. Sheridan GW, Matsen FA. Fasciotomy in the treatment of the acute compartment syndrome. *Journal of Bone and Joint Surgery* 1976;**58**:112–15.
2. Mubarak SJ, Hargens AR. Acute compartment syndrome. *Surgical Clinics of North America* 1983;**63**:539–64.
3. Lagerstrom CF, Reed RLV II, Rowlands BJ, Fischer RP. Early fasciotomy for acute clinically evident posttraumatic compartment syndrome. *American Journal of Surgery* 1989;**158**:36–9.
4. Matsen FA III, Winquist RA, Krugmire RB Jr. Diagnosis and management of compartmental syndromes. *Journal of Bone and Joint Surgery* 1980;**62**:286–91.
5. Mubarak SJ, Owen CA, Hargens AR, *et al.* Acute compartment syndrome: diagnosis and treatment with the aid of the wick catheter. *Journal of Bone and Joint Surgery* 1978;**60**:1091–5.
6. Blick SS, Brumback RJ, Poka A, *et al.* Compartment syndrome in open tibial fractures. *Journal of Bone and Joint Surgery* 1986;**68**:1348–53.
7. McQueen MM, Court-Brown CM. Compartment monitoring in tibial fractures. *Journal of Bone and Joint Surgery* 1996;**78**:99–104.
8. Tiwari A, Haq AI, Myint F, Hamilton G. Acute compartment syndromes. *British Journal of Surgery* 2002;**89**:397–412.

SECTION 2

Upper extremity fractures and dislocations

SHANMUGANATHAN RAJASEKARAN

21	**Acromioclavicular joint injuries**	285
	Shanmuganathan Rajasekaran, Rishi Mugesh Kanna, Jayaramaraju Dheenadhayalan	
22	**Clavicular fractures**	288
	Shanmuganathan Rajasekaran, Rishi Mugesh Kanna, Jayaramaraju Dheenadhayalan	
23	**Sternoclavicular joint injuries**	291
	Shanmuganathan Rajasekaran, Rishi Mugesh Kanna, Jayaramaraju Dheenadhayalan	
24	**Scapular fractures**	294
	Shanmuganathan Rajasekaran, Rishi Mugesh Kanna, Jayaramaraju Dheenadhayalan	
25	**Dislocations of the glenohumeral joint**	297
	Shanmuganathan Rajasekaran, Rishi Mugesh Kanna, Jayaramaraju Dheenadhayalan	
26	**Fractures of the proximal humerus**	303
	Shanmuganathan Rajasekaran, Rishi Mugesh Kanna, Jayaramaraju Dheenadhayalan	
27	**Humeral shaft fractures**	307
	Shanmuganathan Rajasekaran, Rishi Mugesh Kanna, Jayaramaraju Dheenadhayalan	
28	**Fractures of the distal humerus**	311
	Shanmuganathan Rajasekaran, Rishi Mugesh Kanna, Jayaramaraju Dheenadhayalan	
29	**Fractures and dislocations of the elbow**	316
	Shanmuganathan Rajasekaran, Rishi Mugesh Kanna, Jayaramaraju Dheenadhayalan	
30	**Fractures of the shaft of the radius and ulna**	322
	Shanmuganathan Rajasekaran, Rishi Mugesh Kanna, Jayaramaraju Dheenadhayalan	
31	**Fractures of the distal radius**	327
	Shanmuganathan Rajasekaran, Rishi Mugesh Kanna, Jayaramaraju Dheenadhayalan	

21

Acromioclavicular joint injuries

SHANMUGANATHAN RAJASEKARAN, RISHI MUGESH KANNA, JAYARAMARAJU DHEENADHAYALAN

Introduction	285	Classification	286
Anatomy	285	Treatment	286
Mechanism of injury	285	Complications	286
Clinical evaluation	285	Summary	287
Radiographic evaluation	285	References	287

NATIONAL BOARD STANDARDS

- Revise knowledge of the anatomy of the shoulder
- Understand the pathophysiology of acromioclavicular joint injury
- Diagnose and classify the injury
- Be able to advise a patient on the prognosis

INTRODUCTION

Acromioclavicular (AC) joint injuries are common because of the vulnerable position of the joint on the lateral aspect of the shoulder, and because the joint absorbs direct forces with any blow to the shoulder or falls on the outstretched hand or elbow.[1] AC joint injuries are very common in young males involved in contact sports and, depending on the injury velocity, they can be a simple ligamentous strain or complex dislocation. Management depends on the severity of injury, ranging from supportive care to surgical stabilization.

ANATOMY

The AC joint is a diarthrodial joint, with fibrocartilage-covered articular surfaces, located between the lateral end of the clavicle and the medial acromion. It is covered by a thin capsule. The AC and coracoclavicular (CC) ligaments provide the main support. The AC joint capsule is strongest at its superior and posterior margins and helps to prevent upward dislocation of the joint. Fibres of the deltoid and trapezius muscles blend superiorly to strengthen the joint.

MECHANISM OF INJURY

Direct injury due to a fall onto the shoulder accounts for most injuries. Indirect injuries through a fall on the outstretched arm can also cause an AC joint strain. The injury is usually purely ligamentous, but can be associated with fractures of the clavicle, acromion process or coracoid process.

CLINICAL EVALUATION

The patient presents with pain and swelling over the joint and frequently supports the upper limb by cupping the elbow with the opposite hand. Tenderness can be elicited over the AC joint. The characteristic anatomic feature is 'downward sag of the shoulder and arm'. A visual step-off deformity or tenting of the skin overlying the distal clavicle indicates a severe deformity with instability.

RADIOGRAPHIC EVALUATION

A standard anteroposterior radiograph of the shoulder usually exhibits the injury well, but visualization of both

Table 21.1 Classification of acromioclavicular (AC) joint injury[4]

Type	AC joint	AC ligament	Coracoclavicular ligament	Deltoid and trapezoid muscles
I	Intact	Sprain	Intact	Intact
II	Displaced	Torn	Sprain/intact	Intact
III	Disrupted	Torn	Torn	Usually intact
IV	Disrupted	Torn	Torn	Detached
V	Disrupted	Torn	Torn	Detached
VI	The AC joint is dislocated with the clavicle displaced inferiorly (extremely rare)			

AC joints on a single large film helps to identify and evaluate the displacement better. Stress radiographs (performed with 4.5–7 kg (10–15 lb) weights held in both hands) help to differentiate severe injuries from partial grade I or II injuries and to evaluate the separation of the joint better.

CLASSIFICATION

The injury is classified (Table 21.1 and Fig. 21.1) depending on the degree and direction of displacement of the distal clavicle. Type I injuries indicate a simple strain with minimal or no displacement. Type II injuries have superior displacement of less than one-half of the diameter of the clavicle and are associated with disruption of the AC ligaments but sparing of the CC ligaments. Type III injuries have complete disruption of both CC and AC ligaments and are associated with greater superior displacement of the clavicle. In type IV injuries the dislocation is complete and the clavicle is displaced posteriorly into the trapezius, which is well visualized in an axillary view of the shoulder. In type V injuries, the clavicle buttonholes through the trapezius and is palpable subcutaneously. Type VI injuries are a rare form of injury in which the clavicle is dislocated inferiorly under the acromion or the coracoid.

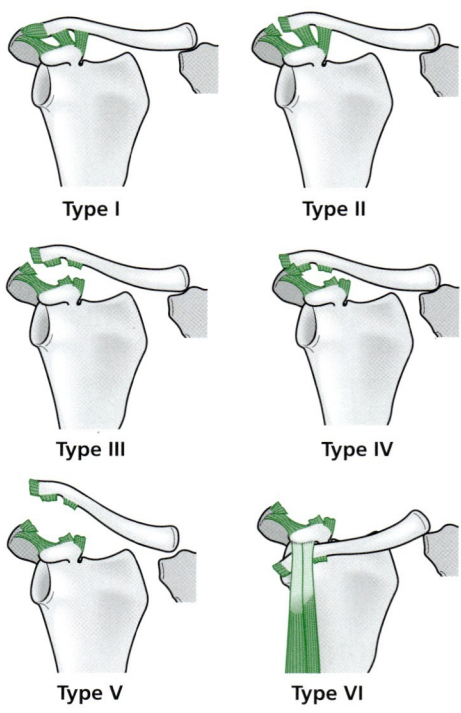

Figure 21.1 Six different types of acromioclavicular joint injury (see text for details).

TREATMENT

Non-operative

Type I and II injuries should be treated non-operatively, and a good functional result can be obtained. In type III and more severe injuries, operative treatment is usually advocated, although the results are controversial. Surgical treatment is preferred in manual labourers and overhead-throwing athletes who have sustained a type III AC joint injury.

Operative

Surgical procedures aim at preventing superior migration, either by fixing the distal clavicle directly to the acromion or by augmenting the CC ligaments, or a combination of both.[2,3] Current treatment is the use of the AC Joint Tightrope to reduce and hold the dislocation. In neglected cases (chronic AC joint dislocation) the preferred treatment is Tightrope fixation augmented with autograft hamstring tendon.

COMPLICATIONS

Symptomatic post-traumatic arthritis or osteolysis of the AC joint is relatively rare and will require resection of the distal clavicle. Postoperative complications include failure of fixation, causing chronic symptomatic instability, and hardware failure with a slippage of the wires or cut-out of metalwork.

SUMMARY

AC joint injuries represent varying degrees of disruption of the ligamentous attachments between the clavicle and scapula. Treatment principles focus on the potential for these injuries to have persistent displacement and instability of the clavicle. Non-operative treatment is favoured and is successful in most patients with type I, II or III injuries.

> **KEY LEARNING POINTS**
>
> - Acromioclavicular joint injuries are common in young adults following high-velocity injuries.
> - The severity of damage to the supporting acromioclavicular and coracoclavicular ligaments determines the type of injury.
> - Type I and II injuries are treated conservatively.
> - Type III–VI injuries may require surgical treatment.

REFERENCES

● = Key primary paper
◆ = Major review article

● 1. Cadenat FM. The treatment of dislocations and fractures of the outer end of the clavicle. *International Clinics* 1917;**1**:145–69.
◆ 2. Weaver JK, Dunn HK. Treatment of acromioclavicular injuries, especially complete acromioclavicular separation. *Journal of Bone and Joint Surgery (American)* 1972;**54**:1187–94.
3. Tossy JD, Mead NC, Sigmond HM. Acromioclavicular separations: useful and practical classification for treatment. *Clinical Orthopaedics and Related Research* 1963;**28**:111–19.
4. Williams GR, Nguyen VD, Rockwood CR. Classification and radiographic analysis of acromioclavicular dislocations. *Applied Radiology* 1989;**18**:29–34.

22

Clavicular fractures

SHANMUGANATHAN RAJASEKARAN, RISHI MUGESH KANNA, JAYARAMARAJU DHEENADHAYALAN

Introduction	288	Treatment	289
Anatomy	288	Complications	289
Clinical evaluation	288	Summary	290
Radiographic evaluation	288	References	290
Classification	289		

NATIONAL BOARD STANDARDS

- Know the uniqueness of clavicular anatomy
- Diagnose and classify clavicular fractures
- Know the significance of lateral clavicle injuries

INTRODUCTION

The clavicle is the most commonly fractured bone, accounting for up to 12% of all adult fractures. The clavicle is entirely superficial and transmits all the force absorbed by the upper extremity to the thorax, which explains its vulnerability to injury. More than 85% of fractures occur as a result of either a direct fall onto the shoulder or a direct hit. The fracture is highly amenable to conservative treatment with a brace, and surgery is required in only selected patients.

ANATOMY

The clavicle is an 'S'-shaped long bone placed horizontally. It forms an important stabilizer between the axial and appendicular skeleton. Although the subclavian vessels and brachial plexus are in close proximity to the bone, they are rarely injured in a fracture of the clavicle. The medial end articulates with the sternum, and the lateral end articulates with the acromion process of the scapula. The coracoclavicular (CC) ligaments are attached to the lateral clavicle and provide vertical stability to the acromioclavicular (AC) joint.

CLINICAL EVALUATION

Patients present with localized pain, swelling and deformity over the fractured bone. Being a subcutaneous bone, ecchymosis and tenting of the skin are also frequently present. In fractures of the middle third, the proximal (medial) fragment is often pulled up by the sternocleidomastoid muscle, and the weight of gravity on the upper extremity pulls downward on the lateral fragment, accentuating the deformity. A careful neurovascular examination of the ipsilateral upper limb and auscultation of the chest is necessary, especially in high-energy injuries, because of the presence of vital structures in close proximity.

RADIOGRAPHIC EVALUATION

Standard anteroposterior radiographs are usually adequate to confirm the presence of a clavicular fracture. Comminution, displacement and the degree of overriding of the fractured fragments should be noted as they decide the nature of treatment. A chest radiograph may be ordered in patients with suspected pneumothorax. In this film, also look for injuries of the scapula and ribs.

CLASSIFICATION[1]

Clavicular fractures can be classified based on the level of the fracture:[1]

- *Fracture of the proximal third (5%)*. Usually, displacement is minimal because of the presence of strong costoclavicular ligaments. In children and teenagers, it may represent an epiphyseal injury.
- *Fractures of the middle third (80%)*. This is the most common level of fracture in both children and adults. The fragments are secured by ligamentous and muscular attachments.
- *Fracture of the distal third (15%)*. This is subclassified according to the location of the fracture with respect to the attachment of the CC ligaments (Fig. 22.1):[2]
  - type 1: fractures lateral to the CC ligament attachment
  - type 2: fractures medial to the CC ligament attachment
  - type 3: fractures through the distal clavicular articular surface
  - type 4: paediatric fractures with a thick periosteal sleeve
  - type 5: comminuted, unstable fractures.

TREATMENT

Non-operative treatment

Most clavicular fractures can be successfully treated non-operatively, with comfort and pain relief being the goals of treatment as nature heals the fracture.[3] A sling has been shown to give the same results as a figure-of-eight bandage but provides more comfort and fewer skin problems. A certain degree of shortening and deformity can result, but patient satisfaction is good and functional results are excellent. In general, immobilization for 2–3 weeks in children and 4–6 weeks in adults is all that is necessary to achieve union. Active movements of the other joints of the limb, including the shoulder, must be started as early as possible especially in elderly patients.

Operative treatment

There are a few but definite indications for operative treatment:

- Open fractures require operative intervention with debridement, irrigation and stabilization.
- Fractures lateral to the coracoid with torn CC ligaments may be associated with gross displacement of more than 1–2 cm, leading to non-union.
- Although rare, fractures associated with neurovascular injuries will require stabilization following neurovascular repair.
- Combined injuries of the neck of the scapula and clavicle are termed 'floating shoulder' and represent a double disruption of the superior shoulder suspensory complex. Stabilization of the clavicular fracture is advocated to stabilize the shoulder complex.
- Established non-unions due to either gross comminution or soft-tissue interposition will need operative intervention.

Operative fixation may be accomplished usually by plate fixation or rarely by the use of intramedullary pins. Plates are placed, either on the superior or the anteroinferior aspect of the clavicle.[4] Extreme care must be exercised in inserting the screws because of the presence of underlying neurovascular structures. Plate and screw fixation require extensive exposure. The resultant scar can be unsightly and the plate can also be quite prominent beneath the skin, necessitating removal later on. Intramedullary pins (Hagie pin or Rockwood pin) are placed by opening the fracture site and inserting the nail in antegrade fashion through the lateral fragment and then in retrograde fashion into the medial fragment. These patients require regular radiological follow-up since there is a possibility of wire migration or breakage.

COMPLICATIONS

- *Malunion*. Malunions are common and, although they do not cause functional problems, they may cause a lump and prominence. It is better that patients are counselled about this. Surgery is rarely required as the appearance improves as a result of remodelling over a period of time.
- *Non-union*. The incidence of non-union in clavicular fractures varies from 0.1% to 13.0%. Various factors such as the severity of the initial trauma, displaced fragments, presence of soft-tissue interposition, open injuries and primary open reduction and internal

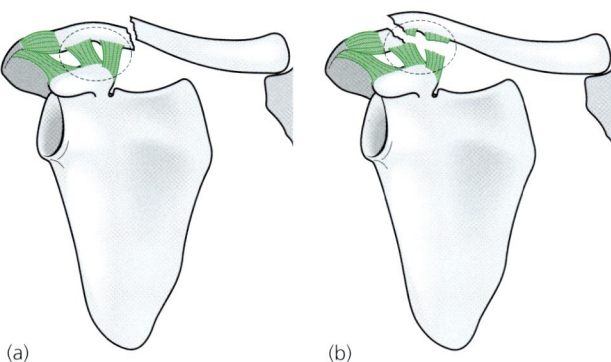

Figure 22.1 Neer's classification of distal third clavicular fractures. The coracoclavicular ligament is highlighted by the dotted circle. Note the position of the fracture line with respect to the ligament in the two types.

fixation have been implicated. Management depends on the functional impairment of the particular patient and, if required, open reduction and internal fixation with bone grafting is advised.
- *Neurovascular injury.* Although rare, it can occur acutely during either the initial injury or surgery and chronically secondary to compression by callus or deformity.

SUMMARY

Fracture of the clavicle is one of the very common orthopaedic injuries. Because of its inherent reparative capacities, it has rapid healing properties. Despite the proximity of major vascular, nervous and cardiopulmonary structures, associated injury is uncommon. Treatment is predominantly conservative with selective surgical indications. Malunion occurs frequently with non-operative care but the ensuing deformity does not affect the functional results.

KEY LEARNING POINTS

- Fractures of the clavicle are the most common long-bone injuries.
- Diagnosis is quick and straightforward because of its subcutaneous location.
- Lateral end clavicular fractures deserve special attention and management as it forms part of the acromioclavicular joint.
- With conservative care, most fractures heal with good functional outcome.
- Surgery is reserved for special situations.

REFERENCES

- ● = Key primary paper
- ◆ = Major review article

●1. Allman Jr FL. Fractures and ligamentous injuries of the clavicle and its articulation. *Journal of Bone and Joint Surgery (American)* 1967;**49**:774–84.
●2. Neer CS. Fractures of the distal third of the clavicle. *Clinical Orthopaedics and Related Research* 1968;**58**:43–50.
◆3. Robinson CM. Fractures of the clavicle in the adult. Epidemiology and classification. *Journal of Bone and Joint Surgery (British)* 1998;**80**:476–84.
4. Shen WJ, Liu TJ, Shen YS. Plate fixation of fresh displaced midshaft clavicle fractures. *Injury* 1999;**30**:497–500.

23

Sternoclavicular joint injuries

SHANMUGANATHAN RAJASEKARAN, RISHI MUGESH KANNA, JAYARAMARAJU DHEENADHAYALAN

Introduction	291	Treatment	292
Anatomy	291	Complications	292
Mechanism of injury	291	Summary	292
Clinical evaluation	291	References	293
Radiographic evaluation	292		

NATIONAL BOARD STANDARDS

- Understand the mechanism of sternoclavicular joint injury
- Diagnose and classify the injury
- Know the significance of posterior dislocations
- Be able to conduct closed reductions

INTRODUCTION

Injuries to the sternoclavicular (SC) joint are rare, accounting for less than 3% of shoulder injuries, and are usually associated with high-velocity injuries.[1] Mild sprains respond very well to conservative treatment. Dislocations require reduction manoeuvres and a short period of immobilization. It is important to identify posterior dislocations; these are frequently missed but can cause compression of the vital mediastinal structures.

ANATOMY

The SC joint is a diarthrodial joint and is the major articulation between the axial and appendicular skeleton. Less than 50% of the clavicular end articulates with the manubrium sterni. The poor osseous stability is compensated by the costoclavicular ligaments, disc ligament, interclavicular ligament and the thick joint capsule. The medial clavicle physis ossifies late and unites with the shaft in the third decade of life. Therefore, some of the sternoclavicular joint dislocations can be true physeal separations.

MECHANISM OF INJURY

SC joint injuries are high-energy events and are frequently associated with other injuries. They can be a direct injury to the joint or as a consequence of indirect force applied over the shoulder joint. Most of them are anterior dislocations, in which the medial end of the clavicle displaces anteriorly, lying in the subcutaneous plane. The rest are posterior dislocations, in which the clavicle is pushed into the mediastinum. Posterior dislocations are uncommon but may need emergency treatment because of the proximity to important structures such as the great vessels, trachea, oesophagus and the phrenic nerve.

CLINICAL EVALUATION

Pain, swelling, ecchymosis and tenderness over the SC joint are common. In anterior dislocation, palpation reveals the prominent medial end of the clavicle near the manubrium sterni. There may be puckering of the overlying skin with a sense of fluctuation in posterior dislocations. Patients with posterior dislocations may present critically with shortness of breath, venous engorgement

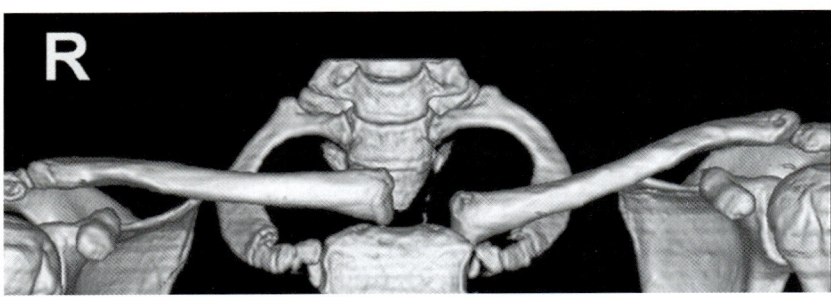

Figure 23.1 Three-dimensional reconstructed CT scan of both of the sternoclavicular joints shows an anterior dislocation on the right side.

and a choking sensation due to pressure on mediastinal structures, and need to be treated expediently.[2] The importance of a proper neurovascular assessment and chest auscultation need not be overemphasized.

RADIOGRAPHIC EVALUATION

Anteroposterior chest radiographs show asymmetry of the clavicles. The radiograph should be thoroughly scrutinized for the presence of pneumothorax. Dislocations are more clearly seen in a *serendipity view* in which the X-ray beam is tilted 40° cephalad and aimed at the manubrium.[3] With an anterior dislocation, the medial clavicle lies above the interclavicular line; with a posterior dislocation, the medial clavicle lies below this line. A CT scan is helpful to document subtle unrecognized subluxations and helps in doubtful cases to differentiate fractures of the medial clavicle from dislocations (Fig. 23.1).

TREATMENT

Non-operative treatment

The majority of anterior dislocations can be effectively treated by non-operative methods in the form of ice packs, sling immobilization for a week and gradual return to activities. Attempts at closed reduction are not warranted as reductions will not remain reduced and there is no effective brace available that will hold a reduction in position.

Operative treatment

Posterior dislocations, however, need intervention owing to the concern that acute or chronic impingement of critical structures will lead to late sequelae. Under general anaesthesia, the medial clavicular head can be grabbed using a pointed instrument such as a towel clip and pulled back into position. A roll between the shoulder blades along with lateral traction of the abducted arm will help in reduction. In general, no stabilization of the joint is required.

COMPLICATIONS

Posterior dislocations are frequently missed because of the paucity of clinical signs and because they usually occur in a polytrauma setting. However, they can be associated with a variety of serious sequelae such as pneumothorax, laceration of the superior vena cava, venous congestion of the neck, oesophageal or tracheal rupture, subclavian and carotid artery injury, and thoracic outlet syndrome. Chronic unreduced anterior dislocations can be associated with cosmetic disfigurement because of an enlarged medial prominence of the clavicle. Arthritic symptoms due to an unstable SC joint can occur, and this can be treated by resection of the clavicular head.[4]

SUMMARY

Injuries to the SC joint are unusual. The ligaments that stabilize the joint are so strong that a substantial force is necessary to dislocate it. The most common sources of SC dislocation are motor vehicle accidents and sports injuries. Anterior dislocations are much more common than posterior dislocations and are treated conservatively. Posterior dislocations, although rare, can be quite catastrophic and require emergency management.

> ### KEY LEARNING POINTS
>
> - Injuries to the sternoclavicular joint are uncommon.
> - Anterior dislocations are uncomplicated and are best treated non-operatively.
> - Posterior dislocations, which can be fatal, should be promptly diagnosed and reduced.
> - Special radiographs, such as the serendipity view, or CT scan may be required to make the diagnosis.

REFERENCES

● = Key primary paper
◆ = Major review article

●1. Nettles JL, Linscheid R. Sternoclavicular dislocations. *Journal of Trauma* 1968;**8**:158–64.
●2. Heinig CF. Retrosternal dislocation of the clavicle: early recognition, x-ray diagnosis, and management. *Journal of Bone and Joint Surgery (American)* 1968;**50A**:830.
◆3. Rockwood Jr CA. Dislocations of the sternoclavicular joint. *Instructional Course Lectures* 1975;**24**:144.
4. Lunseth PA, Chapman KW, Frankel VH. Surgical treatment of chronic dislocation of the sternoclavicular joint. *Journal of Bone and Joint Surgery (British)* 1975;**57**:193–6.

24

Scapular fractures

SHANMUGANATHAN RAJASEKARAN, RISHI MUGESH KANNA, JAYARAMARAJU DHEENADHAYALAN

Introduction	294	Treatment	295
Anatomy	294	Complications	295
Mechanism of injury	294	Scapulothoracic dissociation	295
Clinical evaluation	294	Summary	296
Radiographic evaluation	294	References	296
Classification	295		

NATIONAL BOARD STANDARDS

- Revise your knowledge of scapula anatomy
- Diagnose scapular fractures
- Look for associated injuries
- Understand management principles

INTRODUCTION

Fractures of the scapula are relatively uncommon injuries, accounting for 0.5–1% of all fractures.[1] They are commonly seen in young males as a result of direct trauma in high-velocity motor vehicle accidents. Hence, a thorough evaluation, looking for associated vital organ injuries, is important in these patients. The presence of a scapular fracture should alert the surgeon to the presence of other serious injuries because 30–95% of scapular fractures are associated with injuries of the head, neck, chest and spine.

ANATOMY

The scapula is a flat, triangular bone connecting the upper extremity to the axial skeleton. It is well covered by the attachment of muscles on both the dorsal and ventral sides, which usually prevents gross displacement of the fragments following fractures.

MECHANISM OF INJURY

Significant direct trauma is usually required to fracture the scapula. However, fractures of the scapular neck and glenoid and intra-articular fractures can occur through axial loading on the outstretched arm.

CLINICAL EVALUATION

A thorough primary survey is indicated, with special attention to airway, breathing and circulation before the scapular fracture is attended to. These fractures are usually associated with severe contusion over the upper back with painful restriction of shoulder movements, especially abduction.

RADIOGRAPHIC EVALUATION

Initial radiographs (Fig. 24.1) consist of a true anteroposterior view, an axillary view and a scapular Y view (true scapular lateral). A chest radiograph is an essential part of

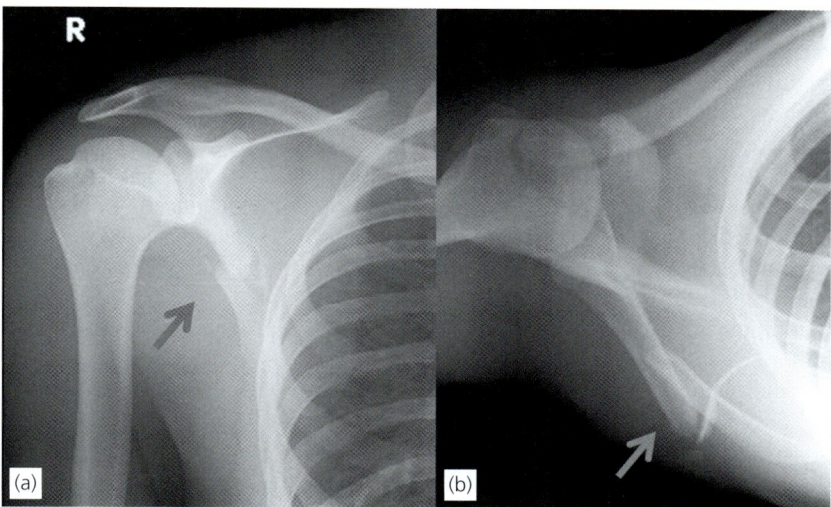

Figure 24.1 Anteroposterior (a) and lateral (b) radiographs of the scapula with the shoulder joint show a fracture of the lateral scapular border (arrows). This fracture can be treated conservatively.

the evaluation to rule out associated injuries to thoracic structures. CT may be useful for further characterizing intra-articular fractures of the glenoid.

CLASSIFICATION

An anatomical classification has been proposed by Zdravkovic and Damholt:[2]

Type I   Fractures of the scapular body
Type II Apophyseal fractures, including the acromion and coracoid
Type III Fractures of the superolateral angle, including the scapular neck and glenoid

TREATMENT

Most scapular fractures are amenable to non-operative treatment, consisting of sling use and early range of shoulder motion.[3] Operative indications are limited and include displaced intra-articular glenoid fractures involving greater than 25% of the articular surface; scapular neck fractures with more than 40° angulation and 9 mm medial displacement; scapular neck fractures with an associated displaced clavicular fracture; and fractures of the acromion that impinge on the subacromial space and when the fracture occurs as a part of floating shoulder.

Floating shoulder

This consists of double disruptions of the superior shoulder suspensory complex (SSSC).[4] The SSSC is a bone/soft-tissue ring that includes the glenoid process, the coracoid process, the coracoclavicular ligaments, the distal clavicle, the acromioclavicular joint and the acromion process.

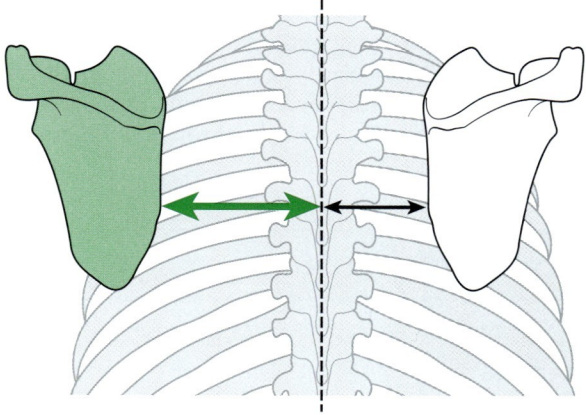

Figure 24.2 A right scapulothoracic dissociation. In the anteroposterior radiograph of the chest, the difference in the distances between the medial borders of the scapula on either side of the midline should not be more than 2.5 cm. In a scapulothoracic dissociation, this distance is more than 2.5 cm.

Traumatic disruption of two or more components of the SSSC, usually secondary to high-energy injury, is frequently described as a floating shoulder. These injuries usually require operative stabilization.

COMPLICATIONS

Associated injuries account for most serious complications, because of the high-energy nature of these injuries. Malunion and non-union are extremely rare.

SCAPULOTHORACIC DISSOCIATION

Scapulothoracic dissociation (Fig. 24.2) is a traumatic disruption of the scapula from its muscular attachments of the posterior chest wall, frequently resulting in an 'internal' forequarter amputation. The mechanism is a violent traction and rotation force. It can be associated with fracture or dislocation involving the clavicle or scapula, or without bony injury. Associated injury to the neurovascular structures to varying degrees is the rule. This injury is associated with a poor outcome and leads to a flail extremity in 52%, early amputation in 21% and death in 10%. Diagnosis is based on clinical features of severe swelling around the shoulder, a pulseless arm and varying degrees of neurological deficits. Radiologically there is lateral displacement of the scapula on a chest radiograph. Treatment involves resuscitation, vascular repair and exploration of the brachial plexus as indicated, and stabilization of bone and joint injuries.

SUMMARY

The scapula plays a vital role in the effective functioning of the arm. It stabilizes the upper extremity against the thorax through the glenoid, the acromioclavicular joint, the clavicle and the sternoclavicular joint, supported by the strong muscles of pectoral girdle. Fractures of the scapula occur infrequently. Diagnosis is made through radiographs. Treatment is mainly conservative.

KEY LEARNING POINTS

- Fractures of the scapula are rare injuries (0.5–1% of all fractures).
- Fractures of the scapula usually occur in young males following motor vehicle accidents.
- Always look for other vital organ injuries as up to 85% of these injuries have been associated with injuries to the chest, head and abdomen.
- Conservative treatment in a sling with early shoulder rehabilitation gives good results in most patients.

REFERENCES

- ● = Key primary paper
- ◆ = Major review article

● 1. Ideberg R. Unusual glenoid fractures: a report on 92 cases. *Acta Orthopaedica Scandinavica* 1987;**58**:191–2.
2. Zdravkovic D, Damholt VV. Comminuted and severely displaced fractures of the scapula. *Acta Orthopaedica Scandinavica* 1974;**45**:60–65.
3. Rockwood CA. Management of fractures of the scapula. *Orthopaedic Transactions* 1986;**10**:219.
4. Williams Jr GR, Naranja J, Klimkiewicz J, *et al*. The floating shoulder: a biomechanical basis for classification and management. *Journal of Bone and Joint Surgery (American)* 2001;**83A**:1182–7.

25

Dislocations of the glenohumeral joint

SHANMUGANATHAN RAJASEKARAN, RISHI MUGESH KANNA, JAYARAMARAJU DHEENADHAYALAN

Introduction	297	Recurrent shoulder instability: TUBS and AMBRI	300
Pathoanatomy of the shoulder dislocation	297	Posterior dislocation of the shoulder	300
Mechanism of injury	298	Inferior glenohumeral dislocation (luxatio erecta)	301
Clinical evaluation	298	Superior glenohumeral dislocation	301
Radiographic evaluation	298	Summary	301
Treatment	299	References	302
Complications	299		

NATIONAL BOARD STANDARDS

- Understand the anatomy of the shoulder joint
- To know the important shoulder stabilizers
- Pathoanatomy of shoulder dislocations
- Know the types of dislocations
- Be able to conduct closed reductions
- Know the indications and principles of surgical treatment

INTRODUCTION

Dislocations of the shoulder joint are very common injuries, accounting for up to 45% of all dislocations.[1] Anterior dislocations occur more frequently than posterior dislocations while inferior and superior dislocations are rare. The high incidence of shoulder dislocation is related to the fact that the shoulder joint is a totally unconstrained joint and thus allows the greatest range of motion of any articulation in the body. The glenoid fossa articulates with only 25% of the articular surface of the humeral head and, although it is augmented by the labrum, it contributes little to the stability of the joint. The labrum, joint capsule, glenohumeral ligaments (superior, middle and inferior) and adhesive–cohesive forces owing to the presence of synovial fluid provide passive stability while the deltoid, long head of biceps and the rotator cuff provide active stability to the shoulder joint. So the ligaments serve as static restraints and the muscles serve as dynamic stabilizers (Fig. 25.1). The rotator cuff muscles (supraspinatous, infraspinatous and teres minor) with the subscapularis and the long head of biceps are the important muscular stabilizers. The neurovascular bundle lies close to the lower body of the glenohumeral joint and can be injured in anteroinferior dislocations.

PATHOANATOMY OF THE SHOULDER DISLOCATION

Shoulder dislocations are usually traumatic events and are always associated with stretching and tearing of the capsule. See fig. 25.2 for the anatomy. In younger patients, the anterior capsule and labrum are avulsed from the glenoid (Bankart's lesion) and this may also occasionally include a small fragment of the bone (bony Bankart's lesion). The soft-tissue avulsion is usually off the glenoid, but occasionally it can be off the humerus with avulsion of glenohumeral ligaments (HAGL lesion). When the humeral head dislocates anterior to the glenoid fossa, a compression fracture can occur on the posterolateral part of the humeral head owing to the force of impaction of the head on the anterior edge of the glenoid (Hill–Sachs lesion). This is seen in 27% of acute anterior dislocations and 74% of recurrent anterior dislocations. In more elderly patients beyond the age of 40, associated rotator cuff tears can occur. There is considerable discussion on the pathology that predisposes to recurrent dislocation. It is usually a combination of factors, as studies have shown that sectioning of the anterior capsule alone does not lead to instability.

Dislocations are commonly classified by direction (anterior, inferior, posterior or multidirectional), onset (acute, recurrent or chronic) and aetiology (traumatic, minimally traumatic, atraumatic or microanterior instability). Anterior dislocation of the shoulder is the most common, accounting for about 90% of shoulder dislocations.

MECHANISM OF INJURY

Anterior glenohumeral dislocation may occur as a result of either direct or indirect trauma.[2] Indirect trauma to the upper extremity with the shoulder in abduction, extension and external rotation is the most common mechanism. Direct, anteriorly directed impact to the posterior shoulder may produce an anterior dislocation. Recurrent dislocations with minimal trauma may occur in patients with congenital or acquired ligamentous laxity.

CLINICAL EVALUATION

The patient typically presents with the dislocated shoulder held in slight abduction and external rotation with the arm supported with the opposite hand. Any attempt at movements produces severe pain. There is flattening of the roundness of the shoulder owing to a relative prominence of the acromion, a hollow beneath the acromion laterally and a palpable mass anteriorly.

A careful neurovascular examination is important to assess the integrity of the axillary nerve (sensation over the deltoid) and the musculocutaneous nerve (sensation on the anterolateral forearm). Sometimes patients may present after spontaneous reduction. Here, a typical history and apprehension of the patient to abduct or extensively rotate the shoulder must raise suspicion of a dislocation.

RADIOGRAPHIC EVALUATION

Anteroposterior and trans-scapular lateral ('Y') views are adequate to confirm the diagnosis (Fig. 25.3). Only if the direction of the dislocation is not clearly evident should an axillary view be obtained as this may produce pain and severe spasm to the patient. Radiographs must be examined for associated tuberosity fractures and other bony injuries. Special views of the shoulder such as the

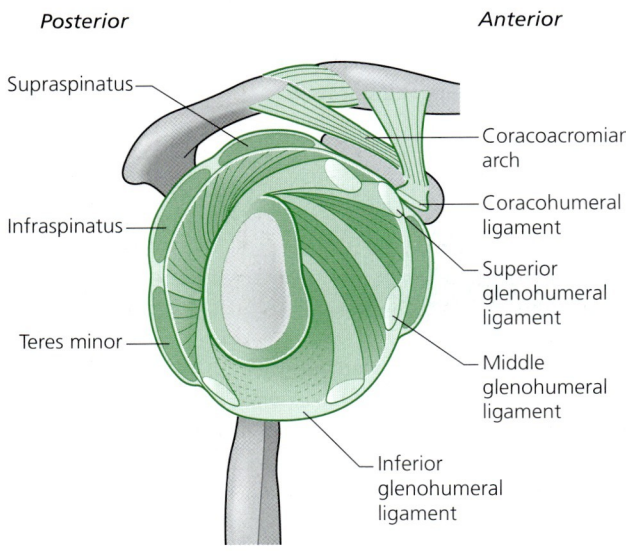

Figure 25.1 Anatomy of the shoulder joint as viewed from the humeral articular surface. The static and dynamic stabilizers of the shoulder joint are shown.

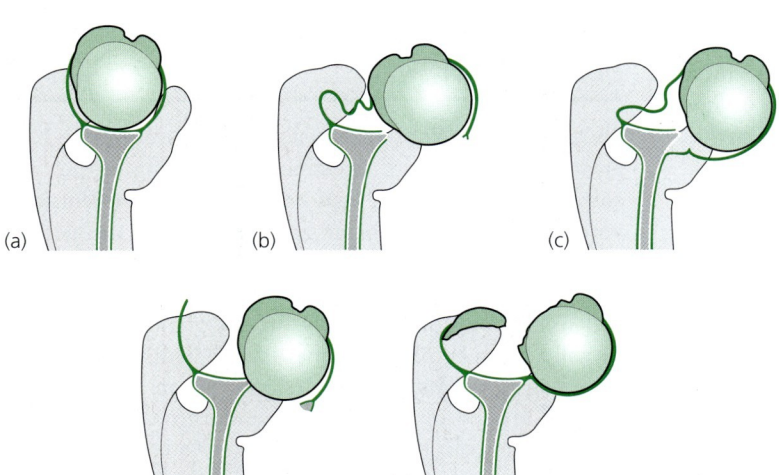

Figure 25.2 (a–e) The normal shoulder anatomy and the various pathological lesions in an anterior shoulder dislocation. (a) Normal anatomy of the shoulder. (b) Anterior capsular tear. (c) Capsular Bankart's lesion (avulsion of the capsule from the anterior glenoid). (d) Bony Bankart's lesion. (e) Hill–Sachs lesion (fracture of the posterolateral surface of the humeral head).

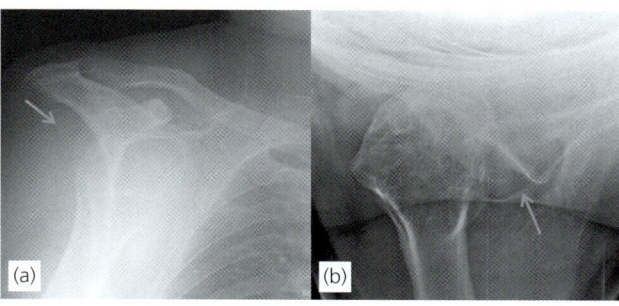

Figure 25.3 (a,b) Anterior glenohumeral dislocation. (a) The anteroposterior radiograph of the shoulder shows the dislocated humeral head lying anteroinferiorly under the coracoid process. (b) The axillary view shows the humeral head lying anterior to the glenoid fossa. Note the empty glenoid fossa in both the views (arrows).

Hill–Sachs view (tangential view of the anteroinferior glenoid rim), West Point axillary view and Stryker notch view (to visualize a posterolateral humeral head defect) are not mandatory in the acute setting.

CT may be useful in defining humeral head or glenoid impression fractures, and anterior labral bony injuries. MRI may be used to identify rotator cuff, capsular and glenoid labral lesions. Both CT and MRI are usually not required in the evaluation of acute dislocations.

TREATMENT

Treatment of the first episode of dislocation

Reduction of the dislocation must be performed at the earliest as it provides prompt relief of pain. This can usually be achieved even without full anaesthesia, provided the reduction is done gently with good muscle relaxation.

Numerous techniques of reduction have been described. *Hippocrates* proposed a method of reduction in which one foot is placed across the axillary fold and onto the chest wall to provide countertraction, with traction and gentle internal rotation of the affected upper extremity. Later *Kocher* proposed a technique using traction and external rotation and gently levering the humeral head on the anterior glenoid to effect reduction. These methods are rarely followed now as they are associated with increased risk of humeral fracture. The two commonly performed methods are either the *Stimson* prone reduction technique or the reduction by traction with abduction and external rotation (*Milch technique*). In the Stimson technique, after injection of 10–20 mL of 1% lidocaine into the glenohumeral joint, the patient is placed prone on an examination table with the involved arm hanging in a dependent position from the edge of the table. Eventually, with sufficient fatigue in the shoulder musculature, the joint can be easily reduced into normal position.

In the more commonly performed method of reduction by traction, the patient lies supine with analgesia obtained either by intravenous sedation or, preferably, by a subclavian perivascular block regional anaesthesia. An assistant applies countertraction by holding the two ends of a sheet passed around the thorax near the axilla and the forearm is gently pulled in a line of 30° of abduction, 20° of forward flexion and gradually externally rotated. The traction must be gentle and sustained, avoiding sudden and forceful attempts as this may lead to a fracture, especially in the elderly. Once sustained gentle traction has been given, as the shoulder muscles fatigue, the shoulder is adducted and gently internally rotated to reduce the joint.

In the rare event of inability to reduce an acute anterior dislocation, soft-tissue interposition must be suspected. This may require open reduction. Other indications for operative intervention are a grossly displaced greater tuberosity fracture that does not fall into position or a glenoid fracture that is greater than 5 mm in size.

Post-reduction treatment

The shoulder is usually immobilized for a brief period in a sling until pain relief is achieved, but the length of immobilization has no effect on the susceptibility for further recurrent dislocations. A range of motion and rotator cuff strengthening exercises should be initiated at the earliest but abduction and external rotation should be avoided.

COMPLICATIONS

Early complications

These include nerve injuries involving the axillary and/or musculocutaneous nerves in approximately 5–14% of dislocations. These are usually neurapraxia and almost always recover spontaneously. Both neural and vascular injuries can occur in young adults involved in high-velocity injuries. The greater tuberosity may shear off during the dislocation; however, it usually falls into place during reduction. If it remains displaced, internal fixation is required. Vascular injuries involve the axillary artery and typically can occur in elderly patients with atherosclerosis. They can also occur at the time of an open or closed reduction.

Late complications

Recurrent anterior dislocation is the most common complication after dislocation and the incidence is related to the age at the time of initial dislocation – the lower the age, the higher the incidence of recurrence. Susceptibility for redislocation is unrelated to the type or length of post-reduction immobilization. Recurrent dislocation is related to ligament and capsular changes and occasionally to large bony lesions such as the Hill–Sachs or the bony Bankart lesion. Patients may also have pain as a result of recurrent subluxation or instability without an actual dislocation. Shoulder stiffness can also occur because of prolonged immobilization and is more common in patients over the age of 40 years.

RECURRENT SHOULDER INSTABILITY: TUBS AND AMBRI

There are two different types of recurrent shoulder instability, one that follows a previous traumatic shoulder dislocation and the other that presents without any history of previous trauma.[3] The aetiology, presenting features, pathology and management principles are different for both these conditions.

After an acute traumatic dislocation, the type of recurrent instability observed is termed TUBS (*t*raumatic, *u*nidirectional, *B*ankart lesion; *s*urgery is often necessary). These patients have no problems of generalized ligament laxity and the dislocation is purely secondary to the disturbances caused by the previous trauma. They are usually young patients and have excellent results following surgery. Different types of surgical repair have been described. At present both open and arthroscopic Bankart repairs are in vogue.[4] Arthroscopic repair is technically difficult but the redislocation rates are comparable to open Bankart repairs. We prefer the inferior capsular shift reconstruction, which addresses the Bankart's lesion and also the laxity of the capsule and has a very high success rate.

The other type of recurrent instability presents without any previous history of trauma and is termed AMBRI (*a*traumatic, *m*ultidirectional, *b*ilateral, *r*ehabilitation is the primary mode of treatment; *i*nferior capsular shift is performed only rarely).[5] Often the shoulder may show instability in two or more directions, and patients demonstrate signs of general systemic laxity. The typical patient is a 'double-jointed' adolescent demonstrating a sulcus sign and apprehension when stress is applied in both the anterior or posterior directions. By strengthening the dynamic stabilizers, it should be possible to overcome the inherent glenohumeral joint laxity. Non-operative treatment is the treatment of choice because operative management is associated with a high failure rate. If physical rehabilitation fails to provide adequate improvement, however, these patients often require surgical tightening of the entire shoulder capsule with the inferior capsular shift procedure.[6]

POSTERIOR DISLOCATION OF THE SHOULDER

Posterior dislocation (Fig. 25.4) accounts for less than 10% of all shoulder dislocations.[7] A high degree of suspicion is necessary as up to 60% of posterior dislocations are missed on initial examination.

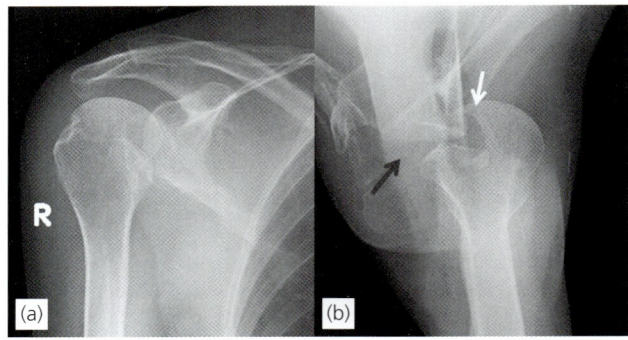

Figure 25.4 Anteroposterior (a) and axillary lateral (b) radiographs of a neglected posterior dislocation of the shoulder. The anterolateral aspect of the humeral head has a defect (reverse Hill–Sachs lesion; white arrow) that would prevent a stable reduction of the dislocation. The empty glenoid fossa is shown by the black arrow.

Mechanism of injury

A fall onto an adducted and forward flexed arm may result in a posterior dislocation. But, more often, posterior dislocations occur as a result of indirect injury that produces marked internal rotation and adduction, such as during a convulsion or an electrocution. A direct trauma applied to the anterior shoulder may also result in a posterior translation of the humeral head.

Clinical evaluation

A posterior glenohumeral dislocation does not present with striking deformity and the symptoms can be minimal, leading to frequently missed diagnosis. The shoulder typically is in the position of adduction, flexion and internal rotation. Limited forward elevation (often <90°) with restricted external rotation should raise suspicion of the diagnosis. In thinner individuals, a palpable mass posterior to the shoulder and flattening of the anterior shoulder may be obvious.

Radiographic evaluation

The findings in the standard anteroposterior views may often appear normal unless carefully examined. The humeral head, because it is medially rotated, loses its normal contour and is shaped like an electric light bulb. The glenoid appears partially vacant (space between anterior rim and humeral head >6 mm) – 'vacant glenoid' sign. There is absence of the normal elliptic overlap of the humeral head on the glenoid. The 'trough' sign is an impaction fracture of the anterior humeral head caused by the posterior rim of glenoid, which is more visible on the lateral view. Posterior dislocations are most readily recognized on the axillary view. CT scans will also show clearly the posterior dislocation and the percentage of the humeral head impacted during the dislocation.

Treatment

Closed reduction is best done under general anaesthesia. With the patient supine, traction should be applied to the adducted arm in the line of the deformity with gentle lifting of the humeral head into the glenoid fossa. The shoulder should never be forced into external rotation, as this may result in a humeral head fracture if an impaction fracture is locked on the posterior glenoid rim. If the head is locked, axial traction should be accompanied by lateral traction on the upper arm to unlock the humeral head from the glenoid.

Post reduction, a radiograph should be done to confirm reduction. If the shoulder is stable, a sling immobilization is adequate. However if the shoulder subluxates or redislocates, the shoulder is immobilized in a shoulder spica in mild abduction and lateral rotation for a period of 3 weeks.

External rotation and deltoid isometric exercises may be performed during the period of immobilization. After discontinuation of immobilization, an aggressive internal and external rotator strengthening programme is instituted.

Open reduction is indicated if dislocation is irreducible (impaction fracture on the posterior glenoid preventing reduction). Major displacement of an associated lesser tuberosity fracture or a fractured large posterior glenoid fragment will require fixation. If the shoulder is unstable secondary to a large humeral impaction fracture, a transfer of the lesser tuberosity with attached subscapularis into the defect (modified McLaughlin procedure) or a hemiarthroplasty (>40% involvement) is indicated.

Complications

Missed posterior dislocations are quite common and the management has to be individualized depending on the age of the patient, the duration since dislocation and the presence of any fracture. They will invariably require surgery and good results can be obtained even when the intervention is done as late as 6 months.

Recurrent dislocation may occur with large anteromedial humeral head defects and large posterior glenoid rim fractures. They may require surgical stabilization to prevent recurrence.

INFERIOR GLENOHUMERAL DISLOCATION (LUXATIO ERECTA)

This very rare injury results from a hyperabduction force causing impingement of the neck of the humerus on the acromion, which levers the humeral head out inferiorly. The patient typically presents in a characteristic 'salute' fashion, with the humerus locked in abduction and forward elevation. Pain is usually severe; the humeral head is palpable on the lateral chest wall and axilla.

Injury to the axillary artery or brachial plexus is common and must be looked for. Associated rotator cuff tears, pectoralis injury and proximal humeral fracture are also common. Anteroposterior and axillary views are typically diagnostic, with inferior dislocation of the humeral head and superior direction of the humeral shaft along the glenoid margin.

Closed reduction may be accomplished by the use of traction–countertraction manoeuvres. Axial traction in line with the humeral shaft, with a gradual decrease in shoulder abduction and countertraction applied with a sheet around the patient's thorax, usually achieves reduction. Failure of closed reduction is due to the humeral head 'buttonholing' through the inferior capsule and soft-tissue envelope. Open reduction is then indicated.

SUPERIOR GLENOHUMERAL DISLOCATION

This very rare injury occurs with extreme anterior and superior directed force applied to the adducted upper extremity, such as a fall from a height onto the upper extremity. The humeral head is forced superiorly from the glenoid fossa. Typically it is accompanied by fractures of the acromion, clavicle, coracoid and humeral tuberosities, as well as by soft-tissue injury to the rotator cuff, glenohumeral capsule, biceps tendon and surrounding musculature.

The patient typically presents with a foreshortened upper extremity held in adduction and a palpable humeral head above the level of the acromion. The anteroposterior radiograph is typically diagnostic, with dislocation of the humeral head superior to the acromion process. Closed reduction with axial traction applied in an inferior direction and lateral traction applied to the upper arm achieves reduction. Irreducible dislocations may require open reduction.

SUMMARY

The wide range of motion allowed by the shoulder joint enables us to keep the upper limb at various positions in space. However, in order to achieve such mobility, the bony stability of the joint is reduced and depends mainly on various static and dynamic soft-tissue stabilizers. As such, the shoulder is one of the most commonly dislocated joints in the human body. Most traumatic dislocations are anterior and are treated efficiently by closed methods of reduction. Late instability is a potential complication that may require surgical stabilization procedures, either open or arthroscopic. With the increasing interest in recreational and sporting activities, the incidence of glenohumeral instability may be increasing. Effective shoulder rehabilitation techniques are available for these multidirectional instabilities and surgery is reserved for select patients only.

KEY LEARNING POINTS

- The glenohumeral joint is the most mobile and most commonly dislocated major joint.
- The tremendous range of motion is achieved at the expense of intrinsic skeletal stability. Various dynamic muscular and static ligamentous stabilizers provide the main stability.
- Although glenohumeral dislocations are commonly associated with the young and athletic, they occur at all ages.
- Patient age is the most important determinant of the anatomical pathology, complications and prognosis of glenohumeral dislocations. Young patients are more prone to recurrent dislocations and older individuals have a higher incidence of acute complications.
- Older patients can sometimes have an associated rotator cuff injury and, if present, surgical treatment should be considered.
- The vast majority of glenohumeral dislocations are anterior. Subcoracoid dislocations are the most common, followed by subglenoid, subclavicular and intrathoracic.
- Closed reduction under anaesthesia is successful in most cases.
- Patients with late instability either have TUBS (*t*raumatic, *u*nidirectional, *B*ankart lesion; *s*urgery is often necessary) or AMBRI (*a*traumatic, *m*ultidirectional, *b*ilateral, *r*ehabilitation is the primary mode of treatment; *i*nferior capsular shift is performed only rarely). Patients with TUBS require surgical treatment, usually a Bankart's repair. Although AMBRI lesions are treated with physiotherapy effectively, they may rarely require surgical intervention.
- Posterior dislocations are uncommon whereas inferior and superior dislocations are very rare.

REFERENCES

● = Key primary paper
♦ = Major review article

●1. Hippocrates. The classic: Injuries of the shoulder: dislocations. *Clinical Orthopaedics and Related Research* 1989;**246**:4–7.
●2. McLaughlin HL, Cavallaro WU. Primary anterior dislocation of the shoulder. *American Journal of Surgery* 1950;**80**:615–21.
♦3. Rowe CR, Sakellarides HT. Factors related to recurrences of anterior dislocations of the shoulder. *Clinical Orthopaedics and Related Research* 1961;**20**:40–7.
4. Bankart AS. The pathology and treatment of recurrent dislocation of the shoulder joint. *British Journal of Surgery* 1939;**26**:23–9.
♦5. Neer C. II. Involuntary inferior and multidirectional instability of the shoulder etiology, recognition and treatment. *Instructional Course Lectures* 1985;**34**:232–8.
6. Pollock RG, Owens JM, Flatow EL, *et al*. Operative results of the inferior capsular shift procedure for multidirectional instability of the shoulder. *Journal of Bone and Joint Surgery (American)* 2000;**82**:919–28.
●7. McLaughlin HL. Posterior dislocation of the shoulder. *Journal of Bone and Joint Surgery (American)* 1952;**34**:584–90.

26

Fractures of the proximal humerus

SHANMUGANATHAN RAJASEKARAN, RISHI MUGESH KANNA, JAYARAMARAJU DHEENADHAYALAN

Introduction	303	Treatment	304
Mechanism of injury	303	Complications	305
Clinical evaluation	303	Summary	306
Radiographic evaluation	304	References	306
Fracture classification	304		

NATIONAL BOARD STANDARDS

- Understand the anatomy of the proximal humerus
- Understand the significance of vascular anatomy of the humeral head
- Be able to diagnose and classify the proximal humerus fractures
- Be aware of management principles

INTRODUCTION

Fractures of the proximal humerus account for up to 45% of all humeral fractures. The proximal humerus comprises four main osseous segments, namely the humeral head, the lesser tuberosity, the greater tuberosity and the humeral shaft. The humeral head is connected to the shaft through the anatomical neck. Fractures of the anatomical neck are uncommon, but they have a poor prognosis because of the interference with the vascular supply to the humeral head. The surgical neck of the humerus distal to the tuberosities is a common site for fractures. The blood supply to the proximal humerus depends on the anterior and posterior circumflex humeral vessels and through the muscular attachments of the tuberosities.

Once a fracture occurs, the osseous segments may be displaced by the pull of the muscles attached to the fragment. The greater tuberosity is displaced superiorly and posteriorly by the supraspinatus. The lesser tuberosity is displaced medially by the subscapularis. The humeral shaft is adducted medially by the pectoralis major, and the proximal fragment is usually abducted by the fibres of the deltoid.

MECHANISM OF INJURY

Fractures of the proximal humerus have a bimodal age distribution. They occur following high-energy motor vehicle accidents in young patients and as the result of a fall on the outstretched hand in elderly patients. Pathological fractures, electrocution and sudden muscular contraction are less common causes.

CLINICAL EVALUATION

Patients present with pain, swelling and tenderness over the shoulder, and attempted shoulder movement is painful. The injured extremity is usually supported by the contralateral hand. A careful neurovascular examination is essential as neurovascular injury can occur in fractures with a medially displaced shaft of the humerus. Axillary nerve injury can be diagnosed by the absence of sensation on the lateral aspect of the proximal arm (referred as the 'regiment badge area').

RADIOGRAPHIC EVALUATION

A set of radiographs (shoulder trauma series) is necessary to assess the fracture planes and displacement. This consists of anteroposterior and lateral views in the scapular plane as well as an axillary shoulder view. CT scans are helpful in evaluating articular involvement, the degree of fracture displacement, impression fractures of the head and glenoid rim fractures.

FRACTURE CLASSIFICATION

Neer's classification system (Fig. 26.1), the most commonly used, is based on the four-part anatomy of the proximal humerus: the humeral head, the lesser and greater tuberosities, and the proximal humeral shaft.[1] A part is defined as 'displaced' if a displacement of more than 1 cm or an angulation of more than 45° is present. The classification depends on the number of displaced fragments and not on the fracture lines. Thus, however many fracture lines may be there, if the fragments are undisplaced, it is regarded as a one-part fracture (Table 26.1).

TREATMENT

Minimally displaced fractures

Up to 85% of fractures of the proximal humerus are minimally displaced or non-displaced. Sling immobilization or swathe is used for comfort.[2] The patient is followed up radiologically to detect loss of fracture reduction. Early pendulum exercises and active shoulder mobilization can be started.

Two-part fractures

- *Anatomical neck fractures* are rare and difficult to treat by closed reduction. Because of the precarious blood supply, they are associated with a high incidence of osteonecrosis. They require open reduction and internal fixation (ORIF) in younger patients or a prosthesis in elderly patients (shoulder hemiarthroplasty).
- *Surgical neck fractures* can be treated with open reduction and fixation with pins, intramedullary nails with or without a supplemental tension band, or plate and screws.
- *Greater tuberosity fractures*, if they are displaced more than 5–10 mm, require ORIF with screws or tension band wires. Rotator cuff repair will be required in the presence of cuff injury (Fig. 26.2).
- *Lesser tuberosity fractures* may be treated conservatively unless the fragment displaces and blocks rotation.

Table 26.1 Neer's classification of fractures of the proximal humerus

Type	Fracture type	Subtype
1	One-part fractures (no displaced fragments regardless of the number of fracture lines)	
2	Two-part fractures	1 Anatomic neck 2 Surgical neck 3 Greater tuberosity 4 Lesser tuberosity
3	Three-part fractures	1 Surgical neck with greater tuberosity 2 Surgical neck with lesser tuberosity
4	Four-part fractures	
5	Fracture dislocations	
6	Articular surface fracture	

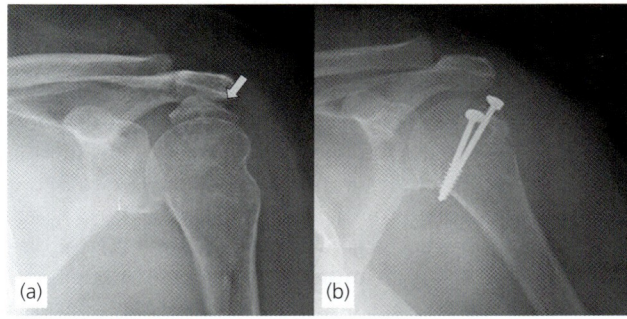

Figure 26.2 Avulsion fracture of the greater tuberosity of the humerus. (a) Pre-operative radiograph shows an avulsion fracture of the greater tuberosity migrated posterosuperiorly (arrow). (b) The fragment has been reduced anatomically and fixed with two partially threaded 4.5 mm cancellous screws.

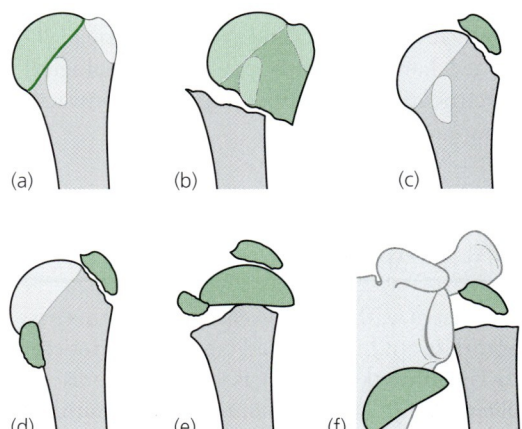

Figure 26.1 (a–f) The different types of fractures of the proximal humerus. (a) One-part fracture (none of the fragments are displaced). (b) Two-part anatomical neck fracture. (c) Greater tuberosity fracture. (d) Three-part fracture. (e) Four-part fracture. (f) Fracture dislocation.

Three-part fractures

These are unstable fractures owing to wide displacement of the fragments as a result of opposing muscle forces. Displaced fractures in younger individuals require operative fixation with locking plate and screws. Preservation of the vascular supply is of paramount importance during surgical reduction. Older patients benefit from primary prosthetic replacement (hemiarthroplasty) and early shoulder mobilization.

Four-part fractures

The incidence of avascular necrosis is high (15–35%).[3] ORIF may be attempted in young patients if the humeral head is located within the glenold fossa. Fixation may be achieved with multiple Kirschner wires, screw fixation, or plate and screw.[4] Primary prosthetic replacement of the humeral head (hemiarthroplasty) is the procedure of choice in the elderly.

Fracture dislocations

Two-part fracture dislocations may be treated closed after shoulder reduction, once the fragments fall back into position. In three- and four-part fracture dislocations, because of the high incidence of osteonecrosis, hemiarthroplasty is advised, especially in the elderly (Fig. 26.3). ORIF can be attempted in younger individuals (Fig. 26.4). Articular surface fractures are often associated with dislocations. Patients with >40% of humeral head involvement may require hemiarthroplasty.[5] Screw fixation can be considered in young patients, if possible.

COMPLICATIONS

The most common chronic complication is stiffness and loss of movement of the affected shoulder. Abduction and internal rotation are especially lost and this can be as a result of malunion and persistent displacement of the greater tuberosity. Stiffness can be prevented by early rehabilitation and motivation of the patient to perform physical therapy at home frequently. Delayed union and non-union are also common, especially with three- and four-part fractures. If this is associated with pain and severe restriction of movements, then treatment is either an internal fixation with bone grafting or a hemiarthroplasty. Osteonecrosis of the fragments is another common complication in displaced three- or four-part fractures and fracture dislocations. In the acute setting, displaced fractures may have associated nerve and vascular damage and the involvement of axillary, median, radial and ulnar nerves has been reported with equal frequency.

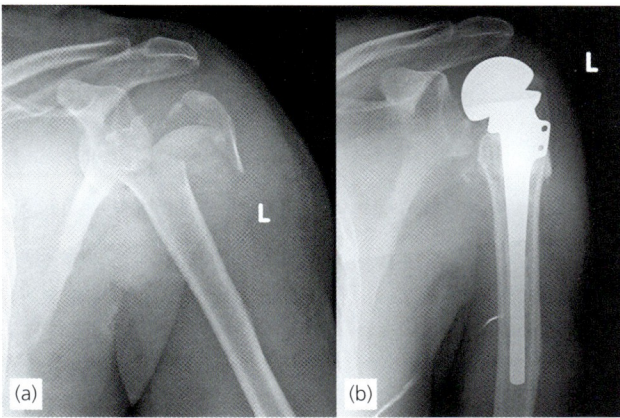

Figure 26.3 Pre-operative (a) and postoperative (b) radiographs of an elderly patient who has sustained a fracture dislocation of the proximal humerus. A hemiarthroplasty has been performed because of the high risk of avascular necrosis and post-traumatic stiffness in these patients.

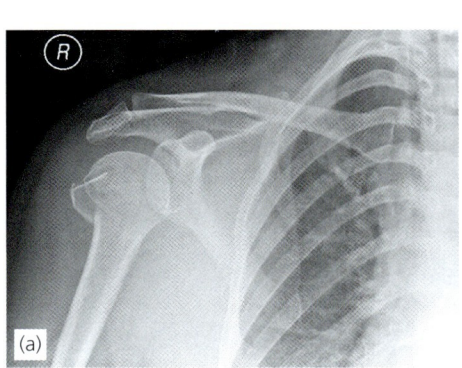 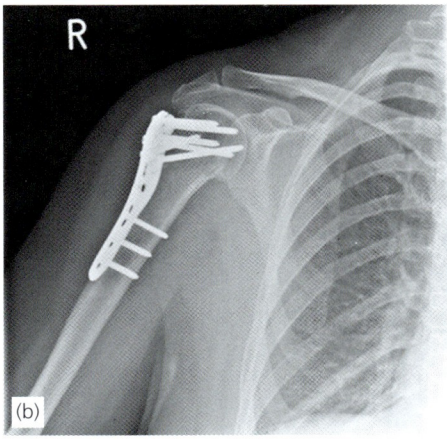

Figure 26.4 (a) Valgus impacted fracture of the proximal humerus. (b) The injury has been treated by open reduction and internal fixation with a locking plate.

SUMMARY

Next to shoulder dislocation, fractures of the proximal humerus account for most of the traumatic skeletal shoulder girdle injuries. Apart from radiographs, CT scans may be required to assess the fracture anatomy and morphology, which would help in surgical planning. Thorough three-dimensional anatomy of the shoulder, the blood supply of the proximal humerus and knowledge about fracture healing are vital for the operating surgeon.

KEY LEARNING POINTS

- The proximal humerus is the most common site for humeral fractures (45%).
- Depending upon the number of fractured fragments and their displacement, fractures of the proximal humerus are classified as one-part to four-part fractures.
- The options of surgical management range from K-wire fixation, tension band cerclage wires and intramedullary nails to various kinds of plates. Fractures in elderly patients need rigid fixation for early shoulder rehabilitation.
- Four-part fractures and fracture dislocations affect the blood supply of the humerus and can cause avascular necrosis. These fractures are better managed by hemiarthroplasty.

REFERENCES

● = Key primary paper
◆ = Major review article

● 1. Neer CS. I. Displaced proximal humeral fractures. II. Treatment of three-part and four-part displacement. *Journal of Bone and Joint Surgery (American)* 1970; **52**:1090–103.
◆ 2. Stewart MJ, Hundley JM. Fractures of the humerus: a comparative study in methods of treatment. *Journal of Bone and Joint Surgery (American)* 1955;**37**:681–92.
◆ 3. Szyszkowitz R, Seggl W, Schleifer P, et al. Proximal humeral fractures: management techniques and expected results. *Clinical Orthopaedics and Related Research* 1993;**292**:13.
4. Kristiansen B, Christensen SW. Plate fixation of proximal humeral fractures. *Acta Orthopaedica Scandinavica* 1986;**57**:320–3.
5. Paavolainen P, Bjorkenheim JM, Slatis P, et al. Operative treatment of severe proximal humeral fractures. *Acta Orthopaedica Scandinavica* 1983;**54**:374–9.

27

Humeral shaft fractures

S RAJASEKARAN, RISHI MUGESH KANNA, J DHEENADHAYALAN

Introduction	307	Classification	308
Anatomy	307	Treatment	308
Mechanism of injury	307	Complications	308
Clinical evaluation	307	References	310
Radiographic evaluation	307		

NATIONAL BOARD STANDARDS

- Know the surgical anatomy of the humerus
- Understand the relationship of neurovascular structures with the bone
- Be familiar with the principles of management
- Know the importance of distal humeral shaft fractures

INTRODUCTION

Humeral shaft fractures are relatively common injuries (3–5% of all fractures). Most of them occur after direct blows. The radial nerve is prone to damage, either during the initial injury or during fracture reduction. Conservative treatment gives good results in the majority of patients.

ANATOMY

The humeral shaft has a rich vascular supply, being densely covered with muscular attachments. By definition, the humeral shaft extends from the insertion of pectoralis major to the supracondylar ridge. The radial nerve along with the profunda brachii artery winds around the humeral shaft posteriorly in the spiral groove. At the region where it travels from the posterior to the anterior compartment, it is transfixed to the bone by the lateral intermuscular septum and is prone to injury by fractures in this region. Depending on the level of fracture, the fracture fragments are displaced by the strong muscular attachments into different positions.

MECHANISM OF INJURY

Direct trauma to the arm is the most common mode of injury and results in transverse or comminuted fractures. In elderly patients, indirect injury through a fall on an outstretched arm results in spiral or oblique fractures.

CLINICAL EVALUATION

Patients with humeral shaft fractures typically present with pain, swelling, deformity and shortening of the affected arm. A careful neurovascular examination is done with particular attention to radial nerve function and is documented.

RADIOGRAPHIC EVALUATION

Anteroposterior and lateral radiographs of the humerus, including the shoulder and elbow joints, are the only imaging studies usually required.

CLASSIFICATION

These fractures can be descriptively classified based on the location (proximal third, middle third, distal third), degree of displacement or the fracture anatomy (transverse, oblique, spiral, segmental, comminuted).

TREATMENT

The principles of treatment are to achieve union with an acceptable alignment and to restore the patient quickly to pre-injury functional status. This is usually achieved by conservative measures in the majority of patients.

Non-operative treatment

> It is perhaps the easiest of the major long bones to treat by conservative methods.
>
> Sir John Charnley

Most humeral shaft fractures (>90%) will heal with non-surgical management. About 20° of angulation and up to 3 cm of apposition do not cause functional disability in the upper limb.[1]

The methods of conservative care are:[2]

- *Hanging cast.* This utilizes gravity-dependent traction by the weight of the cast and arm to effect fracture reduction. It is useful in displaced midshaft humeral fractures, particularly spiral or oblique patterns.
- *Coaptation splint.* This utilizes dependency traction to effect fracture reduction. It is indicated for the acute treatment of humeral shaft fractures with minimal shortening and for short oblique or transverse fracture patterns that may displace with a hanging arm cast.
- *Thoracobrachial immobilization (Velpeau dressing).* This is used in elderly patients or children who are unable to tolerate other methods of treatment and in whom comfort is the primary concern. It is indicated for minimally displaced or non-displaced fractures that do not require reduction.
- *Functional bracing.*[3] This utilizes hydrostatic soft-tissue compression to effect and maintain fracture alignment while allowing motion of adjacent joints. It is typically applied 1–2 weeks after injury, after the patient has been initially placed in a hanging arm cast or coaptation splint and swelling has subsided. It consists of an anterior and posterior shell held together with Velcro straps. Success depends on an upright patient and tightening the brace daily. The functional brace is usually needed for a period of 8 weeks after fracture or until there is radiographic evidence of union. The treating orthopaedic surgeon should be wary of distraction in transverse humeral fractures, thus posing an increased risk of non-union.

Operative treatment

Although most humeral shaft fractures can be managed by non-operative methods, with 100% expected union rates, there are a few instances when surgical stabilization would be prescribed. The indications for operative treatment are polytraumatized patients, inadequate closed reduction, pathological fracture, associated vascular injury, floating elbow injury, segmental fractures, fractures with intra-articular extension, bilateral humeral fractures, open fractures, neurological loss following penetrating trauma, radial nerve palsy occurring after fracture manipulation and non-union. The anterolateral approach is usually preferred for proximal third humeral shaft fractures. The posterior approach also provides an excellent exposure of the entire humerus and is preferred for distal third humeral fractures and whenever there is a need to explore the radial nerve.

METHODS OF OPERATIVE STABILIZATION

Operative stabilization can be performed by a compression plate device, by intramedullary fixation or, rarely, by external fixation.[4] Open reduction and internal fixation with a compression plate gives the best functional results and is the usual preferred method of fixation (Fig. 27.1). One should take care to preserve soft-tissue attachments of butterfly fragments during exposure and fixation. Intramedullary fixation is indicated in segmental fractures, fractures in extremely osteopenic bone and pathological humeral fractures. Either flexible nails or rigid interlocked nails are used. Multiple flexible nails inserted antegrade or retrograde fill the canal to achieve an interference fit. They are primarily reserved for humeral shaft fractures with minimal comminution. Interlocked nails have proximal and distal interlocking facilities and are able to provide rotational and axial fracture stability. Antegrade nailing methods are associated with a high incidence of shoulder pain and efforts must be taken to avoid damage to the rotator cuff to minimize postoperative shoulder problems. The proximal aspect of the nail should also be countersunk to prevent subacromial impingement. External fixation is indicated in special situations such as infected non-unions and open fractures with extensive soft-tissue loss.

COMPLICATIONS

Radial nerve injury occurs in up to 18% of cases. It is commonly seen with middle third fractures. *Holstein–Lewis syndrome* refers to spiral distal third humeral fractures, which may entrap or lacerate the nerve as it passes through

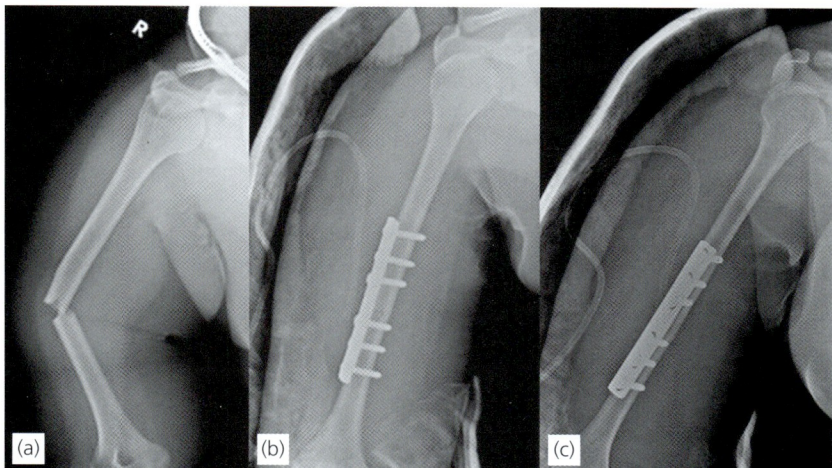

Figure 27.1 A transverse midshaft humeral fracture in a polytrauma patient treated by open anatomical reduction and internal fixation with dynamic compression plate and screws.

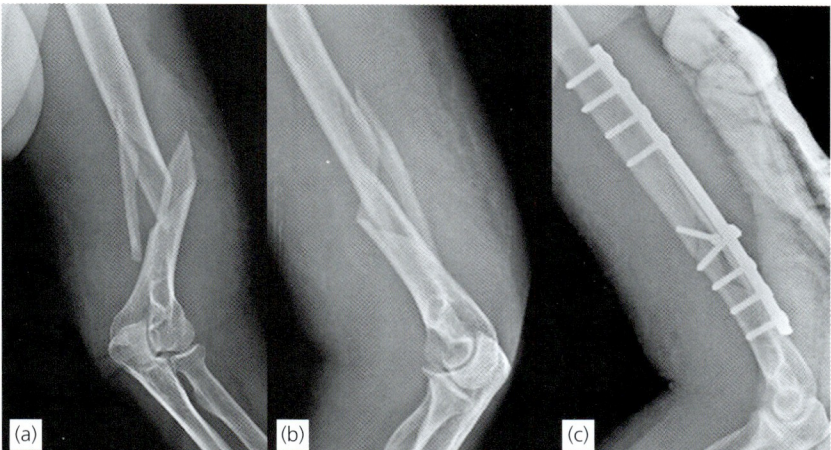

Figure 27.2 Anteroposterior (a) and lateral (b) radiographs of a distal third humeral fracture. In these spiral fractures, the radial nerve can be entrapped by the lateral intermuscular septum (Holstein–Lewis syndrome). In this case, the fracture has been stabilized through a posterior approach by a dynamic compression plate and interfragmentary screws (c).

the lateral intermuscular septum (Fig. 27.2).[5] The neurological injury can also occur during manipulation of the fracture. Most injuries are neurapraxia with spontaneous recovery within 5 months. Neurological recovery is assessed clinically by Tinel's sign, electromyography and nerve conduction studies. If there is no recovery even after 6 months, tendon transfers to correct the wrist drop and loss of extension at the metacarpophalangeal joints of the fingers and thumb can be performed with good functional results. Vascular injury is uncommon in closed injuries but can occur in open injuries. The brachial artery has the greatest risk for injury in fractures at the junction of the proximal and distal third of the arm. Malunion is frequent after conservative fractures but usually does not produce functional disability. Non-unions may occur with overdistraction during conservative treatment or following internal fixation due to decreased vascularity of the fractured ends or poor surgical techniques.

KEY LEARNING POINTS

- Fractures of the humeral shaft are common injuries and account for 3–5% of all fractures.
- Neurovascular examination of the injured limb is vital before initiating treatment.
- Diagnosis is straightforward and fracture anatomy can be assessed by radiographs.
- Most fractures will heal with appropriate conservative care.
- Owing to the wide range of motion of the shoulder and elbow and the minimal effect of shortening, a larger degree of radiographic malunion can be accepted with little functional deficit.
- Surgery is indicated in specific situations.

REFERENCES

● = Key primary paper
◆ = Major review article

◆1. Mast JW, Spiegal PG, Harvey JP, *et al*. Fractures of the humeral shaft. *Clinical Orthopaedics and Related Research* 1975;**12**: 254–62.
2. Holm CL. Management of humeral shaft fractures. Fundamental nonoperative techniques. *Clinical Orthopaedics and Related Research* 1970;**91**:132–9.
◆3. Sarmiento A, Zagorski JB, Zych G, *et al*. Functional bracing for the treatment of fractures of the humeral diaphysis. *Journal of Bone and Joint Surgery (American)* 2000;**82**:478–86.
4. Vander Griend RA, Tomasin J, Ward EF. Open reduction and internal fixation of humeral shaft fractures: results using AO plating techniques. *Journal of Bone and Joint Surgery (American)* 1986;**68**:430–3.
●5. Holstein A, Lewis GB. Fractures of the humerus with radial nerve paralysis. *Journal of Bone and Joint Surgery (American)* 1963;**45**:1382–8.

28

Fractures of the distal humerus

SHANMUGANATHAN RAJASEKARAN, RISHI MUGESH KANNA, JAYARAMARAJU DHEENADHAYALAN

Introduction	311	Treatment	312
Classification	311	Complications	313
Anatomy	311	Transcondylar fractures	313
Mechanism of injury	312	Capitellum fractures	313
Clinical evaluation	312	Trochlear fractures	314
Radiographic evaluation	312	Epicondylar fractures	314
Intercondylar fractures	312	References	315

NATIONAL BOARD STANDARDS

- Know the three-dimensional anatomy of the distal humerus
- Understand the relationship of neurovascular structures with the bone
- Be familiar with the types of fracture
- Know the importance of early, anatomical reduction and mobilization

INTRODUCTION

Fractures of the adult distal humerus are uncommon injuries, and constitute only 2% of all fractures.[1] However, they are important as most of them are peri-articular fractures and have a risk of associated neurovascular injury. Extension of the fracture line into the articular surface in these fractures mandates a rigid anatomical reduction so that secondary arthritis and stiffness can be avoided. The close proximity of major neurovascular elements demands a thorough neurovascular examination.

CLASSIFICATION

Based on the location of the fracture line and involvement of articular elements, these fractures can be broadly classified as supracondylar, transcondylar intercondylar, condylar, capitellum, trochlear, lateral epicondylar and medial epicondylar fractures. Intercondylar fractures of the distal humerus are the most common fracture pattern in adults. Mehne and Matta have descriptively classified bicolumnar fractures based on the configuration of fracture lines[2] (Fig. 28.1). The other types are predominantly seen in children and will be discussed in detail in the paediatric section.

ANATOMY

The distal humerus is roughly triangular in shape, with the medial and lateral columns forming the two sides and the base formed by the articular elements (trochlea and the capitellum). The corners of the triangle are formed by the condyles. The capitellum articulates with the radius and the trochlea with the ulna. Their articulating surfaces project distally and anteriorly at an angle of 45°. The centres of the arcs of rotation of each condyle lie on the same horizontal axis, and relative malalignment between them interferes with the flexion–extension arc. The longitudinal axis of the forearm is placed at 4–8° of valgus compared with the arm (carrying angle).

Fractures of the distal humerus

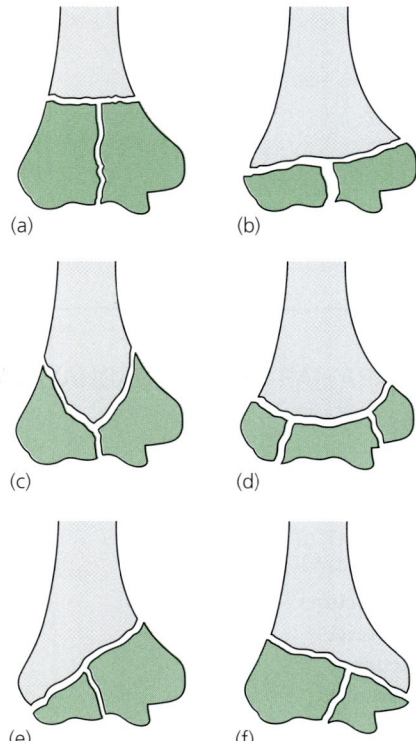

Figure 28.1 Mehne and Matta classification of bicolumnar distal humeral fractures. (a) High T fracture; (b) low T fracture; (c) Y fractures; (d) H fractures; (e) medial L fracture; (f) lateral L fractures.

MECHANISM OF INJURY

The majority of these fractures are seen in younger individuals following high-velocity road traffic accidents. They can also be a part of a shattered elbow as a result of a direct blow when the elbow is injured by approaching vehicles (side swipe injuries). Most low-energy distal humeral fractures result from a simple fall onto the elbow in elderly persons.

CLINICAL EVALUATION

Diagnosis is usually straightforward as most patients with these fractures present with a clear history of injury associated with pain, swelling, displacement and crepitus. High-velocity injuries can be associated with extensive soft-tissue damage. A careful neurovascular evaluation is essential because of the close proximity of the brachial artery and the median, ulnar and radial nerves. Severe swelling can cause an increase in forearm compartment pressure with the risk of compartment syndrome, resulting in Volkmann's ischaemic contracture. Serial neurovascular examinations with compartment pressure monitoring may be necessary in such patients.

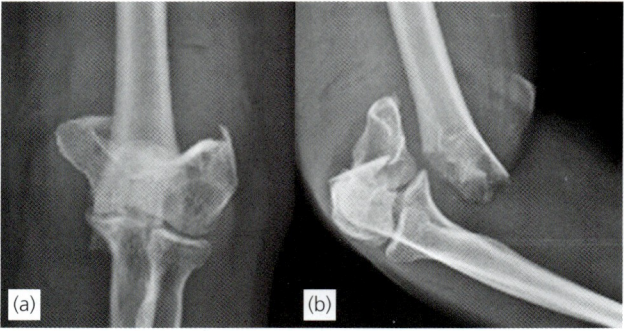

Figure 28.2 Anteroposterior (a) and lateral (b) radiographs of a distal humerus fracture. This is a Y type distal humeral metaphyseal fracture with minimal intra-articular extension.

RADIOGRAPHIC EVALUATION

Standard anteroposterior and lateral views of the elbow are usually sufficient, and additional oblique radiographs may be helpful for further fracture definition (Fig. 28.2). In undisplaced fractures, the presence of effusion or haemarthrosis causes displacement of the adipose layer overlying the joint capsule, and this is seen in the lateral radiograph as a radiolucent line (fat pad sign). In complex fractures, CT helps in defining the fracture fragments clearly and is useful in preoperative planning.

INTERCONDYLAR FRACTURES

These are the most common type of fractures of the adult distal humerus. Comminution is common in these fractures. Fracture fragments are often displaced by unopposed muscle pull at the medial (flexor mass) and lateral (extensor mass) epicondyles, which rotate the articular surfaces.

TREATMENT

Treatment must be individualized according to the patient's age, bone quality and degree of comminution. As most of these fractures involve the joint, operative treatment for anatomical reduction and stable fixation of the fragments is usually required. Restoration of articular surface alignment and a stable internal fixation that allows early mobilization of the joint are vital to achieve good functional outcomes.

Non-operative treatment is indicated only when the fractures are undisplaced, in elderly patients with severe osteopenia and comminution and in patients with significant comorbid conditions precluding operative management.[3] Non-operative options for displaced fractures include cast immobilization, traction with an olecranon pin or the 'bag of bones' technique,[4] in which the arm is placed in a collar and cuff with as much flexion as possible after initial reduction. Early active mobilization is started once pain subsides.

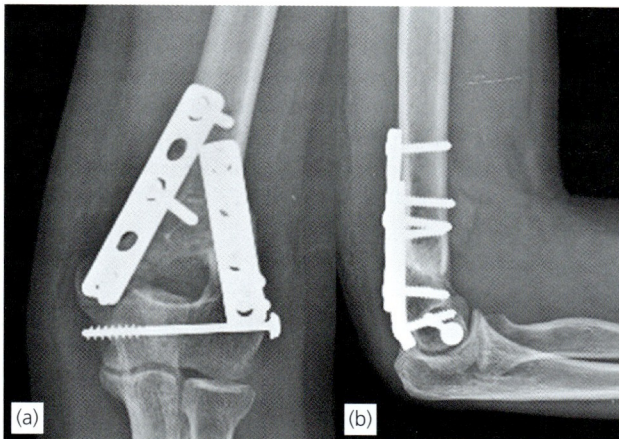

Figure 28.3 Postoperative anteroposterior (a) and lateral (b) radiographs of the fracture shown in Fig. 28.2. A lag cancellous screw has been used to secure the intercondylar fracture. Dual 3.5 mm dynamic compression plates have been used to stabilize the medial and lateral columns. For maximum biomechanical strength of the construct, there should be one posterior plate and one medial plate. The use of locking plates further enhances the strength of the construct.

The goals of operative treatment are to restore articular congruity and to secure the supracondylar component.[5,6] The fracture anatomy can be exposed either by elevating the triceps tendons as a tongue or by an olecranon osteotomy and reflecting the triceps. Usually, dual plate fixation with one plate to stabilize the medial and lateral columns is required (Fig. 28.3). Reduction of intercondylar elements and interfragmentary screw fixation is achieved, followed by alignment of the reconstructed articular fragments with the metaphyseal segment with dual plate fixation. In patients with severe comminution or osteoporosis, specially designed locking plate constructs give good results. A total elbow arthroplasty (semiconstrained) may be considered in markedly comminuted fractures and in fractures in osteoporotic bone.

COMPLICATIONS

Post-traumatic arthritis can occur in fractures in which the articular congruity has not been established. Failure of fixation can also occur as a result of a comminuted fracture pattern, leading to pain and stiffness of the joint. The other common complications of operative treatment are iatrogenic neurovascular injury and infection.

TRANSCONDYLAR FRACTURES

These occur primarily in elderly patients with osteopenic bone following a fall onto an outstretched hand or a force applied to a flexed elbow. Non-operative treatment with an above-elbow cast immobilization is indicated for non-displaced or minimally displaced fractures in elderly patients who are debilitated. Range of motion exercises should be initiated as soon as the patient is able to tolerate therapy. Operative treatment should be undertaken for open fractures, unstable fractures or displaced fractures. Open reduction and internal fixation with a single or a double plate is usually done.

CAPITELLUM FRACTURES

These represent <1% of all elbow fractures and usually occur in the coronal plane, parallel to the anterior humerus.[7] Most of them occur after a fall onto an outstretched hand with the elbow in varying degrees of flexion and are occasionally associated with radial head fractures. Since the fracture fragment does not have a soft-tissue attachment, it can displace and interfere with joint motion. Hence, displaced fractures require surgical stabilization (Fig. 28.4).

Classification

Type I	The fracture involves a large osseous component of capitellum, sometimes with trochlear involvement (Hahn–Steinthal fragment).
Type II	The fracture involves mainly the articular cartilage with a minimal amount of subchondral bone (Kocher–Lorenz fragment).
Type III	The entire capitellum is markedly comminuted.

Treatment

Undisplaced fractures can be treated non-operatively with immobilization in a posterior splint for 3 weeks followed by range of elbow motion exercises. Operative treatment is indicated in displaced fractures in which open reduction and internal fixation of the displaced fragment is achieved with screws (Fig. 28.5). Excision is indicated for severely comminuted type I fractures, type II fractures and in chronic untreated fractures with limited elbow motion.

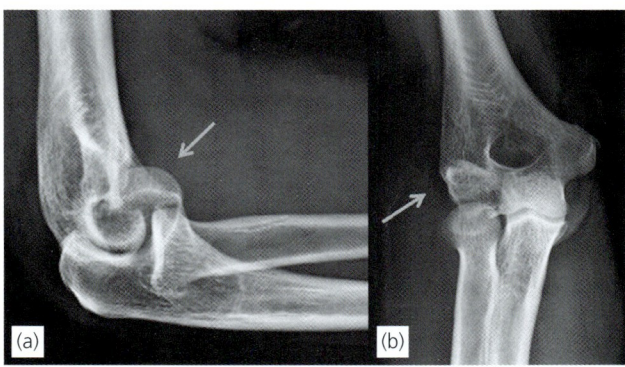

Figure 28.4 Lateral (a) and anteroposterior (b) radiographs reveal a displaced capitellum fracture (arrows).

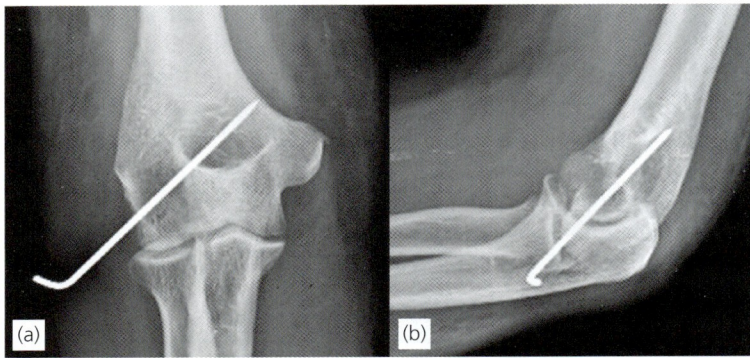

Figure 28.5 Postoperative anteroposterior (a) and lateral (b) radiographs of the fracture shown in Fig. 28.2. The fracture has been reduced and a 2.5 mm Kirschner wire inserted to hold the fracture reduction. Alternatively, a headless screw, which can be buried inside the articular surface, can be used as well.

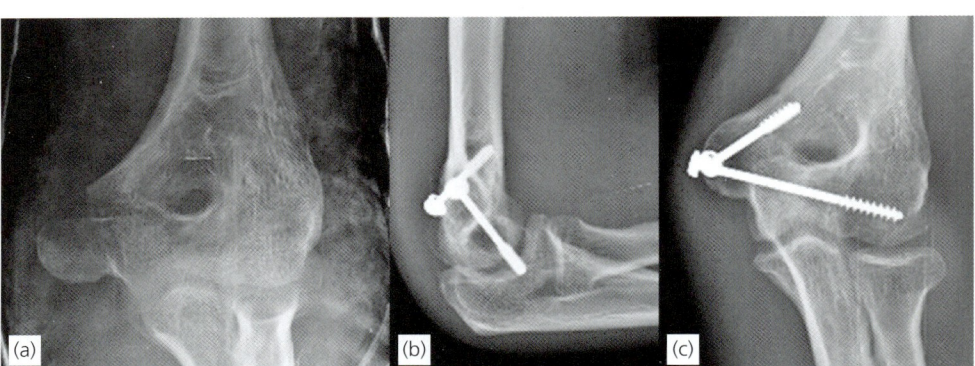

Figure 28.6 Fracture of the medial epicondyle. (a) Anteroposterior view shows a displaced medial condyle fracture. Lateral (b) and anteroposterior (c) views showing open reduction and internal fixation of the fragment with cancellous lag screws.

Complications

Complications include avascular necrosis of the fragment, leading to post-traumatic arthritis with pain and restriction of movements. In some patients, especially children, a cubitus valgus deformity may slowly develop.

TROCHLEAR FRACTURES

These are extremely rare fractures and are mostly seen in association with elbow dislocation. Non-displaced fractures may be managed with posterior splinting for 3 weeks followed by range of motion exercises. Displaced fractures should receive open reduction and internal fixation with a Kirschner wire or screw fixation. Fragments not amenable to internal fixation should be excised. Post-traumatic arthritis and stiffness can occur if there is incongruity of articular surfaces.

EPICONDYLAR FRACTURES

Isolated medial and lateral epicondylar injuries are extremely rare in adults. Most of them are avulsion fractures due to either sudden muscular contraction or direct injuries. A short period of immobilization in a posterior splint followed by active mobilization is sufficient in most patients. Operative reduction and fixation is advised in patients with displaced fragments in the presence of ulnar nerve symptoms, elbow instability to valgus stress, wrist flexor weakness and symptomatic non-union of the displaced fragment (Fig. 28.6). Fragments interfering with elbow motion can be excised.

KEY LEARNING POINTS

- Fractures of the distal humerus are complex injuries and remain a challenge to the orthopaedic surgeon.
- These injuries often are comminuted, involve the articular surface and many occur in elderly patients with osteoporosis.
- Most fractures of the distal humerus in adults require operative treatment aiming at anatomical articular surface reduction and rigid stabilization.
- Even with good surgical techniques, a 'normal' elbow is rarely the outcome, and functional results are compromised by stiffness, pain and weakness.
- Rarely in elderly patients with osteoporosis and significant medical comorbidities, non-operative treatment with the 'bag of bones' technique may be reasonable.

REFERENCES

- ● = Key primary paper
- ◆ = Major review article

◆1. Ring D, Gulotta L, Jupiter J. Articular fractures of the distal part of the humerus. *Journal of Bone and Joint Surgery (American)* 2003;**85A**:232–8.

●2. Mehne DK, Matta J. Bicolumn fractures of the adult humerus. Presented at the 53rd Annual Meeting of the American Academy of Orthopaedic Surgeons, 1986, New Orleans, LA.

◆3. Garcia JA, Mykula R, Stanley D. Complex fractures of the distal humerus in the elderly. *Journal of Bone and Joint Surgery (British)* 2001;**84B**:812–16.

◆4. Robinson CM, Hill RM, Jacobs N, *et al.* Adult distal humeral metaphyseal fractures: epidemiology and results of treatment. *Journal of Orthopaedic Trauma* 2003;**17**:38–47.

◆5. McKee MD, Wilson TL, Winston L, *et al.* Functional outcome following surgical treatment of intra-articular distal humeral fractures through a posterior approach. *Journal of Bone and Joint Surgery (American)* 2000;**82A**:1701–7.

●6. Miller WE. Comminuted fractures of the distal end of the humerus in the adult. *Journal of Bone and Joint Surgery (American)* 1964;**46**:644–57.

7. Collert S. Surgical management of fracture of the capitulum humeri. *Acta Orthopaedica Scandinavica* 1977;**48**:603–6.

29

Fractures and dislocations of the elbow

SHANMUGANATHAN RAJASEKARAN, RISHI MUGESH KANNA, JAYARAMARAJU DHEENADHAYALAN

Elbow dislocation	316	Fractures of radial head	319
Fractures of the olecranon	318	References	321

NATIONAL BOARD STANDARDS

- Revise your knowledge of elbow anatomy
- Know the important stabilizing ligaments and articular geometry
- Diagnose and classify the various peri-articular fractures
- Be familiar with indications and principles of surgical management
- Be able to advise a patient on the prognosis

ELBOW DISLOCATION

Introduction

Elbow dislocation accounts for up to 25% of elbow injuries.[1] Most of them occur in the adolescent population as a result of a direct injury by a fall on the outstretched arm. In uncomplicated dislocations, conservative treatment is usually successful.

Anatomy

The elbow is a complex of three joints, the *ulnohumeral*, *radiohumeral* and *proximal radioulnar joints*, which together provide a flexion range of 0–150° and a pronation–supination arc of 85° from the neutral. The stability of the joint is provided by the congruity of bony structures, surrounding muscles and ligamentous constraints. The medial collateral ligament (MCL) is the main medial stabilizer resisting a valgus stress, whereas the lateral stability is provided by the lateral ulnar collateral ligament and the anconeus muscle along with the radial head (Fig. 29.1).

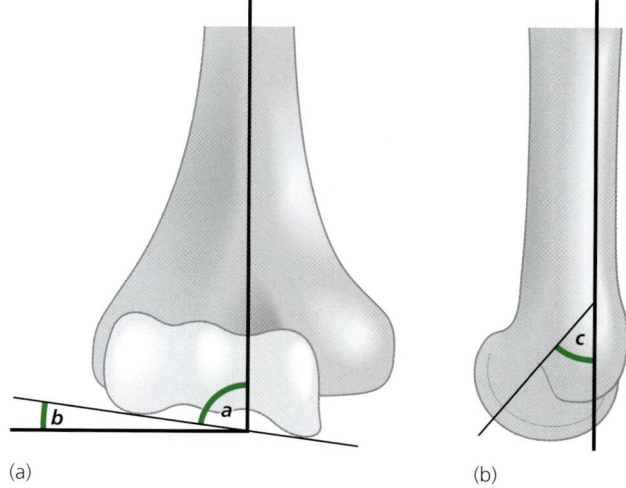

Figure 29.1 The various angular relationships between the distal humeral articular surface and the humeral shaft. (a) The distal humeral articular surface is placed at an angle of 4–8° of valgus, which results in the carrying angle of the elbow (angle b). (b) The articular segment projects forward from the line of the shaft at an angle of 40° (angle c) and behaves as a tie arch at the level of distal humeral flare.

Mechanism of injury

The more common posterior dislocation occurs as a result of a fall on the outstretched arm when the olecranon is driven back out of the trochlear fossa. The less common anterior dislocation occurs as a result of a direct blow on the olecranon when the elbow is in a partially flexed position.

Clinical examination

The dislocated elbow is unstable, swollen and painful and the patient typically supports the injured extremity with the opposite hand. In a posterior dislocation, the olecranon is very prominent and posteriorly displaced with a taut biceps tendon. A careful examination for neurovascular injury must be done, both before and after reduction of the dislocation. Care must be taken to identify associated fractures of the olecranon, radial head and coronoid process of the ulna.

Radiographic evaluation

The standard anteroposterior and lateral radiographs of the elbow will reveal the type of dislocation and should be scrutinized for other associated fractures (Fig. 29.2). Based on the direction of the displacement of the ulna relative to the humerus, the dislocation is termed posterior, anterior, lateral, medial and divergent. Patients with suspected intra-articular fractures, persistent instability and incongruous reduction need to be further evaluated with a CT scan.

Treatment principles

Dislocations without associated fractures are usually treated by reducing the joint under a regional block or a short intravenous regional anaesthesia. The neurovascular status should be reassessed, followed by evaluation of stability. The elbow is splinted for 2–3 weeks, following which active physiotherapy is started. The associated ligamentous injuries will heal spontaneously, restoring the stability of the joint. Post-reduction instability or an incongruent reduction must raise suspicion of associated fractures, loose bodies and severe ligamentous injuries. Operative treatment is indicated in complex fracture dislocations and when the elbow cannot be held in a concentrically reduced position, when it re-dislocates or when the dislocation is deemed unstable. Here stability is achieved by open reduction and internal fixation and repair of soft tissues.

Fracture dislocations of the elbow joint

Elbow dislocations can be associated with fractures around the joint. The radial head is fractured in 10% of patients, and the medial or lateral epicondyle can be avulsed in 15–20% of patients. In children, the medial epicondyle can become trapped in the joint space during the process of reduction and result in an incongruent reduction. The coronoid process can be fractured by avulsion of the brachial muscle or, rarely, by a direct injury of the coronoid over the trochlear notch. Elbow dislocations that are associated with one or more intra-articular fractures are at a greater risk for recurrent or chronic instability. Patients in whom excision of the radial head is performed in the acute stage have a risk of re-dislocation. They must be stabilized in such cases either by cross-pinning the joint or by an external fixator. Posterior elbow dislocation with fractures of the radial head and coronoid process and disruption of the MCL is called the 'terrible triad injury' (*Hotchkiss*)[2] and such patients have very unstable elbows. This condition is managed surgically with fixation of the coronoid, repair or replacement of the radial head, and medial collateral ligament repair.

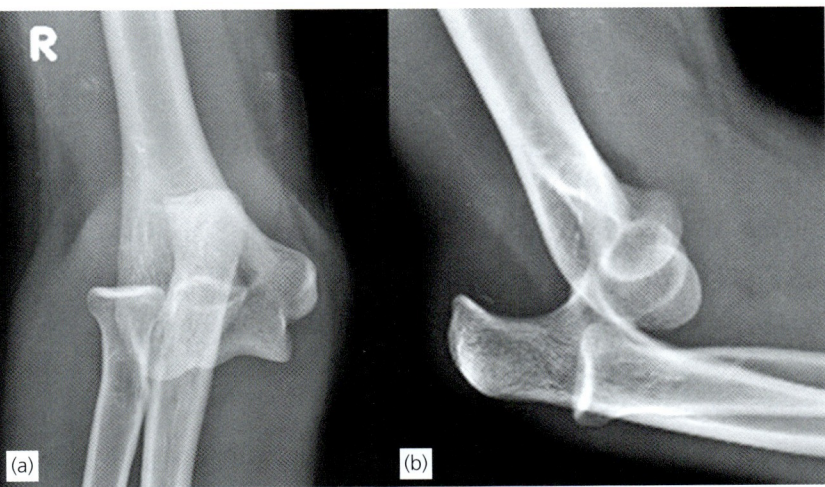

Figure 29.2 Anteroposterior (a) and lateral (b) radiographs of a case of posterior elbow dislocation. Note that, in the anteroposterior views, it is more of a 'posterolateral' dislocation than a simple posterior dislocation.

Complications

Loss of a few degrees of extension can occur, especially in dislocations associated with soft-tissue injuries. In severe cases and in patients with associated head injuries, formation of heterotopic bone leading to myositis ossificans is a potential complication. Owing to the close proximity of vital neurovascular structures, acute dislocations can be associated with injuries to the brachial artery and the median nerve.

FRACTURES OF THE OLECRANON

Introduction

Fractures of the olecranon assume clinical importance as they are invariably intra-articular fractures and, when displaced, result in a disruption of the triceps mechanism, leading to loss of elbow extension.[3] Avulsion fractures due to sudden contraction of the triceps are noted in the elderly, whereas fractures due to direct injuries are more common in younger patients. Direct injuries are often associated with open wounds as the olecranon is a subcutaneous bone. High-energy injuries causing elbow dislocation can be associated with comminuted olecranon fractures (Fig. 29.3).

Anatomy

The upper end of the ulna has its articulating surface, *the sigmoid notch*, formed by the olecranon and the coronoid process. The articulation between the sigmoid notch and the humeral trochlea is purely a hinge joint, allowing motion only about the flexion–extension axis and providing intrinsic stability to the elbow joint. Injuries of the olecranon or the coronoid process compromise anteroposterior stability of the elbow.

Clinical evaluation

Patients typically present with the upper extremity supported by the contralateral hand with the elbow in slight extension. Palpation reveals a defect in the olecranon. Direct injuries are often associated with severe swelling and open wounds.

Radiographic evaluation

Standard anteroposterior and lateral radiographs of the elbow should be obtained. Patients with comminuted fractures and those associated with trochlear fractures may require additional investigation with a CT scan.

Classification

Based on fracture pattern, Schatzker *et al.* classified (Table 29.1) the olecranon fractures into six types.[4]

Treatment

Non-operative treatment is indicated only for undisplaced fractures and displaced fractures in elderly patients with

Table 29.1 Schatzker's classification of distal radius fractures

Type	Description
Transverse	Represents an avulsion fracture from a sudden pull of the triceps muscle
Transverse impacted	A direct force sometimes leads to a transverse fracture with comminution and depression of the articular fragments
Oblique	This results from a hyperextension injury as the olecranon tip is impacted in the olecranon fossa. The fracture line begins at the midpoint of the sigmoid notch and runs distally
Comminuted	This results from direct high-energy trauma. Associated ligamentous injuries or fractures of the coronoid process can make the elbow unstable
Oblique distal	Fractures extend distal to the coronoid and compromise elbow stability
Fracture dislocation	This is usually associated with severe high-energy trauma and is often a compound injury

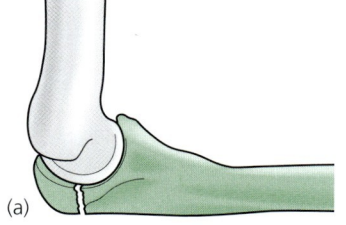 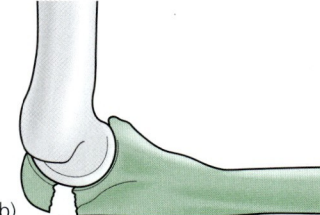 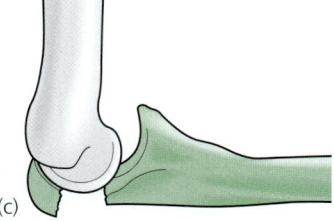

Figure 29.3 The Mayo classification of fractures of the olecranon. The fracture is divided into three main types as type 1, undisplaced (a); type 2, displaced (b); and type 3, unstable (c) fractures. Each type can be further subdivided into non-comminuted (A) and comminuted (B) fractures.

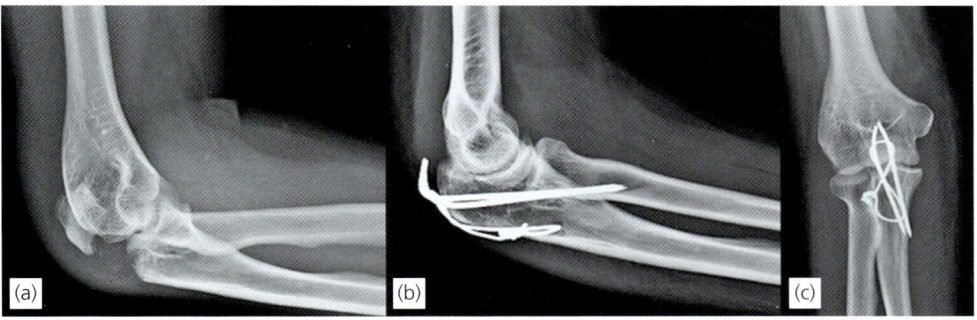

Figure 29.4 (a–c) Lateral radiographs of a type 2A olecranon fracture. The fracture has been treated by open anatomical reduction and internal fixation with two parallel Kirschner wires and figure-of-eight tension band wiring.

significant comorbidities. Immobilization in a long arm cast with the elbow in about 45° of flexion is advised. In general, there is adequate fracture stability at 3 weeks to remove the cast and initiate range of motion exercises.

The standard treatment is an open reduction followed by internal fixation, the type of which is decided by the pattern of the fracture. Tension band wiring with stainless steel cerclage wires is used in combination with two parallel Kirschner wires (Fig. 29.4). The Kirschner wires help to keep the fragments in position and the tension band counteracts the tensile forces, converting them to compressive forces. Intramedullary fixation with a single 6.5 mm cancellous lag screw can be used in transverse fractures. This may be used in conjunction with tension band wiring also. Plates and screws are used for comminuted olecranon fractures, fractures with distal extension of the fracture line, associated coronoid fractures, Monteggia fractures and fracture dislocations.

Complications

The fracture being intra-articular, pain and early degeneration may occur if accurate reduction is not established. Irritation of the skin owing to prominent hardware is common as the bone is subcutaneous. Removal of tension band wires after fracture union is sometimes necessary because of loosening and backing out of the Kirschner wires.

FRACTURES OF RADIAL HEAD

Introduction

The radial head articulates with the capitellum and is involved in the transmission of the force across the joint at all angles. Apart from its importance in pronation and supination movements, it also plays a pivotal role in the valgus stability of the elbow. Retaining the radial head is important in younger patients, in patients with associated injuries to the elbow such as dislocation or fracture of the coronoid, and in patients who are sports professionals or with high-demand jobs involving the upper limb.[5]

Mechanism of injury

The most common mode of injury is a fall onto the outstretched hand. The radial head fractures as it collides with the capitellum. This is frequently associated with injury to the ligamentous structures of the elbow.

Clinical evaluation

Patients present with pain, tenderness over the radial head, and limited elbow and forearm motion. The medial collateral ligament should be examined for injury by checking for valgus instability. In patients with a radial head fracture dislocation, there can be an associated interosseous ligament and distal radioulnar joint disruption (Essex-Lopresti lesion), which can be clinically diagnosed by associated swelling and tenderness over the wrist. This is a very unstable injury and requires surgical stabilization at both the elbow and the wrist.

Radiographic evaluation

Standard anteroposterior and lateral radiographs of the elbow usually reveal the fracture. In patients with undisplaced fractures, a positive fat pad sign is often present on the lateral views. Visualization of the radiocapitellar articulation is best obtained by a *Greenspan view*, which is taken with the forearm in neutral rotation and the radiographic beam angled 45° cephalad. It is prudent to include the wrist and the forearm while taking the radiographs when there is clinical evidence of wrist pain and tenderness.

Classification

Mason has proposed a classification based on the type and extent of displacement of the fracture (Fig. 29.5).[6] Johnston later added a type IV injury to this classification for injuries which were associated with dislocation of the elbow.

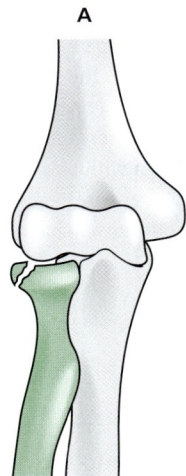 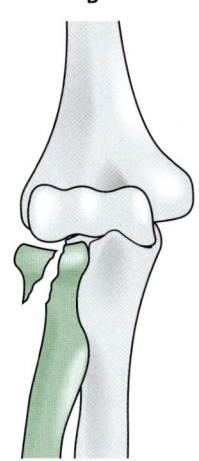 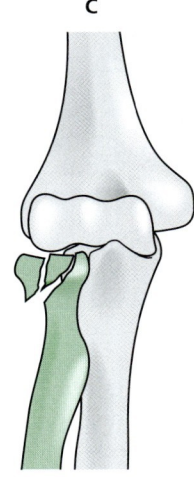

Figure 29.5 Mason's classification of radial head fractures. A, non-comminuted fracture; B, displaced partial radial head fracture; C, comminuted radial head fracture.

Treatment

Most undisplaced isolated fractures of the radial head and small fractures displaced less than 2 mm can be treated non-operatively. Symptomatic management consists of a sling or a posterior supportive splint and early range of motion.

Open reduction and internal fixation with mini-screws is indicated for isolated partial radial head fractures causing restriction of elbow motion and instability. Partial radial head fractures with displacement more than 2 mm and involving more than 30% of the articular surface are best treated by internal fixation. Fractures involving the entire head of the radius are reconstructed and stabilized with the radial neck with mini-plates. If they are not reconstructable, a radial head excision is performed.

Prosthetic replacement is indicated in irreparable comminuted fractures of the radial head associated with instability. The rationale for use is to prevent proximal migration of the radius. Silicone rubber prostheses were previously used but lost their popularity as they did not provide stability and often caused destructive synovitis. Metallic radial head implants are now being used with increasing frequency and are the prosthetic implants of choice in the unstable elbow.

Excision of the radial head is indicated in irreparable comminuted fractures of the radial head without much instability. Results following excision are generally good with only a few patients experiencing mild pain and discomfort. Associated ligamentous injuries and an Essex-Lopresti lesion[7] (Box 29.1) should be ruled out before attempting a radial head excision. The management of radial neck fractures is different (Box 29.2).

Complications

In patients with severe comminution, severe post-traumatic osteoarthritis with pain and stiffness of the elbow can occur.

> **BOX 29.1: Essex-Lopresti lesion**
>
> This is defined as a radial head fracture with longitudinal disruption of the forearm interosseous ligament, with or without a dislocation of the distal radioulnar joint. As this can be frequently overlooked, it is important to enquire and look for associated wrist pain or tenderness. Radial head excision in this injury will result in proximal migration of the radius. Treatment is repair or replacement of the radial head with stabilization of the distal radioulnar joint.

> **BOX 29.2: Fractures of the radial neck**
>
> Fractures of the neck of the radius are classified similar to fractures of the radial head, into three types. The fracture is usually clearly seen in the standard radiographic views of the elbow. Undisplaced fractures without significant angulation and displacement are treated conservatively in a posterior elbow splint. Displaced fractures are treated by fixing the radial head and the neck with a mini-plate and 2.7 mm screws. Long oblique neck fractures can be repaired directly with small cortical screws using an interfragmentary technique. Comminuted fractures not suitable for internal fixation are treated by excising the radial head.

Chronic wrist pain from unrecognized injuries to the forearm interosseous ligament, distal radioulnar joint or triangular fibrocartilage complex can occur. Valgus instability of the elbow is a problem in patients with associated ligament injuries and in patients in whom an excision has been done before skeletal maturity.

KEY LEARNING POINTS

- The elbow joint complex has three separate articulations – the radiocapitellar, the ulnotrochlear and the proximal radioulnar joints – all housed inside one capsule. The joint connects the arm to the forearm and hand, moving them in space, and serves a vital load-carrying function.
- Most elbow dislocations can be treated conservatively. Look for associated ligament injuries and fractures, which define the need for surgical treatment.
- Fractures of the olecranon affect the lever arm of elbow extension. Displaced and comminuted fractures can affect the articular congruity and hence require open anatomical reduction and internal fixation.
- Fractures of the head of the radius are relatively common injuries of the elbow. It is an important secondary stabilizer of the elbow. Surgical treatment is indicated for displaced, comminuted fractures and unstable elbow injuries. In irreparable fractures, a radial head excision can be done. In injuries with coexisting damage to the primary elbow stabilizers, an internal fixation with plate or prosthetic joint replacement is required.

REFERENCES

- ● = Key primary paper
- ◆ = Major review article

◆1. Ring D, Jupiter JB. Fracture-dislocation of the elbow. *Journal of Bone and Joint Surgery (American)* 1998;**80A**:566–80.

◆2. Morrey BF. Current concepts in the treatment of fractures of the radial head, the olecranon, and the coronoid. *Journal of Bone and Joint Surgery (American)* 1995;**77A**:316–27.

3. Regan W, Morrey BF. Fractures of the coronoid process of the ulna. *Journal of Bone and Joint Surgery (American)* 1990;**71A**:1348–54.

●4. Schatzker J. Fractures of the olecranon. In: *The Rationale of Operative Fracture Care*. Berlin, Germany: Springer-Verlag, 1991.

5. Hotchkiss RN. Displaced fractures of the radial head: Internal fixation or excision. *Journal of the American Academy of Orthopaedic Surgeons* 1997;**5**:1–10.

●6. Mason ML. Some observations on fractures of the head of the radius with a review of one hundred cases. *British Journal of Surgery* 1959;**42**:123–132.

●7. Essex-Lopresti P. Fractures of the radial head with distal radioulnar dislocation. *Journal of Bone and Joint Surgery (British)* 1951;**33B**:244–7.

30

Fractures of the shaft of the radius and ulna

SHANMUGANATHAN RAJASEKARAN, RISHI MUGESH KANNA, JAYARAMARAJU DHEENADHAYALAN

Introduction	322	Fractures of the radial shaft	324
Fractures of both forearm bones	322	References	326
Fractures of the ulnar shaft	323		

NATIONAL BOARD STANDARDS

- Revise your knowledge of anatomy of the forearm
- Know the various muscular attachments to the bones and the different muscle planes
- Diagnose and classify the fractures
- Be familiar with indications and principles of surgical management

INTRODUCTION

Forearm fractures are common injuries seen in young males following motor vehicle accidents and contact sports. This also explains the higher incidence of open fractures in the forearm, being next only to tibial fractures. The radius and ulna are bound together by the interosseous membrane and articulate at the superior and the inferior radioulnar joints. The ulna, which is relatively straight, acts as an axis around which the radius rotates in supination and pronation. Attaining the perfect anatomical relationship between the forearm bones and the perfect anatomical shape (angulation and rotation) of the individual bones is important to achieve good functional results.

Several muscles are attached to the forearm bones that affect the position of the fracture fragments after injury and tend to displace the fractures being treated conservatively. The biceps and the supinator muscles are attached to the forearm bones proximally and they exert rotational forces in fractures of the proximal third of the radius. Distally the pronator teres, inserting on the midshaft, and the pronator quadratus, on the distal quarter of the radius, exert both angulatory and rotational forces. Fractures of the ulna usually do not undergo rotation and are rather displaced by angulatory forces.

It is important that the relative length and rotation of both the bones are accurately restored as a loss of supination and pronation can otherwise result. Injuries of the forearm usually result in fractures of both the ulna and radius. Isolated fractures of either the radius or the ulna usually result in a dislocation of the other forearm bone at either the proximal or distal radioulnar joint. Fractures due to direct injury of the ulna with minimal displacement (nightstick fractures) are an exception.

FRACTURES OF BOTH FOREARM BONES

Clinical evaluation

Patients present with pain, swelling, deformity of the involved forearm and loss of forearm function. A careful neurovascular examination is essential. Excruciating, unremitting pain, tense forearm compartments, or pain on passive stretch of the fingers should raise suspicion of impending or established compartment syndrome. An urgent fasciotomy may be required.[1]

Radiographic evaluation

Anteroposterior and lateral views of the forearm should be obtained (Fig. 30.1). Radiographic evaluation should

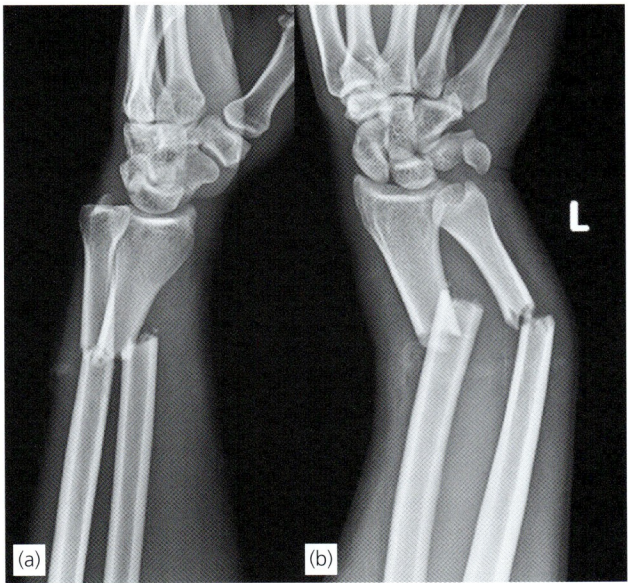

Figure 30.1 Anteroposterior (a) and lateral (b) radiographs of a patient with fracture of both the radius and ulna at the level of the distal third of the forearm.

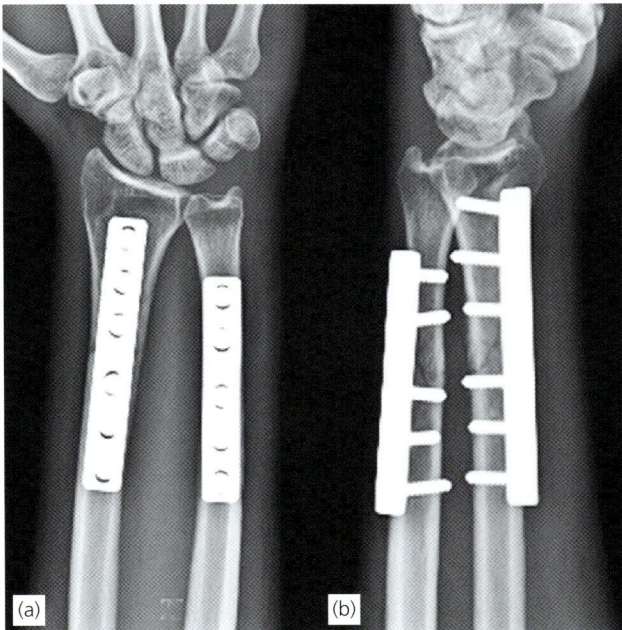

Figure 30.2 Anteroposterior (a) and lateral (b) radiographs of the forearm show open anatomical reduction and internal fixation with a low-contact dynamic compression plate. A minimum of four cortical purchases on either side of the fracture is enough for the stability of the construct in a simple non-comminuted fracture.

include the ipsilateral wrist and elbow to rule out the presence of associated fracture or dislocation.

Classification

The fractures are predominantly classified descriptively based on skin integrity (closed or open), location (proximal, middle, distal), severity of surgery (comminuted, segmental, multifragmented) and displacement of fracture fragments.

Treatment

The rare, non-displaced fracture of both the radius and the ulna may be treated with a well-moulded, long arm cast in neutral rotation with the elbow flexed to 90°. The patient should have frequent follow-up to evaluate for possible loss of fracture reduction. In patients in whom a good reduction is achieved using closed methods, conservative treatment is appropriate. In the majority of adults, open reduction and internal fixation is the procedure of choice for displaced forearm fractures involving the radius and ulna. Internal fixation involves the use of compression plating (3.5 mm dynamic compression plate) with or without bone grafting (Fig. 30.2).[2] Restoration of ulnar and radial length, rotational alignment and the anatomical lateral bow of the radius are important aims of fracture fixation. External fixation may be used in patients with severe bone or soft-tissue loss, gross contamination or infected non-union or in patients with open fracture dislocations.

Complications

Because of the peculiar anatomy of the forearm bones and the nature of muscle attachment, malunions are common with conservative treatment. Non-union following operative treatment is generally the result of improper fracture fixation techniques, bone loss at the fracture site owing to comminution and open injuries. Forearm fractures are rarely associated with neurovascular injuries, but the radial artery, superficial radial nerve and the posterior interosseous nerve can be injured iatrogenically during surgery. Post-traumatic radioulnar synostosis can occur, especially in fractures of the proximal one-third that are treated by internal fixation and in which bone grafting has been done along the interosseous membrane. Compartment syndrome is common in patients following high-velocity or crush injuries. Clinical suspicion should immediately warrant a prompt fasciotomy to avoid Volkmann's ischaemic contracture.

FRACTURES OF THE ULNAR SHAFT

These can occur as a result of direct trauma to the ulna (nightstick fractures). A Monteggia fracture denotes a fracture of the ulna accompanied by radial head dislocation, in which the mechanism of injury differs depending according to the type (Fig. 30.3).

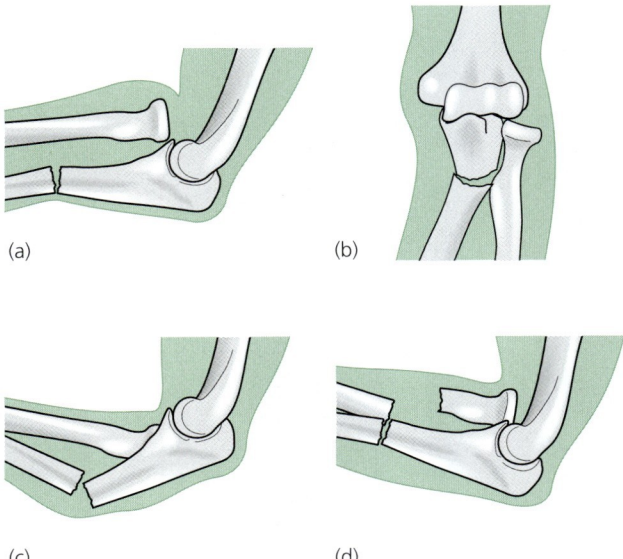

Figure 30.3 Bado's classification of a Monteggia fracture dislocation. (a) Type 1. Anterior dislocation of the radial head with fracture of the ulnar diaphysis at any level with anterior angulation. (b) Type 2. Posterior/posterolateral dislocation of the radial head with fracture of the ulnar diaphysis with posterior angulation. (c) Type 3. Lateral/anterolateral dislocation of the radial head with fracture of the ulnar metaphysis. (d) Type 4. Anterior dislocation of the radial head with fractures of both the radius and ulna within the proximal third at the same level.

Table 30.1 Bado's classification of Monteggial fracture dislocations

Type	Fracture dislocation
Type I	Anterior dislocation of the radial head with fracture of the ulnar diaphysis at any level with anterior angulation
Type II	Posterior/posterolateral dislocation of the radial head with fracture of the ulnar diaphysis with posterior angulation
Type III	Lateral/anterolateral dislocation of the radial head with fracture of the ulnar metaphysis
Type IV	Anterior dislocation of the radial head with fractures of both the radius and ulna within the proximal third at the same level

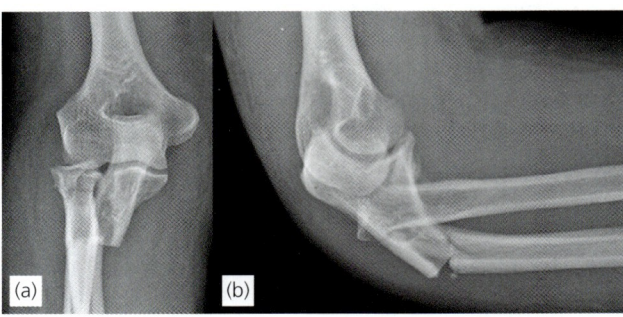

Figure 30.4 Anteroposterior (a) and lateral (b) radiographs of a type 2 Monteggia fracture dislocation. The radial head is dislocated posteriorly and the proximal ulnar fracture is angulated posteriorly.

Nightstick fractures

Patients with nightstick fractures present with local swelling, pain, tenderness, abrasions and bruising at the site of injury. Radiographs of the forearm show the fracture anatomy. Undisplaced or minimally displaced ulnar fractures may be treated with plaster immobilization followed by active range of motion exercises for the elbow, wrist and hand at 8 weeks. Displaced fractures should be treated with open reduction and internal fixation using a 3.5 mm dynamic compression plate.

Monteggia fracture

Patients with Monteggia fractures present with elbow swelling, deformity, crepitus and painful range of elbow motion, especially supination and pronation.[3] A careful neurovascular examination is essential because nerve injury, especially to the radial or posterior interosseous nerve, can occur. Anteroposterior and lateral views of the elbow and forearm, including the wrist, reveal the fracture type and the direction of radial head dislocation. Depending on this, Bado classified Monteggia fractures into four types[4] (Table 30.1 and Fig. 30.4).

TREATMENT

Closed reduction and casting of Monteggia fractures should be reserved only for the paediatric population. A careful radiological surveillance both in the immediate post-reduction and follow-up period is essential to ensure complete reduction of the radial head. Adult Monteggia fractures usually require open reduction and internal fixation of the ulnar shaft with a plate (Fig. 30.5). Restoration of ulnar length usually results in spontaneous reduction of the radial head. In the rare event that an open reduction is required for the radial head, the annular ligament should be repaired.

FRACTURES OF THE RADIAL SHAFT

Fractures of the proximal two-thirds of the radius without associated injuries are considered to be truly isolated but are very rare. Usually they occur following a fall onto an outstretched hand. A Galeazzi fracture refers to a fracture of the radial diaphysis at the junction of the middle and distal thirds with associated disruption of the distal

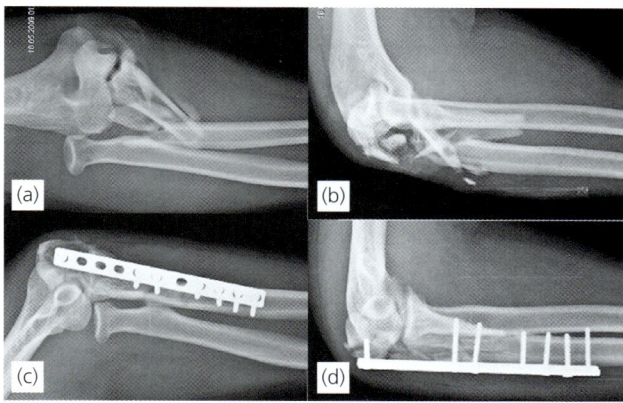

Figure 30.5 (a,b) Type 3 Monteggia fracture dislocation. Note that the radial head is dislocated anterolaterally with significant comminution of the ulnar metaphysis. (c,d) Postoperative anteroposterior and lateral radiographs show that the ulnar fracture has been reduced and fixed with a dynamic compression plate. In these comminuted fractures, reduction of the radial head dislocation helps in aligning the fragments and achieving the correct ulnar length.

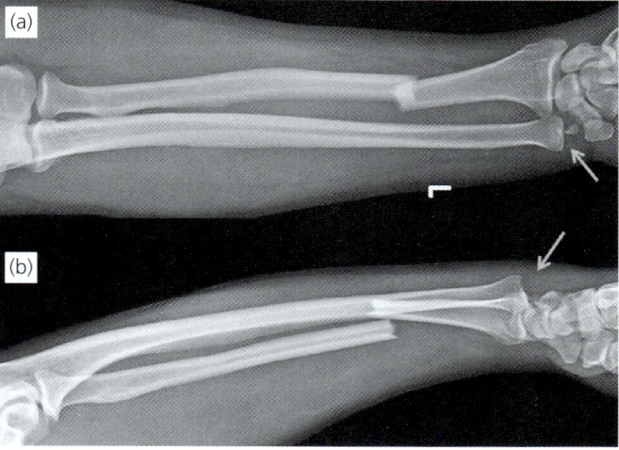

Figure 30.6 Anteroposterior (a) and lateral (b) radiographs of the forearm showing a Galeazzi fracture dislocation. The radius is fractured with disruption of the distal radioulnar joint. The ulnar styloid is fractured and the distal ulna is dislocated dorsally.

radioulnar joint.[5] A reverse Galeazzi fracture denotes a fracture of the distal ulna with associated disruption of the distal radioulnar joint.

Clinical evaluation

Pain, swelling and tenderness over the fracture site are typically present. Galeazzi fractures typically present with wrist pain and midline forearm pain in addition to the radial shaft fracture. Neurovascular injury is rare.

Radiographic evaluation

Anteroposterior and lateral radiographs of the forearm, elbow and wrist should be obtained (Fig. 30.6). Radiographic signs of distal radioulnar joint injury are a fracture at the base of the ulnar styloid, a wide distal radioulnar joint, a subluxed ulna and radial shortening of more than 5 mm.

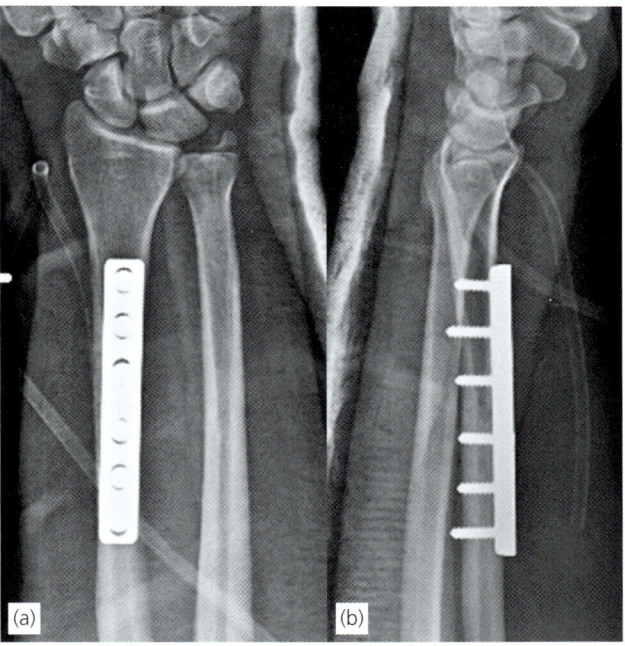

Figure 30.7 (a,b) The fracture shown in Fig. 4010.6 has been reduced and fixed with a dynamic compression plate. Once the radial fracture is reduced and aligned, the distal ulna falls back in place automatically.

Treatment

Galeazzi fractures are referred to as the 'fracture of necessity' because of the need for open reduction and internal fixation in all the patients. Internal fixation by 3.5 mm dynamic compression plates by a volar approach is the treatment of choice[6] (Fig. 30.7). Kirschner wire fixation of the distal radioulnar joint may be necessary only rarely in patients with gross instability of the distal radioulnar joint.

Complications

Distal radioulnar joint instability with clinical disability may occur in patients with malunions and non-unions. Neurovascular injury is usually iatrogenic. There is a risk of superficial radial nerve injury (beneath the brachioradialis) with anterior radius approaches. The posterior interosseous nerve (beneath the supinator) can be injured with proximal radius approaches.

KEY LEARNING POINTS

- Fractures of the forearm are commonly seen in young males involved in road traffic accidents.
- The forearm bones are bound together by the interosseous membrane and articulate with each other at the superior and inferior radioulnar joints. Forearm injuries can be considered as 'intra-articular' fractures since they can potentially affect supination and pronation movements.
- The goals of treatment of forearm fractures should be to attain anatomical reduction of the skeleton, restoring bone length, rotation and the interosseous space, and to secure fixation of the skeleton to enable early soft-tissue rehabilitation.
- Almost all adult forearm fractures are best treated by open reduction and internal fixation with dynamic compression plating. More than 95% union rates can be achieved only by internal fixation.
- Inadequate attainment of goals of fracture treatment can lead to loss of motion, muscle imbalance and disability of hand function.

REFERENCES

- ● = Key primary paper
- ◆ = Major review article

●1. Whitesides TE, Haney TC, Morimoto K, *et al*. Tissue pressure measurements as a determinant for the need of fasciotomy. *Clinical Orthopaedics and Related Research* 1975;**113**:43–51.
2. Chapman MW, Gordon JE, Zissimos AG. Compression-plate fixation of acute fractures of the diaphyses of the radius and ulna. *Journal of Bone and Joint Surgery (American)* 1989;**71**:159–69.
●3. Monteggia GB. *Instituzioni Chirurgiche*, vol. 5. Milan, Italy: Maspero, 1814.
●4. Bado JL. The Monteggia lesion. *Clinical Orthopaedics and Related Research* 1967;**50**:71–86.
●5. Galeazzi R. Ueber ein besonderes Syndrom bei Verletzungen im Bereich der Unterarm knochen. *Archiv für Orthopädische und Unfall-Chirurgie* 1934;**35**:557–62.
6. Thompson JE. Anatomical methods of approach in operations on the long bones of the extremities. *Annals of Surgery* 1918;**68**:309.

31

Fractures of the distal radius

SHANMUGANATHAN RAJASEKARAN, RISHI MUGESH KANNA, JAYARAMARAJU DHEENADHAYALAN

Introduction	327	Classification	328
Anatomy	327	Treatment	329
Mechanism of injury	327	Complications	330
Clinical evaluation	327	References	330
Radiographic evaluation	328		

NATIONAL BOARD STANDARDS

- Know the anatomy of the wrist and distal radius
- Understand injury mechanism and fracture anatomy
- Diagnose and classify the fractures
- Know the indications and principles of surgical management

INTRODUCTION

Distal radius fractures account for up to 20% of all emergency orthopaedic admissions and are the most common fractures of the upper extremity. The incidence of distal radius fractures is high in elderly female patients because of osteoporosis.

ANATOMY

The metaphysis of the distal radius is composed primarily of cancellous bone, which is one of the primary sites of osteoporosis in the elderly. The distal radius articulates with the scaphoid and lunate, as well as with the distal ulna. About 80% of the axial load transmitted from the hand through the wrist is borne by the distal radius, and the rest is borne by the ulna via the triangular fibrocartilage complex (TFCC). The TFCC is a thick triangular ligament which connects the distal radius and ulna and can be frequently injured in fractures of the distal radius. The distal radius gives attachments to the palmar and dorsal radiocarpal ligaments, which often remain intact in a distal radius fracture, facilitating reduction through 'ligamentotaxis'.

MECHANISM OF INJURY

The most common mechanism of injury is a fall onto an outstretched hand with the wrist in dorsiflexion. During the injury, the volar cortex of the radius first fails in tension with the fracture propagating dorsally. With further force transmission, bending forces induce compression stresses across the dorsal cortex, resulting in comminution. Cancellous impaction of the metaphysis leads to radial shortening. High-energy injuries seen in polytraumatized young patients may result in significantly comminuted and displaced unstable fractures to the distal radius.

CLINICAL EVALUATION

Patients present with pain, swelling and the classical wrist deformity (dorsal in Colles-type or dorsal Barton-type fractures and volar in Smith-type fractures). Carpal tunnel compression symptoms are common (20%) owing to direct trauma from fracture fragments, haematoma formation or increased compartment pressure. Younger patients sustaining injury in high-velocity accidents have a higher incidence of open injuries.

RADIOGRAPHIC EVALUATION

Posteroanterior and lateral views of the wrist should be obtained, with oblique views reserved for further fracture definition (Fig. 31.1). The normal radiographic parameters of the distal radius are as follows:

- radial inclination of 22°
- radial length (distal to the ulnar articular surface) of 11 mm
- palmar radial tilt of 12° (Fig. 31.2). Reversal of the normal palmar tilt following a radial fracture results in load transfer onto the ulna and TFCC; the remaining load is then borne eccentrically by the distal radius and is concentrated on the scaphoid fossa. This may lead to radiocarpal arthritis if not anatomically reduced in the younger patient.

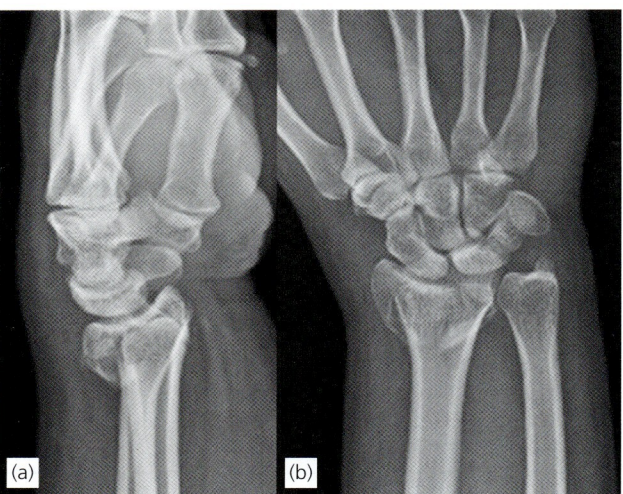

Figure 31.1 Lateral (a) and anteroposterior (b) radiographs of the wrist shows an extra-articular fracture of the distal radius with typical displacement: proximal migration, dorsal angulation and radial deviation.

CLASSIFICATION

Many classification systems have been proposed for distal radius fractures. The Frykman[1] classification of distal radius fractures is based on the pattern of intra-articular involvement (Table 31.1).

Fernandez has proposed a mechanism-based classification system that addresses the potential for ligamentous injury and helps in planning treatment options[2,3] (Table 31.2).

Colles fracture

More than 90% of distal radius fractures fall into this group. Abraham Colles from Dublin, Ireland, initially gave this description for pure extra-articular fractures of the distal radius.[4] The classic 'dinner fork' deformity is a combination of dorsal angulation (apex volar), dorsal displacement, radial shift and radial shortening. The mechanism of injury is a fall onto a hyperextended, radially deviated wrist with the forearm in pronation.

Smith fracture (reverse Colles fracture)

This is an extra-articular fracture with volar angulation (apex dorsal) of the distal radius with a 'garden spade'

Table 31.1 Frykman classification of distal radius fractures

Fracture	Distal ulnar fracture	
	Absent	Present
Extra-articular	I	II
Intra-articular involving the radiocarpal joint	III	IV
Intra-articular involving the DRUJ	V	VI
Intra-articular involving the radiocarpal joint and DRUJ	VII	VIII

DRUJ, distal radioulnar joint.

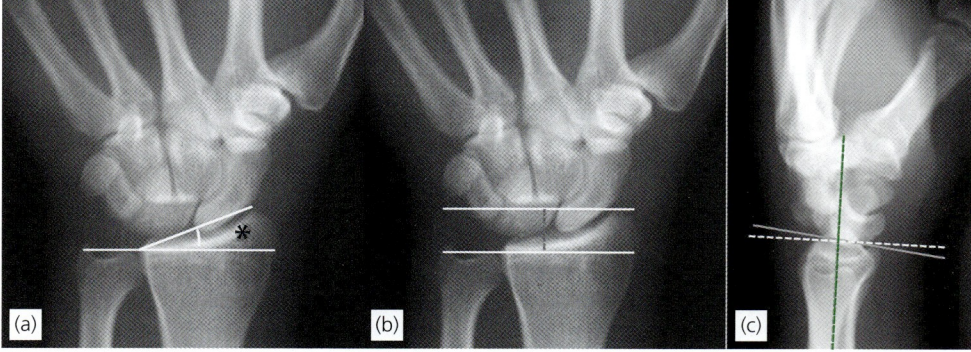

Figure 31.2 The normal radiographic measurements of the distal radius. (a) The radial inclination (asterisk) is measured between the horizontal and the distal radial articular surface. (b) The radial length (dashed line) is measured between two horizontal lines drawn parallel to each other at the level of the distal radial and ulnar ends. The palmar (volar) tilt is measured in the lateral radiograph between a perpendicular (dashed green line) to the radial axis and a line drawn along the articular surface (solid line).

Table 31.2 Fernandez mechanism-based classification of distal radius fractures

Type	Mechanism of injury
Type I	Metaphyseal bending fracture with the inherent problems of loss of palmar tilt and radial shortening relative to the ulna (DRUJ injury)
Type II	Shearing fracture requiring reduction and often buttressing of the articular segment
Type III	Compression of the articular surface without the characteristic fragmentation
Type IV	Avulsion fracture or radiocarpal fracture dislocation
Type V	Combined injury with significant soft-tissue involvement owing to high-energy injury

DRUJ, distal radioulnar joint.

deformity. The mechanism of injury is a fall onto a flexed wrist with the forearm fixed in supination. This is a potentially unstable fracture pattern and almost always requires open reduction and internal fixation with plate and screws.

Barton fracture

This is a type of intra-articular fracture dislocation of the wrist in which the dorsal or volar rim of the distal radius is displaced with the carpal bones. Accordingly the fracture is classified as either a volar or a dorsal Barton fracture. Volar involvement is more common. The mechanism of injury is a fall onto a dorsiflexed wrist with the forearm fixed in pronation because of a shearing force. Being an unstable injury involving the articular surface, it requires open reduction and internal fixation to achieve a stable and anatomical reduction.

Radial styloid fracture (chauffeur's fracture, Hutchinson fracture)

This is an avulsion fracture of the radial styloid process with extrinsic ligaments remaining attached to the styloid fragment. It may involve the entire styloid or a portion of it. It is often associated with intercarpal ligamentous injuries. Internal fixation is often required, by either open or closed methods. A Kirschner wire can be used as a joystick to manipulate the fragment into alignment and then fixed with the main shaft.

TREATMENT

Management depends on various factors such as the fracture pattern, quality of bone, soft-tissue injury, fracture comminution, fracture displacement, injury velocity and patient factors, e.g. age, associated medical conditions, injuries and compliance. Acceptable radiographic parameters for a 'reduced' fracture of the radius would include radial length within 2–3 mm of the contralateral wrist, neutral palmar tilt, minimal articular step-off (less than 2 mm) and less than 5° loss of radial inclination.

All fractures should have attempted closed reduction, even if it is expected that surgical management may be needed. Fracture reduction helps to reduce post-traumatic swelling and provides pain relief. Cast immobilization is sufficient for undisplaced or minimally displaced fractures and displaced fractures that are stable after reduction. The cast should be worn for approximately 6 weeks until the fracture has healed. It is important to look for secondary displacement of fracture fragments within the cast, so the patient is usually asked to come back after 1 week for a follow-up radiograph to ensure that the fracture has not displaced. In the first week the initial post-traumatic swelling subsides and the cast may become loose, thus predisposing to this particular complication. Early shoulder, elbow and finger range of movement exercises are important to avoid stiffness.

Operative indications include secondary loss of reduction, instability, articular comminution, metaphyseal comminution or bone loss, and distal radioulnar joint incongruity. Various methods of fracture fixation are available and are selected depending on the type of fracture, displacement, involvement of articular surface, extent and degree of fracture comminution.

Percutaneous pinning using two or three Kirschner wires placed across the fracture site is primarily used for extra-articular fractures or two-part intra-articular fractures (Fig. 31.3). It is supplemented with a cast. The pins are removed at 3–4 weeks postoperatively and mobilization

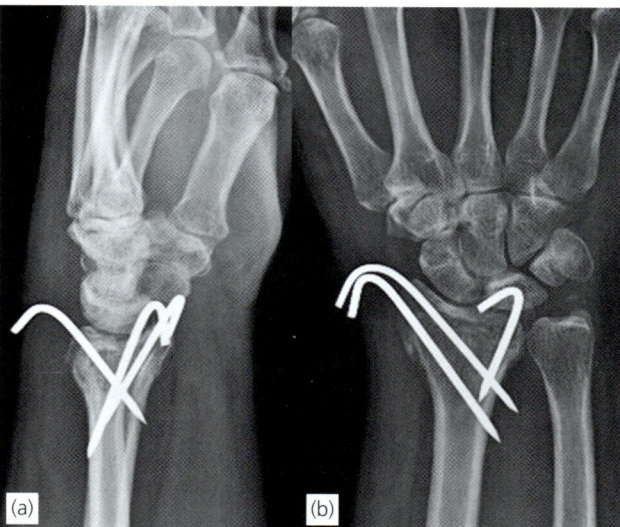

Figure 31.3 Lateral (a) and anteroposterior (b) radiographs of the distal radius fracture shown in Fig. 31.1. The fracture fragments have been reduced by closed manipulation and fixed with percutaneous Kirschner wires. The ends of the wires are bent and kept outside the skin to facilitate removal.

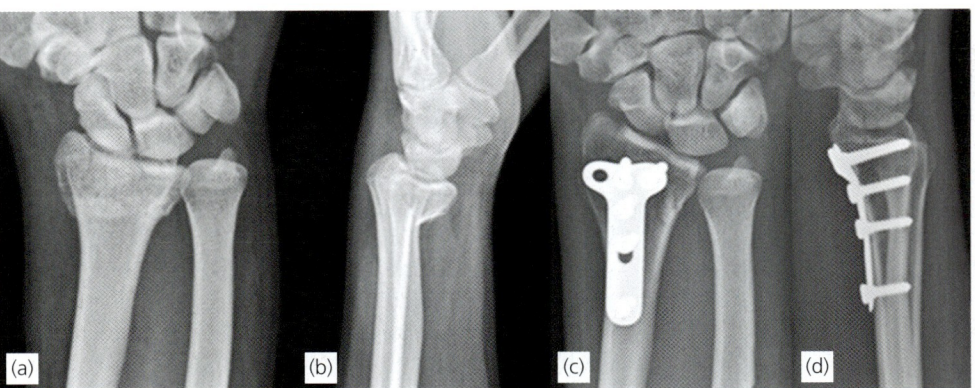

Figure 31.4 Pre-operative (a,b) and postoperative (c,d) lateral radiographs of a volar Barton's fracture treated by open reduction and internal fixation with an Ellis buttress plate.

started at 6 weeks. *Kapandji 'intrafocal' pinning* is a special technique of pinning in which Kirschner wires are inserted through the fracture site to trap the fracture fragments and driven into the proximal opposite intact cortex.[5] *Transarticular external fixation* is based on the integrity of ligaments around the radius, which, when stretched, pulls the fragments into position.[6] Two Schanz pins are placed on either side of the fracture; the distal pins are usually inserted in the second metacarpal bone. This fixation can be supplemented with percutaneous Kirschner wiring. Pins may be removed at 3–4 weeks, followed by cast application for a further 3 weeks. *Open reduction and internal fixation* with a buttress plate or volar locking plate allows anatomical reduction of fragments, bone grafting to elevate the articular surface and immediate stability to initiate early range of motion exercises. The plate can be applied on either the dorsal or the volar surfaces (Fig. 31.4). Dorsal plating is associated with extensor tendon complications and is best avoided. Recent developments in the surgical management of distal radius fractures include the use of specially contoured locking plates, artificial bone substitutes and cement,[7] and use of arthroscopy for intra-articular reduction of fractures.

COMPLICATIONS

Malunion is a common problem, especially after conservative management. The patient can be asymptomatic with a residual deformity alone or symptomatic with pain and restriction of movements. The TFCC can also be injured in up to 50% of distal radial fractures and can result in chronic disabling wrist pain.[8] Peripheral nerve dysfunction can occur and the median nerve is most commonly affected. The median nerve can be injured by direct trauma during the fracture or displacement, injury through a proximal radial fragment and injury from displacement of a volar fragment. Injury to the radial artery rarely occurs with open fractures. It can also occur with markedly displaced fractures and with dislocations of the radius and ulna. Carpal fractures and intercarpal ligament injuries may accompany radial fractures and can cause chronic intercalated segmental instabilities of the wrist. Other complications of distal radial fractures include carpal tunnel syndrome, post-traumatic radiocarpal osteoarthritis with limitation of wrist range of motion, reflex sympathetic dystrophy, rupture of the extensor pollicis longus tendon owing to attrition over a malunited fracture and, rarely, non-union.

KEY LEARNING POINTS

- Fractures of the distal radius are common, especially in elderly women.
- Even with a residual deformity, most patients with low functional requirements have excellent functional results with conservative treatment.
- More aggressive treatment with surgical methods (wires, external fixation, plates) is appropriate in higher demand, younger individuals.
- Treatment must be individualized based on the fracture pattern, injury mechanism and force, associated medical problems, quality of bone, functional requirements of the patient and patient compliance.
- In high-demand individuals, the restoration and maintenance of articular and distal radial anatomy with respect to the ulna enhances the potential for a full functional recovery.

REFERENCES

- ● = Key primary paper
- ◆ = Major review article

●1. Frykman GK. Fractures of the distal radius including sequelae-shoulder-hand-finger syndrome, disturbance in the distal radio-ulnar joint and impairment of nerve function. *Acta Orthopaedica Scandinavica* 1967;**Suppl. 108**:7–153.

2. Fernandez DL, Geissler WB. Treatment of displaced articular fractures of the radius. *Journal of Hand Surgery* 1991;**16**:375–84.
3. Fernandez DL. Fractures of the distal radius: operative treatment. *Instructional Course Lectures* 1993;**42**:73–88.
●4. Colles A. On the fracture of the carpal extremity of the radius. *Edinburgh Medical and Surgical Journal* 1814;**10**:182–6.
5. Walton NP, Brammar TJ, Hutchinson J, *et al*. Treatment of unstable distal radial fractures by intrafocal, intramedullary K-wires. *Injury* 2000;**32**:383–9.
6. Edwards Jr GS. Intra-articular fractures of the distal part of the radius treated with the small AO external fixator. *Journal of Bone and Joint Surgery (American)* 1991;**73**:1241–50.
7. Sanchez-Sotelo J, Munuera L, Madero R. Treatment of fractures of the distal radius with remodellable bone cement. *Journal of Bone and Joint Surgery (British)* 2000;**82**:856–63.
◆8. Jupiter JB, Fernandez DL. Complications following distal radial fractures. *Journal of Bone and Joint Surgery (American)* 2001;**83**:1244–65.

SECTION 3

Lower extremity fractures and dislocations

SHANMUGANATHAN RAJASEKARAN

32	Dislocations and fracture dislocations of the hip *Shanmuganathan Rajasekaran, Vijay Kamath, Jayaramaraju Dheenadhayalan*	335
33	Femoral neck fractures *Shanmuganathan Rajasekaran, Vijay Kamath, Jayaramaraju Dheenadhayalan*	340
34	Intertrochanteric fractures *Shanmuganathan Rajasekaran, Vijay Kamath, Jayaramaraju Dheenadhayalan*	346
35	Subtrochanteric fractures *Shanmuganathan Rajasekaran, Vijay Kamath, Jayaramaraju Dheenadhayalan*	350
36	Femoral shaft fractures *Shanmuganathan Rajasekaran, Vijay Kamath, Jayaramaraju Dheenadhayalan*	353
37	Distal femoral fractures *Shanmuganathan Rajasekaran, Vijay Kamath, Jayaramaraju Dheenadhayalan*	358
38	Patellar dislocation *Shanmuganathan Rajasekaran, Rishi Mugesh Kanna, Jayaramaraju Dheenadhayalan*	363
39	Knee dislocations *Shanmuganathan Rajasekaran, Rishi Mugesh Kanna, Jayaramaraju Dheenadhayalan*	365
40	Patellar fractures and extension mechanism injuries *Shanmuganathan Rajasekaran, Rishi Mugesh Kanna, Jayaramaraju Dheenadhayalan*	368
41	Tibial plateau fractures *Shanmuganathan Rajasekaran, Vijay Kamath, Jayaramaraju Dheenadhayalan*	372
42	Fractures of the tibia and fibula *Shanmuganathan Rajasekaran, Rishi Mugesh Kanna, Jayaramaraju Dheenadhayalan*	377
43	Tibial plafond fractures *Shanmuganathan Rajasekaran, Vijay Kamath, Jayaramaraju Dheenadhayalan*	382
44	Injuries of the ankle joint *Shanmuganathan Rajasekaran, Rishi Mugesh Kanna, Jayaramaraju Dheenadhayalan*	386
45	Talar fractures and dislocation *Sureshan Sivananthan, Shanmuganathan Rajasekaran*	394
46	Calcaneum fractures *Sureshan Sivananthan, Shanmuganathan Rajasekaran*	398
47	Fractures of the midfoot *Shanmuganathan Rajasekaran, Vijay Kamath, Jayaramaraju Dheenadhayalan*	403
48	Injuries of the tarsometatarsal (Lisfranc) joint *Shanmuganathan Rajasekaran, Rishi Mugesh Kanna, Jayaramaraju Dheenadhayalan*	407
49	Fractures of the forefoot *Shanmuganathan Rajasekaran, Rishi Mugesh Kanna, Jayaramaraju Dheenadhayalan*	411
50	Metatarsophalangeal joint, phalangeal and interphalangeal joint injuries *Shanmuganathan Rajasekaran, Rishi Mugesh Kanna, Jayaramaraju Dheenadhayalan*	414

32

Dislocations and fracture dislocations of the hip

SHANMUGANATHAN RAJASEKARAN, VIJAY KAMATH, JAYARAMARAJU DHEENADHAYALAN

Introduction	335	Anterior dislocations	338
Posterior dislocations	335	References	339

NATIONAL BOARD STANDARDS

- Revise your knowledge of hip joint anatomy
- Understand the pathophysiology of hip dislocation
- Know the methods of closed reduction
- Be able to advise a patient on the prognosis and complications

INTRODUCTION

Hip dislocations almost always result from high-energy trauma, such as motor vehicle accident or fall from a height. The direction of the pathological force and the position of the lower extremity at the time of impact determines whether the hip dislocates anteriorly or posteriorly. Posterior dislocations constitute 85–90% of traumatic dislocations, with anterior dislocations accounting for the remainder.[1]

POSTERIOR DISLOCATIONS

Mechanism of injury

Posterior dislocations result from trauma to the flexed knee (e.g. dashboard injury) with the hip in varying degrees of flexion. A neutral or an adducted hip will result in a dislocation without an acetabular fracture. If the hip is in slight abduction at the time of injury, an associated fracture of the posterior–superior rim of the acetabulum will occur.

Clinical evaluation

The typical presentation in a posterior dislocation is a shortened, slightly flexed, internally rotated and adducted limb. This presentation may be altered by injuries to the ipsilateral extremity and acetabulum. Approximately 50% of patients sustain concomitant fractures and major organ or other musculoskeletal injuries, and they should be carefully looked for. Ipsilateral knee, patellar and femur fractures are the commonly associated injuries. Sciatic nerve injury is present in 10–20% of posterior dislocations; therefore, a neurovascular examination of the ipsilateral limb is essential.

Radiographic evaluation

An anteroposterior radiograph of the pelvis with a cross-table lateral view of the affected hip is mandatory. In a dislocated hip, the Shenton's line is broken and the joint space is asymmetric. In a posterior dislocation the affected femoral head will appear smaller than the normal hip with the femoral shaft in adduction, while, in an anterior dislocation, the femoral head will appear slightly larger than the normal with the shaft in abduction. The relative appearance of the greater and lesser trochanters may indicate pathological internal or external rotation of the hip. The lateral view will help distinguish a posterior from an anterior dislocation.

Associated fractures of the femoral neck or acetabulum must be carefully ruled out. Judet (45° oblique) views of the hip may be helpful to ascertain the presence of osteochondral fragments, the integrity of the acetabulum and the congruence of the joint spaces. CT scans are usually obtained following closed reduction of a dislocated hip. If closed reduction is not possible and an open reduction is planned, a CT scan should be obtained to detect associated femoral head and acetabular fractures and the presence of intra-articular fragments.

Classification

The most commonly followed classification of posterior dislocation is the Thompson and Epstein classification[2] (Table 32.1 and Fig. 32.1).

Treatment

The treatment of a dislocation or fracture dislocation of the hip depends primarily on the type of injury. The dislocated hip should be reduced on an emergency basis to relieve pain and to decrease the risk of osteonecrosis of the femoral head as the incidence increase when reduction is delayed for more than 12 hours. Following reduction, the hip should be placed in traction if unstable, and definitive treatment of femoral head and acetabular fractures can be deferred to the subacute phase.

TYPE I POSTERIOR DISLOCATION

Closed reduction should be performed preferably under general anaesthesia, and reduction under intravenous sedation is attempted only rarely. Only one or two attempts at closed reduction should be made, failing which open reduction is indicated to prevent further damage to the femoral head. Many methods of closed reduction have been described, namely the *Stimson prone gravity technique*, *Allis method*, *Bigelow manoeuvre* and the *East Baltimore lift*. Described below are the Bigelow manoeuvre and the East Baltimore lift.

Bigelow manoeuvre (Fig. 32.2)

With the patient supine, the surgeon applies longitudinal traction on the limb in the line of deformity and the hip is flexed to at least 90°. The femoral head is then levered into the acetabulum by abduction, external rotation and extension of the hip. An audible 'clunk' is a sign of a successful closed reduction.

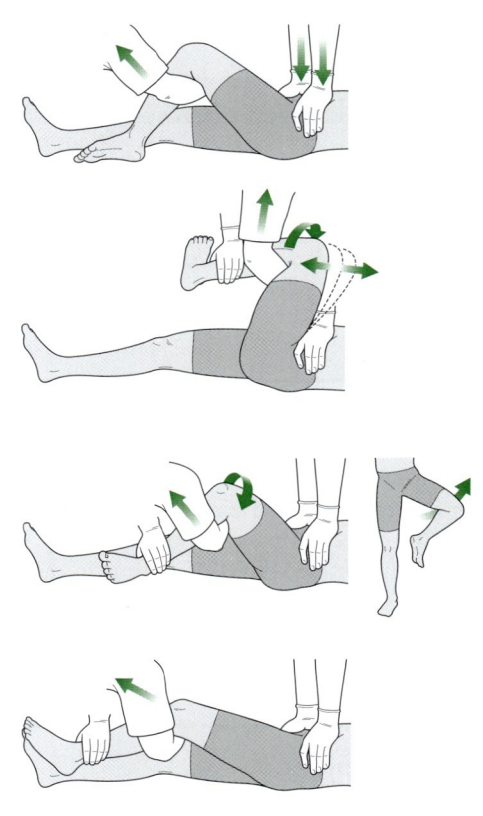

Figure 32.2 Bigelow reduction manoeuvre for posterior dislocation of hip.

Table 32.1 Thompson and Epstein classification of posterior hip dislocations

Type	Description
Type I	Simple dislocation with or without an insignificant posterior wall fragment
Type II	Dislocation associated with a single large posterior wall fragment
Type III	Dislocation with a comminuted posterior wall fragment
Type IV	Dislocation with fracture of the acetabular floor
Type V	Dislocation with fracture of the femoral head

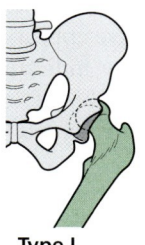 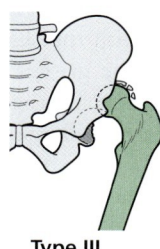 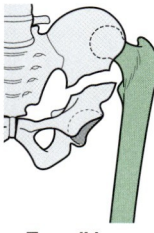 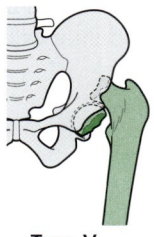

Type I Type II Type III Type IV Type V

Figure 32.1 Thompson and Epstein classification of posterior dislocation of the hip.

East Baltimore lift[3]

With the patient supine, the surgeon stands on the affected side with an assistant on the opposite side. The patient's leg is flexed so that the hip and knee are at 90°. The surgeon places his or her arm that is closest to the patient's head under the proximal calf of the patient, cradling the leg in his or her elbow with his or her hand resting on the shoulder of the assistant. The surgeon's other hand grips the patient's ankle. The assistant's arm passes under the proximal calf of the patient (similar to the surgeon's) and rests on the surgeon's shoulder. The surgeon and assistant squat slightly with knees bent. They straighten up together to apply traction to the hip without straining their backs. The surgeon rotates the leg at the ankle. A second assistant stabilizes the pelvis.

Radiographs should be obtained to confirm the adequacy of reduction. Persistent widening of the distance between the radiographic teardrop and the femoral head compared with the normal hip indicates entrapment of osteocartilaginous fragments or the acetabular labrum. Thin slice CT scan evaluation should be performed in such patients. Closed reduction is followed by immobilization in Buck's traction, an abduction pillow or Thomas splint.

Failure of closed reduction may be due to (1) buttonholing of the femoral head through the posterior capsule; (2) interposition of the piriformis, obturator and gemelli muscles; (3) a torn acetabular labrum; or (4) osteochondral acetabular fragments and fracture fragments from the femoral head. An open reduction should be performed immediately.

TYPE II, III AND IV POSTERIOR DISLOCATIONS

The hip is reduced as an emergency procedure and the acetabular fracture can be treated within the next few days according to the guidelines laid down for the management of isolated acetabular fractures.

In type II dislocations following closed reduction, the hip stability should be evaluated while the patient is still under anaesthesia. In patients who have an acetabular fracture that involves more than half of the articular surface of the posterior wall the stability test is avoided as these hips are assumed to be inherently unstable. All patients with a failed stability test and type III or IV dislocations require surgical intervention for the acetabular fracture.

Open reduction of posterior dislocations is usually performed through a Kocher–Langenbeck approach. In the presence of an associated femoral head fracture, an anterior Smith-Petersen approach maybe preferred.

TYPE V POSTERIOR FRACTURE DISLOCATION WITH FEMORAL HEAD FRACTURE

Fractures of the femoral head occur as a shearing injury as the flexed hip is driven across the posterior wall of the acetabulum during dislocation. Small inferior fragments of the femoral head tend to be free of soft-tissue attachments, whereas larger fragments frequently are still connected to the acetabulum by the ligamentum teres.

Pipkin subclassified Epstein–Thomas type V fracture dislocations into four additional subtypes[4] (Table 32.2 and Fig. 32.3).

Treatment

Factors that determine the nature of treatment include (1) the concentricity of the reduced femoral head in the acetabulum, (2) the accuracy of the reduction of the displaced femoral head fragment, (3) the size of the femoral

Table 32.2 Pipkin classification of posterior dislocation of the hip with femoral head fracture

Type	Description
Type I	Posterior dislocation of the hip with fracture of the femoral head caudad to the fovea capitis
Type II	Posterior dislocation of the hip with fracture of the femoral head cephalad to the fovea capitis
Type III	Type I or II posterior dislocation with associated fracture of the femoral neck
Type IV	Type I, II or III posterior dislocation with associated fracture of the acetabulum

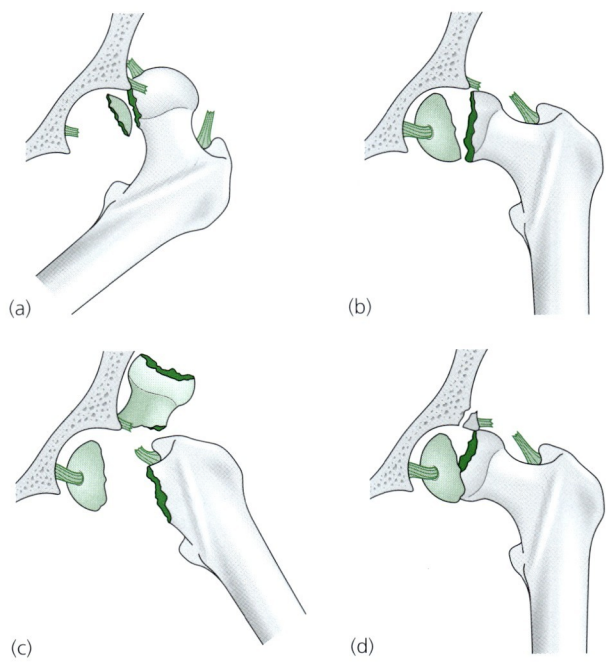

Figure 32.3 Pipkin classification of posterior dislocation of the hip with femoral head fracture. (a) Type I; (b) type II; (c) type III; (d) type IV.

head fragment, (4) the stability of the reduction and (5) the age of the patient.

Management after closed or open reduction ranges from short periods of bed rest to various durations of skeletal traction (Table 32.3). No correlation exists between early weight bearing and osteonecrosis. Therefore, partial weight bearing is advised. If reduction is concentric and stable, a short period of bed rest is followed by protected weight bearing for 4–6 weeks.

Special situations

In the case of an ipsilateral displaced or non-displaced femoral neck fracture, closed reduction of the hip should not be attempted. The fracture should be provisionally stabilized through a lateral approach. A gentle reduction is then performed, followed by definitive fixation of the femoral neck.

Prognosis

The outcome following hip dislocation ranges from an essentially normal hip to a slow deterioration to a severely painful and degenerated joint. Most authors report a 70–80% good or excellent outcome in simple posterior dislocations. When posterior dislocations are associated with a femoral head or acetabular fracture, however, the nature of the associated fractures dictates the outcome.

Complications

Sciatic nerve injury occurs in 10–20% of hip dislocations. Sciatic nerve injury may occur by stretch of the nerve over the posteriorly dislocated femoral head, laceration by the posterior acetabular fracture fragments or nerve ischaemia from pressure on it by the head. Usually, the peroneal portion of the nerve is affected, with little if any dysfunction of the tibial nerve. The prognosis is unpredictable and most authors report only 40–50% full recovery. If a sciatic nerve injury occurs following a closed reduction, then entrapment of the nerve is likely and surgical exploration is indicated. Osteonecrosis of varying degree is observed in 5–40% of injuries. The incidence increases with delay in reduction and repeated attempts at closed reduction, and the condition may become clinically apparent only after a few years. Post-traumatic osteoarthritis is the most frequent long-term complication and the incidence is higher with associated acetabular fractures or transchondral fractures of the femoral head. Heterotopic ossification occurs in 2% of patients and is related to the initial muscular damage and haematoma formation.

ANTERIOR DISLOCATIONS

Anterior dislocations result from forced external rotation and abduction of the hip. If the hip is in flexion during dislocation, it results in an inferior (obturator) dislocation, and if in extension a superior (pubic) dislocation occurs.

Classification

Anterior hip dislocations were classified by Epstein (Table 32.4).

Table 32.3 Management guidelines for posterior fracture dislocations of hip

Type	Description
Type I	If closed reduction results in a concentric stable reduction minor malalignment of the fragment is acceptable. If closed reduction is not concentric or is impossible, open reduction with excision of small fragments should be done immediately. Large fragments also are removed, provided that they do not alter the post-reduction stability
Type II	Immediate closed reduction is attempted. Anatomical reduction of the superior head fragments is crucial and this should be assessed in the post-reduction radiographs and CT. If the reduction is non-anatomical and non-concentric, open reduction should be done. Any soft-tissue attachments to the fragment, including the ligamentum teres, should be preserved if possible. Internal fixation of the fragments is easily performed through an anterior Smith-Petersen approach. In elderly patients a replacement is indicated because of the high rate of osteonecrosis and post-traumatic arthritis
Type III	In young patients, open reduction and internal fixation of the fracture is indicated, while in older patients or in a hip with pre-existing disease a replacement is indicated
Type IV	The treatment is dictated by the type of acetabular fracture. In young patients, if concentric reduction with reasonable joint congruity cannot be obtained by closed means, open reduction and internal fixation of all major fragments is performed. In older patients or in a hip with pre-existing disease a replacement is indicated

Table 32.4 Epstein classification of anterior hip dislocations

Type	Description
Type I	Superior dislocations, including pubic and subspinous
IA	No associated fractures
IB	Associated fracture or impaction of the femoral head
IC	Associated fracture of the acetabulum
Type II	Inferior dislocations, including obturator and perineal
IIA	No associated fractures
IIB	Associated fracture or impaction of the femoral head
IIC	Associated fracture of the acetabulum

Clinical evaluation

Clinically, the hip is in marked external rotation with mild flexion and abduction. Injury to the femoral artery, vein or nerve may occur as a result of an anterior dislocation and must be looked for.

Treatment

Closed reduction is achieved by longitudinal traction on the thigh with a lateral force on the proximal thigh while simultaneously pushing the femoral head to the acetabulum. The reverse Bigelow manoeuvre may also be used. Here the traction is applied in the line of the deformity, the hip is then adducted, internally rotated and extended. If closed reduction fails, open reduction is performed thorough a Smith-Petersen approach.

Anterior dislocations of the hip have a high incidence of associated femoral head injuries. This ranges from 25% to 75% and may be transchondral or indentation types. Patients without an associated femoral head injury usually have a good outcome.

KEY LEARNING POINTS

- Hip dislocations are the result of high-energy trauma and up to 50% of patients have concomitant injuries.
- Irrespective of the type of dislocation, the hip should be reduced on an emergency basis.
- Post-reduction radiographs must be evaluated for a congruent reduction. If in doubt, a CT scan is necessary to rule out intra-articular fragments of labrum or bone.
- Sciatic nerve injury occurs in 10–20% of hip dislocations. The prognosis is unpredictable, with only 40–50% of patients having full recovery
- Osteonecrosis is observed in 5–40% of injuries and may present as late as 5 years after the injury.

REFERENCES

- ● = Key primary paper
- ◆ = Major review article

◆1. Sahin V, Karakas ES, Aksu S, et al. Traumatic dislocation and fracture-dislocation of the hip: a long term follow-up study. *Journal of Trauma* 2003;**54**:520-9.

◆2. Thompson VP, Epstein HC. Traumatic dislocation of the hip: a survey of two hundred and four cases covering a period of twenty-one years. *Journal of Bone and Joint Surgery (American)* 1951;**33A**:746.

3. Schafer SJ, Anglen JO. The East Baltimore lift: a simple and effective method for reduction of posterior hip dislocations. *Journal of Orthopaedic Trauma* 1999;**13**:56.

◆4. Stannard JP, Harris HW, Volgal DA, et al. Functional outcome of patients with femoral head fractures associated with hip dislocations. *Clinical Orthopaedics and Related Research* 2000;**377**:44.

Femoral neck fractures

SHANMUGANATHAN RAJASEKARAN, VIJAY KAMATH, JAYARAMARAJU DHEENADHAYALAN

Introduction	340	Treatment	342
Mechanism of injury	340	Complications	344
Clinical evaluation	340	Fatigue/stress fractures	345
Radiographic evaluation	341	References	345
Classification	341		

NATIONAL BOARD STANDARDS

- Revise your knowledge of vascular and osseous anatomy of the femoral head and neck
- Understand treatment decision-making and the treatment algorithm
- Know the methods of closed reduction and fixation
- Be able to advise a patient on the prognosis and complications

INTRODUCTION

Femoral neck fractures account for 50% of hip fractures and are common in the elderly beyond the age of 70 years. About 80% of neck fractures occur in women, and the incidence doubles every 5–6 years in women above the age of 30 years. The incidence in younger patients is low and is associated mainly with high-energy trauma. Risk factors include female sex, increasing age, poor health, tobacco and alcohol use, a previous fracture and a low oestrogen level.

Fractures of the neck of the femur (NOF) occur in an area with a thin or absent periosteum and are intracapsular,[1] where the synovial fluid prevents haematoma consolidation, predisposing these fractures to non-union. In displaced fractures, the precarious femoral head blood supply may be impaired or entirely lacking, predisposing to osteonecrosis and secondary degenerative changes of the femoral head.

MECHANISM OF INJURY

In elderly patients NOF fractures are mostly low-energy injuries occurring as a result of an indirect twisting injury causing a forced external rotation of the lower extremity. This impinges the osteoporotic neck onto the posterior lip of the acetabulum, resulting in a fracture of the neck with posterior comminution. A fall with direct impact on the greater trochanter can result in a valgus impaction fracture. In the younger age group NOF fractures occur secondary to high-energy trauma and can be associated with severe comminution and other associated injuries.

CLINICAL EVALUATION

Patients with displaced NOF fractures are non-ambulatory, with the lower limb typically shortened and externally rotated. However, patients with an impacted fracture have no deformity and may be able to bear weight. Anterior hip tenderness and pain with bi-trochantric compression and hip movements are however present. The presence of prior hip pain should alert the physician to the possibility of a pathological fracture. About 10% of these patients have associated upper limb osteoporotic fractures in the wrist and shoulder.

The pre-injury ambulatory status should be determined as it is critical in determining optimal treatment.

RADIOGRAPHIC EVALUATION

An anteroposterior view of the pelvis and a cross-table lateral view of the involved hip should be performed. An internal rotation view of the injured hip helps to evaluate the fracture pattern. If a fracture is suspected and the radiographs fail to confirm the diagnosis, bone scanning, CT scan or MRI may be used. Thin slice CT cuts with three-dimensional reformations are used to look for a crack in the cortex or trabecular discontinuity. T_1-weighted MRI has been found to be 100% sensitive in patients with equivocal radiographic findings. It is important to note that the technetium bone scan may not be positive until at least 3 days have passed since the injury.

CLASSIFICATION

Fractures of the NOF were initially classified depending on the anatomical location as (a) subcapital, (b) transcervical or (c) basicervical (Fig. 33.1). In 1928 Pauwels classified NOF fractures into three types depending upon the degree of the angle that the fracture line makes with the horizontal (Fig. 33.2). This classification is based on the biomechanical basis that an increasing angle leads to increasing shear forces across the fracture types, leading to increased incidence of non-union.

The Garden classification[2] is based on the degree of displacement and its influence on stability and incidence of avascular necrosis. The relationship of the medial compression trabeculae in the head and pelvis is used as an index of displacement (Table 33.1 and Fig. 33.3).

Table 33.1 Garden's classification of fracture of the neck of the femur

Type	Description
Type I	Incomplete, impacted fracture in valgus malalignment (generally stable)
Type II	Complete and non-displaced on anteroposterior and lateral views
Type III	Complete with partial displacement; trabecular pattern of the femoral head does not line up with that of the acetabulum
Type IV	Completely displaced; trabecular pattern of the head assumes a parallel orientation with that of the acetabulum

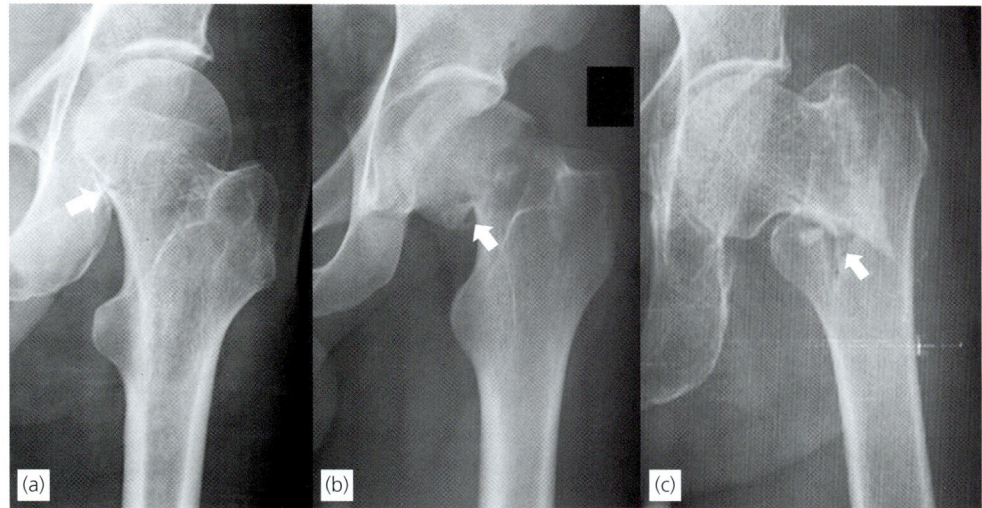

Figure 33.1 Anatomical classification of neck of femur fractures. (a) Subcapital, (b) transcervical, (c) basicervical.

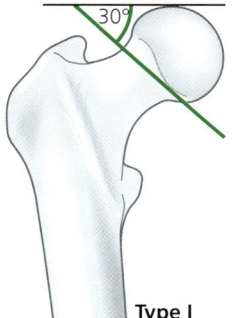 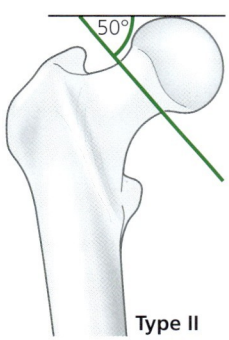 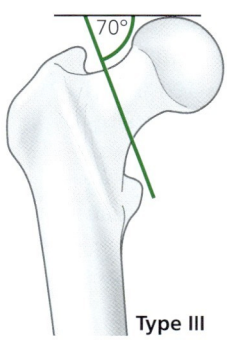

Figure 33.2 Pauwels' classification of fracture of the neck of the femur. (a) Type I, 30°. (b) Type II, 50°. (c) Type III, 70°. Increasing shear forces with increasing angle leads to more fracture instability and non-union.

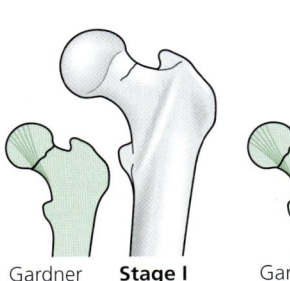 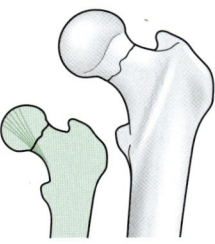 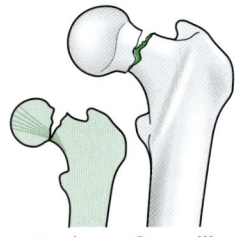 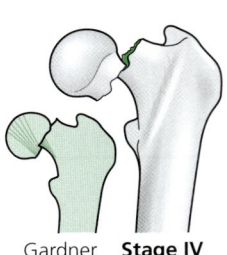

Gardner type I — **Stage I** ; Gardner type II — **Stage II** ; Gardner type III — **Stage III** ; Gardner type IV — **Stage IV**

Figure 33.3 Garden's classification of fracture of the neck of the femur. The classification is based on the relationship of the medial (compression) trabeculae in the head and pelvis. (See Table 33.1 for a description.)

The Comprehensive Classification of Fractures (Müller) divides the fractures of the NOF into three groups, based on the level of the fracture in the neck, the stability of the fracture and its displacement. Thus, B1 are neck fractures, subcapital, with slight displacement; B2 are transcervical fractures; and B3 are subcapital fractures with marked displacement. This classification is very detailed in its characterization of the fracture morphology and is more useful for research purposes than in routine clinical application.

Irrespective of the classification, the extent of displacement is of clinical importance. Non-displaced fractures include truly non-displaced fractures and impacted valgus femoral neck fractures and they have a much lower incidence of both non-union and avascular necrosis than displaced fractures.

TREATMENT

It is important to splint the injured limb early to protect it from additional damage, as well as to minimize the patient's discomfort. The goal of treatment is early ambulation by obtaining early anatomical reduction and stable internal fixation or prosthetic replacement. This is essential to avoid the complications of prolonged recumbency such as poor pulmonary atelectasis, venous stasis and pressure ulceration. Non-operative treatment for traumatic fractures is indicated only rarely for patients who are at extreme medical risk for surgery.

Impacted/non-displaced fractures

Impaction fractures are generally stable; however, approximately 8–33% of 'impacted' fractures will displace without internal stabilization. *In situ* fixation with three cancellous screws has a union rate of up to 100% and hence it is safer to fix these fractures. Up to 10% of patients may develop osteonecrosis, and this is attributed to secondary kinking of the lateral epiphyseal vessels, tethering of the medial vessels in a valgus position or intracapsular hypertension. The presence of a pathological fracture, pre-existing arthritis and other metabolic conditions requires prosthetic replacement.

Displaced fractures

All displaced subcapital fractures require surgical treatment. The decision that the surgeon must make is whether to treat the fracture with reduction and internal fixation or whether to carry out a primary arthroplasty.

In young patients with normal bone, emergency closed/open reduction with internal fixation is required. Fractures of the NOF in young patients are associated with high rates of osteonecrosis and non-union.[3] Outcomes depend on the *severity of the injury*, including the amount of displacement, comminution and the extent of vascular compromise to the femoral head, as well as the *timing and adequacy of the reduction and fixation*. Even when surgery has been performed satisfactorily, 10–15% of patients develop complications of avascular necrosis and non-union.[4] The surgeon unfortunately has less control over osteonecrosis because the blood supply to the femoral head after femoral neck fracture is quite precarious.

In elderly patients the treatment depends on the age, pre-injury functional status, quality of bone and life expectancy. In patients up to the age of 75 years who are ambulatory with high functional demand and good bone quality, early reduction and rigid internal fixation is recommended. If the patient has low functional demand or the bone quality is poor then a modular bipolar hemiarthroplasty or total hip arthroplasty is preferred. To achieve early ambulation and to avoid the possible problems of non-union and osteonecrosis, many surgeons recommend primary prosthetic replacement in elderly ambulatory patients. In patients over the age of 75 years a cemented bipolar hemiarthroplasty is advocated.

Irrespective of age, patients with pathological fractures, poor ambulatory status before fracture, pre-existing hip arthritis, poor bone quality and neurological conditions such as dementia, ataxia, hemiplegia and Parkinsonism require a primary arthroplasty.

OPERATIVE TREATMENT PRINCIPLES

Closed/open reduction and internal fixation

Reduction

Emergency anatomical reduction is a priority, as early reduction reduces the risk of osteonecrosis and anatomical reduction improves union rates. Closed reduction techniques have been described by Whitman[5] (reduction in extension) and Leadbetter[6] (reduction in flexion). The aim should be for an anatomical reduction or one with the head in slight valgus and neutral version or minimally anteverted. Any degree of residual varus or retroversion is unacceptable, as it leads to a high incidence of loss of fixation and redisplacement. Reduction should be checked fluoroscopically and satisfactory reduction can be evaluated by the Garden alignment index. If satisfactory reduction cannot be obtained by closed methods, open reduction using a Watson-Jones anterolateral approach to the hip is indicated. The interval between the tensor fasciae latae and the abductors is bluntly developed, and the vastus lateralis is elevated off the intertrochanteric ridge. The capsule is divided anteriorly along the axis of the neck of the femur and transversely released from its insertion into the proximal part of the femur. With sutures as retracting aids, the fracture can be visualized. A bone hook can be used to disimpact the fracture by applying a laterally directed force, and a blunt instrument can be inserted to improve the reduction (i.e. lift the proximal fragment anteriorly). The insertion area for internal fixation devices on the lateral aspect of the proximal end of the femur is easily exposed.

Fixation

Once reduction is achieved, fixation with three parallel screws in an inverted triangular configuration is usually adequate for most femoral neck fractures (Fig. 33.4). The screws should be inserted parallel to the axis of the neck and parallel to each other so that they act together as lag screws and also do not block the head from settling down on the neck if there is any resorption at the fracture. Screws positioned along the posterior femoral neck resist retroversion forces and screws along the calcar resist varus forces. Alternately, in basicervical fractures, in presence of osteopenia or comminution of the lateral cortex, a dynamic hip screw with an additional anti-rotation screw can be done.

Prosthetic replacement

Prosthetic replacement compared with internal fixation has the advantages of earlier ambulation with full weight bearing and eliminates the risks of non-union, osteonecrosis and failure of stabilization. However, it is a more extensive procedure associated with increased blood loss, longer surgical duration and greater infection rates. There is also increased mortality and morbidity when salvage procedures are needed. Prosthetic replacement can be a hemiarthroplasty (Fig. 33.5) or total hip arthroplasty depending on the individual case. The indications and contraindications for hemiarthroplasty are in Table 33.2.

The hemiarthroplasty prosthesis may be a bipolar or unipolar implant. The advantages of bipolar over the unipolar prosthesis include reduced risk of acetabular erosion, lower risk of postoperative dislocation and easy conversion to a total hip replacement as it is modular. The disadvantages of a bipolar prosthesis include the risk of polyethylene debris and, over time, the bipolar prosthesis may lose motion at its inner bearing and functionally become unipolar. In the presence of osteopenia and porosis, better functional results are obtained with use of polymethylmethacrylate cement; however, there is a small risk of intra-operative hypotension and increased infection with the use of cement.

Primary total hip arthroplasty is indicated in patients with significant pre-existing joint disease such as rheumatoid arthritis, osteonecrosis and osteoarthritis. Although good results are reported, the complication rate is higher than with hemiarthroplasty with increased risk for dislocation and infection. Patient selection must be carefully done as a total hip replacement is a considerably larger and longer procedure in this elderly population.

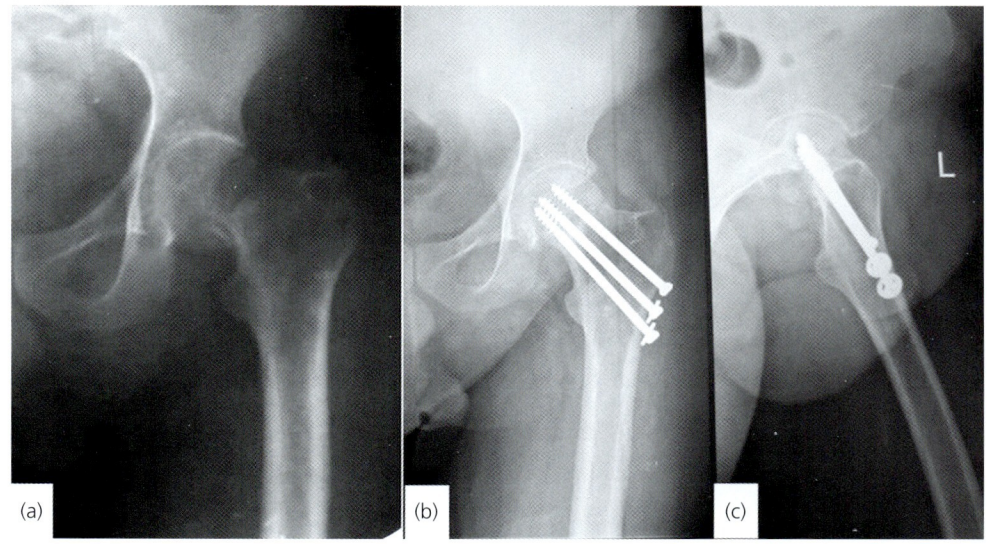

Figure 33.4 (a) Garden type III fracture. (b,c) Healed after stabilization with multiple cannulated screws.

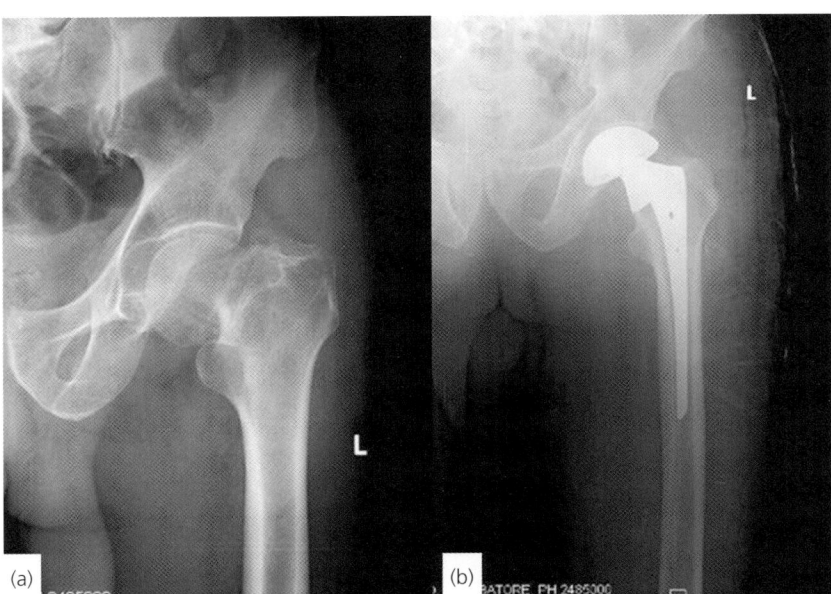

Figure 33.5 (a) Garden type III fracture in a 70 year old patient. (b) Managed with a bipolar hemiarthroplasty.

Table 33.2 Indications and contraindications for hemiarthroplasty

Indications	Contraindications
Comminuted, displaced femoral neck fracture in the elderly	Active sepsis
Pathological fracture	Active young person
Poor medical condition	Pre-existing acetabular disease (e.g. rheumatoid arthritis)
Poor ambulatory status before fracture	
Associated neurological conditions (dementia, ataxia, hemiplegia, Parkinsonism)	

COMPLICATIONS

Non-union following internal fixation is observed in up to 5% of non-displaced fractures and up to 25% of displaced fractures. Young patients are treated with proximal femoral realignment osteotomy (Fig. 33.6) or muscle pedicle graft whereas elderly patients are treated with arthroplasty.

Avascular necrosis occurs in 10–15% of patients with impacted or non-displaced fractures and in 30–35% of patients with displaced fractures. Fracture displacement with damage to the arteriolar supply, as well as intracapsular tamponade, plays a causative role. Following fracture union, the symptoms of avascular necrosis may be delayed up to 2 years. Patients usually present with groin or proximal thigh pain and progressive limp and limb shortening. Treatment is guided by symptoms and a total hip replacement is usually necessary in very symptomatic patients.

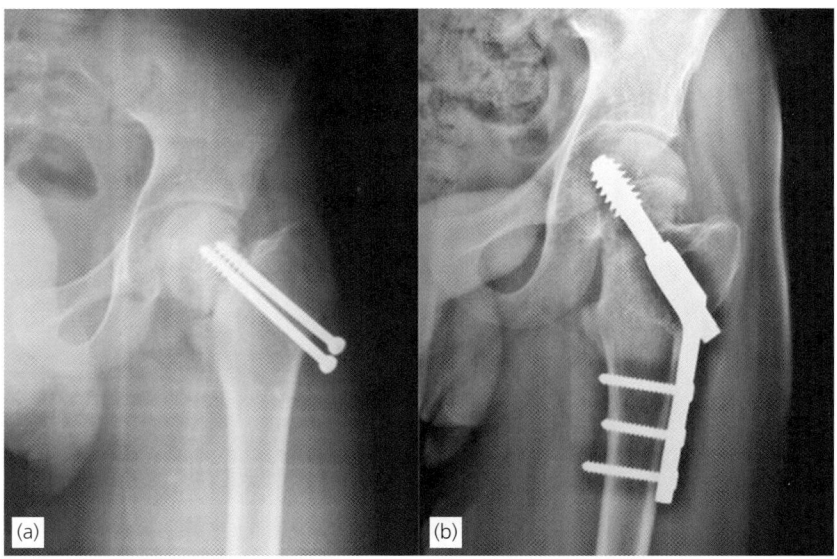

Figure 33.6 (a) Non-union fracture of the neck of the femur after inadequate fixation with two cancellous screws. (b) Femoral realignment osteotomy and stabilization with a dynamic hip screw resulted in union.

Failure of internal fixation is usually related to technical problems (malreduction, poor implant insertion), non-union, osteonecrosis, infection or poor quality osteoporotic bone. It may be managed with repeat internal fixation or prosthetic replacement.

FATIGUE/STRESS FRACTURES

These are seen in athletes, military recruits and ballet dancers, and are attributed to cyclical loading. Patients with osteoporosis and osteopenia are at particular risk. Tension-sided stress fractures (seen at the superior lateral neck on an internally rotated anteroposterior view) are at significant risk for displacement and *in situ* screw fixation is recommended. Compression-sided stress fractures (seen as a haze of callus at the inferior neck) are at lesser risk for displacement without additional trauma. A protective crutch ambulation is recommended until asymptomatic.

> ### KEY LEARNING POINTS
>
> - Femoral neck fractures are orthopaedic emergencies and urgent reduction and rigid fixation is the default line of management. In elderly, low-demand, poor ambulators with poor bone quality, a hemireplacement is advised.
> - Outcomes of displaced neck of femur fractures depend on the severity of the injury and the timing and adequacy of the reduction and fixation. Even when surgery has been performed satisfactorily, 10–15% of patients develop complications of avascular necrosis and non-union.
> - Avascular necrosis occurs in 10–15% of patients with impacted or non-displaced fractures and in 30–35% of patients with displaced fractures.

REFERENCES

- ● = Key primary paper
- ◆ = Major review article

●1. Chung SMK. The arterial supply of the developing proximal end of the human femur. *Journal of Bone and Joint Surgery (American)* 1976;**58A**:961.

●2. Garden RS. Low-angle fixation in fractures of the femoral neck. *Journal of Bone and Joint Surgery (British)* 1961;**43B**: 647–63.

◆3. Ly TV, Swiontkowski MF. Treatment of femoral neck fractures in young adults. *Journal of Bone and Joint Surgery (American)* 2008;**90A**:2254–66.

◆4. Lu-Yao GL, Keller RB, Littenberg B, *et al*. Outcomes after displaced fractures of the femoral neck: a meta-analysis of one hundred and six published reports. *Journal of Bone and Joint Surgery (American)* 1994;**76A**:15.

●5. Whitman R. The abduction method: considered as the exponent of a treatment for all forms of fracture at the hip in accord with surgical principles. *American Journal of Surgery* 1933;**21**:335–338.

●6. Leadbetter GW. Closed reduction of fractures of the neck of the femur. *Journal of Bone and Joint Surgery* 1938;**20**:108–113.

34

Intertrochanteric fractures

SHANMUGANATHAN RAJASEKARAN, VIJAY KAMATH, JAYARAMARAJU DHEENADHAYALAN

Introduction	346	Treatment	347
Mechanism of injury	346	Complications	349
Clinical evaluation	346	Greater trochanteric fractures	349
Radiological evaluation	346	Lesser trochanteric fractures	349
Classification	347	References	349

NATIONAL BOARD STANDARDS

- Revise your knowledge of trochanteric anatomy and biomechanics
- Understand the classification of trochanteric fractures
- Know the methods of treatment for these fractures
- Be able to advise a patient on the prognosis and complications

INTRODUCTION

Intertrochanteric fractures, more correctly referred to as pertrochanteric fractures, occur in the region between the greater and lesser trochanters of the proximal femur, occasionally extending into the subtrochanteric region. They account for nearly 50% of all fractures of the proximal femur, with reported mortality rates ranging from 15% to 30%. Intertrochanteric fractures occur more commonly in women (2:1 to 8:1) in the sixth or seventh decade.

Intertrochanteric fractures differ from fractures of the neck of femur in the following respects:

- The deforming muscle forces produce greater shortening and more external rotation of the lower limb than in fractures of the neck of femur.
- Extracapsular fractures occur in cancellous bone with an abundant blood supply. As a result, non-union and osteonecrosis are not major problems; however, malunion is a complication.

MECHANISM OF INJURY

Ninety per cent of intertrochanteric fractures in the elderly result from a simple fall, whereas in younger individuals they are usually the result of a high-energy injury.

CLINICAL EVALUATION

Patients with displaced intertrochanteric fractures present with the injured lower extremity shortened and externally rotated, whereas those with undisplaced fractures present with painful ambulation, deep trochantric tenderness and painful hip movements.

RADIOLOGICAL EVALUATION

An anteroposterior view of the pelvis and an anteroposterior and a cross-table lateral view of the involved proximal femur are adequate to assess the fracture morphology.

CLASSIFICATION

Among the earliest classifications was that proposed by Boyd and Griffin,[1] who classified fractures in the peritrochanteric area of the femur into four types (Table 34.1 and Fig. 34.1); this classification, however, does not aid in treatment planning.

Newer classification systems have been developed to aid in treatment decision-making. Most of the classifications of trochanteric fractures are based on the number of fragments and whether or not the lesser trochanter is split off as a separate fragment. Thus, the two-part fracture is one in which the fracture follows extracapsularly the course of the intertrochanteric crest. With further force the lesser trochanter and the greater trochanter can split off, creating the three- and four-part fractures. The lesser trochanter and surrounding bone are posteromedial and this is an area that is subjected to very large compressive stresses and is important to the load-bearing capacity of the femur. The presence of a fracture of the lesser trochanter and adjacent bone has led to the classification of these three- and four-part fractures as unstable and the two-part fracture as stable. This is the scheme followed in the classification by Kyle and Gustilo.[2] It recognizes four types: type I, the stable non-displaced fracture without comminution; type II, which is stable with minimal comminution; type III, which is unstable and has a large posteromedial comminuted area; and type IV, which has a subtrochanteric extension and is highly unstable and difficult to treat.

The Evans classification is based on pre-reduction and post-reduction stability, i.e. the convertibility of an unstable fracture configuration to a stable reduction.[3] Fracture stability is determined by the presence of posteromedial bony contact, which acts as a buttress against fracture collapse. In stable fracture patterns, the posteromedial cortex remains intact or has minimal comminution, making it possible to obtain and maintain a stable reduction. Unstable fracture patterns are characterized by greater comminution of the posteromedial cortex. Although they are inherently unstable, these fractures can be converted to a stable reduction if medial cortical opposition is obtained.

Reverse obliquity fractures

Reverse obliquity intertrochanteric fractures are inherently unstable fractures characterized by an oblique fracture line extending from the medial cortex proximally to the lateral cortex distally. The location and direction of the fracture line result in a tendency to medial displacement from the pull of the adductor muscles. These are best treated as subtrochanteric fractures.

TREATMENT

Rigid internal fixation with early mobilization of the patient is the standard method of treatment of intertrochanteric fractures. A mortality rate of 34.6% for trochanteric fractures treated by traction has been reported compared with 17.5% for fractures treated by internal fixation. Non-operative treatment is rarely indicated and is reserved only for patients who are at extreme medical risk for surgery. These patients are at increased risk for complications of prolonged recumbency. Malunion is to be expected and accepted.

The aim of surgery is a stable internal fixation to allow early ambulation. Stability of fracture fixation depends on bone quality, fracture pattern, fracture reduction, implant design and implant placement. The surgeon has control over the reduction, implant choice and its placement.

Table 34.1 Boyd and Griffin classification of peritrochanteric fractures

Type	Description
Type 1	Fractures that extend along the intertrochanteric line from the greater to the lesser trochanter
Type 2	Comminuted fractures, the main fracture being along the intertrochanteric line, but with multiple fractures in the cortex
Type 3	Fractures that are basically subtrochanteric with at least one fracture passing across the proximal end of the shaft just distal to or at the lesser trochanter. Varying degrees of comminution are associated
Type 4	Fractures of the trochanteric region and the proximal shaft, with fracture in at least two planes, one of which usually is the sagittal plane

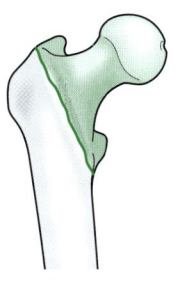
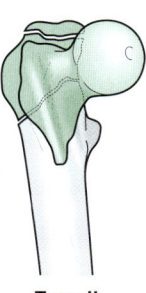
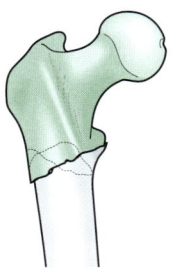
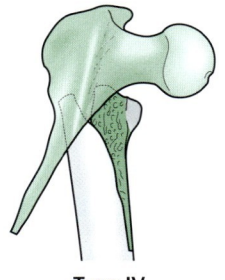

Type I Type II Type III Type IV

Figure 34.1 Boyd and Griffin classification of trochanteric fractures. Reproduced with permission from Boyd HB, Griffin LL. Classification and treatment of trochanteric fractures. *Archives of Surgery* 1949;**58**:853.

Reduction of the fracture

The goal is to achieve a stable reduction, i.e. posteromedial cortical contact. The reduction of the fracture is carried out on the fracture table with the aid of image intensification. The limb is placed in traction and in slight abduction and internal rotation. This is usually sufficient to align the femoral head and neck fragment with the shaft and recreate the patient's normal neck shaft angle. It is important to check on the lateral projection that the shaft has not sagged posteriorly. After the reduction manoeuvre, fracture stability should be checked fluoroscopically. In the anteroposterior view look for contact of the medial cortex, and in the lateral view for posterior cortical contact. If stability cannot be achieved by closed manoeuvres then open reduction should be performed. Often, the distal shaft fragment is found to be sagging posteriorly and this needs to be corrected to achieve stability. In the rare instance that anatomical reduction cannot be achieved by open means then a non-anatomical but stable reduction should be obtained by osteotomy and medial displacement techniques described by Sarmiento and Diamon-Hughston.[4]

Implant choice and implant positioning

SLIDING HIP SCREWS

Sliding hip screws include the compression (dynamic) hip screw (Fig. 34.2) that provides compression in the intertrochantric plane and compression plates (Medoff plate) that provide additional compression axially.

The most important technical aspects of screw insertion are (1) placement within 1 cm of subchondral bone to provide secure fixation and (2) central or posterior–inferior position in the femoral head. Baumgaertner *et al.* described the tip–apex distance (Fig. 34.3) that can be used to determine the lag screw position within the femoral head.[5] It is the sum of the distances from the apex of the femoral head to the tip of the lag screw on anteroposterior and lateral radiographs, correcting for magnification. The sum should be <25 mm to minimize the risk of lag screw cutout.

A 4–12% incidence of loss of fixation is reported, most commonly with unstable fracture patterns. Most failures of fixation are attributable to technical problems of screw placement and/or fracture reduction. In younger individuals with a large posteromedial fragment, after fixation of the sliding hip screw, a lag screw through the proximal hole of the plate may be used to fix the posteromedial fragment.

The Medoff bi-axial compression plate allows for compression of the proximal fracture fragment to the femoral shaft in addition to the compression achieved by the compression hip screw.

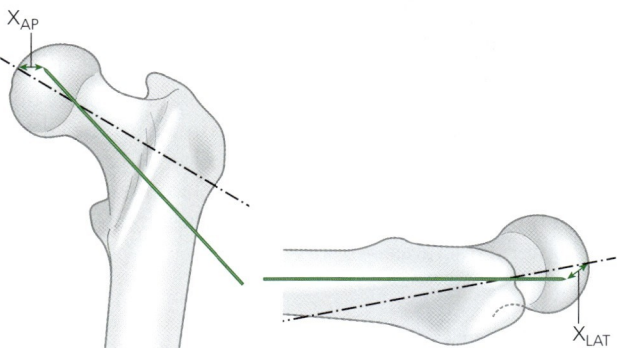

Figure 34.2 Calculation of the tip–apex distance. Distances from the tip of the implant to the apex of the femoral head on anteroposterior (a) and lateral (b) views are summed ($X_{AP} + X_{Lat}$). A tip–apex distance of less than 25 mm should be achieved. Redrawn from Baumgaertner MR, Curtin SL, Lindskog DM, *et al*. The value of the tip–apex distance in predicting failure of fixation of peritrochanteric fractures of the hip. *Journal of Bone and Joint Surgery (American)* 1995;**77A**:1058.

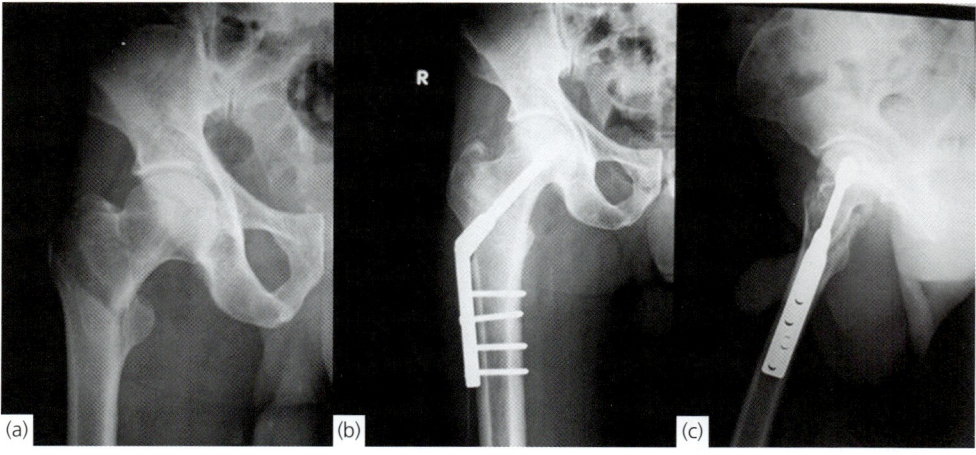

Figure 34.3 (a) Stable intertrochantric fracture. (b,c) Stabilized with a dynamic hip screw.

INTRAMEDULLARY HIP SCREW

These include the Gamma nail and the antegrade femoral nail. This implant combines the features of a sliding hip screw and an intramedullary nail. The advantages of the intramedullary hip screw is that it can be inserted in a closed manner with limited fracture exposure, decreased blood loss and less soft-tissue injury than a sliding hip screw. In addition, these devices are subjected to a lower bending moment than the sliding hip screw owing to their intramedullary location. However, the procedure is more technically demanding, and fracture at the distal locking screw has been reported to occur in 3–6% of patients.

The intramedullary hip screw limits the amount of fracture collapse, compared with an sliding hip screw, and is hence preferred in unstable comminuted intertrochanteric fractures, intertrochanteric fractures with subtrochanteric extension and in reverse obliquity fractures.[6]

PROSTHETIC REPLACEMENT

Primary prosthetic replacement is recommended only for severely comminuted unstable intertrochanteric fractures in elderly patients with significant osteoporosis which would compromise fixation. A calcar replacement hemiarthroplasty is needed because of the level of the fracture. Disadvantages include morbidity associated with a more extensive operative procedure and the risk of postoperative prosthetic dislocation.

COMPLICATIONS

Loss of fixation most commonly results from varus collapse of the proximal fragment with cutout of the lag screw from the femoral head. Lag screw cutout is usually due to technical errors of lag screw placement within the femoral head, inability to obtain a stable reduction and osteoporosis, which precludes secure fixation. Non-union occurs in less than 2% of patients, especially in patients with unstable fracture patterns.

GREATER TROCHANTERIC FRACTURES

Isolated greater trochanteric fractures, although rare, typically occur in older patients as a result of a direct blow. Treatment of greater trochanteric fractures is usually non-operative.

Operative management can be considered in younger, active patients who have a widely displaced greater trochanter. Tension band wiring of the displaced fragment and the attached abductor muscles is the preferred technique.

LESSER TROCHANTERIC FRACTURES

These are most common in adolescence, typically secondary to forceful iliopsoas contracture.

In the elderly, isolated lesser trochanter fractures are pathognomonic for pathological lesions of the proximal femur.

KEY LEARNING POINTS

- Trochantric fractures constitute 50% of all fractures of the proximal femur with reported mortality rates ranging from 15% to 30%.
- Unstable fracture patterns comprise those with comminution of the posteromedial cortex, subtrochanteric extension or a reverse obliquity pattern.
- Surgical stabilization is the default line of management.
- The lag screw should be placed centrally or posteroinferiorly.
- Tip–apex distance <25 mm is crucial when using a sliding hip screw or intramedullary nailing to prevent cutout and loss of reduction.

REFERENCES

- ● = Key primary paper
- ◆ = Major review article

●1. Boyd HB, Griffin LL. Classification and treatment of trochanteric fractures. *Archives of Surgery* 1949;**58**:853.

●2. Kyle RF, Gustilo RB, Premer RF. Analysis of six hundred and twenty-two intertrochanteric hip fractures. *Journal of Bone and Joint Surgery (American)* 1979;**61**:216–221.

●3. Evans E. The treatment of trochanteric fractures of the femur. *Journal of Bone and Joint Surgery* 1949;**31B**:190–203.

●4. Zuckerman JD. *Comprehensive Care of Orthopaedic Injuries in the Elderly*. Baltimore, MD: Urban and Schwarzenberg, 1990.

5. Baumgaertner MR, Curtin SL, Lindskog DM, *et al*. The value of the tip-apex distance in predicting failure of fixation of peritrochanteric fractures of the hip. *Journal of Bone and Joint Surgery (American)* 1995;**77A**:1058.

◆6. Pajarinen J, Lindahl J, Michelsson O, *et al*. Pertrochanteric femoral fractures treated with a dynamic hip screw or a proximal femoral nail: a randomised study comparing post-operative rehabilitation. *Journal of Bone and Joint Surgery (British)* 2005;**87B**:76.

Subtrochanteric fractures

SHANMUGANATHAN RAJASEKARAN, VIJAY KAMATH, JAYARAMARAJU DHEENADHAYALAN

Introduction	350	Treatment	351
Mechanism of injury	350	Choice of implants	351
Clinical evaluation	350	Complications	352
Radiological evaluation	350	References	352
Classification	350		

NATIONAL BOARD STANDARDS

- Understand the classification of subtrochantric fractures
- Know the methods of treatment
- Be able to advise a patient on the prognosis and complications

INTRODUCTION

A subtrochanteric fracture is a fracture between the lesser trochanter and the isthmus of the femoral diaphysis. They account for 10–34% of hip fractures and have a higher potential for non-union as the bone is mainly cortical and the fragments are displaced by muscle forces which abduct the proximal fragment and adduct the distal fragments considerably.

MECHANISM OF INJURY

In young adults subtrochanteric fractures are the result of high-energy trauma, whereas in the elderly they can occur even with low-energy trauma. The subtrochanteric region is also a frequent site for pathological fractures, accounting for 17–35% of all subtrochanteric fractures. A history of previous pain at the site even before the fracture and a transverse fracture with sclerosed or irregular margins must arouse suspicion of a pre-existing pathology.

CLINICAL EVALUATION

Subtrochanteric fractures are high-energy injuries, and associated major organ and skeletal injuries should be looked for. Significant haemorrhage may occur into the thigh, and frequently these patients are haemodynamically unstable. The fracture must be splinted immediately and early definitive fixation should be performed to limit further soft-tissue damage and haemorrhage.

RADIOLOGICAL EVALUATION

Standard anteroposterior and lateral radiographs are adequate to evaluate fracture morphology and plan treatment. The hip and knee joints should also be included in the study.

CLASSIFICATION

The *Fielding* classification is based on the location of the primary fracture line in relation to the lesser trochanter[1] and the *Seinsheimer* classification is on the number of major bone fragments and the location and shape of the fracture lines.[2] Both of them are less useful as they do not guide management of the fracture. The presently popular classification system is the *Russell–Taylor*[3] classification (Table 35.1 and Fig. 35.1), which evolved in response to the development of second-generation interlocked nails. The classification is based on lesser trochanteric continuity and fracture extension into the piriformis fossa, the two major variables influencing the treatment. This classification is useful as it guides the choice of implant to stabilize the fracture according to its morphology.

Table 35.1 Russell–Taylor classification of subtrochanteric fractures

Type	Description
Type I	Fractures with an intact piriformis fossa in which:
IA	The lesser trochanter is attached to the proximal fragment
IB	The lesser trochanter is detached from the proximal fragment
Type II	Fractures that extend into the piriformis fossa and:
IIA	Have a stable medial construct (posteromedial cortex)
IIB	Have comminution of the piriformis fossa and lesser trochanter, associated with varying degrees of femoral shaft comminution.

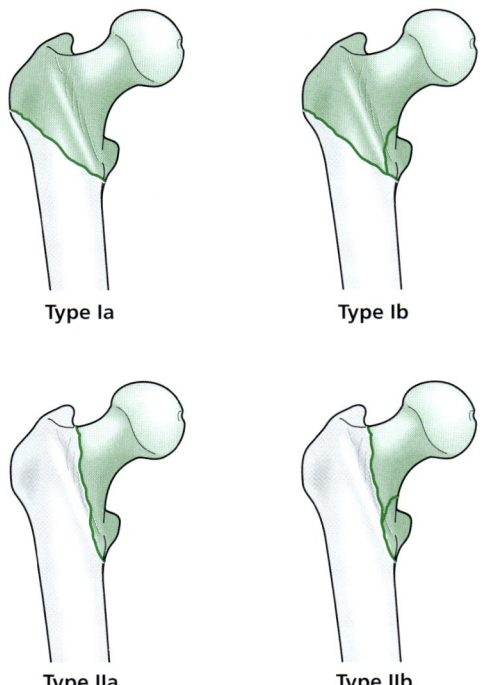

Figure 35.1 Russell–Taylor classification of subtrochanteric fracture of the femur based on involvement of piriformis fossa. (See text for a description.)

TREATMENT

Operative treatment is indicated in all subtrochanteric fractures, and non-operative treatment is reserved only for those elderly individuals who are high-risk candidates for surgery and for children. This involves skeletal traction in the 90°/90° position followed by cast bracing. Non-operative treatment results in increased morbidity and mortality owing to complications associated with prolonged bed rest, as well as in non-union, delayed union and malunion with varus angulation, rotational deformity and shortening.

Subtrochanteric fractures may be stabilized with intramedullary nails, compression hip screws or 95° fixed angle devices. The recommendations for the choice of implant based on the Russell–Taylor classification of subtrochantric fractures are given in Table 35.2.

CHOICE OF IMPLANTS

An intramedullary device such as the interlocked nail is preferred because of the advantages of less disruption of the fracture environment, retained blood supply to bone fragments and less operative blood loss than when plate–screw devices are used.[4] First-generation centromedullary nails are indicated for subtrochanteric fractures with both trochanters intact (type IA). However, in the presence of loss of the posteromedial cortex (type IB), a second-generation cephalomedullary reconstruction nail is indicated (Fig. 35.2). Reconstruction nails allow length and rotational control, even when the lesser trochanter is not intact. Involvement of the piriformis fossa (type IIA or IIB) does not contraindicate its use, but does increase the technical difficulty of placement.

Compression hip screw and 95° fixed angle plates (Fig. 35.3) are best suited for fractures involving both trochanters.[5] An accessory screw can be inserted beneath the fixed angle blade or screw into the calcar to increase proximal fixation. A dynamic condylar screw is technically

Table 35.2 Management recommendations based on the Russell–Taylor classification

Fracture type		Description
IA	Piriformis fossa and lesser trochanter intact	Standard interlocking nail
IB	Piriformis fossa intact, lesser trochanter fractured	Reconstruction nail
IIA	Piriformis fossa fractured, lesser trochanter intact	Sliding hip screw or reconstruction nail
IIB	Piriformis fossa and lesser trochanter fractured	Sliding hip screw with bone graft or reconstruction nail

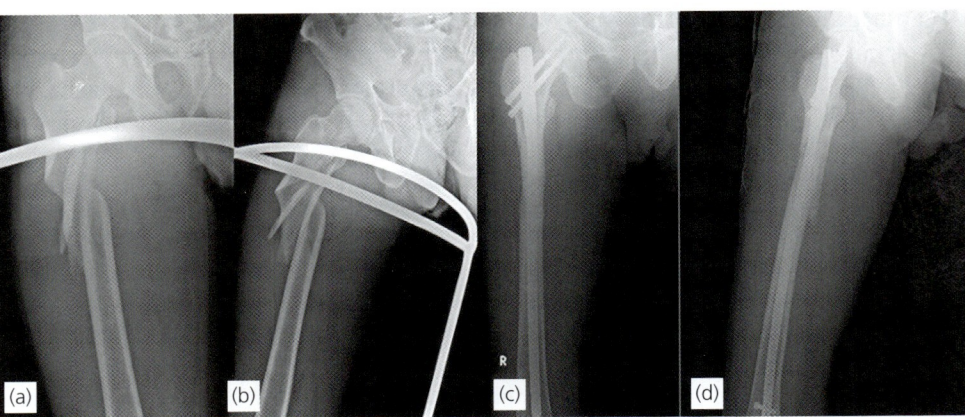

Figure 35.2 (a,b) Russell–Taylor type IB fracture. (c,d) Stabilized with a reconstruction nail.

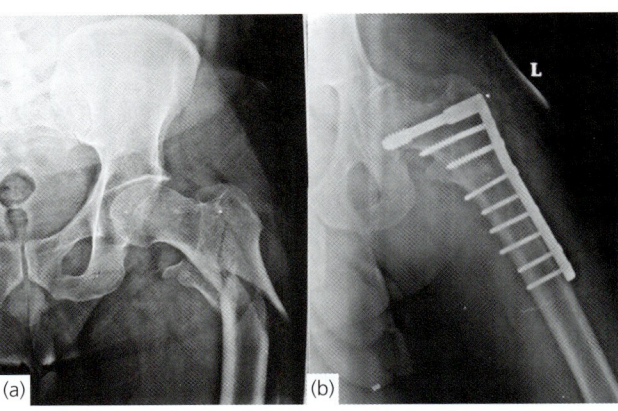

Figure 35.3 (a) Comminuted subtrochantric fracture (Russell–Taylor type IIB). (b) Healed after stabilization with a 95° fixed angle plate.

easier to insert than a blade plate. One must take care not to devitalize the fracture fragments during fracture reduction and fixation. If medial dissection is necessary to achieve reduction, primary autogenous iliac bone grafting should be used.

COMPLICATIONS

In comminuted fractures, non-union usually occurs in the femoral shaft portion of the fracture. Non-unions that develop following intramedullary nailing can be treated by exchange nailing using a larger diameter intramedullary nail. Bone grafting of the non-union site and additional stabilization with a plate over the nail may also be performed. Loss of fixation with compression hip screw devices occurs either because of screw cutout from the femoral head or because of neck or plate breakage. With interlocked nails, loss of fixation is commonly related to failure to lock the device statically, comminution of the entry portal or use of smaller diameter nails. Treatment involves removal of hardware, revision internal fixation and bone grafting. Coxa varus may occur as result of the uncorrected abduction deformity of the proximal segment caused by the hip abductors.

> ### KEY LEARNING POINTS
>
> - High biomechanical stress, poor vascularity and lack of cancellous bone predispose subtrochantric fractures to non-union, malunion and implant failure.
> - Surgery is the default pathway of treatment except in the rare situation of high risk of medical complications for surgery.
> - The Russell–Taylor classification aids in choosing the implant for fracture stabilization.
> - Generally, fixation with intramedullary nails offers better results than extramedullary fixations with plate and screws.

REFERENCES

- ● = Key primary paper
- ◆ = Major review article

● 1. Fielding JW, Magliato HJ. Subtrochanteric fractures. *Surgery, Gynecology and Obstetrics* 1966;**122**:555–569.
● 2. Seinsheimer III F. Subtrochanteric fractures of the femur. *Journal of Bone and Joint Surgery (American)* 1978;**60A**:300.
  3. Russell TA, Taylor JC. Subtrochanteric fractures of the femur. In: Browner BD, Jupiter JB, Levine AM, Trafton PG (eds) *Skeletal Trauma*, 2nd edn. Philadelphia, PA: W.B. Saunders, 1997.
◆ 4. Barquet A, Francescoli L, Rienzi D, Lopez L. Intertrochanteric-subtrochanteric fractures: treatment with the long Gamma nail. *Journal of Orthopaedic Trauma* 2000;**14**:324–8.
◆ 5. Vaidya SV, Dholakia DB, Chatterjee A. The use of a dynamic condylar screw and biologic reduction techniques for subtrochanteric femur fractures. *Injury* 2003;**34**:123–8.

Femoral shaft fractures

S RAJASEKARAN, VIJAY KAMATH, J DHEENADHAYALAN

Introduction	353	Treatment	354
Clinical evaluation	353	Complications	356
Radiological evaluation	353	References	356
Classification	353		

NATIONAL BOARD STANDARDS

- Revise your knowledge of femur anatomy and muscular attachments
- Know the different treatment methods, including the advantages and disadvantages of each
- Be able to advise a patient on the prognosis and complications

INTRODUCTION

A fracture of the femoral diaphysis occurring between 5 cm distal to the lesser trochanter and 5 cm proximal to the adductor tubercle is termed a shaft fracture. Femoral shaft fractures occur most frequently in young men after high-energy trauma and elderly women after a low-energy fall. Pathological fractures commonly occur at the relatively weak metaphyseal–diaphyseal junction. A fracture that is inconsistent with the degree of trauma should arouse suspicion for pathological fracture.

CLINICAL EVALUATION

The diagnosis is usually obvious with a swollen thigh and a shortened and rotated limb. These patients may be haemodynamically unstable as, often, more than 1000 mL blood loss may occur into the thigh. These fractures are the result of high-energy trauma, and associated musculoskeletal and major organ injury is seen in 5–15% of cases. About half of these patients also have ipsilateral knee ligamentous and meniscal injuries, and hence stability of the knee should be evaluated with the patient under anaesthesia immediately after bony stabilization.

RADIOLOGICAL EVALUATION

Anteroposterior and lateral radiographs including the joint above and below are evaluated to determine the fracture pattern and comminution, bone quality, presence of bone loss and the presence of air in the soft tissues. Associated hip dislocations and femoral neck and intertrochanteric fractures should be ruled out. Associated femoral neck fractures, although found in only 2.5–6% of patients, are missed in 30% of patients. The proximal segment of the femur is normally in abduction and the appearance of the femoral shaft in adduction should alert the surgeon to the possibility of an associated posteriorly dislocated hip (Fig. 36.1).

CLASSIFICATION

Femoral shaft fractures may be classified descriptively based on the location (proximal, middle or distal one-third),

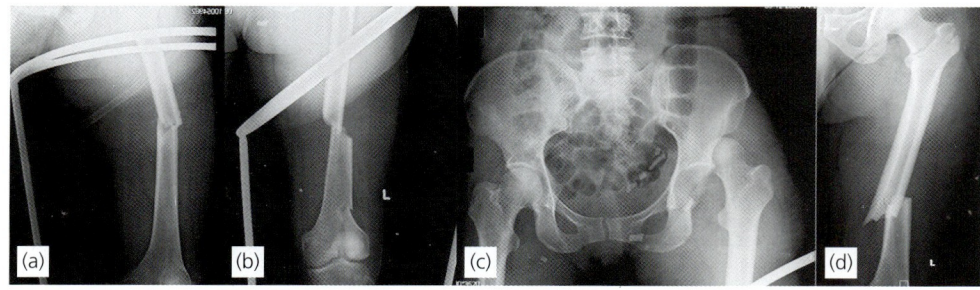

Figure 36.1 (a) Isolated fracture of the shaft of femur showing abduction of the proximal fragment owing to the muscular forces acting on it. (b,c) In this case, the proximal fragment is in adduction owing to the presence of a coexisting hip dislocation. (d) Another example of proximal fragment adduction owing to a displaced trochanteric fracture.

Table 36.1 Winquist and Hansen classification system for femoral shaft fractures

Type	Description
Type I	Minimal or no comminution
Type II	Cortices of both fragments at least 50% intact
Type III	50–100% cortical comminution
Type VI	Circumferential comminution with no cortical contact

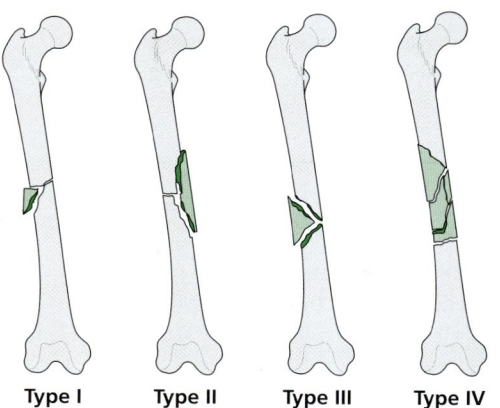

Figure 36.2 Winquist and Hansen classification of femoral shaft fractures. Redrawn with permission from Browner BD, Jupiter JB, Levine AM, et al. *Skeletal Trauma*. Philadelphia, PA: W.B. Saunders, 1992:1537.

pattern of the fracture geometry (spiral, oblique or transverse), amount of displacement (shortening, translation, angulation or rotational deformity), extent of comminution (comminuted, segmental or butterfly fragment) and status of soft-tissue envelope (open or closed). The Winquist and Hansen classification based on the diameter of bone that is comminuted was commonly used prior to the introduction of statically locked intramedullary nails[1] (Table 36.1 and Fig. 36.2). Type I and II fractures are axially stable, whereas type III and IV fractures are both axially and rotationally unstable. Rotational stability for less comminuted fractures is determined by the amount of comminution and obliquity of the fracture, with more transverse fracture patterns being less rotationally stable. Axially stable fractures are more amenable to earlier weight bearing after intramedullary nailing.

TREATMENT

Emergency treatment consists of the immediate application of a Thomas splint before radiographs are obtained as this decreases pain, further soft-tissue injury and bleeding and also the incidence of fat embolism. Operative stabilization is the standard of care for most femoral shaft fractures. Non-operative management as definitive treatment is rarely indicated and is limited to patients with significant medical comorbidities in whom surgery is contraindicated. In these patients, lower femoral or upper tibial skeletal traction is used for 6 weeks followed by cast–brace application. The problems with non-operative treatment include knee stiffness, limb shortening, prolonged hospitalization, respiratory and skin ailments, and malunion.

Principles of operative care

Surgical stabilization should be performed as early as possible and is particularly important in the multiply injured patient. Skeletal traction must be used if a delay in surgical treatment is expected to be greater than 12–24 hours.

Choice of implant

INTRAMEDULLARY NAILING

Reamed locked antegrade intramedullary nailing through the piriformis fossa is the gold standard for treatment of femoral shaft fractures.[2] Healing rates as high as 99%, with low complication rates, have been achieved with this treatment. Intramedullary location of the implant results in lower tensile and shear stresses on the implant than plate fixation. Other benefits of intramedullary nailing over plate fixation include less extensive exposure and dissection, lower infection rate and less quadriceps scarring.

Closed intramedullary nailing in closed fractures has the advantage of maintaining both the fracture haematoma and the attached periosteum. If reaming is performed, the reamed products provide a combination of osteoinductive and osteoconductive materials to the site of the fracture. Locking of the nail also allows restoration of length and alignment with comminuted fractures, early functional use of the extremity, rapid and high union rates of more than 95% and low re-fracture rates (Fig. 36.3).

The role of unreamed intramedullary nailing for the treatment of femoral shaft fractures is controversial.[3] The potentially negative effects of reaming for insertion of intramedullary nails include elevated intramedullary pressures, elevated pulmonary artery pressures, increased fat embolism and increased pulmonary dysfunction. The potential advantages of reaming include the ability to place a larger implant, increased union and decreased hardware failure. Evidence indicates that the clinical relevance of marrow content embolization during the reaming process is negligible and is outweighed by the benefits of reaming on the healing process. Nonetheless, sharp reamers, proper reamer design and slow passage of the reamer can decrease intramedullary pressures and fat embolization. Care in reaming is important in patients with associated chest or lung injury. Reaming across segmental fracture fragments should be done with great care to avoid spinning of the fragments, which can lead to stripping of these fragments and neurovascular injury.

The timing of femoral nailing and reaming in a polytraumatized patient is controversial.[4] Early intramedullary nailing is associated with elevation of certain proinflammatory markers, and this may place the patient at high risk for developing complications. In patients with polytrauma or multiple long bone fractures, early stabilization by external fixation followed by delayed intramedullary nailing is recommended.

Recently, implants for retrograde locked nailing have been developed. Indications for retrograde nailing include severe obesity, pregnancy, bilateral fractures and fractures of the ipsilateral tibia, as well as patellar or acetabular fractures (which require repair via a posterior hip approach). The ease of identifying the starting point makes it the preferred choice in morbidly obese patients. Its use is contraindicated in the presence of an associated open traumatic wound around the knee, and in patients with restricted knee motion of less than 60°.

PLATE FIXATION

Plate fixation is no longer the first choice in femoral shaft fractures because of the potential disadvantages of increased blood loss, stress shielding of the bone, increased risk of infection, additional soft-tissue injury and decreased vascularization beneath the plate. The present role of plates is in the management of fractures with an extremely narrow or obliterated (because of previous pathology) medullary canal in which intramedullary nailing is difficult and in fractures that have associated proximal or distal extension into the pertrochanteric or condylar regions. Minimally invasive methods such as indirect reduction techniques and submuscular plating have been advocated to reduce soft-tissue disruption and maximize healing potential during plating of femoral shaft fractures. In patients with an associated vascular injury, the exposure for the vascular repair frequently involves a wide exposure of the medial femur. If femoral stabilization is desired, a plate can be applied quickly medially through the open exposure.

EXTERNAL FIXATION

External fixation is most often used as a temporary stabilizing device, and its use as definitive treatment for femoral shaft fractures is restricted to the paediatric population. Temporary external fixation has a role in the stabilization of fractures in multiply injured patients and in open fractures where repeated debridement is expected (Fig. 36.4). The disadvantages of using external fixation as a definitive treatment are pin tract infection, a higher incidence of nonunion, loss of knee motion as a result of muscle impalement and limited ability to adequately stabilize the femoral shaft resulting in angular malunion and femoral shortening.

Special situations

ASSOCIATED NECK OF FEMUR FRACTURES

The method of internal fixation must be carefully chosen in each patient. Options for operative fixation include a reconstruction nail, retrograde femoral nailing for the

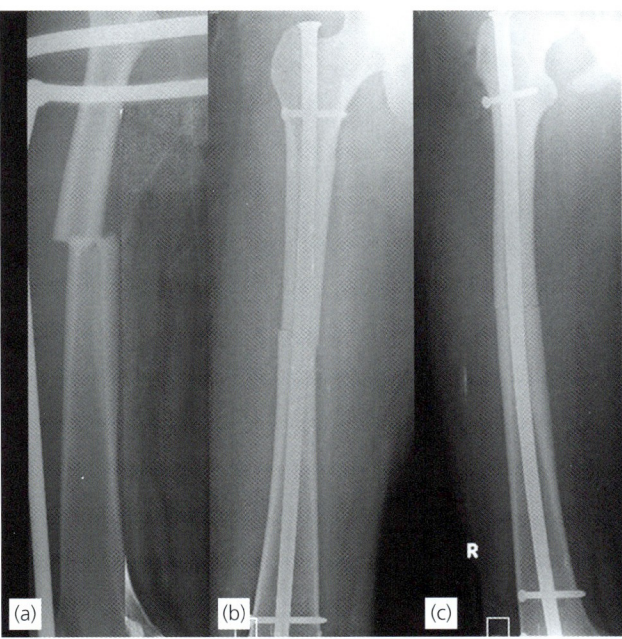

Figure 36.3 (a) Transverse femoral shaft fracture managed by dynamic intramedullary interlocked nailing (b,c).

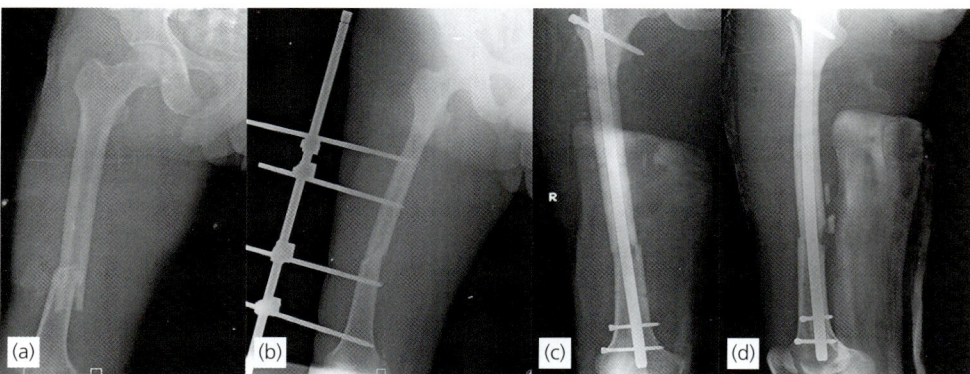

Figure 36.4 (a,b) A Gustilo grade IIIB open femoral shaft fracture was debrided and temporarily stabilized with an external fixator. (c,d) Interlocked intramedullary nailing has been performed once the wound was healthy and adequate soft-tissue cover was achieved.

shaft fracture with multiple screw fixation for the femoral neck, and compression plating of the shaft fracture with screw fixation of the femoral neck.

OPEN INJURIES

Between 5% and 20% of femoral shaft fractures are open injuries. Treatment is emergency debridement with skeletal stabilization. Wounds should be extended for evaluation of the deeper tissues and all non-viable soft tissue and bone should be debrided. Serial debridements at 24–48 hour intervals are indicated with higher grade open injuries. Although closure of contaminated wounds should be avoided, there is controversy on whether clean wounds should be left open or closed between serial debridements. Immediate intramedullary nailing of open femoral shaft fractures can be performed in clean wounds. Initial external fixation is useful when repeat irrigation and debridement of a contaminated intramedullary canal is necessary and in the most severely injured patients. Intravenous antibiotics should be initiated when the patient presents for treatment and should be continued until definitive wound closure takes place.

FLOATING KNEE (IPSILATERAL ASSOCIATED TIBIAL FRACTURE)

Good results, similar to those found after high-energy isolated injury, have been obtained with retrograde nailing of the femur followed by antegrade nailing of the tibia through a single anterior knee approach. These patients have a high incidence of closed degloving on the skin around the knee, and this should be carefully looked for to avoid skin necrosis and complications.

COMPLICATIONS

Vascular injury may result in fractures of the middle and lower one-thirds from injury of the femoral artery at the adductor hiatus. Compartment syndrome occurs only with significant bleeding. It presents as pain out of proportion, tense thigh swelling, numbness or paraesthesias in the medial thigh (saphenous nerve distribution), or painful passive quadriceps stretch. Fat embolism is a potentially fatal complication of femoral shaft fractures and is discussed separately in a different chapter. Non-union occurs in approximately 1–5% of fractures treated with nailing. Healing complications are more common when small diameter unreamed nails are used. Non-union is usually managed with nail removal, reaming and exchange nailing with a larger diameter nail with additional bone grafting procedures in fractures with bone loss or atrophic non-unions. Malunions are usually in conservatively treated patients and the fracture usually unites in varus, internal rotation and shortening owing to muscular deforming forces.

> **KEY LEARNING POINTS**
>
> - Diaphyseal femur fractures are the result of high-energy trauma and are associated with considerable soft-tissue damage and blood loss.
> - Unless there is gross comminution or the patient is not a surgical candidate, fractures of the shaft of the femur should be treated by closed reamed antegrade interlocking nailing.
> - Unless contraindicated stabilization should be performed within 24 hours. The more severely injured the patient, the more critical stable fixation of the femur fracture becomes. Early fixation has been shown to be associated with decreased narcotic use, reduced pulmonary complications (e.g. adult respiratory distress syndrome) and a decreased mortality rate.

REFERENCES

● = Key primary paper
◆ = Major review article

●1. Winquist RA, Hansen ST, Clawson DK. Closed intramedullary nailing of femoral fractures. *Journal of Bone and Joint Surgery (American)* 1984;**66**:529–39.

2. Kempf I, Grosse A: Beck G. Closed locked intramedullary nailing: its application to comminuted fractures of the femur. *Journal of Bone and Joint Surgery (American)* 1985;**67**:709–20.

◆3. Bhandari M, Guyatt GH, Tong D, *et al.* Reamed versus nonreamed intramedullary nailing of lower extremity long bone fractures: a systematic overview and meta-analysis. *Journal of Orthopaedic Trauma* 2000;**14**:2–9.

◆4. Bone LB, Johnson KD, Weigelt J, *et al.* Early versus delayed stabilization of femoral fractures: a prospective randomized study. *Journal of Bone and Joint Surgery (American)* 1989;**71**:336–40.

37

Distal femoral fractures

S RAJASEKARAN, VIJAY KAMATH, J DHEENADHAYALAN

Introduction	358	Treatment	359
Clinical evaluation	358	Complications	361
Radiographic evaluation	358	References	362
Classification	358		

NATIONAL BOARD STANDARDS

- Revise your knowledge of distal femur anatomy and muscular attachments
- Know the different treatment methods
- Be able to advise a patient on the prognosis and complications

INTRODUCTION

Distal femoral fractures account for about 7% of all femur fractures. A bimodal age distribution exists, with a high incidence in young adults from high-energy trauma and a second peak in the elderly from minor falls. Open fractures occur in 5–10% of all distal femur fractures.

CLINICAL EVALUATION

In patients with distal femoral fractures assessment of neurovascular status is mandatory as the proximity of the neurovascular structures to the fracture is an important anatomical consideration. The incidence of vascular disruption with isolated supracondylar fractures is between 2% and 3%; however, in the presence of a knee dislocation this approaches up to 40%. A pulseless pale limb with a tense swelling in the popliteal area or severe ecchymosis would suggest rupture of a major vessel. When a distal femoral fracture is associated with an overlying laceration, care must be taken during debridement to determine whether the wound has connection with the knee joint.

RADIOGRAPHIC EVALUATION

In addition to the anteroposterior and lateral views, two 45° oblique radiographs help to determine the fracture pattern. Traction views are helpful to determine the fracture pattern better. Complex intra-articular fractures and osteochondral lesions may require CT for accurate assessment of fracture geometry and pre-operative planning. MRI may be of value in evaluating associated injuries to ligamentous or meniscal structures. In the presence of a suspected vascular injury an arteriogram or MR angiography is indicated.

CLASSIFICATION

The classification of distal femoral fractures described by Müller et al.[1] (Fig. 37.1 and Table 37.1) and expanded in the AO classification is useful in determining treatment and prognosis. It is based on the location and pattern of the fracture and considers all fractures within the transepicondylar width of the knee.

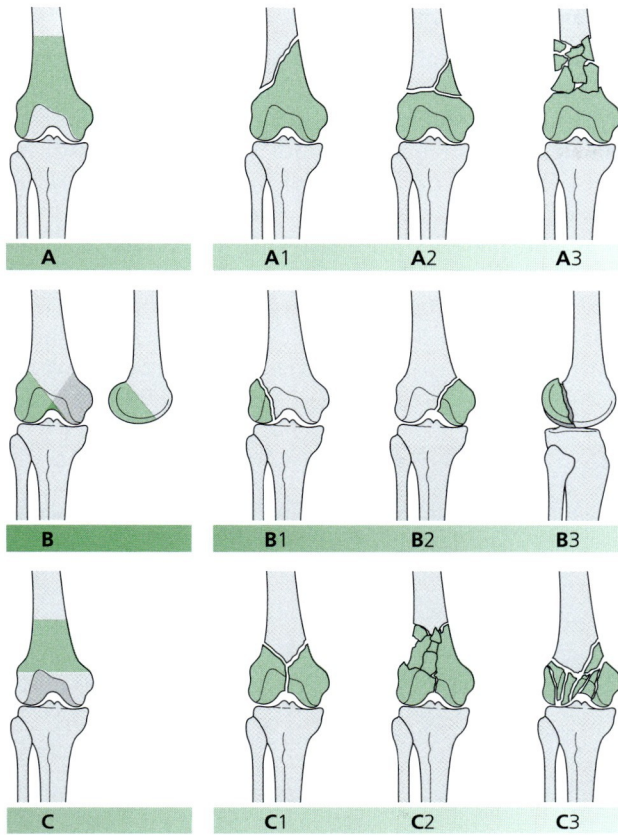

Figure 37.1 The Müller classification system of supracondylar/intracondylar femur fractures. Reproduced with permission from Müller ME, Nazarian S, Koch P, Schatzker J (eds). *The Comprehensive Classification of Fractures of Long Bones*. Berlin, Germany: Springer-Verlag, 1990.

Table 37.1 Müller classification of distal femoral fractures

Type	Description
Type A	Fractures involve the distal shaft only with varying degrees of comminution
Type B	Condylar fractures:
B1	A sagittal split of the lateral condyle
B2	A sagittal split of the medial condyle
B3	A coronal plane fracture (Hoffa fracture)
Type C	T-condylar and Y-condylar fractures
C1	No comminution
C2	A comminuted shaft fracture with two principal articular fragments
C3	Fractures have intra-articular comminution

TREATMENT

Distal femoral fractures may be managed surgically or non-operatively depending on the fracture pattern and displacement.[2]

Non-operative

Non-operative management is indicated in incomplete or undisplaced fractures, impacted stable fractures in elderly patients, in the presence of severe osteopenia and in patients with significant medical comorbidities. Stable, undisplaced fractures are managed in a hinged knee brace, with partial weight bearing. Displaced distal femoral fractures are best managed by surgical stabilization; however, if surgery is contraindicated, a 6–12 week period of skeletal traction is followed by bracing. The objective is not absolute anatomical reduction, but restoration of the knee joint axis to a normal relationship with the hip and ankle. Complications include knee stiffness, varus and internal rotation deformity and the complications associated with prolonged recumbency.

Operative treatment

Most displaced supracondylar and intercondylar distal femur fractures are amenable to surgical fixation with either plate osteosynthesis or intramedullary nailing.

PRINCIPLES OF THE MANAGEMENT OF INTRA-ARTICULAR FRACTURES

- Anatomical reconstruction of the articular surface and stabilization with interfragmentary lag screws.
- Reattachment of the articular segment to the proximal segment, with an effort to restore the normal anatomical relationships.
- The fixation must be stable enough to allow early knee mobilization and prevent knee stiffness.
- A correct choice of implant must be made to suit the fracture anatomy.

CHOICE OF IMPLANT

The various implants used for stabilizing these fractures include intramedullary nails, plates of various designs and screws only.

Screws

Fixation by interfragmentary lag screws alone is indicated in non-comminuted, unicondylar fractures in young adults with good bone stock.

Plates

Plates that offer a fixed angle construct, such as 95° blade plates, 95° condylar screws and locking plate devices, are indicated when treating fractures with metaphyseal comminution. These constructs minimize the risk of varus collapse seen with traditional non-fixed angle devices such as condylar buttress plates. The *95° condylar blade plate* was one of the first plate and screw devices to gain wide acceptance for treatment of distal femur fractures. This provides

excellent fracture fixation but is technically demanding as accurate insertion in three planes simultaneously is required.
- *Dynamic condylar screw (DCS)*. A minimum of 4 cm of uncomminuted bone in the femoral condyles above the intercondylar notch is necessary for successful fixation. This is technically easier to insert than a condylar blade plate, and interfragmentary compression is also possible through its lag screw design. Overall, results are similar to the results obtained with blade plates. Disadvantages of the DCS are the bulkiness of the device and the poorer rotational control than with the blade plate.
- *Condylar buttress plates* are commonly used in fractures with less than 3–4 cm of intact femoral condylar bone and in fractures with a large amount of articular comminution. The numerous holes in the distal end of the plate allow multiple screws to be directed into comminuted fragments. The screw, however, may toggle within the plate holes, and in highly comminuted medial buttress fractures this may lead to loss of fixation and varus malunion. In the presence of medial instability after application of a lateral buttress plate, an additional medial buttress plate is recommended. This, however, entails extensive soft-tissue damage.
- *Locking plates* (Fig. 37.2) with fixed angle screws provide increased stability of the construct and are an alternative to the DCS and blade plate. The screws lock to the plate and therefore provide angular stability to the construct. These plates offer multiple distal and proximal locking options. The less invasive stabilization technique plate, which uses locked screws and percutaneous fixation after indirect reduction of the fracture, may be used. This has the advantages of reduced soft-tissue injury and biological fixation but the procedure is technically demanding. With such minimally invasive techniques, the use of bone grafts, even in the presence of metaphyseal comminution, is not routinely necessary.[3]

Intramedullary nails

These devices obtain more 'biological' fixation than plates because they are load-sharing, rather than load-sparing, implants. They offer greater soft-tissue preservation, and bone grafting is required less often.[4] The major disadvantage of nail fixation is that it provides less rigid stabilization of distal femoral fractures than plate fixation.

A retrograde intramedullary nail (supracondylar nail) inserted through the intercondylar notch can be used to treat type A and many type C1 and type C2 fractures (Fig. 37.3) that are within 4–5 cm of the intercondylar notch. Intra-articular type C1 and type C2 fractures with non-displaced

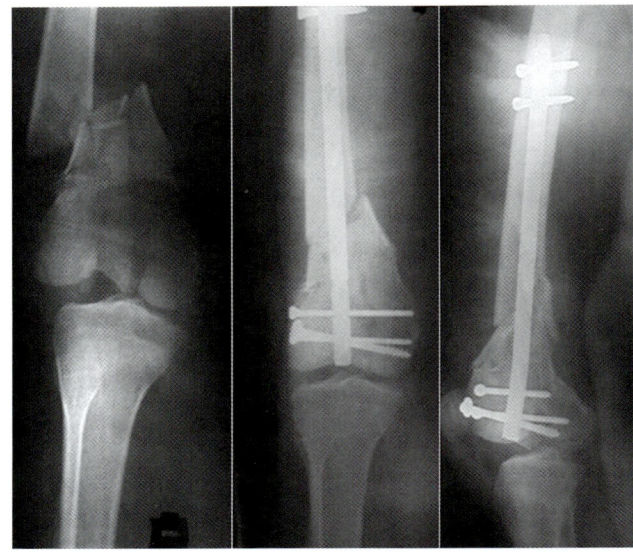

Figure 37.3 AO type C2 fracture stabilized with a supracondylar nail. The intercondylar fragments were stabilized with interfragmentary lag screws prior to passage of the supracondylar nail.

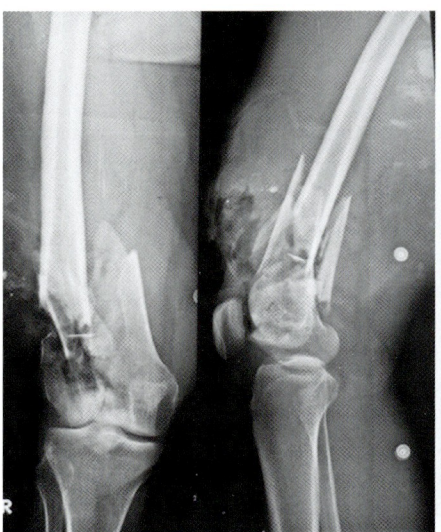

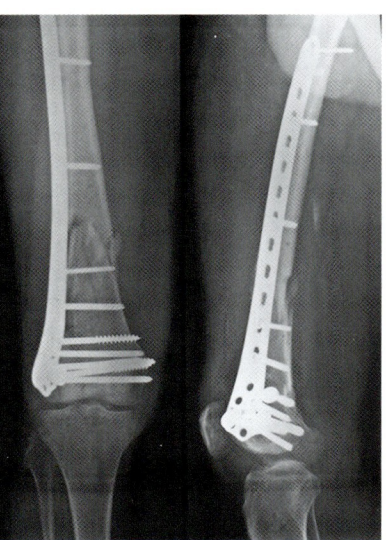

Figure 37.2 AO type C2 fracture stabilized with a locking plate.

intercondylar splits can be converted to type A patterns with percutaneous screw fixation of the condyles, usually with 6.5 mm cannulated screws before intramedullary nailing.[5] The screws are placed such that they do not interfere with subsequent retrograde nailing. The disadvantages of this device include knee stiffness, patellofemoral problems and the potential for knee sepsis in the event of postoperative infection. Antegrade intramedullary nails have limited use owing to the wide canal in this region, and are usually associated with a higher incidence of malunions and non-unions.

External fixation

In patients whose medical condition requires rapid fracture stabilization, fractures associated with vascular injury or in patients with major soft-tissue lesions, external fixation allows for rapid fracture stabilization while still allowing access to the limb and patient mobilization. Definitive treatment by external fixation (unilateral half-pin fixator or a hybrid frame) is rarely used because of the problems of pin tract infection, quadriceps scarring, delayed or non-union, and loss of reduction after device removal.

Special situations

Vascular injury is encountered in 2% of cases of distal femoral fractures. Arteriography or MR angiography helps to confirm the diagnosis and site of injury. If arterial reconstruction is necessary, temporary fixation with an external fixator should be performed prior to the vascular repair. Definitive fracture management can proceed after the vascular procedure is completed. Fasciotomy of the lower leg should be considered in all cases requiring vascular reconstruction to avoid compartment syndrome.

Condylar fractures

Unicondylar fractures (AO type B) are rare. If suspected a CT scan is often helpful to describe the fracture in more detail. Undisplaced fractures can be treated non-operatively, but must be followed closely for loss of reduction. Displaced unicondylar fractures require surgical fixation to prevent the complications of axial malalignment, post-traumatic arthritis, knee stiffness and instability frequently reported after non-operative treatment. These fractures can often be stabilized with interfragmentary screws, and in the presence of osteoporotic bone additional support with a buttress plate is indicated.

Postoperative management (Table 37.2)

In the immediate postoperative period, if the condition of the skin and soft tissues allows, the injured limb should be mobilized on a continuous passive motion device. Active range of motion exercises and partial weight bearing with crutches is started 2–3 days after stable fixation. Weight bearing is allowed with radiographic evidence of healing, which usually occurs by 6–12 weeks.

Table 37.2 Summary of management strategies for supracondylar and intercondylar femur fractures

Situation	Treatment option
Unicondylar fractures: undisplaced or displaced less than 1 mm (AO type B)	A hinged knee brace or cast-brace with regular follow-up; alternatively, percutaneous screw fixation
Displaced unicondylar fractures (AO type B)	Open reduction and internal fixation with screws or locked plates
Extra-articular distal femur fractures (AO type A)	Retrograde supracondylar nails or locking plates
T- and Y-condylar fractures (AO type C)	Internal fixation with locking plates or fixed angle 95° condylar blade plate or dynamic condylar screw

COMPLICATIONS

The common complications include failure of fixation, malunion, non-union, post-traumatic osteoarthritis and knee stiffness. Loss of knee motion is the most common complication and occurs as a result of scarring, quadriceps damage or articular disruption during injury. Failure of fixation occurs because of poor bone stock, inadequate fracture stabilization and patient non-compliance during postoperative care. Malunion usually results from unstable fixation. Varus deformity is common but malunion may occur in hyperextension or -flexion also. Non-union is less frequent because of the rich vascular supply to this region and the predominance of cancellous bone, but may occur in open injuries with bone loss or poor surgical technique with periosteal and soft-tissue damage. Post-traumatic osteoarthritis is common when the articular congruity is not restored. It may also reflect chondral injury at the time of trauma.

KEY LEARNING POINTS

- The incidence of vascular injury with isolated supracondylar fractures is between 2% and 3%, and up to 40% in the presence of a knee dislocation. Hence immediate and serial vascular status evaluation is mandatory.
- Displaced fractures, especially if involving the articular surface, require surgical stabilization, whereas non-operative management is restricted for undisplaced unicondylar or impacted supracondylar fractures.
- Fixed angle constructs, such as 95° blade plates, 95° condylar screws and locking plate devices, are preferred when treating fractures with metaphyseal comminution as these prevent varus collapse.

REFERENCES

- ● = Key primary paper
- ◆ = Major review article

●1. Müller ME, Nazarian S, Koch P, Schatzker J (eds). *The Comprehensive Classification of Fractures of Long Bones.* Berlin, Germany: Springer-Verlag, 1990.

●2. Stewart MJ, Sisk TD, Wallace SL. Fractures of the distal third of the femur: a comparison of methods of treatment. *Journal of Bone and Joint Surgery (American)* 1966;**48A**:784.

●3. Kregor PJ. Distal femur fractures with complex articular involvement: management by articular exposure and submuscular fixation. *Orthopedic Clinics of North America* 2002;**33**:153–75.

◆4. Leung KS, Shen WY, So WS, et al. Interlocking intramedullary nailing for supracondylar and intracondylar fractures of the distal part of the femur. *Journal of Bone and Joint Surgery (American)* 1991;**73**:333–40.

5. Zehntner MK, Marohesi DG, Burch H, et al. Alignment of supracondylar/intracondylar fractures of the femur after internal fixation by AO/ASIF technique. *Journal of Orthopaedic Trauma* 1992;**6**:318–26.

38

Patellar dislocation

SHANMUGANATHAN RAJASEKARAN, RISHI MUGESH KANNA, JAYARAMARAJU DHEENADHAYALAN

Introduction	363	Treatment	364
Mechanism of injury and classification	363	Complications	364
Clinical evaluation	363	References	364
Radiographic evaluation	363		

NATIONAL BOARD STANDARDS

- Understand the anatomy of the patellar retinaculum
- Able to diagnose clinically and confirmit radiologically
- Able to reduce the dislocation and explain the prognosis

INTRODUCTION

Only acute post-traumatic dislocation of the patella is discussed in this chapter. Patellar dislocation is more common in women owing to physiological laxity and in patients with connective tissue disorders (e.g. Ehlers–Danlos or Marfan syndrome).

MECHANISM OF INJURY AND CLASSIFICATION

Patellar dislocations are classified as lateral, medial, intra-articular and superior, depending on the direction of dislocation, which depends on the mechanism of the injury. Lateral dislocation is the most common, with other types seen only rarely. Lateral dislocation occurs with forced internal rotation of the femur on an externally rotated and planted tibia with the knee in flexion. Medial instability is rare and usually iatrogenic, congenital, traumatic or associated with atrophy of the quadriceps musculature.[1] Superior dislocation usually occurs in elderly individuals from forced hyperextension injuries to the knee with the patella locked on an anterior femoral osteophyte.

Intra-articular dislocations of the patella are of two types.[2] The most common type is a horizontal intra-articular dislocation of the patella with detachment of the quadriceps tendon where the articular surface of the patella is directed towards the tibial articular surface. In the other type, the patella also is dislocated horizontally, but its inferior pole is detached from the patellar tendon, and the articular surface faces proximally.

CLINICAL EVALUATION

Patients typically cannot bear weight and are unable to flex the knee. There is an associated haemarthrosis and a displaced patella is evident on palpation. Lateral dislocations have medial joint tenderness as they have medial retinacular tears at the femoral insertion of the medial patellofemoral ligament.

RADIOGRAPHIC EVALUATION

Radiographic evaluation includes anteroposterior and lateral views of the knee. A 39–71% incidence of osteochondral or chondral injury after acute patellar dislocation has been reported. An MRI of the knee is useful to identify these lesions as well as any associated medial soft-tissue injury.

TREATMENT

Acute dislocations of the patella are usually managed by closed methods.[3] Lateral dislocations are reduced by extension of the flexed knee with pressure applied to the lateral margin of the patella. The patient can ambulate in a cylindrical cast with the knee locked in extension for 3 weeks, after which time progressive flexion is instituted with physical therapy for quadriceps strengthening. Surgical intervention for acute dislocations is rarely indicated; however, any displaced osteochondral fragments should be removed, and the disrupted medial tissues, including the vastus medialis muscle, repaired. Surgical reduction is also required for intra-articular dislocations to repair the extensor mechanism.

COMPLICATIONS

The most common complication is redislocation. Young patients and those with inherent ligamentous laxity have an increased incidence of redislocation. Prolonged immobilization may result in loss of knee motion and it is important to institute early range of motion exercises. Patellofemoral pain may occur from chondral injury.

> **KEY LEARNING POINTS**
>
> - Acute patellofemoral dislocations are traumatic injuries and the patella usually dislocates laterally.
> - Diagnosis is made on clinical examination and confirmed in radiographs.
> - The dislocation can usually be reduced by manipulation and the knee joint is immobilized until the soft tissues are healed.

REFERENCES

● = Key primary paper
◆ = Major review article

◆1. Sallay PI, Poggi J, Speer KP, *et al*. Acute dislocation of the patella: a correlative pathoanatomic study. *American Journal of Sports Medicine* 1996;**24**:52.
◆2. Nsouli AZ, Nahabedian AM. Intraarticular dislocation of the patella. *Journal of Trauma* 1988;**28**:256.
◆3. Cash JD, Hughston JC. Treatment of acute patellar dislocation. *American Journal of Sports Medicine* 1988;**16**:244.

39

Knee dislocations

SHANMUGANATHAN RAJASEKARAN, RISHI MUGESH KANNA, JAYARAMARAJU DHEENADHAYALAN

Introduction	365	Classification	366
Mechanism of injury	365	Treatment	366
Clinical evaluation	365	Complications	367
Radiographic evaluation	366	References	367

NATIONAL BOARD STANDARDS

- Understand the neurovascular anatomy around the knee joint
- Know the associated ligamentous injuries
- Be able to plan treatment and explain the prognosis

INTRODUCTION

Traumatic knee dislocation is an uncommon injury but may be limb threatening as a result of associated vascular injury and hence it is managed as an orthopaedic emergency.[1] The true incidence is probably underreported as 20–50% of dislocations spontaneously reduce. Significant soft-tissue injury is necessary for a knee dislocation to occur, including rupture of at least three or four major ligamentous structures of the knee. The anterior and posterior cruciate ligaments (ACL and PCL) are disrupted in most cases, with a varying degree of injury to the collateral ligaments, capsular elements and menisci.[2] Common peroneal nerve and popliteal vessel injury may occur. Associated fractures of the tibial eminence, tibial tubercle, fibular head or neck, and capsular avulsions are also common.

MECHANISM OF INJURY

Most knee dislocations are high-energy injuries. The direction of the dislocation is determined by the abnormal force vector (Table 39.1).

CLINICAL EVALUATION

The diagnosis of a dislocated knee is usually obvious; however, as many dislocations reduce spontaneously the patient may have a relatively normal-appearing knee. Subtle signs of injury such as mild abrasions, a minimal effusion or complaints of knee pain may be the only abnormalities. In the presence of an obvious dislocation, immediate reduction should be undertaken.

Arterial injury occurs in up to 32% of dislocations and is commonly associated with posterior dislocations. A cold cyanotic foot with absence of pulses in the pedal vessels along with tenderness, swelling and ecchymosis in the popliteal fossa are signs of arterial injury and require prompt arterial evaluation and management. Repeat neurovascular examinations should be performed after any reduction manoeuvre because vasospasm or thrombosis resulting from an unsuspected intimal tear may cause delayed ischaemia hours or even days after reduction. Injury to the popliteal vein is rare. Nerve injuries occur in 16–43% of dislocations and are commonly associated with the posterolateral type. The peroneal nerve is injured more often than the tibial component. The injury usually is a neurapraxia but can also be rarely a complete transection. The extent of ligamentous injury is related

Table 39.1 Mechanism of injury and reduction manoeuvres for knee dislocations

Type of dislocation	Mechanism of injury	Reduction manoeuvres
Anterior	Forceful knee hyperextension beyond −30° with or without varus/valgus stress	Axial limb traction is combined with lifting of the distal femur
Posterior	Posteriorly directed force against the proximal tibia of a flexed knee as in a 'dashboard' injury	Axial limb traction is combined with extension and lifting of the proximal tibia
Medial/lateral	Varus force disrupts lateral supporting structures/valgus force disrupts medial supporting structures	Axial limb traction is combined with lateral/medial translation of the tibia
Rotatory	Varus/valgus with rotatory component	Axial limb traction is combined with derotation of the tibia

to the degree of displacement, with injury occurring with displacement greater than 10–25% of the resting length of the ligament. Gross instability after reduction indicates extensive soft-tissue disruption.

RADIOGRAPHIC EVALUATION

A knee dislocation is a potentially limb-threatening condition, hence immediate reduction is sometimes recommended even before radiographic evaluation. Following reduction, anteroposterior (AP) and lateral views of the knee should be obtained to assess the reduction and evaluate associated injuries. Irregular and asymmetric joint spaces, lateral capsular avulsions of the ligaments and osteochondral defects (Segond sign–avulsion fracture of the lateral tibial plateau) may be observed on the radiographs. Widened knee joint spaces may indicate soft-tissue interposition and the need for open reduction. After the initial reduction, MRI is useful for evaluation of ligament and meniscus injuries, occult fractures, articular cartilage lesions and capsular disruption. MRI gives essential information for pre-operative planning for ligament reconstruction, such as the number of allografts that will be needed.[3]

CLASSIFICATION

Knee dislocation is classified primarily by the direction of the dislocated tibia in relation to the femur (anterior, posterior, medial, lateral and rotatory). Rotary dislocations are designated further as anteromedial, anterolateral, posteromedial or posterolateral. The description should include open vs closed and reducible vs irreducible. It may be classified as occult, indicating a knee dislocation that has spontaneously reduced.

TREATMENT

Immediate closed reduction is essential even at the site of the accident. Direct pressure on the popliteal space should be avoided during or after reduction. Reduction manoeuvres for specific dislocations are given in Table 39.1. After reduction, the haemarthrosis is aspirated and the knee immobilized in full extension. The neurocirculatory status should be checked frequently for 5–7 days.

Posterolateral dislocations are often 'irreducible' owing to buttonholing of the medial femoral condyle through the medial capsule, resulting in a dimple sign over the medial aspect of the limb. This requires an open reduction.

After reduction, the ligamentous injuries can be managed non-operatively or by surgical repair. Non-operative management entails immobilization in extension in a brace for 6 weeks. External fixation is indicated if the reduction is unstable or subluxes during immobilization in a brace, in obese patients, in open injuries, polytrauma patients with or without head injury and if vascular repair has been performed. Alternatively a large transarticular pin can be placed through the intercondylar notch of the femur into the intercondylar eminence of the tibia to provide immediate stability. Most authors recommend repair of the torn structures as non-operative treatment has been associated with poorer outcomes than operative treatment.

Indications for emergency surgery after knee dislocation include vascular injury, open fractures, open dislocations, irreducible dislocation and compartment syndrome. Restoration of vascular integrity takes precedence over other injuries. Vascular injuries require external fixation and vascular repair with a reverse saphenous vein graft from the contralateral leg. Amputation rates as high as 86% have been reported when there is a delay beyond 8 hours in restoration of circulation. A fasciotomy should be performed at the time of vascular repair for limb ischaemia to prevent compartment syndrome.

There is debate over the timing of ligamentous repair procedures after a knee dislocation. Two reasons cited for delaying surgery include allowing a period of vascular monitoring and reducing the risk of arthrofibrosis. Current literature however favours acute repair of posterolateral structures, capsular structures and avulsion fractures as soon as the condition of the patient and limb allow. A combined ACL and PCL reconstruction and meniscal injury management can be performed in a delayed fashion with acceptable results. Postoperative rehabilitation programmes after a knee dislocation should allow range-of-motion exercises as soon as the integrity of soft-tissue repair, vascular repair and ligament reconstruction permit.

COMPLICATIONS

Limited range of motion of the knee joint is the most common complication and is related to scar formation and capsular tightness. Vascular compromise may result in atrophic skin changes, hyperalgesia, claudication and muscle contracture.

> ### KEY LEARNING POINTS
>
> - Knee dislocations have potential for vascular complications and hence are true orthopaedic emergencies.
> - Immediate reduction and prompt evaluation and repair of any vascular damage in the injured extremity are mandatory.
> - Repeat vascular examination is of paramount importance because vasospasm or thrombosis resulting from an unsuspected intimal tear may cause delayed ischaemia hours or even days after reduction.
> - Surgical repair of the ligament injuries is recommended as the long-term outcomes are better than non-operative management.

REFERENCES

- ● = Key primary paper
- ◆ = Major review article

●1. Conwell HE, Alldredge RH. Complete dislocations of the knee joint: a report of 7 cases with end-results. *Surgery, Gynecology and Obstetrics* 1937;**64**:94.

◆2. Roman PD, Hopson CN, Zenni EJ Jr. Traumatic dislocation of the knee: a report of 30 cases and literature review. *Orthopedic Reviews* 1987;**16**:917.

◆3. Twaddle BC, Hunter JC, Chapman JR, *et al.* MRI in acute knee dislocation: a prospective study of clinical, MRI, and surgical findings. *Journal of Bone and Joint Surgery (British)* 1996;**78B**:573.

40

Patellar fractures and extension mechanism injuries

SHANMUGANATHAN RAJASEKARAN, RISHI MUGESH KANNA, JAYARAMARAJU DHEENADHAYALAN

Introduction	368	Complications	369
Clinical features	368	Osteochondral fractures	370
Radiographic evaluation	368	Knee extensor mechanism injuries	370
Classification	369	References	371
Treatment	369		

NATIONAL BOARD STANDARDS

- Revise your knowledge of patellar anatomy
- Know the different treatment methods
- Be able to advise a patient on the prognosis and complications

INTRODUCTION

Patellar fractures represent 1% of all skeletal injuries and are commonly seen in the age group of 20–50 years.[1] Patellar fractures may occur from direct or indirect trauma to the knee. Direct trauma produces comminuted or stellate fractures and may produce chondral injury to the distal femur or patella. Displacement is typically minimal owing to preservation of the medial and lateral retinacular expansions. More commonly, the fracture results from an abrupt quadriceps contraction, which results in an avulsion of the inferior or superior pole or a transverse fracture. Transverse fractures may be associated with tears of the medial and lateral retinacular expansions and the degree of fragment displacement suggests the extent of retinacular disruption. Most patellar fractures, however, are caused by a combination of direct and indirect forces.

CLINICAL FEATURES

Patients present with pain, swelling and tenderness of the involved knee with a feeling of giving way on attempted walking. A defect in the patella may be palpable. Inability of the patient to extend the affected knee actively usually indicates an associated disruption of the extensor mechanism and a torn retinaculum.

In direct injuries with an overlying wound, it is imperative to confirm that an open fracture or traumatic arthrotomy has not occurred. Confirmation can be achieved with a *saline retention test* by injecting 30–60 mL of 0.9% normal saline into the knee and observing extravasation of fluid from the wound. This test may not be 100% reliable in open fractures with very small traumatic arthrotomies and a thorough exploration is needed during surgery.

RADIOGRAPHIC EVALUATION

Anteroposterior (AP), lateral and axial views of the knee should be obtained. Transverse fractures usually are best seen on a lateral view, whereas vertical fractures, osteochondral fractures and articular incongruity are best evaluated on axial views. A bipartite patella, seen in 8% of the population, may be mistaken for a fracture. It usually occurs in the superolateral position, has smooth margins and is bilateral in 50% of individuals.

CLASSIFICATION

Fractures may be classified as either undisplaced or displaced or on a morphological fracture pattern as stellate, comminuted, transverse, vertical (marginal), polar or osteochondral types (Fig. 40.1).

TREATMENT

Non-operative treatment

Undisplaced or minimally displaced (2–3 mm) fractures with minimal articular disruption (1–2 mm) may be treated non-operatively in a cylinder cast for 4–6 weeks. Early weight bearing is encouraged, advancing to full weight bearing with crutches as tolerated by the patient.

Surgical treatment

OPEN REDUCTION AND INTERNAL FIXATION

Fractures with more than 3 mm of displacement or articular incongruity and open fractures are best treated operatively. Internal fixation techniques include Magnusson wiring, modified tension banding (using parallel longitudinal Kirschner wires), tension band through cannulated compression screws and circumferential cerclage wiring. The most secure fixation is obtained with modified tension band wiring (Fig. 40.2). The retinacular disruption should be repaired at the time of surgery and fixation should be secure enough to allow early motion.

PATELLECTOMY

If the amount of comminution and articular damage preclude salvage of the entire patella, a partial or total patellectomy may be indicated. Total patellectomy impairs the efficiency of the quadriceps mechanism and every effort should be made to save all of the patella or at least its proximal or the distal third, if practical (the largest fragment is preserved).[2] The extensor mechanism is reattached to the patella through drill holes. If patellar tendon advancement is performed, care is taken to reattach the tendon to the remaining central portion of the patella to maintain an extensor mechanism that is congruous in the patellofemoral articulation. In the presence of an extensively comminuted fracture, a total patellectomy may be required. Postoperatively, if stable internal fixation is achieved, gentle active-assisted and passive flexion exercises are initiated after 7–10 days. Active extension is delayed for 6 weeks. When a partial patellectomy has been done or less stable constructs are achieved, the knee joint is maintained in extension for approximately 6 weeks before initiating flexion.

COMPLICATIONS

Common complications associated with patellar fractures are post-traumatic osteoarthritis, loss of knee motion and decreased extensor strength with a lag. Rare complications include refracture, non-union (2%) and osteonecrosis.

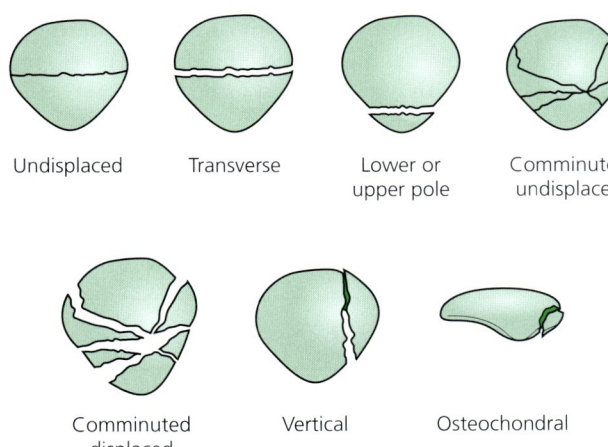

Figure 40.1 Classification of patellar fractures.

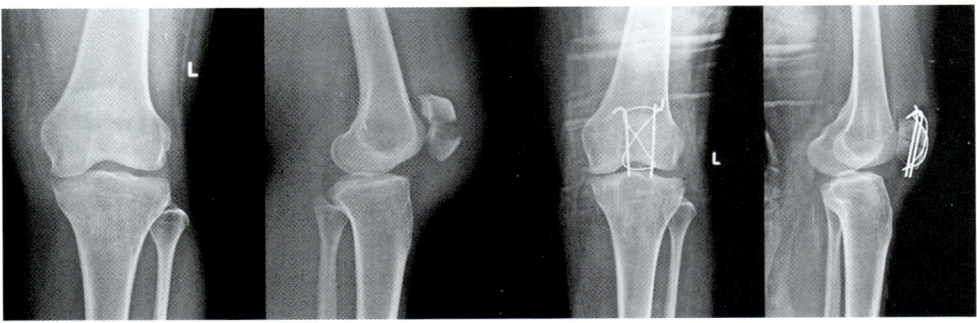

Figure 40.2 Anteroposterior and lateral radiographs of a patient with a displaced transverse patellar fracture. The fracture has been treated by open reduction and internal fixation with tension band wiring.

OSTEOCHONDRAL FRACTURES

This is often the result of a patellar dislocation. If an osteochondral fracture is suspected, an arthroscopy to inspect the joint and remove small fragments of bone and cartilage may be of benefit. A large osteochondral fragment can have an adequate osseous layer and may be amenable for open or arthroscopic fixation. Cartilage injuries predispose to early arthritic changes.[3]

KNEE EXTENSOR MECHANISM INJURIES

The extensor mechanism consists of the quadriceps muscle complex, quadriceps tendon, patella, patellar tendon and patellar tendon insertion into the tibial tubercle. Disruption of the extensor mechanism occurs during a sudden eccentric contraction of the quadriceps muscles with the foot planted and the knee flexed. Extensor mechanism disruptions commonly occur in patients with systemic illness such as diabetes or renal failure, or with the use of exogenous steroids. Corticosteroid injections for treatment of patellar tendinitis are associated with an increased incidence of rupture. Early recognition of this injury is crucial because results of early surgical repair of both quadriceps and patellar tendon ruptures are more favourable than late repair or reconstruction.[4]

Quadriceps tendon rupture

The quadriceps tendon usually ruptures within 2 cm proximal to the superior pole of the patella. In patients less than 40 years of age, ruptures are most often mid-substance, whereas in those over the age of 40 years rupture usually occurs at the bone–tendon junction. Patients usually present with sensation of a sudden 'pop' while stressing the extensor mechanism and pain in the knee. There is usually tenderness and a palpable defect proximal to the superior pole of the patella. With a complete rupture, the patient will be unable to perform a straight leg-raising effort. A partial tear frequently results in the patient's ability to lift his or her leg, but with a considerable lag.

Anteroposterior and lateral radiographs with the knee in 30° of flexion is obtained. Distal displacement of the patella (patella baja) may be observed. On the flexion lateral radiograph, the lower pole of the patella should be at the level of the line projected anteriorly from the intercondylar notch (*Blumensaat line*). In cases of an unclear diagnosis, an MRI or an ultrasound may be obtained.

An incomplete tear with active full knee extension is managed with immobilization of the knee in extension for 4–6 weeks. Complete ruptures require repair. The quadriceps tendon is reapproximated to bone using non-absorbable sutures passed through bone tunnels. The tendon is repaired close to the articular surface to avoid patellar tilting. Mid-substance tears are treated with end-to-end repair. A distally based partial-thickness quadriceps tendon turned down across the repair site (Codivilla technique) helps to reinforce the repair. Chronic tears require a V–Y advancement of a retracted quadriceps tendon.

Patellar tendon rupture

Patellar tendon rupture is usually associated with degenerative changes of the tendon. The proximal and distal insertion areas are relatively avascular and hence are common sites of rupture. Rupture occurs most commonly at the inferior pole of the patella.

Patients usually present with a sensation of a sudden 'pop' while stressing the extensor mechanism, an inability to bear weight or extend the knee against gravity and pain in the knee. There is usually a palpable defect with pain during passive knee flexion and partial or complete loss of active extension. Anteroposterior and flexion lateral radiographs are obtained similar to when assessing a quadriceps tendon rupture. A *patella alta* (proximal displacement of patella) will be observed.

Partial tears with active full knee extension are managed with limb immobilization in extension for 3–6 weeks. In complete ruptures, the patellar tendon is reattached to the patella with non-absorbable sutures passed through longitudinal bone tunnels and the retinacular tear repaired.[5] The repair may be reinforced with wire or cable. Postoperatively the knee is immobilized in a hinged knee brace locked at 20° with active flexion, and passive extension exercises are initiated after 2 weeks. Active extension is allowed after 3 weeks.

KEY LEARNING POINTS

- Patellar fracture can occur by both direct and indirect trauma.
- It is important to identify and treat injuries to the retinacular expansions.
- Undisplaced fractures can be treated through non-operative methods with an above-knee plaster cast.
- In displaced fractures, operative treatment is advantageous for the following reasons: improved fracture reduction, maintenance of reduction until union, re-establishment of soft-tissue continuity and restoration of the functional integrity of the knee joint.
- Open reduction and wire fixation is the operative treatment of choice for patellar fractures.
- Quadriceps and patellar tendon ruptures are treated by operative methods as chronic unhealed tendon ruptures have a poor prognosis.

REFERENCES

● = Key primary paper
◆ = Major review article

◆1. Boström A. Fracture of the patella: a study of 422 patellar fractures. *Acta Orthopaedica Scandinavica* 1972;**143**:1.
◆2. Saltzman CL, Goulet JA, McClellan T, *et al*. Results of treatment of displaced patellar fractures by partial patellectomy. *Journal of Bone and Joint Surgery (American)* 1990;**72A**:1279.
◆3. Mandelbaum BR, Seipel PR, Teurlings L. Articular cartilage lesions: current concepts and results. In: Arendt E (ed.) *Orthopaedic Knowledge Update*. Rosemont, IL: American Academy of Orthopaedic Surgeons, 1999:19–28.
◆4. Siwek CW, Rao JP. Ruptures of the extensor mechanism of the knee joint. *Journal of Bone and Joint Surgery (American)* 1981;**63A**:932.
◆5. Marder RA, Timmerman LA. Primary repair of patellar tendon rupture without augmentation. *American Journal of Sports Medicine* 1999;**27**:304.

ID
Tibial plateau fractures

SHANMUGANATHAN RAJASEKARAN, VIJAY KAMATH, JAYARAMARAJU DHEENADHAYALAN

Introduction	372	Treatment	373
Mechanism of injury	372	Complications	375
Clinical evaluation	372	Tibial spine fractures	375
Radiographic evaluation	373	References	376
Classification	373		

NATIONAL BOARD STANDARDS

- Revise your knowledge of tibial plateau anatomy
- Understand the mechanism of injury
- Know the different types and the treatment principles
- Be able to advise a patient on the prognosis and complications

INTRODUCTION

Tibial plateau fractures constitute 1% of all fractures. Bicondylar fractures account for 10–30%, whereas isolated medial and lateral plateau injuries account for the remaining injuries. Although only 3% of these fractures are open injuries, many of them have closed degloving, deep abrasions or severe soft-tissue injuries which require careful consideration in deciding the timing and nature of surgery.[1]

MECHANISM OF INJURY

Tibial plateau fractures have a bimodal age distribution. In young individuals with strong bones, these fractures follow high-energy injuries and are often split fractures with associated ligamentous disruption. In elderly patients with osteopenic bone, these may occur after a simple fall. Here depression and split depression fractures are common without any ligamentous injury.

Fractures of the tibial plateau occur as a result of varus or valgus forces coupled with axial loading. The direction and magnitude of the generated force, age of the patient, bone quality and amount of knee flexion at impact determine the size, location and displacement of the fragments (Fig. 41.1).

CLINICAL EVALUATION

The knee is usually swollen, painful with some deformity. Haemarthrosis occurs frequently and aspiration may reveal marrow fat, indicating a fracture. The extent of injury to the overlying soft tissues must be carefully assessed and even small lacerations must be suspected to have a communication with the joint. Intra-articular instillation of 50–75 mL of normal saline may be necessary to evaluate possible communication with overlying lacerations. There may be associated meniscal tears in up to 50% and cruciate or collateral ligamentous injury in up to 30% of tibial plateau fractures.

Neurovascular injury and compartment syndrome must be ruled out, particularly with high-energy injuries. The trifurcation of the popliteal artery is tethered posteriorly between the adductor hiatus proximally and the soleus complex distally. Hence tibial plateau fractures are often associated with neurovascular injuries. Arterial

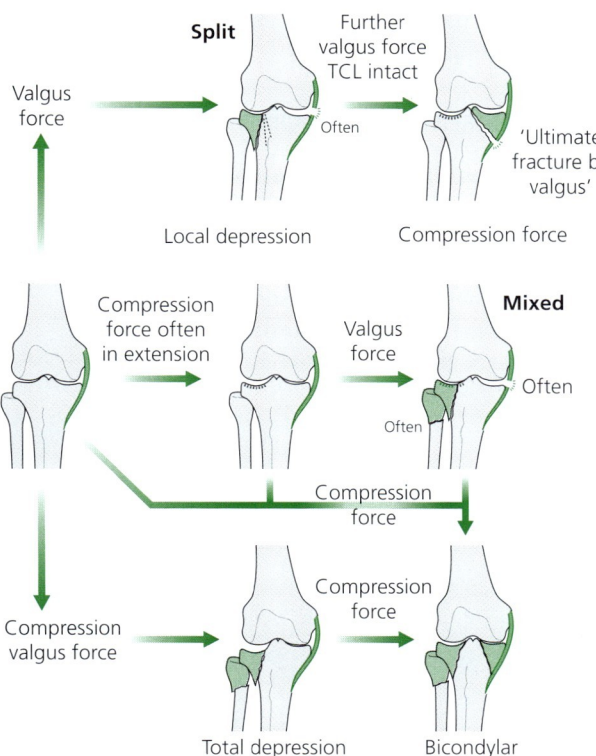

Figure 41.1 Relationship of force to tibial condylar fractures. Tibial collateral ligament (TCL) injuries commonly occur in split and mixed fractures of lateral plateau. In mixed fractures, the fibula is often fractured. In total depression fractures, proximal fibular fracture or proximal tibiofibular diastasis occurs. Redrawn with permission from Schulak DJ, Gunn DR. Fractures of the tibial plateaus: a review of the literature. *Clinical Orthopedic and Related Research* 1975;**109**:166.

injuries are usually traction-induced intimal damage presenting as thrombosis and only rarely do lacerations occur. The peroneal nerve is similarly tethered laterally as it courses around the fibular neck and can be injured due to stretching (neurapraxia).

RADIOGRAPHIC EVALUATION

Anteroposterior and lateral radiographs supplemented by 40° internal and external rotation oblique projections for lateral and medial plateau visualization should be obtained. A 10–15° caudally tilted plateau view can be used to assess articular step-off. Avulsion of the fibular head, the Segond sign (lateral capsular avulsion) and Pellegrini–Steada lesion (calcification along the insertion of the medial collateral ligament) are all signs of associated ligamentous injury. Stress views with fluoroscopic image intensification with the patient under mild sedation are useful for the detection of collateral ligament injuries.

Table 41.1 Schatzker classification of tibial plateau fractures

Type	Description
Type I	Lateral plateau, split fracture
Type II	Lateral plateau, split depression fracture
Type III	Lateral plateau, depression fracture
Type IV	Medial plateau fracture
Type V	Bicondylar plateau fracture
Type VI	Plateau fracture with separation of the metaphysis from the diaphysis

The degree of fragmentation or depression of the articular surface is better delineated with CT with three-dimensional reconstructed images. MRI is useful for evaluating injuries to the menisci, the cruciate and collateral ligaments, and also the soft-tissue envelope. CT or MRI angiography is required in the setting of suspected vascular injury.

CLASSIFICATION

Tibial plateau fractures have been classified by Schatzker into six types (Table 41.1). Types I–III are low-energy injuries while types IV–VI are high-energy injuries (Fig. 41.2).

TREATMENT

Principles of management

NON-SURGICAL TREATMENT

Non-surgical treatment is recommended for low-energy tibial plateau fractures which are stable to varus–valgus stress and include undisplaced or minimally displaced fractures. Non-surgical treatment is also indicated in non-ambulatory patients and those not medically fit for surgery. Treatment includes the use of a hinged knee brace and mobilization. Active-assisted and passive range of motion exercises are initiated immediately and weight bearing is typically delayed for 8–12 weeks. Alternatively, an above-knee cast may be used.

SURGICAL TREATMENT

Surgery is indicated in the following situations:

- articular depression of >5 mm or instability of >10° (because of depression or condyle subluxation) compared with the contralateral side
- high-energy injuries involving the metaphyseal–diaphyseal junction or unstable bicondylar fractures

- open fractures, associated compartment syndrome and vascular injuries
- floating knees injuries with associated lower femoral fractures.

Current surgical treatment strategies include open reduction and internal fixation (ORIF) with adjunctive techniques such as limited open reduction, arthroscopically assisted reduction and fixation,[2] and augmented internal fixation with resorbable bone cements. External fixation including temporary spanning fixators, hybrid and/or fine-wire fixation, and combined limited ORIF are acceptable techniques, particularly for patients with significant soft-tissue injury (Fig. 41.3).

OPERATIVE TREATMENT PRINCIPLES

1. Soft-tissue injuries should heal prior to surgical stabilization as this avoids wound dehiscence and infection.
2. Reconstruction of the articular surface and re-establishment of tibial alignment is the goal. Guidelines for fixation according to the fracture pattern are given in Table 41.2.

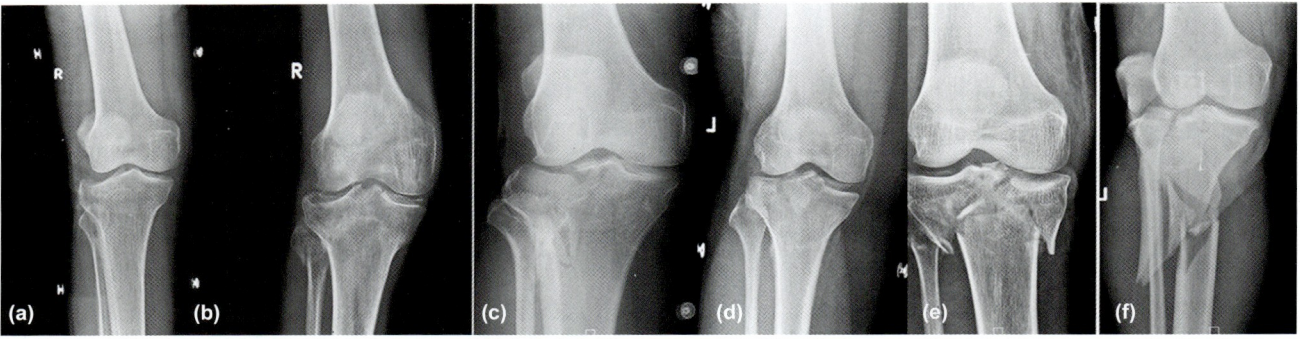

Figure 41.2 (a–f) The six types of tibial plateau injuries (Schatzker classification).

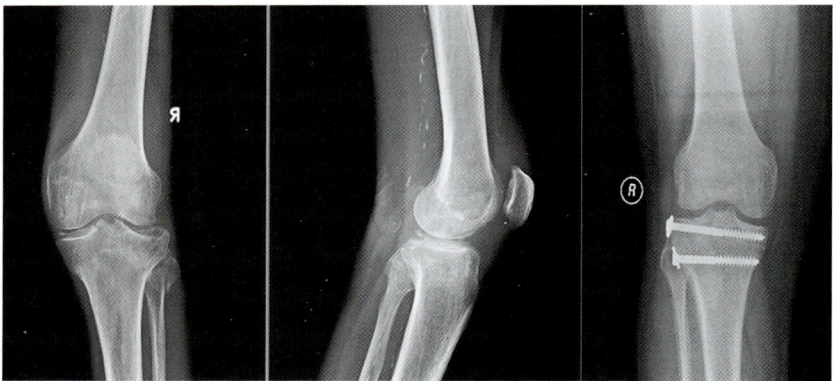

Figure 41.3 Schatzker type II tibial plateau fracture treated with open reduction, impaction bone grafting and fixation with cancellous screws.

Table 41.2 Guidelines for fixation according to the fracture pattern

Type	Description
Type I	Displaced uncomminuted fragments can be fixed with two transverse cancellous screws. Open reduction and fixation with a buttress or locked plate is generally done if there is a significant widening
Type II	Open reduction, elevation of the depressed plateau 'en masse', bone grafting of the metaphysis with fixation of the fracture with cancellous screws in the subchondral region: 'raft' screws, and buttress plating of the lateral cortex (Fig. 41.4)
Type III	Elevation of the articular fragments, bone-grafting, and buttress plating of the lateral cortex
Type IV	Open reduction and fixation with a medial buttress plate and cancellous screws (Fig. 41.5)
Type V	Fracture reduction is similar to type II injuries. Both condyles can be fixed with buttress plates; however, dual plating has a high incidence of soft-tissue healing problems and infection rates. Alternatively, the most unstable condyle (usually lateral) is selected for the buttress fixation via an anterolateral approach and the other condyle is stabilized by percutaneous screw fixation. Fractures of the posterior medial plateau may require a posteromedial incision for fracture reduction and plate stabilization
Type VI	Treatment is similar to type V fractures. Alternatively hybrid external fixation may also be used

3. The menisci should never be excised to facilitate exposure.
4. Injuries to the meniscus as well as intra-articular and extra-articular ligamentous structures should be addressed. Avulsed anterior cruciate ligament or posterior cruciate ligament with a large bony fragment should be repaired. Reconstruction of intrasubstance cruciate ligament tears should be delayed.
5. Arthroscopy may be used to evaluate the adequacy of reduction of articular surfaces, the menisci and the cruciate ligaments. Arthroscopic-assisted reduction and fixation is a useful tool for accurate reduction of articular surfaces.
6. Biological plate fixation and percutaneous screw fixation reduce soft-tissue damage and wound-healing complications.
7. Use of locked plates eliminates the need for double plating of bicondylar tibial plateau fractures and is also useful in osteoporotic bone.
8. Postoperative continuous passive motion and active range of motion exercises are important to achieve a good range of joint motion (Table 41.2, Figs 41.4 and 41.5).

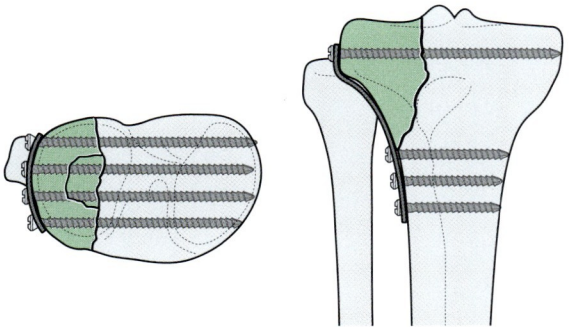

Figure 41.4 Peri-articular tibial plateau fixation with 'raft' or subchondral screws. The screws maintain the articular reduction, but offer no stability for the metadiaphyseal component of the injury.

COMPLICATIONS

The most common complication is knee stiffness. This occurs as a result of trauma from injury and surgical dissection, extensor retinacular injury, scarring of soft tissues and prolonged postoperative immobility. Malunion or non-union is commonly seen in Schatzker VI fractures at the metaphyseal–diaphyseal junction and this is related to the extent of comminution, unstable fixation, implant failure or infection. Post-traumatic osteoarthritis results from articular incongruity, chondral damage at the time of injury or malalignment of the mechanical axis. Infection may occur as a result of incisions through compromised soft tissues with extensive dissection for implant placement and is more common when dual plating is employed.

TIBIAL SPINE FRACTURES

Tibial spine or tibial eminence fractures are terms used to describe an injury to the intercondylar region of the tibial plateau. The tuberculum intercondylare mediale is the site of insertion of the ACL. No ligamentous insertions occur on the lateral portion of the tibial eminence. Tibial spine fractures often follow a simple, low-energy fall onto an outstretched leg. The ACL, although intact, is typically avulsed at the insertion and may become functionally incompetent. Occasionally, the fracture will extend into the weight-bearing portion of the articular surface of the medial tibial plateau.

The fractures are classified into three types based on the extent of displacement. Type I fractures are undisplaced, type II fractures are partially displaced or hinged and type III fractures are completely displaced. A fourth type, the comminuted tibial eminence fracture, has also been described.

Surgical intervention is preferable for type III and IV fractures as a high incidence of ACL incompetence has been reported with non-surgical treatment. An open surgical technique with a parapatellar arthrotomy and internal fixation with lag screws is usually done. The current favoured techniques include arthroscopically assisted reduction and internal fixation.[3] This technique

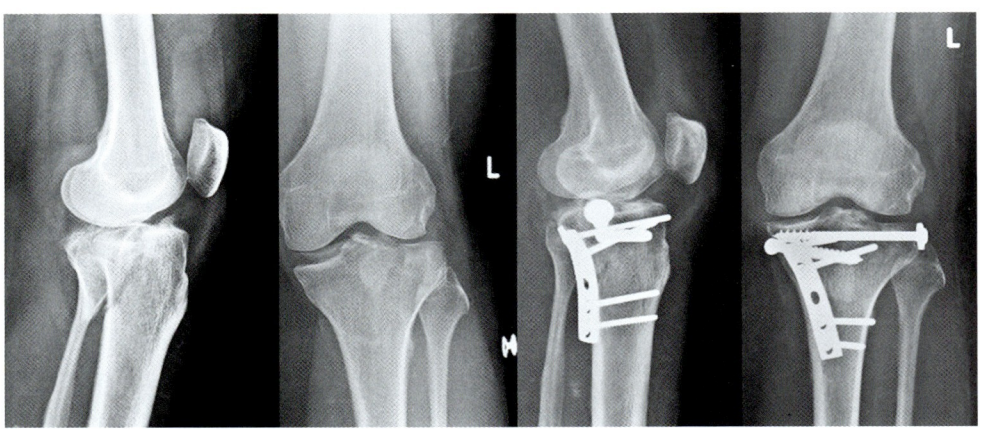

Figure 41.5 Schatzker type IV fracture treated by open reduction and internal fixation with medial buttress plating and lateral lag screws.

is accomplished using standard arthroscopic portals with an accessory portal placed high anterolaterally or anteromedially to manipulate the fracture. The fracture is reduced and secured with percutaneous Kirschner wires followed by cannulated screw fixation. Postoperatively, active-assisted range of motion is initiated immediately in a hinged brace. A rehabilitation protocol, similar to that used for an ACL injury is followed.

KEY LEARNING POINTS

- In young patients, these injuries are high-energy injuries and are often associated with significant oedema, soft-tissue injury and/or neurovascular injury.
- CT scans are helpful for assessment of displacement of the fragments and for surgical planning.
- It is important to wait for soft-tissue healing prior to undertaking internal fixation to avoid skin necrosis and wound complications.
- Indications for surgical stabilization include articular incongruence of 5–8 mm and more than 10° of joint instability.
- Locking fixed-angle plates provide the option of stabilizing various fracture patterns with the use of a single device and are especially useful in osteoporotic bones.

REFERENCES

- ● = Key primary paper
- ◆ = Major review article

◆●1. Schatzker J, McBroom R. Tibial plateau fractures: The Toronto experience 1968–1975. *Clinical Orthopaedics and Related Research* 1979;**138**:94–104.

◆2. Hung SS, Chao EK, Chan YS, *et al.* Arthroscopically assisted osteosynthesis for tibial plateau fractures. *Journal of Trauma* 2003;**54**:356–63.

◆3. Reynders P, Reynders K, Broos P. Pediatric and adolescent tibial eminence fractures: arthroscopic cannulated screw fixation. *Journal of Trauma* 2002;**53**:49–54.

42

Fractures of the tibia and fibula

SHANMUGANATHAN, VIJAY KAMATH, JAYARAMARAJU DHEENADHAYALAN

Introduction	377	Treatment	378
Anatomy	377	Special situations	380
Mechanism of injury	377	Complications	380
Clinical evaluation	378	Stress fractures	380
Radiographic evaluation	378	Isolated fibular shaft fractures	380
Classification	378	References	380

NATIONAL BOARD STANDARDS

- Revise your knowledge of anatomy of the leg and its compartments
- Know the injury mechanism
- Be able to carry out initial management of tibial open injuries
- Know the different treatment methods including advantages and disadvantages
- Be able to advise a patient on the prognosis and complications

INTRODUCTION

The tibia is the most commonly fractured long bone with an approximate incidence of 26 diaphyseal fractures per 100 000 population per year. There is a high incidence of open fractures as one-third of the tibial surface is subcutaneous.

ANATOMY

The tibia is a long tubular bone with a triangular cross-section and is responsible for 85% of weight-bearing load, whereas the fibula transmits the remaining. The endosteal blood supply is from the nutrient artery that arises from the posterior tibial artery, and the bulk of the periosteal blood supply arises from the anterior tibial artery. The distal third is supplied by periosteal anastomoses around the ankle with branches entering the tibia through ligamentous attachments. There is a watershed area at the junction of the middle and distal thirds where the blood supply is reduced. If the nutrient artery is disrupted, there is reversal of flow through the cortex, and the periosteal blood supply becomes more important. It is important to preserve the periosteal attachments during fracture fixation.

MECHANISM OF INJURY

Fractures may occur as a result of direct or indirect trauma. Direct injuries are usually high-energy injuries and result in transverse or comminuted fractures with displacement and a high incidence of associated soft-tissue injury. Indirect injuries on the other hand occur as a result of torsion and result in spiral, minimally displaced fractures and little soft-tissue damage. Bending forces give rise to short oblique fractures. Crush injuries result in highly comminuted or segmental fracture patterns and are associated with extensive soft-tissue injury. Isolated fibular shaft fractures result from direct trauma to the lateral aspect of the leg. Tibial fractures associated with segmental fibular fractures usually indicate severe energy or violence.

CLINICAL EVALUATION

The diagnosis is usually obvious and evaluation of the neurovascular status in every patient is imperative. The extent of soft-tissue injury dictates the line of management. The presence of fracture blisters may contraindicate early open reduction. Compartment syndrome is a devastating complication of tibial fractures.[1] The limb must be monitored for compartment syndrome as it may present late. The classical clinical features are pain out of proportion to the injury, a tense limb and pain on gentle passive dorsiflexion of the foot (Fig. 42.1). Any patient with persistent and severe pain even after splinting and paraesthesia in the foot must be suspected to have compartment syndrome. It is important to remember that the pulse can be normally felt in the early stages, and a pale, pulseless paralytic limb are late signs of established compartment syndrome. If compartment syndrome is suspected, compartment pressures should be monitored at regular intervals. Compartment pressures higher than 30 mmHg and/or pressure within 30 mmHg of diastolic pressure are considered indications for four-compartment (anterior, lateral, superficial posterior and deep posterior) fasciotomy. Deep posterior compartment syndrome may be missed because of uninvolved overlying superficial compartment, and can result in claw toes. Tibial fractures can also be associated with a high incidence of knee ligament injuries. Following stabilization of the fracture, the presence of ligamentous instability must be checked intra-operatively.

RADIOGRAPHIC EVALUATION

Radiographic evaluation must include anteroposterior and lateral views that include the entire tibia with visualization of the ankle and knee joints. The radiographs must also be assessed for the presence of secondary fracture lines that may cause displacement during operative treatment, osseous defects and for gas in the soft tissues. Gas in the soft tissues is usually secondary to open injuries but may also signify the presence of gas gangrene, necrotizing fasciitis or other anaerobic infections. CT or magnetic resonance angiography is indicated if an arterial injury is suspected.

CLASSIFICATION

Tibial shaft fractures may be classified descriptively based on the location (proximal, middle or distal one-third), pattern (spiral, oblique or transverse), extent of displacement (shortening, translation, angulation or rotational deformity and percentage of cortical contact), extent of comminution (comminuted, segmental or butterfly fragment) and status of soft-tissue envelope (open or closed).

The Arbeitsgemeinschaft für Osteosynthesefragen (AO) classification advocates a higher level of classification for an increasing severity of injury. Type A fractures are simple fractures that are spiral, oblique or transverse. Type B fractures result from higher energy dissipation at the level of the injury and are classified as spiral, bending or fragmented wedges. Type C fractures are complex fractures with multiple spiral fractures, segmental fractures or highly comminuted fractures.

TREATMENT

The treatment depends on the morphology of the fracture, status of the soft-tissue envelope, the neurovascular status, associated skeletal and other major organ injuries and the general medical status of the patient. Most of the tibial fractures may be treated operatively or non-operatively. Surgical treatment is generally the preferred method of treatment as it allows early mobilization and avoids complications of prolonged immobilization.

Non-operative treatment

This is generally reserved for isolated, closed, low-energy fractures with minimal displacement and comminution. Union rates as high as 97% have been reported.

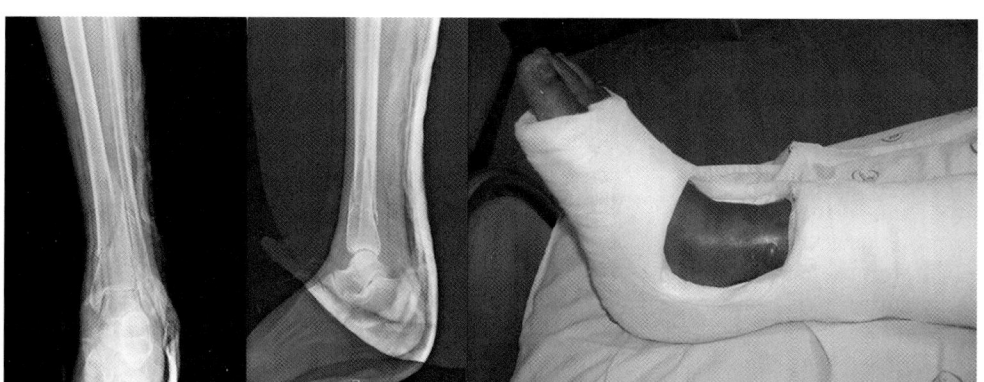

Figure 42.1 Anteroposterior and lateral radiographs of a patient who had sustained a fracture of both bones of the leg. The clinical picture shows the presence of a compromised skin condition and the presence of blisters.

Non-operative treatment involves achieving an acceptable reduction and immobilization in a long leg cast with partial weight bearing with crutches as soon as tolerated by the patient. Advancement to full weight bearing can begin by the second to fourth week. After 4–6 weeks, the long leg cast may be exchanged for a patella-bearing cast or fracture brace. The average time to union depends on the pattern of fracture and soft-tissue injury, and is generally about 16 weeks.

Recommendations for acceptable fracture reduction are less than 5° of varus–valgus angulation, less than 10° of anteroposterior angulation, less than 10° of rotation (with external rotation better tolerated than internal rotation), and less than 15 mm of shortening. More than 50% cortical contact is recommended. A rough guide to alignment of the limb is that the anterior superior iliac spine, centre of the patella and base of the second proximal phalanx should be in the same linear axis.

Operative treatment

Depending on the personality of the fracture, intramedullary nails, plates or an external fixator may be used to stabilize these fractures. Intramedullary (IM) nailing – interlocking nails or flexible IM nails (Enders, rush rods) have numerous advantages over plates. They preserve the periosteal blood supply and limit the soft-tissue damage. Interlocking nails also have the advantages of being able to control alignment, translation and rotation and are therefore recommended for most fracture patterns. Locking provides rotational control, prevents shortening in the presence of comminution and bone loss and hence it is the preferred method of internal fixation (Fig. 42.2).

The debate over the use of reamed *vs* unreamed nails is now resolved in favour of reaming. Reaming allows for the use of a larger diameter, stronger nail and gives better results in both closed and open fractures. Unreamed nails preserve the intramedullary blood supply in open fractures where the periosteal supply has been destroyed and are currently reserved mainly for higher grade open fractures. It is however significantly weaker than the larger reamed nails and is associated with a higher incidence of non-unions, loss of reduction and implant failures.[2] With the success of interlocking nails, flexible nails are rarely used. They are recommended only in children and adolescents with open physes. The significant advantage of 'biological fixation' with IM nails and the attendant complications of infection and wound breakdown associated with the use of plates have decreased their use as the primary mode of stabilization. These are generally reserved for fractures extending into the metaphysis or epiphysis. Union rates of up to 97% are reported.[3]

Plating usually requires open surgery and the location of the incision and careful handling of the soft tissues are vital in order to minimize complications. However, a certain amount of soft-tissue damage and periosteal stripping is inevitable, and this is a particular problem in comminuted or open fractures. In recent years, plates have been developed that have less periosteal contact (low-contact dynamic compression plates).

Biological plating refers to a subcutaneous plating technique in which the plate is placed in position using image guidance after fracture reduction and screws are inserted percutaneously.[4] The recent development of locking plates has potentially increased the scope of biological plating. These plates will mainly be used for extra-articular proximal tibial plateau and distal tibial plafond fractures rather than for diaphyseal fractures. They undoubtedly provide superior fixation in osteopenic bone, as all the screws have to loosen for the plate to fail. They are therefore particularly useful in treating proximal tibial fractures in older patients. The plates can be used with unicortical or bicortical screws.

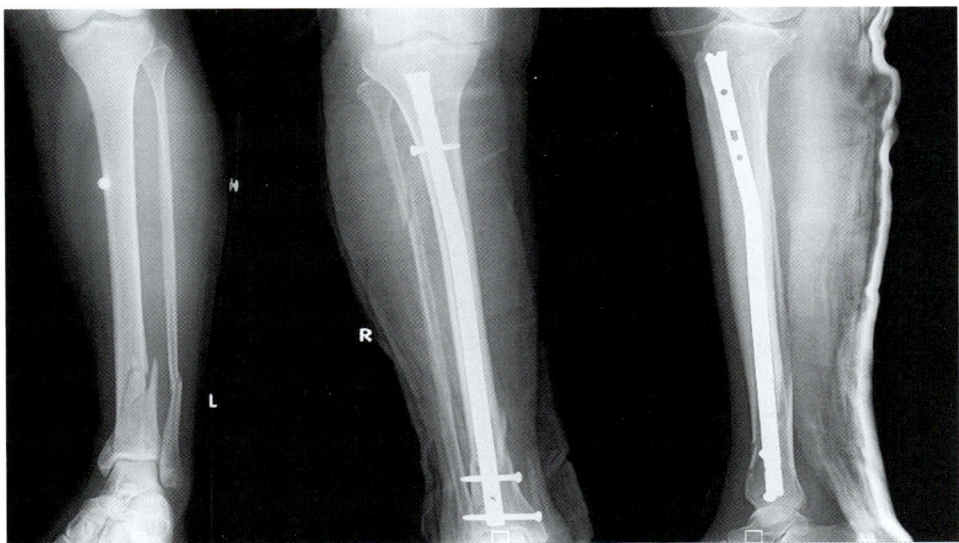

Figure 42.2 Anteroposterior radiograph of a patient who had sustained a fracture of both bones of the leg. The fracture has been reduced and fixed with an intramedullary nail as shown in the postoperative radiographs.

Currently, tibial plating is not advocated for the routine management of diaphyseal fractures. Not only does it cause unnecessary soft-tissue damage, but it is also inappropriate in comminuted fractures, as long plates are required. The only circumstances in which it might be used are when there is a proximal tibial diaphyseal fracture and when there is a combination of a proximal diaphyseal fracture and a tibial plateau fracture. Under these circumstances, the use of locking plates is preferred.

External fixation is primarily used as a temporary stabilization to treat severe open fractures. It is also indicated in closed fractures complicated by compartment syndrome and in polytrauma situations where rapid stabilization of fractures is required. Conversion to IM nails is preferably carried out within 2–3 weeks as otherwise the pin tracts may get colonized, increasing the rate of infection. Although high union rates of up to 90% have been reported, external fixators are rarely used as a definitive method of treatment owing to the high incidence of pin tract infections and poor patient tolerance.[5]

SPECIAL SITUATIONS

- Fractures of the tibial diaphysis with an intact fibula can be treated non-operatively if the tibial fracture is non-displaced. However, if it is displaced, operative treatment in the form of IM nailing is recommended.
- In tibial fractures treated non-operatively, frequent radiographic evaluation is necessary as these fractures have a tendency to develop varus deformity.
- Proximal tibia fractures near the metaphyseal–diaphyseal junction account for about 7% of all tibia diaphyseal fractures. IM nailing of these fractures is technically difficult as they tend to malalign, the commonest deformities being valgus and apex anterior angulation. The proximal fragment is difficult to control while attempting reduction. A blocking screw or a percutaneously inserted small reduction plate prior to IM nailing would help to maintain fracture reduction during nail insertion.[6]
- Distal tibia fractures treated with IM nails tend to align into valgus angulation. In such cases, a small distal fibular plate can be used to stabilize the usually coexisting fibular fracture to prevent malalignment.

COMPLICATIONS

Non-union is associated with high-velocity injuries and open fractures resulting in extensive periosteal stripping, fractures complicated by infection, the presence of an intact fibula which keeps the tibial fracture distracted, inadequate fracture fixation and improper surgical techniques.[7] In fractures complicated by compartment syndrome, the resulting ischaemia is associated with scarring of extensor tendons and posterior compartment muscles. This results in a claw toe deformity. Reflex sympathetic dystrophy is most common in patients unable to bear weight early and with prolonged cast immobilization.

STRESS FRACTURES

Stress fractures of the tibia are commonly seen in military recruits. These injuries occur most commonly at the metaphyseal–diaphyseal junction. It is characterized by the presence of sclerosis at the posteromedial cortex. In ballet dancers, these fractures are commonly seen in the middle third. They are insidious in onset and occur because of overuse.

Radiographic findings may be delayed by several weeks. Technetium bone scanning, CT and MRI scans are useful in the early diagnosis of stress fractures. Treatment primarily consists of cessation of the offending activity such as jogging and patients with acute symptoms require a short-leg walking cast.

ISOLATED FIBULAR SHAFT FRACTURES

Isolated fibular shaft fractures are treated non-operatively and this consists of weight bearing as tolerated. Although not necessary for healing, a short period of immobilization may be advised to minimize pain. Non-union is rare because of the extensive muscular attachments.

> ### KEY LEARNING POINTS
>
> - Fractures of the tibia are one of the most common serious skeletal injuries. They are slow to heal and can result in permanent sequelae.
> - The subcutaneous location of the anteromedial surface of the tibia predisposes to severe bone and soft-tissue injury, and there is a high incidence of open fractures.
> - Intramedullary locking nails are the preferred means of fracture stabilization.
> - Both acute complications, such as open injuries, compartment syndrome, neurovascular injury, and chronic sequelae, e.g. non-union, malunion, delayed union, are common with tibial fractures.

REFERENCES

- ● = Key primary paper
- ◆ = Major review article

◆1. McQueen MM, Gaston P, Court-Brown CM. Acute compartment syndrome: who is at risk? *Journal of Bone and Joint Surgery (British)* 2000;**82**:200–3.

♦2. Bhandari M, Tornetta P III, Sprague S, *et al*. Predictors of reoperation following operative management of fractures of the tibial shaft. *Journal of Orthopedic Trauma* 2003;**17**:353–61.

♦3. Keating JF, O'Brien PI, Blachut PA, *et al*. Reamed interlocking intramedullary nailing of open fractures of the tibia. *Clinical Orthopaedics and Related Research* 1997;**338**:182–91.

♦4. Collinge CA, Sanders RW. Percutaneous plating in the lower extremity. *Journal of the American Academy of Orthopaedic Surgeons* 2000;**8**:211–16.

♦5. Ricci WM, O'Boyle M, Borrelli J, *et al*. Fractures of the proximal third of the tibial shaft treated with intramedullary nails and blocking screws. *Journal of Orthopedic Trauma* 2001;**15**:264–70.

♦6. Henley MB, Chapman JR, Agel J, *et al*. Treatment of type II, IIIA, and IIIB open fractures of the tibial shaft: A prospective comparison of unreamed interlocking intramedullary nails and half-pin external fixators. *Journal of Orthopedic Trauma* 1998;**12**:1–7.

♦7. Bhandari M, Guyatt GH, Tong D, *et al*. Reamed versus nonreamed intramedullary nailing of lower extremity long bone fractures: a systematic overview and meta-analysis. *Journal of Orthopedic Trauma* 2000;**14**:2–9.

43

Tibial plafond fractures

SHANMUGANATHAN RAJASEKARAN, VIJAY KAMATH, JAYARAMARAJU DHEENADHAYALAN

Introduction	382	Classification	383
Mechanism of injury	382	Treatment	383
Clinical evaluation	382	Complications	385
Radiographic evaluation	382	References	385

NATIONAL BOARD STANDARDS

- Knowledge of the unique anatomy of the distal tibia
- Understand the mechanisms of injury
- Know the treatment principles
- Know the potential complications, their prevention and management

INTRODUCTION

The terms *tibial plafond fracture*, *pilon fracture* and *distal tibial explosion fracture* have all been used to describe intra-articular fractures of the distal tibia. These fractures account for 7–10% of all tibial fractures.

MECHANISM OF INJURY

Tibial plafond fractures can occur as a result of a variety of injury mechanisms. Falls from a height produce axial compression forces and can cause impaction of the articular surface with significant comminution. Plantarflexion or dorsiflexion of the ankle at the time of injury results in either a primarily posterior or anterior plafond injury respectively. Skiing accidents produce torsion combined with a varus or valgus stress. They often result in a fracture with two or more large fragments and minimal articular comminution. Injuries producing combined compression and shear forces result in complex fracture patterns with components of both compression and shear.

CLINICAL EVALUATION

Patients typically present with pain, swelling and deformity of the distal leg. The tibia is subcutaneous in this region and therefore there is the danger of displaced fracture fragments producing excessive skin pressure converting a closed injury into an open one. The swelling can increase, rapidly necessitating serial neurovascular examinations and assessment of skin integrity, necrosis and fracture blisters. Meticulous assessment of soft-tissue damage is of paramount importance as the thin soft-tissue envelope surrounding the distal tibia can be severely damaged. This may result in inadequate healing of surgical incisions with wound necrosis and skin slough if not treated appropriately. In high-energy violence, it is prudent to wait for a few days for swelling to reduce before planning surgery. Most pilon fractures are often associated with injuries to the calcaneus, tibial plateau, pelvis and the vertebra.

RADIOGRAPHIC EVALUATION

Anteroposterior, lateral and mortise radiographs should be obtained to analyse the fracture morphology. A CT scan with three-dimensional reconstruction is often required to evaluate the fracture pattern.

CLASSIFICATION

The Rüedi and Allgöwer classification (Table 43.1, Fig. 43.1) is the most commonly used classification and is based on the severity of comminution and the displacement of the articular surface.[1]

Prognosis depends on the severity of injury. Rüedi and Allgöwer type I and type II, and AO (Arbeitsgemeinschaft für Osteosynthesefragen) type A fractures yield much better functional results with fewer complications than the more severe fracture patterns (Fig. 43.2).

TREATMENT

Pilon fractures are usually high-energy injuries with significant comminution and displacement of fragments and hence most often require operative management. Non-operative management is used primarily for undisplaced fracture patterns (such as AO types A1, B1 and C1) or in severely debilitated patients. Treatment involves a long leg cast for 6 weeks followed by bracing that allows early range-of-motion exercises. Loss of reduction is commonly encountered. Limited fixation with 3.5 mm or 4 mm screws, inserted after either percutaneous or limited open reduction, combined with plaster immobilization may be adequate treatment for AO types B1, B2, and stable C1 fractures.

For displaced pilon fractures, operative treatment gives superior results to non-operative treatment. A variety of surgical options including lag screw fixation, open reduction and internal fixation with plates, and external fixation with or without limited internal fixation are available (Figs 43.3 and 43.4).

The status of the soft tissues takes precedence. Surgery may be delayed for several days to allow reduction of ankle swelling, resolution of fracture blisters and demarcation of compromised soft tissues. External fixation can be used temporarily to provide skeletal stabilization, restoration of length and partial fracture reduction while waiting for definitive surgery.

Open reduction of fracture and plate fixation may be the best way to achieve a precisely reduced articular surface but one has to be aware of the complication of skin breakdown.[2] The use of low-profile implants, indirect reduction techniques, avoiding incisions over the anteromedial tibia and the use of biological fixation (minimally invasive) techniques minimize the complications of plating. The principles of surgery include maintenance of fibular length and stability, restoration of tibial articular surface, bone grafting of metaphyseal defects and buttressing of the distal tibia. The increased soft-tissue complications of this procedure have led to the use of a two-stage protocol where initially the fibula is fixed and the tibia is maintained in an external fixator. After the soft-tissue swelling has subsided, the tibia is fixed with or without bone grafting.[3] Postoperative management consists of initial immobilization in neutral dorsiflexion and early ankle motion exercises. Non-weight bearing for 12–16 weeks is necessary and gradual weight bearing is allowed once there is radiographic evidence of healing.

External fixators with or without minimal internal fixation are commonly used. Joint-spanning external fixation may be used in patients with significant soft-tissue compromise or open fractures. Reduction is maintained via distraction and ligamentotaxis. If adequate reduction is obtained, external fixation may be used as the definitive treatment in the presence of severe soft-tissue injury. Potential disadvantages include pin tract infection, pin loosening and ankle stiffness. Articulating spanning fixators may theoretically avoid tibiotalar stiffness.

Hybrid external fixation is a type of non-spanning external fixator and is most appropriate for AO type A, type C1 and type C2 fractures. Fracture reduction is enhanced using thin wires with or without olives to restore the articular surface and maintain bony stability. Tensioned wires in the epiphyseal fragment of the tibia are connected to half-pins

Table 43.1 Rüedi and Allgöwer classification of pilon fractures

Type I	Non-displaced cleavage fracture of the ankle joint
Type II	Displaced fracture with minimal impaction or comminution
Type III	Displaced fracture with significant articular comminution and metaphyseal impaction

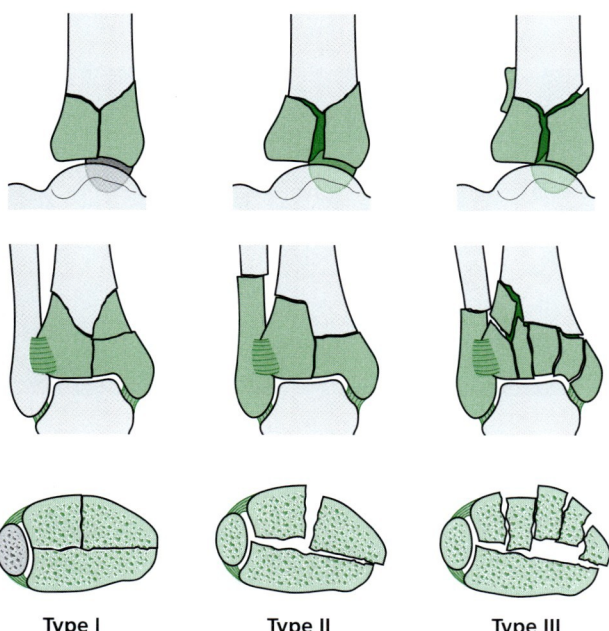

Figure 43.1 Rüedi and Allgöwer classification of distal tibia fractures. Adapted with permission from Rüedi Tg Allgöwer M, Schneider R, et al. Manual of Internal Fixation, 2nd en. New York, NY: Springer-Verlag, 1979.

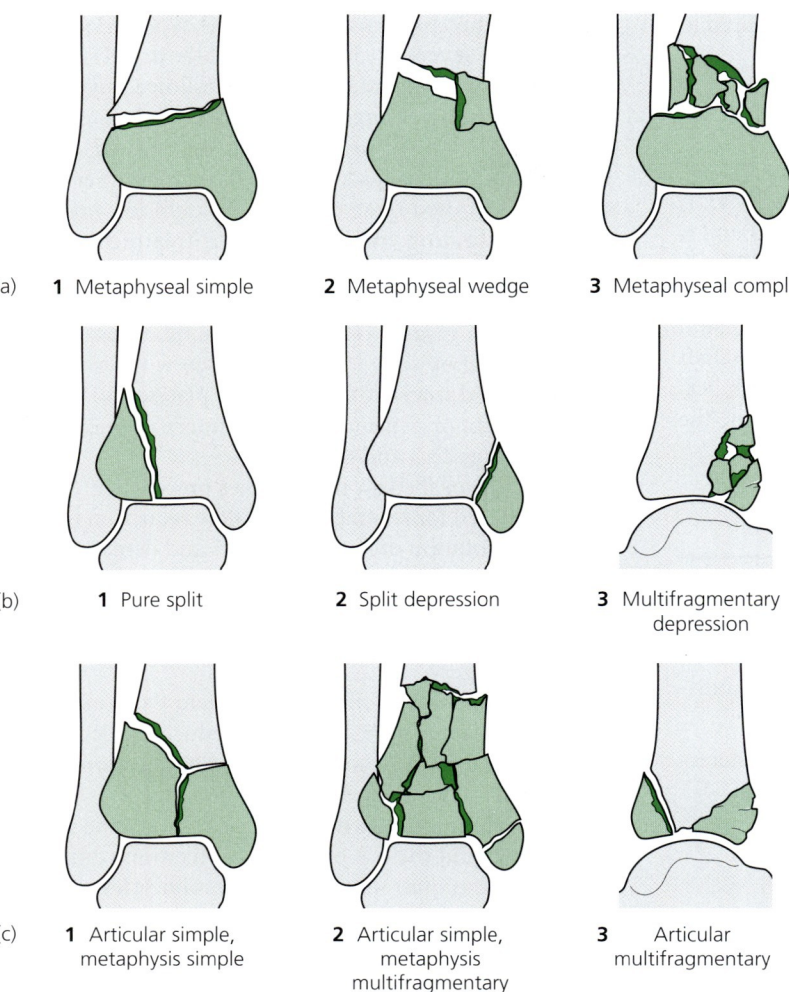

Figure 43.2 Orthopaedic Trauma Association (OTA) classification. The three types and nine groups of the AO/OTA classification of distal tibia fractures are illustrated. The three types of fractures are extra-articular, partial articular and total articular, and they are divided into nine groups based on the amount of comminution, as shown. (a) Tibia/fibula, distal extra-articular. (b) Tibia/fibula, distal, partial articular. (c) Tibia/fibula complete articular. Reproduced with permission from Orthopaedic Trauma Association Committee for Coding and Classification. Fracture and dislocation compendium, *Journal of Orthopaedic Trauma* 1996;**10**(Suppl 1):1.

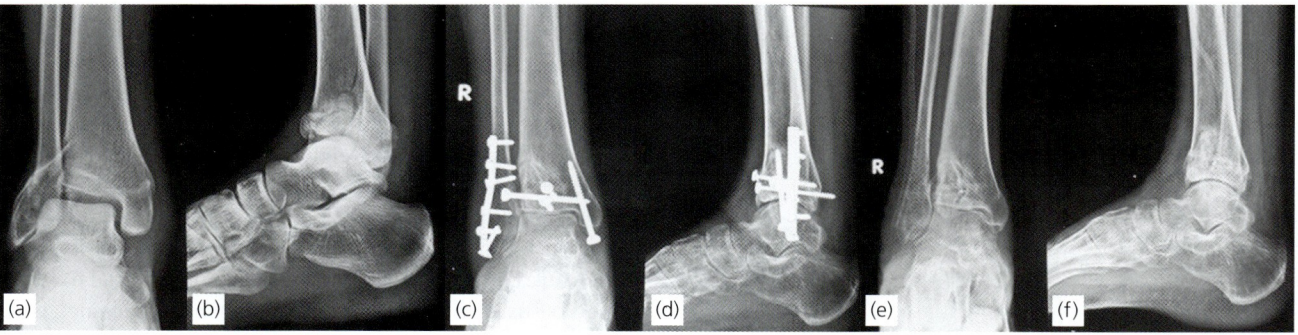

Figure 43.3 (a, b) Rüedi and Allgöwer type III pilon fracture. (c, d) Open reduction and stabilization with lag screws and stabilization of the fibula with a semi-tubular plate. (e, f) Two years post-surgery, following implant removal.

placed in the diaphysis. It is especially useful when internal fixation of any kind is contraindicated.

Reports of external fixation combined with limited internal fixation for tibial pilon fractures have shown a decreased incidence of infection compared with similar fractures treated with plate and screw devices. The articular surface is reduced percutaneously, under fluoroscopic guidance, or through limited incisions made directly over fracture lines and stabilized with screws and the fracture is stabilized with a spanning fixator.

Arthrodesis of the ankle joint is generally performed as a salvage procedure after other treatments have failed and post-traumatic arthritis has ensued. Primary arthrodesis may be performed in selected severe open fractures with extensive articular comminution and talar injury. In these patients, functional results are likely to be poor with mere internal

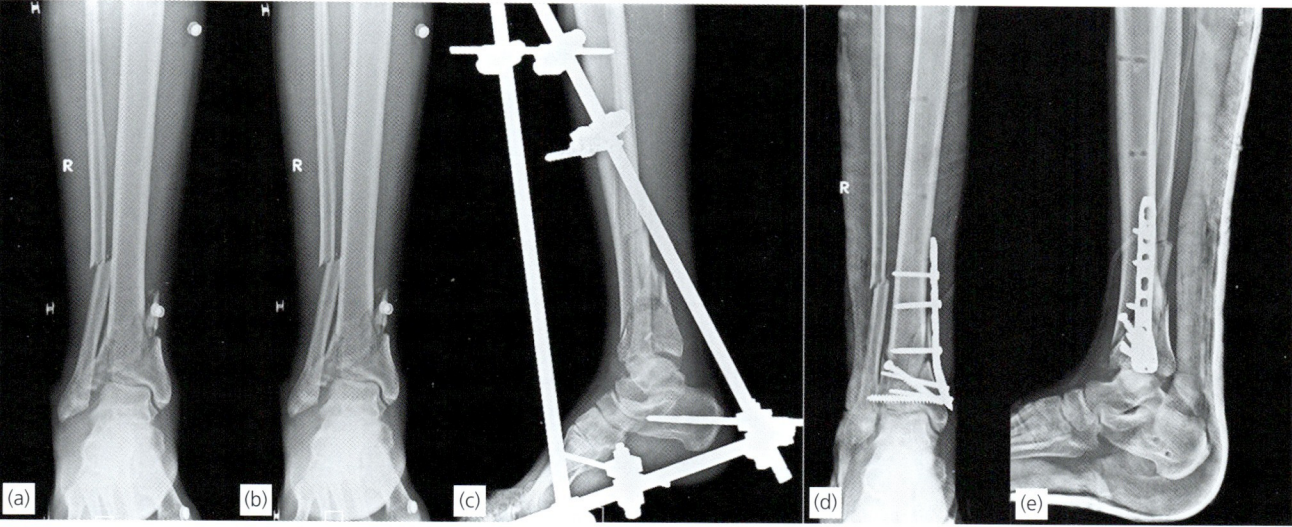

Figure 43.4 (a, b) Rüedi and Allgöwer type III pilon fracture; (c) temporary stabilization was performed with a spanning external fixator as the soft-tissue condition was poor; (d, e) stabilization with locking plate and lag screws through a minimally invasive approach was performed when the skin condition improved.

fixation. This procedure is best done after fracture comminution has consolidated and soft tissues have recovered.

COMPLICATIONS

Poor prognosis is associated with severe articular comminution (AO C3 and Rüedi–Allgöwer type III fracture), associated talar injury, severe soft-tissue injury, poor reduction of the articular surface, unstable fixation and postoperative wound infection.[4] The reported incidence of non-union is 5%, regardless of treatment method. Non-union occurs at the diaphyseal–metaphyseal junction and is common in fractures with plated or intact fibula, unrecognized bone loss or comminution of the tibia that was not bone grafted. Infection is associated with open injuries and soft-tissue devitalization secondary to poor surgical technique. Infections may lead to osteomyelitis, malunion or non-union. Post-traumatic arthritis is common with intra-articular irregularity, thus emphasizing the need for anatomic restoration of the articular surface.

KEY LEARNING POINTS

- Most fractures require surgical stabilization as these fractures have a high tendency for displacement, malalignment, delayed union and articular incongruity.
- Do not operate through compromised soft tissue in a tibial plafond fracture.
- The surgeon must achieve a balance between the goals of anatomical reduction and prevention of wound complications.

REFERENCES

- ● = Key primary paper
- ◆ = Major review article

●1. Rüedi T, Allgöwer M. Fractures of the lower end of the tibia into the ankle joint. *Injury* 1969;**1**:92.

◆2. Etter C, Ganz R. Long-term results of tibial plafond fractures treated with open reduction and internal fixation. *Archives of Orthopaedic and Trauma Surgery* 1991;**11**:227.

◆3. Dickson KF, Montgomery S, Field J. High energy plafond fractures treated by a spanning external fixator initially and followed by a second stage open reduction internal fixation of the articular surface: Preliminary report. *Injury* 2001;**32**(Suppl 4):SD92–8.

◆4. Wyrsch B, McFerran MA, McAndrew M, et al. Operative treatment of fractures of the tibial plafond: A randomized, prospective study. *Journal of Bone and Joint Surgery (American)* 1996;**78**:1646–57.

44

Injuries of the ankle joint

S RAJASEKARAN, RISHI MUGESH KANNA, J DHEENADHAYALAN

Introduction	386	Complications	391
Mechanism of injury	386	Ankle sprains	391
Clinical evaluation	386	Syndesmosis sprains	391
Radiographic evaluation	387	Achilles tendon rupture	393
Classification	387	References	393
Treatment	388		

NATIONAL BOARD STANDARDS

- Understand the complex anatomy of the ankle joint
- Know the principles of classification
- Be able to classify injury based on radiographs and recommend appropriate treatment

INTRODUCTION

The ankle is a complex hinge joint comprising articulations of the fibula, tibia and talus along with a complex ligamentous system. Isolated malleolar fractures account for two-thirds of fractures, with bimalleolar fractures occurring in one-quarter of patients and trimalleolar fractures occurring in the remaining 5–10%. Open fractures are rare, accounting for just 2% of all ankle fractures. As ankle fractures are intra-articular injuries, accurate reduction is required for a satisfactory long-term result. It must be emphasized that fractures around the ankle have associated ligamentous ruptures that can determine the functional outcome.

MECHANISM OF INJURY

The pattern of ankle injury is dependent on many factors, including the age of the patient, bone quality, mechanism of injury, position of the foot at the time of injury, and the magnitude, direction and rate of loading. Specific mechanisms and the resultant injuries are discussed in the section on classification.

CLINICAL EVALUATION

Patients present with pain, swelling, tenderness, a variable amount of deformity and inability to bear weight. The extent of soft-tissue injury and neurovascular status should be evaluated. A grossly dislocated ankle should be reduced and splinted immediately even before radiographs are taken to prevent neurovascular compromise and potential skin necrosis. The entire length of the fibula should be palpated for tenderness because associated fibular fractures may be found proximally as high as the proximal tibiofibular articulation. A 'squeeze test' may be performed approximately 5 cm proximal to the intermalleolar axis to assess possible syndesmotic injury.

RADIOGRAPHIC EVALUATION

Anteroposterior (AP), lateral and mortise views (taken with the foot in 15–20° of internal rotation to offset the intermalleolar axis) are essential for evaluating any ankle injury. A tibiofibular overlap of <10 mm and tibiofibular clear space *(the distance between the medial wall of the fibula and the incisural surface of the tibia is called the tibiofibular clear space)* of >5 mm in the AP view is abnormal and implies syndesmotic injury. A talar tilt difference in width of the medial and lateral aspects of the superior joint space of >2 mm indicates medial or lateral disruption. On the lateral view, the dome of the talus should be centred under the tibia and congruous with the tibial plafond. Posterior tibial tuberosity fractures and avulsion fractures of the talus by the anterior capsule may also be found.

On the mortise view (Fig. 44.1), a medial clear space >4–5 mm is abnormal and indicates lateral talar shift. The talocrural angle should be normally between 8° and 15°. A tibiofibular overlap <1 cm indicates syndesmotic disruption.

CLASSIFICATION

Ankle fractures may be classified by mechanistic or radiographic criteria. The Lauge-Hansen classification (Figs 44.2 and 44.3) consists of four hyphenated descriptions of the fracture mechanism (supination–external rotation (SER), supination–adduction (SA), pronation–external rotation (PER), pronation–abduction (PA)).[1] The first term describes the position of the foot at the time of injury and the second term describes the direction of the deforming force on the foot.

SER force accounts for 40–75% of malleolar fractures. The first stage consists of a tear of the anterior capsule and anterior tibiofibular ligament. In stage II, the injury progresses laterally, resulting in an oblique or spiral fracture of the fibula at the level of the plafond. Stage III involves a tear of the posterior capsule or posterior malleolus fracture. Stage IV consists of a transverse medial malleolus fracture or tear of the deltoid ligament.

SA force accounts for 10–20% of malleolar fractures. This is the only type associated with medial displacement of the talus. The first stage consists of a rupture of the lateral collateral ligaments or a transverse avulsion fracture of the lateral malleolar tip. This is followed by an oblique, shear-type fracture of the medial malleolus caused by medial translation of the talus.

PA force accounts for 5–20% of malleolar fractures. PA injuries initially place stress on the medial structures, resulting in either a deltoid ligament failure or avulsion of the distal tip of the medial malleolus. The second stage involves injury to the posterior complex, and the third stage involves an oblique fracture of the distal fibula caused by shear of the abducted talus.

PER force accounts for 5–20% of malleolus fractures. The PER injury pattern begins medially, with transverse fracture of the medial malleolus or a rupture of the deltoid ligament. The second stage is characterized by disruption of the anterior tibiofibular ligament with or without avulsion fracture at its insertion sites. The third stage results in a spiral fracture of the distal fibula at or above the level of the syndesmosis running from anterosuperior to posteroinferior. Stage IV produces either a rupture of the posterior tibiofibular ligament or an avulsion fracture of the posterolateral tibia.

Danis–Weber classification

The Danis–Weber/AO (Arbeitsgemeinschaft für Osteosynthesefragen) classification (Table 44.1, Fig. 44.3) is based on the level of the fibular fracture: the more proximal the fracture, the greater the risk of syndesmotic disruption and associated instability. Three types of fractures are described.

- *Maisonneuve fracture* is an external rotation-type of ankle injury in which the fracture of the fibula is in the proximal third.

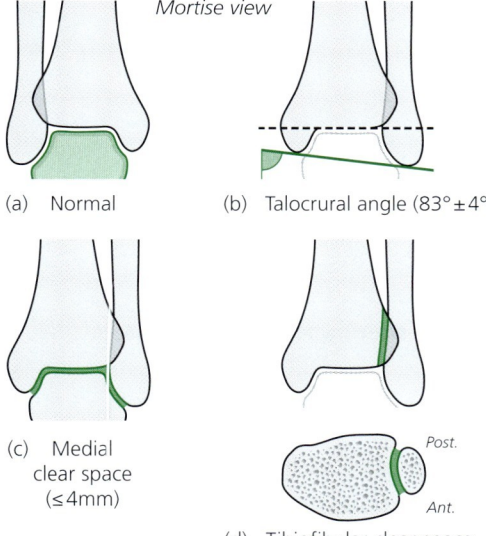

Figure 44.1 Radiographic appearance of the normal ankle on mortise view. (a) The condensed subchondral bone should form a continuous line around the talus. (b) The talocrural angle should be approximately 83°. When the opposite side can be used as a control, the talocrural angle of the injured side should be within a few degrees of the non-injured side. (c) The medial clear space should be equal to the superior clear space between the talus and the distal tibia and ≤4 mm on standard radiographs. (d) The distance between the medial wall of the fibula and the incisural surface of the tibia, the tibiofibular clear space, should be less than 6 mm.

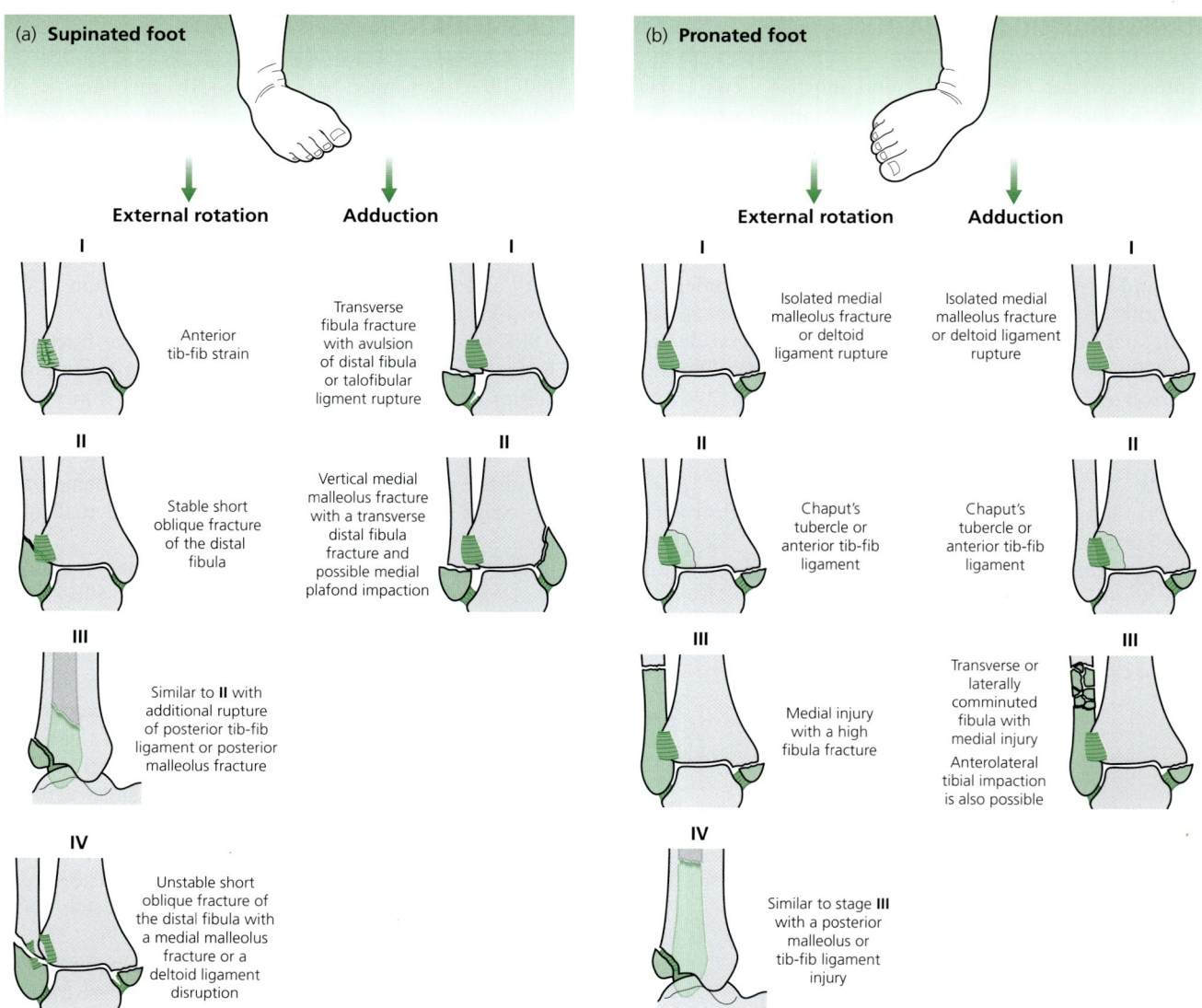

Figure 44.2 (a) Lauge-Hansen supination–external rotation and supination–adduction ankle fractures. (b) Lauge-Hansen pronation–external rotation and pronation–abduction ankle fractures.

- *LeForte–Wagstaffe fracture* is an avulsion fracture of the anterior fibular tubercle by the anterior tibiofibular ligament and is usually associated with Lauge-Hansen SER-type fracture patterns.
- *Tillaux–Chaput fracture* is an avulsion of the anterior tibial margin by the anterior tibiofibular ligament and is the tibial counterpart of the LeForte–Wagstaffe fracture.

Chondral injuries commonly accompany ankle fractures but are often unrecognized. Loren and Ferkel[3] reported that 63% of ankle fractures showed chondral injury which was more frequently on the medial aspect of the talus. PER fractures had a higher incidence of injury (70%) than SER fractures (46%). Seventy-five per cent of fractures with syndesmotic disruption also have chondral damage.

TREATMENT

Severely displaced fractures and dislocated ankles should be reduced immediately to minimize swelling, reduce articular cartilage damage, lessen the risk of skin breakdown, and minimize pressure on the neurovascular structures. Following fracture reduction, the ankle should be immobilized in a well-padded posterior splint and post-reduction radiographs should be obtained for fracture assessment.

Non-displaced, stable fracture patterns with an intact syndesmosis may be treated non-operatively in a short leg cast and allowed weight bearing as tolerated. Displaced fractures for which stable anatomic reduction is achieved are treated by placing the limb in a long leg cast to maintain rotational control for 4–6 weeks. Serial radiographic evaluation is necessary to ensure maintenance of reduction and healing. If adequate healing is demonstrated, the patient is placed in a short leg cast. Weight bearing is restricted until fracture healing is demonstrated. Postreduction radiographs are assessed for the normal relationships of the ankle mortise, and the weight-bearing alignment of the ankle should be at a right angle to the longitudinal axis of the leg. The contours of the articular surface must also be congruous as the best functional outcomes are obtained by anatomical joint restoration.

Open reduction and internal fixation (ORIF) is indicated following failure to achieve or maintain closed reduction, unstable fractures that may result in talar displacement or widening of the ankle mortise and in open fractures. Soft-tissue status is important and internal fixation should be performed only when the swelling around the ankle has subsided. Occasionally, a closed fracture with severe soft-tissue injury or massive swelling may require reduction and stabilization with an external fixator to allow soft-tissue management before definitive fixation.

Isolated medial malleolus fractures

Non-displaced medial malleolus fractures are usually treated non-operatively. However, internal fixation may be appropriate in certain cases to hasten healing and rehabilitation. Displaced fractures should be stabilized as persistent displacement allows the talus to tilt into varus with poor functional results (Fig. 44.4).

Larger fractures can usually be stabilized with two 4 mm cancellous screws and fractures with smaller fragments with a figure-of-eight tension band wire fixation. Although stainless steel implants are commonly used, bioabsorbable screws made of polyglycolic acid or polylactic acid may also be used.[4]

Isolated lateral malleolus fractures

Minimally displaced (2–3 mm) isolated lateral malleolar fractures distal to the syndesmosis may be treated non-operatively. Fractures with more than 3 mm displacement should be stabilized using a lag screw or tension band wiring. For fractures at or above the syndesmosis, restoration of fibular length and rotation using a combination of lag screws and plate is essential to achieve normal mortise anatomy.

Bimalleolar fractures

Closed reduction often can be accomplished, but the fracture can displace when the swelling subsides. Nonunion and frequent malunions are seen in bimalleolar

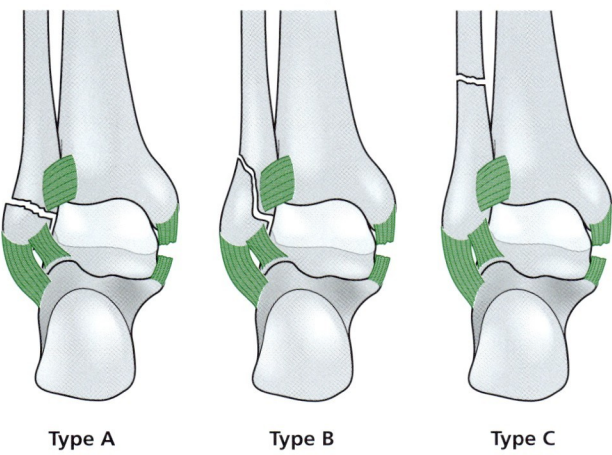

Figure 44.3 Weber/Arbeitsgemeinschaft für Osteosynthesefragen fractures. The staging is completely determined by the level of fibular fracture. Type A occurs below the plafond, whereas type C starts above the plafond. Reproduced with permission from Michelson JD. Ankle fractures resulting from rotational injuries. *Journal of the American Academy of Orthopaedic Surgeons* 2003;**11**:403–12.

Table 44.1 Danis–Weber/AO (Arbeitsgemeinschaft für Osteosynthesefragen) classification of ankle fractures

Type A	This involves a fracture of the fibula below the level of the tibial plafond, an avulsion injury that results from supination of the foot and that may be associated with an oblique or vertical fracture of the medial malleolus. This is equivalent to the Lauge-Hansen supination–adduction injury
Type B	This oblique or spiral fracture of the fibula is caused by external rotation occurring at or near the level of the syndesmosis; 50% have an associated disruption of the anterior syndesmotic ligament, whereas the posterior syndesmotic ligament remains intact and attached to the distal fibular fragment. There may be an associated injury to the medial structures or the posterior malleolus. This is equivalent to the Lauge-Hansen supination–eversion injury
Type C	This involves a fracture of the fibula above the level of the syndesmosis causing disruption of the syndesmosis almost always with associated medial injury. This category includes Maisonneuve-type injuries and corresponds to Lauge-Hansen pronation–eversion or pronation–abduction stage III injuries

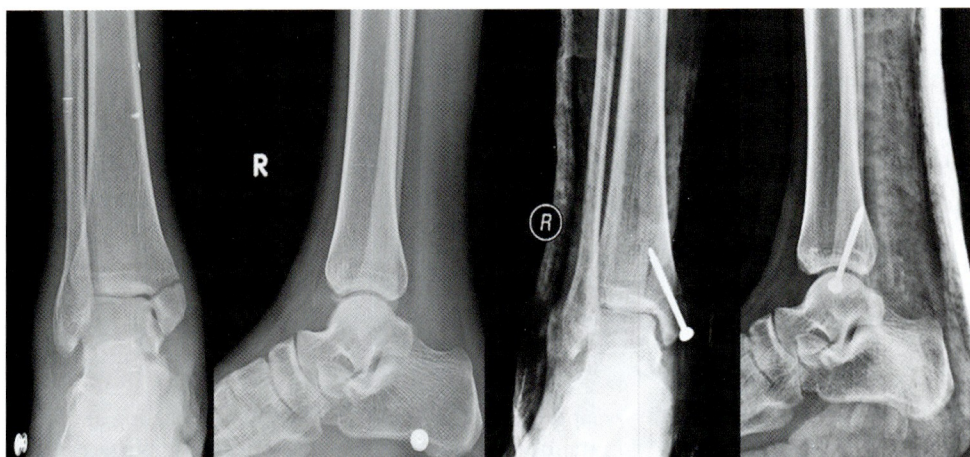

Figure 44.4 Isolated displaced medial malleolar fracture treated by anatomical reduction and internal fixation with a malleolar screw.

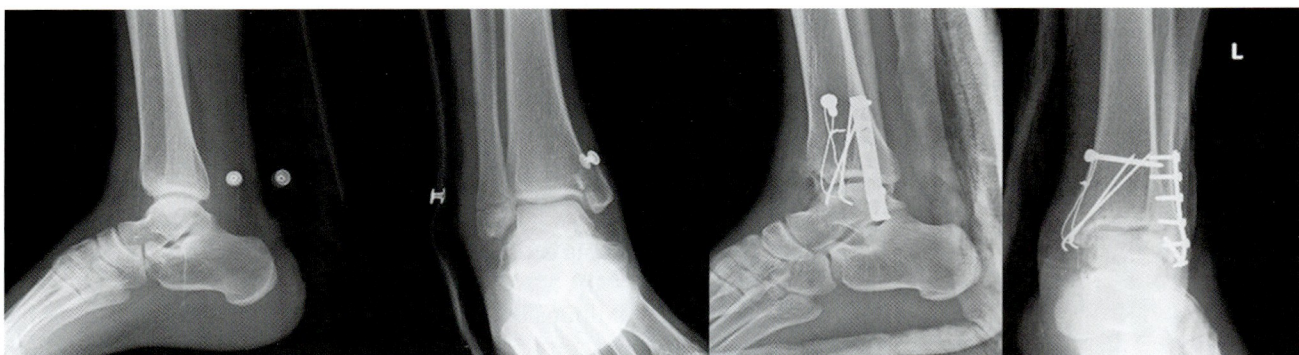

Figure 44.5 A Weber's type A fracture treated by open reduction and internal fixation with tension band wiring of the medial malleolus and plating for the fibula.

fractures treated by closed methods, and hence ORIF of both malleoli is recommended. The lateral malleolar fracture is first stabilized achieving normal length and rotation with plate and screw fixation (Fig. 44.5). An antiglide technique (plate on the posterior aspect of the fibula) may be used to avoid prominent hardware. Simple oblique lateral malleolar fractures with minimal comminution may be stabilized with lag screws. The medial malleolar fracture is then stabilized with lag or malleolar screws. Achieving perfect reduction is important because the talus tends to shift in the mortise. A 1 mm lateral shift of the talus reduces the effective weight-bearing area of the talotibial articulation by 20–40%, and a 5 mm shift reduces it by almost 80%.

A deltoid ligament tear and lateral malleolar fracture can occur from the same mechanism of injury as bimalleolar injuries. The optimal treatment of this injury consists of ORIF of the fibula, medial exploration and repair of the deltoid ligament if needed.

Fibular fractures above the plafond may often require syndesmotic stabilization. After fixation of the medial and lateral malleoli is achieved, the syndesmosis should be stressed intra-operatively by lateral pull on the fibula with a bone hook or by stressing the ankle in external rotation. Syndesmotic instability can then be recognized clinically and under image intensification. The syndesmosis is stabilized with a syndesmotic screw inserted from the fibula to the tibia, placed 2–3 cm proximal to the tibial plafond, directed parallel to the joint surface, and angled 30° anteriorly. Both three- and four-cortex fixation has been advocated, with four-cortex fixation offering greater stability, but no study has shown superior results with either method of fixation. Traditionally the syndesmotic screw is placed with the ankle in a neutral position or 10° of dorsiflexion so as not to affect the postoperative range of dorsiflexion. Weight bearing is not permitted for 8 weeks to allow for sufficient syndesmotic healing. Recommendations in the literature range from routine removal of the screw before weight bearing to allow for restoration of normal distal fibular motion to removal after the fracture has healed only if symptoms develop.[5] Very proximal fibular fractures with syndesmosis disruption can usually be treated with syndesmosis fixation without direct fibular reduction and stabilization. One must however achieve correct fibular length and rotation before performing syndesmotic fixation.

Trimalleolar (Cotton) fractures

The same principles and indications for open reduction outlined for bimalleolar fractures also apply to trimalleolar fractures. The posterior fragment usually falls into place once the fibula has been anatomically reduced. Indirect reduction and stabilization with an anterior to posterior lag screw, or a posterior to anterior lag screw, is indicated if the fracture of the posterior malleolus involves more than 25% of the articular surface, has a step-off or gap of more than 3 mm, or is associated with persistent posterior subluxation of the talus.

Open fractures

These fractures require emergency debridement in the operating room. Immediate internal fixation after surgical debridement is recommended as stable fixation helps to prevent infection and aids soft-tissue healing. If the wound is severely contaminated, a temporary external fixator can be placed spanning the ankle, and open reduction can be done when the wound is judged to be clean and swelling has decreased. Antibiotic prophylaxis should be continued postoperatively. Wounds with skin loss may require an immediate soft-tissue cover as exposed bone and articular cartilage dry and necrose rapidly.

COMPLICATIONS

Non-union is rare and is more commonly associated with conservative treatment of medial malleolus fractures. It commonly follows residual fracture displacement, interposed soft tissue or associated lateral instability resulting in shear stresses across the deltoid ligament. Post-traumatic arthritis can occur secondary to articular damage at the time of injury or due to altered biomechanics as a result of poor reduction of the fracture. Reflex sympathetic dystrophy and malunion commonly of the lateral malleolus are other complications reported.

ANKLE SPRAINS

Most ankle sprains are caused by a twisting injury to the ankle. The most common ankle sprain consists of an inversion injury of the foot with some degree of plantarflexion. Here the period of recovery is relatively short and uneventful. A more relevant injury with a completely different period of recovery is the injury while the foot is in eversion, the so-called 'high ankle sprain'. It accounts for 1–15% of the total ankle sprains. Therefore, the first issue when approaching a patient with an ankle sprain should be directed to identifying the mechanism of injury.

Mechanism of injury

The mechanism of injury and the exact ligaments injured depend on the position of the foot and the direction of the stress. With the ankle in *plantarflexion*, inversion injuries first strain the anterior talofibular ligament and then the calcaneofibular ligament. However, with the ankle in dorsiflexion and inversion, the injury is usually isolated to the calcaneofibular ligament. With ankle dorsiflexion and external rotation, the injury will more probably involve the syndesmotic ligaments. The syndesmotic ligaments, and in particular the posterior and inferior tibiofibular ligament, can also be injured with the ankle dorsiflexed and the foot internally rotated. Figure 44.6 shows the anatomic location of the ligaments. Fractures can occur with simple inversion injuries.

Evaluation

Patients with mild sprains complain of pain but are usually ambulant whereas patients with severe sprains present with swelling around the ankle and difficulty with weight bearing secondary to pain. Physical findings may include swelling, ecchymosis, tenderness, instability, crepitus, vascular status, muscle dysfunction and deformity. The location of the tenderness helps to delineate the involved ligaments.

Patients should undergo radiographic examination to rule out occult foot and ankle injuries with a radiographic series of the foot and ankle (AP, lateral and mortise views). In the acute setting, pain is quite limiting. It is very difficult to stress the ankle joint or obtain ankle stress radiographs to confirm which ligaments are intact.

Treatment

The traditional principles of rest, immobilization, compression, elevation, icing and protected weight bearing should be applied. For mild sprains, one can start early mobilization and range-of-motion, isometric exercises. For moderate or severe sprains, one can immobilize the ankle in neutral position or slight dorsiflexion for the first 10–14 days and then initiate mobilization, range-of-motion and isometric exercises. For more severe sprains, taping or bracing programmes are continued during sports activities for 6 months, and a supervised rehabilitation programme used. Patients who continue to have pain in the ankle that does not decrease with time should be evaluated again for an occult osseous or chondral injury.

SYNDESMOSIS SPRAINS

Syndesmotic sprains account for approximately 1% of all ankle sprains and may occur without a fracture or frank diastasis. Tibiofibular syndesmotic ligamentous injuries are slower to recover than other ankle ligamentous injuries

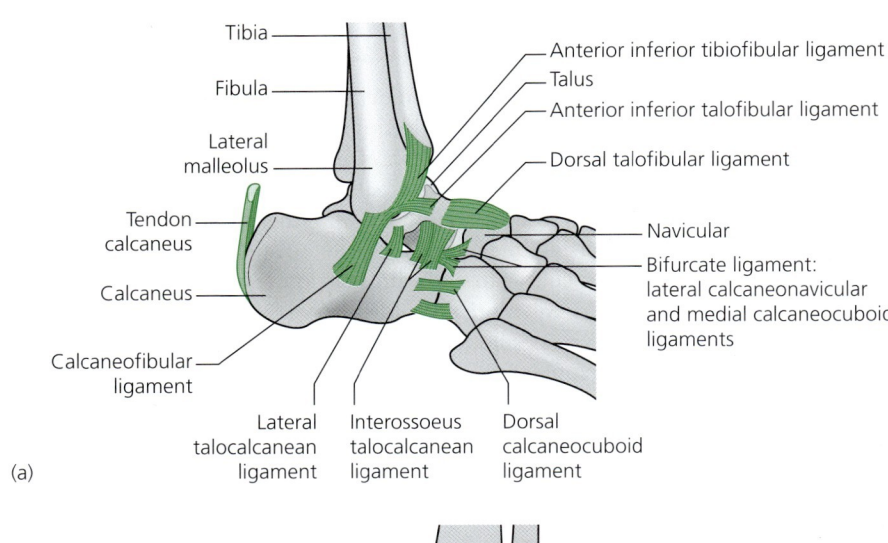

Figure 44.6 Anatomic description of the most significant ligaments and bones of the ankle and midfoot area.

and may benefit from a more restrictive approach to initial management.

Immediately after a syndesmotic ankle sprain, the patient will have well-localized tenderness in the area of the sprain, but soon thereafter, with ensuing swelling and ecchymosis, the precise location of the sprain often becomes obscured. On palpation, there will be tenderness along the most anterior and distal aspect of the syndesmosis of the ankle. Clinical tests that can be used to isolate syndesmotic ligament injury include: the *squeeze test*, described by Hopkinson et al.,[6] which involves squeezing the fibula at the mid-calf. If this manoeuvre reproduces distal tibiofibular pain, it is likely that the patient has sustained some injury to the syndesmotic region.

The external rotation stress test

Any degree of external rotation, which stresses the ankle mortise, will increase or reproduce the pain. The external rotation can be applied directly by the examiner holding the lower leg with one hand and torque on the foot with the opposite hand while keeping the ankle in a neutral position, so the talus is locked in the ankle mortise.

If the patient can tolerate weight bearing, a more sensitive test for a syndesmosis injury consists of standing on the injured leg and applying an external rotation force to the ankle with an internal turn of the pelvis with the knee fully extended. If the patient can stand and perform some degree of external rotation, the suspicion for an unstable mortise should be low.

The radiographic evaluation of a syndesmotic injury, in an acute setting, involves an attempt at weight-bearing radiographs of the ankle and, if negative, an external rotation stress view. The best projection to assess the stability of the syndesmosis is the mortise view. In the weight-bearing mortise view, a competent syndesmosis should show no widening of the medial clear space (between the medial malleolus and the medial border of the talus) and a tibiofibular clear space of 6 mm or less. If the syndesmosis appears intact on routine radiograph, but suspicion for syndesmotic injury remains high, consider stress views of the ankle while applying external rotation to the foot. The patient has to be either sedated or injected with local anaesthetic along the syndesmosis prior to its evaluation. The radiographs are assessed for widening of the medial joint space and tibiofibular clear space on the mortise view and for posterior displacement of the fibula relative to the tibia on the lateral view. An MRI evaluation of the syndesmosis may also help to delineate injury to the syndesmotic ligaments.

If the syndesmosis is stable or in the absence of fractures, the patient is immobilized in a walking cast or boot for 6–8 weeks followed by a functional return to activities of daily living and sports. If the syndesmosis is unstable or in the presence of a proximal fibular fracture, the patient will require fixation of the syndesmosis with screws followed by immobilization for 6–8 weeks.

ACHILLES TENDON RUPTURE

Most Achilles tendon problems are related to overuse injuries and are multifactorial. The principal factors include host susceptibility and mechanical overload. The spectrum of injury ranges from paratenonitis to tendinosis to acute rupture. In a trauma setting, a true rupture is the most common presentation.

Patients typically experience sudden severe pain behind the ankle. With a partial rupture, physical examination may only reveal a localized, tender area of swelling. With complete rupture, examination normally reveals a palpable defect in the tendon. In this setting, the Thompson test is generally positive (i.e. squeezing the calf does not cause active plantarflexion), and the patient usually is incapable of performing a single heel raise. In case of doubt, an ultrasound will demonstrate a gap within the tendon fibres. If ultrasound is not available, an MRI will be diagnostic.

There is significant controversy regarding the choice of treatment for an acute Achilles tendon rupture. Proponents of surgical repair indicate lower recurrent rupture rates, improved strength and a higher percentage of patients who return to sports activities. Proponents of non-operative treatment stress the high surgical complication rates resulting from wound infection, skin necrosis and nerve injuries. Most doctors tend to treat active patients who are interested in continuing athletic endeavours with operative treatment and inactive patients or those with other comorbid medical factors with non-operative approaches.

In non-operative treatment, the foot is immobilized in equinus for 8 weeks in a short leg cast. Progressive weight bearing is generally permitted at 2–4 weeks after injury. After removal of the cast, a heel lift is used while making the transition back to wearing normal shoes. Progressive resistance exercises for the calf muscles are started at 8–10 weeks, with a return to athletic activities at 4–6 months.

Different operative techniques, including percutaneous and open approaches, have been described. Percutaneous approaches, have the advantage of decreased dissection but carry the disadvantages of potential entrapment of the sural nerve and an increased chance of inadequate tendon capture. With distal ruptures, reattachment of the tendon to the calcaneus is performed with transosseous suture fixation.

KEY LEARNING POINTS

- The ankle is a complex hinge, weight-bearing joint in which both bones and ligaments play vital roles.
- Normal function depends significantly on precise structural integrity.
- The ankle is not intrinsically stable and requires support from the ligaments, muscles and tendons of the foot that cross it.
- The overlying skin is thin with a tenuous blood supply. Only tendons and neurovascular structures cross the joint and provide no significant coverage for it.
- An injury of the ankle region can affect the bone, articular surface, ligaments, tendons, nerves or blood vessels that cross it.
- Management of ankle injuries requires a thorough evaluation identifying the anatomic structures involved and the severity and extent of damage to articular structures.
- Once the injuries have been defined, ideal treatment necessitates an anatomical repair, to provide stability without compromising the surrounding structures.

REFERENCES

- ● = Key primary paper
- ◆ = Major review article

●1. Lauge-Hansen N. Fractures of the ankle, II: combined experimental-surgical and experimental-roentgenologic investigations. *Archives of Surgery* 1950;**60**:957.

◆2. Michelson JD. Ankle fractures resulting from rotational injuries. *Journal of the American Academy of Orthopaedic Surgeons* 2003;**11**:403–12.

◆3. Loren GJ, Ferkel RD. Arthroscopic assessment of occult intra-articular injury in acute ankle fractures. *Arthroscopy* 2002;**18**:412–21.

◆4. Böstman OM, Hirvensalo E, Vainionpaa S, *et al.* Ankle fractures treated using biodegradable internal fixation. *Clinical Orthopaedics and Related Research* 1989;**238**:195.

◆5. Boden SD, Labropoulos PA, McCowin P, *et al.* Mechanical considerations for the syndesmosis screw. *Journal of Bone and Joint Surgery (American)* 1989;**71A**:1548.

●6. Hopkinson WJ, St. Pierre P, Ryan JB, Wheeler JH. Syndesmotic sprains of the ankle. *Foot and Ankle* 1990;**10**:325–30.

45

Talar fractures and dislocation

SURESHAN SIVANANTHAN, SHANMUGANATHAN RAJASEKARAN

Introduction	394	Posterior process fractures	396
Talar neck fractures	394	Talar body fractures	397
Talar head fractures	396	Subtalar dislocation (peritalar dislocation)	397
Lateral process fractures	396	References	397

NATIONAL BOARD STANDARDS

- Revise your knowledge of talar anatomy, especially the blood supply
- Know the different injury types and the treatment methods
- Be able to advise a patient on the prognosis depending on the injury

INTRODUCTION

The talus acts as a link between the ankle, subtalar and transverse tarsal joints. Talus fractures account for 2% of all lower extremity injuries and 5–7% of all foot injuries. About 70% of the talar surface is covered by articular cartilage along its five weight-bearing surfaces and hence almost any talar fracture involves a joint. It is devoid of muscle or tendon attachments and its vascular supply is dependent entirely on fascial structures.[1] As a result, capsular disruptions can result in osteonecrosis. Fractures are classified according to the anatomic location as lateral process fractures, posterior process fractures, talar head fractures, talar body fractures and talar neck fractures.

TALAR NECK FRACTURES

Talar neck fractures occur commonly with forced dorsiflexion and were historically known as the 'aviator's astragalus' as it was common when planes impacted the ground and the rudder bar forcefully dorsiflexed the foot resulting in a talar neck fracture.

Mechanism of injury

The talar neck fractures by forced impaction on the anterior margin of the tibia during hyperdorsiflexion. This is most commonly seen with motor vehicle accidents or a fall from a height.

Clinical evaluation

Patients present with swelling of the ankle with tenderness of the talus and subtalar joint and painful foot movements. About 15–25% of fractures are open and due to high-energy mechanism injuries. Prolonged dislocation with tenting of the skin may result in pressure necrosis on the overlying soft tissues, compromising soft-tissue integrity and resulting in possible infection. Emergency reduction of the talus under sedation prior to sending the patient for radiographs is recommended. Foot compartment syndrome is rare but possible and must be carefully looked for in patients with severe swelling.

Radiological evaluation

In addition to the standard anteroposterior (AP) and lateral radiographs of the ankle, a Canale view (Fig. 45.1) is obtained. This provides an optimum view of the talar neck. CT is helpful to delineate the fracture morphology and assess articular involvement. Fractures that appear non-displaced on plain radiographs may show unrecognized comminution or articular step-off on CT scan.

Classification

The original classification of talar neck fractures by Hawkins had three types of fractures,[2] and Canale and Kelley added a fourth type[3] (Table 45.1).

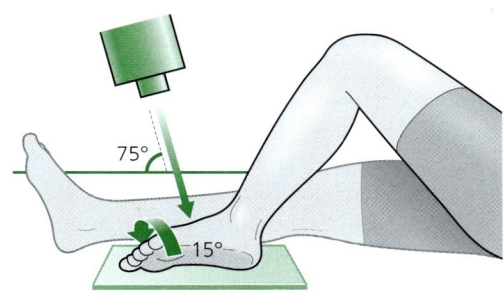

Figure 45.1 Canale and Kelly view of the foot. Taken with the ankle in maximum equinus, the foot is placed on a cassette, pronated 15°, and the radiographic source is directed cephalad 15° from the vertical. From Bucholz RW, Heckman JD, Court-Brown C, et al. (eds) *Rockwood and Green's Fractures in Adults*, 6th edn. Philadelphia, PA: Lippincott Williams & Wilkins, 2006.

Table 45.1 Talar neck fractures (Hawkins classification)

Type I	Non-displaced
Type II	Associated subtalar subluxation or dislocation
Type III	Associated subtalar and ankle dislocation
Type IV	Type III with associated talonavicular subluxation or dislocation

Types II, III and IV are associated with progressive severity in disruption of vascular supply to the fracture fragments. In type I fractures, the incidence of osteonecrosis is 0–15%, in type II it is 20–50%, in type III it is 20–100% and in type IV it is usually 100% (Fig. 45.2).[4]

Treatment

The management depends on the degree of displacement.[5] Type I fractures can be treated with a short leg cast for 8–12 weeks. The patient should remain non-weight bearing for 6 weeks until clinical and radiographic evidence of fracture healing is present. Many surgeons however prefer surgical treatment to avoid the risk of late displacement. This fracture pattern is amenable to percutaneous internal fixation with 'lag screws' from a posterolateral insertion site.

Displacement greater than 2 mm requires surgical management to avoid further vascular and soft-tissue compromise. Immediate closed reduction is indicated, with emergency open reduction and internal fixation (ORIF) for all open or irreducible fractures, particularly those with residual subluxation, dislocation or pressurized soft tissues. If open reduction is necessary, all major fragments should be salvaged. Primary arthrodesis is usually avoided.

Surgical approaches include the anteromedial, posterolateral, anterolateral and the combined anteromedial–anterolateral. The combined approach is used only when greater visualization of the talar neck is needed.

Internal fixation is usually accomplished with two interfragmentary lag screws or headless screws placed perpendicular to the fracture line. The screws can be inserted in antegrade or retrograde fashion. Posterior-to-anterior directed screws have been demonstrated to be biomechanically stronger. Medial comminution may require bone grafting and medial plating to prevent subsequent varus malunion. Titanium screws may offer an advantage if postoperative MRI is to be considered for evaluation of postoperative osteonecrosis. A short leg cast or removable boot should be placed postoperatively for 8–12 weeks, and the patient should be kept non-weight bearing (Fig. 45.3).

The Hawkins sign represents osteopenia that is seen beneath the subchondral surface of the talar dome and is seen at 6–8 weeks after the fracture, indicating talar revascularization. Absence of this sign in radiographs performed at 6 weeks indicates possible avascular necrosis. If osteonecrosis is suspected, MRI may be useful in making an early diagnosis.

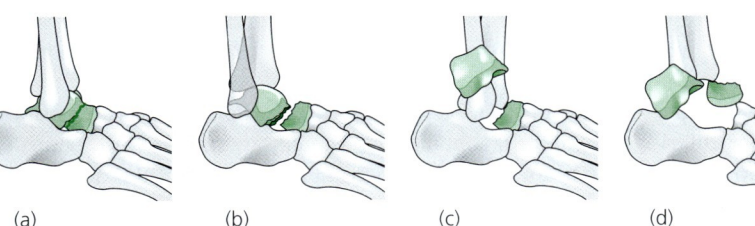

Figure 45.2 (a) Type I talar neck fracture; (b) type II; (c) type III; (c) type IV. From Canale ST, Kelly FB Jr. Fractures of the neck of the talus: long-term evaluation of 71 cases. *Journal of Bone and Joint Surgery (American)* 1978;**60A**:143.

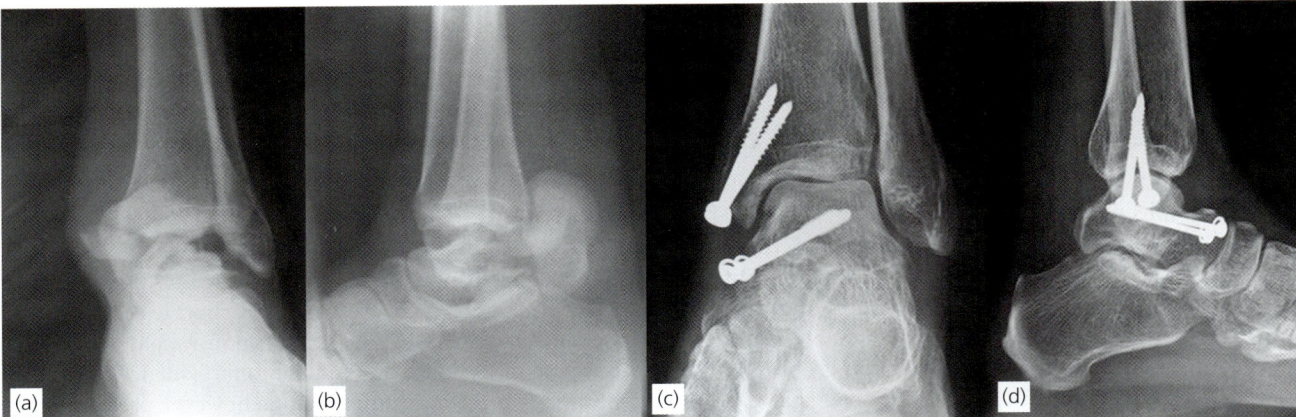

Figure 45.3 (a, b) Canale type III talar neck fracture with medial malleolus fracture: (c, d) Open reduction and stabilization of the medial malleolus with malleolar screws and the talar neck with lag screws was performed; both fractures healed. No osteonecrosis is seen at 4 years

If the fracture has healed and no cystic changes or collapse are noted, progressive, protected weight bearing can be instituted at 8 weeks, with regular clinical and radiographic re-evaluation.

Complications

Post-traumatic arthritis occurs in 40–90% of cases and is due to chondral injury at the time of fracture or persistent articular incongruity. This may occur in either the ankle or subtalar joints. The rates of arthritis in the subtalar joint, ankle joint or both the joints are 50%, 30% and 25%, respectively. Osteonecrosis is common and is related to initial fracture displacement as mentioned above. Delayed union (>6 months) may occur in up to 15% of cases. It may be treated by open reduction and bone grafting.

TALAR HEAD FRACTURES

Fractures of the head of the talus constitute 5–10% of talar injuries. Two mechanisms of injury have been suggested: axially directed loading and compression of the talar head and a dorsal compression fracture on the anterior tibial plafond. Plain radiographs may define the fracture clearly, but a CT scan is often necessary for definitive diagnosis and evaluation of displacement. The fracture of the head with loss of support of the talonavicular joint may be associated with clinical instability of the triple joint complex. Injuries to the calcaneocuboid and subtalar joints are common with this injury.

Displaced fractures of the head of the talus should be treated with open reduction and internal fixation with cancellous lag screws using an anteromedial approach. Care should be taken to not strip any remaining vascular supply of the head. Early motion can be started from approximately 2 weeks after surgery and delayed weight bearing is initiated at a minimum of 6 weeks. Osteonecrosis of the fractured segment of the head has been reported to be 10%, and, if degenerative arthrosis occurs, talonavicular arthrodesis may be indicated.

LATERAL PROCESS FRACTURES

Lateral process fractures, also described as *snowboarder fractures*, are created by forced dorsiflexion and external rotation of the foot. This fracture is commonly missed on initial presentation on plain radiographs of the ankle. CT is helpful to ascertain the extent of the fracture, which may encompass a significant portion of the lateral aspect of the posterior facet. Fractures with less than 2 mm displacement are treated nonoperatively in a short leg cast for 6 weeks, followed by 6 weeks in a removable weight-bearing cast. Fractures with more than 3–4 mm displacement or involving >10% of the articular surface should be fixed using lag screws.

POSTERIOR PROCESS FRACTURES

Fractures of the posterior process involve the posterior 25% of the articular surface and include the posteromedial and posterolateral tubercles. They occur during forced ankle inversion whereby the posterior talofibular ligament avulses the lateral tubercle or by forced equinus and direct compression. The posterolateral tubercle is more frequently involved, and flexion and extension of the hallux may exacerbate symptoms because of the close proximity of the flexor hallucis longus tendon in its posterior groove.

Diagnosis of fractures of the posterior process of the talus can be difficult, and should be suspected when a patient previously diagnosed to have an ankle sprain does not improve by 6 weeks.

Non-displaced or minimally displaced fractures without significant subtalar involvement are treated with a short leg cast for 6 weeks whereas displaced fractures are treated operatively. If the fragment is large with significant subtalar joint involvement, it should be fixed. If the fragment is small or diagnosed late, primary excision is performed.

TALAR BODY FRACTURES

It is important to distinguish talar body fractures from talar neck fractures. Inokuchi et al.[6] identified these injuries as talar body fractures if the inferior fracture line was proximal to the lateral process of the talus and as talar neck fractures if the inferior fracture line was distal to the lateral process of the talus. Although the incidence of osteonecrosis is similar between talar neck and talar body fractures, a higher incidence of post-traumatic subtalar osteoarthrosis has been noted after talar body fractures. Non-displaced talar body fractures have a reported incidence of osteonecrosis of 25%; however, with displacement, the rate increases to 50%.[7]

Diagnosis should be made by a plain radiograph, and CT may be indicated for complete evaluation of the fracture pattern and displacement. Displaced fractures should be treated with ORIF. An 88% incidence of osteonecrosis or post-traumatic arthritis has been reported, with worse results occurring in comminuted and open fractures. Comminuted fractures of the body of the talus with gross displacement are difficult to treat with uniformly poor long-term results. Accurate replacement of the fragments is often impossible and procedures such as talectomy or calcaneotibial fusion are required. As the results of talectomy are usually poor, calcaneotibial fusion combined with talectomy is preferred. The foot is painless and stable, and enough compensatory movement usually develops in the midtarsal joints to enable the patient to walk with a fairly elastic gait.

SUBTALAR DISLOCATION (PERITALAR DISLOCATION)

Subtalar dislocation refers to the simultaneous dislocation of the distal articulations of the talus at the talocalcaneal and talonavicular joints. The dislocations are closed in approximately 75% of patients. Most (85%) of the dislocations are medial (the foot is dislocated medial to the talus), although lateral, anterior and posterior dislocations have been reported. Forced inversion of the foot results in a medial subtalar dislocation, whereas eversion produces a lateral subtalar dislocation.

All subtalar dislocations require closed reduction. Under adequate analgesia with knee flexion and longitudinal foot traction, the foot deformity is accentuated to 'unlock' the calcaneus. The deformity is then reversed and reduction occurs with a 'clunk'.

Post-reduction CT should be performed to fully ascertain the extent of associated osteochondral injuries and congruency of reduction of the subtalar joint. Intra-articular fragments blocking congruent reduction require surgical excision.

Irreducible dislocations occur in 32% of patients owing to entrapment of bone or soft-tissue structures. With medial dislocations, the talar head can become trapped by the capsule of the talonavicular joint, the extensor retinaculum or extensor tendons, or the extensor digitorum brevis muscle. With a lateral dislocation, the posterior tibial tendon may be entrapped. Open reduction is required in such instances and is usually performed through a longitudinal anteromedial incision for medial dislocations and a sustentaculum tali approach for lateral dislocations.

KEY LEARNING POINTS

- The vascular supply to the talus reaches it via the fascial attachments and hence capsular disruption (either traumatic or surgical) leads to osteonecrosis. The incidence of osteonecrosis with neck fractures increases with the severity of injury.
- Type I talar neck fractures can be managed non-operatively; types II, III and IV require open reduction and internal fixation with cancellous 'lag' screws.
- A high index of suspicion is required to diagnose lateral and posterior tubercle fractures, as these fractures are easily missed on radiographs and hence a CT scan may be required.
- Subtalar dislocations should be reduced on an emergency basis, and failure of closed reduction requires open reduction. The presence of bone fragments in the subtalar joint is an indication for surgery.

REFERENCES

- ● = Key primary paper
- ◆ = Major review article

● 1. Mulfinger GL, Trueta J. The blood supply of the talus. *Journal of Bone and Joint Surgery (British)* 1970;**52**:160.

● 2. Hawkins LG. Fractures of the neck of the talus. *Journal of Bone and Joint Surgery (American)* 1970;**52**:991.

● 3. Canale ST, Kelly FB Jr. Fractures of the neck of the talus: long-term evaluation of seventy-one cases. *Journal of Bone and Joint Surgery (American)* 1978;**60**:143–56.

◆ 4. Vallier HA, Nork SE, Barei DP, et al. Talar neck fractures: results and outcomes. *Journal of Bone and Joint Surgery (American)* 2004;**86**:1616.

◆ 5. Sanders DW, Busam M, Hattwick E, et al. Functional outcomes following displaced talar neck fractures. *Journal of Orthopaedic Trauma* 2004;**18**:265.

◆ 6. Inokuchi S, Ogawa K, Usami N. Classification of fractures of the talus: clear differentiation between neck and body fractures. *Foot and Ankle International* 1996;**17**:748–50.

● 7. Vallier HA, Nork SE, Benirschke SK, et al. Surgical treatment of talar body fractures. *Journal of Bone and Joint Surgery (American)* 2004;**86**:180.

46

Calcaneus fractures

SURESHAN SIVANANTHAN

Introduction	398	Classification	399
Mechanism of injury	398	Treatment	400
Clinical evaluation	398	Complications	401
Radiographic evaluation	398	References	402

NATIONAL BOARD STANDARDS

- Know the three-dimensional anatomy of the calcaneus
- Understand the mechanism of injury
- Know the different fracture types and the treatment principles

INTRODUCTION

The calcaneus is the most frequently fractured tarsal bone and accounts for approximately 2% of all fractures. About 60–75% of calcaneal fractures are intra-articular and bilateral calcaneal fractures are present in 5–10% of cases. Intra-articular calcaneal fractures have significant importance as poor outcomes of treatment are associated with poor overall health status.

MECHANISM OF INJURY

Most intra-articular fractures occur as a result of axial loading as in falls from a height. The talus is driven down into the calcaneus, which is composed of a thin cortical shell surrounding cancellous bone. Twisting forces are associated with extra-articular calcaneal fractures, which include fractures of the anterior and medial processes or the sustentaculum tali. In elderly diabetic patients, there is an increased incidence of tuberosity fractures from avulsion by the Achilles tendon.

CLINICAL EVALUATION

Patients present with heel pain, ecchymosis, swelling, and widening of the heel associated with tenderness. Careful evaluation of soft tissues and neurovascular status is essential. About 10% of calcaneal fractures have an associated compartment syndrome of the foot and this must be ruled out. Massive swelling may result in blistering around the foot and ankle. Up to 50% of patients with calcaneal fractures may have other associated injuries, including lumbar spine fractures (10%) and fractures of the lower extremities (25%).

RADIOGRAPHIC EVALUATION

Radiographic evaluation of the patient with a suspected calcaneal fracture should include a lateral view of the hindfoot, a Harris axial view, Brodén view and an anteroposterior (AP) and oblique view of the foot. The lateral radiograph (Fig. 46.1) is used to assess height loss (loss of Böhler angle, Gissane angle) and rotation of the posterior facet. The Harris view is made to assess varus position of the tuberosity and width of the heel. AP and oblique views of the foot are made to assess the anterior process and calcaneocuboid involvement. A single Brodén view, obtained by internally rotating the leg 40° with the ankle in neutral, then angling the beam 10–15° cephalad, is made to evaluate congruency of the posterior facet. A CT scan helps to further characterize the fracture and position of the peroneal and flexor hallucis tendons. This helps to plan further management.

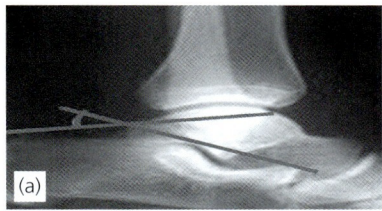
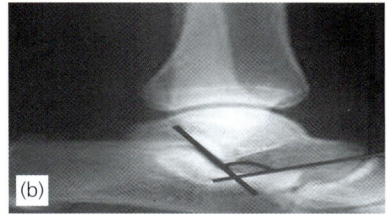

Figure 46.1 Böhler's tuber joint angle is composed of a line drawn from the highest point of the anterior process of the calcaneus to the highest point of the posterior facet and a line drawn tangential from the posterior facet to the superior edge of the tuberosity. The angle is normally between 20° and 40°; a decrease in this angle indicates that the weight-bearing posterior facet of the calcaneus has collapsed, thereby shifting body weight anteriorly. (b) The Gissane (crucial) angle is formed by two strong cortical struts extending laterally, one along the lateral margin of the posterior facet and the other extending anterior to the beak of the calcaneus. These cortical struts form an obtuse angle usually between 95° and 105° and are visualized directly beneath the lateral process of the talus; an increase in this angle indicates collapse of the posterior facet.

CLASSIFICATION

Calcaneal fractures can be extra-articular (not involving the subtalar joint) or intra-articular (involving the subtalar joint).

Extra-articular fractures

Extra-articular fractures constitute 25–30% of calcaneal fractures and include the following.

1. *Anterior process fractures* that result from strong plantarflexion and inversion, which tighten the bifurcate and interosseous ligaments leading to avulsion fracture.
2. *Posterior tuberosity fractures* may result from avulsion by the Achilles tendon.
3. *Medial process fractures* are vertical shear fractures that occur due to loading of the heel in valgus.
4. *Sustentacular fractures* that occur with heel loading accompanied by severe foot inversion.
5. *Body fractures* not involving the subtalar articulation. These are caused by axial loading. Significant comminution, widening, and loss of height may occur along with a reduction in the Böhler angle without posterior facet involvement.

Intra-articular fractures

Intra-articular fractures are traditionally classified using the Essex-Lopresti classification[1] or the Sanders classification,[2] which is based on CT scan.

ESSEX–LOPRESTI CLASSIFICATION (FIG. 46.2)

With axial loading, the posterolateral edge of the talus splits the calcaneus obliquely through the posterior facet, producing two main fragments: an anteromedial fragment,

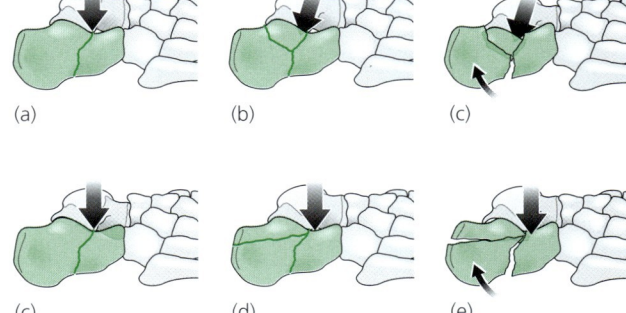

Figure 46.2 Mechanism of injury according to Essex-Lopresti. (a–c) Joint depression. (d–f) Tongue.

which consists of the sustentaculum ('constant' fragment), and a posterolateral fragment, which has an intra-articular component. The ensuing fracture (primary fracture line) is almost always present and extends from the proximal, medial aspect of the calcaneal tuberosity, through the anterolateral wall, usually in the vicinity of the crucial angle of Gissane. The most variable aspect of this fracture line is its position through the posterior facet of the calcaneus. It can be located in the medial third near the sustentaculum tali, the central third or the lateral third near the lateral wall.

In addition to the primary fracture line, a secondary fracture component may be created, based on additional energy imparted and the position of the foot at the time of injury. As the axial force continues, the medial spike attached to the sustentaculum is pushed further towards the medial heel skin. Often an anterior fracture extends towards the anterior process and may exit into the calcaneocuboid joint. The additional fractures of the posterior facet can be divided into two types. If the fracture line producing the posterior facet fragment exits behind the posterior facet and anterior to the attachment of the Achilles tendon, the injury is called a *joint depression type*. If it exits distal to the Achilles tendon insertion, it is called a *tongue type*.

SANDERS CLASSIFICATION (FIG. 46.3)

This CT scan classification is based on the number and location of articular fragments. The posterior facet of the calcaneus is divided into three fracture lines (A, B and C, corresponding to the lateral, middle and medial fracture lines on the coronal image). Thus, there can be a total of four potential pieces: lateral, central, medial, sustentaculum tali. A displacement of greater than 2 mm is considered significant. The Sanders classification has become more widely accepted in evaluation of these fractures owing to its precision regarding the location and number of fracture lines through the posterior facet (Table 46.1).

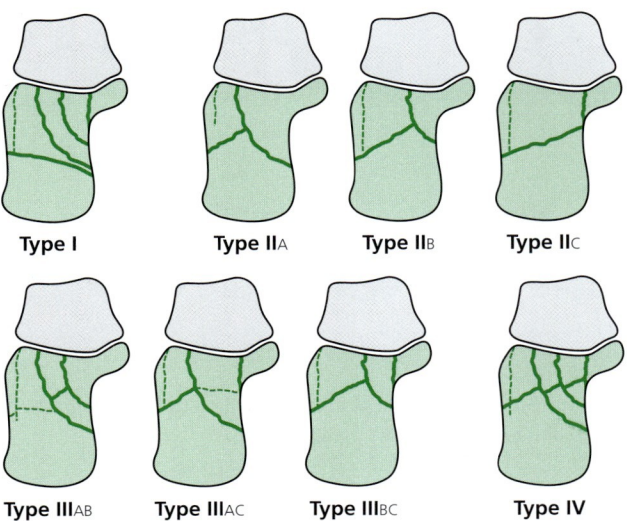

Figure 46.3 Schematic diagram of Sanders classification. Reproduced with permission from Sanders R, Fortin P, Pasquale T, et al. Operative treatment in 120 displaced intra-articular calcaneal fractures: Results using a prognostic computed tomography scan classification. *Clinical Orthopaedics and Related Research* 1993;**290**:87–95.

Table 46.1 Sanders CT scan-based classification of intra-articular fractures

Type	Description
Type I	All non-displaced fractures regardless of the number of fracture lines
Type II	Two-part fractures of the posterior facet; subtypes IIA, IIB, IIC, based on the location of the primary fracture line
Type III	Three-part fractures with a centrally depressed fragment; subtypes IIIAB, IIIAC, IIIBC
Type IV	Four-part articular fractures; highly comminuted

TREATMENT

Despite adequate reduction and treatment, fractures of the calcaneus may be severely disabling injuries, with variable prognosis and degrees of functional debilitation. Treatment remains controversial, with no clear indication for operative *vs* non-operative treatment.

Extra-articular fractures

All non-displaced or minimally displaced extra-articular calcaneal fractures can be managed non-operatively. The management guidelines are summarized in Table 46.2.

Non-operative treatment consists of a well-padded supportive splint to allow resolution of the initial fracture haematoma. A well-moulded plaster cast with the ankle in neutral position is applied. Early subtalar and ankle joint range-of-motion exercises are initiated, and non-weight-bearing restrictions are maintained for approximately 10–12 weeks, until radiographic union. Fractures in patients with severe peripheral vascular disease, insulin-dependent diabetes or with other medical comorbidities prohibiting surgery may also be treated non-operatively.

Intra-articular fractures

Non-displaced intra-articular fractures are managed non-operatively. The management of displaced fractures is controversial with strong proponents for both non-operative and operative management.[3] There is no solid evidence to suggest that patients who have open reduction and internal fixation (ORIF) have better functional results.[4] The Canadian Orthopaedic Trauma Society trial comparing operative and non-operative treatment of displaced intra-articular calcaneal fractures found that, as a whole, without stratification into various demographic classes, the outcomes after non-operative treatment were not different from the outcomes after operative treatment. However, with operative treatment significantly better results occurred in certain fracture groups such as women, younger adults, patients with a lighter workload, patients not receiving worker's compensation, patients with a higher initial Böhler angle (less severe initial injury) and those with an anatomic reduction on postoperative CT evaluation. Those having non-operative treatment of their fracture were 5.5 times more likely to require a subtalar arthrodesis for post-traumatic arthritis than those undergoing operation. ORIF of intra-articular calcaneal fractures can be expected to benefit patients only if near-anatomical reconstruction is achieved. Most authors agree that the inability to surgically obtain and maintain an anatomical reduction of the posterior facet is probably associated with a worse outcome than closed non-operative treatment.

The goals of surgery are restoration of congruity of the subtalar articulation, normal width and height of the

Table 46.2 Management guidelines for calcaneal fractures

Fracture	Morphology	Treatment
Anterior process	Non-displaced/minimally displaced/fractures with <<25% involvement of the calcaneal–cuboid articulation	Non-operative
	>25% involvement of the calcaneal–cuboid articulation	Fixation with small/mini-fragment screw
Tuberosity (avulsion) fractures	Non-displaced	Non-operative
	Displaced	
	(1) Gastrocnemius–soleus complex is incompetent	Fixation with a lag screw
	(2) Fragment involves the articular surface of the joint	
	(3) Posterior skin is at risk from pressure from the displaced tuberosity	
	(4) Bone is extremely prominent and will affect shoe wear	
Medial and lateral process fractures	Non-displaced	Non-operative
	Displaced	Closed manipulation and cast
Body fractures (not involving the subtalar joint)	Non-displaced/<1 cm displacement	Non-operative
	(1) Significant displacement resulting in varus/valgus deformity	
	(2) Lateral impingement	
	(3) Translation of the posterior tuberosity	Open reduction and internal fixation

calcaneus and the Böhler angle. Maintenance of the normal calcaneocuboid articulation, decompression of the subfibular space available for the peroneal tendons and neutralization of the varus deformity of the fracture are all important. Surgery should not be attempted until swelling in the foot and ankle has adequately subsided. However, it should not be delayed beyond 3 weeks. Open reduction can be obtained through a medial approach, combined medial and lateral approach or a lateral approach alone. Open reduction has complications including wound dehiscence, calcaneal osteomyelitis and sural nerve injury. Postoperative management includes non-weight bearing for 8–12 weeks with early institution of subtalar range-of-motion exercises.

Occasionally a tongue-type fracture may present without any additional fracture lines, widening of the lateral wall or significant displacement at the primary fracture line. These cases can be treated by closed reduction by the axial pin fixation of Gissane, which was popularized by Essex-Lopresti (Fig. 46.4).

COMPLICATIONS

Fracture blisters and complications of primary or secondary skin loss can occur. Post-traumatic arthritis of either the subtalar or calcaneocuboid joint and loss of subtalar motion are common due to articular damage, especially in displaced and comminuted fractures. Problems with

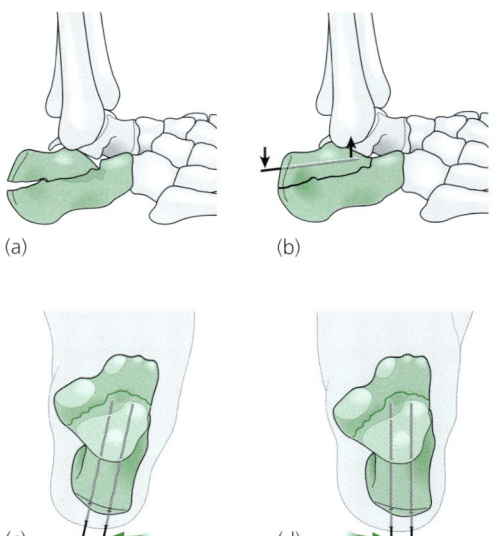

Figure 46.4 Essex-Lopresti technique as modified by Tornetta. Once guide pins are correctly positioned, they are exchanged for 6.5–8.0 mm cannulated cancellous lag screws.

shoe fitting occur because of heel widening and varus. Increased heel width also results in lateral impingement on the peroneal tendons on the fibula. Reflex sympathetic dystrophy may also occur with operative or non-operative management.

KEY LEARNING POINTS

- Although different types of radiographic views have been described, CT imaging provides the most complete, reliable assessment of these fractures.
- Compartmental syndrome of the foot can occur in 2–5% of patients and must be treated with urgent decompression.
- Isolated avulsion fractures do not usually involve the subtalar joint. If minimally displaced, they may be treated by a short-leg, non-weight-bearing cast with the ankle in neutral position for 4–6 weeks. Tongue-type avulsion fractures with major displacement require reduction and internal fixation of the displaced bone to reattach the Achilles tendon.
- Treatment recommendations for intra-articular fractures are (1) conservative treatment for non-displaced or minimally displaced fractures with early range of motion, (2) axial fixation with a metallic pin for tongue-type fractures and (3) open reduction and internal fixation for joint depression fractures.
- Surgical reduction for intra-articular fractures is advocated only if the fracture can be anatomically reduced and held in that reduced position, as only near-anatomical reconstruction will benefit the patient.

REFERENCES

- ● = Key primary paper
- ◆ = Major review article

●1. Essex-Lopresti P. The mechanism, reduction technique, and results in fractures of the os calcis. *British Journal of Surgery* 1952;**39**:395.

●2. Sanders R. Current concepts review: displaced intra-articular fractures of the calcaneus. *Journal of Bone and Joint Surgery (American)* 2000;**82**:233

◆3. Buckley R, Tough S, McCormack R, *et al.* Operative compared with nonoperative treatment of displaced intra-articular calcaneal fractures: a prospective, randomized, controlled multicenter trial. *Journal of Bone and Joint Surgery (American)* 2002;**84**:1733.

◆4. Sanders R. Current concepts review: displaced intra-articular fractures of the calcaneus. *Journal of Bone and Joint Surgery (American)* 2000;**82**:233.

47

Fractures of the midfoot

SHANMUGANATHAN RAJASEKARAN, VIJAY KAMATH, JAYARAMARAJU DHEENADHAYALAN

Introduction and relevant anatomy	403	Tarsal navicular	405
Clinical evaluation	404	Navicular dislocation	405
Radiographic evaluation	404	Cuboid fractures	405
Classification	404	Cuneiform fractures	405
Treatment	404	References	406
Complications	405		

INTRODUCTION

The midfoot is the section of the foot distal to the Chopart joint line and proximal to the Lisfranc joint line[1] (Fig. 47.1). It consists of the navicular, cuboid, the medial, middle and lateral cuneiforms, as well as the metatarsal–cuneiform articulations. The midfoot has constrained motion because of multiple recessed articulations as well as strong ligamentous and capsular attachments. The midtarsal joint consists of the calcaneocuboid and talonavicular joints, which act in concert with the subtalar joint during inversion and eversion of the foot. The cuboid acts as a linkage across the three naviculocuneiform joints, allowing only minimal motion. Ligamentous attachments include the plantar calcaneonavicular (spring) ligament, bifurcate ligament, dorsal talonavicular ligament, dorsal calcaneocuboid ligament, dorsal cuboidonavicular ligament and long plantar ligament (Fig. 47.2a,b).

The navicular bone is the keystone of the medial longitudinal arch of the foot. It articulates with the cuneiforms, cuboid, calcaneus and talus. Coupled motion between these structures (transverse tarsal joint) provides inversion and eversion of the midfoot and forefoot relative to the hindfoot. The navicular has extensive articular surfaces with a poor blood supply and a relatively avascular central portion. Thick ligaments on its plantar and dorsal aspect support the navicular cuneiform joints. The spring ligament and superficial

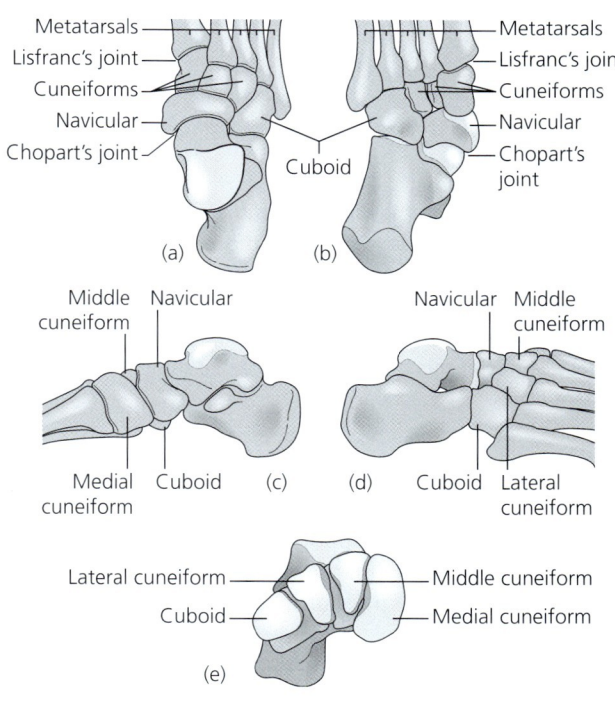

Figure 47.1 Bony anatomy of the midfoot. (a) Dorsal view. (b) Plantar view. (c) Medial view. (d) Lateral view. (e) Coronal view.

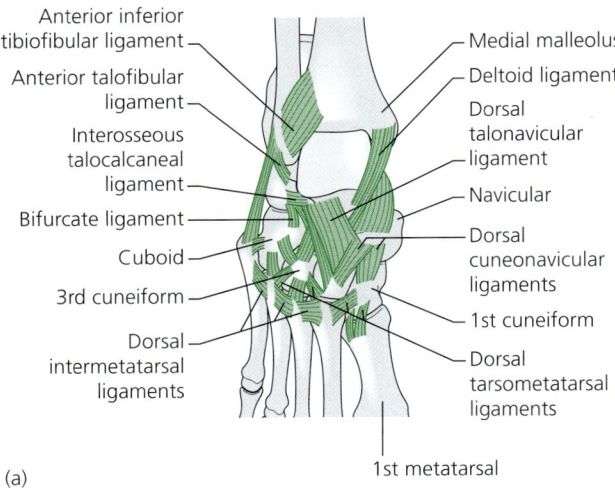

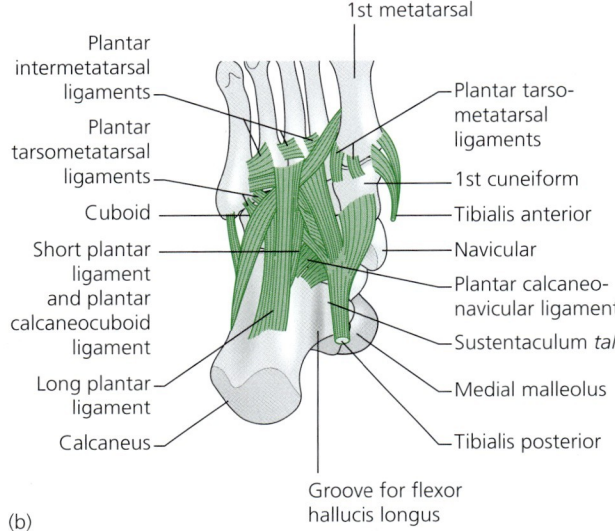

Figure 47.2 Ligamentous structure of the midfoot. (a) The dorsal view shows extensive overlap of the interosseous ligaments. (b) The plantar ligaments are thicker than their dorsal counterparts and are dynamically reinforced by the tibialis anterior, tibialis posterior and peroneus longus tendons. Note the extensive attachments of the tibialis posterior throughout the midfoot bones.

deltoid provide strong support to the plantar and medial aspects of the talonavicular joint. Accessory navicular (os tibiale externum) are present in 15% of patients and are bilateral in 70–90%.

Injuries to the midfoot are relatively rare. Most injuries are due to high-energy trauma and may result from direct impact or a combination of axial loading and torsion. Low-energy trauma may result in a sprain with injury to the ligaments.

CLINICAL EVALUATION

Depending on the extent of injury, patients present with swelling, tenderness, ecchymosis and deformity. In mild injuries, stress manoeuvres consist of forefoot abduction, adduction, flexion and extension and may result in reproduction of pain and instability. In severe cases, serial examinations may be warranted to evaluate the possibility of foot compartment syndrome.[2]

RADIOGRAPHIC EVALUATION

Anteroposterior (AP), lateral and oblique radiographs of the foot should be obtained. Stress views or weight-bearing radiographs may help to delineate subtle injuries. CT may be helpful in characterizing fracture dislocation injuries with articular comminution. MRI may be used to evaluate ligamentous injury.

CLASSIFICATION

The injuries are classified based on the direction of applied force to the foot.

- *Medial stress injury.* Inversion injury occurs with adduction of the midfoot on the hindfoot.
- *Longitudinal stress injury.* Here the force is transmitted through the metatarsal heads proximally along the rays with resultant compression of the midfoot between the metatarsals and the talus with the foot plantarflexed. Longitudinal forces pass between the cuneiforms and fracture the navicular typically in a vertical pattern.
- *Lateral stress injury.* This commonly results in an avulsion fracture of the navicular with a comminuted compression fracture of the cuboid. The 'nutcracker fracture of the cuboid' is due to the crushing of the cuboid between the calcaneus and the fourth and fifth metatarsal bases when the forefoot is driven laterally.
- *Plantar stress injury.* This may result in sprains to the midtarsal region with avulsion fractures of the dorsal lip of the navicular, talus, or anterior process of the calcaneus.

TREATMENT

Sprains are treated with non-rigid dressings with protected weight bearing for 4–6 weeks. Non-displaced fractures may be treated with a short leg cast or boot with initial non-weight bearing for 6 weeks. Displaced fracture patterns often require open reduction and internal fixation (e.g. with Kirschner wires or lag screws) and/or external fixation. Bone grafting of the cuboid may be necessary in lateral stress injuries. Severe crush injuries with extensive comminution may require arthrodesis to restore the longitudinal arch of the foot.

COMPLICATIONS

Post-traumatic osteoarthritis may occur as a result of residual articular incongruity or chondral injury at the time of trauma.

TARSAL NAVICULAR

Isolated fractures of the navicular bone are rare and it is important to rule out concomitant injuries to the midtarsal joint complex. These injuries occur most often due to axial loading of the foot. Direct impaction, although uncommon, can cause avulsions to the periphery or crush injury in the dorsal plantar plane.

Patients typically present with a painful foot and dorsomedial swelling and tenderness. It is important to rule out associated ankle and foot injuries. AP, lateral, medial oblique and lateral oblique views should be obtained to ascertain the extent of injury to the navicular as well as to detect associated injuries. A CT scan may be obtained to better characterize the fracture.

Navicular fractures are classified as cortical avulsion fractures (40–50%), tuberosity fractures (20–25%) and body fractures (30%). Body fractures have been subclassified by Sangeorzan[3] (Fig. 47.3).

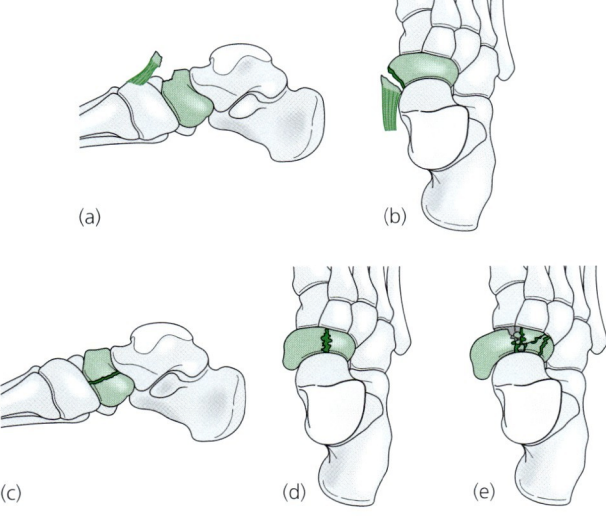

Figure 47.3 Classification of navicular fractures.
(a) Avulsion-type fracture; (b) tuberosity fractures; (c) type I body fracture; (d) type II body fracture; (e) type III body fracture From Bucholz RW, Heckman JD, Court-Brown C, et al. (eds.) Rockwood and Green's Fractures in Adults, 6th edn. Philadelphia, PA: Lippincott Williams & Wilkins, 2006.

Most avulsion fractures are small and can be managed by immobilization in a non-weight-bearing cast until symptoms resolve. Open reduction and internal fixation is indicated if a fragment includes more than 25% of the articular surfaces and fragment displacement more than 3 mm. Primary talonavicular fusion is considered if more than 40% of the articular surface cannot be reconstructed.

NAVICULAR DISLOCATION

Isolated dislocation or subluxation of the navicular is rare. The mechanism is hyperplantarflexion of the forefoot with subsequent axial loading. Open reduction is usually necessary to restore both navicular position and articular congruity.

CUBOID FRACTURES

Isolated cuboid injuries are rare and are usually seen in association with injuries to the talonavicular joint or other midfoot structures. Direct trauma to the dorsolateral aspect of the foot may result in fractures of the cuboid. Indirect injuries due to torsional stress or forefoot abduction result in impaction of the cuboid between the calcaneous and the lateral metatarsals ('nutcracker injury'). Patients typically present with pain, swelling and tenderness to palpation at the dorsolateral aspect of the foot. Apart from routine radiographic views, CT scan may be necessary to assess the extent of injury and instability.

Isolated fractures of the cuboid with no evidence of loss of osseous length or interosseous instability can be treated by non-weight-bearing cast for 4–6 weeks. Open reduction and internal fixation is indicated if there is more than 2 mm of joint surface disruption or any evidence of longitudinal compression. Severe comminution and residual articular displacement may necessitate calcaneocuboid arthrodesis.

CUNEIFORM FRACTURES

These usually occur in conjunction with tarsometatarsal injuries. The usual mechanism is indirect axial loading of the bone. Localized tenderness over the cuneiform region, pain in the midfoot with weight bearing, or discomfort with motion through the tarsometatarsal joints can signify injury to these bones. AP, lateral and oblique views should be obtained. These should be weight bearing if possible. Coronal and longitudinal CT scans of the midfoot can be used to better define the extent of the injury.

KEY LEARNING POINTS

- The midfoot is the section of the foot distal to the Chopart joint line and proximal to the Lisfranc joint line.
- These injuries are often missed and need a high index of suspicion.
- Most injuries can be managed by conservative methods and the treatment of coexisting other fractures take precedence.
- Displaced fractures and those involving the articular surface need reduction and internal fixation.

REFERENCES

- ● = Key primary paper
- ◆ = Major review article

◆1. Heckman JD. Fractures and dislocations of the foot. In: Rockwood CA, Green DP, Bucholtz RW, Heckman JD (eds) *Rockwood and Green's Fractures in Adults*, 4th edn. Philadelphia, PA: Lippincott-Raven; 1996:2267–405.

◆2. Myerson M. Management of crush injuries and compartment syndromes of the foot. In: Meyerson M. (ed.) *Foot and Ankle Disorders*, Vol. 2. Philadelphia, PA: W.B. Saunders, 2000:1223–44.

●3. Sangeorzan BJ, Benirschke SK, Mosca V, *et al.* Displaced intraarticular fractures of the tarsal navicular. *Journal of Bone and Joint Surgery (American)* 1989;**71**:1504–10.

48

Injuries of the tarsometatarsal (Lisfranc) joint

SHANMUGANATHAN RAJASEKARAN, RISHI MUGESH KANNA, JAYARAMARAJU DHEENADHAYALAN

Introduction	407	Classification	408
Clinical evaluation	407	Treatment	408
Radiographic evaluation	407	References	410

NATIONAL BOARD STANDARDS

- Understand the complex anatomy of the tarsometatarsal joints
- Able to diagnose clinically and confirm the different injury types radiologically
- Able to plan treatment and explain prognosis

INTRODUCTION

The Lisfranc joint complex consists of the tarsometatarsal, intermetatarsal and intertarsal joints.[1] Injuries of the tarsometatarsal articulation range from mild sprains to widely displaced debilitating injuries. The incidence of Lisfranc injuries is rare, but approximately 20% of Lisfranc injuries are initially overlooked.[2]

Injuries of the Lisfranc joint complex result from either direct or indirect mechanisms. Direct injuries result from a dorsally applied force. This results in either plantar metatarsal displacement if the force is applied to the metatarsal base, or dorsal metatarsal displacement if the force is applied to the cuneiforms. There is a high incidence of associated tarsal fracture, significant soft-tissue destruction and compartment syndrome. Indirect injuries occur from a combination of axial loading and twisting on an axially loaded, plantarflexed foot. Because of the mechanism of injury, relatively weaker dorsal ligaments and greater mobility between the first and second metatarsals, the displacement is typically dorsal with diastasis between the first and second metatarsals and their corresponding cuneiforms.

CLINICAL EVALUATION

Patients present with pain, variable swelling, foot deformity and tenderness on the dorsum of the foot. Neurovascular examination is essential, as Lisfranc joint dislocation may be associated with impingement on or laceration of the dorsalis pedis artery. Severe foot swelling is common with high-energy injuries and serial neurovascular examination or compartment pressure monitoring is required to evaluate for compartment syndrome.

RADIOGRAPHIC EVALUATION

Anteroposterior, internal oblique and lateral foot radiographs are obtained to evaluate the tarsometatarsal articulations (Fig. 48.1). Despite normal radiographs, if injury is suspected, a CT scan can be used to assist in the diagnosis. A CT scan will show the osseous structures as well as the amount of intra-articular comminution. Associated fractures of the cuneiforms, cuboid and/or metatarsals are common and should be looked for.

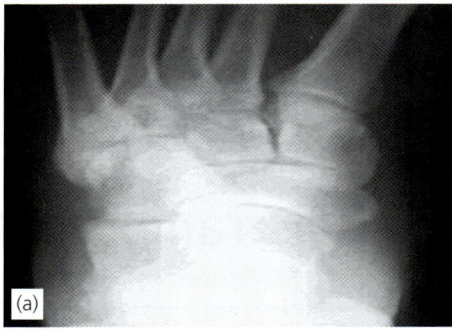
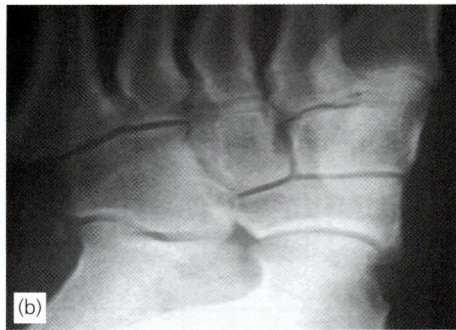

Figure 48.1 Anteroposterior and medial oblique view of the normal tarsometatarsal joint. Normal radiographs include collinearity of the medial aspect of the second metatarsal base and medial cuneiform on the anteroposterior view, the medial aspect of the fourth metatarsal base with the medial aspect of the cuboid and the medial aspect of the third metatarsal with the lateral cuneiform on the oblique view. Any incongruity is pathological, as is any dorsal displacement of the metatarsals seen on a lateral radiograph. Diastasis of 2 mm between the medial and middle cuneiforms is considered pathological. The 'fleck' sign represents an avulsion of the Lisfranc ligament off the base of the second metatarsal.

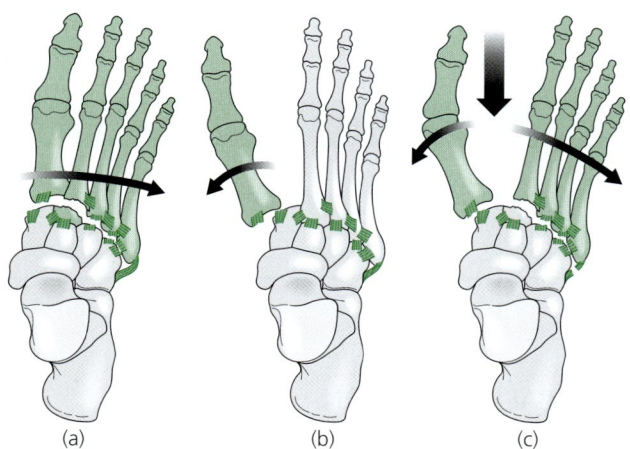

Figure 48.2 The classification by Quenu and Kuss. (a) Homolateral–all five metatarsals displaced in the same direction. (b) Isolated–one or two metatarsals displaced from the others. (c) Divergent–displacement of the metatarsals in both the sagittal and coronal planes. Further subdivisions are used to identify the direction of dislocation in the homolateral pattern (medial or lateral) and the partial disruption (first or lesser).

CLASSIFICATION

Classification schemes for Lisfranc injuries guide the clinician in defining the extent and pattern of injury, although they are of little prognostic value. The *Quenu and Kuss* classification (Fig. 48.2) is based on commonly observed patterns of injury.[3] The *Myerson* classification (Fig. 48.3 and Table 48.1) is based on the observed patterns of injury with regard to treatment.[4]

TREATMENT

Non-surgical treatment is used for patients with ligamentous injuries with or without small plantar avulsion fractures of the metatarsal/tarsal bones and non-displaced fractures. This consists of a non-weight-bearing well-moulded short leg cast for 8 weeks, followed by gradual weight bearing in a removable boot brace. Repeat radiographs are necessary once the swelling decreases to detect osseous displacement.

Surgery is performed for injuries with >2 mm displacement of the tarsometatarsal joint. If anatomic reduction can be obtained by closed means, percutaneous internal fixation can be performed. But an interposed

Table 48.1 Myerson classification

Type A injuries	Total incongruity	Displacement of all five metatarsals with or without fracture of the base of the second metatarsal. The usual displacement is lateral or dorsolateral, and the metatarsals move as a unit
Type B injuries	Partial incongruity	One or more articulations remain intact. Type B1 injuries are medially displaced, sometimes involving the intercuneiform or naviculocuneiform joint. Type B2 injuries are laterally displaced and may involve the first metatarsal–cuneiform joint
Type C injuries	Divergent	Divergent injuries and can be partial (C1) or complete (C2). These generally are high-energy injuries, associated with significant swelling, and prone to complications, especially compartment syndrome

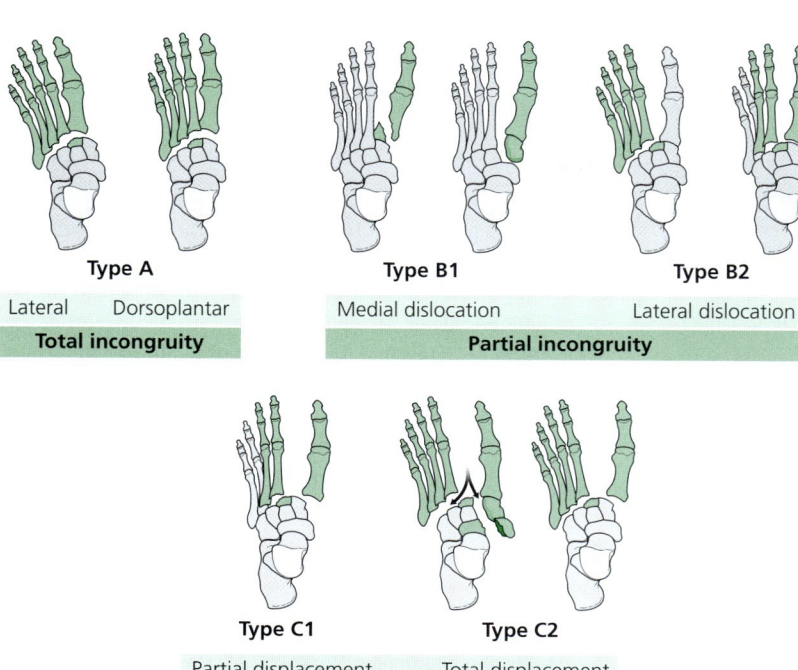

Figure 48.3 Myerson classification of Lisfranc fracture dislocations. Adapted with permission from Myerson MS, Fisher RT, Burgess AR, et al. Fracture-dislocations of the tarsometatarsal joints: end results correlated with pathology and treatment. *Foot and Ankle* 1986;**6**:225–42.

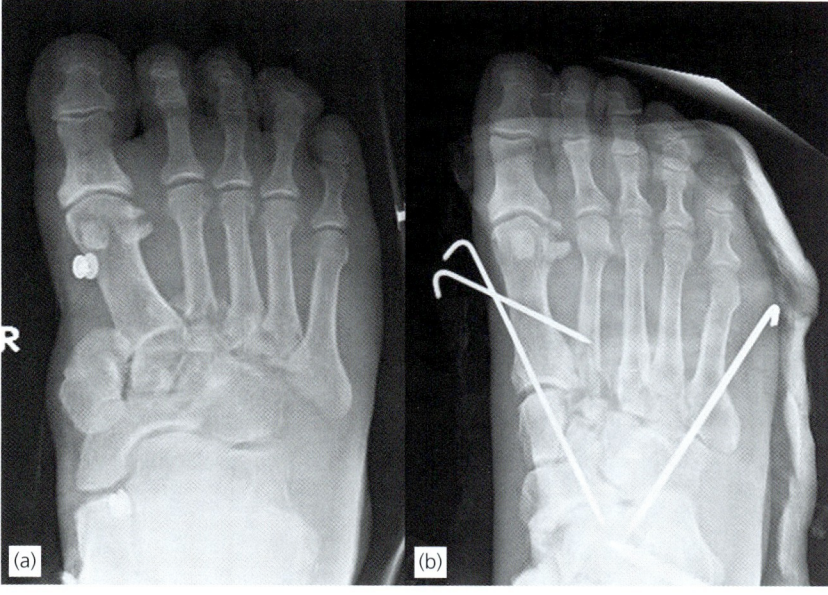

Figure 48.4 (a) Homolateral type of Lisfranc dislocation; (b) open reduction and stabilization with Kirschner wires.

Lisfranc ligament remnant can frequently block reduction and result in the joint springing open, once internal fixation is removed. Therefore, open reduction is frequently necessary through a single or dual longitudinal incision as dictated by the injury pattern. The key to reduction is correction of the fracture dislocation of the second metatarsal base. Fixation is achieved with 4.0 mm screws for the medial (first tarsometatarsal joint) and middle (second, third tarsometatarsal joints) columns and Kirschner wires for the lateral (fourth, fifth tarsometatarsal joints) column. A severe abduction mechanism may result in compression of the cuboid, which may require lateral plating and bone grafting to avoid residual abduction. Fixation allows arthrofibrosis of the injured joints, which preserves the normal slope of the foot. Patients should not bear weight for 8 weeks, followed by gradual weight bearing in a removable boot brace.[5]

Implant removal is usually performed to avoid breakage and to restore tarsometatarsal motion. Lateral column stabilization can be removed at 6–12 weeks; however, medial fixation should not be removed for 4–6 months. Some authors advocate that, although screw breakage can occur, it is preferable to leave the screws in place as removal can lead to planovalgus deformity. Immediate complete arthrodesis of the midfoot has been associated with poor results, although partial arthrodesis tends to have better results than complete arthrodesis (Fig. 48.4).[6]

KEY LEARNING POINTS

- The incidence of Lisfranc injuries is rare but increasing because of motor vehicle crashes.
- The tarsometatarsal joints of the foot are very stable and immobile structures and hence Lisfranc injuries result from high-energy forces.
- Lisfranc injury can be caused by direct or indirect mechanisms. Most are usually a component of multiple injuries and may be caused by high-energy motor vehicle or industrial accidents.
- The injuries vary from being pure fractures and fracture dislocations to pure ligamentous disruptions and have a progressively worsening prognosis. Severe, displaced injuries require open reduction and internal fixation.

REFERENCES

● = Key primary paper
◆ = Major review article

◆1. Peicha G, Labovitz J, Seibert FJ, *et al*. The anatomy of the joint as a risk factor for Lisfranc dislocation and fracture-dislocation: an anatomical and radiological case control study. *Journal of Bone and Joint Surgery (British)* 2002;**84**:981–5.
●2. Aitken AP, Poulson D. Dislocations of the tarsometatarsal joint. *Journal of Bone and Joint Surgery (American)* 1963;**45**:246.
3. Quenu E, Kuss G. Etude sur les luxations du metatarse du diastasis entre le 1er et le 2^{e} metatarsien. *Revue de Chirurgie* 1909;**39**:281–336.
●4. Myerson M, Fisher R, Burgess A, *et al*. Dislocations of the tarsometatarsal joints: end results correlated with pathology and treatment. *Foot and Ankle* 1986;**6**:225.
◆5. Teng AL, Pinzur MS, Lomasney L, *et al*. Functional outcome following anatomic restoration of tarsal-metatarsal fracture-dislocation. *Foot and Ankle International* 2002;**23**:922–6.
◆6. Mulier T, Reynders P, Dereymaeker G, Broos P. Severe Lisfrancs injuries: primary arthrodesis or ORIF? *Foot and Ankle International* 2002;**23**:902–5.

49

Fractures of the forefoot

SHANMUGANATHAN RAJASEKARAN, RISHI MUGESH KANNA, JAYARAMARAJU DHEENADHAYALAN

FIRST TO FOURTH METATARSAL FRACTURES	411	Complications	412
Introduction	411	FIFTH METATARSAL INJURIES	412
Clinical evaluation	411	Introduction	412
Radiographic evaluation	411	Treatment	412
Treatment	411	References	413
Fractures of the metatarsal necks	412		

FIRST TO FOURTH METATARSAL FRACTURES

INTRODUCTION

This is a common injury. Fractures of the central metatarsals are much more common than first metatarsal fractures and can be isolated or part of a more significant injury pattern.[1] Acute metatarsal fractures may occur as a result of a direct blow, which usually results in a transverse fracture, or as a result of an indirect twisting or avulsion mechanism. Metatarsal base fractures are usually associated with midfoot injury. Stress fractures may occur especially at the necks of the second and third metatarsals and the proximal fifth metatarsal.

CLINICAL EVALUATION

Patients typically present with pain, swelling and tenderness over the site of fracture. Neurovascular evaluation is important. Compartment syndrome can be seen in patients with more severe fractures, particularly those resulting from a direct blow.

RADIOGRAPHIC EVALUATION

In isolated injuries to the foot, weight-bearing films should be obtained in the anteroposterior and lateral planes. The lateral radiographic view of the metatarsals is important for judging sagittal plane displacement of the metatarsal heads. Oblique views can be helpful to detect minimally displaced fractures. Radiographs should be evaluated for other metatarsal/tarsal injuries. MRI and technetium bone scans may aid in the diagnosis of an occult stress fracture.

TREATMENT

As a rule, the soft-tissue injury is more severe than the fracture. Initial treatment should include a compression dressing and elevation to control swelling.

First metatarsal shaft fractures

Any displacement of fracture fragments in a metatarsal fracture should be least tolerated in the first ray. The best way to determine operative or non-operative treatment for isolated first metatarsal fractures is with stress radiographs. Displacement of the position of the first metatarsal through the joint or fracture site on stress films represents instability that requires fixation. If there is not much instability, these fractures can be managed in a short leg cast with weight bearing as tolerated for 4–6 weeks.

Second to fourth metatarsal shaft fractures

Non-surgical treatment is indicated if displacement is less than 3 mm or angulation is less than 10°. Treatment can vary from the use of a cast with weight bearing as tolerated for a stable fracture to casting and non-weight bearing for an unstable fracture pattern prone to displacement. Surgery is indicated for displacement of greater than 3–4 mm or sagittal displacement of greater than 10°. If metatarsal fractures are associated with a Lisfranc ligamentous injury at the tarsometatarsal junction, surgical stabilization is necessary because of inherent instability.

FRACTURES OF THE METATARSAL NECKS

These may be associated with displacement of the metatarsal head towards the weight-bearing surface of the foot, which disrupts the normal mechanics of proper weight bearing. Fractures of the first metatarsal neck or of multiple metatarsal necks must be reduced and stabilized with percutaneous K-wire fixation because they are often unstable. An isolated metatarsal neck fracture should be grossly aligned to avoid abnormal pressure of the metatarsal head on the sole of the foot (transfer metatarsalgia) and to avoid forcing the toe against the top of the shoe. The foot must be immobilized in a short leg walking cast for 6–10 weeks.

COMPLICATIONS

Malunion, non-union and arthritic degeneration of the tarsometatarsal and metatarsophalangeal joints are possible complications of first metatarsal fractures. Transfer metatarsalgia to the lesser toes can occur with shortening of the metatarsal length.

FIFTH METATARSAL INJURIES

INTRODUCTION

Fractures of the fifth metatarsal are separated roughly into two groups, proximal base fractures and distal spiral fractures. Proximal fifth metatarsal fractures are further divided by the location of the fracture (Fig. 49.1). Each implies a separate causality, location, treatment and prognosis.[2]

Zone I fractures (93%) are avulsion injuries of the cancellous tuberosity, which occur secondary to contraction of the long plantar ligament and peroneus brevis insertion. Although most are extra-articular, some may involve the metatarsocuboid joint. Zone II fractures (Jones fracture) occur at the metaphyseal–diaphyseal junction. They result from adduction or inversion of the forefoot. The fracture is caused by tensile stress along the lateral border of the metatarsal. This is a circulatory watershed region that is subject to potential non-union secondary to poor blood supply. Zone III fractures occur in the proximal 1.5 cm of the diaphyseal shaft of the metatarsal and are typically stress fractures. These are relatively rare and seen mainly in athletes, who usually present with prodromal symptoms before complete fracture. Possible aetiological factors include low arches and associated first metatarsal hypermobility, as well as cavovarus deformities, both of which can result in abnormally high stresses placed on the lateral foot. Poor blood supply in this region may also predispose an individual to impaired injury healing, resulting in non-union.

TREATMENT

Zone I fractures

These are treated with a stiff-soled shoe and weight bearing as tolerated once symptoms diminish. If there is a large intra-articular fragment with displacement or if the base fragment has retracted proximally, indicative of peroneus brevis retraction, internal fixation is necessary. Continued symptoms after non-surgical treatment are rare and may necessitate removal of the non-union fragment, with reattachment of the peroneus brevis.

Zone II fractures

A non-displaced fracture is managed initially in a short leg non-weight bearing cast worn for a few weeks followed by a weight-bearing cast till union has been achieved. Fractures with displacement and comminution can be

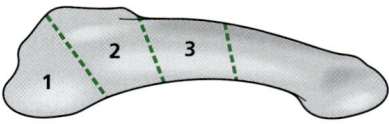

Figure 49.1 Three zones of proximal fifth metatarsal fracture. Zone I: avulsion fracture of the cancellous tuberosity. Zone II: fracture at the metaphyseal–diaphyseal junction (Jones fracture). Zone III: proximal diaphyseal stress fracture.

treated similarly; however, in a high-performance athlete, consideration should be given to early open reduction and internal fixation with an intramedullary screw, which allows for earlier mobilization.[3,4]

Zone III fractures

Initial treatment is by a non-weight-bearing cast for a few weeks. Strict adherence to non-weight bearing is necessary until radiographic evidence of fracture healing. If sclerosis is noted at the fracture site, this indicates circulatory compromise, and surgical intervention is necessary to remove avascular fibrous tissue, graft the area and compress the fracture with an intramedullary screw.

Spiral fractures of the distal fifth metatarsal are common and occur frequently in dancers and professional athletes. They usually occur because of a rotational force being applied to the foot while axially loaded in a plantarflexed position. Treatment is symptomatic, with a hard-soled shoe.

> ### KEY LEARNING POINTS
>
> - Isolated second to fourth metatarsal fractures can be treated non-surgically if displacement is <3 mm or angulation is <10°. Surgical stabilization is advocated if displacement is >3 mm and angulation is >10° or if associated with midfoot injuries.
> - After reduction of a first metatarsal fracture, if the great toe remains cocked up or the first web space remains widened then the reduction is incomplete or unstable and surgery may be required.
> - Treatment of proximal fifth metatarsal injuries is dependent on the zone of fracture. Zone I fractures should be treated symptomatically unless there is gross (>3 mm) displacement, in which case the treatment of choice is open reduction and internal fixation. Jones fractures may be managed non-operatively in a non-weight bearing cast for 8–12 weeks in most cases; however, surgery should be considered in elderly people and high-performance athletes.

REFERENCES

- ● = Key primary paper
- ◆ = Major review article

◆1. Alepuz ES, Carsi VV, Alcántara P, et al. Fractures of the central metatarsal. *Foot and Ankle International* 1996;**17**:200.

●2. Torg JS, Balduini FC, Zelko RR, et al. Fractures of the base of the fifth metatarsal distal to the tuberosity. *Journal of Bone and Joint Surgery (American)* 1984;**66**:209–14.

◆3. Josefsson PO, Karlsson M, Redlund-Johnell I, et al. Jones fracture: surgical versus nonsurgical treatment. *Clinical Orthopaedics and Related Research* 1994;**299**:252.

◆4. Rosenberg GA, Sferra JJ. Treatment strategies for acute fractures and nonunions of the proximal fifth metatarsal. *Journal of the American Academy of Orthopaedic Surgeons* 2000;**8**:332.

50

Metatarsophalangeal joint, phalangeal and interphalangeal joint injuries

SHANMUGANATHAN RAJASEKARAN, RISHI MUGESH KANNA, JAYARAMARAJU DHEENADHAYALAN

First metatarsophalangeal joint	414	Phalangeal fractures	415
Fractures and dislocations of the lesser metatarsophalangeal joints	415	Dislocation of the interphalangeal joint	416
		References	416
Sesamoids	415		

NATIONAL BOARD STANDARDS

- Understand the complex anatomy of the forefoot joints
- Able to diagnose clinically and demonstrate fractures radiologically
- Able to plan treatment and explain prognosis

FIRST METATARSOPHALANGEAL JOINT

Introduction

Injuries to the first metatarsophalangeal (MTP) joint are relatively common, especially following athletic activities or ballet dancing.[1] These injuries occur primarily because of varying grades of hyperextension of the first MTP joint and range from a sprain to frank dislocation with disruption of the plantar capsule and plate. The head of the first metatarsal becomes trapped between the flexor hallucis brevis and abductor hallucis tendons medially, and the lateral head of the flexor hallucis brevis and adductor tendons laterally.

Anatomically, the metatarsal head is held by the plantar plate and the deep transverse metatarsal ligament on the dorsal aspect. On the plantar surface, the plantar aponeurosis prevents further reduction. The flexor hallucis longus tendon usually lies lateral to the metatarsal head.

Clinical and radiographic evaluation

Patients typically present with pain, swelling and tenderness of the first MTP joint. Most dislocations are dorsal with the proximal phalanx cocked up and displaced dorsally and proximally producing a dorsal prominence and shortening of the toe. Anteroposterior, lateral and oblique views of the foot may demonstrate capsular avulsion.

Classification

Bowers and Martin classified first MTP joint injuries as in Table 50.1.[2] Jahss[3] classified first MTP joint dislocations based on the integrity of the sesamoid complex (Table 50.2).

Treatment

First MTP joint sprains are managed with protective taping with gradual return to activity. Temporary use of a

Table 50.1 Bowers and Martin classification

Grade	Description
Grade I	Strain at the proximal attachment of the volar plate from the first metatarsal head
Grade II	Avulsion of the volar plate from the metatarsal head
Grade III	Impaction injury to the dorsal surface of the metatarsal head with or without an avulsion or chip fracture

Table 50.2 Jahss classification

Type	Description
Type I	Volar plate avulsed off the first metatarsal head, proximal phalanx displaced dorsally; intersesamoid ligament remaining intact and lying over the dorsum of the metatarsal head
Type IIA	Rupture of the intersesamoid ligament
Type IIB	Longitudinal fracture of either sesamoid

hard-soled shoe with a rocker bottom is recommended for comfort. Operative intervention is indicated in cases of displaced intra-articular fractures and significant valgus instability.

For Jahss type I dislocations, closed reduction may be initially attempted. However, soft-tissue interposition commonly prevents reduction and open reduction is required. Jahss type IIA and IIB dislocations are easily reduced by longitudinal traction with or without hyperextension of the first MTP joint. After reduction, the patient should be placed in a short leg walking cast with a toe extension for 3–4 weeks to allow capsular healing. Displaced avulsion fractures of the base of the proximal phalanx should be stabilized. Small osteochondral fractures may be excised; however, large fragments require fixation.

Complications

Post-traumatic osteoarthritis, hallux rigidus and recurrent dislocation can be a sequela in a small group of patients.

FRACTURES AND DISLOCATIONS OF THE LESSER METATARSOPHALANGEAL JOINTS

'Stubbing' injuries are very common and may result in dislocation or avulsion fractures. Comminuted intra-articular fractures may occur by direct trauma. The incidence is higher for the fifth MTP joint because its lateral position renders it more vulnerable to injury.[4] Patients typically present with tenderness and deformity of the involved digit. Dislocation of the MTP joint typically manifests as dorsal prominence of the base of the proximal phalanx.

Simple dislocations or non-displaced fractures are managed by reduction with longitudinal traction and 'buddy strapping' for 4 weeks and a rigid shoe orthosis to limit MTP joint motion. Intra-articular fractures of the metatarsal head or the base of the proximal phalanx may be treated by excision of a small fragment or more usually by benign neglect, especially in the presence of comminution. An open reduction and internal fixation (ORIF) with Kirschner wires or screw fixation can be carried out when there is a large fragment.

SESAMOIDS

The sesamoids are an integral part of the capsuloligamentous structure of the first MTP joint. They function within the joint complex as both shock absorbers and fulcrums in supporting the weight-bearing function of the first toe. A high incidence of sesamoid fractures is seen in ballet dancers and runners secondary to repetitive hyperextension at the MTP joints.

These fractures are usually the result of a direct force applied to this area of the foot either from a fall with landing on the metatarsal heads or from a weight being dropped on the foot. Occasionally, these injuries occur as avulsion fractures from forceful hyperextension of the great toe or from traction injuries to the flexor hallucis brevis.

The patient presents with localized pain over the area, with accentuation of symptoms with passive extension or active flexion of the MTP joint.

Anteroposterior, lateral and oblique views of the forefoot are usually sufficient to demonstrate a transverse fracture of the sesamoids. Occasionally, a tangential view of the sesamoids is necessary to visualize a small osteochondral or avulsion fracture. This must be differentiated from a congenital bipartite sesamoid which is seen in 10–30% of people with an 85% bilateral occurrence. Local pain and irregularity on the radiograph are the distinguishing features for a fracture. It is sometimes difficult to visualize on plain radiographs and a CT may be needed. Technetium bone scanning or MRI may be used to identify stress fractures not apparent by plain radiography.

Non-operative management should initially be attempted, with soft padding combined with a short leg walking cast for 4 weeks followed by a shoe with a metatarsal pad for 4–8 weeks. If pain persists, a sesamoid resection with reconstitution of the tendon is indicated.

PHALANGEAL FRACTURES

Phalangeal fractures are the most common injury to the forefoot. The first and fifth digits are in especially vulnerable

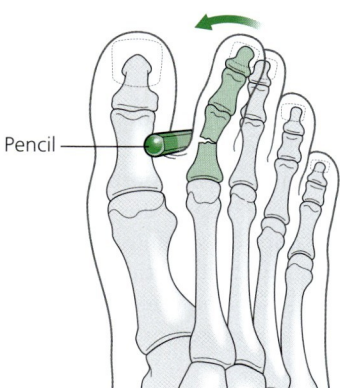

Figure 50.1 A method of closed reduction for displaced proximal phalanx fractures. A hard object, such as a pencil, is placed in the adjacent web space and is used as a fulcrum for reduction.

positions for injury because they form the medial and lateral borders of the distal foot.

Phalangeal fractures may occur due to a 'stubbing' injury (axial loading with secondary varus or valgus force) that results in spiral or oblique fracture, or due to a 'direct blow' (heavy object dropped onto the foot) resulting in a transverse or comminuted fracture.

Patients typically present with pain, swelling and variable deformity of the affected digit. Anteroposterior, lateral and oblique views of the foot should be obtained.

Phalanx fractures are classified descriptively depending on their location (proximal, middle or distal), angulation and displacement and the presence of comminution, intra-articular extension or a fracture dislocation.

Surgical treatment of phalangeal fractures of the toes is rarely required because most phalangeal fractures can be treated successfully by conservative measures. Non-displaced fractures irrespective of articular involvement can be treated with 'buddy strapping' and protected weight bearing in a stiff-soled shoe. Fractures with clinical deformity require reduction. Closed reduction is usually adequate and stable (Fig. 50.1). Operative reduction is reserved for fractures with gross instability or persistent intra-articular discontinuity.

DISLOCATION OF THE INTERPHALANGEAL JOINT

Dislocation of the interphalangeal joint of the hallux usually is caused by hyperextension, with the distal phalanx positioned dorsal to the proximal phalanx. Closed reduction under digital block should be attempted. Longitudinal traction is applied in the axial plane of the deformity, followed by flexion when the distal phalanx is level with the articular surface of the proximal phalanx. Once reduced, the interphalangeal joint is usually stable and can be adequately treated with buddy strapping and progressive activity as tolerated. If a post-reduction radiograph shows persistent widening of the joint space, open reduction is indicated even if the toe rests in the proper position clinically. The plantar plate or a sesamoid bone is usually found to be interposed in the joint. Irreducible dislocations warrant open reduction.

Interphalangeal joint dislocations of the lesser toes are usually due to an axial load applied at the terminal end of the digit. Closed reduction by longitudinal traction and buddy strapping to the adjacent toe for 3 weeks is usually adequate as once reduced they are stable. In the rare event of irreducibility, open reduction is indicated.

KEY LEARNING POINTS

- Metatarsophalangeal joint injuries occur as a result of hyperextension and soft-tissue interposition may occur as in type I Jahss injuries.
- For Jahss type I dislocations, closed reduction is attempted; if irreducible, open reduction is performed. Jahss type II dislocations can usually be managed non-operatively.
- The majority of phalangeal fractures can be managed non-operatively with closed reduction and strapping. Fractures with gross instability or persistent intra-articular discontinuity require surgical stabilization.

REFERENCES

- ● = Key primary paper
- ◆ = Major review article

● 1. Brunet JA. Pathomechanics of complex dislocations of the first metatarsophalangeal joint. *Clinical Orthopaedics and Related Research* 1996;**332**:126.
● 2. Bowers Jr KD, Martin RB. Turf-toe: a shoe surface related football injury. *Medicine and Science in Sports and Exercise* 1976;**8**:81.
◆ 3. Jahss MH. Traumatic dislocations of the first metatarsophalangeal joint. *Foot and Ankle* 1980;**1**:15.
◆ 4. Brunet JA, Tubin S. Traumatic dislocation of lesser toes. *Foot and Ankle International* 1997;**18**:406.

SECTION 4

51 Acetabular fractures   419
Anish Potty, Sureshan Sivananthan

52 Pelvic fractures   425
Anish Potty

53 Spinal fractures   439
S Rajasekaran, Rishi Mugesh Kanna, Ajoy Prasad Shetty

54 Head and face trauma   466
Patrick H Warnke

55 Paediatric fractures and dislocations   481
Dorien Schneidmueller, Christoph Nau, Ingo Marzi

56 Compartment syndrome   503
Ashish K Sharma, Edward T Mah

57 Management of fracture complications   515
Robert B Simonis, Andrew M Richards, David S Elliott

Acetabular fractures

ANISH POTTY, SURESHAN SIVANANTHAN

Anatomy of the acetabulum	419	Non-operative treatment	423
Clinical presentation	420	Operative management	423
Radiology	420	Surgical approaches	423
Fracture classification	421	Results	423
CT and its role	422	Summary	424
Surgical indications	422	Reference	424

ANATOMY OF THE ACETABULUM

The acetabulum is the socket component of the ball and socket joint of the hip. The socket is formed by confluence of the ilium, the ischium and the pubis by the age of 12–14 years. The articulating surface is made up of 2–3 mm thick hyaline cartilage and is oriented inferiorly, laterally and anteriorly.

The *inferior orientation* can be measured by the centre edge angle (angle of Wiberg) using a line connecting the lateral rim of the acetabulum and the centre of the femoral head and the vertical, which should not be less than 10° at 1–4 years of age, and within the range 15–20° at 5 years of age.[1] The *transverse angle* normally measures 51° at birth and 40° at maturity and is the angle between a line passing from the superior to the inferior acetabular rim and the horizontal plane, which affects the acetabular lateral coverage of the femoral head and several other parameters.[1] The magnitude of the *anterior orientation*, or acetabular anteversion angle, is the angle between the axis of the femoral neck and the axis of the femoral condyles and affects the internal or external rotation of the leg. A normal angle is approximately 12°; an increased angle (toeing-in) is called coxa anteverta and a decreased angle (toeing-out) coxa retroverta.[1]

Letournel's column concept

The supporting structures of the acetabulum can be illustrated by Letournel's column concept.[2] He described it as being held by an inverted Y made up of the anterior and posterior columns of bone.

The anterior column (Fig. 51.1a) consists of the bone in the anterior iliac wing, the anterior wall, the superior pubic ramus and the pelvic brim. The posterior column (Fig. 51.1b) consists of the bone along the posterior border of the pelvis between the greater and lesser sciatic notch, the posterior of the acetabulum and the ischial ramus.

CLINICAL PRESENTATION

Most are the result of high-energy mechanisms, especially in younger individuals. Low-energy fractures are seen in elderly people with severe osteoporosis. Fractures occur following a direct blow to the acetabulum through the trochanter or indirectly through the knee or foot. Patients may complain of hip or groin pain and an inability to walk or to use the leg but most commonly they arrive with shock and polytrauma. On physical examination, there may be bruising

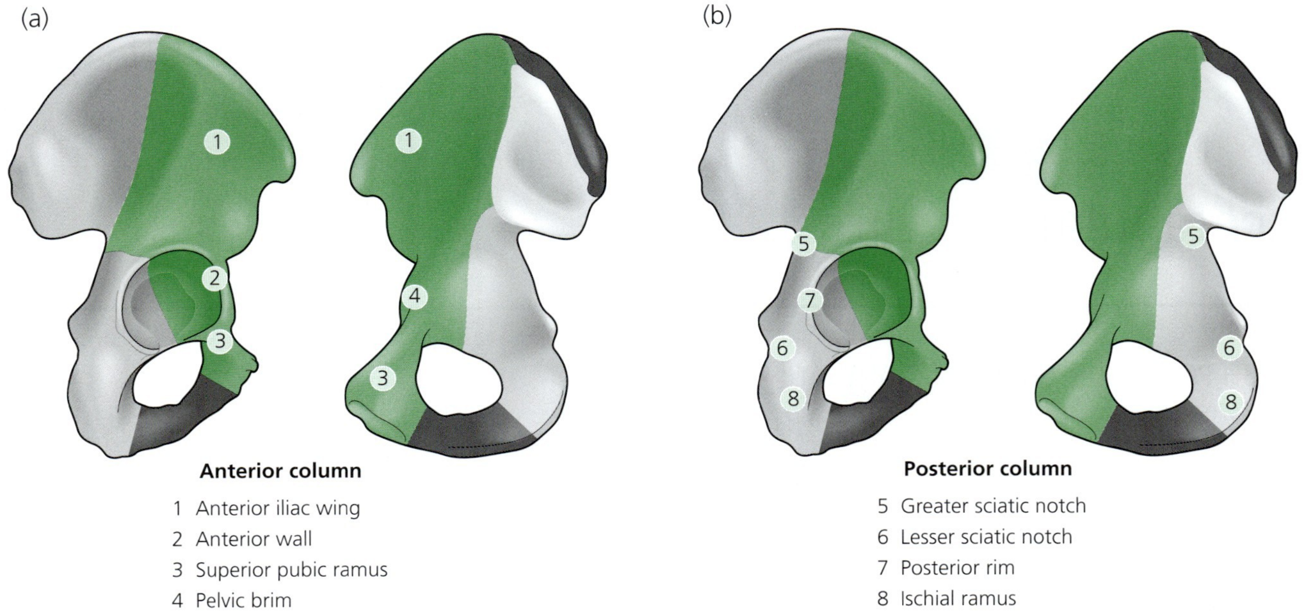

Figure 51.1 Letournel's column: (a) anterior column; (b) posterior column.

Anterior column
1. Anterior iliac wing
2. Anterior wall
3. Superior pubic ramus
4. Pelvic brim

Posterior column
5. Greater sciatic notch
6. Lesser sciatic notch
7. Posterior rim
8. Ischial ramus

around the pelvis, perineum and genitals. Haematuria and bleeding per rectum or per vagina should be suspected with pelvic fractures. All suspected pelvic and acetabular fractures in a trauma setting should be treated according to ATLS (advanced trauma life support) guidelines (Chapter 15).

Dislocation associated with an acetabulum fracture represents an orthopaedic emergency, and can occur in up to 30% of fractures. Most are posterior, with some occurring centrally. Urgent relocation may have long-term outcome implications. Most patients will have associated injuries, most commonly to the head or extremities. One out of 10 individuals will present with injuries to the urological system, peripheral nervous system or have an associated pelvic ring injury (Table 51.1).

RADIOLOGY

On the anteroposterior radiograph, Judet described six lines that represent a portion of acetabular anatomy.[3] A clear understanding of these specific lines will aid in diagnosing the particular fracture type. The definitive diagnosis of the type of fracture is made using three standard radiographic views: the anteroposterior view, and two 45° oblique views or Judet's views, which include the obturator and iliac oblique radiographs (Table 51.2).

The obturator oblique radiograph is obtained with the injured side rotated 45° towards the radiographic beam. The obturator oblique radiograph allows for evaluation of the anterior column and the posterior wall of the acetabulum. The iliac oblique, conversely, allows for evaluation of the posterior column and the anterior wall of the acetabulum.

Table 51.1 Incidence of associated injuries with acetabular fractures

Associated injuries	56–77%
Head injury	12–42%
Extremity	35–45%
Urological	6–11%
Neurological	12–13%
Pelvic	10–15%

Table 51.2 Six lines of Judet in anteroposterior pelvis radiographs

Six lines of Judet	Corresponding areas in the hemipelvis
Iliopectineal line	Anterior column
Ilioischial line	Posterior column
Radiographic roof	Superior articular surface
Anterior rim	Anterior wall
Posterior rim	Posterior wall
Tear drop	Quadrilateral surface

The adequacy of the obliques is determined by the position of the tip of the coccyx near the medial border of the femoral head (Fig. 51.2).

FRACTURE CLASSIFICATION

Judet and Letournel described 10 fracture patterns defined by the three standard radiographic films.[3] They subdivid-

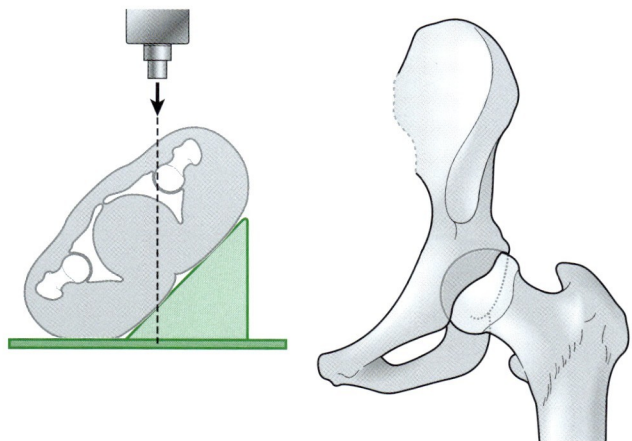

Figure 51.2 Obturator oblique view.

ed these into five elementary fractures and five associated fractures based on extensive anatomical and radiological studies. Accurate interpretation of the radiographs and classification of fracture patterns will help to determine the surgical approach and pre-operative planning of these complex fractures.

The elementary fracture patterns are diagnosed when a part or all of a supporting column of the acetabulum has been detached from the remaining pelvis. These include fractures of the posterior wall (Fig. 51.3a), the posterior column (Fig. 51.3b), the anterior wall (Fig. 51.3c) and the anterior column (Fig. 51.3d). They included one fracture, the transverse (Fig. 51.3e), which involved both columns. This was included in the elementary patterns because of the simplicity or purity of the fracture pattern.

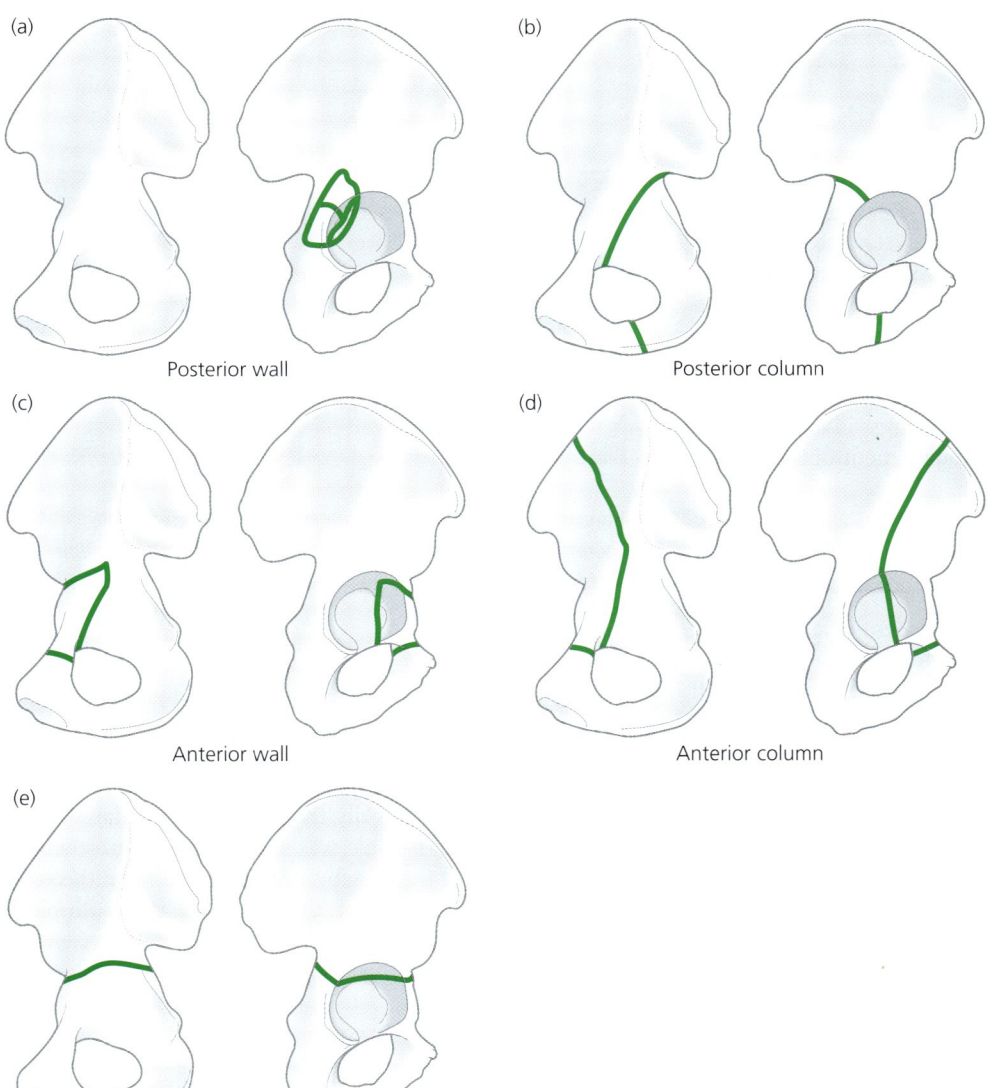

Figure 51.3 Elementary fracture patterns.

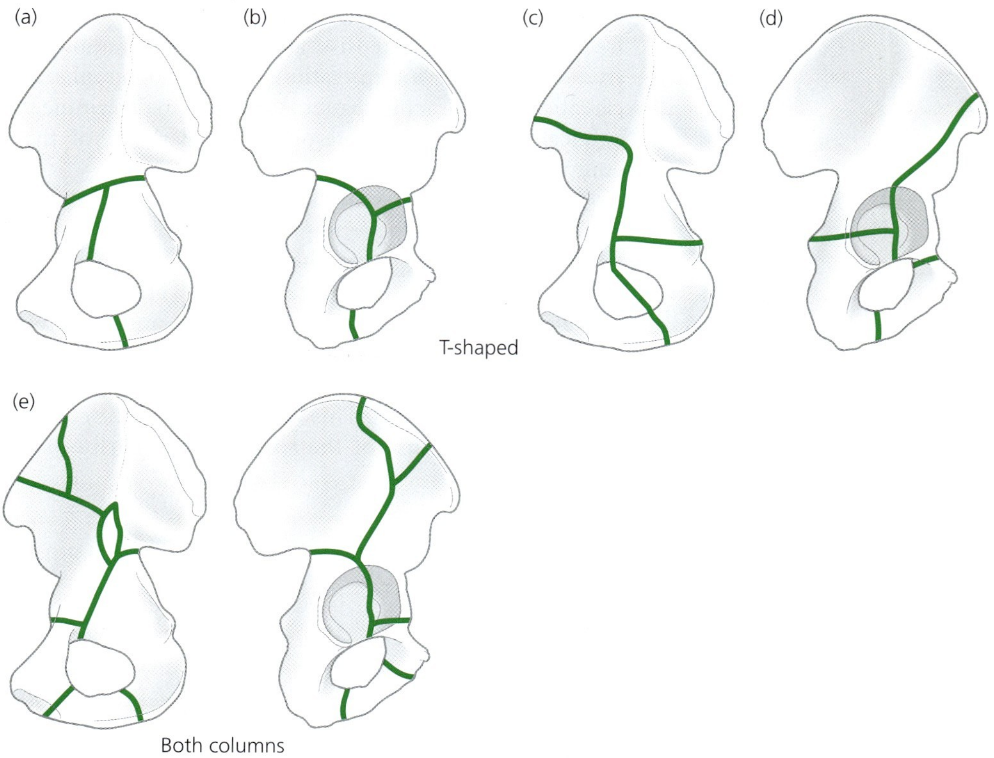

(a) (b) (c) (d)

T-shaped

(e)

Both columns

Figure 51.4 Associated fracture patterns.

Five associated fracture patterns included at least two of the elementary forms. These are the posterior column/posterior wall (Fig. 51.4a), the transverse posterior wall (Fig. 51.4b), the T-shaped fracture (Fig. 51.4c, identified by the vertical separation between the anterior and posterior columns), the anterior plus posterior hemi-transverse fracture (Fig. 51.4d) and the associated both-column fracture (Fig. 51.4e). The associated both-column fracture is distinguished from the other fractures involving both columns of bone by a complete detachment of the acetabulum from the intact iliac wing.

CT AND ITS ROLE

CT is an indispensable tool and provides critical information such as rotational displacement of each fracture component. It helps to define anatomic structures; it will better define the fracture lines in the pelvis, an articular segment which has been rotated and impacted into the surrounding cancellous bone or a free incarcerated fragment. Posterior pelvic ring or femoral head fractures which may significantly alter the outcome are identified.

Roof arch angle

In order to better understand surgical indications, a better understanding of the superior articular surface or weight-bearing portion of the acetabulum has been attempted. This has been defined traditionally by the roof arch angle as described by Matta.[4] A fracture was deemed to involve the superior articular surface if the fracture line entered

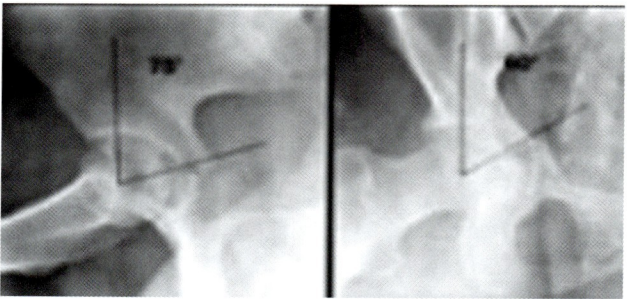

Figure 51.5 Superior articular surface. Roof arch angle >45°; therefore, the fracture does not involve the superior articular surface.

the joint at less than 45° from the perpendicular that passes through the centre of the acetabulum on any of the three views obtained with the patient out of traction (Fig. 51.5).

Olson attempted to better define this superior roof by using CT.[5] Mathematically the superior articular surface or the 45° roof arch angle was shown to be equivalent to the top 10 mm of the acetabulum evaluated from the subchondral condensation of the superior acetabulum. A fracture which enters the top 10 mm is thought to involve the superior articular surface.

SURGICAL INDICATIONS

The surgical indications for fractures of the acetabulum are loss of joint congruence or joint symmetry on any of the three radiographic views. This represents joint instability and therefore is an indication for surgery. A fracture of the posterior wall that consists of >20–30% of the posterior articular surface as determined by CT, or any fracture or dislocation with retained intra-articular fracture fragments.

Subluxation of the femoral head is typically seen in the direction of fracture displacement. It can be secondary to intra-articular bone and may be an indication for traction pre-operatively to diminish wear on the femoral head and acetabular cartilage.

NON-OPERATIVE TREATMENT

Non-operative treatment has traditionally included bed rest for 5–8 weeks with or without traction. Tornetta has also described the use of intra-operative stress radiographs to determine if occult instability exists.[6] Using this as an additional determination of non-operative treatment he showed that 91% of these patients went on to have excellent results in 3 years. The study identified that fractures associated with additional pelvic ring pathology were unstable or more likely to displace. Non-operative treatment is therefore indicated if the femoral head remains congruent to the acetabulum on all three views, if a fracture within the superior articular surface is displaced <2 mm or if a fracture is displaced greater than this with roof arc angles >45° on all three views.

OPERATIVE MANAGEMENT

The principles of operative fixation include anatomic reduction of the joint surface with stable fixation to allow early mobilization.

The approach, timing and ultimate treatment should be influenced by the condition of the soft tissues. Open fractures are rare, and abraded skin may be in the area of the preferred approach; soft-tissue degloving injuries may occur in up to 10–15%. Degloving of the skin and fat from the underlying fascia may cause ecchymosis, decreased sensation and fluctuance over the injured area (Morel–Lavalle lesions). This has a significant impact on wound management and the infection rate. Up to 30% of the operative sites may be colonized at the time of surgery.

SURGICAL APPROACHES

With regards to surgical approach, traditionally a single approach is preferred. This can be in the form of the Kocher–Langenbeck approach, which may be extended with the use of a trochanteric flip, the ilioinguinal approach or more extensile approaches. The use of simultaneous or sequential combined approaches may be advantageous for certain fracture patterns.

Kocher–Langenbeck approach

The Kocher–Langenbeck (Fig. 51.6) approach is typically utilized to access bone of the posterior aspect of the acetabulum. Digital evaluation of the anterior portion of the acetabulum can be obtained. Typically, treatment indications for the Kocher–Langenbeck approach are a posterior wall or column fracture, transverse fractures with or without an associated posterior wall, a posterior column/posterior wall fracture or T-shaped fractures.

Ilioinguinal approach

The ilioinguinal approach allows access to the anterior portions of the pelvis. Indirect digital evaluation of the posterior portions can be performed. This approach is typically used to approach fractures of the anterior wall and column, anterior posterior hemi-transverse fractures, both-column fractures and rarely transverse fractures (Fig. 51.7).

Extended iliofemoral approach

This allows access to the majority of the innominate bone, including both anterior and posterior columns. Its indications are for specific associated both-column fractures, T-shaped fractures and very high transverse/posterior wall fractures. Its particular usefulness is in fractures greater than 3 weeks of age involving both columns of the acetabulum (Fig. 51.8).

RESULTS

The results following open reduction and internal fixation of acetabular fractures have been shown to be highly

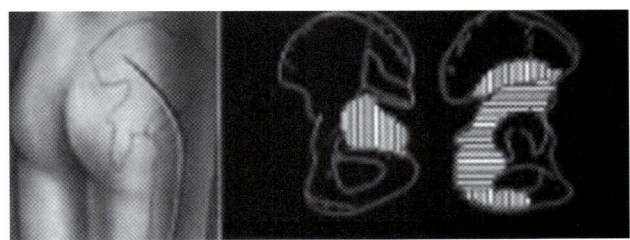

Figure 51.6 Kocher–Langenbeck (K-L) approach.

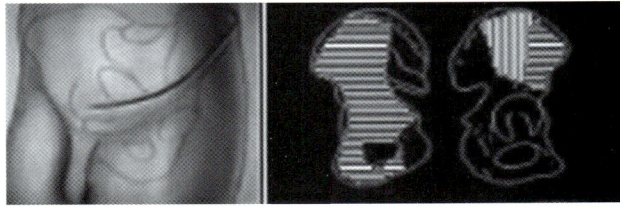

Figure 51.7 The ilioinguinal approach.

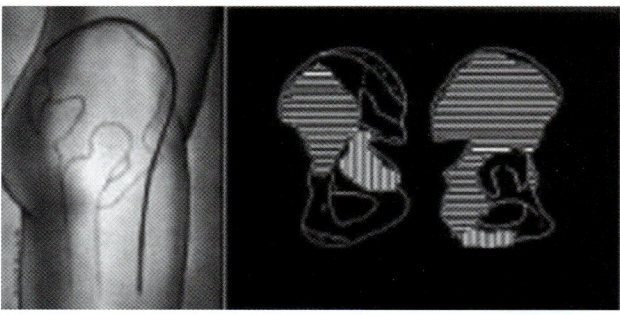

Figure 51.8 Extended iliofemoral approach.

dependent upon experience and expertise of the surgeon. Good to excellent results in large single-surgeon series by Letournel, Matta and Mayo are reported to occur in 75% and 80% of complex patterns. In other studies with multiple surgeons caring for fewer fractures, good to excellent results have been seen in less than 50% of those treated operatively. This validates a documented learning curve as described by Letournel for acetabular fracture surgery.

Typically, the clinical results correlate with the adequacy of reduction and avoidance of complications. The results appeared to deteriorate in patients who are older than 40 years. There have been no sign ificant differences noted in outcome for specific fracture patterns. Although posterior wall fracture may seem easier to approach and treat, only 75–80% of these fractures in large single-surgeon series have been associated with good to excellent results.

SUMMARY

In summary, radiographic evaluation allows diagnosis and determination of surgical indications. Fracture type determines approach. Outcome is dependent on the commitment of the surgeon. Joint preservation and satisfactory outcome are possible in the majority of patients treated appropriately.

REFERENCE

1. Schuenke M, Schulte E, Schumacher U and Ross L. *Thieme Atlas of Anatomy: General Anatomy and Musculoskeletal System.* Stuttgart: Thieme, 2006:365–89.
2. Letournel E. Fractures of the cotyloid cavity, study of a series of 75 cases. *Journal of Chronic Diseases* 1961; **82**: 47-87.
3. Judet R, Judet J and Letournel E. Fractures of the Acetabulum: Classification and Surgical Approaches for Open Reduction: Preliminary report. *Journal of Bone and Joint Surgery American* 1964; **46**:1615-1675.
4. Matta JM. Fractures of the Acetabulum: Early Results of a Prospective Study. *Current Orthopaedic Practice* 1986; **205**: 2-312.
5. Olson SA. The computerized tomography subchondral arc: a new method of assessing acetabular articular continuity after Fracture (A preliminary report). *Journal of Orthoapedic Trauma* 1993; **7**: 402-13.
6. Tornetta P. Non-operative management of acetabular fractures: The use of dynamic stress views. *Journal of Bone and Joint Surgery (British)* 1999; **81-B**:67-70.

52

Pelvic fractures

ANISH POTTY

Introduction	425	Treatment	430
Problems	425	Pre-operative details	433
Frequency	426	Intra-operative details	434
Aetiology	426	Postoperative details	434
Presentation	426	Follow-up	434
Relevant anatomy	428	Complications	434
Pelvis as a conduit for neurovascular structures	428	Outcome and prognosis	435
Neurological structures	429	Future and controversies	436
Muscles groups around the pelvis	429	References	437
Work-up	429		

NATIONAL BOARD STANDARDS

- Know the features of pelvic fractures, including the work-up
- Understand the surgical treatment and outcomes
- Be aware of the controversies around stability

INTRODUCTION

Pelvic fractures have historically been treated non-operatively. The earliest management of pelvic fractures consisted of prolonged bed rest followed by mobilization as fracture healing occurred and symptoms abated. Other methods also used to treat pelvic fractures included closed reduction under general anaesthesia, traction, spica casts, pelvic slings and turnbuckles.[1–4]

Operative management of unstable pelvic injuries has increased recently because of several factors. Improved and coordinated treatment of polytraumatized patients, improved anaesthetic techniques, including blood salvage systems, advances in intra-operative fluoroscopic imaging techniques, standardized pelvic implant systems, and better understanding of injury and deformity patterns have allowed for successful operative treatment of patients with pelvic ring injuries. Operative management of unstable pelvic ring injuries allows for earlier patient mobilization, thereby decreasing complications associated with bed rest. Operative management also allows for correction and prevention of significant pelvic deformities, thus improving clinical outcomes.

PROBLEMS

Unstable pelvic fractures typically occur as a result of high-energy injuries. Associated organ system injuries are commonly observed with pelvic fractures because of the energy imparted to the patient. Head, chest and abdominal injuries frequently occur in association with pelvic fractures. Fractures of the extremities and spinal column also can occur in patients with pelvic fractures.

Haemorrhage may accompany pelvic fractures. Most haemorrhage associated with pelvic fractures occurs as a result of bleeding from exposed fractures, soft-tissue injury, and local venous bleeding.[5] Arterial injuries also may contribute to haemorrhage, albeit less commonly than venous bleeding.[6]

Unstable and displaced pelvic ring disruptions cause significant deformity, pain and disability. Deformities resulting from pelvic ring injuries include any combination of rotational and translational deformities. Significant permanent (sustained) pelvic deformities have been identified with poorer patient outcomes and decreased activity levels.[7–9]

FREQUENCY

The incidence of pelvic fractures in the USA has been estimated to be 37 cases per 100 000 person-years.[10] The incidence of pelvic fractures is greatest in people aged 15–28 years. In people younger than 35 years, males sustain more pelvic fractures than females; whereas in people older than 35 years, women sustain more pelvic fractures than men.[11] Most pelvic fractures that occur in younger patients result from high-energy mechanisms, whereas pelvic fractures sustained in the elderly population occur from minimal trauma, such as a low fall.[11]

AETIOLOGY

Pelvic fractures occur after both low-energy and high-energy events. Low-energy pelvic fractures occur commonly in two distinct age groups: adolescents and elderly people. Adolescents typically present with avulsion fractures of the superior or inferior iliac spines or apophyseal avulsion fractures of the iliac wing or ischial tuberosity resulting from an athletic injury. Low-energy pelvic fractures in elderly people frequently result from falls while ambulating, which are highlighted by stable fractures of the pelvic ring. Elderly patients also may present with insufficiency fractures, typically of the sacrum and anterior pelvic ring.[12]

High-energy pelvic fractures most commonly occur after motor vehicle crashes. Other mechanisms of high-energy pelvic fractures include motorcycle crashes, motor vehicles striking pedestrians and falls.

PRESENTATION

Because most unstable and displaced pelvic ring injury fractures occur as the result of high-energy mechanisms, many patients present with associated primary organ system injuries. A careful assessment of the patient must begin with an examination for immediate life-threatening injuries. Assessment should begin in an orderly fashion to avoid missing injuries. The American College of Surgeons has popularized advanced trauma life support (ATLS), a programme that provides a systematic and orderly treatment protocol for traumatized patients under the direction of a general surgeon or trauma surgeon.[13] This protocol has been used successfully at many trauma centres and is recommended by the authors.

Soft-tissue injuries provide an indirect measurement of the energy sustained by the patient. Scrotal, labial, flank and inguinal haematomata commonly accompany pelvic ring injuries and are indicative of intrapelvic haemorrhage.[14] Soft-tissue injury is observed along a continuum from superficial abrasions and lacerations to closed internal degloving injuries,[15] to open wounds. Lacerations of the perineum must be carefully sought during the initial physical examinations and secondary surveys. Rectal and vaginal lacerations may be overlooked because the initial examination concentrates on more obvious injuries. Rectal, vaginal and perineal lacerations are indicative of severe injuries and indicate an open fracture contaminated by urine, stool or other environmental contaminants.

A Morel-Lavallee lesion is a post-traumatic soft-tissue degloving injury, originally described by French surgeon Victor Auguste Francois Morel-Lavallee in 1863.[15,16] These lesions result from direct or tangential shearing forces that separate the skin and subcutaneous tissues from the underlying fascia. These shearing forces can disrupt perforating vessels and nerves, creating a potential space that fills with blood, lymph, debris and fat (necrotic and/or viable). Closed degloving injuries are most commonly found adjacent to osseous protuberances, and have been described along the greater trochanter, flank, buttock, lumbar spine, scapula and knee.[13,17–19] If therapy is insufficient, large areas of necrosis can form, which will negatively influence operative measures.

Clinical presentation

Morel-Lavallee lesions are frequently identified within hours to days after the inciting trauma, but one-third of patients present months or years after the initial trauma.[20] Morel-Lavallee lesions can be isolated, but they are frequently associated with underlying fractures. These lesions are most often unilateral, but bilateral lesions have been described.[21,22] Patients complain of pain, swelling and stiffness. On physical examination, patients often have a soft fluctuant area of contour deformity, with or without skin discoloration and skin hypermotility. Skin sensation is frequently decreased because of shearing injuries to the cutaneous nerves. Skin necrosis can occur acutely or in a delayed fashion.

MRI is the imaging modality of choice in the evaluation of Morel-Lavallee lesions.[13] Morel-Lavallee lesions are well-defined oval, fusiform or crescentic lesions and may have tapering margins that fuse with adjacent fascial planes. Morel-Lavallee lesions may show fluid–fluid levels, septations and variable internal signal intensity dependent on the concentration of haemolymphatic fluid and the acuity of the lesion.

Conservative treatment with compression can be utilized for small acute lesions that have not developed a capsule.[23] The presence of a capsule suggests that conservative or percutaneous treatment will be unsuccessful and the lesion will recur if not treated surgically. Tseng and Tornetta[16] successfully managed lesions with early percutaneous drainage, debridement, irrigation and suction drainage. Percutaneous drainage and sclerodesis have been effective, utilizing agents such as talc and doxycycline.[19] Some physicians perform open debridement with delayed closure or closure by secondary intention for all lesions, but others feel that this can be reserved for those lesions that have a peripheral capsule or failed conservative treatment. Infection is a potential complication, necessitating the use of antibiotic therapy.

Manual palpation of the pelvis should be included in assessing patients with pelvic ring injuries. Palpation must be undertaken carefully to avoid harming the patient. Manual palpation can reveal crepitus from fractures and assists with determination of pelvic stability. Manual compression along the iliac crests provides a tactile assessment of pelvic ring stability. Contralateral push–pull examinations of the lower extremities are rarely necessary to identify instability.

Blood at the external urethral meatus is indicative of a urethral disruption. Perineal and genital swelling also reflect urethral disruption. Digital rectal examination may reveal a high-riding prostate gland in the male, which also is suggestive of a urethral disruption. Bladder disruptions occur frequently with pelvic fractures and may be intraperitoneal, extraperitoneal or both. Gross haematuria is the most common clinical finding supporting a diagnosis of a bladder disruption.[24] The presence of gross haematuria demands evaluation of the lower genitourinary (GU) system under the direction of a urologist.

Axial and appendicular skeletal injuries are frequently associated with pelvic ring injury fractures. Careful examination of the spine and extremities is indicated as part of complete patient evaluation. Particular attention to the lower extremities may demonstrate limb length discrepancies associated with superior hemipelvic translations. Internal and/or external rotational deformities resulting from deformities of the pelvis may be noted by similar deformities in the lower extremities.

Injuries to the pelvic ring may cause injury to any of the neurovascular structures that traverse the pelvis. Vascular injuries are usually lacerations of venous structures.[5] Arterial injuries also occur but much less frequently than venous injuries.[6] The source of bleeding, venous or arterial, may contribute to haemorrhage and demands urgent management.

Neurological injuries typically occur as injuries to the L5 or S1 nerve roots.[5,25] L4 nerve root injuries also may occur with severe pelvic ring injuries. Sacral fractures frequently accompany pelvic ring fractures and may have S2–S5 sacral nerve root injuries. Lower sacral nerve root injuries may lead to bowel and bladder incontinence and sexual dysfunction. Detection of these nerve injuries is difficult in the acute setting, but careful examination may demonstrate perineal numbness and decreased rectal tone in the acute period.

Management

Management of pelvic fractures in the immediate setting is centred on controlling life-threatening injuries, particularly severe haemorrhage. Several techniques have been used to control haemorrhage; these techniques are based on decreasing the volume of the pelvis, thereby limiting the amount of blood that can escape into the pelvic cavity.

Perhaps the simplest method to decrease pelvic volume is securely wrapping a sheet around the patient's pelvis. External fixators and other external pelvic clamps have been advocated to control pelvic volume, with the added benefit of providing bony stability, thereby preventing fracture movement and dislodgment of clots.[26] Pneumatic antishock garments also have been used to control haemorrhage associated with pelvic fractures. Care must be taken when using pneumatic antishock garments as they increase intramuscular and intrathoracic pressure, potentially leading to compartment syndrome and respiratory compromise distress. Pneumatic antishock garments are contraindicated in patients with pulmonary oedema and/or diaphragmatic rupture.[13]

The primary goal for the treatment of pelvic fractures in the acute setting is to provide early stable fixation to allow for patient mobilization. Several studies have demonstrated beneficial effects with early pelvic fracture treatment such as decreased blood transfusion requirements, decreased systemic complications, decreased hospital stays and improved patient survival.[27,28] Secondary considerations for operative management of pelvic fractures in the acute setting are the correction or prevention of significant pelvic translational and rotational deformities that have been associated with poorer clinical outcomes.[8,26,29]

Several classification systems have been developed to assist with injury pattern recognition and management decisions; perhaps the best known are those described by Tile[30] and Burgess et al.[31] Both of these classification schemes provide recommendations for management of pelvic fractures based on the function of the posterior ligamentous structures to support the pelvic ring. Others prefer to describe injuries based on the anatomic location of the pelvic ring injuries and the associated displacements and instabilities.[32]

Pennal and Tile developed a classification scheme for pelvic fractures, which described injuries to the pelvic ring based on the vector of the deforming force and divided these into lateral compression (LC) injuries, anteroposterior compression (APC) injuries and vertical shear injuries.[33] Tile further modified this classification scheme to include radiographic signs of pelvic stability or instability. Type A injuries are classified as those that are rotationally and vertically stable. Type B injuries are categorized as those injuries that are rotationally unstable but vertically stable. Type C injuries are rotationally and vertically unstable.[30]

The Tile classification scheme for pelvic fractures is as follows:[30]

- Type A – Rotationally and vertically stable
  - A1 – Avulsion fractures
  - A2 – Stable iliac wing fractures or minimally displaced pelvic ring fractures
  - A3 – Transverse sacral or coccyx fractures.
- Type B – Rotationally unstable and vertically stable
  - B1 – Open-book injuries
  - B2 – LC injuries
  - B3 – Bilateral type B injuries.
- Type C – Rotationally unstable and vertically unstable
  - C1 – Unilateral injury
  - C2 – Bilateral injuries in which one side is a type B injury and the contralateral side is a type C injury
  - C3 – Bilateral injury in which both sides are type C injuries.

Young and Burgess further expanded the classification of Tile by adding a combined mechanism category in recognition that many pelvic fractures result from a combination of vectors. Their classification divided LC and APC fractures into subgroups I, II and III, which are based on the amount of disruption based on anteroposterior (AP), inlet and outlet pelvic radiographs. This classification facilitates stratification of the amount of energy imparted to the patient.[19,31] This classification also has been demonstrated to be predictive of associated injury patterns based on the type of pelvic ring deformity.[34]

Vertical shear fractures are characterized by vertical rami fractures or a diastasis of the symphysis pubis anteriorly and vertical displacement of the posterior pelvic ring through the sacroiliac (SI) joint, sacrum or ilium. Combined mechanism fractures are characterized by a combination of the above-mentioned injury patterns.

RELEVANT ANATOMY

The pelvic ring consists of two innominate bones connected anteriorly at the symphysis pubis and posteriorly to the sacrum at the SI joints. Anatomically, the pelvis is divided into the false pelvis and the true pelvis. The false pelvis is defined as that portion of the pelvis from the iliac crests superiorly to the pelvic brim inferiorly. The true pelvis is defined from the pelvic brim inferiorly to the pelvic floor.

Pelvic ligaments

The bones of the pelvis are held together by strong ligaments and can be divided into four groups: those connecting the sacrum and ilium; those connecting the sacrum and ischium; those connecting the two pubic bones at the symphysis pubis; and those uniting the sacrum and coccyx.[19] The anterior and posterior SI ligaments link the iliac bones to the sacrum. Two distinct bands demarcate the posterior SI ligaments. The short posterior interosseus ligaments consist of fibres running from the ridge of the sacrum to the posterior superior and posterior inferior iliac spines. The long posterior SI ligament consists of fibres originating from the posterior superior iliac spine, which then intermingle with originating fibres of the sacrotuberous ligament, covering the short posterior SI ligament and attaching to the lateral sacrum. The anterior SI ligaments consist of fibrous bands that join the anterior surface of the sacrum to the adjacent anterior ilium.[19]

The sacrospinous and sacrotuberous ligaments connect the sacrum to the ischium. The sacrospinous ligament, originating from the lateral margin of the inferior sacrum and attaching at the ischial spine, assists in resisting external rotation forces of the pelvis.[31] The sacrotuberous ligament has a broad origin from the posterior superior and posterior inferior iliac spines and the entire lateral margin of the posterior sacrum. The sacrotuberous ligament courses posteriorly to the sacrospinous ligament, inserting on the ischial tuberosity. The sacrotuberous ligament resists sagittal plane rotational deformities and vertical shearing of the pelvis.[31]

The symphysis pubis is a movable articular joint without a synovial membrane. An interpubic disc, the superior pubic ligaments and the arcuate ligaments inferiorly connect the pubic bones. The remainder of the ligaments that surround the pelvis are ligaments that do not have significant stabilizing roles for the pelvis, including ligaments connecting the sacrum and coccyx, the lateral lumbosacral ligaments originating at the L5 transverse processes and attaching to the sacral ala, and the iliolumbar ligaments, running from the L5 transverse processes to the iliac crests.[31]

PELVIS AS A CONDUIT FOR NEUROVASCULAR STRUCTURES

The pelvis acts to connect the axial skeleton with the appendicular skeleton of the lower extremities and, in this role, serves as a conduit for neurovascular structures.

Vascular structures

The common iliac blood vessels enter into the false pelvis, in which the division into the external and internal iliac vessels occurs. The external iliac vessels continue through the false pelvis atop the pubic rami medial to the iliopectineal eminence. The internal iliac vessels dive into the pelvis, where they divide into somatic branches, visceral branches, and limb and perineal branches. Other vessels of the pelvis include the terminal branch of the aorta, the median sacral artery and the superior rectal artery, a continuation of the inferior mesenteric artery.[19]

The somatic segmental branches[19] are as follows:

- iliolumbar
- lateral sacral.

The visceral branches are as follows:

- umbilical
- inferior vesicle
- superior vesicle
- middle rectal.

The limb and perineal branches are as follows:

- superior gluteal
- inferior gluteal
- internal pudendal
- obturator.

NEUROLOGICAL STRUCTURES

The neurological contents of the pelvis collectively have been referred to as the lumbosacral plexus. This consists of what are individually known as the lumbar plexus and the sacral plexus. Anatomically, the lumbar plexus is an abdominal structure whose branches enter the pelvis. Conversely, the sacral plexus is entirely pelvic in origin. The lumbar plexus consists of nerve roots from L1 to L4. The sacral plexus consists of those more caudal nerve roots. Each plexus can be divided into ventral and dorsal branches. The larger nerves of the pelvis originate from the sacral plexus.

The most cephalic of the nerves of the pelvis are the ilioinguinal and iliohypogastric nerves. These originate from the L1 nerve root. Both enter the pelvis on the surface of the psoas muscle, which they cross obliquely as they travel distally. They penetrate the abdominal wall muscles to serve as cutaneous innervation of the areas surrounding the pelvis. The iliohypogastric nerve supplies the skin of the posterolateral buttock, while the ilioinguinal nerve supplies the root of the penis and scrotum.[19]

The lumber plexus can be divided into nerves consisting of dorsal or ventral branches. The psoas muscle anatomically separates these nerves. The femoral and lateral femoral cutaneous nerves are the primary dorsal branches of the lumbar plexus. The femoral nerve (L2, 3, 4) lies lateral to the psoas between the psoas and the iliacus muscles as it enters the pelvis over the iliac wing.[19] It innervates the iliacus muscle then exits the pelvis beneath the inguinal ligament to supply both motor as well as sensory fibres to the anterior compartment of the thigh.[20] The lateral femoral cutaneous nerve also emerges lateral to the psoas. It travels over the iliacus and becomes superficial to supply sensation to the lateral thigh.[19]

The ventral branches of the lumbar plexus are represented in the obturator nerve (L2, 3, 4). The obturator nerve appears medial to the psoas just above the pelvis; it then enters the pelvis, with the vertebral column on its medial side and the psoas lateral to it. The obturator nerve travels with the internal iliac vessels and the ureter on the lateral pelvic wall. Running along the surface of the obturator internus muscle, the obturator nerve then leaves the pelvis through the obturator canal.[19] Its main function is to provide motor innervation to the adductors of the thigh.[20]

The branches of the sacral plexus originate in the pelvis, in which the sacral plexus lies anterior to the piriformis muscle. The nerves of the plexus can be divided into ventral and dorsal branches, all of which exit the pelvis through the greater sciatic foramen notch. All branches pass below the piriformis muscle except the superior gluteal nerve (L4, 5, S1), which exits above the piriformis.[19] The dorsal branches of the plexus include the superior (L4–S1) and inferior (L5–S2) gluteal nerves and the common peroneal portion of the sciatic nerve (L4–S2). The anterior or ventral divisions supply the calf, plantar foot and thigh through the tibial nerve (L4–S3).[35]

MUSCLES GROUPS AROUND THE PELVIS

Several important muscle groups are around the pelvis. The muscles of the pelvic floor, the levator ani muscle and the coccygeus muscles are composed of voluntary muscles, which support the pelvic viscera and control the voluntary sphincters of the rectum and urethra.[36] Additionally, the muscles of the pelvic floor have been noted to impart stability to the pelvic ring.[26] Another muscle around the pelvis includes the piriformis muscle, which is an important anatomic landmark demarcating the division of the superior and inferior gluteal vessels and assisting with identification of the sciatic nerve. Many other muscles originate and insert on the bones of the pelvis, a discussion of which is beyond the scope of this chapter and can be referenced from anatomy textbooks.

WORK-UP

Laboratory studies

A complete blood cell count, renal panel, coagulation profile and toxicology screens usually are obtained in the emergency department upon patient presentation. Serial haematocrits are helpful in the acute setting to monitor resuscitation efforts.

Imaging studies

- An AP pelvic radiograph
  - is obtained as a component of the initial trauma evaluation
  - highlights most major pelvic disruptions.[37]

- When looking at an AP pelvis radiograph be sure to evaluate the 'six lines':
  1. the iliopectineal line to evaluate the anterior column
  2. the ilioischial line to evaluate the posterior column
  3. the dome of the acetabulum
  4. the 'tear drop' to evaluate the anteroinferior portion of the acetabular fossa
  5. the anterior rim of the acetabulum
  6. the posterior rim of the acetabulum.

It is also, of course, important to evaluate the rest of the bony structures visible on the radiograph, including the pubic rami, the SI joints, the neck of each femur, the visualized lumbar spine and sacrum and the pubic symphysis.

Fractures in the pelvis can be difficult to visualize and, if there is doubt, one can order additional views, including inlet and outlet views, to further evaluate for rami fractures. The inlet view will allow for evaluation of the superior rami for fractures and the pelvis for AP displacement of the pelvis. Outlet views will allow for evaluation of the inferior rami for fractures and for determination of superoinferior displacement of the pelvis. Judet views are one additional study that can be ordered to evaluate the acetabulum. These views are taken at a 45° angle to the pelvis. The obturator oblique radiograph will allow for evaluation of the anterior column and the posterior wall of the acetabulum. The iliac oblique, conversely, will allow for evaluation of the posterior column and the anterior wall of the acetabulum.

- Inlet pelvic radiograph[33]
  - X-ray tube angled 45° caudad and centred on the umbilicus
  - Highlights AP and mediolateral translations, and internal and external rotatory deformities.
- Outlet pelvic radiograph[33]
  - X-ray tube angled 45° cephalad and centred on the symphysis pubis
  - Highlights superior and inferior translations abduction and/or adduction, and flexion and/or extension rotational deformities.
- Lateral sacral radiograph[38,39]
  - Indicated in injuries sustained from falls and when bilateral sacral fractures are noted on plain radiographs or CT scans
  - Demonstrates transverse fracture of the sacral body and/or kyphosis of the sacrum.
- Pelvic CT scans
  - Useful to confirm plain film findings and more to document sacral morphology when planning percutaneous iliosacral screw placement[40]
  - Often can be included with abdominal CT scans
  - Five-millimetre axial images from iliac crests to acetabular dome, then 3 mm axial images including all acetabular articular segments, then 5 mm slices through the remainder of the caudal pelvis[32]
  - Remember that a normal CT of the pelvis will take 5 mm cuts, which may lead one to miss subtle fractures. The musculoskeletal pelvis will allow for full and detailed evaluation of all of the osseous structures of the pelvis and assist in the determination of what pathology is present, if any. It is important to remember, however, that all classification systems for pelvic fractures are based on plain radiographs, and, as such, are necessary for operative planning
  - Three-dimensional reformatted pelvic CT scans also may be beneficial to highlight pelvic ring injuries and associated deformity patterns.
- Pelvic angiograms
  - Indicated in patients with ongoing haemorrhage after adequate intravenous fluid resuscitation and provisional pelvic ring stabilization
  - Useful in patients who have pelvic ring or acetabular injuries involving the greater sciatic notch to detect obvious or occult injury to the superior gluteal artery
  - Embolization of lacerated arterial vessels may be performed at the same setting, as can manipulative reductions using the angiography fluoroscopic imaging system.
- Retrograde urethrogram
  - Indicated in patients suspected of having urethral tears
  - Recommended to be performed under the direction of a urologist.
- Cystogram
  - Indicated in patients suspected of having a urinary bladder injury
  - Recommended to be performed under the direction of a urologist.

TREATMENT

Medical therapy

Initial therapy in the acutely injured patient centres on the ABCs as recommended by ATLS protocols published by the American College of Surgeons.[13] The following mnemonic defines the specific, ordered, prioritized evaluations and interventions that should be followed in injured patients:[13]

A. Airway with cervical spine control
B. Breathing
C. Circulation
D. Disability or neurological status
E. Exposure (undress) with temperature control

After initial resuscitation and stabilization, other non-life-threatening injuries are evaluated and managed appropriately. Following these guidelines, under the direction of a trauma surgeon or general surgeon, patient treatment is optimized.

Surgical therapy

SYMPHYSIS PUBIS DISRUPTIONS

Disruptions of the symphysis pubis are typically described as resulting from an anterior or posterior force impacting on the pelvis; however, laterally directed compressive forces also have been implicated in creating symphyseal disruptions.[26,32] Indications to operatively stabilize symphysis pubis disruptions are determined by the amount of instability between the pubic bones. Several authors have recommended operative stabilization when the pubic diastasis is greater than 2.5 cm, based on experimental evidence demonstrating that pubic bone displacement greater than 2.5 cm implies rupture of the anterior sacroiliac, the sacrospinous and the sacrotuberous ligaments, rendering the pelvis rotationally unstable.[26,31]

Letournel[41] recommended operative stabilization of symphyseal disruptions when the pubic diastasis measured greater than 1.5 cm. Routt *et al.*[32] also noted that children and people of smaller stature may demonstrate rotational pelvic instability with pubic diastases less than 2.5 cm. It has been observed that a symphysis pubis diastasis may increase after administration of general anaesthesia, implying that plain radiographs may underestimate the actual deformity due to associated muscle spasm.

Treatment options for symphyseal disruptions consist of external fixation or more mechanically sound open reduction with internal fixation. Anterior pelvic external fixation can be used in patients with small symphyseal disruptions with incomplete posterior ligamentous injury.[32,41,42] The use of an anterior external fixator is potentially beneficial because it avoids operative exposures, potential bleeding from venous plexus injuries and bladder perforation associated with open stabilization.[42] The external fixator is also useful to avoid wound contamination when suprapubic catheters are in place for the treatment of urinary bladder disruptions. The external fixator should remain in place until healing is demonstrated, which usually occurs between 6 and 12 weeks postoperatively.[41,42] External pelvic fixation is cumbersome for patients and is associated with pintrack infections and even osteomyelitis.

Open reduction and internal fixation is preferred for unstable symphyseal injuries. Open reduction and internal fixation avoids the inconvenience of wearing and removing an external fixator. Surgical stabilization is performed through a Pfannenstiel surgical exposure, or an extension of a midline exposure may be used. Tenaculum clamps, Farabeuf clamps and pelvic reduction clamps may be used to reduce the pubic diastasis. Implants commonly used to stabilize symphyseal disruptions are 3.5 mm reconstruction plates, 4.5 mm reconstruction plates, 3.5 mm low-contact dynamic compression plates and 4.5 mm low-contact dynamic compression plates. Regardless of the plate used, at least two screws should be placed on each side of the defect to prevent subsequent rotatory deformities. The larger plates do not fit the symphyseal area well and for this reason 3.5 mm pelvic reconstruction plates are preferred.

PUBIC RAMUS FRACTURES

Pubic ramus fractures occur as parasymphyseal fractures, midramus fractures and pubic root fractures in association with distraction and compression injuries of the pelvis.[32] Displacement of pubic rami fractures may cause impingement or laceration of the bladder, vagina and perineum, and, for these reasons, operative management may be considered. Operative treatment of pubic rami fractures is indicated to provide additional pelvic ring stability in association with posterior pelvic ring fixation. Stabilization of pubic rami fractures also may be considered in fractures involving the obturator neurovascular canal with accompanying neurological injury.

Treatment options for pubic rami fractures include external fixation, percutaneous screw fixation, and open reduction and internal fixation. External fixation with either multiple pins[42] or single pins in each hemipelvis may be used successfully in conjunction with stabilization of posterior ring injuries to impart additional stability to the pelvic fixation construct. External fixation for pubic ramus fractures is indicated to impart additional stability after posterior pelvic ring repair and also when percutaneous or open treatment is contraindicated.

Intramedullary fixation has been described for treatment of pubic rami fractures.[39,44] Intramedullary pubic ramus fixation with a 4.5 mm cortical screw has demonstrated fixation strength equivalent to plate fixation and has demonstrated good results in clinical settings.[40,44] Intramedullary stabilization of ramus fractures may be performed with either a percutaneous or open technique with either antegrade or retrograde screw placement in the pubic ramus. Extramedullary plate fixation is another option to stabilize pubic rami fractures after open reduction and usually is achieved with 3.5 mm pelvic reconstruction plates.

ILIAC WING FRACTURES

Iliac wing fractures are caused by forces applied directly to the iliac wing. Simple fracture patterns without associated pelvic ring instability are managed with non-operative measures. Comminuted iliac wing fractures are caused by high-energy injuries, and severe soft-tissue injury, including open wounds, frequently accompany these injuries.[45]

Indications for operative management of iliac wing fractures include associated skin abnormalities, significant closed degloving injuries and open wounds. Severely displaced or comminuted iliac wing fractures, unstable iliac fractures that preclude adequate pulmonary function secondary to pain, bowel herniation or incarceration within the fracture, and fractures associated with unstable pelvic ring injuries are other indications for open reduction and internal fixation.[32,45] Pre-operative pelvic angiograms are recommended for fractures involving the greater sciatic notch.

The lateral window of the ilioinguinal surgical exposure is used to access iliac wing fractures. After fracture exposure, tenaculum clamps, Farabeuf clamps and Schanz pins used as joysticks are used to obtain fracture reduction. Fracture reduction is maintained with medullary lag screws in combination with pelvic reconstruction plates for definitive stabilization. For patients with open iliac fractures, the fixation construct should rely on medullary screws in order to seclude the implants from contamination.

Crescent fractures

Crescent fractures are actually fractures of the posterior ilium extending from the iliac crest into the greater sciatic notch and are associated with an articular dislocation of the anterior sacroiliac joint and commonly result after LC injuries to the iliac wing[31] but also may occur secondary to anteriorly or posteriorly directed forces.[32] Crescent fractures typically result in a stable posterior iliac fragment and a rotationally unstable iliac component. The posterior iliac fragment is stable owing to the attachment of the intact posterior SI ligaments, whereas the iliac component is rotationally unstable.[17] When viewed laterally, the posterior iliac stable segment is crescent shaped, hence the terminology. Surgical stabilization is indicated owing to the inherent instability of the iliac wing component of the fracture and the dislocation of the SI joint.

Crescent fractures may be treated with the patient positioned either prone or supine, depending upon associated pelvic ring injuries, acetabular fractures, soft-tissue injuries and the location of the crescent fracture. Fractures treated from the prone position are exposed with a vertical paramedian dorsal surgical approach, allowing direct reduction of the iliac fracture and indirect reduction of the SI joint. The iliac fracture is visualized directly, reduced with clamps, and stabilized with lag screws and 3.5 mm reconstruction plates along the iliac wing.[17] Percutaneously placed iliosacral screws also may be used to supplement fixation.

Treatment of crescent fractures with the patient in the supine position allows for direct reduction of the SI joint and indirect reduction of the iliac fracture.[46] The lateral window of the ilioinguinal surgical exposure is used to access the SI joint. After the SI joint is visualized and debrided, reduction is performed under direct visualization using a combination of clamps, external fixators, and, occasionally, a femoral distractor used in compression. The SI joint is stabilized with iliosacral screws, 3.5 mm reconstruction plates placed perpendicular to one another, or both used in combination.[32]

Isolated percutaneous treatment of crescent fractures using iliosacral screw fixation can be used if the posterior iliac fracture fragment is small, the unstable iliac wing component can be reduced with closed manipulative means, and the sacral safe zone is large enough to accommodate an iliosacral screw.[40] This technique can be used with either prone or supine positioning using well-described techniques for placement of iliosacral screws.[32,47]

Sacroiliac joint disruptions

SI joint disruptions occur as a result of an anteriorly or posteriorly directed force to the pelvis associated with symphysis pubis disruptions or rami fractures.[8,7,25] Incomplete disruptions of the SI joint typically are characterized by rupture of the anterior SI ligaments with a concurrent symphyseal disruption of less than 2.5 cm.[26] These injuries are not associated with vertical instability and may be managed non-operatively, with an external fixator or open reduction and internal fixation.[26,42]

Complete disruptions or dislocations of the SI joint are associated with rupture of the anterior and posterior SI joint ligaments. A rotationally and/or vertically unstable pelvis characterizes these injuries. Because of the poor results with persistent SI joint subluxations and dislocations, surgical reduction and stabilization is recommended.

Open treatment of SI joint disruptions can be performed from either the supine or prone position. Stabilization in the supine position usually is achieved using the lateral window of the ilioinguinal surgical exposure. After debridement of the joint space, the dislocation is reduced. Care must be taken with exposure across the SI joint to avoid excessive medial dissection to prevent injury to the L5 nerve root. Distal ipsilateral femoral traction, Schanz pins within the ilium, tenaculum clamps, Farabeuf clamps, pelvic reduction clamps and a femoral distractor used in compression may all be helpful in reducing SI joint disruptions.[48]

Stabilization is achieved with either 3.5 or 4.5 mm pelvic reconstruction plates placed perpendicular to one another across the SI joint. Plates should be contoured carefully to avoid distraction at the inferior portion of the SI joint.[49] The S1 nerve root is at risk when drilling and inserting a screw within the sacral ala, and fluoroscopic guidance is recommended.

Stabilization of SI disruptions from the prone position uses a vertical paramedian dorsal surgical exposure; however, one must be wary of significant wound problems that may develop using posterior exposures in a compromised soft-tissue envelope.[27,42] Unlike anterior surgical exposures, reduction of the SI joint is performed indirectly because visualization is compromised as the joint is brought into reduction. Reduction is verified manually by palpation of the anterior aspect of the SI joint through the greater sciatic notch and radiographically with intra-operative fluoroscopic imaging. Reduction of the dislocated ilium to the sacrum may be assisted with clamps placed through the greater sciatic notch clamping the posterior iliac wing to the sacral ala.[47,50] Stabilization is obtained with combinations of transiliac plates using either pelvic reconstruction or dynamic compression plates, transiliac screws and iliosacral screws.

Use of iliosacral screws has gained popularity for stabilization of SI joint disruptions. Percutaneously placed iliosacral screws have been used after both open and closed reduction of SI joint disruptions. Iliosacral screws may be placed in either the prone[47] or supine position[49] with good results. When using percutaneous techniques for posterior ring stabilization, it is helpful to reduce and stabilize the anterior pelvic ring injuries, which indirectly reduce the posterior ring, thereby allowing for safe iliosacral screw placement.[40]

Careful examination of plain radiographs and CT scans is essential in evaluating sacral morphology and planning for safe iliosacral screw placement.[40] Cannulated iliosacral screws are inserted under fluoroscopic guidance using inlet, outlet and lateral sacral images.[40,51] Others prefer solid iliosacral screw placement, with which the tactile sensation of the drill bit engaging into the sacral ala and sacral body is used to assist with fluoroscopic imaging in safe placement of iliosacral screws.[47,52] Still others favour CT scan-guided placement of iliosacral screws.[53,54] Each technique has its advantages and associated potential problems but each demands that the surgeon understand the local anatomy and achieve accurate reductions.

Sacral fractures

Sacral fractures frequently occur with pelvic ring injuries. Sacral fractures commonly are classified by the location of the sacral fracture. Type I fractures involve the sacral ala, type II fractures involve the sacral foramina and type III fractures involve the central portion of the sacrum.[55] Roy-Camille et al.[39] have further subclassified central sacral fractures. Operative stabilization of sacral fractures is indicated in those fractures that are displaced, those that lend themselves to pelvic ring instability and those sacral fractures with foraminal debris causing a neurological deficit.

Sacral fractures usually are treated by indirect reduction techniques unless a need for foraminal decompression is present or an acceptable reduction cannot be obtained by closed manipulative means. Open treatment is performed in the prone position using a vertical paramedian dorsal surgical exposure. Direct access to the posterior sacrum is achieved by elevating the paraspinal muscles from the sacrum, whereby decompression of the sacral foramina may be accomplished. After fracture reduction, stabilization is obtained with transiliac bars, transiliac screws, transiliac plates or iliosacral screws. Despite the implant, care must be taken not to overcompress the sacral fractures and potentially create an iatrogenic sacral nerve root injury.

Iliosacral screws may be placed in the supine or prone position to stabilize sacral fractures after closed manipulative means. Reduction and stabilization of associated anterior fractures facilitate reduction of sacral fractures, allowing for safe iliosacral screw placement.[40] Contraindications to a percutaneous iliosacral screw technique are an inability to obtain a reduction of the sacral fracture, sacral dysmorphism or fractures of the neural foramina requiring debridement. Neurodiagnostic monitoring should be considered when foraminal debris is present and/or foraminal decompression is undertaken. Several different types of monitoring have been used with good results, including somatosensory-evoked potentials, continuous electromyographic monitoring and stimulus-evoked electromyography.[50,56,57] Neurodiagnostic monitoring does not protect the patient from a surgeon with poor understanding of the anatomy and its radiographic correlations.

PRE-OPERATIVE DETAILS

Pre-operative traction is a consideration for patients with displaced pelvic fractures to prevent large pelvic translations and provide patient comfort. Skeletal traction is preferred in the ipsilateral distal femur if not contraindicated. Ten to 30 pounds (4.5–13.5 kg) of traction is sufficient to meet the goals of provisional stabilization.

Deep venous thrombosis (DVT) prophylaxis is recommended in the pre-operative setting. Both mechanical and pharmacological methods are available for DVT prophylaxis. Subcutaneous heparin, low molecular weight heparin, warfarin and aspirin are all used for DVT prophylaxis. Compression hose and sequential compression devices also are used in combination with pharmacological methods to prevent DVT formation. Internal venal caval filters are used occasionally when pharmacological prophylaxis is contraindicated or a DVT has been detected. Consideration should be given to pre-operative duplex ultrasonography, especially in patients with prolonged bed rest prior to surgery.

A screening haematocrit must be obtained, and the patient must have a type and cross-match prior to surgery. Cellsavers are valuable tools to decrease the need for blood transfusions.

Patients with neurological injuries require special consideration in the pre-operative period. Sciatic nerve palsies must be recognized, and splinting of the ankle is required to prevent equinus contractures. Injuries to all, or portions, of the lumbosacral plexus may occur with pelvic ring injuries. When possible, these injuries should be clearly documented in the pre-operative setting to avoid confusion about potential iatrogenic injuries. Neurodiagnostic monitoring may be desirable, and should be arranged pre-operatively if necessary.

If intra-operative fluoroscopy is to be used and the patient has ingested oral contrast, an AP pelvic radiograph is recommended pre-operatively to ensure that fluoroscopic visualization is adequate. Residual contrast should be evacuated prior to surgery and a repeat AP pelvic radiograph performed after bowel evacuation.

Pre-operative templating of plates to a skeletal model may prove beneficial by decreasing operative time and increasing operative efficiency. For example, transiliac plates are easily contoured to a skeletal model and after sterilization may be applied to the ilium with possible minor modifications.

INTRA-OPERATIVE DETAILS

The operating table usually is chosen to allow for intra-operative fluoroscopic imaging, and a radiolucent table is recommended. For supine positioning, the patient is placed elevated on a lumbosacral support beneath the back along the axis of the spine, which allows iliosacral screw insertions if needed. The arms are placed at 90° to the body on padded arm boards to allow for proper positioning of the C-arm. If traction is to be used, a traction apparatus from the table can be used, or traction may be applied by hanging the weights over the side of the table.

Prone positioning is performed on the same table using padded chest rolls, which relieve abdominal pressure and allow ventilation. Pads are placed anterior to the knees, and pillows are placed anterior to the legs to elevate the toes off the table. The arms are placed in a flying position with 45° of shoulder abduction and neutral shoulder elevation. The elbows are flexed to 90°, and the hands are positioned pronated on the arm board.

If neurological monitoring is used, the set-up should be performed pre-operatively. The technician should establish the workings of the set-up, and baseline values should be obtained. An understanding should exist between the examiner and the anaesthetist regarding the type of anaesthetic agents because neurological recordings vary with certain anaesthetics.

POSTOPERATIVE DETAILS

Portable postoperative AP, inlet and outlet pelvic radiographs are taken in the recovery room to assess pelvic ring reconstruction and implant safety. If radiographic imaging is inferior using a portable technique, then consideration should be given to taking radiographs in the radiology department on discharge from the recovery room. Postoperative CT scanning is recommended to assess pelvic ring reduction and implant safety, particularly when iliosacral screws are used.

Pain control is important in the postoperative period to assist with patient mobilization. Epidural narcotics provide excellent pain relief in the acute postoperative period; however, one must be aware of potential epidural bleeding with concurrent anticoagulation. Patient-controlled analgesic machines work well to alleviate postoperative pain, and patients do not depend on nursing administration of narcotic analgesics. Long-acting oral narcotic medications may be useful as an adjunct to patient-controlled analgesia to provide sustained pain control. After discontinuation of intravenous narcotic medications, both long-acting and short-acting oral narcotics are used to manage postoperative pain.

DVT prophylaxis is important postoperatively and should be managed aggressively. Mechanical methods, such as supportive stockings, work to decrease venous stasis, thereby decreasing the risk of DVT formation. Sequential compression devices also work to decrease venous stasis, but they also may have a role in stimulating the fibrinolytic system and stimulation of tissue factor pathway inhibitor release.[58]

Pharmacological prophylaxis consists of subcutaneous heparin, low molecular weight heparin, warfarin and aspirin. The particular agent to choose is beyond the scope of this discussion, but evidence suggests that combined mechanical and pharmacological prophylaxes may result in greater protection than either alone.[58] Inferior vena caval filters may be placed in the peri-operative setting for patients in whom pharmacological DVT prophylaxis and treatment is contraindicated and also in patients with documented DVTs.

FOLLOW-UP

Patients are mobilized based on their particular injury pattern, with a goal of full weight bearing by 3 months postoperatively. After discharge from the hospital, patients are seen at follow-up 2 weeks postoperatively for a wound check. Patients are seen again 6 weeks postoperatively for repeat clinical and radiographic examination. Further postoperative visits are scheduled at 3, 6 and 12 months postoperatively.

COMPLICATIONS

Muscle ruptures and hernias

Muscle ruptures and hernias have been reported infrequently with pelvic ring injuries. Ryan[59] noted that APC injuries were associated with avulsion of the medial portion of the rectus abdominus muscle, which could give rise to ventral hernias. Ryan[59] also noted an association of direct inguinal hernias with pubic rami fractures occurring after disruption of the posterior wall of the inguinal canal. These are avoided when open reduction/internal fixation is selected for these fractures because the associated soft-tissue injuries are repaired at the time of closure. Bowel perforation, bowel entrapment and bowel herniation also have been documented with comminuted iliac wing fractures.[45]

Neurological injury

Approximately 10% of all patients who sustain pelvic fractures also sustain neurological injury. Most neurological injuries involve the L5 and S1 nerve roots of the lumbosacral plexus; however, a significant number of patients also can experience sexual dysfunction secondary to nerve injury of the lower sacral nerves.[25,60] Associated sacral fractures account for many neurological deficits with pelvic ring injuries. Denis et al.[55] reported a 28% incidence of nerve injury in patients after transforaminal sacral fractures and a 56% incidence of nerve injuries if the central sacrum was fractured.

Femoral nerve palsies may develop secondary to iliac haematoma and pubic ramus or certain acetabular pattern fracture displacements. Fractures of the pubic ramus at the superolateral aspect of the obturator foramen may cause obturator nerve injury. Lateral femoral cutaneous nerve injuries also may occur as a result of a direct blow to the lateral pelvic region in proximity to the anterior superior iliac spine and fracture displacement of this area.

Postoperative wound infection

The incidence of postoperative wound infection is low after anterior surgical exposures to the pelvis; however, the incidence increases with indwelling suprapubic catheters, colostomy or drains in the region of the surgical incisions.[30] Posterior surgical exposures are associated with higher instances of postoperative wound infection related to the soft-tissue injury, particularly those injuries associated with closed internal degloving injuries.[15,42] Postoperative wound infections after percutaneous fixation techniques are very low, occurring only infrequently.[61]

Non-union after a pelvic fracture is uncommon, whereas malunion is more common. Pennal and Massiah[62] evaluated 42 patients with delayed union and non-union after pelvic fractures. The authors found that the patients who were treated surgically with stabilization and bone grafting demonstrated union in 15 of 16 patients. Non-unions in patients treated non-operatively did not heal; these patients had poorer outcomes than the surgically treated group. Matta and Tornetta[63] treated 37 patients with pelvic malunions and non-unions. They highlighted the need for multiple-staged procedures to achieve satisfactory results, which were demonstrated in 32 patients, although 19% of the patients suffered complications.

Proximal DVTs

Proximal DVTs have been reported in as many as 61% of pelvic fracture patients without prophylaxis.[64] Magnetic resonance venography has documented a 34% incidence of proximal DVT in patients with acetabular fractures who were treated prophylactically with low-dose heparin and mechanical compression devices.[58] Documentation of proximal DVTs is important because these are most likely to embolize to the lungs. The incidence of pulmonary emboli is 2–12% in patients with pelvic fractures, whereas fatal pulmonary embolism has been reported in 0.5–10% of patients sustaining pelvic fractures.[58] Detection of proximal DVTs with venography or magnetic resonance venography is expensive and often impractical in the polytraumatized patient; therefore, the most effective treatment of patients with pelvic fractures is adequate prophylaxis.

Genitourinary

GU complications occur in up to 37% of patients with pelvic ring injuries.[21] The most common GU complications occurring with pelvic ring injuries are bladder disruptions and ureteral disruptions, particularly in male patients. Less commonly, the ureters and kidneys may be injured.[24] Dyspareunia and erectile dysfunction occur in approximately 29% of patients with pelvic ring injuries.[21,22] Dyspareunia usually is caused by a displaced ramus fracture, causing pressure on the vaginal vault. Erectile dysfunction can have many causes, including vascular injury, neurological injury and psychological stress. A patient with erectile dysfunction should be referred to a urologist for evaluation and treatment.

OUTCOME AND PROGNOSIS

Early stabilization of pelvic ring injuries has demonstrated improved outcomes in patients with pelvic fractures. Stabilization of pelvic fractures immobilizes bleeding cancellous surfaces, thereby decreasing overall blood loss.[5] Goldstein et al.[27] noted decreased operative time, blood transfusions and hospital stays for patients who were treated within 24 hours of hospital admission. Similarly, Latenser et al.[28] noted decreased complications, blood loss, hospital stays, long-term disability and better survival for patients treated within 8 hours of hospital admission.

Injury pattern and reduction of fracture-related displacements have been correlated with outcome results. Patients with injuries involving the SI joint have poorer results than patients with either sacral fractures or iliac wing fractures.[2,6,26] Posterior pelvic displacement of 5 mm has been identified as leading to poorer patient outcomes.[9] Another study noted that pelvic displacement greater than 1 cm in any plane led to increased levels of pain compared with patients with less than 1 cm of displacement. Limb length discrepancy greater than 2.5 cm also has been implicated in poor results.[26]

Permanent neurological injury contributes to poorer patient outcomes after pelvic ring injury and is present in approximately 20% of patients with unstable pelvic ring injuries.[30,65] Tile[30] noted that permanent nerve damage led to unsatisfactory results in 12 of 248 patients. Templeman et al.[61] also noted that neurological injury was associated with compromised outcome in patients with sacral fractures. Most neurological injuries after pelvic ring injuries involve the L5 and S1 nerve roots, although injury may occur along any portion of the lumbosacral trunk. Management of neurological injuries is expectant, as neurological recovery has been documented as long as 4 years after injury.[66]

FUTURE AND CONTROVERSIES

Controversies in treating pelvic fractures revolve around the issue of pelvic stability. Definitions of pelvic stability are vague and hard to quantify in a clinical setting. As a result of a nebulous definition of pelvic stability, determining the type and amount of pelvic stabilization is also controversial. Perhaps Bucholtz and Peters[18] best state the problem, as follows:

> as a general rule, if a posterior ring injury is nondisplaced or impacted, the pelvis is probably stable. If there is a superior or AP displacement of the hemipelvis of 1 cm or more, the pelvis is clearly unstable. All injuries between these two extremes may or may not be stable, and must be evaluated and treated individually.

Most clinicians responsible for the care of patients with pelvic ring injuries will base instability on the physical examination. Instability is defined as the inability to resist deformation with physiological loading.

The future of pelvic fracture management will probably involve advances in imaging techniques. Except for major pelvic disruptions, the state of the posterior ligamentous structures is inferred from clinical examination, plain radiographs and CT scans.[67] MRI may have a role one day in visualizing the posterior ligamentous structures, allowing for these injuries to be better defined.

Computer-assisted surgery is being developed and studied at various locations. Computer-assisted surgery comprises robotics, image-guided surgical devices, surgical navigation systems, pre-operative planners and simulators, and augmented reality or hybrid reality computer interfaces.[66] Computer-assisted surgery has been used successfully around the pelvis to assist with pelvic osteotomies.[68] As the technology improves and familiarity grows with these techniques, computer-assisted surgery will probably be used in the management of pelvic fractures. Surgeons should not assume that computer-assisted surgery and robotics substitute for their personal knowledge of pelvic injuries and radiographic correlations. The pelvic anatomy, its injury patterns, and their treatments are to date best directed by knowledgeable humans rather than computer software.

KEY LEARNING POINTS

- Operative management of unstable pelvic injuries has increased.
- Unstable pelvic fractures typically are a result of high-energy injuries and may be associated with primary organ system injuries.
- Soft-tissue injuries provide an indirect measurement of the energy sustained by the patient.
- A Morel-Lavallee lesion is a post-traumatic soft-tissue degloving.
- Injuries to the pelvic ring may cause injury to any of the neurovascular structures that traverse the pelvis.
- Neurological injuries typically occur as injuries to the L5 or S1 nerve roots.
- First management is centred on controlling life-threatening injuries and to provide early stable fixation.
- Pennal and Tile developed a very useful classification scheme for pelvic fractures.
- The bones of the pelvis are held together by strong ligaments and can be divided into four groups.
- Radiographs include anteroposterior pelvis, inlet and outlet views, lateral sacral and CT (obturator and iliac obliques for the acetabulum).
- Letournel recommended operative stabilization of symphyseal disruptions when the pubic diastasis measured greater than 1.5 cm.
- Indications for operative management of iliac wing fractures include associated skin abnormalities, significant closed degloving injuries and open wounds.
- Crescent fractures are actually fractures of the posterior ilium extending from the iliac crest into the greater sciatic notch.
- Complete disruptions or dislocations of the sacroiliac joint are associated with rupture of the anterior and posterior sacroiliac joint ligaments.
- Sacral fractures usually are treated by indirect reduction techniques unless a need for foraminal decompression is present or an acceptable reduction cannot be obtained by closed manipulative means.
- Approximately 10% of all patients who sustain pelvic fractures also sustain neurological injury.
- The incidence of postoperative wound infection is low after anterior surgical exposures to the pelvis; however, the incidence increases with indwelling suprapubic catheters, colostomy or drains in the region of the surgical incisions.
- Proximal deep vein thromboses have been reported in as many as 61% of pelvic fracture patients without prophylaxis.
- Genitourinary complications occur in up to 37% of patients with pelvic ring injuries.
- Early stabilization of pelvic ring injuries has demonstrated improved outcomes.
- Controversies in treating pelvic fractures revolve around the issue of pelvic stability.

REFERENCES

- ● = Key primary paper
- ◆ = Major review article

◆1. Dunn AW, Morris HD. Fractures and dislocations of the pelvis. *Journal of Bone and Joint Surgery (American)* 1968;**50**:1639-48.

◆2. Holdsworth F. Dislocation and fracture-dislocation of the pelvis. *Journal of Bone and Joint Surgery (British)* 1948;**30B**:461-6.

◆3. Holm CL. Treatment of pelvic fractures and dislocations. Skeletal traction and the dual pelvic traction sling. *Clinical Orthopaedics and Related Research* 1973;**97**:97-107.

◆4. Watson-Jones R. Dislocations and fracture-dislocations of the pelvis. *British Journal of Surgery* 1938;**25**:773-81.

●5. Huittinen VM, Slätis P. Postmortem angiography and dissection of the hypogastric artery in pelvic fractures. *Surgery* 1973;**73**:454-62.

◆6. Schield DK, Tile M, Kellam JF. Open reduction internal fixation of pelvic ring fractures. *Journal of Orthopaedic Trauma* 1991;**5**:226.

◆7. Failinger MS, McGanity PL. Unstable fractures of the pelvic ring. *Journal of Bone and Joint Surgery (American)* 1992;**74**:781-91.

●8. McLaren AC, Rorabeck CH, Halpenny J. Long-term pain and disability in relation to residual deformity after displaced pelvic ring fractures. *Canadian Journal of Surgery* 1990;**33**:492-4.

9. Pohlemann T, Bosch U, Gansslen A, Tscherne H. The Hannover experience in management of pelvic fractures. *Clinical Orthopaedics and Related Research* 1994;**Aug**:69-80.

10. Gansslen A, Pohlmann T, Paul C, Lobenhoffer P. Epidemiology of pelvic ring injuries. *Injury* 1996;**27**(Suppl. 1):13-20.

●11. Melton LJ 3rd, Sampson JM, Morrey BF, Ilstrup D. Epidemiologic features of pelvic fractures. *Clinical Orthopaedics and Related Research* 1981;**Mar**:43-7.

◆12. Gotis-Graham I, McGuigan L, Diamond T, et al. Sacral insufficiency fractures in the elderly. *Journal of Bone and Joint Surgery (British)* 1994;**76**:882-6.

◆13. American College of Surgeons' Committee on Trauma. *Advanced Trauma Life Support (Course for Physicians)*. Chicago, IL: American College of Surgeons 1993.

◆14. Peltier LF. Complications associated with fractures of the pelvis. *Journal of Bone and Joint Surgery (American)* 1965;**47**:1060-9.

●15. Hak DJ, Olson SA, Matta JM. Diagnosis and management of closed internal degloving injuries associated with pelvic and acetabular fractures: the Morel-Lavallee lesion. *Journal of Trauma* 1997;**42**:1046-51.

●16. Tseng S, Tornetta P. Percutaneous management of Morel-Lavallee lesions. *Journal of Bone and Joint Surgery* 2006;**88**:92-6.

●17. Borrelli J Jr, Koval KJ, Helfet DL. The crescent fracture: a posterior fracture dislocation of the sacroiliac joint. *Journal of Orthopaedic Trauma* 1996;**10**:165-70.

◆18. Bucholtz RW, Peters P. Assessment of pelvic stability. In: Bassett FH (ed.) *Instructional Course Lectures*. Rosemont, IL: American Academy of Orthopaedic Surgeons, 1988:119-27.

◆19. Burgess A, Jones A. Fractures of the pelvic ring. In: Rockwood C Jr, Green DP, Bucholtz R, Heckman J (eds) *Fractures in Adults*. Philadelphia, PA: Lippincott-Raven, 1996:1575-615.

20. Clemente C. *Anatomy: A Regional Atlas of the Human Body*, 2nd edn. Baltimore, MD: Urban and Schwarzenberg, 1981.

●21. Cole JD, Blum DA, Ansel LJ. Outcome after fixation of unstable posterior pelvic ring injuries. *Clinical Orthopaedics and Related Research* 1996;**Aug**:160-79.

●22. Copeland CE, Bosse MJ, McCarthy ML, et al. Effect of trauma and pelvic fracture on female genitourinary, sexual, and reproductive function. *Journal of Orthopaedic Trauma* 1997;**11**:73-81.

◆23. Dalinka MK, Arger P, Coleman B. CT in pelvic trauma. *Orthopaedic Clinics of North America* 1985;**16**:471-80.

◆24. Watnik NF, Coburn M, Goldberger M. Urologic injuries in pelvic ring disruptions. *Clinical Orthopaedics and Related Research* 1996;**Aug**:37-45.

●25. Huittinen VM, Slätis P. Nerve injury in double vertical pelvic fractures. *Acta Chirurgica Scandinavica* 1972;**138**:571-5.

◆26. Tile M. Pelvic ring fractures: should they be fixed? *Journal of Bone and Joint Surgery (British)* 1988;**70**:1-12.

◆27. Goldstein A, Phillips T, Sclafani SJ, et al. Early open reduction and internal fixation of the disrupted pelvic ring. *Journal of Trauma* 1986;**26**:325-33.

●28. Latenser BA, Gentilello LM, Tarver AA, et al. Improved outcome with early fixation of skeletally unstable pelvic fractures. *Journal of Trauma* 1991;**31**:28-31.

29. Slatis P, Huittinen VM. Double vertical fractures of the pelvis. A report on 163 patients. *Acta Chirurgica Scandinavica* 1972;**138**:799-807.

◆30. Tile M. Anatomy. In: Tile M (ed.) *Fractures of the Pelvis and Acetabulum*. Baltimore, MD: Williams & Wilkins, 1995:12-21.

◆31. Burgess AR, Eastridge BJ, Young JW, et al. Pelvic ring disruptions: effective classification system and treatment protocols. *Journal of Trauma* 1990;**30**:848-56.

◆32. Routt ML Jr, Simonian PT, Swiontkowski MF. Stabilization of pelvic ring disruptions. *Orthopaedic Clinics of North America* 1997;**28**:369-88.

◆33. Pennal GF, Tile M, Waddell JP, Garside H. Pelvic disruption: assessment and classification. *Clinical Orthopaedics and Related Research* 1980;**151**:12-21.

◆34. Dalal SA, Burgess AR, Siegel JH, et al. Pelvic fracture in multiple trauma: classification by mechanism is key to pattern of organ injury, resuscitative requirements, and outcome. *Journal of Trauma* 1989;**29**:981-1000; discussion 1000-2.

35. Hollinshead W. Pelvis. In: *Anatomy for Surgeons: The Back and Limbs*, 3rd edn. Philadelphia, PA: Harper Rowe, 1982.

36. Anson B (ed.). *Morris' Human Anatomy*. New York, NY: McGraw-Hill, 1966.

◆37. Young J, Burgess A. *Radiologic Management of Pelvic Ring Fractures*. Baltimore, MD: Urban and Schwarzenberg, 1987.

●38. Nork SE, Jones CB, Harding SP, et al. Percutaneous stabilization of U-shaped sacral fractures using iliosacral screws: technique and early results. *Journal of Orthopaedic Trauma* 2001;**15**:238-46.

39. Roy-Camille R, Saillant G, Gagna G, Mazel C. Transverse fracture of the upper sacrum. Suicidal jumper's fracture. *Spine* 1985;**10**:838–45.
●40. Routt ML Jr, Nork SE, Mills WJ. Percutaneous fixation of pelvic ring disruptions. *Clinical Orthopaedics and Related Research* 2000;**375**:15–29.
◆41. Letournel E. Pelvic fractures. *Injury* 1978;**10**:145–8.
◆42. Kellam JF. The role of external fixation in pelvic disruptions. *Clinical Orthopaedics and Related Research* 1989;**Apr**:66–82.
●43. Simonian PT, Routt ML Jr, Harrington RM, Tencer AF. Internal fixation of the unstable anterior pelvic ring: a biomechanical comparison of standard plating techniques and the retrograde medullary superior pubic ramus screw. *Journal of Orthopaedic Trauma* 1994;**8**:476–82.
44. Simonian PT, Routt ML Jr, Harrington RM, Tencer AF. Box plate fixation of the symphysis pubis: biomechanical evaluation of a new technique. *Journal of Orthopaedic Trauma* 1994;**8**:483–9.
45. Switzer JA, Nork SE, Routt ML Jr. Comminuted fractures of the iliac wing. *Journal of Orthopaedic Trauma* 2000;**14**:270–6.
46. Lange R, Webb L, Mayo K. Efficacy of the anterior approach for fixation of sacroiliac dislocations and fracture-dislocations. *Journal of Orthopaedic Trauma* 1990;**4**:220–1.
◆47. Matta JM, Saucedo T. Internal fixation of pelvic ring fractures. *Clinical Orthopaedics and Related Research* 1989;**329**:83–97.
48. Simpson LA, Waddell JP, Leighton RK, et al. Anterior approach and stabilization of the disrupted sacroiliac joint. *Journal of Trauma* 1987;**27**:1332–9.
49. Routt ML Jr, Simonian PT, Mills WJ. Iliosacral screw fixation: early complications of the percutaneous technique. *Journal of Orthopaedic Trauma* 1997;**11**:584–9.
50. Moed BR, Ahmad BK, Craig JG, et al. Intraoperative monitoring with stimulus-evoked electromyography during placement of iliosacral screws. An initial clinical study. *Journal of Bone and Joint Surgery (American) and Related Research* 1998;**80**:537–46.
51. Routt ML Jr, Simonian PT, Agnew SG, Mann FA. Radiographic recognition of the sacral alar slope for optimal placement of iliosacral screws: a cadaveric and clinical study. *Journal of Orthopaedic Trauma* 1996;**10**:171–7.
52. Templeman D, Schmidt A, Freese J, Weisman I. Proximity of iliosacral screws to neurovascular structures after internal fixation. *Clinical Orthopaedics and Related Research* 1996;**Aug**:194–8.
●53. Ebraheim NA, Rusin JJ, Coombs RJ, et al. Percutaneous computed-tomography-stabilization of pelvic fractures: preliminary report. *Journal of Orthopaedic Trauma* 1987;**1**:197–204.
54. Nelson DW, Duwelius PJ. CT-guided fixation of sacral fractures and sacroiliac joint disruptions. *Radiology* 1991;**180**:527–32.
55. Denis F, Davis S, Comfort T. Sacral fractures: an important problem. Retrospective analysis of 236 cases. *Clinical Orthopaedics and Related Research* 1988;**227**:67–81.
◆56. Vrahas M, Gordon RG, Mears DC, et al. Intraoperative somatosensory evoked potential monitoring of pelvic and acetabular fractures. *Journal of Orthopaedic Trauma* 1992;**6**:50–8.
57. Webb LX, Araujo WD, Donofrio P. Continuous EMG monitoring for placement of percutaneous iliosacral screws. *Orthopaedic Transactions* 1996;**20**:134.
◆58. Montgomery KD, Geerts WH, Potter HG, Helfet DL. Practical management of venous thromboembolism following pelvic fractures. *Orthopaedic Clinics of North America* 1997;**28**:397–404.
59. Ryan EA. Hernias related to pelvic fractures. *Surgery, Gynecology & Obstetrics* 1971;**133**:440–6.
60. Weis EB Jr. Subtle neurological injuries in pelvic fractures. *Journal of Trauma* 1984;**24**:983–5.
◆61. Templeman D, Goulet J, Duwelius PJ, et al. Internal fixation of displaced fractures of the sacrum. *Clinical Orthopaedics and Related Research* 1996;**Aug**:180–5.
◆62. Pennal GF, Massiah KA. Nonunion and delayed union of fractures of the pelvis. *Clinical Orthopaedics and Related Research* 1980;**Sep**:124–9.
◆63. Matta JM, Tornetta P 3rd. Internal fixation of unstable pelvic ring injuries. *Clinical Orthopaedics and Related Research* 1996;129–40.
●64. Geerts WH, Code KI, Jay RM, et al. A prospective study of venous thromboembolism after major trauma. *New England Journal of Medicine* 1994;**331**:1601–6.
◆65. Reilly MC, Zinar DM, Matta JM. Neurologic injuries in pelvic ring fractures. *Clinical Orthopaedics and Related Research* 1996;**Aug**:28–36.
66. DiGioia AM 3rd. What is computer assisted orthopaedic surgery? *Clinical Orthopaedics and Related Research* 1998;**Sep**:2–4.
67. Gill K, Bucholz RW. The role of computerized tomographic scanning in the evaluation of major pelvic fractures. *Journal of Bone and Joint Surgery (American)* 1984;**66**:34–9.
◆68. Langlotz F, Bachler R, Berlemann U, et al. Computer assistance for pelvic osteotomies. *Clinical Orthopaedics and Related Research* 1998;**Sep**:92–102.

53

Spinal fractures

SHANMUGANATHAN RAJASEKARAN, RISHI MUGESH KANNA, AJOY PRASAD SHETTY

GENERAL CONCEPTS OF SPINAL INJURIES	439	Radiographic evaluation	445
Introduction	439	Injuries to the occiput–C1–C2 complex	446
Epidemiology	439	SUBAXIAL CERVICAL SPINE INJURIES	453
Socioeconomic burden of spinal cord injury	440	Introduction	453
Pre-hospital care	440	Classification of subaxial injuries	453
Pathophysiology of spinal cord injury	440	Gunshot injuries	458
Neural injury in spinal fractures	440	INJURIES OF THE THORACOLUMBAR SPINE	459
Evaluation in the emergency department	442	Introduction	459
Radiographic evaluation	444	Radiographic evaluation	459
Principles of treatment	444	Classification	460
INJURIES OF THE CERVICAL SPINE	445	References	465
Introduction	445		

NATIONAL BOARD STANDARDS

- To understand the mechanism of different types of vertebral injuries
- To understand the pathophysiology of spinal cord injury
- To classify injuries enabling to develop a management plan
- To order appropriate radiological investigation and interpret them
- To understand the principles of early and definite management of spinal injuries

GENERAL CONCEPTS OF SPINAL INJURIES

INTRODUCTION

Spinal injuries assume importance for several reasons. First, the spinal cord is housed and protected by the vertebral column and hence injuries of the spinal column endanger the function of the spinal cord. Second, the stability of the vertebral column is vital for a comfortable upright posture and for one's ability to move without pain. Third, the normal sagittal and coronal alignment of the spinal column can be disturbed by an injury. Spinal alignment is important to establish a normal centre of gravity for the body during ambulation. A thorough knowledge and understanding of these basic principles of spinal injuries is essential for the successful evaluation and management of individual spinal injuries.

EPIDEMIOLOGY

Acute traumatic spinal cord injury (SCI) occurs worldwide with an estimated annual incidence of 15–40 cases per million.[1] Although injury to the vertebral column (6%) occurs much less frequently than injuries to the appendicular skeleton, half of these injuries (2.6%) can be associated with a neurological injury. SCI occurs with the greatest frequency in the 20–30 year age group with a male-to-female ratio of 4:1. The presence of a SCI dramatically affects a patient's chances of surviving the initial period of hospitalization. For patients with a SCI, the overall mortality during the initial hospitalization is 17%. In those who survive, it is associated with severe physical, psychological, social and economic burdens on patients and their families.

SOCIOECONOMIC BURDEN OF SPINAL CORD INJURY

SCI poses significant economic problems to the patient and society. It is the worst survivable injury a person can incur in an accident. Since most patients who sustain these injuries are in their productive age group, the loss of many years of good quality of life causes the greatest loss to society. This is especially important as improvements in rehabilitation have resulted in nearly normal life expectancy for many young individuals with a SCI. In the USA, the lifetime direct medical cost of SCI is estimated to be from $630 000 to $970 000 per injured person.[2] The aggregate annual direct medical cost of traumatic SCI is estimated at $7.74 billion. High-level tetraplegia accounts for 80% of the direct medical cost of SCI. Paraplegia accounts for 4% and incomplete injuries account for approximately 15% of the total aggregate costs.

PRE-HOSPITAL CARE

It has been observed that 20% of SCI patients die en route to the hospital and up to 3–25% of patients can have worsening of spinal cord damage during transport. Overall, 85% of patients with a SCI who survive the first 24 hours are still alive 10 years later compared with 98% of patients of similar age and sex without SCI.[3] Therefore, effective pre-hospital care executed in a quick and timely manner through organized paramedics helps in reducing the morbidity and mortality of SCI during the 'golden hour'. With the development of regional trauma centres and increased training of paramedics and emergency medical technicians, the chances of survival after serious SCI have increased.

The important goals of pre-hospital management include a rapid and accurate assessment, identification of shock and hypoxaemia, initiation of intervention techniques and rapid and safe transportation to the definitive centre. The Advanced Trauma Life Support (ATLS) protocol mandates that all injured patients are assumed to have a spinal injury and one must anticipate the worst case scenario. Any suspicion of spinal injury mandates rigid spinal immobilization. Some situations in which spinal immobilization would be indicated are evidence of neurological deficit, spinal pain or tenderness, high-velocity trauma, head and maxillofacial injury, unconscious patient, diving injury and the presence of distracting injuries such as major limb fractures.

PATHOPHYSIOLOGY OF SPINAL CORD INJURY

The pathophysiology of SCI is considered to be biphasic, consisting of a primary and a secondary phase of injury. Primary injury refers to physical disruption of the spinal cord, i.e. axons, blood vessels and cell membranes, caused by mechanical forces. This occurs during the initial trauma, when mechanical forces disrupt the integrity of the vertebral column. The extent of neural tissue damage is determined by the rate of force application, the degree of neural tissue compression and the duration of neural tissue compression. Secondary injury refers to additional neural tissue damage resulting from the biological response initiated by the physical tissue disruption. The secondary injury phase occurs as a result of vascular dysfunction, oedema, ischaemia, electrolyte shifts, free radical production, inflammation and delayed apoptotic cell death. The secondary injury phase results in a protracted period of tissue destruction. The secondary injury cascade results in rapid damage to the neural tissue owing to a variety of inflammatory responses that are profound in the first 8 hours after injury. So the initial 3–8 hours after injury provide a potential window of opportunity in which the secondary phase of SCI can be mitigated by various measures such as immobilizing the spinal column, maintaining adequate saturation and blood pressure and administering pharmacological agents. In animal studies, it has been found that surgical decompression of the spinal cord within the first 3 hours after injury helps in reducing the magnitude of neurological injury. However, this would be highly impractical in SCIs in humans.

NEURAL INJURY IN SPINAL FRACTURES

The most common site of SCI is the cervical region, accounting for 50–64% of traumatic SCIs. In the lumbar region, 20–24% of patients sustain neurological deficits. Approximately half of the patients with an acute SCI have a complete injury with no preservation of motor or sensory function in the sacral cord segments. At present, the patient's neurological status after the period of spinal shock is the only factor that can predict the chances of neurological recovery. Any patient who still has a complete neurological deficit at 72 hours after the injury has a very poor chance of neurological recovery. Therefore, an accurate and detailed neurological evaluation of the motor power, sensory and reflex functions should be performed at the time of the initial evaluation. This examination should be repeated at intervals and documented. An important element of neurological examination is the evaluation of sacral sparing. Sacral sparing is represented by the presence of perianal sensation, voluntary rectal motor function and great toe flexor activity; it indicates at least partial continuity of spinal cord tracts. It signifies an incomplete cord injury, with the potential for a greater return of cord function following resolution of spinal shock.

However, in approximately 50% of patients immediately after injury, there occurs a brief period of physiological spinal cord 'shutdown' in response to injury. This phase is described as the 'spinal shock' characterized by a state of flaccid paralysis, areflexia and lack of sensation below the level of injury. This occurs most commonly in cervical and upper thoracic injuries. Resolution of spinal shock may be recognized when reflex arcs caudal to the level of injury begin to function again, usually within 24–48 hours of injury. These caudal reflex arcs include the bulbocavernosus reflex (S3–4) and the anal wink (S2–4). The bulbocavernosus reflex refers to contraction of the anal sphincter in response to stimulation of the trigone of the bladder with either a squeeze on the glans penis, a tap on the mons pubis or a pull on a urethral catheter. The anal wink is a contraction of the external anal sphincter in response to a perianal pinprick. The absence of these reflexes indicates the phase of spinal shock. The return of these reflexes generally within 24–48 hours of the initial injury marks the end of spinal shock. The absence of motor or sensory function below the level of injury after spinal shock has resolved indicates a complete injury with a poor prognosis for neurological recovery. These sacral reflexes, however, are not prognostic for lesions involving the conus medullaris or the cauda equina.

To ascertain and document clearly the neurological status, the American Spinal Injury Association (ASIA) form is used (Fig. 53.1). ASIA has also provided definitions of terminologies commonly used to document SCI and for communication between health personnel (Table 53.1). The ASIA grades severity of SCIs from A to E on the ASIA impairment scale. The definitions of each grade and the steps involved in classifying a patient are given in Fig. 53.2.

Classification of spinal cord injuries

SCI occurs in various patterns depending on the type and extent of injury to the spinal cord. As explained above, it can be broadly classified into complete and incomplete injuries. A complete injury is one which does not have any motor or sensory function in the sacral segments. Any spinal injury with the presence of sacral sparing is considered to be incomplete. This classification is made after the period of spinal shock and is required to help in prognosticating neurological recovery and the functional consequences of SCI. An incomplete spinal cord syndrome may be a Brown–Séquard syndrome, central cord syndrome, anterior cord syndrome, posterior

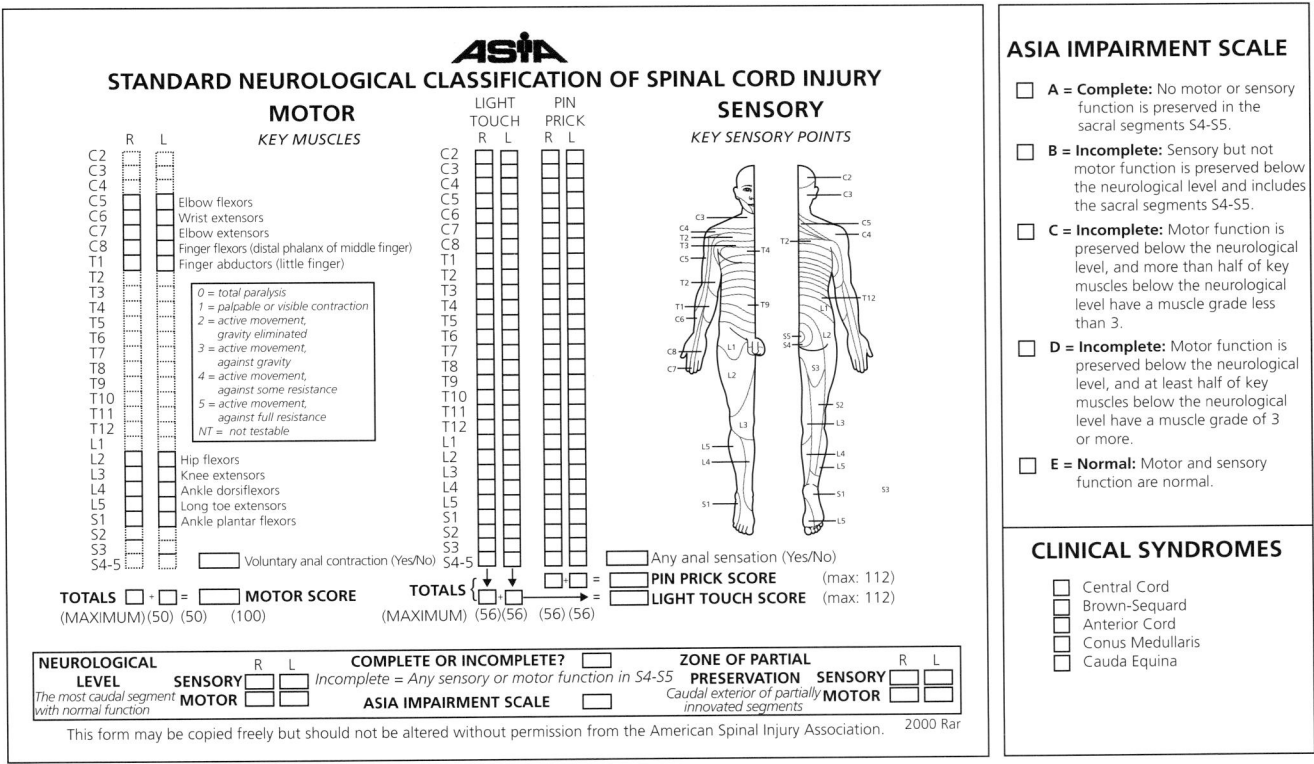

Figure 53.1 American Spinal Injury Association (ASIA) form for standard neurological classification of spinal cord injury. For functional scoring, 10 key muscle segments corresponding to innervation by C5, C6, C7, C8, T1, L2, L3, L4, L5 and S1 are each given a functional score of 0–5 out of 5. For sensory scoring, both right and left sides are graded for a total of 100 points. For the 28 sensory dermatomes on each side of the body, sensory levels are scored on a 0–2 point scale, yielding a maximum possible pinprick score of 112 points for a patient with normal sensation. Reproduced with permission from American Spinal Injury Association.

cord syndrome or, rarely, monoparesis of one extremity (Table 53.2).

EVALUATION IN THE EMERGENCY DEPARTMENT

In the emergency department, every patient should be assessed and resuscitated according to the ATLS guidelines of: airway, breathing, circulation, disability and exposure (ABCDE). The emphasis is on avoiding hypoxia and hypotension. Loss of spinal cord microcirculation, loss of autoregulation, hypoxaemia and ischaemia play important roles in the pathogenesis of secondary spinal cord damage. Quadriplegic patients are able to inspire only using their diaphragm, because their abdominal and intercostal muscles are paralysed. Positive pressure or mechanical ventilation may be required for adequate pulmonary function. Early and appropriate medical management (maintain mean arterial blood pressure >90 mmHg and 100% oxygen saturation) of a patient with acute SCI optimizes the potential for neurological recovery.

Protection of the spine and spinal cord is another important management aspect during all stages of treatment, including the pre-hospital care and primary survey. It should be assumed that all trauma patients have a cervical spine injury until proven otherwise, especially those with altered mental status or following blunt head or neck trauma. Through every stage of management, it is essential to maintain rigid cervical immobilization with a hard cervical collar. The head-tilt and the 'chin-lift' manoeuvre are avoided in patients with cervical spine injury. If orotracheal intubation is required, manual in-line stabilization should be maintained throughout the intubation process.

The patient's history is ascertained and details regarding the mechanism of injury, witnessed head trauma, movement of extremities and level of consciousness immediately following trauma are documented. Chest and abdominal injuries are common with fractures in the thoracic and lumbar region. Therefore, evaluation of injuries to the head, chest, abdomen, pelvis and extremities is important. The patient is log-rolled to evaluate the spine and the skin for bruising and abrasions. The spinous processes are palpated for tenderness and abnormal widening. The vertebral injury can also occur at multiple non-contiguous levels in 15–20% of patients sustaining a spinal injury. Calenoff[4] found a 5% incidence of multiple non-contiguous vertebral injuries with

Table 53.1 American Spinal Injury Association definition of terms used for describing spinal cord injury

Term	Definition
Neurological level	The most caudal segment with normal sensory and motor function on both sides
Sensory level	The most caudal segment with normal sensory function on both sides
Motor level	The most caudal segment with normal motor function on both sides
Skeletal level	Radiographic level of greatest vertebral damage
Sensory score	Numeric summary value of sensory impairment
Motor score	Numeric summary value of motor impairment
Incomplete injury	Partial preservation of sensory and/or motor function below the neurological level AND sensory and/or motor preservation of the lowest sacral segment
Complete injury	Absence of sensory and motor function in the lowest sacral segment
Zone of partial preservation	Dermatomes and myotomes caudal to the neurological level that remain partially innervated. Only used in complete injuries

From American Spinal Injury Association. *Standards for Neurological Classification of Spinal Injury*. Chicago, IL: ASIA, 2006, with permission.

- Determine sensory levels on both sides
- Determine motor levels on both sides
- Determine single neurological level

(lowest segment where motor and sensory function is normal on both sides, and is the cephalad of the levels determined in steps 1 and 2)

- Determine injury is complete or incomplete

(based on sacral sparing)

- Determine ASIA grade

Is injury incomplete? → YES, then it is ASIA A

↓ NO

Is motor injury incomplete? → NO, then it is ASIA B

↓ YES

Are at least half of key muscles below injury are of grade ≥3?

↓ NO, it is ASIA C   ↳ YES, it is ASIA D

Is sensation and motor function normal in all segments?

↓

YES, it is ASIA E

Figure 53.2 Steps in classifying spinal cord injury. Reproduced with permission from American Spinal Injury Association. *Standards for Neurological Classification of Spinal Injury*. Chicago, IL: ASIA, 2006. ASIA, American Spinal Injury Association.

Table 53.2 Descriptions of incomplete cord injury patterns

Syndrome	Lesion	Clinical presentation
Brown–Séquard syndrome	Hemicord injury with ipsilateral motor, light touch sensation and proprioception loss and contralateral pain and temperature sensory loss	The result of a unilateral laminar or pedicle fracture, penetrating injury or rotational injury resulting in a subluxation The prognosis is good, with >90% of patients regaining bowel and bladder function and ambulatory capacity
Central cord syndrome	Incomplete cervical white matter injury The centrally located arm tracts in the cortical spinal area are the most severely affected, and the leg tracts are affected to a lesser extent	Associated with an extension injury to an osteoarthritic spine in a middle-aged patient and presents with flaccid paralysis of the upper extremities and spastic paralysis of the lower extremities Radiographs frequently demonstrate no fracture or dislocation, because the lesion is created by a pincer effect between anterior osteophytes and posterior infolding of the ligamentum flavum The prognosis is fair, and more than 50% of patients have return of bowel and bladder control, become ambulatory and have improved hand function
Anterior cord syndrome	The lesion involves the anterior grey matter with preservation of dorsal columns	The patient presents with variable motor and pain/temperature loss with preserved light touch and proprioception The prognosis is good if recovery is evident and progressive within 24 hours of injury
Posterior cord syndrome	This is a rare injury with isolated involvement of the posterior column	Loss of deep pressure, deep pain and proprioception with full voluntary power, pain and temperature sensation
Conus medullaris syndrome	This is seen in T12–L1 injuries and results in an areflexic bladder and bowel and weak lower extremities	A pure lesion involves a loss of voluntary bowel and bladder control with preserved lumbar root function. The irreversible nature of this injury to the sacral segments is evidenced by the absence of the bulbocavernosus reflex and the perianal wink
Cauda equina	Injury to the lumbosacral nerve roots within the spinal canal	Bilateral radicular pain, numbness, weakness, hyporeflexia or areflexia in lower limbs, saddle anaesthesia and loss of voluntary bowel and bladder function
Root injury	Avulsion or compression injury to single or multiple nerve roots (brachial plexus avulsion)	Dermatomal sensory loss, myotomal motor loss and absent deep tendon reflexes

half of the secondary lesions having been initially missed. Therefore, it is mandatory to evaluate other regions of the spine to look for tenderness, abrasions and interspinous widening.

Patients with cervical and thoracic SCIs can present with hypotension and bradycardia. This is called neurogenic shock and it occurs secondary to sympathetic outflow disruption ('functional sympathectomy') with resultant unopposed vagal (parasympathetic) tone. Initial tachycardia and hypertension immediately after injury are followed by hypotension accompanied by bradycardia and venous pooling. Hypotension from neurogenic shock may be differentiated from cardiogenic, septic and hypovolaemic shock by the presence of bradycardia, as opposed to tachycardia. Recognizing neurogenic shock as distinct from haemorrhagic shock (Table 53.3) is critical for safe initial resuscitation of a trauma patient.

Table 53.3 Differentiating neurogenic from hypovolaemic shock

Neurogenic shock	Hypovolaemic shock
Hypotension	Hypotension
Bradycardia	Tachycardia
Warm extremities	Cold extremities
Normal urine output	Low urine output

Intravenous replacement therapy should maintain systolic blood pressure between 80 and 100 mmHg. Treatment of bradycardia should begin with atropine 0.2–0.5 mg intravenously. Volume expansion is used judiciously to increase intravascular supply and stroke volume. If hypotension persists, vasopressors such as dopamine or dobutamine can be used.

RADIOGRAPHIC EVALUATION

Emergency radiological evaluation of the patient's spine requires consideration of other aspects of the patient's condition. The initial ATLS series of radiographs for a trauma patient should include a lateral view of the cervical spine (ideally down to T1) and anteroposterior views of the chest and pelvis. A lateral cervical radiograph obtained in the emergency room is the minimum requirement in assessing the patient's spine. Complete spine films are performed at the earliest convenient point of time, remembering that 10–15% of patients with a spinal fracture have a non-contiguous spinal injury. Patients complaining of neck pain should undergo complete radiographic evaluation of the cervical spine, including anteroposterior and odontoid views. Lateral radiographic examination of the entire spine is recommended in patients with spine fractures when complete clinical assessment is impaired by neurological injury or other associated injuries.

CT scans may be necessary for cervical spine clearance in patients with questionable or inadequate plain radiographs and also to better delineate fracture morphology (Fig. 53.3). MRI aids in evaluating spinal cord or root injury, intervertebral discs, supporting ligamentous structures as well as degree of canal compromise. The use of MRI is limited, however, to patients who are stable enough to be taken to the imaging area without significant life-support equipment. Immediate MRI scanning is indicated in unexplained neurological deficit, discordant skeletal and neurological levels of injury, and worsening neurological status.

Clearing the spine in trauma patients

A cleared spine in a patient implies that diligent spine evaluation is complete and the patient does not have a spinal injury requiring treatment. The necessary elements for a complete spine evaluation are a good history to assess for high-risk events and high-risk factors, a thorough physical examination to check for physical signs of spinal injury or neurological deficit and appropriate imaging studies based on initial evaluation.

Asymptomatic trauma patients without neck pain or midline tenderness who are awake, alert and not intoxicated, and have no 'distracting' non-spinal injuries may be cleared without cervical spine radiographs. Patients with neck pain, midline tenderness, pain with active range of movements, neurological deficit, altered mental status or 'distracting' non-spinal injuries require radiographic evaluation of the cervical spine. A cervical spine series consisting of an anteroposterior, lateral and open-mouth view is recommended. Supplemental CT examination is recommended to provide more detail of inadequately visualized levels, especially the cervicothoracic and occipitocervical junction. However, despite the absence of apparent osseous injury, instability can exist from spinal soft-tissue disruption of ligaments, facet capsules and disc tissue. MRI is sensitive for acute soft-tissue injury and may be an option, but the incidence of MRI abnormalities has been shown to be between 25% and 40%, suggesting that MRI may be over-sensitive. Moreover, MRI is only reliable for identifying soft-tissue injury within 48 hours of the traumatic event.

PRINCIPLES OF TREATMENT

The treatment is divided into the initial management and definitive management of the fracture. The definitive management of specific fractures of the cervical and thoracolumbar spine will be covered in their respective sections.

The initial management of a spine-injured patient includes the following.

Resuscitation and haemodynamic stabilization of the patient

The primary and secondary surveys provide the trauma team with the opportunity to recognize life-threatening head, chest, abdomen and pelvic injuries, and to institute

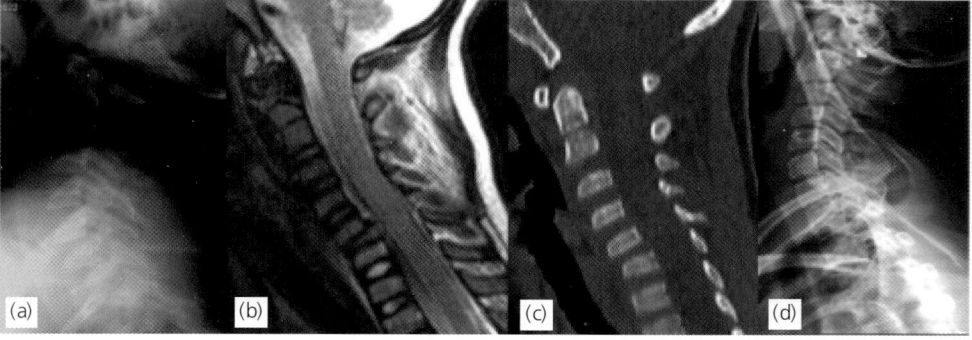

Figure 53.3 (a) Lateral cervical radiograph of a child who presented with neck pain after a road traffic accident. The radiograph does not reveal any obvious pathology. (b,c) Sagittal MRI and CT images show subluxation at the C5–6 level with disc disruption and cord contusion. (d) In such situations, a swimmer's view, taken by hyperabducting one arm and pulling the other arm down, also helps in visualizing the lower cervical spine.

life- and limb-saving interventions. Throughout resuscitation, all efforts must be taken to immobilize these patients safely, as though they had an associated spinal injury. It is essential to catheterize patients with a neurological deficit as early as possible. This serves to avoid damage to the intrinsic bladder wall neural structures from overdistension as well as to monitor urine output. Haemorrhagic gastritis is a common early complication thought to be the result of unopposed vagal tone resulting in increased gastric activity. Gastroprotective agents should be used as prophylaxis against this potential complication.

Immobilization and realignment of the spine

The number and quality of surviving neurons traversing the injured site play an essential role in recovery after SCI. Therefore, an important concept in the acute phase of management is the prevention of injury to the surviving neural structures. Stabilization of unstable injured motion segments itself plays an important role in preventing reinjury. In addition, it is widely accepted that early realignment of the spine and therefore indirect decompression of the spinal canal may also optimize functional recovery. All patients with a spinal injury should be placed on a spine board; however, they should be removed from the spine board (by log-rolling) as soon as possible to minimize pressure sore formation. A special backboard with a head cut-out must be used for children to accommodate their proportionally larger head size and prominent occiput.

For the cervical spine, immobilization with a cervical orthosis (for stable fractures) or Gardner–Wells tong traction (for unstable injuries) should be maintained in the emergency setting. Cervical dislocations and severe compression fractures are frequently considered for reduction by means of axial traction. Traction may be initiated as soon as a malalignment is noted on emergency lateral cervical radiography and this is supported by reports of patients improving in neurological function after the application of cervical traction. Traction is contraindicated in distractive cervical spine injuries, type IIA Hangman's fracture and in patients with pre-existing spinal deformity, such as ankylosing spondylitis.

Pharmacological management of acute spinal cord injury

Secondary tissue damage after SCI is time dependent and, therefore, potentially treatable. Numerous pharmacological agents thought to mitigate the secondary effects of SCI have been extensively studied and widely debated in recent years. These include naloxone (opiate receptor antagonist), calcium channel blockers, free radical scavengers, neurotropic compounds and, most notably, steroids and gangliosides.

According to the recommendations of the National Acute Spinal Cord Injury Studies (NASCIS) III, a 30 mg/kg bolus of intravenous methylprednisolone is given over 15 minutes. After a 45 minute gap, a 23 hour infusion of 5.4 mg/kg of methylprednisolone is given, if administered within 3 hours of injury, or a 47 hour infusion if administered within 3–8 hours after injury[5]. Methylprednisolone has no benefit if started more than 8 hours after injury. Patients with penetrating SCI, those with injuries below the T12 vertebra and those with pure root lesions do not benefit from treatment with methylprednisolone. Such a high dose of steroids is also associated with potential complications such as sepsis, respiratory infections, wound-healing complications and gastritis. Given the modest improvement in functional recovery and the significant complications associated with the use of methylprednisolone, there is much debate regarding the risk–benefit ratio of methylprednisolone use in SCI. Other pharmacological agents have not demonstrated any significant benefit in terms of functional neural recovery in well-designed prospective human trials.

INJURIES OF THE CERVICAL SPINE

INTRODUCTION

Cervical spine injuries occur secondary to high-energy mechanisms, including motor vehicle accident (45%) and fall from a height (20%) and less commonly during athletic participation (15%). Forced flexion or extension resulting from unrestrained deceleration forces is the mechanism for most cervical spine injuries. Neurological injury occurs in 40% of patients with cervical spine fractures and is more frequently associated with lower cervical spine injuries.

RADIOGRAPHIC EVALUATION

The standard radiographic evaluation of the cervical spine includes the lateral, open-mouth (odontoid) and anteroposterior plain films. The lateral view will detect up to 85% of significant cervical spine injuries provided that the occiput–C1, all seven cervical vertebrae and the C7–T1 junctions are visualized. In patients with a short neck, it is necessary to obtain a swimmer's view to visualize the cervicothoracic junction. To obtain a swimmer's view, the upper extremity proximal to the X-ray beam is abducted 180° with axial traction on the contralateral upper extremity, and the beam directed 60° caudad. Important points to consider in interpreting plain radiographs of the occipitocervical spine are shown in Box 53.1.

Stress flexion/extension radiographs rarely if ever should be performed if instability is suspected; they should be performed in the awake and alert patient only. In a patient with neck pain, they are best delayed until spasm has subsided, which can mask instability. Passive flexion and extension stressing of the cervical spine, performed by an experienced physician under fluoroscopy, has a reported sensitivity of 92.3% and specificity of 98.8% for detecting significant ligamentous injuries and instability of the cervical spine.

CT scanning can provide rapid and detailed assessment of the spine. It is a cost-effective primary screening tool in patients at high or moderate risk for cervical injuries. It is valuable to assess the upper cervical spine or the cervicothoracic junction, especially if it is inadequately visualized by plain radiography and in intubated patients (plain films can miss up to 17% of injuries of the upper cervical spine). CT scans with reconstructions may be obtained to characterize the fracture pattern and degree of canal compromise more clearly.

MRI is extremely sensitive and specific for evaluation of the paravertebral soft tissues, including the spinal cord, intervertebral discs and ligamentous structures. Patients with abnormal neurological findings, particularly incomplete injuries, should undergo MRI scanning of the relevant spinal segment(s) to visualize the spinal cord and nerve roots. However, MRI is less sensitive, less specific and less cost-effective than the plain film series or screening CT for the identification and evaluation of cervical fractures.

INJURIES OF THE OCCIPUT–C1–C2 COMPLEX

In this section, injuries are discussed from rostral to caudal, including occipital condyle fractures, occipitocervical dislocations, axis fractures, atlantoaxial ligamentous injury, odontoid fracture, traumatic spondylolisthesis of the axis and C2-body fractures. The craniocervical junction is highly susceptible to injury because of the large lever arm induced cranially by the skull and the relative freedom of movement of the craniocervical junction, which relies predominantly on ligamentous structures rather than on intrinsic bony stability.

Occipital condyle fractures

Occipital condyle fractures should be considered a marker for potentially lethal trauma, with an 11% mortality rate from associated injuries. The incidence of associated cervical spine injury at another level is 31%. The mechanism of injury involves compression and lateral bending; this causes either compression fracture of the condyle as it presses against the superior facet of C1 or avulsion of the alar ligament with extremes of atlanto-occipital rotation. Cranial nerve palsies may develop days to weeks after injury and most frequently affect cranial nerves IX, X and XI. The sensitivity of plain radiography for diagnosis is as low as 3% and a CT scan is frequently necessary for diagnosis.

Occipital condyle fractures have been classified by Anderson and Montesano[6] (Fig. 53.4). Type I fractures (3% of occipital condyle fractures) are comminuted impaction

> **BOX 53.1: Things to note while observing plain radiographs of the occipitocervical spine**
>
> - **Wackenheim line** is drawn as a continuation from the clivus caudally. The tip of the odontoid should be within 1–2 mm of this line
> - **Powers ratio.** The basion to posterior C1 arch distance divided by the anterior arch to opisthion distance (BD/AC) should be <1. A ratio greater than 1 suggests possible anterior dissociation
> - The anterior cortex of the odontoid should be parallel to the posterior cortex of the anterior ring of the atlas. Any kyphotic or lordotic deviation may indicate an odontoid fracture or transverse atlantal ligament disruption
> - The atlantodens interval should be less than 3 mm in an adult (5 mm in a child)
> - The space available for the cord is measured as the distance from the posterior cortex of the odontoid to the anterior cortex of the posterior arch of the atlas and should amount to more than 13 mm
> - Widening of the pre-vertebral soft tissue (normal is <10 mm at C1)

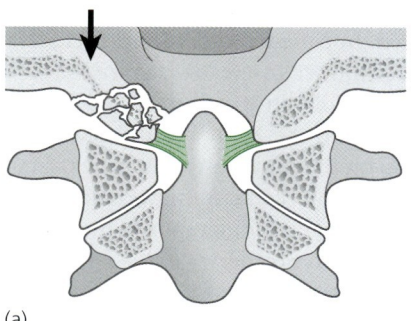
(a)

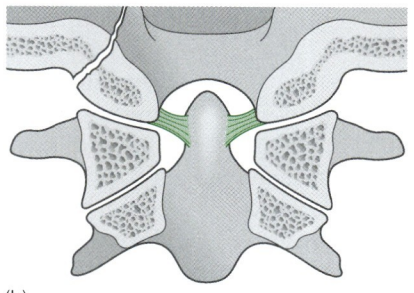
(b)

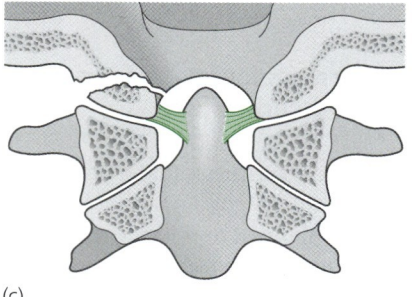
(c)

Figure 53.4 Anderson and Montesano classification of occipital condyle fractures. (a) Type I, comminuted impaction fractures. (b) Type II, condyle fractures extending into the base of the skull. (c) Type III, avulsion fractures. Reproduced with permission from Anderson PA, Montesano PX. Morphology and treatment of occipital condyle fractures. *Spine* 1988;**13**:731.

condyle fractures resulting from an axial load and are usually stable. Type II fractures (22%) involve extension of a basilar skull fracture into the condyle and these are also stable. Type III fractures (75%) are condylar avulsion fractures; they are potentially unstable and should raise clinical suspicion for an underlying occipitocervical dissociation. Type I and II fractures are stable and managed nonoperatively in a rigid cervical collar or halo vest for 8 weeks. Type III fractures are unstable and immobilization for 12 weeks in a halo vest is recommended. After the period of immobilization, if instability is observed on flexion and extension films, an occipital-to-C2 fusion may be necessary.

Occipitocervical dislocation

Occipitocervical dislocations, also known as craniovertebral dissociations, are high-energy injuries resulting from a combination of hyperextension, distraction and rotation at the craniocervical junction. It is twice as common in children, owing to the inclination and shallowness of the condyles and the large head. Most instances of traumatic occipitocervical dislocation are lethal and survivors may demonstrate a wide range of neurological injuries.

Diagnosis of occipitocervical dislocation can be challenging because of the poorly visualized osseous detail on plain radiographs of this region. The most frequently described measurement is the Powers ratio, which divides the basion to posterior arch distance by the anterior arch to opisthion distance (Fig. 53.5). A ratio greater than 1 suggests possible anterior dissociation. The Harris basion–axial interval (BAI)/basion–dental interval (BDI) method measures the distance from the basion to a line drawn tangentially to the posterior border of C2 (a distance greater than 12 mm or less than 4 mm is abnormal) and the distance from the basion to the odontoid (greater than 12 mm is abnormal). This is considered by some to be the most sensitive measurement. Overall, the sensitivity of plain radiographs for occipitocervical dislocation is approximately 57%. The sensitivity of CT and MRI has been estimated to be 84% and 86%, respectively, and one or both of these adjunctive studies is recommended for patients with suspected occipitocervical dissociation injuries. Occipitocervical dislocation injuries have been classified by Traynelis, based on the position of the occiput in relation to C1 (Fig. 53.6). Immediate treatment includes halo vest application with strict avoidance of traction. Early surgical stabilization of the atlanto-occipital joint is recommended as ligamentous healing in a halo vest is unpredictable, and many of these injuries are so unstable that displacement may occur even in the halo vest.

Atlas fractures

Fractures of the atlas constitute approximately 7% of cervical spine fractures and are rarely associated with neurological injury. This is because of the large amount of space available for the cord. Fifty per cent of these injuries are associated with other cervical spine fractures, especially odontoid fractures and spondylolisthesis of the axis. The mechanism of injury is axial compression with elements of

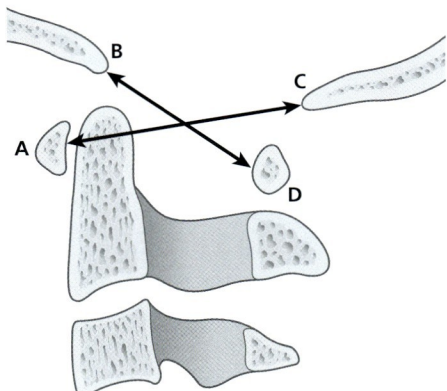

Figure 53.5 Powers ratio. The ratio is derived from basion to posterior arch distance (BD) by the anterior arch to opisthion distance (AC).

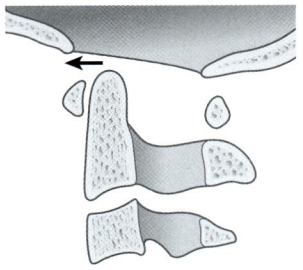

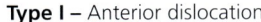

Type I – Anterior dislocation

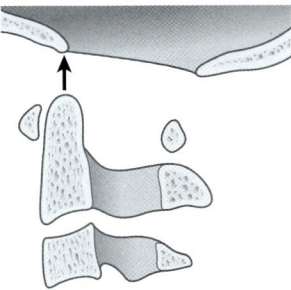

Type II – Distraction separation

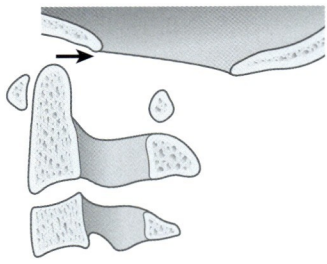

Type III – Posterior dislocation

Figure 53.6 Classification of occipitocervical dislocation. (a) Type I, occipital condyles anterior to the atlas; most common. (b) Type II, condyles longitudinally dissociated from atlas without translation (result of pure distraction). (c) Type III, occipital condyles posterior to the atlas.

hyperextension and asymmetric loading of the condyles causing variable fracture patterns.

Clinical symptoms include headache and suboccipital pain with limitation of movement. Cranial nerve lesions of VI–XII and neurapraxia of the suboccipital and greater occipital nerves may be associated. Damage to the spinal cord is uncommon because a significant cord injury at this level causes immediate death. Vertebral artery injuries may cause symptoms of basilar insufficiency such as vertigo, blurred vision and nystagmus.

Anteroposterior films, including an open-mouth view and a lateral view, and CT scanning are performed. The common fracture sites are the anterior arch, either midline or just lateral to the midline, and the posterior arch at its narrowest portion just posterior to each lateral mass.

Levine and Edwards[7] (Fig. 53.7) classified atlas fractures into three types: (1) isolated posterior arch fractures, (2) lateral mass fractures and (3) burst fractures (Jefferson fracture). Other fractures that occur include isolated transverse process fracture, isolated anterior arch fracture and anterior tubercle.

Fracture stability is based on the integrity of the transverse ligament. If the transverse ligament is disrupted, the C1 injury is considered unstable. It is important to recognize this instability as the management is different from stable burst fractures. In open-mouth radiographs, if the combined lateral mass overhang is 7 mm or more, rupture of the transverse ligament has probably occurred. The integrity of the ligament can also be evaluated by measuring the atlantodens interval on the lateral view. An atlantodens interval >3 mm in adults is indicative of a ligament insufficiency. Transverse ligament insufficiency may also be diagnosed directly by identifying bony avulsion on CT scan or ligament rupture on MRI.

Isolated anterior or posterior arch fractures, transverse process fractures and undisplaced/minimally displaced lateral mass fractures can be treated conservatively with 6–12 weeks of immobilization in a rigid cervical collar. Stable burst fractures (intact transverse ligament) can be treated in a rigid cervical collar or a halo vest. Unstable burst fractures (disruption of the transverse ligament) should be reduced with halo traction. Halo traction should be maintained for 3–6 weeks before application of a halo vest, which is worn for a further period of 6 weeks. These injuries can also be treated surgically through a posterior C1–2 fusion.

Pure transverse ligament injuries (traumatic C1–2 instability)

Pure transverse ligament injuries most commonly result from a fall with a blow to the back of the head. Dickman et al[8]. classified injuries of the transverse atlantal ligament

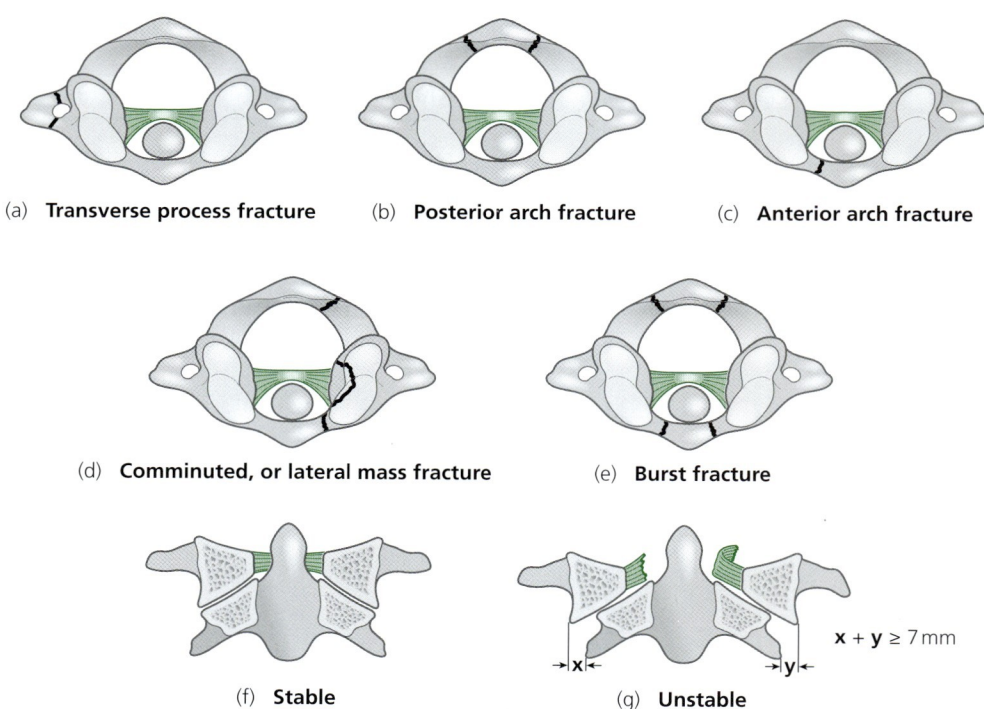

Figure 53.7 Classification of atlas fractures. (a) Isolated transverse process fracture. (b) Isolated posterior arch fracture. (c) Isolated anterior arch fracture. (d) Comminuted or lateral mass fracture. (e) Burst fracture (Jefferson type). (f,g) Jefferson fractures. When a comminuted fracture of C1 shows bilateral overhang of the lateral masses that totals 7 mm or more, rupture of the transverse ligament has probably occurred, rendering the spine unstable.

into two types. Type I injuries are midsubstance ruptures, which are least likely to heal, and hence early surgical treatment with C1–2 fusion may be necessary. Initial treatment consists of immobilization through skull traction and then posterior stabilization of the C1–2 complex with a Gallie-type fusion. Type II injuries are avulsions involving the insertion of the transverse ligament on the lateral masses of C1. Because of higher rates of healing, an initial attempt at external immobilization using a halo vest is a reasonable treatment option in these patients.

Atlantoaxial rotary subluxation and dislocation

The atlantoaxial joint is stabilized by the transverse ligament and the alar ligaments. The transverse ligament prevents excessive anterior shift of the atlas on the axis, whereas the alar ligaments prevent excessive rotation; the right alar ligament limits left rotation and vice versa. Hence, excessive rotation beyond physiological limits can lead to ligament insufficiency.

Rotary subluxation of C1 on C2 is uncommon in adults and is a different entity from rotary subluxation seen in children. Adults usually present with rotary subluxation secondary to trauma, whereas, in children, the aetiology is varied, including tonsillitis, following an upper respiratory tract infection, minor head injury or induction of general anaesthesia. Children are predisposed to suffer from rotary injuries because their relatively larger head exerts a greater moment at the C1–2 joint, ligamentous laxity is greater and the articular surface of the C1–2 joints is more horizontally inclined in children than in adults.

Patients present with neck pain, torticollis (characteristic 'cock robin' position), decreased neck movement and, occasionally, symptoms of vertebrobasilar insufficiency. Neurological involvement is fortunately uncommon. The mechanism of injury is flexion/extension with a rotational component, although in some cases it can occur spontaneously with no reported history of trauma.

Open-mouth radiographs may show asymmetry of C1 lateral masses with unilateral facet joint narrowing or overlap (wink sign). The lateral mass of the atlas, which is rotated anteriorly, appears wider and closer to the midline than its counterpart on the opposite side. The C2 spinous process may be rotated from the midline on an anteroposterior view. CT scanning is excellent in visualizing the dislocation, determining whether it is unilateral or bilateral, and identifying fractures.

Fielding and Hawkins[9] classified atlantoaxial rotary fixation into four types (Table 53.4 and Fig. 53.8). The importance of the classification is the increasing risk of spinal instability with potential neurological compromise and a higher likelihood of recurrent deformity with the more severe types.

Table 53.4 The Fielding and Hawkins classification of rotary displacement

Type/incidence	Classification characteristics	Additional points
Type I (47%)	Simple rotary displacement without anterior shift, odontoid acts as the pivot	ADI <3 mm, transverse ligament intact
Type II (30%)	Rotary displacement with anterior displacement (ADI) of 3–5 mm, opposite facet acts as the pivot	Transverse ligament insufficient
Type III	Rotary displacement with both joints anteriorly displaced, one side is rotated further forward than the other	ADI >5 mm, transverse and alar ligaments incompetent
Type IV (rare)	Rotary displacement with a posterior displacement of one or both lateral masses of the atlas	–

ADI, atlantodens interval.

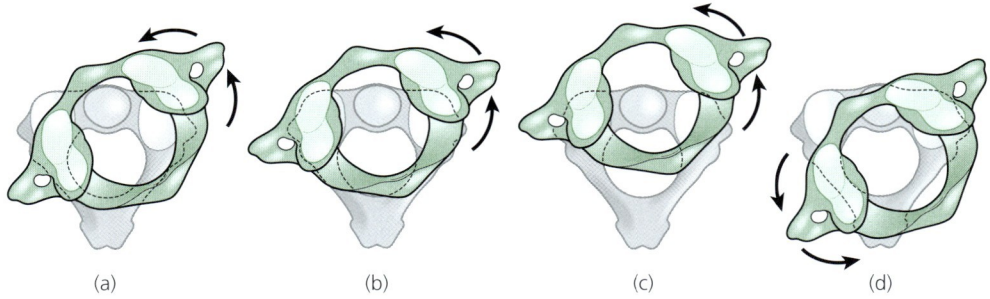

Figure 53.8 The Fielding and Hawkins classification of rotary displacement. (a) Type I; (b) type II; (c) type III; (d) type IV. Redrawn from Fielding JW, Hawkins RJ. Atlanto-axial rotatory fixation: fixed rotatory subluxation of the atlanto-axial joint. *Journal of Bone and Joint Surgery (American)* 1977;**59A**:37.

The treatment options include conservative care, immobilization, traction, manual reduction and surgery. If the trauma is minor, cervical traction or manipulation may allow reduction of the dislocation. The choice between conservative treatment and C1–2 fusion is directly dependent on whether or not the transverse ligament is torn or avulsed. With an intact transverse ligament, management is usually conservative. Surgery is advised for patients who have spinal instability or neural involvement or who fail to achieve or maintain reduction by conservative measures. The surgical treatment is C1–2 fusion with a C1–2 transarticular screw, C1–2 screw rod construct or a Gallie/Brooks–Jenkins procedure.

Fractures of the odontoid process

Odontoid fractures constitute 8–18% of all cervical fractures, with neurological deficits occurring in 10–20% of cases. High-velocity trauma such as motor vehicle accidents account for most odontoid fractures in young adults, whereas low-velocity injuries, such as falls, account for the injuries in the elderly (osteoporotic fractures) and children. The mechanism of injury includes avulsion of the apex of the dens by the alar ligament or lateral/oblique forces that cause fracture through the body and base of the dens. Posteriorly displaced fractures are the result of hyperextension whereas anteriorly displaced fractures are due to a hyperflexion force.

The vascular supply of the C2 vertebra is from the apex, via a periapical plexus that is supplied by a branch of the basilar artery, and from the base, via the vertebral artery with a watershed area in the neck of the odontoid. This watershed area of poor vascularity, lack of periosteum and cancellous bone results in high non-union rates of type II odontoid fractures.

Symptoms can be minimal, but severe pain behind the ears and neck stiffness are frequent. Patients often report a feeling of instability at the base of the skull and present holding their head with both hands.

Odontoid fractures are one of the most commonly missed spinal fractures; hence, radiographs should be critically evaluated for odontoid fractures. Subtle signs such as retropharyngeal swelling may alert the physician to the presence of a fracture. Fine-section CT with sagittal and coronal reformations should be considered if the open-mouth view is obscured, if a high index of suspicion for a fracture exists clinically or on radiographs, or if the patient has altered mental status. A CT should also be obtained to fully characterize the fracture morphology to assist in management decision-making.

Odontoid fractures have been classified by Anderson and D'Alonzo[10] into three types, with Hadley adding a fourth type – type IIA (Table 53.5 and Fig. 53.9).

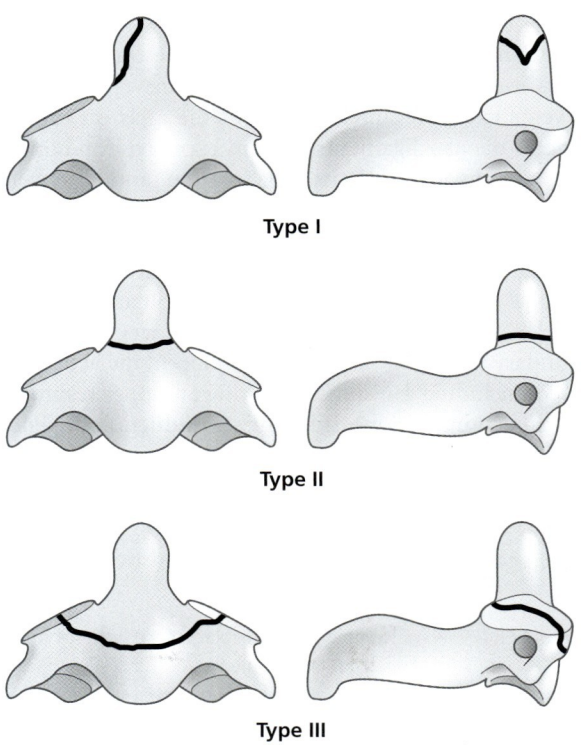

Figure 53.9 The Anderson and D'Alonzo classification of odontoid fractures. Redrawn from Anderson LD, D'Alonzo RT. Fractures of the odontoid process of the axis. *Journal of Bone and Joint Surgery (American)* 1974;**56A**:1663.

Table 53.5 Classification of odontoid fractures

Type/incidence	Fracture characteristic	Important facts
Type I (5%)	Oblique avulsion fracture of the apex	Represents an avulsion of the alar and apical ligaments, Rule out atlanto-occipital dislocation
Type II (60%)	Fracture at the junction of the dens with the body of C2	High non-union rate. Rule out associated transverse atlantal ligament injury
Type IIA (Hadley)	Comminuted injury extending from the waist of the dens into the body of the axis	Highly unstable
Type III (30%)	Fracture extending into the cancellous portion of the body of C2 and possibly involving one or both of the superior articular facets	High likelihood of union owing to the cancellous bed of the fracture site

Type I fractures can be immobilized in an external orthosis for 6–8 weeks once the possibility of an associated occipitocervical dissociation has been excluded. Type III fractures have been reported to have a sufficiently high healing rate with rigid external immobilization in a halo vest.

Treatment of type II fractures is controversial and depends largely on specific patient and fracture characteristics. Treatment options include halo vest immobilization, anterior odontoid screw stabilization or a posterior C1–2 fusion. While undisplaced or minimally displaced fractures that are easily reduced may be treated with halo vest immobilization for 6–12 weeks, non-union rates ranging from 10% to 77% have been reported for displaced fractures.

A number of risk factors associated with an increased incidence of non-union for type II odontoid fractures have been identified. These include initial fracture displacement of >4 mm, >10° angulation, posterior displacement, fracture comminution, elderly patients, delayed treatment, smoking and inability to achieve or maintain a reduction. Early surgical treatment is an option for patients with any of these risk factors. Elderly patients tolerate halo vest immobilization poorly, demonstrate decreased healing rates and should be considered for early surgical management.

Anterior fixation is indicated for most type II and shallow type III fractures in patients older than 7 years (Fig. 53.10). The procedure is contraindicated in fractures with an oblique pattern, disruption of the atlantal transverse ligament, non-unions, pathological fractures and osteoporosis. Patients with a short neck, a rigid neck or cervical kyphosis and thoracic kyphosis/barrel chest are not suitable for this procedure as there is a technical difficulty associated with passage of the screw. Posterior C1–2 fusion is then indicated. Studies comparing one- versus two-screw techniques show that there is no difference between the two in terms of load to failure and hence a single anterior screw is adequate.

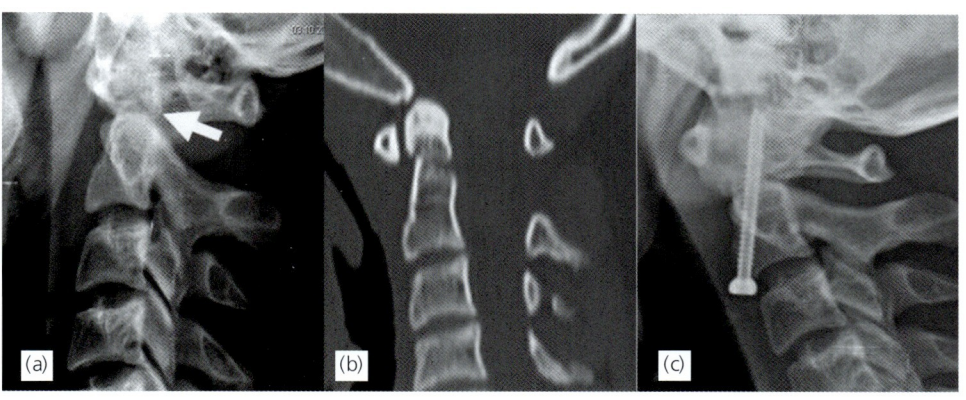

Figure 53.10 (a,b) Preoperative lateral view and sagittal CT scan of cervical spine showing displaced fracture of odontoid process. (c) Postoperative radiograph shows good reduction of the odontoid fracture and ideal position of a single screw inserted through an anterior approach.

Table 53.6 Classification of traumatic spondylolisthesis of the axis (according to Effendi, modified by Levine)

Type/incidence	Fracture characteristics	Stability	Mechanism of injury
Type I (29%)	Non-displaced or minimally displaced (translation <3 mm) fractures with no angulation	Relatively stable as the C2–3 disc is intact and only minimal ligamentous injury	Result from hyperextension and axial loading with failure of the neural arch in tension
Type II (56%)	Type II fractures have more than 3 mm of anterior translation and significant angulation at the C2–3 disc. Predominantly vertical fracture line	Unstable as the C2–3 disc is disrupted	Result from hyperextension and axial load followed by rebound flexion
Type IIA (6%)	Variant of type II fractures that have severe angulation between C2 and C3 with minimal translation. Usually have a more horizontal than vertical fracture line	Unstable owing to extensive discoligamentous injury	Result from a flexion–distraction injury. Avulsion of the entire C2–3 intervertebral disc in flexion with injury to the posterior longitudinal ligament, leaving the anterior longitudinal ligament intact
Type III (9%)	A pars interarticularis fracture with posterior facet injuries; severe angulation and translation with unilateral or bilateral facet dislocation of C2–3	Unstable owing to extensive discoligamentous and facet dislocation injury	Result from flexion–distraction followed by hyperextension; initial anterior facet dislocation of C2 on C3 followed by extension injury fracturing the neural arch

Traumatic spondylolisthesis of C2 (hangman's fracture)

This injury, characterized by bilateral fractures of the pars interarticularis with varying degrees of intervertebral disc disruption, is commonly termed a hangman's fracture. The mechanism of injury includes motor vehicle accidents and falls with flexion, extension and axial loads. Hanging mechanisms involve hyperextension and distraction injury, in which the patient may experience bilateral pedicle fractures and complete disruption of the disc and ligaments between C2 and C3.

SCI in patients who survive the initial trauma is relatively uncommon, so the patient may complain of little more than local pain and stiffness. There is, however, tenderness over the spinous process of C2. Anteroposterior and lateral radiographs and a CT scan are essential. The retropharyngeal space may be widened on the lateral view. There is a 30% incidence of concomitant cervical spine fractures.

The commonly used classification scheme is Levine and Edwards' modification of the Effendi and Francis classification[7] (Table 53.6 and Fig. 53.11).

Type I injuries are stable and heal with 12 weeks of immobilization in a rigid cervical orthosis. Type II injuries usually require skull traction with slight extension of the neck over a rolled up towel for 3–6 weeks to maintain anatomical reduction. Serial radiographic confirmation of maintenance of reduction is required. The patient can be mobilized in a halo vest for the rest of the 3 month period. In type IIA injuries, traction may exacerbate the condition; therefore, a halo vest with slight compression is applied under image intensification to achieve and maintain anatomical reduction for 12 weeks until union occurs. Anterior interbody fusion and plating of the C2–3 interspace for a type IIA injury may be performed as an alternative to halo immobilization. Bilateral C2 pars screw osteosynthesis is an option to stabilize type II injuries after reduction (Fig. 53.12). For type III injuries, surgery is required because of the inability to obtain or maintain reduction of the C2–3 facet dislocation. Initial halo traction is followed by open reduction and fusion. Surgical options include an anterior C2–3 interbody fusion or a posterior C1–3 fusion.

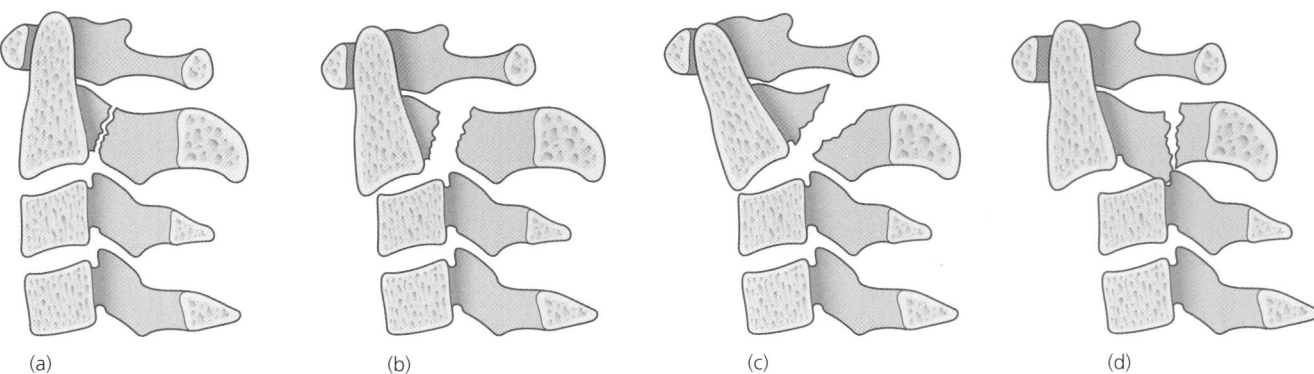

Figure 53.11 Classification of traumatic spondylolisthesis of the axis (according to Effendi, modified by Levine). (a) Type I, non-displaced fracture of the pars interarticularis. (b) Type II, displaced fracture of the pars interarticularis. (c) Type IIa, displaced fracture of the pars interarticularis with disruption of the C2–3 discoligamentous complex. (d) Type III, dislocation of C2–3 facet joints with fractured pars interarticularis.

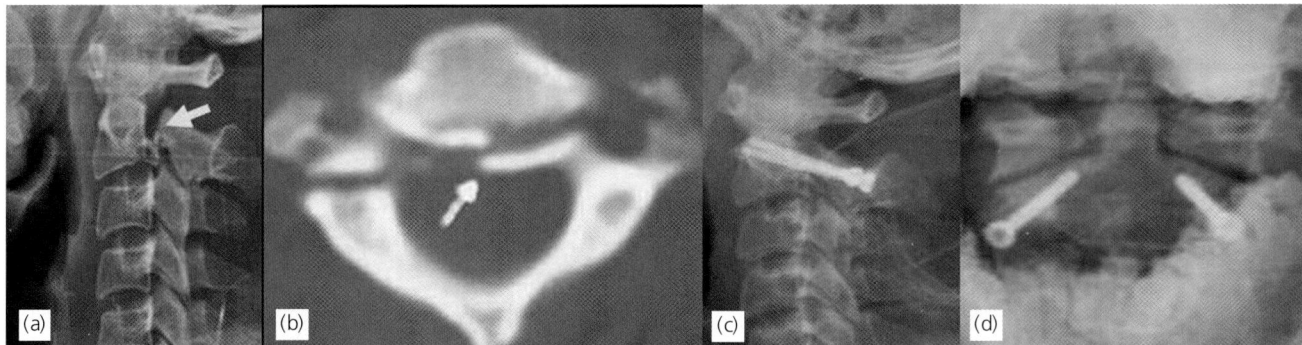

Figure 53.12 (a,b) Pre-operative lateral radiograph and CT scan showing bilateral fracture of pars interarticularis of C2 with extension into the vertebral artery foramen. (c,d) Postoperative anteroposterior and lateral radiographs showing good reduction of the fracture and bicortical purchase of the screws on both the pedicles.

SUBAXIAL CERVICAL SPINE INJURIES

INTRODUCTION

The subaxial spine (C3–7) can be conceptualized as a three-column system (Denis) and this is important for a good understanding of spinal stability. The bony structures counteract compression and the ligamentous complexes resist distractive forces (Fig. 53.13). The stability of the subaxial spine may be assessed using the criteria by White and Punjabi[11] (Box 53.2).

The mechanism of injury includes motor vehicle accidents, falls, diving accidents and blunt trauma. Radiographic evaluation usually consists of anteroposterior and lateral views; oblique views may be requested to visualize the pedicles, foramen and facet joints. Interpretation of a subaxial cervical spine radiograph has been described earlier in the chapter under radiographic evaluation of the cervical spine (Box 53.3 and Fig. 53.14).

CLASSIFICATION OF SUBAXIAL INJURIES

Many classifications of subaxial spine injuries have been formulated, but the most commonly used is the system developed by Allen and Ferguson.[12] Six distinct phylogenies were described based on the mechanism of injury, including the direction of the injury force and the position of the neck at the time of the injury. Each phylogeny is subdivided into stages of progressive severity. The three commonly observed categories are compression–flexion (CF), distraction–flexion (DF), and compression–extension (CE).

Compression–flexion injuries (Fig. 53.15)

CF injuries are defined by compressive failure of the anterior half of the vertebral body (anterior column) without disruption of the posterior body cortex and without retropulsion into the spinal canal. They occur most commonly at C4, C5 and C6 and account for 20% of subaxial spine fractures. Owing to the stability of CF stage I and II injuries they can be treated in a cervical orthosis for a period of 10–12 weeks. CF stage III and IV injuries without posterior element fracture, ligament disruption, facet dislocation or neurological injury are stable fractures that heal with 8–12 weeks of halo vest immobilization. The stability of the posterior ligamentous structures should be verified by the criteria of White and Panjabi, using CT and MRI in conjunction with examination findings of the patient. Should instability in a CF stage III or IV injury be

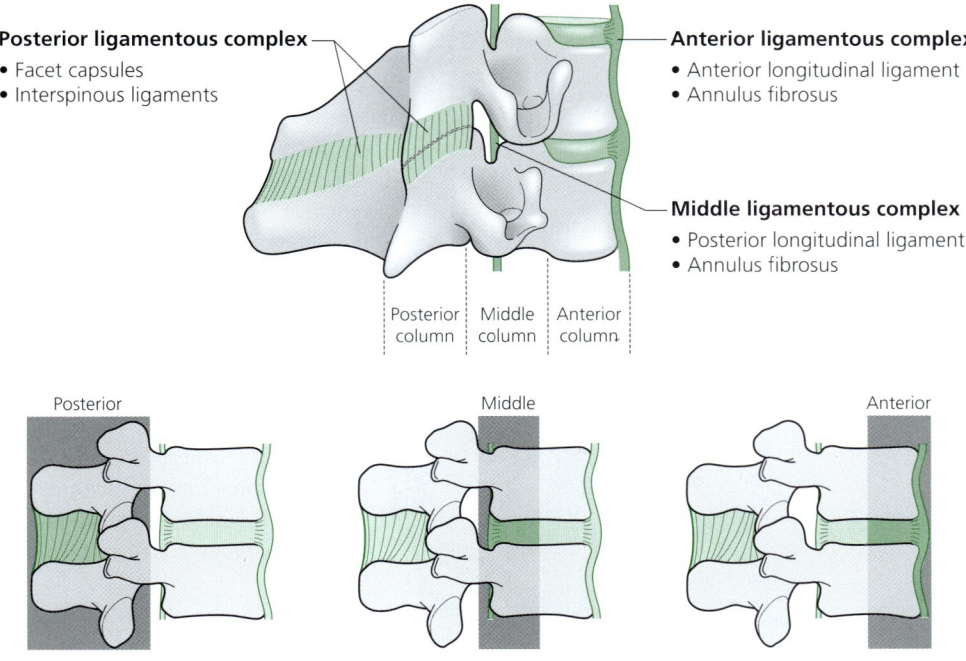

Figure 53.13 The components of the three columns of the cervical spine. In the anterior column, the anterior vertebral body and intervertebral disc resist compressive loads, while the anterior longitudinal ligament and annulus fibrosis are the most important check reins to distractive forces (extension). In the middle column, the posterior vertebral body and uncovertebral joints resist compression, while the posterior longitudinal ligament and annulus fibrosis limit distraction. In the posterior column, the facet joints and lateral masses resist compressive forces, while the facet joint capsules, interspinous ligaments and supraspinous ligaments counteract distractive forces. A similar concept is followed in the thoracolumbar spine as well (the shaded areas indicate the respective columns, i.e. posterior, middle and anterior).

of concern, either an anterior corpectomy and fusion (preferred if anterior neural compression is present) or a posterior cervical fusion may be performed. CF stage V fractures with posterior element disruption and incompetent posterior ligaments are three-column unstable injuries and require an anterior decompression and plate fixation followed by a supplemental posterior stabilization if required.

Vertical compression fractures (burst fractures) (Fig. 53.16)

Burst fractures are characterized by compressive failure of the vertebral body with fracture extension through the posterior body cortex and some degree of bone retropulsion into the spinal canal. Burst fractures have a significantly higher rate of instability than compression fractures and are frequently associated with SCI. Vertical compression (VC) fractures account for 15% of subaxial injuries and occur most commonly at the C6/C7 level.

The initial treatment of these injuries with neurological deficits is longitudinal skull traction to realign the spinal canal and indirectly decompress the canal via ligamento-

---

BOX 53.2 Checklist for diagnosis of clinical instability in lower cervical spine (White and Panjabi criteria)

Element	Point value
Anterior elements destroyed or unable to function	2
Posterior elements destroyed or unable to function	2
Relative sagittal plane translation >3.5 mm	2
Relative sagittal plane rotation >11°	2
Positive stretch test	2
Medullary (cord) damage	2
Root damage	1
Abnormal disc narrowing	1
Dangerous loading anticipated	1

A total of 5 or more is considered to indicate an unstable spine.

BOX 53.3 Important points to observed while assessing plain radiographs of the subaxial cervical spine

- Continuity of radiographic lines: anterior vertebral line, posterior vertebral line, spinolaminar line and spinous process line
- Widening or narrowing of disc spaces
- Increased distance between spinous processes or facet joints
- Any fracture lines in the bodies or in the posterior elements
- Any displacement of the spinous process on the anteroposterior film
- Any antero- or retrolisthesis on the lateral radiograph
- Acute kyphosis or loss of lordosis
- Any increase in the width of the retropharyngeal space in front of the vertebral bodies (>4 mm at C3, C4; <15 mm at C5, C6, C7)
- Radiographic markers of cervical spine instability (on the lateral view) include:
  - Compression fractures with >25% loss of height
  - Angular displacements >11° between adjacent vertebrae
  - Translation >3.5 mm on flexion–extension view
  - Intervertebral disc space separation >1.7 mm (while performing the 'stretch test')

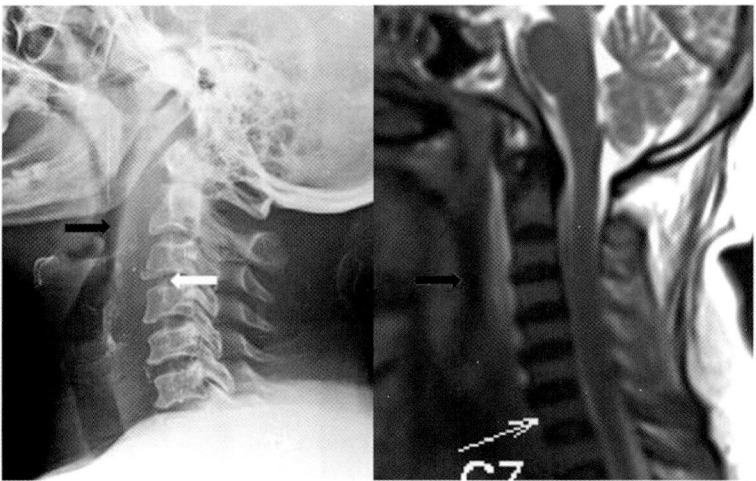

Figure 53.14 Lateral radiographs and sagittal MRI of a 50 year old patient with a stable C3 fracture (dashed arrow). Lateral radiograph shows a widened prevertebral space due to haematoma (arrows), which is clearly demonstrated in the MRI.

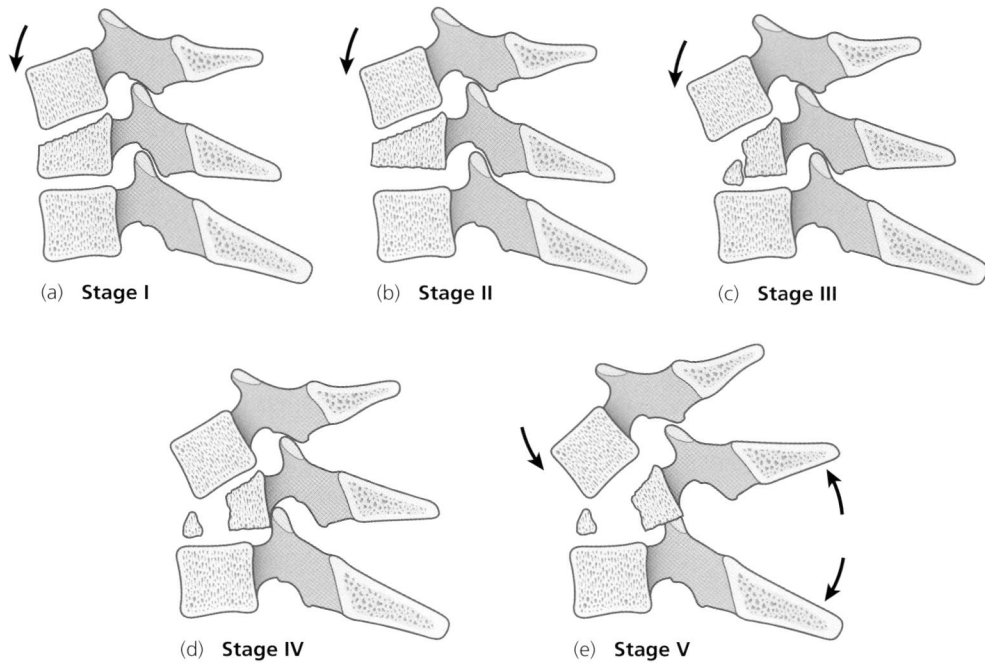

Figure 53.15 (a–e) The five stages of compression–flexion injuries. (a) Stage I. Blunting of anterior body; posterior elements intact. (b) Stage II. 'Beaking' of the anterior body; loss of anterior vertebral height. (c) Stage III. Fracture line passing from the anterior body through the inferior subchondral plate. (d) Stage IV. Deformation of the centrum and fracture of the beak with the inferoposterior margin displaced <3 mm into the neural canal. (e) Stage V. 'Teardrop' fracture; bony injuries as in stage 3, but with more than 3 mm of displacement of inferoposterior margin into the neural canal. From Bucholz RW, Heckman JD, Court-Brown C, et al. (eds). *Rockwood and Green's Fractures in Adults*, 6th edn. Philadelphia, PA: Lippincott Williams & Wilkins, 2006.

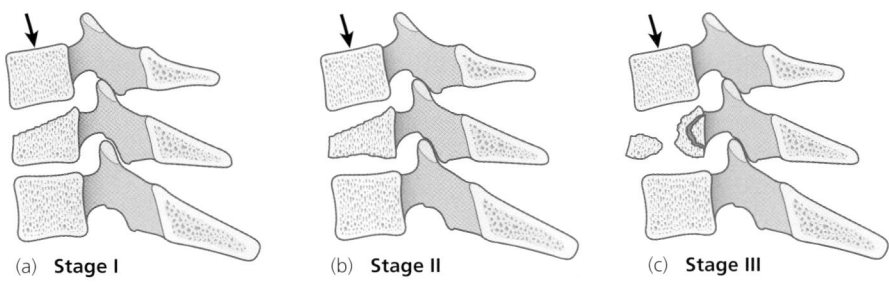

Figure 53.16 (a–c) The three stages of vertical compression injuries. (a) Stage I. Fracture through the superior or inferior endplate with no displacement. (b) Stage II. Fracture through both endplates with minimal displacement. (c) Stage III. Burst fracture; displacement of fragments peripherally and into the neural canal. From Bucholz RW, Heckman JD, Court-Brown C, et al. (eds). *Rockwood and Green's Fractures in Adults*, 6th edn. Philadelphia, PA: Lippincott Williams & Wilkins, 2006.

taxis. VC stage I is a stable fracture and is managed in a rigid cervical orthosis for a period of 6–12 weeks. VC stage II without deficits is managed in a rigid cervical orthosis or a halo vest. VC stage III injuries are similar to VC stage II injuries except for displacement of the vertebral body into the canal. These injuries may be treated in a halo vest; however, in the presence of SCI anterior surgical decompression and instrumented fusion is required (Fig. 53.17). In the presence of disrupted posterior elements, supplemental posterior instrumented fusion should be considered.

Distraction–flexion injuries (Fig. 53.18)

DF injuries account for 15% of subaxial cervical injuries. Bilateral facet dislocations are often associated with significant SCIs (Fig. 53.19). Unilateral facet dislocations are commonly associated with a monoradiculopathy (Fig. 53.20). Unilateral or bilateral facet injuries are associated with disruption of the disc, which may herniate into the spinal canal. Failure to recognize the herniated disc may result in a neurological deficit when realignment of the spine with skull traction is attempted.

456 Spinal fractures

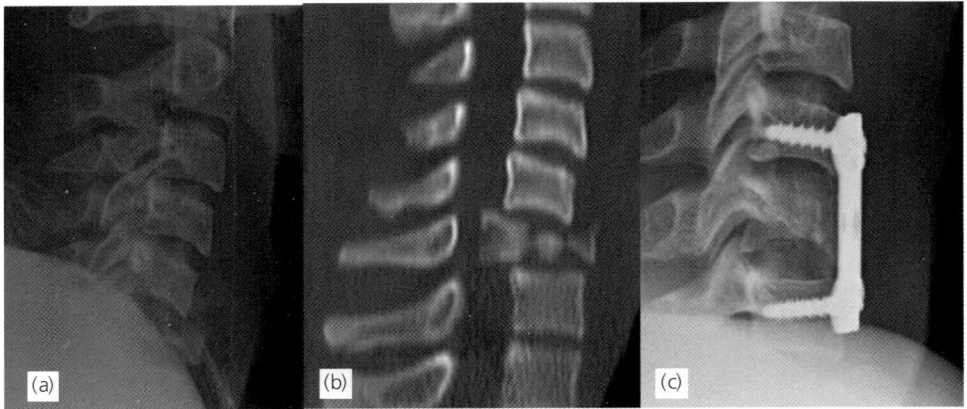

Figure 53.17 (a,b) Lateral radiographs and CT scan of the cervical spine showing a burst fracture of the C6 vertebral body with retropulsion of a bony fragment into the canal. (c) Postoperative lateral radiographs shows complete corpectomy of C6 with the anterior cervical plate and screws in a good position.

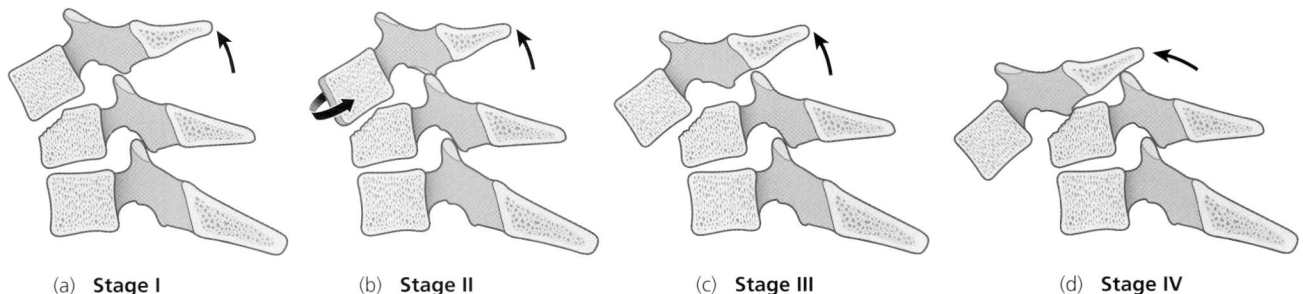

(a) Stage I (b) Stage II (c) Stage III (d) Stage IV

Figure 53.18 (a–d) The four stages of distraction flexion injuries. (a) Stage I. Failure of the posterior ligaments, divergence of the spinous processes and facet subluxation. (b) Stage II. Unilateral facet dislocation; translation always <50%. (c) Stage III. Bilateral facet dislocation; translation of 50% and 'perched' facets. (d) Stage IV. Bilateral facet dislocation with 100% translation (giving the appearance of a 'floating' vertebra). From Bucholz RW, Heckman JD, Court-Brown C, et al. (eds). *Rockwood and Green's Fractures in Adults*, 6th edn. Philadelphia, PA: Lippincott Williams & Wilkins, 2006.

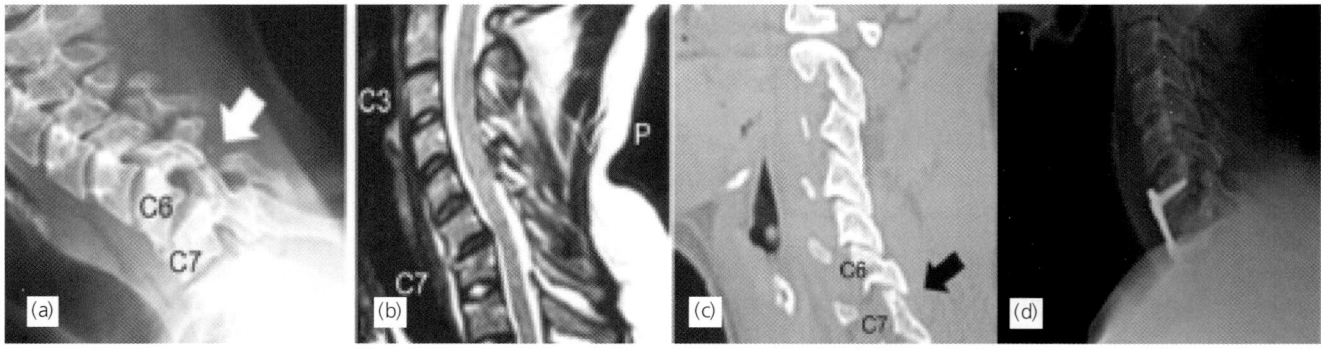

Figure 53.19 (a) Lateral radiograph of the cervical spine showing a perched C6–7 facet due to a flexion–distraction injury (arrow). (b,c) Mid-sagittal T_2-weighted MRI and CT scan of the same patient showing a C6 on C7 bifacetal subluxation (arrow in c). (d) Following an anterior cervical discectomy complete reduction could be achieved. Stabilization by instrumented fusion with a tricortical iliac bone graft and locking plate was performed.

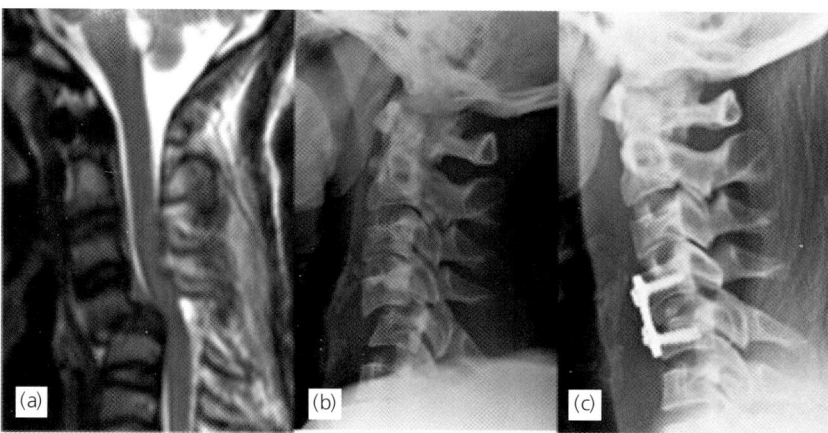

Figure 53.20 A C4–5 bifacetal dislocation with a disrupted disc. Manipulative reduction by traction could produce a neurological deficit in this patient. An anterior cervical discectomy followed by reduction and anterior cervical plating was the treatment of choice.

Patients with cervical facet dislocations should undergo timely reduction. Whether or not a pre-reduction MRI to assess the status of the disc is required is debatable. Some authors advocate that awake, alert and cooperative patients can safely undergo closed reduction with serial neurological examinations and plain radiographic assessment following the placement of each additional weight.[13] Development of new or worsening neurological deficits is an indication to cease attempts at closed reduction and obtain an MRI scan to rule out herniated disc material. They suggest a pre-reduction MRI only for patients who are obtunded or who cannot be easily examined to avoid the risk of further neurological injury during the reduction process and for failed closed reductions. A post-reduction MRI is advised to evaluate for the presence of a herniated disc and epidural haematoma to guide the approach of surgical treatment. On the contrary, Arena et al.[14] reported that 8.8% of patients with cervical facet subluxations or dislocations had an associated cervical disc extrusion and recommended routine pre-operative evaluation with MRI. If the disc is herniated, anterior discectomy and fusion should be performed to avoid neurological deterioration. A supplementary posterior fusion is optional.

It is prudent to be sure that disc material has not been displaced into the spinal canal with a pre-reduction MRI, especially with bilateral facet dislocations in a neurologically intact individual. It is emphasized that closed reduction of obtunded patients should be undertaken only after an MRI scan. A treatment algorithm is shown in Fig. 53.21.

Overall, as many as 26% of patients with cervical facet dislocations will fail attempted closed reduction, with higher failure rates observed for patients with unilateral facet dislocations. In this group of patients, open reduction and fusion is required. Following successful closed reduction, prolonged halo vest immobilization is a treatment option as healing with spontaneous anterior interbody fusion may occur. However, this is unpredictable and posterior instrumented fusion is recommended. This is especially so in the presence of extensive neurological deficit, to aid in nursing care. Unilateral facet dislocations that are reduced in traction may be immobilized in a halo vest for 8–12 weeks with the possibility that stability would be obtained by spontaneous

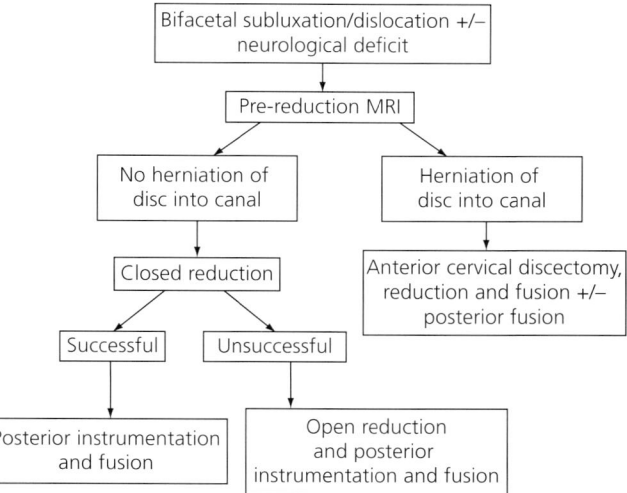

Figure 53.21 Treatment algorithm for bifacetal dislocations.

fusion. Failure of closed reduction mandates open reduction and instrumented fusion, either anteriorly or posteriorly.

Compression–extension injuries (Fig. 53.22)

CE injuries are typically described as posterior element fractures but may involve the anterior bony elements depending on the degree of force imparted to the spine. CE stage I and II are successfully treated in a cervical orthosis or a halo vest. CE stage III may be managed in a halo vest or by posterior instrumented fusion. CE stage IV and V are best treated with posterior reduction, decompression and instrumented fusion. In the presence of significant anterior column injury, an adjunctive anterior stabilization may be performed.

Distraction–extension injuries (Fig. 53.23)

Distraction–extension (DE) injuries account for 22% of subaxial cervical injuries and are commonly seen in elderly patients with ankylosing spondylitis and diffuse

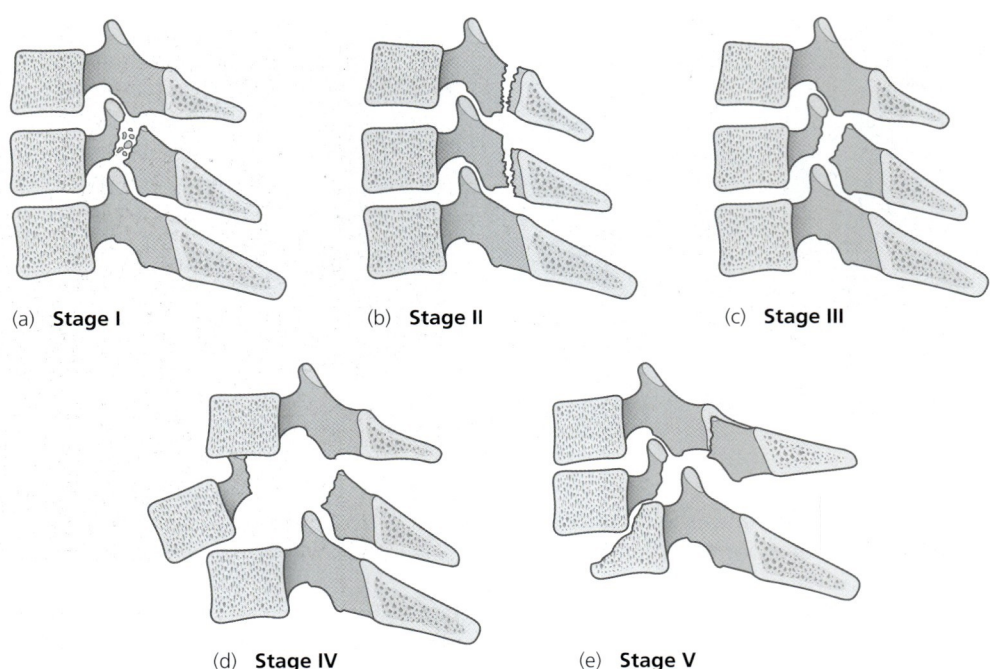

Figure 53.22 (a–e) The five stages of compression extension injuries. (a) Stage I. Unilateral vertebral arch fracture with or without anterior rotatory vertebral displacement. (b) Stage II. Bilateral laminar fracture without other tissue failure. (c) Stage III. Bilateral vertebral arch fractures with fracture of the articular processes, pedicles, lamina or some bilateral combination, without vertebral body displacement. (d) Stage IV. Bilateral vertebral arch fractures with partial vertebral body width displacement anteriorly. (e) Stage V. Bilateral vertebral arch fracture with full vertebral body displacement anteriorly; ligamentous failure at the posterosuperior and anteroinferior margins. From Bucholz RW, Heckman JD, Court-Brown C, et al. (eds). *Rockwood and Green's Fractures in Adults*, 6th edn. Philadelphia, PA: Lippincott Williams & Wilkins, 2006.

idiopathic skeletal hyperostosis (Fig. 53.24). Often, these injuries appear benign, but if neglected they can be associated with significant neurological morbidity. DE stage I injuries can be managed in a halo vest. However, because of the potential for displacement, especially in injuries involving the disc space, many authors advocate an anterior fusion. DE stage II injuries are extremely unstable (three-column injuries) and hence require anterior cervical instrumented fusion.

Lateral flexion injuries (Fig. 53.25)

Lateral flexion (LF) injuries account for 20% of subaxial cervical spine injuries. Although SCI is rare with LF injuries, spinal nerve root and brachial plexus injuries do occur. LF stage I injuries are managed in a rigid cervical orthosis. LF stage II injuries require reduction via skeletal traction followed by a posterior stabilization. If SCI, nerve root injury or anterior instability is present, an anterior decompressive procedure may be necessary.

GUNSHOT INJURIES

Missile impact against bony elements may cause high-velocity fragmentation associated with gross instability

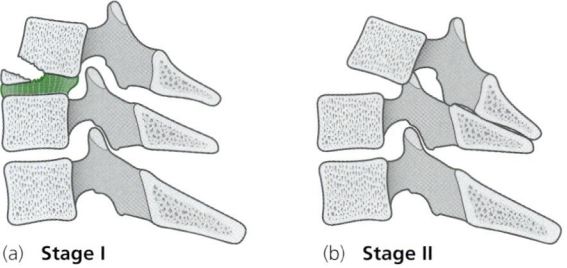

Figure 53.23 (a,b) The two stages of distraction extension injuries. (a) Stage I. Failure of the anterior ligamentous complex or transverse fracture of the body; widening of the disc space and no posterior displacement. (b) Stage II. Failure of the posterior ligament complex and superior displacement of the body into the canal. From Bucholz RW, Heckman JD, Court-Brown C, et al. (eds). *Rockwood and Green's Fractures in Adults*, 6th edn. Philadelphia, PA: Lippincott Williams & Wilkins, 2006.

and complete SCI. Surgical extraction of missile fragments is rarely indicated in the absence of canal compromise. Missiles that traverse the oesophagus or pharynx should be removed, with aggressive exposure and debridement of the missile tract as these injuries carry high incidences of abscess formation, osteomyelitis and mediastinitis.

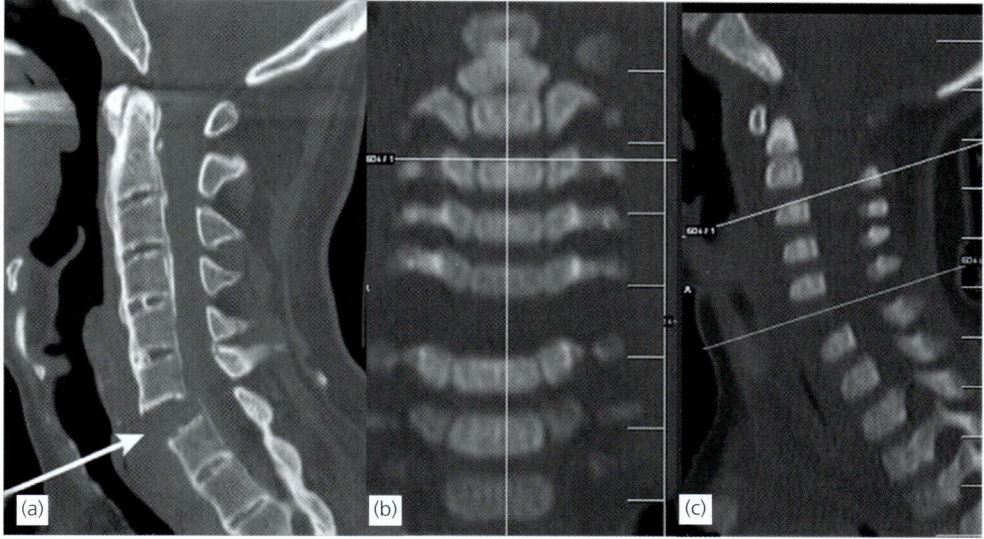

Figure 53.24 Distraction injuries of the cervical spine. (a) Sagittal CT image shows a C6–7 extension–distraction three-column injury in a patient with ankylosing spondylosis. This is a highly unstable injury with an increased risk of neurological deficit. (b,c) Coronal and sagittal CT images of a 6 month old child who sustained a spinal injury in a vehicular accident. The child sustained a distractive injury at the level of the C5–6 vertebrae evident by significant widening of the C5–6 intervertebral space. These are highly unstable injuries and traction is contraindicated in both these injuries.

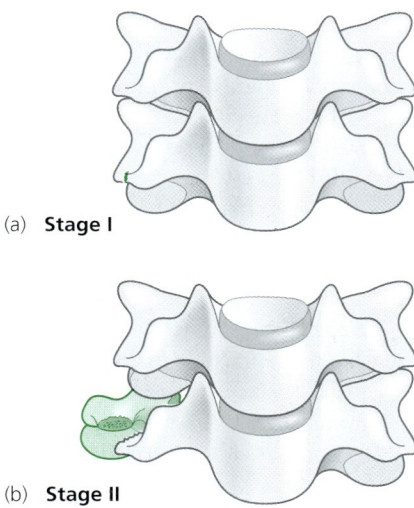

Figure 53.25 Lateral flexion injuries. Blunt trauma from the side places the ipsilateral spine in distraction while compressing the contralateral spine. (a) Stage I. Asymmetric centrum fracture with a unilateral arch fracture. (b) Stage II. Displacement of the body and contralateral ligamentous failure. Adapted from Rizzolo SJ, Cotler JM. Unstable cervical spine injuries: specific treatment approaches. *Journal of the American Academy of Orthopaedic Surgeons* 1993;**1**:57–66.

INJURIES OF THE THORACOLUMBAR SPINE

INTRODUCTION

Injuries to the thoracolumbar spine are usually the result of high-energy blunt trauma. Sixty-five per cent of thoracolumbar fractures occur as a result of motor vehicle trauma or fall from a height, with the remainder caused by athletic participation and assault. Approximately 50% of all thoracic and lumbar fractures occur at thoracolumbar junction, with 16% occurring in the thoracic spine. The increased incidence of fractures to the thoracolumbar junction is the result of its location at the transition point between the rigid thoracic rib cage and the more mobile lumbar spine. In addition, the sagittal alignment of the spine changes from kyphosis to lordosis, which distributes more stress on the anterior and middle columns. The facet alignment changes from a coronal orientation in the thoracic spine to a sagittal alignment in the lumbar spine, allowing for greater flexion and extension motion. Also, the intervertebral discs are taller than in the thoracic spine, decreasing anterior column stiffness. Neurological injury complicates 15–20% of fractures at the thoracolumbar junction.

RADIOGRAPHIC EVALUATION

Anteroposterior and lateral views of the thoracic and lumbar spine are obtained. Most fractures of the thoracolumbar spine are obvious on radiographs; however, it is essential to accurately classify the fracture as this has a direct bearing on the management and outcomes.

Radiographic evaluation should include assessment of the kyphosis angle, loss of anterior vertebral height and interspinous diastasis on lateral radiographs as well as rotation and translation on the anteroposterior radiographs as this provides information regarding the status of the posterior osseoligamentous complex (POLC).

Disruption of the POLC implies a three-column injury; these are unstable injuries requiring surgical management.

CT and/or MRI of the injured area may be obtained to characterize the fracture further, to assess for canal compromise and to evaluate the degree of neural compression. CT scans provide finer detail of the bony involvement, the extent of canal compromise and occult posterior element fractures. Approximately 25% of burst fractures are misdiagnosed as compression fractures if radiographs alone are evaluated; hence, it is important to evaluate significant thoracic and lumbar fractures with a CT scan. MRI is required for patients with a neurological deficit to identify possible spinal cord, cauda equine or root injury, cord oedema and haemorrhage, or epidural hematoma. MRI can be used to evaluate for soft-tissue injury to the intervertebral discs and posterior ligamentous disruption.

CLASSIFICATION

Numerous classification systems have been proposed. These are mostly based on the mechanism of injury or the extent of ligamentous and neurological injury.

The commonly used classification systems include the Denis classification,[15] the AO comprehensive classification,[16] the McAfee classification,[17] and the thoracolumbar injury classification and severity score by Vaccaro et al.[13]

The **Denis classification** is a three-column concept of spinal injury developed using a series of more than 400 CT scans of thoracolumbar injuries. Denis noted that one or more of the three columns predictably failed in axial compression, axial distraction or translation from combinations of forces in different planes. Instability exists with disruption of any two of the three columns. Thoracolumbar stability usually follows the middle column: if it is intact, then the injury is usually stable.

McAfee's classification

McAfee's classification (Fig. 53.26) is based on the mechanism of failure of the middle osteoligamentous complex (posterior longitudinal ligament, posterior half of the vertebral body and the posterior annulus fibrosus) and is divided into six patterns. The six patterns are wedge–compression fracture, stable burst fracture, unstable burst fracture, Chance fracture, flexion–distraction injury and translational injuries.

COMPRESSION FRACTURES

Compression fractures result from forward flexion and cause isolated failure of the anterior column. These can be anterior (89%) or lateral (11%). Radiographs demonstrate a wedge-shaped defect in the vertebral body that results in varying degrees of kyphosis. They are rarely associated with neurological compromise except when multiple adjacent vertebral levels are affected. They are generally stable injuries; neurologically intact patients with less than 30° of kyphosis and less than 50% loss of vertebral body height can be treated with a hyperextension thoracolumbar spinal orthosis (TLSO). They are considered unstable if associated with loss of >50% vertebral body height and angulation >20°. This would suggest the possibility of posterior ligament complex disruption, and hence there is a tendency

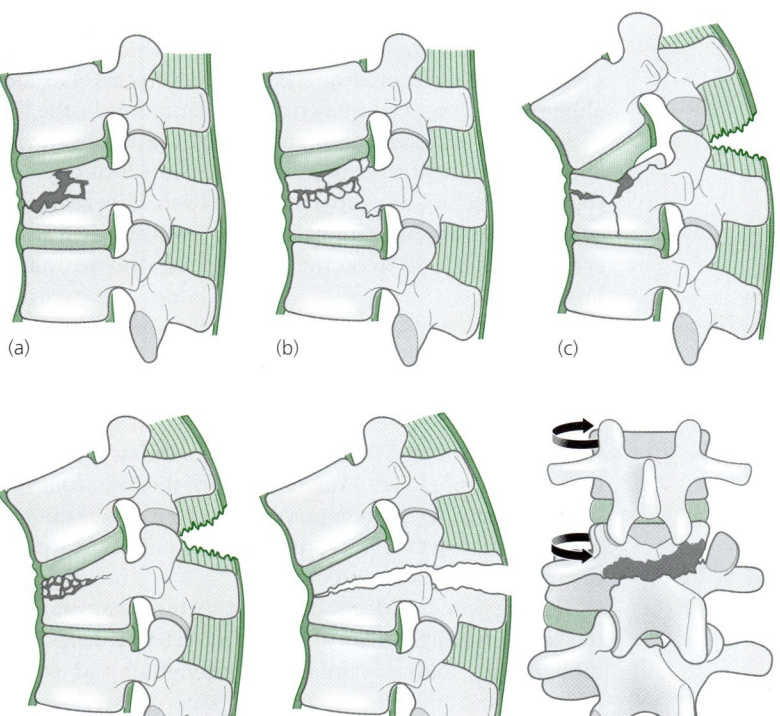

Figure 53.26 (a) Wedge compression fracture. (b) Stable burst fracture. (c) Unstable burst fracture. (d) Flexion– distraction injury. (e) Chance fracture. (f) Translational injury. Reproduced with permission from Hansen ST, Swiontkowski MF. *Orthopaedic Trauma Protocols*. New York, NY: Raven, 1993:222.

for post-traumatic kyphosis and progressive neural symptoms because of instability in these patients. Unstable fractures or multiple adjacent compression fractures may require spinal stabilization with or without cement augmentation.

BURST FRACTURES (FIG. 53.27)

The mechanism is compression failure of the anterior and middle columns under an axial load with or without failure of the POLC. McAfee described burst fractures as being stable or unstable. In *stable burst fractures*, the anterior and middle columns fail in compression, with no loss of integrity of the POLC. In *unstable burst fractures*, the anterior and middle columns fail in compression, and the POLC is disrupted. The posterior column can fail in compression, lateral flexion or rotation. McAfee noted that unstable fractures were associated with early progression of neurological deficits and spinal deformity as well as late onset of neurological deficits and mechanical back pain. Factors indicative of instability in burst fractures included >50% canal compromise, >15–25° of kyphosis and >40% loss of anterior body height.

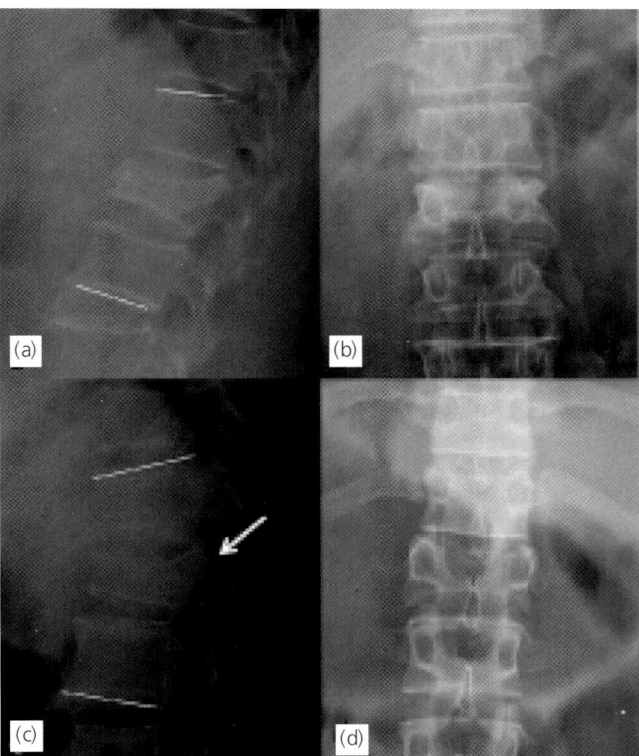

Figure 53.27 (a,b) Anteroposterior and lateral radiographs of a stable burst fracture. (c,d) Anteroposterior and lateral radiographs of an unstable burst fracture. Factors indicative of instability in burst fractures included fragment retropulsion (white arrow), >50% canal compromise, >15–25° of kyphosis (measured between the proximal and distal vertebra; white lines) and >40% loss of anterior body height.

Characteristic radiographic features of a burst fracture include loss of posterior vertebral body height, posterior vertebral body angle >100°, a break in the posterior aspect of the vertebral body with narrowing of the spinal canal on the lateral view and widening of the interpedicular distance on anteroposterior view.

Patients with stable burst fractures who are neurologically intact can be managed in a TLSO or with hyperextension casting. Unstable burst fractures with intact neurology should be considered for a surgical stabilization. These injuries can be stabilized either posteriorly with indirect decompression or interiorly by direct decompression and stabilization. The load sharing classification by McCormack et al.[19] helps to decide between an anterior and a posterior procedure. A point value is assigned to the degree of vertebral body comminution, fracture fragment apposition and kyphosis. Injuries with scores greater than 6 would be better treated with the addition of anterior column reconstruction to posterior stabilization. Greater than 50% canal compromise, even if the patient is neurologically intact, is often mentioned as a criterion for surgery. But in recent years, there has been growing evidence to suggest that these injuries may be managed non-operatively with equivalently good radiological and clinical outcomes.[20] The fact that the patient remains neurologically intact is evidence enough that the degree of canal compromise is not sufficient to cause neural damage and hence the need for surgical decompression of the canal is not present.

In patients who are neurologically incomplete or with cauda equina injury an anterior decompression, reconstruction and stabilization are advocated. In the presence of a compromised posterior ligamentous complex, the anterior vertebral reconstruction may require augmentation with a posterior stabilization. Posterior decompression (indirect decompression via ligamentotaxis or posterior/posterolateral decompression) and fixation is an alternative procedure for these injuries. Posterior surgery avoids the morbidity of anterior exposure in patients who have concomitant pulmonary or abdominal injuries; it also has shorter operative times and decreased blood loss. The anterior procedure, however, is preferred as most authors are of the opinion that posterior decompression is not as effective in ensuring optimal neural decompression as an anterior decompression. In the presence of a complete neurological injury decompression to regain neurological function is generally felt to be of little or no benefit. Hence, surgical treatment is limited to a posterior approach aimed at stabilization and realignment.

DISTRACTION–FLEXION INJURIES (CHANCE FRACTURES, 'SEAT BELT'-TYPE INJURIES)

DF injuries result from a flexion moment with the fulcrum located at varying distances from the anterior portion of the vertebral column. The resulting injury can involve bone, ligament, or a combination of bone and ligament. When the fulcrum is located adjacent to the vertebral body

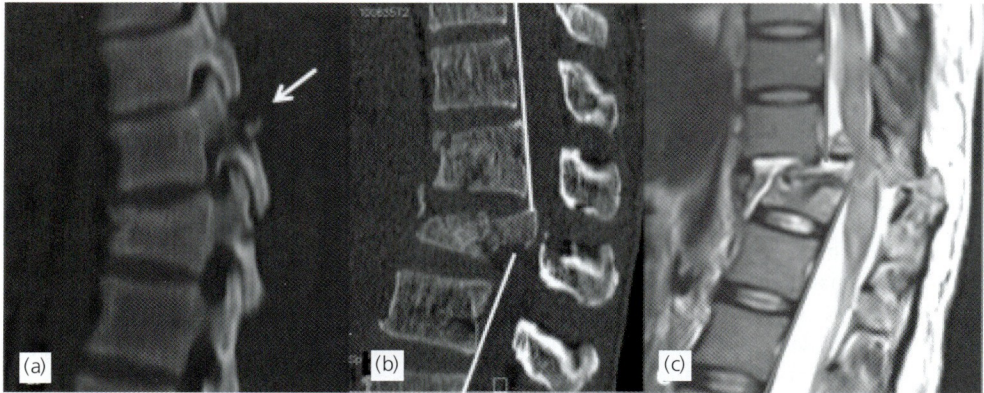

Figure 53.28 Unstable spinal injuries. (a) Chance fracture. The white arrow indicates a distractive failure of the posterior column. (b) Flexion–distraction injury. The fulcrum is at the anterior column; the middle and posterior column fail in distraction. (c) Fracture dislocation. All the three columns fail in translational shear.

(posterior to the anterior longitudinal ligament), the anterior column fails in compression and the middle and posterior columns fail in tension (McAfee DF injury) (Fig. 53.28). As the fulcrum moves more anterior (axis anterior to the anterior longitudinal ligament), the deforming forces become purely distractive and all three columns will fail in tension (McAfee–Chance fracture). Patients are usually neurologically intact; however, up to 50% may have associated abdominal injuries because the lap belt provides the fulcrum against the abdominal wall.

Patients with a purely bony injury can be managed with hyperextension casting because of the healing properties of bone. However, those with pure ligamentous and combined bony and ligamentous injuries should undergo a posterior short-segment spinal fusion (in compression) because of involvement of all three columns and the poor healing properties of ligaments. In the presence of an incomplete neurological injury an initial posterior reduction for alignment and stability is recommended followed by a posterolateral or anterior decompression in the presence of residual canal compromise. Most often, however, realignment may itself serve to relieve any neurological compression.

FRACTURE DISLOCATIONS (TRANSLATIONAL INJURIES)

All three columns fail under compression, tension, rotation or shear, with translational deformity. There is malalignment of the neural canal in the transverse plane and up to 90% of these injuries are associated with a SCI, most commonly complete. Because all three spinal columns are involved, these fractures are very unstable and hence require surgical stabilization. Posterior surgery is most useful for achieving reduction and stability in these injuries and can be performed once the clinical condition is optimized. In patients with complete neurological injury, surgery allows for early mobilization and helps to minimize the morbidity and mortality associated with these injuries.

Minor spinal injuries

These injuries do not affect the stability of the spinal column and are rarely associated with neurological deficits. Transverse process fractures are most common. These fractures can result from different mechanisms of injury and should be treated symptomatically. Patients tend to have significant pain and require heavier analgesia. Transverse process fractures of the lumbar spine are mostly innocuous but sometimes may indicate missed fractures in the vertebral bodies.

AO FRACTURE CLASSIFICATION SYSTEM

The **AO comprehensive classification** system has been proposed for thoracic and lumbar fractures based on their radiographic morphology. In 1994 Magerl[16] analysed 1445 cases of thoracolumbar injuries from five institutions in Europe and presented a comprehensive classification of the thoracolumbar fracture based on mechanism of injury and morphological pattern of the fracture. The classification implemented AO concepts that had been originally applied to extremity fractures, with categorization of the severity of the injury on a progressive scale from Type A to Type C, and has been adopted as AO classification. The primary types of fracture depend on the mechanism of injury and include Type A – compression, Type B – distraction, and Type C – rotation and/or shear injuries. Each of the three main fracture types is divided into three subtypes (1, 2 and 3), which in turn are separated into three subgroups, depending on the mechanism of injury (flexion or extension) and morphology of the fracture. According to the AO classification, Type A1 indicates the most simple and Type C3 indicates the most severe forms of injuries, and the magnitude of instability and risk of neurological deficit increase with the ascending category of the fracture types. Despite being a comprehensive classification system, with an ordinal scale from A1 to C3, this system had two big deficiencies. The AO classification system failed to offer a clear definition of instability. Also, this system did not consider the presence of neurological deficit, which is often a very important determinant in clinical decision making.

THE THORACOLUMBAR INJURY SEVERITY SCORE (TLISS) AND THORACOLUMBAR INJURY CLASSIFICATION AND SEVERITY SYSTEM (TLICS)

The TLISS/TLICS was developed by an international group of spine surgeons, 'the Spine Trauma Study Group' (Fig. 53.29).[18] The TLISS is based on three major injury characteristics:

- mechanism of injury,
- integrity of the posterior ligamentous complex (PLC)
- neurological status.

Based on the severity scores within these three categories, a total score is calculated that can be used to guide treatment. The mechanisms of injury in the TLISS system are identical to those proposed by the AO group (axial compression, distraction, rotation/shear) and these were scored with greater points for more unstable injury mechanism. Although technically a severity score, the TLISS meets the criteria for a classification system. TLISS also provides a scheme that seeks to uniformly categorize injuries and indicate uniform treatment.[21]

Gunshot wounds

In general, fractures associated with low-velocity gunshot wounds are stable fractures. This is the case with most handgun injuries. They are associated with a low infection rate and can be prophylactically treated with 48 hours of a broad-spectrum antibiotic. Transintestinal gunshot wounds require special attention. In these cases, the bullet passes through the colon, intestine or stomach before passing through the spine. These injuries carry a significantly higher rate of infection. Broad-spectrum antibiotics should be continued for 7–14 days. High-energy wounds, as caused by a rifle or military assault weapon, require open debridement and stabilization. Neural injury is often secondary to a blast effect in which the energy of the bullet is absorbed and transmitted to the soft tissues. Because of this unique mechanism, decompression is rarely indicated. One exception is when a bullet fragment is found in the spinal canal between the level of T12 and L5 in the presence of a neurological deficit. Rarely, delayed bullet extraction may be indicated for lead toxicity or late neurological deficits owing to migration of a bullet fragment.

Sacral fractures

Sacral fractures are usually the result of high-energy trauma; 80–90% are associated with pelvic fractures and are often overlooked. Neurological injuries of the lower sacral roots (S2–4) are often missed because only L5 and S1 can be evaluated by manual muscle testing. Perianal sensory changes and absence of a bulbocavernosus reflex should be sought in patients with this type of injury.

Sacral fractures are generally classified according to the direction of the fracture line. Fractures may be vertical, transverse or oblique, although vertical fractures are the most common. The Denis classification system divides the sacrum into three zones[22] (Table 53.7). Zone 1 (alar zone) spans the sacral ala to the lateral border of the neural foramen. Zone 2 (foraminal) represents the neural foramen (Fig. 53.30). Zone 3 (central canal) involves the central sacrum and canal. The direction of the fracture line and type of fracture determine the likelihood of a neurological injury.

TLISS classification

Morphology of Injury		Nerological status		PLC status	
Type	Points	Involvement	Points	Involvement	Points
Compression	1	Intact	0	Intact	0
Burst	1	Root injury	2	Indeterminate	2
Translation	3	Cord/conus – Complete	2	Disrupted	3
Distraction	4	InComplete	3		
		Cauda equina	3		

Score < 3 Non-operative management
Score = 4 Non-operative or operative (Surgeon Preference)
Score > 5 Operative management

PLC, posterior ligament complex

Figure 53.29 The Thoraco-lumbar injury severity system and management guidelines.

Table 53.7 Denis classification of sacral fractures

Zone	Fracture characteristics	Neurological deficit
Zone I	*Fractures thorough the lateral ala* Commonly associated with lateral compression pelvic injuries	5.9% incidence of neural injury. Usually an injury to the L5 nerve root or the sciatic nerve
Zone II	*Fracture line through one or more foramina* May include ala, but does not extend into the central canal	28.4% incidence of neural injury. Commonly unilateral in nature. Important as patients with unilateral sacral root injuries usually have normal bowel and bladder function
Zone III	*Fracture line through the central canal* but frequently extends in zone I and II Transverse fractures, burst fractures and fracture dislocations of the sacrum. Usually occur at S2–3 as this is the apical kyphotic angulation between the upper and lower aspects of the sacrum	50% incidence of neurological injuries. Commonly bilateral sacral root involvement with bowel, bladder and sexual dysfunction

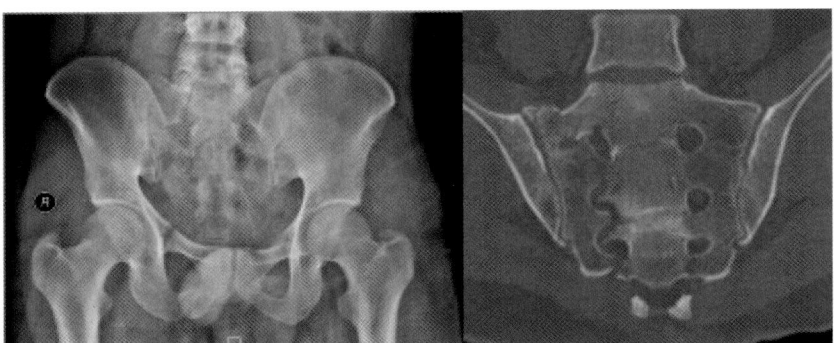

Figure 53.30 Denis type 2 sacral fracture in a 30 year old man. The anteroposterior view of the pelvis shows a bilateral pubic ramus fracture along with a sacral fracture. The coronal CT section reveals the fracture through the right sacral foramina.

Indications for surgical management of sacral fractures include bowel and bladder dysfunction in the setting of an unstable fracture with substantial coronal or sagittal deformity. Vertical fractures can typically be treated with posterior sacroiliac plating or percutaneously placed sacroiliac screws. Placement of percutaneous sacroiliac screws can be technically demanding, and the L5 and S1 nerve roots are at risk during the procedure. If this technique is used to treat a zone 2 injury, the screw should not be loaded in compression to avoid neural injury. Patients with displaced transverse or oblique fractures may undergo bilateral plating. Neural decompression via laminectomy may be indicated in patients with neurological deficits and canal compromise, and recovery of bowel and bladder function may be seen. In patients without neurological injury who have minimally displaced fractures, bracing is usually sufficient. Much of the sacrum distal to the S1–2 level can be disrupted (including the lower half of the sacroiliac joint) without significantly weakening the pelvic ring. For sacral fractures associated with other pelvic ring fractures, anterior external fixation of the injured ring indirectly stabilizes the fractured sacrum.

KEY LEARNING POINTS

- The severity of neurological deficit is determined by the extent of neural tissue damage and it depends on the rate of force application, the degree and duration of neural tissue compression.
- The pathophysiology of spinal cord injury (SCI) is biphasic, consisting of a primary and a secondary phase of injury. The first 3–8 hours after injury is a potential window of opportunity in which the secondary phase of SCI could be mitigated.
- The Advanced Trauma Life Support principles of management of a trauma patient should be followed during pre-hospital resuscitation and emergency room management.
- It is essential to maintain rigid cervical immobilization and to keep the patient on a backboard during initial evaluation.
- Craniocervical dissociation should be considered with any occipital condyle fracture.

- The transverse ligament is important for the stability of the atlantoaxial joint. Its integrity should always be evaluated in fractures of the atlas, dens and rotary subluxations.
- Patients with unilateral and bilateral facet dislocations require MRI before reduction to evaluate for a herniated disc. This is more important, especially if a patient is not awake and alert, and is unable to cooperate with serial examinations during reduction manoeuvres.
- The morphology of the injury, the neurological condition of the patient, and the integrity of the posterior ligaments are most important in dictating treatment in subaxial spinal injuries.
- Independent of neurological status or integrity of the posterior ligaments, distraction and translation injuries are managed optimally with an initial posterior approach for realignment and stabilization, followed, if necessary, by an anterior decompression and/or stabilization.

REFERENCES

- ● = Key primary paper
- ◆ = Major review article

1. Kraus JF, Franti CE, Riggins RS, et al. Incidence of traumatic spinal cord lesions. *Journal of Chronic Diseases* 1975;**28**:471.
2. DeVivo MJ. Causes and costs of spinal cord injury in the United States. *Spinal Cord* 1997;**35**:809-813.
3. Wood II GW. Chapter 35 – Fractures, Dislocations, and Fracture-Dislocations of the Spine, Canale & Beaty: Campbell's Operative Orthopaedics, 11th edn. 1761-1831.
4. Calenoff L, Chessare JW, Rogers LF, et al. Multiple level spinal injuries: importance of early recognition. *AJR American Journal of Roentgenology* **130**:665, 1978.
5. Bracken MB, Shepard MJ, Holford TR, et al. Administration of methylprednisolone for 24 or 48 hours or tirilazad mesylate for 48 hours in the treatment of acute spinal cord injury. Results of the third national acute spinal cord injury randomized controlled trial. National Acute Spinal Cord Injury Study. JAMA 1997;**277**:1597-604.
6. Anderson PA, Montesano PX. Morphology and treatment of occipital condyle fractures. *Spine* 1988;**13**:731.
7. Levine AM, Edwards CC. Treatment of injuries in the C1-C2 complex. *Orthopaedic Clinics of North America* 1986;**17**:31.
8. Dickman CA, Greene KA, Sonntag VK. Injuries involving the transverse atlantal ligament: classification and treatment guidelines based upon experience with 39 injuries. *Neurosurgery* 1996;**38**:44.
9. Fielding JW, Hawkins RJ. Atlanto-axial rotatory fixation: fixed rotatory subluxation of the atlanto-axial joint. *Journal of Bone and Joint Surgery (American)* 1977;**59A**:37.
10. Anderson LD, D'Alonzo RT. Fractures of the odontoid process of the axis. *Journal of Bone and Joint Surgery (American)* 1974;**56A**:1663.
11. White AA, Southwick WO, Panjabi MM. Clinical instability in the lower cervical spine: a review of past and current concepts, *Spine* 1976;**1**:15.
12. Allen Jr BL, Ferguson RL, Lehmann R, et al. Mechanistic classification of closed indirect fractures and dislocations of the lower cervical spine. *Spine* 1982;**7**:1.
13. Vaccaro AR, Falatyn SP, Flanders AE, et al. Magnetic resonance evaluation of the intervertebral disc, spinal ligaments, and spinal cord before and after closed traction reduction of cervical spine dislocations. *Spine* 1999;**24**:1210.
14. Eismont FJ, Arena MJ, Green BA. Extrusion of an intervertebral disc associated with traumatic subluxation or dislocation of cervical facets: case report. *J Bone Joint Surg Am* 1991;73:1555-60.
15. Denis F. The three-column spine and its significance in the classification of acute thoracolumbar spinal injuries. *Spine* 1983;**8**:817-31.
16. Magerl F, Aebi M, Gertzbein SD, et al. A comprehensive classification of thoracic and lumbar injuries. *European Spine Journal* 1994;**3**:184-201.
17. McAfee PC, Yuan HA, Lasda NA. The unstable burst fracture. *Spine* 1982;**7**:365-73.
18. Vaccaro AR, Lim MR, Hurlbert RJ, et al. Surgical decision making for unstable thoracolumbar spine injuries: results of a Consensus Panel Review by the Spine Trauma Study Group. *Journal of Spinal Disorders and Techniques* 2006;**19**:1-7.
19. McCormack T, Karaikovic E, Gaines RW. The load sharing classification of spine fractures. *Spine* 1994;**19**:1741-4.
20. Boerger TO, Limb D, Dickson RA. Does 'canal clearance' affect neurological outcome after thoracolumbar burst fractures? *Journal of Bone and Joint Surgery (British)* 2000;**82B**:629-35.
21. Sethi MK, Schoenfeld AJ, Bono CM, et al. The evolution of thoracolumbar injury classification systems. *Spine J.* 2009;**9**:780-8.
22. Denis F, Davis S, Comfort T. Sacral fractures: an important problem. Retrospective analysis of 236 cases. *Clinical Orthopaedics and Related Research* 1988;**227**:67-81.

54

Head and face trauma

PATRICK H WARNKE

Introduction	466	Midfacial fractures	473
Clinical diagnosis of head and maxillofacial trauma	467	Classification of skull fractures	478
Classification of maxillofacial fractures	471	References	479
Mandible fractures	472		

NATIONAL BOARD STANDARDS

- Describe common clinical patterns of head and face trauma and important diagnostic findings
- Be familiar with required diagnostic tools and necessary imaging/radiographic plains for common maxillofacial fracture types
- Be able to explain treatment options and management pathways for common maxillofacial fractures

INTRODUCTION

Head and face injuries involving the maxillofacial skeleton are common and can be a challenge for orthopaedic surgeons involved in emergency services if access to maxillofacial expertise is limited. Apart from the aesthetic appearance of the patient, the maxillofacial region is associated with a number of important functions of daily life, including sight, smell, mastication, breathing and speaking. Wrong treatment or delayed decision-making may therefore severely affect the future lifestyle of the patient.

This chapter outlines general descriptions of common head and face injuries and its associated treatment options.

General considerations

Overlooked injuries and delayed diagnoses are still common problems in the treatment of polytrauma or multitrauma patients even though improved diagnostic tools such as multislice CT scans may have led to a decreased incidence.[1] Each year, physicians in Canadian and United States emergency departments treat more than 8 million patients with head injury, representing approximately 6.7% of the 120 million total emergency department visits.[2] Therefore, head and maxillofacial skeletal injuries are not uncommon and often occur in polytrauma patients. Lin et al.[3] investigated 111 010 patients admitted and hospitalized because of trauma injuries during the years 2000–2004, in which 5.3% were maxillofacial or dental injuries. Most of these injuries were traffic related (54.5%), followed by events at home (18.7%). Facial injuries combined with injuries to other organs occurred in 63.2% of the patients. In another series of 729 patients with multitrauma as a result of traffic accidents, 11% had facial bone fractures, of which fractures of the mandible appeared to be the most common (61%).[4]

If a patient presents with multiple injuries, adequate consultation and examinations must be carried out by experienced practitioners or specialists before entering the operating theatre[5] (Box 54.1). Often it might be possible for different specialists to treat multitrauma patients simultaneously, thereby shortening the overall operating time. Some diagnostic tricks will be explained in this chapter to lead the way for fast identification of skull and maxillofacial fractures on first inspection.

> **BOX 54.1: Indications for consultation in patients with head and maxillofacial trauma**
>
> Ophthalmologist
> - Blindness or impaired vision
> - Eyeball trauma or large eyelid laceration
> - Impaired eyeball movement (diplopia)
> - Orbital/retrobulbar haemorrhage
> - Asymmetric pupils, missing light reaction
>
> Maxillofacial surgeon
> - Large soft-tissue defects in the head and face
> - Fractures of the midface, mandible, orbits and/or frontal sinus
> - Visible deformity, abnormal mobility
> - Dental malocclusion, dental fracture
> - Impaired mouth opening/closure
> - Extraoral haematoma around orbits (monocle or raccoon sign)
> - Intraoral haematoma
> - Impaired eyeball movement (diplopia)
> - Facial anaesthesia or nerve palsies
>
> ENT surgeon
> - Post-traumatic hearing problems
> - Vertigo
> - Large defects in external ear, bleeding from external canal (meatus acusticus)
> - Cerebrospinal fluid otorrhoea/rhinorrhoea ('tramlines')
> - Laryngeal/pharyngeal trauma
> - Facial nerve palsy
>
> Neurosurgeon
> - Intracranial problems: bleeding and/or air in intracranial space (CT scan)
> - Skull fracture
> - Fracture of dorsal wall of frontal sinus
> - Cerebrospinal fluid otorrhoea/rhinorrhoea ('tramlines')
> - Nerve palsy of unknown origin
> - Blindness or impaired vision
> - Asymmetric pupils, missing light reaction
> - Reduced Glasgow Coma Scale score

> **BOX 54.2: Management of unconscious patients with head injury**
>
> As in most emergency situations, history taking, examination and initial management are carried out simultaneously. Note that over 50% of patients with severe head injuries have associated systemic injuries. Do not allow an apparently isolated head injury to divert you from carrying out a full assessment of the airway, breathing and circulation (ABC) of your patient. Identify and treat other life-threatening injuries as you go. Stay on alert to resuscitate as necessary. Keep in mind that inadequate resuscitation may exacerbate secondary brain injury.
> - Call for experienced help
> - Clear the airway (suck out debris and insert an oropharyngeal airway)
> - Administer high-flow oxygen
> - Apply a rigid cervical collar
> - Your patient needs intubating if his/her gag reflex is reduced or absent
> - Ensure that breathing is adequate, with bilateral air entry. If not, consider chest trauma as a cause
> - Attach a cardiac monitor and record heart rate, blood pressure, respiratory rate and temperature
> - Is circulation adequate or is your patient in shock? Hypotension in patients with brain injuries is unlikely to have an intracranial cause. Search for a source of blood loss (chest, abdomen, pelvis)
> - Watch out for bradycardia and hypertension. These indicate rising intracranial pressure
> - Treat hypotension with crystalloids, but be cautious: too much fluid can exacerbate cerebral oedema. Stop fluids when your patient is normotensive
> - Send blood for cross-match (and full blood count, urea and electrolytes, and glucose). Check the blood concentrations of glucose with a blood glucose testing stick and give intravenous glucose if it is low
> - Take an arterial blood gas sample
> - Be aware of both *hypercapnia*, which causes cerebral vasodilation and increases intracranial pressure, and *hypoxia*, which may cause ischaemic brain damage. If PaO_2 is less than 9 kPa on air or $PaCO_2$ greater than 5.3 then your patient needs ventilating
>
> From Turner K, Jones A, Handa A. Emergency management of head injuries. *Student BMJ* 2000;**8**:131-74.[6]

CLINICAL DIAGNOSIS OF HEAD AND MAXILLOFACIAL TRAUMA

The first examination should eliminate immediate problems such as airway obstruction, excessive bleeding and severe ocular injuries. These must be attended to first and the clinical examination continued later. Unconscious patients with head injuries are generally in a critical situation, as life-threatening airway obstructions may occur instantly at any time. If cervical spine injury in a high-impact trauma cannot be excluded as radiographs are not available on primary examination, a rigid cervical collar should be attached.

Box 54.2 shows a simple guide for management of unconscious patients with head injuries by Turner et al.[6]

Neurological examination

The neurological examination should begin with an overall impression of the patient. The Glasgow Coma Scale score gives a rough impression of neurological status (Table 54.1). Especially changes in the score are important as they give first evidence of improvement or deterioration of the patient. The British Society of Rehabilitation Medicine[7] has defined the scale of head injuries as

- mild (Glasgow Coma Scale score 13–15)
- moderate (9–12)
- severe (<9).

After moderate head injuries 63% of patients remain disabled 1 year after their accident and after severe injuries the figure rises to 85%. Surprisingly, minor head injuries also have a poor prognosis with 79% suffering severe headaches, 59% suffering memory problems and 34% unemployed 3 months after the injury. Only 45% of patients who have suffered a minor head injury are fully recovered a year later.[6,8] The neurological examination also includes testing of cranial nerves, which can be checked during the extraoral examination.

Extraoral examination

INSPECTION

Start the extraoral examination by carefully *inspecting* the face and scalp for lacerations, bruising, asymmetries and deformity. Accurate exploration and manual palpation of lacerations is important prior to wound closure as foreign bodies such as fragments of crushed car glass often remain in subcutaneous tissue after traffic accidents. Scalp injuries may be concealed by hair and clotted blood, so that wound cleaning and rinsing with saline or peroxide and additional brushing may be helpful at this time. Check for evidence of a cerebrospinal fluid (CSF) leakage often from the nose or ears (rhinorrhoea, otorrhoea), typically seen as a flow of clear watery fluid running between lines of clotted blood ('tramlines').[5] Bleeding from the ear or nose in cases of suspected CSF leak, when dabbed on a tissue paper, shows a clear ring of wet tissue beyond the blood stain, called a 'halo' or 'ring' sign. A CSF leak can also be revealed by analysing the glucose level and by measuring tau-transferrin.

The examination of the orbits and periorbital region plays a pivotal role. Haematoma and/or swelling around the orbits after trauma are often a reliable sign to identify a fracture of the orbits and require further radiological examination (Fig. 54.1).

Midfacial fractures are usually associated with fractured orbital walls and most frequently the orbital floor (see fracture patterns in Fig. 54.8). In Le Fort 2 and 3 fractures

Table 54.1 Glasgow coma scale

		Score
Eye opening	Spontaneously	4
	To speech	3
	To pain	2
	None	1
Verbal response	Orientated	5
	Confused	4
	Inappropriate	3
	Incomprehensible	2
	None	1
Motor response	Obeys commands	6
	Localizes to pain	5
	Withdraws from pain	4
	Flexion to pain	3
	Extension to pain	2
	None	1
Maximum score		15

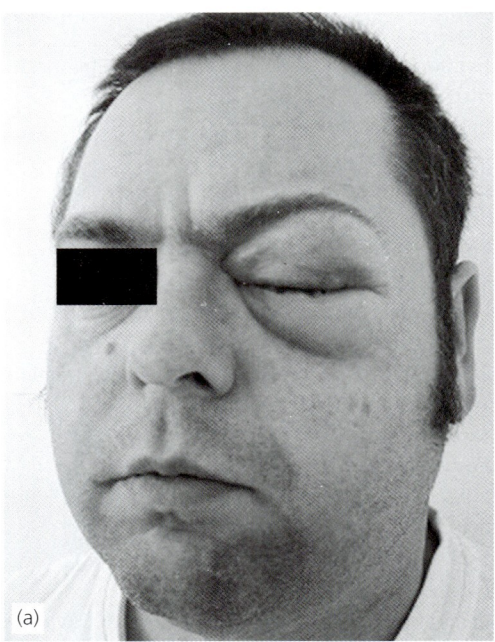
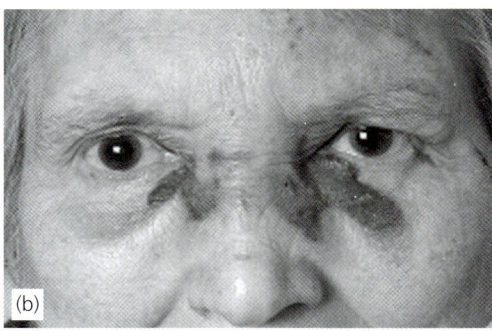

Figure 54.1 (a) Unilateral *monocle haematoma* with swelling around the left orbit. The eyelids are swollen because of trauma and air emphysema. Air was blown from the maxillary sinus via fracture gaps along the left orbital floor into the orbital soft tissues. (b) The bilateral *raccoon sign/haematoma* might be moderate with only mild swelling in some cases even though a Le Fort 2 fracture is present as in this patient. Note: Radiograph examination is mandatory if orbital haematoma is present to rule out any hidden fracture!

both orbits are injured and haematoma often occurs on both sides ('raccoon sign'). If haematoma only occurs on one side (monocle haematoma or 'black eye') it is often associated with a hidden single fracture of the orbital wall ('blow-out fracture') or with the orbital floor in a zygoma ('tripod') fracture. If swelling occurs around the orbit and inside the eyelids after blowing the nose then fracture is highly likely, as air has been blown from the sinus via fracture gaps into the orbit (Fig. 54.1). Air in subcutaneous soft tissue may be palpable as crepitation.[5]

Also eyeball movement may be impaired on the fractured site or direct trauma to the eyeball is evident. The eye inspection should start with checking the integrity of the eyeball and ability to see for both eyes. Then check for shape/size differences of the pupils on both sides and their corresponding response to light. Any abnormalities require an immediate consultation of an ophthalmologist and a neurosurgeon (Box 54.1). The eyeball movement can be checked by holding up a pen 50 cm in front of the patient. The patient should focus on the pen, which is then alternately moved up/downwards and to both sides. If the patient sees the pen twice (diplopia), dysfunction of the extraocular muscles is often the reason due to fragments trapped inside the fractured orbit. Diplopia may also be the result of altered globe positions due to severely fractured orbits. Another reason could be due to contusion of the central nervous system or even injury of the cranial nerves.

A critical complication of the fractured orbit is retrobulbar haematoma, which can lead to irreversible blindness of the eye due to compression of the optic nerve. Retrobulbar haematoma may also emerge after orbit surgery and fracture reduction, especially when the patient is on anticoagulation medication. It always requires immediate action at the time to release the pressure and to prevent blindness. See Box 54.3 for signs and symptoms.[5]

PALPATION

Further *palpation* should elicit any tenderness, crepitation, depressed or penetrating bone fragments or contour irregularities. Palpate all contours of the skull, midface and mandible. Start from top to bottom and from lateral to medial. Ask the patient to report pain and anaesthesia/paraesthesia while palpating.

Note the function of the trigeminal nerve. Fractures along the orbital floor frequently cause anaesthesia or paraesthesia on the infraorbital cheek or lateral maxilla (infraorbital nerve/trigeminus maxillary division V2). Mandibular fractures with severe dislocation may cause anaesthesia along the lateral chin (mental nerve/trigeminus mandibular division V3).

Check for any tenderness or tangible fracture lines in key areas:[5]

- zygomatic arch
- frontozygomatic sutures (lateral upper orbital rims)
- nasofrontal area (nasal base and septum)
- infraorbital rims
- base of the mandible
- temporomandibular joint (TMJ) areas (with open and closed mouth).

A simple method of detecting mandibular fractures extraorally is to press carefully but firmly at both angles of the mandible.[5] This should produce medial compression and flex the whole mandible, producing motion and discomfort in any fracture site. Additionally press on the chin with the mouth open for detection of condylar neck or TMJ fractures. Compression of the zygomatic arch should cause discomfort in zygomatic fractures. If the first radiographic image shows clear maxillofacial fractures, then painful palpation can be abandoned and the patient may be sent straight for CT imaging.

NOTE

- Do not forget tetanus prophylaxis, if any extraoral wounds are present.
- Remove all incorporated dirt from facial skin wounds and scratches prior to wound closure as otherwise visible intimidating dirt tattooing will stay.
- Haematoma and/or swelling around the orbit require radiological examination as these are frequently associated with hidden fractures of the orbital walls.
- Pain relievers may camouflage severe pain in retrobulbar haematoma.

Intraoral examination

Intraoral examination starts usually with inspection. Haematomas in the buccal or labial sulcus as well as mucosal lacerations are indirect signs of fractures,[5] whereas a lingual haematoma in the floor of the mouth is highly likely to be a result of a mandibular fracture and can practically be seen as a direct diagnostic sign of fracture.

Check the occlusion and ask the patient if anything has changed with the trauma. Even in non-displaced fractures

---

BOX 54.3: Signs and symptoms of retrobulbar haematoma

1. Severe pain!
2. Progressive loss of vision (pupil becomes fixed and dilated)
3. Proptosis/ptosis
4. Subconjunctival haemorrhage
5. Swelling of the eyelids

Note: Pain relievers may camouflage the important symptom of pain and should not be administered in orbital trauma or after orbital surgery if stringent regular eyeball inspection cannot be provided by trained staff.

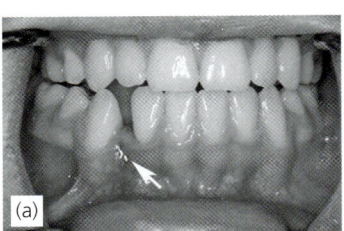
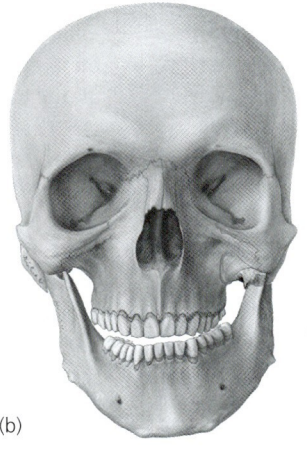
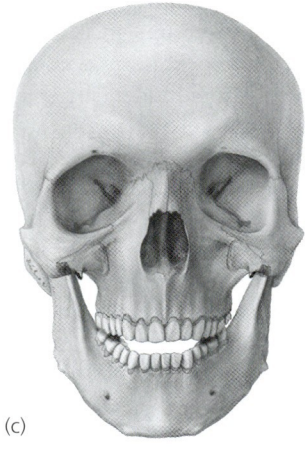

Figure 54.2 Malocclusion in mandibular fractures. (a) A step in the occlusion with disrupted gingiva on the alveolar crest (arrow). (b) Unilateral left condylar neck fracture with deviation of the mandible to the left. An open bite between the right molars may occur too. (c) Bilateral condylar neck fracture with open bite in front. Images (b) and (c) copyright Andreas Reinhardt and Franz Haerle. Reproduced from ref. 21 with permission from the artists and Thieme Medical Publishers, Inc.

the patient often will report slight malocclusion. A step, deviation or discontinuity in the occlusion often together with disrupted alveolar crest gingiva is a reliable sign of fracture (Fig. 54.2). Condylar neck fractures of the mandible often result in a frontal open bite situation (non-occlusion) or a lateral malocclusion or deviation (Fig. 54.2).

Le Fort fractures usually lead to an unstable maxilla or midface. A frontal open-bite situation with non-occlusion of the incisors is often present. To check for Le Fort fractures it is best to place one hand on the patient's forehead and rest the fingers on the nasal base and both lateral orbital rims. Use your other hand to grab the frontal maxillary alveolar crest and push back and forth to test for instability (Fig. 54.3). Then palpate along the alveolar crest to the maxillary molar region and press onto the zygomatic maxillary buttress from intraorally. A zygomatic complex fracture or Le Fort fracture (1 and 2) will often cause a tangible step along the zygomatic buttresses and the patient will express discomfort.

You may also tap with a metal instrument against the maxillary teeth. If a high and sharp click is apparent the maxilla is highly likely to be stable. A hollow or dull sound is frequently associated with a Le Fort fracture.

Ask the patient to open the mouth. If any functional impairment or discomfort along the lateral cheek is present, then a zygoma/zygomatic arch or a mandibular condylar process fracture needs to be taken into account.

Loose teeth should stay in the alveolus or should be immediately reinserted. When impossible to reinsert, keep dislocated teeth in sterile saline and instantly request consultation of a maxillofacial surgeon or dentist. Do not add disinfectants or mechanical force (cleaning) to extruded teeth as the fragile desmodontal tissue covering the roots might be irreversibly damaged. Successful tooth replantation requires a viable desmodont.

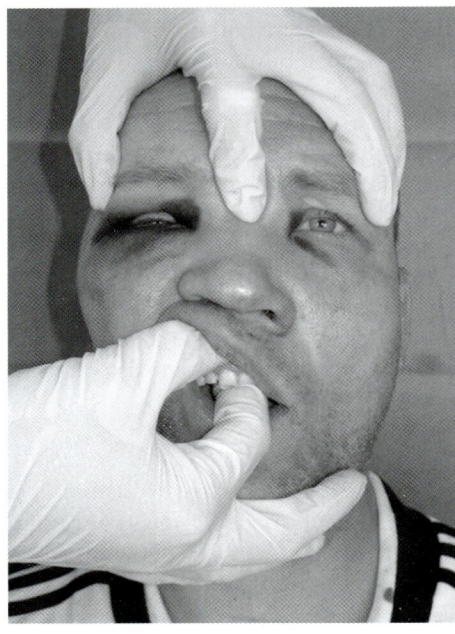

Figure 54.3 Bimanual palpation for instability of the midface in Le Fort fractures. Grab the maxillary alveolar crest while placing the fingers of the other hand on the nasal base and the lateral orbital rims. Beware of loose teeth, which should stay in the alveolus until fixation.

NOTE

- New malocclusion after trauma is a direct sign of fracture.
- If post-traumatic haematoma on the floor of the mouth is present, fracture of the mandible is highly likely.
- Loose teeth should stay in the alveolus, be immediately reinserted or at least kept in sterile saline. Do not add disinfectants or mechanical force (cleaning).

Radiological examination

The indication for radiological examination is based on the clinical checks. In case you identify signs of fracture or if you cannot rule out the presence of fracture a radiological examination should be performed. A golden rule is if any new impaired function, malocclusion or haematoma in the maxillofacial region occurs after trauma, further radiological examination is indicated. Always check whether accurate radiographs have already been performed if you are not the first doctor to see the patient.

Plain radiographs are the foundation of imaging. They may be sufficient on their own or may need to be complemented by other modalities, such as CT scanning or the latest cone beam digital volume tomography (DVT) scans. The last are more expensive and a higher radiation dosage might be applied if a CT scan is the primary diagnostic tool.

Fractures should be imaged in at least two planes, preferably at right angles to one other.[9] Practical combinations of planes for the most common fractures are given in the following paragraphs. A CT scan is of high value if fractures along the orbits or the skull are suspected. Also, nonbony intracranial post-traumatic disorders such as free air or bleeding can be detected with CT. These require immediate consultation of a neurosurgeon (Box 54.1). In addition, retrobulbar haemorrhage or incarceration of extraocular muscles can be easily identified with CT and it should be performed when these are suspected.

However, in severely injured or polytrauma patients the decision to perform CT is obvious. It may be ambivalent to send the patient to the CT unit if only mild trauma occurred and the Glasgow Coma Scale score has not reduced.

The New Orleans Criteria include seven items (Box 54.4) that were developed as a decision-making tool regarding CT scans for patients with minor head injury and a Glasgow Coma Scale score of 15.[10]

CLASSIFICATION OF MAXILLOFACIAL FRACTURES

Several different classifications have been used in the past, especially for midfacial fractures. Some of them are internationally respected and suitable for clinical work and treatment planning. Some definitions are required in relation to maxillofacial fractures.[5]

Relations to the overlying tissues

Whether a fracture is covered by soft tissue or not plays an important role in orthopaedic surgery. For a rough description of maxillofacial fractures the following three terms may be applied:[5]

- *Closed*: The fracture is not situated in the dentate area. No rupture or cut of oral mucosa or skin is present that would have direct contact to the fracture site. For example, the majority of mandibular condylar neck fractures and single zygomatic arch fractures are closed. Skull fractures may also be closed without skin laceration as long as skull base fractures do not involve the sinuses.
- *Open*: All fractures in the dentate area! Additionally, fractures where lacerations of the skin or oral mucosa have direct contact to the fracture site. Le Fort and zygomatic complex fractures always involve the sinuses. The sinusoidal mucosa is disrupted and the fractures have contact to nasal air ventilation. Thus fractures involving the sinuses shall be classified as open even though there is often no skin or mucosa laceration visible.
- *Complicated*: Open fractures with a considerable injury of the overlying soft tissues. For example high-impact fractures or gunshot wounds.

Open and contaminated fractures of the extremities are always a challenge for the orthopaedic surgeon as the risk for development of an osteomyelitis is likely and well reported.[11] However, in maxillofacial surgery most of the fractures are open fractures and are usually contaminated by oral flora, for example if the dentate areas are involved. Surprisingly, open maxillofacial fractures have a low infection rate, which would mainly affect the soft tissues. Also, minor operations such as tooth extractions can be performed without antibiotic cover. Osteomyelitis is also rare in long-term operations such as orthognathic surgery and has been reported by only 0.2%.[12] One reason for the low infection rate of maxillofacial bone may be a recently detected innate immune system in oral bone.[13] Oral bone produces human beta defensins: antimicrobial peptides that can ward off invading bacteria (Fig. 54.4). These peptides are also detectable in long bones, but at a much a lower level. Research is ongoing on this field.

Mode of fracture

Several different modes of fractures can be defined.[5]

- *Greenstick*: This fracture involves one cortical wall, while the opposite cortical side is bent only. The periosteum

> **BOX 54.4: New Orleans Criteria**
>
> Cranial CT is required for patients with minor head injury with any one of the following findings. The criteria apply only to patients who also have a Glasgow Coma Scale score of 15.
>
> 1. Headache
> 2. Vomiting
> 3. Older than 60 years
> 4. Drug or alcohol intoxication
> 5. Persistent anterograde amnesia (deficits in short-term memory)
> 6. Visible trauma above the clavicle
> 7. Seizure

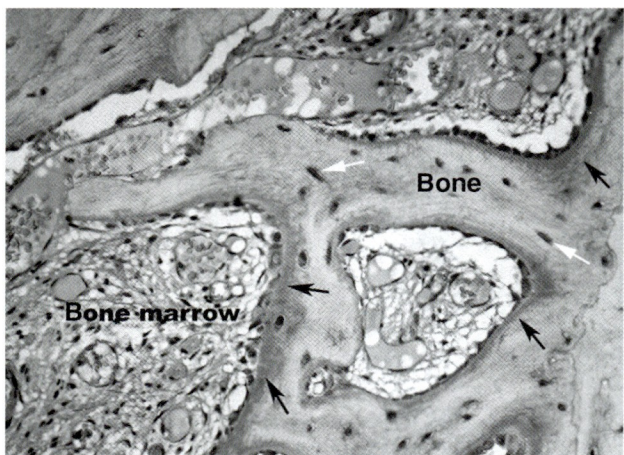

Figure 54.4 Oral bone might be protected by an innate immune system of human beta defensins (HBD), antimicrobial peptides, to ward off bacterial invasion. The figure shows immunostaining of HBS type 3 in oral bone (black arrows). Osteocytes show positive immunoreaction on HBD-3 (white arrows). Thus, osteomyelitis following surgery in the contaminated maxillofacial region is relatively uncommon.

stays mainly intact. These kinds of fractures are often found in children or young teenagers.
- *Single*: A single fracture line in the same bone.
- *Multiple*: Two or more fracture lines in the same bone.
- *Comminuted*: Two or more fracture lines that communicate with each other. Multiple bone fragments are often visible on radiographs and are often dislocated.
- *A defect*: Bone fragments are missing and a gap is present. A critical size defect will not heal by local bone regeneration only and in the maxillofacial region is defined as a gap about 1 cm or more. Bone grafts or alternatives are required for reconstruction.

Additional characteristics of the fracture

Additional terms are often applied when describing the nature of the fracture.[5]

- *Direct or indirect*: The area of the initial trauma and the relation to the fracture is important. Direct fractures are associated with the area of impact. Indirect fractures are in the same bone, but are due to biomechanical reasons further away from the initial trauma and are often located at insubstantial fragile areas of the bone. For example, a direct fracture next to the midline of the mandible is often associated with an indirect fracture of the condylar process (or even both condylar processes).
- *Blow out*: The classic blow-out fracture is an indirect fracture and involves the orbital walls. For example, a punch or tennis ball impact on the eyeball often leads to an instant pressure increase in the orbit and to a fracture of the orbital wall. Thus, fragments of the orbital floor plus soft tissue are 'blown out' into the maxillary sinus.
- *Pathological*: There is a pathological process involving the bone, predisposing to a fracture due to a minor trauma. For example, a mandibular tumour/metastasis or large dentogenous cyst that has destabilized the mandible.
- *Spontaneous*: A fracture in the atrophic bone. Atrophy often in combination with osteoporosis is predisposing to fracture due to a minor trauma. For example, the edentulous mandible may be severely atrophic in older patients (sometimes less than 10 mm height). Thus, mastication forces can lead to fracture.
- *Impacted*: One fragment is firmly impacted into another. For example, the zygomatic complex may be impacted after trauma.

Anatomic site of the fracture

The anatomic location should also be taken into account when describing the fracture. This is especially important when a fracture must be classified for description, for example as a Le Fort-type fracture (see following paragraphs).

MANDIBLE FRACTURES

Mandible fractures are often combined direct and indirect fractures (Box 54.5). The direct fractures are mainly found in the anterior mandible (including symphysis and parasymphysis). These fracture lines are anterior to the mental nerve foramina or go through the foramen. A step in the occlusion between the canine and the first premolar may be a clinically visible sign. If you detect a direct fracture around the canine or the premolar region, there will often be an indirect condylar fracture (or angle fracture) on the opposite side (Fig. 54.5).[5] Classical anatomic sites of mandibular fracture lines are described in Figs 54.6 and 54.7.[5]

BOX 54.5: Important clinical signs for mandibular fracture

- Step in occlusion with ruptured attached gingiva (often in canine/premolar region)
- Malocclusion with deviation or frontal open-bite situation (frontal non-occlusion)
- Haematoma on floor of mouth

Required plain radiographs

1. Panoramic view (orthopantomography)
2. Intraoral occlusal film
3. Posterior anterior projection of mandible with opened mouth (Clementschisch's view) to detect condylar fractures

Midfacial fractures 473

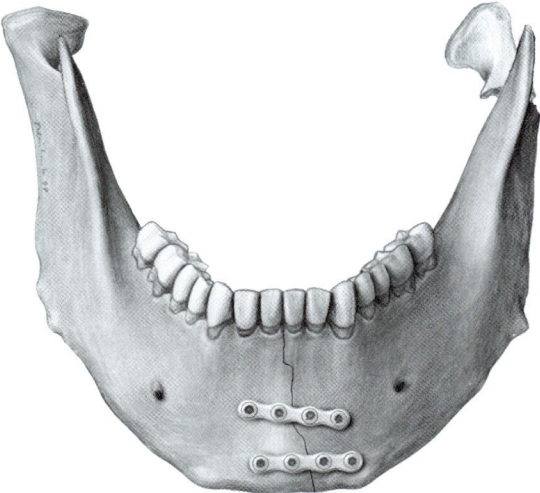

Figure 54.5 A direct fracture next to the midline of the mandible or in the canine/premolar region is often associated with an indirect fracture of the condylar process (here the patient's left condyle). Therefore, always check for an additional indirect fracture of the condylar necks when you diagnose a fracture in the anterior mandible! Here two osteosynthesis plates have already been placed in the preferred biomechanical positions. Image copyright Andreas Reinhardt and Franz Haerle. Reproduced from ref. 21 with permission from the artists and Thieme Medical Publishers, Inc.

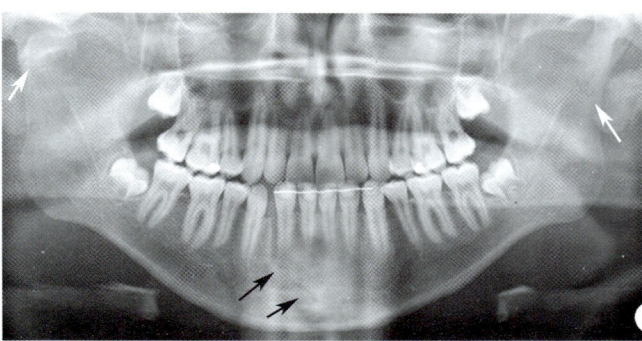

Figure 54.6 Combined direct and indirect mandibular fractures frequently occur. Panoramic view illustrating a direct anterior parasymphyseal fracture (black arrows) of the anterior mandible and indirect bilateral condylar neck fractures (white arrows). Clementschisch's view and a mandibular occlusal film are suggested additional radiographic planes.

MIDFACIAL FRACTURES

The classification of midfacial fractures is mainly based on the classification of two French surgeons.[14] In 1886 the Parisian Alphonse Guerin[15] described fractures of the dentate area of the maxilla without displacement, a special condition still bearing his name today. In 1901 René Le Fort from Lille investigated fracture patterns of the facial skeleton from 35 cadaver skulls that he subjected to a variety of traumas and subsequently dissected.[16] Thus, he identified the innate lines of weakness of the midfacial bone that form typical fracture patterns known as Le Fort I, II and III (Fig. 54.8) fracture levels today. Important clinical signs for Le Fort fractures can be found in Box 54.6. However, the Le Fort classification does not take into account any degree of comminution or displacement. In high-energy trauma other fracture lines, especially in the

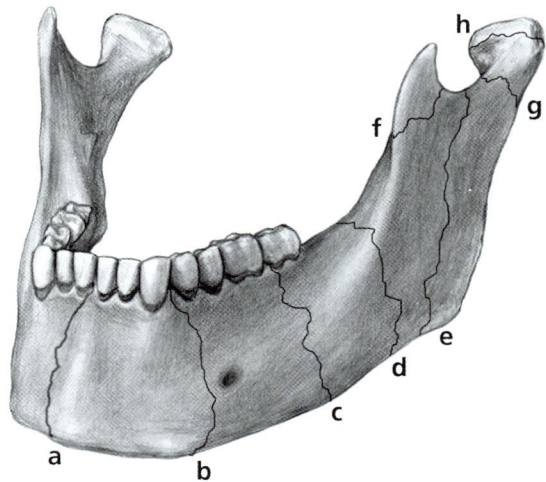

Figure 54.7 Anatomic sites of mandibular fractures. (a) Midline (symphysis); (b) parasymphysis; (c) body (behind the mental foramen and anterior to the masseter muscle); (d) angle (posterior to the anterior masseter line and inferior to the mandibular foramen); (e) ramus; (f) coronoid; (g) condylar; (h) intracapsular of the temporomandibular joint. Image copyright Andreas Reinhardt and Franz Haerle. Reproduced from ref. 21 with permission from the artists and Thieme Medical Publishers, Inc.

> **BOX 54.6: Important clinical signs for Le Fort fractures**
>
> - Unstable maxilla/midface
> - Malocclusion with deviation or frontal open-bite situation (non-occlusion)
> - Hollow sound when clicking on upper teeth
> - Raccoon sign (Le Fort II and III)
> - Blood in maxillary sinus (haematosinus) on radiographs (Le Fort I and II, often also in Le Fort III)
> - Unstable nasal bridge (Le Fort II and III)
> - Tangible steps along: zygomatic maxillary buttress (Le Fort I and II), infraorbital rims (Le Fort II), lateral orbital rims (Le Fort III)
> - Impaired eyeball motion (Le Fort II and III)
>
> Required plain radiographs (CT scan in axial and coronal planes is preferred when available)
>
> 1. Occipitomental projection
> 2. Axial view of zygomatic arch
> 3. Panoramic view (orthopantomography)

naso-ethmoid complex, with severe displacement of fragments may appear. To give you an internationally well-accepted tool to describe midface fractures the following paragraphs may act as common all-purpose classifications. More distinct descriptions may be used by specialized maxillofacial surgeons, but may be less useful in general communication.

Le Fort I fracture

The Le Fort I fracture level (horizontal) describes the separation of the complete maxilla from the rest of the midfacial skeleton (Fig. 54.8a). Le Fort I fractures may result from a force of injury directed low on the maxillary alveolar rim in a downward direction. The fracture extends from the nasal septum to the lateral pyriform rims, travels horizontally above the teeth apices, crosses below the zygomaticomaxillary junction and traverses the pterygomaxillary junction to interrupt the pterygoid plates.[17]

Le Fort II fracture

The Le Fort II fracture level (pyramidal) describes the separation of the maxilla together with the medial face complex up to the nasal bridge from the rest of the midfacial skeleton, thus forming a pyramidal shape (Fig. 54.8b). A Le Fort II fracture may be the result of a blow to the lower or mid-maxilla. The fracture pattern extends from the nasal bridge at or below the nasofrontal suture through the frontal processes of the maxilla, inferolaterally through the lacrimal bones and inferior orbital floor and rim through or near the inferior orbital foramen, and inferiorly through the anterior wall of the maxillary sinus; it then travels under the zygoma, across the pterygomaxillary fissure and through the pterygoid plates.[17]

Le Fort III fracture

The Le Fort III fracture level (transversal) describes the complete separation of the midfacial skeleton from the neurocranium (Fig. 54.8c). Le Fort III fractures, also termed craniofacial disjunctions, may follow impact to the nasal bridge or upper maxilla. These fractures start at the nasofrontal and frontomaxillary sutures and extend posteriorly along the medial wall of the orbit through the nasolacrimal groove and ethmoid bones. The thicker sphenoid bone posteriorly usually prevents continuation of the fracture into the optic canal. Instead, the fracture continues along the floor of the orbit along the inferior orbital fissure and continues superolaterally through the lateral orbital wall, through the zygomaticofrontal junction and the zygomatic arch. Intranasally, a branch of the fracture extends through the base of the perpendicular plate of the ethmoid, through the vomer and through the interface of the pterygoid plates to the base of the sphenoid.[17]

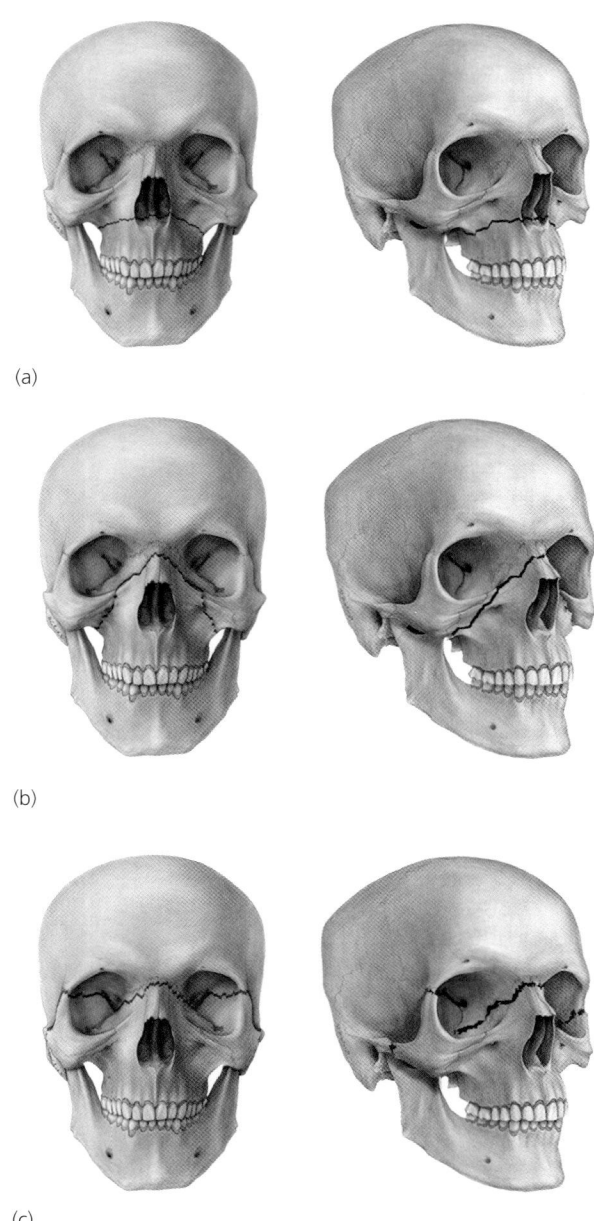

(a)

(b)

(c)

Figure 54.8 Le Fort fracture classification: the Le Fort fracture lines represent inherent lines of weakness in the midfacial skeleton. (a) Le Fort I fracture; (b) Le Fort II fracture; (c) Le Fort III fracture. Images (b) and (c) copyright Andreas Reinhardt and Franz Haerle. Reproduced from ref. 21 with permission from the artists and Thieme Medical Publishers, Inc.

Zygoma fractures

The integrity of the zygoma and its related anatomical structures is important in the maintenance of normal facial width and prominence of the cheek. The zygoma also constitutes the anterior orbital floor and forms a major part of the maxillary sinus. In addition, by making up the anterior lateral floor, it is a major contributor to the orbit.[18,19]

Zygoma fractures are often called 'tripod' fractures in clinical language, even though from a frontal view the zygoma can be seen to articulate with four bones. Superiorly the zygoma is connected to the frontal bone at the lateral orbital rim, medially by the maxilla and posteriorly by the greater wing of the sphenoid bone within the orbit. From a lateral view, the temporal process of the zygoma fuses with the zygomatic process of the temporal bone to form the zygomatic arch. If you only focus on the maxillary base, the lateral orbital rim and the zygomatic arch, the zygomatic corpus is placed on these three pods (tripod).

Fracture lines in a sole zygoma fracture typically run from the maxillary sinus walls through the infraorbital rim, involve the orbital floor and extend to the inferior orbital fissure (Fig. 54.9). The fracture line then continues to the zygomatic sphenoid suture area and on to the frontozygomatic suture line.[18,19] The zygomatic arch is always fractured, which may lead to dysfunction of the underlying temporal muscle, so that mouth opening is impaired. Note that all zygomatic complex fractures involve the orbit, making visual complications such as diplopia a frequent occurrence as the inferior rectus muscle of the eyebulb is often incarcerated in the fracture gaps (Box 54.7). A retrobulbar haematoma is a severe complication in a zygoma fracture (Box 54.3) and often leads to blindness in that eye.

The intraorbital branch of the fifth cranial nerve runs within the orbital floor. Thus fractures of the orbital floor often cause paraesthesia in the infraorbital region and cheek on the compromised side. Maxillary teeth may also be numb on that side. But note that zygoma fractures never involve the dentate maxilla, so that malocclusion is not evident in a sole zygomatic fracture (Fig. 54.9).

Other clinical signs for zygoma fractures are a monocle haematoma (black eye), especially when it is associated with emphysema of the eyelids (Fig. 54.1a). The fracture lines in the orbital floor and maxillary sinus walls often lead to a haematosinus, which is a clearly visible indirect fracture sign on radiographs (Fig. 54.10). The occipitomental

BOX 54.7: Important clinical signs for zygoma fractures

- Monocle haematoma (often together with emphysema)
- Diplopia
- Paraesthesia along infraorbital nerve
- Impaired mouth opening
- Haematosinus and hanging drop sign (radiograph)

Required plain radiographs (CT scan is preferred when available)

1. Occipitomental cranial projection
2. Submental vertical projection (SMV view)
3. Panoramic view

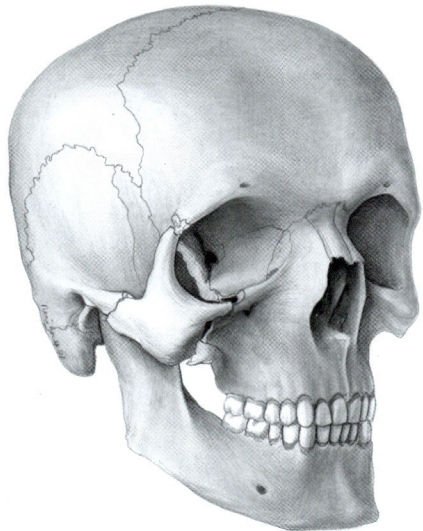

Figure 54.9 Zygoma fracture of the right lateral midface, which always involves the orbit. Image copyright Andreas Reinhardt and Franz Haerle. Reproduced from ref. 21 with permission from the artists and Thieme Medical Publishers, Inc.

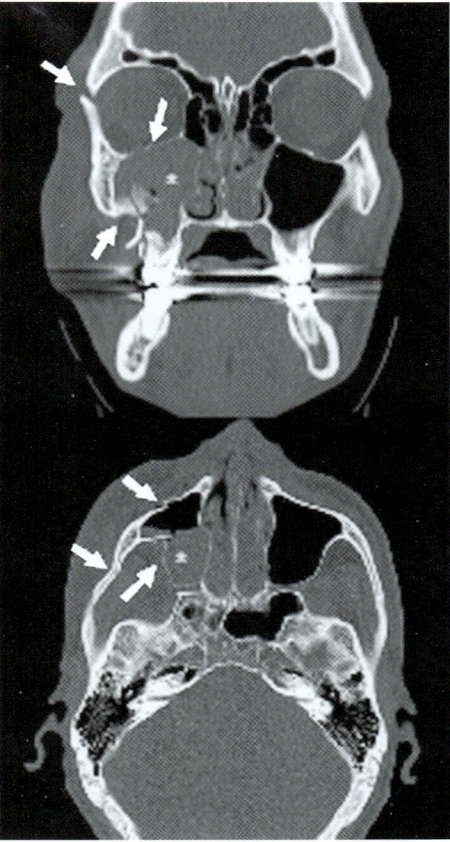

Figure 54.10 CT scans of the midface showing a right zygomatic fracture. Typical fracture lines (arrows) can be identified. Note the unilateral haematosinus (*) that is often detectable and an indirect sign for zygomatic fractures.

projection of the skull is a good radiographical plane to detect fracture lines in the intra-orbital rim, lateral orbital rim and zygomaticomaxillary buttress. Besides a haematosinus a prolapse of incarcerated orbital soft tissue hanging from the orbital floor into the maxillary sinus may be visible ('hanging drop sign') (Fig. 54.11). A submental vertical radiographic projection (SMV view) as a second plane will show fractures of the zygomatic arch.

Reduction and fixation of midfacial and mandibular fractures

In facial skeletal fractures the goal of fracture treatment is reduction and fixation of unstable fracture segments. This simple general concept in surgical fracture treatment becomes increasingly complex in patients with extensive or panfacial fractures.

In particular, besides the integrity of the support bolsters of the facial skeleton, the midfacial height and projection, especially the correct dental occlusion needs to be renormalized. Even minimal changes in the dental occlusion lead to discomfort and masticatory dysfunction in the patient. Thus, occlusion is the first base when attempting correct fixation of fracture segments. Once the proper occlusal plane is restored, definitive reduction and fixation of the fractures may be undertaken.

Fractures of the midface are often overlooked in polytrauma patients, if typical fracture signs are not obvious or other injuries distract the examiner. In general, midfacial fractures are treated surgically if they produce malocclusion, enophthalmos, diplopia, infraorbital nerve anaesthesia or unacceptable aesthetic deformity. Surgical treatment usually consists of internal stabilization using mini/microplate and screw osteosynthesis. Low-profile non-compression titanium plates secured with monocortical self-tapping screws are preferred. Accurate contouring of the plates is essential for precise reduction and fixation. Plates must be positioned in areas of robust bone (i.e. buttresses). All plates and screws are usually removed in a second surgical procedure after 4–6 months. However, discussion of whether metal removal is necessary is ongoing.

Open reduction and osteosynthesis can often be delayed until swelling decreases, particularly if the indication for surgery is not clear or if other life-threatening injuries have to be treated first. Anticoagulation medication of the patient may also delay surgery, especially when the orbit is involved. To reduce the risk of retrobulbar haemorrhage it may be important to change anticoagulation therapy until surgery is performed. If malocclusion is present and surgery must be delayed, it is important to insert a maxillo-mandibular fixation (wiring the teeth to keep the jaw shut) to stabilize the segments until surgery (Fig. 54.12) to prevent infection. In edentulous jaws the dental prostheses can be reinserted to find the occlusion position and the jaws can be fixed via inserted screw-hooks and elastic rubber bands.[14]

Mandible fracture treatment

For a simple fractured mandible or simple Le Fort I maxillary fracture, treatment ranges from a conservative maxillomandibular fixation alone to restore the occlusal

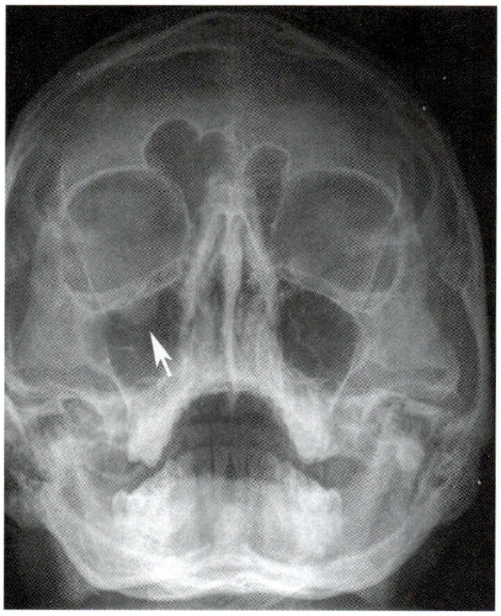

Figure 54.11 'Hanging drop' sign (occipitomental view): if a haematosinus is not visible an orbital floor fracture might also be identified by incarcerated soft tissue prolapsing into the sinus mimicking a hanging drop (arrow).

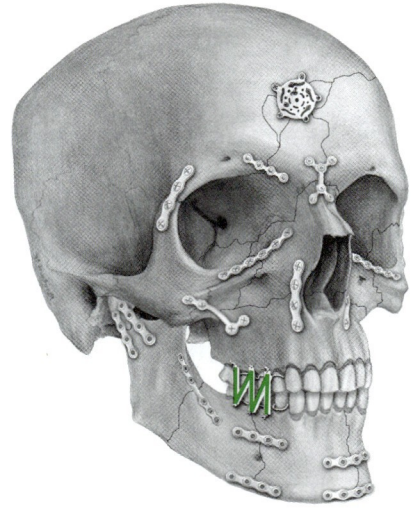

Figure 54.12 Placing of mini- and microplates along typical fractures lines respecting biomechanically favourable positions. The correct occlusion position is found through dental wiring combined with intermaxillary elastics (green). Image copyright Andreas Reinhardt and Franz Haerle. Reproduced from ref. 21 with permission from the artists and Thieme Medical Publishers, Inc.

plane up to an open reduction and stable osteosynthesis, or both.

To perform maxillomandibular fixation, metal bars (arch bars) are wired to the buccal surface of the upper and lower teeth and then connected to each other after correct occlusion has been established. For intermaxillary connection multiple elastic rubber bands or wires can be used. A more elegant method is the insertion of tiny ligatures around the premolars and first molars (Stout–Obwegeser ligatures).[14] These can be connected by elastics or wires (Fig. 54.12). Fixation may need to last up to 6 weeks if no osteosynthesis is performed. Also, in cases of open reduction a maxillomandibular fixation shall be made to find the correct occlusion before plates are inserted. All metal bars and wiring can be removed at the end of surgery.

Exposure of mandible bone and fracture lines is performed via a marginal, submarginal or alveolar rim mucosal incision. Preparation is performed subperiosteally with special attention to the mental nerves. The fracture line must be exposed completely on the vestibular side. In the dentate parts of the mandible, two parallel miniplates below the dental roots are preferred. A single plate is sufficient in the jaw angle (Fig. 54.12).

Patients with maxillomandibular fixation should permanently carry wire cutters for reopening in case of emergency. Food consumption is restricted to liquids or puréed foods. Tooth brushing is reduced, especially when full metal arch bars have been inserted. To control plaque formation and to prevent infection and halitosis, mouth rinses with chlorhexidine 0.1% can be used two or three times a day.

Simple condylar fractures may require only 2 weeks of maxillomandibular fixation, followed by a soft diet and physiotherapy. Severely displaced condyles with over 15° of displacement from the ramus axis or fractures in the lower and mid-section areas of the ramus may require open reduction and osteosynthesis for a better functional outcome. Two miniplates are preferred for fixation of a condylar fracture (Fig. 54.12).

Condylar fractures in children should not be rigidly immobilized because ankylosis and abnormal facial development may result. Flexible elastic maxillomandibular fixation over 1 week is often sufficient followed by orthodontic apparatuses.

Le Fort I fracture treatment

For stable, non-displaced Le Fort I fractures, 6 weeks of maxillomandibular fixation alone may be sufficient to allow for correct reduction (see 'Mandible fractures' section). Unstable fractures require an osteosynthesis, which has the advantage of early removal of metal bars and wiring. Exposure of the maxillary bone and fracture lines is performed via a marginal, submarginal or alveolar rim mucosal incision. Preparation is performed below the periosteum up to the infraorbital nerves. Disimpaction forceps may be used for reduction. Four miniplates are required in the Le Fort I plane. Before plating the maxillomandibular fixation to reconstruct, the occlusal plane must be in position. Plates are placed along the zygomaticomaxillary buttress and next to the nasal apertura piriformis on the nasomaxillary buttress (Fig. 54.12).

Le Fort II fracture treatment

Exactly as for Le Fort I fractures, disimpaction, maxillomandibular fixation, intraoral incisions and exposure of maxillary bone and fracture lines are performed. The fracture lines along the inferior orbital rims are displayed via subciliary or transconjunctival incisions. Disimpaction can be achieved with disimpaction forceps, but with careful attention to the nasolacrimal duct, inferior orbital nerve and extraocular muscles, which may be involved in middle and high maxillary fractures. Always perform maxillomandibular fixation prior to plate insertion. In general, the pyramidal midfacial segment is stabilized to the intact zygoma along the zygomaticomaxillary buttress and at the inferior orbital rim. Thinner microplates instead of miniplates are preferred at the inferior orbital rim (Fig. 54.12).[14] In severely displaced orbital floor fractures resorbable PDS foils might be an option to reconstruct the orbital walls.

Le Fort III fracture treatment

The occlusal plane of the stable mandible and the cranium lead the way for correct reduction of a Le Fort III fracture. Disimpaction can be performed with disimpaction forceps followed by maxillomandibular fixation. In some cases with only minor or no displacement a simple maxillomandibular fixation over 6 weeks is sufficient.

In open reduction, fracture lines along the inferior orbital rims and orbital floor are displayed via subciliary or transconjunctival incisions. Lateral brow or upper eyelid incisions or bicoronal scalp flaps may be used additionally for exposure to the frontozygomatic buttress and the glabellar nasal base.[14] Miniplates are placed on the lateral orbital rim or frontozygomatic buttress, whereas smaller microplates are used at the inferior orbital rim and the frontonasal base (X-shaped plate). In severely displaced orbital walls resorbable polydioxanone (PDS) foils may be used to reconstruct the orbit in primary surgery.

Zygoma fracture treatment

Zygoma fractures do not involve the dentate maxilla. Thus, no malocclusion is evident and no maxillomandibular fixation necessary. Disimpaction can be achieved through a percutaneous hook placed below the zygomatic buttress. The zygoma complex can be manually repositioned when pulling outwards.[14] In other techniques a retractor can be placed below the zygomatic arch via a superior auricular incision.[14] In some cases the zygoma is stable after simple repositioning and no further osteosynthesis is required. If the zygoma is unstable or severely displaced an open reduction is performed. The inferior orbital rim is exposed through a subciliary or transconjunctival incision, whereas the lateral orbital rim is displayed via a lateral brow or upper eyelid incision. A miniplate is placed on the lateral orbital rim and a microplate on the inferior orbital rim. In comminuted zygoma fractures an additional third miniplate may be placed on the zygomaticomaxillary buttress (Fig. 54.12).[14] In displaced orbital floor fractures resorbable PDS foils may be used to reconstruct the orbit.

CLASSIFICATION OF SKULL FRACTURES

Skull fractures affect the neurocranium, which envelops the brain, and are not classified as maxillofacial skeletal fractures, even though skull fractures may communicate with maxillofacial fractures in severely injured patients. Thus, skull fractures are normally treated by neurosurgeons. Maxillofacial or mandible fractures go to maxillofacial surgeons. A basic overview of skull fractures and their typical signs important for orthopaedic surgeons is discussed in the following paragraphs. (For further reading and more detailed classification see Qureshi et al.[19])

The brain is an exceptionally fragile organ surrounded by CSF, enclosed in a meningeal covering and protected inside the skull. CSF plays a key role in coup and contrecoup injuries to the brain.[19] A blow to a stationary but moveable head causes acceleration, and the brain floating in CSF lags behind, sustaining an injury directly underneath the point of impact (coup injury). When a moving head hits the floor, sudden deceleration results in an injury to the brain on the opposite side (contrecoup injury).[19]

The skull has several condensed areas, such as the mastoid processes, the glabella, the external occipital protuberance and the external angular process. The skull is joined by three arches on either side.[19]

The skull vault is composed of cancellous bone (diploë) sandwiched between two tablets, the lamina externa (1.5 mm) and the lamina interna (0.5 mm).[19]

Fractures of the skull may also follow typical patterns at certain anatomic sites. The thin squamous temporal and parietal bones over the temples and the sphenoid sinus, the foramen magnum, the petrous temporal ridge, and the inner parts of the sphenoid wings at the skull base are often included in the fracture lines. The middle cranial fossa is the weakest area, because of thin bones and several foramina. Other sites prone to fracture include the cribriform plate and the roof of orbits in the anterior cranial fossa and the areas between the mastoid and dural sinuses in the posterior cranial fossa.[19]

Skull fractures can be roughly classified as linear or depressed.[19] Simple linear fracture is by far the most common type of fracture, especially in children younger than 5 years. Temporal bone fractures represent 15–48% of all skull fractures. Basilar skull fractures represent 19–21% of all skull fractures. Depressed fractures are frontoparietal (75%), temporal (10%), occipital (5%) and other (10%). Most of the depressed fractures are open fractures (75–90%).[19]

Linear skull fractures

Low-energy or blunt trauma over a broad plane of the skull may result in linear fractures. These fractures are often without consequence. Patients with uncritical linear skull fractures are frequently clinically asymptomatic. Often only swelling occurs at the site of impact, and the skin may or may not be ruptured. But linear fractures could possibly cause significant problems when they run through vascular foramina, the venous sinus grooves or a suture. Under these circumstances severe epidural haematoma, venous sinus thrombosis and occlusion or sutural diastasis may develop and a neurosurgeon should be consulted.

Basilar fractures are at the base of the skull and are mostly linear fractures. They are regularly associated with a dural tear.[19] The majority of linear skull base fractures run into the temporal bone. It is important to subdivide temporal basilar fractures into petrous and non-petrous fractures; the latter include fractures that involve mastoid air cells. These fractures do not present with cranial nerve deficits.[19]

Patients with petrous temporal bone fractures may present with CSF otorrhoea and bruising over the mastoids. Anterior cranial fossa fractures are often associated with midfacial fractures and could result in CSF rhinorrhoea. Loss of consciousness and Glasgow Coma Scale score may vary depending on an associated intracranial pathological condition. Longitudinal temporal bone fractures can result in conductive deafness of greater than 30 dB due to ossicular chain disruption. Deafness lasts longer than 6 weeks. Temporary deafness that resolves in less than 3 weeks is due to haemotympanum and mucosal oedema in the middle ear fossa. Facial palsy, nystagmus and facial numbness are secondary to involvement of the seventh, sixth and fifth cranial nerves, respectively. Transverse temporal bone fractures involve the eighth cranial nerve and the labyrinth, resulting in nystagmus, ataxia and permanent neural hearing loss.[19]

Depressed skull fractures

High-energy trauma to a small surface area of the skull often causes depressed skull fractures (e.g. blow with a hammer). Comminution of fragments starts from the point of maximum impact and spreads centrifugally.[19] Bone fragments should be depressed greater than the adjacent inner table of the skull to be of clinical significance, requiring operation and elevation.[19] Neurological signs such as loss of consciousness and reduced Glasgow Coma Scale score are more frequent in depressed fractures and may vary depending on other associated intracranial injuries such as epidural haematoma, dural tears and seizures. Open fractures may be identified by skin lacerations above the fracture and often lead to contamination. Fractures running through the orbit, the paranasal sinuses and middle ear structures can also produce an open fracture, when air enters the cranial cavity. In these situations trapped air is detectable between the fractured bones and the brain silhouette on CT scans. Consultation with a neurosurgeon is important.

If a skull fracture is suspected or cannot be ruled out radiographic examination must be performed. A posterior–anterior and lateral cranial view of the skull gives a first impression. A CT scan is the preferred option. In plain radiographs the distinction between fracture lines and sutures may be difficult for the inexperienced viewer. The differences according to Qureshi et al.[19] are summarized in Box 54.8.

Surgical treatment

The role of surgery is limited in the management of skull fractures. Adults with simple linear skull fractures and absence of neurological symptoms may not require any intervention at all. Infants with simple linear fractures need at least overnight observation regardless of neurological status.[19] Surgery is often not necessary, but treatment decisions should be made according to a neurosurgeon's advice.

Uncomplicated depressed fractures in neurologically intact infants often heal well and smooth out with time, without elevation or surgical intervention.[19] Problematical open depressed fractures in infants and children must be forwarded to a neurosurgeon as surgical intervention is required.

Many neurosurgeons favour elevation of depressed skull fractures if the displaced segment is more than 5 mm below the inner table of the adjacent fracture segments.[19]

Open fractures with severe contamination, dural tear, trapped intracranial air (pneumocephalus), intracranial haematoma or unstable occipital condylar spine fracture require immediate surgical treatment.[20] Another indication for surgical treatment is a persistent CSF leak. An atlantoaxial arthrodesis can be attained with an inside–outside fixation.

Craniectomy with resection of skull segments is performed if the underlying brain is damaged and swollen. In these instances, cranioplasty is required at a later date.[19]

REFERENCES

- ● = Key primary paper
- ◆ = Major review article

◆1. Pfeifer R, Pape HC. Missed injuries in trauma patients: A literature review. *Patient Safety in Surgery* 2008;**2**:20.
2. McCaig LF, Ly N. National Hospital Ambulatory Medical Care Survey: 2000 emergency department summary. *Advance Data* 2002;**327**:1–27.
3. Lin S, Levin L, Goldman S, Sela G. Dento-alveolar and maxillofacial injuries: a 5-year multi-center study. Part 2: severity and location. *Dental Traumatology* 2008;**24**:56–8.
4. Oikarinen VJ, Lindqvist C. The frequency of facial bone fractures in patients with multiple injuries sustained in traffic accidents. *Proceedings of the Finnish Dental Society* 1975;**71**:53–7.
5. Paatsama J, Suuronen R, Lindqvist C. Establishing a clinical diagnosis and surgical treatment plan. In: Booth PW, Schendel S, Hausamen J-E (eds) *Maxillofacial Surgery*. St Louis, MO: Churchill Livingstone, 1999.
6. Turner K, Jones A, Handa A. Emergency management of head injuries. *Student BMJ* 2000;**8**:131–74.
7. The British Society of Rehabilitation Medicine. *Rehabilitation after Traumatic Brain injury*. London, UK: British Society of Rehabilitation Medicine, 1998.
8. Royal College of Surgeons of England. *Report of the Working Party on the Management of Patients with Head Injuries*. London, UK: Royal College of Surgeons of England, 1999.
●9. Bowley NB. Radiology for maxillofacial trauma. In: Booth PW, Schendel S, Hausamen J-E (eds) *Maxillofacial Surgery*. St Louis, MO: Churchill Livingstone, 1999.
10. Haydel MJ, Preston CA, Mills TJ, et al. Indications for computed tomography in patients with minor head injury. *New England Journal of Medicine* 2000;**343**:100–5.
11. Harley BJ, Beaupre LA, Jones CA, et al. The effect of time to definitive treatment on the rate of nonunion and infection in open fractures. *Journal of Orthopaedic Trauma* 2002; **16**:484–90.
12. Teltzrow T, Kramer FJ, Schulze A, et al. Perioperative complications following sagittal split osteotomy of the mandible. *Journal of Craniomaxillofacial Surgery* 2005;**33**:307–13.
13. Warnke PH, Springer IN, Russo PA, et al. Innate immunity in human bone. *Bone* 2006;**38**:400–8.
●14. Härle F. Surgical management of maxillary fractures. In: Booth PW, Schendel S, Hausamen J-E (eds) *Maxillofacial Surgery*. St Louis, MO: Churchill Livingstone, 1999.

BOX 54.8: Differences between skull fractures and sutures on plain radiographs (e.g. posteroanterior and lateral cranial view)

Fractures
- Greater than 3 mm in width
- Widest at the centre and narrow at the end
- Run through both the outer and the inner lamina of bone, hence appear darker
- Usually over temporoparietal area
- Usually run in a straight line
- Angular turns

Sutures
- Less than 2 mm in width
- Same width throughout
- Lighter on radiographs than fracture lines
- At specific anatomic sites
- Do not run in a straight line
- Curvaceous

Qureshi et al.[19]

- 15. Guérin A. Des fractures du maxillaire superieur. *Archives Géneraux de Médicine* 1886;**6**:5–13.
- 16. Le Fort R. Etude expérimentale sur les fractures de la máchoire supérieure. *Revue Chirurgique de Paris* 1901;**23**:208–27, 360–79, 479–507.
  17. Kim DW, Egan KK, Tawfilis AR, *et al.* Facial trauma, maxillary and Le Fort fractures. http://www.emedicine.com/plastic/TOPIC481.HTM
  18. Segal Z, McDonald WS, Thaller SR. Facial trauma, zygomatic complex fractures. http://www.emedicine.com/plastic/TOPIC531.HTM
♦ 19. Qureshi N, Harsh G 4th. Skull fractures. http://www.emedicine.com/med/TOPIC2894.HTM
  20. Pait TG, Al-Mefty O, Boop FA, *et al.* Inside-outside technique for posterior occipitocervical spine instrumentation and stabilization: preliminary results. *Journal of Neurosurgery* 1999;**90**(1 Suppl.):1–7.
- 21. Haerle F, Champy M, Terry B. *Atlas of Craniomaxillofacial Osteosynthesis: Microplates, Miniplates, and Screws.* Stuttgart, Germany: Thieme Publishing.

55

Paediatric fractures and dislocations

DORIEN SCHNEIDMUELLER, CHRISTOPH NAU, INGO MARZI

Introduction	481	Epiphyseal separation of the distal femur	495
Epidemiology of fractures in children	481	Osseous metaphyseal ligament ruptures	496
Skeletal development and fracture healing	482	Epiphyseal fractures of the distal femur	496
Characteristics of injuries to the immature skeleton	483	Epiphyseal fractures of the proximal tibia	496
Diagnosis	484	Avulsions of the tibial tuberosity	497
Treatment	485	Intercondylar eminence avulsions	497
Specific fracture types	486	Fractures of the patella	497
Distal humerus	488	Fractures of the proximal tibial metaphysis	498
Proximal forearm	490	Fractures of the tibial diaphysis	498
Forearm	491	Fractures of the ankle	498
Proximal femur	493	Fracture classifications	499
Diaphyseal femur	494	The multiply injured child	499
Distal femur	495	Further reading	502
Fractures around the knee	495		

NATIONAL BOARD STANDARDS

- Know the anatomy and growth of immature bones including remodelling
- Understand the physiology and biomechanics of bone remodelling in childhood
- Know the Salter–Harris classification of growth plate injuries and be able to relate the prognosis of injuries to the classification
- Know the specific features of the multiply injured child
- Know the indications for radiological imaging in the child, including CT and MRI
- Be able to spot children's fractures which may give rise to long term problems and manage appropriately
- Be aware of the legal framework related to child safeguarding and understand the statutory responsibilities of the orthopaedic surgeon
- Know the risk factors and specific injury patterns associated with non-accidental injuries

INTRODUCTION

Children are not just small adults. Differences in anatomy, physiology and biomechanics lead to different fracture patterns and different problems in diagnosis and therapeutic management compared to the adult.

EPIDEMIOLOGY OF FRACTURES IN CHILDREN

The knowledge of fracture incidence and age-specific distribution constitute the basis of adequate treatment and for developing accident prevention strategies. Paediatric trauma constitutes 13–32% of all registered injuries.

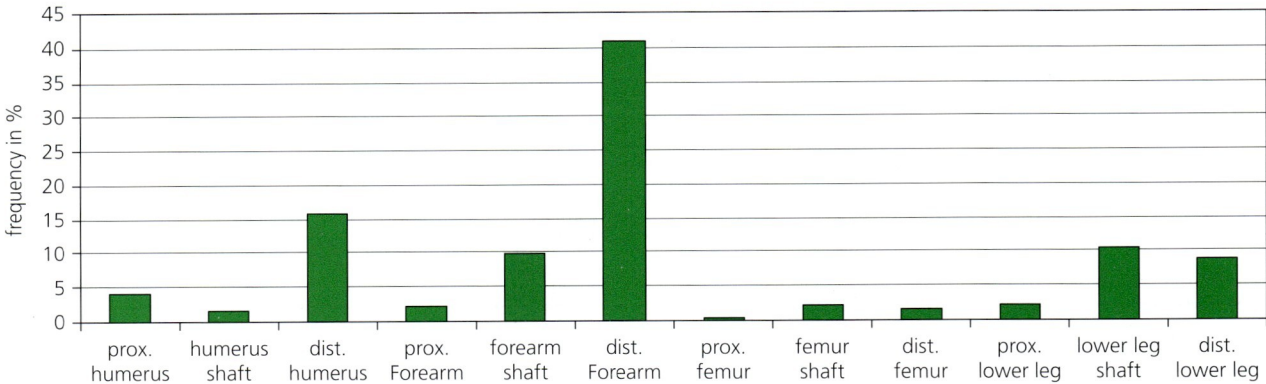

Figure 55.1 Distribution of the frequency of fractures of the long bones in children (n = 678).

Fractures constitute 10–25% of all injuries. During the last 50 years fracture incidence has increased with an increasing number of sports-related injuries and a broader spectrum of sports activities. Ninety per cent of all fractures occur at the extremities, whereas fractures of the trunk constitute only 10%. The risk of sustaining a fracture increases with age until approximately age 13 years. The overall annual incidence is about 21–25 fractures per 1000 children. Boys have a 1.2–1.6 higher risk to sustain a fracture than girls. While in younger children the proportion is nearly balanced, after the age of 8 years boys are disproportionately more often involved in accidents than girls. Fractures of the long bone in the upper extremity are observed two to three times more often than fractures in the lower extremity. The main area is the metaphysis with 65% followed by the diaphysis with 25%. Injuries of the epiphysis are less frequent with a rate of 10%. The predominating injury is fracture of the distal forearm, which constitutes nearly 25% of all fractures, followed by fractures of the hand. Considering the long bones, the most common injury is fracture of the distal radius (40%), followed by fractures of the distal humerus (16%), the tibial shaft (10%) and the distal tibia (9%) (Fig. 55.1). Significant patterns are observed: first, the fractures of the distal humerus in infants are mainly caused by playground accidents or at home; second, fractures of the lower leg in older children and adolescents are associated with a high rate of road traffic accidents; and, third, fractures of the distal forearm in all age groups are caused by sports-related trauma.

SKELETAL DEVELOPMENT AND FRACTURE HEALING

Bone development is from the physis, which is responsible for the longitudinal growth of the skeleton, and by the periosteal and endosteal system, which provides diameter growth (see Chapter 59).

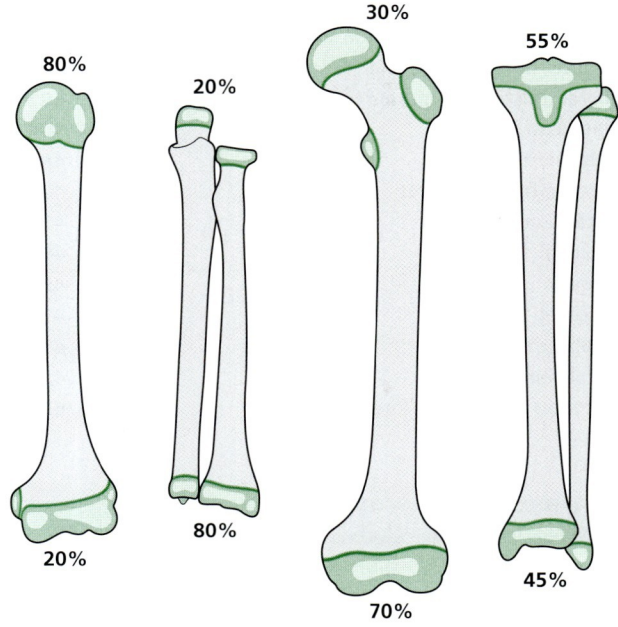

Figure 55.2 Percentage of the longitudinal growth of each physis of the long bone.

Periosteally mediated appositional bone formation with concomitant endosteal bone resorption leads to enlargement of the overall diameter of the long bones. This system provides fracture healing, remodelling of callus formations and post-traumatic deformities.

Longitudinal growth of the long bone takes place in the physis, although each physis has a different specific portion of the overall length of the particular long bone. Depending on gender and maturity of the skeleton, humoral and hormonal factors lead to closure of the physis in adolescents, and therefore to an end of longitudinal growth.

The contribution of each physis to longitudinal growth is different. The highest growth potential at the upper extremity is located at the proximal humerus and the distal forearm, whereas the physis located around the elbow only contributes to a small extent to longitudinal growth. The physis with the greatest part of the longitudinal growth at the lower extremity is located centrically around the knee joint, whereas the physis with the lowest growth potential is located at the proximal femur and the distal lower leg (Fig. 55.2) ('Towards the elbow I grow and away from the knee I flee').

CHARACTERISTICS OF INJURIES TO THE IMMATURE SKELETON

Metaphysis and diaphysis

BUCKLE FRACTURE

This fracture occurs in the area of the metaphysis where the bone offers the highest porosity.

GREENSTICK FRACTURES

A greenstick fracture occurs as a result of the bowing above the border of elasticity. The energy of the trauma is not sufficient to break the bone completely. It is characterized by a full fracture on one side with an intact opposite cortex. Because of the faster fracture healing and callus building of the opposite side, a danger of refracture exists in the diaphysis if fracture healing is absent in the area of the fracture gap (Fig. 55.3).

Epiphysis and physis

The physis separates the metaphysis from the epiphysis and is the area in which growth in length takes place. Please see Chapter 5 for a more complete description of the physis.

The Salter–Harris classification of the fractures of the physis is widely accepted worldwide.

This classification is easy to use and has a good prognostic value. One disadvantage is that it is difficult to distinguish Salter–Harris V fractures (rare) from Salter–Harris I fractures at initial presentation, and type V may progress to growth arrest later on. Fracture types I–V were described by Robert Salter and Robert Harris from Toronto in 1963 (Fig 55.4).

Type 1 is characterized by physeal separation; type II by a fracture that traverses the physis and exits through the metaphysis; type III by a fracture that traverses the physis before exiting through the epiphysis; and type IV by a fracture that traverses the epiphysis, physis and metaphysis. Type V describes a crush injury of the physis.

The mnemonic 'SALTR' can be used to help remember the first five types. This mnemonic requires the reader to imagine the bones as long bones, with the epiphyses at the base.

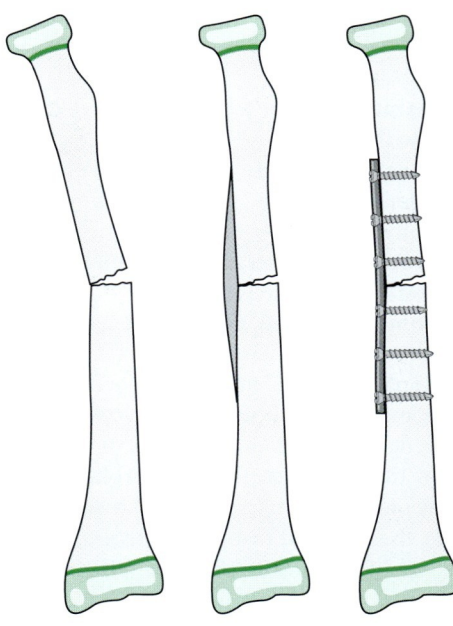

Figure 55.3 Development of a partial pseudarthrosis in a diaphyseal greenstick fracture: the faster callus formation on the convex side has a blocking effect similar to an incorrectly implanted plate osteosynthesis, so that equal fracture healing is not possible.

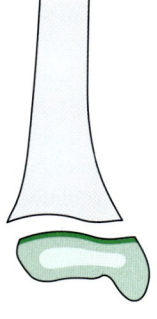 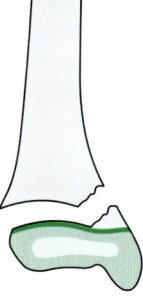 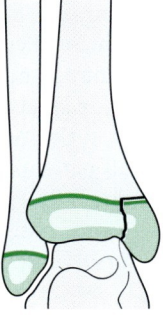 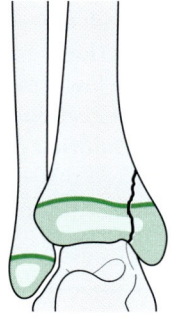

Salter-Harris I   Salter-Harris II   Salter-Harris III   Salter-Harris IV

Figure 55.4 Salter and Harris classification of fractures that included the physis. I, epiphyseal loosening; II, epiphyseal loosening with a metaphyseal wedge; III, epiphyseal fracture; IV, epiphyseal fracture with metaphyseal participation.

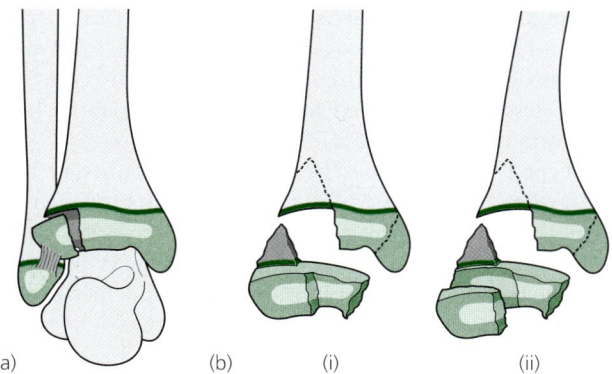

Figure 55.5 Transition fractures of the distal tibia. (a) Two-plane fracture/Tilleaux fracture: epiphyseal fracture in a physis already beginning to close. (b) Triplane fracture: epiphyseal fracture in a physis already beginning to close with a dorsal, metaphyseal (triplane I) or epimetaphyseal (triplane II) wedge.

I–S = **Separation**. Injury to the cartilage of the physis (growth plate).
II–A = **Above**. The fracture lies above the physis.
III–L = **Lower**. The fracture is below the physis in the epiphysis.
IV–T = **Through**. The fracture is through the metaphysis, physis and epiphysis.
V–R = **Rammed (crushed)**. The physis has been crushed.

Transitional fractures most often occur in the distal tibia; they can, however, also appear elsewhere. The affecting force deflects to the joint by means of the already ossified part of the physis, so that a ventrolateral epiphyseal fragment is produced analogous to an osseous syndesmosis rupture, the so-called *two-plane fracture*, which is related to the size of the closure of the physis that has already taken place. Additional torsional forces can lead to further dorsal fragments, corresponding to a Volkmann triangle, the so-called *tri-plane fracture* (Fig. 55.5). If the metaphyseal fracture line ends in the physis, it is called a tri-plane I or two-part fracture; if it runs through the metaphysis and epiphysis into the joint, it is called a tri-plane II or three-part fracture. Compared with fractures of a wide, open physis, the fracture line often runs oblique; the Salter–Harris III and IV injury is usually perpendicular to the physis, and mostly lies medial beyond the weight-bearing part of the joint, whereas a transitional fracture usually lies within the zone. Because of the low remaining growth potential of these children, reconstruction of the joint surface is the primary aim in these injuries; growth disorders are not usually expected in adolescents.

Dislocations

The frequency of dislocations rises with a decrease in ligament stability. Therefore, joint dislocations are mostly found in adolescents. They present as an emergency and should be brought back into the correct position as quickly as possible to minimize secondary damage.

Ligament injury

Bony ligament ruptures can often be found in children under 10 years old because of the high stability of the ligaments. They can occur inside as well as outside the articulation. Ruptures inside the ligament mostly appear in adolescents.
Common examples are:

- bony rupture of the anterior cruciate ligament; intercondylar eminence rupture
- rupture of the ulnar styloid process
- rupture of the volar plate at the fingers.

Osteochondral fractures

Osteochondral fragments can often be found in connection with joint dislocations at the distal femur, patella, head of the radius and the capitellum of the humerus. They can cause other problems such as a free joint body and should always be fixed, if possible, to reconstruct the joint surface. Small fragments can be removed.

Apophyseal injuries

Apophyseal separations can result from increasing muscular stress and hormonal influences, predominantly during adolescence. Most of these injuries are found in the elbow (ulnar epicondyle) and in the pelvis and femur (lesser and greater trochanter; anterior, inferior and superior iliac spine). They are not associated with the epiphysis joints and therefore they are not involved in longitudinal growth of the bone. Growth disturbances can, however, affect the shaping of the particular bones.

DIAGNOSIS

Clinical examination

The first part of the clinical investigation is the history, which identifies the site of the injury, the energy of the trauma and whether the trauma could have been caused by child abuse or pathological fractures.

A thorough inspection is followed by careful palpation; all patients should be given age-appropriate information about the procedure. The peripheral blood circulation, motor function and sensory function have to be evaluated in all cases.

More detailed functional tests are mostly unnecessary in the acute stage and can cause additional pain for the child.

Diagnostic imaging

Radiographic diagnosis represents a special challenge. Radiation exposure should always be strictly minimized and all possible means should be used to reduce the radiation dose. Because of the large portion of X-ray-permeable cartilage tissue and the characteristics of the ossification centres, knowledge of age-dependent diagnostic findings is essential for the examiner. Comparative images of the opposite side in the diagnosis of fresh injuries does not replace this knowledge and has been found to be inefficient and unnecessary. For the protection of the child, if surgery is indicated by the first radiograph, a second plane is unnecessary. If required, the second plane can be obtained intra-operatively under anaesthesia. For all other fractures, radiographs in two planes (anteroposterior and lateral), including the adjacent joint, are standard. Radiographs should be centred over the injury, and overview pictures in two planes should be avoided. In special cases, such as a transitional fracture, additional diagonal images are helpful.

Owing to the X-ray-permeable cartilage tissue, some injuries can only be recognized by an increased distance of the physis or a deviation of the adjoining bone. Additional imaging modalities are covered in Chapter 11.

TREATMENT

The aim of treatment is to achieve rapid healing of a fracture without complications, bearing in mind any related costs. Patients' needs and wishes can be taken into account with the knowledge of the growth prognosis and possibilities of complications. This is mainly relevant for the shaft; the nearer the fracture is to the joint, the more the treatment is determined by the fracture. Adequate pain therapy should always be included in the primary treatment. For example, splinting can be used for immobilization and/or pain relief prior to further diagnostic procedures.

Non-surgical treatment

It is the aim of the therapy to achieve fast fracture healing without complications

Adequate pain therapy should always belong to the primary therapy. Therefore, it may be necessary to accomplish splinting for immobilization and/or pain relief prior to further diagnostic procedures.

In a predominant number of cases, children's injuries can be treated adequately by conservative techniques. Usually immobilization, e.g. with a cast, is sufficient. At certain localizations, immobilization in small children takes place using special bandages, e.g. the Desault bandage at the proximal humerus, the backpack bandage at the clavicle.

CAST WEDGING

Axis deviations in the frontal and sagittal plane of the shaft can be corrected by cast wedging in a circular cast. It is predominantly indicated in distal forearm fractures and tibia shaft fractures with a malposition in the frontal and/or sagittal plane. It is usually performed 8 days after primary cast immobilization. The primary swelling should have reduced up to that point so that a secondary dislocation is not to be expected. Relative stability is given by the already generated callus, which reduces the pain; however, the remaining plastic deformability allows for correction of the malposition.

The main risk with this procedure is that the patient may develop a compression ulcer on the opposite side of the wedging. If pain occurs on the opposite side, a window can be cut out of the cast and additional cushioning can be used. See box 55.1 for technical advice.

> **BOX 55.1: T-cast wedging: key points**
>
> T-cast wedging is performed by hemicircular opening using a saw and successive extending. The wedge always has to be placed in the transverse section of the extremity at the concavity's deepest point of the axis deviation (Fig. 55.6). In fractures at the shaft's centre, the wedge is located directly over the fracture zone. The further distal the fracture is located the further proximal the wedging has to be placed to achieve an effective lever arm and to impact enough force on the distal fragment. If enough correction is achieved, the wedge will be filled, e.g. with cork and a new cast will be made.

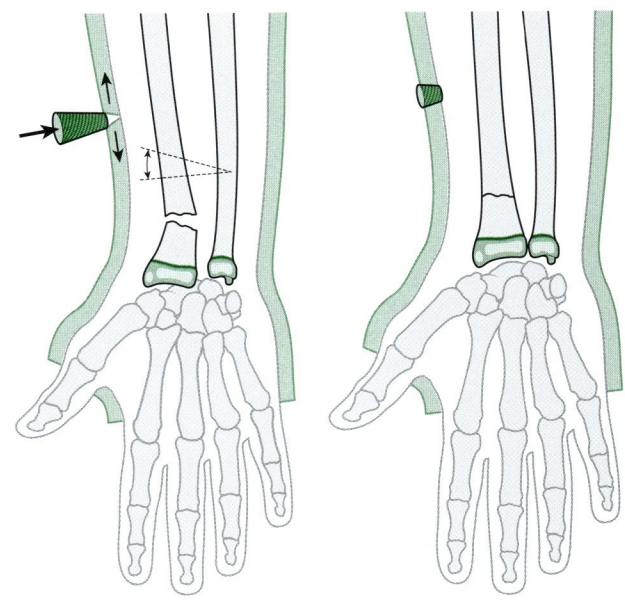

Figure 55.6 Cast wedging in the concavity of the dislocation.

TRACTION

Traction therapy, either traditional or gallows, plays a role in the treatment of femoral shaft fractures in infants. The disadvantages is the long period of immobilization.

A collar and cuff is used for a dynamic correction of a slightly dislocated humerus fracture. Adjustment of the bandage to gradually bring the elbow to the maximum possible acute-angle position, leads to slow correction of the malposition.

Surgical treatment

Completely dislocated or unstable fractures that cannot be converted into a stable fracture by closed reduction are an indication for surgery. The aim is to achieve a stable situation to avoid further reductions or changes in treatment. Factors such as further surgery (e.g. secondary removal of metal), costs, available resources and personal experience play a role in the choice of method of osteosynthesis.

Reduction

Dislocations have to be reduced. In order to avoid unnecessary pain and fear, this should be performed under general anaesthesia with a surgical team on standby that can proceed to open reduction if necessary. An open reduction should be performed in any joint fractures with a dislocation of the joint surface >2 mm, defect fractures and partial open fractures. Generally, the first reduction should be the only reduction. In fractures of the phalanxes with significant deviation, a reduction under local anaesthesia can be performed.

Surgical treatment concepts

- *Kirschner-wire osteosynthesis.* Wires can be placed percutaneously using a minimally invasive procedure. This is indicated in metaphyseal fractures It can also be used in epiphyseal fractures in small children or in patients with small fracture fragments. Removal of the percutaneously placed and above-skin wires can usually be performed without anaesthesia. However, immobilization with a cast is necessary to maintain stability. The disadvantages of this technique are that percutaneous, protruding wires should not be in direct contact with the cast; this can be prevented either by sufficient cushioning or by a cast-free zone.
- *Screw osteosynthesis.* This is especially indicated in joint fractures, since the fracture gap can be compressed, but it is also useful in joint separations with a sufficient metaphyseal wedge. Protection with a cast is usually necessary.
- *Elastic stable intramedullary nailing (ESIN).* This is a minimally invasive, movement- and partial load-stable procedure in the treatment of diaphyseal and metaphyseal shaft fractures. The principle of this procedure is based on three-point support with two pre-twisted flexible titanium nails inserted within the bone shaft. The ideal fracture is a diaphyseal transverse fracture, but diagonal and spiral fractures can also be treated by ESIN using the basic biomechanical principles. Examples include femur shaft fractures, forearm shaft fractures, proximal humerus fractures, radius neck fractures and supracondylar fractures.
- For other methods of fixation please refer to Chapter 19.

SPECIFIC FRACTURE TYPES

Proximal humerus

In the majority of cases, fractures of the proximal humerus mostly concern subcapital fractures followed by epiphyseal separations with or without a metaphyseal wedge. Epiphyseal injuries are rare. The peak age is between 11 and 12 years. Owing to the large growth potential of the proximal epiphysis joint, substantial angulation can be tolerated and left to spontaneous correction (Fig. 55.7). For children younger than 10 years, varus, either anteversion or retroversion, deviation up to 50° depending on the age of the patient and a valgus deviation up to 10° are the limits of tolerance; in children older than 10 years, these tolerance limits are 20° and 10° respectively. Treatment is usually conservative with immobilization in a Gilchrist or Desault bandage for 3–4 weeks. If the correction limits are exceeded, a reduction needs to be performed, which mostly can be achieved closed. If soft tissue is entrapped and impairs a proper reduction, an open procedure is required. The preferred osteosynthesis procedure is retrograde ESIN. Alternatively, a percutaneous K-wire osteosynthesis can be performed; however, this requires additional immobilization for 4 weeks until the wires are removed.

Diaphyseal humerus

Humerus shaft fractures usually arise as a result of birth trauma or in adolescence. The remodelling potential of humerus shaft fractures is clearly less than that of more proximal fractures. Nevertheless, malpositions can be adjusted because of the large functional compensation potential of the closely related shoulder joint. However, axis deviations greater than 10° often lead to a cosmetic impairment, so these should not be left. Side-to-side malpositions can be easily corrected and shortenings up to 2 cm can be tolerated. In all fractures within the correction limits, treatment is conservative by immobilization in a Gilchrist or a Desault bandage, if necessary followed by a brace. All other fractures can usually be reduced closed and stabilized by antegrade or retrograde ESIN.

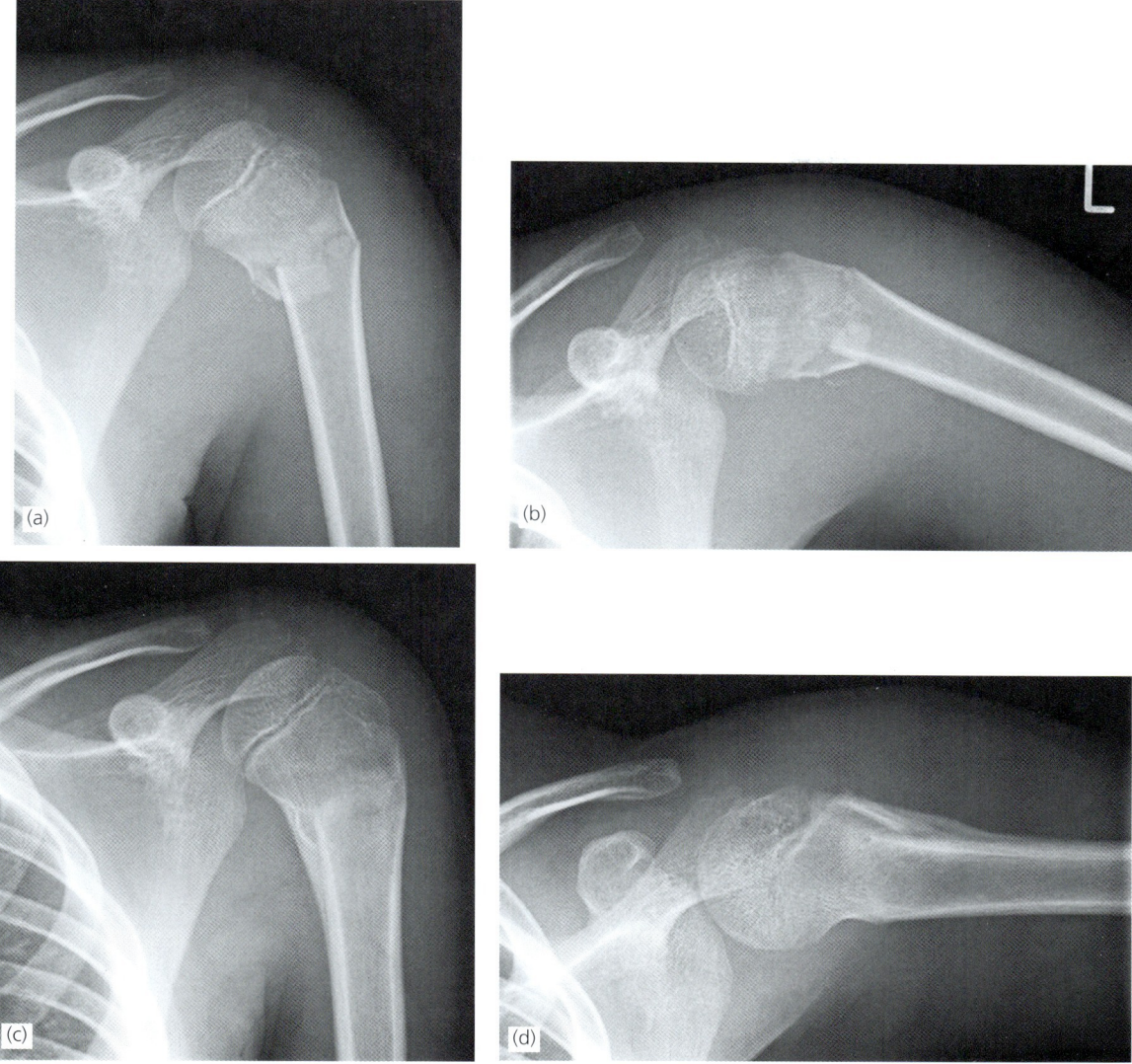

Figure 55.7 Conservative therapy of a proximal humerus fracture in a 12 year old. Development after 8 weeks with already beginning remodelling.

As an alternative method, external fixation can be used in multifragment fractures or those with extensive tissue damage; however, there is a higher risk of radial nerve injury. Birth trauma-related injuries also heal with complete remodelling, even with larger malpositions. In this case, pain therapy with an individually adapted bandage is indicated for a few days (Fig. 55.8).

Fractures around the elbow

In order to correctly identify fractures (or the lack thereof) in this area, it is important to know the order of appearance of centres of ossification around the elbow, and this can be remembered using the mnemonic CRITOL (Table 55.1)

In the distal humerus it is important to know that the anterior humeral line should run through the middle third of the capitellum on the true lateral radiograph, and also that the Baumann angle should be 78–85°. The Baumann angle is the angle subtended by a line perpendicular to the long axis of the humerus and a line along the lateral condylar physis and is used to assess the adequacy of supracondylar humerus fracture reduction in the coronal plane. Also the radius should be pointing at the capitellum in all views.

It is also important to be aware of the anterior and posterior fat pads in the supracondylar region, which are normally not visible on radiographs, but with fracture and resultant haematoma formation they are elevated and become visible on the lateral radiograph as radiolucent 'sails'; this is known as the fat pad sign, and with careful clinical correlation can signify an occult fracture in the distal humerus.

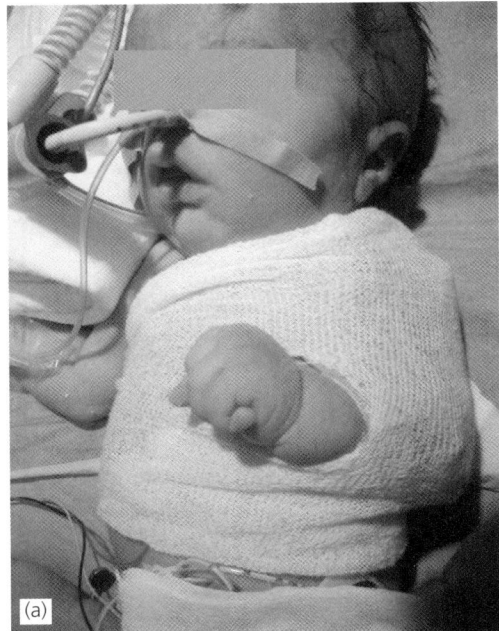
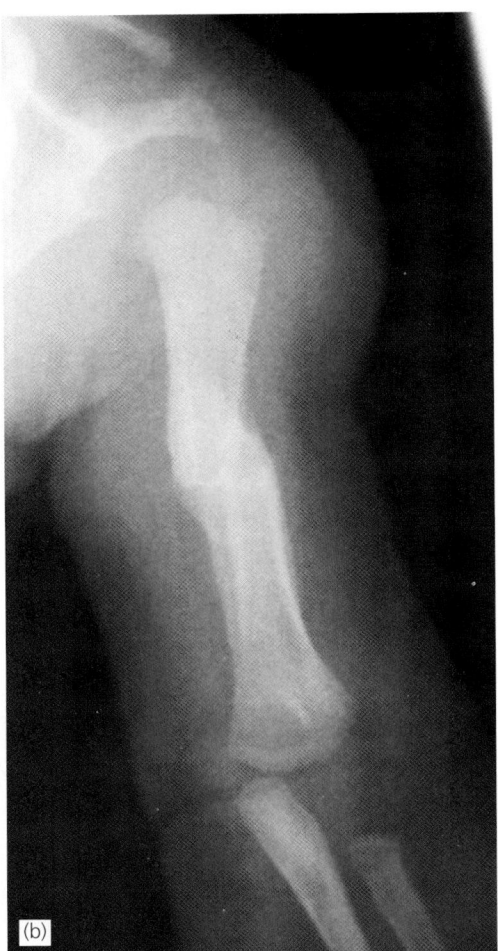
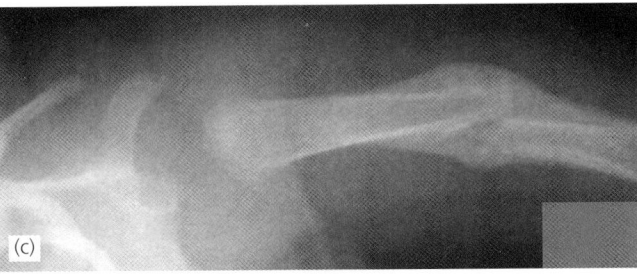

Figure 55.8 Birth traumatic humerus shaft fracture. Immobilization by individually adjusted Desault bandage. Development after 6 weeks.

Table 55.1 Order of appearance of ossification centres around the elbow

Ossification centre	Age of appearance in girls (years)
Capitellum	1
Radial Head	3
Internal (medial) epicondyle	5
Trochlea	7
Olecranon	9
Lateral epicondyle	11

There is a 2 year delay in boys for all centres except for the capitellum.

DISTAL HUMERUS

Supracondylar fractures

The supracondylar fracture of the humerus (SCH) accounts for the majority of paediatric elbow fractures and is therefore mentioned first. 95% of SCH fractures are extension type injuries. This fracture has been classified by Gartland, who in 1959 noted 'the trepidation with which men, otherwise versed in the management of trauma, approach a fresh supracondylar fracture'.

Kaye Wilkins modified the Gartland classification but kept the basis of three types. Type I is an undisplaced fracture where the anterior humeral line still passes through the ossification centre of the capitellum. Type II fractures are displaced but have an intact hinge of bone located posteriorly in extension type fractures. Type II can be further subdivided into A (without rotation) or B (with rotation). Type III fractures are completely displaced with no cortical contact.

Furthermore, in 2006, Leitch *et al.* retrospectively reviewed 297 extension type III fractures and found that 3% of these had multidirectional instability, with instability in both flexion and extension. This instability was found with the patient under anaesthesia and therefore they proposed a type IV addition to the Gartland system. However, only time will tell if this addition is widely adopted. In any case, many surgeons today eschew the Gartland classification because of only moderate interobserver agreement and opt to treat SCH fractures based on an assessment of the degree of displacement. In addition, von Laer has also described a four-type classification taking the rotational instability into account.

TREATMENT

The management of these fractures remains controversial. Neurovascular injury can occur in these patients and one must be fully cognizant of this possibility and thus take special care to document the neurovascular status upon admission.

Nerve injuries associated with SCH fractures are (in decreasing order of frequency) as follows: (1) anterior interosseous nerve, (2) median nerve (in posterolateral displacement), (3) radial nerve (in posteromedial displacement) and least frequently (4) ulnar nerve. Ulnar nerve injury is rarely due to the fracture but most usually due to iatrogenic injury from K-wire placement.

Vascular injury can occur in up to 1% of SCH fractures and the radial pulse should be monitored. If the radial artery pulse is absent after reduction, an open revision has to be performed. In these cases, injury to the vessel wall or entrapment of the vessel–nerve bundle in the fracture gap is usually found. However, if there is no pulse but the hand is warm and well perfused, the patient might be critically observed for 24–48 hours. Preoperative angiography is not indicated in a pulseless limb as it delays fracture reduction, which usually corrects the vascular problem. However, if the pulse is lost after reduction and K wiring or if there is a cool pulseless hand (rare), this is an indication for exploration of the brachial artery.

Type I fractures are treated in an above-elbow cast in 90° of elbow flexion. Type II fractures can be treated with closed reduction if there is no swelling, the anterior humeral line bisects the capitellum and if there is no medial cortical impaction. The above-elbow cast can be removed at 3 weeks.

The majority of type II and all type III fractures are treated with closed reduction and K wiring. There is a lot of discussion regarding K-wire configuration: in summary, crossed wires have been found to be more stable biomechanically in the laboratory than lateral wires alone. However, use of a medial wire is associated with a 3–8% risk of iatrogenic ulnar nerve injury. Therefore, open localization and digital protection of the ulnar nerve is mandatory prior to the insertion of K-wires.

COMPLICATIONS

The main complications of treatment include the risk of Volkmann ischaemic contracture due to compression of the brachial artery from casting at greater than 90° of flexion and more rarely due to injury from the fracture itself.

A recent small retrospective series reported that significant swelling at presentation and a delay in fracture reduction may be important warning signs for the development of compartment syndrome. Another much talked about complication is cubitus varus or 'gunstock deformity', which is usually a cosmetic deformity with little functional problem. The rate of cubitus varus is lower with closed reduction and wiring than with closed reduction and casting. Cast treatment can also result in recurvatum, and this is due to the limited growth potential of the distal humerus. Finally, stiffness is a complication that can be avoided with early mobilization and pin removal soon after fracture healing at 3–4 weeks.

Lateral condyle fractures

The most widely used classification is based on the amount of displacement of the fracture. Type I fractures are displaced less than 2 mm with an intact articular surface; type II fractures are displaced 2–4 mm with a displaced articular surface; and type III fractures are displaced more than 4 mm and rotated as well.

TREATMENT

Type I fractures are treated with an above-elbow cast for 3–4 weeks. Up to 10% of these fractures can displace sufficiently with cast treatment to require subsequent reduction and pinning. Type II fractures are treated operatively with closed reduction and percutaneous K wiring or screw osteosynthesis but may require open reduction if joint congruity cannot be obtained with closed methods. Type III fractures require open reduction and fixation with K-wires or screws. The K-wires must be divergent to minimize the risk of subsequent fracture displacement and the distal K-wire must engage the ossified distal humeral metaphysis. It is important to insert the screws from the dorsoradial metaphysis in order to protect the physis. If open reduction is necessary, the soft tissues must never be dissected off the lateral condyle because this will lead to decreased blood supply and potential osteonecrosis of the lateral condyle. Also, the joint line should be visualized to ensure anatomic reduction.

COMPLICATIONS

The main specific complications of treatment include stiffness, osteonecrosis and non-union or malunion. Stiffness is minimized by mobilizing the elbow early, as soon as fracture healing is complete. Cubitus valgus is the frequent result of non-union and this should be managed with bone grafting and screw fixation because tardy ulnar nerve palsy is a common sequelae of non-union and cubitus valgus which manifests itself years after the initial injury (if ever). Tardy ulnar nerve palsy is treated by ulnar nerve transposition.

Y-type and medial condyle fractures

Y-type and medial condyle fractures are very rare and should be reduced and stabilized with K-wires and screws, similar to the procedure for lateral condyle fractures.

Epicondylar fractures

This fracture predominantly appears at the ulnar side together with a (sub)luxation of the elbow. Therefore, coexisting injuries have to be considered and lateral ligamentous stability has to be controlled. Fractures with a deviation up to a maximum of 0.5 cm can be treated conservatively; fractures with larger deviation, mostly combined with subluxation of the elbow, should be fixed, preferably with a cannulated screw osteosynthesis, or K-wires in smaller children. Growth disturbances are not to be expected since these are apophyseal injuries. A specific complication after conservative therapy is the development of a pseudarthrosis, which, however, is rarely symptomatic.

Dislocation of the elbow

In many cases, a displacement of the ulnar epicondyle, followed by radial as well as ulnar- side ligament lesions, radius head fractures, radial condylar fractures, coronoid process or olecranon fractures are combined. Isolated elbow luxation usually occurs in older children and remains mostly stable after reduction.

If a radial or ulnar instability is left untreated, there is a risk of re-luxation; this is also the case if the ulnar condyle is displaced. Thus, surgery is indicated by instability as well as by coexisting injuries. All other fractures are immobilized in an upper arm cast for 2–3 weeks after the initial reposition and stability examination.

PROXIMAL FOREARM

Radial neck fractures

An actual epiphyseal radius head fracture is rare in infancy. More common are radial neck fractures, with metaphyseal fractures in approximately two-thirds of cases and epiphyseal separations in one-third of cases. These usually arise from a fall on the outstretched arm or in association with luxation of the elbow or as a Monteggia-like lesion. Because of the large correction potential, relatively large malpositions can be left. As a limit, tilting of 45° in under 10 year olds is considered acceptable, whereas in older children 20° tilting is the limit. Functional therapy should be started as early as possible, and the time for immobilization for pain therapy should be kept as short as possible (approximately 1–2 weeks). Because there is only a metaphyseal blood supply to the radial epiphysis, there is a risk of post-traumatic disturbance of the blood circulation, with necrosis and deformation of the radial head. Dislocated fractures should be reduced in a closed manner in order not to endanger the blood circulation to the radius head. The reduction can be fixed and indirectly reduced by a retrograde elastic nail from the distal radius.

Fracture of the proximal ulna

Intra- and extra-articular fractures of the olecranon can be differentiated. Very often there is a combination injury with, for example, a radius neck fracture, radius head subluxation as a Monteggia injury or fractures of the distal humerus. Undislocated fractures can be treated conservatively in an upper arm cast for approximately 3–4 weeks. The traction powers of the triceps muscle can easily lead to a dislocation, which should be anatomically reduced by an open procedure and stabilized by tension wiring or screw osteosynthesis. Extra-articular fractures frequently present a varus malposition, which are usually poorly adjusted with spontaneous correction and can lead to disturbances of rotation.

Dislocation of the radial head/Monteggia lesion

Isolated subluxations of the radius head are extremely rare after trauma. Usually, there is accompanying pathology of the ulna as a Monteggia injury, which can easily be missed if there is bowing of the ulna. The classical Monteggia fracture consists of an ulnar shaft fracture with a simultaneous subluxation of the radius head. We characterize functionally equivalent injuries in which the ulna is fractured more proximally as Monteggia-like lesions, up to an olecranon fracture. In addition, a luxation and/or fracture of the radius head can occur as a result of trauma. If an allegedly isolated radius head luxation is visible, a radiograph of the entire lower arm can be used to exclude a fracture of the ulnar shaft, especially a bowing injury. In contrast, for an isolated ulnar fracture in the lower arm, a radiograph of the elbow can be used to exclude a luxation of the radius head. The proximal radius axis must extend to the core of the humeral capitellum in all planes (Fig. 55.9). If recognized and treated as part of the primary diagnosis, the prognosis is good. With reduction of the ulnar fracture, a reduction of the radial head can be easily achieved. The ulna is stabilized either with ESIN or, in proximal fractures, with a mini-plate osteosynthesis.

The later the injury is recognized, the worse the prognosis. Significant malfunctions can result from extension and clumping of the radial head. Usually a complex angulation-distraction osteotomy of the ulna is necessary to bring back the radial head into its original position. In addition, congenital dysplasia of the radial head (e.g. oblique) and pre-existing dislocations have to be kept in mind.

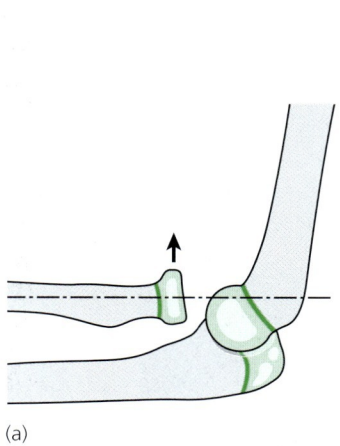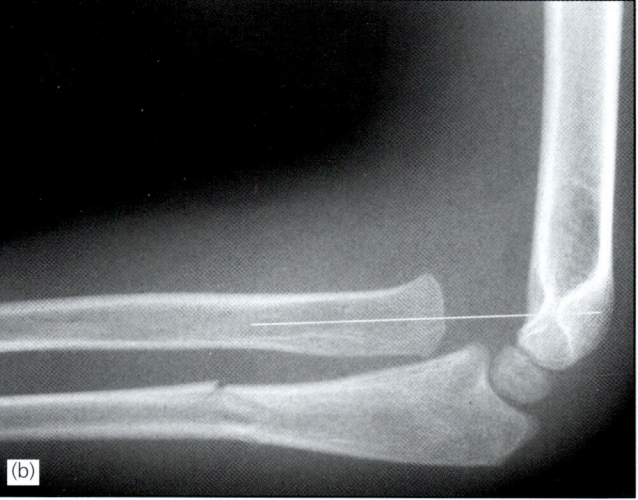

Figure 55.9 Radial head luxation: the elongation of the proximal radius axis has to project itself to the core of the humeral capitellum in all radiographic planes.

Nursemaid's elbow (pulled elbow syndrome)

The pulled elbow syndrome is one of the most common injuries in the emergency room in the young child under the age of 5 years. After the age of 5 years, the attachment of the annular ligament to the neck of the radius strengthens and prevents displacement and radial head subluxation.

This injury occurs with longitudinal traction on the outstretched arm of the child, causing the orbicular ligament to subluxate over the radial head. The child classically presents with the elbow extended and the forearm pronated. Radiographs are not necessary and treatment consists of supination of the forearm and flexion of the elbow past 90° with the examiners' thumb over the radial head to feel for a snap that accompanies reduction of the radial head.

FOREARM

Forearm fractures are categorized according to their location and degree of displacement and/or angulation. Greenstick fractures are usually rotational injuries. The majority of fractures can be treated with closed reduction and above-elbow casting. Apex volar fractures are casted in pronation, and apex dorsal fractures (due to pronation) are casted in supination to neutralize the deforming muscle forces.

The indications for operative intervention include unacceptable alignment following closed reduction (see Table 55.2). The parameters are as follows:

1. greater than 10° deformity in children over the age of 8;
2. greater than 15° deformity in children younger than 8;
3. Significantly displaced fractures.

Table 55.2 Acceptable angular correction in degrees

Age (years)	Lateral: boys (°)	Lateral: girls (°)	Anteroposterior radiograph (°)
>9	20	15	15
9–11	15	10	5
11–13	10	10	0
>13	5	0	0

Adapted from Rockwood and Green 2006.

Operative techniques include flexible intramedullary nails, or in the older child open reduction and plating. Advantages of an intramedullary device include a small dissection, use of a load-sharing device with the resultant decrease in stress risers and easier removal of metalwork.

Complications include re-fracture (5%), risk of malunion, compartment syndrome (commoner with intramedullary fixation) and stiffness (which is rare).

Distal radius

In contrast to the shaft centre the distal metaphyseal forearm is able to correct axis deviations up to 30°. In children over 12 years, no malpositions should be left. The reduction should take place under general anaesthesia and a surgical team on stand-by. Unstable metaphyseal fractures and epiphysiolysis are best fixed with a percutaneous K-wire osteosynthesis after mostly closed reduction (Fig. 55.10). Fractures at the transition of the very distal shaft are often not adequately supplied by K-wire osteosynthesis or intramedullary splinting, so that an external fixation might

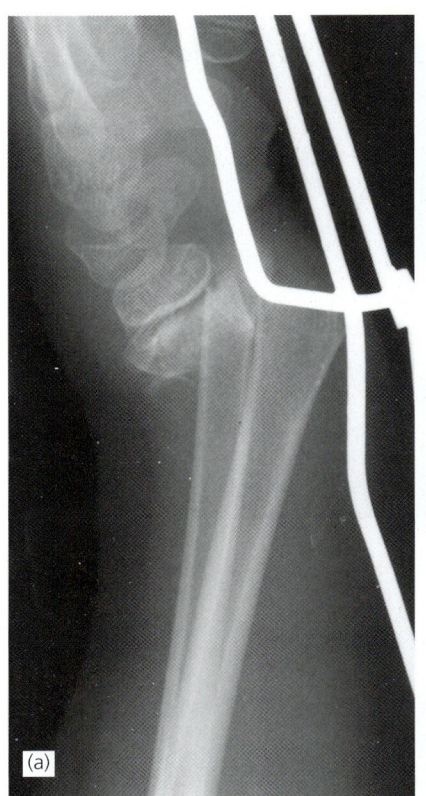
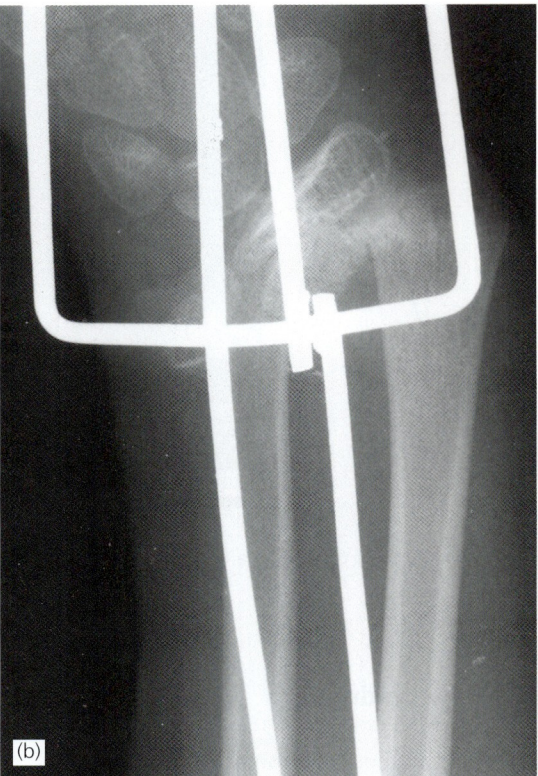
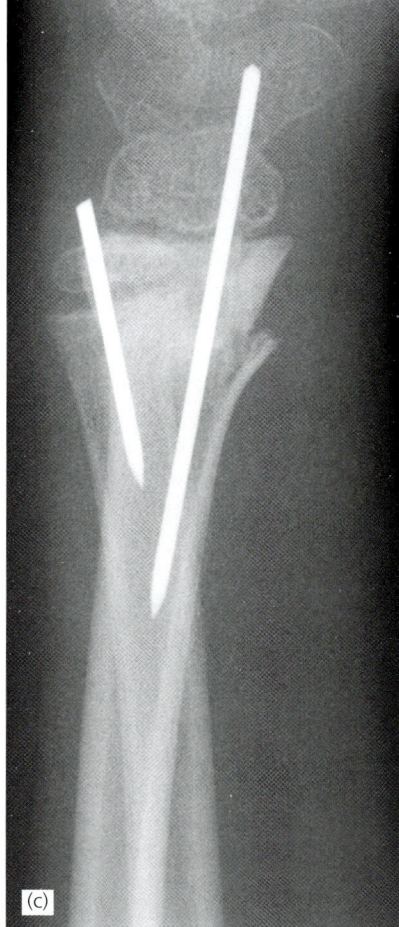
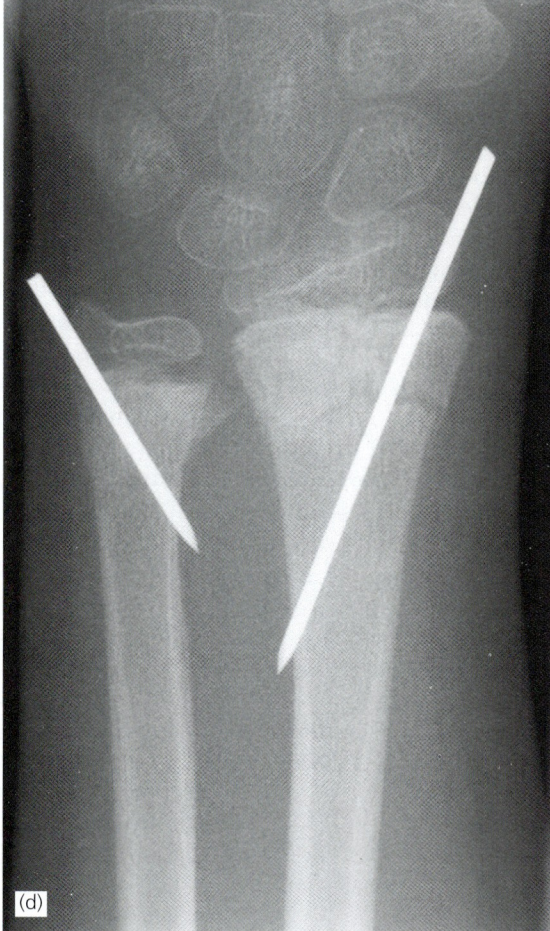

Figure 55.10 Salter II injury of the distal radius of an 11-year-old girl. Closed reduction and percutaneous K-wire stabilization if unstable.

be used. Buckle fractures or greenstick fractures are considered to be stable and can be treated with a forearm cast for 2–3 weeks until the fracture heals. Closed reduction and casting is generally successful in treating most of these fractures. For physeal fractures the reduction has to be achieved in one step, and multiple manoeuvres have to be avoided.

Completely displaced or 'off ended' distal radius fractures in a child should be treated with closed reduction and percutaneous K wiring to decrease the incidence of re-displacement, as up to 30% of these fractures which appear stable after closed reduction will displace at 1 or 2 weeks after closed reduction and casting.

Complications include malunion, which often remodels spontaneously, and growth arrest, which is rare. One complication of K wiring is damage to the superficial radial nerve, and this is best avoided using the 'nick and spread' technique, in which a haemostat is used to spread the soft tissues until bone is exposed through a small nick in the skin.

GALEAZZI LESION

A radius shaft fracture with simultaneous ulnar head luxation in the distal radioulnar joint (DRUJ) is called a classical Galeazzi fracture. This injury rarely occurs in infancy.

In a complete luxation of the DRUJ, an injury of the triangular fibrocartilaginous complex must always be excluded. Unstable fractures, particularly deviations of the radius >10°, require surgery with reduction and stabilization of the radius fracture.

Pelvic fractures

Pelvic fractures are rare injuries in childhood and adolescence, with an incidence between 2.4% and 7.5%. Because of the high elasticity of paediatric bone, the thick periosteum and the strong ligament apparatus, large forces are necessary to cause fractures of the pelvis. Road traffic accidents are the main cause of pelvic fractures. In addition, the anatomically flatter pelvis in children provides less protection for intrapelvic organs. Therefore, concomitant injuries must always be expected, and can increase morbidity and mortality. This has to be considered in the diagnosis. Generally, a spiral CT, which will show the pelvic fracture clearly, is carried out after Advanced Trauma Life Support (ATLS) in the severely wounded child. Because of the different anatomy from adults, a different injury patterns can be observed. Fractures of the acetabulum are seen much more rarely in children than in adults.

Pelvic fractures are often stable in children, so the majority can be treated conservatively. Dislocated and unstable fractures should be reduced and stabilized in a similar way to those in adults.

Recent investigations have shown that the potential for spontaneous correction in children has been frequently overrated, and pelvic fractures that heal in malposition are associated with significant long-term consequences such as lower back pain, limping and leg length discrepancies.

Avulsion injuries have to be distinguished from high-energy injuries. Avulsion injuries usually occur in sporty, active adolescents. The apophyseal muscle insertion is torn out because of sudden muscle tension, usually at the anterior inferior iliac spine or at the anterior superior iliac spine and at the iliac tuberosity. Usually, conservative treatment is sufficient. Only badly dislocated fractures or painful pseudarthrosis require surgical intervention.

PROXIMAL FEMUR

Injuries of the proximal femur are extremely rare in infancy and are usually associated with severe trauma and accompanying injuries. Because of the blood supply to the head of the femoral neck there is a higher risk of femoral head necrosis; therefore, growth disturbance with subsequent femoral neck shortening may take place in all injuries.

For this reason, all dislocated fractures have to be treated as an emergency and must be reduced as quickly as possible. Relief of the intracapsular haematoma is recommended and stabilization should be performed in order not to endanger the blood supply to the proximal femur. Therefore, treatment is conservative in only exceptional cases, with a pelvic leg cast in babies and infants. Otherwise, a closed or open reduction and stabilization are performed, preferably with cannulated screws; alternatively, a plate and/or ESIN can be used in type III fractures. Epiphyseal fractures are rare, and traumatic epiphyseal separation is extremely rare and appears mostly as a birth trauma. This rare injury has to be distinguished from non-traumatic epiphyseal separations in the adolescent

The classification follows the AO Paediatric Comprehensive Classification.

E/1	Epiphyseal separation
E/2	Epiphyseal separation with metaphyseal wedge
M/1	Transcervical femoral neck fracture
M/2	Cervicobasal femoral neck fracture
M/3	Intertrochanteric fracture of the femur

Traumatic hip subluxation also occurs as a result of high-speed traumas in adolescents. It may also occasionally appear in infants as a result of bagatelle traumas. It should be reduced as rapidly as possible under general anaesthesia as later reductions (>6 hours after trauma) have a worse prognosis. A CT scan after reduction can be used to exclude accompanying bony injuries of the pelvis or the femoral head. If there is any suspicion of femoral head necrosis, MRI should be carried out.

DIAPHYSEAL FEMUR

Femoral shaft fractures are usually the result of high-energy trauma. Therefore, accompanying injuries have to be expected. In radiographic diagnosis, one plane is sufficient for all dislocated fractures; however, a complete set of radiographs must be obtained, at the latest in the operating theatre, to show the adjacent joints. The more distal a fracture is located, the greater the likelihood of a spontaneous correction of the dislocation. Since a significant increase in leg length has to be expected as a result of increased growth stimulation during the remodelling process, an anatomical reduction should be attempted in order to limit leg length discrepancies.

The choice of treatment method is mainly related to the age of the child. Although conservative treatment by overhead traction and/or pelvis–leg cast is more common in children up to 3 years old, surgical treatment is preferred in older children. This provides good pain relief and enables a rapid recovery with only a short hospital stay.

The preferred method for simple diaphyseal transverse fractures is stabilization by ESIN. However, diagonal fractures can also be stabilized by means of this three-point support (Fig. 55.11). By introduction of the so-called end caps (Synthes), lengthwise-unstable diagonal fractures can also be made stable, without requiring secondary compression. External fixation offers a good alternative in all unstable fractures, whereas plate osteosynthesis is usually only required in exceptional cases, e.g. as a bridging plate in long compound fractures. Fixation by a solid intramedullary nail has to be considered in large and heavy adolescents if ESIN is unsuitable. In this case, there is a risk of vessel lesions at the entrance of the nail with subsequent head necrosis. Other complications include the risk of limb length discrepancy, and patients and their parents should be informed about this. Angular malunion is a complication associated with traction and spica casting and can be minimized by using careful technique and regular monitoring. Delayed union and non-union are rare complications.

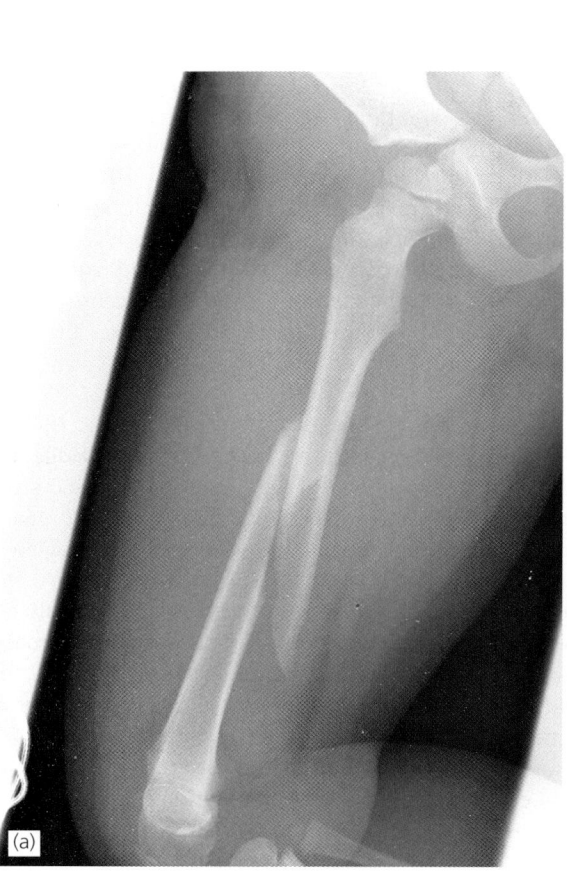
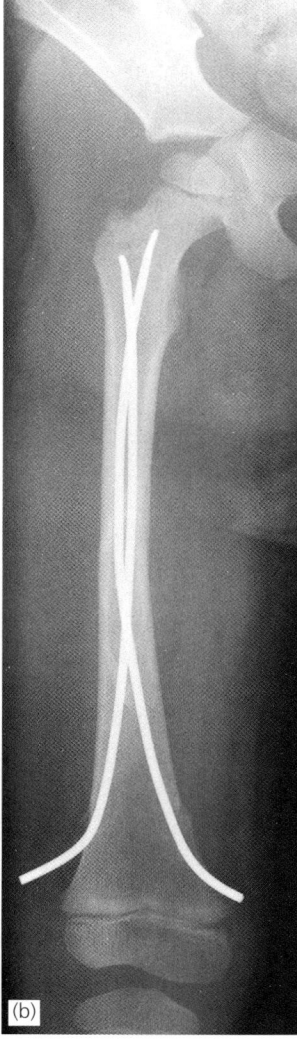

Figure 55.11 Multiple injured 5-year-old girl: closed reduction and stabilization with elastic stable intramedullary nailing.

DISTAL FEMUR

Metaphyseal buckle fractures can be separated from complete fractures in this area since they are impacted and stable and need only cast immobilization. In complete fractures a radiograph is recommended after 8 days to exclude a secondary dislocation. Unstable or dislocated fractures are reduced as a closed procedure and fixed with percutaneous crossed K-wires (Fig. 55.12). In these cases, additional immobilization in an upper leg cast is necessary. Alternatively, these fractures can be fixed by descending ESIN.

The closer the fracture is to the physis, the more often growth disturbances have to be expected. These are usually a partial dorsal closure of the physis with resulting antecurvature. Stimulation of growth that affects leg length has to be expected according to the patient's age and the amount of the remodelling required.

FRACTURES AROUND THE KNEE

Fractures in the region of the knee mainly arise in the context of sports injuries. The diagnosis can be hindered because of irregular centres of ossification. In unclear cases, MRI is helpful to exclude intra-articular injuries. The reduction should always be performed under general anaesthesia with definitive stabilization to avoid further complications caused by secondary dislocations. The following fractures can be differentiated in the knee:

Extra-articular fractures	Epiphyseal separation of the distal femur and the proximal tibia (Salter–Harris I and II injuries) Metaphyseal osseous ligament avulsions Extra-articular avulsions of the tuberosity
Intra-articular fractures	Epiphyseal fracture of the distal femur and the proximal tibia (Salter–Harris III and IV injuries) Patellar fracture Intercondylar eminence avulsion Intra-articular avulsion of the tuberosity

EPIPHYSEAL SEPARATION OF THE DISTAL FEMUR

Epiphyseal separations are the most common injuries of the distal femur. Mostly, growth plate slippage with a small metaphyseal wedge is found. In many cases this fracture results from birth trauma, or maltreatment in infants. A lesion of the blood vessel–nerve bundle can occur because of a dorsal deviation; therefore, angiography should be performed in uncertain cases to exclude a vessel lesion. Undislocated fractures can be treated conservatively in an upper leg cast for 5–6 weeks. All fractures with an axis deviation as well as a side-to-side deviation of the metaphyseal width should be reduced under general anaesthesia because spontaneous correction of axis deviation is limited. If this does not succeed because of, for example, tissue interposition, this must be carried out as an open procedure.

To secure the reduction, crossed, solid percutaneous K-wires are inserted in addition to a cast. If the metaphyseal wedge is large enough it can be fixed by a screw osteosynthesis. Partial blocking growth disturbances often occur, so that patients must be followed up regularly until completion of growth or until 2 years after the trauma.

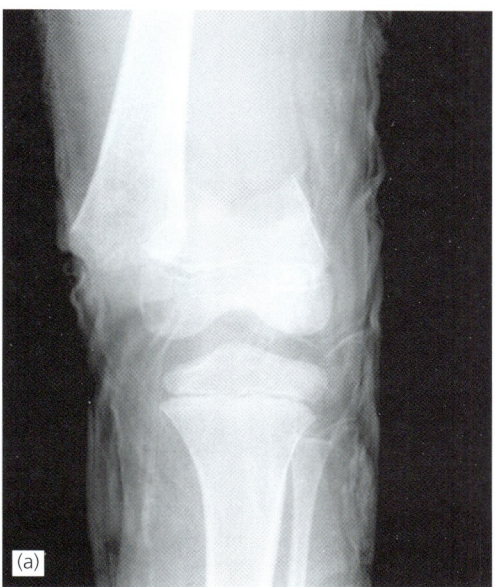
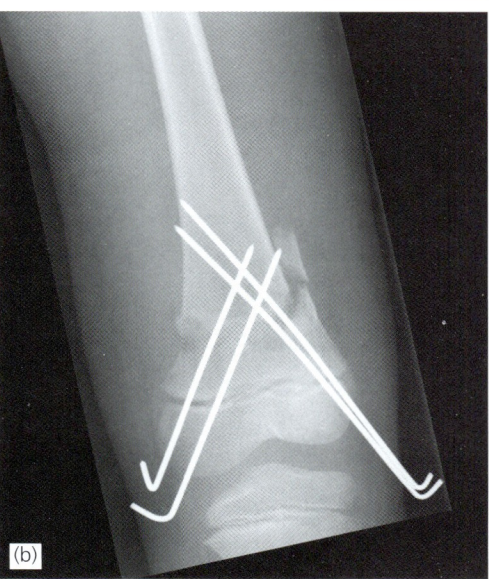

Figure 55.12 Eight-year-old boy with fracture of the distal femur. Closed reduction and percutaneous K-wire stabilization.

OSSEOUS METAPHYSEAL LIGAMENT RUPTURES

These appear primarily in the still open physis. The diagnosis is made radiologically, but, in small undislocated fractures, a haematoma and pain may indicate this injury. Excessive stability tests of the side ligament apparatus should be avoided so as not to provoke a secondary dislocation.

Undislocated avulsions can be treated conservatively in an upper leg cast for 4 weeks. Post-traumatic knee joint instabilities are rare. Dislocated fragments are reduced open and are fixed by screw osteosynthesis, which reduces the risk of the physis overlapping periosteal bridging with resultant partial growth disturbance. If this occurs, an arthroscopy of the knee should follow to exclude intra-articular knee joint lesions. Follow-up of patients is essential to detect growth disturbances with resulting varus or valgus deformity. This could appear as a bone bridge or as a so-called necrosis bridge caused by lesions of the blood vessels supplying the physis.

EPIPHYSEAL FRACTURES OF THE DISTAL FEMUR

In epiphyseal injuries in which the physis is still open, epiphyseal fractures (Salter–Harris III) and epimetaphyseal fractures (Salter–Harris IV) can be differentiated from the so-called transition fractures in adolescents, in whom the physis is beginning to close. Usually, severe trauma is the cause of the injury. A vessel lesion has to be excluded because of the proximity of the vessel–nerve bundle. If there is suspicion of an inner knee injury or an inconclusive radiological result, MRI can be helpful. Reconstruction of the articular surface is the aim of treatment. All fractures with an articular step or a fracture gap of >2 mm require surgical intervention. Undislocated fractures can be treated in an upper leg cast for 4–5 weeks, and radiological follow-up should be performed to exclude a secondary dislocation after 1 week. Dislocated fractures are reduced, for example arthroscopically, and are stabilized by screw osteosynthesis under compression of the fracture gap. Clinical follow-up is necessary to detect possible post-traumatic growth disturbances.

EPIPHYSEAL FRACTURES OF THE PROXIMAL TIBIA

Separations of the physis with (Salter–Harris II) or without (Salter–Harris I) metaphyseal involvement are extremely rare. Owing to the proximity of the vessel–nerve bundle, deviations can lead to vessel lesions with severe circulation disturbances analogous to knee joint luxations in adults. Axis deviations, especially in the frontal plane, are usually corrected insufficiently and can lead to an extreme genu valgum or varum position. Also, blocking growth disturbances can lead to axis deviations because of early physis closure (Fig. 55.13). Undislocated fractures can be treated conservatively in an upper leg cast. Dislocated fractures can mostly be reduced as a closed procedure and retained in an upper leg cast if stable; in cases of instability, a percutaneous K-wire osteosynthesis is performed.

The axis should be documented radiologically after reduction and should be measured by an epiphyseal angle if necessary (Fig. 55.14), as small deviations can lead to relevant axis deviations.

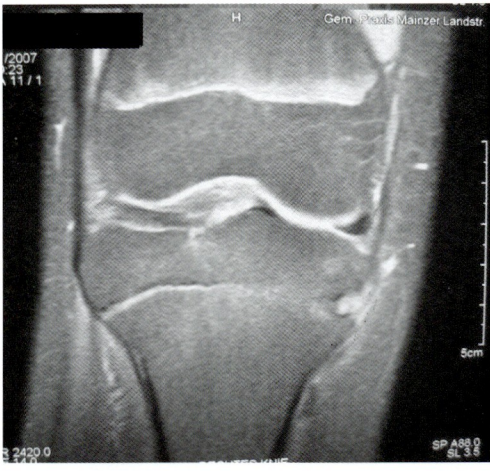

Figure 55.13 Early closure of the medial physis of the proximal tibia after epiphyseal deviation and conservative therapy in a 14-year-old girl.

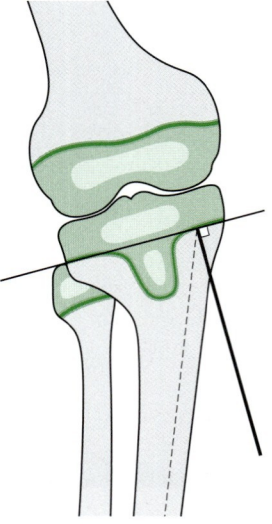

Figure 55.14 Epiphyseal axis angle.

AVULSIONS OF THE TIBIAL TUBEROSITY

Avulsions of the tibial tuberosity usually occur in adolescent males. A predisposition as a result of Osgood–Schlatter disease has been suggested. Sudden tension of the quadriceps muscle during sporting activity, with resulting inability to stretch and local pressure pain and a haematoma, is the reason in most cases. Intra- and extra-articular fractures are differentiated according to the treatment. The Watson–Jones classification differentiates these fractures into three types: types I and II are extra-articular fractures, whereas type III is an intra-articular fracture. The aim of therapy is to reconstruct the extension apparatus and to reconstruct the tibial articular surface anatomically.

Undislocated fractures are rare because of the muscle tension at the tibial tuberosity. Undislocated injuries, i.e. types I and II (<5 mm deviation), can be treated conservatively in an upper leg cast for 6 weeks with partial weight bearing. All intra-articular and dislocated fractures are reduced openly and stabilized by screw osteosynthesis. In adolescence, the physis may be crossed since closure of the physis has already started. Growth disturbances are rare in adolescence. A recurvature of the knee can result in younger children because of early physis closure. Growths in the zone of the tuberosity can occur because of callus formation and because of large bone fragments, which can be problematic especially in kneeling activities and which have to be removed.

INTERCONDYLAR EMINENCE AVULSIONS

While intraligamentary ruptures of the cruciate ligaments occur most often in adolescents and adults, osseous ligament avulsions occur mostly in children under the age of 12 years following trauma. In these cases the anterior cruciate ligament is usually involved as an intercondylar eminence avulsion. Concomitant intra-articular injuries such as lesions of the meniscus and cartilage have to be considered.

Rarely, chronic knee joint pain and chronic instability is the result of congenital aplasia of the intercondylar eminence in which the anterior cruciate ligament is absent.

The classification follows Meyers and McKeever according to the grade of deviation:

Type I   Little ventral deviation
Type II   Obvious ventral deviation; the dorsal part is still in contact with the epiphysis of the tibia
Type III   Complete avulsion

The aim of treatment is to restore the stability of the cruciate ligament. In these cases undislocated fractures (type I) and reduced fractures (type II) can be treated conservatively in an upper leg cast in 15° flexion. The reduction usually succeeds by extension of the knee joint under radiological control. Immobilization starting in extension can be done in order to ensure the reduction result, which can be shifted to a 15° flexion after 3 weeks. If necessary, puncture of any haemarthrosis can be performed.

A continuous haematoma has to be considered after a puncture injury. We use prophylactic measures such as immobilization in an upper leg cast splint, elastic bandaging underpacked with a cut-out foam cushion, manual cooling by icepacks and raising the limb, as well as walking on forearm crutches.

Dislocated injuries (types II and III) are reduced and fixed under arthroscopic control. There are many types of osteosynthesis procedures. Usually, we perform retrograde screwing or transosseous suturing with polydioxanone sutures (PDS) in small bony fragments. In these cases, an iatrogenic lesion of the physis of the proximal tibia should be avoided. Growth disturbances are rare because epiphyseal injuries do not affect the physis and, if they do occur, they are likely to be iatrogenic.

Note that the anterior horn of the meniscus can wedge in and block the reduction in Meyers and McKeever type II and III injuries.

The stability of the cruciate ligament determines the prognosis. A persisting instability leads to a high rate of meniscus and cartilage lesions with the risk of developing early arthrosis. Therefore, follow-up of the stability of the cruciate ligament is necessary because a secondary anterior cruciate ligament insufficiency can occur. Interestingly, the rate of intraligamentous anterior cruciate ruptures increases steadily in childhood, which might be due to increasing sports activities. In these cases and if there is clinical instability, detected by MRI and a tendency for the joint to give way, early reconstruction with semitendinosus or quadriceps femur tendon is indicated. New techniques for fixation have been established in order to prevent relevant growth plate injury.

FRACTURES OF THE PATELLA

Fractures of the patella are much rarer in childhood than in adults because of the mainly cartilaginous patella and the more lax ligaments. Osteochondral fractures as concomitant injuries to a patellar luxation occur more often. Transverse fractures can be differentiated from longitudinal fractures, from osteochondral avulsion fractures and from central osteochondral defects.

Note that, in some cases, additional ossification centres arise. If there is incomplete fusion of all cores, a 'patella partita' will develop (mostly bipartite), which is usually asymptomatic.

The aim of treatment is the reconstruction of the extension apparatus, as well as the reconstruction of the articular surface. Undislocated fractures with uninjured extension apparatus (mainly longitudinal fractures) can be treated conservatively in an upper-leg cast. Dislocated fractures are reduced open or as an arthroscope-assisted procedure and are supported by tension band or screw osteosynthesis. Proximal or distal avulsion fractures can be fixed by a transosseous suture, and osteochondral fragments can be stabilized by resorbable pins.

The main risks are of a continuance of a joint incongruence, which can lead to a femoropatellar arthrosis. Pseudarthrosis results only in insufficient osteosynthesis.

FRACTURES OF THE PROXIMAL TIBIAL METAPHYSIS

Non-problematic compression fractures have to be differentiated from bending fractures in the proximal metaphyseal area. Compression fractures usually heal without complication, whereas bending fractures tend to heal with an increasing valgus dislocation because of partial growth stimulation.

Note that an already visible medial fracture gap in the anteroposterior plane radiograph indicates a valgus dislocation.

Therefore, dislocations must be treated with a reduction with compression of the medial fracture gap to decrease the risk of a later valgus deformity. Slightly dislocated (<10°) or undislocated fractures can be treated conservatively in an upper leg cast. A cast wedging can be performed on day 8 to achieve a medial compression. Dislocated fractures are reduced closed and are fixed by compression osteosynthesis, e.g. plate osteosynthesis or external fixation.

It is important that iatrogenic lesions of the apophysis of the tibial tuberosity are avoided.

FRACTURES OF THE TIBIAL DIAPHYSIS

Lower leg fractures are among the most common fractures of the lower extremity. In two-thirds of cases only the tibia is affected; in one-third of cases there is a complete fracture.

Depending on remaining deviation and the necessary remodelling a leg length distraction of approximately 0.5–1 cm can occur as a result of growth stimulation. Because of this, no significant deviations should be left to spontaneous correction. For children younger than 10 years, a varus of 5°, antecurvature or recurvature of 10°, and no valgus or rotation deviations are the limits to guide treatment.

Isolated tibia fractures are considered as stable and can be treated conservatively in an upper-leg cast. They tend to a varus deviation because of muscle tension and the blocking effect of the intact fibula, so that a radiograph to check the position should be performed after 8 days. A cast wedging can antagonize the varus deviation.

Complete lower leg fractures are mostly unstable, so we recommend surgical stabilization by ESIN or external fixation axis control and earlier mobilization. However, in young children, conservative treatment is possible, but a secondary valgus deviation due to muscle tension and the absence of the stabilizing effect of the fibula must be assessed radiologically.

Stress fractures are a special type of fracture. Stress reactions, including stress fractures, occur most often in the tibia as a result of an increase in sporting activities in children. The so-called 'toddler's fracture' is a special type of stress fracture. The toddler's fracture appears in infants because of unaccustomed stress when the child begins to walk, without trauma, and can be recognized by a corresponding callus formation on the radiograph.

FRACTURES OF THE ANKLE

The Dias–Tachdjian classification is used for paediatric ankle fractures, and this system is similar to the Lauge-Hansen classification used in adults. In most straightforward distal tibial physeal fractures (Salter–Harris I and II) closed reduction is sufficient, and acceptable reduction is within 2–3 mm of anatomic alignment and less than 10° of angulation. Operative treatment is needed in fractures that cannot be reduced due to interposed periosteum or soft tissues and in complex fractures involving the joint. Salter–Harris III and IV fractures with displacement need mostly closed reduction and cannulated screw fixation without crossing or impairing the physis. The most severe complication of the later injuries are physeal arrest.

TRANSITIONAL FRACTURES

It is important to mention two specific types of ankle fractures that involve adolescents with physes that are beginning to but not completely closed. The first unique fracture is the Tillaux fracture of the anterolateral tibial epiphysis that occurs with a supination external rotation (SER) injury. The second unique fracture is a triplane fracture that includes an anterolateral fragment of the distal tibial epiphysis (like a Tillaux fracture) but in addition includes a metaphyseal fracture. These may be two- or three-part fractures. The reason these types of fracture occur in this location is that the distal tibial physis starts to close centrally, then medially and last laterally.

These fractures can be treated by closed reduction and casting if there is less than 2 mm of joint incongruity. Although mostly closed, in Tillaux fractures often open reduction and internal fixation are indicated if there is greater than 2 mm of displacement. Fixation is usually with one or two cannulated screws. These screws can be placed parallel to the physis in the epiphysis, but in Tillaux fractures they are usually placed oblique towards the metaphyhsis, since physis arrest has already started.

The complications of this latter unique injury include the risk of joint incongruity. If the fracture is not reduced to within 2 mm of anatomic alignment, ankle pain and degenerative changes are common in later years.

FRACTURE CLASSIFICATIONS

Classification systems are widely used in orthopaedic and trauma surgery. Standardized, accessible and easy-to-use documentation plays a key role in reporting clinical and epidemiological data and allows comparison and documentation of different conditions. Such systems provide a common language for defining and categorizing pathology in both retrospective and prospective clinical studies. This is becoming increasingly important for implementing quality control in diagnostic and therapeutic measures. Therefore, a practical standardized form of documentation is necessary, which is accessible to everyone and easy to use.

Numerous fracture classification systems have been proposed in orthopaedics, but specific paediatric classifications are rare. They mostly describe specific single fractures. Fracture classifications of the long bones were adapted from the well-known fracture scheme of the AO into a so-called AO Child Survey with 10 additional child-specific items. The growing bone is capable of spontaneously correcting remaining deviations but there is a risk of growth disturbances. In contrast to adult classifications, a hierarchical order of paediatric fracture types by severity, diagnostic or therapeutic management, or prognosis is not possible because these parameters are influenced by many different factors.

- Injury patterns in children seem to be much more dependent on the maturity of the physis than on the mechanism of the injury; this is the reason that complicated articular fractures, as seen in adults, are not found in children as long as the epiphyseal plate is still wide open.
- In addition to factors such as site and displacement, the choice of treatment type is mainly influenced by the patient's age. The prognosis of growth depends on the patient's age, the contribution to growth of the growth plates, the maturity of the growth plates, the extent of displacement, and the site of the fracture in the bone and in the skeleton.
- While the epiphyseal growth plates are open, growth disturbances can occur; however, this also depends on the fracture site, the displacement and the age of the child.

These considerations have led to the development of classification systems of paediatric long bone fractures. Please refer to the AO Website and Chapter 19 for more details regarding the AO Pediatric Comprehensive Classification of long bone fractures.

THE MULTIPLY INJURED CHILD

Accident-related injuries still remain the main cause of death in childhood and adolescence. The knowledge of child-specific differences in the cause of the injury, the injury pattern in comparison to adults and the physiological specialties in childhood are essential for an adequate therapy.

Road traffic accidents are the main cause of death, peaking between the ages of 6 and 12 years. Compared with adults, children are significantly more frequently involved in accidents as pedestrians and cyclists. Regarding the injury pattern, head injuries dominate against all other localizations. The traumatic brain injury (TBI) is the highest cause of death in the childhood, with a peak in the under 5 year olds and a second peak in the over 15 year olds. The relation of the big and heavy head in comparison to the body leads to a special injury sensitivity. Besides the calvarium is still thin and provides little protection, so that small traumas lead to significant injuries at that age. The paediatric Glasgow Coma Scale (GCS) (Table 55.3) is commonly used to evaluate head injury in children. A GCS score less than 8 at presentation indicates a higher risk of mortality. The GCS motor score 72 hours after injury predicts the risk of permanent disability following TBI. The two most important prognostic indicators of long- term neurological recovery and function are (1) oxygen saturation at the time of presentation and (2) GCS score 72 hours after injury.

Extremity injuries are the second highest localization of injuries. The lower extremity is more often involved than the upper extremity. The pelvis and spine are significantly less frequently involved than in the adult. Injuries of the thoracolumbar transition come to the fore at the spine. Most of them are compression injuries that can be treated conservatively. The younger the child is the more probable is an injury of the cervical spine. The cervical spine presents the highest injury localization at the spine in the under 10 year olds. The atlas and axis are extremely fragile and complex injuries are often lethal. The diagnosis of discoligamentary injuries may be difficult because of the increased physiological laxity. A special type of infantile spine injury is the SCIWORA syndrome (spinal cord injury without radiographic abnormalities). In this case we observe spinal cord damage due to tension, because the tension is much higher in the spine than in the spinal cord.

The pelvis is very flexible because of the high amount of cartilage, so that strong forces can act upon without osseous injuries. Therefore, injuries of the genitourinary system have to be excluded even without the existence of a pelvis fracture. The risks of genitourinary injuries are greatest in patients with anterior pelvic fractures. Pelvis ring fractures are rare; pelvic avulsion fractures are more frequent, but usually do not need an operational intervention. Massive bleeding, intra-abdominal or retroperitoneal, mainly from the pre- sacral vein plexus, can lead to early death through haemorrhagic shock if it is not treated.

In contrast to that, more abdominal injuries occur in children. This can be ascribed to a physiological lower position of the diaphragm with less osseous covering of the spleen and the liver, as well as the relative size of the

Table 55.3 Paediatric Glasgow Coma Scale

Score	Older than 5 years	Age 1–5 years	Younger than 1 year
Best motor response			
6	Obeys commands	Obeys commands	
5	Localizes pain	Localizes pain	Localizes pain
4	Withdrawal	Withdrawal	Abnormal withdrawal
3	Flexion to pain	Abnormal flexion	Abnormal Flexion
2	Extensor rigidity	Extensor rigidity	Abnormal extension
1	None	None	None
Best verbal response			
5	Oriented	Appropriate words	Smiles/cries appropriately
4	Confused	Inappropriate words	Cries
3	Inappropriate words	Cries/screams	Cries inappropriately
2	Incomprehensible	Grunts	Grunts
1	None	None	None
Eye opening			
4	Spontaneous	Spontaneous	Spontaneous
3	To speech	To speech	To shout
2	To pain	To pain	To pain
1	None	None	None

parenchymatous organs comparison with the rest of the trunk. The distance between the body surface and the organs is less than in the adult, which leads to a greater likelihood of injuries.

In European countries, thoracic injuries and abdominal injuries are mainly caused by blunt trauma. The thorax of the child is very flexible so that severe intrathoracic injuries have to be expected even without osseous injuries like rib fractures. The assessment of injury severity mainly follows the injury severity score (ISS), which estimates the severity of the injuries using a point system (Abbreviated Injury Scale, AIS). The Paediatric Trauma Score (PTS) is the most common scoring system for the multiply injured child. The advantage of the PTS is fast adaptability at the site of the accident or in the trauma room. A PTS of 0 correlates with a mortality of 100%

Children can compensate for the loss of blood to a great extent and respond late with signs of a shock. Therefore, a persisting tachycardia with coexisting cold peripheries should be classified as an imminent decompensation.

The complication rate in the polytraumatized child is much lower than in adults. Organ failure, like acute respiratory distress syndrome, is rare in childhood. Lethality rises significantly with an ISS ≥25, a GCS <8 and an emergency blood transfusion of ≥20 mL/kg bodyweight. The outcome of the TBI followed by impairment of extremity injuries is crucial for long-term prognosis.

TREATMENT

Surgical treatment of fractures is more common in the multiply injured child as surgical fixation of fractures facilitates patient care and mobilization, and thus decreases the risk of pressure sores. Treatment of open fractures is discussed in Chapter 17 and the management of polytrauma is further discussed in Chapter 15 Treatment of the polytraumatized child should follow ATLS guidelines.

NON-ACCIDENTAL INJURY

The concept of non-accidental injury (NAI) was first introduced by Caffey in 1946.

Child abuse should be suspected in any fracture before walking age. Other presentations which raise suspicion include multiple injuries in a child without a witnessed or reasonable explanation, a child with both long bone and head injuries, significant delays before seeking medical attention, multiple fractures at various stages of healing and evasive or aggressive parental responses to questioning. Features of outright neglect may be apparent. A good birth and past medical history must also be obtained. However, it is also important for the surgeon not to alienate the parents by making ill-worded comments about child abuse. It is best to refer these patients to the child protection team, which is present in any hospital.

Lower socioeconomic class, special needs children, preterm children and unplanned pregnancies are at increased risk. The majority of fractures in NAI occur in children under 2 years of age and 25–56% in children under the age of 1 year. In a systematic review published in the *British Medical Journal*, rib fractures were shown to have the highest probability for abuse followed by humeral, femoral and skull fractures. The long bones most frequently injured in abuse are the femur, tibia and humerus. Femoral fractures are traditionally associated with NAI, and systematic reviews suggest that they occur more commonly in abuse than tibial or fibular fractures, with the mid-shaft being the commonest site. The spiral fracture pattern of the femur is most commonly related to abuse in children under 15 months. Other classic fracture patterns described in NAI include the 'corner' and bucket handle fracture patterns.

Corner fractures and bucket handle fractures are similar in aetiology despite their different names. A small bucket handle fracture may appear as a corner fracture on the radiograph depending on the angle of the radiograph. A true corner fracture is still similar to a small bucket handle fracture. Post mortem analysis has shown that these transmetaphyseal fractures occur through the weak zone of provisional calcification in the physis.

Spinal injuries occur in less than 1% of cases of NAI and include rupture of spinal ligaments and vertebral fractures. The mechanism of injury is usually due to vigorous shaking or direct blows. Since the infant head is relatively large, the cervical spine may be subject to large forces in flexion–extension type injuries. Digital injuries may also be present and are the result of squeezing or forced hyperextension.

Simple investigations to rule out NAI include biochemical profile for metabolic bone disease as well as genetic testing for osteogenesis imperfecta. Full skeletal surveys are recommended in children under the age of 2 years to diagnose occult fractures. The orthopaedic surgeon should reassess the cases which are unclear and be proactive in surveillance, for example by repeating radiographs and skeletal survey in 10–14 days when calcification previously not visible may appear. Additional imaging modalities such as CT or bone scanning may be used when necessary according to local guidelines.

In summary, reporting of suspected NAI is mandatory and failure to report these cases puts the child at a 50% risk of repeat abuse and up to 10% risk of death. In addition, a thorough examination by a paediatrician is necessary to rule out other injuries due to abuse.

KEY LEARNING POINTS

- The contribution of each physis to longitudinal growth is different; good growth potential is located at the physis of the proximal humerus, the distal radius, the distal femur and the proximal tibia.
- The child is able to compensate the remaining post-traumatic deformities to a certain extent by epiphyseal and periosteal correction mechanisms. The amount of correction potential depends on the age of the child, the growth reserves of the corresponding physis and the location and direction of the deviation.
- Growth stimulation happens after every fracture. The degree depends on the age of the child, the extent and direction of deviation, the number and the timing of the repositioning attempts and the degree of necessary remodelling.
- Inhibitory growth disorders can be caused by damage of the physis, which leads to a partial or full growth arrest. The degree depends on the age and the maturity of the child, the location within the skeleton, the proximity to the physis and the degree of the deviation.
- In children, the fracture pattern is stereotypical and mainly depends on the maturity of the physis and age.
- Physeal fractures are classified by Salter–Harris; prognostically and therapeutically Salter–Harris I and II have to be differentiated from Salter–Harris III and IV
- Epiphyseal fractures in adolescents with a closed physis have a special fracture pattern and are called transitional fractures. Reconstruction of the joint surface is the primary aim in these injuries; growth disorders are not expected.
- Radiographs: comparative images of the opposite side are inefficient and not recommended.
- Supracondylar fracture of the humerus: the Rogers line has been shown to help define the degree of deviation. Instability often leads to a cubitus varus.
- Stable fractures of the radial condylus of the humerus have to be differentiated from instable fractures by taking an radiograph 4–6 days after trauma.
- Radial neck: spontaneous correction is best with early functional therapy.
- Monteggia fracture: early diagnosis is essential for the outcome. The proximal radius axis must extend to the core of the humeral capitellum in all planes. The head of the radius can be reduced with certainty only if any pathology of the ulna is eliminated.
- Greenstick fracture of the forearm: with asymmetrical compression they have the tendency to refracture.
- Fractures of the proximal femur have a high risk of developing a head necrosis.
- Intercondylar eminence avulsion: the anterior horn of the meniscus can wedge in and block the reduction in Meyers and McKeever type II and III injuries.
- Fractures of the proximal tibial metaphysis: this fracture tends to heal with an increasing valgus which leads to a genu valga. A visible medial fracture gap in the anteroposterior plane radiograph indicates a valgus dislocation, which indicates reduction with medial compression.

FURTHER READING

Aitken AP. The end results of the fractured distal tibial epiphysis. *Journal of Bone and Joint Surgery* 1936;**18**:685–91.

Beaty JH. Fractures of the proximal humerus and shaft in children. *Instructional Course Lectures* 1992;**41**:369.

Beaty JH, Kasser JR. *Rockwood and Wilkin's Fractures in Children*, 6th edn. Riverwoods IL: Lippincott Williams and Wilkins, 2005.

Cramer KE. The pediatric polytrauma patient. *Clinical Orthopaedics and Related Research* 1995;**318**:125–35.

Ertl JP, Barrack RL, Alexander AH, Van Buecken K. Triplane fracture of the distal tibial epiphysis: Long term follow up. *Journal of Bone and Joint Surgery (American)* 1988;**70**:967–76.

Gartland JJ. Management of supracondylar fractures of the humerus in children. *Surgery, Gynecology & Obstetrics* 1959;**109**:145–54.

Green NE. Tibia valga caused by asymmetrical overgrowth following a nondisplaced fracture of the proximal tibial metaphysis. *Journal of Pediatric Orthopaedics* 1983;**3**:235–7

Heal J, Bould M, Livingstone J, et al. Reproducibility of the Gartland classification for supracondylar humeral fractures in children. *Journal of Orthopaedic Surgery* 2007;**15**:12–14.

Houshian S, Holst AK, Larsen MS, Torfing T. Remodeling of Salter-Harris type II epiphyseal plate injury of the distal radius. *Journal of Pediatric Orthopaedics* 2004;**24**:472–6.

Jayakumar P, Barry M, Ramachandran M. Orthopaedic aspects of paediatric non-accidental injury. *Journal of Bone and Joint Surgery (British)* 2010;**92**:189–95.

Kemp AM, Dunstant F, Harrison S et al. Patterns of skeletal fractures in child abuse: systematic review. *British Medical Journal* 2008;**337**:1518.

Leitch KK, Kay RM, Femino JD, et al. Treatment of multidirectionally unstable supracondylar humeral fractures in children. A modified Gartland type IV fracture. *Journal of Bone and Joint Surgery (American)* 2006;**88**:980–5.

Loder RT, Feinberg JR. Orthopaedic injuries in children with nonaccidental trauma: demographics and incidence from the 2000 kids' inpatient database. *Journal of Pediatric Orthopaedics* 2007;**27**:421–6.

Marzi I. *Kindertraumatologie*, 2nd edn. Heidelberg, Germany: Springer, 2010.

Metaizeau JP, Lascombes P, Lemelle JL, et al. Reduction and fixation of displaced radial neck fractures by closed intramedullary pinning. *Journal of Pediatric Orthopaedics* 1993;**13**:355–60.

Metaizeau JP. Stable elastic intramedullary nailing for fractures of the femur in children. *Journal of Bone and Joint Surgery (British)* 2004;**86**:954–7.

Meyers MH, McKeever FM. Fracture of the intercondylar eminence of the tibia. *Journal of Bone and Joint Surgery (American)* 1959;**41**:209–22.

Mirsky EC, Karas EH, Weiner LS. Lateral condyle fractures in children: evaluation of classification and treatment. *Journal of Orthopaedic Trauma* 1997; **11**:117–20.

Omid R, Choi PD, Skaggs DL. Supracondylar Humeral Fractures in Children. *Journal of Bone and Joint Surgery (American)* 2008;**90**:1121–32.

Ramachandran M, Skaggs DL, Crawford HA, et al. Delaying treatment of supracondylar fractures in children. Has the pendulum swung too far? *Journal of Bone and Joint Surgery (British)* 2008;**90**:1228–33.

Salter RB, Harris WR. Injuries involving the epiphyseal plate. *Journal of Bone and Joint Surgery (American)* 1963;**45**:587–622.

Skaggs DL. Elbow fractures in children: Diagnosis and Management. *Journal of the American Academy of Orthopaedic Surgeons* 1997;**5**: 303–12.

Slongo TF. Ante- and retrograde intramedullary nailing of humerus fractures. *Operative Orthopädie und Traumatologie* 2008;**20**:373–86.

Slongo TF. Correction osteotomy of neglected 'Monteggia' lesion with an external fixator. *Operative Orthopädie und Traumatologie* 2008;**20**:435–49.

Sullivan JA. Fractures of the lateral condyle of the humerus. *Journal of the American Academy of Orthopaedic Surgeons* 2006;**14**:58–62.

Till H, Huttl B, Knorr P, Dietz HG. Elastic stable intramedullary nailing (ESIN) provides good long-term results in pediatric long-bone fractures. *European Journal of Pediatric Surgery* 2000;**10**:319–22.

Von Laer L. *Pediatric Fractures and Dislocations*. New York, NY: Thieme, 2004.

Von Laer L. The supracondylar fracture of the humerus in children. *Archives of Orthopaedic and Trauma Surgery* 1979;**95**:123–40.

Von Laer L. Fracture of condylus radialis humeri during skeletal growth. *Archives of Orthopaedic and Trauma Surgery* 1981;**98**:275–83.

Wilkins KE. The operative management of supracondylar fractures. *Orthopedic Clinics of North America* 1990;**21**:269–89.

56

Compartment syndrome

ASHISH K SHARMA, EDWARD T MAH

Introduction	503	Management	508
History	503	General principles of treatment of compartment syndrome	510
Anatomic considerations	505	References	512
Aetiology	506		
Pathogenesis	506		

NATIONAL BOARD STANDARDS

- Understand the pathophysiology of compartment syndrome
- Know the key presenting features and able to diagnose it
- Know how to manage this important complication
- Know when to perform fasciotomy

INTRODUCTION

Compartment syndrome is a complex and challenging orthopaedic emergency with potential to cause one of the most destructive complications after a limb injury – Volkmann's ischaemic contracture (VIC). Although there have been significant advances in the diagnosis, prevention and management of acute compartment syndrome, it still remains a relatively common clinical problem, especially in trauma centres and acute care facilities. Although there has been a significant drop in the incidence of subsequent VIC in developed countries with well-managed trauma facilities and adequate protocols for management of compartment syndrome, it continues to occur and can result in a challenging clinical presentation.

Compartment syndrome is defined as raised interstitial tissue pressure within a confined space in the body (an osseofascial compartment) leading to inadequate tissue perfusion and eventually leading to tissue necrosis within the compartment.[1]

Compartment syndrome most commonly involves the forearm and leg, and rarely the hand, foot, thigh, arm, shoulder and buttocks. Often the usual cause of compartment syndrome of the forearm is traumatic interruption of the arterial blood flow, leading to ischaemia of the forearm muscles, mainly the forearm flexor muscles. Also often affected are the forearm nerves, mainly the median nerve and to a lesser extent the ulnar nerve. The radial nerve is rarely involved. Muscles of the volar compartment of the forearm, especially the flexor digitorum profundus and flexor pollicis longus, may get necrosed and even totally degenerated depending on the severity of the ischaemia.

HISTORY

Skeletal muscle ischaemia was first described by Hildebrand[2] in 1869, quoting Hamilton's cases of 1850, without giving reference. So far, Hamilton's account has not been found.

Richard von Volkmann[3] of Halle first described the condition in 1869 and later again in 1875 as 'a deformity of the hand and wrist resulting from an interference of some nature with the blood supply of the muscles of the forearm. This condition was preceded by the application of tight splints or bandages for the fracture of the humerus in the region of the elbow joint'.

Again in his classic article published in 1881, Volkmann[3] said that he believed that the affection was due to ischaemia caused by muscular tissue being deprived of arterial blood, in consequence of which the muscles perished from want of oxygen. He pointed out that the contracture comes on sometime after the initial paralysis and it becomes more marked as more repair tissue is laid down. He said that, from the onset of the condition, there is considerable rigidity, which is increased as more scar tissue is laid down. This concept of external pressure most commonly from tight bandages, ultimately leading to paralytic contracture, became accepted generally, but, in the subsequent 50 years, opinions changed.

Littlewood,[4] in 1900, drew attention to the soft-tissue effusion that occurred in an injured limb and thought that it was pressure of this swelling beneath the deep fascia that occluded the circulation.

Thomas,[5] in 1909, after studying 107 paralytic contractures, found that some paralytic contractures followed severe contusion of the forearm alone. In these, fractures were absent and a splint or bandage was not applied to the limb. The idea thus established that extrinsic pressure was not necessarily the sole cause of the ischaemia.

Murphy,[6] in 1914, in a comprehensive résumé on the subject proposed that VIC was caused by an internal pressure due to haemorrhage and oedema within the muscle that is surrounded by unyielding deep fascial compartments of the forearm, with subsequent obstruction of venous return. He advised slitting the deep fascia in front of the elbow within the first 36 hours after injury.

During the First World War, the problems of arterial injuries focused on the phenomenon of arterial spasm.

Jepson,[7] in 1926, was the first investigator to successfully reproduce ischaemic contracture in animals (dogs) by bandaging an extremity and preventing venous return. He demonstrated that these contractures might be prevented by prompt surgical decompression. This led him to conclude that contracture is due to a combination of factors, most important of which are impairment of venous flow, extravasations of blood and serum, and swelling of the tissues with consequent pressure on the blood vessels and nerves in the involved area.

Sir Robert Jones,[8] in 1928, concluded that VIC could be caused by pressure from within, from without or from both.

Leriche,[9] in 1928, proposed that a nervous reflex mediated through the sympathetic nervous system causes an arterial spasm, occluding both the main vessel and the collateral branches. Treatment of impending VIC was therefore directed towards interruption of this reflex arc by synaptic block or arterial stripping aiming to manage the arterial spasm.

Lloyd Griffiths,[10] in 1940, in his Hunterian lecture on the subject, said that VIC was solely due to an arterial injury, with reflex spasm of the collateral vessels. He dismissed all considerations of venous occlusion or subfascial haematoma. He thought that tight splintage was 'merely contributory'. His conclusions were generally accepted and repeated in almost every paper on the subject for the next 25 years.

Fontaine et al.,[11] in 1950, demonstrated experimentally that interruption of the blood supply as well as a cerebrospinal reflex mechanism are both equally important in the aetiopathogenesis of VIC and that compression produced by tight plaster casts only aggravated the previously existing circulatory disturbance.

Blount,[12] Ruth et al.[13] and Cregan[14] pointed out that constriction or division of a main vessel does not invariably lead to ischaemic necrosis and that absence of radial pulsations alone does not indicate impending VIC. Ruth et al.[13] pointed out that the vulnerability of certain muscles to vascular damage is partly related to the intramuscular vascular pattern in the forearm and that certain muscles are involved so much more often in VIC than the remaining muscles of the forearm.

As suggested by Cohen[15] and Brooks,[16] and supported by Lipscomb,[17] arterial spasm, which accompanies injury to a major vessel, must extend far enough to involve the vessels on which the collateral circulation depends if ischaemic necrosis is to occur, and necrosis is massive if the spasm is sufficiently prolonged.[17] The vascular pattern of the flexor and pronator muscles in the forearm probably explains why these structures are so much more often involved in Volkmann's contracture than are the remaining muscles in the forearm.[13]

Lipscomb[17] concluded that (1) arterial injury with associated vascular spasm is the most important cause of VIC and (2) in the upper extremity, major arterial obstruction is not so important in the production of the contracture as is the associated spasm of the collateral blood vessels.

Seddon,[18] in 1966, challenged the arterial injury theory. He noticed that all his patients had early and gross swelling and 50% had peripheral pulses palpable. He recommended early fasciotomy as a general rule for management of early compartment syndrome.

Eaton and Green,[19] in 1972, described a traumatic ischaemia–oedema cycle, which leads to compartment syndrome. They said that most commonly the anterior compartment is involved, but, rarely, the posterior or even the intrinsic compartments can be involved in addition. They advised surgical decompression from proximal forearm to the wrist, with secondary wound closure and additional split skin grafts if required. Whitesides et al.[20] advised the surgical decompression to extend from distal arm to the carpal tunnel release. Gelberman et al.[21] advocated the volar extensile single longitudinal curvilinear incision for decompression of the forearm, which included incising the palmar antebrachial fascia, forearm neurovascular structures, carpal tunnel as well as the mobile wad.

Holden,[22] in 1979, took the ischaemia–oedema cycle theory further and described two types of ischaemia. Type 1 is when the major vessels are impaired proximal to the elbow, resulting in secondary ischaemia of the flexors distal to the injury. Type 2 is when direct trauma causes ischaemia at the site of injury. In both situations, an osseofascial compartment syndrome develops.

Mubarak and Carroll,[23] in 1979, advanced the concept of tissue fluid pressure build-up in closed osseofascial compartments because of complex symptoms caused by circulatory disturbances of muscles and nerves. Their studies suggested that the normal range of intracompartmental pressure (ICP) is 0–8 mmHg. In compartment syndrome, it reaches 30–50 mmHg or sometimes even as high as 80 mmHg.

The importance of measuring the ICPs was demonstrated by Mubarak et al.[24] and Hargens et al.[25] Matsen et al.[26] showed that, as ICP rises, venous pressure rises. When venous pressure rises to more than the capillary perfusion pressure, the capillaries collapse. The ICPs at which this occurs and mandates intervention is generally agreed to be more than 30 mmHg.

Tsuge[27] concluded that Holden[22] type 1 is more severe in extent and degree than type 2, and the former develops in small children and assumes a typical contracture, whereas the latter is seen in youths or adults and tends to develop into a selective type of ischaemia.

Many opinions have thus been expressed, but the main point is that compartment syndrome and VIC are caused by a complex interplay of multiple factors: venous stasis in addition to disturbance of arterial flow, followed by ischaemic degeneration of muscle. The resulting oedema within the specially structured deep fascia in turn further impairs the circulation, and, during the repetition of this cycle, necrosis of muscles progresses.

ANATOMIC CONSIDERATIONS

Compartment syndrome may occur in varied locations, even in the anterior or posterior compartments of the leg, but the classic location is the flexor compartment of the forearm. This location has several unique anatomic features that predispose it to developing compartment syndrome. It has a strong fascial roof, and at its entrance lie two potential obstructions.[19] First and lying most superficial is the lacertous fibrous fascia, which fans medially from the biceps tendon as the latter inserts on the proximal radius. The second is the bulky pronator teres muscle, which arises from the medial epicondyle and passes obliquely beneath the inelastic *lacertous fibrosus* to create a V-shaped sphincter beneath which the brachial artery and the median nerve must pass to enter the flexor compartment. Oedema, haematoma or intramuscular haemorrhage in this crucial region may cause sufficient compression of these neurovascular structures to precipitate the ischaemia–oedema cycle. Also, this yoke-like restraint of the biceps tendon and its lacertous fibrous fascia fixes these vessels to the distal fragment, preventing their displacement away from the sharp anterior edge of the proximal fragment.

In the classical aetiopathogenesis of compartment syndrome when there is unreduced supracondylar fracture of the humerus, the forearm is displaced backwards, the fold of deep fascia kinking the brachial artery and the veins around the lower end of the humerus. Also, because of backward displacement and swelling about the flexed elbow, the skin is drawn across the tight antecubital space, compressing off the main venous return of the forearm that is subcutaneous and at the anterior aspect of the elbow. The contents within the closed compartment of the deep fascia swell, raising the ICP to such a high level that blood cannot circulate in this closed compartment. Thus, the contents undergo varied degrees of necrosis and eventually fibrosis.

The course of the brachial artery and its branches makes it vulnerable to injury and compression at several levels. At the supracondylar level, since its distal course is fixed by the biceps tendon and the lacertous fibrosus, the brachial artery may be lacerated, contused or angulated across the fracture edge in supracondylar fractures of the humerus. Just beyond the lacertous fibrous fascia, the brachial artery divides into the more superficial radial artery and the deeper ulnar artery. The radial artery courses more superficially and is not crossed transversely by another structure in the forearm. The ulnar artery, with its major branch, the interosseous artery, however, passes deep to the pronator teres and is the sole blood supply of the flexor digitorum profundous and flexor pollicis longus. These are the muscles most severely involved in Volkmann's contracture.

Eaton and Green[19] described how the median nerve is also anatomically vulnerable to compression. It accompanies the brachial artery beneath the biceps tendon–lacertous fibrosus arch and then enters the substance of the pronator teres, usually passing beneath its superficial (humeral) and deep (ulnar) heads. As it emerges, it passes beneath a thickened band of fascia that connects the humeral and ulnar origins of the flexor digitorum superficialis muscle. The median nerve is commonly compressed at this point – diffusely by the swollen, contracted or fibrotic pronator teres muscle and locally by the sharp unyielding edge of the conjoined origin of the flexor digitorum superficialis muscle.

Collateral vessels serving the flexor compartment are minimal. Adequate collaterals exist around the elbow, but these do not enter the antebrachial compartment. Instead, they join the brachial or radial arteries proximal to the pronator teres. A single exception is the posterior interosseous artery, a branch of the ulnar artery, which has a recurrent branch anastomosing with the lateral elbow collateral vessels. The posterior interosseous artery, however, lies in the dorsal compartment and can shunt blood to the volar compartment only when the common interosseous artery is patent and the pressure gradient is sufficient to produce flow to this compartment. In patients with severe VIC, the arterial spasm affects all branches of the common interosseous artery, including the posterior interosseous. Therefore, this recurrent collateral vessel is rendered ineffective. Evidence of posterior interosseous insufficiency in VIC is the presence of fibrosis of and loss of function of deep extensor muscles, e.g. the abductor pollicis longus, extensor pollicis longus and extensor pollicis brevis.

AETIOLOGY

Compartment syndrome is most commonly seen after injuries to the leg[28–30] and forearm,[31] but it can also occur in the arm, thigh, foot, hand, buttock and abdomen. Traumatic injury is the most common cause: 40% of all compartment syndromes being caused after fractures of the tibia shaft[32] and the incidence in tibia shaft fractures being 1–10%.[32–37] Twenty-three per cent of compartment syndromes are caused by soft-tissue injuries without fractures, and 18% are caused by fractures of the forearm. It can also occur after non-traumatic causes (Box 56.1). Subclinical compartment syndromes may be responsible for some postoperative disabilities following intramedullary nailing of long-bone fractures.[38]

BOX 56.1: Causes of acute compartment syndrome

Increased compartment volume
- Fracture
  - supracondylar humerus
  - forearm bones
  - distal radius
- Soft-tissue injury
  - crush syndrome
  - severe contusion
  - muscle tear
  - wringer injuries
  - gunshot wounds
- Iatrogenic (postoperative inflammation, fracture fixation with oversize implants)
- Exertion (intensive muscle use)
- Strenuous exercise
- Tetany
- Eclampsia
- Seizures
- Bleeding
- Bleeding or coagulation disorder (e.g. haemophilia)
- Anticoagulant therapy
- Postoperative vascular injury
- Traumatic rupture of vascular malformation
- Fluid extravasations into soft tissues
- Ruptured cysts/ganglia
- During arthroscopy with fluid extravasation
- Infection (acute haematogenous osteomyelitis)
- Increased capillary permeability or pressure
- Venous obstruction/ligation
- After prolonged ischaemia/tourniquet
- Arterial bypass grafting
- Ergotamine ingestion
- Thermal injury
- Electrical injury
- Frostbite
- Snakebite
- Intra-arterial drug injection
- Reimplantation
- Cardiac catheterization and angiography
- Embolectomy
- Nephrotic syndrome
- Viral myositis
- Leukaemic infiltration
- Miscellaneous
- Metastasis to skeletal muscle
- High-pressure injection injury
- Transfusion infiltration into soft tissues

Decreased compartmental volume
- Tight casts/splints
- Prolonged limb pressure (e.g. lengthy surgeries, anaesthesia, comatose patient)
- Excessive traction on fractured limb

PATHOGENESIS

The increased tissue pressure in compartment syndrome occurs because of the uncertain effect of trauma or other causes on the small vessels – arterioles, capillaries or veins.

Different theories have been proposed for the pathogenesis of compartment syndrome.

The critical closing pressure theory[39]

Transmural pressure (TM) is the pressure difference across the vessel wall between the intravascular (P_{in}) and extravascular (P_{out}) tissue (Fig. 56.1). This is balanced by the vessel wall tension (T) consisting of vessel tissue elasticity and active contractility of vessel smooth muscle. According to Laplace's law, the pressure gradient across the vessel wall is given by:

$$TM = T/r$$

where r is the radius of the vessel.

Rising tissue pressure leads to a dropping of the transmural pressure, and at a critical point the vessel wall elasticity is lost. At this point, when T/r is more than TM, the vessels collapse and blood flow will be decreased or may temporarily stop.[40] However, flow may resume after 30–60 seconds from ischaemia-induced local release of vasodilators depending on vasomotor tone and the amount of tissue pressure.

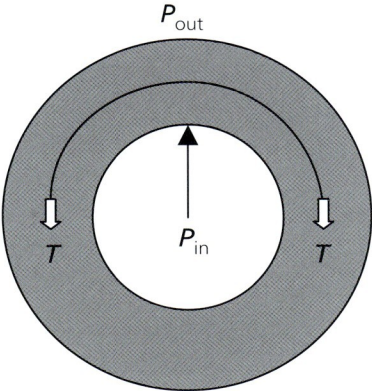

Figure 56.1 Transmural pressure.

The arteriovenous gradient theory[41]

This theory has gained the most popularity recently.[42,43] Blood flow (BF) in vascular channels of tissues is directly proportional to the arteriovenous pressure gradient (AV) [difference between the local arterial pressure (P_a) and the local venous pressure (P_v)] and inversely proportional to the local vascular resistance (R) and expressed by the equation:

$$BF = P_a - P_v/R$$

Increased tissue pressure in acute compartment syndrome causes the veins to collapse. This leads the AV gradient and thus the BF to fall, causing reduced tissue perfusion. Ischaemia begins when local blood flow cannot meet the metabolic demands of the tissues. Reduced venous drainage causes the interstitial tissue pressure to rise, leading to tissue oedema. Rising interstitial fluid pressure causes lymphatic drainage to increase, but, after it reaches its maximum, the lymphatic vessels collapse too. Swelling and oedema continue to rise until the arterial flow is compromised in the late stages of compartment syndrome (Fig. 56.2).

The microvascular occlusion theory[44]

Capillary occlusion has been proposed as the main factor in reducing blood flow in acute compartment syndrome. This theory suggests that, whenever the tissue pressure values approach the capillary pressure levels, capillaries are occluded. This increases the capillary membrane permeability to plasma proteins. This in turn further increases the tissue oedema, which eventually leads to lymphatic obstruction. Evidence from animal experiments has been reported showing that increasing compartment pressure reduces the number of perfused capillaries per unit area, and that there is complete cessation of muscle capillary blood flow when the compartment pressure is within about 25 mmHg of the mean arterial pressure (Fig. 56.3).[45]

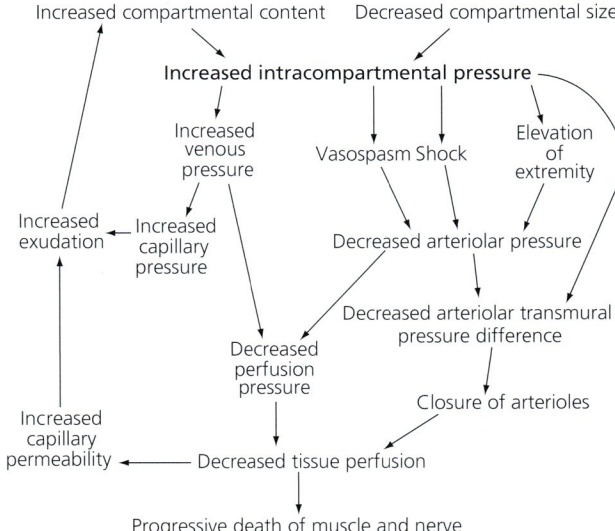

Figure 56.2 Matsen's unified concept of compartment syndrome.

Normal resting intramuscular pressure is usually less than 6 mmHg. In compartment syndrome, the intramuscular pressure can increase to more than 100 mmHg. The initial insult causes haemorrhage, oedema or both in the closed fascial compartments of the extremities. Rising compartment pressure ultimately leads to compartmental tamponade, microcirculatory impairment and sustained ischaemia. This vicious cycle of increasing ischaemia was originally described by Matsen and Clawson[46] and further expanded by Hargens et al.[44] When the compartmental pressure is left untreated and allowed to increase, a reduction in blood flow occurs leading to muscle and nerve ischaemia, which can be irreversible.[47–49] The extent of tissue injury depends on compartmental pressure and time.[48,49]

Effect on muscle

Raised compartmental pressure leads to reduced blood flow to skeletal muscle. Skeletal muscle is the most vulnerable to ischaemic damage. The duration of ischaemia influences the amount of muscle necrosis, with increasing irreversible changes occurring more with increased periods of ischaemia.[50–52]

The centre of the muscle belly undergoes more severe necrotic damage than the periphery, although the vulnerability of muscles to ischaemia varies depending on the muscle fibre type. *Type 1 aerobic fibres* (red/slow-twitch fibres), which depend on oxidative metabolism of triglycerides, are more vulnerable to ischaemia than *type 2 anaerobic fibres* (white/fast-twitch fibres).[53] That explains why some muscle groups are more vulnerable to ischaemic damage than others.

Normal resting intramuscular tissue pressure is usually less than 6 mmHg. Any inciting event of compartment syndrome raises this pressure due to the resulting oedema or haemorrhage and causes muscle ischaemia due to a decrease

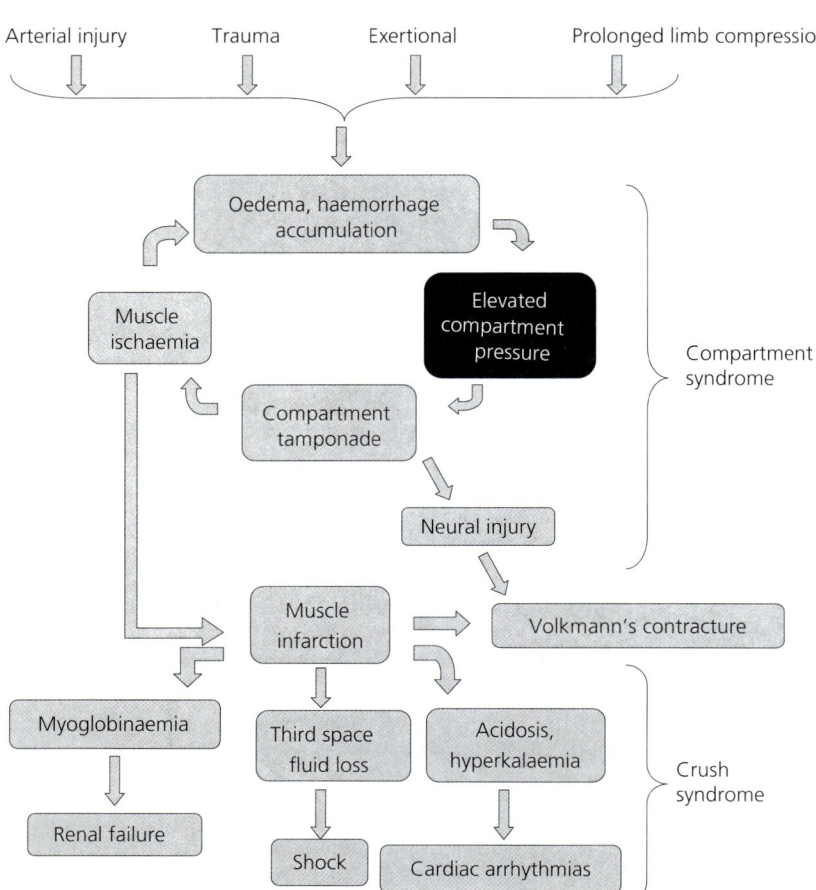

Figure 56.3 Hargen's and Akenson's[44] concept of pathophysiology of compartment syndrome, including crush syndrome.

in capillary flow. The critical tissue pressure threshold is 10–20 mmHg below the diastolic blood pressure or 25–30 mmHg below the mean arterial blood pressure.[54–57] Animal studies have shown that compartmental pressures more than 30 mmHg maintained for more than 8 hours can cause irreversible muscle damage.

Effect on nerve

Peripheral nerve conduction block by high muscle compartment pressure occurs from an as yet unclear complex interplay of ischaemia, compression, toxic free radicals and acidosis.[58] Both the *duration* and *magnitude* of compartmental pressure elevation are important in producing neuromuscular deficits. Pressures that are benign for a few hours may be detrimental if allowed to persist for longer periods.[59–61] Thus, continuous monitoring of tissue pressure is important in tracking the ICP trend. However, there is considerable variation of tolerance to pressure among different individuals.[58]

Effect on bone

Compartment syndrome reduces the healing capacity of long bones, by possibly reducing the extra-osseous blood supply and non-union can be a possible complication.[62–65]

MANAGEMENT

Diagnosis

The first step in the successful management of acute compartment syndrome is prompt diagnosis. Acute compartment syndrome is a medical emergency and any delay in its diagnosis is the single most important cause of morbidity,[29,66,67] with potential to cause disastrous consequences including amputation and even death. The end result of unchecked acute compartment syndrome can be loss of neuromuscular function of a limb due to muscle and nerve damage, ischaemic contracture, infection and delayed union of a fracture.

Clinical examination

Diagnosis of acute compartment syndrome is made clinically and confirmed by actual measurement of compartmental tissue fluid pressure. Initially, a high index of suspicion is important to make a diagnosis. Compartment syndrome can occur after any injury pattern, from varied aetiology, velocity of impact or degree of comminution of the fracture. It can also occur after an open fracture, often when small, transverse fascial tears fail to adequately decompress the compartment.

Clinical diagnosis is made from the presenting physical symptoms and signs, which include increasing pain, pain on passively stretching the muscle of the affected compartment, altered sensation, muscle weakness and palpable tenseness of the compartment which may or may not be tender.

Pain is often the first and most important symptom and usually out of proportion to the clinical picture. The nursing record may show the patient's need for more frequent doses of pain relief or switching over to stronger analgesics, but the pain is often unremitting irrespective of the amount of analgesics given. Constricting casts and dressings often exacerbate the pain and their release may give a transient but often minimal relief from pain. However, pain itself is an unreliable and variable indicator.[26] It can range from being very mild to severe with subjective variations. Passive stretching of the overlying non-ischaemic muscles in limb trauma (e.g. fracture or blunt trauma) may cause pain. Moreover, pain of injury may mask that of impending compartment syndrome. Pain if used as a diagnostic indicator of acute compartment syndrome has a high proportion of missed or false negative cases (sensitivity of 19%), but a low proportion of false positive cases (specificity of 97%).[68] It cannot be elicited in unconscious patients and is an unreliable indicator in small children in whom clinical suspicion is raised by manifested agitation, anxiety and restlessness.

Pain on passively stretching the muscles of the affected compartment (e.g. passively extending the fingers in acute compartment syndrome affecting the volar compartment of the forearm) is a recognized symptom, but this is also an unreliable sign.[24] Passive stretching of the overlying non-ischaemic muscles in limb trauma (e.g. fracture or blunt trauma) too may cause pain.

Altered sensations (paraesthesia, hypoaesthesia or anaesthesia) may be manifested in the area distal to the compartment, in the sensory distribution of the nerves traversing the compartment involved. However, sensory changes may be late and often the last clinical finding to develop as the compartment syndrome progresses.[29] Simultaneous nerve injury not related to the development of the compartment syndrome may also manifest sensory changes. Paraesthesias have a high proportion of false negative cases (sensitivity of 13%), but a low proportion of false positive cases (specificity of 98%).[68]

Weakness of the muscle groups affected in acute compartment syndrome occurs late,[68] but is also of low diagnostic value since this can also result from associated nerve injury, direct injury to the muscle or inhibition of muscle function from pain. Moreover, frank muscle weakness is often late to appear; so to wait for this to manifest can be a disaster.

Palpable tenseness of the swollen affected compartment is often the earliest sign and palpating reproduces the patient's pain. However, it is difficult to determine how much pain is from the fracture or the injury itself and how much from the tenderness of the swollen compartment syndrome. The compartment may feel very hard depending on the ICP and the overlying skin often appears shiny. Occasionally, the tenseness of the compartment affected may not be obvious, particularly in the deep flexor compartment of the forearm (or the deep posterior compartment of the leg) where the compartment is completely buried under the superficial muscle compartments and may lead to delay in diagnosis.

Peripheral pulses are almost always present in acute compartment syndrome, unless the injury involves damage to vessels, or in peripheral shutdown in shock or when it is difficult to palpate pulses because of the overlying swelling. Compartment syndrome involves shutdown of small thin-walled vessels within the compartment affected. Thus capillary return in the periphery is usually intact except in the very advanced stage. However, if pulses are present, it does not exclude the diagnosis of compartment syndrome. Doppler studies or arteriography are indicated in acute compartment syndrome with absent pulses and a suspicion of arterial damage but are not for the diagnosis of compartment syndrome.

Clinical signs and symptoms if used in combination may increase the diagnostic ability. The probability of compartment syndrome with one clinical finding is about 25%, but rises to 93% if three clinical findings are present.[68]

Hargens and Mubarak's six Ps characteristic of acute compartment syndrome are:

- high *p*ressure
- *p*ain (especially with passive stretch)
- *p*araesthesias
- *p*aresis
- *p*ink skin colour
- *p*ulse (distal pulse present).

Intracompartmental pressure measurement and monitoring

Although compartment syndrome is diagnosed clinically, it is confirmed by measuring the ICP. This is the most important investigation in acute compartment syndrome. Several methods are available to measure the ICP:

1. needle manometer method[69]
2. wick or slit catheter technique[24]
3. continuous monitoring infusion technique[70]
4. hand-held transducers (Stryker Intra-compartmental Pressure System).

The Whitesides straight needle manometer method is the least accurate method[71] and is not appropriate for clinical use. Side-port needles and slit catheters are more accurate than straight needles. The arterial line manometer and the Stryker manometer device are the most accurate devices if used with either the side-port needle or the slit catheter.[71] Newer devices with the transducer placed at the tip of the catheter do not depend on the fluid column and so do not have the problem of fluid patency.

Although the recently available new devices are easier to use and are perhaps more reliable, these still have their limitations and have potential measurement error. Thus, clinical findings and judgement should always have an upper hand in making the diagnosis and treatment plan.

Near-infrared spectroscopy (NIRS) is a promising non-invasive technique for the continuous monitoring of tissue oxygen delivery. NIRS involves placing a probe on the skin and it detects light absorbance of haemoglobin chromophores to determine tissue oxygen saturation (StO_2). This correlates to tissue pressures, as proven in experimental studies and those involving healthy human volunteers, but needs to be validated in human volunteers with injury. However, there are recent reports that the NIRS device fails to register tissue saturation values at some point in half the individuals. This occurs more often in individuals with darker skin, possibly because melanin clearly interferes with the quality of the reflected NIRS signal.[72]

Radiographs

These are required to investigate for possible underlying fractures and fracture dislocation, their reduction and possible radio-opaque foreign bodies.

Doppler flowmetry and arteriography

Doppler flowmetry and arteriography are valuable in verifying a suspected arterial injury, but not for diagnosis of acute compartment syndrome. These investigations should not delay fasciotomy. Arteriography can be performed in the operating room, so that vascular repair, if needed, can be done in the same sitting, without delaying fasciotomy.

MRI, CT and ultrasound

MRI, CT and ultrasound can be helpful in delineating the necrotic areas of the muscle compartment, but these are really not necessary, and the process of getting them done is often time-consuming and may delay the surgical management of acute compartment syndrome. These can be a choice in chronic or exertional compartment syndrome.

Delay in diagnosis of compartment syndrome

Diagnosis of compartment syndrome is likely to be delayed in patients with concomitant central or peripheral nervous system involvement, multiple trauma, alcohol or drug intoxication, patients who are unable to communicate or patients with burns (Box 56.2).[73]

Differential diagnosis

ARTERIAL INJURY OR OCCLUSION

Pulses are absent or diminished in arterial injury or occlusion, but intact in compartment syndrome. Passive muscle stretch causes pain. Motor or sensory deficit may be present.

NERVE INJURY

Motor or sensory deficit may be present, but passive muscle stretch does not cause any pain unless muscle is also injured. Pulses are usually normal.

BOX 56.2: Patients prone to delay in diagnosis of compartment syndrome

- Head injury
- Cerebrovascular accident
- Spinal cord injury
- Peripheral nerve injury
- Anaesthetized patients (general/local)
- Alcoholic/drug-overdosed patients
- Mentally disabled patients
- Burn patients
- Infants/young patients

GENERAL PRINCIPLES OF TREATMENT OF COMPARTMENT SYNDROME

Goals for the management of acute compartment syndrome are to restore tissue perfusion to the affected muscles and nerves of the compartment affected, to prevent or minimize the injury and to avoid any residual loss of function. Treatment may be non-operative for impending compartment syndrome or surgical for established compartment syndrome.

Non-operative treatment

Non-operative treatment may be an option if the stage is of *impending* compartment syndrome. All tight circumferential bandages and casts are removed down to skin. Exaggerated flexion or extension of the wrist should be repositioned to reduce intracarpal interstitial fluid pressures. Alternative methods of immobilization or fixation should be chosen if necessary to maintain fracture reduction. Excessive flexion of the elbow, if corrected to a more extended position, often corrects the compartmental pressures to a certain extent. Avoid excessive elevation of the limb. If symptoms persist, fasciotomy is indicated. There is no role of elevation, ice compresses or sympathetic blocks in symptomatic compartment syndrome. Borderline symptomatic patients may be monitored with an indwelling catheter. Persistently borderline or doubtful patients should preferably have a fasciotomy rather than delay treatment. Delay in treatment can have devastating consequences. Hyperbaric oxygen is still experimental in non-operative management of compartment syndrome and cannot be recommended as an established treatment method.

Fasciotomy

Open and extensive fasciotomies of all the compartments within the part of the limb affected by compartment syndrome is the treatment of choice.[26,36,67,74,75]

Fasciotomy not only relieves compartmental pressure, but also helps in re-establishing tissue perfusion if done timely enough and if there is no arterial injury or compromise.

For the leg, all four compartments must be decompressed, usually via two long, longitudinal incisions. It will be necessary to debride necrotic tissue, sometimes several times. In the other common site, the forearm, the three compartments (the mobile wad of three, the volar and extensor) can be released via two incisions (one curvilinear volar incision across the elbow and straight to the wrist to include releasing the carpal tunnel and one straight incision along the extensor ulna border). The hand has 10 compartments (requiring five incisions); similarly, the foot. Compartment syndrome is most common in the lower leg and forearm. In the leg the anterior compartment is the most frequently involved.

Critical compartmental pressure for fasciotomy

There is no universal agreement on the compartmental pressures beyond which fasciotomy should be performed. Varied methods of pressure measurement are partly responsible for the disagreement. With needle manometer techniques, with or without continuous infusion, relatively higher values are acceptable. Fasciotomy is generally indicated when compartmental pressures rise to within 10–30 mmHg of the patient's diastolic blood pressure if the patient is symptomatic.[69] With wick, slit or Stryker intracompartmental pressure system (STIC) methods, where continuous infusion is not used, relatively lower critical pressures are generally acceptable. There is a significant individual variation among different individuals for their tolerance to raised ICP.[30,76] Whitesides et al.[69] were the first to suggest that the variation in tolerance to raised ICP among different individuals is due to variations in systemic blood pressures, and that inadequate tissue perfusion results when tissue pressures rise to within 10–30 mmHg of the diastolic pressures. This concept of differential pressure (difference between the diastolic blood pressure and the ICP) of 30 mmHg as a threshold for decompression in acute compartment syndrome has been proven in clinical studies as a safe threshold.[65,77,78] The threshold differential pressures in children may be less than 30 mmHg as they have lower diastolic pressures than adults. Thus, for children, the use of mean arterial pressure has been recommended instead of the diastolic pressure.[74]

Another important variable in ICP measurement is the distance from the fracture at which the compartment pressure is recorded.[56] The 'zone of peak pressure' is within a few centimetres of the fracture and failure to measure tissue pressure from the zone of peak pressure can result in serious underestimation of the maximal compartmental pressure.

Continuous ICP monitoring is more useful than a single pressure reading, since the trend in change of ICP is probably more significant. Except for extreme cases, fasciotomy should not be performed based on an odd single high ICP reading. If the ICP shows a downward trend in continuous monitoring and differential pressure is rising, it is justified to still observe the patient in anticipation of the differential pressure returning to within the safe limit and relatively quickly.

KEY LEARNING POINTS

- Compartment syndrome is a complex and challenging orthopaedic emergency with potential to cause one of the most destructive complications after a limb injury – Volkmann's ischaemic contracture.
- Compartment syndrome may occur in varied locations, such as the anterior or posterior compartments of the leg, and the classic location is the flexor compartment of the forearm.
- The increased tissue pressure in compartment syndrome occurs because of the uncertain effect of trauma or other causes on the small vessels – arterioles, capillaries or veins.
- Acute compartment syndrome is a medical emergency and any delay in its diagnosis is the single most important cause of failure.
- Diagnosis of acute compartment syndrome is made clinically and confirmed by actual measurement of compartmental tissue fluid pressure.
- Pain is often the first symptom, usually ischaemic in nature and out of proportion to the clinical picture.
- The six Ps are: high pressure; pain (especially with passive stretch); paraesthesias; paresis; pink skin colour; pulse (distal pulse present).
- Diagnosis of compartment syndrome is likely to be delayed in patients with concomitant central or peripheral nervous system involvement, multiple trauma, alcohol or drug intoxication, patients who are unable to communicate or patients with burns.
- Non-operative treatment may be an option if the stage is of impending compartment syndrome.
- Open and extensive fasciotomies of all the compartments within the part of the limb affected by compartment syndrome is the treatment of choice.

REFERENCES

● = Key primary paper
♦ = Major review article

●1. Mubarak SJ, Hargens AR, Owen CA, et al. The wick catheter technique for measurement of intramuscular pressure. *Journal of Bone and Joint Surgery (American)* 1976;**58A**:1016–20.
2. Hildebrand O. Die Lehre von den ischmischen Muskellahmungen und Kontrakturen. *Zeitschrift Chirurgie* 1906;**108**:201.
●3. Volkmann R. Die ischaemischen Muskellähmungen und Kontrakturen. *Zentralblatt für Chirurgie* 1881;**8**:801.
●4. Leonards D, Littlewood H. Volkmann's contracture. *Lancet* 1902;**159**:193.
●5. Thomas JJ. Nerve involvement in the ischaemic paralysis and contracture of Volkmann. *Annals of Surgery* 1909;**49**:330.
6. Murphy JB. Myositis. *Journal of the American Medical Association* 1914;**63**:1240.
7. Jepson PN. Ischaemic contracture: experimental study. *Annals of Surgery* 1926;**84**:785–95.
●8. Jones R. Address on Volkmann's contracture with specific reference to treatment. *British Medical Journal* 1928;**2**:639.
9. Leriche R. Surgery of the sympathetic system: indications and results. *Annals of Surgery* 1928;**883**:449–69.
●10. Griffiths DL. Volkmann's ischaemic contracture. *British Journal of Surgery* 1940;**28**:239–60.
11. Fontaine R, Kayser C, Klein M, et al. Physiological and morphological modifications of the striated muscle following intra-arterial injections of iodo-organic product into the humeral artery of the dog–experimental Volkmann's contracture. *Revue de Chirurgie* 1950;**69**:15–36.
●12. Blount WP. Editorial. Volkmann's ischemic contracture. *Surgery, Gynecology and Obstetrics* 1950;**90**:244–6.
13. Ruth E, Bowden M, Gutmann E. The fate of voluntary muscle after vascular injury in man. *Journal of Bone and Joint Surgery (British)* 1949;**31B**:356–68.
●14. Cregan JCF. Prolonged traumatic arterial spasm after supracondylar fracture of the humerus. *Journal of Bone and Joint Surgery (British)* 1951;**33B**:363–4.
15. Cohen SM. Traumatic arterial spasm. *Guy's Hospital Reports* 1940;**20**:201–16.
16. Brooks B. Surgical applications of therapeutic venous obstruction. *Archives of Surgery* 1929;**19**(Pt 1):1–23.
♦17. Lipscomb PR. The etiology and prevention of Volkmann's Ischemic contracture. *Surgery, Gynecology and Obstetrics* 1956;**103**:353–61.
♦18. Seddon HJ. Volkmann's ischaemia in the lower limb. *Journal of Bone and Joint Surgery (British)* 1966;**48**:627–36.
●19. Eaton RG, Green WT. Epimysiotomy and fasciotomy in the treatment of Volkmann's ischemic contracture. *Orthopedic Clinics of North America* 1972;**3**:175.
20. Whitesides TE Jr, Harada H, Morimoto K. Compartment syndromes and the role of fasciotomy, its parameters and techniques. *Instructional Course Lectures* 1977;**26**:179.
21. Gelberman RH, Szabo RM, Williamson RV, et al. Tissue pressure threshold for peripheral nerve viability. *Clinical Orthopaedics* 1983;**178**:285–91.
♦22. Holden CEA. The pathology and prevention of Volkmann's ischaemic contracture *Journal of Bone and Joint Surgery (British)* 1979;**61**:296–300.
♦23. Mubarak SJ, Carroll NC. Volkmann's contracture in children: aetiology and prevention, *Journal of Bone and Joint Surgery (British)* 1979;**61B**:285.
♦24. Mubarak SJ, Owen CA, Hargens AR, et al. Acute compartment syndrome: diagnosis and treatment with the aid of the Wick catheter. *Journal of Bone and Joint Surgery (American)* 1978;**60A**:1091.
♦25. Hargens AR, Mubarak SJ, Akeson WH, et al. Critical pressure and time relationships in compartment syndromes. International Research Society for Orthopaedics and 7. Traumatology (SIROT), First Meeting, Program and Abstracts, 15–20 October 1978, Kyoto, Japan, p. 21.
♦26. Matsen FA, Winquist RA, Krugmire RB. Diagnosis and management of compartmental syndromes. *Journal of Bone and Joint Surgery (American)* 1980;**62A**:286.
♦27. Tsuge K. Treatment of established Volkmann's ischemic contracture. *Plastic and Reconstructive Surgery* 1986;**77**:80.
28. Bradley EL III. The anterior tibial compartment syndrome. *Surgery, Gynecology and Obstetrics* 1973;**136**:289–97.
♦29. Rorabeck CH, Macnab L. Anterior tibial compartment syndrome complicating fractures of the shaft of the tibia. *Journal of Bone and Joint Surgery (American)* 1976;**58**:549–50.
30. Halpern AA, Nagel DA. Anterior compartment pressure in patients with tibial fracture. *Journal of Trauma* 1980;**20**:786–90.
31. Gelberman RH. Upper extremity compartment syndromes. In: Mubarak SJ, Hargens AR (eds) *Compartment Syndromes and Volkmann's Contracture*. Philadelphia, PA: W.B. Saunders, 1981.
32. McQueen MM, Gaston P, Court-Brown CM. Acute compartment syndrome. Who is at risk? *Journal of Bone and Joint Surgery (British)* 2000;**82B**:200.
●33. Court-Brown CM, Byrnes T, McLaughlin G. Intramedullary nailing of tibial diaphyseal fractures in children with open physes. *Injury* 2003;**34**:781–5.
34. Blick SS, Brumback PJ, Poka A, et al. Compartment syndrome in open tibial fractures. *Journal of Bone and Joint Surgery (American)* 1986;**68**:1348–53.
35. Williams J, Gibbons M, Trindle H, et al. Complications of nailing in closed tibial fractures. *Journal of Orthopedic Trauma* 1995;**9**:476–81.
36. McQueen MM, Court-Brown CM. Compartment monitoring in tibial fractures: the pressure threshold for decompression. *Journal of Bone and Joint Surgery (British)* 1996;**78**:99–104.
●37. Finkemeier CG, Schmidt AH, Kyle RF, et al. A prospective randomised study of intramedullary nails inserted with and without reaming for the treatment of open and closed fractures of the tibial shaft. *Journal of Orthopedic Trauma* 2000;**14**:187–93.

- 38. Robinson CM, O'Donnell J, Will E, Keating JF. Dropped hallux after the intramedullary nailing of tibial fractures. *Journal of Orthopedic Trauma (British)* 1999;**81B**:481–4.
39. Burton A. On the physical equilibrium of small blood vessels. *Journal of Biomechanics* 1971;**4**:155–8.
40. Ashton H. Critical closing pressure in human peripheral vascular beds. *Clinical Science* 1962;**22**:79–87.
41. Matsen FA, Krugmire RB. Compartmental syndromes. *Surgery, Gynecology and Obstetrics* 1978;**147**:943–9.
- ♦42. Elliott KGB, Johnstone AJ. Diagnosing acute compartment syndrome. *Journal of Bone and Joint Surgery (British)* 2003;**85**:625.
43. Vollmar B, Westermann S, Menzer M. Microvascular response to compartment syndrome-like external pressure elevation: an in vivo fluorescence microscopic study in the hamster striated muscle. *Journal of Trauma* 1999;**46**:91–6.
44. Hargens AR, Akeson WH, Mubarak SJ, et al. Fluid balance within the canine anterolateral compartment and its relationship to compartment syndromes *Journal of Bone and Joint Surgery (American)* 1978;**60**:499–505.
45. Hartsock LA, O'Farrell D, Seaber AV, et al. Effect of increased compartment pressure on the microcirculation of skeletal muscle. *Microsurgery* 1998;**18**:67–71.
46. Matsen FA, Clawson DK. The deep posterior compartmental syndrome of the leg. *Journal of Bone and Joint Surgery (American)* 1975;**57**:34–9.
47. Heppenstall RB, Scott R, Sapiga A, et al. A comparative study of the tolerance of skeletal muscle to ischemia. *Journal of Bone and Joint Surgery (American)* 1986;**68**:820.
- •48. Rorabeck CH, Clarke KM. The pathophysiology of the anterior tibial compartment syndrome. An experimental investigation. *Journal of Trauma* 1978;**18**:299–304.
- •49. Rorabeck CH, Castle GSP, Hardie R, et al. Compartmental pressure measurements: an experimental investigation using the slit catheter. *Journal of Trauma* 1981;**21**:446–9.
50. Labbe R, Lindsay T, Walker PM. The extent and distribution of skeletal muscle necrosis after graded periods of complete ischaemia. *Journal of Vascular Surgery* 1987;**6**:152–7.
51. Petrasek PF, Homer-Vanmasinkam S, Walker PM. Determinants of ischaemic injury to skeletal muscle. *Journal of Vascular Surgery* 1994;**19**:623–31.
52. Hayes G, Liauw S, Romaschin AD, et al. Separation of reperfusion injury from ischaemia induced necrosis. *Surgical Forum* 1988;**39**:306–8.
53. Lindsay TF, Liauw S, Rouraschin AD, et al. The effect of ischaemia/reperfusion on adenosine nucleotide metabolism and xanthine oxidase production in skeletal muscle. *Journal of Vascular Surgery* 1990;**12**:8–15.
54. Hartsock LA, O'Farrell D, Seaber AV, et al. Effect of increased compartment pressure on the microcirculation of skeletal muscle. *Microsurgery* 1998;**18**:670–1.
55. Heppenstall RB, Sapega AA, Scott R, et al. The compartment syndrome: an experimental and clinical study of muscular energy metabolism using phosphorus nuclear magnetic resonance spectroscopy. *Clinical Orthopaedics* 1988;**226**:138–55.
56. Heckman MM, Whitesides TE, Greve SR, et al. Histologic determination of the ischaemic threshold of muscle in the canine compartment syndrome model. *Journal of Orthopaedic Trauma* 1993;**7**:199–210.
57. Matava MS, Whitesides TE, Seiler JG, et al. Determination of the compartment pressure threshold of muscle ischaemia in a canine model. *Journal of Trauma* 1994;**37**:50–8.
58. Matsen FA, Mayo KA, Krugmire RB, et al. A model compartment syndrome in man with particular reference to the quantification of nerve function. *Journal of Bone and Joint Surgery (American)* 1978;**59**:648–53.
59. Sheridan GW, Matsen FA, Krugmire RB. Further investigations on the pathophysiology of the compartmental syndrome. *Clinical Orthopedics* 1977;**123**:266–70.
60. Rorabeck CH, Clarke KM. The pathophysiology of the anterior tibial compartment syndrome: an experimental investigation. *Journal of Trauma* 1978;**18**:299–304.
61. Hargens AR, Romine JS, Sipe JC, et al. Peripheral nerve conduction block by high muscle compartment pressure. *Journal of Bone and Joint Surgery (American)* 1979;**61**:192–200.
62. Delee JC, Stiehl JB. Open tibia fracture with compartment syndrome. *Clinical Orthopedics* 1981;**160**:175–84.
63. Court-Brown CM, McQueen MM. Compartment syndrome delays tibial union. *Acta Orthopaedica Scandinavica* 1987;**58**:249–52.
64. Turen CH, Burgess AR, Vanco B. Skeletal stabilization for tibial fractures associated with acute compartment syndrome. *Clinical Orthopedics* 1995;**315**:163–8.
65. McQueen MM, Christie J, Court-Brown CM. Acute compartment syndrome in tibial diaphyseal fractures. *Journal of Bone and Joint Surgery (British)* 1996;**78**:95–8.
66. Matsen FA, Clawson DK. The deep posterior compartmental syndrome of the leg. *Journal of Bone and Joint Surgery (American)* 1975;**57**:34–9.
- ♦67. Rorabeck CH. The treatment of compartment syndromes of the leg. *Journal of Bone and Joint Surgery (British)* 1984;**66**:93–7.
68. Ulmer T. The clinical diagnosis of compartment syndrome of the lower leg: are clinical findings predictive of the disorder? *Journal of Orthopaedic Trauma* 2002;**16**:572–7.
- •69. Whitesides TE Jr, Haney TC, Morimoto K, Hirada H. Tissue pressure measurements as a determinant for the need of fasciotomy. *Clinical Orthopedics* 1975;**113**:43.
70. Matsen FA, Mayo KY, Sheridan GW, et al. Monitoring of intramuscular pressure. *Surgery* 1976;**79**:702–9.
71. Boody AB, Wongworawat MD. Accuracy in the measurement of compartment pressures: a comparison of three commonly used devices. *Journal of Bone and Joint Surgery (American)* 2005;**87**:2415–22.
72. Wassenaar EB, Van den Brand JGH. Reliability of near-infrared spectroscopy in people with dark skin pigmentation *Journal of Clinical Monitoring and Computing* 2005;**19**:195–9.

- 73. Ouellette EA. Compartment syndromes in obtunded patients. *Hand Clinics* 1998;**14**:33.
- 74. Mars M, Hadley GP. Raised compartmental pressure in children: a basis for management. *Injury* 1998;**29**:183–5.
- 75. Sheridan GW, Matsen FA. Fasciotomy in the treatment of acute compartment syndrome. *Journal of Bone and Joint Surgery (American)* 1976;**58A**:112.
- 76. Matsen FA, Wyss CR, Krugmire RB, *et al*. The effect of limb elevation and dependency on local arteriovenous gradients in normal human limbs with particular reference to limbs with increased tissue pressure. *Clinical Orthopedics* 1980;**150**:187–95.
- 77. White TO, Howell GED, Will EM, *et al*. Elevated intramuscular compartment pressures do not influence outcome after tibial fracture. *Journal of Trauma* 2003;**55**:1133–8.
- 78. Øvre S, Hvaal K, Holm I, *et al*. Compartment pressure in nailed tibial fractures: A threshold of 30 mmHg for decompression gives 29% fasciotomies *Archives of Orthopaedic Trauma Surgery* 1998;**118**:29–31.

57

Management of fracture complications

ROBERT B SIMONIS, ANDREW M RICHARDS, DAVID S ELLIOTT

Introduction	515	Malunion	527
Non-union	515	Psychosocial aspects of fracture complications	528
Management of fracture non-union	520	References	530

NATIONAL BOARD STANDARDS

- Revise the basic science of bone healing
- Classify non-union and understand its aetiology
- Rationalize the surgical management of non-union
- Understand the management of infected non-union
- Describe malunion and advise on surgical options
- Counsel a patient for complex limb reconstruction
- Understand the psychosocial effects of fracture complications

INTRODUCTION

The long-term complications of fractures include non-union, infected non-union and malunion.

Their management is time-consuming with frequent hospital admissions. These complications may lead to long-term dysfunction with chronic pain, disability and clinical depression.

NON-UNION

Non-union was historically defined as 'painless movement at a non-healed fracture'. It is now defined as 'when the fracture healing process has ceased to progress'.[1] The diagnosis is made on clinical and radiological findings.

In delayed union, the fracture-healing process is slowed, but the fracture may still go on to unite without surgical intervention. The treatment of delayed union is expectant; surgical intervention is indicated only when healing has ceased.

Perkins' rules (Table 57.1) for the normal time to fracture union remain a useful guide.[2] They illustrate that different bones and different fracture patterns vary in their time to union.

Diagnosis of non-union

To judge whether a fracture has united on radiographs is difficult. Even experienced trauma surgeons will disagree. The two classic radiological views (anteroposterior and lateral) often give inadequate information. If the patient is still symptomatic and the two standard radiographs appear to show union, two additional radiographs, taken at 45° obliquity, should be obtained (Fig. 57.1). One of these four views should be collinear with the plane of the fracture (Fig. 57.2), and the probability of showing a non-union is significantly increased.[3]

Table 57.1 Perkins' rules for normal time to fracture union

	Oblique fracture	Transverse fracture
Arm	6 weeks	12 weeks
Leg	12 weeks	24 weeks

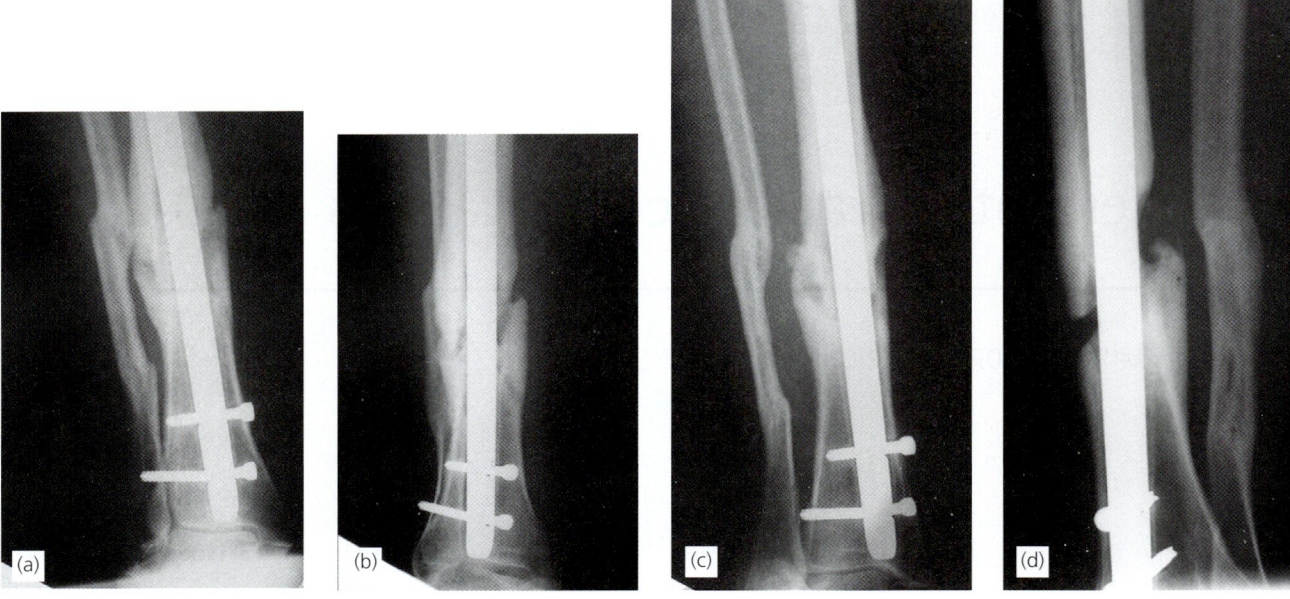

Figure 57.1 (a–d) 'Four-view radiographs' should be acquired to confirm non-union.

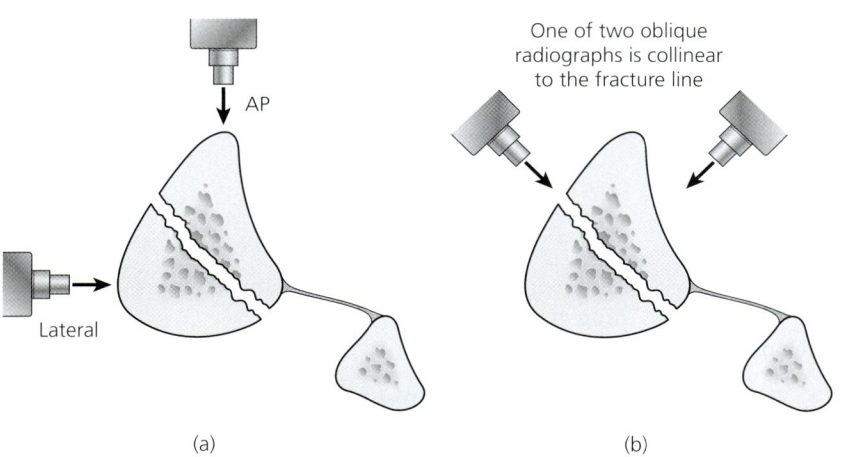

Figure 57.2 Radiographs collinear with the fracture line on additional oblique views. AP, anteroposterior.

When one fragment of a transverse non-union is buried inside the other, like a peg and socket, it will not be shown on these four views. In these rare cases, a CT scan will be necessary to demonstrate the fracture line (Fig. 57.3).[4,5]

The Weber–Cech non-union classification[6]

This radiological classification implies a correlation with fracture biology and suggests treatment methods, as follows.

HYPERTROPHIC NON-UNION (ELEPHANT'S FOOT)

This shows prolific callus formation and is thought to be vascular with good healing potential. Excess motion at the fracture site results in non-union.

ATROPHIC NON-UNION (RAT'S TAIL)

Characterized by an absence of callus. The atrophic bone ends are tapered and may be osteopenic or sclerotic. Bone vascularity is believed to be deficient.

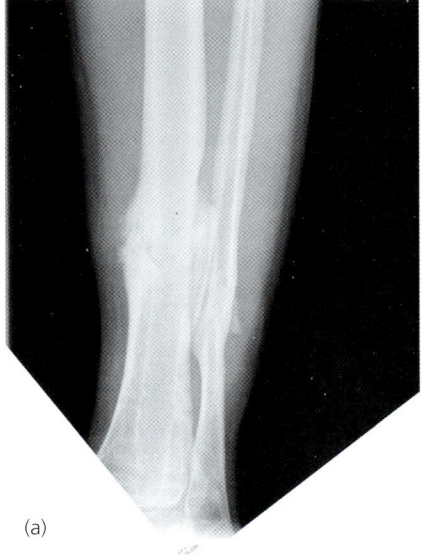
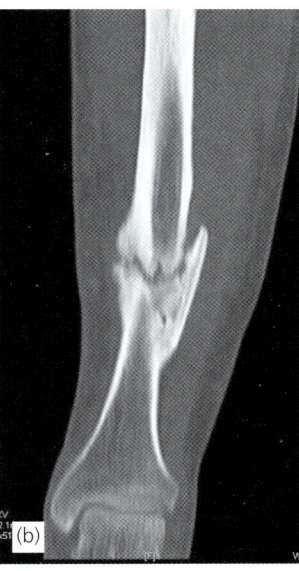

Figure 57.3 (a and b) A 'peg and socket' pattern non-union clearly shown on CT scan but not on plain radiograph.

SYNOVIAL PSEUDARTHROSIS

A freely mobile non-union that features a fibrous capsule around a cavity filled with viscous fluid, creating a false joint. They are most commonly found in the humerus.

The bone-healing organ

When a bone is fractured the free ends are surrounded by blood. Clot surrounds the bone ends as a fusiform swelling; it is also present within the medullary canal. This clot then differentiates into the various tissues seen in the callus formation of healing bone. Conceptually this differentiated clot can be viewed as a bone-healing organ (BHO). The function of the BHO is to produce callus that will mature into new bone and unite the fracture.

The ability of the BHO to create new bone is dependent on:

- pluripotent mesenchymal stem cells with a blood supply, nutrients and growth factors
- an appropriate mechanical strain environment.

An understanding of this concept of the BHO enables us to classify non-union and assists in management.

Classification of non-union based on biology and mechanics

A fracture fails to unite because of failure of the BHO. Either the biology or the mechanical environment is wrong, or a combination of both. Classifying non-union according to its aetiology enables the surgeon to rationalize treatment options (Table 57.2).

Table 57.2 Aetiology of non-union

Biological causes	Mechanical causes
Poor blood supply	Incorrect strain environment
	Inappropriate fixation
Open fractures	Excess shear strain
	Malalignment
	Fracture morphology
High-energy injury	Lack of stimulus
	Non-weight bearing
Vascular disease	
Diabetes	
Infection	
Drugs	
Non-steroidal anti-inflammatory drugs	
Steroids	
Immunosuppressants	
Smoking	

Biological factors affecting bone healing[7]

BLOOD SUPPLY

A reduced blood supply to the BHO will impair delivery of oxygen, inflammatory cells, stem cells and nutrients. A build-up of carbon dioxide and other metabolites produces an acid environment that is detrimental to bone healing.

Vessel injury

In a high-energy injury the periosteum with its blood supply is stripped from the bone. Segmental fractures in addition also damage the endosteal blood supply, resulting in loss of blood supply to whole fragments. Segments of dead bone are interposed between potential healing bone ends.

Microvascular disease

Chronic microvascular disease, most commonly as a result of diabetes, reduces blood supply to a non-union. A reduced provision of essential nutrients leads to failure of ossification with the formation of only fibrous or cartilaginous tissue.

INFECTION

Infected non-union results from an open fracture or infected internal fixation. Infection causes necrosis at the ends of the fracture fragments. This dead bone leads to instability with increased motion at the fracture site and consequently to non-union. Infection also leads to prosthetic loosening and failure of fixation.

SMOKING

Only for the last 20 years have we known the deleterious effects of tobacco smoking on fracture healing: 60% of patients in our non-union practice smoke. Fractures of the tibial shaft take longer to unite and have a higher incidence of non-union in the smoker. Hypothetical modes of action include a reduced blood supply, high levels of reactive oxygen intermediates, low concentration of antioxidant vitamins and the direct effect of nicotine on arteriole endothelial receptors and osteoblasts. The clinician should offer a stern warning when a non-union patient admits to smoking. To stop smoking improves the chance of successful surgery. Evidence as to whether nicotine patch supplementation is better than smoking is contradictory.

DRUGS

Non-steroidal anti-inflammatory drugs

Non-steroidal anti-inflammatory drugs (NSAIDs) inhibit cyclo-oxygenase activity, inhibiting the production of prostaglandins. Clinical studies have shown a marked association between non-union and NSAIDs in long-bone fractures.

Steroids

Long-term steroid therapy is detrimental to fracture repair. Patients on steroids should be given longer estimates of the time their fracture will take to heal.

OTHER BIOLOGICAL CAUSES

Other factors that have a deleterious effect on fracture healing are diabetes, old age, anaemia, nutrition and alcohol.

Mechanobiology of bone healing

The science of how tissue differentiation depends on the physical stress imparted upon it is termed 'mechanobiology'. Pauwels[8] introduced this concept in his book *Biomechanics of Fracture Healing*. He hypothesized that when mesenchymal tissue was placed under tension it would become ligament or tendon. The same tissue when compressed would change to cartilage and then ossify to bone.

The mechanical environment dictates whether a fracture is going to unite.

PERREN'S INTERFRAGMENTARY STRAIN THEORY

Perren's interfragmentary strain theory[9-11] postulates that the nature of tissues formed in a BHO is dependent on the magnitude of strain. Interfragmentary strain (ε) is defined as the relative displacement of the fracture gap ends (d) divided by the initial fracture gap width (G). Calculated as:

$$\varepsilon = d/G.$$

Strain is therefore altered by changes in the size of the initial fracture gap and by the amount of movement at the fracture site (Fig. 57.4):

- $\varepsilon > 100\%$: non-union
- $\varepsilon > 10\%$ and $< 100\%$: fibrous tissue
- $\varepsilon > 2\%$ and $< 10\%$: cartilage/endochondral ossification
- $\varepsilon < 2\%$: direct bone union.

Both insufficient and excessive strain in the fracture gap will prevent bone formation. A certain level of strain produces fibrous tissue. This new fibrous tissue reduces interfragmentary movement and hence reduces strain (Fig. 57.5), thus allowing the formation of cartilage. Increasing stiffness of the BHO allows endochondral ossification and finally bone.

CARTER'S STRAIN THEORIES

In Carter's theory of mechanobiology[12,13] not only the magnitude but also the vector of the mechanical force (tension/compression/shear) affects tissue differentiation.

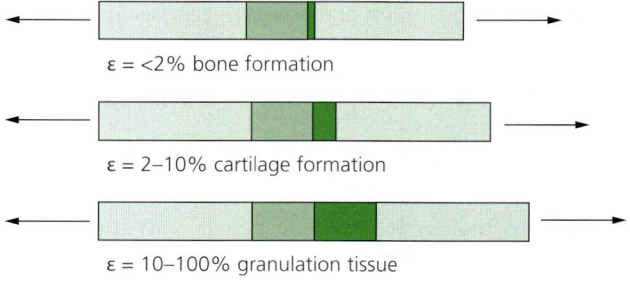

Figure 57.4 Greater displacement increases strain. Mid-green: initial fracture gap; dark green: displacement.

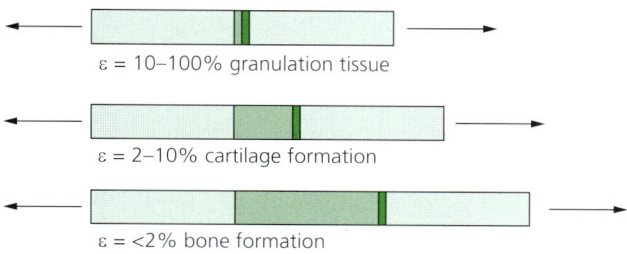

Figure 57.5 A larger initial fracture gap will reduce strain. Mid-green: initial fracture gap; dark green: displacement.

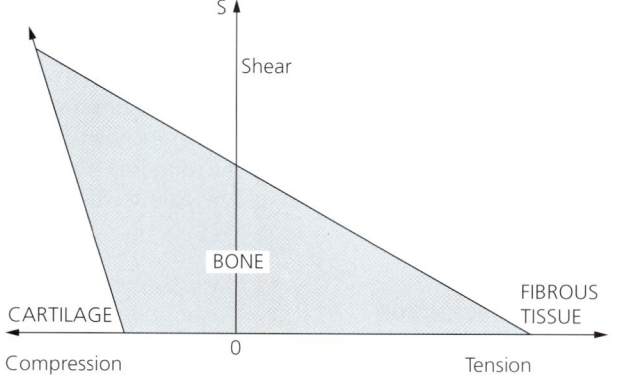

Figure 57.6 The effect of shear stress on bone healing.

Carter shows how detrimental shear is to bone formation; increasing shear decreases the chances of bone formation and union (Figs 57.6 and 57.7). The ideal bone-healing environment has zero shear. The cells within the BHO form bone with the correct mechanical environment. The surgeon manipulates this environment to achieve union.

DIRECT BONE HEALING (PRIMARY)

Direct or primary bone healing[14] occurs when a fracture is anatomically reduced and held rigidly. The bone is deceived into believing that a fracture has not occurred and no BHO is formed. The normal remodelling process of 'cutting cones' crossing the fracture continues. This process lays down lamellar bone and knits the two ends of the fracture together. For this to occur there must be bone contact and absolute stability, providing a very low strain environment. As the fracture gap (G) is very small, almost no displacement (d) is tolerated. Any displacement creates high strain inhibiting bone formation. We do not regard primary or direct bony healing as a healing process. The bone is simply remodelling.

INDIRECT BONE HEALING (SECONDARY)

When direct bone contact or rigidity is not achievable a BHO is formed, with the production of callus.[10] This is

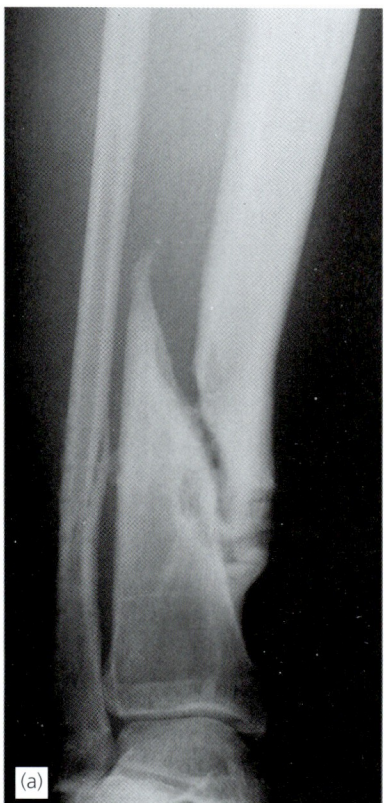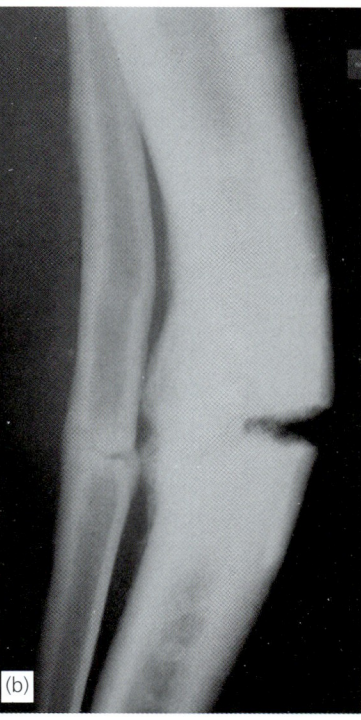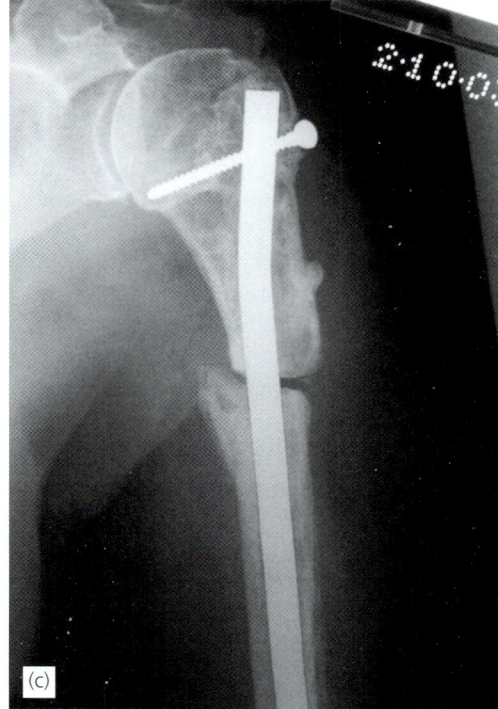

Figure 57.7 Three types of shear. (a) Simple; (b) bending; (c) rotational.

called indirect or secondary bone healing. Anatomical reduction is not required and movement is beneficial; so-called relative stability. As there is a large fracture gap (G), some displacement (d) is needed to produce an appropriate strain environment to form bone from the fracture haematoma. Absolute stability in the presence of a large fracture gap will cause non-union.

MANAGEMENT OF FRACTURE NON-UNION

A non-union occurs when the *biology* around the fracture is deficient or the *mechanical environment* of the fixation is wrong. Both of these factors must be addressed.

Biological causes are difficult to correct; one should try to improve the blood supply and reduce the effect of any coexisting disease. Unfavourable mechanics must be addressed surgically with correction of alignment and appropriate fixation.

At the first consultation, realistic expectations of outcome with the patient should be established. Some non-unions are not treatable and amputation may be the best option.

Biological treatment

The principles of biological treatment of a non-union are:

- increase the blood supply to stimulate bone healing
- diagnose and eradicate infection
- bone graft
- use of osteoinductive agents.

INCREASE THE BLOOD SUPPLY

A satisfactory blood supply to the non-union site is the single most important biological factor in achieving bone union.

Various surgical techniques can improve the circulation to a limb, and therefore the non-union site; these include intramedullary reaming and both tibial and fibular osteotomies. A surgical intervention to one limb may even increase the blood supply to other limbs by hormonal control.[15–17]

DIAGNOSE AND ERADICATE INFECTION

The presence of infection dramatically alters the treatment of a non-union. It is sometimes extremely difficult to determine whether infection is present. A balanced judgement using experience, the clinical picture, imaging and pathological information should be made. Once bacteria have been cultured appropriate long-term antibiotics should be commenced as an adjunct to surgical management.

BONE GRAFT

The authors rarely use bone grafting to augment bone healing in cases of non-union. However, bone grafting can be a useful addition to appropriate fixation in atrophic non-union and synovial pseudarthrosis.

Autologous bone graft gives the best chance of success. Allograft or calcium phosphate substitutes are not as effective as autograft and are probably not indicated when this surgery is the last chance for limb salvage.

Use a large quantity of cancellous bone taken from the posterior iliac crest. The adherence of periosteum over the non-union site provides a useful guide to the location of the non-union. Incise this periosteum longitudinally, and peel it back using a sharp osteotome taking with it adherent small slivers of bone. One develops an envelope of periosteum with petals of cortical bone around the non-union. Croutons of cancellous bone are then packed under this layer, circumferentially surrounding the non-union. Meti-culous attention should be paid to this simple procedure.

PAPINEAU TECHNIQUE

The Papineau technique may be used in cases of septic non-union with soft-tissue defects. Although time-consuming (several months), it is a reliable method of limb salvage. It is an alternative to bone transport if an Ilizarov frame is not available.[18]

The Papineau technique:

- infected bone and sequestra are excised
- the remaining bone fragments are stabilized with a simple external fixator
- the defect is irrigated daily until macroscopically clean
- a large volume of cancellous bone graft is then packed into the bony defect, contained by the soft-tissue envelope
- the graft should extend 2 cm beyond the ends of the remaining bone fragments
- daily irrigation continues until granulation tissue covers the bone graft, allowing split skin grafting.

AUGMENTING FRACTURE HEALING

Bone morphogenetic proteins

There is current interest in the use of osteoinductive factors in the treatment of non-union. There is little clinical evidence to date that bone morphogenetic proteins augment fracture healing.

Recently, there has been an explosion of commercial products claiming to enhance or accelerate fracture healing. These include demineralized bone matrix, calcium phosphate substitutes, hydroxyapatite in bovine collagen and platelet-rich plasma. So far, there have been no controlled trials on their efficacy, only individual case reports.[19,20]

Physical treatments

Electricity in various forms has been shown to improve bone healing. Pulsed electromagnetic fields have been effective in treating hypertrophic non-unions. High-intensity ultrasound has been shown to accelerate fracture healing in animals, although there is no evidence that it successfully treats non-union.

All these treatments, although promising, cannot address the issue of deformity. Their clinical effectiveness and cost-effectiveness is yet to be proven.[21,22]

Optimizing the mechanical environment

The treatment of the mechanical causes of non-unions is more straightforward. Surgery restores anatomical alignment and stabilizes the non-union, creating an optimal strain environment for bone healing. The surgeon must create an appropriate strain environment to promote bone healing. This can be achieved with anatomical reduction and absolute stability, causing direct bone healing (a low-strain environment). If this is not possible then with relative stability and indirect bone healing with callus formation in a moderate strain environment.

Shear in any form should be avoided. The method of fixation should be carefully planned and executed to achieve this. Sometimes just altering the strain environment, by changing the method of fixation, is enough to produce union.

Method of fixation

The choice of fixation takes into account the following variables: presence of infection; location; fracture morphology; condition of soft tissues; experience of the surgeon; and availability of fixation methods.

PRESENCE OF INFECTION

Bone infection is a spectrum of diseases.[23] The severity of the infection dictates treatment.

Quiescent infection

This is characterized by a watery discharge, with no obvious sequestra and no significant bacterial culture. This resolves with rigid stabilization and compression using an external fixator. The discharge usually stops within 12 weeks and the fracture goes on to unite within a further few months. Compression should be increased each month in the outpatient clinic.

Active infection

Active infection is indicated by a constant purulent discharge, dead bone, sequestra and poor soft tissues. Active infection requires radical resection of dead and infected bone and excision of infected soft tissue. This is followed by a complex limb reconstruction using bone transport.

A circular frame providing rigid stability is essential for treating infection. It is not uncommon for an infected tibial non-union to require 12 months and an infected femur 18 months of treatment with a frame.

Avoiding bone resection can reduce treatment time by a year. The decision on whether just to stabilize and compress or to resect and commit the patient to bone transport is difficult. It can only be learnt from clinical experience. If simple stabilization with compression fails, the treatment must start over again with resection and bone transport. This 'misjudgement' can result in up to 30 months wearing a frame. Most patients cannot tolerate such an extended treatment. It is not uncommon for the patient to opt for an amputation, even though the limb may still be salvageable.

LOCATION OF NON-UNION

Lower limb

Weight bearing produces axial compression at the non-union. Weight bearing is a powerful stimulus for bone healing and should be encouraged after non-union surgery.

Standard plate fixation is not durable enough to treat non-union of the femur. It is rarely strong enough for non-union of the tibia. Fixation with an intramedullary nail or a circular frame will allow axial compression while neutralizing shear forces. Metaphyseal fractures, close to a joint, are best treated with fine wire frames or fixed-angle locking plates.

When treating a tibial non-union, the counterproductive effect of an intact fibula should be considered. An intact fibula provides a static distraction force holding the two ends of a tibial non-union apart. It also creates a cantilever–bending force pushing the tibia into varus, creating a bending shear force at the non-union site.

If this is the case, a fibula osteotomy is beneficial: it

- allows the tibia to be load bearing
- allows axial compression of the tibia
- allows reduction of the tibia
- reduces shear force at the non-union
- increases blood supply to the limb.

Upper limb

The weight of the arm creates a tension force across the non-union. A compressive force can be achieved by plating or with a circular fine wire frame. Intramedullary nailing cannot produce compression and we advise against its use in cases of non-union of the humerus. There is never a place for exchange nailing in humeral non-union. The arm does not bear full body weight; therefore, plates are durable enough and are our recommended surgical treatment for non-unions in the upper limb.

FRACTURE MORPHOLOGY

Non-unions have only one fracture gap. A multifragmentary fracture starts with many fracture lines; most unite leaving the strain to be concentrated through one fracture line, resulting in a uniplanar non-union.

Non-unions have three types of morphology:

1. *Transverse*: caused by an excessive bending shear force that can be neutralized with plates, nails or circular frames.
2. *Spiral*: caused by an excessive rotational shear force. This is best controlled by an intramedullary nail or with a circular frame.
3. *Oblique*: caused by an excessive axial or simple shear force. This pattern is the most difficult to treat. Axial compression of an oblique non-union leads to the creation of greater shear forces. To oppose this shear the two parts of the non-union should be distracted, but this creates a potentially unhelpful tension force across the non-union. The shearing forces need to be neutralized by compression at right angles to the fracture. In the arm this can be achieved by lag screws and neutralization plate fixation. However, this type of fixation is not durable enough to allow weight bearing in the leg. Intramedullary nails are poor at stabilizing this fracture pattern. Circular fine wire frames are able to compress these oblique non-unions but complex frame designs are required (Fig. 57.8). These oblique non-unions remain a very difficult surgical problem.

CONDITION OF THE SOFT TISSUES

Internal fixation is contraindicated when there is poor vascularity, infection or soft-tissue deficiency. The Ilizarov technique can be used to treat all these problems, usually without the need for flap coverage from a plastic surgeon. During bone transport soft tissue is pulled down along with bone and this often fills in skin defects.

EXPERIENCE OF THE SURGEON

The surgeon should choose a technique with which he has experience. If a particular case requires a different approach or specific surgical equipment is not available, referral to an appropriate institution should be made. This is the last chance to save the limb; limited opportunities should not be wasted by inappropriate surgery.

AVAILABLE FIXATION TECHNIQUES

Internal fixation can be achieved with intramedullary nails, and by locking and non-locking plating systems. They must provide stability, be appropriate to the fracture pattern and be durable enough to last until union. Non-unions take longer to heal than fresh fractures and metalwork failure is a real possibility.

PLATE FIXATION

Traditional plate fixation relies on the friction between screws, the plate and the bone to maintain rigidity of construct. If there is no progression to union, traditional plating will eventually fail. This method of fixation still has a role to play in non-union surgery especially in the upper limb. Locking plate fixation acts as an internal type of external fixator. It provides durable fixation in weaker bone, as found in osteoporosis or metaphyseal cancellous bone. It is especially useful for treating periarticular non-union.

INTRAMEDULLARY NAILS

Diaphyseal non-unions of the tibia and femur respond well to exchange nailing; it is important to insert the largest possible nail. This will allow axial compression while neutralizing shear. The latest generation nails with their multiple locking options, combined with 'Poller' screws, can treat metaphyseal non-union successfully.

EXTERNAL FIXATION

External fixation has long been the mainstay of the non-union surgeon. Circular fine wire frame techniques give excellent fixation in all types of non-union and in all parts of the bone. Deformity can be addressed and the mechanical environment can be manipulated throughout the treatment. The circular fine wire frame is a very powerful and effective tool. However, it is not popular with patients, especially in the Western world.

Specific site non-union

We will now consider non-union of some specific bones.

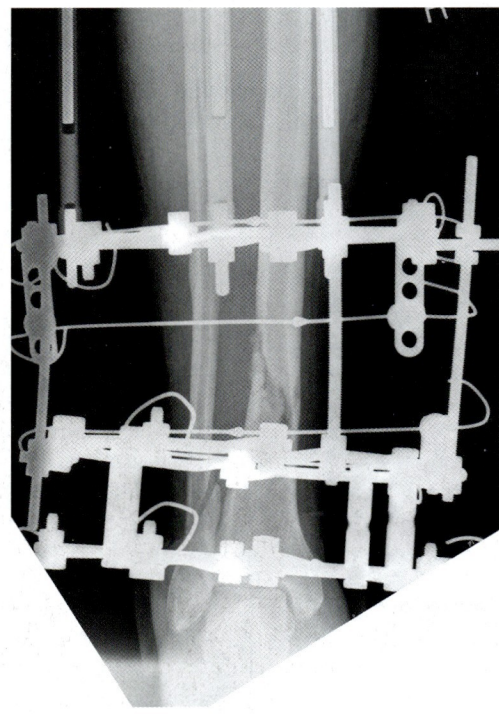

Figure 57.8 Complex frame and wire combinations are needed to oppose shear in an oblique non-union.

FEMUR

The rate of non-union of fractures in the trochanteric region of the femur is higher when the fracture is fixed in varus. Treatment consists of revision fixation with a valgus osteotomy. Salvage is with a calcar-replacing prosthetic replacement. See Figs 57.9 and 57.10.

TIBIA

Over the last 100 years the tibia has become the most common bone to develop non-union possibly because of the invention of the motorcycle. Non-union of the shaft is estimated to be up to 10% of all tibial fractures. The rate is higher in high-energy injuries with soft-tissue damage. See Figs 57.11–57.13.

HUMERUS

Non-union of the shaft occurs in 2–5% of all humeral fractures.[24] This incidence is second only to the tibia. Shaft fractures treated with intramedullary nails have a higher incidence of non-union than those treated with plate fixation. See Figs 57.14–57.17.

FOREARM

Non-union of the radius or ulna produces a length discrepancy, which must be corrected to allow forearm rotation. An interposition graft of cancellous bone from the iliac crest is held rigidly in compression with a plate. Up to 6 cm of bone can be replaced with this technique. Creeping substitution allows assimilation of the bone block over the following few months.[25,26] See Fig. 57.18.

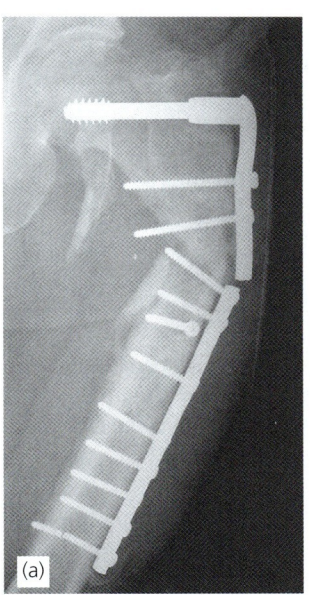
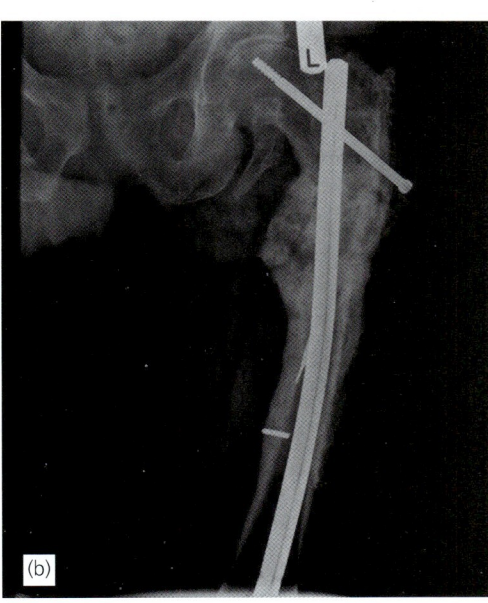

Figure 57.9 (a and b) For non-union of the femur intramedullary fixation is more durable than a plate.

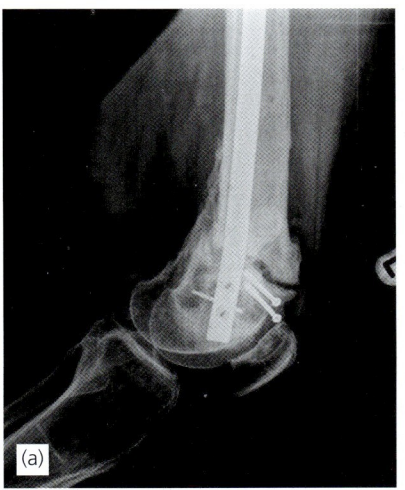
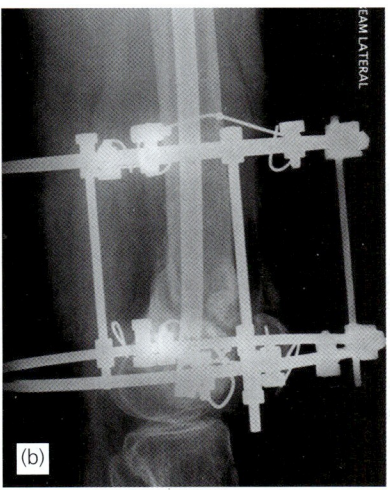
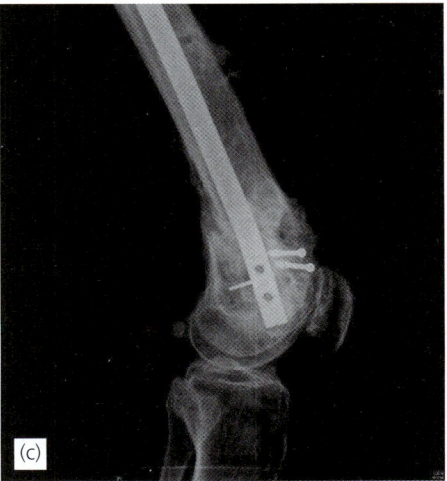

Figure 57.10 (a–c) This very distal transverse metaphyseal femoral fracture failed to unite after treatment with a retrograde nail. Stabilization with a two-ring frame over the nail produces union.

524 Management of fracture complications

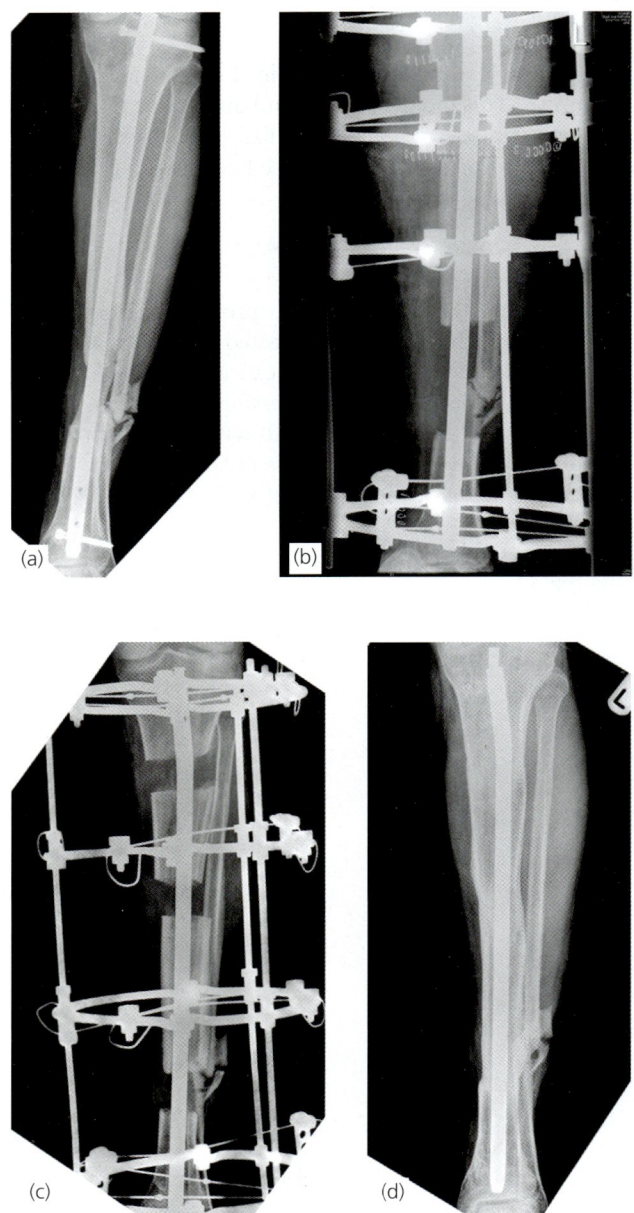

Figure 57.11 (a–d) Dead bone has been excised back to normal bleeding bone. Bone loss is addressed with bone transport, performed over a nail to maintain alignment; a double osteotomy reduces transport time.

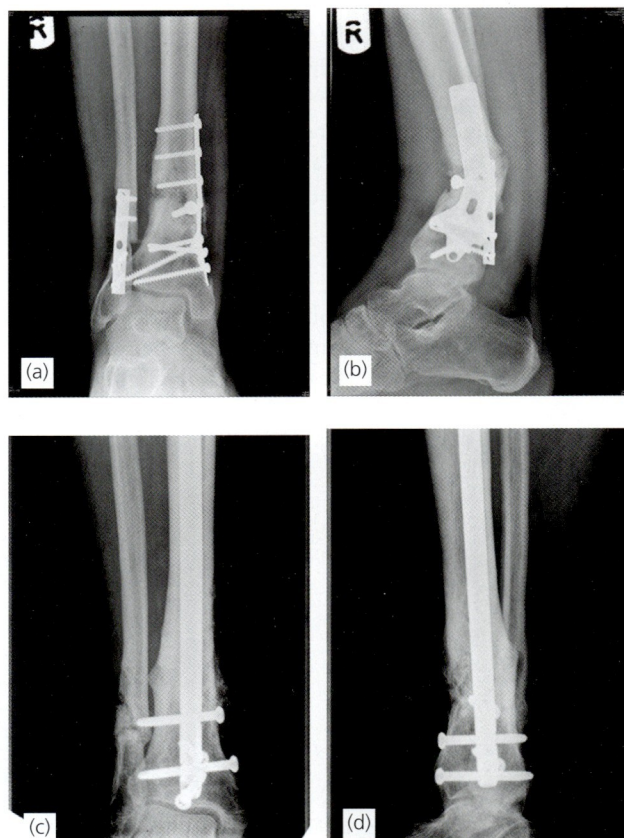

Figure 57.12 (a–d) Malalignment and inappropriate fixation results in non-union. The metalwork is removed with a percutaneous technique to keep the bone-healing organ intact. Intramedullary fixation in anatomical alignment produces union.

Amputation

The simplest treatment of a non-union is amputation; it gives a guaranteed end result. We always discuss the possibility of amputation with the patient and family at their first consultation. They must realize that if complex limb reconstruction fails, amputation is then the only available option.

The indications for amputation include the following.

INFECTED NON-UNION WITH SIGNIFICANT BONE LOSS

Distraction osteogenesis can realistically produce no more than 6 cm of new bone regeneration at each osteotomy site; 12 cm at a double osteotomy. Reconstruction of more than 10–12 cm is not usually a realistic option and the patient should be offered an amputation.

ASSOCIATED NEUROLOGICAL DAMAGE

A flail useless limb is not worth saving. Sciatic nerve palsy associated with a femoral non-union nearly always leads to amputation.

POOR VASCULARITY AND HEAVY SMOKER

These patients have a very poor success rate for union.

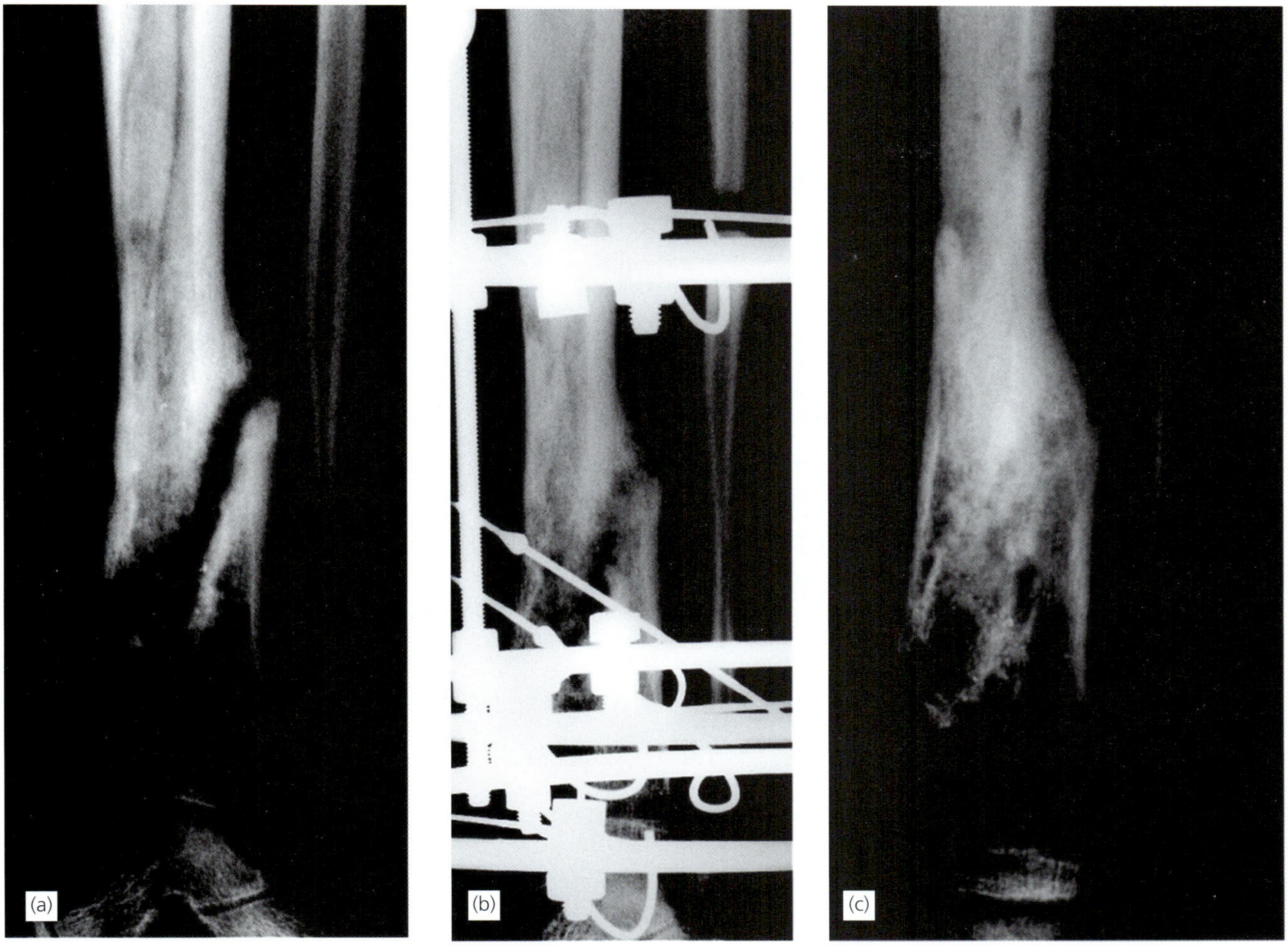

Figure 57.13 (a–c) An oblique fracture of the distal tibia fails to unite because of excessive shear. Appropriately placed olive wires neutralize this shear force.

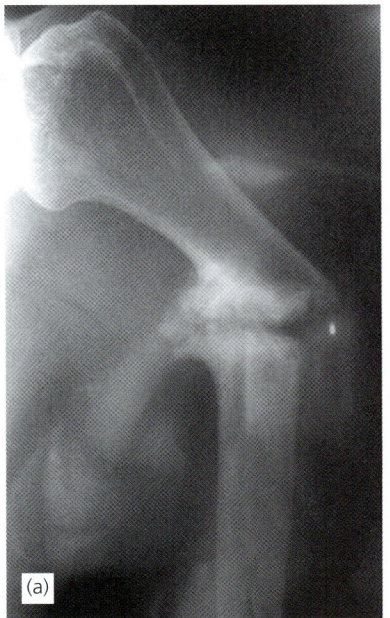

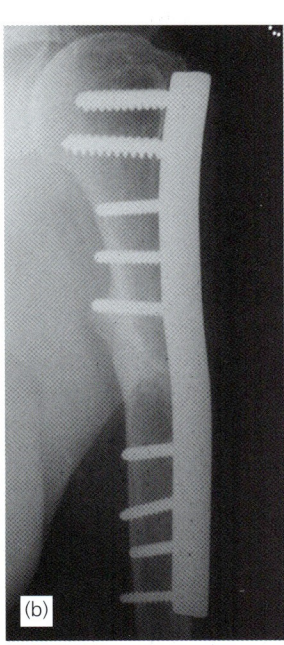

Figure 57.14 (a and b) A humeral non-union successfully treated with compression plating.

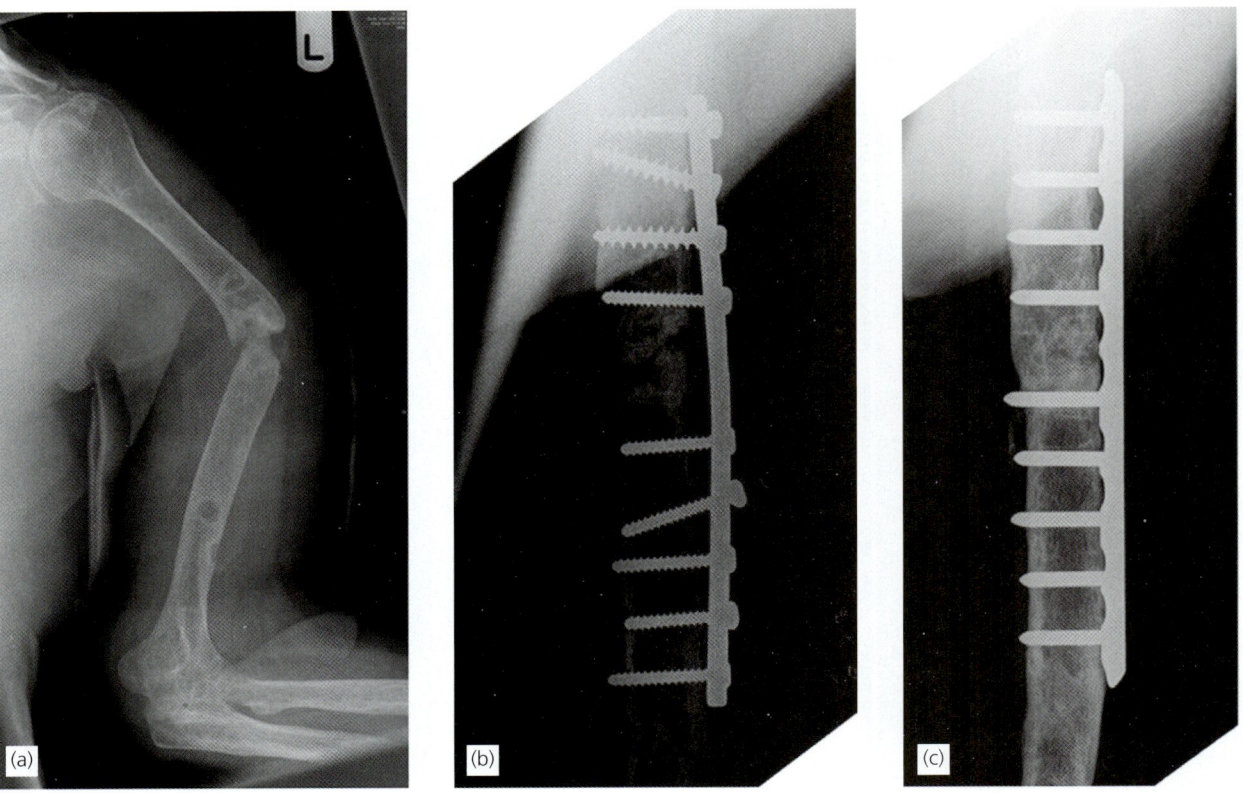

Figure 57.15 (a–c) A humeral non-union treated initially with a traditional plating technique fails to unite and the plate loosens. A locking plate provides a more robust fixation and leads to union.

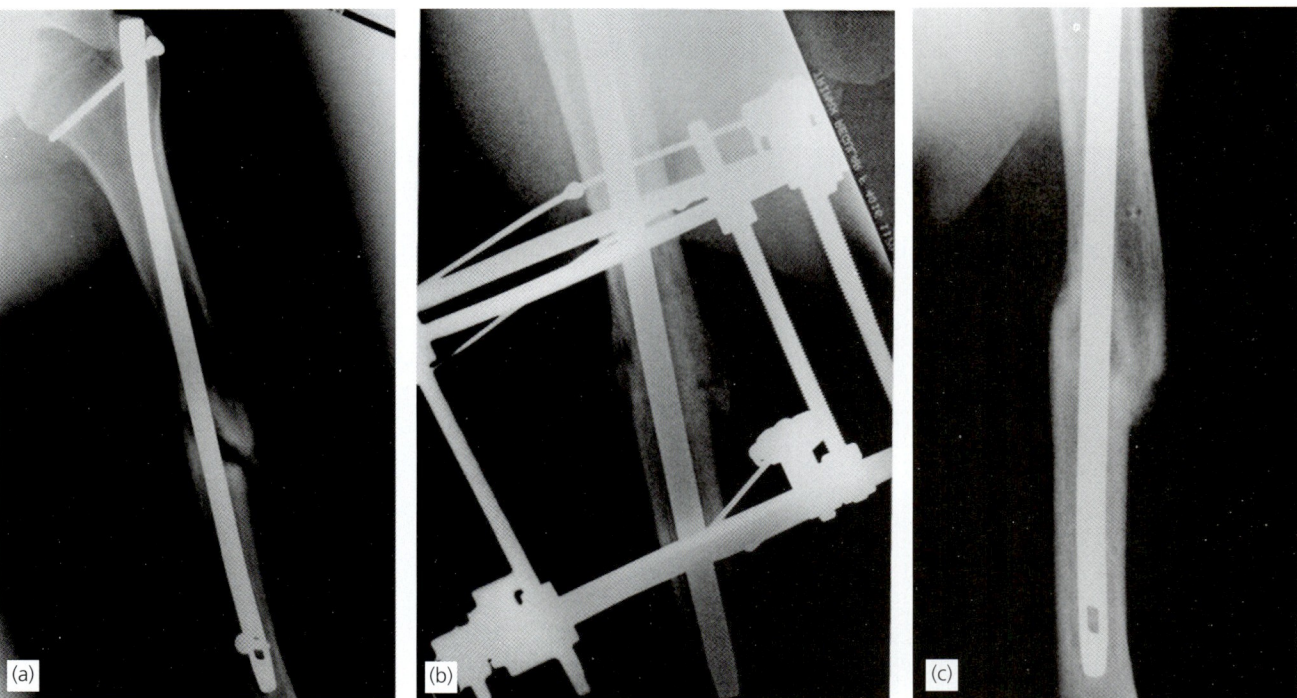

Figure 57.16 (a–c) An intramedullary humeral nail does not provide compression nor does it stop rotational shear. Both can be corrected with a frame over the nail. Locking screws have to be removed.

FRAME ACOPIA

Those living alone, alcoholics, drug addicts, the depressed, the self-employed and the elderly all cope badly with a frame.

MALUNION

Malunion occurs when a fracture has united but in a non-anatomical position.

Deformity, like displacement in a fresh fracture, may occur in four ways:

- translation
- angulation
- rotation
- axial shortening.

Malunion may cause loss of function and cosmetic problems. In the lower limb malunion changes the biomechanics, leading to secondary degenerative changes in the knee and ankle. Minor deformity should probably be accepted. The decision on whether to operate is difficult and each case is unique. The decision to treat a malunion of any bone should be made on symptoms or to correct a malalignment that would eventually develop into arthritis. Surgery should not be an attempt to improve the cosmetic clinical or radiological appearance.

Femoral malunion

Rotational deformity of the femur may follow intramedullary nailing. Internal rotation causes a patient to trip over his own feet. External rotation leads to a chronic strain of the medial collateral ligament of the knee. Unless mild, both deformities would benefit from a corrective osteotomy.

Tibial malunion

Varus malunion is often symptomatic and leads to medial compartment osteoarthrosis of the knee. A varus deformity of 10° or more should probably be corrected. Patients have a higher tolerance to valgus deformity. There is less evidence that it produces degeneration in the knee or ankle.[27]

Tibial pilon malunion

Intra-articular fractures of the distal tibia may lead to an incongruent deformity of the ankle joint. Secondary arthritis can set in within 1 year of the accident. Symptomatic patients are best served with an ankle arthrodesis, performed with either a circular frame or an ankle arthrodesis nail.

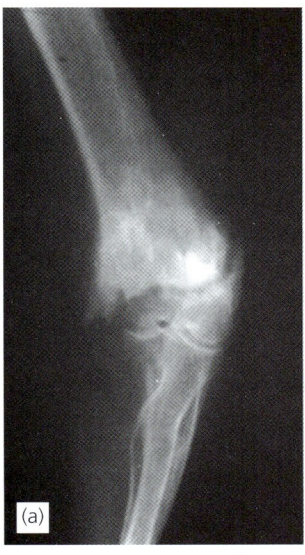
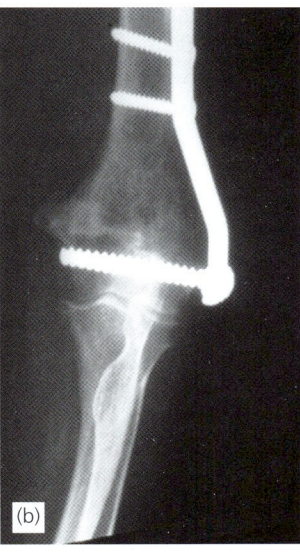

Figure 57.17 (a and b) Extremely distal supracondylar fractures of the humerus have a high rate of non-union. The small articular fragment can be purchased with a single large cancellous screw. Fixation and compression to the shaft is achieved with a dynamic compression plate.

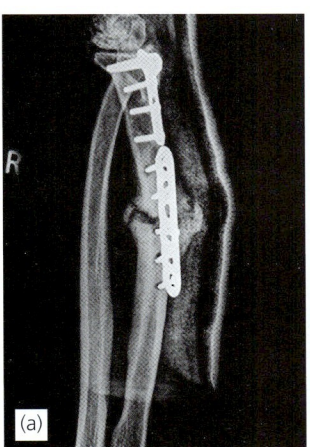
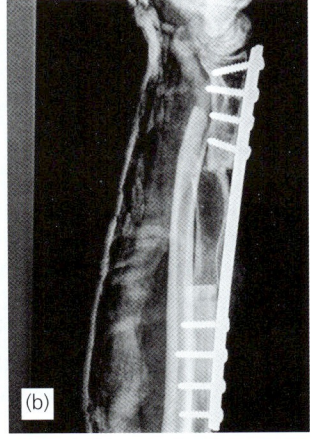
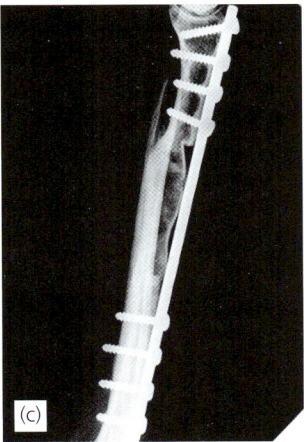

Figure 57.18 (a–c) An interposition cancellous graft treats segmental bone loss in a non-union of the radius.

Lengthening

Impaction of a femoral or tibial fracture leads to shortening of the leg. A leg length discrepancy produces a limp and later low lumbar back pain. How much leg length discrepancy merits surgical correction depends upon the patient and the surgeon. The enormity of the surgical lengthening procedure, and a high rate of complications, leads us to favour a shoe raise for less than 4 cm. The surgeon may be tempted into lengthening with a lesser degree of discrepancy especially in the younger patient. Caution should be exercised as complications of lengthening include joint stiffness, chronic pain, non-union and complex regional pain syndrome.

Gradual femoral or tibial lengthening can be performed using the distraction osteogenesis technique of Ilizarov at a metaphysis. Care must be taken to align the frame correctly or an angular deformity will be produced. Distal femoral lengthening often leads to a stiff knee, and hence we prefer subtrochanteric lengthening. The frame is more cumbersome, but we have experienced fewer complications with proximal femoral lengthening.

Tibiocalcaneal fusion

Until recently avascular necrosis of the talus would inevitably lead to below knee amputation (Fig. 57.19). Nowadays the talus can be excised and the tibia fused to the os calcis. The resulting 5 cm of shortening is corrected by distraction osteogenesis of an osteotomy of the proximal tibia. The treatment is complex and prolonged but the limb can be saved.[28]

Ilizarov technique for deformity

The correction of a simple angular deformity can be achieved with a closing wedge osteotomy, but this produces shortening. The Ilizarov technique provides a workable solution for all types of deformity and length can be maintained.

We no longer calculate the design of the Ilizarov frame from radiographs taken pre-operatively. The frame is constructed on the operating table, with the assistance of C-arm image intensification. The limb is rotated under the image intensifier until the deformity is maximal. This image enables the surgeon to understand the deformity and calculate the centre of rotation of angulation (CORA). An appropriate frame is then assembled.[29]

An Ilizarov frame for deformity can be constructed as follows:

- An upper transverse reference wire is passed parallel to the knee joint. A two-ring Ilizarov box is constructed using this wire as a reference.
- A similar distal two-ring box is constructed parallel to the ankle joint.
- These two boxes provide a magnified illustration of the deformity outside the leg (Fig. 57.20).
- The 'driver' (a distraction rod) is attached at the narrowest position between these two rings.
- Two hinged rods are placed equidistant (the same number of holes) from the driver. This dictates that the two hinges are placed in the same orientation perpendicular to the plane of maximal deformity.
- The tibia is divided at the site of deformity with a low-energy Gigli saw.
- If these two hinges are placed at the CORA a simple correction will be made.
- Place them on the opposite side of the bone to the driver and lengthening will be achieved. Proximal or distal placement to the CORA will produce translation.

The Taylor spatial frame fixator, an alternative to the Ilizarov frame, consists of two rings connected by six telescopic struts at special universal joints. The Taylor spatial frame fixator is capable of correcting six axes of deformity either acutely or gradually in the outpatient clinic. A specific computer program is required to calculate the correction.

PSYCHOSOCIAL ASPECTS OF FRACTURE COMPLICATIONS

Fortunately the majority of fractures proceed to union without complication. A non-union, infected or not, causes pain and loss of function. By the time patients reach the non-union specialist they will have had several unsuccessful operations and will be sceptical of all surgeons. They may also have developed the psychological and social problems that occur with long-term pain and disability. Many patients will be clinically depressed, may have lost their job and may have become dependent on those around them. Those closest to the patient will also be feeling the strain of the constant support they are expected to provide.

At this point the non-union surgeon will have to engage carefully with the patient and prepare them for further surgery, more pain and the possibility of wearing a frame for over a year. All this is done in an attempt to save a limb that will never again be normal.

It is important that the surgeon communicates effectively with the patient and their family. Only when the patient takes responsibility for their injury and cooperates fully with the treatment process is there any chance of a positive outcome. Patients must learn to accept that their life is never going to be the same as it was before their accident.

Psychosocial aspects of fracture complications 529

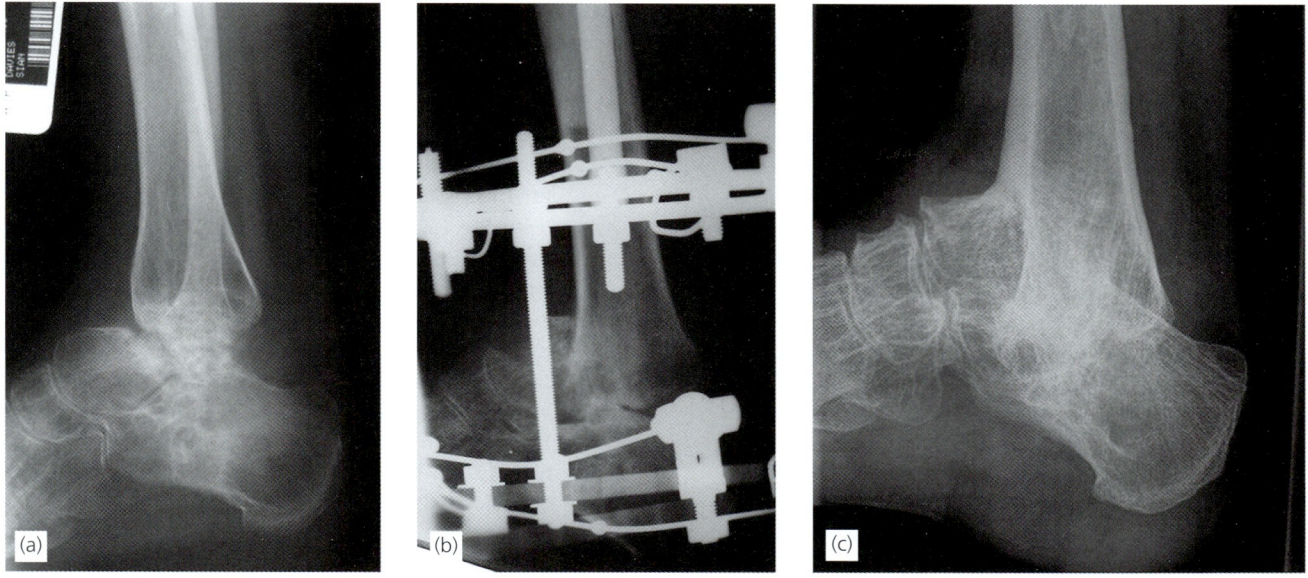

Figure 57.19 (a–c) Avascular necrosis of the talus successfully treated with a tibiocalcaneal fusion and proximal bone lengthening.

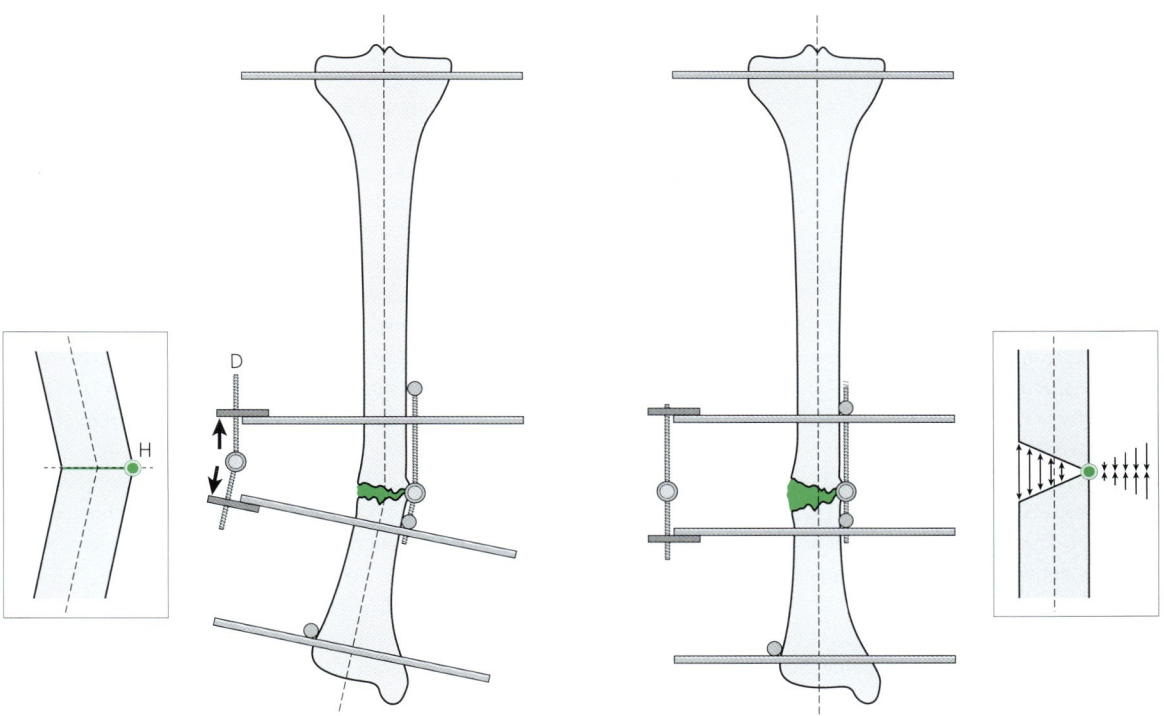

Figure 57.20 Example of a two-box/four-ring frame constructed to correct a malunion of the tibia. H, center of rotation of angulation. Position of the hinge if no lengthening is required. D, driver.

> **KEY LEARNING POINTS**
>
> - A non-union is classified according to its aetiology.
> - Non-union will result if either the biological environment or the mechanical environment is wrong.
> - The biological environment should be optimized by eradicating infection, improving the blood supply and by stopping smoking and non-steroidal anti-inflammatory drugs.
> - The mechanical environment is corrected by restoring alignment and holding this with a robust fixation; an appropriate strain environment allows new bone formation and union.
> - Malunion should be corrected if it is symptomatic or will predictably cause premature degeneration of an adjacent joint.
> - A circular fine wire frame provides a workable solution for many types of non-union and malunion.

REFERENCES

- ● = Key primary paper
- ◆ = Major review article

1. Wiss DA, Stetson WB. Tibial nonunion: treatment alternatives. *Journal of the American Academy of Orthopaedic Surgeons* 1996;**4**:249–57.
2. Perkins G. The care of fractures in plaster of Paris. *Practitioner* 1958;**180**:321–3.
3. Ebraheim NA, Savolaine ER, Patel A, *et al*. Assessment of tibial fracture union by 35–45 degrees internal oblique radiographs. *Journal of Orthopaedic Trauma* 1991;**5**:349–50.
4. Bhattacharyya T, Bouchard KA, Phadke A, *et al*. The accuracy of computed tomography for the diagnosis of tibial nonunion. *Journal of Bone and Joint Surgery (American)* 2006;**88**:692–7.
5. Kuhlman JE, Fishman EK, Magid D, *et al*. Fracture nonunion: CT assessment with multiplanar reconstruction. *Radiology* 1988;**167**:483–8.
6. Weber BG, Cech O. *Pseudoarthrosis: Pathology, Biomechanics, Therapy, Results*. Berne, Switzerland: Hans Huber Medical Publisher, 1976.
◆7. Gaston MS, Simpson AH. Inhibition of fracture healing. *Journal of Bone and Joint Surgery (British)* 2007;**89**:1553–60.
8. Pauwels F. Grundriß einer Biomechanik der Fracturheilung. In *34e Kongress der Deutschen Orthopädischen Gesellschaft*. Stuttgart: Ferinand Engke, 1941:464–508. (Transl. by Manquet P, Furlong R. *Biomechanics of the Locomotor Apparatus*. New York, NY: Springer-Verlag, 1980:106–37.)
◆9. Perren SM, Matter P, Rüedi R, Allgöwer M. Biomechanics of fracture healing after internal fixation. *Surgery Annual* 1975;**7**:361–90.
◆10. Perren SM. Physical and biological aspects of fracture healing with special reference to internal fixation. *Clinical Orthopaedics and Related Research* 1979;**138**:175–96.
◆11. Perren SM. Evolution of the internal fixation of long bone fractures. The scientific basis of biological internal fixation: choosing a new balance between stability and biology. *Journal of Bone and Joint Surgery (British)* 2002;**84**:1093–110.
12. Carter DR, Blenman PR, Beaupré GS. Correlations between mechanical stress history and tissue differentiation in initial fracture healing. *Journal of Orthopaedic Research* 1988;**6**:736–48.
13. Blenman PR, Carter DR, Beaupré GS. Role of mechanical loading in the progressive ossification of a fracture callus. *Journal of Orthopaedic Research* 1989;**7**:398–407.
14. Danis R. *Theorie et Pratique de l'Osteosynthese*. Paris, France: Masson and Cie Editeurs, 1949.
●15. Ilizarov GA. The tension-stress effect on the genesis and growth of tissues. Part I. The influence of stability of fixation and soft-tissue preservation. *Clinical Orthopaedics and Related Research* 1989;**238**:249–81.
●16. Ilizarov GA. The tension-stress effect on the genesis and growth of tissues. Part II. The influence of the rate and frequency of distraction. *Clinical Orthopaedics and Related Research* 1989;**239**:263–85.
◆17. Bedi A, Karunakar MA. Physiologic effects of intramedullary reaming. *Instructional Course Lectures* 2006;**55**:359–66.
●18. Archdeacon MT, Messerschmitt P. Modern Papineau technique with vacuum-assisted closure. *Journal Orthopaedic Trauma* 2006;**20**:134–7.
●19. Friedlaender GE, Perry CR, Cole JD, *et al*. Osteogenic protein-1 (bone morphogenetic protein-7) in the treatment of tibial nonunions. *Journal of Bone and Joint Surgery (American)* 2001;**83A**(Suppl. 1):S151–8.
◆20. Novicoff WM, Manaswi A, Hogan MV, *et al*. Critical analysis of the evidence for current technologies in bone-healing and repair. *Journal of Bone and Joint Surgery (American)* 2008;**90**(Suppl. 1):85–91.
21. Brighton CT, Shaman P, Heppenstall RB, *et al*. Tibial nonunion treated with direct current, capacitive coupling, or bone graft. *Clinical Orthopaedics and Related Research* 1995;**321**:223–34.
◆22. Busse JW, Bhandari M, Kulkarni AV, Tunks E. The effect of low-intensity pulsed ultrasound therapy on time to fracture healing: a meta-analysis. *Canadian Medical Association Journal* 2002;**166**:437–41.
◆23. Motsitsi NS. Management of infected nonunion of long bones: the last decade (1996–2006). *Injury* 2008;**39**:155–60.

24. Christensen S. Humeral shaft fractures, operative and conservative treatment. *Acta Chirurgica Scandinavica* 1967;**133**:455–60.
●25. Nicoll EA. The treatment of gaps in long bones by cancellous insert grafts. *Journal of Bone and Joint Surgery (British)* 1956;**38B**:70–82.
●26. Davey PA, Simonis RB. Modification of the Nicoll bone-grafting technique for nonunion of the radius and/or ulna. *Journal of Bone and Joint Surgery (British)* 2002;**84**:30–3.
●27. Milner SA, Davis TR, Muir KR, *et al.* Long-term outcome after tibial shaft fracture: is malunion important? *Journal of Bone and Joint Surgery (American)* 2002;**84A**:971–80.
28. Dennison MG, Pool RD, Simonis RB, Singh BS. Tibiocalcaneal fusion for avascular necrosis of the talus. *Journal of Bone and Joint Surgery (British)* 2001;**83**:199–203.
◆29. ASAMI Group. Basic principles of operative technique. In: Maiocchi A, Aronson J. (eds) *Operative Principles of Ilizarov*. Baltimore, MD: Williams and Wilkins, 1991:65–77.

PART 5

PAEDIATRIC ORTHOPAEDIC SURGERY

BENJAMIN JOSEPH

58	**Clinical assessment of the paediatric patient**	535
	Michael P Horan, Forest Walker, Todd A Milbrandt	
59	**Developmental disorders of human skeleton**	541
	Chezhiyan Shanmugam, Umile Giuseppe Longo, Nicola Maffulli	
60	**Normal and pathological gait in children**	563
	Richard Beauchamp	
61	**Developmental diseases of the skeleton**	570
	Sunil Bajaj, Sanjeev S Madan	
62	**Bone and joint infections in children**	578
	Vrisha Madhuri, Hamish Crawford, James Huntley	
63	**Juvenile idiopathic arthritis**	589
	Tracy V Ting, Brent Graham	
64	**Neuromuscular disorders**	598
	Kishore Mulpuri, Sanjeev Madan, Uni Narayanan, Nick Nicolaou, Shahryar Noordin, Renjit A Varghese, Janet Walker	
65	**Spinal disorders in children**	626
	Stephen Tredwell, Christopher Reilly	
66	**Hip disorders in children**	642
	Hamish Crawford, James A Fernandes, James HP Hui, Arjandas Mahadev, Kishore Mulpuri, Kiran AN Saldanha, Jean-Claude Theis, Simon P Kelley	
67	**Knee disorders in children**	666
	Kevin Lim, James HP Hui, Andrew Lim, Azura Mansor, Ismail Munajat, Kishore Mulpuri, Simon P Kelley	
68	**Disorders of the leg in children**	675
	Stanley Jones, Sunil Bajaj, Nicolas Nicolaou, James A Fernandes, Kiran AN Saldanha	
69	**Disorders of the foot in children**	690
	Haemish A Crawford, James S Huntley, Benjamin Joseph	

58

Clinical assessment of the paediatric patient

MICHAEL P HORAN, FOREST WALKER, TODD A MILBRANDT

Introduction	535	The hip examination	539
The lower extremity screen	536	The spine screen	540
The foot examination	538	References	540

NATIONAL BOARD STANDARDS

- Be aware of the difference between dealing with paediatric patients and their families, and adult patients
- Know the growth patterns and development of paediatric patients
- Understand the age-related changes to the paediatric physical exam
- Be able to assess a parent's concerns about their child
- Assess the paediatric hip for pathology or pain
- Assess normal growth versus pathological growth

INTRODUCTION

As in most areas of paediatric medicine, the orthopaedic physical examination of a child is unique compared with that of the adult patient. The paediatrician's often repeated phrase 'children are not just small adults' is especially pertinent in the orthopaedic realm as the growth and development of the child present a dynamic situation that changes as the child gets older. Knowledge of normal development and pathological conditions is required to accurately assess the child.

The patient and the family also present unique challenges. The patient's age and previous experience with other physicians will dictate the course of the examination. Even a very young child may have already associated the doctor's office visit with getting a shot and naturally be very apprehensive. Dealing with the family often presents more challenges than dealing with the nervous child. Parents may have their own predetermined notions and fears as to what could be wrong with their child, and skilfully assuaging their concerns is one of the most important aspects of the encounter.

A good deal of the physical examination takes place prior to actually laying hands on the patient. Anyone who has examined a child knows the error in immediately approaching the patient to start the examination. The result is at best an apprehensive child, and at worst the patient in a flood of tears and hiding behind the mother or father. Instead, when entering the room, the examiner needs to immediately begin to develop rapport with the patient and parents by introducing him- or herself to everyone. Paying special attention to something about this child is very important, such as a toy he or she has, a unique piece of clothing, the child's name, or some other personal characteristic. Children like to feel important and, younger children especially, like to talk about themselves. Showing interest builds trust. It is also important to view the world from the child's eyes, i.e. to see it on their level. Crouching down or sitting down on the floor where the child is playing shows a willingness to be on the child's level and, in one simple step, further builds trust. Performing the examination while the child sits on one of the parent's lap can create a level of comfort for the child and the parents (Fig. 58.1).

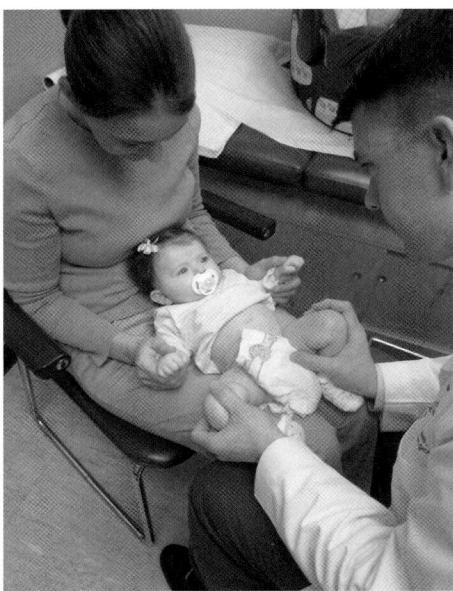

Figure 58.1 Examining the child in the parent's lap can ease the anxiety of both the child and the parent.

During the first minute or so of the encounter, you are building your rapport and, at the same time, keenly observing the child's behaviour and abilities. It takes only a few seconds to watch the patient playing with a toy, moving around the room, climbing on the table, or even running behind his or her parent to hide to develop a quick assessment of the child's overall function. During this initial encounter is when the chief complaint and brief history can be elicited. While the parent or patient, depending on the child's age, is relaying the reason for the visit, observing the patient's demeanour is important in assessing his or her objectives. The overbearing parents of an overworked 16 year old competitive swimmer with a sore shoulder may be arriving with a different expectation from the first-time mother who is concerned about her healthy baby's feet and who simply needs reassurance. The art of the encounter is perceiving the subtle differences and addressing the concerns.

The physical examination itself will include the same basic elements for all ages with specific areas of focus depending on the patient's age and development. Certainly the extremity and spine alignment, range of motion and neurological examination will be performed on all patients, but special focus on areas such as the newborn's hips, the toddler's extremity alignment and the teenager's spine will be necessary owing to the typical chief complaint at various ages.

After the initial assessment and relationship building, the patient should be asked to sit on the examination table. Babies and apprehensive children may be more apt to comply with an examination sitting on the parent's lap. A bottle may calm a crying baby, who will relax and yield a better musculoskeletal examination when calm. If the child is still apprehensive, examining a stuffed animal or even a parent first may calm his or her nerves and even encourage their interest.

The following sections will address specific areas of examination for the paediatric orthopaedic patient based on age and clinical concern. The topics covered here are applicable to most settings except for acute trauma.

THE LOWER EXTREMITY SCREEN

One of the most common presentations to the paediatric orthopaedist is for concern of in-toeing, out-toeing, bowlegs or knock-knees. Parents or grandparents usually have great concern that 'something doesn't look right' and have been seen by their primary care doctor, who has then sent them on to the orthopaedist. The age varies at presentation from infant to toddler, and the concern is usually correlated to the patient's stage of development.

An important aspect of the paediatric screen, and specifically the lower extremity examination, is observational gait analysis. Having the child walk down the hallway or even just across the room can quickly reveal rotation, alignment or neurological abnormalities. The chapters that follow in this Paediatric Orthopaedic section of the book deal with more specific aspects of gait analysis, pathology and implications.

Examination of the child in a standing position to view his or her clinical lower extremity alignment is often all that is needed to quickly assess whether the child falls within the age-appropriate alignment of the tibia and femur. The intercondylar distance and the intermalleolar distance can also be measured for reference for follow-up visits. The concern is typically about the tibial and femoral alignment at the knee, but it is also important to assess the overall coronal alignment of the ankle and, if needed, an assessment of the hip.[1] As a rule of thumb in terms of tibiofemoral alignment, the child should reach 0° by 2 years of age, and progress towards a valgus alignment with further growth. Adult valgus is typically reached by the age of 7 years. Children who are close to this or beyond this age with residual varus warrant radiographs to evaluate for more precise measurement. Many practitioners will choose to order a set of films at initial presentation, then ask the child to return for a follow-up visit to look for resolution of the concern with growth. Often the best clinical experience for the patient with a normal examination is that of one in which the examiner spends adequate time explaining to the family about normal development. The aid of a preprinted chart or photographs is useful in this regard, as is using an older or younger sibling who might be present to show the changes of alignment with age.

While the child is standing, assess leg length discrepancies by checking for a level pelvis (Fig. 58.2).[2] Combine this examination with the spine screen mentioned below for efficiency. Ascertain whether one side of the pelvis appears higher than the other with the patient standing flatfooted. Checking for leg length with the patient supine by comparing the anterior superior iliac spine to the medial malleolar distance can also be performed. If a discrepancy is noted,

The lower extremity screen 537

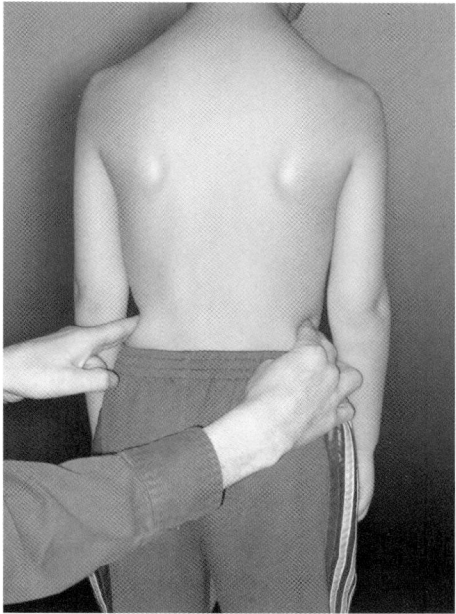

Figure 58.2 By palpating the iliac crests bilaterally one can make a determination of a leg length difference.

small blocks (Coleman blocks) of known height can be placed under the shorter side until the pelvis is level and will yield a clinical assessment of the discrepancy.[2]

The in-toeing and out-toeing concern is one of rotation of the lower extremity.[3] The easiest way to assess this is by determination of the rotational profile of the legs. The hip, tibia and forefoot rotation make up the components of the rotational profile. Determination of femoral anteversion, tibial torsion and forefoot-to-hindfoot alignment will help elucidate any pathological alignment. To assess the hip, the child should be examined with the hips in extension by asking him or her to lie prone with the knee flexed at 90°. Internal and external rotation, with a hand placed on the ipsilateral pelvis to stabilize pelvis motion, should be assessed in this manner (Fig. 58.3). To assess tibial rotation, the alignment of the transmalleolar axis should be determined.[4] While the child is lying prone, hold the knee in 90° of flexion and the ankle in neutral plantar/dorsiflexion. Place your thumb and index finger on the malleoli and look down the axis of the tibia from above in relation to the hindfoot (Fig. 58.4). This will give you an estimate of the tibial rotation. While you have the foot in this position, a quick assessment of the adduction of the lateral border of

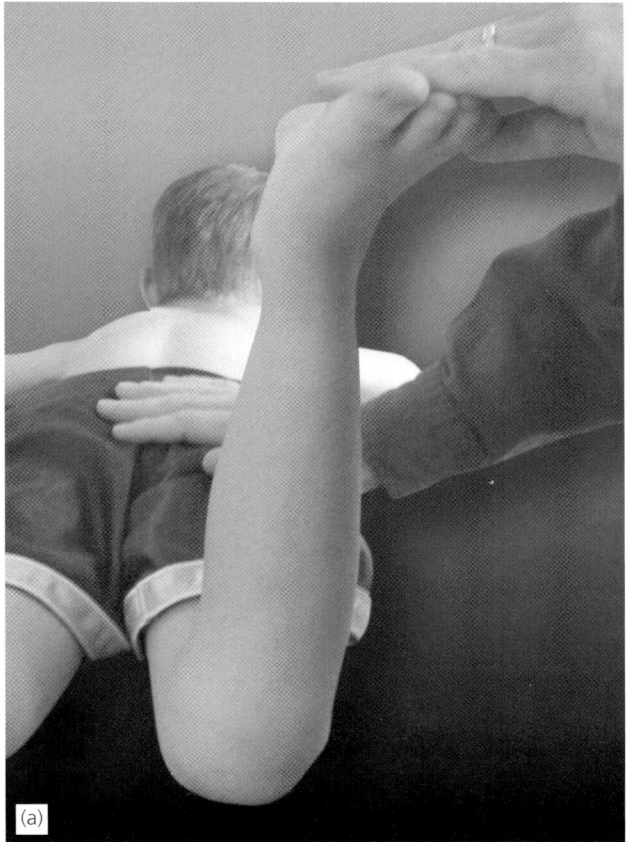
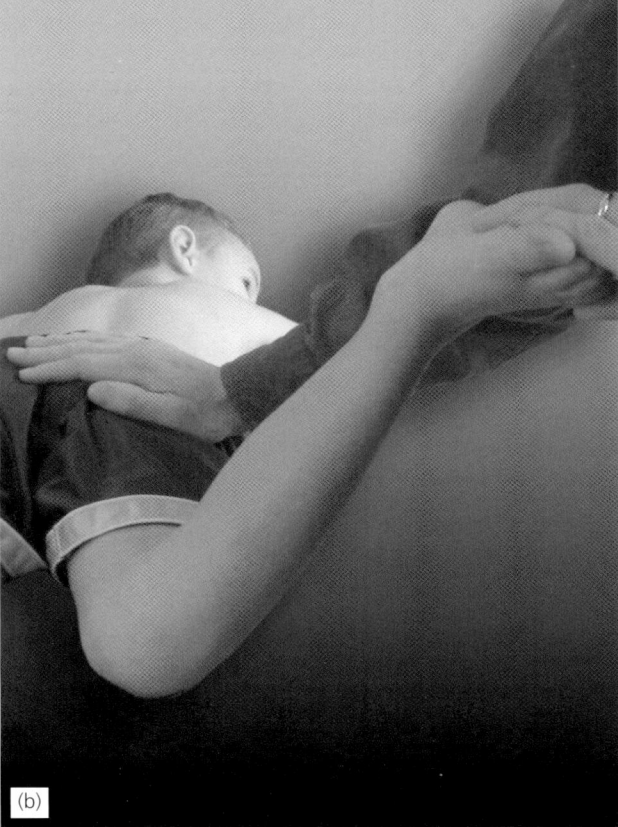

Figure 58.3 With the patient prone, the rotational profile of the femurs may be accessed. Internal (a) and external (b) rotation of the femur will be evaluated. A hand placed on the ipsilateral pelvis will stabilize the pelvis.

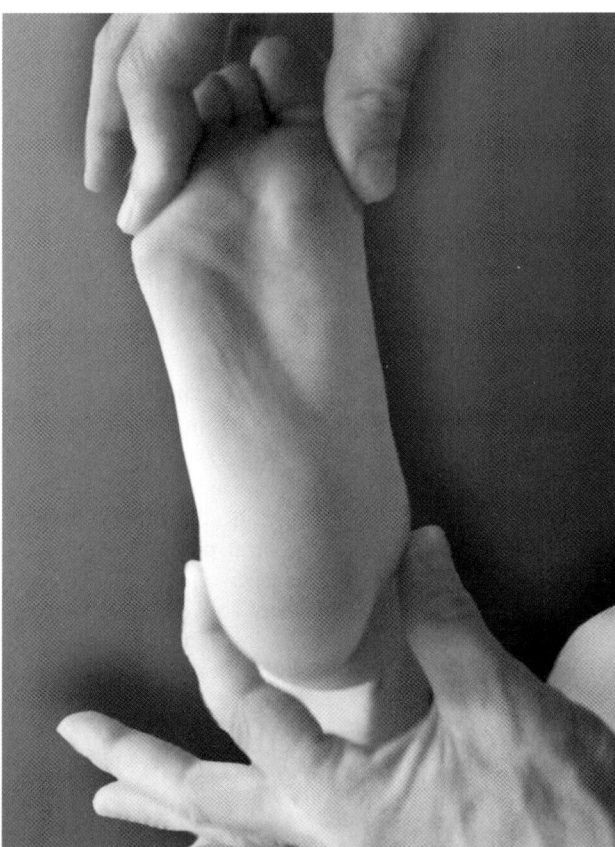

Figure 58.4 To evaluate the rotation of the tibia, place the patient prone and flex the knees. By placing your fingers on the medial and lateral malleoli and comparing that axis with the axis of the tibia, the transmalleolar axis can be established.

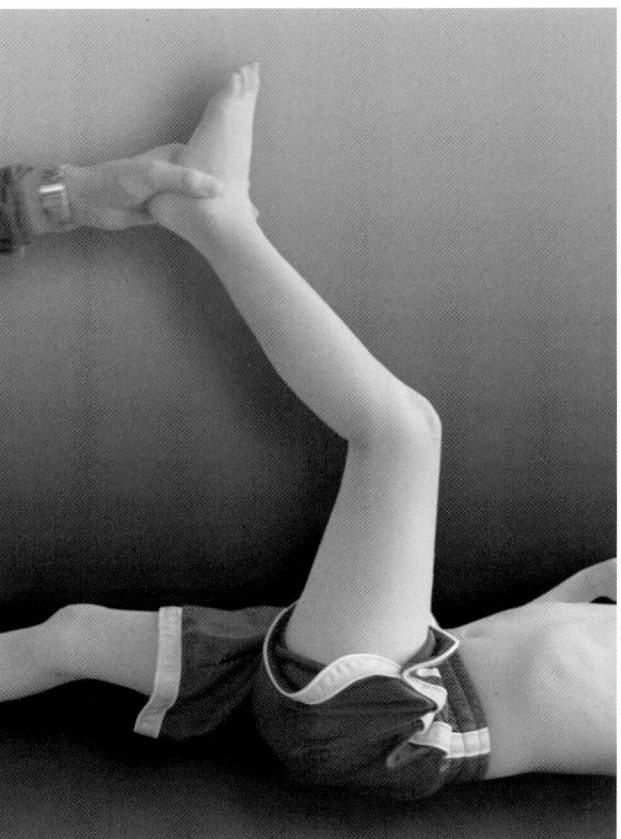

Figure 58.5 The flexibility of the hamstrings can be evaluated by placing the child supine and flexing the hip to 90°. By extending the knee in this position, an angle between the vertical line and the angle of the leg will determine the popliteal angle.

the foot will yield forefoot-to-hindfoot alignment.[4] This can be a very quick process and can be performed in one patient position.

The child should also be checked for contractures of the lower extremity while on the examination table. Documentation of ankle dorsiflexion and plantarflexion is performed with the knee flexed and extended. The gastrocnemius and soleus muscles can be elucidated as the source of a contracture by checking the dorsiflexion in knee flexion and knee extension. Both examinations should be performed with the foot locked in supination to ensure that ankle motion is being examined and that subtalar motion or a midfoot break is not contributing to the apparent range of motion. Not being able to dorsiflex the foot to neutral because of contracture is concerning and should be examined further.

Lower extremity flexibility and contractures can also be assessed by examination of the hamstrings and hip flexors. The hamstrings can be assessed through measuring the popliteal angle. Ask the patient to lie supine and flex one hip up to 90°. With the hip flexed, slowly extend the knee until the hamstrings are taught. The distance between a vertical line and the angle of the lower leg is the popliteal angle (Fig. 58.5). Angles greater than 45° indicate a contracture. Hip flexion is measured by having the patient in the same supine position and flexing one hip up past 90°. The contralateral hip should remain extended and may indicate a flexion contracture otherwise.

THE FOOT EXAMINATION

A common presentation to the paediatric orthopaedist is for examination of the foot for flat feet, foot pain or other pathology such as clubfoot.[5] Again, the presentation is typically related to the age of the patient and often there is a family history of similar complaints. The infant should be checked for a supple, flexible foot that is correctable to a neutral position. Positional changes are common in infants, and those that are not correctable may point to underlying pathology. Syndactyly or hemimelic structures should be noted as well as these may also point towards an underlying disorder. Toes that overlap or are hyperflexed (curly toes) should be noted as this may also be a family concern.

The toddler's foot presentation is usually one concerned with alignment as mentioned previously.

Examination of the lateral border of the foot will yield information about forefoot adduction.

The adolescent and teenage patient may be brought to the paediatric orthopaedist for evaluation of foot pain or flat feet.[5] In addition to the above examinations, observe the patient's foot position while standing. Note the foot arch and the ankle alignment. A patient with a flat arch and a valgus-appearing ankle should be asked to stand on his or her tiptoes. In a flexible flat foot, the arch should reconstitute when the first metacarpal phalangeal joint is flexed through the windlass effect of the plantar fascia. The ankle should fall into a varus position as well. Feet that are not flexible may have an underlying pathology such as a tarsal coalition that needs further study. Having a cavus deformity to the foot, or an abnormally high arch, may also point towards an underlying disorder especially if unilateral.

THE HIP EXAMINATION

The paediatric hip examination can be extensive, and thus should be tailored according to the patient's age. In infants, the physician is mostly concerned with developmental dysplasia of the hip (DDH).[6] While adolescents may also have a subluxed or dislocated hip, this is not a common finding. They more often report a painful limp, hip or knee that may be indicative of problems such as slipped capital femoral epiphysis, Legg–Calvé–Perthes disease or, if presenting with systemic symptoms, transient synovitis or septic arthritis, among others.[7,8]

Infants

The diagnosis of DDH in infants can initially be made via positive Barlow or Ortolani tests (Fig. 58.6),[6] and, if necessary, verified with imaging studies. Both examinations should be performed with the patient supine, and on each leg independently. A quiet, calm child is imperative for an adequate hip examination. If this is not possible then another attempt in a different setting is recommended. The Barlow examination tests for a subluxable or dislocatable hip (Use the mnemonic Barlow = dislocataBle). The examination is performed by grasping the thigh of the leg being tested with the thumb on the lesser trochanter and the fingers on the greater trochanter while at the same time using the other hand to stabilize the contralateral pelvis and leg. With the hip in flexion, apply pressure posteriorly while adducting the hip – this motion will result in a palpable, and sometime audible, 'clunk' for a dislocatable hip, with a somewhat milder result for subluxable hips. The Ortolani manoeuvre tests for a reducible hip (Ortolani = Out). Using the same hand placement and stabilization of the pelvis, apply upwards pressure on the greater trochanter while abducting the hip. Again, a 'clunk' will indicate a dislocated hip with relocation of the femoral head to the acetabulum. Finally, a positive Galeazzi sign may also be useful in diagnosing DDH (Fig. 58.7).[6] In this test, the patient is supine, with the hips and knees flexed, with the feet flat on the table. If the knees are not level with one another in this position, it may be indicative of a dislocated or subluxed hip (alternatively, a positive Galeazzi sign could indicate a femoral length discrepancy). However, it should be noted that, if the dislocation is bilateral, this will yield a false-negative Galeazzi sign (Fig. 58.7).

Adolescents

A range of motion (ROM) examination of the hip and radiographs will be useful in diagnosing the adolescent presenting with a painful hip, knee (referred pain from obturator, femoral or sciatic nerve) or limp.[7,8] As with the rotational profile examination, ask the patient to lie prone with the knees flexed to 90° while moving the ankles inwards and outwards and stabilizing the pelvis. With the

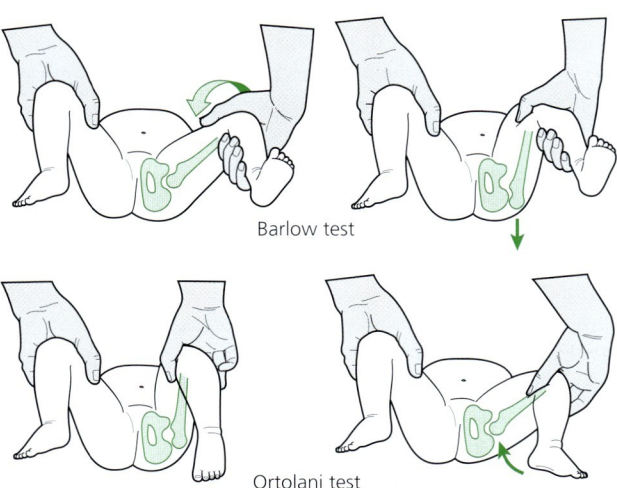

Figure 58.6 The Barlow and Ortolani tests will evaluate the presence of a dislocated or dislocatable hip.

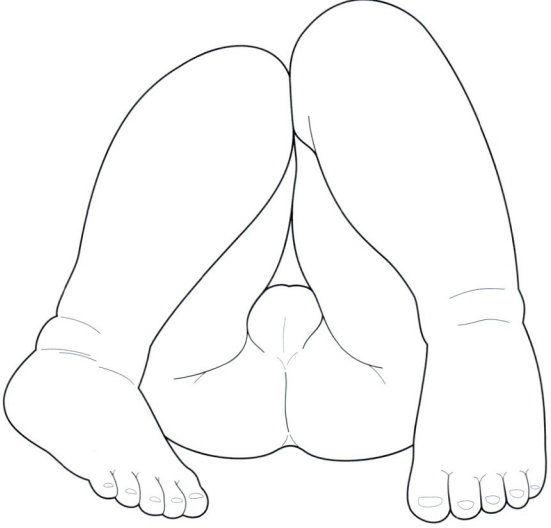

Figure 58.7 The Galleazi sign, or apparent inequality of femoral lengths, can be seen in a dislocated hip.

patient supine, evaluate the symmetry of hip adduction and abduction, flexion and extension, being sure to stabilize the pelvis at all times to prevent compensation for limited ROM with pelvic tilt.

THE SPINE SCREEN

The paediatric orthopaedist will be asked to evaluate many patients for possible spinal pathology, including back pain, scoliosis, kyphosis and associated conditions.[9-11] The spine screen is straightforward. The patient should be in a gown or loose shorts that can be adjusted so the shoulders, top of the pelvis and spine can be visualized. Also, the feet must be out of socks and shoes as the spine screen is not complete without examination of the feet for possible unilateral differences in contractures as mentioned above.[9]

First, examine the patient standing to assess shoulder height, clinical alignment of the spine, and whether the pelvis is level. Placing a fingertip on each iliac crest is useful if the crests cannot be visualized, as is often the case in heavyset patients. Next, ask the patient to bend forward at the waist and let his or her arms hang forward in Adam's forward bend test position (Fig. 58.8).[9] Note the alignment of the spine while observing the patient from the back as the patient bends forward. Also make note of any rotational deformities manifested by a protrusion of one side of the rib cage or lumbar spine. Palpate the spine to find any spots of tenderness and ask the patient to flex and extend the cervical spine to assess for any neck pain.[11] Finally, perform a thorough neurological examination. A quick and complete neurological examination will address upper and lower extremity reflexes and muscle strength. It should also include abdominal reflexes to assess for thoracic pathology.[9,10]

To perform this, stroke each of the four quadrants of the abdomen with the patient relaxed and lying on the examination table. The umbilicus should twitch towards the quadrant that is being stimulated. Unilateral differences in reflexes or strength should be further assessed.

KEY LEARNING POINTS

- The paediatric examination is unique with respect to dealing with young patients, families and parents who all have different concerns at the time of the visit.
- It is important to build rapport and put the patient and family at ease.
- An infant may be most comfortable on a parent's lap.
- Lower limb rotation, alignment, and length discrepancies are common reasons for evaluation.
- The spine examination also requires a neurological examination and examination of the feet.

REFERENCES

1. Sass P, Hassan G. Lower extremity abnormalities in children. *American Family Physician* 2003;**68**:461–8.
2. Sabharwal S, Kumar A. Methods for assessing leg length discrepancy. *Clinical Orthopaedics and Related Research* 2008;**466**:2910–22.
3. Lincoln TL, Suen PW. Common rotational variations in children. *Journal of the American Academy of Orthopaedic Surgeons* 2003;**11**:312–20.
4. Karol LA. Rotational deformities in the lower extremities. *Current Opinion in Pediatrics* 1997;**9**:77–80.
5. Houghton KM. Review for the generalist: evaluation of pediatric foot and ankle pain. *Pediatric Rheumatology Online Journal* 2008;**6**:6.
6. Vitale MG, Skaggs DL. Developmental dysplasia of the hip from six months to four years of age. *Journal of the American Academy of Orthopaedic Surgeons* 2001;**9**:401–11.
7. Flynn JM, Widmann RF. The limping child: evaluation and diagnosis. *Journal of the American Academy of Orthopaedic Surgeons* 2001;**9**:89–98.
8. Houghton KM. Review for the generalist: evaluation of pediatric hip pain. *Pediatric Rheumatology Online Journal* 2009;**7**:10.
9. Asher MA. Scoliosis evaluation. *Orthopaedic Clinics of North America* 1988;**19**:805–14.
10. Diab M. Physical examination in adolescent idiopathic scoliosis. *Neurosurgery Clinics of North America* 2007;**18**:229–36.
11. Houghton KM. Review for the generalist: evaluation of low back pain in children and adolescents. *Pediatric Rheumatology Online Journal* 2010;**8**:28.

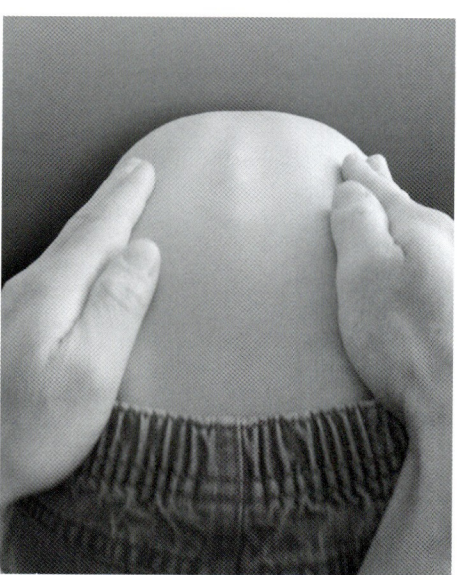

Figure 58.8 The Adams forward bend test can evaluate for the rotation associated with scoliosis. Any increase in the prominence of one side of the spine necessitates further evaluation.

59

Developmental disorders of human skeleton

CHEZHIYAN SHANMUGAM, UMILE GIUSEPPE LONGO, NICOLA MAFFULLI

Introduction	541	Molecular pathogenesis	544
Epidemiology	541	International nosology and classification	549
Limb morphogenesis	542	Diagnostic considerations	549
Skeletal morphogenesis	543	Management of the skeletal dysplasias	556
Growth plate histology	544	References	558

NATIONAL BOARD STANDARDS

- Understand the classification of different types of dwarfism
- Know the genetic basis of the common skeletal dysplasias
- Understand the molecular basis of common dysplasias
- Understand the management of common skeletal dysplasias
- Know about the prognosis of common developmental disorders

INTRODUCTION

Developmental disorders of bone comprise a large heterogeneous group of genetic disorders, and they are very rare. However, depictions in ancient figurines and sculptures signify their prevalence for many centuries.

The disorders are known by various terms such as skeletal dysplasia, osteochondrodysplasia and chondrodysplasia for those affected by disturbance in endochondral ossification, and as dysostoses for those affected by disturbance in membranous ossification. The terms 'skeletal dysmorphology syndrome' and 'constitutional disorders of bone' are synonyms of developmental disorder of bone, and they are used in a wider context.

Developmental disorders of the human skeleton are divided into two broad groups: the osteochondrodysplasias and the dysostoses. The osteochondrodysplasias are not apparent at birth and they continue to evolve throughout life; they may become obvious at a later stage as a result of gene expression.[1] The dysostoses are static and their malformations occur during blastogenesis (the first 8 weeks of embryonic life).[2]

For individual descriptions of osteochondrodysplasias and the dysostoses, see Chapter 33.

EPIDEMIOLOGY

Males and females are equally affected by developmental disorders, as most of them are autosomal dominantly inherited. Some enzyme deficiency disorders are autosomal recessive. Usually, structural abnormalities tend to be autosomal dominant, whereas enzyme disorders tend to be autosomal recessive. Males are primarily affected in X-linked recessive disorders. X-linked dominant disorders may be lethal in males. There are no racial predilections.

Incidence

Developmental disorders affect 2–5 per 10 000 livebirths.[3]

Prevalence

Prevalence rates vary for different skeletal dysplasias, between populations and between studies. The crude prevalence rate is 2.3/10 000 births.[4] In a large study conducted in the west of Scotland by Connor et al.,[5] the prevalence of lethal neonatal skeletal dysplasias was 1.1/10 000 births.

The most frequently diagnosed lethal conditions were thanatophoric dysplasia (0.24/10 000), osteogenesis imperfecta (0.18/10 000), rhisomelic chondrodysplasia punctata (0.12/10 000), campomelic syndrome (0.1/10 000) and achondrogenesis (0.1/10 000).[5] Achondroplasia is the most common non-lethal skeletal dysplasia.[6] Patients affected with mild forms of skeletal dysplasia may never attend hospital. Therefore, the real prevalence rate is normally twice that of the observed rate.

LIMB MORPHOGENESIS

The skeletal system develops from paraxial and lateral plate mesoderm and from neural crest. Paraxial mesoderm forms somitomeres on each side of the neural tube in the head region, and somites from the occipital region caudally. Somites differentiate into sclerotome (ventromedially) (Fig. 59.1) and dermomyotome (dorsolaterally). During the fourth week of embryogenesis, limb buds appear from the ventrolateral body wall (Fig. 59.2). The limb bud consists of a sclerotome (mesenchymal core) covered by a layer of ectoderm. By the fifth week, the mesenchymal tissue migrates at genetically predetermined sites, condenses and differentiates into chondroblast that forms hyaline type II cartilage template (anlagen).[7] Ectoderm at the distal border of the limb thickens and forms the apical ectodermal ridge (AER).[8] The AER restricts the adjacent mesenchyme to differentiate and retains as rapidly proliferating cells, which allow the limb to grow proximodistally. Cells further from the influence of the AER begin to differentiate into cartilage and muscle. The handplates and footplates are formed from flattening of the terminal portion of the limb buds at 6 weeks. Fingers and toes are formed by programmed cell death in AER that cleaves the ridge into five parts (Fig. 59.3).

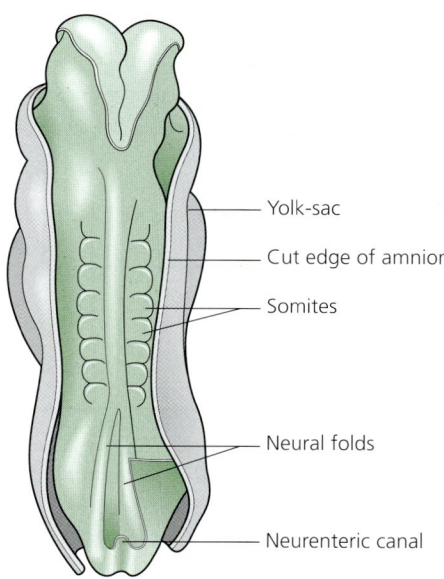

Figure 59.1 Somites, rich in pleuripotent mesodermal tissues distributed on either side of the neural tube. The mesoderm tissues eventually differentiate into dermis (dermatome), skeletal muscle (myotome) and vertebrae (sclerotome).

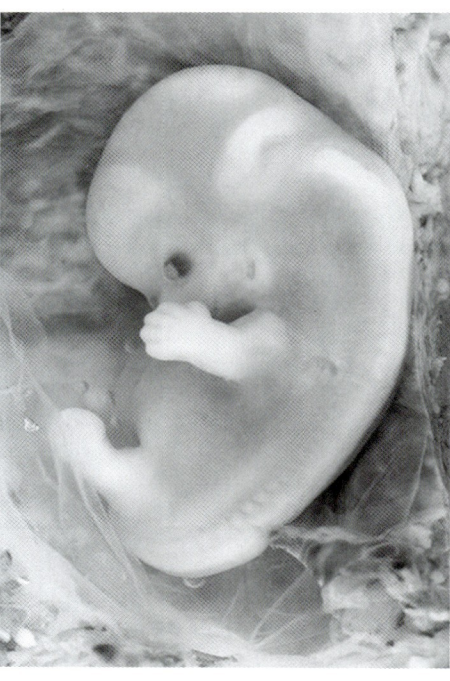

Figure 59.2 A rare image of a 9 week human embryo from an ectopic pregnancy. Formation of limb buds is almost complete by 9 weeks. The somites can be clearly seen through the transparent skin on the side of the neural canal. Courtesy of Ed Uthman MD; http://www.flickr.com/photos/euthman/548063929

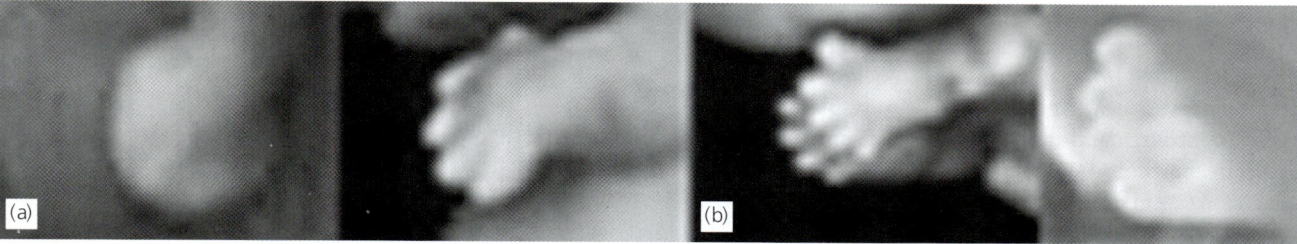

Figure 59.3 (a) Apoptosis at the apical ectodermal ridge creates a separate ridge for each digit. (b) Digit separation is almost complete at 56 days.

SKELETAL MORPHOGENESIS

The complex genetic process determines the skeletal patterning and architectural arrangement that guides the number, size, and shape of the future skeletal elements (Fig. 59.4).[9] Bones are formed by two types of ossification: endochondral and intramembranous ossification.

Endochondral ossification

Endochondral ossification is a highly complex temporally and spatially coordinated process.[10] Most human bones are developed by this method, e.g. long bones, vertebrae, pelvis and the base of the skull.

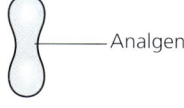
Analgen

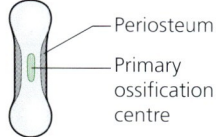
Periosteum
Primary ossification centre

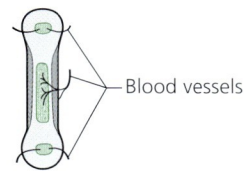
Blood vessels

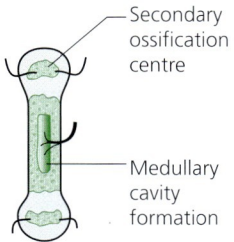
Secondary ossification centre
Medullary cavity formation

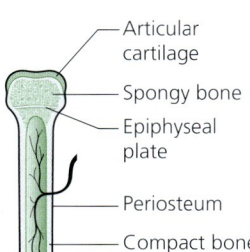
Articular cartilage
Spongy bone
Epiphyseal plate
Periosteum
Compact bone

Figure 59.4 Skeletal morphogenesis.

The primary centre of ossification starts in the middle of the diaphysis. Then, the following steps occur:

- *Periosteum formation*: the perichondrium surrounding the anlagen transforms into periosteum, which gains osteogenic potential after it is vascularized. It begins near birth and continues for 18–19 years. The mesenchymal cells in the anlagen and inner cambium layer of periosteum differentiate into osteoblasts.
- *Bone collar formation*: the osteoblasts lay osteoid to form a collar of compact bone replacing the anlagen. This serves as a scaffold for further new bone formation.
- *Matrix formation and mineralization*: the chondrocytes enlarge and resorb the surrounding cartilage, forming perforated trabeculae of cartilage matrix. They stop secreting collagen, and begin secreting alkaline phosphatase, an enzyme essential for mineralization of cartilage matrix. The chondrocytes subsequently die owing to incarceration and lack of diffusion of nutrients in a tight calcified matrix. This creates large interconnecting spaces (lacunae) within the bone.
- *Bone marrow formation*: a periosteal bud rich in blood vessels, lymphatics and nerves invades the lacunae. The vascularization process carries haemopoietic cells, osteoblasts and osteoclasts into the lacunae that later form the bone marrow.
- *Trabeculae formation*: the osteoblasts lay osteoid over the calcified matrix to form the bone trabecula. The osteoclasts dissolve the spongy bone to form the medullary cavity.
- *Growth plate*: the secondary ossification centres develop in the epiphyses, which expand outwards and to the centre, while the primary ossification continues along the diaphysis towards the epiphyses. The anlagen becomes trapped between the growing primary and secondary ossification centres, forming growth or epiphyseal plates.

The genes that encode for matrix components and enzymes may play a role in regulating the normal developmental processes of growth plate chondrocytes.[11] The alterations in sex hormone level during puberty may halt cartilage proliferation, and the growth plates disappear. Nonetheless, the mechanism behind the cessation of bone growth is yet to be determined.[12]

Intramembranous ossification

The mesenchymal tissues in the dermis differentiate directly into bone. The typical examples are flat bones of the skull, the maxilla and most of the mandible.

Joint formation

The Wnt-4, -14 and -59, and beta-catenin signalling pathways induce synovial joint formation.[13] Joints are formed in the cartilaginous condensations when chondrogenesis is arrested. They are delimited by areas of higher cell density called interzones. Surrounding cells differentiate into a joint capsule.

GROWTH PLATE HISTOLOGY

During endochondral ossification, the transition between epiphyseal cartilage and new bone formation occurs in six functional and morphological stages (Fig. 59.5).[14]

1. *Reserve cartilage zone* (R). This layer consists of typical hyaline cartilage with the chondrocytes arranged in small clusters. They exhibit only occasional cell divisions.
2. *Proliferation zone* (P). The cartilage cells undergo successive mitotic divisions to form columns of chondrocytes separated by matrix rich in proteoglycans.
3. *Maturation zone* (M). The chondrocytes cease their cell division, and enlarge in size.
4. *Hypertrophic and calcification zone* (H). The chondrocytes become greatly enlarged and vacuolated and the matrix becomes calcified. The hypertrophic cells either differentiate into osteoblasts or enter into programmed cell death.[15]
5. *Cartilage degeneration zone* (CD). The dying or dead chondrocytes form lacunae. Lacunae are filled with haemopoietic cells and capillaries forming bone marrow.
6. *Osteogenic zone* (O). This is a transitional zone in which the osteogenic cells differentiate into osteoblasts, which ossify on the spicules of calcified cartilage matrix. Any disturbances to one or more zones of chondrocytes may contribute to the development of skeletal dysmorphology syndrome.

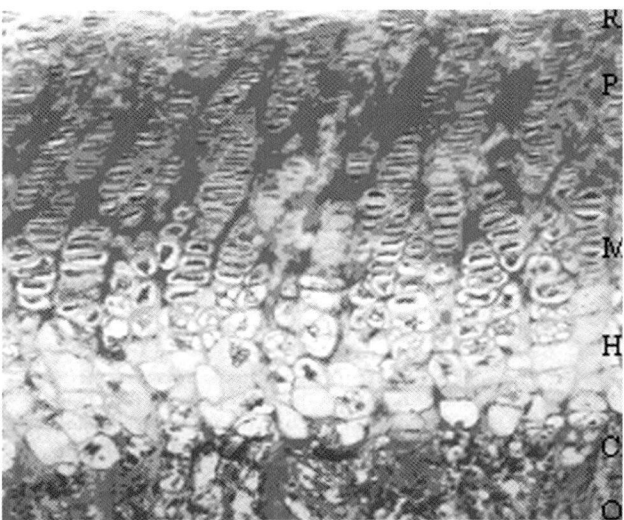

Figure 59.5 Epiphyseal plate histology; haematoxylin and eosin/Alcian blue, ×120. Reproduced with permission from Young B, Heath JW. *Wheater's Functional Histology: A Text and Colour Atlas*, 4th edn. Edinburgh, UK: Churchill Livingstone, 2000:186. Copyright © 2000 Elsevier Inc.

MOLECULAR PATHOGENESIS

Osteochondrodysplasias are caused by a disruption of skeletal patterning and endochondral ossification[59] (Fig. 59.6). Genetic mutations involved in the synthesis of structural proteins and in metabolic pathways, degradation of macromolecules, growth factors and receptors and transcription factors cause disturbances in endochondral ossification that may result in various spectrums of constitutional disorders of bone.[17]

Limb-patterning defects

Early patterning events in fetal skeletogenesis are regulated by a complex signalling system involving members of the

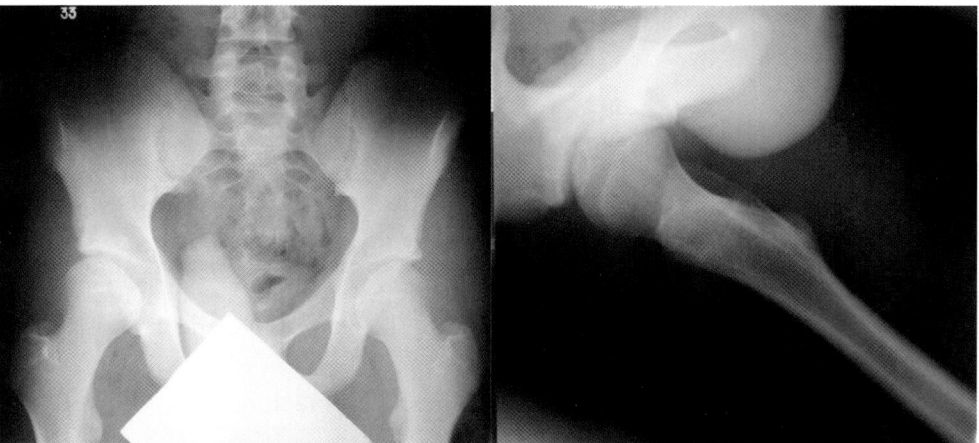

Figure 59.6 Osteochondrodysplasia of the hips. Mild deformation of the femoral heads is seen.

Indian hedgehog (IHH), bone morphogenetic protein (BMP) and Gli families.[18]

- IHH proteins act through both short-range and long-range signalling to pattern tissues during invertebrate and vertebrate development. Bellaiche et al.[19] identified a new *Drosophila* gene, named tout-velu, that encodes an integral transmembrane protein that belongs to the *EXT* gene family. IHH requires tout-velu for diffusion through membranes for long-range signalling to pattern tissues.[19] IHH is possibly a direct regulator of joint development. The distribution and function of Gdf5-expressing interzone-associated cells are affected, thereby producing abnormal joints. However, their patterning at prospective joint sites still occurs.[20]
- Wnt proteins are indispensable for primitive streak formation,[21] mesoderm cell movement,[22,23] generation of the tail organizer,[24] posterior patterning and somitogenesis. Wnt signalling is regulated by antagonistic Sfrp1 and Sfrp2 proteins. They are required for normal anteroposterior (AP) axis elongation and somitogenesis. Abnormal Wnt signalling leads to developmental defects.[25]
- Haycraft et al.[26] found that mutations disrupting the intraflagellar transport process in a cell result in midgestation lethality, associated with skeletal anomalies and abnormal neural tube patterning. Cytochrome P450 oxidoreductase is absolutely necessary for molecular patterning of the brain, abdominal/caudal region and limbs. It also regulates retinoic acid levels and tissue distribution during both early and late stages of embryonic morphogenesis.[27]
- Hyaluronan (HA) is a structural component of extracellular matrices of the distal subapical mesenchymal cells of the developing limb bud. Lack of HA affects cell proliferation, migration and intracellular signalling, and patterning in response to the apical ectodermal ridge.[8] Overexpression of Has2 in limb buds results in skeletal dysmorphology syndrome. However, HA downregulation is required at times to trigger cartilage differentiation during condensation.[28]

Transcription factor defects

Cell-to-cell communication is essential for embryogenesis with respect to cell fate specification, cell polarity, cell behaviour and embryonic patterning.[29] Transcription factors coordinate this complex process.[30] These include ligand–receptor pairs and their antagonists. Most of the transcription networks during skeletogenesis still remain to be elucidated.[30] The roles of some of the transcription factors in skeletal morphogenesis are:

- Missense mutations in core binding factor α1 (*CBFA1*)/runt-related gene 2 (*Runx2*) may cause cleidocranial dysplasia (CCD). *Cbfa1* encodes an osteoblast-specific transcription factor (*OSF2*) that determines osteoblast differentiation and skeletal morphogenesis. CCD is an autosomal dominant disorder of generalized defects in ossification. It is characterized by hypoplastic or absent clavicles, large fontanelles, dental anomalies and delayed skeletal development. It is one of the most common skeletal dysplasias not associated with disproportionate stature. Studies using *OSF2/CBFA1* knock-out mice have provided direct genetic evidence that skeletal dysmorphogenesis results from an alteration in osteoblast differentiation.[31]
- *BMP-7* induces osteoblast differentiation from mesenchymal precursor stem cells both *in vitro* and *in vivo* by upregulating *Runx2/Cbfa1* gene expression.[32]
- *SOX9* encodes a putative transcription factor located on chromosome 17. *Sox9* is structurally related to the testis-determining factor *SRY* and is expressed predominantly in mesenchymal condensations throughout the embryo before and during the deposition of cartilage, consistent with a primary role in skeletal formation.[33] A haploinsufficiency of *SOX9* may cause both skeletal dysmorphology syndrome, e.g. campomelic dysplasia, and autosomal XY sex reversal.[34] The skeletal manifestations include bowing and angulation of the long bones, most often femur, small scapulae, a deformed pelvis and spine, missing ribs and a small thoracic cage.
- The *Pax* family of genes (*Pax1–Pax9*) encodes nuclear transcription factors. They possess a paired domain and a conserved amino acid motif with DNA-binding activity. The primary developmental action may possibly be by signal transduction during tissue interactions, which may lead to a position-specific regulation of cell proliferation.[35] *Pax9* and *Pax1* may act in parallel during morphogenesis of the vertebral column.[36]
- Homeobox (*HOX*) genes control the specification of a limb primordium's outgrowth, organization and differentiation into a functional appendage.[37] Mutations in *Hox* genes may result in skeletal dysmorphology syndrome. A haploinsufficiency of short stature homeobox gene (*SHOX*) has been implicated in idiopathic short stature and short stature phenotype in Turner syndrome. The homozygous mutations of *SHOX* at the dyschondrosteosis locus result in Leri–Weill dyschondrosteosis, and Madelung deformity of the forearm.[38,39]

Proliferative chondrocyte defects

In normal growth plates, parathyroid hormone-related peptide (PTHrP) delays the hypertrophic differentiation of proliferating chondrocytes, whereas *IHH* promotes chondrocyte proliferation.[40] The *IHH*-responsive gene also encodes PTHrP. Mutations of the PTH/PTHrP type I receptor constitutively overstimulate the hedgehog signals. In a study of PTHrP null mice, growth plate histology showed a small proliferative zone and non-hypertrophic cells within the hypertrophic zone of the growth plate.[41] It affects endochondral ossification, leaving intramembranous ossification undisturbed.

- Mutations in *PTHrP* cause various skeletal dysplasias, such as Blomstrand lethal osteochondrodysplasia,[42,43] Jansen-type metaphyseal dysplasia[44] and enchondromatosis.[40] In 1881, Angelo Maria Maffucci, Professor of Pathology at the University of Catania, Italy, described enchondromatosis with multiple angiomas (plebolithis), popularly remembered as 'Maffucci syndrome'.[45] Mutations in the *IHH* gene cause brachydactyly type A, a dominant condition characterized by absent terminal phalanges.[46]
- Growth hormone (GH) stimulates the multiplication of reserve chondrocytes in the epiphyseal plate.[47] It acts both directly and indirectly via insulin-like growth factor (IGF-1). Systemic IGF-1 is a major regulator of proliferation of resulting chondrocytes, which determines the linear growth of bone.[48,49] Nonsense mutations of the GH-releasing hormone receptor cause proportionate short stature.[50] Fibroblast growth factor may influence the actions of IGF-I at the growth plate by altering the number of receptors in chondrocytes.[48]

Any disturbances in the proliferation of chondrocytes may lead to reduced bone size, but not altered shape or structure.

- Fibroblast growth factor receptor 3 gene (*FGFR3*) normally has a negative regulatory effect on bone growth, proliferation and differentiation in the growth plate (Fig. 59.7). Recurrent point mutations in the *FGFR3* gene result in receptor hyperactivation and subsequent amplification of signals, thereby preventing transition of chondrocytes to the proliferative phenotype.[51] The mutated form of the receptor produces the achondroplasia spectrum of disorders. These disorders are characterized by a continuum of severity ranging from mild forms, such as hypochondroplasia,[52] through achondroplasia[53] to lethal neonatal thanatophoric dysplasia.[54] The most characteristic radiological and phenotypic features among this group of disorders are rhisomelic shortening of long tubular bones and spine growth disturbances. The horizontal growth of long bone is unaffected as periosteal ossification remains normal.
- Mutations of *FGF23*, which encodes a phosphaturic protein, may cause autosomal dominant hypophosphataemic rickets. Mutations in the *PEX* proteinase, which is a cleavage of *FGF23*, causes X-linked hypophosphataemic rickets.[55,56]

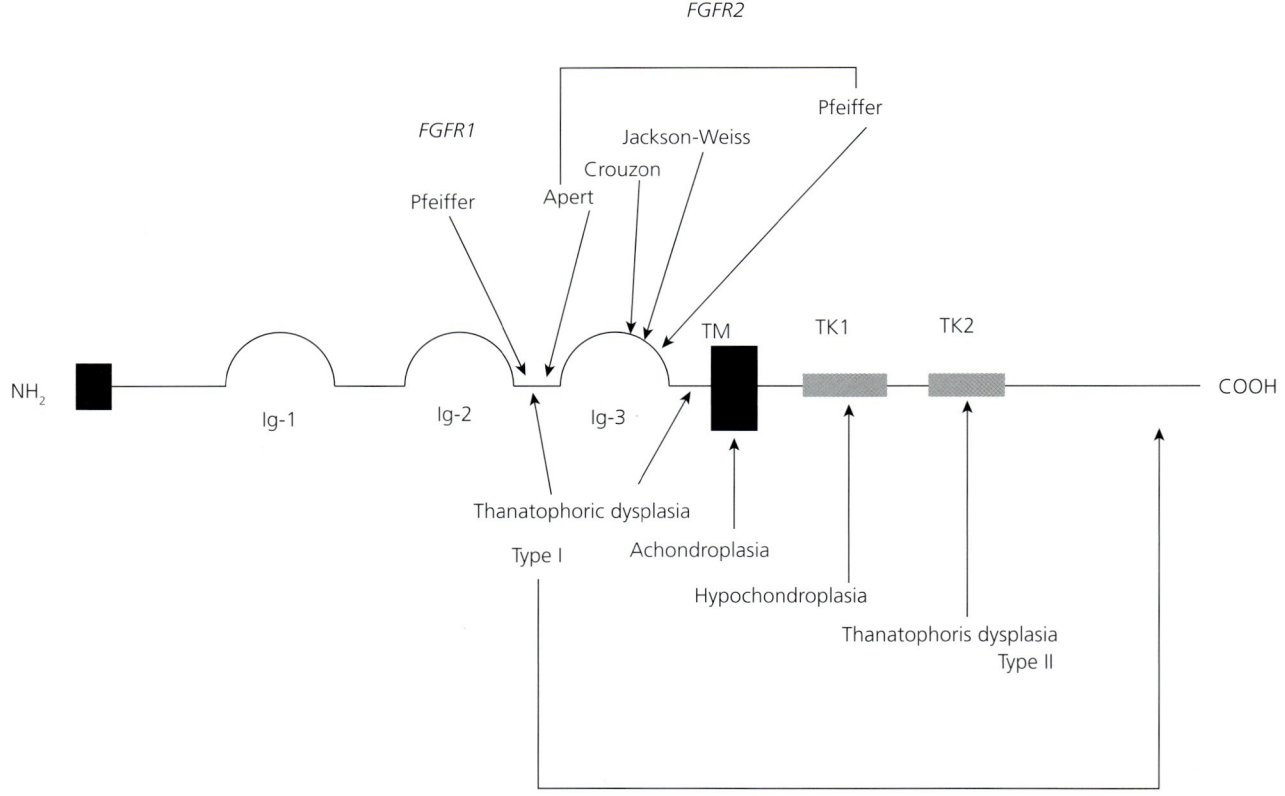

Figure 59.7 Schematic representation of fibroblast growth factor receptor protein. The three loops indicate immunoglobulin (Ig)-like domains, located on the extracellular surface that is responsible for ligand binding. The locations of *FGFR1–FGFR3* mutations are shown by arrows. TM, transmembrane domain; TK1 and TK2, tyrosine kinase domains containing the ATP binding site.

Chondrocyte maturation defects

Calcium/calmodulin-dependent kinase II (CaMKII) is an essential component of intracellular signalling pathways regulating chondrocyte maturation.[57] In chick experiments, using replication-competent retroviruses, a reduction in endogenous CaMKII activity by overexpressing an inhibitory peptide resulted in shortening of the skeletal elements that was associated with a delay in chondrocyte maturation.

Hypertrophic chondrocyte defects

The hypertrophic chondrocytes can transdifferentiate or dedifferentiate and redifferentiate into osteocytes or enter a programmed cell death.[15,58] They are functionally coupled to the recruitment of osteoblasts, vascular cells and osteoclasts during endochondral bone formation. Calcitropic hormones, morphogenic steroids and local tissue factors regulate this process. In addition to osteoblasts, the hypertrophic chondrocytes produce osteocalcin, osteopontin and bone sialoprotein.[15] Various genes regulate them, as follows.

- *Spry1* gene. The excessive expression of the *Spry1* gene has caused decreased chondrocyte proliferation in the presumptive reserve and proliferating zones and increased apoptosis of hypertrophic chondrocytes.[59]
- *Bag1* gene. SOX-9 expresses the *Bag1* gene, which has an anti-apoptotic role in chondrocytic cells.[58]
- *MGP* gene. Human *MGP* is a skeletal extracellular matrix (ECM) protein, and a member of the Gla protein family. Gla proteins contain γ-carboxyglutamic acids[8] that have a high affinity for calcium, phosphate and hydroxyapatite crystals, and the mineral components of the skeletal ECM. They regulate ECM calcification. MGP null mutation results in Keutel syndrome.[59]

Structural protein defects

Bone is a complex tissue and an organ, made of organic and inorganic materials. The organic materials of bone include collagen and a series of non-collagenous proteins and lipids. The inorganic material consists of the mineral hydroxyapatite. There are more than 20 collagen types.[60]

Type 1 collagen is primarily found in bone, skin and tendons, and contributes 85–90% of the total collagenous substance in bone. Types 2, 9, 10 and 11 are found mostly in cartilage.[60] More than 1000 mutations, so far, have been identified in 22 genes governing 12 out of more than 20 collagen types.[60]

TYPE 1 COLLAGEN DEFECTS

Osteogenesis imperfecta is a heritable disorder caused by mutations in the *COL1A1* or *COL1A2* genes encoding the chains of type I collagen.[61] It is characterized by extremely fragile bones, blue sclerae, dentinogenesis imperfecta, hearing loss and scoliosis. Sillence et al.[62] classified osteogenesis imperfecta into four types based on genetic and clinical criteria:

- type I: autosomal dominant inheritance of osteoporosis leading to fractures and distinctly blue sclerae
- type II: autosomal recessive transmission, and a perinatal lethal form
- type III: a progressively deforming type with less scleral blueness
- type IV: a dominantly inherited condition similar to type I with normal sclerae.

More recently, a case of prenatal infantile cortical hyperostosis (Caffey disease) due to missense mutation (3040C→T) in exon 41 of the gene encoding the α_1 chain of type I collagen has been reported (Fig. 59.8). Previously, neither the severe form nor the mild form of prenatal cortical hyperostosis was thought to be related to collagen I mutations.[63]

TYPE 2 COLLAGEN DEFECTS

- Mutations in the *COL2A1* gene coding for type II collagen may cause a continuum of severity ranging from very mild conditions, such as Stickler arthro-ophthalmopathy and familial precocious osteoarthropathy, through spondyloepiphyseal dysplasia, spondyloepimetaphyseal dysplasia and Kniest dysplasia, to perinatally lethal, achondrogenesis type II and hypochondrogenesis (Fig. 59.9).[64,65]
- Mutations in the carboxypropeptide domain of *COL2A1* lead to biosynthesis of an altered collagen chain, seen in platyspondylic lethal skeletal dysplasia, torrance type, and spondyloperipheral dysplasia. They have characteristic metaphyseal changes, platyspondyly and brachydactyly, which distinguishes them from other

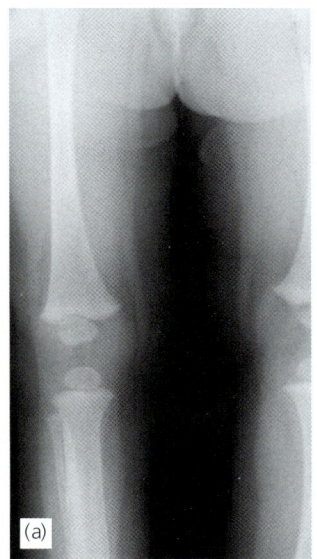 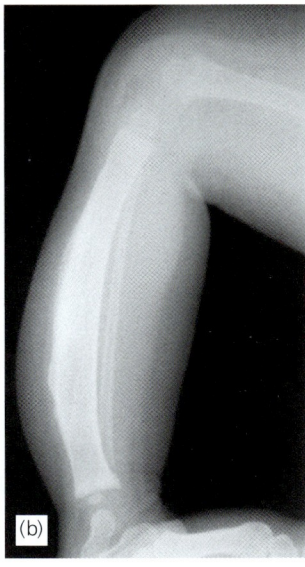

Figure 59.8 Infantile cortical hyperostosis (Caffey–Silverman disease). (a) Tibia varum deformity in the left leg; (b) lateral views of the right leg showing anterior bowing and a pile-up of periosteal bone encasing the shafts of the long bones.

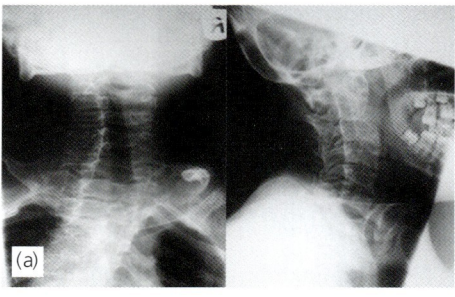
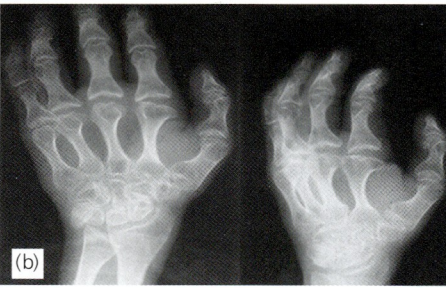
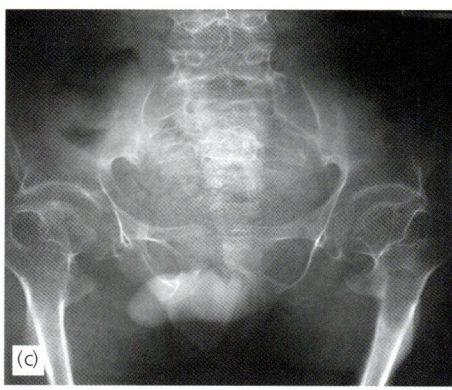
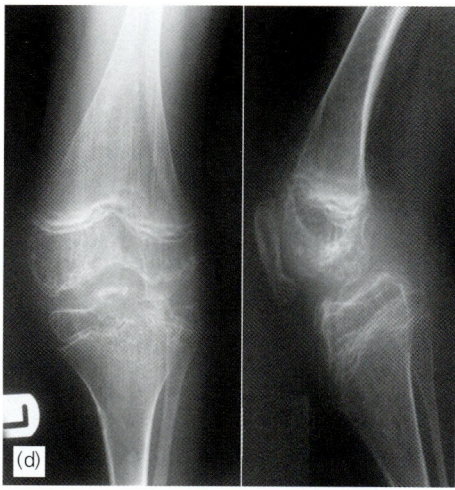

Figure 59.9 Spondyloepiphyseal dysplasia tarda, X-linked. (a) Generalized flattening of the vertebral bodies with a hump-shaped build-up of bone in the upper and lower plate of the vertebrae; (b) flattened epiphysis of the metacarpal bones; (c and d) dysplastic epiphysis of hips and knees with osteoarthritic changes.

type 2 collagenopathies caused by mutations in the triple-helix domain of COL2A1.[66]

- Zankl et al.[67] have described 'spondyloperipheral dysplasia', which is an unusual combination of platyspondyly and brachydactyly. Type II and type XI collagenopathies may sometime overlap to extend the phenotypic spectrum of type II collagenopathy, e.g. oto-spondylomega-epiphyseal dysplasia.[68]

TYPE 9 COLLAGEN DEFECTS

Type IX collagen regulates growth plate width. A study of TSP3/5/Col9 combinatorial knock-out mice demonstrated a 20% reduction in limb length. Singled out TSP5 knock-out mice had no obvious skeletal abnormalities, suggesting that TSP5 is not essential in the growth plate provided other TSPs compensate. In contrast, Col9 knock-out mice have diminished matrillin-3 levels in the ECM and early-onset osteoarthritis.[69] Col9 in combination with TSP3, and TSP5 contribute to growth plate organization. TSP1 defines the timing of growth plate closure when other extracellular proteins are absent.[69] TSP stands for thrombospondin, also known as COMP, is a major component of the extracellular matrix (ECM) of the musculoskeletal system.

TYPE 10 COLLAGEN DEFECTS

Type X collagen is encoded by the COL10A1 gene. It is synthesized specifically and transiently by hypertrophic chondrocytes at sites of endochondral ossification. Point mutations and deletions in the region of the COL10A1 gene encoding the α_1 (X) carboxyl-terminal domain can cause metaphyseal chondrodysplasia, Schmid type (MCDS). Polymerase chain reaction studies of MCDS subjects have revealed unexplained mutation underlying this phenotype.[70,71]

EXTRACELLULAR MATRIX PROTEIN DEFECTS

- *Perlecan*. This is a heparan sulphate proteoglycan that maintains the integrity of all basement membranes, cartilage and several other mesenchymal tissues during development.[72] Functional null mutations of the HSPG2 gene cause dyssegmental dysplasia, Silverman–Handmaker type. It is characterized by anisospondylic micromelia.[73] Missense and splicing mutations cause Schwartz–Jampel syndrome (SJS1).[74] SJS1 is characterized by permanent myotonia, short stature, kyphoscoliosis, bowing of the diaphyses and irregular epiphyses.
- *Aggrecan*. This is a complex proteoglycan core protein rich in keratin sulphate and chondroitin sulphate domains. Aggrecan binds to hyaluronic acid to form huge complexes with type II collagen, stabilized by a link protein.[75] Genetic defects may cause short staturedness.[76,77]
- *Thrombospondin-5 and matrilin-3*. Accumulation of these proteinaceous materials in the rough endoplasmic reticulum compromises cellular function and leads to premature chondrocyte death, e.g. pseudoachondroplasia and multiple epiphyseal dysplasia.[69,78,79]

Metabolic pathway defects

SULPHATE TRANSPORT

- Chondrocytes need inorganic sulphate for proteoglycan sulphation.[80] Sulphate is a hydrophilic anion that cannot passively cross the lipid bilayer of cell membranes. The sulphate–chloride antiporter gene on chromosome 5 encodes sulphate transporter that assists in optimum sulphate influx and efflux.[81–83] Defects in sulphate transport in chondrocytes produces the diastrophic dysplasia (DTD) group of disorders.[84] The disorders range from the mildest form of multiple epiphyseal dysplasia, through Desbuquois dysplasia and the most common DTDs, to perinatally lethal atelosteogenesis type II and achondrogenesis 1B.[80,83,84]
- Carbohydrate sulphotransferase 3 (also known as chondroitin-6-sulphotransferase (C6S)). Defects in C6S cause a phenotypic spectrum ranging from recessive Larsen syndrome, through humerospinal dysostosis, to spondyloepiphyseal dysplasia, Omani type. The clinical features include congenital dislocation of the knees, elbow joint dysplasia with subluxation and limited extension, hip dysplasia or dislocation, clubfoot, short stature and kyphoscoliosis developing in late childhood.[85]
- Arylsulphatase E. A vitamin K-dependent steroid sulphatase that may have a role in bone and cartilage formation.[86] Nonetheless, the exact function is unknown.[83] Mutations in the arylsulphatase E gene located at Xp22.3 result in X-linked recessive chondrodysplasia punctata (CDPX1).[87] CDPX1 is characterized by chondrodysplasia and punctate calcification of cartilage, and often presents with severe spinal cord compression by dysplastic vertebrae.[88]

Enzyme defects

Deficiencies in lysosomal enzymes result in accumulation of glycosaminoglycans which collect in cells, blood and connective tissues. The result is permanent and progressive cellular damage to bone, skeletal structure and connective tissues. To date, 40 different lysosomal storage disorders have been identified according to the accumulated macromolecules.[89] They have been classified as mucopolysaccharidoses (MPS), oligosaccharidoses and glycoproteinoses depending on the type of stored material. They are collectively described as dysostosis multiplex. Table 59.3 is a summary of the common mucopolysaccharidoses along with the complex sugars characteristically found in patients' urine.

- Cathepsin K is a lysosomal cysteine protease critical for bone remodelling by osteoclasts. Various mutations of the cathepsin K gene may cause pyknodysostosis, an autosomal recessive osteosclerotic skeletal dysplasia.[90]
- Sedlin is a 140 amino acid protein with a putative role in endoplasmic reticulum-to-Golgi vesicular transport.[91] Spondyloepiphyseal dysplasia tarda (SEDT) is a progressive skeletal disorder caused by several missense mutations and deletion mutations in the *SEDL* gene at Xp22.12–p22.31.[8,92] The radiographic findings include a hump-shaped deformity of vertebral bodies and mild epiphyseal dysplasia of the femoral head associated with early signs of hip arthrosis. SEDT should be a differential diagnosis in men presenting with early primary bilateral osteoarthrosis.[92]

INTERNATIONAL NOSOLOGY AND CLASSIFICATION

The nomenclature and classification of these disorders are too large to remember. The rapid advances in molecular biology have led to the creation of new subdivisions in the existing classification. The classification and nomenclature need to be regularly updated in view of these increasing discoveries.

The International Working Group on Constitutional Diseases of Bone, which first met in Paris in 1969, created the International Nosology and Classification of Constitutional Diseases of Bone. The purpose of this classification is to unify the terminology used to describe these disorders in different parts of the world.[93] Members of the International Dysplasia Group meet regularly to update and clarify the nomenclature.[1] The 9th International Skeletal Dysplasia Society experts most recently met in Boston, Massachusetts on July 2009 and revised nosology and classification of genetic skeletal disorders and published online on in March 2011.They have classified skeletal disorders into 40 groups, defined by molecular, biochemical and/or radiographic criteria. Four hundred and fifty-six conditions have been included so far in 2010 revision. Out of 456 conditions, 316 were associated with mutations in one or more of 226 different genes, ranging from common recurrent mutations to "private" found in single families or individuals; see reference 94 for the current list.

DIAGNOSTIC CONSIDERATIONS

Clinical evaluation

HISTORY

A proper family history should be taken to identify the pedigree chain of any genetically determined diseases. Many skeletal dysplasias have a prenatal onset and manifest at birth. Therefore, birth length, weight and head circumference should be documented. Careful observation may reveal a Mendelian inheritance pattern. Careful recognition of the milder forms of disorders is needed because they may be easily overlooked, e.g. hypochondroplasia. Review of photographs, radiographs and medical records of family members may be helpful.

A reproductive history such as previous stillbirths, unexplained fetal deaths and other abnormal pregnancy outcomes may provide a clue to skeletal dysplasia in the family. An antenatal history of polyhydramnios or reduced fetal movements should raise suspicion, as most lethal forms of skeletal dysplasias can cause them. Even though most of the skeletal dysplasias are genetic in origin, there may not be a family history of the disorder at all. However, consanguinity, and other family members with short stature or early arthritis may provide additional clues to the possible mode of inheritance.

Random new mutations are commonly seen in most of the autosomal dominant skeletal dysplasias, e.g. achondroplasia and thanatophoric dysplasia. Germ cell mosaicism also induces some dominant disorders. Autosomal recessive disorders usually will have a negative family history. A close consanguineous marriage may increase the chances of autosomal recessive disorders. A male-to-male transmission is possible in X-linked skeletal dysplasia. The rise in mean paternal age has shown an increase in the rates of achondroplasia and osteogenesis imperfecta.

PHYSICAL EXAMINATION

Careful physical examination of the patient and family members and pedigree analysis may help to provide a definitive diagnosis. A growth chart will give vital clues on the longitudinal growth pattern and the timing of onset of the growth disturbance.[95] The anthropometric measurements recorded should include the upper-to-lower segment ratio (U/L), sitting height and arm span.[96] This indicates whether there is disproportionate or proportionate shortening of the trunk and limbs. Assessment should include ascertaining the segment of shortening in the case of short limbs. Skeletal dysplasia may affect proximal (rhisomelic), middle (mesomelic) or distal (acromelic) segments or a combination of these (Table 59.1).

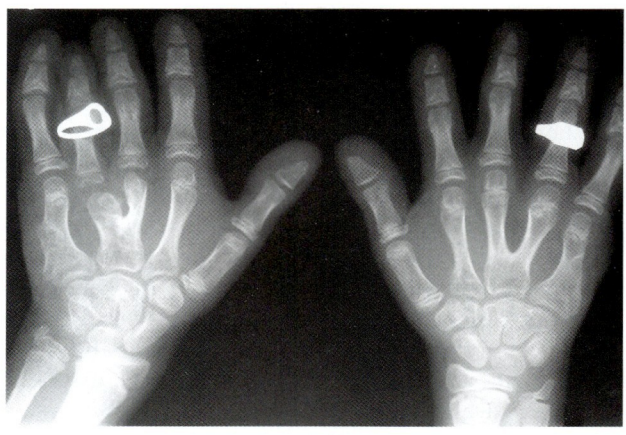

Figure 59.10 Ellis–van Creveld syndrome. Post-axial or axial hexadactyly of fingers with or without fusion of metacarpals. This patient had his sixth digit removed surgically.

Cardiovascular examination can rule out cardiac defects that are associated with oral–facial–skeletal syndromes, such as short rib polydactyly and oral–facial–digital syndrome.[99] Congenital heart defects are occasionally seen in hypochondrogenesis[100] and spondyloepiphyseal dysplasia congenita.[100] More specifically, atrioventricular canal defects are observed in Ellis–van Creveld syndrome (chondroectodermal dysplasia) (Fig. 59.10).[101,102]

Abdominal examination will reveal any organomegaly. Hepatosplenomegaly may be a feature of mucopolysaccharidoses. In Dyggve–Melchior–Clausen dysplasia, mental retardation is an additional finding.[103]

Bone and joint examination may reveal patellar involvement in approximately 90% of patients, and patellar aplasia in 20% of them. General hyperextension of the joints can be seen in type II collagen disorders (Fig. 59.11). Arthrodysplasia of the elbows is reported in approximately 90% of patients.[104] In pseudoachondroplasia, angular

Table 59.1 The diagnosis of skeletal dysplasia based on the segment of bone affected in the shortened limb[97,98]

Rhisomelic (proximal segment)	Mesomelic (middle segment)	Acromelic (distal segment)	Acromesomelic (short middle and distal segment)	Micromelic (overall limb shortening)
Achondroplasia	Langer and Nievergelt types of mesomelic dysplasias	Acrodysostosis	Acromesomelic dysplasia	Achondrogenesis, Fibrochondrogenesis
Hypochondroplasia		Peripheral dysostoses		Kniest dysplasia
Rhisomelic type of chondrodysplasia punctata				Dyssegmental dysplasia
Jansen type of metaphyseal dysplasia	Robinow syndrome			Roberts syndrome
Thanatophoric dysplasia	Reinhardt syndrome			
Atelosteogenesis				
Diastrophic dysplasia				
Spondyloepiphyseal dysplasia				

Diagnostic considerations 551

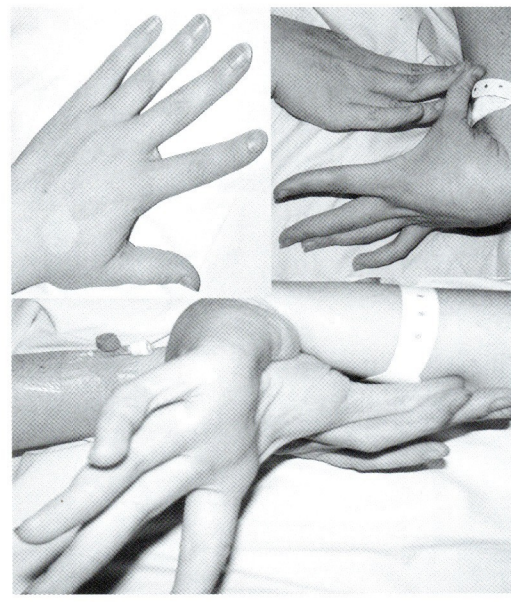

Figure 59.11 Generalized hyperextension of the joints that can be seen in type II collagen disorders.

deformity (genu varum and valgum deformity), rotational deformity (femoral or tibial torsion) or a combination of these is associated with ligamentous laxity.[105] In nail–patella syndrome (NPS), dysplastic nails with triangular lunulae and iliac horns are pathognomonic (Fig. 59.12). The iliac horns are frequently palpable and found in 80% of patients.[106] Urine examination may reveal asymptomatic proteinuria, which may be the only manifestation of NPS in some cases.[107]

Table 59.2 provides a comprehensive compilation of clinical stigmatas in addition to short staturedness that may help in identifying various osteochondral dysplasias and dysostoses.

Imaging

ULTRASONOGRAPHY

Ultrasonography is highly specific for predicting lethal outcome, but is of limited value in accurate diagnosis of the constitutional disorders of bone. At the Cedars–Sinai Medical Center, Los Angeles, CA, USA, where an

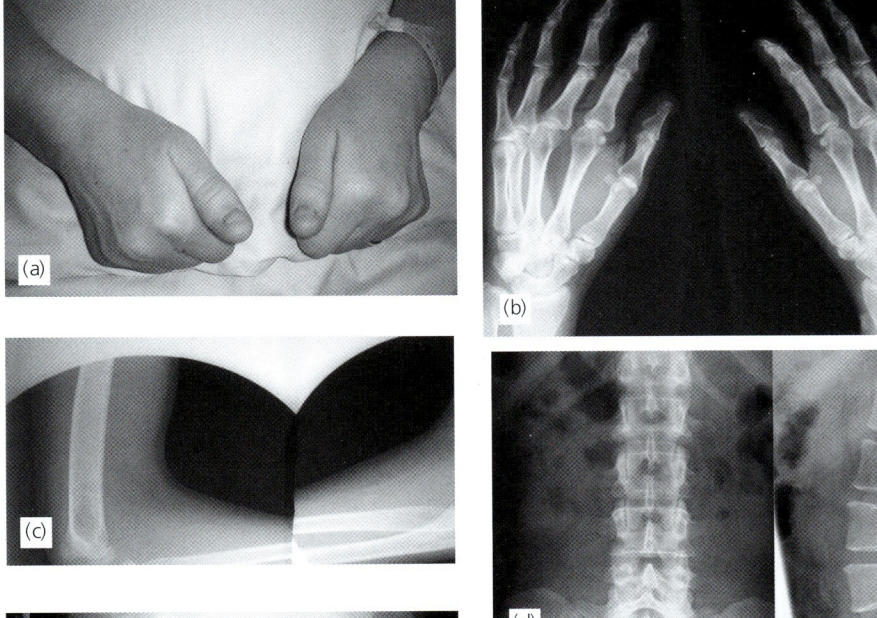

Figure 59.12 Nail–patella syndrome. (a) Dysplastic nails showing longitudinal ridges and onycholysis; (b) sideways bent fingers; (c) webbed appearance at the elbow joint; (d) a rare combination of spondylolytic spondylolisthesis at L5–S1 and 40° fixed flexion deformity of the hips; (e) pelvis showing bilateral iliac horns; (f) knee joints showing bilateral hypoplastic patellas, with the skyline view confirming the dislocated hypoplastic patella.

Table 59.2 Clinical signs, which may help in diagnosing various skeletal dysplasias[97,98]

Skull	Eyes	Mouth	Ears	Thorax/ribs/clavicle	Hands, feet, digits and nails
Disproportionately large head Achondroplasia, Achondrogenesis thanatophoric dysplasia	**Congenital cataract** Chondrodysplasia punctata	**Bifid uvula and high arched or cleft palate** Kniest dysplasia, SED congenita, Diastrophic dysplasia, Metatrophic dysplasia, Camptomelic dysplasia	**Cystic swelling of the pinnae** Diastrophic dysplasia	**Long or narrow thorax** Asphyxiating thoracic dysplasia, Chondroectodermal dysplasia, Metatrophic dysplasia	**Hitchhiker thumb** Diastrophic dysplasia
Clover leaf skull Thanatophoric dysplasia, Apert syndrome, Carpenter syndrome, Crouzon syndrome, Pfeiffer syndrome	**Myopia** Kniest dysplasia and spondyloepiphyseal dysplasia (SED) congenita		**Recurrent fibrous tumour of pinnae** Melnick–Needles osteodysplasty	**Funnel-shaped chest and clavicle hypoplasia** Cleidocranial dysostoses	**Clubfoot** Diastrophic dysplasia, Kniest dysplasia, Osteogenesis imperfecta
Caput membranaceum Hypophosphatasia, Osteogenesis imperfecta congenita				**Pear-shaped chest** Thanatophoric dysplasia, Short-rib polydactyly syndromes, Homozygous achondroplasia	**Polydactyly** *Preaxial* Chondroectodermal dysplasia, Short rib (-polydactyly) syndromes Types 1. Saldino–Noonan syndrome and Verma–Naumoff. 2. Majewski. 3. Beemer–Langer.

Table 59.2 (continued)

Skull	Eyes	Mouth	Ears	Thorax/ribs/clavicle	Hands, feet, digits and nails	
Multiple wormian bones	Cleidocranial dysplasia Osteogenesis imperfecta				*Postaxial*	Chondroectodermal dysplasia Short rib (-polydactyly) syndromes
Craniosynostosis	Apert syndrome Crouzon syndrome Carpenter syndrome Craniosynostosis syndromes Hypophosphatasia			Jeune syndrome	*Pre- and post-axial type of poly-dactyly*	Short rib (-polydactyly) syndromes (50% of types 2 and 3 have these defects, and rarely in type 1
					Nails *Hypoplastic nails with V-shaped triangular lunulae*	Nail–patella syndrome
					Hypoplastic nails *Short and broad nails*	Chondroectodermal dysplasia McKusick metaphyseal dysplasia

International Skeletal Dysplasia Registry has been maintained, a diagnostic accuracy of 81.5% was reported in 1993.[108] Despite this diagnostic accuracy, 7% of fetuses and stillbirths were found to have no evidence of either a bone dysplasia or an obvious dysmorphic syndrome.[108]

Ultrasonography can reveal:

- hypoplastic thorax
- spinal abnormalities such as hemivertebrae, scoliosis and platyspondylia; digital anomalies such as polydactyly, missing digits, hitchhiker thumbs and clubfoot
- craniofacial defects such as ocular hypertelorism, retrognathia/micrognathia, cleft lip, frontal bossing and cloverleaf skull deformity
- decreased fetal movements, which are seen in lethal forms of skeletal dysplasia.

Routine prenatal well-being scans have gained wide acceptance as a diagnostic tool to screen for skeletal dysplasia. Prenatal diagnosis can be made as early as 14 weeks. The prenatal diagnosis of skeletal dysplasia is often initiated by the knowledge of a previous familial history of skeletal dysplasia, or by a short femoral length in the mid-trimester ultrasonograph. However, serial ultrasonographs will be required from the beginning of the second trimester to plot the femoral length growth curves to rule out heterozygous achondroplasia, which may not manifest until the second trimester.[109] It will also distinguish individuals with homozygous (lethal) and heterozygous (non-lethal) achondroplasia from unaffected individuals.[110]

Rhisomelic shortening can be determined by abnormal femur length for a given gestational age. Comparisons of femur length-to-abdominal circumference ratio[111] and limb dimensions-to-head perimeter of the fetus[97] are used in mothers presenting with unknown gestational age. Pradhan and Sankar[112] reported a short humerus as an additional antenatal sonographic feature of oral–facial–digital syndrome type II. A long-bone measurement of less than –4 standard deviations is a definitive indication of skeletal dysplasia, whereas measurements between –2 and –4 standard deviations warrant detailed sonographic examination for other associated anomalies to arrive at a diagnosis.[112] The associated anomalies include maternal hydramnios, fetal hydrops, increased nuchal translucency thickness, congenital heart defects and cystic renal malformation. However, repeat ultrasonography examinations are usually required.

RADIOGRAPHY

Radiographs are the single most powerful tool in evaluating the skeletal dysplasia.[95] In prenatal ultrasonography-confirmed skeletal dysplasias, fetal radiographs may help in reaching an accurate diagnosis or at least in identifying the probable lethal disorders.[108] In children younger than 6 months, an infantogram (AP and lateral radiographs of the whole body) and separate AP films of both hands and a lateral radiograph of the skull can be performed to make an accurate diagnosis. In children older than 6 months, request a skeletal survey.

A typical skeletal survey should include:

- skull (AP, lateral and Towne views)
- thoracolumbar spine (AP and lateral)
- chest (AP)
- pelvis (AP)
- one upper limb (AP and lateral)
- one lower limb (AP and lateral)
- left hand (bone age).

A systematic (ABCD) approach should be followed to interpret the skeletal survey.[1] ABCD stands for: A, **a**natomical localization; B, characteristics of **b**ones; C, **c**omplications; D, **d**ead/alive. The knowledge of the timing and appearance of ossification centres is essential to delineate delayed or deficient ossification of the skeleton, e.g. achondrogenesis (severe disturbance in ossification) or atelosteogenesis ('incomplete' ossification) (Table 59.3).

CT AND MRI SCAN

CT and MRI scan of the skull and brain will be helpful to study the craniospinal anomalies associated with skeletal dysplasias and craniosynostosis. MRI scan has an added advantage in helping to visualize the spinal cord oedema and gliosis that is secondary to bony compression resulting from progressive spinal deformities and scoliosis. Three-dimensional reconstruction will give a spatial orientation while planning reconstructive cosmetic surgery.

Histopathological examination

Post-mortem radiography and histopathological examination may confirm a suspected diagnosis by recognizing specific histological features. These investigations will help in pinpointing the subtype of the genetic disorder, and mode of inheritance. Thereby, effective genetic counselling can be offered to parents. Histological and electron microscopic findings in physeal tissues of various skeletal dysplasias are shown in Table 59.5.

Molecular analyses

Commercially available DNA testing kits can be used to detect *FGFR3* mutations. These kits can be used to diagnose achondroplasia, hypochondroplasia, thanatophoric dysplasia and craniosynostosis syndromes (Apert, Crouzon, Pfeiffer, Jackson–Weiss and Beare–Stevenson syndromes).

Table 59.3 Radiographic findings specific to various dysplasias

Radiological signs	Skeletal dysplasias
Oval translucent area in proximal femur and humerus	Achondroplasia
Dumbbell-shaped appearance of femur	Kniest dysplasia Metatrophic dysplasia
Calcified projections (spikes) at lateral femoral metaphyses	Thanatophoric dysplasia and achondrogenesis types I and II
Cupping of the ends of the rib and long bones and metaphyseal flaring	Achondroplasia Metaphyseal dysplasias Asphyxiating thoracic dysplasia Chondroectodermal dysplasia
Hypoplastic/absent patella and iliac horns	Nail–patella syndrome
Long-bone fractures	Osteogenesis imperfecta syndromes Hypophosphatasia Osteopetrosis Achondrogenesis type I (Parenti–Fraccaro syndrome)
Absence of epiphyseal ossification centres	Spondyloepiphyseal dysplasia (SED) congenita Multiple epiphyseal dysplasia Other SED (unspecified)
Cone-shaped epiphyses	Acrodysostosis Cleidocranial dysplasia Trichorhinophalangeal dysplasia
Stippling of the epiphyses	Chondrodysplasia punctata Multiple epiphyseal dysplasia SED Normal variant hypoparathyroidism
Rib shortening	Short rib–polydactyly syndromes Asphyxiating thoracic dysplasia Chondroectodermal dysplasia Metaphyseal dysplasia Metatrophic dysplasia
Absence of calcification of vertebral bodies	Achondrogenesis types I and II
Severe platyspondylia	Metatrophic dysplasia Lethal perinatal osteogenesis imperfecta Thanatophoric dysplasia Short rib–polydactyly syndromes SED congenita Other types of SED Kniest dysplasia
Abnormal pelvic configuration (small sacrosciatic notches)	Achondroplasia Ellis–van Creveld syndrome Metatrophic dysplasia Thanatophoric dysplasia Jeune syndrome
Severe hypoplasia of the scapula	Camptomelic dysplasia Antley–Bixler syndrome
Double layer patella	Multiple epiphyseal dysplasic
Erlenmeyer flask distal femur	Gaucher diesease

Table 59.4 Histological and electron microscopic findings characteristic of various skeletal dysplasias is often a diagnostic clue

Histopathological findings	Skeletal dysplasia
Densely fibrous collagenous matrix[113]	Fibrochondrogenesis
Large chondrocyte lacunae in the physis and deficient cartilage matrix[114]	Achondrogenesis type II
Ballooned chondrocytes[114]	Hypochondrogenesis (achondrogenesis type III)
'Cottage cheese'[114] or 'Swiss cheese' appearance[115,159] and inclusion bodies of cartilage	Kniest dysplasia Distinct chondrodysplasia
Puddles (lakes) of mucoid material[114]	Dyssegmental dysplasia, Silverman–Handmaker type
Small foci of myxoid degeneration and multinucleated giant cells in resting cartilage[114]	Atelosteogenesis
Transverse plates of lamellar bone indicating cessation of endochondral ossification[114]	Thanatophoric dysplasia
Cytoplasmic inclusions in resting chondrocytes[97]	Type I achondrogenesis, Kniest dysplasia, pseudoachondroplastic spondyloepiphyseal dysplasia (SED), type III short rib–polydactyly syndrome, and SED congenita

Commercial DNA testing kits are not available for all disorders. However, molecular analysis is possible for genetically determined skeletal dysplasias, e.g. *SOX9* mutations in patients with camptomelic dysplasia and Antley–Bixler syndrome. Karyotyping will help in camptomelic dysplasia, as autosomal sex reversal occurs (i.e. female external genitalia with a male karyotype, 46,XY).[117]

MANAGEMENT OF THE SKELETAL DYSPLASIAS

Achondroplasia has been chosen here as an example for the purpose of discussion of management. Achondroplasia is the most common non-lethal, short-statured skeletal dysplasia[6] (Fig. 59.13). Cardinal features include rhisomelic (disproportionate) short stature, prominent frontal bossing, midface hypoplasia, saddle nose, short limbs and hands with long trunk, lordotic lumbar spine, thoracolumbar kyphosis and lumbar spinal stenosis. The fingers are splayed (trident or starfish hand).[118] Joint laxity is commonly seen. Patients often have strong feelings of inferiority psychologically because of their unusual appearance. Obesity is often seen. Children often have otitis media and overcrowding of the teeth owing to the abnormal skull structure.

Follow the diagnostic considerations elaborated above to confirm the diagnosis.

Treatment

MEDICAL TREATMENT

- Medical care includes growth monitoring, controlling weight to prevent obesity, managing frequent middle ear infections and dental crowding, and performing careful neurological examinations. GH and IGF-1 or IGF-2 therapy are found useful in improving severe growth retardation at early stages of bone development.[119,120]
- Drugs may prove successful by blocking extracellular ligand binding or by regulating FGF signalling pathways. The resurrection of normal bone growth may be achieved by promulgation of *FGFR3* signalling in the appropriate cells within the growth plate.[121]

SURGICAL CARE

Short stature

- Leg-lengthening procedures by the crossing method, which means one-stage lengthening of the femur and the tibia of the contralateral limb using distraction osteogenesis, have been proved to be successful.[51]
- Shadi and Koczewski[122] successfully achieved a mean of 8.5 cm lengthening in the humerus with an index of 0.8–1.1 months cm^{-1}. This represents lengthening of more than 50% of the primary segmental length.
- Yasui et al.[123] achieved a mean lengthening of 7.2 cm (range 4.5–12 cm) in the femur and 7.1 cm (range 4.5–13 cm) in the tibia in 35 patients with achondroplasia and seven patients with hypochondroplasia. The mean follow up was 14.5 years. A callus distraction (callotasis) method was used in all patients. The overall functional results are better in limb-lengthened achondroplastics than before lengthening.[123]
- Aldegheri[124] achieved good results in the tibia and fibula with fewer complications using the Orthofix Garches lengthening device by performing additional procedures such as percutaneous tenotomy of the achilles tendon and fixation of the distal segment of the fibula to the tibia to maintain the integrity of the tibiotalar articulation and the alignment of the foot. Soft-tissue neogenesis took place in the central region of the leg after achieving 30% distraction in leg length.[125]
- Anticipate nerve conduction delay at the end of the distraction period.[126] Perform a clinical assessment of

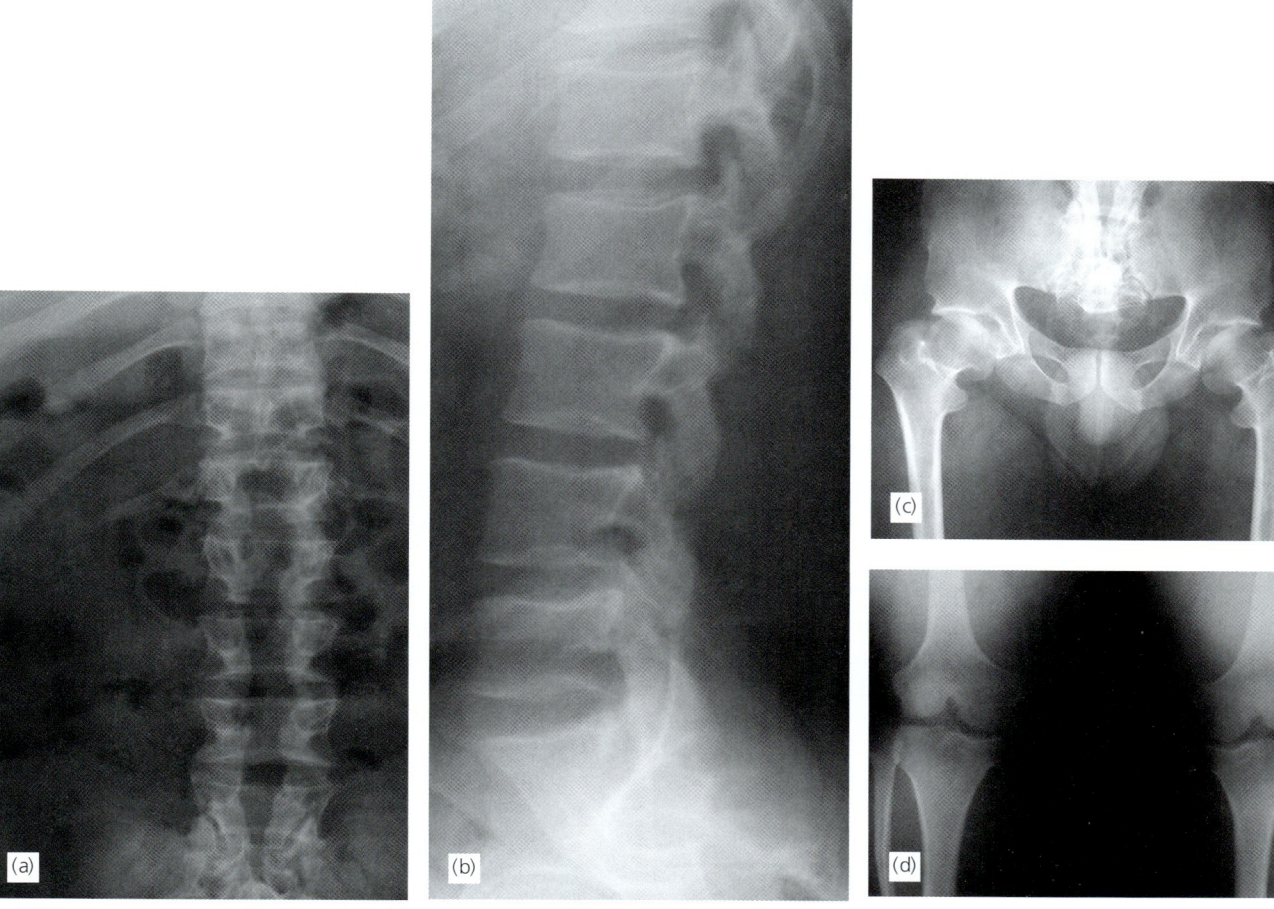

Figure 59.13 Achondroplasia. (a) Vertebral bodies appear flat. The interpediculate distance decreases from the upper to lower lumbar spine. This patient had multilevel spinal decompression. The anterior ends of the ribs are cupped. (b) Posterior aspects of the vertebral bodies are concave. (c) Squared iliac bones with rounding of the corners and lack of flaring. The greater sciatic notch is narrow. The sacrum articulates low in relation to the iliac crest. The iliac and pubic bones are broad and short, and a characteristic oval area of radiolucency is seen in the proximal femur. (d) The articular surface of the distal femur is irregular, and the growth plates are relatively straight.

peripheral nerve function and, if needed, an electrophysiological study to confirm.
- Care should be taken to reduce the distraction period, as weakness of foot dorsiflexion has been reported.
- Consider a new technique of cell therapy, transplanting culture-expanded bone marrow cells and platelet-rich plasma at the corticotomy site. This technique significantly reduces the overall treatment period by accelerating new bone regeneration, especially in femoral lengthening.[127]

Spinal symptoms

- In early adulthood, bracing and modification of the sitting position may be helpful during the initial phases of claudication symptoms due to thoracolumbar kyphosis and spinal stenosis. Surgery is indicated only if there is worsening of neurological symptoms. A one-stage procedure of anterior fusion and posterior decompression with posterolateral fusion using pedicle screw instrumentation has been found to be safe and effective.[128]
- In children with signs of craniomedullary compression, surgical decompression may help to improve neurological, cognitive and respiratory functions.[129] Lower limb hyper-reflexia or clonus on examination, central hypopnoea demonstrated by polysomnography and foramen magnum measurements lower than the mean are some of the indications for the possible need for suboccipital decompression.[130]

MULTIDISCIPLINARY CARE

For comprehensive management of this disorder, the multidisciplinary team should include the following:[129]

- paediatric neurologist or paediatric neurosurgeon
- ear, nose and throat surgeon
- orthopaedist
- psychiatrist
- pulmonologist
- physical therapist
- geneticists and genetic counsellors.

Patients affected by achondroplasia and their families may experience a variety of psychosocial challenges throughout their lives.[131,132] In 2003, Hill et al.[131] conducted a study on parental experiences at the time of diagnosis of their child with a bone dysplasia resulting in short stature. The data revealed that the manner in which the diagnosis was conveyed to the parents played a significant role in their adjustment and acceptance.[131] Parents expect a multidisciplinary team approach in the bone dysplasia clinic in the continued management of the families.

ACKNOWLEDGEMENT

We extend our heartiest thanks to Dr Gavin Stoddart, Consultant Radiologist with special interest in musculoskeletal radiology, Weston General Hospital, Weston-super-Mare, UK, for his incredible contribution of radiographs.

REFERENCES

1. Offiah AC, Hall CM. Radiological diagnosis of the constitutional disorders of bone. As easy as A, B, C? *Pediatric Radiology* 2003;**33**:53–61.
2. Hall CM. International nosology and classification of constitutional disorders of bone (2001). *American Journal of Medical Genetics* 2002;**113**:65–77.
3. Rasmussen SA, Bieber FR, Benacerraf BR, et al. Epidemiology of osteochondrodysplasias: changing trends due to advances in prenatal diagnosis. *American Journal of Medical Genetics* 1996;**61**:49–58.
4. Orioli IM, Castilla EE, Barbosa-Neto JG. The birth prevalence rates for the skeletal dysplasias. *Journal of Medical Genetics* 1986;**23**:328–32.
5. Connor JM, Connor RA, Sweet EM, et al. Lethal neonatal chondrodysplasias in the West of Scotland 1970–1983 with a description of a thanatophoric, dysplasialike, autosomal recessive disorder, Glasgow variant. *American Journal of Medical Genetics* 1985;**22**:243–53.
6. Baujat G, Legeai-Mallet L, Finidori G, et al. Achondroplasia. *Best Practice and Research: Clinical Rheumatology* 2008;**22**:3–18.
7. Kosher RA, Kulyk WM, Gay SW. Collagen gene expression during limb cartilage differentiation. *Journal of Cell Biology* 1986;**102**:1151–6.
8. Gedeon AK, Tiller GE, Le Merrer M, et al. The molecular basis of X-linked spondyloepiphyseal dysplasia tarda. *American Journal of Human Genetics* 2001;**68**:1386–97.
9. Zelzer E, Olsen BR. The genetic basis for skeletal diseases. *Nature* 2003;**423**:343–8.
10. Erlebacher A, Filvaroff EH, Gitelman SE, Derynck R. Toward a molecular understanding of skeletal development. *Cell* 1995;**80**:371–8.
11. Hunziker EB, Schenk RK, Cruz-Orive LM. Quantitation of chondrocyte performance in growth-plate cartilage during longitudinal bone growth. *Journal of Bone and Joint Surgery (American)* 1987;**69**:592–73.
12. Cancedda R, Descalzi Cancedda F, Castagnola P. Chondrocyte differentiation. *International Review Cytology* 1995;**159**:265–358.
13. Guo X, Day TF, Jiang X, et al. Wnt/beta-catenin signaling is sufficient and necessary for synovial joint formation. *Genes and Development* 2004;**18**:2404–17.
14. Barbara Y, John WH. Skeletal tissues. In: Barbara Y, Heath JW (eds) *Wheater's Functional Histology: A Text and Colour Atlas*. Edinburgh, UK: Churchill Livingstone, 2000:186.
15. Gerstenfeld LC, Shapiro FD. Expression of bone-specific genes by hypertrophic chondrocytes: implication of the complex functions of the hypertrophic chondrocyte during endochondral bone development. *Journal of Cellular Biochemistry* 1996;**62**:1–9.
59. Newman B, Wallis GA. Skeletal dysplasias caused by a disruption of skeletal patterning and endochondral ossification. *Clinical Genetics* 2003;**63**:241–51.
17. Tuysuz B. A new concept of skeletal dysplasias. *Turkish Journal of Pediatrics* 2004;**46**:197–203.
18. Hui CC, Joyner AL. A mouse model of greig cephalopolysyndactyly syndrome: the extra-toesJ mutation contains an intragenic deletion of the Gli3 gene. *Nature Genetics* 1993;**3**:241–6.
19. Bellaiche Y, The I, Perrimon N. Tout-velu is a Drosophila homologue of the putative tumour suppressor EXT-1 and is needed for Hh diffusion. *Nature* 1998;**394**:85–8.
20. Koyama E, Ochiai T, Rountree RB, et al. Synovial joint formation during mouse limb skeletogenesis: roles of Indian hedgehog signaling. *Annals of the New York Academy of Sciences* 2007;**1159**:100–12.
21. Liu P, Wakamiya M, Shea MJ, et al. Requirement for Wnt3 in vertebrate axis formation. *Nature Genetics* 1999;**22**:361–5.
22. Heisenberg CP, Tada M, Rauch GJ, et al. Silberblick/Wnt11 mediates convergent extension movements during zebrafish gastrulation. *Nature* 2000;**405**:76–81.
23. Ulrich F, Concha ML, Heid PJ, et al. Slb/Wnt11 controls hypoblast cell migration and morphogenesis at the onset of zebrafish gastrulation. *Development* 2003;**130**:5375–84.
24. Agathon A, Thisse C, Thisse B. The molecular nature of the zebrafish tail organizer. *Nature* 2003;**424**:448–52.
25. Yang Y. Wnts and wing: Wnt signaling in vertebrate limb development and musculoskeletal morphogenesis. *Birth Defects Research Part C Embryo Today* 2003;**69**:305–17.

26. Haycraft CJ, Zhang Q, Song B, et al. Intraflagellar transport is essential for endochondral bone formation. *Development* 2007;**134**:307–59.
27. Ribes V, Otto DM, Dickmann L, et al. Rescue of cytochrome P450 oxidoreductase (Por) mouse mutants reveals functions in vasculogenesis, brain and limb patterning linked to retinoic acid homeostasis. *Developmental Biology* 2007;**303**:66–81.
28. Li Y, Toole BP, Dealy CN, Kosher RA. Hyaluronan in limb morphogenesis. *Developmental Biology* 2007;**305**:411–20.
29. Satoh W, Gotoh T, Tsunematsu Y, et al. Sfrp1 and Sfrp2 regulate anteroposterior axis elongation and somite segmentation during mouse embryogenesis. *Development* 2006;**133**:989–99.
30. Hermanns P, Lee B. Transcriptional dysregulation in skeletal malformation syndromes. *American Journal of Medical Genetics* 2001;**106**:258–71.
31. Lee B, Thirunavukkarasu K, Zhou L, et al. Missense mutations abolishing DNA binding of the osteoblast-specific transcription factor OSF2/CBFA1 in cleidocranial dysplasia. *Nature Genetics* 1997;**59**:307–10.
32. Tou L, Quibria N, Alexander JM. Transcriptional regulation of the human Runx2/Cbfa1 gene promoter by bone morphogenetic protein-7. *Molecular and Cellular Endocrinology* 2003;**205**:121–9.
33. Wright E, Hargrave MR, Christiansen J, et al. The Sry-related gene Sox9 is expressed during chondrogenesis in mouse embryos. *Nature Genetics* 1995;**9**:15–20.
34. Wagner T, Wirth J, Meyer J, et al. Autosomal sex reversal and campomelic dysplasia are caused by mutations in and around the SRY-related gene SOX9. *Cell* 1994;**79**:1111–20.
35. Dahl E, Koseki H, Balling R. Pax genes and organogenesis. *Bioessays* 1997;**19**:755–65.
36. Neubuser A, Koseki H, Balling R. Characterization and developmental expression of Pax9, a paired-box-containing gene related to Pax1. *Developmental Biology* 1995;**170**:701–59.
37. Morgan BA, Tabin CJ. The role of homeobox genes in limb development. *Current Opinion in Genetics and Development* 1993;**3**:668–74.
38. Belin V, Cusin V, Viot G, et al. SHOX mutations in dyschondrosteosis (Leri-Weill syndrome). *Nature Genetics* 1998;**19**:67–9.
39. Clement-Jones M, Schiller S, Rao E, et al. The short stature homeobox gene SHOX is involved in skeletal abnormalities in Turner syndrome. *Human Molecular Genetics* 2000;**9**:695–702.
40. Hopyan S, Gokgoz N, Poon R, et al. A mutant PTH/PTHrP type I receptor in enchondromatosis. *Nature Genetics* 2002;**30**:306–10.
41. Karaplis AC, Luz A, Glowacki J, et al. Lethal skeletal dysplasia from targeted disruption of the parathyroid hormone-related peptide gene. *Genes and Development* 1994;**8**:277–89.
42. Jobert AS, Zhang P, Couvineau A, et al. Absence of functional receptors for parathyroid hormone and parathyroid hormone-related peptide in Blomstrand chondrodysplasia. *Journal of Clinical Investigation* 1998;**102**:34–40.
43. Loshkajian A, Roume J, Stanescu V, et al. Familial Blomstrand chondrodysplasia with advanced skeletal maturation: further delineation. *American Journal of Medical Genetics* 1997;**71**:283–8.
44. Schipani E, Kruse K, Juppner H. A constitutively active mutant PTH-PTHrP receptor in Jansen-type metaphyseal chondrodysplasia. *Science* 1995;**268**:98–100.
45. Ciranni R, Giuffra V, Marinozzi S, Fornaciari G. [Angelo Maria Maffucci (1845–1903) and the beginning of pathological anatomy in Pisa]. *Medicina nei Secoli* 2004;**59**:31–41.
46. Gao B, Guo J, She C, et al. Mutations in IHH, encoding Indian hedgehog, cause brachydactyly type A-1. *Nature Genetics* 2001;**28**:386–8.
47. Baker J, Liu JP, Robertson EJ, Efstratiadis A. Role of insulin-like growth factors in embryonic and postnatal growth. *Cell* 1993;**75**:73–82.
48. Hutchison MR, Bassett MH, White PC. Insulin-like growth factor-I and fibroblast growth factor, but not growth hormone, affect growth plate chondrocyte proliferation. *Endocrinology* 2007;**148**:3122–30.
49. Ohlsson C, Nilsson A, Isaksson O, Lindahl A. Growth hormone induces multiplication of the slowly cycling germinal cells of the rat tibial growth plate. *Proceedings of the National Academy of Sciences of the USA* 1992;**89**:9826–30.
50. Wajnrajch MP, Gertner JM, Harbison MD, et al. Nonsense mutation in the human growth hormone-releasing hormone receptor causes growth failure analogous to the little (lit) mouse. *Nature Genetics* 1996;**12**:88–90.
51. Koczewski P, Shadi M. Surgical treatment of short stature of different etiology by the Ilizarov method. *Endokrynologia, Diabetologia i Choroby Przemiany Materii Wieku Rozwojowego* 2007;**13**:143–6.
52. Bellus GA, McIntosh I, Smith EA, et al. A recurrent mutation in the tyrosine kinase domain of fibroblast growth factor receptor 3 causes hypochondroplasia. *Nature Genetics* 1995;**10**:357–9.
53. Shiang R, Thompson LM, Zhu YZ, et al. Mutations in the transmembrane domain of FGFR3 cause the most common genetic form of dwarfism, achondroplasia. *Cell* 1994;**78**:335–42.
54. Tavormina PL, Shiang R, Thompson LM, et al. Thanatophoric dysplasia (types I and II) caused by distinct mutations in fibroblast growth factor receptor 3. *Nature Genetics* 1995;**9**:321–8.
55. ADHR-Consortium. Autosomal dominant hypophosphataemic rickets is associated with mutations in FGF23. *Nature Genetics* 2000;**26**:345–8.
56. Sabbagh Y, Jones AO, Tenenhouse HS. PHEXdb, a locus-specific database for mutations causing X-linked hypophosphatemia. *Human Mutation* 2000;**59**:1–6.
57. Taschner MJ, Rafigh M, Lampert F, et al. Ca^{2+}/Calmodulin-dependent kinase II signaling causes skeletal overgrowth and premature chondrocyte maturation. *Developmental Biology* 2008;**317**:132–46.

58. Tare RS, Townsend PA, Packham GK, et al. Bcl-2-associated athanogene-1 (BAG-1): a transcriptional regulator mediating chondrocyte survival and differentiation during endochondral ossification. *Bone* 2008;**42**:113–28.
59. Yang X, Harkins LK, Zubanova O, et al. Overexpression of Spry1 in chondrocytes causes attenuated FGFR ubiquitination and sustained ERK activation resulting in chondrodysplasia. *Developmental Biology* 2008;**321**:65–76.
60. Myllyharju J, Kivirikko KI. Collagens and collagen-related diseases. *Annals of Medicine* 2001;**33**:7–21.
61. Burnei G, Vlad C, Georgescu I, et al. Osteogenesis imperfecta: diagnosis and treatment. *Journal of the American Academy of Orthopaedic Surgeons* 2008;**59**:356–66.
62. Sillence DO, Rimoin DL. Classification of osteogenesis imperfect. *Lancet.* 1978;**1(8072)**:1041–2. Epub 1978/05/13.
63. Kamoun-Goldrat A, Martinovic J, Saada J, et al. Prenatal cortical hyperostosis with COL1A1 gene mutation. *American Journal of Medical Genetics A* 2008;**146A**:1820–4.
64. Mortier GR, Wilkin DJ, Wilcox WR, et al. A radiographic, morphologic, biochemical and molecular analysis of a case of achondrogenesis type II resulting from substitution for a glycine residue (Gly691→Arg) in the type II collagen trimer. *Human Molecular Genetics* 1995;**4**:285–8.
65. Spranger J, Winterpacht A, Zabel B. The type II collagenopathies: a spectrum of chondrodysplasias. *European Journal of Pediatrics* 1994;**153**:56–65.
66. Zankl A, Neumann L, Ignatius J, et al. Dominant negative mutations in the C-propeptide of COL2A1 cause platyspondylic lethal skeletal dysplasia, torrance type, and define a novel subfamily within the type 2 collagenopathies. *American Journal of Medical Genetics A* 2005;**133A**:61–7.
67. Zankl A, Zabel B, Hilbert K, et al. Spondyloperipheral dysplasia is caused by truncating mutations in the C-propeptide of COL2A1. *American Journal of Medical Genetics A* 2004;**129A**:144–8.
68. Miyamoto Y, Nakashima E, Hiraoka H, et al. A type II collagen mutation also results in oto-spondylo-megaepiphyseal dysplasia. *Human Genetics* 2005;**118**:175–8.
69. Posey KL, Hankenson K, Veerisetty AC, et al. Skeletal abnormalities in mice lacking extracellular matrix proteins, thrombospondin-1, thrombospondin-3, thrombospondin-5, and type IX collagen. *American Journal of Pathology* 2008;**172**:5964–74.
70. Wallis GA, Rash B, Sykes B, et al. Mutations within the gene encoding the alpha 1 (X) chain of type X collagen (COL10A1) cause metaphyseal chondrodysplasia type Schmid but not several other forms of metaphyseal chondrodysplasia. *Journal of Medical Genetics* 1996;**33**:450–7.
71. Lachman RS, Rimoin DL, Spranger J. Metaphyseal chondrodysplasia, Schmid type. Clinical and radiographic delineation with a review of the literature. *Pediatric Radiology* 1988;**18**:93–102.
72. Costell M, Gustafsson E, Aszodi A, et al. Perlecan maintains the integrity of cartilage and some basement membranes. *Journal of Cell Biology* 1999;**147**:1109–22.
73. Arikawa-Hirasawa E, Wilcox WR, Yamada Y. Dyssegmental dysplasia, Silverman-Handmaker type: unexpected role of perlecan in cartilage development. *American Journal of Medical Genetics* 2001;**106**:254–7.
74. Nicole S, Davoine CS, Topaloglu H, et al. Perlecan, the major proteoglycan of basement membranes, is altered in patients with Schwartz-Jampel syndrome (chondrodystrophic myotonia). *Nature Genetics* 2000;**26**:480–3.
75. Mundlos S, Meyer R, Yamada Y, Zabel B. Distribution of cartilage proteoglycan (aggrecan) core protein and link protein gene expression during human skeletal development. *Matrix* 1991;**11**:339–46.
76. Watanabe H, Kimata K, Line S, et al. Mouse cartilage matrix deficiency (cmd) caused by a 7 bp deletion in the aggrecan gene. *Nature Genetics* 1994;**7**:154–7.
77. Li H, Schwartz NB, Vertel BM. cDNA cloning of chick cartilage chondroitin sulfate (aggrecan) core protein and identification of a stop codon in the aggrecan gene associated with the chondrodystrophy, nanomelia. *Journal of Biological Chemistry* 1993;**268**:23504–11.
78. Posey KL, Yang Y, Veerisetty AC, et al. Model systems for studying skeletal dysplasias caused by TSP-5/COMP mutations. *Cellular and Molecular Life Sciences* 2008;**65**:687–99.
79. Klatt AR, Nitsche DP, Kobbe B, et al. Molecular structure and tissue distribution of matrilin-3, a filament-forming extracellular matrix protein expressed during skeletal development. *Journal of Biological Chemistry* 2000;**275**:3999–4006.
80. Maeda K, Miyamoto Y, Sawai H, et al. A compound heterozygote harboring novel and recurrent DTDST mutations with intermediate phenotype between atelosteogenesis type II and diastrophic dysplasia. *American Journal of Medical Genetics A* 2006;**140**:1143–7.
81. Markovich D. Physiological roles and regulation of mammalian sulfate transporters. *Physiological Reviews* 2001;**81**:1499–533.
82. Rossi A, Cetta G, Piazza R, et al. In vitro proteoglycan sulfation derived from sulfhydryl compounds in sulfate transporter chondrodysplasias. *Pediatric Pathology and Molecular Medicine* 2003;**22**:311–21.
83. Superti-Furga A, Rossi A, Steinmann B, Gitzelmann R. A chondrodysplasia family produced by mutations in the diastrophic dysplasia sulfate transporter gene: genotype/phenotype correlations. *American Journal of Medical Genetics* 1996;**63**:144–7.
84. Miyake A, Nishimura G, Futami T, et al. A compound heterozygote of novel and recurrent DTDST mutations results in a novel intermediate phenotype of Desbuquois dysplasia, diastrophic dysplasia, and recessive form of multiple epiphyseal dysplasia. *Journal of Human Genetics* 2008;**53**:764–8.
85. Hermanns P, Unger S, Rossi A, et al. Congenital joint dislocations caused by carbohydrate sulfotransferase 3 deficiency in recessive Larsen syndrome and humero-spinal

85. dysostosis. *American Journal of Human Genetics* 2008;**82**:1368-74.
86. Wolpoe ME, Braverman N, Lin SY. Severe tracheobronchial stenosis in the X-linked recessive form of chondrodysplasia punctata. *Archives of Otolaryngology – Head and Neck Surgery* 2004;**130**:1423-6.
87. Nino M, Matos-Miranda C, Maeda M, et al. Clinical and molecular analysis of arylsulfatase E in patients with brachytelephalangic chondrodysplasia punctata. *American Journal of Medical Genetics A* 2008;**146A**:997-1008.
88. Garnier A, Dauger S, Eurin D, et al. Brachytelephalangic chondrodysplasia punctata with severe spinal cord compression: report of four new cases. *European Journal of Pediatrics* 2007;**596**:327-31.
89. Reismann P, Tulassay Z. Treatment prospects of lysosomal storage disorders. *Orvosi Hetilap* 2008;**149**:1171-9.
90. Hou WS, Bromme D, Zhao Y, et al. Characterization of novel cathepsin K mutations in the pro and mature polypeptide regions causing pycnodysostosis. *Journal of Clinical Investigation* 1999;**103**:731-8.
91. Gedeon AK, Colley A, Jamieson R, et al. Identification of the gene (SEDL) causing X-linked spondyloepiphyseal dysplasia tarda. *Nature Genetics* 1999;**22**:400-4.
92. Fiedler J, Bergmann C, Brenner RE. X-linked spondyloepiphyseal dysplasia tarda: molecular cause of a heritable disorder associated with early degenerative joint disease. *Acta Orthopaedica Scandinavica* 2003;**74**:737-41.
93. Special report: International nomenclature of constitutional diseases of bone. *AJR American Journal of Roentgenology* 1978;**131**:352-4.
94. Superti-Furga A, Unger S. Nosology and classification of genetic skeletal disorders: 2006 revision. *American Journal of Medical Genetics A* 2007;**143**:1-18.
95. Savarirayan R, Rimoin DL. Skeletal dysplasias. *Advances in Pediatrics* 2004;**51**:209-29.
96. Hall JG, Froster-Iskenius UG, Allanson JE. Special measurements for special conditions. In: Hall J (ed.) *Handbook of Normal Physical Measurements*. New York, NY: Oxford University Press, 1995:445-7.
97. Chen H. Skeletal dysplasia. *Pediatrics: Genetics and Metabolic Disease*. Available from: http://www.emedicine.com/PED/topic625.htm
98. Spranger JW, Brill PW, Poznanski A. Bone dysplasias. In: Spranger JW, Brill PW, Poznanski A (eds) *An Atlas of Genetic Disorders of Skeletal Development*. Munich, Germany, and New York, NY: Urban & Fischer and Oxford University Press, 2002:3-425.
99. Digilio MC, Marino B, Ammirati A, et al. Cardiac malformations in patients with oral-facial-skeletal syndromes: clinical similarities with heterotaxia. *American Journal of Medical Genetics* 1999;**84**:350-6.
100. Potocki L, Abuelo DN, Oyer CE. Cardiac malformation in two infants with hypochondrogenesis. *American Journal of Medical Genetics* 1995;**59**:295-9.
101. Baujat G, Le Merrer M. Ellis-van Creveld syndrome. *Orphanet Journal of Rare Diseases* 2007;**2**:27.
102. Kurian K, Shanmugam S, Harsh Vardah T, Gupta S. Chondroectodermal dysplasia (Ellis van Creveld syndrome): a report of three cases with review of literature. *Indian Journal of Dental Research* 2007;**18**:31-4.
103. Cohn DH, Ehtesham N, Krakow D, et al. Mental retardation and abnormal skeletal development (Dyggve-Melchior-Clausen dysplasia) due to mutations in a novel, evolutionarily conserved gene. *American Journal of Human Genetics* 2003;**72**:419-28.
104. Norton LA, Mescon H. Nail-patella-elbow syndrome. *Archives of Dermatology* 1968;**98**:372-4.
105. Li QW, Song HR, Mahajan RH, et al. Deformity correction with external fixator in pseudoachondroplasia. *Clinical Orthopaedics and Related Research* 2007;**454**:174-9.
106. Goshen E, Schwartz A, Zilka LR, Zwas ST. Bilateral accessory iliac horns: pathognomonic findings in Nail-patella syndrome. Scintigraphic evidence on bone scan. *Clinical Nuclear Medicine* 2000;**25**:476-7.
107. Zuppan CW, Weeks DA, Cutler D. Nail-patella glomerulopathy without associated constitutional abnormalities. *Ultrastructural Pathology* 2003;**27**:357-61.
108. Sharony R, Browne C, Lachman RS, Rimoin DL. Prenatal diagnosis of the skeletal dysplasias. *American Journal of Obstetrics and Gynecology* 1993;**599**:668-75.
109. Bulas DI, Fonda JS. Prenatal evaluation of fetal anomalies. *Pediatric Clinics of North America* 1997;**44**:537-53.
110. Park JHG. Achondroplasia. *Pediatrics: Genetics and Metabolic Disease*. Available from: http://www.emedicine.com/ped/TOPIC12.HTM
111. Ramus RM, Martin LB, Twickler DM. Ultrasonographic prediction of fetal outcome in suspected skeletal dysplasias with use of the femur length-to-abdominal circumference ratio. *American Journal of Obstetrics and Gynecology* 1998;**179**:1348-52.
112. Pradhan M, Sankar H. Short humerus: an additional antenatal sonographic feature of OFDS type II. *Journal of Clinical Ultrasound* 2007;**35**:390-4.
113. Eteson DJ, Adomian GE, Ornoy A, et al. Fibrochondrogenesis: radiologic and histologic studies. *American Journal of Medical Genetics* 1984;**19**:277-90.
114. Gilbert-Barness E, Debich-Spicer DE. Skeletal system. In: Breaugh MJ (ed.) *Handbook of Paediatric Autopsy Pathology*. Totowa, NJ: Humana Press, 2005:384-90.
115. Lachman RS, Rimoin DL, Hollister DW, et al. The Kniest syndrome. *American Journal of Roentgenology, Radium Therapy and Nuclear Medicine* 1975;**123**:805-14.
159. Sconyers SM, Rimoin DL, Lachman RS, et al. A distinct chondrodysplasia resembling Kniest dysplasia: clinical, roentgenographic, histologic, and ultrastructural findings. *Journal of Pediatrics* 1983;**103**:898-904.
117. Meyer J, Sudbeck P, Held M, et al. Mutational analysis of the SOX9 gene in campomelic dysplasia and autosomal sex reversal: lack of genotype/phenotype correlations. *Human Molecular Genetics* 1997;**6**:91-8.
118. Tachdjian MO. Achondroplasia. In: Tachdjian MO (ed.) *Pediatric Orthopaedics*. Philadelphia, PA: W.B. Saunders Company, 1990:721.

119. Seino Y, Yamanaka Y, Shinohara M, *et al*. Growth hormone therapy in achondroplasia. *Hormone Research* 2000;**53** (Suppl. 3): 53–6.
120. Wang Y, Spatz MK, Kannan K, *et al*. A mouse model for achondroplasia produced by targeting fibroblast growth factor receptor 3. *Proceedings of the National Academy of Sciences of the USA* 1999;**96**:4455–60.
121. Aviezer D, Golembo M, Yayon A. Fibroblast growth factor receptor-3 as a therapeutic target for Achondroplasia: genetic short limbed dwarfism. *Current Drug Targets* 2003; **4**:353–65.
122. Shadi M, Koczewski P. [Humeral lengthening with a monolateral external fixator in achondroplasia]. *Endokrynologia, Diabetologia i Choroby Przemiany Materii Wieku Rozwojowego* 2007;**13**:121–4.
123. Yasui N, Kawabata H, Kojimoto H, *et al*. Lengthening of the lower limbs in patients with achondroplasia and hypochondroplasia. *Clinical Orthopaedics and Related Research* 1997;**344**:298–306.
124. Aldegheri R. Distraction osteogenesis for lengthening of the tibia in patients who have limb-length discrepancy or short stature. *Journal of Bone and Joint Surgery* (*American*) 1999;**81**:624–34.
125. Hiraki S, Nakamura I, Okazaki H, *et al*. Skin behavior during leg lengthening in patients with achondroplasia and hypochondroplasia: a short-term observation during leg lengthening. *Journal of Orthopaedic Science* 2006;**11**:267–71.
126. Polo A, Aldegheri R, Zambito A, *et al*. Lower-limb lengthening in short stature. An electrophysiological and clinical assessment of peripheral nerve function. *Journal of Bone and Joint Surgery* (*British*) 1997;**79**:1014–18.
127. Kitoh H, Kitakoji T, Tsuchiya H, *et al*. Distraction osteogenesis of the lower extremity in patients with achondroplasia/hypochondroplasia treated with transplantation of culture-expanded bone marrow cells and platelet-rich plasma. *Journal of Pediatric Orthopaedics* 2007;**27**:629–34.
128. Liao JC, Chen WJ, Lai PL, Chen LH. Surgical treatment of achondroplasia with thoracolumbar kyphosis and spinal stenosis: a case report. *Acta Orthopaedica* 2006;**77**:541–4.
129. Germaine L Defendi. Achondroplasia. Available from: http://www.emedicine.com/ped/TOPIC12.HTM
130. Pauli RM, Horton VK, Glinski LP, Reiser CA. Prospective assessment of risks for cervicomedullary-junction compression in infants with achondroplasia. *American Journal of Human Genetics* 1995;**56**:732–44.
131. Hill V, Sahhar M, Aitken M, *et al*. Experiences at the time of diagnosis of parents who have a child with a bone dysplasia resulting in short stature. *American Journal of Medical Genetics A* 2003;**122A**:100–7.
132. Links. Skeletal dysplasia support groups. Available from: http://www.lpaonline.org/mc/page.do?sitePageId=84636&orgId=lpa

60

Normal and pathological gait in children

RICHARD BEAUCHAMP

Introduction	563
The physical setting	564
The gait cycle	564
Instrumented three-dimensional gait analysis	564
Observational gait analysis	565
Pathological gait	566
References	568

INTRODUCTION

Gait refers to animal locomotion. Bipedal movement with reciprocal support and propulsion stages typifies human gait. Normally, gait is a very fluid and efficient process that expends the least amount of energy. The gait pattern must ensure safety for the walker as well as provide energy absorption to prevent injuries. It must also provide stability to allow propulsion through the efficient deployment of lever arms. Normal walking has several attributes, as proposed by Gage[1] (Box 60.1). Saunders and Inman[2] have described five determinants of gait that produce a dampening down of excessive vertical and lateral movements of the trunk seen with normal gait (Box 60.2). Pathological gait, on the other hand, is inefficient, laborious and often painful. There are many conditions that can lead to the development of pathological gait, and examples of these will be described.

Scientists have been studying human gait patterns for many years.[3] The observational gait analysis theme is one that is put into practice every time a physical examination of the human body takes place. Anyone can do an observational examination without the need for expensive, complicated tools or instruments but, to be accurate and effective in describing gait, one needs experience and understanding.

Observational gait analysis is useful clinically with the naked eye, but it is particularly useful in conjunction with a video recorder that has slow motion and freeze frame capabilities. Observational gait analyses, however, have limited *quantitative* value, tending to concentrate on *descriptive* characteristics instead.[4–6]

Numerous studies have been conducted to rate the reliability of observational compared with instrumented three-dimensional (3D) gait analyses. Although there still is some concordance with instrumented 3D analyses, there is much less reliability with observational analyses alone.[7–12]

When done, it is best to perform the observational gait analysis in a systematic way. There is no 'correct' method, but observers should be consistent in their

---

BOX 60.1: Attributes of gait[1]

1 Stability in stance
2 Sufficient foot clearance during swing
3 Pre-positioning of foot in swing phase
4 Adequate step length
5 Energy conservation

BOX 60.2: The determinants of gait[2]

- Pelvic rotation
- Pelvic tilt
- Knee flexion after heel strike in stance phase
- Foot and ankle motion
- Lateral displacement of the pelvis

approach so as not to miss important events. There are several reference scales that have been published describing gait. Usually, these scales assign numbers to certain gait variables, and then a total 'gait score' is obtained. Most of these scales have not been validated but do serve a useful purpose in training the observer in a systematic, thorough manner. The Physician Rating Scale is one popular method (Table 60.1).[13-20]

Table 60.1 Physician Rating Scale[16]

Dynamic function	Score
1. Crouch	
Severe (>20° hip, knee, ankle)	0
Moderate (5–20° hip, knee, ankle)	1
Mild (>5° hip, knee, ankle)	2
None	3
2. Equinus foot	
Constant (fixed contracture)	0
Constant (dynamic contracture)	1
Occasional heel contact	2
Heel-to-toe gait	3
3. Hind foot	
Varus at foot strike	0
Valgus at foot strike	1
Occasional neutral at foot strike	2
Neutral at foot strike	3
4. Knee	
Recurvatum >5°	0
Recurvatum 0–5°	1
Neutral (no recurvatum)	2
5. Speed of gait	
Only slow	0
Variable (slow-fast)	1
6. Gait	
Toe–toe	0
Occasional heel–toe	1
Heel–toe	2
Total	

THE PHYSICAL SETTING

When assessing a patient's gait, it should be conducted in an area large enough that the patient can move freely and comfortably. Ideally, there should be few distractions to the observer's vision, so that he or she can concentrate on one portion of the patient's gait cycle at a time and then repeat for another. Obviously, if one must assess joint kinematics, then having the patient in shorts and bare feet would be necessary. If the observer is not using a video recorder then the patient must make several 'passes' while they are being observed.[21]

THE GAIT CYCLE

Gait is divided into two main segments. The stance phase, which occupies about 60% of the gait cycle, begins when the advancing leg strikes the ground. This is termed 'heel strike'. In some pathological conditions, e.g. spastic hemiplegia, there is no heel strike, and this term is then replaced with 'weight acceptance' or 'initial contact'. When the leading leg strikes the floor and the trailing leg has not yet begun to lift off, this represents the stage of 'initial double support'. This is what separates walking from running – when running there is no double support phase (Table 60.2). The contralateral leg then lifts off the floor and enters the swing phase (40%) of the cycle. When this leg strikes the ground and again there are two legs on the floor, this is called 'terminal double limb' support.

The gait cycle can be further described as loading response, mid-stance, terminal stance, pre-swing, initial swing, mid-swing and terminal swing (Fig. 60.1). One step length is the distance between the initial contact of each foot. A stride length is the distance between the first and second contact of the same foot. Hence, there are two steps in each stride.

Table 60.2 Support phases

Support phase	Percentage
Stance phase	60%
Initial double support	10%
Mid-stance single limb	40%
Terminal double support	10%
Swing phase	40%

INSTRUMENTED THREE-DIMENSIONAL GAIT ANALYSIS

Some centres have access to 3D instrumented gait laboratories to assess a patient's gait more objectively. This involves the use of very highly technical equipment to view kinematics, kinetics, electromyography and other parameters. These facilities are rarely available to everyone, so will only be referred to for clarification of some of the kinematics (movement).

OBSERVATIONAL GAIT ANALYSIS

Most observations made concerning gait are done on the coronal or frontal plane. However, the observer should make an effort to view the subject from the side as well.

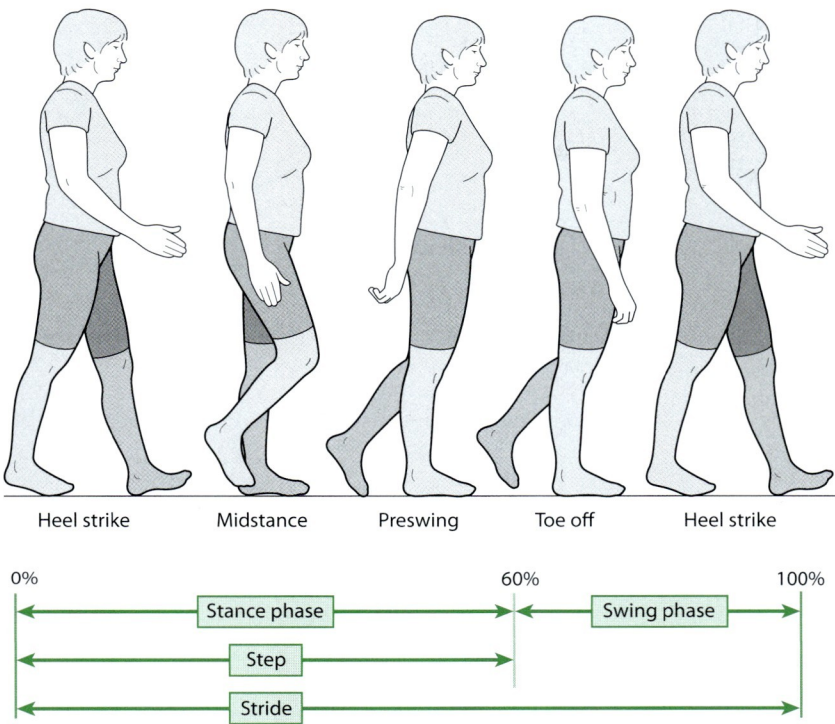

Figure 60.1 The gait cycle.

There are many sagittal plane changes that are very important. Ask the patient to walk at a self-selected speed and then ask him or her to run. Running may exaggerate and even illuminate some pathological conditions not apparent with standard walking velocity. Remember, gait is occurring in three dimensions, so also observe the line of progression for excessive in-toeing or out-toeing (Fig. 60.2). Look for any asymmetry in shoulders, pelvis or arm swing. Notice the cadence or timing of the individual steps. Children's gait does not mature into a heel–toe pattern until at least 3½ years, and they often do not form a consistent mature walking pattern until age 6 or 7 years.[22,23] Hence, there will be some variability, especially in dealing with stride lengths and velocity with different age groups. Sometimes asymmetrical cadence can be heard as well as seen. A limp is defined as an asymmetrical gait with unequal time spent on the legs. Look for the smoothness of the gait and try to formulate an overall impression, e.g. laboured, smooth, jerky, in your description. Take note of any exaggerated up and down oscillation of the patient's centre of mass. Normally, the pelvis oscillates vertically a few centimetres and the trunk leans a few degrees during stance phase.[24] Slower walking velocity can exaggerate lateral trunk sway.

Once the observer has overviewed the patient from both the frontal and sagittal planes, he or she can begin systematically to look at the trunk and pelvis, hip, then the knee, ankle and foot.

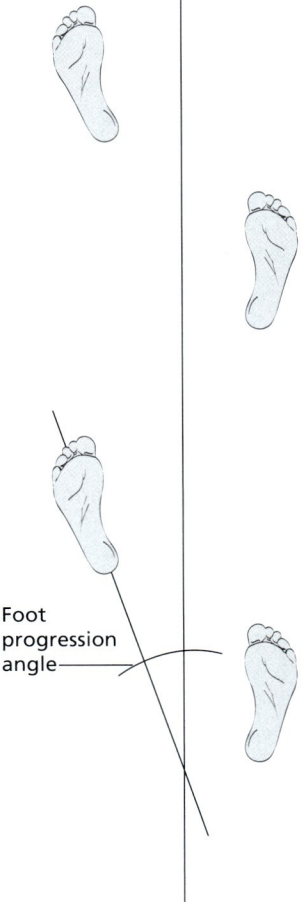

Figure 60.2 The line of progression.

Hip joint

FRONTAL VIEW

Assess for a level pelvis (leg length discrepancy), presence of a Trendelenburg sign (abductor weakness), limb circumduction (femoral torsion) and hip vaulting (leg length discrepancy).

SAGITTAL VIEW

Estimate the amount of hip flexion/extension in swing and in stance, and whether there is increased lumbar lordosis seen with an anterior pelvic tilt or a flat back seen with a posterior pelvic tilt. Normally, the hip is in maximum flexion at mid-swing and achieves maximum extension in terminal stance prior to toe-off (Fig. 60.3).

Knee joint

FRONTAL VIEW

Observe for any static or dynamic malalignment (e.g. genu vara or valga). Knee instability may be seen with varus or valgus thrust during stance. Look for the location of the patella. Squinting or inward-pointing patellae may indicate femoral anteversion/torsion.

SAGITTAL VIEW

Look for maximum knee flexion in mid-swing (as in hip). Heel strike occurs with the knee in almost full extension. About 10° of knee flexion then occurs. This serves as a 'shock absorber' to reduce the transmission of forces across the kinetic chain. There should be complete knee extension prior to toe-off (as in the hip). Observe for knee hyperextension or increased knee flexion in stance, both of which can be seen in pathological conditions (Fig. 60.4).

Ankle and foot

FRONTAL VIEW

Notice the overall line of progression (in-toeing or out-toeing). Rotational issues can occur from hip (anteversion) or shank (tibial torsion) problems. Look for heel

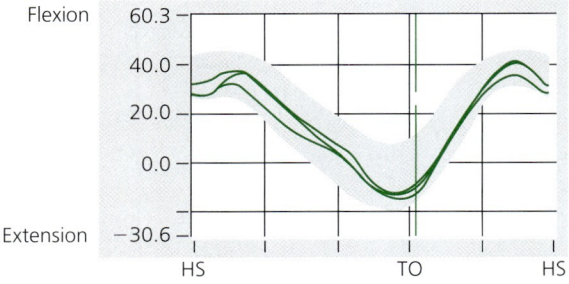

Figure 60.3 Sagittal plane kinematic graph of normal hip. HS, heel strike; TO, toe off.

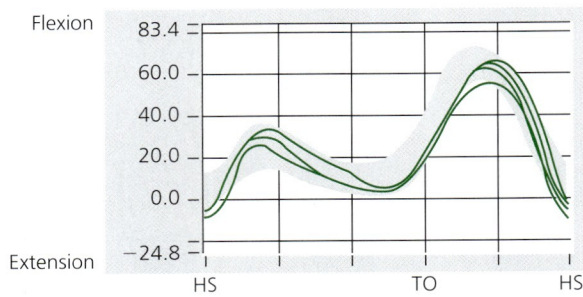

Figure 60.4 Sagittal plane kinematic graph of a normal knee. HS, heel strike; TO, toe off.

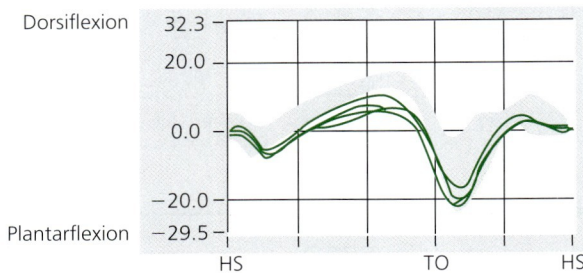

Figure 60.5 Sagittal plane kinematic graph of a normal ankle. HS, heel strike; TO, toe off.

valgus or varus in both swing and stance. One may appreciate metatarsus adductus during the stance phase of the foot. Observe step width.

SAGITTAL VIEW

Look for the weight acceptance pattern of the foot. This is usually heel–toe but may occur as toe–heel, toe only or plantigrade. Try and appreciate the ankle dorsiflexing in swing to help achieve toe clearance from the ground. Watch for any adaptive changes to accommodate leg length discrepancy, equinus, etc. (Fig. 60.5).

If the ankle is in plantarflexion in terminal stance and the knee goes into hyperextension, this is known as the 'ankle plantarflexion/knee extension couple'.[1] The pattern of weight acceptance has been described as having three rockers. The first rocker occurs with heel strike as the foot goes into plantarflexion (the tibialis anterior in this phase contracts eccentrically, decelerating transition into plantarflexion and avoiding foot flap as seen in drop-foot gait when the tibialis anterior is weak or absent). The second rocker occurs when the foot goes into relative dorsiflexion as the tibia glides over the talus. The third rocker is when the foot and ankle plantar flex in preparation for toe-off (Fig. 60.6).

PATHOLOGICAL GAIT

Any deviations from the normal gait patterns described above can be due to several factors, some of more significance than others. They can include conditions due to mechanical factors, weakness, pain and/or joint stiffness. Regardless of the aetiology, the gait patterns will generally

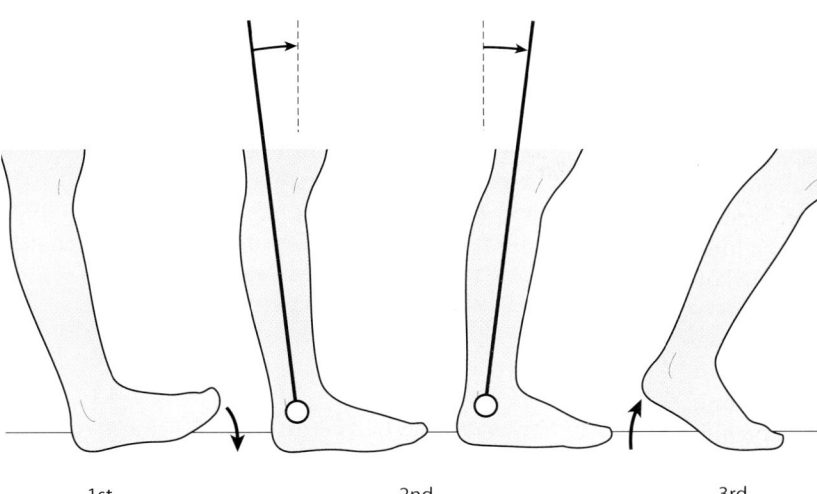

Figure 60.6 The three ankle rockers.

be typified by asymmetry between the right and left sides and decreased or even increased velocity and cadence. The pathological process may lead to the development of compensatory changes in the contralateral limb, trunk or pelvis, which, over time, may lead to their persistence.

Mechanical

In order for the skeleton (body) to generate movement for walking, there needs to be a mechanical advantage for the muscles and tendons to work. This means having strong muscles, and strong attachments for those muscles to the skeleton. It requires stable joints for those muscles to work across. Conditions such as hip instability/dysplasia from developmental dysplasia of the hip, Down syndrome, meningomyelocele or cerebral palsy can lead to altered lever arms at the hip, resulting in a Trendelenburg gait which can remain *uncompensated*, when there is no associated opposite trunk shift, or *compensated*, when the ipsilateral lateral trunk flexion overcomes the pelvic weakness. There may be a shortened stance phase on the affected limb because of the instability. The walking velocity may be slow and the step length asymmetrical. Exaggerated trunk sway or lateral flexion may be seen.

Crouch gait (increased knee flexion in stance) (>30° in stance) may be seen in certain cases of cerebral palsy, especially in spastic diplegia.[25] This can lead to patella alta, which weakens the patellofemoral lever arm, making stance phase very short. This may actually increase the patient's walking velocity, but can lead to eventual deterioration in gait because of knee pain. Stiff-knee gait results when there is abnormal muscle activity in both the knee flexors (hamstrings) and the knee extensors (rectus femoris) in cerebral palsy. This will be seen best on the sagittal plane with diminished peak-knee flexion in swing, and may need to be addressed through either hamstring lengthening or rectus femoris transfer.

Leg length discrepancy is a common condition, but does not produce mechanical alterations in gait until the difference is more than 5.5% of the leg length.[26] Compensatory changes are often seen in the longer leg with increased knee flexion at double limb stance; hip 'hike' may be seen when the patient must 'lift up' their longer leg in swing in order to clear the ground. Other adaptive changes can be increased hip flexion or circumduction in swing of the longer leg or 'early heel-rise' on the shorter limb to allow the longer limb ground clearance.

Antalgic gait

The term 'antalgia' is derived from the word 'analgesia' – to relieve pain. An antalgic gait is a compensatory method that the patient uses to decrease pain during walking. Whether this is from a stress fracture, infection, arthritis, muscle sprain or any other injury, the typical antalgic pattern is a very shortened stance phase. This relieves any excess force being carried through that limb by reducing the vertical ground reaction force. At times a Trendelenburg gait may, in fact, be a form of antalgia secondary to hip joint pathology.

Weakness

Secure muscle attachments to bone to ensure strong lever arms are essential for an efficient gait. However, if the muscles are weak or dysfunctional (e.g. spastic) then there may not be enough power to allow the normal muscle control of the limb. A drop-foot gait, in which there is insufficient dorsiflexion in swing, will produce gait abnormalities that can include high steppage, circumduction and contralateral early heel-rise, which are all done to produce sufficient ground clearance during swing. Equinus at stance phase, if associated with heel contact, will result in the development of an 'ankle plantarflexion/knee extension couple'. Swing phase or initial loading at weight acceptance, if the foot is in varus, may be due to spasticity of the posterior tibial muscle, as seen in cerebral palsy–spastic hemiplegia.

Neurological

Weakness and deficient selective motor control are often associated with neurological conditions. More importantly, however, is the presence of abnormal muscle tone or ataxia. Cerebellar, aural and ophthalmological conditions can lead to ataxia typified by an unsteady gait that is wide based and perhaps has increased velocity. Abnormal muscle tone can manifest as hypotonia or hypertonia. Low tone – hypotonia – can result in slower velocity with prolonged stance phase duration. More frequently, one sees patients with increased tone – hypertonicity. There are various types of hypertonia, including spasticity, dystonia or rigidity. Spasticity is an increased muscle tone typified by an increased stretch reflex, which is velocity dependent. Dystonia produces abnormal limb movement such as athetosis. Most cases of hypertonicity will result in altered temporal/spatial parameters and overall reduce joint excursion and range of movement.

The various forms of cerebral palsy can produce many different pathological gait patterns that are not always pathognomonic to the particular type. Some generalities can be developed, such as the internal rotation of the foot seen in hemiplegia, the equinus typical of most cases of cerebral palsy and the crouch gait seen with spastic diplegia.

> **KEY LEARNING POINTS**
>
> - Observational gait analysis is an essential tool as part of a physical examination.
> - Observational gait analysis has more qualitative (subjective) benefit than quantitative (objective).
> - A systematic approach to observational gait analysis should always be used.
> - The Physician Rating Scale is one of several useful tools to score gait.
> - Pathological conditions often affect a person's gait.

REFERENCES

1. Gage JR. *Gait Analysis in Cerebral Palsy*. London, UK: MacKeith Press, 1991.
2. Saunders JDM, Inman VT, Eberhart HD. The major determinants in normal and pathological gait. *Journal of Bone and Joint Surgery* 1953;**35A**:543–58.
3. Baker R. The history of gait analysis before the advent of modern computers. *Gait & Posture* 2007;**26**:331–42.
4. Harris GF, Westch JJ. Procedures for gait analysis. *Archives of Physical Medicine and Rehabilitation* 1994;**75**:216–25.
5. McGinley JL, Goldie PA, Greenwood KM, Olney SJ. Accuracy and reliability of observational gait analysis data: judgements of push-off in gait after stroke. *Physical Therapy* 2003;**83**:146–60.
6. Toro B, Nester C, Farren P. A review of observational gait assessment in clinical practice. *Physical Therapy and Practice* 2003;**19**:137–49.
7. Eastlock ME, Arvidson J, Snyder-Mackler L, et al. Interrater reliability of videotaped observational gait analysis assessments. *Physical Therapy* 1991;**71**:472–95.
8. Krebs DE, Edelstein JE, Fishman S. Reliability of observational gait analysis. *Physical Therapy* 1985;**65**:1027–33.
9. Mackey AH, Lobb GL, Walt SE, Stott NS. Reliability and validity of the observational gait scale in children with spastic diplegia. *Developmental Medicine & Child Neurology* 2003;**45**:4–11.
10. Narayanan UG. The role of gait analysis in the orthopaedic management of ambulatory cerebral palsy. *Current Opinion in Orthopaedics* 2007;**19**:38–43.
11. Pearson OR, Busse ME, Van Deursen RWM, Wiles CM. Quantification of walking mobility in neurological disorders. *The Quarterly Journal of Medicine* 2004;**97**:463–75.
12. Saleh M, Murdoch G. In defence of gait analysis. Observation and measurement in gait assessment. *Journal of Bone and Joint Surgery* 1985;**67B**:237–41.
13. Boyd RN, Graham HK. Objective measurement of clinical findings in the use of botulinum toxin type A for the management of children with cerebral palsy. *European Journal of Neurology* 1999;**6S**:S23–S35.
14. Brunnekreff JJ, van Uden CJ, van Moorsel S, Kooloos JG. Reliability of videotaped observational gait analysis in patients with orthopaedic impairments. *BMC Musculoskeletal Disorders* 2005;**6**:17.
15. Coutts F. Gait analysis in the therapeutic environment. *Manual Therapy* 1999;**4**:2–10.
16. Koman LA, Mooney JF, Smith BP, et al. Management of spasticity in cerebral palsy with botulinum-A: report of a preliminary randomized double-blind trial. *Journal of Pediatric Orthopaedics* 1994;**14**:299–303.
17. Lord E, Halligan PW, Wade DT. Visual gait analysis: the development of a clinical assessment and scale. *Clinical Rehabilitation* 1998;**12**:107–19.
18. Maathuis KG, van der Schans CP, van Iperen A, et al. Gait in children with cerebral palsy: observer reliability of Physician Rating Scale and Edinburgh Visual Gait Analysis Interval Testing Scale. *Journal of Pediatric Orthopaedics* 2005;**25**:268–72.
19. Read HS, Hillman SJ, Hazelwood ME, Robb JE. The Edinburgh Visual Gait score. *Journal of Pediatric Orthopaedics* 2003;**23**:296–301.
20. Hsueh CL, Hsueh IP, Mao HF. Validity and responsiveness of the Rivermead Mobility Index in stroke patients. *Scandinavian Journal of Rehabilitation Medicine* 2000;**32**:140–2.

21. Sutherland D, Hagy J. Measurement of gait movements from motion picture film. *Journal of Bone and Joint Surgery* 1972;**54A**:787–97.
22. Inman VT, Ralston HJ, Todd F. *Human Walking*. Baltimore, MD: Williams & Wilkins, 1981.
23. Sutherland D, Olsen R, Cooper L, Woo L. The development of mature gait. *Journal of Bone and Joint Surgery* 1980;**62**:336–53.
24. Perry J. *Gait Analysis: Normal and Pathological Function*. New York, NY: McGraw-Hill, 1992.
25. Rodda JM, Graham HK, Nattrass GR, *et al*. Correction of severe crouch gait in patients with spastic diplegia with use of multilevel orthopaedic surgery. *Journal of Bone and Joint Surgery* 2006;**88**:2653–64.
26. Song KM. The effect of leg length discrepancy on gait. *Journal of Bone and Joint Surgery* 1997;**79**:1690–8.

61

Developmental diseases of the skeleton

SUNIL BAJAJ, SANJEEV S MADAN

| Introduction | 570 | Classification of skeletal dysplasia | 570 |
| Pathophysiology | 570 | References | 575 |

INTRODUCTION

Skeletal dysplasias are a heterogeneous group of bone and cartilage disorders resulting in limb deformities and short stature. The short stature (defined as a height that is two or more standard deviations below the mean height for age) could be proportionate or disproportionate depending on the trunk-to-limb length ratio. Disproportionate short stature could result from short limbs or a short trunk. Shortening in a limb could affect the proximal limb segment (rhizomelic), e.g. the arm in the upper limb; the middle segment (mesomelic), e.g. the forearm in the upper limb; or the distal segment (acromelic), e.g. the hand in the upper limb.

PATHOPHYSIOLOGY

Skeletal dysplasias are caused by genetic mutations and there may be several mutations of the individual gene producing a variation in clinical expression of the same condition. There are over 30 known mutations of *COL2A1* gene, all of which result in spondyloepiphyseal dysplasia (SED) with varying expression from severe spinal involvement to precocious osteoarthritis with minimal or no spinal involvement. Similarly, around 100 specific genomic defects have been described in the *COL1A1* and *COL1A2* genes, involved in the formation of type I collagen. They produce a wide clinical spectrum of disease ranging from osteogenesis imperfecta to a form of Ehlers–Danlos syndrome.

These gene defects result in structural or functional protein abnormalities such as specific collagen abnormalities, defective enzyme function, defects in carrier proteins or functional defects such as abnormal bone resorption or tumour suppression (Table 61.1).

CLASSIFICATION OF SKELETAL DYSPLASIA

Sir Thomas Fairbank[1] was the first to make an attempt to classify the skeletal dysplasias. Later, Rubin[2] proposed a classification by grouping them according to the anatomical distribution of bone changes as epiphyseal, physeal, metaphyseal and diaphyseal dysplasia. An international nomenclature of constitutional disorders of the bone was first developed in Paris in 1969 and revised[3–8] in 1977 (Table 61.2).

Achondroplasia

Achondroplasia is the most common form of dysplasia resulting in disproportionate dwarfism, with a reported prevalence of 1.3 per 1000 live births.[9] It is caused by defects in the *FGFR3* (glycine-to-arginine substitution) gene located on chromosome 4p.[10] Although it is inherited as a fully penetrant autosomal dominant trait, 90% of the cases are sporadic as a result of point mutation in the gene.[11] FGFR3 acts on growth plate chondrocytes to regulate linear growth.[12] Achondroplasia is characterized by a defect in endochondral ossification; intramembranous and periosteal ossification are not affected. Consequently, the lengths of long bones are reduced while the diameter is normal.

Table 61.1 Genetic defects that cause skeletal dysplasias

Genetic defect	Type of skeletal dysplasia
Defect in structural cartilage protein	
Type II collagen defects	Spondyloepimetaphyseal dysplasia, spondyloepiphyseal dysplasia, Kniest dysplasia, Stickler syndrome, achondrogenesis II, hypochondrogenesis
Type XI collagen defects	Stickler syndrome
Type IX collagen defects	Multiple epiphyseal dysplasia
Type X collagen defects	Schmid type of metaphyseal dysplasia
Enzyme or carrier protein defects	
Diastrophic dysplasia sulphate transporter	Diastrophic dysplasias
Arylsulphatase E	Chondrodysplasia punctata (X-linked)
Lysosomal enzyme defects	Mucopolysaccharidoses and mucolipidoses
Transmembrane receptor defects	Achondroplasia, hypochondroplasia, thanatophoric dysplasia, metaphyseal dysplasia (Jansen type)
Transcription factor disorders	Camptomelic dysplasia, cleidocranial dysplasia, nail–patella syndrome
Defect in bone resorption	Osteopetrosis, osteopoikilosis, osteopathia striata, melorheostosis, pyknodysostosis
Tumour suppression	Multiple exostosis (mutation in *EXT1* and *EXT2* leads to increased risk of malignancy)

Table 61.2 Outline of the international classification of constitutional disorders of bone

Group		Examples (not complete list)
Osteochondrodysplasias	Identifiable at birth	**Achondroplasia**, achondrogenesis, thanatophoric dysplasia, chondrodysplasia punctata, diastrophic dysplasia, chondroectodermal dysplasia (Ellis–van Creveld)
	Identifiable in later life	Hypochondroplasia, dyschondrosteosis, spondyloepiphyseal dysplasia tarda
Disorganized development of cartilage and fibrous components		Dysplasia epiphysealis hemimelica, **multiple hereditary exostosis**, enchondromatosis, **fibrous dysplasia (usual form = Jaffe–Lichtenstein; with skin pigmentation and precocious puberty = McCune–Albright), neurofibromatosis**
Abnormalities of density of cortical diaphyseal structure and/or metaphyseal modelling		**Osteogenesis imperfecta**, juvenile osteoporosis, osteopetrosis, **osteopuikilusis** melorheostosis
Dysostoses with cranial and facial involvement		Craniostenosis, **cleidocranial dysostosis**, acrocephalosyndactyly (Apert syndrome), mandibulofacial dysostosis
Dysostoses with predominant axial involvement		Vertebral segmentation defects including Klippel–Feil syndrome, Sprengel anomaly
Dysostoses with predominant involvement of extremities		Acheiria, apodia, ectrodactyly, familial radioulnar synostosis, symphalangism, polydactyly, syndactyly
Idiopathic osteolyses		Phalangeal, tarsocarpal, multicentric
Chromosomal aberrations		
Primary metabolic abnormalities	Calcium and/or phosphorus	**Hypophosphataemic rickets**, idiopathic hypercalciuria, hypophosphatasia, pseudohypoparathyroidism
	Complex carbohydrates	**Mucopolysaccharidoses, Marfans**
	Lipids	Niemann–Pick disease, **Gaucher disease**
	Nucleic acids	Adenosine deaminase deficiency
	Amino acids	Homocystinuria
	Metals	Menkes kinky hair syndrome

Modified from Horan F, Beighton P. *Orthopaedic Problems in Inherited Skeletal Disorders.* New York, NY: Springer-Verlag, 1982.
Key examples in bold.

CLINICAL FEATURES

Achondroplasia is characterized by rhizomelic disproportionate short stature that is recognizable even in the antenatal period by ultrasonography.[13] The child has a disproportionately large head, short limbs and a trunk of normal length. The arm span is diminished and the fingertips reach only to the greater trochanters. The hands are short and broad with all of the digits of equal length and an increased web space between the middle and ring fingers – the trident hand.[14] Flexion contractures of the elbows, radial head dislocation, genu varum with mild femoral bowing and internal tibial torsion may occur. Kyphosis of the thoracolumbar spine is often seen in infants; this is superseded by a rigid exaggerated lumbar lordosis in the walking child. The facial features include a prominent forehead, flattened nasal bridge and prominent mandibles.

RADIOGRAPHIC FEATURES

Radiographs of the limbs reveal normal diaphyseal diameter but reduced length. There is flaring of the metaphysis and the epiphysis is usually normal. The pelvis is short and wide with small sciatic notches. Hip radiographs show an apparent coxa vara with short femoral necks and trochanteric overgrowth. In the anteroposterior view of the lumbar spine there is progressive narrowing of the transverse interpedicular distance from L1 to L5.

Orthopaedic and neurosurgical management in achondroplasia mainly focuses on the spinal problems. Stenosis of the foramen magnum leading to brainstem and cervical cord compression can occur in infancy, which may necessitate posterior surgical decompression. Hydrocephalus due to a Chiari malformation at the craniovertebral junction may require urgent shunting. Progressive thoracolumbar kyphosis and kyphosis may require surgery. Lumbar canal stenosis with neurogenic claudication may become symptomatic in the adolescent. Symptoms include leg and back pain brought on by walking and relieved by bending forward, which tends to reduce lumbar lordosis and produces more space in the spinal canal. MRI is useful to visualize the extent of stenosis and planning treatment in the form of laminectomy and posterior decompression.

Multiple epiphyseal dysplasia

Multiple epiphyseal dysplasia (MED) includes a group of disorders with epiphyseal involvement of the tubular bones leading to short stature and early arthritis. The epiphyses are usually symmetrically involved. This entity was first described by Fairbank,[15,16] who called it dysplasia epiphysealis multiplex. There are many forms of MED, the two most common being type I, or the Fairbank form, and the milder type II described by Ribbing.[17] MED has a prevalence of nine per 100 000.[18]

GENETICS

Both autosomal dominant and autosomal recessive forms of transmission are seen in MED, the former being the more common transmission.

It is probably the most genetically heterogeneous dysplasia caused by mutations in several genes: the *COMP* gene,[19] genes coding for type IX collagen (*COL9A1*, *COL9A2* and *COL9A3*),[20–23] the gene coding for extracellular matrix protein matrilin 3 (*MATN3*)[24] and the *DTDST* gene.[25] The gene that codes for COMP is located on chromosome 19 and is the same gene that is abnormal in pseudoachondroplasia. The gene encoding for the α_2 polypeptide chain of type IX collagen is located on chromosome 1.[26,27] Patients with this gene defect tend to have more knee involvement with relative sparing of the hips,[28] in contrast to defects in the gene encoding another which results in hip dysplasia.

PATHOLOGY

Disorganized endochondral ossification and irregularity of cartilage cells is seen in the epiphysis; metaphyseal remodelling is not affected. The misshapen epiphyses lead to early degenerative arthritis, especially in the weight-bearing joints.

Electron microscopy shows intracytoplasmic inclusions in the chondrocytes; these inclusions represent dilation of the rough endoplasmic reticulum.

CLINICAL FEATURES

The condition is not recognizable at birth. Early signs include delay in walking, limp and a waddling gait. Joint pain, stiffness or contractures especially at elbows and knees are not uncommon. Epiphyseal deformity at the elbow can cause ulnar nerve entrapment, requiring nerve transposition. Although short stature is common, true dwarfism is not associated with this condition because many patients are above the third percentile for height.

RADIOGRAPHIC FINDINGS

Changes are predominantly seen in the epiphysis and include delay in the appearance of the ossification centres and small, fragmented, mottled and flattened epiphyses. Epiphyseal height (measured at the distal femur) and carpal height are decreased and may assist in reaching an early diagnosis before degenerative arthritis begins.[29–31]

The radiographic changes in the proximal femur may be confused with Perthes disease; however, the two conditions can be differentiated on closer scrutiny (Table 61.3).

Other changes in the hips include coxa vara (not necessarily bilateral) and short femoral necks. Squared-off distal femoral condyles and a shallow intercondylar notch may be seen and genu varum or valgum may be present. In the lateral radiograph of the knee a double-layered patella that is characteristic of MED may be present. Irregular epiphyses may be seen in the hands with short metacarpals and phalanges. The spine is normal in MED.

ORTHOPAEDIC MANAGEMENT

In young patients who are symptomatic, proximal femoral osteotomies to improve hip biomechanics may be needed. Valgus proximal femoral osteotomy may improve congruency if hinge abduction is present on arthrography; shelf acetabular augmentation has been done in some patients with MED to improve coverage of the misshapen femoral head. Angular deformities in lower extremities may be corrected by hemiepiphysiodesis or osteotomies. Total joint arthroplasty may be needed in young adults with severe joint disease.

Spondyloepiphyseal dysplasias

Spondyloepiphyseal dysplasia (SED) includes a group of allelic chondrodysplasias caused by different mutations in the gene coding for type II collagen. SED congenita, SED tarda and Stickler syndrome (a very rare hereditary arthro-ophthalmopathy) are included in this group.

Table 61.3 Features that help to differentiate multiple epiphyseal dysplasia from Perthes disease

Multiple epiphyseal dysplasia	Perthes disease
Always bilateral	Bilateral in a small proportion
Symmetric involvement	If bilateral, usually metachronous findings with both hips at different stages of the disease
Acetabular changes are usually seen	Acetabular changes uncommon
Metaphyseal cysts absent	Metaphyseal cysts are common
Changes in other joints like shoulders and knees	Other joints are normal

GENETICS

SED is characterized by type II collagenopathies[32–34] resulting from mutation of the *COL2A1* gene located on chromosome 12. As over 30 different mutations of the *COL2A1* gene may occur, there could be a wide range of phenotypic expression in SED.

SED congenita is inherited as an autosomal dominant trait, although most cases are a result of sporadic mutations. SED tarda inheritance is either autosomal recessive or X-linked recessive.

CLINICAL FEATURES

Short trunk disproportionate dwarfism with rhizomelic and mesomelic shortening is seen in SED. SED tarda presents a milder clinical picture and manifests later in childhood. The child presents with progressive coxa vara and tibia vara with internal tibial torsion. Spinal deformities include thoracic kyphoscoliosis with an exaggerated lumbar lordosis. Atlantoaxial instability or cervical myelopathy may develop. Children with SED congenita require periodic ophthalmic review as they can have severe myopia and develop retinal detachment and cataracts. A rare form of SED congenita is associated with nephrotic syndrome.

RADIOGRAPHIC FINDINGS

Delayed appearance of the epiphyses[35] is typical in SED. On appearing, the epiphyses become flattened and irregular. Radiographs of the spine show platyspondyly. Odontoid hypoplasia or os odontoideum may be present. Since atlantoaxial instability may be present in these children flexion–extension cervical radiographs must be obtained before any anaesthetic procedure.

ORTHOPAEDIC MANAGEMENT

Orthopaedic management would include spinal stabilization surgery or arthroplasty for precocious osteoarthritis. Osteotomies around hip and knee may be needed for correction of angular malalignment.

Mucopolysaccharidoses

These are lysosomal storage disorders characterized by intracellular accumulation of semidegraded glycosaminoglycans caused by a lack of lysosomal enzymes. The overall incidence of the mucopolysaccharidoses is one in 25 000 live births.[36]

The glycosaminoglycans that accumulate include heparin sulphate, keratin sulphate, dermatan sulphate and

Table 61.4 Different types of mucopolysaccharidosis (MPS) and the enzyme deficiency in each

Name	Inheritance	Enzyme defect	MPS excreted in urine	Facial features	Cornea
MPS I Hurler syndrome	Autosomal recessive	α-L-iduronidase	Dermatan sulphate Heparan sulphate	Grotesque	Cloudy
MPS II Hunter syndrome	Sex-linked recessive	Sulphoiduronate sulphatase	Heparan sulphate Dermatan sulphate	Grotesque	Clear
MPS III Sanfilippo syndrome	Autosomal recessive	N-heparan sulphatase or α-acetylglucosaminidase	Heparan sulphate	Not coarse	Clear
MPS IV Morquio syndrome	Autosomal recessive	N-acetylgalactosamine-6-sulphate sulphatase	Keratan sulphate	Not coarse	Cloudy
MPS I-S/MPS V Scheie syndrome	Autosomal recessive	α-L-iduronidase	Heparan sulphate Dermatan sulphate	Coarse	Cloudy
MPS VI Maroteaux–Lamy syndrome	Autosomal recessive	N-acetylgalactosamine-4-sulphate sulphatase	Dermatan sulphate	Coarse	Cloudy

chondroitin sulphate, causing impaired cellular function. These are excreted in the urine.

Mucopolysaccharidoses are subdivided into different types depending on the enzyme deficiency and the type of substance that accumulates as result of the deficiency. The most common among these subtypes are Morquio syndrome and Hurler syndrome.

CLINICAL FEATURES

The abnormalities may be apparent at birth or may develop later in childhood. The common clinical features are short stature, enlarged skull and thickened calvarium and abnormal facies. Spinal deformities (scoliosis and kyphosis) and angular malalignment at the hips and knees are common. The hands are short and wide, with typical shapes of the metacarpals and phalanges. The second to fifth metacarpals are pointed at their proximal ends, and the phalanges are bullet shaped. The pelvis exhibits flared iliac bones with dysplastic acetabula.

Although there are many phenotypic similarities between the different mucopolysaccharidoses, some features do differ between the different subtypes.

Different types of mucopolysaccharidosis (MPS) and the enzyme deficiency in each is shown in Table 61.4.

DIAGNOSIS OF MUCOPOLYSACCHARIDOSIS

In addition to the clinical and radiological features, the diagnosis can be made from biochemical tests on the urine for the various gycosaminoglycans. Enzyme assays from fibroblasts, leucocytes and serum also help to establish the type of enzyme deficiency. Prenatal amniotic cell and chorionic villous sampling can diagnose MPS in the affected fetus.

MANAGEMENT

Recent molecular genetic and transplantation research has improved the prognosis for MPS patients. Bone marrow transplantation or umbilical cord blood transplantation from unrelated donors (in children without suitable bone marrow transplant) has been done in Hurler syndrome, with encouraging results.

Both gene therapy and enzyme replacement therapy are under investigation.

Multiple hereditary exostosis

Hereditary multiple exostosis, also known as multiple hereditary osteochondromatosis, cartilaginous exostosis and diaphyseal aclasis, is the most common tumour-like skeletal dysplasia with a prevalence of one in 50 000 live births. It is characterised by multiple osteochondromas throughout the skeleton.

GENETICS

It is inherited as an autosomal dominant condition with variable penetrance and expressivity. Anomalies have been found in the *EXT1* gene on chromosome 8, the *EXT2* gene on chromosome 11 and the *EXT3* gene on chromosome 19. Mutations of the *EXT1* and *EXT2* genes cause disorders of proteoglycan synthesis (and, thus, abnormal cell signalling), leading to chondrocyte disorganization in the growth plate, which results in the development of the exostoses. Mutation in the *EXT1* gene is asso-ciated with malignant transformation of exostoses to chondrosarcomas.

CLINICAL FEATURES

Cartilaginous exostoses or osteochondromata arising from the metaphyses are found throughout the skeleton, predominantly involving the long bones, iliac crests, scapulae and ribs. They extend down the diaphysis during growth. In the long bones, 70% have involvement of the distal femur, 70% the proximal tibia and 30% the proximal fibula. They cease growing at skeletal maturity.

The exostosis may result in a leg length discrepancy or angular malalignment, depending on the type of growth inhibition at the adjacent physis. Patients with MME generally have short, thick femoral necks. MHE is not to be confused with Gardner syndrome, which is a colonic polyposis syndrome with associated osteomas.

RADIOLOGY

The exostosis is seen as a pedunculated or sessile bony excrescence at the metaphysis. The trabecular and cortical bone of the osteochondroma is continuous with that of the metaphysis on AP pelvis radiographs. Trumpeting of distal femur may be seen owing to lack of remodelling. Irregular zones of calcification may be seen in the cartilage caps of the osteochondroma. Extensive calcification and an increase in the thickness (>1 cm) and shape of the cartilage cap suggest malignant transformation.

MALIGNANT TRANSFORMATION

This is suggested by a sudden increase in size of the exostosis or onset of pain. Malignant transformation results in a chondrosarcoma. Osteochondromas arising from pelvic and shoulder girdles are more prone to malignant transformation. Also *EXT1* mutations are more frequently associated with malignant transformation. The risk of malignant transformation is reported to be 0.9–5%.[37–39]

TREATMENT

Excision of the exostosis is needed only if there are complications such as pressure effects producing pain or nerve entrapment. Occasionally, excision may be needed to correct angular malalignment of limb length discrepancy.

Multiple enchondromatosis (Ollier disease)

This condition was described by Ollier in 1889. It is characterized by the presence of unilateral asymmetric hyaline cartilage islands in the metaphyses and diaphyses of the long bones, which are continuous with the growth plates. These may expand, resulting in deformity or growth inhibition. The common bones affected are the phalanges, femur and tibia.

If the enchondromatosis is associated with multiple soft-tissue haemangiomas the condition is called Maffucci syndrome.

Malignant transformation into low-grade chondrosa comas by 40 years of age is likely to occur in 25–30% of patients with Ollier disease. However, malignant transformation rates are much higher (up to 100%).

ORTHOPAEDIC MANAGEMENT

Fixation of pathological fracture, curettage and bone grafting, corrective osteotomy or hemiepiphysiodesis for angular corrections and epiphysiodesis or limb lengthening may be needed to correct limb length discrepancy.

> **KEY LEARNING POINTS**
>
> - Once MHE has been diagnosed, make sure patient understands the significance of their disorder and inform them that they are on a life-long surveillance program.
> - Any pain or growth in a lesion once the physes have closed is suspicious for malignant transformation.

REFERENCES

1. Fairbank HAT. *An Atlas of General Affections of the Skeleton*. Edinburgh, UK: Livingstone, 1951.
2. Rubin P. *Dynamic Classification of Bone Dysplasias*. Chicago, IL: Mosby Year Book, 1964.
3. Bergsma D (ed.). Limb malformations. *Birth Defects Original Article Series*, vol. 10, no. 5. The National Foundation, March of Dimes. New York, NY: Intercontinental Medical Book Corp., 1974.
4. Bergsma D (ed.). Malformation syndromes. *Birth Defects Original Article Series*, vol. 10, no. 7. The National Foundation, March of Dimes. New York, NY: Intercontinental Medical Book Corp., 1974.
5. Bergsma D (ed.). Skeletal dysplasias. *Birth Defects Original Article Series*, vol. 10, no. 12. The National Foundation, March of Dimes. New York, NY: Intercontinental Medical Book Corp., 1974.
6. Bergsma D (ed.). Disorders of connective tissue. *Birth Defects Original Article Series*, vol. 11, no. 6. The National Foundation, March of Dimes. New York, NY: Intercontinental Medical Book Corp., 1975.

7. Bergsma D (ed.). Morphogenesis and malformation of the limb. *Birth Defects Original Article Series,* vol. 13, no. 1. The National Foundation, March of Dimes. New York, NY: Intercontinental Medical Book Corp., 1975.
8. Bergsma D (ed.). The genetics of hand malformations. *Birth Defects Original Article Series,* vol. 14, no. 3. The National Foundation, March of Dimes. New York, NY: Intercontinental Medical Book Corp., 1978.
9. Ain MC, Elmaci I, Hurko O, et al. Reoperation for spinal restenosis in achondroplasia. *Journal of Spinal Disorders* 2000;**13**:168.
10. Francomano CA, Ortiz de Luna RI, Hefferon TW, et al. Localization of the achondroplasia gene to the distal 2.5 Mb of human chromosome 4p. *Human Molecular Genetics* 1994;**3**:787.
11. Rousseau F, Bonaventure J, Legeai-Mallet L, et al. Mutations in the gene encoding fibroblast growth factor receptor-3 in achondroplasia. *Nature* 1994;**371**:252.
12. Horton WA. Fibroblast growth factor receptor 3 and the human chondrodysplasias. *Current Opinion in Pediatrics* 1997;**9**:437.
13. Kurtz AB, Filly RA, Wapner RJ, et al. In utero analysis of heterozygous achondroplasia: variable time of onset as detected by femur length measurements. *Journal of Ultrasound in Medicine* 1986;**5**:137.
14. Marie P. L'achondroplasie dans l'adolescence et l'age adult. *La Presse Médicale* 1900;**8**:17.
15. Fairbank HAT. Dysplasia epiphysialis multiplex. *Proceedings of the Royal Society of Medicine* 1946;**39**:315.
16. Fairbank HAT. Dysplasia epiphysialis multiplex. *British Journal of Surgery* 1947;**34**:225.
17. Ribbing S. Studien uber hereditare multiple Epiphysenstorungen. *Acta Radiologica Supplement* 1937;**34**:77.
18. Andersen Jr PE, Hauge M. Congenital generalised bone dysplasias: a clinical, radiological, and epidemiological survey. *Journal of Medical Genetics* 1989;**26**:37.
19. Briggs MD, Hoffman SMG, King LM, et al. Pseudoachondroplasia and multiple epiphyseal dysplasia due to mutations in the cartilage oligomeric matrix protein gene. *Nature Genetics* 1995;**10**:330–6.
20. Annunen S, Paassilta P, Lohiniva J, et al. An allele of COL9A2 associated with intervertebral disc disease. *Science* 1999;**285**:409–12.
21. Czarny-Ratajczak M, Lohiniva J, Rogala P, et al. A mutation in COL9A1 causes multiple epiphyseal dysplasia: Further evidence for locus heterogeneity. *American Journal of Human Genetics* 2001;**69**:969–80.
22. Muragaki Y, Mariman ECM, van Beersum SEC, et al. A mutation in the gene encoding the [alpha]2 chain of the fibril-associated collagen IX, COL9A2, causes multiple epiphyseal dysplasia (EDM2). *Nature Genetics* 1996;**12**:103–5.
23. Paassilta P, Lohiniva J, Annunen S, et al. COL9A3: A third locus for multiple epiphyseal dysplasia. *American Journal of Human Genetics* 1999;**64**:1036–44.
24. Chapman KL, Mortier G, Chapman K, et al. Mutations in the region encoding the von Willebrand factor A domain of matrilin-3 are associated with multiple epiphyseal dysplasia. *Nature Genetics* 2001;**28**:393–6.
25. Prinster C, Del Maschio M, Beluffi G, et al. Diagnosis of hypochondroplasia: the role of radiological interpretation. Italian Study Group for Hypochondroplasia. *Pediatric Radiology* 2001;**31**:203.
26. Briggs MD, Choi H, Warman ML, et al. Genetic mapping of a locus for multiple epiphyseal dysplasia (EDM2) to a region of chromosome 1 containing a type IX collagen gene. *American Journal of Human Genetics* 1994;**55**:678.
27. Muragaki Y, Mariman EC, van Beersum SE, et al. A mutation in the gene encoding the alpha 2 chain of the fibril-associated collagen IX, COL9A2, causes multiple epiphyseal dysplasia (EDM2). *Nature Genetics* 1996;**12**:103.
28. Unger SL, Briggs MD, Holden P, et al. Multiple epiphyseal dysplasia: radiographic abnormalities correlated with genotype. *Pediatric Radiology* 2001;**31**:10.
29. Ramaswami U, Hindmarsh PC, Brook CG. Growth hormone therapy in hypochondroplasia. *Acta Paediatrica Supplement* 1999;**88**:116.
30. Paassilta P, Lohiniva J, Annunen S, et al. COL9A3: A third locus for multiple epiphyseal dysplasia. *American Journal of Human Genetics* 1999;**64**:1036–44.
31. Hastbacka J, de la Chapelle A, Mahtani MM, et al. The diastrophic dysplasia gene encodes a novel sulfate transporter: positional cloning by fine-structure linkage disequilibrium mapping. *Cell* 1994;**78**:1073.
32. Anderson IJ, Goldberg RB, Marion RW, et al. Spondyloepiphyseal dysplasia congenita: genetic linkage to type II collagen (COL2AI). *American Journal of Human Genetics* 1990;**46**:896.
33. Chan D, Rogers JF, Bateman JF, et al. Recurrent substitutions of arginine 789 by cysteine in proalpha 1 (II) collagen chains produce spondyloepiphyseal dysplasia congenita. *Journal of Rheumatology Supplement* 1995;**43**:37.
34. Cole WG, Hall RK, Rogers JG. The clinical features of spondyloepiphyseal dysplasia congenita resulting from the substitution of glycine 997 by serine in the alpha 1(II) chain of type II collagen. *Journal of Medical Genetics* 1993;**30**:27.
35. Crossan JF, Wynne-Davies R, Fulford GE. Bilateral failure of the capital femoral epiphysis: bilateral Perthes disease, multiple epiphyseal dysplasia, pseudoachondroplasia, and spondyloepiphyseal dysplasia congenita and tarda. *Journal of Pediatric Orthopaedics* 1983;**3**:297.
36. Nelson J. Incidence of the mucopolysaccharidoses in Northern Ireland. *Human Genetics* 1997;**101**:355.
37. Garrison RC, Unni KK, McLeod RA, et al. Chondrosarcoma arising in osteochondroma. *Cancer* 1982;**49**:1890.

38. Philippe C, Porter DE, Emerton ME, *et al.* Mutation screening of the EXT1 and EXT2 genes in patients with hereditary multiple exostoses. *American Journal of Human Genetics* 1997;**61**:520.

39. Wicklund CL, Pauli RM, Johnston D, *et al.* Natural history study of hereditary multiple exostoses. *American Journal of Human Genetics* 1995;**55**:43.

62

Bone and joint infections in children

VRISHA MADHURI, HAMISH CRAWFORD, JAMES HUNTLEY

SEPTIC ARTHRITIS	578	Aetiology and pathogenesis	582
Introduction	578	Clinical features	583
Pathogenesis and pathological anatomy	578	Clinical investigations	584
History	579	Management	584
Physical examination	579	CHRONIC OSTEOMYELITIS	586
Investigations	579	Chronic osteomyelitis: primary types	586
Differential diagnosis	580	Chronic pyogenic osteomyelitis: secondary type	587
Treatment	580	References	588
Complications and sequelae	582	Further reading	588
ACUTE HAEMATOGENOUS OSTEOMYELITIS	582		
Introduction	582		

NATIONAL BOARD STANDARDS

- Knowledge of immature bone and joint anatomy and pathological process of infection in a child; common causative organisms and special circumstances clinical findings, risk factors, indications for investigations – blood investigations plain radiographs, ultrasounds, CT scan, MRI and bone scan in infection – and their interpretation; differential diagnosis from irritable hip and other conditions
- Detailed knowledge of treatment for bone and joint infections

SEPTIC ARTHRITIS

INTRODUCTION

Bacterial infection of a joint is referred to as septic arthritis; although, strictly speaking, *any* bacterial infection might qualify, in practice the term is restricted to joint infections caused by pyogenic bacteria. Septic arthritis is more common in infants and toddlers than in older children. In infants the hips, knees, shoulders and ankles are the usual sites and often more than one joint is affected. The infection can cause permanent damage and disability if treatment is delayed; hence early recognition with prompt medical and surgical treatment is imperative.

PATHOGENESIS AND PATHOLOGICAL ANATOMY

Septic arthritis may result from haematogenous infection of the synovium, spontaneous decompression of a contiguous osteomyelitis (Fig. 62.1) or direct inoculation of a joint following trauma. In the neonate metaphyseal blood vessels extend into the epiphysis across the physis, facilitating spread of infection to the joint by this route.

In 1874 Sir Thomas Smith described patterns of joint destruction in an infant that led to partial or complete loss of the joint and resulted in a flail and weak joint with shortening of the limb. This is eponymously referred to as Tom Smith arthritis.[1] The two distinct types of destruction are:

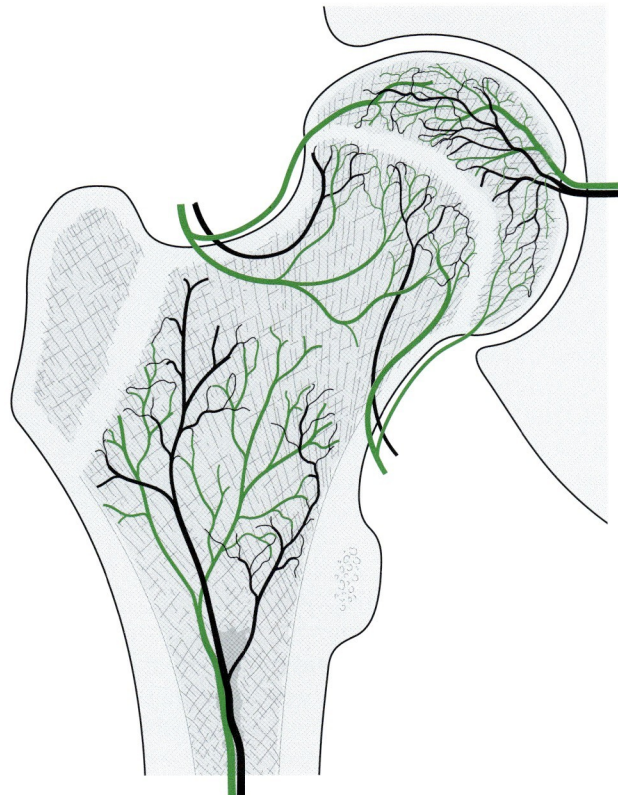

Figure 62.1 The infection is started by bacteria settling in the hairpin arterial loops and venous sinusoids at the metaphysis. The metaphyseal abscess thus formed bursts through the thin metaphyseal bone into the hip joint capsule, leading to septic arthritis.

1. destruction starting from the joint surface and proceeding inwards with rapid loss of the articular end of the bone
2. destruction originating in a subarticular bone abscess that bursts into the joint by a small opening near the margin of the articular cartilage; the knee, hip, ankle and shoulder joints are vulnerable to this process as the metaphyses of the concerned bones lie within the joint capsule.

The potential for damage in the hip is higher than in other joints owing to its anatomical peculiarity and the susceptibility of the capital femoral epiphysis to ischaemia, physeal damage and instability.

HISTORY

The presentation is acute with pain, high fever and swelling of the affected joint accompanied by irritability, malaise, anorexia and bodyache. Other features include limp, inability to weight bear and (at a later stage) refusal to move the limb. In neonates fever may not be prominent and failure to feed and immobility of the limb (pseudoparalysis) may be the only symptoms. There may be a history of trauma, a recent or concurrent illness such as chickenpox, or a focus of infection in the ear, skin or throat. Antibiotic usage can mask symptoms. Risk factors are prematurity, low birth weight, multiple invasive procedures in an intensive care unit, septicaemia, birth asphyxia, neonatal jaundice and impaired immunity.

PHYSICAL EXAMINATION

The salient features are (1) fever; (2) local warmth, erythema and oedema; (3) tender swelling of the joint; (4) positioning of the joint to accommodate more fluid, for example, flexion at the knee, flexion abduction and external rotation at the hip, and abduction at the shoulder (Fig. 62.2); (5) inability to weight bear; and (6) spasm and pain on passive joint movement.

Associated septicaemia may result in generalized constitutional disease which can be severe enough to mask local signs. Since septic arthritis can be multifocal, joints other than the affected one should also be examined, particularly those that are less accessible such as the spinal and sacroiliac joints.

INVESTIGATIONS

A white blood cell (WBC) count, erythrocyte sedimentation rate (ESR) and C-reactive protein (CRP) level should be done as preliminary investigations. WBC counts are elevated

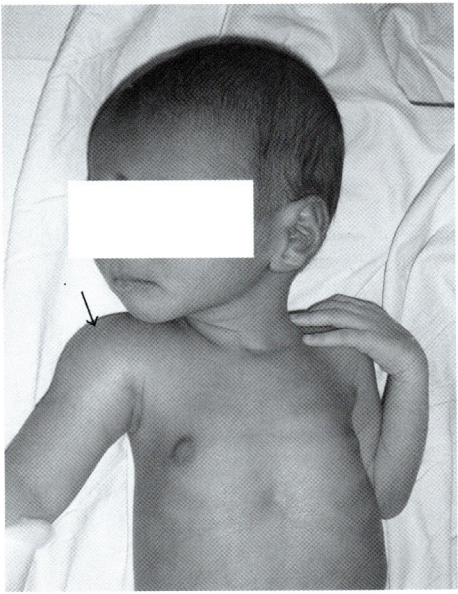

Figure 62.2 A 2 week old neonate with shoulder septic arthritis. Note the abducted attitude and circumferential swelling (arrow).

in one- to three-quarters of cases with polymorphonuclear leucocytosis and a shift to the left in more than half. ESR is very sensitive and elevated in 90% of cases but may take 3–5 days to peak and more than 3 weeks to normalize. CRP begins to rise in 6 hours; it peaks after 1–2 days and normalizes within 6–9 days and is therefore better suited for monitoring the progress of the disease. The fall of ESR and CRP is slower when there is an associated osteomyelitis. Both make good negative predictors of septic arthritis.

A plain radiograph may demonstrate early abnormalities such as joint space widening, soft-tissue oedema and obliteration of fat planes. Later in the disease joint destruction, subluxation, dislocation and adjacent osteomyelitis may be evident.

An ultrasound examination is useful as, in expert hands, it is 100% sensitive in diagnosing an effusion (Fig. 62.3). Although echogenic debris may be seen in the effusion, ultrasound cannot conclusively distinguish a sterile effusion from a septic effusion. Sonography also provides additional information such as spread in tissue planes outside the joint, a metaphyseal focus of infection or physeal separation. In deeper joints sonographic guidance can aid aspiration.

Culture of synovial fluid is key to establishing a diagnosis, but is positive in less than two-thirds of cases. *Staphylococcus aureus* is the most common pathogen found, followed by streptococci. *Haemophilus influenzae* type b used to be a frequent offender in children under 4 years but infection with this organism is declining as a result of vaccination. Neonates are more likely to have infection with Gram-negative bacilli and group B *Streptococcus*, and those with sickle cell anaemia are predisposed to *Salmonella* infection. *Kingella kingae*, a normal commensal of the oropharynx, has also been implicated in septic arthritis and osteomyelitis, especially in children younger than 4 years.[2]

A synovial WBC count of >40 000 mm^{-3} with 90% polymorphs has been regarded as indicating septic arthritis; however, the sensitivity of this criterion is only 61%, which is too low for this to be a useful screening tool. The role of bone scan, CT and MRI (Fig. 62.5) in the diagnosis of septic arthritis in children is limited, but these tools are helpful in confirming or excluding concomitant osteomyelitis.[3]

DIFFERENTIAL DIAGNOSIS

Septic arthritis needs to be differentiated from other causes of joint effusion. In older children rheumatoid arthritis and seronegative spondyloarthropathy should be excluded by looking for polyarthritis, systemic disease, eye lesions, urethritis and human leucocyte antigen B27. Other joint diseases in this age group are toxic synovitis, irritable hip and post-infectious arthritis. The Boston Children's Hospital treatment algorithm using fever, non-weight bearing ESR of at least 40 mm/hour and serum WBC count of at least 12 000 mm^{-3} found the probability of septic arthritis to be 3.0%, 40%, 93.1% and 99.6% when one, two, three or all four predictors were present. Reactive arthritis following *Yersinia*, *Salmonella* and *Chlamydia* infections (the last particularly in adolescent males) should also be considered.[4] When distinguishing septic arthritis from transient synovitis Caird *et al.*[5] found an elevation in CRP of more than 2.0 mg dL^{-1} to be a strong independent risk factor for septic arthritis of the hip.

Rheumatic fever may present as monoarthritis but can be distinguished by its flitting and fleeting arthropathy with high anti-streptolysin O titres and echocardiographic changes. Haemarthrosis can be ruled out by history, aspiration and an appropriate coagulation work-up, if indicated.

Osteomyelitis causing adjacent sympathetic effusion and joint pain can usually be ruled out by ultrasound examination. Rare differentials are acute leukaemia, viral arthritis, Henoch–Schönlein purpura and Lyme disease.

TREATMENT

Septic arthritis is a surgical emergency. Joint damage can occur as early as 8 hours after the onset of arthritis and hence bacteria and exudates must be removed without

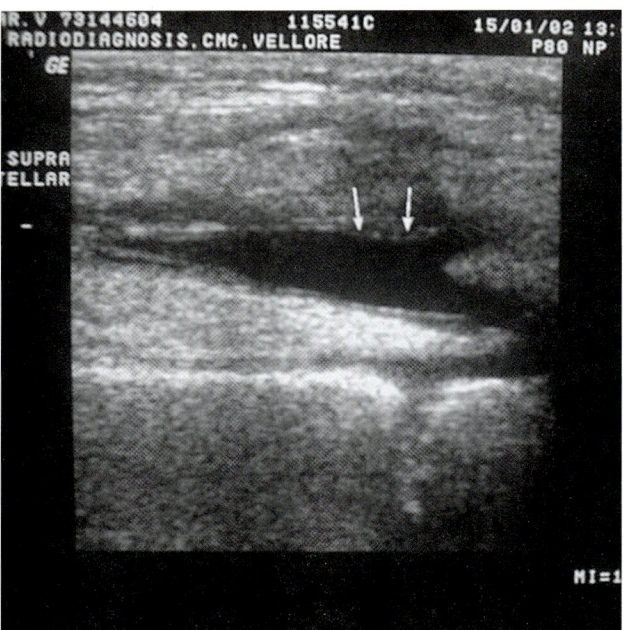

Figure 62.3 Knee joint effusion in the suprapatellar pouch (arrows) seen on ultrasound. Articular margins are well-defined echogenic surfaces with no penetration of the ultrasound waves; the physis is visualized. The synovium is visualized as a hypoechoic band of tissue. Fluid within the joint appears as anechoic. The joint capsule appears as a well-defined echogenic margin, which allows the sound beam to pass through.

delay by arthrotomy, drainage and appropriate intravenous antibiotics. If the initial joint aspiration yields pus or turbid fluid an immediate arthrotomy is indicated. Arthrotomy opens up loculated sepsis and achieves thorough drainage including that of associated soft-tissue and bone infection. A closed suction drain is inserted and removed after drainage ceases. Arthrotomy and drainage give consistently good results, especially in the first week before significant joint damage has occurred. If the joint aspirate is clear the result of a Gram-stained smear (or bacterial culture if smear examination is negative) should be awaited.

Some authors have reported lower morbidity and faster return of joint function with arthroscopy and lavage, especially in patients who have presented very early after the onset of symptoms. There also are advocates of multiple aspirations of the hip under ultrasound guidance as an alternative to surgical drainage in children presenting within 24 hours. These forms of management do not have wide acceptance as yet, require considerable judgement and need to be applied selectively if utilized.

Choice of antibiotic

Empirical antibiotic therapy is started after aspiration for culture. The antibiotic chosen should provide therapy for *Staphylococcus* and group A *Streptococcus* in all age groups as well as Gram-negative organisms in infants. In children between 6 months and 4 years the drug should also cover *H. influenzae*. In those with sickle cell anaemia, *Salmonella* organisms should be sensitive to the administered antibiotic. When dealing with patients who have received antibiotic therapy elsewhere and those who have been on chemotherapy for malignancy, there may be a higher incidence of methicillin-resistant *S. aureus* or multidrug-resistant organisms and the antibiotic protocol may need appropriate modification. Some of the recommended regimes are detailed in Table 62.1.

Mode and duration of administration

Parenteral therapy is indicated until the pathogen is isolated and its sensitivity has been determined. After this, oral medication can be commenced provided there has been an initial clinical response and the patient has no malabsorption or known abnormal drug distribution or metabolism. Compliance of oral antibiotic therapy must be monitored at least once weekly. Rapid resolution of clinical signs and symptoms coupled with normalization of CRP in 1 week in a patient who presents early indicate a 3 week course of treatment. Otherwise a 4 week course of treatment is required. If arthritis has become chronic treatment needs to be continued until the CRP level returns to normal.

A third important component of management is to rest the joint during the acutely inflamed stage and after

Table 62.1 Septic arthritis in children: the organisms and recommended antibiotics

Age	Organisms	Recommended antibiotics (first-line drugs)	Recommended antibiotics (when resistance is likely: immunocompromised, oncology patients; prolonged hospitalization; partially treated patients)
<6 months	Staphylococci Streptococci Gram-negative bacteria	Cloxacillin 200 mg kg^{-1} day^{-1} + Gentamicin 7.5 mg kg^{-1} day^{-1}	Vancomycin HCl 50 mg kg^{-1} day^{-1} + rifampicin 15 mg kg^{-1} day^{-1} or teicloplanin 12 mg kg^{-1} day^{-1} + amikacin 15 mg kg^{-1} day^{-1}
6 months–2 years	*Haemophilus influenzae* type B *Staphylococcus aureus** Streptococci	2nd and 3rd generation cephalosporins (e.g. cefuroxime 75–100 mg kg^{-1} day^{-1}, cefotaxime, ceftriaxone)	4th generation cephalosporins (e.g. cefapime) or imipenem or meropenem
>2 years	*Staphylococcus aureus* Streptococci	Cloxacillin 200 mg kg^{-1} day^{-1}	Vancomycin HCl 50 mg kg^{-1} day^{-1} + rifampicin 15 mg kg^{-1} day^{-1} or teicloplanin 12 mg kg^{-1} day^{-1}

*Methicillin-resistant *Staphylococcus aureus*: vancomycin HCl 50 mg kg^{-1} day^{-1} + (rifampicin 15 mg kg^{-1} day^{-1} or teicloplanin 12 mg kg^{-1} day^{-1}).

drainage. This can be by traction, splinting or (in an infant hip) Pavlik harness. The Pavlik harness is comfortable and allows the joint good containment, stability and mobility in a safe range.

COMPLICATIONS AND SEQUELAE

Complications are due to delay in treatment or inadequate surgical drainage. In children under 4 years weakened flail joints may occur as a consequence of Tom Smith arthritis. Other complications following septic arthritis of the hip are growth disturbances resulting in coxa breva, coxa valga or coxa vara, loss of the capital physis and joint dislocation.[6] In extreme cases, when both hip and knee are involved, the physeal damage can result in severe limb length discrepancy.[7] There may also be physeal or metaphyseal fracture and avascular necrosis of the epiphysis in those with associated osteomyelitis. Damage to the articular surface results in fibrosis, stiffness and, in extreme cases, bony ankylosis. Physeal bars, often central, are seen, and are surprisingly amenable to treatment by resection and interposition (Fig. 62.4). In patients treated early the only sequela may be coxa magna with no functional limitation.

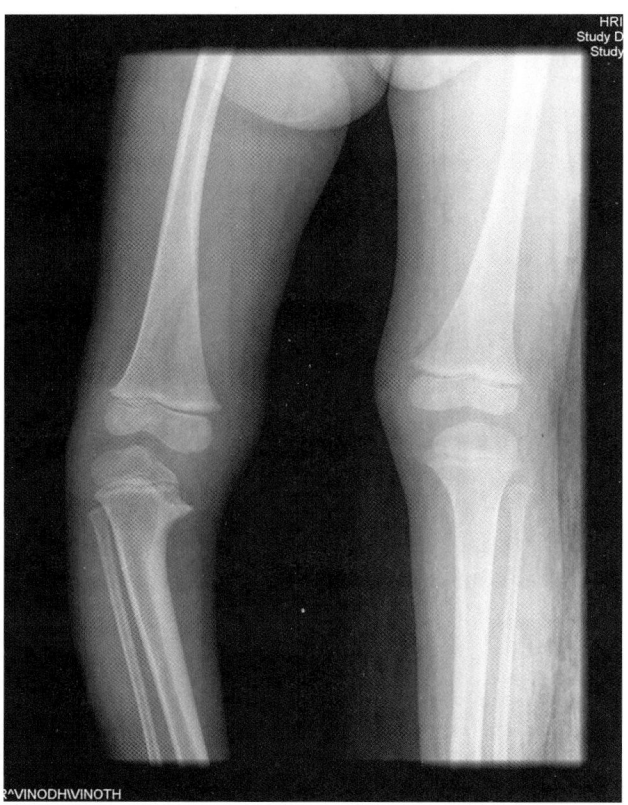

Figure 62.4 Physeal arrest medial aspect with tibia vara deformity following septic arthritis in infancy.

ACUTE HAEMATOGENOUS OSTEOMYELITIS

INTRODUCTION

The incidence of acute haematogenous osteomyelitis (AHO) in children has declined markedly in certain regions,[8] but remains common elsewhere. In the pre-antibiotic era, AHO had a mortality of 36%.[9] Today, early diagnosis and treatment with intravenous antibiotics are essential to the vastly improved outcome. The predominant organism remains *S. aureus*. In infants there has been a decrease in infantile infections due to *H. influenzae* but the number of *K. kingae* infections is increasing. In some regions, methicillin-resistant *S. aureus* (MRSA) is a significant cause.[10] Key points in the management are given in Box 62.1.

> **BOX 62.1: Key points in the management of acute haematogenous osteomyelitis (AHO)**
>
> - Suspect AHO in a child who is systemically unwell (especially fever) with bone pain or a limp
> - Early referral and prompt diagnosis and treatment of patients with probable AHO improves outcomes
> - Aggressive parenteral antibiotic; choice based on:
>   – the age of the child
>   – the most likely organisms
> - Imaging, especially MRI, to assess site of infection/collections and delineate any surgical approach
> - Treatment with intravenous antibiotics may need to be prolonged: until the clinical symptoms and signs have improved

AETIOLOGY AND PATHOGENESIS

AHO usually develops in the metaphysis of long bones (most commonly the tibia and femur) after a bacteraemia. Trauma is an important predisposing factor.[9,11] Acute infection in metaphyseal cancellous bone may progress through the cortex, forming a subperiosteal abscess. This can breach the periosteum to track externally. Alternatively, a subperiosteal collection may deprive some cortical bone of blood supply – with dead cortical bone forming a sequestrum. In joints having an intra-articular metaphysis (the hip, shoulder, elbow and knee), osteomyelitis can easily progress to a septic arthritis. In the neonate, transphyseal blood vessels allow infection to spread to the epiphysis. A high proportion (60–100%) of neonates with septic arthritis have an associated osteomyelitis.[12]

Panton–Valentine leucocidin (PVL) is an exotoxin, secreted by some *S. aureus* strains, toxic to neutrophils. PVL may be responsible for increased severity of musculoskeletal

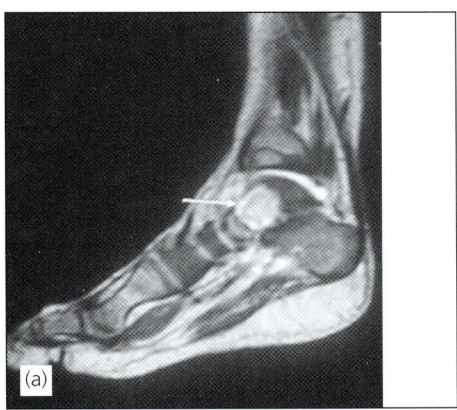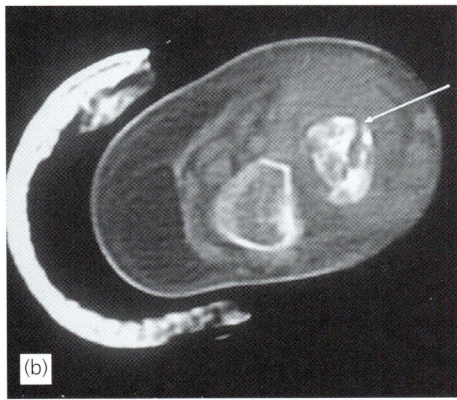

Figure 62.5 This child with acute lymphatic leukaemia was diagnosed with septic arthritis of the ankle. The talus osteomyelitis was picked up 6 weeks later on radiographs. At that stage: (a) T_2 density MRI shows increased signal density and anterior cortical breech and minimal fluid in the ankle; (b) CT scan shows a cortical break with high density and low signal intensity around, indicating an abscess.

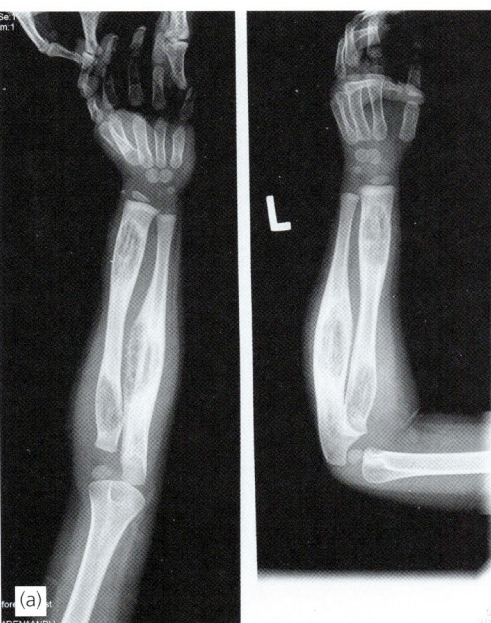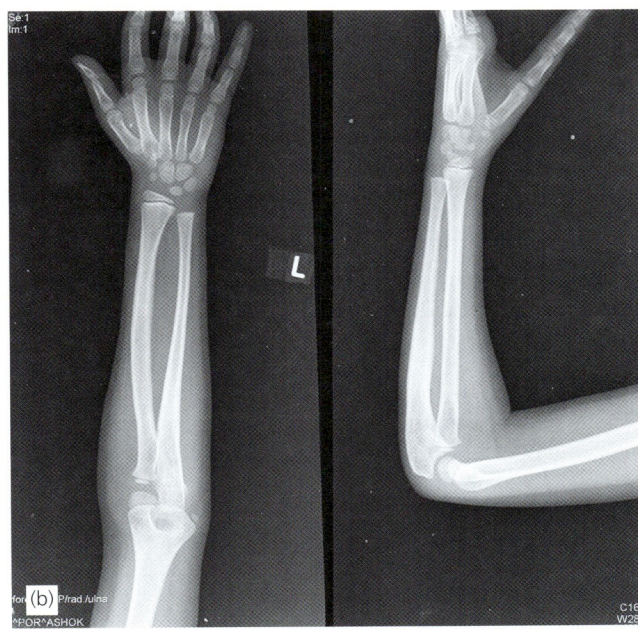

Figure 62.6 (a) Spina ventosa lesions in the forearm of a 4 year old show fusiform expansion with ballooning of the forearm shaft, dense periosteal reaction and destruction of underlying bone (*spina*, short bone; *ventosa*, filled with air). (b) The forearm bones show excellent remodelling after healing.

sepsis.[13,14] In practice, we have not yet found PVL status to be a helpful guide to management.

CLINICAL FEATURES

Bone pain, tenderness and fever indicate osteomyelitis until investigations show another cause (Box 62.2). Antalgic gait and general malaise are other features. However, in immunocompromised and neonatal patients there may be few features until the condition is well advanced. Bone pain is an indication to investigate and treat aggressively for presumed osteomyelitis. Pelvic osteomyelitis has a large differential, including psoas abscess, urinary tract infection, septic arthritis hip, appendicitis and gynaecological conditions.

BOX 62.2: Acute osteomyelitis: differential diagnosis

- Septic arthritis
- Non-septic arthritis, including juvenile idiopathic arthritis
- Transient synovitis
- Neoplasia: Ewing's sarcoma, osteosarcoma, leukaemia (Fig. 62.5), metastatic neuroblastoma
- Langerhan's cell histiocytosis
- Sickle cell disease
- Fracture (especially in the neuromuscular patient)
- Avascular necrosis: Perthes disease, haemophilia, infarct
- Gaucher disease
- Haemarthrosis, e.g. haemophilia

CLINICAL INVESTIGATIONS

These include blood tests (CRP, ESR, WBC count and blood cultures) and imaging (plain films, MRI, bone scan and ultrasound) (Box 62.3).

> **BOX 62.3: Investigation and management of suspected acute osteomyelitis**
>
> - Investigations:
>   — Blood tests: full blood count, erythrocyte sedimentation rate, C-reactive protein, cultures
>   — Imaging: plain radiographs
>   — Consider bone aspiration
>   — Further imaging: consider MRI/bone scan
> - Management:
>   — Intravenous antibiotics
>   — Rest/elevation
>   — Reassessment
>   — Further imaging if deterioration
>   — Consider surgical drainage
>   — Adjust antibiotics in light of clinical changes and culture results

1. *CRP.* This is raised in 98% of patients at admission.[15] A value in the normal range does not preclude infection, especially in neonates and patients with comorbidities (e.g. immunocompromise, anaemia, sickle cell disease).
2. *ESR.* This is >20 mm h^{-1} in approximately 80% of cases,[10] but is non-specific.
3. *WBC count.* The differential may show a left shift, but is an unreliable indicator of bone infection, being elevated in only 35–40% of cases.[16] Leukaemia must be considered as a potential diagnosis in a young child with bone pain and fever. The blood film and WBC count will help with this diagnosis.
4. *Blood cultures.* These are only positive in 30–50% of patients with AHO.[16]
5. *Plain radiographs.* These are usually normal in the first 7–10 days of AHO, but are useful in the differential diagnosis. Later, periosteal elevation with resorption and/or new bone formation may occur.
6. *Bone scan.* This is useful if the infection is multifocal, or the site is hard to localize.[17] A cold scan may indicate either that the disease process is not well advanced or that there is hypoperfusion, as in osteonecrosis.
7. *MRI* (Fig. 62.7). This is the most sensitive test for osteomyelitis (97–100%) and has a specificity of 73–92%. It defines (1) soft-tissue extension, (2) intra-osseous collection, (3) joint involvement and (4) planning for the surgical approach.[18,19]
8. *Bone aspiration.* This accurately identifies the infecting organism in 75–80% of cases.[16] Some surgeons advocate aspiration before starting the parenteral antibiotics. However, aspiration usually involves sedation or a general anaesthetic, which delays the start of treatment. We do not routinely aspirate bone before starting antibiotics but start antibiotics as soon as the diagnosis is suspected – and then image the child with either MRI or bone scan. If an abscess is present that requires surgical drainage, specimens are attained at that stage, with the proviso that antibiotics may make isolation of the organism impossible. Conversely, in regions where MRSA is a significant cause of AHO, bone aspiration may be useful; initial treatment can be with vancomycin, and this can be changed when other organisms are found to be responsible.

MANAGEMENT

The aims of treatment are:

1. to prevent overwhelming sepsis
2. to cure the local disease as rapidly as possible
3. to prevent complications (growth plate damage, pathological fracture, osteonecrosis, deep vein thrombosis and chronic osteomyelitis).

Prompt diagnosis and appropriate intravenous antibiotics can lead to complete resolution with no further sequelae. However, AHO can be awkward to treat as its presentation and manifestations are so variable. Three factors to consider are: (1) the patient, (2) the organism and (3) the bone.

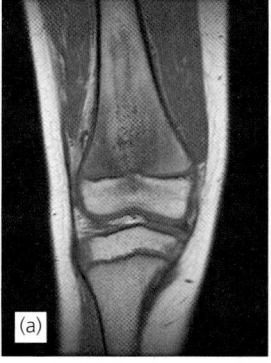
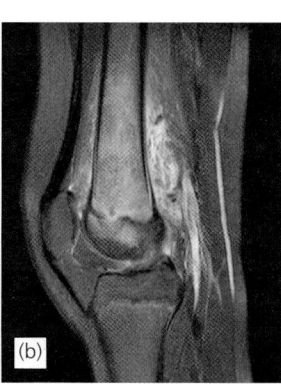
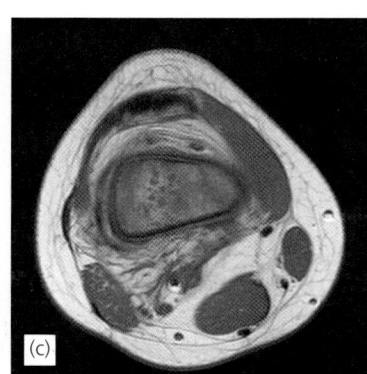

Figure 62.7 (a–c) Non-contrast magnetic resonance scans in a 5 year old boy presenting with a 24 hour history of limp, fever and distal thigh pain.

The patient

Bone infection occurs predominantly in lower socioeconomic classes, and delayed presentation in this group is common. As a result, the infection is well established before treatment has started. Complications (Box 62.4) are therefore more likely. Other patients presenting late are the immunocompromised (e.g. on steroids), the neuromuscular group ('bone pain' misdiagnosed as a fracture) and the neonate (clinical signs can be few; also often present with a pseudoparalysis). If there are significant comorbidities, the clinical course is less predictable – patients with diabetes mellitus, haemoglobinopathies, chronic renal disease or rheumatoid arthritis will often require intravenous antibiotics for 2–3 months.

> **BOX 62.4: Acute haematogenous osteomyelitis: complications**
>
> - Overwhelming sepsis
> - Deep vein thrombosis
> - Septic thrombus and pulmonary septic emboli
> - Pathological fracture
> - Antibiotic complications: neutropenia
> - Chronic osteomyelitis
> - Growth disturbance

Patients with sickle disease have an increased risk of osteomyelitis, and are more prone to complications.[20] It can be difficult to distinguish a sickle crisis from AHO, but fever and raised ESR suggest infection. *S. aureus* remains the most common pathogen, but *Salmonella* must also be covered.

The organism

S. aureus is the commonest infecting organism (Table 62.2). Other organisms should be considered in certain age groups and patient groups; this knowledge is paramount

Table 62.2 Common pathogens by age, and appropriate antibiotic

	Organism	Antibiotic
Neonate	*Streptococcus*	Cefotaxime, or oxacillin and gentamicin
	Staphylococcus aureus	
	Coliforms: Gram-negative bacilli	
Infant/child	*Staphylococcus aureus*	Oxacillin and ampicillin
Sickle cell disease	*Salmonella*	Cefotaxime or chloramphenicol

to appropriate antibiotic selection. If the patient is slow to improve, other organisms such as *H. influenzae* and *K. kingae* need to be considered. In some areas, community-acquired MRSA is a significant cause.

The bone

Infection of the metaphysis of proximal tibia and distal femur (most common sites) is relatively straightforward to diagnose and treat. Diaphyseal extension is uncommon if AHO is treated early; therefore, whole bone osteomyelitis and its sequelae are rare. AHO of the pelvis, clavicle and calcaneus/talus is less common, so diagnosis is often delayed. These bones are also largely cancellous, which may make eradication awkward and treatment prolonged.

Antibiotics should be given early, on the assumption of AHO. The patient needs to be monitored closely with assessment of vital signs, range of movement and pain. Deterioration or lack of response requires consideration of repeat imaging, debridement or a change in antibiotics. A repeat MRI is useful to identify further collections (intraosseus or subperiosteal) or spread of infection. Infected deep vein thromboses may be visualized in vessels abutting AHO, which may result in septic embolization and require anticoagulation.[21]

C-REACTIVE PROTEIN

Values during treatment can be useful to monitor control of infection.[9] With concordant clinical findings, a declining CRP indicates when a change from intravenous to oral antibiotics is appropriate (Box 62.5). For uncomplicated AHO, the CRP is likely to have normalized by day 9. Antibiotic treatment should be continued orally for a total of at least 3–4 weeks, although intravenous antibiotics may be discontinued after clinical normalization (often <1 week).

> **BOX 62.5: Factors to consider for switching from parenteral to oral antibiotics**
>
> - The patient: immunocompromised *vs* healthy
> - The organism: *Staphylococcus aureus vs Escherichia coli*, *Pseudomonas*, methicillin-resistant *Staphylococcus aureus*
> - The bone: proximal tibia *vs* pelvis, clavicle, calcaneus
> - The clinical response: rapid clinical improvement *vs* repeat surgical debridement

LENGTH OF TREATMENT

The clinical course must be closely monitored, with surgical interventions and antibiotics used appropriately. In resistant/intractable cases and compromised hosts, intravenous antibiotics should be continued until all clinical features are resolved (antibiotic treatment time may need to be extended to between 6 and 12 weeks).

SURGICAL INTERVENTION

If an abscess is localized by MRI, then surgical debridement is mandatory. The surgical approach is guided by the imaging. Occasionally, small abscesses in difficult locations can be drained percutaneously with the help of ultrasound guidance or CT scanning, e.g. pelvic osteomyelitis. The bone does not usually need to be 'drilled' as part of the debridement, as usually the intraosseous collection has decompressed into a subperiosteal collection. We leave large drains in the wounds following debridement and close the skin edges loosely with sutures. The patient returns to the operating room 24–48 hours later, for a repeat washout/debridement. Definitive closure is performed only when the infection is controlled. If a large amount of pus is still present at the 'second look', the wound is left open and a suction dressing applied.

OUTPATIENT REVIEW

We generally review patients at 3, 6 and 12 weeks, for clinical examination, plain radiography and blood investigations (WBC count, ESR and CRP). Patients on home flucloxacillin have weekly liver function tests and neutrophil counts, as there is a high rate of flucloxacillin-associated neutropenia.

CHRONIC OSTEOMYELITIS

The term chronic is applied to osteomyelitis in two situations: (1) when an acute (pyogenic) infection becomes persistent and (2) when the inflammation is of low grade from the outset. The former may be termed *secondary* chronic osteomyelitis whereas the latter can be regarded as *primary*.

CHRONIC OSTEOMYELITIS: PRIMARY TYPES

Brodie's abscess

This is an insidiously developing chronic pyogenic osteomyelitis often occurring in the upper tibial metaphysis. Since it is a localized form of suppuration it may also be termed a chronic bone abscess. Although often referred to as a subacute form of osteomyelitis the lesion may persist for many years. In fact the case described by Sir Benjamin Brodie in 1832 had a 12 year history. It is the result of infection by organisms of low virulence in immunocompetent hosts.[1]

Usually trivial trauma draws the patient's attention to the lesion and intermittent mild to severe pain and mild swelling are the presenting features. The ESR and WBC count are often normal. The usual radiographic picture is that of a circumscribed lytic lesion with a sclerotic margin. The latter typically has a sharp inner border and a hazy outer zone. Bone scan shows increased localized uptake.

Because of these findings the most important aspect of Brodie's abscess is the differential diagnosis, which includes benign tumours or tumour-like conditions such as osteoid osteoma, eosinophilic granuloma, non-ossifying fibroma, enchondroma and unicameral bone cyst as well as malignancies such as leukaemia and Ewing's sarcoma. Investigation with CT and MRI as for tumours is required. The penumbra sign, a hyperintense rim around the main cavity on T_1-weighted MRI, helps to distinguish infection from other lesions. The diagnosis can be confirmed on biopsy when clinical and radiographic findings are non-specific. Treatment is by curettage and appropriate antibiotics.

Sclerosing osteomyelitis

In chronic osteomyelitis, destructive (necroinflammatory) and reparative (new bone formation) processes are usually present side by side. However, in some cases, the latter markedly predominate, resulting in a form of osteomyelitis whose main, if not sole, feature is osteosclerosis. This type is difficult to diagnose with confidence because cultures are often negative. The lack of inflammation means that biopsy is also often unhelpful in this regard. The differential diagnosis includes osteoid osteoma and other bone lesions associated with marked sclerosis.

Chronic recurrent multifocal osteomyelitis

This is a chronic osteomyelitis of uncertain cause. Bone pains and fever are the presenting features and there is an association with inflammatory processes of the skin (usually palmoplantar pustulosis or psoriasis vulgaris) and gastrointestinal tract (most often Crohn disease or ulcerative colitis). Laboratory findings are non-diagnostic. Plain radiographs show metaphyseal or diaphyseal osteolytic lesions surrounded by sclerosis. Biopsies are consistent with osteomyelitis, but cultures are almost always negative. Similar lesions in children may receive the diagnosis of SAPHO (synovitis, acne, pustulosis, hyperostosis and osteitis) syndrome. Although the clinical pictures are different, these two diseases are part of the same spectrum. A genetic component is implicated.

Tuberculous osteomyelitis

Tuberculosis is a major cause of skeletal infection in the developing world. In the developed world there is a resurgence of this disease because of AIDS, homelessness, a decline in tuberculosis control programmes and immigration. The causative organism is *Mycobacterium tuberculosis*, a slowly dividing acid-fast bacillus.

PATHOLOGY

The source is often unknown, a concurrent pulmonary focus being seen in less than 50% of cases. The sparse bacilli in the lesion are engulfed by macrophages, which cluster together and transform into epithelioid granulomas. The latter undergo necrosis and a continuation of this process results in gradual destruction of the affected bone and eventual extension of granulomatous inflammation into the surrounding soft tissues. Sequestra are not often seen in tuberculosis, but when present are coarse and sandy.

CLINICAL FEATURES AND INVESTIGATIONS

Systemic features of low-grade fever and loss of weight and appetite are coupled with local pain, tenderness, swelling and decreased range of motion. However, the lesion may remain asymptomatic and be unmasked only by minor trauma. Solitary involvement is the usual presentation, but multifocal and disseminated bone involvement can occur. The metaphysis of long bones is commonly involved. A cold abscess, muscle wasting and enlarged regional matted lymph nodes may also be seen.

Relevant investigations include a local radiograph, chest radiograph and a Mantoux test. Radiographically, four basic patterns of bony lesions are described: cystic, infiltrative, focal erosions and spina ventosa (Fig. 62.6) or tuberculous dactylitis (*spina*, short bone; *ventosa*, filled with air). There are no pathognomonic features on radiographs, but osteopenia and a soft-tissue shadow are common, and periosteal reactions may be seen in the spina ventosa (Fig. 62.6) and infiltrative varieties.[22] Lesions can cross the physis but may not cause growth arrest.

The ESR is mildly elevated and the tuberculin test is usually positive. Biopsy of the lesion is the most valuable diagnostic test, the best area for biopsy being from a cystic lesion. Direct identification of mycobacteria with the Ziehl–Neelsen stain is usually not possible as bacilli are frequently scanty. However, in endemic areas the presence of epithelioid granulomas, particularly if accompanied by caseation, can be regarded as consistent with tuberculosis. Polymerase chain reaction is another sensitive and specific test that can be used for diagnosis. Culture of the organism is the most sensitive and specific but takes up to 6 weeks.

DIFFERENTIAL DIAGNOSIS

Tuberculosis mimics a number of other diseases in children, such as subacute and chronic pyogenic osteomyelitis, fungal infections, cartilaginous tumours, osteoid osteoma, eosinophilic granuloma, non-ossifying fibroma, metastatic neuroblastoma, desmoplastic fibroma and Ewing's sarcoma. These are usually excluded by biopsy of the lesion.

TREATMENT

Multiagent chemotherapy is the mainstay. Using four agents for 2 months for the intensive phase and two agents for 4 months for the maintenance phase is recommended, and the prognosis is good with modern chemotherapy. The World Health Organization has recommended a regime for the treatment of skeletal tuberculosis.[23] Curettage and drainage may be required as an ancillary treatment and speeds up the healing process.

CHRONIC PYOGENIC OSTEOMYELITIS: SECONDARY TYPE

Introduction

In infants and children this form of chronic osteomyelitis is the result of failed/delayed diagnosis or treatment. It is unusual in developed countries but is common where resources are limited. Early and adequate surgical drainage and excision of any sequestra combined with early appropriate antibiotic therapy is key to preventing acute osteomyelitis from becoming chronic. If there is persistent elevation of CRP 14 days after institution of therapy, chronic osteomyelitis is likely. Radiographs at this stage also show changes such as periosteal elevation, lytic areas and sequestrum formation.

Pathological anatomy and clinical presentation

The hallmark of chronicity is the *sequestrum* – a portion of bone, usually cortical, which has undergone necrosis as a result of septic infarction. Its size varies markedly and in severe cases the entire shaft of a long bone may become necrotic. The sequestrum is often surrounded by a sleeve of sclerotic, relatively avascular, reactive new bone (termed the *involucrum*), which in turn is covered by thickened periosteum, scarred muscle and subcutaneous tissue. Holes in the involucrum (called cloacae) lead into draining sinuses within the soft tissues. Small sequestra or fragments thereof may be discharged through the sinuses. Recurrent fever and pain ensue when these sinuses are periodically blocked by granulation tissue.

Management

Thorough surgical debridement, saucerization of bone to ensure adequate drainage of any cavity, and appropriate antibiotic therapy are the mainstays of treatment. In children, management along these lines usually produces clinical improvement because of their excellent bone-healing capacity. Rarely, restoration of a well-vascularized soft-tissue envelope by local or distant muscle/myocutaneous/cutaneous flaps may be necessary.

Sequelae

These include growth arrest, deformity, pathological fracture, limb length discrepancy, scarring of skin, recurrent ulceration and stiffness of adjacent joints. Squamous cell carcinoma (arising from a chronic sinus) and amyloidosis are well-recognized late complications.

REFERENCES

1. Rang M. *The Story of Orthopaedics*. Philadelphia, PA: W.B. Saunders, 2000: 203–20.
2. Ryan MJ Kavanagh R, Wall PG, Hazleman BL. Bacterial joint infections in England and Wales: analysis of bacterial isolates over a four year period. *British Journal of Rheumatology* 1997;**36**:370–3.
3. McGillicuddy DC, Shah KH, Friedberg RP, *et al*. How sensitive is the synovial fluid WBC count. *American Journal of Emergency Medicine* 2007;**7**:749–52.
4. Kocher MS, Mandiga R, Zurakowski D, *et al*. Validation of a clinical prediction rule for the differentiation between septic arthritis and transient synovitis of the hip in children. *Journal of Bone and Joint Surgery (American)* 2004;**86**:1629–35.
5. Caird MS, Flynn JM, Leung YL, *et al*. Factors distinguishing septic arthritis from transient arthritis of the hip in children. *Journal of Bone and Joint Surgery (American)* 2006;**88A**:1251–7.
6. Eyre-Brook AL. Septic arthritis of the hip and osteomyelitis of the upper end of the femur in infants. *Journal of Bone and Joint Surgery (British)* 1960;**42B**:11–20.
7. Choi H, Yoo WJ, Cho TJ, Chung CY. Operative reconstruction for septic arthritis of the hip. *Orthopaedic Clinics of North America* 2006;**37**:173–83.
8. Blyth MJG, Kincaid R, Craigen MAC, Bennet GC. The changing epidemiology of acute and subacute haematogenous osteomyelitis in children. *Journal of Bone and Joint Surgery (British)* 2001;**83B**:99–102.
9. White M, Dennison WM. Acute haematogenous osteomyelitis in childhood. *Journal of Bone and Joint Surgery (British)* 1952;**34B**:608–23.
10. Arnold SR, Elias D, Buckingham SC, *et al*. Changing patterns of acute hematogenous osteomyelitis and septic arthritis: emergence of community-associated methicillin-resistant Staphylococcus aureus. *Journal of Pediatric Orthopaedics* 2006;**26**:703–8.
11. Whalen JL, Fitzgerald Jr RH, Morrissy JT. A histological study of acute hematogenous osteomyelitis following physeal injuries in rabbits. *Journal of Bone and Joint Surgery (American)* 1988;**70A**:1383–92.
12. Shaw BA, Kasser JR. Acute septic arthritis in infancy and childhood. *Clinical Orthopaedics and Related Research* 1990;**257**:212–25.
13. Dohin B, Gillet Y, Kohler R, *et al*. Pediatric bone and joint infections caused by Panton-Valentine leukocidin-positive Staphylococcus aureus. *Pediatric Infectious Disease Journal* 2007;**6**:1042–8.
14. Mitchell PD, Hunt DM, Lyall H, *et al*. Panton-Valentine leukocidin-secreting Staphylococcus aureus causing severe musculoskeletal sepsis in children. A new threat. *Journal of Bone and Joint Surgery (British)* 2007;**89B**:1239–42.
15. Unkila-Kallio L, Kallio MJ, Eskola J, Peltola H. Serum C-reactive protein, erythrocyte sedimentation rate, and white blood cell count in acute haematogenous osteomyelitis of children. *Pediatrics* 1994;**93**:59–62.
16. Karwowska A, Davies HD, Jadavji T. Epidemiology and outcome of osteomyelitis in the era of sequential intravenous-oral therapy. *Pediatric Infectious Disease Journal* 1998;**17**:1021–6.
17. Jaramillo D, Treves ST, Kasser JR, *et al*. Osteomyelitis and septic arthritis in children: appropriate use of imaging to guide treatment. *AJR American Journal of Roentgenology* 1995;**165**:399–403.
18. Unger E, Moldofsky P, Gatenby R, *et al*. Diagnosis of osteomyelitis by MR imaging. *AJR American Journal of Roentgenology* 1988;**150**:605–10.
19. Mazur JM, Ross G, Cummings J, *et al*. Usefulness of magnetic resonance imaging for the diagnosis of acute musculoskeletal infections in children. *Journal of Pediatric Orthopaedics* 1995;**15**:144–7.
20. Epps CH, Bryant D'OD, Coles MJM, Castro O. Osteomyelitis in patients who have sickle-cell disease. Diagnosis and management. *Journal of Bone and Joint Surgery (American)* 1991;**81A**:1029–34.
21. Hollmig ST, Copley LA, Browne RH, *et al*. Deep venous thrombosis associated with osteomyelitis in children. *Journal of Bone and Joint Surgery (American)* 2007;**65A**:431–7.
22. Rasool MN. Osseous manifestations of tuberculosis in children. *Journal of Pediatric Orthopaedics* 2001;**21**:749–55.
23. World Health Organization. *Treatment of Tuberculosis: Guidelines for National Programmes*. Geneva, Switzerland: WHO, 2003:27–39.

FURTHER READING

Nade S. Bone and joint infections in childhood. *Current Paediatrics* 1996;**6**:9–15.

//

Juvenile idiopathic arthritis

TRACY V TING, BRENT GRAHAM

Introduction	589
Definition	589
Epidemiology	589
Aetiology	590
Pathophysiology	590
Clinical manifestations	591
Laboratory findings	593
Radiography	594
Treatment	594
Prognosis and outcomes	595
References	595

INTRODUCTION

Juvenile idiopathic arthritis (JIA) is one of the most common chronic autoimmune disorders in children. It is the most common childhood rheumatic disease. Formerly known as juvenile rheumatoid arthritis (JRA) and juvenile chronic arthritis (JCA), JIA is now the widely accepted terminology. Under the new criteria, JIA consists of seven different subtypes: oligoarticular (persistent or extended), polyarticular (rheumatoid factor (RF) negative and positive), systemic, enthesitis-related, psoriatic and other (Box 63.1).[1,2]

DEFINITION

JIA occurs in children with at least 6 weeks' duration of persistent arthritis with symptom onset occurring at <16 years old. Arthritis is defined as swelling or, in the absence of swelling, limitation of motion accompanied by pain with motion, tenderness or warmth.[3] JIA is diagnosed by both clinical history and examination. Onset of symptoms is often insidious and painless (relative to other types of arthritis); therefore, a high level of suspicion must be maintained in order to make the diagnosis in a timely manner. Several patients will present initially to the orthopaedist for evaluation of limp, swelling, joint contracture or joint pain. JIA is a group of highly heterogeneous disorders requiring a thorough knowledge of the signs and symptoms of the disease and the course and progression of each subtype in order to correctly make a diagnosis.

EPIDEMIOLOGY

JIA has an incidence of approximately 3–10 cases per 100 000 per year.[4,5] The prevalence is reported at ~1 per 1000 children.[4,6] Sex and age of onset differ by subtype, but overall girls are affected twice as often as boys with an average age of onset at 4 years for girls and 10 years for boys.[7] Girls tend to develop anterior eye disease (uveitis) associated with arthritis more commonly than boys (8:1).[8] With regard to racial differences, JIA seems to occur more commonly in Caucasians, with a lower prevalence in African American and Asian populations.[9] Phenotypic differences also occur across racial groups, with African American children having a lower incidence of antinuclear antibodies (ANAs) and uveitis but a higher rate of RF positivity and older age at onset than Caucasian children.[10] Seasonal variation has not been consistently seen across all subtypes, but may occur with systemic JIA.[11]

AETIOLOGY

The aetiology of JIA remains unknown. It has been hypothesized to be due to a combination of genetic factors, environmental triggers and dysregulated immune mechanisms. There often is a recent history of viral illness at the onset of symptoms. Proposed environmental triggers include common infections of the upper respiratory tract

> **BOX 63.1: Classification criteria for juvenile idiopathic arthritis (International League of Associations for Rheumatology, Durban, 1997)**
>
> By definition: arthritis of ⩾1 joint of >6 weeks' duration with onset occurring in a child <16 years old
> 1. Oligoarticular
>   A. A Persistent arthritis: ⩽4 joints involved
>   B. B Extended arthritis: initial presentation with ⩽4 joints involved, but after 6 months of disease extends to include ⩾5 joints
> 2. Polyarticular (RF negative)
>   C. Arthritis involves ⩾5 joints within first 6 months of presentation; RF testing is negative
> 3. Polyarticular (RF positive)
>   D. Arthritis involves ⩾5 joints within first 6 months of presentation; RF testing is positive on at least two occasions (over 3 months)
> 4. Systemic-onset arthritis
>   Arthritis associated with daily fevers of ⩾2 weeks' duration with at least one of the following:
>   E. A Generalized lymphadenopathy
>   F. B Maculopapular (salmon-coloured) evanescent, non-fixed rash
>   G. C Hepatosplenomegaly
>   H. D Serositis
> 5. Enthesitis-related arthritis
>   Arthritis and enthesitis or either arthritis or enthesitis with two of the following:
>   I. A Presence of HLA-B27
>   J. B Sacroiliac joint pain or inflammatory spinal pain
>   K. C HLA-B27-associated disease (IBD, spondyloarthropathy, painful anterior uveitis) in a first-degree relative
>   L. D Acute red, painful anterior uveitis associated with photophobia
>   M. E Onset of arthritis in a boy >8 years old
> 6. Psoriatic arthritis
>   Arthritis and psoriasis or arthritis with two of the following:
>   N. A Nail changes (onycholysis or pitting)
>   O. B Dactylitis (typically great MTP)
>   P. C Psoriasis in first-degree relative
> 7. Undifferentiated
>   Q. A Patients who do not fit any of the specific subtypes above
>   R. B Patients who fit criteria for more than one subtype
>
> HLA, human leucocyte antigen; IBD, inflammatory bowel disease; MTP, metatarsal phalanges; RF, rheumatoid factor.
> Adapted from Petty et al.[2]

or gastrointestinal system, although these have not been proven to be causal. Epstein–Barr virus (EBV), rubella, influenza A and chlamydial infections have been implicated as possible triggers associated with the onset of JIA.[12–15] Also, parvovirus B19 has been isolated from synovial fluid in patients with JIA.[16]

While there are reported cases of familial disease, JIA is often an isolated process and infrequently occurs among siblings.[17,18] However, there does appear to be a greater recurrence risk for developing JIA in first-degree relatives.[19] Furthermore, there is a strong familial history of other autoimmune disorders.[20] Recent studies have revealed the role of multiple human leucocyte antigen (HLA) loci and non-HLA-associated genes in the complexity of genetic involvement in JIA.[21–25]

PATHOPHYSIOLOGY

Over time (~2 years), chronic inflammation and accumulation of synovial fluid and synovial thickening can lead to progressive bony changes and erosions, if left untreated. It has been found that an increase in cytokine production, including tumour necrosis factor α (TNF-α) and interleukin 15 (IL-15), appears to play a major role in the pathogenesis of JIA.[26,27] In systemic JIA, cytokines IL-1, IL-6 and TNF-α are markedly elevated and are currently areas targeted for medication therapy.[28]

Synovial fluid in patients with JIA is notably thin compared with the normal thick, yellow fluid, with little mucin clotting. It contains abundant neutrophils, plasma cells, dendritic cells, T cells, cytokines and complement cleavage products. In the acute stage, synovium is hypervascular with abundant lymphocyte and polymorphonuclear leucocyte production. Pannus production, inflammatory cell induction of synoviocyte proliferation and invasion of the synovial tissue, leads to significant destruction of the cartilage. Rice bodies are small, white pieces of fibrin that occasionally can be found within the joint fluid.

Pannus destruction of cartilage is followed by subchondral bone loss. Osteopenia is also a potential complication. Bony erosions are secondary to aggressive osteoclast activity and occur primarily at synovial attachment sites. Patients with polyarticular and systemic JIA tend to be most commonly affected with more aggressive bony involvement. Bony erosion is rare in prepubertal children.

Increased vascularity of affected joints leads to alteration of linear growth, with the involved joint/limb growing at an accelerated rate in prepubertal and pubertal children with open physes. This phenomenon is most commonly seen about the knee. Aggressive medical treatment of the arthritis minimizes this complication.[29] With long-term and poorly controlled disease, accelerated maturation occurs over time and leads to early closure of the physis. Thus, the affected bones are shorter. This result is most commonly seen in the forearm and digits. The mandibular bone grows by enchondral ossification. Consequently, temporomandibular joint arthritis leads to mandibular undergrowth.

Table 63.1 Recommendations for eye screening of uveitis in juvenile idiopathic arthritis

Age at onset (years)	Type	ANA	Duration	Frequency of eye examination (risk)
≤6	Oligo or poly	+	≤4 years	Every 3 months (high)
		+	>4 years	Every 6 months (moderate)
		+	>7 years	Every 12 months (low)
		−	≤4 years	Every 6 months (moderate)
		−	>4 years	Every 12 months (low)
	Systemic		Any	Every 12 months (low)
>6	Oligo or poly	+	≤4 years	Every 6 months (moderate)
		+	>4 years	Every 12 months (low)
		−		Any	Every 12 months (low)
	Systemic		Any	Every 12 months (low)

ANA, anti-nuclear antibody; oligo, oligoarticular juvenile idiopathic arthritis; poly, polyarticular juvenile idiopathic arthritis.
Adapted from Cassidy et al.[31]

CLINICAL MANIFESTATIONS

Oligoarticular JIA

PERSISTENT OLIGOARTICULAR ARTHRITIS

This is the most common subtype of JIA, representing ~40–60% of JIA cases. It typically occurs in girls (5:1) aged 1–3 years old, with fair skin and light eye colour. Oligoarticular disease involves arthritis in four or fewer joints, with the large joints (knees, ankles, wrists and elbows) most commonly affected. Children rarely present with hip involvement.

The history of presentation is common for the insidious onset of a limp or abnormal gait. There are often complaints of mild swelling or tenderness and warmth. Erythema is not typical. A history of trauma might be present but may be coincidental. Parental report of morning stiffness is also typical. Septic arthritis should be ruled out. Typically, urgent joint aspiration is not required if the patient presents insidiously and does not have fever, leucocytosis, severely painful motion or significantly elevated inflammatory markers (erythrocyte sedimentation rate (ESR) of >40 mm h^{-1}). However, in unclear cases, joint aspiration should be undertaken to rule out a septic joint.

Patients with oligoarthritis more commonly (than other subtypes) have a positive ANA test (of at least 1:80 dilution) associated with the development of uveitis (inflammatory eye disease), which occurs in ~20–30% of patients.[30] Uveitis is a serious complication of oligoarticular JIA that requires routine screening and evaluation with a slit-lamp examination (Table 63.1).[31]

Patients with monoarticular disease should have symptoms of at least 3 months' duration, with exclusion of other aetiologies including a septic joint, reactive arthritis, Lyme disease, pigmented villonodular synovitis, osteomyelitis, osteochondritis dissecans, discoid lateral meniscus, synovial chondromatosis, haemophilia and malignancy.

Some cases of oligoarticular disease are relatively benign, respond well to intra-articular corticosteroid injections (see Treatment), and resolve within 6–12 months from onset. Besides uveitis, other morbidities associated with oligoarticular disease include the risk of leg length discrepancy (which results from hypervascularity of chronic inflammation) and recurrent disease (occurring in ~20%, typically within the first year following inactive disease).

EXTENDED OLIGOARTICULAR ARTHRITIS

Patients with extended oligoarticular JIA initially present with four or fewer involved joints in the initial 6 months of presentation; however, additional joints later become affected (to include five or more total joints). These patients are classified as having extended disease (with evolution of symptoms after 6 months' duration). This subtype typically has a prolonged course similar to polyarticular disease.

Polyarticular JIA (RF negative)

This occurs in 20–30% of all patients with JIA with a slight female predilection (3:1). Polyarticular RF-negative JIA involves five or more joints within the first 6 months of disease onset. Typically, symmetric arthritis of the small joints of the hands and feet as well as larger joints of the wrists, knees, elbows and ankles are affected. Asymmetry of arthritis does occur, although less commonly. Additionally, cervical and temporomandibular joint involvement is more typical of polyarticular disease. Unlike RF-positive patients, those who are RF negative are at a slightly lower risk for aggressive disease. There is generally a lower risk of inflammatory eye disease than in those children with oligoarticular JIA, but routine screening is still required, particularly for young girls with a positive ANA test.

Polyarticular disease seems to occur in two peaks, with the first at 2–5 years old and the second at 10–14 years old. The latter group is more likely to be found with RF positivity (see below). On rare occasions, systemic symptoms of fever, anorexia, organomegaly and lymphadenopathy are seen with polyarticular disease.

Polyarticular JIA (RF positive)

This occurs in ~10% of all JIA patients. RF-positive polyarticular JIA affects five or more joints within the first 6 months of presentation (small, medium and large joints; symmetrical or asymmetrical). RF testing is considered to be positive if present on two different occasions, at least 3 months apart. Patients who are RF positive are at higher risk for severe, aggressive disease with a greater potential for the development of subcutaneous nodules and erosive joint disease that persists into adulthood. This subtype closely resembles the chronic course of early-onset, adult rheumatoid arthritis, with a low likelihood of drug-free remission. Patients with polyarticular JIA tend to have a lower risk of inflammatory eye disease than those with oligoarticular JIA, but do require regular screening.

The differential diagnosis of arthritis by presentation for oligoarthritis and polyarthritis is given in Table 63.2.

Systemic-onset JIA

Systemic disease is one of the most difficult subtypes of JIA to diagnose. The diagnosis is made by excluding other causes of fever and recognizing the characteristic clinical features of the disease. Systemic JIA occurs in ~10–20% of all patients with JIA and, likewise, is often difficult to treat. Classic systemic symptoms include a quotidian or bi-quotidian fever (one or two daily spikes with rapid return to normal or subnormal temperature), a diffuse, salmon-coloured, non-fixed, non-pruritic, macular rash that wors-

Table 63.2 Differential diagnosis of arthritis by presentation

Disease	Clues
A. Oligoarthritis	
1. *Acute presentation*	
Septic arthritis/osteomyelitis	Fever, exquisitely painful joint
Reactive arthritis (post-streptococcal, EBV, parvovirus, enteric infection)	Preceding illness (URI, sore throat, diarrhoea)
Lyme disease	History of tick bite and/or travel to Lyme endemic area
Acute rheumatic fever	Migratory arthritis, preceding streptococcal infection
Haemophilia	Male, family history for haemophilia
Trauma	History of trauma
Malignancy (leukaemia, neuroblastoma)	Fatigue, anorexia, severe (night-time) pain
Mechanical derangement (e.g. discoid lateral meniscus, osteochondritis dissecans)	Lack of warmth or synovial thickening
2. *Chronic presentation*	
JIA (oligo, psoriatic, ERA)	>6 weeks' duration, minimal pain
Infection (fungal, TB)	Immunosuppressed, history of contact with TB
Pigmented villonodular synovitis	Abnormal MRI findings (blooming on gradient echo sequences)
Sarcoidosis	± Hilar lymphadenopathy on radiograph
B. Polyarthritis	
JIA (poly, psoriatic, ERA)	>6 weeks' duration, minimal pain
Reactive arthritis	Preceding illness (URI, sore throat, diarrhoea), typically resolves in <6 weeks
Gonococcal arthritis	Sexually active, rash on palms/soles
Lyme disease	History of tick bite and/or travel to Lyme endemic area
SLE	Malar rash, photosensitivity
IBD-associated arthritis	Bloody stools, anorexia
Sarcoidosis	± Hilar lymphadenopathy on radiograph
Immunodeficiency syndromes	Recurrent infections, poor growth
Mucopolysaccharidoses	

EBV, Epstein–Barr virus; ERA, enthesitis-related arthritis; IBD, inflammatory bowel disease; JIA, juvenile idiopathic arthritis; oligo, oligoarticular JIA; poly, polyarticular JIA; SLE, systemic lupus erythematosus; TB, tuberculosis; URI, upper respiratory infection.

ens during fever, lymphadenopathy and serositis (~10%). Arthritis is often polyarticular and symmetrical with erosions occurring rapidly in ~25%. Patients can present at any age (but by definition must be <16 years old), and there is no obvious sex predilection. Symptoms can range from mild to severe, with symptom onset occurring in no specific order. Symptoms of anorexia and fatigue are commonly present. Laboratory findings typically include elevated acute-phase reactants (ESR and C-reactive protein (CRP)), a normo- to microcytic anaemia, and thrombocytosis.[32] Hyperferritinaemia is also frequently present.[33] Additional studies to evaluate for serositis (chest radiograph and echocardiography for pleural and pericardial effusions) may be helpful. In the diagnostic phases for systemic JIA, a strong suspicion for malignancy should also be present. Children occasionally undergo bone marrow aspiration to further clarify the diagnosis prior to onset of immunosuppressant treatment. Historically, approximately 25% of patients will develop aggressive polyarticular disease that is unresponsive to therapy;[34] however, recent advances in therapy will probably improve this number. A serious and potentially life-threatening complication, macrophage activation syndrome (MAS), is commonly associated with systemic-onset JIA and should always be considered in these patients who are acutely ill. MAS is associated with hyperferritinaemia, hypofibrinogenaemia with a falsely normal ESR, thrombocytopenia and hepatic dysfunction. An association with EBV has been recognized, but MAS can occur precipitously without an obvious infectious trigger.

Enthesitis-related arthritis

Older boys (12–14 years old) are the group most commonly affected by enthesitis-related arthritis (ERA). A diagnosis of ERA requires either (1) both arthritis and enthesitis or (2) arthritis *or* enthesitis with at least two of the following: arthritis or enthesitis of the sacroiliac joint and/or spinal involvement; HLA-B27 positive and/or a family history of a first-degree relative with an HLA-B27-associated disease (ankylosing spondylitis, inflammatory bowel disease with sacroiliitis, ERA, Reiter syndrome or acute anterior uveitis); painful, acute anterior uveitis; or onset of arthritis in males >8 years old. Usual sites of complaints include pain in the entheses (ligament, tendon or fascial insertions) surrounding the patella, tibial tuberosity, iliac crest and Achilles tendon, heel pain and/or lower back or sacroiliac pain. Anterior eye disease is typically of sudden onset, painful and associated with erythema and photophobia, in contrast to the insidious-onset uveitis associated with other JIA subtypes. Uveitis in this subtype is strongly related to the presence of the HLA-B27 antigen (occurring in ~50%).[35] Patients classified as having the ERA subtype include not only those patients with juvenile ankylosing spondylitis and undifferentiated spondyloarthritis, but also those with inflammatory bowel disease-associated arthritis and reactive arthritis (including Reiter syndrome of arthritis, urethritis and conjunctivitis that is associated commonly with preceding bloody diarrhoea or *Chlamydia trachomatis* infection). Patients with psoriasis or a history of psoriasis in self or family, presence of RF or systemic features are excluded from this subtype.

Psoriatic arthritis

A diagnosis of psoriatic arthritis in children requires the presence of at least two of the following: (1) presence of psoriasis or a family history of a first-degree relative with psoriasis, (2) dactylitis or sausage digit (often seen in the toes), (3) nail changes, including onycholysis or pitting, and (4) exclusion of other diseases or features (RF positive, systemic features, family history of HLA-B27-associated diseases, and/or arthritis beginning after age 8 years in a boy who is HLA-B27 positive). Overall, psoriatic arthritis accounts for 2–15% of patients with JIA. Children may present with an asymmetric, large or small joint arthritis long before skin changes and vice versa.[36,37] Patients with psoriatic arthritis are at risk for inflammatory eye disease, which occurs in ~10–20% but can be somewhat more difficult to treat. Presence of ANAs in these patients is also associated with an increased risk of uveitis. Bony changes are often not erosive, except in association with the presence of HLA-B27 and spinal/axial involvement.[36–38]

Undifferentiated

In rare cases, classification of chronic arthritis in children is unclear and cannot be defined by any of the above subtypes. Patients who have overlapping features of more than one subtype are also classified in this category. With time, most patients are categorized within one of the more clearly defined subtypes.

LABORATORY FINDINGS

In general, laboratory findings can be useful screening tools but lack specificity. Inflammatory markers, including ESR (30–40 mm^{-3}) and CRP, are elevated in the majority of cases, but not all. In systemic-onset JIA, anaemia, leucocytosis (30 000–50 000 mm^{-3}) and thrombocytosis are common. Hyperferritinaemia is also found. A positive ANA test (titre >1:80) is found primarily in oligoarticular JIA. A positive ANA test in patients with oligoarticular or polyarticular JIA has a direct association with the risk of uveitis. Testing to rule out other infectious causes can be helpful if the clinical history and examination are unclear; these include Lyme titres (enzyme-linked immunosorbent assay screening with western blot confirmation), both anti-streptolysin antibodies and anti-DNAse B antibodies (for recent streptococcal infection), EBV titres and parvovirus titres.

Synovial fluid analysis can be helpful to rule out a septic joint. Total white blood cells in inflammatory synovial fluid of JIA ranges from 2000 to 60 000, with a predominance of neutrophils. Biopsy of the synovium is rarely performed unless the diagnosis remains uncertain.

RADIOGRAPHY

Imaging is useful in the guidance of treatment and evaluation of progression of disease. In early disease, plain radiographic films may reveal early features of arthritis: osteopenia, joint space widening (from synovial hypertrophy) and periarticular soft-tissue swelling. Late features of arthritis of periosteal reaction and osteopenia, bony erosions causing 'notching', and joint space narrowing can also be visualized on plain films. Epiphyseal overgrowth may be seen. Subluxation of the metacarpal joints, wrists and hips can occur in late disease. Ankylosis appears in the final stages of destruction.

Additional imaging, including CT and MRI, may be helpful in the diagnostic phases of JIA, particularly when the presentation is atypical or other illnesses cannot be ruled out. A CT scan is particularly useful for ruling out tarsal coalition and demonstrating bony changes in the sacroiliac and temporomandibular joints. MRI (with gadolinium contrast) is useful in detecting synovitis, extent of involvement, and cartilage and bony destructive changes, and ruling out other causes of joint pain or limitation of motion (pigmented villonodular synovitis, osteochondritis dissecans or discoid lateral meniscus).

TREATMENT

Medications

A multidisciplinary team approach is best for the management of JIA, including specialists from rheumatology, ophthalmology, physical and occupational therapy, nursing, social work, nutrition and orthopaedics. Initial medical treatment of JIA includes a non-steroidal anti-inflammatory drug (NSAID), such as naproxen (15–20 mg kg^{-1} day^{-1} divided twice daily) or meloxicam (0.125 mg kg^{-1} day^{-1}; maximum 7.5 mg day^{-1}). Addition of an H2 blocker or proton pump inhibitor may be required for prevention of NSAID-induced gastritis and peptic ulcer disease.

Patients with oligoarticular disease often respond well to intra-articular corticosteroid injection, which effectively reduces pannus formation. Triamcinolone hexacetonide (~1 mg kg^{-1} per large joint; ~0.5 mg kg^{-1} per medium joint) is preferred because of its low lipid solubility, which allows for delayed resorption and prolonged local effectiveness. Treatment often provides resolution of symptoms for 6 months to 2 years. Subcutaneous atrophy can occur at the injection site, particularly in smaller joints. Fluoroscopy or ultrasound guidance is often helpful, as is injecting normal saline through the needle as it is withdrawn from the joint.

Oral corticosteroids (prednisone) are less commonly used in the routine treatment of patients with JIA. However, in severe polyarticular disease or systemic disease, prednisone is often necessary. In systemic JIA, a dose of 1–2 mg kg^{-1} day^{-1} (daily or divided twice daily) can be initiated at presentation; however additional steroid-sparing agents should also be recommended early on because of the significant side-effects of prolonged daily corticosteroid use (Cushingoid appearance, weight gain, mood changes, osteopenia and inhibition of linear growth). Patients with systemic JIA may have difficulty weaning off corticosteroids owing to the severity of the inflammatory response in this subtype of disease. In polyarticular disease, often low-dose prednisone (approximately 0.1–0.2 mg kg^{-1} day^{-1}) can have significant and rapid benefit and may be used as a bridging agent until other therapies take effect. Uveitis is also treated by topical glucocorticoids with the potential for iatrogenic complications of glaucoma and cataracts.

Most of the subtypes (excluding oligoarticular without uveitis, which typically responds well to NSAID treatment and corticosteroid injections alone) will require more aggressive treatment with advanced, second-line agents. A disease-modifying anti-rheumatic drug such as methotrexate (MTX), an anti-folate metabolite and anti-inflammatory, is the first choice of second-line agents. It is effective at a weekly dose of 10–15 mg m^{-2} dispensed either orally or via injection.[39,40] Absorption rates vary with oral dosing; therefore, subcutaneous injection is often preferred. Full effectiveness is not seen until at least 6 weeks after the initiation of MTX. Folic acid (1 mg daily) is given to aid in minimizing the adverse side-effects of mouth sores, nausea and elevation of transaminases. Other side-effects that require monitoring with routine blood tests include neutropenia and hepatic transaminase elevation. Liver toxicity is rare and biopsy is typically unnecessary. Rarely, children can develop pulmonary symptoms following initiation of treatment that requires monitoring. Some children develop a psychological reaction or aversion to MTX, with significant nausea. This side-effect can sometimes be remedied with behavioural feedback.

TNF inhibitors are newer biological agents that are being utilized in the treatment of JIA (primarily polyarticular disease). Randomized, placebo-controlled trials have shown that etanercept is effective in the treatment of polyarticular JIA when given as a subcutaneous injection once or twice weekly.[41,42] It is approved by the US Food and Drug Administration for the treatment of polyarticular JIA in children as young as 2 years.[43] Adalimumab (subcutaneous injection every 2 weeks) has also recently been approved for use in JIA. Infliximab appears to have similar findings, although monthly infusions are less convenient.[44,45] The treatment of ERA and severe uveitis consists primarily of these last two agents.[46-48]

Another biological agent, Abatacept, a selective co-stimulation modulator, has also been approved for use in polyarthritis in children aged 6 years and older in the United States.[49,50] Other slower acting, second-line medications such as hydroxychloroquine, sulfasalazine and leflunomide have been utilized in the treatment of JIA, with less compelling results.

An anti-IL-1 receptor antagonist, anakinra, has been used (off-label) in the treatment of systemic JIA with often dramatic results in responders.[51–53] A daily subcutaneous injection, anakinra has proven to be a highly effective steroid-sparing agent in systemic-onset disease. Other biological agents targeting key cytokines (IL-6, IL-1) are currently in testing in systemic JIA.[54,55] Tocilizumab (an anti-IL-6 agent) was recently approved by the US Food and Drug Administration for systemic JIA in children aged 2 years and older.[56]

With all immunosuppressant medications, one must monitor patients closely for infection, as there is a slightly higher risk for illness. Live virus vaccines cannot be safely given. Prior to the use of biological agents, all patients should have a purified protein derivate test to screen for latent tuberculosis which has been reactivated following the use of TNF-blocking agents.

Physical and occupational therapy

The goals of physical and occupational therapy are to increase the range of motion and flexibility, improve physical conditioning and strengthening, maintain a healthy joint position, decrease pain and educate patients about joint protection. After several months of disease, muscle atrophy can occur. Physical strengthening is key to improving muscle bulk. Additionally, serial casting and/or intermittent splinting may be necessary in severe joint flexion contractures (particularly about the knee) to preserve or improve the range of motion. Cock-up wrist splinting, particularly at night, is very important with active wrist synovitis and can prevent subluxation.

Surgical therapy

With the recent advances in medical treatment, surgical intervention is rarely necessary. However, in certain cases, such as cervical instability, mandibular hypoplasia with instability, and severe bony erosion and destruction, surgical intervention may be necessary. In the event of significant leg length discrepancy, epiphysiodesis may be useful to limit asymmetric growth; however, this procedure is almost never required with appropriate medical management. One should remain aware that accelerated maturation also means early closure of the physis, with the potential for correction without surgical intervention. Total joint arthroplasty is most common for the hip and knees, but infrequently performed in childhood.

PROGNOSIS AND OUTCOMES

Morbidity in JIA has declined in the past decade, particularly with the introduction of biological agents, with success similar to that seen in adult patients with rheumatoid arthritis. Previously seen morbidities, such as severe deformities and decreased ambulation (complete wheelchair dependence), are rare. Additional long-term studies on treatment and disease outcomes will continue to be needed in the field of paediatric JIA.

KEY LEARNING POINTS

- Juvenile idiopathic arthritis is the most common rheumatic disease of childhood and one of the most common chronic diseases of childhood.
- Juvenile idiopathic arthritis is a chronic arthritis occurring for ≥6 weeks in a child <16 years old.
- A high index of suspicion is needed to aid in the diagnosis of these particularly heterogeneous diseases.
- The most common subtypes include oligoarticular, polyarticular (rheumatoid factor positive or negative) and systemic arthritis.
- Routine screening for eye disease (uveitis) is necessary.
- Newer medications such as methotrexate and biological agents have changed the outlook of juvenile idiopathic arthritis.
- The treatment approach is multidisciplinary, with primary goals of preservation of function and range of motion and prevention of aggressive bony erosions.

REFERENCES

- ● = Key primary paper
- ◆ = Major review article

1. Fink CW. Proposal for the development of classification criteria for idiopathic arthritides of childhood. *Journal of Rheumatology* 1995;**22**:1566–9.
●2. Petty RE, Southwood TR, Baum J, *et al.* Revision of the proposed classification criteria for juvenile idiopathic arthritis: Durban, 1997. *Journal of Rheumatology* 1998;**25**:1991–4.
3. Cassidy JT, Levinson JE, Bass JC, *et al.* A study of classification criteria for a diagnosis of juvenile rheumatoid arthritis. *Arthritis and Rheumatism* 1986;**29**:274–81.
4. Cassidy JT, Petty RE, Laxer RM, Lindsley CB. *Textbook of Pediatric Rheumatology*, 5th edn. Philadelphia, PA: Elsevier Saunders, 2005:209–10.

5. Kaipiainen-Seppänen O, Savolainen A. Incidence of chronic juvenile rheumatic diseases in Finland during 1980–1990. *Clinical and Experimental Rheumatology* 1996;**14**:441–4.
6. Peterson LS, Mason T, Nelson AMO, et al. Juvenile rheumatoid arthritis in Rochester, Minnesota 1960–1993. Is the epidemiology changing? *Arthritis and Rheumatism* 1996;**39**:1385–90.
7. Schaller JG. Juvenile rheumatoid arthritis: series 1. *Arthritis and Rheumatism* 1977;**20**(2 Suppl.):165–70.
8. Cassidy JT, Sullivan DB, Petty RE. Clinical patterns of chronic iridocyclitis in children with juvenile rheumatoid arthritis. *Arthritis and Rheumatism* 1977;**20**(2 Suppl.):224–7.
9. Lawrence RC, Helmick CG, Arnett FC, et al. Estimates of the prevalence of arthritis and selected musculoskeletal disorders in the United States. *Arthritis and Rheumatism* 1998;**41**:778–99.
10. Schwartz MM, Simpson P, Kerr KL, Jarvis JN. Juvenile rheumatoid arthritis in African Americans. *Journal of Rheumatology* 1997;**24**:1826–9.
11. Feldman BM, Birdi N, Boone JE, et al. Seasonal onset of systemic-onset juvenile rheumatoid arthritis. *Journal of Pediatrics* 1996;**129**:513–18.
12. Ogra PL, Chiba Y, Ogra SS, et al. Rubella-virus infection in juvenile rheumatoid arthritis. *Lancet* 1975;**1**:1157–61.
13. Chantler JK, Tingle AJ, Petty RE. Persistent rubella virus infection associated with chronic arthritis in children. *New England Journal of Medicine* 1985;**313**:1117–23.
14. Albani S. Infection and molecular mimicry in autoimmune diseases of childhood. *Clinical and Experimental Rheumatology* 1994;**12**(Suppl. 10):S35–41.
15. Pritchard MH, Matthews N, Munro J. Antibodies to influenza A in a cluster of children with juvenile chronic arthritis. *British Journal of Rheumatology* 1988;**27**:176–80.
16. Lehman HW, Knoll A, Küster RM, Modrow S. Frequent infection with a viral pathogen, parvovirus B19, in rheumatic diseases of childhood. *Arthritis and Rheumatism* 2003;**48**:1631–8.
17. Moroldo MB, Chaudhari M, Shear E, et al. Juvenile rheumatoid arthritis in affected sibpairs: extent of clinical phenotype concordance. *Arthritis and Rheumatism* 2004;**50**:1928–34.
18. Moroldo MB, Tauge BL, Shear ES, et al. Juvenile rheumatoid arthritis in affected sibpairs. *Arthritis and Rheumatism* 1997;**40**:1962–6.
19. Prahalad S, O'Brien E, Fraser AM, et al. Familial aggregation of juvenile idiopathic arthritis. *Arthritis and Rheumatism* 2004;**50**:4022–7.
20. Prahalad S, Shear ES, Thompson SD, et al. Increased prevalence of familial autoimmunity in simplex and multiplex families with juvenile rheumatoid arthritis. *Arthritis and Rheumatism* 2002;**46**:1851–6.
●21. Rossen RD, Brewer EJ, Sharp RM, et al. Familial rheumatoid arthritis: linkage of HLA to disease susceptibility locus in four families where proband presented with juvenile rheumatoid arthritis. *Journal of Clinical Investigation* 1980;**65**:629–42.
22. Nepom B. The immunogenetics of juvenile rheumatoid arthritis. *Rheumatic Disease Clinics of North America* 1991;**17**:825–42.
23. Prahalad S, Ryan MH, Shear ES, et al. Juvenile rheumatoid arthritis: linkage to HLA demonstrated by allele sharing in affected sibpairs. *Arthritis and Rheumatism* 2000;**43**:2335–8.
24. Thompson SD, Moroldo MB, Guyer L, et al. A genome-wide scan for juvenile rheumatoid arthritis in affected sibpair families provides evidence of linkage. *Arthritis and Rheumatism* 2004;**50**:2920–30.
25. Rosen P, Thompson S, Glass D. Non-HLA gene polymorphisms in juvenile rheumatoid arthritis. *Clinical and Experimental Rheumatology* 2003;**21**:650–6.
26. Grom AA, Murray KJ, Luyrink L, et al. Patterns of expression of tumor necrosis factor alpha, tumor necrosis factor beta, and their receptors in synovia of patients with juvenile rheumatoid arthritis and juvenile spondyloarthropathy. *Arthritis and Rheumatism* 1996;**39**:1703–10.
27. Scola MP, Thompson SD, Brunner HI, et al. Interferon-gamma:interleukin 4 ratios and associated type 1 cytokine expression in juvenile rheumatoid arthritis synovial tissue. *Journal of Rheumatology* 2002;**29**:369–78.
♦28. Müller K, Herner EB, Stagg A, et al. Inflammatory cytokines and cytokine antagonists in whole blood cultures of patients with systemic juvenile chronic arthritis. *British Journal of Rheumatology* 1998;**37**:562–9.
29. Sherry DD, Stein LD, Reed AM, et al. Prevention of leg length discrepancy in young children with pauciarticular juvenile rheumatoid arthritis by treatment with intraarticular steroids. *Arthritis and Rheumatism* 1999;**42**:2330–4.
♦30. Saurenmann RK, Levin AV, Feldman BM, et al. Prevalence, risk factors, and outcome of uveitis in juvenile idiopathic arthritis: a long-term followup study. *Arthritis and Rheumatism* 2007;**56**:647–57.
31. Cassidy J, Kivlin J, Lindsley C, Nocton J. Ophthalmologic examinations in children with juvenile rheumatoid arthritis. *Pediatrics* 2006;**117**:1843–5.
32. Koerper MA, Stempel DA, Dallman PR. Anemia in patients with juvenile rheumatoid arthritis. *Journal of Pediatrics* 1978;**92**:930–3.
33. Pelkonen P, Swanljung K, Siimes MA. Ferritinemia as an indicator of systemic disease activity in children with systemic juvenile rheumatoid arthritis. *Acta Paediatrica Scandinavica* 1986;**75**:64–8.
34. Schneider R, Lang BA, Reilly BJ. Prognostic indicators of joint destruction in systemic-onset juvenile rheumatoid arthritis. *Journal of Pediatrics* 1992;**120**:200–5.
35. Ansell BM. Spondyloarthropathy in childhood: a review. *Journal of the Royal Society of Medicine* 1981;**73**:205–9.
36. Southwood TR, Petty RE, Malleson PN, et al. Psoriatic arthritis in children. *Arthritis and Rheumatism* 1989;**32**:1007–13.
37. Roberton DM, Cabral DA, Malleson PN, Petty RE. Juvenile psoriatic arthritis: followup and evaluation of diagnostic criteria. *Journal of Rheumatology* 1996;**23**:166–70.
38. Shore A, Ansell BM. Juvenile psoriatic arthritis: an analysis of 60 cases. *Journal of Pediatrics* 1982;**100**:529–35.

●39. Giannini EH, Brewer EJ, Kuzmina N, et al. Methotrexate in resistant juvenile rheumatoid arthritis. Results of the U.S.A-U.S.S.R double-blind, placebo-controlled trial. The Pediatric Rheumatology Collaborative Study Group and The Cooperative Children's Study Group. New England Journal of Medicine 1992;326:1043-9.

●40. Ruperto N, Murray KJ, Gerloni V, et al. A randomized trial of parental methotrexate comparing an intermediate dose with a higher dose in children with juvenile idiopathic arthritis who failed to respond to standard doses of methotrexate. Arthritis and Rheumatism 2004;50:2191-201.

●41. Lovell DJ, Giannini EH, Reiff A, et al. Etanercept in children with polyarticular juvenile rheumatoid arthritis. Pediatric Rheumatology Collaborative Study Group. New England Journal of Medicine 2000;16:763-9.

●42. Lovell DJ, Reiff A, Jones OY, et al. Long-term safety and efficacy of etanercept in children with polyarticular-course juvenile rheumatoid arthritis. Arthritis and Rheumatism 2006;54:1987-94.

43. Lovell DJ, Ruperto N, Goodman S, et al. Adalimumab with or without methotrexate in juvenile rheumatoid arthritis. New England Journal of Medicine 2008;359:810-20.

●44. Ruperto N, Lovell DJ, Cuttica R, et al. A randomized, placebo-controlled trial of infliximab plus methotrexate for the treatment of polyarticular-course juvenile rheumatoid arthritis. Arthritis and Rheumatism 2007;56:3096-106.

45. Lovell DJ, Ruperto N, Goodman S, et al. Adalimumab is safe and effective during long-term treatment of patients with juvenile rheumatoid arthritis: results from a 2-year study. Arthritis and Rheumatism 2007;21(Suppl.):S292.

46. Saurenmann RK, Levin AV, Rose JB, et al. Tumour necrosis factor alpha inhibitors in the treatment of childhood uveitis. Rheumatology (Oxford) 2006;45:982-9.

47. Biester S, Deuter C, Michels H, et al. Adalimumab in the therapy of uveitis in childhood. British Journal of Ophthalmology 2007;91:319-24.

48. Tynjälä P, Kotaniemi K, Lindahl P, et al. Adalimumab in juvenile idiopathic arthritis-associated chronic anterior uveitis. Rheumatology (Oxford) 2008;47:339-44.

49. Giannini EH, Ruperto N, Prieur AM, et al. Efficacy of abatacept in different sub-populations of juvenile idiopathic arthritis (JIA): results of a randomized withdrawal study. Arthritis and Rheumatism 2007;21(Suppl.):S291.

50. Lovell DJ, Ruperto N, Prieur AM, et al. Abatacept treatment of juvenile idiopathic arthritis (JIA): safety report. Arthritis and Rheumatism 2007;21(Suppl.):S292.

51. Verbsky JW, White AJ. Effective use of the recombinant interleukin 1 receptor antagonist anakinra in therapy resistant systemic onset juvenile rheumatoid arthritis. Journal of Rheumatology 2004;31:2071-5.

52. Pascual V, Allantaz F, Arce E, et al. Role of interleukin-1 (IL-1) in the pathogenesis of systemic onset juvenile idiopathic arthritis and clinical response to IL-1 blockade. Journal of Experimental Medicine 2005;201:1479-86.

53. Lequerré T, Quartier P, Rosellini D, et al. Interleukin-1 receptor antagonist (anakinra) treatment in patients with systemic-onset juvenile idiopathic arthritis or adult onset Still disease: preliminary experience in France. Annals of Rheumatic Diseases 2008;67:302-8.

54. Yokota S, Miyamae T, Imagawa T, et al. Therapeutic efficacy of humanized recombinant anti-interleukin-6 receptor antibody in children with systemic-onset juvenile idiopathic arthritis. Arthritis and Rheumatism 2005;52:687-93.

55. Yokota S, Imagawa T, Mori M, et al. Efficacy and safety of tocilizumab in patients with systemic-onset juvenile idiopathic arthritis: a randomised, double-blind, placebo-controlled, withdrawal phase III trial. Lancet 2008;371:998-1006.

56. Lovell DJ, Giannini EH, Kimura Y, et al. Preliminary evidence for sustained bioactivity of IL-1 Trap (Rilonacept), a long-acting IL-1 inhibitor, in systemic juvenile idiopathic arthritis (SJIA). Arthritis and Rheumatism 2007;21(Suppl.):S514.

64

Neuromuscular disorders

KISHORE MULPURI, SANJEEV MADAN, UNI NARAYANAN, NICK NICOLAOU, SHAHRYAR NOORDIN, RENJIT A VARGHESE, JANET WALKER

CEREBRAL PALSY	598	Incidence and aetiology	608
Definition	598	General considerations	608
Epidemiology and aetiology	598	Orthopaedic management	609
Pathophysiology of musculoskeletal abnormalities	599	Regional assessment	609
Classification of cerebral palsy	599	MUSCULAR DYSTROPHIES AND HEREDITARY NEUROPATHIES	610
Priorities and goals of treatment in cerebral palsy	600	Muscular dystrophy	610
Evaluation of children with cerebral palsy	600	Hereditary motor and sensory neuropathies	613
Treatment of musculoskeletal problems	602	OBSTETRIC BRACHIAL PLEXUS PALSY	615
Orthopaedic procedures at the hip	602	Introduction	615
Orthopaedic procedures at the knee	603	Incidence	615
Orthopaedic procedures at the calf, ankle and foot	604	Theories of causation	615
Postoperative rehabilitation following multilevel surgery	605	Risk factors	616
Orthopaedic procedures in non-ambulatory cerebral palsy	606	Classification, sites of involvement and frequency	616
Hip instability in cerebral palsy	606	Natural history	616
Spinal deformities in cerebral palsy	607	Clinical features	617
The upper extremity in cerebral palsy	607	Diagnosis	617
Summary	608	Treatment	617
MYELOMENINGOCELE	608	References	618
Introduction	608		

CEREBRAL PALSY

DEFINITION

Cerebral palsy (CP) is the term applied to a heterogeneous group of permanent disorders of the development of movement and posture, causing limitation of activity, that are attributable to **non-progressive** disturbances that occurred in the developing fetal or infant brain. The motor disorders are often accompanied by disturbances of sensation, perception, cognition, communication and behaviour, epilepsy and secondary musculoskeletal problems.[1,2]

EPIDEMIOLOGY AND AETIOLOGY

CP constitutes the most common cause of chronic childhood disability, with the prevalence estimated to be between two and three per 1000 live births.[3] The aetiology includes congenital brain malformations (5–15%); prenatal causes (50–70%), such as intra-uterine infections, placental malformations, complications of prematurity, brain haemorrhages and stroke (pre- or neonatal); perinatal causes such hypoxic–ischaemic encephalopathy (10%); and post-natal causes (10–25%), such as head injury, metabolic encephalopathy, hyperbilirubinaemia and infections. CP may result from the interaction of multiple risk factors, and, in some cases, there may not be an identifiable cause. Prematurity is the most common risk factor for CP owing to the fragile cerebral vasculature, immature autoregulation of cerebral blood flow and the vulnerable cerebral parenchyma. Other risk factors include low birth weight, multiple births, intra-uterine infections, Apgar scores <5 at 5 minutes, post-natal hyperbilirubinaemia and maternal disorders (e.g. diabetes). A number of genetic disorders (Rett syndrome, fragile X syndrome, familial or hereditary spastic paraparesis) and metabolic disorders (mucopolysaccharidoses, phenylketonuria, etc.) can masquerade as CP.

PATHOPHYSIOLOGY OF MUSCULOSKELETAL ABNORMALITIES

The lesion in the brain produces specific abnormalities of tone and movement depending on the location of the lesion (in decreasing order of incidence: spastic; dyskinetic: dystonia, athetoid; or mixed patterns). Associated with the upper motor neurone disorder are the features of hypertonia, hyper-reflexia and co-contractions. In addition, owing to loss of connections to the lower motor neurone, other features include weakness, loss of selective motor control and deficits in balance and coordination.[4] There is a delay in developmental motor milestones. The interaction between spasticity and weakness leads to both neural and mechanical changes in muscle and progressive musculoskeletal pathology (Fig. 64.1). Hypertonicity creates dynamic muscle contractures. Usual muscle growth occurs in response to the stimulus of stretch arising from typical physical activities of a normally developing child. The decreased physical activities associated with developmental delay, along with the hypertonia that impedes muscle stretch, impairs muscle growth relative to the growing skeleton, resulting in static or fixed contractures in which the muscles are too short for the distance they are to traverse.[5] The abnormal forces on the growing skeleton also lead to bony deformities and joint instability (lever arm dysfunction),[6] manifested in abnormal and inefficient gait patterns in those who can walk and corresponding limitations in physical function and sometimes pain. For example, the increased femoral anteversion, which is normal in infancy, fails to spontaneously reduce in a developmentally delayed child because of the absence of corrective forces associated with increased hip extension acquired during the normal progression from crawling, pulling up to stand, to walking, and may be further exacerbated in the face of contractures about the hip. Although the primary lesion in the brain is not progressive, the secondary musculoskeletal consequences become worse with growth.[7–10]

CLASSIFICATION OF CEREBRAL PALSY

An international multidisciplinary group proposed a new classification system that has at its core the Gross Motor Functional Classification System (GMFCS).[2] The GMFCS is a five-level ordinal system that has become the standard for categorizing individuals based on the severity of their motor disability.[11] The GMFCS has been shown to be reliable and valid[12] and its prognostic utility has been established in a prospective longitudinal population-based cohort study of 657 children.[13] Levels I–III are ambulatory. Children in GMFCS level I can perform all the activities of their age-matched peers, albeit with some difficulties with their speed, balance and coordination. In level II, children have similar functional abilities on flat and familiar surfaces, but require support on uneven surfaces or when climbing stairs. Children in level III are also independent walkers but require an assistive device such as a crutch or a

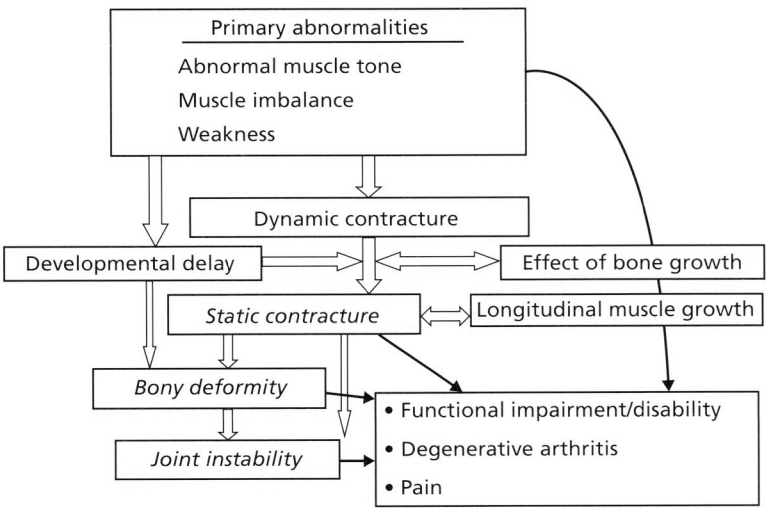

Figure 64.1 Effects of musculoskeletal abnormalities.

walker, and may use wheelchairs for longer distances. Children in levels IV and V are non-ambulatory. In level IV they may weight bear for transfers and use a walker for exercise purposes, whereas in level V children cannot achieve any functional weight bearing and are usually totally dependent on caregivers. The GMFCS provides an excellent basis for stratification of patients in outcome evaluations.

In addition to the GMFCS, the proposed new classification system also considers four additional dimensions[2] to provide a comprehensive description of each child with CP. These dimensions are (1) nature and typology of the motor disorder based on the dominant type of tone and movement abnormality (spastic, ataxic, dystonic, athetoid); (2) accompanying impairments that may have a greater impact on the functional abilities of the individual than the primary motor abnormality (e.g. seizure disorders, hearing and visual problems, cognitive and attention deficits, emotional and behavioural issues and secondary musculoskeletal problems); (3) anatomical distribution (limb, truncal and bulbar involvement) and neuroimaging findings: the terms diplegia, hemiplegia and quadriplegia are being replaced by the terms unilateral or bilateral CP; and (4) cause and timing, to the extent that this is determinable, since these are likely to influence the presentation and natural history.

PRIORITIES AND GOALS OF TREATMENT IN CEREBRAL PALSY

It is important to separate the goals of treatment for ambulatory and non-ambulatory children. For ambulatory children with CP, the goals are primarily to preserve or improve gait efficiency (decrease energy consumption) and physical function in order to increase activities and participation, and secondarily to improve the appearance of gait.[14] The severely involved non-ambulatory children with CP (GMFCS levels IV and V) often have a number of other comorbid conditions such as seizure disorders, visual and hearing impairments, cognitive delay, communication difficulties, swallowing difficulties, drooling, aspiration, gastro-oesophageal reflux, constipation and incontinence. Many of these children are at risk for aspiration pneumonias and for malnutrition requiring gastrostomy or gastrojejunostomy tubes for safe feeding. Additionally, they experience the musculoskeletal consequences of contractures and deformities of the upper and lower limbs and trunk. These children are at high risk of developing progressively increasing hip instability and scoliosis, which can cause pain and interfere with positioning, seating and caregiving. These children rely on caregivers for much of their activities of daily living. For these children the goals of treatment are to prevent or relieve pain, facilitate caregiving and preserve or improve the quality of life.[15]

EVALUATION OF CHILDREN WITH CEREBRAL PALSY

Each clinical encounter begins with an elicitation of concerns of the parents and the child (whenever possible). This not only allows one to generate a list of problems and priorities on which to focus, but also provides an opportunity to understand and educate families about their expectations. The physical examination that follows attempts to understand where the source of the problems might lie, which in turn influences decision-making about potential solutions.

Visual observation of gait

For ambulatory children, the physical examination begins with a visual observation of the gait, both barefoot and in the child's usual orthotics and footwear. This is done from the front/back and the side using a systematic approach to look for abnormalities at each level: foot and ankle, the knee, hip and pelvis, the trunk and upper extremities, with due consideration of the sagittal, transverse and coronal planes. Look for specific gait patterns. A useful framework to evaluate gait abnormalities is to assess the five priorities of gait:[16,17] (1) stability in stance; (2) (foot) clearance in swing; (3) correct pre-positioning of foot for the next step; (4) adequate step length; and (5) energy efficiency (minimizing the excursion of the body's centre of mass during walking). The source of each problem identified during the visual observation of gait is assessed during the static examination of the child.

Static physical examination

The static examination (on the table) includes assessment of muscle length and tone, bony alignment, muscle strength and selective control. Muscle length is assessed indirectly by the joint range of motion of different muscle groups at each segment. For the lower extremities, this includes hip flexion/extension (Thomas test); hip abduction (with knees flexed and extended to assess the additional contribution of the gracilis); the popliteal angle; ankle dorsiflexion; prone knee flexion (Duncan–Ely sign for rectus femoris tightness), etc. Range of motion is assessed passively with both a fast and a slow stretch; the fast stretch elicits a catch (R_1) often well before the maximal passive range obtained by the slow, sustained stretch (R_2). This feature of spasticity is velocity dependent. The larger gap between the R_1 and R_2 represents the dynamic component of the contracture, and is more amenable to spasticity management. R_2 represents the static assessment of muscle length. As R_2 approaches R_1, there is increasing static contracture or true shortening of the muscle tendon unit (in addition to tightness), which may require serial casting when the magnitude of the contracture is mild or surgical lengthening when the contracture is severe. Often, biarticular muscles are more involved than muscles that cross only one joint. It is therefore important to separately test the length of both groups of muscles (when possible) that contribute to range in order to intervene selectively on the biarticular muscles (e.g. medial hamstrings from short head of biceps (unilateral vs bilateral popliteal angle), gastrocnemius from soleus (Silfverskiöld test). Document the presence of fixed contractures at the hip (flexion, adduction or windswept); the knee (flexion or extension contractures); and the ankle (equinus, equinovalgus, equinovarus). Bony alignment includes assessment of the torsional profile in the prone position to evaluate for excessive femoral anteversion (based on the arc of internal and external rotation and the trochanteric palpation test)[18,19] and tibial torsion (based on thigh–foot angle and the transmalleolar axis). Examination of the spine is to detect any spinal deformity in the coronal/transverse (scoliosis) and sagittal (kyphosis/hyperlordosis) planes. In non-ambulatory children it is important to assess the impact of any spinal deformity on sitting balance and seating.

Examination of the upper extremity is particularly important in unilaterally (hemiplegic) involved children in whom upper extremity limitations may affect bimanual activities; and in more severe bilaterally involved children in whom upper extremity contractures may interfere with caregiving. An assessment of active range of motion, sensation and selective control of muscles is important for decision-making regarding the likely effectiveness of surgical lengthening and/or tendon transfers for functional gain.

Gait analysis

Gait analysis is often used in the assessment of children with ambulatory CP to refine clinical decision-making.[20] Three-dimensional gait analysis generated in a motion laboratory provides kinematic data that describe the motion of each limb segment in three planes, kinetic data that include moments and powers about the joints, and dynamic electromyography that documents the timing of individual muscle activation during the gait cycle. Three-dimensional gait analysis provides insight beyond what is derivable from observational analysis alone, and has the potential to influence or alter treatment decisions for at least some patients. Gait analysis can help distinguish primary abnormalities (which might benefit from treatment) from secondary abnormalities (which represent coping responses and which require no treatment).[21] Gait analysis has identified recognizable gait patterns that can be classified and used for making treatment decisions, the effectiveness of which can be assessed using gait analysis as a measure of gait outcomes. There are many sources of variability, however, including patients themselves, the gait laboratories and testing processes, interpretation of data and surgeons' surgical recommendations.[20] Although gait analysis has been shown to alter decision-making,[22–24] the evidence to date that the decisions based on gait analysis lead to better outcomes remains to be seen, and randomized controlled trials are currently under way to address this area of controversy.[20]

Abnormal gait patterns in cerebral palsy

Understanding pathological gait requires an understanding of normal gait. There are recognizable gait patterns associated with bilateral and unilateral CP. In bilateral CP, there are four main patterns.[25] These are (1) true equinus (equinus ankle, extended knee, extended hip) characterized by a toe–toe gait; (2) jump gait (equinus ankle, flexed knee, flexed hip); (3) apparent equinus (up on toes despite neutral ankle to accommodate flexed knee and flexed hip); and (4) crouch gait (dorsiflexed foot segment relative to tibial shank occurring either because of calcaneus at the ankle or because of midfoot break; flexed knee and hip). Crouch gait might be iatrogenic in children who have had overlengthened Achilles tendons, or may indeed be a consequence of the natural history in children with more severe bilateral CP (GMFCS level III). Each of these patterns can be associated with a stiff knee pattern and abnormal rotation. A stiff knee gait is characterized by limited flexion in initial swing because of tightness of the rectus femoris, which affects clearance of the foot in swing phase. Internal (or external) rotation gait can arise from above the knee (increased femoral anteversion or medial torsion) and/or below the knee (abnormal internal or external tibial torsion), and is inferred from the foot and knee progression angles.

In unilateral CP (hemiplegia) four types of gait have been described.[26] Type 1 is characterized by equinus in swing phase only (drop-foot pattern); type 2 has equinus in swing and stance phase (toe–toe or toe–heel gait); in type 3, the knee is involved as well, showing abnormal flexion (jump) or stiff knee pattern; and in type 4, there is additional proximal involvement at the hip.

Although these patterns of gait are recognizable, the distinctions are not always clear with many permutations and combinations involving one or both lower extremities.

TREATMENT OF MUSCULOSKELETAL PROBLEMS

The principles of musculoskeletal treatments include (1) prevention of joint contractures and skeletal deformities by muscle stretching, spasticity reduction and muscle strengthening; and (2) correction of significant contractures and bony deformities when these have already occurred. These objectives and indeed the overall management of CP are best achieved using a multidisciplinary approach.

Early intervention includes complementary strategies used sequentially or in combination, including physical therapy, orthotics (braces) and serial casting to stimulate the stretch that would normally be derived from usual physical activity in order to stimulate muscle growth and to prevent contractures. These are often accompanied by measures to reduce muscle tone by local or systemic pharmacological (botulinum toxin A (BTX-A), phenol injections) or neurosurgical (selective dorsal rhizotomy (SDR), intrathecal baclofen) methods. These facilitate the stretch from therapy and serial casting, and improve tolerance of brace wear, which in turn might prevent or delay the onset of static contractures and bony deformities.[27,28]

Dynamic deformities are managed by intramuscular injections of BTX-A,[28,29] which results in a temporary paralysis of muscle that facilitates stretch obtained from physiotherapy or serial casting. The local reduction of spasticity improves joint range of motion, delays the progress or onset of fixed contractures and might enhance function,[29] and delays or decreases the need for orthopaedic surgery.[30] BTX-A injections are superior to placebo injections in reducing calf muscle spasticity and increasing ankle dorsiflexion in the short term, but have only equivalent efficacy in the short term when compared with serial casting, with mixed evidence regarding the combination of serial casting plus BTX-A.[31–39] However, there is only limited evidence in the literature to support that BTX-A potentiates the effect of therapy interventions to reduce the mechanical aspects of hypertonicity,[27,40–44] and even less evidence that these effects translate into measurable functional benefits in terms of activities and participation.[45]

Severe spasticity involving bilateral lower extremities in children with good balance and muscle strength and selective control might benefit from more extensive spasticity control such as SDR. A meta-analysis of three randomized trials confirmed that, for children aged 4–8 years with spastic CP, SDR plus physiotherapy (PT) does produce a clinically significant reduction in spasticity at 12 months, and a statistically significant but relatively small functional benefit when compared with PT alone.[46–49] Despite the effectiveness of SDR in the short term, the question remains whether these small benefits are worth the time, effort and expense involved. There is little evidence that SDR reduces the need for or the amount of subsequent orthopaedic surgery,[50–52] and the long-term effects and benefits of SDR have yet to be elucidated.

Baclofen is a γ-aminobutyric acid (GABA) agonist that can reduce generalized spasticity. However, oral baclofen is poorly absorbed, and the large doses required for any meaningful effect can cause undesirable side-effects. Intrathecal administration of baclofen by an implantable pump allows for very small doses (micrograms) to directly reach the target tissue, can be a very effective way to control severe generalized hypertonia due to spasticity or dystonia, and is usually reserved for more severely involved children (GMFCS level V), as it is expensive and associated with significant complications.[53–55]

Established musculoskeletal problems are best addressed with simultaneous (single event) multilevel orthopaedic surgery, including fractional muscle or tendon lengthening, tendon transfers and corrective osteotomies to address bony deformities and joint instability that contribute to lever arm dysfunction.[56,57] Addressing all deformities simultaneously avoids the 'birthday syndrome' of staged isolated procedures,[14] and limits the interventions to one hospitalization and one period of rehabilitation. Surgery is best delayed until the child is 8–10 years old, which also reduces the likelihood of recurrence of contractures with further growth.[21] Some believe that early surgical interventions during childhood development will enhance function and allow further improvement of motor skills, with further surgery as needed when the child is older.[58] This approach also uses multilevel procedures as needed and has been referred to as 'staged multilevel interventions in the lower extremity'. There is some evidence from small case series that children with spastic diplegia who underwent staged orthopaedic procedures had unpredictable results.[59] There are few published studies that evaluate the long-term effects of multilevel orthopaedic surgery at skeletal maturity let alone into adulthood.[60,61]

Based on the physical examination, the gait assessment, imaging studies (where appropriate) and the intraoperative examination under anaesthesia, there are a number of specific orthopaedic soft-tissue procedures and osteotomies at the surgeon's disposal.

ORTHOPAEDIC PROCEDURES AT THE HIP

Psoas lengthening

The indication for psoas lengthening in ambulatory children is controversial because much of the power generated during walking in children with CP comes from the hip pulling up.[62,63] A selective lengthening of the psoas (sparing the iliacus) done over the brim of the pelvis[64,65] can be considered when there is a hip flexion contracture >30°, confirmed under anaesthesia, with reduced hip extension in terminal stance. In non-ambulatory children, a psoas lengthening is performed as part of the routine release when dealing with hip instability. For this indication, a distal iliopsoas tenotomy at the level of insertion into the lesser trochanter is acceptable.

Adductor lengthening

In ambulatory children adductor lengthening is seldom necessary. Adductor surgery is usually restricted to

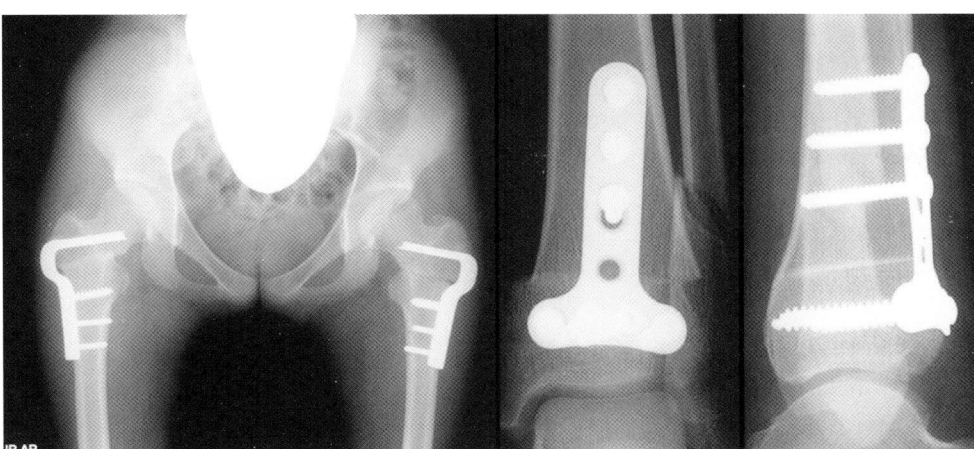

Figure 64.2 Blade plate fixation.

percutaneous or open release of adductor longus alone.[21] More extensive adductor releases to include the adductor brevis and the proximal gracilis are indicated in non-ambulant children with significant adduction contractures in order to regain an acceptable range of abduction to facilitate perineal hygiene and diapering, or as part of the reconstructive procedure for hip instability to facilitate the concomitant proximal femoral varus derotational osteotomy.

Femoral derotational or varus derotational osteotomies

Increased femoral anteversion leads to an internal rotation gait and may be the cause of scissoring with the medially rotated knee striking the contralateral side during swing. The corresponding foot progression angle may be internal, normal or even external if accompanied by increased external tibial torsion. This combination of internal rotation of the hip and external rotation of the tibial segment creates a pseudovalgus appearance at the knee. Radiographs of hips with excessive anteversion show increases in the apparent neck shaft angle (coxa valga), although true coxa valga is commonly present as well. Excessive anteversion can be addressed with proximal (intertrochanteric) or distal femoral osteotomies, with no clear evidence of one being superior to the other.[66,67] The advantage of the proximal osteotomy is that it allows for the addition of varusization, since excessive femoral anteversion when there is true coxa valga can cause some subluxation.[68] Additionally, since the osteotomy is performed proximal to the insertion of the iliopsoas on the lesser trochanter, some functional lengthening of the psoas occurs with the derotation. The proximal osteotomy can be done supine or prone, the latter having the advantage of providing reliable (bilateral) intra-operative assessment of the torsional profile. Internal fixation with a blade plate provides sufficient stability, obviating the need for any external immobilization.[69] Supported weight bearing is permissible after 3–4 weeks (Fig. 64.2).

Periacetabular pelvic osteotomies

The hip in CP is typically flexed, adducted and internally rotated. This leads to a gradual displacement of the femoral head in a posterolateral direction. Acetabular dysplasia develops over time owing to the mechanical pressure of the subluxating femoral head. Since the acetabular deficiency is usually posterolateral, the reconstructive pelvic osteotomy should improve posterolateral coverage. This is best accomplished with a Dega-type periacetabular osteotomy (or one of its adaptations), which is a lateral opening wedge osteotomy that hinges on the triradiate cartilage and spares the inner table.[70,71] Local bone graft from the anterior iliac crest can be divided into trapezoidal wedges, wider posteriorly than anteriorly, to achieve the posterolateral coverage. The procedure is indicated for the reconstruction of subluxated or dislocated hips in children over 6 years in combination with the proximal femoral varus derotational osteotomy.

ORTHOPAEDIC PROCEDURES AT THE KNEE

Hamstring lengthening

The medial hamstrings are more commonly involved than the lateral and as such are more appropriate for lengthening in ambulatory children.[62,72] Functional hamstring length is assessed by the unilateral and bilateral popliteal angle, the latter performed with the contralateral side flexed at the hip and knee to neutralize the anterior pelvic tilt.[73] In the presence of a significant anterior pelvic tilt (e.g. because of a hip flexion contracture) the hamstring length may be normal, and indiscriminate lengthening might result in further anterior pelvic tilt and a compensatory lumbar lordosis.[62] The intramuscular tenotomies of gracilis and semitendinosus and fractional lengthening of semimembranosus aponeurosis can be performed through a posteromedial or midline posterior approach just above the knee. Lateral hamstrings (biceps femoris) are less frequently lengthened in ambulatory children for fear of knee hyperextension and weak hip extension.[74] Some recommend tenotomy of the semitendinosus, which is then transferred to the adductor tubercle to prevent increased anterior pelvic tilt proximally. In non-ambulatory children both medial and lateral hamstrings may be lengthened using a single midline posterior incision or two (postero-medial and posterolateral) incisions.

Distal femoral extension osteotomy

In crouch gait, if there are significant knee flexion contractures (15–30°) and the hamstring length is relatively normal, a distal femoral extension osteotomy is an effective way to achieve 'full' extension of the knee.[75] The osteotomy is done through a lateral incision using a subvastus approach to the supracondylar aspect of the distal femur. An anteriorly based closing wedge osteotomy is performed using a blade plate for stable internal fixation. All structures posterior to the femur are effectively put on stretch, including the sciatic/peroneal nerve, so attempts to hyperextend the knee (especially with the hip flexed) intra-operatively or in the immediate postoperative period (if there is an indwelling epidural catheter for analgesia) are associated with an increased risk of nerve stretch injury, which can result in extended periods, sometimes lasting months, of hypersensitivity in the feet. Postoperative immobilization in some flexion is recommended for a few days following surgery before the knee is passively extended fully.

Anterior epiphysiodesis, using staples or eight-plates to gradually correct fixed flexion deformities in children who have sufficient growth remaining, has been reported but the longer term effectiveness of these procedures remains to be seen.[21]

Patellar tendon shortening or advancement

This is usually done in combination with the distal femoral extension osteotomy to address the patella alta that is commonly present in crouch gait. This is accomplished either by an infrapatellar shortening procedure of the patellar tendon[21] or by a patellar tendon advancement by a distal transfer of the tibial tubercle (the anterior section of the apophysis in a skeletally immature child).

Rectus femoris transfer

The transfer of the rectus femoris to the medial hamstrings is indicated when there is co-contraction of the rectus femoris and the hamstrings,[17,76,77] which causes a stiff-knee gait pattern characterized by the limited amount of knee flexion in early swing phase resulting in poor foot clearance (drag).[76] The Duncan–Ely sign is positive on the physical examination. Gait kinematics show decreased amplitude and delay of peak knee flexion in swing. Dynamic electromyography shows abnormal activation of the rectus femoris throughout swing. The procedure is indicated to improve knee flexion in early swing in order to improve foot clearance. The rectus femoris tendon is separated from the underlying vasti and the detached tendon is tenodesed to the semitendinosus, gracilis or sartorius. Early postoperative range of motion (immediate CPM (continuous passive motion)) is important to prevent adhesions. Postoperative rehabilitation, including strengthening, is crucial for the success of this procedure. Rectus transfers to the semitendinosus have been shown to increase knee flexion during swing.[76] However, overall outcomes are mixed and this procedure is best reserved for higher functioning ambulatory children (GMFCS levels I, II and some III) who are motivated and capable of participating in a rehabilitation programme.[76,78,79]

ORTHOPAEDIC PROCEDURES AT THE CALF, ANKLE AND FOOT

Gastrocnemius and soleus lengthening

In bilateral CP, the soleus muscle is often spared and does not contribute to the equinus contracture, as manifested by the normal dorsiflexion achieved with the knee flexed. Under these circumstances, lengthening of the gastrocnemius (Strayer recession) alone,[80] separate from the soleus, is necessary to avoid unduly weakening the plantarflexors and creating an iatrogenic crouch gait, a well-recognized complication of tendo-Achilles lengthening in diplegics.[81–84] Delaying surgery until 8 years old reduces the risks of recurrence and overcorrection.[10] The gastrocnemius lengthening is performed at the junction of the proximal and mid-calf, just distal to the inferior ends of the muscle bellies of the medial and lateral heads of the gastrocnemius, where the aponeurosis of gastrocnemius is separable from the underlying soleus.[80] In older children with longstanding equinus, there may be additional, although milder, contracture of the soleus. In these children, it is possible to obtain additional dorsiflexion by dividing the aponeurosis of the soleus immediately deep to the divided gastrocnemius, while preserving the underlying muscle fibres of the soleus. This allows for a differential lengthening of both gastrocnemius and soleus.[21] In unilaterally involved children (hemiplegics), both gastrocnemius and soleus are tight and therefore a tendo-Achilles lengthening is appropriate. This can be performed by a percutaneous or mini-open sliding technique (Hoke or White) or open z-lengthening.[85] The most common complication of tendo-Achilles lengthening in a hemiplegic is recurrence of equinus if the procedure is done when the child is young.

Tibialis posterior split tendon transfer or lengthening

Equinovarus deformities (more common in unilateral CP or hemiplegia) can be addressed with intramuscular lengthening of the tibialis posterior tendon if the contracture is fixed or a split tibialis posterior tendon transfer to the peroneus brevis if the hindfoot varus is flexible.[86] Transfers are more likely to be effective and last longer when done in younger children with dynamic rather than fixed contractures.

Split tibialis anterior tendon transfers to the cuboid are preferred by some if the hindfoot varus deformities are primarily in the swing phase of gait.[87] The precise indications for these transfers, and their comparative effectiveness, remains controversial. Some combine tibialis posterior tendon lengthening with split tibialis anterior tendon transfers in combination with tendo-Achilles lengthening to achieve the desired outcome.[88] The common goal is to achieve a braceable plantigrade foot both in stance phase, so that weight bearing is evenly distributed (not along the lateral border), and in swing phase to prevent difficulties with foot clearance.

Distal tibial (supramalleolar) derotational osteotomies

The external foot progression angle associated with increased external torsion results in malorientation and shortening of the lever arm of the foot for push-off. Distal tibial derotational osteotomies (Fig. 64.3) can be performed to correct excessive external tibial (or internal) torsion and stabilized with internal fixation.[89] A concomitant osteotomy of the fibula is not necessary for most distal tibial derotational osteotomies.

Calcaneal osteotomies

A number of hindfoot osteotomies have been described to tackle fixed hindfoot varus or valgus deformities. Equinovalgus deformities, which are more common in bilaterally involved children with CP, are addressed with lateral column lengthening through the calcaneus proximal to the anterior process, using bone graft (iliac crest or allograft), along with peroneal tendon lengthening and gastrocnemius–soleus recessions to address the accompanying equinus, which will be unmasked when the valgus is corrected.[90] Although this procedure provides excellent correction of the hindfoot valgus and restores a medial arch, there is a high rate of recurrence, which can be reduced by adding medial procedures, such as capsulodesis of the talonavicular joint and tibialis posterior tendon advancement. If, following the correction of the hindfoot valgus, mid/forefoot supination is apparent, this should be addressed with a plantarflexion osteotomy of the first ray to restore the normal tripod of the weight-bearing plantigrade foot. Calcaneal (tuberosity) osteotomies using closing wedge or sliding osteotomies are reserved for more severe rigid varus or valgus deformities of the hindfoot.

Subtalar (extra-articular) arthrodesis can be combined with the calcaneal osteotomies described above in order to correct and hold the deformity permanently.[91]

Other foot procedures include plantar fascial release and extension osteotomies of the first ray (base of first metatarsal or medial cuneiform) to address midfoot cavus, which is often a component of equinovarus deformities. Tenotomy of the peroneus longus with tenodesis to the peroneus brevis can be a useful adjunct. Painful hallux valgus deformities require arthrodesis of the first metatarsophalangeal joint, but this is recommended only if the equinovalgus deformity (and external tibial torsion if present) are addressed at the same time.

POSTOPERATIVE REHABILITATION FOLLOWING MULTILEVEL SURGERY

The success of multilevel orthopaedic surgery is closely linked with the rehabilitation necessary.[17] In the first 3 weeks, postoperative pain should be minimized effectively in order to initiate an early physiotherapy programme of range of motion/stretch followed by weight bearing from 4 to 6 weeks and gait training and strengthening thereafter.[92] Casts are usually removed at between 4 and 6 weeks and measurements made for supportive braces (ankle–foot orthoses). From 6 weeks to 3 months after surgery, there is a focus on strengthening and reduction of walking aids. Overall function can be expected to deteriorate from the baseline pre-operative state for 3 months, with recovery to baseline function by 6 months and progressively greater improvements noted at 12 and even up to 24 months following surgery.[93]

ORTHOPAEDIC PROCEDURES IN NON-AMBULATORY CEREBRAL PALSY

Non-ambulatory children with CP (GMFCS levels IV and V) are prone to develop lower and upper extremity contractures that can interfere with positioning and caregiving, progressive hip instability that can become

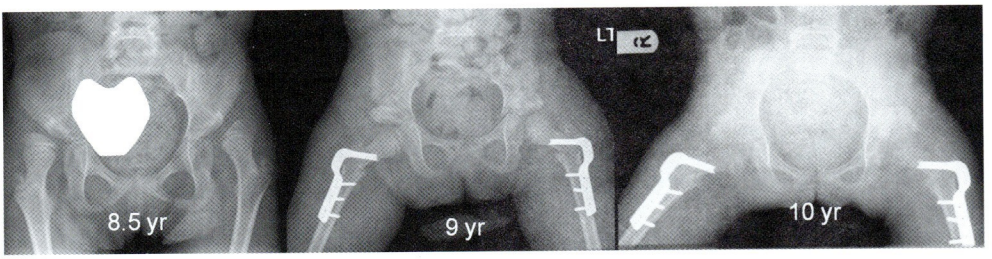

Figure 64.3 Distal tibial derotational osteotomies.

painful, and spinal deformities that affect positioning, sitting comfort, balance and endurance. All interventions for these children are directed at facilitating caregiving, promoting comfort, and maximizing health and quality of life.[15]

HIP INSTABILITY IN CEREBRAL PALSY

The hip is at risk for progressive instability in direct relation to the severity of CP (0% in GMFCS level I; 15% in GMFCS level II; 39% in GMFCS level III; 70% in GMFCS level IV; and 90% in GMFCS level V).[94,95] The time of maximum risk is between 4 and 12 years.[96] Left untreated, a hip dislocation is likely to become painful, but also interfere with dressing and perineal care.[97] Untreated hip dislocations in adults with CP have been associated with increased risk of sitting comfort, pressure sores and femoral fractures.[98,99] For these reasons, management of hip instability in childhood is a worthwhile endeavour to prevent these complications. The principles of management are similar to those outlined previously. Clinical and/or radiographic surveillance is recommended for the more involved children.[95,100,101] In children younger than 4 years, the use of BTX-A injections along with abduction bracing does reduce the adduction contractures and can delay surgery, which might minimize the risk of recurrence and repeat surgery.[102,103] There is some controversy whether early prophylactic surgery is superior to reconstructive surgery at the first signs of symptoms (contracture interfering with caregiving or pain).[104] Early prophylactic surgery (when the migration percentage has increased >30–40% without symptoms) has the theoretical benefit of lesser surgery but at the greater risk of repeat surgery, which might include the same operations being done if primary surgery was carried out later. Systematic reviews of soft-tissue (adductor releases alone) surgery have shown very high recurrence rates.[105] Adductor and psoas lengthening alone can be sufficient if, following the soft-tissue releases, the femoral head lies centred within the acetabulum with the hip held in neutral abduction. If the hip needs to be abducted at all to reduce the femoral head, a corresponding varusization of the proximal femur is indicated.[106] When these guidelines are applied, very few children meet the criteria for soft-tissue releases alone. Proximal femoral varus derotational osteotomy is performed and stabilized with a fixed-angle device (e.g. 90° blade plate). An open reduction of the femoral head is only necessary if the femoral head is dislocated or if the migration percentage is in excess of 60–70°. A periacetabular pelvic osteotomy (Dega or variant) is added if there is significant acetabular dysplasia in children over 6 years (Fig. 64.4).[70,71,107] As general rule, it is better to perform bilateral surgery including proximal femoral osteotomies in children with severe bilateral CP, as the risk of the contralateral side dislocating following unilateral surgery is high.

Hip reconstructions are preferable to salvage operations. If an adolescent has a longstanding untreated hip dislocation in which the femoral head has lost its sphericity and is severely deformed (owing to its exposure to the forces of the overlying abductors), thereby precluding a reliable reconstruction, it is better to wait until there are symptoms. For these children an effective salvage procedure is a proximal femoral head resection at the base of the neck, along with a subtrochanteric valgus osteotomy of the femur, tenodesis of the ligamentum teres to the lesser trochanter, and capsular closure, in addition to the adductor and psoas lengthening.[108] This combination effectively provides sufficient abduction for perineal hygiene and pain relief from the previous dislocation. This procedure is seldom associated with heterotopic ossification and proximal migration, which were complications of other salvage procedures that involved more extensive proximal femoral resections.

Patients with windswept deformity of the hips require an asymmetrical approach to the deformity based on a careful assessment. On the adducted and internally rotated side, the adductors, flexors and medial hamstrings are released along with an external derotational osteotomy of the femur. On the abducted and externally rotated side, the abductors, iliotibial band and lateral hamstrings may have to be released, and derotational osteotomies of the femur based on whether the femur is anteverted or not. Sometimes the 'abducted' side is just less adducted and requires similar procedures to those on the more adducted side.[109]

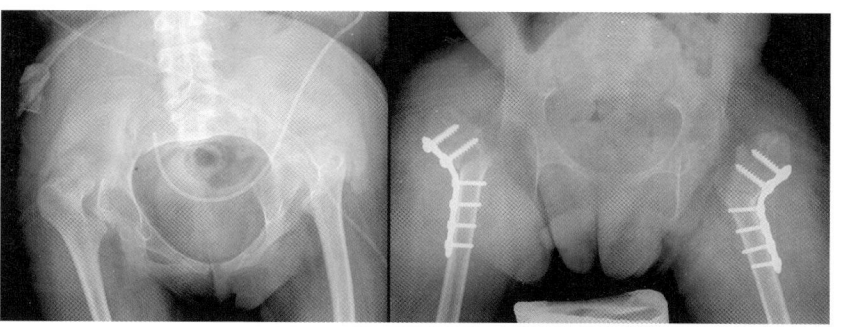

Figure 64.4 Treatment for acetabular dysplasia.

Hip reconstructive surgery is often accompanied by medial and lateral hamstring lengthening to address severe knee flexion contractures if they are interfering with positioning, dressing or caregiving.

SPINAL DEFORMITIES IN CEREBRAL PALSY

Spinal deformity is common in more severely involved children (GMFCS levels IV and V). These have been classified into: type 1, predominantly thoracic or thoracolumbar scoliosis with no pelvic obliquity; type 2, long C-shaped curves extending to the sacropelvis; and type 3, collapsing type of kyphosis with no coronal plane deformity.[110] Thoracolumbar curves tend to progress more than thoracic or lumbar curves, and the larger a curve at presentation, the more likely it is to get worse. Many of the spinal deformities remain flexible, allowing the child to be positioned comfortably in a wheelchair with appropriate lateral supports and back tilt to keep the child upright. External bracing is not often tolerated because these children are often fed by a gastrostomy tube. There is also little evidence that braces prevent progression in neuromuscular curves. More rigid curves that are creating discomfort and pressure-related problems may require custom seating with moulded backs instead, to accommodate and support the child in an upright position. There is little evidence to support whether a prophylactic surgical approach is necessary. A reactive approach may be just as effective once seating modifications have failed to be effective. The standard surgical intervention is a long instrumented posterior spinal fusion to include the upper thoracic levels to the pelvis. This can be accomplished with unit rods and sublaminar wires or with more modern, stronger but more expensive pedicle screw constructs. The latter, in combination with intra-operative traction, obviates the need for anterior releases for larger curves. The objectives of the surgery are to level the pelvis, to improve the truncal balance in order to improve sitting comfort and endurance, and to prevent pulmonary problems associated with a large curve.

THE UPPER EXTREMITY IN CEREBRAL PALSY

The classic appearance is of internal rotation and adduction at the shoulder, flexion of the elbow, flexion of the wrist with or without pronation and/or ulna deviation, flexion of fingers and a thumb in palm deformity. In addition to contractures, sensory impairments are common. The impact of these deformities may be functional (limiting the use for bimanual activities, such as keyboarding, communication devices, switches), positional (affecting dressing and hygiene), pain or cosmesis (appearance). Treatments should be tailored to address these issues where applicable, and include selective injections (guided by ultrasound or muscle stimulation) of BTX-A, splinting and surgery in select cases after non-operative interventions have failed. Sensory deficits are more significant than deformity in limiting hand function. The value of early stretching, splinting and casting is controversial. Operative indications are based on discriminatory sensibility, intelligence, motivation and overall function. Operative intervention might best be delayed until late childhood, when patient cooperation, functional needs, motivation and disability can better be ascertained.

Internal rotation and adduction of the shoulder seldom warrants surgery, but, when the deformity prevents adequate hand placement or hygiene and fails to respond to non-operative interventions, restoration of shoulder range may be achieved by lengthening of the subscapularis and pectoralis major with transfers of the latissimus dorsi or the teres major to the greater tuberosity and external derotational osteotomy.[111]

Flexion contractures of the elbow can be addressed surgically with lengthening of the elbow flexors (biceps, brachialis and brachioradialis) and, if necessary, an anterior elbow capsular release.

The position of the wrist is key to hand function. A flexed wrist leads to extension of the fingers by the effect of tenodesis and puts the finger flexors at a biomechanical disadvantage. Fingers in a flexed position may preclude grasp. With the wrist held extended, the flexed fingers may prevent active extension necessary for release. Musculoaponeurotic lengthening (e.g. flexor–pronator mass), intramuscular tendon lengthening, flexor–pronator slide and a variety of tendon transfers have been described to reduce wrist flexor strength and augment wrist extension (e.g. flexor carpi ulnaris to the extensor carpi radialis brevis, or flexor carpi radialis to the extensor carpi radialis brevis); finger extension augmentation (e.g. flexor digitorum superficialis transfer), improved supination (pronator teres transfer). Wrist arthrodesis may be required in patients with severe spasticity associated with significant problems of hygiene, cosmesis or pain. Proximal row carpectomy with adjunctive soft-tissue releases may be necessary to achieve a neutral position.

Treatment decisions for thumb in palm deformity are based on the House classification of the deformity and include flexor pollicis longus lengthening, first web and intrinsic release with a four-flap z-plasty, and stabilization of the metacarpophalangeal joint as needed.[112]

SUMMARY

The musculoskeletal consequences of CP are significant in both ambulant and non-ambulant children with CP. The priorities and goals for these two groups are quite distinct. The management of the musculoskeletal consequences are most effectively accomplished using a multidisciplinary approach. Orthopaedic surgery plays an important role in the management of these children. However, evidence to support the effectiveness of many of these interventions in terms of outcomes that are meaningful to this population remains to be established.[15,113–115] Where differences have been made, the longevity of these outcomes up to and beyond skeletal maturity into adulthood is less clear.[60] Basic science research about the biology of the brain development and epidemiological research might eventually provide the means to prevent CP in the first place or reverse the impact of brain injury, thereby reducing the need for orthopaedic surgery, which we must recognize deals with the peripheral consequences of CP and does nothing for the primary problem.

MYELOMENINGOCELE

INTRODUCTION

Myelomeningocele, also known as *spina bifida* and *myelodysplasia*, is the most common major birth defect and one of a group of conditions constituting *spinal dysraphism*.

These disorders result from failure of the normal sequence by which the spine and its overlying elements form. Embryonic ectoderm within the first 4 weeks of life develops into the neural tube, the structure ultimately responsible for producing the central nervous system (CNS) including the spinal cord, overlying vertebrae, paraspinal muscles and skin.[120] Failure of this tube to form correctly gives rise to spinal dysraphism. If the defect arises at the rostral end of the neural tube the brain and skull fail to form properly, producing *anencephaly*.

At the caudal end the degree of failure of formation in myelomeningocele allows the spinal cord and nerve roots with their surrounding meninges to prolapse at the level of the defect, giving the appearance of a thin sac through which the neural elements can be seen. The sac itself is devoid of skin and varies in size according to the volume of cerebrospinal fluid present.

Lesions occur most commonly in the lumbosacral area, although they can arise more proximally. There is associated dysplasia of the cord, with the level of the lesion giving rise to neurological symptoms that often correspond to a higher level.[121]

Variations in the severity give rise to two other less common disorders. In *spina bifida occulta* there is failure of the posterior arch to form but affected individuals in most cases have normal function of the cord. Clinical findings may include abnormal hair distribution over the affected area, or the presence of a dimple, lipoma or a haemangioma, but often the abnormality is an incidental finding. A *meningocele* occurs when the meninges without any neural tissue prolapse in a sac covered by normal-looking skin.

INCIDENCE AND AETIOLOGY

Rates vary from 0.6 to 0.9 per 1000 live births, with a slight predilection for females in a number of studies. There are racial variations with high rates reported in some parts of the world and geographical variations within countries.[122–124]

Rates are gradually declining in the developed world owing in part to pre-natal diagnosis and dietary supplementation with folic acid. Supplementation with 0.4 mg folate during early pregnancy and prior to conception has been shown to reduce the incidence.[125,126]

The use of ultrasound has allowed early identification of affected pregnancies.[127] Measuring levels of α-fetoprotein also assists. This fetal protein remains detectable in maternal serum and amniotic fluid with the presence of a neural tube defect, as well as with abdominal wall closure defects. Both of these methods have been successfully used as population screening tests.[128]

Different socioeconomic class may also play a role, as does a family history, which accounts for an increased risk in siblings. Despite all of these associations the exact cause in most cases is not understood.

GENERAL CONSIDERATIONS

The major problems facing the neonate born with myelomeningocele relate to the presence of the sac and the potential for overwhelming sepsis from CNS infection to occur. Pre-natally diagnosed neonates are delivered by caesarean section to avoid trauma to the sac and underlying neural elements, and early neurosurgical intervention for closure of the sac is carried out in most cases within 48 hours. This involves closure of the dura and overlying skin with or without the use of flaps depending on the size of the lesion. The role of fetal surgery for sac closure with the potential to reduce damage to the neural tissues and improve outcome is the subject of current investigation and is not widespread practice.[129]

After closure of the defect, hydrocephalus may ensue as a result of the Arnold–Chiari malformation in which displacement of the cerebellum and medulla oblongata into the foramen magnum obstructs cerebrospinal fluid. This is associated with developmental delay and can lead to death; treatment requires insertion of a ventriculoperitoneal shunt with subsequent long-term monitoring to ensure correct functioning until the tendency decreases after a number of years.

Other neurological abnormalities may also be present, including tethered cord syndrome, diastematomyelia and hydromyelia. These can sometimes be the cause of deterioration in the neurological status later in life.

Renal failure remains the commonest cause of death after the first year of life and is a consequence of the paralysed bladder. Reflux and hydronephrosis with frequent infections lead to this, and require active management and observation, with self-catheterization often required. Early surgical repair of the myelomeningocele may alter the complications.[130]

ORTHOPAEDIC MANAGEMENT

The role of the orthopaedic surgeon is as part of a multidisciplinary team dealing with a wide range of pathology in what is a complex and demanding condition.

The key aims of orthopaedic involvement are to assist in establishing the prognosis for mobility and independence, maximizing potential and identifying any deterioration in function that may arise from the disease associations of the condition.

This begins with a proper clinical assessment of the affected child, which often follows in the first few weeks of life after neurosurgical intervention to close the sac. The examination involves identifying the level of preserved motor and sensory function by clinical observation for muscle contraction and response to sensory stimulation in a dermatomal distribution. Key motor function to determine includes the presence of contraction of the quadriceps, iliopsoas and gluteus medius.[131] These muscle groups, and in particular quadriceps power, are important as they allow prediction of the potential for independent ambulation. The majority of those with normal quadriceps strength maintain strength and mobility into adulthood.

Lesions below L4 mean that most affected individuals will be independently able to mobilize. Lesions at L3 and higher rarely allow ambulation. A strict pattern is not always followed and there can be considerable variation in function with the same level of lesion between affected individuals. Scoring systems do exist for neurological assessment.[132]

Periodic assessment is also critical to assess for deterioration in function, developing deformities, changing requirements for orthoses and intact skin.

Associated orthopaedic problems

A spectrum of additional factors make management of the patient with myelomeningocele more complicated. When considering surgical intervention one should be aware that the risk of postoperative infection is much higher. Loss of protective sensation predisposes to pressure sores that can be difficult to treat. Pathological fractures can occur, and the presentation may not be accompanied by pain or a history of trauma. There is also an increased risk of significant allergy to latex in up to 15%.[133]

REGIONAL ASSESSMENT

Spine

Spinal deformity can be congenital, arising as a direct result of the myelomeningocele or malformations such as hemivertebrae and intrathecal anomalies.[134]

The underlying degree of neuromuscular imbalance predisposes to the development of scoliosis. With sacral lesions the risk of scoliosis is around 5%, but with lesions at L1 and above the risk increases to greater than 90%.[135] Moderate curves can be treated initially with bracing while the child continues to grow.[136] Continued regular review is necessary to identify the 80% with curve progression. When occurring rapidly, this may be due to the presence of a tethered cord. Complications of surgery are high, and the best results are obtained by combined anterior and posterior fusion, with fusion to the pelvis carried out for coexisting pelvic obliquity.[137]

Kyphosis provides a significant challenge; it does not respond to bracing, progresses with time and contributes to pulmonary dysfunction, poor sitting balance and local skin pressure necrosis. It can be congenital or acquired and requires complex surgical intervention.[138] This involves kyphectomy or vertebral subtraction with instrumented fusion. Complication rates are high both peri- and postoperatively.

In all cases treatment should be individualized, depending on the age, degree of deformity and general health of the patient.

Hip

Problems encountered include hip subluxation, dislocation and contractures. Treatment aims to allow flexion and therefore sitting, and stable hip extension for supported standing in appropriate cases.[139] Difficulties in management exist mainly for lower lesions, in which imbalance produces various contractures.

Flexion contractures are often the main problem, and are caused by unopposed spasticity of the iliopsoas. In wheelchair-bound patients it is less of a concern, but, in those who have the potential to walk, greater than 20–30° of contracture may inhibit gait. These patients benefit from flexor releases.[140]

Abduction contractures are also common and can be associated with external rotation of the hip. Proper positioning, stretching exercises and splinting may help prevent this, but surgical release is sometimes indicated, requiring release of the tensor fasciae latae, gluteus medius and minimus, rectus femoris and sartorius.

Hip dislocation is most commonly seen in those with a lesion at the L3–4 level. Management of this remains highly controversial. Intervention depends on the functional demand and in most is not required. The general trend is towards non-operative management of hip dislocation, particularly as hip pain is rare. Late dislocation may follow from tethering of the cord.

The constant imbalance in muscle power drives the hip to an 'at risk' position, meaning that most interventions practised for other conditions fail in this group of patients. Historically, muscle-balancing procedures and bony realignment of the femur and acetabulum have been used. Muscle balancing involves transfer of the iliopsoas tendon with part of the lesser trochanter via a trough cut in the ilium to the greater trochanter (Mustard transfer)[141] or to the posterior greater trochanter through a window in the ilium with iliacus transferred to the outer wall of the pelvis (Sharrard transfer)[142]. Both of these procedures have been shown to have variable results, with recurrence of subluxation a common problem, particularly when surgery is performed on older children.

Knee

Flexion contractures are the most common knee problem, although they rarely require any treatment in the wheelchair-bound patient. In the ambulatory, difficulty with walking can occur, with additional energy expended with increasing contractures. It often develops with growth. Treatment can involve initial splinting and stretching, lengthening of the hamstrings, sometimes with posterior capsular release necessary. Occasionally, extension osteotomy of the distal femur is required for correction.[143]

Extension contractures are far less common, but can again be treated by serial casting and splintage, with quadriceps lengthening for resistant cases. Congenital hyperextension, dislocation and recurvatum of the knee have also been described.

Torsional deformities of the tibia can require intervention in the form of a supramalleolar osteotomy in which foot position interferes with gait or causes pressure problems with orthoses, leading to sores.[144]

Foot and ankle

Deformities of the foot present as congenital anomalies or develop with time. More than two-thirds of deformities in patients with low lesions require surgical intervention. Treatment aims to allow orthotic fitting and a plantigrade foot free of pressure sores.

Talipes equinovarus (clubfoot) occurs in one-third of patients. Treatment is much more complicated by the rigidity of the foot, making conservative management more complicated with a higher rate of recurrence of deformity and an increased risk of fracture and pressure sores. Recent data suggest that use of the Ponseti method in clubfeet in myelomeningocele achieves good correction, albeit with a higher rate of recurrence requiring further casting.[145] For resistant cases, good results have been obtained with surgical correction, mirroring the techniques used in idiopathic clubfeet.[146,147]

Congenital vertical talus occurs more commonly in these patients, causing a planovalgus foot, and, because of the lack of protective sensation, the prominent talus leads to ulceration of the skin in this area. Surgical management is the frequent outcome, often after the age of 3 years. Casting and manipulation are ineffective.[148]

Equinus deformity can occur independently, and is managed with manipulation and later with lengthening procedures of the Achilles tendon.

Calcaneal deformity is thought in part to be related to muscle imbalance around the foot and ankle, although this is not evident clinically in all cases. It can present at birth or develop with growth. The position of the heel makes orthotic use difficult and predisposes to heel ulceration. Lesions at L4 or lower are the frequent association, and deformity frequently progresses. Treatment involves addressing the imbalance; in those with voluntary and involuntary dorsiflexion (but not spasticity) the tibialis anterior tendon can be re-routed via the interosseous membrane to the heel, with additional anterior structure releases as needed.[149,150]

Valgus deformity of the ankle is also common, particularly in lesions at the L4–5 level.[151] Skin problems around the medial malleolus require intervention to realign the ankle. In younger patients screw hemiepiphysiodesis can be performed; in older patients a supramalleolar closing wedge osteotomy will achieve the same desired correction. Hindfoot valgus can be managed with a sliding calcaneal osteotomy.[152]

MUSCULAR DYSTROPHIES AND HEREDITARY NEUROPATHIES

MUSCULAR DYSTROPHY

Dystrophinopathies

By far the most common of the muscular dystrophies is Duchenne muscular dystrophy (DMD). It is an X-linked recessive disorder that occurs in two or three per 10 000 boys.[153] It is due to a mutation in the dystrophin gene, which codes for a protein involved in the cell membrane calcium transport. The gene is expressed in all muscles and the brain. In most cases, DMD has an out-of-frame deletion or duplication that results in a non-functional dystrophin protein. This causes a loss of muscle cells with progressive proximal-to-distal muscle weakness. Despite advances in medical management, it continues to be fatal in the second or third decade of life. Becker muscular dystrophy results from less extensive mutations in the same gene and produces a partially functional dystrophin protein. The clinical disease is less severe with later onset and less profound weakness.

CLINICAL PICTURE

The diagnosis of DMD can be suspected in boys with a serum creatine kinase level that is 200–300 times that of the normal level. Genetic testing can be confirmatory in two-thirds of those patients who have large abnormalities in the dystrophin gene.[154] Muscle biopsy is needed for the diagnosis in the remaining one-third. Histology will show muscle fibre degeneration with increased cellularity. There is proliferation of the interstitial connective tissue with adipose replacement. Special staining with antidystrophin antibodies shows complete lack of staining in the sarcolemma in DMD, and only partial staining in Becker muscular dystrophy. Electromyography will show low-amplitude, short duration, polyphasic motor unit action potentials.

Early symptoms such as flatfeet and mild motor delay may present as early as age 2–3 years. The average age of walking is 18 months. Frequently, however, the diagnosis is not suspected until age 4–5 years, when tiptoe walking, waddling and tripping become more pronounced. The pseudohypertrophy of the calf results from fatty replacement of the muscle tissue (Fig. 64.5a). The proximal-to-distal progression of weakness results in gait abnormalities and contractures as boys try to maintain erect posture. The Gower manoeuvre of quadruped stance and walking up the legs with the hands to get up off the floor and the slip through of underarm lifting are signs of proximal muscle weakness (Fig. 64.5b). Increased lordosis and tiptoe walking are efforts to maintain the body's centre of gravity posterior to the hip and anterior to the knee to utilize unaffected joint capsules as the proximal hip extensors and quadriceps weaken first. It is made possible by the fact that the gastrocnemius weakness occurs later in the disease process. Short leg bracing to prevent tiptoe walking will often make walking impossible.

As quadriceps weakness progresses to the point of an extension lag of 15° or more of knee extension against gravity when sitting, walking may become impossible without bracing above the knee. Often, by this point, bracing is complicated by hip abduction contractures of the tensor fascia lata due to wide-based gait and equinovarus foot deformities due to late occurring weakness in the gastrocnemius and posterior tibialis. A surgical strategy of hip abductor releases, tendo-Achilles lengthening and posterior tibialis tendon transfer to the dorsolateral foot, followed by ischial-bearing knee–ankle–foot orthoses with knee-drop locks, may be used in selected patients to prolong walking ability. As with any surgery, illness or injury in patients with muscular dystrophy, aggressive management to get the child upright and walking is paramount. They have so little muscle reserve that any disuse atrophy from bed rest may result in permanent loss of function. Owing to progressive upper extremity weakness, assistive devices for walking are of little use.

The disease progression usually results in wheelchair dependence by age 10–14 years. At this point, the progressive truncal weakness begins to produce progressive kyphoscoliosis and pelvic obliquity in 85% of patients and screening radiographs should be performed.[154] Spinal orthoses and seating systems have not been demonstrated to prevent curve progression and may compromise pulmonary function. Therefore, early spinal fusion is preferred to manage spinal deformity before progressive pulmonary and cardiac muscle dysfunction preclude such surgery. Fusion of the entire thoracic and lumbar spine with or without the pelvis is recommended because additional curves will develop in the unfused segments.

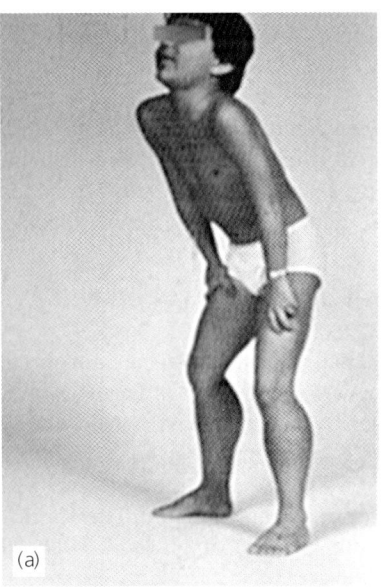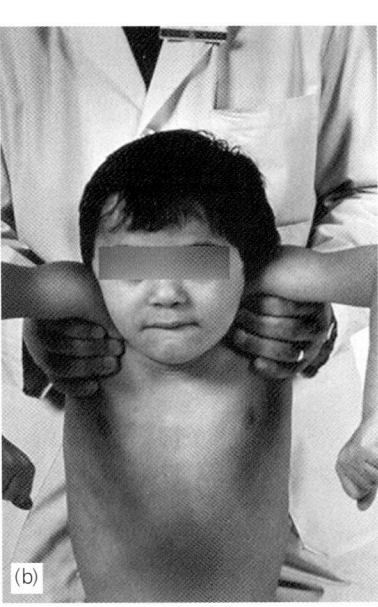

Figure 64.5 (a) Pseudohypertrophy of the calf is seen in Duchenne muscular dystrophy. Accessory use of the hands on the thigh supplements for the weak quadriceps muscles. (b) Slip-through is seen due to weakness of the proximal muscles of the shoulder girdle.

REHABILITATION

Early therapy should be geared toward maintaining muscle strength and the prevention of contractures. Strengthening exercises should not be overly aggressive as this could result in an increased rate of muscle destruction. Passive stretching of the tensor fascia lata, hamstrings, gastrocnemius and posterior tibialis may help prevent contractures along with part-time bracing. Contractures progress rapidly once walking ceases, and wheelchair modifications such as hip adductor pads, trunk and head supports, and foot rests become important for positioning. Because of upper extremity weakness, powered wheelchair mobility with adapted living spaces and transportation must be planned for, as these children will spend half their life in wheelchairs. Equipment for transfers and self-feeding may facilitate home care.

Respiratory exercises and pulmonary toilet are necessary to maintain breathing function and prevent infection. Sleep apnoea is also common and pressure support at night may become necessary. Ninety per cent of children with DMD have abnormal electrocardiograms. Cardiomyopathy and arrhythmias may interfere with the ability to exercise, especially late in the disease. Intellectual development is impaired, with an average IQ of 70 in patients with DMD.

CORTICOSTEROID MANAGEMENT

The beneficial effect of steroids in DMD was first reported in 1974.[155] Since then, six class I randomized controlled trials have concluded that steroids improve muscle strength and functional outcome. These studies have looked at prednisone/prednisolone or deflazacort. The mechanism of the steroid effect in DMD is unclear. DMD is associated with inflammation and fibrosis of the muscle tissue. Steroids affect signal transduction regulation with a direct nuclear effect on T cells.

Most clinical studies of steroid treatment demonstrate improvements or stabilization of declining muscle function. One study demonstrated a 1 year prolongation of walking.[156] Others have shown preservation of lung and cardiac function. Studies with higher steroid doses overall had better functional results and a lower rate of scoliosis but higher rates of side-effects, particularly weight gain and cataracts. Boys with DMD have reduced bone mineral density and increased fracture rates, probably because of inactivity. This is made worse by steroid therapy. Deflazacort reportedly has less effect on vertebral bone mass than prednisone. Some studies with prednisone have shown similar effect on bone mass but possibly less risk of weight gain.

GENE THERAPY

Obstacles to gene therapy in DMD are the large size of the gene and its expression in all muscles and the brain.[157,158] Replacement of the complete dystrophin gene by viral vectors has been complicated by its large size. A phase I/IIa trial involving administration of a microversion of the gene with an adeno-associated viral vector is ongoing. Potential limitations include immune response to the virus and the fact that the vector rarely incorporates into chromosomes so the vector's genome will be lost with subsequent cell divisions.

Antisense oligonucleotides are used to redirect splicing and induce exon skipping. By targeting an out-of-frame deletion in DMD, an antisense oligonucleotide can restore the reading frame and allow dystrophin to be produced. The limitations are that different deletions will require different antisense oligonucleotides, and the treatment effect is limited by its persistence in the tissue, the half-life for the skipped mRNA and the resultant protein.

The final strategy under investigation involves read-through of stop codons. Aminoglycosides have been shown to suppress stop codons. In DMD this could allow read-through of the premature stop codon and production of a functional protein. Because of the potential toxicity of gentamicin, a small molecule, PTC124, was developed which allows ribosomes to bypass the nonsense mutations in mRNA. The theoretical risk is that this strategy may result in global mistranslation and clinical trials are in progress.

Limb girdle muscular dystrophy

Limb girdle muscular dystrophies (LGMDs) are progressive myopathies that affect the muscles around the scapula and pelvic girdles.[159] There is a wide spectrum of severity developing from childhood to adulthood. Initial motor milestones may be normal or slightly delayed with toe walking. Pelvic muscle weakness precedes shoulder girdle involvement. Muscle weakness is progressive but variable and may result in wheelchair dependence and scoliosis. Clinically, there is associated calf and tongue hypertrophy, selective skeletal muscle involvement and late-stage cardiac complications. They are classified by the inheritance pattern of autosomal dominant LGMD1 and autosomal recessive LGMD2. These two classes are then subdivided further by the gene locus that is involved. Nineteen different genes have been identified. They involve both structural proteins and enzymes acting in the cell nucleus, cytosol, cytoskeleton or sarcolemma. Adeno-associated viral-mediated *LCMD2C* gene transfer is being studied.

Facioscapulohumeral muscular dystrophy

Facioscapulohumeral muscular dystrophy is an autosomal dominant disease with a variable severity and age of onset, from infancy to adulthood.[160] There is 95% penetrance by age 20 years. This is linked to chromosome 4q35, resulting in a reduced number of repeats in a sequence termed D4Z4. Facial muscle atrophy results in incomplete eye closure, transverse smile and absence of eye and forehead wrinkling. Shoulder girdle weakness results in horizontal

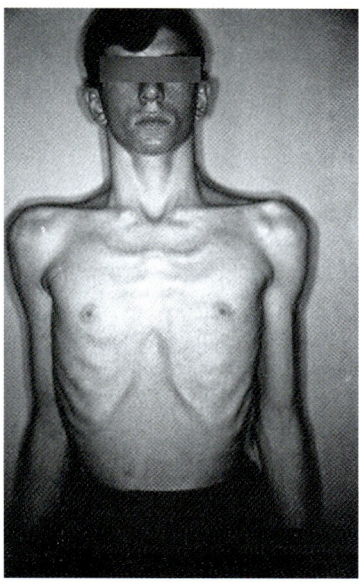

Figure 64.6 Transverse smile, horizontal clavicles and sparing of the deltoid muscles are seen in facioscapulohumeral muscular dystrophy.

clavicles and winging of the scapulae with relative sparing of the deltoid muscles (Fig. 64.6). Anterior tibialis and pelvic girdle muscle involvement may occur. Sensorineural hearing loss is common. Cardiac involvement is not seen and life expectancy is normal. Serum creatine kinase levels are normal and muscles do not show the inflammatory response seen DMD.

Emery–Dreifuss muscular dystrophy

Emery–Dreifuss-type muscular dystrophy is inherited by a sex-linked recessive pattern.[161] It results from mutations in the *X-EMD* gene on the long arm of chromosome X at Xq28. It is characterized by progressive muscle weakness in the upper arm, calf and neck flexors, resulting in elbow flexion and equinus contractures and spinal stiffness. There is no pseudohypertrophy and serum creatine kinase levels are only mildly elevated. This form of muscular dystrophy is associated with heart block and should be managed with a pacemaker.

Congenital muscular dystrophy

Presenting with neonatal weakness, hypotonia and developmental delay, congenital muscular dystrophy may be associated with arthrogryposis at birth or progressive joint contractures.[162] Congenital muscular dystrophy is autosomal recessive in inheritance. The evolution pattern is variable and in most cases mental development is normal. Serum creatine kinase may be elevated in the first years of life and tends to decrease with time. Electromyography shows a myopathic pattern and muscle biopsy shows muscle fibre necrosis and regeneration.

HEREDITARY MOTOR AND SENSORY NEUROPATHIES

The inherited peripheral neuropathies represent a heterogeneous group of disorders with varying motor, sensory and autonomic dysfunction. The widely used clinical and electrophysiological classification of Dyck and Lambert[163,164] has given way to an ever-expanding classification based on genetic testing. More than 30 causative genes have been identified. To make things more confusing, the same phenotype can be caused by different genes, and the same gene defect can result in different phenotypes.

Charcot–Marie–Tooth disease

These neuropathies affect both the Schwann cell (neuronal) and the axonal components of the peripheral nerve. During nerve development there is a complex interplay between these two components. Different genetic defects within the same gene can affect either the Schwann cell, resulting in demyelination, or the axon, resulting in an axonal phenotype. In general, 70% of patients with classical demyelinating Charcot–Marie–Tooth (CMT) disease type 1A have duplication of the gene coding for peripheral myelin protein 22 (PMP22) on chromosome 17.[165] However, many other causative genes have been identified and, in the case of the different clinical types of CMT disease, the same gene(s) may be involved in several types. This brings into question the separation of demyelinating CMT1 disease and axonal CMT2 disease, which was originally based on electrophysiological testing. Complicating the matter further are molecular genetic classifications which are difficult to interpret in clinical practice because of wide-ranging phenotypes. Table 64.1 shows causative genes identified so far in CMT disease.[165]

CLINICAL FEATURES

Features of CMT disease types 1 and 2 are often similar and difficult to distinguish clinically.[166] They result in a chronic progressive neuropathy beginning distally and working proximally, with lower extremity symptoms preceding those of the upper extremity. Even within families, there is considerable variation in the age of onset, rapidity of progression and severity of disease. There is atrophy of involved muscles and diminished reflexes. Muscle imbalance results in foot deformities, usually cavovarus. Weakness in anterior tibialis function results in foot drop, accessory overpull of the long toe extensors and fixed equinus. Proximal weakness contributes to hip dysplasia and progressive spinal deformities and patients should be evaluated with screening radiographs. Upper extremity weak-

Table 64.1 Causative genes in Charcot–Marie–Tooth (CMT) disease

CMT1		CMT2		X-linked	Intermediate	
Autosomal dominant	Autosomal recessive	Autosomal dominant	Autosomal recessive		Dominant intermediate	Others
PMP22	GDAP1	MFN2	GDAP1	GJ 1	DMN2	GJ 1
MPZ	MTMR2	KIF1B	LMNA		YARS	NEFL
LITAF	MTMR13	RAB7	MED25			MPZ
EGR2	KIAA1985	GARS				
NEFL	NDRG1	NEFL				
	EGR2	HSP27				
	PRX	HSP22				
	CTDP1	MPZ				
	PMP22					
	MPZ					

PMP22, peripheral myelin protein 22; *MPZ*, myelin protein zero; *LITAF*, lipopolysaccharide-induced tumour necrosis factor; *EGR2*, early growth response 2; *GJ 1*, gap junction protein beta 1; *GDAP1*, ganglioside-induced differentiation-associated protein 1; *MTMR2*, myotubularin-related protein 2; *MTMR13*, myotubularin-related protein 13; *KIAA1985*, KIAA 1985; *NDRG1*, N-*myc* downstream-regulated gene 1; *PRX*, periaxin; *CTDP1*, CTD phosphatase subunit 1; *KIF1B* , kinesin family member 1B-β ; *MFN2*, mitofusin 2; *RAB7*, RAS-associated protein RAB7; *GARS*, glycyl-tRNA synthetase; *NEFL*, neurofilament light polypeptide 68 kDa; *HSP27*, heat shock 27 kDa protein 1; *HSP22*, heat shock 22 kDa protein 8; *LMNA*, lamin A/C; *MED25*, mediator of RNA polymerase II subunit 25; *DMN2*, dynamin 2; *YARS*, tyrosyl-tRNA synthetase.

ness presents with hand cramping with writing and typing, dropping things because of weakness of thumb opposition and intrinsic wasting and contractures. Sensory loss is a later finding than motor loss and can be most often detected with vibratory sense testing.

Pes cavus and/or varus are frequent presenting symptoms of CMT disease. CMT disease is also the most common cause of pes cavus in 45% of cases.[167] Patients presenting with bilateral cavus feet have a 78% chance of having CMT disease.[168] The foot deformities result because of the initial involvement of the foot intrinsics and peroneal muscles before the tibial muscles. The plantar fascia is the main stabilizer of the longitudinal arch. At toe-off, the dorsiflexion of the metatarsal phalangeal joints tightens the plantar fascia, stabilizing and elevating the medial arch. The unopposed function of the long toe extensors leads to an exaggerated windlass effect on the plantar fascia. This results in cavus and toe clawing. The relatively strong peroneus longus results in depression of the first metatarsal, adding to the cavus and the initially pronated forefoot deformity. The strong posterior tibialis, unopposed by the peroneus brevis, results in hindfoot varus and the persistent heel inversion leads to subsequent forefoot supination. In planning treatment of the foot deformity, the progressive nature of the disease needs to be considered as the muscle imbalance pattern may change. Initially, these deformities are flexible and may be amenable to bracing with foot orthotics to control the varus. Foot drop may require bracing in an ankle–foot orthosis with hindfoot moulds to control the foot deformity.

As the deformities persist and progress, they become more rigid. Surgical treatment is used for those foot deformities that cannot be braced. The surgery needed is based on the particular muscle imbalances and deformities present and the flexibility of those deformities. The flexibility of the hindfoot varus can be assessed by weight bearing on a lateral forefoot block.[169] This concentrates a valgus force on the hindfoot and creates a relief for the plantarflexed first metatarsal to allow forefoot pronation. The hindfoot flexibility can also be assessed in the prone position.[170] Those deformities which are flexible can be managed by soft-tissue procedures such as plantar fascial releases for cavus, posterior tibialis lengthenings or transfers to the dorsolateral foot for varus, and peroneus longus transfers to prevent plantarflexion of the first metatarsal. Additionally, toe extensor transfers, Hibbs/Jones type, can be used to address the clawtoe deformities. More rigid deformities require osteotomies, such as first metatarsal dorsiflexion for forefoot varus, midfoot osteotomies for cavus and calcaneal osteotomies for hindfoot varus. Arthrodeses for deformity correction should be a last resort because of the high rate of adjacent joint degeneration, especially as the sensory component of the disease progresses.[171,172]

Hip dysplasia has been found in 6% of patients with CMT disease and associated pain may add to difficulty in walking during later life.[173] It is more common in females and in those with CMT1 disease. Osteotomies have been reported to improve symptoms but are also associated with a higher than expected rate of nerve palsies. These observations were based on older diagnostic criteria for CMT disease and may represent overlap clinically with the newer diagnosis of hereditary neuropathy with liability to pressure palsies. Spinal deformities are seen in 10–38% of patients with CMT disease, usually scoliosis or kyphoscoliosis.[174,175] They are usually mild to moderate in magnitude and may not respond to bracing. They are more frequent in females and in those with CMT1 disease based on the older clinical and electrophysiological classification.

Recent genetic studies have shown that spinal deformity may be predictive of CMT4C and is especially severe with Src homology 3 domain and tetratricopeptide repeat-containing protein 2 (KIAA 1985) mutations.[176]

MEDICAL AND GENE TREATMENTS

There is still no effective treatment in CMT disease. Overexpression of *PMP22* is part of the disease mechanism in CMT1A and progesterone is known to increase *PMP22* expression.[177] The progesterone antagonist onapristone has been shown in animal trials to improve the CMT phenotype by improving the axonal support function of the Schwann cells. While this improves our understanding of the disease mechanism, onapristone is toxic to humans. Ascorbic acid is a promoter of myelination and has been shown to inhibit *PMP22* expression in a dose-dependent fashion, requiring at least 3 g per day. Since ascorbic acid is well tolerated by humans, it is being used in clinical trials. Neurotrophin 3 is secreted by the Schwann cells to promote axonal regeneration. Improved axonal regeneration in animal models has been demonstrated with neurotrophin 3 treatment, and patients with CMT disease given neurotrophin 3 showed improvements in sensory changes.

Dejerine–Sottas syndrome

Dejerine–Sottas syndrome, also known as hereditary motor sensory neuropathy III, is a very aggressive autosomal recessive demyelinating polyneuropathy with onset in infancy and young childhood.[178] It is associated with pes cavus, dropfoot and delayed motor milestones. The children frequently become wheelchair dependent and develop significant spinal deformity. Sensory loss is present in a stocking–glove distribution. There is profound, <12 m s^{-1}, slowing of nerve conduction velocity and elevated protein levels in cerebrospinal fluid. Recent genetic studies show similar genes involved in both Dejerine–Sottas syndrome and CMT1, suggesting that they may indeed be variants of the same disease.[165]

OBSTETRIC BRACHIAL PLEXUS PALSY

INTRODUCTION

Obstetric brachial plexus birth palsy (OBPP) refers to the paralysis of the upper extremity secondary to a traction or compression injury to the brachial plexus during birth.[179,180] OBPP was originally described by Smellie[181] in 1765; the findings were further substantiated by the works of Duchenne[182] and Erb[183] in the 1870s. Klumpke[184] in 1885 described a lesion of the C8–T1 nerve roots of the brachial plexus. Although the majority of infants demonstrate spontaneous recovery, some have persistent neurological deficits with upper limb impairment.[181–184]

INCIDENCE

The incidence of OBPP varies from 1.51 to 3.3 per 1000 live births.[185–188]

THEORIES OF CAUSATION

The mechanical theory of causation is the most widely accepted with traction on the neural elements being responsible for the actual lesions of obstetrical brachial plexus paralysis. OBPP results from excessive lateral traction on the head away from the shoulder.[184,186] This force on the brachial plexus can cause varying degrees of injury to the nerves, including traction preserving the continuity of the nerve (neuropraxia) or rupture of the nerve roots or trunks (axontemesis or neurotemesis) and avulsion of the nerve roots from the spinal cord.

In addition, cross-innervations can occur in cases of complete root rupture where the gaps are short, such that nerve regeneration is possible but produces misdirection of the regenerating motor axons. This results in co-contraction of synergistic and antagonistic muscles and prevents full excursion of the muscles such that they develop secondary contractures.[189]

RISK FACTORS

The two most important risk factors are high birth weight and shoulder dystocia.[185–187] In general, two patterns of association are seen: the high birth weight baby with normal vertex presentation and the normal birth weight baby with breech presentation. Risk factors associated with OBPP are outlined in Box 64.1.

> **BOX 64.1: Risk factors**
>
> - High birth weight (average vertex brachial plexus palsy (BPP), 3.8–5.0 kg; average breech BPP, 1.8–3.7 kg; average unaffected, 2.8–4.5 kg)[185–187]
> - Shoulder dystocia[185–187]
> - Breech delivery
> - Prolonged labour[186]
> - Multiparity
> - Assisted delivery (e.g. use of mid/low forceps, vacuum extraction; forceful downward traction on the head during delivery)[185–187]
> - Maternal diabetes
> - Previous child with obstetric brachial plexus palsy

CLASSIFICATION, SITES OF INVOLVEMENT AND FREQUENCY

The original classification of OBPP was based on nerve root involvement (Table 64.2).

Gilbert and Tassin[190] and Narakas[191] proposed a new classification of OBPP (Table 64.3) to replace earlier regional classifications. This classification is useful as it provides a clear definition of the extent of injury to the brachial plexus and offers a broad guide to prognosis.

NATURAL HISTORY

The natural history of OBPP depends on the underlying pattern of nerve injury and root involvement. The vast majority of upper plexus lesions do tend to resolve and improve with time. Avulsions of nerve roots from the spinal cord, however, are associated with very poor chance of recovery.

Gilbert and Tassin[190] suggested that recovery of antigravity biceps and deltoid function by 3 months of age was predictive of complete spontaneous recovery. This finding has been widely accepted,[188] but also challenged by Michelow et al.[192] and others.[193] Michelow et al.[192] noted a 12% error rate in predicting outcome using Gilbert and Tassin's method and suggested using a more comprehensive assessment that took into account elbow flexion and extension, wrist extension and thumb extension (the Toronto scale). Smith and colleagues[193] noted that patients with a C5–6 injury and absent biceps muscle function at 3 months old often have good long-term shoulder function without brachial plexus surgery. Those with more extensive levels of injury had more prolonged recovery times.

Failure of return of function by 3–6 months,[190] evidence of proximal nerve root injury, i.e. Horner syndrome, phrenic nerve palsy, presence of winging of the scapula and evidence of root avulsion from the spinal cord, i.e. spasticity in the lower limbs and awkward gait, are poor prognostic indicators (Box 64.2).[194]

In patients who do not have complete spontaneous recovery, the initial presentation is that of varying degrees of muscle weakness related to the nerves involved in the brachial plexus. The muscle imbalance around the joints of the upper extremity can then progress over time, resulting in decreasing range of motion and joint contractures (Table 64.4). Over time, secondary bony deformities develop along with joint instability and dislocation, especially around the shoulder.[201] The secondary changes around the shoulder are akin to changes occurring in a paralytic hip dislocation.

BOX 64.2: Prognostic indicators of obstetric brachial plexus palsy

- Good prognostic indicators
  - Recovery of antigravity elbow flexion and shoulder abduction at 3 months
- Poor prognostic predictors
  - Failure of return of antigravity elbow flexion and shoulder abduction by 3–6 months
  - Evidence of proximal nerve root injury
  - Horner syndrome
  - Phrenic nerve palsy
  - Long thoracic nerve palsy (paralysis of serratus anterior — winging of scapula)
  - Dorsal scapular nerve palsy (paralysis of rhomboids)
  - Evidence of root avulsion from spinal cord
  - Spasticity in ipsilateral lower limb
  - Awkward gait and urinary problems

Table 64.2 Original classification of obstetric brachial plexus palsy (OBPP)

Type of OBPP	Nerve roots involved
Erb–Duchenne palsy	C5, C6
Total plexus palsy	C5–T1
Klumpke palsy	C8, T1

Table 64.3 New classification of obstetric brachial plexus palsy (OBPP)

Group	Nerve roots involved	Clinical presentation	Rate of full recovery (%)
Group I	C5, C6	Paralysis of deltoid and biceps. Good hand function	90%
Group II	C5, C6, C7	Paralysis of deltoid, biceps and elbow, wrist and hand extensors. Normal long finger flexors	65%
Group III	C5–T1 (incomplete)	Incomplete paralysis of entire brachial plexus (all weak except some finger flexion)	<50%
Group IV	C5–T1 (complete); sympathetics	Complete paralysis (all atonic); Horner syndrome	None

Table 64.4 Muscle contractures, bony deformities and joint instabilities in obstetric brachial plexus palsy

Region	Muscle contractures	Bony deformity and Joint instability
Shoulder	Adduction: medial rotation contractures; isolated abduction contractures Abduction: lateral rotation contractures	Glenohumeral instability, posterior dislocation of shoulder Glenoid fossa shallow and flattened Elevated hypoplastic scapula Coracoid process directed inferiorly[195,196]
Elbow	Flexion, extension contractures	
Forearm	Pronation, supination contractures	Increases ulna curvature, radial head dislocation, conical deformity of radial head[197]
Wrist	Flexion, extension contractures	
Hand	Flexion contractures	

CLINICAL FEATURES

At birth, the infant presents with a limp upper extremity. No spontaneous movement of the extremity may be noted. Swelling may be present in the shoulder girdle. Any movement may be associated with pain. Over the next few days the swelling resolves and sensitivity of the limb improves.

With Erb palsy, the paralysis involves the shoulder abductors and elbow flexors and supinators of the forearm, resulting in the waiter tip position, with the shoulder held in adduction and internal rotation, the elbow extended and forearm pronated.

With complete brachial plexus paralysis, the entire arm and hand is flail with no movement. A Horner syndrome (eyelid ptosis and pupillary miosis) may be noted, suggesting avulsion of the lower brachial plexus. Phrenic nerve palsy is also suggestive of a very severe avulsion injury.

DIAGNOSIS

Supplementary investigations are shown in Table 64.5.

Table 64.5 Supplementary investigations[194]

Supplementary investigation	Purpose
Myelography and CT myelography[198]	For detecting avulsions of nerve roots from the spinal cord
MRI, fast spin echo MRI[199,200]	To detect preganglionic nerve root injuries
Electrodiagnostic studies: nerve conduction and electromyography	

TREATMENT

Non-surgical

An essential component of treatment of OBPP is joint mobilization and range of movement exercises to minimize the development of contractures and maintain a stable, congruent glenohumeral joint.[194] This is instituted early in OBPP, preferably by the parents with appropriate guidance from occupational or physical therapists.

Surgical

EARLY

Infants who do not initiate recovery until after 3 months old may be candidates for microsurgery.[190] Other indications for microsurgery include Toronto Scale score <3.5 and total brachial plexopathy with Horner syndrome. The optimal timing of surgery is debated. Microsurgery involves brachial plexus exploration, neurolysis, resection of the neuroma and nerve grafting and/or nerve transfer procedures in the case of root avulsions.[202–204]

In patients with early muscle contractures in the absence of joint instability, early muscle release and appropriate transfers maybe indicated to maximize the range of motion, maintain a congruent joint and avoid secondary bony changes. Posterior shoulder dislocation before the age of 1 year has been noted in neonatal brachial plexus palsy.[205] These patents require early surgery to reduce the joint and maintain congruency.

LATE

When muscle recovery is incomplete, contractures and joint subluxation can occur over time. In the shoulder, the most common deformity is an adduction internal rotation contracture. In the presence of good elbow and hand function, these patients may benefit from late soft-tissue reconstruction. Surgical options include release of the adductors – pectoralis major and subscapularis[180] – with release and transfer of the internal rotators – the latissmus dorsi and teres major[206–209] – to the outside of the humerus to function as external rotators.

These operations can be done even in patients with mild to moderate glenohumeral dysplasia as remodelling of the glenohumeral joint has been shown to occur.[194,210] The presence of glenohumeral dislocation or severe glenohumeral deformity (humeral head flattening, loss of normal glenoid architecture) is a contraindication for soft-tissue surgery. In these situations, the patient may benefit from external rotation osteotomy of the humerus that reorients the shoulder arc of rotation into a more functional range.[211]

For cases in which paralysis of the elbow does not permit elbow flexion, a number of tendon transfers involving the pectoralis major, triceps, latissimus dorsi and flexor pronator mass of the forearm have been described.

Arthrodesis of the shoulder may be an option in patients with a flail unstable shoulder with useful hand and elbow function.

KEY LEARNING POINTS

- Obstetric brachial plexus birth palsy is a paralysis of the upper extremity secondary to a traction or compression injury to the brachial plexus during birth.
- The two most important risk factors are high weight at birth and shoulder dystocia.
- The classification of obstetric brachial plexus birth palsy proposed by Narakas[191] is useful as it provides a clear definition of the extent of injury and offers a broad guide to prognosis. Narakas group I is associated with a 90% recovery rate, whereas Narakas group IV is associated with a poor chance of spontaneous recovery.
- Recovery of antigravity biceps and deltoid function by 3 months old or a Toronto scale score >3.5 was predictive of complete spontaneous recovery.
- Early brachial plexus exploration and nerve repair is indicated in patients with poor biceps recovery at 3 months old and total brachial plexopathy with root avulsion. Early muscle release and appropriate transfers can maximize the range of motion, maintain a congruent joint and avoid secondary bony changes. They can also lead to remodelling of mild to moderate glenohumeral dysplasia.
- Late reconstructive surgery helps to optimize upper limb function when selected appropriately.

REFERENCES

1. Bax M, Goldstein M, Rosenbaum P, et al. Proposed definition and classification of cerebral palsy, April 2005. *Developmental Medicine and Child Neurology* 2005;**47**:571–6.
2. Rosenbaum P, Paneth N, Leviton A, et al. A report: the definition and classification of cerebral palsy April 2006. *Developmental Medicine and Child Neurology Supplement* 2007;**109**:8–14.
3. Stanley F, Blair E, Alberman E. *Cerebral Palsies: Epidemiology and Causal Pathways.* London: MacKeith Press, 2000.
4. Gage JR. The neurological control system for normal gait. In: Gage JR (ed.) *Gait Analysis in Cerebral Palsy.* London, UK: MacKeith Press, 1991:37–60.
5. Ziv I, Blackburn N, Rang M, Koreska J. Muscle growth in normal and spastic mice. *Developmental Medicine and Child Neurology* 1984;**26**:94–9.
6. Gage JR, Schwartz M. Pathologic gait and lever arm dysfunction. In: Gage JR (ed.) *The Treatment of Gait Problems in Cerebral Palsy.* London, UK: MacKeith, 2004:180–204.
7. Bell KJ, Ounpuu S, DeLuca PA, Romness MJ. Natural progression of gait in children with cerebral palsy. *Journal of Pediatric Orthopaedics* 2002;**22**:677–82.
8. Johnson DC, Damiano DL, Abel MF. The evolution of gait in childhood and adolescent cerebral palsy. *Journal of Pediatric Orthopaedics* 1997;**17**:392–6.
9. Murphy KP, Molnar GE, Lankasky K. Medical and functional status of adults with cerebral palsy. *Developmental Medicine and Child Neurology* 1995;**37**:1075–84.
10. Bottos M, Feliciangeli A, Sciuto L, et al. Functional status of adults with cerebral palsy and implications for treatment of children. *Developmental Medicine and Child Neurology* 2001;**43**:516–28.
11. Palisano R, Rosenbaum P, Walter S, et al. Development and reliability of a system to classify gross motor function in children with cerebral palsy. *Developmental Medicine and Child Neurology* 1997;**39**:214–23.
12. Wood E, Rosenbaum P. The gross motor function classification system for cerebral palsy: a study of reliability and stability over time. *Developmental Medicine and Child Neurology* 2000;**42**:292–6.
13. Rosenbaum PL, Walter SD, Hanna SE, et al. Prognosis for gross motor function in cerebral palsy: creation of motor development curves. *JAMA Journal of the American Medical Association* 2002;**288**:1357–63.
14. Rang M, Cerebral palsy In: Morrissy RT (ed.) *Lovell and Winter's Pediatric Orthopaedic.* Philadelphia, PA: Lippincott, 1990:465–506.
15. Narayanan UG, Fehlings D, Weir S, et al. Initial development and validation of the Caregiver Priorities and Child Health Index of Life with Disabilities (CPCHILD). *Developmental Medicine and Child Neurology* 2006;**48**:804–12.

16. Gage JR. The role of gait analysis in the treatment of cerebral palsy. *Journal of Pediatric Orthopaedics* 1994;**14**:701–2.
17. Gage JR. *Gait Analysis in Cerebral Palsy*. London, UK: MacKeith Press, 1991:102–7.
18. Davids JR, Benfanti P, Blackhurst DW, Allen BL. Assessment of femoral anteversion in children with cerebral palsy: accuracy of the trochanteric prominence angle test. *Journal of Pediatric Orthopaedics* 2002;**22**:173–8.
19. Ruwe PA, Gage JR, Ozonoff MB, DeLuca PA. Clinical determination of femoral anteversion. A comparison with established techniques. *Journal of Bone and Joint Surgery (American)* 1992;**74**:820–30.
20. Narayanan UG. The role of gait analysis in the orthopaedic management of ambulatory cerebral palsy. *Current Opinion in Pediatrics* 2007;**19**:38–43.
21. Bache CE, Selber P, Graham HK. The management of spastic diplegia. *Current Orthopaedics* 2003;**17**:88–104.
22. DeLuca PA, Davis 3rd RB, Ounpuu S, et al. Alterations in surgical decision making in patients with cerebral palsy based on three-dimensional gait analysis. *Journal of Pediatric Orthopaedics* 1997;**17**:608–14.
23. Cook RE, Schneider I, Hazlewood ME, et al. Gait analysis alters decision-making in cerebral palsy. *Journal of Pediatric Orthopaedics* 2003;**23**:292–5.
24. Kay RM, Dennis S, Rethlefsen S, et al. The effect of preoperative gait analysis on orthopaedic decision making. *Clinical Orthopaedics and Related Research* 2000;**372**:217–22.
25. Rodda J, Graham HK. Classification of gait patterns in spastic hemiplegia and spastic diplegia: a basis for a management algorithm. *European Journal of Neurology* 2001;**8**(Suppl. 5):98–108.
26. Winters Jr TF, Gage JR, Hicks R. Gait patterns in spastic hemiplegia in children and young adults. *Journal of Bone and Joint Surgery (American)* 1987;**69**:437–41.
27. Dumas HME, O'Neil M, Fragala MA. Expert consensus on physical therapist intervention after botulinum toxin A injection for children with cerebral palsy. *Pediatric Physical Therapy* 2001;**13**:122–32.
28. Boyd RN, Pliatsios V, Starr R, et al. Biomechanical transformation of the gastroc-soleus muscle with botulinum toxin A in children with cerebral palsy. *Developmental Medicine and Child Neurology* 2000;**42**:32–41.
29. Thompson NS, Baker RJ, Cosgrove AP, et al. Musculoskeletal modelling in determining the effect of botulinum toxin on the hamstrings of patients with crouch gait. *Developmental Medicine and Child Neurology* 1998;**40**:622–5.
30. Molenaers G, Desloovere K, De Cat J, et al. Single event multilevel botulinum toxin type A treatment and surgery: similarities and differences. *European Journal of Neurology* 2001;**8**(Suppl. 5):88–97.
31. Ubhi T, Bhakta BB, Ives HL, et al. Randomised double blind placebo controlled trial of the effect of botulinum toxin on walking in cerebral palsy. *Archives of Disease in Childhood* 2000;**83**:481–7.
32. Koman LA, Mooney JF, Smith BP, et al. Botulinum toxin type A neuromuscular blockade in the treatment of lower extremity spasticity in cerebral palsy: a randomized, double-blind, placebo-controlled trial. BOTOX Study Group. *Journal of Pediatric Orthopaedics* 2000;**20**:108–15.
33. Sutherland DH, Kaufman KR, Wyatt MP, et al. Double-blind study of botulinum A toxin injections into the gastrocnemius muscle in patients with cerebral palsy. *Gait & Posture* 1999;**10**:1–9.
34. Cardoso ES, Rodrigues BM, Barroso M, et al. Botulinum toxin type A for the treatment of the spastic equinus foot in cerebral palsy. *Pediatric Neurology* 2006;**34**:106–9.
35. Boyd RN, Hays RM. Current evidence for the use of botulinum toxin type A in the management of children with cerebral palsy: a systematic review. *European Journal of Neurology* 2001;**8**(Suppl. 5):1–20.
36. Corry IS, Cosgrove AP, Duffy CM, et al. Botulinum toxin A compared with stretching casts in the treatment of spastic equinus: a randomised prospective trial. *Journal of Pediatric Orthopaedics* 1998;**18**:304–11.
37. Flett PJ, Stern LM, Waddy H, et al. Botulinum toxin A versus fixed cast stretching for dynamic calf tightness in cerebral palsy. *Journal of Paediatrics and Child Health* 1999;**35**:71–7.
38. Kay RM, Rethlefsen SA, Fern-Buneo A, et al. Botulinum toxin as an adjunct to serial casting treatment in children with cerebral palsy. *Journal of Bone and Joint Surgery (American)* 2004;**86A**:2377–84.
39. Ackman JD, Russman BS, Thomas SS, et al. Comparing botulinum toxin A with casting for treatment of dynamic equinus in children with cerebral palsy. *Developmental Medicine and Child Neurology* 2005;**47**:620–7.
40. Ade-Hall RA, Moore AP. Botulinum toxin type A in the treatment of lower limb spasticity in cerebral palsy. *Cochrane Database of Systematic Reviews* 2000;(2):CD001408.
41. Bjornson K, Hays R, Graubert C, et al. Botulinum toxin for spasticity in children with cerebral palsy: a comprehensive evaluation. *Pediatrics* 2007;**120**:49–58.
42. Lannin N, Scheinberg A, Clark K. AACPDM systematic review of the effectiveness of therapy for children with cerebral palsy after botulinum toxin A injections. *Developmental Medicine & Child Neurology* 2006;**48**:533–9.
43. Desloovere K, Molenaers G, Jonkers I, et al. A randomized study of combined botulinum toxin type A and casting in the ambulant child with cerebral palsy using objective outcome measures. *European Journal of Neurology* 2001;**8**(Suppl. 5):75–87.
44. Scholtes VA, Dallmeijer AJ, Knol DL, et al. The combined effect of lower-limb multilevel botulinum toxin type a and comprehensive rehabilitation on mobility in children with cerebral palsy: a randomized

45. Gough M, Fairhurst C, Shortland AP. Botulinum toxin and cerebral palsy: time for reflection? *Developmental Medicine and Child Neurology* 2005;**47**:709–12.
46. McLaughlin J, Bjornson K, Temkin N, et al. Selective dorsal rhizotomy: meta-analysis of three randomized controlled trials. *Developmental Medicine and Child Neurology* 2002;**44**:17–25.
47. McLaughlin JF, Bjornson KF, Astley SJ, et al. Selective dorsal rhizotomy: efficacy and safety in an investigator-masked randomized clinical trial. *Developmental Medicine and Child Neurology* 1998;**40**:220–32.
48. Wright FV, Sheil EM, Drake JM, et al. Evaluation of selective dorsal rhizotomy for the reduction of spasticity in cerebral palsy: a randomized controlled trial. *Developmental Medicine and Child Neurology* 1998;**40**:239–47.
49. Steinbok P, Reiner AM, Beauchamp R, et al. A randomized clinical trial to compare selective posterior rhizotomy plus physiotherapy with physiotherapy alone in children with spastic diplegic cerebral palsy. *Developmental Medicine and Child Neurology* 1997;**39**:178–84.
50. Hägglund G, Andersson S, Düppe H, et al. Prevention of severe contractures might replace multilevel surgery in cerebral palsy: results of a population-based health care programme and new techniques to reduce spasticity. *Journal of Pediatric Orthopaedics B* 2005;**14**:269–73.
51. Thomas SS, Buckon CE, Piatt JH, et al. A 2-year follow-up of outcomes following orthopedic surgery or selective dorsal rhizotomy in children with spastic diplegia. *Journal of Pediatric Orthopaedics B* 2004;**13**:358–66.
52. Steinbok P. Outcomes after selective dorsal rhizotomy for spastic cerebral palsy. *Child's Nervous System* 2001;**17**(1–2):1–18.
53. Butler C, Campbell S. Evidence of the effects of intrathecal baclofen for spastic and dystonic cerebral palsy. AACPDM Treatment Outcomes Committee Review Panel. *Developmental Medicine and Child Neurology* 2000;**42**:634–45.
54. Albright AL. Intrathecal baclofen in cerebral palsy movement disorders. *Journal of Child Neurology* 1996;**11**(Suppl. 1):S29–S35.
55. Campbell W, Ferrel A, McLaughlin JF, et al. Long-term safety and efficacy of continuous intrathecal baclofen. *Developmental Medicine and Child Neurology* 2002;**44**:660–5.
56. Nene AV, Evans GA, Patrick JH. Simultaneous multiple operations for spastic diplegia. Outcome and functional assessment of walking in 18 patients. *Journal of Bone and Joint Surgery (British)* 1993;**75**:488–94.
57. Norlin R, Tkaczuk H. One session surgery on the lower limb in children with cerebral palsy. A five year follow-up. *International Orthopaedics* 1992;**16**:291–3.
58. Sussman MD, Aiona MD. Treatment of spastic diplegia in patients with cerebral palsy. *Journal of Pediatric Orthopaedics B* 2004;**13**:S1–12.
59. Fabry G, Liu XC, Molenaers G. Gait pattern in patients with spastic diplegic cerebral palsy who underwent staged operations. *Journal of Pediatric Orthopaedics B* 1999;**8**:33–8.
60. Saraph V, Zwick EB, Auner C, et al. Gait improvement surgery in diplegic children: how long do the improvements last? *Journal of Pediatric Orthopaedics* 2005;**25**:263–7.
61. Gough M, Eve LC, Robinson RO, et al. Short-term outcome of multilevel surgical intervention in spastic diplegic cerebral palsy compared with the natural history. *Developmental Medicine and Child Neurology* 2004;**46**:91–7.
62. DeLuca PA, Ounpuu S, Davis RB, et al. Effect of hamstring and psoas lengthening on pelvic tilt in patients with spastic diplegic cerebral palsy. *Journal of Pediatric Orthopaedics* 1998;**18**:712–18.
63. Novacheck TF, Trost JP, Schwartz MH. Intramuscular psoas lengthening improves dynamic hip function in children with cerebral palsy. *Journal of Pediatric Orthopaedics* 2002;**22**:158–64.
64. Sutherland DH, Zilberfarb JL, Kaufman KR, et al. Psoas release at the pelvic brim in ambulatory patients with cerebral palsy: operative technique and functional outcome. *Journal of Pediatric Orthopaedics* 1997;**17**:563–70.
65. Patrick JH. Techniques of psoas tenotomy and rectus femoris transfer: 'new' operations for cerebral palsy diplegia – a description. *Journal of Pediatric Orthopaedics B* 1996;**5**:242–6.
66. Kay RM, Rethlefsen SA, Hale JM, et al. Comparison of proximal and distal rotational femoral osteotomy in children with cerebral palsy. *Journal of Pediatric Orthopaedics* 2003;**23**:150–4.
67. Pirpiris M, Trivett A, Baker R, et al. Femoral derotation osteotomy in spastic diplegia. Proximal or distal? *Journal of Bone and Joint Surgery (British)* 2003;**85**:265–72.
68. Bobroff ED, Chambers HG, Sartoris DJ, et al. Femoral anteversion and neck-shaft angle in children with cerebral palsy. *Clinical Orthopaedics and Related Research* 1999;**364**:194–204.
69. Ounpuu S, DeLuca P, Davis R, Romness M. Long-term effects of femoral derotation osteotomies: an evaluation using three-dimensional gait analysis. *Journal of Pediatric Orthopaedics* 2002;**22**:139–45.
70. McNerney NP, Mubarak SJ, Wenger DR. One-stage correction of the dysplastic hip in cerebral palsy with the San Diego acetabuloplasty: results and complications in 104 hips. *Journal of Pediatric Orthopaedics* 2000;**20**:93–103.
71. Karlen JW, Skaggs DL, Ramachandran M, Kay RM. The Dega osteotomy: a versatile osteotomy in the treatment of developmental and neuromuscular hip pathology. *Journal of Pediatric Orthopaedics* 2009;**29**:676–82.
72. Thometz J, Simon S, Rosenthal R. The effect on gait of lengthening of the medial hamstrings in cerebral palsy. *Journal of Bone and Joint Surgery (American)* 1989;**71**:345–53.
73. Hoffinger SA, Rab GT, Abou-Ghaida H. Hamstrings in cerebral palsy crouch gait. *Journal of Pediatric Orthopaedics* 1993;**13**:722–6.

74. Kay RM, Rethlefsen SA, Skaggs D, Leet A. Outcome of medial versus combined medial and lateral hamstring lengthening surgery in cerebral palsy. *Journal of Pediatric Orthopaedics* 2002;**22**:169-72.
75. Rodda JM, Graham HK, Nattrass GR, et al. Correction of severe crouch gait in patients with spastic diplegia with use of multilevel orthopaedic surgery. *Journal of Bone and Joint Surgery (American)* 2006;**88**:2653-64.
76. Chambers H, Lauer A, Kaufman K, et al. Prediction of outcome after rectus femoris surgery in cerebral palsy: the role of cocontraction of the rectus femoris and vastus lateralis. *Journal of Pediatric Orthopaedics* 1998;**18**:703-11.
77. Gage JR, Perry J, Hicks RR, et al. Rectus femoris transfer to improve knee function of children with cerebral palsy. *Developmental Medicine and Child Neurology* 1987;**29**:159-66.
78. Rethlefsen S, Tolo VT, Reynolds RA, Kay R. Outcome of hamstring lengthening and distal rectus femoris transfer surgery. *Journal of Pediatric Orthopaedics B* 1999;**8**:75-9.
79. Saw A, Smith PA, Sirirungruangsarn Y, et al. Rectus femoris transfer for children with cerebral palsy: long-term outcome. *Journal of Pediatric Orthopaedics* 2003;**23**:672-8.
80. Strayer LM. Recession of the gastrocnemius. An operation to relieve spastic contracture of the calf muscles. *Journal of Bone and Joint Surgery* 1950;**32A**:671-6.
81. Dietz FR, Albright JC, Dolan L. Medium-term follow-up of Achilles tendon lengthening in the treatment of ankle equinus in cerebral palsy. *Iowa Orthopaedic Journal* 2006;**26**:27-32.
82. Rose SA, DeLuca PA, Davis 3rd RB, et al. Kinematic and kinetic evaluation of the ankle after lengthening of the gastrocnemius fascia in children with cerebral palsy. *Journal of Pediatric Orthopaedics* 1993;**13**:727-32.
83. Steinwender G, Saraph V, Zwick EB, et al. Fixed and dynamic equinus in cerebral palsy: evaluation of ankle function after multilevel surgery. *Journal of Pediatric Orthopaedics* 2001;**21**:102-7.
84. Borton DC, Walker K, Pirpiris M, et al. Isolated calf lengthening in cerebral palsy. Outcome analysis of risk factors. *Journal of Bone and Joint Surgery (British)* 2001;**83**:364-70.
85. Graham HK, Fixsen JA. Lengthening of the calcaneal tendon in spastic hemiplegia by the White slide technique. A long-term review. *Journal of Bone and Joint Surgery (British)* 1988;**70**:472-5.
86. Green NE, Griffin PP, Shiavi R. Split posterior tibial-tendon transfer in spastic cerebral palsy. *Journal of Bone and Joint Surgery (American)* 1983;**65**:748-54.
87. Hoffer MM, Barakat G, Koffman M. 10-year follow-up of split anterior tibial tendon transfer in cerebral palsied patients with spastic equinovarus deformity. *Journal of Pediatric Orthopaedics* 1985;**5**:432-4.
88. Barnes MJ, Herring JA. Combined split anterior tibial-tendon transfer and intramuscular lengthening of the posterior tibial tendon. Results in patients who have a varus deformity of the foot due to spastic cerebral palsy. *Journal of Bone and Joint Surgery (American)* 1991;**73**:734-8.
89. Dodgin DA, De Swart RJ, Stefko RM, et al. Distal tibial/fibular derotation osteotomy for correction of tibial torsion: review of technique and results in 63 cases. *Journal of Pediatric Orthopaedics* 1998;**18**:95-101.
90. Mosca VS. Calcaneal lengthening for valgus deformity of the hindfoot. Results in children who had severe, symptomatic flatfoot and skewfoot. *Journal of Bone and Joint Surgery (American)* 1995;**77**:500-12.
91. Dennyson WG, Fulford GE, Subtalar arthrodesis by cancellous grafts and metallic internal fixation. *Journal of Bone and Joint Surgery* 1976;**58B**:507.
92. Dodd KJ, Taylor NF, Damiano DL. A systematic review of the effectiveness of strength-training programs for people with cerebral palsy. *Archives of Physical Medicine and Rehabilitation* 2002;**83**:1157-64.
93. Graham HK, Selber P. Musculoskeletal aspects of cerebral palsy. *Journal of Bone and Joint Surgery (British)* 2003;**85B**:157-66.
94. Soo B, Howard JJ, Boyd RN, et al. Hip displacement in cerebral palsy. *Journal of Bone and Joint Surgery (American)* 2006;**88**:121-9.
95. Scrutton D, Baird G, Smeeton N. Hip dysplasia in bilateral cerebral palsy: incidence and natural history in children aged 18 months to 5 years. *Developmental Medicine and Child Neurology* 2001;**43**:586-600.
96. Miller F, Bagg MR. Age and migration percentage as risk factors for progression in spastic hip disease. *Developmental Medicine and Child Neurology* 1995;**37**:449-55.
97. Graham HK. Painful hip dislocation in cerebral palsy. *Lancet* 2002;**359**:907-8.
98. Cooperman DR, Bartucci E, Dietrick E, Millar E. Hip dislocation in spastic cerebral palsy: long term consequences. *Journal of Pediatric Orthopaedics* 1987;**7**:268-76.
99. Noonan KJ, Jones J, Pierson J, et al. Hip function in adults with severe cerebral palsy. *Journal of Bone and Joint Surgery (American)* 2004;**86A**:2607-13.
100. Dobson F, Boyd RN, Parrott J, et al. Hip surveillance in children with cerebral palsy. Impact on the surgical management of spastic hip disease. *Journal of Bone and Joint Surgery (British)* 2002;**84**:720-6.
101. Gordon GS, Simkiss DE. A systematic review of the evidence for hip surveillance in children with cerebral Palsy. *Journal of Bone and Joint Surgery (British)* 2006;**88B**:1492-6.
102. Mall V, Heinen F, Siebel A, et al. Treatment of adductor spasticity with BTX-A in children with CP: a randomized, double-blind, placebo-controlled study. *Developmental Medicine and Child Neurology* 2006;**48**:10-3.
103. Graham HK, Boyd R, Carlin JB, et al. Does botulinum toxin a combined with bracing prevent hip displacement in children with cerebral palsy and 'hips at risk'? A randomized, controlled trial. *Journal of Bone and Joint Surgery (American)* 2008;**90**:23-33.

104. Hagglund G, Andersson S, Düppe H, et al. Prevention of dislocation of the hip in children with cerebral palsy. The first ten years of a population-based prevention programme. *Journal of Bone and Joint Surgery (British)* 2005;**87**:95–101.
105. Stott NS, Piedrahita L. Effects of surgical adductor releases for hip subluxation in cerebral palsy: an AACPDM evidence report. *Developmental Medicine and Child Neurology* 2004;**46**:628–45.
106. Miller F, Girardi H, Lipton G, et al. Reconstruction of the dysplastic spastic hip with peri-ilial pelvic and femoral osteotomy followed by immediate mobilization. *Journal of Pediatric Orthopaedics* 1997;**17**:592–602.
107. Gordon JE, Capelli AM, Strecker WB, et al. Pemberton pelvic osteotomy and varus rotational osteotomy in the treatment of acetabular dysplasia in patients who have static encephalopathy. *Journal of Bone and Joint Surgery (American)* 1996;**78**:1863–71.
108. McHale KA, Bagg M, Nason SS. Treatment of the chronically dislocated hip in adolescents with cerebral palsy with femoral head resection and subtrochanteric valgus osteotomy. *Journal of Pediatric Orthopaedics* 1990;**10**:504–9.
109. Emery DFG, Wedge JH. Orthopaedic management of children with total body involvement cerebral palsy. *Current Orthopaedics* 2003;**17**:81–7.
110. Lonstein JE, Akbarnia A. Operative treatment of spinal deformities in patients with cerebral palsy or mental retardation. An analysis of one hundred and seven cases. *Journal of Bone and Joint Surgery (American)* 1983;**65**:43–55.
111. Saeed W. Cerebral palsy of the upper extremity: the surgical perspective. *Current Orthopaedics* 2003;**17**:105–16.
112. House JH, Gwathmey FW, Fidler MO. A dynamic approach to the thumb-in palm deformity in cerebral palsy. *Journal of Bone and Joint Surgery (American)* 1981;**63**:216–25.
113. Goldberg MJ. Measuring outcomes in cerebral palsy. *Journal of Pediatric Orthopaedics* 1991;**11**:682–5.
114. Paul SM, Siegel KL, Malley J, et al. Evaluating interventions to improve gait in cerebral palsy: a meta-analysis of spatiotemporal measures. *Developmental Medicine and Child Neurology* 2007;**49**:542–9.
115. Butler C, Goldstein M, Chambers H, et al. Evaluating research in developmental disabilities: a conceptual framework for reviewing treatment outcomes. AACPDM Treatment Outcomes Committee Report 1998–1999. Available from: http://www.aacpdm.org/index?service=page/treatmentOutcomesReport.
116. Adolfsen SE, Ounpuu S, Bell KJ, et al. Kinematic and kinetic outcomes after identical multilevel soft tissue surgery in children with cerebral palsy. *Journal of Pediatric Orthopaedics* 2007;**27**:658–67.
117. Cuomo AV, Gamradt SC, Kim CO, et al. Health-related quality of life outcomes improve after multilevel surgery in ambulatory children with cerebral palsy. *Journal of Pediatric Orthopaedics* 2007;**27**:653–7.
118. Novacheck TF, Gage JR. Orthopedic management of spasticity in cerebral palsy. *Child's Nervous System* 2007;**23**:1015–31.
119. Andersson C, Mattsson E. Adults with cerebral palsy: a survey describing problems, needs, and resources, with special emphasis on locomotion. *Developmental Medicine and Child Neurology* 2001;**43**:76–82.
120. Banta JV. The team approach in the care of the child with myelomeningocoele. *Journal of Pediatric Orthopaedics* 1990;**2**:263–73.
121. Fletcher JM, Copeland K, Frederick JA, et al. Spinal lesion level in spina bifida: a source of neural and cognitive heterogeneity. *Journal of Neurosurgery* 2005;**102**(3 Suppl.):268–79.
122. Williams LJ, Rasmussen SA, Flores A, et al. Decline in the prevalence of spina bifida and anencephaly by race/ethnicity: 1995–2002. *Pediatrics* 2005;**116**:580–6.
123. EUROCAT Working Group. Prevalence of neural tube defects in 20 regions of Europe and the impact of prenatal diagnosis, 1980–1986. *Journal of Epidemiology and Community Health* 1991;**45**:52–8.
124. McDonnell RJ, Johnson Z, Delaney V, Dack P. East Ireland 1980–1994: Epidemiology of neural tube defects. *Journal of Epidemiology and Community Health* 1999;**53**:782–8.
125. Oakley GP. The scientific basis for eliminating folic acid-preventable spina bifida: a modern miracle from epidemiology. *Annals of Epidemiology* 2009;**19**:226–30.
126. Centres for Disease Control and Prevention. Spina bifida and anencephaly before and after folic acid mandate: United States, 1995–1996 and 1999–2000. *Morbidity and Mortality Weekly Report (MMWR)* 2004;**53**:362–5.
127. Nicolaides KH, Campbell S, Gabbe SG, Guidetti R. Ultrasound screening for spina bifida: cranial and cerebellar signs. *Lancet* 1986;**2**:72–4.
128. Shaer CM, Chescheir N, Schulkin. Myelomeningocele: a review of the epidemiology, genetics, risk factors for conception, prenatal diagnosis, and prognosis for affected individuals. *Obstetrical and Gynecological Survey* 2007;**62**:471–9.
129. Johnson MP, Gerdes M, Rintoul N, et al. Maternal-fetal surgery for myelomeningocele: neurodevelopmental outcomes at 2 years of age. *American Journal of Obstetrics and Gynecology* 2006;**194**:1145–50; discussion 1150–2.
130. Tarcan T, Onol FF, Ilker Y, et al. The timing of primary neurosurgical repair significantly affects neurogenic bladder prognosis in children with myelomeningocele. *Journal of Urology* 2006;**176**:1161–5.
131. Mazur JM, Menelaus MB. Neurologic status of spina bifida patients and the orthopedic surgeon. *Clinical Orthopaedics and Related Research* 1991;**264**:54–64.
132. Oi S, Matsumoto S. A proposed grading and scoring system for spina bifida: Spina Bifida Neurological Scale (SBNS). *Child's Nervous System* 1992;**8**:337–42.
133. Tosi LL, Slater JE, Shaer C, et al. Latex allergy in spina bifida patients: prevalence and surgical implications. *Journal of Pediatric Orthopaedics* 1993;**13**:709.

134. Trivedi J, Thomson JD, Slakey JB, et al. Clinical and radiographic predictors of scoliosis in patients with myelomeningocele. *Journal of Bone and Joint Surgery (American)* 2002;**84**:1389.
135. Carstens C, Paul K, Niethard FU, et al. Effect of scoliosis surgery on pulmonary function in patients with myelomeningocele. *Journal of Pediatric Orthopaedics* 1991;**11**:459.
136. Muller EB, Nordwall A. Brace treatment of scoliosis in children with myelomeningocele. *Spine* 1994;**19**:151.
137. Banta JV. Combined anterior and posterior fusion for spinal deformity in myelomeningocele. *Spine* 1990;**15**:946.
138. Carstens C, Koch H, Brocai DR, Niethard FU. Development of pathological lumbar kyphosis in myelomeningocele. *Journal of Bone and Joint Surgery (British)* 1996;**78**:945–50.
139. Broughton NS, Menelaus MB, Cole WG, et al. The natural history of hip deformity in myelomeningocele. *Journal of Bone and Joint Surgery (British)* 1993;**75**:760.
140. Correll J, Gabler C. The effect of soft tissue release of the hips on walking in myelomeningocele. *Journal of Pediatric Orthopaedics B* 2000;**9**:148.
141. Mustard WT. A follow-up study of iliopsoas transfer for hip instability. *Journal of Bone and Joint Surgery (British)* 1959;**41**:289.
142. Sharrard WJ. Posterior iliopsoas transplantation in the treatment of paralytic dislocation of the hip. *Journal of Bone and Joint Surgery (British)* 1964;**46**:426.
143. Zimmerman MH, Smith CF, Oppenheim WL. Supracondylar femoral extension osteotomies in the treatment of fixed flexion deformity of the knee. *Clinical Orthopaedics and Related Research* 1982;**171**:87–93.
144. Fraser RK, Menelaus MB. The management of tibial torsion in patients with spina bifida. *Journal of Bone and Joint Surgery (British)* 1993;**75**:495.
145. Gerlach DJ, Gurnett CA, Limpaphayom N, et al. Early results of the Ponseti method for the treatment of clubfoot associated with myelomeningocele. *Journal of Bone and Joint Surgery (American)* 2009;**91**:1350–9.
146. de Carvalho Neto J, Dias LS, Gabrieli AP. Congenital talipes equinovarus in spina bifida: treatment and results. *Journal of Pediatric Orthopaedics* 1996;**16**:782.
147. Flynn JM, Herrera-Soto JA, Ramirez NF, et al. Clubfoot release in myelodysplasia. *Journal of Pediatric Orthopaedics B* 2004;**13**:259.
148. Frawley PA, Broughton NS, Menelaus MB. Incidence and type of hindfoot deformities in patients with low-level spina bifida. *Journal of Pediatric Orthopaedics* 1998;**18**:312.
149. Georgiadis GM, Aronson DD. Posterior transfer of the anterior tibial tendon in children who have a myelomeningocele. *Journal of Bone and Joint Surgery (American)* 1990;**72**:392.
150. Broughton NS, Graham G, Menelaus MB. The high incidence of foot deformity in patients with high-level spina bifida. *Journal of Bone and Joint Surgery (British)* 1994;**76**:548.
151. Malhotra D, Puri R, Owen R. Valgus deformity of the ankle in children with spina bifida aperta. *Journal of Bone and Joint Surgery (British)* 1984;**66**:381.
152. Torosian CM, Dias LS. Surgical treatment of severe hindfoot valgus by medial displacement osteotomy of the os calcis in children with myelomeningocele. *Journal of Pediatric Orthopaedics* 2000;**20**:226.
◆153. Darras BT, Menache CC, Kunkel LM. Dystrophinopathies. In: Jones H, DeVivo D, Darras B (eds) *Neuromuscular Disorders of Infancy, Childhood, and Adolescence: a Clinician's Approach.* New York, NY: Butterworth Heinemann, 2003:649–99.
154. Karol LA. Scoliosis in patients with Duchenne muscular dystrophy. *Journal of Bone and Joint Surgery* 2007;**89A**(Suppl. 1): 155–62.
155. Angelini C. The role of corticosteroids in muscular dystrophy: a critical appraisal. *Muscle and Nerve* 2007;**364**:424–35.
156. Angelini C, Pegoraro E, Turella E, et al. Deflazacort in Duchenne dystrophy: study of long-term effect. *Muscle and Nerve* 1994;**17**:386–91.
157. Rodino-Klapac LR, Chicoine LG, Kaspar BK, Mendell JR. Gene therapy for Duchenne muscular dystrophy: expectations and challenges. *Archives of Neurology* 2007;**64**:1236–41.
158. Muntoni F, Wells D. Genetic treatments in muscular dystrophies. *Current Opinion in Neurology* 2007;**20**:590–4.
◆159. Daniele N, Richard I, Bartoli M. Ins and outs of therapy in limb girdle muscular dystrophies. *International Journal of Biochemistry and Cell Biology* 2007;**39**:1608–24.
160. Orrell RW, Darras BT, Griggs RC. Facioscapulohumeral dystrophy, scapuloperoneal syndromes, and distal myopathies. In: Jones H, DeVivo D, Darras B (eds) *Neuromuscular Disorders of Infancy, Childhood, and Adolescence: a Clinician's Approach.* New York, NY: Butterworth Heinemann, 2003:701–9.
161. Deymeer F. Emery-Dreifuss muscular dystrophy. In: Jones H, DeVivo D, Darras B (eds) *Neuromuscular Disorders of Infancy, Childhood, and Adolescence: a Clinician's Approach.* New York, NY: Butterworth Heinemann, 2003:753–63.
162. Jones K, North K. Congenital muscular dystrophies. In: Jones H, DeVivo D, Darras B (eds) *Neuromuscular Disorders of Infancy, Childhood, and Adolescence: a Clinician's Approach.* New York, NY: Butterworth Heinemann, 2003:633–47.
●163. Dyck PJ, Lambert EH. Lower motor and primary sensory neuron diseases with peroneal muscular atrophy. I. Neurologic, genetic, and electrophysiologic findings in hereditary polyneuropathies. *Archives of Neurology* 1968;**18**:603–18.
●164. Dyck PJ, Lambert EH. Lower motor and primary sensory neuron diseases with peroneal muscular atrophy. II. Neurologic, genetic, and electrophysiologic findings in various neuronal degenerations. *Archives of Neurology* 1968;**18**:619–25.

165. Reilly MM. Sorting out the inherited neuropathies. *Practical Neurology* 2007;**7**:93–105.
166. Chance PF, Escolar DM, Redmond A, *et al*. Hereditary neuropathies in late childhood and adolescence. In: Jones H, DeVivo D, Darras B (eds) *Neuromuscular Disorders of Infancy, Childhood, and Adolescence: a Clinician's Approach*. New York, NY: Butterworth Heinemann, 2003:389–406.
167. Schwend RM, Drennan JC. Cavus foot deformity in children. *Journal of the American Academy of Orthopaedic Surgery* 2003;**11**:201–11.
168. Nagai MK, Chan G, Guille JT, *et al*. Prevalence of Charcot-Marie-Tooth disease in patients who have bilateral cavovarus feet. *Journal of Pediatric Orthopaedic Surgery* 2006;**26**:438–43.
169. Coleman SS, Chesnut WJ. A simple test for hindfoot flexibility in the cavovarus foot. *Clinical Orthopaedics and Related Research* 1977;**123**:60–2.
170. Price BD, Price CT. A simple demonstration of hindfoot flexibility in the cavovarus foot. *Journal of Pediatric Orthopaedics* 1997;**17**:18–19.
171. Wetmore RS, Drennan JC. Long-term results of triple arthrodesis in Charcot-Marie-Tooth disease. *Journal of Bone and Joint Surgery* 1989;**71**:417–22.
172. Wukich DK, Bowen JR. A long-term study of triple arthrodesis for correction of pes cavovarus in Charcot-Marie-Tooth disease. *Journal of Pediatric Orthopaedics* 1989;**9**:433–7.
173. Walker JL, Nelson KR, Heavilon JA, *et al*. Hip abnormalities in children with Charcot-Marie-Tooth disease. *Journal of Pediatric Orthopaedics* 1994;**14**:54–9.
174. Walker JL, Nelson KR, Stevens DB, *et al*. Spinal deformity in Charcot-Marie-Tooth disease. *Spine* 1994;**19**:1044–7.
175. Karol LA, Elerson E. Scoliosis in patients with Charcot-Marie-Tooth disease. *Journal of Bone and Joint Surgery* 2007;**89**:1504–10.
176. Azzedine H, Ravise N, Verny C, *et al*. Spine deformities in Charcot-Marie-Tooth 4C caused by SH3TC2 gene mutations. *Neurology* 2006;**67**:602–6.
177. Shy ME. Charcot-Marie-Tooth disease: an update. *Current Opinion in Neurology* 2004;**17**:579–85.
178. Gabreels-Festen A, Gabreels F. Congenital and early infantile neuropathies. In: Jones H, DeVivo D, Darras B (eds) *Neuromuscular Disorders of Infancy, Childhood, and Adolescence: a Clinician's Approach*. New York, NY: Butterworth Heinemann, 2003:361–88.
179. Metaizeau JP, Gayet C, Plenat F. Les lésions obstétricales du plexus brachial. [Brachial plexus birth injuries. An experimental study]. *Chirurgiue Pediatrique* 1979;**20**:159–63.
180. Sever JW. Obstetric paralysis: its etiology, pathology, clinical aspects and treatment, with report of four hundred and seventy cases. *American Journal of Diseases of Children* 1916;**12**:541–78.
181. Smellie W. *A Collection of Cases and Observations in Midwifery*, 4th edn. Dublin, Ireland: T. and J. Whitehouse, 1764:446.
182. Duchenne GBA. *De L'Electrisation Localisee et de son Application a la Pathologie et a la Therapeutique*, 2nd edn [French]. Paris, France: J.B. Bailiere, 1872:357–62.
183. Erb W. Ueber eine eigenthümliche Localisation von Lähmungen im Plexus brachialis. *Verhandlungen des naturhistorisch-medicinischen Vereins zu Heidelberg* 1874;**2**:130–7.
184. Klumpke A. Contribution a l'étude des paralysies radiculaires du plexus brachial [French]. *Revue de Médecine (Paris)* 1885;**5**:591–3.
185. Levine MG, Holroyde J, Woods JR, *et al*. Birth traumas: incidence and predisposing factors. *Obstetrics and Gynecology* 1984;**63**:792–5.
186. Mollberg M, Wennergren M, Bager B, *et al*. Obstetric brachial plexus palsy: a prospective study on risk factors related to manual assistance during the second stage of labor. *Acta Obstetrica et Gynecologica* 2007;**86**:198–204.
187. Foad SL, Mehlman CT, Ying J. The epidemiology of neonatal brachial plexus palsy in the United States. *Journal of Bone and Joint Surgery (American)* 2008;**90A**:1258–64.
188. Kondo T. Reconstruction of shoulder function. Presented at the 10th Symposium on the Brachial Plexus. Lausanne, 19–22 January 1992.
189. Lagerkvist AL, Johansson U, Johansson A, *et al*. Obstetric brachial plexus palsy: a prospective, population-based study of incidence, recovery, and residual impairment at 18 months of age. *Developmental Medicine and Child Neurology* 2010;**52**:529–34.
190. Gilbert A, Tassim JL. Surgical repair of the brachial plexus in obstructive paralysis [French]. *Chirurgie* 1984;**110**:70–5.
191. Narakas A. Obstetrical brachial plexus injuries. In: Lamb DW (ed.) *The Paralysed Hand*. Edinburgh, UK: Churchill Livingstone, 1987:116–35.
192. Michelow BJ, Clarke HM, Curtis CG, *et al*. The natural history of obstetric brachial plexus palsy. *Plastic and Reconstructive Surgery* 1994;**93**:675–80; discussion 681.
193. Smith NC, Rowan P, Benson LJ, *et al*. Neonatal brachial plexus palsy. Outcome of absent biceps function at three months of age. *Journal of Bone and Joint Surgery (American)* 2004;**86A**:2163–70.
194. Waters PM. Update on the management of pediatric brachial plexus palsy. *Journal of Pediatric Orthopaedics* 2005;**25**:116–26.
195. Kattan K, Spitz HB. Roentgen findings in obstetrical injuries to the brachial plexus. *Radiology* 1968:**91**:462–7.
196. Pollock AN, Reed MH. Shoulder deformities from obstetrical brachial plexus paralysis. *Skeletal Radiology* 1989;**18**:295–7.
197. Aitken J. Deformity of the elbow joint as a sequel to Erb's obstetrical paralysis. *Journal of Bone and Joint Surgery (British)* 1952;**34B**:352–65.
198. Kawai H, Tsuyuguchi Y, Masada K. Identification of the lesion in brachial plexus injuries with root avulsion: a comprehensive assessment by means of preoperative

198. findings, myelography, surgical exploration and intraoperative electrodiagnosis. *Neuro-Orthopaedics* 1989;**7**:15–23.
199. Yilmaz K, Caliskan M, Oge E, *et al*. Clinical assessment, MRI, and EMG in congenital brachial plexus palsy. *Pediatric Neurology* 1999;**21**:705–10.
200. Van Ouwerkerk WJ, van der Sluijs JA, Nollet F, *et al*. Management of obstetric brachial plexus lesions: state of the art and future developments. *Child's Nervous System* 2000;**16**:638–44.
201. Birch R, Bonney G, Wynn Parry CB. Birth lesions of the brachial plexus. In: Birch R, Bonney G, Wynn Parry CB (eds) *Surgical Disorders of the Peripheral Nerves: Shoulder*, vol. 3. New York, NY: Churchill Livingstone, 1998:209–33.
202. Kawabata H, Kawai H, Masatomi T, Yasui N. Accessory nerve neurotisation in infants with brachial plexus palsy. *Microsurgery* 1994;**15**;768–72.
203. Kawabata H, Shibata T, Matsui Y, Yasui N. Use of intercostal nerves for neurotisation of the musculocutaneous nerve in infants with birth related brachial plexus palsy. *Journal of Neurosurgery* 2001;**94**:386–91.
204. Terzis JK, Papakonstantinou KC. Management of obstetric brachial plexus palsy. *Hand Clinics* 1999;**15**:717–36.
205. Moukoko D, Ezaki M, Wilkes D, Carter P. Posterior shoulder dislocation in infants with neonatal brachial plexus palsy. *Journal of Bone and Joint Surgery (American)* 2004;**86A**:787–93.
- 206. L'Episcopo J. Tendon transplantation in obstetrical paralysis. *American Journal of Surgery* 1934;**25**:122–5.
207. Phipps GJ, Hoffer MM. Latissimus dorsi and teres major transfer to rotator cuff for Erb's palsy. *Journal of Shoulder and Elbow Surgery* 1995;**4**:124–9.
208. Zancolli E, Zancolli E. Palliative surgical procedures in sequellae of obstetrical palsy. In: Tubiana R (ed.) *The Hand*, vol. IV. Philadelphia, PA: W.B. Saunders, 1991:602–23.
209. Nath RK, Paizi M. Improvement in abduction of the shoulder after reconstructive soft-tissue procedures in obstetric brachial plexus palsy. *Journal of Bone and Joint Surgery (British)* 2007;**89B**:620–6.
210. Waters PM, Bae DS. The early effects of tendon transfers and open capsulorrhaphy on glenohumeral deformity in brachial plexus birth palsy. *Journal of Bone and Joint Surgery (American)* 2008;**90A**:2171–9.
211. Waters PM, Bae DS. The effect of derotational humeral osteotomy on global shoulder function in brachial plexus birth palsy. *Journal of Bone and Joint Surgery (American)* 2006;**88A**:1035–42.

65

Spinal disorders in children

STEPHEN TREDWELL, CHRISTOPHER REILLY

Introduction	626	Sagittal plane deformity	637
Post-natal growth and development of the spinal column	626	Adolescent postural kyphosis: evaluation and management	637
Congenital vertebral anomalies: overview	627	Scheuermann's kyphosis: evaluation and management	639
Juvenile idiopathic scoliosis	634	References	639
Adolescent idiopathic scoliosis	635		

NATIONAL BOARD STANDARDS

- Understand the development of the spinal column
- Be aware of the types of vertebral anomalies and know how to assess children with these anomalies
- Know the details of assessment of a child with idiopathic scoliosis and the treatment options
- Be aware of the common causes of kyphosis and their management

INTRODUCTION

The bony spinal column is the central element of the axial trunk; it is responsible for protection of the enclosed neural elements and the paradoxically dual role of trunk flexibility and trunk stability. Pathological states that compromise any or all of these three major tasks will reduce the patient's overall ability to function.

The superimposition of growth onto a compromised spine can significantly increase the resulting disability. The treating physician therefore must not only know the natural history of the disease state but also the impact of the patient's remaining growth on that disease state (Fig. 65.1a,b).

POST-NATAL GROWTH AND DEVELOPMENT OF THE SPINAL COLUMN

The growth of the spinal column must contend with the spinal cord, the spinal canal and the bony vertebrae themselves.[1]

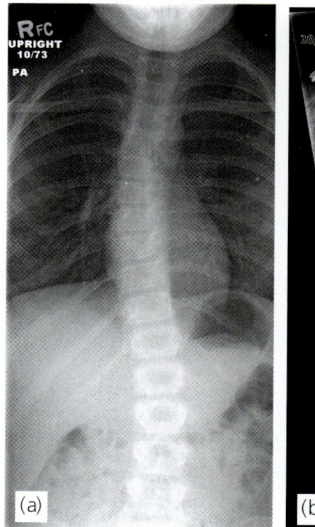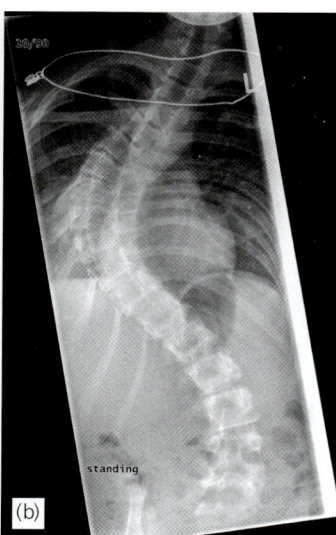

Figure 65.1 A radiographic example of a case of rapid progression of curve magnitude. A 10° curve at age 9 years is shown in (a) Progression was rapid to approximately 75° by age 13 (b).

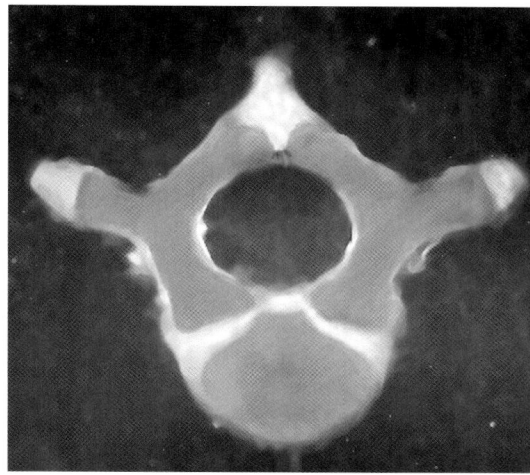

Figure 65.2 Mid-thoracic vertebra at 26 weeks' gestation. The primary ossification centres for the centrum and the pedicle–posterior element complex are well formed. The neurocentric junction separates the centrum from the pedicle–posterior element complex. The neurocentric junction will close in early adolescence. The secondary centres of ossification have not yet appeared and are seen as their cartilaginous precursors: those for the tips of the transverse processes and the spinous process are seen here; the two ring apophyses at either end of the centrum are not seen on this view.

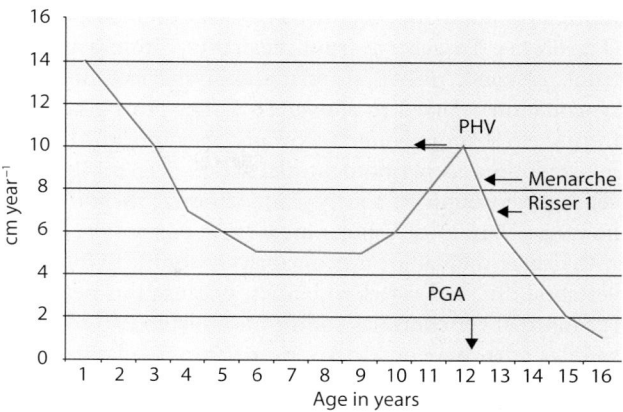

Figure 65.3 Peak height velocity (PHV) and peak growth age (PGA) precede both menarche and the appearance of the iliac apophysis (Risser 1).

Although the spinal cord occupies the full length of the spinal column in the embryo, by birth the conus has ascended to the level of the third or fourth lumbar vertebra and by adulthood to lumbar vertebra 1 or 2.[1] Conditions that interfere with the ability of the cord to ascend, such as a 'tethered cord' secondary to a hypertrophied filum terminale or lipomeningocele can present during the rapid trunk growth of the first 2 years of life with neurological problems.

The vertebral canal develops early and by 6–8 years has reached adult diameter.[1] The growth of the bony vertebrae is from three primary and five secondary centres of ossification as shown in Fig. 65.2.

Over the growing years, the thoracic vertebrae average 0.8 and the lumbar vertebrae 1.0 mm of longitudinal growth per year.[2]

This growth is not at a constant rate. There are two major peaks in spinal growth velocity: the first is from birth to 2 years, and the second in early adolescence. It is during these times of rapid growth that spinal deformity can also progress rapidly.

It becomes necessary therefore to be able to identify spine maturity indicators in the individual patient in order to manage deformity. Maturity indicators may be historical (e.g. menarche in young women), may come from longitudinal clinical measurement of standing or sitting height, or may be derived from clinical or radiographic examination.

The patient population with the greatest challenge to the clinician in determining maturity is the adolescent group. Sanders[3] divides peri-pubertal growth into adrenarche and gonadarche; he notes that adrenarche occurs first, is marked by adrenal cortex maturity and heralds the adolescent growth spurt. Sanders emphasizes the important link between gonadarche, which he defines as the 'maturing of ovaries and testes with concomitant gonadal steroid production and rapid growth'. During gonadarche, the fine light axillary and pubic hair of adrenarche coarsens and darkens, testicular enlargement occurs in males and breast development and menarche in females.

The maximum growth rate is termed peak height velocity (PHV),[3] and the age at PHV is termed peak growth age (PGA). PHV and PGA occur later in males than in females and are not as closely linked to sexual maturity as they are in females.[3] Fig. 65.3 shows a stylized trunk growth velocity curve with maturity indicator markers. Note that in the adolescent female the menarche occurs after both PHV and PGA.

The discussion that follows will focus on congenital vertebral anomalies (scoliosis and kyphosis) and the idiopathic scoliosis group. Other aetiologies of spinal deformity will be presented in summary form (Table 65.1).

CONGENITAL VERTEBRAL ANOMALIES: OVERVIEW

The duality of trunk stability and mobility conferred by a mobile vertebral column, by way of its major functional advantage, spawned the subphylum of the vertebrates. This duality is achieved by way of a complex embryological syncopation, the genetic control of which has been largely retained from fish to mammal.

The basic embryological segmental building blocks of the axial trunk are the somites, which form in humans between the 25th and 35th day following fertilization.[4] By the 32nd day, there are about 30 somite pairs, each of which contains a sclerotome (skeletal primordium), a myotome (segmental muscle primordium) and a dermatome (dermal primordium). At this stage, muscle primordia do not bridge segments but are confined to them (Fig. 65.4a). To achieve trunk flexibility within a unified trunk a second, 'off set', segmentation is needed; this is the syncopation referred to above. To achieve this goal, cells from the sclerotome migrate towards the notochord forming a continuous perinotochordal sheath (Fig. 65.4b). The cell concentration of the peri-notochordal sheath is not homogeneous; loose cellular areas from one somite merge with denser cellular areas of an adjacent somite to form the vertebral disc and vertebral bodies. Because this new unit (primordial vertebra) has contributions from two adjacent somites, the myotome-derived trunk musculature now bridges vertebral segments, allowing controlled mobility of the derived bony elements (Fig. 65.4c). Segmental arteries and nerves now lie at the mid-portion of the embryonic vertebrarather than between segments.[4]

The complexity of segmentation is under the control of a novel biological 'somite clock' in one of the Notch signalling pathways.[5] Disturbances of genes in the Notch pathway in mouse models can cause somite segmentation defects that result in vertebral anomalies. Given the very strong conservation of genetic signalling pathways related to spine formation throughout mammals, disturbance of the Notch signalling pathway is the most likely cause of vertebral anomalies in humans as well. Early evidence to support this theory can be found in studies that have identified Notch pathway mutations in spondylocostal dysplasia type 1 (*DLL3* gene);[5,6] spondylocostal dysplasia type 2 (*MESP2*

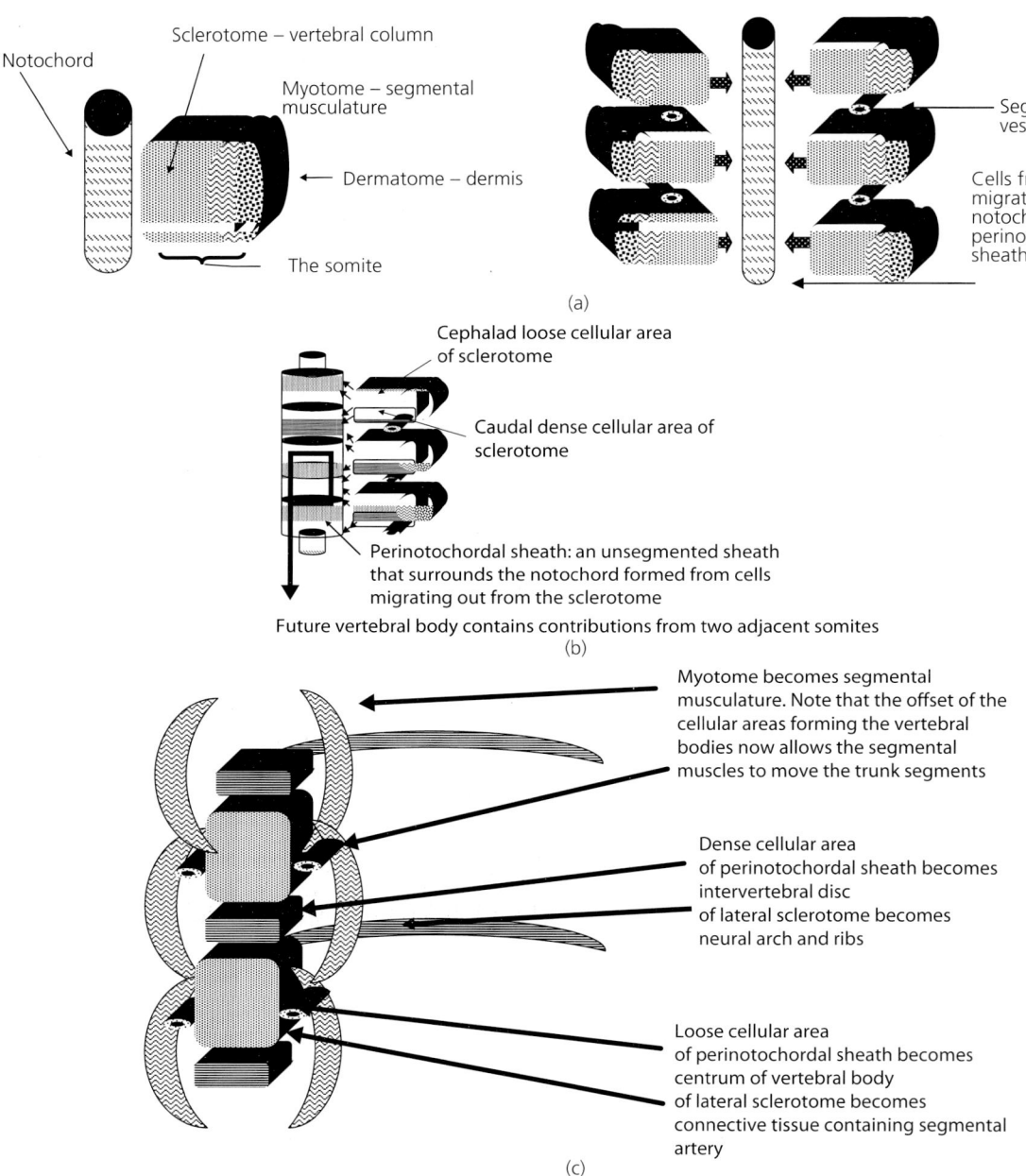

Figure 65.4 (a-c) Schematic of the basic embryological building blocks of the axial trunk.

gene);[7] and spondylocostal dysplasia type 3 (*LNFG* gene).[8] Genetic mutation, sporadic, syndromic or teratogenic, that affects the Notch pathway during segmentation can therefore produce a resultant vertebral malformation.

Clinical expression of vertebral malformation may be syndromic, e.g. spondylocostal dysplasia, Klippel–Feil anomaly, Jarco–Levin syndrome or, more commonly, sporadic: the familiar hemivertebra or unsegmented bar.

Winter *et al.*[9] popularized classification of the radiographic phenotype into failures of formation (hemivertebrae), failures of segmentation (unsegmented bar) or mixed anomalies (combinations of formation and segmentation defects) (Fig. 65.5).

Spinal deformity in general is a three-dimensional pathology, its division into coronal plane deformity (scoliosis) and sagittal plane deformity (kyphosis) aids in the conception of pathology and in communication but is usually an oversimplification of the clinical reality. The plane of maximum deformity is rarely truly coronal or sagittal. As the plane of maximum deformity moves from coronal to sagittal, the prognosis and the natural history change.

Congenital vertebral anomalies: patient evaluation

Patients with congenital vertebral anomalies flow into an orthopaedic evaluation stream from many directions. An increasing number of consultations are triggered before delivery because of an abnormal fetal ultrasound; chest or abdominal radiographs that are carried out early in life for other medical pathology trigger others. The commonest reason for referral remains clinical concern with obvious deformity.

History is the major component of the initial assessment. Syndromic spinal deformity must be separated from sporadic. Possible teratogenic aetiologies are important for mother, child and future pregnancies (e.g. maternal diabetes, drugs, both medically indicated and recreational, and environmental toxins).[10,11]

The child's growth history is important: abnormal developmental milestones focus one's attention on possible neural axis deformity, a history of rapid progression of deformity may dictate an earlier intervention, and failure to thrive may underscore thoracic insufficiency with feeding difficulties.[12]

Physical examination is divided into axial and extra-axial. Axial examination will include location: cervical, thoracic and lumbar. It is important to identify junctional curves (cervicothoracic, thoracolumbar and lumbosacral); the natural histories of these curves tend to be more severe and the treatment strategies more complex. The plane of maximum deformity is also important. Those curves with a major coronal component (congenital scoliosis) can be associated with trunk imbalance, thoracic insufficiency, head tilt (secondary to bony torticollis), and shoulder or pelvic tilt (usually secondary to a junctional deformity). Those curves with a major sagittal component (congenital kyphosis) have increased risk of compromise of the spinal canal and therefore also of the spinal cord. Axial examination should also look for mid-line skin pigmentation or hair patches as well as a gluteal cyst or sinus; all as possible signs of underlying neural malformation.

Extra-axial physical examination should start with the patient's height and weight as the beginning of a continuous prospective record of growth. Record anomalies, especially those that may be associated with neural abnormality (e.g. vertical talus, unilateral cavus foot or hemiatrophy).

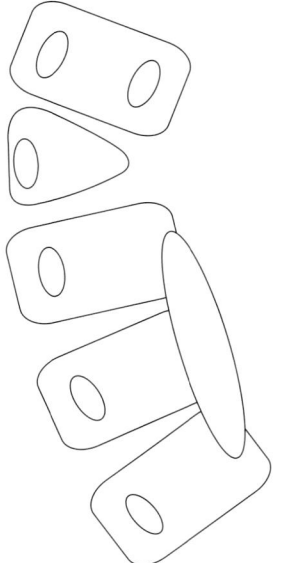

Figure 65.5 Congenital vertebral anomalies.[9]

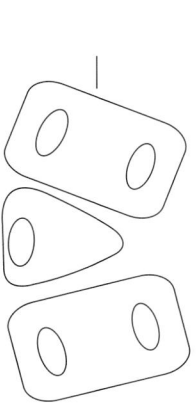
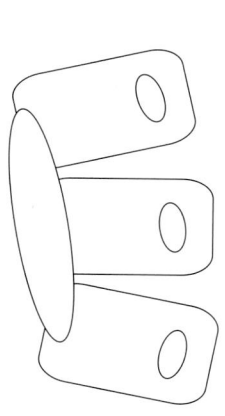

Failure of formation (hemivertebra)

Failure of segmentation (unsegmented bar)

Mixed lesion

Neurological examination should be repeated at least yearly, including recording of abdominal reflexes (often the only clinical finding in syringo- or hydromyelia).

Imaging studies begin with plain radiographs of the entire spine both anteroposterior (AP) and lateral. The plain radiograph substantiates diagnosis and can serve as a monitor of progression. The plain radiograph also serves as a context within which more sophisticated studies such as MRI and CT scans are referenced. Depending on clinical findings, severity and progression, the MRI and/or CT may be postponed until the child can tolerate the examination without the need for sedation. The association with extra spinal anomalies, genitourinary (20–40%),[13] cardiac (20–25%)[13] and neural axis (up to 35%),[14] dictates imaging of these systems as well (ultrasound, MRI, cardiogram).[15]

The goal of imaging studies of the bony anomalies is to precisely describe the abnormality and therefore to forecast the natural history and to plan intervention if needed. Growth plays a major role in the progression of all deformities of the immature spine but nowhere is it as important as in congenital scoliosis and kyphosis. The nature of these deformities is their potential to induce asymmetrical growth at the segmental level (Fig. 65.6). Unsegmented bars produce deformity by tethering growth on one side so that the growth on the other side of the vertebra creates the deformity. The severity of deformity relates positively to the number of unsegmented levels and negatively to the extent of the lack of segmentation across the vertebra. Vertebral anomalies where the lack of segmentation crosses the midline towards the normal side have lesser progression and deformity than do the more peripheral bars.

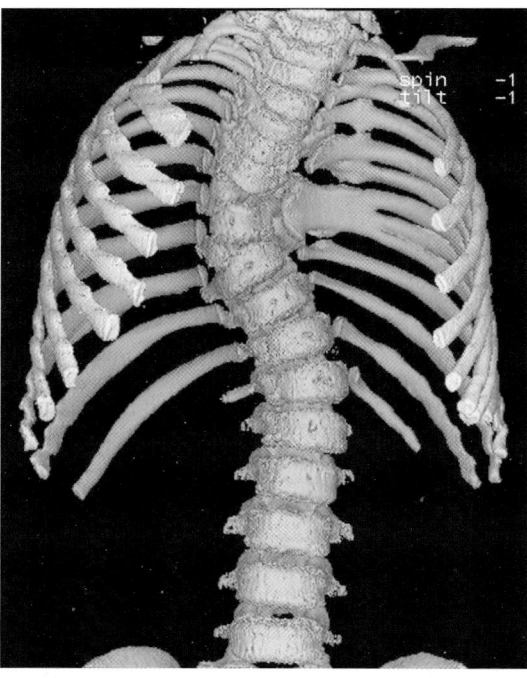

Figure 65.6 A three-dimensional CT reconstruction of a female patient showing rib fusions; failure of formation; and failure of segmentation of vertebral bodies.

Rib formation is also somite derived (Fig. 65.4c), and therefore fused ribs can be part of the radiographic phenotype and contribute to the tethering effect. Early in life, the vertebral bar may be cartilaginous or not easily seen; in the infant seemingly isolated rib fusions plus deformity should be interpreted as having associated vertebral segmentation anomalies.

Simple failures of formation (wedge vertebrae) in the coronal plane do not have the same potential for aggressive progression as do the peripheral segmentation defects. When the major deformity is in the sagittal plane, however, the sharp angular kyphosis caused by failures of formation ('wedge' or hemivertebra) can cause spinal canal compromise and secondary neurological defect.

Mixed lesions, both segmentation error and failure of formation, have a natural history that is an algebraic sum of the deformities; some will cancel each other out to produce a short but relatively straight trunk, some will be additive and produce severe deformity. (Fig. 65.6). The combination of a peripheral unsegmented bar with a contralateral hemivertebra produces one of the most aggressive patterns.

Congenital vertebral anomalies: treatment

In patients with congenital scoliosis and kyphosis the goals of treatment are to alter those natural histories that can produce harm, or to reconstruct those deformities that have already progressed to a harmful state. When one has the advantage of seeing the child early in life, rigorous work-up and meticulous follow-up can predict curve patterns that will progress and allow early and less hazardous intervention. There are five treatment options. (Box 65.1)

> **BOX 65.1: Treatment options for congenital vertebral anomalies**
>
> 1. Accept deformity that will not progress to cause harm; these children should be followed to maturity (as should all patients who require surgical intervention).
> 2. Fuse deformities *in situ* where the predicted end deformity will be unacceptable but the present state is acceptable.
> 3. Partial fusion ('convex hemiarthrodesis') in the presence of a congenital anomaly in the coronal plane (scoliosis) where the involved area is short and predicted progression is significant. The extension of the convex surgically fused area by one or two levels plus growth has the potential to correct the curve.
> 4. Vertebral excision plus or minus osteotomy to reconstruct major deformity.
> 5. Lateral extra-axial distraction realignment (vertical expanding prosthetic titanium rib (VEPTR)) to hold the spine corrected during growth.

Bracing has a limited role in congenital spine deformity. Bracing cannot influence bony deformity nor offset asymmetrical vertebral growth, but it can control secondary curves that arise in compensation to the induced trunk imbalance of the primary congenital deformity.

Fusion *in situ* is the least hazardous surgical intervention and is indicated in the presence of a mild to moderate curve with documented progression. Curves with a Cobb angle of over 40° are unlikely to benefit from *in situ* fusion. While simple this intervention is not without problems: slow progression of the curve in the face of a solid posterior fusion can occur as can variations on the so-called 'crankshaft' phenomenon (see below under Infantile idiopathic scoliosis).

Partial fusion to offset the influence of unbalanced growth is intellectually appealing. The theory is that by creating a surgical fusion on the side contralateral to the anomaly the deforming growth will cease; by extending the fusion an additional level, the remaining growth on the pathological side will act to correct the deformity. This approach, termed convex hemiarthrodesis, was popularized by Winter and colleagues.[16,17]

The indications are relatively narrow: short curves (2–3 abnormal vertebral levels), moderate (<35°) curvatures and significant growth potential remaining (age 5 years or less). Major reconstructive surgery in this group includes any or all of vertebrectomy, osteotomy, anterior and posterior releases, or fusions plus or minus instrumentation. These curves are stiff and the spinal canal is often compromised; correction is therefore often less than one would like and the complication rates higher. Lateral, extra-axial distraction realignment of complex and progressive congenital deformity by way of a vertically expanding titanium strut or VEPTR was introduced by Campbell in the mid-1990s and the early results reported in 2003[18] (Fig. 65.7).

Campbell's early results suggest that, following expansion thoracoplasty and serial expansions of the VEPTR, complex curves can be controlled with thoracic spine growth of up to 8 mm per year (normal thoracic spine growth age 5–9 years is 6 mm per year). He also noted positive changes in pulmonary function and coined the term thoracic insufficiency to identify the clinical state where 'the thorax is unable to support normal respiration or lung growth'.[12] The procedure is complex, and further operations are frequently required for serial expansions, wound complications and implant migration.

The idiopathic scoliosis group

Although the idiopathic scoliosis group represents the commonest clinical diagnosis in North American and European orthopaedic practice, as the name suggests the

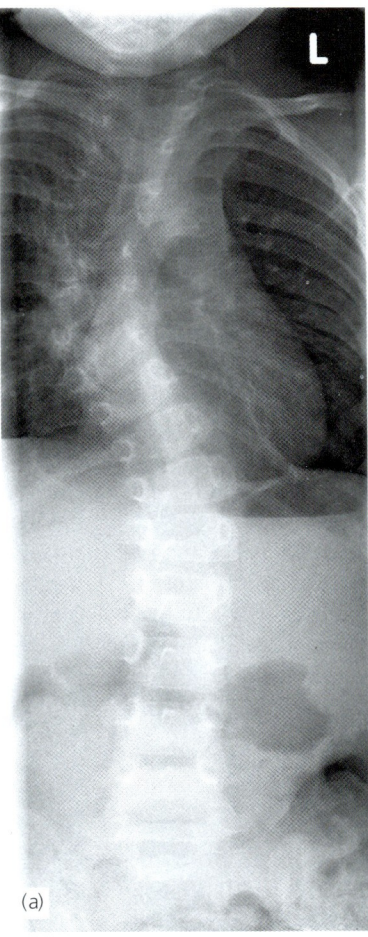
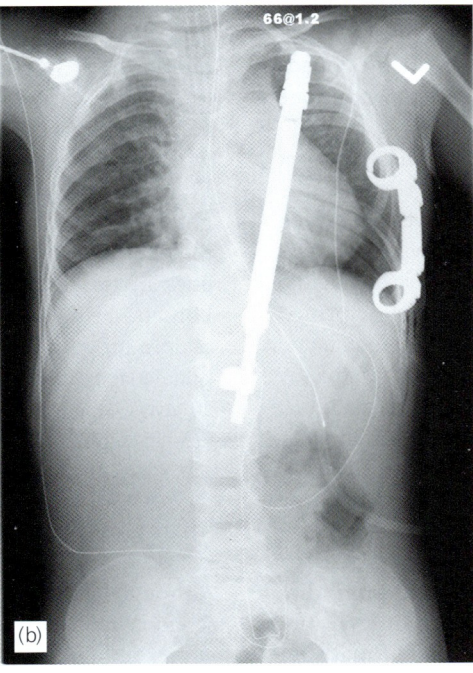

Figure 65.7 Radiographs of the patient in Fig. 65.6 with a congenital deformity (a) that was treated with a vertical expanding prosthetic titanium rib (b).

cause is unknown. Various authors have attributed the idiopathic group to errors in connective tissue, neurological control, muscle control, hormone balance (melatonin) or bony growth.[19–22] Other authors have attributed curve formation in this group as a response to pre-existing sagittal deformity.[23] Although clinical evidence suggests a genetic influence, to date no gene-based hypothesis has been robust enough to explain either the familial occurrences or the variations in phenotype.

The theories of aetiology do allow some overlap of one on the other with a scoliosis as the result. Examples are genetic influence on neurological control of balance (Friedrich's ataxia), on connective tissue strength (Marfan syndrome) or on muscle strength (Duchenne's muscular dystrophy). All of these syndromes may result in scoliosis, many mimic the appearance of an idiopathic curve on radiographs and none is idiopathic scoliosis. Scoliosis then becomes a more general diagnosis representing a final common pathway of structural response to challenges to axial stability. It is likely that the idiopathic group contains more than one syndrome; the challenge to the clinical investigator is to split off the known aetiological groups from the heterogeneous whole rather than to claim to have found a common aetiology for the whole group.

Classically the idiopathic group has been divided into three: infantile (onset birth to age 3), juvenile (onset >age 3–8) and adolescent (onset age 10 to the completion of growth). With the above comments concerning aetiology in mind, this chapter will consider the classical construct acknowledging that in the near future subgroups may split off as aetiologies that are more concrete are described.

The morbidity of idiopathic scoliosis

The morbidity of idiopathic scoliosis is best viewed through three different lenses: of cosmetic deformity, of cardiopulmonary compromise and of mechanical back pain. Other aetiologies of curvature add their own unique comorbidities to the above list.

The largest group of idiopathic scoliosis has its onset during the pre-pubertal adolescent growth spurt; the majority of the patients with significant curves are young women. The onset of the curve coincides with development of body image of self as an independent sexual being. The superimposition of a self concept of being deformed during this maturing process can be very damaging. Payne et al.[24] found that scoliosis was a significant risk factor for psychological issues and health-compromising behaviour. Fowles et al.[25] reported on women in their thirties who had had no treatment for significantly large curvatures (>40°). Many women took jobs away from the public eye, over half did not marry and most had asked for significant time off for back pain.

The most serious and least well-understood morbidity is the impact of curvature on pulmonary function. A recurring theme in this chapter is the importance of maturity (or lack of it) on the prognosis of spinal curvature. This concept is most important for the understanding of the impact of curve on the lung. At birth, the infant has a full compliment of pulmonary alveoli, many have not yet opened to functional status and exist as alveolar 'buds'. These buds open and become functional as the child grows and the thoracic cage expands. By 7–9 years the alveoli are open and the potential for full pulmonary function exists. Curves that progress early in life have the potential to distort thoracic cage growth, inhibit alveolar maturation and therefore impact significantly on lung function. Later onset curves can also inhibit lung function by interfering with the mechanics of chest wall function, producing both a stiffer construct than is normal as well as a reduction in thoracic volume; this aetiology relates positively to curve size[26] and/or thoracic lordosis.

Clinical observations support the above concepts. Nachemson[27] in 1968 reported that pulmonary death in patients with scoliosis related strongly to age of onset; adolescent idiopathic scoliosis in this series was not a contributing factor to pulmonary death, but infantile and early juvenile cases were. Weinstein et al.[28] in 1981 reported on a 50 year follow-up of untreated idiopathic scoliosis and found that pulmonary pathology in the adult related to curve size and to thoracic curves. In his series, only curves greater than 100° Cobb showed an increased risk for cor pulmonale.

Pulmonary function loss shows a restrictive pattern with decrease in vital capacity and FEV_1 (forced expiratory volume in 1 second). In adolescent-onset curves, restriction is not common in curvatures less than 80° without other comorbidities such as lordosis. (Fig. 65.8a,b).

Back pain from degenerative change, spinal stenosis or curve-induced listhesis is seen in the adult with significant curvature and also seems related to size of curve as well as location of curve (lumbar spine). Weinstein et al.'s[28] series reported pain as a minor component of the follow-up but did equate it to curve size. Gremeaux et al.[29] noted that lumbar curves, curve size and rotatory listhesis related to pain intensity. Haefeli et al.[30] noted a positive correlation with curve size.

The morbidity of scoliosis relates to curve size and to the potential for the curve to increase. Again, we are indebted to the work of Weinstein for long-term follow-up and guidelines in this area. In the 1983 paper by Weinstein and Ponseti[31] he notes that curves of 30° Cobb or less at maturity seldom progress and that curves of 50–70° Cobb at maturity have a significant risk of increase that averages 30° over 20 years (Fig. 65.5). The results for the smaller curves (25–40° Cobb) are also supported by Gabos et al.[32]

Infantile idiopathic scoliosis

Although recognized as a clinical problem for many years, scoliosis in the very young was usually lumped in with other curves until described as a discrete group by J. I. P. James

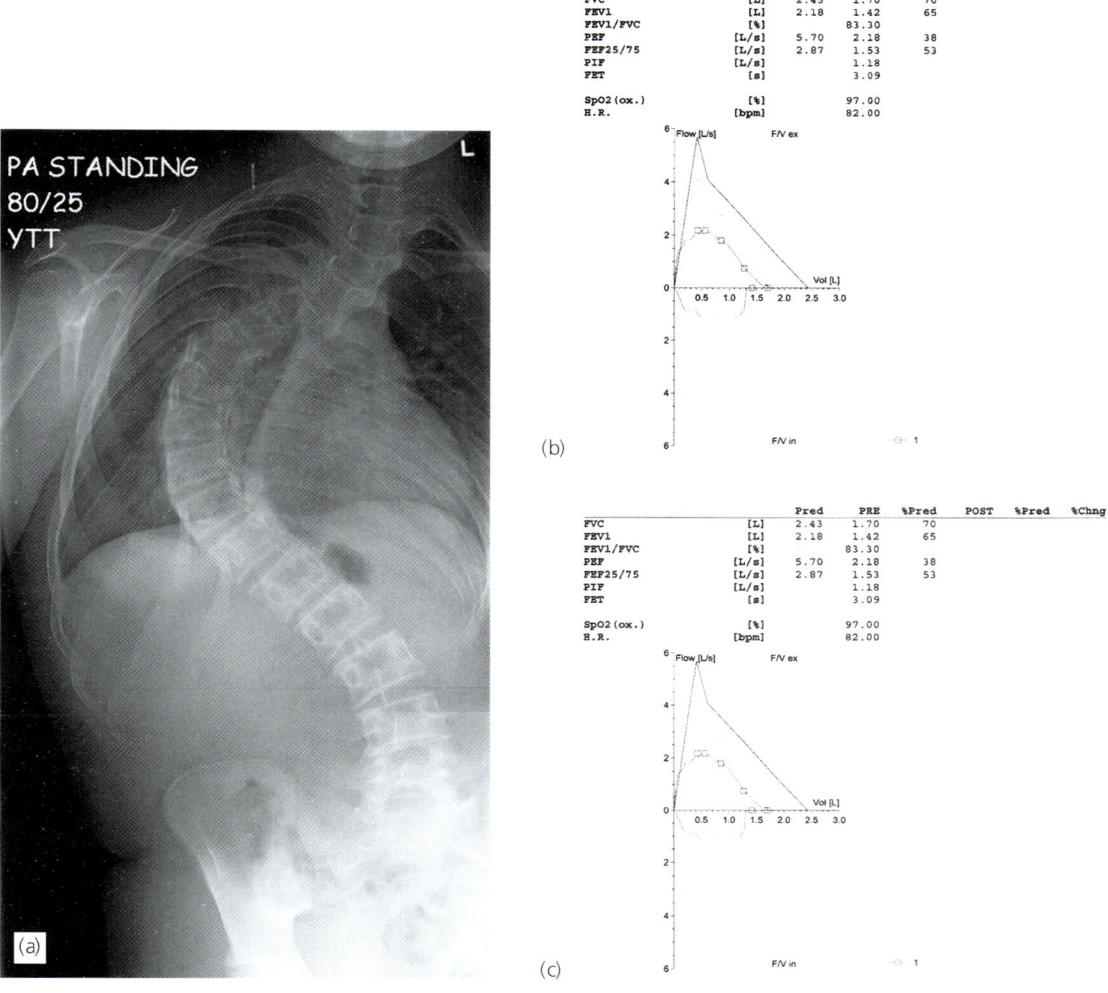

Figure 65.8 A young female with a very large curve and significant lordosis. Her associated decreased pulmonary function is superimposed upon a normal pulmonary function curve (c). Her forced expiratory volume over 1 second (FEV_1) is 65% of normal and the forced vital capacity (FVC) is 70% of predicted.

of Edinburgh.[33] The hallmarks of this group are onset within the first 3 years of life, a gender preference for males, a curve preference to the left side and a strong association with plagiocephaly (Box 65.2). The natural history of the curvature shows that a significant number will be non-progressive or resolve and a smaller number will progress. The progressive curves in the infantile group are among the most difficult management problems in paediatric spinal deformity.[33]

> **BOX 65.2: Common features of infantile idiopathic scoliosis**
>
> - Onset within the first 3 years of life
> - A gender preference for males
> - A curve preference to the left side
> - A strong association with plagiocephaly

Fernandez and Weinstein[34] in 2007 cited the common features of 906 patients with infantile-onset scoliosis as reported by 12 different authors. Not all features were reported in each series: in the group as a whole 36% of the curves were progressive and 64% were non-progressive or resolving. The mean age of onset was 12 months for the progressive group and 5.5 months for the non-progressive or resolving group.

Gender was not reported for just over 22% of the group; when reported however there was a slight male predominance (progressive 54.7%, and non-progressive 57.9%). The side of involvement was also not reported in just over 22%, but when reported the curve was to the left in 74.6% of progressive curves and 81.3% of non-progressive curves. A rib vertebral angle difference (RVAD) of less than 20° was seen in 72.5% of the progressive group and in 9% of the non-progressive curves. This later measurement was introduced by Mehta[35] and describes the relationship of the ribs to the vertebral body at the apex of the curve as a prognostic indicator of progression.[36]

As clinical series of the infantile group have accumulated, several authors have observed that most true infantile scoliosis has onset before age 2 rather than age 3.

INFANTILE IDIOPATHIC SCOLIOSIS: CLINICAL EXAMINATION

Patient history is again important; the age at which the curve was obvious should be noted, as should the rapidity of curve progression. A history of failure to thrive is likewise notable; Mehta[35] observed that many of the patients with progressive curves appeared undernourished. Family history of connective tissue disorder or neurological problems may suggest other causes than idiopathic especially in the child with onset after age 2.

Physical examination should note the direction of the curve (convex left or convex right) and curve flexibility. Plagiocephaly is very common in this group;[36] its absence while not ruling out the diagnosis should be a stimulus to explore other aetiologies. Infantile idiopathic scoliosis has also been associated with developmental hip dysplasia.[36]

Because of the possibility of other aetiologies, accurate and repeated neurological examinations are important. Routine MRI examinations of all infantile curves over 20° Cobb angle have been recommended by Dobbs and Lenke,[37] who reported an incidence of neural axis abnormalities of 21% in a series of 46 patients. One might contend that, with a demonstrated neural axis deformity, the positive cases are not true infantile idiopathic curves and that the curves should be reclassified as neurogenic. This is a valid point and only underscores the importance of accurate diagnosis and also supports the authors' contention that MRI studies are integral to the work-up of curves in the very young that are more than 20°.

INFANTILE IDIOPATHIC SCOLIOSIS: MANAGEMENT

The obvious first goal of management is to separate the progressive curves from the non-progressive. This will only truly be accomplished with adequate clinical follow-up. Even though a small percentage of curves with a RVAD of greater than 20° will prove to be non-progressive, all curves within this group that measure over 25° Cobb should be considered for bracing. All curves with a RVAD of over 20° and demonstrated progression of over 5° Cobb should be braced. The goal of bracing needs patient explanation to the family. Most progressive infantile idiopathic curves will eventually need surgery, but the longer the curve can be controlled with a brace the lesser will be the surgical intervention both in extent of surgery and in surgical risk (Fig. 65.9).

Surgical intervention is either temporizing or definitive. Curves that progress to greater than 50° despite bracing where the patient has significant trunk and thoracic cage growth remaining may benefit from one of the so-called 'growing rod' systems.[38] The concept of this intervention is

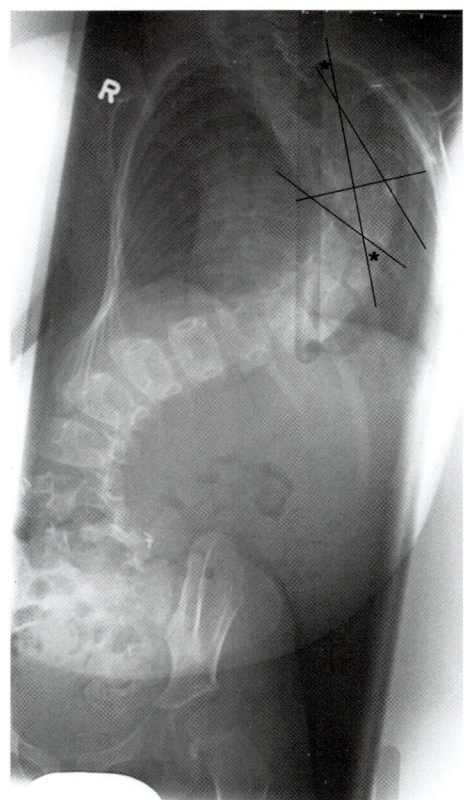

Figure 65.9 A radiograph of a young boy with a progressive infantile idiopathic curve. Rib vertebral angles (Mehta) are shown as asterisks. Rib vertebral angle difference in this case is 30°.

to insert a posterior distraction device that can be serially lengthened as the patient grows. The curve is controlled and trunk growth facilitated. A definitive instrumentation is performed when the patient reaches peak growth age. In the infantile idiopathic curve and in some of the juvenile idiopathic patients, persistence with a simple posterior system through the peak growth period will tether growth posteriorly and induce a 'crank-shaft' phenomenon. The crank-shaft phenomenon was described by Dubousset[39] and refers to the deformity produced by continued or accelerated anterior growth of vertebral bodies in the presence of a posterior fusion or tether. When this occurs in the presence of a pre-existing scoliotic curvature, the anterior growth twists the spine around the posterior tether much like the stairs on a spiral staircase. Posterior spinal fusion preformed before peak growth age has a significant risk of subsequent crank-shaft deformity.[39]

JUVENILE IDIOPATHIC SCOLIOSIS

Juvenile idiopathic scoliosis is usually defined as an idiopathic curve with onset between the ages of 3 and 8 years. Conceptually it is a curve that arises during the plateau phase of trunk growth velocity. The importance of this curve group lies in the potential for significant worsening during the adolescent growth spurt. The juvenile group shows a similar curve pattern and female preponderance with adolescent idiopathic scoliosis.

Juvenile idiopathic scoliosis: clinical examination

Because of the potential for the curve to increase rapidly as the child approaches PHV, longitudinal follow-up is essential in this group. If the treating clinic has the facility to provide Tanner staging,[36] it is very useful. Tanner staging is more accurate than radiographic or growth chart measurements in charting maturity and in predicting PHV.[36] The difficulty with Tanner staging is the intimate nature of the examination. Success revolves around patient and family education as to the value and goals of the examination, trained sensitive personnel and appropriate examination settings.

As in all scoliosis management, search for aetiologies other than idiopathic is important. The neurological examination is especially important, and within this examination the documentation of the abdominal reflex is essential. The unilateral absence of this reflex is often the only abnormality in curves induced by cervical syrinx or by Arnold Chiari malformation. Spinal curvature plus unilateral absence of the abdominal reflex is an indication for MRI examination even if there are no other findings (Fig. 65.10).

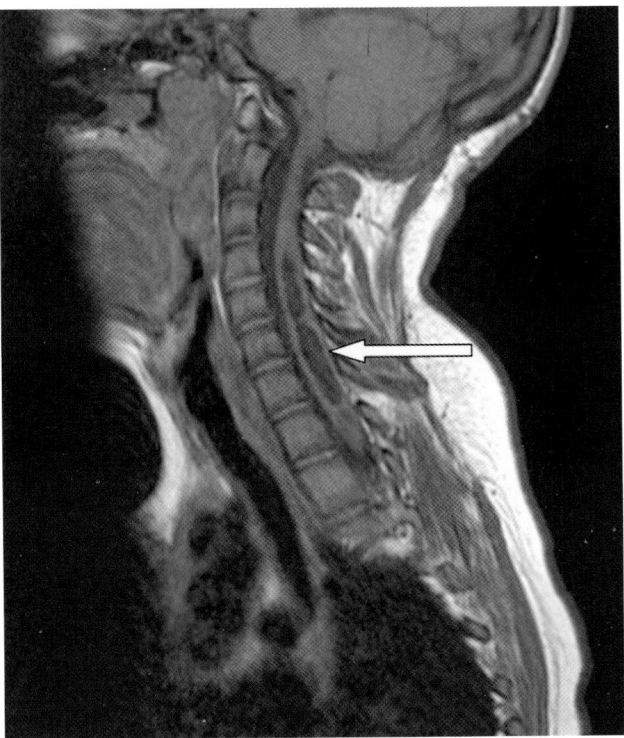

Figure 65.10 A sagittal MRI slice showing a syrinx (arrow). An abnormal clinical finding of an absent abdominal reflex may indicate a syrinx.

Juvenile idiopathic scoliosis: management

The patient with juvenile idiopathic scoliosis will usually come to bracing. Curves below 25° Cobb may be followed closely, but curves larger than this should be considered for bracing. As in the infantile group bracing may be a strategy to allow trunk growth in cases where the definitive answer will be surgery, although in a small number of cases bracing may be definitive care and be able to control the curve to the cessation of growth.

Because of the risk of crank-shaft deformity, some authors[40] recommend both anterior and posterior fusions in this group if surgery is carried out before PHV. Because of this, in curves that are in the lower surgical range, a strategy that employs bracing until after peak growth age and then utilizes posterior instrumentation can reduce the extent of surgery by avoiding an anterior procedure. Surgery is a decision that must be individualized to each patient. Given that curves in the 50–60° Cobb range at maturity progress an average of 30° during adult life,[24] surgery is considered at 50° and is recommended at 60° if the patient is mature (2 years past menarche). For the juvenile group, a curve that reaches 45–50° before PGA will almost inevitably progress to surgery and it is in this group that persistence with bracing to PGA would be recommended. Those curves that progress in the brace to over 60° before PGA would be operated on in the immature state and an anterior fusion (usually thoracoscopic) would be carried out to prevent crank-shaft deformity.

ADOLESCENT IDIOPATHIC SCOLIOSIS

Adolescent idiopathic scoliosis (AIS) is the largest subsection of the idiopathic group and the largest subgroup of scoliosis to present clinically in Europe and North America (scoliosis secondary to poliomyelitis, however, remains the leading presentation worldwide). The management of adolescent idiopathic scoliosis brings together many of the themes discussed above such as prevalence, natural history, maturity indices, non-surgical and surgical management.

If one includes all adolescent idiopathic curvatures greater than 10° Cobb the prevalence of AIS approaches 20 per 1000 population and a gender ratio of female to male of 2:1. Neither the gender ratio nor the prevalence of AIS is linear. Curves of greater than 20° Cobb have a prevalence of 3–5 per 1000 population and a gender ratio female to male of 5:1; curves greater than 30° Cobb have a prevalence of 1–3 per 1000 population and a gender ratio of 10:1[41].

The tendency for AIS curves to progress is relative to both curve magnitude and skeletal maturity. A combination of a large curve and immaturity is a clinical challenge; most of these curves will progress. The combination of a small to modest curve with maturity will often be a stable situation requiring no intervention other than follow-up.

Fortunately, the later combination is the most common. The clinical challenge is to translate 'large curve' and 'immaturity' as it relates to large populations to the specific case in the clinic. Little et al.[40] noted that in females curves of less than 30° Cobb at PHV had only a 4% chance of progressing to surgery. Clinically it may be difficult to chart PHV, especially on the initial visit. Recalling that menarche (a marker easily obtained at history) occurs after PHV a patient with a curve of less than 30° Cobb who is post menarche can be safely monitored. Conversely, Little et al.[40] also reported that females who had not achieved PHA and who had a curve of more than 30° Cobb carried a risk for subsequent surgery of 83%.

Adolescent idiopathic scoliosis: clinical examination

As with all curvatures the history and clinical examination focuses on establishing the diagnosis to rule in or out other possible causes of curvature. Not all syndromes are blatant in their clinical expression. The pigmentation of neurofibromatosis can be limited to axillary or inguinal freckling, the neurological findings of cervical syrinx causing spinal curvature to an absent abdominal reflex. Marfan syndrome exists on a clinical spectrum from the obvious to patients with minor findings only.

Adolescent idiopathic curvatures tend to be convex to the right in the thoracic spine and convex to the left in the lumbar. Curves of other aetiologies do not have side preferences and therefore left-sided thoracic curves have an increased chance of having a different aetiology. Adolescent idiopathic curvatures of over 30° Cobb have a gender ratio of 10:1 favouring females. Large curves in adolescent boys can also be diagnosed as idiopathic but only after other causes are excluded.

All structural causes of scoliosis have a three-dimensional aspect that is clinically expressed as trunk rotation. Lack of rotation suggests a secondary cause of curvature, e.g. tumour, disc protrusion, infection, syrinx or tethered cord. The forward bending test of Adams (Fig. 65.11a,b) displays the rotation of the structural curve as well as allowing description of the degree of rib prominence.

The second major theme of clinical examination in the adolescent group is maturity. As we have emphasized above, knowledge of the patient's maturity is essential to the planning of rational management. No one component can fully satisfy a maturity assessment; therefore, overlapping observations are best. Does the patient look her stated age? Is there a growth history (growth spurt, family height records)? Is she pre- or post menarche? If the clinic is suited to Tanner staging, this information should be recorded. A standing height measure should be part of every visit.

Radiographic assessment of skeletal maturity is attractive but also has drawbacks. Truly accurate assessment of skeletal age assessment and its relationship to PHV is difficult.[3] One of the more accurate indicators of the patient having yet to attain PHV is the presence of open triradiate cartilages in the acetabulum. Radiographic examination of this area however includes the risk of gonadal exposure

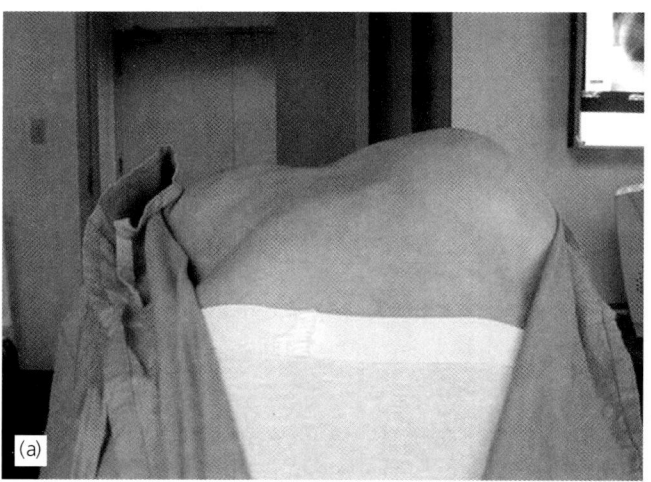
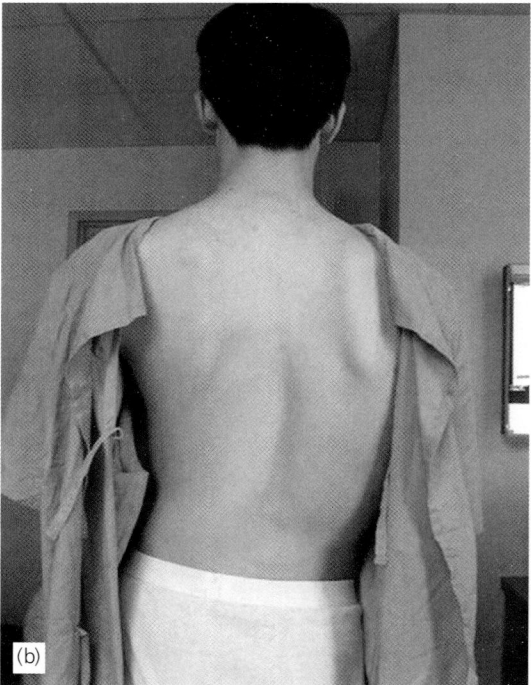

Figure 65.11 Clinical images demonstrating the Adams forward bend test (a). Note the patient's prominent rib hump is not evident on the posterior standing view (b).

and has not, therefore, gained wide popularity. Markers of wrist and elbow maturity relate to peak height[42] and are less radiographically invasive.

Adolescent idiopathic scoliosis: management

The goal of management is to achieve a balanced axial skeleton that retains flexibility and can support normal function into adult life. Curves that are small and non-progressive (<30° Cobb) need no aggressive treatment, although the patient may need counselling and follow-up. Patients with curves that are at risk to progress with projected trunk growth but where the curve is still relatively small (<40° Cobb) can be considered for bracing. Bracing as definitive management for progressive curves over 40° Cobb is not effective. The ability of bracing to manage progressive curves in the 25–40° range remains an area of contention. Studies that have favoured bracing[43–45] observed results better than the natural history of the curves left alone and better than other modalities, such as electrical stimulation. In all series however some braced curves progressed and some required surgery.

Studies that have not noted brace success[46,47] could find no difference between braced and non-braced groups. Current clinical practice leans toward bracing curves between 25° and 40° Cobb when there is trunk growth remaining. Each clinical situation is unique and the broad guidelines can be modified to fit the patient and her family's needs and desires.

Surgical intervention is also strongly influenced by patient and family views as well as by knowledge of the natural history. Armed with the knowledge that curves over 50° Cobb at maturity progress 30° on average in adult life,[28] and that those curves that do progress have difficulties that are primarily in the areas of self-image and degenerative arthritic pain, surgical discussion can begin at curves of 50° (Fig. 65.12). In the adolescent group, surgery can be introduced as an option at 50° Cobb and encouraged as an option at 60°. Note that PHA does not equate with the spine maturity of the adult nor does the cessation of vertical growth. Most progression algorithms are directed at curves in the 20–35° range, it is not unusual for a curve that measures 55° Cobb at age 13 and 18 months post menarche to present at age 16 in the 60–65° range.

The choice of surgical approach varies from centre to centre and also varies over time. This variation will continue into the future; excellent results can be achieved by either anterior (Fig. 65.13a,b) or posterior surgical approaches and by a variety of implant designs (Fig. 65.14a,b).

SAGITTAL PLANE DEFORMITY

Sagittal plane pathology results from an exaggeration or diminution of the physiological sagittal curvatures. In late fetal and early infant life the sagittal plane is a

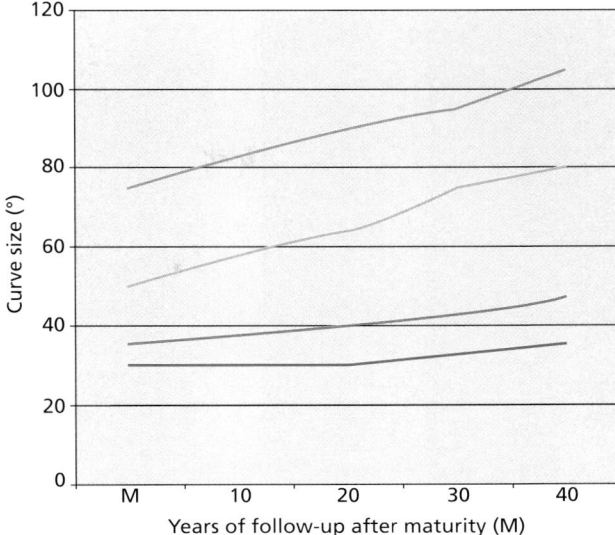

Figure 65.12 Progression of thoracic idiopathic curves after maturity. Graph is based on data from Weinstein and Ponseti (1983).[31]

smooth kyphotic curve. As the trunk and neck muscles mature, secondary sagittal curves appear. The secondary cervical and lumbar lordotic curvatures now balance the primary thoracic and sacral curvatures of infancy; the resultant trunk is now well suited to upright posture and function.

The normal adult thoracic kyphosis is between 20° and 40° Cobb; the range of normal in the developing adolescent is probably broader than this.[48] Hyperkyphosis ('kyphosis') refers to thoracic spine kyphosis over 40°; hypokyphosis to kyphosis of 0–20° and true lordosis to those thoracic spines whose sagittal curve is less than 0° Cobb.

The diagnosis of hyperkyphosis in the younger child suggests either congenital bony anomaly or trunk muscle weakness. In the adolescent two additional clinical entities are important: postural kyphosis and Scheuermann's kyphosis.

ADOLESCENT POSTURAL KYPHOSIS: EVALUATION AND MANAGEMENT

As discussed in the section on idiopathic scoliosis, the adolescent growth period is marked by a surge in trunk growth velocity. Trunk muscle development follows growth and therefore a period of relative trunk weakness is common. This relative weakness can be accentuated or ameliorated by lifestyle.

The patient with postural kyphosis presents with a cosmetic complaint; pain if present is generally vague and aching. When viewed from the side the patient will show a flexible, smooth exaggeration of the normal thoracic

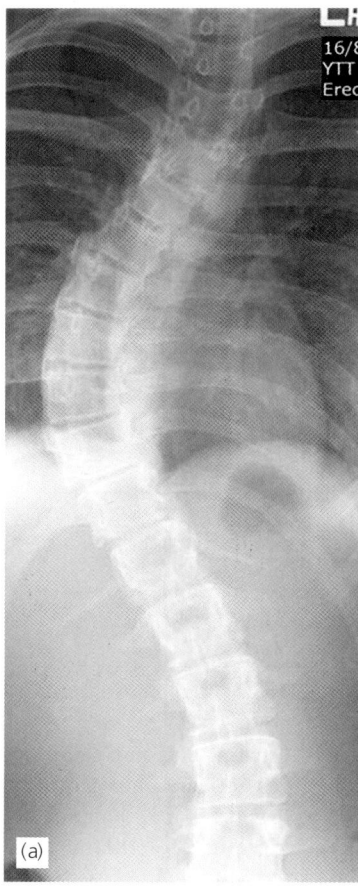 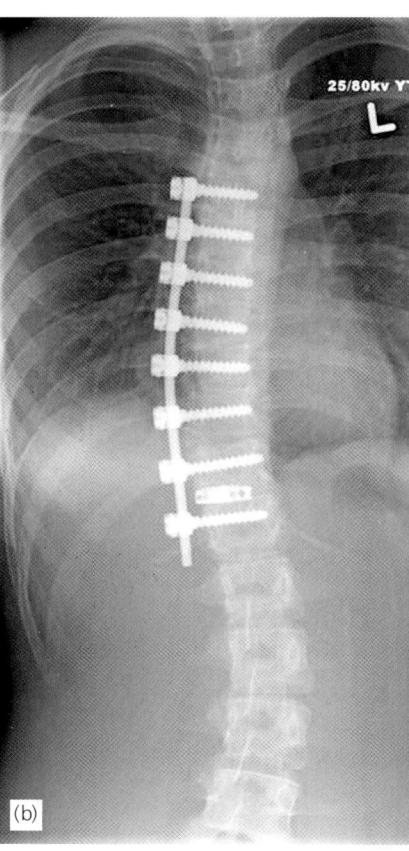

Figure 65.13 A radiographic example of an anterior approach to surgical correction of an adolescent idiopathic curve showing a pre-operative curve of approximately 60° (a) and the anterior instrumentation *in situ* (b).

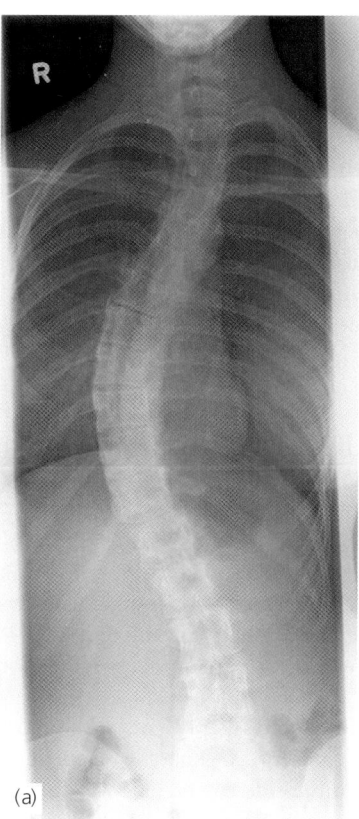 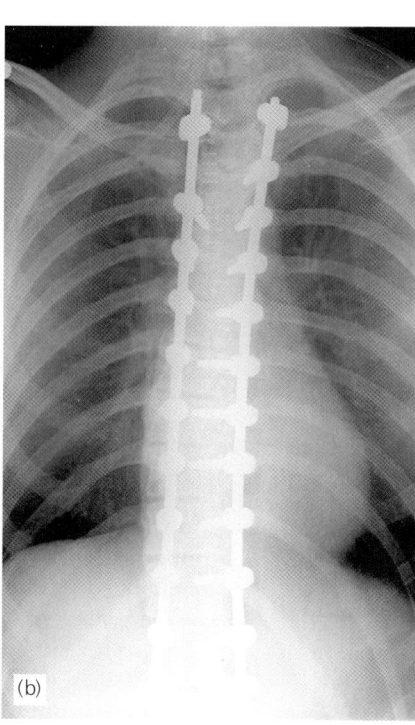

Figure 65.14 A radiographic example of a posterior approach to surgical correction of an adolescent idiopathic curve showing a pre-operative curve of approximately 50° (a) and the posterior instrumentation *in situ* (b).

kyphosis, the shoulders are rounded forward into adduction, the cervical spine is 'shot forward' so that the mandible is anterior to the sternum. Radiographic examination shows a long-segment kyphosis with a smooth arc and no bony pathology.

Although improving core trunk strength is one of the major goals of therapy it will often fail unless head and neck posture is also corrected by teaching 'chin retraction' to realign the head and neck over the trunk. Bracing is rarely indicated.

SCHEUERMANN'S KYPHOSIS: EVALUATION AND MANAGEMENT

In contradistinction to the postural kyphosis patients those with Scheuermann's kyphosis present with a stiff kyphotic segment, pain can be absent or relatively well localized and severe. The so-called 'forward shot neck' of the postural group is usually absent, exaggerated lumbar lordosis is often present. Physical examination reveals tightness of both hamstring and pectoral muscle groups; straight-leg raising is usually restricted. Radiographic examination will show a long segment kyphosis with apical changes of the vertebral end plates that produce an erosive picture with resultant vertebral body wedging. To fit the syndrome one should see wedging of more than 5° over three or more levels (Fig. 65.15).

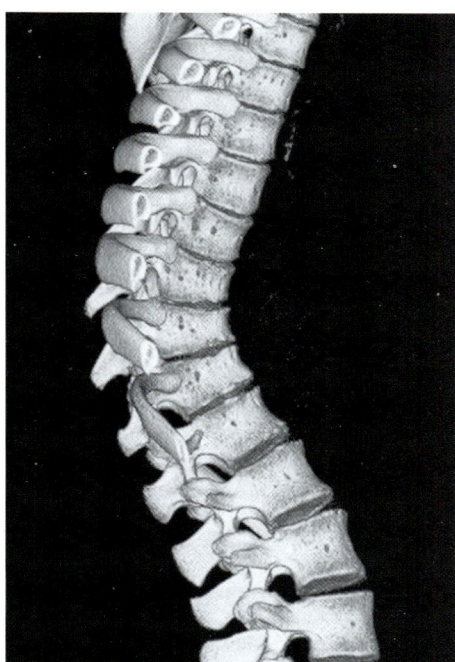

Figure 65.15 A three-dimensional CT reconstruction of the spine of an 18 year old boy with Scheuermann's kyphosis presenting with vertebral wedging.

In addition, unlike postural kyphosis, intervention may not stop at physiotherapy. Bracing can be effective especially to control both pain and curve progression. Surgery is rarely indicated except in larger curves. Function in the untreated adult is generally good.[49] In the adult cardiac and pulmonary problems are rare when the kyphosis is less than 100°; mechanical back pain is more intense than age-matched controls,[49] but is usually responsive to non-operative treatments.

REFERENCES

● = Key primary paper
◆ = Major review article

●1. Labrom RD. Growth and maturation of the spine from birth to adolescence. *Journal of Bone and Joint Surgery* 2007;**89**:3–7.

2. Sarwark JF. Growth considerations of the immature spine. *Journal of Bone and Joint Surgery* 2007;**89**:8–13.

●3. Sanders JO. Maturity indicators in spinal deformity. *Journal of Bone and Joint Surgery* 2007;**89A**:14–20.

4. O'Rahilly R, Muller, F. *Human Embryology and Teratology*, 3rd edn. New York, NY: Wiley-Liss, 2001.

5. Kusumi K, Turnpenny PD. Formation errors of the vertebral column. *Journal of Bone and Joint Surgery* 2007;**89A**:64–71.

6. Bulman MP KK, *et al.* Mutations in the human delta homologue, DLL3, cause axial skeletal defects in spondylocostal dysostosis. *Nature Genetics* 2000;**24**:438–41.

7. Whittock NV, Dea S. Mutated MESP2 causes spondylocostal dysostosis in humans. *American Journal of Human Genetics* 2004;**74**:1249–54.

8. Sparrow DB, *et al.* Mutation of the LUNATIC FRINGE gene in humans causes spondylocostal dysostosis with a severe vertebral phenotype. *American Journal of Human Genetics* 2006;**78**:28–37.

◆9. Winter RB, Leonard LJE, AS, Smith DE. *Congenital Deformities of the Spine*. New York, NY: Thieme-Stratton Inc, 1983.

10. Aberg A WL, Kallen B. Congenital malformations among infants whose mothers had gestational diabetes or preexisting diabetes. *Early Human Development* 2001;**61**:85–95.

11. Wide KWB, Kallen B. Major malformations in infants exposed to antiepileptic drugs in utero, with emphasis on carbamazepine and valproic acid: a nation-wide, population-based register study. *Acta Paediatrica* 2004;**93**:174–6.

●12. Campbell RMJ, Smith MD, *et al.* The characteristics of thoracic insufficiency syndrome associated with fused ribs and congenital scoliosis. *Journal of Bone and Joint Surgery* 2003;**85**:399–408.

13. Hensinger R, Basu PS, Elsebaie H, Noordeen MH. Congenital spinal deformity: a comprehensive assessment at presentation. *Spine* 2002;**27**:2255-9.
14. Prahinski JR, Polly DW, McHale KA, et al. Occult intraspinal anomalies in congenital scoliosis. *Journal of Pediatric Orthopedics* 2000;**20**:59-63.
15. Hedequist D, Emans, J. Congenital scoliosis: a review and update. *Journal of Pediatric Orthopedics* 2007;27:106-16.
16. Winter RB. Convex anterior and posterior hemiarthrodesis and hemieipiphyseodesis in young children with progressive congenital scoliosis. *Journal of Pediatric Orthopedics* 1981;**1**:361-6.
17. Winter RB LJ, Denis F, Sta-Ana de la Rosa H. Convex growth arrest for progressive congenital scoliosis due to hemivertebrae. *Journal of Pediatric Orthopedics* 1988;**8**:633-8.
18. Campbell RMJ, Hell-Vocke, AM. Growth of the thoracic spine in congenital scoliosis after expansion thoracoplasty. *Journal of Bone and Joint Surgery* 2003;**85**:409-20.
19. Nordwall A. Studies in idiopathic scoliosis: Relevant to etiology, conservative and operative treatment. *Acta Orthopaedica Scandinavica* 1973;**150**(Suppl.):18-70.
20. Bylund P, Jansson E, Dahlberg E, Eriksson E. Muscle fiber types in thoracic erector spinae muscles. *Clinical Orthopaedics and Related Research* 1987;**241**:222-8.
21. Qiu XS TN, Yeung HY, Lee KM, et al. Melatonin receptor 1B (MTNR1B) gene polymorphism is associated with the occurrence of adolescent idiopathic scoliosis. *Spine* 2007;**32**:1748-53.
22. Alexander MA BW, Ebbesson SDE. Can experimental dorsal rhisotomy produce scoliosis? *Journal of Bone and Joint Surgery* 1972;**54**:1509-13.
23. Dickson RA, Lawton JO, Archer IA, Butt WP. The pathogenesis of idiopathic scoliosis. Biplanar asymmetry. *Journal of Bone and Joint Surgery* 1984;**66B**:8-15.
24. Payne WK, Ogilvie JW, Rsnick MD, et al. Does scoliosis have a psychological impact and does gender make a difference? *Spine* 1997;**22**:1380-4.
25. Fowles JV, Drummond DS, L'Ecuyer S, et al. Untreated scoliosis in the adult. *Clinical Orthopaedics and Related Research* 1978;**134**:212-17.
26. Pehrsson K, Bake B, Larsson S, Nachemson A. Lung function in adult idiopathic scoliosis: a 20 year follow up. *Thorax* 1991;**46**:474-8.
●27. Nachemson A. A long term follow-up study of non-treated scoliosis. *Acta Orthopaedica Scandinavica* 1968;**39**:466-76.
●28. Weinstein SL, Zavala DC, Ponseti IV. Idiopathic scoliosis: long-term follow-up and prognosis in untreated patients. *Journal of Bone and Joint Surgery* 1981;**63A**:702-12.
29. Gremeaux V, Casillas J-M, Fabbro-Peray P, et al. Analysis of low back pain in adults with scoliosis. *Spine* 2008;**33**:402-5.
30. Haefeli M, Elfering A, Kilian R, et al. Nonoperative treatment for adolescent idiopathic scoliosis: a 10- to 60-year follow-up with special reference to health-related quality of life. *Spine* 2006;**31**:355-66.
●31. Weinstein SL, Ponseti IV. Curve progression in idiopathic scoliosis. *Journal of Bone and Joint Surgery* 1983;**65A**:447-55.
32. Gabos PG, Bojescul JA, Bowen JR, et al. Long-term follow-up of female patients with idiopathic scoliosis treated with the Wilmington orthosis. *Journal of Bone and Joint Surgery* 2004;**86A**:1891-9.
33. James JIP. Idiopathic scoliosis; the prognosis, diagnosis, and operative indications related to curve patterns and the age at onset. *Journal of Bone and Joint Surgery (British)* 1954;**36**:36-40.
34. Fernandez P, Weinstein SL. Natural history of early onset scoliosis. *Journal of Bone and Joint Surgery* 2007;**89**(Suppl. 1):21-33.
●35. Mehta MH. The rib-vertebra angle in the early diagnosis between resolving and progressive infantile scoliosis. *Journal of Bone and Joint Surgery (British)* 1972;**54B**:230-43.
36. Ceballos T, Ferrer-Torrelles, Castillo F, Fernandez-Paredes E. Prognosis in Infantile idiopathic scoliosis. *Journal of Bone and Joint Surgery* 1980;**62A**:863-75.
37. Dobbs MD, Lenke LG. Prevalence of neural axis abnormalities in patients with infantile idiopathic scoliosis. *Journal of Bone and Joint Surgery* 2002;**84**:2230-4.
38. Akbarnia BA. Management themes in early onset scoliosis. *Journal of Bone and Joint Surgery* 2007;**89A**:42-54.
●39. Dubousset J, Herring A, shufflebarger H. The Crankshaft Phenomenon. *Journal of Pediatricorthopedics* 1989;**9**:541-50.
●40. Little DG, Song KM, Katz D, Herring JA. Relationship of peak height velocity to other maturity indicators in idiopathic scoliosis in girls. *Journal of Bone and Joint Surgery* 2000;**82A**:685-93.
41. Lonstein JE, Carlson JM. The prediction of curve progression in untreated idiopathic scoliosis during growth. *Journal of Bone and Joint Surgery* 1984;**66A**:1061-71.
42. Dimeglio A, Charles YP, Daures JP, et al. Accuracy of the Sauvegrain method in determining skeletal age during puberty. *Journal of Bone and Joint Surgery* 2005;**87A**:1689-96.
43. Nachemson AL, Peterson LE. Effectiveness of treatment with a brace in girls who have adolescent idiopathic scoliosis. A prospective, controlled study based on data from the Brace Study of the Scoliosis Research Society. *Journal of Bone and Joint Surgery* 1995;**77A**:815-22.
44. Rowe DE, Bernstein SM, et al. A meta-analysis of the efficacy of non-operative treatments for idiopathic scoliosis. *Journal of Bone and Joint Surgery* 1997;**79A**:664-74.
●45. Lenssinck M-LB, Frijlink, AC, Berger M, et al. Effect of bracing and other conservative interventions in the treatment of idiopathic scoliosis in adolescents: a systematic review of clinical trials. *Physical Therapy* 2005;**85**:1329-39.

46. Goldberg C, Dowling F, *et al.* A statistical comparison between natural history of idiopathic scoliosis and brace treatment in skeletally immature adolescent girls. *Spine* 1993;**18**:902–8.
47. Noonan KJ, Weinstein SL, *et al.* Use of the Milwaukee brace for progressive idiopathic scoliosis. *Journal of Bone and Joint Surgery* 1996;**78A**:557–67.
48. Boseker E, Moe J, *et al.* Determination of 'normal' thoracic kyphosis: a roentgenographic study of 121 'normal' children. *Journal of Pediatric Orthopedics* 2000;**20**:796–8.
●49. Murray PM, Weinstein SL, Spratt KF. The natural history and long-term follow-up of Scheuermann kyphosis. *Journal of Bone and Joint Surgery* 1993;**75A**:236–48.

66

Hip disorders in children

HAMISH CRAWFORD, JAMES A FERNANDES, JAMES HP HUI, YI-JIA LIM, ARJANDAS MAHADEV, KISHORE MULPURI, KIRAN AN SALDANHA, JEAN-CLAUDE THEIS, SIMON P KELLEY

SCREENING FOR DEVELOPMENTAL DYSPLASIA OF THE HIP	642	DEVELOPMENTAL COXA VARA	652
Introduction	642	Introduction	652
Clinical screening	643	Diagnosis	652
Ultrasound screening	643	PERTHES DISEASE	653
Radiography	645	Introduction	653
DEVELOPMENTAL DYSPLASIA OF THE HIP	645	Aetiology and epidemiology	653
Introduction	645	Pathology	653
Normal embryology and development of the hip	645	Clinical features and natural history	653
Pathoanatomy of developmental dysplasia of the hip	646	Differential diagnosis	653
Natural history of untreated developmental dysplasia of the hip	647	Prognostic factors	654
Treatment	647	Treatment	655
The neglected developmental dysplasia of the hip in older childhood	649	SLIPPED CAPITAL FEMORAL EPIPHYSIS	657
Conclusion	650	Introduction and epidemiology	657
PROXIMAL FOCAL FEMORAL DEFICIENCY	650	Pathogenesis and aetiology	657
Introduction	650	Classification	657
Classification	650	Natural history	658
Clinical features	650	Clinical presentation	658
Treatment	651	Diagnostic imaging	658
		TRANSIENT SYNOVITIS	659
		References	663

SCREENING FOR DEVELOPMENTAL DYSPLASIA OF THE HIP

INTRODUCTION

Developmental dysplasia of the hip (DDH) in infancy and childhood remains a common condition in orthopaedic practice. Early diagnosis relies on a well-organized screening programme mainly based on clinical, ultrasound and radiological examination.

The aim of a screening programme for DDH is to identify abnormal hips early in the neonatal period in order to avoid long-term morbidity as a result of remaining undetected.

DDH represents a spectrum of clinically hidden anatomical abnormalities which lead to various degrees of hip instability (from subluxation to dislocation) and growth disturbance of the acetabulum and femoral head (dysplasia). The precise definition and aetiology of DDH remains controversial. Untreated, these abnormalities can lead to premature degenerative joint disease, impaired walking and chronic pain.

Estimates of the incidence of DDH in newborns has been reported between 1.5 and 20 per 1000 births. The incidence varies widely worldwide and is influenced by genetic and racial factors.

Screening is based on the systematic clinical assessment of all newborns in areas where there is a high incidence.

CLINICAL SCREENING

The clinical examination should be carried out by orthopaedic surgeons experienced in paediatric hip disorders and is based on assessment of risk factors and hip examination looking for hip instability.

The following risk factors are strongly associated with DDH: breech position, family history of DDH and female sex. Additional risk factors may include maternal primiparity, high birthweight, oligohydramnios and congenital anomalies. However, only a minority of infants diagnosed with DDH have risk factors (10–27% excluding female gender), and among those with risk factors only 1–10% will have DDH. This means that the majority of infants diagnosed with DDH are female and have no risk factors. Therefore, a selective screening based on risk factors is ineffective.

The most common screening methods involve the physical examination of the hips and lower extremities. Provocative testing looking for hip instability includes the Ortolani and Barlow tests. The Ortolani test (Fig. 66.1) involves adduction of the flexed hip with a gentle posterior force followed by abduction of the flexed hip with a gentle anterior force. An exit and entry clunk is normally felt as the hip moves from a reduced to a dislocated position and vice versa. Whereas the Ortolani test attempts to identify a dislocatable hip, the Barlow test will identify a subluxable hip by carrying out a posterior drawer with the hip flexed and adducted in order to detect hip laxity without dislocation. These two tests have been shown to have a high degree of operator dependence with a high rate of false positives and negatives. In addition, confusion between a 'click' and a 'clunk' when performing these tests, and the significance of each of these tests, can lead to significant interobserver variation.

Measuring the sensitivity and specificity of both these clinical tests in a prospective study is almost impossible, but assessing the impact of a screening programme on the incidence of late diagnosis of DDH provides an indirect measure of sensitivity if one believes that neonatal hip instability and late dislocation are the same condition. There is increasing evidence that this might not be the case and that late diagnosed DDH is actually a true developmental problem rather than the result of a missed dislocation at birth.

Over time, the Ortolani and Barlow tests become less sensitive as the infant increases in size and bulk. A hip adduction contracture develops, leading to a lack of abduction, and eventually the hip becomes unreducable. In the case of a unilateral hip dislocation asymmetrical abduction will draw attention to the abnormality, but bilateral dislocations are more difficult to detect as the abduction of both hips is symmetric but reduced. Other signs such as asymmetrical gluteal and thigh skin folds have been shown to have very poor sensitivity and specificity. Leg length discrepancy is difficult to assess until the child starts walking. Finally, a limp and gait abnormality will draw attention to a dislocated hip after the walking age.

The degree of training and experience of the examiner has been shown to be a strong predictor of the effectiveness of a hip screening programme. Although paediatricians and orthopaedic surgeons are normally involved in the screening, other non-medical practitioners such as physiotherapists and neonatal nurse practitioners have been shown to perform as well.

ULTRASOUND SCREENING

In addition to clinical examination hip ultrasound is used to enhance screening for DDH. The use of ultrasound, however, remains controversial mainly because of reports of high false-positive rates leading to potentially harmful follow-up and interventions. Despite this, hip ultrasound has been widely accepted as a useful tool in the diagnosis of DDH and is widely used in many countries.

Hip ultrasound was introduced by Graf in the 1980s. It allows imaging of the cartilaginous acetabulum and capital epiphysis of the hip in a static as well as in a dynamic fashion. It can be used as a universal screening tool for all newborns, but this requires significant resources and is probably not cost-effective.

Selective use of ultrasound to image the hips of newborns who are clinically stable but have significant risk factors associated with DDH has been shown to be ineffective in reducing the incidence of late cases.

After the neonatal period the concern is not so much instability but dysplasia. Ultrasound in this situation has a lot to offer as a static examination allowing visualization of the hip joint development without the harmful effect of radiation.

Once the capital epiphysis starts to ossify around 4–6 months radiological imaging of the hip becomes the gold standard.

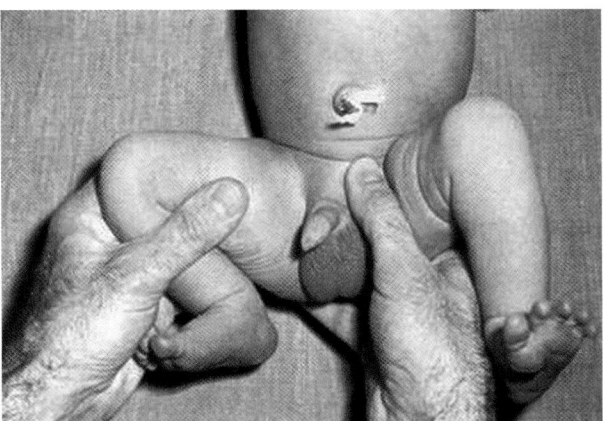

Figure 66.1 Ortolani test for routine screening of hip instability.

Ultrasound technique

The hip can be examined in the coronal and transverse planes (Figs 66.2 and 66.3) and in a static or dynamic mode. A linear array transducer (5 or 7.5 MHz) is recommended for imaging the neonatal hip, and this is normally carried out by a sonographer.

Graf's sonographic classification of hip types is based on static acetabular morphology mainly. He used the osseous acetabular roof (alpha angle) and the cartilaginous acetabular roof (beta angle) to quantify acetabular development. Based on this and the position of the femoral head in relation to the acetabulum, he described different types of hip morphology from immature to dislocated hips.

Later on, Novik described a static and dynamic transverse scan allowing for assessment of hip stability on ultrasound for the first time. Morin introduced the concept of femoral head coverage (FHC), which is the percentage value of femoral head covered by the bony acetabular roof. This was later further developed by Terjesen, who reported that a normal FHC was around 55%. He also described a transverse scan from a lateral approach with the hips flexed and a medial approach with the hip abducted.

The advantage of dynamic hip screening has been recognized for some time, and this certainly adds another dimension to ultrasound as it allows direct visualization of hip instability and makes it more relevant to clinical examination and management.

Various other ultrasound techniques have been used, and some centres seem to use it beyond the time when the capital epiphysis has appeared to reduce the number of radiographs taken in these children.

Reliability of ultrasound in the diagnosis of DDH

One of the criticisms of ultrasound has been that it is operator dependent and that interpretation of the findings is difficult and can lead to overtreatment. Inter- and intra-observer reliability has been studied extensively, especially in relation to Graf's classification. Intra-observer agreement has been reported as good, but agreement between radiologists looking at the same ultrasound is only moderate. There are also significant differences in agreement between what is normal or abnormal and this can have clinical consequences.

Dias showed that the alpha and beta angle measurements had only a fair degree of reproducibility. Other studies have found that the alpha angle and FHC were the most reliable measurements.

Rosendahl looked at the reliability of static and dynamic images. She found a high degree of intra-observer and a moderate degree of interobserver agreement in the classification of hip morphology and a moderate degree of interobserver agreement in determining the stability of the hip. She also reported that there was operator-dependent variation in the quality of scans and that, as a result, substantial training and attention to detail were necessary when carrying out hip ultrasound and interpreting the results.

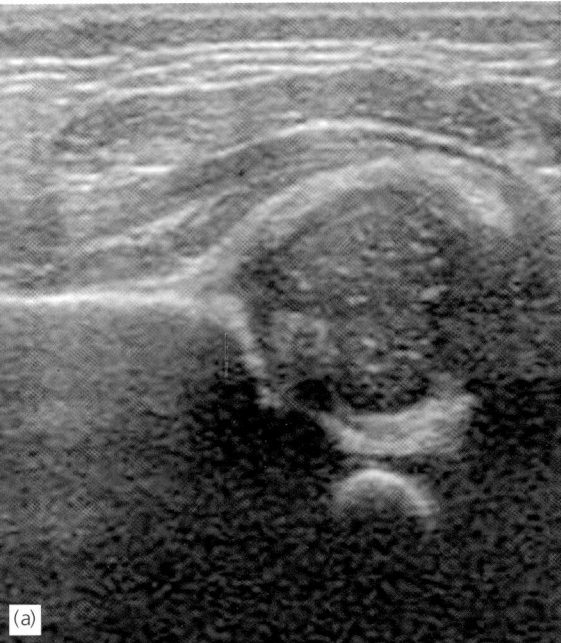

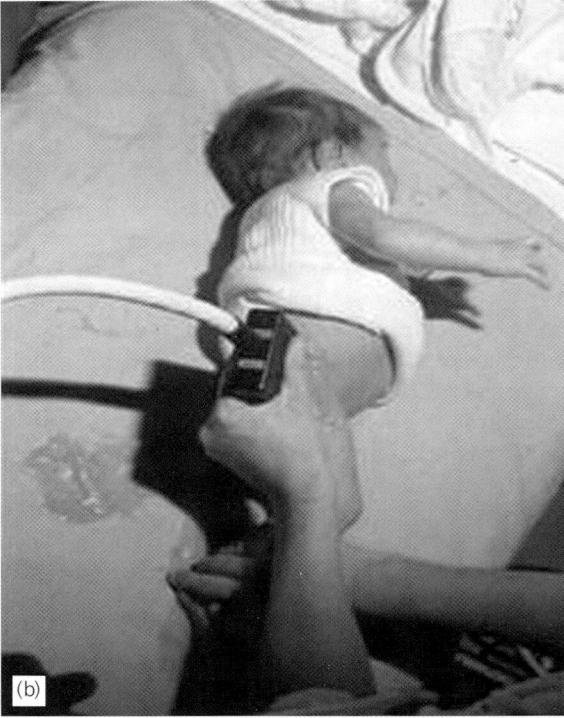

Figure 66.2 Coronal ultrasound scan.

Normal embryology and development of the hip 645

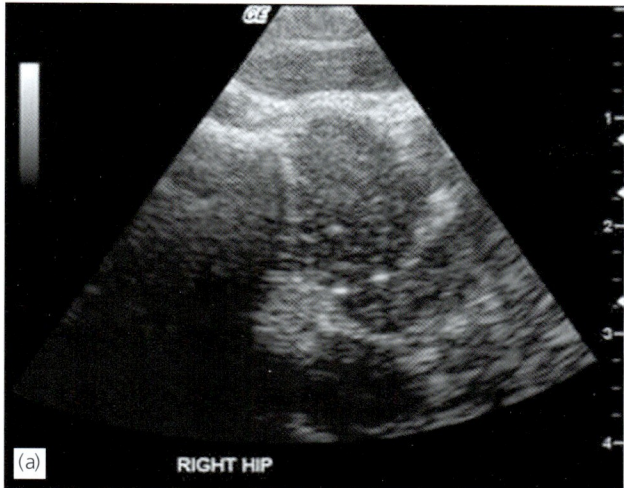

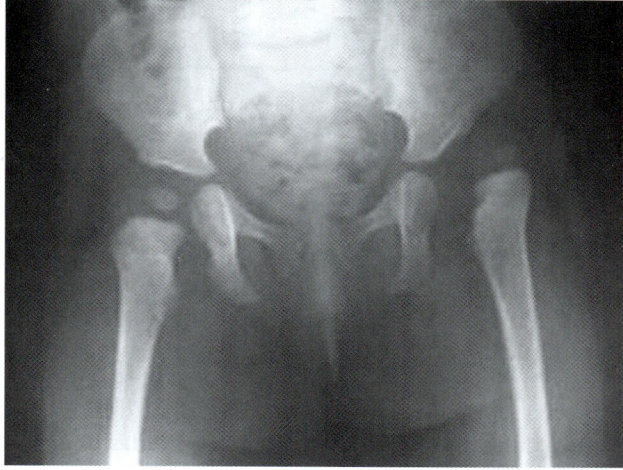

Figure 66.4 Radiograph of left hip dislocation.

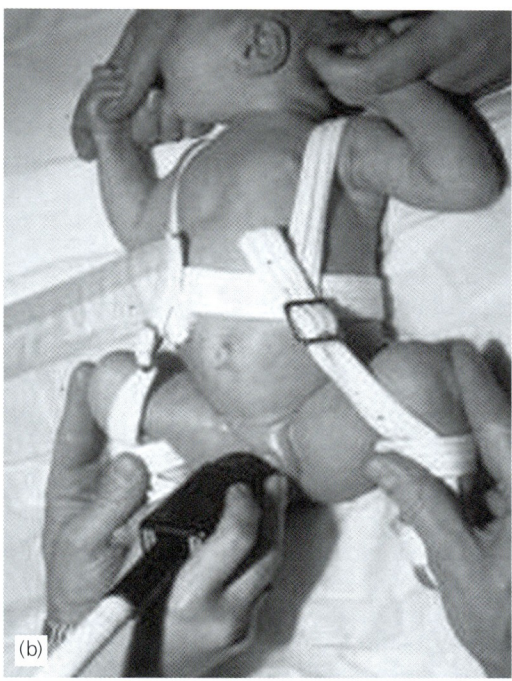

Figure 66.3 Transverse ultrasound scan.

RADIOGRAPHY

Once the capital epiphysis has started to ossify (4–6 months) an anteroposterior and lateral hip radiograph is recommended and will show the position of the hip as well as the acetabular development. Serial acetabular angle measurements (Fig. 66.4) are used to monitor hip development. Radiography should not be used for routine screening.

Screening for DDH will identify most abnormal hips in the neonatal period by clinical and ultrasound examination. The question of whether it will eliminate late cases and lead to improved outcomes in the long term remains unclear. Routine clinical hip examination by well-trained health practitioners in combination with ultrasound and radiography remains the gold standard in DDH screening.

DEVELOPMENTAL DYSPLASIA OF THE HIP

INTRODUCTION

In order to effectively manage DDH one needs to understand the normal embryology of the hip joint, the pathoanatomical factors that lead to DDH and its consequent natural history.

NORMAL EMBRYOLOGY AND DEVELOPMENT OF THE HIP

The components of the hip joint, the acetabulum and femoral head, arise from the same cluster of mesenchymal cells in which a cleft develops at about the seventh week of gestation. The development of the immature hip joint is complete by the eleventh week of gestation.

The subsequent normal development of the hip requires a well-centred femoral head in an adequately formed acetabulum. The final shape of the acetabulum is largely determined by the age of 8 years; this age serves as a good prognostic landmark in the management of DDH.

The final increase in the depth of the acetabulum occurs during the adolescent growth spurt by ossification of the secondary growth centres. Thus, any surgical disturbance of these secondary growth centres, especially at the periphery of the acetabulum, can lead to hip dysplasia in adulthood.

PATHOANATOMY OF DEVELOPMENTAL DYSPLASIA OF THE HIP

At birth, there is a tight fit between the femoral head and acetabulum created by the surface tension of synovial fluid. As demonstrated in post-mortem dissections, it is very difficult to dislocate the hip even after the capsule is divided. In DDH, this tight fit is lost and the femoral head is then able to glide in and out over the acetabular edge.

At birth, the pathological findings can range from mild capsular laxity to severe dysplasia. The dysplastic hip typically has a ridge of hyaline cartilage at the margin of the acetabulum called the neolimbus. The femoral head glides over this ridge when the Ortolani manoeuvre is performed. In the normal hip, the labrum is everted and contributes to the acetabular coverage and hip stability.

Fortunately, in the majority of instances, all the pathological changes can be reversed if treatment is instituted early.

Epidemiology and risk factors

The aetiology of DDH is known to be due to both genetic and environmental factors. The risk of DDH is higher in babies with some factors that are identifiable at birth; they include:

- breech presentation
- oligohydramnios
- female
- first born
- positive family history
- ethnic background (e.g. Native American)
- presence of torticollis or foot deformity (calcaneovalgus, metatarsus varus, clubfeet).

Diagnosis

The most effective diagnostic tool at birth remains clinical examination with the Ortolani and Barlow manoeuvres. These tests are most useful before the age of 3 months.

Ultrasound is used to diagnose the more subtle dysplastic hips which are not overtly dislocated as well as for follow-up to ascertain effectiveness of treatment.

Radiographs, although not useful at birth owing to the lack of ossification of the hip, are used after the age of 3 months to assist in diagnosis and follow-up.

CLINICAL

At birth

Both the examiner and the baby should be calm and the amount of force used to grip the child's limbs should be similar to that used to pick up an egg. Both hips are flexed beyond 90°, grasping both thighs with the thumb on the medial aspect of the thigh just above the knee and the fingers over the greater trochanter over the lateral aspect. Both legs are grasped together but each is examined one at the time with the other keeping the pelvis stable. The hips, initially in the abducted position, are then adducted one at a time.

To perform the Ortolani manoeuvre, upon abducting the affected hip, a dislocated hip would ride over the ridge of the acetabulum formed by the neolimbus as the hip reduces with a 'clunk'. This would then be a positive Ortolani test. Thus, the Ortolani manoeuvre is a test of reducibility.

To perform the Barlow manoeuvre, the affected hip, which is initially reduced, is adducted with a gentle posterior force. This force is applied without turning the child's knee or the examiner's knee white. If the hip is dysplastic, it will dislocate. A positive Barlow sign, therefore, is a reduced but dislocatable hip. Thus, the Barlow manoeuvre is a test of dislocatability.

Occasionally, no obvious 'clunk' is felt, but, instead, what seems like a certain looseness. This then is called hip laxity. This could be due to laxity of immaturity or due to acetabular dysplasia with or without femoral head subluxation.

In summary, the possible clinical variants of a newborn hip examination based on Ortolani and Barlow manoeuvres are:

- normal stable and reduced hip
- a lax hip.
- a reduced but dislocatable hip (Barlow positive)
- a dislocated but reducible hip (Ortolani positive).

OLDER INFANT AND CHILDREN

The reliability of the Ortolani and Barlow tests is best before of the age of 3 months.

After this age, a unilateral dislocation is suspected when there is an apparent shortening of the thigh demonstrated with the child lying supine with the hips and knees flexed. The knees will be at different levels – a sign referred to as the Galeazzi sign. Other signs that are often present are asymmetric gluteal and thigh skin folds and limited passive abduction of the affected hip. Bilateral dislocations are more difficult to diagnose in the infant, and the clinician must have a high index of suspicion especially if risk factors are present.

A unilateral dislocation in the ambulant child usually manifests as a painless limp, which is characteristically a Trendelenburg gait, whereas children with bilateral dislocations present with a hyperlordotic waddling gait.

Radiographs are the modality of choice after this age for both diagnosis and follow-up.

When reading the radiographs of an infant the following lines are important guides with regards to the assessment of DDH:

- The Hilgenreiner line is a line joining both triradiate cartilages.
- The Perkins line is a line drawn perpendicular to the Hilgenreiner line and running through the lateral edge of

the acetabulum. The ossification centres of the reduced femoral head are situated in the lower medial quadrant of the intersection of the Perkins and Hilgenreiner lines.
- The acetabular index is the angle obtained by inserting a line along the bony acetabular roof and the Hilgenreiner line. This angle changes as the infant grows, as noted by Caffey.
- The Shenton line is a continuous curved line drawn by tracing the inferior border of the superior ramus continuing onto the arched medial border of the femoral neck and metaphysis. This line is non-continuous when the affected hip is subluxed or dislocated.
- The medial gap is the gap between the medial border of the metaphysis of the femur and the acetabular tear drop. This distance in the affected hip is increased compared with the normal hip.
- In the older age group when the centre of the femoral ossific centre can accurately be determined, the centre–edge angle can be measured. This angle is made with a line passing the centre of the femoral ossific centre and the lateral acetabular edge and a line perpendicular to the Hilgenreiner line passing through the centres of the femoral ossific centre. The normal angle is greater than 20°.

NATURAL HISTORY OF UNTREATED DEVELOPMENTAL DYSPLASIA OF THE HIP

If the diagnosis of DDH is missed at birth, the resultant scenarios of the affected hip are as follows:

- it can become normal
- it can become subluxed
- it can become completely dislocated
- it can remain reduced with acetabular dysplasia.

Because it is not possible to determine the course of development once a DDH is diagnosed, all cases are subjected to treatment.

In the long term, the natural history of early hip degenerative disease will depend on:

- Presence or absence of a false acetabulum. The presence of a false acetabulum predisposes the 'joint' to early degenerative changes, which in turn produces pain and reduced range of motion. Without the presence of a false acetabulum, the hip can maintain a good range of painless motion.
- Bilaterality. Generally bilateral dislocations have better range of motion with less gait abnormality. They, however, develop hyperlordosis, which can lead to lower back pain. Unilateral dislocation can develop limb length inequality, ipsilateral valgus knee deformity with a laxity of the medial collateral ligament, degenerative changes in the lateral compartment of the ipsilateral knee, gait disturbances and secondary scoliosis.
- Hip congruency. Subluxed hips will develop early degenerative disease in all patients by the third or fourth decade of life. Even in hips that are well reduced but show acetabular dysplasia, this will eventually lead to subluxation and its consequences as described above. Although dislocated hips with a false acetabulum can also develop degenerative changes, it is less severe with a later onset than those with subluxed hips.

TREATMENT

DDH must be treated early in order to change the natural history for the better.

The goal of treatment of DDH at any age is to ensure a congruently reduced hip in a well-covered acetabulum by maintaining an optimal environment for development of the acetabulum and femoral head.

Treatment of the newborn

The normal stable and reduced hip does not need any further treatment. Those with risk factors and those found to be lax would have an ultrasound at 6 weeks to ascertain whether there is any acetabular dysplasia with or without subluxation. Six weeks is also a good time to exclude laxity due to immaturity.

If the hip findings are found to be normal, no further treatment is required. However, if there is any doubt, treatment should be started as described below.

The dislocatable hip, dislocated hip and those found to be dysplastic at the sixth week will undergo treatment in the form of the use of the Pavlik harness. Excellent results have been widely reported when used appropriately.

PAVLIK HARNESS

The Pavlik harness was first described by Arnold Pavlik in the 1950s. It consists of a chest strap, shoulder straps with anterior and posterior straps which control flexion and abduction of the hips, respectively, while restricting extension and adduction of the hips. This results in the hip being in the human position, which is about 100° of hip flexion and 100° of combined abduction. The kicking motion allowed in this position stretches the contracted parts, which, as a consequence, promotes and maintains the spontaneous reduction of the subluxed or dislocated hip.

The contraindications to the use of the Pavlik harness are as follows:

- in congenital stiff joints such as arthrogryposis
- congenital ligamentous laxity such Ehlers–Danlos syndrome
- children older than 10 months
- poor family compliance.

Once in a Pavlik harness, which is worn 23 hours a day, weekly ultrasounds are recommended until the hips are found to be stably and concentrically reduced, which usually takes about 3 weeks. After that, the harness is worn until the ultrasound and radiographs (done from the age of 3 months onwards) show normal findings. This will take at least 3 months for children less than 3 months old, and approximately double their age for those who present when they are older.

The child is usually weaned off the harness in the last 2 months for night-time wear. If the child begins to ambulate during the treatment, abduction braces will be required.

Follow-up will depend on how stably reduced the hip is. If it remains well reduced, radiographs at 3, 6, 12 and 18 months would be a good guide. In general, if the hip remains concentrically reduced with good acetabular coverage by the age of 18 months, it is very unlikely to dislocate or be subluxed.

After 3 weeks, if stable reduction cannot be achieved with Pavlik harness or if the hip redislocates during the follow-up period, then the next stage of treatment is instituted.

It is important to recognize the pitfalls of the use of Pavlik harness, including:

- inappropriate use in contraindicated cases resulting in persistent dislocation
- inferior dislocation of the hip as a result of excessive flexion
- femoral neuropathy
- avascular necrosis due to excessive abduction.

Besides poor harness fit, poor compliance or poor understanding with regards to the use Pavlik harness is largely the cause of these pitfalls. Therefore, in populations where compliance or understanding are deemed to be problems, a simpler form of plastic abduction splint is best used. These can be used in older children and modified accordingly to allow for ambulation.

Treatment up to age of 6 months

This group would represent those who present before the age of 6 months and failed Pavlik harness as outlined above.

As the child gets older, the unreduced hip will produce other secondary changes (such as tight adductors and flexors, hypertrophy of ligamentum teres, hourglass contracture of capsule, inverted limbus, the acetabulum becoming filled with fibrous tissue) make occurence of spontaneous reduction difficult, and can account for the failure of treatment with Pavlik harness or abduction splints.

The next stage would then be a close reduction, usually after a percutaneous adductor tenotomy has been performed under general anaesthesia. It is recommended that this be preceded by a period of traction of about 2–3 weeks, which can be carried out at home if the proper support is available. Traction stretches out tight structures and allows for safe reduction with minimal risk of AVN; it is less of a priority in patients for whom soft-tissue releases and open reduction with femoral and/or acetabular surgery will be deemed necessary.

Post-reduction, an intra-operative arthrography is recommended to ensure concentric reduction before a hip spica is applied in the human position. The cast is then changed every 6 weeks to allow for growth. Usually, a casting period of 3 months will suffice. This is then followed by an abduction brace until there is clinical and radiological evidence of a stable, concentrically reduced hip with good acetabular cover.

Beyond the age of 6 months, closed reduction, although it might be attempted, is less likely to be successful.

Treatment in patients aged 6–18 months

This group will also include patient younger than 6 months who failed closed reduction and adductor tenotomy.

The anatomical blocks to a closed reduction would be:

- Extra-articular blocks:
  – adductor longus
  – iliopsoas.
- Intra-articular blocks (in order of decreasing importance):
  – the hourglass joint capsule
  – the hypertrophied ligamentum teres
  – transverse acetabular ligament.
  – inverted labrum
  – pulvinar.

The neolimbus previously thought to be an important block is rarely so; in fact, it is important in the formation of the secondary ossification centres, which allow for better acetabular cover. Therefore, it should not be surgically disturbed.

As mentioned above, closed reduction becomes less successful in this age group and thus the goals of treatment should be to:

- remove the blocks of reduction with releases of the adductor longus and the iliopsoas for the extra-articular blocks and address the intra-articular blocks listed above by opening the hip joint
- openly reduce the hip; it is important that the reduction is carried out without any tension as it may result in AVN
- maintain the reduction; this can be achieved with a good capsulorrhaphy.

Acetabular surgery is usually not performed as it is believed that, once the femoral head is concentrically reduced before the age of 18 months, the development of the acetabulum will follow.

There are several approaches described to achieve the above goals, but two options are usually discussed:

- The anterior approach (Smith–Peterson approach).
  - This begins with a modified bikini incision. The hip is then approached by developing a plane between the sartorius and tensor fascia lata, being careful not to injure the lateral cutaneous nerve of the thigh. The reflected head of the rectus femoris is the next landmark, and another plane is developed between the rectus head and the gluteus medius. Once the reflected head of the rectus is released, the extracapsular fat will be the guide to the capsule underneath. Blunt dissection is carried out all around the capsule to visualize it as much as possible to allow for the release of the hourglass capsule. The joint is opened by creating flaps for a good capsulorrhaphy. The intra-articular blocks are then identified and released, keeping in mind that the neolimbus or labrum should not be excised.
  - The adductor longus is released via a separate transverse inguinal incision.
  - The tendinous part of iliopsoas is sectioned at the level of the pelvic brim by entering the iliopsoas fascia below the inguinal line, medial to the sartorius. It is important to identify and preserve the femoral nerve with this approach.
- The medial approach.
  - This starts with a transverse groin incision. Once the adductor longus is visualized and released, a plane is developed between the pectineus and adductor brevis. The iliopsoas tendon is visualized and released, after which the capsulotomy is performed and the transverse acetabular ligament is transected. The ligamentum teres and pulvinar are identified and removed. The medial circumflex femoral artery must be visualized and preserved in order to avoid AVN of the femoral head.

The medial approach is more direct with regards to releasing the blocks to reduction. However, owing to its limited exposure, a capsulorrhaphy cannot be done. Coupled with the lack of familiarity with this approach, the anterior approach is usually preferred.

The postoperative management will be described below.

Treatment for patients older than 18 months

It is believed that acetabular growth is favourably influenced when the femoral head is concentrically reduced within the acetabulum. However, above the age of 18 months, acetabular remodelling is limited, leaving a dysplastic acetabulum even after concentric reduction of the femoral head. In these cases, there is a need for acetabular surgery.

The most distinguished and successful methods in terms of clinical outcome remain to be the Salter osteotomy. The Salter osteotomy involves the redirection of the acetabulum to a more anterolateral position, as it is believed that in DDH the acetabular insufficiency is mainly over the anterolateral aspect. The osteotomy is maintained with a wedge of bone taken from the iliac crest and fixed with threaded pins. It is important to note that this is a redirectional osteotomy and therefore the shape and capacity of the acetabulum does not change.

The prerequisites of a Salter osteotomy are as follows:

- ability to bring the femoral head to the level of the acetabulum without any tension as in the open reduction described above
- release of contracture of the adductors and iliopsoas
- complete and concentric reduction
- reasonable congruity of the hip joint surface
- good range of hip joint motion
- correct age of patient (Salter quoted 6 years as the upper limit for complete dislocation secondary to DDH).

The postoperative immobilization for the open reduction with and without Salter osteotomy is similar.

Postoperative immobilization

Postoperatively, the child is placed in a hip spica cast when the hips are about 20° of flexion and 30° of abduction on each side. This cast is kept on for about 6 weeks, after which follow-up radiographs are taken. In most cases of open reduction only, a further 6 weeks is required to stabilize the hip and ensure strength of the capsulorrhaphy. If the radiographs show good healing of the osteotomy site, the cast can be removed and the child allowed to ambulate as tolerated. This has the added advantage of avoiding hip stiffness, which is sometimes seen after a Salter osteotomy.

Occasionally, the child can be weaned off with a plastic abduction splint or Petrie cast after cast removal if the stability of the hip is in question.

THE NEGLECTED DEVELOPMENTAL DYSPLASIA OF THE HIP IN OLDER CHILDHOOD

The upper age limit for treatment of DDH depends largely on the likelihood of complications from surgery versus the natural history of the condition if left untreated. Surgical complications of AVN, redislocation and resubluxation are more common in older children. Also, if an initially dislocated hip become subluxed as a result of surgery, the child then has a worse prognosis with regards to early osteoarthritis.

With these issues in mind, the upper limit for surgery for unilateral dislocations and subluxation has been quoted to be 8 years. Beyond this, there is no further remodelling of both the femoral head and the acetabulum. However, with improved techniques, this upper limit is constantly being challenged by centres that specialize in this surgery and therefore are able to minimize the complications.

As patients with bilateral involvement have a better prognosis, the upper limit of about 5 years old is more accepted. Once again, however, this age limit is continuously increasing in specialized centres.

CONCLUSION

DDH is a spectrum of hip conditions that are rooted in a dysplastic acetabulum. It is imperative that this condition is diagnosed as early as possible, as treatment in the early stages is fairly straightforward and with exceedingly good results and prognosis. The treatment becomes increasingly more complicated with age and is fraught with many surgical complications. One must be cautious in treating older children and weigh the benefits of surgery versus natural history complications.

PROXIMAL FOCAL FEMORAL DEFICIENCY

INTRODUCTION

The term proximal focal femoral deficiency has been mainly used to describe dysplasia of the proximal femur with an apparent discontinuity between the femoral neck and shaft. In many cases, the defect in the proximal femur ossifies as the child grows older but it is difficult to predict how much and to what extent the cartilage will ossify. The term has also been used to include congenital short femur with less severe femoral deficiency in which the femur is short but without a defect in the neck.[1] More recently, the term congenital longitudinal deficiency of the femur has been used.

The cause of femoral deficiency is not known, and the disorder normally does not have a genetic link.

CLASSIFICATION

The Aitken classification system has been widely used[2] (Table 66.1).

Various other classifications based on radiographic appearances include those of Amstutz, Pappas, Hamanishi, Fixsen and Lloyd-Roberts. Gillespie and Torode[3] proposed a classification based on clinical features and treatment. In group I, the foot on the affected side reaches the mid-tibia on the normal side or lower with the legs extended. These patients are considered suitable candidates for limb-lengthening procedures. In group II, there is severe shortening of the femur and the foot reaches above the mid-tibia on the normal side, often being at the level of the normal knee. These patients are best treated with amputation or rotationplasty followed by prosthetic management. Gillespie later modified this classification to include three groups. Paley[4] also proposed a treatment-based classification to aid in planning reconstructive lengthening procedures.

CLINICAL FEATURES

The affected thigh is short, the hip is flexed and abducted, and the limb is externally rotated. Flexion contractures of

Table 66.1 Aitken classification of proximal focal femoral deficiency

Type	Femoral head	Acetabulum	Femoral segment	Relationship among components of femur and acetabulum at skeletal maturity
A	Present	Normal	Short	A defect in the subtrochanteric region that ossifies as the child grows and resolves by skeletal maturity, but a subtrochanteric varus deformity of varying severity may persist
B	Present	Adequate or moderately dysplastic	Short, usually proximal bony tuft	As the child matures the femoral head develops, but at maturity there is no bony continuity between the femoral shaft and head
C	Absent or represented by ossicle	Severely dysplastic	Short, usually proximally tapered	No ossification of the upper portion of the femur and no articular relationship between femur and acetabulum
D	Absent	Absent; obturator foramen enlarged	Extremely short and deformed or absent	None

the hip and knee make the limb appear shorter than it actually is. Other associations include ipsilateral fibular hemimelia in 45% of cases, acetabular dysplasia even when the head of femur is present, genu valgum due to lateral femoral condylar hypoplasia, absent or hypoplastic cruciate ligaments in the knee, equinovalgus deformity of the foot, and absent lateral rays of the foot.[5] The disorder may be accurately diagnosed prenatally with sonography. Most children with femoral deficiencies are able to compensate for their deformities and do not experience a delay in achieving developmental milestones. They usually start walking at the expected age.

TREATMENT

Treatment has to be individualized depending on the predicted limb length discrepancy at maturity and stability of the hip and knee. Two strategies of reconstruction are possible: one is biological lengthening reconstruction; the other is an ablative option with prosthetic reconstruction. Limb reconstruction by limb-lengthening methods is indicated when the femur is predicted to be at least half as long as the normal femur at maturity, a predicted discrepancy of less than 17–20 cm and one that can be corrected with no more than three separate equalization procedures with or without contralateral epiphysiodesis of the knee. The prerequisites for lengthening are a stable hip (rendered stable by reconstruction) and a knee that is reasonably stable.

When the predicted length of affected limb at maturity is less than 50% of the contralateral limb and the hip is stable, prosthetic fitting can be facilitated by knee fusion accompanied by either a Syme's or Boyd's amputation or a Van Nes rotationplasty. Although rotationplasty[6] allows better function, as documented by clinical observation, gait analysis and oxygen consumption studies, it has the disadvantages of derotation over time, cosmetic problems and is quite often not accepted by parents.

When the hip is unstable (when the femur has no continuity with the hip joint and there is a dysplastic acetabulum), the abductor–extensor lurch results in a significant functional and cosmetic problem. Iliofemoral stabilization can be achieved by reconstructive osteotomies of the upper femur and acetabulum. Other methods of achieving stabilization are Steel's iliofemoral or Brown's iliofemoral fusion with rotationplasty and Ilizarov's pelvic support osteotomy.

Rarely, proximal focal femoral deficiency can be bilateral, resulting in short stature and a waddling gait. In these cases surgical treatment such as amputation is contraindicated. Extension equinus prostheses are used to enhance height. This spectrum of disorder is generally dealt with in specialist centres with expertise in both surgical and prosthetic reconstruction. Realistic expectations need to be given to the child's caregiver and complete restoration of the affected limb is rarely possible.

DEVELOPMENTAL COXA VARA

INTRODUCTION

Coxa vara refers to a deformity of the proximal femur where the neck shaft angle measures significantly less than its normal value on an anteroposterior radiograph, typically less than 110°.[7]

The coxa vara deformity may be identified in many diseases, which are classified into three main types: congenital, acquired and developmental.[8]

Developmental coxa vara is considered a rare but distinct disease entity manifested by specific clinical and radiographic features with an incidence of one in 25 000 children.[9] It may be bilateral in 30–50% of cases. It has no predilection for sex, side or race.[10]

Developmental coxa vara is not present at birth and is not associated with other skeletal manifestations. It usually presents after walking age in the second or third year with a painless limp or mild limb length discrepancy in unilateral cases. In bilateral cases a progressive waddling (Trendelenburg) gait can be seen secondary to abductor insufficiency. Clinical examination also reveals a limitation of hip abduction and internal rotation.

Rather than being the uniplanar deformity that its name would suggest, coxa vara is in fact a complex three-dimensional deformity that includes not only increased varus but also significant retroversion of the proximal femur,[11,12] a widened and more vertical proximal femoral growth plate, a short femoral neck[13,14] and a characteristic triangular bone fragment in the inferior medial corner of the neck. This has been compared to a Salter–Harris type II defect.[11]

The cause is unknown but it has been theorized that there is a defect in endochondral ossification in the femoral neck and physis; the columnar structure of the physis is disordered with reduced numbers of cartilage cells.[13,15] Other less popular theories are that it could be secondary to a vascular insult[13] or increased intrauterine pressure.

DIAGNOSIS

Plain radiographs of the hip are the investigation of choice.[14] Characteristic of this condition is a bony defect resembling an inverted Y shape in the inferior portion of the neck, the two diverging limbs of the Y formed by the physis and an area of abnormal metaphyseal ossification. The neck–shaft angle is typically less than 110°. On the anteroposterior view the most useful measurement to monitor progression and determine treatment is the Hilgenreiner epiphyseal (HE) angle[16] (Fig. 66.5). CT can be used to determine further detail about the particular features of individual deformities to assist with preoperative planning.

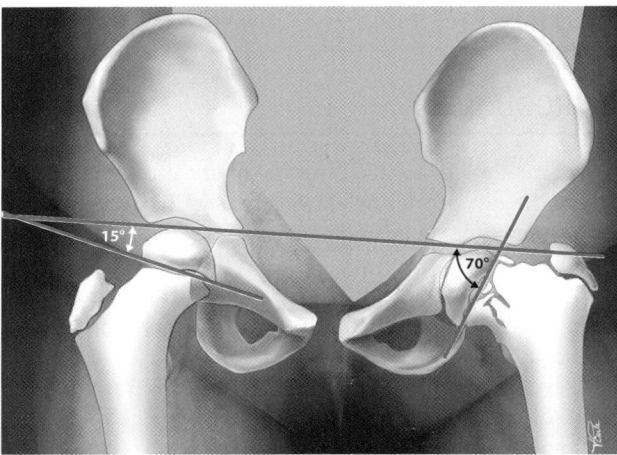

Figure 66.5 Normal right hip showing the Hilgenreiner epiphyseal (HE) angle of 15°. Left hip shows features of developmental coxa vara including proximal femoral varus, widened and more vertical physis, short femoral neck and characteristic triangular bone fragment in the inferior medial corner of the neck. The HE angle measures 70°.

Treatment

Non-operative management has little to offer in the management of a progressive or severe deformity, being unable to affect the natural history.[17–19] Untreated coxa vara can lead to acetabular dysplasia, hip subluxation and degenerative arthritis.[16]

Hips with an HE angle <45° can be managed expectantly as they are unlikely to develop progressive deformity. Those with an HE angle >60° are candidates for surgical correction, whereas those with an HE angle of between 45° and 60° should be carefully monitored with serial radiographs for signs of disease progression.[10,12,16,20,21]

A range of different proximal femoral osteotomies and methods of fixation have been proposed for the correction of coxa vara.[10,12,20–26] More important than the particular osteotomy is that the goals of surgery are achieved. These include correction of the abnormal proximal femoral varus and retroversion, restoration of the articulotrochanteric distance and abductor lever arm, and creating an HE angle of <40°. Attainment of these goals will improve the mechanics of the hip joint, converting abnormal sheer stress at the femoral neck into favourable compression. This will give an excellent chance of a rapidly healing osteotomy and cervicometaphyseal defect with a minimal chance of recurrence and improved function.[12,20,21,25,26]

A severe or rapidly progressive coxa vara is also best treated as soon as it is deemed that the proposed surgery is technically feasible so that the normal development can commence at the earliest opportunity.[21,24] This must be balanced against the fact that older children tend to have a lower recurrence rate and less chance of implant failure because of a more robust proximal femur.[16]

PERTHES DISEASE

INTRODUCTION

Perthes disease is a form of osteochondrosis that affects the capital femoral epiphysis in children. The blood supply to the epiphysis is interrupted and the epiphysis undergoes avascular necrosis. Although the disease is self-limiting in that the blood supply to the epiphysis gets restored eventually, the consequences of the disease can be permanent and far reaching. It normally affects boys aged between 4 and 7.

AETIOLOGY AND EPIDEMIOLOGY

The cause for the vascular insult is unknown; various theories of causation have been proposed but there is insufficient evidence to prove any of them. Genetic and several environmental factors have been implicated. Currently, there is some suggestion that children with Perthes disease have a disorder of the clotting mechanism, with deficiency of factors such as protein C or S and factor V Leiden mutation.[27,28]

The prevalence of the disease varies profoundly between and within countries. In the UK, the disease is common in Merseyside.[29] In India, a very high prevalence of the disease has been noted in the southwest coastal plain, but it is uncommon in other parts of the country.[30] The age at onset of the disease varies: the mean age is around 6 years in Caucasian children,[31] whereas it is around 8 years in south Asian children.[30] In Merseyside, the disease tends to affect children from inner city areas where overcrowding and undernutrition is common,[29] but this trend is not seen in south India.[30]

PATHOLOGY

The pathology of Perthes disease has been studied from few necropsy specimens[32–34] and the data from these studies suggest that the disease may develop following repeated infarcts. The entire epiphysis or a part of it may undergo necrosis depending on the extent of the vascular insult. Apart from features of aseptic avascular necrosis of the epiphysis, changes in the articular cartilage, growth plate and the synovium have been noted. Articular cartilage hypertrophy and growth plate irregularities occur. Once the disease is established, a reactive synovitis may ensue and this may be mediated by immune mechanisms.[35,36]

CLINICAL FEATURES AND NATURAL HISTORY

The clinical onset of the disease is heralded by hip pain and a limp. The onset is usually insidious and there are no constitutional symptoms. In most affected children there is mild to moderate restriction of abduction and internal rotation movements of the hip; the remaining movements are often unaffected. Occasionally, severe restriction of movements may be encountered with fixed deformities.[37] Subtle anthropometric abnormalities have been noted in affected children with reduction of stature and disproportionate growth retardation of the appendicular skeleton, the terminal segments being most affected.[38,39]

The blood supply to the epiphysis does get restored spontaneously except if the onset is in adolescence.[40] As the blood supply gets restored the avascular necrotic bone is gradually resorbed and new bone is laid down by a process of creeping substitution. Over a period of 2–4 years the entire epiphysis is reconstituted with new bone. The evolution of the disease can be followed quite clearly on sequential plain radiographs and the disease can be classified on the basis of the stage of evolution as the stage of avascular necrosis, the stage of fragmentation, the stage of regeneration and the healed stage (stages I–IV; see Fig. 66.6).

In a proportion of children complete revascularization and reconstitution of the epiphysis occurs without any deformation of the shape of the femoral head and these hips function normally through adult life. However, in the remaining children, varying degrees of deformation of the femoral head occurs and these children are prone to develop degenerative arthritis in early adult life[41] (Fig. 66.7). Apart from frank irregularity of the femoral contour, varying degrees of coxa magna frequently occur. Premature closure of the capital femoral physis and greater trochanteric overgrowth may also occur. If the tip of the greater trochanter grows beyond the centre of the femoral head a Trendelenburg gait will develop.

DIFFERENTIAL DIAGNOSIS

Transient synovitis may present with similar clinical findings; the radiographs however show no changes within the femoral epiphysis and a radioisotope bone scan will show an increased uptake in the region of the hip. Narrowing of the joint space may be noted in pauciarticular juvenile chronic arthritis. Gaucher disease and sickle cell disease may all present with similar radiological findings. Haemoglobin electrophoresis will help to identify sickle cell disease. Some children with epiphyseal dysplasia and children with hypothyroidism may have radiological appearances akin to Perthes disease, but the changes are bilateral whereas bilateral involvement in Perthes disease is not common.

PROGNOSTIC FACTORS

Several factors appear to influence the likelihood of the femoral head getting deformed during the evolution of the disease. Among them, the most important are the age at onset of the disease, the extent of epiphyseal involvement,

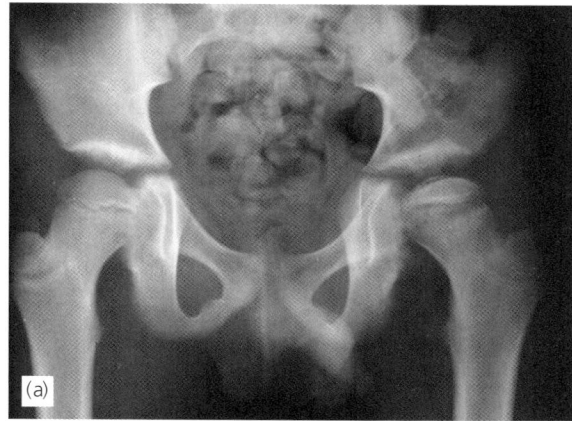

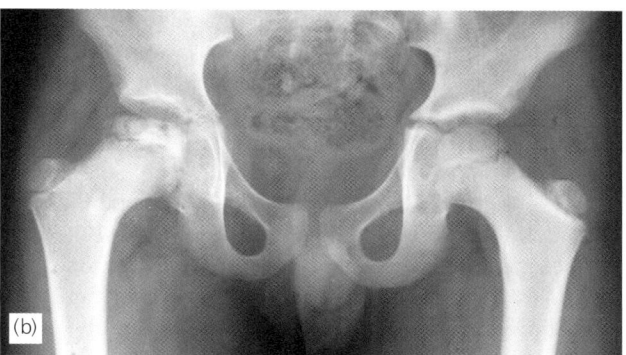

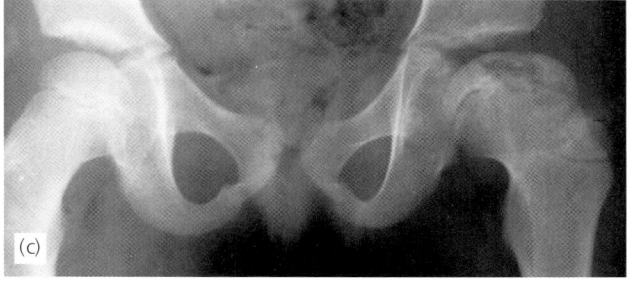

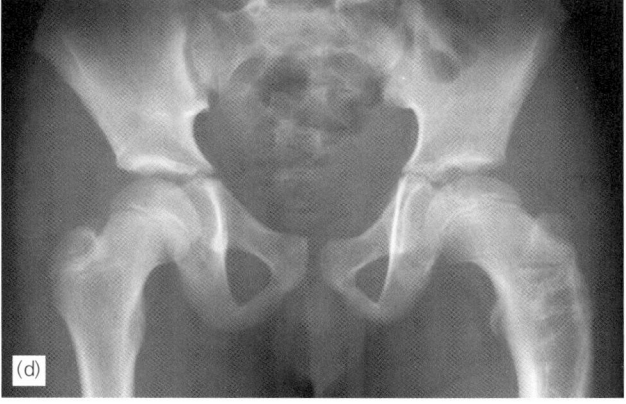

Figure 66.6 The evolution of Perthes disease can be seen on sequential plain radiographs of a child with this disease. The disease passes through stages of avascular necrosis (a), fragmentation (b), regeneration (c) and final healing (d).

the extent of epiphyseal collapse and epiphyseal extrusion. Several other radiological changes in the proximal femur and the acetabulum have also been identified as poor prognostic factors. Some of these were included as 'head-at-risk' signs,[42] but subsequent studies have shown that not all of these reliably predict the prognosis.

The prognosis is better when the age at onset of the disease is lower; children under the age of 5 years at onset tend to have a good prognosis (although not invariably so). If the disease onset is in adolescence, the prognosis is very poor.[40]

The extent of epiphyseal involvement may be estimated early in the course of the disease (stage of avascular necrosis) if the plain radiograph shows a subchondral fracture that runs parallel to the articular surface of the femoral head. Salter and Thompson[43] classified hips into two groups on the basis of whether the fracture line extended to less than half the width of the epiphysis or beyond half the width of the epiphysis. Not all patients present early in the disease with a clearly visible subchondral fracture line, and, as a consequence, this method of estimation of the extent of epiphyseal involvement will be possible in only about one-third of children with Perthes disease.

Catterall[42] classified hips into four groups on the basis of the extent of involvement assessed from anteroposterior and frog lateral views during the stage of fragmentation and showed that the prognosis was best in group I and poorest in group IV (Box 66.1).

> **BOX 66.1: Catterall's classification of epiphyseal involvement in Perthes disease**
>
> - Group I: less than half the epiphysis (the anterior part) is avascular
> - Group II: half the epiphysis is avascular
> - Group III: more than half the epiphysis (but not the entire epiphysis) is avascular
> - Group IV: the entire epiphysis is avascular

The extent of epiphyseal collapse was shown to have a bearing on the outcome by Herring et al.;[44] the greater the collapse the poorer the prognosis (Fig. 66.7). Herring et al.[44] suggested that collapse of the lateral part of the epiphysis (the lateral pillar) was the most important and went on to classify hips assessed in the stage of fragmentation into three groups based on the degree of collapse of the lateral pillar. A fourth group, called B–C border, was introduced more recently[45] (Box 66.2).

Epiphyseal extrusion predisposes to epiphyseal collapse and deformation of the femoral head. When epiphyseal extrusion exceeds 20%, there is a high risk of permanent femoral head deformation.[46] This is arguably the most important prognostic factor and the only one that may be modified by treatment. Epiphyseal extrusion almost invariably develops in children over the age of 7 (Fig. 66.8).

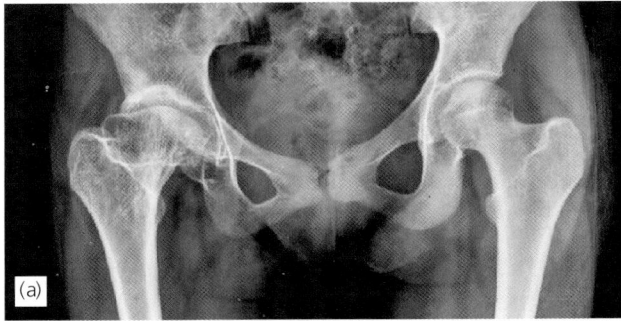
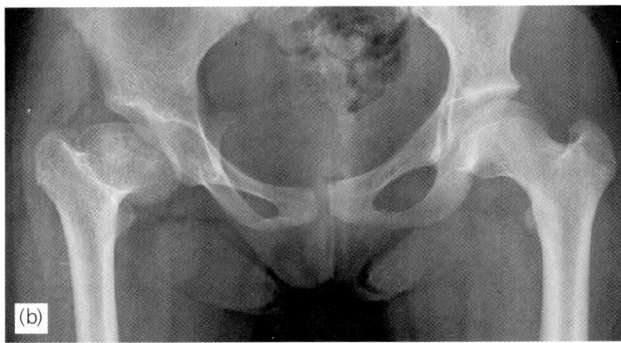
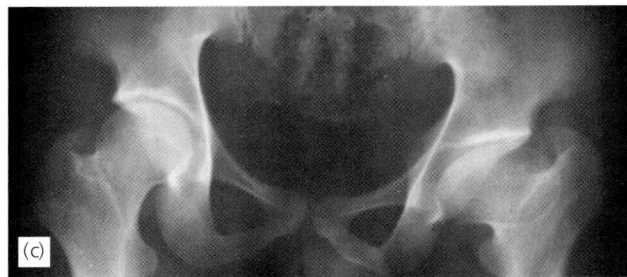

Figure 66.7 Sequelae of Perthes disease include frank irregularity of the femoral head (a), coxa magna (b) and coxa breva with trochanteric overgrowth (c).

> **BOX 66.2: Herring's lateral pillar classification of epiphyseal collapse**
>
> - A: no collapse of the height of the lateral pillar
> - B: less than 50% collapse of the height of the lateral pillar
> - B–C border: 50% collapse of the height of the lateral pillar
> - C: greater than 50% collapse of the height of the lateral pillar

TREATMENT

The primary aim of treatment is to prevent the femoral head from getting deformed. In order to succeed, one needs to be aware of the pathogenesis and the timing of femoral head deformation so that appropriate timely intervention can be instituted.

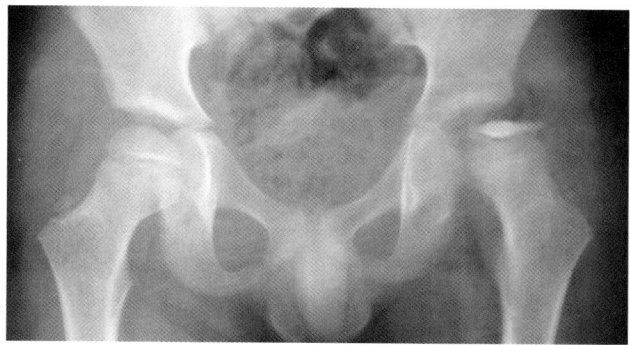

Figure 66.8 Epiphyseal extrusion can be clearly seen in this child with Perthes disease; the medial joint space is increased and there is uncovering of the epiphysis.

side the acetabular margin. Extrusion tends to increase as the disease progresses and may exceed 20% during the latter part of the stage of fragmentation. Weight-bearing stresses and muscular forces transmitted across the acetabular margin can deform the extruded femoral head at two stages. The trabeculae of the avascular bone are more susceptible to fracture and collapse and this often occurs during the stage of fragmentation. During the stage of regeneration, new woven bone grows over the necrotic epiphysis from the periphery. This new woven bone is vulnerable to deformation as the bone trabeculae are not aligned so as to resist deforming stresses (as in lamellar bone), and, if extrusion is present at this stage, the femoral head can be irreparably deformed. There is evidence to suggest that irreversible deformation of the femoral head occurs either during the latter part of the stage of fragmentation or in the early stage of regeneration.[47]

Pathogenesis and timing of femoral head deformity

Following the vascular insult, synovitis and articular cartilage hypertrophy occurs. The cartilage hypertrophy is most marked on the medial aspect of the hip, and this initiates extrusion of the lateral part of the avascular epiphysis out-

Treatment options

Prolonged bed rest and weight relief that was advocated in the past is not favoured currently. The trend is to try to prevent and correct femoral head extrusion, i.e. achieve femoral head 'containment'. Since it is the anterolateral

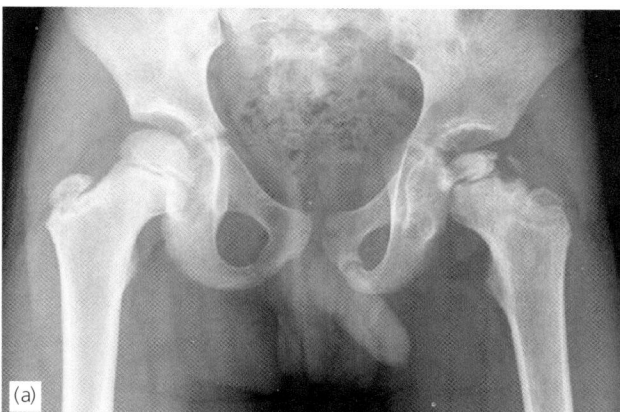
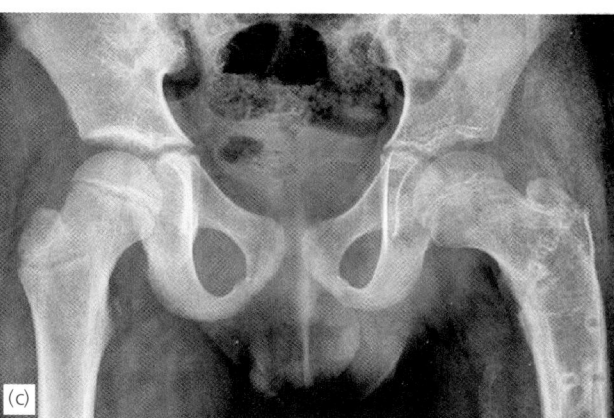
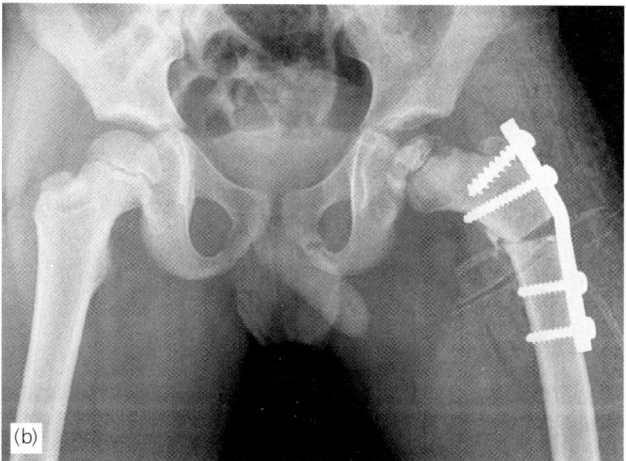
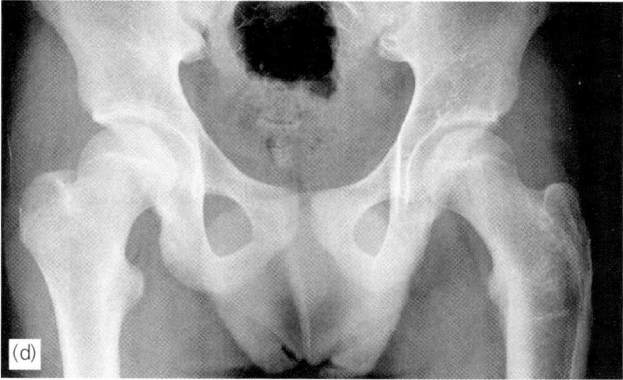

Figure 66.9 A varus derotation osteotomy was performed in this 8 year old boy with Perthes disease (a), early in the fragmentation stage (b). The final outcome is very satisfactory with a spherical femoral head at healing (c) and at skeletal maturity (d).

part of the epiphysis that extrudes, containment attempts to ensure that this part of the epiphysis remains covered by the acetabulum. This can be achieved in the following ways:[48–50]

- Keep the hip abducted and internally rotated (or abducted and flexed):
  - in a splint till the disease heals
  - by performing a femoral varus derotation (or varus extension) osteotomy (Fig. 66.9).
- Cover the anterolateral part of the femoral epiphysis:
  - by an innominate osteotomy that rotates the acetabulum anterolaterally (e.g. Salter osteotomy)
  - by creating a shelf over the anterolateral aspect of the femoral head.

Irrespective of the method adopted it is imperative that containment be achieved sufficiently early in the course of the disease, before the femoral head gets irreversibly deformed. It follows that containment must be achieved before the late fragmentation stage.

Factors to consider before planning treatment

- The age of the patient.
- The extent of epiphyseal involvement.
- The presence of epiphyseal extrusion.
- The range of hip motion.
- The stage of evolution of the disease.

Recommended treatment

An outline of treatment based on these factors is presented in the Table 66.2.

In the older child, if surgical containment is undertaken, prophylactic trochanteric epiphysiodesis may also be performed to prevent trochanteric overgrowth and a Trendelenburg gait.[50,51]

SLIPPED CAPITAL FEMORAL EPIPHYSIS

INTRODUCTION AND EPIDEMIOLOGY

Slipped capital femoral epiphysis (SCFE) is the most common adolescent hip disorder. If diagnosis and treatment is delayed there is a high risk of complications.

The incidence varies quite profoundly between different ethnic populations. The highest incidence in the USA is seen among the blacks. The disease is common among Polynesians, but relatively uncommon in Asians.

SCFE is more common in boys than in girls.

PATHOGENESIS AND AETIOLOGY

SCFE occurs because of a dehiscence through the hypertrophic zone of the capital femoral physis. Close to adolescence, the physis widens with diminution of the perichondral ring and, at this stage, there is an inherent weakness of the physis. The name 'slipped epiphysis' is inaccurate as it is not the epiphysis that moves; the femoral neck displaces superiorly and into external rotation off the epiphysis, which itself remains in the acetabulum.

The causes for SCFE are multifactorial, both genetic and environmental. While the inheritance pattern of SCFE is considered to be autosomal dominant with variable penetrance, there remains a possibility that the inheritance may be polygenetic in nature.

Table 66.2 Indications and contraindications for containment in Perthes disease

Variable	Indications for containment	Contraindications for containment
Age	In children under 7 years at onset if there is demonstrable extrusion In children over 7 years contain early (even before any extrusion is evident) as extrusion almost invariably occurs in these older children	In children under 7 years without any extrusion
Extent of involvement	If half or more than half of the epiphysis is avascular	If less than half of the epiphysis is avascular
Stage of the disease	Stage of avascular necrosis or the stage of fragmentation	Stage of regeneration or healed stage
Extrusion	If extrusion is present (in child under 12 years at onset of disease) OR Even if extrusion is absent in children aged between 7 and 12 years	If extrusion is absent (in children under 7 years at onset of disease)
Range of hip motion	Normal	Restricted

The environmental factors that predispose to SCFE include trauma, mechanical factors (e.g. obesity and retroversion of the physis), endocrine abnormalities, renal failure and irradiation.

Apart from contributing to increased sheer stress across the physis, obesity may also be responsible for producing imbalance in a humoral regulator of chondrocyte apoptosis. Femoral retroversion has also been shown to increase shear stress across the physis.

Endocrine abnormalities such as panhypopituitarism, hypothyroidism and growth hormone deficiency have all been associated with SCFE. A very high proportion of children with untreated hypothyroidism may eventually develop SCFE. Thyroid hormone (T3) stimulates proliferation and differentiation of chondrocytes into their hypertrophic form. Thyroid hormone deficiency adversely affects the maturation of chondrocytes, leading to eventual defective mineralization. In patients with growth hormone deficiency, SCFE often develops during or after hormone replacement therapy because of inhibition of chondrocyte differentiation. The chondrocytes remain in the proliferative stage for a long duration, destabilizing the physis in the process.

CLASSIFICATION

A classification system based on the onset of symptoms divides SCFE into acute, acute-on-chronic and chronic slips. An acute slip is one with symptoms of less than 3 weeks' duration whereas a chronic slip has symptoms for more than 3 weeks. An acute-on-chronic slip is one in which there is a sudden exacerbation of symptoms owing to acute displacement of an already chronically slipped epiphysis.

Currently, the classification suggested by Loder et al.[52] is popular because of its prognostic significance. They classified slips into stable and unstable slips on the basis of ability to bear weight on the limb. Stable slips are those in which the patient can weight bear with or without crutches, whereas unstable slips are those in which the patient is unable to bear any weight in the limb.

NATURAL HISTORY

The unstable SCFE is akin to a displaced Salter–Harris type I fracture, with a high risk of subsequent avascular necrosis. In stable SCFE, the slow process of slippage over time allows remodelling to take place. Concomitant bone resorption occurs anteriorly, with deposition of new bone posteriorly. As the femoral neck slips anteriorly and superiorly, femoral retroversion develops. Untreated SCFE, especially if severe, will eventually lead to secondary osteoarthritis in most cases.

CLINICAL PRESENTATION

Although most patients are adolescents, SCFE can occur in younger children, and this is referred to as juvenile SCFE. The usual presenting symptom is pain in the groin or knee. Failure to recognize that the knee pain may be referred from the hip can lead to a delay in diagnosis. This emphasizes the need to mandatorily examine the hip in a child complaining of pain in the knee. The patient with an acute, unstable SCFE will not be able to weight bear at all, and often there may be a history of trauma. A chronic, stable SCFE can occasionally present with a mere gait abnormality without significant hip pain.

Physical examination will reveal that the patient walks with an antalgic gait with the affected limb in external rotation. There is usually a fixed external rotation deformity and associated loss of internal rotation of the affected hip.

DIAGNOSTIC IMAGING

Radiographs should include anteroposterior and frog-leg lateral views of the pelvis, and both hips must be visualized in order to exclude bilateral involvement. If a frog-leg lateral view is unattainable because of severe hip pain, a true lateral or cross-table lateral of the hip will suffice for the initial assessment (Figs. 66.10 and 66.11). On the anteroposterior view, a line drawn along the superior cortex of the femoral neck (Klein's line) should

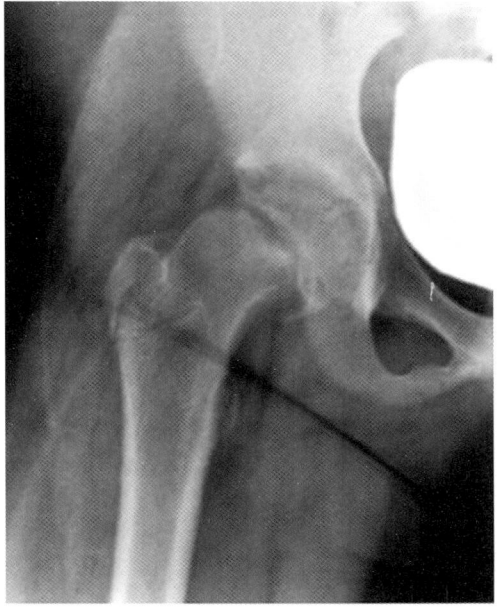

Figure 66.10 An anteroposterior view of the right hip showing the slipped capital femoral epiphysis with metaphyseal remodelling.

transect the femoral epiphysis in normal hips. However, in the presence of a slipped epiphysis, Klein's line fails to do so, and lies above the epiphysis instead (Fig. 66.12).

The severity of the slip may be assessed on the anteroposterior or frog-leg lateral views. The slip may be graded as mild, moderate or severe based on whether the epiphysis has slipped less than one-third, between one-third and two-thirds or more than two-thirds of the width of the femoral neck, respectively, as assessed on the anteroposterior view. Alternatively, the slip angle can be measured from the frog-lateral view. A slip angle less than 30° is regarded as a mild slip whereas an angle greater than 60° is regarded as severe.

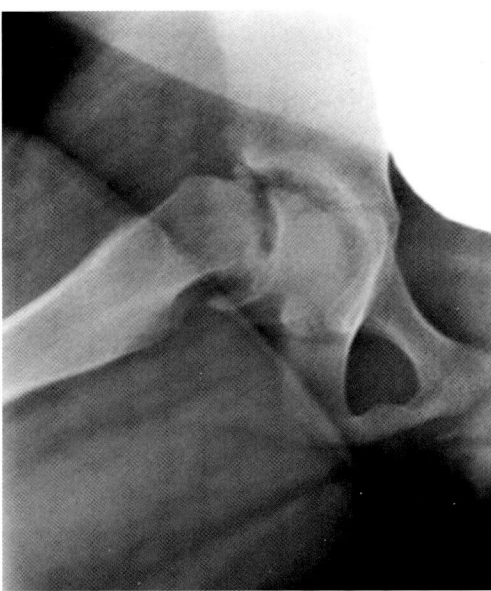

Figure 66.11 The lateral view of the right hip of the same child as in Fig. 66.10 showing the posterior slip of the capital femoral epiphysis.

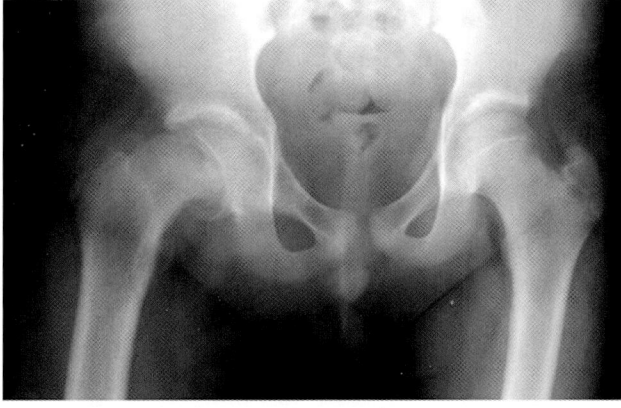

Figure 66.12 The anteroposterior view of the hips of the same child as in Fig. 66.10 shows that Klein's line on the right hip is not transecting the lateral aspect of the capital epiphysis, which is diagnostic of slipped capital femoral epiphysis.

Treatment

The management of SCFE remains controversial in the following areas:

- the timing of surgery and the role of manipulation in unstable SCFE
- fixation methods
- the role of femoral osteotomy
- the role of prophylactic pinning.

UNSTABLE SLIPPED CAPITAL FEMORAL EPIPHYSIS

Although the exact management of the unstable SCFE is still controversial, the goals of treatment are generally agreed upon:

- prevention of further slippage and promotion of physeal closure
- prevention of avascular necrosis and chondrolysis
- maintaining hip function.

Options for treatment of unstable SCFE include:

- percutaneous internal fixation (*in situ* or with deliberate closed manipulation and reduction)
- epiphysiodesis
- proximal femoral osteotomy
- open reduction and internal fixation.

Current trends in Europe, the UK and the USA favour percutaneous *in situ* fixation of unstable SCFE.

There is some evidence in the literature to suggest that there may be an 'unsafe window' between 24 and 72 hours from the onset of symptoms, with an increased risk of avascular necrosis during this period. Consequently, it is recommended that surgery should be performed either within 24 hours after the onset of pain; if this is not possible, surgery should be deferred for 1 week.

The role of deliberate, gentle manipulation and reduction of an unstable SCFE is controversial as well. While some authors have reported favourable results following manipulative reduction, there is still concern regarding the possibility of an increased risk of avascular necrosis with any attempt at manipulation. Fortunately, gentle preoperative traction and intra-operative positioning on the traction table often results in reduction of the unstable slip, obviating the need for any deliberate manipulation, and this is what is recommended.

Whether an arthrotomy for decompression of the joint would reduce the risk of avascular necrosis is still not confirmed. However, it is believed that this may help reduce intracapsular pressure in unstable slips, and help improve the blood supply to the epiphysis.

While two screws afford more rotational stability, a single screw has been shown to be sufficient for fixation even in unstable SCFE. Limiting the number of implants inserted and proper, accurate placement of screws or pins also reduces the risk of postoperative complications of avascular necrosis and chondrolysis.

STABLE SLIPPED CAPITAL FEMORAL EPIPHYSIS

There is less controversy with regards to management of stable slips. In general, a single percutaneous screw is sufficient to fix the epiphysis[53] (Fig. 66.13).

The role of proximal femoral osteotomy

A proximal femoral osteotomy to realign the head and neck may be performed at the level of the physis, through the femoral neck or in the intertrochanteric or subtrochanteric region; the more proximal the osteotomy the greater the potential for correction. An osteotomy through the physis restores the normal anatomy without creating a fresh deformity; all other osteotomies create a more distal deformity to compensate for the deformity at the level of the physis. A subtrochanteric osteotomy can make future hip arthroplasty technically more difficult. However, the main concern with more proximal osteotomies relates to a higher incidence of avascular necrosis and chondrolysis, and for this reason an intertrochanteric or subtrochanteric osteotomy may be more advisable.

The recommended timing of the osteotomy in the literature ranges from early osteotomy (cuneiform osteotomy of the femoral neck), to correct severe, unstable slips, to delayed osteotomy (at any of the previously mentioned levels), to correct residual deformity after physeal closure. Early osteotomy to correct deformity in severe, unstable slips should be performed only by experienced surgeons. A safer option would be to perform *in situ* screw fixation in the final position achieved after initial traction and positioning on a traction table, followed by a delayed osteotomy after physeal closure if required.

The role of prophylactic pinning

The reported incidence of bilateral involvement ranges from 23% to 65%, with an average of 46%. Prophylactic pinning of the uninvolved hip is recommended for children who are prepubertal with a bone age of 12 or less for girls and 13 or less for boys, and in children with known endocrine disorders irrespective of their age at presentation.

Management of complications of slipped capital femoral epiphysis

AVASCULAR NECROSIS

Once avascular necrosis develops, management is aimed at optimizing function and delaying the onset of secondary osteoarthritis (Fig. 66.14). Unfortunately, avascular

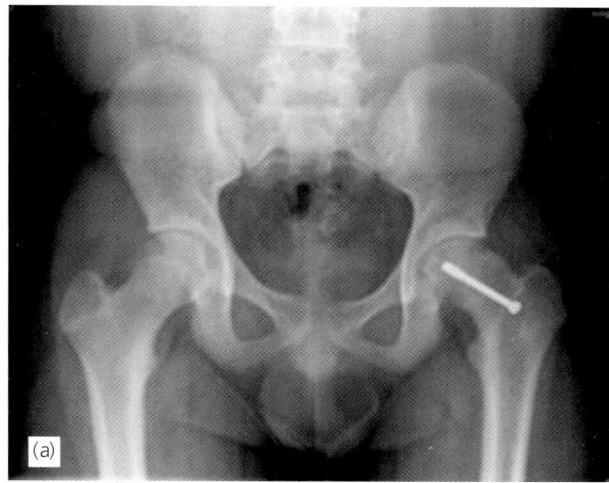

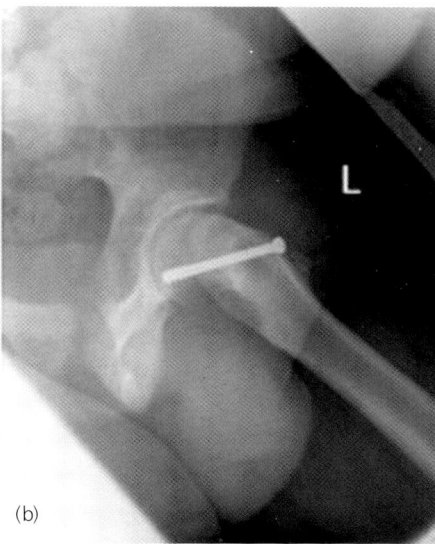

Figure 66.13 (a and b) The postoperative radiographs of a patient with acute slip of the capital femoral epiphysis treated with single percutaneous screw fixation directed to the centre of the capital epiphysis perpendicular to the physis in both anteroposterior and lateral views.

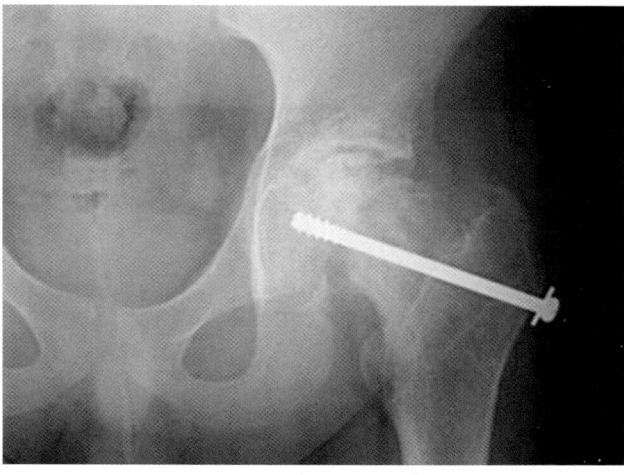

Figure 66.14 The late complication of slip of the capital femoral epiphysis with avascular necrosis of the femoral head in the child previously treated with percutaneous screw fixation (Fig. 66.15).

necrosis is not always recognized early and progressive collapse of the femoral head with pin or screw protrusion can further damage the hip. As soon as avascular necrosis is recognized, weight bearing is strictly avoided. Any implant protrusion is dealt with by removal of hardware if the physis has closed or by screw exchange to a shorter implant if the physis is still open. Analgesics and physiotherapy to maintain joint range of motion are also instituted.

If the loss of blood supply is segmental, and gross deformity does not occur, this treatment may suffice and a reasonable outcome may be anticipated. However, if the entire epiphysis is avascular and gross collapse of the epiphysis occurs the outcome will be poor. An appropriate proximal femoral osteotomy can be considered to improve joint congruency and improve the range of motion of the hip in a few selected cases.

CHONDROLYSIS

Chondrolysis or acute cartilage necrosis often follows penetration of the implant into the joint. It manifests weeks or months later as a painful or painless reduction in range of motion often with fixed deformities. A 50% reduction in joint space, as compared with the normal hip, is diagnostic. In a proportion of cases, the chondrolysis may resolve spontaneously with progressive improvement of range of motion over a period of time. Often, it progresses to painless or painful ankylosis of the hip.

Prevention of implant penetration into the hip joint is the best way to minimize the risk of chondrolysis. The risk of implant penetration may be reduced by using the minimal number of pins or screws possible, and by placing the implants in the centre of the epiphysis using the approach–withdrawal technique using fluoroscopy.

If the condition has been chronic and hip contractures have developed, surgical release of the soft tissues can be considered if stretching and splinting fail. If all else fails after protracted therapy, hip joint fusion may be one good option in young active patients.

With improvements in joint replacement techniques, state-of-the-art implants and better tribology, surface replacement may become a preferred option for secondary osteoarthritis following SCFE in young adults.

TRANSIENT SYNOVITIS

Transient synovitis is an acute, self-limiting inflammatory process of the synovial lining, most commonly affecting the hip. By definition, symptoms should be transient and function should return to normal, usually within 7–10 days.[54] Typically, there are no long-term sequelae, although mild, asymptomatic coxa magna has been described in up to 33%.[55] It should be differentiated from the term 'irritable hip', which has been defined as any abnormality of the hip found on history or clinical examination, but with no pathology noted on assessment by imaging.[56]

The aetiology is not well understood, although it may be thought of as a reactive condition that most often affects the hip.[57] Trauma, antecedent systemic bacterial or viral infection (especially upper respiratory tract) and allergic reaction have been suggested as potential causes and may all lead to a final common clinical syndrome.[58,59]

The incidence of transient synovitis is approximately 3% in a child's lifetime. Up to 40% of children presenting to emergency departments with a limp are diagnosed with transient synovitis, followed by 'overuse' and idiopathic causes.[56] It occurs most commonly in children aged 3–8 years, although it can occur into the teenage years. The peak incidence is roughly 5–6 years, which is similar to Perthes disease. Boys are affected twice as often as girls. Seasonal variation has been shown in one study in the northern hemisphere with a peak in the autumn, but this has not been well demonstrated in other, larger, series.[60] The frequency of this condition and its similarity to other more serious diseases (e.g. septic arthritis, juvenile rheumatoid arthritis, Perthes disease) make thorough knowledge of this condition essential for practising primary care providers.[61]

Patients present with pain in the groin, thigh or knee along with a limp. Because of the pain and the reactive effusion, internal rotation, extension and abduction are limited. The hip is usually held in a position of flexion and external rotation so that the hip capsule is relaxed as much as possible and the elevated intracapsular pressure is relieved.[62] Symptoms are usually unilateral, with less than 5% being bilateral.[61]

Temperature is normal to slightly elevated (rarely over 38°C). Serological markers of inflammation are typically normal or mildly elevated. Radiographs are often normal unless slight widening of the medial joint space is present secondary to the effusion.[54,60,61,63] Bone scans are not useful in distinguishing between transient synovitis and septic arthritis.[63] Patients with transient synovitis have an effusion, synovial thickening or both on ultrasound or MRI. The effusion is typically non-echogenic on ultrasound, although the usefulness of this in making a definitive diagnosis is debated.[63] Up to 25% have synovial swelling or effusion on the contralateral side on MRI or ultrasound.[64]

Given a similar presentation to more potentially devastating conditions, such as septic arthritis, the diagnosis of transient synovitis must be one of exclusion (see Box 66.3). A delay in diagnosis of septic arthritis has been shown to lead to worse outcome, and so a timely diagnosis is prudent.[65] Patients with septic arthritis usually present with more severe pain and spasm, fever and are generally more toxic appearing. The serological markers are also often consistently elevated.[61,66–69]

Because no single laboratory test or imaging modality is able to definitively differentiate between transient synovitis and septic arthritis, multiple clinical algorithms have been proposed combining various presentation variables

> **BOX 66.3: Differential diagnosis**
>
> - Septic arthritis
> - Perthes disease
> - Rheumatic fever
> - Juvenile rheumatoid arthritis
> - Slip of the capital femoral epiphysis
> - Trauma/fracture
> - Osteomyelitis
> - Idiopathic
> - Reactive arthritis
> - Neoplasia
> - Haemophilia
> - Sickle cell disease

(see Box 66.4).[66–69] While they are simple to use, they have not been found to be reliable or valid when applied to different patient populations.[66] Although they give guidance to clinicians in the face of difficult diagnostic dilemmas, they should be used with caution.

If there is sufficient clinical suspicion of septic arthritis, an aspiration under general anaesthetic or sedation should

> **BOX 66.4: Predicted probability of septic arthritis**
>
> | No. of factors present | Predicted probability of septic arthritis (%) |
> | --- | --- |
> | 0 | 16.9 |
> | 1 | 36.7 |
> | 2 | 62.4 |
> | 3 | 82.6 |
> | 4 | 93.1 |
> | 5 | 97.5 |
>
> *The factors:*
> - Fever: >38.5°C
> - Refusal to bear weight
> - Serum white blood cell count: $>12.0 \times 10^9 \, L^{-1}$
> - Erythrocyte sedimentation rate: >40 mm h^{-1}
> - Serum C-reactive protein level: >20.0 mg L^{-1}
>
> Adapted from Caird *et al*.[67]

be performed. The gold standard for ruling out a diagnosis of septic arthritis remains aspiration of joint fluid for cell count, Gram stain, culture and sensitivity. In transient synovitis a joint aspiration will yield serous and sterile fluid with a low cell count.[61]

Optimal treatment is rest, avoidance of weight bearing and anti-inflammatory therapy.[70] Because of the risk of Reye syndrome, aspirin should be avoided. Traction with the hip in extension has fallen out of favour given that the position of extension combined with distraction of the femoral head within the acetabulum increases intracapsular pressure, increasing pain and theoretically decreasing perfusion of the femoral epiphysis.[55,60] The recurrence rate is up to 10% in 6 months, but one must consider the possibility of other diagnosis if a patient re-presents with significant symptoms.[71]

> **KEY LEARNING POINTS**
>
> - Developmental coxa vara is not present at birth or associated with other skeletal manifestations.
> - It is a complex three-dimensional deformity of proximal femoral varus and retroversion.
> - The Hilgenreiner epiphyseal angle is the mainstay of monitoring progress.
> - Surgery is indicated for a Hilgenreiner epiphyseal angle of >60°.
> - Results of surgery are dependent on restoration of hip biomechanics.
> - Perthes disease is a self-limiting osteochondrosis of the capital femoral epiphysis.
> - The aetiology of Perthes disease remains unclear.
> - In a proportion of children with Perthes disease, the femoral head can become deformed.
> - The prognosis is poor in the older child with Perthes disease and when the entire epiphysis is avascular.
> - Extrusion of the femoral head is the most important factor that can lead to femoral head deformation.
> - Femoral head deformation occurs in the latter part of the stage of fragmentation or in the early phase of regeneration.
> - Treatment aimed at preventing femoral head deformation should be instituted before the latter part of the stage of fragmentation.
> - Containment, if achieved early, offers a good chance of preventing femoral head deformation.

REFERENCES

- ● = Key primary paper
- ◆ = Major review article

1. Hamanishi C. Congenital short femur: clinical, genetic and epidemiological comparison of the naturally occurring condition with that caused by thalidomide. *Journal of Bone and Joint Surgery (British)* 1980;**62B**:307–20.
2. Aitken GT. Proximal femoral focal deficiency: definition, classification and management. In: Aitken GT (ed.) *A Symposium on Proximal Femoral Focal Deficiency: A Congenital Anomaly*. Washington, DC: National Academy of Sciences, 1969:1–22.

3. Gillespie R, Torode IP. Classification and management of congenital abnormalities of the femur. *Journal of Bone and Joint Surgery (British)* 1983;**65B**:557–68.
4. Paley D. Lengthening reconstruction surgery for congenital femoral deficiency. In: Herring JA, Birch JG (eds) *The Child with a Limb Deficiency*. Rosemont, IL: American Academy of Orthopaedic Surgeons, 1998:113–32.
5. Koman LA, Meyer LC, Warren FH. Proximal femoral focal deficiency: a 50-year experience. *Developmental Medicine and Child Neurology* 1982;**24**:344.
6. McClenaghan BA, Krajbich JL, Pirone AM, et al. Comparative assessment of gait after limb salvage procedures. *Journal of Bone and Joint Surgery (American)* 1989;**71A**:1178–82.
7. Amstutz HC, Wilson Jr PD. Dysgenesis of the proximal femur (coxa vara) and its surgical management. *Journal of Bone and Joint Surgery (American)* 1962;**44A**:1–24.
8. Fairbank HA. Coxa vara due to congenital defect of the neck of the femur. *Journal of Anatomy* 1928;**62** (Pt 2):232–7.
9. Beals RK. Coxa vara in childhood: evaluation and management. *Journal of the American Academy of Orthopedic Surgery* 1998;**6**:93–9.
10. Serafin J, Szulc W. Coxa vara infantum, hip growth disturbances, etiopathogenesis, and long-term results of treatment. *Clinical Orthopaedics and Related Research* 1991;**272**:103–13.
11. Kim HT, Chambers HG, Mubarak SJ, Wenger DR. Congenital coxa vara: computed tomographic analysis of femoral retroversion and the triangular metaphyseal fragment. *Journal of Pediatric Orthopaedics* 2000;**20**:551–6.
12. Carroll K, Coleman S, Stevens PM. Coxa vara: surgical outcomes of valgus osteotomies. *Journal of Pediatric Orthopaedics* 1997;**17**:220–4.
13. Chung SM, Riser WH. The histological characteristics of congenital coxa vara: a case report of a five year old boy. *Clinical Orthopaedics and Related Research* 1978;**132**:71–81.
14. Pavlov H, Goldman AB, Freiberger RH. Infantile coxa vara. *Radiology* 1980;**135**:631–40.
15. Bos CF, Sakkers RJ, Bloem JL, et al. Histological, biochemical, and MRI studies of the growth plate in congenital coxa vara. *Journal of Pediatric Orthopaedics* 1989;**9**:660–5.
●16. Weinstein JN, Kuo KN, Millar EA. Congenital coxa vara. A retrospective review. *Journal of Pediatric Orthopaedics* 1984;**4**:70–7.
17. Le Mesurier AB. Developmental coxa vara. *Journal of Bone and Joint Surgery (British)* 1948;**30B**:595–605.
18. Barr J. Congenital coxa vara. *Archives of Surgery* 1929;**18**:1909.
19. Zadek I. Congenital coxa vara. *Archives of Surgery* 1935;**30**:62.
20. Cordes S, Dickens DR, Cole WG. Correction of coxa vara in childhood. The use of Pauwels' Y-shaped osteotomy. *Journal of Bone and Joint Surgery (British)* 1991;**73**:3–6.
21. Desai SS, Johnson LO. Long-term results of valgus osteotomy for congenital coxa vara. *Clinical Orthopaedics and Related Research* 1993;**294**:204–10.
22. Burns KA, Stevens PM. Coxa vara: another option for fixation. *Journal of Pediatric Orthopaedics* B 2001;**10**:304–10.
23. Sabharwal S, Mittal R, Cox G. Percutaneous triplanar femoral osteotomy correction for developmental coxa vara: a new technique. *Journal of Pediatric Orthopaedics* 2005;**25**:28–33.
24. Weighill FJ. The treatment of developmental coxa vara by abduction subtrochanteric and intertrochanteric femoral osteotomy with special reference to the role of adductor tenotomy. *Clinical Orthopaedics and Related Research* 1976;**116**:116–24.
25. Widmann RF, Hresko MT, Kasser JR, Millis MB. Wagner multiple K-wire osteosynthesis to correct coxa vara in the young child: experience with a versatile 'tailor-made' high angle blade plate equivalent. *Journal of Pediatric Orthopaedics B* 2001;**10**:43–50.
26. Pauwels F. *Biomechanics of the Normal and Diseased Hip*. New York, NY: Springer-Verlag, 1976.
27. Glueck CJ, Crawford A, Roy D, et al. Association of antithrombotic factor deficiencies and hypofibrinolysis with Legg-Perthes disease. *Journal of Bone and Joint Surgery (American)* 1996;**78A**:3–14.
28. Glueck CJ, Brandt G, Gruppo R, et al. Resistance to activated protein C and Legg-Perthes disease. *Clinical Orthopaedics and Related Research* 1997;**338**:139–52.
29. Hall AJ, Barker DJ, Dangerfield PH, Taylor JF. Perthes' disease of the hip in Liverpool. *British Medical Journal* 1983;**287**: 1757–9.
30. Joseph J, Chacko V, Rao BS, Hall AJ. The epidemiology of Perthes' disease in south India. *International Journal of Epidemiology* 1988;**17**:603–7.
31. Catterall A. *Legg-Calve-Perthes' Disease*. Edinburgh, UK: Churchill Livingstone, 1982:60–1.
32. Jensen OM, Lauritzen J. Legg-Calve-Perthes' disease: morphological studies in two cases examined at necropsy. *Journal of Bone and Joint Surgery (British)* 1976;**58B**:332–8.
33. Ponseti IV. Legg-Perthes' disease: observations on pathological changes in two cases. *Journal of Bone and Joint Surgery (American)* 1956;**38A**:739–50.
34. Catterall A, Pringle J, Byers PD, et al. Perthes' disease: is the epiphyseal infarction complete? *Journal of Bone and Joint Surgery (British)* 1982;**64B**: 276–81.
35. Joseph B. Serum immunoglobulin in Perthes' disease. *Journal of Bone and Joint Surgery (British)* 1991;**73**:509–10.
36. Joseph B, Pydisetty RKV. Chondrolysis and the stiff hip in Perthes disease. *Journal of Pediatric Orthopaedics* 1996;**16**:15–19
37. Chacko V, Joseph B, Seetharam B. Perthes' disease in south India. *Clinical Orthopaedics and Related Research* 1986;**209**:95–9.
38. Burwell RG, Dangerfield PH, Hall DJ, et al. Perthes' disease. An anthropometric study revealing impaired and

disproportionate growth. *Journal of Bone and Joint Surgery (British)* 1978;**60B**:46–77.

39. Hall AJ, Barker DJ, Dangerfield PH, et al. Small feet and Perthes' disease. A survey in Liverpool. *Journal of Bone and Joint Surgery (British)* 1988;**70B**:611–13.

40. Joseph B, Mulpuri K, Verghese G. Perthes' disease in the adolescent. *Journal of Bone and Joint Surgery (British)* 2001;**83**:715–20.

41. Stulberg SD, Cooperman DR, Wallensten R. The natural history of Legg-Calve-Perthes' disease. *Journal of Bone and Joint Surgery (American)* 1981;**63**:1095–108.

42. Catterall A. The natural history of Perthes' disease. *Journal of Bone and Joint Surgery (British)* 1971;**53B**:37–53.

43. Salter RB, Thompson GH. Legg-Calve-Perthes disease: the prognostic significance of the subchondral fracture and the two-group classification of the femoral head involvement. *Journal of Bone and Joint Surgery (American)* 1984;**66A**:479–89.

44. Herring JA, Neustadt JB, Williams JJ, et al. The lateral pillar classification of Legg-Calve-Perthes disease. *Journal of Pediatric Orthopaedics* 1992;**12**:143–50.

45. Herring JA, Kim HT, Browne R. Legg-Calve-Perthes disease. Part I. Classification of radiographs with use of the modified lateral pillar and Stulberg classifications. *Journal of Bone and Joint Surgery (American)* 2004;**86**:2103–20.

46. Green NE, Beuchamp RD, Griffin PP. Epiphyseal extrusion as a prognostic index in Legg-Calve-Perthes disease. *Journal of Bone and Joint Surgery (American)* 1981;**63**:9000–5.

47. Joseph B, Varghese G, Mulpuri K, et al. The natural evolution of Perthes' disease: a study of 610 children under 12 years of age at disease onset. *Journal of Pediatric Orthopaedics* 2003;**23**:590–600.

48. Daly K, Bruce C, Catterall A. Lateral shelf acetabuloplasty in Perthes' disease: a review at the end of growth. *Journal of Bone and Joint Surgery (British)* 1999;**81**:380–4.

49. Salter RB. The present status of surgical treatment for Legg-Perthes' disease. *Journal of Bone and Joint Surgery (American)* 1984;**66**:961–6.

50. Matan AJ, Stevens PM, Smith JT, Santora SD. Combination trochanteric arrest and intertrochanteric osteotomy for Perthes' disease. *Journal of Pediatric Orthopaedics* 1996;**16**:10–14.

51. Shah H, Siddesh ND, Joseph B, Nair SN. Effect of trochanteric epiphyseodesis in older children with Perthes' disease. *Journal of Pediatric Orthopaedics* 2009;**29**:889–95.

52. Loder RT, Arbor A, Richards BS. Acute slipped capital femoral epiphysis: the importance of physeal stability. *Journal of Bone and Joint Surgery (American)* 1993;**75**:1134–40.

53. Koval KJ, Lehman WB, Rose D, et al. Treatment of slipped capital femoral epiphysis with a cannulated screw technique. *Journal of Bone and Joint Surgery (American)* 1989;**71**:1370–7.

54. Macnicol MF. The irritable hip in childhood. *Current Orthopaedics* 2004;**18**:284–90.

55. Kallio P, Ryoppy S, Kunnamo I. Transient synovitis and Perthes' disease. *Journal of Bone and Joint Surgery (British)* 1986;**68**:808–11.

56. Fischer SU, Beattie TF. The limping child: epidemiology, assessment and outcome. *Journal of Bone and Joint Surgery (British)* 1999;**81**:1029–34.

57. Diab M. The limping child: transient synovitis. In: Abel MF (ed.) *Orthopaedic Knowledge Update. Pediatrics 3*. Rosemont, IL: American Academy of Orthopaedic Surgeons, 2006:13–14.

58. Edwards E. Transient synovitis of hip joint in children. *JAMA* 1952;**148**:30–4.

59. Jacobs BW. Synovitis of the hip in children and its significance. *Pediatrics* 1971;**47**:558–66.

60. Landin L, Danielsson L, Wattsgard C. Transient synovitis of the hip. Its incidence, epidemiology, and relationship to Perthes. *Journal of Bone and Joint Surgery (British)* 1987;**69**:238–42.

61. Do T. Transient synovitis as a cause of painful limps in children. *Current Opinion in Paediatrics* 2000;**12**:48–51.

62. Vegter J. The influence of joint posture on intra-articular pressure. A study of transient synovitis and Perthes' disease. *Journal of Bone and Joint Surgery (British)* 1987;**69**:71–4.

63. Zamzam M. The role of ultrasound in differentiating septic arthritis from transient synovitis of the hip in children. *Journal of Pediatric Orthopaedics B* 2006;**15**:418–22.

64. Ehrendorfer S, LeQuesne G, Penta M, et al. Bilateral synovitis in symptomatic unilateral transient synovitis of the hip: an ultrasonographic study in 56 children. *Acta Orthopaedica Scandinavica* 1996;**67**:149–52.

65. Gillespie R. Septic arthritis of childhood. *Clinical Orthopaedics and Related Research* 1973;**96**:152–9.

66. Luhmann SJ, Jones A, Schootman M, et al. Differentiation between septic arthritis and transient synovitis of the hip in children with clinical prediction algorithms. *Journal of Bone and Joint Surgery (American)* 2004;**86**:956–62.

67. Caird MS, Flynn JM, Leung YL, et al. Factors distinguishing septic arthritis from transient synovitis of the hip in children. *Journal of Bone and Joint Surgery (American)* 2006;**88**:1251–7.

68. Kocher MS, Zurakowski D, Kasser JR. Differentiating between septic arthritis and transient synovitis of the hip in children: an evidence-based clinical prediction algorithm. *Journal of Bone and Joint Surgery (American)* 1999;**81**:1662–70.

69. Jung ST, Rowe SM, Moon ES, et al. Significance of laboratory and radiologic findings for differentiating between septic arthritis and transient synovitis of the hip. *Journal of Pediatric Orthopaedics* 2003;**23**:368–72.

70. Hart J. Transient synovitis of the hip in children. *American Family Physician* 1996;**54**:1587–91.

71. Illingworth CM. Recurrences of transient synovitis. *Archives of Disease in Childhood* 1983;**58**:620–3.

67

Knee disorders in children

JAMES HP HUI, KEVIN LIM, ANDREW LIM, AZURA MANSOR, ISMAIL MUNAJAT, KISHORE MULPURI, SIMON P KELLEY

CONGENITAL DISLOCATION OF THE KNEE	664	Radiographic evaluation	667
Introduction	664	Treatment options	667
Classification	664	GENU VARUM AND VALGUM	667
Aetiology	665	Introduction	667
Clinical features	665	Causes of pathological genu varum and valgum	668
Treatment	665	Consequences of genu varum and valgum	668
CONGENITAL AND ACQUIRED DISLOCATION OF THE PATELLA	665	Assessment of a child with genu varum or valgum	669
		Treatment	669
Anatomy and biomechanics	665	BLOUNT DISEASE	670
Mechanism of dislocation	666	Introduction	670
Classification of patellar dislocations	666	References	671

CONGENITAL DISLOCATION OF THE KNEE

INTRODUCTION

Congenital dislocation of the knee (CDK) is a dramatic birth abnormality. The newborn's knee is in recurvatum and the foot may present at the infant's mouth or shoulders. Hyperflexion of the hips should raise the suspicion of associated hip dislocation. Referral to the orthopaedic surgeon is therefore made shortly after birth. It is the most severe form of knee hyperextension in the newborn.

CDK is a rare disorder and is believed to be about 50–80 times less frequent than developmental dislocation of the hip.

CLASSIFICATION

Congenital knee dislocation must be distinguished from congenital subluxation of the knee or congenital hyperextension of the knee. In all three variations there is hyperextension of the knee. The distinguishing features are outlined in Table 67.1.

An ultrasound or a lateral radiograph of the knee may help differentiate among the three. Fluoroscopy can provide a dynamic assessment in equivocal cases. Arthrography and MRI have also been used to aid in diagnosis.

AETIOLOGY

Bilateral CDK is almost always syndromic, and a search for associated syndromes should be made at the initial evaluation. Associated syndromes are typically the laxity syndromes, such as Larsen, Ehlers–Danlos or Beals syndromes. Ipsilateral hip dislocation has been reported to occur 70% of the time, and ipsilateral clubfoot 50% of the time.

Unilateral CDK can occur in isolation or as part of a neurological syndrome such as arthrogryposis or spinal dysraphism.

Table 67.1 Classification of congenital knee dislocation

Abnormality	Grade	Clinical features	Additional remarks
Congenital hyperextension	I	Passive flexion beyond neutral possible	
Congenital subluxation	II	Passive flexion to neutral possible	Femoral and tibial epiphysis in contact
Congenital dislocation	III	Passive flexion to neutral not possible	Tibia is anteriorly translated on the femur

CDK is the result of abnormal fetal positioning. Once the abnormal position occurs, lack of fetal movement from neuromuscular conditions or laxity from associated syndromes results in persistent dislocation. Quadriceps atrophy and fibrosis follow. Patellar hypoplasia and iliotibial band contracture and fibrosis may also be the result of decreased *in utero* movement.

CLINICAL FEATURES

Children with CDK usually present with a hyperextended knee that may or may not be reducible. Pes calcaneovalgus may be associated with CDK and may be quite severe. When a knee dislocation is present, the hips must always be evaluated.

Absence of the cruciate ligaments is more frequent in bilateral cases associated with laxity syndromes. In unilateral cases, the knee is usually relatively stable once the knee is reduced. In true CDK, anterior subluxation of the posteromedial and posterolateral structures can sometimes occur, including the hamstring tendons and the iliotibial band. Dense adhesions between the atrophic quadriceps muscle complex, the femur and, occasionally, the iliotibial band make closed reduction impossible.

TREATMENT

The treatment of CDK depends on the severity of the abnormality.

Non-operative treatment

In a child with a congenital hyperextension of the knee or mild knee subluxation, a Pavlik harness can be used. The posterior straps are gradually tightened to provide more knee flexion as treatment progresses. Alternatively, serial manipulations and casting can be employed and removable splints can be used to maintain knee flexion. Manipulation or closed reductions must be performed gently as there is a risk of iatrogenic physeal separation of the distal femur. A lateral knee radiograph is therefore important to document restoration of the tibiofemoral joint. Once more than 90° of knee flexion is obtained, it is unlikely that further treatment is required.

Knees with more severe subluxation or dislocation do not respond to stretching or splinting. Traction has been used to achieve gradual reduction. Closed reduction should be abandoned if appropriate reduction of the tibia cannot be achieved.

Operative treatment

Complete dislocations that are not amenable to splinting or casting in progressive flexion will require surgical treatment. These can range from a simple V–Y advancement of the quadriceps tendon through to a more extensive lengthening of the quadriceps mechanism. An anterior capsulotomy may be necessary, while releases of the medial hamstrings, iliotibial band and lateral intermuscular septum may be necessary to correct valgus and external rotation deformity.

A cast is used for immobilization, with the knee held in about 45° of flexion, to prevent recurrent subluxation of the tibia. Pressure on the skin on the anterior aspect of the knee may make it necessary to bring the patient back for further manipulation until the knee can be flexed to 90°.

CONGENITAL AND ACQUIRED DISLOCATION OF THE PATELLA

ANATOMY AND BIOMECHANICS

The knee joint is formed by articulation of the femur, tibia and patella. The patella is the largest sesamoid bone in the body and is located within the quadriceps tendon. The lateral articular facets of the patella are larger than the medial ones. The most medial facet is called the odd facet, making contact with the femoral condyle only in flexion. The medial border of the patella receives fibres of the vastus medialis, the lowest fibres of which form the vastus medialis obliquus aligned at 65° to the vertical axis. They are important medial stabilizers of the patella. The patellar tendon inserts laterally on the tibial tubercle and the quadriceps alignment along the femoral shaft produces a valgus pull on the patella. This lateral pull is countered by the higher lateral femoral trochlea, the medial patellofemoral ligament and the oblique fibres of the vastus medialis. The quadriceps angle (Q angle) is formed from the intersection of a line joining the anterior superior iliac spine to the patella and a line from the centre of the patella to the tibial tubercle. The normal Q angle is 14–20° and measures more in females.

The femoral condyles are unequal in size and are asymmetric, the medial condyle being larger. In progressing from extension to flexion, the patella articulates inferiorly, following which the contact area moves superiorly. After 30°, the trochlea is the major stabilizer of the patella. At 90°, the contact reaches the superior patella and, in full flexion, the complete load is taken by both of the facets.

One of the functions of the patella is to increase the mechanical advantage of the extensor apparatus and act as a lever to increase the extension capacity of the quadriceps. This produces significant forces across the patellofemoral articular surfaces with 60% the force across the lateral facet.

MECHANISM OF DISLOCATION

Dislocations of the patella are usually lateral, and the factors which increase the susceptibility to dislocation include the following bony and soft-tissue factors:

- an increased Q angle due to
  – a laterally inserted patellar tendon
  – excessive tibial external rotation
  – genu valgum
  – femoral anteversion
- patella alta
- trochlear hypoplasia or shallow patellofemoral groove
- insufficiency of the vastus medialis and the medial patellofemoral ligament
- genu recurvatum
- patellar hypermobility owing to hypermobile joint syndrome
- contracture of the vastus lateralis.

CLASSIFICATION OF PATELLAR DISLOCATIONS

Patellar dislocations can be broadly classified into congenital (the spectrum includes habitual dislocation) and acquired (traumatic dislocation), which is commonly sports related.

Congenital patellar dislocation

PERSISTENT TYPE

Congenital dislocation of the patella is often familial and affects both knees. The dislocation occurs antenatally or shortly after birth and, once the dislocation occurs, it is irreducible. The patella is often small and misshapen and there may be abnormalities of the quadriceps mechanism such as congenital absence of the vastus lateralis. The laterally dislocated patella may be attached to the iliotibial band.

The diagnosis should be made as early as possible after birth, but this is not easy in clinical practice. The patella can be clearly felt in a normal infant only when knee is in an extended position. A dislocated patella is smaller and often may not be palpable until the child is 3–4 years old.

The characteristic features of congenital patellar dislocation include: inability to extend the knee either actively or passively, a fixed flexion deformity of the knee and absence of the patella from the trochlear fossa. Congenital dislocation of the knee must be suspected if a flexion contracture of the knee joint is present since birth. There may be associated foot anomalies such as club feet, calcaneovalgus or congenital vertical talus.

A delay in walking upright may be noted if the diagnosis is not made in infancy, although the child may kneel-walk. If the flexion contracture is mild the child may walk with a near normal gait.

HABITUAL TYPE

This type of dislocation occurs during childhood or the adolescent years and may be associated with conditions such as nail–patella syndrome, Down syndrome and chondrodysplasia.[6]

Lateral dislocation of the patella occurs each time the knee is flexed between 20° and 60°. Less commonly, the habitual dislocation can also occur during knee extension. The patella may be normal or hypoplastic. Genu valgum, external rotatory deformity of the tibia or a hypoplastic lateral femoral condyle all predispose to this condition.

- Patients <20 years:
  – late childhood to adolescent period.
- Lateral dislocation during each knee flexion:
  – 20–60°
  – can also occur during knee extension.

Acquired patellar dislocation

ACUTE TRAUMATIC TYPE

Acute traumatic dislocation is usually a consequence of a twisting injury to the knee. The child may describe it as a medial dislocation instead of lateral because of the prominence of the uncovered medial femoral condyle. The tendency to redislocate is significantly greater in adolescents than in those over the age of 20 years at the time of the primary dislocation. Acute unreduced dislocations may present with pain, swelling and a flexed attitude of the knee. More often, the patella either spontaneously reduces or is reduced straight after the injury.

Examination of the knee will demonstrate a large effusion and medial patellar tenderness. A defect in the medial patellar retinaculum may be felt. An osteochondral fracture occurring either at the time of dislocation or at reduction and loose fragments may or may not be visible on a radiograph. If present, they can cause symptoms of mechanical blocking or knee locking. Associated injuries such as anterior cruciate ligament rupture and medial meniscal injury have been reported and these should be assessed carefully.

RECURRENT TYPE

With recurrent subluxation, the intensity of pain and swelling is less than at the time of the initial injury. Quadriceps wasting is common and the patellar apprehension test is positive. This is elicited by pushing the patella laterally, which causes the patient anxiety and is often resisted. Patellar tracking should be assessed with the knee flexed over the edge of the examination couch. Other joints should be assessed for hyperlaxity.

RADIOGRAPHIC EVALUATION

The role of imaging the knee after an acute patellar dislocation serves two important functions in assisting management. First, it serves to detect intra-articular injuries such as osteochondral fractures and tears of the medial patellofemoral ligament (MPFL). In addition, it provides information on factors which may have predisposed the knee to injury, such as patella alta or trochlear dysplasia.

Plain radiography has been the traditional standard form of initial assessment. A standard four-view knee series, including a skyline or Merchant view, is recommended.

A true lateral radiograph is useful in the assessment of the Insall–Salvati index, which is the ratio of the patellar tendon length to the greatest diagonal length of the patella.

The axial Merchant view at 45° of flexion provides measurements of medial–lateral displacement such as the patellofemoral congruence angle.

CT scanning can be performed as a dynamic study and is highly effective in detecting patellar tracking anomalies, lateral patellar tilt and patellar subluxation in varying degrees of early knee flexion.

MRI provides a more accurate assessment of patellofemoral congruence than radiographs because of the difference between osseous and cartilaginous contours of the patella. MRI is also more sensitive in detecting chondral and osteochondral lesions as well as soft-tissue lesions such as injury to the MPFL.

TREATMENT OPTIONS

Acute dislocation

Conservative methods should be used whenever possible, which includes closed reduction, control of pain and swelling, physiotherapy and functional retraining.

Current indications for early operative treatment are controversial but an asymmetrical, subluxed patella or evidence of an intra-articular fragment are indications for operative treatment with repair of medial ligaments, lateral release and excision or internal fixation of the osteochondral fragment. Larger fragments, especially those involving the articular surfaces, should be fixed with biodegradable implants. Repair of the medial patellofemoral ligament and torn retinaculum should be performed anatomically with avoidance of overtensioning to prevent medial dislocation of the patella. The repair should be evaluated through a full range of movement to ensure stability, normal patellar tracking and proper tensioning of the repair.

Recurrent dislocation

Various surgical procedures have been described for recurrent dislocation; no single procedure has been shown to be superior to another. Factors such as the patient's age, functional needs, extent of malalignment and joint condition are important aspects to be considered prior to operative intervention.

Lateral retinacular release in isolation is inadequate and should always be accompanied by another procedure. Proximal realignment for patellofemoral instability specifically should include repair or reconstruction of the medial patellofemoral ligament.

Correcting dysplastic factors, in particular tibial tubercle transfers (such as the Roux–Goldthwait or Elmslie–Trillat procedures) and trochleoplasties, is best reserved for situations in which more minimal surgery has failed as it does not always yield better results. Arthroscopic procedures such as lateral release and a medial structure repair, as well as proximal realignment procedures, have been described.[7]

The subjective result of operative treatment is better and the redislocation rate is lower if the mechanism of injury is traumatic rather than non-traumatic and if there is no family history of patellar dislocation.

GENU VARUM AND VALGUM

INTRODUCTION

The normal anatomical alignment of the lower limb in a skeletally mature individual is such that the mechanical axis (that runs from the centre of the femoral head to the centre of the ankle joint) bisects the knee when the person stands erect with the patellae facing forwards. However, in normal young children, this is not the case as, with growth, the alignment of the limb deviates considerably from this adult pattern (Table 67.2).

It is important to be aware of the fact that the limb alignment changes in this manner in normal children and that the varus or valgus deformities noted at these specified ages should be regarded as physiological.Co

Rarely, without any demonstrable underlying pathology, physiological genu varum or valgum may not resolve and then some treatment may be needed.

CAUSES OF PATHOLOGICAL GENU VARUM AND VALGUM

Angular deformities at the knee may develop on account of pathology in the epiphysis, the physis or the metaphysis of the femur, the tibia or both (Table 67.3). It is important that the site of the deformity is identified in order to correct it as close to the site as possible. Occasionally, genu valgum may be encountered in the older child or adolescent without any obvious underlying cause (Fig. 67.1).

CONSEQUENCES OF GENU VARUM AND VALGUM

Genu varum and valgum result in abnormal loading of the joint and, if uncorrected, can predispose to degenerative arthritis. More severe degrees of deformity can cause the collateral ligament on the convex side of the deformity to stretch and this in turn will result in joint instability. Genu valgum also predisposes to patellar instability.

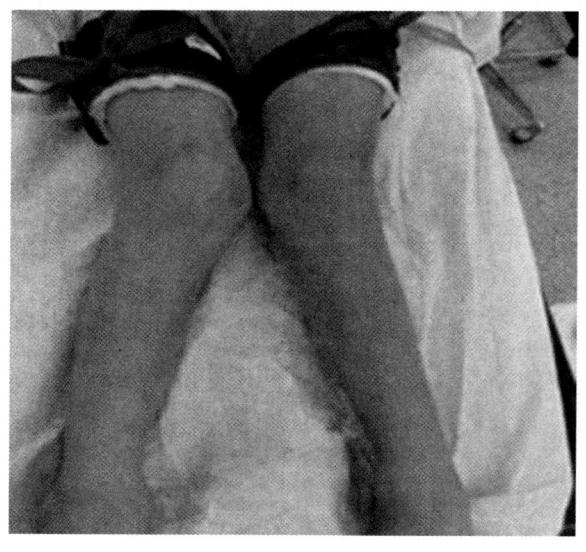

Figure 67.1 Appearance of a child with bilateral genu valgum.

Table 67.2 Normal lower limb alignment in children

Age	Normal knee alignment
At birth	Varus angulation of 10–15°
At 18 months to 2 years	Neutral alignment
At 3–4 years	Valgus angulation of 10–15°
At 10–12 years	Adult femorotibial alignment achieved (7° valgus)

Table 67.3 Aetiology of genu varum and valgum

Site	Pathology	Deformity	
		Genu varum	Genu valgum
Epiphysis	Partial destruction owing to septic arthritis in infancy	If medial half of femoral or tibial epiphysis is destroyed	If lateral half of the femoral or tibial epiphysis is destroyed
	Abnormal epiphysis in skeletal dysplasia		e.g. Ellis–van Creveld syndrome
	Abnormal epiphysis in association with congenital anomaly		e.g. hypoplastic lateral femoral condyle in association with fibular hemimelia (post- axial deficiency)
Physis	Rickets	Frequently seen	Frequently seen
	Blount disease	Commonly, abnormal growth of the medial side of the tibial physis	Rarely, the lateral side of the tibial physis may be affected
	Physeal bar following infection or trauma	Peripheral bar located on the medial side of the femur or tibia	Peripheral bar located on the lateral side of the femur or tibia
Metaphysis	Abnormal growth in skeletal dysplasia	e.g. metaphyseal chondrodysplasia	
	Tether in the metaphyseal region	Focal fibrocartilaginous dysplasia	e.g. osteochondroma, metaphyseal fracture (Cozen's fracture)
	Pathological bone in the metaphysis		e.g. fibrous dysplasia, Ollier disease

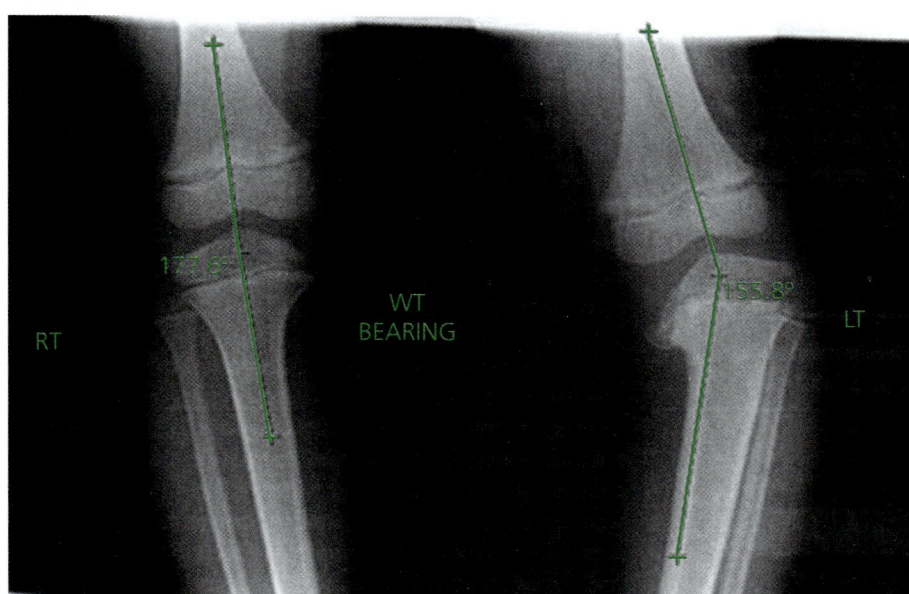

Figure 67.2 Anteroposterior view of the knee showing the genu varum of the left knee with medial tibial plateau depression in a child with Blount disease.

Abnormal loading of the knee in a child with genu varum due to early Blount disease can impair normal development of the epiphysis and physis. This contributes to progression of the deformity with the tibial condyle getting depressed (Fig. 67.2).

ASSESSMENT OF A CHILD WITH GENU VARUM OR VALGUM

If the underlying cause for the deformity is not evident, a careful clinical examination can help to elucidate the possible cause. Unilateral deformities are almost always pathological and the cause is likely to be local pathology in the femur or tibia. Bilateral symmetrical deformities are more likely to be the result of metabolic disorders or skeletal dysplasia, especially if associated with reduced stature.

The progression or resolution of bilateral deformity can be monitored on each visit by measuring the intercondylar distance for genu varum and the intermalleolar distance for genu valgum, without having to resort to radiographs on each visit. However, if surgery is being contemplated, a full-length weight-bearing radiograph is needed to plot the mechanical axis of each limb and to plan the corrective surgery.

Genu varum is often associated with internal tibial torsion, and this torsional deformity needs to be measured especially in unilateral cases as it would need to be addressed while correcting the angular deformity.

If a metabolic abnormality such as rickets is diagnosed, appropriate medical treatment must be instituted before embarking on any surgical intervention.

TREATMENT

Bracing

Bracing with a knee–ankle–foot orthosis may be effective in the young child with unresolved physiological genu varum and in very early Blount disease. It may also be effective in correcting mild deformities associated with active rickets while medical treatment for rickets is under way.

Physeal surgery

PHYSEAL BAR EXCISION

If a physeal bar occupies less than 25% of the surface area of the total physis, an attempt can be made to excise the bar provided there is sufficient growth left. Excision of the bar and interposition with fat may prevent progression of the deformity. Correction of the deformity may also be anticipated if the deformity is not severe to begin with. This procedure will not be effective if the child is very close to skeletal maturity.

TEMPORARY ARREST OF GROWTH

Temporary arrest of growth of the convex side of the deformity can be achieved by inserting staples or a small two-holed plate (8 plate) astride the physis and retaining the fixation until adequate correction of the deformity has been achieved. A screw placed across the physis can also have the same effect. Once the implants are removed, the physis resumes its growth.

PERMANENT EPIPHYSIODESIS

In children with large physeal bars that are not resectable, permanent epiphysiodesis of the viable part of the physis may be needed to prevent recurrence of the deformity after correction. This would result in limb length inequality which would then need to be addressed.

Corrective osteotomy

- Acute correction: with a closed-wedge osteotomy is the preferred treatment for bilateral deformities.
- Gradual correction.

BLOUNT DISEASE

INTRODUCTION

Blount disease,[8] or tibia vara, is a developmental condition characterized by disordered endochondral ossification of the medial part of the proximal tibial physis resulting in multiplanar deformities of the lower limb, including proximal tibial varus, procurvatum and internal rotation.[9]

Two major forms of this disease are recognized based on age of onset:[8,10] infantile tibia vara occurs before 4 years of age; late-onset tibia vara typically occurs after 6–8 years of age. Because of the inconsistency of descriptions of late-onset disease, Thompson and Carter[11] reclassified the late-onset group into juvenile onset (4–10 years) and adolescent onset (>10 years) to cover all age groups.

Infantile-onset tibia vara is more common than late-onset disease.[12] Bilateral cases are common in the infantile group.[13] There is significant racial variance with a predilection for obese Black children and Scandinavian children.[10,14]

Histopathologically, all forms of Blount disease share the same characteristics, the major differences between the groups being the age of onset, the amount of remaining growth and the magnitude of the medial compression forces across the proximal tibial physis which directly affects the options for treatment and outcome potential. Abnormalities of the proximal medial tibial physis include hypertrophic chondrocytes, acellular cartilage and abnormal groups of capillaries. This indicates that the asymmetric compression and shear forces acting across the proximal tibial physis result in suppression and deviation of normal endochondral ossification, thus leading to the deformities described.[11,15,16]

The first clinical issue is to discriminate which children with genu varum are normal physiological variants and which have a pathological cause for their deformity, as the former are most likely to correct spontaneously. Other differential diagnoses that must be considered are hypophosphataemic rickets, focal fibrocartilaginous dysplasia, metaphyseal chondrodysplasia and post-traumatic deformity. Blount disease is suspected in those children who are obese, often above the 95th percentile for weight, have a sharp angular deformity based at the medial proximal tibia and a lateral thrust when they walk. The rotational profile shows internal tibial torsion. Physiological genu varum, which is by far the most common of the differential diagnoses, tends to show a less angular deformity with a smoother transition from femur to tibia in the frontal plane without the lateral thrust. Imaging is critical in the diagnostic process.

A standing frontal plane radiograph of both legs with the patellae pointing forwards is the minimum standard of imaging required to correctly diagnose Blount disease.[13] Further radiographic analysis can then be undertaken with anteroposterior and lateral views of both tibiae and a scanogram. Characteristic features on radiograph demonstrate sharp varus angulation in the metaphysis, a widened and irregular physeal line medially, a medially sloped and irregularly ossified epiphysis and a prominent beaking of the medial metaphysis with lucent cartilage islands within the beak (Fig. 67.3).[12] The magnitude of the deformity can be calculated using the metaphyseal–diaphyseal angle of Levine and Drennan,[17] which can assist in identifying children at risk of developing infantile Blount disease. Levine and Drennan noted that a measurement of greater than 11° was indicative of an increased likelihood of progression. Other authors have made more detailed analyses of the usefulness of this measurement;[18] however, no radiographic measurement should be used in isolation. More importantly, clinical decisions should be made based on a combination of careful serial clinical and radiographic examinations.[9]

In 1952 Langenskiold[10] developed a six-stage classification system for infantile tibia vara based on a description of radiographic changes at the proximal tibia. This must also be interpreted with caution as it does not signify a natural history, sequential progression or prognostic indicator of

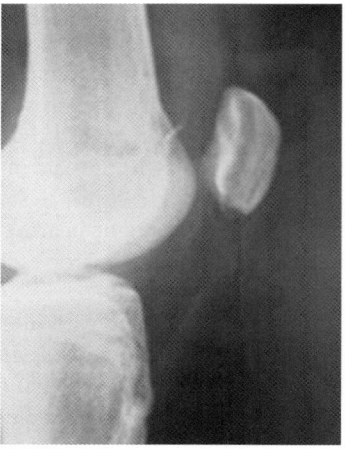

Figure 67.3 Lateral radiograph of the knee showing an osteochondral fragment at the distal femur.

the disease. Clinical deformity does not necessarily correlate to the Langenskiold stage.[19]

Untreated Blount disease produces a severe and progressive complex proximal tibial deformity of increasing varus, procurvatum, internal tibial torsion and growth retardation with associated joint deformity.[12]

The use of orthotics in infantile Blount disease is controversial.[9] An appropriate brace is a knee–ankle–foot orthosis locked in extension to unload the pathological medial physis. There are retrospective studies showing good results from this modality,[20,21] and also studies showing no improvement over the natural history.[22] The best results tend to occur in those in whom bracing is started early.[14,21] Inherent difficulties with a bracing programme for Blount disease include compliance with the orthosis, and, in the young age group in which a brace may be most successful, it may be difficult to distinguish physiological genu varum from true Blount disease. There is no place for the use of orthotics in late-onset disease.

For infantile Blount disease a variety of surgical treatments have been proposed, including resection of the physeal bar,[23] hemiepiphysiodesis,[24] guided growth[25] and medial plateau elevation.[26,27] The best evidence, however, is for a proximal tibial valgus and external rotational osteotomy with 10° of overcorrection performed before the age of 4 years (Fig. 67.4a,b).[12,28–30]

In late-onset disease the surgical procedures are more complex and the results less certain. After a full analysis of the three-dimensional deformity with respect to angulation, rotation and length, a reconstruction can be performed using a selection or combination of medial tibial plateau elevation,[26,27] completion proximal tibial epiphysiodesis, hemiepiphyseal stapling,[31] an acute or gradual proximal tibial multiplanar corrective osteotomy and lengthening using axial or circular external fixation.[9,11,28,32–38] A compensatory distal femoral deformity may be treated with hemiepiphysiodesis, guided growth or osteotomy.[39] Consideration may be given to the use of contralateral epiphysiodesis for the equalization of leg lengths.

KEY LEARNING POINTS

- There are two major groups of Blount disease: infantile and late onset.
- It is more common in obese Black children and Scandinavian children.
- The deformity occurs secondary to abnormal pressure over the medial proximal tibial physis.
- Radiographs are required for differentiation from physiological bowing.
- The natural history tends to a progressive deformity.
- Orthotic use is controversial.
- The surgical management depends on comprehensive deformity analysis.

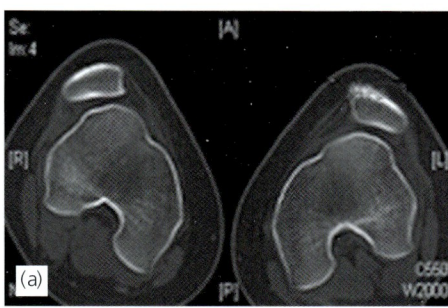
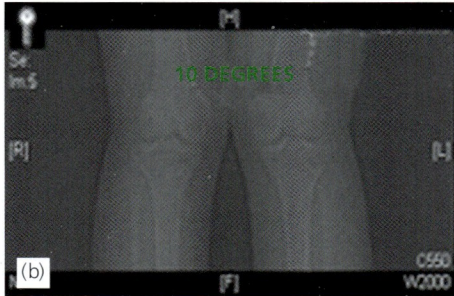

Figure 67.4 (a and b) Axial view CT scans of the knees in 10° flexion showing bilateral subluxation of the patella.

REFERENCES

- ● = Key primary paper
- ◆ = Major review article

1. Parsch K. [Ultrasound diagnosis of congenital knee dislocation]. *Der Orthopäde* 2002;**31**:306–7.
2. Kamata N, Takahashi T, Nakatani K, Yamamoto H. Ultrasonographic evaluation of congenital dislocation of the knee. *Skeletal Radiology* 2002;**31**:539–42.
3. Iwaya T, Sakaguchi R, Tsuyama N. The treatment of congenital dislocation of the knee with the Pavlik harness. *International Orthopaedics* 1983;**7**:25–30.
4. Bensahel H, Dal Monte A, Hjelmstedt A, et al. Congenital dislocation of the knee. *Journal of Pediatric Orthopaedics* 1989;**9**:174–7.
5. Schoenecker P, Rich M. The lower extremity. In: Morrissy R, Weinstein S (eds) *Lovell & Winter's Pediatric Orthopaedics*, 6th edn 2005, Philadelphia: Lippincott, Williams and Wilkins.
6. Gao GX, Lee EH, Bose K. Surgical management of congenital and habitual dislocation of the patella. *Journal of Pediatric Orthopaedics* 1990;**10**:255–60.
7. Roux C. Recurrent dislocation of the patella: operative treatment. *Clinical Orthopaedics and Related Research* 1979;**144**:4–8.

8. Blount W. Osteochondrosis deformans tibiae. *Journal of Bone and Joint Surgery* 1937;**19**:1–29.
9. Sabharwal S. Blount disease. *Journal of Bone and Joint Surgery (American)* 2009;**91**:1758–76.
10. Langenskiold A. Tibia vara (osteochondrosis deformans tibiae); a survey of 23 cases. *Acta Chirurgica Scandinavica* 1952;**103**:1–22.
11. Thompson GH, Carter JR. Late-onset tibia vara (Blount's disease). Current concepts. *Clinical Orthopaedics and Related Research* 1990;**255**:24–35.
12. Johnston 2nd CE. Infantile tibia vara. *Clinical Orthopaedics and Related Research* 1990;**255**:13–23.
13. Sabharwal S, Lee Jr J, Zhao C. Multiplanar deformity analysis of untreated Blount disease. *Journal of Pediatric Orthopaedics* 2007;**27**:260–5.
14. Loder RT, Johnston 2nd CE. Infantile tibia vara. *Journal of Pediatric Orthopaedics* 1987;**7**:639–46.
15. Trueta J, Trias A. The vascular contribution to osteogenesis. IV. The effect of pressure upon the epiphysial cartilage of the rabbit. *Journal of Bone and Joint Surgery (British)* 1961;**43B**:800–13.
16. Wenger DR, Mickelson M, Maynard JA. The evolution and histopathology of adolescent tibia vara. *Journal of Pediatric Orthopaedics* 1984;**4**:78–88.
17. Levine AM, Drennan JC. Physiological bowing and tibia vara. The metaphyseal-diaphyseal angle in the measurement of bowleg deformities. *Journal of Bone and Joint Surgery (American)* 1982;**64**:1158–63.
18. Feldman MD, Schoenecker PL. Use of the metaphyseal-diaphyseal angle in the evaluation of bowed legs. *Journal of Bone and Joint Surgery (American)* 1993;**75**:1602–9.
19. Langenskiold A. Tibia vara: osteochondrosis deformans tibiae. Blount's disease. *Clinical Orthopaedics and Related Research* 1981;**158**:77–82.
20. Zionts LE, Shean CJ. Brace treatment of early infantile tibia vara. *Journal of Pediatric Orthopaedics* 1998;**18**:102–9.
21. Raney EM, Topoleski TA, Yaghoubian R, et al. Orthotic treatment of infantile tibia vara. *Journal of Pediatric Orthopaedics* 1998;**18**:670–4.
22. Shinohara Y, Kamegaya M, Kuniyoshi K, Moriya H. Natural history of infantile tibia vara. *Journal of Bone and Joint Surgery (British)* 2002;**84**:263–8.
23. Andrade N, Johnston CE. Medial epiphysiolysis in severe infantile tibia vara. *Journal of Pediatric Orthopaedics* 2006;**26**:652–8.
24. Westberry DE, Davids JR, Pugh LI, Blackhurst D. Tibia vara: results of hemiepiphyseodesis. *Journal of Pediatric Orthopaedics B* 2004;**13**:374–8.
25. Stevens PM. Guided growth for angular correction: a preliminary series using a tension band plate. *Journal of Pediatric Orthopaedics* 2007;**27**:253–9.
26. Schoenecker PL, Johnston R, Rich MM, Capelli AM. Elevation of the medial plateau of the tibia in the treatment of Blount disease. *Journal of Bone and Joint Surgery (American)* 1992;**74**:351–8.
27. Jones S, Hosalkar HS, Hill RA, Hartley J. Relapsed infantile Blount's disease treated by hemiplateau elevation using the Ilizarov frame. *Journal of Bone and Joint Surgery (British)* 2003;**85**:565–71.
28. Miller S, Radomisli T, Ulin R. Inverted arcuate osteotomy and external fixation for adolescent tibia vara. *Journal of Pediatric Orthopaedics* 2000;**20**:450–4.
29. Rab GT. Oblique tibial osteotomy for Blount's disease (tibia vara). *Journal of Pediatric Orthopaedics* 1988;**8**:715–20.
30. Schoenecker PL, Meade WC, Pierron RL, et al. Blount's disease: a retrospective review and recommendations for treatment. *Journal of Pediatric Orthopaedics* 1985;**5**:181–6.
31. Park SS, Gordon JE, Luhmann SJ, et al. Outcome of hemiepiphyseal stapling for late-onset tibia vara. *Journal of Bone and Joint Surgery (American)* 2005;**87**:2259–66.
32. Gordon JE, Heidenreich FP, Carpenter CJ, et al. Comprehensive treatment of late-onset tibia vara. *Journal of Bone and Joint Surgery (American)* 2005;**87**:1561–70.
33. Price CT, Scott DS, Greenberg DA. Dynamic axial external fixation in the surgical treatment of tibia vara. *Journal of Pediatric Orthopaedics* 1995;**15**:236–43.
34. van Huyssteen AL, Hastings CJ, Olesak M, Hoffman EB. Double-elevating osteotomy for late-presenting infantile Blount's disease: the importance of concomitant lateral epiphysiodesis. *Journal of Bone and Joint Surgery (British)* 2005;**87**:710–15.
35. Stanitski DF, Dahl M, Louie K, Grayhack J. Management of late-onset tibia vara in the obese patient by using circular external fixation. *Journal of Pediatric Orthopaedics* 1997;**17**:691–4.
36. Alekberov C, Shevtsov VI, Karatosun V, et al. Treatment of tibia vara by the Ilizarov method. *Clinical Orthopaedics and Related Research* 2003;**409**:199–208.
37. Feldman DS, Madan SS, Ruchelsman DE, et al. Accuracy of correction of tibia vara: acute versus gradual correction. *Journal of Pediatric Orthopaedics* 2006;**26**:794–8.
38. Feldman DS, Madan SS, Koval KJ, et al. Correction of tibia vara with six-axis deformity analysis and the Taylor Spatial Frame. *Journal of Pediatric Orthopaedics* 2003;**23**:387–91.
39. Gordon JE, King DJ, Luhmann SJ, et al. Femoral deformity in tibia vara. *Journal of Bone and Joint Surgery (American)* 2006;**88**:380–6.

68

Disorders of the leg in children

STANLEY JONES, SUNIL BAJAJ, NICOLAS NICOLAOU, JAMES A FERNANDES, KIRAN AN SALDANHA

TORSIONAL AND BOWING DEFORMITIES OF THE TIBIA	673	LIMB LENGTH INEQUALITY	677
Tibial torsion	673	Introduction	677
Congenital posteromedial bowing of tibia	674	Aetiology	678
CONGENITAL PSEUDARTHROSIS OF THE TIBIA	675	Assessment of leg length discrepancy	678
Introduction	675	Imaging	679
Incidence and aetiology	675	Prediction of leg length discrepancy	679
Clinical features	675	Treatment	680
Classification	675	References	685
Treatment	676		

NATIONAL BOARD STANDARDS

- Learn torsional and bowing deformities of the tibia
- Know congenital posteromedial bowing of the tibia
- Understand congenital pseudarthrosis of the tibia

TORSIONAL AND BOWING DEFORMITIES OF THE TIBIA

TIBIAL TORSION

Rotational problems of the lower extremity in children are a common cause of parental anxiety, causing them to seek a consultation with the orthopaedic surgeon. It is important to realize that the majority of them are physiological or postural problems, affecting both lower extremities in a symmetrical fashion.

The rotational profile in toddlers and children shows a great degree of variation. Variations within 2 standard deviations (SD) of the mean are referred to as version, whereas variations more than 2SD from the mean are called torsion.

Tibial torsion or version is measured as the angle between the transmalleolar axis of the ankle and the bicondylar axis of the knee. Tibial torsion can be external or internal.[1–3] Internal tibial torsion is more commonly seen in infants, whereas external tibial torsion is more common in older children.

Aetiology of tibial torsion

- Intra-uterine malposition: abnormal internal tibial torsion in infants is thought to be the result of intra-uterine malposition as preterm infants do not exhibit internal tibial torsion.
- There is an undocumented relationship between abnormal sitting (sitting in the W position) or sleeping posture (prone sleeping) with tibial torsion.
- Neuromuscular conditions such as myelodysplasia or poliomyelitis are associated with tibial torsion.
- Tibial torsion can result from traumatic causes such as malunited tibial fractures.

- Tibial torsion may be familial, stressing the need to obtain a proper family history and conduct a parental examination in all such cases.

Examination of a child with tibial torsion

- Tibial torsion presents as in-toeing (internal tibial torsion) or out-toeing (external tibial torsion).
- Examination starts with a good history, especially enquiring about any rotational problems in the family.
- A rotational profile examination should be undertaken in any child with tibial torsion.

Examination starts by observing the child walk, looking for abnormalities in gait and foot progression angle (the angle created by the long axis of the foot in relation to the line of progression when walking). It ranges from −5° to 20°. Tibial torsion would result in values outside this range.

With the child lying prone and the knee flexed to 90°, the feet can be examined for metatarsus adductus and the thigh–foot angle can be measured (angle between the long axis of the femur and the heel bisector line). The thigh–foot angle is a measure of tibial version and normal values range from 0° to 20°. Examination of the child prone is the best way to determine the site of torsional deformity.[2,4]

The transmalleolar axis is measured with the child in a sitting position by comparing the transcondylar axis of the tibia with the bimalleolar axis.

Femoral anteversion is then assessed by examining the range of rotation at the hip joint. This is also best done with the child prone. Internal rotation of more than 70° and external rotation of less than 20° indicates excessive femoral anteversion. The Gages test also helps to determine femoral anteversion.

Radiology

A single anteroposterior radiograph of the pelvis is advisable to exclude other conditions such as developmental dysplasia of the hip and slipped upper femoral epiphysis, which can also present with rotational problems.

CT scans to measure the amount of tibial torsion may be helpful if surgery is considered, as these have been shown to be more accurate than clinical examination.[5]

Treatment

The natural history of rotational variation in long bones is spontaneous correction by 5–6 years in the vast majority of children.[6] The mainstay of treatment is observation and parental education. Orthoses, insoles and positioning devices are of no benefit. Instead, they increase parental anxiety[6] and frustration or may result in a secondary deformity.[7]

Surgical correction is rare and is indicated when there is a significant persistent rotational abnormality in children 8 years and older.[1,2,8] A tibial derotation osteotomy, preferably at the supramalleolar level, may be undertaken. An osteotomy of the fibula may not be necessary if the correction required is less than 20°.

CONGENITAL POSTEROMEDIAL BOWING OF TIBIA

Congenital posteromedial bowing of the tibia is a non-dysplastic benign condition which usually resolves spontaneously with time. It must be differentiated from two other forms of tibial bowing, namely anterolateral bowing commonly seen in neurofibromatosis and anteromedial bowing typical of fibular hemimelia.

Clinical features

The tibial deformity (posteromedial bow) is usually unilateral and recognizable at birth. It is associated with a calcaneovalgus deformity of the foot. The calf of the affected leg is usually smaller in size, with weakness of the triceps surae. A dimple may be seen at the apex of the angulation. In addition to the angulation, the affected limb may be shorter.

Natural history

There is a tendency towards spontaneous resolution of the deformity (especially the posterior bow) with time. Resolution is rapid within the first 6 months and slows down after 1 year. Tibial angulation usually corrects by the age of 2 years. The foot deformity resolves earlier and resolution may be complete by 9 months.

However, residual angular deformity may persist in children with severe bowing with shortening of the limb. The amount of shortening varies, and average shortening is 13% of the total limb length.[9,10] An association between the degree of shortening and the severity of the medial bow has been suggested by Shah et al.[11]

Radiological features

Radiographs of the affected leg show posteromedial bowing of the tibia and fibula. The bone structure is normal without any abnormal fibrocystic lesions or medullary sclerosis, but there may be increased thickness of the cortex on the concave side of the bow, in keeping with Wolff's law.

Abnormalities of fibular length, eccentric ossification and abnormal wedging of distal tibial epiphysis have been reported by Shah et al.[11]

Treatment

Initial treatment in the newborn involves gentle stretching of the ankle to overcome the dorsiflexion contracture and stretch out the tight lateral ankle structures. This can be done by the parents.

If the deformity is more severe, serial casting of the ankle into plantarflexion may be tried. Once a plantigrade position is achieved, the correction is maintained by splints, until the child starts weight bearing.

Corrective osteotomy may be needed if there is no resolution of the bowing by 4 years old. Bone healing after osteotomy is normal without the risk of pseudarthrosis.

Leg length discrepancy of more than 2 cm (2–5 cm) may be managed by epiphysiodesis of the longer limb. Limb length discrepancy of more than 5 cm should be managed by lengthening of the shorter limb.

Residual valgus angulation of the ankle due to a wedge-shaped distal tibial epiphysis may require medial hemiepiphysiodesis. This is achieved by percutaneous insertion of a screw across the medial malleolar physis.

CONGENITAL PSEUDARTHROSIS OF THE TIBIA

INTRODUCTION

The term congenital pseudarthrosis of the tibia (CPT) is in itself misleading. A pseudarthrosis is defined as a 'false joint' occurring at the site of a fracture. In this condition, there is an underlying abnormality within the tibia itself that predisposes to fracture within the first 2 years of life, subsequently forming a pseudarthrosis. This is one of the most difficult lesions to treat surgically and it is exceedingly difficult to achieve union.

INCIDENCE AND AETIOLOGY

CPT is a rare condition affecting approximately 1 in 200 000 live births.[12–15] The cause remains elusive, but the underlying defect may be due to defective tibial periosteum.[16] Alteration in perfusion leads to the poor healing characteristics of the bone. An example of this theory comes from congenital constriction band syndrome,[17–19] in which pseudarthrosis has been successfully treated with excision of the constricting band, restoring the periosteal blood supply.

Around 50% of patients with CPT will have neurofibromatosis (NF),[12] although less than 10% of those with neurofibromatosis will have CPT. The strong association of CPT with NF may be explained by observations in mouse models. The *NF1* tumour suppressor gene produces neurofibromin. This gene is altered in neurofibromatosis, leading to changes in osteoblast, osteoclast, vascular endothelial cell and fibroblast function.[20–22] This may also explain the association that exists between fibrous dysplasia and CPT.

CLINICAL FEATURES

At birth, a fracture is rarely present; the classical finding is a bowed tibia with the apex lying anterolaterally. The deformity may be associated with a skin dimple, limb shortening and dysplasia of the fibula or fifth ray and ankle valgus. It is usually unilateral. The presence of café-au-lait spots should raise the suspicion of neurofibromatosis, although their absence does not exclude this diagnosis as the spots may appear later.

Radiographs are performed to identify the nature and site of the pseudarthrosis, which is normally in the middle to distal third; in addition, mechanical axis views identify associated shortening and deviation from the normal axis. Many different features may be seen, some of which form the basis of classification.

CLASSIFICATION

Various classification systems based on the radiographic morphology exist.[13,14,23,24] There is no universally agreed system based on both the clinical features and radiographic findings. Of the available systems, the Boyd and Andersen classifications are most frequently used, each having six categories. The different systems do not give a guide as to the best form of treatment and so have limited value. The radiographic appearances described can also change during the course of the disease. The dysplastic types identified in all three of the classification systems described are associated with poorer results of treatment (Table 68.1).

Table 68.1 Classification of congenital pseudarthrosis of the tibia

Crawford classification	Andersen classification	Boyd classification
Non-dysplastic type I. Anterolateral bowing with increased density and sclerosis of medullary canal *Dysplastic type* II. Anterolateral bowing with failure of tubularization III. Cystic changes IV. Frank pseudarthrosis	I. Club foot II. Cystic III. Late IV. Fibular V. Dysplastic VI. Angulated	I. Fracture present at birth II. Hourglass constriction of tibia III. Bone cysts IV. Sclerotic segment of tibia V. Dysplastic fibula VI. Intra-osseous neurofibroma

TREATMENT

For a relatively rare condition, there is a large number of treatment options described. Few disorders cause so much difficulty in obtaining union and as a result success rates for many described techniques in CPT are poor. The complexity is compounded by the risk of re-fracture after obtaining union. This re-fracture risk does fall with increasing age, although a re-fracture can occur even after skeletal maturity. Added challenges include the associated risk of damage to the physis, leading to further deformity and the difficulty of internal and external fixation of small bones in the skeletally immature patient. In essence, a number of factors in addition to the poor healing quality of bone need to be taken in to consideration.

Principles of treatment

The principal aim of treatment of anterolateral bowing prior to fracture and development of a pseudarthrosis is to prevent or delay their occurrence for as long as possible. Splinting has been shown to be effective in some instances if continued until skeletal maturity.

The first goal for an established pseudarthrosis is to obtain bony union. Other goals are to prevent re-fracture, minimize subsequent skeletal deformity, optimize lower limb function and prevent symptomatic leg length discrepancy. There is controversy regarding the age at which surgery should be carried out once the fracture occurs, with some authors suggesting that delaying treatment improves union rates.[12]

The pathological bone and the associated hamartomatous material at the site of the pseudarthrosis must be fully excised if treatment is to be successful. At the same time, it is important to balance this principle with preservation of as much bone stock as possible to facilitate reconstruction.

Free vascularized fibular grafting

This form of treatment utilizes a free fibular graft, normally from the contralateral limb,[25] or in some cases from the same side.[26] The graft is harvested with an intact vascular pedicle, and, using microsurgical techniques, is anastomosed to the local blood supply with internal fixation and with or without stabilization using external fixation. This form of surgery is complicated and requires long operating times and two surgical teams to prepare both the graft and the pseudarthrosis. Donor site morbidity must also be considered, and for technical reasons it is difficult to perform in small children. Union rates with this technique are reportedly as high as 95%.[27,28]

Intramedullary fixation and grafting

This approach has the advantage of being relatively easy to perform and allows internal splintage of the affected tibia, thereby preventing re-fracture after union (Figs 68.1–68.3). Its use can be applied in children less than 3 years old,[29] and by promoting early union lessens the risk of deformity occurring with growth. The procedure requires excision of the pseudarthrosis and shortening of the bone with subsequent intramedullary fixation.[30–32] To stimulate union, cortical or cancellous grafts are used, with cortical grafts recommended. More recently, bone metalloproteinases have been used with good results.[33]

Many techniques require transfixing of the ankle joint, which can be associated with significant stiffness, but this transfixion may prevent later ankle deformity. The rods used require changing to a larger size as growth occurs or by using elongating rods. Union rates with this technique are high, in some series 85% or more; this remains the initial treatment of choice in most centres.[34]

External fixation and distraction osteogenesis

Some of the best results published come from use of this complicated and time-consuming technique,[35–38] which

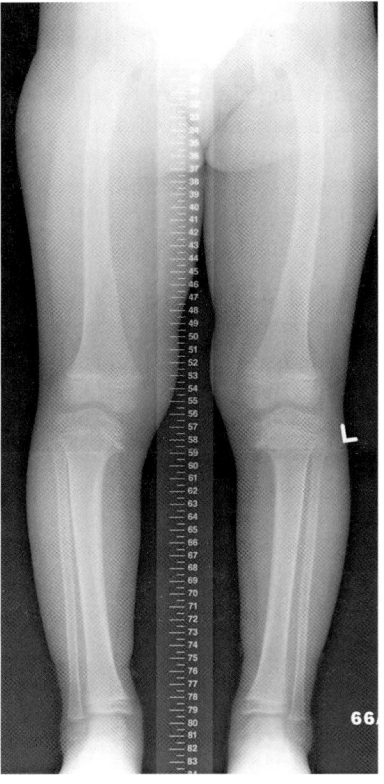

Figure 68.1 Dysplastic congenital pseudarthrosis of the tibia.

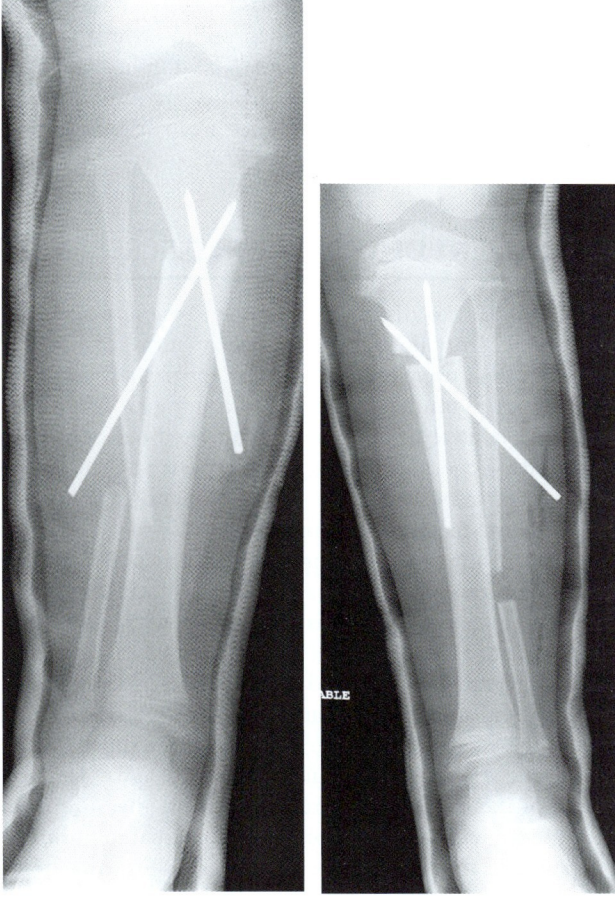

Figure 68.2 Intramedullary fixation and grafting.

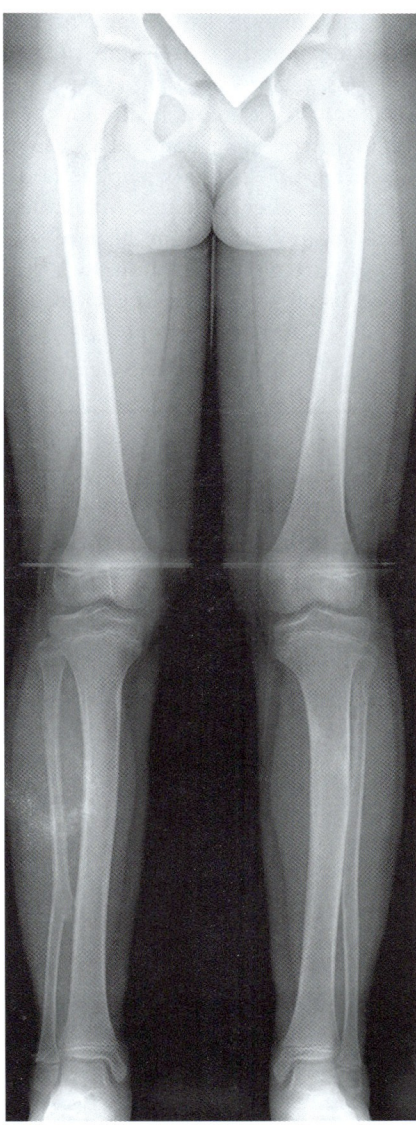

Figure 68.3 Union after intramedullary fixation and grafting.

has the added advantage of allowing concomitant lengthening and deformity correction. The pseudarthrosis is excised; the bone ends compressed; and lengthening performed via a proximal osteotomy. Re-fracture is a problem;[39] rates are higher in younger patients.

Treatment outcomes

Some patients will respond poorly to treatment, and amputation must always be considered in severe cases where multiple operations have already failed. In such cases disarticulation at the ankle gives good results as opposed to amputation through the pseudarthrosis.

At skeletal maturity, 67% of patients will be unlimited in walking distance, 40% will require bracing of the affected extremity and only 30% will have normal ankle function. Despite the numerous techniques available, this highlights the difficulty in obtaining good results in this complicated condition.[40]

LIMB LENGTH INEQUALITY

INTRODUCTION

Minor discrepancies in leg length between 0.5 and 1.5 cm can be found in one-third of the normal asymptomatic population.[41,42] Leg length inequality or discrepancy (LLD) less than 2 cm, if symptomatic, is best treated by a small heel raise or shoe raise. There is no consensus regarding the threshold beyond which treatment is indicated. While discrepancies less than 2.3 cm result in slight gait asymmetry,[43] discrepancies of 2.5 cm or more will result in postural imbalance and uneven gait, generally characterized by increased loading on the longer limb. LLD has been implicated in excessive stress on hip or knee joints, resulting in osteoarthritis of these joints in the longer leg. There are reports of an increased incidence of leg length inequality in patients with chronic low-back pain,[44,45] and also amelioration of back pain after leg length equalization procedures. LLD has also been implicated in the development of scoliosis and lower extremity dysfunction, such as stress fractures, plantar fasciitis or parapatellar knee pain.

AETIOLOGY

Causes of LLD can be congenital, developmental or acquired. Congenital causes are those in which the discrepancy is apparent at birth. They include congenital longitudinal lower limb deficiencies (i.e. proximal femoral focal deficiency, fibular deficiency, tibial hemimelia), idiopathic hemihypertrophy or hemiatrophy (anisomelia) and secondary to myelomeningocele and spinal dysraphism (Fig. 68.4).

Developmental causes in which the discrepancy evolves with growth include congenital clubfoot deformity, enchondromatosis, osteochondromatosis, neurofibromatosis with gigantism, congenital pseud-arthrosis of the tibia, melorheostosis or vascular anomalies such as Klippel–Trénaunay–Weber syndrome. Acquired causes include physeal growth disturbance from trauma, infection, tumour and irradiation.

ASSESSMENT OF LEG LENGTH DISCREPANCY

It is important to distinguish between true and apparent shortening. In true shortening, one or more of the segments in the lower limb is short. In apparent shortening, there is an asymmetry in the positioning of one lower extremity relative to the other due to fixed deformities of the joints. True shortening is due to structural causes, whereas apparent shortening is due to functional (postural) causes. Some patients may have both.

The amount of shortening can be estimated by having the patient stand with graduated blocks (block test) under the shorter leg until the pelvis is level (Fig. 68.5). When the patient is not able to stand, it can be assessed in the supine position by drawing the child's legs parallel in an extended position and noting the relative levels of the soles of the feet or the medial malleoli or by flexing the hips 90° and noting the relative knee height (Galeazzi's sign). The true length of the limb is measured with a tape measure from the anterior superior iliac spine to the medial joint line of the knee and to the tip of the medial malleolus while hold-

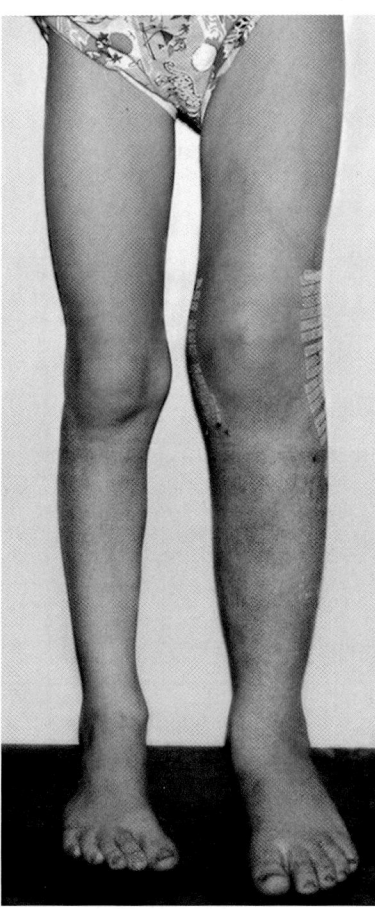

Figure 68.4 Left-sided syndromic hemihypertrophy secondary to neurofibromatosis.

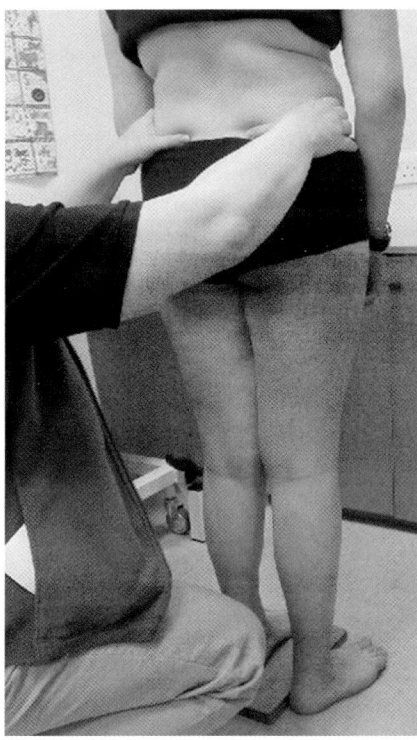

Figure 68.5 Block test to measure limb length inequality.

ing the legs in symmetric positions at the hips, knees and feet. Apparent length is measured from the umbilicus to the medial malleolus.

When the patient walks, compensatory mechanisms such as circumduction of the long leg, vaulting over the long leg, excessive flexion of the hip and knee of the long leg, or toe-walking on the short leg are noted.[46]

IMAGING

Accurate measurements of the limbs and the individual femoral and tibial segments can be done by radiographic methods. One should not forget to take into account discrepancy of length in the pelvic and submalleolar segments. The following methods are used.

- *Teleroentgenograph.* With the patient supine, a radiograph of the entire lower extremity is obtained on a long film under the patient using a single exposure centred on the limbs.
- *Orthoroentgenograph.* A long film is placed under the patient and three exposures are made centred at the hip, knee and ankle level without moving the patient or the film.[47] This reduces the magnification error that can occur with a single exposure in a teleroentgenograph. This technique can also be used in a weight-bearing position so that angular deformities, mechanical axis deviations and limb length can be assessed simultaneously.[48]
- *Scanogram.* Scanogram differs from orthoroentgenograph in that, in addition to the radiographic tube being moved over the patient for three exposures, the film is moved under the patient, thus reducing the size of the film required (Fig. 68.6).
- *CT.* This can be performed with lower radiation exposure and greater accuracy.[49] It can be used also when there are positioning difficulties secondary to joint contractures or in the presence of external fixators.

PREDICTION OF LEG LENGTH DISCREPANCY

In a skeletally immature child, eventual leg length discrepancy at maturity depends on the rate at which each bone is growing. Prediction of leg length discrepancy at maturity can be made using one of the several methods.

Anderson–Green–Messner growth-remaining charts

Anderson, Green and Messner examined longitudinal growth data obtained in 100 children (50 boys and 50 girls), who were assessed at least once a year in the 8 years before their growth terminated, and published data on the longitudinal growth of the femur and tibia.[50,51] The annual rate of

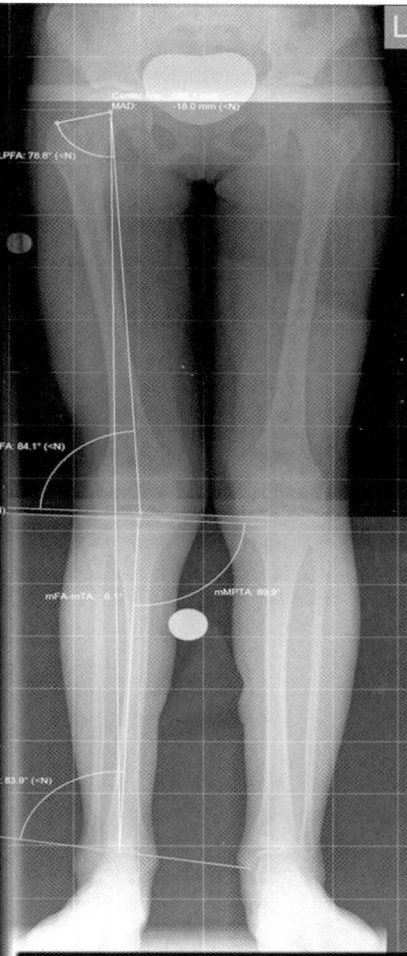

Figure 68.6 Scanogram to measure leg lengths and deformity planning.

overall growth (stature) rapidly decreased from birth to age 6 years, and was stable from age 6 to age 9 years (average stature increment 5.7 cm). Femoral length increased at an average annual rate of 2.0 cm, and tibial length increased at an average annual rate of 1.6 cm. A pubertal growth spurt typically occurred sometime after age 9 (usually reaching a maximum between 10 and 12 years of age in girls and between 12 and 14 years of age in boys). This was followed by a final 4 year period of rapid decline in the rate of growth until cessation of growth. The age at which the growth spurt occurred varied from one child to the next.

In general, growth continued for 2 years after the adolescent growth spurt, irrespective of the age at which it occurred. By noting the length of each of the 100 femora and tibiae at specific equally spaced skeletal ages, Anderson and colleagues derived increments of growth of the entire femur and tibia and the growth at the specific physes using figures for the proportional contribution of growth obtained from the semilongitudinal study of sharply delineated growth arrest lines on consecutive radiographs. They found that 71% of femoral growth occurred distally and 57% of tibial growth occurred proximally. These results were then used to compile the growth-remaining charts for boys and girls in the distal femur and proximal tibia.

Menelaus method

West and Menelaus[52] modified the previously reported White and Stubbins[53] method. This method (rule of thumb) is based on the assumptions that the distal femur and proximal tibia grow at the rate of 9 mm and 6 mm per year, respectively, and that the cessation of growth in boys occurs at age 16 and in girls at age 14.

Moseley straight-line graph

Moseley[54] constructed a graph based on a mathematical reanalysis of Anderson and colleagues' chronological growth data on the length of the femur and tibia. He represented the growth of the legs by straight lines by a suitable manipulation of the scale of the abscissa. As a consequence, with the nomogram of skeletal age to correct for percentile growth, the growth of the short leg is represented as a straight line and the leg length inequality is represented as the vertical distance between the lines; the line indicating the growth of the shorter leg has a less steep slope than that of the longer leg.

Paley multiplier method

Paley and co-workers[55] identified an arithmetic factor (multiplier) by dividing femoral and tibial lengths at skeletal maturity by the femoral and tibial lengths at different ages during growth for each percentile group using a variety of available leg length databases. The length of each leg and the difference in leg length at maturity (assuming constant growth inhibition) can be calculated by multiplying these measurements by the appropriate multiplier for the subject's age and gender.

There are potential inaccuracies in using these methods to calculate growth remaining. Identifying the cause of leg length inequality in children is important for determining the ultimate discrepancy at skeletal maturity. Shapiro[56] pointed out that not all growth inhibition in growing children is linear (i.e. results in a constant percentage of growth inhibition or acceleration in the affected limb). He described five basic patterns of leg length inequality development based on an assessment of discrepancy development in 803 patients. Type 1 is an upward slope pattern, implying a stable percentage of growth inhibition compared with the normal leg, e.g. proximal femoral focal deficiency, Ollier disease (enchondromatosis), congenital femoral deficiency with more than 6 cm of shortening, physeal obliteration from any cause, and poliomyelitis. Type 2 is characterized by an upward slope–deceleration pattern, e.g. some patients with congenital femoral deficiency with less than 6 cm of shortening or with poliomyelitis. Type 3 is characterized by an upward or downward slope–plateau pattern, most typical of post-femoral shaft fracture overgrowth. Type 4 is an upward slope–plateau–upward slope pattern and was seen only in abnormalities involving the proximal femur, such as septic arthritis, Legg–Perthes disease and avascular necrosis (AVN) associated with the treatment of developmental dysplasia of the hip. Type 5 is characterized by an upward slope–plateau–downward slope pattern, meaning that an initially increasing discrepancy actually decreases with subsequent growth.

Anderson and colleagues used skeletal age determined by using the Greulich and Pyle atlas[57] for bone age based on hand and wrist radiographs, but noted that assessments from the elbow, hip, knee and foot can also be used, as well as physical maturation parameters (such as the Tanner stages of development). They suggested that more precise estimates of future growth in an individual child could be made by using skeletal rather than chronological age, particularly in children whose level of maturation was consistently advanced or retarded 2 years or more compared with their chronological age. Little and colleagues[58] found that use of Greulich and Pyle's atlas and either the Anderson–Green–Messner charts or Moseley's straight-line graph did not improve the accuracy of prediction using the Menelaus method alone, which is based on chronological age. The modified Sauvegrain method of assessing skeletal age is also a simple reliable reproducible method,[59] and the TW3 (Tanner Whitehouse) method using hand and wrist radiographs is supposedly quite accurate.[60]

TREATMENT

Leg length discrepancy expected to be greater than 2–2.5 cm at maturity has been traditionally considered an indication for length equalization,[61] whereas most patients with less than 2 cm discrepancy have not needed any treatment. Discrepancy of more than 5% corresponding to approximately 4 cm at skeletal maturity is associated with alterations in gait mechanism and energy consumption.[46] Therefore, this should be considered an absolute level above which limb length equalization by some means should be attempted. The options are use of orthoses, shortening of longer leg and lengthening of shorter leg.

Orthoses

Shoe lifts can be considered for discrepancies more than 2 cm. Although there is no clear upper limit, shoe lifts greater than 8 cm are not well tolerated and may make the ankle unstable. Ankle–foot orthoses incorporating shoe lifts can be used to stabilize the ankle. Extension prosthesis is another alternative in non-surgical management of large leg length discrepancies.

Shortening procedures

Shortening of the long leg in a child is achieved by inducing growth arrest either permanently by epiphysiodesis or temporarily by epiphyseal stapling or plating. In an adult, this is achieved by acute shortening procedures.

INDUCED GROWTH ARREST

Epiphysiodesis

Phemister[62] first described the technique of epiphysiodesis (physiodesis probably more accurate) in which a piece of cortex was removed at the level of the growth plate and replaced with its ends reversed after excising the underlying epiphysis to a depth of 1 cm. More commonly, epiphysiodesis is now performed using Canale et al.'s[63] percutaneous drilling technique.

Growth can also be stopped temporarily or permanently by using epiphyseal stapling, transphyseal screws or '8' plates.

Epiphyseal stapling

Blount and Clark[64] recommended placing three evenly spaced staples extraperiosteally with their tines parallel to the physis. He noted that growth of the physis was the same as the other side after removal. Although, theoretically, removal of staples after correction in a skeletally immature patient should be followed by symmetric normal growth in practice, complications of rebound overgrowth requiring further intervention or the absence of growth, resulting in overcorrection of the leg length inequality, new angular deformity or reverse angular deformity, can occur. Even when the patient reaches skeletal maturity without requiring staple removal or a readjustment in management, staples frequently need to be removed because of soft-tissue irritation from staple prominence, extrusion or displacement into the joint.

Transphyseal screws

Métaizeau and colleagues[65] have described reversible growth arrest using percutaneously inserted transphyseal screws (Fig. 68.7). Cannulated fully or partially threaded cancellous screws can be used in either crossed or uncrossed fashion for the femur and tibia. As with staples, screws can be removed after correction has been achieved, but there is some possibility of permanent growth arrest or rebound effect, especially if done at the younger age.

'8' plates

Stevens[66] described a technique of guided growth using '8' plates across the physis in a similar fashion to staples. Growth can be temporarily stopped using plates on the medial and lateral sides of the physis. Angular deformity can be corrected by using an '8' plate on one side of the physis. Compared with staples, there is a lower possibility of extrusion of '8' plates and the removal of plates is easier.

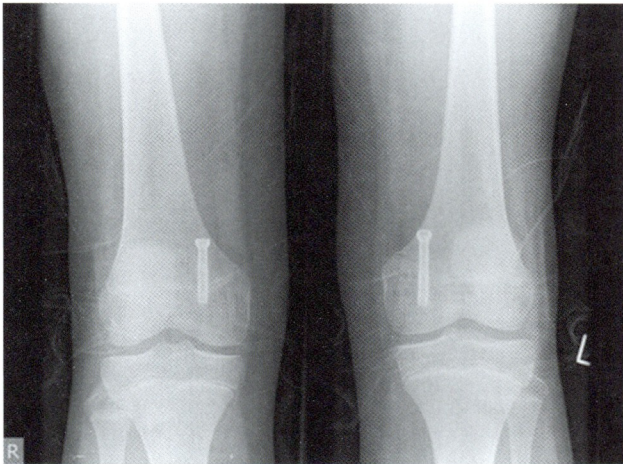

Figure 68.7 Métaizeau technique of hemiepiphysiodesis using screws, final corrected result.

ACUTE SHORTENING

If the height is adequate, acute shortening of bone is a reasonable option for length equalization in skeletally mature patients.

Acute femoral shortening is preferable when the discrepancy is localized to the femur in order to maintain symmetric knee height. Shortening can be undertaken in the proximal femur at subtrochanteric level using either a blade plate or contoured compression screw plate, in the mid-diaphyseal level using a plate or intramedullary rod and in the distal metaphyseal level using a compression screw plate. Closed intramedullary shortening can be performed using an intramedullary saw or by a percutaneous method with diaphyseal osteotomies (Fig. 68.8), splitting of the intercalary segment and insertion of a locked intramedullary rod.[67] Significant technical problems include difficulty completing the osteotomy using the cam-deployed intramedullary saw, particularly posteriorly at the linea aspera; fragmentation and displacement of the intercalary bone segment; and rotational malalignment and distraction at the osteotomy site. AVN of the femoral head after intramedullary rod insertion in the piriformis fossa in skeletally immature patients and fat embolism are other serious potential complications.

Weakness of hamstrings and quadriceps occurs at least temporarily after femoral shortening and limits the extent of shortening that should be undertaken. Significant weakness occurs when the shortening is more than 10% of the original length at mid-diaphyseal level, but at the subtrochanteric level muscle weakness is not a significant problem, even when the shortening is 12–15% of original length. Distal metaphyseal shortening is less desirable because of the incongruity of the bone segments after shortening owing to the funnel shape of the distal femur. Therefore, in the absence of deformity, open or closed

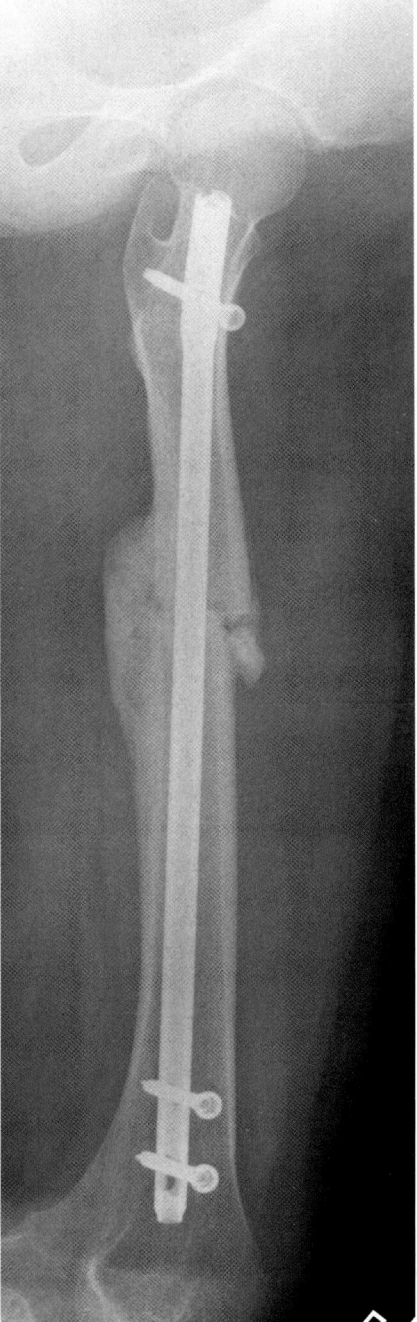

Figure 68.8 Acute femoral shortening using percutaneous diaphyseal osteotomies and stabilization using trochanteric entry locking intramedullary adolescent nail.

subtrochanteric shortening is preferable to either mid-diaphyseal or distal metaphyseal shortening. When there is associated deformity, osteotomy for angular correction and shortening can be performed at the level of the deformity.

Acute tibial shortening has major potential complications, including compartment syndrome, circulatory impediment, foot weakness and non-union. This precludes its common use for limb length equalization. The procedure must be performed in an open fashion because the intercalary bone fragment must be extracted from the leg and the fibula must be osteotomized to allow shortening of the limb segment. Gradual shortening using an external fixator after excising a segment is an option, but this is a prolonged, cumbersome procedure with complications of the fixator and delayed docking site healing.

Limb-lengthening procedures

Despite the improvements in limb-lengthening techniques, the complications of limb lengthening exceed those of epiphysiodesis or acute shortening. Although the parents and patients would usually prefer to focus on methods of lengthening the shorter limb, it is important to counsel them that the purpose of treatment is primarily to maximize function and mobility and secondarily to address cosmetic concerns to the extent possible. The compensatory mechanisms for a short extremity begin to break down with the development of the strategy of toe-walking, which generally occurs when limb shortening reaches 5% of the contralateral limb (approximately 4 cm in a patient with 50th percentile length in the tibia and femur). Thus, an expected limb length inequality of 4 cm can be considered a relative indication for leg lengthening. When the expected shortening approaches 10% (8 cm), leg lengthening should be considered in preference to shortening of the longer leg because attempting to correct discrepancies of this magnitude by shortening procedures may be excessive. Angular deformities requiring correction when associated with ipsilateral shortening can also be considered a relative indication for limb lengthening.

Timing of lengthening depends on the expected limb length discrepancy at maturity. Whenever leg length discrepancy is 10% or less of the contralateral limb, lengthening is best performed around skeletal maturity to avoid any subsequent growth disturbance and to allow for a more precise estimation of the amount of lengthening required. If a greater discrepancy is anticipated, and the expected overall height at maturity is adequate, a combined lengthening with an appropriately timed contralateral epiphysiodesis should be performed. If contralateral epiphysiodesis is not an acceptable option, staged lengthenings of 15–20% of the original length of the bone should be considered.

Historically, Codivilla[68] is credited with the earliest description of limb lengthening using traction on the osteotomized femur, followed by incorporation of the limb in plaster. Others, including Putti, Abbott, Bosworth and Anderson, have reported variations of this technique for limb lengthening. Wagner[69] described a technique using fixation of a lengthening device to bone with Schanz pins, diaphyseal osteotomy and acute lengthening of 1 cm followed by gradual, continued lengthening at a rate of 1–2 mm per day and second stage plating and bone grafting of the osteotomy. Significant advances in the technique of limb lengthening using external fixation were made by Ilizarov[70–72] and De Bastiani et al.[73–75] They recommended gradual distraction either across the physis (chondrodiatasis) or after low-energy osteotomy or corticotomy (callotasis).

The options for limb lengthening are stimulation of natural growth, acute lengthening and gradual lengthening.

STIMULATION OF NATURAL GROWTH

Although various methods of stimulation of growth of the shorter limb have been tried, none of them have been proven to be effective. These include periosteal stripping, insertion of bone pegs or dissimilar metals in the vicinity of the physeal line, lumbar sympathectomy to induce blood flow, interfering with the intramedullary circulation by mechanical blocking of the medullary cavity, creation of an artificial arteriovenous fistula and transplantation of physeal cartilage into areas of deficient or damaged physis. None of these methods has shown any substantial increase in longitudinal growth sufficient to make them clinically applicable. Animal experiments of vascularized total physeal transplants and insertion of a free plug of iliac crest apophyseal cartilage into surgically induced defects have shown some promise; neither technique has been developed enough to have broad clinical applicability.

ACUTE LENGTHENING

Transiliac lengthening of a short limb has been described in patients requiring Salter innominate osteotomy for acetabular dysplasia with an associated ipsilateral shortening of 3 cm or less. A quadrangular iliac crest bone graft is used instead of the traditional triangular graft in order to increase the limb length. Acute lengthening of femur and even tibia has been described where, after osteotomy and extensive soft-tissue release, the bone is acutely distracted, fixed with either intramedullary rod or plate and screws and the gap at the osteotomy site is filled with allograft or autologous iliac crest bone graft. These procedures are associated with major complications, including acute femoral or sciatic nerve injury, femoral artery occlusion, reflex sympathetic dystrophy, intra-operative fracture at a site remote from the osteotomy, implant failure, delayed union or non-union.

GRADUAL LENGTHENING

Chondrodiatasis

Attempts to stimulate longitudinal growth by applying mechanical traction across the physis have been variably referred to as chondrodiatasis, epiphysiolysis, epiphyseal distraction, distraction epiphysiolysis or epiphyseal traction. In animal experiments, before applying distraction across the physis, some authors have deliberately produced a physeal fracture and others have not. Many studies indicate that distraction across the physis produces an epiphyseal separation after a period of a few days to a few weeks, which can be followed by further lengthening. The occurrence of this acute separation depends on the rate and extent of distraction force applied to the physis. De Bastiani and colleagues[74] noted experimentally that lower forces or slower distraction (e.g. 0.5 mm per day) could result in hypertrophy of the cellular layers of the physis without actual acute physeal separation, and introduced the term chondrodiatasis to specifically refer to physeal distraction without separation. The term has now been commonly used for physeal distraction, regardless of whether physeal separation is intended or occurs.

Because most causes of limb length inequality are related to a disturbance of normal physeal function, chondrodiatasis seems to be an appealing option in skeletally immature patients. However, the technique is not commonly used for several reasons. Even with gradual physeal distraction, physeal separation is not always a controllable event and may occur with a painful audible pop despite efforts to avoid it. Segmental fixation of the epiphysis is more difficult than segmental fixation of the metaphysis, and fixation generally being intra-articular carries a risk of pin tract infection, which may lead to septic arthritis. Following distraction, the growth plate can close prematurely or the rate of growth can slow down.

Callotasis

Currently, the more commonly used method of leg lengthening is by gradual distraction (callotasis) of a fracture callus after low-energy percutaneous osteotomy, 'corticotomy', of the long bone. Unlike Wagner's method of diaphyseal lengthening, the corticotomy is performed usually in the metaphysis with careful preservation of the soft-tissue envelope surrounding the bone. There is no initial distraction at the time of corticotomy. Instead, gradual distraction begins only after a 3–21 day latent period during which fracture callus develops at the corticotomy site (Fig. 68.9). Lengthening occurs at a rate that is tolerable to the fracture callus and soft tissues, without interfering with the blood supply – typically 1 mm per day. After the desired length is achieved, the limb is maintained in the lengthened state in the external fixator until adequate consolidation of the new bone has occurred (the consolidation period), to minimize the risk of fracture after removal of the apparatus. Typically, the consolidation period is approximately twice as long as the distraction period.

Ilizarov[70,71] found that, with preservation of the soft-tissue envelope and callotasis techniques, the tension created by gradual distraction stimulated neogenesis not only of bone but also of soft tissues, including skin, blood vessels, peripheral nerves and muscle. He referred to this process as the 'tension–stress effect on the genesis and growth of tissues'. Several authors reported significantly fewer soft-tissue complications, better new bone formation and obviating the need for secondary bone grafting and internal fixation when they replaced the Wagner method using the same external fixation device.

The reported incidence of complications associated with gradual leg lengthening ranges from 14% to 134% (i.e. more than one complication for each segment lengthened). They include nerve or vessel injury during device application, incomplete osteotomy, premature consolidation, poor regenerate bone formation, joint subluxation, neuropraxia, pin site infection and development of ring sequestrum, regenerate bone fracture, subsequent growth disturbance of the lengthened leg and psychological stress. Paley[76] classified these untoward events as *problems* (not requiring operative intervention to resolve), *obstacles* (requiring operative intervention but without permanent

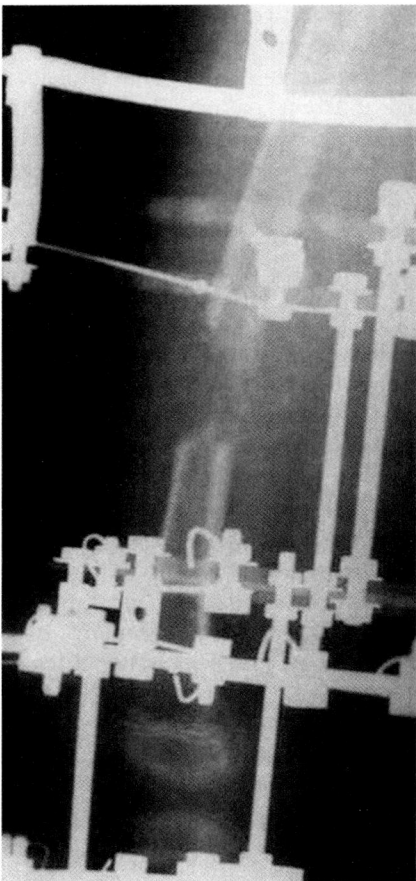

Figure 68.9 Limb lengthening by callotasis or callus distraction; note the early new bone formation.

sequelae) or *complications* (intraoperative injury or anything resulting in permanent sequelae).

Current advances in the knowledge of distraction osteogenesis, concepts of frame and fixator stability, and the precise method of inserting wires and pins have significantly reduced the complications reported in the previous decade in limb-lengthening procedures. Further progress has been made with computer-assisted fixator and frame programmes (Taylor spatial frame, Hexapod) and the evolution of intramedullary lengthening nails: Albizzia,[77] ISKD[78] and Fitbone,[79] which probably have a bright future at least in older adolescents and adults in whom LLD is the predominant deformity. Deformity planning by Paley[76] has now changed the way of analysing limb length discrepancies and deformities of angulation, translation and rotation. This method is now universally used by reconstructive surgeons. Limb lengthening and reconstruction is generally performed by specialist surgeons in centres with a dedicated multidisciplinary team and the key to good outcomes is a well-prepared family and child with intensive pre- and postoperative rehabilitation.

KEY LEARNING POINTS

- Most rotational problems of the lower extremity in children are physiological or postural problems, and symmetrical.
- Examination starts by observing the child walk, looking for abnormalities in gait and foot progression angle.
- A single anteroposterior radiograph of the pelvis is advisable to exclude other conditions such as developmental dysplasia of the hip and slipped upper femoral epiphysis, which can also present with rotational problems.
- The natural history of rotational variation in long bones is spontaneous correction by 5–6 years in the vast majority of children.
- Congenital posteromedial bowing of the tibia is a non-dysplastic benign condition which usually resolves spontaneously with time.
- Congenital pseudarthrosis of the tibia (CPT) is a rare condition affecting approximately 1 in 200 000 live births (50% have neurofibromatosis).
- Few disorders cause so much difficulty in obtaining union and as a result success rates for many described techniques in CPT are poor.
- Leg length inequality or discrepancy discrepancies of 2.5 cm or more will result in postural imbalance and uneven gait, generally characterized by increased loading on the longer limb.
- It is important to distinguish between true and apparent shortening; use the block test; also radiographs, scanograms and computed tomography are useful.
- In a skeletally immature child, eventual leg length discrepancy at maturity depends on the rate at which each bone is growing. Various methods exist to determine this.
- Shortening of the long leg in a child is achieved by inducing growth arrest either permanently by epiphysiodesis or temporarily by epiphyseal stapling or plating. In an adult, this is achieved by acute shortening procedures.
- Despite the improvements in limb-lengthening techniques (can be acute or chronic technique; of the latter, callostasis is now most commonly used), the complications of limb lengthening exceed those of epiphysiodesis or acute shortening.

REFERENCES

- ● = Key primary paper
- ◆ = Major review article

◆1. Staheli LT. Rotational problems in children. *Journal of Bone and Joint Surgery (American)* 1993;**75**:939.

◆2. Staheli LT, Corbett M, Wyss C, et al. Lower extremity rotational problems in children – Normal values to guide treatment. *Journal of Bone and Joint Surgery (American)* 1985;**67**:39.

◆3. Staheli LT. Lower positional deformity in infants and children: a review. *Journal of Pediatric Orthopaedics* 1990;**10**:559.

◆4. Kling TF, Hensinger RN. Angular and torsion deformities of the lower limbs in children. *Clinical Orthopaedics and Related Research* 1983;**176**:136.

●5. Murphy SB, Simon SR, Kijewski PK, et al. Femoral anteversion. *Journal of Bone and Joint Surgery (American)* 1987;**69**:1169.

◆6. Staheli LT. Footwear for children. In: Schafer M (ed.) *AAOS Instructional Course Lectures*, vol. 43. Rosemont, IL: American Academy of Orthopaedic Surgery, 1994:193.

●7. Fabry G, MacEwan GD, Shands Jr AR. Torsion of the femur. a follow up study in normal and abnormal conditions. *Journal of Bone and Joint Surgery (American)* 1973;**55**:1726.

◆8. Tachdjian MO. Disorders of the leg. In: Tachdjian MO (ed.) *Paediatric Orthopaedics*, 4th edn. Philadelphia, PA: W.B. Saunders, 2008:1006.

●9. Hofmann A, Wenger DR. Posteromedial bowing of the tibia. Progression of discrepancy in leg lengths. *Journal of Bone and Joint Surgery (American)* 1981;**63**:384.

10. Pappas AM. Congenital posteromedial bowing of the tibia and fibula. *Journal of Pediatric Orthopaedics* 1984;**4**:525.

●11. Shah HH, Doddabasappa SN, Joseph B. Congenital posteromedial bowing of the tibia: a retrospective analysis of growth abnormalities in the leg. *Journal of Pediatric Orthopaedics B* 2009;**18**:120-8.

◆12. Hefti F, Bollini G, Dungl P, et al. Congenital pseudarthrosis of the tibia: history, etiology, classification and epidemiologic data. *Journal of Pediatric Orthopaedics B* 2000;**9**:11-15.

◆13. Crawford AH, Schorry EK. Neurofibromatosis in children: the role of the orthopaedist. *Journal of the American Academy of Orthopaedic Surgeons* 1999;**7**:217-30.

●14. Andersen KS. Radiological classification of congenital pseudarthrosis of the tibia. *Acta Orthopaedica Scandinavica* 1973;**44**:719-27.

●15. Heikkinen ES, Poyhonen MH, Kinnunen PK, et al. Congenital pseudarthrosis of the tibia: treatment and outcome at skeletal maturity. *Acta Orthopaedica Scandinavica* 1999;**70**:275-82.

16. Hermanns-Sachweh B, Senderek J, Alfer J, et al. Vascular changes in the periosteum of congenital pseudarthrosis of the tibia. *Pathology, Research and Practice* 2005;**201**:305-12.

●17. Magee T, Mackay DR, Segal LS. Congenital constriction band with pseudarthrosis of the tibia: a case report and literature review. *Acta Orthopaedica Belgica* 2007;**73**:275-8.

18. Zionts LE, Osterkamp JA, Crawford TO, Harvey JP. Congenital annular bands in identical twins. A case report. *Journal of Bone and Joint Surgery* 1984;**66A**:450-3.

- 19. Tanguy AF, Dalens BJ, Boisgard S. Congenital constricting band with pseudarthrosis of the tibia and fibula. *Journal of Bone and Joint Surgery (American)* 1995;**77**:1251–4.
- 20. Schindeler A, Little DG. Recent insights into bone development, homeostasis and repair in type I neurofibromatosis. *Bone* 2008;**42**:616–22.
- 21. Leslela HV, Kuorilehto T, Risteli J, et al. Congenital pseudarthrosis of neurofibromatosis type 1: impaired osteoblast differentiation and function and altered NF1 gene expression. *Bone* 2009;**44**:243–50.
- 22. Cho TJ, Seo JB, Lee HR, et al. Biologic characteristics of fibrous hamartoma from congenital pseudarthrosis of the tibia associated with neurofibromatosis type I. *Journal of Bone and Joint Surgery (American)* 2008;**90**:2735–44.
- 23. Boyd HB. Pathology and natural history of congenital pseudarthrosis of the tibia. *Clinical Orthopaedics and Related Research* 1982;**166**:5.
- 24. Andersen KS. Congenital pseudarthrosis of the leg. Late results. *Journal of Bone and Joint Surgery (American)* 1976;**74**:161.
- 25. Gilbert A, Brockman R. Congenital pseudarthrosis of the tibia. Long term follow up of 29 cases treated by microvascular bone transfer. *Clinical Orthopaedics and Related Research* 1995;**314**:37.
- 26. Coleman SS, Coleman DA. Congenital pseudarthrosis of the tibia: treatment by transfer of the ipsilateral fibula with vascular pedicle. *Journal of Pediatric Orthopaedics* 1994;**14**:156.
- 27. Weiland AJ, Weiss AP, Moore JR, Tolo VT. Vascularized fibular grafts in the treatment of congenital pseudarthrosis of the tibia. *Journal of Bone and Joint Surgery (American)*. 1990;**72**:654–62.
- 28. Romanus B, Bollini G, Dungl P, et al. Free vascular fibular transfer in congenital pseudarthrosis of the tibia: results of the EPOS multicenter study. *Journal of Pediatric Orthopaedics B* 2000;**9**:90–3.
- 29. Joseph B, Somaraju W, Shetty SK. Management of congenital pseudarthrosis of the tibia in children under 3 years of age: effect of early surgery on union of the pseudarthrosis and growth of the limb. *Journal of Pediatric Orthopaedics B* 2003;**2**:740–6.
- 30. Fern ED, Stockley I, Bell MJ. Extending intramedullary rods congenital pseudarthrosis of the tibia. *Journal of Bone and Joint Surgery (British)* 1990;**72**:1073–5.
- 31. Anderson DJ, Schoenecker PL, Sheridan JJ, Rich MM. Use of an intramedullary rod for the treatment of congenital pseudarthrosis of the tibia. *Journal of Bone and Joint Surgery (American)* 1992;**74**:161–8.
- 32. Joseph B, Mathew G. Management of congenital pseudarthrosis of the tibia by excision of the pseudarthrosis, onlay grafting and intramedullary nailing. *Journal of Pediatric Orthopaedics B* 2000;**9**:16–23.
- 33. Lee FY, Sinicropi SM, Lee FS, et al. Treatment of congenital pseudarthrosis of the tibia with recombinant human bone morphogenic protein: a report of 5 cases. *Journal of Bone and Joint Surgery (American)* 2006;**88**:627–33.
- 34. Grill F, Bollini G, Dungl P, et al. Treatment approaches for congenital pseudarthrosis of the tibia: results of the EPOS multi-center study. *Journal of Pediatric Orthopaedics B* 2000;**9**:75–89.
- 35. Boero S, Catagni M, Donzelli O, et al. Congenital pseudarthrosis of the tibia associated with neurofibromatosis 1: treatment with Ilizarov's device. *Journal of Pediatric Orthopaedics* 1997;**17**:675.
- 36. Ghanem I, Damsin JP, Carlioz H. Ilizarov technique in the treatment of congenital pseudarthrosis of the tibia. *Journal of Pediatric Orthopaedics* 1997;**17**:685.
- 37. Guidera KJ, Raney EM, Ganey T, et al. Ilizarov treatment of congenital pseudarthroses of the tibia. *Journal of Pediatric Orthopaedics* 1997;**17**:668.
- 38. Paley D, Catagni M, Argnani F, et al. Treatment of congenital pseudarthrosis of the tibia using the Ilizarov technique. *Clinical Orthopaedics and Related Research* 1992;**280**:81–93.
- 39. Cho TJ, Choi IH, Lee SM, et al. Refracture after Ilizarov osteosynthesis in atrophic-type congenital pseudarthrosis of the tibia. *Journal of Bone and Joint Surgery (British)* 2008;**90**:488–93.
- 40. Weintroub S, Grill F. Congenital pseudarthrosis of the tibia: part I (Editorial). *Journal of Pediatric Orthopaedics B* 2000;**9**:1–2.
- 41. Hellsing AL. Leg length inequality: A prospective study of young men during their military service. *Uppsala Journal of Medical Sciences* 1988;**93**:245.
- 42. Soukka A, Alaranta H, Tallroth K, et al. Leg-length inequality in people of working age: the association between mild inequality and low-back pain is questionable. *Spine* 1991;**16**:429.
- 43. Liu XC, Fabry G, Molenaers G, et al. Kinematic and kinetic asymmetry in patients with leg-length discrepancy. *Journal of Pediatric Orthopaedics* 1998;**18**:187.
- 44. Gofton JP. Persistent low back pain and leg length disparity. *Journal of Rheumatology* 1985;**12**:747.
- 45. ten Brinke A, van der Aa HE, van der Palen J, et al. Is leg length discrepancy associated with the side of radiating pain in patients with a lumbar herniated disc? *Spine* 1999;**24**:684.
- 46. Song KM, Halliday SE, Little DG. The effect of limb-length discrepancy on gait. *Journal of Bone and Joint Surgery (American)* 1997;**79**:1690.
- 47. Green WT, Wyatt GM, Anderson M. Orthoentgenography as a method of measuring the bones of the lower extremity. *Journal of Bone and Joint Surgery (American)* 1946;**28**:60.
- 48. Saleh M, Milne A. Weight-bearing parallel beam scanography for the measurement of leg length and joint alignment. *Journal of Bone and Joint Surgery (British)* 1994;**76**:156.
- 49. Kogutt MS. Computed radiographic imaging: use in low-dose leg length radiography. *AJR American Journal of Roentgenology* 1987;**148**:1205.
- 50. Anderson M, Green WT, Messner MB. Growth and predictions of growth in the lower extremities. *Journal of Bone and Joint Surgery (American)* 1963;**45**:1.

♦51. Anderson M, Messner MB, Green WT. Distribution of lengths of the normal femur and tibia in children from one to eighteen years of age. *Journal of Bone and Joint Surgery (American)* 1964;**46**:1197.

●52. Westh RN, Menelaus MB. A simple calculation for the timing of epiphyseal arrest: a further report. *Journal of Bone and Joint Surgery (British)* 1981;**63**:117.

●53. White JW, Stubbins SG. Growth arrest for equalizing leg lengths. *JAMA* 1944;**126**:1146.

●54. Moseley CF. A straight-line graph for leg-length discrepancies. *Journal of Bone and Joint Surgery (American)* 1977;**59**:174.

●55. Paley D, Bhave A, Herzenberg JE, et al. Multiplier method for predicting limb-length discrepancy. *Journal of Bone and Joint Surgery (American)* 2000;**82**:1432.

●56. Shapiro F. Developmental patterns in lower-extremity length discrepancies. *Journal of Bone and Joint Surgery (American)* 1982;**64**:639.

♦57. Greulich WW, Pyle SI. *Radiographic Atlas of Skeletal Development of the Hand and Wrist.* Stanford, CA: Stanford University Press, 1959.

♦58. Little DG, Nigo L, Aiona MD. Deficiencies of current methods for the timing of epiphysiodesis. *Journal of Pediatric Orthopaedics* 1996;**16**:173.

59. Dimeglio A, Charles YP, Daures JP, et al. Accuracy of the Sauvegrain method in determining skeletal age during puberty. *Journal of Bone and Joint Surgery (American)* 2005;**87**:1689–96.

♦60. Tanner JM, Healy MJR, Goldstein H, Cameron N. *Assessment of Skeletal Maturity and Prediction of Adult Height (TW3 Method)*, 3rd edn. London, UK: Saunders, 2002.

61. Stanitski DF. Limb-length inequality: assessment and treatment options. *Journal of the American Academy of Orthopaedic Surgeons* 1999;**7**:143.

62. Phemister DB. Operative arrestment of longitudinal growth of bones in the treatment of deformities. *Journal of Bone and Joint Surgery (American)* 1933;**15**:1.

●63. Canale ST, Russell TA, Holcomb RL. Percutaneous epiphysiodesis: experimental study and preliminary clinical results. *Journal of Pediatric Orthopaedics* 1986;**6**:150.

●64. Blount WP, Clark GR. Control of bone growth by epiphyseal stapling: preliminary report. *Journal of Bone and Joint Surgery (American)* 1949;**31**:464.

●65. Métaizeau JP, Wong-Chung J, Bertrand H, et al. Percutaneous epiphysiodesis using transphyseal screws (PETS). *Journal of Pediatric Orthopaedics* 1998;**18**:363.

66. Stevens PM. Guided growth for angular correction: a preliminary series using a tension band plate. *Journal of Paediatrics* 2007;**27**:253–9.

♦67. Winquist RA, Hansen Jr ST, Pearson RE. Closed intramedullary shortening of the femur. *Clinical Orthopaedics and Related Research* 1978;**136**:54–61.

♦68. Codivilla A. On the means of lengthening in the lower limbs, the muscles and the tissues which are shortened through deformity. *American Journal of Orthopedic Surgery* 1905;**2**:353.

♦69. Wagner H. Operative lengthening of the femur. *Clinical Orthopaedics and Related Research* 1978;**136**:125–42.

70. Ilizarov GA. The tension-stress effect on the genesis and growth of tissues. Part I. The influence of stability of fixation and soft-tissue preservation. *Clinical Orthopaedics and Related Research* 1989;**238**:249–81.

●71. Ilizarov GA. The tension-stress effect on the genesis and growth of tissues. Part II. The influence of the rate and frequency of distraction. *Clinical Orthopaedics and Related Research* 1989;**239**:263–85.

●72. Ilizarov GA. Clinical application of the tension-stress effect for limb lengthening. *Clinical Orthopaedics and Related Research* 1990;**250**:8–26.

●73. De Bastiani G, Aldegheri R, Renzi Brivio L, et al. Chondrodiatasis-controlled symmetrical distraction of the epiphyseal plate: limb lengthening in children. *Journal of Bone and Joint Surgery (British)* 1986;**68**:550.

74. De Bastiani G, Aldegheri R, Renzi Brivio L, et al. Limb lengthening by distraction of the epiphyseal plate: a comparison of two techniques in the rabbit. *Journal of Bone and Joint Surgery (British)* 1986;**68**:545.

75. De Bastiani G, Aldegheri R, Renzi-Brivio L, et al. Limb lengthening by callus distraction (callotasis). *Journal of Pediatric Orthopaedics* 1987;**7**:129.

♦76. Paley D. Problems, obstacles, and complications of limb lengthening by the Ilizarov technique. *Clinical Orthopaedics and Related Research* 1990;**250**:81–104.

♦77. Guichet JM, Deromedis B, Donnan LT, et al. Gradual femoral lengthening with the Albizzia intramedullary nail. *Journal of Bone and Joint Surgery (American)* 2003;**85**:838.

78. Hankemeier S, Pape HC, Gosling T, et al. Improved comfort in lower limb lengthening with the intramedullary skeletal kinetic distractor: principles and preliminary clinical experiences. *Archives of Orthopaedic and Trauma Surgery* 2004;**124**:129.

●79. Baumgart R, Betz A, Schweiberer L. A fully implantable motorized intramedullary nail for limb lengthening and bone transport. *Clinical Orthopaedics and Related Research* 1997;**343**:135.

69

Disorders of the foot in children

HAEMISH A CRAWFORD, JAMES S HUNTLEY, BENJAMIN JOSEPH

Congenital clubfoot	688	References	693
Other common disorders of the foot in children	691		

NATIONAL BOARD STANDARDS

- Be aware of details of the non-operative method of treatment of idiopathic congenital talipes equinovarus
- Know the indication and scope of surgical intervention for idiopathic congenital talipes equinovarus
- Distinguish self-limiting disorders of the infant's foot from deformities that persist
- Distinguish flexible flatfoot from rigid flatfoot

CONGENITAL CLUBFOOT

Introduction

Congenital talipes equinovarus (CTEV) is a lower limb condition present at birth in which there is (to varying extents and stiffness) cavus, forefoot adductus, heel varus, ankle equinus and internal tibial torsion.

Epidemiology

There is a marked variation in incidence according to geography and race: it is just over 1 per 1000 for European Caucasian live births. The rate is lower in Japan (0.5/1000), and higher for South Pacific populations (6–7/1000). The male–female ratio is 2.5:1, and 50% of cases are bilateral. Left and right feet are equally affected. Most cases are 'isolated' but approximately 20% are 'syndromic', occurring with other anomalies, e.g. spina bifida, cerebral palsy and arthrogryposis.

Aetiology

Club foot may result from an osseous, muscular or neuropathic error, or may be termed idiopathic of these the last is by for the most frequent. Many theories have been advanced,

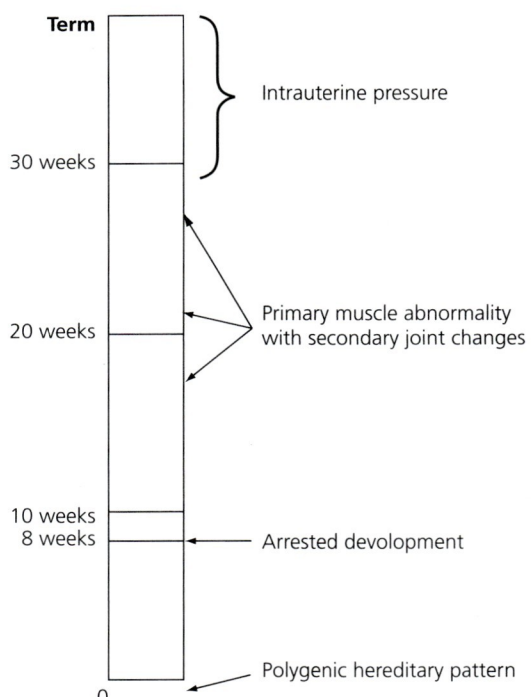

Figure 69.1 The four major factors which may produce a club foot deformity. (Reproduced, with permission, from Fuller, D. J. and Duthie, R. B. (1974) *AAOS Instructional Course Lectures* **23**, 53-61)

including intrauterine moulding, developmental defects and anomalies of other systems (neurogenic, myogenic, vascular). Both genetic and environmental factors (especially maternal smoking) have been implicated. Almost one-quarter of CTEV patients have a positive family history – a sibling of an affected patient has a 2–4% risk. There are many tissue abnormalities in CTEV, including deficiency of calf muscle bulk, changes in muscle histology, bone and joint deformities (e.g. talus and calcaneocuboid joint) and vascular hypoplasia.

Anatomy

The deformity is complex and involves the Chopart, subtalar and ankle joints. The primary bony deformity is thought to be the talus, which is short, angled medially and plantarflexed. The navicular is medially subluxated. The calcaneus is short, wide, adducted and passes into varus. The cavus occurs because of a 'pronation-twist' – a relatively greater flexion of the first metatarsal in relation to the hindfoot. This is the key to Ponseti's argument that the cavus must be corrected first by supination of the forefoot.[1]

Examination

This includes the hip and spine as associated anomalies are common. If toes are absent then consideration must be given to tibial dysplasia. The hands should also be examined – if the fingers are stiff then distal arthrogryposis is possible; if there is symphalangism then tarsal coalitions of genetic basis should be considered.

Classification

There have been several attempts at classification systems for CTEV – the early ones were dogged by the problems of poor inter- and intra-observer reliability. The two systems that have achieved pre-eminence are the DiMeglio[2] and Pirani classifications[3] (Table 69.1). The Pirani system[3,4] is shorter and is now applied almost universally. It is easy to use and of prognostic relevance. The deformity is graded according to six components: posterior crease, empty heel and rigid equinus (hindfoot group); and medial crease, lateral border curvature and position of the talar head (midfoot group). Each component is given a score of 0, 0.5 or 1. Each foot therefore can be assigned a rating from 0 (normal) to 6 (severe).

Prenatal ultrasound

Prenatal diagnosis of talipes may allow the future parents to plan ahead and come to terms with their child having a deformity that is likely to require active treatment, and be made aware of what that treatment is likely to entail. The expectation is of a good functional outcome and this needs to be identified. Local figures should be available for advice concerning possible diagnoses, e.g. on our unit, we advise that (1) the possibility of a false positive (i.e. normal feet or postural variant) is about 5% and (2) the risk of undiagnosed congenital anomalies – for which management is more complex and outcome is more guarded – is about 20%.

Treatment

The aim is to achieve a pain-free, supple and plantigrade foot.

Conservative treatments involve stretching, manipulation, strapping, plasters and percutaneous tenotomies. Other manipulative treatments (including the current French – or 'functional' method) continue to have many advocates. Generally, the Ponseti method has superseded other regimens, such as Kite's method, in which a different and erroneous sequence of deformity correction was used.

Table 69.1 Pirani classification

Assigned		Normal	Moderately abnormal	Severely abnormal
Score		0	0.5	1
Hindfoot	Posterior crease	Fine creases that do not alter the contour	One or two deep creases that do not alter the contour	Deep creases that change the contour
	Rigidity equinus (maximal dorsiflexion)	Normal	Less than normal but >90°	>90°
	Empty heel	Calcaneal tuberosity is easily palpable	Heel pad somewhat empty	No bony prominence palpable in heel pad
Midfoot	Curve of lateral border	Ruler from hindfoot touches head of fifth metatarsal	Ruler from hindfoot touches base of fifth metatarsal	Ruler from hindfoot touches hindfoot only
	Medial crease (in corrected position)	Fine creases that do not alter the contour	One or two deep creases that do not alter the contour	Deep creases that change the contour
	Talar head coverage	Navicular is completely reducible	Partial reduction	Easily palpable talar head with medial subluxation of the navicular

THE PONSETI METHOD

The technique involves manipulation and serial casting.[5] Cast application is a skilled process. After manipulation/stretching, a below-knee cast is applied and moulded. After setting, the cast is extended above the thigh, maintaining hyperabduction of the foot. In most cases, a correction can be obtained after five casts. The Pirani score should be evaluated at each casting for a more objective evaluation of progress. (High-quality Ponseti handbooks are available online.)

1. In the first cast, the cavus is reduced by supinating the forefoot (elevating the first ray) to align it properly with the hind foot. This makes the deformity more marked!
2. Thereafter, the hindfoot varus, inversion and adduction deformities are corrected simultaneously, by simultaneous lateral shift of the navicular, cuboid and calcaneus. This is performed by abducting the foot against counter-pressure exerted at the lateral talar head. Pressure must not be exerted at the calcaneocuboid joint against a stabilized heel; this was termed 'Kite's error' by Ponseti.
3. The Achilles tendon may require percutaneous lengthening (see below) before application of the last cast (which is left on for 3 weeks). It is necessary that the heel varus is corrected before this stage.
4. A foot-abduction brace is a critical feature of the protocol.[6] The bar (length equal to the child's shoulder width) has shoes attached at both ends. Some dorsiflexion is built into the boots/bar construct. These are rotated externally 40° (normal side) and 70° (CTEV side). The brace should be worn full time for at least 3 months and then at night and naptimes (at least 10 hours per day) for 3–4 years.
5. There is a possibility of a requirement for later surgery, especially a tibialis anterior tendon transfer.

ACHILLES TENOTOMY

Over 80% patients require a percutaneous Achilles tenotomy. This cannot be performed until the heel varus has been corrected. Usually this procedure is performed under local anaesthesia. The percutaneous tenotomy is performed in a medial to lateral direction (to minimize neurovascular risk) with the tendon under tension. A small beaver cataract blade is our preferred implement.

TIBIALIS ANTERIOR TENDON TRANSFER

This procedure is the commonest used to treat for dynamic supination in swing, which is a feature of early recurrence. The aim is to negate the tendency to oversupination and rebalance the foot. Any fixed deformity must be corrected first, and usually this can be done with a Ponseti casting regimen. We recommend the tibialis anterior tendon transfer (TATT) as described by Ponseti and Smoley,[7] in which the whole tendon is rerouted deep to the extensor retinaculum through the lateral cuneiform.

Surgical treatments

Our approach is derived from that of Turco.[8] Although undercorrection may allow relapse/recurrence, overcorrection may lead to a valgus heel and stiff/painful foot. Surgery should be tailored to the particular patient – the 'à la carte' approach as advocated by Bensahel et al.[9] – e.g. some patients may require only the posterior part of the posteromedial release.

POSTERIOR/POSTEROMEDIAL RELEASES

Our posteromedial release is derived from Turco.[8] The incision (8–9 cm) runs from the base of the first metatarsal posteriorly, inferior to the medial malleolus and on to the lateral side of the Achilles tendon.

There are five potential stages:

1. *Posterior release.* Initially we define the posterolateral corner, identifying the sural nerve, peroneal tendon sheath and posterior talofibular ligament. The Achilles tendon is Z-lengthened. Flexor hallucis longus and the neurovascular bundle are identified and retracted medially. Similarly, the peroneal tendons and sural nerve are retracted laterally. Reflecting (superiorly and inferiorly) the two limbs of the Z-lengthened Achilles allows clearance of the fibrofatty tissue on the posterior capsule. Full capsulotomies of the posterior ankle and subtalar joints are performed.
2. *Medial release.* The abductor hallucis is defined and the tendon sheaths of tibialis posterior and flexor digitorum longus are opened. Much fibrotic tissue may have to be removed. The knot of Henry is divided to free flexor hallucis longus and flexor digitorum longus. The neurovascular bundle is mobilized and tibialis posterior is Z-lengthened just above the medial malleolus.
3. *Subtalar release.* The tendon sheath of flexor hallucis longus is released to allow its retraction with the neurovascular bundle away from the medial subtalar joint, which is divided under direct vision. The medial subtalar joint can be followed around to the talar neck, and the spring ligament divided. Retraction of the navicular tuberosity distally and flexor digitorum longus proximally allows the medial side of the calcaneocuboid joint to be reached with rongeurs and cleared of fibrofatty material before incision of the medial side of the joint. The lateral side of the calcaneocuboid joint is broken down with a MacDonald's dissector.
4. *Forefoot release.* Abductor hallucis, plantar fascia and toe flexors are all assessed and released if appropriate.

5. *Reassembly.* Talonavicular fixation is secured with a K-wire, and the Achilles tendon sutured in its lengthened position. Tibialis posterior and its sheath are repaired. It is important to leave the tibiotalar component of the deltoid ligament intact – otherwise fixed valgus of the hindfoot may result.

Postoperative care involves casting for 12 weeks with cast changes at 2 and 6 weeks (wire removal at 6 weeks).

Secondary surgery

There is a risk of approximately 25% that a relapse (or overcorrection) will occur post surgery, of such a degree that secondary surgery is required.

Conclusion

The recommendations are limited because the evidence base is small, but initially all treatment should be conservative, involving one of the modern regimens such as Ponseti.

OTHER COMMON DISORDERS OF THE FOOT IN CHILDREN

Introduction

Congenital and acquired deformities of the foot are commonly encountered in paediatric orthopaedic practice; several require no treatment at all but some do need to be treated energetically. The structure of the foot changes from infancy to adolescence and often what appears to be pathological resolves with time as the child grows.

Self-limiting disorders of the infant's foot

INFANTILE FLAT FOOT

The vast majority of infants have no visible medial longitudinal arch because in infancy there is fat in the instep and consequently the foot print resembles that of a child with flat foot. In addition, ligament laxity is more pronounced in infancy. The fat in the instep decreases as the child grows, and, with tightening of the ligaments and improved muscular tone, the medial longitudinal arch develops. A well-formed arch is present by the age of 6 years, although the arch may fail to form in the presence of obesity and generalized ligament laxity.

CONGENITAL CALCANEOVALGUS

Congenital calcaneovalgus deformity is a deformity that develops on account of intrauterine moulding. The baby may be born with the dorsum of the foot in contact with the shin (Fig. 69.2). This seemingly severe deformity

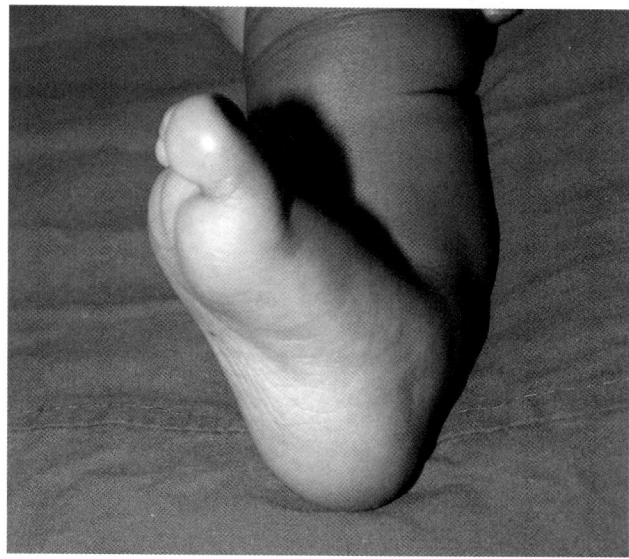

Figure 69.2 Appearance of the foot of a newborn with calcaneovalgus deformity of the right foot. The dorsum of the foot is almost in contact with the shin.

improves quite dramatically within days of birth. The deformity may be more severe when seen in association with congenital posteromedial bowing of the tibia. Passive manipulation of the foot into plantarflexion and inversion will facilitate early resolution of the deformity. In the occasional severe case a few serial casts may be needed.

Congenital deformities that persist

CONGENITAL CONVEX PES VALGUS (CONGENITAL VERTICAL TALUS)

Congenital convex pes valgus is a complex deformity that affects the hindfoot and the forefoot – the hindfoot is in equinus and valgus, whereas the forefoot is abducted and dorsiflexed. The talonavicular joint is dislocated with the navicular sitting on the dorsum of the neck of the talus. The talus is markedly plantarflexed and the head of the talus that is unsupported by the spring ligament is palpable in the sole of the foot. The Achilles tendon, the ankle and toes dorsiflexors and the peronei are all contracted to varying degrees. The medial longitudinal arch is completely reversed giving rise to the characteristic 'rocker bottom' appearance of the foot (Fig. 69.3).

The condition is much rarer than congenital clubfoot and, though it can occur as an isolated deformity, it is often associated with chromosomal defects such as trisomy 18, arthrogryposis (multiple congenital contractures) or neural tube defects.

Until recently, extensive soft-tissue release surgery, reduction of the talonavicular dislocation and K-wire fixation was the recommended treatment.[10,11] More recently,

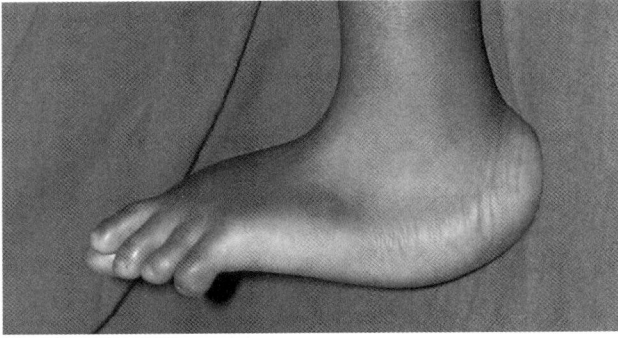

Figure 69.3 Congenital vertical talus in an infant with trisomy 18. The convex contour of the sole of the foot with total reversal of the longitudinal arch is clearly seen.

sequential serial manipulations followed by limited soft-tissue surgery have been shown to be effective.[12] The foot is manipulated into inversion and adduction and, after the forefoot deformity is corrected, limited tendon releases and percutaneous K-wire fixation of the talonavicular joint is performed. After obtaining correction, bracing through infancy and a thermoplastic ankle–foot orthosis for 2 years after the child has started walking is recommended.[3]

The results are likely to be poorer in children with arthrogryposis and spina bifida. In children with spina bifida, muscle imbalance may need to be corrected by appropriate tendon transfers to avoid the risk of recurrence of the deformity.

METATARSUS ADDUCTUS AND SKEWFOOT

Metatarsus adductus is a common deformity characterized by an adduction deformity at the tarsometatarsal joints (Lisfranc joint) of the foot.[13] Metatarsus is a relatively innocuous deformity but may be associated with developmental dysplasia of the hip.[14] Children with an adducted forefoot at birth must be carefully examined to exclude the more serious hip pathology. Metatarsus adductus needs to be differentiated from forefoot adduction of clubfoot; the site of the deformity in the latter situation is the mid-tarsal joint (Chopart joint).

In the majority of instances metatarsus adductus improves as the child grows but may not completely correct. The mild residual deformity causes no functional disability and usually is not noticeable. In a small proportion of children the deformity does not resolve and then shoe wearing may become difficult. For this reason surgery may be needed and this involves osteotomies of the bases of all the metatarsals and release of the tight abductor hallucis muscle.[15]

Skewfoot is a rare complex deformity that is difficult to treat.[16] The metatarsals are adducted at the tarsometatarsal joints but the mid-foot is abducted at the mid-tarsal joint and the hindfoot is in valgus and equinus. This gives rise to a serpentine appearance of the foot. Treatment of this deformity is difficult and may entail osteotomies of the hindfoot and midfoot.[17]

Foot deformities in the older child

FLAT FOOT

Flat foot, pes planus and pes planovalgus are terms used to describe a foot deformity where the medial longitudinal arch is low or totally collapsed. The hind foot is in valgus and the forefoot is abducted at the mid-tarsal joint (Fig. 69.4).

The flat foot deformity may be flexible (the arch can be restored) or rigid and this differentiation is important as the prognosis and treatment differ for these two forms of flat foot. If the medial longitudinal arch can be restored when the child stands on tiptoes or when the great toe is passively dorsiflexed by the examiner (Jack's test), the flat foot is flexible.[18] On the other hand, if the arch does not get restored by either of these manoeuvres the deformity is considered to be rigid.[19]

Flexible flat foot is common in pre-school children and is totally asymptomatic in the vast majority of instances.[20] On account of the valgus position of the heel, the sole of

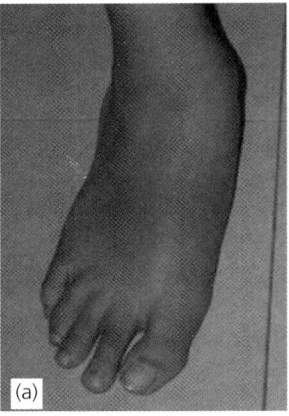
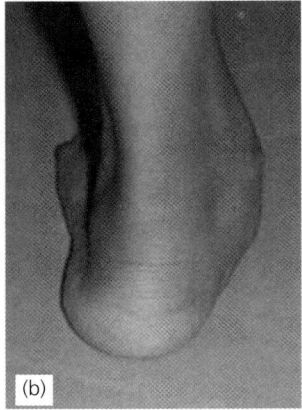

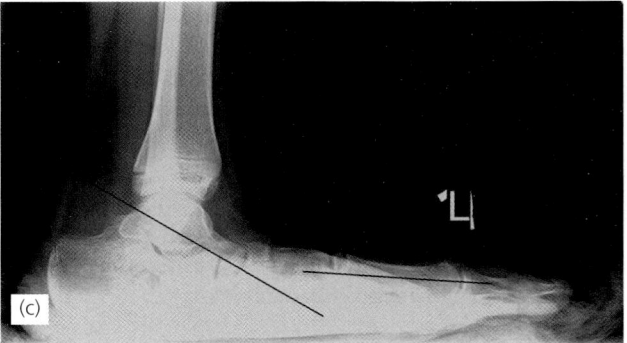

Figure 69.4 Clinical and radiographic appearances of flat foot in an adolescent. The hindfoot is in valgus and the forefoot is abducted (a,b). The weight-bearing lateral radiograph (c) shows that the talus is plantarflexed and its long axis is not in line with the long axis of the first metatarsal.

footwear tends to wear down fast on the medial side and the heel counter of shoes becomes distorted. Apart from this inconvenience, most flexible flat feet function well. A small proportion of children complain of foot strain after prolonged physical activity. Very few children complain of pain on normal walking.

Since the majority of flat feet are symptomatic and function normally, treatment is not required. Use of orthotics and shoe inserts may reduce the wearing down of shoes and offer some relief of foot strain.[21,22] However, there is no evidence to suggest that prolonged use of orthoses and shoe inserts in any way alters the natural history of flat foot.[23] The shoe inserts that have been used include arch supports, Helfet heel cups and UCBL (University of California Biomechanics Laboratory) inserts. In the rare instance of pain on normal walking surgical intervention may be justified.

Surgery for symptomatic flat foot falls into three categories: operations that try to restore the arch, operations that correct the hindfoot valgus and operations that correct the forefoot abduction.[24–29] Interestingly, correction of the forefoot abduction or the hindfoot valgus does improve the arch of the foot. If these measures fail, fusion of the subtalar joint may be needed.

RIGID FLAT FOOT

Rigid flat foot is usually seen in children with tarsal coalition. The underlying condition is due to failure of separation of the tarsal bones during intrauterine development. Though the anomaly is present from birth symptoms appear in late childhood or early adolescence. The two most common sites of coalition are the middle facets of the talus and calcaneum (talocalcaneal coalition) and the anterior end of the calcaneum and the lateral aspect of the navicular (calcaneonavicular coalition). The involved bones may be connected by a bony bar, cartilage or dense fibrous tissue. If left uncorrected, arthritis may develop in the subtalar or mid-tarsal joints.

If, on clinical examination of a symptomatic rigid flat foot, limited motion of the subtalar or mid-tarsal joints is noted, anteroposterior, oblique and lateral view radiographs of the foot must be obtained. Calcaneonavicular bars show up well in the oblique film. If a coalition is not visible on the plain radiographs, fine cut CT scans should be done. Talocalcaneal coalitions are best visualized in CT scans. The size of the coalition can also be mapped from the scans and this helps to decide the treatment.[30,31] If the coalition involves less than 33% of the area of the total subtalar articular surface, resection of the coalition may be considered (provided arthritic changes have not developed). Fat or muscle is interposed after the bar is resected to minimize the chances of recurrence of the bar. Resection of the bar often alleviates pain and some motion at the subtalar and mid-tarsal joints is also restored following resection.[32–34]

> **KEY LEARNING POINTS**
>
> - Conservative treatment of idiopathic congenital talipes equinovarus (CTEV) should be started soon after birth.
> - The initial grade of severity is predictive of outcome and predicts the need for tenotomy.
> - Current conservative methods (including Ponseti) show improved results over earlier methods.
> - Non-compliance with the foot-abduction bar is an important cause of failure in the Ponseti method.
> - Forced manipulation and casting may lead to oedema and later fibrosis, making surgery more difficult.
> - 'À la carte' surgery is justified in resistant CTEV.
> - Infantile flat foot and congenital calcaneovalgus usually resolve spontaneously.
> - Congenital convex pes valgus and the more severe forms of metatarsus adductus will require surgical intervention.
> - The vast majority of flexible flat feet need no treatment.
> - Symptomatic rigid flatfoot is often associated with tarsal coalition, and resection of the coalition, if performed, early yields good results.

REFERENCES

1. Ponseti IV. Treatment of congenital club foot. *Journal of Bone and Joint Surgery (American)* 1992;**74**:448–54.
2. Dimeglio A, Bensahel H, Souchet P, *et al*. Classification of clubfoot. *Journal of Pediatric Orthopaedics B* 1995;**4**:129–36.
3. Pirani S, Outerbridge H, Moran M, Sawatsky B (eds). *A Method of Evaluating the Virgin Clubfoot with Substantial Interobserver Reliability: The Original Description of the Classification*. Miami, FL: Pediatric Orthopaedic Society of North America, 1995.
4. Scher DM, Feldman DS, van Bosse HJ, *et al*. Predicting the need for tenotomy in the Ponseti method for correction of clubfeet. *Journal of Pediatric Orthopaedics* 2004;**24**:349–52.
5. Ponseti I. *Congenital Clubfoot: Fundamentals of Treatment*. Oxford, UK: Oxford University Press, 1996.
6. Morcuende JA, Dolan LA, Dietz FR, Ponseti IV. Radical reduction in the rate of extensive corrective surgery for clubfoot using the Ponseti method. *Pediatrics* 2004;**113**:376–80.
7. Ponseti IV, Smoley EN. Congenital clubfoot: The results of treatment. *Journal of Bone and Joint Surgery* 1963;**45**:261–75.

8. Turco VJ. Resistant congenital club foot – one-stage posteromedial release with internal fixation. A follow-up report of a fifteen-year experience. *Journal of Bone and Joint Surgery (American)* 1979;**61**:805–14.
9. Bensahel H, Csukonyi Z, Desgrippes Y, Chaumien JP. Surgery in residual clubfoot: one-stage medioposterior release 'a la carte'. *Journal of Pediatric Orthopaedics* 1987;**7**:145–8
10. Lloyd-Roberts GC, Spence AJ. Congenital vertical talus. *Journal of Bone and Joint Surgery (British)* 1958;**40**:33–41.
11. Kodros SA, Dias LS. Single-stage surgical correction of congenital vertical talus. *Journal of Pediatric Orthopaedics* 1999;**19**:42–8.
12. Dobbs MB, Purcell DB, Nunley R, Morcuende JA. Early results of a new method of treatment for idiopathic congenital vertical talus. Surgical technique. *Journal of Bone and Joint Surgery (American)* 2007;**89**(Suppl. 2):111–21.
13. Ponseti IV, Becker JR. Congenital metatarsus adductus: the results of treatment. *Journal of Bone and Joint Surgery (American)* 1966;**48**:702–11.
14. Kumar SJ, MacEwen GD. The incidence of hip dysplasia with metatarsus adductus. *Clinical Orthopaedics and Related Research* 1982;**164**:234–5.
15. Berman A, Gartland JJ. Metatarsal osteotomy for correction of adduction of the fore part of the foot in children. *Journal of Bone and Joint Surgery (American)* 1971;**53**:498–506.
16. Berg EE. A reappraisal of metatarsus adductus and skewfoot. *Journal of Bone and Joint Surgery (American)* 1986;**68**:1185–96.
17. Mosca VS. Flexible flatfoot and skewfoot. *Journal of Bone and Joint Surgery (American)* 1995;**77**:1937–45.
18. Bordelon RL. Hypermobile flatfoot in children. Comprehension, evaluation, and treatment. *Clinical Orthopaedics and Related Research* 1983;**181**:7–14.
19. Jack EA. Naviculo-cuneiform fusion in the treatment of flat foot. *Journal of Bone and Joint Surgery (British)* 1953;**35**:75–82.
20. Pfeiffer M, Kotz R, Ledl T, et al. Prevalence of flat foot in preschool-aged children. *Pediatrics* 2006;**118**:634–9.
21. Bleck EE, Berzins UJ. Conservative management of pes valgus with plantar flexed talus, flexible. *Clinical Orthopaedics and Related Research* 1977;**122**:85–94.
22. Helfet AJ. A new way of treating flat feet in children. *Lancet* 1956;**i**:262–4.
23. Wenger DR, Mauldin D, Speck G, et al. Corrective shoes and inserts as treatment for flexible flatfoot in infants and children. *Journal of Bone and Joint Surgery (American)* 1989;**71**:800–10.
24. Fraser RK, Menelaus MB, Williams PF, Cole WG. The Miller procedure for mobile flat feet. *Journal of Bone and Joint Surgery (British)* 1995;**77**:396–9.
25. Mosca VS. Calcaneal lengthening for valgus deformity of the hindfoot. Results in children who had severe, symptomatic flatfoot and skewfoot. *Journal of Bone and Joint Surgery (American)* 1995;**77**:500–12.
26. Ragab AA, Stewart SL, Cooperman DR. Implications of subtalar joint anatomic variation in calcaneal lengthening osteotomy. *Journal of Pediatric Orthopaedics* 2003;**23**:79–83.
27. Koutsogiannis E. Treatment of mobile flat foot by displacement osteotomy of the calcaneus. *Journal of Bone and Joint Surgery (British)* 1971;**53**:96–100.
28. Marcinko DE, Lazerson A, Elleby DH. Silver calcaneal osteotomy for flexible flatfoot: a retrospective preliminary report. *Journal of Foot Surgery* 1984;**23**:191–8.
29. GE Phillips. A review of elongation of os calcis for flat feet. *Journal of Bone and Joint Surgery (British)* 1983;**65**:15–18.
30. Wilde PH, Torode IP, Dickens DR, Cole WG. Resection for symptomatic talocalcaneal coalition. *Journal of Bone and Joint Surgery (British)* 1994;**76**:797–801.
31. Comfort TK, Johnson LO. Resection for symptomatic talocalcaneal coalition. *Journal of Pediatric Orthopaedics* 1998;**18**:283–8.
32. Mosier KM, Asher M. Tarsal coalitions and peroneal spastic flat foot. *Journal of Bone and Joint Surgery (American)* 1984;**66**:976–84.
33. Danielsson LG. Talo-calcaneal coalition treated with resection. *Journal of Pediatric Orthopaedics* 1987;**7**:513–17.
34. Scranton Jr PE. Treatment of symptomatic talocalcaneal coalition. *Journal of Bone and Joint Surgery (American)* 1987;**69**:533–8.

PART 6

SPORTS MEDICINE

MARK D MILLER

70 Exercise physiology, epidemiology and special considerations — 697
Chealon D Miller, Joseph M Hart

71 Essential arthroscopic skills — 712
Kimberly A Turman, Mark D Miller

72 Head and spine injuries in sport — 720
James Brezina, Dino Samartzis, Francis H Shen

73 The evaluation and treatment of glenohumeral instability, superior labrum anterior to posterior tears and rotator cuff tears — 729
Matthew T Provencher, Allison McNickle, Janeth Kim, Brian J Cole, Neil Ghodadra

74 Athletic injuries of the elbow, wrist and hand — 750
A Bobby Chhabra, Jesse Seamon

75 Pelvis, hip and thigh — 772
Benjamin G Domb, JW Thomas Byrd

76 Diagnosis and treatment of non-ligamentous knee injuries — 782
Samir G Tejwani, Jessica E Ellerman, Freddie H Fu

77 Diagnosis and management of ligamentous injuries of the knee — 805
Randy Mascarenhas, Eric J Kropf, Christopher D Harner

78 Leg, ankle and foot injuries — 821
John E Femino, Ned Amendola

70

Exercise physiology, epidemiology and special considerations

CHEALON D MILLER, JOSEPH M HART

Exercise physiology	697	Special considerations: nutrition	705
Epidemiology: injuries and prevention	705	References	709

NATIONAL BOARD STANDARDS

- Understand skeletal muscle physiology to include form and function
- Describe energy metabolism
- Define cardiopulmonary considerations with exercise
- Describe muscle injury to include prevention
- Understand nutrition and ergogenic aids

EXERCISE PHYSIOLOGY

Exercise physiology requires an understanding of the intimate relationship among cardiovascular, pulmonary and muscle physiology. The orthopaedic surgeon must use his or her knowledge of skeletal muscle structure and function and implement energy metabolism and exercise performance to gain an understanding of how skeletal muscle responds to exercise. This information can be used to guide athletes in maximizing training and obtaining proper nutrition to enhance performance. This chapter will concentrate on skeletal muscle physiology, focusing on types of muscle fibres, muscle contractions and neuronal input. This chapter will also include a brief description of the biochemical pathways involved in muscle metabolism and how multiple organ systems interact for maximum exercise performance. Furthermore, understanding the physiology of muscle damage and the benefits of proper nutrition for maximal athletic performance will be discussed.

Skeletal muscle physiology

THE BUILDING BLOCKS OF SKELETAL MUSCLE

Skeletal muscle is the largest tissue mass in the body and constitutes approximately 40–45% of an individual's total body weight. The basic structural element of skeletal muscle is the muscle fibre, and each fibre consists of numerous cells that have multiple nuclei fused together. There are various types of muscle fibres, each with varying fatigue, tension and contractile profiles.[1] Descriptions of each type are included in later sections. Each muscle fibre is a long cell, but can be shorter than the length of the muscle because of its arrangement. Arrangements range from parallel to oblique and the types of oblique orientation range from pennate, bipennate, fusiform and multipennate (Fig. 70.1).[2,3]

Muscle fibres are arranged into fascicles, which are the building blocks of functional muscle groups. Each layer of muscle is surrounded by connective tissue layers that

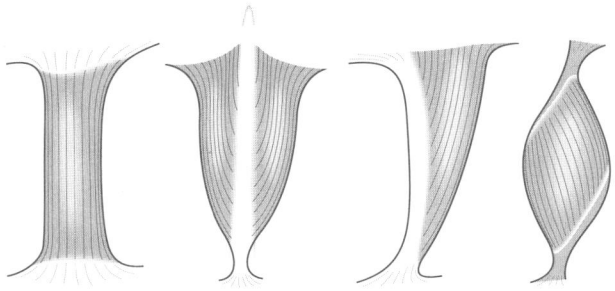

Figure 70.1 Arrangement of muscle fibres. Reproduced with permission from Buckwalter et al.[2]

further stabilize organization of the functional muscle groups. Those connective tissue layers include the endomysium, perimysium and epimysium. Endomysium is a membrane that surrounds individual fibres, arranging them into distinct fascicles. Finally, perimysium surrounds individual fascicles while epimysium surrounds the whole muscle (Fig. 70.2).[2]

Two muscles of the same tissue mass can be arranged in different ways for a given effect. The maximal force that a muscle can produce is proportional to its cross-sectional area, while the amount of shortening and the speed of shortening are both directly related to the fibre length. Therefore, a muscle needed more for strength will have a larger quantity of shorter fibres (Fig. 70.3b), whereas a muscle needed more for shortening will have fewer fibres that are longer to accommodate (Fig. 70.3a).[2] Resistance training will enhance the cross-sectional area of a specific fibre type, while endurance training will increase the maximal shortening velocity of an unloaded muscle.[4]

MUSCLE FIBRE TYPES

There are three basic types of muscle fibres: type I, type IIA and type IIIB.[5] Types I and II are determined by their time to peak tension, while the difference between type IIA and type IIB is dependent upon their mode of energy utilization. Type I fibres are slow-twitch, high-oxidative fibres. They are fatigue resistant and are usually recruited for low-level endurance exercises. Because of their endurance capabilities, they are found predominately in postural muscles and are known to have high amounts of mitochondria and myoglobin. In addition to their slow rate of contraction, type I fibres have a relatively low strength of contraction.[2,6]

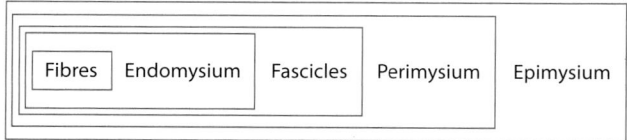

Figure 70.2 Macrostructure of skeletal muscle.

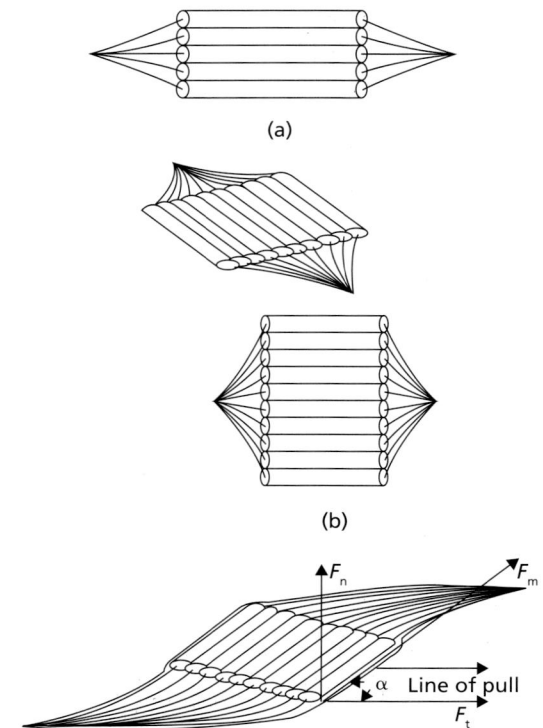

Figure 70.3 Skeletal muscle arrangement. Reproduced with permission from Buckwalter et al.[2]

Type II fibres have a high glycolytic capacity, with a fast rate of contraction (fast-twitch fibres) and a high strength of contraction. For this reason, they are recruited for short bursts of quick, heavy work. Type II fibres are subcategorized into either A or B, based on energy use. Type IIA fibres have an intermediate aerobic capacity whereas type IIB fibres are anaerobic. Type IIB fibres are functionally limited by their ability to sustain activity for long periods of time because of lactic acid accumulation.[2,6] The triceps is composed mainly of type I fibres, whereas the biceps is an example of a muscle with predominately type II fibres (Table 70.1).

Most human muscle is a mixture of fibre types. Muscle fibre type distributions have been shown to influence many aspects of physiology from low back pain to athletic performance.[7] Studies of athletes have shown that sprinters have more type II fibres whereas long distance runners have more type I fibres. Whether nature or nurture is responsible for an individual's ability to participate in activities that require endurance versus high-intensity and short duration activities favours nature; however, the answer continues to evolve in research studies.[8,9]

STRUCTURE OF SKELETAL MUSCLE

Skeletal muscle is composed of various proteins responsible for contraction when calcium is present. Histological sections of skeletal muscle fibres show that there are repeating structural patterns within the fibres called

Table 70.1 Characteristics of human skeletal muscle types.

	Type I	Type IIa	Type IIB
Other names	Red, slow twitch (ST)	White, fast twitch (FT)	Fast glycolytic (FG)
	Slow oxidative (SO)	Fast oxidative glycolytic (FOG)	
Speed of contraction	Slow	Fast	Fast
Strength of contraction	Low	High	High
Fatigability	Fatigue resistant	Fatigable	Most fatigable
Aerobic capacity	High	Medium	Low
Anaerobic capacity	Low	Medium	High
Motor unit size	Small	Larger	Largest
Capillary density	High	High	Low

myofibrils. Myofibrils have a banding pattern that exact a striated appearance upon muscle fibres, giving skeletal muscle its descriptive term 'striated muscle'.[10]

Myofibrils within skeletal muscle fibres have alternating light and dark band structures regularly arranged in a repeating pattern called sarcomeres. Both dark and light bands contain a darkly staining line that bisects them. The dark band is also called the A-band and consists of myosin proteins arranged in parallel with interconnecting filaments called the M-line. Myosin also contains two globular proteins that project from its longitudinal axis to form cross-bridges with the thin filaments in proximity to the larger, thick myosin molecules (Fig. 70.4).[10] Creatine kinase is known to be associated with thick filaments at the M-line and is believed to be involved in the phosphorylation of adenosine diphosphate (ADP) to adenosine triphosphate (ATP), a critical step in supplying energy molecules to muscle cross-bridges.[11]

The light band of sarcomeres is called the I-band and consists of thin filaments. Thin filaments consist of actin, troponin and tropomyosin, three proteins important in skeletal muscle structure and function. The Z-line is the darkly staining line that bisects the I-band and connects the thin filaments. A-bands and I-bands are interwoven and will interact in a manner to cause a muscle contraction that will be discussed later in the chapter (Fig. 70.4).[12]

Muscle fibres are individually surrounded by a plasma membrane known as the sarcolemma. Within the contents of the sarcolemma is the muscle fibre sarcoplasm. The sarcoplasm is equivalent to the cytoplasm of other cell types. The sarcoplasm can be thought of as the contents of the sarcolemma minus the nuclei. Just beneath the sarcolemma at the periphery of an individual muscle fibre are the nuclei and stem cells of the fibre. Just superficial to the sarcolemma is a connective tissue known as endomysium, which has many capillaries needed for blood supply to muscle.

MOTOR UNIT

Muscle contraction occurs as a result of input from nerve fibres at the neuromuscular junction. The force of the muscular contraction depends on the number of motor units firing. A motor unit is ultimately defined as a single alpha motor neurone axon and the muscle fibres it innervates. The motor unit size is dependent upon the number of muscle fibres that are innervated by the nerve fibre.[6]

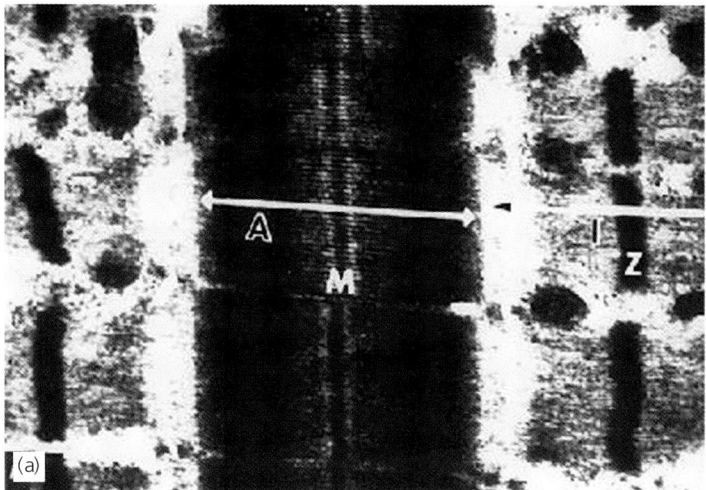
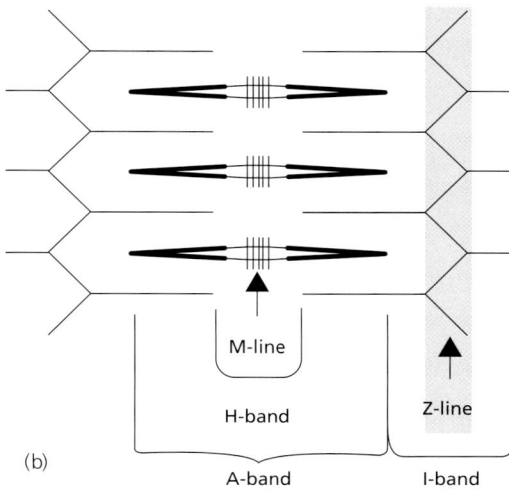

Figure 70.4 (a) Muscle microstructure. (b) The basic structural unit of skeletal muscle, the sarcomere. Reproduced with permission from Buckwalter et al.[2]

Muscle fibres have contact with one nerve terminal, but one nerve terminal can innervate several muscle fibres. The production of force by a skeletal muscle can be increased or decreased through the recruitment of more or fewer motor units.[1] Each motor fibre type is dependent upon the motor nerve it interacts with.[13] Motor unit types include the type I, type IIA and type IIB motor unit types previously mentioned.

Motor units are stimulated to contract by the action potential, an electrical impulse originating from the cell body of the nerve. During a contraction, motor units undergo coordinated steps that are described by the Henneman principle.[14] The Henneman size principle states that smaller motor units (those with few muscle fibres innervated by a single motor axon) will be recruited before larger motor units (those with more muscle fibres innervated by a single motor axon).[14] Nerves form contact with the muscle fibres via a specialized synapse known as the motor end plate. The motor end plate includes the terminal portion of the nerve and the muscle membrane in which the nerve will interact. Electrical impulses are propogated via the axon of the neurone to the nerve terminal. At the nerve terminal, the electrical impulse allows release of chemical transmitters that can react on the muscle membrane receptors. There is a small gap, known as the gap junction, that separates the nerve from the muscle at the motor end plate (Fig. 70.5).[15,16]

Acetylcholine (Ach) is a key neurotransmitter that acts at the motor end plate. It is stored in the presynaptic axon in membrane-encased compartments called vesicles. When an electrical impulse reaches the terminal end of the axon near the motor end plate, calcium ions flow into the cell via channels. The increase in calcium concentration causes the vesicles to fuse with the presynaptic membrane, releasing Ach into the synapse.[17] Ach diffuses across the synaptic cleft and binds to Ach-specific receptors on the surface of the muscle membrane. The muscle membrane consequently depolarizes, resulting in muscle contraction. Acetylcholinesterase deactivates the neurotransmitter, and the by-products of this reaction are reabsorbed and repackaged in the presynaptic nerve terminal (Fig. 70.6).[2]

Numerous synthetic and naturally present substances have an effect at the neuromuscular junction. Examples include curare, a naturally occurring agent that was historically used in warfare. Curare binds Ach receptors and disallows Ach-induced impulse transmission. Succinylcholine inhibits impulse transmission by binding to the receptor and depolarizing the receptor; this prevents the further depolarization of the receptor by Ach. Acetylcholinesterase itself is the target of many drug interventions as well. Examples include neostigmine and edrophonium that block acetylcholinesterases reversibly, while certain insecticides have irreversible effects with grave consequences.[18] Understanding the occurrences at the neuromuscular junction has allowed for investigators to target these processes as well as treat pathological conditions that occur at the junction. For example, myasthenia gravis, a muscle fatigue disorder characterized by autoimmune attack of Ach receptors, is

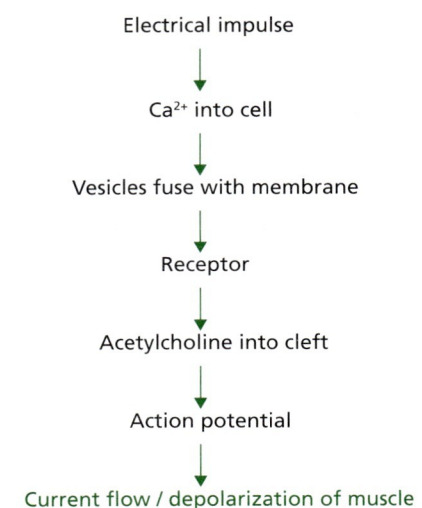

Figure 70.6 Flow of nerve signal.

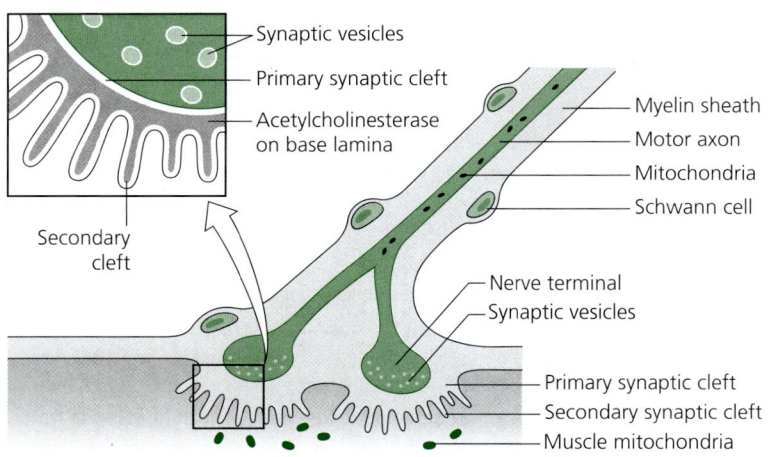

Figure 70.5 Nerve synapse. Reproduced with permission from Buckwalter et al.[2]

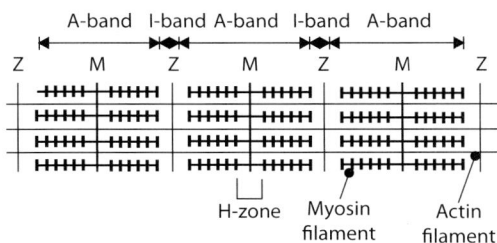
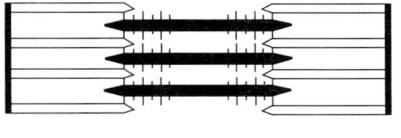
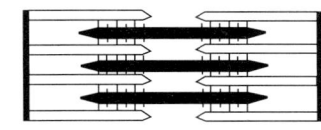

Figure 70.7 Skeletal muscle contraction. Reproduced with permission from Buckwalter et al.[2]

typically treated with agents such as acetylcholinesterase inhibitors that provide excess Ach available for muscle contraction.[19]

MUSCLE CONTRACTION

Gross muscle contraction has been studied on a microstructural level and is the result of links made between the thick and thin filaments mentioned in section Skeletal muscle structure. Cross-bridges from thick to thin filaments allow sliding motions through conformational changes powered by ATP. These conformational changes can cycle multiple times. Troponin and tropomyosin molecules are linked to actin. Tropomyosin is linked to troponin and prevents the formation of cross-bridges. When calcium is available, it interacts with troponi, allowing for changes in the troponin–tropomyosin complex and permitting cross-bridge formation and shortening (Fig. 70.7).

Muscle contraction has been studied under various conditions with the discovery of three labelled periods of muscle function: isometric, isotonic and isokinetic. Isometric muscle contraction is the production of muscle tension without changes in muscle length or joint movement. Isometric contraction is a measure of static strength and can be demonstrated when one pushes against an immovable object, such as a wall. The rotator cuff and its ability to compress the humerus into the glenoid surface is another example of isometric contraction. In both examples, muscle contraction producing tension is present, but there is no change in the length of the muscle.

In isotonic contraction, muscle is shortened against a constant tension or load. Biceps curls and bench presses are both examples of isotonic contraction in which muscle is contracting against a constant load. The constant load can also be one's own body mass, as in squatting exercises against gravity. Isotonic contraction can be demonstrated in two phases: concentric contraction and eccentric contraction (isokinetic exercise also contains these two subcategories). In concentric contraction, a generation of force leads to muscle contraction and shortening if the load on the muscle is less than the force the muscle creates. On the other hand, the load on the muscle can be greater than the force generated on the muscle and this is known as eccentric muscle action.[2] During muscle training eccentric contractions involve controlled lengthening of a muscle while contracting against a load. Bicep curls exhibit both concentric and eccentric contraction. During flexion, the biceps is undergoing concentric contraction, and, during controlled extension, the biceps is undergoing eccentric contraction (Fig. 70.8). It is important to have controlled motion during eccentric contracting, to maximize strengthening and decrease the likelihood of muscle injury. Recent studies have shown that eccentric muscle contractions cause greater oxidative stress than concentric exercises, which may cause increased stress in muscles undergoing eccentric contraction.[20] Also, eccentric muscle contraction has been implicated in the occurrence of delayed onset of muscle soreness (DOMS), which will be described later.

Isokinetic contraction involves keeping the speed (distance per unit time) constant on an actively contracting muscle while the load is changed in order to maintain a constant velocity. Isokinetic exercises require special exercise equipment and are a measure of dynamic strength.[21] The exercises are best used for rehabilitation protocols and functional assessment and are not observed in most muscles during normal ambulation or activity.

The force generated by muscle fibres is transmitted across the myotendinous junction. This area is the weak link and the primary site of injury that occurs during muscle injury. The area is composed of highly folded membranes that increase the surface area, decrease the stresses and change those stresses from tensile to shear because of the

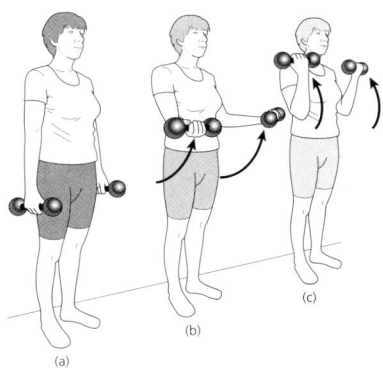

Figure 70.8 (a) Extension during biceps curl (eccentric contraction). (b) Flexion during biceps curl (concentric contraction).

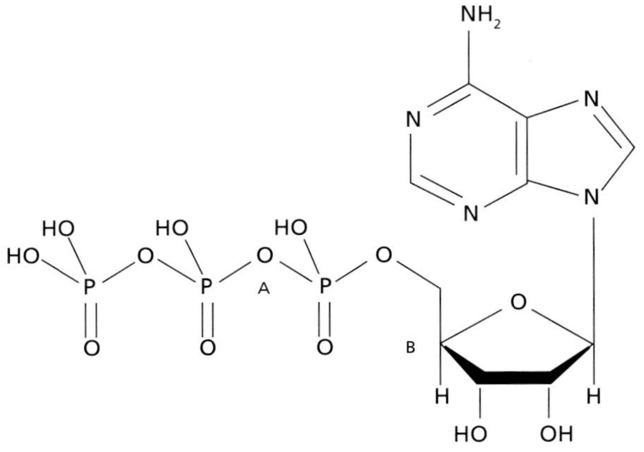

Figure 70.9 Adenosine triphosphate molecule.

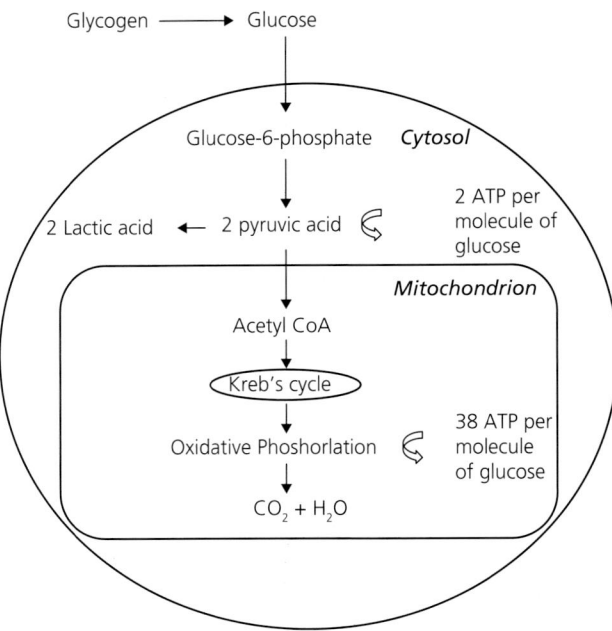

Figure 70.10 Adenosine triphosphate (ATP) yield of anaerobic and aerobic metabolism.

parallel arrangement of the membranes. Also at the junction are numerous cytoskeletal proteins that allow for a special affinity between the muscle fibre membranes and the collagen fibres of the tendon.[22]

Energy metabolism

ENERGETICS OF MUSCLE

The immediate chemical energy source for muscle is ATP. This molecule is composed of an adenosine molecule attached to three serial inorganic phosphate molecules. The three phosphate molecules are attached to the adenosine molecule in a chain (Fig. 70.9). The energy necessary for muscle metabolism occurs through cleavage of the bonds in the ATP molecule, with cleavage of the last two bonds releasing the highest amount of energy. Although ATP is constantly being used, the human body is able to maintain relatively constant levels of high-energy phosphates even under conditions of increased use.

Another source of high-energy phosphates in muscle is the molecule creatine phosphate (CP). However, CP cannot be used directly by the muscle cell and must use ADP to form ATP via the enzyme creatine kinase:

$$ADP + CP \circledR ATP + creatine$$

This reaction creates an ATP molecule that the cell can use. There is also another enzyme found in muscle, myokinase, which maintains ATP concentration by combining two ADP molecules to create ATP and adenosine monophosphate (AMP):[2]

$$ADP + ADP \circledR ATP + AMP$$

Athletic activity requires the replenishment of phosphagens, and the production of ATP is usually the factor that limits one's level of athletic performance. Other phosphagens, such as CP, are not in adequate supply to maintain energy levels during athletic performance. The human body relies on two metabolic pathways to replenish ATP: the aerobic (oxygen present) and anaerobic (oxygen not present) pathways. Aerobic metabolism is the primary source of ATP replenishment when oxygen is available. Aerobic metabolism uses the breakdown products of glucose molecules. The glucose molecules are broken down into two pyruvate molecules that enter the Kreb cycle, yielding 38 (34 net) ATP molecules (Fig. 70.10). Skeletal muscle glucose uptake can increase as much as 28-fold with exercise.[23] However, glucose is available in only limited amounts as glucose-6-phosphate or stored as glycogen. Liver has the ability to store glycogen at higher concentrations; however, because of its mass, skeletal muscle has the highest quantity of glycogen in the body.[24] Nevertheless, glycogen is stored in liver and skeletal muscle in limited quantities overall. Sedentary lifestyles can predispose one to lower glycogen stores, possibly secondary to decreased muscle mass.[25]

Anaerobic metabolism is the primary source of ATP when oxygen is not available and is a less efficient system. It is the primary form of metabolism during strenuous, high-intensity, short exercises. It results in two ATP molecules and lactic acid.[26] Lactic acid accumulation leads to acidosis and is thought to be the primary cause of muscle fatigue during exercise (Fig. 70.10).[27]

Glucose is considered to be the primary energy source, but fats and proteins can also be used as energy sources in the oxidative (oxygen present) pathway of energy production. Fats are potentially the largest energy store in the body. It is usually in the form of triglycerides (three fatty acids on a glyceraldehyde molecule), which can be cleaved to free fatty acids that undergo β-oxidation into acetyl

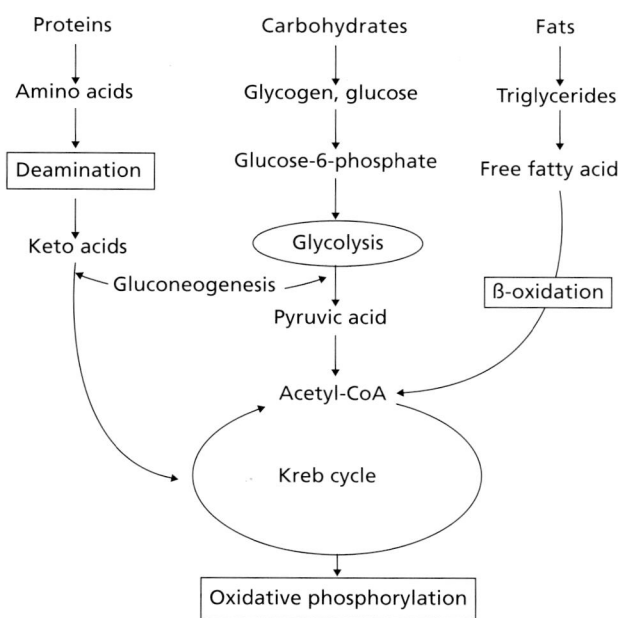

Figure 70.11 Sources of energy production. Reproduced with permission from Buckwalter et al.[2]

Co-A. Acetyl Co-A has the ability to enter the Kreb cycle as well. The amount of energy made depends on the length of the fatty acid chain. While the body has a preference for glucose and fat for adequate energy source, proteins are usually metabolized as a last resort. They are not used during rest or exercise of any intensity unless one's nutritional status is compromised.[28] They can be broken down into amino acids, which can be deaminated to ketoacids that can be used in the Kreb cycle. Ketoacids can also undergo gluconeogenesis in instances of severe glucose depletion (Fig. 70.11).[2]

At the beginning of an exercise course, ATP is supplied via the ATP-CP (ATP–phosphocreatine system) mentioned above. This system can also supply energy for very short duration, high-intensity bursts of exercise, but only lasts for a few seconds. The use of energy sources usually begins with stored phosphagens. As the duration of an exercise increases and the intensity remains high, anaerobic systems replenish ATP, producing lactate and inducing fatigue. Anaerobic systems can act and allow for ATP replenishment for about 1–2 minutes. As the intensity falls, aerobic systems can meet demands and begin to replenish ATP. Therefore, aerobic systems allow for lower intensity exercises lasting longer durations. The rate of acidosis caused by anaerobic systems is dependent on the cardiovascular system's ability to supply oxygen and the metabolic capacity of the muscle fibres (type I vs type II). During times of high intensity and short exercise, glucose is preferentially used because its oxidation requires less oxygen per mole than that of fatty acids.[29] During prolonged aerobic exercises, there is a shift from carbohydrate use to fatty acid oxidation to preserve carbohydrate stores.[2,30]

Exercise performance

TRAINING AND MUSCLE

Muscle is capable of adaptation, and the type of training regimen will affect the tissue response. The overload and specific adaptations to imposed demands (SAID) principles are theories on how muscle adapts to change. In simple terms the overload principle states that muscle will adapt to its extrinsic stresses, and applies to resistance training. The SAID principle is more involved and describes how a certain exercise or type of training will produce adaptations specific to the activity performed and only in the muscles that are stressed by that activity. Therefore, runners will gain strength in their legs and not their arms. Application of this principle is essential for training because, in order for one to increase their performance in a given activity, they must do training exercises that influence muscles involved in that activity.[31–33]

Endurance training exercises involve relatively low tension and increased repetitions. On a cellular level, this type of exercise increases the number of mitochondria per cell and the capillary density supplying those cells, and decreases the muscle cross-sectional area to allow for improved oxygen delivery to tissues.[34] The goal of endurance training is to improve aerobic performance. Endurance training can lead to the conversion of type II fibres to type I fibres and allows for the increased use of fat for energy.[2]

Strength training involves decreased repetitions and increased resistance. This leads to an increase in muscle size that experimental evidence has revealed is mostly due to muscle hypertrophy as opposed to muscle hyperplasia. The strength gains obtained during the first few weeks of strength training are mostly the result of neuromuscular adaptations. The nervous system recruits larger motor units with higher frequencies of stimulation when faced with increased exercise intensity and muscle fatigue.[1]

CARDIOPULMONARY SYSTEMS AND EXERCISE

The primary responsibility of the cardiovascular system is to supply oxygen-rich blood to exercising skeletal muscle. The ability to both provide ample oxygen to tissues and remove the build-up of metabolic by-products, such as lactate, are thought to be limiting factors in exercise performance.

The Fick equation is used to determine one's oxygen consumption (VO_2) during a particular period of time.[35–37] It is measured by multiplying cardiac output (CO) by the difference between arterial and venous oxygen content or concentration ($C_a - C_v$):

$$VO_2 = CO \times (C_a - C_v)$$

The Fick equation represents the 'oxygen reserve', or the balance between oxygen delivery and consumption.

During exercise, oxygen consumption increases until a plateau is reached and no further uptake of oxygen occurs despite continued exercise intensity, limiting exercise performance.[38] There is also exercise performance limited by lactate production. The lactate threshold is defined as the point in oxygen uptake where pyruvate levels exceed metabolic capacity, leading to increased serum lactic acid levels.[30] Endurance athletes have been shown to improve their ability to increase both their oxygen consumption and their lactate threshold.

CO is equal to heart rate multiplied by stroke volume (CO = HR × SV). Since the supply of oxygen-rich arterial blood to skeletal muscle and other tissues is needed for exercise performance, CO is the determining factor in exercise performance. The equation has two variables that affect CO and therefore oxygen supply. Studies have shown that increases in oxygen demand are accommodated by increases in SV in early exercise and increases in heart rate in later exercise.[29] The heart rate in young individuals can increase to as much as 200 beats per minute, but this ability to increase diminishes with age, and can be calculated by the maximum heart calculation during exercise target:[39]

$$\text{Maximum heart rate} = 220 - \text{age}$$

The vascular system responds to exercise by vasodilation. leading to increased blood flow and only moderate increases in blood pressure. As skeletal muscle demands more blood, the visceral system volunteers portions of its blood supply and decreased visceral perfusion is observed.[38]

In conjunction with increased cardiovascular function, respiratory rates can increase from normal levels of 12–20 breaths per minutes to 50 breaths per minute with heavy exercise.[40] Much attention has centred on improving cardiopulmonary function with high-altitude training. High-altitude training increases one's oxygen-carrying capacity by increasing renal secretion of erythropoietin and subsequent increase in red blood cell production. However, some studies show that the changes seen at high altitudes correct themselves quickly upon return to sea level. Moreover, oxygen consumption and exercise intensity can decrease with increases in atmosphere. Therefore, the benefits of high-altitude training may be offset by its risks, including pulmonary hypertension, cerebral hypoperfusion and right heart failure. Newer training regimens at lower elevations should be considered and researched as alternatives to high-altitude training.[41]

HORMONES AND SKELETAL MUSCLE

Insulin and glucagon are two very important hormones in skeletal muscle physiology. Insulin is primarily an anabolic hormone that allows for the increased storage of glucose, fatty acids and amino acids. Insulin levels decrease with all forms of exercise as skeletal muscle increases its consumption of glucose, thereby lowering the circulating serum glucose levels and suppressing insulin release.[42] On the other hand, glucagon has a reciprocal effect. It is the primary catabolic hormone and will allow for the mobilization of various energy molecules from their storage sites. There are increases in serum levels of glucagon during exercise in order to maintain serum levels of glucose via gluconeogenesis and glycogenolysis.

Pituitary hormones, such as growth hormone, have varying effects on muscle and exercise. Growth hormone exerts anabolic effects on muscle and shows increased serum levels during exercise.[43] It increases the amino acid transport into cells for protein incorporation leading to an increase in skeletal muscle synthesis.

Adrenal hormones are also affected by exercise. Since dehydration is a concern during exercise, it is no surprise that many of the water regulatory hormones are affected during strenuous exercise. Aldosterone levels increase during increased physiological energy expenditure and serve to prevent the loss of water and sodium during exercise.[44] Cortisol, a glucocorticoid, also increases during exercise, leading to increases in gluconeogenesis in the liver, lipolysis, and protein degradation in liver and in muscles. Hormones secreted by the adrenal medulla, epinephrine and norepinephrine, also increase during exercise.[45] With prolonged exercise, basal levels of catecholamines decrease, leading to lower resting and exercise-related heart rates and blood pressures. As a result of this physiological response, athletes have increased ability to perform intense exercise.[46]

MUSCLE DAMAGE AND DISUSE

Strenuous activity predisposes the athlete to a continuum of muscle injury, from simple soreness to more complicated tears. Muscle soreness usually occurs 24–72 hours after intense exercise and resolves 5–7 days after exercise.[47,48] Since it does not occur immediately after exercise it has been termed DOMS. It is probably secondary to inflammation and is associated mostly with eccentric exercise.[49] Patients will demonstrate reduced activity and display firm, swollen muscles. Strength loss is common and mechanical forces are largely responsible for decreased muscle length and other physiological manifestations. If high enough tensile stresses are present, structural abnormalities will result, including Z-band streaming, A-band disruption, and myofibril misalignment and structural damage.[2,50] Myofibrils themselves experience an influx of calcium that causes increased pressure and oedema. Recent studies have shown that skeletal muscle injury causes fibrosis and scar at the endomysium. Formation of those cells can propagate other inflammatory mediators and lead to continued skeletal muscle injury.[51] At the same time, cellular membranes are damaged, allowing for the leakage of intracellular proteins such as the enzyme creatine kinase. Inflammatory mediators then allow for increased capillary wall permeability, leading to rising serum levels of creatine kinase days after injury.[52] The overall effect of DOMS is decreased muscle endurance and decreased force production, and can lead to decreased athletic performance.[53]

Muscle strains are thought to occur at the myotendinous junction. Muscle fatigue is the reduced ability of a muscle to produce force during and/or after exercise that leads to an impairment of performance.[54] Fatigue can be a result of a combination of peripheral and central fatigue. Peripheral fatigue occurs at or distal to the neuromuscular junction while central fatigue may be physiological or psychological.[55] Peripheral muscle fatigue is most often caused by accumulation of metabolic by-products such as lactic acid and inorganic phosphates. Central fatigue can be affected by motivation and reduced alpha motor neurone excitability secondary to spine pathology.[56] Fatigue increases muscle susceptibility to strain by reducing the muscle's ability to absorb energy. Therefore, as there is an onset of fatigue, one is more likely to experience muscle strain.[2]

Muscle tears usually result from direct trauma. After muscle tears, the normal muscle tissue heals with a dense connective tissue scar. Models of muscle tears show that muscle that has undergone a tear in its mid-substance will regain only one-half of its motor strength after healing.[2]

Although strenuous activity can lead to muscle damage, non-use or immbolization can also have damaging effects on muscle. Immobilization causes a series of events that have been noted on the molecular level. First, change that occurs with immobilization is exponential muscle loss. Loss of strength then occurs with loss of muscle mass. Next, muscle has a decreased ability to use fats in aerobic metabolic pathways, which leads to increased fatigability. As a result, muscles should be immobilized in order to improve maintenance of strength.

EPIDEMIOLOGY: INJURIES AND PREVENTION

Injuries

In an effort to systematize reporting of athletic injuries, the US National Collegiate Athletic Association (NCAA) compiled reports of 180 000 injuries and roughly 1 million exposure histories in collegiate sports from 1988 to 2004.[57] Injuries were compiled from 16 sports activities: men's baseball, women's softball, women's and men's basketball, women's field hockey, men's American football (autumn and spring), women's and men's lacrosse, women's and men's soccer, men's and women's gymnastics, and men's wrestling.

Pre-season games were shown to have a lower injury rate than in-season games; however, pre-season training and practices were two to three times more likely to have injuries than those in-season. Poorly conditioned athletes, multiple practices in a single day with little recovery time, and stress of competition as players try out for starter positions all contributed to a higher rate of injury in pre-season practice. Furthermore, player-to-player contact accounts for the majority of injuries: roughly 58% during games and 41% in practice. There is no surprise then that men's football dominated all of the sport activities in the number of ankle ligament sprains, anterior cruciate ligament injuries and concussions given the required contact. Lower extremities sustained the greatest injury, accounting for 50% of reported injuries.

Prevention

Injury prevention has been shown to increase player productivity and to decrease the likelihood of long-term limitations. For example, knee injury, especially cruciate ligament injuries, has long been linked to osteoarthritis of the knee in young adults.[58] Regulations have been set in motion by the NCAA to increase awareness and prevention of injury, such as requiring eye protection for women's lacrosse or preventing clipping in men's football.[57] In 2000, the National Athletic Trainer's Association released guidelines for the medical care of the intercollegiate athlete.[59] The increase in medical awareness and even the 86% increase in the number of certified athletic trainers (from 1995 to 2005) are also promising movements towards better injury prevention.

The NCAA Injury Surveillance System recommends focusing on the implementation and enforcement of existing policies and rules developed for competition. Phased-in practices in the pre-season may help to condition the athletes better and allow the time needed for recovery. Pre-season physical examinations may identify old injuries that may worsen with practice, or that are in need of rehabilitation, before attempting training to reduce long-term mechanical risks.[60]

SPECIAL CONSIDERATIONS: NUTRITION

In 2000, the American Dietetic Association, American College of Sports Medicine and Dieticians of Canada released a joint statement offering nutritional recommendations for athletes. The selection of food and fluids, the timing of intake and the supplement choices can directly affect health and exercise performance. Athletes should strive to maintain energy balance, which is defined as when energy intake (such as food, fluids and nutritional supplementation) equals energy expenditure (including resting metabolic rate, thermic effect of food and physical activity expenditure). If athletes intentionally or unintentionally limit energy intake, the body then uses fat and muscle stores as a means of energy. Consequently, muscle loss hurts performance by a reduction in strength and endurance.

Energy demands are met by oxidation of fat and carbohydrates. Body glucose stores, primarily in the form of glycogen in muscle and in the liver, are small relative to what can be used for exercise. Carbohydrate intake is necessary to maintain blood glucose levels during exercise and replenish muscle glycogen stores. It takes approximately 24–48 hours for muscle and liver stores to be replenished, if adequate carbohydrates are available, after exercise.[61] Diets should therefore have at least 60% of total caloric intake allotted to carbohydrates,[62] or 8–10 g kg^{-1} of carbohydrates per day. Furthermore, timing of intake is equally important, since glycogen resynthesis is most rapid immediately following exercise; 1–2 g kg^{-1} should be consumed within the first hour of completing exercise.[61] High carbohydrate intake may be achieved by consuming frequent small meals and snacks, by using a food exchange system by decreasing the intake of fat and, in some cases, by consuming foods with a high glycaemic index (Table 70.2).

Protein's roles include the formation of muscle protein, haemoglobin (to transport oxygen) and enzymes (for energy metabolism), and catabolism.[63] Furthermore, eight of the 20 essential amino acids must be obtained from the diet. High-protein foods include meat, eggs and fish, which contain all the essential amino acids. Therefore, vegetarian diets should pay special attention to foods with a higher protein value, as discussed later. Protein may constitute 12–15% of total energy intake, which translates to a daily protein intake of 1.2–1.7 g kg^{-1} of body weight per day.[64] The suggested protein intake can usually be met with normal diet and does not require supplementation. Calorie restriction in the setting of hard physical exercise can result in an increased rate of protein catabolism and an increase in cortisol and catecholamines that can compromise immune function (Table 70.2).

Triglycerides serve as a major energy reserve for exercise. Lipid stores are found in adipose tissue, muscle and in the circulation; 1 kg of adipose tissue can supply energy for approximately 10–20 hours of exercise.[65] Furthermore, increased aerobic exercise leads to an increased utilization of triglycerides for energy.[63] Fat is essential for energy, fat-soluble vitamins and essential fatty acids, and there is no performance benefit to consuming a diet with less than 15% fat. High-fat diets immediately preceding exercise have not been shown to enhance performance,[64,65] and studies still favour carbohydrate loading before endurance activity. The supplemental use of omega-3 fatty acids, such as eicosapentaenoic and docosahexaenoic fatty acids from fish oils, has been postulated to increase oxygen delivery to muscles by increasing vasodilation from its by-product, prostaglandin E1.[63] However, few studies have addressed this assumption (Table 70.2).

Since water and electrolytes cannot be stored, failing to consume electrolyte-balanced fluids before and during exercise may result in dehydration.[66] Therefore, 2 hours before exercise, athletes should consume 400–600 mL (14–22 oz) of fluid. Athletes should also consume 150–350 mL (6–12 oz) of fluid every 15–20 minutes during exercise depending on tolerance. Furthermore, when competing in warm, humid conditions, sweating becomes non-functional, since it drips off the body as opposed to being evaporated and cooling the body. Athletes are encouraged not only to maintain hydration before and during exercise but also to consume a meal or snack low in fat and fibre to facilitate gastric emptying and minimize gastrointestinal distress and with adequate carbohydrate content to maintain blood glucose levels.

Ergogenic aids

The popularity of ergogenic aids may be problematic in counselling athletes regarding nutritional supplementation. Ergogenic aids are aimed at enhancing performance, by enhancing energy metabolism, reducing body fat or enhancing muscle production.[62] Ergogenic aids may be problematic because manufacturers can make even unsubstantiated claims regarding performance enhancement as long as no claims are made regarding the ability of the supplements to 'diagnose, mitigate, treat, cure and prevent' disease.[67] Unfortunately, there is limited evidence to support the vast array of ergogenic aids available for purchase. The Joint Committee recommends not only scientifically validating claims made by the manufacturers of ergogenic aids but also evaluating the legality and safety of these aids in counselling athletes.

Creatine is one ergogenic aid that has been studied and shown to have an impact on muscle growth and performance enhancement. Creatine is endogenously produced by amino acid precursors arginine, glycine and methionine for the role of energy metabolism. The storage form, creatine phosphate, is broken down by creatine kinase during exercise, releasing the phosphate

Table 70.2 Joint statement nutritional recommendations for athletes

Energy source	Suggested intake	Special considerations
Carbohydrates	55–58%	1–2 g kg^{-1} consumed in hour after exercise
		Depends on sex, environmental conditions and sport type
Protein	12–15%	Achieved with meat, eggs and dairy products
		Vegetarian diets can be sustained with appropriate intake
Fat	25–30%	No benefit to fat intake less than 15%

Position of the American Dietetic Association, Dietitians of Canada, and the American College of Sports Medicine: nutrition and athletic performance. *Journal of the American Dietetic Association* 2000;**100**:1543-56.

group for the formation of ATP, thus producing energy. Elevated muscle creatine levels increase the rate by which creatine phosphate is resynthesized following exercise. Harris et al.[68] found that high doses of creatine resulted in a 15-fold increase in blood circulating creatine concentrations. The results were discernible after 2 days of 1–2 kg day^{-1} creatine intake. Gain in muscle mass most probably results from increased protein synthesis in response to creatine ingestion, perhaps as a result of cell swelling.

Words such as 'doping' have been commonplace in sports as the desire to improve performance and win competitions may motivate athletes to use banned substances. As a sports medicine physician, management of such athletes is especially problematic because use is surreptitious and many athletes may periodically discontinue use to evade detection.[69] Formal drug testing, instituted by both the International Olympic Committee and the NCAA, may help to discourage use of banned substances.[70] However, the sports medicine physician should be aware of the possible use of banned substances by athletes.

Androgens and their precursors, including testosterone esters, androstenedione and dehydroepiandrosterone (DHEA), are commonly used as a means to increase muscle mass and muscle strength. Furthermore, some athletes may use human chorionic gonadotrophin, which increases endogenous release of androgens from Leydig cells, making them more difficult to detect.[69] Testosterone esters have been shown to increase serum testosterone levels and muscle strength whereas the efficacy of androgen precursors is somewhat questionable. Wallace et al.[71] found a slight increase in lean muscle mass in men who were given androstenedione and DHEA; however, the results were not statistically significantly different from the placebo group. Androgen use is not benign; rather, the side-effects can become quite hazardous. The elevation of exogenous testosterone decreases spermatogenesis, increases gynecomastia, leads to aggressive behaviour, and can cause virilization of female athletes.[69] Furthermore, lipid disturbances (e.g. decreased serum high-density lipoproteins), hepatotoxicity and cardiac disease have been associated with the use of 17-alpha-alkylated androgens and DHEA (Table 70.3).[69,70]

Nutritional considerations for specific groups

VEGETARIANS

Given the proposed dietary recommendations for protein and fats, vegetarian diets may seem to be insufficient. However, vegetarian diets can certainly meet the energy requirements of the athlete. Endurance athlete groups, such as triathletes, runners and cyclists, may adopt vegetarian diets to meet increased carbohydrate needs or weight control. Furthermore, vegetarian diets may be undertaken for religious customs or to enjoy the overall benefits in cardiovascular health. Vegetarian diets have limitations that, if appropriately recognized, can be addressed to meet the needs of athletes.

Vegetarian diets high in fibre may not adequately meet the energy needs of competing athletes given the non-metabolizable form of the carbohydrates.[72] However, vegetarian athletes may attain appropriate levels of energy by consuming more meals and snacks and meat alternatives, including textured vegetable protein tofu, avocados, nuts, dried fruit, and honey and jams.[73] Because plant proteins are not as easily digested as animal proteins, vegetarian athletes should increase their protein intake by roughly 10%.[74] Furthermore, proteins derived from eggs and textured vegetable (e.g. tofu) and dairy products provide essential amino acids and can meet the protein needs of vegetarian athletes.

Vegetarians also have lower muscle creatine levels than non-vegetarian competitors, and may benefit from creatine supplementation.[73] Furthermore, vegetarian athletes are at risk for deficiencies in vitamins B12 and D, riboflavin, iron, calcium and zinc, since many of these micronutrients are highly available in animal products. For example, plant-based iron has a lower bioavailability

Table 70.3 Additional substances

Substance	Mechanism	Findings
Stimulants (e.g. caffeine, amphetamines)	Heightened energy, appetite suppression, reduced need for sleep	Arrhythmias, anxiety, agitation
Recombinant erythropoietin	Increased red blood cell production, thereby increasing oxygen-carrying capacity	Haematocrit >50 in men Haematocrit >47 in women
Insulin	Anabolic effects on muscle	Hypoglycaemia
Growth hormone	Increased muscle mass, reduced fat	Peripheral oedema, paraesthesias, arthralgias, carpal tunnel syndrome
β-blockers	Reduction of tremors	Reduced heart rate

Other drugs that may be used to enhance physiological performance include stimulants (e.g. caffeine and amphetamines), recombinant erythropoietin, which increases red blood cell production and hence increases oxygen-carrying capacity, and growth hormone.
Snyder PJ. Use of androgens and other drugs by athletes. *UpToDate*.

than haem iron found in animal products. Therefore, vegetarians may have overall lower iron stores despite intakes equal to or higher than those of their omnivore counterparts. Soya products and fibre itself can inhibit non-haem iron absorption.[75] Vitamin C (ascorbic acid) intake may play a role in counteracting these effects.[67]

WOMEN

While nutrition recommendations for male and female athletes are relatively similar, subtle differences in the metabolism of energy substrates require some attention when counselling female athletes. For example, women tend to utilize more lipid and carbohydrate energy sources than their male counterparts, as influenced by oestrogen and progesterone levels that enhance lipolysis and decreased glucose utilization.[76] Unfortunately, many female athletes adopt calorie-restricted diets, especially by minimizing lipid contributions, as a means to modify body physique secondary to societal pressures to maintain low body fat composition and preoccupation with body image.[77] The female athlete triad – disordered eating, amenorrhoea and osteoporosis – was first identified by the American College of Sports Medicine in 1992.[78] The female athlete triad is characterized by dieting with the desire to lose weight, which, if severe enough, results in disordered eating. Low energy intake in conjunction with high energy expenditure has been shown to alter the secretion of luteinizing hormone and follicle-stimulating hormone, resulting in amenorrhoea and loss of bone mass in young women.[78] Since oestrogen plays a role in calcium absorption and bone formation, low oestrogen levels may result in lower peak bone masses in young female athletes. These athletes are more susceptible to decreased mineral bone density as well as to increased risk of musculoskeletal injury (i.e. increased susceptibility to skeletal stress fractures because of altered mineralization).[79] Complaints of fatigue, irritation and, consequently, poor athletic performance may result.[77,80]

Calorie restriction is also frequently associated with poor vitamin and mineral intake, particularly calcium, iron, zinc, magnesium, zinc and B complex vitamins (e.g. folate).[81] For example, female athletes tend to have a poor iron intake, which is attributable to avoidance of foods with haem iron, such as meat and poultry, and restricted energy intakes.[77] Fortunately, these micronutrients can be attained in adequate amounts by encouraging the use of vitamin supplementation or by consuming fortified foods.

If weight loss is desired, increasing energy expenditure rather than reducing energy intake is most effective in protecting resting metabolic rate, which can be lower in severely calorie-restricted diets. Moderate decreases of intake, such as 300–500 kcal, may facilitate weight loss, but should be avoided if intense training is already under way.[77] Decreases in intake can be accomplished by altering food choices and serving sizes. Furthermore, increases in food consumption during and after exercise may be beneficial as exercising skeletal muscles are particularly sensitized to glucose and amino acids.[80] Coordination of caloric intake and exercise may serve to optimize physical performance. Carbohydrate intake should be matched to the type of athletic activity performed. Female endurance athletes may benefit from high-carbohydrate diets since they maximize glycogen stores.

CHILDREN

The involvement of children and adolescents in organized athletics produces lasting benefits, notably healthier nutritional habits as adults.[82] Nutrition is especially important in these populations because of the interplay of daily nutritional requirements for sports participation and those for continuing growth and development. In particular, children's hydration needs differ from those of adults as children are more likely to absorb heat from their environments, creating an increased risk of heat exhaustion and increasing fluid requirements before and after activity.[83] Child athletes should aim to drink an additional 0.5–1.0 L day^{-1} of fluid.[83]

Adequate protein intake of at least 12–15% of daily dietary energy is also necessary to prevent the metabolism of growing muscle reserves for energy. While carbohydrates are necessary components of energy intake for children and adolescents, glycolytic pathways are not as well developed in children as they are in adolescents and adults. Therefore, child athletes may rely on fat as much as carbohydrates to support exercise and activity.[83] Petrie et al.[83] recommend that at least 50% of daily caloric intake comprises carbohydrates, specifically grain-based foods and fruit. Unsaturated fats should constitute roughly 25% of energy intake in young athletes. The added benefit is increased absorption of fat-soluble vitamins and minerals. Young athletes who restrict fat calories for weight control should attempt this only if their baseline weight is in excess of what is needed for health. However, such attempts should be done with caution as the risks include growth impairment.[84]

Calcium and iron have both been identified among the micronutrients as being deficient in adolescents, having lasting effects on peak bone mass and resulting in anaemia in adolescent girls. Calcium deficiencies not only limit bone growth but also may influence the risk of stress fractures.[83] Even iron deficiencies not producing overt anaemia can negatively affect athletic and cognitive performance. Simply increasing iron intake is not adequate; rather, the intake of absorbable forms of iron, such as hemin, which is found in animal products, should be increased, and iron intake should be coupled with absorption facilitators, such as protein.

OLDER ADULTS

While ageing may bring about declines in energy expenditure and resting metabolic rate, remaining physically active

Table 70.4 Estimated energy requirements for older adults who are active

Age group in years	Men (kcal day^{-1})	Women (kcal day^{-1})	Diet composition
50–59	2757	2186	Carbohydrate: 45–65%
60–69	2657	2116	Fat: 20–35%
70–79	2557	2046	
80–89	2457	1967	

Institute of Medicine. *Dietary Reference Intakes For Energy, Carbohydrates, Fiber, Fat, Protein, And Amino Acids (Macronutrients)*. Washington, DC: National Academy Press, 2002.

attenuates these changes. The benefits of participation in athletics by masters athletes (athletes older than 50 years) include better lipid profiles, bone health, glucose tolerance and mood states than in age-matched sedentary controls.[85,86] Ageing is associated with a decline in lean muscle mass. Physical activity, such as resistance training, helps to maintain muscle mass and an adequate intake of small amounts of protein (0.1–0.2 g kg^{-1} h^{-1}) can enhance muscle anabolism during recovery of endurance and resistance exercise. This can be delivered with milk, eggs, cheese, yogurt, lean meat, fish, and poultry. A decline in activity corresponds to a decline in health benefits brought about by exercise and remaining physically active (Table 70.4).[87]

> **KEY LEARNING POINTS**
>
> - There are three types of muscle fibres: Type I, Type IIA and Type IIB.
> - The immediate chemical energy source for muscle is ATP, which can come from the anaerobic and aerobic system.
> - The anaerobic system supplies 2 ATP per molecule of glucose while the aerobic system supplies 38 ATP per molecule of glucose.
> - Muscle strains are thought to occur at the myotendinous junction.

REFERENCES

1. Lorenz T, Campello M. Biomechanics of skeletal muscle. In: Nordin M, Frankel V (eds) *Basic Biomechanics of the Musculoskeletal System*. Baltimore, MD: Lippincott Williams and Wilkins, 2001:148–75.
2. Buckwalter JA, Einhorn TA, Simon SR (eds). *Orthopaedic Basic Science: Biology and Biomechanics of the Musculoskeletal System*. Rosemont, IL, American Academy of Orthopaedic Surgeons, 2000.
3. Tortora SR, Grabowski GJ (eds). *Principles of Anatomy and Physiology*. Hoboken, NJ: John Wiley & Sons, 2006.
4. Malisoux L, Francaux M, Theisen D. What do single-fiber studies tell us about exercise training? *Medicine and Science in Sports and Exercise* 2007;**39**:1051–60.
5. Pette D. Metabolic heterogeneity of muscle fibres. *Journal of Experimental Biology* 1985;**115**:179–89.
6. Vaccaro AR (ed.). *OKU 8: Home Study Syllabus*. Rosemont, IL: American Academy of Orthopaedic Surgeons, 2005.
7. Mannion AF, Dumas GA, Stevenson JM, Cooper RG. The influence of muscle fiber size and type distribution on electromyographic measures of back muscle fatigability. *Spine* 1998;**23**:576–84.
8. Adams GR, Hather BM, Baldwin KM, Dudley GA. Skeletal muscle myosin heavy chain composition and resistance training. *Journal of Applied Physiology* 1993;**74**:911–15.
9. Aloisi M. [Intra-tissue specialization of skeletal muscle]. *Rivista di Istochimica, Normale e Patologica* 1975;**19**(1–4):43–9.
10. Huxley AF. Muscle structure and theories of contraction. *Progress in Biophysics and Biophysical Chemistry* 1957;**7**:255–318.
11. Lee CS, Nicholson GA, O'Sullivan WJ. Some properties of human skeletal muscle creatine kinase. *Australian Journal of Biological Sciences* 1977;**30**:507–17.
12. Huxley HE. Electron microscope studies on the structure of natural and synthetic protein filaments from striated muscle. *Journal of Molecular Biology* 1963;**7**:281–308.
13. Beardwell A. The spatial organization of motor units and the origin of different types of potential. *Annals of Physical Medicine* 1967;**9**(4):139–57.
14. Henneman E, Somjen G, Carpenter DO. Functional significance of cell size in spinal motoneurons. *Journal of Neurophysiology* 1965;**28**:560–80.
15. Buckley GA. The structure and development of the motor end-plate. *Physiotherapy* 1972;**58**:274–6.
16. Seid D, Cole WV. The investigation of the ultramorphologic structure of the motor end-plate. *Journal of the American Osteopathic Association* 1968;**67**:1029–30.
17. Engel AG, Lambert EH, Santa T. Study of long-term anticholinesterase therapy. Effects on neuromuscular transmission and on motor end-plate fine structure. *Neurology* 1973;**23**:1273–81.
18. Cannard K. The acute treatment of nerve agent exposure. *Journal of the Neurological Sciences* 2006;**249**:86–94.
19. Kalamida D, Poulas K, Avramopoulou V, *et al*. Muscle and neuronal nicotinic acetylcholine receptors. Structure, function and pathogenicity. *FEBS Journal* 2007;**274**:3799–845.
20. Kon M, Tanabe K, Lee H, *et al*. Eccentric muscle contractions induce greater oxidative stress than concentric contractions in skeletal muscle. *Applied Physiology Nutrition and Metabolism* 2007;**32**:273–81.
21. Laird Jr CE, Rozier CK. Toward understanding the terminology of exercise mechanics. *Physical Therapy* 1979;**59**:287–92.

22. Noonan TJ, Garrett Jr WE. Muscle strain injury: diagnosis and treatment. *Journal of the American Academy of Orthopaedic Surgeons* 1999;**7**:262-9.
23. Katz A, Broberg S, Sahlin K, Wahren J. Leg glucose uptake during maximal dynamic exercise in humans. *American Journal of Physiology* 1986;**251**(1 Pt 1):E65-70.
24. Karlsson J, Nordesjo LO, Saltin B. Muscle glycogen utilization during exercise after physical training. *Acta Physiologica Scandinavica* 1974;**90**:210-17.
25. Costill DL, Fink WJ, Hargreaves M, et al. Metabolic characteristics of skeletal muscle during detraining from competitive swimming. *Medicine and Science in Sports and Exercise* 1985;**17**:339-43.
26. Matthews CK, Van Holde KE, Ahern KG (eds). *Biochemistry.* San Francisco, CA: Benjamin/Cummings, 2000.
27. Holloszy JO, Coyle EF. Adaptations of skeletal muscle to endurance exercise and their metabolic consequences. *Journal of Applied Physiology* 1984;**56**:831-8.
28. Krogh A, Lindhard J. The relative value of fat and carbohydrate as sources of muscular energy: with appendices on the correlation between standard metabolism and the respiratory quotient during rest and work. *Biochemistry Journal* 1920;**14**:290-363.
29. Hasson S (ed.). *Clinical Exercise Physiology.* St. Louis, MO: Mosby, 1994.
30. Putman CT, Jones NL, Lands LC, et al. Skeletal muscle pyruvate dehydrogenase activity during maximal exercise in humans. *American Journal of Physiology* 1995;**269**(3 Pt 1):E458-68.
31. Hellebrandt FA. Application of the overload principle to muscle training in man. *American Journal of Physical Medicine* 1958;**37**:278-83.
32. Kraemer WJ, Ratamess NA. Fundamentals of resistance training: progression and exercise prescription. *Medicine and Science in Sports and Exercise* 2004;**36**: 674-88.
33. Wathen D, Roll F. Training methods and modes. In: Baechle TR (ed.) *Essentials of Strength Training and Conditioning.* Champaign, IL: Human Kinetics, 1994.
34. Trappe S, Harber M, Creer A, et al. Single muscle fiber adaptations with marathon training. *Journal of Applied Physiology* 2006;**101**:721-7.
35. Barstow TJ, Mole PA. Simulation of pulmonary O_2 uptake during exercise transients in humans. *Journal of Applied Physiology* 1987;**63**:2253-61.
36. Fick A. Poggendorff's Annalen. *Philosophical Magazine* 1855;**10**:30-9.
37. Weissman C, Abraham B, Askanazi J, et al. Effect of posture on the ventilatory response to CO_2. *Journal of Applied Physiology* 1982;**53**:761-5.
38. Laughlin MH. Cardiovascular response to exercise. *American Journal of Physiology* 1999;**277**(6 Pt 2):S244-59.
39. Astrand P, Rodahl K, Dahl H, Stromme S. *Textbook of Work Physiology,* 4th edn. Champaign, IL: Human Kinetics, 2003.
40. Wasserman K, Whipp BJ. Exercise physiology in health and disease. *American Review of Respiratory Disease* 1975;**112**:219-49.
41. Hainsworth R, Drinkhill MJ, Rivera-Chira M. The autonomic nervous system at high altitude. *Clinical Autonomic Research* 2007;**17**:13-19.
42. Naveri H, Kuoppasalmi K, Harkonen M. Metabolic and hormonal changes in moderate and intense long-term running exercises. *International Journal of Sports Medicine* 1985;**6**: 276-81.
43. VanHelder WP, Casey K, Radomski MW. Regulation of growth hormone during exercise by oxygen demand and availability. *European Journal of Applied Physiology and Occupational Physiology* 1987;**56**:628-32.
44. Montain SJ, Laird JE, Latzka WA, Sawka MN. Aldosterone and vasopressin responses in the heat: hydration level and exercise intensity effects. *Medicine and Science in Sports and Exercise* 1997;**29**:661-8.
45. Hartley LH, Mason JW, Hogan RP, et al. Multiple hormonal responses to graded exercise in relation to physical training. *Journal of Applied Physiology* 1972;**33**:602-6.
46. Hull EM, Young SH, Ziegler MG. Aerobic fitness affects cardiovascular and catecholamine responses to stressors. *Psychophysiology* 1984;**21**:353-60.
47. Cleak MJ, Eston RG. Delayed onset muscle soreness: mechanisms and management. *Journal of Sports Sciences* 1992;**10**:325-41.
48. Gulick DT, Kimura IF, Sitler M, et al. Various treatment techniques on signs and symptoms of delayed onset muscle soreness. *Journal of Athletic Training* 1996;**31**:145-52.
49. Smith LL. Acute inflammation: the underlying mechanism in delayed onset muscle soreness? *Medicine and Science in Sports and Exercise* 1991;**23**:542-51.
50. Stauber WT, Clarkson PM, Fritz VK, Evans WJ. Extracellular matrix disruption and pain after eccentric muscle action. *Journal of Applied Physiology* 1990;**69**:868-74.
51. Shu B, Shen Y, Wang AM, et al. Histological, enzymohistochemical and biomechanical observation of skeletal muscle injury in rabbits. *Chinese Journal of Traumatology* 2007;**10**:150-3.
52. Newham DJ, Jones DA, Ghosh G, Aurora P. Muscle fatigue and pain after eccentric contractions at long and short length. *Clinical Science (London)* 1988;**74**:553-7.
53. Cheung K, Hume P, Maxwell L. Delayed onset muscle soreness: treatment strategies and performance factors. *Sports Medicine* 2003;**33**:145-64.
54. Hunter SK, Duchateau J, Enoka RM. Muscle fatigue and the mechanisms of task failure. *Exercise and Sports Sciences Reviews* 2004;**32**(2):44-9.
55. Nordlund MM, Thorstensson A, Cresswell AG. Central and peripheral contributions to fatigue in relation to level of activation during repeated maximal voluntary isometric plantar flexions. *Journal of Applied Physiology* 2004;**96**:218-25.
56. Gandevia SC. Spinal and supraspinal factors in human muscle fatigue. *Physiological Reviews* 2001;**81**:1725-89.
57. Hootman J, Dick R, Agel J. Epidemiology of collegiate injuries for 15 sports: summary and recommendations for injury prevention initiatives. *Journal of Athletic Training* 2007;**442**:311-19.

58. Gelber AC, Hochberg MC, Mead LA, *et al.* Joint injury in young adults and risk for subsequent knee and hip osteoarthritis. *Annals of Internal Medicine* 2000;**133**:321–8.
59. National Athletic Trainers Association. *Recommendations and Guidelines for Appropriate Medical Coverage of Intercollegiate Athletics.* Dallas, TX: National Athletic Trainers Association, 2003.
60. Hergenroeder AC. Prevention of sports injuries. *Pediatrics* 1998;**101**:1057–63.
61. Ivy JL, Katz AL, Cutler CL, *et al.* Muscle glycogen synthesis after exercise: effect of time of carbohydrate ingestion. *Journal of Applied Physiology* 1988;**64**:1480–5.
62. Maughan R. The athlete's diet: nutritional goals and dietary strategies. *Proceedings of the Nutrition Society* 2002;**61**:87–96.
63. Williams MH. Nutritional ergogenic aids/supplements and exercise performance. In: Harries M, Williams C, Stanish WD, Micheli L J (eds). *Oxford Textbook of Sports Medicine.* Oxford, UK: Oxford University Press, 1998.
64. Williams C. Diet and sports performance. In: Harries M, Williams C, Stanish WD, Micheli L J (eds) *Oxford Textbook of Sports Medicine.* Oxford, UK: Oxford University Press, 1998.
65. Bjorntop P. Importance of fat as a support nutrient for energy: metabolism of athletes. *Journal of Sports Sciences* 1991;**9**:71–6.
66. Economos CD, Bortz SS, Nelson ME. Nutritional practices of elite athletes. Practical recommendations. *Sports Medicine* 1993;**16**(6): 381–99.
67. Position of the American Dietetic Association, Dietitians of Canada, and the American College of Sports Medicine: nutrition and athletic performance. *Journal of the American Dietetic Association* 2000;**100**:1543–56.
68. Harris RC, Soderlund K, Hultman E. Elevation of creatine in resting and exercised muscle of normal subjects by creatine supplementation. *Clinical Science (London)* 1992;**83**:367–74.
69. Snyder P. Use of androgens and other drugs by athletes. Retrieved March, 2009, from www.uptodate.com.
70. Armsey TD, Hosey RG. Medical aspects of sports: epidemiology of injuries, preparticipation physical examination, and drugs in sports. *Clinics in Sports Medicine* 2004;**23**:255–79.
71. Wallace MB, Lim J, Cutler A, Bucci L. Effects of dehydroepiandrosterone vs androstenedione supplementation in men. *Medicine and Science in Sports and Exercise* 1999;**31**:1788–92.
72. American Dietetic Association; Dietitians of Canada. Position of the American Dietetic Association and Dietitians of Canada: vegetarian diets. *Journal of the American Dietetic Association* 2003;**103**:748–65.
73. Venderley AM, Campbell WW. Vegetarian diets: nutritional considerations for athletes. *Sports Medicine* 2006;**36**:293–305.
74. National Research Council. *Recommended Dietary Allowances*, 10th edn. Washington, DC: National Academy Press, 1989.
75. Shaw NS, Chin CJ, Pan WH. A vegetarian diet rich in soybean products compromises iron status in young students. *Journal of Nutrition* 1995;**125**:212–19.
76. Braun B, Horton T. Endocrine regulation of exercise substrate utilization in women compared to men. *Exercise and Sports Sciences Reviews* 2001;**29**:149–54.
77. Manore MM. Nutritional needs of the female athlete. *Clinics in Sports Medicine* 1999;**18**:549–63.
78. American College of Sports Medicine. Position stand: the female athlete triad. *Medicine Science Sports Exercise* 1997;**29**:i–ix.
79. Lloyd T, Triantafyllou SJ, Baker ER, *et al.* Women athletes with menstrual irregularity have increased musculoskeletal injuries. *Medicine and Science in Sports and Exercise* 1986;**18**:374–9.
80. Volek JS, Forsythe CE, Kraemer WJ. Nutritional aspects of women strength athletes. *British Journal of Sports Medicine* 2006;**40**:742–8.
81. Beals KA, Manore MM. Nutritional status of female athletes with subclinical eating disorders. *Journal of the American Dietetic Association* 1998;**98**:419–25.
82. Cavadini C, Decarli B, Grin J, *et al.* Food habits and sport activity during adolescence: differences between athletic and non-athletic teenagers in Switzerland. *European Journal of Clinical Nutrition* 2000;**54**(Suppl. 1): S16–20.
83. Petrie HJ, Stover EA, Horswill CA. Nutritional concerns for the child and adolescent competitor. *Nutrition* 2004;**20**:620–31.
84. Butte NF. Fat intake of children in relation to energy requirements. *American Journal of Clinical Nutrition* 2000;**72**(5 Suppl.):1246S–52S.
85. Morgan WP, Costill DL. Selected psychological characteristics and health behaviors of aging marathon runners: a longitudinal study. *International Journal of Sports Medicine* 1996;**17**:305–12.
86. Seals DR, Hagberg JM, Allen WK, *et al.* Glucose tolerance in young and older athletes and sedentary men. *Journal of Applied Physiology* 1984;**56**:1521–5.
87. Rosenbloom CA, Dunaway A. Nutrition recommendations for masters athletes. *Clinics in Sports Medicine* 2007;**26**:91–100.

71

Essential arthroscopic skills

KIMBERLY A TURMAN, MARK D MILLER

Introduction	712	Ankle arthroscopy	716
Arthroscopic equipment and instrumentation	712	Elbow arthroscopy	716
Arthroscopic concepts	713	Wrist arthroscopy	717
Knee arthroscopy	713	Complications of arthroscopy	718
Shoulder arthroscopy	714	Conclusion	718
Hip arthroscopy	715	References	718

NATIONAL BOARD STANDARDS

- Understand the concept of triangulation
- Know about hypotensive anaesthesia
- Know the standard portals for knee and shoulder arthroscopy
- Understand the commonly used arthroscopic knots and suture techniques
- Know the commonly used graft materials
- Understand the possible complications that may arise

INTRODUCTION

Arthroscopy dates back to 1918 when the Japanese surgeon Takagi used a cystoscope to evaluate a knee joint.[1] Watanabe, another Japanese surgeon, later refined the arthroscope and developed the concept of triangulation.[1] Since that time, arthroscopy has continued to evolve with expanding indications and surgical techniques. To best apply the arthroscopic technique, a thorough knowledge of basic arthroscopic concepts and skills is essential. As with all surgical procedures, a successful outcome is dependent upon a careful patient assessment, including history and physical examination with confirmatory imaging studies. Accurate diagnoses and patient selection are crucial. When used appropriately, arthroscopy can result in improved efficiency, fewer complications and quicker recovery times than many open techniques. The surgeon must also, however, be aware of the limitations of arthroscopic surgery.

ARTHROSCOPIC EQUIPMENT AND INSTRUMENTATION

Specialized equipment and instruments are required to perform arthroscopy. As such, it is useful to have theatre staff who are familiar with the arthroscopic technique. The cornerstone of arthroscopy is the arthroscope, a fibreoptic instrument inserted through a cannula to allow direct visualization of joints. A fibreoptic cable attached to the arthroscope displays the view onto a screen, and a camera in the arthroscope allows for recording and printing of images. Arthroscopes are classified by their diameter and viewing angle. The most commonly used arthroscope is 4 mm with a 30° viewing angle.

In addition to the basic arthroscopic equipment, a variety of specialized arthroscopic instruments are available. Both hand-operated (e.g. probes, baskets, grabbers) and motorized (e.g. shavers, burrs) instruments are utilized. These instruments are available in a variety of shapes and sizes. Radiofrequency devices are also available and may be used for tissue ablation and electrocautery purposes. Specialized instruments are continually developed in conjunction with the development of new arthroscopic techniques. A variety of implants must also be available and include meniscal repair devices, suture anchors and fixation strategies for cruciate ligament reconstruction to name a few. All of these instruments and implants are again ideally stored in or near the arthroscopy suite.

Irrigation fluid is another important component of arthroscopy. It allows for distension of joints to improve visualization and operative access as well as aiding in removal of debris. Lactated Ringer's solution is more physiological than normal saline and is the preferred irrigation fluid.[2] Epinephrine may be added to decrease bleeding. Hypotensive anaesthesia will also promote improved visualization, particularly in the shoulder. The irrigation system is typically attached to the arthroscopic cannula and joint distension is maintained with use of commercially available pumps or gravity.

Finally, a variety of positioning and traction devices are available to aid the surgeon performing arthroscopy. These are particularly helpful when an assistant is not available. Tourniquets may be utilized in certain circumstances. Specialized drapes help promote a sterile operative environment. An operating room of sufficient size must be available to accommodate the arthroscopic equipment.

ARTHROSCOPIC CONCEPTS

To be a successful arthroscopist, several fundamental concepts must be understood. First, as mentioned, the typical arthroscope has a 30° viewing angle. This allows for a greater field of vision and improved control. With the arthroscope held stationary, a 60° field of vision is achieved by simply rotating the viewing angle. It should also be remembered that the degree of magnification is related to the distance of the object from the lens of the arthroscope. Relative measurements may be determined by comparison with a standardized or calibrated probe.

Triangulation is another fundamental arthroscopic concept described in detail by DeHaven.[3] It involves placing the arthroscope through one portal and the working instruments through a separate portal. The instruments are then brought into the field of view of the arthroscope. The view of the arthroscope and the tip of the working instrument form the apex of a triangle. Triangulation allows for independent movements of the arthroscope and the working instruments while keeping both in perspective. If one becomes disoriented, the arthroscope should be retracted slightly to create a larger field of vision. If the arthroscopic instrument still cannot be located, it may be brought into contact with the arthroscope and then advanced off the end of the arthroscope, subsequently bringing it back into the field of vision.

Arthroscopic knot tying is a skill that must be mastered by the arthroscopic surgeon. Suture management is of prime importance during many cases. A number of sliding and locking knots are described for arthroscopic use. The Samsung Medical Center (SMC) knot in particular is an excellent locking, sliding knot with inherent security and low profile.[4] Arthroscopic knot pushers and other instruments are available to assist the surgeon with knot tying.

The arthroscopic surgeon must also be proficient in harvesting autografts for use in arthroscopic reconstructions. The most commonly used grafts are patellar tendon and hamstring autografts. The surgeon should be familiar with available allografts as an alternative.

Care and attention to detail must be used when positioning extremities for arthroscopy to avoid complications such as neuropraxias. Positioning devices may aid with this endeavour. Tourniquets should be utilized only when necessary and the inflation time minimized as much as possible. One must be cognizant that some leg holder positioning devices can have a tourniquet effect even without a tourniquet inflated.

While arthroscopy may be used for diagnostic purposes, a thorough clinical and imaging evaluation will typically establish a diagnosis. Arthroscopy may then be used to confirm the diagnosis and carry out a variety of therapeutic tasks. An examination under anaesthesia should be conducted at the initiation of any arthroscopic procedure. A thorough knowledge of anatomy is crucial to successful arthroscopy and will be further addressed in the following sections.

KNEE ARTHROSCOPY

Indications

The knee is the most common joint examined by the arthroscopic surgeon. Indications for knee arthroscopy are numerous and diverse. Meniscal pathology is one of the most common applications of arthroscopy and accounts for approximately 50% of knee injuries requiring surgery.[5] Partial meniscectomy is perhaps the most common procedure, although techniques for meniscal repair continue to evolve. The indications for meniscal transplantation are also being explored. Focal chondral lesions are commonly addressed arthroscopically with a variety of techniques, including shaving chondroplasty, microfracture, osteochondral autograft and allograft transfers, and autologous chondrocyte implantation. Reconstruction of the cruciate ligaments is performed with an arthroscopically assisted technique. Synovial biopsies may be obtained to help establish diagnoses in rheumatological disorders, and synovectomy may be used to treat a variety of synovial disorders as well as to resect pathological plicae. Arthroscopy may form a portion of the treatment for patellar disorders with lateral release and to assist medial patellofemoral ligament reconstructions. Other indications for knee arthroscopy include irrigation and debridement for septic arthritis, loose body removal, patellar clunk syndrome, and to aid with fracture reduction and fixation in some tibial plateau and tibial eminence fractures.

Positioning

Two forms of positioning are commonly used for knee arthroscopy depending on surgeon preference. First, the patient may be placed supine with the foot of the operating table extended. A lateral post is used to help provide valgus stress and the leg is brought off the side of the table to achieve flexion. The lateral compartment is easily entered by placing the extremity into a figure-of-four position. Alternatively, commercially available leg holders may be used. The non-operative extremity is typically placed into a well-leg holder while the operative extremity is placed into a leg holder that fits around the tourniquet. The foot of the operating table is lowered to allow the operative extremity to hang freely. The well-leg holder must be well padded to prevent compression on the peroneal nerve.

Portal placement and associated anatomy

Several arthroscopic portals can be established for knee arthroscopy. Standard portals include an anterolateral portal placed initially as a viewing portal and an anteromedial portal created as a working portal. These portals are positioned just above the joint line on the lateral and medial sides of the patellar tendon. The arthroscope and instruments may be alternated between these portals to improve visualization and access to the intra-articular pathology. An additional superolateral or superomedial portal may be used to aid in fluid management based on surgeon preference.

Several accessory portals may also be utilized. A posteromedial portal may help in visualizing the posterior horn of the medial meniscus and posterior cruciate ligament. A posterolateral portal located between the iliotibial band and biceps tendon may at times be helpful, although care must be taken to protect the peroneal nerve. A proximal superomedial portal located 4 cm proximal to the medial edge of the patella may be useful in evaluating patellar tracking. Other potential portals include the far medial, far lateral and midpatellar portals.

Diagnostic arthroscopy

A systematic examination of the joint should be carried out at the initiation of any arthroscopic procedure. With regards to the knee, the arthroscope is first placed into the anterolateral portal to complete the diagnostic evaluation. A probe may be placed into the anteromedial portal to assist. All regions of the knee joint should be examined, including the patellofemoral articulation, suprapatellar pouch, medial and lateral gutters, medial and lateral compartments, and intercondylar notch. Additional portals are established as needed and all surgical pathology subsequently addressed.

SHOULDER ARTHROSCOPY

Indications

The indications for shoulder arthroscopy continue to evolve as improved techniques and results comparable to open procedures are achieved. The most common shoulder afflictions treated with arthroscopy include rotator cuff pathology and impingement syndromes, shoulder instability and labral pathology, and conditions of the distal clavicle. Arthroscopic capsular release may be a component of the treatment for recalcitrant adhesive capsulitis. Other indications include irrigation and debridement for septic arthritis and removal of loose bodies.

Positioning

Two positioning methods exist for shoulder arthroscopy. The first is lateral decubitus and requires a traction system to suspend the operative arm in 45° abduction and 15° forward flexion. Careful positioning is necessary to prevent complications such as transient neuropraxias.[6,7] Other potential disadvantages of the lateral position include distorted anatomy if unfamiliar with the technique, poor toleration of regional anaesthesia and difficulty in converting to open procedures. In efforts to overcome some of these potential disadvantages, the beach chair position was developed.[8] In this position the patient is kept supine and elevated into a sitting position. Care again must be taken in appropriate positioning with particular focus on maintaining cervical spine alignment. While both positioning techniques are effective, one may be preferred over the other in certain situations. For example, the beach chair position may be preferable in rotator cuff repairs, particularly if there is concern for a potential need to convert to a mini-open procedure. In contrast, instability repairs, and in particular posterior labral repairs, are often best approached in the lateral position. Thus, a well-trained arthroscopist is familiar and competent in both techniques.

Portal placement and associated anatomy

Numerous portals have been described for shoulder arthroscopy and portal selection is based on the requisites of the case. Bony landmarks should be palpated and outlined to aid proper portal placement. The posterior portal, located 2 cm medial and 2–3 cm inferior to the posterolateral corner of the acromion, is the most commonly used viewing portal. A 'soft spot' in this region corresponds to the interval between the infraspinatus and teres minor. The arthroscopic cannula and trocar should be directed towards the coracoid to successfully enter the glenohumeral joint space. Distension of the joint with saline prior to establishing the portal may allow an easier entry. When placing the arthroscope in the subacromial space from the posterior portal, it should be directed more superiorly and towards the anterolateral corner of the acromion.

The standard anterior portal, located lateral to the coracoid and just distal to the anterior edge of the acromion, is the most commonly used working portal. This portal is created under direct visualization from the posterior portal. A spinal needle is first introduced into the rotator interval and into a triangle bounded by the biceps tendon superiorly, the humeral head laterally and the subscapularis tendon inferiorly. An arthroscopic cannula is then placed into this position and the outflow connected to the cannula to improve visualization.

A standard lateral portal is created when working in the subacromial space to aid with bursectomy, decompression and cuff repair. This portal is located approximately 2 cm distal to the lateral edge of the acromion in line with the posterior clavicular line. A spinal needle is again utilized to confirm proper orientation prior to formally creating the portal. The location of the axillary nerve in correlation to the lateral edge of the acromion has been documented.[9] It is commonly accepted that the average distance from the acromion to the axillary nerve is 5 cm.[10] This distance must also be remembered when converting an arthroscopic case into an open procedure.

A variety of accessory portals may also be established as necessary to gain access to the intra-articular pathology. An anteroinferior (5 o'clock) portal located approximately 2 cm below the anterosuperior portal and just above the subscapularis tendon is useful in the setting of arthroscopic Bankart repairs.[11] A posterolateral portal (portal of Wilmington) is beneficial in superior labral (i.e. SLAP – superior labral tear from anterior to posterior) repairs and is located 1 cm anterior and just off the lateral edge of the posterolateral corner of the acromion.[12] Another posterolateral (7 o'clock) portal may facilitate access to the posterior glenoid labrum and axillary pouch.[13] This portal is created approximately 2 cm inferior to the standard posterior portal. A superior (supraspinatus or Neviaser) portal is located in the notch between the posterior acromioclavicular joint and scapular spine and may also be useful in superior labral and biceps pathology.[14] Finally, a superolateral portal has been described just lateral to the acromion on a line drawn from the acromion to the coracoid and may be of benefit in suture management for cuff repairs.[15]

In general, the posterior portals place the suprascapular artery and nerve at risk and the axillary nerve at lesser risk. Anterior portals risk injury to the cephalic vein, axillary artery and nerve, and musculocutaneous nerve if one drifts inferior and medial. Superior portals risk the suprascapular artery and nerve and lateral portals the axillary nerve as discussed above.[16,17]

Diagnostic arthroscopy

Diagnostic evaluation of the glenohumeral joint is typically carried out through the posterior viewing portal at the initiation of the case. It is also helpful to create the anterior working portal such that a probe may be used to further evaluate the intra-articular structures. Structures that should be visualized and palpated include the biceps tendon and its anchor, labrum circumferentially, articular surfaces of the humeral head and glenoid, glenohumeral ligaments and capsule, rotator cuff, and axillary recess for loose bodies. The biceps and its superior labral attachment are visualized first to gain orientation. A normal variation of the superior labrum may exist with separation from the glenoid and confluence with the middle glenohumeral ligament (Buford complex) or a sublabral recess with simple detachment.[18] The glenohumeral ligaments are thickenings of the capsule. The anterior band of the inferior glenohumeral ligament is of prime importance and is typically addressed with Bankart repairs.

In the subacromial space, the bursal side of the rotator cuff, undersurface of the acromion and acromioclavicular joint should be visualized. Brisk bleeding while working in the subacromial space may be due to injury to the acromial branch of the thoracoacromial artery that runs in the coracoacromial ligament.

HIP ARTHROSCOPY

Indications

The indications and uses for hip arthroscopy are more limited and continue to be defined. Currently, the most common indications include labral tears, femoroacetabular impingement, loose bodies, chondral lesions, synovial conditions, rupture or impingement of the ligamentum teres, septic arthritis and unexplained intractable hip pain.[19]

Positioning

Once again, there are two basic positions utilized for hip arthroscopy. The lateral position was first popularized by Glick et al.[20] Traction is applied through use of a modified fracture table or commercially available distractor and the operative extremity is placed in 45° abduction and 10° flexion. Alternatively, the patient may be placed supine as described by Byrd.[21] This technique makes use of a standard fracture table with padded peroneal post and traction. The operative extremity is positioned in extension and 25° of abduction. Pudendal nerve palsies are possible with inappropriate use of traction and positioning. In either setting, fluoroscopy is recommended to assist entry into the joint. Cannulated obturators also assist placement of the arthroscopic cannulas into the joint over a guidewire. Owing to the thick soft-tissue envelope, extra long instruments are required.[22]

Portal placement and associated anatomy

Three primary portals are utilized in hip arthroscopy and include the direct anterior, anterolateral or anterior trochanteric, and the posterolateral or posterior trochanteric portals. The direct anterior portal is created at the intersection of a line drawn distal from the anterior superior iliac spine and a line drawn medial from the superior edge of the greater trochanter. The lateral femoral cutaneous nerve lies lateral and branches proximal to this portal, although the branches remain at risk.[23] The femoral nerve is an average of 3.2 cm medial to the portal.[23] The trochanteric portals are created at the anterior and posterior borders of the superior edge of the greater trochanter. The superior gluteal nerve is in proximity to both trochanteric portals with an average distance of 4.4 cm from each.[23] The sciatic nerves are an average of 2.9 cm inferior to the posterolateral portal.[23]

Diagnostic arthroscopy

The anterolateral portal is established as the initial viewing portal. Structures that may be visualized and subsequently addressed include the labrum, articular surfaces, ligamentum teres and pulvinar, and transverse acetabular ligament. The arthroscope must ultimately be repositioned among portals to ensure optimal visualization of all structures.

ANKLE ARTHROSCOPY

Indications

Ankle arthroscopy can also be a very useful technique in the surgeon's arsenal. A common procedure is debridement of synovial or osteophytic impingement. Other indications include the removal of loose bodies, management of osteochondral lesions of the talus, arthroscopically assisted ankle arthrodesis, and synovial biopsy or synovectomy for rheumatological conditions. Arthroscopy at the initiation of lateral ankle stabilization procedures is often beneficial in identifying commonly associated intra-articular pathology.

Positioning

Ankle arthroscopy is performed with the patient supine. A number of commercially available ankle distractors are available to aid in joint distraction and visualization.

Manual or invasive distraction may also be used.[24] While a standard arthroscope is often adequate, it is helpful to have a smaller diameter (2.7 mm) arthroscope available. Smaller diameter shavers may also be necessary to prevent iatrogenic chondral injury.

Portal placement and associated anatomy

Two portals are typically sufficient for ankle arthroscopy. These include the anteromedial and anterolateral portals. The anteromedial portal is located adjacent to the tibialis anterior tendon at the level of the ankle joint. If this portal drifts too far medial, the saphenous vein may be injured. It lies an average of 7.4 mm medial.[25] The anterolateral portal is located just lateral to the peroneus tertius tendon. Injury to the superficial peroneal nerve is avoided with a nick and spread technique. The nerve is located an average of 6.2 mm from the portal.[25] A posterolateral portal may also be created to gain access to the posterior joint. This portal is created just lateral to the Achilles tendon and places the sural nerve, which lies within 6.0 mm, at risk.[25] Alternatively, a 70° arthroscope may be used from the anterior portals to view posteriorly. Posteromedial portals are not recommended because of the high risk of injury to the posterior tibial artery and tibial nerve. Similarly, a central anterior portal may injure the dorsalis pedis artery and deep peroneal nerve.

Diagnostic arthroscopy

The ankle joint is first insufflated with saline. The anterior portals are then created. Structures visualized include the lateral sulcus, tip of the fibula, articular surfaces of the distal tibia and talus, medial sulcus, and tip of the medial malleolus. Identified pathology may then be addressed.

ELBOW ARTHROSCOPY

Indications

While the indications for elbow arthroscopy are again less well defined than knee and shoulder arthroscopy, it is very useful in certain circumstances. These include the removal of loose bodies, synovectomy, osteophytic debridement, irrigation and debridement of a septic joint, and capsular release or excision.

Positioning

The patient may be placed supine,[26] prone[27] or lateral[28] for elbow arthroscopy. The supine position requires suspension of the involved extremity and access to the posterior elbow is limited. The prone position may allow easier visualization and arthroscopic instrumentation. An arm board is placed under the upper arm and the forearm is allowed to hang freely with the elbow in 90° of flexion. Because the arm is free, manipulation of the elbow is possible throughout the case. The main disadvantages of prone positioning are related to anaesthesia and airway concerns. The lateral decubitus position avoids many of the disadvantages of the other two positions.

Portal placement and associated anatomy

Multiple portals have been described for elbow arthroscopy and may be divided into medial, posterior and lateral portals. Prior to establishing portals, the joint is distended with saline through the lateral soft spot (anconeus triangle), defined as the centre of a triangle formed by the radial head, tip of the olecranon and lateral epicondyle. All elbow arthroscopic portals should be created with the nick and spread method owing to the proximity of surrounding neurovascular structures.

The proximal anteromedial portal is located 2 cm proximal to the medial epicondyle and just anterior to the intermuscular septum.[27] It is a primary viewing portal. An anteromedial portal is also described 2 cm distal and 2 cm anterior to the medial epicondyle; however, it is less favoured than the proximal portal because of an increased risk of injury to the medial antebrachial cutaneous nerve and median nerve.

The direct lateral portal is created in the anconeus triangle as previously described. This portal is useful for fluid management as well as for viewing the posterior joint. A direct posterior portal may be created as an accessory portal to instrument the posterior joint. It is located 2–3 cm proximal to the tip of the olecranon and traverses the triceps tendon. An additional posterolateral portal may be created 3 cm proximal to the olecranon tip overlying the lateral condylar ridge.

The anterolateral portal is located 3 cm distal and 1 cm anterior to the lateral epicondyle with the elbow flexed 90°.[26,29] The radial nerve is at particular risk with this portal. A proximal anterolateral portal has been suggested as an alternative to the standard anterolateral portal to lessen the risk to neurovascular structures.[30] It is located 2 cm proximal and 1 cm anterior to the lateral epicondyle. This portal provides excellent visualization of the anterior compartment and may be developed as the initial portal.

Diagnostic arthroscopy

The proximal anteromedial portal is commonly established first and allows visualization of the anterior compartment including the radiocapitellar articulation, coronoid process and fossa, and the anterior and lateral joint capsule. The lateral portal is established to better visualize the ulnohumeral articulation and medial capsule as well as the coronoid process and fossa. Creation of a direct lateral or posterolateral portal allows visualization of the posterior compartment including the olecranon tip and fossa, medial and lateral gutters, and posterior elbow articulations.

WRIST ARTHROSCOPY

Indications

Wrist arthroscopy may be indicated for both diagnostic as well as therapeutic means. As many injuries to the wrist have become better understood, arthroscopy has taken a larger role. The evaluation of carpal instability and treatment of injuries to the wrist ligaments and triangular fibrocartilage complex (TFCC) are enhanced with wrist arthroscopy. Arthroscopy is also frequently employed as an adjunct in the management of intra-articular distal radius fractures. Other potential uses include debridement of chondral lesions, loose body removal, synovectomy, irrigation and debridement of the septic joint, and to assist management of ulnar impaction syndrome.

Positioning

Wrist arthroscopy is performed with the patient supine and the upper extremity placed on an arm board. Commercial traction devices are available to provide the necessary distraction of the joint. Owing to the smaller joint size, instruments of reduced size are required, including the use of a 2.7 mm arthroscope.

Portal placement and associated anatomy

Wrist arthroscopy portals are designated in reference to the dorsal wrist compartments. The nick and spread method should be utilized for portal establishment. The 3–4 portal is the primary viewing portal and is located between the extensor pollicis longus and extensor digitorum communis tendons. It is approximately 1 cm distal to Lister's tubercle. The 4–5 portal, located between the extensor digitorum communis and extensor digiti minimi tendons, is a primary working portal. The 6R portal is another good working portal and is just radial to the extensor carpi ulnaris tendon.

A variety of additional portals are available, but their use is more limited because of their proximity to neurovascular structures. The 6U portal places the dorsal ulnar nerve at risk. It is located an average of 4.5 mm from the portal.[31] The 1–2 portal is also used infrequently as the radial artery and sensory branch of the radial nerve are within 3–5 mm.[31] A distal radioulnar joint portal may be created as an accessory portal without significant risk.

Midcarpal portals include the radial and ulnar midcarpal and scaphotrapeziotrapezoid (STT) portals. The radial midcarpal is typically used for visualization. It is located 1 cm distal to the 3–4 portal. The ulnar midcarpal portal is 1 cm distal to the 4–5 portal.

Inflow is typically through the arthroscope. Outflow is possible through an 18 gauge catheter placed in the 1–2, 6R or 6U portal location. Establishing outflow is important to prevent fluid extravasation and potential compartment syndrome.[32]

Diagnostic arthroscopy

The joint is insufflated through the 3–4 portal location and this portal is then created. Outflow is established and the 4–5 portal is created under direct visualization for placement of a probe. The intra-articular structures of the wrist and midcarpal joints are numerous and complex. With regards to the wrist, the TFCC, articular surfaces, intrinsic carpal ligaments, and extrinsic carpal ligaments may be visualized arthroscopically. From radial to ulnar these structures are the radial styloid, radioscaphocapitate ligament, long radiolunate ligament, scaphoid proximal pole, radius scaphoid facet, scapholunate interosseous ligament, radioscapholunate ligament of Testut, lunate proximal pole, radius lunate facet, short radiolunate ligament, TFCC, ulnolunate ligament, ulnotriquetral ligament, lunatotriquetral interosseous ligament, and the triquetrum proximal pole. In the midcarpal joint from radial to ulnar the structures include the STT, capitate proximal pole, scaphoid distal pole, scapholunate interval stability, lunate distal pole, lunatotriquetral interval stability, triquetrum distal pole, capitohamate interval and the hamate proximal pole.

COMPLICATIONS OF ARTHROSCOPY

As with all surgical procedures, arthroscopy has inherent risks. The most common complication is probably iatrogenic injury to intra-articular structures, particularly the chondral surfaces. The risk of this procedure is related to the experience of the surgeon and attention to technique. Proper placement of portals is also crucial to lessen this risk as well as the risk of iatrogenic neurovascular injury. A thorough knowledge of the surrounding anatomy is essential. In areas at high risk, the nick and spread method of portal placement should be routinely utilized. This involves incising only the skin, then using a blunt haemostat to create a pathway for the arthroscopic instruments. Complications secondary to tourniquet use may be minimized by using wide cuffs and minimizing the inflation time.[33] Fluid extravasation has been reported and is likely to be more common in the setting of trauma (fractures, knee dislocations).[34] In this setting, one must be aware of potentially inducing a compartment syndrome. Synovial fluid fistula formation is a rare complication due to poor portal closure. Treatment consists of immobilization and occasionally delayed closure. Infection is another rare complication of arthroscopy and is treated with antibiotics. Irrigation and debridement may be required in severe cases. Lastly, lower extremity deep venous thrombosis and pulmonary embolism are rare complications of knee arthroscopy. While routine prophylaxis is not recommended, a high index of suspicion and low threshold to obtain appropriate studies (e.g. ultrasound) will minimize the consequences of this complication.

CONCLUSION

Arthroscopy as a technique continues to evolve and new applications will continue to be developed. It is a very useful tool for the orthopaedic surgeon. Proper patient selection remains of utmost importance and arthroscopy should not replace an appropriate evaluation. Arthroscopy should rarely be used solely for diagnostic means, but rather to confirm and treat intra-articular afflictions.

> ### KEY LEARNING POINTS
>
> - Arthroscopic applications abound for the knee and shoulder. Other commonly treated joints include the hip, ankle, elbow and wrist.
> - Specialized arthroscopic equipment and instruments are required.
> - Triangulation, fluid management and arthroscopic visualization are fundamental concepts.
> - A thorough understanding of the associated anatomy is essential for portal placement and management of intra-articular pathology.
> - Arthroscopy should not replace a complete patient evaluation and proper patient selection is paramount.

REFERENCES

1. Jackson RW. Quo venis quo vadis: the evolution of arthroscopy. *Arthroscopy* 1999;**15**:680–5.
2. Reagan BF, McInery VK, Treadwell BV, *et al*. Irrigating solutions for arthroscopy: a metabolic study. *Journal of Bone and Joint Surgery (American)* 1983;**65**:629–31.
3. DeHaven KE. Principles of triangulation for arthroscopic surgery. *Orthopedic Clinics of North America* 1982;**13**:329–36.
4. Kim SH, Ha KI. The SMC knot: a new slip knot with locking mechanism. *Arthroscopy* 2000;**16**:563–5.
5. Jensen JE, Conn RR, Hazelrigg G, *et al*. Symptomatic evaluation of acute knee injuries. *Clinics in Sports Medicine* 1985;**4**:295–312.
6. Hennrikus WL, Mapes RC, Bratton MW, *et al*. Lateral traction during shoulder arthroscopy: its effect on tissue perfusion measured by pulse oximetry. *American Journal of Sports Medicine* 1995;**23**:444–6.

7. Klein AH, France JC, Mutschler TA, *et al.* Measurement of brachial plexus strain in arthroscopy of the shoulder. *Arthroscopy* 1987;**10**:255–8.
8. Warner JP. Shoulder arthroscopy in the beach chair position: basic setup. *Operative Techniques in Orthopaedics* 1991;**1**:147–54.
9. Hoppenfeld S, deBoer P. *Surgical Exposures in Orthopaedics*, 2nd edn. Philadelphia, PA: J.B. Lippincott, 1994:25–9.
10. Beals TC, Harryman DT, Lazarus MD. Useful boundary of the subacromial bursa. *Arthroscopy* 1998;**14**:465–70.
11. Davidson PA, Tibone JE. Anterior inferior (5 o'clock) portal for shoulder arthroscopy. *Arthroscopy* 1995;**11**:519–25.
12. Morgan CD, Burkhart SS, Palmeri M, *et al.* Type II SLAP lesions: three subtypes and their relationships to superior instability and rotator cuff tear. *Arthroscopy* 1998;**14**:553–5.
13. Morrison DS, Schafer RK, Friedman RL. The relationship between subacromial space pressure, blood pressure, and visual clarity during arthroscopic subacromial decompression. *Arthroscopy* 1995;**11**:557–60.
14. Neviaser TJ. Arthroscopy of the shoulder. *Orthopedic Clinics of North America* 1987;**3**:361–72.
15. Laurencin CT, Detsh A, O'Brien SJ, *et al.* The superior lateral portal for arthroscopy of the shoulder. *Arthroscopy* 1994;**10**:255–8.
16. Meyer M, Graveleau N, Hardy P, *et al.* Anatomic risks of shoulder arthroscopy portals: anatomic cadaveric study of 12 portals. *Arthroscopy* 2007;**23**:529–36.
17. Nottage WM. Arthroscopic portals: anatomy at risk. *Orthopedic Clinics of North America* 1993;**24**:19–26.
18. Williams MM, Snyder SJ, Buford D. The Buford complex – the 'cord-like' middle glenohumeral ligament and absent anterosuperior labrum complex: a normal anatomic capsulolabral variant. *Arthroscopy* 1994;**10**:241–7.
19. Khanduja V, Villar RN. Arthroscopic surgery of the hip. *Journal of Bone and Joint Surgery (British)* 2006;**88**:1557–66.
20. Glick J, Sampson T, Gordon R, *et al.* Hip arthroscopy by the lateral approach. *Arthroscopy* 1987;**3**:4–12.
21. Byrd JWT. Hip arthroscopy utilizing the supine position. *Arthroscopy* 1994;**10**:275–80.
22. Monllau JC, Solano A, Leon A, *et al.* Tomographic study of the arthroscopic approaches to the hip joint. *Arthroscopy* 2003;**29**:368–72.
23. Byrd JWT, Pappas JN, Pedley MJ. Hip arthroscopy: an anatomic study of portal placement and relationship to the extra-articular structures. *Arthroscopy* 1995;**11**:418–23.
24. Yates C, Grana W. A simple distraction technique for ankle arthroscopy. *Arthroscopy* 1988;**4**:103–5.
25. Feiwell LA, Frey C. Anatomic study of arthroscopic portal sites of the ankle. *Foot & Ankle* 1993;**14**:142–7.
26. Andrews JR, Carson WG. Arthroscopy of the elbow. *Arthroscopy* 1985;**1**:97–107.
27. Poehling GG, Whipple TL, Sisco L. Elbow arthroscopy: a new technique. *Arthroscopy* 1989;**5**:222–4.
28. O'Driscoll SW, Morrey BF. Arthroscopy of the elbow: diagnostic and therapeutic benefits and hazards. *Journal of Bone and Joint Surgery (American)* 1992;**74**:84–94.
29. Andrews JR, Baumgarten TE. Arthroscopic anatomy of the elbow. *Orthopedic Clinics of North America* 1995;**26**:671–7.
30. Stothers K, Day B, Reagan WR. Arthroscopy of the elbow: anatomy, portal sites, and a description of the proximal lateral portal. *Arthroscopy* 1995;**11**:449–57.
31. Abrams RA, Petersen M, Botte MJ. Arthroscopic portals of the wrist: an anatomic study. *Journal of Hand Surgery* 1994;**19**:940–4.
32. Botte MJ, Cooney WP, Linscheid RL. Arthroscopy of the wrist: anatomy and technique. *Journal of Hand Surgery* 1989;**14**:313–16.
33. Sapega AA, Heppenstall RD, Chance B, *et al.* Optimizing tourniquet application and release times in extremity surgery: a biomechanical and ultrastructural study. *Journal of Bone and Joint Surgery (American)* 1985;**67**:303–14.
34. Noyes FR, Spievack ES. Extraarticular fluid dissection in tissues during arthroscopy: a report of clinical cases and a study of intraarticular and thigh pressures in cadavers. *American Journal of Sports Medicine* 1982;**10**:346–51.

72

Head and spine injuries in sport

JAMES BREZINA, DINO SAMARTZIS, FRANCIS H SHEN

Introduction	720	Cervical spine injuries	724
Concussion in sport	720	References	727
Cervical neuropraxia ('stinger')	722		

INTRODUCTION

Direct trauma in athletes can lead to neurological injuries related to the head and cervical spine. Common neurological presentations are concussions, cervical nerve pinch syndrome or 'stingers' as well as other less common injuries such as fractures and dislocations, herniated cervical discs with radiculopathy and transient quadriplegia associated with spinal stenosis. Debate exists over the incidence and long-term risks of repeated neurological insults to the central and peripheral nervous system. Universal guidelines for evaluation of these injuries and return to play criteria are lacking. This chapter will review the clinical presentations, management and return to play criteria for the neurological presentations of concussions and stingers, as well as cervical sprains and fractures in the athlete.

CONCUSSION IN SPORT

Concussion is a common yet serious injury in the athletic population. A useful definition proposed by the Committee on Head Injury Nomenclature of the Congress of Neurological Surgeons defines a concussion as 'a clinical syndrome characterized by immediate and transient posttraumatic impairment of neural function, such as alteration of consciousness, disturbance of vision, equilibrium, etc., due to brainstem involvement'. A more general definition is any trauma-induced alteration in mental status that *may or may not* include loss of consciousness.[1] Many athletes feel a pressure to return to play quickly and therefore may not be as forthcoming regarding injuries or symptoms related to a head injury. Long-term deficits in the form of the post-concussion syndrome have been described after a single event;[2] however, if identified and properly managed, most concussive injuries result in a good prognosis with minimal deleterious effects.

Pathophysiology

The pathophysiology of head injury is not well understood, and several mechanisms of injury have been proposed.[3,4] It is likely that a combination of these proposed mechanisms leads to the concussive syndrome. Animal models have been developed which demonstrate axonal shear damage (axotomy) with acceleration and deceleration forces on the brain.[5] A coup injury results from a forceful blow to the resting mobile head, typically producing a brain injury deep to the point of cranial impact, whereas the contrecoup injury produces maximal brain injury opposite to the side of cranial impact as the brain rebounds within the confines of the calvarium. Vascular aetiology may also play a role in traumatic brain injury. Loss of autoregulation of the blood supply to the brain can lead to vascular engorgement, increased intracranial pressure and, in severe cases (second impact syndrome), brain herniation.[6]

History and physical examination

Variable presentations of a traumatic brain injury are not uncommon; therefore, a high index of suspicion and careful serial neurological examinations may be required. In some instances, the athlete may be obviously down and injured on the field, but, more likely, the athlete will report to you on the sidelines complaining of a 'ding' or having their 'bell rung'. The signs and symptoms of a concussion must be addressed at this time (Box 72.1).[3] Signs of a concussion are observed by the staff and may include confusion, amnesia, clumsy movements, change in speech patterns, loss of consciousness and behaviour and personality abnormalities. The symptoms reported by the athlete may include, but are not limited to, headache, nausea, alterations in balance or concentration and memory loss. Headache is the most commonly reported symptom and may be seen in up to 70% of athletes who sustain a concussion.[7]

Evaluation of the athlete with a suspected concussion begins with standard trauma protocols (ABCs), including cervical spine clearance. A systematic physical examination must include vital signs, evaluation of peripheral sensation and strength, cranial nerve evaluation and examination of cognition (Box 72.2).[8] The physical examination should be repeated after exertional testing before an athlete is cleared to return to play.[9]

BOX 72.1: Signs and symptoms of concussion

- Signs observed by the clinician
  - Confusion about assignment
  - Forgets play
  - Appears dazed or confused
  - Unsure of game, score, opponent
  - Loss of consciousness
  - Clumsy movements
  - Answers questions slowly
  - Shows behaviour or personality changes
  - Retrograde amnesia: forgetting events prior to injury
  - Antegrade amnesia: forgetting events after the time of injury
- Symptoms reported by the athlete
  - Nausea
  - Headache
  - Balance problems or dizziness
  - Double vision
  - Hypersensitivity to light and noise
  - Feelings of fatigue
  - Changes in sleep patterns
  - Feeling 'foggy' or groggy

Initial management

Always suspect a cervical spine injury in an athlete with a concussion. In the unconscious athlete on the field, airway, breathing and circulation (ABCs) should be the first priority. The cervical spine should be immobilized in the unconscious athlete until it can be cleared clinically, or radiographically. Initial management involves removing the player from the game, and performing a careful neurological examination. The athlete should be observed and repeat examinations performed as needed. It is important to remember that exertional testing is an important component in the evaluation of the patient.

Return to play

The decision to allow a player to return to play is a difficult one. Currently, no universally accepted algorithm

BOX 72.2: Head injury evaluation

- ABCs: evaluate and maintain an airway!
- LOC: evaluate level of consciousness (LOC) before moving. Clear cervical spine
- Vital signs: increased intracranial pressure leads to increased blood pressure and decreased pulse
- Orientation: person, place, time
- Memory: before and after injury. What happened? Score? Opponent?
- Balance: Romburg test – stand with feet together and eyes closed. Maintain balance for 20 seconds
- Cranial nerves:
  I   Smell
  II   Visual acuity
  III Pupil reflex
  IV Lateral eye movement
  V   Sensation to face
  VI Eye movement
  VII Facial expression
  VIII Hearing
  IX Swallowing
  X   Pulse
  XI Shrug shoulders
  XII Stick out tongue
- Strength, coordination and sensation
- Standardized assessment of concussion
- Exertional testing: all testing should be repeated after exertion before an athlete is cleared to return to play
- The athlete should not return to play if there is any loss of consciousness, disorientation or persisting symptoms

exists,[10] and the decision should be individualized to each athlete, the circumstances surrounding the injury and serial neurological examinations. Table 72.1 outlines examples of recent concussion grading symptoms[3] whereas Table 72.2 outlines return to play criteria.[11] The more severe the grade of the concussion, the more cautious one must be before allowing the athlete to return to sport.

Post-concussion syndrome

The true incidence of post-concussion syndrome is unknown. Symptoms consist of headache, especially with exertion, labyrinthine disturbance, fatigue, irritability and impaired cognitive function. The symptoms often correlate with the duration of the post-traumatic amnesia.[12] Consideration for advanced imaging with CT may be necessary in cases where symptoms persist or are more severe.

Second impact syndrome

Second impact syndrome is defined as a rapid brain swelling and herniation following a second brain injury. This well-described syndrome can result in rapid death.[13,14] Typically, the athlete is still symptomatic from the first injury and returns to play prior to complete resolution of the concussion. Often, the second injury is a relatively minor head injury that occurs shortly after a previous head injury. It is important to note that second impact syndrome may occur without loss of consciousness after either of the injuries.

CERVICAL NEUROPRAXIA ('STINGER')

The stinger or 'burner' was initially described in 1965 and was eventually given the name 'cervical nerve pinch syndrome'.[15] The reported incidence among collegiate contact football players is 49–65%, and it has been shown to be the most common symptomatic upper extremity nerve injury in athletes.[16] The injury may result from a traction or compression of the brachial plexus or the cervical nerve roots. Although most symptoms of cervical neuropraxia are transient, some athletes may suffer from prolonged symptoms with recurrent episodes.[17] It is important to consider other aetiologies, such as cervical cord injuries, structural spine injuries, herniated cervical discs with radicular symptoms, congenital defects and cervical stenosis, when evaluating the athlete with a stinger.

Mechanism of injury, signs and symptoms

Activities which cause extreme forceful lateral neck flexion combined with shoulder depression can lead to compression of the ipsilateral nerve roots of a stretch of the contralateral plexus. This most commonly leads to injuries of the upper trunk of the brachial plexus or injuries to the cervical 5th and 6th roots. Brachial plexus injuries most commonly affect high school American football players whereas cervical root injuries are found more often in collegiate and professional athletes.[18] This higher incidence of root injury may be related to a history of recurrent stingers, foraminal stenosis, cervical disc disease or congenital canal stenosis.[17,18] Bilateral symptoms or lower extremity symptoms should raise the suspicion for a spinal cord injury.

Symptoms usually involve a single upper extremity and are characterized by burning pain and paraesthesias radiating from the neck to the supraclavicular area into the shoulder and may involve the hand.[15,17,18] These symptoms often resolve within seconds to minutes but may persist for hours or even days. As the C5–6 myotomes are most commonly affected, the patient may demonstrate

Table 72.1 Recent concussion grading scales

Guideline	Grade 1	Grade 2	Grade 3
Cantu	No LOC	LOC lasts >5 minutes OR	LOC lasts >5 minutes OR
	Post-traumatic amnesia <30 minutes	Post-traumatic amnesia lasts >30 minutes	Post-traumatic amnesia lasts >24 hours
Colorado	Confusion without amnesia No LOC	Confusion with amnesia No LOC	LOC (of any duration)
American Academy of Neurology	Transient confusion No LOC Concussion symptoms resolve <5 minutes	Transient confusion No LOC Concussion symptoms last >15 minutes	LOC (of any duration)

LOC, loss of consciousness.

Table 72.2 Concussion management

Classification	Grade	Signs/symptoms	1st concussion	2nd concussion	3rd concussion
Colorado Medical Society	I	(+) Confusion (−) Amnesia (−) LOC	Return to play if symptoms resolve within 20 minutes	Terminate contest; return to play if without symptoms for 1 week	Terminate contest; return to play if without symptoms for 3 months
	II	(+) Confusion (+) Amnesia (−) LOC	Terminate contest; return to play if without symptoms for 1 week	Terminate contest; return to play if without symptoms for 1 month	Terminate season; return to play if without symptoms next season
	III	(+) LOC	Terminate contest; hospital evaluation; return to play in 1 month after 2 consecutive weeks without symptoms	Terminate season; return to play if without symptoms next season	Terminate season; strongly discourage return to contact or collision sports
Cantu grading system	I	(+) Amnesia <30 minutes' duration (−) LOC	Return to play if asymptomatic for 1 week*	Return to play in 2 weeks after 1 week without symptoms	Terminate season; return to play next season if asymptomatic
	II	(+) LOC <5 minutes' duration OR (+) Amnesia >30 minutes but <24 hours' duration	Return to play if asymptomatic for 2 weeks*	Return to play in 1 month (consider season) after 1 week without symptoms	Terminate season; return to play next season if asymptomatic
	III	(+) LOC >5 minutes' duration OR (+) Amnesia >24 hours' duration	Return to play in 1 month after 1 week without symptoms*	Terminate season; return to play next season if asymptomatic	Consider no further contact sports
American Academy of Neurology	I	(+) Confusion is transient (−) LOC †Symptoms <15 minutes duration	May return to play if symptoms clear within 15 minutes	Terminate contest; may return to play if without symptoms on exertion for 1 week	
	II	(+) Confusion is transient (−) LOC †Symptoms >15 minutes' duration	Terminate contest; may return to play if without symptoms on exertion for 1 week	Terminate contest; may return to play if without symptoms on exertion for 2 weeks; terminate season with any CT/MRI scan abnormalities	
	III	(+) LOC	Terminate contest; hospital evaluation if LOC persists or neurological abnormality; if LOC brief, return to play in 1 week if no symptoms on exertion; if LOC prolonged (>1 minute), return in 2 weeks if no symptoms on exertion	Terminate contest; return to play after 1 month without symptoms*	

*CT or MRI scans if signs or symptoms persist.
LOC, loss of consciousness. Data from Bailes JE, Cantu RC. Head injuries in athletes. *Neurosurgery* 2001;48:26–46.

weakness of shoulder abduction, elbow flexion and arm external rotation.[19]

Initial management

Evaluation on the field begins with establishing the mechanism of injury (lateral flexion/shoulder depression or extension/compression). The patient should be asked to describe the location of the pain and the duration of the symptoms, even if they have resolved. Physical examination should include evaluation of the cervical spine for tenderness, evidence of muscle spasm or other indications of structural damage. Once a structural cervical spine injury has been ruled out, examination of the upper extremity, including active and passive range of motion, a sensory examination and deep tendon reflex testing, is carried out. Examination of the contralateral arm is used as a control.

If there is a suspicion of a cervical spine injury, as indicated by midline tenderness, bilateral upper extremity involvement or lower extremity involvement, immobilization and spine precautions should be implemented with appropriate transport to a facility capable of evaluating and treating cervical spine injuries.

Treatment and return to play

For those stingers lasting more than a few minutes or those associated with midline cervical tenderness or limited neck range of motion, an MRI of the cervical spine is indicated prior to allowing the athlete to return to play.[20] Cervical disc disease with herniations and neural foraminal stenosis have been documented in patients with recurrent stingers. The MRI will also provide information on accessing fractures, ligamentous disruption, congenital malformations or canal stenosis. Electromyographic studies may be of value if symptoms persist for more than 2–3 weeks.[17,19] They are most helpful in delineating between a brachial plexus injury and a cervical root injury, and to follow changes over time; however, most authors recommend that complete normalization of the physical examination and a lack of contraindications on imaging studies guide the time frame for return to play clearance.[19] As with concussion injuries, no universally accepted return to play criteria have been established, but useful evidence-based algorithms have been proposed that may assist in the physician's decision-making process (Box 72.3).[21]

CERVICAL SPINE INJURIES

Cervical spine injuries in sports are uncommon but they can lead to significant and long-term disability.

BOX 72.3: Return to play

- No contraindications
  - Fewer than three episodes of a prior burner/stinger lasting <24 hours, with full range of cervical motion without evidence of neurological deficits
  - One episode of transient quadriplegia with full cervical range of motion, no evidence of residual neurological deficit and no evidence of disc herniation or instability
- Relative contraindications
  - Prolonged symptomatic stinger/burner or transient quadriparesis lasting >24 hours
  - Three or more previous episodes of stinger/burner or two episodes of transient quadriparesis; the patient must have full cervical range of motion and strength without neck discomfort
- Absolute contraindication
  - More than two episodes of transient quadriparesis/quadriplegia
  - Clinical history, physical examination findings or imaging confirmation of cervical myelopathy/myelomalacia
  - Continued cervical neck discomfort, decreased range of motion or evidence of neurological deficit after any cervical spine injury

---

Normally, excessive axial loads applied to the head are dissipated through the paravertebral muscles, intervertebral discs and normal lordosis of the cervical spine. The cervical spine is at greatest risk when the normal lordotic curve is straightened, at approximately 30° of flexion. Injuries of the cervical spine are often divided into upper cervical injuries (occiput, atlas, axis) and lower cervical injuries (C3–7).

History, physical examination and imaging

As always, evaluation of the cervical spine at the time of injury begins with stabilization and advanced trauma life support protocols. Helmets and shoulder pads generally should not be removed prior to arrival at a medical facility unless urgent airway access is required. Spinal cord injury should be assumed in all unconscious patients, or in those patients who complain of axial neck pain or have evidence of neurological injury. A detailed history from the patient and witnesses will need to be documented, including the mechanism of injury and the subsequent status of the patient. Physical examination should include neurological assessments performed on the field and repeated upon arrival at the medical facility. The cervical spine examination should make note of tenderness, range of motion (if radiographically cleared) and a detailed neurological examination. Neurological examination must access each spinal level with regards to muscle strength grading, sensation and appropriate deep tendon reflexes for both the upper and lower extremities.

Initial radiographic evaluation for suspected cervical injuries includes anteroposterior (AP), lateral, oblique and odontoid views. The lateral radiograph must include all seven cervical vertebrae as well as the C7–T1 disc space. The lateral radiograph should be examined for any prevertebral soft-tissue swelling, fractures or malalignment. Abnormal soft-tissue swelling on the lateral radiograph suggests underlying cervical spine injury. In adults, soft-tissue swelling greater than 7 mm at C2 and greater than 22 mm at C4 suggests cervical injury.[22] The AP view provides information on spinous process alignment, whereas odontoid views allow for visualization of the C1 lateral masses as well as the odontoid. In the presence of adequate and normal plain radiographs with continued midline cervical pain or tenderness, flexion–extension cervical spine films are useful to access ligamentous disruption. Instability is present on the flexion–extension radiographs if there is more than 3.5 mm of translation or greater than 11° of angulation at adjacent segments.[22] Alternatively, an MRI provides information on the integrity of the ligaments and discs of the cervical spine. When a fracture is present on the plain radiographs, CT scans with three-dimensional reconstruction provide additional information regarding fracture pattern and displacement.

Upper cervical injuries

OCCIPITAL CONDYLE FRACTURES

Occipital condyle fractures are rare but may be associated with other spine fractures in up to one-third of cases. Cranial nerve deficiencies my be noted on the physical examination (most commonly cranial nerves IX, X, XI and XII). CT imaging is useful to identify and classify these fractures. Type I fractures are non-displaced impaction fractures, type 2 fractures are basilar skull fractures extending into the foramen magnum, whereas type 3 fractures are ligamentous avulsion fractures of the alar ligament. Management of type 1 and 2 fractures is with a hard cervical collar for 1–2 months. Type 3 fractures are considered unstable and are best managed with halo immobilization or with occipitocervical fusion.[21]

ATLANTO-OCCIPITAL DISLOCATION

Atlanto-occipital dislocation is a rare injury resulting from hyperextension, translation, rotation and distraction.[24] These injuries often result in serious neurological injury and death. Several radiographic measurements have been developed to access atlanto-occipital alignment. Classification of these injuries is based upon the direction of displacement: Type 1 is longitudinal distraction without displacement, type 2 injuries are most common and are characterized by anterior displacement of the occiput, whereas type 3 injuries demonstrate posterior displacement of the occiput. Management of these injuries is surgical occipitocervical fusion.[25]

ATLAS FRACTURES

Atlas fractures result from axial loading, and the fracture pattern correlates with the position of the head during impaction. Approximately 50% of these injuries are associated with other cervical spine fractures. As the space available for the cord is relatively large at this level, isolated fractures of the atlas are usually not associated with neurological symptoms. Fracture stability is dependent on the integrity of the transverse atlantal ligament. Incompetence of the transverse ligament is noted when the atlanto-dens interval is greater than 4 mm on the lateral radiograph, there is lateral mass widening greater than 6.9 mm on the open mouth odontoid radiograph, or a bony avulsion or tear of the ligament is noted on plain films, CT or MRI.[23] Isolated, stable C1 fractures are treated with hard cervical collar immobilization. Unstable fractures are treated with halo immobilization. The presence of malunion, non-union or persistent instability necessitates occipitocervical fusion.

ODONTOID FRACTURES

Fractures of the odontoid typically arise from a flexion moment, although extension and rotation may also lead to a fracture. Classification[26] of odontoid fractures is divided into three types: type I fractures are an avulsion of the distal tip of the odontoid and are stable if there is less than 2 mm of displacement; type II fractures are located at the base of the dens and are the most common fracture pattern; and type III fractures extend into the body of the axis. Treatment of stable type I fractures is immobilization in a rigid cervical collar for 2–3 months with flexion–extension radiographs on follow-up. Type II fractures with less than 6 mm of displacement can be managed with halo immobilization for 2–3 months. Surgical intervention for type II odontoid fractures is considered with fracture displacement greater than 6 mm, angulation greater than 10°, non-union, persistent instability or inability to maintain reduction. Type III fractures are best managed with closed reduction and halo immobilization for 2–3 months.

AXIS ISTHMUS FRACTURES (HANGMAN'S FRACTURES)

This injury results from hyperextension, axial load and rebound flexion. Neurological injury is uncommon in minimally displaced hangman's fractures. Classification is based upon the amount of displacement of the fracture. Type I fractures are vertical fractures with less than 3 mm of displacement and no angulation. These fractures are treated with a rigid orthosis for 2–3 months. Type II fractures have more than 3 mm of anterolisthesis and angulation. Type IIa fractures are those with angulation but no anterolisthesis, suggesting a three-column ligamentous injury. Traction should not be applied for these injures. Treatment of type II injuries involves reduction and halo immobilization. Type III fractures are vertical fractures with a significant amount of anterolisthesis and have the highest risk of neurological deficits. Type III injuries are often treated with open reduction with stabilization.[27]

Lower cervical injuries

COMPRESSION–FLEXION AND COMPRESSION–EXTENSION INJURIES

Compression–flexion injuries account for 20% of subaxial cervical spine fractures and are characterized by anterior vertebral compression with posterior element distraction.[28] Stable compression flexion injuries may be treated with a rigid cervical orthosis for 2–3 months. Unstable compression–flexion injuries, with disruption of the posterior ligamentous complex (two-column injuries), may be managed with halo immobilization. Compression flexion injuries with all three columns of the spine involved, or those with neurological compromise, require anterior decompression, fusion and instrumentation.[29] Compression–extension injuries are characterized by failure of the posterior ligament that progresses from posterior arch fractures (stages I and II) through increasing degrees of vertebral body anterolisthesis (stages III–V). Stable compression–extension (stages I and II) can usually be managed with a hard cervical collar, while unstable injuries (stages III–V) usually require reduction and fusion. Vertical compression fractures make up 15% of subaxial cervical spine fractures and most often involve the C5–6 level.[29] Minimal fracture deformity can be treated with a collar whereas fractures with displacement or neurological injury necessitate anterior decompression and fusion.

DISTRACTION INJURIES

Distraction cervical spine injuries are classified according to flexion or extension type injuries. Distraction–flexion injuries account for 10% of lower cervical fractures and are commonly managed by reduction and skeletal traction. If instability is present following reduction, instrumented fusion should be considered. MRI should be performed prior to surgical intervention to evaluate the integrity of the intervertebral disc. A compromised disc often necessitates an anterior discectomy and fusion. Distraction–extension injuries result from tensile failure of the spinal elements in extension. Brace treatment in distraction–extension injuries is difficult and reduction with halo immobilization or surgical fusion is often necessary.[30]

CERVICAL SPRAINS AND STRAINS

Cervical strains are injuries to the muscle–tendon unit whereas cervical sprains are defined as ligamentous injuries and are potentially unstable. Patients will present with pain, tenderness and decreased range of motion. Radiographs may demonstrate a loss of normal cervical lordosis secondary to muscle spasm. Initial treatments are conservative and may include collar immobilization and analgesics. If initial radiographs are negative, flexion–extension radiographs may be helpful to evaluate for ligamentous injury and instability. MRI studies should be considered for patients with persistent symptoms.

TRANSIENT QUADRIPLEGIA

Transient quadriplegia is an axial load injury to a stenotic cervical spine which leads to temporary loss of motor and/or sensory function of the extremities. It is estimated to occur in approximately seven per 10 000 college football players. A pincer-like mechanism of injury is proposed that leads to acute compression of the cervical spinal cord between cervical segments and the posterior ligamentum flavum in a narrow spinal canal. Complaints of bilateral burning dysaesthesias, paraesthesias, weakness of the extremities and temporary paralysis may occur. Klippel–Feil syndrome, intervertebral disc disease and congenital or acquired cervical stenosis are predisposing factors to this condition. Return to play criteria have been suggested (Box 72.3) but no universal guidelines have been adopted. Patients with structural causes of cervical stenosis and an episode of transient quadriplegia should be prohibited from participating in contact sports.[30]

> **KEY LEARNING POINTS**
>
> - Concussions and stingers result from direct trauma to the neurological system in athletes.
> - The lack of universally accepted guideless for evaluation and return to play criteria makes management of these conditions particularly challenging to the clinician.
> - Return to play criteria: most authors recommend that complete normalization of the physical examination and a lack of contraindications on imaging studies guide the time frame for return to play clearance.

- Evaluation of the cervical spine at the time of injury begins with stabilization and advanced trauma life support protocols. Helmets and shoulder pads generally should not be removed prior to arrival at a medical facility unless urgent airway access is required.
- Spinal cord injury should be assumed in all unconscious patients, or in those patients who complain of axial neck pain or have evidence of neurological injury.

REFERENCES

1. American Academy of Neurology. Practice parameter: the management of concussion in sports (summary statement). Report of the Quality Standards Subcommittee of the American Academy of Neurology. *Neurology* 1997;**48**:581–5.
2. McCrea M, Guskiewicz KM, Marshall SW, et al. Acute effects and recovery time following concussion in collegiate football players: the NCAA Concussion Study. *JAMA Journal of the American Medical Association* 2003;**290**:2556–63.
3. Lovell MR, Collins MW, Iverson GL, et al. Grade 1 or 'ding' concussions in high school athletes. *American Journal of Sports Medicine* 2004;**32**:47–54.
4. Covassin T, Swanick CB, Sachs ML. Epidemiological consideration of concussions among intercollegiate athletes. *Applied Neuropsychology* 2003;**10**:12–22.
5. Ucar T, Tanriover G, Gurer I, et al. Modified experimental mild traumatic brain injury model. *Journal of Trauma* 2006;**60**:558–65.
6. Cantu RC. Second-impact syndrome. *Clinics in Sports Medicine* 1998;**17**:37–44.
7. Collins MW, Field M, Lovell MR, et al. Relationship between post-concussion headache and neuropsychological test performance in high school athletes. *American Journal of Sports Medicine* 2003;**31**:168–73.
8. Shen FH. Concussion in sports. In: Miller MD, Sekiya J (eds) *Sports Medicine Core Knowledge in Orthopaedics.* Philadelphia, PA: Mosby, 2006.
9. McCrea M, Kelly JP, Randolph C, et al. Standardized assessment of concussion: on site mental status evaluation of the athlete. *Journal of Head Trauma Rehabilitation* 1998;**13920**:27–35.
10. Standaert CJ, Herring SA, Cantu RC. Expert opinion and controversies in sports and musculoskeletal medicine: concussion in the young athlete. *Archives of Physical Medicine and Rehabilitation* 2007;**88**:1077–9.
11. Asthagiri AR, Dumont AS, Sheehan JM. Acute and long-term management of sports-related closed head injuries. *Clinics in Sports Medicine* 2003;**22**:559–79.
12. Bleiberg J, Cernich AN, Cameron K, et al. Duration of cognitive impairment after sports concussion. *Neurosurgery* 2004;**54**:1073–8.
13. Mueller FO, Cantu RC. Catastrophic injuries and fatalities in high school and college sports, fall 1982–spring 1988. *Medicine & Science in Sports & Exercise* 1990;**22**:737–41.
14. Mueller FO. Catastrophic head injuries in high school and college sports. *Journal of Athletic Training* 2001;**36**:312–15.
15. Chrisman OD, Snook GA, Stanitis JM, et al. Lateral-flexion neck injuries in athletic competition. *Journal of the American Medical Association* 1965;**192970**:117–19.
16. Clancy Jr WG, Brand RL, Bergfield JA. Upper trunk brachial plexus injuries in contact sports. *American Journal of Sports Medicine* 1977;**5**:209–16.
17. Hershman EB. Brachial plexus injuries. *Clinics in Sports Medicine* 1990;**9**:311–29.
18. Levitz CL, Reilly PJ, Torg JS. The pathomechanics of chronic recurrent cervical nerve root neuropraxia. The chronic burner syndrome. *American Journal of Sports Medicine* 1997;**25**:73–6.
19. Di Benedetto M, Markey K. Electrodiagnostic localization of traumatic upper trunk brachial plexopathy. *Archives of Physical Medicine and Rehabilitation* 1984;**65**:15–17.
20. Dimberg EL, Burns TM. Management of common neurologic conditions in sport. *Clinics in Sports Medicine* 2005;**24**:638–57.
21. Vaccaro AR, Watkins B, Albert TJ, et al. Cervical spine injuries in athletes: current return-to-play criteria. *Orthopaedics* 2001;**24**:699–703.
22. White AA, Panjabi M. *Clinical Biomechanics of the Spine*, 2nd edn. Philadelphia, PA: Lippincott Williams & Wilkins, 1990.
23. Buholz RW, Burkhead WZ. The pathologic anatomy of fatal atlanto-occipital dislocations. *Journal of Bone and Joint Surgery (American)* 1979;**61**:248–50.
24. Powers B, Miller MD, Kramer RS, et al. Traumatic anterior atlanto-occipital dislocation. *Neurosurgery* 1979;**4**:12–17.
25. Vaccaro AR, Cotler JM. Traumatic injuries of the adult upper cervical spine. In: An HS, Simpson MJ (eds) *Surgery of the Cervical Spine.* Baltimore, MD: Williams & Wilkins, 1994.
26. Anderson LD, D'Alonzo RT. Fractures of the odontoid process of the axis. *Journal of Bone and Joint Surgery (American)* 1974;**56**:1663–74.
27. Levine AM, Edwards CC. The management of traumatic spondylolisthesis of the axis. *Journal of Bone and Joint Surgery (American)* 1985;**67**:217–26.
28. Shen FH. Cervical spine injuries. In: Miller MD, Sekiya, J (eds) *Sports Medicine Core Knowledge in Orthopaedics.* Philadelphia, PA: Mosby, 2006.

29. Allen BL, Ferguson RL, Lehman TR, O'Brien RP. A mechanistic classification of closed, indirect fractures and dislocations of the lower cervical spine. *Spine* 1982;**7**:1–27.

30. Simpson MJ, Sutton D, Rizolo SJ, Cotler JM. Traumatic injuries of the adult lower cervical spine. In: An HS, Simpson MJ (eds) *Surgery of the Cervical Spine*. Baltimore, MD: Williams & Wilkins, 1994.

73

The evaluation and treatment of glenohumeral instability, superior labrum anterior to posterior tears and rotator cuff tears

MATTHEW T PROVENCHER, ALLISON McNICKLE, JANETH KIM, BRIAN J COLE, NEIL GHODADRA

Introduction	729	Rotator cuff tears and repair	741
Shoulder instability	729	References	745
Superior labrum anterior to posterior tears and repair	739		

NATIONAL BOARD STANDARDS

- To understand the history, examination and pathology associated with shoulder instability
- To understand reliable surgical principles for repair of shoulder instability
- To learn how to diagnose a SLAP (superior labrum anterior poster) tear of the shoulder, and understand history, examination and imaging characteristics of SLAP tears
- To understand surgical management principles for SLAP tears
- To learn the key diagnostic features and treatment options for rotator cuff tears.

INTRODUCTION

Glenohumeral instability, superior labrum anterior to posterior (SLAP) tears and rotator cuff tears are among the most commonly encountered shoulder diagnoses. Through a combination of patient history, physical examination and well-selected radiographic studies, each of these may be accurately diagnosed and subsequently treated. This chapter describes the diagnosis and surgical management of several important shoulder conditions, and highlights surgical management techniques and technical pearls.

SHOULDER INSTABILITY

The stability of the glenohumeral joint depends on a complex balance between the static anatomy of the capsular restraints and the dynamic mechanics of its surrounding muscles, tendons and proprioceptive components. Intrinsically, the static stabilizers of the shoulder include the bony glenoid, the humerus and its articular version, the negative intra-articular pressure, the labrum, the glenohumeral ligaments, the capsule and the rotator interval. The dynamic stabilizers, which include the rotator cuff, scapular rotator muscles, biceps tendon, superior labrum and proprioceptive receptors, play even a greater role in the shoulder's stability when there is injury to the static stabilizers.[1,2] In addition, because only one-third of the humeral head is in contact with the glenoid at any time, the dynamic stabilizers play a critical role in the stability of the joint.[3]

Static stabilizers

Excessive glenoid or humeral head retroversion is thought to predispose one to posterior instability. The average glenoid version is 7° of retroversion and the proximal humerus retroversion averages 30° with a neck–shaft angle of between 130° and 140°.[1,4,5] The labrum is a fibrocartilaginous ring that serves to increase the glenoid's depth and deepen the concavity of the joint, which increases the surface area of contact for the humeral head. It acts like a wedge preventing anterior or posterior excessive translation.[6–8] The labrum also serves as an anchor for the glenohumeral ligaments and capsule. During rotator cuff contraction, the labrum facilitates a concavity compression mechanism as the humeral head is compressed into the glenoid. Transection of the labrum has reduced resistance to translation by 20%.[9,10] Concavity compression is important for stability as the rotator cuff provides dynamic compression and facilitates the efficacy of the static stabilizers.[3,11,12] The *Bankart* tear of the anteroinferior labrum and associated inferior capsular injury is the 'essential lesion' for anterior instability.[13–15] An *ALPSA lesion*, or anterior labral periosteal sleeve avulsion, can cause the same instability pattern as the capsule is detached from the glenoid, healing in a medially displaced position. A humeral avulsion of the glenohumeral ligament (HAGL) lesion[16–18] is when the capsule is injured and detached from the humerus instead of the glenoid, and is a rarer, but important, aspect of instability pathology to recognize.

The *capsule and glenohumeral ligaments*, which are distinct thickenings of capsular tissues, restrain motion mostly at the extremes of motion. With the arm at the side up to mid-ranges of rotation, these structures are relatively lax. The anterior capsule tightens in extension and the posterior capsule during flexion. The inferior glenohumeral ligament (IGHL) complex is the primary static check against anterior, posterior and inferior translation between 45° and 90° of glenohumeral elevation.[5,19–22] As the arm approaches adduction, the superior glenohumeral ligament (SGHL) and middle glenohumeral ligament (MGHL) limit inferior translation in the lower ranges of elevation and external rotation in the middle ranges of elevation, respectively.[23,24] The SGHL, coracohumeral ligament and IGHL function together to limit inferior translation of the adducted shoulder and act as secondary restraints against posterior translation.[22–26]

Within the capsular joint, there exists a relative *negative pressure gradient* as high osmotic pressures of the interstitial surrounding tissues draw water out of the joint.[27] Negative pressure increases as the glenoid and humerus separate, causing a suction-like effect and increasing the stability of the joint. Any pathological condition that causes 'venting' of the normal negative intra-articular pressure, such as a rent in the capsule, a labral tear or an enlarged rotator interval defect, significantly increases anteroposterior translation and external rotation.[24,28,29]

The *rotator interval* is the region between the subscapularis and supraspinatus and is composed of the coracohumeral ligament and the superior glenohumeral ligament. A tear or laxity in this region may cause instability inferiorly in the adducted position, and increased anteroposterior translation.[26,30]

Dynamic stabilizers

Both the *rotator cuff* and the *biceps tendon*[31–33] stabilize the shoulder actively as they increase compression across the glenohumeral joint requiring more load to translate the humeral head during active contraction. *Scapulothoracic stabilizers* are also important as they centre the glenoid under the humerus; some patients who present with shoulder instability may have associated scapular dyskinesis, further contributing to their instability.[1,20,22,28,34–38] Finally, proprioception is an important feedback mechanism derived from receptors in the joint capsule to provide accurate perception of the joint in space.[39–42]

The normal shoulder has some inherent 'laxity', or passive translation of the humeral head with shoulder motion, which should not be confused with pathological instability. Laxity is defined as *painless* translation that is decreased by static and dynamic restraints of the shoulder at the extremes of motion.[12,25,43] Instability, however, is defined as symptomatic laxity, which reproduces the patient's symptoms owing to excessive translation of the glenohumeral joint.[44] There is a spectrum to the degree of instability, which can present merely as pain with subtle instability, or voluntary or involuntary subluxation, to frank dislocation. The shoulder can be unstable in one direction from a traumatic episode, or it can become increasing unstable in more than one direction, referred to as multidirectional instability.

Glenohumeral instability can be the result of a traumatic episode (i.e. tackle injury), cumulative microtrauma (i.e. bench pressing) and/or increasing laxity with the development of pain and a sensation of instability in atraumatic, ligamentously lax patients. Voluntary instability in the anterior direction may be associated with an underlying psychiatric diagnosis; however, this is not universally the case with posterior instability.

Anterior instability

CLINICAL PRESENTATION

The aetiology of anterior shoulder instability is from trauma, high-energy repetitive stress and overuse, or atraumatic instability as a component of multidirectional instability. The most common mechanism of traumatic initial anterior dislocation is an indirect force with the arm in the externally rotated abducted position. The anteriorly dislocated patient will present with an adducted and internally rotated arm and may not be able to externally rotate or fully abduct the arm. The posterior aspect of the shoulder will appear hollow as the anterior aspect will look full with the humeral head visible.

Young patients under 30 years old have an 80–90% chance of recurrent instability and will complain about 'dead arm syndrome' and recurrent subluxations.[18,45–47] Patients complain of feelings of instability, clicking or catching in provocative manoeuvres, or sometimes just pain. In one study of acute anterior shoulder dislocations,

97% had Bankart lesions, or complete detachment of the capsulolabral complex from the anteroinferior glenohumeral rim and neck; 90% had a Hill–Sachs lesion; and 10% had a SLAP tear; rotator cuff tears were not seen.[18] Patients older than 40 years frequently suffer concomitant rotator cuff tears with the initial dislocation, causing weakness and the inability to lift the arm overhead, and are important to recognize in the setting of an instability event.[48]

PHYSICAL EXAMINATION FINDINGS

Visual inspection may reveal deltoid atrophy because shoulder dislocations can injure the axillary nerve. Patients with anterior subluxations often have tenderness over the posterior capsule, and those with secondary impingement may have tenderness to palpation over the greater tuberosity or biceps tendon. The range of motion may be limited, so it is important to rule out continued shoulder subluxation or dislocation. Many overhead athletes will present with excessive external rotation with reduced internal rotation, signifying a tight posterior capsule. Specific tests for anterior instability include the apprehension[49] and relocation examination[50,51] and the load and shift manoeuvre. A positive sulcus sign – symptomatic inferior translation of the shoulder – indicates multidirectional instability of the shoulder.[52,53]

The load and shift manoeuvre is best done with the patient supine. The examiner positions the patient's arm in the plane of the scapula, at 45–60° of abduction and neutral rotation. The examiner then grasps the proximal humerus at the level of the deltoid insertion with the thumb posterior and fingers on the anterior joint. Using the other arm, the examiner provides an anterior or anteroinferior force and assesses the amount of humeral head translation. While maintaining an axial load, the patient's arm can be gradually rotated into external rotation, and the IGHL should become tight, decreasing anterior translation. Grade 1 signifies the humeral head is just over the anterior glenoid rim and rides up onto the labrum. Grade 2 translation occurs when the entire humeral head translates over the glenoid rim but spontaneously reduces with the removal of force, and grade 3 is complete dislocation which does not reduce.

The apprehension examination is performed with the patient both seated and lying down. The examiner abducts the patient's arm to 90° and gradually externally rotates the humerus. The hand of the examiner is placed over the humeral head and is pushing the shoulder forward. With increasing external rotation, the patient will have an apprehensive feeling and either guard or communicate the feelings of instability.

The relocation test is done immediately after the apprehension manoeuvre; replicating the same abduction and external rotation, except with a posteriorly directed force on the proximal humerus. This should stabilize the joint from translating anteriorly, and both the apprehension and pain should disappear.

IMAGING

Plain radiographs should be obtained in all patients who present with symptoms and signs of instability. It is also imperative that an axillary lateral be obtained in order to ensure that the humerus is contained by the glenoid. The standard radiographic series consists of anteroposterior, scapular-Y view and axillary lateral. A true anteroposterior film may also be obtained (the beam is oriented 20° internally) to determine the presence of glenoid fractures or avulsions. Additional lateral images to better evaluate glenoid fractures and bone loss include the apical oblique[54] and the West Point[55] views. In the setting of chronic instability, three-dimensional CT both with and without the humeral head digitally subtracted provides important information regarding any glenoid bone loss and the extent of Hill–Sachs (humeral head compression injury) deformity. Both MRI and magnetic resonance arthrogram (MRA) provide information on tears of the glenoid labrum, capsular injuries (HAGL lesion), and other associated injuries such as SLAP and rotator cuff tears.

SURGICAL INDICATIONS

Indications for surgical treatment include irreducible, open or recurrent dislocation, failure of non-operative treatment, and the revision situation – failed procedures with significant glenoid or humeral bone defects. Patients under 30 years old who are athletic have been shown to have up to a 92% recurrence rate after initial anterior dislocation of the shoulder.[47] Surgical decision-making for the first-time dislocator remains controversial, although several randomized studies[56,57] have demonstrated better outcomes with operative stabilization than with non-operative sling management. It is generally well accepted that younger, athletic patients will benefit most from a stabilization procedure, and those who are older and more sedentary will benefit most from a comprehensive rehabilitation programme assuming that the rotator cuff is uninjured. Although the gold standard for operative treatment has been an open capsular shift, arthroscopic treatment continues to evolve and results are increasingly encouraging and offer the benefit of subscapularis preservation.[58,59] Both open and arthroscopic approaches have been shown to be effective in preventing recurrence,[60] although open repair should be strongly considered in the setting of significant glenoid bone loss (greater than 25%),[61–63] capsular insufficiency,[12,60] large Hill–Sachs injuries and in certain revision situations.[64]

SURGICAL TECHNIQUES

Preferred technique for arthroscopic capsulolabral repair

Either the beach chair or lateral decubitus position may be utilized to perform a capsulolabral repair, although, if there is any pathology that extends posteriorly, the lateral position facilitates access to this area of the glenohumeral joint. In the lateral position, general anaesthesia is used

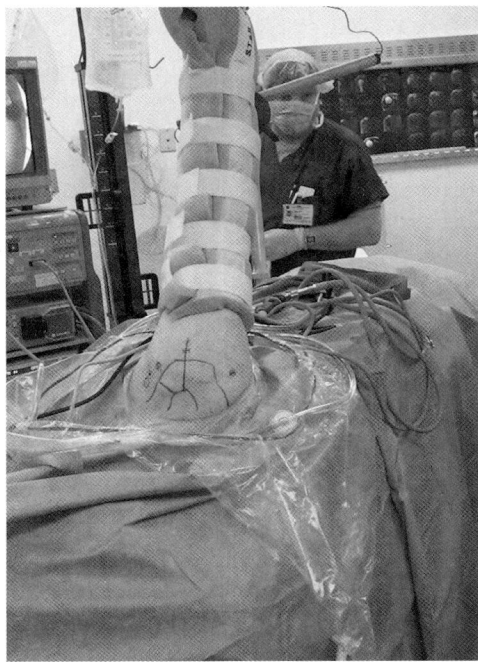

Figure 73.1 Operating room set-up for the lateral decubitus position. The arm is placed in approximately 50° of abduction and 15° of forward flexion.

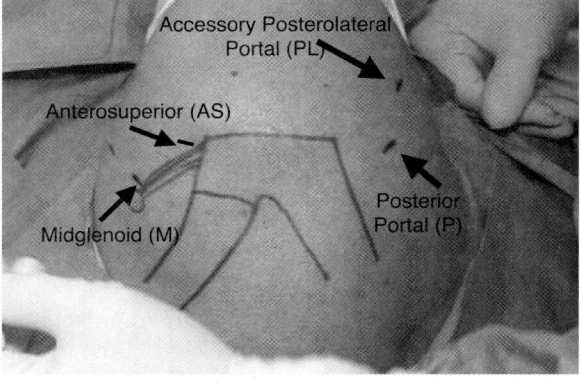

Figure 73.2 Arthroscopic portals utilized during instability procedure. Portals are labelled (P, posterior; AS, anterosuperior; MG, mid-glenoid; PL, posterolateral – o'clock portal).

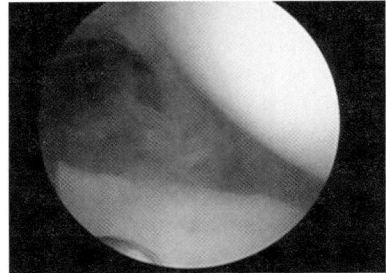

Figure 73.3 Establishing the mid-glenoid portal.

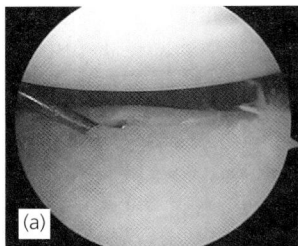 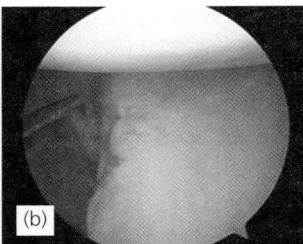

Figure 73.4 Glenohumeral joint as viewed from the anterosuperior portal for (a) a patient with no glenoid bone loss and (b) another with glenoid bone loss of approximately 15%.

and may be supplemented with a regional block. A bean-bag positioner is utilized, ensuring that all bony prominences are well padded. The arm is placed in an abduction traction device that provides about 50° of abduction and 15° of forward flexion during the operation (Fig. 73.1). The table is generally turned 90° in order to facilitate access to the anterior aspect of the glenohumeral joint. The beach chair is inclined approximately 50° to allow access to the anterior aspect of the shoulder.

A standard posterior portal is made approximately 1 cm inferior and just medial to the lateral edge of the acromion, and a 4 mm arthroscope is inserted. An arthroscopic pump with low-pressure or gravity inflow is utilized, and an anterosuperior portal established in the superior aspect of the rotator interval (Fig. 73.2) with an outside-in technique using an 18 gauge spinal needle; the skin incision is made just inferior to the anterolateral aspect of the acromion and is made large enough to accommodate a 5 mm cannula. A mid-glenoid portal is also established just superior to the subscapularis tendon, and inclined down to the glenoid 20°; the skin incision is just lateral to the coracoid and is large enough to accommodate an 8.25 mm cannula (Fig. 73.3).

The diagnostic portion of the arthroscopy is completed ensuring that the glenoid labrum, SLAP area, rotator cuff and posterosuperior humeral head (Hill–Sachs area) are fully evaluated. An engaging Hill–Sachs lesion usually indicates significant bone loss (assess with internal and external rotation of the humerus). At this point, the arthroscope is switched to the anterosuperior portal and the anterior labrum, capsule and any glenoid bone loss evaluated. Glenoid bone loss should be carefully evaluated and the amount of loss referenced off the bare spot. A measurement of less than 6 mm from the bare spot to the anterior glenoid suggests deficiency of greater than 25% and open augmentation (Latarjet, iliac crest bone graft) should be strongly considered (Fig. 73.4). Acute bony Bankart injuries generally have a small bony fracture that may be incorporated into the arthroscopic repair.[62,65] The capsular attachments should also be assessed to ensure that a HAGL lesion is not present, as failure to address the HAGL lesion either with open surgery or arthroscopically may lead to early failure.

The arthroscope may be maintained in the anterosuperior portal or returned to the posterior portal for capsule and labrum preparation. Not infrequently, an anterior labral periosteal sleeve avulsion lesion is encountered,

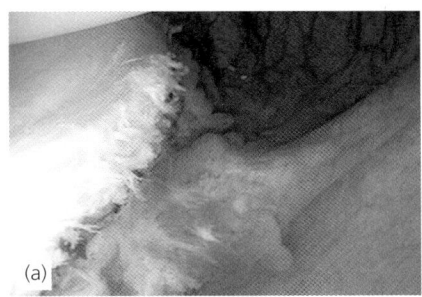 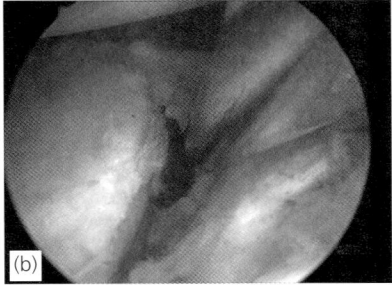 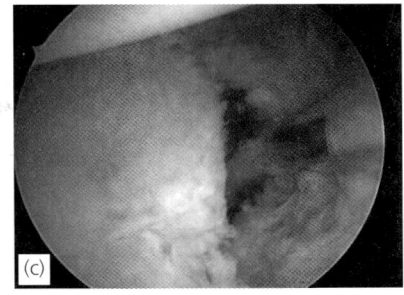

Figure 73.5 Anterior labral tear (a), healed medially down the neck of the glenoid in an anterior labral periosteal sleeve avulsion configuration. The labral tear has to be elevated (b) off the glenoid until just the most posterior fibres of the subscapularis muscle are visible (c).

which is when the labrum and capsule are ruptured off the glenoid and healed medially down the glenoid neck. The glenoid will appear as though there is 'no labrum', when, in fact, it is healed in a medially displaced position on the glenoid. It is crucial to fully 'liberate' the labrum directly off the glenoid and ensure that it is fully mobile from the most inferior aspect of the tear (where the labrum once again becomes competent inferiorly or slightly posteriorly) to the superior extent. Usually this is from 3 o'clock to 6 o'clock in a right shoulder. An arthroscopic elevator device is utilized to fully 'liberate' the labrum from the glenoid, and this step is complete once the most posterior fibres of the subscapularis tendon are visualized (Fig. 73.5).

Once the labrum is fully mobilized, it should 'float' easily back up to the level of the glenoid rim. The capsule is gently abraded with a rasp and the glenoid is also gently burred (on reverse) to remove all soft tissue and provide a fresh bony bed for labral healing. Several portals may be utilized for capsulolabral repair and anchor placement. The midglenoid portal is the workhorse for the anterior anchors; however, the trajectory of this portal may not allow for anchor placement in the most inferior aspect of the glenoid, which is an important aspect of the capsulolabral repair. A 7 o'clock portal may be utilized to obtain inferior and posteroinferior anchor and repair instrumentation access to the most inferior part of the joint.[66,67] The 7 o'clock (accessory posterolateral) portal is made with an outside-in technique using an 18 gauge spinal needle, approximately 2 cm lateral and 1 cm anterior to the original posterior portal. Anchors and repair instrumentation may be passed through a cannula inserted from this position (Fig. 73.6).

In general, a total of three or four anchors should be utilized for the capsulolabral repair, keeping in mind that 'three below three' (three anchors well placed below 3 o'clock) are necessary for a solid repair. A variety of anchors may be utilized: metal, bioabsorbable, biocomposite and also non-absorbable plastic are all available and are up to surgeon preference. The majority are approximately 3.0 mm in diameter and are preloaded with a no. 2 stitch, many of which are available in high-strength suture.

Anchors are progressively placed, starting inferiorly, first through either the 7 o'clock portal or the anterior mid-glenoid portal. Suture management is critical for success, and an additional portal across the glenohumeral joint facilitates

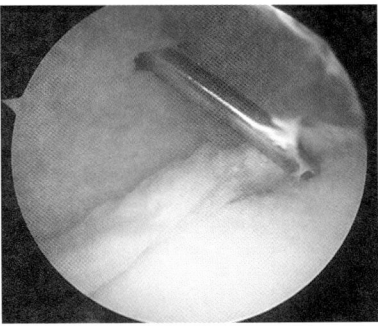

Figure 73.6 Establishing the posterolateral (7 o'clock) portal.

suture shuttling. The first anchor should be placed at the inferior aspect of the tear, right on the glenoid rim (2 mm on the glenoid rim) to allow for the capsulolabral tissue to be repaired back up to the glenoid. Once the anchor is in place, a variety of capsulolabral repair devices are available to obtain a plication of capsular tissue (generally 1 cm)[68] and to ensure that the entire labrum is included in the repair. There are many shuttling techniques to accomplish the repair, and these necessitate proficiency with the repair instrumentation. It should be noted that an optimal repair strategy is to shift the capsular tissue and IGHL from an inferior to superior position; thus, the capsulolabral repair is started inferior to the placement of the anchor in order to shift the tissue superiorly. This addresses the anteroinferior and stretch component of instability. The sutures may be placed in simple vertical or horizontal repair configurations; none has demonstrated superiority. The sutures are tied with either a sliding–locking knot or a non-sliding knot, backed up with a minimum of three alternating half-hitches for optimal loop and knot security (Fig. 73.7).

Anchors are progressively placed anteriorly until the 2 or 3 o'clock position to accomplish the repair. The final repair should reproduce a glenoid bumper anteroinferiorly, with all anchors providing sufficient tension and dimpling of the tissue (Fig. 73.8). Postoperatively, patients wear an abduction sling for 6 weeks, during which passive Codman exercises are instituted for the first 1–2 weeks, followed by passive range of motion in the scapular plane up to 6 weeks (flexion 120°, abduction 120°, external rotation 30° at the side). Aggressive external rotation at the side and

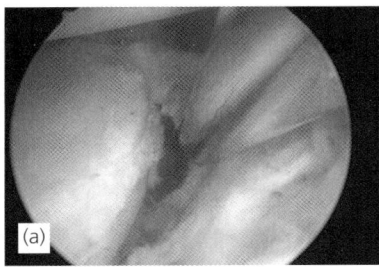 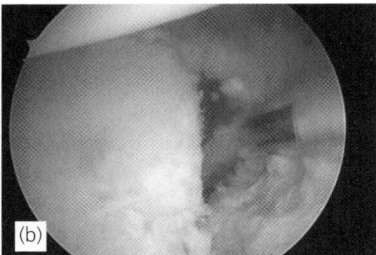 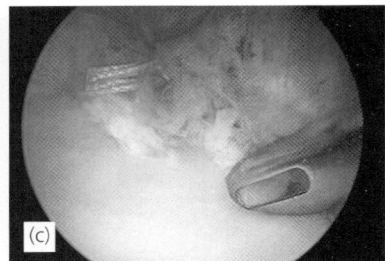

Figure 73.7 Arthroscopic repair steps for an anterior instability case. Once the labrum is prepared, glenoid anchors are inserted on the glenoid rim starting inferiorly (a). A capsulolabral repair device is utilized to perform the repair (b), and the sutures are appropriately shuttled (c).

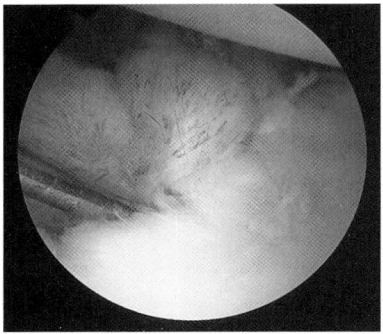

Figure 73.8 The final anterior repair as viewed from the anterosuperior portal.

in abduction is avoided for 6 weeks, then progressive stretching, full range of motion and an active range of motion plan is emphasized from week 6 to week 16. Participation in most sports is delayed at least 4 months, with no contact sports until 6 months.

Preferred technique for open anterior capsulorrhaphy

Exposure

With the patient in the beach chair position, the axillary fold is identified by internal rotation of the arm. Subcutaneous marcaine and epinephrine may be utilized prior to the incision. The incision is made in this fold from the inferior border of the pectoralis major tendon extending superiorly for 5 cm. A subcutaneous dissection is then meticulously performed, retracting the cephalic vein and deltoid muscles laterally while retracting the pectoralis major muscle medially. There may be a leash of vessels that can be ligated for better exposure. The clavipectoral fascia is then incised lateral to the coracobrachialis and the short head of the biceps tendon, and these structures are retracted medially, protecting the musculocutaneous nerve.

The subscapularis tendon is then identified and incised 1 cm medial to the musculotendinous junction from the uppermost portion of the subscapularis. Blunt dissection then must be performed to identify the interval between the muscle and capsule. This is easier at the medial and inferior portion of the subscapularis. The plane in between the muscle and capsule is developed with an elevator. The superior portion of the tendon and capsule are then incised laterally. The entire anterior capsule is exposed by retracting the tendon medially and retracted with a Hohmann retractor. The axillary nerve resides in the inferior capsular pouch, and caution is taken with retraction.

Capsulotomy

The patient's arm is then positioned in 45° of abduction and 45° of external rotation. This tightens the anterior capsule, which facilitates the incision 5–10 mm medial to its insertion of the humeral neck from the rotator interval to the anteroinferior capsular pouch. The humeral head is retracted with a ring retractor and the capsule is retracted medially, allowing inspection of the entire labrum, articular surfaces and the undersurface of the supraspinatus tendon.

Labral repair

After a Bankart lesion is identified, the torn capsulolabral complex is elevated off the glenoid rim to the glenoid neck. The glenoid is then decorticated to bleeding bone and suture anchors are placed at the osteochondral rim of the glenoid. Approximately three to five anchors are placed on the most anterior aspect of the glenoid rim; the capsule is pulled laterally, and both limbs of the suture are passed through the capsulolabral complex so that, when they are tied, the labrum is reapproximated anatomically and firmly back onto the glenoid. Suture passers and penetrators facilitate suture passage through the capsule.

Closure

After repair of the labral tear, the lateral capsulotomy and rotator interval are closed with non-absorbable sutures. This should be done with the patient's arm in 45–60° of abduction and 45–60° of external rotation. If there is capsular redundancy, then an anteroinferior capsular superior shift can be performed at the rotator interval and sutured. For excessive capsular redundancy, the rotator interval is closed and the capsule is incised in between the MGHLs and IGHLs. This creates two flaps. The inferior flap is shifted superiorly, obliterating the inferior capsular pouch. The arm is then changed to 20° of abduction and 35° of external rotation, and the superior flap is shifted inferiorly. The capsular shift is accomplished with non-absorbable sutures.

The subscapularis is then closed without any shortening in a side-to-side repair. A drain is generally placed in the subdeltoid space, and the subcutaneous tissues are closed with absorbable sutures and the skin is closed with a non-absorbable monofilament suture in a subcutaneous running fashion. The postoperative regimen is similar to the arthroscopic repair except that the subscapularis repair is protected for up to 6 weeks, avoiding internal rotation contraction or strengthening.

Posterior instability

BIOMECHANICAL CONSIDERATIONS

The most important static stabilizers to posterior instability is the posterior band of the IGHL complex, coracohumeral ligament and posterior capsule, especially when the arm is forward flexed, adducted and internally rotated.[69] Posterior instability may also result from excessive glenoid or humeral retroversion,[70,71] glenoid hypoplasia, posterior glenoid bone loss and loss of chondrolabral containment – through excessive retroversion and loss of posteroinferior labral height.[72,73] The posterior capsule is also biomechanically different from the anterior capsule – the anterior capsule and the anterior IGHL are thicker with different strain patterns from the posterior capsule and posterior IGHL.[74] However, posterior shoulder stability still relies on the integrity of the capsule and IGHL; posterior instability only results after significant posterior capsular stretch, injury and/or subsequent redundancy.

The subscapularis has been identified as the primary dynamic stabilizer preventing posterior translation;[21] however, all of the rotator cuff musculature stabilizes the joint during active motion by providing concavity compression of the joint and properly orienting the humeral head on the glenoid.

CLINICAL PRESENTATION

Many times patients with posterior instability will present with generalized shoulder pain or pain at the posterior aspect of the shoulder. Pain from subluxation may be from rotator cuff tendinitis from excessive stretching as the static stabilizers fail. These patients may also have elements of multidirectional instability – they will have multiple non-specific complaints of shoulder pain, weakness, paraesthesias and problems carrying weight at their sides.[62,75–77]

PHYSICAL EXAMINATION FINDINGS

Patients with posterior instability may have tenderness with palpation at the posterior glenohumeral joint line.[75,76] Range of motion is usually normal and symmetric. Altered scapulothoracic motions resulting from scapular winging is common.[78,79] The posterior apprehension or stress test may reproduce the specific shoulder pain;[76,80,81] apprehension is not usually present in posteriorly unstable patients. If the patient is positive on the apprehension manoeuvre, this may alert the physician that the patient is unstable anteriorly. Additional posterior instability tests include the jerk test,[75,76] the Kim test[82] and the load and shift test.[44] These tests may be positive for pain only. Subluxation is not as commonly seen in the posterior unstable patient as in the anteriorly unstable patient. Patients with a painful jerk test demonstrated a higher failure rate with non-operative treatment.[75,76] Finally, some patients with posterior instability will also have a symptomatic inferior sulcus; they are best classified and treated as multidirectional instability.

RADIOGRAPHIC EVALUATION

An axillary view is essential to diagnose posterior dislocations or subluxations. Occasionally patients who experience a traumatic posterior dislocation will have a reverse Hill–Sachs lesion, which is an impaction fracture of the anterosuperior humeral head found at the level of the lesser tuberosity.[75,76] Posterior rim defects such as fractures, erosions and calcifications, fractures of the humeral tuberosities, calcification of the capsule or of the tendons and formation of osteophytes should all be noted on plain films of the shoulder. Glenoid hypoplasia (a shallow or irregular glenoid fossa), prominent coracoid process, enlarged acromion, distal clavicle abnormalities, hypoplasia of the upper ribs and flattening of the humeral head[83] can also be seen on standard radiographs. CT is an excellent study to assess the glenoid for hypoplasia, bone loss and degree of retroversion.

MRI and magnetic resonance arthrogram (MRA) offer valuable additional information to visualize the posterior

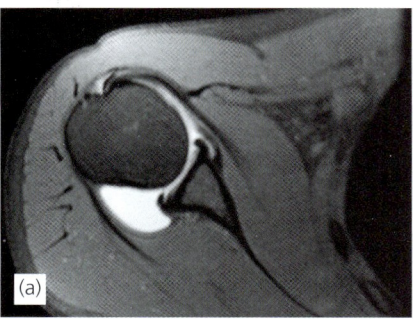
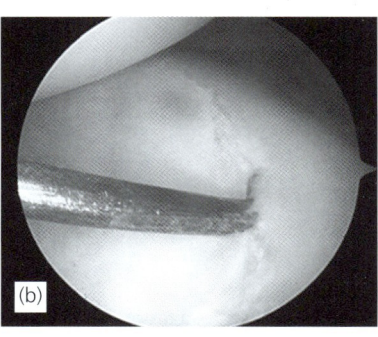

Figure 73.9 Magnetic resonance arthrogram axial image of a posterior labral tear (a). A Kim lesion, or marginal crack in the posterior labrum (b).

and inferior capsulolabral structures, the rotator interval, the biceps labral anchor and the rotator cuff. MRA findings of a Kim lesion,[72] which is an incomplete avulsion of the posterior labrum, are shown in Fig. 73.9.

SURGICAL DECISION-MAKING

Patients with a history of traumatic subluxation or dislocation or instability resulting from cumulative microtrauma are less likely to respond to non-operative treatment.[40,84,85] Operative stabilization is considered for patients who continue to have limited function secondary to pain and/or instability, who are psychologically stable and who have failed an adequate trial of conservative therapy. Open procedures include bone blocks, glenoid osteotomy and or rotational osteotomy of the proximal humerus, open posterior capsular shifts, posterior capsular plication, infraspinatus advancement, reverse Putti–Platt plication and reverse Bankart repair. However, the open posterior shoulder approach has shown various outcomes, including up to an overall recurrence rate of 50% utilizing three different open posterior procedures.[75,76,86–88]

Arthroscopic procedures are reserved for patients without significant bone loss or fracture. These procedures include arthroscopic capsulolabral repair, capsular plication and rotator interval closure.

SURGICAL TECHNIQUE

Positioning

Both the beach chair and lateral decubitus positions have been used for the arthroscopic treatment of posterior capsulolabral repair and/or capsulorrhaphy. The lateral decubitus position has been shown to open the inferior and posterior quadrants more effectively and allows for easy access to these areas. The arm is usually abducted 50° and flexed approximately 15° by an arm-traction sleeve. An axillary traction device or pillow bump placed in the axilla further opens up the posteroinferior area of the shoulder.

Portal placement

A standard diagnostic arthroscopy is performed, starting from the standard posterior portal. An anterior superior portal is made in the rotator interval; the camera is then inserted in this portal to address the posterior structures.

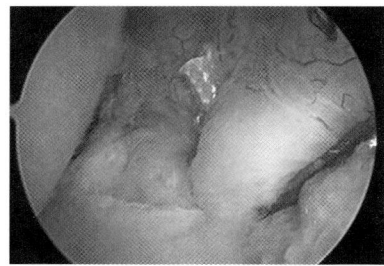

Figure 73.10 The posterior repair is performed from the 7 o'clock posterolateral portal.

An accessory posterolateral portal (7 o'clock portal) is made for instrumentation and anchor placement, and facilitates posterior repair.[66,67] The 7 o'clock enters the joint inferiorly about 1 cm anterior and 2 cm lateral to the standard posterior portal (Fig. 73.10). A clear 8.25 mm cannula is inserted to accommodate all instruments needed for repair and/or capsulorrhaphy.

Preparation of the labrum

Preparation of the chondrolabral junction in a posterior labral tear is easier through the anterior portal instead of through the posterior or posterolateral portal[89] (Fig. 73.11). The labrum should be meticulously probed, and, if a Kim lesion is present, the labrum should be completely elevated off the glenoid and an anchor repair should be performed. An incomplete tear or crack of the posterior labrum, such as a Kim lesion, is a common reason for failure of capsulorrhaphy without the use of anchors (Fig. 73.12).

Capsulolabral repair

With the camera in the anterosuperior portal, the two posterior working portals are utilized to accomplish the posterior capsulolabral repair. Depending upon the examination under anaesthesia and clinical instability findings, usually a 1 cm capsular plication is utilized, along with the labral repair (if the labrum is torn or compromised). Glenoid anchors are utilized to perform the repair with either vertical or horizontal mattress sutures, tied with a reliable arthroscopic knot. Up to four anchors may be

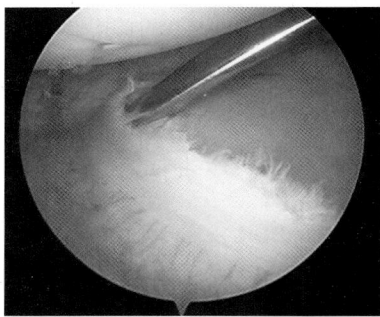

Figure 73.11 Preparation of the posterior labrum is facilitated with an elevator device inserted from the mid-glenoid portal.

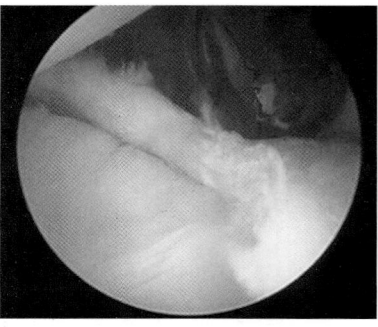

Figure 73.12 Arthroscopic view of a posterior labral tear.

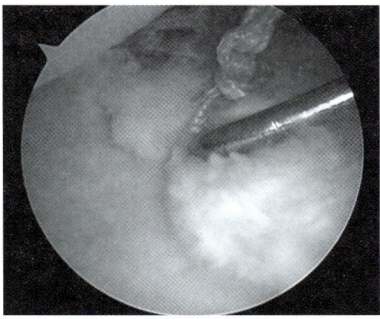

Figure 73.13 Arthroscopic view from the anterosuperior portal of the final posterior capsulolabral repair.

necessary from most inferiorly at 6 o'clock up to approximately 10 or 11 o'clock posterosuperiorly (Fig. 73.13).

Rotator interval closure

This procedure remains controversial. The rotator interval has been shown in some studies to be an important posterior and inferior stabilizer of the shoulder. Too vigorous a closure causes loss of external rotation, especially with the arm at the side.[90–92] Some studies[26] of open rotator interval closures have shown that posterior and inferior instability was improved after an open, medial to lateral, imbrication of the rotator interval structures, especially the coracohumeral ligament. Recent biomechanical studies have suggested that the arthroscopic rotator interval closure, which does not address the coracohumeral ligament, is not as beneficial to improve posterior and/or inferior shoulder stability; however, it may improve anterior stability.[90–92] If desired, one or two interval closure sutures are utilized from the SGHL to the MGHL with an inferior to superior shift, usually blindly tying the knot over the capsule while gently backing out the cannula.[93,94]

POSTOPERATIVE MANAGEMENT

Postoperatively, the patients are immobilized in a 30° abduction pillow in neutral rotation for 4–6 weeks. Patients may perform passive pendulum exercises, gentle passive motion and active elbow and wrist motion. Restriction of internal rotation and adduction is maintained for 6 weeks. After 4–6 weeks, active motion is started, and range of motion is increased and a strengthening programme of the rotator cuff and scapular stabilizing exercises are started. At the 6 month point, patients are allowed unrestricted return to full activities after a sports-specific training programme.

Multidirectional instability

The definition of multidirectional instability is increased symptomatic glenohumeral laxity in more than one direction (anterior, posterior and/or inferior).[95] Shoulders that are unstable in two or three directions usually have a com-

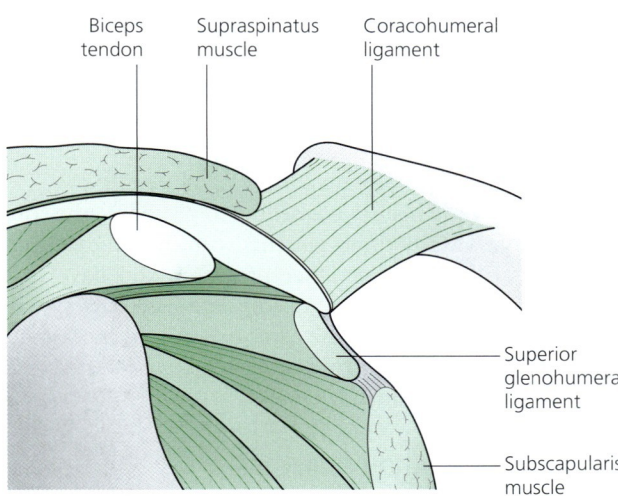

Figure 73.14 Coronal view of the anatomy of the rotator interval.

ponent of inferior instability and a large, redundant capsule. A positive sulcus sign, however, is not pathological unless it reproduces instability symptoms of pain, weakness or early fatigue. It is critical to differentiate normal laxity and pathological instability that reproduces symptoms of instability.

BIOMECHANICAL CONSIDERATIONS

Bony anatomy, the labrum and scapular inclination are static stabilizers against inferior instability. The inferior capsule and the IGHL are also important inferior stabilizers. The coracohumeral ligament contained in the rotator interval helps prevent inferior subluxation in external rotation (Fig. 73.14). Dynamic inferior stability of the shoulder joint is maintained by the supraspinatus and the long head of the biceps. A 'circle' concept has been introduced that if the posteroinferior capsule is under tension, there is a reciprocal load-sharing injury in the anterosuperior capsule;[96] however, this is highly debated.[97]

CLINICAL PRESENTATION

Patients with multidirectional instability will often present with repetitive and/or cumulative microtrauma and progressive episodes of instability, such as that seen in baseball or volleyball players, or with progressive bidirectional instability from a discrete traumatic event. The most frequent aetiology of recurrent multidirectional instability is repetitive microtrauma. This is seen in sporting activities that involve repetitive loading of the shoulder in front of the body, as seen in baseball, softball, kayaking, volleyball, rowing, swimming and American football. The shoulder is usually flexed, adducted and internally rotated, stretching out the posterior band of the IGHL. These activities repetitively injure the posterior and inferior capsulolabral complex. This damage of the static stabilizers puts increasing stress on the rotator cuff, and tendinitis or secondary impingement is common in these athletes.

Patients with multidirectional instability will present with non-specific complaints of pain, decreased athletic performance and loss of strength. In addition, complaints of paraesthesias, neuritic or radicular-type pain that mimics thoracic outlet syndrome, and feelings of instability or subluxation during sleep are common.

Eliciting a good history is essential to providing the correct diagnosis. Many times patients with multidirectional instability will have seen other providers and have had failed surgery. It is important to correlate subjective symptoms with the position of the arm. It is also important to ask about any family history of collagen disorders, such as Ehlers–Danlos syndrome.

PHYSICAL EXAMINATION FINDINGS

Both shoulders should be examined, and any obvious dislocation, subluxation, asymmetry, abnormal motion, muscle atrophy, swelling and scapular winging should be noted. Wide-shaped scars may suggest a collagen disorder. Range of motion is usually normal, and the shoulder should be tested for anterior, posterior and inferior instability. Multidirectionally unstable patients will have a positive inferior sulcus test, which should reproduce some of the patient's symptoms.[95] The test is performed by placing a force inferiorly on the humerus in neutral to 20° of abduction. The distance between the anterior margin of the acromion and the superior humeral head is recorded. The test can be done with the arm in 90° of abduction as well, applying a downward force on the proximal humerus to cause inferior displacement. A positive test is when pain and symptoms of instability are reproduced with observed increased inferior translation (usually >2 cm).

Patients with multidirectional instability will also present with apprehension during range of motion manoeuvres and will commonly have tenderness along the medial angle of the scapula and anterior rotator cuff. Many times internal rotation strength is decreased and anterior impingement occurs as the humerus rides high and stretches the rotator cuff tendons.

Atraumatic patients with increasing instability will often present with generalized ligamentous laxity. Hyperextension of the elbows greater than 5°, the ability to touch the thumb to the ipsilateral forearm, hyperextension of the metacarpophalangeal joints more than 90°, and touching the palm of each hand to the floor while keeping the knees extended are all indicative of generalized ligamentous laxity. This entity has been documented in 40–75% who had surgery for multidirectional instability and has been associated with decreased success with surgical intervention.

RADIOGRAPHIC EVALUATION

Plain films may reveal an inferior subluxation of the humerus in the glenoid. MRI and MRA are valuable to assess the capsule, integrity of the labrum, the rotator

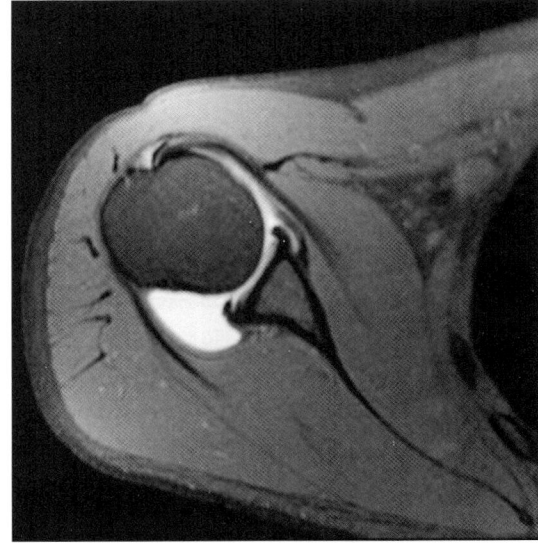

Figure 73.15 Magnetic resonance arthrogram of a large, patulous capsule in a patient with multidirectional shoulder instability.

interval and the rotator cuff. The capsular area has been shown to be increased with MRA evaluation[98] (Fig. 73.15).

SURGICAL DECISION-MAKING

Rehabilitation remains the initial treatment of choice, especially in patients with atraumatic instability, those with generalized ligamentous laxity and those with instability secondary to repetitive microtrauma. Patients with a traumatic event or a capsulolabral tear are less likely to respond to non-operative treatment. Operative stabilization is reasonable in those with limited function secondary to pain and continued symptoms and those who have failed non-operative treatments (usually greater than 6 months).

Open procedures include capsular shifts, subscapularis tendon transfer and capsular plication with infraspinatus advancement. The results of open procedures have been mixed, with 40–91% successful. Open treatment of multidirectional instability is still considered the gold standard, especially when inferior capsular pathology is addressed. Arthroscopic procedures include arthroscopic capsulolabral repairs and capsular plication.

SURGICAL TECHNIQUES

Position

The patient should be placed in the lateral decubitus position with a traction sleeve.

Diagnostic arthroscopy with standard portals

There is usually a positive 'drive-through' sign with a 'sky box'[99] view (Fig. 73.16), with excessive laxity of the

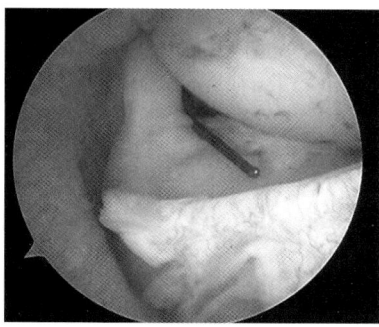

Figure 73.16 A large patulous capsule posteroinferiorly, demonstrating a 'sky-box' view from the posterior portal.

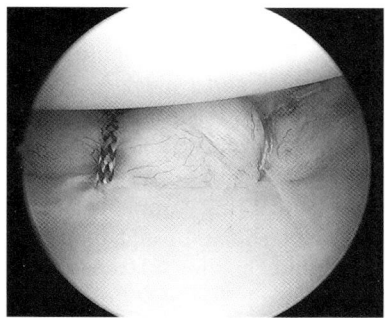

Figure 73.17 Technique of capsular plication to an intact labrum in a multidirectional instability case.

posteroinferior capsule. Multidirectional instability may also be associated with a 'triple labral lesion', which is a circumferential labral tear causing multidirectional instability.[100]

Sequence of repair

The inferior and posteroinferior pathology is first addressed with suture anchors and capsulolabral repair, then any anterior labral tears are addressed, and finally the superior (SLAP) region as the shoulder volume diminishes with each repair.

Capsular plication

Usually, a 1 cm plication adequately addresses the capsular deformation; however, the exact amount should be specific to the patient and to the instability finding. The posteroinferior and inferior aspects of the capsulolabral complex are repaired with three to five plication sutures (Fig. 73.17). Anchors should be utilized for repair if the labrum is torn or cracked; if it is in good condition, then the labrum has excellent holding strength for a capsulolabral repair.[101] In a cadaveric model, an isolated posteroinferior plication of 1 cm resulted in a 9° loss of internal rotation and an 11° loss of abduction; 1 cm plication of the entire posterior capsule resulted in a 15° loss of abduction and a 21° loss of internal rotation.[68] The axillary nerve is at risk inferiorly; placing the arm in abduction/external rotation with perpendicular traction decreases the risk of injury.[102–104] An anteroinferior and direct inferior 1 cm plication is 12.5 mm away from the nerve; posteroinferior plication is 24.1 mm away.

SUPERIOR LABRUM ANTERIOR TO POSTERIOR TEARS AND REPAIR

The superior labrum is meniscoid in shape and is loosely attached to the glenoid rim, especially near the supraglenoid tubercle. Approximately 50% of the long biceps tendon arises from the superior labrum; thus, SLAP lesions are classified by the extent of labral and biceps involvement.[105] Type I is characterized by labral fraying without detachment from the glenoid or biceps disruption. In type II, the most common, the biceps origin is detached in addition to labral fraying. An intact (type III) or disrupted (type IV) biceps anchor is associated with a bucket-handle tear of the labrum in the final two classes, with type IV comprising intratendinous tears. Conventionally, a type I is treated typically with debridement, and a type 2 with surgical repair. Traditionally, a type III SLAP tear is treated with either debridement and resection of the displaced bucket-handle tear or surgical repair, and treatment of a type IV is by biceps tenotomy with or without proximal biceps fixation (tenodesis). The incidence of SLAP tears is estimated to be 6% in the general population.[106]

Clinical presentation

The typical presentation of a SLAP lesion includes deep, poorly localized shoulder pain and 'catching', 'snapping' or 'popping' with forward flexion or abduction.[107] Traumatic SLAP lesions result from compression or traction injuries, such as a fall on an outstretched arm or catching a heavy, falling object. However, SLAP tears in the overhead athlete frequently lack a single event aetiology and may result from poor throwing mechanics. They are typically seen in overhead athletes such as in baseball, volleyball, tennis and weight lifting.

Physical examination

For patients with a symptomatic SLAP tear, tenderness is localized anteriorly near the bicipital groove and worsens with stressing of the biceps anchor complex. Physical testing attempts to compress and challenge the superior labral complex; thus the Speed and Yergason tests are usually positive (generate anterior pain) in SLAP lesions. However, these patients may also have positive Neer or Hawkins signs, misguiding the clinician towards impingement or rotator cuff pathology. In evaluating tests designed for SLAP lesion detection – active compression (O'Brien's active compression test), pain provocation and rotation compression – the positive predictive value (PPV) varies widely, with most studies reporting 50–75%.[107,108] Kim's biceps load test is reported to have greater than 90% sensitivity and specificity with a PPV of 83%, although these results have not been verified independently or in a large study population.[109] Physical examination findings and history create an index of suspicion, yet imaging studies can assist in diagnostic suspicion. Arthroscopy remains the gold standard for definitive diagnosis.

Imaging

For the diagnosis of SLAP tears, the current standard is MRI, occasionally supplemented with intra-articular contrast (gadolinium). The sensitivity and specificity of MRI for detecting labral lesions are reported at approximately 90%,[110] both of which are increased by the use of an arthrogram series. Increased signal is indicative of damage and, if contrast is utilized, a frayed labrum appears cloudy or fuzzy. Proper diagnosis depends upon familiarity with normal labral variants and the appearance of shoulder anatomy on MRI. The typical finding for a SLAP type II tear is fluid clearly separating the biceps anchor point from the superior labral fibrous complex. This is best visualized on a coronal image (Fig. 73.18), as either fluid or contrast demonstrating a tear between the superior glenoid margin and the biceps anchor. Occasionally, the sagittal oblique images demonstrate contrast between the glenoid and superior labrum as well.

Management and surgical indications

Initial treatment of SLAP tears is conservative, including rest, physical therapy and non-steroidal anti-inflammatory drugs (NSAIDs). The goal of physical therapy is capsular stretching, rotator cuff strengthening and stabilization of the scapula. Conservative management is generally unsuccessful; thus, it is frequently omitted in athletes or high-demand patients. Surgical intervention is not indicated for patients who are unwilling or unable to complete the rehabilitation protocol or the diagnosis of SLAP pathology is uncertain.

Surgical technique

Initially, a diagnostic arthroscopy is performed through a standard, posterior glenohumeral portal. The glenohumeral articular cartilage and undersurface of the rotator cuff are inspected for concomitant pathology; then attention is focused on the labrum to identify the location and type of lesion. Daluga and Daluga[111] have reported successful repair through a single anterior portal, while O'Brien et al.[112] have proposed a combination of superolateral and transrotator cuff portal for lesion repair posterior to the biceps anchoring complex. If an anterior portal is utilized, placement should be high enough in the rotator interval to facilitate anchor placement. Percutaneous anchor placement through the rotator cuff musculotendinous junction may be utilized to avoid cannula placement through the cuff.

The frayed regions of the labrum and the bony site of repair should be debrided with a shaver to optimize repair interface contact. The extent of tearing is evaluated to determine the number of anchors needed to secure the repair (Fig. 73.19). After pilot hole tapping, glenoid anchors loaded with a no. 2 suture are inserted into the glenoid margin at a 45° angle. A labral repair device is utilized to pass the suture through the labrum, prior to arthroscopic knot tying with standard techniques (Fig. 73.20). The authors' preferred technique for SLAP type II repairs includes the placement of two anchors – one anterior and one posterior to the biceps tendon (Fig. 73.21). Domb et al.[113] demonstrated that double anchor (simple) and single anchor mattress suture configurations had a higher load to failure value than one simple suture repair in a cadaveric

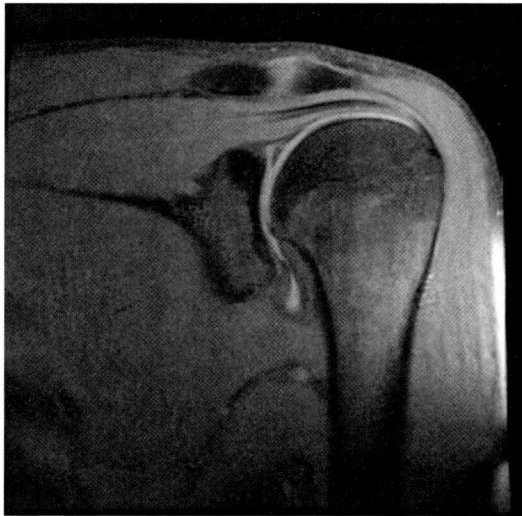

Figure 73.18 Coronal magnetic resonance arthrogram image of a superior labrum anterior to posterior tear with gadolinium dye extending superiorly under the biceps anchor.

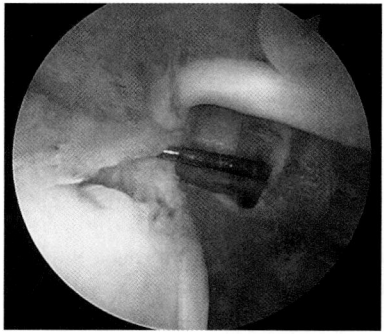

Figure 73.19 Arthroscopic view from the posterior portal of a superior labrum anterior to posterior type 2 tear.

study. With this technique, however, it is critical to avoid non-anatomical placement of the proximal aspect of the biceps tendon at the level of the insertion. Furthermore, more posterior tears may require more anchors or anchors placed more central and posterior along the top of the glenoid rim.

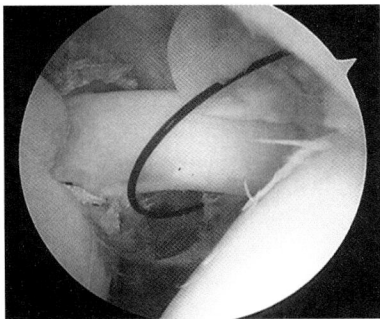

Figure 73.20 The superior labrum anterior to posterior repair anchor is inserted posteriorly, and the superior labrum repaired posteriorly.

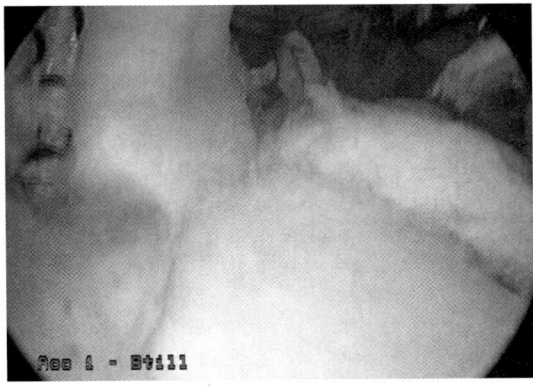

Figure 73.21 Final superior labrum anterior to posterior type 2 repair construct.

Outcomes

Positive outcomes are reported for up to 4 years; long-term follow-up studies have yet to be completed. Reports of improvement in pain, instability and function as early as 6–8 weeks after surgery are consistent across numerous studies. On the other hand, studies of labral debridement have failed to demonstrate long-term pain and functional improvement with less than half of patients able to return to their previous activity level.[114] Conflicting reports exist as to whether outcomes are better in isolated SLAP repair or combined procedures. Coleman et al.[115] reported that, while combined and isolated SLAP repairs had similar American Shoulder and Elbow Society (ASES) and L'Insalata scores, subjective assessment of outcomes was significantly less for isolated repairs. In athletes, the return to play rate is consistently over 50% with a few reports of greater than 90%.[116,117] Overall, repair of SLAP type II lesions has been validated in the short term; however, additional studies are needed to evaluate long-term outcomes, modes of failure and the rate of revision surgery. The repair of SLAP lesions in relatively older patients remains controversial, and may be associated with higher failure rates because of diminished blood supply and mechanical considerations. A summary of outcomes in given in Table 73.1.

ROTATOR CUFF TEARS AND REPAIR

Presentation

Rotator cuff tears occur in patients of all ages. Chronic impingement syndromes and degenerative changes contribute to the high incidence of tears in middle-aged patients. Tears are less common in younger individuals with predominantly traumatic or sports-related aetiologies. The most common symptom is shoulder pain, which localizes to the acromion or diffuses over the deltoid. Typically, pain occurs at night and is exacerbated by overhead and lifting activities. Additionally, patients complain of weakness and decreased range of motion.

Table 73.1 Recent clinical studies on surgical intervention for SLAP tears.

Author (date)	Patients	Lesion	Follow-up	Results
Enad and Kurtz[118] (2007)	36	Type II	29 months	16/18 SLAP only; good/excellent UCLA score
				17/18 combined; good/excellent UCLA score
Coleman et al.[115] (2007)	50	Type II	3.4 years	65% SLAP only; good/excellent satisfaction
				81% combined; good/excellent satisfaction
Funk and Snow[116] (2007)	18	14 type II	6 months	Average return to play 2.6 months
		3 type III		Average playing at previous level 94%
		1 type IV		
Paxinos et al.[117] (2006)	24	22 type II	2 years	22/24 returned to pre-injury activity level
		1 type III		
		1 type IV		

SLAP, superior labrum anterior to posterior; UCLA, University of California at Los Angeles.

Physical examination

Severe atrophy of the supraspinatus or infraspinatus will result in visual asymmetry and a sunken appearance to the posterior shoulder. Palpation reveals tenderness over the acromion, possibly accompanied by subacromial crepitation. Classically, the patient's active range of motion is restricted with intact passive range of motion. Testing of external rotation, abduction and forward elevation will demonstrate decreased strength in comparison with the contralateral side. Specific clinical tests attempt to replicate impingement. Park et al.[119] reported that the Neer sign and Hawkins–Kennedy sign are most sensitive (75%) for partial thickness tears, whereas the painful arc sign is best for predicting full thickness tears. Although provocative tests are not diagnostic, positive results will increase the index of suspicion for a rotator cuff tear.

Radiographic findings

Patients with suspected rotator cuff tears generally undergo a five-view series of radiographs: anterior to posterior at neutral, internal and external rotation, plus axillary and supraspinatus outlet view. Radiographic findings of interest include bony changes of the greater tuberosity, acromion type and presence of glenohumeral arthritis. Decreased distance between the humeral head and acromion is indicative of a massive tear; however, plain radiographs do not identify the location, type and size of lesions. With accuracy greater than 90%, MRI facilitates evaluation of muscle fatty infiltration and tendon retraction in addition to the size and location of the tear.

Surgical management

Surgical repair is indicated for symptomatic full thickness tears after conservative treatment – physical therapy, NSAIDs and cortisone injections – have failed. In the case of functional tears in low-demand patients (i.e. the elderly), debridement of the torn cuff and subacromial decompression may suffice.

Successful arthroscopic rotator cuff repair is contingent upon the surgeon's skill and proficiency. Bursal and capsular tissue swells with arthroscopic irrigation, limiting the optimal window for repair to approximately 2 hours. Efficient evaluation of tear characteristics as well as timely completion of ancillary procedures will permit adequate time for rotator cuff repair. If all procedures cannot be completed within the time frame, the surgeon should be prepared to convert to a mini-open repair.

Positioning and portal placement

The patient is placed in the beach chair position with bony prominences padded so that the medial border of the scapula is just off the edge of the table. Range of motion is evaluated, especially internal and external rotation at neutral and 90° of abduction. The patient is sedated and receives analgesia via an intrascalene block plus 30 mL of 0.5% bupivicaine (with epinephrine) injected into the subacromial space. After sterile preparing and draping, the coracoid process, acromioclavicular joint and scapular spine are palpated and marked. With the index finger in the notch between the acromioclavicular joint and the scapular spine and the middle finger on the coracoid process, the posterior portal placement – between the infraspinatus and teres minor muscles – is indicated by the thumb, approximately 2 cm inferior and 1 cm medial to the posterolateral acromion. From a 1 cm skin incision, a trocar is advanced, aiming towards the coracoid process until it 'pops' through the posterior capsule. If resistance is encountered, the arm is rotated or abducted to localize the joint space. The glenohumeral joint, labrum and undersurface of the cuff are inspected for pathology, with tearing marked with a no. 1 polydioxanone suture (Fig. 73.22).

The arthroscope is redirected to the subacromial space and a spinal needle is used to establish the location for two additional portals. An anterior portal is placed just lateral to the coracoid process, entering the subacromial space within a triangle bordered by the long head of the biceps brachii (superior), humeral head (laterally) and the subscapularis tendon (inferiorly). The standard lateral portal is established 2 cm lateral to the midpoint of the acromion, as indicated by the notch between the clavicle and the spine of the scapula. Additional accessory portals – such as the superolateral, Neviaser or posteromedial – are useful for suture parking and tying, especially at the distal margins of the tendon[120,121] (Fig. 73.23).

A thorough bursectomy and debridement of the subacromial space removes excess and inflamed tissue that swells to impair visualization. From the lateral portal, fibrous, whitish tissue is removed with a shaver while avoiding the well-vascularized fatty tissue. In order to

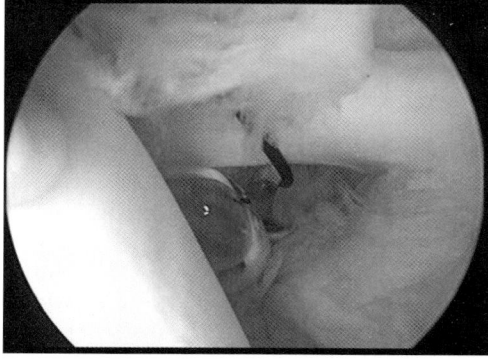

Figure 73.22 A marker stitch (blue no. 1 polydioxanone) is placed to mark a supraspinatus tear in the glenohumeral joint, and is utilized to locate the tear in the subacromial space.

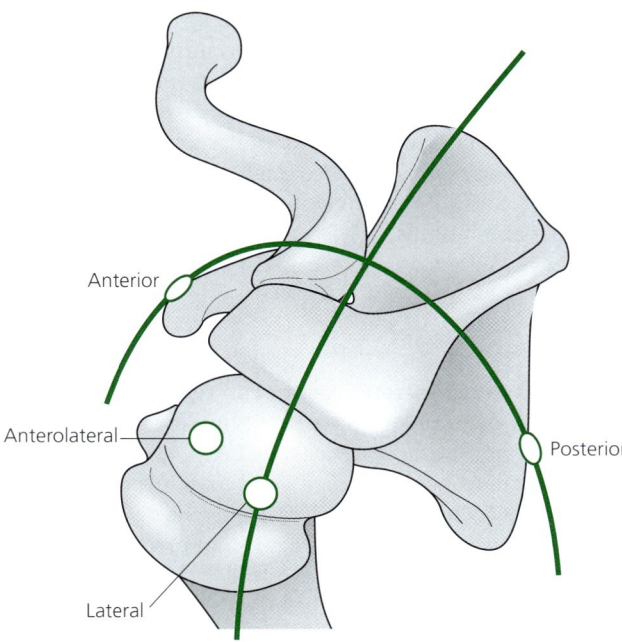

Figure 73.23 Shoulder portals that are commonly used during a rotator cuff repair.

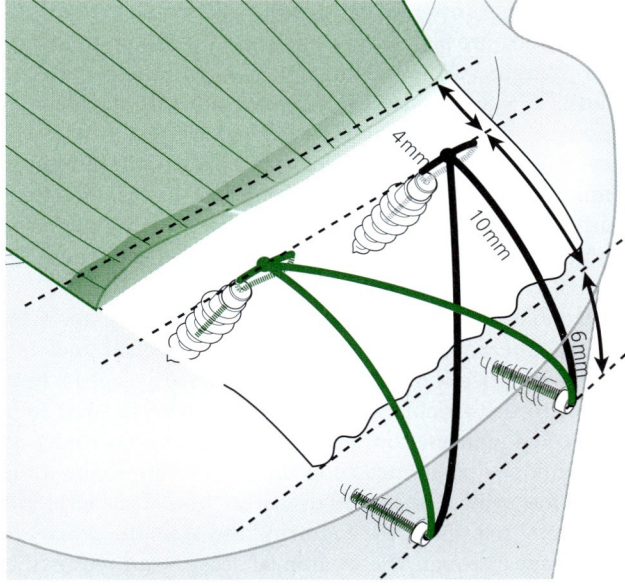

Figure 73.24 Diagram of the rotator cuff footprint, and measurements to accomplish double row repair construct.

complete the bursectomy posteriorly, placements are reversed with the lateral portal providing a global view of the subacromial space. If impingement is a factor in the rotator cuff pathology, the acromion is converted to a type 1 (flat) profile via acromioplasty. The coracoacromial ligament is ablated with an electrocautery device, followed by burring to smooth and reduce the acromial profile.

Rotator cuff repair

Evaluation of the rotator cuff tear should include: (1) size, (2) pattern and (3) mobility. Reapproximation to the greater tuberosity is attempted by pulling parallel to the muscle fibre axis with a tendon grasper. If the tear is not reducible, a single or double rotator interval slide and release of the coracohumeral ligament are used to increase tendon mobility.[122] U-shaped or L-shaped tear configurations necessitate an initial side-to-side repair prior to bony reapproximation. Frayed margins are debrided, then the longitudinal aspect repaired from medial to lateral, with one suture for every 5 mm of tearing. Numerous devices exist for side-to-side suture passing, including antegrade (direct bite of the tendon with the suture passed via a needle) and retrograde (rotator cuff penetrated first and then the suture retrieved) suture passers.[123] It is critical to assess the repair reduction while performing the rotator cuff repair in order to avoid improper tissue reapproximation to the rotator cuff footprint. Knot tying is delayed until all sutures are placed to facilitate subsequent passing. If multiple sutures are necessary, pairs are separated with suture saver devices or isolated through different portals to prevent fouling. Knots are tied from medial to lateral using half-hitches on alternating posts.

There is a growing interest in double-row and transosseous equivalent repairs.[120,123,124] The supraspinatus footprint is roughly trapezoidal, lying between the bicipital groove and bare area. Beginning approximately 1 mm from the cartilage surface, the insertion is approximately 25 mm anterior to posterior and 12–16 mm medial to lateral[125,126] (Fig. 73.24). To optimize healing, a bleeding bony surface is created with a shaver and small burr. Violation of the cortical layer should be avoided to maintain the integrity of suture anchor placement. Numerous anchor configurations exist involving single row, double row and transosseous equivalent fixation. Compared with single row designs, double row anchoring with mattress sutures provides better reapproximation of the supraspinatus footprint.[124,126–131] No single method is appropriate for all tears; thus, familiarity with multiple techniques is vital to successful repair.

Crescent tears without retraction, either full or partial thickness, are amenable to single row repair, while double row or transosseous equivalent provides better attachment and retention for retracted L-shaped or U-shaped tears after side-to-side repair.[120] Anchors are placed at the 'dead man's angle' (45°)[132] such that the superior edge of the eyelet is at bone level. Deeper placement increases the likelihood of suture failure due to chafing, while shallow placement results in a proud eyelet and difficult suture tensioning.

For single row repairs, double-loaded anchors with a no. 2 suture are placed approximately 1 cm from the articular margin, with one anchor per centimetre of tear width.[129,133] Sutures are passed retrograde through the tendon 5–10 mm from the torn margin using a penetrator device. After all suture passing is completed, the tendon is reduced and the knots are tied with half-hitches on alternating posts. Reapproximation to the greater tuberosity and suture tying are done in 10° of forward flexion and 10° of abduction to limit tension on the repair.

Double row techniques are useful in U-shaped or L-shaped tears subsequent to longitudinal repair and sufficient mobilization. One or two anchors are placed 2 mm lateral to the articular surface, with sutures secured in a horizontal mattress configuration. Thus, the remainder of the tendon is positioned to facilitate the reapproximation of the footprint. The second row of anchors is placed along the lateral margin of the footprint and the sutures passed retrograde through the tendon at least 5 mm from the edge. Exact positioning of the suture may replicate a Mason–Allen configuration, a mattress suture or a simple suture depending on the requirements for replicating the footprint (Fig. 73.25).

Transosseous equivalent constructs have gained favour as a method to maximize tendon–bone contact and evenly distribute load across the repair. For transosseous equivalent repairs, one or two anchors (medial row) are placed 2 mm lateral from the articular margin. The tendon is reapproximated and medial sutures passed at the musculotendinous junction, 10–15 mm from the free edge. At each anchor, the suture is tied in a horizontal mattress configuration to medial load the repair. The remaining suture is brought laterally to form a suture bridge or compression construct. Sutures are loaded into one of several repair devices (PushLock, Arthrex, Naples, FL; Versalok, Mitek, Norwood, MA) for performing a transosseous equivalent repair; these are inserted at the lateral margin of the greater tuberosity[134] (Fig. 73.26). Suture ends and extra suture are trimmed and the subacromial space is irrigated prior to instrument removal. Incision closure is done in three layers with absorbable suture.

The shoulder is immobilized in an abduction sling for 6 weeks after surgery. The day after surgery, the patient begins pendulum and passive range of motion exercises. At week 6 postoperatively, active range of motion and shoulder – rotator cuff, deltoid and scapular stabilizers – strengthening exercises started. Light sports activity is permitted at about 3 months with return to full work and activities at 6 months.

Results

Outcomes of arthroscopic rotator cuff repair are comparable to mini-open and open repair.[135] Grading via University of California at Los Angeles (UCLA), ASES and other scoring systems has quantified good to excellent results in more than 85% of patients. The current re-tear rate is 25–40%; however, repair failure does not preclude symptomatic relief. Cummins and Murrell[136] identified suture pull-out from the tendon as the major site (86%) of failure, although failure may also occur at the anchor–bone interface or the suture itself. Advanced patient age and chronic tears are associated with increased risk of failure as a result of fatty infiltration, retraction and poor tendon quality. Although double row fixation has better structural outcomes, no significant difference has been noted in subjective patient outcomes.[133]

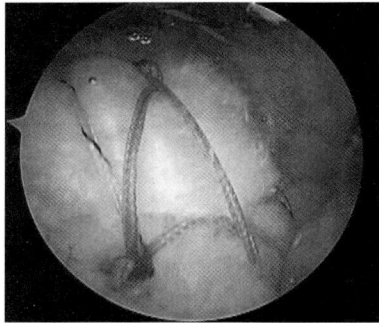

Figure 73.26 Transosseous equivalent final repair construct.

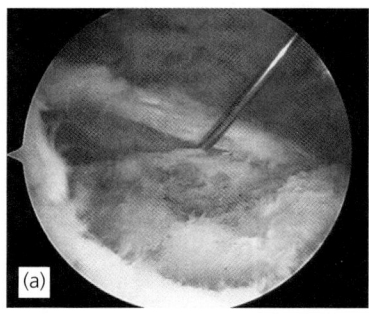 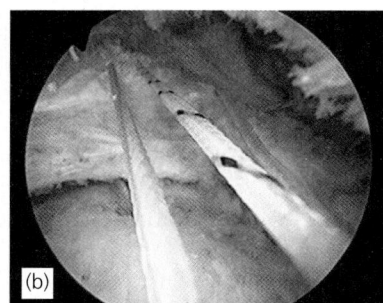 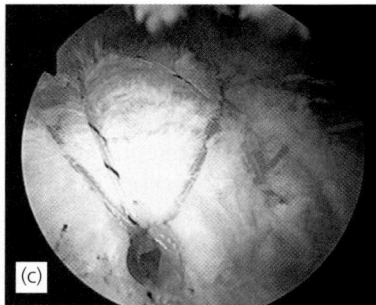

Figure 73.25 Rotator cuff repair, demonstrating rotator cuff repair (a), medial row anchor placement (b) and final transosseous equivalent lateral row repair (c).

KEY LEARNING POINTS

- Instability
  - Shoulder instability comprises a spectrum of pathological laxity; unidirectional instability is frequently anterior, occasionally posterior.
  - Multidirectional instability includes a symptomatic (reproduces patient's symptoms) inferior sulcus component.
  - Instability includes some component of capsular injury and stretch, especially the anterior band of the inferior glenohumeral ligament for anterior instability.
  - Arthroscopic capsulolabral repair is an effective treatment for all types of shoulder instability.
  - Knowledge of glenoid anchor fixation devices, repair and shuttling techniques is paramount.
  - Recommended treatment for glenohumeral instability is capsulolabral repair, ensuring that the capsule and labrum are both repaired after adequate glenoid bone preparation.
- Superior labrum anterior to posterior (SLAP) tears
  - The most common SLAP tears are type I (frayed bicipital anchor site) and type II (complete detachment).
  - Provocative physical examination tests are not entirely specific for SLAP tears.
  - Patient history and symptoms of deep glenohumeral pain with overhead activities coupled with provocative testing manoeuvres helps confirm the diagnosis.
  - SLAP tears may extend posterior and/or anteriorly.
  - Recommended treatment is an arthroscopic debridement of type I tears and labral repair of type II tears.
- Rotator cuff tears
  - A variety of tear patterns should be recognized; partial versus complete tears, as well as tear type: crescent, L-shaped, reverse L-shaped, massive and retracted.
  - Knowledge of the rotator cuff footprint is important.
  - The supraspinatus is approximately 14–16 mm medial to lateral and 25 mm anterior to posterior, and attaches medially at the glenoid articular margin. The infraspinatus is similar in size, but is not against the articular margin.
  - Arthroscopic repair techniques continue to evolve, including double row and transosseous equivalent methods.
  - Recommended treatment is an arthroscopic subacromial debridement and/or decompression with rotator cuff repair of any significant partial thickness (>50% medial to lateral width) or full thickness tears.
  - A variety of techniques including single row, double row and transosseous equivalent may be utilized. Familiarity with repair devices is essential.

REFERENCES

1. Saha A. Dynamic stability of the glenohumeral joint. *Acta Orthopaedica Scandinavica* 1971;**42**:491–505.
2. Speer K, Deng X, Torzilli P, et al. A biomechanical evaluation of the Bankart lesion. *Transactions of the Orthopaedic Research Society* 1993;**39**:315.
3. Levine WN, Flatow EL. The pathophysiology of shoulder instability. *American Journal of Sports Medicine* 2000;**28**:910–17.
4. Soslowsky L, Flatow E, Bigliani L. Articular geometry of the glenohumeral joint. *Clinical Orthopaedics and Related Research* 1992;**285**:181–90.
5. Warner JJ, Deng X-H, Warren RF, Torzilli PA. Static capsuloligamentous restraints to superior-inferior translation of the glenohumeral joint. *American Journal of Sports Medicine* 1992;**20**:675–85.
6. Cooper D, Arnoczky S, O'Brien S. Anatomy, histology, and vascularity of the glenoid labrum: an anatomical study. *Journal of Bone and Joint Surgery (American)* 1992;**74**:46–52.
7. Prodromos C, Ferry J, Schiller A. Histological studies of the glenoid labrum from fetal life to old age. *Journal of Bone and Joint Surgery (American)* 1990;**72**:1344–8.
8. Soslowsky LJ, Malicky DM, Blasier RB. Active and passive factors in inferior glenohumeral stabilization: a biomechanical model. *Journal of Shoulder and Elbow Surgery* 1997;**6**:371–9.
9. Itoi E, Hsu HS, An KN. Biomechanical investigation of the glenohumeral joint. *Journal of Shoulder and Elbow Surgery* 1996;**5**:407–24.
10. Lippitt S, Matsen F. Mechanisms of glenohumeral joint stability. *Clinical Orthopaedics and Related Research* 1993;**291**:20.
11. Bowen M, Deng X, Warner J, et al. The effect of joint compression on stability of the glenohumeral joint. *Transactions of the Orthopaedic Research Society* 1992;**38**:289.
12. Matsen 3rd FA. The biomechanics of glenohumeral stability. *Journal of Bone and Joint Surgery (American)* 2002;**84A**:495–6.
13. Bankart A. The pathology and treatment of recurrent dislocation of the shoulder joint. *British Journal of Surgery* 1938;**26**:23–9.

14. Rowe C, Patel D, Southmayd W. The Bankart procedure: a long-term end-result study. *Journal of Bone and Joint Surgery (American)* 1978;**60**:1–16.
15. Speer KP, Deng X, Borrero S, et al. Biomechanical evaluation of a simulated Bankart lesion. *Journal of Bone and Joint Surgery (American)* 1994;**76**:1819–26.
16. Bach BR, Warren RF, Fronek J. Disruption of the lateral capsule of the shoulder. *Journal of Bone and Joint Surgery (British)* 1988;**70**:274–6.
17. Nicola T. Anterior dislocation of the shoulder. The role of the articular capsule. *Journal of Bone and Joint Surgery (American)* 1942;**24**:614–16.
18. Taylor DC, Arciero RA. Pathologic changes associated with shoulder dislocations. Arthroscopic and physical examination findings in first-time, traumatic anterior dislocations. *American Journal of Sports Medicine* 1997;**25**:306–11.
19. Basmajian JV, Bazant FJ. Factors preventing downward dislocation of the adducted shoulder joint. *Journal of Bone and Joint Surgery (American)* 1959;**41A**:1182–6.
20. Ovesen J, Nielsen S. Stability of the shoulder joint. Cadaver study of stabilizing structures. *Acta Orthopaedica Scandinavica* 1985;**56**:149–51.
21. Turkel SJ, Panio MW, Marshall JL, Girgis FG. Stabilizing mechanisms preventing anterior dislocation of the glenohumeral joint. *Journal of Bone and Joint Surgery (American)* 1981;**63**:1208–17.
22. Warner J, Micheli L, Arslanian L, et al. Scapulothoracic motion in normal shoulders and shoulders with glenohumeral instability and impingement syndrome: a study using Moire topographic analysis. *Clinical Orthopaedics and Related Research* 1992;**285**:191–9.
23. Helmig P, Sojbjerg JO, Sneppen O, et al. Glenohumeral movement patterns after puncture of the joint capsule: an experimental study. *Journal of Shoulder and Elbow Surgery* 1993;**2**:209–15.
24. Warner J, Deng X, Warren R. Superior-inferior translations in the intact and vented glenohumeral joint. *Journal of Shoulder and Elbow Surgery* 1993;**2**:99–125.
25. Harryman 2nd DT, Sidles JA, Harris SL, Matsen 3rd FA. Laxity of the normal glenohumeral joint: a quantitative in vivo assessment. *Journal of Shoulder and Elbow Surgery* 1992;**1**:66–7.
26. Harryman 2nd DT, Sidles JA, Harris SL, Matsen 3rd FA. The role of the rotator interval capsule in passive motion and stability of the shoulder. *Journal of Bone and Joint Surgery (American)*. 1992;**74**:53–66.
27. Browne A, Hoffmeyer P, An KN. The influence of atmospheric pressure on shoulder stability. *Orthopaedic Transactions* 1990;**14**:259.
28. Kumar V, Balasubramaniam P. The role of atmospheric pressure in stabilizing the shoulder. An experimental study. *Journal of Bone and Joint Surgery (British)* 1985;**67**:719–21.
29. Wuelker N, Brewe F, Sperveslage C. Passive glenohumeral joint stabilization: a biomechanical study. *Journal of Shoulder and Elbow Surgery* 1994;**3**:129–34.
30. Cole BJ, Rodeo SA, O'Brien SJ, et al. The anatomy and histology of the rotator interval capsule of the shoulder. *Clinical Orthopaedics and Related Research* 2001;**390**:129–37.
31. Glousman R, Jobe F, Tibone J, et al. Dynamic electromyographic analysis of the throwing shoulder with glenohumeral instability. *Journal of Bone and Joint Surgery (American)* 1988;**70**:220–6.
32. Itoi E, Kuechle D, Newman S, et al. Stabilizing function of the biceps in stable and unstable shoulders. *Journal of Bone and Joint Surgery (British)* 1993;**75**:834–6.
33. Itoi E, Motzkin NE, Morrey BF, An KN. Stabilizing function of the long head of the biceps in the hanging arm position. *Journal of Shoulder and Elbow Surgery* 1994;**3**:135–42.
34. Clark J, Sidles J, Matsen F. The relationship of glenohumeral joint capsule to the rotator cuff. *Clinical Orthopaedics and Related Research* 1990;**254**:29–34.
35. Ferrari D. Capsular ligaments of the shoulder: anatomical and functional study of the anterior-superior capsule. *American Journal of Sports Medicine* 1990;**18**:20–4.
36. McMahon P, Debski R, Thompson W, et al. Shoulder muscle forces and tendon excursions during glenohumeral abduction in the scapular plane. *Journal of Shoulder and Elbow Surgery* 1995;**4**:199–208.
37. McMahon PJ, Jobe FW, Pink MM, et al. Comparative electromyographic analysis of shoulder muscles during planar motions: anterior glenohumeral instability versus normal. *Journal of Shoulder and Elbow Surgery* 1996;**5**:118–23.
38. Ovesen J, Nielsen S. Experimental distal subluxation in the glenohumeral joint. *Archives of Orthopaedic and Trauma Surgery* 1985;**104**:78–81.
39. Blasier R, Soslowsky L, Malicky D, Palmer M. Posterior glenohumeral subluxation: active and passive stabilization in a biomechanical model. *Journal of Bone and Joint Surgery (American)* 1997;**79A**:433–40.
40. Burkhead W, Rockwood C. Treatment of instability of the shoulder with an exercise program. *Journal of Bone and Joint Surgery (American)* 1992;**74**:890–6.
41. Jerosch J, Clahsen H, Grosse-Hackmann A. Effects of proprioceptive fibers in the capsule tissue in stabilizing the glenohumeral joint. *Orthopaedic Transactions* 1992;**16**:773.
42. Vangsness CT, Ennis M, Taylor JG, Atkinson R. Neural anatomy of the glenohumeral ligaments, labrum, and subacromial bursa. *Arthroscopy* 1995;**11**:180–4.
43. Hawkins RJ, McCormack RG. Posterior shoulder instability. *Orthopedics* 1988;**11**:101–7.
44. Gerber C, Ganz R. Clinical assessment of instability of the shoulder. With special reference to anterior and posterior drawer tests. *Journal of Bone and Joint Surgery (British)* 1984;**66**:551–6.
45. Arciero RA, Wheeler JH, Ryan JB, McBride JT. Arthroscopic Bankart repair versus nonoperative treatment for acute, initial anterior shoulder dislocations. *American Journal of Sports Medicine* 1994;**22**:589–94.
46. Henry JH, Genung JA. Natural history of glenohumeral dislocation: revisited. *American Journal of Sports Medicine* 1982;**10**:135–7.

47. Wheeler JH, Ryan JB, Arciero RA, Molinari RN. Arthroscopic versus nonoperative treatment of acute shoulder dislocations in young athletes. *Arthroscopy* 1989;**5**:213–17.
48. Neviaser RJ, Neviaser TJ, Neviaser JS. Anterior dislocation of the shoulder and rotator cuff rupture. *Clinical Orthopaedics and Related Research* 1993;**291**:103–6.
49. Rowe CR, Zarins B. Recurrent transient subluxation of the shoulder. *Journal of Bone and Joint Surgery (American)* 1981;**63**:863–72.
50. Lo IKY, Nonweiler B, Woolfrey M, et al. An evaluation of the apprehension, relocation, and surprise tests for anterior shoulder instability. *American Journal of Sports Medicine* 2004;**32**:301–7.
51. Silliman J, Hawkins R. Classification and physical diagnosis of instability of the shoulder. *Clinical Orthopaedics and Related Research* 1993;**291**:7–19.
52. Altcheck DW. T-Plasty modification of the Bankart procedure for multidirectional instability of the anterior and inferior types. *Journal of Bone and Joint Surgery (American)* 1991;**73**:105–12.
53. Neer C, Foster C. Inferior capsular shift for involuntary inferior and multidirectional instability of the shoulder. *Journal of Bone and Joint Surgery (American)* 1980;**62**:897–908.
54. Garth WP, Slappey CE, Ochs CW. Roentgenographic demonstration of instability of the shoulder: the apical oblique projection. *Journal of Bone and Joint Surgery (American)* 1984;**66**:1450–3.
55. Roukos JR, Feagin JA. Modified axillary roentgenogram: a useful adjunct in the diagnosis of recurrent instability of the shoulder. *Clinical Orthopaedics and Related Research* 1972;**82**:84–6.
56. Bottoni CR, Smith EL, Berkowitz MJ, et al. Arthroscopic versus open shoulder stabilization for recurrent anterior instability: a prospective randomized clinical trial. *American Journal of Sports Medicine* 2006;**34**:1730–7.
57. Kirkley A, Werstine R, Ratjek A, Griffin S. Prospective randomized clinical trial comparing the effectiveness of immediate arthroscopic stabilization versus immobilization and rehabilitation in first traumatic anterior dislocations of the shoulder: long-term evaluation. *Arthroscopy* 2005;**21**:55–63.
58. Sachs RA, Williams B, Stone ML, et al. Open Bankart repair: correlation of results with postoperative subscapularis function. *American Journal of Sports Medicine* 2005;**33**:1458–62.
59. Scheibel M, Tsynman A, Magosch P, et al. Postoperative subscapularis muscle insufficiency after primary and revision open shoulder stabilization. *American Journal of Sports Medicine* 2006;**34**:1586–93.
60. Armstrong A, Boyer D, Ditsios K, Yamaguchi K. Arthroscopic versus open treatment of anterior shoulder instability. *Instructional Course Lectures* 2004;**53**:559–63.
61. Burkhart SS, De Beer JF. Traumatic glenohumeral bone defects and their relationship to failure of arthroscopic Bankart repairs: significance of the inverted-pear glenoid and the humeral engaging Hill-Sachs lesion. *Arthroscopy* 2000;**16**:677–94.
62. Mologne TS, Provencher MT, Menzel KA, et al. Arthroscopic stabilization in patients with an inverted pear glenoid: results in patients with bone loss of the anterior glenoid. *American Journal of Sports Medicine* 2007;**35**:1276–83.
63. Sugaya H, Moriishi J, Kanisawa I, Tsuchiya A. Arthroscopic osseous Bankart repair for chronic recurrent traumatic anterior glenohumeral instability. *Journal of Bone and Joint Surgery (American)* 2005;**87**:1752–60.
64. Stein DA, Jazrawi L, Bartolozzi AR. Arthroscopic stabilization of anterior instability: a review of the literature. *Arthroscopy* 2002;**18**:912–24.
65. Sugaya H, Kon Y, Tsuchiya A. Arthroscopic repair of glenoid fractures using suture anchors. *Arthroscopy* 2005;**21**:635.
66. Difelice GS, Williams 3rd RJ, Cohen MS, Warren RF. The accessory posterior portal for shoulder arthroscopy: description of technique and cadaveric study. *Arthroscopy* 2001;**17**:888–91.
67. Goubier JN, Iserin A, Duranthon LD, et al. A 4-portal arthroscopic stabilization in posterior shoulder instability. *Journal of Shoulder and Elbow Surgery* 2003;**12**:337–41.
68. Gerber C, Werner C, Macy J, et al. Effect of selective capsulorrhaphy on the passive range of motion of the glenohumeral joint. *Journal of Bone and Joint Surgery (American)* 2003;**85A**:48–55.
69. Inui H, Sugamoto K, Miyamoto T, et al. Glenoid shape in atraumatic posterior instability of the shoulder. *Clinical Orthopaedics and Related Research* 2002;**403**:87–92.
70. Metcalf MH, Duckworth DG, Lee SB, et al. Posteroinferior glenoplasty can change glenoid shape and increase the mechanical stability of the shoulder. *Journal of Shoulder and Elbow Surgery* 1999;**8**:205–13.
71. Weishaupt D, Zanetti M, Nyffeler RW, et al. Posterior glenoid rim deficiency in recurrent (atraumatic) posterior shoulder instability. *Skeletal Radiology* 2000;**29**:204–10.
72. Kim SH, Ha KI, Yoo JC, Noh KC. Kim's lesion: an incomplete and concealed avulsion of the posteroinferior labrum in posterior or multidirectional posteroinferior instability of the shoulder. *Arthroscopy* 2004;**20**:712–20.
73. Kim SH, Noh KC, Park JS, et al. Loss of chondrolabral containment of the glenohumeral joint in atraumatic posteroinferior multidirectional instability. *Journal of Bone and Joint Surgery (American)* 2005;**87**:92–8.
74. Bey MJ, Hunter SA, Kilambi N, et al. Structural and mechan-ical properties of the glenohumeral joint posterior capsule. *Journal of Shoulder and Elbow Surgery* 2005;**14**:201–6.
75. Hawkins R, Koppert G, Johnston G. Recurrent posterior instability (subluxation) of the shoulder. *Journal of Bone and Joint Surgery (American)* 1984;**66A**:169–74.
76. Hawkins R, McCormack R. Posterior shoulder instability. *Orthopedics* 1988;**11**:101–7.
77. Kim SH, Kim HK, Sun JI, et al. Arthroscopic capsulolabroplasty for posteroinferior multidirectional instability of the shoulder. *American Journal of Sports Medicine* 2004;**32**:594–607.
78. Petersen SA. Posterior shoulder instability. *Orthopedic Clinics of North America* 2000;**31**:263–74.

79. Warner JJ, Micheli LJ, Arslanian LE, et al. Patterns of flexibility, laxity, and strength in normal shoulders and shoulders with instability and impingement. *American Journal of Sports Medicine* 1990;**18**:366-75.
80. Bigliani L, Pollock R, McIlveen S, et al. Shift of the posteroinferior aspect of the capsule for recurrent posterior glenohumeral instability. *Journal of Bone and Joint Surgery (American)* 1995;**77**:1011-120.
81. Pollock RG, Bigliani LU. Recurrent posterior shoulder instability. Diagnosis and treatment. *Clinical Orthopaedics and Related Research* 1993;**291**:85-96.
82. Kim S, Park J, Jeong W, Shin S. The Kim test: a novel test for posteroinferior labral lesion of the shoulder – a comparison to the jerk test. *American Journal of Sports Medicine* 2005;**33**:1188-92.
83. Wirth MA, Groh GI, Rockwood Jr CA. Capsulorrhaphy through an anterior approach for the treatment of atraumatic posterior glenohumeral instability with multidirectional laxity of the shoulder. *Journal of Bone and Joint Surgery (American)* 1998;**80**:1570-8.
84. Fronek J, Warren RF, Bowen M. Posterior subluxation of the glenohumeral joint. *Journal of Bone and Joint Surgery (American)* 1989;**71A**:205-16.
85. Kiss J, Damrel D, Mackie A, et al. Non-operative treatment of multidirectional shoulder instability. *International Orthopaedics* 2001;**24**:354-7.
86. Hawkins RH. Glenoid osteotomy for recurrent posterior subluxation of the shoulder: assessment by computed axial tomography. *Journal of Shoulder and Elbow Surgery* 1996;**5**:393-400.
87. Hawkins RJ, Janda DH. Posterior instability of the glenohumeral joint. A technique of repair. *American Journal of Sports Medicine* 1996;**24**:275-8.
88. Tibone JE, Bradley JP. The treatment of posterior subluxation in athletes. *Clinical Orthopaedics and Related Research* 1993;**291**:124-37.
89. Provencher MT, Romeo AA, Solomon DJ, et al. Arthroscopic preparation of the posterior and posteroinferior glenoid labrum. *Orthopedics* 2007;**30**:904-5.
90. Plausinis D, Bravman JT, Heywood C, et al. Arthroscopic rotator interval closure: effect of sutures on glenohumeral motion and anterior-posterior translation. *American Journal of Sports Medicine* 2006;**34**:1656-61.
91. Provencher MT, Mologne TS, Hongo M, et al. Arthroscopic versus open rotator interval closure: biomechanical eval-uation of stability and motion. *Arthroscopy* 2007;**23**:583-92.
92. Yamamoto N, Itoi E, Tuoheti Y, et al. Effect of rotator interval closure on glenohumeral stability and motion: a cadaveric study. *Journal of Shoulder and Elbow Surgery* 2006;**15**:750-8.
93. Cole BJ, Mazzocca AD, Meneghini RM. Indirect arthroscopic rotator interval repair. *Arthroscopy* 2003;**19**:E28-31.
94. Taverna E, Sansone V, Battistella F. Arthroscopic rotator interval repair: the three-step all-inside technique. *Arthroscopy* 2004;**20**:105-9.
95. Neer 2nd CS. Involuntary inferior and multidirectional instability of the shoulder: etiology, recognition, and treatment. *Instructional Course Lectures* 1985;**34**:232-8.
96. Warren RF, Kornblatt IB, Marchand R. Static factors affecting posterior shoulder stability. *Orthopaedic Transactions* 1984;**8**:89.
97. Weber SC, Caspari RB. A biomechanical evaluation of the restraints to posterior shoulder dislocation. *Arthroscopy* 1989;**5**:115-21.
98. Dewing CB, McCormick F, Bell SJ, et al. An analysis of capsular area in anterior, posterior, and multidirectional instability. *American Journal of Sports Medicine* 2008;**36**:515-22.
99. Wolf EM, Eakin CL. Arthroscopic capsular plication for posterior shoulder instability. *Arthroscopy* 1998;**14**:153-63.
100. Lo IK, Burkhart SS. Triple labral lesions: pathology and surgical repair technique: report of seven cases. *Arthroscopy* 2005;**21**:186-93.
101. Provencher MT, Verma N, Obopilwe E, et al. A biomechanical analysis of capsular plication versus anchor repair of the shoulder: can the labrum be used as a suture anchor? *Arthroscopy* 2007;**24**:210-16.
102. Eakin CL, Dvirnak P, Miller CM, Hawkins RJ. The relationship of the axillary nerve to arthroscopically placed capsulolabral sutures. An anatomic study. *American Journal of Sports Medicine* 1998;**26**:505-9.
103. Price MR, Tillett ED, Acland RD, Nettleton GS. Determining the relationship of the axillary nerve to the shoulder joint capsule from an arthroscopic perspective. *Journal of Bone and Joint Surgery (American)* 2004;**86A**:2135-42.
104. Uno A, Bain GI, Mehta JA. Arthroscopic relationship of the axillary nerve to the shoulder joint capsule: an anatomic study. *Journal of Shoulder and Elbow Surgery* 1999;**8**:226-30.
105. Vangsness Jr CT, Jorgenson SS, Watson T, Johnson DL. The origin of the long head of the biceps from the scapula and glenoid labrum. An anatomical study of 100 shoulders. *Journal of Bone and Joint Surgery (British)* 1994;**76**:951-4.
106. Mileski RA, Snyder SJ. Superior labral lesions in the shoulder: pathoanatomy and surgical management. *Journal of the American Academy of Orthopaedic Surgeons* 1998;**6**:121-31.
107. Nam EK, Snyder SJ. The diagnosis and treatment of superior labrum, anterior and posterior (SLAP) lesions. *American Journal of Sports Medicine* 2003;**31**:798-810.
108. Jones GL, Galluch DB. Clinical assessment of superior glenoid labral lesions: a systematic review. *Clinical Orthopaedics and Related Research* 2007;**455**:45-51.
109. Kim SH, Ha KI, Han KY. Biceps load test: a clinical test for superior labrum anterior and posterior lesions in shoulders with recurrent anterior dislocations. *American Journal of Sports Medicine* 1999;**27**:300-3.
110. Bencardino JT, Beltran J, Rosenberg ZS, et al. Superior labrum anterior-posterior lesions: diagnosis with MR arthrography of the shoulder. *Radiology* 2000;**214**:267-71.

111. Daluga DJ, Daluga AT. Single-portal SLAP lesion repair. *Arthroscopy* 2007;**23**:321.
112. O'Brien SJ, Allen AA, Coleman SH, Drakos MC. The trans-rotator cuff approach to SLAP lesions: technical aspects for repair and a clinical follow-up of 31 patients at a minimum of 2 years. *Arthroscopy* 2002;**18**:372–7.
113. Domb BG, Ehteshami JR, Shindle MK, et al. Biomechanical comparison of 3 suture anchor configurations for repair of type II SLAP lesions. *Arthroscopy* 2007;**23**:135–40.
114. Cordasco FA, Steinmann S, Flatow EL, Bigliani LU. Arthroscopic treatment of glenoid labral tears. *American Journal of Sports Medicine* 1993;**21**:425–30.
115. Coleman SH, Cohen DB, Drakos MC, et al. Arthroscopic repair of type II superior labral anterior posterior lesions with and without acromioplasty: a clinical analysis of 50 patients. *American Journal of Sports Medicine* 2007;**35**:749–53.
116. Funk L, Snow M. SLAP tears of the glenoid labrum in contact athletes. *Clinical Journal of Sport Medicine* 2007;**17**:1–4.
117. Paxinos A, Walton J, Rutten S, et al. Arthroscopic stabilization of superior labral (SLAP) tears with biodegradable tack: outcomes to 2 years. *Arthroscopy* 2006;**22**:627–34.
118. Enad JG, Kurtz CA. Isolated and combined type II SLAP repairs in a military population. *Knee Surgery, Sports Traumatology, Arthroscopy* 2007;**15**:1382–9.
119. Park HB, Yokota A, Gill HS, et al. Diagnostic accuracy of clinical tests for the different degrees of subacromial impingement syndrome. *Journal of Bone and Joint Surgery (American)* 2005;**87**:1446–55.
120. Cole BJ, ElAttrache NS, Anbari A. Arthroscopic rotator cuff repairs: an anatomic and biomechanical rationale for different suture-anchor repair configurations. *Arthroscopy* 2007;**23**:662–9.
121. Glenn Jr RE, McCarty LP, Cole BJ. The accessory posteromedial portal revisited: utility for arthroscopic rotator cuff repair. *Arthroscopy* 2006;**22**:1133.
122. Lo IK, Burkhart SS. Arthroscopic repair of massive, contracted, immobile rotator cuff tears using single and double interval slides: technique and preliminary results. *Arthroscopy* 2004;**20**:22–33.
123. Yanke A, Provencher MT, Cole BJ. Arthroscopic double-row and 'transosseous-equivalent' rotator cuff repair. *American Journal of Orthopedics* 2007;**36**:294–7.
124. Park MC, Elattrache NS, Ahmad CS, Tibone JE. 'Transosseous-equivalent' rotator cuff repair technique. *Arthroscopy* 2006;**22**:1361–5.
125. Curtis AS, Burbank KM, Tierney JJ, et al. The insertional footprint of the rotator cuff: an anatomic study. *Arthroscopy* 2006;**22**:609.
126. Ruotolo C, Fow JE, Nottage WM. The supraspinatus footprint: an anatomic study of the supraspinatus insertion. *Arthroscopy* 2004;**20**:246–9.
127. Ahmad CS, Stewart AM, Izquierdo R, Bigliani LU. Tendon-bone interface motion in transosseous suture and suture anchor rotator cuff repair techniques. *American Journal of Sports Medicine* 2005;**33**:1667–71.
128. Ma CB, Comerford L, Wilson J, Puttlitz CM. Biomechanical evaluation of arthroscopic rotator cuff repairs: double-row compared with single-row fixation. *Journal of Bone and Joint Surgery (American)* 2006;**88**:403–10.
129. Mazzocca AD, Millett PJ, Guanche CA, et al. Arthroscopic single-row versus double-row suture anchor rotator cuff repair. *American Journal of Sports Medicine* 2005;**33**:1861–8.
130. Smith CD, Alexander S, Hill AM, et al. A biomechanical comparison of single and double-row fixation in arthroscopic rotator cuff repair. *Journal of Bone and Joint Surgery (American)* 2006;**88**:2425–31.
131. Tuoheti Y, Itoi E, Yamamoto N, et al. Contact area, contact pressure, and pressure patterns of the tendon-bone interface after rotator cuff repair. *American Journal of Sports Medicine* 2005;**33**:1869–74.
132. Burkhart SS. The deadman theory of suture anchors: observations along a south Texas fence line. *Arthroscopy* 1995;**11**:119–23.
133. Sugaya H, Maeda K, Matsuki K, Moriishi J. Functional and structural outcomes after arthroscopic full-thickness rotator cuff repair: single-row versus dual-row fixation. *Arthroscopy* 2005;**21**:1307–16.
134. Lafosse L, Brozska R, Toussaint B, Gobezie R. The outcome and structural integrity of arthroscopic rotator cuff repair with use of the double-row suture anchor technique. *Journal of Bone and Joint Surgery (American)* 2007;**89**:1533–41.
135. Severud EL, Ruotolo C, Abbott DD, Nottage WM. All-arthroscopic versus mini-open rotator cuff repair: a long-term retrospective outcome comparison. *Arthroscopy* 2003;**19**:234–8.
136. Cummins C, Murrell G. Mode of failure for rotator cuff repair with suture anchors identified at revision surgery. *Journal of Shoulder and Elbow Surgery* 2003;**12**:128–33.

74

Athletic injuries of the elbow, wrist and hand

A BOBBY CHHABRA, JESSE SEAMON

| Elbow injuries | 750 | Hand injuries | 762 |
| Wrist injuries | 755 | References | 768 |

NATIONAL BOARD STANDARDS

- Ability to utilize clinical history, physical exam and diagnostic studies to appropriately evaluate and identify injuries to the elbow, wrist and hand
- Understand the treatment options for common injuries of the elbow, wrist and hand in athletes
- Become skillful at performing the physical exam manoeuvre necessary to diagnose dynamic instability of the elbow and wrist
- Understand the rationale and evidence for both surgical and non-surgical treatment of injuries to the elbow, wrist and hand in athletes

ELBOW INJURIES

Lateral epicondylitis

Lateral epicondylitis, also called 'tennis elbow', is one of the most common causes of elbow pain in the general population and the athlete.[1] The incidence of lateral epicondylitis has been reported to be four to seven times greater than medial epicondylitis.[2] Many theories have been proposed as to the aetiology of lateral epicondylitis. These include inflammatory processes involving the radiohumeral bursa, annular ligament and periosteum.[3] Other proposed theories have included decreased vascularity of the lateral epicondylar region and fluoroquinolone antibiotics.[2] The most accepted theory focuses on the idea that repetitive wrist extension leads to cumulative microtears in the tendinous origin of the ECRB with the proliferation of fibrotic hypervascular healing (angiofibroblastic hyperplasia).[3,4]

Patients present with a complaint of pain in the lateral elbow that radiates down the forearm. In many cases that pain has a gradual and insidious onset, and may be associated with decreased grip strength.[2] On examination, patients have point tenderness 1–2 cm distal to the lateral epicondyle. Pain is made worse with passive wrist flexion and active wrist extension.[1] Additional provocative manoeuvres include resisted long finger extension and resisted forearm supination. The 'chair test' is performed by asking the patient to lift a chair with the shoulder adducted, the wrist pronated and the elbow extended. The reproduction of symptoms in considered a positive test. Grip strength can be assessed with a dynamometer, and is often weaker on the affected side.[4] Plain films are usually negative, although in some cases calcifications may be present at the lateral epicondyle.[1] CT may be useful for better delineating the presence of calcifications or lateral epicondylar spurs, and MRI has limited indications for lateral epicondylitis.[2]

The initial treatment of lateral epicondylitis is conservative, and this can be effective up to 90% of the time.[2] Conservative measures consist of modification of activities, non-steroidal anti-inflammatory drugs (NSAIDs), ice and local steroid injections.[1–3] The use of counterforce bracing, which limits contractile expansion of the extensor mass, can help relieve symptoms associated with activities of daily life.[2,3] Rehabilitation of the extensor muscle mass and technique modification are critical to preventing recurrent injury.[3]

Surgical intervention is indicated if aggressive conservative treatment fails to relieve symptoms of lateral epicondylitis.[1,2,4] Current surgical treatment of lateral epicondylitis includes excision of degenerative tissue with anatomical repair, tendon lengthening, drilling of the lateral epicondyle and arthroscopic ECRB release.[2,4] Excellent results have been obtained with both tendon lengthening and excision of diseased tissue with anatomical repair, in regard to symptomatic relief.[2,5,6] In patient groups studied by Goldberg et al.[6] and Rosenberg et al.[5] good to excellent results were obtained approximately 90% of the time. Cortical drilling of the lateral epicondyle with the goal of increasing vascularity to the region does not appear to increase the effectiveness of surgery, and may be associated with increased pain, stiffness and wound complications.[7] The lateral collateral ligament should be protected during the procedure to prevent iatrogenic injury. Arthroscopy may offer advantages over open techniques because it allows for examination of intra-articular structures, preservation of the common extensor origin and shorter rehabilitation times.[4]

Medial epicondylitis

Medial epicondylitis of the elbow accounts for 10–20% of all epicondylitis diagnoses.[1] Baseball pitchers are most susceptible to medial epicondylitis, although it may be seen in athletes participating in golf, tennis, bowling, racquetball, American football, javelin, archery and weight lifting.[8,9]

The mechanism of injury is repetitive stress and overuse of the flexor–pronator muscle group, resulting in chronic microtears at the musculotendinous junction of the pronator teres, flexor carpi radialis and, less commonly, flexor carpi ulnaris, palmaris longus and flexor digitorum superficialis muscles.[8] Over time, the microtears fail to heal normally, resulting in the loss of the parallel orientation of collagen fibres and fibroblast invasion with the formation of granulation tissue.[10]

These athletes present with complaints of pain and swelling of the medial elbow made worse with exacerbating activities such as throwing, overhead serving and the golf swing.[1] On examination there is often pain with palpation of the medial epicondyle in the region of the flexor–pronator muscle group tendinous origin.[9] This pain may radiate approximately 1 cm distally into the forearm, and decreased range of motion may be present if flexion contracture has occurred.[10] Pain is often made worse with resisted wrist flexion and forearm pronation. A Tinel's sign may be elicited at the cubital tunnel if associated ulnar neuropathy is present. The integrity of the ulnar collateral ligament (UCL) should be assessed by performing a valgus stress test, and a milking test (see section on Ulnar collateral ligament disruption for more information).[3] Plain films may reveal the presence of calcifications approximately 25% of the time.[10] MRI and ultrasound can be effective in ruling out damage to the underlying UCL and in assessing for gross tears of the flexor–pronator muscle group.[8]

The initial treatment for medial epicondylitis is conservative, with the aim of relieving pain and inflammation with gradual rehabilitation of the flexor–pronator muscle group.[1,3,8,9] These measures include rest, NSAIDs, ice, local steroid injections and counterforce bracing.[3,8] Rehabilitation of the flexor–pronator mass and technique modification are important to prevent reinjury.[3] Failure of conservative treatment is an indication for surgical intervention.[8] Current surgical treatment recommendations are excision of the pathological portion of tendon, enhancement of local vascularity to promote healing by placing drill holes in the medial epicondyle, reattachment of elevated tendon back to the epicondyle and repair of any resultant defect.[8,10] During surgery, any ulnar nerve or UCL pathology should be identified and treated if present.[3,8,9] Reports in the literature indicate that good to excellent results are obtained with surgical intervention approximately 85% of the time.[8,10–13]

Ulnar collateral ligament disruption

Rupture of the UCL can be both an acute and a chronic process, and is seen most commonly in athletes who participate in sports requiring overhead throwing, especially baseball pitchers.[14] Injury to the UCL has been reported in other athletes as well, including javelin throwers, water polo players, hockey players, tennis players, arm wrestlers, weight lifters and gymnasts.[15]

The throwing athlete is exposed to extreme and repetitive valgus stresses across the elbow joint. The load across the medial elbow joint of an elite baseball pitcher when throwing has been estimated to equal the tensile force of the UCL.[16]

Attenuation and rupture of the UCL leads to a number of associated problems with the elbow, which include valgus extension overload syndrome, ulnar neuritis, medial epicondylitis and radiocapitellar overload syndrome.[15] Sports requiring rapid extension of the elbow with pronation and valgus stress leave the athlete most susceptible to injury from these chronic forces. Injury occurs from three mechanisms: (1) valgus stress along the medial elbow joint, (2) compression of the lateral side of the elbow and (3) medially directed sheer of the posterior elbow. Valgus stress applied to the elbow during the overhead throwing motion or overhead tennis serve exceed 60 N m, whereas the estimated ultimate tensile strength of the UCL is 33 N m based on cadaveric studies.[15] Approximately 120 N m of varus force must be developed within the arm to resist these forces from valgus stress.[16] Chronic tensile forces applied to the medial elbow are responsible for the development of medial epicondylitis as a result of repeated microtears of the flexor–pronator mass, as discussed above. Increased valgus stress also predisposes the ulnar nerve to traction, compression and friction injury, which leads to chronic irritation and swelling, often called ulnar neuritis. Valgus extension overload syndrome occurs from these valgus stresses as attenuation of the UCL allows for increased medial shearing and impingement of the olecranon in the posteromedial

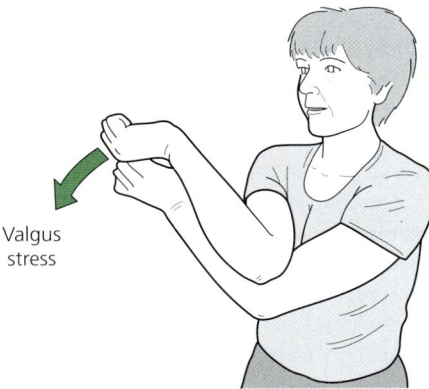

Figure 74.1　Milking manoeuvre.

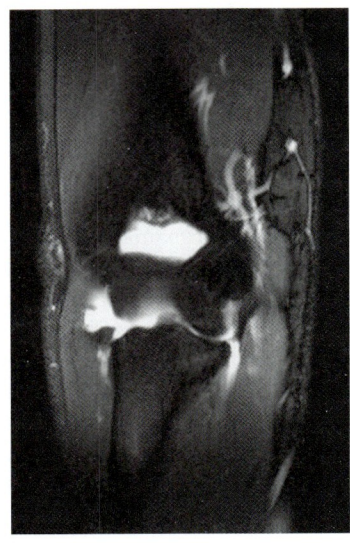

Figure 74.2　Ulnar collateral ligament tear on MRI.

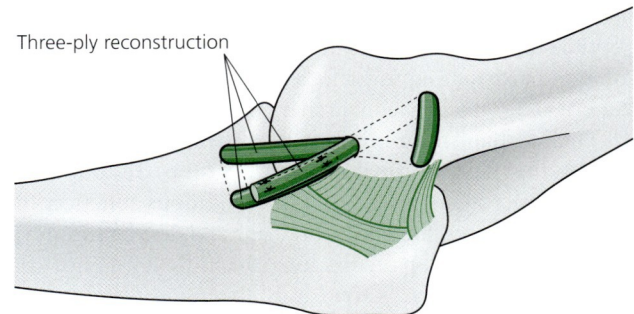

Figure 74.3　Ulnar collateral ligament reconstruction.

olecranon fossa (see Valgus extension overload syndrome).[15] Radiocapitellar overload syndrome occurs from compression of the joint because of inability to properly handle valgus stresses from an attenuated UCL. This results in compression of the radial head against the capitellum, which can result in chondromalacia and radiocapitellar joint degeneration. Subsequent osteophyte formation can lead to the presence of loose bodies within the joint.[1,15]

The key to diagnosis is examination of the UCL to determine functional integrity of the ligament.[15] One option is the valgus stress test, performed with the elbow in 30° and 70° of flexion with the forearm in neutral.[14] A positive test is indicated by increased joint opening or lack of rebound at the end of joint opening compared with the other extremity.[14] The milking manoeuvre can be performed by flexing the elbow past 90° with the forearm in supination and asking the patient to use the uninvolved arm to grasp the thumb, thus imparting a valgus stress (Fig. 74.1) The examiner can palpate for tenderness and joint space opening.[14,15] A moving valgus stress test can be performed by abducting and externally rotating the shoulder of the involved extremity while applying a valgus force through the elbow during the full range of flexion and extension. A painful arc should be reproduced at 80–120° if a UCL tear is present.[14,16] Both MRI and CT arthrograms are effective for diagnosing complete tears of the UCL with very high sensitivity (Fig. 74.2).[17] MRI offers the additional advantage of allowing for better analysis of the surrounding neuromuscular structures.[16] Partial tears are considerably more difficult to detect with MRI or CT arthrogram.[17]

Non-operative treatment of UCL injuries is indicated for non-throwing athletes and the general lower demand population as the intact flexor–pronator mass will provide for elbow stability.[18] At best, half of athletes can be expected to return to sport at the previous level of competition with non-operative treatment.[14,19,20] Partial UCL injuries should be treated initially with a period of 3 months of rest (no throwing), flexor–pronator strengthening, followed by a gradual progressive throwing programme.

Surgical treatment is indicated for overhead throwing athletes with complete rupture of the anterior bundle of the UCL or in athletes who have failed conservative measures and an adequate period of rest and rehabilitation.[18] Surgical options include primary repair of the UCL versus reconstruction of the UCL with a free tendon graft. The results of primary repair have not been as promising as those from UCL reconstruction, and the only indication for primary repair is complete ligament avulsion from the proximal attachment on the medial epicondyle (assuming the ligament is not calcified).[16]

The first UCL reconstruction was described by Jobe et al.[21] in 1986 and consisted of replacing the ruptured anterior bundle of the UCL with a free tendon graft passed in a figure-of-eight fashion through tunnels created in both the ulna and medial epicondyle, followed by suturing the graft to itself (Fig. 74.3). Many modifications have been made to this procedure, including the use of a muscle-splitting approach,[22] a muscle-splitting approach without ulnar nerve transposition[23] and a non-figure-of-eight method described by Altcheck and colleagues as the 'docking technique'.[16,24] Altcheck and colleagues[24] reported a 92% rate of return to the previous level of competition with the docking procedure in a series of 36 patients. The more conventional figure-of-eight method of reconstruction has been associated with a return to previous level of competition or higher in approximately 80% of a group of 67 patients in a study by Azar et al.,[25] and Thompson et al.[23] performed a similar procedure without transposition of the ulnar nerve and found that all 83 athletes were able to return to competitive play. Rehabilitation after surgery is prolonged, and unrestricted throwing is not allowed until approximately 1 year.

Valgus extension overload syndrome

Valgus extension overload syndrome is seen in athletes who participate in throwing and racquet sports and is the most common reason for surgery among baseball players.[14,18]

During the throwing motion, large tensile forces develop along the medial side of the elbow which are resisted by the UCL in concert with the olecranon fossa, flexor–pronator mass and radiocapitellar joint. As the arm decelerates at the end of the throwing motion, the elbow flexors are relied upon to provide eccentric contractions which control full extension at the elbow. When this fails, the olecranon is forcefully jammed into the olecranon fossa.[26] The combination of this powerful extension force with increased valgus forces transmitted to the olecranon and olecranon fossa from an attenuated UCL allows the posteromedial olecranon to undergo repetitive impingement and shearing within the medial olecranon fossa. This results in the development of chondromalacia, osteophyte formation and the presence of loose bodies.[1,14,15,18,26]

Initial treatment of valgus extension overload syndrome is conservative with rest, rehabilitation with strengthening of the flexor–pronator muscle groups, NSAIDs and ice.[1,14,18] For those who fail conservative treatment, surgical intervention is indicated with osteophyte excision and removal of loose bodies.[1,14,18,26] UCL reconstruction may be required as well during this procedure. Although this can be accomplished with arthrotomy, arthroscopy is less invasive and allows for complete diagnostic assessment of the elbow including the integrity of the UCL.[26] Elbow arthroscopy will allow for return to pre-operative function in approximately three-quarters of throwing athletes.[14,18,27,28]

Osteochondritis dissecans

Osteochondritis dissecans (OCD) of the humeral capitellum is a common cause of lateral elbow pain in children aged between 11 and 16 (Fig. 74.4a–c).[29]

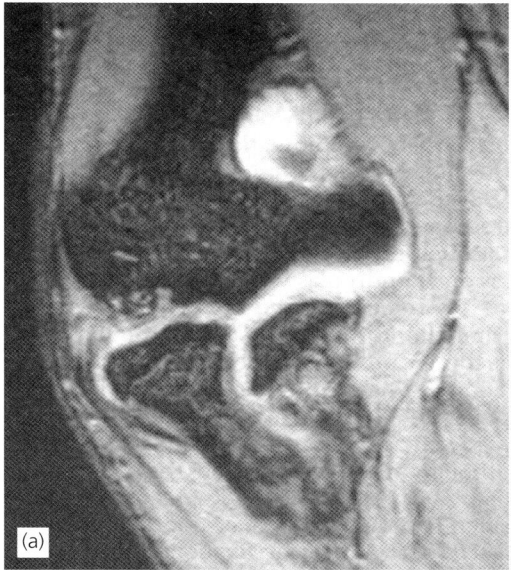
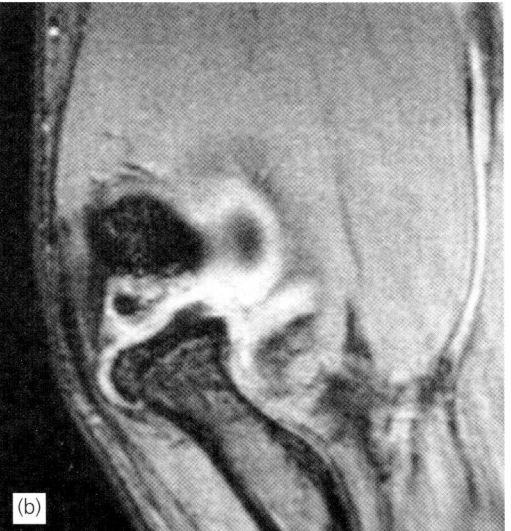
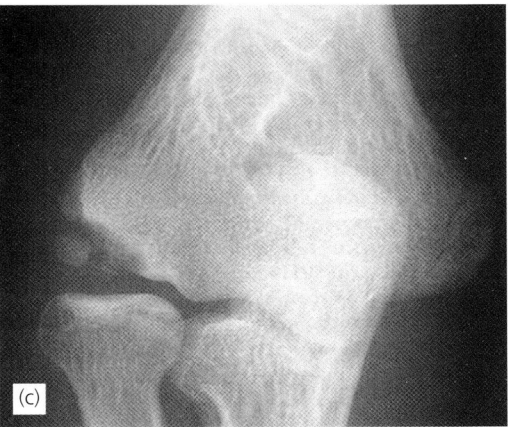

Figure 74.4 Osteochondritis dissecans. (a) Radiograph. (b) MRI. (c) Advanced OCD lesion of the numeral capitellum with articular surface collapse and loose body. Reproduced with permission from Miller MD, Cole BJ (eds). *Textbook of Arthroscopy*. Philadelphia, PA: Saunders, 2004:308–9.

Although OCD is seen in non-athletes, the incidence is highest in the dominant arms of throwers, and it can also be seen in young gymnasts as well.[1,29,30] Current theories on pathogenesis centre on the idea that compression forces of the radiocapitellar joint, from either valgus stress or direct compression, result in disruption of the already tenuous blood supply of the capitellar epiphysis, leading to osteonecrosis.[18] During the early phases of the disease the overlying articular cartilage is hyperaemic and oedematous. With time, the necrotic portion of injured bone at the articular cartilage interface undergoes resorption and is replaced by vascular granulation tissue. Once this occurs, one of two events can take place. Either the articular cartilage remains intact and the bony defect is eventually healed, or the necrotic segment detaches completely and forms a loose body within the joint.[31]

Early on in OCD the changes in the humeral capitellum may not be obvious on plain films.[1] However, as the OCD progresses, the plain films will often show flattening of the capitellar subchondral bone and islands of subchondral bone surrounded by a zone of rarefaction.[30] Advanced cases of OCD may have articular surface collapse, loose bodies, osteophytes, subchondral cysts and radial head enlargement on plain films.[29] Imaging with T_1-weighted MRI can be especially helpful in diagnosing OCD early in the process when plain films may be normal.[31] Ultrasound can be used to detect capitellar flattening in the early stages of OCD.[30]

There is no universally accepted guideline for the treatment of OCD, although four factors play a role in determining treatment. These include patient symptoms, radiographic appearance, articular cartilage status and whether or not the involved segment is detached. The detachment of the involved segment is most important for determining treatment plans.[31] If the articular cartilage remains intact overlying a completely attached capitellar lesion, non-operative treatment is recommended with a period of immobilization and refraining from athletics for an extended period of time (6 months or greater).[31] Surgery can be performed arthroscopically to evaluate the OCD lesion to confirm whether the articular cartilage is intact and to debride symptomatic synovitis. Surgery is indicated for those patients who fail non-operative treatment, those who have mechanical symptoms or those in whom loose bodies are present.[18] Additional indications may include evidence of fracture of the surface of the articular cartilage or displacement of the capitellar lesion.[31] Arthroscopic surgery with debridement, fragment excision, loose body excision (if present) and abrasion chondroplasty is recommended.[14] Fixation of unstable capitellar fragments has not been shown to offer any significant advantage over simple excision.[18,31] Outcomes of surgery are variable, and patients often have a loss of range of motion of the elbow and a predisposition to early arthritic changes.

Posterolateral rotatory instability of the elbow

Posterolateral rotatory instability (PLRI) of the elbow occurs as a result of damage to the lateral ligament complex of the elbow.[32] This damage usually occurs from three mechanisms: elbow dislocation, a varus elbow stress or iatrogenic causes.[33]

Elbow dislocation is the most common cause of PLRI of the elbow. The ligamentous damage during an elbow dislocation has been subdivided into three stages (Fig. 74.5). In stage I, the damage occurs only to the lateral ulnar collateral ligament (LUCL complex). In stage II, the damage extends to the posterior and anterior elbow capsule. In stage IIIa damage extends to the posterior bundle of the UCL, in stage IIIb the damage extends to the anterior bundle of the UCL and in stage IIIc all soft tissue has been stripped off the medial side of the distal humerus.[33] The most common mechanism of action for elbow dislocation in athletes is a fall on an outstretched hand.[1] Initial treatment of stable ligamentous elbow dislocations is urgent reduction and protected range of motion for the first 6 weeks. PLRI results after elbow dislocations when the LUCL complex fails to heal adequately.

Patients present with non-specific elbow complaints. They may complain of poorly defined pain with symptoms of snapping, locking or clunking of the elbow during motion.[1] There is usually a history of antecedent trauma to the elbow, especially in the under-20 population in which over 75% of these injuries are due to elbow dislocation.[32] A routine physical examination of these patients is often unremarkable.[1] However, it is important to test these patients for valgus instability with the forearm in both pronation and supination. Those who have valgus instability with the forearm supinated have PLRI of the elbow, whereas those who

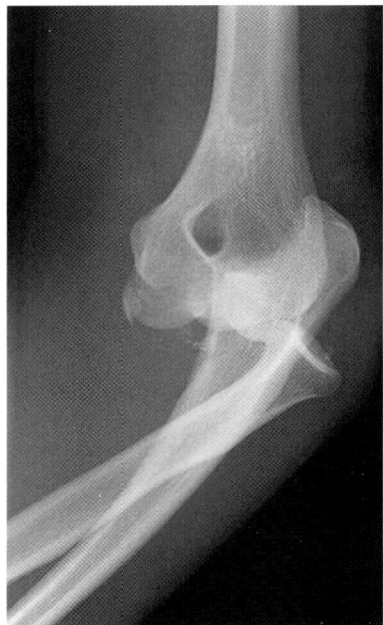

Figure 74.5 Elbow dislocation.

have valgus instability with the forearm pronated have UCL injuries.[32] Several tests have been described to evaluate for PLRI. The lateral pivot shift test is performed by placing the patient in a supine position with the shoulder joint flexed in such a way that their arm is over their head. The shoulder is then maximally externally rotated, the humerus is stabilized by the examiner and the elbow is placed in flexion. The forearm is supinated and a valgus force is applied along with a slight axial force to the elbow joint. As the elbow is extended with application of the valgus force a guarding response may be noted.[33] The posterior skin of the elbow may dimple as the radial head subluxes posteriorly. Once flexion exceeds 40° the radial head will reduce and an audible clunk may be heard[32] (Fig. 74.6). Unless the patient is anaesthetized, guarding and apprehension usually prevent any of the above signs from being obvious and thus constitute a positive test.[32,33] Plain films of the elbow are usually normal, unless the ligament damage is associated with an avulsion fracture.[32] MRI with contrast may be used as an adjuvant to diagnosis, but ultimately the diagnosis of PLRI is a clinical one.[33] Arthroscopy is reliable in diagnosing PLRI.

Treatment for patients with functional impairments from PLRI is with surgical intervention.[1,32,33] Surgery typically consists of reconstruction of the lateral ligament complex of the elbow with a free tendon graft or direct repair if the ligament is stretched or avulsed directly from the bone.[1,32] Good or excellent results have been obtained about 85% of the time using reconstructive techniques as described above.[32]

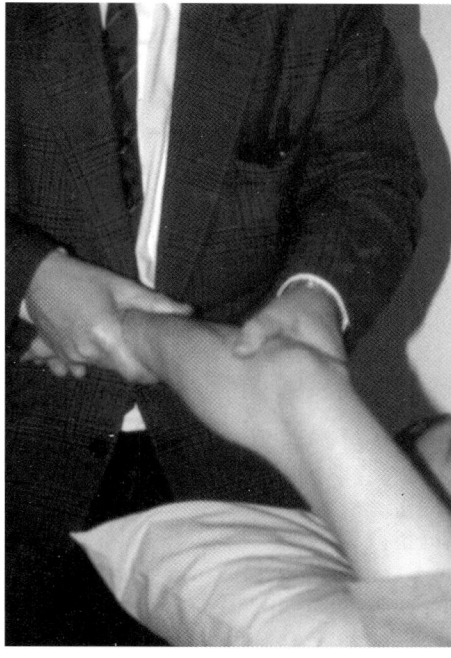

Figure 74.6 Posterolateral rotatory instability test. Reproduced with permission from Mehta JA, Bain GI. Posterolateral rotatory instability of the elbow. *Journal of the American Academy of Orthopaedic Surgeons* 2004;**12**:409.

WRIST INJURIES

Scaphoid fractures

The scaphoid is the most commonly injured carpal bone in athletes, accounting for up to 60–70% of carpal bone fractures.[34,35] Scaphoid fractures are susceptible to complications, including malunion, non-union and early-onset wrist arthritis. Accordingly, prompt diagnosis and appropriate treatment are essential to providing the athlete with a healthy and functional wrist.[36] The mechanism of injury for a scaphoid fracture is a fall on an outstretched hand with the wrist in radial deviation and extension.[34–37]

Patients present with a primary complaint of wrist pain and have tenderness and swelling in the anatomic snuff box.[35] Pain can be elicited by axial compression at the tip of the thumb, dorsiflexion of the wrist and forced ulnar deviation with the forearm pronated.[34,35] In patients presenting with a chronic or late scaphoid fracture, radial-sided wrist pain, decreased grip strength and inability to do push-ups are common findings.[36] Initial work-up consists of anteroposterior, lateral and scaphoid views of the wrist (30° of dorsiflexion and 20° of ulnar deviation). Frequently, the initial radiographs are negative, especially for non-displaced scaphoid fractures. Options at this point include further imaging with CT or MRI, a thumb spica for 2 weeks, followed by repeat radiographs, or a bone scan 3 days after injury.[34–37] In athletes with radial-sided wrist pain and clinical suspicion of scaphoid fracture with negative radiographs, further imaging is indicated at the time of presentation.[34] MRI is the most reliable study for diagnosing acute scaphoid fractures and is the preferred study for the professional or collegiate athlete if cost is not an issue (Fig. 74.7).[34,36,38]

The main treatment goal for scaphoid fractures is to obtain union of the fracture site.[34] The natural progression

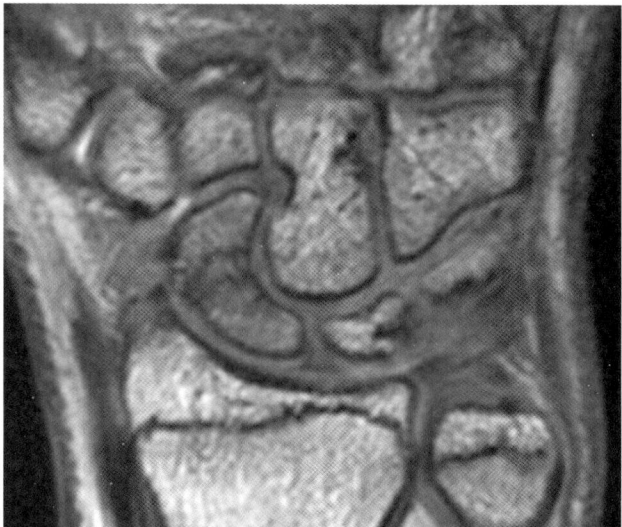

Figure 74.7 Scaphoid fracture on MRI.

of the untreated scaphoid fracture is non-union followed by progressive radiocarpal arthritis.[34,36] Risk factors for non-union include smoking, displacement greater than 1 mm, vertical oblique fractures, proximal pole fractures and osteonecrosis.[35]

The optimal treatment of scaphoid fractures depends on the location of the fracture, the stability of the fracture, the sport and the desire of the athlete. Treatment options typically consist of immobilization with no return to sports until healed, immobilization with return to sports and open reduction and internal fixation (ORIF) of the scaphoid fracture.[34,36] The traditional treatment for the completely non-displaced middle one-third scaphoid fracture is with casting, typically in a thumb spica in radial deviation and wrist flexion.[37] Alternatively, a long arm cast (Munster type) can be worn for 4 weeks, followed by a short arm cast.[34] This method has been shown to result in union of 90–100% of fractures of the scaphoid within 9–12 weeks.[34,39] Above-elbow casts are indicated for fractures involving the proximal two-thirds of the scaphoid to prevent forearm pronation, whereas below-elbow casts are appropriate for distal scaphoid fractures owing to the improved blood supply and higher healing potential.[37] Typically, treatment with immobilization alone involves missing 3 months of sports participation.[34]

Indications for ORIF of scaphoid fractures include displacement greater than 1 mm (with a scapholunate angle >60° and a radiolunate angle >15°), non-union, carpal instability and involvement of the proximal pole.[34–38] K-wires are often necessary to manipulate the fracture fragments into proper position.[35,36] Internal fixation should be performed with a cannulated compression screw for maximum rigidity.

Established scaphoid non-union may be treated by non-vascularized or vascularized bone grafts with screw fixation as long as no significant arthritis or degenerative change is present. Chronic scaphoid non-unions result in progressive arthritis because of changes in the kinematics of the proximal row (scaphoid non-union advanced collapse wrist). In those patients with significant degenerative change, treatment options include anterior/posterior interosseous neurectomy, limited or total wrist arthrodesis and proximal row carpectomy.[38]

Fractures of the middle third of the scaphoid that are non-displaced or minimally displaced may be treated with either casting as described above or internal fixation.[34,36] Inoue and Shionoya[40] found that, in workers treated with internal fixation versus those with cast treatment, return to work was 4 weeks earlier (6 vs 10 weeks). The union rates were 100% for the internal fixation group and 98% for the casted group.[34,36,40] In the athlete, the advantage of internal fixation is earlier rehabilitation and return to protected activities and range of motion, and this is the preferred treatment method in this population (Fig. 74.8).[36] Athletes in contact sports should not be allowed to return to unrestricted activities until healing is confirmed. CT scans are often required to evaluate healing.

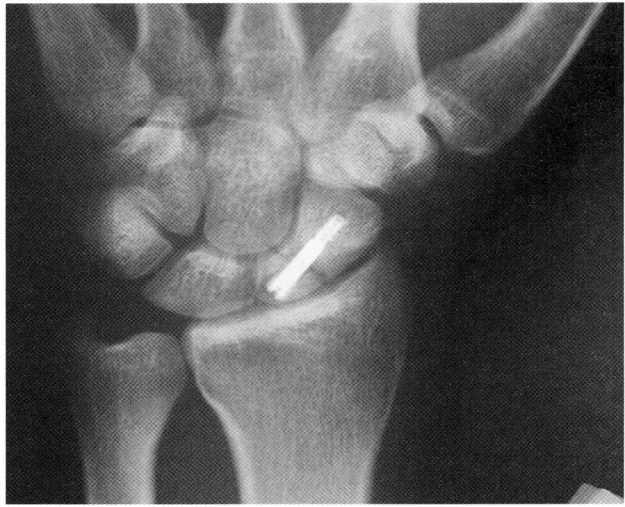

Figure 74.8 Open reduction and internal fixation: scaphoid fracture.

Hook of hamate fractures

Fractures of the hamate account for approximately 2–4% of carpal bone fractures.[34,37,41] Fractures involving the hook of the hamate typically affect athletes involved in racquet sports, golf and baseball.[34,42] Long-term complications of untreated hook of hamate fractures include rupture of the digital flexor tendons, carpal tunnel syndrome, non-union and ulnar neuropathies.[41] Fractures of the hook of the hamate run a high risk of non-union.[42] The mechanisms of injury include direct forces as in a fall or crush, shearing forces from the attached flexor digiti minimi and opponens digiti minimi muscles, or a combination of the two.[41] In some cases, chronic microtrauma may be to blame.[42]

The usual presentation is an athlete who plays golf, racquet sports or baseball with ulnar-sided wrist pain.[34] These fractures tend to present late, with associated ulnar nerve paraesthesias and weakened grip strength.[37] On examination, there is pain over the hook of the hamate at the base of the hypothenar eminence made worse by flexion of the ring and little fingers. Pain is also noted with dorsoulnar deviation. Capillary refill should be assessed to rule out damage to the ulnar artery, and neurological integrity should be checked with two-point discrimination.[34,37,40,41] Oblique, anteroposterior and lateral radiographs rarely demonstrate fractures of the hook of the hamate.[37,42] Instead, carpal tunnel and supinated oblique views should be obtained.[34] CT scan has been shown to be 100% sensitive and can be used to confirm the diagnosis (Fig. 74.9).[34,42]

Treatment options for hook of hamate fractures vary from immobilization with casting to ORIF and bony excision.[34] Minimally displaced acute fractures can be treated with immobilization for 6 weeks.[42] For acute displaced fractures both ORIF and hook excision are treatment options, although excision is the most frequently recommended treatment with ORIF being reserved for

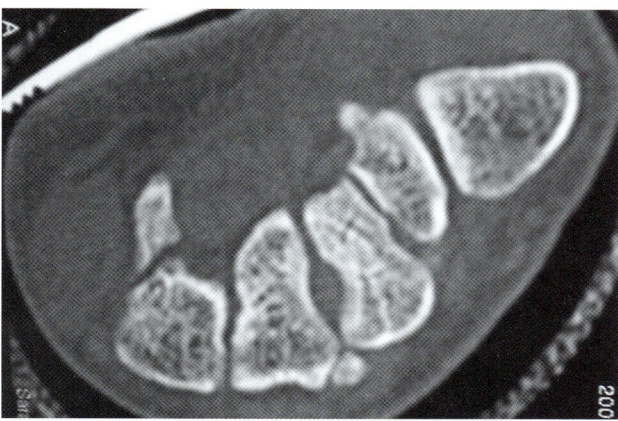

Figure 74.9 Hook of hamate fracture on CT.

those patients who have an excellent chance of healing.[34,41] ORIF has a high complication rate and is not the preferred treatment option. Excision of the hook of the hamate allows for accelerated rehabilitation and minimal immobilization. Return to sports is usually possible in 4–10 weeks.[34]

Scapholunate instability

The scapholunate interosseous ligament (SLIL) is the most commonly injured ligament of the wrist.[43–45] Injuries to the SLIL are common in football and other contact sports secondary to collisions with other athletes.[44]

The mechanism of injury for SLIL tears is wrist hyperextension with ulnar deviation and intracarpal supination.[45] This mechanism is reproduced in sports when an athlete falls on an outstretched and pronated hand.[43–45] This axial compression force can wedge the capitate between the scaphoid and lunate as the extension of the distal carpal row places an extension moment on the scaphoid via the volar midcarpal ligaments. The combination of these forces causes rupture and avulsion of the SLIL.[44] The degree of disruption of the SLIL determines both the severity of symptoms and the clinical findings. The disruption of the SLIL results in volar flexion of the scaphoid with concurrent extension of the lunate (dorsal intercalated segmental instability deformity).[44,45] These injuries occur as part of a spectrum of instability seen in perilunate injuries as described by Mayfield. In stage I the scapholunate ligament is disrupted; in stage II the captiate dislocates dorsally from the lunate as the space of Poirier is violated; in stage III the lunotriquetral ligament is disrupted; and in stage IV the lunate dislocates volarly from the remaining carpal bones.

The severity of the SLIL injury varies depending on the degree of disruption of the ligament. Small tears may be associated with mild weakness, pain and dynamic instability. More substantial tears are often associated with rotary subluxation of the scaphoid, causing an obvious 'snap' on provocative motions with a palpable dorsal pole of the scaphoid. Complete tears lead to scapholunate dissociation and static instability visible on standard plain films.[45,46] Instability may be confirmed with a Watson's test by placing

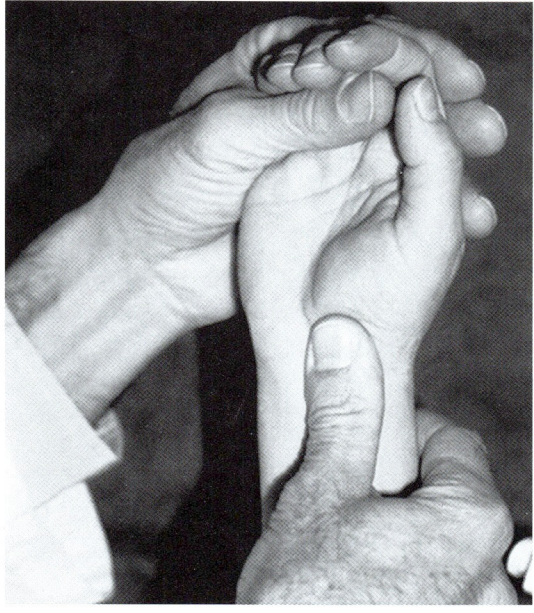

Figure 74.10 Watson's manoeuvre. Reproduced with permission from Green D, Hotchkiss R, Pederson W (eds). *Green's Operative Hand Surgery*, vol. 1, 5th edn. Philadelphia, PA: Elsevier Churchill Livingstone, 2005:493.

the forearm in pronation while placing pressure on the volar distal pole of the scaphoid and the dorsal lip of the radius as the wrist is moved back and forth in ulnar and radial deviation.[43,44] A painful 'snap' or 'pop' with radial deviation is considered a positive test so long as it is not present on the contralateral wrist (Fig. 74.10).[44]

Plain films play an important role in the diagnosis of SLIL injuries. On the posteroanterior radiograph the flexed posture of the scaphoid secondary to SLIL rupture makes it appear shortened and the prominent outer cortex is visualized; this is often called the cortical ring sign. Additionally, a scapholunate gap of greater than 2–3 mm may be present on the posteroanterior film and is called the Terry Thomas sign.[43–45] The lateral view usually reveals a scapholunate angle of greater than 70°, compared with the normal 30–60° (Fig. 74.11).[43,45] In a situation where there is high clinical suspicion of a SLIL injury in the absence of radiographic evidence on plain films, an MRI with intra-articular contrast is the next appropriate imaging study (Fig. 74.12).[44] Wrist arthroscopy evaluation of the ligament allows for direct visualization and is used to make a definitive diagnosis.[43]

Athletes with dynamic instability associated with partial tears can be managed with immobilization in a short arm cast for 2–6 weeks followed by the use of a removable splint for rehabilitation exercises and range of motion. Arthroscopic evaluation and debridement of partial injuries is often necessary to confirm the diagnosis. Return to sports is possible with an approved short arm playing cast.[44] The use of thermal shrinkage of partial SLIL tears has been attempted but long-term results are pending.[43] Injuries to the SLIL that have occurred within 6 months and are associated with complete tears and static pathological scaphoid flexion.[44,45] The treatment of the chronic SLIL injury in the athlete can be challenging, as many procedures for correction involve significant loss of range of motion at the wrist.[43,46] Primary repair can be attempted as late as 9 months after injury.[43] If scapholunate ligament disruptions are not treated, the kinematics of the wrist are disrupted, leading to progressive arthrosis of the wrist (scapholunate advanced collapse wrist). The key to treatment is early diagnosis of the extent of the injury and early surgical treatment if indicated.

Triangular fibrocartilage complex injuries of the distal radioulnar joint

The triangular fibrocartilage complex (TFCC) is the primary stabilizer of the distal radioulnar joint (DRUJ).[47] Accordingly, injuries to the TFCC affect the underlying stability of the DRUJ. TFCC injuries are common in athletes and can result from acute trauma, falls, overuse and repetitive microtrauma.[43] These injuries are common in gymnastics, racquet sports, golf, pole-vaulting and boxing.[43] The TFCC consists of the triangular fibrocartilage (called the articular disc), a meniscus homologue, the dorsal and volar radioulnar ligaments, the UCL, the ulnar triquetral ligament, the ulnolunate ligament, and the sheath of the extensor carpi ulnaris tendon (Fig. 74.13).[43,47,48] Classification of TFCC injuries is based on the Palmer method, which divides TFCC injuries into traumatic and degenerative classes.[47-49] Class 1 injuries are subdivided into four separate subcategories denoted by letters A–D. A class 1A injury involves injury to the avascular triangular fibrocartilage. A class 1B injury involves TFCC peripheral

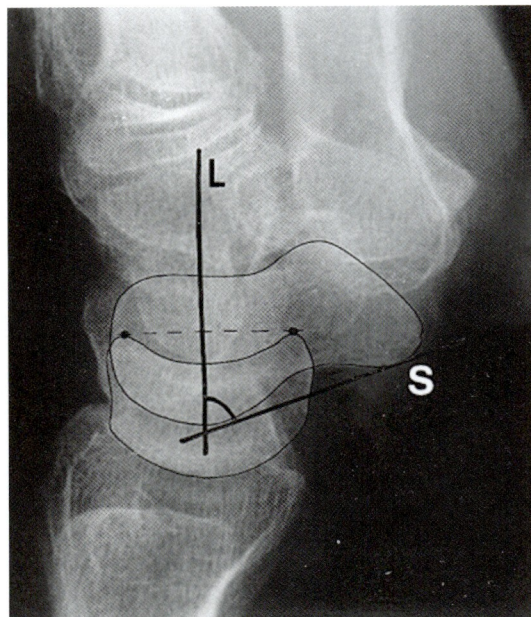

Figure 74.11 Scapholunate angle. Reproduced with permission from Green D, Hotchkiss R, Pederson W (eds). *Green's Operative Hand Surgery*, vol. 1, 5th edn. Philadelphia, PA: Elsevier Churchill Livingstone, 2005:558.

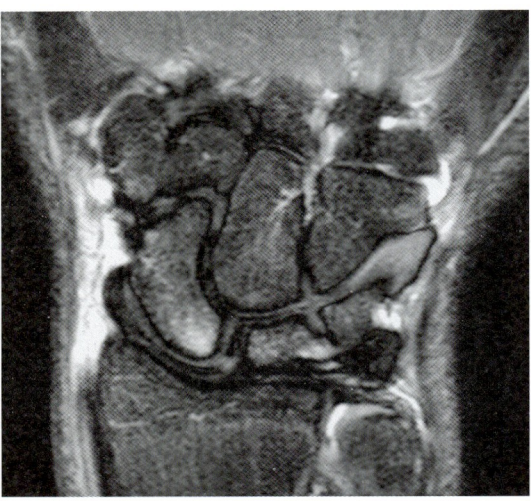

Figure 74.12 Scapholunate ligament tear on MRI.

instability should be treated with operative intervention.[44] Surgical intervention involves a dorsal approach with the use of bone anchors or pull-out sutures to reattach the SLIL along with pinning of the scaphoid and lunate to maintain anatomic reduction and a dorsal capsulodesis procedure to augment the ligament repair. Alternatively, arthroscopic reduction with percutaneous pinning may be used for surgical treatment of the acute tear. A dorsal capsulodesis is often done to augment the repair as it tethers the dorsal pole of the scaphoid and prevents

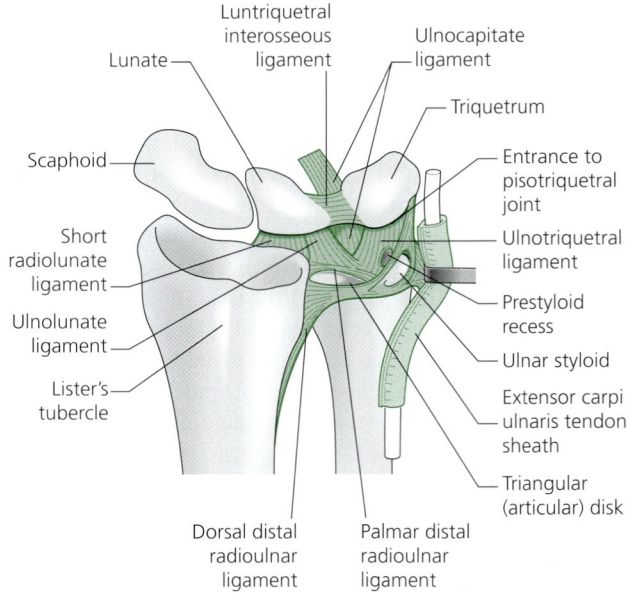

Figure 74.13 Anatomy of the triangular fibrocartilage complex. Reproduced with permission from Miller MD. *Review of Orthopaedics*, 4th edn. Philadelphia, PA: Saunders, 2004:393.

tears at the base of the ulnar styloid and may be associated with a distal ulnar fracture. A class 1C injury involves injury to the distal portions of the ulnolunate and ulnotriquetral ligaments resulting in avulsion from the respective carpal bones. A class 1D injury involves avulsion of the TFCC from the distal radius.[47,48] Degenerative changes are class 2 injuries and represent a spectrum of ulnocarpal impaction with each subclass adding a layer of injury to the other.[48] Type 2A injuries involve thinning of the triangular fibrocartilage; type 2B injuries involve a 2A injury plus lunate or ulnar chondromalacia; type 2C injuries have additional perforation of the central portion of the TFCC; and type 2D injuries have all the components of 2A–C with lunotriquetral ligament disruption. Lastly, the type 2E injury has the components of 2A–D with ulnocarpal arthritis (Fig. 74.14a,b).[47,48] Athletic injuries are more frequently class 1 injuries and acute in nature. Class 2 injuries are more chronic in presentation.

Patients present with a chief complaint of ulnar-sided wrist pain with associated clicking or popping sensations on pronation/supination movements.[48] Assessing for DRUJ instability is a critical part of the physical examination as TFCC tears can be associated with partial or complete instability of the DRUJ.[47] A 'piano key test' is performed by asking the patient to press the palm of the pronated forearm on the examining table while the examiner attempts to move the ulna in the volar and dorsal direction. A positive test occurs when there is obvious volar and dorsal translation of the ulna with or without pain.[43,47] The DRUJ 'shuck' or 'ballottement' test is performed by grinding the distal radius and ulna against one another in the neutral position. Abnormal tests occur when laxity or crepitus is present and are indicative of both instability and degeneration.[47]

Diagnostic work-up following physical examination begins with plain radiographs of the wrist. Both zero rotation posteroanterior views and lateral views of the wrist should be obtained.[48] There are four signs on the radiograph that may indicate injury to the TFCC and associated DRUJ instability. These include an ulnar styloid base fracture, widening of the DRUJ space on the posteroanterior view, dislocation on the lateral view, and more than 5 mm radial shortening relative to the ulna.[47,50]

Additional diagnostic studies include triple arthrography, MRI and arthroscopy.[48,51] Triple arthrography may miss approximately half of TFCC injuries and demonstrates only 11% of all wrist pathology.[48,51–54] Factors that influence the effectiveness of MRI include the quality of the MRI machine and the skill of the musculoskeletal radiologist interpreting the film.[48] Arthroscopy has become the gold standard technique used to diagnose TFCC tears.[43,51]

Treatment for high-level athletes with TFCC tears often begins with arthroscopy to help confirm the diagnosis and treat the underlying injury.[43] Surgical repair of the TFCC injury is determined by the type of TFCC injury present.[48] Type 1A injuries can be repaired with simple debridement of the articular disc.[43,48] Type 1B injuries can be treated with arthroscopic or open primary

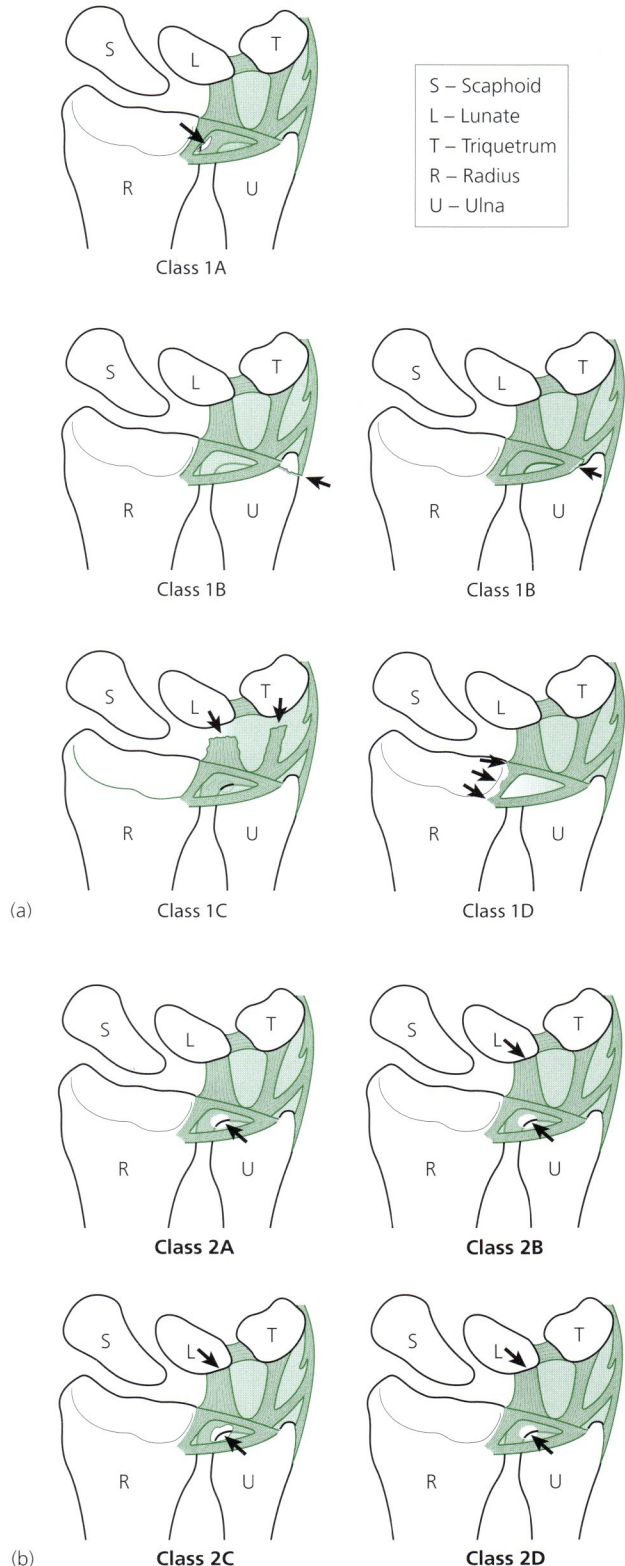

Figure 74.14 Palmer's classification of triangular fibrocartilage complex tears. (a) Class 1. (b) Class 2. Reproduced with permission from Green D, Hotchkiss R, Pederson W (eds). *Green's Operative Hand Surgery*, vol. 1, 5th edn. Philadelphia, PA: Elsevier Churchill Livingstone, 2005:614–15.

ligament repair to facilitate quicker return to activity.[43,47,48] Peripheral TFCC repairs have an excellent healing potential because of enhanced vascularity in this region. Type 1C injuries are treated similarly to type 1B injuries in that, acutely, immobilization is acceptable treatment, but failure to heal necessitates arthroscopic or open repair of the ulnolunate and ulnotriquetral ligaments.[47,48] Treatment for 1D injuries is under debate, but debridement of the radial attachment of the TFCC and direct arthroscopic repair are both being used with some success.[48] For type 2 degenerative injuries treatment options centre around arthroscopic debridement and extra-articular ulnar shortening or intra-articular wafer resection, as described by Feldon et al.,[50] so long as positive ulnar variance is less than 3 mm.[43,48] If associated ulnocarpal arthritis is present, salvage distal ulnar arthroplasty procedures are considered (Darrach, Bowers and Sauve–Kapandji operations).[48]

Handlebar palsy

Handlebar palsy is the compression of the ulnar nerve in Guyon's canal secondary to repetitive static hyperextension of the wrist. It is commonly seen in athletes participating in cycling, martial arts and racquet sports.[55]

Patients present with paraesthesias of the ring and small fingers and variable degrees of decreased grip strength. Pain is most often noted in the small finger only.[55] On examination there may be a positive Tinel's sign over Guyon's canal. Aside from assessing sensation to light touch over the ring and small fingers with two-point discrimination, the strength of the intrinsic muscles of the hand should be determined. The examiner should attempt to elicit a Froment's sign (flexor pollicis longus activation to substitute for a weakened adductor pollicis), a Wartenberg sign (maintenance of the small finger in abduction) and grip strength should be tested. These signs are present in chronic compression neuropathy situations and indicate denervation of intrinsic musculature. If there is a history of trauma, a fracture to the hook of the hamate should be ruled out by radiograph.[56] Electromyography and nerve conduction studies are helpful in the diagnosis.

Conservative treatment includes rest, NSAIDs and splinting. Failure to improve with these measures or evidence of intrinsic muscle weakness is an indication for surgical decompression of Guyon's canal.[55,56]

Hypothenar hammer syndrome

Hypothenar hammer syndrome occurs secondary to repetitive trauma to the ulnar–volar portion of the hand and is commonly seen in martial arts athletes, baseball catchers and air hammer operators. Trauma occurs to the ulnar artery within or distal to Guyon's canal, causing internal damage to the artery, thrombus formation and, in some case, aneurysms leading to vasospasm.[55]

Patients present with complaints of cold intolerance and pain in the palm. Symptoms are worse with activities such as catching a ball; in severe cases digital ulceration may be present.[55,56] On physical examination there may be findings suggestive of handlebar palsy secondary to ulnar nerve compression from aneurysm formation. An Allen's test will be positive and allows the clinician to delineate hypothenar hammer syndrome from simple ulnar nerve compression as a positive Tinel's sign will be found in both conditions.[56] Arteriography may be required to make the diagnosis.

Treatment is usually conservative, with rest and padding of the palm often being adequate for relief of symptoms. Vasolytic and sympatholytic pharmacological agents can play a role in treatment. In some circumstances, surgery is required to restore normal flow dynamics to the injured artery and should be preceded by an arteriogram. When surgery is required, it involves removal of the aneurysm or thrombus followed by vein graft reconstruction of the ulnar artery.[55,56]

de Quervain's tenosynovitis

de Quervain's tenosynovitis is a stenosing tenosynovitis of the tendons of the first dorsal compartment, namely the abductor pollicis longus and extensor pollicis brevis.[57,58] This represents the most common tendinopathy of the wrist in athletics.[59] The mechanism of injury is repetitive gliding of the extensor pollicis brevis and abductor pollicis longus tendons through the sheath of the first dorsal compartment just superficial to the radial styloid, resulting in shear stresses that, over time, cause inflammation of the tenosynovium.[57–59] Sports that require repetitive ulnar deviation coupled with a forceful grasp, such as golf, fly fishing, racquet sports and javelin and discus throwing, put the athlete at increased risk.[57]

Patients present with a chief complaint of pain over the radial styloid that is made worse with grip and ulnar deviation. On examination, tenderness and swelling over the styloid are the most common findings, although some athletes may have crepitus or triggering of the thumb.[57] A Finklestein's test should be performed by having the patient flex the thumb in the palm followed by ulnar deviation of the wrist. A test is considered positive if the patient's symptoms are reproduced.[58]

Treatment for early stages of de Quervain's tenosynovitis may consist of rest, immobilization in a thumb spica and the use of NSAIDs with complete cure expected 25–72% of the time.[57,59] A corticosteroid injection may also be used for the initial management of this condition or for more advanced cases, with reported cure rates of 80%.[58–60] Surgical management is the treatment of choice if conservative measures fail, and consists of decompression of the first dorsal compartment.[57,58,59,61]

Intersection syndrome

Intersection syndrome is an inflammatory condition that occurs at the intersection of the abductor pollicis longus and extensor pollicis brevis of the first dorsal compartment with the ECRB and extensor carpi radialis longus (ECRL) of the second dorsal compartment approximately 4–6 cm proximal to the wrist joint.[59] While no one cause for the pathophysiology has been identified, theories include friction between the intersecting tendons resulting in development of an additional adventitial bursa, tenosynovitis of the ECRB and ECRL, and hypertrophy of the muscles of the first dorsal compartment leading to increased pressure on the ECRB and ECRL.[57,58] The condition is seen most commonly in athletes who participate in sports requiring repetitive wrist extension such as rowing, racquet sports and weight lifting.[58,59]

Athletes present with pain over the dorsum of the distal forearm. On examination crepitus, swelling and pain to palpation are appreciated approximately 4–6 cm proximal to Lister's tubercle.[57–59] Initial management consists of rest, NSAIDs, corticosteroid injections and immobilization. While conservative management is usually successful, surgery is indicated if these measures fail to provide adequate relief.[62] Surgical intervention includes decompression of the second dorsal compartment, debridement of the bursa and fasciotomy of the first dorsal compartment muscles.[58,59,62]

Extensor carpi ulnaris tendinitis and subluxation

Extensor carpi ulnaris tendinitis is the second most frequent tendinitis of the wrist after de Quervain's tenosynovitis.[57,59] Tendinitis of the extensor carpi ulnaris results from repetitive friction of the extensor carpi ulnaris tendon through the sixth dorsal compartment, resulting in pain and inflammation. This is commonly seen in racquet sports, rowing, baseball and golf.[57–59,62] In some cases, the extensor carpi ulnaris tendon may sublux through its subsheath and retinaculum owing to rupture of these structures after an acute force resulting in supination, volar flexion and ulnar deviation of the wrist.[57,58] This injury has been reported in tennis players most commonly, but it has also occurred in weight lifters, golfers and rodeo riders.[59]

Athletes with extensor carpi ulnaris tendinitis present with ulnar-sided wrist pain made worse with activities that require resisted or forceful wrist extension.[57,58] On examination pain is reproduced with resisted wrist extension and point tenderness over the sixth dorsal compartment. In patients with subluxation of the extensor carpi ulnaris, supination and ulnar deviation of the affected wrist will often reproduce symptoms and be associated with an audible snap.[57–59]

Treatment of extensor carpi ulnaris tendinitis is conservative and consists of splinting, rest, NSAIDs and corticosteroid injections into the tendon sheath as needed.[59,62] In chronic cases of extensor carpi ulnaris tendinitis associated with fibrosis of the tendon sheath, surgical decompression is warranted for relief of symptoms.[58,62] In patients who do not respond to conservative measures, TFCC injury should be ruled out by arthroscopy.[62]

In acute cases of extensor carpi ulnaris subluxation, treatment options consist of immobilization for 6 weeks or surgical intervention. In athletes, early surgical intervention is advisable as it allows for a more aggressive rehabilitation programme.[58,59,62] The extensor carpi ulnaris can be stabilized surgically by creating a sling of retinaculum, using a free retinacular graft, or, if satisfactory subsheath tissue is present, it may be sutured directly to the ulnar groove.[58,62] TFCC injury is associated with disruption of the extensor carpi ulnaris retinaculum and subsheath and should be evaluated and treated concomitantly.

Gymnast's wrist and dorsal wrist syndromes

Dorsal wrist syndromes are common in all sports in which repetitive axial loads are absorbed by the hyperextended wrist.[59] Gymnastics in particular is associated with wrist pain, with up to 45% of gymnasts reporting wrist pain of at least 6 months' duration.[63]

Causes of chronic wrist pain in the gymnast include distal radial physeal stress fractures, scaphoid impaction syndrome, dorsal impingement syndrome and occult ganglionic cysts.[59,63] Rarer causes of pain include avascular necrosis of the capitate and stress fractures of the scaphoid.[63] This pain is exacerbated by repetitive hyperextension and axial loading and is often localized to the dorsum of the wrist.

In the paediatric gymnast distal radial physeal stress fractures are a common cause of chronic dorsal wrist pain.[63] The fractures are diagnosed based on three stages. In stage 1 there is clinical evidence of injury in the absence of radiographic evidence and return to sports is possible in approximately 4 weeks. Stage 2 injuries are associated with radial growth plate changes including cystic change and physeal widening. Return to sports is delayed for 2–4 months in these patients. In a stage 3 injury, ulnar positive variance from physeal growth arrest of the radius is noted along with cystic change and physeal widening.[59] MRI may be required to confirm the diagnosis (Fig. 74.15).

Scaphoid impaction syndrome presents with pain, weakness and tenderness at the dorsal and radial aspect of the wrist. Symptoms are exacerbated by hyperextension of the wrist, and tenderness to palpation over the dorsal portion of the scaphoid is evident on physical examination. Plain films may show hypertrophy of the scaphoid dorsal rim or the presence of a small osteophyte on lateral views with the wrist in slight flexion. Conservative measures such as rest and splinting with corticosteroid injections can be used as initial treatment. For chronic cases that have not responded to conservative therapy, surgical intervention is indicated and includes removal of hypertrophic bone and synovial debridement.[64]

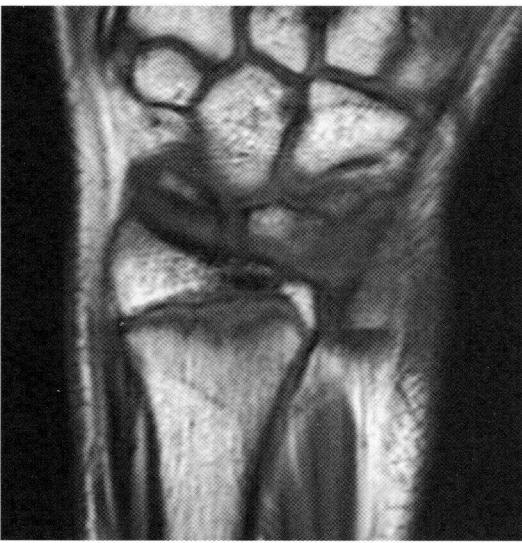

Figure 74.15   Epiphysiolysis (gymnast's wrist).

Dorsal impingement syndrome results from chronic dorsal capsulitis that leads to synovial thickening of the dorsal wrist capsule. CT scan may reveal the presence of osteophytes along the dorsal distal radius and adjacent carpal bones, which are usually not evident on plain film. Treatment consists of rest, splinting, NSAIDs and steroid injections. Failure to respond to conservative measures is an indication for surgical intervention, which may include debridement of inflamed synovial tissue, removal of osteophytes and posterior interosseous neurectomy.[59]

Occult dorsal ganglion cysts can result from athletic activity involving repetitive wrist hyperextension and axial loading and often present as a dorsal wrist pain syndrome.[59,64] The ganglion develops from the scapholunate ligament and is a reactive change in response to repetitive trauma.[64] Immobilization, rest and corticosteroid treatment is the first-line treatment, with surgical excision of the ganglion and resection of the distal posterior interosseous nerve reserved for refractory cases.[59,64] Scapholunate ligament injury should be ruled out as it is in the differential diagnosis.

HAND INJURIES

Jersey finger

The forceful disruption of the flexor digitorum profundus (FDP) insertion at the base of the volar distal phalanx is called a jersey finger injury.[65] Most commonly, this injury is seen in football players following a tackle in which the actively flexed distal interphalangeal joint is forced into hyperextension. The bony insertion of the FDP tendon is the most common site of rupture and the ring finger is involved in over three-quarters of injuries (Fig. 74.16).[65–68]

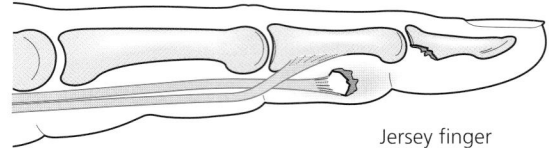

Figure 74.16   Jersey finger (flexor digitorum profundus avulsion fracture). Reproduced with permission from Greene WB. *Netter's Orthopaedics*. Philadelphia, PA: Saunders, 2006:357.

Leddy and Packer[66] have classified jersey finger injuries into three categories. In a type I injury the tendon retracts into the palm with subsequent loss of the vincular blood supply. The tendon must be reinserted within 7–10 days to prevent muscle contracture.[65,69–71] MRI and ultrasound are helpful in determining the level of retraction of the FDP tendon.

In type II injuries, the FDP tendon retracts to the level of the proximal interphalangeal joint, thus maintaining blood supply from the long vinculum.[65,67,69] Typically, a small piece of bone attached to the FDP allows it to get stuck at the level of the proximal interphalangeal joint in the chiasm of the flexor digitorum superficialis.[5] The window for reinsertion is 6 weeks for these injuries, but surgical repair is still recommended in the acute phase.[65,67–69]

In a type III injury there is avulsion of the FDP with an associated large bony fragment that is often caught in the A4 pulley.[68] Repair should be attempted in the acute setting with ORIF of the avulsed fragment.[67,68] Rarely, the FDP may rupture separately from the fracture fragment; these so-called type IIIb (also called type IV) injuries are treated in a two-stage manner. First, the avulsion fracture is corrected with ORIF, followed by flexor tendon repair.[65,67–69]

For patients who present with chronic jersey finger injuries treatment options are varied and include flexor digitorum superficialis tendon grafts, arthrodesis of the distal interphalangeal joint, tendon stump excision and observation without surgical intervention.[65,67–69]

Mallet finger

The disruption of the terminal tendon of the extensor mechanism insertion at the base of the dorsal distal phalanx is known as a mallet finger injury. It is the most common closed tendon injury among athletes and is seen among baseball players, football wide receivers and basketball players.[65,69]

The mechanism of injury is an acute force causing hyperflexion of the extended distal phalanx at the distal interphalangeal joint, as in a blow to the fingertip while attempting to catch a ball.[65,69] In some cases, the injury is caused by a fracture at the base of the dorsal distal phalanx with concomitant loss of the extensor mechanism at the fracture site. Rarely, a twisting-type injury to the distal interphalangeal joint can cause a tear in one of the merging lateral bands, leading to a mallet finger injury.[67] Untreated mallet finger injuries will often progress to swan neck deformities with hyperextension of the proximal interphalangeal joint and loss of grip strength.[72]

On physical examination patients have an extensor lag across the distal interphalangeal joint that can vary from 15° to more than 60°, although this deformity may take several days to develop.[72] Radiographs are recommended to rule out an associated fracture or joint subluxation.[72,73]

Treatment of closed acute mallet finger injuries is usually undertaken by splinting the distal interphalangeal joint in extension for 8 weeks while leaving the proximal interphalangeal joint free to move normally. Following 8 weeks of splinting in this fashion, the splint may be worn at night for an additional 4 weeks and during athletic activities for 2 months.[65,69,74] Even patients presenting as late as 1–3 months may be treated with splinting successfully.[65,67,69,72]

Mallet finger injuries that involve more than one-third of the articular surface with volar dislocation of the distal interphalangeal joint, or injuries associated with avulsion of large bony fragments, may be treated with surgical intervention.[65,74] This is achieved via ORIF of the avulsed fragment and reduction of the dislocated distal interphalangeal joint aided by longitudinal placement of a single K-wire.[65]

Mallet deformities of the thumb are rare injuries, accounting for approximately 3% of mallet finger injuries. Current treatment recommendations are to splint the interphalangeal joint of the thumb in extension for 6–8 weeks.[69]

Chronic mallet finger deformities (defined as >4 weeks) are often treated successfully with additional splinting for up to 10–18 weeks followed by 2 weeks of night splinting.[67,75]

Bennett's fracture

A Bennett's fracture is an oblique fracture dislocation at the ulnar base of the first metacarpal, which extends into the first carpometacarpal joint.[76] The larger distal fragment is displaced proximally, radially and dorsally by the pull of the abductor pollicis longus muscle, whereas the proximal fragment remains tethered to the joint because of strong volar beak ligament attachment.[76,77] The mechanism of injury is typically an axial load to an adducted and flexed thumb.[69,78]

The diagnosis can be made with both anteroposterior and lateral radiographs (Fig. 74.17). CT scan can be helpful as well for more complex-appearing fractures.[69,76] Treatment is closed reduction with percutaneous pinning for fractures involving less than 20% of the first carpometacarpal joint.[78] Fragments larger than 20%, fractures associated with greater than 1 mm of articular incongruity or fractures associated with soft-tissue interposition should be treated with ORIF with lag screw stabilization.[76–79] It is critical to properly reduce a Bennett's fracture as failure to

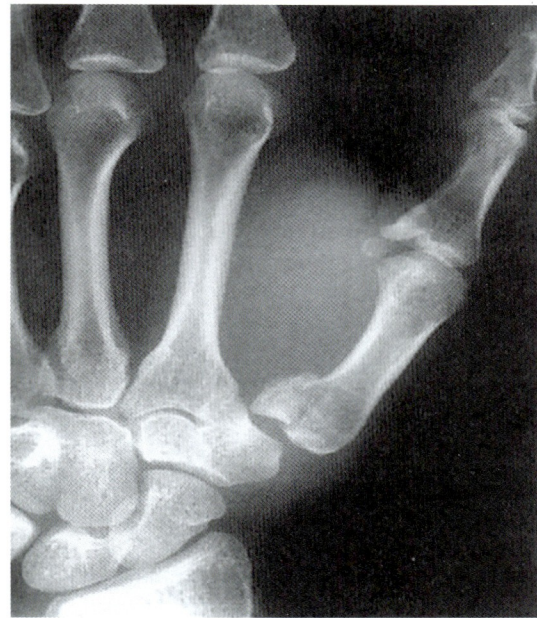

Figure 74.17 Bennett's fracture.

do so can lead to malunion with chronic subluxation and the development of early arthritis.[69] Reduction can be achieved by applying longitudinal traction to the first metacarpal, followed by extension, abduction and pronation.[77]

A Rolando fracture is a more severe variant of a thumb base fracture in which there is a comminuted intra-articular fracture of the carpometacarpal joint in a 'T' or 'Y' arrangement.[76] Most commonly these fractures occur from powerful axial loading across the first carpometacarpal joint, allowing for sufficient force to provide a comminuted fracture of the articular surface.[78] Treatment is surgical intervention with ORIF that usually requires multiple K-wires, or screw and plate fixation.[76]

Skier's and gamekeeper's thumb

Gamekeeper's thumb refers to chronic lateral laxity of the ulnar collateral ligament of the thumb, whereas skier's thumb refers to the acute disruption of the ulnar collateral ligament. The terms are often used interchangeably.[80]

The mechanism of injury is a forceful radial deviation of the proximal phalanx at the metacarpophalangeal joint and is most often seen in skiers, basketball players and other ball-handling athletes.[69,80–82] The majority of the time, the UCL is avulsed from its distal insertion with or without an accompanying portion of bone.[69,81,82] It is often the case that the avulsed portion of the UCL folds back on itself and relocates proximal and dorsal to the adductor pollicis aponeurosis, allowing it to become interposed between the distal ligamentous end and the insertion at the base of the proximal phalanx and making healing difficult.[83,84] This is often noted on physical examination

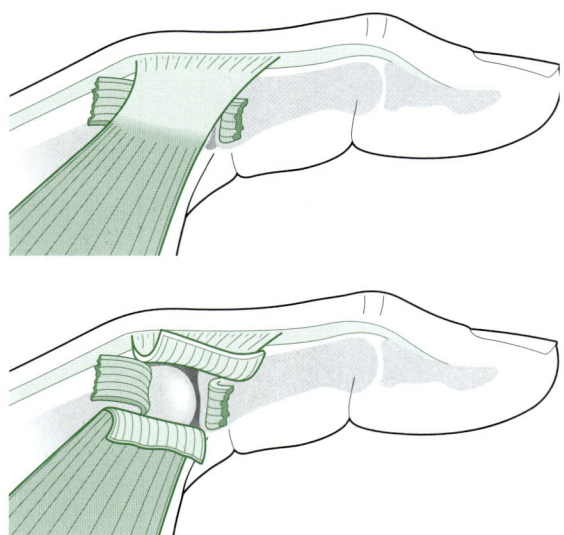

Figure 74.18 Stener's lesion. Reproduced with permission from Miller MD. *Review of Orthopaedics*, 4th edn. Philadelphia, PA: Saunders, 2004:250.

as a palpable lump and is referred to as a Stener's lesion, after the physician who first described it (Fig. 74.18).[69,83,85]

Patients present with tenderness and swelling of the metacarpophalangeal joint that is mostly localized to the ulnar side on palpation. Instability of the metacarpophalangeal joint may be assessed by passive radial deviation of the thumb at the metacarpophalangeal joint in full extension and in 30° of flexion. Increased opening of the metacarpophalangeal joint compared with the contralateral side can be considered a positive test. Additionally, stress radiographs can be taken for clinical documentation.[69,81] A complete tear is evidenced by a greater than 30° difference in angulation compared with the contralateral side or palpable subluxation of the proximal phalanx relative to the metacarpal head (Fig. 74.19).[69,81]

Treatment depends on the severity of the UCL injury. Partial tears can be managed with simple immobilization in a thumb spica with the thumb in palmar abduction for 4–6 weeks, or alternatively with 20° of thumb flexion and a free interphalangeal joint for 3–4 weeks followed by application of a removable splint for an additional 3 weeks.[81,82] Indications for surgery include a complete tear, 33% subluxation of the proximal phalanx relative to the metacarpal head, and the presence of a Stener lesion.[69]

Surgery with primary repair of the UCL through bone tunnels or with suture anchors is advocated for acute complete ruptures.[69,82,83] ORIF becomes necessary for large avulsed bony fragments with greater than 3 mm of separation and concurrent rotation.[69,83] Controversy exists about the optimum treatment for chronic injuries of the UCL as success has been obtained with free tendon grafting and secondary ligament repair.[83,86] Joint fusion should be reserved for cases with visible articular damage, failed reconstruction/ligament repair, and in individuals not willing to cooperate with the rehabilitation programme necessary for full recovery postoperatively.[86]

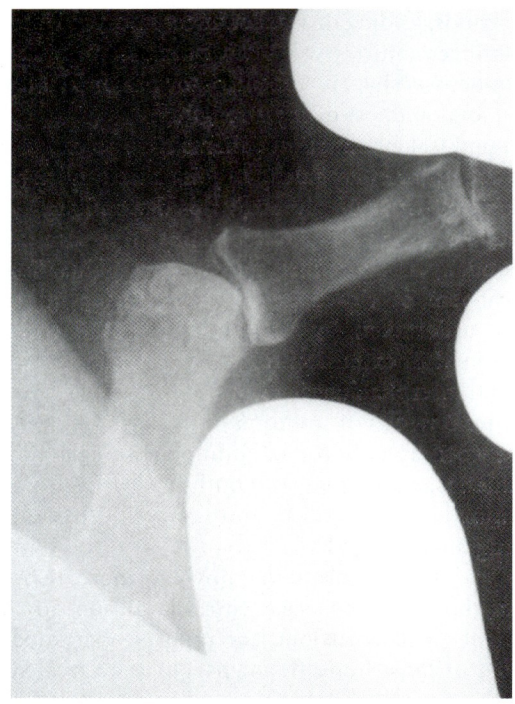

Figure 74.19 Ulnar collateral ligament: stress view.

Proximal interphalangeal joint dislocations

Dislocation of the proximal interphalangeal joint is a very common injury in ball-handling sports. Dislocations of the proximal interphalangeal joint are usually dorsal, with lateral and volar dislocations also occurring but not as frequently. The most common mechanism of injury is an axial force causing hyperextension of the joint (Fig. 74.20a,b).[81]

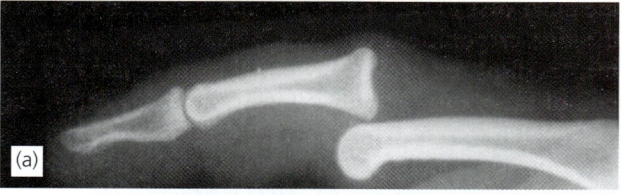
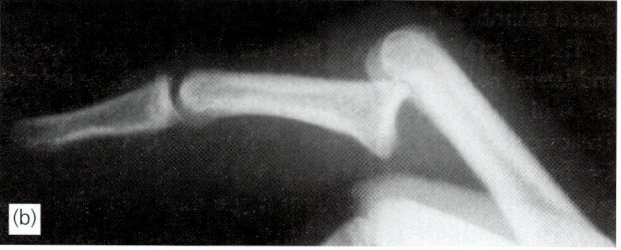

Figure 74.20 Proximal interphalangeal dislocation. (a) Dorsal. (b) Volar.

In a dorsal dislocation of the proximal interphalangeal joint the middle phalanx is displaced dorsal relative to the proximal phalanx.[87] Typically, these injuries are reducible and stable.[87] Reduction is accomplished by applying axial traction to the finger with proximal interphalangeal flexion to reduce the joint.[81]

Dorsal dislocations can be classified into three categories. In type I dislocations there is avulsion of the volar plate from the middle phalanx and a small longitudinal tear in the collateral ligaments, but the articular surfaces remain in contact.[76,81,87] Treatment for a type I dislocation is buddy taping with early range of motion until resolution of symptoms.[81]

Type II injuries are defined by avulsions of the volar plate from the middle phalanx with large longitudinal splits in the collateral ligaments and dorsal dislocation of the middle phalanx so that it rests on the dorsal condyle of the proximal phalanx. These dislocations are reduced as described above and treated with buddy taping for 3 weeks.[88]

Lastly, a type III injury involves a fracture dislocation. Fracture dislocations may be either volar or dorsal, although dorsal fracture dislocations are much more common.[88] Dorsal fracture dislocations occur when the base of the middle phalanx is driven proximally and dorsally into the proximal phalanx, resulting in a palmar base fracture of the middle phalanx and a dorsal dislocation of the proximal interphalangeal joint.[88] Because this area of the middle phalanx serves as an attachment for collateral ligaments and the volar plate, instability can become severe with relatively small avulsion fractures of the palmar articular surface.[69,76] A stable type III dislocation involves less than 30% of the articular surface, allowing a portion of the collateral ligament to remain intact on the middle phalanx. In an unstable type III dislocation injury, greater than 40% of the articular surface is involved, leading to complete separation of the volar plate and collateral ligaments from the middle phalanx.[76,88] Unsupported lateral finger radiographs are critical to making the diagnosis and examination with fluoroscopy may be utilized if lateral radiographs provide an unclear picture of the extent of bony involvement.[69] Stable fracture dislocations can be reduced and splinted in a dorsal extension block splint with the proximal interphalangeal joint in flexion for 4–6 weeks. The patient is seen weekly and radiographs obtained to confirm maintenance of reduction. Flexion can be slowly decreased after 2 weeks.[69] For unstable type III injuries or difficult to reduce stable injuries, treatment recommendations vary. Fracture dislocations with minimally comminuted fragments can be treated by ORIF of the large bony fragment, closed reduction with percutaneous pinning and a dorsal extension blocking splint, and the use of a dorsal extension blocking splint alone if the proximal interphalangeal joint is stable in flexion.[69,76,88] For comminuted and chronic fracture dislocations volar plate arthroplasty, as described by Eaton and Malerich,[89] may be necessary.[69]

Lateral dislocations occur because of avulsion (partial or complete) of the volar plate from the middle phalanx and rupture of one collateral ligament.[87] Treatment is controversial for lateral dislocations. Kahler and McCue[81] advocate surgical repair of ruptured collateral ligaments and associated volar plate injuries for lateral dislocations in athletes. Frieberg et al.[87] advocate treatment with simple buddy taping to the adjacent finger for 3 weeks.

Volar dislocation of the proximal interphalangeal joint is a rare injury and can be classified as straight volar, lateral volar or rotatory.[69] The most common mechanism of injury is a longitudinally directed compression force with concurrent rotation of the semiflexed middle phalanx along the proximal interphalangeal joint.[76] This leads to rupture of one collateral ligament, followed by volar dislocation of the middle phalanx and disruption of the central slip. Partial disruption of the transverse retinacular ligaments and volar plate can also occur.[81] Initial treatment is closed reduction followed by splinting of the proximal interphalangeal joint in extension for 6 weeks to prevent the formation of a boutonnière deformity.[69] In most rotatory-type volar dislocations, closed reduction is not possible because the dorsal condyle of the proximal phalanx buttonholes between the central slip and lateral band.[76] Open reduction is the preferred treatment in these cases with open repair of the central slip and transarticular pinning of the proximal interphalangeal joint for 3 weeks.[69] Failure to appropriately recognize and treat a volar dislocation of the proximal interphalangeal joint can result in the formation of a chronic boutonnière deformity.[87]

Boutonnière deformity

Boutonnière deformity is caused by the disruption of the central slip of the extensor mechanism at the base of the dorsal middle phalanx. Three main mechanisms are responsible for the boutonnière deformity. They are acute forceful hyperflexion of the proximal interphalangeal joint, volar and lateral dislocation of the proximal interphalangeal joint and deep contusion along the proximal middle phalanx.[74] Volar lateral dislocations of the proximal interphalangeal joint are believed to be the most common mechanism of injury.[65] When the central slip ruptures, the lateral bands gradually migrate volar to the proximal interphalangeal joint axis, which stretches the triangular ligament and concentrates the force of the lateral bands across the distal interphalangeal joint, causing extension with concurrent flexion of the proximal interphalangeal joint (Fig. 74.21).[65,69,74,81]

Treatment for acute closed boutonnière deformities is with immobilization of the proximal interphalangeal and metacarpophalangeal joint in extension, allowing for free motion of the distal interphalangeal joint for 6–8 weeks.[65,69] Night splinting should be continued for an additional 2–3 weeks following continuous splinting.[81]

The window for treatment of acute closed central slip ruptures in this fashion is 3 weeks. After 3 weeks, signs of

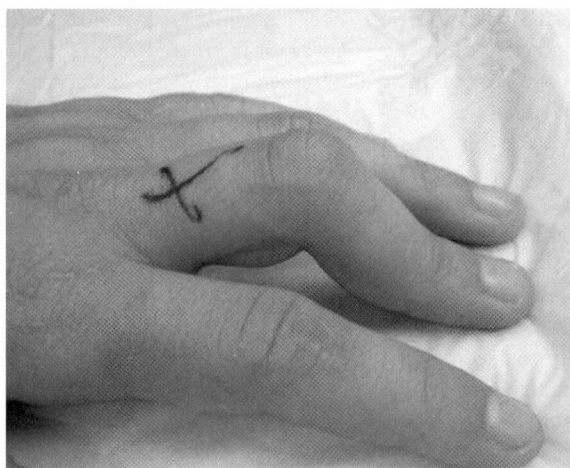

Figure 74.21 Boutonnière deformity.

fixed deformity may already be present and splinting should be attempted for at least 3 months, as described previously, so long as the joint is supple.[81] If the proximal interphalangeal joint is not passively correctable, a dynamic splint is used until the proximal interphalangeal joint deformity has resolved, followed by splinting as described previously.[75] Failure of a boutonnière deformity to correct with conservative measures is an indication for surgical intervention. This may include repair and shortening of the central slip, anatomical relocation of the lateral bands, free tendon grafting and release of associated adhesions.[65,75]

Pseudoboutonnière deformity

While clinically similar to the boutonnière deformity, the pseudoboutonnière deformity occurs by a different mechanism and has different treatment from the classic boutonnière deformity. A hyperextension injury to the distal interphalangeal joint causes a proximal disruption of the proximal interphalangeal volar plate, with subsequent scar tissue formation causing flexion contracture of the proximal interphalangeal joint.[69] Distal interphalangeal hyperextension is caused by contracture of the lateral bands and oblique retinacular ligament. Unlike a classic boutonnière deformity, the central slip is intact. Clinically, the injury can be differentiated from a true boutonnière deformity by slight rather than fixed hyperextension of the proximal interphalangeal joint, a history of a hyperextension injury, radiographic evidence of calcification around the volar plate and lack of tenderness over the dorsal proximal interphalangeal joint.[81] Treatment consists of a trial of conservative management with splinting of the proximal interphalangeal if the angle of deformity is less than 45°. Surgical intervention in the form of a capsular release with K-wire placement across the proximal interphalangeal joint for 3 weeks is the recommended treatment if greater than 45° of angulation is present.[65] Early recognition and conservative treatment of this injury is successful.

Hand fractures

Phalangeal fractures are a common injury in athletes and are classified as comminuted, transverse, oblique or spiral in nature.[90] Direct blows to the phalanges are likely to cause transverse or comminuted fractures, whereas twisting forces often result in spiral or oblique fracture patterns. In many cases, phalangeal fractures display angular deformity and displacement secondary to the pull of the intrinsic hand musculature on the associated fracture fragments and the initial mechanism of injury.[91]

Phalangeal fractures which are non-displaced can be treated conservatively with buddy taping and splinting.[90] Following reduction, any phalangeal fracture with greater than 6 mm of shortening, greater than 15° of angular deformity or any rotational deformity should be treated surgically with percutaneous pinning or ORIF.[91,92] In many cases spiral and oblique fractures must be treated with ORIF or percutaneous pinning to prevent rotational malalignment.[91] ORIF is commonly performed in athletes to accelerate rehabilitation and allow for early range of motion. Athletes should not be allowed to return to contact activities without protection or until there is adequate radiographic healing (4–6 weeks).

Proximal phalanx fractures tend to displace with apex volar orientation secondary to the pull of the interossei on the proximal fragment of the phalanx.[93] Fractures of the middle phalanx are relatively uncommon.[93] Fractures distal to the flexor digitorum superficialis insertion display apex volar angulation whereas more proximal fractures may display dorsal angulation secondary to the pull of the central slip of the extensor mechanism (Fig. 74.22a,b).[91]

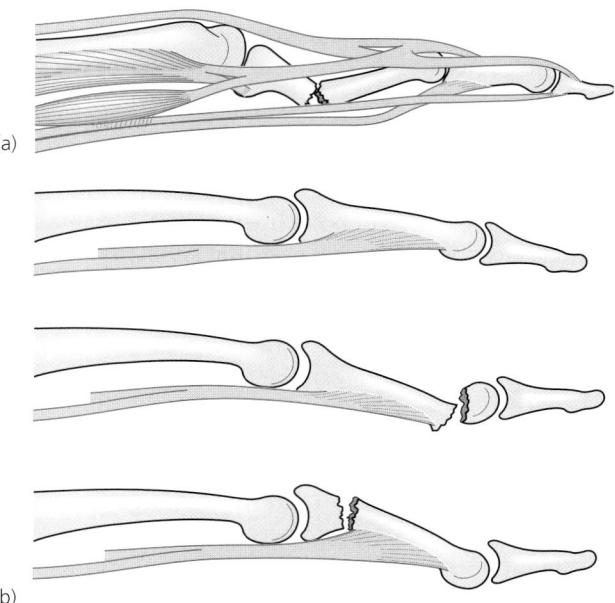

Figure 74.22 (a) Proximal phalanx fracture with volar angulation. (b) Middle phalanx fracture with dorsal and volar angulation.

Fractures of the distal phalanx constitute over half of all hand fractures and occur from crushing or axially directed forces.[91,93] Fracture tends to occur at the tuft of the distal phalanx from a crushing force or at the base from an axially directed force.[91] Avulsion fractures of the dorsal and volar lip can occur secondary to mallet and jersey finger-type injuries, respectively.[65,92] Associated nail bed injuries are common with distal phalanx fractures and should be appropriately treated.[94]

Metacarpal fractures are common injuries, accounting for over 33% of all hand fractures.[95,96] The fifth metacarpal is the most commonly fractured of the metacarpal bones, accounting for roughly half of all metacarpal fractures and 20% of all hand fractures.[96,97] Metacarpal fractures are subdivided into neck fractures, base fractures, shaft fractures and distal fractures.[95] Fractures of the metacarpal shaft can be further subdivided as transverse, oblique/spiral and comminuted.[98]

Fractures of the metacarpal neck most commonly involve the fourth and fifth metacarpal.[97] Fractures of the neck of the fifth metacarpal are often referred to as boxer's fractures.[95] These fractures often occur just below the metacarpal head, and lead to volar displacement of the metacarpal head relative to the proximal fracture fragment.[95] Following closed reduction and splinting, radiographs are taken to assess the degree of angular deformity of the fracture. Lee and Jupiter[96] reported that approximately 30° of flexion deformity is acceptable at the fifth metacarpal neck, 20° of flexion deformity is acceptable at the fourth metacarpal neck, and only 10° of flexion deformity is acceptable at the necks of the second and third metacarpals. In many patients a flexion deformity of up to 45° of the fifth metacarpal neck can be tolerated with adequate functional results. Nevertheless, reduction and splinting should be attempted to improve angulation. If adequate reduction cannot be attained, percutaneous pinning becomes necessary to maintain the reduction.[69,98] ORIF is reserved for soft-tissue entrapment, multiple metacarpal fractures, high-energy trauma, open fractures and pathological fractures.[96,97,99] Surgical intervention for metacarpal neck fractures, particularly the fifth metacarpal neck, is rarely needed. High-performance athletes may require surgical treatment to accelerate rehabilitation and allow for early range of motion.

Metacarpal shaft fractures can be transverse, oblique/spiral and comminuted.[97] Transverse fractures that are non-displaced may be treated with splinting alone.[96,97] Unstable fractures are managed with percutaneous pinning, intramedullary pinning, compression plating or lag screw fixation (Fig. 74.23a–c).[97]

Oblique and spiral fractures of the metacarpal result in both shortening and rotational malalignment.[97,100] In general, shortening of 3–4 mm is acceptable for these fractures, but no malrotation is acceptable.[100] For oblique/spiral fractures in which the fracture length is at least twice the length of the metacarpal shaft, stabilization can be achieved with several interfragmentary lag screws.[97,99,100] Short oblique/spiral fractures are treated with a combination of an

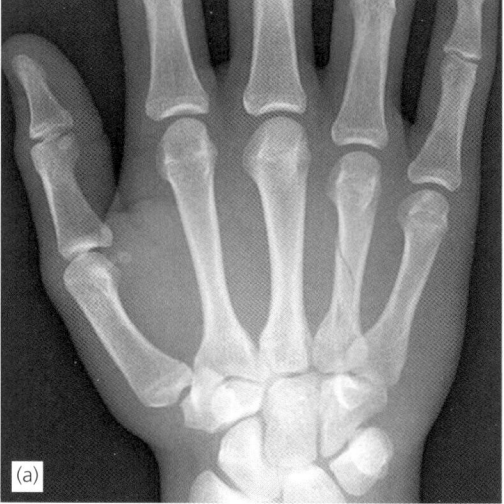
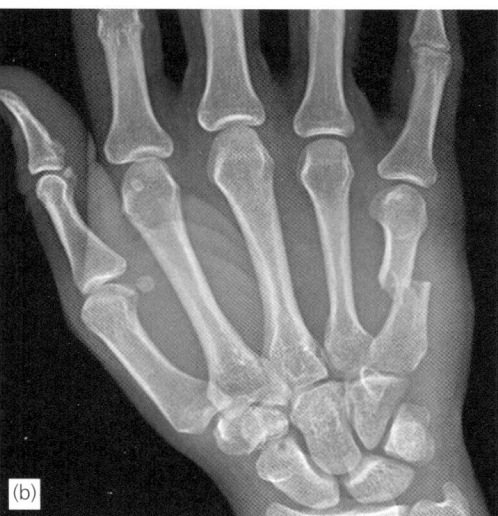
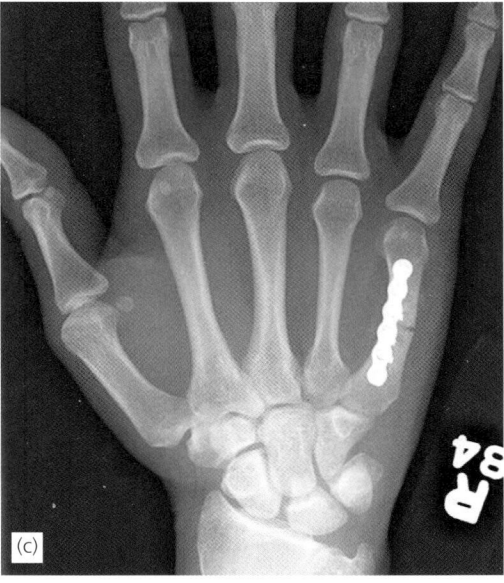

Figure 74.23 (a) Stable fourth metacarpal shaft spiral fracture. (b) Unstable displaced fifth metacarpal shaft fracture. (c) Open reduction and internal fixation fifth metacarpal shaft fracture.

interfragmentary lag screw and a dorsal neutralization plate to counteract shear and rotational stresses.[96,97]

Comminuted fractures of the metacarpal are almost always due to high-energy trauma. Associated soft-tissue injury is common, and swelling around the injury may be extensive. Typically, open reduction and rigid fixation are required for these injuries, with bone grafting becoming necessary for fractures involving more than one-third of the bone.[97]

Fractures occurring at the base of the metacarpal require careful examination to rule out intra-articular involvement.[95] The fourth and fifth metacarpals are the most commonly involved.[95] The pull of the wrist extensor tendons can act as deforming forces, leading to proximal retraction of the attached fracture fragment.[95] Fractures at the base of the fifth metacarpal may become unstable owing to the relative mobility of the joint and the pull of the extensor carpi ulnaris.[101] In these fractures, the displaced metacarpal fragment subluxes in a proximal and dorsal direction while the remaining portion of the metacarpal (usually the radial one-third) maintains its articulation with the hamate, resulting in a fracture dislocation of the fifth carpometacarpal joint.[76] This fracture is often called a 'baby Bennett's' fracture. These fractures tend to be unstable, and accordingly percutaneous pin fixation is usually required to maintain reduction.[76] Ligamentous dislocations of the fourth and fifth carpometacarpal joint occur in athletes and require urgent reduction and surgical stabilization with pin fixation.[76]

KEY LEARNING POINTS

- Lateral epicondylitis is caused by chronic repetitive micro tears of the Extensor Carpi RadialisBrevis muscle *tendon origin* resulting in healing with hypervascular fibrotic tissue.
- Medial epicondylitis is much less common than lateral epicondylitis and usually occurs from repetiviemicrotears at the musculotendinous junction of the flexor pronator mass in throwing athletes and golfers.
- Complete disruption of the ulnar collateral ligament of the elbow is seen in overhead throwing athletes. Surgical treatment *for complete tears of the ulnar collateral ligament* with reconstruction of the anterior band provides for the most reliable return to sport.
- Valgus extension overload syndrome occurs from medial side elbow laxity as the posteromedial olecranon impinges in the olecranon fossa during the deceleration phase of the throwing motion.
- Osteochondritis Dissecans lesions of the humeral articular surface should *initially* be managed conservatively unless there is completely detached articular cartilage and loose bodies.
- Posterolateral rotatory instability of the elbow (PLRI) occurs from attenuation of the Lateral ulnar collateral ligament (LUCL), most frequently from a posterolateral dislocation event.
- The scaphoid is the most commonly injured carpal bone and has an extremely tenuous blood supply to the proximal 2/3. Consideration should be given to treating even non-displaced fractures with screw fixation to prevent later displacement and promote earlier return to activity and wrist ROM.
- Hook of the hamate fractures are seen in individuals participating in racquet sports, golf, or baseball/softball. When conservative treatment fails, excision is a better treatment option than ORIF.

REFERENCES

- ● = Key primary paper
- ◆ = Major review article

◆1. Safran MR. Elbow injuries in athletes: a review. *Clinical Orthopaedics and Related Research* 1995;**310**:257–77.
2. Whaley AL, Baker CL. Lateral epicondylitis. *Clinics in Sports Medicine* 2004;**23**:677–92.
◆3. Ciccotti MG, Charlton WPH. Epicondylitis in the athlete. *Clinics in Sports Medicine* 2001;**20**:77–94.
4. Bradley JP, Petrie RS. Osteochondritis dissecans of the humeral capitellum: diagnosis and treatment. *Clinics in Sports Medicine* 2001;**20**:565–90.
5. Rosenberg N, Henderson I. Surgical treatment of resistant lateral epicondylitis. Followup study of 19 patients after excision, release, and repair of the proximal common extensor origin. *Archives of Orthopaedic and Trauma Surgery* 2002;**122**:514–17.
6. Goldberg EJ, Abraham E, Siegel I. The surgical treatment of chronic lateral humeral epicondylitis by common extensor release. *Clinical Orthopaedics and Related Research* 1988;**233**:208–12.
7. Khashaba A. Nirschl tennis elbow release with or without drilling. *British Journal of Sports Medicine* 2001;**35**:200–1.
◆8. Ciccotti MC, Schwarts MA, Ciccotti MG. Diagnosis and treatment of medial epicondylitis of the elbow. *Clinics in Sports Medicine* 2004;**23**:693–706.
9. Field LD, Savoie FH. Common elbow injuries in sport. *Sports Medicine* 1998;**26**:193–205.
10. Grana W. Medial epicondylitis and cubital tunnel syndrome in the throwing athlete. *Clinics in Sports Medicine* 2001;**20**:541–8.
11. Vangsness C, Jobe FW. Surgical technique of medial epicondylitis: results in 35 elbows. *Journal of Bone and Joint Surgery (American)* 1991;**73**:409–11.

12. Gabel GT, Morrey BT. Operative treatment of medial epicondylitis: the influence of concomitant ulnar neuropathy at the elbow. *Journal of Bone and Joint Surgery (American)* 1995;**77**:1065-9.
13. Wittenberg RH, Schaal S, Muhr G. Surgical treatment of persistent elbow epicondylitis. *Clinical Orthopaedics and Related Research* 1992;**278**:73-80.
14. Eygendaal D, Safran MR. Postero-medial elbow problems in the adult athlete. *British Journal of Sports Medicine* 2006;**40**:430-4.
◆15. Safran MR. Ulnar collateral ligament injury in the overhead athlete: diagnosis and treatment. *Clinics in Sports Medicine* 2004;**23**:643-64.
◆◆16. Hyman J, Breazeale NM, Altchek DW. Valgus instability of the elbow in athletes. *Clinics in Sports Medicine* 2001;**20**:25-46.
17. Wills AA, Thornton SJ, Altchek DA. Reconstruction of elbow ligaments in athletes. *Atlas of the Hand Clinics* 2006;**11**:125-36.
◆18. Cain EL, Dugas JR, Wolf RS, Andrews JR. Elbow injuries in throwing athletes: a current concepts review. *American Journal of Sports Medicine* 2003;**31**:621-35.
19. Barnes DA, Tullos HS. An analysis of 100 symptomatic baseball players. *American Journal of Sports Medicine* 1978;**6**:62-7.
20. Rettig AC, Sherrill C, Snead DS, et al. Nonoperative treatment of ulnar collateral ligament injuries in throwing athletes. *American Journal of Sports Medicine* 2001;**29**:7-15.
●21. Jobe FW, Stark H, Lomabrdo SJ. Reconstruction of the ulnar collateral ligament in athletes. *Journal of Bone and Joint Surgery (American)* 1986;**68A**:1158-63.
●22. Smith GR, Altchek DW, Pagnani, et al. A muscle-splitting approach to the ulnar collateral ligament of the elbow. Neuroanatomy and operative technique. *American Journal of Sports Medicine* 1996;**24**:575-80.
23. Thompson WH, Jobe FW, Yocum LA, Pink MM. Ulnar collateral ligament reconstruction in athletes: muscle splitting approach without transposition of the ulnar nerve. *Journal of Shoulder and Elbow Surgery* 2001;**10**:152-7.
●24. Rohrbough JT, Altcahek DW, Hyman J, et al. Medial collateral ligament reconstruction of the elbow using the docking technique. *American Journal of Sports Medicine* 2002;**30**:541-8.
25. Azar FM, Andrews JR, Wilk KE, Groh D. Operative treatment of ulnar collateral ligament injuries of the elbow in athletes. *American Journal of Sports Medicine* 2000;**28**:16-23.
26. Ahmad CS, ElAttrache NS. Valgus extension overload syndrome and stress injury of the olecranon. *Clinics in Sports Medicine* 2004;**23**:665-76.
27. Fideler BM, Kvitne RS, Jordan S. Posterior impingement of the elbow in professional baseball players. *Journal of Shoulder and Elbow Surgery* 1997;**6**:169-70.
28. Reddy AS, Kvitne RS, Yocum LA, et al. Arthroscopy of the elbow: a long-term clinical review. *Arthroscopy* 2000;**16**:588-94.
◆29. Rudzki JR, George AP. Juvenile and adolescent elbow injuries in sports. *Clinics in Sports Medicine* 2004;**23**:581-608.
30. Bradley JP, Petrie RS. Osteochondritis dissecans of the humeral capitellum: diagnosis and treatment. *Clinics in Sports Medicine* 2001;**20**:565-90.
31. Stubbs MJ, Field LD, Savoie FH. Osteochondritis dissecans of the elbow. *Clinics in Sports Medicine* 2001;**20**:1-10.
32. Smith JP, Savoie FH, Field LD. Posterolateral rotatory instability of the elbow. *Clinics in Sports Medicine* 2001;**20**:47-58.
33. Singleton SB, Conway JE. PLRI: posterolateral rotatory instability of the elbow. *Clinics in Sports Medicine* 2004;**23**:629-42.
◆34. Rettig AC. Athletic injuries of the wrist and hand. Part I. Traumatic injuries of the wrist. *American Journal of Sports Medicine* 2003;**31**:1038-48.
35. Haisman JM, Rohde RS, Weilan AJ. Acute fractures of the scaphoid. *Journal of Bone and Joint Surgery (American)* 2006;**88**:2750-8.
36. Rettig AC. Management of acute scaphoid fractures. *Hand Clinics* 2000;**16**:381-96.
37. Geissler WB. Carpal fractures in athletes. *Clinics in Sports Medicine* 2001;**20**:167-88.
38. Steinman SP, Adams JE. Scaphoid fractures and nonunions: diagnosis and treatment. *Journal of Orthopaedic Science* 2006;**11**:424-31.
39. Cooney WP, Dobyns JH, Linschfield RL. Nonunion of the scaphoid: analysis of the results from bone grafting. *Journal of Hand Surgery* 1980;**5**:343-54.
40. Inoue G, Shionoya K. Herbert screw fixation by limited access for acute fractures of the scaphoid. *Journal of Bone and Joint Surgery (American)* 1997;**79**:418-22.
41. Walsh IV JJ, Bishop AT. Diagnosis and management of hamate hook fractures. *Hand Clinics* 2000;**16**:397-403.
42. Vigler M, Aviles A, Lee SK. Carpal fractures excluding the scaphoid. *Hand Clinics* 2006;**22**:501-16.
◆43. Rettig AC. Athletic injuries of the wrist and hand. Part I. Traumatic injuries of the wrist. *American Journal of Sports Medicine* 2003;**31**:1038-48.
44. Lewis DM, Osterman AL. Scapholunate instability in athletes. *Clinics in Sports Medicine* 2001;**20**:131-40.
45. Cohen MS. Ligamentous injuries of the wrist in the athlete. *Clinics in Sports Medicine* 1998;**17**:533-52.
46. Linschfield RL, Dobyns JH. Athletic injuries of the wrist. *Clinical Orthopedics and Related Research* 1985;**198**:141-51.
47. Nicolaidis SC, Hildreth DH, Lichtman DM. Acute injuries of the distal radioulnar joint. *Hand Clinics* 2000;**16**:449-60.
48. Ahn AK, Chang D, Plate A. Triangular fibrocartilage complex tears. *Bulletin of the NYU Hospital of Joint Diseases* 2006;**64**:114-18.
●49. Palmer AK. Triangular fibrocartilage cartilage complex lesions: a classification. *Journal of Hand Surgery* 1989;**14**:594-606.
●50. Feldon P, Terrono AL, Belsky MR. Wafer distal ulna resection for triangular fibrocartilage tears and/or ulna impaction syndrome. *Journal of Hand Surgery* 1992;**17A**:731-7.
51. Nagle DJ. TFCC tears in athletes. *Clinics in Sports Medicine* 2001;**20**:155-66.

52. Chung CK, Zimmerman ND, Travis TT. Wrist arthrography versus arthroscopy: a comparative study of 150 cases. *Journal of Hand Surgery* 1996;**21**:591–4.
53. Schers TJ, Van Heusden HA. Evaluation of chronic wrist pain. Arthroscopy superior to arthrography: comparison in 39 patients. *Acta Orthopaedica Scandinavica* 1995;**66**:540–2.
54. Nagle DL, Benson LS. Wrist arthroscopy: indications and results. *Arthroscopy* 1992;**8**:198–203.
♦55. Nuber GW, Assenmacher J, Bowen MK. Neurovascular problems in the forearm, wrist, and hand. *Clinics in Sports Medicine* 1998;**17**:585–610.
♦56. Rettig AC. Wrist and hand overuse syndromes. *Clinics in Sports Medicine* 2001;**20**:591–611.
57. Plancher KD, Peterson RK, Steichen JB. Compressive neuropathies and tendinopathies in the athletic elbow and wrist. *Clinics in Sports Medicine* 1996;**15**:331–72.
58. Rettig AC. Wrist and hand overuse syndromes. *Clinics in Sports Medicine* 2001;**20**:591–612.
♦59. Rettig AC. Athletic injuries of the wrist and hand. Part II. Overuse injuries of the wrist and traumatic injuries to the hand. *American Journal of Sports Medicine* 2004;**32**:262–73.
60. Osterman AL, Moskow L, Low D. Soft-tissue injuries of the hand and wrist in racquet sports. *Clinics in Sports Medicine* 1988;**7**:329–48.
61. Jackson WT, Wiegas SF, Coon T. Anatomical variations in the first extensor compartment of the wrist. *Journal of Bone and Joint Surgery (American)* 1986;**68**:923–6.
62. Kiefhaber TR, Stern PJ. Upper extremity tendinitis and overuse syndromes in the athlete. *Clinics in Sports Medicine* 1992;**11**:39–56.
63. DiFiori JP, Caine DJ, Malina RM. Wrist pain, distal radial physeal injury, and ulnar variance in the young gymnast. *American Journal of Sports Medicine* 2006;**34**:840–9.
64. Linschfield RL, Dobyns JH. Athletic injuries of the wrist. *Clinical Orthopedics and Related Research* 1985;**198**:141–51.
65. Aronowitz ER, Leddy JP. Closed tendon injuries of the hand and wrist in athletes. *Clinics in Sports Medicine* 1998;**17**:449–67.
66. Leddy JP, Packer JW. Avulsion of the profundus tendon insertion in athletes. *Journal of Hand Surgery* 1977;**2**:66.
67. Tuttle HG, Olvey SP, Stern PJ. Tendon avulsion injuries of the distal phalanx. *Clinical Orthopaedics and Related Research* 2006;**445**:157–68.
68. Stamos BD, Leddy JP. Closed flexor tendon disruption in athletes. *Hand Clinics* 2000;**16**:359–65.
♦69. Rettig AC. Athletic injuries of the wrist and hand. Part II. Overuse injuries of the wrist and traumatic injuries to the hand. *American Journal of Sports Medicine* 2004;**32**:262–73.
70. Steinberg DR. Acute flexor tendon injuries. *Orthopedic Clinics of North America* 1992;**23**:25–40.
71. Boyer MI, Strickland JW, Engles DR, et al. Flexor tendon repair and rehabilitation: state of the art in 2002. *Journal of Bone and Joint Surgery* 2002;**84**:1684–706.
72. Patel MR, Shekhar SD, Bassini-Lipson L. Conservative management of chronic mallet finger. *Journal of Hand Surgery* 1986;**11**:570–3.
73. Craig EV. *Clinical Orthopaedics*. Philadelphia, PA: Lippincott Williams and Wilkins, 1999.
74. Blair WF, Steyers CM. Extensor tendon injuries. *Orthopedic Clinics of North America* 1992;**23**:141–8.
75. Scott SC. Closed injuries to the extensor mechanism of the digits. *Hand Clinics* 2000;**16**:367–73.
76. Palmer RE. Joint injuries of the hand in athletes. *Clinics in Sports Medicine* 1998;**17**:513–31.
♦77. Lee SG, Jupiter JB. Phalangeal and metacarpal fractures of the hand. *Hand Clinics* 2000;**16**:323–32.
78. Peterson JJ, Bancroft LW. Injuries of the fingers and thumbs in athletes. *Clinics in Sports Medicine* 2006;**25**:527–42.
79. Edmunds OJ. Traumatic dislocation and instability of the trapeziometacarpal joint of the thumb. *Hand Clinics* 2006;**22**:365–92.
80. Newland CC. Gamekeepers thumb. *Orthopedic Clinics of North America* 1992;**23**:41–8.
81. Kahler DM, McCue III FC. MP and PIP joint injuries of the hand including the thumb. *Clinics in Sports Medicine* 1992;**11**:57–76.
82. Garret EW, Speer KP, Kirkendall DT. *Principles and Practice of Orthopaedic Sports Medicine*. Philadelphia, PA: Lippincott Williams and Wilkins, 2000.
83. Melone CP, Beldner S, Basuk RS. Thumb collateral ligament injuries: an anatomic basis for treatment. *Hand Clinics* 2000;**16**:345–57.
84. Baskies MA, Tuckman D, Paksima N, Posner MA. A new technique for reconstruction of the ulnar collateral ligament of the thumb. *American Journal of Sports Medicine* 2007;**35**:1321–5.
●85. Stener B. Displacement of the ruptured ulnar collateral ligament of the metacarpophalangeal joint. *Journal of Bone and Joint Surgery (British)* 1962;**44B**:869–79.
86. Fairhurst M, Hansen L. Treatment of 'gamekeeper's thumb' by reconstruction of the ulnar collateral ligament. *Journal of Hand Surgery (British)* 2002;**27B**:542–5.
87. Freiberg A, Pollard BA, Macdonald MR, Duncan MJ. Management of proximal interphalangeal joint injuries. *Hand Clinics* 2006;**22**:235–42.
88. Glickel SZ, Barron OA. Proximal interphalangeal joint fracture dislocations. *Hand Clinics* 2000;**16**:333–44.
●89. Eaton RG, Malerich MM. Volar plate arthroplasty of the proximal interphalangeal joint: a review of ten years of experience. *Journal of Hand Surgery* 1980;**5**:250–68.
90. Peterson JJ, Bancroft LW. Injuries of the fingers and thumbs in athletes. *Clinics in Sports Medicine* 2006;**25**:527–42.
91. Lee SG, Jupiter JB. Phalangeal and metacarpal fractures of the hand. *Hand Clinics* 2000;**16**:323–32.
92. Culver JE, Anderson TE. Fractures of the hand and wrist in the athlete. *Clinics in Sports Medicine* 1992;**11**:101–28.
93. Capo JT, Hastings H. Metacarpal and phalangeal fractures in athletes. *Clinics in Sports Medicine* 1998;**17**:491–511.
94. Hart RG, Kleinert HE. Fingertip and nail bed injuries. *Emergency Medicine Clinics of North America* 1993;**11**:755–65.

95. Peterson JJ, Bancroft LW. Injuries of the fingers and thumbs in athletes. *Clinics in Sports Medicine* 2006;**25**:527–42.
96. Lee SG, Jupiter JB. Phalangeal and metacarpal fractures of the hand. *Hand Clinics* 2000;**16**:323–32.
◆97. Capo JT, Hastings H. Metacarpal and phalangeal fractures in athletes. *Clinics in Sports Medicine* 1998;**17**:491–511.
98. Culver JE, Anderson TE. Fractures of the hand and wrist in the athlete. *Clinics in Sports Medicine* 1992;**11**:101–28.
99. Freeland AE, Orbay JL. Extraarticular hand fractures in adults. *Clinical Orthopaedics and Related Research* 2006;**445**:133–45.
100. Kawamura K, Chung KC. Fixation choices for closed simple unstable oblique phalangeal and metacarpal fractures. *Hand Clinics* 2006;**22**:243–51.
◆101. American Society for Surgery of the Hand. *The Hand*. Rosemount, IL: American Society for Surgery of the Hand, 1990.

75

Pelvis, hip and thigh

BENJAMIN G DOMB, JW THOMAS BYRD

Introduction	772	Syndromes	775
Anatomy of the pelvis, hip and thigh	772	Disorders of bone	776
Contusions	773	Intra-articular disorders	778
Muscle strains	774	Arthroscopy	779
Bursitis	775	References	779
Nerve entrapment	775		

NATIONAL BOARD STANDARDS

- Understand important anatomical structures of the hip joint
- Describe the diagnostic and therapeutic features of soft tissue injuries of the hip
- Identify bony lesions of the hip
- Describe portals and procedures for hip arthroscopy

INTRODUCTION

Traditionally, athletic injuries of the thigh, hip and pelvis have received relatively minor attention. This is probably because of three factors. First, injuries in this area may be less common than in other areas. Second, our investigative skills including clinical assessment and imaging techniques for the hip have been less sophisticated than for other joints. Finally, until recently, there have been fewer interventional methods, both conservative and surgical, available to treat the hip.

With the advent of hip arthroscopy we have become aware of a plethora of intra-articular disorders that previously went unrecognized and largely untreated. This development, combined with improved clinical skills and advanced imaging technology, has added immensely to our understanding of the spectrum of disorders in this area.

ANATOMY OF THE PELVIS, HIP AND THIGH

Of all major joints in the body, the hip comes closest to being a true ball-and-socket joint (Fig. 75.1). Its constrained bony architecture provides it with greater stability, but less mobility, than the shoulder. The horseshoe or lunate articular surface of the acetabulum surrounds the acetabular fossa. The inferior portion of the fossa contains the acetabular attachment of the ligamentum teres. Above this is a small fat pad encased in synovium that collectively forms the pulvinar. The articular surface of the acetabulum is encompassed by the fibrocartilaginous labrum, which is contiguous with the transverse acetabular ligament bridging the fossa inferiorly.[1] In comparison with the shoulder, the labrum in the hip is of lesser importance to joint stability. Nonetheless, it is likely to be important in distributing weight-bearing forces across the joint surfaces, maintaining the suction seal of the joint and facilitating normal joint lubrication. The abduction angle of the acetabulum relative to the horizontal plane averages 35° with 20° of forward flexion.[2]

The femoral head forms two-thirds of a sphere. Medially is a bare spot, the fovea capitis, which is the femoral attachment site of the ligamentum teres. The neck shaft angle averages 130° and the femoral neck is anteverted 14° relative to the bicondylar axis at the knee.

The hip capsule comprises the stout iliofemoral ligament anteriorly, the ischial femoral ligament posteriorly

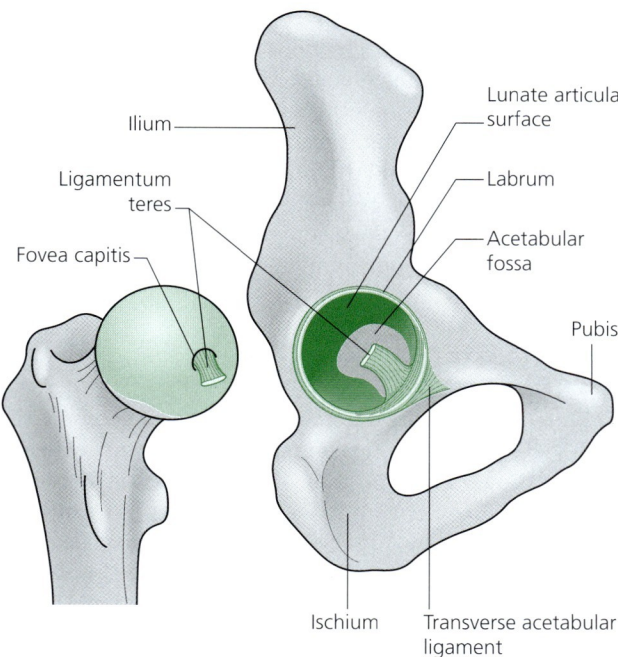

Figure 75.1 Formed from portions of the ilium, ischium and pubis, the lunate-shaped articular surface of the acetabulum surrounds the fossa containing the acetabular attachment of the ligamentum teres and fat, both encased in synovium. The labrum effectively deepens the socket and is contiguous with the transverse acetabular ligament inferiorly. The articular surface of the femoral head forms approximately two-thirds of a sphere. Medially, the ligamentum teres attaches at the fovea capitis. The diameter of the femoral neck is only 65% of the diameter of the femoral head, which allows for freer range of motion without marginal impingement. Reprinted with permission from Delilah Cohn, The Medical Illustration Studio, Nashville, TN, USA.

and the relatively weak pubofemoral ligament inferiorly. The spiralling nature of the ligamentous configuration makes the capsule taut in extension with internal rotation and relaxed when the hip is slightly flexed and externally rotated.

The intricacies of dynamic muscle function across the hip joint are quite complex. The action of individual muscles may change depending on joint position. However, conceptually understanding the relevant anatomy of the region is simplified by viewing the muscle groups as a superficial and a deep layer.[3]

The superficial layer consists of the tensor fascia lata, sartorius and gluteus maximus. The fascia lata covers the entire hip region and splits to encase both the deep and superficial surfaces of the tensor fascia lata and gluteus maximus. The tensor fascia lata and gluteus maximus distally become the iliotibial band. The gluteus maximus also has a separate insertion to the proximal femur. This fibromuscular sheath was termed the 'pelvic deltoid' by Henry,[4] reflecting how it covers the hip much as the deltoid muscle covers the shoulder. The gluteus maximus is the largest muscle in the body while the sartorius is the longest.

The gluteus medius is transitional between the superficial and deep layers with its origin superficial on the iliac crest covered by the fascia lata and its insertion deep on the greater trochanter.

The deep layer includes posterior, lateral, anterior and medial groups. Posteriorly are the piriformis, obturator internus, superior and inferior gemella, obturator externus and quadratus femoris. Laterally is the gluteus minimus. Anteriorly, the origin of the rectus femoris covers the capsule and anterior to this is the iliopsoas tendon. Medially are the adductor longus, magnus and brevis, pectineus and gracilis.

The lower extremity receives its innervation from the lumbosacral plexus, which forms the sciatic, femoral and obturator nerves as well as various smaller branches. The hip receives innervation from L2 to S1 of the plexus, but principally from L3. This explains the presence of medial thigh pain often accompanying hip pathology as symptoms may be referred to the L3 dermatome.

The femoral neurovascular structures (nerve, artery and vein) exit the pelvis under the midportion of the inguinal ligament. At the level of the hip joint, these structures lie on the anterior surface of the iliopsoas muscle, which separates them from the hip. The lateral femoral cutaneous nerve, providing sensation to the lateral thigh, exits the pelvis under the inguinal ligament, close to the anterosuperior iliac spine.

Posteriorly, 10 neurovascular structures exit the sciatic notch, including the sciatic nerve, superior and inferior gluteal nerves, and arteries. An intricate vascular anastomosis has been described providing perfusion to the femoral head that includes the ascending branch of the first perforating artery, the descending branch of the inferior gluteal artery and the transverse branches of the medial and lateral circumflex femoral arteries. However, it is the lateral retinacular vessels which are the termination of the medial circumflex femoral artery that appear to be the most essential component of the femoral head vascularity. Also contributing to the vascularity are terminal branches of the medullary artery from the shaft of the femur and, to a variable extent, the artery of the ligamentum teres, which arises from a posterior division of the obturator artery. Owing to its intra-articular isolation, the femoral head is highly dependent on this tenuous vascular supply.

CONTUSIONS

Contusions represent the most common injury of the pelvis, hip and thigh region. The severity is widely variable, but most contusions resolve with minimal intervention. The key to treatment is proper diagnosis, as some contusions may have lasting consequences if neglected or mismanaged.[5,6]

Iliac crest contusion

This is referred to as a 'hip pointer' in American football. The injury occurs from a direct blow incurred from a fall or collision. Occasionally, periostitis or exostosis may develop. In adolescents, radiographs should be carefully inspected to rule out avulsion of the iliac apophysis.

The common principles of treatment are to reduce swelling and pain and then gently implement range of motion followed by strengthening. Occasional judicious use of local corticosteroid injection has sometimes been advocated. The criterion for return to sports is full pain-free function. Additional padding over the affected area may also be helpful to prevent recurrence.

Quadriceps contusions

Common in contact and collision sports, these injuries result from a direct blow to the thigh with resultant haemorrhage and muscle fibre disruption. Myositis ossificans may also develop as a consequence of this injury.

Acute treatment consists of modalities to reduce swelling, including cold, compression, elevation and rest. Resting and immobilization with the knee in flexion maintains tension on the quadriceps muscle, which may help reduce pooling and lessen the likelihood of contracture and scar.[7] Also, during the acute phase, it is important to monitor for compartment syndrome of the thigh.[8,9] Crutches should be used as necessary until the athlete can achieve a painless, normal gait. Once the acute phase has passed, formal quadriceps rehabilitation begins with gentle range of motion and progressive strengthening.

MUSCLE STRAINS

Most commonly, strains develop from a violent eccentric force while the muscle is attempting to contract.[10,11] As with contusions, early treatment focuses on reducing pain and swelling with compression, ice, elevation and rest while maintaining normal muscle length. After subsidence of the acute symptoms, gentle flexibility followed by conditioning is implemented. Return to sport is mostly dictated by the athlete's functional performance. General guidelines include full pain-free range of motion and 90% strength. In general, reinjuries tend to be more severe and require longer recovery. Therefore, good judgement is necessary in determining when the athlete should return to play.

Hamstring strain

The hamstrings serve as hip extensors and knee flexors and are one of the most frequently injured muscle groups. A common mechanism of injury is sprinting with hip flexion and knee extension. Because of the variable locations of the musculotendinous junctions in this group, strain can occur anywhere along the posterior thigh.

Complete avulsion of the tendinous origin of the hamstrings from the ischium can also occur. For cases with chronic symptoms and dysfunction, surgical repair of the tendinous origin may result in significant improvement.[12] Some have suggested that acute repair may provide a superior functional outcome in high-level athletes.[12]

Adductor strain

Adductor injuries are especially common in soccer and ice hockey.[13] The adductor longus is the most frequently injured (Fig. 75.2). Location of the injury can be determined by careful palpation and the presence of pain with resisted adduction. Adductor involvement may also be a component of a more complex lesion reflecting breakdown of the pelvic stabilizers discussed in section Athletic pubalgia.

Rectus femoris strain

As a two-joint muscle, it is the most injury prone of the quadriceps group (Fig. 75.2). Accompanying pain will usually be elicited with either resisted hip flexion or knee extension. In general, acute injuries tend to occur distally in the thigh and chronic injuries more often near the origin at the hip. Avulsion of the anteroinferior iliac spine may also occur, especially in adolescence.[14]

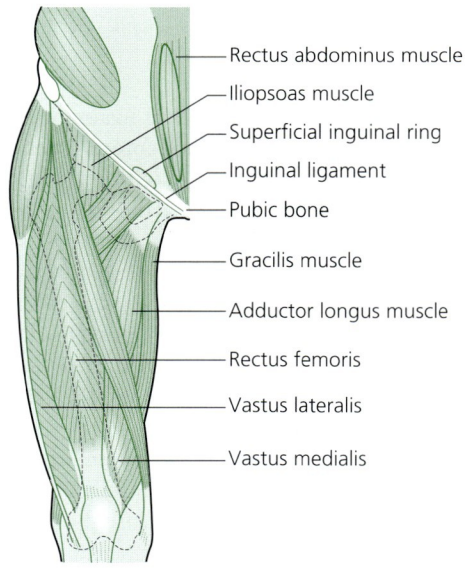

Figure 75.2 Anterior view illustrates the geographic location of the anterior and medial thigh musculature. Reprinted with permission from Brunet ME, Hontas RB. The thigh. In: DeLee JC, Drez Jr D (eds) *Orthopaedic Sports Medicine*. Philadelphia, PA: W.B. Saunders, 1994:1086–112.

Iliopsoas strain

Injury to this powerful muscle can occur but is probably not common. Careful assessment is necessary to differentiate the numerous structures that exist anterior to the hip. This can usually be distinguished from strain of the origin of the rectus femoris, which could also elicit pain with resisted hip flexion, because pain is absent with resisted knee extension.

BURSITIS

There are at least 13 consistent bursae around the hip region and numerous others that are variously present.[15] Bursitis can be a significant source of pain. This may be difficult to differentiate from other types of soft-tissue inflammation and may coexist with tendinitis/tendinosis or other friction syndromes. Inflammation of the larger bursa are usually the most clearly recognized.

Trochanteric bursitis

This condition is characterized by lateral pain and tenderness to palpation of the bursa overlying the greater trochanter. This is commonly seen in association with friction of the overlying iliotibial band, particularly in runners. More commonly encountered in females, the wide pelvis and prominent trochanter are implicated. Treatment includes oral anti-inflammatory medication, modification of the offending activities and stretching to reduce the tension of the overlying abductor mechanism. Judicious use of corticosteroid injection of the bursa is appropriate for recalcitrant cases. Rarely, bursectomy may be indicated.[16]

Iliopsoas bursitis

A common cause of anterior hip pain in athletes, this bursitis often coexists with mechanical irritation of the iliopsoas tendon. MRI may show excessive fluid within this bursa. Bursography and concomitant injection of anaesthetic and corticosteroid is diagnostic and may be therapeutic for cases unresponsive to conventional conservative treatment. When necessary, surgery is usually directed at the offending iliopsoas tendon.[17]

Ischial bursitis

This condition may be caused by direct trauma or prolonged sitting. It can be difficult to differentiate from disorders of the hamstring origin. Conservative treatment is the standard, and judicious injection may be appropriate.

NERVE ENTRAPMENT

Any nerve arising from the lumbosacral plexus may become entrapped. These disorders may present with confusing symptoms in the absence of motor or sensory deficits.[18] Treatment is sometimes controversial, but an understanding of these entities is important for an accurate assessment. A few of the more common are discussed.

Lateral femoral cutaneous nerve

This is the most easily recognized of the nerve conditions around the hip. The nerve is susceptible to compression as it exits underneath the anterior superior iliac spine and becomes superficial. This can occur from tight belts or pads or long periods of hip flexion. The condition is referred to as 'meralgia paraesthetica'. Relief from the offending activity may be helpful. Surgical release is rarely necessary.

Obturator nerve

Obturator nerve entrapment among athletes has been reported as a result of a fascial band compressing the nerve as it exits the obturator canal. Surgical release has been successfully reported in properly selected cases.[19]

Pudendal nerve

Compression of the pudendal nerve has been reported among cyclists with neuropraxia characterized by sensory loss to the perineum and impotency in severe cases.[20] The condition is usually transient, although recovery may be incomplete. This has also been reported as a complication of hip arthroscopy and other fracture management necessitating distraction on a fracture table.[21,22]

Sciatic nerve

Entrapment of the sciatic nerve may potentially occur anywhere along its course from the abdomen to the knee.[23] One recognized site is at the level of the ischial tuberosity from the fibrous edge of the biceps femoris origin. Another entity is compression of the sciatic nerve by the piriformis muscle, referred to as 'piriformis syndrome' (see below).

SYNDROMES

Snapping iliopsoas tendon

Snapping of the iliopsoas tendon is caused as it transiently lodges against the anterior femoral head and capsule or pectineal eminence while the tendon is gliding across the front of the hip and pelvic brim. The characteristic 'clunk' occurs as the hip comes from a flexed, abducted, externally rotated position towards extension with internal rotation.[24]

Most cases can be managed conservatively with a stretching programme, anti-inflammatory medications and modification of offending activities.[17] Bursography may be useful in the diagnosis, and simultaneous injection of the bursa may potentially be therapeutic. Ultrasonography is another diagnostic tool that may substantiate snapping of the tendon. Successful surgical treatment has been reported for recalcitrant cases.[25] Partial lengthening can be performed by relaxing incisions placed at the myotendinous junction. Several arthroscopic methods have been described with the advantage of addressing associated intra-articular pathology present in many cases.

Snapping iliotibial band

A snapping iliotibial band is visually quite prominent and can usually be actively demonstrated by the patient while standing. The patient may feel like the hip is subluxing, and this may be suggested by the visual appearance, but it is rarely the case. Treatment focuses on conservative measures including stretching, conditioning, modalities to reduce inflammation, and modification of the offending activities. Failing these measures, selective corticosteroid injection within the trochanteric bursa may be appropriate. Success has been described with a variety of surgical procedures for recalcitrant cases.[26–28] The common principle is relaxation of the tendinous portion directly overlying the greater trochanter.

Piriformis syndrome

This relatively uncommon condition is thought to result from compression of the sciatic nerve by the piriformis muscle.[29] Typically, this results in sciatica-type symptoms that may culminate in an unrewarding work-up of the lumbar spine. The term piriformis syndrome is often inaccurately used to describe many causes of poorly defined posterior hip pain. Many other posterior soft-tissue structures can be injured or painful in the absence of involvement of the piriformis.

Palpation for posterior tenderness is performed and symptoms may be provoked with either resisted external rotation or passive internal rotation of the extended hip. The most characteristic examination finding is when symptoms are elicited by direct palpation of the piriformis muscle against the anterior sacrum on either rectal or vaginal examination.

Treatment is conservative but surgical release of the piriformis tendon and decompression of the sciatic nerve has been reported with successful results in properly selected cases.[30,31] With surgery, it is important to be aware of the numerous anomalous variations that exist between the piriformis and sciatic nerve, including interdigitation of the two, which requires careful exploration both to ensure adequate decompression and to avoid iatrogenic injury.

Athletic pubalgia

This condition results from either acute macrotrauma or repetitive microtrauma to the region constituting the insertion of the rectus abdominis and the origin of the hip abductors at the pubis.[32] This entity is increasingly diagnosed in ice hockey and soccer, as well as other elite-level sports in which the typical mechanism of injury is common.

The diagnosis is usually based on a high index of suspicion when pain localized to this area remains unresponsive to conservative treatment. Investigative studies are usually unrevealing, although MRI is becoming more sensitive at detecting signal changes within the substance of the tendon.

For recalcitrant cases, surgical exploration with repair of the pelvic floor, including the rectus abdominis and release of the adductor longus, has met with successful results in high-performance athletes.[33] The results in lower demand individuals have been less predictable.

DISORDERS OF BONE

Fractures

Proximal femoral fractures which are common in an elderly population have distinct characteristics in an active younger adult population. More violent force is necessary to sustain the injury. Consequently, there is greater associated soft-tissue trauma and concern for complications, including avascular necrosis and non-union. Anatomic reduction and rigid fixation of these fractures is paramount to achieving a good outcome.[34]

Hip fractures in children are uncommon and result only from severe trauma unless a pathological process is present. A unique entity is the slipped capital femoral epiphysis, which may occur spontaneously or with a relatively minor precipitating injury. Prompt and accurate assessment is essential to an optimal outcome. The hip should always be considered as a potential source of referred symptoms in any child with thigh or knee pain. Another condition which may coincidentally present in active young children is Legg–Calvé–Perthes disease.

Dislocation/subluxation

Similarly to femoral fractures in athletes, dislocation of the hip usually requires a very violent force. The importance of prompt treatment and assurance of a concentric reduction is well documented. Avascular necrosis, a recognized consequence of this injury, may also occur with traumatic subluxation in the absence of a complete dislocation episode.[35,36]

Stress fractures

Femoral neck stress fractures are, in general, the most concerning because of the risk of propagating a displaced fracture. Stress fractures of this region may initiate from the medial or lateral side and the treatment strategy differs. Stress fractures of the lateral neck involve the tensile surface and represent a fracture at risk. Early surgical stabilization is recommended because of the high risk of displacement.[37,38] Medial neck stress fractures are on the compressive surface of the bone and inherently more stable. Conservative treatment is an appropriate option. It is imperative that the patient be kept below the threshold of symptoms, which may obligate protected weight bearing with crutches for a period of time. Surgical fixation is generally reserved for patients with symptoms that do not respond promptly to conservative measures. Healing will typically require 3–6 months before activity modifications can be lifted.

Stress fractures of the femoral shaft can usually be managed conservatively, but still require some caution because of potential displacement.[39] Again, whether the lesion involves the compressive or tensile cortex will partially determine the necessary precautions. Stress fractures of the pelvis can occur, including the sacrum and pubis. The diagnosis can be easily made with clinical suspicion and imaging studies. Caution is sometimes necessary not to misinterpret these as neoplastic lesions.

Avulsion fractures

These injuries are most commonly seen in adolescent males. At this age, these apophyseal avulsion injuries occur because the physis is the weakest site, having not yet closed, while muscle power has markedly increased in conjunction with the appearance of androgenous hormones. As with musculotendinous strains, the injury is usually the result of a sudden ballistic manoeuvre with accompanying eccentric loading of the tendinous insertion site to bone. The diagnosis is usually evident based on the clinical assessment and radiographic findings. The amount of initial displacement rarely widens over time, although follow-up radiographs may be prudent. Sites of involvement, in order of decreasing frequency, include the antero superior iliac spine, ischium, lesser trochanter, antero inferior iliac spine, iliac crest and greater trochanter. Treatment of these injuries is generally non-operative with an excellent prognosis for return to unrestricted activities.[40] Surgery has occasionally been advocated for severely displaced fractures, but there is no evidence of a superior outcome over conservative management. Crutches are often necessary to develop a painless gait. Gentle range of motion and conditioning are implemented as symptoms allow. Return to unrestricted sports can be anticipated within 6–10 weeks, depending on location, severity of injury and age of the athlete.

Apophysitis

Apophysitis may occur anywhere within the hip girdle, but the most common site of involvement is the iliac crest. This generally represents an overuse phenomenon, although the onset of symptoms may be acute, or associated with a period of intense activity. The diagnosis may be purely clinical, characterized by pain and tenderness to palpation along the iliac crest in a skeletally immature patient. With chronic involvement, radiographs may demonstrate slight asymmetrical physeal widening on the side of involvement. Treatment is symptomatic, principally modifying offending activities while the discomfort subsides.

Osteonecrosis

Osteonecrosis (avascular necrosis) of the femoral head may be causally related to trauma, especially dislocation or subluxation of the hip.[36] However, it may also occur coincidentally in active individuals. It may be idiopathic, but a search should be made for other causative factors (i.e. alcohol abuse, catabolic steroids, decompression sickness, etc.) Radiographs will vary from normal to advanced collapse depending on the stage of the disease. MRI is important for both diagnosis and accurate staging.

Osteitis pubis

This disorder of the symphysis pubis occurs as a consequence of repetitive trauma. It may occur with any intense activity, but is seen with greatest frequency in soccer, hockey and running. Examination is characterized by tenderness localized to the region of the symphysis but there may be accompanying tenderness or spasm within the adductor musculature. With chronic cases, radiographs will show irregularities around the symphysis, including both cystic formation and sclerosis. Radionuclide scanning will reveal increased activity and MRI may show surrounding oedema. However, some degree of caution is necessary, as all of these findings may be variously present, in minimally symptomatic individuals. Treatment includes rest, anti-inflammatory medication and local modalities. Occasional judicious use of local corticosteroid injection has been advocated for recalcitrant conditions.[41] Resolution can be expected in most cases, but the period of morbidity may be several months. Surgery may be considered as a salvage situation for chronic intractable symptoms.

Various techniques have been described but only with small series and variable results.

Tumours

The pelvis and hip account for about 10–15% of all primary musculoskeletal tumours. Secondary malignancies have a similar predilection for this area, but the overall likelihood of metastatic disease is exceedingly greater, especially among older adults. Although benign and malignant neoplasms around the hip are uncommon, they must be considered in cases of unexplained pain or circumstances in which the episode of trauma may seem trivial or coincidental. Because of the deeply situated anatomy of this area, lesions may gain considerable size before they are noticed by the patient or are discernible on examination. Thus, a high index of suspicion is always important, and early and prompt referral to an experienced musculoskeletal oncologist is warranted.

INTRA-ARTICULAR DISORDERS

Loose bodies

Symptomatic loose bodies may occur as a result of trauma or disease such as synovial chondromatosis. The importance of removal has been well documented by Epstein[42] in order to slow the secondary damage incurred by third-body wear. Most sizeable loose bodies can be diagnosed with various imaging techniques, especially with CT or MRI arthrography. Arthroscopic removal represents an excellent alternative to traditional open methods.[43]

Labral tears

Labral tears represent a significant source of mechanical hip pain (Fig. 43.3a,b). Tears may be degenerative or traumatic. Even in the presence of a clear history of trauma, suspect that there may have been some predisposition to tearing such as the morphology of the labrum or underlying degeneration. There is a particularly high incidence of labral anomalies and tearing in the presence of acetabular dysplasia. Arthroscopic debridement of labral tears can produce gratifying results and labral repairs are starting to find a role.[44–46] However, sometimes the response may be more modulated by accompanying degenerative disease or uncertain circumstances. Surgically addressing underlying bony abnormalities may be important in preventing return of symptoms. Both high-resolution MRI and gadolinium MRI are steadily improving at recognizing this diagnosis.

Femoroacetabular impingement

Increasingly recognized as a source of pain in athletes and as a potential cause of labral tears and cartilage degeneration, femoroacetabular impingement takes two main forms: cam and pincer impingement. In cam impingement, an aspherical femoral head causes abnormal forces and eventually damage to the labrum and peripheral cartilage of the acetabulum. In pincer impingement, the femoral neck abuts an overhanging acetabular rim during joint motion, leading to tears of the labrum.[47,48] Open and arthroscopic means of correcting these deformities have met with successful relief of symptoms and return to sport.[49–52]

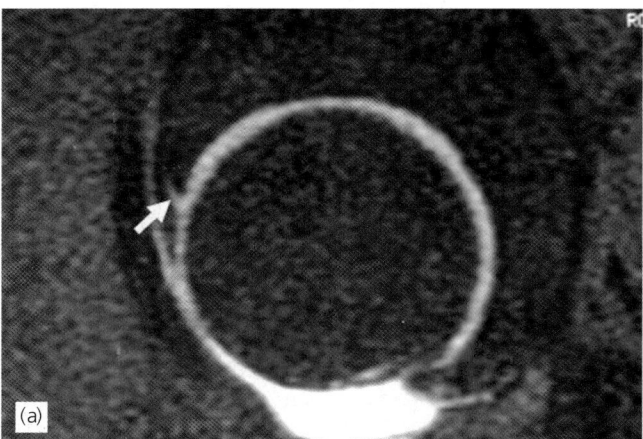
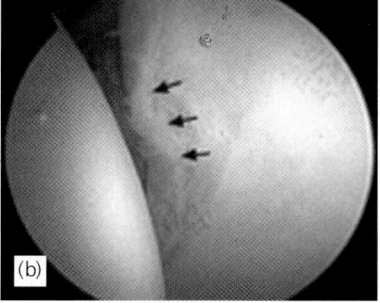

Figure 75.3 A 27 year old woman with pain and catching of the left hip. (a) Sagittal image MRI with gadolinium arthrography reveals a tear of the anterior labrum (arrow). (b) Arthroscopic view illustrates the tear of the anterior labrum at the articular labral junction (arrows). Reprinted with permission from Byrd JWT. Thigh, hip and pelvis. In: Miller MD, Cooper DE, Warner JJP (eds) *Review of Sports Medicine and Arthroscopy* 2nd edn. Philadelphia, PA: W.B. Saunders, 2005:114–39.

Chondral injuries

Chondral injuries exist on a spectrum from acute isolated fragments to diffuse degenerative disease. Current MRI technology will occasionally reveal articular surface defects, but in general is poor at discerning the extent of articular involvement. Acute traumatic fragments are increasingly recognized as a cause of recalcitrant mechanical hip pain and respond well to excision. The long-term prognosis of these lesions is still concerning. Microfracture of the subchondral bone may be effective for focal lesions.[53]

Ruptured ligamentum teres

Rupture of the ligament uniformly accompanies dislocation of the hip. However, rupture can also occur as a consequence of a twisting injury or subluxation episode in the absence of dislocation.[54] The ruptured portion can catch within the joint and be a significant source of mechanical hip pain. MRI may suggest involvement of the ligamentum teres, but is rarely conclusive. Arthroscopic debridement of the ruptured portion can result in pronounced symptomatic improvement.[55] The vessel of the ligamentum teres may contribute to the vascularity of the femoral head. However, it is unlikely that debridement of the ruptured portion would have any adverse effect on the head's viability.

ARTHROSCOPY

Arthroscopy of the hip is a well-established method with numerous reports highlighting its efficacy. The constrained ball-and-socket architecture of the joint, the dense surrounding soft-tissue envelope and the thick capsule with limited compliance provide unique challenges for arthroscopy. Nonetheless, these challenges can be overcome by adherence to the basic principles of the technique.

For obvious forms of pathology, such as symptomatic loose bodies, arthroscopy offers an excellent alternative to traditional open techniques necessary in the past. Perhaps more importantly, arthroscopy offers a less invasive method of treatment for many elusive forms of intra-articular pathology that previously went untreated and often unrecognized.

KEY LEARNING POINTS

- Anatomy of the pelvis, hip and thigh, including bony, soft-tissue and neurovascular anatomy.
- Conservative treatment of common sites of contusions including the iliac crest and quadriceps.
- Mechanism and treatment options for muscles most commonly involved in strain injuries including hamstring, adductors, rectus femoris and, iliopsoas.
- Signs and symptoms of trochanteric, iliopsoas and ischial bursitis.
- Syndromes involving the pelvis, hip and thigh such as internal and external snapping hip, piriformis syndrome and athletic pubalgia.
- Common disorders of bone in the athletic population including fracture, stress fracture and osteitis pubis.
- Spectrum of intra-articular hip disorders involved in sports medicine including labral tears and FAI.
- Basic principles for application of arthroscopy in the hip region.

REFERENCES

- ● = Key primary paper
- ◆ = Major review article

1. Agur AMR. *Grant's Atlas of Anatomy*, 10th edn. Baltimore: Williams & Wilkins, 1999.
2. Byrd JWT. Gross anatomy. In: Byrd JWT (ed.) *Operative Hip Arthroscopy*. New York, NY: Thieme, 1998;69–82.
3. Hoppenfeld S, deBoer P. *Surgical Exposures in Orthopaedics: The Anatomic Approach*, 2nd edn. Philadelphia, PA: J.B. Lippincott, 1994.
4. Henry AK. *Extensile Exposure*, 2nd edn. New York, NY: Churchill Livingstone, 1973.
●5. Crisco JJ, Jokl P, Heinen GT, *et al*. A muscle contusion injury model. Biomechanics, physiology, and histology. *American Journal of Sports Medicine* 1994;**22**:702–10.
●6. Jackson DW, Feagin JA. Quadriceps contusions in young athletes. Relation of severity of injury to treatment and prognosis. *Journal of Bone and Joint Surgery (American)* 1973;**55**:95–105.
◆7. Ryan JB, Wheeler JH, Hopkinson WJ, *et al*. Quadriceps contusions. West Point update. *American Journal of Sports Medicine* 1991;**19**:299–304.
●8. Rooser B, Bengtson S, Hagglund G. Acute compartment syndrome from anterior thigh muscle contusion: a report of eight cases. *Journal of Orthopaedic Trauma* 1991;**5**:57–9.
9. Winternitz Jr WA, Metheny JA, Wear LC. Acute compartment syndrome of the thigh in sports-related injuries not associated with femoral fractures. *American Journal of Sports Medicine* 1992;**20**:476–7.
10. Best TM. Muscle-tendon injuries in young athletes. *Clinics in Sports Medicine* 1995;**14**:669–86.
11. Gross RH. Acute musculotendinous injuries. In: Stanitski CL, DeLee JC, Drez DJ (eds) *Pediatric and Adult Sports Medicine*. Philadelphia, PA: W.B. Saunders, 1994:131–43.
12. Cohen S, Bradley J. Acute proximal hamstring rupture. *Journal of the American Academy of Orthopaedic Surgeons* 2007;**15**:350–5.

- 13. Merrifield HH, Cowan RF. Groin strain injuries in ice hockey. *Journal of Sports Medicine* 1973;**1**(2):41-2.
14. Hughes 4th CT, Hasselman CT, Best TM, *et al.* Incomplete, intrasubstance strain injuries of the rectus femoris muscle. *American Journal of Sports Medicine* 1995;**23**:500-6.
15. Gross ML, Nasser S, Finerman GAM. Hip and pelvis. In: DeLee JC, Drez Jr D (eds) *Orthopaedic Sports Medicine*. Philadelphia, PA: W.B. Saunders, 1994:1063-85.
- 16. Baker Jr CL, Massie RV, Hurt WG, Savory CG. Arthroscopic bursectomy for recalcitrant trochanteric bursitis. *Arthroscopy* 2007;**23**:827-32.
- 17. Byrd JW. Evaluation and management of the snapping iliopsoas tendon. *Instructional Course Lectures* 2006;**55**:347-55.
18. McCrory P, Bell S. Nerve entrapment syndromes as a cause of pain in the hip, groin and buttock. *Sports Medicine* 1999;**27**:261-74.
19. Bradshaw C, McCrory P, Bell S, *et al.* Obturator nerve entrapment. A cause of groin pain in athletes. *American Journal of Sports Medicine* 1997;**25**:402-8.
20. Weiss BD. Clinical syndromes associated with bicycle seats. *Clinics in Sports Medicine* 1994;**13**:175-86.
- 21. Hofmann A, Jones RE, Schoenvogel R. Pudendal-nerve neurapraxia as a result of traction on the fracture table. A report of four cases. *Journal of Bone and Joint Surgery (American)* 1982;**64**:136-8.
- 22. Clarke MT, Arora A, Villar RN. Hip arthroscopy: complications in 1054 cases. *Clinical Orthopaedics and Related Research* 2003;**406**:84-8.
23. Puranen J, Orava S. The hamstring syndrome. A new diagnosis of gluteal sciatic pain. *American Journal of Sports Medicine* 1988;**16**:517-21.
- 24. Allen WC, Cope R. Coxa saltans: the snapping hip revisited. *Journal of the American Academy of Orthopaedic Surgeons* 1995;**3**:303-8.
- 25. Ilizaliturri Jr VM, Villalobos FE Jr, Chaidez PA, *et al.* Internal snapping hip syndrome: treatment by endoscopic release of the iliopsoas tendon. *Arthroscopy* 2005;**21**:1375-80.
26. Brignall CG, Stainsby GD. The snapping hip. Treatment by Z-plasty. *Journal of Bone and Joint Surgery (British)* 1991;**73**:253-4.
27. Byrd JWT. Snapping hip. *Operative Techniques in Sports Medicine* 2005;**13**:46-54.
28. Ilizaliturri VM, Martinez-Escalante FA, Chaidez PA, Camacho-Galindo J. Endoscopic iliotibial band release for external snapping hip syndrome. *Arthroscopy* 2006;**22**:505-10.
- 29. Parziale JR, Hudgins TH, Fishman LM. The piriformis syndrome. *American Journal of Orthopedics* 1996;**25**:819-23.
- 30. Benson ER, Schutzer SF. Posttraumatic piriformis syndrome: diagnosis and results of operative treatment. *Journal of Bone and Joint Surgery (American)* 1999;**81**:941-9.
31. Byrd JWT. Piriformis syndrome. *Operative Techniques in Sports Medicine* 2005;**13**:71-9.
- 32. Taylor DC. Abdominal musculature abnormalities as a cause of groin pain in athletes. *American Journal of Sports Medicine* 1991;**19**:421.
- 33. Meyers WC, Foley DP, Garrett WE, *et al.* Management of severe lower abdominal or inguinal pain in high-performance athletes. PAIN (Performing Athletes with Abdominal or Inguinal Neuromuscular Pain Study Group). *American Journal of Sports Medicine* 2000;**28**:2-8.
34. Canale ST, Beaty JH, Pelvic and hip fractures. In: Rockwood Jr CA, Wilkins KE, Beaty JH (eds) *Fractures in Children*, 4th edn. Philadelphia, PA: Lippincott-Raven, 1996:1109-93.
35. Moorman CT, Warren RF, Hershman EB, *et al.* Traumatic posterior hip subluxation in American football. *Journal of Bone and Joint Surgery (American)* 2003;**85A**:1190-6.
- 36. Cooper DE, Warren RF, Barnes R. Traumatic subluxation of the hip resulting in aseptic necrosis and chondrolysis in a professional football player. *American Journal of Sports Medicine* 1991;**19**:322-4.
37. Boden BP, Speer KP. Femoral stress fractures. *Clinics in Sports Medicine* 1997;**16**:307-17.
38. Fullerton Jr LR, Snowdy HA. Femoral neck stress fractures. *American Journal of Sports Medicine* 1988;**16**:365-77.
39. Johnson AW, Weiss Jr CB, Wheeler DL. Stress fractures of the femoral shaft in athletes: more common than expected. A new clinical test. *American Journal of Sports Medicine* 1994;**22**:248-56.
40. Paletta Jr GA, Andrish JT. Injuries about the hip and pelvis in the young athlete. *Clinics in Sports Medicine* 1995;**14**:591-628.
- 41. Holt MA, Keene JS, Graf BK, *et al.* Treatment of osteitis pubis in athletes. Results of corticosteroid injections. *American Journal of Sports Medicine* 1995;**23**:601-6.
42. Epstein HC. Posterior fracture-dislocations of the hip; long-term follow-up. *Journal of Bone and Joint Surgery (American)* 1974;**56**:1103-27.
- 43. Byrd JW. Hip arthroscopy for posttraumatic loose fragments in the young active adult: three case reports. *Clinical Journal of Sport Medicine* 1996;**6**:129-33; discussion 133-4.
- 44. Robertson WJ, Kadrmas WR, Kelly BT. Arthroscopic management of labral tears in the hip: a systematic review of the literature. *Clinical Orthopaedics and Related Research* 2007;**455**:88-92.
- 45. Byrd JW, Jones KS. Prospective analysis of hip arthroscopy with 2-year follow-up. *Arthroscopy* 2000;**16**:578-87.
46. Farjo LA, Glick JM, Sampson TG. Hip arthroscopy for acetabular labral tears. *Arthroscopy* 1999;**15**:132-7.
47. Beck M, Kalhor M, Leunig M, Ganz R. Hip morphology influences the pattern of damage to the acetabular cartilage: femoroacetabular impingement as a cause of early osteoarthritis of the hip. *Journal of Bone and Joint Surgery (British)* 2005;**87B**:1012-18.

◆48. Lavigne M, Parvizi J, Beck M, et al. Anterior femoroacetabular impingement. Part I. Techniques of joint preserving surgery. *Clinical Orthopaedics and Related Research* 2004;**418**:61–6.

●49. Beck M, Leunig M, Parvizi J, et al. Anterior femoroacetabular impingement. Part II. Midterm results of surgical treatment. *Clinical Orthopaedics and Related Research* 2004;**418**:67–73.

●50. Ganz R, Gill TJ, Gautier E, et al. Surgical dislocation of the adult hip a technique with full access to the femoral head and acetabulum without the risk of avascular necrosis. *Journal of Bone and Joint Surgery (British)* 2001;**83**:1119–24.

51. Beaule PE, Le Duff MJ, Zaragoza E. Quality of life following femoral head-neck osteochondroplasty for femoroacetabular impingement. *Journal of Bone and Joint Surgery (American)* 2007;**89**:773–9.

52. Philippon M, Schenker M, Briggs K, Kuppersmith D. Femoroacetabular impingement in 45 professional athletes: associated pathologies and return to sport following arthroscopic decompression. *Knee Surgery, Sports Traumatology, Arthroscopy* 2007;**15**:908–14.

53. Enseki KR, Martin RL, Draovitch P, et al. The hip joint: arthroscopic procedures and postoperative rehabilitation. *Journal of Orthopaedic and Sports Physical Therapy* 2006;**36**:516–25.

●54. Gray AJ, Villar RN. The ligamentum teres of the hip: an arthroscopic classification of its pathology. *Arthroscopy* 1997;**13**:575–8.

●55. Byrd JW, Jones KS. Traumatic rupture of the ligamentum teres as a source of hip pain. *Arthroscopy* 2004;**20**:385–91.

76

Diagnosis and treatment of non-ligamentous knee injuries

SAMIR G TEJWANI, JESSICA E ELLERMAN, FREDDIE H FU

Introduction	782	Meniscus injury	785
Synovial disease	782	Cartilage injury	788
Pathological plica	783	Extensor mechanism	791
Synovial chondromatosis	783	References	797
Pigmented villonodular synovitis	784		

NATIONAL BOARD STANDARDS

- Define synovial lesions of the knee and describe treatment techniques
- Describe the key diagnostic tests and treatment principles for meniscal injuries
- Understand different treatment options for articular cartilage injuries
- Describe key findings for extensor mechanism injuries and define treatment goals

INTRODUCTION

Non-ligamentous knee injuries represent a large variety of intra-articular and extra-articular pathologies, which often present with similar subjective complaints and symptoms, but differ significantly in examination findings and management. The focus of this chapter will be to review conditions within this group, including synovial disease, cartilage injury, meniscus injury, extensor mechanism problems and closed degloving injury.

SYNOVIAL DISEASE

Mature synovial membrane is pale pink and lines all surfaces of the joint space, excluding articular cartilage and fibrocartilaginous structures.[1,2] Synovium is composed of a thin layer of synovial cells, or synoviocytes, known as the intimal layer, above a fibrovascular subintimal layer, which contains arterioles, fat and connective tissue cells.[1,3] The intimal layer consists of cells with macrophage function (synovial A cells) and those with a synthesizing function (synovial B cells).

Synovial disease can be present in both traumatic and atraumatic situations, leading to gross and microscopic morphological changes. Synovium can become opaque (osteoarthritis), reddish brown (pigmented villonodular synovitis (PVNS), haemophilia, haemarthrosis) or villous (inflammatory arthritides, osteoarthritis, septic arthritis). White foci or soft-tissue calcifications can be present in synovial chondromatosis, gout and crystalline pyrophosphate deposition. Diagnosing synovial disease can be difficult due to the overlap of symptoms such as diffuse pain, effusion, locking and instability with those of mechanical derangements such as meniscal and ligament tears. Thus, a meticulous history, physical examination, radiographs and often MRI are required in the work-up in order to make an accurate diagnosis.

PATHOLOGICAL PLICA

Plicae represent normal variants of knee synovium. As remnants of the mesenchymal tissue occupying the space between the distal femoral and proximal tibial epiphyses, their incomplete resorption can leave synovial pleats in any area of the knee.[4] Most commonly, plicae present in the superior and inferior aspect of the knee (50–65%), without clinical relevance. Lateral plicae are rare (1–3%), whereas medial plicae are present in autopsies in 25–33% of knees.[5–7] In most knees plicae are asymptomatic. However, chronic inflammation secondary to direct trauma, repetitive activity, kneeling or pathological synovial conditions can result in focal pain, oedema and loss of normal synovial elasticity.

Medial plica syndrome is most common in young adults, typically occurring after blunt trauma to the knee.[5] In these cases the plica becomes fibrotic, thickened and eventually symptomatic as it abrades the femoral condyle in extension and the patella in flexion. This ultimately can lead to secondary symptomatic inflammatory synovitis and articular cartilage wear.[4,5,8,9] Patients with medial plica syndrome typically report medial peri-patellar pain located above the joint line, most commonly exacerbated by repeated flexion and extension. Non-specific history and examination findings include crepitus, popping, snapping, catching, pseudolocking and effusion. Clinical findings can mimic those of medial meniscus tear, chondral injury or patellar instability, and therefore the knee should be carefully evaluated for these conditions.[10] A superficial, palpable, painful cord medial to the patella, when present, is essentially pathognomonic for this pathological condition.[5]

MRI and arthroscopy can aid in the diagnosis of a plica, although a thorough history and physical examination are needed to elucidate the clinical significance. Axial multiplanar gradient-recalled MRI images have a sensitivity and specificity of 73% and 78%, respectively, in identifying the lesion. Sagittal T_2-weighted images have a sensitivity and specificity of 71% and 83%, and combining the two techniques increases the sensitivity to 95%.[8]

The clinical significance of plicae in other locations is unclear. Suprapatellar plica syndrome has been described as chronic, intermittent dull pain at the superior portion of the knee, aggravated by climbing stairs or prolonged sitting. Additional findings can include local tenderness, a palpable superomedial band and audible snapping, potentially representing a variant of medial plica syndrome.[5,11] Similarly, physical examination often cannot accurately diagnose the cause of these non-specific symptoms and thus MRI and arthroscopy are valuable in making the diagnosis. Signs and symptoms common to a lateral patellar plica include pain above the lateral joint line and snapping, resulting in examination findings of lateral tenderness and occasionally a palpable cord.[5] In general, lateral peri-patellar plicae are typically thin and asymptomatic.

Once the diagnosis of a symptomatic plica is confirmed based upon history, physical examination and possibly MRI, initial non-surgical treatment is generally preferable. Options include activity modification, oral anti-inflammatory medications, massage, cryotherapy, ultrasound, hamstring stretching, physiotherapy and electrophoresis.[4] Additionally, combination injection of anaesthetic mixed with steroid directly into the plica intra-articularly can be performed for diagnostic and therapeutic purposes.[4,12] Refractory cases are treated with arthroscopic resection of the plica to its base, and generally result in symptomatic relief within days[4,13,14] (Fig. 76.1a,b). Simply incising the plica fold, as opposed to complete resection, should be avoided, as plicae have a tendency to heal and cause persistent symptoms.[4,5,12]

SYNOVIAL CHONDROMATOSIS

First described by Jaffe in 1958, synovial chondromatosis, also known as synovial osteochondromatosis, is a monoarticular condition affecting men and women equally from the third to fifth decade of life, most commonly in the knee.[15] As a dynamic tissue, the synovium is capable of proliferation, and, in some cases, of undergoing metaplasia to cartilage.[16] As part of the disease process, metaplastic foci typically remain fixed as part of the joint capsule; however, these bodies may vary in number and detach.[15,17] The three temporal phases of synovial chondromatosis include (1) active intrasynovial disease without loose bodies, (2) transitional lesions with both active intrasynovial

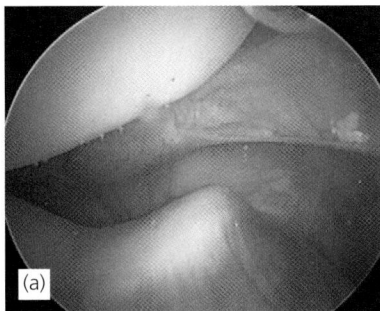 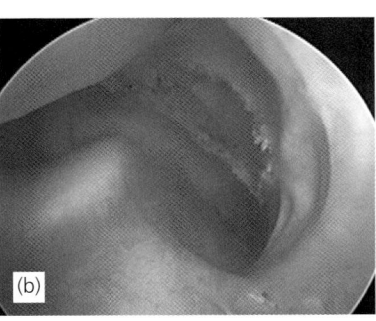

Figure 76.1 Right knee medial plica. (a) A 70° arthroscope placed in the superolateral portal reveals a prominent medial plica interposed between the patella (above) and femoral trochlea (below). (b) The medial plica has been resected with an arthroscopic shaver to its synovial base.

proliferation and free loose bodies, and (3) multiple free osteochondral bodies with no evidence of intrasynovial disease.[17,18]

Patients with synovial chondromatosis tend to present without a history of trauma or overuse.[18,19] Diagnosis can be difficult due to a multitude of non-specific complaints, including swelling, pain and stiffness. Flexion contracture may be present, along with findings of tenderness, effusion and crepitus.[18] Radiographs may reveal multiple radiopaque loose bodies; however, definitive diagnosis has traditionally required histological confirmation from synovial biopsy.[18,20] In the setting of normal radiographs, patterns of lobulated intra-articular signals consistent with hyaline cartilage are discernable on MRI, suggesting the diagnosis.[18,21] Three distinct MR patterns have been described: (a) lobulated homogeneous intra-articular masses isointense to muscle on T_1-weighted and hyperintense on T_2-weighted images, (b) pattern a plus foci of signal void on all pulse sequences representing the calcification, (c) patterns a and b plus foci of peripheral low signal surrounding fat-like signal corresponding to ossification.[22,23]

Coolican and Dandy[24] described three distinct arthroscopic appearances of synovial chondromatosis: deep lesions (normal synovium overlying lesions), superficial lesions (cartilage fragments attached to synovial fringes or partly covered by synovium) and free cartilage fragments (normal synovium, only fragments). For the benefit of symptomatic relief and increased function, complete synovectomy and removal of loose bodies are mainstay treatment options. Arthroscopic debridement is generally effective; however, large masses may develop in the posterior capsule that are amenable only to open surgical excision. Although isolated loose bodies rarely recur, extensive multifocal synovial involvement is difficult to eradicate. Rates of recurrence caused by inadequate removal of loose bodies have been estimated to be as high as 15%, with repeat arthroscopic synovectomy generally being successful.[18,25]

It is important to note that, although rare, dedifferentiation of synovial chondromatosis to a low-grade chondrosarcoma is possible.[22,26,27] In these cases, tissue biopsy demonstrates loss of growth patterns typical of synovial chondromatosis, myxoid matrix changes, necrosis and peripheral spindling of chondroid lobules, suggestive of malignancy.[26] Because there is a large sampling error with needle biopsy, malignant transformation should be suspected in chronic stable cases with a sudden exacerbation of symptoms. Treatment of chondrosarcoma should be performed in conjunction with an oncology team; specific management is beyond the scope of this chapter.

PIGMENTED VILLONODULAR SYNOVITIS

Pigmented villonodular synovitis (PVNS) is a synovial proliferative disorder characterized by hypertrophic villous and/or focal nodular changes, in addition to haemosiderin deposition.[22,28] PVNS is typically monoarticular or found in tendon sheaths, with the knee being the most commonly affected joint.[29] Granowitz et al.[30] first classified PVNS into two distinct clinical forms, diffuse and localized, in 1976. Additional subtypes have since been described, including loose body, localized pedunculated nodule, aggregates of nodules confined to one compartment, diffuse synovial involvement and synovial disease extending into the bursa.[16,31]

The annual incidence of PVNS as a whole remains rare at 1.8 per million persons.[32,33] Men and women are equally affected, with disease onset typically occurring in the third or fourth decade of life.[34] The more common diffuse form of PVNS (75%) characteristically involves the entire synovial lining of the affected joint, whereas the localized form (25%) consists of nodules or pedunculated masses of synovial lining.[35] While its exact pathophysiology remains unknown, PVNS is thought to be a benign neoplastic process, an inflammatory hyperplasia or a reaction to repeated trauma or haemorrhage.[22] Atypical variants of PVNS have been observed, including primary malignant and transformed benign PVNS, substantiating the neoplastic capacity of the lesion. Additionally, recent studies on ultrastructural and cytogenetic analysis have led to a present theory heavily weighted towards a neoplastic aetiology.[36]

Although frequently asymptomatic, diffuse PVNS can present with mild pain and limitation of range of motion due to effusion.[36] Patients with localized PVNS may present with pain, locking, instability, swelling and the sensation of a mass; range of motion is typically preserved.[29,32,37,38] Thus, PVNS must be included in the differential diagnosis of internal derangement of the knee.

The exact diagnosis of PVNS is based on the histological presence of intracellular and subsynovial haemosiderin pigments, predominance of nodular structures compared with villi, presence of macrophage multinucleate cells, production of collagen and mitotic cellular elements. Plain radiographs are usually normal, but bony changes such as increased synovial density or radiolucent cystic defects may be detectable.[39] Plain radiographic clues of focal PVNS in the infrapatellar fat pad include loss of fat density with the absence of calcification.[40–42] MRI remains a useful tool in the characterization of PVNS, as haemosiderin is a magnetic material.[43] Proliferative synovial tissue deposits result in a spotty low signal or extensive low signal area on T_1- and T_2-weighted images, and are best seen on fast field echo sequence MRI images. T_2 fast spin echo and gradient echo images in particular show heterogeneity with multiple signal voids due to the presence of haemosiderin.[22] Fat-suppressed sequences obscure deposits, strengthening the diagnosis of PVNS[44] (Fig. 76.2a).

The most widely accepted treatment for PVNS is synovectomy, and both open and arthroscopic approaches have been performed with success (Fig. 76.2b). Comparisons of open versus arthroscopic techniques have revealed many advantages of arthroscopic treatment,

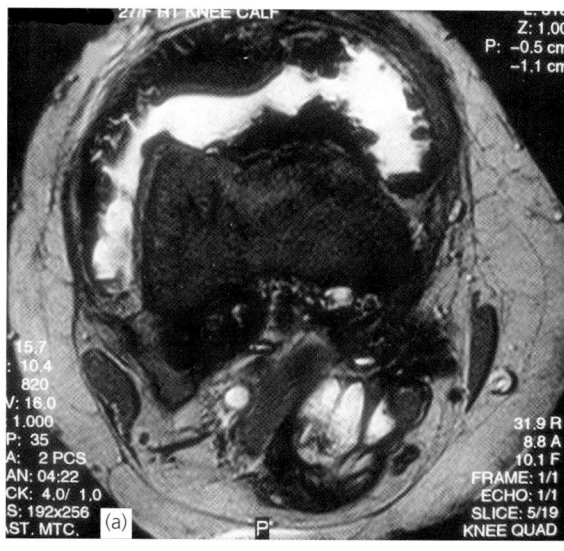
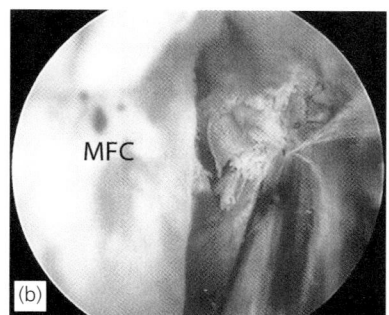

Figure 76.2 Right knee pigmented villonodular synovitis (PVNS). (a) Axial fat-suppressed MRI section demonstrates diffuse PVNS involving the medial gutter, lateral gutter, and peri-patellar synovium. (b) An arthroscopic shaver is placed in the medial gutter to perform a synovectomy.

including improved accuracy of evaluation of the knee joint, the ability to treat other pathology, faster recovery through more rapid rehabilitation, decreased risk of joint stiffness and less pain.[45] Open synovectomy is indicated in cases of posterior extra-articular extension or extreme fibrosis, the presence of which increases the risk of vascular or neurological injury if the procedure is performed arthroscopically.[36,46–48] Although partial synovectomy is beneficial for focal disease, total synovectomy must be performed to achieve maximal clinical results in diffuse PVNS.[37,49,50] Owing to the predilection of localized PVNS for the anterior compartment, disease foci in these cases are typically accessible with standard arthroscopy without the need for accessory portals.[32,38,40,51]

Although attempted total synovectomy can result in subjective, clinical and radiographic eradication of diffuse PVNS, recurrence is not uncommon due to incomplete microscopic resection.[45] Recurrence rates ranging from 10% to 56% have been reported, anytime from the first month to many years postoperatively.[34,36,52–54] To reduce the risk of disease recurrence, complete arthroscopic synovectomy combined with radiation therapy in anti-inflammatory doses has been suggested.[55,56] Additional indications for adjuvant radiotherapy include the possibility to treat inaccessible or hidden disease sites and small foci of residual disease.[55–57] Adjuvant radiotherapy is applied via external beam radiation or intra-articular radio-colloid injections, and should be typically reserved for recurrent lesions since post-radiation fibrosis, swelling and healing problems can result.[36,58] Even more troublesome is the risk of malignant transformation, as patients with malignant PVNS and a history of radiation therapy have been identified.[36,59,60] For these reasons, the role of radiotherapy remains controversial in the treatment of diffuse PVNS. In patients with PVNS refractory to treatment with open surgical synovectomy, alternative treatment with intra-articular etanercept to block tumour necrosis factor α has recently been utilized with promising results.[61,62]

MENISCUS INJURY

Meniscal injury and repair

The medial and lateral menisci play a critical role in load transmission, shock absorption, secondary stabilization, proprioception, joint lubrication and articular cartilage nutrition.[63–71] Surgical meniscectomy or meniscal injuries which result in damage or loss of meniscus function can lead to accelerated degenerative changes in the knee.[72–78]

When possible, repair of meniscal tear is generally preferred over resection, as numerous studies have demonstrated that restoration of meniscus function can prevent future degenerative changes.[79–84] Open meniscal repair via an arthrotomy has been successful, but with associated surgical morbidity.[80] The first reported arthroscopic meniscal repair was in Japan by Ikeuchi.[86] Arthroscopically assisted repair has been found to be equivalent to open repair[82–84] and is the current standard of care.[85–88] The three most common techniques are inside-out, outside-in and all-inside.

Unfortunately, not all meniscal tears are amenable to repair. Certain parameters have been defined to help guide which injury patterns should be addressed by repair as opposed to meniscectomy.[85,87] First, the tear should be in a well-vascularized area, within the peripheral 10–25% of the meniscus. This 'red–red' zone, as described by Arnoczky and Warren,[89] is supplied by a peri-meniscal capillary plexus, and thus has a higher potential for healing than the 'red–white' (middle third) and 'white–white' (inner third) zones. Second, longitudinal tears have a higher rate of healing than radial, horizontal cleavage or complex tears; this includes bucket-handle tears. Third, the knee must be stable, as meniscal repairs tend to fare poorly in ligament-deficient knees.[88,89] Fourth, most candidates for repair are under the age of 40, who, compared with an older population, are less likely to have articular cartilage wear, poor tissue quality, inferior blood supply or difficulty with rehabilitation.[85,87]

The inside-out meniscal repair technique was popularized by Charles Henning in North America in 1980 and is our preferred method of repair.[81,90] For medial repairs, a skin incision is made vertically just posterior to the superficial medial collateral ligament (MCL), measuring 3–4 cm in length, with one-third extending above the medial joint line and two-thirds below. Superficial dissection is carried out through the sartorial fascia, with care taken to avoid injury to the overlying infrapatellar branch of the saphenous nerve. Deep dissection is performed between the posterior oblique ligament (POL) and the superficial MCL, which lies anteriorly.[91] A Henning retractor is then placed superficial to the capsule. For lateral repairs, the incision is made vertically just posterior to the lateral collateral ligament (LCL), measuring 3–4 cm in length, with one-third extending above the medial joint line, and two-thirds below. Dissection is carried out through the superficial fascia, and then between the iliotibial band and biceps femoris muscle. The lateral head of the gastrocnemius muscle is elevated medially along its lateral border and the Henning retractor is placed superficial to the capsule. For tears amenable to repair, zone-specific cannulas (ConMed, Largo, FL) are typically utilized to place vertical mattress sutures using prepackaged 2-0 braided non-absorbable sutures on double-armed straight flexible needles. Prior to suture placement, a rasp is used to abrade the tear surfaces to clear fibrous tissue and stimulate blood flow. The needles are retrieved individually through the corresponding incision and the paired sutures are tied over the capsule to complete the repair. Vertical mattress sutures are biomechanically superior to horizontal mattress sutures and therefore we place them whenever possible.[92]

Augmentation of the meniscal repair can be performed with synovial abrasion using a rasp or with fibrin clot. A fibrin clot can be obtained from 40–60 mL of blood drawn from the patient during surgery and placed in a beaker. Coagulation can be expedited by rolling a frosted stirring rod in the beaker. Prior to tying the sutures, a cannula can be used to deliver the clot into the meniscal repair site; the sutures are then pulled tight and tied.

Occasionally, a meniscus tear is associated with a peri-meniscal cyst, which lies in communication with the joint space adjacent to the capsule. Meniscal cysts most commonly arise on the lateral side of the knee secondary to a horizontal cleavage lateral meniscus tear.[93–95] Cysts associated with medial meniscus tears are also well recognized, although occasionally medial cysts have been reported to occur in the absence of obvious meniscal pathology.[96,97] Patients generally present with tenderness over the joint line and a palpable mass. Definitive management consists of cyst decompression and treatment of the underlying meniscal pathology. Good results have been reported with arthroscopic or open cyst decompression combined with partial meniscectomy.[93,94,96,98] When possible, we perform cyst decompression using a probe or shaver placed through the meniscal tear directly into the cyst, followed by manipulation of the cyst contents into the joint space; cases of inadequate decompression are addressed with open cyst excision via an incision made directly over the cyst. Subsequently, we perform meniscal repair of most horizontal cleavage tears utilizing an arthroscopic inside-out technique, or partial meniscectomy when repair is not feasible (Fig. 76.3a–d). An outside-in technique combined with decompression has also been reported with success.[99] Both techniques are reliable, safe and result in minimal morbidity. As a temporizing measure for those in whom surgery is not an option due to medical or temporal reasons, ultrasound-guided percutaneous cyst drainage has

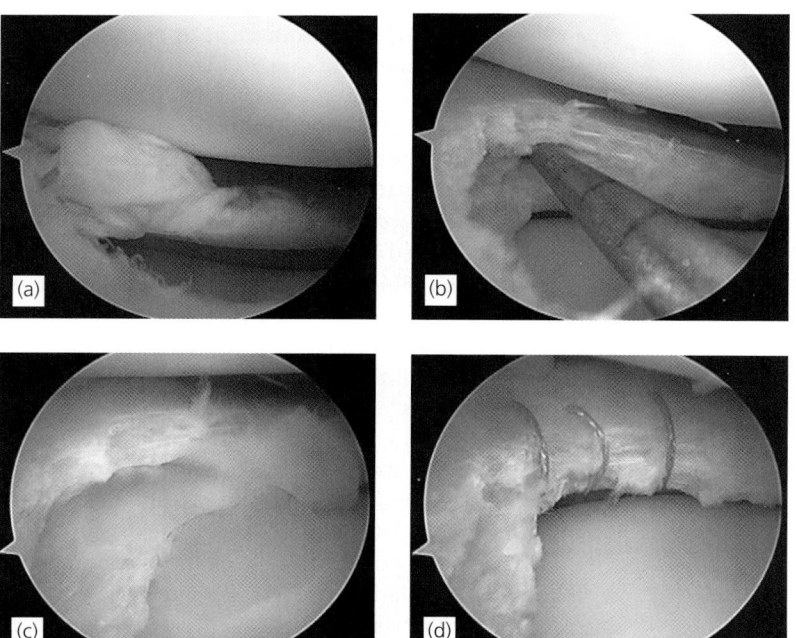

Figure 76.3 Right knee lateral meniscal tear with peri-meniscal cyst. (a) Complex lateral meniscus tear. (b) The unstable portion of the lateral meniscus has been resected to reveal a horizontal cleavage component in the peripheral rim. A probe is placed through the tear into the peri-meniscal cyst to decompress it. (c) The cyst contents are expressed into the joint space and evacuated with a shaver. (d) Inside-out lateral meniscus repair with vertical mattress sutures. Additional sutures are placed into the anterior horn to complete the repair.

been reported to be safe with variable efficacy; although some patients were able to return to competitive sport at 10 month follow-up, recurrence of symptoms was reported in as early as 1 week in others.[100]

We have found the outside-in technique to be most beneficial for anterior meniscus tears.[101,102] Although we seldom use this technique, generally good results have been reported.[103] The principles of this technique include outside-in needle passage across the meniscal tear site, followed by suture passage into the joint space, and some form of knot tying to achieve a mattress suture.

All-inside meniscal repair is predicated on the utilization of small inert or bioabsorbable implants to achieve fixation across meniscal tear sites without the use of accessory skin incisions. The first implants used were predominantly arrows, darts or screws. Problems have been reported with those implants involving poor fixation, high failure rates, intra-articular implant migration with loose body-type chondral injury, extra-articular implant migration and adverse reaction to biomaterials.[104–108] These devices have generally been replaced with a newer generation of implants that are easier to use, potentially with fewer complications.[109] Newer all-inside meniscus repair products require the placement of a buttress at the meniscocapsular junction, which is linked via suture to an intra-articular buttress that rests against the meniscal surface.[110] Special cannulas are required for sequential deployment of each portion of the device. Tensioning across the repair site is possible, and sutures can be placed in vertical, horizontal or oblique mattress configurations. At early follow-up, clinical results have demonstrated a decrease in failures and complications compared with earlier generation all-inside implants.[111] Further study is warranted.

Medial meniscus posterior root injury and repair

A less commonly recognized but problematic injury that deserves special mention is meniscal root injury. In 1991, Pagnani et al.[112] described a posterior horn medial meniscus root tear (PHMMRT) with meniscal extrusion in a 20-year-old football player; surgical repair was deferred due to inability to mobilize the chronically extruded meniscus. PHMMRT results in loss of meniscal circumferential hoop stress, and is biomechanically equivalent to a total meniscectomy.[113] Sequelae of untreated PHMMRT include medial joint compartment overload, accelerated cartilage degeneration and osteoarthritis. The diagnosis may be overlooked, as radiographs are often negative, MRI findings are typically subtle, and arthroscopic visualization is limited by difficult access to the root insertion in the posterior aspect of the knee.[114,115] In cases of isolated PHMMRT with an intact MCL, a 70° arthroscope in the Gillquist view or a 30° arthroscope placed in a posteromedial portal are typically needed to adequately visualize the root insertion (Fig. 76.4a–c).

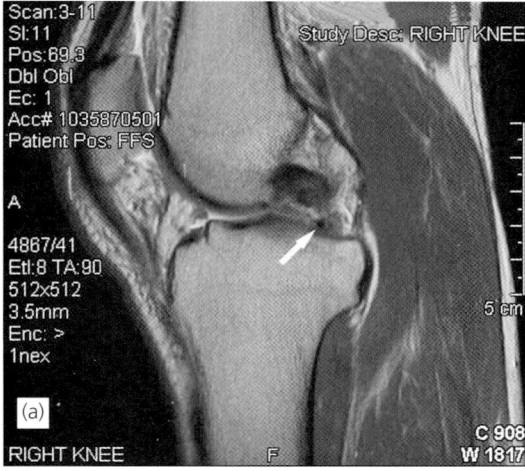
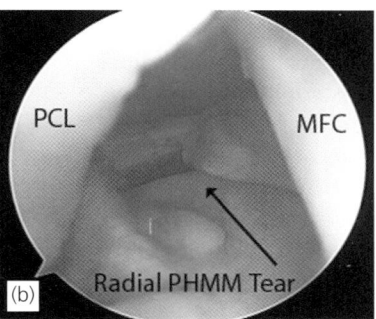
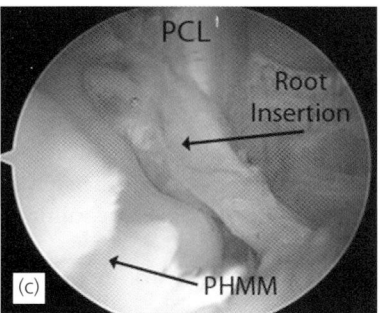
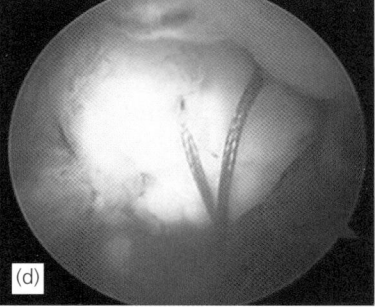

Figure 76.4 Right knee posterior horn medial meniscus root tear (PHMMRT). (a) Sagittal MRI section demonstrates subtle finding of attenuation of the medial meniscus posterior root (arrow). (b) A 70° arthroscope placed in the Gillquist view, underneath the posterior cruciate ligament (PCL) and adjacent to the medial femoral condyle (MFC), reveals a radial tear in the medial meniscus posterior root extending to the capsule (arrow). (c) A 30° arthroscope placed in a posteromedial portal clearly visualizes the radial PHMMRT, with lateral excursion of the remaining meniscus (foreground) from its root insertion. (d) Final suture repair of the PHMMRT to a new, more medial, tibial insertion site, as seen with a 70° arthroscope placed in the Gillquist view. Images courtesy of Christopher D. Harner, MD.

T_2 MRI images and technetium bone scan can detect increased medial compartment metabolic activity, suggestive of joint overload. Early diagnosis is critical for joint preservation and is best made by a meticulous arthroscopic examination.

In a clinical review, 31 patients with PHMMRT had a mean age 41 years and mean body mass index of 30. They were most often male (65%), had a specific mechanism of injury (74%) and had isolated meniscal pathology with or without degenerative changes (61%).[115] Biomechanical cadaveric study has demonstrated that, under axial loading, PHMMRT and total medial meniscectomy result in comparable increases in peak medial compartment contact force, external tibial rotation and lateral tibial translation.[113] In the same study, PHMM root repair was found to restore the loading and kinematic profiles of the knee to the intact state, strongly supporting the role of repair as a treatment option. Thus, the goal of surgical management is to re-establish the stability and function of the PHMM root, thereby restoring the joint-protective mechanical properties of the medial meniscus.

Biomechanical cadaveric study has analysed the fixation strength of various repairs for PHMMRTs, using 2-0 braided suture in a tibial tunnel.[116] The mean ultimate load to failure for the native PHMM root insertion was 643 N. For root repair, the modified Kessler stitch (132 N) was shown to provide a greater strength of fixation than both the horizontal mattress stitch (91 N, $P = 0.039$) and the simple stitch (70 N, $P = 0.003$).

PHMM root repair involves an adaptation of current medial meniscus transplant methods.[117] Arthroscopically assisted PHMM root repair has been described using a small arthrotomy in the interval between the superficial MCL and POL, which allows for horizontal mattress no. 0 non-absorbable suture placement.[118] This approach was preferred as it enabled maximum manual control of the suture, direct visualization of the posterior root insertion and the strongest suture configuration possible. It was found to enable a reliable, secure and accurately placed repair, with negligible morbidity. A modified, oblique notchplasty is performed along the posterior aspect of the medial femoral condyle, to increase access to the tear. In subacute or chronic cases with insufficient meniscal excursion, it is generally not possible to fix the lateral meniscal rim to the native root insertion site. Accordingly, a new tibial insertion site is created more medially with the use of a rasp and shaver. Decortication of the tibial plateau must be performed in order to expose a vascular osseous bed for healing to the overlying meniscus. A suture tunnel bridge at the lateral tibial cortex, just distal to the metaphyseal flare, is created through a 2 cm incision for suture passage and definitive fixation. An anterior cruciate ligament (ACL)-tip guide is used to place one 3/32'K-Wire in the new tibial insertion; the wire is subsequently exchanged with a Hewson suture passer (Smith and Nephew, Memphis, TN). A posteromedial arthrotomy along the posterior border of the superficial MCL is next performed for suture placement. Three no. 2 Silky Polydek Sutures (Teleflex Medical, Research Triangle Park, NC) are placed in horizontal mattress fashion along the anterior border of the POL to allow for later repair to the MCL. Two no. 0 Silky Polydek sutures with a small tapered needle are placed into the lateral extent of the PHMM under direct visualization, 1 cm apart, in horizontal mattress fashion. Each set of sutures is then retrieved to the lateral tibial cortex with the suture passer. Tension is applied to the sutures to seat the meniscal root in the new tibial bed, and they are subsequently tied over a 14 mm polypropylene button (Ethicon, Somerville, NJ) or a 4.5 mm bicortical screw-post with washer (Fig. 76.4d). Closure of the POL window is performed in 10° of knee extension with care taken not to advance the POL onto the superficial MCL. The rehabilitation protocol is similar to that for meniscal repair, with clinical and radiographic healing observed at short-term follow-up. In a modification of this technique, arthroscopic PHMM root repair using two no. 2 non-absorbable sutures ina simple stitch fashion has also been reported with success.[119]

CARTILAGE INJURY

Osteochondritis dissecans

In 1888 König originally described osteochondritis dissecans (OCD) of the knee, a condition in which a segment of articular cartilage and subchondral bone become fragmented and potentially displaced from the underlying bone.[120] Although the exact aetiology of OCD is unclear, possible causes include ischaemia, repetitive microtrauma, genetic predisposition and endocrine disorders associated with epiphyseal abnormalities. The incidence of OCD of the knee based upon arthroscopic examinations is estimated at 1.2%, most commonly in children between 10 and 15 years of age.[121] There is a slight male preponderance, with cases occurring bilaterally in up to 30% of patients.[122,123] The lateral aspect of the medial femoral condyle is most commonly affected, followed by the lateral femoral condyle and rarely the patella.[124]

In early cases of OCD without displacement, patients often report non-specific pain and variable activity-related effusion. In later cases of OCD with unstable or displaced lesions, patients can complain of mechanical symptoms as well. Lesions can be stratified into juvenile and adult forms, based upon the skeletal age of the patient, which has been found to be a significant prognostic factor in healing.[122,125] Patients with open physes and increased activity on bone scan are more likely to heal their OCD lesions than those with closed growth plates or minimal metabolic activity.[126]

Standard radiographs obtained in the work-up of OCD include posteroanterior flexion weight bearing at 45°, lateral weight bearing at 30°, and Merchant views. Bone scan can be utilized to assess the probability of healing in a lesion, or monitor healing of a lesion. The stage of OCD lesions can be classified based on radiographic or surgical findings. Cahill and Berg[127] have described a system based on anteroposterior and lateral radiographs. An accurate T_2 MRI-based system has also been developed; it emphasizes the importance of identifying fluid deep to the subchondral fragment, which is indicative of an unstable lesion.[128] At the time of arthroscopy, the classification system created by Guhl can be utilized to assist in decision-making; type I lesions are intact with cartilage softening, type II are stable with breached cartilage, type III are hinged fragments, and type IV are completely displaced, resulting in a loose body.[129]

Non-operative treatment, consisting of activity modification with or without protected crutch weight bearing, can be used initially for patients with stable lesions. These patients can be followed with serial physical examinations, radiographs and bone scans to assess for healing. Poor prognosis is associated with signs of loosening or displacement, sclerosis on plain radiographs, lesions greater than 2 cm, overlying chondromalacia and closed physes.[123] Operative treatment of OCD is generally elected for symptomatic stable lesions which fail to heal, hinged or displaced fragments, and loose bodies. In skeletally mature patients, a shorter course of non-operative treatment may be elected for unstable non-displaced lesions, given the lower likelihood of these lesions to heal than in patients with open physes.

For stable OCD lesions, arthroscopically assisted antegrade transchondral drilling can be performed in the skeletally immature to stimulate vascular ingrowth and healing. In the skeletally mature patient with an OCD lesion, retrograde transosseous drilling can be done with a Kirschner wire, or with a larger drill bit to allow bone grafting of the subchondral bed.[130]

Management of unstable lesions is dependent upon the degree of displacement and amount of fragment deformation. Hinged or displaced fragments with good congruency to their subchondral bed can be treated with internal fixation, with or without bone drilling or bone grafting. Options for internal fixation include cannulated metal or bioabsorbable headed screws, cannulated headless screws, variable pitch headless screws, bioabsorbable darts or pins, and bone pegs. Autograft, when needed, can be obtained from the region of Gerdy's tubercle in the proximal tibia or the iliac crest. Alternatively, corticancellous allograft can be used. In one study, Miniaci and Tytherleigh-Strong[131] reported on the successful use of multiple 4.5 mm osteochondral dowel grafts to fix unstable OCD lesions in 20 knees. The dowels were harvested from the edges of the femoral trochlea and passed through the centre and periphery of the fragments; MRI demonstrated healing in all cases by 6 months.

Large OCD fragments or fragments with poor congruency to their subchondral bed often necessitate an open surgical approach with curettage and bone grafting of the subchondral bed, followed by fragment fixation. OCD lesions without a repairable fragment can be treated by salvage procedures, which include microfracture, osteochondral autograft or allograft, and autologous chondrocyte implantation (ACI).

Microfracture

The microfracture technique is generally indicated for full-thickness loss of articular cartilage in either a weight-bearing area between the femur and tibia or an area of contact between the patella and trochlear groove. Unstable cartilage that overlies the subchondral bone is also an indication. The surgical technique and clinical results of microfracture for full-thickness chondral defects has been well described by Steadman et al.[132,133] Non-operative treatment is typically recommended for at least 12 weeks after clinical diagnosis of a chondral lesion. Initial management can include activity modification, physical therapy, non-steroidal anti-inflammatory drugs, intra-articular injections and possibly dietary supplements that may have cartilage-stimulating properties. Contraindications to microfracture include axial malalignment (greater than 5° of increased varus or valgus than the contralateral knee), patient unwillingness to follow a strict and rigorous rehabilitation protocol, partial-thickness defects, inability to use the opposite leg for weight bearing during the protected weight-bearing time, systemic immune-mediated disease and cartilage disease.

To perform the microfracture technique, a shaver or curette is first used to debride all loose or marginally attached cartilage from the surrounding rim of articular cartilage, in order to form a stable perpendicular edge of healthy viable cartilage around the defect. This rim functions to hold in the clot as it forms. Next, the cartilage cap that remains over many lesions is removed with a curette. Finally, an awl is used to make multiple holes, or 'microfactures', in the exposed subchondral bone plate. The awl, which is typically available in 30°, 45° and 90° angles, must be directed perpendicular to the bone as it is advanced, to a depth of 2–4 mm. Fat droplets can usually be seen coming from the marrow cavity after penetration of the bone. Generally, microfracture holes are created around the periphery of the defect first, immediately adjacent to the healthy stable cartilage rim. Additional holes are placed 3–4 mm apart towards the centre. Penetration of the subchondral bone disrupts the subchondral vessels, leading to a fibrin clot and granulation tissue formation in the defect. Undifferentiated mesenchymal cells migrate into the defect and proliferate, forming fibrocartilage repair tissue which can cover the defect.[134–136] One notable disadvantage of the microfracture technique is that this fibrocartilage lacks type II collagen and thus the durability and strength of normal hyaline cartilage are not restored.

Osteochondral autograft/allograft transfer

For larger full-thickness chondral lesions, osteochondral autograft transplantation (OATS) can be performed to fill the defect. OATS entails open or arthroscopic harvesting of cylindrical plugs of cartilage with the underlying subchondral bone, and transplanting them directly into the osteochondral defect. Donor sites which have been found to have the least contact pressure are the superolateral ridge of the lateral femoral condyle proximal to the sulcus terminalis, and the periphery of the intercondylar notch.[137] Generally, the harvester is seated to a depth of 15 mm for chondral defects and 25 mm for osteochondral defects, although some variability exists depending on the system used. Orienting the plugs to restore articular congruency is of the utmost importance, as excessive prominence or countersinking of as little as 0.5 mm can result in increased contact forces or accelerate degeneration of adjacent cartilage.[138] Grafts 6–8 mm in diameter are generally optimal for creating a congruent articular surface with high a graft fill percentage. Optimal graft filling is greater than 70%, and can reach between 90% and 100% when variable diameter grafts are used simultaneously.[139]

Advantages of OATS include the direct transfer of intact hyaline cartilage with its subchondral plate and attached bone, no risk of disease transmission and only one surgical procedure needed. Disadvantages are limitations in donor source tissue, difficulty addressing lesions greater than 2 cm^2, donor site morbidity, and inability to always completely fill lesions due to plug–lesion or plug–plug mismatch. In one study, Chow et al.[140] reported on midterm results on OATS performed on 30 full-thickness chondral lesions on the femoral condyles between 10 and 25 mm in diameter. Excellent outcomes were achieved in 87% of patients, and histological examination revealed viable chondrocytes and normal hyaline cartilage in the completely healed cases.

As opposed to autograft, osteochondral allograft has also been used, with success rates between 63% and 77% reported at up to 10 year follow-up.[141,142] Concerns regarding diminishing chondrocyte viability with time, cost, disease transmission and immunological reaction have limited widespread utilization of allograft.[143]

Ideal lesions for OATS are small, focal, unipolar full-thickness chondral or osteochondral defects measuring 10–20 mm^2 in diameter.[144] Age limitations are typically 15–50 years old, and body mass index below 30 is preferable. It has been shown that the knee can provide sufficient donor tissue to address defects 30–40 mm^2 in diameter without significant morbidity, and some use OATS in these more challenging cases.[145] An advantage of OATS is that it can be used in cases of bone loss, as in OCD lesions, of up to 6–8 mm in depth. Contraindications for OATS include diffuse osteoarthritis, rheumatoid or other inflammatory arthritis, patient non-compliance, adjacent neoplasm, infection, lack of appropriate donor site and bipolar lesions. Lesions greater than 40 mm^2 in diameter, particularly on the weight-bearing surfaces of the joint, are better suited for size-matched bulk osteochondral allograft or ACI.

Autologous chondrocyte implantation

Restoration of osteochondral defects greater than 25–30 mm^2 in diameter, up to 150 mm^2, can be performed with ACI, which was first reported clinically in 1994.[146] ACI is currently typically employed for symptomatic, unipolar, full-thickness, or near full-thickness chondral or shallow osteochondral lesions. Smaller lesions can be treated first with microfracture, while some consider ACI a first-line option in larger symptomatic lesions in high demand patients. In the knee, approved usage is for the trochlea and femur, although success has been observed in off-label usage on the tibia and patella as well.

ACI is performed in two stages. First, articular cartilage cells are arthroscopically harvested from the knee and expanded ex vivo in cell cultures. For bony defects greater than 8 mm in depth, bone grafting can be performed at this time. At the second surgery an arthrotomy is performed and the chondral defect prepared in a manner similar to that for microfracture. A periosteal tissue flap is harvested from the anteromedial tibia, and sutured to the cartilage rim of the defect. A watertight seal is created around the periphery with fibrin glue. The cultured chondrocytes are implanted into the cavity and the flap is closed completely. Advantages of ACI are the ability to treat larger lesions and no risk of disease transmission. Disadvantages of ACI include the cost, need for a second procedure, risk of infection, need for an arthrotomy and the potentially heterogeneous nature of the repair tissue that is formed.

Fu et al.[147] performed a comparison between ACI and debridement for symptomatic, large, full-thickness chondral defects of the knee. Although patients treated with debridement had some functional improvement at follow-up, patients who received ACI obtained a higher level of knee function and had greater relief from pain and swelling at 3 years. In the adolescent population, Micheli et al.[148] reported on 37 full-thickness cartilage lesions of the distal femur treated with ACI. Defects had a mean diameter of 54 mm and patients had a mean age of 16 years. At 4.3 year mean follow-up, all patients had improvements in overall condition, pain and swelling, suggesting efficacy for ACI in these cases. Similarly, Brittberg et al.[149] found good or excellent results after ACI in 83% of 61 patients at 5–11 year follow-up.

A prospective, randomized controlled comparison of mosaicplasty and ACI demonstrated superiority with ACI in 100 patients based upon outcome scores, clinical measurement and arthroscopic examination.[150] Conversely, a randomized study comparing microfracture with ACI in 80 patients concluded that microfracture was superior based upon clinical evaluation and outcome scores at 2 year follow-up; it should be noted that a postoperative rehabilitation protocol which included early partial weight bearing in the ACI group may have had some deleterious effects on the healing in those cases.[151] Overall, accurate assessment of the efficacy of various cartilage restoration techniques is difficult given the number of concomitant injuries and previous procedures, but each approach has demonstrated promise in the clinical setting. Further study is warranted to determine a comprehensive treatment algorithm.

EXTENSOR MECHANISM

Patellar tendon rupture

Patellar tendon rupture typically results from an eccentric quadriceps muscle contraction against resistance. Knee position is often variable, as is the amount of force involved. For isolated traumatic rupture of the patellar tendon, 80% occur in patients below 40 years of age.[152] Most commonly, these patients have a history of patellar tendinitis, 'jumper's knee', or other systemic pathology.[153] Physical examination typically reveals a palpable defect inferior to the patella, associated swelling and ecchymosis, and an inability to actively extend the knee or perform a straight leg raise.[154] However, in some cases of patellar tendon rupture active straight leg raise with or without lag is still possible, due to an intact patellar retinaculum. On examination, the patella may rest more proximally than the uninjured side and is seen to migrate proximally with active quadriceps contraction.[152] Less frequently, the tendon is ruptured at its insertion on the tibial tubercle; in these cases history may reveal prior trauma, steroid injection, or previous Osgood–Schlatter disease.[152] Midsubstance rupture is often correlated with systemic disease, although cases have been observed in young, healthy athletes. Diabetes, rheumatoid arthritis, gout, obesity, hyperparathyroidism, systemic lupus erythematosus (SLE), osteomalacia and systemic steroid use have all been shown to cause tendon necrosis, fibrosis, and/or microscopic vascular damage.[155–163] Most commonly, the tendon ruptures off the inferior pole of the patella, and may be accompanied by a bony fragment that is visible radiographically. A lateral knee radiograph may reveal resultant patella alta due to the unopposed pull of the quadriceps muscle[152] (Fig. 76.5a).

Neither MRI nor sonography can easily distinguish intrasubstance tears from tendon degeneration, but both methods can accurately distinguish partial from full-thickness tears.[164,165] (Fig. 76.5b). Although MRI is typically preferred for surgical planning, sonography has the advantage of dynamic imaging.

Early surgical repair produces the optimal clinical outcomes. The patellar tendon, along with the medial and lateral retinacula, should be primarily repaired for midsubstance ruptures, or repaired through a transosseous technique for proximal and distal ruptures (Fig. 76.5c,d). Depending on tissue quality and tissue excursion, repair can be augmented with a cerclage wire, hamstring autograft, or hamstring allograft passed through the patella and tibial tuberosity, tightened in approximately 60° of knee flexion.[166,167] Wire removal should be performed at 6–8 weeks.[154]

In the setting of chronic patellar tendon rupture, primary repair can be difficult or impossible due to contracture of the quadriceps muscle, which often must be freed from the femur to allow for adequate distal mobilization of the patella. When necessary, the gracilis and semitendinosus tendons can be used as autograft substitution for the native patellar tendon; multiple alternative reconstructive techniques have been described, which all aim to recreate a functional tendinous attachment between the patella and tibial tubercle.[154]

In children 8–12 years old, a patellar 'sleeve fracture' can occur. In these cases, the distal osseous pole of the patella plus a patellar periosteal sleeve is avulsed with an intact patellar tendon. Repair of the disrupted extensor mechanism is performed utilizing a transosseous suture technique, with tension band wiring utilized for larger fragments.

Rupture of the patellar tendon may also occur in association with knee dislocation, and its timely repair is essential for long-term knee function.[168] Combined ruptures of the patellar tendon and ACL have also been reported, particularly with forceful eccentric contraction of the quadriceps against a fixed foot. In these cases, primary augmented repair of the patellar tendon along with ACL reconstruction has been successful.[169]

Adequate rehabilitation postoperatively is critical to the success of patellar tendon repair. Cast immobilization regimens following surgery ranging from 6 to 11 weeks have been reported with overall favourable results.[153,170–174] However, accompanying weakness, stiffness and patella baja are undesirable and can potentially be reduced by early mobilization.[153,174] Research has demonstrated that postoperative immobilization in a cast is unnecessary following suture repair of the patellar tendon and retinacula, when protected by a cerclage wire.[153] Current rehabilitation protocols vary, but in general incorporate early mobilization. In general, a continuous passive motion (CPM) device begins on postoperative day 1, from 0° to 60°. Weight bearing as tolerated is permitted immediately, with crutches and a hinged knee brace locked in extension. From 2 to 6 weeks, under the supervision of a physical therapist, flexion can be incrementally increased to 90°, with the incorporation of quadriceps sets and straight leg raising exercises. Crutches are discontinued at 6 weeks, and ambulation with the brace unlocked is permitted. At 6–10 weeks, if present, cerclage wire removal should be performed. Biking and running are permitted between 2 and 3 months, with pivoting allowed at 4–6 months, depending on the severity of the initial injury and nature of the repair.

Larsen and Lund[172] reported excellent or good results in seven of ten patients after repair of patellar tendon rupture. Marder and Timmerman[175] reported that primary repair of

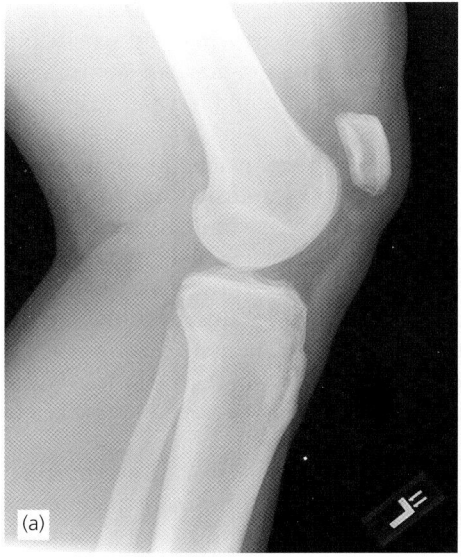
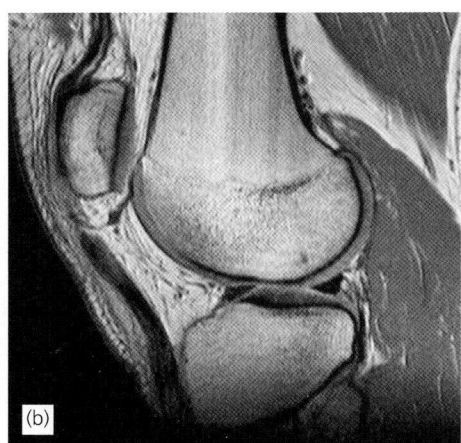
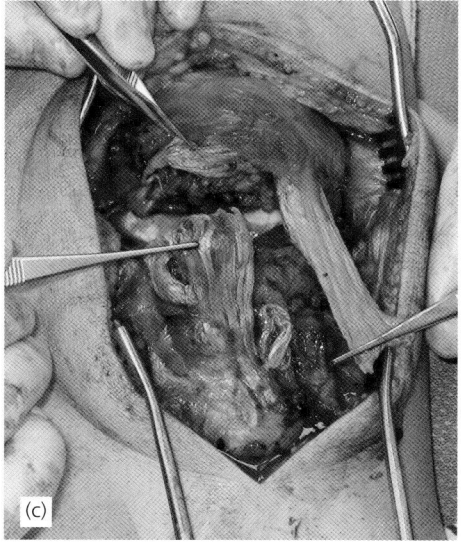
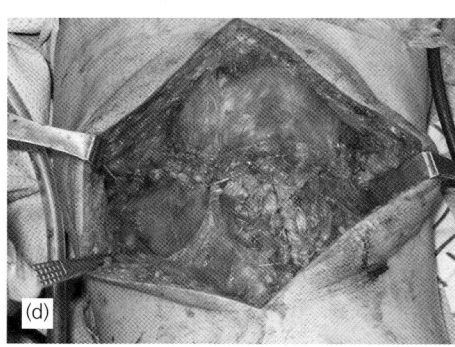

Figure 76.5 Left knee acute patellar tendon rupture in a collegiate football player. (a) Lateral knee radiograph demonstrating patella alta. (b) Sagittal MRI section demonstrates a gap between the patellar tendon and the inferior pole of the patella. (c) Complex rupture pattern of the patellar tendon involving the patellar attachment, midsubstance, tibial attachment, medial retinaculum, and lateral retinaculum. (d) Final repair of the patellar tendon using a transosseous technique in the patella and tibial tubercle. Suture repair of the medial and lateral retinacula to the mid-coronal plane, and the tendon midsubstance, was also performed. Images courtesy of Jon K. Sekiya, MD.

acute patellar tendon rupture without augmentation allowed return to full activity in 12 of 14 cases; strength was 92% of the contralateral knee, patellofemoral symptoms occurred in 30% and knee flexion was limited 5° on average.

Quadriceps tendon rupture

Quadriceps tendon rupture most commonly occurs in patients older than 40 years of age, and is often associated with degenerative changes of the tendon due to concurrent systemic medical disease.[152,176,177] Approximately 75% of the tendon fibres must generally be severed for functionally incapacitating rupture to occur, demonstrating the strength and durability of this structure under normal conditions.[163] Normal ageing creates numerous intratendinous changes which can lead to weakness, including cystic and myxoid degeneration, microangioblastic dysplasia, decreased collagen, and calcification.[163] A spectrum of pathology can affect the quadriceps tendon to varying degrees, including tendinosis, partial rupture, acute unilateral rupture, and bilateral rupture.

Quadriceps tendon rupture typically occurs when the quadriceps muscle contracts eccentrically with the knee held in a slightly flexed position, most often during attempts to regain balance or avoid a fall.[163,177,178] Quadriceps tendon rupture has also been reported from weight lifting, falls from height, or simple stumbling.[179] Ruptures may be confined to the tendon, or may extend to the distal aponeurosis of the vastus muscles. Most tears are incomplete and involve the rectus femoris tendon. Rupture typically occurs 1–2 cm proximal to the upper patellar pole, corresponding to the avascular region of the rectus.[180] One-third of ruptures occur bilaterally, most often in patients with diabetes, SLE, rheumatoid arthritis, gout, prolonged systemic steroid use, hyperparathyroidism, or end-stage renal disease; all of these conditions have been shown to cause tendon necrosis, fibrosis, or microscopic vascular damage.[155–163,181,182] In cases of unilateral rupture, one-fifth present with additional systemic medical conditions such as renal disease and uraemia, which accelerate tendon ageing by weakening the quadriceps mechanism through associated muscle fibre atrophy.[163,183,184]

Physical examination findings include acute pain, ecchymosis, lack of active knee extension, and preservation of passive knee extension.[163] A suprapatellar gap may or may not be palpable, depending on the extent of the tear and the presence of absence of haematoma. With an incomplete rupture, the patient may be able to perform a straight leg raise from a supine position, but unable to extend the knee from a flexed position. With active quadriceps contraction a suprapatellar defect may become palpable and the patella will not migrate proximally.

Plain radiographs are often of limited value, but may reveal patella baja or an avulsed bony fragment from the superior pole of the patella. Calcification may be seen at the site of quadriceps insertion on the patella, representing areas of previous microtrauma. Although ultrasound is an inexpensive and accurate method to diagnose complete quadriceps tendon rupture, extensive technician experience is required.[185–187] MRI is the most reliable tool to distinguish partial and complete tendon rupture.[188]

Incomplete or partial (<50%) quadriceps tendon ruptures are treated with immobilization in full extension for 4–6 weeks.[152,189] In borderline cases for which surgery is chosen, partial and more proximal lesions can be addressed with tendon-to-tendon primary suture repair. Complete tears require repair preferably within 72 hours of the injury in order to avoid proximal migration and scarring of the quadriceps musculature. Augmentation with local tissue transfer, allograft, or synthetic material can be performed as needed based upon tissue quality, retraction, size of defect, and chronicity of tear. Early repair or reconstruction typically results in good or excellent functional results, while later reconstruction may result in residual quadriceps weakness.[152] For rupture near the patella, repair can be performed via a transosseous technique or using suture-anchors in the proximal patellar pole. Both approaches utilize no. 2 or larger non-absorbable suture to reapproximate the tendon to its patellar origin. Tendoplasty can be required if scarring or retraction of the quadriceps muscle occurs. For both unilateral and bilateral rupture, prompt surgical repair has been found to result in equally successful outcomes when assessed by physical examination, Lysholm and Tegner scores, a functional questionnaire, quadriceps isokinetic testing, and radiographs.[184]

The principles of postoperative rehabilitation are to protect the repair while regaining full range-of-motion and quadriceps strength. Immediate postoperative hinged-knee brace placement, with touch-down crutch weight bearing with the brace locked in extension permitted. Quadriceps sets are initiated immediately, while prone active flexion exercises out of the brace can start at 3 weeks. Weigh bearing can be progressed to full at 6 weeks, at weight time the brace can be unlocked. Flexion should be regained gradually, at approximately 10–15° per week. Typically 45° of flexion can be attained by week 4, 90° by week 8 and full flexion by 12 weeks. Eventually, closed chain exercises and biking can be done at 4 months, with progressive strengthening and jogging thereafter. Return to sport usually requires 9–12 months of continuous rehabilitation, but can take up to 18 months.[170] Most patients with bilateral simultaneous and unilateral tendon repairs can expect good range of motion and return to their previous occupation, but many have persistent weakness and difficulty returning to a higher level of sporting activities.[184,190]

Patellar instability

Patellofemoral instability is defined as the inability of the patella to stay within the confines of the trochlea from 0° to 20° of knee flexion, and was first recognized by Hughston as a significant cause of disability in athletes.[191] Predisposing factors to patellar instability include patella alta, generalized ligamentous laxity, patellar hypoplasia, trochlear hypoplasia, lateral femoral condyle hypoplasia, excessive femoral anteversion, genu recurvatum and excessive Q angle. Patellar instability is a disabling condition that can be unilateral or bilateral, and typically affects young patients with a female preponderance.[192]

A thorough understanding of the soft-tissue and osseous anatomy of the patellofemoral joint is necessary to understand the pathophysiology, diagnosis and treatment of patellar instability. There are three patellar facets – lateral, medial, and odd – and two trochlear facets – medial and lateral. Axial view of the patellofemoral articulation demonstrates a wider lateral aspect. Two retinacula, one medial and a larger lateral one, attach to the femur to provide stability as they become confluent with the capsule. Biomechanical research has demonstrated that the medial patellofemoral ligament (MPFL), a thickening of the medial retinaculum, is the primary restraint to lateral patellar motion.[193,194] Acute lateral patellar dislocation or chronic repetitive patellar subluxation can result in damage to the MPFL and associated medial supporting structures, resulting in lateral patellar instability.[195–198]

A decision to proceed with surgical management of patellar instability must be based upon a careful history, physical examination and radiographic studies. Salient physical examination findings include vastus medialis obliquus (VMO) atrophy or dysplasia, vastus lateralis hyperplasia, patella alta, lateral patellar displacement, excessive Q angle, lateral pull sign, passive patellar lateral hypermobility, and a positive apprehension sign. Examination of patients with isolated lateral patellar compression syndrome without instability, on the other hand, would demonstrate restriction of medial patellar glide, limitation of passive patellar tilt, peripatellar lateral retinacular tenderness, and a normal Q angle.[199]

Standard radiographs obtained in the work-up of patellar instability include a 45° posteroanterior flexion weight-bearing view, a lateral view in 30° of flexion, and a Merchant view at 45° of flexion. If present, a hypoplastic lateral femoral condyle or trochlear dysplasia can manifest as the 'crossing sign', as described by Dejour *et al.*[200] To assess for patellar alta, the Insall and Salvati Index can be calculated from the lateral radiograph, using the ratio between the patellar tendon length and the greatest diagonal length of the patella; normal values are approximately 0.9–1.2.[201] An abnormal congruence angle of greater than 16° signifies lateral patellar subluxation on the Merchant view.[202] MRI is useful to identify MPFL injury, characteristic bone bruise patterns along the lateral femoral condyle, as well as chondral injuries, which most typically affect the medial patellar facet after acute dislocation (Fig. 76.6a–c). Some have advocated the use of kinematic MRI in assessing patellar instability, with a focus on quantifying parameters such as the tibial tubercle–femoral notch distance, femoral sulcus angle, femoral sulcus depth, lateral patellar angle, patellar lateralization, and patella–patellar tendon ratio.[203] Potentially, this could aid in more accurate identification of causative pathology in patellar instability, and thus lead to optimal surgical management.[204] Further study is warranted.

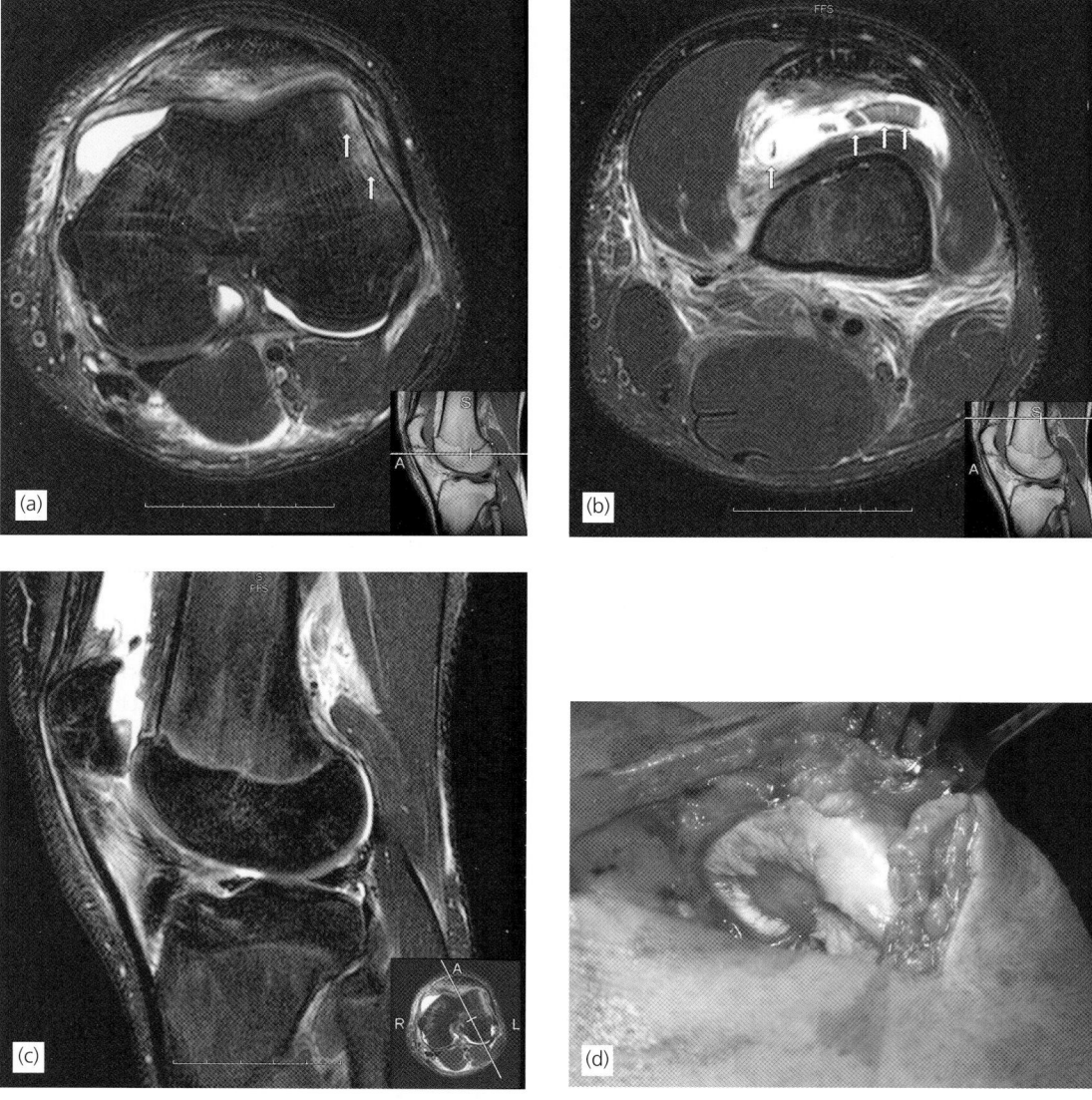

Figure 76.6 Left knee acute patellar dislocation with patellar osteochondral injury in a high school football player. (a) T_2 axial MRI section demonstrates characteristic oedema in the lateral femoral condyle after acute lateral patellar dislocation (arrows). (b) T_2 axial MRI section demonstrates a larger displaced osteochondral fragment present in the patellofemoral joint (arrows). (c) T_2 sagittal MRI section demonstrates a large osteochondral defect on the undersurface of the patella. (d) Medial peri-patellar arthrotomy reveals a large full-thickness patellar chondral injury with some loss of subchondral bone.

Non-operative treatment is typically the first-line treatment for patellar instability; however, up to 53% of patients report persistent symptoms.[205–208] After acute dislocation, initial treatment is focused on minimizing stretch of the elongated medial structures with taping or bracing, gaining full range of motion, and strengthening of the quadriceps and hamstrings.[209] Training of the gluteal musculature to control femoral position and limb alignment also results in improvement of patellar seating in the trochlea; however, in patients lacking sufficient bony restraint, muscles, even when well trained, cannot control forces placed on the patellofemoral joint. In refractory cases surgical management is ultimately necessary to improve passive and dynamic patellofemoral stability.

Regarding historical treatment, in 1888 Roux[210] addressed recurrent patellar dislocation with a lateral release, medial reefing and distalization of the patellar tendon insertion. In 1904, Goldthwait[211] modified the distal portion of this procedure, by transferring the lateral half of the patellar tendon medial to the pes anserine insertion. The distal portion of the procedure was again modified in 1938, by Hauser, who transferred the entire patellar insertion and associated tibial bone block medially, distally and posteriorly along the medial slope of the proximal tibia. This technique has fallen out of favour due to the increased patellofemoral contact forces and the resultant accelerated chondrosis that occurs from posteriorization of the bone block. The Roux–Elmslie–Trillat procedure, as modified by Cox, entails a medial capsular reefing, lateral retinacular release and medial displacement of the tibial tuberosity utilizing an intact distal periosteal hinge, making it useful for both patella alta and an increased Q angle.[212] For more progressive disease, Fulkerson et al.[213] later described an anteromedial tibial transfer for patients with patellar malalignment and patellofemoral arthrosis; the procedure decreases patellofemoral contact force and shifts load to the more proximal, healthier chondral surfaces on the patella.

Primary indications for surgical intervention include acute lateral patellar dislocation with osteochondral fragment, or persistent disability and symptomatic instability after a supervised rehabilitation programme (Fig. 76.6d). Lateral patellar compression syndrome without instability is typically addressed by isolated arthroscopic lateral release, with care taken to preserve the vastus lateralis insertion on the patella. Patellar instability can be treated with the modified Roux–Elmslie–Trillat reconstruction, except in the presence of excessive patellofemoral chondrosis, for which a Fulkerson distal realignment and a proximal reconstruction can be performed. Options for proximal procedures include medial reefing, lateral release, and MPFL reconstruction. For patellar instability with normal alignment, Miller et al.[214] reported favourable results with isolated arthroscopic medial reefing. In the skeletally immature patient with an open tibial growth plate distal realignment procedures are contraindicated, and thus management is focused on proximal procedures.

In patients with underlying femoral trochlear dysplasia, trochlear osteotomy has been attempted to correct the bony deficiency. Koëter et al.[215] reported that anterior lateral femoral condyle open wedge osteotomy was found to be effective in preventing recurrent dislocation in 17 knees at mean 51 month follow-up. In these cases, the deficient articular surface of the lateral femoral condyle was restored by lateral elevation. It should be noted that osteotomy carries the risk of damage to the articular cartilage, the creation of an incongruent patellofemoral articulation, and elevated patellofemoral contact pressures.[216,217] To avoid these risks, as well as those associated with tibial tubercle osteotomy, MPFL reconstruction has been explored as an anatomic-based option to restore patellofemoral instability.

MPFL reconstruction can be performed with or without lateral retinacular release, using semitendinosus, gracilis, quadriceps tendon, or synthetic grafts.[218–222] At 5 year minimum follow-up after MPFL reconstruction using a transferred semitendinosus tendon, Deie et al.[223] reported no recurrent dislocations in 68 knees; there was an improvement in postoperative Kujala score, as well as radiographic correction of patellar tilt and congruence angle. Schöttle et al.[224] reported on 15 knees at mean 47 month follow-up after MPFL reconstruction using semitendinosus autograft. Tibial tubercle medialization was performed in eight patients, who had a tibial tubercle to trochlear groove distance greater than 15 mm, signifying patella alta. Overall Kujala scores increased significantly and patellar tilt was decreased; one patient suffered recurrent dislocation and three had residual apprehension on examination. Nomura et al.[225] reported on the long-term efficacy of MPFL reconstruction, with or without lateral release, in preventing recurrent patellar dislocation and the progression of knee osteoarthritis. In their series, 24 knees were analysed at mean 11.9 year follow-up. Based on Crosby/Insall criteria, 88% of knees were excellent or good, with further lateral subluxation or dislocation occurring in only two knees. Mean Kujala scores improved significantly and only two knees had definite radiographic progression of patellofemoral arthritis from 'none to mild' pre-operatively to 'moderate' postoperatively. Multiple additional series have reported good to excellent results of MPFL reconstruction for patellar instability utilizing varying graft sources, fixation techniques and tensioning methods.[226–230] Depending on the surgical technique, notable risks of MPFL reconstruction include patellar fracture, abductor tubercle fracture, patellar overconstraint with resultant patellofemoral arthrosis, and persistent instability.

Morel–Lavallee lesion of the knee

The Morel–Lavallee lesion (MLL) is an injury most commonly described in the region of the hip joint after blunt trauma. Deforming forces of pressure and shear result in a closed soft-tissue degloving lesion, in which the skin and subcutaneous tissue are separated from the underlying fascia, disrupting the perforating vessels. The space created can fill with blood, lymph and necrotic fat, potentially leading to bacterial colonization and infection. Pseudocysts can form at the site of the original lesion, resulting in recurrent fluid accumulation.[231–234]

Recently, MLL has been reported to occur in the knee as a result of shearing trauma in the National Football League.[235] In these cases, MLL was found to be a distinct lesion from prepatellar bursitis and quadriceps contusion, with 81% occurring from a shearing blow on the playing surface (Fig. 76.7). The most common motion deficit was active knee flexion, and the average time for resolution of the fluid collection and achievement of full active flexion was 16 days. Approximately half of the knees were treated successfully with compression wrap, cryotherapy and motion exercises, while half required at least one aspiration. In cases where three aspirations failed to resolve recurrent serosanguinous fluid collections, the MLL was successfully treated with doxycycline sclerodesis with minimal morbidity and immediate return to play. The diagnosis of the lesion was often subtle, with an insidious progression of symptoms and potentially subtle physical examination findings of an extra-articular fluid collection extending to the mid-coronal plane. Thus, a thorough history and high index of suspicion was necessary to make the diagnosis. The authors concluded that MLL should be included in the differential diagnosis of intra-articular knee pathology, particularly in the setting of effusion after blunt trauma.

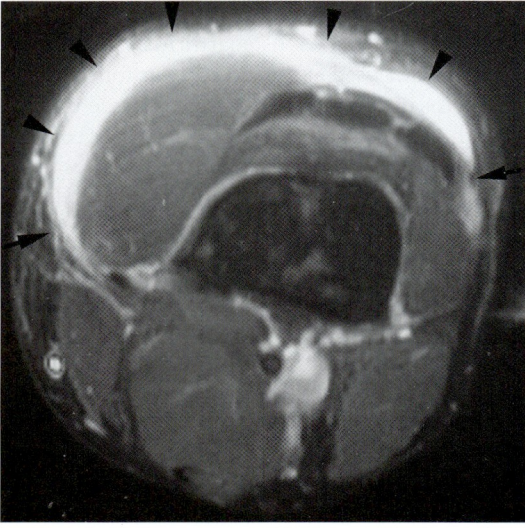

Figure 76.7 Right knee Morel–Lavallee lesion in a professional football player. Axial MRI section at the level of the femoral metaphysis, proximal to the patella, demonstrates a confluent fluid collection between the vastus musculature and the subcutaneous fat (arrowheads). The delamination plane of dissection can be visualized at the periphery of the lesion (arrows), extending to the mid-coronal plane medially.

KEY LEARNING POINTS

- Synovial disease of the knee can present with non-specific symptoms such as generalized pain, effusion, locking and instability, mimicking meniscal, chondral and ligamentous injury. Meticulous history and physical examination along with appropriate radiographs and MRI are typically necessary to make an accurate diagnosis. Conditions such as symptomatic medial plica, synovial chondromatosis, and pigmented villonodular synovitis (PVNS) can be safely and successfully treated arthroscopically in a majority of cases.
- The medial and lateral menisci play a critical role in load transmission, shock absorption, secondary stabilization, proprioception, joint lubrication and articular cartilage nutrition. Meniscal root tear results in loss of meniscal circumferential hoop stress, and is biomechanically equivalent to a total meniscectomy. Meniscal injuries which result in loss of meniscus function can lead to accelerated degenerative changes in the knee. When possible, meniscal tears should be repaired; arthroscopic techniques with vertical mattress sutures and direct root repair are the current standard of care.
- Osteochondritis dissecans of the knee most commonly affects males between 10 and 15 years of age, at the lateral aspect of the medial femoral condyle. Stable lesions, particularly in patients with open physes, can often be treated successfully with protected weight bearing, while unstable lesions often require internal fixation. Cases of incongruent fragments or large bone defects can be addressed by microfracture, osteochondral autograft or allograft, autologous chondrocyte implantation, or a combination of techniques.
- Microfracture is indicated for full-thickness loss of articular cartilage in either a weight-bearing area between the femur and tibia or an area of contact between the patella and trochlear groove, including areas underneath unstable cartilage flaps. Salient points in the technique include the creation of a stable peripheral chondral rim, curettage of the cartilage cap over the osseous base of the lesion, and the perpendicular placement of multiple subchondral holes with an awl to a depth of 2–4 mm.
- Osteochondral autograft transplantation (OATS), particularly when performed to achieve greater than 90% fill, is an efficacious one-stage procedure for treating small, focal, unipolar full-thickness chondral or osteochondral defects measuring 10–40 mm^2 in diameter. Autologous chondrocyte implantation (ACI) is a two-stage surgical procedure that can be used to treat symptomatic,

unipolar, full-thickness or near full-thickness chondral or shallow osteochondral lesions greater than 25 mm^2 in diameter, up to 150 mm^2.
- Unilateral patellar tendon rupture most commonly occurs in patients under 40 years of age as a result of eccentric quadriceps muscle contraction, while bilateral cases often occur in the setting of systematic disease such as diabetes, rheumatoid arthritis, gout, obesity, hyperparathyroidism, systemic lupus erythematosus, osteomalacia and systemic steroid use. Transosseous repair in conjunction with retinacular repair yields good healing rates.
- Quadriceps tendon rupture most commonly occurs in patients older than 40 years of age due to eccentric muscle contraction, and is often associated with degenerative changes of the tendon due to concurrent systemic medical disease. One-third of ruptures occur bilaterally, most often in patients with diabetes, systemic lupus erythematosus, rheumatoid arthritis, gout, prolonged systemic steroid use, hyperparathyroidism, or end-stage renal disease. Incomplete or partial (<50%) quadriceps tendon rupture is treated with immobilization in full extension for 4–6 weeks, while more extensive rupture can be successfully treated via a transosseous technique or using suture-anchors in the proximal patellar pole.
- Patellofemoral instability is defined as the inability of the patella to stay within the confines of the trochlea from 0° to 20° of knee flexion, and can be due to patella alta, generalized ligamentous laxity, patellar hypoplasia, trochlear hypoplasia, lateral femoral condyle hypoplasia, excessive femoral anteversion, genu recurvatum and excessive Q angle. First-time dislocation can be successfully treated with rehabilitation in approximately 50% of cases. Surgical options for refractory cases include medial patellofemoral ligament reconstruction, medial reefing, lateral release, tibial tubercle transfer, or a combination of techniques.
- Morel–Lavallee lesion (MLL) of the knee is a closed-degloving injury which most commonly occurs in athletes due to blunt, shearing trauma, and is a distinct lesion from prepatellar bursitis and quadriceps contusion. Physical examination and MRI typically reveal decreased active knee flexion and a large suprapatellar area of palpable fluctuance. In elite athletes approximately 50% of cases can be treated successfully with compression wrap, cryotherapy and motion exercises. In cases where multiple aspirations fail to resolve recurrent serosanguinous fluid collections, MLL can be successfully treated with doxycycline sclerodesis with minimal morbidity.

REFERENCES

- ● = Key primary paper
- ◆ = Major review article

◆1. Vigorita VJ. The synovium: normal and pathological conditions. In: Insall JN, Scott WN (eds) *Surgery of the Knee*, vol. 2, 3rd edn. Philadelphia, PA: Churchill Livingston, 2001:1103–8.

◆2. O'Rahilly R, Gardner E. The embryology of moveable joints. In: Sokoloff L (ed.) *The Joints and Synovial Fluid*, vol. 1. New York, NY: Academic Press, 1978:49–103.

3. Hasselbacher P. Structure of the synovial membrane. *Clinics in Rheumatic Diseases* 1981;**7**:57.

◆4. Dupont JY. Synovial plicae of the knee. Controversies and review. *Clinics in Sports Medicine* 1997;**16**:87–122.

5. García-Valtuille R, Abascal F, Cerezal L, et al. Anatomy and MR imaging appearances of synovial plicae of the knee. *Radiographics* 2002;**22**:775–84.

●6. Jouanin T, Dupont JY, Halimi P, Lassau JP. The synovial folds of the knee joint: anatomical study. *Anatomia Clinica* 1982;**4**:47–53.

7. Boles CA, Martin DF. Synovial plicae in the knee. *AJR American Journal of Roentgenology* 2001;**177**:221–7.

8. Jee WH, Choe BY, Kim JM, et al. The plica syndrome: diagnostic value of MRI with arthroscopic correlation. *Journal of Computer Assisted Tomography* 1998;**22**:814–18.

●9. Hardaker WT, Whipple TL, Bassett FH. Diagnosis and treatment of the plica syndrome of the knee. *Journal of Bone and Joint Surgery (American)* 1980;**62**:221–5.

10. Tindel NL, Nisonson B. The plica syndrome. *Orthopedic Clinics of North (American)* 1992;**23**:613–18.

11. Bae DK, Nam GU, Sun SD, Kim YH. The clinical significance of the complete type of suprapatellar membrane. *Arthroscopy* 1998;**14**:830–5.

12. Ewing JW. Plica: pathologic or not? *Journal of the American Academy of Orthopaedic Surgeons* 1993;**1**:117–21.

13. Hansen H, Boe S. The pathological plica in the knee. Results after arthroscopic resection. *Archives of Orthopaedic and Trauma Surgery* 1989;**108**:282–4.

14. Tearse DS, Clancy WG, Gersoff WK. The symptomatic lateral synovial plica of the knee. Presented at the 7th Annual Meeting of the Arthroscopy Association of North America, Washington, DC, 1998.

●15. Jaffe HL. *Tumors and Tumorous Conditions of the Bones and Joints*. London, UK: Henry Kimpton, 1958.

◆16. Vigorita VJ. The synovium: normal and pathological conditions. In: Insall JN, Scott WN (eds) *Surgery of the Knee*, vol. 2, 3rd edn. Philadelphia, PA: Churchill Livingston, **2001**:1126–9.

●17. Milgram JW. Synovial osteochondromatosis: a histopathologic study of thirty cases. *Journal of Bone and Joint Surgery (American)* 1977;**59**:792.

18. Iyengar J, Luke A, Ma CB. An unusual presentation of synovial chondromatosis of the knee: a case report. *Clinical Journal of Sport Medicine* 2007;**17**(2):157–9.

19. Crotty JM, Monu JU, Pope TL Jr. Synovial osteochondromatosis. *Radiology Clinics of North America* 1996;**34**:327-42.
20. Goldman AB, DiCarlo EF. Pigmented villonodular synovitis. Diagnosis and differential diagnosis. *Radiology Clinics of North America* 1988;**26**:1327-47.
21. Ryan RS, Harris AC, O'Connell JX, Munk PL. Synovial osteochondromatosis: the spectrum of imaging findings. *Australasian Radiology* 2005;**49**:95-100.
◆22. Helpert C, Davies A, Evans N, Grimer RJ. Differential diagnosis of tumours and tumour-like lesions of the infrapatellar (Hoffa's) fat pad: pictorial review with an emphasis on MR imaging. *European Radiology* 2004;**14**:2337-46.
23. Kramer J, Recht M, Deely DM, et al. MR appearance of idiopathic synovial osteochondromatosis. *Journal of Computer Assisted Tomography* 1993;**17**:772-6.
24. Coolican MR, Dandy DJ. Arthroscopic management of synovial chondromatosis of the knee. Findings and results in 18 cases. *Journal of Bone and Joint Surgery (British)* 1989;**71**(3):498-500.
◆25. Davis RI, Hamilton A, Biggart JD. Primary synovial chondromatosis: a clinicopathologic review and assessment of malignant potential. *Human Pathology* 1998;**29**(7):683-8.
●26. Bertoni F, Unni KK, Beabout JW, Sim FH. Chondrosarcomas of the synovium. *Cancer* 1991;**67**:155-62.
27. Kenan S, Abdelwahab IF, Klein MJ, Lewis MM. Case report 817: Synovial chondrosarcoma secondary to synovial chondromatosis. *Skeletal Radiology* 1993;**22**:623-6.
28. Masih S, Antebi A. Imaging of pigmented villonodular synovitis of the knee. Arthroscopic treatment. *Clinics in Orthopedic Surgery* 2003;**271**:218-24.
29. Parikh SN, Chen AL, Ergas E. Localized pigmented villonodular synovitis: arthroscopic diagnosis and management of an 'invisible' lesion. *Arthroscopy* 2002;**18**:e31.
●30. Granowitz SP, D'Antonio J, Mankin HJ. The pathogenesis and long-term end results of pigmented villonodular synovitis. *Clinics in Orthopedic Surgery* 1976;**114**:335-51.
31. Abdul-Karim FW, el-Naggar AK, Joyce MJ, et al. Diffuse and localized tenosynovial giant cell tumor and pigmented villonodular synovitis: a clinicopathologic and flow cytometric DNA analysis. *Human Pathology* 1992;**23**:729-35.
32. Kim SJ, Shin SJ, Choi NH, Choo ET. Arthroscopic treatment for localized pigmented villonodular synovitis of the knee. *Clinics in Orthopedic Surgery* 2000;**379**:224-30.
◆33. Myers BW, Masi AT, Feigenbaum SL. Pigmented villonodular synovitis and tenosynovitis: A clinical epidemiologic study of 166 cases and literature review. *Medicine* 1980;**59**:223-8.
●34. Byers PD, Cotton RE, Deacon OW, et al. The diagnosis and treatment of pigmented villonodular synovitis. *Journal of Bone and Joint Surgery (British)* 1968;**50**:290-305.
35. Kim RS, Kang JS, Jung JH, et al. Clustered localized pigmented villonodular synovitis. *Arthroscopy* 2005;**21**:761.
36. Ofluoglu O. Pigmented villonodular synovitis. *Orthopedic Clinics of North America* 2006;**37**(1):23-33.
37. Ogilvie-Harris DJ, McLean J, Zarnett ME. Pigmented villonodular synovitis of the knee. The results of total arthroscopic synovectomy, partial, arthroscopic synovectomy, and arthroscopic local excision. *Journal of Bone and Joint Surgery (American)* 1992;**74**(6):952.
38. Moskovich R, Parisien JS. Localized pigmented villonodular synovitis of the knee. Arthroscopic treatment. *Clinics in Orthopedic Surgery* 1991;**271**:218-24.
39. Bouali H, Deppert EJ, Leventhal LJ, et al. Pigmented villonodular synovitis: a disease in evolution. *Journal of Rheumatology* 2004;**31**:1659-62.
40. Palumbo RC, Matthews LS, Reuben JM. Localized pigmented villonodular synovitis of the patellar fat pad: a report of two cases. *Arthroscopy* 1994;**10**:400-3.
41. Delcogliano A, Galli M, Menghi A, Belli P. Localized pigmented villonodular synovitis of the knee: report of two cases of fat pad involvement. *Arthroscopy* 1998;**14**:527-31.
42. Choi NH. Localized pigmented villonodular synovitis involving the fat pad of the knee: case report. *American Journal of Knee Surgery* 2000;**13**:117-19.
43. Muscolo DL, Makino A, Cost-Paz M, Ayerza M. Magnetic resonance imaging evaluation and arthroscopic resection of localized pigmented villonodular synovitis of the knee. *Orthopedics* 2000;**23**:367-9.
44. Cheng XG, You YH, Liu W, et al. MRI features of pigmented villonodular synovitis (PVNS). *Clinical Rheumatology* 2004;**23**:31-4.
45. Zvijac JE, Lau AC, Hechtman KS, et al. Arthroscopic treatment of pigmented villonodular synovitis of the knee. *Arthroscopy* 1999;**15**:613-17.
46. Chin KR, Brick GW. Extraarticular pigmented villonodular synovitis. *Clinics in Orthopedic Surgery* 2002;**404**:330-8.
47. Kramer DE, Frassica FJ, Cosgarea AJ. Total arthroscopic synovectomy for pigmented villonodular synovitis of the knee. *Techniques in Knee Surgery* 2004;**3**:36-45.
48. Ogilvie-Harris DJ, Al Thani S. Complications of surgery on synovium and soft tissues. *Sports Medicine and Arthroscopy Review* 2004;**12**:167-71.
49. De Ponti A, Sansone V, Malcherè M. Result of arthroscopic treatment of pigmented villonodular synovitis of the knee. *Arthroscopy* 2003;**19**(6):602-7.
50. Akgün I, Ogüt T, Kesmezacar H, Dervisoglu S. Localized pigmented villonodular synovitis of the knee. *Orthopedics* 2003;**26**:1131-5.
51. Beguin J, Locker B, Vielpeau C, Souquieres G. Pigmented villonodular synovitis of the knee: Results from 13 cases. *Arthroscopy* 1989;**5**:61-4.
●52. Jaffe HL, Lichtenstein L, Sutro CJ. Pigmented villonodular synovitis, bursitis and tenosynovitis. A discussion of synovial and bursal equivalents of tenosynovial lesion commonly denoted as xanthoma, xanthogranuloma, giant cell tumor, or myeloplaxoma of tendon sheath, with some considerations of this tendon sheath lesion itself. *Archives of Pathology* 1941;**31**:731-65.

53. Gonzalez Della Valle A, Piccaluga F, Potter HG, et al. Pigmented villonodular synovitis of the hip. 2- to 23-year followup study. *Clinics in Orthopedic Surgery* 2001;**388**:187–99.
●54. Johansson JE, Ajjoub S, Coughlin LP, et al. Pigmented villonodular synovitis of joints. *Clinics in Orthopedic Surgery* 1982;**163**:159–66.
55. Blanco CE, Leon HO, Guthrie TB. Combined partial arthroscopic synovectomy and radiation therapy for diffuse pigmented villonodular synovitis of the knee. *Arthroscopy* 2001;**17**:527–31.
56. Chin KR, Barr SJ, Winalski C, et al. Treatment of advanced primary and recurrent diffuse pigmented villonodular synovitis of the knee. *Journal of Bone and Joint Surgery (American)* 2002;**84A**:2192–202.
●57. Atmore WG, Dahlin DC, Ghormley RK. Pigmented villonodular synovitis: a clinical and pathological study. *Minnesota Medicine* 1956;**39**:196–202.
58. Brien EW, Sacoman DM, Mirra JM. Pigmented villonodular synovitis of the foot and ankle. *Foot and Ankle International* 2004;**25**:908–13.
◆59. Layfield LJ, Meloni-Ehrig A, Liu K, et al. Malignant giant cell tumor of synovium (malignant pigmented villonodular synovitis): a histologic and fluorescence in situ hybridization analysis of 2 cases with review of the literature. *Archives of Pathology and Laboratory Medicine* 2000;**124**:1636–41.
60. Kalil RK, Unni KK. Malignancy in pigmented villonodular synovitis. *Skeletal Radiology* 1998;**27**:392–5.
61. Fiocco U, Sfriso P, Oliviero F, et al. Intra-articular treatment with the TNF-alpha antagonist, etanercept, in severe diffuse pigmented villonodular synovitis of the knee. *Reumatismo* 2006;**58**:268–74.
62. Kroot EJ, Kraan MC, Smeets TJ, et al. Tumour necrosis factor alpha blockade in treatment resistant pigmented villonodular synovitis. *Annals of the Rheumatic Diseases* 2005;**64**:497–9.
●63. Walker PS, Erkman MJ. The role of the meniscus in force transmission across the knee. *Clinics in Orthopedic Surgery* 1975;**109**:184–92.
64. Lee SJ, Aadalen KJ, Malaviya P, et al. Tibiofemoral contact mechanics after serial medial meniscectomies in the human cadaveric knee. *American Journal of Sports Medicine* 2006;**34**:1334–44.
●65. Markolf KL, Mensch JS, Amstutz HC. Stiffness and laxity of the knee—the contribution of the supporting structures. *Journal of Bone and Joint Surgery (American)* 1976;**58A**:583–94.
●66. Fukubayashi T, Kurosawa H. The contact area and pressure distribution pattern of the knee: a study of normal and osteoarthritic knee joints. *Acta Orthopaedica Scandinavica* 1980;**51**:871–9.
●67. Hsieh HH, Walker PS. Stabilizing mechanisms of the loaded and unloaded knee joint. *Journal of Bone and Joint Surgery (American)* 1976;**58A**:87–93.
●68. Levy IM, Torzilli PA, Warren RF. The effect of medial meniscectomy of anterior posterior motion of the knee. *Journal of Bone and Joint Surgery (American)* 1982;**64A**:883–7.

69. Petrosini AV, Sherman OA. A historical perspective on meniscal repair. *Clinics in Sports Medicine* 1996;**15**:445–53.
●70. Kusayama T, Harner CD, Carlin GJ, et al. Anatomical and biomechanical characteristics of human meniscofemoral ligaments. *Knee Surgery, Sports Traumatology, Arthroscopy* 1994;**2**:234–7.
71. Allen CR, Wong EK, Livesay GA, et al. Importance of the medial meniscus in the anterior cruciate ligament-deficient knee. *Journal of Orthopaedic Research* 2000;**18**:109–15.
●72. King D. The function of semilunar cartilages. *Journal of Bone and Joint Surgery (British)* 1936;**18B**:1069–76.
●73. King D. The healing of semilunar cartilages. *Journal of Bone and Joint Surgery (British)* 1936;**18B**:333–42.
●74. Fairbank T. Knee joint changes after meniscectomy. *Journal of Bone and Joint Surgery (British)* 1948;**30B**:664–70.
75. Allen PR, Denham RA, Swan AV. Late degenerative changes after meniscectomy: factors affecting the knee after the operation. *Journal of Bone and Joint Surgery (British)* 1984;**66B**:666–71.
●76. Appel H. Late results after meniscectomy in the knee joint. A clinical and roentgenologic follow-up investigation. *Acta Orthopaedica Scandinavica* (Suppl.) 1970:133.
●77. Johnson RJ, Kettlekemp DB, Clark W, Leaverton P. Factors affecting late results after meniscectomy. *Journal of Bone and Joint Surgery (American)* 1974;**56A**:719–29.
●78. Tapper EM, Hoover NW. Late results after meniscectomy. *Journal of Bone and Joint Surgery (American)* 1969;**69A**:517–26.
79. Sgaglione NA, Steadman JR, Shaffer B, et al. Current concepts in meniscus surgery: resection to replacement. *Arthroscopy* 2003;**19**(Suppl. 1):161–88.
80. DeHaven KE, Lohrer WA, Lovelock JE. Long-term results of open meniscal repair. *American Journal of Sports Medicine* 1995;**23**:524–30.
81. Cannon WD. Arthroscopic meniscal repair. In: Insall JN, Scott WN (eds) *Surgery of the Knee,* vol. 1, 3rd edn. Philadelphia, PA: Churchill Livingstone, 2001:521–37.
82. Baratz ME, Rehak DC, Fu FH, Rudert MJ. Peripheral tears of the meniscus. The effect of open versus arthroscopic repair on intraarticular contact stresses in the human knee. *American Journal of Sports Medicine* 1988;**16**:1–6.
83. Steenbrugge F, Verdonk R, Verstraete K. Long-term assessment of arthroscopic meniscus repair: a 13-year follow-up study. *Knee* 2002;**9**:181–7.
84. Johnson MJ, Lucas GL, Dusek JK, Henning CE. Isolated arthroscopic meniscal repair: a long-term outcome study (more than 10 years). *American Journal of Sports Medicine* 1999;**27**:44–9.
85. Elkousy HA, Sekiya JK, Harner CD. Broadening the indications for meniscal repair. *Sports Medicine and Arthroscopy Review* 2002;**10**:270–5.
86. Ikeuchi H. Arthroscopic peripheral meniscus repair. *Sports Medicine and Arthroscopy Review* 1993;**1**:103.
87. Rispoli DM, Miller MD. Options in meniscal repair. *Clinics in Sports Medicine* 1999;**18**:77–91.

88. Cooper DE, Arnoczky SP, Warren RF. Arthroscopic meniscal repair. *Clinics in Sports Medicine* 1990;**9**:589–607.
89. Arnoczky SP, Warren RF. Microvasculature of the human meniscus. *American Journal of Sports Medicine* 1982;**10**:90–5.
90. Schulte KR, Fu FH. Meniscal repair using the inside-to-outside technique. *Clinics in Sports Medicine* 1996;**15**:455–67.
•91. Warren LF, Marshall JL. The supporting structures and layers on the medial side of the knee: an anatomical analysis. *Journal of Bone and Joint Surgery (American)* 1979;**61**:56–62.
92. Post WR, Akers SR, Kish V. Load to failure of common meniscal repair techniques: effects of suture technique and suture material. *Arthroscopy* 1997;**13**:731–6.
93. Ryu RK, Ting AJ. Arthroscopic treatment of meniscal cysts. *Arthroscopy* 1993;**9**:591–5.
94. Hulet C, Souquet D, Alexandre P, *et al.* Arthroscopic treatment of 105 lateral meniscal cysts with 5-year average follow-up. *Arthroscopy* 2004;**20**:831–6.
95. Parisien JS. Arthroscopic treatment of cysts of the menisci. A preliminary report. *Clinics in Orthopaedic Surgery and Related Research* 1990;**257**:154–8.
96. Mills CA, Henderson IJ. Cysts of the medial meniscus. Arthroscopic diagnosis and management. *Journal of Bone and Joint Surgery* 1993;**75**:293–8.
97. Erginer R, Tucel I, Ogut T, *et al.* Medial meniscus anterior horn cyst: arthroscopic decompression. *Arthroscopy* 2004;**20**(Suppl 2):9–12.
98. Seger BM, Woods GW. Arthroscopic management of lateral meniscal cysts. *American Journal of Sports Medicine* 1986;**14**:105–8.
99. Lu KH. Arthroscopic meniscal repair and needle aspiration for meniscal tear with meniscal cyst. *Arthroscopy* 2006;**22**:1367.e1–4.
100. Macmahon PJ, Brennan DD, Duke D, *et al.* Ultrasound-guided percutaneous drainage of meniscal cysts: preliminary clinical experience. *Clinical Radiology* 2007;**62**:683–7.
101. Cohen DB, Wickiewicz TL. The outside-in technique for arthroscopic meniscal repair. *Operative Techniques in Sports Medicine* 2003;**11**:91–103.
102. Chong KC, Chan BK, Chang HW. A simple method of meniscus repair using the arthroscopic outside-in technique. A technical note. *Arthroscopy* 2006;**22**:794.e1–e5.
103. Morgan CD, Wojtys EM, Casscells CD, Casscells SW. Arthroscopic meniscal repair evaluated by second-look arthroscopy. *American Journal of Sports Medicine* 1991;**19**:632–7.
104. Otte S, Klinger HM, Beyer J, Baums MH. Complications after meniscal repair with bioabsorbable arrows: two cases and analysis of the literature. *Knee Surgery, Sports Traumatology, Arthroscopy* 2002;**10**:250–3.
105. Anderson K, Marx RG, Hannafin J, Warren RF. Chondral injury following meniscal repair with a biodegradable implant. *Arthroscopy* 2000;**16**:749–53.
106. Hechman KS, Uribe JW. Cystic hematoma formation following use of a biodegradable arrow for meniscal repair. *Arthroscopy* 1999;**15**:207–10.
107. Siebold R, Dehler C, Boes L, Ellermann A. Arthroscopic all-inside repair using the Meniscus Arrow: long-term clinical follow-up of 113 patients. *Arthroscopy* 2007;**23**:394–9.
108. Kurzweil PR, Tifford CD, Ignacio EM. Unsatisfactory clinical results of meniscal repair using the meniscus arrow. *Arthroscopy* 2005;**21**:905.
109. Diduch DR, Poelstra KA. The evolution of all-inside meniscal repair. *Operative Techniques in Sports Medicine* 2003;**11**:83–90.
110. Miller MD, Hart JA. All-inside meniscal repair. *Instructional Course Lectures* 2005;**54**:337–40.
111. Haas AL, Schepsis AA, Hornstein J, Edgar CM. Meniscal repair using the FasT-Fix all-inside meniscal repair device. *Arthroscopy* 2005;**21**:167–75.
•112. Pagnani MJ, Cooper DW, Warren RF. Extrusion of the medial meniscus. *Arthroscopy* 1991;**7**:297–300.
•113. Allaire RB, Muriuki MG, Chauhan C, *et al.* Meniscal root tear alters joint contact and kinematics. Orthopaedic Research Society, Annual Meeting, San Diego, CA, 2007, Poster no.157.
114. Jones AO, Houang MT, Low RS, Wood DG. Medial meniscus posterior root attachment injury and degeneration: MRI findings. *Australasian Radiology* 2006;**50**:306–13.
•115. Beasely L, Robertson D, Armfield D, *et al.* Medial meniscus root tears: an unsolved problem—demographic, radiographic and arthroscopic findings. *Pittsburgh Orthopaedic Journal* 2005;**16**:155.
•116. Papalia R, Muriuki MG, Hefferman MJ, Harner CD. An in vitro evaluation of meniscal root insertion strength and repair techniques. Orthopaedic Research Society, Annual Meeting, San Diego, CA, 2007, Poster no. 797.
117. Yoldas EA, Sekiya JK, Irrgang JJ, *et al.* Arthroscopically assisted meniscal allograft transplantation with and without combined anterior cruciate ligament reconstruction. *Knee Surgery, Sports Traumatology, Arthroscopy* 2003;**11**:173–82.
118. Tejwani SG, Harner CD. Arthroscopically-assisted posterior horn medial meniscus root repair. *Pittsburgh Orthopaedic Journal* 2007;**18**:284–7.
119. Kim YM, Rhee KJ, Lee JK, *et al.* Arthroscopic pullout repair of a complete radial tear of the tibial attachment site of the medial meniscus posterior horn. *Arthroscopy* 2006;**22**:795.e1–4.
•120. König F. Ueber freie Korper in den Glenken. *Zeitschrift Chirurgie* 1888;**27**:90–109.
121. Bradley J, Dandy D. Osteochondritis dissecans and other lesions of the femoral condyles. *Journal of Bone and Joint Surgery (British)* 1989;**71**:518–22.
122. Cahill B. Osteochondritis dissecans of the knee: treatment of juvenile and adult forms. *Journal of the American Academy of Orthopaedic Surgeons* 1995;**3**:237–47.

123. Hefti F. Osteochondritis dissecans: a multicenter study of the European Pediatric Orthopaedic Society. *Journal of Pediatric Orthopaedics* 1999;**8**:231–45.
124. Yoshida S, Ikata T, Takai H, *et al*. Osteochondritis dissecans of the femoral condyle in the growth stage. *Clinics in Orthopedic Surgery* 1998;**346**:162–70.
125. Mubarak S, Carrol M. Familial osteochondritis dissecans of the knee. *Clinics in Orthopedic Surgery* 1979;**140**:130–6.
126. Paletta G, Bednarz P, Stanitski CL, *et al*. The prognostic value of quantitative bone scan in knee osteochondritis dissecans. *American Journal of Sports Medicine* 1998;**26**:7–14.
127. Cahill B, Berg B. 99m-technetium phosphate compound scintigraphy in the management of juvenile osteochondritis dissecans of the femoral condyles. *American Journal of Sports Medicine* 1983;**11**:329–35.
128. O'Connor MA, Palaniappan M, Kahn N, Bruce CE. Osteochondritis dissecans of the knee in children: a comparison of MRI and arthroscopic findings. *Journal of Bone and Joint Surgery (British)* 2002;**84B**:258–62.
129. Guhl JF. Arthroscopic treatment of osteochondritis dissecans. *Clinics in Orthopedic Surgery* 1982;**167**:65–74.
130. Lebolt JR, Wall EJ. Retroarticular drilling and bone grafting of juvenile osteochondritis dissecans of the knee. *Arthroscopy* 2007;**23**:794.e1–4.
131. Miniaci A, Tytherleigh-Strong G. Fixation of unstable osteochondritis dissecans lesions of the knee using arthroscopic autogenous osteochondral grafting (mosaicplasty). *Arthroscopy* 2007;**23**:845–51.
132. Steadman JR, Rodkey WG, Rodrigo JJ. 'Microfracture': surgical technique and rehabilitation to treat chondral defects. *Clinics in Orthopedic Surgery* 2001;**391**(Suppl):S362–9.
133. Steadman JR, Rodkey WG, Singleton SB, Briggs KK. Microfracture technique for full-thickness chondral defects: techniques and clinical results. *Operative Techniques in Orthopaedics* 1997;**7**:300–4.
●134. Campbell CJ. The healing of cartilage defects. *Clinics in Orthopedic Surgery* 1969;**64**:45–63.
●135. DePalma AF, McKeever CD, Subin SK. Process of repair of articular cartilage demonstrated by histology and autoradiography with tritiated thymidine. *Clinics in Orthopedic Surgery* 1966;**48**:229–42.
136. Shapiro F, Koide S, Glimcher MJ. Cell origin and differentiation in the repair of full thickness defects of articular cartilage. *Journal of Bone and Joint Surgery (American)* 1993;**75**:532–53.
137. Simonian PT, Sussmann PS, Wickiewicz TL, *et al*. Contact pressures at osteochondral donor sites in the knee. *American Journal of Sports Medicine* 1998;**26**:491–4.
138. Koh J, Wirsing K, Lautenschlager E, Zhang LO. The effect of graft height mismatch on contact pressure following osteochondral grafting. *American Journal of Sports Medicine* 2004;**32**:317–20.
139. Hangody L, Rathonyi GK, Duska Z, *et al*. Autologous osteochondral mosaicplasty: surgical technique. *Journal of Bone and Joint Surgery (American)* 2004;**86**:65–72.
140. Chow JC, Hantes ME, Houle JB, Zalavras CG. Arthroscopic autogenous osteochondral transplantation for treating knee cartilage defects: a 2- to 5-year follow-up study. *Arthroscopy* 2004;**20**:681–90.
141. Beaver RJ, Gross AE. Fresh small-fragment osteochondral allograft in the knee joint. In: Aichroth PM, Cannon WD Jr (eds) *Knee Surgery. Current Practice.* Cologne, Germany: Deutscher Arzte-Verlag, 1992:464–71.
142. Meyers MH, Akeson W, Convery FR. Resurfacing of the knee with fresh osteochondral allograft. *Journal of Bone and Joint Surgery (American)* 1989;**71**:704–13.
◆143. Czitrom AA, Langer F, VcKee N, Gross AE. Bone and cartilage allotransplantation: a review of 14 years of research and clinical studies. *Clinics in Orthopedic Surgery* 1986;**208**:141–5.
144. Bobic V, Morgan C, Carter T. Osteochondral autologous graft transfer. *Operative Techniques in Sports Medicine* 2000;**8**:168–78.
145. Hangody L, Fules P. Autologous osteochondral mosaicplasty for the treatment of full-thickness defects of weight-bearing joints. *Journal of Bone and Joint Surgery (American)* 2003;**85**(Suppl 2):25–32.
146. Brittberg M, Lindahl A, Nilsson A, *et al*. Treatment of deep cartilage defects in the knee with autologous chondrocyte implantation. *New England Journal of Medicine* 1994;**331**:889–95.
147. Fu FH, Zurakowski D, Browne JE, *et al*. Autologous chondrocyte implantation versus debridement for treatment of full-thickness chondral defects of the knee: an observational cohort study with 3-year follow-up. *American Journal of Sports Medicine* 2005;**33**:1658–66.
148. Micheli LJ, Browne JE, Erggelet C, *et al*. Autologous chondrocyte implantation of the knee: multicenter experience and minimum 3-year follow-up. *Clinical Journal of Sport Medicine* 2001;**11**:223–8.
◆149. Brittberg M, Peterson L, Sjogren-Jansson E, *et al*. Articular cartilage engineering with autologous chondrocyte transplantation: a review of recent developments. *Journal of Bone and Joint Surgery (American)* 2003;**85A**(Suppl 3):109–15.
150. Bentley G, Biant LC, Carrington RW, *et al*. A prospective, randomised comparison of autologous chondrocyte implantation versus mosaicplasty for osteochondral defects in the knee. *Journal of Bone and Joint Surgery (British)* 2003;**85**:223–30.
151. Knutsen G, Engebretsen L, Ludvigsen TC, *et al*. Autologous chondrocyte implantation and compared with microfracture in the knee: a randomized trial. *Journal of Bone and Joint Surgery (American)* 2004;**86A**:455–64.
152. Fu FH, Stone DA. *Sports Injuries, Mechanisms, Prevention Treatment,* 2nd edn. Philadelphia, PA: Lippincott, Williams, Wilkins, 2001:1112.
153. Bhargava S. Traumatic patella tendon rupture: early mobilisation following surgical repair. *Injury* 2004;**35**:76–9.
◆154. McMahon P, Kaplan L. Sports medicine. In: Skinner HB (ed.) *Current Diagnosis and Treatment in Orthopedics,* 4th edn. 2006: Chapter 4.

◆155. MacEachern AG, Plewes JL. Bilateral simultaneous spontaneous rupture of the quadriceps tendons: Five case reports and a review of the literature. *Journal of Bone and Joint Surgery (British)* 1984;**66**:81–3.

156. Bhole R, Flynn JC, Marbury TC. Quadriceps tendon ruptures in uremia. *Clinics in Orthopedic Surgery* 1985;**195**:200–6.

157. Stern RE, Harwin SF. Spontaneous and simultaneous rupture of both quadriceps tendons. *Clinics in Orthopedic Surgery* 1980;**147**:188–9.

158. Lombardi LJ, Cleri DJ, Epstein E. Bilateral spontaneous quadriceps tendon rupture in a patient with renal failure. *Orthopedics* 1995;**18**:187–91.

159. Razzano CD, Wilde AH, Phalen GS. Bilateral rupture of the infrapatellar tendon in rheumatoid arthritis. *Clinics in Orthopedic Surgery* 1973;**91**:158–61.

160. Wener JA, Schein AJ. Simultaneous bilateral rupture of the patellar tendon and quadriceps expansions in systemic lupus erythematosus: A case report. *Journal of Bone and Joint Surgery (American)* 1974;**56**:823–4.

161. Preston ET. Avulsion of both quadriceps tendons in hyperparathyroidism. *Journal of the American Medical Association* 1972;**221**:406–7.

162. Levy M, Seelenfreund M, Maor P, et al. Bilateral spontaneous and simultaneous rupture of the quadriceps tendons in gout. *Journal of Bone and Joint Surgery (British)* 1971;**53**:510–13.

163. Ilan DI, Tejwani N, Keschner M, Leibman M. Quadriceps tendon rupture. *Journal of the American Academy of Orthopaedic Surgeons* 2003;**11**:192–200.

164. Peace KA, Lee JC, Healy J. Imaging the infrapatellar tendon in the elite athlete. *Clinical Radiology* 2006;**61**:570–8.

165. Yu JS, Petersilge C, Sartoris DJ, et al. MR imaging of injuries of the extensor mechanism of the knee. *Radiographics* 1994;**14**:541–51.

166. Ramseier LE, Werner CML, Heinzelmann M. Quadriceps and patellar tendon rupture. *Injury* 2006;**37**:516–19.

167. Ahrberg A, Josten C. Augmentation of patella fractures and patella tendon ruptures with the McLaughlin-Cerclage. *Unfallchirurg* 2007;**110**:685–90.

168. Ozkan C, Kalaci A, Tan I, Sarpel Y. Bilateral dislocation of the knee with rupture of both patellar tendons. A case report. *Knee* 2006;**13**:333–6.

169. Futch LA, Garth WP, Folsom GJ. Acute rupture of the anterior cruciate ligament and patellar tendon in a collegiate athlete. *Arthroscopy* 2007;**23**:112.e1–4.

170. Kuechle DK, Stuart MJ. Isolated rupture of the patellar tendon in athletes. *American Journal of Sports Medicine* 1994;**22**:692–5.

171. Kuo-yao H, Kun-chuang W, Wei-pin H, Wen-wei Hsu R. Traumatic patellar tendon ruptures: a follow-up study of primary repair and neutralisation wire. *Journal of Trauma* 1994;**36**:658–60.

172. Larsen E, Lund PM. Ruptures of the extensor mechanism of the knee joint: clinical results and patellofemoral articulation. *Clinics in Orthopedic Surgery* 1986;**213**:150–3.

173. Noyes FR, Torvik PJ, Hyde WB. Biomechanics of ligament failure. *Journal of Bone and Joint Surgery (American)* 1974;**56A**:1406–18.

174. Siwek CW, Rao JP. Ruptures of the extensor mechanism of the knee joint. *Journal of Bone and Joint Surgery (British)* 1981;**63A**:932–7.

175. Marder RA, Timmerman LA. Primary repair of patellar tendon rupture without augmentation. *American Journal of Sports Medicine* 1997;**27**:304–7.

176. Kelly DW, Carter VS, Jobe FW, Kerlan RK. Patellar and quadriceps tendon ruptures—jumper's knee. *American Journal of Sports Medicine* 1984;**12**:375.

●177. Scuderi C. Ruptures of the quadriceps tendon. *American Journal of Surgery* 1958;**95**:626–35.

●178. McMaster PE. Tendon and muscle ruptures: clinical and experimental studies on the causes and location of subcutaneous ruptures. *Journal of Bone and Joint Surgery* 1933;**15**:705–22.

179. Neubauer T, Wagner M, Potschka T, Riedl M. Bilateral, simultaneous rupture of the quadriceps tendon: a diagnostic pitfall? *Knee Surgery, Sports Traumatology, Arthroscopy* 2007;**15**:43–53.

180. Zanetti M, Hodler J. Ultrasonography and magnetic resonance tomography (MRI) of tendon injuries. *Orthopade* 1995;**24**:200–8.

181. Peiro A, Ferrandis R, Garcia L, Alcazar E. Simultaneous and spontaneous bilateral rupture of the patellar tendon in rheumatoid arthritis. *Acta Orthopaedica Scandinavica* 1975;**46**:700–3.

182. Barasch E, Lombardi U, Arena L, Epstein E. MRI visualization of bilateral quadriceps tendon-rupture in a patient with secondary hyperparathyroidism: implications for diagnosis and therapy. *Computing Medical Imaging* 1989;**13**:407–10.

◆183. Walker LG, Glick H. Bilateral spontaneous quadriceps tendon ruptures: A case report and review of the literature. *Orthopedic Reviews* 1989;**18**:867–71.

184. Konrath GA, Chen D, Lock T, et al. Outcomes following repair of quadriceps tendon ruptures. *Journal of Orthopaedic Trauma* 1998;**12**:273–9.

185. Mahlfeld K, Franke J, Schaeper O, Grasshoff H. Simultaneous bilateral rupture of the quadriceps tendon, a diagnostical problem? *Ultraschall in der Medizin* 2000;**21**:226–8.

186. Heyde CE, Mahlfeld K, Stahel PF, Kayser R. Ultrasonography as a reliable diagnostic tool in old quadriceps tendon ruptures: a prospective multicenter study. *Knee Surgery, Sports Traumatology, Arthroscopy* 2005;**13**:564–8.

187. Wick M, Muller EJ, Ekkernkamp A, Muhr G. Misdiagnosis of a late simultaneous and bilateral rupture of the quadriceps tendon. *Unfallchirurg* 1997;**100**:320–3.

188. Sagiv P, Gepstein R, Amdur B, Hallel T. Bilateral spontaneous rupture of the quadriceps tendon misdiagnosed as a 'neurological condition'. *Journal of the American Geriatrics Society* 1989;**37**:750–2.

189. Blazina ME, Kerlan RK, Jobe FW, et al. Jumper's knee. *Orthopedic Clinics of North America* 1973;**4**:665–78.

190. De Baere T, Geulette B, Manche E, Barras L. Functional results after surgical repair of quadriceps tendon rupture. *Acta Orthopaedica Belgica* 2002;**68**:146-9.
191. Hughston JC. Subluxation of the patella. *Journal of Bone and Joint Surgery (American)* 1968;**50A**:1003-26.
◆192. Fu, FH, Stone, DA. *Sports Injuries,* 2nd edn. Philadelphia, PA: Lippincott, Williams, and Wilkins, 2001:229-31.
●193. Conlan T, Garth WP Jr, Lemons JE. Evaluation of the medial soft-tissue restraints of the extensor mechanism of the knee. *Journal of Bone and Joint Surgery (American)* 1993;**75A**:682-93.
194. Desio SM, Burks RT, Bachus KN. Soft tissue restraints to lateral patellar translation in the human knee. *American Journal of Sports Medicine* 1998;**26**:59-65.
195. Fithian DC, Paxton EW, Cohen AB. Indications in the treatment of patellar instability. *Journal of Knee Surgery* 2004;**17**:47-56.
196. Kujala UM, Osterman K, Kvist M, et al. Factors predisposing to patellar chondropathy and patellar apicitis in athletes. *International Orthopaedics* 1986;**10**:195-200.
197. Kolowich PA, Paulos LE, Rosenberg TD, Farnsworth S. Lateral release of the patella: indications and contraindications. *American Journal of Sports Medicine* 1990;**18**:359-65.
198. Hautamaa PV, Fithian DC, Kaufman KR, et al. Medial soft tissue restraints in lateral patellar instability and repair. *Clinics in Orthopedic Surgery* 1998;**349**:174-82.
199. Fu FH, Maday MG. Arthroscopic lateral release and the lateral patellar compression syndrome. *Orthopedic Clinics of North America* 1992;**23**:601-12.
200. Dejour H, Walch G, Nove-Josserand L, Guier C. Factors of patellar instability: an anatomic radiographic study. *Knee Surgery, Sports Traumatology, Arthroscopy* 1994;**1**:19-26.
●201. Insall J, Salvati E. Patellar position in the normal knee. *Radiology* 1971;**101**:101-4.
●202. Merchant AC, Mercer RL, Jacobsen RH, Cool CR. Roentgenographic analysis of patellofemoral congruence. *Journal of Bone and Joint Surgery (American)* 1974;**56A**:1391-6.
203. Shellock FG, Stone KR, Crues JV. Development and clinical application of kinematic MRI of the patellofemoral joint using an extremity MR system. *Medicine and Science in Sports and Exercise* 1999;**31**:788-91.
204. McNally EG, Ostlere SJ, Pal C, et al. Assessment of patellar maltracking using combined static and dynamic MRI. *European Radiology* 2000;**10**:1051-5.
205. Cofield RH, Bryan RS. Acute dislocation of the patella: results of conservative treatment. *Journal of Trauma* 1977;**17**:526-31.
206. Larsen E, Lauridsen F. Conservative treatment of patellar dislocations: influence of evident factors on the tendency to redislocation and the therapeutic result. *Clinics in Orthopedic Surgery* 1982;**171**:131-6.
207. Cash JD, Hughston JC. Treatment of acute patellar dislocation. *American Journal of Sports Medicine* 1988;**16**:244-9.
●208. Hawkins RJ, Bell RH, Anisette G. Acute patellar dislocations. The natural history. *American Journal of Sports Medicine* 1986;**14**:117-20.
209. McConnell J. Rehabilitation and nonoperative treatment of patellar instability. *Sports Medicine and Arthroscopy* 2007;**15**:95-104.
210. Roux C. Recurrent dislocation of the patella: operative treatment. *Revista Chirurgie* 1888;**8**:682-9.
211. Goldthwait HE. Slipping or recurrent dislocation of the patella: with the report of eleven cases. *Boston Medical and Surgical Journal* 1904;**150**:169-74.
212. Cox JS. Evaluation of the Roux-Elmslie-Trillat procedure for knee extensor realignment. *American Journal of Sports Medicine* 1982;**10**:303-10.
213. Fulkerson JP, Becker GJ, Meaney JA, et al. Anteromedial tibial tubercle transfer without bone graft. *American Journal of Sports Medicine* 1990;**18**:490-7.
214. Miller JR, Adamson GJ, Pink MM, et al. Arthroscopically assisted medial reefing without routine lateral release for patellar instability. *American Journal of Sports Medicine* 2007;**35**:622-9.
215. Koëter S, Pakvis D, van Loon CJ, van Kampen A. Trochlear osteotomy for patellar instability: satisfactory minimum 2-year results in patients with dysplasia of the trochlea. *Knee Surgery, Sports Traumatology, Arthroscopy* 2007;**15**:228-32.
216. Steiner TM, Torga-Spak R, Teitge RA. Medial patellofemoral ligament reconstruction in patients with lateral patellar instability and trochlear-dysplasia. *American Journal of Sports Medicine* 2006;**34**:1254.
217. Kuroda R, Kambic H, Valdevit A, Andrish J. Disruption of patellofemoral joint pressures after femoral trochlear osteotomy. *Knee Surgery, Sports Traumatology, Arthroscopy* 2002;**10**:33-7.
218. Burks RT, Luker MG. Medial patellofemoral ligament reconstruction. *Techniques in Orthopaedics* 1997;**12**:185-91.
219. Schock EJ, Burks RT. Medial patellofemoral ligament reconstruction using a hamstring graft. *Operative Techniques in Orthopaedic Surgery* 2001;**9**:169-75.
220. LeGrand AB, Greis PE, Dobbs RE, Burks RT. MPFL reconstruction. *Sports Medicine and Arthroscopy Review* 2007;**15**:72-7.
221. Nomura E, Inoue M, Suqiura H. Ultrastructural study of the extraarticular Leeds-Keio ligament prosthesis. *Journal of Clinical Pathology* 2005;**58**:665-6.
222. Chassaing V, Tremoulet J. Medial patellofemoral ligament reconstruction with gracilis autograft for patellar instability. *Revue de Chirurgie Orthopédique et Réparatrice de l'Appareil Moteur* 2005;**91**:335-40.
223. Deie M, Ochi M, Sumen Y, et al. A long term follow up study after medial patellofemoral ligament reconstruction using the transferred semitendinosus tendon for patellar dislocation. *Knee Surgery, Sports Traumatology, Arthroscopy* 2005;**13**:522-8.

224. Schöttle PB, Fucentese SF, Romero J. Clinical and radiological outcome of medial patellofemoral ligament reconstruction with a semitendinosus autograft for patella instability. *Knee Surgery, Sports Traumatology, Arthroscopy* 2005;**13**:516–21.
225. Nomura E, Inoue M, Kobayashi S. Long-term follow-up and knee osteoarthritis change after medial patellofemoral ligament reconstruction for recurrent patellar dislocation. *American Journal of Sports Medicine* 2007;**35**:1851–8.
226. Mikashima Y, Kimura M, Kobayashi Y, *et al*. Clinical results of isolated reconstruction of the medial patellofemoral ligament for recurrent dislocation and subluxation of the patella. *Acta Orthopaedica Belgica* 2006;**72**:65–71.
227. Gomes JLE, Marczyk LRS, Cesar de Cesar P, Jungblut CF. Medial patellofemoral ligament reconstruction with semitendinosus autograft for chronic patella instability: a follow-up study. *Arthroscopy* 2004;**20**:147–51.
228. Drez D, Edwards TB, Williams CS. Results of medial patellofemoral ligament reconstruction in the treatment of patellar dislocation. *Arthroscopy* 2001;**17**:298–306.
229. Nomera E, Motoyasu I. Hybrid medial patellofemoral ligament reconstruction using the semitendinosus tendon for recurrent patellar dislocation: minimum 3 year's followup. *Arthroscopy* 2006;**22**:787–93.
230. Fernandez E, Sala D, Castejon M. Reconstruction of the medial patellofemoral ligament for patellar instability using a semitendinosus autograft. *Acta Orthopedica Belgica* 2005;**71**:303–8.
231. Hak DJ, Olson SA, Matta JM. Diagnosis and management of closed internal degloving injuries associated with pelvic and acetabular fractures: the Morel-Lavallee lesion. *Journal of Trauma* 1997;**42**:1046–51.
232. Kottmeier SA, Wilson SC, Born CT, *et al*. Surgical management of soft tissue lesions associated with pelvic ring injury. *Clinics in Orthopaedic Surgery and Related Research* 1996;**329**:46–53.
●233. Kudsk KA, Sheldon GF, Walton RL. Degloving injuries of the extremities and torso. *Journal of Trauma* 1981;**21**:835–9.
◆234. Letournel E, Judet R. *Fractures of the Acetabulum,* 2nd edn. Elson RA (ed.) (trans.). Berlin, Germany: Springer, 1993:337–97.
235. Tejwani SG, Cohen SB, Bradley JP. Management of Morel-Lavallee lesion of the knee: twenty-seven cases in the National Football League. *American Journal of Sports Medicine* 2007;**35**:1162–7.

77

Diagnosis and management of ligamentous injuries of the knee

RANDY MASCARENHAS, ERIC J KROPF, CHRISTOPHER D HARNER

Introduction	805	Posterolateral corner injuries	812
Medial collateral ligament injury	805	Multiligamentous knee injury (knee dislocation)	813
Anterior cruciate ligament tears	807	References	815
Posterior cruciate ligament injury	811		

NATIONAL BOARD STANDARDS

- Describe diagnostic and therapeutic options for ligamentous injuries of the knee to include ACL, PCL, MCL, and LCL
- Understand the anatomy and function of the posteromedial and posterolateral corners of the knee
- Explain key treatment principles for multiple ligamentous knee injuries

INTRODUCTION

Knee ligament injuries commonly occur during athletic participation or high-energy trauma such as motor vehicle accidents. Initial presentation typically consists of a history of trauma followed by knee swelling, pain and early or late instability. Appropriate management of such injuries is dependent upon accurate and complete diagnosis, which stems from thorough patient history and systematic physical examination of the knee.

MEDIAL COLLATERAL LIGAMENT INJURY

Medial collateral ligament (MCL) sprain is the most common knee ligament injury. Injuries most commonly occur via a direct valgus blow to the knee during activities such as American football, soccer, skiing or hockey.[1] The patient typically relays a history of a blow to the outside of the knee followed by pain, swelling and limited motion.

Relevant anatomy

The MCL is composed of both a superficial and deep portion. Three distinct layers have been described on the medial side of the knee, with the superficial MCL and posterior oblique ligament (POL) located in layer two.[2,3] The deep MCL and posteromedial capsule form layer three and serve as an important anchor for the medial meniscus. The proximal origin of the MCL is found on the medial femoral epicondyle, with the distal insertion site on the medial metaphyseal tibia under the pes anserinus. Since it is a large fan-shaped structure, some portion of the MCL is taut during all degrees of knee flexion. The anterior fibres tighten as the posterior fibres relax during flexion.

Biomechanical studies have shown the MCL to be the primary stabilizer to valgus stress,[2,4] with the ligament providing 78% of restraint in 25° of flexion and 57% restraint at 5° of flexion.[1] The POL, a thickening of the deep posterior capsule in layer two, lies posterior and deep to the MCL.[5] The POL tenses in extension and prevents medial opening with valgus loading when the knee is in full extension. Together, the MCL and POL resist abnormal external tibial rotation.[2,6]

Physical examination

To maximize the diagnostic value of physical examination, the patient should be relaxed, and the uninjured knee used as a control. To perform a valgus stress test, secure the ankle with one hand and place the other hand around the knee with the thenar eminence abutting the fibular head. Valgus stress is applied at 30° of flexion to isolate the superficial MCL. The degree of opening as well as quality of endpoint is determined and compared with the uninjured knee and graded as follows:[3]

Grade I   pain along the MCL, but less than 5 mm of detectable opening
Grade II 5–10 mm of laxity with a firm endpoint
Grade III greater than 10 mm of opening without a firm endpoint.

In cases of suspected MCL injury, the knee should also be tested in full extension. The capsule, anterior cruciate ligament (ACL), POL, medial meniscus and semimembranosus all contribute to valgus restraint in full extension. Accordingly, asymmetric medial opening to valgus force in full extension indicates combined MCL and POL damage and suggests potential ACL/PCL (posterior cruciate ligament) injury.[6,7] With combined MCL/ACL injury, the haemarthrosis may be less impressive than typically seen with isolated ACL injury because of extravasation of blood into the soft tissue through tears in the medial capsular ligament. Pain, swelling and muscle spasm can sometimes hinder performance of a complete physical examination. In these cases, the patient should be splinted and re-examined in a few days when pain and swelling have subsided.

Imaging

Plain radiographs should be obtained in the setting of any acute knee injury, and are necessary to rule out associated lateral tibial plateau fracture. However, MRI is the gold standard with suspected MCL injury. MRI (Fig. 77.1) can determine the site and extent of injury to the MCL while also providing valuable information regarding the ACL, meniscus and other structures.[8]

Treatment

The treatment of MCL injury continues to evolve over time. Historically, protocols advocated immediate, direct suture repair of the torn MCL and POL,[5,9,10] but more recent studies have shown excellent results with non-operative management of isolated MCL and combined ACL/MCL injuries.[11–14]

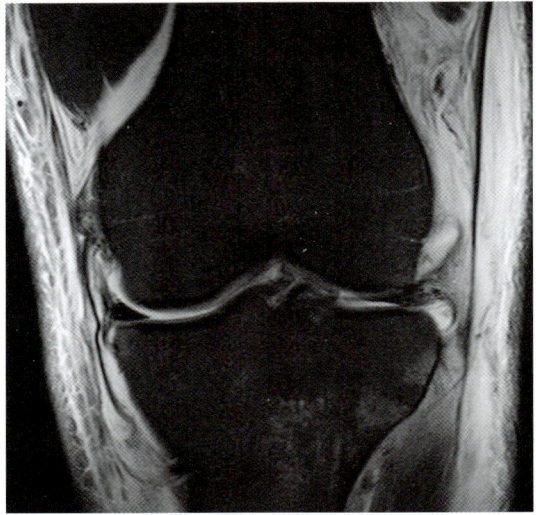

Figure 77.1 Single coronal T_2-weighted MRI of the left knee. There is evidence of significant (grade II) medial collateral ligament injury at its tibial insertion.

GRADE I AND II MCL INJURY

Isolated partial MCL tears (grades I and II) typically do well with non-operative management. Temporary immobilization and protected weight bearing with crutches is used for early pain control, followed by isometric, isotonic and isokinetic strengthening programmes as soon as the pain begins to subside. Early weight bearing is encouraged with the joint held in full extension in a knee immobilizer. When a comfortable range of motion is achieved, the immobilizer is removed and progressive weight bearing is allowed. Crutch-free ambulation is not permitted until the patient is limp free. Persistent or intermittent knee effusion during rehabilitation indicates the possibility of associated meniscal or articular cartilage injury and warrants further investigation. Return to sport or full activity is allowed when the full range of motion and at least 80% strength compared with the contralateral side is achieved. Grade I injuries generally return to unrestricted activity in 2 weeks, whereas grade II usually take 3 weeks. Bracing is usually not needed and the long-term prognosis for these partial tears is generally excellent.[15]

GRADE III MCL INJURY

Although once advocated for complete MCL tears,[9,10] more recent studies do not support early surgical repair for isolated MCL injuries unless there is severe debilitating instability.[6] The non-operative management of grade III tears has shown excellent results even in highly competitive athletes who returned to contact sports.[11–13,16,17] The injured leg is splinted in full extension for 2 weeks, after which motion through a comfortable range is started and the patient is allowed to bear weight as tolerated. The splint is usually discontinued between 3 and 4 weeks, and crutch-free walking is limited until the patient is limp free. An agility programme begins when isokinetic testing reveals at least 80% strength/power/endurance compared with the uninjured leg. Bracing is recommended for return to contact sports in the same season, with discontinuation the following season.

COMBINED MCL/ACL INJURIES

Repair of combined MCL/ACL injuries remains controversial. The ACL is the primary restraint to anterior tibial displacement, but also serves as a secondary restraint to valgus instability along with the PCL. Injury to the ACL and MCL will thus result in anterior and valgus instability. With complete and incomplete MCL injury, surgical reconstruction of the ACL alone has shown good functional results.[7,18,19]

Operative repair of the MCL is generally only considered with a grade III MCL injury that is grossly unstable both in 30° of flexion and full extension.[1] The knee is initially immobilized in extension for 3–4 weeks to allow the MCL to potentially heal. Rehabilitation to recover range of motion follows. ACL reconstruction is performed when the patient has recovered the full range of motion, and the knee is examined for residual medial laxity intraoperatively after ACL reconstruction is complete. If still grossly unstable, particularly in full extension, MCL repair is warranted. If an avulsion of the ligament from the femur or tibia is identified, it can be repaired with suture anchors. The POL can be tightened with suture anchors as well. Hughston and colleagues[6,9] have emphasized the importance of anterior advancement of the POL to restore medial stability to the knee. If repair of medial structures is performed, the risk of postoperative arthrofibrosis is high. An aggressive rehabilitation programme focusing on regaining full extension should be implemented in these patients.[20]

CHRONIC MCL LAXITY

Chronic medial laxity in the setting of ACL or PCL injury can lead to later failure of the cruciate reconstruction. In such cases, multiple techniques have been described for MCL reconstruction. The posterior capsule and POL can be plicated to the posterior aspect of a retensioned MCL. Also, reconstruction of the MCL with Achilles allograft has been described if the native MCL is thin and attenuated.

ANTERIOR CRUCIATE LIGAMENT TEARS

ACL injury is extremely common in a young active population, with over 100 000 ACL reconstruction procedures performed in the USA annually. ACL ruptures commonly result from non-contact cutting, rotational or deceleration mechanisms. Patients will classically report an audible 'pop' followed by pain, swelling and an inability to continue activity. ACL injuries can also occur with combined multiligamentous injuries, as in the dislocated knee. Chronic ACL-deficient patients will present with complaints of continued instability and pain.

Anatomy

The ACL is the primary restraint to anterior translation of the tibia, measuring approximately 33 mm in length with a mid-substance diameter of 11 mm.[21,22] The ligament originates from the posterior aspect of the medial wall of the lateral femoral condyle and inserts on the tibia between the tibial spines. Both insertion sites are broad and are of far greater area than that of the mid-substance ligament.[23] The ACL comprises two distinct functional bundles (posterolateral and anteromedial) named for their relative insertion points on the tibial footprint. The anteromedial bundle is tight in flexion, whereas the posterolateral bundle tightens in extension.[24]

Physical examination

General observation of patient body habitus, gait and alignment should be noted as unrecognized malalignment can later be a cause for failure following ACL reconstruction. A generalized knee examination is performed, including inspection, palpation, active and passive range of motion testing, and distal neurovascular testing. Range of motion may be limited in the acute setting because of pain and effusion, but the examiner should suspect potential mechanical blocks to extension such as displaced bucket-handle meniscal tears, ACL stump remnants or loose osteochondral fragments. A dedicated ligamentous knee examination is then performed, using the contralateral uninjured knee for comparison.

Several tests are performed to specifically test the integrity of the ACL. The Lachman test is the most sensitive test,[25] and is performed at neutral rotation with the knee flexed 20–30°. An anterior translation force is applied to the tibia with one hand while the other hand stabilizes the femur (Fig. 77.2). The degree of anterior translation of the tibia and the presence or absence of an endpoint is assessed compared with the opposite knee and graded as follows:

Grade I   less than 5 mm displacement
Grade II 5–10 mm displacement
Grade III 10 mm of displacement.

The anterior drawer test is performed with the knee flexed to 90°. While the foot is stabilized by the hip of the examiner, an anterior directed force is applied to the proximal tibia. The extent of anterior tibial translation is again compared with the opposite leg. Finally, the pivot shift test is performed with the hip in slight abduction as a valgus

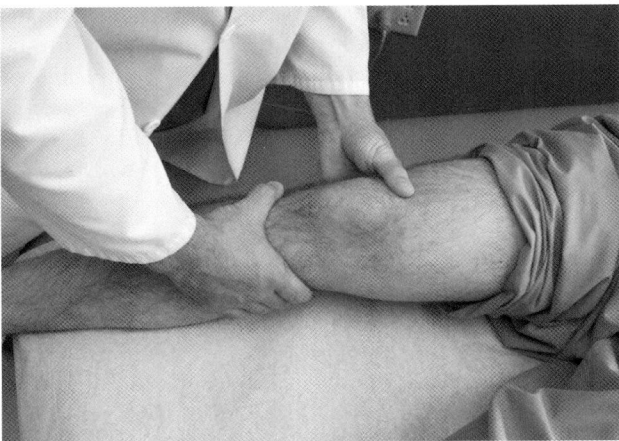

Figure 77.2 The Lachman test is performed with the knee in 20–30° of flexion. The examiner places one hand on the femur and stabilizes it, while the other hand imparts an anterior translational force to the proximal tibia. The degree of translation and quality or absence of an endpoint is noted.

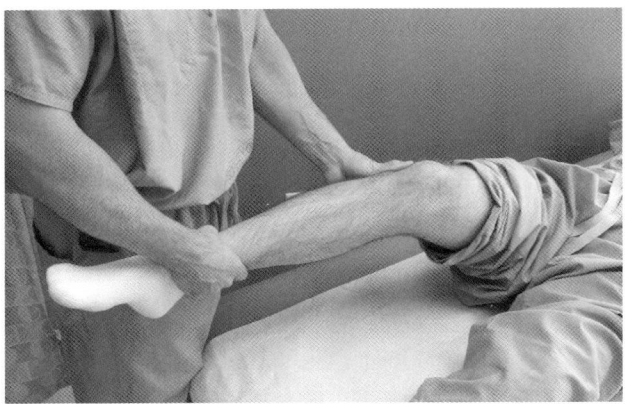

Figure 77.3 The pivot shift test. With the hip in slight abduction, the examiner externally rotates the foot and applies a valgus force to the extended knee. In the anterior cruciate ligament-deficient knee, the tibia will reduce as the knee is brought into approximately 20° of flexion. The test is hard to perform in the clinical setting secondary to patient guarding.

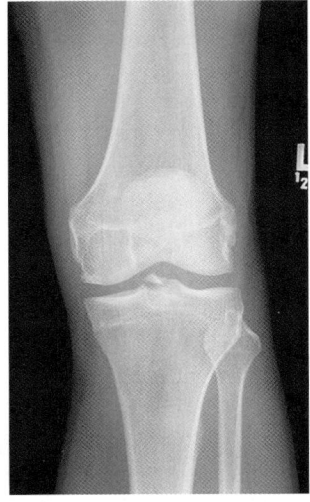

Figure 77.4 Posteroanterior plain radiograph of an acutely injured knee reveals a classic tibial spine avulsion fracture.

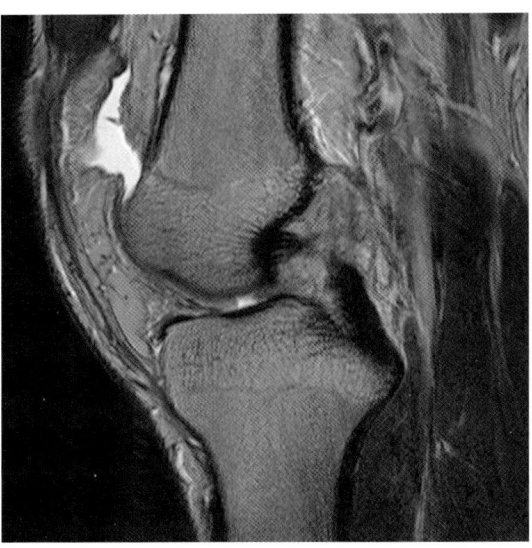

Figure 77.5 Sagittal plane T_2-weighted MRI. An acute anterior cruciate ligament rupture is visualized.

force is applied to the extended knee (Fig. 77.3). In the ACL-deficient knee, the tibia rests in an internally rotated and anteriorly subluxed position. As the knee is flexed to 20°, the tibia reduces resulting in the 'pivot shift'. The degree of 'shift' is graded as grade I or pivot glide, grade II or shift and grade III or transiently locked out. This test can be difficult to perform in the awake patient because of guarding, but is highly sensitive and specific during the examination under anaesthesia.[25,26]

Imaging

Plain radiographs should be obtained to evaluate any acutely injured knee. Standard posteroanterior flexion, 30° lateral and Merchant views are typically adequate. In the paediatric patient, it is particularly important to assess physes and to suspect tibial spine avulsion fractures (Fig. 77.4). The Segond fracture[27] represents a posterolateral capsular avulsion from the tibia and is considered pathognomonic for ACL injury. Degenerative changes may be radiographically evident in the setting of chronic ACL deficiency. Lower extremity alignment can be more accurately assessed with longstanding cassette views. MRI is the gold standard in suspected ACL injury (Fig. 77.5), with sensitivities reported to be greater than 90%.[28] In the acutely injured ACL, a pathognomonic bone bruise pattern is typically seen, involving the posterior third of the lateral tibial plateau and the middle third of the lateral

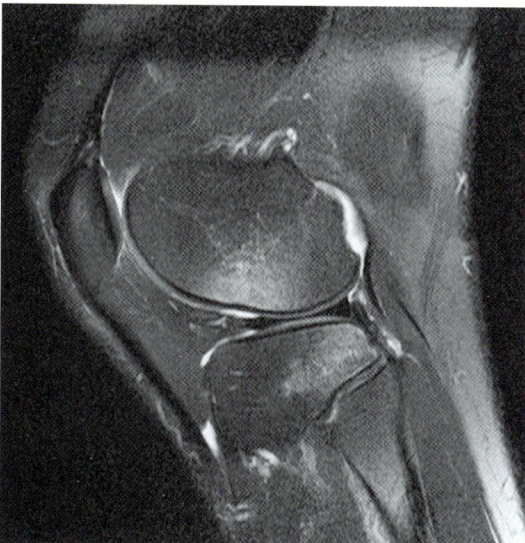

Figure 77.6 Sagittal plane T_2-weighted MRI. In this image, a typical 'bone bruise' pattern is seen, involving the posterior third of the lateral tibial plateau and the middle third of the lateral femoral condyle. This pattern is considered pathognomonic of acute anterior cruciate ligament injury.

femoral condyle (Fig. 77.6). It is crucial to assess the integrity of both bundles of the ACL[29] and to evaluate for associated collateral/cruciate ligament, meniscal or articular cartilage injury. These data are vital to the development of an appropriate operative plan.

Treatment

The natural history of ACL injury is not fully understood.[30] With so many confounding variables, including patient age, activity level and extent of associated injuries, the direct comparison of operative and non-operative management is extremely difficult. Age and activity level are important considerations in the management of ACL injury. Generally, poor results and recurrent episodes of instability have been reported with non-operative management of young, active patients who attempt to return to pre-injury activity levels.[31,32] Specifically, Shelton et al.[33] found that 70% of athletes were able to complete their season in a brace after acute ACL injury, but 61% suffered recurrent instability and 62% had meniscal and/or chondral injuries at the time of ACL reconstruction. As a result, surgery is considered the gold standard for active patients who want to return to their previous level of activity.

NON-OPERATIVE MANAGEMENT

Initial treatment of all isolated ACL injuries begins with protected weight bearing and early range of motion, followed by closed-chain quadriceps and hamstring strengthening exercises. If non-operative treatment is pursued, the goals of

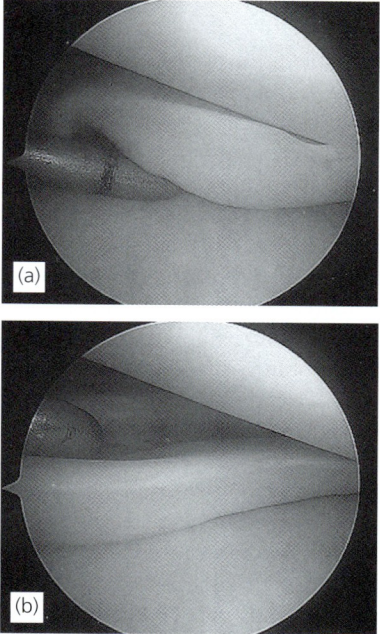

Figure 77.7 Arthroscopic images of the right knee. A bucket-handle medial meniscal tear is visualized. (a) The tear is easily displaced with an arthroscopic probe and (b) extends to the red–white zone of the meniscus. The patient depicted chose to delay surgery and had multiple repeat episodes of instability prior to definitive anterior cruciate ligament reconstruction and meniscal repair.

functional stability and prevention of further injury must be appreciated by the patient. Activity modification with avoidance of high-energy cutting movements is important. Functional bracing is controversial, as it has been shown to decrease anterior translation with minimal stress but not at physiological loading. ACL-deficient knees have historically been associated with a high incidence of recurrent instability, complex meniscal tears and late degenerative changes (Fig. 77.7a,b).[34–36] Patients who elect for non-operative treatment should be made aware of these concerns.

OPERATIVE MANAGEMENT

Techniques of ACL reconstruction have evolved tremendously over the past 30 years. Even as graft choices and fixation devices and methods continue to evolve and improve, several principles remain integral to successful ACL reconstruction. These include surgical technique, tunnel placement, timing of surgery and postoperative rehabilitation protocols. ACL reconstruction performed in the immediate post-injury period has been associated with a high incidence of arthrofibrosis and knee stiffness.[37] Preoperative rehabilitation is performed until full range of motion and quadriceps strength returns. This typically takes 3–6 weeks and allows time for the acute inflammatory reaction to subside.

GRAFT SELECTION

There are multiple graft options available for the patient undergoing ACL reconstruction. All possess unique advantages and disadvantages, and can be compared using various criteria, including biomechanical properties, biology of healing, ease of harvest, associated graft morbidity, fixation strength and 'return to play' guidelines. Factors such as patient age, activity level, associated injury and comorbidities definitely influence final graft choice.

Patellar tendon autograft tissue yields greater stiffness and a higher energy to failure[38] and an ability to revascularize[39] than other graft options. Mean strength is reported as 168% of the native ACL[38] and stable initial fixation is achieved via bone plugs. Patellar tendon autograft is contraindicated in patients with pre-existing patellofemoral chondrosis, extensor mechanism malalignment and narrow-width patellar tendon.[40] Reported intra-operative complications include patellar fracture,[41] incorrect tunnel placement[42] and violation of the posterior femoral cortex.[43] Potential postoperative complications with patellar tendon autograft include extensor mechanism disruption,[44] arthrofibrosis and limited range of motion.[37] Patellofemoral pain and quadriceps weakness[45,46] are also more common with this graft choice.

Another commonly employed option is hamstring autograft tissue. The quadruple-stranded hamstring autograft has been shown to be 240% stronger than the native ACL and 138% stronger than patellar tendon autografts.[47] Other advantages include the large cross-sectional area which maximizes vascular ingrowth[48] and the avoidance of trauma to the extensor mechanism. The principal disadvantage to using hamstring grafts lies in difficulty with fixation[49] and the relative lack of tendon to bone healing[50] when compared with patellar tendon grafts. Hamstring autograft is generally avoided in sprinting athletes, patients with prior history of hamstring injury and in cases of associated MCL or posteromedial capsular injury. Reported complications after hamstring autograft ACL reconstruction include loss of fixation,[50,51] persistent hamstring weakness,[52,53] tunnel expansion[54] and early graft failure.[55]

Allograft tissue as a graft option offers the advantages of smaller incisions, lack of donor site morbidity, shorter operative time, reduced postoperative pain and tensile strength equal to or exceeding all autogenous graft options.[56,57] However, although extremely uncommon, the potential for viral disease transmission exists.[58] Immune reaction to foreign tissue,[59] lack of tissue availability, high costs and potentially higher failure rates[60,61] are all additional concerns with the use of allograft tissue.

Postoperative rehabilitation

Following ACL reconstruction, the patient is placed in a hinged knee brace for 6 weeks, initially locked in full extension for the first week. Continuous passive motion is started immediately after surgery from 0° to 45° of flexion, increasing by 10° per day. The patient is allowed to bear weight as tolerated from the first postoperative day with crutches. Crutches are gradually weaned at 1 month postoperatively. Non-cutting and non-twisting sports are allowed at 12 weeks from surgery, and typically include swimming, cycling and straight-line running. Return to unrestricted activity generally occurs at 6 months postoperatively.

Special considerations in ACL reconstruction

THE SKELETALLY IMMATURE PATIENT

ACL reconstruction in the skeletally immature patient remains a controversial topic. As an increasing number of adolescents continue to engage in high-level sporting activities, the incidence of complete intrasubstance ACL tears has risen dramatically.[62] One study in particular revealed that 65% of adolescents (13–18 years) who suffered a knee injury with an acute haemarthrosis had some injury to the ACL.[63] As in the adult population, neglected ACL injury is associated with recurrent episodes of instability, and associated meniscal and chondral injury.[64] However, surgical treatment options are complicated by the risks of lower extremity shortening and/or angular deformity that may result from direct trauma to the immature physis.[65]

Entirely extraphyseal procedures are non-anatomic and therefore yield poor clinical outcomes.[66] As a result, these techniques should be reserved only for very young patients with significant growth remaining. It should also be understood that the need for later revision in this patient population is extremely high. For the slightly more mature patient, the literature supports partial transphyseal ACL reconstruction. The femoral side can be fixed in the 'over the top' position while a small transphyseal tunnel is drilled on the tibial side. To reduce the risk of growth disturbance, the tibial tunnel should be drilled vertically through the physis and a soft-tissue graft is utilized in these patients.[67,68] The graft can be fixed with a standard post on both sides in an extraphyseal fashion. Careful follow-up should ensue to monitor growth and plan for intervention if early physeal closure occurs.[69]

THE FEMALE ATHLETE

The risk of ACL injury in non-contact cutting sports (basketball, soccer) is greater in female athletes.[70] Proposed predisposing factors for female athletes include anatomic factors such as increased varus alignment of the hip, increased valgus alignment of the knee and smaller intercondylar notch size. Hormonal factors, proprioceptive factors and neuromuscular factors, including excessive joint laxity, poor relative hamstring strength and jump/landing mechanics, have all been implicated as potential causes of this increased risk as well.[70–74]

DOUBLE-BUNDLE ACL RECONSTRUCTION

Recently, double-bundle ACL reconstruction has begun to gain popularity. Multiple biomechanical studies have provided evidence to suggest that single-bundle reconstruction does not effectively restore normal knee kinematics. Specifically, rotational instability often persists despite surgery.[75–79] Anatomic double-bundle reconstruction affords at least the theoretical advantage of more favourable restoration of normal knee kinematics.[76] Clinical outcomes studies are limited, with the longest follow-up averaging 2 years. In these studies, little or no clinical difference can be seen at this time interval.[80,81] Long-term follow-up and randomized controlled trials are necessary to more accurately define the role of anatomic double-bundle ACL reconstruction.

POSTERIOR CRUCIATE LIGAMENT INJURY

PCL injury is far less common than ACL injury. Most injuries occur during athletics or in high-energy trauma such as motor vehicle accidents. Typically, a posteriorly directed blow to the proximal tibia results (dashboard injury), but PCL injury may also occur with falls onto a flexed knee while the foot is plantarflexed.[82] Hyperextension mechanisms typically cause combined injury to the PCL and posterolateral corner complex.[83] Suspicion for multiligamentous knee injury should be high in the setting of such high-energy trauma.[82]

Anatomy

The PCL is an intravascular structure contained within its own synovial layer. It originates from a broad area on the anterolateral aspect of the medial femoral condyle[84] and inserts below the articular surface on the posterior tibia in the fovea between the medial and lateral tibial plateaus.[85] The ligament is composed of anterolateral and posteromedial bundles and receives some contribution from variable meniscofemoral ligaments. The larger anterolateral bundle tightens in knee flexion and is the primary restraint to posterior tibial displacement at 90° of flexion. The posteromedial bundle becomes taut in extension. The meniscofemoral ligaments are variable in distribution and originate from the posterior horn of the lateral meniscus and insert into the PCL. These ligaments (anterior, Humphrey; posterior, Wrisberg) have been found to contribute as much as 28% of resistance to posteriorly directed forces with the knee at 90° of flexion.[86] The PCL functions as the primary restraint to posterior translation when the knee is flexed beyond 30°. In the PCL-deficient knee, posterior translation is minimal with the knee fully extended and most pronounced at 90° of flexion.[87] The PCL is also a secondary restraint to varus/valgus stress and aids the posterolateral corner (PLC) complex in resisting external tibial rotation.[88,89]

Clinical evaluation

The posterior drawer test is the most specific test for detecting PCL injury.[90] To perform the test, a posteriorly directed force is applied to the anterior proximal tibia with the knee flexed 90° (Fig. 77.8). In the uninjured knee, the medial tibial plateau should rest 1 cm anterior to the medial femoral condyle. With grade I injury (0–5 mm translation), a step-off is still felt but diminished while the posterior force is applied. In grade II injury (5–10 mm translation), the medial plateau will be flush with the condyle. In grade III injury (>10 mm translation), the medial tibial plateau can be displaced posterior to the medial femoral condyle.

If the tibia can be displaced more than 10 mm, combined injury should be suspected. Most commonly, the PLC will be involved. It is vital to assess the status of the PLC as multiple studies have shown that reconstruction of the PCL alone in the setting of unrecognized PLC injury is prone to high rates of failure.[87,91]

The posterior sag test can provide further information about the status of the PCL. With the patient supine, the hip and knee are flexed to 90°, and the examiner supports the weight of the limb at the foot. With a complete PCL tear, the pull of gravity will displace the tibia posterior to the femur.

Imaging

Standard posteroanterior flexion, 30° lateral and Merchant views are typically obtained, with particular attention paid to possible PCL avulsion fractures, posterior tibial subluxation, and associated tibial plateau fractures. In the chronic PCL-deficient knee, posteroanterior flexion weight-bearing views and patellar views may help evaluate degenerative changes. Lateral stress radiographs may be useful to evaluate for tibial–femoral step-off.[92]

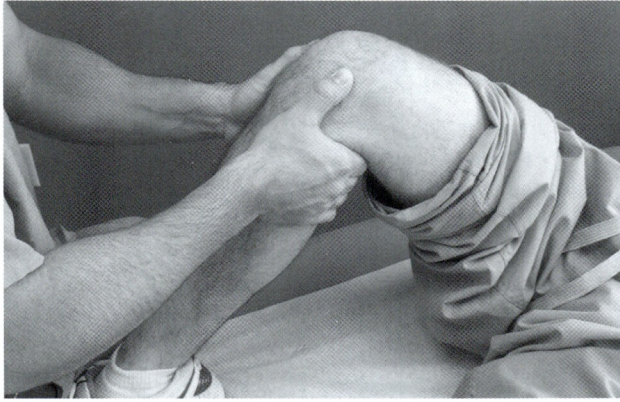

Figure 77.8 Posterior drawer test. The knee is positioned in 90° of flexion and the examiner palpates the medial femoral condyle in relation to the medial plateau. In an uninjured knee, the medial condyle should rest 1 cm anterior to the tibial plateau. As a posteriorly directed force is applied, the examiner grades the change in step-off and feels for the presence or absence of an endpoint.

MRI is highly sensitive and specific in the diagnosis and description of acute PCL tears and associated injuries.[93] However, given the healing potential of an injured PCL, the ligament may have a near normal appearance on MRI over time.[94]

Treatment

The natural history of PCL-injured knees remains to be determined. Unfortunately, most studies to date are retrospective only, and include a variety of patients both acute and chronic in duration with isolated and multiligamentous injuries.[95–99] Clearly, better prospective outcome studies are needed to determine the true natural history of PCL-deficient knees.

Non-operative management

The treatment of isolated PCL injury is controversial. Several studies have shown good short-term outcomes with conservative management of isolated PCL injuries.[82,96,100] Most authors generally agree that grade I and II PCL injuries can be treated non-operatively[82,90,91,97] with initial immobilization, protected weight bearing in extension and progressive quadriceps-strengthening exercises.[87] However, this does not mean that the PCL-deficient knee treated non-operatively is entirely normal. PCL deficiency alters knee biomechanics, resulting in increased posterior translation, abnormal chondral wear and associated pain.[98,99,101] Multiple studies with long-term follow-up have shown the development of significant, progressive degenerative changes in the medial and patellofemoral compartments of PCL-deficient knees treated conservatively.[97,102]

Operative treatment

ISOLATED PCL INJURIES

The decision to pursue operative treatment is generally based upon the age and activity level of the patient, the severity and timing of the injury and the symptoms currently displayed by the patient. Current recommendations advocate non-operative management for isolated, asymptomatic PCL injuries with less than 10 mm of posterior translation appreciable on examination.[87,103] Treatment begins with 4 weeks of immobilization followed by aggressive quadriceps strengthening while limiting hamstring loading in order to prevent posterior tibial subluxation. The treatment of isolated grade III PCL injuries (10–15 mm translation) is more complicated and controversial. Most authors agree with surgical intervention in cases of severe tibial subluxation and multiligamentous knee injury. Surgical management is recommended for isolated chronic grade III PCL injuries with recalcitrant pain or instability despite an appropriate rehabilitation programme. In the unique case of PCL bony avulsion, early screw fixation has shown good results.[104]

Generally, combined injuries are treated at 2 weeks post injury. Early reconstruction avoids capsular scarring while still allowing for anatomic repair.[105,106] Both transtibial and tibial inlay techniques are widely used in PCL reconstruction. Both can be performed with single- and double-bundle techniques. The tibial inlay technique was developed to avoid graft passage around the sharp angle of the articular margin of the tibia[107] and has been shown to result in less graft laxity with cyclic loading.[108] However, patient positioning and risks associated with a posterior incision make this technique difficult. The double-bundle technique is thought to provide superior restoration of knee kinematics through flexion and extension when compared with single-bundle approaches.[91,109,110] Short-term results are promising but longer term follow-up is needed.

It is well documented that reconstruction of the PCL alone with an unrecognized PLC injury has an extremely high potential for graft failure.[91] Varus malalignment and thrust should be evaluated, and a proximal tibial osteotomy should be performed to correct varus deformity and reduce posterior tibial translation if appropriate.[103]

Rehabilitation

Postoperatively, the knee is immobilized in full extension for 2–4 weeks. Prone passive flexion exercises are performed in the early postoperative period to minimize hamstring activation. Partial weight-bearing and quadriceps exercises are begun immediately. Closed kinetic chain exercises are started at 6 weeks, and hamstring strengthening is generally delayed until about 4 months. Patients usually return to full activities at 9–12 months after surgery.

POSTEROLATERAL CORNER INJURIES

Isolated PLC injuries are rare and generally result from a posterolateral or varus force to the proximal part of the tibia with the knee at or near full extension.[111] Such injuries are often seen in athletic trauma, falls and motor vehicle accidents.[112] PLC–PCL injury can occur through similar mechanisms, but also when a flexed knee receives a posterior force on the tibia while in external rotation.[113] Gross knee dislocations typically cause severe PLC injury in association with other ligamentous injuries.[114] Combined ACL and PLC injury may occur and results in increased anterior and posterior tibial translation, varus laxity, and coupled posterolateral and anterolateral rotatory instability.[115]

Anatomy

Three distinct lateral knee anatomic layers have been identified on the lateral side of the knee.[116] Layer one includes the superficial fascia, iliotibial band, biceps femoris tendon and peroneal nerve. Layer two is the lateral collateral ligament (LCL), and layer three consists of the popliteus, popliteofibular ligament, arcuate ligament, fabellofibular ligament, coronary ligament and posterolateral capsule. The structures in layers two and three make up the PLC complex and resist anterolateral and posterolateral tibial rotation.[117] Collectively, the PLC and LCL resist posterolateral rotation and varus displacement of the tibia, with the PLC playing a greater role in resisting posterolateral rotation and the LCL resisting varus displacement of the tibia.[118]

Diagnosis

The majority of PLC injuries occur in conjunction with injuries to other ligaments, often complicating the physical examination.[119] Injury to the PLC is suggested by ecchymosis, oedema, induration and tenderness over the PLC of the knee and fibular head.[112] Additionally, patients with PLC injuries typically walk with a varus thrust gait.[120]

To detect LCL injury, varus stress testing is performed in 30° of flexion and full extension. Increased lateral widening at 30° indicates LCL injury while laxity in full extension is consistent with combined LCL/cruciate ligament injury. The posterior drawer test is performed at 30° and 90° of knee flexion with particular attention paid to the degree of posterolateral rotation. Normal posterior translation at 90° with an increase at 30° suggests isolated PLC injury.[121] The tibial external rotation test (dial test) is performed at 30° and 90° (Fig. 77.9). With the patient prone, an external rotation force is applied and the foot–thigh angle is measured and compared with the contralateral side. Increased side-to-side differences in external rotation at 30° but not 90° suggest isolated PLC injury, whereas increased external rotation in both positions suggests combined PCL–PLC injury.[122] MRI is the gold standard in suspected PLC injuries, with thin slice coronal oblique views providing the greatest diagnostic value.[123]

Treatment

Truly isolated LCL injury is rare and should raise suspicion of associated injury. With that said, non-operative management is indicated for isolated grades I and II LCL injuries.[124,125] Partial tears will heal following 6 weeks of early motion and protected weight bearing. If the athlete returns to sport in the same season, a brace should be worn.

Non-operative management has shown good to excellent results in grades I and II PLC injuries, but poor outcomes and residual laxity with grade III injuries.[124–126] Acute grade III isolated or combined PLC injury is best treated early with direct repair when possible. Otherwise, augmentation or reconstruction of all injured ligaments is indicated. Chronic PLC injuries are best treated with PLC reconstruction and associated cruciate reconstruction as indicated. Surgical options for PLC injuries include various partial and complete tendon transfers, as well as anatomic reconstruction and/or augmentation using both autograft and allograft tissue.[120,122,126–132] Failure to diagnose and treat PLC injury in a patient undergoing ACL or PCL reconstruction greatly increases the likelihood of graft failure after cruciate reconstruction.[91]

Rehabilitation

Rehabilitation emphasizes range of motion, quadriceps strengthening and patellofemoral joint protection. After surgery, patients are weight bearing as tolerated with continuous passive motion and heel slides. Quadriceps strengthening is important with early straight leg raises being the key exercise. No resisted flexion or extension exercises are performed, and patients progress to non-impact sliding/gliding exercises as tolerated. Swimming and stationary cycling begin by the end of the second postoperative week.

MULTILIGAMENTOUS KNEE INJURY (KNEE DISLOCATION)

Knee dislocations are devastating injuries with potentially limb-threatening complications. Dislocations result predominantly from motor vehicle accidents, but can also occur during athletic participation.[133] Prompt accurate diagnosis, stabilization and treatment are vital as up to 13% of injuries can ultimately result in amputation secondary to

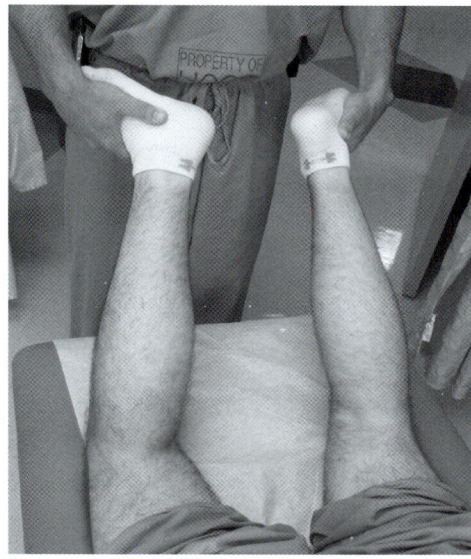

Figure 77.9 Dial test. With the patient lying prone, the examiner externally rotates the tibia and measures the thigh–foot angle at both 30° and 90° of flexion. Side-to-side difference of greater than 10° is considered abnormal, suggestive of posterolateral corner injury with or without posterior cruciate ligament injury.

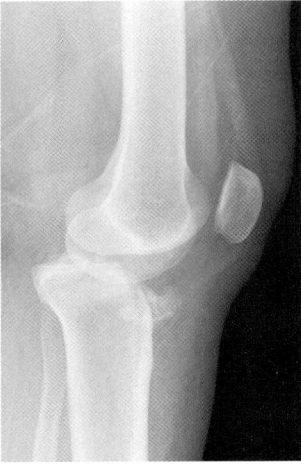

Figure 77.10 Lateral radiograph (pre-reduction) in acute posterior knee dislocation with associated tibial plateau fracture.

vascular injury.[134] The true incidence of knee dislocations is difficult to determine because up to 50% of patients will present after spontaneous reduction.[135] As a general rule, instability of two or more ligaments following trauma should raise suspicion for knee dislocation, even with normal radiographs.[133]

Classification

The descriptive classification system is based on direction of dislocation. Anterior dislocations are most common and generally occur in both high- and low-energy hyperextension injuries. Posterior dislocations are second most common and are usually associated with high-energy trauma (Fig. 77.10).[136] The PCL and ACL are commonly injured, whereas injury to the collaterals is variable. Medial and lateral dislocations are extremely uncommon.[134] Rotatory knee dislocations are the rarest of all dislocations.[134] and often result in injury to both collateral and cruciate ligaments. They are most commonly posterolateral in direction, and are often irreducible, necessitating prompt operative intervention (Figs 77.11 and 77.12).

Vascular and neurological injury

Reported incidence of popliteal artery injury following knee dislocation ranges from 4.6% to 80%.[133] Timing of vascular repair is critical, as a tremendous decline in limb salvage rates is seen with delays of more than 8 hours.[134] Popliteal artery injuries occur across a spectrum from intimal tears to complete transections, with anterior dislocations more commonly resulting in intimal injuries and posterior dislocations more commonly associated with complete tears of the artery.[136] Vascular injury can occur in all types of dislocations and can present in a delayed fashion, so serial vascular examination is needed for at least

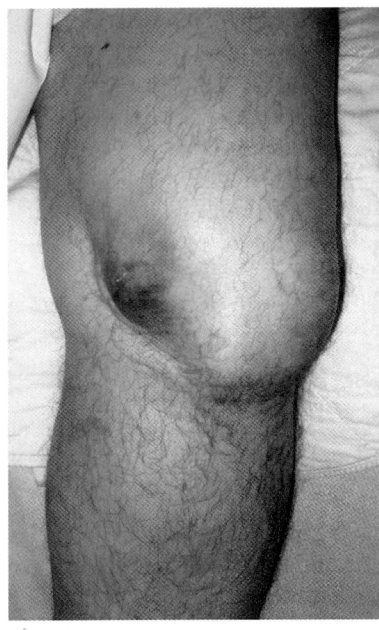

Figure 77.11 Photograph of left knee following a high-energy fall from height. Note the medial-sided ecchymoses and 'dimple' sign pathognomonic for irreducible posterolateral knee dislocation. In this case, the medial femoral condyle had 'button-holed' the vastus medialis and required open reduction.

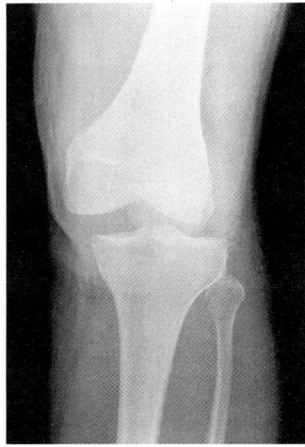

Figure 77.12 Anteroposterior radiograph of the knee depicted in Fig. 77.10. Note the significantly widened medial joint space and the laterally subluxed tibia and patella.

24 hours after surgery.[137] Many surgeons advocate arteriography to evaluate vascular injury in the setting of all knee dislocations, but others call for more selective choice, citing ankle brachial indexes[138] and clinical examination[139,140] as being valid options to direct towards choosing angiography. Neurological injury is reported in 16–50% of knee dislocations,[141] with the peroneal and posterior tibial nerves being most commonly injured. Such injuries are most frequently seen with posterolateral dislocations.

Clinical evaluation and treatment

After evaluation by a dedicated trauma service to rule out or treat life-threatening injuries, a thorough history and physical examination is performed. If the knee remains dislocated at the time of presentation, reduction under conscious sedation with traction/counter-traction should be performed. It is important to assess and document both pre- and post-reduction neurovascular status. Following reduction, the limb should be stabilized with a long leg splint. Posterior tibial and dorsalis pedis pulses should be palpated or assessed with a Doppler ultrasound machine and compared with the opposite side. However, the presence of pulses does not rule out vascular injury. Ankle brachial indexes and/or arteriography should be obtained if there is even the slightest clinical suspicion of vascular injury.[142] If delays are present, arteriography should be performed in the operating room with early intervention by a vascular surgeon as necessary.

Immediate surgical intervention is warranted in cases of irreducible dislocation or vascular injury. The orthopaedic surgeon may need to perform external fixation in order to provide stability to the limb prior to or during vascular grafting. In addition, fasciotomies are routinely performed at the time of revascularization. Therefore, the vascular and orthopaedic surgeons need to develop a cohesive, coordinated operative plan. Open dislocations should be serially irrigated and debrided with the administration of intravenous antibiotics and soft-tissue coverage procedures if required.[143]

Numerous studies have reported more favourable outcomes with operative treatment of multiligamentous knee injuries.[143–146] In the past, authors advocated for a staged ligamentous repair/reconstruction with early PCL reconstruction followed by repair of the ACL and collaterals several months later.[147–149] They cited decreased postoperative stiffness and full range of motion with no varus/valgus instability as advantages of this course of treatment. Most authors now believe that combined reconstruction of the ACL and PCL with repair or reconstruction of the collaterals and the PLC can be performed in the acute setting (less than 3 weeks) with no increase in rates of arthrofibrosis.[150–153] Tissue quality, severity of the injury and knee stability dictate whether repair or reconstruction of the collaterals and PLC is performed at the time of cruciate reconstruction.

KEY LEARNING POINTS

- The medial collateral ligament (MCL) is a broad ligament that attaches to the medial femoral epicondyle and to the medial aspect of the tibia under the pes anserinus. The ligament primarily resists valgus stress, and lateral clipping injuries or twisting mechanisms are the primary causes of injury to the MCL.
- The anterior cruciate ligament (ACL) is composed of two distinct functional bundles (anteromedial and posterolateral). The posterolateral bundle is tight in extension and the anteromedial bundle tightens in flexion.
- Non-operative management of complete ACL injury predisposes the patient to recurrent instability, associated meniscal and chondral injury and subsequent degenerative changes in the knee. ACL reconstruction is indicated in the young, active patient who wishes to return to a pre-injury level of activity.
- The posterior cruciate ligament (PCL) is the primary restraint to posterior tibial translation, and, like the ACL, consists of two bundles. The anterolateral bundle makes up the bulk of the PCL and is tight in flexion and loose in extension. The posteromedial bundle is tight in extension and loose in flexion. PCL injuries often occur in combination with other ligamentous injury during high-energy trauma.
- Posterolateral corner injuries (PLC) injuries may present in isolation or as a component of combined injuries. The PLC must always be examined with ligamentous knee injuries, as cruciate ligament reconstruction without attention to the PLC has shown poor results and a high incidence of subsequent graft failure.
- Knee dislocation should always be suspected following trauma with evidence of injury to two or more ligaments. More than 50% of patients with knee dislocations will present following spontaneous reduction. The presence of pulses does not rule out vascular injury. Serial examination and/or angiography should be performed when vascular injury is suspected.

REFERENCES

- ● = Key primary paper
- ◆ = Major review article

1. Pressman A, Johnson DH. A review of ski injuries resulting in combined injury to the anterior cruciate ligament and medial collateral ligaments. *Arthroscopy* 2003;**19**:194–202.
2. Warren LA, Marshall JL, Girgis F. The prime static stabilizer of the medial side of the knee. *Journal of Bone and Joint Surgery (American)* 1974;**56**:665–74.
●3. Warren LF, Marshall JL. The supporting structures and layers on the medial side of the knee: an anatomical analysis. *Journal of Bone and Joint Surgery (American)* 1979;**61**:56–62.
4. Grood ES, Noyes FR, Butler DL, Suntay WJ. Ligamentous and capsular restraints preventing straight medial and lateral laxity in intact human cadaver knees. *Journal of Bone and Joint Surgery (American)* 1981;**63**:1257–69.

- 5. Hughston JC, Eilers AF. The role of the posterior oblique ligament in repairs of acute medial (collateral) ligament tears of the knee. *Journal of Bone and Joint Surgery (American)* 1973;**55**:923–40.
- 6. Frank C, Woo SL, Amiel D, et al. Medial collateral ligament healing. A multidisciplinary assessment in rabbits. *American Journal of Sports Medicine* 1983;**11**:379–89.
7. Hillard-Sembell D, Daniel DM, Stone ML, et al. Combined injuries of the anterior cruciate and medial collateral ligaments of the knee: Effect of treatment on stability and function of the joint. *Journal of Bone and Joint Surgery (American)* 1996;**78**:169–76.
8. Nakamura N, Horibe S, Toritsuka Y, et al. Acute grade III medial collateral ligament injury of the knee associated with anterior cruciate ligament tear: The usefulness of magnetic resonance imaging in determining a treatment regimen. *American Journal of Sports Medicine* 2003;**31**:261–7.
- 9. Hughston JC, Barrett GR. Acute anteromedial rotatory instability. Long-term results of surgical repair. *Journal of Bone and Joint Surgery (American)* 1983;**65**:145–53.
10. O'Donoghue DH. Surgical treatment of fresh injuries to the major ligaments of the knee. 1950. *Clinical Orthopaedics and Related Research* 2007;**454**:23–6; discussion 14.
11. Ellsasser JC, Reynolds FC, Omohundro JR. The non-operative treatment of collateral ligament injuries of the knee in professional football players. An analysis of seventy-four injuries treated non-operatively and twenty-four injuries treated surgically. *Journal of Bone and Joint Surgery (American)* 1974;**56**:1185–90.
12. Fetto JF, Marshall JL. Medial collateral ligament injuries of the knee: a rationale for treatment. *Clinical Orthopaedics and Related Research* 1978;**132**:206–18.
- 13. Indelicato PA. Non-operative treatment of complete tears of the medial collateral ligament of the knee. *Journal of Bone and Joint Surgery (American)* 1983;**65**:323–9.
14. Millett P, Pennock A, Sterett W, Steadman J. Early reconstruction in combined ACL-MCL injuries. *Journal of Knee Surgery* 2004;**17**:94–8.
15. Lundberg M, Messner K. Long-term prognosis of isolated partial medial collateral ligament ruptures. A ten-year clinical and radiographic evaluation of a prospectively observed group of patients. *American Journal of Sports Medicine* 1996;**24**:160–3.
16. Indelicato PA, Hermansdorfer J, Huegel M. Nonoperative management of complete tears of the medial collateral ligament of the knee in intercollegiate football players. *Clinical Orthopaedics and Related Research* 1990;**July**:174–7.
17. Reider B, Sathy MR, Talkington J, et al. Treatment of isolated medial collateral ligament injuries in athletes with early functional rehabilitation. A five-year follow-up study. *American Journal of Sports Medicine* 1994;**22**:470–7.
18. Noyes FR, Barber-Westin SD. The treatment of acute combined ruptures of the anterior cruciate and medial ligaments of the knee. *American Journal of Sports Medicine* 1995;**23**:380–9.
19. Sims WF, Jacobson KE. The posteromedial corner of the knee: medial-sided injury patterns revisited. *American Journal of Sports Medicine* 2004;**32**:337–45.
20. Robins AJ, Newman AP, Burks RT. Postoperative return of motion in anterior cruciate ligament and medial collateral ligament injuries. The effect of medial collateral ligament rupture location. *American Journal of Sports Medicine* 1993;**21**:20–5.
- 21. Girgis FG, Marshall JL, Monajem A. The cruciate ligaments of the knee joint. Anatomical, functional and experimental analysis. *Clinical Orthopaedics and Related Research* 1975;**106**:216–31.
22. Amis AA. Anterior cruciate ligament replacement. Knee stability and the effects of implants. *Journal of Bone and Joint Surgery (British)* 1989;**71**:819–24.
- 23. Harner CD, Baek GH, Vogrin TM, et al. Quantitative analysis of human cruciate ligament insertions. *Arthroscopy* 1999;**15**:741–9.
24. Amis AA, Dawkins GP. Functional anatomy of the anterior cruciate ligament. Fibre bundle actions related to ligament replacements and injuries. *Journal of Bone and Joint Surgery (British)* 1991;**73**:260–7.
- 25. Malanga GA, Andrus S, Nadler SF, McLean J. Physical examination of the knee: A review of the original test description and scientific validity of common orthopedic tests. *Archives of Physical Medicine and Rehabilitation* 2003;**84**:592–603.
26. Bach BR, Warren RF, Wickiewicz TL. The pivot shift phenomenon: Results and description of a modified clinical test for anterior cruciate ligament insufficiency. *American Journal of Sports Medicine* 1988;**16**:571–6.
27. Dietz GW, Wilcox DM, Montgomer JB. Segond tibial condyle fracture: lateral capsular ligament avulsion. *Radiology* 1986;**159**:467–9.
28. Munshi M, Davidson M, MacDonald PB, et al. The efficacy of magnetic resonance imaging in acute knee injuries. *Clinical Journal of Sport Medicine* 2000;**10**:34–9.
29. Starman JS, Vanbeek C, Armfield DR, et al. Assessment of normal ACL double bundle anatomy in standard viewing planes by magnetic resonance imaging. *Knee Surgery, Sports Traumatology, Arthroscopy* 2007;**15**:493–9.
30. Fithian DC, Paxton LW, Goltz DH. Fate of the anterior cruciate ligament-injured knee. *Orthopedic Clinics of North America* 2002;**33**:621–6.
31. Daniel DM, Stone ML, Dobson BE, et al. Fate of the ACL-injured patient. A prospective outcome study. *American Journal of Sports Medicine* 1994;**22**:632–44.
32. Hawkins RJ, Misamore GW, Merritt TR. Followup of the acute nonoperated isolated anterior cruciate ligament tear. *American Journal of Sports Medicine* 1986;**14**:205–10.
33. Shelton WR, Barrett GR, Dukes A. Early season anterior cruciate ligament tears: A treatment dilemma. *American Journal of Sports Medicine* 1997;**25**:656–8.
34. Gillquist J, Messner K. Anterior cruciate ligament reconstruction and the long-term incidence of gonarthrosis. *Sports Medicine* 1999;**27**:143–56.

- 35. Neyret P, Donell ST, Dejour H. Results of partial meniscectomy related to the state of the anterior cruciate ligament. Review at 20 to 35 years. *Journal of Bone and Joint Surgery (British)* 1993;**75**:36–40.
36. Buss DD, Min R, Skyhar M, et al. Nonoperative treatment of acute anterior cruciate ligament injuries in a selected group of athletes. *American Journal of Sports Medicine* 1995;**23**:160–5.
37. Harner CD, Irrgang JJ, Paul J, et al. Loss of motion after anterior cruciate ligament reconstruction. *American Journal of Sports Medicine* 1992;**20**:499–506.
- 38. Noyes FR, Butler DL, Grood ES, et al. Biomechanical analysis of human ligament grafts used in knee-ligament repairs and reconstructions. *Journal of Bone and Joint Surgery (American)* 1984;**66**:344–52.
39. Arnoczky SP, Tarvin GB, Marshall JL. Anterior cruciate ligament replacement using patellar tendon. An evaluation of graft revascularization in the dog. *Journal of Bone and Joint Surgery (American)* 1982;**64**:217–24.
40. Noyes FR, Barber SD, Mangine RE. Bone-patellar ligament-bone and fascia lata allografts for reconstruction of the anterior cruciate ligament. *Journal of Bone and Joint Surgery (American)* 1990;**72**:1125–36.
41. Christen B, Jakob RP. Fractures associated with patellar ligament grafts in cruciate ligament surgery. *Journal of Bone and Joint Surgery (British)* 1992;**74**:617–19.
42. Franco MG, Bach BR Jr, Bush-Joseph CA. Intraarticular placement of Kurosaka interference screws. *Arthroscopy* 1994;**10**:412–17.
43. Bush-Joseph CA, Bach BR Jr, Bryan J. Posterior cortical violation of the femoral tunnel during endoscopic anterior cruciate ligament reconstruction. *American Journal of Knee Surgery* 1995;**8**:130–3.
44. Marumoto JM, Mitsunaga MM, Richardson AB, et al. Late patellar tendon ruptures after removal of the central third for anterior cruciate ligament reconstruction: A report of two cases. *American Journal of Sports Medicine* 1996;**24**:698–701.
- 45. Aglietti P, Buzzi R, D'Andria S, Zaccherotti G. Patellofemoral problems after intraarticular anterior cruciate ligament reconstruction. *Clinical Orthopaedics and Related Research* 1993;**288**:195–204.
46. Sachs RA, Daniel DM, Stone ML, Garfein RF. Patellofemoral problems after anterior cruciate ligament reconstruction. *American Journal of Sports Medicine* 1989;**17**:760–5.
47. Butler DL, Grood ES, Noyes FR, Sodd AN. On the interpretation of our anterior cruciate ligament data. *Clinical Orthopaedics and Related Research* 1985;**June**:26–34.
48. Noyes FR, Butler DL, Paulos LE, Grood ES. Intra-articular cruciate reconstruction. I: Perspectives on graft strength, vascularization, and immediate motion after replacement. *Clinical Orthopaedics and Related Research* 1983;**Jan–Feb**:71–7.
49. Noyes FR, Grood ES. The strength of the anterior cruciate ligament in humans and Rhesus monkeys. *Journal of Bone and Joint Surgery (American)* 1976;**58**:1074–82.
50. Ishibashi Y, Rudy TW, Livesay GA, et al. The effect of anterior cruciate ligament graft fixation site at the tibia on knee stability: evaluation using a robotic testing system. *Arthroscopy* 1997;**13**:177–82.
- 51. Uchio Y, Ochi M, Adachi N, et al. Determination of time of biologic fixation after anterior cruciate ligament reconstruction with hamstring tendons. *American Journal of Sports Medicine* 2003;**31**:345–52.
52. Ellera Gomes JL, Marczyk LR. Anterior cruciate ligament reconstruction with a loop or double thickness of semitendinosus tendon. *American Journal of Sports Medicine* 1984;**12**:199–203.
53. Goradia VK, Rochat MC, Grana WA, Egle DM. Strength of ACL reconstructions using semitendinosus tendon grafts. *Journal of the Oklahoma State Medical Association* 1998;**91**:275–7.
54. Clatworthy MG, Annear P, Bulow JU, Bartlett RJ. Tunnel widening in anterior cruciate ligament reconstruction: a prospective evaluation of hamstring and patella tendon grafts. *Knee Surgery, Sports Traumatology, Arthroscopy* 1999;**7**:138–45.
55. Toritsuka Y, Shino K, Horibe S, et al. Second-look arthroscopy of anterior cruciate ligament grafts with multistranded hamstring tendons. *Arthroscopy* 2004;**20**:287–93.
- 56. Rihn JA, Harner CD. The use of musculoskeletal allograft tissue in knee surgery: Instructional Course 105. *Arthroscopy* 2003;**19**(Suppl. 1):51–66.
57. Pearsall AW 4th, Hollis JM, Russell GV Jr, Scheer Z. A biomechanical comparison of three lower extremity tendons for ligamentous reconstruction about the knee. *Arthroscopy* 2003;**19**:1091–6.
- 58. Asselmeier MA, Caspari RB, Bottenfield S. A review of allograft processing and sterilization techniques and their role in transmission of the human immunodeficiency virus. *American Journal of Sports Medicine* 1993;**21**:170–5.
59. Malinin TI, Levitt RL, Bashore C, et al. A study of retrieved allografts used to replace anterior cruciate ligaments. *Arthroscopy* 2002;**18**:163–70.
60. Jackson DW, Windler GE, Simon TM. Intraarticular reaction associated with the use of freeze-dried, ethylene oxide-sterilized bone-patella tendon-bone allografts in the reconstruction of the anterior cruciate ligament. *American Journal of Sports Medicine* 1990;**18**:1–10; discussion 10–1.
61. Jackson DW, Grood ES, Goldstein JD, et al. A comparison of patellar tendon autograft and allograft used for anterior cruciate ligament reconstruction in the goat model. *American Journal of Sports Medicine* 1993;**21**:176–85.
62. Dorizas JA, Stanitski CL. Anterior cruciate ligament injury in the skeletally immature. *Orthopedic Clinics of North America* 2003;**34**:355–63.
63. Stanitski CL, Harvell JC, Fu FH. Observations on acute knee hemarthrosis in children and adolescents. *Journal of Pediatric Orthopaedics* 1993;**13**:506–10.
- 64. Millett PJ, Willis AA, Warren RF. Associated injuries in pediatric and adolescent anterior cruciate ligament tears: Does a delay in treatment increase the risk of meniscal tear? *Arthroscopy* 2002;**18**:955–9.

65. Paletta GA Jr. Special considerations: Anterior cruciate ligament reconstruction in the skeletally immature. *Orthopedic Clinics of North America* 2003;**34**:65–77.
66. Aronowitz ER, Ganley TJ, Goode JR, et al. Anterior cruciate ligament reconstruction in adolescents with open physes. *American Journal of Sports Medicine* 2000;**28**:168–75.
67. Stadelmaier DM, Arnoczky SP, Dodds J, Ross H. The effect of drilling and soft tissue grafting across open growth plates. A histologic study. *American Journal of Sports Medicine* 1995;**23**:431–5.
68. Shelbourne KD, Patel DV, McCarroll JR. Management of anterior cruciate ligament injuries in skeletally immature adolescents. *Knee Surgery, Sports Traumatology, Arthroscopy* 1996;**4**:68–74.
69. Simonian PT, Metcalf MH, Larson RV. Anterior cruciate ligament injuries in the skeletally immature patient. *American Journal of Orthopedics* 1999;**28**:624–8.
♦70. Arendt E, Dick R. Knee injury patterns among men and women in collegiate basketball and soccer. NCAA data and review of literature. *American Journal of Sports Medicine* 1995;**23**:694–701.
71. Harner CD, Paulos LE, Greenwald AE, Rosenberg TD, Cooley VC. Detailed analysis of patients with bilateral anterior cruciate ligament injuries. *American Journal of Sports Medicine* 1994;**22**:37–43.
72. LaPrade RF, Burnett QM 2nd. Femoral intercondylar notch stenosis and correlation to anterior cruciate ligament injuries. A prospective study. *American Journal of Sports Medicine* 1994;**22**:198–202; discussion 203.
73. Shelbourne KD, Facibene WA, Hunt JJ. Radiographic and intraoperative intercondylar notch width measurements in men and women with unilateral and bilateral anterior cruciate ligament tears. *Knee Surgery, Sports Traumatology, Arthroscopy* 1997;**5**:229–33.
74. Wojtys EM, Huston LJ, Lindenfeld TN, et al. Association between the menstrual cycle and anterior cruciate ligament injuries in female athletes. *American Journal of Sports Medicine* 1998;**26**:614–19.
75. Logan MC, Williams A, Lavelle J, et al. Tibiofemoral kinematics following successful anterior cruciate ligament reconstruction using dynamic magnetic resonance imaging. *American Journal of Sports Medicine* 2004;**32**:984–92.
♦76. Chhabra A, Starman JS, Ferretti M, et al. Anatomic, radiographic, biomechanical, and kinematic evaluation of the anterior cruciate ligament and its two functional bundles. *Journal of Bone and Joint Surgery (American)* 2006;**88**(Suppl 4):2–10.
●77. Tashman S, Collon D, Anderson K, et al. Abnormal rotational knee motion during running after anterior cruciate ligament reconstruction. *American Journal of Sports Medicine* 2004;**32**:975–83.
78. Brandsson S, Karlsson J, Sward L, et al. Kinematics and laxity of the knee joint after anterior cruciate ligament reconstruction: pre- and postoperative radiostereometric studies. *American Journal of Sports Medicine* 2002;**30**:361–7.
79. Bush-Joseph CA, Hurwitz DE, Patel RR, et al. Dynamic function after anterior cruciate ligament reconstruction with autologous patellar tendon. *American Journal of Sports Medicine* 2001;**29**:36–41.
80. Adachi N, Ochi M, Uchio Y, et al. Reconstruction of the anterior cruciate ligament. Single- versus double-bundle multistranded hamstring tendons. *Journal of Bone and Joint Surgery (British)* 2004;**86**:515–20.
81. Yasuda K, Kondo E, Ichiyama H, et al. Anatomic reconstruction of the anteromedial and postero lateral bundles of the anterior cruciate ligament using hamstring tendon grafts. *Arthroscopy* 2004;**20**:1015–25.
82. Fowler PJ, Messieh SS. Isolated posterior cruciate ligament injuries in athletes. *American Journal of Sports Medicine* 1987;**15**:553–7.
83. Kannus P, Bergfeld J, Jarvinen M, et al. Injuries to the posterior cruciate ligament of the knee. *Sports Medicine* 1991;**12**:110–31.
●84. Harner CD, Baek GH, Vogrin TM, et al. Quantitative analysis of human cruciate ligament insertions. *Arthroscopy* 1999;**15**:741–9.
●85. Girgis FG, Marshall JL, Monajem A. The cruciate ligaments of the knee joint. Anatomical, functional and experimental analysis. *Clinical Orthopaedics and Related Research* 1975;**Jan–Feb**:216–31.
86. Gupte CM, Bull AM, Thomas RD, Amis AA. The meniscofemoral ligaments: secondary restraints to the posterior drawer. Analysis of anteroposterior and rotary laxity in the intact and posterior-cruciate-deficient knee. *Journal of Bone and Joint Surgery (British)* 2003;**85**:765–73.
87. Harner CD, Hoher J. Evaluation and treatment of posterior cruciate ligament injuries. *American Journal of Sports Medicine* 1998;**26**:471–82.
88. Veltri DM, Deng XH, Torzilli PA, et al. The role of the cruciate and posterolateral ligaments in stability of the knee. A biomechanical study. *American Journal of Sports Medicine* 1995;**23**:436–43.
89. White LM, Miniaci A. Cruciate and posterolateral corner injuries in the athlete: Clinical and magnetic resonance imaging features. *Seminars in Musculoskeletal Radiolology* 2004;**8**:111–31.
90. Covey CD, Sapega AA. Injuries of the posterior cruciate ligament. *Journal of Bone and Joint Surgery (American)* 1993;**75**:1376–86.
●91. Harner CD, Vogrin TM, Hoher J, et al. Biomechanical analysis of a posterior cruciate ligament reconstruction. Deficiency of the posterolateral structures as a cause of graft failure. *American Journal of Sports Medicine* 2000;**28**:32–9.
92. Hewett TE, Noyes FR, Lee MD. Diagnosis of complete and partial posterior cruciate ligament ruptures. Stress radiography compared with KT-1000 arthrometer and posterior drawer testing. *American Journal of Sports Medicine* 1997;**25**:648–55.

93. Gross ML, Grover JS, Bassett LW, et al. Magnetic resonance imaging of the posterior cruciate ligament. Clinical use to improve diagnostic accuracy. *American Journal of Sports Medicine* 1992;**20**:732–7.
94. Shelbourne KD, Jennings RW, Vahey TN. Magnetic resonance imaging of posterior cruciate ligament injuries: assessment of healing. *American Journal of Knee Surgery* 1999;**12**:209–13.
95. Cross MJ, Powell JF. Long-term followup of posterior cruciate ligament rupture. A study of 116 cases. *American Journal of Sports Medicine* 1984;**12**:292–7.
96. Dandy DJ, Pusey RJ. The long-term results of unrepaired tears of the posterior cruciate ligament. *Journal of Bone and Joint Surgery (British)* 1982;**64**:92–4.
97. Keller PM, Shelbourne KD, McCarroll JR, Rettig AC. Nonoperatively treated isolated posterior cruciate ligament injuries. *American Journal of Sports Medicine* 1993;**21**:132–6.
98. Parolie JM, Bergfeld JA. Long-term results of nonoperative treatment of isolated posterior cruciate ligament injuries in the athlete. *American Journal of Sports Medicine* 1986;**14**:35–8.
99. Torg JS, Barton TM, Pavlov H, Stine R. Natural history of the posterior cruciate ligament-deficient knee. *Clinical Orthopaedics and Related Research* 1989;**246**:208–16.
100. Geissler WB, Whipple TL. Intraarticular abnormalities in association with posterior cruciate ligament injuries. *American Journal of Sports Medicine* 1993;**21**:846–9.
◆101. Shelbourne KD, Davis TJ, Patel DV. The natural history of acute, isolated, nonoperatively treated posterior cruciate ligament injuries: A prospective study. *American Journal of Sports Medicine* 1999;**27**:276–83.
102. Boynton MD, Tietjens BR. Long-term followup of the untreated isolated posterior cruciate ligament-deficient knee. *American Journal of Sports Medicine* 1996;**24**:306–10.
◆103. Miller MD, Bergfeld JA, Fowler PJ, et al. The posterior cruciate ligament injured knee: principles of evaluation and treatment. *Instructional Course Lectures* 1999;**48**:199–207.
104. Kim SJ, Shin SJ, Cho SK, Kim HK. Arthroscopic suture fixation for bony avulsion of the posterior cruciate ligament. *Arthroscopy* 2001;**17**:776–80.
105. Fanelli GC, Edson CJ. Posterior cruciate ligament injuries in trauma patients: Part II. *Arthroscopy* 1995;**11**:526–9.
●106. Hoher J, Harner CD, Vogrin TM, et al. In situ forces in the posterolateral structures of the knee under posterior tibial loading in the intact and posterior cruciate ligament-deficient knee. *Journal of Orthopedic Research* 1998;**16**:675–81.
107. Berg EE. Posterior cruciate ligament tibial inlay reconstruction. *Arthroscopy* 1995;**11**:69–76.
108. Bergfeld JA, McAllister DR, Parker RD, et al. A biomechanical comparison of posterior cruciate ligament reconstruction techniques. *American Journal of Sports Medicine* 2001;**29**:129–36.
109. Giffin JR, Haemmerle MJ, Vogrin TM, Harner CD. Single- versus double-bundle PCL reconstruction: a biomechanical analysis. *Journal of Knee Surgery* 2002;**15**:114–20.
110. Cain EL Jr, Clancy WG Jr. Posterior cruciate ligament reconstruction: two-bundle technique. *Journal of Knee Surgery* 2002;**15**:108–13.
111. Hughston JC, Andrews JR, Cross MJ, Moschi A. Classification of knee ligament instabilities. Part II. The lateral compartment. *Journal of Bone and Joint Surgery (American)* 1976;**58**:173–9.
112. Baker CL Jr, Norwood LA, Hughston JC. Acute posterolateral rotatory instability of the knee. *Journal of Bone and Joint Surgery (American)* 1983;**65**:614–18.
113. Wascher DC, Markolf KL, Shapiro MS, Finerman GA. Direct in vitro measurement of forces in the cruciate ligaments. Part I: The effect of multiplane loading in the intact knee. *Journal of Bone and Joint Surgery (American)* 1993;**75**:377–86.
114. Grana WA, Janssen T. Lateral ligament injury of the knee. *Orthopedics* 1987;**10**:1039–44.
115. Veltri DM, Deng XH, Torzilli PA, et al. The role of the cruciate and posterolateral ligaments in stability of the knee. A biomechanical study. *American Journal of Sports Medicine* 1995;**23**:436–43.
●116. Seebacher JR, Inglis AE, Marshall JL, Warren RF. The structures of the posterolateral aspect of the knee. *Journal of Bone and Joint Surgery (American)* 1982;**64**:536–41.
117. Markolf KL, Wascher DC, Finerman GA. Direct in vitro measurement of forces in the cruciate ligaments. Part II: The effect of section of the posterolateral structures. *Journal of Bone and Joint Surgery (American)* 1993;**75**:387–94.
118. Nielsen S, Ovesen J, Rasmussen O. The posterior cruciate ligament and rotatory knee instability. An experimental study. *Archives of Orthopaedic and Trauma Surgery* 1985;**104**:53–6.
119. Noyes FR. PCL & posterolateral complex injuries. Overview. *American Journal of Knee Surgery* 1996;**9**:171.
120. Noyes FR, Barber-Westin SD. Surgical reconstruction of severe chronic posterolateral complex injuries of the knee using allograft tissues. *American Journal of Sports Medicine* 1995;**23**:2–12.
121. Hughston JC, Norwood LA Jr. The posterolateral drawer test and external rotational recurvatum test for posterolateral rotatory instability of the knee. *Clinical Orthopaedics and Related Research* 1980;**Mar–Apr**:82–7.
◆122. Veltri DM, Warren RF. Posterolateral instability of the knee. *Instructional Course Lectures* 1995;**44**:441–53.
123. Yu JS, Salonen DC, Hodler J, et al. Posterolateral aspect of the knee: improved MR imaging with a coronal oblique technique. *Radiology* 1996;**198**:199–204.
124. Covey DC. Injuries of the posterolateral corner of the knee. *Journal of Bone and Joint Surgery (American)* 2001;**83A**:106–18.

125. Kannus P. Nonoperative treatment of grade II and III sprains of the lateral ligament compartment of the knee. *American Journal of Sports Medicine* 1989;**17**:83–8.
126. Hughston JC, Jacobson KE. Chronic posterolateral rotatory instability of the knee. *Journal of Bone and Joint Surgery (American)* 1985;**67**:351–9.
127. Latimer HA, Tibone JE, El Attrache NS, McMahon PJ. Reconstruction of the lateral collateral ligament of the knee with patellar tendon allograft. Report of a new technique in combined ligament injuries. *American Journal of Sports Medicine* 1998;**26**:656–62.
128. Wascher DC, Grauer JD, Markoff KL. Biceps tendon tenodesis for posterolateral instability of the knee. An in vitro study. *American Journal of Sports Medicine* 1993;**21**:400–6.
129. Fanelli GC, Larson RV. Practical management of posterolateral instability of the knee. *Arthroscopy* 2002;**18**(Suppl. 1):1–8.
130. Lee MC, Park YK, Lee SH, et al. Posterolateral reconstruction using split Achilles tendon allograft. *Arthroscopy* 2003;**19**:1043–9.
131. Kim SJ, Shin SJ, Jeong JH. Posterolateral rotatory instability treated by a modified biceps rerouting technique: technical considerations and results in cases with and without posterior cruciate ligament insufficiency. *Arthroscopy* 2003;**19**:493–9.
132. Pavlovich RI, Nafarrate EB. Trivalent reconstruction for posterolateral and lateral knee instability. *Arthroscopy* 2002;**18**:E1.
133. Shelbourne KD, Porter DA, Clingman JA, et al. Low-velocity knee dislocation. *Orthopedic Reviews* 1991;**20**:995–1004.
◆134. Green NE, Allen BL. Vascular injuries associated with dislocation of the knee. *Journal of Bone and Joint Surgery (American)* 1977;**59**:236–9.
135. Montgomery JB. Dislocation of the knee. *Orthopedic Clinics of North America* 1987;**18**:149–56.
136. Kennedy JC. Complete dislocation of the knee joint. *Journal of Bone and Joint Surgery (American)* 1963;**45**:889–904.
137. Treiman GS, Yellin AE, Weaver FA, et al. Examination of the patient with a knee dislocation. The case for selective arteriography. *Archives of Surgery* 1992;**127**:1056–62; discussion 1062–3.
138. Klineberg EO, Crites BM, Flinn WR, et al. The role of arteriography in assessing popliteal artery injury in knee dislocations. *Journal of Trauma* 2004;**56**:786–90.
139. Mills WJ, Barei DP, McNair P. The value of the ankle-brachial index for diagnosing arterial injury after knee dislocation: a prospective study. *Journal of Trauma* 2004;**56**:1261–5.
140. Stannard JP, Sheils TM, Lopez-Ben RR, et al. Vascular injuries in knee dislocations: the role of physical examination in determining the need for arteriography. *Journal of Bone and Joint Surgery (American)* 2004;**86-A**:910–15.
141. Wascher DC, Dvirnak PC, DeCoster TA. Knee dislocation: initial assessment and implications for treatment. *Journal of Orthopaedic Trauma* 1997;**11**:525–9.
◆142. Rihn JA, Groff YJ, Harner CD, Cha PS. The acutely dislocated knee: evaluation and management. *Journal of the American Academy of Orthopaedic Surgeons* 2004;**12**:334–46.
143. Taylor AR, Arden GP, Rainey HA. Traumatic dislocation of the knee. A report of forty-three cases with special reference to conservative treatment. *Journal of Bone and Joint Surgery (British)* 1972;**54**:96–102.
144. Henshaw RM, Shapiro MS, Oppenheim WL. Delayed reduction of traumatic knee dislocation. A case report and literature review. *Clinical Orthopaedics and Related Research* 1996;**330**:152–6.
145. Petrie RS, Trousdale RT, Cabanela ME. Total knee arthroplasty for chronic posterior knee dislocation: report of 2 cases with technical considerations. *Journal of Arthroplasty* 2000;**15**:380–6.
146. Simonian PT, Wickiewicz TL, Hotchkiss RN, Warren RF. Chronic knee dislocation: reduction, reconstruction, and application of a skeletally fixed knee hinge. A report of two cases. *American Journal of Sports Medicine* 1998;**26**:591–6.
147. Ohkoshi Y, Nagasaki S, Shibata N, et al. Two-stage reconstruction with autografts for knee dislocations. *Clinical Orthopaedics and Related Research* 2002;**May**:169–75.
148. Almekinders LC, Dedmond BT. Outcomes of the operatively treated knee dislocation. *Clinical Sports Medicine* 2000;**19**:503–18.
149. Fanelli GC, Giannotti BF, Edson CJ. Arthroscopically assisted combined anterior and posterior cruciate ligament reconstruction. *Arthroscopy* 1996;**12**:5–14.
150. Sisto DJ, Warren RF. Complete knee dislocation. A follow-up study of operative treatment. *Clinical Orthopaedics and Related Research* 1985;**198**:94–101.
151. Thomsen PB, Rud B, Jensen UH. Stability and motion after traumatic dislocation of the knee. *Acta Orthopaedica Scandinavica* 1984;**55**:278–83.
152. Harner CD, Waltrip RL, Bennett CH, et al. Surgical management of knee dislocations. *Journal of Bone and Joint Surgery (American)* 2004;**86A**:262–73.
153. Liow RY, McNicholas MJ, Keating JF, Nutton RW. Ligament repair and reconstruction in traumatic dislocation of the knee. *Journal of Bone and Joint Surgery (British)* 2003;**85**:845–51.

78

Leg, ankle and foot injuries

JOHN E FEMINO, NED AMENDOLA

EXERCISE-INDUCED LEG PAIN	821	Flexor hallucis longus stenosis and posterior ankle impingement	839
Tibial stress fractures	821	Lateral ankle ligamentous instability	840
Medial tibial stress syndrome	824	Syndesmotic sprains	842
Exertional compartment syndrome	825	Deltoid ligament sprains	843
Common peroneal nerve entrapment	826	MIDFOOT AND FOREFOOT PAIN	843
Superficial peroneal nerve entrapment	828	Lisfranc sprains	843
TENDON PROBLEMS	829	Navicular stress fractures	845
Achilles tendon ruptures	829	Fifth metatarsal fractures	846
Achilles tendon tendinopathy	831	Lateral and medial plantar nerve entrapment	847
Peroneal tendon problems	834	Stress fractures of the first metatarsophalangeal joint sesamoid bones	848
Posterior tibial tendon tenosynovitis and tears	835	References	849
ANKLE PROBLEMS	836		
Osteochondral lesions of the talus	836		
Anterior ankle and subtalar joint impingement	838		

NATIONAL BOARD STANDARDS

- Describe diagnostic tests and treatment principles for stress fractures of the foot and ankle
- Identify key soft tissue injuries of the ankle to include treatment options
- Explain the diagnosis and treatment of ankle sprains and other injuries of the ankle
- Describe soft tissue injuries of the foot and their treatment

EXERCISE-INDUCED LEG PAIN

Exercise-induced leg pain is a common presenting complaint among athletes. Previously, the general term of 'shin splints' was used to describe the common complaints of exercise-induced leg pain. Over time, study of this problem has led to the description of specific clinical syndromes associated with this common complaint. A systematic approach to diagnosis can be aided by thinking of the different pathologies and the associated tissue types. For instance, nerve-related pain may present at a site remote from the actual pathology due to the longitudinal nature of the structure of a nerve, whereas pain and tenderness from a tibial stress fracture will be very focal. A list of the common causes of exercise-induced leg pain and the associated tissues is provided in Table 78.1.

TIBIAL STRESS FRACTURES

Aetiology

Tibial stress fractures are one of the most common stress fractures seen in athletes and military recruits, and may account for up to 20% of injuries in track athletes.[1–5]

Table 78.1 Aetiology and differential

Tissue of origin	Examples of pathology
Bone	Tibial stress fracture, fibular stress fracture
Periosteum	Periostitis (medial tibial stress syndrome)
Muscle or fascia	Exertional compartment syndrome, fascial herniation
Tendon	Achilles, peroneal, or tibialis posterior tendinopathy
Nerve	Common or superficial peroneal nerve entrapment
Blood vessel	Popliteal artery entrapment, intermittent claudication, or other insufficiency, venous insufficiency
Distant (referred)	Spinal radiculopathy

Predisposing factors that have been reported can be both gender specific and general. They include narrow medullary canal and poor conditioning, menstrual disturbance and restrictive eating habits.[1,6,7] For example one study found that female athletes with a history of oligomenorrhoea were six times more likely to have had a stress fracture.[8] A study of military recruits found that both genders were at greater risk for sustaining a stress fracture due to poor physical conditioning and relative smaller thigh muscles than control subjects without stress fractures. Male cases had narrower external bone diameters than control subjects, whereas female cases had decreased cortical thickness and bone mineral density.[1] Another possible aetiology is gait asymmetry. Recent investigation found that in female runners levels of gait asymmetry ranged from 3.1% for peak vertical ground reaction force to 49.8% for lateral ground reaction force in the group with no previous stress fracture. They did not find statistically significant difference in gait asymmetry between the groups. However, the authors found that the group with previous stress fractures did have higher overall lateral ground reaction forces. The authors concluded that previously injured subjects train closer to the fracture threshold and that asymmetry may dictate which side may be injured.[9] Fracture location may be related to specific aetiological factors. One study found that in 29 unilateral tibial stress fractures 10 were anterior and 19 were posteromedial. Nine of the 10 anterior mid-diaphyseal fractures occurred in the push-off/landing leg whereas no difference was found in the posteromedial distal fracture group.[10] Ekenman et al.[11] found in a later study that the in vivo strain at the posteromedial distal tibia was greatest during forefoot landing as opposed to heel landing. The greatest strain on the anterior mid-diaphyseal tibia was at ground contact after voluntary vertical drop.[11] This further suggests that different mechanical aetiologies may exist for different sites.

Pathology

Mechanical and biological factors as noted above can predispose bone to injury during periods of sharply increased activity as seen during athletic training or in military recruits. The increased strain leads to initial bone resorption as a part of the remodelling response and the bone is temporarily weak. Accumulated stress can overcome the rate of bone hypertrophy and stress fractures can ensue.[12]

As alluded to above, there are different sites of tibial stress fractures. Proximal and distal third metaphyseal fractures usually occur medial or posteromedial, are on the compression side of the bone and heal with conservative treatment. Mid-diaphyseal stress fractures occur on the anterior tension side of the cortex and have the propensity for slower healing and delayed union with conservative treatment. One study found seven of 151 tibial stress fractures that were anterior mid-diaphyseal stress fractures that presented and were found to be biopsy-proven non-unions.[13] Therefore, in athletes these fractures are often best treated with intramedullary fixation.

Evaluation

A high index of suspicion for tibial stress fracture should arise when an athlete complains of leg pain and difficulty training or bearing weight that is not relieved with rest. This is particularly true in the setting of a relatively sudden increase in the intensity of training. Unlike medial tibial stress syndrome, rest alone will not relieve the pain. Symptoms of neurovascular abnormalities such as with peripheral nerve entrapments or exertional compartment syndrome should be excluded.

Physical examination

The most important physical finding is localized tenderness over the site of the fracture. This differs from medial tibial stress syndrome, which presents with diffuse longitudinal tenderness. A thorough neurovascular examination should be performed in any athlete presenting with exercise-induced leg pain; however, this should be normal in an athlete with an isolated tibial stress fracture.

Imaging studies

Plain radiographs can show evidence of bone response such as periosteal reaction, cortical thickening or fracture lucency. When the troublesome anterior mid-diaphyseal fractures are present one may see 'the dreaded black line',[14] where the fracture presents as a radiographic non-union (Fig.). In cases where obvious findings are not present on plain radiographs, then MRI is the preferred choice of imaging.[15–17] Specifically, a wide zone of high signal across the entire bone as seen on the short tau inversion–recovery (STIR) sequence was found to be the most sensitive portion of the MRI examination for diagnosing tibial stress fractures. By comparison, periostitis revealed longitudinal high signal along the cortical bone but not the medullary bone.[16] A bone scan can also be helpful but is less specific, since it does not necessarily differentiate from medial tibial stress syndrome[18] and does not provide the anatomic detail of an MRI. CT scan can also provide more detailed information of cortical such as osteopenia[17] but cannot show the early signs of marrow oedema.

Treatment

OBJECTIVES

The objectives of treatment are to decrease the repeated stress on the bone and allow it to rest and heal. Most tibial stress fractures can be healed with non-operative treatment of immobilization and varying degrees of rest, but some may require operative treatment with intramedullary nailing.[19]

Non-operative treatment consists of varying degrees of rest and immobilization for non-displaced fractures. In some cases, up to 8 weeks of cast immobilization may be necessary (Figs 78.1 and 78.2), but for many athletes relative rest and mobilization with a cast or brace may be all that is needed.[20] In a study of soldiers, the use of a pneumatic brace did not improve healing time or function. Pulsed low-intensity ultrasound has been suggested as an aid to healing tibial stress fractures,[21] but in one prospective randomized double-blinded study of tibial stress fractures in military recruits, the use of pulsed ultrasound did not show any significant difference in time to healing in two similar groups.[22]

OPERATIVE TREATMENT

Intramedullary tibial nailing (Figs 78.3) has become the operative treatment of choice for non-healing anterior tibial diaphyseal stress fractures that do not respond to the usual non-operative treatments of rest and immobilization with casting or bracing.[6,23] Anterior mid-diaphyseal fractures account for all of the 16 stress fractures in the 12 patients reported in the studies of Chang and Harris[6] and Varner et al.[23]

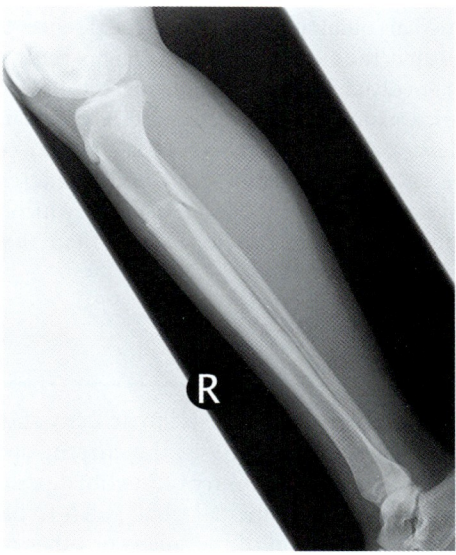

Figure 78.2 Anteroposterior and lateral radiographs 5 months later, after casting and functional bracing, with good alignment and mature healed fracture. The patient went on to record personal best times in competition several months later.

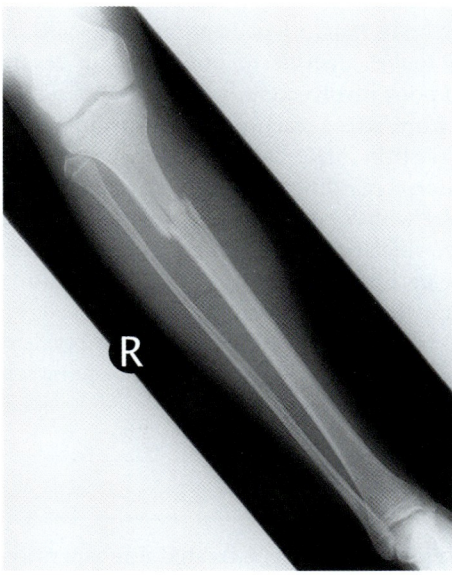

Figure 78.1 Anteroposterior and lateral radiographs of proximal tibial stress fracture in a 17 year old female long distance runner.

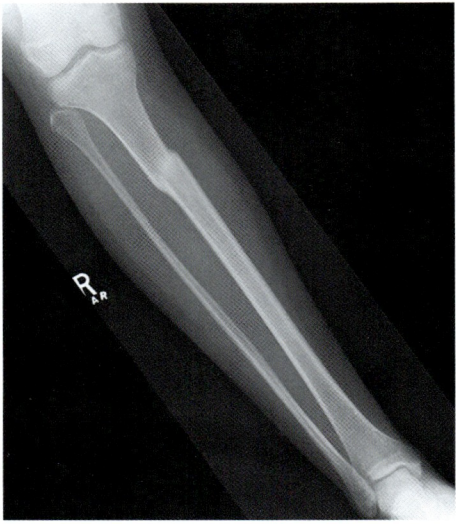

Figure 78.3 Intramedullary tibial nailing

MEDIAL TIBIAL STRESS SYNDROME

Aetiology

Medial tibial stress syndrome (MTSS) is the most common cause of exertional leg pain in athletes. It presents as exercise-related pain at the posteromedial border of the mid-tibia, which resolves with cessation of activity and rest. It is particularly seen in athletes who perform repetitive jumping and running activities. MTSS is considered to be a periostitis of the posterior medial border of the tibia. It was once thought to be due to traction at the origin of the posterior tibialis muscle; however, it is now thought to be due primarily to traction of the soleus muscle fascia on the posteromedial tibial periosteum.[24–26] Evidence has also suggested that the flexor digitorum longus muscle origin may also involved.[24] Foot posture, specifically varus foot alignment, was found in one study to be associated with the incidence of MTSS.[27] Others have suggested a pronated foot type to be a risk factor.[25,28] Gender difference was shown in one study of military recruits in which females were twice as likely to develop MTSS than their male counterparts.[28]

Pathology

Although few scientific data exist to actually show what the pathophysiology of MTSS is, the current opinion is that it is due to a traction injury of the tibial periosteum. Periostitis of the posteromedial tibial is felt to be due to the repetitive contraction of the soleus or other posterior leg muscles and the traction generated at the periosteal attachment of the musculature and associated fascia. This is commonly seen in sports with repetitive jumping and running, suggesting a similar spectrum of overuse as seen in stress fractures. Support for this concept is mostly indirect from bone scan and MRI findings in athletes with this problem, suggesting an inflammatory response at the site of pain. Abnormally decreased local bone density has been shown with MTSS in one study comparing athletes with long-term symptoms and both athletic and non-athletic control subjects. The symptomatic legs demonstrated 15% and 23% lower bone density than in non-athletic and athletic controls respectively. The overall bone density was higher than non-athletic controls but lower than athletic controls at comparable sites.[29] Another study found histological evidence of decreased bone density in athletes who underwent surgery for MTSS. In this study, the authors compared bone scan findings with histological samples of periosteum and bone taken at the time of surgery. They found variable histological findings of periosteum, including fibrous thickening, increased vascularity and occasionally chronic inflammatory cells, haemosiderin staining and acid mucopolysaccharide deposition. Histological findings in local bone included loss of osteocytes, enlargement of some lacunae and lamellar disorganization. Although they did not find correlation between bone scan findings and histology, they did make two interesting observations. Cases with periosteal thickening demonstrated normal bone scans whereas those with little loss of osteocytes had an abnormal bone scan.[30] Whether this reflects a continuum of the disease process or suggests a failure of successful healing in individuals with loss of osteocytes and bone quality remains to be seen.

Evaluation

The diagnosis of MTSS is made by systematic evaluation and involves the same thought process as when ruling out tibial stress fracture. Patients presenting with history of exertional leg pain in the absence of chronic exertional compartment syndrome (CECS) and stress fracture will have focal pain and tenderness at the posteromedial border of the tibia at the mid-tibia. The pain will worsen with exercise activity and may diminish with cessation of exercise, but does not completely go away. This distinguishes MTSS from CECS because in CECS cessation of exercise brings complete relief of symptoms.

Imaging studies

Both three-phase bone scan and MRI have been suggested for helping to evaluate patients with exertional leg pain, and specific findings for MTSS have been described to help differentiate it from tibial stress fracture. Bone scan findings when positive reveal focal or linear uptake at the posteromedial border of the tibia.[15,30–33] MRI demonstrates periosteal oedema and can differentiate frank cortical fracture and bone marrow oedema as well. MRI has been reported to be superior to bone scan in resolving the degree of bone involvement.[15] MRI can differentiate stress fracture from stress reaction in the medullary bone and from periostitis. MRI has been shown to also provide information regarding muscle inflammation in MTSS specifically with a contrast-enhanced T_1-weighted image sequence, which revealed enhancement of the posterior leg musculature in the region of periostitis.[32] Mattila et al.[32] also found that, while the contrast-enhanced T_1 images were also best for demonstrating periosteal oedema, STIR images were better for demonstrating oedema within the marrow (Fig. 78.4).

Treatment

Most cases of MTSS can be treated non-operatively with modification of training or a period of absolute rest in some cases. When the symptoms do not resolve with reasonable measures of rest, then surgical treatment may

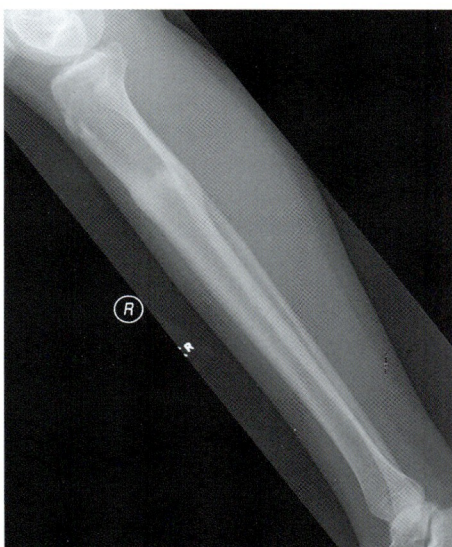

Figure 78.4 Oedema within the bone marrow.

provide relief of pain and allow resumption of athletic activity.[26,34–36] Results of surgery in these retrospective studies are not universally promising however. Fasciotomy is the most common procedure recommended, and good or excellent results have been reported in approximately 80% of patients with periostitis.[26,35] One study found that, while pain relief was improved by 72% in 46 of 78 patients who returned for re-evaluation, only 41% of those patients returned to presymptom sports activity.[36] Patients who fail non-operative measures and are considering surgery should be cautioned against overly optimistic expectations of pain relief and return to sports.

EXERTIONAL COMPARTMENT SYNDROME

Aetiology

CECS of the leg is a well-documented clinical problem in which the muscle compartments of the leg develop increasing pressure with exercise, leading to pain. In addition, this elevation of pressure has been shown to resolve after fasciotomy in patients with CECS,[37] and can be debilitating for an athlete who is affected. Although much has been written about this condition, there is still no clear understanding of the pathophysiology of it.[38,39] The presentation is typical although not specific and involves the onset of leg pain with increasing activity that is more diffuse than that usually seen in MTSS. It is generally thought to be due to increased muscle compartment pressures. However, many possible factors have been suggested, including increased muscle bulk, fascial thickness and stiffness, stimulation of fascial stretch receptors, poor venous return, micromuscular injury and small myopathic abnormalities.[39]

Pathology

The actual cause of elevated muscle compartment pressure in CECS is not known. One thought is that increased muscle compartment pressure impairs the normal capillary blood flow and exchange of oxygen and metabolites, thus producing an ischaemic type of pain. The idea of fascial stiffness as a cause was examined by subjecting CECS patients and controls to the same exercise protocol and measuring the muscle size of the anterior tibialis by ultrasound. It was found that muscle size increased by 8% in both groups whereas pain was induced only in the CECS group.[38] The authors concluded that the fascial stiffness was the same in both groups. The onset of CECS symptoms has been correlated with muscle relaxation pressure and blood flow during monitored exercise testing. With the onset of symptoms in nine CECS patients, the muscle relaxation pressure increased and blood flow to the muscles decreased. This observation was not found at 8 months after fasciotomy, and patients experienced no symptoms with exercise testing.[40] It was concluded that muscle ischaemia due to increased muscle relaxation pressure was the cause of pain in CECS. Experimental evidence has shown that in patients with documented CECS there is a decrease in the muscle production of phosphofructase after compartment release. Phosphofructase is a marker of glycolytic metabolism that rises during anaerobic muscle activity. This provides further evidence that fasciotomy improves muscle blood flow allowing a shift to a more aerobic muscle activity after fasciotomy.[41] Another study using nuclear blood flow monitoring in five patients with diagnosed CECS and five normal volunteers did not show any difference in blood flow between these two groups.[42] In summary, while muscle function may become more anaerobic and result in an ischaemic type of pain as a result of increased compartment pressure, it has not been clearly demonstrated that this phenomenon is due to a lack of blood flow to the involved muscles.

Evaluation

The patient history and physical examination are critical in diagnosing CECS and have been described as local leg pain associated with swelling, sometimes paraesthesias, and occasionally transient motor findings such as drop-foot. These symptoms evolve predictably during exercise and usually subside with cessation of exercise.

Unlike MTSS or a stress fracture, patients with CECS do not have focal tenderness along the tibia. The definitive test for diagnosing CECS is intramuscular pressure measurement before, during and after a defined exercise protocol, usually running on a treadmill. Values that have been suggested for diagnosis of CECS are pre-exercise resting pressure >15 mmHg, a 1 minute post-exercise pressure of >30 mmHg or a 5 minute post-exercise pressure of >20 mmHg.[43] This protocol was determined after review of 131 patients, of whom 45 were diagnosed with CECS. In that study the only significant difference found between the two groups was a much higher incidence of muscle herniation in the CECS group.

Imaging studies and other tests

MRI, MRI spectroscopy and nuclear-medicine blood flow studies have all shown only limited success.[42] Electromyography and nerve conduction studies have been shown to reveal a lack of increase in potentiation of the peroneal motor amplitude post exercise in CECS patients compared with controls who did show increased motor potentiation after exercise. Additionally, the CECS subjects demonstrated decreased vibratory sensation post exercise as well.[44]

Treatment

OBJECTIVES

Although the pathophysiology of CECS remains unclear, it is well accepted that there are two means to alleviate symptoms. Common non-operative treatments for many sport-related injuries such as physical therapy, non-steroidal anti-inflammatory drugs (NSAIDs) and orthosis are generally ineffective. Activity modification to avoid symptoms has been discussed;[45,46] however, the only method of treatment that may allow for return to sports activity is surgical release of the involved compartments.[45–53] This however does not guarantee a return to the level of performance that an athlete may desire, and patients should be counselled carefully to convey realistic expectations. The surgical technique of fasciotomy in CECS does not require the release of the skin in addition to the fascia, as is often the case in acute compartment syndrome due to severe trauma and crush injuries. Therefore, the release of the compartments of the leg for CECS can be done with limited incision fasciotomy. It is essential however that complete release of the involved compartments be achieved regardless of the specific technique. Treatment of anterior compartment involvement alone,[52,54,55] anterior and lateral compartments,[56,57] the anterior and deep posterior compartments[49,58] and deep posterior compartment alone[59] have all been described. One study comparing those with anterior and lateral compartment release alone and posterior compartment release found that they had 95% good results in the anterolateral group but only 65% good results in the group who underwent deep posterior compartment release. Another study of patients with deep posterior compartment release showed similar findings, and the authors felt that patients' residual symptoms were probably due to the posterior tibialis muscle alone and the authors recommended that this muscle specifically be released.[49] Rorabeck[60] had previously suggested that the posterior tibialis muscle functions as a fifth compartment of the leg. One report showed that the outcome of anterior compartment release alone resulted in 95% good results whereas subjects who underwent anterior and lateral compartment release had 65% good results. The authors concluded that single compartment release for isolated anterior compartment pathology was favourable.[57]

Minimally invasive techniques can be done with one or two incisions. The risk to the superficial peroneal nerve or its branches should be kept in mind when releasing the anterior and lateral compartments. The anatomy of the superficial peroneal nerve can be quite variable and several different patterns have been well described.[61–64] Injury to the nerve has been reported.[55] More recently the use of endoscopic visualization to aid with minimal incision compartment release has been reported and may have the promising benefit of decreasing the risk of damage to peripheral nerves.[51,65–67] Caution with this technique should be applied, particularly in release of the deep posterior compartment where postoperative haematoma has been reported.[66]

COMMON PERONEAL NERVE ENTRAPMENT

Aetiology

Common peroneal nerve compression or injury has been shown to have a plethora of causes, including masses, anatomic variations, complications of surgery about the knee, weight loss, inversion injuries and trauma such as posterolateral corner knee injuries and knee dislocations.[68–74] In addition, positional problems associated with abdominal, thoracic or pelvic surgery, such as the lithotomy position for prolonged periods, have been implicated.[68,75,76] Sports-specific nerve entrapment has been reported most commonly in runners[77–79] but can be seen in any athlete where repetitive compression or stretch to the nerve occurs.[78,80,81] Although sensory or motor neuropathy may be part of the presenting complaints, common peroneal nerve entrapment should be considered a possible diagnosis in any athlete presenting with exercise-induced leg pain.

Pathology

The anatomy of the structures surrounding the peroneal nerve as it passes around the neck of the fibula is implicated as the main reason for the susceptibility of the nerve to injury or compression in this location. The unyielding fascia that creates the 'fibular tunnel' comprises the attachment of the peroneus longus muscle (Fig. 78.5), which blends with the crural fascia anteriorly and the fibular neck and fascia of the soleus muscle posteriorly.[82] The dynamic contraction of these muscles probably adds to the cumulative forces acting on the nerve during repetitive exercise. The proximity to the fibular head and neck places the nerve at risk for injury due to subluxation or dislocation of the proximal fibula with the nerve firmly constrained by the fascial sling of the peroneus longus muscle.[83–90] Cases of generalized ligamentous laxity may predispose to instability at this joint.[87,91] Study of the vascular supply of the peroneal nerve has shown that this region of the nerve is relatively hypovascular as it wraps around the fibular neck, which probably contributes to its vulnerability at this location.[92] The pathophysiology of nerve compression is discussed below in the section on lateral and medial plantar nerve entrapment.

Evaluation

The presentation of exercise-induced leg pain can include a number of pathologies, including entrapment of the common peroneal nerve, particularly CECS.[78,93] As with all cases of exercise-induced leg pain a thorough history and physical examination will help guide the examiner towards the diagnosis. Complaints of muscle weakness such as drop-foot or sensory disturbance, particularly on the dorsum of the foot, suggest the possibility of common peroneal nerve entrapment. Pain may present either local to the proximal fibula or more diffusely down the leg, suggesting CECS. Palpation of the peroneal nerve over the fibular neck will usually reproduce pain and in some cases may generate distal symptoms as well. Neurophysiological studies have been recommended by many, but may not be positive in cases of exercise-induced pain alone.[77–79,81,94] MRI has been recommended, especially to rule out masses such as ganglion cysts.[95–97] The high resolution of ultrasound and the superficial location of the peroneal nerve have been shown to be helpful in diagnosing masses around the peroneal nerve in this location.[98] Ultrasound has the additional advantage of allowing for dynamic examination with muscle contraction, joint motion and palpation of the tender area.[99]

Physical examination

The key physical examination findings can include hypoaesthesia over the dorsum of the foot, weakness of the anterior or lateral compartment muscles or both, a positive Tinel sign over the nerve may be rendered with or without radiation, and direct palpation may reproduce symptoms especially of pain.[78,79,93,94] Examination immediately after running with symptoms present is the ideal time to elicit abnormal physical examination findings.[78,94] It cannot be overemphasized that multiple aetiologies for exercise-induced leg pain may be present and can coexist.[78,93,94]

Treatment

Once common peroneal nerve entrapment has been established as the cause of exercise-induced leg pain in an athlete, it is unlikely that conservative measures will resolve the pain and allow return to the previous competitive level. In cases of idiopathic peroneal nerve palsy, conservative treatment has been recommended;[100] however, in an athlete desiring to return to competition, it is unlikely that a period of relative rest will resolve the problem. Surgical release of the common peroneal nerve entrapment in athletes has been reported by several authors with overall good results.[79,81,94] The overlap of other causes of exercise-induced leg pain can be a reason for failure of pain relief with nerve release alone; therefore, the accuracy of diagnosis is critical to obtaining a good outcome. As has been shown with other nerve entrapments in the leg, incomplete release could be another reason for failure to relieve pain.

SUPERFICIAL PERONEAL NERVE ENTRAPMENT

Aetiology

Entrapment of the superficial peroneal nerve has been reported as a cause of activity-related leg pain. The anatomy of the terminal portion of the superficial peroneal nerve has been shown to have highly variable branching patterns and locations of fascial exit from the muscle compartments.[64,101–104] Symptomatic nerve compression is due to entrapment at the fascial exit of the superficial peroneal

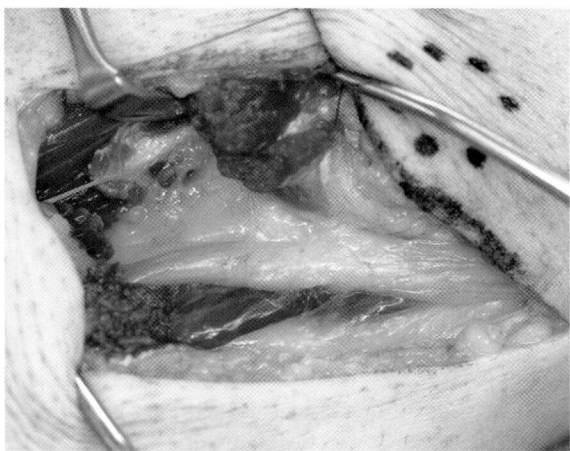

Figure 78.5 Operative photograph of the common peroneal nerve after release of the superficial head of the peroneus longus muscle. Note the narrowing of the nerve as it passes the fibular neck in this location as a result of chronic compression.

nerve or one of the branches. Repetitive ankle and foot motion can lead to cumulative traction on the nerve, and thus exercise-associated onset of pain and sometimes numbness.

Pathology

Two different scenarios have been described that explain superficial peroneal entrapment and both are based on a different type of anatomic fascial exit. One described way in which the nerve exits the fascia is via a simple defect in the fascia overlying the muscle of the anterior or lateral compartment.[105,106] The onset of pain is associated with activity as the underlying muscle swells and bulges through the fascial defect, thus trapping the nerve against the unyielding edge of the fascia. The other anatomic variation is a fascial exit that is formed by a tunnel of fascia which can exist in the septum between the anterior and lateral compartments.[102,104] This tunnel has been shown to approach 7 cm in surgical cases where nerve release was performed.[107] Entrapment is not just a static phenomenon however. Once the nerve has been entrapped, it can no longer glide with the motion of the ankle and foot during activity. This tethering effect leads to excessive traction on the nerve, especially with ankle plantarflexion and inversion. In cadavers, this has been shown to require 1–3 mm of glide with physiological motion of the ankle and hindfoot in inversion. The strain on the nerve as well as the excursion are significantly increased with sectioning of the lateral ligaments, simulating an inversion injury or chronic instability.[108] Reports of symptomatic nerve entrapment after ankle inversion injuries have supported this concept.[109,110] The pathophysiology of nerve compression is discussed below in the section on lateral and medial plantar nerve entrapment.

Evaluation

As with common peroneal nerve entrapment, there can be overlap with CECS and with entrapment of the common peroneal nerve as well.[111,112] A history of severe ankle inversion injury or chronic instability would also suggest consideration of the diagnosis in the setting of anterolateral leg pain with exertion. Complaints of dorsal foot numbness may not be present. Neurophysiological tests can demonstrate conduction delay with nerve conduction testing.[106,107,113] However, abnormal nerve conduction tests have been shown in asymptomatic runners[77] and normal findings have been reported in surgically proven cases of nerve entrapment.[110]

Physical examination

Physical findings can include pain with direct palpation over an area of entrapment. This may be visualized by a muscle herniation seen bulging beneath the skin. In most cases the superficial peroneal nerve can be visualized beneath the skin of the dorsolateral foot and ankle and can be traced by palpation to the fascial exit. This is particularly helpful in cases where the nerve originates from the lateral compartment along the anterior border of the fibula. Palpation of such a superficial structure can elicit symptoms and help to rule out deeper sources of pain. Pressure at the location of entrapment can elicit the symptoms of sensory change and pain. A Tinel's sign may be present but the absence of it does not exclude the diagnosis, nor should the presence of this sign be considered a definitive confirmation of diagnosis. The most reliable finding is to have the patient's pain reproduced on palpation. Since the symptoms typically occur with the repetitive activities that involve running, prolonged pressure by the examiner may be required to reproduce the cumulative nerve irritation that the athlete experiences with activity. Decreased sensation on the dorsum of the foot with sparing of the first web space should usually help exclude involvement of the deep peroneal nerve and help to rule out a more proximal nerve injury of the common peroneal nerve.

Treatment

NON-OPERATIVE TREATMENT

The objective of treatment is clearly to relieve pain by decreasing or eliminating the traction and tethering effects on the nerve. In cases of more acute pain after an inversion injury, the use of a night splint to keep the ankle at neutral rather than the usual resting equinus position of the ankle can provide a prolonged period of rest for the nerve and allow it to heal. Activity modification for a period of 4–8 weeks might also prove to be helpful. Neuropathic symptoms consistent with autonomic instability such as with chronic regional pain syndrome may require evaluation by a chronic pain specialist for medical treatment or in some cases sympathetic blockade. Physiotherapy to help with nerve desensitization may also prove helpful.

OPERATIVE TREATMENT

In cases where the presentation is more chronic and presumably pain is due to either muscle herniation or perineural fibrosis within a fascial tunnel, then non-operative treatments typically do not provide long-lasting pain relief to allow return to sport. In the case of entrapment due to muscle herniation, release and local fasciotomy have been useful in relieving pain and allowing return to sport in most cases.[105,106] When the nerve is entrapped within a fascial tunnel which is typically adjacent to the intermuscular septum between the anterior and lateral compartments

(Fig. 78.6), then surgical release of the tunnel with fasciotomy can be equally useful.[103,107,110] Patients must be cautioned that pain relief may not be sufficient to allow return to the desired sport activity, and surgery can worsen the pain in some cases.[103] This is a concern in the patient with signs of autonomic dysfunction in addition to clear signs of entrapment. Referral to a chronic pain consultant in order to maximize medical management before surgery should always be considered in such cases before proceeding with surgical release. In some cases, release of the nerve entrapment may lead to resolution of the sympathetic mediated nerve pain.[110]

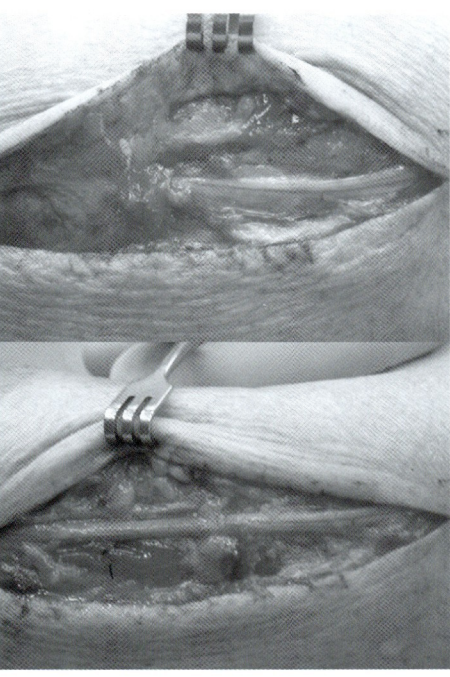

Figure 78.6 Operative photographs of a superficial peroneal nerve before and after release at the fascial exit from the lateral compartment of the leg. Note the narrowing and hyperaemia over several centimetres where the nerve was stenosed within the fibrous tunnel.

TENDON PROBLEMS

ACHILLES TENDON RUPTURES

Aetiology

The incidence of Achilles tendon rupture has been studied,[114,115] with a peak in the fourth decade. Men are affected significantly more often than women. Although most ruptures occur during sports activities,[116] intrinsic biological and biochemical factors may play a predisposing significant role.[117]

The aetiology of Achilles tendon rupture is not completely clear, but several predisposing factors exist: chronic, subclinical degeneration is commonly present in the area of rupture, possibly altering the biomechanical characteristics;[118,119] hypovascularity in the area where the Achilles tendon most frequently ruptures (2–6 cm proximal to its insertion);[120,121] also, eccentric loads may exceed the tensile strength of the tendon.[122,123]

Pathophysiology

The Achilles tendon connects the gastrosoleus unit to the calcaneus. Proximally, the aponeurosis of the gastrocnemius (ventrally) and of the soleus (dorsally) merge into each other, undergoing rotation during development to form the Achilles tendon. The Achilles tendon is enveloped by a paratenon along its whole length. The paratenon can itself be a cause of pain when it becomes inflamed.[124] The Achilles tendon is the most commonly injured tendon with complete or partial tears.[117] This tendon is one of the high tensile stress areas in the human body, supporting between two and five times body weight during every step.[125] If the tendon is lengthened more than 3–4% of its normal length, it starts to disrupt[126] and fails at 8% of its physiological length. Subclinical microtears or injury probably occur during physiological activity, but there is a propensity to heal.[127]

Although normal tendons can rupture under extreme loads, it appears that tendons with areas of degeneration are commonly injured and this has been confirmed at the time of repair.[128] In one small study of 14 ruptured Achilles tendons, only five showed areas of degeneration.[129] In the study by Jacobs et al.[130] more than 50% of the Achilles tendons examined showed signs of degeneration. Fox et al.[131] found that, of the 22 patients with Achilles tendinopathy, 10 subsequently suffered a complete tear. Intratendinous degeneration may be a feature of ageing, and more than 90% of patients operated for an Achilles tendon rupture within 48 hours from the injury showed a degenerative tendinopathy.[117]

At the time of repair the tendon injury may extend for several centimetres proximal to the actual gap. Distally the stump is usually very good-quality tissue for repair techniques.

The gap distance at the site of the tear may vary with the position of the foot, and some authors have treated these based on the apposition of the ruptured tendon ends.[132–139] The healing response begins immediately after rupture, and even days after the injury one encounters oedematous tissue, fibrinous reaction and haemorrhage. Arner and Lindholm[120] identified four stages in the reparative process of unoperated ruptured Achilles tendons. Most importantly, by 2 weeks from the time of the tear, there is formation of fibrous tissue, at various phases of differentiation and reorganization. This has been confirmed by electron microscopy[133]

Evaluation

PHYSICAL EXAMINATION

If a rupture of the Achilles tendon is suspected, the diagnosis should not be difficult.

First, a patient with an acute rupture usually presents to the hospital emergency department with the classic history of sudden pain with an audible pop and a sensation of being struck directly on the calf. Often significant forces are described. More chronic ruptures may have a typical history that is more insidious, with a minor traumatic event followed by decreased functional ability.

In addition, ruptures are not completely disabling and patients can still weight bear and walk with minor difficulty, usually from accessory flexors and using a flat-footed gait.[140] Therefore, rupture may not completely become apparent until the patients try more strenuous activity. This may be one of the reasons for a delayed presentation.

Missed diagnosis generally occurs because of lack of clinical suspicion.[140] When examined soon after the injury, a gap, indicative of a tear in the substance of the tendon, can be seen and palpated. With increased time after the tear, the gap can be obliterated by oedema and healing and palpation becomes unreliable. In general, in the acute situation, if a gap is not palpable, with some resistance along the tendon with resisted plantarflexion, then a complete tear in unlikely and one is probably dealing with a partial or a proximal intramuscular tear. In this situation, the squeeze test (below) will also demonstrate some plantarflexion.

The best way to further assess the Achilles tendon is with the patient in the prone position and feet hanging off the end of the examining table. This allows a systematic assessment of mechanical alignment, such as palpation of areas of tenderness and nodules, palpation of defects in the tendon in dorsiflexion and crepitus, which are all hallmarks of Achilles pathology.

Specialized tests include the Simond's calf squeeze test,[141] later described by and accredited to Thompson and Doherty.[142] This involves squeezing the patient's calf muscles while examining for a lack of plantarflexion compared with the contralateral side, a finding suggestive of Achilles rupture. Matles' test[143] is where the patient is placed in a prone position while actively flexing their knee to 90°. If the foot on the affected side falls into neutral or a dorsiflexed position, then an Achilles tendon rupture may be diagnosed. The needle test and the Copeland test are not commonly used, and are somewhat painful as well, and in the authors' opinion are usually not required. The needle test[144] entails inserting a hypodermic needle through the skin and calf, medial to the midline approximately 10 cm proximal to tendon insertion. The ankle is then alternately planter flexed and dorsiflexed. If the tip of the needle lies in the substance of the tendon it should point distally if an intact tendon distal to the needle exists. If it points proximal, there is a loss of continuity between the tendon insertion and the needle. Copeland[145] described inflating (100 mmHg) a sphygmomanometer cuff around the mid-calf of the affected leg with the patient prone. The foot is then dorsiflexed, and if the pressure rises to 140 mmHg then the tendon is intact; however, no increase in pressure may be suggestive of discontinuity.

Imaging

Although the history and physical examination are most important to diagnosing Achilles pathology, imaging studies may be helpful. It is the author's opinion that imaging studies are most useful to help in the diagnosis of the progression of tendinopathy, not for acute rupture, and are discussed in more detail in the next section.

With an acute Achilles tear, radiographs should be performed to assess for a distal avulsion (i.e. Haglund's with calcification of the tendon insertion).

Ultrasound may be useful, but subject to interpretation, for partial versus complete ruptures, and for tendon degeneration. In addition it can be a quick evaluation of the gap distance or approximation of the ends.

MRI is the gold standard for imaging musculoskeletal tissues, and will give information on the extent of tendon involvement, but in the acute tendon rupture will probably not affect treatment decisions. In the chronic rupture, MRI is very useful for pre-operative planning.

Treatment

OBJECTIVES

The Achilles tendon is one of the most commonly ruptured tendons in the human body because of acute and chronic stress overload. Normal Achilles function in the active individual is essential in walking, running and other sporting activities. Obviously, the level of activity is a spectrum among patients, and therefore operative versus non-operative treatment continues to be utilized with variable indications. In addition, open versus percutaneous surgical techniques are described without much concrete evidence about which method is superior. Investigation continues into determining the optimal treatment of Achilles tendon rupture.

Non-operative treatment

Partial Achilles tendon rupture

Partial Achilles tendon rupture will usually respond to non-operative treatment outlined below. These tears are often at the musculotendinous junction, and heal very well without surgical intervention. However, if this fails one may consider a primary repair or a reconstructive procedure if chronic or a significant defect exists.

Complete Achilles tendon rupture

Complete rupture of the Achilles may be treated operatively or non-operatively. The proponents of operative treatment cite the rerupture rate as the main disadvantage of non-operative treatment. This ranges from 0% to 5% as reviewed by various authors.[123,146]

The proponents of non-operative treatment cite the complication rate as the main disadvantage of operative treatment. This ranges from 4.9% to 26.8%, again reviewed by Waterston et al.[123]

In a recent meta-analysis by Lo et al.[146] it was concluded that operative treatment reduces the rerupture rate over non-operative treatment with the minor and moderate complication rates being 20 times greater. Thus, a tailored approach considering the concerns and health of the patient was recommended.

Based on the above literature, it is reasonable to suggest that an operative treatment plan may be recommended for the experienced surgeon with an active young healthy patient who desires to return to activity quickly.

OPERATIVE TREATMENT

Operative treatment may be subdivided into a primary repair versus reconstruction. Primary repair is the best option in the acute setting where ample tendon is preserved suitable for repair. Reconstruction is better reserved for the more chronic cases with excessive tendonosis or acute cases without ample adequate tendon that is repairable. More specifically, one should be able to approximate healthy tendon without excessive plantarflexion to consider a primary repair otherwise we would recommend a reconstruction such as that of Wapner et al.[147]

The percutaneous techniques may be becoming more popular given the development of safer and user-friendlier surgical instrumented devices. Although there is low-level evidence with these techniques one must consider the possible or theoretical complications of sural nerve injury and a weaker repair leading to a higher rerupture rate.[148,149]

Acute open repair is our method of choice with end-to-end approximation of the tendon utilizing a suture technique similar to that of Jaakkola et al.[150] Others have reinforced these repairs using a collagen tendon prosthesis,[151] Marlex mesh,[152,153] fascial turn downs[154] or carbon fibre composites.[155] We prefer not to utilize these methods unless a primary repair is not possible.

ACHILLES TENDON TENDONOPATHY

Aetiology and pathology

The most comprehensive study on tendon pathology and rupture was performed by Kannus and Jozsa[118] where 891 tendon ruptures were examined for histopathology as were 445 aged-matched controls. The pathological changes in these Achilles tendons include hypoxic degeneration (45%), mucoid degeneration (19%), tendolipomatosis (6%), calcifying tendonopathy (3%) and multiple changes (23%). Other histological studies showed degenerative changes in the tendons that ruptured.[120,131,156–158] Jozsa et al.[159] showed that the types of collagen were different in normal versus pathological tendons. Normal Achilles tendons had greater quantities of collagen type 1 than ruptured Achilles tendons, which had more collagen type 3. This is consistent with the findings of increased collagen type III in scar tissue, equine tendon scar[160] and human hypertrophic tissue.[156] The presence of this type III collagen probably makes the tendon less resistant to tensile forces and therefore more likely to rupture.[159]

With respect to inflammatory changes seen in Achilles pathology it is interesting to note that none of the ruptured tendons in the studies of Kannus and Jozsa[118] and Jozsa et al.[161] showed inflammatory cell infiltrate. In the study by Kvist et al.,[162] they showed persistent histological signs of inflammation in patients afflicted with chronic paratenonitis and suggested this to be a 'different mechanism of inflammation'. In general, the histology of the more chronic tedon injury shows little or no inflammation.

The presence of symptoms (pain) of the Achilles prior to tendon rupture range from about 10% to 30%.[117,118,131] Thus, one must question whether it is tendonitis or more accurately tendonopathy which makes a tendon more susceptible to rupture. Indeed, it may be that the early stages of tendonitis may represent the clinical phase associated with pain and weakness curtailing an individual's ability to participate and thus less opportunity for rupture. Further, it may be the later stages of tendon disease where the pathological changes render the tendon less resistant to tensile forces and more prone to rupture.

Classification

Achilles pathology may be categorized as insertional tendonitis involving the tendon–bone junction or non-insertional tendonitis involving the tendon proximal to its insertion.[163] Non-insertional tendonitis may involve the paratenon and/or the tendon itself. Involvement of either of these two components may occur in isolation or in combination as classified by Puddu et al.[158]

1. *Peritendinitis* consists of thickening of the peritendon that was adherent to normal tissue. The histology shows capillary proliferation with production of inflammatory cells within the peritendinous tissue.
2. *Tendonosis* describes the degenerative process occurring within the tendon itself. Pathological changes include hyaline degeneration with a decrease in the normal cell population, mucoid degeneration with chondroid metaplasia of tenocytes, fatty degeneration of tenocytes, lipomatous infiltration of large areas of

tendon, an increase in matrix mucopolysaccharides and fibrillation of collagen fibres.
3. *Peritendinitis with tendonosis* is the most common type of process with acute and chronic changes present both in the tendon and the paratenon in varying degrees. The paratenon changes usually occur at the same level as the tendonosis.

Insertional tendonitis may also be subdivided.

1. *Insertional calcific tendonitis* is more a pathological entity associated with the various tendonopathies often in the pathological insertional Achilles tendonosis.
2. *Haglund's deformity* refers to a prominent posterior superior tuberosity of the calcaneus, which acts as an irritative focus (below). Pavlov et al. described this as significant if the tuberosity projects above the upper parallel pitch line where 70% of subjects with heel pain demonstrated this compared with 32% who were asymptomatic. Another measurement, the Phillip and Fowler angle, is considered to be suggestive of Haglund's if greater than 69°.[164] Retrocalcaneal bursitis refers to inflammation of the deep subfascial synovial bursa anterior to the Achilles tendon insertion.
3. *Precalcaneal bursitis* refers to inflammation of the subcutaneous and subfascial bursal structures at the posterior aspect of the Achilles insertion. This inflammation is often caused by localized shoe pressure.
4. *Retrocalcaneal bursitis* refers to inflammation of the subcutaneous and subfascial bursal structures at the anterior aspect of the Achilles insertion.
5. *Calcaneal exostosis* refers to a localized protuberance or growth of bone usually localized posterolateral to the Achilles tendon. This inflammation is often caused by localized shoe pressure and has been coined 'pump bump'.[165] This problem often becomes prominent in skaters (hockey and figure skaters) or in ski boots that rub on the prominence. The exostosis with an inflamed bursa over the top of it is often called 'skaters heel'. This condition, in contrast to the older patient population with Haglund's syndrome, is generally found in younger athletes and patients and is usually only a mechanical irritation of the posterolateral exostosis resulting from shoe wear.
6. *Severe osteochondrosis* is a paediatric condition best described as a calcaneal apophysitis with a symptomatic tendon, which is only listed here for completeness.

Smart et al.[166] considered partial Achilles rupture and total rupture as two additional categories of Achilles pathology. Curwin and Stanish[167] divided symptoms of tendonitis into six levels alluding to a continuum of degenerative disease.

Evaluation

HISTORY AND PHYSICAL EXAMINATION

When approaching the patient with Achilles pathology, it may be best to consider the continuum of pathology similar to that proposed by Puddu et al.[158] In the early phases, patients will complain of pain following strenuous activities; this will usually progress to pain with regular activities and sometimes at rest.

With respect to sporting activities, specifically one should gather information regarding warm-up, mileage, intensity, running surface and shoe wear.

Patients with an acute rupture generally present to the hospital emergency department with the classic history of sudden pain with an audible pop and a sensation of being struck by a fellow sportsman. More chronic ruptures also tend to have a typical history that is more insidious, with a minor traumatic event followed by decreased functional ability.

The physical examination begins with inspection of the patient's footwear and then lower limb alignment, non-weight-bearing (anterior, posterior and lateral), standing in and out of footwear. Gait analysis should be performed as well.

The best way to further assess the Achilles tendon is with the patient in the prone position and feet hanging off the end of the examining table. This allows a systematic assessment of mechanical alignment, palpation of areas of tenderness, nodules, defects in the tendon and crepitus, all hallmarks of Achilles pathology.

IMAGING

Although the history and physical examination are most important to diagnosing Achilles pathology, imaging studies are often utilized and very helpful in tendonopathy.

Plain radiographs confirm any bony prominence such as an exostosis visualized best on an axial view of the heel as a posterolateral prominence, i.e. Haglund's. Distal calcification should be identified and important for pre-operative considerations.

Ultrasound is useful for demonstrating bursal inflammation and any tendon degeneration. It does not give a morphological picture but is useful to study biomechanical properties[134] or assess structure post surgical repair.[168]

Lastly, MRI is the gold standard for imaging musculoskeletal tissues, being more sensitive than conventional radiographs.[120] This will give more detailed information about the mid-substance of the tendons and surrounding structures. Paratendonitis is detected as a layer of fluid surrounding the tendon.[169] Weinstabl et al.[139] describe four specific categories of lesions seen on MRI.

1. Thickening of the tendon without structural change of the tendon tissue.
2. Degeneration, thickening of the tendon with central signal changes.
3. Incomplete rupture: thickening of the tendon with structural changes longitudinally and horizontally, including the partatenon.
4. Complete rupture

Treatment

OBJECTIVES

Most patients with Achilles pathology excluding rupture may be successfully managed with non-operative treatment. Taunton et al.[170] showed that 75% of runners with Achilles tendonitis were managed successfully, with 15% remaining recalcitrant to treatment. Aetiological factors should be addressed. A multifaceted approach to reduce pain, rehabilitate and prevent overload is essential in treatment.

Non-operative treatment

IMMOBILIZATION

It is recommended that only short periods (2–4 weeks) of immobilization be utilized, since total immobilization has been shown to be detrimental to tendon and muscle strength, and articular cartilage and worsens joint stiffness.[117] This treatment is useful as the first phase of a broader treatment plan including other modalities below, particularly if the patient has pain with everyday walking.

ORTHOTICS

Use of customized orthotics may relieve symptoms and provide a more biomechanical favourable condition to halt or reverse progression. As a generalized principle, shoe wear with a good sole and solid heel counter should be recommended to prevent excessive heel movement during stance. The orthotics should also correct flexible hindfoot malalignment in the coronal plane. Pump bump spacers may be utilized to unload pressure areas in the heel posteriorly. Also, a heel lift may unload the Achilles to some extent through a decreased dorsiflexion angle at the ankle.

MEDICATIONS

Although commonly used, injected or oral anti-inflammatory medications have not proven to effective in clinical trials. Also, one should be aware of the potential deleterious affects of Achilles injection and they are generally not recommended.

STRETCHING AND STRENGTHENING

Stretching is a very important part of non-operative treatment regimes. An excellent daily routine would include static rather than ballistic stretching for 5 minutes before going to bed and upon rising in the morning. Commercial splints for stretching such as Prostretch serve as an excellent adjunct for stretching. Night splints, although cumbersome, will provide one with a continuous minor stretch that reduces morning pain and stiffness.

STRENGTHENING

Once the inflammatory processes are under control with appropriate rest and stretching one may concentrate more on a strengthening programme such as an eccentric exercise programme proposed by Curwin and Stanish in 1984.[167] Eccentric strengthening causes a greater overall reduction in pain than the traditional concentric exercises.[171]

OPERATIVE TREATMENT

Indications and pre-operative planning

Indications for surgery will vary depending on the severity of pathology and medical condition of the patient. In general, one must consider all non-surgical treatment modalities before surgery for one can always operate at any time. Although non-hard data exist on negative prognostic patient factors specifically for outcomes in Achilles tendon surgery one must take factors such as diabetes mellitus, smoking, malnourishment and generalized poor medical condition into account before embarking on a surgical course.

Since Achilles pathology may present at any stage from simple tendonitis to frank rupture one must use all clinical information to make an accurate diagnosis, which will dictate surgical options. Thus, careful pre-operative planning is essential to determine surgical fitness of the patient and the actual surgical procedure to be performed.

OPERATIVE TECHNIQUES

Paratendonitis and tendonosis

In the earlier stages of paratendonitis alone with no tendinosis, non-operative measures are usually successful. If resistant to non-operative treatment then debridement of the paratenon alone is indicated. If the pre-operative work-up indicates that there is tendonosis in the mid-substance of the tendon then it should be incised longitudinally and areas of degeneration should be debrided. Although no randomized studies comparing operative debridement with ongoing non-operative treatment exist, there are several case series which report fair results after surgical treatment.[172–176]

Insertional disorders

In these common problems surgical treatment is indicated if non-operative treatment failed and the patient continues to be symptomatic. In these cases, a bony prominence, which is prominent medially and laterally and posteriorly, a retrocalcaneal bursitis, and calcification of the tendon often coexist. Surgical treatment has been described with a lateral incision, medial and lateral, J incision, and a midline posterior. The authors' preference is to use a posterior midline approach. This allows for splitting and debridement of the tendon, excision of the prominence, and repair or reconstruction of the tendon insertion.

PERONEAL TENDON PROBLEMS

Aetiology

Peroneal tendon pathology is a spectrum of disorders that can cause pain and disability prohibiting athletic activity. Injuries such as calcaneal fractures and severe ankle inversion injuries can lead to acute peroneal tendon, avulsion or tear of the superior peroneal retinaculum and fracture of the os peroneum with complete rupture of the peroneus longus.[99,177–185] These injuries can subsequently lead to chronic problems of pain, instability of the peroneal tendons or both. Underlying anatomic features have also been suggested as causes of peroneal tendon pathology. The mass effect of a hypertrophied low-lying peroneus muscle belly or the presence of an accessory peroneus quartus muscle with its attachment on the lateral calcaneal wall have been associated with chronic peroneal tendon pain, longitudinal tears and attenuation of the retinaculum, which can lead to subluxation of the tendons.[186–188] A flat or convex posterior fibular surface has been associated with chronic tendon instability;[189–192] large or irregular peroneal tubercle and varus or cavovarus foot shape have also been implicated.[99,178,183–185]

Pathology

Tears of the peroneal tendons usually involve longitudinal splits of the tendon with or without chronic degenerative changes, depending upon the duration of the problem. The superior peroneal retinaculum may be avulsed with bone or cartilage and has been likened to a Bankart lesion in the shoulder. The retinaculum may also be attenuated.[178,181,184,185,193] Chronic dislocation of the tendons is associated with a pseudo-pouch that the tendons remain in lateral to the fibula.[194] Complete tendon rupture is rare and is most likely with a fracture of the os peroneum.[179] Owing to the mechanism of injury, inversion injury of the ankle probably being most common, the lateral ankle ligaments may frequently be injured and incompetent as well.[177,181,195,196] Accessory muscles and hypertrophied low-lying brevis muscles create a mass effect and stenosis of the tendons behind the fibula and can lead to attenuation of the retinaculum and instability.[99,186–188]

Evaluation

Plain radiographs are generally not very helpful for diagnosing anatomical pathology of the peroneal tendons. A rim fracture from a superior peroneal retinacular avulsion can provide evidence for such an injury, but this is acutely apparent upon inspection and examination in most cases. A large peroneal tubercle is also clinically evident. Separation or retraction of an os peroneum more than 6 mm can be found by radiographs and should always be looked for on the lateral foot radiograph.[179] MRI and ultrasound have been widely reported for the evaluation of peroneal tendon and retinaculum evaluation.[99,179,197–204] The benefits of each have been described, and the primary limitation of MRI is in evaluating structures that pass obliquely around the ankle because they are not within any of the three orthogonal planes of MRI. Ultrasound has the advantage of being infinitely adjustable to capture tendons as they course obliquely, and can provide dynamic information such as subtle instability.[99]

Physical examination

Physical examination for instability can be performed with the ankle in a dorsiflexed position with resisted hindfoot eversion. The examiner's hand should be placed behind the ankle with the finger tips on the posterior border of the fibula while the other hand resists eversion. Gross or subtle instability can be palpated and often corresponds to reproduction of the patient's symptoms. A snapping noise may or may not be heard. Tenderness over the superior peroneal retinacular attachment on the fibula may be present, and correspond to the patient's pain. Tenderness over the tendons behind the fibula, at the peroneal tubercle or distally at the beginning of the cuboid tunnel of the peroneus longus may be present. Tenderness over the base of the fifth metatarsal may be associated with acute peroneus brevis tendonitis or an avulsion fracture of the fifth metatarsal. One must be careful to not mistake tenderness of the sural nerve, or lateral subtalar joint tenderness, for peroneal tendon pathology since different structures may be over or under the peroneal tendons.

Treatment

Conservative treatment of acute peroneal tendon injuries can be tried and has been reported to work well about 50% of the time.[177,181,205] This could include immobilization for up to 6 weeks followed by physiotherapy to regain strength, balance and conditioning. However, for athletes with acute injury, patients with acute fractures such as the calcaneus who have a fixed dislocation, or any patient with chronic pain and instability operative treatment is necessary for improving pain and function.[178,182,183,185,194–196,205–211] Among these reports various techniques have been described for reattachment of the superior peroneal retinaculum, including direct repair through drill holes, the use of suture anchors, fibular groove deepening, reduction of the attenuated retinaculum with repair, transposition beneath the calcaneofibular ligament, fibular osteotomy to create a bone block and the use of free tendon graft such as a portion of the peroneus brevis or gracilis autograft. Recently, some authors have reported using endoscopic techniques to evaluate and treat peroneal tendon pathology.[212,213] Debridement and repair of the tendon is probably the best treatment as long as 50% of the tendon can be salvaged, although no objective data exist to guide this decision. Sometimes the brevis tendon may be hypertrophied and widened so that debridement with tubularization is necessary. Tendon transfers and allograft and autograft techniques have been described.[185]

POSTERIOR TIBIAL TENDON TENOSYNOVITIS AND TEARS

Aetiology

The posterior tibialis muscle is the most important inverter of the hindfoot originating in the deep posterior compartment of the leg and terminating distally with its tendon passing behind and below the medial malleolus and then inserting on the navicular and plantar aspect of the cuneiforms. The region of the tendon behind and below the medial malleolus is a relatively avascular area and this has been suggested as a possible aetiological factor in the development of tendon problems at this location[214] and undergoes concentric contraction during heel-off and eccentric contraction from heel strike to foot flat stance. During cutting and jumping sports, repetitive high mechanical stress is placed on the tendon. Posterior tibial tendon tenosynovitis is an inflammation of the lining of the tendon sheath and is seen with some frequency, although the true incidence is not known and probably depends on a variety of factors, including foot posture, training regimen, specific sport and footwear.[215] Posterior tibial tendon tendinosis or tendon tears in young athletes (<30 years of age) are an uncommon problem and few series have reported on this.[216–218] In contrast to the common problem of posterior tibial tendon dysfunction seen in middle-aged adults which typically presents with a valgus foot deformity, most of these cases in young athletes did not involve a valgus foot deformity. Biomechanical models that simulate a flat foot have shown an increase in the excursion and resistance to gliding in the posterior tibial tendon.[219,220] Although these findings may suggest that an underlying flat foot deformity can play a major role in the development of posterior tibial tendon pathology, this has only been associated in a couple of the described cases of posterior tibial tendon pathology in young athletes.[216,217] It would seem then that, at least in the operative cases reported, the athletic injury to posterior tibial tendon is more likely due to repetitive trauma than underlying foot posture. However, it is also likely that if left untreated this condition would probably lead to an acquired flat foot eventually.[215,217] Dynamic evaluation of gait, landing and push-off in affected athletes might help to shed light on this. Rupture after steroid injection to the tendon has been described in a 20 year old athlete.[218]

Pathology

In cases where the operative pathology has been described, the tendon pathology can include tenosynovitis of the lining of the tendon sheath, stenosis paratendinitis, longitudinal split tears and partial rupture, early tendinosis, and in one case an associated tear of the anterior portion of the anterior deltoid ligament.[216–218] Systemic inflammatory disorders such as rheumatoid arthritis can also afflict young athletes and should be considered a possible diagnosis.[215] Other related problems that can affect the posterior tibial tendon are damage due to ankle fractures, avulsion of the flexor retinaculum and subluxation/dislocation of the tendon from behind the medial malleolus, and injury to the insertion on the navicular with or without an associated type II accessory navicular.[215]

Evaluation

Plain radiographs can help to evaluate alignment and may help to rule out stress fractures. Also, plain radiographs can demonstrate an accessory navicular and rarely bony irregularity of the medial malleolus, suggesting an avulsion of the flexor retinaculum attachment on the posteromedial border of the medial malleolus. Helpful views include weight-bearing anteroposterior (AP) and lateral foot radiographs, AP and oblique ankle views and a hindfoot alignment view to assess the degree of valgus at the heel.[221]

Other diagnostic modalities for evaluating the posterior tibial tendon include MRI and ultrasound.[222,223] Typical MRI findings that have been described include fluid within the tendon sheath surrounding the tendon indicating tenosynovitis, thickening of the tendon indicating tendinosis, heterogeneous signal within the tendon indicating partial tear, and fluid filling the tendon sheath indicating complete tear.[222] Ultrasound has been used to detect the same pathologies, and due to the higher resolution of ultrasound may be better at detecting intratendinous pathology.[99,223]

Physical examination

Physical examination findings in acute tenosynovitis include swelling and tenderness over the course of the posterior tibial tendon behind and below the medial malleolus. The normal concavity behind the medial malleolus may be obliterated. Pain localized to the medial ankle and hindfoot with resisted inversion or with a single toe-rise test will usually reproduce the patient's pain. The resisted inversion test should be carried out, beginning with the hindfoot in an everted position and the ankle plantarflexed, which isolates the posterior tibial tendon. In the inverted position, the anterior tibialis can strongly hold the foot in an inverted position, although with elevation of the first ray and dorsiflexion of the ankle. The one-foot toe-rise test should be performed with minimal upper extremity support, which can invalidate the test. The examiner looks from the back and normal function should demonstrate heel elevation and inversion. In cases of more chronic tendon pathology, swelling and tenderness may be less significant, but pain and weakness with resisted inversion and an abnormal single toe-rise test will still be present.

Treatment

Treatment of acute tenosynovitis should be prompt in order to avoid the sequelae of tendon degeneration and acquired deformity. The goal of treatment is to calm the inflamed tenosynovium, restore normal strength and protect the tendon from further injury. If deformity is present, it must be either corrected with surgery or controlled with orthoses.

NON-OPERATIVE TREATMENT

Early diagnosis and aggressive implementation of non-operative treatment has been highly recommended in order to prevent the more severe long-term consequences of ongoing posterior tibial tendon dysfunction.[224] In cases of early and mild tenosynovitis, relative rest with decreased training and cross-training with the use of an offloading semirigid orthosis may be enough to allow for recovery. Gentle stretching and focal strengthening can be implemented once the acute inflammation is calmed. The use of NSAIDs and icing can also be considered. In cases where more severe inflammation is present, immobilization with a cast or cast boot for 3–4 weeks can be tried with transition to rigid ankle stirrup.[225] A supportive orthosis can be used for long-term support and may include a medial heel post, a moderate arch support or a medial forefoot post, depending on the morphology of the foot.

OPERATIVE TREATMENT

In cases that do not respond to non-operative treatment, surgical tenosynovectomy can be beneficial. The use of tendoscopy for debridement around the posterior tibial tendon has been recently reported and promises quicker recovery with a low complication rate.[226] Stenosing paratendonitis may be present and requires debridement of the adherent tissues. If possible, a portion of the flexor retinaculum at the distal posterior margin of the medial malleolar attachment should be preserved or surgical reattachment will be necessary.[215,216] When tendon stability behind the medial malleolus is a concern, then deepening of the retromalleolar groove can be considered. If a longitudinal split in the tendon is encountered, it should be debrided and repaired. When partial ruptures are found, debridement and repair are reasonable if the remaining tendon is visibly healthy and is not attenuated. If the tendon is too severely attenuated, a tendon transfer of the flexor digitorum longus should be considered, and if deformity is present imbrication of the spring ligament and possibly a medial sliding calcaneal osteotomy might be indicated. Retaining the posterior tibial tendon when tendinosis is advanced is a matter of some controversy. Factors that might lead one to excise the tendon when performing a tendon transfer would include loss of normal elasticity of the posterior tibialis muscle and extensive tendinosis.[215] Postoperatively a casting for 4–8 weeks with return to sport between 8 and 16 weeks has been reported with synovectomy and debridement.[215–218] Tendon transfers and osteotomies should be protected in a cast for 6 weeks. Tendon transfers should be casted in slight plantarflexion and inversion initially.

ANKLE PROBLEMS

OSTEOCHONDRAL LESIONS OF THE TALUS

Aetiology and pathology

The current understanding of osteochondral lesions (OCLs) of the talus is based on the classic work of Bernt and Harty.[227] They indicated for the first time that these lesions are more often transchondral fractures than spontaneous necrosis of bone. Since that time much has been written regarding these lesions and they are now understood to be a spectrum of pathology and thus the term 'osteochondral lesions'. The most common locations of these lesions have frequently been described as being in the posteromedial and central-lateral or anterolateral regions of the talar body as described by Loomer et al.[228] using CT scanning. Loomer et al.[228] also described a type V lesion which is a subchondral cyst beneath an intact cartilage surface. The presence of an intact cartilage surface allows for retrograde techniques of debridement and grafting without violation of the cartilage surface.[229] A more recent report describes a novel MRI grid system of mapping the talar dome. The authors felt that in the 428 lesions evaluated by their unique grid system that the most common sites were at the middle of the medial talar dome (62%) and the middle of the lateral talar dome (34%).[230] This is essentially a descriptive change, since the clinical approaches to these lesions clearly demonstrate that the lateral lesions are more easily accessed from anterior, and the medial lesions almost always require more posterior exposure. Whereas osteotomy of the medial malleolus is usually necessary for medial lesions, most lateral lesions can be accessed anteriorly without osteotomy.[231] Lateral lesions are generally thought to be due to inversion and dorsiflexion leading to a shallow osteochondral chip off the lateral talar ridge due to an oblique impaction against the fibula as the lateral ligaments give way. Medial lesions are thought to be due to the more common mechanism of inversion with plantarflexion, which would explain the more posterior location and the slightly higher incidence. The more direct axial impaction with these injuries might explain the more common subchondral bone necrosis and greater depth of these lesions.

Evaluation

A history of an inversion injury is common but not a requisite for the finding of an OCL. Patient complaints may consist of pain with weight bearing, swelling, catching and locking if the lesion has become a loose fragment. In general, physical examination is not very specific in diagnosing OCL of the talus, but the finding of a painful swollen joint in the setting of a previous inversion injury should lead one to further investigation.[232] However, in cases without history of trauma and no other easily identified cause of pain, suspicion should also be high. Standard radiographs are an important first step in the evaluation of ankle and hindfoot pain but a negative plain radiograph series does not rule out the possibility of an OCL. Loomis et al. have shown a sevenfold increase in the detection of OCLs with CT scanning compared with plain radiographs.[228] Bone scan has been shown to be very sensitive for OCL but does not provide the detailed information of CT or MRI, making it less helpful than these newer techniques.[233,234] A prospective study comparing helical CT, MRI and diagnostic arthroscopy with history and physical examination revealed that CT and MRI were significantly better than history, physical examination and plain radiographs in detecting OCL. There was no statistical difference between helical CT and MRI, but diagnostic arthroscopy was inferior to both.[232] In addition to the radiographic staging system of Bernt and Harty, and the CT staging system of Loomer et al., other authors have suggested the use of MRI for staging of OCL.[235] The added benefit of MRI is the ability to evaluate the integrity of the articular cartilage and differentiate lesions with intact cartilage from those without.

Treatment

There is no clear evidence that OCLs progress over time or that they lead to a higher incidence of degenerative joint disease of the ankle. Therefore, treatment should be based on symptoms rather than on natural history. A recent study of the longitudinal behaviour of OCLs evaluated by MRI found that of 29 lesions 13 progressed, seven improved and nine were unchanged.[236] A recent systematic review of electronic databases from 1966 to 2000 found 14 studies that reported on non-operative treatment and on average had a 45% chance of success. However, it is generally accepted that initial non-operative treatment for undisplaced lesions is reasonable. There is no definitive protocol but cast immobilization for 4–6 weeks with initial non-weight bearing for 2–3 weeks is what the authors consider reasonable. Functional rehabilitation can be started after removal of the cast with clinical symptoms to monitor progress. If symptoms recur then a repeat MRI is helpful in pre-operative planning to see if the lesion has progressed. For lesions that are displaced, operative treatment should be performed either to excise the fragment and debride and drill the base of the lesion or to perform reduction and fixation if sufficient bone is present on the osteochondral fragment and the underlying bone is healthy and not cystic.

Operative treatment

The above-mentioned systematic review identified four reports of excision alone, 10 of excision and curettage, and 21 of excision, curettage and drilling of the lesion. The success of debridement and drilling was superior to the other two methods with an 86% rate of success compared with 78% for excision and curettage and 38% for excision alone. Thus excision, curettage and drilling remains the most recommended first-line surgical treatment of OCL of the talus, in the absence of a repairable lesion.[237] In one study, the similar technique of microfracture has been reported to have 93% good to excellent results.[238] More research is needed to conclude that this technique is actually superior to drilling.

The recent advances in autologous tissue transfer as well as allograft transfer for OCL has led to growing enthusiasm for alternatives when debridement and drilling fail to relieve symptoms. Although there is evidence that repeat arthroscopic debridement can yield favourable results, the published results of osteochondral tissue transfer are more encouraging, with many authors reporting favourable results and low morbidity of donor knee sites.[239–246] However, one recent study suggested that the risk of donor site morbidity is greater than previously thought.[247] As noted above, the approach for medial lesions almost always requires a medial malleolar osteotomy while most lateral lesions can be approached through an anterior capsulotomy. When lateral lesions are more posterior in the central dome, a Chaput osteotomy can be used to gain excellent access to the lesion.[231] Type V lesions can be approached through a retrograde transosseous technique, allowing preservation of the cartilage surface.[229]

ANTERIOR ANKLE AND SUBTALAR JOINT IMPINGEMENT

Aetiology

Ankle and subtalar joint impingement in athletes can be due to either bony or soft-tissue impingement. A history of previous inversion injury of the ankle and hindfoot are common in these cases. Inversion injuries involve varying degrees of plantarflexion and not only place excessive tension on the soft tissues of the anterolateral ankle but also on the anteromedial ankle and lateral subtalar joint.[248-252] In extreme plantarflexion posterior impingement lesions can also develop as described elsewhere in this chapter.[253] Tears of ankle and subtalar joint ligaments and tears of the capsular tissues may occur, and can lead to soft-tissue impingement lesions which become entrapped within the ankle and/or subtalar joint during dorsiflexion or in the case of the subtalar joint eversion and dorsiflexion.

Pathology

The anterior ankle synovial fold of the ankle has been shown to be a triangular band of tissue consisting of synovium, fat and collagen connective tissues which lies across the anterior ankle.[254] This fold of tissue normally has an intimate relationship with the tibiotalar articulation anteriorly. Tearing of the anterior capsule and synovial tissues leads to loose ends of tissue that can become repetitively entrapped within the anterior ankle with dorsiflexion. This loose tissue is found to consist of hypertrophied synovium and scar tissue and histologically has been shown to have changes consistent with chronic inflammation.[249,255] The most distal fascicle of the anterior syndesmotic ligaments has also been described as a cause of anterolateral ankle soft-tissue impingement and has been associated with a history of inversion injury.[256-258] This is commonly associated with synovial soft-tissue impingement as seen as the time of arthroscopy. The subtalar joint soft-tissue impingement has been associated with hypertrophic synovial soft-tissue impingement and torn anterior subtalar and interosseous subtalar ligament tears.[248,250,251] Associated bony lesions can also contribute to the impingement, particularly of the ankle.[259-261] These may be associated with degenerative changes in the ankle, but it has also been suggested that they may result from repetitive contact with the ball in soccer players.[262] It should also be remembered that a number of different injuries can result from inversion injuries and multiple problems such as lateral ankle instability may exist in any given patient.[263]

Evaluation

Radiological studies have been described for aiding in the diagnosis of anterior ankle or sinus tarsi impingement. At best these are an adjunct to the history and physical examination findings that have been shown to be most effective in diagnosing these lesions.[264] CT arthrography, MRI arthrography and enhanced sequence three-dimensional fat-suppressed imaging have been recommended with a high degree of sensitivity.[265-267] Other authors have suggested that MRI alone is a poor predictor of ankle soft-tissue impingement.[264,268] Thus it appears that the key factor in using CT or MRI is to use intra-articular contrast in order to demonstrate the soft-tissue abnormality. These studies can be helpful in evaluation of sinus tarsi subtalar impingement as well.[250,269] Ultrasound may be of benefit, especially because of the ability to dynamically visualize impingement, especially when bony spurs may be involved.[270,271] When anteromedial ankle and medial gutter osteophytes are present, it has been shown that an oblique foot radiograph is essential for detecting these lesions, which are not demonstrated on a lateral ankle radiograph.[272,273]

Physical examination

The key physical examination finding for any of these impingement lesions is to reproduce the impingement dynamically.[264,274] This is accomplished by placing mild digital pressure over the area of suspected impingement and dorsiflexion the ankle, thus recreating the impingement event. The pain associated with this manoeuvre will distinctly reproduce the patient's symptoms and will be markedly more painful than the tenderness generated by static palpation alone (Fig. 78.7). For the subtalar joint,

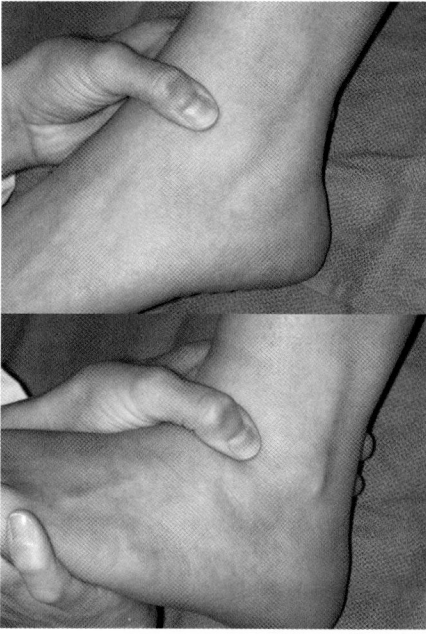

Figure 78.7 Impingement test for anterolateral soft-tissue impingement of the ankle. Gentle digital pressure is placed over the anterolateral recess and the examiner dorsiflexes the ankle. This will reproduce pain due to soft-tissue impingement.

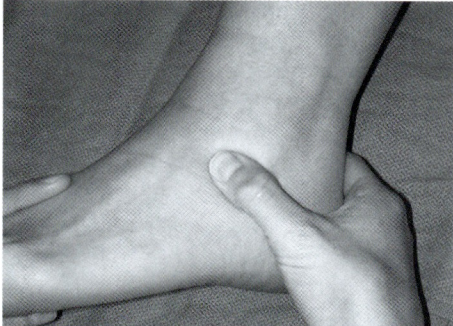

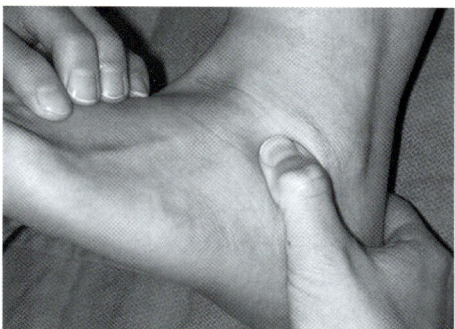

Figure 78.8 Impingement test for subtalar soft-tissue impingement. Here the digital pressure is gently applied over the sinus tarsi while the examiner dorsiflexes the ankle and everts the subtalar joint.

pressure is applied over the sinus tarsi and dorsiflexion and eversion will reproduce the pain due to soft-tissue impingement (Fig. 78.8).

Treatment

OBJECTIVES

The objectives of treatment are to reduce the occurrence of the impingement and address any associated problems such as lateral ankle instability. Therefore, physiotherapy to address either dynamic or mechanical instability may be tried with anti-inflammatory medications to try and decrease inflammation, and theoretically decrease the size of the lesion. An injection of corticosteroids into the soft tissues but not into the joint may be tried, but this is not reported for ankle impingement. Steroid injection of subtalar impingement has been reported in one study, indicating that this might be useful for this condition in some patients.[269]

NON-OPERATIVE TREATMENT

There is no recommended programme of non-operative treatment for anterior impingement, and this is understandable since most of these cases involve either redundant scar tissue and chronically inflamed synovium or additional bony spurs. There is probably little chance of non-operative treatment leading to a long-term resolution of these problems and will probably only delay patients' eventual return to play.

OPERATIVE TREATMENT

There are numerous reports of arthroscopic debridement of soft-tissue and bony impingement lesions of the ankle and subtalar joint.[248–253,255,259–261,275–279] The results are generally good with return to play or full activity in 2–4 months. Results in cases where there is radiographic evidence of degenerative joint disease tend to do less well, but most will still benefit when pain is due primarily to the impingement lesion.[260,261]

FLEXOR HALLUCIS LONGUS STENOSIS AND POSTERIOR ANKLE IMPINGEMENT

Aetiology and pathology

Posterior ankle pain can be a difficult problem to diagnose because the causes of pain can be due to various anatomic structures, all of which are intimately approximated. The trigonal process of the talus creates the lateral side of the entrance to the fibro-osseous tunnel that the flexor hallucis longus (FHL) tendon passes through on its way to the foot. The trigonal process can be of various sizes and can also exist as a separate ossicle from an ununited secondary ossification centre. This process or os is susceptible to trauma with extreme plantarflexion and can be fractured or the fibrous junction can become unstable, and become painful. The motion of the ankle and the FHL can aggravate this problem. The FHL muscle can extend so far distally that it inhibits the normal excursion of the tendon with ankle and toe dorsiflexion and creates a stenosis effect at the entrance to the fibro-ossoeous tunnel.[280] In addition, injury to the posterior tibial–fibular ligaments can lead to torn ligamentous tissue that can become a source of soft-tissue impingement at the posterior ankle joint. A condition of posteromedial soft-tissue impingement due to tear of the posterior deep deltoid ligament has also been described.[281] Of course, more than one of these problems can coexist.[282–285]

Evaluation

Lateral radiographs of the ankle can plainly show the presence of a large trigonal process or os trigonum.[286] However, MRI (Fig. 78.9) can prove more helpful in detailing the presence of bone marrow oedema or surrounding inflammation of the FHL tendon, or abnormalities of the posterior ligamentous structures.[287–291] Although bone scanning can indicate a fracture or perhaps an unstable os trigonum, it will not provide the information about the soft tissues that MRI will. Musculoskeletal

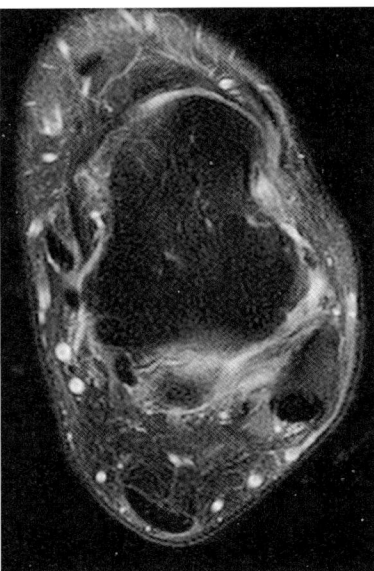

Figure 78.9 Axial and sagittal T_2-weighted MRI of an American football lineman with posterior ankle impingement syndrome. There is a large os trigonum with bone marrow oedema and clinical irritation of the flexor hallucis longus tendon. Note the soft-tissue impingement lesion of the posterior ankle seen on the sagittal MRI. This represents the deep portion of the posterior tibial–fibular ligament that courses behind the ankle joint, which is torn and unstable.

ultrasound has also been helpful in the evaluation of posterior ankle impingement and has been shown to be a useful tool in guiding injections into this area.[289,291] Fluoroscopically guided injection of local anaesthetic has been reported for diagnosing symptomatic unstable os trigonum.[292]

Physical examination

Physical examination for posterior ankle pain should first rule out the presence of Achilles tendon or calcaneal problems. Evaluation should also include a good sensory and vascular examination particularly looking for signs of tarsal tunnel syndrome, which can coexist. Typically, patients will have increased pain with passive plantarflexion of the ankle to maximal plantarflexion, at which point the mechanical impingement occurs in the case of symptomatic os trigonum or bony impingement. In cases of soft-tissue impingement, an augmentation to this manoeuvre is to put mild pressure over the posteromedial and posterolateral soft tissues of the ankle and then passively plantar flex the ankle. This will reproduce the pain from soft-tissue impingement by placing the unstable soft tissues into the joint, thus reproducing what is an otherwise dynamic problem. Tenderness of the FHL can be elicited best by putting direct pressure over the FHL at the level of the talus, approaching it from behind the neurovascular bundle and just medial to the Achilles tendon. This can be augmented by dorsiflexing the ankle and hallux, which places the FHL under tension. The action of dorsiflexion can also lend evidence to the presence of FHL stenosis due to a hypertrophied low-lying muscle belly. First the examiner places the ankle in neutral while supporting the first metatarsal head to simulate the ground. Then the hallux is dorsiflexed. In cases of FHL stenosis the hallux will be limited to little or no dorsiflexion in this position. Allowing the ankle to passively plantar flex in resting equinus and then retesting the hallux dorsiflexion will demonstrate supple and full motion of the first metatarsophalangeal (MTP) joint. While this may provide evidence for FHL stenosis, this manoeuvre does not reliably induce symptoms without associated palpation.

Treatment

Non-operative treatment of posterior ankle impingement can be tried with a period of relative rest, avoiding jumping or plantarflexion exercises, NSAIDs, or even a brief trial of immobilization in a walking boot. Ultrasound-guided injections have been shown to be effective in some cases, allowing return to activity in a relatively short time.[291] Surgical treatment of posterior ankle impingement can include release of the FHL, excision of an os trigonum or painful trigonal process, and debridement of posterior ligamentous soft-tissue impingement. Both open and endoscopic techniques for these procedures have been reported.[280,282–285,293–299]

LATERAL ANKLE LIGAMENTOUS INSTABILITY

Aetiology

The lateral ankle ligament complex comprises three ligaments, which all arise from the distal fibula. The anterior talofibular ligament (ATFL), calcaneofibular ligament (CFL) and the posterior talofibular ligament (PTFL) each contribute to the control of lateral ankle stability in different ankle positions. The ankle is maximally stable to inversion stresses in ankle neutral and dorsiflexion when the joint surface is maximally congruent. As the ankle is plantarflexed, the ATFL and CFL contribute increasingly towards providing lateral ankle stability, and are vulnerable to injury with excessive inversion in plantarflexion.[300,301] The PTFL helps to control translation of the tibia on the talus at heel strike and is not commonly injured with most inversion injuries.

Lateral ankle instability is a term that should be used for true mechanical deficiency of the normal ligamentous constraints of the lateral ankle joint. This is a chronic condition which should be differentiated from the complaint of the ankle 'giving way', which can result from other causes of ankle pain and lead an athlete to quickly off-load the ankle to avoid pain. The patient history is typically one of 'giving way' and then the onset of pain. True lateral ankle instability is manifested by the ankle rolling into excessive inversion during routine activity and then becoming painful because of an inversion injury. Lateral instability is often found after one or more inversion injuries as a lasting sequela once the acute injury has resolved. It represents a failure of a torn ligament to heal sufficiently and provide normal ligamentous stability. The degree of relative instability at the time of an acute injury is not of consequence as most acute inversion injuries are treated non-operatively with functional rehabilitation regardless of the degree of ligament injury.[302]

In addition to the gross mechanical laxity or incompetence of the ligaments, it has been shown that the reaction times of the peroneal muscles is prolonged in subjects with previous inversion injury, suggesting a delayed or abnormal proprioception response related to the ligament injury.[303] Also, the pattern of muscle activation for the entire leg in subjects with chronic ankle instability has been shown to be abnormal and slower than in controls.[304] Finally, the mechanical effect of a varus heel posture has been associated with an increased likelihood of inversion injury and lateral ankle instability.[305,306]

Pathology

In addition to the mechanical incompetence of the lateral ankle ligaments, other associated injuries have been described. As expected, excessive inversion can place many structures at risk for injury besides the lateral ankle ligaments. Arthroscopic examination prior to lateral ligament reconstruction in a series of 21 patients revealed 95% of cases had associated intra-articular pathology.[307] Others have reported associated injury of the peroneal tendons and retinaculum, anterolateral soft-tissue impingement due to capsular tears or tears of the inferior bundle of the anterior tibial–fibular ligament, synovitis, loose bodies and OCLs of the talus among 77% of a series of 61 patients undergoing lateral ligament reconstruction.[308] In another study of 30 patients who underwent ankle arthroscopy prior to lateral ligament reconstruction, there were chondral lesions of the tibial plafond and talus in 63% of patients. Another study of 180 ankles in 160 patients undergoing lateral ankle ligament reconstruction noted 63% incidence of associated pathologies. The authors noted that in the 20 revision cases hindfoot varus (28%) and undiagnosed peroneal tendon pathology (25%) were seen in addition to the underlying lateral ligament pathology.[309]

Evaluation

Diagnostic studies that have been used for confirming injury of the lateral ankle ligaments include MRI arthrography, musculoskeletal ultrasound, and stress radiographs with either manual or mechanical stress forces applied.[302,310–313] However, the diagnosis of clinically significant instability can be difficult to determine by tests alone because of the wide range of normal ligamentous laxity among individuals.

Physical examination

The physical examination of the ankle in a patient with complaints of instability should be comprehensive and the examiner should be aware of the other associated diagnoses listed above. The specific tests used to assess for ligamentous insufficiency are the anterior drawer (AD) and talar tilt (TT) tests. The AD test is performed by stabilizing the tibia with one hand and then grasping the foot from the calcaneus and dorsal hindfoot with the other hand. The foot is then drawn anteriorly relative to the tibia to assess the excursion and endpoint of the stress on the joint. Since the lateral instability is partly rotatory, this can be enhanced by internally rotating the foot at the same time that the anterior force is applied. The TT test is performed by stabilizing the tibia medially and with the opposite hand controlling the calcaneus and hindfoot and inverting the heel. Again, the application of some internal rotation recreates the true motion of instability. The hand that stabilizes the tibia can be used to palpate the lateral gutter and feel for any abnormal gapping of the interval between the anterior distal fibula and the lateral talar process. This space should not normally open with an intact ATFL.

It has been shown by systematic review that the wide variability in published AD and TT values with stress radiographs precludes the use of any normal values with these tests for predicting clinically significant laxity.[302] Therefore, the main value of these manoeuvres for diagnosing clinical instability is the reproduction of patient symptoms by the generation of apprehension and/or pain.

Treatment

NON-OPERATIVE TREATMENT

Acute inversion injuries are typically treated with functional rehabilitation focusing on decreasing inflammation, preserving motion (especially avoiding equinus contracture), and redeveloping motor strength, balance and proprioception. In chronic ankle instability these same principles apply, and a course of physiotherapy with the focus on eliminating equinus and improving strength, balance and proprioception should be the first line of treatment.[314] Orthoses with lateral heel posting for hindfoot varus or forefoot posting for a depressed first ray may be helpful. Assessment for underlying varus heel alignment and/or cavus foot posture with a depressed first ray can be carried out with a Coleman block test. Radiographic evaluation for alignment should include a hindfoot alignment view. The use of ankle braces has been shown to be helpful in preventing recurrent inversion injuries in male and female football players.[315,316]

OPERATIVE TREATMENT

The operative treatment for chronic lateral ligament instability has been extensively written about. In general, the many described procedures can be grouped into two types of lateral ligament reconstruction procedures: anatomic and non-anatomic tenodesis stabilizations. The non-anatomic procedures such as the Watson–Jones, Evans or Christman–Snook rely upon sacrifice of part or all of the peroneus brevis, which is generally considered to be an important motor unit for normal ankle and hindfoot function. These procedures can reduce lateral instability effectively but in turn lead to abnormal subtalar stiffness.[317] Long-term results with tenodesis repairs have shown that although stability is restored up to 50% of patients are in pain, perhaps due to the effects of abnormal limitation of subtalar motion.[318–321]

The anatomic procedures described by Brostrom, Gould and Karlsson repair the ATFL and CFL by either imbrication or direct repair to bone and overlapping periosteal flaps.[318,322,323] Gould's modification added the stem of the inferior extensor retinaculum to the ATFL repair, which augments the effect of repairing the CFL by adding another structure connecting the talus and calcaneus.[323,324] These procedures as a group should preserve normal ankle and subtalar motion while restoring lateral stability. Results reported with these types of repair have been good or excellent in 80–95% of cases.[307,324–329] Augmentation of these techniques with free tendon autograft, allograft or split peroneus brevis Evans-type augmentation have been described for cases where there is insufficient native tissue as in some revision cases, patients with hyperlaxity, and large or high-demand patients such as athletes.[327,330–333]

In cases of heel varus associated with lateral ligament instability or hyperlaxity, the addition of a valgus-producing calcaneal osteotomy should be strongly considered and may be more important to outcome than tendon augmentation in some cases.[305,334–336] The effect of heel alignment and the application of a valgus Dwyer osteotomy to improve lateral instability has been reported with good results.[337]

In summary, the evaluation of lateral ankle ligament instability can be a complex process to assess for the many associated pathologies that can result from inversion injuries. Assessment must be comprehensive to identify other causes of pain, and specific attention should be given to the evaluation of overall ligamentous laxity and foot alignment. Non-operative treatments including problem-specific physiotherapy, orthoses and bracing can be tried, but the long-term results of non-operative treatment when instability persists may be deleterious to the ankle and hindfoot.[338] When surgical reconstruction is considered, a well-thought-out plan should be devised, which may include tendon augmentation, associated surgical repairs such as for peroneal tendon tears or instability, arthroscopic evaluation and treatment of intra-articular pathologies, and realignment procedures such as calcaneal osteotomy.

SYNDESMOTIC SPRAINS

Aetiology

The syndesmosis is a strong ligament complex that joins the distal tibia and fibula at the ankle, and resists external rotation of the talus. Syndesmotic sprains are much less common than ankle sprains affecting the lateral ankle ligaments.[263,339] Syndesmotic sprains in the absence of fracture have been noted to cause significant disability and time lost to injury in athletes compared with lateral ankle sprains.[339–343]

Pathology

The syndesmosis is a complex ligamentous structure and has three main sets of ligaments making up the anterior and posterior tibial–fibular ligaments and the interosseous tibial–fibular ligaments (Fig. 78.10). It is not known which of these are injured in most cases, nor what the severity of ligament injury is for specific cases. It also remains to be shown what pathology exists in cases where patients have residual pain, which is particularly evident with push-off on the affected side.[342]

Evaluation

Evaluation of any ankle injury should include examination for syndesmotic injury. Diagnosis of syndesmotic sprains is primarily based on physical examination and an inability to fully weight bear on the affected leg. Tenderness over the anterior syndesmosis above the ankle joint line has been indicated as one strong predictor of syndesmotic injury.[344] The 'squeeze test', which is pressure applied proximally to compress the fibula and tibia together,

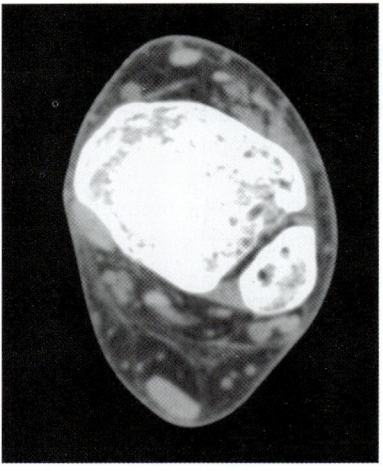

Figure 78.10 An axial CT scan with soft-tissue technique showing the anterior and posterior tibial–fibular ligaments of the syndesmosis, which have intermediate signal on this image.

has been recommended and has been shown in both cadaver and clinic reports to be effective in stressing the syndesmosis.[341,345] MRI has been suggested as a diagnostic tool, and it can reveal many abnormalities of specific anatomic structures. In one study the MRI findings in 21 patients were compared with intra-operative findings for patients with ankle trauma and showed good diagnostic accuracy using a prescribed protocol for reading the studies.[346] How this information can be applied to syndesmotic sprains and whether it can help to guide the best course of treatment remains to be seen. As with joint instability problems elsewhere, the static nature of MRI findings may not provide insight into the presence of dynamic joint instability.

Treatment

Most cases reported have been of non-operative treatment for isolated syndesmotic sprains, and a recent systematic review revealed only two cases of operative treatment in qualifying reports.[347] Additionally no consistent method of non-operative rehabilitation and treatment has been described, and return to play is generally based upon the player reporting pain with activity. Treatment modalities that have been described include limitation of activity, immobilization, ice, anti-inflammatory medications and graduated strengthening and conditioning as tolerated.

DELTOID LIGAMENT SPRAINS

The deltoid ligament of the ankle comprises two parts: superficial and deep components. Both of these have named bundles, but it is the deep portion of the deltoid ligament that is considered the most important medial ankle stabilizer. The main function of the deep deltoid ligament is to prevent external rotation of the ankle. Thus it is excessive external rotation force that can affect the deep deltoid and syndesmotic ligaments. Deltoid ligament sprains are an infrequently recognized isolated injury, and in the absence of a fracture are usually seen with syndesmotic ligament injuries.[347,348] Occurrences of deltoid ligament sprains have also been found by MRI in a series of patients presenting with inversion injuries of the ankle.[349] The deltoid ligament is placed under strain with external rotation forces to the ankle similar to those that also injure the syndesmosis; however, the deltoid ligament is also strained by excessive hindfoot valgus, and chronic deltoid ligament injury has been recognized in association with valgus foot deformity.[350] Treatment of deltoid ligament injury is usually provided by the reduction and fixation of displaced ankle fractures and syndesmotic ligament injuries. The maintenance of a reduced ankle seems to provide a satisfactory setting for subsequent healing of the deltoid ligament. It has been noted however that medial gutter or posteromedial ankle impingement lesions can result from the scarring of torn deep components of the deltoid ligament.[281,351] As noted elsewhere in this chapter, arthroscopic debridement can be useful for the treatment of this chronic problem.

MIDFOOT AND FOREFOOT PAIN

LISFRANC SPRAINS

Aetiology

Sprains of the Lisfranc joint typically occur as the result of low-energy indirect trauma whereby the foot is typically in a plantarflexed position and an axial load is applied to the foot either by an opponent falling on the posterior heel or by one's own body weight. The line of force is directed plantar to the midfoot joints and thus negates the usual mechanical protection of the plantar fascia and plantar ligaments. This reversal of the normal mechanics of the midfoot leads to failure under tension of the relatively weak dorsal ligaments and eventual disruption of the stronger plantar ligaments as the midfoot buckles. Another described mechanism is forced abduction of a foot where the forefoot is anchored, such as in sailboarding.[352] In direct trauma such as in a crush injury, a force is applied to the foot dorsally and thus much higher injury is required to overcome the tensile strength of the plantar ligaments[353,354] and plantar fascia which normally protect the bony arch from collapse.

Pathology

Subtle injuries of the Lisfranc ligaments are typically seen in indirect injuries such as in athletes. These injuries typically involve the second metatarsal base or the first metatarsal and cuneiform. The three ligaments that anchor the second metatarsal base in its mortise between the three cuneiforms are the dorsal Lisfranc ligament, the interosseous Lisfranc ligament (Fig. 78.11) and the plantar ligament between the first cuneiform and the second and third metatarsals. The last two are much stronger than the dorsal ligament. It has recently been shown that if all three ligaments are torn, then gross instability of the second metatarsal base is created.[355] Injury of the dorsal ligament alone leaves the joint stable with weight-bearing stress. It is not clear how often injury to the dorsal and interosseous ligaments alone might lead to clinical instability. The first ray is stabilized by the same three ligaments as well as the interosseous ligament between the first two cuneiforms. Proximally the plantar capsular ligament of the first naviculocuneiform ligament provides some stability as well, but not enough to maintain sagittal plane stability once the other ligaments are torn.

Evaluation

Evaluation of indirect Lisfranc injuries is focused on diagnosing an unstable injury, as these usually require surgical intervention. Different radiographic tests have been recommended by different authors for determining whether an injury is unstable. Gross findings include any step-off of the line of the medial border of the second metatarsal and the second cuneiform on an AP radiograph. The medial border of the fourth metatarsal and medial border of the cuboid has also been noted as a fairly constant finding, but can vary up to 2 mm in some normal specimens. The relationship of the base of the fifth metatarsal to the cuboid is too variable to be of any benefit. An additional recommendation has been that the space between the bases of the first and second metatarsal should not be more than 2 mm apart. In cases where a patient is unable to bear weight but the initial radiographs are not abnormal, several different recommendations have been suggested. Some authors recommend a weight-bearing AP or a weight-bearing lateral radiograph.[356,357] The inferior border of the first cuneiform should be at least 1.5 mm higher than the inferior border of the fifth metatarsal on a standing lateral radiograph. If it is less than that, it may indicate an unstable injury of the Lisfranc joint. Others have recommended stress radiographs[358,359]. A recent cadaver study showed that injury-specific stress radiographs for the transverse and longitudinal injuries were superior to a weight-bearing AP radiograph with 22.5 kg (50 lb) of weight.[355]

In subtle injuries (Fig. 78.12) where the diagnosis of instability is not clear, it may be prudent to carry out examination under anaesthesia. If instability is present, surgical stabilization is indicated.

Physical examination

Physical findings may include inability to bear weight, swelling and plantar ecchymosis, tenderness over the Lisfranc joint and pain with either active or passive motion of these joints. Injuries with severe displacement are at risk for development of compartment syndrome and tearing of the perforating branch of the dorsalis pedis leading to forefoot amputation in severe cases in one report. This would be rare for any athletic injury.

Treatment

OBJECTIVES

The objectives of treatment are to allow healing of the ligaments in an anatomic fashion. This can require obtaining and maintaining anatomic reduction in any displaced or unstable injury. Better outcomes with maintenance[354,360–363] of an anatomic reduction have been reported.

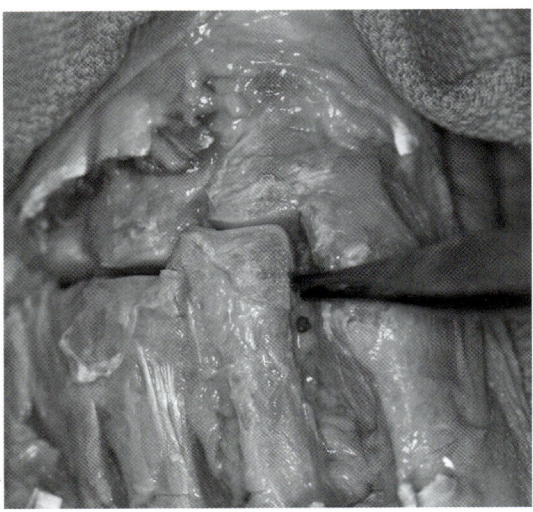

Figure 78.11 The instrument is in the interspace between the base of the second metatarsal and the medial cuneiform. The dorsal, interosseous and plantar ligaments between these two bones have been cut. The result is lateral displacement of the second metatarsal base.

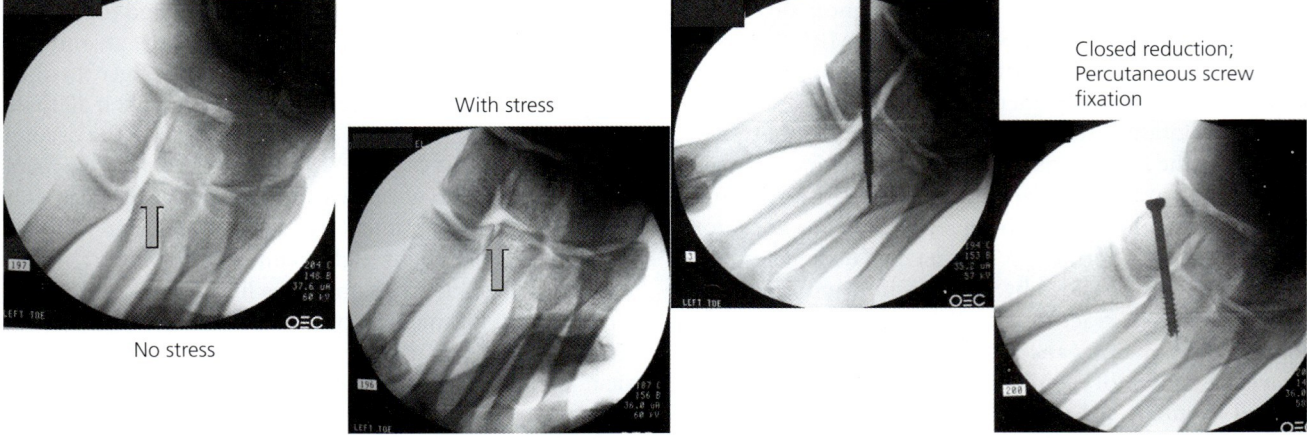

Figure 78.12 Twenty-one-year-old male football player, unable to weight bear following twisting midfoot injury.

NON-OPERATIVE TREATMENT

Non-operative treatment can be used successfully in cases where no instability exists. There remains some concern that our present efforts at determining instability are not ideal as some patients with presumed stable injuries do end up with long-term pain and loss of function (Myerson, Albright).

OPERATIVE TREATMENT

It is important to distinguish subtle injuries as described above, common in athletes, from gross tarsometatarsal instability or dislocation (Fig. 78.13).

In these types of subtle injury one must clearly make the diagnosis. Stabilization should be considered with the presence of diastasis or instability. In these subtle cases fixation can be percutaneous with fixation across the area of the Lisfranc ligament (shown above).

In the past, for more severe injuries, either closed or open reduction with percutaneous wires was recommended by many authors, but more recent reports have shown that temporary transarticular screw fixation allows more reliable maintenance of reduction and no apparent long-term tendency to develop degenerative changes related to the use of screws. Primary fusion of these injuries has been discussed and recommended but should be reserved for severe injuries with either multidirectional instability or articular comminution[364]. Although no consensus exists as to how long to keep a patient non-weight bearing or how long to leave screws in place, most authors would keep a patient non-weight bearing for at least 6 weeks and keep the screws in place for 6–12 weeks, although the trend seems to be towards leaving the screws in for longer if there are concerns of losing reduction before sufficient soft-tissue healing occurs. Technical points include careful handling of soft tissues as the deep peroneal and superficial nerves are at risk. Most authors recommend longitudinal incisions, usually between the first two rays and the third and fourth rays if needed. Screws placed axially across the tarsometatarsal joints should be recessed into the dorsal metarsal bases with the creating of pocket holes using a burr. The will avoid the undesirable comminution of the dorsal cortex and loss of fixation. Joint reduction should be anatomic and static (non-compressive) fixation is preferred, but if this does not allow for maintaining anatomic reduction then compression can be considered.

NAVICULAR STRESS FRACTURES

Aetiology

Stress fractures of the navicular bone are reported to range from 15% to 35% of lower extremity stress fractures.[2,4,365,366] They are considered to be one of the more high-risk stress fractures for possible non-union and injury time away from sports. The most common sports in most series are track and long-distance running.[2,367–369] Sprinting, hurdles and jumping events seem to be more likely to cause navicular stress fracture than middle and long distance running according to one study of track and field athletes.[4] In a study of tennis players, navicular stress fractures were the most common type of stress fracture, and junior players were significantly more likely to sustain stress fractures than senior players.[366] Gender differences have been noted in military populations but the same has not been shown in athletes.[4,367]

Pathology

Navicular stress fractures tend to be vertically oriented in the sagittal plane and begin dorsally and propagate towards the plantar cortex. The navicular is considered to

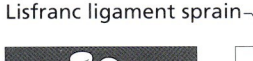
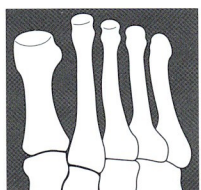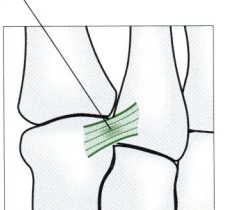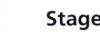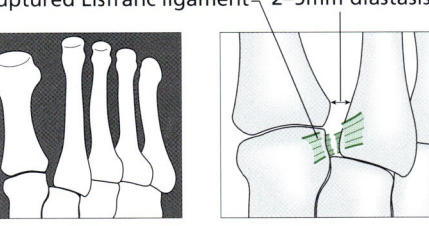

Stage I No diastasis   **Stage II** Diastasis, no arch height loss

Figure 78.13 Lisfranc injuries.

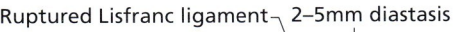
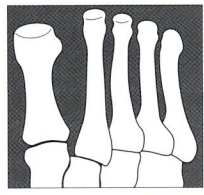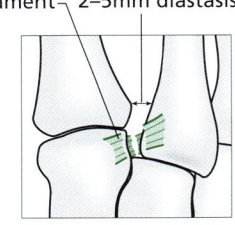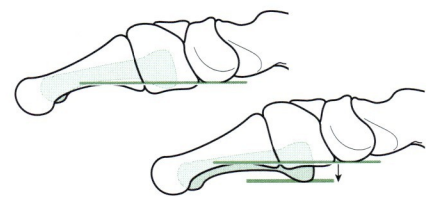

Stage III   Diastasis and loss of longitudinal arch height

be a bone with limited blood supply and the location of the fracture tends to be in the watershed area of the bone.[370]

Evaluation

Navicular stress fractures may be difficult to detect and the examiner may find focal tenderness over the navicular, but diagnosis usually depends upon having a high level of clinical suspicion. Although these fractures can be seen by plain radiographs, bone scan, CT or MRI, or multiple radiological studies may be required as plain radiographs will often fail to demonstrate a navicular stress fracture or its extent.[365,371–377] A high level of clinical suspicion should lead one to have a low threshold for ordering auxiliary tests when the diagnosis is considered. Bone scans are sensitive and can be used as a screening test, but they do not offer the anatomic information necessary for planning treatment.[378] CT scanning has been used to demonstrate navicular stress fractures as incomplete or complete and to reveal the presence of sclerosis or cystic changes. A CT classification has been suggested and three types demonstrate dorsal beaking, fracture to the mid-portion of the body, and complete fracture of both the dorsal and plantar cortex.[376,379] Since complete fractures fare the worst, this classification may be useful in guiding treatment and patient counselling.

Treatment

The treatment of navicular stress fractures is difficult and recovery is long, even in successful cases. In fractures that have minimal propagation through the navicular and in the absence of sclerosis and cystic changes, non-operative treatment with a non-weight-bearing cast can be used for 6–8 weeks. If overpronation is noted, then a medially posted orthosis may be a reasonable consideration. Radiographic healing may not be seen for 4 or more months and the absence of complete radiographic healing may be seen in clinically successful cases.[365,372,376,379–381]

Surgical intervention is usually performed with lag screw fixation across the fracture line either from medial to lateral or from lateral to medial.[365,368,373,375,376,379,380] Debridement and bone grafting can be considered in cases where non-union and notable sclerosis and cystic changes are seen.[382] Overall return to activity takes at least 3–4 months in cases of successful healing. Some athletes may not be able to recover and return to their regular activity, and this possibility should be discussed early in the treatment course.

FIFTH METATARSAL FRACTURES

Aetiology

Four types of fifth metatarsal fracture have been described, and the location of the fracture has significance for treatment. The most proximal fractures have been delineated into three types.[383] The first type are avulsion type fractures which occur proximal to the intermetatarsal joint between the bases of the fourth and fifth metatarsals. These are also the most common type of fifth metatarsal fracture, and are associated with inversion ankle injuries.[384] The second type are the acute fractures that enter the fourth–fifth intermetatarsal joint, and have been coined 'Jones' fractures, originally described by Sir Robert Jones in 1902, who included himself in a series of four cases. His elegant recounting of his own fracture described how it occurred during dancing.[385] The third type is stress fractures, which occur in the proximal metadiaphyseal region and exit the bone medially distal to the proximal intermetatarsal joint.[386] Both Jones fractures and stress fractures probably result from excessive medial–lateral forces and are not due to an inversion injury alone.[387] A fourth type of fifth metatarsal fracture has been called a 'dancer's' fracture and is usually a spiral or oblique fracture of the diaphysis.[388]

Pathology

The avulsion fracture of the fifth metatarsal is the most common type of fifth metatarsal fracture.[384] The fifth metatarsal base lends attachment to both the insertions of the peroneus brevis and peroneus tertius, and also the lateral band of the plantar fascia. The peroneus brevis has been thought to be the cause of these fractures, but it has been shown in a cadaveric model that the lateral band of the plantar fascia is more likely to be the structure that causes these fractures.[389] The diaphyseal 'dancer's' fracture can occur with inversion type injuries have been described in and usually heal without complication.[388]

Jones-type fractures, as described above, are acute fractures and should be clearly differentiated from the more distal stress fractures. The fifth metatarsal stress fracture occurs more distally than the Jones-type fracture and has been linked to cavovarus foot deformity with altered biomechanical loading of the lateral border of the foot.[390,391] Both Jones fractures and stress fractures can be difficult to treat and have a higher incidence of non-union and refracture. This has been attributed to the less robust blood supply in this location, which lies in a watershed area between the nutrient artery and the proximal metaphyseal blood supply. Mechanical factors can also be a hindrance to healing and, in addition to cavovarus foot posture, torsional strains due to the effect of the peroneal muscle attachments on the proximal fragment have been implicated.[392]

Evaluation

Presentation of fifth metatarsal fractures is associated with acute injury, with the exception of stress fractures, which may have a more indolent course, and complaints may be of a more nagging pain without a memorable injury. When stress fractures present acutely they may or may not have a history of prodromal symptoms, but the radiographs will show signs of periosteal healing or in some cases a clear non-union and sclerosis of the fracture site. Plain radiographs in the AP, oblique and lateral views are helpful for diagnosis and assessment of the fracture pattern, and can help with evaluation of the biomechanical alignment of the foot. In the case of prodromal pain without radiographic evidence of a fracture, then an MRI or bone scan might be indicated, although this is not common.

Physical examination

Physical examination is typically straightforward with tenderness being elicited at the site of the fracture. Since these fractures often present with an acute injury, typically an inversion injury, it is important to perform a thorough examination to diagnose any other associated injuries. Assessment of the biomechanical alignment of the foot, again looking for subtle cavus or metatarsus adductus tendencies in the case of stress fractures, is important for subsequent treatment.[390,391]

Treatment

The objectives of treatment are to obtain healing and return to play, but the treatment must be guided by the classification of the fracture.[393] In the case of avulsion fractures and diaphyseal 'dancer's' fractures functional treatment with weight-bearing cast boots is often all that is required until satisfactory healing is observed by radiographic assessment and clinical resolution of pain with weight bearing, usually in 6–8 weeks.[388,393,394] In some cases where significant displacement is present, or in avulsion fractures with significant articular step-off, surgical reduction and fixation may be indicated.[388,393]

In the case of Jones fractures, both non-operative and operative treatments have been recommended for Jones fractures. The trend towards operative treatment in athletes should not preclude discussion of the risks and benefits of both treatment options with a patient.[383,384,387,393–400] Non-operative treatment for a Jones-type fracture should consist of 6 weeks of non-weight bearing in a cast, followed by a period of protection using a stiffened shoe with a full-length carbon fibre or steel plate. The chance of refracture and non-union must be weighed against the risks of surgery, which can include failed treatment or pain due to injury to the sural nerve, which has been shown to be at risk.[401] Although the goal of early return to play is more likely to be achieved with operative treatment, the risk of refracture is also diminished with operative treatment.[383,384,387,393–400] In any displaced Jones fracture, operative treatment in an athlete should be the treatment of choice.

With non-operative treatment non-weight bearing in a cast for 6–8 weeks is followed by a walking cast if healing is being shown on radiographs. If lack of radiographic healing is present at 8 weeks, then consideration of intramedullary screw fixation should be strongly considered in an athlete. With operative treatment using an intramedullary lag screw such as a 4.5 mm malleolar screw, healing usually occurs by 12 weeks, with progression of activity in a stiff-soled shoe.[383,384,393,397]

The metadiaphyseal stress fracture has been classified by Torg et al.[386] based on radiographic appearance of the fracture. The Torg type I fracture is a stress fracture treated the same as a Jones fracture with the assumption that the biological potential for healing is the same as that for an acute fracture. Torg types II and III have progressive evidence of non-union and do not respond well to non-operative treatment. Operative intervention should include some type of stimulation of the fracture non-union site with over-drilling of the non-union prior to screw placement or open debridement and bone grafting with intramedullary screw placement.[391,393] Again, in such cases, careful evaluation to detect underlying predisposing mechanical causes should lead to addressing deformities with either offloading orthoses or, in some cases, consideration of surgical realignment.

LATERAL AND MEDIAL PLANTAR NERVE ENTRAPMENT

Aetiology

The aetiology of entrapment of the medial and lateral plantar nerves or their branches is multifactorial and can be an extension of tarsal tunnel syndrome (compression of the posterior tibial nerve) or exist with concomitant nerve compression at the level of the lumbosacral spine.[402] Heel pain is common and is usually associated with pathology of the plantar fascia; however, plantar nerve entrapment can mimic or coexist with plantar fascial pathology.[403] The specific sports-related occurrence of nerve compression near the heel can be due to direct mechanical trauma and foot morphology such as pes cavus or pes planus and the degree of pronation that occurs with weight-bearing activity. It has been shown that the position of hindfoot eversion or inversion, which components of the dynamic motion of pronation and supination, significantly increases the pressure within the tarsal tunnel and affects the plantar branches of the posterior tibial nerve as well.[404–406]

Pathology

Peripheral nerve compression can occur with a number of causes, and begins with damage to the capillary flood flow through the connective tissue sleeve of the nerve fibres.

Direct trauma due to landing on a hard object or an ill-fitting shoe or orthosis can lead to inflammation, oedema and vascular insufficiency due to inhibition of epineural and endoneural blood flow. Intermittent or chronic compression can have the same effect, and over time can lead to epineurial fibrosis, which adds to the vascular insufficiency of the nerve. Many causes of chronic compression have been reported and can include: vascular leashes, tight fascial bands, accessory muscles, hypertrophied muscles and masses. Pain associated with nerve compression is probably due to this local dysvascular state. Intermittent compression and choking of the capillary blood flow can occur with excessive or constrained excursion of the nerves which must normally glide over many millimetres with normal joint motion. Excessive excursion can occur with over-pronation and constrained excursion can occur with epineural fibrosis that results from ongoing nerve compression. Damage to the neural cells leads to impaired axonal transport and nerve dysfunction, which manifests as motor and sensory changes which can be detected with electrodiagnostic testing.[407–409]

Evaluation

Evaluation of medial and lateral plantar nerve entrapment should begin with a careful history and physical examination. A history of activity-related heel pain or arch pain with or without sensory changes should alert the examiner to the possibility of these problems. A careful physical examination including looking for proximal sites of nerve compression from the lumbosacral spine to the tarsal tunnel should be performed both to rule out other sites as the main problem and to detect a double crush scenario. The more typical cause of heel pain related to plantar fasciitis usually manifests with palpation of the central band of the plantar fascia with the toes dorsiflexed in ankle neutral position activating the windlass mechanism. Tenderness may be elicited either in the mid-arch or at the insertion of the plantar fascia on the calcaneus. With lateral plantar nerve entrapment, tenderness will usually be more lateral at the proximal origin of the abductor hallucis fascia, although tenderness can extend to the plantar heel or be referred there due to the sensory branch of the lateral plantar nerve, which supplies the periosteum in this location. If the lateral nerve is irritated at the plantar heel, which could be due to a large bone spur, tenderness will be increased with relaxation of the plantar fascia and decreased with tension placed on the plantar fascia, which would then shield the nerve. Tenderness of the medial plantar nerve is found beneath the navicular where the nerve passes deep to the naviculocalcaneal ligament, which also acts as a part of the deep fascia of the abductor hallucis. This inserts on the medial wall of the calcaneus, creating a tunnel for the medial plantar neurovascular bundle. This Y-shaped attachment then continues posteriorly, creating the tunnel for the lateral plantar bundle deep to the abductor hallucis, where the lateral plantar nerve is typically found to be tender. Atrophy of the abductor hallucis can be seen with longstanding nerve compression of the medial plantar nerve.[403,406,410–416] Plain radiographs can reveal unusually large calcaneal spurs and weight-bearing lateral, AP foot views can help detect a tendency towards overpronation. An MRI of the ankle and heel can help to evaluate for masses.[417] Electrodiagnostic tests can detect both sensory and motor dysfunction of the plantar nerves. Sensory changes are more easily detected. The target muscle for the medial plantar nerve is the abductor hallucis and the abductor digiti quinti is the target muscle for EMG evaluation of the lateral plantar nerve.[402,406,407,410,416,418] A negative electrodiagnostic examination does not rule out these diagnoses and should not be used to exclude patients from treatment.

Principles of treatment

Treatment should include measures to relieve pressure on the heel and arch, which involves careful examination of the shoes and any orthoses. Overpronation should be addressed with an orthosis that provides a post beneath the first and second rays at the forefoot to help support the medial column of the foot, and avoid any enhancement in the arch which is very likely to increase pain due to direct pressure.[406,410,416] In cases where fibrosis leads to limitation of normal nerve excursion, hand therapists have developed techniques for mobilizing the median nerve in carpal tunnel syndrome, but similar techniques have not been reported for the foot and ankle.[409] Operative treatment involves surgical release of the abductor fascia over the involved nerve and if any indication of tarsal tunnel involvement is present, then a full tarsal tunnel release with release of both plantar nerves is indicated. Referral to a spine specialist should be considered before surgery in any patient who has suggestion of a double crush injury due to proximal nerve root compression.

STRESS FRACTURES OF THE FIRST METATARSOPHALANGEAL JOINT SESAMOID BONES

Aetiology

Stress fractures of the sesamoids of the first MTP joint are difficult problems to treat in athletes, and often lead to prolonged disability and loss of time from play. These fractures are most common in athletes with repetitive forefoot loading such track and field athletes and gymnasts.[419] The onset of pain is typically insidious and the time to diagnosis can be delayed. There may be a tendency for the medial sesamoid to be more commonly affected, but only small series have been reported.[419,420] The sesamoid bones can develop as bipartite bones with a fibrous junction that performs well in most patients, but may become injured and present in a similar fashion. Other than repetitive trauma, there has not been any clear aetiology of these fractures shown.

Evaluation

Physical examination typically demonstrates direct tenderness over the affected sesamoid bone, which is increased with passive dorsiflexion of the hallux. Radiological evaluation can include plain radiographs, which should include an AP view that can demonstrate the fracture in many cases. A dorsiflexion lateral view may show separation of the fragments if complete diastasis is present; however, this is more likely with an acute fracture and requires tearing of the strong surrounding soft tissues consisting of the flexor hallucis brevis, plantar plate and capsule. A sesamoid view, which is taken in an axial position with the hallux dorsiflexed, can demonstrate joint space narrowing, which may be seen with longstanding pathology. Bone scan, CT and MRI have been recommended for additional evaluation.[419,421,422] Bone scan is sensitive but has been shown to have some positive findings in 29% of asymptomatic infantry recruits and 26% of sedentary adults.[423] MRI can reveal other pathologies such as avascular necrosis of the sesamoids, adjacent tendonitis and overlying bursitis.[424]

Treatment

Treatment in cases of intact bone segments can be started with cast immobilization for 4–6 weeks followed by limited training for up to 4 months in stiff-soled shoes or with carbon fibre inserts to shield the first MTP joint. If degenerative joint changes or avascular necrosis are present, then early excision can be considered. If pain is not improved excision of the involved sesamoid has shown good results in small series.[419,420,424,425] Return to training can begin usually 6–8 weeks after excision.[420] The surgical technique should include meticulous repair of the flexor hallucis brevis tendon and capsule, and careful handling of the plantar digital nerves, which are adjacent to the sesamoids. The medial sesamoid is best approached through a longitudinal medial incision, which can allow for mobilization of the plantar skin laterally to approach the sesamoid through a longitudinal tendon-splitting incision, thus avoiding a plantar scar in a weight-bearing location, which is more likely to be painful. The lateral sesamoid can be safely approached through a plantar incision placed longitudinally beneath the first webspace. This again will allow for a direct tendon-splitting approach and a good anatomic repair of the plantar soft tissues. In cases where the fragments are unequal in size the larger of the two fragments may be maintained if the remaining joint surface is intact.

REFERENCES

1. Beck TJ, Ruff CB, Shaffer RA, et al. Stress fracture in military recruits: gender differences in muscle and bone susceptibility factors. *Bone* 2000;**27**:437–44.
2. Brukner P, Bradshaw C, Khan KM, et al. Stress fractures: a review of 180 cases. *Clinical Journal of Sport Medicine* 1996;**6**:85–9.
3. Milgrom C, Giladi M, Stein M, et al. Stress fractures in military recruits. A prospective study showing an unusually high incidence. *Journal of Bone and Joint Surgery* 1985;**67**:732–5.
4. Bennell KL, Malcolm SA, Thomas SA, et al. The incidence and distribution of stress fractures in competitive track and field athletes. A twelve-month prospective study. *American Journal of Sports Medicine* 1996;**24**:211–17.
5. Matheson GO, Clement DB, McKenzie DC, et al. Stress fractures in athletes. A study of 320 cases. *American Journal of Sports Medicine* 1987;**15**:46–58.
6. Chang PS, Harris RM. Intramedullary nailing for chronic tibial stress fractures. A review of five cases. *American Journal of Sports Medicine* 1996;**24**:688–92.
7. Giladi M, Milgrom C, Simkin A, et al. Stress fractures and tibial bone width. A risk factor. *Journal of Bone and Joint Surgery* 1987;**69**:326–9.
8. Bennell KL, Malcolm SA, Thomas SA. Risk factors for stress fractures in female track-and-field athletes: a retrospective analysis. *Clinical Journal of Sport Medicine* 1995;**5**:229–35.
9. Zifchock RA, Davis I, Hamill J. Kinetic asymmetry in female runners with and without retrospective tibial stress fractures. *Journal of Biomechanics* 2006;**39-15**:2792–7.
10. Ekenman I, Tsai-Fellander L, Westblad P, et al. A study of intrinsic factors in patients with stress fractures of the tibia. *Foot and Ankle International* 1996;**17**:477–82.
11. Ekenman I, Halvorsen K, Westblad P, et al. Local bone deformation at two predominant sites for stress fractures of the tibia: an in vivo study. *Foot and Ankle International* 1998;**19**:479–84.
12. Milgrom C, Finestone A, Novack V, et al. The effect of prophylactic treatment with risedronate on stress fracture incidence among infantry recruits. *Bone* 2004;**35**:418–24.
13. Orava S, Hulkko A. Stress fracture of the mid-tibial shaft. *Acta Orthopaedica Scandinavica* 1984;**55**:35–7.
14. Batt ME, Kemp S, Kerslake R. Delayed union stress fractures of the anterior tibia: conservative management. *British Journal of Sports Medicine* 2001;**35**:74–7.
15. Fredericson M, Bergman AG, Hoffman KL, Dillingham MS. Tibial stress reaction in runners. Correlation of clinical

symptoms and scintigraphy with a new magnetic resonance imaging grading system. *American Journal of Sports Medicine* 1995;**23**:472–81.
16. Aoki Y, Yasuda K, Tohyama H, *et al*. Magnetic resonance imaging in stress fractures and shin splints. *Clinical Orthopaedics and Related Research* 2004;**421**:260–7.
17. Gaeta M, Minutoli F, Scribano E, *et al*. CT and MR imaging findings in athletes with early tibial stress injuries: comparison with bone scintigraphy findings and emphasis on cortical abnormalities. *Radiology* 2005;**235**:553–61.
18. Matheson GO, Clement DB, McKenzie DC, *et al*. Scintigraphic uptake of 99mTc at non-painful sites in athletes with stress fractures. The concept of bone strain. *Sports Medicine* 1987;**4**:65–75.
19. Young AJ, McAllister DR. Evaluation and treatment of tibial stress fractures. *Clinical Sports Medicine* 2006;**25**:117.
20. Whitelaw GP, Wetzler MJ, Levy AS, *et al*. A pneumatic leg brace for the treatment of tibial stress fractures. *Clinical Orthopaedics and Related Research* 1991;**270**:301–5.
21. Brand JC, Brindle T, Nyland J, *et al*. Does pulsed low intensity ultrasound allow early return to normal activities when treating stress fractures? A review of one tarsal navicular and eight tibial stress fractures. *Iowa Orthopedic Journal* 1999;**19**:26–30.
22. Rue JP, Armstrong DW, Frassica FJ, *et al*. The effect of pulsed ultrasound in the treatment of tibial stress fractures. *Orthopedics* 2004;**27-11**:1192–5.
23. Varner KE, Younas SA, Lintner DM, Marymont JV. Chronic anterior midtibial stress fractures in athletes treated with reamed intramedullary nailing. *American Journal of Sports Medicine* 2005;**33**:1071–6.
24. Beck BR, Osternig LR. Medial tibial stress syndrome. The location of muscles in the leg in relation to symptoms. *Journal of Bone and Joint Surgery (American)* 1994;**76**:1057–61.
25. Michael RH, Holder LE. The soleus syndrome. A cause of medial tibial stress (shin splints). *American Journal of Sports Medicine* 1985;**13**:87–94.
26. Detmer DE. Chronic shin splints. Classification and management of medial tibial stress syndrome. *Sports Medicine* 1986;**3**:436–46.
27. Sommer HM, Vallentyne SW. Effect of foot posture on the incidence of medial tibial stress syndrome. *Medicine and Science in Sports and Exercise* 1995;**27**:800–4.
28. Yates B, White S. The incidence and risk factors in the development of medial tibial stress syndrome among naval recruits. *American Journal of Sports Medicine* 2004;**32**:772–80.
29. Magnusson HI, Westlin NE, Nyqvist F, *et al*. Abnormally decreased regional bone density in athletes with medial tibial stress syndrome. *American Journal of Sports Medicine* 2001;**29**:712–15.
30. Bhatt R, Lauder I, Finlay DB, *et al*. Correlation of bone scintigraphy and histological findings in medial tibial syndrome. *British Journal of Sports Medicine* 2000;**34**:49–53.
31. Allen MJ, O'Dwyer FG, Barnes MR, *et al*. The value of 99Tcm-MDP bone scans in young patients with exercise-induced lower leg pain. *Nuclear Medicine Communications* 1995;**16**:88–91.
32. Mattila KT, Komu ME, Dahlstrom S, *et al*. Medial tibial pain: a dynamic contrast-enhanced MRI study. *Magnetic Resonance Imaging* 1999;**17**:947–54.
33. Samuelson DR, Cram RL. The three-phase bone scan and exercise induced lower-leg pain. The tibial stress test. *Clinical Nuclear Medicine* 1996;**21**:89–93.
34. Holen KJ, Engebretsen L, Grontvedt T, *et al*. Surgical treatment of medial tibial stress syndrome (shin splint) by fasciotomy of the superficial posterior compartment of the leg. *Scandinavian Journal of Medicine and Science in Sports* 1995;**5**:40–3.
35. Jarvinnen M, Aho H, Niittymaki S. Results of the surgical treatment of the medial tibial syndrome in athletes. *International Journal of Sports Medicine* 1989;**10**:55–7.
36. Yates B, Allen MJ, Barnes MR. Outcome of surgical treatment of medial tibial stress syndrome. *Journal of Bone and Joint Surgery (American)* 2003;**85-A-10**:1974–80.
37. Puranen J, Alavaikko A. Intracompartmental pressure increase on exertion in patients with chronic compartment syndrome in the leg. *Journal of Bone and Joint Surgery (American)* 1981;**63**:1304–9.
38. Birtles DB, Minden D, Wickes SJ, *et al*. Chronic exertional compartment syndrome: muscle changes with isometric exercise. *Medicine and Science in Sports and Exercise* 2002;**34-12**:1900–6.
39. Lecocq J, Isner-Horobeti ME, Dupeyron A, *et al*. [Exertional compartment syndrome]. *Annales de Réadaptation et de Médecine Physique* 2004;**47**:334–45.
40. Styf J, Korner L, Suurkula M. Intramuscular pressure and muscle blood flow during exercise in chronic compartment syndrome. *Journal of Bone and Joint Surgery* 1987;**69**:301–5.
41. Embree MJ. *Chronic Compartment Syndrome: an Analysis at the Cellular Level*. London, Ontario: The University of Western Ontario, 1996.
42. Amendola A, Rorabeck CH, Vellett D, *et al*. The use of magnetic resonance imaging in exertional compartment syndromes. *American Journal of Sports Medicine* 1990;**18**:29–34.
43. Pedowitz RA, Hargens AR, Mubarak SJ, Gershuni DH. Modified criteria for the objective diagnosis of chronic compartment syndrome of the leg. *American Journal of Sports Medicine* 1990;**18**:35–40.
44. Rowdon GA, Richardson JK, Hoffmann P, *et al*. Chronic anterior compartment syndrome and deep peroneal nerve function. *Clinical Journal of Sport Medicine* 2001;**11**:229–33.
45. Fronek J, Mubarak SJ, Hargens AR, *et al*. Management of chronic exertional anterior compartment syndrome of the lower extremity. *Clinical Orthopaedics and Related Research* 1987;**220**:217–27.
46. Tzortziou V, Maffulli N, Padhiar N. Diagnosis and management of chronic exertional compartment syndrome (CECS) in the United Kingdom. *Clinical Journal of Sport Medicine* 2006;**16**:209–13.

47. Detmer DE, Sharpe K, Sufit RL, Girdley FM. Chronic compartment syndrome: diagnosis, management, and outcomes. *American Journal of Sports Medicine* 1985;**13**:162–70.
48. Rorabeck CH, Bourne RB, Fowler PJ. The surgical treatment of exertional compartment syndrome in athletes. *Journal of Bone and Joint Surgery (American)* 1983;**65**:1245–51.
49. Rorabeck CH, Fowler PJ, Nott L. The results of fasciotomy in the management of chronic exertional compartment syndrome. *American Journal of Sports Medicine* 1988;**16**:224–7.
50. Slimmon D, Bennell K, Brukner P, et al. Long-term outcome of fasciotomy with partial fasciectomy for chronic exertional compartment syndrome of the lower leg. *American Journal of Sports Medicine* 2002;**30**:581–8.
51. Stein DA, Sennett BJ. One-portal endoscopically assisted fasciotomy for exertional compartment syndrome. *Arthroscopy* 2005;**21**:108–12.
52. Styf JR, Korner LM. Chronic anterior-compartment syndrome of the leg. Results of treatment by fasciotomy. *Journal of Bone and Joint Surgery (American)* 1986;**68**:1338–47.
53. Wood ML, Almekinders LC. Minimally invasive subcutaneous fasciotomy for chronic exertional compartment syndrome of the lower extremity. *American Journal of Orthopedics* 2004;**33**:42–4.
54. Almdahl SM, Samdal F. Fasciotomy for chronic compartment syndrome. *Acta Orthopaedica Scandinavica* 1989;**60**:210–11.
55. de Fijter WM, Scheltinga MR, Luiting MG. Minimally invasive fasciotomy in chronic exertional compartment syndrome and fascial hernias of the anterior lower leg: short- and long-term results. *Military Medicine* 2006;**171**:399–403.
56. Mouhsine E, Garofalo R, Moretti B, et al. Two minimal incision fasciotomy for chronic exertional compartment syndrome of the lower leg. *Knee Surgery, Sports Traumatology, Arthroscopy* 2006;**14**:193–7.
57. Schepsis AA, Gill SS, Foster TA. Fasciotomy for exertional anterior compartment syndrome: is lateral compartment release necessary? *American Journal of Sports Medicine* 1999;**27**:430–5.
58. Schepsis AA, Martini D, Corbett M. Surgical management of exertional compartment syndrome of the lower leg. Long-term followup. *American Journal of Sports Medicine* 1993;**21**:811–17.
59. Biedert RM, Marti B. Intracompartmental pressure before and after fasciotomy in runners with chronic deep posterior compartment syndrome. *International Journal of Sports Medicine* 1997;**18**:381–6.
60. Rorabeck CH. Exertional tibialis posterior compartment syndrome. *Clinical Orthopaedics and Related Research* 1986;**208**:61–4.
61. Sarrafian SK. Nerves. In: Sarrafian SK (ed.) *Anatomy of the Foot and Ankle: Descriptive, Topographic, Functional*, 2nd edn. Philadelphia, PA: J.B. Lippincott Co., 1993:356–65.
62. Aktan Ikiz ZA, Ucerler H. The distribution of the superficial peroneal nerve on the dorsum of the foot and its clinical importance in flap surgery. *Foot and Ankle International* 2006;**27**:438–44.
63. Kurtoglu Z, Aktekin M, Uluutku MH. Branching patterns of the common and superficial fibular nerves in fetus. *Clinical Anatomy* 2006;**19**:621–6.
64. Ucerler H, Ikiz AA. The variations of the sensory branches of the superficial peroneal nerve course and its clinical importance. *Foot and Ankle International* 2005;**26–11**:942–6.
65. Kitajima I, Tachibana S, Hirota Y, et al. One-portal technique of endoscopic fasciotomy: Chronic compartment syndrome of the lower leg. *Arthroscopy* 2001;**17**:33.
66. Lohrer H, Nauck T. Endoscopically assisted release for exertional compartment syndromes of the lower leg [In Process Citation]. *Archives of Orthopaedic and Trauma Surgery* 2007;**127**:827–34.
67. Leversedge FJ, Casey PJ, Seiler JG, Xerogeanes JW. Endoscopically assisted fasciotomy: description of technique and in vitro assessment of lower-leg compartment decompression. *American Journal of Sports Medicine* 2002;**30**:272–8.
68. Aprile I, Caliandro P, Giannini F, et al. Italian multicentre study of peroneal mononeuropathy at the fibular head: study design and preliminary results. *Acta Neurochir Suppl* 2005;**92**:63–8.
69. Bottomley N, Williams A, Birch R, et al. Displacement of the common peroneal nerve in posterolateral corner injuries of the knee. *Journal of Bone and Joint Surgery* 2005;**87**:1225–6.
70. Fansa H, Plogmeier K, Gonschorek A, Feistner H. Common peroneal nerve palsy caused by a ganglion. Case report. *Scandinavian Journal of Plastic and Reconstructive Surgery and Hand Surgery* 1998;**32**:425–7.
71. Krivic A, Stanec S, Zic R, et al. Lesion of the common peroneal nerve during arthroscopy. *Arthroscopy* 2003;**19**:1015–18.
72. Montgomery AS, Birch R, Malone A. Entrapment of a displaced common peroneal nerve following knee ligament reconstruction. *Journal of Bone and Joint Surgery* 2005;**87**:861–2.
73. Stoff MD, Greene AF. Common peroneal nerve palsy following inversion ankle injury: a report of two cases. *Physical Therapy* 1982;**62–10**:1463–4.
74. Vieira RL, Rosenberg ZS, Kiprovski K. MRI of the distal biceps femoris muscle: normal anatomy, variants, and association with common peroneal entrapment neuropathy. *AJR American Journal of Roentgenology* 2007;**189**:549–55.
75. Liu YH, Wang JJ, Chang CF. Common peroneal nerve palsy following a surgical procedure—a case report. *Acta Anaesthesiologica Sinica (China)* 1999;**37**:101–3.
76. Nonthasoot B, Sirichindakul B, Nivatvongs S, Sangsubhan C. Common peroneal nerve palsy: an unexpected complication of liver surgery. *Transplantation Proceedings* 2006;**38**:1396–7.
77. Colak T, Bamac B, Gonener A, et al. Comparison of nerve conduction velocities of lower extremities between runners

77. and controls. *Journal of Science and Medicine in Sport* 2005;**8**:403–10.
78. Leach RE, Purnell MB, Saito A. Peroneal nerve entrapment in runners. *American Journal of Sports Medicine* 1989;**17**:287–91.
79. Moller BN, Kadin S. Entrapment of the common peroneal nerve. *American Journal of Sports Medicine* 1987;**15**:90–1.
80. Lorei MP, Hershman EB. Peripheral nerve injuries in athletes. Treatment and prevention. *Sports Medicine* 1993;**16**:130–47.
81. Mitra A, Stern JD, Perrotta VJ, Moyer RA. Peroneal nerve entrapment in athletes. *Annals of Plastic Surgery* 1995;**35**:366–8.
82. Ryan W, Mahony N, Delaney M, et al. Relationship of the common peroneal nerve and its branches to the head and neck of the fibula. *Clinical Anatomy* 2003;**16**:501–5.
83. Sijbrandij S. Instability of the proximal tibio-fibular joint. *Acta Orthopaedica Scandinavica* 1978;**49**:621–6.
84. Thomason PA, Linson MA. Isolated dislocation of the proximal tibiofibular joint. *Journal of Trauma* 1986;**26**:192–5.
85. Levy M. Peroneal nerve palsy due to superior dislocation of the head of the fibula and shortening of the tibia (Monteggia-like fracture dislocation of the calf). *Acta Orthopaedica Scandinavica* 1975;**46**:1020–5.
86. Ishikawa H, Hirohata K. Bilateral peroneal nerve palsy secondary to posterior dislocation of the proximal tibiofibular joint in rheumatoid arthritis. *Rheumatology International* 1984;**5**:45–7.
87. Sekiya JK, Kuhn JE. Instability of the proximal tibiofibular joint. *Journal of the American Academy of Orthopaedic Surgeons* 2003;**11**:120–8.
88. O'Rourke SK, McManus F. Dislocation of the proximal tibio-fibular joint—a soccer injury? *Irish Journal of Medicine Sciences* 1982;**151**:53–4.
89. Turco VJ, Spinella AJ. Anterolateral dislocation of the head of the fibula in sports. *American Journal of Sports Medicine* 1985;**13**:209–15.
90. Ogden JA. Subluxation of the proximal tibiofibular joint. *Clinical Orthopaedics and Related Research* 1974;**101**:192–7.
91. Ogden JA. Subluxation and dislocation of the proximal tibiofibular joint. *Journal of Bone and Joint Surgery (American)* 1974;**56**:145–54.
92. Kadiyala RK, Ramirez A, Taylor AE, et al. The blood supply of the common peroneal nerve in the popliteal fossa. *Journal of Bone and Joint Surgery* 2005;**87**:337–42.
93. McCrory P, Bell S, Bradshaw C. Nerve entrapments of the lower leg, ankle and foot in sport. *Sports Medicine* 2002;**32**:371–91.
94. Fabre T, Piton C, Andre D, et al. Peroneal nerve entrapment. *Journal of Bone and Joint Surgery (American)* 1998;**80**:47–53.
95. Iverson DJ. MRI detection of cysts of the knee causing common peroneal neuropathy. *Neurology* 2005;**65-11**:1829–31.
96. Kim S, Choi JY, Huh YM, et al. Role of magnetic resonance imaging in entrapment and compressive neuropathy – what, where, and how to see the peripheral nerves on the musculoskeletal magnetic resonance image: part 1. Overview and lower extremity. *European Radiology* 2007;**17**:139–49.
97. Loredo R, Hodler J, Pedowitz R, et al. MRI of the common peroneal nerve: normal anatomy and evaluation of masses associated with nerve entrapment. *Journal of Computer Assisted Tomography* 1998;**22**:925–31.
98. Visser LH. High-resolution sonography of the common peroneal nerve: detection of intraneural ganglia. *Neurology* 2006;**67**:1473–5.
99. Femino JE JJ, Craig CL, Kuhns LR. Dynamic ultrasound of the foot and ankle: adult and pediatric applications. *Techniques in Foot and Ankle Surgery* 2007;**6**:50–61.
100. Pigott TJ, Jefferson D. Idiopathic common peroneal nerve palsy—a review of thirteen cases. *British Journal of Neurosurgery* 1991;**5**:7–11.
101. Blair JM, Botte MJ. Surgical anatomy of the superficial peroneal nerve in the ankle and foot. *Clinical Orthopaedics and Related Research* 1994;**305**:229–38.
102. Ducic I, Dellon AL, Graw KS. The clinical importance of variations in the surgical anatomy of the superficial peroneal nerve in the mid-third of the lateral leg. *Annals of Plastic Surgery* 2006;**56**:635–8.
103. Styf J. Entrapment of the superficial peroneal nerve. Diagnosis and results of decompression. *Journal of Bone and Joint Surgery* 1989;**71**:131–5.
104. Williams EH, Dellon AL. Intraseptal superficial peroneal nerve [In Process Citation]. *Microsurgery* 2007;**27**:477–80.
105. McAuliffe TB, Fiddian NJ, Browett JP. Entrapment neuropathy of the superficial peroneal nerve. A bilateral case. *Journal of Bone and Joint Surgery* 1985;**67**:62–3.
106. Sridhara CR, Izzo KL. Terminal sensory branches of the superficial peroneal nerve: an entrapment syndrome. *Archives of Physical Medicine and Rehabilitation* 1985;**66-11**:789–91.
107. Styf J, Morberg P. The superficial peroneal tunnel syndrome. Results of treatment by decompression. *Journal of Bone and Joint Surgery* 1997;**79**:801–3.
108. O'Neill PJ, Parks BG, Walsh R, et al. Excursion and strain of the superficial peroneal nerve during inversion ankle sprain. *Journal of Bone and Joint Surgery (American)* 2007;**89**:979–86.
109. Acus RW, Flanagan JP. Perineural fibrosis of superficial peroneal nerve complicating ankle sprain: a case report. *Foot and Ankle* 1991;**11**:233–5.
110. Johnston EC, Howell SJ. Tension neuropathy of the superficial peroneal nerve: associated conditions and results of release. *Foot and Ankle International* 1999;**20**:576–82.
111. Raikin SM, Rapuri VR, Vitanzo P. Bilateral simultaneous fasciotomy for chronic exertional compartment syndrome. *Foot and Ankle International* 2005;**26-12**:1007–11.
112. Schepsis AA, Fitzgerald M, Nicoletta R. Revision surgery for exertional anterior compartment syndrome of the lower

113. Izzo KL, Sridhara CR, Rosenholtz H, Lemont H. Sensory conduction studies of the branches of the superficial peroneal nerve. *Archives of Physical Medicine and Rehabilitation* 1981;**62**:24–7.
114. Leppilahti J, Puranen J, Orava S. Incidence of Achilles tendon rupture. *Acta Orthopaedica Scandinavica* 1996;**67**:277–9.
115. Nillius SA, Nilsson BE, Westlin NE. The incidence of Achilles tendon rupture. *Acta Orthopaedica Scandinavica* 1976;**47**:118–21.
116. Landvater SJ, Renstrom PA. Complete Achilles tendon ruptures. *Clinical Sports Medicine* 1992;**11**:741–58.
117. Jozsa L, Balint JB, Kannus P, et al. Distribution of blood groups in patients with tendon rupture. An analysis of 832 cases. *Journal of Bone and Joint Surgery* 1989;**71**:272–4.
118. Kannus P, Jozsa L. Histopathological changes preceding spontaneous rupture of a tendon. A controlled study of 891 patients. *Journal of Bone and Joint Surgery (American)* 1991;**73-10**:1507–25.
119. Strocchi R, De Pasquale V, Guizzardi S, et al. Human Achilles tendon: morphological and morphometric variations as a function of age. *Foot and Ankle* 1991;**12**:100–4.
120. Arner O, Lindholm A. Subcutaneous rupture of the Achilles tendon; a study of 92 cases. *Acta Chirurgica Scandinavica Supplementum* 1959;**116**(Suppl.):1–51.
121. Langerrgren C, Lindholm A. Vascular distribution in the Achilles tendon: Angiographic and micrographic study. *Acta Chirurgica Scandinavica* 1959;**116**:491–5.
122. Viidik A. Tensile strength properties of Achilles tendon systems in trained and untrained rabbits. *Acta Orthopaedica Scandinavica* 1969;**40**:261–72.
123. Waterston SW, Maffulli N, Ewen SW. Subcutaneous rupture of the Achilles tendon: basic science and some aspects of clinical practice. *British Journal of Sports Medicine* 1997;**31**:285–98.
124. Kvist H, Kvist M. The operative treatment of chronic calcaneal paratenonitis. *Journal of Bone and Joint Surgery* 1980;**62**:353–7.
125. Scott SH, Winter DA. Internal forces of chronic running injury sites. *Medicine and Science in Sports and Exercise* 1990;**22**:357–69.
126. Williams JG. Achilles tendon lesions in sport. *Sports Medicine* 1986;**3**:114–35.
127. Parry DA, Craig AS. Collagen fibrils and elastic fibers in rat-tail tendon: an electron microscopic investigation. *Biopolymers* 1978;**17**:843–5.
128. Williams JG. Achilles tendon lesions in sport. *Sports Medicine* 1993;**16**:216–20.
129. Kvist M, Jarvinen M. Clinical, histochemical and biomechanical features in repair of muscle and tendon injuries. *International Journal of Sports Medicine* 1982;**3**(Suppl.) 1:12–14.
130. Jacobs D, Martens M, Van Audekercke R, et al. Comparison of conservative and operative treatment of Achilles tendon rupture. *American Journal of Sports Medicine* 1978;**6**:107–11.
131. Fox JM, Blazina ME, Jobe FW, et al. Degeneration and rupture of the Achilles tendon. *Clinical Orthopaedics and Related Research* 1975;**107**:221–4.
132. Bleakney RR, Tallon C, Wong JK, et al. Long-term ultrasonographic features of the Achilles tendon after rupture. *Clinical Journal of Sport Medicine* 2002;**12**:273–8.
133. Enwemeka CS. The effects of therapeutic ultrasound on tendon healing. A biomechanical study. *American Journal of Physical Medicine and Rehabilitation* 1989;**68**:283–7.
134. Fukashiro S, Itoh M, Ichinose Y, et al. Ultrasonography gives directly but noninvasively elastic characteristic of human tendon in vivo. *European Journal of Applied Physiology and Occupational Physiology* 1995;**71**:555–7.
135. Knobloch K, Thermann H, Huefner T. Dynamic ultrasound as a selection tool for reducing Achilles tendon reruptures. *American Journal of Sports Medicine* 2007;**35**:150; author reply.
136. Kotnis R, David S, Handley R, et al. Dynamic ultrasound as a selection tool for reducing achilles tendon reruptures. *American Journal of Sports Medicine* 2006;**34**:1395–400.
137. Majewski M, Lehmann M, Dick W, Steinbruck K. [Value of sonography to monitor the course of Achilles tendon rupture after treatment—comparison of conservative therapy, percutaneous tendon adaptation, and open suture]. *Unfallchirurg* 2003;**106**:556–60.
138. Thermann H, Frerichs O, Holch M, Biewener A. Healing of Achilles tendon, an experimental study: part 2—Histological, immunohistological and ultrasonographic analysis. *Foot and Ankle International* 2002;**23**:606–13.
139. Weinstabl R, Stiskal M, Neuhold A, et al. Classifying calcaneal tendon injury according to MRI findings. *Journal of Bone and Joint Surgery* 1991;**73**:683–5.
140. Maffulli N. Clinical tests in sports medicine: more on Achilles tendon. *British Journal of Sports Medicine* 1996;**30**:250.
141. Simonds FA. The diagnosis of the ruptured achilles tendon. *Practitioner* 1957;**179**:56–8.
142. Thompson TC, Doherty JH. Spontaneous rupture of tendon of Achilles: a new clinical diagnostic test. *Journal of Trauma* 1962;**2**:126–9.
143. Matles AL. Rupture of the tendo Achilles. Another diagnostic sign. *Bulletin of the Hospital for Joint Diseases* 1975;**36**:48–51.
144. O'Brien T. The needle test for complete rupture of the Achilles tendon. *Journal of Bone and Joint Surgery (American)* 1984;**66**:1099–101.
145. Copeland SA. Rupture of the Achilles tendon: a new clinical test. *Annals of the Royal College of Surgeons of England* 1990;**72**:270–1.
146. Anderson MW, Ugalde V, Batt M, Gacayan J. Shin splints: MR appearance in a preliminary study. *Radiology* 1997;**204**:177–80.

147. Wapner KL, Pavlock GS, Hecht PJ, et al. Repair of chronic Achilles tendon rupture with flexor hallucis longus tendon transfer. *Foot and Ankle* 1993;**14**:443–9.
148. Klein J, Tiling T. [Tendon injuries in sports.] *Langenbecks Archiv für Chirurgie Supplement Kongressband* 1991:473–6.
149. Rowley DI, Scotland TR. Rupture of the Achilles tendon treated by a simple operative procedure. *Injury* 1982;**14**:252–4.
150. Jaakkola JI, Hutton WC, Beskin JL, Lee GP. Achilles tendon rupture repair: biomechanical comparison of the triple bundle technique versus the Krakow locking loop technique. *Foot and Ankle International* 2000;**21**:14–17.
151. Kato YP, Dunn MG, Zawadsky JP, et al. Regeneration of Achilles tendon with a collagen tendon prosthesis. Results of a one-year implantation study. *Journal of Bone and Joint Surgery (American)* 1991;**73**:561–74.
152. Hosey G, Kowalchick E, Tesoro D, et al. Comparison of the mechanical and histologic properties of Achilles tendons in New Zealand white rabbits secondarily repaired with Marlex mesh. *Journal of Foot Surgery* 1991;**30**:214–33.
153. Ozaki J, Fujiki J, Sugimoto K, et al. Reconstruction of neglected Achilles tendon rupture with Marlex mesh. *Clinical Orthopaedics and Related Research* 1989;**238**:204–8.
154. Soma CA, Mandelbaum BR. Repair of acute Achilles tendon ruptures. *Orthopedic Clinics of North America* 1995;**26**:239–47.
155. Parsons JR, Rosario A, Weiss AB, Alexander H. Achilles tendon repair with an absorbable polymer-carbon fiber composite. *Foot and Ankle* 1984;**5**:49–53.
156. Bailey AJ, Bazin S, Sims TJ, et al. Characterization of the collagen of human hypertrophic and normal scars. *Biochimica et Biophysica Acta* 1975;**405**:412–21.
157. Perugia L, Pollini PTR, Ippolito E. Ultrastructural aspects of degenerative tendinopathy. *International Orthopaedics* 1978;**1**:303–7.
158. Puddu G, Ippolito E, Postacchini F. A classification of Achilles tendon disease. *American Journal of Sports Medicine* 1976;**4**:145–50.
159. Jozsa L, Balint BJ, Reffy A, Demel Z. Fine structural alterations of collagen fibers in degenerative tendinopathy. *Archives of Orthopaedic and Trauma Surgery* 1984;**103**:47–51.
160. Williams IF, Heaton A, McCullagh KG. Cell morphology and collagen types in equine tendon scar. *Research in Veterinary Science* 1980;**28**:302–10.
161. Jozsa L, Balint BJ, Reffy A, Demel Z. Hypoxic alterations of tenocytes in degenerative tendinopathy. *Archives of Orthopaedic and Trauma Surgery* 1982;**99**:243–6.
162. Kvist MH, Lehto MU, Jozsa L, et al. Chronic achilles paratenonitis. An immunohistologic study of fibronectin and fibrinogen. *American Journal of Sports Medicine* 1988;**16**:616–23.
163. Clain MR, Baxter DE. Achilles tendinitis. *Foot and Ankle* 1992;**13**:482–7.
164. Fowler A, Phillip JF. Abnormalities of the calcaneus as a cause of painful heel: its diagnosis and operative treatment. *British Journal of Surgery* 1942;**32**:494–8.
165. Keck SW, Kelly PJ. Bursitis of the posterior part of the heel; evaluation of surgical treatment of eighteen patients. *Journal of Bone and Joint Surgery (American)* 1965;**47**:267–73.
166. Smart GW, Taunton JE, Clement DB. Achilles tendon disorders in runners—a review. *Medicine and Science in Sports and Exercise* 1980;**12**:231–43.
167. Curwin SL, Stanish WD. *Tendonitis: Its Etiology and Treatment.* Lexington, Toronto: Collamore Press, 1984.
168. Maffulli N, Dymond NP, Regine R. Surgical repair of ruptured Achilles tendon in sportsmen and sedentary patients: a longitudinal ultrasound assessment. *International Journal of Sports Medicine* 1990;**11**:78–84.
169. Panageas E, Greenberg S, Franklin PD, et al. Magnetic resonance imaging of pathologic conditions of the Achilles tendon. *Orthopedic Reviews* 1990;**19–11**:975–80.
170. Taunton JE, Clement DB, Smart GW, et al. A triplanar electrogoniometer investigation of running mechanics in runners with compensatory overpronation. *Canadian Journal of Applied Sport Sciences* 1985;**10**:104–15.
171. Niesen-Vertommen SL, Taunton JE, Clement DB, Mosher RE. The effect of eccentric versus concentric exercise in the management of Achilles tendonitis. *Clinical Journal of Sports Medicine* 1992;**2**:109–13.
172. Amiel D, Woo SL, Harwood FL, Akeson WH. The effect of immobilization on collagen turnover in connective tissue: a biochemical-biomechanical correlation. *Acta Orthopaedica Scandinavica* 1982;**53**:325–32.
173. Denstad TF, Roaas A. Surgical treatment of partial Achilles tendon rupture. *American Journal of Sports Medicine* 1979;**7**:15–17.
174. Leach RE, Schepsis AA, Takai H. Long-term results of surgical management of Achilles tendinitis in runners. *Clinical Orthopaedics and Related Research* 1992;**282**:208–12.
175. Nelen G, Martens M, Burssens A. Surgical treatment of chronic Achilles tendinitis. *American Journal of Sports Medicine* 1989;**17**:754–9.
176. Schepsis AA, Leach RE. Surgical management of Achilles tendinitis. *American Journal of Sports Medicine* 1987;**15**:308–15.
177. Bonnin M, Tavernier T, Bouysset M. Split lesions of the peroneus brevis tendon in chronic ankle laxity. *American Journal of Sports Medicine* 1997;**25**:699–703.
178. Brage ME, Hansen ST. Traumatic subluxation/dislocation of the peroneal tendons. *Foot and Ankle* 1992;**13**:423–31.
179. Brigido MK, Fessell DP, Jacobson JA, et al. Radiography and US of os peroneum fractures and associated peroneal tendon injuries: initial experience. *Radiology* 2005;**237**:235–41.
180. Ebraheim NA, Zeiss J, Skie MC, Jackson WT. Radiological evaluation of peroneal tendon pathology associated with calcaneal fractures. *Journal of Orthopaedic Trauma* 1991;**5**:365–9.

181. Ferran NA, Oliva F, Maffulli N. Recurrent subluxation of the peroneal tendons. *Sports Medicine* 2006;**36–10**:839–46.
182. Karlsson J, Eriksson BI, Sward L. Recurrent dislocation of the peroneal tendons. *Scandinavian Journal of Medicine and Science in Sports* 1996;**6**:242–6.
183. Redfern D, Myerson M. The management of concomitant tears of the peroneus longus and brevis tendons. *Foot and Ankle International* 2004;**25–10**:695–707.
184. Sammarco GJ. Peroneal tendon injuries. *Orthopedic Clinics of North America* 1994;**25**:135–45.
185. Squires N, Myerson MS, Gamba C. Surgical treatment of peroneal tendon tears [Record Supplied By Publisher]. *Foot and Ankle Clinics* 2007;**12**:675–95.
186. Geller J, Lin S, Cordas D, Vieira P. Relationship of a low-lying muscle belly to tears of the peroneus brevis tendon. *American Journal of Orthopedics* 2003;**32–11**:541–4.
187. Hammerschlag WA, Goldner JL. Chronic peroneal tendon subluxation produced by an anomalous peroneus brevis: case report and literature review. *Foot and Ankle* 1989;**10**:45–7.
188. Sobel M, Bohne WH, O'Brien SJ. Peroneal tendon subluxation in a case of anomalous peroneus brevis muscle. *Acta Orthopaedica Scandinavica* 1992;**63**:682–4.
189. Kollias SL, Ferkel RD. Fibular grooving for recurrent peroneal tendon subluxation. *American Journal of Sports Medicine* 1997;**25**:329–35.
190. Porter D, McCarroll J, Knapp E, Torma J. Peroneal tendon subluxation in athletes: fibular groove deepening and retinacular reconstruction. *Foot and Ankle International* 2005;**26**:436–41.
191. Title CI, Jung HG, Parks BG, Schon LC. The peroneal groove deepening procedure: a biomechanical study of pressure reduction. *Foot and Ankle International* 2005;**26**:442–8.
192. Zoellner G, Clancy W. Recurrent dislocation of the peroneal tendon. *Journal of Bone and Joint Surgery (American)* 1979;**61**:292–4.
193. Zammit J, Singh D. The peroneus quartus muscle. Anatomy and clinical relevance. *Journal of Bone and Joint Surgery* 2003;**85**:1134–7.
194. Adachi N, Fukuhara K, Tanaka H, et al. Superior retinaculoplasty for recurrent dislocation of peroneal tendons. *Foot and Ankle International* 2006;**27–12**:1074–8.
195. Mason RB, Henderson JP. Traumatic peroneal tendon instability. *American Journal of Sports Medicine* 1996;**24**:652–8.
196. Miyamoto W, Takao M, Komatu F, Uchio Y. Reconstruction of the superior peroneal retinaculum using an autologous gracilis tendon graft for chronic dislocation of the peroneal tendons accompanied by lateral instability of the ankle: technical note. *Knee Surgery, Sports Traumatology, Arthroscopy* 2007;**15**:461–4.
197. Grant TH, Kelikian AS, Jereb SE, McCarthy RJ. Ultrasound diagnosis of peroneal tendon tears. A surgical correlation. *Journal of Bone and Joint Surgery (American)* 2005;**87**:1788–94.
198. Khoury NJ, el-Khoury GY, Saltzman CL, Kathol MH. Peroneus longus and brevis tendon tears: MR imaging evaluation. *Radiology* 1996;**200**:833–41.
199. Magnano GM, Occhi M, Di Stadio M, et al. High-resolution US of non-traumatic recurrent dislocation of the peroneal tendons: a case report. *Pediatric Radiology* 1998;**28**:476–7.
200. Major NM, Helms CA, Fritz RC, Speer KP. The MR imaging appearance of longitudinal split tears of the peroneus brevis tendon. *Foot and Ankle International* 2000;**21**:514–19.
201. Mota J, Rosenberg ZS. Magnetic resonance imaging of the peroneal tendons. *Topics in Magnetic Resonance Imaging* 1998;**9**:273–85.
202. Neustadter J, Raikin SM, Nazarian LN. Dynamic sonographic evaluation of peroneal tendon subluxation. *AJR American Journal of Roentgenology* 2004;**183**:985–8.
203. Rosenberg ZS, Bencardino J, Astion D, et al. MRI features of chronic injuries of the superior peroneal retinaculum. *AJR American Journal of Roentgenology* 2003;**181**:1551–7.
204. Schweitzer ME, Eid ME, Deely D, et al. Using MR imaging to differentiate peroneal splits from other peroneal disorders. *AJR American Journal of Roentgenology* 1997;**168**:129–33.
205. Safran MR, O'Malley D, Fu FH. Peroneal tendon subluxation in athletes: new exam technique, case reports, and review. *Medicine and Science in Sports and Exercise* 1999;**31–7**(Suppl.):S487–S92.
206. Das De S, Balasubramaniam P. A repair operation for recurrent dislocation of peroneal tendons. *Journal of Bone and Joint Surgery* 1985;**67**:585–7.
207. Martens MA, Noyez JF, Mulier JC. Recurrent dislocation of the peroneal tendons. Results of rerouting the tendons under the calcaneofibular ligament. *American Journal of Sports Medicine* 1986;**14**:148–50.
208. Saxena A, Cassidy A. Peroneal tendon injuries: an evaluation of 49 tears in 41 patients. *Journal of Foot and Ankle Surgery* 2003;**42**:215–20.
209. Slatis P, Santavirta S, Sandelin J. Surgical treatment of chronic dislocation of the peroneal tendons. *British Journal of Sports Medicine* 1988;**22**:16–18.
210. Steel MW, De Orio JK. Peroneal tendon tears: return to sports after operative treatment. *Foot and Ankle International* 2007;**28**:49–54.
211. Steinbock G, Pinsger M. Treatment of peroneal tendon dislocation by transposition under the calcaneofibular ligament. *Foot and Ankle International* 1994;**15**:107–11.
212. Lui TH. Endoscopic peroneal retinaculum reconstruction. *Knee Surgery, Sports Traumatology, Arthroscopy* 2006;**14**:478–81.
213. van Dijk CN, Kort N. Tendoscopy of the peroneal tendons. *Arthroscopy* 1998;**14**:471–8.
214. Petersen W, Hohmann G, Stein V, Tillmann B. The blood supply of the posterior tibial tendon. *Journal of Bone and Joint Surgery* 2002;**84**:141–4.
215. Conti SF. Posterior tibial tendon problems in athletes. *Orthopedic Clinics of North America* 1994;**25**:109–21.
216. McCormack AP, Varner KE, Marymont JV. Surgical treatment for posterior tibial tendonitis in young

competitive athletes. *Foot and Ankle International* 2003;**24**:535–8.
217. Porter DA, Baxter DE, Clanton TO, Klootwyk TE. Posterior tibial tendon tears in young competitive athletes: two case reports. *Foot and Ankle International* 1998;**19**:627–30.
218. Woods L, Leach RE. Posterior tibial tendon rupture in athletic people. *American Journal of Sports Medicine* 1991;**19**:495–8.
219. Arai K, Ringleb SI, Zhao KD, et al. The effect of flatfoot deformity and tendon loading on the work of friction measured in the posterior tibial tendon. *Clinical Biomechanics (Bristol)* 2007;**22**:592–8.
220. Uchiyama E, Kitaoka HB, Fujii T, et al. Gliding resistance of the posterior tibial tendon. *Foot and Ankle International* 2006;**27**:723–7.
221. Saltzman CL, el-Khoury GY. The hindfoot alignment view. *Foot and Ankle International* 1995;**16**:572–6.
222. Khoury NJ, el-Khoury GY, Saltzman CL, Brandser EA. MR imaging of posterior tibial tendon dysfunction. *AJR American Journal of Roentgenology* 1996;**167**:675–82.
223. Miller SD, Van Holsbeeck M, Boruta PM, et al. Ultrasound in the diagnosis of posterior tibial tendon pathology. *Foot and Ankle International* 1996;**17**:555–8.
224. Ross JA. Posterior tibial tendon dysfunction in the athlete. *Clinics in Podiatric Medicine and Surgery* 1997;**14**:479–88.
225. Raikin SM, Parks BG, Noll KH, Schon LC. Biomechanical evaluation of the ability of casts and braces to immobilize the ankle and hindfoot. *Foot and Ankle International* 2001;**22**:214–9.
226. Bulstra GH, Olsthoorn PG, Niek van Dijk C. Tendoscopy of the posterior tibial tendon. *Foot and Ankle Clinics* 2006;**11**:421–iii.
227. Bernt AL, Harty, M. Transchondral fractures (osteochondritis dissecans) of the talus. *Journal of Bone and Joint Surgery* 1959;**41–A**:988.
228. Loomer R, Fisher C, Lloyd-Smith R, et al. Osteochondral lesions of the talus. *American Journal of Sports Medicine* 1993;**21**:13–19.
229. Taranow WS, Bisignani GA, Towers JD, Conti SF. Retrograde drilling of osteochondral lesions of the medial talar dome. *Foot and Ankle International* 1999;**20**:474–80.
230. Raikin SM, Elias I, Zoga AC, et al. Osteochondral lesions of the talus: localization and morphologic data from 424 patients using a novel anatomical grid scheme. *Foot and Ankle International* 2007;**28**:154–61.
231. Tochigi Y, Amendola A, Muir D, Saltzman C. Surgical approach for centrolateral talar osteochondral lesions with an anterolateral osteotomy. *Foot and Ankle International* 2002;**23–11**:1038–9.
232. Verhagen RA, Maas M, Dijkgraaf MG, et al. Prospective study on diagnostic strategies in osteochondral lesions of the talus. Is MRI superior to helical CT? *Journal of Bone and Joint Surgery* 2005;**87**:41–6.
233. Sisler J. Radiographic imaging of the post traumatic chronic tarsal pain. *Clinical Journal of Sports Medicine* 1989;**1**:67–70.
234. Stroud CC, Marks RM. Imaging of osteochondral lesions of the talus. *Foot and Ankle Clinics* 2000;**5**:119–33.
235. Mintz DN, Tashjian GS, Connell DA, et al. Osteochondral lesions of the talus: a new magnetic resonance grading system with arthroscopic correlation. *Arthroscopy* 2003;**19**:353–9.
236. Elias I, Jung JW, Raikin SM, et al. Osteochondral lesions of the talus: change in MRI findings over time in talar lesions without operative intervention and implications for staging systems. *Foot and Ankle International* 2006;**27**:157–66.
237. Barnes CJ, Ferkel RD. Arthroscopic debridement and drilling of osteochondral lesions of the talus. *Foot and Ankle Clinics* 2003;**8**:243–57.
238. Thermann H, Becher C. [Microfracture technique for treatment of osteochondral and degenerative chondral lesions of the talus. 2-year results of a prospective study]. *Unfallchirurg* 2004;**107**:27–32.
239. Al-Shaikh RA, Chou LB, Mann JA, et al. Autologous osteochondral grafting for talar cartilage defects. *Foot and Ankle International* 2002;**23**:381–9.
240. Assenmacher JA, Kelikian AS, Gottlob C, Kodros S. Arthroscopically assisted autologous osteochondral transplantation for osteochondral lesions of the talar dome: an MRI and clinical follow-up study. *Foot and Ankle International* 2001;**22**:544–51.
241. Giannini S, Buda R, Grigolo B, Vannini F. Autologous chondrocyte transplantation in osteochondral lesions of the ankle joint. *Foot and Ankle International* 2001;**22**:513–17.
242. Hangody L. The mosaicplasty technique for osteochondral lesions of the talus. *Foot and Ankle Clinics* 2003;**8**:259–73.
243. Hangody L, Kish G, Karpati Z, et al. Treatment of osteochondritis dissecans of the talus: use of the mosaicplasty technique—a preliminary report. *Foot and Ankle International* 1997;**18–10**:628–34.
244. Hangody L, Kish G, Modis L, et al. Mosaicplasty for the treatment of osteochondritis dissecans of the talus: two to seven year results in 36 patients. *Foot and Ankle International* 2001;**22**:552–8.
245. Kreuz PC, Steinwachs M, Erggelet C, et al. Mosaicplasty with autogenous talar autograft for osteochondral lesions of the talus after failed primary arthroscopic management: a prospective study with a 4-year follow-up. *American Journal of Sports Medicine* 2006;**34**:55–63.
246. Lee CH, Chao KH, Huang GS, Wu SS. Osteochondral autografts for osteochondritis dissecans of the talus. *Foot and Ankle International* 2003;**24–11**:815–22.
247. Reddy S, Pedowitz DI, Parekh SG, et al. The morbidity associated with osteochondral harvest from asymptomatic knees for the treatment of osteochondral lesions of the talus. *American Journal of Sports Medicine* 2007;**35**:80–5.
248. Frey C, Feder KS, Di Giovanni C. Arthroscopic evaluation of the subtalar joint: does sinus tarsi syndrome exist? *Foot and Ankle International* 1999;**20**:185–91.
249. Meislin RJ, Rose DJ, Parisien JS, Springer S. Arthroscopic treatment of synovial impingement of the ankle. *American Journal of Sports Medicine* 1993;**21**:186–9.

250. Oloff LM, Schulhofer SD, Bocko AP. Subtalar joint arthroscopy for sinus tarsi syndrome: a review of 29 cases. *Journal of Foot and Ankle Surgery* 2001;**40**:152–7.
251. Tasto JP. Arthroscopy of the subtalar joint and arthroscopic subtalar arthrodesis. *Instruction Course Lectures* 2006;**55**:555–64.
252. Tol JL, van Dijk CN. Anterior ankle impingement. *Foot and Ankle Clinics* 2006;**11**:297.
253. Henderson I, La Valette D. Ankle impingement: combined anterior and posterior impingement syndrome of the ankle. *Foot and Ankle International* 2004;**25**:632–8.
254. Tol JL, van Dijk CN. Etiology of the anterior ankle impingement syndrome: a descriptive anatomical study. *Foot and Ankle International* 2004;**25**:382–6.
255. Ferkel RD, Karzel RP, Del Pizzo W, et al. Arthroscopic treatment of anterolateral impingement of the ankle. *American Journal of Sports Medicine* 1991;**19**:440–6.
256. Akseki D, Pinar H, Bozkurt M, et al. The distal fascicle of the anterior inferior tibio-fibular ligament as a cause of anterolateral ankle impingement: results of arthroscopic resection. *Acta Orthopaedica Scandinavica* 1999;**70**:478–82.
257. Bassett FH, Gates HS, Billys JB, et al. Talar impingement by the anteroinferior tibiofibular ligament. A cause of chronic pain in the ankle after inversion sprain. *Journal of Bone and Joint Surgery (American)* 1990;**72**:55–9.
258. van den Bekerom MP, Raven EE. The distal fascicle of the anterior inferior tibiofibular ligament as a cause of tibiotalar impingement syndrome: a current concepts review. *Knee Surgery, Sports Traumatology, Arthroscopy* 2007;**15**:465–71.
259. Nihal A, Rose DJ, Trepman E. Arthroscopic treatment of anterior ankle impingement syndrome in dancers. *Foot and Ankle International* 2005;**26–11**:908–12.
260. Tol JL, Verheyen CP, van Dijk CN. Arthroscopic treatment of anterior impingement in the ankle. *Journal of Bone and Joint Surgery* 2001;**83**:9–13.
261. van Dijk CN, Tol JL, Verheyen CC. A prospective study of prognostic factors concerning the outcome of arthroscopic surgery for anterior ankle impingement. *American Journal of Sports Medicine* 1997;**25**:737–45.
262. Tol JL, Slim E, van Soest AJ, van Dijk CN. The relationship of the kicking action in soccer and anterior ankle impingement syndrome. A biomechanical analysis. *American Journal of Sports Medicine* 2002;**30**:45–50.
263. Fallat L, Grimm DJ, Saracco JA. Sprained ankle syndrome: prevalence and analysis of 639 acute injuries. *Journal of Foot and Ankle Surgery* 1998;**37**:280–5.
264. Liu SH, Nuccion SL, Finerman G. Diagnosis of anterolateral ankle impingement. Comparison between magnetic resonance imaging and clinical examination. *American Journal of Sports Medicine* 1997;**25**:389–93.
265. Hauger O, Moinard M, Lasalarie JC, et al. Anterolateral compartment of the ankle in the lateral impingement syndrome: appearance on CT arthrography. *AJR American Journal of Roentgenology* 1999;**173**:685–90.
266. Lee JW, Suh JS, Huh YM, et al. Soft tissue impingement syndrome of the ankle: diagnostic efficacy of MRI and clinical results after arthroscopic treatment. *Foot and Ankle International* 2004;**25–12**:896–902.
267. Robinson P, White LM, Salonen DC, et al. Anterolateral ankle impingement: MR arthrographic assessment of the anterolateral recess. *Radiology* 2001;**221**:186–90.
268. Haller J, Bernt R, Seeger T, et al. MR-imaging of anterior tibiotalar impingement syndrome: agreement, sensitivity and specificity of MR-imaging and indirect MR-arthrography. *European Journal Radiology* 2006;**58**:450–60.
269. Zwipp H, Swoboda B, Holch M, et al. [Sinus tarsi and canalis tarsi syndromes. A post-traumatic entity]. *Unfallchirurg* 1991;**94–12**:608–13.
270. Robinson P. Impingement syndromes of the ankle [epub ahead of print] [Record Supplied By Publisher]. *European Radiology* 2007.
271. Shetty M, Fessell DP, Femino JE, et al. Sonography of ankle tendon impingement with surgical correlation. *AJR American Journal of Roentgenology* 2002;**179**:949–53.
272. Tol JL, Verhagen RA, Krips R, et al. The anterior ankle impingement syndrome: diagnostic value of oblique radiographs. *Foot and Ankle International* 2004;**25**:63–8.
273. van Dijk CN, Wessel RN, Tol JL, Maas M. Oblique radiograph for the detection of bone spurs in anterior ankle impingement. *Skeletal Radiology* 2002;**31**:214–21.
274. Molloy S, Solan MC, Bendall SP. Synovial impingement in the ankle. A new physical sign. *Journal of Bone and Joint Surgery* 2003;**85**:330–3.
275. De Berardino TM, Arciero RA, Taylor DC. Arthroscopic treatment of soft-tissue impingement of the ankle in athletes. *Arthroscopy* 1997;**13**:492–8.
276. Hassan AH. Treatment of anterolateral impingements of the ankle joint by arthroscopy [In Process Citation]. *Knee Surgery, Sports Traumatology, Arthroscopy* 2007;**15**:1150–4.
277. Kim SH, Ha KI. Arthroscopic treatment for impingement of the anterolateral soft tissues of the ankle. *Journal of Bone and Joint Surgery* 2000;**82**:1019–21.
278. Liu SH, Raskin A, Osti L, et al. Arthroscopic treatment of anterolateral ankle impingement. *Arthroscopy* 1994;**10**:215–18.
279. Urguden M, Soyuncu Y, Ozdemir H, et al. Arthroscopic treatment of anterolateral soft tissue impingement of the ankle: evaluation of factors affecting outcome. *Arthroscopy* 2005;**21**:317–22.
280. Michelson J, Dunn L. Tenosynovitis of the flexor hallucis longus: a clinical study of the spectrum of presentation and treatment. *Foot and Ankle International* 2005;**26**:291–303.
281. Paterson RS, Brown JN. The posteromedial impingement lesion of the ankle. A series of six cases. *American Journal of Sports Medicine* 2001;**29**:550–7.
282. Gould N. Stenosing tenosynovitis of the flexor hallucis longus tendon at the great toe. *Foot and Ankle* 1981;**2**:46–8.
283. Hamilton WG. Stenosing tenosynovitis of the flexor hallucis longus tendon and posterior impingement upon the os trigonum in ballet dancers. *Foot and Ankle* 1982;**3**:74–80.

284. Kolettis GJ, Micheli LJ, Klein JD. Release of the flexor hallucis longus tendon in ballet dancers. *Journal of Bone and Joint Surgery (American)* 1996;**78**:1386–90.
285. Sammarco GJ, Cooper PS. Flexor hallucis longus tendon injury in dancers and nondancers. *Foot and Ankle International* 1998;**19**:356–62.
286. Mouhsine E, Crevoisier X, Leyvraz PF, et al. Post-traumatic overload or acute syndrome of the os trigonum: a possible cause of posterior ankle impingement. *Knee Surgery, Sports Traumatology, Arthroscopy* 2004;**12**:250–3.
287. Bureau NJ, Cardinal E, Hobden R, Aubin B. Posterior ankle impingement syndrome: MR imaging findings in seven patients. *Radiology* 2000;**215**:497–503.
288. Fiorella D, Helms CA, Nunley JA. The MR imaging features of the posterior intermalleolar ligament in patients with posterior impingement syndrome of the ankle. *Skeletal Radiology* 1999;**28-10**:573–6.
289. Masciocchi C, Catalucci A, Barile A. Ankle impingement syndromes. *European Journal Radiology* 1998;**27**(Suppl. 1):S70–3.
290. Peace KA, Hillier JC, Hulme A, Healy JC. MRI features of posterior ankle impingement syndrome in ballet dancers: a review of 25 cases. *Clinical Radiology* 2004;**59-11**:1025–33.
291. Robinson P, Bollen SR. Posterior ankle impingement in professional soccer players: effectiveness of sonographically guided therapy. *AJR American Journal of Roentgenology* 2006;**187**:W53–8.
292. Jones DM, Saltzman CL, El-Khoury G. The diagnosis of the os trigonum syndrome with a fluoroscopically controlled injection of local anesthetic. *Iowa Orthopedic Journal* 1999;**19**:122–6.
293. Abramowitz Y, Wollstein R, Barzilay Y, et al. Outcome of resection of a symptomatic os trigonum. *Journal of Bone and Joint Surgery (American)* 2003;**85-A-6**:1051–7.
294. Hedrick MR, McBryde AM. Posterior ankle impingement. *Foot and Ankle International* 1994;**15**:2–8.
295. Jourdel F, Tourne Y, Saragaglia D. [Posterior ankle impingement syndrome: a retrospective study in 21 cases treated surgically]. *Revue de Chirurgie Orthopédique et Réparatrice de l'Appareil Moteur* 2005;**91**:239–47.
296. Marumoto JM, Ferkel RD. Arthroscopic excision of the os trigonum: a new technique with preliminary clinical results. *Foot and Ankle International* 1997;**18-12**:777–84.
297. Phisitkul P JJ, Femino JE, Saltzman CL, Amendola A. Technique of prone ankle and subtalar arthropscopy. *Techniques in Foot and Ankle Surgery* 2007;**6**:30–7.
298. van Dijk CN, Scholten PE, Krips R. A 2-portal endoscopic approach for diagnosis and treatment of posterior ankle pathology. *Arthroscopy* 2000;**16**:871–6.
299. Hamilton WG, Geppert MJ, Thompson FM. Pain in the posterior aspect of the ankle in dancers. Differential diagnosis and operative treatment. *Journal of Bone and Joint Surgery (American)* 1996;**78-10**:1491–500.
300. Fujii T, Kitaoka HB, Luo ZP, et al. Analysis of ankle-hindfoot stability in multiple planes: an in vitro study. *Foot and Ankle International* 2005;**26**:633–7.
301. Rasmussen O, Tovborg-Jensen I. Anterolateral rotational instability in the ankle joint. An experimental study of anterolateral rotational instability, talar tilt, and anterior drawer sign in relation to injuries to the lateral ligaments. *Acta Orthopaedica Scandinavica* 1981;**52**:99–102.
302. Frost SC, Amendola A. Is stress radiography necessary in the diagnosis of acute or chronic ankle instability? *Clinical Journal of Sport Medicine* 1999;**9**:40–5.
303. Lofvenberg R, Karrholm J, Sundelin G, Ahlgren O. Prolonged reaction time in patients with chronic lateral instability of the ankle. *American Journal of Sports Medicine* 1995;**23**:414–17.
304. Van Deun S, Staes FF, Stappaerts KH, et al. Relationship of chronic ankle instability to muscle activation patterns during the transition from double-leg to single-leg stance. *American Journal of Sports Medicine* 2007;**35**:274–81.
305. Fortin PT, Guettler J, Manoli A. Idiopathic cavovarus and lateral ankle instability: recognition and treatment implications relating to ankle arthritis. *Foot and Ankle International* 2002;**23-11**:1031–7.
306. Larsen E, Angermann P. Association of ankle instability and foot deformity. *Acta Orthopaedica Scandinavica* 1990;**61**:136–9.
307. Ferkel RD, Chams RN. Chronic lateral instability: arthroscopic findings and long-term results. *Foot and Ankle International* 2007;**28**:24–31.
308. Digiovanni BF, Fraga CJ, Cohen BE, Shereff MJ. Associated injuries found in chronic lateral ankle instability. *Foot and Ankle International* 2000;**21-10**:809–15.
309. Strauss JE, Forsberg JA, Lippert FG. Chronic lateral ankle instability and associated conditions: a rationale for treatment [In Process Citation]. *Foot and Ankle International* 2007;**28-10**:1041–4.
310. Helgason JW, Chandnani VP. MR arthrography of the ankle. *Radiologic Clinics of North America* 1998;**36**:729–38.
311. Kanbe K, Hasegawa A, Nakajima Y, Takagishi K. The relationship of the anterior drawer sign to the shape of the tibial plafond in chronic lateral instability of the ankle. *Foot and Ankle International* 2002;**23**:118–22.
312. Kemen M, Ernst R, Bauer KH, et al. [Sonographic versus radiological assessment of chronic outer ligament instability of the upper ankle joint]. *Unfallchirurg* 1991;**94-12**:614–18.
313. Seligson D, Gassman J, Pope M. Ankle instability: evaluation of the lateral ligaments. *American Journal of Sports Medicine* 1980;**8**:39–42.
314. Mohammadi F. Comparison of 3 preventive methods to reduce the recurrence of ankle inversion sprains in male soccer players. *American Journal of Sports Medicine* 2007;**35**:922–6.
315. Surve I, Schwellnus MP, Noakes T, Lombard C. A fivefold reduction in the incidence of recurrent ankle sprains in soccer players using the Sport-Stirrup orthosis. *American Journal of Sports Medicine* 1994;**22**:601–6.

316. Sharpe SR, Knapik J, Jones B. Ankle braces effectively reduce recurrence of ankle sprains in female soccer players [Record Supplied By Publisher]. *Journal of Athletic Training* 1997;**32**:21–4.
317. Fujii T, Kitaoka HB, Watanabe K, et al. Comparison of modified Brostrom and Evans procedures in simulated lateral ankle injury. *Medicine and Science in Sports and Exercise* 2006;**38**:1025–31.
318. Karlsson J, Bergsten T, Lansinger O, Peterson L. Lateral instability of the ankle treated by the Evans procedure. A long-term clinical and radiological follow-up. *Journal of Bone and Joint Surgery* 1988;**70**:476–80.
319. Korkala O, Sorvali T, Niskanen R, et al. Twenty-year results of the Evans operation for lateral instability of the ankle. *Clinical Orthopaedics and Related Research* 2002;**405**:195–8.
320. Lucht U, Vang PS, Termansen NB. Lateral ligament reconstruction of the ankle with a modified Watson-Jones operation. *Acta Orthopaedica Scandinavica* 1981;**52**:363–6.
321. Krips R, van Dijk CN, Halasi PT, et al. Long-term outcome of anatomical reconstruction versus tenodesis for the treatment of chronic anterolateral instability of the ankle joint: a multicenter study. *Foot and Ankle International* 2001;**22**:415–21.
322. Brostrom L. Sprained ankles. VI. Surgical treatment of 'chronic' ligament ruptures. *Acta Chirurgica Scandinavica* 1966;**132**:551–65.
323. Gould N, Seligson D, Gassman J. Early and late repair of lateral ligament of the ankle. *Foot and Ankle* 1980;**1**:84–9.
324. Hamilton WG, Thompson FM, Snow SW. The modified Brostrom procedure for lateral ankle instability. *Foot and Ankle* 1993;**14**:1–7.
325. Ahlgren O, Larsson S. Reconstruction for lateral ligament injuries of the ankle. *Journal of Bone and Joint Surgery* 1989;**71**:300–3.
326. Ajis A, Younger AS, Maffulli N. Anatomic repair for chronic lateral ankle instability. *Foot and Ankle Clinics* 2006;**11**:539–45.
327. Caprio A, Oliva F, Treia F, Maffulli N. Reconstruction of the lateral ankle ligaments with allograft in patients with chronic ankle instability. *Foot and Ankle Clinics* 2006;**11**:597–605.
328. Karlsson J, Bergsten T, Lansinger O, Peterson L. Reconstruction of the lateral ligaments of the ankle for chronic lateral instability. *Journal of Bone and Joint Surgery (American)* 1988;**70**:581–8.
329. Karlsson J, Eriksson BI, Bergsten T, et al. Comparison of two anatomic reconstructions for chronic lateral instability of the ankle joint. *American Journal of Sports Medicine* 1997;**25**:48–53.
330. Coughlin MJ, Schenck RC, Grebing BR, Treme G. Comprehensive reconstruction of the lateral ankle for chronic instability using a free gracilis graft. *Foot and Ankle International* 2004;**25**:231–41.
331. Girard P, Anderson RB, Davis WH, et al. Clinical evaluation of the modified Brostrom-Evans procedure to restore ankle stability. *Foot and Ankle International* 1999;**20**:246–52.
332. Sammarco GJ, Di Raimondo CV. Surgical treatment of lateral ankle instability syndrome. *American Journal of Sports Medicine* 1988;**16**:501–11.
333. Sammarco GJ, Idusuyi OB. Reconstruction of the lateral ankle ligaments using a split peroneus brevis tendon graft. *Foot and Ankle International* 1999;**20**:97–103.
334. Kuhn MA, Lippert FG. Revision lateral ankle reconstruction. *Foot and Ankle International* 2006;**27**:77–81.
335. Van Bergeyk AB, Younger A, Carson B. CT analysis of hindfoot alignment in chronic lateral ankle instability. *Foot and Ankle International* 2002;**23**:37–42.
336. Vienne P, Schoniger R, Helmy N, Espinosa N. Hindfoot instability in cavovarus deformity: static and dynamic balancing. *Foot and Ankle International* 2007;**28**:96–102.
337. Csizy M, Hintermann B. [Dwyer osteotomy with or without lateral stabilization in calcaneus varus with lateral ligament insufficiency of the upper ankle joint]. *Sportverletz Sportschaden* 1996;**10**:100–2.
338. Lofvenberg R, Karrholm J, Lund B. The outcome of nonoperated patients with chronic lateral instability of the ankle: a 20-year follow-up study. *Foot and Ankle International* 1994;**15**:165–9.
339. Gerber JP, Williams GN, Scoville CR, et al. Persistent disability associated with ankle sprains: a prospective examination of an athletic population. *Foot and Ankle International* 1998;**19–10**:653–60.
340. Boytim MJ, Fischer DA, Neumann L. Syndesmotic ankle sprains. *American Journal of Sports Medicine* 1991;**19**:294–8.
341. Hopkinson WJ, St Pierre P, Ryan JB, Wheeler JH. Syndesmosis sprains of the ankle. *Foot and Ankle* 1990;**10**:325–30.
342. Taylor DC, Englehardt DL, Bassett FH. Syndesmosis sprains of the ankle. The influence of heterotopic ossification. *American Journal of Sports Medicine* 1992;**20**:146–50.
343. Wright RW, Barile RJ, Surprenant DA, Matava MJ. Ankle syndesmosis sprains in national hockey league players. *American Journal of Sports Medicine* 2004;**32**:1941–5.
344. Nussbaum ED, Hosea TM, Sieler SD, et al. Prospective evaluation of syndesmotic ankle sprains without diastasis. *American Journal of Sports Medicine* 2001;**29**:31–5.
345. Teitz CC, Harrington RM. A biochemical analysis of the squeeze test for sprains of the syndesmotic ligaments of the ankle. *Foot and Ankle International* 1998;**19**:489–92.
346. Vogl TJ, Hochmuth K, Diebold T, et al. Magnetic resonance imaging in the diagnosis of acute injured distal tibiofibular syndesmosis. *Investigative Radiology* 1997;**32**:401–9.
347. Williams GN, Jones MH, Amendola A. Syndesmotic ankle sprains in athletes. *American Journal of Sports Medicine* 2007;**35**:1197–207.
348. Lin CF, Gross ML, Weinhold P. Ankle syndesmosis injuries: anatomy, biomechanics, mechanism of injury, and clinical guidelines for diagnosis and intervention. *Journal of Orthopaedic and Sports Physical Therapy* 2006;**36**:372–84.

349. Tochigi Y, Yoshinaga K, Wada Y, Moriya H. Acute inversion injury of the ankle: magnetic resonance imaging and clinical outcomes. *Foot and Ankle International* 1998;**19–11**:730–4.
350. Song SJ, Lee S, O'Malley MJ, et al. Deltoid ligament strain after correction of acquired flatfoot deformity by triple arthrodesis. *Foot and Ankle International* 2000;**21**:573–7.
351. Egol KA, Parisien JS. Impingement syndrome of the ankle caused by a medial meniscoid lesion. *Arthroscopy* 1997;**13**:522–5.
352. Curtis MJ, Myerson M, Szura B. Tarsometatarsal joint injuries in the athlete. *American Journal of Sports Medicine* 1993;**21**:497–502.
353. de Palma L, Santucci A, Sabetta SP, Rapali S. Anatomy of the Lisfranc joint complex. *Foot and Ankle International* 1997;**18**:356–64.
354. Myerson M, Fisher RT, Brugess AR, Kenzora JE. Fracture dislocations of the tarsometatarsal joints: end results correlated with pathology and treatment. *Foot and Ankle* 1986;**6**:225–42.
355. Kaar S, Femino J, Morag Y. Lisfranc joint displacement following sequential ligament sectioning [In Process Citation]. *Journal of Bone and Joint Surgery (American)* 2007;**89-10**:2225–32.
356. Nunley JA, Vertullo CJ. Classification, investigation, and management of midfoot sprains: Lisfranc injuries in the athlete. *American Journal of Sports Medicine* 2002;**30**:871–8.
357. Faciszewski T, Burks RT, Manaster BJ. Subtle injuries of the Lisfranc joint. *Journal of Bone and Joint Surgery (American)* 1990;**72-10**:1519–22.
358. Goossens M, De Stoop N. Lisfranc's fracture-dislocations: etiology, radiology, and results of treatment. A review of 20 cases. *Clinical Orthopaedics and Related Research* 1983;**176**:154–62.
359. Coss HS, Manos RE, Buoncristiani A, Mills WJ. Abduction stress and AP weightbearing radiography of purely ligamentous injury in the tarsometatarsal joint. *Foot and Ankle International* 1998;**19**:537–41.
360. Granberry WM LP. Dislocation of the tarsometatarsal joints. *Surgery, Gynecology and Obstetrics* 1962;**114**:467–9.
361. Hardcastle PH, Reschauer R, Kutscha-Lissberg E, Schoffmann W. Injuries to the tarsometatarsal joint. Incidence, classification and treatment. *Journal of Bone and Joint Surgery* 1982;**64**:349–56.
362. Arntz CT HS. Dislocations and fracture dislocations of the tarsometatarsal joints. *Orthopedic Clinics of North America* 1987;**18**:105–14.
363. Willpppula E. Tarsometatarsal fracture-dislocation. *Acta Orthopaedica. Scandinavica.* 1973;**44**:335–45.
364. Coetzee JC, Ly TV. Treatment of primarily ligamentous Lisfranc joint injuries: primary arthrodesis compared with open reduction and internal fixation. Surgical technique. *Journal of Bone and Joint Surgery (American)* 2007;**89**(Suppl. 2 Pt.1):122–7.
365. Jones MH, Amendola AS. Navicular stress fractures. *Clinical Sports Medicine* 2006;**25**:151.
366. Maquirriain J, Ghisi JP. The incidence and distribution of stress fractures in elite tennis players. *British Journal of Sports Medicine* 2006;**40**:454–9.
367. Bennell KL, Brukner PD. Epidemiology and site specificity of stress fractures. *Clinical Sports Medicine* 1997;**16**:179–96.
368. Boden BP, Osbahr DC. High-risk stress fractures: evaluation and treatment. *Journal of the American Academy of Orthopaedic Surgeons* 2000;**8**:344–53.
369. Goergen TG, Venn-Watson EA, Rossman DJ, et al. Tarsal navicular stress fractures in runners. *AJR American Journal of Roentgenology* 1981;**136**:201–3.
370. Di Giovanni CW. Fractures of the navicular. *Foot and Ankle Clinics* 2004;**9**:25–63.
371. Bojanic I, Pecina MM. [Conservative treatment of stress fractures of the tarsal navicular in athletes]. *Rev Chir Orthop Reparatrice Appar Mot* 1997;**83**:133–8.
372. Burne SG, Mahoney CM, Forster BB, et al. Tarsal navicular stress injury: long-term outcome and clinicoradiological correlation using both computed tomography and magnetic resonance imaging. *American Journal of Sports Medicine* 2005;**33-12**:1875–81.
373. Khan KM, Brukner PD, Kearney C, et al. Tarsal navicular stress fracture in athletes. *Sports Medicine* 1994;**17**:65–76.
374. Pavlov H, Torg JS, Freiberger RH. Tarsal navicular stress fractures: radiographic evaluation. *Radiology* 1983;**148**:641–5.
375. Saillant G, Noat M, Benazet JP, Roy-Camille R. [Stress fractures of the tarsal navicular. Apropos of 20 cases]. *Revue de Chirurgie Orthopédique et Réparatrice de l'Appareil Moteur* 1992;**78**:566–73.
376. Saxena A, Fullem B, Hannaford D. Results of treatment of 22 navicular stress fractures and a new proposed radiographic classification system. *Journal of Foot and Ankle Surgery* 2000;**39**:96–103.
377. Kiss ZS, Khan KM, Fuller PJ. Stress fractures of the tarsal navicular bone: CT findings in 55 cases. *AJR American Journal of Roentgenology* 1993;**160**:111–15.
378. Lee S, Anderson RB. Stress fractures of the tarsal navicular. *Foot and Ankle Clinics* 2004;**9**:85–104.
379. Saxena A, Fullem B. Navicular stress fractures: a prospective study on athletes. *Foot and Ankle International* 2006;**27–11**:917–21.
380. Khan KM, Fuller PJ, Brukner PD, et al. Outcome of conservative and surgical management of navicular stress fracture in athletes. Eighty-six cases proven with computerized tomography. *American Journal of Sports Medicine* 1992;**20**:657–66.
381. Potter NJ, Brukner PD, Makdissi M, et al. Navicular stress fractures: outcomes of surgical and conservative management. *British Journal of Sports Medicine* 2006;**40**:692–5.
382. Fitch KD, Blackwell JB, Gilmour WN. Operation for non-union of stress fracture of the tarsal navicular. *Journal of Bone and Joint Surgery* 1989;**71**:105–10.

383. Quill GJ. Fractures of the proximal fifth metatarsal. *Orthopaedic Clinics of North America* 1995;**26**:353-61.
384. Lawrence SJ, Botte MJ. Jones' fractures and related fractures of the proximal fifth metatarsal. *Foot and Ankle* 1993;**14**:358-65.
385. Jones R. Fracture of the base of the fifth metatarsal bone by indirect violence. *Annals of Surgery* 1902;**35**:697-700.
386. Torg JS, Balduini FC, Zelko RR, et al. Fractures of the base of the fifth metatarsal distal to the tuberosity. Classification and guidelines for non-surgical and surgical management. *Journal of Bone and Joint Surgery (American)* 1984;**66**:209-14.
387. Kavanaugh JH, Brower TD, Mann RV. The Jones fracture revisited. *Journal of Bone and Joint Surgery (American)* 1978;**60**:776-82.
388. O'Malley MJ, Hamilton WG, Munyak J. Fractures of the distal shaft of the fifth metatarsal. 'Dancer's fracture'. *American Journal of Sports Medicine* 1996;**24**:240-3.
389. Richli WR, Rosenthal DI. Avulsion fracture of the fifth metatarsal: experimental study of pathomechanics. *AJR American Journal of Roentgenology* 1984;**143**:889-91.
390. Theodorou DJ, Theodorou SJ, Boutin RD, et al. Stress fractures of the lateral metatarsal bones in metatarsus adductus foot deformity: a previously unrecognized association. *Skeletal Radiology* 1999;**28-12**:679-84.
391. Weinfeld SB, Haddad SL, Myerson MS. Metatarsal stress fractures. *Clinical Sports Medicine* 1997;**16**:319-38.
392. Vertullo CJ, Glisson RR, Nunley JA. Torsional strains in the proximal fifth metatarsal: implications for Jones and stress fracture management. *Foot and Ankle International* 2004;**25**:650-6.
393. Rosenberg GA, Sferra JJ. Treatment strategies for acute fractures and nonunions of the proximal fifth metatarsal. *Journal of the American Academy of Orthopaedic Surgeons* 2000;**8**:332-8.
394. De Lee JC, Evans JP, Julian J. Stress fracture of the fifth metatarsal. *American Journal of Sports Medicine* 1983;**11**:349-53.
395. Josefsson PO, Karlsson M, Redlund-Johnell I, Wendeberg B. Closed treatment of Jones fracture. Good results in 40 cases after 11-26 years. *Acta Orthopaedica Scandinavica* 1994;**65**:545-7.
396. Lehman RC, Torg JS, Pavlov H, De Lee JC. Fractures of the base of the fifth metatarsal distal to the tuberosity: a review. *Foot and Ankle* 1987;**7**:245-52.
397. Porter DA, Duncan M, Meyer SJ. Fifth metatarsal Jones fracture fixation with a 4.5-mm cannulated stainless steel screw in the competitive and recreational athlete: a clinical and radiographic evaluation. *American Journal of Sports Medicine* 2005;**33**:726-33.
398. Portland G, Kelikian A, Kodros S. Acute surgical management of Jones' fractures. *Foot and Ankle International* 2003;**24-11**:829-33.
399. Sarimo J, Rantanen J, Orava S, Alanen J. Tension-band wiring for fractures of the fifth metatarsal located in the junction of the proximal metaphysis and diaphysis. *American Journal of Sports Medicine* 2006;**34**:476-80.
400. Zelko RR, Torg JS, Rachun A. Proximal diaphyseal fractures of the fifth metatarsal – treatment of the fractures and their complications in athletes. *American Journal of Sports Medicine* 1979;**7**:95-101.
401. Donley BG, McCollum MJ, Murphy GA, Richardson EG. Risk of sural nerve injury with intramedullary screw fixation of fifth metatarsal fractures: a cadaver study. *Foot and Ankle International* 1999;**20**:182-4.
402. Schon LC, Glennon TP, Baxter DE. Heel pain syndrome: electrodiagnostic support for nerve entrapment. *Foot and Ankle* 1993;**14**:129-35.
403. Oztuna V, Ozge A, Eskandari MM, et al. Nerve entrapment in painful heel syndrome. *Foot and Ankle International* 2002;**23**:208-11.
404. Barker AR, Rosson GD, Dellon AL. Pressure changes in the medial and lateral plantar and tarsal tunnels related to ankle position: a cadaver study. *Foot and Ankle International* 2007;**28**:250-4.
405. Bracilovic A, Nihal A, Houston VL, et al. Effect of foot and ankle position on tarsal tunnel compartment volume. *Foot and Ankle International* 2006;**27**:431-7.
406. Baxter DE, Thigpen CM. Heel pain – operative results. *Foot and Ankle* 1984;**5**:16-25.
407. Lundborg G, Dahlin LB. Anatomy, function, and pathophysiology of peripheral nerves and nerve compression. *Hand Clinics* 1996;**12**:185-93.
408. Rempel D, Dahlin L, Lundborg G. Pathophysiology of nerve compression syndromes: response of peripheral nerves to loading. *Journal of Bone and Joint Surgery (American)* 1999;**81-11**:1600-10.
409. Mackinnon SE. Pathophysiology of nerve compression. *Hand Clinics* 2002;**18**:231-41.
410. Baxter DE, Pfeffer GB. Treatment of chronic heel pain by surgical release of the first branch of the lateral plantar nerve. *Clinical Orthopaedics and Related Research* 1992;**279**:229-36.
411. Johnson ER, Kirby K, Lieberman JS. Lateral plantar nerve entrapment: foot pain in a power lifter. *American Journal of Sports Medicine* 1992;**20**:619-20.
412. Louisia S, Masquelet AC. The medial and inferior calcaneal nerves: an anatomic study. *Surgical and Radiologic Anatomy* 1999;**21**:169-73.
413. Oh SJ, Kwon KH, Hah JS, et al. Lateral plantar neuropathy. *Muscle and Nerve* 1999;**22**:1234-8.
414. Rask MR. Medial plantar neurapraxia (jogger's foot): report of 3 cases. *Clinical Orthopaedics and Related Research* 1978;**134**:193-5.
415. Rondhuis JJ, Huson A. The first branch of the lateral plantar nerve and heel pain. *Acta Morphologica Neerlando-Scandinavica* 1986;**24**:269-79.
416. Schon LC, Baxter DE. Neuropathies of the foot and ankle in athletes. *Clinical Sports Medicine* 1990;**9**:489-509.

417. Farooki S, Theodorou DJ, Sokoloff RM, *et al.* MRI of the medial and lateral plantar nerves. *Journal of Computer Assisted Tomography* 2001;**25**:412–16.
418. Kaplan PE, Kernahan WT. Tarsal tunnel syndrome: an electrodiagnostic and surgical correlation. *Journal of Bone and Joint Surgery (American)* 1981;**63**:96–9.
419. Biedert R, Hintermann B. Stress fractures of the medial great toe sesamoids in athletes. *Foot and Ankle International* 2003;**24**:137–41.
420. Hulkko A, Orava S, Pellinen P, Puranen J. Stress fractures of the sesamoid bones of the first metatarsophalangeal joint in athletes. *Archives of Orthopaedic and Trauma Surgery* 1985;**104**:113–17.
421. Biedert R. Which investigations are required in stress fracture of the great toe sesamoids? *Archives of Orthopaedic and Trauma Surgery* 1993;**112**:94–5.
422. Karasick D, Schweitzer ME. Disorders of the hallux sesamoid complex: MR features. *Skeletal Radiology* 1998;**27**:411–18.
423. Chisin R, Peyser A, Milgrom C. Bone scintigraphy in the assessment of the hallucal sesamoids. *Foot and Ankle International* 1995;**16**:291–4.
424. Richardson EG. Injuries to the hallucal sesamoids in the athlete. *Foot and Ankle* 1987;**7**:229–44.
425. Van Hal ME, Keene JS, Lange TA, Clancy WG. Stress fractures of the great toe sesamoids. *American Journal of Sports Medicine* 1982;**10**:122–8.

PART 7

MUSCULOSKELETAL ONCOLOGY

PAUL COOL

79	**Clinical evaluation, principles of biopsy and staging** *Theodore W Parsons III, Scot E Campbell*	863
80	**Principles of chemotherapy and radiotherapy** *Hamid Sheikh, Michael Leahy, James Wylie*	874
81	**Bone tumours** *David C Mangham and Paul Cool*	882
82	**Soft-tissue sarcomas** *Gillian L Cribb*	912
83	**Skeletal metastases and pathological fractures** *Jonathan James Gregory, Paul Cool*	925
84	**Limb reconstruction for musculoskeletal tumours** *Emma K Reay and Craig H Gerrand*	940
85	**Amputations, prosthetics and orthotics** *Frank Gottschalk, Ruth M O'Sullivan, Daniel Porter*	954

79

Clinical evaluation, principles of biopsy and staging

THEODORE W PARSONS III, SCOT E CAMPBELL

Introduction	865	Staging	870
Clinical evaluation	865	Summary	871
Imaging studies	866	References	871
Biopsy	870		

NATIONAL BOARD STANDARDS

- Understand the staging system and what factors impact prognosis
- Be familiar with patterns of bone destruction on plain radiographs
- Recognize periosteal reaction patterns and how they relate to tumor activity
- Understand why bone scintigraphy demonstrates uptake, and what lesions may not be detected on scintigraphy
- Understand the role of computed tomography in identifying lesions of bone
- Recognize basic MRI appearance patterns for tumors of soft tissue and bone
- Understand the importance of pre-procedural planning for biopsies

INTRODUCTION

Musculoskeletal neoplasia is relatively rare, and thus is not commonly encountered by the practising orthopaedic surgeon. Most radiographic lesions noted in the clinical setting are associated with prior trauma, an inflammatory or infectious condition or, less commonly, represent metastases from an underlying carcinoma. Skeletal lesions are often noted serendipitously, and these serendipitous discoveries frequently include developmental conditions such as osteochondroma.

Benign lesions are, fortunately, far more common than malignant lesions, but the initial clinical presentation of any lesion may be confusing. Tumours are generally missed by practising physicians, either because they are simply not recognized or because they are felt to be so uncommon as to not merit any consideration in the differential diagnosis. Given that musculoskeletal lesions appear in virtually all age groups and in all anatomical parts of the body, consideration of an underlying neoplasm is important in patients presenting with unexplained pain, pathological fracture, the presence of a mass or when the clinical history and the clinical presentation 'don't quite add up'.[1] Careful attention to the presenting patient's history, complaints, pain pattern and clinical examination should alert the clinician to the potential presence of a neoplastic process.

CLINICAL EVALUATION

Appropriate evaluation of the patient with a suspected musculoskeletal neoplasm includes careful history, physical examination, imaging studies and biopsy as necessary.[2] Synthesizing this information allows the patient to be placed into an appropriate staging category, which ultimately assists in identification of the lesion, helps delineate the lesion's anatomical extent, and provides information that allows the physician to formulate an appropriate treatment strategy and determine the expected prognosis.

History

Obtaining a complete history of every patient, including an appropriate past medical history, family history and review of systems, is not only important but provides useful information. Noting any antecedent trauma and documenting the onset and location of any symptoms is helpful. Given that many patients present with pain, ascertaining the type of pain, how long it has been present, what if anything exacerbates the pain and what may relieve the pain is an important component of the initial evaluation. For example, a soft-tissue mass that waxes and wanes in size and changes with activity levels often indicates a vascular lesion. The patient with an identified bone lesion who claims to have minimal pain except with impact-loading activity probably indicates a structural or mechanical problem associated with the bone lesion, possibly even an impending pathological fracture. (A simple stress fracture would also present in a similar fashion.) A patient who initially claims to have minimal and adequately controlled pain, but subsequently admits to using narcotics in order to keep the pain at a minimum level, would suggest a more aggressive, potentially destructive bone lesion. Such a history of narcotic use for pain control, or the presence of night pain, pain at rest and/or the presence of constitutional symptoms are of particular concern, and should serve as 'red flags'.

Noting the patient's age is another important piece of information, given that many neoplasms have a predilection for certain age groups.[3]

In the rare circumstance where a pathological fracture through a bone lesion has occurred, it is important to note whether or not symptoms of pain or discomfort were present prior to the time of fracture. A history of symptoms that pre-date the fracture typically indicates a more aggressive process, which generally will require a biopsy as part of the workup. Care should always be exercised in the evaluation and treatment of these particular patients. The goal in this circumstance is to avoid contamination of the surrounding tissues caused by an exposure or treatment plan that is found to be inappropriate if an underlying malignancy is ultimately identified.[4]

Physical examination

Following an appropriate history, a careful and thorough examination of the patient should be performed. Such examination includes documentation of any deformities; the presence of any skin changes; the size, location and characteristics of any soft tissue or bony masses; abnormal or painful joint motion and any associated effusion; and the presence or absence of regional adenopathy. A careful assessment of the motor/sensory examination, along with an appropriate vascular examination, should also be included. If the possibility of metastatic carcinoma is entertained, examination of such primary sites as prostate, breast, thyroid, etc. should either be performed as part of the initial evaluation, or arrangements made for an additional examination of these areas by the appropriate specialist.

Laboratory studies

Although typically non-specific, laboratory studies can be helpful in evaluation of patients with suspected neoplasia, particularly in the case of multiple lesions. For example, an elevated prostate-specific antigen (PSA) in the male patient with one or more blastic lesions of bone is highly suspicious for metastatic prostate carcinoma. Abnormalities in serum or urine electrophoresis levels, in association with multiple lytic lesions, are typically diagnostic of multiple myeloma. Micro-haematuria in the patient with lytic lesions of bone may be the first indication of metastatic renal cell carcinoma.

In general, laboratory tests should include a complete blood count, C-reactive protein, sedimentation rate and simple serum chemistries. Such tests may help to distinguish between lesions that are a result of infection from other primary neoplasia, although marrow-packing lesions (e.g. Ewing's sarcoma, multiple myeloma) may result in anaemia and elevated sedimentation rates. Malignant bone-forming lesions may demonstrate elevated levels of alkaline phosphatase.

IMAGING STUDIES

Following an appropriate clinical evaluation, obtaining appropriate imaging studies provides important information that allows further characterization of the lesion in question and often establishes the definitive diagnosis. It is important to obtain these imaging studies prior to the performance of any biopsy, as the results of these studies can be significantly altered or degraded as a result of any invasive procedure.

Standard radiography

For tumours of bone, plain film radiography remains the diagnostic gold standard and is the imaging method of choice because of the inherent contrast from calcium hydroxyapatite crystal within the bone.[5] For soft-tissue tumours, radiographs should similarly be obtained, as the location of the lesion and the presence of any associated periosteal reaction or soft-tissue mineralization are helpful for characterization. Orthogonal radiographic views of any lesion are mandatory. Careful scrutiny of plain radiographs can provide significant information about the lesion and often results in an appropriate differential diagnosis.

While characterizing the lesion, identifying the bone of involvement, longitudinal location, relationship to the physis and transverse location (central, eccentric, cortical, juxtacortical) often narrows the differential diagnosis. For example, chondroblastoma and giant cell tumour typically occur in the epiphyses or apophyses of long bones.[6,7] Osteofibrous dysplasia and adamantinoma are classically tibial lesions.[8,9] Non-ossifying fibroma is

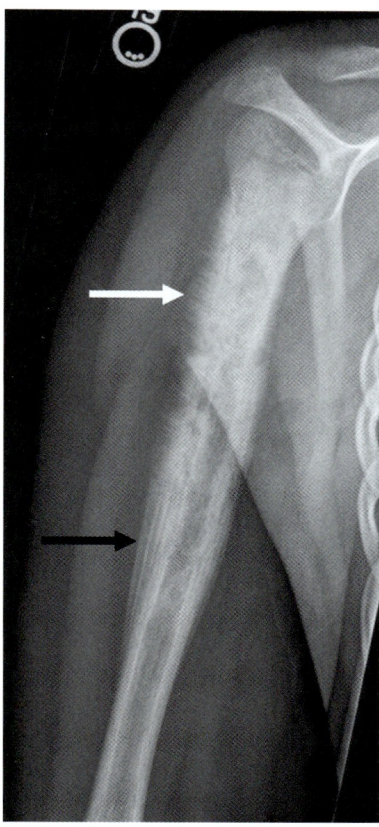

Figure 79.1 Seven-year-old girl with arm pain. Anteroposterior radiograph of the humerus demonstrates a large lytic/sclerotic lesion with permeative pattern of bone destruction in the proximal humerus. Note the spiculated (white arrow) and 'onion-skin' (black arrow) patterns of periosteal new bone formation. Ewing sarcoma.

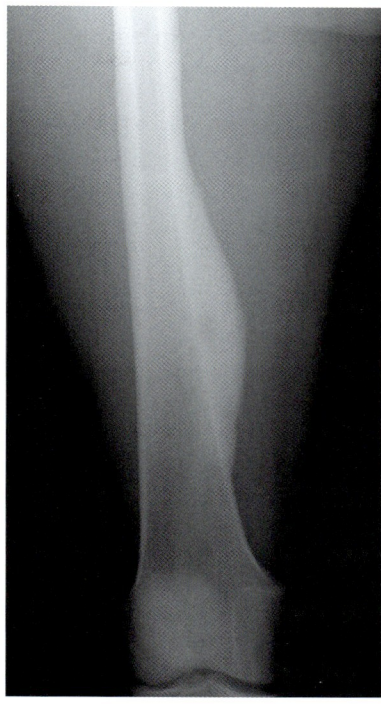

Figure 79.2 Twenty-eight-year old man with thigh pain, worsening for 3 years. Smooth, thick periosteal new bone formation at the distal medial femur with central lucent nidus. Osteoid osteoma.

cortically based and occurs in the metaphysis of long bones, typically in the lower extremity,[10] whereas simple bone cysts are centrally located, often in the proximal humerus or femur.

Large lesions often result from either aggressive lesions, or those with longstanding, slowly progressive growth.[11] In chondroid tumours, large size significantly favours chondrosarcoma over enchondroma.[12,13]

The pattern of bone destruction reveals the growth rate or aggressiveness of the lesion.[14] Permeative and 'moth-eaten' patterns of destruction result from aggressive, usually malignant (or infectious) lesions[14] (Fig. 79.1), whereas indolent lesions result in a well-circumscribed 'geographic' pattern of destruction.[5,14] A sclerotic rim indicates that the surrounding bone has responded with osteoblastic repair,[5] and is more often associated with benign, latent lesions of bone. Endosteal scalloping is typically indicative of a more active lesion, although such a finding may slowly develop over a prolonged period of time.

The periosteum is sensitive to trauma or pressure, responding by depositing new bone. The pattern of periosteal new bone formation often reveals the aggressiveness of the lesion. Slowly growing tumours cause smooth, solid periosteal new bone formation (Fig. 79.2), whereas aggressive lesions (e.g. osteosarcoma, Ewing's sarcoma) result in a lamellated ('onion skin') or spiculated ('sun-burst') pattern of periosteal new bone formation[5] (Fig. 79.1). Rapid cortical destruction may result in detachment of the periosteum, causing an appearance of an acute angle, with the open end toward the tumour (Codman's triangle).[5]

When present, matrix mineralization in a lesion can be a very helpful clue to the diagnosis. Stippled or 'arc and ring' calcifications indicate a chondroid tumour. Amorphous, 'cloud-like' mineralization is typical of osteosarcoma or blastic metastases such as prostate carcinoma. Fibrous dysplasia typically demonstrates a 'ground-glass' appearance, while bone infarcts often reveal a swirling, 'smoke up the chimney' mineralized pattern.[11]

Bone scintigraphy

Bone scintigraphy (BS) is particularly useful in determining whether a bone lesion is active or indolent. Slowly growing or inactive lesions typically demonstrate minimal radiopharmaceutical uptake, whereas actively bone-forming lesions, both benign and malignant, typically demonstrate

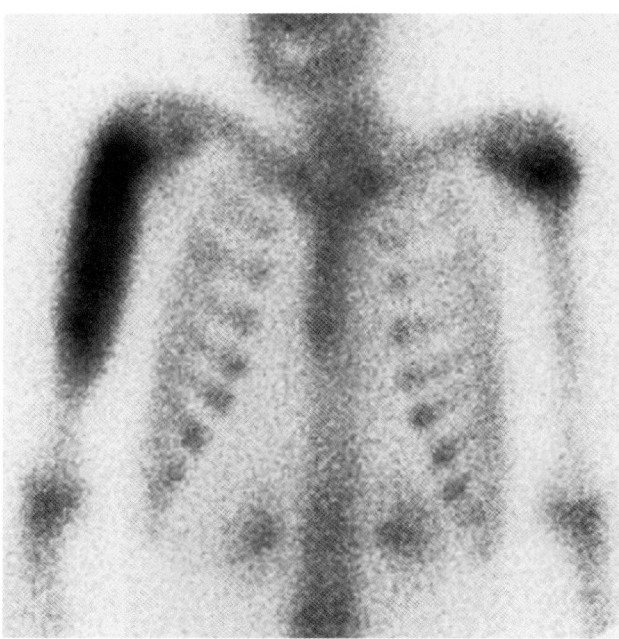

Figure 79.3 Seven-year-old girl with arm pain (same case as in Fig. 79.1). Four hour delayed phase image from Tc-99m HDP (hydroxymethylene diphosphonate) bone scan demonstrates intense radiopharmaceutical uptake in the proximal humerus in this Ewing's sarcoma.

intense radiopharmaceutical uptake[15,16] (Fig. 79.3). A transition from mild radiopharmaceutical uptake to intense uptake is an ominous sign suggestive of malignant transformation.[17] Bone scintigraphy also provides a sensitive evaluation for the presence and extent of metastatic disease, although notable exceptions include multiple myeloma, renal cell carcinoma and thyroid carcinoma, in which metastases often demonstrate little if any abnormal radiopharmaceutical uptake.[18,19] In addition, the radiopharmaceutical uptake at bone scintigraphy may be helpful to identify a radiographically occult lesion, lesions causing increased risk for pathological fracture or the most active lesion (or portion of a lesion) for biopsy.[17]

Computed tomography

Essentially all CT scanners today are helical (spiral) scanners capable of rapidly producing cross-sectional imaging with high spatial resolution. CT is inferior to MRI in characterizing soft-tissue tumours[20] but has similar accuracy in staging.[21] Because of its high spatial resolution, CT is useful in identifying lytic or sclerotic lesions in small flat bones.[20] CT is superior to MRI in characterizing matrix mineralization and identifying cortical destruction[22,23] (Fig. 79.4). CT is useful in both detecting and guiding percutaneous ablative therapies of osteoid osteoma.[24,25] Needle biopsy of musculoskeletal malignancies using CT guidance is accurate and safe if performed appropriately and after consultation with the musculoskeletal oncologist.[26,27]

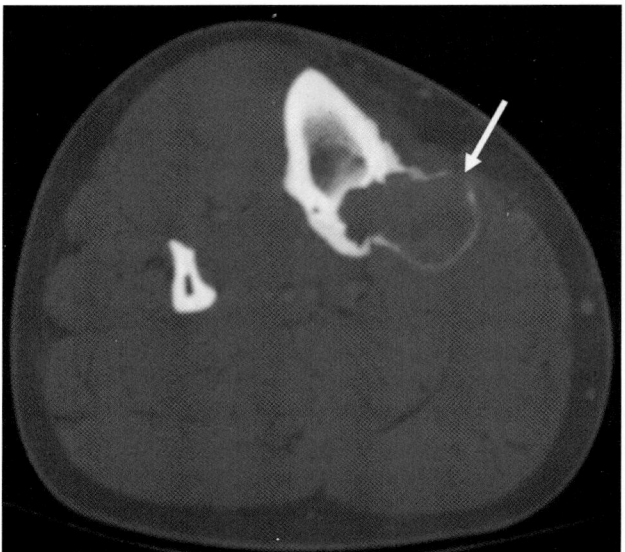

Figure 79.4 Twenty-year-old man with palpable mass at medial aspect of calf. Axial CT image demonstrates an expansile, cortically based lesion of the medial tibia with a thin rim and focal cortical disruption (arrow). Aneurysmal bone cyst.

Magnetic resonance imaging

MRI has improved our ability to characterize and stage musculoskeletal tumours, and plan appropriate limb-sparing surgery,[28] because of superior soft-tissue contrast. Although many different sequence parameters are in use, knowledge of a few imaging characteristics may be helpful for the orthopaedic surgeon evaluating a lesion. For example, entities that demonstrate high signal intensity on T_1-weighted images include fat, blood product, gadolinium contrast, proteinaceous material, melanin and particulate calcium.[29–31] Reduced or obstructed venous flow, surgical packing material or haemostatic agents may also demonstrate high T_1 signal intensity.[29,32] On the other hand, T_2-weighted images demonstrate high signal intensity in most musculoskeletal tumours, as well as cystic lesions, joint or synovial fluid and oedema. When a cystic lesion has blood product, cellular debris or fat within it, the settling of materials of different density will produce a 'fluid–fluid level', or layered appearance on T_2-weighted images (Fig. 79.5). Notable tumours that often demonstrate this appearance include aneurysmal bone cyst, telangiectatic osteosarcoma and synovial sarcoma.[33] Contrast enhancement typically indicates increased blood flow and/or vascular permeability, and can differentiate viable tumour from cyst or reactive oedema.[34] Some lesions demonstrate characteristic patterns of enhancement, such as the serpentine and lobulated enhancement in a soft-tissue haemangioma[34] (Fig. 79.6). Gradient recalled echo (GRE) sequences may be used to confirm the presence of subtle calcification or chronic blood product (e.g. pigmented villonodular synovitis), because of its sensitivity to signal loss from these tissues ('bloom artefact').[35,36]

T_1-weighted images are also useful for evaluation of bone marrow. As a general rule, infiltrative processes such as haematopoietic marrow demonstrate mildly decreased signal intensity (lighter than adjacent muscle), whereas marrow replacement from tumour or infection appears at least as dark as adjacent muscle on T_1-weighted images.[37–39] Rarely, myeloma or acute myelogenous leukaemia may have a 'faint' pattern of marrow infiltration.[40,41]

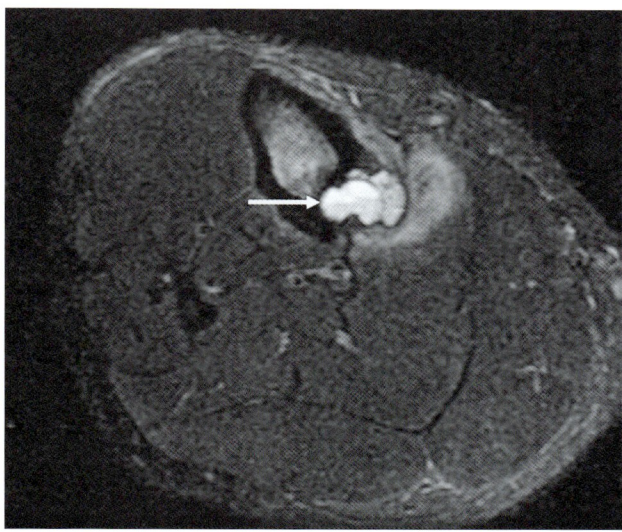

Figure 79.5 Twenty-year-old man with palpable mass (same case as in Fig. 79.3). Axial T_2-weighted image demonstrates high signal intensity and fluid–fluid levels in this aneurysmal bone cyst (arrow). Note surrounding soft tissue hyperintensity.

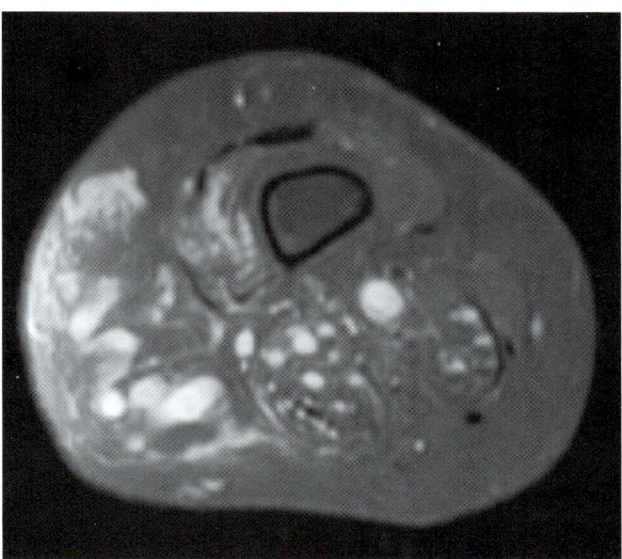

Figure 79.6 Thirty-year-old woman with a known soft-tissue haemangioma of the thigh. Axial contrast enhanced T_1-weighted image with fat suppression demonstrates large, contrast filled vessels with a serpentine and lobulated appearance, extending through fascial planes, muscles and subcutaneous fat.

MRI is particularly useful in identifying the anatomical location and boundaries of a lesion, and its relationship to surrounding structures, which is vital in surgical planning. MRI is inferior to CT for characterizing matrix mineralization and identifying cortical penetration[22,23] (compare Figs. 79.4 and 79.5).

Positron emission tomography

Positron emission tomography (PET) imaging most commonly utilizes ^{18}F-fluorodeoxyglucose (FDG) as radiotracer, and provides evaluation of tissue metabolism.[42] When combined with CT, anatomical localization of lesions is obtained along with physiological information (Fig. 79.7). PET is sensitive in detecting small tumours and skin

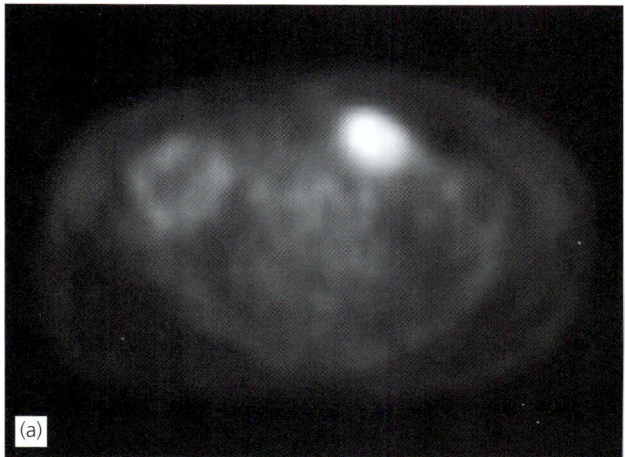

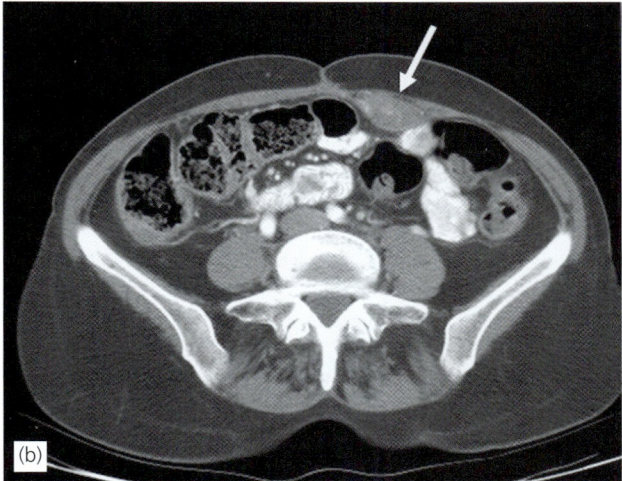

Figure 79.7 Fifty-eight-year-old woman with history of gastrointestinal stromal tumour. (a) Axial image through the lower abdomen from an ^{18}F-fluorodeoxyglucose positron emission tomography scan reveals a focus of intense radiopharmaceutical uptake anteriorly. (b) Corresponding axial CT image reveals the location of the metastatic lesion to be within the left rectus abdominis muscle (arrow).

lesions,[43] and the degree of uptake on PET has been shown to correlate with the aggressiveness of the lesion.[44] Also, the relative decrease in radiopharmaceutical uptake after chemotherapy, compared with the pre-chemotherapy uptake, has been shown to correlate histologically with the percentage of necrosis of the tumour.[45]

PET is more sensitive than BS for detection of metastases from Ewing sarcoma or multiple myeloma, and for detection of osteolytic or mixed lytic/blastic osseous metastases.[46,47] PET is inferior to BS for osteoblastic metastases, and less sensitive than CT for lung metastases from osteogenic sarcoma.[48,49] PET is relatively non-specific, since some benign lesions can have high uptake,[50] and some sarcomas, particularly those with largely acellular matrix, can exhibit a 'dilution effect' with relatively low uptake.[42] The precise role for the use of PET in the staging of neoplasia is still in evolution.

BIOPSY

Once clinical and imaging evaluations are complete, establishing an appropriate differential diagnosis is generally possible. In certain instances (such as lipoma, osteochondroma, etc.) a definitive diagnosis can be established and no further workup is necessary. Such benign lesions can typically be observed. However, when uncertainty remains as to the definitive diagnosis or aggressiveness of a lesion, biopsy is the appropriate final step in the staging process. Although the biopsy is a technically simple procedure, it must be planned very carefully by the treating surgeon. Unnecessary or inadvertent contamination of structures surrounding the biopsy site, inappropriate placement of the biopsy site or excessive post-biopsy haemorrhage can seriously threaten the success of the definitive surgical procedure.[51]

The biopsy may be accomplished via closed techniques (fine needle aspiration or core needle biopsy) or by an open incisional (or rarely excisional) technique, depending upon lesion location, the institution and the experience of the surgeon/pathologist.[52] Advantages of a closed technique include reduced tissue contamination and the ability to perform this procedure outside the operating room, with accuracy nearing that of open procedures in many institutions. Where larger amounts of tissue are required for diagnostic testing, open techniques are generally required.

STAGING

Most orthopaedic surgeons utilize the staging system described by Enneking and his colleagues. This system incorporates clinical, radiographic (anatomical) and histological data to categorize lesions based upon their aggressiveness.[53] Benign lesions are designated using Arabic numerals and are identified as latent, active or aggressive, depending upon their radiographic presentation (Table 79.1). Whereas latent benign lesions often only require observation and serial radiographs, some active and most aggressive (and virtually all potentially malignant) lesions require complete staging studies and biopsy to establish a definitive diagnosis.

Malignant lesions, which are designated using Roman numerals, are divided into either histologically low-grade lesions (I), histologically high-grade lesions (II) or lesions of any histological grade that have regional or distant metastasis (III) (Table 79.2). Each category is further divided into intracompartmental (A) or extracompartmental (B) lesions, depending on the anatomical spread of the tumour. Consequently, higher stages reflect more aggressive tumour behaviour.

Table 79.1 Enneking system for staging benign tumours of bone

Stage	Definition	Behaviour	Example
1	Latent	Remains static, may heal spontaneously	Enchondroma
2	Active	Progressive growth, limited by natural barriers	Chondroblastoma
3	Aggressive	Progressive growth, not limited by natural barriers	Giant cell tumour

Adapted from Enneking WF, Spanier SS, Goodman MA. A system for the surgical staging of musculoskeletal sarcomas. *Clinical Orthopaedics* 1980;**153**:106–20.

Table 79.2 Enneking system for staging malignant tumours of bone

Stage	Grade	Site	Metastases
I-A	G1 (low)	T1 intracompartmental	M0 (none)
I-B	G1 (low)	T2 extracompartmental	M0 (none)
II-A	G2 (high)	T1 intracompartmental	M0 (none)
II-B	G2 (high)	T2 extracompartmental	M0 (none)
III	G1 (low) or G2 (high)	T1 or T2 intra/extracompartmental	M1 (regional or distant)

Adapted from Enneking WF, Spanier SS, Goodman MA. A system for the surgical staging of musculoskeletal sarcomas. *Clinical Orthopaedics* 1980;**153**:106–20.

The American Joint Committee on Cancer (AJCC) devised a somewhat different staging system that grades tumours based upon histological diagnosis in a four-stage system which similarly considers the presence of metastases.[54] Although this system is not as commonly used among practising orthopaedic surgeons, some familiarity is useful, particularly when communicating with other medical specialties. The AJCC system for bone lesions includes size (greater or less than 8 cm), histological grade, location and presence/absence of metastases as classification variables. The soft-tissue system variables include size (greater or less than 5 cm) and depth (superficial or deep) in addition to histological grade and presence/absence of metastases.

Because staging is based upon several parameters (histological grade, the presence or absence of metastatic disease and the anatomical extent of the tumour) the application of this information ultimately allows for a reasonable estimate of overall prognosis and the construction of a definitive treatment plan. Generally speaking, the higher the stage of the lesion, the worse the overall prognosis and potential for survival. Of all the staging variables, the most important prognostic indicator is the presence of metastases, followed by histological grade.[55]

SUMMARY

Utilizing a systematic approach in the evaluation of musculoskeletal neoplasia not only simplifies the diagnostic process, it is essential for appropriate staging and classification. A careful history and physical examination followed by appropriate imaging studies facilitates the formation of a reasonable differential diagnosis. If necessary, tissue can be obtained for histological diagnosis and, ultimately, the tumour can be categorized as malignant or benign and the staging complete. Through this consistent approach to tumour evaluation, patient care can be optimized as an accurate diagnosis is established and an appropriate treatment plan formulated.

Finally, it is important to remember that lesions suspected of being malignant, or any lesion where the diagnosis is uncertain but which might include malignancy, should be referred to a musculoskeletal oncologist for definitive care. Failure to do so in a timely fashion may compromise patient care and have devastating consequences on the ultimate outcome.

KEY LEARNING POINTS

- The possibility of neoplasia should be considered in patients with a mass, unexplained pain, pathological fracture or discordant history and examination.
- Clinical evaluation of patients with musculoskeletal neoplasia includes a careful history, examination and appropriate imaging studies.
- Plain film radiography remains the gold standard for diagnostic imaging of bone tumours.
- CT is superior for characterizing matrix mineralization and identifying bone destruction.
- MRI is superior for evaluating anatomical locations and relationships, lesional boundaries and in assisting surgical planning.
- Biopsy, when necessary, requires careful planning to avoid contamination of surrounding structures and potential serious treatment complications.
- Staging includes tumour histological grade, anatomical location/size and presence or absence of metastases; it provides prognostic information and aids in planning definitive treatment.

REFERENCES

- ● = Key primary paper
- ◆ = Major review article

◆1. Ward WG. Orthopaedic oncology for the non-oncologist orthopaedist: introduction and common errors to avoid. In: Zuckerman JD (ed.) *Instructional Course Lectures*, vol. 48. Rosemont, IL: American Academy of Orthopaedic Surgeons, 1999:577–86.

2. Parsons TW, Filzen TW. Evaluation and staging of musculoskeletal neoplasia. *Hand Clinics* 2004;**20**:137–45.

3. Peabody TD. Clinical presentation and recommended evaluation of a patient with a suspected bone tumor. In: Fitzgerald RH, Kaufer H, Malkani AL (eds) *Orthopaedics*. St. Louis, MO: Mosby, 2002:1014–27.

4. Frassica FJ, Weber KL. Evaluation and staging of benign bone tumors. In: Schwartz HS (ed.) *Orthopaedic Knowledge Update: Musculoskeletal Tumors 2*. Rosemont, IL: American Academy of Orthopaedic Surgeons, 2007:75–80.

5. Dorfman HD, Czerniak B. *Bone Tumors*. St. Louis, MO: Mosby, 1998.

6. Ramappa AJ, Lee FY, Tang P, et al. Chondroblastoma of bone. *Journal of Bone and Joint Surgery America* 2000;**82A**:1140–5.

●7. Campanacci M, Baldini N, Boriani S, Sudanese A. Giant-cell tumor of bone. *Journal of Bone and Joint Surgery America* 1987;**69**:106–14.

8. Park YK, Unni KK, McLeod RA, Pritchard DJ. Osteofibrous dysplasia: clinicopathologic study of 80 cases. *Human Pathology* 1993;**24**:1339–47.

●9. Keeney GL, Unni KK, Beabout JW, Pritchard DJ. Adamantinoma of long bones: a clinicopathologic study of 85 cases. *Cancer* 1989;**64**:730–7.

10. Moser RP Jr, Sweet DE, Haseman DB, Madewell JE. Multiple skeletal fibroxanthomas: radiologic-pathologic correlation of 72 cases. *Skeletal Radioliology* 1987;**16**:353–9.
◆11. Parsons TW, Frink SJ, Campbell SE. Musculoskeletal neoplasia: helping the orthopaedic surgeon establish the diagnosis. *Seminars in Musculoskeletal Radiology* 2007;**11**:3–15.
12. Kendell SD, Collins MS, Adkins MC, et al. Radiographic differentiation of enchondroma from low-grade chondrosarcoma in the fibula. *Skeletal Radiology* 2004;**33**:458–66.
13. Geirnaerdt MJ, Hermans J, Bloem JL, et al. Usefulness of radiography in differentiating enchondroma from central grade 1 chondrosarcoma. *AJR American Journal of Roentgenology* 1997;**169**:1097–104.
14. Lodwick GS, Wilson AJ, Farrell C, et al. Determining growth rates of focal lesions of bone on radiographs. *Radiology* 1980;**134**:577–83.
15. Gilday DL, Ash JM. Benign bone tumors. *Seminars in Nuclear Medicine* 1976;**6**:33–46.
16. Mankin HJ. Chondrosarcoma of bone. In: Menendez LR (ed.) *Orthopaedic Knowledge Update: Musculoskeletal Tumors*. Rosemont, IL: American Academy of Orthopaedic Surgeons, 2002:187–94.
17. Bouvier JF, Chassard JL, Brunat-Mentigny M, et al. Radionuclide bone imaging in diaphyseal aclasis with malignant change. *Cancer* 1986;**57s**:2280–4.
18. Bataille R, Chevalier J, Rossi M, Sany J. Bone scintigraphy in plasma-cell myeloma: a prospective study of 70 patients. *Radiology* 1982;**145**:801–4.
19. Otsuka N, Fukunaga M, Morita K, et al. Photon-deficient finding in sternum on bone scintigraphy in patients with malignant disease. *Radiation Medicine* 1990;**8**:168–72.
20. Tehranzadeh J, Mnaymneh W, Ghavam C, et al. Comparison of CT and MR imaging in musculoskeletal neoplasms. *Journal of Computer Assisted Tomography* 1989;**13**:466–72.
◆21. Panicek DM, Gatsonis C, Rosenthal DI, et al. CT and MR imaging in the local staging of primary malignant musculoskeletal neoplasms: Report of the Radiology Diagnostic Oncology Group. *Radiology* 1997;**202**:237–46.
22. Lee YY, Van Tassel P, Nauert C, et al. Craniofacial osteosarcomas: plain film, CT, and MR findings in 46 cases. *AJR American Journal of Roentgenology* 1988;**150**:1397–402.
23. Collins MS, Koyama T, Swee RG, Inwards CY. Clear cell chondrosarcoma: radiographic, computed tomographic, and magnetic resonance findings in 34 patients with pathologic correlation. *Skeletal Radiology* 2003;**32**:687–94.
24. Assoun J, Richardi G, Railhac JJ, et al. Osteoid osteoma: MR imaging versus CT. *Radiology* 1994;**191**:217–23.
25. Holsaker HS, Garg S, Moroz L, et al. The diagnostic accuracy of MRI versus CT imaging for osteoid osteoma in children. *Clinical Orthopedics and Related Research* 2005;**433**:171–7.
●26. Dupuy DE, Rosenberg AE, Punyaratabandhu T, et al. Accuracy of CT-guided needle biopsy of musculoskeletal neoplasms. *AJR American Journal of Roentgenology* 1998;**171**:759–62.
27. Shin HJ, Amaral JG, Armstrong D, et al. Image-guided percutaneous biopsy of musculoskeletal lesions in children. *Pediatric Radiology* 2007;**37**:362–9.
28. Cheng EY, Thompson RC. New developments in the staging and imaging of soft-tissue sarcomas. *Instructional Course Lectures* 2000;**49**:443–51.
29. Bonneville F, Cattin F, Marsot-Dupuch K, et al. T1 signal hyperintensity in the sellar region: spectrum of findings. *Radiographics* 2006;**26**:93–113.
30. de Kerviler E, Cuenod CA, Clement O, et al. What is bright on T1 MRI scans? *Journal of Radiology* 1998;**79**:117–26.
31. Bangert BA, Modic MT, Ross JS, et al. Hyperintense disks on T1-weighted MR images: correlation with calcification. *Radiology* 1995;**195**:437–43.
32. Spiller M, Tenner MS, Couldwell WT. Effect of absorbable topical hemostatic agents on the relaxation time of blood: an in vitro study with implications for postoperative magnetic resonance imaging. *Journal of Neurosurgery* 2001;**95**:687–93.
33. Van Dyck P, Vanhoenacker FM, Vogel J, et al. Prevalence, extension and characteristics of fluid-fluid levels in bone and soft tissue tumors. *European Radiology* 2006;**16**:2644–51.
34. May D, Good R, Smith D, et al. MR imaging of musculoskeletal tumors and tumor mimickers with intravenous gadolinium: experience with 242 patients. *Skeletal Radiology* 1997;**26**:2–15.
35. Eckhardt BP, Hernandez RJ. Pigmented villonodular synovitis: MR imaging in pediatric patients. *Pediatric Radiology* 2004;**34**:943–7.
36. Rand T, Trattnig S, Male C, et al. Magnetic resonance imaging in hemophilic children: value of gradient echo and contrast-enhanced imaging. *Magnetic Resonance Imaging* 1999;**17**:199–205.
●37. Vande Berg BC, Malghem J, Lecouvet FE, Maldague B. Classification and detection of bone marrow lesions with magnetic resonance imaging. *Skeletal Radiology* 1998;**27**:529–45.
38. Petren-Mallmin M. Clinical and experimental imaging of breast cancer metastases in the spine. *Acta Radiologica Supplementum* 1994;**391**:1–23.
39. Ruzal-Shapiro C, Berdon WE, Cohen MD, Abramson SJ. MR imaging of diffuse bone marrow replacement in pediatric patients with cancer. *Radiology* 1991;**181**:587–9.
40. Takagi S, Tanaka O, Miura Y. Magnetic resonance imaging of femoral marrow in patients with myelodysplastic syndromes or leukemia. *Blood* 1995;**86**:316–22.
41. Baur-Melnyk A, Buhmann S, Durr HR, Reiser M. Role of MRI for the diagnosis and prognosis of multiple myeloma. *European Journal of Radiology* 2005;**55**:56–63.

42. Hicks RJ, Toner GC, Choong PFM. Clinical applications of molecular imaging in sarcoma evaluation. *Cancer Imaging* 2005;**5**:66-72.
43. Messa C, Landoni C, Pozzato C, Fazio F. Is there a role for FDG PET in the diagnosis of musculoskeletal neoplasms? *Journal of Nuclear Medicine* 2000;**41**:1702-3.
44. Adler LP, Blair HF, Makley JT, *et al*. Noninvasive grading of musculoskeletal tumors using PET. *Journal of Nuclear Medicine* 1991;**32**:1508-12.
45. Hawkins DS, Rajendran JG, Conrad EU, *et al*. Evaluation of chemotherapy response in pediatric bone sarcomas by [F-18]-fluorodeoxy-D-glucose positron emission tomography. *Cancer* 2002;**94**:3277-84.
●46. Peterson JJ, Kransdorf MJ, O'Connor MI. Diagnosis of occult bone metastases: positron emission tomography. *Clinical Orthopaedics and Related Research* 2003;**415S**:S120-8.
47. Kneisl JS, Patt JC, Johnson JC, Zuger JH. Is PET useful in detecting occult nonpulmonary metastases in pediatric bone sarcomas? *Clinical Orthopaedics and Related Research* 2006;**450**:101-4.
48. Fogelman I, Cook G, Israel O, Van der Wall H. Positron emission tomography and bone metastases. *Seminars in Nuclear Medicine* 2005;**35**:135-42.
49. Iagaru A, Chawla S, Menedez L, Conti PS. 18F-FDG PET and PET/CT for detection of pulmonary metastases from musculoskeletal sarcomas. *Nuclear Medicine Communications* 2006;**27**:795-802.
50. Aoki J, Endo K, Watanabe H, *et al*. FDG-PET for evaluating musculoskeletal tumors: a review. *Journal of Orthopedic Science* 2003;**8**:435-41.
51. Mankin HJ, Mankin CJ, Simm MA. The hazards of biopsy revisited. *Journal of Bone and Joint Surgery* 1996;**78A**:656-63.
52. Aboulafia AJ, Levine AM, Schmidt DP. Biopsy. In: Schwartz HS (ed.) *Orthopaedic Knowledge Update: Musculoskeletal Tumors 2*. Rosemont, IL: American Academy of Orthopaedic Surgeons, 2007:3-11.
●53. Enneking WF, Spanier SS, Goodman MA. A system for the surgical staging of musculoskeletal sarcomas. *Clinical Orthopaedics and Related Research* 1980;**153**:106-20.
54. Green FL, Page DL, Fleming ID, *et al*. (eds) *AJCC Cancer Staging Handbook*, 6th edn. New York, NY: Springer-Verlag, 2002:213-5.
55. Wunder JS. Musculoskeletal tumors: staging systems. In: Menendez LR (ed.) *Orthopaedic Knowledge Update: Musculoskeletal Tumors*. Rosemont, IL: American Academy of Orthopaedic Surgeons, 2002:21-7.

80

Principles of chemotherapy and radiotherapy

HAMID SHEIKH, MICHAEL LEAHY, JAMES WYLIE

Introduction	874
General principles of radiotherapy	874
Side-effects of radiotherapy	875
Principles of radiotherapy specific to sarcoma	876
General principles of chemotherapy	878
Principles of chemotherapy specific to sarcoma	880
References	881

NATIONAL BOARD STANDARDS

- Understand basic principles of radiotherapy and chemotherapy
- Understand common side-effects of radiotherapy and chemotherapy
- Basic knowledge of the role of chemotherapy and radiotherapy in sarcoma

INTRODUCTION

The optimal management of any patient with a malignancy relies on a well coordinated multidisciplinary team (MDT) to optimize the use of surgery, chemotherapy and radiotherapy (RT). The treatment of patients with soft-tissue and bone sarcomas is an excellent example of this. To operate effectively each member of the MDT should understand the principles of the treatments provided by the other members of the team, including the selection of patients for multimodal therapy, and they should have an understanding of how the effects of one treatment can affect the delivery and the outcome of other treatments to be given.

In general orthopaedic practices, the commonest clinical scenario involving cancer patients will be in the diagnosis and management of secondary metastatic disease involving the skeleton. This section explores the general principles behind RT and chemotherapy that can be applied to the metastatic setting where the intent of treatment is palliative. Later sections focus principally on the role of these modalities in the multidisciplinary radical treatment of primary malignancies of bone or soft tissue (i.e. sarcomas). Relevant review articles are listed in the references.[1–5]

GENERAL PRINCIPLES OF RADIOTHERAPY

Radiotherapy involves the controlled delivery of ionizing radiation to tumour-bearing tissues producing cancer cell death through direct DNA damage. Cancer cells have inherently less ability to repair this damage than normal cells. Treatment is typically delivered via a linear accelerator and involves multiple daily treatments (fractions) of equal dose. This approach is designed to maximize tumour cell death while minimizing damage to normal tissues. *Palliative RT* is typically delivered in 1–10 fractions aiming to improve symptoms rather than cure cancer. Possible indications for palliative RT include improving bone pain, shrinking soft-tissue masses, drying fungating tumours and obtaining haemostasis in bleeding tumours. *Radical* RT refers to treatment given with curative intent, which is typically given over 4–7 weeks and involves higher total doses. In these situations RT may be employed as an organ preservation strategy as an alternative to ablative surgery. Different tumours have different sensitivity to RT, and management algorithms vary accordingly. The treatment of less radiosensitive tumours often requires initial surgery to remove the macroscopic tumour followed by *adjuvant* RT to try and kill off any remaining microscopic disease, e.g. breast, rectal cancer, sarcoma. Alternatively

Table 80.1 Different radiotherapy characteristics

Radiation type	Delivery	Physical characteristics	Advantages/uses
Megavoltage (4–20 MV)	Via linear accelerator	Able to deliver high doses deep into tissues. Often employed with multiple static shaped beams (3D conformal radiotherapy) or multiple separate beam segments within a single beam (IMRT). Dose decreases with increasing depth	Widely available. Using computer planning permits good dose coverage of complex tumour volumes. Commonly employed in all cancer treatments
Kilovoltage (80–300 kV)	Via smaller superficial unit	Able to deliver dose from a few millimetres to several centimetres beneath skin depending on energy used. Employed as a single field	Simple treatment. Most commonly used to treat tumours confined to skin. 300 kV can treat deeper tumours
Electrons	Via linear accelerator	Dose delivered near skin surface. Employed as single field. Relatively rapid fall off in dose with depth.	Simple treatment. Superficial tumours only. Used when there is a need to avoid excessive dosage to a deeper sensitive normal structure
Protons	Via cyclotron	Very abrupt/reproducible fall off in dose at depth. Often employed using multiple static beams	Not available in UK. Several centres in Europe. Used to treat tumours lying close to critical structures (e.g. chordoma at skull base)
Brachytherapy	Radiation source placed directly into tumour via needles/tube	Very rapid fall off in dose away from radiation source	Standard approach for soft-tissue sarcoma in some institutes. Considerable expertise needed

neo-adjuvant RT can be given prior to surgical resection, which has the added advantage of potentially downsizing the tumour prior to resection. In more radiosensitive tumours radical RT alone may be curative, e.g. lymphoma, plasmacytoma, and head and neck cancer.

Lymphoma, germ cell tumours
Squamous cell carcinoma
Adenocarcinoma
Sarcoma, melanoma, renal cell carcinoma

Increasing sensitivity ↑

Different types of radiation exist and the clinical oncologist exploits their different physical characteristics with the aim of delivering a uniform dose to the tumour while minimizing the dose to the unaffected normal tissues (Table 80.1).

SIDE-EFFECTS OF RADIOTHERAPY

Side-effects depend on the particular tissue and volume irradiated and the dose of RT received. They are typically divided into early (during and immediately post treatment) and late effects (can occur months/years after treatment).

Table 80.2 Radiotherapy side-effects

Tissue	Acute effects	Late effects
Skin	Erythema leading to moist desquamation if severe	Skin and subcutaneous atrophy and fibrosis. Telangectasia
Gastrointestinal	Mucositis, enteritis, colitis, proctititis	Diarrhoea, bleeding, stricture, fistula, incontinence
Neurological	Rare	Plexopathy, neuropathy
Lymphatic	Rare	Lymphoedema
Bone/joint	Rare	Fracture, joint stiffness, osteonecrosis

Acute side-effects are relatively common and are generally due to acute inflammation of the affected organ and may escalate throughout treatment. They normally settle soon after completing treatment unless serious tissue damage has occurred. Late effects are rarer but often permanent and are therefore more serious. Careful treatment delivery means late effects, if they occur, are generally manageable. Examples of commoner side-effects are listed in Table 80.2.

PRINCIPLES OF RADIOTHERAPY SPECIFIC TO SARCOMA

Radiotherapy has a minor role to play in the management of bone sarcomas but is a commonly used modality in the multidisciplinary treatment of soft-tissue sarcomas (STSs). In the 1960s RT texts advocated radical surgery as the only curative treatment for STSs and that there was no role for RT as sarcomas were regarded as radioresistant tumours. These observations were largely based on patients treated solely by RT, when doses of radiation were low, tumours were large and the available RT techniques were rudimentary.

Although very wide radical resection or amputation is effective in achieving local control, there can be significant functional and cosmetic consequences. In the 1970 to 1980s, in an effort to reduce the magnitude of surgery and thereby improve function, single centres started to report acceptable local control rates by combining marginal excisions with RT. The rationale was that surgery removed the macroscopic tumour and RT treated any possible residual microscopic disease within the remaining reactive zone. A small National Cancer Institute trial, which randomized 43 patients with high-grade extremity sarcoma to amputation or a limb-sparing resection plus adjuvant RT, concluded that there was no statistical difference in disease-free survival or overall survival in each arm.

In 1985 the US National Institute of Health convened a Consensus Development Conference on limb sparing, and recommended a combined modality limb-sparing approach as the new standard of care.

Randomized trials have since provided evidence that adjuvant RT (Table 80.3) using either standard external beam RT (EBRT) or brachytherapy (BRT) techniques following marginal excision can lead to improved local control compared to surgery alone. BRT has no effect in low grade tumours.

Not all STSs require additional RT. Several single institutional reports have shown good local control in selected patients treated with surgery alone. These reports have generally included tumours less than 5 cm resected with negative margins and are summarized in Table 80.4.

Once a diagnosis of STS is reached, collaboration between the specialist surgeon and oncologist is crucial before any attempt at definitive surgery is undertaken. The role of additional chemotherapy is discussed below. Once the decision has been reached that RT is required in a limb-conserving approach, the timing of RT relative to surgery needs to be decided taking into account dose and volume constraints, anatomical location, size of primary and whether skin grafts are needed.

Table 80.3 Randomized trials of wide excision with or without adjuvant radiotherapy in management of soft-tissue sarcomas

Institution (author)	Treatment group	RT dose (Gy)	No. patients	Local failure rate (%)	Overall survival (%)	
High grade						
MSKCC (Pisters)	Surgery + BRT	45	56	9	67	At 5 years
	Surgery alone	-	63	30	67	
NCI (Yang)	Surgery + chemo + EBRT	45 + 18 (boost)	47	0	75	At 10 years
	Surgery + chemo	-	44	22	74	
Low grade						
MSKCC (Pisters)	Surgery + BRT	45	22	36	96	At 5 years
	Surgery alone	-	23	26	95	
NCI (Yang)	Surgery + EBRT	45 + 18 (boost)	26	5	NR	At 10 years
	Surgery alone	-	24	36	NR	

BRT, Brachytherapy; EBRT, external beam radiotherapy; NR, not recorded.

Table 80.4 Published series of surgery alone for soft-tissue sarcomas

Institution (author)	Year of publication	No. of patients	Selection criteria	Local failure rate (%) at 5 years	Distant failure rate (%) at 5 years
MDACC (Pisters)	2007	88	T1 primary R0 excision	8	4
Mayo (Fabrizio)	2000	34	Not specified	20	14
Harvard (Baldini)	1999	74	Not specified	7	12
Roswell Park (Karakousis)	1995	116	2 cm margin	10	NR
MSKCC (Geer)	1992	117	T1 primary	8	5
Lund (Rydholm)	1991	56	'Contained' clear margin	7	NR

T1, <5 cm tumour; NR, not recorded; R0, microscopic negative margin.

Table 80.5 A proposed treatment algorithm for radiotherapy combined with limb sparing surgery

	Principal treatment modality	Treatment algorithm
Primary, low-grade, superficial	Surgery: wide excision	Aim to achieve ⩾1 cm margin and deep fascia
Primary, low-grade, deep and ⩽5 cm	Surgery: wide excision	Aim to achieve ⩾1 cm margin or intact fascial layer
Primary, low-grade, deep and >5 cm	Surgery: wide excision	Aim to achieve ⩾1 cm margin or intact fascial layer. Consider adjuvant RT if smaller margin achieved
Primary, high-grade, superficial	Surgery: wide excision	Aim to achieve 1–2 cm margin and deep fascia. Adjuvant RT if smaller margin achieved
Primary, high-grade, deep, ⩽5 cm	Surgery: wide excision + adjuvant RT (pre- or postop)	Consider avoiding RT if ⩾2 cm margin or intact fascia
Primary, high-grade, deep, >5 cm	Surgery: wide excision + adjuvant radiation therapy (pre- *or* postop)	Consider amputation if more than one compartment involved. *Isolated limb perfusion may also be considered

*Neoadjuvant and adjuvant chemotherapy practices vary widely and are not included. RT, radiotherapy.

The advantages of postoperative RT are

- no delay in the definitive surgical treatment
- accurate pathological staging is possible on the main specimen guiding future treatments
- RT is selectively given to those with inadequate surgical margins
- pre-operative RT can incur complications in wound healing. A Canadian trial randomized 190 patients to pre-operative RT or postoperative RT following excision. The dose given pre-operatively was slightly lower than the postoperative dose. The primary endpoint was the rate of wound complications. The trial was stopped early as a significant difference emerged with 35% of pre-operative patients having complications as opposed to 17% of postoperative patients. However, later follow-up revealed less subcutaneous fibrosis and limb swelling in the pre-operative group in which a lower RT dose was employed but the rates of local control and overall were not statistically different at a median follow-up of 7 years.

The advantages to pre-operative RT are

- smaller irradiated volume because of better tumour definition
- lower total doses of RT used pre-operatively achieve identical levels of local control to higher doses used postoperatively
- larger inoperable tumours may sometimes be downstaged, which can facilitate achieving clear surgical margins without the need for resecting large volumes of normal tissue
- tumours requiring extensive split-skin grafts or reconstruction might best be irradiated beforehand as a large skin graft tolerates RT poorly and planning postoperative RT after flap reconstruction can result in a very large irradiated volume
- some body sites are limited by adjacent nearby sensitive tissues which tolerate the higher doses of postoperative RT poorly, e.g. tumours adjacent to the brachial plexus, spinal cord, bowel or kidney.

Principles of radiotherapy planning in sarcoma

Most RT is planned after obtaining a CT scan through the affected area. The starting point is to define the gross tumour volume (GTV), which represents the radiologically defined tumour (pre-operative) or tumour bed (postoperative) taken to include areas of oedema.

The clinical target volume (CTV) comprises the GTV plus a margin to encompass potential microscopic spread taking into account routes of tumour spread. In the postoperative setting, this includes all tissues handled during surgery, all scars and drain sites. Intracompartmental axial margins of at least 2 cm are required but bone, interosseous membranes and fascial planes act as barriers to microscopic dissemination and so tighter margins can be employed in areas where these structures intervene. The preferential spread of tumour cells longitudinally along muscle fibres means longer margins are employed in this direction, typically 5 cm beyond the GTV or at least 1 cm beyond the scar. It is common practice to use a shrinking field, with 50 Gy in the first phase, and a reduced 2–3 cm margin to 60–66 Gy for the second phase of treatment. Ongoing trials are exploring the optimal margin which should be placed around the tumour (Fig. 80.1).

By convention, the CTV is usually expanded all round by a further margin of 5 mm to make the planning target volume (PTV), to allow for daily variation and errors in patient set-up and organ motion.

Tighter margins can be employed pre-operatively and the total dose is typically 50 Gy.

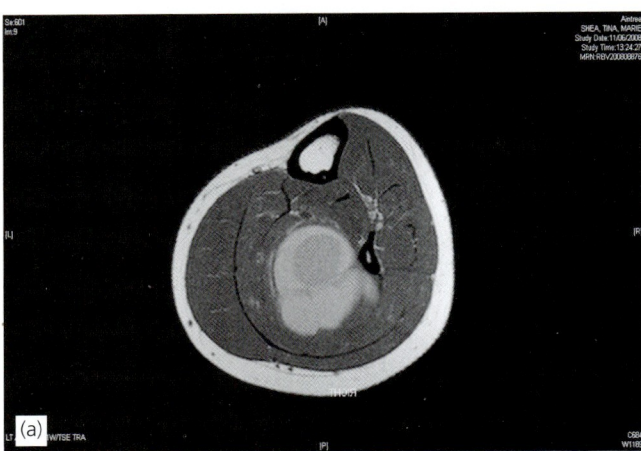 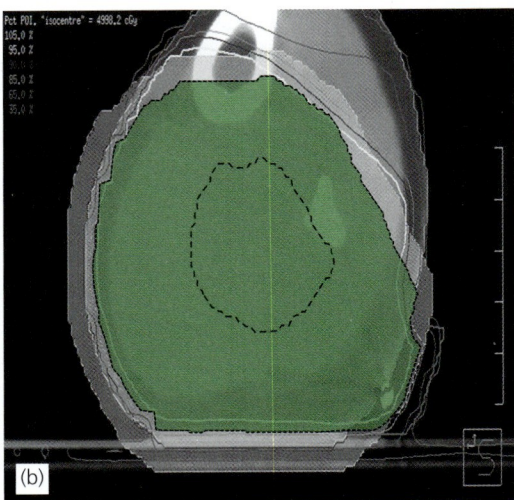

Figure 80.1 (a) MRI axial image of soft-tissue sarcoma in hamstring compartment of right lower leg. (b) Radiotherapy CT plan illustrating gross tumour volume (dashed contour), clinical target volume (dotted contour) and PTV (green colourwash) and minimum coverage by the required 95% dose level (bold white contour).

Table 80.6 Benign diseases treated with radiotherapy

Condition	Treatment plan	Mechanism of action
Keloid	Excision followed immediately by RT	Preventing fibroblast proliferation
Heterotopic ossification	Immediate prophylactic RT in high-risk patients	Killing of pluripotential mesenchymal cells
Bursitis/plantar fasciitis/tendonitis	Controversial. RT may improve symptoms in some refractory patients	Possible anti-inflammatory effect
Pigmented villonodular synovitis (PVNS)	Synovectomy and excision of extracapsular disease followed by RT once wounds healed	Direct cell kill
Fibromatosis (desmoid)	Usually inoperable cases. Occasionally as adjuvant after excision	Probable direct cell kill

Principles of radiotherapy in benign disease

Radiotherapy may occasionally be employed in orthopaedic practices to treat benign disease. In these situations the advantages of RT must be balanced against the small risk of inducing a second cancer 10–20 years after treatment. Examples of such treatments are shown in Table 80.6.

GENERAL PRINCIPLES OF CHEMOTHERAPY

Chemotherapy is an increasingly broad term potentially referring to any systemic anti-cancer therapy. Approximately 100 compounds are available that could be considered as traditional *cytotoxics* and these drugs cause cell death through direct damage to DNA, inhibition of DNA synthesis and interruption of key elements of cell division such as the mitotic spindle. More recently, drugs targeting specific enzymes in critical pathways of proliferation have been developed and are termed *targeted therapies*.

The *rationale* for using systemic therapies in cancer management is that the main threat to life from most tumours is from metastatic disease and therefore whereas surgery and RT may deal effectively with the primary tumour, these therapies are ultimately limited in improving survival since many (perhaps most) patients who die of their cancer have had micrometastatic disease present at the outset that is not clinically detectable.

Conversely, the limitation of using systemic therapy is that unless total cell kill can be achieved the therapy will not be curative and although notable exceptions exist where this is achieved (for example germ cell cancer, lymphoma and leukaemia) for most patients with clinically detectable metastatic disease systemic therapies are insufficiently effective to achieve a sustained complete remission.

The term *adjuvant chemotherapy* is used when systemic therapy is added to optimal local tumour control (surgical excision and/or RT) when there is no clinically detectable metastatic disease. The rationale for using chemotherapy in this way is that the drugs may be more effective when used against minimal residual disease or micrometastatic disease than when used against overt metastatic disease. It should be noted that unless highly predictive markers exist to identify those patients with micrometastatic disease, using adjuvant chemotherapy almost always means that a proportion of the patients treated have derived no added benefit from such treatment as they have no distant spread of their cancer and have already been cured by the local therapy. This is important because all chemotherapy carries risk of morbidity and even mortality from both acute toxicity and also from late effects. Therefore, to have an overall benefit, adjuvant chemotherapy has to reduce cause-specific mortality to a larger extent than the treatment-specific mortality for which it is responsible. This means that it is vital that 'all-cause' mortality is the endpoint measured when assessing the benefit of adjuvant chemotherapy.

The term *neoadjuvant* is used to mean treatment given before the local therapy. There are a number of reasons why this may be beneficial.

- It reduces delay in the treatment of the patient with the systemic therapy.
- If the therapy is successful in causing tumour involution it may allow a smaller, less mutilating operation.
- It allows assessment of the chemosensitivity of the tumour.

The disadvantages of neoadjuvant chemotherapy include:

- If it is ineffective, it delays removal of the primary tumour which may allow metastatic spread to occur if it has not already.
- If the tumour progresses during this delay it may render a patient inoperable.
- If the tumour was operable and non-metastatic at presentation then it is unnecessary therapy.

For this reason, unless a cancer that is particularly sensitive to chemotherapy is being treated, neoadjuvant chemotherapy is usually avoided unless the tumour is already locally advanced and inoperable.

Palliative chemotherapy is the term given to chemotherapy used when cure is not the goal. In most cases where the cancer is metastatic, therapy will be palliative in intent. Selecting patients for palliative chemotherapy requires careful assessment of the potential toxicity of therapy and how this would be tolerated by the patient with its consequent detriment to their quality of life compared with the chance that there will be a substantial change in the patient's symptoms or survival.

Side-effects of chemotherapy

Chemotherapy side-effects are drug specific and depend on both the dose and frequency of administration. Most side-effects occur around the time of drug delivery but late effects such as infertility, second malignancy and organ damage can develop many years later (Table 80.7).

Drug resistance

Ultimately chemotherapy failure in any given patient is due to the development of chemotherapy drug resistance. Even if the majority of the cell population is sensitive to the agent used, each successive dose will kill the sensitive cells while the resistant clones survive. This leads to an increasing fraction of the cell population being made up of resistant cells. Drug resistance may be passive (due for example to failure of the chemotherapy to penetrate ischaemic areas with poor blood supply) or active (e.g. because of upregulation of cell membrane ion pumps such as *p*-glycoprotein that transport the chemotherapy drug out of the cell).

Combination regimens *vs* single agents

A principle established early in the development of chemotherapy is that drug resistance can be minimized by using combinations of drugs with different mechanisms

Table 80.7 Chemotherapy side-effects

Toxicity	Comments	Treatment
Haematological	Bone marrow suppression common. Dose limiting for many cytotoxics. Typically occurs 10–14 days after treatment	Blood product support. Prompt diagnosis and treatment of neutropenic sepsis
Alopecia	Reversible	Wigs. Can be minimized by scalp cooling before/during and following bolus chemotherapy administration
Gastrointestinal	Nausea and vomiting typically worst for first 48 hours. Mucositis occurs with some drugs	Prophylactic 5HT3-receptor antagonists. Maintain good oral hygiene
Pulmonary/cardiac/renal	Rare. Can be dose related. Confirm adequate function prior to starting treatment	Vigilance and early discontinuation if symptoms develop
Neurological	Rare. Peripheral neuropathy commonest	Vigilance and early discontinuation if symptoms develop. Usually reversible

of action. Typically, new agents are first tested for single agent activity in a given disease and then combination regimens designed where multiple active drugs can be given together. This has been successful in improving cure rates in those chemo-curable cancers mentioned above. In the palliative setting, however, the disadvantage of greater toxicity inherent in combination regimens needs careful consideration.

PRINCIPLES OF CHEMOTHERAPY SPECIFIC TO SARCOMA

Cytotoxic chemotherapy is now regarded as standard of care in the multimodal primary treatment of embryonal rhabdomyosarcoma, Ewing's sarcoma and osteosarcoma because of convincing evidence of an improvement in overall survival following the introduction of this modality to a purely surgical approach. Such evidence has been lacking in most other sarcoma histology subtypes despite a number of randomized trials and meta-analyses of these trials and if there is any benefit from conventional cytotoxic drugs, it is not likely to be large. International practice varies.

For the reasons described above, the chemotherapy for those highly responsive sarcomas (embryonal rhabdomyosarcoma, Ewing's and osteosarcoma) is typically started pre-operatively as a neoadjuvant therapy. Where complex endoprostheses (EPR) are required there is also a practical benefit as it allows time for the construction of the EPR (Table 80.8).

International practice varies considerably for most other soft tissue sarcomas. In the UK and much of Europe neo-adjuvant therapy would likely be reserved for locally advanced tumours where good response might lead to limb salvage surgery, whereas in some US centres it is more universally applied. It is generally agreed that combination regimens with two or more drugs are preferable and have also been used interdigitated with pre-operative RT. Treatment-related toxicity can be pronounced, and concurrent use of both chemotherapy and RT limits the ability to deliver adequate doses of either modality.

Recently, considerable interest has been generated by the results obtained from several centres using *isolated limb perfusion*. In this treatment, patients are usually selected with large peripheral tumours which would require amputation for a radical excision. The procedure involves placing a tourniquet around the limb, and transferring the circulation to a bypass machine in which the infusate can be heated to above body temperature (usually 42°C) and cytotoxic drugs introduced. The advantage of this procedure is that much higher concentration of drugs can be achieved in the isolated limb than would be tolerable in the systemic circulation. For soft tissue sarcomas the combination of busulphan and TNF has been found to be highly synergistic and result in an 80% limb salvage rate. Randomized controlled trial results confirming this observation are awaited.

Table 80.8 Chemotherapy used in sarcoma

Sarcoma	Commonest drugs used	Neoadjuvant/adjuvant	Palliative	Research developments
Ewing Sarcoma of bone and soft tissue (PPNET)	Vincristine Ifosfamide Doxorubicin Etoposide	Pre-op chemo is standard of care. Definite survival benefit	Useful palliation with salvage chemotherapy	Targeted therapies
Osteosarcoma	Cisplatin Doxorubicin Methotrexate Ifosfamide Etoposide	Pre-op chemo is standard of care. Definite survival benefit	Some benefit in salvage therapy, rarely curative	Targeted therapies
Chondrosarcoma	None known to be reliably effective	Not used	Rarely used	Urgently required
Leiomyosarcoma/ liposarcoma/synovial sarcoma/pleomorphic undifferentiated sarcoma/angiosarcoma	Doxorubicin Ifosfamide (Dacarbazine)	No evidence of improvement in overall survival. May improve local control. Not routinely used in UK	~25% of patients will get a modest response lasting on average 9 months with single therapy regimens	Combination therapies. Newer drugs: gemcitabine, paclitaxel. Specific subtypes may be sensitive to particular drugs, e.g. angiosarcoma and paclitaxel; myxoid liposarcoma and trabectidin

Metastatic disease

For most patients with most cancers, the detection of metastatic disease means a poor prognosis. For sarcoma patients, average survival is about 12 months. Exceptions to this include those highly sensitive sarcomas already mentioned. Palliative therapy may provide a modest benefit to some patients and considerable debate exists regarding the best choice of regimen. In view of the rarity of these tumours and the lack of good clinical trial data, a high priority should be given to ensuring such patients have the opportunity to be entered into available clinical trials, and this is another good reason supporting referral to specialist teams.

> ### KEY LEARNING POINTS
>
> - Radiotherapy and chemotherapy have a key palliative role in many solid cancers.
> - Surgery and radiotherapy have key roles in the majority of soft tissue sarcoma.
> - Except for some highlighted exceptions, chemotherapy has a palliative role in the majority of soft tissue sarcoma.
> - Surgery and chemotherapy have key roles in the majority of bone sarcomas.

REFERENCES

- ● = Key primary paper
- ◆ = Major review article

- ●1. O'Sullivan B, Davis AM, Turcotte R, et al. Preoperative versus postoperative radiotherapy in soft-tissue sarcoma of the limbs: a randomised trial. Lancet 2009; **359**:2235–41.
- ◆2. NICE. *Improving Outcomes for People with Sarcoma*. London: National Institute for Health and Clinical Excellence, 2006.
- ◆3. O'Sullivan B, Wylie J, Catton C, *et al.* The local management of soft tissue sarcoma. *Seminars in Radiation Oncology* 1999;**9**:328–48.
- ◆4. Misra A, Mistry N, Grimer R, Peart F. The management of soft tissue sarcoma. *Journal of Plastic Reconstructive and Aesthetic Surgery* 2009;**62**:161–74.
- ◆5. Clark MA, Fisher C, Judson I, Thomas JM. Soft-tissue sarcomas in adults. *New England Journal of Medicine* 2005;**353**:701–11.

81

Bone tumours

DAVID C MANGHAM AND PAUL COOL

Introduction	882	Chondroblastoma	894
Epidemiology	883	Enchondroma and chondrosarcoma	896
Clinical presentation of bone neoplasms	884	Osteosarcoma	898
Basics of bone structure and remodelling	885	Parosteal osteosarcoma	901
Radiological diagnosis	885	Ewing's sarcoma	902
Pathology of bone neoplasms	887	Malignant fibrous histiocytoma	904
Simple bone cyst/unicameral bone cyst	887	Chordoma	904
Aneurysmal bone cyst	888	Myeloma	906
Giant cell tumour of bone	889	Lymphoma	907
Eosinophilic granuloma	890	Conclusion	908
Fibrous dysplasia	891	Acknowledgement	909
Osteoid osteoma and osteoblastoma	891	References	909

NATIONAL BOARD STANDARDS

- Learn the warning signs of malignant bone tumours
- To understand the principles in the assessment of bone tumours
- To understand the principles of biopsy of bone tumours
- To understand the pathology of bone tumours
- Learn the epiphyseal, diaphyseal and metaphyseal bone tumours
- To understand the principles of management of primary bone tumours

INTRODUCTION

This chapter is concerned with the pathological aspects of benign and primary malignant bone neoplasms. Developmental or tumour-like lesions will only be mentioned in the differential diagnoses. Recently, the historical distinction of gross tissue dysplasias and hamartomas from neoplasms has become progressively blurred. The classification of certain mass-forming cellular proliferations as gross tissue dysplasias and hamartomas was based on gross and microscopic morphology, but in large part due to the advent of molecular biological technologies the genetic bases of these lesions have been discovered causing many of them to be reconsidered as neoplastic processes. In particular, the discovery of specific mutations and the demonstration of monoclonality in lesions such as aneurysmal bone cyst, fibrous dysplasia and osteochondroma support the view that these are all true neoplasms rather than the variably held historical views that these were developmental abnormalities, dysplasias and hamartomas respectively. As such, these lesions will be considered in this chapter as true neoplasms. This chapter will only consider primary bone tumours, and will not concern itself with the clinically important field of metastatic bone disease. Detailed discussion of treatment options is discussed in subsequent

Table 81.1 The WHO Classification of Bone Tumours (2002)

Cartilage tumours
Osteochondroma*
Chondroma
    Enchondroma*
    Periosteal chondroma
    Multiple chondromatosis*
Chondroblastoma*
Chondromyxoid fibroma
Chondrosarcoma
    Central, primary and secondary*
    Peripheral
    Dedifferentiated*
    Mesenchymal
    Clear cell

Osteogenic tumours
Osteoid osteoma*
Osteoblastoma*
Osteosarcoma
    Conventional*
        chondroblastic
        fibroblastic
        osteoblastic
    Telangiectatic
    Small cell
    Low grade central
    Secondary
    Parosteal*
    Periosteal
    High grade surface

Fibrogenic tumours
Desmoplastic fibroma
Fibrosarcoma

Fibrohistiocytic tumours
Benign fibrous histiocytoma
Malignant fibrous histiocytoma*

Ewing's sarcoma/primitive neuroectodermal tumour
Ewing's sarcoma*

Haematopoietic tumours
Plasma cell myeloma*
Malignant lymphoma, NOS*

Giant cell tumour
Giant cell tumour*
Malignancy in giant cell tumour

Notochordal tumour
Chordoma*

Vascular tumours
Haemangioma
Angiosarcoma

Smooth muscle tumours
Leiomyoma
Leiomyosarcoma

Lipogenic tumour
Lipoma
Liposarcoma

Neural tumour
Neurilemmoma

Miscellaneous tumours
Adamantinoma
Metastatic malignancy

Miscellaneous lesions
Aneurysmal bone cyst*
Simple cyst*
Fibrous dysplasia*
Osteofibrous dysplasia
Langerhans cell histiocytosis*
Erdheim–Chester disease
Chest wall hamartoma

Joint lesion
Synovial chondromatosis

*Tumours discussed in this chapter are marked with an asterisk.

chapters. This chapter is limited to the pathology of the more common benign and malignant primary bone tumours. Table 81.1 lists the bone tumour classification accepted recently by the World Health Organization (WHO).[1] The tumours that are discussed in this chapter are marked with an asterisk. Before specific entities are described, brief overviews of the epidemiology, clinical presentation and radiological features and staging of bone tumours is merited, as well as a consideration of the histology of bone structure and remodelling.

EPIDEMIOLOGY

The incidence of malignant bone neoplasms is well established through various national data collection programmes. In the USA, the National Cancer Institute's (NCI) Surveillance Epidemiology and End Result (SEER) programme (www.seer.cancer.gov) collects high-quality epidemiological data from approximately 10% of the US population. The programme has been running since 1975, and the latest available incidence data cover 2002–6 (http://seer.cancer.gov/statfaicts/html/bones.html). In the NCI monograph 'Cancer incidence and survival among children and adolescents: SEER program 1975–1995' there is additional detailed statistical information on childhood and adolescent bone cancer (http://seer.cancer.gov/publications/childhood/). The age adjusted incidence rate for primary malignant bone tumours was 0.9 per 100 000 per year. The incidence is slightly higher in men than in women (1.0 per 100 000 per year and 0.7 per 100 000 per year, respectively). This makes primary malignant bone tumours among the rarest of cancers, accounting for only 0.2% of all cancer types. There was no significant trend in primary bone cancer incidence over the period 2002–6. The given median age of primary bone cancer was 39 years of age; this means little without breaking down the age distribution into cancer subtypes (http://seer.cancer.gov/publications/childhood/). Indeed, the three commonest malignant bone tumours show distinctively different age distributions.

The majority of malignant primary bone tumours arise *de novo* and are primary. However, precursors for malignancy have been described[1] and are divided into high-, moderate- and low-risk precursors.

High-risk precursors include

- Ollier's disease
- Maffucci syndrome
- familial retinoblastoma.

Moderate-risk precursors are

- diaphyseal aclasia (multiple osteochondromas)
- Paget's disease
- radiation osteitis.

Low-risk precursors include

- fibrous dysplasia
- osteonecrosis
- chronic osteomyelitis.

Osteosarcoma is the commonest primary malignant bone tumour and shows a bimodal age distribution (children and elderly people). The peak in elderly people is largely accounted for by osteosarcoma secondary to Paget's disease or radiation treatment. The second commonest bone cancer, chondrosarcoma, almost exclusively affects adults and becomes progressively more common with age. Ewing's sarcoma of bone is the third commonest bone cancer. It affects children and young adults and becomes progressively rare with age. There is a slight male preponderance in incidence, except in younger children. A striking racial difference is seen for Ewing's sarcoma. This tumour, in several series, has been shown to be up to six times more common in white children than in black children. There are no significant racial differences for the other primary malignant bone tumours. In contrast, the incidence of benign bone tumours is very difficult to establish because the majority of them are clinically silent. Only when a benign bone tumour produces pain, swelling, deformity or fracture does it come to medical attention and have any chance of accessing a registry. Benign surface bone tumours, such as osteochondroma, are likely to be symptomatic due to swelling and/or nerve compression. In contrast, benign medullary bone tumours may produce no symptoms and remain undetected. With the advent of more sophisticated and more commonly performed radiographic imaging (especially MRI) we may soon learn the true incidence of benign bone tumours, but we are unaware of any systematic radiological or autopsy report on the incidence of benign bone tumours. Nevertheless, it is fair to say that symptomatic benign bone tumours (i.e. defined as those that come to medical attention) are more common than malignant bone tumours.

CLINICAL PRESENTATION OF BONE NEOPLASMS

Essentially, bone tumours present with only a limited range of symptoms and signs. It is worth considering the pathological correlates with each sign or symptom in turn. In particular, it is useful to consider the rate of growth of the mass, its infiltrative or non-infiltrative nature and the response of the host bone to the presence of the neoplasm.

- *Fracture is due to* extensive replacement of functional bone by tumour.
- *Pain is due to* stimulation of the richly innervated nerve periosteum by tearing (i.e. due to fracture) or infiltration and/or pressure by growing tumour.

Non-mechanical symptoms and pain at night are concerning symptoms, especially around the knee in an adolescent. These symptoms do warrant urgent further investigations.

- *Swelling is due to* mass of the tumour or haematoma following pathological fracture.
- *Deformity is due to* slowly evolving abnormal bone remodelling influenced by the presence of the tumour.
- *Distant symptoms or signs are due to* the presence of metastatic deposits (most commonly in the lung).
- *Generalized symptoms, e.g. tiredness/weakness/weight loss, are due to* metabolic effects of the tumour.

All treatment options are dependent on an accurate histopathological diagnosis. This is established in the clinicoradiological context of the individual case and it is imperative that all bone tumour diagnoses are considered by a multidisciplinary medical team that must include experienced surgeons, pathologists, radiologists and oncologists.[2]

The diagnostic input should include the following.

- A review of the clinical presentation and past medical history. In particular, the patient's age, site of lesion, duration of symptoms, particular events (e.g. pathological fracture) and history of previous tumours (e.g. past history of carcinoma of breast, prostate, etc.). Certain previous or coexistent tumours (e.g. retinoblastoma, soft-tissue neurofibroma, osteochondroma, enchondroma, etc.) that might indicate a tumour syndrome.
- A thorough clinical examination, not only of the diseased part but generally, e.g. evidence of hyperparathyroidism, neurofibromatosis, osteochondromatosis, primary malignancy, etc.
- Laboratory investigations including erythrocyte sedimentation rate, C-reactive protein, calcium, phosphate, alkaline phosphatase, serum electrophoresis and urinalysis for Bence–Jones proteins.
- Comprehensive radiological imaging of the diseased area, and, where indicated, imaging of other areas, e.g. bone scan, skeletal survey. Imaging of abdomen and chest for detection of possible primary sites and presence of possible metastases.
- A decision whether or not to establish a tissue diagnosis. Biopsies should be planned in an attempt to gain the maximum information, e.g. biopsy should sample the most aggressive area of the tumour and/or the interface between the tumour and adjacent bone.

Many bone tumour types affect limited/characteristic age groups and most tumours have predilections for certain bones as well as for certain regions within bones. It follows that the patient's age and the site of the tumour are often important aids in establishing the diagnosis. An accurate working diagnosis can often be made before a lesion has been biopsied. For example, a purely lytic, eccentrically placed tumour involving the epiphysis and metaphysis of the distal radius in a 35-year-old patient is almost certainly a giant cell tumour of bone. Certain musculoskeletal diseases, including bone tumours, show strong ethnic links (e.g. Ewing's sarcoma and Pagetic sarcoma are essentially diseases of Caucasians). Some other non-neoplastic bone diseases that may enter the differential diagnosis of bone tumours include Gaucher's disease (Ashkenazi Jews) and sickle cell anaemia (Afro-Caribbean).

BASICS OF BONE STRUCTURE AND REMODELLING

In order to better understand the radiological and pathological features of bone tumours, it is useful to give a brief overview of the nature of bone and the fundamentals of bone remodelling, as well as to clarify the precise meaning of some of the descriptive terms commonly employed. We can define types of bone by anatomical location – i.e. cortical and medullary – as well as by gross and microscopic architecture. Architecturally, there are two important bone types: compact bone and trabecular bone. In addition, bone can be defined by its nature, i.e. lamellar and woven types.

Compact bone is defined as bone that possesses an internal blood supply, and, conversely, trabecular (also known as cancellous or spongy) bone is bone that lacks an internal blood supply. Normal cortical bone is of compact type and normal medullary bone is of trabecular type. However, in pathological conditions, compact bone may be present within the medulla (e.g. sclerosis around a Brodie's abscess) and trabecular bone may exist in a subperiosteal location (e.g. as part of the periosteal response to fracture).

As mentioned, the bone can also be defined by its nature: lamellar or woven. The coordinated production of bone by a sheet of cooperative osteoblasts will deposit a plate (or lamella) of bone. In terms of functional attributes, this is high-quality bone and forms the entire normal adult skeleton. Conversely, the hurried, slightly disorganized production of bone by sheets of osteoblasts produces so-called 'woven bone'. Compared with lamellar bone, woven bone lacks the internal plate structure and has more irregularly distributed and slightly larger osteocytes at a higher density. As a consequence, woven bone lacks the high functional performance of lamellar bone. The presence of woven bone, in its many shapes and forms, indicates rapid bone production and is seen in growing, reparative and diseased states.

Bone matrix is mineralized osteoid, and can only be resorbed by one cell type, the osteoclast, and formed by one cell type, the osteoblast. Significant bone resorption and formation can only occur at the bone surface, and there is a maximum rate at which this can occur. It follows that, for a tumour to expand in this rigid environment, it must be either at the expense of resorbing bone or by permeative growth through host bone. Histologically, tumour permeative growth is defined as that which occurs around lamellar bone trabeculae in the medulla or through lamellar bone Haversian canals in the cortex. If an intramedullary bone tumour is non-permeative and static or slow growing, the host bone has an opportunity to respond to its presence by producing a sclerotic rim of compact bone. Therefore, the presence of a confining rim of sclerotic, compact bone around an intramedullary lesion is an indication that the lesion is benign. On the other hand, the absence of a sclerotic rim indicates that the tumour is growing faster than the rate at which the host bone is able to respond. Tumour permeative growth is a histological feature of malignancy (with the notable exceptions of eosinophilic granuloma and haemangioma).

RADIOLOGICAL DIAGNOSIS

Obtaining a plain radiograph of the clinically suspected area is an essential early step in establishing a diagnosis. The radiological diagnosis of bone tumours is primarily made on the basis of the plain radiographs. Further investigations are performed to narrow down the differential diagnosis and for a better assessment of the extent of the lesion.

Further imaging modalities, namely CT imaging, MRI and bone scintigraphy, are often necessary to refine a radiological diagnosis or differential diagnosis. Radiological assessment of a bone lesion will yield several important features of a bone tumour:

- its presence (i.e. normal or abnormal radiograph)
- its location, in particular which bone as well as where in the bone (e.g. epiphyseal/metaphyseal/diaphyseal and surface/intra-cortical/intra-medullary)
- its size and shape, and whether it is confined to bone or has extended into soft tissue.

The majority of bone tumours are metaphyseal in location. However, some tumours tend to be epiphyseal or diaphyseal.

Epiphyseal tumours are

- giant cell tumour (physes closed)
- chondroblastoma
- intra-articular osteoid osteoma (atypical)
- clear cell chondrosarcoma.

Apart from clear cell chondrosarcoma, all other epiphyseal tumours are benign.

Tumours that tend to be located in the diaphysis are

- eosinophilic granuloma
- osteoid osteoma
- fibrous dysplasia
- adamantinoma (tibia)
- Ewing's sarcoma.

Further useful radiographic observations are

- whether the lesion is ill-defined or sharply circumscribed (i.e. permeative or not)
- whether the lesion is lytic (pure bone resorption), sclerotic (bone formation), or both
- whether the lesion *per se* has radiographically apparent properties (especially matrix mineralization).

Full radiological assessment of a patient with a suspected malignant primary bone tumour includes

- radiographs of the whole affected bone in two planes
- MRI scan of the lesion
- CT scan of the lesion
- chest radiographs
- CT scan of the chest
- radioisotope bone scan or whole body MRI scan
- ultrasound scan/CT scan of abdomen to exclude a primary renal tumour (if the lesion is lytic).

Further imaging will establish whether the lesion is solitary or multifocal. Lesions within the same bone are classed as satellite or skip lesions. Satellite lesions are distant from the tumour, but occur within the reactive zone. Skip lesions are outside the reactive zone.

A radioisotope bone scan is a sensitive scan to detect distant bone metastases. However, certain tumours, such as multiple myeloma, are usually cold on bone scan and a whole body MRI scan can be more sensitive and specific to detect distant disease.[3]

If the tumour breaches the cortex or is a surface tumour, it will interact with the periosteum. The relatively quiescent periosteum can be activated in a number of ways.

A slowly growing subperiosteal lesion will slowly peel the periosteum off the bone cortex and stimulate it to form new, usually compact, bone.

More rapid elevation of the periosteum by tumour or haematoma associated with pathological fracture will stimulate a less organized, more trabecular bone production.[2] Some malignant tumours (e.g. Ewing's sarcoma and lymphoma) will cause some elevation of the periosteum, but will also permeate straight through the periosteum to produce an ill-defined soft-tissue mass. In such cases, periosteal reaction may be quite subtle and associated with a significant periosteal mass.

If the periosteum is elevated in the diaphyseal part of a bone, it tends to be symmetrical and fusiform. Therefore, the periosteal reaction in Ewing's sarcoma has often a characteristic multilayered 'onion skin' appearance.

However, the periosteum is firmly attached near the physis. Consequently, a Codman's triangle occurs if the periosteum is elevated in the metaphyseal area (as in osteosarcoma).

Osteoblastic and chondroblastic tumours often mineralize their matrix product, permitting a radiological assessment of the tumour's nature. Cartilage matrix calcifies to give a speckled, indistinct appearance, whereas mineralized bone matrix has a sharper, 'harder' and often more dense appearance. In the case of cartilaginous neoplasms, the extent of calcification often correlates to the benignity of the tumour, since enchondromas are more likely than chondrosarcomas to produce a hyaline-type, well-differentiated matrix similar to that seen in the physeal growth plate (a normal tissue counterpart that undergoes cellular hypertrophy and matrix calcification).

Following staging, a decision should be taken whether the lesions require a biopsy. The biopsy should be taken by the bone tumour unit that will be responsible for the surgical care of the patient.[4–6] The biopsy should be positioned so that it can be excised 'en block' with the resection specimen at the time of definitive surgery to reduce the risk of recurrence. The biopsy site should be in line with an extensile approach to the affected bone. A tourniquet can be used, but the limb should not be exsanguinated (although the limb can be elevated). Bone biopsies are usually taken with a Jamshidi needle under image guidance, either fluoroscopy or CT, depending on the nature and position of the lesion. The Jamshidi needle has a bevelled edge, allowing a core of bone to be harvested for histological analysis without crushing it. Most bone tumour treatment centres agree that cytological fine needle aspiration (FNA) is insufficient to make a histological diagnosis of bone tumour.

An open bone biopsy may be required. This should be done via a longitudinal incision in line with the extensile approach required for the definitive surgery to remove the tumour.

Following histological analysis, the case should be discussed in a multidisciplinary meeting to discuss the diagnosis and plan treatment.[1,2,7–9]

PATHOLOGY OF BONE NEOPLASMS

The entities recognized in the recent WHO classification of bone tumours[1] are listed in Table 81.1. Only a selection of the most commonly encountered entities can be discussed in this chapter.[1,2,7–9] The genetic analysis of neoplasia is an important field that has revolutionized our understanding of the pathogenesis of tumours. Furthermore, the discovery of specific genetic mutations in tumour types and subtypes that were originally classified by morphological criteria has validated the original morphological approach to tumour classification. The key molecular discoveries for each tumour type will be described where appropriate.

SIMPLE BONE CYST/UNICAMERAL BONE CYST

A simple, unicameral or solitary bone cyst is an intramedullary cyst that is usually unilocular and filled with serous or serosanguineous fluid.[1] The age, sex and site distribution are shown in Fig. 81.1.

Clinically, unicameral bone cysts are often asymptomatic, but they can produce pain. These cysts often present with a pathological fracture.

Radiologically, the cyst is usually located in the meta-diaphyseal region and grows away from the physis. There may be minimal cortical expansion, and the cortex is usually thin (allowing pathological fracture). Sclerosis around the lesion is usually absent. CT and MRI confirm the presence of fluid within the cyst cavity.[10] There may be septation within the cyst. A 'fallen leaf' sign is pathognomonic for a simple bone cyst and is the result of cortical fracture (Fig. 81.2). Usually a confident radiological diagnosis can be made and a biopsy may not be required. However, this should be performed if there is any diagnostic doubt.

Macroscopically, the cavity of the cyst is filled with serous or serosanguineous fluid. The cavity is lined with a membrane and there may be some septae.

Microscopically, the lining of the cyst is a fibrous membrane that may contain foci of reactive new bone formation or cementum-like material.

The cyst may resolve spontaneously or sometimes following fracture.[11] A number of treatments have been described for simple bone cysts. All these treatments rely on the puncture or removal of the fibrous membrane lining of the cyst. A biopsy in itself can be curative if the lining of the cyst is punctured and the cyst wall collapses. Other treatments that have been described include injection with steroid or bone marrow, the insertion of a unicortical screw and curettage of the lining of the cyst. If a pathological fracture has occurred, the fracture can usually be treated conservatively and the cyst may resolve if the membrane has been punctured by the fracture. Otherwise, the cyst can be curetted after the fracture has united. However, internal fixation may be necessary (i.e. in a hip fracture).

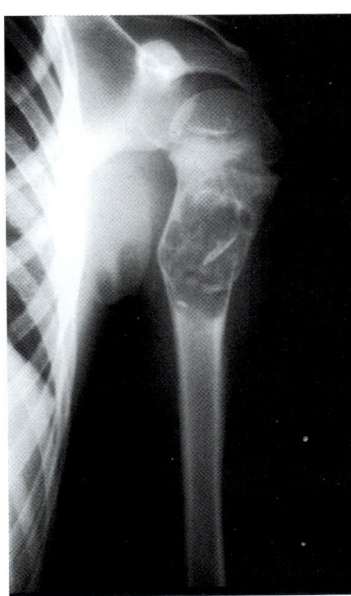

Figure 81.2 Simple bone cyst (SBC): radiograph of a typical simple bone cyst in the proximal humerus, showing the 'fallen leaf sign' that is pathognomonic for a simple bone cyst.

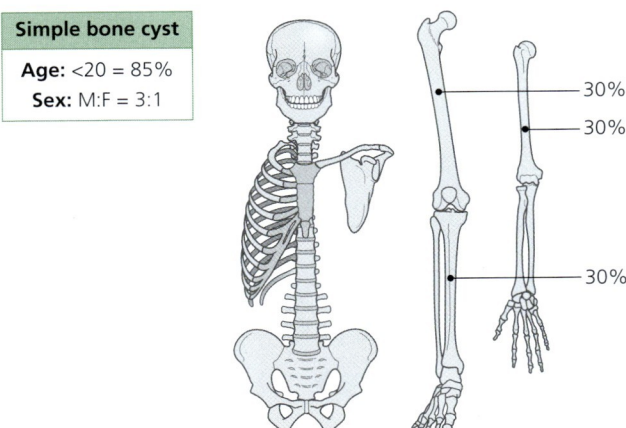

Figure 81.1 Simple bone cyst/unicameral bone cyst.

Recurrence rates of up to 20% have been reported.[1] Retarded growth, malunion and avascular necrosis of the femoral head following treatment of pathological fracture can occur.[12]

ANEURYSMAL BONE CYST

Aneurysmal bone cyst (ABC) is traditionally divided into primary (i.e. de novo) and secondary (i.e. intimately associated with a distinct bone tumour) ABC. In recent years it has been demonstrated that primary, but not secondary, ABC has a characteristic translocation, namely chromosomal rearrangement of the short arm of chromosome 17.[13] This is usually present as a balanced translocation with the long arm of chromosome 16, although other chromosomal partners have been described that may exchange genetic material with chromosome 17. The 17p oncogene upregulated by these translocations is the ubiquitin protease *USP6* gene sited at 17p13. The age distribution at clinical presentation, sites of involvement and sex ratio for primary ABC are given in Fig. 81.3.

Clinically, patients usually present with a painful bony swelling or (less commonly) a pathological fracture. In the spine the patient may have neurological symptoms.

Radiologically, ABC most often affects the metaphyseal regions of long bones and the posterior elements of vertebrae in the immature skeleton (Fig. 81.4). The lesion is closely associated with the physis and primary ABC is rare in the skeletally mature. It is a purely lytic and eccentrically located 'expansile' lesion that is sharply demarcated from adjacent normal bone and usually lacks peripheral sclerosis. The uneven scalloping of the endosteum gives a trabeculated appearance. The extracortical component has an intact, thin, subperiosteal reactive bone shell. On MRI, there are usually so-called fluid–fluid levels due to sedimentation of erythrocytes in the stagnant blood-filled spaces.[14] It is important to note that this is not a specific feature to ABC, and can be seen in any blood filled cavity,

e.g. telangiectatic osteosarcoma. Also look for an associated primary lesion because, as noted above, ABC can be secondary.[15]

Macroscopically, ABC is well demarcated from surrounding bone, and is a boggy, haemorrhagic, 'expansile' mass. Variably sized, blood-filled cavities are present as well as solid areas.

Microscopically, ABC has a characteristic low-power appearance of variably sized, blood-filled spaces separated by cellular septa containing spindle cells, histiocytes, osteoclasts, reactive osteoblasts producing trabeculae of woven bone. Reflecting the haemorrhagic nature of the tumour, deposition of haemosiderin pigment is common (Fig. 81.4). Uncommonly, and causing some terminological confusion, ABCs can be solid.[16] Such cases are composed of identical cellular and matrical elements to those seen in

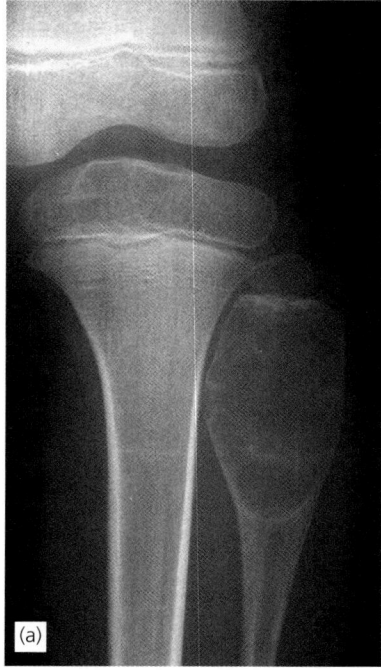
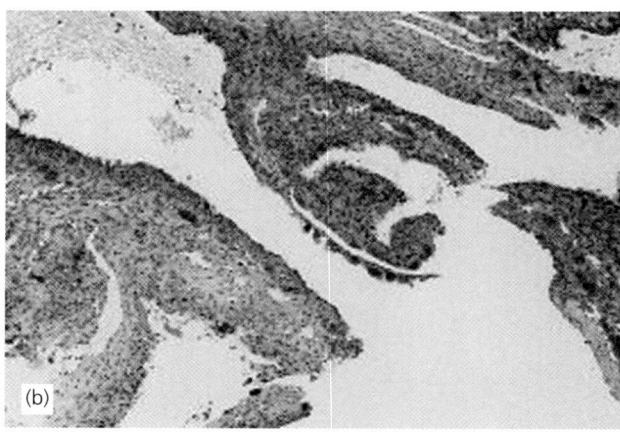

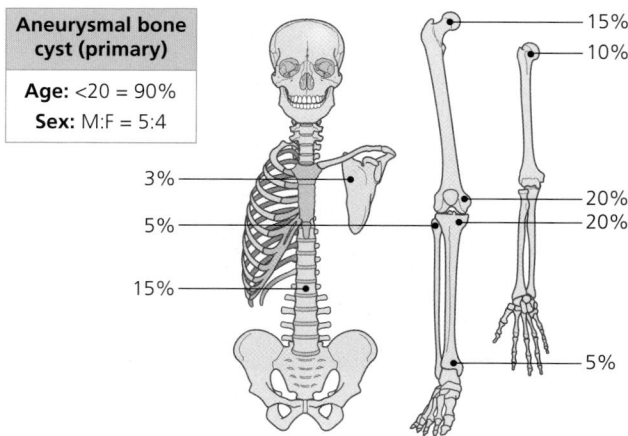

Figure 81.3 Aneurysmal bone cyst: age range and sex ratio.

Figure 81.4 Aneurysmal bone cyst (ABC): plain radiograph and haematoxylin and eosin section of aneurysmal bone cyst.

the septa of the cystic variant. The vast majority of secondary ABCs occur in association with benign bone tumours, most commonly giant cell tumour of bone and chondroblastoma.[14]

Aneurysmal bone cysts are usually treated by curettage. The recurrence rate following curettage is between 20% and 70% (significantly higher than simple bone cyst).

GIANT CELL TUMOUR OF BONE

Giant cell tumour (GCT) of bone is a benign, locally destructive tumour composed histologically of neoplastic, ovoid mesenchymal cells and, characteristically evenly dispersed, often very large, multinucleate osteoclast-like giant cells. The age range, site distribution and sex ratio of GCT is given in Fig. 81.5. It accounts for around 5% of all primary bone tumours.[1]

Patients usually present with pain, swelling or joint stiffness. Up to 10% of patients present with a pathological fracture. Histologically, GCTs are indistinguishable from 'brown tumours' in hyperparathyroidism. It is therefore essential that all patients have their calcium and phosphate levels checked, particularly if there are multiple lesions.

Radiologically, GCT almost exclusively affects the epiphysis and the metaphysis in skeletally mature individuals. The lesion is often quite large (7–15 cm), eccentric and purely lytic with a sharp interface with normal bone. It almost always abuts the articular cartilage (Fig. 81.6). GCT can show a thin, intact rim of often 'expanded' cortical bone, or a breach in the cortex and periosteum with soft tissue extension.[17] A 'soap-bubble' appearance has been described.

Macroscopically, GCT involves the parts of bone described radiologically, and has a sharply defined edge with a haemorrhagic, redcurrant jelly-like cut surface. Histologically, the classic appearance is of sheets of monotonous, ovoid, mesenchymal cells with active, but benign, cytological features, and evenly distributed, often extremely large, multinucleate osteoclast-like giant cells (Fig. 81.6). However, in different areas, other features are often seen. In particular, haemorrhagic areas, sometimes with cavitations resembling ABCs, i.e. secondary ABC. Also commonly seen are benign fibrohistiocytic areas, often with clusters of foamy histiocytes – presumably

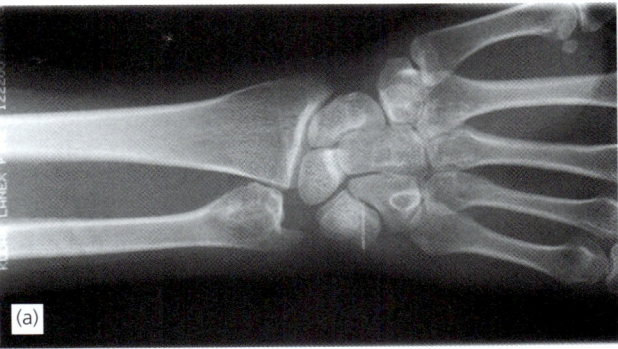

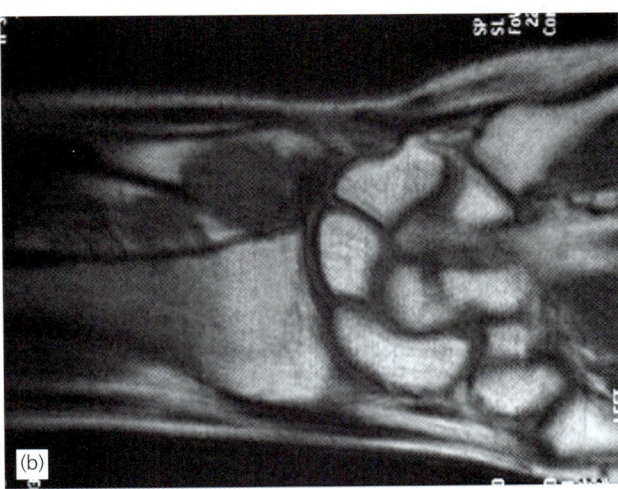

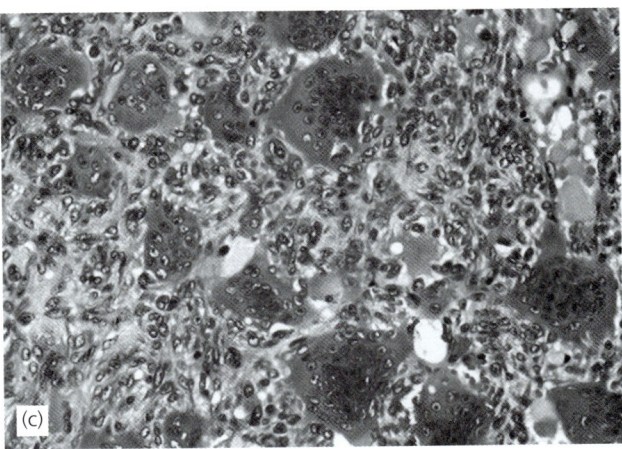

Figure 81.6 Giant cell tumour of bone (GCT): (a, b) Plain radiograph and MR scan of a distal ulnar GCT that extends to the undersurface of the articular cartilage. (C) High power haematoxylin and eosin section of a typical area of a GCT showing large, multinucleate osteoclast-like giant cells set against a background sheet of mononuclear stromal cells.

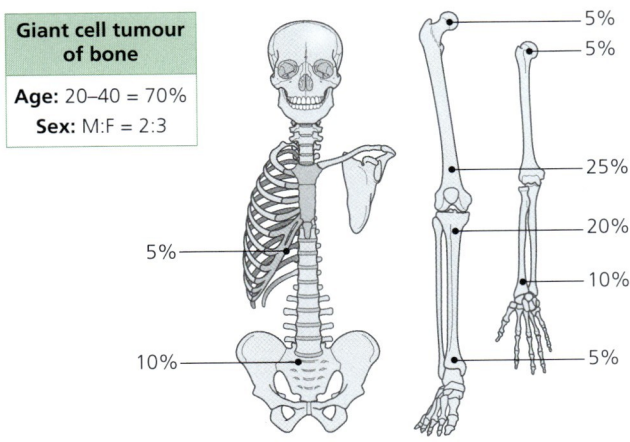

Figure 81.5 Giant cell tumour of bone: age range and sex ratio.

an organizing process secondary to extensive haemorrhage. It is not uncommon to see poorly formed, osteoid-like trabeculae; indeed, it has been repeatedly demonstrated that the neoplastic stromal cells of GCT have a limited osteoblastic phenotype. The most commonly reported genetic abnormality is shortened telomeres affecting multiple chromosomes.[18] The behaviour of most GCTs is of a non-metastasizing, locally aggressive neoplasm that is usually treated by thorough curettage.[19] Occasionally, where local disease is extensive and involves soft tissues, and/or there is a pathological fracture, excision with surgical reconstruction is performed. The recurrence rate following curettage with adjuvant treatment (burr down, argon beam coagulation, cryotherapy, phenol) is approximately 25% and usually occurs within the first 2 years.[1] Excision of the lesion has a lower recurrence rate.

Rarely, GCTs with benign histological features can generate so-called benign, pulmonary implants. These are not true metastases by virtue of their self-limiting growth potential.

Rare cases of malignant (sarcomatous) transformation in GCT have been described.[20] More commonly these are giant cell-rich bone sarcomas.

EOSINOPHILIC GRANULOMA

Eosinophilic granuloma (EG) is generally regarded as a neoplasm. The key constituent cell is the Langerhan's cell, a type of histiocyte that is most commonly seen in the epidermis, is involved in antigen presentation and can be defined by its characteristic grooved nucleus, immunohistochemically detectable CD1a and its cytoplasmic Birbeck granules visible under the electron microscope. The lesion is usually solitary (disseminated forms have been labelled Hand–Schuller–Christian disease and Letterer Siwe disease) and the sites of involvement, age range and sex ratio are shown in Fig. 81.7.[21,22]

Patients usually present with pain or swelling.

Radiologically, EG may appear aggressive. The lesion is lytic and usually well demarcated with peripheral sclerosis and a variable periosteal reaction (Fig. 81.8). Spinal body involvement may result in vertebra plana and/or neurological involvement. The differential diagnosis often

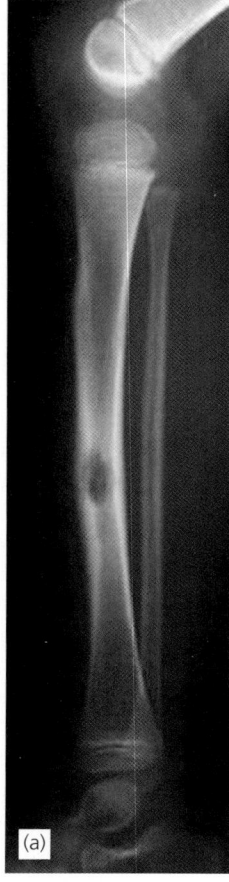

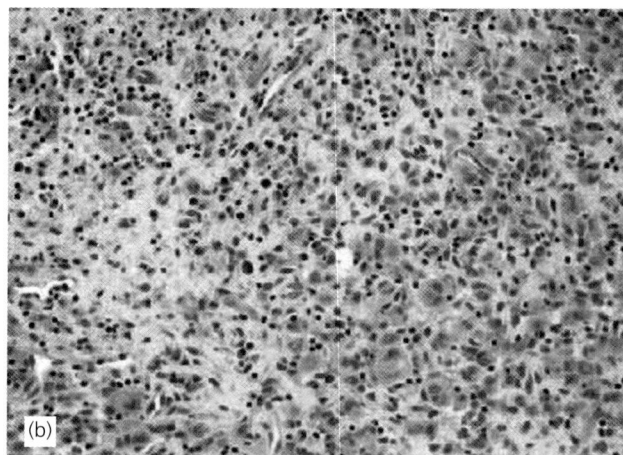

Figure 81.8 Eosinophilic granuloma (EG): (a) lateral plain radiograph showing the lytic eosinophilic granuloma affecting the diaphysis. (b) High power haematoxylin and eosin section showing the typical appearance of eosinophilic granuloma.

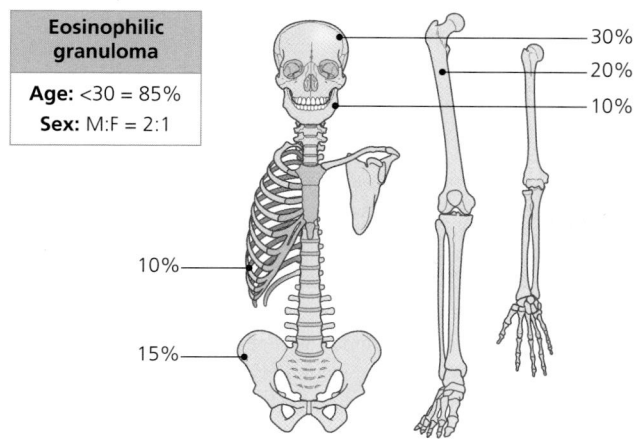

Figure 81.7 Eosinophilic granuloma: age range and sex ratio.

includes Ewing's sarcoma and a biopsy is required to confirm the diagnosis.

Macroscopically, lesional tissue is soft and red/brown. Microscopically, there is typically a mixed inflammatory cell infiltrate dominated by an eosinophil infiltrate and medium-sized, so-called Langerhan's histiocytic cells with a characteristic nucleus: ovoid in shape with finely dispersed chromatin and a nuclear membrane fold that gives the impression of a nuclear groove (Fig. 81.8). Other cells often present are lymphocytes, plasma cells and a variable number of neutrophils. Neutrophils, although often not mentioned in standard texts, are commonly present as a minor feature, but may be quite numerous giving a mixed osteomyelitis/EG appearance. In such cases, it is often wise to treat the patient with antibiotics. Solitary EG is usually treated expectantly and may resolve spontaneously. Treatment with steroid injection and curettage have also been described.

The diagnosis of EG relies on the demonstration of scattered, often clustered, Langerhan's cells aided by the immunohistochemical demonstration of CD1a expression. If this is performed, it is no longer necessary to demonstrate the presence of cytoplasmic Birbeck granules by more expensive and time-consuming electron microscopy. X chromosome inactivation study has demonstrated that the Langerhan's cells in EG are monoclonal.[23] EG is usually monostotic and has a favourable prognosis. If the disease process is disseminated, especially with visceral involvement, then the prognosis is usually very poor.

FIBROUS DYSPLASIA

Fibrous dysplasia is a benign fibro-osseous lesion that, until recently, has been considered to be a developmental abnormality. With the demonstration of monoclonality and the involvement of a mutated gene that encodes the α-subunit of the G protein (Gs alpha) that stimulates cAMP production, it now seems clear that it is a neoplastic process with a fibro-osseous histogenesis.[24] The age distribution at clinical presentation, sites of involvement and sex ratio are given in Fig. 81.9. Fibrous dysplasia may be monostotic or polyostotic.[25] Where polyostotic, it may be associated with skin pigmentation and precocious puberty (McCune–Albright syndrome) or intramuscular myxoma (Mazabraud syndrome).[26] The polyostotic form is usually confined to one extremity or side but can be more extensive.

Clinically, fibrous dysplasia may be asymptomatic or present with pain or pathological fracture.[27] Longstanding lesions, particularly in the femoral neck, may give rise to bone deformity (i.e. shepherd's crook deformity of the hip) (Fig. 81.10).

Radiologically, fibrous dysplasia has a non-aggressive, often 'expansile' appearance with a ground glass internal appearance. There is no soft-tissue component and this slowly evolving lesion lacks a discernible periosteal reaction. Fibrous dysplasia, like many bone tumours, can be associated with a secondary aneurysmal bone cyst.

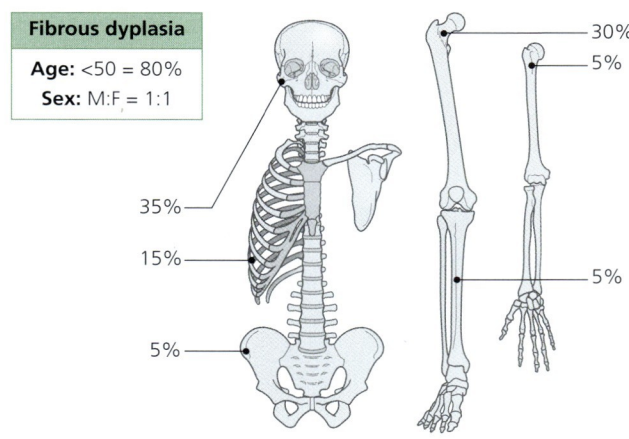

Figure 81.9 Fibrous dysplasia: age range and sex ratio.

Macroscopically, the host bone is often expanded to accommodate the lesion, which is well defined with a tan/grey colour and a firm, sometimes gritty, texture. Because fibrous dysplasia develops in the growing skeleton, it may become intimately associated with the physis. The physeal cartilage can become disrupted and incorporated into the lesion to give an enchondromatous appearance. Where this happens, the gross macroscopic (and radiological) appearance may be modified, especially if the cartilage matrix calcifies.

Microscopically, the classic appearance of fibrous dysplasia is a disorganized fibrous stroma from which irregular, malshaped and apparently purposeless bone trabeculae emanate. The background fibroblast-like spindle cells are cytologically bland, and the bone trabeculae characteristically lack a monolayer rim of osteoblasts (although this may not be the case towards the periphery) (Fig. 81.10). On occasion, cementum-like or psammomatous calcifications are produced rather than bony trabeculae. There may be secondary features such as islands of foamy histiocytes or myxoid change.

Malignant transformation of fibrous dysplasia has been described,[1] but is very rare.

OSTEOID OSTEOMA AND OSTEOBLASTOMA

Although listed separately in the WHO classification, these tumours show enough similarities that they will be considered together.[1,28] Osteoid osteoma (OO) and osteoblastoma (OBL) are benign osteoblastic neoplasms that are histologically identical. They are distinguished by an arbitrarily designated difference in their size; lesions 2 cm or less in diameter are classified as OO, and lesions greater than 2 cm in diameter are classified as OBL. This overriding use of size as distinguishing criterion is unique in the classification of human neoplasia. However, once so classified, the skeletal distribution and intra-osseous location of OO and OBL is quite different. OBL more commonly affects the axial skeleton and the medullary bone, and, conversely, OO more commonly affects the appendicular skeleton and is more often cortically sited. It has been suggested that the important underlying difference in these tumours is that the intra-osseous site of origin determines the attainable size. Medullary lesions may achieve a greater size before clinical presentation because they are in a less densely sclerotic environment and further removed from the densely innervated periosteum (i.e. are less likely to produce pain early in their development). This, however, is controversial, and most pathologists continue to view them as separate but closely related lesions.

The age, sex and site distributions of OO and OBL are indicated in Figs 81.11 and 81.12.

Clinically, osteoid osteomas usually present with pain at night (due to periostitis), that is typically relieved by salicylates or anti-inflammatories.[29] However, if the lesion is close to a joint, it can present with synovitis and diagnosis may be more difficult.[30] Osteoblastomas in the spine predilect the posterior elements and the sacrum and may present with scoliosis or nerve root compression.[31,32]

Multicentric OO and/or OBL is excessively rare. For osteoid osteoma, plain radiographs show a dense sclerotic lesion in the cortex with or without a discernible central lucency. CT shows the cortically based

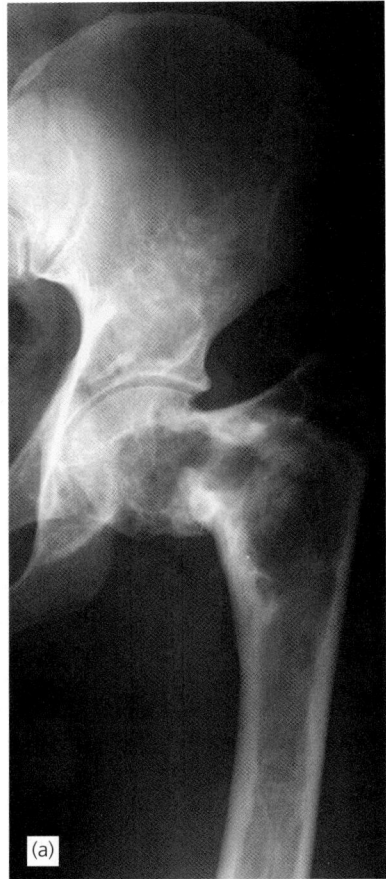

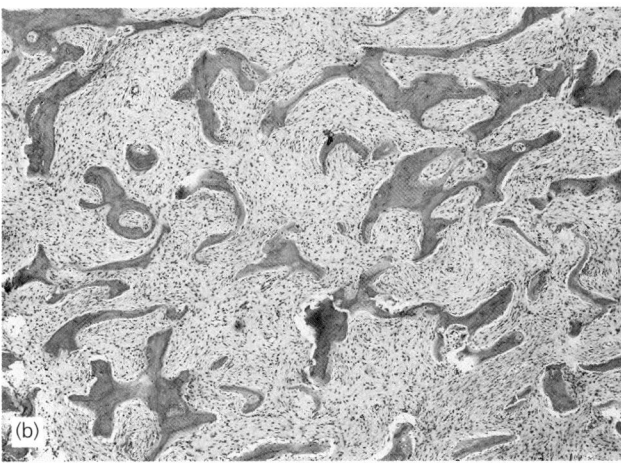

Figure 81.10 Fibrous dysplasia (FD): (a) plain radiograph showing the shepherd's crook deformity due to fibrous dysplasia involving the femoral neck. (b) Low power haematoxylin and eosin section showing irregularly formed and distributed woven bone trabeculae emanating from a background of loose fibrous tissue.

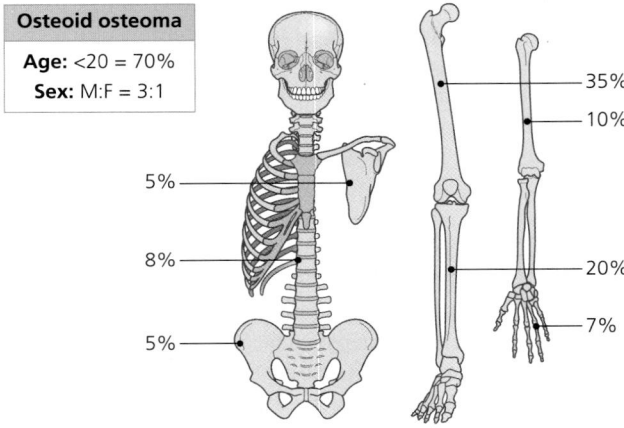

Figure 81.11 Osteoid osteoma: age range and sex ratio.

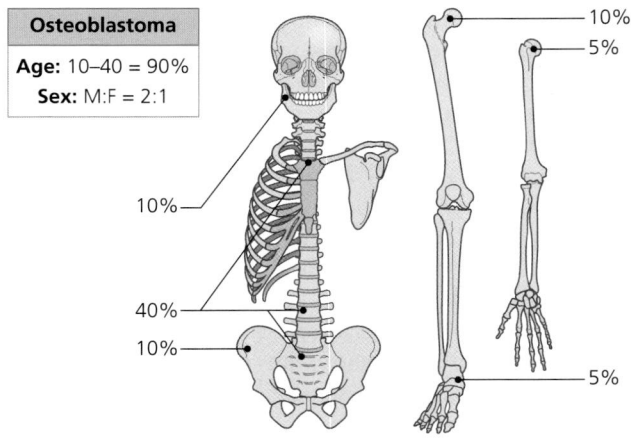

Figure 81.12 Osteoblastoma: age range and sex ratio.

nidus and surrounding sclerosis more clearly (Fig. 81.13). For osteoblastoma, plain radiographs reveal a well-circumscribed, lytic lesion. MRI and CT show the well-defined lytic mass. When the lesion is vertebral, it involves the posterior elements (Fig. 81.14). Macroscopically, both tumours are well defined and red/brown with a gritty consistency. Larger lesions (i.e. OBL) are usually centred on the medulla, and may cause an erosive appearance in the adjacent bone. However, there is always an intact periosteum, which, if closely approached by the tumour, will show reactive new bone formation (Figs 81.13 and 81.14). Nowadays, osteoid osteomas are usually treated with CT-guided radiofrequency thermocoagulation.[33] Osteoblastomas may also be suitable for radiofrequency thermocoagulation, but invasive surgery may be necessary.

Microscopically, both tumours show richly vascularized areas with immature and maturing trabecular bone

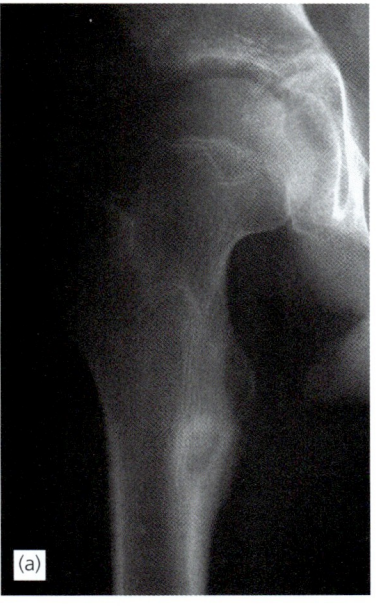
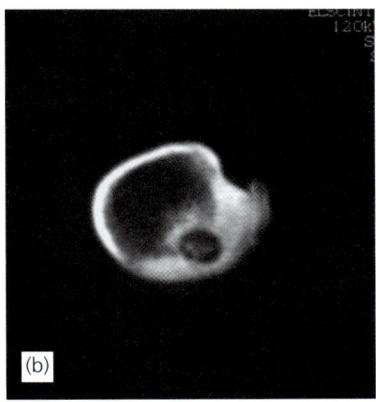
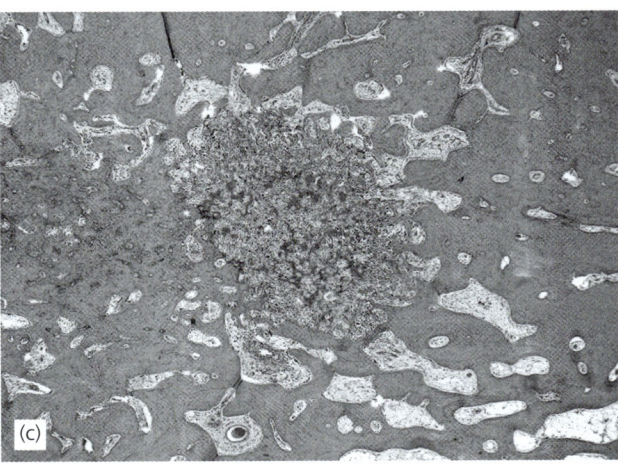

Figure 81.13 Osteoid osteoma (OO): (a, b) plain radiograph and CT scan showing a nidus of osteoid osteoma. (C) Low-power haematoxylin and eosin sections of an osteoid osteoma.

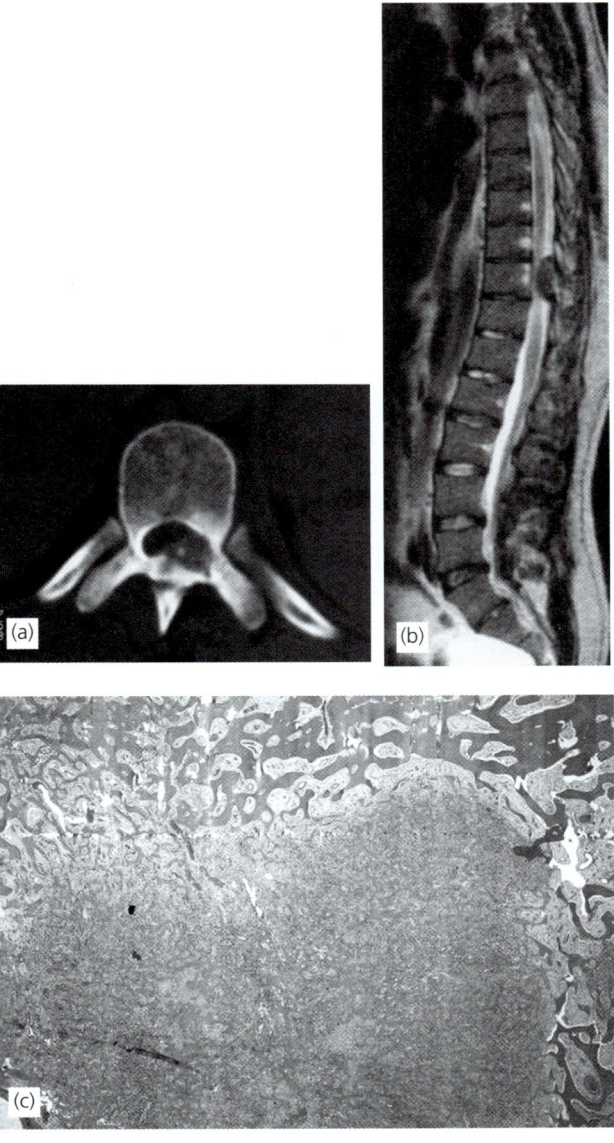

Figure 81.14 Osteoblastoma (OBL): (a, b) CT and MR images of an osteoblastoma arising from the posterior elements of a vertebra and impinging on the spinal canal. (c) Low-power haematoxylin and eosin section of an osteoblastoma.

production.³⁴ The bone trabeculae are disorganized but retain a discernible monolayer of, often very active, surface osteoblasts. This osteoblastic monolayer, with produced bone matrix on one side and a supporting, richly vascular fibroblastic connective tissue on the other, is an important feature in helping distinguish reactive and benign neoplastic osteoblastic activity from malignant osteoblastic tumours (i.e. osteosarcoma). In osteosarcoma, the required degree of cooperation between osteoblasts (and with their supportive fibrovascular stroma) is lost and, hence, so is its morphological manifestation of osteoblast monolayer formation. There is usually extravasation of erythrocytes as well as osteoclast-like giant cell accumulation. Another common feature is the presence of scattered larger cells with smudged nuclei (i.e. degenerative nuclear features). An unusual feature is the well-documented innervation seen in OO. This has recently also been clearly demonstrated in osteoblastoma. Other areas of the tumour can produce a more sclerotic and occasionally fibrillary osteoid matrix, and such areas can closely mimic sclerosing areas of osteoblastic osteosarcoma. OO and OBL do not permeate and entrap surrounding bone. Larger lesions (i.e. OBL) are bone tumours that can be associated with haemorrhagic/'cystic' lesions morphologically indistinguishable from aneurysmal bone cyst – i.e. so-called secondary aneurysmal bone cyst (Figs 81.3 and 81.4). There are reports on genetic abnormalities in OO and OBL,³⁵,³⁶ but, currently, their number is few and no consistent genetic abnormalities have emerged. There are reports of osteoblastomas with more aggressive clinical behaviour, and rare reports of transformation to frank osteosarcoma. Some authors have correlated local clinical aggressiveness with certain histological features, notably plumpness of the osteoblasts and a higher mitotic rate.

The prognosis following treatment is good with a low incidence of recurrence.³³

CHONDROBLASTOMA

Chondroblastoma is a benign, chondroid neoplasm that nearly always arises in the epiphyseal region of bones before physeal closure. The age range, site distribution and sex ratio are given in Fig. 81.15.³⁷,³⁸

Chondroblastoma presents with persistent, often long-standing, joint pain. A joint effusion may be present.

Radiologically, chondroblastoma are lytic, small (average 4 cm diameter), well-demarcated (sometimes with a thin rim of bony sclerosis) lesions that occur in the epiphyseal region of young adolescents/adults (Fig. 81.16). It is not unusual for the lesion to be missed on initial radiographs. A bone scan can help in identifying the lesion. Chondroblastomas can be centrally or eccentrically placed. Generally, the bone is not expanded and there is no periosteal reaction as the lesion is in the epiphysis. There may an effusion due to localized synovitis. A CT scan shows calcifications in one-third of the cases, which can be

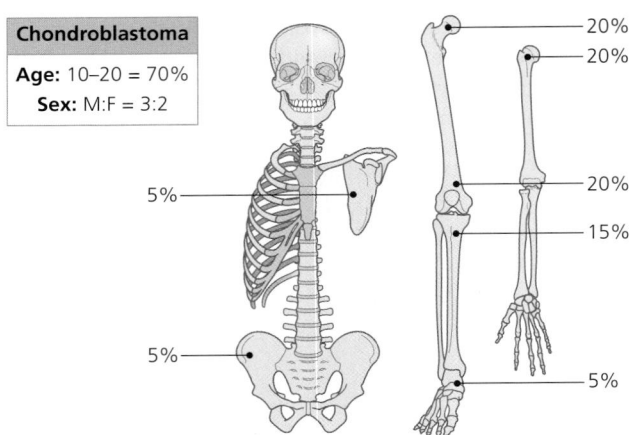

Figure 81.15 Chondroblastoma: age range and sex ratios.

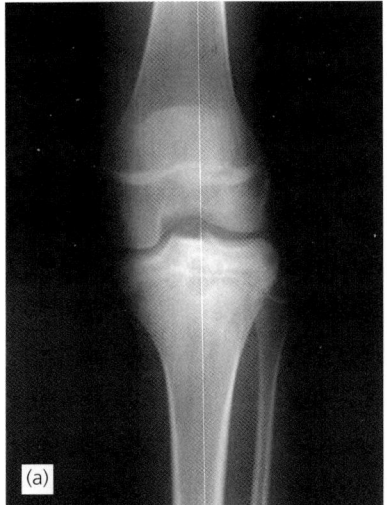

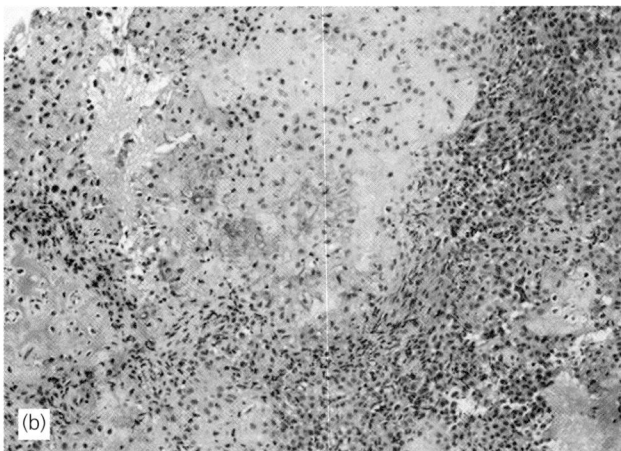

Figure 81.16 Chondroblastoma: (a) plain radiograph showing a proximal tibial epiphyseal chondroblastoma. (b) Medium power haematoxylin and eosin section of a chondroblastoma showing chondroid matrix and adjacent cellular area.

helpful in making the diagnosis.[38] Chondroblastomas may create a secondary aneurysmal bone cyst.

Histologically, the lesion is vaguely, sometimes markedly, lobular due to alternating and merging areas of greater and lesser pale, eosinophilic matrix production. The neoplastic cell is a medium-sized, round to ovoid cell, with distinct cytoplasmic borders and clefted, or sometimes crenated, nuclei. The tumour cell-produced matrix is usually pink and hyaline, and encases the lesional cells in lacunae. This feature gives the tumour its chondroid appearance (Fig. 81.16). True, basophilic, hyaline cartilage is distinctly uncommon in chondroblastoma. So-called 'chicken wire calcification' describes the connected network of pericellular calcification that is quite commonly seen in chondroblastoma. Chromosomal abnormalities involving chromosomes 5 and 8 have been reported.[39] Surgical curettage has been described as the preferred treatment for chondroblastoma. But treatment is difficult as the tumour is epipyseal in location and future joint function is a concern. More recently, radiofrequency thermocoagulation has been reported to have good results.[40]

Rare cases can give rise to so-called pulmonary implants, distinguishable from metastases in that they are non-progressive. Similar pulmonary implants are more commonly seen, although still distinctly rare, in giant cell tumour of bone. The claimed existence of a true malignant chondroblastoma is controversial.

Recurrence rates following treatment have been reported between 14% and 18% and usually occur within the first 2 years.

Osteochondroma

Osteochondroma is a cartilage-covered bony outgrowth and has a marrow-containing medulla that is in continuity with the medulla of the bone from which it arises. These lesions are sometimes referred to as osteocartilaginous exostoses and sometimes, rather loosely, as simply exostoses. They can be multiple, when the condition is referred to as hereditary osteochondromatosis, hereditary multiple exostoses or diaphyseal aclasia (with reference to the associated meta-diaphyseal deformity seen in such cases). Osteochondroma is probably the most common of all primary bone tumours[8,9] and for many years was considered to be a developmental abnormality due to some deficiency in the containment of the physis. However, with the discovery of cytogenetic aberrations involving the *EXT* genes (in both sporadic and hereditary forms, and in solitary as well as multiple lesions) it became clear that this is another developmental bone lesion that is now best regarded as a neoplasm.[41–43] The sites of involvement, age distribution and sex ratios are given in Fig. 81.17.

Clinically, osteochondromas can be asymptomatic and found incidentally. Symptoms are usually related to the size and location of the osteochondroma. The patient may present with symptoms of swelling, neurovascular

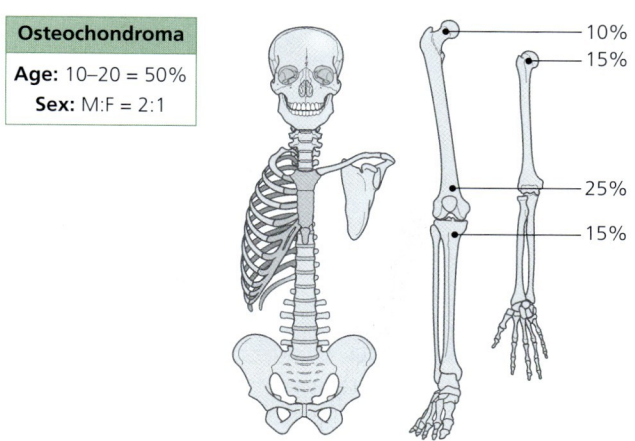

Figure 81.17 Osteochondroma: age range and sex ratio.

obstruction, mechanical irritation, bursa formation, infarction or fracture. The risk of malignant transformation is estimated at 1% in solitary osteochondromas and 1–3% in patients with diaphyseal aclasia.[8,9,44] An increase in size, particularly after the patient has reached skeletal maturity, is of concern and warrants further investigation.

Radiologically, osteochondromas are seen as sessile or pedunculated lesions that flare out from the bone surface with cortical continuity of their stalk (Fig. 81.18). This is often best appreciated on CT. The medulla of the bone of origin is in continuity with the medulla of the lesion. The osteochondroma always grows away from the joint and never has structures attached to it.

A thick cartilage cap (>10 mm) is a radiological concern that the lesion has undergone malignant transformation.[45]

Macroscopically and microscopically, it can be appreciated that the whole lesion is ultimately the product of the cartilage cap, which is originally on the bone surface and from the edge of the physis (Fig. 81.18). The cartilage cap is the neoplastic element. As the benign bone surface cartilage cap grows, it differentiates in the same way as the growth plate from which it originally derived. As such, the under-surface of the cartilage cap produces mineralizing hyaline cartilage matrix that is resorbed by osteoclasts which, in turn, stimulates osteogenesis. This is precisely the process of endochondral ossification that occurs at the metaphyseal aspect of the physis. In time, the cartilage cap may exhaust itself and the entire calcified cartilage matrix is resorbed and replaced by bone. The unevenness of the cartilage cap's growth and resorption gives the characteristic cauliflower-like appearance of the osteochondromatous cap.

Symptomatic osteochondromas can be treated with excision. The neoplastic cartilage cap should be removed completely to avoid recurrence. The recurrence rate is lower in older patients who have a 'burned out' cartilage cap than in younger patients with an active cartilage cap.

Patients with multiple osteochondromas are usually kept under surveillance.

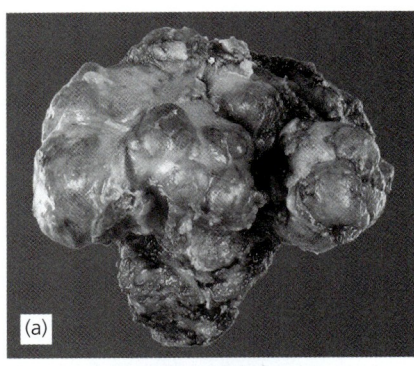
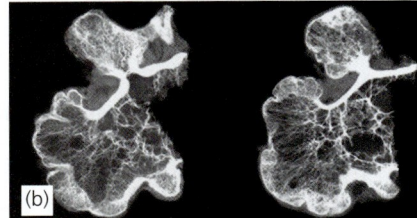
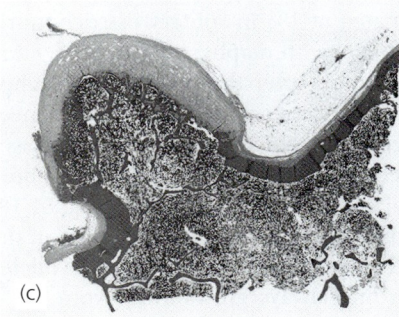

Figure 81.18 Osteochondroma: (a) intact resected multinodular osteochondroma. (b) Radiograph of a whole slice through specimen A. (c) Low-power haematoxylin and eosin section of an osteochondroma with detail of the cartilage cap.

ENCHONDROMA AND CHONDROSARCOMA

Enchondroma is a benign cartilaginous neoplasm occurring within bone. Chondrosarcoma is its malignant counterpart. These tumours are best considered together because their distinguishing features lie along a continuum. Both are usually solitary lesions, but may be multiple (i.e. enchondromatosis or Ollier's disease with or without malignant transformation). When enchondromatosis is associated with soft-tissue haemangiomas, the disease is referred to as Maffucci's disease. Patients with enchondromatosis have an approximately 25% risk of developing malignancy. This is usually a low-grade chondrosarcoma, but high-grade sarcomas such as osteosarcoma and dedifferentiated chondrosarcoma have also been described.[46,47] The common sites of involvement, age distribution and sex ratio for both enchondroma and chondrosarcoma are given in Figs 81.19 and 81.20.[9,48] Enchondroma is one of the more common primary bone tumours, and many are

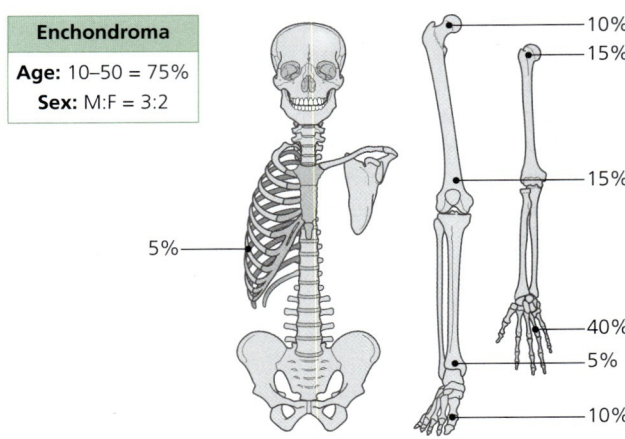

Figure 81.19 Enchondroma: age distribution and sex ratio.

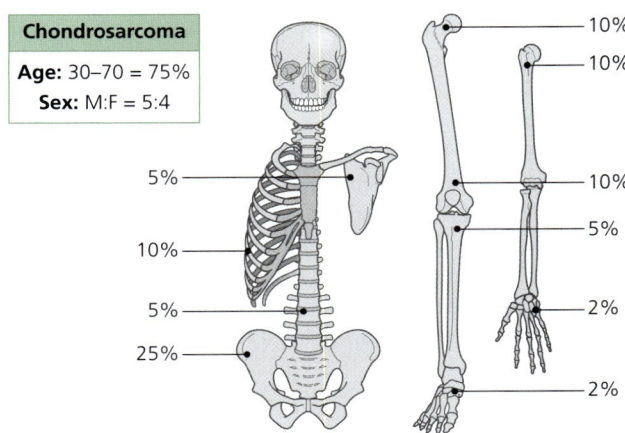

Figure 81.20 Chondrosarcoma: age distribution and sex ratio.'

clinically silent. Chondrosarcoma is the second most common primary bone malignancy (after osteosarcoma). The evidence that these tumours represent points on a continuum is

- when patients with Ollier's disease are monitored closely, there is often temporal progression from a radiologically benign enchondroma to a frankly malignant chondrosarcoma
- when solitary chondrosarcomas are excised, careful study often shows associated, presumably precursor, enchondromatous areas.

The histological spectrum between enchondroma and chondrosarcoma forms a continuum. At the benign end of the spectrum, the lesion is generally hypocellular, composed of hyaline, often mineralized, matrix; it lacks a permeative growth pattern and the chondrocytes show no significant nuclear atypia and mitoses are absent. Conversely, at the fully malignant end of the spectrum, the tumour is cellular, composed of poor-quality, often myxoid matrix, shows a permeative growth pattern, and the chondrocytes display nuclear atypia and mitotic activity.

Cartilaginous tumours display a spectrum of locally aggressive features, and it is sometimes the case that cartilaginous tumours possess radiological and pathological features which are intermediate between enchondroma and chondrosarcoma; such cases can be labelled 'atypical enchondroma' to denote their borderline nature. Because it is common, when examining resected chondrosarcomas, to find small areas that are indistinguishable from enchondroma it is likely that at least some chondrosarcomas arise from a pre-existing enchondroma. Some bone tumour treatment centres recognize the existence of a borderline cartilaginous tumour. These are variously labelled as 'cartilaginous lesion of uncertain malignant potential' (CLUMP), atypical enchondroma or even 'grade half chondrosarcoma'.

Enchondromas may present with a palpable swelling (especially in the hands and feet) or pathological fracture. However, many cartilage tumours are asymptomatic (especially in the long bones) and are often a coincidental finding. Longstanding pain is a concerning symptom and may indicate a chondrosarcoma.

Radiologically, enchondroma is an intra-osseous lytic lesion, often showing an ill-defined, woolly internal calcification, with a variably sclerotic margin. There is often bone 'expansion' as the host bone remodels to accommodate the tumour. Endosteal scalloping is usually present where the medullary lesion abuts the cortex (Fig. 81.21). Compared with enchondroma, chondrosarcoma is, on average, larger, less likely to be calcified, less well defined and often breaches the cortex with a discernible periosteal reaction (i.e. permeates bone and has a significant growth rate) (see Fig. 81.22). Occasionally, an intact enchondroma is discovered incidentally during a post-mortem examination or when a bone has been excised for another tumour type. The bone scan can be 'hot' in enchondromas and chondrosarcomas and is an unreliable distinguishing feature. Further imaging with CT and MRI is essential in the assessment of cartilaginous tumours. MRI defines the extent of the lesion and CT shows calcification and bone destruction (permeation). Both of these investigations are important for the assessment of these cartilage tumours.

The biopsy should be carefully planned and discussed at the multidisciplinary meeting between surgeon, radiologist and pathologist. A biopsy track should be chosen to allow subsequent excision if required.[4–6] The biopsy should be taken with image guidance, preferably CT. Especially in low-grade tumours, the biopsy could be prone to sampling error and it is essential to discuss the biopsy result at the multidisciplinary meeting to make an accurate diagnosis.

Macroscopically, enchondromas are pale blue, glistening, usually small lesions that are sharply circumscribed from the surrounding bone. On the other hand, chondrosarcomas are variably sized, often large, ill-defined tumours that are pale blue or white. Often large tumours cavitate centrally and the soft/semi-fluid central area is commonly pale green (see Fig. 81.22). There may also be areas of intralesional haemorrhage and, especially in necrotic areas, calcification. The cortex is usually significantly eroded and there may be a pathological fracture. The presence of subperiosteal tumour extension is common.

Histologically, the most reliably identified feature of chondrosarcoma (to aid distinction from enchondroma/atypical enchondroma), and, in essence, its defining feature is the presence of permeative growth. This is defined histologically as tumour being present on at least three sides of a lamellar (i.e. pre-existing) bone trabecula (in medullary bone), or permeation through a Haversian canal (in compact bone). Other histological features have been mentioned above in the comparator between enchondroma and chondrosarcoma (Figs 81.21 and 81.22). Cytogenetic analyses of chondrosarcoma have shown a large number of

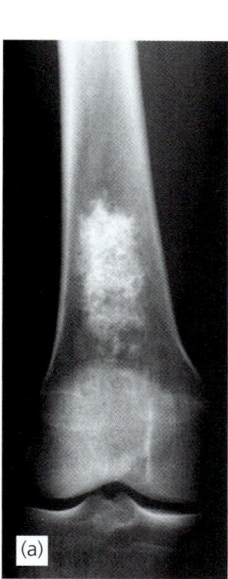
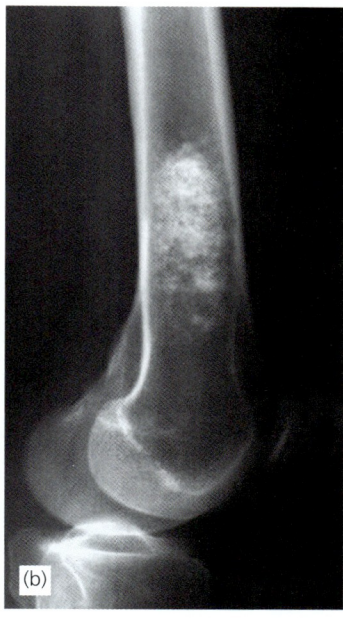
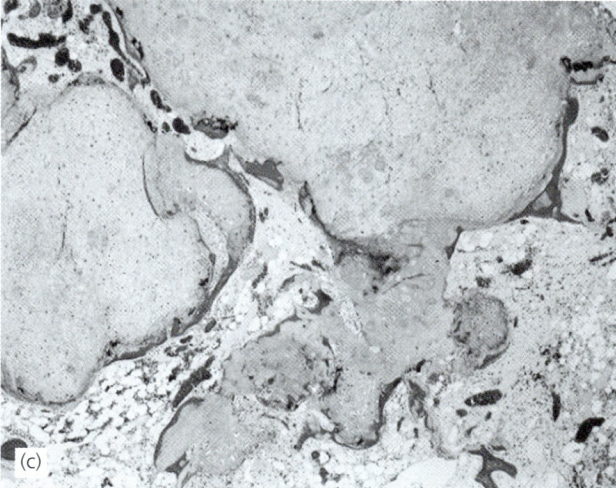

Figure 81.21 Enchondroma: (a, b) plain radiographs of a distal femoral enchondroma. (c) Low-power haematoxylin and eosin section showing lobules of enchondroma encased by reactive 'host' bone.

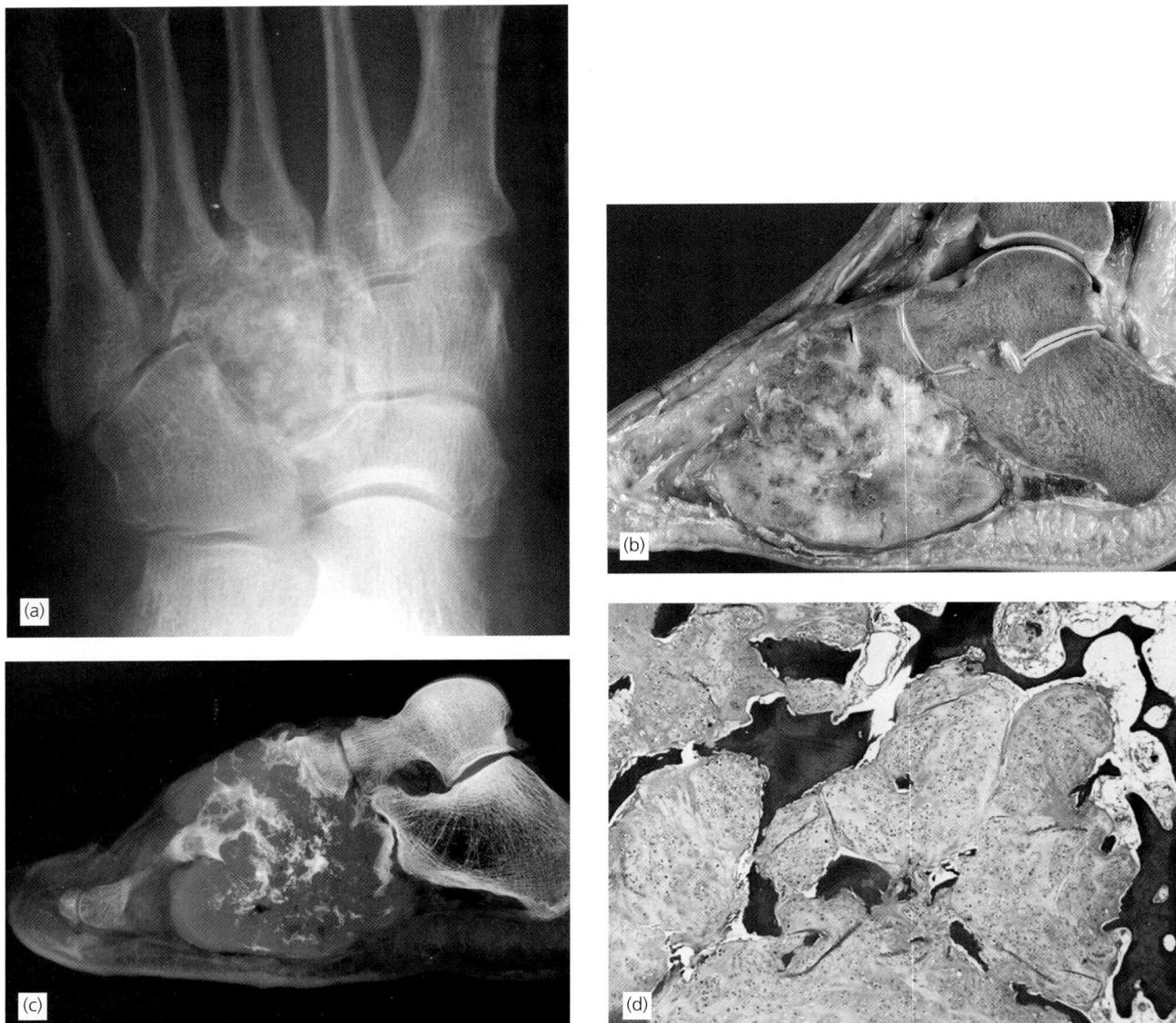

Figure 81.22 Chondrosarcoma. (a) Plain radiograph showing a chondrosarcoma involving the forefoot. (b, c) Sagittal section through the foot showing the chondrosarcoma of the forefoot and a plain radiograph of the specimen. (d) Low power haematoxylin and eosin section showing the permeative growth of the chondrosarcoma through the 'host' bone.

structural abnormalities. The most distinctive abnormalities involve chromosomes 1 and 7. For chondrosarcoma, the risk of metastatic spread correlates closely with tumour size and grade.[49] It is noteworthy that there is a good deal of variability in the grading of chondrosarcomas between sarcoma treatment centres as there is a fairly high degree of subjectivity in the interpretation of published criteria. This is evidenced by the often marked variability in the number of chondrosarcomas assigned to each of the three grades in published series of chondrosarcomas.

Secondary chondrosarcomas are those that arise from an identified pre-existing benign cartilaginous lesion, i.e. an enchondroma or an osteochondroma. Surface cartilaginous tumours, apart from osteochondroma, are distinctly uncommon and will not be discussed here. Dedifferentiated chondrosarcoma refers to a chondrosarcoma in which a high-grade, non-cartilaginous sarcoma has arisen (Fig. 81.23). The prognosis for such tumours is particularly poor.[1]

Histological features of enchondroma and chondrosarcoma are listed in Table 81.2. The radiological correlates of these are also given.

OSTEOSARCOMA

Osteosarcoma is defined as a sarcoma in which there is direct production of osteoid by the malignant cells. The percentage of sarcoma cells producing osteoid may be very

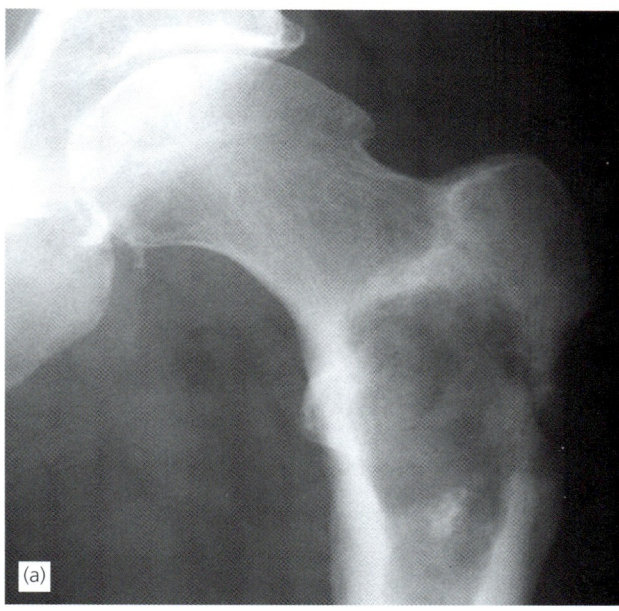
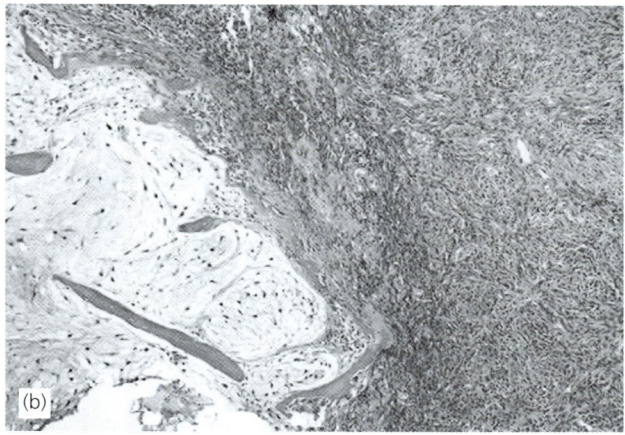

Figure 81.23 Dedifferentiated chondrosarcoma: (a) plain radiographs of a dedifferentiated chondrosarcoma involving the proximal femur. The calcification within the precursor chondrosarcomatous lesion and the purely lytic dedifferentiated sarcomatous element are apparent. (b) Medium-power haematoxylin and eosin sections of dedifferentiated chondrosarcoma showing the collision of the high grade, poorly differentiated pleomorphic sarcoma with the precursor chondrosarcoma.

Table 81.2 Histological and radiological features of enchondroma and chondrosarcoma

Histological features	Radiological features
Enchondroma	
Less cellular	
Less lobular	
More hyaline matrix	More likely to be calcified
No permeative growth	Well defined
Sometimes encased by bone	Well defined, with/without peripheral sclerosis
No or little cytological atypia	
Chondrosarcoma	
More cellular	
More lobular	
More myxoid matrix	Less likely to be calcified
Permeative growth present	Less well-defined
Not usually encased by bone	Lacks peripheral sclerosis (although necrotic tumour can be encased by bone)
Some or marked nuclear atypia	

small. There are a number of different subtypes of osteosarcoma, variably defined on the basis of their histological appearance and/or their site in/on bone. Thus, medullary osteosarcoma can be classified as high or low grade, and high-grade osteosarcoma is further classified as osteoblastic, chondroblastic, fibroblastic, telangiectatic, small cell, giant cell rich or epithelioid, depending on their histological appearance.[9,50–52]

Rarely, osteosarcomas are judged to arise within the cortex ('intra-cortical osteosarcoma'). Bone surface osteosarcomas are uncommon, and are classified as parosteal, periosteal and 'high-grade surface'. Parosteal osteosarcoma shares histological features with low-grade, intramedullary osteosarcoma and is a tumour of adults that most commonly arises on the posterior aspect of the distal femur. Periosteal osteosarcoma is an adult surface tumour with an often dominant chondroblastic component and is of intermediate to high grade.

Additionally, we can classify osteosarcoma into primary and secondary types. Primary osteosarcomas arise de novo, whereas secondary osteosarcomas arise against a background of a different tumour type (e.g. as the dedifferentiated component of a chondrosarcoma), in diseased bone (most commonly in Pagetic bone) or as a late (5–15-year interval) complication of local radiotherapy.

The commonest type of osteosarcoma, and indeed, the commonest primary malignant bone tumour (with an incidence of approximately 4 per million, per year), is high-grade primary intramedullary osteosarcoma (i.e. conventional osteosarcoma).[81] Within this group, most osteosarcomas are either osteoblastic, chondroblastic or fibroblastic (in that order). Owing to the constraints of space, high-grade intramedullary osteosarcoma will be the only type of osteosarcoma discussed in the following paragraphs. The age range, sex ratio and site distribution is in

Fig. 81.24. Osteosarcoma is most common in the fastest growing bones (around the knee). In descending order of growth (and incidence) these are distal femur, proximal tibia, proximal femur and proximal humerus.

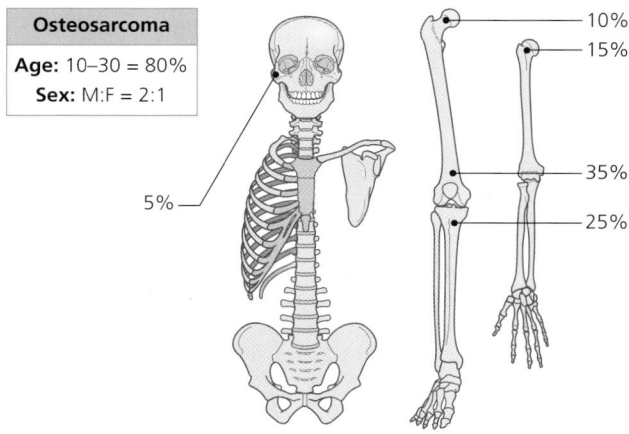

Figure 81.24 Osteosarcoma: age range and sex ratio.

Clinically, patients usually present with pain or swelling. Especially night pain or non-mechanical bone pain in an adolescent or young adult is of clinical concern. There may be a palpable mass or effusion. Pathological fracture is relatively uncommon (up to 10%).[1] Laboratory testing may show an elevated alkaline phosphatase and/or lactic dehydrogenase.

The radiological appearance of conventional osteosarcoma is that of a meta-diaphyseal (only very rarely diaphyseal or epiphyseal)[54] tumour which is ill-defined, destructive, often large, and centred on the medulla. The tumour is variably mineralized (from densely sclerotic to apparently purely lytic)[55] and, commonly, shows cortical destruction and a periosteal reaction. The periosteal reaction at the edge of the tumour sometimes shows the classic Codman's triangle (or, more accurately, 'angle') appearance (Fig. 81.25). Sun-ray spiculae have also been described. A small minority of osteosarcomas can be associated with skip lesions (located outside the reactive zone) or satellite lesions (located within the reactive zone). These are separate tumour

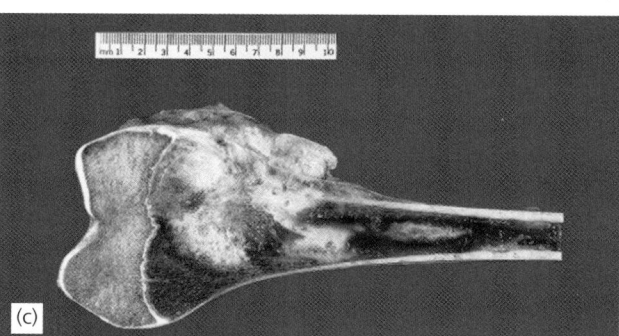

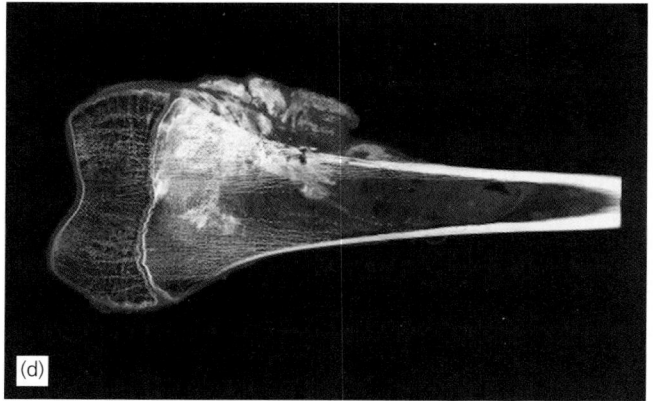

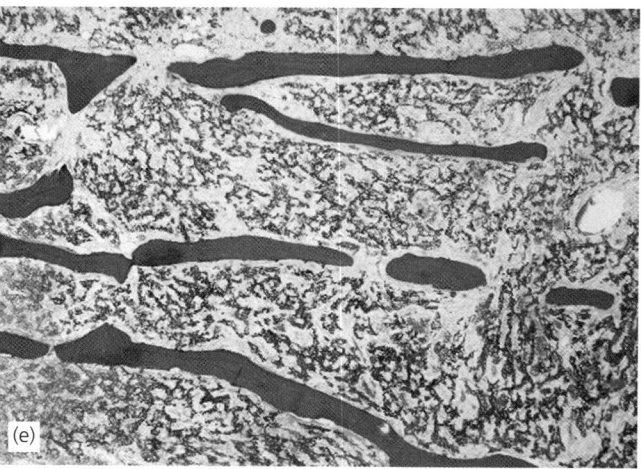

Figure 81.25 Osteosarcoma (high grade, intramedullary type): (a, b) plain radiographs of a distal femoral, high-grade, osteoblastic osteosarcoma showing the classic 'sun ray' appearance. (c, d) Excised osteosarcoma and radiograph of a coronal slice. (e) Low-power haematoxylin and eosin stained sections showing the permeative growth pattern of the residual osteosarcomatous filigree matrix. The specimen is post-chemotherapy and only the tumour matrix has survived.

deposits within the same bone and sited more proximally than the dominant lesion.

Macroscopically, the tumour reflects the radiological appearance, with an often heterogeneous, variably ossified, often focally necrotic or haemorrhagic appearance. There may be a prominent chondroblastic or a bloody, cavitated, telangiectatic component. Wholesale bone destruction is typical. There is usually an extracortical, but subperiosteal, component. Extension beyond the periosteum into the soft tissues proper is quite commonly seen, but is usually only a minor component (Fig. 81.25). Microscopically, there is a wide variety of appearances, but in all cases, by definition, there are sarcomatous cells directly producing osteoid. Osteoid is the non-mineral component of bone matrix and, because histological sections are cut from tissue that has been demineralized in the laboratory, it is osteoid that is seen down the microscope. It is not always easy to distinguish osteoid from simple collagenous matrix. However, whereas collagenous matrix tends to be fibrillar with an ill-defined edge, osteoid is amorphous with a sharp edge and can have a branching or micronodular architecture. This is most striking in the osteoblastic variant where osteoid is laid down by individual cells with no attempt at cooperation or coordination with neighbouring tumour osteoblasts. This lack of cooperation between malignant osteoblasts results in the formation of a filigree, or network, pattern of matrix deposition (Fig. 81.25). As this continues, the individual tumour cells entomb themselves in their own product, starving themselves of nutrients and causing a degree of regression of malignant features (so-called 'normalization'). The end result is a dense, purposeless sheet of osteoid with entrapped malignant osteoblasts in lacunae. Lesser degrees of osteoid production are common. Indeed, other subtypes of osteosarcoma are characterized by the production of cartilage or fibrous matrices. As is common in high-grade sarcomas in general, zones of tumour necrosis and haemorrhage are commonly seen. As was earlier described (and defined) for chondrosarcoma, and as is the case for all malignant bone tumours, osteosarcomas show a permeative growth pattern. Here the infiltrative and rapid growth capability of the tumour results in the entrapment of often partially resorbed, lamellar bone within the tumour substance. Pre-existing host bone is readily recognized by its lamellar appearance, which is a consequence of its slow, orderly, formation by the coordinated activity of sheets of normal osteoblasts. By contrast, rapidly formed bone produced by osteosarcoma cells is woven in nature. Malignant woven bone is distinguished from the rapidly formed woven bone produced by reactive, non-neoplastic osteoblasts (e.g. in fracture callus) by virtue of the purposeful trabecular structure and the lining of a coordinated monolayer of osteoblasts in the latter process. Conventional osteosarcomas show highly complex cytogenetic abnormalities, both quantitatively and qualitatively.[56,57] Although no characteristic or specific diagnostically useful genetic abnormality has been identified, abnormalities in particular chromosomal regions have been identified. 1p11-13, 1q11-12, 1q21-22, 11p14-15, 14p11-13, 15p11-13, 17p and 19q13 are the chromosomal regions most commonly affected by structural abnormalities, and +1, -6q, -9, -10, -13 and -17 are the most common chromosomal imbalances. The development of conventional osteosarcoma is associated with the Li–Fraumeni and hereditary retinoblastoma syndromes. The 5-year survival rate for osteosarcoma improved markedly with the introduction of cytotoxic chemotherapy in the 1970s. However, since then, the 5-year survival rate has stubbornly remained around 70%. Nearly all patients who succumb to their disease develop pulmonary metastases.[58] The most predictive unfavourable prognostic factors are metastases at or after the time of diagnosis, and poor histological response (<90% necrosis) to neoadjuvant chemotherapy.

PAROSTEAL OSTEOSARCOMA

Parosteal osteosarcoma is a low-grade surface osteosarcoma. It is a rare tumour, but is the most common of the surface osteosarcomas and accounts for 4% of all osteosarcomas.[1] The tumour most commonly arises from the posterior aspect of the distal femur, followed by the proximal tibia and proximal humerus. Other locations have been described, but are rare.[59] Females are slightly more affected than males (Fig. 81.26).[59]

Clinically, patients usually present with a painless swelling, but localized symptoms may occur. Radiographs show a bony swelling. In contrast to osteochondromas the intramedullary cavity of the distal femur is not in continuity with the lesion (Fig. 81.27). The MRI and CT scans are performed to evaluate the extent of the intramedullary involvement of the tumour. The peripheral parts of the tumour tend to be less mineralized.[60] It is important to have completed the staging investigations and have these images at the multidisciplinary team meeting to plan the biopsy. Particularly in this tumour it is important to select the biopsy route with care and to have a surgical plan once

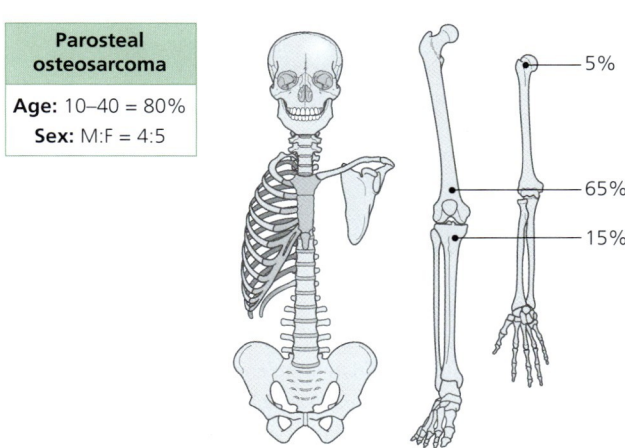

Figure 81.26 Parosteal osteosarcoma: age range and sex ratio.

the diagnosis of parosteal osteosarcoma has been confirmed. If there is little intramedullary involvement in a distal femoral lesion, it may be possible to perform a 'shark bite' excision, in which case a biopsy from lateral or medial may be preferable. However, a 'shark bite' excision is not possible if there is significant intramedullary involvement and a distal femoral resection may be required; in which case the biopsy is usually taken via an anterior approach. Chemotherapy is not usually required for this tumour, unless there is dedifferentiation.

Macroscopically, parosteal osteosarcoma is a hard bony mass that may have nodules of cartilage attached to it. The intramedullary cavity is invaded by the tumour in about 25% of the cases.[1]

Microscopically, the tumour consists of well-formed bony trabeculae (Fig. 81.27) that are arranged in a parallel manner.[61] The stromal spindle cells usually show minimal atypia.[1] There is a spindle cell proliferation between the bony trabeculae. In about 50% of the cases, there is cartilaginous differentiation. But this cartilage does not show the columnar arrangement as in osteochondromas. Approximately 15% of the tumours will dedifferentiate to high-grade spindle cell sarcomas (i.e. to osteosarcoma or malignant fibrous histiocytoma). This is usually at the time of a recurrence, but may be present at the time of diagnosis. Immunohistochemistry is unhelpful in the diagnosis of these tumours.

Parosteal osteosarcoma has a different chromosomal alteration from conventional osteosarcoma. Supernumerary ring chromosomes have been described in parosteal osteosarcoma, often as the only alteration.[62]

The prognosis of parosteal osteosarcoma is much better than that of conventional osteosarcoma, with a 5-year survival of 90%.[59] However, if the tumour dedifferentiates, the prognosis is similar to that of conventional osteosarcoma.

EWING'S SARCOMA

Ewing's sarcoma is a small, round cell sarcoma that principally affects children and young adults. There is a male predominance and the tumour is strikingly less common in patients of Afro-Caribbean descent.[1] It is less common than myeloma, osteosarcoma and chondrosarcoma, accounting for approximately 8% of primary malignant bone tumours. Where there is prominent light microscopical, immunohistochemical and/or electron microscopical evidence of neuroectodermal differentiation, these tumours are often referred to as (peripheral) primitive neuroectodermal tumours (PNET). The age range, site distribution and sex ratio are in Fig. 81.28.

Ewing's sarcoma principally involves the pelvis, femur tibia/fibula and humerus, although any bone may be affected. The tumour is usually diaphyseal in location. As for most primary malignant bone tumours, pain and swelling are the commonest features. Pathological fracture is less common than for other primary malignancies. There are often systemic symptoms and signs, in particular fever, anaemia and a raised erythrocyte sedimentation rate.

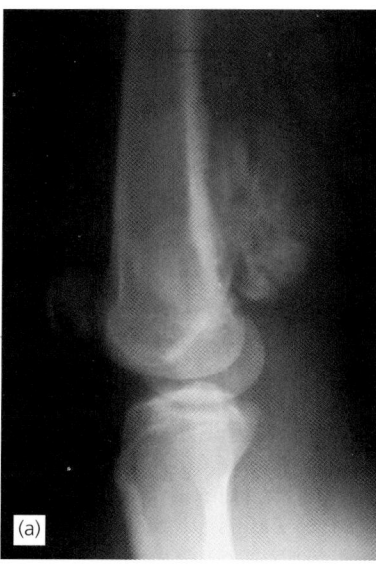

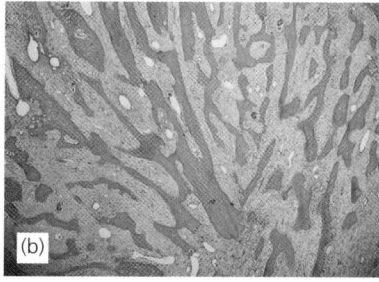

Figure 81.27 Parosteal osteosarcoma: (a) plain radiograph showing a parosteal osteosarcoma arising from the posterior aspect of the distal femur. There is no continuity between the tumour and the intramedullary cavity of the distal femur. The cortex of the distal femur is intact. (b) Haematoxylin and eosin stain showing well formed bony trabeculae with a hypocellular spindle cell stroma.

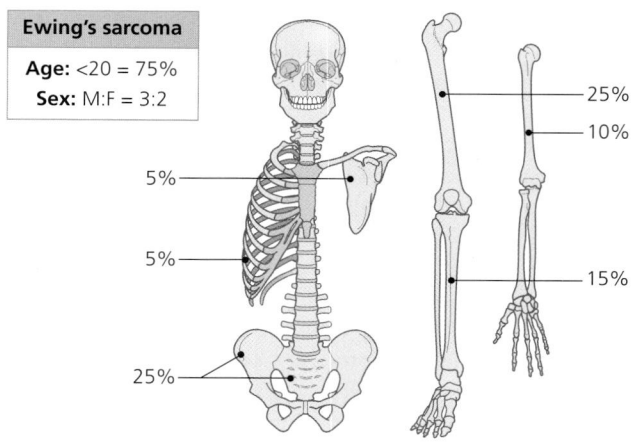

Figure 81.28 Ewing's sarcoma: age range and sex ratio.

Radiologically, the tumour can be quite subtle on plain radiographs. The lesion is usually ill defined and irregularly osteolytic. A common sign is the so-called 'onion skin' appearance due to waves of periosteal elevation followed by periosteal bone formation (Fig. 81.29). There may be either cortical thinning or cortical sclerosis. Very often there is a sizeable soft-tissue mass beyond the elevated periosteum. MRI scans allow the often surprising true extent of the disease (within the marrow and in the soft tissues) to be visualized. Resection specimens are nearly always post chemotherapy. On gross inspection the tumour is almost always centred on the medulla, with an ill-defined advancing edge, a mixed pattern of osteolysis and osteosclerosis, an often prominent onion skin periosteal reaction and, usually a subperiosteal and soft-tissue tumour component (Fig. 81.29). Because the resected samples are nearly always post chemotherapy, the typical grey/tan colour of the viable tumour is often scanty and sometimes not at all apparent. The necrotic tumour has largely been resorbed and replaced by loose, often mildly gelatinous, fibrovascular tissue. This gives a pale yellow, myxoid appearance in the gross specimen. Histologically, the classical experience is of sheets of monotonous appearing small, round cells with scanty cytoplasm and virtually no extracellular matrix (Fig. 81.29). The nuclei are round, or slightly angular, with fine chromatin dispersion and often very small or indiscernible nucleoli. The mitotic rate is highly variable, and is often surprisingly low for such an aggressive tumour. Where the cytoplasm can be discerned, it is often pale due to glycogen accumulation. Very commonly, there are irregularly outlined zones of tumour necrosis. In the Ewing's sarcoma variant of PNET, so-called Homer–Wright rosettes are formed.[63] It is not uncommon to see forme fruste rosettes in otherwise typical Ewing's sarcoma, supporting the now fully established view that Ewing's sarcoma and PNET represent different points on a morphological spectrum. A small, but significant, minority of cases may show striking morphological variations. The tumour cells may be larger and more spindled, may have more prominent nucleoli, and, in rare cases may produce a significant amount of matrix (even osteoid in rare cases). Such cases confirm the importance of carrying out adjunctive tests to properly establish the diagnosis. It is mandatory to use immunohistochemistry with/without molecular diagnostic tests to support the diagnosis of Ewing's sarcoma. This is because Ewing's sarcoma can be mimicked by a variety of other malignant tumours, especially on a small biopsy sample. In particular, metastatic small cell carcinoma (especially in older patients) and lymphoma may, on occasion, mimic Ewing's sarcoma. Primary bone lymphoma (usually high grade, B-cell, non-Hodgkin's lymphoma, but, especially in the young, lymphoblastic lymphoma) is a close mimic clinically (especially in terms of systemic symptoms), radiologically (may be indistinguishable on plain radiographs and MRI scans) and microscopically (especially where the sample is

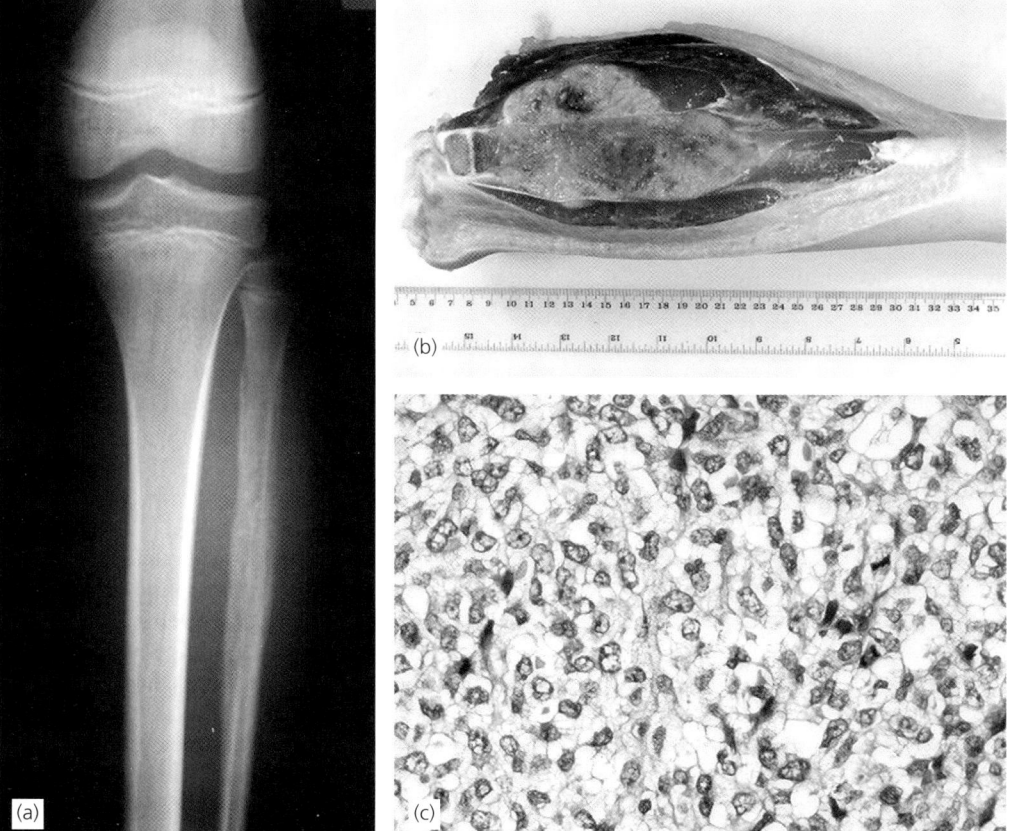

Figure 81.29 Ewing's sarcoma: (a) plain radiograph showing a Ewing's sarcoma affecting the proximal fibular metadiaphysis. (b) Amputated specimen sectioned sagitally through the proximal fibular tumour. Note the elevated periosteum that has been breached by the tan-coloured tumour. (c) High-power haematoxylin and eosin sections of Ewing's sarcoma showing sheets of 'small round blue' cells. In this field cytoplasmic 'clearing' due to glycogen accumulation is prominent.

small and suboptimally prepared). In such a situation, immunohistochemistry will usually allow detection of a lymphoma phenotype. For some lymphoblastic lymphomas, an extended immunohistochemical panel is required. More recently, there are molecular biological methods that can be very usefully applied to paraffin-embedded biopsy tissue samples permitting the positive detection of Ewing's sarcoma-specific genetic translocations. These specific chromosomal translocations involve the 5′ end of the *EWS* gene from chromosome 22q12 fusing to a member of the ETS family of transcription factors, most commonly FLI-1 located at 11q24 (95% of cases).[64,65] Electron microscopy is, nowadays, rarely needed to establish a diagnosis of Ewing's sarcoma. The electron microscopical features of typical Ewing's sarcoma are sheets of small/oval primitive cells, cytoplasmic glycogen accumulations, primitive cell–cell junctions and, less commonly, cytoplasmic neurosecretory granules.

The 5-year survival rate for Ewing's sarcoma improved markedly in the 1970s with the introduction of cytotoxic chemotherapy. However, since then, the 5-year survival rate has stubbornly remained around 50%. Nearly all patients who succumb to their disease develop pulmonary metastases.[58] Bone metastases are not uncommon in Ewing's sarcoma. The most predictive unfavourable prognostic factors are metastases at or after the time of diagnosis, axial skeleton distribution, size, poor histological response (<90% necrosis) to neoadjuvant chemotherapy and, in approximately 10% of cases, tumour p53 gene mutation.

MALIGNANT FIBROUS HISTIOCYTOMA

Malignant fibrous histiocytoma (MFH) of bone is a high-grade, poorly differentiated sarcoma composed of fibroblasts/myofibroblasts and undifferentiated pleomorphic cells.[66] Often these tumours are reported as high-grade, pleomorphic (or pleomorphic/spindle cell) sarcomas of bone. MFH of bone is relatively rare, accounting for less than 2% of all primary bone sarcoma cases. It is generally a tumour of adults, with a peak incidence in the fifth and sixth decades (Fig. 81.30). Rarely, the tumour can arise in the skeletally immature, but, often in such cases, thorough examination of multiple tissue blocks will reveal a minor component of osteosarcoma. Along with osteosarcoma, these tumours can be secondary to Paget's disease of bone, bone infarcts and local radiotherapy.[1,67–69] The skeletal distribution of bone MFH is very similar to that of classic osteosarcoma. There is a male preponderance of cases. The clinical signs and symptoms are the same as for classic osteosarcoma, namely pain, swelling and pathological fracture.

Radiologically, the tumour is a poorly defined, lytic mass, usually with cortical destruction and a subperiosteal or soft-tissue extension. However, a periosteal reaction is uncommon.[70] MFH is nearly always centred on the metaphysis (Fig. 81.31). Grossly, the excised tumour

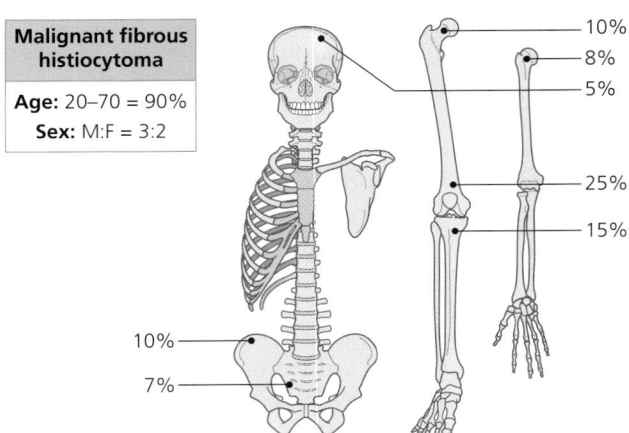

Figure 81.30 Malignant fibrous histiocytoma: age range and sex ratio.

resembles classic osteosarcoma, but, by definition, the tumour lacks the bone matrix production.

The tumour is usually soft, fleshy and tan coloured, and is ill defined. Cortical destruction with periosteal elevation and soft tissue extension is common (Fig. 81.31). Histologically, the tumour is similar to the more common pleomorphic–storiform soft-tissue counterpart. The tumour cells are large with highly malignant nuclear features and may be spindled or large and polygonal. They form sheets or short, disorganised fascicles giving a classical storiform architecture (Fig. 81.31). Particularly in post-chemotherapeutic cases, there may be extensive tumour necrosis. Immunohistochemistry can be useful in the differential diagnosis of metastatic sarcomatoid carcinoma (rarely a practical problem) and metastatic malignant melanoma. Because of the chaotic karyotype of bone MFH and the lack of any identified diagnostic or prognostic marker, molecular biological techniques are currently not particularly clinically useful. The clinical management of MFH is very similar to that of osteosarcoma. The prognosis is marginally worse with approximately 50% 5-year survival. As for osteosarcoma, the histological assessment of necrosis in the resected specimen following neoadjuvant chemotherapy has proven to be prognostically useful.

CHORDOMA

Chordoma is a notochordal sarcoma usually of low/intermediate malignancy.[1] Chordoma is approximately half as common as Ewing's sarcoma, accounting for up to 4% of primary malignant bone tumours. It is a tumour of adults, with a peak incidence in the sixth decade and is more common in males (Fig. 81.32). The distribution of chordoma is spinal, principally the sacrum and base of skull.

The clinical presentation is due to the presence of the slowly destructive mass. In addition to longstanding local

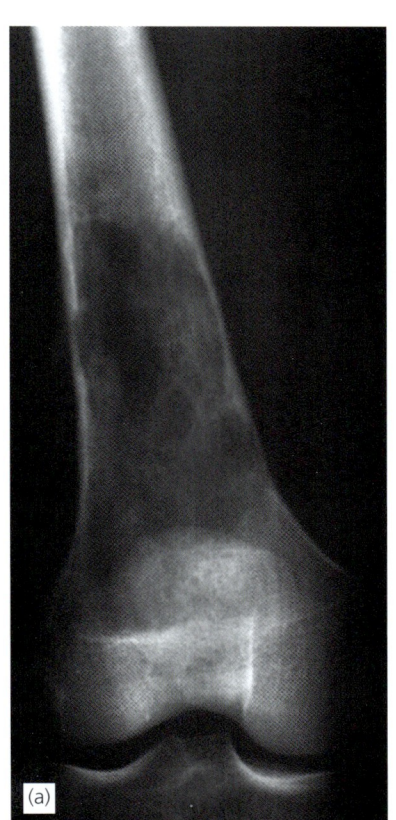
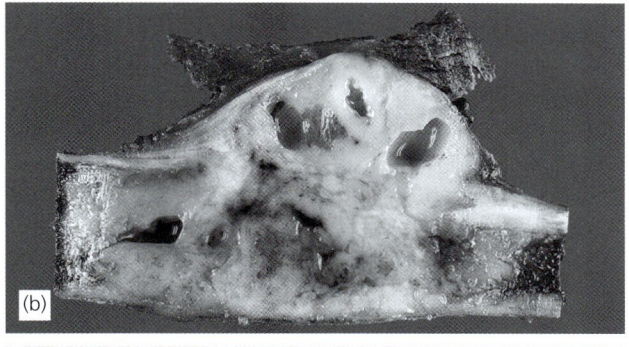
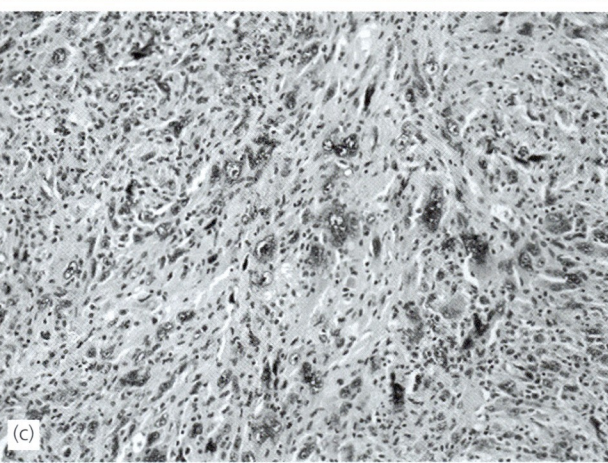

Figure 81.31 Malignant fibrous histiocytoma (MFH) of bone. (a) Plain radiograph of a distal femoral metaphyseal MFH of bone. (b) En bloc excision specimen of an MFH of bone. (c) High-power haematoxylin and eosin section of an MFH of bone showing large, bizarre sarcomatous cells set in a collagenous stroma.

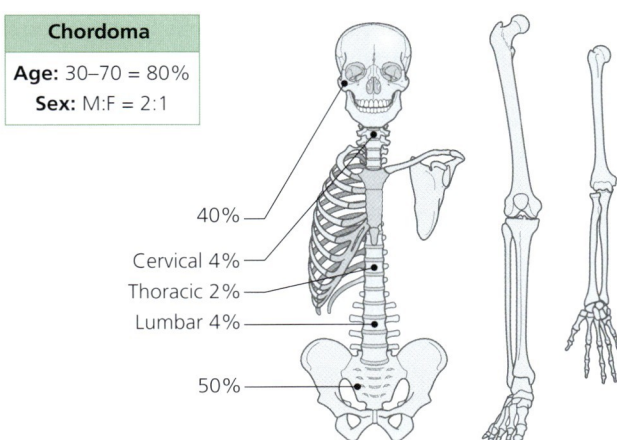

Figure 81.32 Chordoma: age range and sex ratio.

pain, constipation is common for sacrococcygeal tumours. Most of these tumours are palpable by rectal examination. Nerve dysfunction, such as paraesthesia, is usually a late symptom of sacrococcygeal chordomas.

Headaches and cranial nerve compression are common for spheno-occipital tumours. The ocular nerve is most commonly affected and patients may develop endocrine disturbances due to pituitary gland involvement.

Cervico-thoraco-lumbar tumours usually present with pain and nerve root compression.

Radiologically, chordoma is a solitary, central/midline, destructive bone tumour of the axial skeleton that produces a lateral/anterior extra-osseous mass.[71] There may be intralesional calcification. MRI studies show a typically located mass with a high T_2-weighted signal.[72] Grossly, chordoma is an osteo-destructive, lobulated, myxoid mass often grey/tan-coloured with haemorrhagic areas (Fig. 81.33). Sacral tumours are often large at presentation (average 10 cm diameter), whereas base of skull tumours present earlier and are, therefore, usually smaller. Histologically, lobules of tumour are composed of large, cohesive cells with abundant pink, often vacuolated cytoplasm set in a pale blue gelatinous matrix (Fig. 81.33). These are the classic 'physaliphorous cells'. Tumour cells often form branching cords or islands, but may form solid sheets with little matrix production. The degree of nuclear atypia and the mitotic rate are highly variable and are indicative of tumour aggressiveness. Some cases can resemble chondrosarcoma, at least focally, and, in such instances, the use of immunohistochemistry to detect cytokeratin expression is useful in establishing the correct diagnosis. Other tumours that can morphologically resemble chordoma are myxopapillary ependymoma and renal cell carcinoma. Again, immunohistochemistry is useful in aiding distinction. Rarely, chordoma can dedifferentiate to generate a highly aggressive undifferentiated sarcoma with a more aggressive behaviour.[73] Genetic analysis has been performed on a limited number of cases, and the most frequent findings have been loss of material from the short arms of chromosomes 1, 3 and 9, and from the long arms of chromosomes 3 and 17.[74] Gains of chromosomal material have been

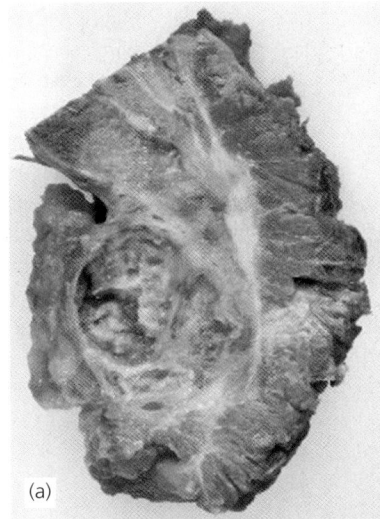

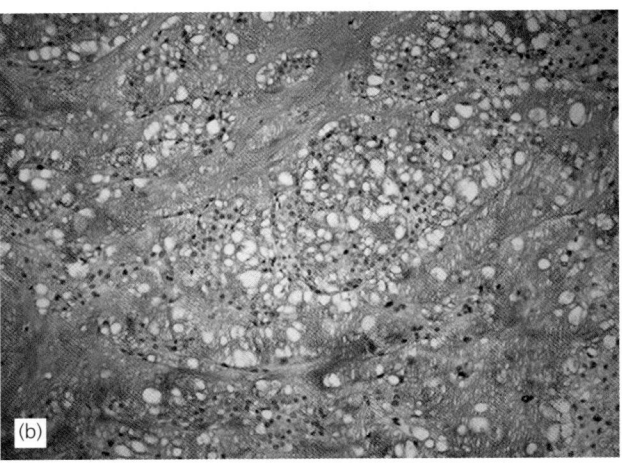

Figure 81.33 Chordoma. (a) Sacral chordoma excision specimen cut sagitally. (b) Medium power haematoxylin and eosin section showing typical appearance of chordoma – cords of large, cohesive cells set in a richly myxoid stroma.

found on the long arms of chromosomes 5 and 7. The natural history of chordoma is progressive local disease, and eventually metastatic spread. Metastases may be widespread and can involve lung, bone, soft tissue, skin and local lymph nodes.

Surgical excision is the only curative treatment, but this is often difficult due to its location or size. Sacral tumours above S2 are difficult to resect without significant functional deficit, including bowel and bladder dysfunction. The tumour is insensitive to chemotherapy or radiotherapy. Some reports have suggested a response to proton therapy and carbon ions.[75,76]

MYELOMA

Plasma cell neoplasms can be divided into multifocal (multiple myeloma) and solitary (plasmacytoma). Multiple myeloma is the most common primary bone

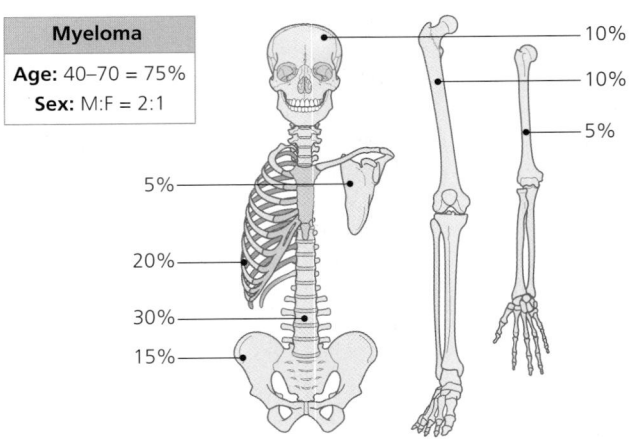

Figure 81.34 Myeloma: age and sex ratios.

neoplastic disease, accounting for nearly half of all cases.[1] It is a disease of late middle life and elderly people, and men are more commonly affected (Fig. 81.34) (http://info.cancerresearchuk.org/cancerstats/types/multiplemyeloma/incidence/). Bone pain, weight loss and weakness are common symptoms. Pathological fractures, especially of vertebrae, are common. Patients are usually anaemic because of marrow destruction. Hypercalcaemia is common. Consequently patients often suffer some degree of renal failure, also due to renal tubular casts of immunoglobulin light chain. In the vast majority of patients a monoclonal gammopathy is detectable, and Bence–Jones protein is found in the serum of 75% of patients.[77] Patients are often immunocompromised due to marrow displacement. The axial skeleton and the proximal appendicular skeleton are the most common sites of involvement.[77]

Radiologically, the changes are often very typical. The classical plain radiographic appearance is of multiple, round, punched-out lytic areas of bone destruction. However, multiple myeloma can also be osteosclerotic.[9] If the bone is expanded by the tumour, lytic and sclerotic areas are usually present giving a soap bubble appearance. Extensive soft-tissue involvement is uncommon at presentation. The differential diagnosis is with metastatic carcinoma. Grossly, the areas of tumour are fleshy, soft and tan coloured or haemorrhagic (Fig. 81.35). Microscopically, if well or moderately differentiated, the tumour can be seen to be composed of sheets of plasma cells (Fig. 81.35). However, it is not uncommon for myeloma to be poorly differentiated; when this is the case immunohistochemistry can be employed to aid the diagnosis. In some cases, extensive immunoglobulin light chain deposition results in sheets of amyloid and renal failure. Multiple cytogenetic abnormalities have been described in myeloma and the karyotype is usually complex.

Solitary plasmacytoma shares the radiological and pathological features described above. Many cases will progress to multiple myeloma, but, not surprisingly, the

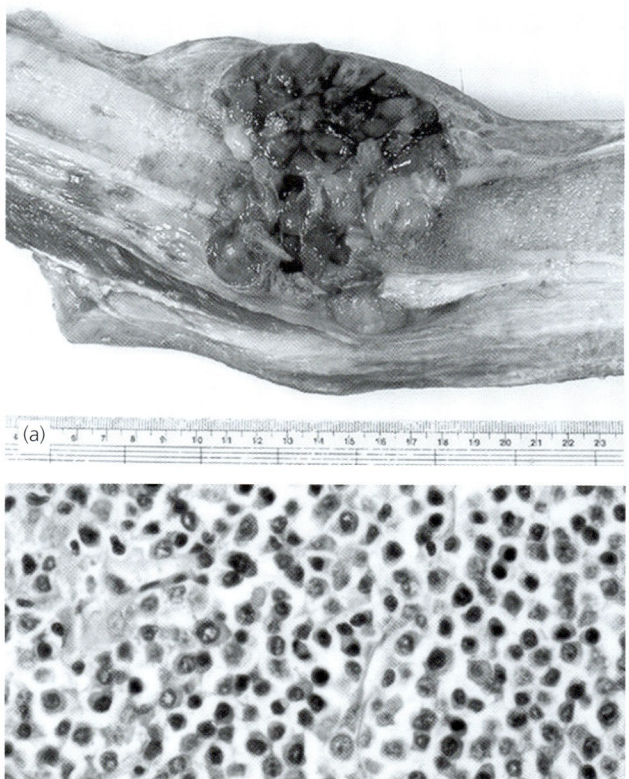

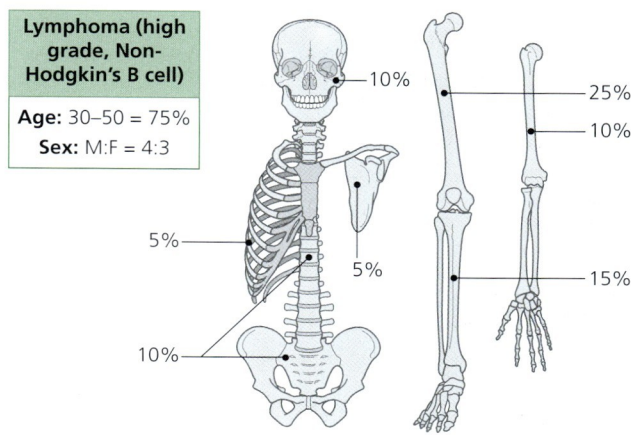

Figure 81.36 Lymphoma (high-grade non-Hodgkin's B cell): age range and sex ratio.

Figure 81.35 Myeloma. (a) Amputated lower limb showing a pathological fracture through a destructive myeloma. (b) High-power haematoxylin and eosin stained sections of myeloma showing sheets of plasma cells with some degree of nuclear pleomorphism.

prognosis is significantly better than multiple myeloma at presentation. Rarely, plasmacytoma or multiple myeloma can induce bony sclerosis.[77] In such cases, the diagnosis may only become apparent following the biopsy.

The role of the orthopaedic surgeon is to aid diagnostically if a biopsy is required and to maintain skeletal integrity. Pathological fractures in patients with myeloma may well heal following haematological treatment and internal fixation is often preferable to surgical excision. However, a solitary plasmacytoma is usually best excised and reconstructed.

LYMPHOMA

Lymphoma of bone accounts for approximately 5% of primary malignant bone tumours.[1] The vast majority (> 90%) are high-grade, B-cell non-Hodgkin's lymphomas with Hodgkin's disease, T-cell lymphomas and lymphoblastic (often null) lymphomas accounting for the rest. From a surgeon's perspective, the importance is in being aware of this differential diagnosis when considering a possible primary sarcoma to avoid a misdiagnosis and unnecessary surgical intervention. Bone lymphoma is slightly more common in males and can affect any age group, with a peak incidence in the fifth decade (Fig. 81.36).[78,79] Any bone may be affected, but the femur is the most common site. Bone lymphoma is usually metadiaphyseal or diaphyseal.

The usual symptoms of localized pain, swelling and, possibly, pathological fracture may be accompanied by systemic symptoms such as fever and night sweats.

The radiological findings show an ill-defined, generally lytic (but often with patchy sclerotic areas) tumour that has usually involved the soft tissues (Fig. 81.37). The process is highly permeative with little periosteal response. MRI often shows surprisingly extensive disease, and a bone scan can show multifocal tumour deposits. Radiologically, the differential diagnosis includes infection and Ewing's sarcoma, as well as metastatic carcinoma. Gross pathological specimens are rare because this is generally not a surgical disease. The role of the orthopaedic surgeon is supportive in making the diagnosis and maintaining skeletal integrity. However, where a pathological fracture has occurred, an excision may be indicated (Fig. 81.37) as healing of these fractures is rare if radiotherapy is required.

The tumour is almost always centred on the medulla of the metadiaphysis or diaphysis, with marked bony destruction and a pathological fracture. The tumour is fleshy, soft and tan coloured and has usually spread to produce a soft-tissue mass. Microscopically, the typical high-grade, non-Hodgkin's B-cell lymphoma is formed of permeative sheets of medium to large cells, with clearly malignant nuclear features, a high mitotic rate, widespread individual cell death (apoptosis) and little or no extracellular matrix (Fig. 81.37). In soft-tissue extensions, islands of tumour

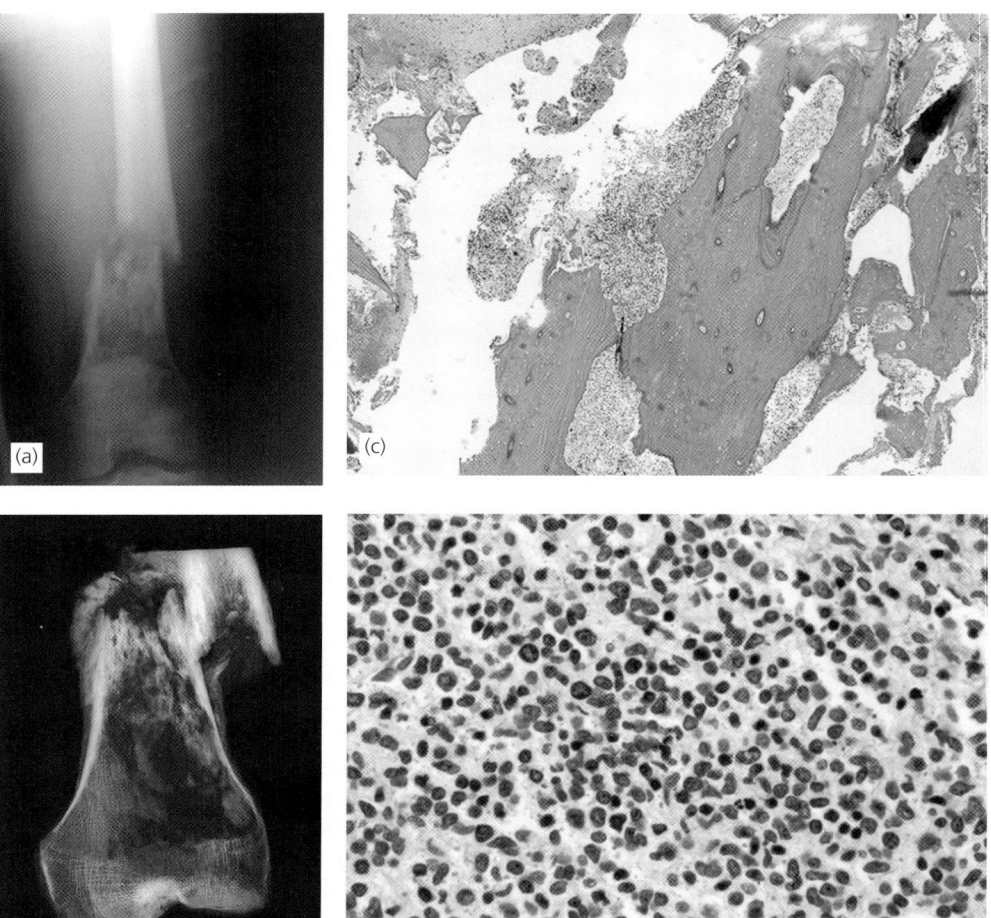

Figure 81.37 Lymphoma. (a) Plain radiograph of a pathological fracture through a distal femoral metaphyseal lymphoma. (b) Radiograph of the coronally sliced resected distal femur. (c, d) Low- and high-power haematoxylin and eosin sections showing the lymphoma permeating through 'moth-eaten' cortical bone and the cytological features of the tumour.

cells readily infiltrate through periosteum, fascia and muscle. Immunohistochemistry is extremely useful to confirm the lymphoma immunophenotype. Most bone lymphomas express leucocyte common antigen (CD45) and B-cell markers (CD20 and CD79a). Importantly, the less common lymphoblastic lymphomas, which affect young patients, can be negative for these markers and additional immunostains are required to confirm the diagnosis (CD10, TdT). Rarely other lymphoma types occur (Hodgkin's disease and T-cell lymphomas). It is important to be aware that in the advanced stages of nodal lymphoma and non-bone extranodal lymphoma, bone can be involved. Obviously, it is also the case that the marrow can be filled with neoplastic cells in lymphocytic, lymphoblastic and myeloid leukaemias. There are no specific genetic abnormalities for lymphomas involving bones rather than other sites. Several specific genetic abnormalities have been described for B-cell lymphomas, often translocations resulting in immunoglobulin rearrangements. Bone lymphoma is generally treated with chemotherapy and prognosis is mainly reliant on the lymphoma subtype and stage.[1]

CONCLUSION

Collectively, primary bone tumours are clinically, radiologically and pathologically diverse. These relatively rare tumours are best dealt with by an experienced multidisciplinary team that, together, can reconcile the clinical and radiological aspects of a case with the interpretation of the pathological tissue generated by biopsy to establish a diagnosis and, hence, guide the treatment. In particular, the radiological and pathological features are complementary, being different modalities to highlight common features. The burgeoning field of molecular biology in neoplastic disease has already delivered much to our understanding of sarcoma pathogenesis, and promises much more for the future. The morphological study of bone tumours by radiological, and gross and microscopical pathological, means has been, and will remain, the platform on which the molecular classification of tumours has been built. The hope is that ever-more sophisticated molecular pathological classification will lead to tailored and more effective treatments in the future.

> **KEY LEARNING POINTS**
>
> - Non-mechanical bone pain and night pain are concerning symptoms and warrant urgent further investigations, especially in adolescents with symptoms around the knee.
> - Plain radiographs are the key to diagnosing bone tumours.
> - Solitary bone lesions require further investigations and a diagnosis, even if the patient is known to have a malignancy.
> - Staging should be completed before biopsy.
> - The biopsy should be performed in the centre that is ultimately responsible for the surgical treatment.
> - The biopsy should be performed via an extensile approach, allowing for the biopsy track to be excised at the time of definitive surgical treatment.
> - Diagnosis should be made before planning treatment.
> - Assessment and management of bone tumours requires a full multidisciplinary team including surgeons, radiologist, pathologists and oncologists.
> - The management of chondrosarcoma is surgical, but other malignant primary bone tumours require a combination of surgical and oncological treatments.

ACKNOWLEDGEMENT

The authors would like to thank Mr A. Jones from the Robert Jones and Agnes Hunt Orthopaedic Hospital in Oswestry, Shropshire for his invaluable help in the preparation of this manuscript.

REFERENCES

- ● = Key primary paper
- ◆ = Major review article

◆1. World Health Organization: Classification of tumours: Pathology and genetics of tumours of soft tissue and bone. Edited by CDM Fletcher, KK Unni, F Mertens. IARC Press, 2002.
◆2. Davies AM, Mangham DC. Bone tumors. In: Gourtsoyiannis N, Ros P (eds) *Radiologic-Pathologic Correlations From Head To Toe*. Berlin, Germany: Springer-Verlag, 2005.
3. Schmidt GP, Reisser MF, Bauer-Melnyk. Whole body MRI for the staging and follow up of patients with metastases *European Journal of Radiology* 2009;**70**:393–400.
●4. Mankin HJ, Lange TA, Spanier SS. The hazards of biopsy in patients with malignant primary bone and soft tissue tumors. *Journal of Bone and Joint Surgery (American)* 1982;**64A**:1121–7.
●5. Mankin HJ, Mankin CJ, Simon MA. The hazards of the biopsy, revisited. *Journal of Bone and Joint Surgery (American)* 1996;**78A**:656–62.
●6. Springfield D, Rosenberg A. Biopsy: Complicated and risky. *Journal of Bone and Joint Surgery (American)* 1996;**78A**:639–43.
7. Dorfman HD, Czerniak B. *Bone Tumors*. St Louis, MO: Mosby.
8. Schajowicz F. *Tumors and Tumor-like Lesions of Bone*. Berlin, Germany: Springer.
9. Unni KK. *Dahlin's Bone Tumors General Aspects And Data On 11,087 Cases*, 5th edn. Philadelphia, PA: Lippincott-Raven.
◆10. Margau R, Babyn P, Cole W, *et al*. MR imaging of simple bone cysts in children: not so simple. *Pediatric Radiology* 2000;**30**:551–7.
11. Ambacher T, Maurer F, Weise K. [Spontaneous healing of a juvenile bone cyst of the tibia after pathological fracture]. *Unfallchirurgie* 1999;**102**:972–4.
12. Stanton RP, Abdel-Mota'al MM. Growth arrest resulting from unicameral bone cyst. *Journal of Pediatric Orthopedics* 1998;**18**:198–201.
13. Panoutsakopoulos G, Pandis N, Kyriazoglou I, *et al*. Recurrent t(16;17)(q22;p13) in aneurysmal bone cyst. *Genes Chromosomes Cancer* 1999;**26**:265–6.
14. Kransdorf MJ, Sweet DE. Aneurysmal bone cyst: concept, controversy, clinical presentation and imaging. *AJR American Journal of Roentgenology* 1995;**164**:573–80.
◆15. Martinez V, Sissons HA. Aneurysmal bone cyst. A review of 123 cases including primary lesions and those secondary to other bone pathology. *Cancer* 1988;**61**:2291–304.
16. Bertoni F, Bacchini P, Capanna R, *et al*. Solid variant of aneurysmal bone cyst. *Cancer* 1993;**71**:729–34.
●17. Campanacci M, Boriani S, Giunti A. Giant cell tumor of bone. *Journal of Bone and Joint Surgery (American)* 1987;**69**:106–14.
18. Schwarts HS, Dahir GA, Butler MG. Telomere reduction in giant cell tumor of bone and with aging. *Cancer* 1993;**71**:132–8.
19. Cribb GL, Cool WP, Hill SO, Mangham DC. Distal tibial giant cell tumour treated with curettage and stabilisation with an Ilizarov frame. *Foot and Ankle Surgery* 2009;**15**:28–32.
20. Nascimento AG, Huvos AG, Marcove RC. Primary malignant giant cell tumor of bone: a study of eight cases and review of the literature. *Cancer* 1979;**44**:1393–402.
●21. Jaffe HL, Lichtenstein L. Eosinophilic granuloma of bone: a condition affecting one, several or many bones, but apparently limited to the skeleton and representing the mildest clinical expression of the peculiar inflammatory histiocytosis also underlying Letterer-Siwe disease and Schuller-Christian disease. *Archives of Pathology* 1944;**37**:99.
22. Lieberman PH, Jones CR, Steinman RM, *et al*. Langerhans cell (eosinophilic) granulomatosis. A clinicopathologic study encompassing 50 years. *American Journal of Surgery and Pathology* 1996;**20**:519–52.
23. Willman CL, Busque L, Griffith BB, *et al*. Langerhans'-cell histiocytosis (histiocytosis X) – a clonal proliferative disease. *New England Journal of Medicine* 1994;**331**:154–60.

24. Cohen MM Jr. Fibrous dysplasia is a neoplasm. *American Journal of Medical Genetics* 2001;**98**:290-3.
●25. Harris WH, Dudley HR, Barry RJ. The natural history of fibrous dysplasia. *Journal of Bone and Joint Surgery (American)* 1962;**44**:207-33.
26. Faivre L, Nivelon-Chevallier A, Kottler ML, et al. Mazabraud syndrome in two patients: clinical overlap with McCune-Albright syndrome. *American Journal of Medical Genetics* 2001;**99**:132-6.
27. Chapurlat RD, Meunier PJ. Fibrous dysplasia of bone. *Baillieres Best Practice and Research Clinical Rheumatology* 2000;**14**:385-98.
28. Jackson RP, Reckling FW, Mants FA. Osteoid osteoma and osteoblastoma. Similar histologic lesions with different natural histories. *Clinical Orthopedics and Related Research* 1977;**Oct**:303-13.
◆29. Healey JH, Ghelman B. Osteoid osteoma and osteoblastoma. Current concepts and recent advances. *Clinical Orthopedics and Related Research* 1986;**Mar**:76-85.
30. Norman A, Abdelwahab IF, Buyon J, Matzkin E. Osteoid osteoma of the hip stimulating an early onset osteoarthritis. *Radiology* 1970;**96**:301-6.
31. Kirwan EO, Hutton PA, Pozo JL, Ransford AO. Osteoid osteoma and benign osteoblastoma of the spine. Clinical presentation and treatment. *Journal of Bone and Joint Surgery (British)* 1984;**66**:21-6.
32. Nemoto O, Moser RP Jr, Van Dam BE, et al. Osteoblastoma of the spine. A review of 75 cases. *Spine* 1990;**15**:1272-80.
33. Cribb GL, Goude WH, Cool P, et al. Percutaneous radiofrequency thermocoagulation of osteoid osteomas; factors affecting therapeutic outcome. *Skeletal Radiology* 2005;**34**:702-6.
34. Jaffe HL. Osteoid osteoma: a benign osteoblastic tumor composed of osteoid and atypical bone. *Archives of Surgery* 1935;**31**:709.
35. Baruffi MR, Volpon JB, Neto JB, Casartelli C. Osteoid osteomas with chromosome alterations involving 22q. *Cancer Genetics and Cytogenetics* 2001;**129**:177-80.
36. Radig K, Schneider-Stock R, Mittler U, et al. Genetic instability in osteoblastic tumors of the skeletal system. *Pathology, Research and Practice* 1998;**194**:669-77.
●37. Bloem JL, Mulder JD. Chondroblastoma: a clinical and radiological study of 104 cases. *Skeletal Radiology* 1985;**14**:1-9.
38. Turcotte RE, Kurt AM, Sim FH, Unni KK, McLeod RA. Chondroblastoma. *Human Pathology* 1993;**24**:944-9.
39. Swarts SJ, Neff JR, Johansson SL, et al. Significance of abnormalities of chromosomes 5 and 8 in chondroblastoma. *Clinical Orthopedics* 1998;189-93.
●40. Tins B, Cassar-Pullicino V, McCall I, et al. Radiofrequency ablation of chondroblastoma using a multi-tined expandable electrode system: initial results. *European Radiology* 2006;**16**:804-10.
41. Bovee JV, Cleton-Jansen AM, et al. EXT-mutation analysis and loss of heterozygosity in sporadic and hereditary osteochondromas and secondary chondrosarcomas. *American Journal of Human Genetics* 1999;**65**:689-98.
42. Bridge JA, Nelson M, Orndal C, et al. Clonal karyotypic abnormalities of the hereditary multiple exostoses chromosomal loci 8q24.1 (EXT1) and 11p11-12 (EXT2) in patients with sporadic and hereditary osteochondromas. *Cancer* 1998;**82**:1657-63.
43. Mertens F, Rydholm A, Kreicbergs A, et al. Loss of chromosome band 8q24 in sporadic osteocartilaginous exostoses. *Genes Chromosomes Cancer* 1994;**9**:8-12.
44. Kivioja A, Ervasti H, Kinnunen J, et al. Chondrosarcoma in a family with multiple hereditary exostoses. *Journal of Bone and Joint Surgery* 2000;**82**:261-6.
45. De Beuckeleer LH, De Schepper AM, Ramon F. Magnetic resonance imaging of cartilaginous tumors: is it useful or necessary? *Skeletal Radiology* 1996;**25**:137-41.
46. Liu J, Hudkins PG, Swee RG, Unni KK. Bone sarcomas associated with Ollier's disease. *Cancer* 1987 **59**:1376-85.
47. Schwartz HS, Zimmerman NB, Simon MA, et al. The malignant potential of enchondromatosis. *Journal of Bone and Joint Surgery (American)* 1987;**69**:269-74.
◆48. Schajowicz F. Cartilage forming tumors. In: Schajowicz F. (ed) *Tumors and Tumor-like Lesions of Bone*. Berlin, Germany: Springer.
49. Bjornsson J, McLeod RA, Unni KK, et al. Primary chondrosarcoma of long bones and limb girdles. *Cancer* 1998;**83**:2105-19.
50. Dahlin DC, Coventry MB. Osteogenic sarcoma. A study of six hundred cases. *Journal of Bone and Joint Surgery (Ameican)* 1967;**49**:101-10.
◆51. Dahlin DC, Unni KK. Osteosarcoma of bone and its important recognizable varieties. *American Journal of Surgical Pathology* 1977;**1**:61-72.
52. Sanerkin NG. Definitions of osteosarcoma, chondrosarcoma, and fibrosarcoma of bone. *Cancer* 1980;**46**;178-85.
53. Dorfman HD, Czerniak B. Bone cancers. *Cancer* 1995; **75**:203-10.
54. Raymond AK, Murphy GF, Rosenthal DI. Case report 425: Chondroblastic osteosarcoma: clear cell variant of femur. *Skeletal Radiology* 1987;**16**:336-41.
55. deSantos LA, Edeiken B. Purely lytic osteosarcoma. *Skeletal Radiology* 1982;**9**:1-7.
56. Fletcher JA, Gebhardt MC, Kozadewich HP. Cytogenetic aberrations in osteosarcomas. Nonrandom deletions, rings, and double-minute chromosomes. *Cancer Genetics and Cytogenetics* 1994;**77**:81-8.
57. Mertens F, Mandahl N, Orndal C, et al. Cytogenetic findings in 33 osteosarcomas. *International Journal of Cancer* 1993;**55**:44-50.
58. Cool P, Grimer RJ, Rees R. Surveillance in patients with sarcoma of the extremities. *European Journal of Surgical Oncology* 2005;**31**:1020-4.
●59. Okada K, Frassica FJ, Sim FH, et al. Parosteal osteosarcoma. A clinicopathological study. *Journal of Bone and Joint Surgery (American)* 1994;**76**:366-78.
60. Bertoni F, Present D, Hudson T, Enneking WF. The meaning of radiolucencies in parosteal osteosarcoma. *Journal of Bone and Joint Surgery (American)* 1985;**67**:901-10.

61. Jaffe JL. *Tumors and Tumorous Conditions of the Bones and Joints*. Philadelphia, PA: Lea & Febiger.
62. Sinovic JF, Bridge JA, Neff JR. Ring chromosome in parosteal osteosarcoma. Clinical and diagnostic significance. *Cancer Genetics and Cytogenetics* 1992;**62**:50–2.
63. Ushigome S, Shimoda T, Nikaido T, *et al*. Primitive neuroectodermal tumors of bone and soft tissue. With reference to histologic differentiation in primary or metastatic foci. *Acta Pathologica Japonica* 1992; **32**:113–22.
64. Aurias A, Rimbaut C, Buffe D, *et al*. Chromosomal translocations in Ewing's sarcoma. *New England Journal of Medicine* 1983;**309**:496–7.
65. Turc-Carel C, Philip I, Berger MP, *et al*. Chromosomal translocations in Ewing's sarcoma. *New England Journal of Medicine* 1983;**309**:497–8.
66. Feldman F, Norman D. Intra- and extraosseous malignant histiocytoma (malignant fibrous xanthoma). *Radiology* 1972;**104**:497–508.
67. Huvos AG, Woodard HQ, Heilweil M. Postradiation malignant fibrous histiocytoma of bone. A clinicopathologic study of 20 patients. *American Journal of Surgical Pathology* 1986;**10**:9–18.
68. McCarthy EF, Matsuno T, Dorfman HD. Malignant fibrous histioctyoma of bone: a study of 35 cases. *Human Pathology* 1979:**10**:57–70.
69. Murphey MD, Gross TM, Rosenthal HG. From the archives of the AFIP. Musculoskeletal malignant fibrous histioctyoma: radiologic-pathologic correlation. *Radiographics* 1994;**14**:807–26.
●70. Capanna R, Bertoni F, Bacchini P, *et al*. Malignant fibrous histioctyoma of bone. The experience at the Rizzoli Institute: report of 90 cases. *Cancer* 1984:**54**:177–87.
71. Sundaresan N, Galicich JH, Chu FC, Huvos AG. Spinal chordomas. *Journal of Neurosurgery* 1979;**50**:312–19.
72. D'Haen B, De Jaegere T, Goffin J, *et al*. Chordoma of the lower cervical spine. *Clinical Neurology and Neurosurgery* 1995;**97**:245–8.
73. Meis JM, Raymond AK, Evans HL, *et al*. 'Dedifferentiated' chordoma. A clinicopathologic and immunohistochemical study of three cases. *American Journal of Surgical Pathology* 1987;**11**:516–25.
74. Tallini G, Dorfman H, Brys P, *et al*. Correlation between clinicopathological features and karyotype in 100 cartilaginous and chordoid tumours. A report from the chromosomes and morphology (CHAMP) collaborative study group. *Journal of Pathology* 2002;**196**:194–203.
75. Schulz-Ertner D, Haberer T, Jäkel O, *et al*. Radiotherapy for chordomas and low-grade chondrosarcomas of the skull base with carbon ions. *International Journal of Radiation Oncology Biology Physics* 2002;**53**:36–42.
76. Hug E, Loredo L, Slater J, *et al*. Proton radiation therapy for chordomas and chondrosarcomas of the skull base. *Journal of Neurosurgery* 1999;**91**(3):432–39.
77. Salmon SE, Cassady JR. Plasma cell neoplasms. In: DeVita VT, Hellman S, Rosenberg S (eds) *Cancer, Principles and Practice of Oncology*. Philadelphia, PA: JB Lippincott, 1954.
78. Braunstein EM, White SJ. Non Hodgkin lymphoma of bone. *Radiology* 1980;**135**:59–63.
●79. Heyning FH, Hogendoorn PC, Kramer MH, *et al*. Primary non-Hodgkin's lymphoma of bone: a clinico-pathological investigation of 60 cases. *Leukemia* 1999;**13**:2094–8.

82

Soft-tissue sarcomas

GILLIAN L CRIBB

Introduction	912	Staging of soft-tissue sarcomas	914
Epidemiology	912	Biopsy	915
Age and location	912	Principles of surgical treatment of soft-tissue tumours	915
Aetiology	912	Adjunctive oncological treatments	916
Clinical characteristics	913	Pathology of soft-tissue tumours	916
Imaging	913	References	921
Classification of soft-tissue tumours	913		

NATIONAL BOARD STANDARDS

- To understand the features suggesting a sarcoma
- Know the different types of soft-tissue tumours
- Learn the workup
- Learn the principles of surgical treatment

INTRODUCTION

Benign soft-tissue tumours are common and malignant soft-tissue sarcomas are relatively rare. It important to recognize features associated with soft-tissue sarcomas so appropriate referral can be made to a specialist centre. The clinical features of a soft-tissue mass that are highly suggestive of malignancy include increasing size and pain, size greater than 5 cm, deep to deep fascia and recurrence of a previously excised mass. Local and distant staging needs to be performed to allow multidisciplinary management. The mainstay of treatment for soft-tissue sarcomas is surgery and radiotherapy.

EPIDEMIOLOGY

Benign mesenchymal tumours occur 100 times more frequently than sarcomas.[1] There are approximately 8700 new cases of soft-tissue sarcoma diagnosed in the USA each year[2] and about 1500 in the UK.[3] Soft-tissue sarcomas account for 0.63% of all new cancer cases and 1.15% of deaths from cancer in the USA.[2]

AGE AND LOCATION

Lipomas are the most common soft-tissue tumour;[4] they are rare in the hand, lower leg and foot, and very uncommon in children.[5] The extremities are the most common site for soft-tissue sarcomas with 40% occurring in the lower limb and girdle and 20% in the upper limb and girdle.[3] Overall soft-tissue sarcomas are more common with advancing age, with the median age for presentation being 65 years;[1] however, the age-related incidences do vary. Embryonal rhabdomyosarcomas occur exclusively in children, synovial sarcomas mostly in young adults and pleomorphic high-grade sarcoma, liposarcoma and leiomyosarcomas are more common in older people.

AETIOLOGY

The aetiology of most benign and malignant soft-tissue tumours is unknown. Radiation exposure has been recognized to induce sarcomas since the 1920s; the risk has been estimated to be up to 0.8% in exposed populations.[6] A recent large series[7] showed the median latency period from radiation exposure to sarcoma development was 8.4 years, and these sarcomas accounted for 2.5% of all soft-tissue sarcomas seen by Cha et al. at their institution. Breast cancer (29%) was the most common malignancy for which radiation was used, followed by lymphoma and prostate cancer.

Some genetic conditions are associated with soft-tissue tumours. Neurofibromas are the most common benign tumour seen in type 1 neurofibromatosis (NF-1); their malignant counterpart malignant peripheral nerve sheath tumour (MPNST) occurs in patients with this autosomal dominant condition, especially where there has been radiation exposure.[8]

Li–Fraumenni syndrome[9] is a rare autosomal dominant disorder caused by mutations in p53, a tumour suppressor gene. Sarcomas (particularly osteosarcoma) develop at a young age (less than age 45), and first-degree relatives are at a higher risk of developing malignancies, including breast cancer and bone and soft-tissue sarcomas.[10] Children who survive hereditary retinoblastoma have an exceptionally high risk of developing both bone and soft-tissue sarcomas, particularly osteosarcoma and leiomyosarcoma.[11,12]

CLINICAL CHARACTERISTICS

Benign soft-tissue tumours outnumber sarcomas by 100 to 1.[1] Symptoms are usually non-specific; 99% of benign soft-tissue tumours are superficial and 95% are less than 5 cm in diameter.[13] The presentation of a sarcoma is often with the accidental finding of a painless mass. The four clinical features that are highly suggestive for malignancy are[14]

- increasing in size
- size greater than 5 cm
- painful
- deep to deep fascia.

In addition any lesion which is recurrent should also be regarded with a high index of suspicion. Patients exhibiting any of these features require referral to a specialist centre to ensure they get optimal treatment.[15]

IMAGING

Pre-treatment imaging is essential in the workup and staging of a soft-tissue tumour.

Plain radiographs

Plain radiographs should be the initial mode of imaging of the mass or region in question; they will most frequently be normal but can provide invaluable information if not. Radiographs can give an initial assessment of the osseous reaction to a soft-tissue tumour such as remodelling, periosteal reaction or overt destruction.[16]

Magnetic resonance imaging

MRI is the imaging modality of choice for detecting, characterizing and staging soft-tissue tumours.[1] Tumours can be distinguished well from normal fat, muscle and neurovascular structures, and MRI is therefore essential in guiding the biopsy and planning surgery. It can also give clues to the nature of the lesion[8] with some benign conditions having very characteristic MR appearances, such as lipomas, haemangioma, ganglion, neurofibromas and pigmented villodular synovitis.[17,18] Most connective tissue sarcomas are dark on T_1- and light on T_2-weighting[8] and are heterogeneous. The use of gadolinium contrast further helps define the extent of the lesion;[8] this can differentiate solid from cystic lesions, evaluate haematomas and haemorrhagic lesions and identify necrosis within a tumour.[16]

Ultrasound scanning

Ultrasound scanning is rarely used as the primary modality in the assessment of a soft-tissue mass;[16] however, it can be useful in differentiating cystic from solid masses[19] and assessing the vascularity of a lesion.[20] Image-guided biopsies of soft-tissue masses can be performed reliably under ultrasound guidance.[21–23]

Computerized tomography

CT scanning is useful in delineation of the osseous architecture and where MRI is contraindicated.[16] CT can be also used to guide biopsies.[24–26] A baseline chest CT scan at the time of diagnosis of a soft-tissue sarcoma for evidence of lung metastasis is essential for accurate staging of patients.

Positron emission tomography

Positron emission tomography (PET) is the gold standard in metabolic imaging; this uses radioisotopes that undergo positron emission decay. Fluorodeoxyglucose PET has been shown to be 95% sensitive and 75% specific in the diagnosis of soft-tissue sarcomas.[27] PET is also of use in pre-treatment grading, guiding biopsies to the most metabolically active areas of the tumour and evaluation of local recurrence and metastases; however, further studies are required to determine how best to use this technique to complement or replace conventional imaging.[28]

CLASSIFICATION OF SOFT-TISSUE TUMOURS

The new WHO classification of soft-tissue tumours[1] classifies soft-tissue tumours into four categories.

Benign

Lesions that usually do not recur and those that do recur do so in a non-destructive fashion and are almost always readily cured by re-excision. They exceedingly rarely metastasize (<1/50 000 cases); this is entirely unpredictable on the basis of conventional histological examination.

Intermediate (locally aggressive)

Lesions that recur locally and are associated with an infiltrative and locally destructive growth pattern. These lesions do not metastasize but typically require wide excision in order to ensure local control, e.g. desmoid fibromatosis.

Intermediate (rarely metastasizing)

Locally aggressive (as intermediate) but in addition show well-documented ability to give rise to distant metastases in occasional cases. This risk is <2% but is not predictable on the basis of histomorphology.

Malignant

Potential for locally destructive growth and recurrence and a significant risk of distant metastases ranging from 20% to almost 100% depending on histological type and grade.

STAGING OF SOFT-TISSUE SARCOMAS

Once all the imaging studies have been performed and the biopsy obtained, it should be possible to stage the tumour, which is essential for treatment planning.[8] Staging is based on clinical and histological parameters and provides information on the extent of the tumour.[1]

The major staging system used for soft-tissue sarcomas was described by the American Joint Committee on Cancer (AJCC);[29] this gives four stages based on histological grade, tumour size and depth, and the presence of distant or nodal metastases (Table 82.1).

Table 82.1 American Joint Committee on Cancer staging for soft-tissue sarcoma (modified from Greene[29])

Primary tumour (T)	Classification				
T1	Tumour ≤5 cm				
	T1a superficial tumour				
	T1b deep tumour				
T2	Tumour >5 cm				
	T2a superficial				
	T2b deep tumour				
Regional lymph nodes					
N0	No regional lymph node metastases				
N1	Regional lymph node metastases				
Distant metastases					
M0	No distant metastases				
M1	Distant metastases				
Histological grade (G)					
Low Grade	Grade 1				
High Grade	Grades 2 or 3				
Stage grouping					
Stage I	T1a,1b,2a,2b	N0	M0	Low grade	
Stage II	T1a,1b,2a	N0	M0	High grade	
Stage III	T2b	N0	M0	High grade	
Stage IV	Any T	N1	M0	Any G	
	Any T	N0	M1	Any G	
5-year survival					
Stage	%				
I	86				
II	72				
III	52				
IV	10–20				

Histological grade

Histological grade of a soft-tissue sarcoma is the most important prognostic factor. Grading is based on histological parameters and evaluates the degree of malignancy and the probability of distant metastases.[1] The two most widely used grading systems are those described by Trojani et al.[30] and the United States National Cancer Institute (NCI);[31] these are both three-grade systems (i.e. grades 1, 2 and 3). The Trojani system is the most used in Europe and is based on tumour differentiation, mitotic count and tumour necrosis. The NCI system uses a combination of histological type, cellularity, pleomorphism and mitotic rate. For the AJCC staging system grade 1 is considered low grade, and grades 2 and 3 are considered high grade.[1]

Size

Size is also an important prognostic factor in soft-tissue sarcoma with less than 5 cm and greater than 5 cm being most commonly used. Grimer[32] has shown that a patient's surgical treatment, likelihood of metastases at diagnosis and overall risk of death are affected by the size of the soft-tissue sarcoma. Patients who underwent limb salvage had smaller tumours (mean 10.2 cm) than those who underwent amputation (mean 12.1 cm); those with smaller tumours were less likely to have metastases at diagnosis (3% in tumours <5 cm, 18% in tumours >25 cm) and the overall risk of death was 8.5 times higher in tumours greater than 25 cm than in those less than 5 cm.

Lymph node metastases

Lymph node metastases in soft-tissue sarcoma of an extremity is uncommon, occurring in less than 5% of patients.[35] In a review of 37 patients with nodal metastases the most common sarcomas were epithelioid sarcoma (20%), rhabdomyosarcoma (19%), clear cell sarcoma (11%) and angiosarcoma (11%).[33]

Distant metastases

Distant metastases are present in one-tenth of patients at the diagnosis of their soft-tissue sarcoma. The lungs are the most common site for distant metastases.

Tumours that are low grade histologically, small in size and confined within a compartment have a good prognosis and may only require surgical excision, whereas those that are high grade histologically and large in size and have metastasized or recurred locally often require adjunctive therapies such as radiotherapy or chemotherapy in addition to surgery.[8]

BIOPSY

Refer to (page 870) for the principles of biopsy

Clinically and radiologically benign-appearing lesions do not have to have a biopsy. However, a biopsy is indicated in benign aggressive, malignant and questionable lesions to establish a histological diagnosis to allow planning of definitive treatment.[34]

PRINCIPLES OF SURGICAL TREATMENT OF SOFT-TISSUE TUMOURS

The principal treatment for soft-tissue sarcomas is surgical, and the biopsy site or track is excised en bloc with the tumour. There are four basic types of excision; each is based on the relationship of the plane of dissection to the tumour and its relationship to the reactive zone or pseudocapsule (Fig. 82.1). When they grow, sarcomas form a solid mass that grows centrifugally, with the periphery of the lesion being the least mature. In contrast to the true capsule that surrounds benign lesions, which is composed of compressed normal cells, sarcomas are generally enclosed by a reactive zone, or pseudocapsule. This consists of compressed tumour cells and a fibrovascular zone of reactive tissue with a variable inflammatory component that interacts with the surrounding normal tissues.[34]

- *Intralesional excision*: within the tumour mass, leaving macroscopic tumour behind.
- *Marginal*: through the reactive zone of the tumour, often leaving macroscopic foci of tumour (appropriate for the majority of benign lesions).
- *Wide*: outside of the reactive zone, leaving no tumour other than skip metastases.
- *Radical*: often including the entire limb and involving the entire compartment in which the tumour was located.

In general most surgeons like to achieve a wide margin if possible for high-grade sarcomas;[8] there is controversy regarding the optimal margin width, but it is generally considered to be a few centimetres.[34] In some circumstances, particularly in cases with neurological or vascular proximity, a marginal margin is accepted. Patients with microscopically positive margins are at increased risk

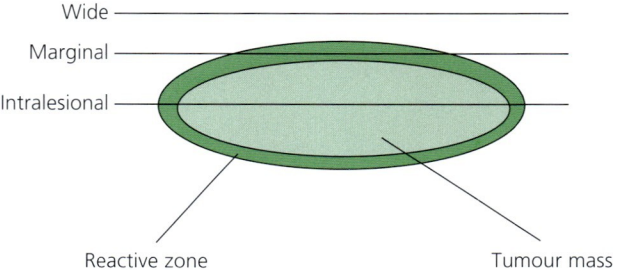

Figure 82.1 Planes of dissection.

of local recurrence and tumour-related mortality.[35] Reconstruction may be required following the excision of the tumour in the form of muscle transfer or skin grafts, vascular grafts or replacement of bone in the form of allograft or metallic implant.

Approximately 5% of soft-tissue sarcomas require amputation.[36] The major indications are where there is anticipated inadequate limb function after wide excision, multicompartmental neurovascular tumour involvement and where there was local tumour contamination from unplanned prior surgery.[37]

ADJUNCTIVE ONCOLOGICAL TREATMENTS

Please refer to page 874.

PATHOLOGY OF SOFT-TISSUE TUMOURS

The *WHO Classification of Soft-tissue Tumours*[1] classifies soft-tissue tumours according to their tissue of origin; this is summarized in Table 82.2. The most common types are described below.

Table 82.2 World Health Organization Classification of Soft Tissue Tumours (from Fletcher et al.[1])

Type	Benign	Intermediate	Malignant
Adipocytic	Lipoma	Atypical lipomatous tumour	Liposarcoma
Fibroblastic/myofibroblastic	Nodular fasciitis	Solitary fibrous tumour	Adult fibrosarcoma
	Proliferative fasciitis and myositis	Haemangiopericytoma	Myxofibrosarcoma
	Myositis ossificans		Low-grade fibromyxoid sarcoma
	Ischaemic fasciitis		Sclerosing epithelioid fibrosarcoma
	Elastofibroma		
	Fibroma of tendon sheath		
	Superficial fibromatoses		
	Desmoid-type fibromatoses		
So-called fibrohistiocytic tumours	Giant cell tumour of tendon sheath		Pleomorphic malignant fibrous histiocytoma/undifferentiated
	Diffuse type giant cell tumour		Giant cell malignant fibrous histiocytoma
	Fibrohistiocytomas		
	Giant cell tumour of tendon sheath		Inflammatory malignant fibrous histiocytoma
Smooth muscle tumours	Angioleiomyoma		
	Leiomyoma of deep soft tissues		Leiomyosarcoma
Pericytic (perivascular) tumours	Glomus tumours		
	Myopericytoma		
Skeletal muscle tumours	Rhabdomyoma	Epithelioid haemangioendothelioma	Rhabdomyosarcoma
Vascular tumours	Haemangiomas		Kaposiform haemangioendothelioma
	Epitheliod haemangioma		Kaposi sarcoma
	Angiomatosis		Angiosarcoma of soft tissue
	Lymphangioma		
Chondro-osseous tumours	Soft-tissue chondroma		Extraskeletal osteosarcoma
Tumours of uncertain differentiation	Intramuscular myxoma		Synovial sarcoma
			Epithelioid sarcoma
			Alveolar soft part sarcoma
			Clear cell sarcoma of soft tissue
			Extraskeletal myxoid chondrosarcoma

Tumours of cranial and spinal nerves
1. Schwannoma (neurinoma, neurilemoma)
   1. cellular, plexiform, and melanotic subtypes
2. Neurofibroma
   1. circumscribed (solitary) neurofibroma
   2. plexiform neurofibroma
3. Malignant peripheral nerve sheath tumour (malignant schwannoma)
   1. epithelioid
   2. divergent mesenchymal or epithelial differentiation
   3. melanotic

Adipocytic tumours

Lipomatous tumours are the largest group of mesenchymal tumours, accounting for 50% of all soft-tissue tumours.[38] Lipomas are the most common benign soft-tissue tumour,[4] and liposarcomas represent the single most common type of soft-tissue sarcoma.[39]

LIPOMA

Lipomas are benign tumours, which usually present as a painless mass. They are most common between ages 40 and 60 years, and approximately 5% of patients have multiple lipomas. Lipomas can occur in the trunk, head and neck, upper and lower extremities. Involvement of the hand and forearm is infrequent.[40] Lipomas may arise in superficial or deep tissues. Deep lipomas can occur between individual muscle fibres (intramuscular) or between muscle groups (intermuscular). Lipomas may be visible on plain radiographs (Fig. 82.2). MRI appearances are characteristic: lipomas are bright on T_1-weighted imaging and moderate to bright on T_2-weighted images. In all sequences, the lesion appears isointense compared with subcutaneous fat.[17] Macroscopically lipomas are well circumscribed and have a yellow, greasy cut surface. Microscopically they are composed of lobules of mature adipocytes.[1]

ANGIOLIPOMA

A benign subcutaneous nodule consisting of mature fat cells intermingled with small and thin-walled vessels.[1] These tumours are more common in males in their teens and early twenties. The forearm is the most common location and lesions may be multiple and painful.

ADIPOCYTIC TUMOURS OF INTERMEDIATE MALIGNANCY

Atypical lipomatous tumour/well-differentiated liposarcoma

This is an intermediate (locally aggressive) malignant mesenchymal neoplasm composed entirely or in part of a mature adipocytic proliferation, showing significant variation in cell size and at least focal nuclear atypia in both adipocytes and stromal cells.[1]

ALT/WDLLL liposarcoma accounts for 40–45% of all liposarcomas, the largest subgroup. The peak incidence is in the sixth decade. The largest series of deep atypical lipomas[41] showed these lesions most commonly occur in the thigh, and are typically large (4–30 cm; mean 18 cm). The local recurrence rate with marginal excision ('shelling out') was 8%, with no alteration in grade of tumour at recurrence. No patients developed metastases or died of their disease.

LIPOSARCOMA

There are five histological subtypes of liposarcoma, well differentiated, dedifferentiated, myxoid, round cell and pleomorphic.[1]

Dedifferentiated liposarcoma

This is a malignant neoplasm showing transition from an atypical lipomatous tumour/well-differentiated liposarcoma to a non-lipogenic sarcoma of variable histological grade.[1] This dedifferentiation can occur in up to 10% of well-differentiated liposarcomas. The risk is higher in deep-seated lesions and as a time-dependent phenomenon.[1] Radiological imaging shows the coexistence of fatty and non-fatty solid components. Local recurrence occurs in at least 40% of patients and distant metastases in 15–20%; overall mortality ranges between 28% and 30% at 5 years.[42–44]

Myxoid/round cell liposarcoma

Myxoid/round cell liposarcomas account for approximately 40% of all liposarcomas[38] and about 10% of all adult soft-tissue sarcomas.[1] These tumours usually occur in the deep tissues of the extremities, with two-thirds occurring in the thigh.[1] Peak incidence is in the fourth and fifth decades. They are prone to recur locally and one-third of patients develop distant metastases. Unlike other sarcomas, myxoid liposarcomas metastasize to extrapulmonary sites such as soft-tissue and bone (often spine). Histologically the tumour is composed of uniform round primitive mesenchymal cells and a variable number of small signet-ring lipoblasts within a prominent myxoid stroma. Myxoid liposarcomas have been shown to be highly radiosensitive with two retrospective reviews showing significant decrease in size after pre-operative radiotherapy.[45,46]

Pleomorphic liposarcoma

Pleomorphic liposarcoma accounts for less than 5% of all liposarcomas and is a high-grade, highly malignant sarcoma seen in elderly people. It contains a variable number of pleomorphic lipoblasts, mitotic activity is high and haemorrhage or necrosis is common.[38] This is a very aggressive sarcoma with a 30–50% metastasis rate and overall tumour-associated mortality of 30–50%.[1]

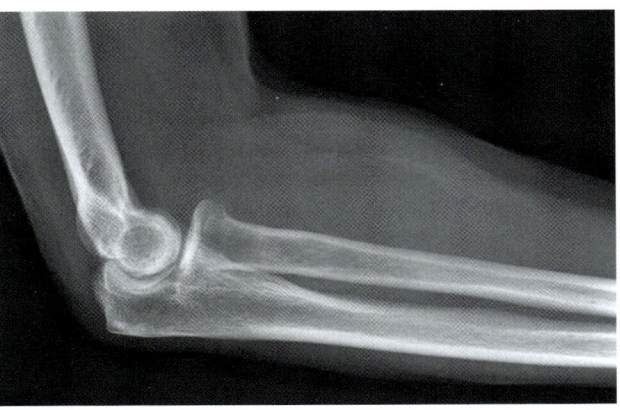

Figure 82.2 Radiograph indicating lipoma

Fibroblastic/myofibroblastic tumours

SUPERFICIAL FIBROMATOSES

Superficial fibromatoses are fibroblastic proliferations that arise in the palmar (Dupuytren's disease), plantar (Ledderhose disease), penile (Peyronie disease) soft-tissues and the dorsum of the proximal interphlangeal joints of the hand (Garrods pads). Histologically these conditions are indistinguishable. Dupuytren's is seen most commonly in patients of northern European extraction and is uncommon in dark-skinned individuals. The prevalence ranges from 2% to 4% in diverse Caucasian populations.[47] The incidence increases with advancing age and is rarely seen in individuals under 30 years; men are 5–15 times more commonly affected than women.[47] Histologically the proliferative phase is by a cellular proliferation of plump, immature spindle cells of varying shapes and sizes. The more mature lesions are much less cellular and contain denser collagen.[1] The lesions have a propensity for local recurrence but are not a malignant or pre-malignant condition.[47]

DESMOID-TYPE FIBROMATOSES

Desmoid-type fibromatoses are clonal fibroblastic proliferations that arise in the deep soft tissues and are characterized by infiltrative growth and a tendency towards local recurrence but an inability to metastasize.[1] They are rare lesions with an incidence of two to four individuals per million per year.[48]

Desmoids occur in three general locations: the extremities (commonly limb girdles and proximal extremity), the abdominal wall (especially in women during and after pregnancy), and the bowel wall and mesentery.[49]

MRI is the imaging modality of choice. On T_1-weighted images, most lesions are near homogeneous and isointense to muscle, whereas on T_2 they are more heterogeneous with an overall signal intensity equal to or slightly lower than fat.[50] Local growth with tissue invasion often results in pain, deformity, organ dysfunction and, rarely, death owing to invasion of vital organs.[51] Macroscopically these lesions are firm and cut with a gritty sensation. The cut surface is glistening white and coarsely trabeculated resembling scar tissue. Microscopically, they are characterized by a proliferation of elongated, slender spindle cells of a uniform appearance set in a collagenous stroma.[1]

Optimal management has not been clearly defined. Surgery, in the form of wide excision, is generally considered the treatment mainstay. However, despite wide surgical margins, a high local recurrence rate is reported by several series, ranging from 24% to 77% at 10 years.[51] Other treatments described include radiotherapy and anti-oestrogen therapies, but there are mixed reports in the literature.

MYXOFIBROSARCOMA

Myxofibrosarcoma, a variant of malignant fibrous histiocytoma (MFH), is one of the most common sarcomas in the elderly population. It occurs predominately in the subcutaneous tissues of the extremities (44% lower extremity and 33% upper extremity), trunk (12%) and head (3%);[52] one-third are deeply located. Local recurrence is frequent and unrelated to histological grade. In contrast, metastases and tumour-associated mortality are closely related to tumour grade.[1] Low-grade tumours do not metastasize; intermediate and high-grade tumours develop metastases in 20–35% of cases. Low-grade lesions can, however, become higher grade lesions with subsequent recurrences.[1]

So-called fibrohistiocytic tumours

GIANT CELL TUMOUR OF TENDON SHEATH (LOCALIZED PIGMENTED VILLONODULAR SYNOVITIS)

Giant cell tumour of the tendon sheath is the most common neoplasm of the hand; other sites affected include the feet, ankle and knee.[53] Men aged 30–50 years are most commonly affected.[54] In the hand most tumours occur in the fingers and are closely related to the tendon sheath or interphalangeal joint. In a recent study of 71 patients[53] 93% of patients presented with a painless swelling, and lesions varied in size from 0.5 cm to 4.5 cm (mean, 1.75 cm). All cases were treated by local marginal excision. Tumour recurrence was seen in three patients (0.04%) and these were re-excised with no further recurrences. Recurrence rates of up to 30% have been reported elsewhere.[1]

DIFFUSE-TYPE GIANT CELL TUMOUR (PIGMENTED VILLONODULAR SYNOVITIS)

Diffuse-type giant cell tumour (DTGCT) is a destructive proliferation of synovial-like mononuclear cells, admixed with multinucleate giant cells.[1] DTGCT is usually monoarticular and arises in the joints, although it may be found in a tendon or bursa.[55] Common intra-articular sites are the knee (75%), hip (15%), ankle, elbow and shoulder, and the average age of presentation is 35 years (range 14–68 years).[56] Patients frequently present with pain, joint effusions and swelling, and the duration of symptoms is variable.[55] MRI findings include a variable extent of nodular synovial proliferation, from mild proliferation to extensive masses, and joint effusions. Haemosiderin is a magnetic material and its deposit on proliferative synovial tissue results in a spotty low signal or extensive low signal area on T_1-and T_2-weighted images. Degenerative joint disease and bone erosions may also be seen.[57] Grossly, DTGCT appears as thickened, reddish-brown synovium (because of haemosiderin deposition) with numerous villous projections. DTGCT is difficult to eradicate and is optimally treated with total synovectomy.[55] Arthroscopic techniques may be useful for diagnostic biopsy, treatment of small local recurrences or nodular pigmented villonodular synovitis; however, an open approach is recommended for advanced disease.[56] Adjuvant treatment modalities include intra-articular instillation of radioactive isotopes or cryosurgical surface spray; these may be considered for patients thought to be at high risk for recurrence. Moderate-dose external beam radiotherapy can be used to control incompletely resected and unresectable disease.[55] Recurrence rates are estimated to be between 18% and 46% in intra-articular lesions and 33% and 50% in extra-articular lesions.[1]

PLEOMORPHIC MALIGNANT FIBROUS HISTIOCYTOMA/UNDIFFERENTIATED HIGH-GRADE PLEOMORPHIC SARCOMA

The term pleomorphic MFH is now reserved for a small group of undifferentiated pleomorphic sarcomas. Historically many sarcomas have been labelled as pleomorphic MFH; however, with advances in immunohistochemistry many of these lesions can be reclassified as other sarcomas, 63% in one series.[58] The group of pleomorphic (MFH-like) sarcomas is the most common type of sarcoma in patients over 40 years, with an overall incidence of one or two cases per 100 000 annually.[1] They are often large, deep-seated tumours of the extremities, which show progressive and often rapid enlargement. Macroscopic appearance is of a well-circumscribed mass, which may appear pseudoencapsulated. High-grade pleomorphic sarcomas are aggressive with an overall 5 year survival rate of 50–60%.[1]

Smooth muscle tumours

LEIOMYOSARCOMA

Leiomyosarcoma is a malignant tumour composed of cells showing smooth muscle features.[1] It most commonly occurs in the uterus, retroperitoneum and abdominal cavity; however, it also occurs at non-visceral sites, where it accounts for 10% of sarcomas. In a recent large study of non-visceral leiomyosarcoma[59] the median age of onset was 70 years (range 20–98 years) with equal gender distribution. The majority of lesions were in the subcutaneous tissues (45%) with 39% deep and 16% cutaneous. Sixty-nine per cent of lesions were in the extremities, and the thigh was the most common site. The vast majority of lesions were high grade with a median size of 4 cm (0.6–35 cm). The 5 and 10 year survival rates were 64% and 46% respectively.

Pericytic (perivascular) tumours

GLOMUS TUMOURS

Glomus tumours are benign neoplasms that account for 1–5% of all soft-tissue tumours of the hand.[60] The normal glomus body is an end-organ apparatus which has a role in controlling blood temperature and blood pressure by regulating peripheral blood flow. The tumours are a result of hyperplasia of one or more of the normal parts of the glomus body and pain develops from contraction of the glomus cells.[60] Patients present with a classic triad of symptoms: (1) hypersensitivity to cold, (2) paroxysmal pain and (3) pinpoint pain in the finger. The tumours mainly occur in women and occur most frequently in the subungal region of the distal phalanx.[61] In a large series[62] bluish discolouration was present in 28% of patients, and pulp nodule or nail deformity occurred in 33% of patients.

MRI is a valuable method of imaging glomus tumours; there is high signal intensity on T_2-weighted images and strong enhancement after gadolinium injection. Dahlin et al.,[61] however, recommend exploration of a clinically suspected glomus tumour even if MRI does not support the diagnosis. Complete surgical excision usually results in permanent relief of symptoms.[60]

Skeletal muscle tumours

RHABDOMYOSARCOMA

Rhabdomyosarcomas are the most common soft-tissue sarcomas among children and young adults. Ninety per cent of rhabdomyosarcomas are diagnosed in individuals under 25 years and they account for 3.5% of malignancies in the 0–14 year age group.[63] Embryonal rhabdomyosarcoma is the most common subtype and occurs in infants and young children; alveolar is the second most common and occurs in adolescents and younger adults;[63] pleomorphic rhabdomyosarcomas occur exclusively in older adults.[64] The major histological feature of rhabdomyosarcomas is their resemblance to developing muscle. All patients require chemotherapy. Surgery involves a wide excision of the primary tumour whenever possible, and incompletely resected tumours are generally treated with radiotherapy. A 5 year survival rate >70% has been achieved in recent trials for patients with localized rhabdomyosarcoma.[65]

Vascular tumours

ANGIOSARCOMA OF SOFT TISSUE

Angiosarcomas account for <1% of sarcomas.[66] They can occur in a previously irradiated field[7] and in a chronically lymphoedematous extremity (Stewart–Treves syndrome).[67] Other characteristics that are unique to angiosarcomas include a propensity for multifocal disease and an ability to spread to lymph nodes and distant bone and soft tissues.[68] Most angiosarcomas present as intermediate- or high-grade lesions and are highly aggressive. Local recurrences develop in about one-fifth of patients and 50% die in the first year after diagnosis of metastatic disease.[1]

Tumours of uncertain differentiation

INTRAMUSCULAR MYXOMA

Intramuscular myxomas are benign soft-tissue tumours characterized by bland spindle-shaped cells embedded in hypocellular, abundantly myxoid stroma.[1] In a study of 51 patients with intramuscular myxomas, the mean age of presentation was 52 years (range 27–89 years) and they were more common in women; the average size of lesions was 5.6 cm (2–15 cm).[69] The large muscles of the thigh, shoulder, buttocks and upper arm are the most frequent sites affected, and the presenting symptom is of a painless mass.[1] On MRI scanning they are homogeneously low signal intensity on T_1-weighted images and high signal intensity on T_2-weighted.[70] Treatment is by local excision and they usually do not recur.

SYNOVIAL SARCOMA

Synovial sarcoma is a mesenchymal spindle cell tumour which displays epithelial differentiation and has a specific chromosomal translocation t(X;18)(p11:q11).[1] Synovial sarcoma accounts for 5–10% of all soft-tissue sarcomas and can occur at any age, including in childhood; however, young adults are most commonly affected.[71] Synovial sarcoma occurs equally in males and females and there are no identifiable aetiological factors. They often develop in para-articular regions of the extremity and almost never arise within the joint and are not associated with normal synovial tissue.[72] There are two histological subtypes: monophasic synovial sarcomas are entirely composed of ovoid-spindle cells, whereas the biphasic subtypes are composed of both spindle cell elements and epithelial components.[72] In a study of 130 patients[73] the median size in the widest diameter was 6 cm (1–25 cm); 4% were low grade, 53% intermediate grade and 43% high grade. As with other soft-tissue sarcomas the mainstay of treatment is surgical, with wide excision and adjuvant radiotherapy. Synovial sarcomas have been found to be particularly chemosensitive and improved disease-specific survival has been seen with ifosfamide-based chemotherapy.[74] Survival rates at 5 years range from 40% to 76%.[73] There is a relatively high rate of late metastases, sometimes up to 30 years after diagnosis.[75] Overall, 40% of tumours metastasize, commonly to lungs, bone and regional lymph nodes. Prognostic factors for survival include tumour size (>5 cm), and status at presentation[73] and invasion of bone and neurovascular structures.[76]

Tumours of neural origin

SCHWANNOMA (NEURILEMOMA)

Schwannomas, are benign peripheral nerve sheath tumours; they occur between the ages of 20 and 50 years and account for 5% of all benign soft-tissue tumours.[77] Schwannomas are well circumscribed and encapsulated. They are composed of two types of tissue known as Antoni A and B. Antoni A areas are cellular and consist of eosinophilic spindle cells with ill-defined cell margins, arranged in random fasicles or whorls. Antoni B tissue comprises small round or spindle-shaped cells set in a copious myxoid matrix. Ultrastructuvally they are composed predominately of schwann cells, the myelin producing cells of peripheral nerve sheath.[4] Sites of involvement include the subcutaneous nerves of the face and neck, extremities and deep tissues of the retroperitoneum and mediastinum. MRI appearances of schwannomas and neurofibromas are similar, and the detection of the nerve running into and out of a fusiform mass oriented along the line of the nerve is pathognomic for a nerve sheath tumour.[78] Nerves tend to be displaced by the eccentric schwannomas, whereas the nerve is central to, or obliterated by, neurofibromas. The 'target sign' is seen in both neurofibromas and schwannomas, i.e. peripheral hyperintensity and central hypointensity on T_2-weighted images, and is due to outer myxoid and central fibrous tissue.[78]

NEUROFIBROMA

Neurofibromas account for slightly more than 5% of benign soft-tissue tumours;[77] they are the most common benign soft-tissue tumour in individuals with NF-1.[80] However, 90% are solitary, occur in young adults and are not associated with NF-1.[78] They may appear as discrete, dermal neurofibromas, focal cutaneous or subcutaneous growths, dumbbell-shaped intraforaminal spinal tumours, or nodular or diffuse plexiform neurofibromas. Impingement on surrounding structures may cause functional compromise, and soft-tissue and bone hypertrophy may occur.[80] In contrast to schwannomas, neurofibromas are poorly circumscribed with ill-defined margins. They consist of a relatively hypocellular proliferation of bland spindle cells.[4]

MALIGNANT PERIPHERAL NERVE SHEATH TUMOUR

Malignant peripheral nerve sheath tumours (MPNSTs) account for approximately 5–10% of all soft-tissue tumours;[75] they are defined as any malignant tumour arising from or differentiating towards cells of the peripheral nerve sheath and have a known association with neurofibromatosis type 1. MPNSTs occur in about 2–5% of NF-1 patients compared with an incidence of 0.001% in the general population.[79] Most NF-1-associated MPNSTs appear to arise within pre-existing plexiform neurofibromas. This observation suggests that individuals with NF-1 and plexiform neurofibromas warrant increased surveillance for development of MPNST, and those with many or very extensive plexiform neurofibromas may have the highest risk.[80] In a series of

205 patients with MPNST,[81] where there were 46 patients with the NF-1 gene, the median age of onset was younger in those carrying the NF-1 gene (27 years; range 18–37 years) than in those without (40 years; range 26–59 years). The majority were located in the trunk (51%) and extremity (45%), with no difference between the groups. The majority of tumours were high grade in both groups. The disease-specific mortality rate was 43% at 10 years. Presentation with either primary or recurrent disease, tumour size or tumour site (trunk vs extremity) were the strongest independent predictors of survival. No significant independent differences between patients with and without NF-1 were observed.

Surveillance strategies

The local recurrence rate in soft-tissue sarcomas is 19% and metastases will develop in 26% of patients.[82] Over two-thirds of local recurrence occur by 2 years and 90% by 4 years.[83] Patients therefore need to carefully followed up with clinical history and examination to identify possible local recurrence after definitive treatment. Regular chest radiography should also be performed, particularly in patients with grade III tumours where 83%, in one series, developed chest metastases.[84] CT and MRI are useful for evaluation of less accessible regions and for assessing equivocal changes found during clinical examination. Cool et al. have shown that their surveillance programme, with clinical examination and chest radiographs, picked up 75% of pulmonary metastases but less that 25% of local recurrences.[85]

KEY LEARNING POINTS

- Benign soft-tissue tumours are common, soft-tissue sarcomas are relatively rare.
- Clinical features highly suggestive of a soft-tissue sarcoma are a history of increasing size, pain, size greater than 5 cm, deep to deep fascia and any recurrent lesion.
- Any patient with these features requires referral to a specialist centre for multidisciplinary management.
- Further workup requires appropriate imaging of the lesion, usually with an MRI scan, and distant staging, usually with a chest CT scan.
- A biopsy is required for histological diagnosis.
- Management of soft-tissue sarcoma requires a combination of surgery and radiotherapy.
- Lipomas are the most common benign soft-tissue tumour and liposarcomas the most common malignant soft-tissue tumour.

REFERENCES

- ● = Key primary paper
- ◆ = Major review article

1. Fletcher CDM, Krishnan K, Mertens F (eds) *World Heath Organization Classification of Tumours: Pathology and Genetics, Tumours of Soft Tissues and Bone*. Lyon, France: IARC Press, 2002.
2. Jemal A, Tiwari RC, Murray T, Ghafoor A, et al. Cancer Statistics 2004. *CA: A Cancer Journal for Clinicians* 2004;**54**:8–29.
◆3. Clark MA, Fisher C, Judson I, Thomas JM. Soft tissue sarcomas in adults. *New England Journal of Medicine* 2005;**353**:701–11.
4. McGee J, Isaacson P, Wright N (eds) *Oxford Textbook of Pathology*, Vol. 2b. Oxford, UK: Oxford University Press, 1992.
5. Rydholm A. Management of patients with soft tissue tumours. strategy developed at a regional oncology center. *Acta Orthopaedica Scandinavica Supplementum* 1983;**203**:13–77.
6. Pierce SM, Recht A, Lingos TI, et al. Long term radiation complications following conservative surgery (CS) and radiation therapy (RT) in patients with early stage breast cancer. *International Journal of Radiation Oncolology Biology Physics* 1992;**23**:915–23.
7. Cha C, Antonescu CR, Quan ML, et al. Long term results with resection of radiation-induced soft tissue sarcomas. *Annals of Surgery* 2004;**239**:903–10.
◆8. Mankin HJ, Hornicek FJ. Diagnosis, classification, and management of soft tissue tumours. *Cancer Control* 2005;**12**:5–21.
9. Li FP, Fraumeni JF Jr. Soft-tissue sarcomas, breast cancer, and other neoplasms. A familial syndrome? *Annals of Internal Medicine* 1969;**71**:747–52.
10. Strong LC, Williams WR, Tainsky MA. The Li-Fraumeni syndrome: from clinical epidemiology to molecular genetics. *American Journal of Epidemiology* 1992;**135**:190–9.
11. Kleinerman R, Tucker MA, Abramson DH, et al. Risk of soft tissue sarcomas by individual subtype in survivors of hereditary retinoblastoma. *Journal of the National Cancer Institute* 2007;**99**:24–31.
12. Wong FL, Boice, JD, Abramson DH, et al. Cancer incidence after retinoblastoma: radiation dose and sarcoma risk. *JAMA* 1997;**278**:1262–7.
13. Myhre-Jensen O. A consecutive 7-year series of 1331 benign soft tissue tumours. Clinicopathologic data. Comparison with sarcomas. *Acta Orthopaedica Scandinavica* 1981;**52**:287–93.
●14. Johnson CJD, Pynsent PB, Grimer RJ. Clinical features of soft-tissue sarcomas. *Annals of the Royal College of Surgeons England* 2001;**83**:203–5.
15. Rydholm A. Improving the management of soft tissue sarcoma. *British Medical Journal* 1998;**317**:93–4.

◆16. Knapp EL, Krandsdorf MJ, Letson GD. Diagnostic imaging update: soft-tissue sarcomas. *Cancer Control* 2005; **12**:22–6.
17. Papp DF, Khanna AJ, McCarthy EF, et al. Magnetic resonance of soft tissue tumours: determinate and indeterminate lesions. *Journal of Bone and Joint Surgery (American)* 2007;**89**:103–15.
◆18. Goodwin RW, O'Donnell P, Saifuddin A. MRI Appearances of common benign soft-tissue tumours. *Clinical Radiology* 2007;**62**:843–53.
19. Lin J, Jacobson JA, Fessell DP, et al. An illustrated tutorial of musculoskeletal sonography: part 4, musculoskeletal masses, sonographically guided interventions, and miscellaneous topics. *AJR American Journal of Roentgenology* 2000; **175**:1711–9.
20. Bodner G, Schocke MF, Rachbauer F, et al. Differentiation of malignant and benign musculoskeletal tumors: combined color and power Doppler US and spectral wave analysis. *Radiology* 2002;**223**:410–16.
21. Konermann W, Wuisman P, Ellermann A, Gruber G. Ultrasonographically guided needle biopsy of benign and malignant soft-tissue and bone tumors. *Journal of Ultrasound Medicine* 2000;**19**:465–71.
22. Soudack M, Nachtigal A, Vladovski E, et al. Sonographically guided percutaneous needle biopsy of soft-tissue masses with histopathologic correlation. *Journal of Ultrasound Medicine* 2006;**25**:1271–7.
23. Torriani M, Etchebehere M, Amstalden E. Sonographically guided core needle biopsy of bone and soft-tissue tumors. *Journal of Ultrasound Medicine* 2002;**21**:275–81.
24. Altuntas AO, Slavin J, Smith PJ, et al. Accuracy of computed tomography guided core needle biopsy of musculoskeletal tumours. *ANZ Journal of Surgery* 2005;**75**:187–91.
25. Hau A, Kim I, Kattapuram S, et al. Accuracy of CT-guided biopsies in 359 patients with musculoskeletal lesions. *Skeletal Radiology* 2002;**31**:349–53.
26. Shin HJ, Amaral JG, Armstrong D. Image-guided percutaneous biopsy of musculoskeletal lesions in children. *Pediatric Radiology* 2007;**37**:362–9.
27. Kransdorf MJ, Murphey MD (ed.) *Imaging of Soft-tissue Tumours*, 2nd edn. Philadelphia, PA: Lippincott, Williams and Wilkins, 2006.
28. Hicks R, Toner GC, Choong PFM. Clinical applications of molecular imaging in sarcoma evaluation. *Cancer Imaging* 2005;**5**:66–72.
29. Greene FL, Page DL, Fleming FD, et al. (eds) *American Joint Committee on Cancer: Cancer Staging Manual*, 6th edn. New York, NY: Springer, 2002.
●30. Trojani M, Contesso G, Coindre JM, et al. Soft-tissue sarcomas of adults: study of pathological prognostic variables and definition of histopathological grading system. *International Journal of Cancer* 1984; **33**:37–42.
31. Fletcher CDM, McKee PH (eds) *Pathobiology of Soft-tissue Tumors*. Edinburgh, UK: Churchill Livingstone 1990.
●32. Grimer RJ. Size matters for sarcomas! *Annals of the Royal College of Surgeons England* 2006;**88**:519–24.
33. Riad S, Griffin AM, Liberman B, et al. Lymph node metastasis in soft-tissue sarcoma of an extremity. *Clinical Othopaedics and Related Research* 2004;**426**:129–34.
34. Malawer M, Sugarbaker PH. *Musculoskeletal Cancer Surgery: Treatment of Sarcomas and Allied Diseases*. Dordrecht, Germany: Kluwer Academic Publishers, 2001.
●35. Pisters PWT, Leung DHY, Woodruff J, et al. Analysis of prognostic factors in 1,041 patients with localized soft-tissue sarcomas of the extremities. *Journal of Clinical Oncology* 1996;**14**:1679–89.
36. Mann GN. Less is (usually) more: When is amputation appropriate for treatment of extremity soft-tissue sarcoma? *Annals of Surgical Oncology* 2005;**12**:1–2.
37. Ghert MA, Abudu A, Driver N, et al. The Indications for and the prognostic significance of amputation as the primary surgical procedure for localized soft-tissue sarcoma of the extremity. *Annals of Surgical Oncology* 2005;**12**:10–17.
38. Dalal KM, Antonescu CR, Singer S. Diagnosis and management of lipomatous tumors. *Journal of Surgical Oncology* 2008;**97**:298–313.
39. Dei Tos AP. Liposarcoma: new entities and evolving concepts. *Annals of Diagnostic Pathology* 2000;**4**:252–66.
40. Cribb GL, Cool WP, Ford DJ, Mangham DC. Giant lipomatous tumours. *Journal of Hand Surgery (British)* 2005;**30**:509–12.
41. Sommerville SMM, Patton JT, Luscombe JC, et al. Clinical outcomes of deep atypical lipomas (well-differentiated lipoma-like liposarcomas of the extremities). *ANZ Journal of Surgery* 2005;**75**:803–6.
42. Weiss SW. Dedifferentiated liposarcoma: a clinicopathological analysis of 155 cases with a proposal for an expanded definition of dedifferentiation. *American Journal of Surgical Pathology* 1997;**21**:271–81.
43. McCormick D, Mentzel T, Beham A, Fletcher CD. Dedifferentiated liposarcoma. Clinicopathologic analysis of 32 cases suggesting a better prognostic subgroup among pleomorphic sarcomas. *American Journal of Surgical Pathology* 1994;**18**:1213–23.
44. Weiss SW, Rao VK. Well-differentiated liposarcoma (atypical lipoma) of deep soft-tissue of the extremities, retroperitoneum, and miscellaneous sites. A follow-up study of 92 cases with analysis of the incidence of 'dedifferentiation'. *American Journal of Surgical Pathology* 1992;**16**:1051–8.
45. Pitson G, Robinson P, Wilke D, et al. Radiation response: An additional unique signature of myxoid liposarcoma. *International Journal of Radiation Oncology Biology Physics* 2004;**60**:522–6.
46. Engstrom K, Bergh P, Cederlund CG, et al. Irradiation of myxoid/round cell liposarcoma induces volume reduction and lipoma-like morphology. *Acta Oncologica* 2007; **46**:838–45.
◆47. Bayat A, McGrouther DA. Management of Dupuytren's disease – clear advice for an elusive condition. *Annals of the Royal College of Surgeons England* 2006;**88**:3–8.

48. Reitamo JJ, Hayry P, Nykyri E, Saxen E. The desmoid tumour. Incidence, sex, age and anatomical distribution in a Finish population. *American Journal of Clinical Pathology* 1982:**77**:665–73.
49. Lewis J, Boland PJ, Leung DHY, *et al*. The enigma of desmoid tumors. *Annals of Surgery* 1999;**229**:866–73.
50. Vandevenne JE, De Schepper AM, De Beuckeleer L. New concepts in understanding evolution of desmoid tumors: MR imaging of 30 lesions. *European Radiology* 1997;**7**:1013–19.
51. Gronchi A, Casali PG, Mariani L, *et al*. Quality of surgery and outcome in extra-abdominal aggressive fibromatosis: a series of patients surgically treated at a single institution. *Journal of Clinical Oncology* 2003;**21**:1390–7.
52. Batra S, Batra M, Sakamuri R, *et al*. High-grade infiltrative myxofibrosarcoma in the forearm presenting as acute carpal tunnel syndrome. *Journal of Hand Surgery* 2008;**33A**:269–72.
53. Monaghan H, Salter DM, Al-Nafussi A. Giant cell tumour of tendon sheath (localized nodular tenosynovitis): clinicopathological features of 71 cases. *Journal of Clinical Pathology* 2001;**54**:404–7.
54. Jones FE, Soule EH, Coventry MB. Fibrous histiocytoma of synovium (giant cell tumour of tendon sheath, pigmented nodular synovitis). *Journal of Bone and Joint Surgery (American)* 1969;**51**:76–86.
55. Durr HR, Stabler A, Maier M, *et al*. Pigmented villonodular synovitis. Review of 20 cases. *Journal of Rheumatology* 2001;**28**:1620–30.
56. Chin KR, Barr SJ, Winalski C, *et al*. Treatment of advanced primary and recurrent diffuse pigmented villonodular synovitis of the knee. *Journal of Bone and Joint Surgery (American)* 2002;**84A**:2192–202.
57. Cheng XG, You YH, Liu W, *et al*. MRI features of pigmented villonodular synovitis (PVNS). *Clinical Rheumatology* 2004;**23**:31–4.
58. Fletcher CD. Pleomorphic malignant fibrous histiocytoma: Fact or fiction? A critical reappraisal based on 159 tumors diagnosed as pleomorphic sarcoma. *American Journal of Surgical Pathology* 1992;**16**:213–28.
59. Svarvar C, Böhling T, Berlin O, *et al*. Clinical course of nonvisceral soft-tissue leiomyosarcoma in 225 patients from the Scandinavian Sarcoma Group. *Cancer* 2007;**109**:282–91.
60. McDermott EM, Weiss A-P. Glomus tumors. *Journal of Hand Surgery* 2006;**31A**:1397–400.
61. Dahlin LB, Besjakov J, Veress B. A glomus tumour: classic signs without magnetic resonance imaging finding. *Scandinavian Journal of Plastic and Reconstructive Surgery and Hand Surgery* 2005;**39**:123–5.
62. Van Geertruyden J, Lorea P, Goldschmidt D, *et al*. Glomus tumors of the hand. A retrospective study of 51 cases. *Journal of Hand Surgery* 1996;**21B**:257–60.
63. Parham DM, Ellison DA. Rhabdomyosarcomas in adults and children: an update. *Archives of Pathology and Laboratory Medicine* 2006;**130**:1454–65.
64. Newton WA, Gehan EA, Webber BL, *et al*. Classification of rhabdomyo-sarcoma and related sarcomas: pathologic aspects and proposal for a new classification—an Intergroup Rhabdomyosarcoma Study. *Cancer* 1995;**76**:1073–85.
65. Walterhouse D, Watson A. Optimal management strategies for rhabdomyosarcoma in children. *Paediatric Drugs* 2007;**9**:391–400.
66. Koch M, Nielsen GP, Yoon SS. Malignant tumors of blood vessels: angiosarcomas, hemangioendotheliomas, and hemangiopericytomas. *Journal of Surgical Oncology* 2008;**97**:321–9.
67. Stewart FW, Treves N. Lymphangiosarcoma in postmastectomy lymphedema. *Cancer* 1949;**1**:64.
68. Abrham JA, Hornicek FJ, Kaufman AM. Treatment and outcome of 82 patients with angiosarcoma. *Journal of Surgical Oncology* 2008;**97**:321–9.
69. Nielsen GP, O'Connell JX, Rosenberg AE. Intramuscular myxoma: a clinicopathologic study of 51 cases with emphasis on hypercellular and hypervascular variants. *American Journal of Surgical Pathology* 1998;**22**:1222–7.
70. Bancroft LW, Kransdorf MJ, Menke DMAJR. Intramuscular myxoma: characteristic MR imaging features. *AJR American Journal of Roentgenology* 2002;**178**:1255–9.
71. Skytting B. Synovial sarcoma. A Scandinavian Sarcoma Group project. *Acta Orthopaedica* 2000;**71**:1–28.
72. Eilber FC, Dry SM. Diagnosis and management of synovial sarcoma. *Journal of Surgical Oncology* 2008;**97**:314–20.
73. Deshmukh R, Mankin HJ, Singer S. Synovial sarcoma: the importance of size and location for survival. *Clinical Orthopaedics and Related Research* 2004;**Feb**:155–61.
74. Eilber FC, Brennan MF, Eilber FR, *et al*. Chemotherapy is associated with improved survival in adult patients with primary extremity synovial sarcoma. *Annals of Surgery* 2007;**246**:105–13.
75. Weiss SW, Goldblum JR. *Enzinger and Weiss's Soft-tissue Tumors*, 4th edn. St Louis, MO: Mosby, 2001.
76. Lewis JJ, Antonescu CR, Leung DHY, *et al*. Synovial sarcoma: a multivariate analysis of prognostic factors in 112 patients with primary localized tumors of the extremity. *Journal of Clinical Oncology* 2000;**18**:2087–94.
77. Kransdorf MJ. Benign soft-tissue tumours in a large referral population: distribution of specific diagnosis by age, sex and location. *AJR American Journal of Roentgenology* 1995;**164**:395–402.
◆78. Goodwin RW, O'Donnell P, Saifuddin A. MRI appearances of common benign soft-tissue tumours. *Clinical Radiology* 2007;**62**:843–53.
79. Ducatman BS, Scheithauer BW, Piepgras DG, *et al*. Malignant peripheral nerve sheath tumors: a clinicopathologic study of 120 cases. *Cancer* 1986;**57**:2006–21.

80. Ferner R, Gutmann DH. International consensus statement on malignant peripheral nerve sheath tumors in neurofibromatosis. *Cancer Research* 2002;**62**:1573–7.
81. Anghileri M, Miceli R, Fiore M, *et al.* Malignant peripheral nerve sheath tumors prognostic factors and survival at a single institution. *Cancer* 2006;**107**:1065–74.
82. Weitz J, Antonescu CR, Brennan MF. localized extremity soft-tissue sarcoma: improved knowledge with unchanged survival over time. *Journal of Clinical Oncology* 2003;**21**:2719–25.
83. Eilber FC, Brennan MF, Riedel E, *et al.* Prognostic factors for survival in patients with locally recurrent extremity soft-tissue sarcomas. *Annals of Surgical Oncology* 2005;**12**:228–36.
84. Lord HK, Salter DM, MacDougall RH, Kerr GR. Is routine chest radiography a useful test in the follow up of all adult patients with soft-tissue sarcoma? *British Journal of Radiology* 2006;**79**:799–800.
85. Cool P, Grimer R, Rees R. Surveillance in patients with sarcoma of the extremities. *European Journal of Surgical Oncology.* 2005;**31**:1020–4.

83

Skeletal metastases and pathological fractures

JONATHAN JAMES GREGORY, PAUL COOL

Introduction	925	Assessment	930
Biology of metastasis	927	Prediction of life expectancy	931
Molecular biology of the tumour–bone interaction	927	Prediction of fracture risk	931
Osteolytic metastasis	927	Treatment	932
Osteoblastic metastasis	928	References	936
Clinical management	929		

NATIONAL BOARD STANDARDS

- Bone and joint disease
- Understand the principles of management of patients with metastatic bone disease in terms of investigation, prophylactic and definitive fixation of pathological fractures and oncological management
- Have knowledge of metastases and principles of management

INTRODUCTION

A pathological fracture occurs through an area of abnormal bone. There is either a reduction in the quantity or quality of bone present. Bone metastases from visceral primary lesions or primary haematopoietic tumours such as myeloma are common and may lead to pathological fracture. There is a complex interaction between the host bone and the invading tumour cells, which influences the behaviour of the lesion. Patients presenting with a bone lesion may be known to have skeletal metastatic disease; it may be the first presentation of a malignancy or a presentation of progression of a previously diagnosed tumour. In patients who present with a lesion with no prior diagnosis of malignancy, a primary bone tumour must be excluded. Investigations are required to stage the lesion locally and distally and to identify the nature of the lesion. This information should then be discussed at a multidisciplinary clinical pathological conference to guide further management.

The prediction of life expectancy is extremely difficult; a patient's prognosis greatly influences the decisions to be made regarding their further management. In the treatment of metastatic disease the goals of surgery are to provide pain relief, preserve or restore function of the limb and to provide an orthopaedic construct that will outlive the patient without the need for further surgery. In patients with limited life expectancy either no surgery or internal fixation may be appropriate. Patients with long life expectancy are more likely to suffer from failure of internal fixation and therefore endoprosthetic replacement is usually performed. The proximal femur is the commonest site of appendicular bone metastases. Most diaphyseal lesions of the femur are treated with intramedullary nailing and proximal femoral lesions managed with prosthetic replacement.

A fracture is described as pathological when it occurs through an area of abnormal bone. There is either a reduction in the quantity or quality of the bone present. The fracture may occur because of a traumatic event or under physiological loads that healthy bone would resist. The majority of pathological fractures are due to metabolic bone disease as a result of osteoporosis. Other metabolic causes of pathological fractures include osteomalacia, Paget's disease and congenital diseases, e.g. osteogenesis imperfecta. Pathological fractures may occur through benign bone lesions, e.g. simple bone cyst, malignant primary bone tumours, skeletal metastases from visceral primary lesions and bone affected by haemopoietic primary tumours, e.g. multiple myeloma.

This chapter will focus on the management of pathological fractures of the extremities due to metastatic bone lesions. Tumours of the spine are covered in the spinal section of this textbook.

The majority of patients who present with a neoplastic pathological fracture will be suffering from metastatic disease. Skeletal lesions may occur many years after the primary tumour has been identified. They may be detected at the same time as the primary tumour is diagnosed, or they may be the presenting complaint that then leads to identification of an underlying primary tumour.

The 'big five' primary tumours responsible for the majority of metastatic bone lesions are breast, prostate, lung, renal and thyroid. At post-mortem, Harrington demonstrated that 84% of patients with breast or prostate cancer had bone metastases.[1] Half of patients with thyroid cancer, 44% with lung cancer and 37% of patients suffering from renal cancer had skeletal lesions. Over 50% of patients with advanced breast or prostate cancer will develop clinically significant bone metastases, and approximately 20% may require orthopaedic intervention.[2] The skeleton is the commonest site of first distant relapse[3] in patients suffering from breast cancer. However, 30% of skeletal metastases do not originate from one of these primary lesions. Less common but still significant sources of skeletal metastases are the bladder, uterus, stomach, colon and malignant melanoma. There are a number of skeletal lesions where the underlying primary tumour is never identified. These are usually adenocarcinomas or squamous cell carcinomas. With modern diagnostic techniques and immunohistochemistry the primary tumour can usually be diagnosed (Fig. 83.1).

The spine is the site most frequently invaded by metastatic disease. Other sites where skeletal metastases are prevalent are the pelvis, proximal femur, proximal humerus and ribs. Within the proximal femur the majority of pathological fractures occur in the femoral neck (50%): 30% in the subtrochanteric region and the remaining 20% in the intertrochanteric region of the proximal femur (Fig. 83.2).

The management of metastatic disease of the skeleton is challenging. Approximately 50% of patients who develop a pathological fracture will die within 6 months of their fracture occurring.[2,4–7] However, patients can survive for years following treatment for metastatic lesions, and they may outlive the orthopaedic implants used to treat them. The challenge for the orthopaedic surgeon is to avoid subjecting patients with a limited life expectancy to massive skeletal reconstruction while not having patients suffer the complications of implant failure with the need for further

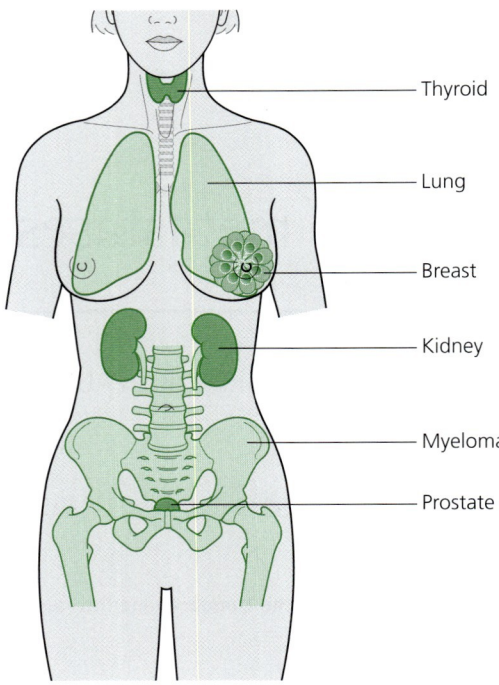

Figure 83.1 Anatomical sites that give rise to the majority of metastatic bone lesions. Myeloma arises from the bone marrow and is not therefore a metastasis per definition.

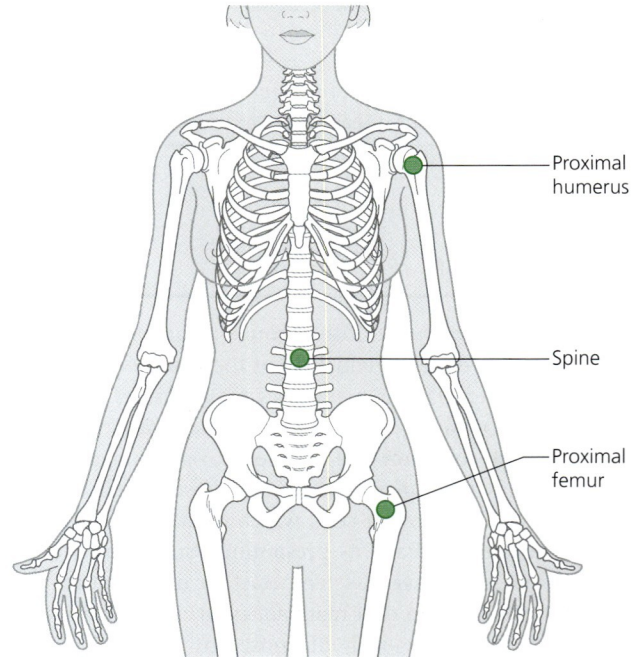

Figure 83.2 The three most common sites for bone metastasis: the spine, proximal femur and the proximal humerus.

surgical intervention. The aim of orthopaedic intervention is to stabilize the skeleton, so providing pain relief and the restoration of mobility. This must be achieved with an orthopaedic construct that will outlive the patient.

The management of pathological fractures and skeletal metastatic disease therefore requires a thorough assessment of the individual patient and management by a multidisciplinary team.

BIOLOGY OF METASTASES

Malignant tumours may spread via haematogenous and lymphatic routes or via direct extension. The vast majority of bone metastases occur due to haematogenous spread. Cells detach from the primary tumour and are carried to a distant site via the vascular system. The tumour cells then attach to and invade at the distant site. Depending upon the nature of the new site and the tumour concerned the metastasis may need to induce local blood vessel formation to allow its survival and further growth. The development of metastatic lesions therefore depends upon systemic, local and tumour factors.

Tumour cells invade the local network of blood vessels and lymphatic channels gaining access to the systemic circulation. The point at which the tumour accesses the circulation has an effect on the location in which metastasis may subsequently develop. The existence of Bateson's paravertebral plexus explains the skeletal distribution of metastases from many visceral primary tumours.[8] The plexus runs from the base of the skull to the sacrum and receives tributaries from the head, neck, breast, retroperitoneum and proximal long bones. It is a low-pressure system of thin-walled, valveless veins. The presence of this valveless system allows retrograde tumour spread and is responsible for the predilection that metastases have for the vertebrae, pelvis, proximal long bones and skull. The persistence of red marrow in the axial skeleton may also contribute to the predilection of metastasis for these sites.

After entering the circulation, the tumour cells have to survive possible recognition and removal by cells of the immune system. The tumour cells require the presence of counter receptors to adhesion molecules expressed at the target organ to enable them to attach at the distant site, e.g. integrins and cadherins. Once they have adhered to and invaded the host tissue, the tumour cells commence cell division, forming a new colony of tumour cells – a metastasis. Traditionally it is believed that as the colony grows in size it has to be able to induce the formation of a local vascular system to keep up with its nutrient requirements. This is certainly a feature of visceral metastases, but whether this is as important in bone metastases has not been proven. Differential expression of angiogenesis-associated genes has been found with prostate cancer metastasis in liver, bone and lymph nodes.[9] Different microvessel densities and distributions were found in the bone metastasis compared with those in the liver, suggesting that angiogenesis is less pronounced in bone metastasis.

Bone metastases may occur within the medullary cavity or within the cortical bone itself. Lung and renal cancers are the most common source of cortical metastases. The blood supply to the cortex via capillaries from the nutrient arteries and periosteal vessels may play a significant role in the development of cortical metastases.

MOLECULAR BIOLOGY OF THE TUMOUR–BONE INTERACTION

Once established within the bone, the metastasis will start to have an effect on the surrounding bone and the bone itself will respond. Classically the radiological appearance of bone lesions are described as osteolytic, osteoblastic and mixed patterns. Purely osteolytic or osteoblastic lesions are uncommon and represent ends of a spectrum. Many lesions are heterogeneous, but with a predominance of osteolytic or osteoblastic processes occurring.[10] Animal models of osteoblastic metastases have shown that initially osteoclast-mediated lytic processes predominate. As the metastasis matures, osteoblastic processes then predominate[11,12] and bone formation occurs. The behaviour of prostate cancer cells may be different within the same metastatic lesion, and there may be heterogeneity between different lesions in the same patient.[13,14]

OSTEOLYTIC METASTASES

Metastases that, on radiographs, appear to cause loss of bone are described as osteolytic. Tumours of renal and thyroid origin as well as multiple myeloma usually produce osteolytic metastasis. Oesophageal and lung carcinoma metastases are highly aggressive and almost exclusively lytic. Breast cancer bone metastases are heterogeneous; most are osteolytic but approximately 20% are osteoblastic. The bone destruction in osteolytic metastasis is due to osteoclast activity rather than direct invasion and removal of bone by the tumour cells[10] or due to hyperaemia causing demineralization. The most marked example of this is in multiple myeloma. There are increased numbers of osteoclasts adjacent to myeloma tumour cells but no changes in osteoclast numbers in areas free of tumour[16] (Fig. 83.3).

The receptor activator of nuclear factor-kappa b ligand (RANK-L) is normally expressed on the surface of osteoblasts and it interacts with the RANK receptor on osteoclast precursors to induce differentiation and activation. This process is modulated by a soluble protein, osteoprotegerin, which acts as a decoy receptor for RANK-L. Osteoprotegerin is produced by osteoblasts as well as other stromal cells. Thus the balance of RANK-L and osteoprotegerin affects osteoclast numbers and activity. Multiple myeloma is associated with profound osteolysis. It has been found that multiple myeloma causes an increase in RANK-L expression and a reduction in osteoprotegerin.[16] These changes may cause increased bone resorption. Treatment with osteoprotegerin has been shown to reduce osteoclast activity, tumour volume within the bone and bone pain in a rat model of bone metastases.[17]

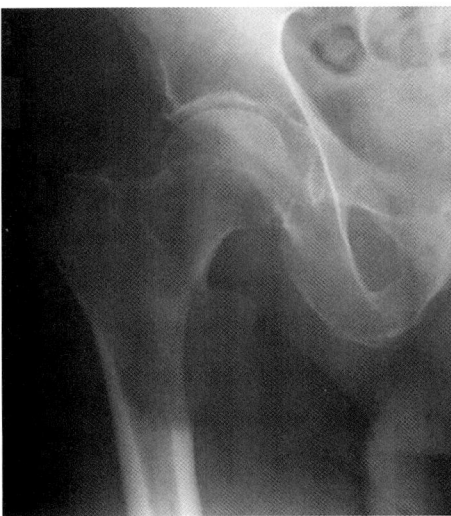

Figure 83.3 An anteroposterior radiograph of the right hip demonstrating an osteolytic metastasis of the proximal femur due to metastatic renal carcinoma. There is almost complete destruction of the lesser trochanter and medial femoral cortex.

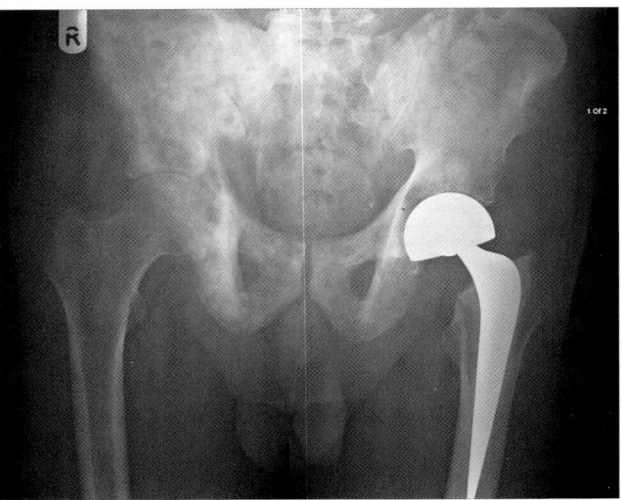

Figure 83.4 Anteroposterior radiograph of the pelvis in a patient suffering from metastatic prostate carcinoma. The patient has previously undergone a bipolar hemiarthroplasty of the left hip for proximal femoral metastasis. The right hemipelvis demonstrates numerous sclerotic metastatic deposits with a pathological fracture of the medial wall of the acetabulum.

The molecular mechanisms of bone destruction due to metastasis are numerous. Parathyroid hormone-related peptide (PTHrP), interleukins 1, 6 and 8, and RANK-L have been shown to be produced by metastasis and to cause osteolysis. There is a self-perpetuating element to the lytic process.[18] As bone is resorbed transforming growth factor β (TGF-β), which is stored within the bone matrix, is released.[19] The TGF-β stimulates PTHrP production by tumour cells, which in turn activates osteoclasts to resorb bone. Expression of PTHrP is greater in metastatic bone lesions than in visceral metastatic sites[20] or in the primary tumour itself. It is unclear if this is due to induction of PTHrP production once the tumour cells settle on bone or whether PTHrP-positive tumours are more likely to metastasize to bone. PTHrP activates osteoclasts by binding to PTHR1 receptors and inducing the expression of RANK-L on bone marrow stromal cells. Osteolysis associated with renal and thyroid metastasis may also be secondary to the hypervascular nature of the tumours. The inorganic matrix of the bone may be 'washed away' by the hyperaemia.

OSTEOBLASTIC METASTASIS

Several pathways are thought to be responsible for tumour-induced bone formation. PTHrP, ET-1, PDGF, IGF and adrenomedullin may all have a role in osteoblastic metastasis. Many of the factors stimulating bone formation act through the final common pathway of RANK-L expression.

ET-1 is a vasoactive peptide that has been shown to act on the endothelin A receptor, inducing bone formation in osteoblastic metastases. *In vitro* it has also been found to inhibit osteoclastic bone resorption and osteoclast mobility.[21] Serum levels of ET-1 are elevated in patients with osteoblastic prostate metastases.[22] An antagonist of ET-1 at the endothelin A receptor has increased the time to progression of bone metastasis and reduced biochemical markers of bone turnover in men suffering from advanced prostate cancer,[23] although it does not improve survival.[24] The final pathway of osteoblast stimulation via endothelin A receptors has not been fully elucidated.

Prostate cancer metastases are usually osteoblastic.[25] There is usually an increase in bone resorption and formation, with an overall net increase in bone mass. In patients with prostate, lung and other solid tumour metastases, high levels of biochemical markers of bone turnover have been shown to correlate with poor prognosis[26,27] and disease progression.[28] High N-telopeptide levels are associated with an increased risk of skeletal related events, disease progression and death compared with patients with low N-telopeptide levels. This is most marked for prostate cancer where high levels are associated with a relative risk of 3.25 for skeletal events and 4.59 for death.[26] N-telopeptide levels also correlated with risk of adverse events and death in patients suffering from breast, prostate and lung cancer or multiple myeloma who were being treated with bisphosphonates[27] (Figs 83.4 and 83.5).

Prostate-specific antigen (PSA) is a kallikrein serine protease and elevated serum levels are found in prostate carcinoma, except where dedifferentiation has occurred. PTHrP is often highly expressed by prostate metastasis. In most tumours high PTHrP levels are associated with osteolysis, thus producing lytic metastases. PSA is able to cleave PTHrP thus inactivating it (A4, A5). This explains why, despite high levels of PTHrP, prostate metastases are not

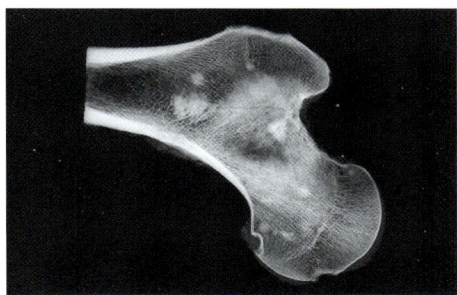

Figure 83.5 A slab radiograph of a proximal femoral resection specimen from a patient with metastatic prostate carcinoma. Note the marked sclerosis in the femoral neck and the vertical fracture line running inferiorly from the base of the femoral neck at the junction with the greater trochanter.

usually osteolytic. It also explains why dedifferentiated prostate carcinoma may produce lytic metastasis, as these tumours produce very little PSA.

PSA appears to modify bone metabolism via several pathways in addition to cleaving PTHrP. *In vitro* it has been shown to be able to induce apoptosis of osteoclast precursor cells in a dose-dependent manner.[31] PSA is also able to act directly on osteoblasts. It appears to promote osteoblast differentiation. It increases osteoprotegerin production and inhibits RANK-L expression.[32] This may act to decrease osteoclast function and contribute to the bone formation associated with prostate metastases. It is unknown which of the mechanisms of PSA action are most significant.

Histologically the bone formed within osteoblastic metastases is woven bone and is therefore biomechanically weaker and more likely to fracture under physiological loads than normal bone. Even if there is no net gain or loss of bone mass, tumours are able to cause disruption in the normal bone remodelling process.[13] Usually in bone remodelling, bone resorption is followed by replacement in the same location. However, metastatic lesions cause bone modelling rather than remodelling, an uncoupling of the normal osteoblast–osteoclast relationship. The temporal relation of bone resorption and replacement is maintained but deposition occurs at different sites to bone resorption, e.g. on opposite sides of trabeculae. The trabecular system is then no longer aligned in the optimal biomechanical configuration, thus reducing the strength of the bone.

The physical nature of the bone microenvironment may contribute to tumour growth. Hypoxia causes induction of hypoxia inducible factor-1, which is associated with increased invasive and metastatic potential.[33–36] Tumour cells often create local areas of acidosis by lactic acid production and reduction in buffering capacity of the host tissue. A fall in pH results in increased osteoclast resorption, osteoclasts being maximally stimulated at pH 6.9 and below.[37] Acidosis also inhibits osteoblast mineralization.[38] Local calcium concentration is another factor in the cycle of self-perpetuation exhibited by bone metastases. Bone resorption leads to increased calcium levels locally within the bone microenvironment as well as systemically. Elevated calcium levels appear to promote tumour growth and stimulate production of PTHrP in breast[39] and prostate[40] metastases, which in turn will cause further osteolysis.

Chemotherapy administered as part of the treatment of malignancy may have adverse effects upon bone. Chemotherapy regimes often produce a premature menopause in women and may also have direct effects on bone. Aromatase inhibitors, which are widely used in the treatment of breast cancer, cause a reduction in bone mineral density.[41,42] Men with prostate cancer have their androgen axis manipulated with gonadotrophin hormone-releasing hormone agents and testosterone antagonists. Androgen deprivation in the treatment of prostate cancer leads to accelerated bone loss in men compared with age-matched controls.[43] The treatment of breast and prostate cancers can therefore lead to a reduction in bone mass, described as cancer treatment-induced bone loss (CTIBL). Women with breast cancer being treated with aromatase inhibitors should have their bone density assessed prior to commencement of therapy. If their bone density is normal no further monitoring is required.[44,45] If the patient has a low baseline bone density then further monitoring is required and treatment with calcium and vitamin D supplementation or bisphosphonates may be required.[46]

CLINICAL MANAGEMENT

The patient history is the most important step in the successful treatment of pathological fractures and metastatic skeletal disease. It must be determined if a patient has any previous history of malignancy and if so whether they are already known to have skeletal metastasis. If there is a previous history of malignancy but no previous history of skeletal metastases what has been their disease-free duration? The answer to these questions allows instigation of the correct management plan.

Patients who are documented to have skeletal metastases and present with a pathological fracture can be treated with surgery without undue delay, unless the primary tumour is renal or thyroid in origin, when pre-operative embolization should be considered. Patients may require adjuvant oncological treatments and these can be discussed with an oncologist, but this does not need to delay surgery.

Patients with a fracture that appears pathological but with no previous history of malignancy need a thorough assessment prior to treatment. The lesion may be a manifestation of metastatic disease, either multiple or solitary, or it may represent a primary bone tumour. If it is a primary bone tumour survival may be significantly compromised by inappropriate orthopaedic intervention. If the patient has a previous history of malignancy but is not known to have skeletal metastases in all probability the lesion is the first presentation of a skeletal metastasis. However, it must be remembered that there are a significant number of patients who are unfortunate enough to suffer from multiple primary malignancies. There are also rare genetic conditions that predispose to multiple primary malignancies which should be borne in mind. For example, Li–Fraumini syndrome causes an almost 100% lifetime risk of breast cancer, and it is also associated with osteosarcoma. Therefore, the first skeletal lesion that is seen in these patients may represent metastatic breast cancer or osteosarcoma. The longer the interval between the primary tumour diagnosis and the appearance of skeletal lesions the less likely it becomes that the lesions relate to the primary tumour. The most common malignancies that present for the first time with a bone lesion are myeloma, lymphoma, lung and renal carcinomas.

ASSESSMENT

Cool and Grimer[47] proposed the following approach to the assessment of a patient who presents with a pathological fracture. There are three phases, the first two phases can be completed at the admitting hospital and if the third phase is required, it is usually preformed at a specialist bone tumour unit.

Phase 1

Enquires regarding medical and surgical past history are made. Special attention should be paid to any previous history of malignancy, family history and risk factors for malignancy. A standard medical examination is performed with emphasis on looking for lymphadenopathy, breast lumps, thyroid lesions and abdominal masses. A rectal examination to check the prostate should be performed in men. Examination of the chest may reveal a malignant effusion.

Radiographs of the full length of the affected bone should be taken in anteroposterior and lateral planes. A chest radiograph should be performed to exclude a primary lung lesion or metastases.

At this stage, blood tests should include a full blood count to examine for anaemia and the white cell count. A C-reactive protein and erythrocyte sedimentation rate should be performed as indices of inflammation. Electrolytes must be checked and hypercalcaemia checked for and, if found, treated promptly. Serum alkaline phosphatase gives an index of bone resorption. Blood should be sent for serum electrophoresis and urine for Bence–Jones protein for the diagnosis of myeloma.

Phase 2

These investigations should be selectively used depending upon clinical suspicion. Blood may be tested for tumour markers. This is most appropriate for prostate-specific antigen (PSA) for diagnosing prostate cancer. If a patient has a PSA below 10 ng mL^{-1} a bone lesion is unlikely to be a metastasis of prostate cancer unless the tumour is dedifferentiated.

Under most circumstances, a technetium-labelled bone scan is the most useful radiological investigation to perform after plain radiographs. It will identify if the lesion is solitary or multiple. It must be remembered however that bone scans may not demonstrate profoundly osteolytic lesions, e.g. myeloma.[48] This is because these tumours induce very little bone formation and so technetium uptake is not increased. In fact metastases from osteolytic renal cell tumours can be diagnosed on bone scans because of the presence of 'cold' spots,[49] as there is an absence of bone formation compared with the rest of the skeleton. An ultrasound scan of the abdomen to examine the kidneys is vital if the bone lesion is osteolytic in order to exclude a renal primary tumour. A CT scan of the abdomen or thorax looking for primary and metastatic lesions can be performed if a primary lesion has not been identified after the other investigations are completed, but CT scanning is not required routinely.

Phases 1 and 2 will provide the diagnosis for most patients who present with a skeletal metastasis or pathological fracture. The phase 1 tests also provide information regarding the medical fitness of the patient for any interventions that may be required. If there is a history of malignancy and there are multiple lesions on the bone scan, treatment is palliative. Further management should centre on treatment of the patient rather than investigation. If the bone scan reveals a solitary lesion with or without a history of malignancy a primary bone tumour is a possible diagnosis and the patient should be discussed with a bone tumour unit. If the patient has a previous history of malignancy and there is a solitary lesion then it could represents a metastasis, but this should not be presumed. Discussion with a bone tumour unit is required.

Rougraff et al.[50] used a similar investigation algorithm when investigating 40 patients with skeletal metastases of unknown origin. History and examination identified the primary site in 3 out of 40 (8%) patients. Plain chest radiographs identified the primary tumour as carcinoma of the lung in 17 out of 40 (43%) patients. CT of the chest, abdomen and pelvis was then performed. These scans revealed six further cases of primary lung cancer (15%), and five intra-abdominal primary tumours (13%). From their study, clinical history, examination and a chest radiograph alone will identify the primary lesion in 51% of cases of skeletal metastases of unknown origin. The most common occult primary tumours in their series were lung (63%) and renal (10%).

In this series, biopsy of the lesion only aided identification of the primary site in three patients (8%) and examination of the biopsy alone without other investigation would not have identified the source of the primary tumour in 65% of cases. This is in disagreement with

Wedin et al.,[51] who suggested that fine needle aspiration cytology (FNAC) should be the initial investigation in patients with skeletal lesions. They reported that this gave the correct diagnosis in 93% of patients. In 48 out of 80 patients presenting with metastatic disease they report that FNAC allowed identification of the primary site. It is not routine practice to perform FNAC in our unit, as many of the radiological investigations are still required to allow local and distal staging of disease and therefore FNAC does not speed up the diagnostic process.

Phase 3

These investigations are usually performed at a specialist bone tumour unit. Further imaging of the lesion itself in the form of CT and MRI may be performed. These allow local staging of tumour extent. If diagnostic uncertainty still exists a biopsy of the lesion should be performed. The biopsy should be performed according to the principles of biopsy discussed in previous chapters, as the lesion may be a primary tumour of bone and survival may be compromised by inadequate thought being given to the biopsy. Positron emission tomography combined with CT (PET/CT) is becoming increasingly available. The use of PET/CT can have a large impact upon clinicians' treatment strategies and can greatly reduce the need for biopsy.[52]

The results of the investigations should then be discussed at a multidisciplinary clinical pathological conference. Close collaboration between the pathologist, radiologist, oncologist and orthopaedic surgeon is required. The aim of the meeting is to define the expected survival of the patient, the likely responsiveness of the tumour to adjuvant treatment, the grade of the lesion, and local and distant extent of any lesions. In light of the information obtained at the multidisciplinary meeting the diagnosis and possible treatment strategies are discussed with the patient and a treatment plan decided upon.

A further consideration when dealing with metastatic skeletal deposits is the responsiveness of the tumour to chemotherapy, radiotherapy or hormonal manipulation. Prostate and breast cancers can be especially hormonally sensitive, which may slow growth of a metastatic deposit as well as prolonging life expectancy. If there is a pathological bone lesion but no fracture oncological manipulation of the tumour may avoid the need for any orthopaedic intervention. This is particularly the case for haematological malignancies, e.g. lymphoma, multiple myeloma.

PREDICTION OF LIFE EXPECTANCY

There have been many attempts to try and accurately predict survival for patients suffering from skeletal metastases. The extent of bony metastases, the presence of soft-tissue metastases and the type of primary lesion have all been suggested to be prognostically significant. The Scandinavian Sarcoma group (2004)[4] concluded that pathological fracture, visceral metastasis, haemoglobin less that 7 mmol L^{-1} and lung cancer being the primary tumour were all independent negative prognostic factors for 1 year survival. In the series from the Scandinavian sarcoma group, 19% of patients died within 6 weeks of surgery. The survival of patients following surgical intervention for bone metastases varies. Several studies have figures of approximately 50% survival at 6 months falling to 10–20% at 2 years.[2,5–7]

Harrington[1] estimated the mean survival after pathological fracture in a series of 289 patients. The estimates were 24.6 months breast, 32.9 prostate, 14.6 renal, 4.1 lung. There have been oncological advances in the management of many of these tumours since this work was published that are likely to have increased the post-fracture survival for some of these tumours.

Recently biochemical markers of bone turnover have been shown to be predictive of death.[26,27] Elevated levels of bone-specific alkaline phosphatase and N-telopeptide were associated with an increased relative risk of dying across a variety of bone metastases. High levels of N-telopeptide were the most prognostically significant. Bone turnover markers may also be used to indicate progression of bone metastases.[53] It remains to be seen if these biochemical markers can be used to guide clinical decision-making.

Scoring systems have been used to try and discriminate between patients with a low or high chance of surviving 1 year after surgery.[54] It is not the practice at our institution to use these scoring systems. Every clinician in this field has treated patients with a good predicted prognosis who have died within months of surgery and conversely patients with very poor predicted prognosis who have done very well. Scoring systems may be a useful audit tool but applied without experience and clinical intuition may lead to inappropriate treatment of patients if followed dogmatically.

PREDICTION OF FRACTURE RISK

The ability to accurately predict which metastatic skeletal lesions will fracture would help prevent patients suffering a fracture or having unnecessary surgery. Several guidelines have been used to try and estimate fracture risk.[55–59] These have considered the geometry of the osseous defect, pain, age of patient, type of tumour and anatomical location. There is very little agreement across these studies about which factors most accurately predict fracture risk. Harrington[1] proposed that there were four risk factors that should lead to prophylactic stabilization. These were cortical destruction greater than 50%, a lesion of more than 2.5 cm in the proximal femur, a pathological avulsion fracture of the lesser trochanter and persisting pain despite irradiation. Mirel[59] developed a score to try and predict fracture risk. A Mirel score is composed of four variables: type of lesion, location of lesion, pain and amount of cortical involvement (Box 83.1). A score of

> **BOX 83.1: Mirel's scoring system to assess the risk of pathological fracture**
>
> Score >8 = high risk of fracture
> Score <7 = low risk of fracture

8 or greater is suggested to equate to a high risk of fracture and prophylactic fixation is proposed. The interobserver reliability of the Mirel score is good (91%), but it has poor specificity (35%).[60]

The Mirel score has several weaknesses. The original paper was based on 78 lesions in 38 patients. Fifty of the lesions were metastases from breast cancer. Eleven cases were due to myeloma, which is not strictly a metastatic lesion. The paper suggests prophylactic fixation at a score of 8 or above. However the fracture risk with a score of 8 was only 15% and a score of 9 had a 33% risk of fracture in the series. Therefore, there is considerable overtreatment of a large number of patients if a score of 8 is used to guide fixation. Only with a score of 10 or above does the risk of fracture become greater than 50%. In fact, pathological fracture through a metastatic lesion is relatively uncommon. Several large series of patients have had fracture rates of approximately 10%,[1] even with proximal femoral lesions.[2,61,62]

There are difficulties assessing the amount of bone involvement on plain radiographs. Approximately 50% of cortical bone has to be missing for a perceptible difference to be visible on plain radiographs. Estimation of defect size is difficult when the zone of transition is broad and ill defined. Keene et al.[61] studied the radiographs of 203 patients with skeletal metastases and felt they were unable to measure the size of 57% of the metastases due to the permeative nature of the lesions. Hipp et al.[63] found that even using radiographs taken of cadaveric bones with no soft-tissue envelope consultant orthopaedic oncologists were unable to accurately size simulated cortical defects or estimate their effect on bone strength. If it were possible to accurately measure defect size there is still the question of how much bone loss can be tolerated before fracture will occur. *In vitro* studies have demonstrated that a diaphyseal defect of 50% leads to strength reductions of 60–90%.[63] The reduction of strength for torsional loads was also related to the longitudinal length of the defect rather than just to the diameter.

It is reported[4,64] that survival after prophylactic fixation is greater than that following treatment for a fracture through a metastasis. This is probably not because of prophylactic surgery but due to confounding factors. Fracture is associated with a more advanced disease state and there is an inherent selection bias as patients treated prophylactically are selected for surgery because they are medically fit enough for the procedure.

Prophylactic fixation is often considered prior to treatment of skeletal metastases with radiotherapy in the belief that the bone is likely to fracture after radiotherapy. There is a great deal of variability in the post-irradiation fracture rates quoted in the literature, with some being as low as 5%.[65] In Mirel's[59] own study it was 35% 6 months after radiotherapy. Although the true risk of fracture after radiotherapy is difficult to predict, the majority of patients will not suffer a post-irradiation fracture and so prophylactic fixation is not always indicated.

TREATMENT

Having established that a patient has multiple metastatic skeletal deposits, all treatment is palliative. Theoretically resection of a solitary skeletal metastasis could be curative, although this is extremely unlikely. The aim of orthopaedic intervention should be to provide pain relief and preserve limb function. Treatment may be needed for a fracture, an impending fracture or for pain relief. Occasionally fractures occur following radiotherapy for metastasis.

Cappanna[66] considered that patients with metastatic tumours of bone could be divided into four groups to aid management. Class 1 patients have a solitary metastasis 3 years or more after being diagnosed with a primary tumour that had a good prognosis. Long-term survival is possible for some of these patients. Class 2 patients have a fracture and therefore require surgical intervention. Class 3 patients have an impending fracture. The Mirel score may be used to guide the decision regarding prophylactic fixation. The difficulty of predicting fracture risk has already been discussed. A class 4 patient has multiple skeletal lesions without fracture. These patients can be managed with oncological therapies. If the treatment or tumour causes a patient who was originally class 4 to be reclassified as class 2 or 3 then orthopaedic intervention may be required (Table 83.1).

Non-operative treatment

The therapeutic benefit of spending time with a patient and their relatives explaining the issues involved in their management should not be underestimated. Fear and anxiety can cause a significant reduction in pain tolerance. The explanation of what is going to happen can go a long way to allaying these fears. Pain should be controlled using the standard analgesic ladder supplemented by traction and local anaesthetic blocks if required. Analgesia should be sufficient to allow the patient to move around in the bed to help reduce the risk of skin breakdown over pressure areas. A pressure-relieving mattress may also provide protection for pressure areas, although this is not always compatible with traction. Thromboprophylaxis should be considered as patients with metastatic carcinoma and a fracture are at high risk for the development of thromboembolic complications. The nutritional status of the patient should be reviewed because of the adverse effect of malnutrition on wound healing and sepsis rate.

Medical conditions require optimization if surgery is being considered. Hypercalcaemia is not only potentially

Table 83.1 Classification of metastatic bone tumours into four classes (Capanna 1999)[66]

Class	Description	Treatment
1	Solitary metastatic lesion Primary with good prognosis and interval after primary more than 3 years Metastasis destroying articular surface	Consider resection of metastasis and reconstruction (e.g. with endoprosthesis)
2	Pathological fracture at any site	Internal fixation; assume fracture will not unite and use appropriate combination of fixation and cementation
3	Impending fracture in a major weight-bearing bone	Decide on risk of pathological facture using Mirel's scoring system
4	Osteoblastic lesions at all sites Osteolytic or mixed lesions in non-structural bones (fibula, rib, sternum, clavicle) Osteolytic lesion with no impending fracture in major weight-bearing bone Lesions of the Iliac wing, anterior pelvis or scapula excluding class 1 patients	Medical/hormonal/radiotherapy in first instance

life threatening, it is also a cause of unpleasant side-effects, e.g. nausea, vomiting, constipation, polydipsia and confusion. Hypercalcaemia is common; it develops in 15% of patients with breast cancer bone metastases.[67] The treatment of hypercalcaemia involves intravenous fluids, bisphosphonates and possibly steroids or diuretics.

In the event that a patient has a very limited life expectancy, involvement of the palliative care team and local hospice services may be appropriate. If the patient can be made comfortable without surgery in the context of a life expectancy of days or weeks, then surgery has little to offer other than the risk of precipitating death.

Bisphosponates have been found to reduce the frequency of skeletally related adverse events and increase the time until the first adverse event in patients suffering from prostate cancer. Adverse skeletal events include fracture, spinal cord compression, requirement for surgery or radiotherapy to a bone.[68] There was also a reduction in bone pain. A meta-analysis of the use of bisphosphonates in prostate cancer supports these findings.[69] There may be differences between bisphosphonates when used in the treatment of metastases. A 20% reduction in skeletal events was reported with zoledronic acid compared with pamidronate in patients with breast cancer metastases, although no difference was found in patients suffering from multiple myeloma.[70] Clodronate was found to cause a decrease in the incidence of bone metastases in patients at high risk of bone metastases from breast cancer during the period of drug administration. More importantly it caused a significant reduction in death rate at 5 years.[71] A meta-analysis of bisphosphonates in breast cancer confirms the reduction in bone pain and skeletal events but doubt is cast on the ability of these agents to reduce the death rate.[72] Bisphosphonates should be considered for the prevention of cancer treatment-induced bone loss (CTIBL) secondary to the hormonal manipulation of breast and prostate cancer.[72,73]

Operative treatment

PRINCIPLES

The surgeon must decide whether internal fixation or endoprosthetic replacement is most appropriate. This decision is guided by the results of the multidisciplinary meeting. Key points are the site and size of the metastasis, life expectancy, possible response to adjuvant therapies and the medical fitness of the patient to tolerate surgery. There is a significant complication rate when operating on patients with metastases. Many series have reoperation rates of approximately 10–15%.[4] However, surgery can provide good levels of pain relief and functional restoration.[74,75] The patient's preoperative function and pain will influence surgical planning. Patients who are bed-bound or in severe pain will accept pain relief and the ability to transfer as surgical aims. If a patient has a proximal humeral lesion without fracture and with full range of movement, then a reduction in function due to endoprosthetic replacement may not be acceptable to the patient.

There is a balance between preservation of function and the risk of implant failure. The functional results of endoprosthetic replacement are often inferior to that of the native joint. There can be a considerable period of rehabilitation following endoprosthesis replacement of the knee, proximal humerus and elbow. There is also the risk of joint subluxation/dislocation with prosthetic replacements. Dislocation rates of 5–10% have been reported.[76] Endoprostheses do have good survivorship in the context of treating metastatic lesions. In a series of endoprostheses for all musculoskeletal tumours, the subgroup of patients treated for metastatic disease had 10 year implant survivorship, with failure defined as any additional surgery, for any cause, of 88%.[77]

Internal fixation has a high failure rate in many series.[74–76] Lesions in the proximal femur treated with internal fixation have an unacceptably high failure rate.[2,74–76] The failure rate of internal fixation is because many pathological lesions do not heal. Union rates of 35% have been found for pathological fractures but this figure varies depending upon the tumour involved.[78] The union rate was also associated with life expectancy, with 75% of lesions healing in patients who lived for more than 6 months. In patients surviving more than 24 months after internal fixation of a pathological fracture more than 25% will experience implant failure.[76] In one series the average survival of patients after surgery who suffered from a failure of fixation was 34.5 months.[75] The average time to implant failure was 17.7 months. The most prudent assumption is that the fracture will never unite and one should use an implant that will be able to outlive the patient (Fig. 83.6).

In locations other than the proximal femur, if predicted survival is less than 1 year or the lesion involves less than a third of the diameter of the bone then internal fixation may be indicated. This may involve the use of plates or nails. Bone defects may be augmented with polymethylmethacrylate cement (Fig. 83.7).

The primary tumour has an enormous influence on the orthopaedic management of a patient. Advice regarding prognosis from the multidisciplinary team is vital. Patients with metastatic lung cancer usually have a very poor prognosis; many die within 3–6 months of presentation with skeletal disease.[1,75] Surgical intervention is usually only indicated if a pathological fracture occurs and internal fixation is usually sufficient as this construct should outlive the patient. Prosthetic replacement is usually only used for the management of proximal femoral lesions in patients with metastatic lung cancer. Patients with breast and renal metastases often have a good life expectancy and therefore there is an increased risk of implant failure if internal fixation is performed. Five-year survivorship in patients with solitary renal bone metastasis can be up to 55%.[79] Many of the patients who suffer failure of internal fixation for pathological lesions have renal metastasis.[76] The life expectancy of these patients exceeds that of the implant used for internal fixation and therefore endoprosthetic replacement may be preferable. Patients suffering from myeloma and prostate

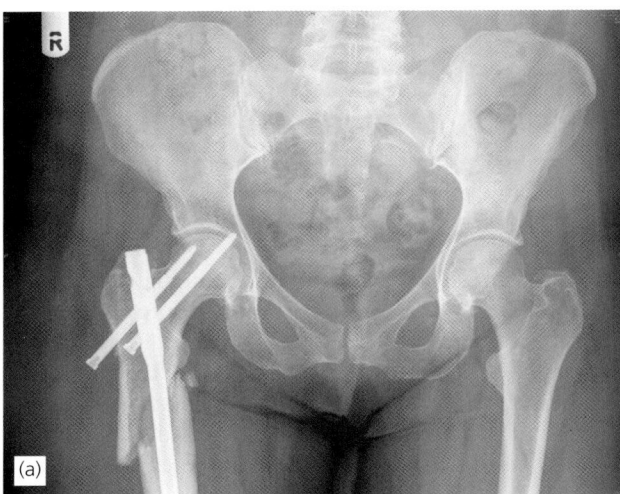

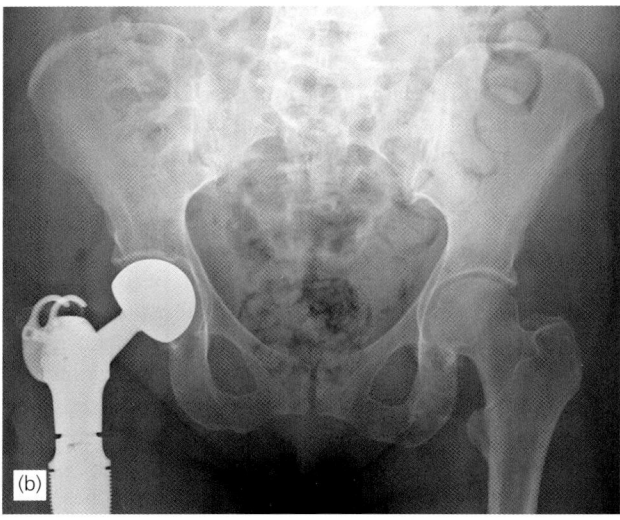

Figure 83.6 A 55-year-old patient with metastatic breast carcinoma presented with a pathological subtrochanteric fracture. This was treated at the receiving hospital with intramedullary fixation (a). The pathological fracture did not heal despite radiotherapy and the patient outlived the orthopaedic construct which failed at 1 year. The internal fixation was revised to a proximal femoral replacement (b).

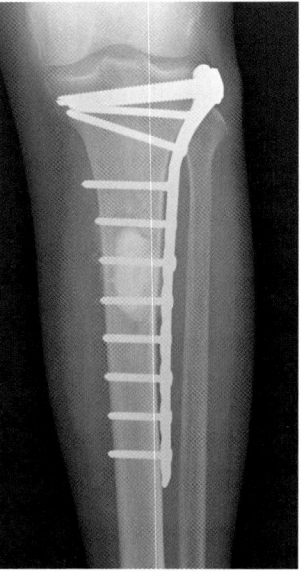

Figure 83.7 A patient presented with pain in their tibia and a solitary lytic lesion in the tibia was identified. After local and distant staging a previously occult gastric carcinoma was diagnosed. Survival was estimated to be less than 6 months and therefore a procedure to maximize mobility with minimal rehabilitation time was required. Internal fixation with a locking plate and cement augmentation was performed followed by adjuvant radiotherapy. The patient quickly regained full mobility. The orthopaedic construct outlived the patient.

metastases have a variable prognosis and therefore surgical planning depends upon the stage of the disease.

In patients who have a solitary metastasis after a long disease-free interval, there is the temptation to try and treat the lesion with curative intent (Cappana class 1). Theoretically the metastatic lesion may be excised en bloc and the defect reconstructed with an endoprosthesis. However, these procedures are rarely curative and before being undertaken meticulous staging of the patient's disease must be performed. In cases of breast cancer, which can have a good prognosis, extensive resection of metastases has not improved survival.[80] Renal metastasis may have a good prognosis[79–82] and there are no oncological treatments that can obtain control of the tumour. Therefore, excision of these lesions with 'curative' intent may be indicated.

Renal and thyroid metastases are hypervascular. It is possible for patients to exsanguinate due to surgery being performed on these lesions. It is therefore imperative that all patients with these lesions have angiography performed pre-operatively with embolization of the main vessels supplying the tumour mass. Surgery should be performed within 48 hours of embolization, otherwise new vessel formation will have occurred and the risk of haemorrhage returned to pre-embolization levels. Reduction in median blood loss following embolization of renal metastases has been shown in several studies[83–85] (Fig. 83.8).

The anatomical location of the lesion is crucial. Lesions in the metaphysis, head and neck of the hip have a greater risk of fracture. Prosthetic replacement of the femoral head and neck with either a total hip replacement or hemiarthroplasty is straightforward and gives good results. Internal fixation of these lesions is not practised because the risk of implant failure is very high (15%).[6,76] The length of the femoral stem should bypass the most distal lesion by two bone diameters to avoid peri-prosthetic fracture occurring.

Obtaining good surgical outcomes with lesions in the metaphysial and peri-articular regions of joints other than the hip is difficult. Periarticular lesions around the knee may be treated with arthroplasty, but this has a longer rehabilitation time than hip arthroplasty. The functional outcome of endoprosthetic replacement of the proximal humerus, distal humerus and distal tibia can be unsatisfactory. In the proximal humerus the rotator cuff is defunctioned by the prosthesis and this compromises function. In these locations internal fixation is considered, especially if life expectancy is short. Intramedullary nailing often fails for metaphyseal lesions as there is insufficient proximal or distal bone stock. Plating may be used for these lesions, especially with the advent of periarticular locking plate fixation[74].

Diaphyseal lesions are usually treated by intramedullary nailing with good results. Intramedullary nailing of the femoral diaphysis for pathological lesions is associated with cardiopulmonary complications.[86,87] Reaming of the intramedullary cavity elevates the intramedullary pressure to levels well above those needed to cause embolization of marrow contents. If the bone is not fractured, the

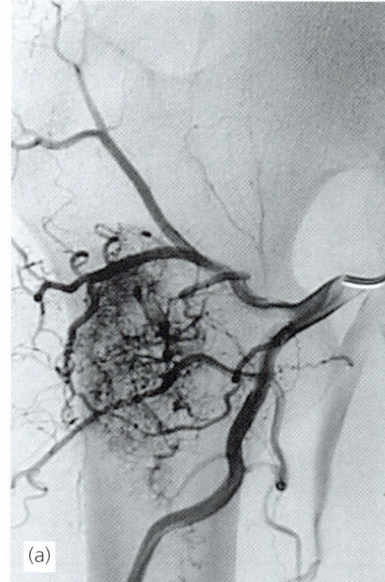

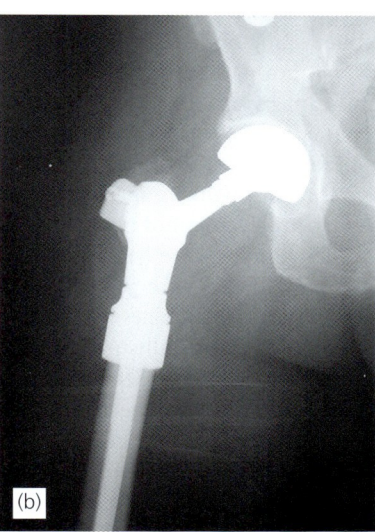

Figure 83.8 Arteriography demonstrating the hypervascular nature of a renal metastasis prior to embolization (a). Within 24 hours of embolization a proximal femoral replacement was performed (b).

bone should have a drill hole made distally to vent the medulla to reduce the risk of embolic phenomena.[88,89] There appears to be no difference in death rate between reamed and unreamed intramedullary nails for the treatment of metastatic lesions.[87] In the femoral diaphysis consideration should be given to using a nail that allows screws to be placed up the femoral neck, e.g. a reconstruction nail. This prevents late femoral neck fracture in the unfortunate patient who suffers from metastatic deposits in the femoral neck at a later date.[90] Intercalary spacers can be used for solitary metastasis in patients with good life expectancy, but they have unpredictable functional outcomes.

Capanna developed a scoring system to aid in the planning of surgical reconstruction of diaphyseal lesions. The patient is assessed with regard to expected survival, the response to adjuvant therapy and the size and site of the lesion. The Karnofsky and Burchenal grading of the patients fitness then modifies this score (Box 83.2). Minimal osteosynthesis is used for a score of <5, reinforced osteosynthesis for a score of 5–10 and an intercalary spacer for a score >10.

> **BOX 83.2: Scoring system and recommended treatment for diaphyseal lesions in Class 2 and 3 patients (Capanna 1999)[66]**
>
> Up to 5 points: minimal or simple osteosynthesis
> 5–10 points: reinforced osteosynthesis
> 10–15 points: endoprosthesis or intercalary spacer

Amputation should be avoided where possible in the treatment of metastatic bone lesions. Amputation will not improve survival in a patient with metastatic disease and there are significant psychological and functional difficulties for the patient to overcome following amputation. Consideration may be given to amputation in the following situations: unremitting pain, fungating lesions, unreconstructable lesions, involvement of neurovascular structures with a functionless limb, severe lymphoedema and failure of previous osteosynthesis with subsequent non-union. Amputation in these circumstances is a challenging procedure. The patients are systemically unwell and there can be profuse bleeding due to hyperaemia secondary to the tumour. Owing to limited life expectancy everything possible should be done to avoid amputation stump complications, as these consume valuable time for a patient with limited life expectancy.

The management of patients suffering from metastatic bone lesions with or without fracture requires multidisciplinary teamwork. The clinical decision-making is difficult, and poor decisions can have disastrous outcomes for the patient. The management of these patients is best undertaken by an orthopaedic surgeon with a special interest in the management of metastatic bone disease and orthopaedic oncology.

> **KEY LEARNING POINTS**
>
> - A pathological fracture occurs through an area of abnormal bone. There is either a reduction in the quantity or quality of the bone present. The majority of pathological fractures are secondary to osteoporosis.
> - 70% of bone metastases are secondary to breast, prostate, thyroid, renal or lung cancer.
> - 50% of patients who sustain a pathological fracture will die within 6 months of fracture; however, some patients may survive for many years. Breast, renal and prostate carcinoma are those most associated with prolonged survival.
> - RANK-L, osteoprotegerin, PTHrP, interleukins and TGF-β are key substrates involved in the metastasis–bone interaction and influence the phenotype of the metastasis.
> - Clinical history, examination and a chest radiograph alone will identify the primary lesion in 51% of cases of skeletal metastasis of unknown origin. The most common occult primary tumour is lung cancer.
> - A bone scan will identify if a lesion is solitary or multiple and can assist in determining prognosis and whether referral to a bone tumour centre is required for biopsy.
> - Determining a patient's prognosis and risk of pathological fracture is difficult and requires discussion at a multidisciplinary clinical pathological conference.
> - Surgical intervention should aim to provide pain relief, preserve or restore mobility/upper limb function and provide an orthopaedic implant that will outlive the patient.

REFERENCES

1. Harrington KD. *Orthopaedic Management of Metastatic Bone Disease.* St Louis, MO: Mosby, 1988.
2. Wedin R, Bauer HC, Rutqvist LE. Surgical treatment for skeletal breast cancer metastasis: a population-based study of 641 patients. *Cancer* 2001;**92**:257–62.
3. Colemann RE, Rubens RD. The clinical course of bone metastasis from breast cancer. *British Journal of Oncology* 1987;**55**:61–6.
4. Hansen BH, Keller J, Laitinen M, et al. The Scandinavian Sarcoma Group Skeletal Metastasis Registry. Survival after surgery for bone metastasis in the pelvis and extremities. *Acta Orthopaedica Scandinavica Supplementum* 2004; **75**:11–15.
5. Wedin R, Bauer HCF, Rutqvist LE. Incidence and outcome of surgical treatment for skeletal breast cancer metastasis:a population based study of 641 patients. *Cancer* 2001; **92**:257–62.
6. Dijstra, S, Wiggers T, van Geel BN and Boxma H. Impending and actual pathological fractures in patients with bone metastasis of long bones. A retrospective study of 233 surgically treated fractures. *European Journal of Surgery* 1994;**160**:535–42.
7. Yazawa Y, frassica F, Chao E, et al. Metastatic bone disease. *Clinical Orthopaedics and Related Research* 1990;**251**:213–19.

8. Batson OV. The function of the vertebral veins and their role in the spread of metastasis. *Archives of Surgery* 1940;**112**:138–49.
9. Morrissey C, True LD, Roudier MP, et al. Differential expression of angiogenesis associated genes in prostate cancer bone, liver and lymph node metastasis. *Clinical Experimental Metastasis* 2008;**25**:377–88.
10. Taube T, Elomaa I, Blomqvist C, et al. Histomorphometric evidence for osteoclast mediated bone resorption in metastatic breast cancer. *Bone* 1994;**15**:161–6.
11. Yonou H, Ochiai A, Goya M, et al. Intraosseous growth of human prostate cancer in implanted adult human bone: relationship of prostate cancer cells to osteoclasts in osteoblastic metastatic lesions. *Prostate* 2004;**58**:406–13.
12. Yi B, Williams PJ, Niewolna M, et al. Tumour derived platelet derived growth factor-BB plays a critical role in osteosclerotic bone metastasis in an animal model of human breast cancer. *Cancer Research* 2002;**62**:917–23.
13. Roudier MP, Vasselle H, True LD, et al. Bone histology at autopsy and matched bone scintigraphy findings in patients with hormone refractory prostate cancer: the effect of bisphosphonate therapy on bone scintigraphy results. *Clinical and Experimental Metastasis* 2003;**20**:171–80.
14. Roudier MP, True LD, Higano CS, et al. Phenotypic heterogeneity of end-stage prostate carcinoma metastatic to bone. *Human Pathology* 2003;**34**:646–53.
15. Bataille R, Chappard D, Basle M. Excessive bone resorption in human plasmacytomas: direct induction by tumour cells *in vivo*. *British Journal of Haematology* 1995;**90**:721–24.
16. Roodman GD. New potential targets for treating multiple myeloma bone disease. *Clinical Cancer Research* 2006;**12**:6270s–3s.
17. Roudier MP, Bain SD, Dougall WC. Effects of RANK-L inhibitor, osteoprotegerin, on the pain and histopathology of bone cancer in rates. *Clinical and Experimental Metastasis* 2006;**23**:167–75.
18. Chirgwin JM, Guise TA. Molecular mechanisms of tumour-bone interactions in osteolytic metastases. *Critical Reviews in Eukaryotic Gene Expression* 2000;**10**:159–78.
19. Dallas SL, Rosser JL, Mundy GR, Bonewald LF. Proteolysis of latent transforming growth factor beta (TGF-beta) binding protein 1 by osteoclasts: a cellular mechanism for release of TGF beta from bone matrix. *Journal of Biological Chemistry* 2002;**277**:21352–60.
20. M. Powell GJ, Southby J, Danks JA, et al. Localization of parathyroid hormone-related protein in breast cancer metastases: increased incidence in bone compared with other sites. *Cancer Research* 1991;**51**:3118–22.
21. Alam AS, Gallagher A, Shankar V, et al. Endothelin inhibits osteoclastic bone resorption by a direct effect on cell motility: implications for the vascular control of bone resorption. *Endocrinology* 1992;**130**:3617–24.
22. Nelson JB, Hedican SP, George DJ, et al. Identification of endothelin-1 in the pathophysiology of metastatic adenocarcinoma of the prostate. *Nature Medicine* 1995;**1**:944–99.
23. Carducci MA, Padley RJ, Breul J, et al. Effect of endothelin-A receptor blockade with Atrasentan on tumor progression in men with hormone refractory prostate cancer: a randomised phase II, placebo-controlled trial. *Journal of Clinical Oncology* 2003;**21**:679–89.
24. Carducci MA, Jimeno A. Targetting bone metastasis in prostate cancer with endothelin receptor antagonists. *Clinical Cancer Research* 2006;**12**:6296s–300s.
25. Charhon SA, Chapuy MC, Delvin EE, et al. Histomorphometric analysis of sclerotic bone metastasis from prostate carcinoma, special reference to osteomalacia. *Cancer* 1983;**51**:918–24.
26. Brown JE, Cook RJ, Major P, et al. Bone turnover markers as predictors of skeletal complications in prostate cancer, lung cancer and other solid tumours. *Journal of the National Cancer Institute* 2005;**97**:59–69.
27. Coleman RE, Major P, Lipton A, et al. Predictice value of bone resorption and formation markers in cancer patients with bone metastasis receiving bisphosphonate Zoledronic acid. *Journal of Clinical Oncology* 2005;**23**:4925–35.
28. Costa L, Demers LM, Gouveia-Oliveira A, et al. Prospective evaluation of the peptide-bound collagen type I cross-links N-telopeptide and C-telopeptide in predicting bone metastases status. *Journal of Clinical Oncologyogy* 2002;**20**:850–56.
29. Cramer SD, Chen Z, Peehl DM. Prostate specific antigen cleaves parathyroid hormone-related protein in the PTH-like domain: inactivation of PTHrP-stimulated cAMP accumulation in mouse osteoblasts. *Journal of Urology* 1996;**156**(2 Pt 1):526–31.
30. Lwamura M, Hellman J, Cockett AT, et al. Alteration of the hormonal bioactivity of parathyroid hormone-related protein (PTHrP) as a result of limited proteolysis by prostate-specific antigen. *Urology* 1996;**48**:317–25.
31. Goya M, Ishii G, Miyamoto S, et al. Prostate specific antigen induces apoptosis of osteoclast precursors: potential role in osteoblastic bone metastases of prostate cancer. *Prostate* 2006;**66**:1573–84.
32. Yonou H, Horiguchi Y, Ohno Y, et al. Prostate specific antigen stimulates osteoprotegerin production and inhibits receptor activator of nuclear factor-kappaB ligand expression by human osteoblasts. *Prostate* 2007;**67**:840–8.
33. Carmeliet P, Dor Y, Herbert JM, et al. Role of HIF-1alpha in hypoxia-mediated apoptosis, cell proliferation and tumour angiogenesis. *Nature* 1998;**394**:485–90.
34. Salnikow K, Costa M, Figg WD, Blagosklonny MV. Hyperinducibility of hypoxia-responsive genes without p53/p21-dependent checkpoint in aggressive prostate cancer. *Cancer Research* 2000;**60**:5630–4.

35. Koshikawa N, Iyozumi A, Gassmann M, Takenaga K. Constitutive upregulation of hypoxia-inducible factor-1alpha mRNA occurring in highly metastatic lung carcinoma cells leads to vascular endothelial growth factor overexpression upon hypoxic exposure. *Oncogene* 2003;**22**:6717–24.
36. Liao D, Corle C, Seagroves TN, Johnson RS. Hypoxia-inducible factor-1alpha is a key regulator of metastasis in a transgenic model of cancer initiation and progression. *Cancer Research* 2007;**67**:563–72.
37. Arnett T. Regulation of bone cell function by acid base balance. *Proceedings of the Nutrition Society* 2003;**62**:511–20.
38. Brandao-Burch A, Utting JC, Orriss IR, Arnett TR. Acidosis inhibits bone formation by osteoblasts *in vitro* by preventing mineralisation. *Calcified Tissue International* 2005;**77**:167–74.
39. Sanders JL, Chattopadhyay N, Kifor O, et al. Extracellular calcium-sensing receptor expression and its potential role in regulating parathyroid hormone-related peptide secretion in human breast cancer cell lines. *Endocrinology* 2000;**141**:4357–64.
40. Sanders JL, Chattopadhyay N, Kifor O, et al. Ca^{2+}-sensing receptor expression and PTHrP secretion in PC-3 human prostate cancer cells. *American Journal of Physiology, Endocrinology and Metabolism* 2001;**281**:E1267–74.
41. Eastell R, Hannon RA, Cuzick J, et al. Effect of an aromatase inhibitor on bone and bone turnover markers: 2-year results of the Anastrozole, Tamoxifen, Alone or in Combination (ATAC) trial (18233230). *Journal of Bone Mineral Research* 2006;**21**:1215–23.
42. Eastell R, Adams JE, Coleman RE, et al. Effect of anastrozole on bone mineral density: 5-year results from the anastrozole, tamoxifen, alone or in combination trial 18233230. *Journal of Clinical Oncology* 2008;**26**:1051–7.
43. Preston DM, Torréns JI, Harding P. Androgen deprivation in men with prostate cancer is associated with an increased rate of bone loss. *Prostate Cancer Prostatic Disease* 2002;**5**:304–10.
44. Coleman RE, Banks LM, Girgis SI, et al. Intergroup Exemestane Study group. Skeletal effects of exemestane on bone-mineral density, bone biomarkers, and fracture incidence in postmenopausal women with early breast cancer participating in the Intergroup Exemestane Study (IES): a randomised controlled study. *Lancet Oncology* 2007;**8**:119–27.
45. Eastell R, Adams JE, Coleman RE, et al. Effect of anastrozole on bone mineral density: 5-year results from the anastrozole, tamoxifen, alone or in combination trial 18233230. *Journal of Clinical Oncology* 2008;**26**:1051–7.
46. Bundred NJ, Campbell ID, Davidson N, et al. Effective inhibition of aromatase inhibitor-associated bone loss by zoledronic acid in postmenopausal women with early breast cancer receiving adjuvant letrozole: ZO-FAST Study results. *Cancer* 2008;**112**:1001–10.
47. Cool P and Grimer R. Pathological fractures of the extremities. *Trauma* 2000;**2**:101–11.
48. Leonard RC, Owen JP, Proctor SJ, Hamilton PJ. Multiple myeloma: radiology or bone scanning? *Clinical Radiology* 1981;**32**:291–5.
49. Kim EE, Bledin AG, Gutierrez C, Haynie TP. Comparison of radionuclide images and radiographs for skeletal metastases from renal cell carcinoma. *Oncology* 1983;**40**:284–6.
50. Rougraff BT, Kneisl JS, Simon MA. Skeletal metastasis of unknown origin. *Journal of Bone and Joint Surgery (American)* 1993;**75A**:1276–81.
51. Wedin R, Henrick CF, Bauer LS, et al. Cytological diagnosis of skeletal lesions. *Journal of Bone and Joint Surgery (British)* 2000;**82B**:673–8.
52. Hillner BE, Siegal BA, Liu D, et al. Impact of positron emission tomography/computer toography and positron emission tomography alone on expected management of patients with cancer: initial results from the National Oncologic PET Registry. *Journal of Clinical Oncology* 2008;**26**:2083–4.
53. Lein M, Wirth M, Miller K, et al. Serial markers of bone turnover in men with metastatic prostate cancer treated with zoledronic acid for detection of bone metastasis progression. *European Urology* 2007;**52**:1381–7.
54. Katagiri H, Takahashi M, Wakai K, et al. Prognostic factors and a scoring system for patients with skeletal metastasis. *Journal of Bone and Joint Surgery* 2005;**87B**:698–703.
55. Beals RK, Lawton GD, Snell WE. Prophylactic internal fixation of the femur in metastatic breast cancer. *Cancer* 1971;**28**:1350–4.
56. Bunting R, Lamont-havers W, Schweon D, Kilman A. Pathologic fracture risk in rehabilitation of patients with bony metastasis. *Clinical Orthopaedics and Related Research* 1985;**192**:222–27.
57. Fidler M: Prophylatic internal fixation of secondary neoplastic deposits in long bones. *British Medical Journal* 1973;**10**:341–43.
58. Fidler M. Incidence of fracture of metastasis in long bones. *Acta Orthopaedica Scandinavica* 1981;**52**:623–7.
59. Mirel H. Metastatic disease in long bones. *Clinical Orthopaedics and Related Research* 1989;**249**;256–64.
60. Damron TA, Morgan H, Prakash, et al. Critical evaluaton of Mirels rating system of impending pathologic fracture *Clinical Orthopaedics and Related Research* 2003;**415**(Suppl):S201–7.
61. Keene JS, Sellinger DS, McBeath AA, Engber WD. Metastatic breast cancer in the femur. A search for the lesion at risk of fracture. *Clinical Orthopaedics and Related Research* 1986;**203**:282.
62. Van der Linden YM, Dijkstra PDS, Kroon HM, et al. Comparative analysis of risk factors for pathological fracture with femoral metastases. *Journal of Bone and Joint Surgery (British)* 2004;**86b**:566–73.
63. Hipp JA, Springfield DS, Hayes WC. Predicting pathologic fracture risk in the management of metastatic bone defects. *Clinical Orthopaedics and Related Research* 1995;**312**:120–35.
64. Bohm P, Huber J. The surgical treatment of bony metastases of the spine and limbs. *Journal of Bone and Joint Surgery (British)* 2002;**84B**:521–9.

65. Cheng DS, Seitz CB, Eyre HJ. Non-operative management of femoral, humeral and acetabular metastasis in patients with breast carcinoma. *Cancer* 1980;**45**:1533–7.
66. Cappana R. The treatment of metastasis in bone. *European Instructional Course Lectures* 1999;**4**:24–34.
67. Colemann RE, Rubens RD. The clinical course of bone metastasis from breast cancer. *British Journal of Oncology* 1987;**55**:61–6.
68. A. Saad F, Gleason DM, Murrey R, et al. A randomised placebo controlled trial of zoledronic acid in patients with hormone refractory prostate carcinoma. *Journal of the National Cancer Institute* 2002;**94**:1458–68.
69. Yuen KK, Shelley M, Sze WM. Bisphosphonates for advanced prostate cancer. *Cochrane Database of Systematic Reviews* 2006;**18**(4) CD006250.
70. Rosen LS, Gordon D, Kaminski M, et al. Long term efficacy and safety of zoledronic acid compared with pamidronate disodium in the treatment of skeletal complications in patients with advanced multiple myeloma or breast carcinoma. A randomised, double blind, multicenter, comparative trial. *Cancer* 2003;**98**:1735–44.
71. Powles T, Paterson S, Kanis JA, et al. Randomized, placebo-controlled trial of clodronate in patients with primary operable breast cancer. *Journal of Clinical Oncology* 2002;**20**:3219–24.
72. Pavlakis N, Schmidt R, Stockler M. Bisphosphonates for breast cancer. *Cochrane Database of Systematic Reviews* 2002;(1):CD003474.
73. Preston DM, Torréns JI, Harding P. Androgen deprivation in men with prostate cancer is associated with an increased rate of bone loss. *Prostate Cancer Prostatic Disease* 2002;**5**:304–10.
74. Gregory JJ, Ockendon M, Cribb GL, Cool WP, Williams DH. The outcome of locking plate fixation for the treatment of periarticular metastases. *Acta Orthopaedica Belgica* 2011; **77**:362–70.
75. Yazawa Y, Frassica F, Chao E, et al. Metastatic bone disease. *Clinical Orthopaedics and Related Research* 1990;**251**:213–19.
76. Wedin R, Bauer HCF, Wersall P. Failures after operation for metastatic lesions of long bones. *Clinical Orthopaedics* 1999;**358**:128–39.
77. Jeys LM, Kulkarni A, Grimer RJ, et al. Endoprosthetic replacement for the treatment of musculoskeletal tumours of the appendicular skeleton and pelvis. *Journal of Bone and Joint Surgery (American)* 2008;**90A**:1265–71.
78. Gainor BJ, Buchert P. Fracture healing in metastatic bone disease. *Clinical Orthopaedics and Related Research* 1983;**178**:297–302.
79. Althausen P, Althausen A, Jennings LC, Mankin HJ. Prognostic factors and surgical treatment of osseous metastases secondary to renal cell carcinoma. *Cancer* 1997;**80**:1103–9.
80. Dürr HR, Müller PE, Lenz T, et al. Surgical treatment of bone metastases in patients with breast cancer. *Clinical Orthopaedics and Related Research* 2002;**396**:191–6.
81. Lin PP, Mirza AN, Lewis VO, et al. Patient survival after surgery for osseous metastases from renal cell carcinoma. *Journal of Bone and Joint Surgery (American)* 2007; **89**:1794–801.
82. Bohm P, Huber J. The surgical treatment of bony metastases of the spine and limbs. *Journal of Bone and Joint Surgery (British)* 2002;**84B**:521–9.
83. Rowe DM, Becker GJ, Rabe FE, et al. Osseous metastases from renal cell carcinoma: embolisation and surgery for restoration of function. *Radiology* 1984;**150**:673–6.
84. Manke C, Bretschneider T, Lenhart M, et al. Spinal metastases from renal cell carcinoma: effect of perioperative particle embolisation on intra-operative blood loss. *American Journal of Neuroradiology* 2001;**22**:997–1003.
85. Roscoe MW, McBroom RJ, St Louis E, et al. Preoperative embolisation in the treatment of osseous metastases from renal cell carcinoma. *Clinical Orthopaedics and Related Research* 1989;**238**:302–7.
86. Barwood SA, Wilson JL, Molnar RR, Choong PF. The incidence of acute cardiorespiratory and vascular dysfunction following intramedullary nail fixation of femoral metastasis. *Acta Orthopaedica Scandinavica* 2000;**71**:147–52.
87. Assal M, Zanone X, Peter RE. Osteosynthesis of metastatic lesions of the proximal femur with a solid femoral nail and interlocking spiral blade inserted without reaming. *Journal of Orthopedic Trauma* 2000;**14**:394–7.
88. Persson EV and Bauer HCCF. Sudden hypotension and profuse bleeding during intra-medullary nailing of the femur in cancer patients: a report of two cases. *Acta Orthopaedica Scandinavica* 1994;**65**:564–7.
89. Choong PF. Cardiopulmonary complications of intramedullary fixation of long bone metastases. *Clinical Orthopaedics and Related Research* 2003; **415**(Suppl):S245–53.
90. Weber KL, O'Connor MI. Operative treatment of long bone metastasis: focus on the femur. *Clinical Orthopaedics and Related Research* 2003;**415**(Suppl):276–8.

84

Limb reconstruction for musculoskeletal tumours

EMMA K REAY AND CRAIG H GERRAND

Introduction, historical perspective and options for limb reconstruction	940	Reconstruction after resection for primary bone sarcomas	942
Assessing limb function after treatment	941	Regional reconstruction	946
The multidisciplinary team	941	Reconstruction in the skeletally immature	950
The role of radiotherapy in local control	941	Reconstruction after resection of soft-tissue sarcomas	951
Biopsy and limb reconstruction	941	Summary	951
Principles of limb-sparing surgery for sarcoma	942	References	951
Limb-sparing surgery for all?	942		

NATIONAL BOARD STANDARDS

- Knowledge of the evidence base for limb preservation and reconstruction
- Understand the surgical options available for limb preservation and reconstruction following resection of musculoskeletal tumours
- Understand the advantages and disadvantages of the different limb reconstruction techniques and their complications
- Outline the surgical principles and techniques for the most common limb reconstruction techniques
- Knowledge of the specific reconstruction options for different anatomical sites, including pelvis, hip, femur, tibia, humerus and in the skeletally immature patient

INTRODUCTION, HISTORICAL PERSPECTIVE AND OPTIONS FOR LIMB RECONSTRUCTION

Over the last 30 years there has been a significant shift in the surgical management of patients with extremity musculoskeletal tumours from amputation to limb-sparing surgery, which is feasible in 90% of patients.[1] Using modern implants and surgical techniques, patients can have functional limbs even following major skeletal and soft-tissue resections.[2] The catalysts of this change were the introduction of effective adjuvant chemotherapy and the development of a clinically useful staging system.

Enneking et al.[3] made a key contribution to the latter by developing the concept of a reactive zone around a tumour, in which there were compressed normal tissues, inflammatory cells and, crucially, tumour cells. Complete resection of a tumour would therefore involve removing the whole of the reactive zone. Allied to this, Enneking et al.[3] described osteofascial compartments in the extremities, the boundaries of which tend to resist the local invasion of tumours. For example, the thigh may be divided into anterior, posterior and medial compartments, with the boundaries being the intermuscular septae. Some sites, such as the popliteal fossa, do not have well-defined osteofascial boundaries and are therefore described as 'extracompartmental'. These concepts led to definitions of surgical margins and a system for tumour staging at a time when cross-sectional imaging was not widely available. By relating the risk of local recurrence to the surgical margins achieved, surgeons could be guided as to what constituted a safe resection margin.[3]

The clinical safety of limb-sparing surgery for extremity osteosarcoma was described in a classic study by Simon et al.,[4] who retrospectively compared limb salvage and amputation for osteosarcoma of the distal femur. Although local recurrence rates were higher in those treated with limb-sparing surgery, this did not have an adverse effect on disease-free or overall survival.[4] Similarly, extremity soft-tissue sarcomas can also be treated successfully with limb-sparing surgery. In a landmark randomized controlled study, Rosenberg et al.[5] showed that, when combined with radiotherapy, limb salvage surgery was not associated with poorer overall survival. However, there were more local recurrences in the group of patients who underwent conservative surgery.[5]

Although debate continues about the relationship between local recurrence and systemic relapse and about the trade-off between limb preservation and control of the malignant tumour, the obvious benefits of a preserved limb mean that limb-sparing surgery has become widely accepted.

The options for major skeletal reconstruction include:

- endoprosthetic reconstruction
- biological reconstruction, using allografts, autografts or both
- an allograft–prosthesis composite.

The selection of a particular reconstructive technique is influenced by the anatomical site, the age and functional demands of the patient, the morbidity associated with the procedure and the risk of complications.

ASSESSING LIMB FUNCTION AFTER TREATMENT

The assessment of limb function after treatment is of great interest to surgeons looking to explore differences between amputation and limb preservation and to compare reconstructive techniques. The two most widely adopted tools for the assessment of function are the Musculoskeletal Tumour Society Score (MSTS) and the Toronto Extremity Salvage Score. The former is a physician-completed measure containing domains relating to pain, function, emotional acceptance, walking stick use, walking ability and gait in the lower extremity and hand positioning, manual dexterity and lifting ability in the upper extremity.[6] The MSTS scale is widely accepted but has been criticized for its poor internal consistency.[7] The Toronto Extremity Salvage Score is a 30-point patient-completed questionnaire measuring attributes which best fit the World Health Organization's definition of disability and which relate to the patient's difficulty in performing specific activities.[8]

THE MULTIDISCIPLINARY TEAM

It is generally accepted that patients with musculoskeletal tumours should be managed by a multidisciplinary team (MDT) comprising specialists from pathology, radiology, medical and clinical oncology, palliative care and rehabilitation medicine, who can determine the most appropriate management strategy for a particular patient. Because sarcomas can present in any anatomical location, the team usually comprises surgeons from plastic surgery, general, thoracic, and head and neck specialties as well as orthopaedic surgery.

THE ROLE OF RADIOTHERAPY IN LOCAL CONTROL

The use of radiotherapy for bone sarcomas is well established for Ewing's tumours, which for many years were treated with radiotherapy alone. However, surgical resection is now considered the treatment of choice unless the morbidity and functional loss associated with surgery is unacceptable, e.g. with large tumours in the spine or pelvis. Adjuvant radiotherapy is used where surgical margins are inadequate. In osteosarcoma, the evidence for adjuvant radiotherapy is low level, consisting of retrospective analyses of heterogeneous groups of patients.[9] In cases in which the surgical margins are inadequate and the response to chemotherapy has been poor, amputation is generally advised.[10]

The use of radiotherapy as an adjuvant treatment for the local control of soft-tissue sarcomas is well established. Most often, external beam radiotherapy is given either pre- or postoperatively. Pre-operative radiotherapy has the benefit that a lower dose (typically 50 Gy vs 66 Gy) can be given, that the area to be treated is readily identified and a lower volume of tissue can be treated, and that, in some tumour types (such as myxoid liposarcoma), the tumour may respond to treatment and reduce in size. However, in some anatomical locations, particularly the thigh, the use of pre-operative radiotherapy is associated with an increase in the risk of wound complications.[11]

BIOPSY AND LIMB RECONSTRUCTION

Sarcomas are highly implantable and therefore the biopsy track is routinely removed during definitive surgery. Errors in biopsy technique can adversely affect the definitive surgical procedure by delaying diagnosis, contaminating the surgical field and, in some cases, making limb-sparing surgery impossible.[12] Therefore, biopsies of musculoskeletal tumours should be carried out by, or in consultation with, the surgical team performing the definitive resection. The principles of biopsy of musculoskeletal tumours are given in Chapter 79.

PRINCIPLES OF LIMB-SPARING SURGERY FOR SARCOMA

In the surgical treatment of bone and soft-tissue sarcoma, the primary aim is to remove all of the tumour. This is usually achieved by obtaining a tumour-free resection margin, the adequacy of which is strongly related to the risk of local recurrence. Conceptually, this margin should be outside the reactive zone (which may contain tumour cells), and thereby be classified as 'wide'.[3] If a tumour is small and surrounded by a sufficient volume of resectable tissue, such as muscle, it may be possible to obtain a truly wide margin. However, most tumours are close to critical anatomical structures such that the resection passes at least in part through what is technically the reactive zone. Surgical margins are often, therefore, described as microscopically positive or negative by the pathologist after an examination of the resection specimen.

Assessing the adequacy of the surgical margin also requires consideration of tumour type, grade and, when neoadjuvant chemotherapy has been given, response to chemotherapy. For example, low-grade lipomatous tumours have a low level of biological activity and are associated with low rates of local and systemic relapse. These can often, therefore, be excised in a deliberately marginal fashion, by shelling out.[13] At the other end of the spectrum, local recurrence in osteosarcoma is associated strongly with systemic relapse. Therefore, the criteria for judging an adequate resection are more rigorous.

In the surgical treatment of extremity sarcoma the surgeon has to balance the benefit of increasing the surgical margin with the subsequent loss of function. Informing this decision is the knowledge that some tissues, such as bone and fascia, are more resistant to tumour invasion than others, such as muscle or fat. Where there is intact fascia, therefore, the surgeon may be confident to leave a narrower margin.

LIMB-SPARING SURGERY FOR ALL?

Although limb-sparing surgery is associated with better functional outcomes than amputation, it is interesting to note that improvements in quality of life scores have not been reliably shown.[2] Reconstructed limbs are cosmetically more acceptable than amputations and provide more function, but they are not normal and patients may feel protective towards them, which in some instances (e.g. physically demanding occupations) may inhibit the patient's ability to participate. Salvaged limbs will often require further surgery. Amputation remains a possibility for the salvaged limb, either early on, because of inadequate surgical margins (particularly in osteosarcoma), or later, following local recurrence or because of complications of the reconstruction. Amputation is usually therefore discussed with patients pre-operatively and may be a reasonable alternative for some faced with the prospect of a complex reconstruction requiring many further procedures.

RECONSTRUCTION AFTER RESECTION FOR PRIMARY BONE SARCOMAS

There are three stages to a limb-sparing procedure.[4] These are:

- tumour resection
- skeletal reconstruction
- soft-tissue coverage and muscle transfers to restore function.

The purpose of the first step is to remove all of the tumour, as previously described. Skeletal reconstruction can be achieved using endoprostheses or biological reconstructions. The final step is an important one. Good soft-tissue reconstruction reduces the risk of implant infection should there be wound necrosis, and a satisfactory soft-tissue repair is likely to improve the function of the salvaged limb.

Relative contraindications to limb-sparing surgery include:

- significant neurovascular involvement
- infection
- situations in which a salvaged limb may be less functional than an amputation (i.e. if there is extensive involvement of the foot).

However, it is possible to reconstruct vessels involved by tumour, and resection of major nerves (e.g. the sciatic) can leave a limb which is still useful to the patient. Limb-sparing surgery is often feasible after pathological fracture.

For some tumours in selected anatomical sites, no skeletal reconstruction is required. Examples include the proximal fibula, the distal ulna and the iliac bone. When, as in the majority of cases, skeletal reconstruction is required, the options include endoprosthetic and/or biological reconstructions. The latter include allografts, autografts and allograft–prosthetic composites. These are discussed in turn below.

Endoprosthetic reconstruction

The use of large endoprostheses for the treatment of bony defects following tumour resection was described as early as 1949 (Stanmore implants were first designed and manufactured in 1949). These early endoprostheses were developed as extensions of joint replacement and were all custom made. By the late 1980s, however, modular systems were introduced which impart more intra-operative flexibility. Endoprostheses have been described in most anatomical locations, but are most frequently used for reconstruction of the proximal femur, distal femur, proximal tibia, humerus and pelvis.

Modern endoprosthetic design aims to provide patients with a long-term, stable reconstruction with minimal complications. Most endoprostheses consist of an articulating component, a body, a stem for skeletal fixation and a collar, with or without a hydroxyapatite coating. Stems for fixation of endoprostheses into diaphyseal bone can be cemented or uncemented and fixation may be augmented by lateral plates if appropriate. Hydroxyapatite extracortical plates have been described for fixation of endoprostheses into short juxta-articular segments of bone.[14] The use of a hydroxyapatite-coated collar on the implant adjacent to host bone has been shown to reduce the rate of aseptic loosening.[15] An example of an endoprosthesis is shown in Fig. 84.1a,b.

COMPLICATIONS OF ENDOPROSTHETIC RECONSTRUCTION

The most common complications of endoprosthetic reconstruction in order of frequency are listed below; overall complication rates vary widely in the literature but occur with a frequency of around 40%:[16–19]

- deep infection
- aseptic loosening
- mechanical failure
- dislocation.

Infection is the most common early complication. Risk factors for infection include radiotherapy, anatomical location, total joint replacement, and reoperation, e.g. for rebushing or secondary patellar resurfacing.[20] Infection rates are highest in the pelvis (25% or higher) followed by the proximal tibia (21%). Novel therapies such as the addition of a silver coating to endoprostheses may lead to lower rates of infection.[21,22]

Aseptic loosening has now become the most common midterm complication in all sites except for the pelvis and proximal tibia. Distal femoral endoprostheses have the highest rate of aseptic loosening at 10 years followed by proximal femur and proximal tibia.[19] The risk of loosening is increased with longer resections, particularly in the femur.[23] Upper limb implants survive longer than lower limb implants.

Mechanical failure in the form of prosthesis fracture is now unusual, but has historically been seen in first-generation Kotz implants, in which holes in the stem for anti-rotation screws often lead to fracture. This is not a problem with modern designs.[24] Rebushing of the moving parts of a hinged knee may be required from time to time, but does not usually require a major revision of the implant.

Dislocation of a hip replaced for tumour is more common than after conventional primary hip replacement because resection of the proximal femur usually requires resection of the anatomical stabilizers of the hip. Strategies to reduce this risk include the use of large diameter bearings along with capsular reconstruction, which can be augmented with an artificial material such as the polyethylene terephthalate mesh tube (Trevira, Implantcast, Buxtehude, Germany).

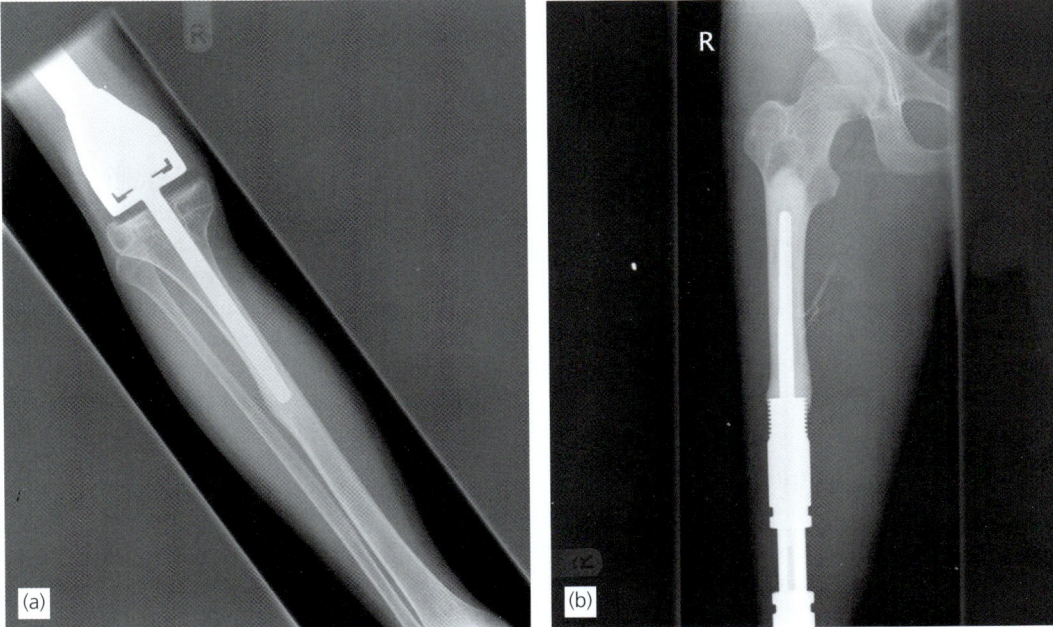

Figure 84.1 (a and b) Reconstruction of the distal femur using a customized, growing implant. The implant is lengthened using an electromagnetic coil. The proximal hydroxyapatite collar shows excellent integration with host bone.

Biological reconstruction

Biological reconstruction can be achieved using the following techniques:

- allograft
- autograft
- irradiated autograft
- distraction osteogenesis.

Reconstructions can be:

- intercalary (replacing a segment of bone but leaving the ends)
- osteochondral (replacing the joint)
- arthrodesis (used across a joint to enable fusion).

ALLOGRAFT

Massive allografts have been used for the reconstruction of large segment bony defects following tumour resection since the early twentieth century.

The advantages of allografts include the ability to shape the graft to the defect at the time of surgery, and that soft tissues attached to the graft can be used in the reconstruction. Allografts may also be useful when resections are performed close to a major joint through metaphyseal bone, in which case it may be difficult to anchor an implant within the resulting short segment, whereas union of allografts to metaphyseal bone may be more reliable.

Once implanted, massive bone allografts tend to incorporate at the ends and, to a lesser extent, on the surface of the graft by a process of creeping substitution. Complete replacement of the graft by host bone is not thought to occur.[25]

Disadvantages of the use of massive bone allografts include the potential for disease transmission, infection, fracture, non-union and reabsorption. There has been some enthusiasm for the use of osteochondral allografts, which include part of the articular surface in an attempt to reconstitute a functioning joint. However, they are currently not commonly used in the UK. In general, allografts are harvested and stored frozen until required. Allografts undergo routine bacteriological and virological analysis and the risk of disease transmission is small. Allografts may be irradiated to destroy viral particles and to reduce the risk of bacteriological infection.

Surgical technique for intercalary structural allograft reconstruction

Pre-operatively, an allograft should be selected that fits the predicted anatomical defect, based on pre-operative radiographs and patient demographics. Once the tumour has been resected, the allograft can be filled with cement if desired, which increases the mechanical strength of the graft, reduces the fracture risk and may reduce the risk of infection. The allograft is fixed to the recipient's bone using long plates which are preferred over intramedullary nails. Plate fixation using implants that span the length of the allograft has the advantage of stabilizing the junctions to allow healing and helps to prevent fracture. The allograft–host junctions may be augmented with morsellized autograft bone (e.g. from the iliac crest) at the time of primary surgery if preferred, or later if the junctions do not unite.

The process of intercalary implantation is as follows:

- tumour resection
- cut the graft to size and swab graft ends for microbiological analysis
- prepare soft tissues for implantation
- on a side table fill the graft with antibiotic-impregnated bone cement, filling from the proximal end
- rigid fixation at the graft–host interface is best achieved with long plates. Screws placed through the graft itself should be unicortical and well spaced to reduce the risk of fracture.
- augment the graft–host interface with autologous cancellous bone graft
- postoperative antibiotics as per the local protocol
- postoperatively, protect weight bearing as appropriate.[26]

An example of this technique used in reconstruction with an irradiated autograft is shown in Fig. 84.2.

Complications of allograft reconstruction

The complications associated with intercalary allograft reconstruction are:

- fracture
- non-union
- infection
- massive resorption.[27]

The majority of complications occur in the first 4 years, indicating that, once the graft is incorporated, it becomes part of a stable and durable reconstruction. Allograft survival rates at 10 years of around 80% have been reported, with limb preservation rates of up to 97% in some studies.[28]

The most common short-term complication is fracture of the allograft, with rates as high as 42%.[26] The risk of fracture may be reduced by using fixation that spans the whole graft and by filling the graft with intramedullary cement.[26] Interestingly, when comparing extracorporeally irradiated autograft with allograft, there were significantly lower rates of non-union in the autograft group.[27]

Functional outcomes following endoprosthetic and allograft reconstructions are similar. Intercalary reconstructions have better outcomes than arthrodeses, which in turn do better than osteochondral reconstructions.[26]

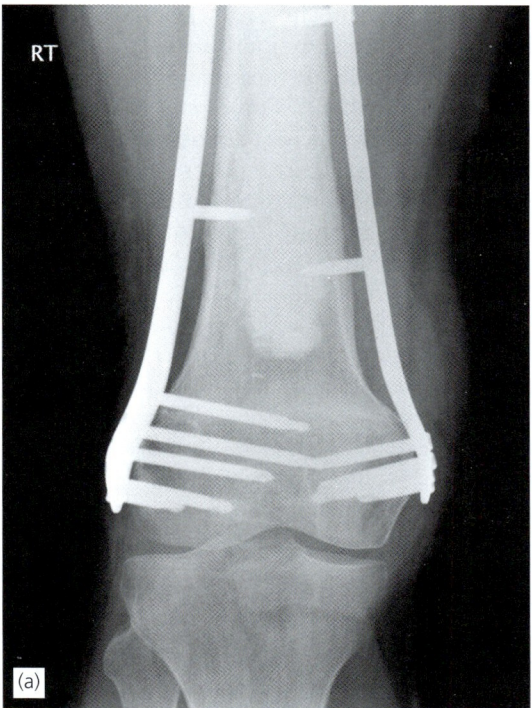 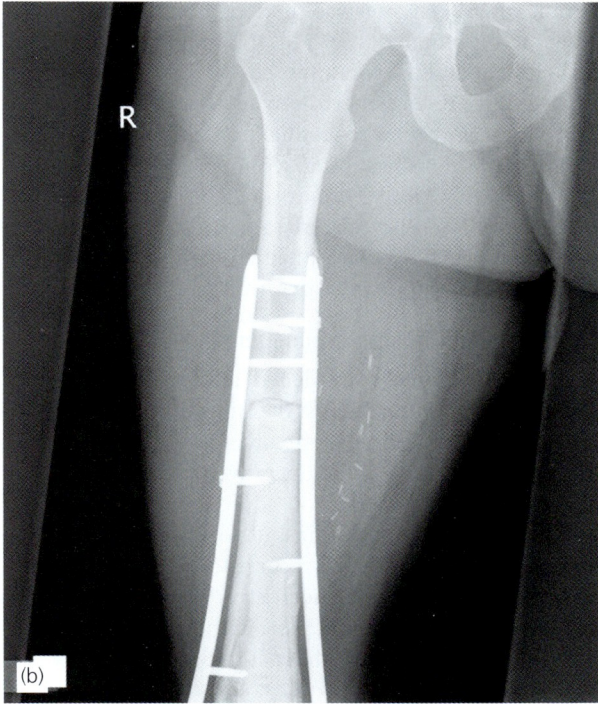

Figure 84.2 (a and b) Postoperative radiographs following reconstruction of the femoral diaphysis with an irradiated autograft. The graft has been filled with methylmethacrylate cement. The radiograph shows good healing at the metaphyseal end of the reconstruction, but poorer healing at the diaphyseal junction, which has subsequently been bone grafted.

Long-term joint deterioration is a recognized complication of osteoarticular allografts and joint resurfacing is occasionally required.

RECONSTRUCTION WITH AUTOGRAFTS

Vascularized fibular grafts

In 1981 Weiland[29] described the first vascularized fibular graft for the treatment of massive bony defects after tumour resection. Vascular fibular grafting has since been described for limb reconstruction in a wide range of anatomical sites, including the distal femur, pelvis, humerus, forearm and proximal tibia. The advantages of vascularized grafts, as compared with non-vascularized grafts, allografts and autografts, include higher union rates, the ability to address soft-tissue defects at the same time using a skin paddle, and the potential for longitudinal growth if the physis is included. Disadvantages include longer operative time, the need to protect the limb while incorporation occurs, and the technically demanding nature of the surgery, which requires microsurgical expertise.

Surgical technique for vascularized fibular grafts

Pre-operative planning includes consideration of the vessels to be anastomosed, the method of anastomosis, the fixation technique and graft alignment. Longer defects may require double barrelling of the graft to improve strength.

Grafts can be fixed with plates, nails or external fixation devices. The last are helpful when graft loading needs to be controlled (such as after tibial reconstruction), until the graft hypertrophies, which can take many months.[30] The technique of using a vascularized graft inside a massive allograft has been described. This has the theoretical benefit of providing good primary stability of the reconstruction with better long-term incorporation.

Complications associated with vascularized fibular grafts

The complications associated with vascularized fibular grafting include those related to the donor site as well as those related to the reconstructed bone:

- pedicle thrombosis
- fracture: 15–40%[30,31]
- non-union
- fixation failure.

The most common early complication is thrombosis of the graft pedicle, which occurs in 10% of patients and affects primarily the vein of the pedicle.[30] The viability of the graft can be monitored if a skin island is taken with the fibula. Care of the postoperative patient with a vascularized graft should include adequate hydration and maintenance of blood pressure. If there is doubt about graft vascularity, early re-exploration can be helpful.

Fracture is often seen after vascularized fibular grafting and is related to the length of the graft, the anatomical location, malalignment and the fixation used.[30,31] Grafts used in the lower extremity often hypertrophy as they are loaded, but this process may rely on sequential fractures. The rates of non-union at the graft–host interface are low, with union rates as high as 95%.[30] Fibular donor site complications are unusual but include sensory disturbances with damage to the common peroneal nerve, flexor hallucis longus contracture and, in children, valgus ankle deformity.

Extracorporeal irradiation and reimplantation

The use of extracorporeally irradiated autograft for the treatment of bone tumours was first described by Spira and Lubin in 1968.[32] The technique involves irradiating the resected segment of bone intra-operatively followed by reimplantation. The advantages of an exact anatomical match and no risk of disease transmission are balanced against the theoretical risks of local recurrence. However, no study has demonstrated an increased risk of tumour recurrence because of reimplantation of bone in this fashion. The process makes it difficult for the pathologist to assess tumour response and surgical margins, and therefore care must be taken in sending the soft-tissue envelope from the specimen for histological examination. This technique may not be suitable where there is significant bone destruction.

The complications of this technique appear to be similar to those seen after the use of allografts, including non-union, infection and fracture.[33]

ALLOGRAFT–PROSTHETIC COMPOSITES

Some authors advocate the use of allograft–prosthetic composites for reconstruction after tumour resection. In this technique, a prosthesis is primarily cemented into a massive allograft before the whole composite is introduced into the patient. The disadvantage of this technique is that the patient is at risk of the complications of allografts, such as non-union and fracture. It has been suggested, however, that in some locations, such as the proximal femur, the soft-tissue attachments of the allograft can lead to improved function.[34]

DISTRACTION OSTEOGENESIS

Distraction osteogenesis has been described for tumour reconstruction, but treatment times are long and there are theoretical concerns about the risk of local recurrence in the regenerate and, for appropriate patients, the effect of chemotherapy on the regenerate.

REGIONAL RECONSTRUCTION

Pelvis

Pelvic reconstruction after tumour resection is a significant surgical challenge. Pelvic tumours are often very large when diagnosed and are usually close to critical anatomical structures. Pelvic tumours are best addressed by surgeons familiar with the anatomy of the region and the reconstructive options. This often benefits from a team approach, including general, plastic and orthopaedic surgeons. Surgical resections are often long and complex, and the risk of complications (e.g. wound necrosis and implant infection) is high. Bony reconstructions should ideally, therefore, be as simple as possible and flexible, given that the procedure and the level of surgical resection may differ from what was planned. Although others are described, all or part of the surgical approach described by Malawer and Sugarbaker[35] can be used to approach the majority of the pelvic ring. The incision begins at the posterior inferior iliac spine and extends across the iliac crest to the anterior superior iliac spine and thence to the pubic tubercle. A vertical iliofemoral component can be developed to gain access to the hip joint.

The extent of the bony pelvic resection can be classified as described by Enneking and Dunham (Fig. 84.3). The resection determines the need for reconstruction. Isolated resections of the iliac crest (PI) or of the anterior pelvis (PIII) may not need reconstruction of the bony pelvis. If a PI resection involves complete removal of the ilioischial bar between the acetabulum and the sacrum, the gap will close over time and may not need reconstruction. However, there is associated limb shortening and some surgeons prefer to reconstruct. Similarly, anterior pelvic resections (PIII) may not require bony reconstruction. The most challenging resections, however, involve the acetabulum, after which some kind of reconstruction is

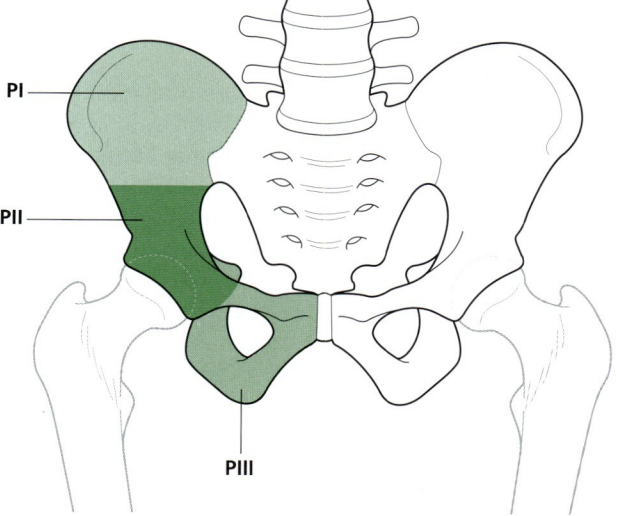

Figure 84.3 Enneking and Dunham classification of pelvic resection. I, iliosacral; II, acetabulum; III, ischiopubic. Reproduced with permission from Hoffmann C, Gosheger G, Gebert C, et al. Functional results and quality of life after treatment of pelvic sarcomas involving the acetabulum. *Journal of Bone and Joint Surgery (American)* 2006;**88**:575–82.

usually required. Reconstruction is particularly demanding when there is little iliac blade remaining.

Reconstructive options include endoprosthesis, massive allograft, autograft and vascularized fibular grafting. Variation in case mix and practice between centres means that the evidence base for choosing one reconstruction over another is small. However, it is clear that reconstruction offers better functional results than hindquarter amputation and that the restoration of pelvic femorosacral continuity is of functional benefit.[36]

Endoprosthetic reconstruction often involves customized implants manufactured to fit the predicted defect. The use of computerised navigation shows considerable promise by making osteotomies more accurate and therefore improving surgical margins and the fit of customised implants. If there is sufficient iliac crest remaining, a saddle prosthesis (a U-shaped prosthesis which articulates with the remaining iliac wing) has the benefit of being straightforward to insert, but it can migrate through the remaining iliac crest. A clinical illustration of the saddle prosthesis is shown in Fig. 84.4. Dislocation may be avoided by securing the implant to the iliac crest using a Trevira tube or vascular graft.[35]

Arthrodesis of the femur to the remaining iliac wing or to the pubis or ischium has been described, and may be of benefit when there has been resection of the hip abductors and the iliopsoas, when the risk of dislocation is high.

Hip and proximal femur

The proximal femur is the second most common site requiring reconstruction. Reconstructive options include endoprosthesis and allograft–prosthesis composites. The latter may be associated with better abductor function.[34] Although hemiarthroplasty has the benefit of retaining the acetabulum, and is the treatment of choice in skeletally immature patients, acetabular pain leads to revision in some patients.

The major challenges in reconstructing the proximal femur are avoiding dislocation and restoring abductor function. When the hip is replaced, large bearings are helpful in avoiding dislocation. However, a good soft-tissue repair, which includes the following, is important:

- Good capsular reconstruction, using the native capsule if present, but otherwise augmented with synthetic mesh. The psoas tendon can often be sutured to the anterior capsule.
- Abductor reconstruction. Attaching the abductors to the implant is sometimes feasible depending on the implant design. However, this repair can be unreliable, and suturing the abductor tendons to the overlying fascia lata leaves a sleeve of muscle with some abductor function.

Postoperative bracing is often useful following reconstruction.

SURGICAL TECHNIQUE

Surgical resection of the proximal femur is usually performed through a posterolateral approach with the patient in the lateral position. However, the more anterior Watson–Jones approach may also be used. The posterolateral approach has the benefit of providing access to the proximal third of the femur and the retrogluteal space. This can be extended to the knee if total femoral replacement is required.

The femoral shaft cut is planned pre-operatively and aims to be 3–4 cm distal to the extent of the tumour in primary sarcomas. The length of the femur, diameter of the femoral canal and size of the femoral head are assessed and a sample is taken from the remaining femoral canal to rule out tumour extension.

A third-generation cementation technique is used to cement the prosthesis *in situ*. Orientation of the prosthesis is crucial: the linea aspera is used as the anatomical guide and the prosthesis is inserted in 5–10° of anteversion.

Soft-tissue reconstruction is then performed with a combination of capsular reconstruction, with native tissue or synthetic augmentation, followed by abductor and vastus repair.

Distal femur

The distal femur is the most common anatomical site for bone sarcomas and is therefore the most commonly reconstructed anatomical site.[19] The reconstruction needs to be able to support weight bearing and to allow adequate function of the lower limb. Reconstructive options include endoprosthetic or allograft–prosthesis composites. An

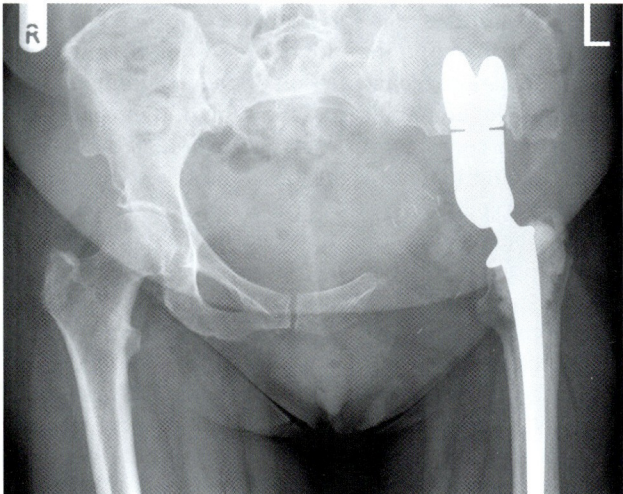

Figure 84.4 Reconstruction of the pelvis using a saddle prosthesis after a type I and II resection for chondrosarcoma.

example of a distal femoral endoprosthesis is shown in Fig. 84.2a,b.

Resection of the distal femur routinely involves excision of all the ligamentous stabilizers of the knee and therefore constrained rotating hinge articulations are usually used. Endoprosthetic reconstruction combines the benefits of rapid reconstruction with early weight bearing. The risk of aseptic loosening has become lower with the introduction of hydroxyapatite-coated stems.[19,37] Good soft-tissue repair and the liberal use of muscle transfers reduce the risk of infection, although this remains a significant risk.

SURGICAL TECHNIQUE

The distal femur can be approached from the medial side, the lateral side or from an anterolateral approach. The medial approach involves taking down the medial hamstring (pes anserinus) tendons to gain access to the neurovascular structures, which can then be dissected in a controlled fashion from the back of the tumour. Most often, resection of the distal femur for primary bone tumour involves resection of a significant proportion of the quadriceps muscle. If a medial biopsy is performed through the vastus medialis muscle, the biopsy track can be resected with the tumour. Following resection of the tumour and implantation of the endoprosthesis, the medial quadriceps can be replaced by a transfer of the medial hamstrings into the quadriceps tendon. Larger defects may require the use of a medial gastrocnemius pedicled flap.

Total femur

Total femoral replacement may be indicated for tumours with extensive involvement of the femur, or when there are skip lesions. Instability is a particular issue for these reconstructions, and a fixed hinge knee may be preferable to a rotating hinge knee, which can permit complete rotation of the implant.[38]

Proximal tibia

Challenges in the reconstruction of the proximal tibia include reconstituting the extensor mechanism and soft-tissue cover. Resections also routinely involve ligation of the anterior interosseous artery, the proximal tibiofibular joint and, on occasion, the lateral popliteal nerve. Historically, high infection rates of proximal tibial implants have been attributed to poor soft-tissue cover. This and the reconstruction of the extensor mechanism have been addressed in recent years by the routine use of a pedicled medial gastrocnemius flap. The patellar tendon can be held out to length using a suture or tape attached to the front of the implant and the whole sutured into the gastrocnemius flap, giving a continuous sleeve through which the quadriceps muscles can work.[37] High rates of mechanical failure and aseptic loosening seen in early devices have been reduced with the introduction of the rotating hinge prostheses and hydroxyapatite coating of the stems.[39]

Distal tibia/foot and ankle

Tumours around the distal tibia and foot are rare, and large case series describing reconstruction techniques do not exist. The challenges facing the surgeon at this site are infection and deformity. Reconstruction around the foot and ankle should aim to provide the patient with local tumour control, restoration of function and a stable foot when standing. After tumour resection, reconstruction of the skeletal and soft-tissue defects is possible using a variety of methods, including custom prostheses, bone transport, limb lengthening with or without a circular frame, bone allografts including osteoarticular grafts or vascularized autografts, arthrodesis and free vascularized musculocutaneous flaps.[40,41] However, a below knee amputation often provides excellent function, and the relative merits of this must be weighed against the need for a complex reconstruction.

Proximal humerus

The aim of humeral reconstruction is to provide a painless upper limb with functional use of the elbow, wrist and hand.[35] Resection of a tumour of the proximal humerus routinely involves removal of the rotator cuff muscles, and so normal function is not to be expected. Furthermore, many tumours require resection of the axillary nerve and the deltoid. A useful classification of shoulder resections is given in Fig. 84.5. A reconstructed shoulder joint is, therefore, often simply a reconstruction for suspending the functioning forearm and hand. However, careful reconstruction of the remaining muscles can improve the stability and function of the reconstruction with a combination of dynamic and static suspension. Scapulohumeral arthrodesis may be the preferred option for patients with particular physical demands, but can be difficult to achieve, particularly if the resection is long.

The surgical options for reconstruction include allografts, endoprosthesis, vascularized fibular grafting and arthrodesis. The implant can be suspended from the remaining scapula using a synthetic mesh tube. The Bayly–Walker shoulder, which is a reverse-polarity implant that screws into the remaining scapula, may also be helpful.

The complications following proximal humeral replacement are similar to those found in other sites and depend on

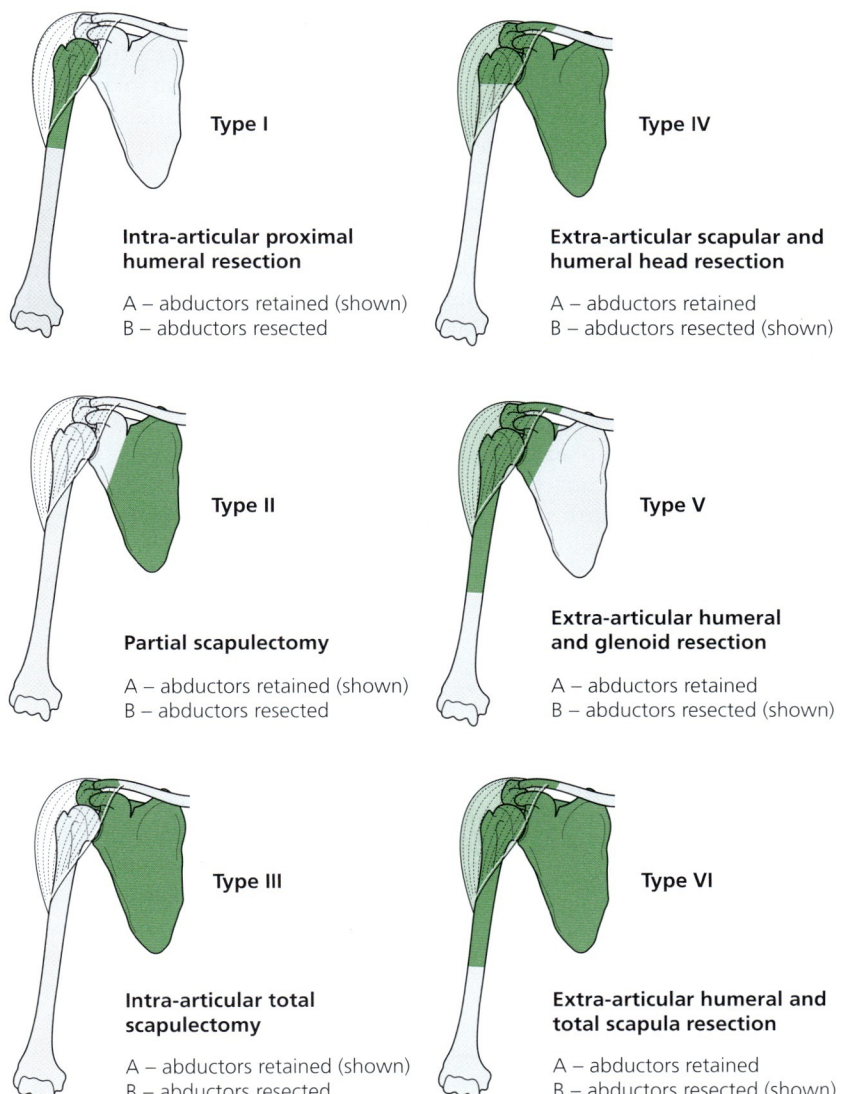

Figure 84.5 Musculoskeletal Tumor Society classification of shoulder girdle resections. S1, the blade or spine of the scapula; S2, the acromion–glenoid complex; S3, proximal epiphysis of the humerus; S4, the proximal metaphysis of the humerus; S5, the proximal part of the diaphysis of the humerus. A, abductor mechanism intact; B, abductor mechanism disrupted. Reproduced with permission from Malawer and Sugarbaker.[35]

the reconstruction method used. Endoprosthetic reconstruction carries a 10 year survival rate of up to 85%.[19]

Distal humerus

Tumours of the distal humerus are rare and account for only 1% of all primary bone lesions. High complication rates, poor functional outcome and instability are common problems following elbow reconstruction. A number of techniques are possible, including arthrodesis, endoprosthetic replacement, excision arthroplasty and allograft reconstruction. The necessity to maintain adequate tumour margins often requires resection of the stabilizing soft tissues around the elbow, with resultant high rates of instability. Care should be taken to protect the ulnar, radial and posterior interosseous nerves around the elbow to ensure a functional limb.[42]

Distal radius

Resection of the distal aspect of the radius is indicated for the treatment of some malignant tumours and for recurrent and locally aggressive benign tumours. The challenge is to maintain the function of the hand by maintaining the length of the radius and thereby the tendons which run over the wrist.[43] Numerous reconstruction techniques have been described, including vascularized fibular grafts, endoprosthetic replacement, autograft, arthrodesis and osteoarticular allografts.[44] The proximity of critical anatomical structures to the distal radius means that wide resections which preserve function are difficult to achieve. Tumours with extra-osseous extensions (such as a giant cell tumour of bone) are therefore associated with high local recurrence rates in this location.

Complications following reconstruction depend upon the type of reconstruction performed. The most commonly used technique of fibular grafting, either vascularized or non-vascularized, benefits from anatomical similarities between the distal radius and proximal fibula, although the reconstructed joint can be subject to early degenerative change. In children, if proximal fibula epiphyseal transfer is performed, articular remodelling can follow.[43] Alternatively, a transplanted fibula can be arthrodesed to the proximal carpal row. Joint stiffness, non-union and fracture are recognized complications.

Hand and wrist

Musculoskeletal tumours of the hand are rare, with reconstruction following tumour resection a significant challenge. The hand has little expendable soft tissue and functionally relies heavily on the preservation of the intrinsic muscles and nerves. Adjuncts such as radiotherapy are also poorly tolerated in the hand, adding to the difficulty in treatment.[45]

RECONSTRUCTION IN THE SKELETALLY IMMATURE

Compensating for future growth remains a major challenge in reconstructing the limbs of children. Primary malignant bone tumours most often occur in areas of greatest growth, e.g. the distal femur, where growth occurs at an average of 10 mm per annum until skeletal maturity (14 years for girls, 16 years for boys). Leg length discrepancy of greater than 2 cm is associated with a significant reduction in physical functioning.[16] Furthermore, amputation in childhood can be associated with excellent long-term outcomes.[46] Decision-making in this group can therefore be challenging, particularly in the very young. Options for limb reconstruction include the following.

Endoprosthetic reconstruction in children

Endoprosthetic reconstructions in children inevitably require revision. If the child survives the initial phase of the malignancy, aseptic loosening will cause failure of the prosthesis because of the radial growth of the bone into which the stem is implanted.

In an attempt to compensate for growth in the salvaged extremity, a number of expandable implants have been developed. Although older designs required a surgical intervention to achieve an increase in length, newer designs can be lengthened non-invasively in an outpatient setting. One such example is the Stanmore Juvenile Tumour System,[47] which uses an armature within the implant to achieve lengthening. The limb is placed inside an electromagnetic coil to activate the device. Lengthening is painless and can be performed in the outpatient clinic. The size of the device means that it may not be suitable for very young patients, but it has made a significant difference to the treatment of these patients. The extendable prosthesis is illustrated in Fig. 84.1a,b.

Biological reconstructions in children

Biological reconstructions in children have the significant advantage that, once healed, further surgical intervention is less likely than for endoprosthetic reconstruction.

ROTATIONPLASTY

Rotationplasty is a technique in which, after distal femoral resection, the remaining limb is rotated through 180° and the ankle becomes the functional equivalent of the knee. Active knee movement then becomes possible. The advantages of a good weight-bearing stump (i.e. the heel) and functional benefit over an above-knee amputation are balanced by the psychological impact of the appearance of the limb. It is likely that these procedures are most successful when there is an active support network for patients and prosthetists are accustomed to dealing with the particular fitting issues involved.

EPIPHYSEAL DISTRACTION

If a primary bone tumour does not involve the epiphysis, epiphyseal distraction is a technique in which the articular surface may be preserved. An external fixator is applied approximately 2 weeks before the surgical window following chemotherapy and distraction is performed. This increases the distance between the tumour and the articular surface and allows a resection to be performed through the physis. The defect can then be reconstructed using an allograft or autograft. This is a complex technique and care has to be taken not to compromise the adequacy of the resection.[48]

VASCULARIZED FIBULAR GRAFT

The use of a vascularized fibular graft has been described in particular anatomical locations, e.g. the proximal humerus. If the physis can be preserved, then some growth of the transplanted bone can be expected.

Table 84.1 Long-term complications of endoprosthetic and biological reconstructions in skeletally immature patients

Endoprosthesis	Biological reconstruction
Deep infection	Implant breakage
Aseptic loosening	Non-union
Implant breakage	Fracture
Dislocation	Superficial infection
	Deep infection

The major complications of endoprosthetic and biological reconstruction in the skeletally immature are listed in Table 84.1.

RECONSTRUCTION AFTER RESECTION OF SOFT-TISSUE SARCOMAS

Principles of resection for soft-tissue sarcoma

Soft-tissue sarcomas are a heterogeneous group of tumours arising from extraskeletal tissues, such as muscle, fascia, nerve and connective and fatty tissues. They rarely involve bone. The treatment of soft-tissue sarcomas is dependent on the histological type and grade of the tumour. The standard local treatment of high-grade sarcomas involves surgical excision and radiotherapy. Radiotherapy may be given pre- or postoperatively, depending on the tumour type and location. Chemotherapy may be indicated for a small number of tumour types, for tumours in children and for patients with metastatic disease. Isolated limb perfusion can reduce the size of the tumour in selected cases.

Many tumours do not require formal reconstruction after resection. However, a multidisciplinary approach including plastic surgeons, general surgeons and vascular surgeons is often helpful, particularly if flap reconstruction or vascular reconstruction are required.

SUMMARY

The contemporary management of primary bone and soft-tissue tumours involves the preservation of the limb in the majority of cases. Reconstructive options following bony reconstruction include endoprostheses, allografts, autografts and composites. Improvements in surgical techniques now give patients the option of long-term functional outcomes exceeding those following amputation in most cases.

> **KEY LEARNING POINTS**
>
> - The rate of limb salvage and reconstruction is 80–90%.
> - Reconstruction can be performed with endoprostheses, allografts or vascularized fibular grafts.
> - The main complication of an endoprosthesis in the longer term is aseptic loosening; the major concern in grafts is fracture.
> - Limb length discrepancy is a major concern in the skeletally immature; >2 cm discrepancy creates a functional disadvantage.

REFERENCES

- ● = Key primary paper
- ◆ = Major review article

1. Wafa H, Grimer RJ. Surgical options and outcomes in bone sarcoma. *Expert Review of Anticancer Therapy* 2006;**6**:239–48.
●2. Davis AM, Devlin M, Griffin AM, et al. Functional outcome in amputation versus limb sparing of patients with lower extremity sarcoma: a matched case-control study. *Archives of Physical Medicine and Rehabilitation* 1999;**80**:615–18.
●3. Enneking WF, Spanier SS, Goodman MA. A system for the surgical staging of musculoskeletal sarcoma. *Clinical Orthopaedics and Related Research* 1980;**153**:106–20.
●4. Simon MA, Aschliman MA, Thomas N, Mankin HJ. Limb-salvage treatment versus amputation for osteosarcoma of the distal end of the femur. *Journal of Bone and Joint Surgery (American)* 1986;**68**:1331–7.
●5. Rosenberg SA, Tepper J, Glatstein E, et al. The treatment of soft-tissue sarcomas of the extremities: prospective randomized evaluations of (1) limb-sparing surgery plus radiation therapy compared with amputation and (2) the role of adjuvant chemotherapy. *Annals of Surgery* 1982;**196**:305–15.
6. Wada T, Kawai A, Ihara K, et al. Construct validity of the Enneking score for measuring function in patients with malignant or aggressive benign tumours of the upper limb. *Journal of Bone and Joint Surgery (British)* 2007;**89**:659–63.
7. Davis AM, Bell RS, Badley EM, et al. Evaluating functional outcome in patients with lower extremity sarcoma. *Clinical Orthopaedics and Related Research* 1999;**358**:90–100.
●8. Davis AM, Wright JG, Williams JI, et al. Development of a measure of physical function for patients with bone and soft tissue sarcoma. *Quality of Life Research* 1996;**5**:508–16.
9. Delaney TF, Park L, Goldberg SI, et al. Radiotherapy for local control of osteosarcoma. *International Journal of Radiation Oncology, Biology, Physics* 2005;**61**:492–8.
10. Bacci G, Forni C, Longhi A, et al. Local recurrence and local control of non-metastatic osteosarcoma of the extremities: a 27-year experience in a single institution. *Journal of Surgical Oncology* 2007;**96**:118–23.

- 11. Davis AM, O'Sullivan B, Bell RS, et al. Function and health status outcomes in a randomized trial comparing preoperative and postoperative radiotherapy in extremity soft tissue sarcoma. *Journal of Clinical Oncology* 2002;**20**:4472-7.
12. Mankin HJ, Mankin CJ, Simon MA. The hazards of the biopsy, revisited. Members of the Musculoskeletal Tumor Society. *Journal of Bone and Joint Surgery (American)* 1996;**78**:656-63.
13. Gerrand CH, Wunder JS, Kandel RA, et al. Classification of positive margins after resection of soft-tissue sarcoma of the limb predicts the risk of local recurrence. *Journal of Bone and Joint Surgery (British)* 2001;**83**:1149-55.
14. Gupta A, Pollock R, Cannon SR, et al. A knee-sparing distal femoral endoprosthesis using hydroxyapatite-coated extracortical plates. Preliminary results. *Journal of Bone and Joint Surgery (British)* 2006;**88**:1367-72.
15. Ward WG, Johnston KS, Dorey FJ, Eckardt JJ. Extramedullary porous coating to prevent diaphyseal osteolysis and radiolucent lines around proximal tibial replacements. A preliminary report. *Journal of Bone and Joint Surgery (American)* 1993;**75**:976-87.
16. Futani H, Minamiszaki T, Nishimoto Y, et al. Long-term follow-up after limb salvage in skeletally immature children with a primary malignant tumor of the distal end of the femur. *Journal of Bone and Joint Surgery (American)* 2006;**88A**:595-603.
17. Ham SJ, Schraffordt KH, Veth RP, et al. Limb salvage surgery for primary bone sarcoma of the lower extremities: Long-term consequences of endoprosthetic reconstructions. *Annals of Surgical Oncology* 1998;**5**:423-36.
18. Torbert JT, Fox EJ, Hosalkar HS, et al. Endoprosthetic reconstructions: results of long-term follow up of 139 patients. *Clinical Orthopaedics and Related Research* 2005;**438**:51-9.
19. Jeys LM, Kulkarni A, Grimer RJ, et al. Endoprosthetic reconstruction for the treatment of musculoskeletal tumors of the appendicular skeleton and pelvis. *Journal of Bone and Joint Surgery (American)* 2008;**90**:1265-71.
20. Jeys LM, Grimer RJ, Carter SR, Tillman RM. Periprosthetic infection in patients treated for an orthopaedic oncological condition. *Journal of Bone and Joint Surgery (American)* 2005;**87**:842-9.
21. Gosheger G, Hardes J, Ahrens H, et al. Silver-coated megaendoprostheses in a rabbit model – an analysis of the infection rate and toxicological side effects. *Biomaterials* 2004;**25**:5547-56.
22. Hardes J, Ahrens H, Gebert C, et al. Lack of toxicological side-effects in silver-coated megaprostheses in humans. *Biomaterials* 2007;**28**:2869-75.
23. Unwin PS, Cannon SR, Grimer RJ, et al. Aseptic loosening in cemented custom-made prosthetic replacements for bone tumours of the lower limb. *Journal of Bone and Joint Surgery (British)* 1996;**78B**:5-13.
24. Mittermyer F, Windhager R, Dominkus M, et al. Revision of the Kotz type of prosthesis for the lower limb. *Journal of Bone and Joint Surgery (British)* 2002;**84B**:401-6.
25. Delloye C, De Nayer P, Allington N, et al. Massive bone allografts in large skeletal defects after tumor surgery: a clinical and microradiographic evaluation. *Archives of Orthopaedic and Trauma Surgery* 1988;**107**:31-41.
26. Gerrand CH, Griffin AM, Davis AM, et al. Large segment allograft survival is improved with intramedullary cement. *Journal of Surgical Oncology* 2003;**84**:198-208.
27. Chen TH, Chen WM, Huang CK. Reconstruction after intercalary resection of malignant bone tumours. *Journal of Bone and Joint Surgery (British)* 2005;**87B**:704-9.
28. Muscolo DL, Ayerza MA, Aponte-Tinao LA, Ranalletta M. Use of distal femoral osteoarticular allografts in limb salvage surgery. *Journal of Bone and Joint Surgery (American)* 2005;**87**:2449-55.
29. Weiland AJ. Vascularised free bone transplants. *Journal of Bone and Joint Surgery (American)* 1981;**63A**:166-9.
30. De Boer HH, Wood MB. Bone changes in the vascularised fibular graft. *Journal of Bone and Joint Surgery (British)* 1989;**71B**:374-8.
31. Minami A, Kasashima T, Iwasaki N, et al. Vascularised fibular grafts. *Journal of Bone and Joint Surgery (British)* 2000;**82B**:1022-5.
32. Spira E, Lubin E. Extracorporeal irradiation of bone tumors. A preliminary report. *Israel Journal of Medical Sciences* 1968;**4**:1015-19.
33. Davidson AW, Hong A, McCarthy SW, Stalley PD. En-bloc resection, extracorporeal irradiation, and re-implantation in limb salvage for bony malignancies. *Journal of Bone and Joint Surgery (British)* 2005;**87**:851-7.
34. Farid Y, Lin PP, Lewis VO, Yasko AW. Endoprosthetic and allograft-prosthetic composite reconstruction of the proximal femur for bone neoplasms. *Clinical Orthopaedics and Related Research* 2006;**442**:223-9.
35. Malawer MM, Sugarbaker PH. *Musculoskeletal Cancer Surgery: Treatment of Sarcoma and Allied Diseases.* Dordrecht, The Netherlands: Kluwer Academic Publishers, 2007.
36. O'Connor MI, Sim FH. Salvage of the limb in the treatment of malignant pelvic tumors. *Journal of Bone and Joint Surgery (American)* 1989;**71**:481-94.
37. Bickels J, Wittig JC, Kollender Y, et al. Reconstruction of the extensor mechanism after proximal tibia endoprosthetic replacement. *Journal of Arthroplasty* 2001;**16**:856-62.
38. Mankin HJ, Hornicek FJ, Harris M. Total femur replacement procedures in tumor treatment. *Clinical Orthopaedics and Related Research* 2005;**438**:60-4.
39. Myers GJ, Abudu AT, Carter SR, et al. The long-term results of endoprosthetic replacement of the proximal tibia for bone tumours. *Journal of Bone and Joint Surgery (British)* 2007;**89**:1632-7.
40. Eralp L, Kocaoglu M, Mohd N, et al. Distal tibial reconstruction with the use of a circular external fixator and an intramedullary nail. The combined technique. *Journal of Bone and Joint Surgery (American)* 2007;**89**:2218-24.

41. Papagelopoulos PJ, Mavrogenis AF, Badekas A, Sim FH. Foot malignancies: a multidisciplinary approach. *Foot and Ankle Clinics* 2003;**8**:751–63.
42. Hanna SA, David LA, Aston WJS, et al. Endoprosthetic replacement of the distal humerus following resection of bone tumours. *Journal of Bone and Joint Surgery (British)* 2007;**89B**:1498–503.
43. Hatano H, Morita T, Kobayashi H, Otsuku H. A ceramic prosthesis for the treatment of tumours of the distal radius. *Journal of Bone and Joint Surgery (British)* 2006;**88B**:1656–8.
44. Kocher MS, Gebhardt MC, Mankin HJ. Reconstruction of the distal aspect of the radius with use of an osteoarticular allograft after excision of a skeletal tumour. *Journal of Bone and Joint Surgery (American)* 1998;**80**:407–19.
45. Pradhan A, Cheung AC, Grimer RJ, et al. Soft tissue sarcomas of the hand. *Journal of Bone and Joint Surgery (British)* 2008;**90B**:209–14.
46. Nagarajan R, Clohisy DR, Neglia JP, et al. Function and quality-of-life of survivors of pelvic and lower extremity osteosarcoma and Ewing's sarcoma: the Childhood Cancer Survivor Study. *British Journal of Cancer* 2004; **91**:1858–65.
47. Gupta A, Meswania J, Pollock R, et al. Non-invasive distal femoral expandable endoprosthesis for limb-salvage surgery in paediatric tumours. *Journal of Bone and Joint Surgery (British)* 2006;**88**:649–54.
48. Canadell J, Forriol F, Cara JA. Removal of metaphyseal bone tumours with preservation of the epiphysis: physeal distraction before excision. *Journal of Bone and Joint Surgery (British)* 1994;**76B**:127–32.

85

Amputations, prosthetics and orthotics

FRANK GOTTSCHALK, RUTH M O'SULLIVAN, DANIEL PORTER

Introduction	954	Prosthetics	963
Gait	954	Orthoses	967
Amputations	957	References	972

NATIONAL BOARD STANDARDS

- To understand gait and the causes of limp
- To understand causes of amputation and when it is indicated
- To know the determinants of wound healing of the stump
- Common levels for amputation
- To request appropriate tests prior to amputation
- Surgical levels of amputations and how they affect energy cost walking
- How to perform an amputation
- To know tissue stabilization
- To learn what a prosthesis is and what an orthosis is
- To know the functional level in spinal cord injury

INTRODUCTION

An understanding of the use of prostheses and orthoses requires knowledge of various aspects of gait, surgery and rehabilitation. Normal gait is the basis for evaluating the amputee and the pathological ambulation. The physician should educate the patient regarding limitations and expectations when a prosthesis is prescribed or when an orthosis is used, and how these appliances may potentially improve patient function.

GAIT

Walking is the repetitive process of sequential lower limb motion to move the body from one location to another, while maintaining upright stability.[1] Walking is a cyclic, energy-efficient activity. It requires that one foot be in contact with the ground at all times – *single-limb support* – with a period when both limbs are in contact with the ground – *double-limb support* (Fig. 85.1). The *step* is the distance between the initial swing and the initial contact of the same limb. *Stride* is the initial contact to initial contact of the same limb (Fig. 85.2). *Velocity* is a function of cadence (steps per unit time) and stride length. *Running* involves a period when neither limb is in contact with the ground. Prerequisites for normal gait include stance-phase stability, swing-phase ground clearance, pre-position of the foot before initial contact, and energy-efficient step length and speed. *Stance phase* occupies 60% of the cycle from initial contact, with progression through loading response, mid-stance, terminal stance and pre-swing. *Swing phase* is 40% of the cycle and starts at initial swing (toe-off), proceeding with limb acceleration to mid-swing, when the limb decelerates at terminal swing before the next cycle (Figs 85.3 and 85.4). During initial swing, the hip and knee flex, and the ankle starts to dorsiflex.

Gait dynamics involve the combined phases of gait and contribute to an energy-efficient process by lessening excursion of the centre of body mass. The head, neck, trunk and arms represent 70% of body weight. The *trunk centre of gravity* of this mass is located just anterior to T10,

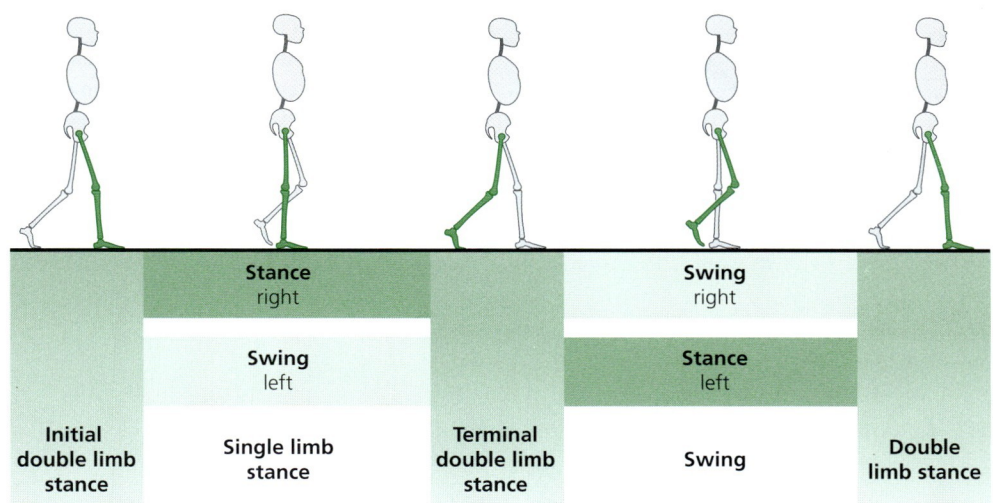

Figure 85.1 Subdivisions of stance and their relationship to bilateral floor contact pattern. Reprinted from Perry J. *Gait Analysis: Normal and Pathological Function.* New York, NY: Slack, 1992, with permission from Slack, Inc.

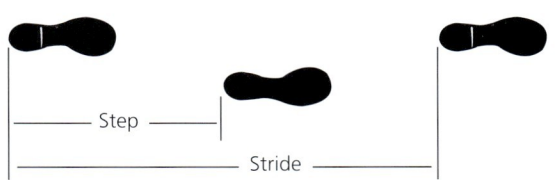

Figure 85.2 Step versus stride. Reprinted from Perry J. *Gait Analysis: Normal and Pathological Function.* New York, NY: Slack, 1992, with permission from Slack, Inc.

which is 33 cm above the hip joints in an individual of average height (184 cm). The body's *line of gravity* is anterior to S2 and provides a reference for the moment arm to the centre of the joint under consideration. The resultant gait pattern resembles a sinusoidal curve.

Determinants of gait (motion patterns)

In mechanical terms, there are six independent degrees of freedom:

1. *Pelvic rotation.* The pelvis rotates about a vertical axis, horizontal rotation, alternately to the left and right of the line of progression, lessening the centre-of-mass deviation in the transverse plane and reducing impact at initial floor contact.
2. *Pelvic list.* The non-weight-bearing contralateral side drops 5°, reducing superior deviation.
3. *Knee flexion at loading.* The stance-phase limb is flexed 15° to dampen the impact of initial loading.
4. *Foot and ankle motion.* Through the subtalar joint, damping of the loading response occurs, leading to stability during mid-stance and efficiency of propulsion at push-off.
5. *Knee motion.* Works together with the foot and ankle to decrease necessary limb motion during walking at a comfortable speed. The knee flexes at initial contact and extends at mid-stance.
6. *Lateral pelvic displacement relates to transfer of body weight onto limb.* The motion is 5 cm over the weight-bearing limb, narrowing the base of support and increasing stance-phase stability.

Muscle action

Agonist and antagonist muscle groups work in concert during the gait cycle to effectively advance the limb through space.[2] The hip flexors advance the limb forward during the swing phase and are opposed during terminal swing before initial contact by the decelerating action of the hip extensors. Most muscle activity is *eccentric*, which is muscle lengthening while contracting, and allows an antagonist muscle to dampen the activity of an agonist and act as a 'shock absorber' (Fig. 85.5). *Isocentric* contraction is muscle length remaining constant during contraction (Table 85.1). Some muscle activity can be *concentric*, in which the muscle shortens to move a joint through space.

Pathological gait involves abnormal gait patterns and is usually caused by multiple factors:[3]

1. Muscle weakness or paralysis decreases the ability to normally move a joint through space. A walking pattern develops based on the specific muscle or muscle group involved and the ability of the individual to achieve a substitution pattern to replace that muscle's action (Table 85.2).
2. Neurological conditions may alter gait by producing muscle weakness, loss of balance, reduced coordination between agonist and antagonist muscle groups (i.e. spasticity) and joint contracture. Hip scissoring is associated with overactive adductors, and knee flexion contracture may be caused by

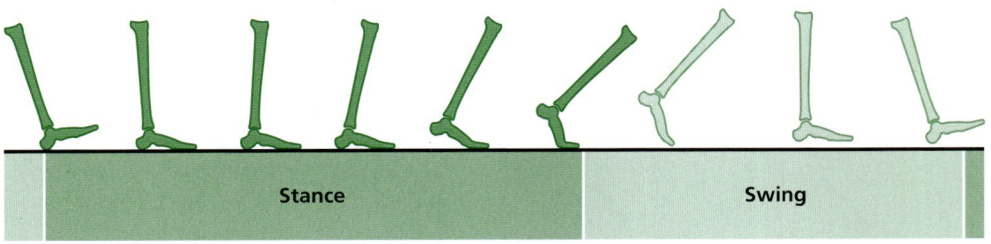

Figure 85.3 Divisions of the gait cycle. Clear and shaded bars represent duration of each phase. Reprinted from Perry J. *Gait Analysis: Normal and Pathological Function.* New York, NY: Slack, 1992, with permission from Slack, Inc.

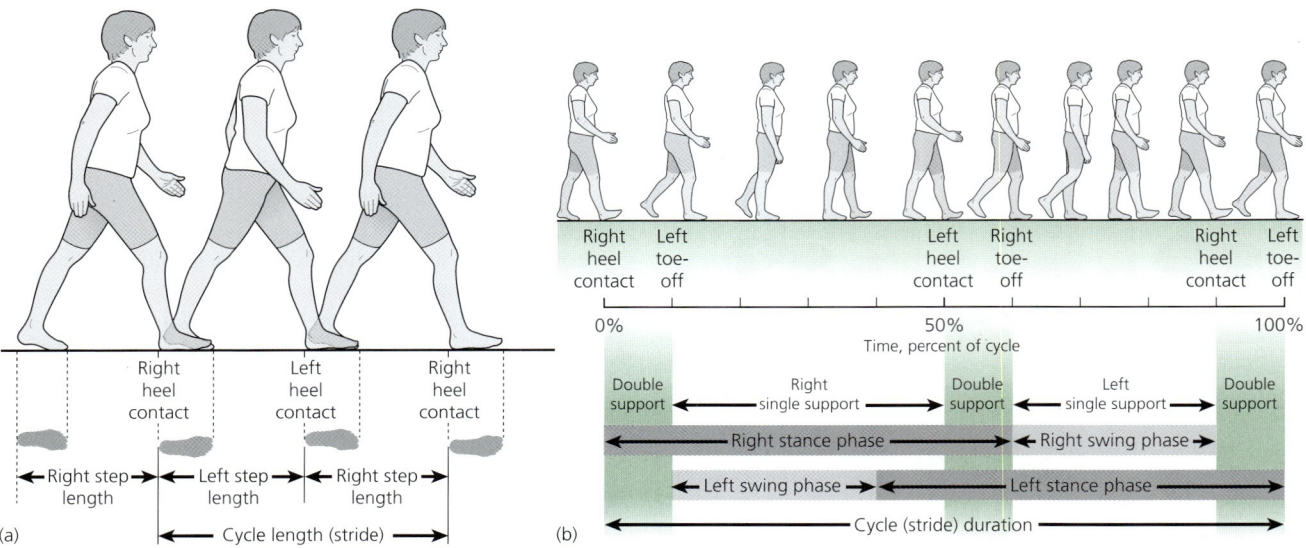

Figure 85.4 Distance and time dimensions of walking cycle. (a) Distance (length). (b) Time. From Inman VT, Ralston H, Todd F. *Human Walking.* Baltimore, MD: Williams & Wilkins, 1981:26.

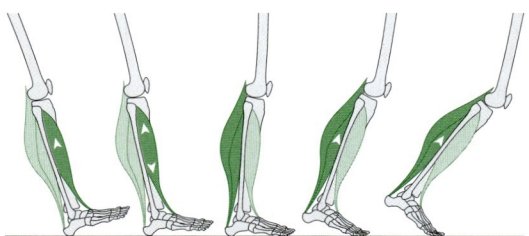

Figure 85.5 Effect of ankle motion, controlled by muscle action, on the pathway of the knee. The smooth and flattened pathway of the knee during stance phase is achieved by forces acting from the leg on the foot. Foot slap is restrained during initial lowering of the foot; afterwards, the plantarflexors raise the heel.

hamstring spasticity. Equinus deformity of the foot and ankle may result in steppage gait and back-setting of the knee.
3. Pain in a limb creates an antalgic gait pattern in which the individual shortens stance phase to lessen the time that the painful limb is loaded. Contralateral swing phase is more rapid.

Table 85.1 Muscle action and function

Muscle	Action	Function
Gluteus medius	Eccentric	Controls pelvic tilt at mid-stance
Gluteus maximus	Concentric	Powers hip extension
Iliopsoas	Concentric	Powers hip flexion
Hip adductors	Eccentric	Control lateral sway (late stance)
Hip abductors	Eccentric	Control pelvic tilt (mid-stance)
Quadriceps	Eccentric	Stabilizes knee at heel strike
Hamstrings	Eccentric	Control rate of knee extension (stance)
Tibialis anterior	Concentric Eccentric[a]	Dorsiflexes ankle at swing Slows plantarflexion rate (initial contact)
Gastrocnemius/ soleus	Eccentric	Slows dorsiflexion rate (stance)

[a] Predominant role.

Table 85.2 Gait abnormalities caused by muscle weakness

Muscle	Phase	Direction	Type of gait	Treatment
Gluteus medius	Stance	Lateral	Abductor lurch	Cane
Gluteus maximus	Stance	Backward	Lurch (hip hyperextension)	
Quadriceps	Stance	Forward	Lurch/back knee gait	AFO
	Swing	Forward	Abnormal hip rotation	
Gastrocnemius/soleus	Stance	Forward	Flat foot (calcaneal) gait	AFO
	Swing	Forward	Delayed heel rise	
Tibialis anterior	Stance	Forward	Foot drop/slap	AFO
	Swing	Forward	Steppage gait	

AFO, ankle–foot orthosis.

4. Joint abnormalities alter gait by changing the range of motion of that joint or by producing pain. Patients with arthritis of the hip and knee may have joint contractures and reduced range of motion. Those with an anterior cruciate-deficient knee have quadriceps avoidance gait, which is a lower than normal net quadriceps moment during mid-stance.
5. Hemiplegia characteristically is the prolongation of stance and double-limb support. Associated problems are ankle equinus, limitation of knee flexion and increased hip flexion. Surgical correction of equinus is usually 1 year after onset. Gait impairment may be excessive plantarflexion, weakness and balance problems.
6. Crutches and canes are walking aids to assist with stability by providing two additional loading points. Canes help shift the centre of gravity to the affected side when the cane is used in the contralateral hand. This decreases the joint reaction forces of the affected lower limb and reduces pain.

Forces across the knee may be four to seven times body weight, and 70% of load across the knee occurs through the medial compartment.

AMPUTATIONS

Amputation surgery should be considered as a reconstructive procedure in those individuals who require an amputation.[4] An amputation is often more appropriate as an option than limb salvage, especially when considering potential activity levels and expected function. There are several indications for an amputation, and the level of the amputation is dependent on the original pathology as well as the underlying general disease processes. The surgeon should be aware that the surgery requires attention to detail and that postoperative care and patient rehabilitation are an integral part of a team concept. The team's focus is centred on the patient, and members of the team consist of the physician, nurses, various therapists and the prosthetist. Optimum function is the goal of rehabilitation and will vary from

Table 85.3 Energy expenditure for amputation

	% energy above baseline	Speed (m min^{-1})	O$_2$ cost level (mL kg^{-1} m^{-1})
Long transtibial	10	70	0.17
Average transtibial	25	60	0.20
Short transtibial	40	50	0.20
Bilateral transtibial	41	50	0.20
Transfemoral	65	40	0.28
Wheelchair	0–8	70	0.16

patient to patient depending on amputation level and cause of the amputation. A reasonable functional goal should be considered at the time of amputation and expectations should be realistic in terms of the overall medical condition of the amputee.

The metabolic cost of walking is increased with proximal-level amputations, and is inversely proportional to the length of the residual limb and the number of functional joints preserved.[5,6] The higher the amputation, the greater the decrease in self-selected, maximum walking speed. Oxygen consumption is increased the higher the amputation (or the shorter the stump); thus the transfemoral amputee with peripheral vascular disease uses close to maximum energy expenditure during normal self-selected velocity walking. Transtibial amputations preserve the knee joint and therefore have less energy expenditure for gait (Table 85.3).

The soft-tissue envelope acts as an interface between the bone of the stump and the prosthetic socket. Ideally, the soft tissue is a mobile, securely attached muscle mass covering the bone end and full-thickness skin that tolerates the direct pressures and pistoning within the prosthetic socket. It is rare for the prosthetic socket to achieve a perfect intimate fit. A non-adherent soft-tissue envelope allows some degree of mobility, or 'pistoning', of the bone within the soft-tissue envelope, thus eliminating the shear forces that produce tissue breakdown and ulceration. Load transfer (i.e. weight bearing) occurs by either end bearing or load distribution over a large area of the stump

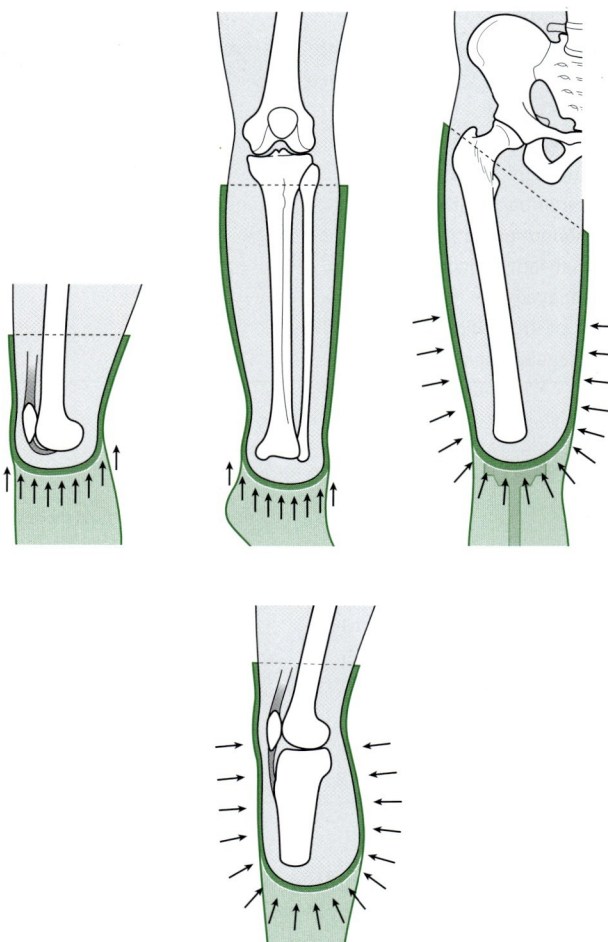

Figure 85.6 End bearing with load transfer is achieved in the knee disarticulation and the ankle disarticulation amputations. Load distribution over a large area is accomplished in transfemoral amputations with either a quadrilateral socket or an adducted narrow medial–lateral socket. The transtibial amputation transfers weight across the whole stump, with the knee flexed approximately 10°.

(Fig. 85.6). End bearing is noted in knee or ankle (Syme's amputation) disarticulations. Intimacy of the prosthetic socket is necessary only for suspension. When the amputation is performed through a long bone (i.e. transfemoral or transtibial), the end of the stump does not take all the weight and the load is transferred by the total contact method. This process requires an intimate prosthetic socket fit and 7–10° of flexion of the knee for transtibial amputation and 5–10° of adduction and flexion of the femur for transfemoral amputation.

Amputation wound healing depends on several factors, which include vascular supply, nutrition and an adequate immune status. Patients with malnutrition or immune deficiency have a high rate of wound failure or infection. A serum albumin level below 3.5 g dL^{-1} indicates a malnourished patient. An absolute lymphocyte count below 1500 mm^{-3} is a sign of immune deficiency. If possible, amputation surgery should be delayed in patients with stable gangrene until these values can be improved by nutritional support, usually in the form of oral hyperalimentation. In severely affected patients, nasogastric or percutaneous gastric feeding tubes are sometimes necessary. When infection or severe ischaemic pain requires urgent surgery, open amputation at the most distal viable level, followed by open wound management, can be accomplished until wound healing can be optimized. Oxygenated blood is absolutely necessary for wound healing and a haemoglobin concentration of more than 10 g dL^{-1} is preferred. Amputation wounds generally heal by collateral flow, so arteriography is rarely useful for predicting wound healing. Doppler ultrasonography has been used as the measure of vascular inflow to predict wound healing in the ischaemic limb. An absolute Doppler pressure of 70 mmHg was originally described as the minimum inflow to support wound healing. The ischaemic index is the ratio of the Doppler pressure at the level being tested to the brachial systolic pressure. It is generally accepted that an ischaemic index of 0.5 or greater at the surgical level is necessary to support wound healing. The ischaemic index at the ankle (i.e. the ankle–brachial index) is the most accepted method for assessing adequate inflow to the ischaemic limb.

Standard Doppler ultrasonography measures arterial pressure. In the normal limb the area under the Doppler waveform tracing is a measure of flow.[7] These values are falsely elevated and not predictive in at least 15% of patients with diabetes and peripheral vascular disease, because of the incompressibility and loss of compliance of calcified peripheral arteries. The toe pressure ischaemic index is more accurate in these patients and, if greater than 0.45, is usually predictive of adequate blood flow. Transcutaneous partial pressure of oxygen has been used as a measure of vascular inflow. It records the oxygen-delivering capacity of the vascular system to the level of contemplated surgery. Values greater than 40 mmHg correlate with acceptable wound-healing rates without the false-positive values seen in non-compliant peripheral vascular diseased vessels. Pressures less than 20 mmHg are predictive for poor healing potential.

Paediatric amputations are usually the result of congenital limb deficiencies, trauma or tumours.[8,9] Congenital amputations are a result of failure of formation of the limb. The present classification system is based on the original work of a 1975 Conference of the International Society for Prosthetics and Orthotics and a subsequent International Organization for Standardization (ISO) standard. Deficiencies are either longitudinal or transverse, with the potential for intercalary deficits. Amputation surgery is rarely indicated in congenital upper limb deficiency; even rudimentary appendages can be functionally useful. In the lower limb, amputation of an unstable segment may allow end bearing and enhanced walking (ankle disarticulation for fibular hemimelia). In the growing child, disarticulations should be performed only when it is necessary to maintain maximal residual limb length and to prevent terminal bony overgrowth. Such overgrowth occurs most commonly in the humerus, fibula, tibia and femur, in that order, and is most common in diaphyseal amputations.[10] Numerous surgical procedures have been described to resolve this problem, but the best method is surgical revision of the stump with adequate resection of bone or autogenous osteochondral capping of the stump.

Indications for amputation

VASCULAR DISEASE

The majority of amputations in the developed countries are for vascular disease and diabetes mellitus. Often, the extremity has developed gangrene or the vascular flow cannot be reconstructed. It has been reported that 90% of amputations are associated with vascular disease. The prevalence of vascular disease is estimated at 8% of the population in persons older than 55 years. There is an increase in the number of persons who have limb-threatening ischaemia because of increased longevity of the population and an increase in the occurrence of diabetes mellitus. Smoking has been shown to be a major risk factor in the development of vascular disease.

Many patients have widespread systemic evidence of vascular impairment that may have an effect on postoperative rehabilitation. The individual's physical reserve is often reduced, affecting the ability to use a prosthesis. Failed bypass operations may result in a higher amputation level and more complications.

For patients to learn to walk with a prosthesis and care for their stump, they must possess certain cognitive capacities. These are (1) memory, (2) attention, (3) concentration and (4) organization. Patients with cognitive deficits or psychiatric disorders have a low probability of becoming successful prosthetic users. A majority of patients are diabetic with inherent immune deficiency. Important risk factors for amputation in diabetic patients are the presence of peripheral neuropathy and the development of deformity and infection. Appropriate consultation with physical therapy, social work and psychology departments is important to determine rehabilitation potential. Medical consultation will help determine cardiopulmonary reserve. The vascular surgeon should determine whether vascular reconstruction is feasible or appropriate. The biological amputation level is the most distal functional amputation level which will support wound healing. This level is determined by the presence of adequate viable local tissue to construct a stump capable of supporting weight bearing, an adequate vascular inflow, and a serum albumin and total lymphocyte count sufficient to aid surgical wound healing. Amputation-level selection is determined by combining the biological amputation level with the rehabilitation potential to determine a level that provides functional independence. Morbidity and mortality rates have remained unchanged for several decades. Thirty per cent of patients die in the first 3 months and nearly 50% within the first year. Overall prosthetic use is 43%.

TRAUMA

Traumatic amputations are done less frequently than those for limb ischaemia, but have seen a small increase with the advent of improved life-saving techniques in severe injuries.[11] Most often, the mangled extremity cannot be salvaged and the decision for amputation is made early. The dilemma is in those extremities that may still be viable and where limb salvage is considered, but ultimate function may be severely compromised. Disability after traumatic amputation may be high and associated with other injuries and post-traumatic stress disorder.

Patients undergoing amputation for trauma are younger than those requiring amputation for disease. The indications for amputation are a combination of soft-tissue, vascular, neurological and bone damage so severe as to preclude limb salvage. Injuries after blasts and explosions cause extensive soft-tissue damage that creates a zone of injury that may be more extensive than initially recognized. Delays in treatment may result in a more proximal amputation because of infection and additional tissue damage. Wounds must always be left open and at least a two-stage procedure is necessary to minimize wound infection and permit additional debridement. Split-thickness skin grafting is permissible provided there is adequate soft tissue (muscle) cover of the bone.

INFECTION

Severe soft-tissue infections occasionally result in the need for amputation to control spread of the problem. Severe osteomyelitis may also not be salvageable and may require an amputation. Two-stage operations are required at a minimum with appropriate antibiotic coverage. Adequate debridement is an absolute requirement prior to wound closure.

TUMOUR

Most often the level of amputation is determined by the site and type of tumour as well as the size at presentation. Amputation is a consideration when limb salvage does not provide adequate functional restoration. There is still controversy in the literature when limb salvage is compared with amputation regarding energy expenditure to ambulate, quality-of-life measures and function with activities of daily living. Expected functional outcome should include the psychosocial and body image values associated with limb salvage. These concerns should be balanced with the apparent improved functional performance and reduced concern for late mechanical injury associated with amputation and prosthetic limb fitting.

General principles

An important principle of amputation surgery is tissue stabilization.[12,13] The creation of a functional stump involves the preservation of muscle function and soft-tissue sensation. Surgery is geared to removal of non-viable tissue and using remaining tissues to create a sensate and functioning stump. Adequate soft-tissue padding is important in the creation of a stable, comfortable stump that is able to provide stability in a prosthetic socket.

When considering the reconstructive aspect of an amputation, whether being done for trauma, ischaemia, infection or tumour, it is important to preserve as much length as is commensurate with the disease process. Bony prominences should be removed and joint function proximal to the amputation site should be near normal. The soft-tissue envelope should be able to withstand normal forces and pressure and provide padding to allow for comfortable socket fit.

SKIN

A sensate stump is important for protection and proprioception. This reduces the potential for skin breakdown when wearing a prosthesis. The presence of proprioception helps when pressure is applied to the prosthesis such as with weight bearing or using an upper limb device. The skin is the interface with the socket and is important for force and load transfer in both directions.

The creation of appropriate skin flaps is important to allow soft-tissue closure without tension and to reduce the risk of wound breakdown. Skin flaps should be created longer than anticipated to avoid the need to shorten the stump unnecessarily. The suture line should be away from any pressure area and should be mobile. Scar placement should be proximal to the end of the stump.

Uncomplicated healing leads to mobile scar and soft tissue over bony areas which is then more durable and pliable. Adherent skin, scar and soft tissue is tender and painful, especially when subject to socket pressure.

To maintain adequate viability of the soft-tissue flaps, one should avoid separating the subcutaneous tissue from the muscle fascia, thus preserving a myocutaneous flap.

MUSCLE

Awareness of the difference between myoplasty and myodesis is important. Myoplasty is the suturing of agonist to antagonist muscles over the end of the bone without anchoring them to the bone. This construct does not provide adequate muscle stability and does not restore resting muscle tension. The construct acts as a sling over the end of the bone and slides back and forth, ultimately creating a bursa at the end of the stump and leading to increased pain and discomfort.

Myodesis is the anchoring of intact or sectioned muscles directly to bone to restore resting muscle tension and to provide a new insertion for those muscles. This provides a stump with good tissue tension and allows for easier prosthetic fitting. The stable soft-tissue foundation allows the patient to be functional with a prosthesis and reduce potential complications related to unstable prosthetic fit. Improved muscle function translates into better stump control and easier prosthetic use.

NERVES

Sectioning of nerves is inevitable in an amputation. The healing response is to form a neuroma and occurs in every nerve that is transected. The end of the nerve should be left deep in muscle and away from any potential pressure area. Painful neuromata may result in difficulty with prosthetic use and be felt as a phantom sensation or pain. Multiple methods of dealing with the nerve at the time of amputation have been tried, all with varied success. The most accepted method of transecting a nerve during amputation is to draw the nerve distally without creating a traction lesion, transect it, and allow retraction away from the end of the stump.

BONE

Most amputations are done through diaphyseal bone, and bone ends should be rounded. The length chosen is that which will allow soft-tissue closure without tension, and still preserve adequate length of the stump. Sufficient bone should be exposed to provide for direct muscle attachment. Whenever possible, a power saw should be used to cut and round the bone. Cooling of the blade is necessary. Periosteal stripping is to be avoided and only that amount necessary to expose bone for cutting should be lifted from the bone.

BLOOD VESSELS

Arteries and veins should be identified individually and ligated separately. It is important to use suture that is secure enough to prevent bleeding. Cauterization should be used for small bleeding points. Bleeding from bone ends can be minimized by pulling muscle over the end of the bone and direct anchoring to bone. Bone wax should be avoided since it remains as a foreign material and is a potential nidus for infection.

Amputation levels: lower limb

Terminology regarding amputation levels is that recommended by the ISO to provide conformity in definitions and procedures. Levels of amputation are shown in Fig. 85.7.

AMPUTATIONS OF THE FOOT

The hallux should be amputated distal to the insertion of the flexor hallucis brevis. Isolated second-toe amputation should be performed just distal to the proximal phalanx metaphyseal flare, so that it acts as a buttress to

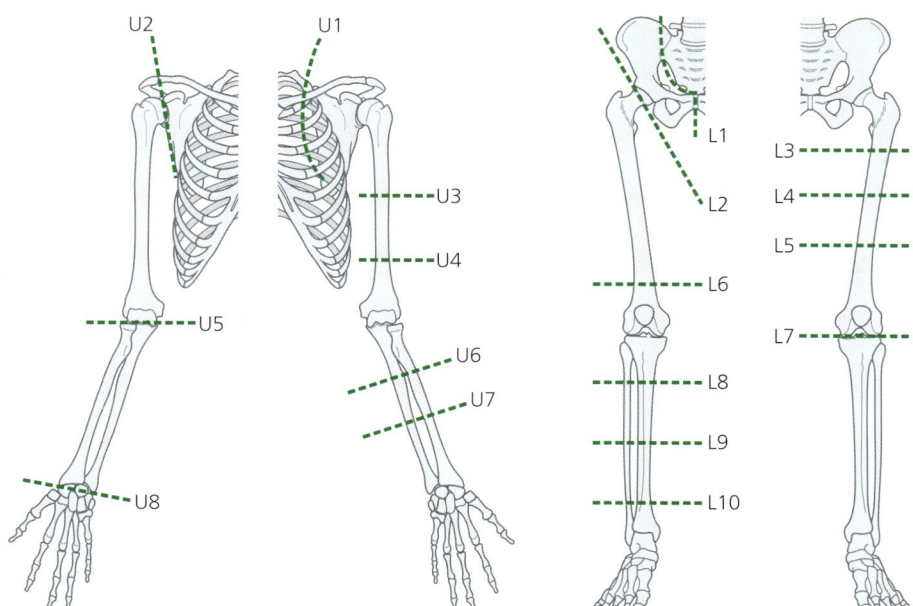

Figure 85.7 Composite illustration of upper (U) limb and lower (L) limb amputations.

prevent late hallux valgus. Single outer (first or fifth) ray resections function well in standard shoes. Resection of more than one ray leaves a narrow forefoot that is difficult to fit in shoes and often results in a late equinus deformity. Central ray resections are complicated by prolonged wound healing and rarely outperform midfoot amputation.

Transmetatarsal and Lisfranc tarsal–metatarsal amputation have little functional difference between them. The long plantar flap acts as a myocutaneous flap and is preferred to fish-mouth dorsal–plantar flaps. Transmetatarsal amputation should be through the proximal metaphyses of the metatarsals to prevent late plantar pressure ulcers under the residual bone ends. Percutaneous tendon Achilles lengthening should be performed with transmetatarsal and Lisfranc amputations to prevent the late development of equinus or equinovarus. Late varus can be corrected with transfer of the tibialis anterior tendon to the neck of the talus.

Some authors have reported reasonable functional outcomes with hindfoot amputation, but most experts recommend avoiding these levels if possible in diabetic and vascular patients. The Chopart amputation is a midtarsal amputation disarticulating the talonavicular and calcaneocuboid joints and is most useful in trauma and tumours. Although children have been reported to function reasonably well, adults retain an inadequate lever arm and are prone to experience fixed equinus of the heel if tendon Achilles lengthening and tibialis anterior tendon transfer are not performed. The Boyd and Pirogoff amputations rely on fusion of the calcaneus to the tibia and thus provide a weight-bearing platform directly on the heel. In general, these amputations are not recommended because of problems with bone healing and poor function.

ANKLE DISARTICULATION

Ankle disarticulation (Syme's amputation) allows direct load transfer and is rarely complicated by late residual limb ulcers or tissue breakdown. It provides a stable gait pattern that rarely requires prosthetic gait training after surgery. Surgery should be performed in one stage, even in ischaemic limbs with insensate heel pads. A patent posterior tibial artery is necessary to ensure healing. The malleoli and metaphyseal flares should be removed from the tibia and fibula, but the remaining tibial articular surface should be retained to provide a resilient end-bearing stump. The heel pad should be secured to the tibia either anteriorly through drill holes or posteriorly by securing the Achilles tendon.

TRANSTIBIAL (BELOW KNEE) AMPUTATION

A long posterior myocutaneous flap is the preferred method of creating a soft-tissue envelope. The tibia should be transected at a level compatible with optimal wound healing. Ideally, the remaining tibia should be between one-third and two-thirds of its original length but not shorter than at least 12–15 cm below the knee joint, provided adequate gastrocnemius or soleus can be used to construct a durable soft-tissue envelope. The fibula is transected at the level of the tibia, but not more than 1 cm shorter. The fibula should be stable and some surgeons have promoted a bone bridge as a method of increasing end bearing. There is no scientific evidence that this occurs, and stability of the fibula is most likely to provide improved fitting of a prosthesis. Posterior muscle should be secured to the bevelled anterior tibia by myodesis through drill holes or to periosteum. Modified soft-tissue flaps may be necessary in trauma and some vascular reconstructions. The skew flap relies on vascular supply of the saphenous and sural vessels and allows for salvage of skin flaps and fascia in patients who have had bypass procedures. Rigid dressings are preferred during the early postoperative period, and early prosthetic fitting may be started 5–21 days after surgery, if the stump is capable of transferring load and the patient has satisfactory physical reserve.

KNEE DISARTICULATION (THROUGH-KNEE AMPUTATION)

The current recommended technique uses a long posterior flap with gastrocnemius muscle as end padding. An alternative is to use sagittal skin flaps and cover the end of the femur with gastrocnemius to act as a soft-tissue envelope end pad. The patellar tendon is sutured to the cruciate ligaments in the femoral condylar notch, leaving the patella on the anterior femur. This level is generally used in the non-walker who can support wound healing at the transtibial or distal level. Knee disarticulation is muscle balanced, provides an excellent weight-bearing platform for sitting and provides a lever arm for transfer. When performed in a potential walker, it provides end bearing for load transfer of the stump.

TRANSFEMORAL (ABOVE KNEE) AMPUTATION

This increases energy cost for walking. Peripheral vascular disease transfemoral amputees are unlikely to become good walkers, so salvaging the limb at the knee disarticulation, or transtibial, level is critical to maintaining functional walking independence. With greater length, the lever arm, suspension and limb advancement are optimized. The optimal transfemoral bone length is 12 cm above the knee joint to accommodate the prosthetic knee (Fig. 85.8). Adductor myodesis is important for maintaining femoral adduction during the stance phase of gait to allow optimal prosthetic function (Fig. 85.9). The major deforming force is into abduction and flexion. Adductor myodesis at normal muscle tension eliminates the problem of adductor roll in the groin. Transecting adductor magnus results in a loss of 70% of adductor pull (Fig. 85.10). Rigid dressings are difficult to apply and maintain at this level. Elastic compression dressings are used and may be suspended about the opposite iliac crest.

HIP DISARTICULATION

Hip disarticulation is infrequently performed, and only an occasional few of these amputees become meaningful prosthetic users because of the high energy requirements for walking. When possible, a gluteal myocutaneous flap is used to cover the hip or pelvis. Post-trauma or tumour patients occasionally use the prosthesis for limited activity. These patients sit in their prosthesis and must use their torso to achieve momentum to 'throw' the limb forward to advance it.

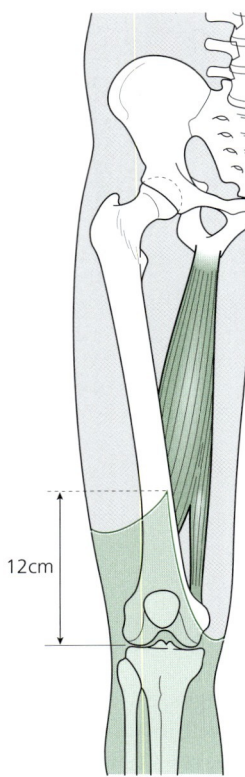

Figure 85.8 Level of amputation and medial myocutaneous flap. Redrawn with permission from Gottschalk F. Transfemoral amputation. In: Bowker J, Michael J (eds). *Atlas of Limb Prosthetics: Surgical, Prosthetic, and Rehabilitation Principles.* St. Louis, MO: Mosby Year Book, 1992:479–86.

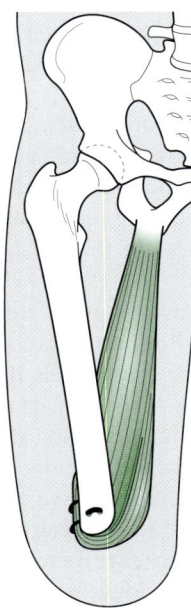

Figure 85.9 Attachment of the adductor magnus to the lateral femur. Redrawn with permission from Gottschalk F. Transfemoral amputation. In: Bowker J, Michael J (eds). *Atlas of Limb Prosthetics: Surgical, Prosthetic, and Rehabilitation Principles.* St. Louis, MO: Mosby Year Book, 1992:479–86.

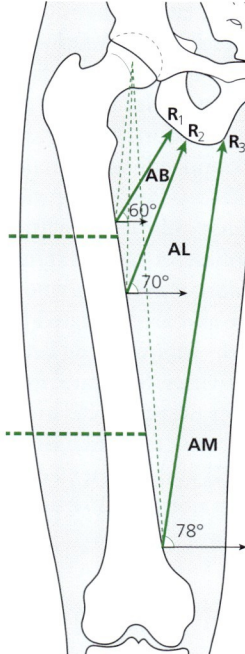

Figure 85.10 Moment arms of the three adductor muscles. Loss of the distal attachment of adductor magnus (AM) will result in a loss of 70% of the adductor pull. R1, R2 and R3 are the resultant forces of the three adductor muscles. AB, adductor brevis; AL, adductor longus. Redrawn with permission from Gottschalk F, Kourosh S, Stills M, et al. Does socket configuration influence the position of the femur in above-knee amputation? *Journal of Prosthetics and Orthotics* 1989;**2**:94–102.

Amputation levels: upper limb

WRIST DISARTICULATION

This level (Fig. 85.7) has two advantages over transradial amputation:

1. preservation of more forearm rotation because of preservation of the distal radioulnar joint
2. improved prosthetic suspension because of the flare of the distal radius.

Wrist disarticulation provides challenges to the prosthetist that may outweigh its benefits since, cosmetically, the prosthetic limb is longer than the contralateral limb and, if myoelectric components are used, the motor and battery cannot be hidden within the prosthetic shank. High levels of function can be obtained at this level of amputation.

TRANSRADIAL AMPUTATION

Forearm rotation and strength are directly related to the length of the transradial (below elbow) amputation stump. The optimal length is the junction of the middle and distal thirds of the forearm, where the soft-tissue envelope can be repaired by myodesis and the components of a myoelectric prosthesis can be hidden within the prosthetic shank. Because function at this level is accomplished by the prosthesis with an opening and closing terminal device, elbow joint retention is essential.

ELBOW DISARTICULATION

The length and shape of elbow disarticulation provide improved suspension and lever-arm capacity. To improve suspension and reduce the need for shoulder harnessing, a 45–60° distal humeral osteotomy is performed. Patients with complete brachial plexus injury and a non-functioning hand and forearm may be best treated by a transradial amputation or elbow disarticulation, which can be fitted with a prosthesis. When not due to Raynaud's or Buerger's disease, gangrene of the upper limb represents end-stage disease, especially in the diabetic patient. These patients experience a high mortality rate and do not survive beyond 24 months. Localized amputations are unlikely to heal. When surgery becomes necessary, amputation should be performed at the trans-radial level to achieve wound healing during the final months of the patient's life.

TRANSHUMERAL AMPUTATION

Muscle anchorage is important and should be directly to bone. The functional impairment of a transhumeral amputation is significant and prosthetic use is cumbersome. As much length of the humerus should be retained as is compatible with adequate soft-tissue closure without tension. Myocutaneous flaps are developed and may be sagittal or anteroposterior. Keeping the humeral head maintains the shoulder contour and makes suspension of clothing easier.

SHOULDER DISARTICULATION AND SCAPULOTHORACIC AMPUTATION

A deltoid myofasciocutaneous flap is advised for shoulder disarticulation and the flap is advanced distally over the axillary area. Axillary skin should be excised. Scapulothoracic amputation is a drastic procedure and may be cosmetically disfiguring. It entails removal of the shoulder girdle and upper limb, leaving the thoracic wall intact.

PROSTHETICS

Upper limb

The shoulder provides the centre of radius of the functional sphere of the upper limb. The elbow acts as the caliper to position the hand at a workable distance from that centre to perform tasks. Multiple joint segment tasks are usually done simultaneously, whereas upper limb prostheses perform these same tasks sequentially; thus, joint and residual limb length salvage is directly correlated with functional outcome. Motion at the retained joints is essential to maximize that function. Residual limb length is important for prosthetic socket suspension and for providing the lever arm necessary to 'drive' the prosthesis through space. Limb salvage is more critical for the upper limb, where sensation is critical to function. An insensate prosthesis provides less function than a partially sensate, partially functional salvaged limb. After amputation, prosthetic fitting should be done as soon as possible, even before complete wound healing has occurred. Outcomes of prosthetic limb use vary from 70% to 85% when prosthetic fitting occurs within 30 days of amputation, for transradial amputation, in contrast with <30% when started late. Myoelectric prostheses provide good cosmetic appearance and are used for sedentary work. They can be used in any position, including overhead activity, and are most successful in the mid-length transradial amputee, in which only the terminal device needs to be activated. Body-powered prostheses are used for heavy labour. The terminal device is activated by shoulder flexion and abduction. Elbow flexion and extension of the prosthesis are controlled by shoulder extension and depression. Optimal mechanical efficiency of figure-of-eight harnesses requires the harness ring to be at the spinous process of C7 and slightly to the non-amputated side.

When the residual forearm is so short as to preclude an adequate lever arm for driving the prosthesis through space, supracondylar suspension (Munster socket) and step-up hinges can be used to augment function. Elbow disarticulation and transhumeral amputations require two motions to develop prehension, making both levels significantly less efficient and the prosthesis heavier than that for amputation at the transradial level. The best function with the least weight at the lowest cost is provided by hybrid prosthetic systems combining myoelectric, traditional body-powered and body-driven switch components. These levels provide minimal function because the patient must sequentially control two joints and a terminal device. When the lever-arm capacity of the humerus is lost in proximal transhumeral or shoulder disarticulation amputations, limited function can be achieved with a manual universal shoulder joint positioned by the opposite hand, combined with lightweight hybrid prosthetic components.

Lower limb

PROSTHETIC FEET

Several designs are available and are divided into five classes:

1. Dynamic response feet which may absorb loads and decrease shear forces to the residual limb. Most dynamic response feet have a flexible keel and are the standard for general use (Fig. 85.11). Correct dynamic prosthetic foot selection requires information about the patient's height, weight, activity level, access to a prosthetist for maintenance, cosmesis and funding. Dynamic response feet may be grouped into articulated and non-articulated feet, which have short or long keels. Articulated dynamic response feet allow inversion and eversion and rotation of the foot and are useful for activities on uneven surfaces.

The keel deforms under load, becoming a spring and allowing dorsiflexion, thereby decreasing the loading on the sound side and providing a spring-like response for push-off. Posterior projection of the keel provides a response at heel strike for smooth transition through stance phase. A sagittal split allows for moderate inversion or eversion. Shortened keels are not as responsive and are indicated for the moderate activity ambulator, whereas long keels are for very high-demand activities. Separate prosthetic feet for running and lower demand activities may be indicated. The dynamic response feet, including the Seattle foot, Carbon Copy II/III and the Flex Foot, allow amputees to undertake most normal activities (Fig. 85.12).

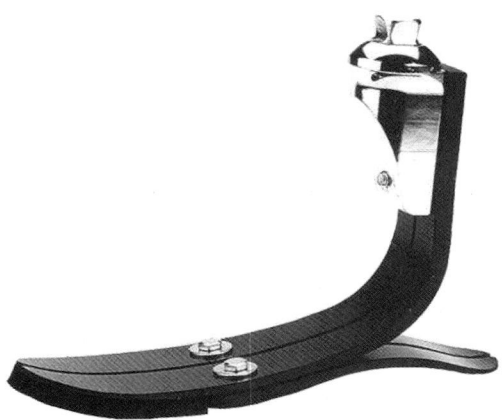

Figure 85.11 Carbon fibre dynamic-response foot with split toe for assistance on uneven ground.

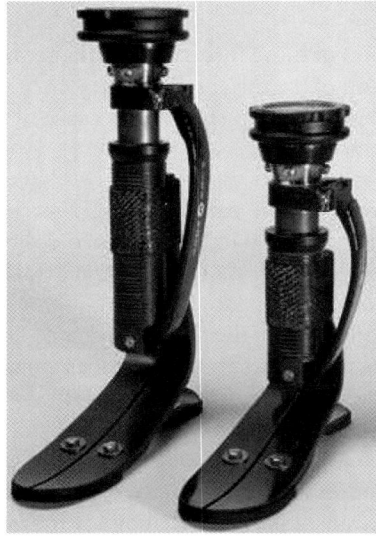

Figure 85.12 Flex Foot with carbon fibre leaf and shock-absorbing leaf spring. Courtesy of Flex Foot, Inc., Aliso Viejo, CA, USA.

2. The elastic keel foot was the earliest of the flexible feet. Known as the SAFE (stationary ankle flexible endoskeletal) foot, it provided a smoother roll over.
3. The multiaxis foot provides inversion, eversion and transverse rotation that is suitable for uneven terrain.
4. The single-axis foot is based on an ankle hinge that provides dorsiflexion and plantarflexion. The disadvantages of the single-axis foot include poor durability and cosmesis.
5. The SACH (solid ankle, cushioned heel) foot has been the standard for decades and was appropriate for general use in low-demand patients. It may lead to overload problems on the non-amputated foot, and its use is being discontinued.

PROSTHETIC SHANKS

The shank is the structural link between prosthetic components. Two varieties exist: endoskeletal, with a soft exterior and load-bearing tubing inside, and exoskeletal, with a hard, load-bearing exterior shell. Rotator units are sometimes added for patients involved in twisting activities (e.g. golf, sitting cross-legged).

PROSTHETIC KNEES

These are used in transfemoral and knee disarticulation prostheses and are chosen based on patient needs. Prosthetic knees provide controlled knee motion in the prosthesis. Alignment stability (the position of the prosthetic knee in relation to the patient's line of weight bearing) is important in the design and fitting of prosthetic knees. Placing the knee centre of rotation posterior to the weight line allows control in the stance phase but makes flexion difficult. Alternatively, with the knee centre of rotation anterior to the weight line, flexion is made easier but at the expense of control. Only the polycentric knee takes advantage of both options by having a variable centre of rotation. Six basic types of knees are available:

1. *Polycentric (four-bar linkage) knee.* This has a moving instant centre of rotation that provides for different stability characteristics during the gait cycle and may allow increased flexion for sitting. It is recommended for patients with transfemoral amputations, patients with knee disarticulations and bilateral amputees (Fig. 85.13).
2. *Stance-phase control (weight activated, or safety) knee.* Functions like a constant-friction knee during the swing phase but 'freezes' by application of a high-friction housing when weight is applied to the limb. Its use is primarily reserved for older patients, high-level amputees or use on uneven terrain.
3. *Fluid-control (hydraulic and pneumatic) knee.* Allows adjustment of cadence response by changing resistance to knee flexion via a piston mechanism. The design prevents excessive flexion and is extended earlier in the gait cycle, allowing a more fluid gait. The knee is best used in active patients who prefer greater utility and variability at the expense of more weight.
4. *Constant-friction knee.* A hinge that is designed to dampen knee swing via a screw or rubber pad that applies friction to the knee bolt. It is a general utility knee and may be used on uneven terrain. It is the most common knee used in childhood prosthetics. Its major disadvantages are that it allows only single-speed walking and relies solely on alignment for stance-phase stability and is therefore not recommended for older, weaker patients.
5. *Variable-friction (cadence control) knee.* Allows resistance to knee flexion to increase as the knee extends by employing a number of staggered friction pads. This knee allows walking at different speeds but is not durable and is not available in endoskeletal systems.
6. *Manual locking knee.* This consists of a constant-friction knee hinge with a positive lock in extension that can be unlocked to allow function similar to that of a constant-friction knee. The knee is often left locked in extension for more stability. The knee has limited indications and is used primarily in weak, unstable patients, those patients just learning to use prostheses and blind amputees.

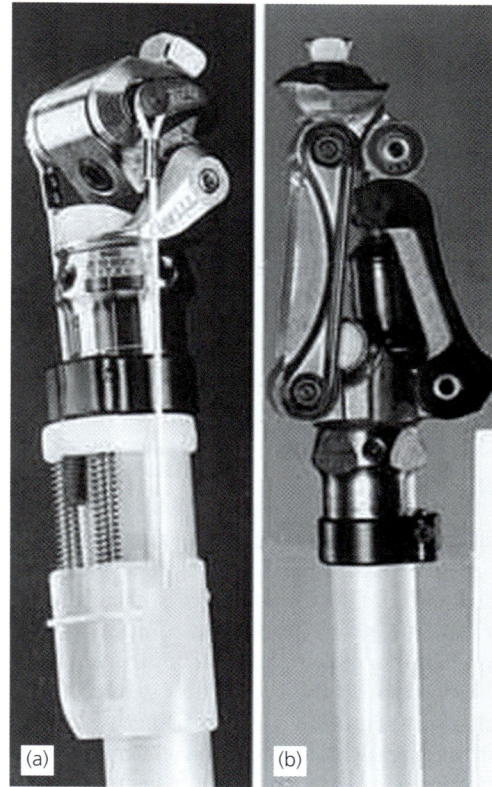

Figure 85.13 (a) Modular endoskeletal polycentric knee with hydraulic swing phase control unit. (b) Microprocessor knee unit for variation in cadence and stair climbing. Courtesy of Otto Bock Orthopaedic Industries, Minneapolis, MN, USA.

Table 85.4 Characteristics of various prosthetic knees

Knee	Action	Advantages	Disadvantages
Constant friction	Limits flexion	Durable, long resistance	Decreased stability
Variable friction	Varies with flexion	Variable cadence	Durability poor
Stance control	Friction brake	Stability during stance	Durability poor, difficult on stairs
Polycentric	Instant centre moves	Stable, increased flexion	Durability poor, heavy
Manual locking	Unlock to sit	Maximum stability	Abnormal gait
Fluid control	Deceleration in swing	Variable cadence	Weight, cost

Information on the various types of prosthetic knees is summarized in Table 85.4.

SUSPENSION SYSTEMS

Suspension is provided in modern lower extremity prosthetics primarily through socket design and suspension sleeves. The use of straps and belts is usually for supplementation. Sockets are prosthetic components designed to provide comfortable functional control and even pressure distribution on the amputated stump. Sockets can be hard (rigid or unlined) or soft (lined with a resilient material and/or flexible shell). In general, suction and socket contour are the primary suspension modalities used. The suction socket provides an airtight seal via a pressure differential between the socket and atmosphere. Total contact support of the residual limb surface prevents oedema formation.

Transtibial suspension

Gel liner suspension systems with a locking pin are the preferred method of suspension. Liners are made from silicone, urethane, or thermoplastic elastomer. The sleeve rolls onto the stump, and the locking pin is then locked into the socket (Fig. 85.14). The liners provide suspension through suction and friction and act as the socket interface. Prosthetic socks worn over the liner accommodate volume fluctuation. This suspension allows unrestricted knee flexion and minimal pistoning.

Prosthetic sleeves use friction and negative pressure for suspension. The sleeves fit snugly to the upper third of the tibial prosthesis and are made from neoprene, latex, silicone or thermoplastic elastomer.

Supracondylar suspension is recommended when the residual limb is less than 5 cm long. The socket is designed to increase the surface area for pressure distribution by raising the medial and lateral socket brim. A wedge may be used in the soft liner.

Supracondylar–suprapatellar suspension encloses the patella in the socket and has a bar proximal to the patella. This design also provides medial–lateral stability, and no additional cuffs or straps are required. Corset-type prostheses can lead to verrucous hyperplasia and thigh atrophy but reduce socket loads, control the direction of swing and provide some additional weight support.

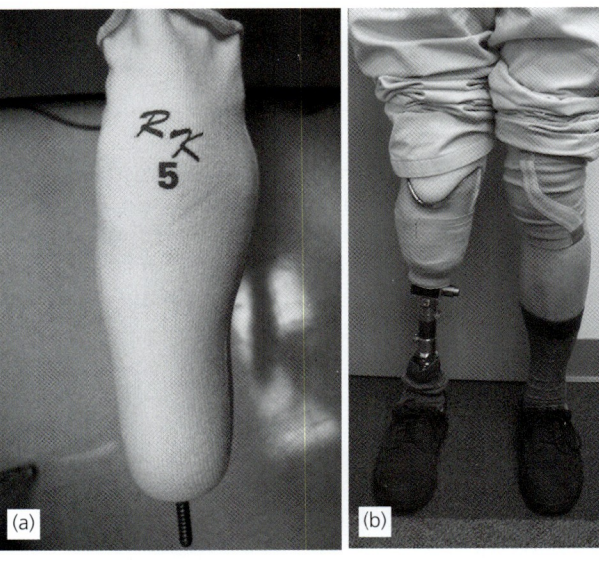

Figure 85.14 (a) Gel liner suspension with locking pin. (b) Transtibial prosthesis with liner locked in place.

Transfemoral suspension

Vacuum (suction) suspension is frequently used. It relies on surface tension, negative pressure and muscle contraction. A one-way expulsion valve helps maintain negative pressure, and no belts or straps are required. Stable body weight is required for this intimate fit. Roll-on silicone or thermoplastic liners may be used with or without locking pins. The total-elastic suspension belt (TES), made of neoprene, fastens around the waist and spreads over a larger surface area (Fig. 85.15). It is an excellent auxiliary suspension. Silesian belts are used to prevent socket rotation in limbs with redundant tissue and are used with the older design systems. Such belts also prevent the socket from slipping off when suction sockets are fitted to short transfemoral stumps and the patient sits.

Transfemoral sockets

Quadrilateral sockets wherein the posterior brim provides a shelf for the ischial tuberosity have been the classic.[14] The design made it difficult to keep the femur in adduction. Ischial containment (narrow medial–lateral) sockets distribute the proximal and medial concentration

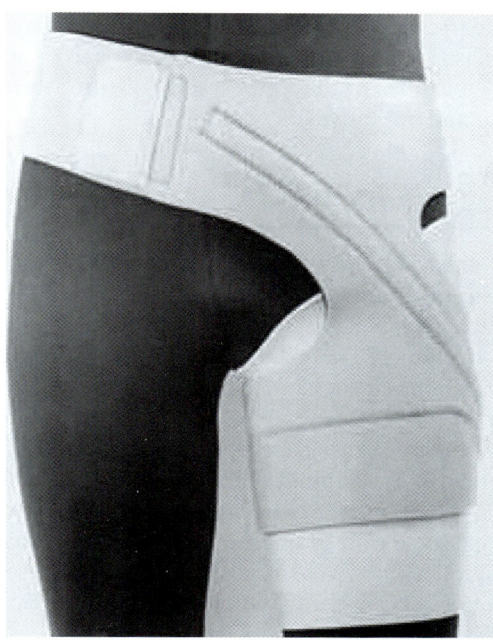

Figure 85.15 Total-elastic suspension belt for suspending a transfemoral socket. Courtesy of Syncor Manufacturers, Green Bay, WI, USA.

Table 85.5 Prosthetic foot gait abnormalities

Foot position	Gait abnormality
Inset	Varus strain, pain (proximedial, distolateral), circumduction
Outset	Valgus strain, pain (proxilateral, distomedial), broad-based gait
Forward placement	Increased knee extension (patellar pain) but stable
Posterior placement	Increased knee flexion/instability
Dorsiflexed foot	Increased patellar pressure
Plantarflexed foot	Drop off, patellar pressure

of forces more evenly as well as enhance socket rotational control. The ischium and ramus are contained within the socket of these more anatomical, comfortable and functional designs. Socket design for a transfemoral prosthesis allows for 10° of adduction of the femur (to stretch the gluteus medius, allowing adequate strength for mid-stance stability) and 5° of flexion (to stretch the gluteus maximus and allow for greater hip extension).

Transtibial sockets

With total surface bearing, pressure is distributed more equally across the entire surface of the transtibial residual limb, and the interface liner material in the socket is important. Urethane liners cope with multidirectional forces by easy material distortion and recovery to original shape. Another liner is made of mineral oil gel with reinforcing fabric. These liners provide good shock-absorbing abilities and reduce skin problems. Total surface bearing is different from total contact, in which different areas have different loads.

Patellar tendon bearing loads all areas of the residual limb that are weight tolerant (i.e. patellar tendon, medial tibial flare, anterior compartment, gastrocnemius and fibular shaft). The anterior wedge shape of the socket helps control rotation of the socket on the limb. Weight-intolerant areas include tibial crest and tubercle, distal fibula and fibular head, peroneal nerve and hamstring tendons. The patellar tendon-bearing supracondylar/suprapatellar socket has proximal extensions over the distal femoral condyles and over the patella. With better shape stumps and improved suspension systems, there is less need for this type of socket.

Common prosthetic problems

TRANSTIBIAL

Pistoning during the swing phase of gait is usually caused by an ineffective suspension system. Pistoning in the stance phase is due to poor socket fit or volume changes in the stump (may require a change in stump sock thickness). Alignment problems are common and are listed in Table 85.5. Pressure-related pain or redness should be corrected with relief of the prosthesis in the affected area. Other problems may be related to the foot: too soft a foot results in excessive knee extension, whereas too hard a foot causes knee flexion and lateral rotation of the toes.

TRANSFEMORAL

Excessive prosthetic length and weak hip abductors or flexors can lead to circumduction, vaulting and lateral trunk bending. Hip flexion contractures and insufficient anterior socket support can lead to excessive lumbar lordosis (compensatory). Inadequate prosthetic knee flexion can lead to terminal knee snap. Medial whip (heel in, heel out) can be caused by a varus knee, excessive external rotation of the knee axis or muscle weakness. Lateral whip (heel out, heel in) is caused by the opposite (valgus knee, internal rotation at the knee and weakness). Table 85.6 summarizes common transfemoral prosthetic gait problems.

STAIR CLIMBING

In general, an amputee will negotiate stairs by leading with their normal limb and descend by leading with their prosthetic limb ('the good goes up and the bad comes down').

ORTHOSES

The primary function of an orthosis is control of motion of certain body segments.[15] Orthoses are used to protect long bones or unstable joints, support flexible deformities and occasionally substitute for a functional task. They may

Table 85.6 Prosthetic gait abnormalities

Gait abnormality	Prosthetic problem
Lateral trunk bending	Short prosthesis, weak abductors, poor fit
Abducted gait	Poor socket fit medially
Circumducted gait	Prosthesis too long, excess knee friction
Vaulted gait	Prosthesis too long, poor suspension
Foot rotation at heel strike	Heel too stiff, loose socket
Short stance phase	Painful stump, knee too loose
Knee instability	Knee too anterior, foot too stiff
Medial/lateral whip	Excessive knee rotation, tight socket
Terminal snap	Quadriceps weakness, unsteady patient
Foot slap, knee hyperextension	Heel too soft
Knee flexion	Heel too hard
Excessive lumbar lordosis	Hip flexion contracture, socket problems

be static, dynamic or a combination of these. With few exceptions, orthoses are not indicated for correction of fixed deformities or for spastic deformities that cannot be easily controlled manually. Orthoses are named according to the joints they control and the method used to obtain/maintain that control (e.g. a short-leg, below-the-knee brace is an ankle–foot orthosis (AFO)).

Shoes

Specific shoes can be used by themselves or in conjunction with foot orthoses. Extra-depth shoes with a high toe box to dissipate local pressures over bony prominences are recommended for diabetic patients. The plantar surface of an insensate foot is protected by use of a pressure-dissipating material. A paralytic or flexible foot deformity can be controlled with more rigid orthoses. The SACH system absorbs the shock of initial loading and lessens the transmission of force to the midfoot as the foot passes through the stance phase. A rocker sole can lessen the bending forces on an arthritic or stiff midfoot during mid-stance as the foot changes from accepting the weight-bearing load to pushing off. It is useful in treating metatarsalgia, hallux rigidus and other forefoot problems. For the rocker sole to be effective, it must be rigid.

Medial heel outflare is used to treat severe flat foot of most causes. Most foot orthoses are used to:

1. align and support the foot
2. prevent, correct or accommodate foot deformities
3. improve foot function.

Three main types of foot orthoses are used: rigid, semi-rigid and soft. Rigid foot orthoses limit joint motion and stabilize flexible deformities. Soft orthoses have best shock-absorbing ability and are used to accommodate fixed deformities of the feet, especially neuropathic, dysvascular and ulcerative disorders.

Ankle–foot orthoses

This is one of the most commonly prescribed lower limb orthoses and is used to control the ankle joint. It may be fabricated with metal bars attached to the shoe or thermoplastic elastomer. The orthosis may be rigid, preventing ankle motion, or it can allow free or spring-assisted motion in either plane.

After hindfoot fusions, the primary orthotic goals are absorption of the ground reaction forces, protection of the fusion sites and protection of the midfoot. The thermoplastic foot section achieves medial–lateral control with high trimlines. When subtalar motion is present, an articulating AFO permits motion by a mechanical ankle joint design. Primary factors in orthotic joint selection include range of motion, durability, adjustability and biomechanical implication on the knee joint. A posterior leaf spring AFO provides stance-phase stability for ankle instability in stance phase.

Knee–ankle–foot orthoses

This orthosis extends from the upper thigh to the foot. It is generally used to control an unstable or paralysed knee joint. It provides mediolateral stability with prescribed amounts of flexion or extension control. A subset of knee–ankle–foot orthoses are knee orthoses. Knee orthoses can be made of elastic for treatment of patellar pathology or of metal and plastic in the case of anterior cruciate ligament instability.

Hip–knee–ankle–foot orthoses

This orthosis provides hip and pelvic stability but is rarely used for the adult paraplegic because of the cumbersome nature of the orthosis and the magnitude of effort in achieving minimal gains. Experimentally, it is being used in conjunction with implanted electrodes and computerized functional stimulation of paraplegics. In children with upper level lumbar myelomeningocele, the reciprocating gait orthoses are modified hip–knee–ankle–foot orthoses that can be used for standing and simulated walking.

Elbow orthoses

Hinged elbow orthoses provide minimal stability in the treatment of ligament instabilities. Dynamic spring-loaded orthoses have been successfully used in the treatment of flexion or extension contractures.

Wrist and hand orthoses

The most common use of wrist and hand orthoses today is for postoperative care after injury or reconstructive surgery. These devices are static or dynamic. The opponens splint is successful in pre-positioning the thumb but impairs tactile sensation. Wrist-driven hand orthoses are used in lower cervical quadriplegics. They may be body powered by tenodesis action or motor driven. Weight and cumbersomeness are the major limiting factors.

Fracture braces

Fracture bracing remains a valuable treatment option for isolated fractures of the tibia and fibula. Prefabricated fracture orthoses can be used in simple foot and ankle fractures, ankle sprains and simple hand injuries.

Paediatric orthoses

Many dynamic orthoses are used in children to control motion without total immobilization. The Pavlik harness has become the mainstay for early treatment of developmental dislocation of the hip. Several dynamic orthoses have been used for containment in Perthes disease.

Spine

CERVICAL SPINE

Numerous orthoses are used to immobilize the cervical spine. Effective immobilization ranges from the various types of collars, to posted orthoses that gain purchase about the shoulders and under the chin, to the halo vest, which achieves the most stability by the nature of its fixation into the skull.

THORACOLUMBAR

Orthoses used for stabilizing mechanical back pain rely on increasing body cavity pressure. Three-point orthoses achieve their control by the length of their lever arm and the subsequent limitation of motion.

Surgery for stroke and closed head injury

The orthopaedic surgeon can play a role in the early management of adult-acquired spasticity secondary to stroke or closed brain injury when the spasticity interferes with the rehabilitation programme. Interventional modalities may include orthotic prescription, serial casting or motor point nerve blocks with short-acting (bupivacaine HCl) or long-acting (phenol 3–4% in glycerol or Botox) agents. Splinting a joint (e.g. the ankle) at neutral is not sufficient to prevent the development of a contracture (e.g. an equinus contracture). When functional joint ranging is insufficient to control deformity, intervention is often indicated. Local anaesthetic injection to the posterior tibial nerve or sciatic nerve before casting relieves pain and allows for maximum correction of the deformity. Open nerve blocks may be warranted to avoid injecting mixed nerves with large sensory contributions. Surgical intervention in adult-acquired spasticity is delayed until the patient achieves maximum spontaneous motor recovery (6 months for stroke and 12–18 months for traumatic brain injury). When patients reach a plateau in functional progress, or when their deformity impedes further progress, intervention may be considered. Invasive procedures in this population should be an adjunct to a standard functional rehabilitation programme, not an alternative. When surgery is considered as a method of improving function, patients should be screened for (1) cognitive deficits, (2) motivation and (3) body-image awareness. Patients should not be confused and must have adequate short-term memory and the capacity for new learning. In addition to specific cognitive strengths, motivation is necessary for patients to utilize functional gains and participate in their rehabilitation programme. Body-image awareness is essential for surgical intervention to become meaningful and potentially beneficial. Patients who lack the awareness of a limb or its position in space should undergo therapy directed towards improving these deficits before embarking on surgical intervention.

LOWER LIMB

Balance is the best predictor of a patient's ability to ambulate after acquired brain injury. The mainstay of treatment for the dynamic ankle equinus component of this gait deviation is to achieve ankle stability in neutral position during initial floor contact (i.e. initial contact and stance) as well as floor clearance during swing phase. An adjustable AFO with ankle dorsiflexion and a plantarflexion stop at neutral is often used during the recovery period, followed by a rigid AFO once the patient has reached a plateau in recovery. When the dynamic equinus overpowers the holding power of the orthosis and patients 'walk out' of their brace, motor-balancing surgery is indicated. The equinus deformity is treated by percutaneous tendon Achilles lengthening. The dynamic varus-producing force in adults is the result of out-of-phase tibialis anterior muscle activity during the stance phase. This dynamic varus deformity is corrected by either split or complete lateral transfer of the tibialis anterior muscle.

UPPER LIMB

There is a paucity of literature dealing with acquired spasticity in the upper limb. Invasive intervention can be considered for functional and non-functional goals. Surgical release of static contracture is generally performed to assist nursing care or hygiene when the fixed contracture and/or spastic component results in skin maceration or breakdown. A functional use of static contracture release is to improve upper extremity 'tracking' (i.e. arm swing) during walking. Most upper extremity surgery performed in this patient population has the goal of increasing prehensile hand function. The goal may be simply to improve placement, enabling use of the hand as a 'paperweight', or to achieve improved fine motor control. In patients with prehensile potential, surgery may allow the 'one-handed' patient to be 'two-handed' by increasing involved hand function from no function to assistive, or from assistive to independent. When the goal of surgery is to improve function, patients must first be screened for cognitive capacity, motivation and body-image awareness. Patients must have the cognitive skills and learning capability to participate in their therapy after surgery and to functionally make use of their newly acquired skills at the completion of their rehabilitation programme. If they are not motivated, they will not participate in the prolonged effort necessary to achieve meaningful functional improvement. Patients with poor stereognosis or neglect (i.e. poor body-image awareness) find that their involved hand 'drifts' in space and is not 'available' for use if they have not been carefully trained in visual compensation techniques. Once it has been determined that the patient has the potential to make functional upper extremity gains with surgery, he or she is graded on the basis of hand placement, proprioception and sensibility, and voluntary motor control. Dynamic electromyography is used when delineation of phasic motor activity is essential. Muscle unit lengthening, by fractional musculotendinous or step-cut methods, of the agonist deforming muscle units is combined with motor-balancing tendon transfers of the antagonists to achieve muscle balance and improved prehensile hand function.

SPINAL CORD INJURY

The functional level in a patient with spinal cord injury is determined by the most distal intact functional dermatome (sensory level) and the most distal motor level where most of the muscles at that level function at least at a 'fair' motor grade.[16,17]

- *Mobility.* The spinal cord injury level determines mobility. C4 and higher levels require high back and head support. At C5, mouth-driven accessories can control a motorized wheelchair. Various body-powered or motor-driven orthoses can assist functional prehension, such as a ratchet wrist hand orthosis. At C6 patients can operate manual wheelchairs and use a flexor hinge wrist and hand orthosis. Transfers are dependent at C4, assisted at C5 and independent at C6 (Table 85.7).
- *Activities of daily living.* Patients at the C6 level can groom and dress themselves. Patients at the C7 level can cut meat. Bowel and bladder function can be controlled via rectal stimulation and intermittent catheterization.
- *Psychosocial factors.* Men may be impotent but can often achieve a reflex erection.
- *Autonomic dysreflexia.* This potentially catastrophic hypertensive event can occur with injuries above T5. It is usually caused by an obstructed urinary catheter or faecal impaction.
- *Surgery.* Spinal fusion is frequently used to expedite rehabilitation and prevent the late development of pain or deformity at the fracture level. Anterior and/or posterior fusion with internal fixation should be performed soon after injury so as to facilitate early rehabilitation. Spasticity and contracture can produce

Table 85.7 Treatment of spinal cord injury by functional level

Functional Level	Working	Not Working	Treatment/Mobility
Above C4	–	Diaphragm, upper extremity muscles	Respirator dependent
C4	Diaphragm/trapezius	Upper extremity muscles	Wheelchair chin/puff
C5	Elbow flexors	Below elbow	Electric wheelchair, rachet
C6	Wrist extensors	Elbow extensors	Wheelchair, flexor hing
C7	Elbow extensor	Grasp	Wheelchair, independent
C8	Finger flexors to middle finger		
T1	Intrinsic muscles	Abdominals/lower extremity muscles	Wheelchair, independent
T2–T12	Upper extremity muscles, abdominals	Lower extremity muscles	Wheelchair, HKAFO (nonfunctional ambulation)
L1	Upper extremity muscles, abdominals, quadriceps	Lower extremity muscles	KAFO; minimum ambulation
L2	Iliopsoas	Knee/ankle	KAFO, household ambulation
L3	Quadriceps	Ankle	AFO, community ambulation
L4	Tibialis anterior	Toe, plantar flexors	AFO, community ambulation
L5	EHL, EDL	Plantar flexors	AFO, independent
S1	Gastrocnemius/soleus	Bowel/bladder	± Metatarsal bar

AFO, ankle-foot orthosis; EDL, extensor digitorum longus; EHL, extensor hallucis longus; HKAFO, hip-knee-ankle-foot orthosis; KAFO, knee-ankle-foot orthosis; ±, with or without.

problems in hygiene or the development of pressure ulcers. Percutaneous, or open, motor nerve blocks with phenol can be used to treat these deformities. When the deformity is a static contracture, muscle release or disarticulation may improve sitting or transfer potential. Tendon transfers can be used in the upper limb to eliminate the need for an orthosis or to allow the patient to achieve function with an orthosis.

Post-polio syndrome

Polio is a viral disease affecting the anterior horn cells of the spinal cord. Post-polio syndrome is not a reactivation of the polio virus. It is an ageing phenomenon whereby more nerve cells become inactive. These patients use a high proportion of their capacity for normal activities of daily living. With ageing and the drop-off of muscle units, they no longer have the reserves to perform their daily activities. Treatment comprises prescribed limited exercise combined with periods of rest, so muscles are maintained but not overtaxed. Standard polio surgery, combining contracture release, arthrodesis and tendon transfer, is indicated when deformity overcomes functional capacity. The use of lightweight orthoses is important in helping patients to remain functionally independent. The syndrome occurs after middle age.

Wheelchairs

Various types of wheelchairs are available for use and their provision depends on the disability that is being treated. Most wheelchairs are manual and a smaller number are power wheelchairs. In a recent review it was noted that the highest rate of wheelchair use was in persons older than 65 years and most of the chairs were manual. Various associated medical problems may affect the type of wheelchair provided. Common conditions include spinal cord injury, multiple sclerosis, Parkinson disease, cerebrovascular accidents, amputations and diabetes mellitus. The patient's cognitive status is important for maintaining safety in the wheelchair. Patients with coexisting arthritis and cardiac/pulmonary conditions may not have the physical reserve to use a manual wheelchair and would be better off with a power chair.

Also to be considered is the environment and activity in which the patient is going to function. Removable arm rests are useful to facilitate transfers to and from the chair. Seating requirements are an important consideration especially in the minimally active person.

Powered wheelchairs are becoming common, especially for those individuals who have difficulty propelling a manual wheelchair. Power chairs may be controlled by hand or by mouth for those individuals who have a high cervical spine injury with quadriplegia and no upper limb function.

KEY LEARNING POINTS

- Gait: walking is a repetitive, sequential, upright, cyclic, energy-efficient activity with one foot on the ground at all times, and can be single or double limb. There is a stance phase (60%) and a swing phase (40%).
- Most muscle activity is eccentric.
- Pathological gait (limp) can be neurological, analgesic or short-leg.
- Most amputations are for vascular disease, diabetes mellitus, infection, trauma or tumour.
- Amputation after trauma is for an ischaemic limb with a vascular injury which cannot be repaired. Gustilo–Anderson grades IIIB and IIIC have high mortality and morbidity.
- In patients with diabetes, the presence of peripheral neuropathy is an important risk factor for amputation.
- For tumours, the decision is between amputation and limb salvage based on expected functional outcome.
- Phantom limb sensation is the feeling that all or part of the amputated limb is present; phantom pain is a burning, painful sensation in the part amputated; complex regional pain syndrome is a common cause of pain.
- Determining the level of an amputation is important (ISO classification). The metabolic cost of walking is increased with proximal-level amputations, and is inversely proportional to the length of the residual limb and the number of functional joints preserved.
- Paediatric amputations are usually the result of congenital limb deficiencies, trauma or tumours.
- Amputation wound healing depends on vascular supply, nutrition and immune status.
- For amputation surgery tissue stabilization (a functional stump, with preservation of muscle function and soft-tissue sensation) is important.
- A prosthetic replaces a lost limb part; an orthosis controls the motion of certain body segments.
- For upper limb amputations, residual limb length is important for prosthetic socket suspension and providing the lever arm necessary to 'drive' the prosthesis through space.
- Myoelectric prostheses provide good cosmetic appearance and are used for sedentary work.
- Pistoning during the swing phase of gait is usually caused by an ineffective suspension system. Pistoning in the stance phase is due to poor socket fit or volume changes in the stump (may require a change in stump sock thickness).
- The best known orthosis is the ankle–foot orthosis.

- Balance is the best predictor of a patient's ability to ambulate after acquired brain injury.
- The functional level in a patient with spinal cord injury is determined by the most distal intact functional dermatome (sensory level) and the most distal motor level where most of the muscles at that level function at least at a 'fair' motor grade.
- Autonomic dysreflexia is a potentially catastrophic hypertensive event that can occur with injuries above T5.
- Post-polio syndrome is not a reactivation of the polio virus.

REFERENCES

- ● = Key primary paper
- ◆ = Major review article

◆1. Inman VT, Ralston H, Todd F. *Human Walking*. Baltimore, MD: Williams & Wilkins, 1981.

◆2. Ounpuu S. The biomechanics of running: a kinematic and kinetic analysis. *Instructional Course Lectures* 1990;**39**:305.

3. Perry J. *Gait Analysis: Normal and Pathological Function*. New York, NY: Slack, 1992.

◆4. Smith D, Bowker J, Michael J (eds). *Atlas of Amputations and Limb Deficiencies: Surgical, Prosthetic, and Rehabilitation Principles*. Rosemont, IL: American Academy of Orthopaedic Surgeons, 2004.

5. Pinzur M, Gold J, Schwartz D, *et al*. Energy demands for walking in dysvascular amputees as related to the level of amputation. *Orthopaedics* 1992;**15**:1033.

●6. Waters RL, Perry J, Antonelli D, *et al*. Energy cost of walking of amputees: the influence of level of amputation. *Journal of Bone and Joint Surgery (American)* 1976;**58**:42.

7. Wyss C, Harrington R, Burgess E, Matsen F. Transcutaneous oxygen tension as a predictor of success after an amputation. *Journal of Bone and Joint Surgery (American)* 1988;**70**:203.

◆8. Gottschalk F (ed.). Symposium on amputation. *Clinical Orthopaedics and Related Research* 1999;**361**:2–115.

●9. Day H. *The Proposed International Terminology for the Classification of Congenital Limb Deficiencies: The Recommendations of a Working Group of ISPO*. London, UK: Spastics International Medical Publications, 1975.

10. Bernd L, Blasius K, Lukoschek M, *et al*. The autologous stump plasty: treatment for bony overgrowth in juvenile amputees. *Journal of Bone and Joint Surgery (British)* 1991;**73**:203–6.

◆11. Gottschalk F. Traumatic amputations. In: Bucholz RW, Heckman JD (eds). *Fractures in Adults*. Philadelphia, PA: Lippincott Williams & Wilkins, 2001:391–414.

12. Gottschalk F, Fisher D. Complications of amputation. In: Conenwett JL, Gloviczki P, Johnston KW, *et al*. (eds). *Rutherford's Vascular Surgery*. Philadelphia, PA: W.B. Saunders, 2000:2213–48.

●13. Lagaard S, McElfresh E, Premer R. Gangrene of the upper extremity in diabetic patients. *Journal of Bone and Joint Surgery (American)* 1989;**71**:257.

14. Gottschalk F, Kourosh S, Stills M, *et al*. Does socket configuration influence the position of the femur in above-knee amputation? *Journal of Prosthetics and Orthotics* 1989;**2**:94–102.

◆15. Goldberg B, Hsu J (eds). *Atlas of Orthoses and Assistive Devices*, 3rd edn. St. Louis, MO: Mosby Year Book, 1997.

●16. Braun R. Stroke and brain injury. In: Green D (ed.) *Operative Hand Surgery*. New York, NY: Churchill Livingstone, 1988:227–54.

●17. Pinzur M, Sherman R, Dimonte-Levine P, *et al*. Adult-onset hemiplegia: changes in gait after muscle-balancing procedures to correct the equinus deformity. *Journal of Bone and Joint Surgery (American)* 1986;**68**:1249–57.

PART 8

THE SPINE

ALEXANDER VACCARO AND STEPHAN BECKER

86	**Pathophysiology of low back pain** Joseph M Hart, Noelle M Selkow, Nicole Cosby, Matthew C Bessette	975
87	**Spinal infections** Shanmuganathan Rajasekaran, P Rishi Mugesh Kanna, T Ajoy Prasad Shetty	982
88	**Degenerative disc disease** Mun Keong Kwan	993
89	**Adult spinal deformity** William C Lauerman, Ryan J Caufield	1007
90	**Surgical options in the osteoporotic spine** Stephan Becker	1024
91	**Spondylolysis and spondylolisthesis** István Hovorka	1048
92	**Tumours of the spine** Stephan Becker, Jason Beng Teck Lim, Volker Schirrmacher, Himanshu Sharma	1058

86

Pathophysiology of low back pain

JOSEPH M HART, NOELLE M SELKOW, NICOLE COSBY, MATTHEW C BESSETTE

Introduction	975
Structure and function of the lumbar spine	975
Anatomical pain generators in low back pain	976
Common diagnoses: non-specific low back pain	976
Common diagnoses: specific lumbar spine injuries	976
Specific lumbar spine injuries: bone	977
Specific lumbar spine injuries: nerve	978
Specific lumbar spine injuries: intervertebral disc	978
Specific lumbar spine injuries: paravertebral musculature	978
Specific lumbar spine injuries: other	979
Summary	979
References	979

NATIONAL BOARD STANDARDS

- Understand the common pain generators
- Know the red flag and yellow flag symptoms
- Understand the common treatment strategies for low back pain
- Know how to counsel and advise patients with low back pain

INTRODUCTION

The prevalence of low back pain (LBP) is disturbingly high with over one-quarter of Americans reporting an episode of LBP lasting at least a day within the past 3 months.[1] Estimates of the prevalence of LBP range from 15% to 30%.[2] The likelihood of experiencing an episode of LBP increases with age, and upwards of 85% of people will have at least one episode in their lifetime. The high cost of medical care,[3] limited activity levels[4] and recurrence of symptoms[5] in people with LBP are of primary concern to clinicians. LBP is a major cause of lost time from work and reductions in normal activity, creating a major burden to society as well as to those individuals who desire to retain normal levels of function.

STRUCTURE AND FUNCTION OF THE LUMBAR SPINE

The lower back plays an important role in structural support and movement in the human body. The bony architecture comprises five lumbar vertebrae joining the thoracic spine and the sacrum. At the sacroiliac joints, the sacrum articulates with the pelvis to connect the axial with the appendicular skeleton. The lumbar vertebrae increase in size from superior to inferior, reflecting progressively increased axial loading. The vertebral bodies are connected cranially and caudally by intervertebral discs. Extending from the bony epiphysial rings and hyaline cartilage end plates of each vertebra, the discs comprise an annulus, a fibrous outer later and a nucleus pulposus, a gelatinous centre. In axial compression and flexion, the discs are the major load-bearing elements of the spine.

The *posterior elements of the spinal column*, including the laminae, transverse processes and spinous process, are connected to the vertebral body by two pedicles at each level. Two zygapophyseal joints, or facet joints, serve as the posterior points of articulation between adjacent segments. These joints control planes of motion of the column, allowing flexion and extension while limiting rotation in the lumbar spine. They accept a higher proportion of compressive loading than other more cranial segments of the spine, particularly during extension. The superior articular process and pedicle are connected to the lamina and inferior articular process on each side of one vertebra by the pars interarticularis.

The *static stability* of the spine is augmented by tensile forces provided by various ligamentous structures. The strong anterior longitudinal ligament (ALL) runs anterior to the vertebral bodies and is attached to the anterior annular fibres of each disc. The posterior longitudinal ligament (PLL) runs posterior to the vertebral bodies and is also continuous with the annular fibres of each disc. It is narrow and weak in the lumbar region. The ligamentum flavum connects adjacent laminae from the interspinous ligaments medially to the facet capsules laterally. The interspinous and supraspinous ligaments bridge the spinous processes at each level. *Dynamic stability* is provided by paravertebral musculature. Numerous muscles in different connective tissue planes with multiple attachments are responsible for movement and the maintenance of posture.

The spinal cord descends between the anterior and posterior elements within the spinal canal. It gives off roots that are named after the vertebral body where they exit just caudally to the pedicles.

ANATOMICAL PAIN GENERATORS IN LOW BACK PAIN

Common pain generators in people with LBP include structures such as ligaments, facet joints, vertebral periosteum, paravertebral musculature and fascia, blood vessels, discs and nerve roots.[6] Both mechanical pressure and chemical mediators are potential sources in people complaining of LBP. Pain can theoretically be derived from any structure with the appropriate innervations. Specific patterns exist, however, to aid the clinician in elucidating the origin of pain. When examining a patient, it is important to remember that lower back pain may be the result of a disease process far removed from the spine.[7] The abdominal viscera, major vascular structures and systemic disease can all manifest as pain in the lumbar region.

The basivertebral nerve is a sensory nerve innervating both end plates.[8] It branches off the sinuvertebral nerve and runs along the basovertebral vein. Studies show increased sprouting of those nerve endings in degenerative disc disease and vertebrae with Modic signs.[9,10] This nerve is currently the focus of clinical studies in the generation of vertebral and discogenic back pain. In the absence of fractures or other pathological processes, vertebral bodies are a rare source of benign chronic LBP.

Intervertebral disc and facet joint pathology is a major contributor to chronic LBP. The nucleus pulposus and deeper layers of the annulus fibrosis are not innervated; however, free and encapsulated nerve endings from the sinuvertebral nerve have been found in the outer annulus of discs. Degenerative changes have been associated with further ingrowth of nerve endings. Pain can also be induced here through disorders in which disruption of the internal structures of the disc expose peripheral (innervated) structures to abnormal internal pressures or tension, thereby generating pain despite maintenance of the structural integrity of the outer annulus.

The joint capsules of the *zygapophyseal (facet) joints* are innervated by medial branches of the posterior rami and contain abundant nociceptive nerve endings. Facet joint degeneration is a common source of lower back pain. Despite its limited range of motion, the *sacroiliac joint* is well innervated and is another common pain generator in the lower back.[11,12]

Chemical irritation and compression of spinal nerve roots can cause radicular pain. Localized back pain can be caused by irritation of the ventral dura, which is innervated by the sinuvertebral nerves along with the posterior annulus and the PLL. LBP can also be caused by compression of the dorsal root ganglia.

Ligaments surrounding the skeletal structure except for the ligamentum flavum are well innervated, but injury can be difficult to diagnose. *Muscular pain* may result from acute strain of a well-innervated muscle.

COMMON DIAGNOSES: NON-SPECIFIC LOW BACK PAIN

Non-specific LBP is a diagnosis given to patients without an identifiable structural or morphological change to correlate to their episode(s) of pain.[13] Non-specific LBP has been defined as a recurring and self-limiting condition that is benign except for the sometimes considerable pain experienced by patients.[14,15] It is one of the most frequent reasons for healthcare consultation and is commonly reported by those presenting with any type of pain. The actual prevalence of non-specific LBP may be difficult to accurately describe, largely due to vague diagnostic definitions as well as the myriad of possible aetiologies and associated comorbidities.[14,16,17] Because by definition a source of pain cannot be identified, it is not surprising that there is a lack of evidence regarding effective treatments.[6] Despite a dearth of proven therapeutic options, the prognosis for an acute episode of non-specific LBP is favourable; resolution of symptoms and resumption of normal activities normally occurs in 4–6 weeks. Ninety per cent of people with non-specific LBP recover within 12 weeks,[13] but those who do not are at an elevated risk of developing long-term, chronic symptoms.

COMMON DIAGNOSES: SPECIFIC LUMBAR SPINE INJURIES

Specific causes of LBP involve a diagnosis that can be attributed to a particular structure or identifiable lesion. In the following text, we have described common low back pathologies by the potential anatomical pain generator: bone/joint, disc, nerve, muscle and other. A structural deformity, traumatic injury, infection, or other disease process may be identified as the specific cause of LBP. Such diagnoses are uncommon in those reporting LBP.

SPECIFIC LUMBAR SPINE INJURIES: BONE

Spondylolysis is a unilateral or bilateral stress fracture through the pars interarticularis (isthmus).[18,19] The defect is thought to be congenital in nature or the result of injury or chronic stress. Defects from stress or injury are precipitated by two different mechanisms. The 'nutcracker' or direct compression mechanism occurs when the inferior articular process of the superior vertebra impacts the pars interarticularis of the inferior vertebra.[18] The 'bony pincers' theory postulates that there is stretching of the pars interarticularis that leads to a stress microfracture. This occurs when the inferior articular process of the vertebra one level above and the superior articular process of the vertebra one level below or the sacrum create tension across the pars interarticularis during extension.[19] The most common injury is sustained at L5, where the posterior elements are subjected to higher physiological loading.[19] Activities involving extension and rotation, such as those regularly carried out by American football linemen and gymnasts, put the patient at greatest risk for injury.[19,20] Of young athletes that present with LBP, up to 47% may have spondylolysis.[18] Patients with spondylolysis usually present with a 'stiff-legged' gait, characterized by stride length shortening due to hamstring stiffness,[20] pain with extension more pronounced in a single-leg stance and pain worsening with activity.[19] Asking for a family history is important, as the incidence is increased up to 69% with hereditary disposition.[19] If this injury is not diagnosed and does not properly heal, it can lead to spondylolithesis.

Spondylolithesis is anterior displacement of the body of one vertebra over that of the inferior vertebra or sacrum in the setting of spondylolysis.[21] This results after bilateral fractures of a pars interacticularis pair. As with spondylolysis, the most common site of injury is the L5 vertebra.[21] Concomitant disc degeneration increases the risk of displacement, and 50–75% of those with spondylolysis eventually develop spondylolithesis.[21] Patients may present with a palpable step-off at the spinous process at the lesion, a shortened trunk, lumbar hyperlordosis, limited range of motion, pain with extension and hamstring tightness.[21] Radicular symptoms may be caused by irritation of nerve roots traversing the step-off between misaligned segments. The prevalence of this injury increases with age. It is most easily visualized on a lateral radiograph of the lumbar spine and is described by the degree of slippage of the superior body over the inferior body.

Vertebral body fractures result from excessive loading of the spine. The characteristics of the force inflicting injury and the state of the bone itself play a significant factor in the type and extent of injury.[22] Low-energy loading results in vertebral end plate fractures and wedging, typically seen in patients with poor bone quality.[22] Radiographic findings of such wedge fractures in the absence of symptoms in older, ostoporotic women is not uncommon, although such injuries can be a source of significant pain. High-energy loading results in a burst fracture,[22] where a compression fracture of the anterior and middle columns can cause retropulsion of the posterior vertebral body into the spinal canal.[23] These burst fractures are typically seen in younger, more active patients.

Acute symptoms may include new or greatly increased back pain, limited mobility and swelling at the fracture site.[24] There may be damage to nerve roots or the spinal cord from protruding vertebral body fragments, which may result in loss of sensory or motor function below the level of the injury. Severe injury may result in full paralysis, bowel and bladder dysfunction, and permanent neurological injury.[24] While this is often caused by automobile and other high-energy trauma, burst fractures have been reported in athletic injuries. The type of treatment indicated is dependent on the stability of the spine and fracture pattern.

Lumbar facet pain results from degenerative changes at the zygapophyseal joint, a common finding in older patients.[11] Facet pathology associated with radicular pain can result from inflammation or disruption of the joints leading to irritation of local nerve roots.[11] Repetitive hyperextension increases the load placed on the facets and stretches the joint capsule, resulting in local pain. Increased frequency and force of loading can lead to microfractures within the joint. While patients are typically neurologically intact in such cases, they may present with pain-inhibited weakness or non-dermatomal sensory loss in the lower extremity.[11] Other signs and symptoms include pain with sitting and pain in the back but not the leg during a straight-leg raise test.

Lumbar spinal stenosis is localized narrowing of the spinal canal due to bony and soft-tissue growth causing back pain and radicular symptoms from nerve root impingement.[25] There are many ways to classify spinal stenosis depending on location and extent. It may be uni- or multisegmental, unilateral or bilateral, and central, lateral or foraminal.[25] Stenosis between L4 and L5 is most common, followed by L3–L4, L5–S1 and L1–L2.[25] Multiple mechanisms lead to stenosis of the canal. Degeneration of the intervertebral disc causes protrusion into the canal leading to ventral or central narrowing. This may lead to intervertebral space height reduction, resulting in narrowing at the neural foramina. Strain at the facets induces joint arthrosis and hypertrophy of the joint capsule, causing further lateral narrowing. The reduction in height of vertebral segments in the axial plane causes the ligamentum flavum to crease, increasing dorsal pressure on the canal.[25] Patients with lumbar stenosis usually present with neurogenic claudication,[25] which is pain radiating into the legs during walking and extension that is relieved by flexion. It is important to differentiate this cause of leg pain from vascular claudication. There are several theories of why the stenosis is symptomatic, including reduced arterial blood flow to the cord, venous congestion leading to compression of the cord and hyperextension increasing direct compression on the cord itself.[25] Patients may report a reduction in their ability to walk certain distances, sensory deficits, hyporeflexia, intermittent paresis, a feeling of 'heavy legs' and a decrease in symptoms with rest.[25] Those over the age of 60 are at greater risk for spinal stenosis.[26]

SPECIFIC LUMBAR SPINE INJURIES: NERVE

Cauda equina syndrome (CES) occurs when there is dysfunction of the sacral and lumbar nerve roots below the conus medularis.[27] This can be caused by a congenitally narrow spinal canal,[27] central or centrolateral disc prolapse, trauma or infection.[28] CES is relatively rare and is a diagnosis for only 2–3% of lumbar disc operations.[29] It occurs most commonly in men aged 40 to 50 secondary to lumbar disc herniation at the L4–L5 and L5–S1 levels. The patient usually describes at least one deficit, including perianal numbness (saddle anaesthesia),[27] lower extremity weakness, or bladder, bowel or sexual dysfunction.[27,28] Other signs and symptoms include back pain with or without referred pain, sensory changes in the lower extremity and decreased reflexes in the lower extremities.[27]

SPECIFIC LUMBAR SPINE INJURIES: INTERVERTEBRAL DISC

Discogenic pain results from injuries to the disc itself, and is more common in patients between the ages of 20 and 50 years. They commonly report predominant back pain that is made worse with prolonged sitting and forward flexion and made better with extension. Physical examination reveals a paucity of findings. There is no evidence of spinal deformity, instability or neural irritation.[30] The disc tissue is rich in nociceptive nerve fibres and neurotransmitters and can become painful if torn. Poor vascular supply and high dynamic compressive loading complicate the process of normal tissue healing.[30] The shape and volume of the patient's disc will change over time as a result of these factors.

Disc degeneration can originate as early as the third decade of life and can be accelerated by obesity, smoking, excessive loading and injury.[31] Gradual dehydration of the nucleus pulposis alters the biomechanical properties of the disc, which can influence the sensitivity of nerve endings due to the release of chemical mediators. It also induces the growth of nervous tissue into the disc, which contributes to increased pain in patients with disc degeneration.[32]

Patients with herniated lumbar intervertebral discs present with dermatomal leg pain (i.e. sciatica) that is worse than pain in the lower back. They may or may not complain of prior episodes of LBP exacerbated by trunk flexion and prolonged sitting or walking and relieved by standing upright or with trunk extension and recumbancy. The specific location of lumbar disc herniations can be elucidated clinically by taking special note of the distribution of pain, numbness, tingling, weakness and altered deep tendon reflexes. Protruded discs occur when the border of a bulging annulus fibrosis is intact but extends beyond the disc's normal anatomical boundaries. Disc extrusions occur when the nuclear material extends beyond damaged or torn annular fibres but still within the confines of the PLL. Sequestered discs occur when nuclear material that is no longer in contact with the remainder of the disc has been forced into the canal and may penetrate the PLL or migrate.

Discitis is an inflammatory process of the intervertebral disc space affecting the lumbar spine. It is most commonly found in children under 10 years of age.[33] The exact aetiology and pathophysiology of the condition is unknown; however, it has been postulated to result from a low-grade viral or bacterial infection.[33] The intervertebral disc and vertebral body surfaces are destroyed by inflammatory processes. Children with discitis often present with a low-grade fever, LBP, and complaints of stiffness in their back. They report difficulty and pain with standing or sitting for prolonged periods of time. Pain usually ceases when the inflammatory process is controlled.

SPECIFIC LUMBAR SPINE INJURIES: PARAVERTEBRAL MUSCULATURE

Muscular pathology is a common cause of lower back pain, especially in athletes and active individuals.[20,34] The paraspinal muscles and ligaments play a key role in the dynamic and static stability of the lower back and greatly increase tolerance to mechanical loading forces. Injuries to these soft-tissue structures are a common cause of both acute and chronic lower back pain. Despite their prevalence, the exact diagnosis of such injuries is difficult and is often made by excluding more serious pathologies.

Forceful elongation, extremes of motion, and unaccustomed activities are all common mechanisms of injury. *Strains* result from tearing within the muscle belly or at the musculotendinous junction leading to inflammation and muscle spasm. *Sprains* result from stretching injuries of the spinal ligaments.

Acute soft-tissue injuries typically cause peak pain levels between 24 and 48 hours after injury that decrease over days to weeks. A patient may suffer from recurrent strains with short asymptomatic intervals between events. Chronic injuries can be more insidious in onset and duration and often lead to extensive workups for other pathology with negative findings. The pain described by patients can be diverse in nature with no specific findings. On examination, muscle spasm of the paraspinal musculature is a common finding. There is localized tenderness to palpation that is exacerbated by certain motions and often relieved with recumbency. Perhaps most importantly, there are no neurological deficits and the pain is not radicular in nature. Imaging is useful only to rule out more serious injury.

Treatment involves a brief period of rest, no more than 1 or 2 days. Bed rest for more than 48 hours is rarely if ever indicated. Cold or heat therapy can be useful to relieve muscle pain or spasm. Non-steroidal anti-inflammatory drugs (NSAIDs) are the first-line choice for pharmacological treatment. After pain relief is achieved, exercises to increase strength and range of motion should be gradually introduced. This is especially important in the case of chronic injuries. Patient education regarding the biomechanics of the lower back as it pertains to their activities is important for avoiding reinjury.

Discrete structural injuries are not the only cause of muscular lower back pain. *Myofascial pain syndrome* is characterized by pain at myofascial trigger points in skeletal muscle. These hypersensitive, discrete areas are nodular and palpable on examination. Patients typically report deep, aching pain in the lower back, buttocks and thighs, along with a restricted range of motion. Palpation of the trigger points reproduces the patient's pain. Treatment of this condition can be difficult and includes multiple mediations and rehabilitation.

Poor strength and endurance of paraspinal muscles predicts LBP occurrence and recurrence.[35–38] Muscles that stabilize the spine can be categorized as local or global. *Global stabilizing muscles* are large torque-producing muscles that provide gross spine movements with little contribution to segmental (intervetrebral) stability. Weakness and imbalance in global stabilizers such as the trunk flexors and extensors have been implicated in the development of LBP.[39,40] *Local stabilizing muscles* attach directly to the vertebrae and cross one or two joints, thereby providing discrete segmental control.[14] Local stabilizing muscles such as the multifidus are commonly atrophied and dysfunctional in patients with LBP.[41–43] In patients with lower back pain or injury, the timing and extent of activation of these different muscle groups can be altered resulting in asynchronous and uncoordinated spinal control.[14] Theoretically, if paravertebral musculature is deficient or unable to stabilize the spine, people may experience abnormal loading on other tissues of the spine such as joint, disc, nerve, etc., which are rich in nociceptive fibres and are common sources of pain.

SPECIFIC LUMBAR SPINE INJURIES: OTHER

Intraspinal cysts are cystic structures of various aetiologies found in the spinal canal. The exact aetiology and prevalence of intraspinal cysts is unknown, although they may become apparent when compression of structures leads to myelopathic or radicular symptoms. Although rare,[44] the majority of symptomatic cysts affect the L2–L5 spinal levels and have been reported in patients between the ages of 19 and 50 years. At this level, their symptoms mimic those of a disc herniation. Dilatation of the structures surrounding the nerve roots may arise as a result of congenital weaknesses in the dura and arachnoid surrounding the root proximal to the dorsal root ganglion.[45] Formation of an intraspinal cyst may also be caused by gas produced in a severely degenerated disc. Pressure from growth of the cyst leads to compression of surrounding structures and neural deficits.

SUMMARY

The variety of possible pain generators around the lumbar spinal column complicates the specific diagnoses of LBP. Non-specific LBP is a common diagnosis that does not implicate a particular offending structure contributing to pain and often carries a favourable prognosis.

Pain during trunk flexion that improves with trunk extension suggests disc or vertebral body related pathology. Pain that is localized to the low back in this sub-group is more likely discogenic whereas pain that radiates to the lower extremity suggests a disc herniation.

Pain during trunk extension that improves with flexion may represent pathology present in the posterior elements of the spinal column. Painful trunk extension that is localized to the low back suggests spondylolysis or spondylolithesis whereas painful extension that radiates down the lower extremity suggests stenosis.

Careful consideration of all potential sources of pain (either involving a specific spine structure or not) in patients complaining of LBP should be included in a thorough examination.

KEY LEARNING POINTS

- Low back pain is prevalent in many populations and has a high impact on quality of life in suffering patients.
- Clinicians should consider pain generators in the lumbar spine when evaluating patients and their treatment options. Surgery is rarely indicated for low back pain alone.
- Pain and or other symptoms may arise from injury or damage to innervated tissues including bone, nerve, disc, muscle and/or ligament.

REFERENCES

1. Deyo RA, Mirza SK, Martin BI. Back pain prevalence and visit rates: estimates from U.S. national surveys, 2002. *Spine* 2006;**31**:2724–7.
2. Andersson GB. Epidemiological features of chronic low-back pain. *Lancet* 1999;**354**:581–5.
3. Frymoyer JW, Cats-Baril WL. An overview of the incidences and costs of low back pain. *Orthopedic Clinics of North America* 1991;**22**:263–71.
4. Verbunt JA, Sieben JM, Seelen HA, et al. Decline in physical activity, disability and pain-related fear in sub-acute low back pain. *European Journal of Pain* 2005;**9**:417–25.
5. MacDonald MJ, Sorock GS, Volinn E, et al. A descriptive study of recurrent low back pain claims. *Journal of Occupational & Environmental Medicine* 1997;**39**:35–43.

6. Deyo RA, Weinstein JN. Low back pain. *New England Journal of Medicine* 2001;**344**:363-70.
7. Sembrano JN, Polly DW, Jr. How often is low back pain not coming from the back? *Spine* 2009;**34**:E27-32.
8. Antonacci MD, Mody DR, Heggeness MH. Innervation of the human vertebral body: a histologic study. *Journal of Spinal Disorders and Techniques* 1998;**11**:526-31.
9. Freemont AJ, Watkins A, Le Maitre C, et al. Nerve growth factor expression and innervation of the painful intervertebral disc. *Journal of Pathology* 2002;**197**:286-92.
10. Ohtori S, Inoue G, Ito T, et al. Tumor necrosis factor-immunoreactive cells and PGP 9.5-immunoreactive nerve fibers in vertebral endplates of patients with discogenic low back Pain and Modic Type 1 or Type 2 changes on MRI. *Spine* 2006;**31**:1026-31.
11. Dreyer SJ, Dreyfuss PH. Low back pain and the zygapophysial (facet) joints. *Archives of Physical Medicine and Rehabilitation* 1996;**77**:290-300.
12. Cavanaugh JM, Lu Y, Chen C, Kallakuri S. Pain generation in lumbar and cervical facet joints. *Journal of Bone and Joint Surgery (American)* 2006;**88**(Suppl 2):63-7.
13. Nordin M, Balague F, Cedraschi C. Nonspecific lower-back pain: surgical versus nonsurgical treatment. *Clinical Orthopaedics and Related Research* 2006;**443**:156-67.
14. Hammill RR, Beazell JR, Hart JM. Neuromuscular consequences of low back pain and core dysfunction. *Clinical Sports Medicine* 2008;**27**:449-62, ix.
15. Keller A, Hayden J, Bombardier C, van Tulder M. Effect sizes of non-surgical treatments of non-specific low-back pain. *European Spine Journal* 2007;**16**:1776-88.
16. Coste J, Spira A, Ducimetiere P, Paolaggi JB. Clinical and psychological diversity of non-specific low-back pain. A new approach towards the classification of clinical subgroups. *Journal of Clinical Epidemiology* 1991;**44**:1233-45.
17. Ozguler A, Leclerc A, Landre MF, et al. Individual and occupational determinants of low back pain according to various definitions of low back pain. *Journal of Epidemiology and Community Health* 2000;**54**:215-20.
18. Sakai T, Sairyo K, Suzue N, et al. Incidence and etiology of lumbar spondylolysis: review of the literature. *Journal of Orthopaedic Science* 2010;**15**:281-8.
19. Leone A, Cianfoni A, Cerase A, et al. Lumbar spondylolysis: a review. *Skeletal Radiology* 2011;**40**:683-700.
20. Lawrence JP, Greene HS, Grauer JN. Back pain in athletes. *Journal of the American Academy of Orthopedic Surgeons* 2006;**14**:726-35.
21. Jones TR, Rao RD. Adult isthmic spondylolisthesis. *Journal of the American Academy of Orthopedic Surgeons* 2009;**17**:609-17.
22. Khan N, Husain S, Haak M. Thoracolumbar injuries in the athlete. *Sports Medicine and Arthroscopy Review* 2008;**16**:16-25.
23. Dai LY, Jiang SD, Wang XY, Jiang LS. A review of the management of thoracolumbar burst fractures. *Surgical Neurology* 2007;**67**:221-31; Discussion 231.
24. Yi L, Jingping B, Gele J, Baoleri X, Taixiang W. Operative versus non-operative treatment for thoracolumbar burst fractures without neurological deficit. *Cochrane Database of Systematic Reviews* 2006:CD005079.
25. Siebert E, Pruss H, Klingebiel R, et al. Lumbar spinal stenosis: syndrome, diagnostics and treatment. *Nature Reviews Neurology* 2009;**5**:392-403.
26. Graw BP, Wiesel SW. Low back pain in the aging athlete. *Sports Medicine and Arthroscopy* 2008;**16**:39-46.
27. Lavy C, James A, Wilson-MacDonald J, et al. Cauda equina syndrome. *British Medical Journal* 2009;**338**:b936.
28. Fraser S, Roberts L, Murphy E. Cauda equina syndrome: a literature review of its definition and clinical presentation. *Archives of Physical Medicine and Rehabilitation* 2009;**90**:1964-8.
29. Gleave JRW, MacFarlane R. Cauda equina syndrome: what is the relationship between timing of surgery and outcome? *British Journal of Neurosurgery* 2002;**16**:325-8.
30. Peng B, Wu W, Hou S, et al. The pathogenesis of discogenic low back pain. *Journal of Bone and Joint Surgery (British)* 2005;**87**:62-7.
31. Zhang YG, Guo TM, Guo X, Wu SX. Clinical diagnosis for discogenic low back pain. *International Journal of Biological Sciences* 2009;**5**:647-58.
32. Biyani A, Andersson GB. Low back pain: pathophysiology and management. *Journal of the American Academy of Orthopedic Surgeons* 2004;**12**:106-15.
33. Fischer GW, Popich GA, Sullivan DE, et al. Diskitis: a prospective diagnostic analysis. *Pediatrics* 1978;**62**:543-8.
34. Bono CM. Low-back pain in athletes. *Journal of Bone and Joint Surgery (American)* 2004;**86A**:382-96.
35. Biering-Sorensen F. A prospective study of low back pain in a general population. I. Occurrence, recurrence and aetiology. *Scandinavian Journal of Rehabilitation Medicine* 1983;**15**:71-9.
36. Biering-Sorensen F. Physical measurements as risk indicators for low-back trouble over a one-year period. *Spine* 1984;**9**:106-19.
37. Biering-Sorensen F. A one-year prospective study of low back trouble in a general population. The prognostic value of low back history and physical measurements. *Danish Medical Bulletin* 1984;**31**:362-75.
38. Biering-Sorensen F, Thomsen CE, Hilden J. Risk indicators for low back trouble. *Scandinavian Journal of Rehabilitation Medicine* 1989;**21**:151-7.
39. Nourbakhsh MR, Arab AM. Relationship between mechanical factors and incidence of low back pain. *Journal of Orthopaedic and Sports Physical Therapy* 2002;**32**:447-60.
40. Lee JH, Hoshino Y, Nakamura K, et al. Trunk muscle weakness as a risk factor for low back pain. A 5-year prospective study. *Spine* 1999;**24**:54-7.
41. Thomas JS, France CR, Sha D, et al. The effect of chronic low back pain on trunk muscle activations in target reaching movements with various loads. *Spine* 2007;**32**:E801-8.

42. Hodges PW, Richardson CA. Delayed postural contraction of transversus abdominis in low back pain associated with movement of the lower limb. *Journal of Spinal Disorders* 1998;**11**:46–56.
43. Hodges PW, Richardson CA. Altered trunk muscle recruitment in people with low back pain with upper limb movement at different speeds. *Archives of Physical Medicine and Rehabilitation* 1999;**80**:1005–12.
44. Chiba KMD, Toyama YMD, Matsumoto MMD, *et al*. Intraspinal cyst communicating with the intervertebral disc in the lumbar spine: discal cyst. *Spine* 2001;**26**:2112–18.
45. Goyal RN, Russell NA, Benoit BG, Belanger JM. Intraspinal cysts: a classification and literature review. *Spine* 1987;**12**:209–13.

87

Spinal infections

SHANMUGANATHAN RAJASEKARAN, P. RISHI MUGESH KANNA, T. AJOY PRASAD SHETTY

Introduction	982
PYOGENIC SPINAL INFECTIONS	982
Introduction	982
Aetiology	983
Pathophysiology	983
Clinical presentation	983
Investigations	983

Differential diagnosis	985
Conservative treatment	985
Surgical treatment	985
Other spinal infections	985
Spinal tuberculosis	987
Further reading	992

INTRODUCTION

Spinal infections can be pyogenic, granulomatous or parasitic. Pyogenic vertebral osteomyelitis is the most commonly encountered form of vertebral infection whereas tuberculosis is more common in the developing countries. Infection develops from haematogenous spread of bacteria, by direct inoculation, by contiguous spread from adjacent structures or from iatrogenic causes. The primary focus of infection in the spine can be in the vertebral body, the intervertebral disc, the epidural space or in the posterior elements. Early diagnosis and management is important, as good results can be obtained even with conservative treatment in the initial stages. But left untreated, these infections can lead to permanent neurological deficits, significant spinal deformity or even death. Management principles in early cases include identification of the organism, appropriate antimicrobial chemotherapy and supportive treatment. Surgical treatment is indicated in patients with extensive vertebral destruction, abscess formation, neurological deficits, deformity and severe pain due to instability. Prognosis depends on the extent of the disease, the type of organism, the severity of neurological and vertebral damage and the general condition of the patient.

PYOGENIC SPINAL INFECTIONS

INTRODUCTION

The current incidence of pyogenic vertebral infection has been reported to be around 3–16% of all osteomyelitis. The population incidence is around one case per 100 000– 250 000 population per year. The incidence is higher in the less developed and developing nations because of malnutrition, immune deficiency states, delayed diagnosis and lack of medical facilities. In the developed nations too, the incidence of spinal infections is on the increase, probably due to increased awareness of the physicians, better diagnostic modalities and the expanding 'at risk' group. This rise has also been attributed to the increased use of vascular devices and spinal instrumentation procedures. A bimodal age distribution has been observed with the first peak occurring in paediatric patients and a second peak in incidence observed at approximately 50–60 years. Because of its rarity and vague initial signs and symptoms, diagnosis is often delayed. It can result in severe compression of the neural structures, and systemic spread of the infection can lead to septicaemia. This can result in significant morbidity and mortality.

AETIOLOGY

Most infections occur due to bacterial spread from a distant site to the spinal column through the bloodstream. The skin, respiratory tract and the genitourinary tract are the common primary foci. But in approximately 30–70% of patients, a primary focus of infection cannot be detected. Several risk factors have been identified for developing vertebral infections (Box 87.1). *Staphylococcus aureus* is by far the most common organism to cause vertebral infection, although any infective organism can potentially cause one. Other pathogens such as *Escherichia coli*, *Proteus* and streptococci have also been isolated.

> **BOX 87.1: Risk factors for acquiring pyogenic vertebral infections**
>
> Advanced age
> Intravenous drug abuse
> Immune deficiency states
> Long-term systemic administration of steroids
> Diabetes mellitus
> Organ transplantation
> Malnutrition
> Malignancy
> Others: infective endocarditis, renal failure, sickle cell disease, chronic alcoholism

PATHOPHYSIOLOGY

The arterial route is the common route of bacterial spread to a vertebra, but retrograde seeding of venous blood via the Batson's venous plexus also plays a role. Whenever intra-abdominal pressure increases, venous blood is shunted from the abdominal and pelvic organs towards the valveless vertebral venous plexus. Rarely, contiguous spread of infection from a nearby infected focus to the vertebra and disc produces infective spondylitis.

About 90–95% of pyogenic spinal infections affect the vertebral body, and the posterior elements of the spine are infrequently involved. This has been attributed to the increased blood supply to the trabecular cancellous bone of the vertebral body and its rich, cellular marrow. Bacteria circulating through the blood may enter a vertebra or a disc space via its arterial or venous blood system. As the blood flow stagnates in the metaphyseal arterial loops just beneath the vertebral endplates, the circulating bacteria readily colonize there. Similarly, blockage of the metaphyseal arteries by septic thrombi may infarct relatively large amounts of bone. Once the subchondral region is infected, the avascular disc is secondarily invaded by bacteria from the endplate region. Communicating arteries and venous plexus allow the spread of septic thrombi from one metaphysis to the other. Most vertebral body infections occur in the lumbar spine because of the high blood flow to this region of the spine. In pyogenic spondylitis, the involvement is usually focal but multiple site involvement can occur in immunocompromised patients. As destruction proceeds, the vertebral canal can be invaded by pus and granulation tissue, which can cause cord compression, meningitis, myelitis and sepsis. A spinal epidural abscess occurs in 5–18% of cases and is most commonly located anteriorly in the epidural space.

CLINICAL PRESENTATION

A precipitous onset with signs of acute pyogenic infection is rare and the usual presentation is one of insidious onset, with back pain being the most common symptom. The pain is initially localized to the level of infection but vague distribution to the paraspinal areas is common. Onset of severe pain usually indicates severe instability due to either gross destruction of the vertebral bodies or involvement of posterior structures, especially the facet joints. Neurological involvement is usually late and is present only when the disease has progressed to the stage of vertebral body collapse with kyphosis or with the development of a large epidural abscess.

Although fever is present only in less than one-third of adult patients, children with vertebral osteomyelitis can present with an abrupt onset of malaise and fever. Young children may not directly complain of back pain but rather present with stiffness of the back, restricted spinal movements and guarded walking. A 'coin test' has been described in children where the child is unable to pick up a coin from the floor because of painful restriction of spinal movements.

Where neurological involvement is suspected, a meticulous neurological examination is a must. This should include a per rectal examination to detect early cauda equina compression. This is important, as early surgical intervention in such cases would be beneficial. Ideally the neurological examination should be repeated and documented at regular intervals, as it gives an idea about the improvement or deterioration of the patient's neurological status over time.

INVESTIGATIONS

Laboratory studies

Leucocytosis can often be absent or minimal (50%) in patients with pyogenic spondylitis. Elevation of the erythrocyte sedimentation rate (ESR), although non-specific, is the most common laboratory abnormality. Unexplained back pain associated with stiffness and an increased ESR should lead the clinician to suspect infective spondylitis as part of the differential diagnosis. C-reactive protein (CRP) is also an excellent indicator of acute inflammation. Rather than single values, serial ESR and CRP values help in predicting infection and also in assessing the response to treatment. In cases of postoperative spondylodiscitis, ESR and CRP values hold more significance. After an uncomplicated spine surgery, the ESR level usually does not exceed 70 mm h^{-1}, does not increase after the second week and returns to normal by the third week. Likewise CRP attains peak levels between 2 and 3 days, followed by an exponential decrease, and normalizes in 10–13 days. If there is a deviation from this pattern (prolonged peak levels, persistent high levels at 2–3 weeks), then it is considered 80% specific for infection. Urine cultures are advised in patients where the genitourinary tract is considered the primary focus. Blood cultures should always be obtained during a febrile episode and prior to administration of antibiotics. But they are not sensitive and are positive in only 60% of patients.

Diagnostic studies

Plain radiographs can be normal in the early stage of the disease as changes in plain radiographs usually lag by a few weeks behind the clinical stage of the disease. Loss of delineation of the trabeculae of the subchondral bone and destruction of the end plates with narrowing of the disc space are usually seen by 2–3 weeks (Fig. 87.1). In advanced disease, destruction of vertebral bodies, collapse with kyphosis and features of spinal instability may be evident. CT is more sensitive in assessing the degree of bone destruction and examining the surrounding soft tissues. It is also used as a guide for accurate placement of the needle while performing a percutaneous biopsy.

MRI is now the investigation of choice because of its ability to depict changes even in the early stages of the disease (Fig. 87.2). It differentiates infected and normal tissues and determines the full extent of the infection. MRI has been shown to have a sensitivity of 96%, a specificity of 92% and an accuracy of 94% in patients with disc space infections. T_1-weighted images show decreased signal intensity changes in the vertebral bodies and disc spaces. In T_2-weighted images, the signal intensity is increased in the vertebral disc and is markedly decreased in the vertebral body. It also clearly documents the location and size of epidural abscess, the presence of sequestrum within the canal, the extent of compromise of the spinal canal, the degree of compression of the spinal cord and also any signal intensity changes in the cord. Asymptomatic multilevel skip lesions are possible and hence MRI investigation must evaluate the whole spine. It is difficult to differentiate between pyogenic and non-pyogenic infections based on MRI alone.

A radionuclear scan with technetium-99m is very sensitive (>90%) for an early diagnosis of pyogenic vertebral osteomyelitis. But it is considered non-specific with only 70% specificity. Although expensive, a radioactive gallium scan is more specific with 80–85% specificity rates. Gallium localizes inflammatory lesions well and when combined with technetium demonstrates virtually all pyogenic vertebral infections. The use of PET-CT in inflammation and infection disorders may be useful in the future and is currently under clinical investigation.

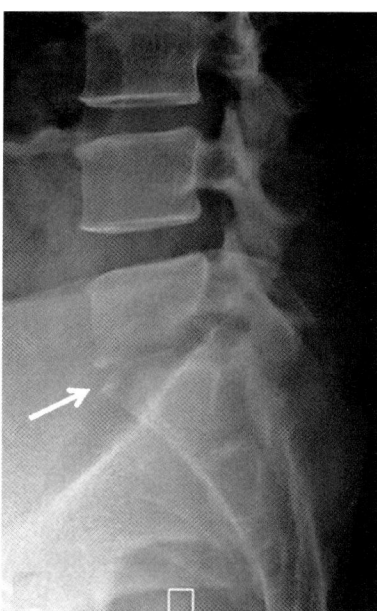

Figure 87.1 Lateral lumbosacral radiograph shows a reduction in disc height, irregularity of the end plates and subchondral osteopenia. These changes are typical of discitis and are observed 2–3 weeks after the onset of the disease.

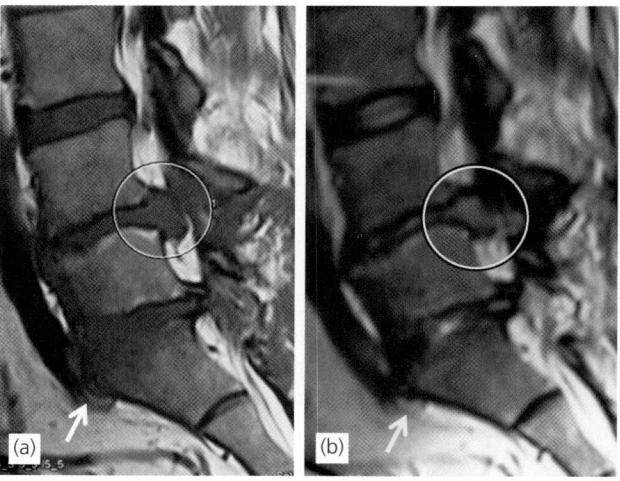

Figure 87.2 Sagittal T_1 and T_2 MRI images of a patient with L5–S1 spondylodiscitis. (a) The T_1 image shows hypointense changes in the disc space and the vertebral body (arrow). (b) The T_2 image shows hyperintense disc space whereas the adjacent vertebral body shows hypointensity.

Histopathology

CT-guided percutaneous biopsy of the infected vertebra or disc is advised, especially in patients without significant neural compression where tissue biopsy is required. Although cultures are positive in only 50–60% of patients, histological findings are invariably confirmative. Trocar biopsies are better than fine needle aspiration because a larger amount of material from the infected area is available for examination. If blood cultures and percutaneous biopsy techniques fail to identify the infecting organism, open surgical biopsy is indicated. An open surgical biopsy has the highest success rate for positive culture findings and diagnostic confirmation. Histological findings are similar to those of any bacterial pyogenic infection. Local destruction of the disc and end plates occurs with infiltration of neutrophils and inflammatory changes in the early stages. Later, a lymphocytic infiltrate predominates.

DIFFERENTIAL DIAGNOSIS

A high degree of suspicion is required for an early diagnosis of spinal infection, especially in patients with risk factors as the presenting symptoms may be vague. The important differential diagnosis is between infection and tumour, although injuries in the osteoporotic spine and spontaneous haematomas may also have similar presentation. In postoperative discitis, the clinical picture and blood investigations are more important than radiological investigations as 'normal' signal intensity changes seen in immediate postoperative period may mimic infection.

CONSERVATIVE TREATMENT

Conservative therapy is usually successful in the early stages of the disease, when the diagnosis is certain, the infective organism is known and appropriate antibiotics can be instituted before the development of severe destruction or neurological complications. Bed rest and intravenous antibiotics are the key features of conservative therapy. Isolation of the organism either from blood culture or through a trocar biopsy of the lesion is preferable before the start of antibiotics. After the harvest of the material, it is prudent to start a first-generation cephalosporin empirically as *Staphylococcus aureus* is the most common organism. Management of comorbid factors such as diabetes mellitus, anaemia, malnutrition and associated diseases is also important.

There is no clear consensus on the duration of antibiotic therapy but generally intravenous antibiotics started based on culture and sensitivity patterns are given for a period of 3–4 weeks followed by an equal period of oral antibiotic therapy. Serial monitoring with ESR and CRP levels is important to judge control of infection, and the antibiotics must be continued for at least a month after the ESR and clinical symptoms have returned to normal. Failure of resolution of clinical symptoms, a persistently high ESR and progressive destruction in radiographs indicate failure of conservative therapy.

SURGICAL TREATMENT

Surgical treatment is required in approximately 10–15% of patients. Persistent symptoms, onset of new symptoms, inability to isolate the organism, ambiguity in diagnosis, onset of neurological deficit or increasing kyphosis are the indications for surgery. Surgery should aim to obtain adequate material for both bacteriological and histological diagnosis, adequately decompress the neural structures and also provide stability with reconstruction of the spinal column. The safety of usage of metallic implants is now well documented and the post-debridement defect can be safely reconstructed with either bone graft or cages. Titanium implants are preferable to stainless steel implants because they allow little biofilm formation with poor bio-adhesive properties, which prevents adhesion of bacteria to the implants. The extent of surgery and the approach must be titrated according to the severity of involvement and the health status of the patient. It should be noted that there is a significant mortality following surgery in the high-risk groups. Laminectomy alone is not to be performed as it invariably produces additional instability. An anterior approach is usually preferred as it provides good access to the area of pathology allowing adequate debridement and reconstruction. Wherever necessary, stability must be achieved by additional posterior instrumentation. In severely debilitated patients, drainage of the abscess by a posterolateral approach may be initially performed. The mortality rate for vertebral osteomyelitis varies from 2–12%. Neurological deficits develop in 15–40% of patients, especially those with comorbidities and multiple risk factors.

OTHER SPINAL INFECTIONS

Postoperative pyogenic infection

Postoperative discitis can potentially occur after any invasive procedure in the disc space. The incidence varies from 1% to 7% depending on the type of surgery and the use of instrumentation. The disc devoid of vascular supply develops discitis even with a small inoculum. Normally in an uncomplicated healing after a disc surgery, the postoperative back pain settles in 2–3 days. Any abnormal back pain starting 2–3 days after surgery, present even at rest, increasing with the movements of the spine should raise the suspicion of discitis. There may be local warmth and tenderness. ESR and CRP levels are raised. As explained before, deviation from the normal postoperative pattern of changes of these inflammatory markers detected from serial measurements help in diagnosis. Initially the radiographs are normal and hence MRI needs to be done if there is a suspicion. It is difficult to differentiate normal postoperative changes and discitis in the MRI. However, presence of hyperintensity changes in the disc space and the vertebral body which enhance with contrast and occurrence of perivertebral abscess confirm the diagnosis (Fig. 87.3). An image-guided biopsy helps in histopathological confirmation of discitis. But an organism is isolatable in only 50% of the patients. Early cases with mild infection do well with rest and appropriate parenteral antibiotic therapy. Usually parenteral antibiotic therapy is given for a period of 3–4 weeks followed by oral antibiotics up to 8 weeks. The duration of therapy depends on various factors such as the severity of infection, type and virulence of the organism, immune status of the patient, presence of comorbid factors, magnitude of surgery performed, etc. Patients who are septic, with abscess formation require thorough debridement. In patients with a large anterior column defect after debridement, a cage or a bone graft should be used to reconstruct the anterior column and provide stability. Instrumentation can be safely used in patients with suspected instability.

Brucella spondylitis

Brucella can affect the spine and mimics tubercular spondylitis. Spinal brucellosis is mainly found in the lumbar region and multiple site infections are also common. The patients present with general constitutional symptoms, polyarthralgia and significant back pain. A strong index of suspicion is required especially in endemic regions and diagnosis is based on radiographs, serology and culture. Radiographic findings include step-like erosions of the margin of the vertebral body, disc space thinning and vertebral segment ankylosis by bridging. The diagnosis usually is confirmed by brucella antibody titres of 1:80 or greater. The usual treatment is chemotherapy for 3 months with tetracycline, rifampicin or streptomycin. Surgical management is reserved for those with neurological compromise or persistent symptoms.

Fungal and parasitic infections

Fungal infections present as granulomatous lesions. They have been observed predominantly in endemic regions. A variety of fungi such as coccidiodomycosis, histoplasmosis, aspergillosis, cryptococcus and blastomycosis has been implicated. Presentation is vague and mimics other chronic granulomatous infections. Histopathology is diagnostic. Chemotherapy with amphotericin B and fluconazole along with surgical debridement gives good results.

Echinococcus granulosus causes large expansile cystic lesions (hydatid cysts) in the vertebra. The vertebra is involved in less than 1% of all hydatidosis but more than 50% of patients with skeletal hydatidosis have vertebral involvement. The most common site is the lower thoracic and upper lumbar vertebral bodies. The discs are relatively resistant to invasion. So the picture of bulging soft-tissue shadows in the paraspinal region (due to confluent cysts) next to destroyed vertebrae with an intact intervening disc is typical of vertebral hydatidosis. The patient presents with localized back pain and varying degrees of neurological features, depending on the extent of canal compromise. Treatment is aimed at near-total radical excision protecting the adjacent vital structures and stabilization with antihelminthal chemotherapy (albendazole or mebendazole for a period of 1 year).

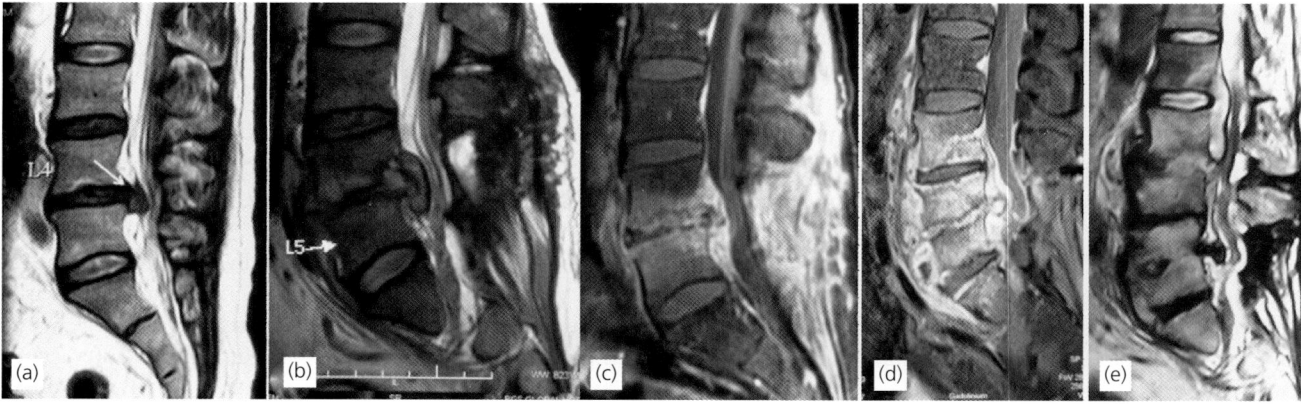

Figure 87.3 Progressive postoperative spondylodiscitis in an immunocompromised patient. (a) Pre-operative sagittal T_2 MR image shows an L4–5 disc prolapse. (b, c) Hyperintense signal and changes in the disc space with perivertebral abscess formation, which enhances with contrast, are seen. (d, e) Progression of lesion to adjacent disc spaces and vertebra with excessive abscess formation and destruction of vertebra. The epidural abscess causes significant thecal sac compression.

SPINAL TUBERCULOSIS

Introduction

Spinal tuberculosis accounts for more than 50% of skeletal tuberculosis and is caused by *Mycobacterium tuberculosis*. Infection results from haematogenous dissemination from a primary focus, usually the lungs, although the associated active focus is identified in less than 10%. The lumbar vertebrae can be involved from infection through the Batson's perivertebral venous plexus. The most common site of infection is the paradiscal type with secondary involvement of the disc. In children, extensive involvement with complete destruction of many adjacent vertebral bodies may be seen. Posterior structures are involved only in about 10% and skip lesions can be identified in 15%. Pathology is one of caseation with progressive destruction of the bone and abscess formation, which may track down along fascial planes according to the region of the involvement (Table 87.1).

Clinical features

Back pain associated with restriction of movements of the spine is the usual presenting feature. Constitutional symptoms of malaise, loss of appetite and weight, evening rise in temperature and night sweats are also common but can be absent in patients with good nutrition. As the disease progresses, collapse of the spine is evident with prominence of the spinous process as a knuckle deformity in the early stages and a very prominent kyphotic deformity in late stages. A cold abscess may be clinically evident, either in the paraspinal area or it may track distally depending on the region of involvement. But it is most often identified in the anteroposterior spine radiographs and MRI scans as a fusiform paraspinal shadow (Fig. 87.4). Neurological involvement occurs in up to 20% of the patients and can occur both in the active phase of the disease and even after complete healing. In active lesions, it is due to the result of direct compression of the cord because of an abscess, inflammatory granulation tissue, a dislodged sequestrum or canal compromise due to instability. In the late stages, it is usually due to stretching of the cord over a bony ridge at the apex of the deformity (Table 87.2). Neurological involvement initially presents as incoordination, clumsiness while walking and slowly progresses to paraplegia in flexion and flaccid paraplegia (Box 87.2).

Differential diagnosis

Tuberculosis is often overdiagnosed in endemic areas and underdiagnosed in developed countries. It should be differentiated from other granulomatous lesions such as fungal spondylitis, metastatic and primary spinal tumours and pyogenic spondylitis. Typical paradiscal involvement, minimal or absent signs of sepsis, presence of a large

Table 87.1 Location of cold abscesses and their pathways of spread from the primary spinal focus

Paths of spread	Presenting region
Cervical spine	
Prevertebral fascia	Retropharyngeal abscesses
Prevertebral fascia	Mediastinum to enter trachea, oesophagus, or pleura
Deep cervical fascia	Posterior to the sternomastoid muscle (posterior triangle of neck)
Thoracolumbar spine	
Intercostal nerves	Chest wall
Ilioinguinal and iliohypogastric nerves	Rectus sheath and lower abdominal wall
Psoas sheath	Thigh
Posterior spinal nerves	Paraspinal region
Superior gluteal nerve	Buttock
Flat muscles of abdominal wall	Petit's triangle
Internal pudendal nerve	Ischiorectal fossa

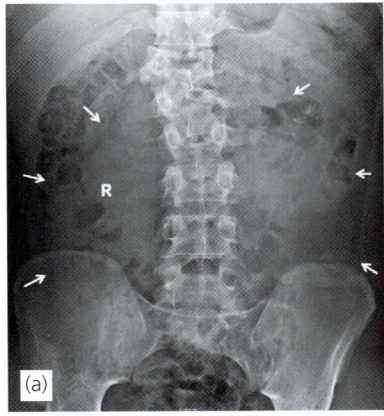

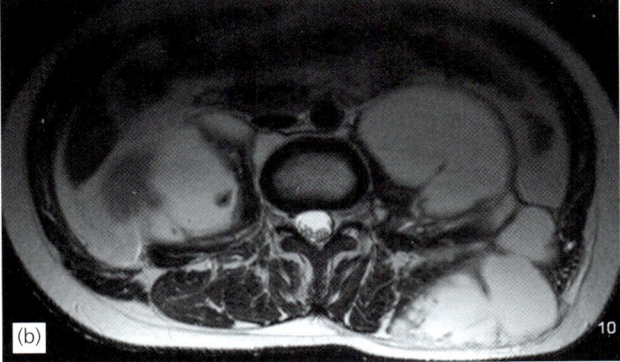

Figure 87.4 Huge bilateral psoas abscess in a patient with thoracolumbar tuberculosis. The anteroposterior radiograph shows paraspinal soft-tissue widening due to the abscess, which is confirmed in the axial MR images.

Table 87.2 Causes of neurological complications in spinal tuberculosis

Cause	Prognosis
Active disease	
Compressive pathology	
Inflammatory oedema	
Granulation and caseous tissue with sequestrated material	Usually responds well to conservative chemotherapy and a middle path regimen can safely be followed
Infective vasculitis	
Spinal tumour syndrome	
Pathological dislocation of spine	
Direct infiltration of tuberculous bacilli into the cord	
Healed disease	
Stretching of cord over the bony ridge at the apex of the deformity (internal gibbus)	
Progressive constriction of cord due to extradural fibrosis	Surgery is essential to relieve mechanical compression. The prognosis is guarded

---

BOX 87.2: Stages of tuberculous paraplegia

Patient is asymptomatic
Neurological examination reveals an extensor plantar response or ankle clonus
↓
Patient has incoordination while walking but can walk with support
↓
Patient is confined to bed due to severe spastic weakness ('paraplegia in extension')
Varying degrees of sensory blunting present
↓
'Paraplegia in flexion' with bladder, bowel involvement and flexor spasms
↓
Flaccid paraplegia

---

abscess and characteristic findings in MRI (see below) help to confirm the diagnosis of spinal tuberculosis.

Workup

BLOOD INVESTIGATIONS

The ESR may be markedly elevated (>70 mm h^{-1}), and serial ESR measurements also help in assessing the response to treatment. The Mantoux skin test is not useful, as a positive test just indicates a previous tuberculous infection. Coexistent infection by human immunodeficiency virus and other immune deficiency conditions can also give a false-negative skin test. The enzyme-linked immunosorbent assay (ELISA) to detect immunoglobulin (Ig) G and IgM antibodies has a reported sensitivity of 60–80%. Polymerase chain reaction (PCR) analysis, especially from tissue samples, is considered very sensitive and specific for the diagnosis of spinal tuberculosis. Tuberculosis PCR from tissue aspirate has a sensitivity of 73.1%, specificity of 93.7% and low false-positivity rates (13.6%). The positive agreement between histopathology and PCR is very good (0.69).

IMAGING STUDIES

The earliest features observed on plain radiographs are vertebral osteoporosis, narrowing of the joint space and indistinct paradiscal margin of vertebral bodies. In the thoracic spine, the cold abscess is visible on plain radiographs as a fusiform or globular radiodense shadow (bird's nest appearance). Longstanding abscesses may produce concave erosions around the anterior surfaces of the vertebral bodies called the *aneurysmal phenomenon*. Wedging of one or two vertebral bodies leads to a kyphotic deformity.

CT and MRI can detect lesions at an earlier stage. CT is useful in assessing accurately the extent of bony destruction and in early identification of posterior element involvement. It also clearly shows spinal lesions of certain regions that are not clearly seen in plain radiographs such as the craniovertebral junction, cervicodorsal region, the sacroiliac joints and the sacrum. CT is also helpful to perform a percutaneous biopsy. MRI is superior to CT scan for demonstrating the extent of disease into the nearby soft tissues, the spread of tuberculous abscess and the degree of neural compression. MRI with contrast is also helpful in differentiating tuberculous lesions from non-infectious diseases. Serial MRI can be used to assess the response to treatment and regression of the disease. A bone scan with Tc-99m is considered to be highly sensitive, but non-specific. It may only aid to localize the site of active disease and to detect multilevel involvement.

HISTOPATHOLOGY AND MICROBIOLOGY

In endemic countries, because of high prevalence, chemotherapy is sometimes started without a definite microbiological diagnosis. This is based on the typical clinical presentation and radiological features in most patients. However, a biopsy is needed in cases of doubtful findings, lack of proper response to drug therapy, suspicion of drug-resistant strains and in patients from non-endemic places. The method most widely used to acquire the sample is CT or fluoroscopy-guided needle/trocar biopsy. The bone tissue or abscess samples obtained are subjected to staining for acid-fast bacilli and culture and sensitivity tests. These microbiological results are positive in only about 50–60% of the cases since skeletal tuberculosis is of paucibacillary variety. So it is important that the tissue should be sent for histopathological examination also. The typical histopathological findings are large caseating necrotizing granulomatous lesions with epithelioid and multinucleated giant cells with lymphocytic infiltration.

Treatment

PRINCIPLES OF MANAGEMENT

General supportive measures include bed rest, external bracing, nutritious diet, vitamins as required, care of bladder, bowels and good nursing care. Modern antitubercular drugs are able to achieve therapeutic levels in caseous tissues and abscesses (isoniazid and rifampicin in bactericidal concentrations, pyrazinamide at fivefold minimum inhibitory concentrations) and excellent clinical cure can be achieved. Hence uncomplicated spinal tuberculosis is considered as a medical disease with selected surgical indications. When surgery is required, the entire anterior tuberculous lesion is thoroughly debrided until bleeding bone surfaces are reached and the defect is reconstructed with grafts/cages. Because of the morbidity of such radical surgeries, many centres prefer to follow the 'middle path regimen'. Ambulant multidrug chemotherapy is advocated for all the patients, and bed rest with external bracing is advised only in the early stages until pain is present. The patient is followed carefully until complete healing of the disease is attained. Surgical treatment is recommended for certain specific indications in these patients (Box 87.3).

ANTITUBERCULAR CHEMOTHERAPY

The currently recommended first-line drug regimen consists of four-drug therapy. This includes isoniazid (H) 5 mg kg^{-1}, rifampicin (R) 10 mg kg^{-1}, pyrazinamide (Z) 20–25 mg kg^{-1}, and ethambutol (E) 15 mg kg^{-1}. In children, ethambutol is replaced by streptomycin, as the former may cause optic neuritis. Studies performed by the British Medical Research Council indicate that tuberculous spondylitis should be treated with combination short-course chemotherapy for 6–9 months. According to the WHO guidelines for the type and duration of antituberculous chemotherapy, spinal tuberculosis is considered to be severe extrapulmonary type (category 1) and treatment is advised for 6 months (2HRZE and 4HR). In cases of relapse or treatment failure, treatment is prescribed according to category 2, i.e. for 8 months (2HRZES, 1HRZE, 5HRE). Some authors prefer to give chemotherapy for 18 months (4HRZE, 14HR), although it has not been proved superior to short-course chemotherapy. Treatment protocol of HIV-positive patients is the same as for HIV-negative patients. HIV patients with lower CD4 counts (<200) have poor prognosis.

BOX 87.3: Indications for surgery in spinal tuberculosis

Neurological deficit
Severe neurological deficits at presentation
Rapidly worsening deficits
New onset or deteriorating deficits during chemotherapy
Unimproved deficits after 6–8 weeks of chemotherapy
Spinal instability
Panvertebral disease
>3 contiguous vertebra involved
Vertebral body loss >1 in thoracic spine and 1.5 in lumbar spine
Children with initial kyphosis >30°
Children with 'spine at risk' signs
Posterior neural arch with pedicular destruction
Clinical instability
Late deformity
Severe kyphosis with late onset neurological deficits
Lack of clinical response to chemotherapy
Failure of clinical improvement after 6 weeks of chemotherapy
Disease recurrence despite chemotherapy
Primary drug resistance

SURGICAL TREATMENT

The aims of surgery in spinal tuberculosis are to obtain tissue samples for biopsy, drain an abscess cavity, achieve debridement of disease focus and to stabilize the spine. These can be achieved either by anterior, posterior or by combined procedures, either as a staged or as a single procedure. The addition of instrumentation in spinal tuberculosis is well accepted and advised especially where instability is present or expected after decompression (Fig. 87.5). A lower threshold for surgery is recommended in case of cervical spine involvement as it is more commonly associated with higher incidence of neurological deficits and compression due to abscess formation (Fig. 87.6). Opinion varies regarding the operative indication for spinal tuberculosis. A large group of surgeons perform debridement and decompression in all cases, irrespective of neurological involvement (radical surgical treatment). Others perform operative decompression only in those patients who do not respond to chemotherapy (middle path regimen). Resources and experience are key factors in the decision to use a surgical approach. The

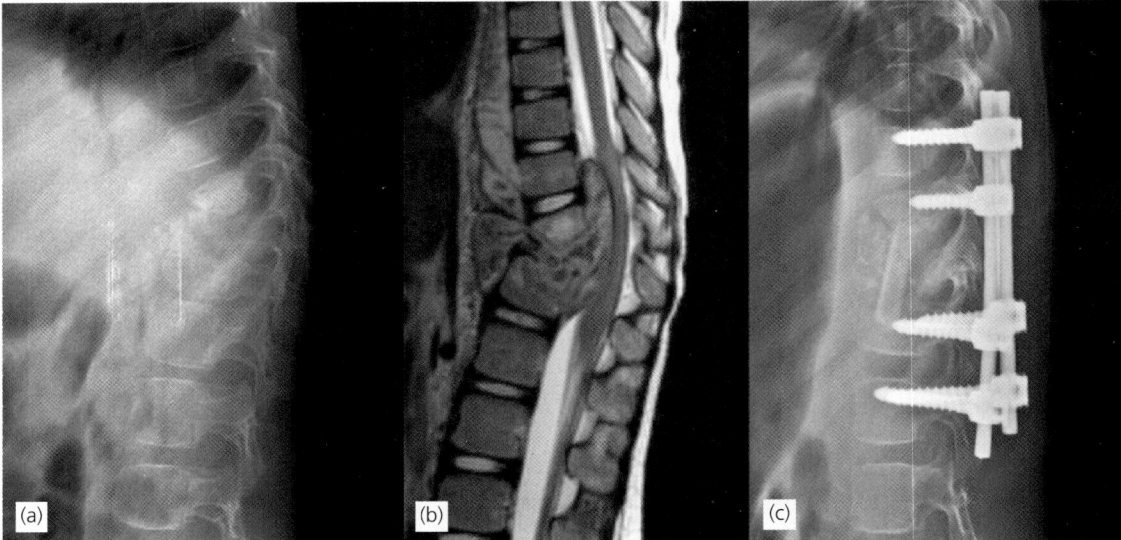

Figure 87.5 Thoracolumbar tuberculosis in a child with positive retropulsion sign on the radiograph and a huge abscess causing cord compression. The lesion has been treated by anterior debridement with fibular strut graft reconstruction and posterior pedicle screw stabilization.

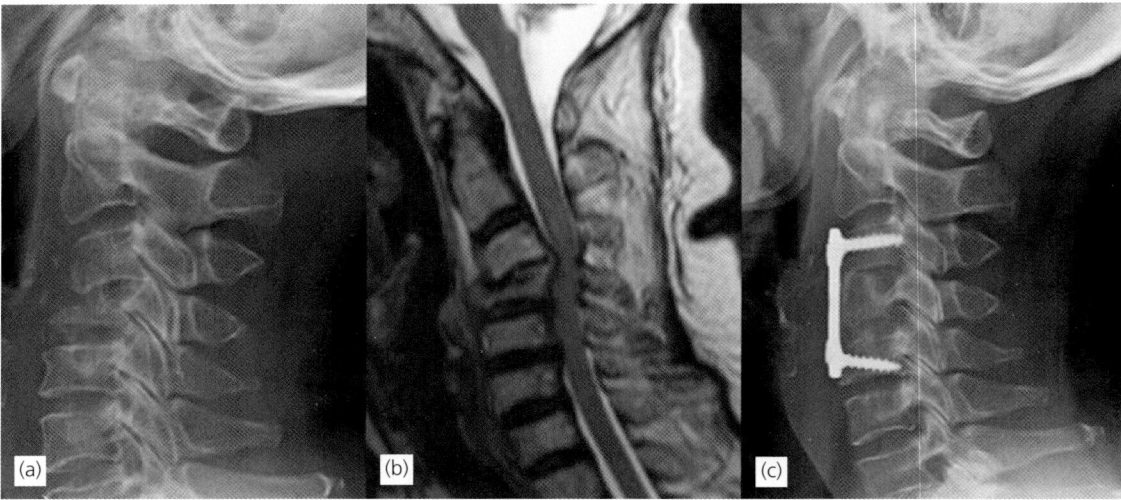

Figure 87.6 C4 vertebral body tuberculosis with kyphosis causing cord compression. The lesion has been treated by anterior debridement, iliac crest autograft reconstruction and stabilization with a plate.

indications for surgery are given in Box 87.3 and shown in Fig. 87.8.

In adults, the indications for surgery to prevent a deformity are less as they tend to collapse less in the active phase and the deformity does not progress after healing and consolidation. In contrast, children can have more and extensive vertebral destruction during the active phase and are also prone to develop late progressive collapse (Fig. 87.7). The possibility of some children developing severe deformity later can be predicted by the presence of certain 'spine at risk' signs in the radiographs (Fig. 87.8). All these lesions indicate subluxation of facet joints at the curve apex leading to instability and curve progression. The presence of more than two signs is associated with significant increase in the deformity (Fig. 87.9).

Prognosis

Current drug regimens are highly effective and achieve excellent cure rates in uncomplicated spinal tuberculosis. Poor prognostic factors in spinal tuberculosis include poor nutritional status, vertebral body loss >2, junctional lesions, neurological deficit of more than 1 year's duration, the presence of myelopathic changes in the cord, coinfection with HIV, poor treatment compliance and drug resistance.

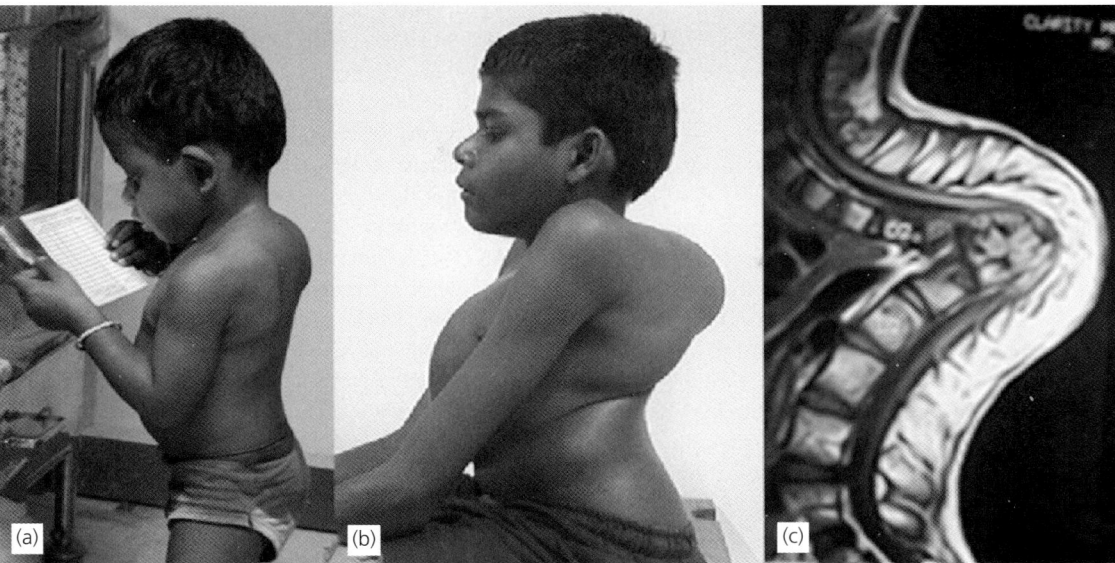

Figure 87.7 Clinical photographs of a child affected by spinal tuberculosis at the age of 4 years. Although the deformity looks minimal at the completion of chemotherapy, it has significantly worsened by adolescence. MRI shows a buckling collapse with cord compression and neurological deficits.

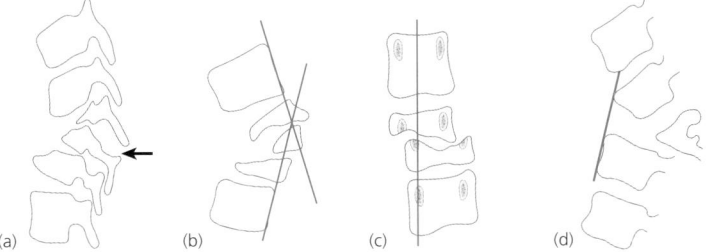

Figure 87.8 (a–d) Diagram of the radiological signs for the 'spine at risk'. (a) Separation of the facet joint. The facet joint dislocates at the level of the apex of the curve, causing instability and loss of alignment. In severe cases the separation can occur at two levels. (b) Posterior retropulsion. This is identified by drawing two lines along the posterior surface of the first upper and lower normal vertebrae. The diseased segments are found to be posterior to the intersection of the lines. (c) Lateral translation. This is confirmed when a vertical line drawn through the middle of the pedicle of the first lower normal vertebra does not touch the pedicle of the first upper normal vertebra. (d) Toppling sign. In the initial stages of collapse, a line drawn along the anterior surface of the first lower normal vertebra intersects the inferior surface of the first upper normal vertebra. 'Tilt' or 'toppling' occurs when the line intersects higher than the middle of the anterior surface of the first normal upper vertebra.

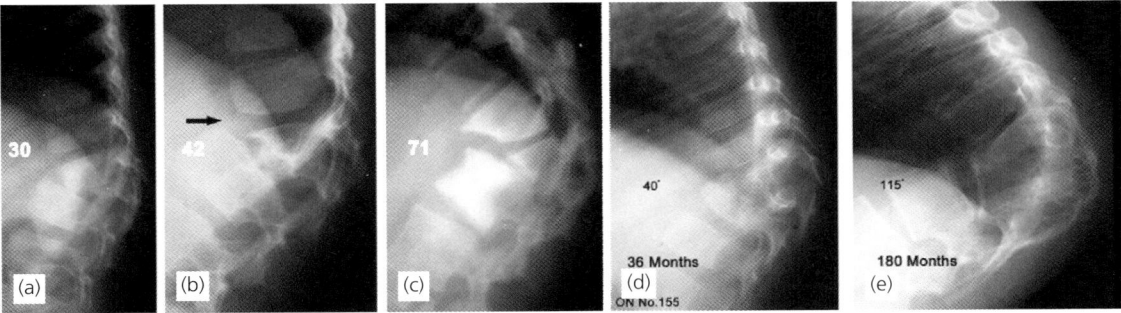

Figure 87.9 Lateral radiograph of thoracolumbar spine of a child with spinal tuberculosis treated by chemotherapy. The kyphosis angle is 30° at the end of treatment, which progressively has worsened to 115° at the end of 15 years. Post-tubercular kyphosis can worsen in children and can be effectively predicted and prevented by looking for the 'spine at risk' signs. This child has had posterior retropulsion and positive toppling sign and hence has worsened.

> **KEY LEARNING POINTS**
>
> **Pyogenic vertebral infections**
>
> - Pyogenic bacterial infections are the most common type of spinal infections.
> - Haematogenous spread of bacteria from a distant primary focus is the common mode of origin.
> - Diagnosis is based on clinical suspicion in high-risk patients, typical radiological findings and by isolating the organism through direct aspiration.
> - Adequate dose of appropriate antibiotics for a period of at least 6–8 weeks is the mainstay of treatment. Surgery is reserved for select indications.
>
> **Spinal tuberculosis**
>
> - *Mycobacterium tuberculosis* infection of the spine is very common in developing countries.
> - Diagnosis is based on typical clinical and radiological features. Histopathological findings are characteristic and show large caseating nectrotizing granulomas with epitheloid cells.
> - Short course ambulant antitubercular chemotherapy is the mainstay of treatment.
> - Surgical debridement, decompression and stabilization are needed in patients with severe neurological deficits, extensive vertebral destruction and deformity.
> - In vertebral infections, titanium implants can be used safely to attain spinal stability.

FURTHER READING

- ● = Key primary paper
- ◆ = Major review article

1. Abbey DM, Turner DM, Warson JS, *et al.* Treatment of postoperative wound infections following spinal fusion with instrumentation. *Journal of Spinal Disorders* 1995;**8**:278.
●2. Collert S. Osteomyelitis of the spine. *Acta Orthopaedica Scandinavica* 1977;**48**:283.
●3. Digby JM, Kersley J. Pyogenic nontuberculous spinal infection. *Journal of Bone and Joint Surgery* 1979;**61B**:47.
4. Krodel A, Kruger A, Lohscheidt K, *et al.* Anterior debridement, fusion, and extrafocal stabilization in the treatment of osteomyelitis of the spine. *Journal of Spinal Disorders* 1999;**12**:17.
●5. Pott P. Remarks on that kind of palsy of the lower limbs which is frequently found to accompany a curvature of the spine. London: J Johnson, 1779.
◆6. Thalgott JS, Cotler HB, Sasso RC, *et al.* Postoperative infections in spinal implants: classification and analysis – a multicenter study. *Spine* 1991;**16**:981.
◆7. Weinstein MA, McCabe JP, Cammisa Jr FP. Postoperative spinal wound infection: a review of 2391 consecutive index procedures. *Journal of Spinal Disorders* 2000;**13**:422.
8. Emery SE, Chan DPK, Woodward HR. Treatment of hematogenous pyogenic vertebral osteomyelitis with anterior debridement and primary bone grafting. *Spine* 1989;**14**:284.
●9. Scoles PV, Quinn TP. Intervertebral discitis in children and adolescents. *Clinical Orthopaedics and Related Research* 1982;**162**:31.
●10. Heusner AP. Nontuberculous spinal epidural infection. *New England Journal of Medicine* 1948;**239**:845.
◆11. Hodgson AR, Skinsnes OK, Leong CY. The pathogenesis of Pott's paraplegia. *Journal of Bone and Joint Surgery* 1967;**49A**:1147.
12. Hodgson AR, Stock FE, Fang HSY, *et al.* Anterior spinal fusion: the operative approach and pathological findings in 412 patients with Pott's disease of the spine. *British Journal of Surgery* 1960;**48**:172.
●13. Rajasekaran S, Shanmugasundaram TK. Prediction of the angle of gibbus deformity in tuberculosis of the spine. *Journal of Bone and Joint Surgery* 1987;**69A**:503.
●14. Rajasekaran S. The natural history of post-tubercular kyphosis in children: Radiological signs which predict late increase in deformity. *Journal of Bone and Joint Surgery* 2001;**83B**:954–62.
◆15. Rajasekaran S. The problem of deformity in spinal tuberculosis. *Clinical Orthopaedics and Related Research* 2002;**398**:85–92.

88

Degenerative disc disease

MUN KEONG KWAN

Introduction	993	Treatment	1001
Definition	993	Future potential therapy in the management	
Aetiology	994	of degenerative disease	1003
Anatomy	994	References	1005
Pathophysiology	995		

NATIONAL BOARD STANDARDS

Theoretical Knowledge
- Understand the pathophysiology of degenerative disc disease
- Symptomatology of the different stages of degenerative disc disease
- Correlation between the clinical findings and the radiological investigation
- Basic principles of the treatments options for different stages of disease

Practical Skills
- Be able to corelate the signs and symptoms with the radiological findings
- Be able to advise a patient on the treatment options

INTRODUCTION

Neck and back pain are one of life's most common presentations in medical practice. It is estimated that up to 80% of people are affected by these symptoms.[1] The lifetime incidence of low back pain is reported to be between 60% and 70%.[2,3] Degenerative disc disease is a main reason for these presentations. These disabilities usually affect the adult working population and result in a significant number of workdays lost. They have become a serious issue worldwide and are associated with a high socioeconomic impact. In the United States, the estimated direct costs of back pain alone in 1990 were approximately 24.3 billion dollars, whereas the indirect costs were reported to be approximately 27.5 billion dollars.[4]

DEFINITION

Degenerative spine disease itself is not a form of disease or pathological condition. It is part of the natural ageing process which involves the spinal column as a result of wear and tear. It encompasses a wide spectrum of conditions ranging from a mild annular injury to severe degenerative deformities.

Most degeneration occurs without any symptoms. Annular tears and disc protrusions are frequently noted on MRI in asymptomatic populations. Only some are symptomatic and present with symptoms such as neck or back pain with or without neurological compression. Jensen et al.[5] reported on the MRI findings in a group of asymptomatic subjects: 64% had one level of intervertebral disc abnormality, and 38% had abnormalities at more than one level. However, the MRI abnormalities included only disc bulges and protrusions but not extrusions. In an autopsy study of 600 human lumbar intervertebral discs, 90% of the discs had evidence of degeneration by age 50 years.[6]

Therefore, the term degenerative disc disease describes progressive deterioration of the spine but not the symptoms. Only when the symptoms of pain and/or neurological compression strike will the patient seek consultation, and then this condition becomes pathological. It is difficult to establish the relationship between symptoms and the degenerative spine, although it is believed to be highly associated.

AETIOLOGY

The underlying aetiology of degenerative disc disease is still unknown. However, studies have shown there are many risk factors which may play a role in the development of this condition. Cigarette smoking has been recognized as one of the important risk factors.[7–9] A degenerated spine occurs usually due to the repetitive injury of the spine (Fig. 88.1).[9,10]

Other risk factors include jobs that require the use of jackhammers and machine tools, prolonged motor vehicle usage, obesity, sagittal malalignment, psychosocial factors such as compensation and psychological stress.[7,9,11,12] Exposure to industrial vibration is also noted to be an important risk factor. Wilder et al.[13] reported that the human spine has a resonance frequency of approximately 5 Hz, which is nearly identical to the dominant frequency in many vehicles. Therefore, this vibration energy will be transmitted and absorbed by the individual spine that works in such environment.

ANATOMY

The intervertebral disc is a structure that links all the vertebrae from C2 to sacrum. The cartilaginous end plates and the intervertebral disc form a structural complex that allows movement between vertebrae, which gives the spine its flexibility and absorbs and distributes the mechanical forces applied to it. The intervertebral disc in adults is relatively avascular, and consists of the central nucleus pulposus surrounded by a tough annulus fibrosus. Both of these structures are made up of collagen and proteoglycans.

The nucleus pulposus is composed of a loose, non-orientated collagen framework (mainly type II collagen), which consists of a sparse population of cells, resembling chondrocytes, that are embedded in a gelatinous matrix of various proteoglycans. Healthy disc cells must be able to synthesize and maintain the extracellular matrix components. The proteoglycan content in the nucleus pulposus is approximately more than 10 times that of the annulus fibrosus content.[14] Proteoglycans attract and hold water in the interverterbral disc to allow the disc to withstand a loading force. The nucleus pulposus contains approximately 80% water. The nucleus pulposus blends in with the inner fibrocartilaginous annulus fibrosus without a clear anatomical demarcation.

The annulus fibrosus consists of a highly orientated densely packed collagen (mainly type I collagen) and becomes progressively more compact and tougher at the periphery. The outer annulus fibrosus forms numerous concentric rings of layers or lamellae. The fibres of each ring cross diagonally to provide greater tensile strength. The outer part of the annulus fibrosus is attached to the adjacent vertebral bodies at the site of the fused epiphyseal ring by Sharpey's fibres and to the anterior and posterior longitudinal ligaments.

Most disc herniations occur in a posterolateral direction because the location of the posterior longitudinal ligament in the middle of the posterior vertebra resists a direct posterior herniation. The annulus fibrosus is most deficient over the posterolateral portion of the disc where a prolapsed disc is likely to occur. The posterior portion of the annulus fibrosus and the posterior longitudinal ligament are innervated by the sinuvertebral nerves (Fig. 88.2).[15] Annular tears involving this complex may be a source of discogenic pain due to exposure of the nerve endings to acidic metabolites of the protruding nucleus pulposus.[16]

Intervertebral disc volume demonstrates a diurnal variation. The disc volume of the lower three lumbar vertebrae reduces in an erect position an average of 16.2% after 7 hours of standing and sitting.[17] The T_2-weighted MRI signal increases as much as 25% after a night's bed rest.[18]

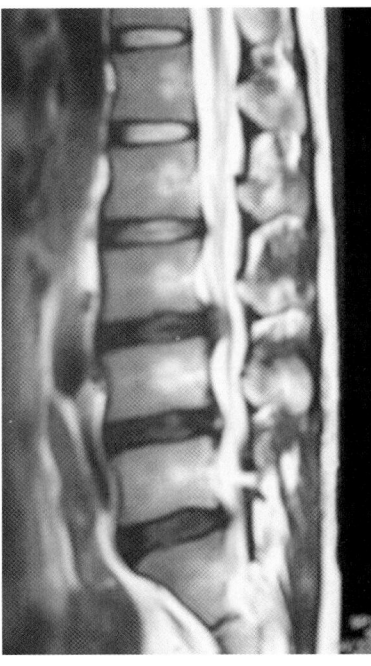

Figure 88.1 Lumbosacral MRI of a 25-year-old man who performed 300 sit-ups daily. He presented with severe back pain associated with right sciatica. MRI showed degenerated L2–L3, L3–L4, L4–L5 and L5–S1 disc levels. The radiculopathy is due to a large protrusion at the L3–L4 level.

PATHOPHYSIOLOGY

With ageing, there are striking structural and biomolecular changes occurring in the intervertebral discs. Structural changes as a result of degenerative disease of the spine especially in relation to the lumbar spine have been well revealed by Kirkaldy-Willis and Farhan.[19] The degenerative changes can be divided into three stages: (1) temporary dysfunction; (2) unstable phase; and (3) stabilization. The duration of each phase varies according to the patient. Different levels of the spine may degenerate at a different rate. In general, a disc herniation is considered a complication within the dysfunction and instability stages, whereas spinal stenosis is a complication of bony outgrowth and/or soft-tissue hypertrophy compressing the neural structure in the late instability and early stabilization stage.[20] With the advent of magnetic resonance imaging, the understanding of disc pathology and treatment has advanced tremendously.

Temporary dysfunction

This stage is seen in patients between the age of 15 and 45 years old. It is characterized by tears in the annulus fibrosus with localized synovitis of the facet joints.

There are three types of annular tears in a degenerated disc.[21] Concentric tears (type I) are caused by rupture of the short transverse fibres connecting the lamellae of the annulus, and are seen as crescentic or oval spaces filled with fluid or mucoid material. In radial tears (type II) the longitudinal fibres are disrupted through all layers of the annulus, from the surface of the annulus to the nucleus. Transverse tears (type III) result from rupture of Sharpey's fibres near their attachment with the ring apophysis, and are imaged as irregular fluid-filled cavities at the periphery of the annulus (Fig. 88.3).

Radial tears of the annulus fibrosus are a potential site for disc herniations.[22] Loss of disc signal does not necessarily occur at this stage. With temporary dysfunction, the patient is incapacitated to varying degrees by acute or subacute low back, pain most likely discogenic in nature or as a result of facet synovitis. The patient can be asymptomatic at this stage as well, despite the above changes.[23,24]

Unstable phase

This stage is seen in patients between the ages of 35 and 70 years old. This stage is characterized by internal disruption of the disc, progressive disc resorption, degeneration of the facet joints with capsular laxity, subluxation and joint erosion.

At this stage, degeneration of the intervertebral disc is accompanied by loss of water content, especially in the nucleus pulposus. T_2-weighted MRI will demonstrate decreased signal changes in the nucleus pulposus of the intervertebral disc.

Further internal disruption of the disc, coupled with the development of annular tears, allows degenerated loose nucleus pulposus fragment(s) to protrude into the defect, resulting in a disc prolapse. At this point, the radiograph may also show the presence of reduced disc height (Fig. 88.4). There are four types of disc prolapse (Fig. 88.5).

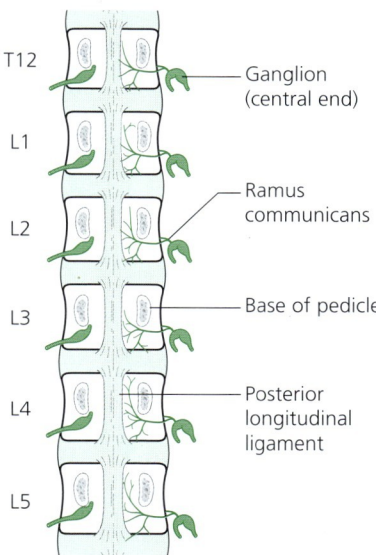

Figure 88.2 Diagram illustrates the sinuvertebral nerve. (From: Pedersen HE, Blunck CFJ, Gardner E. The anatomy of lumbosacral posterior rami and meningeal branches of spinal nerves (sinuvertebral nerves): with an experimental study of their functions. *Journal of Bone and Joint Surgery* 1956;**38A**:377–91).

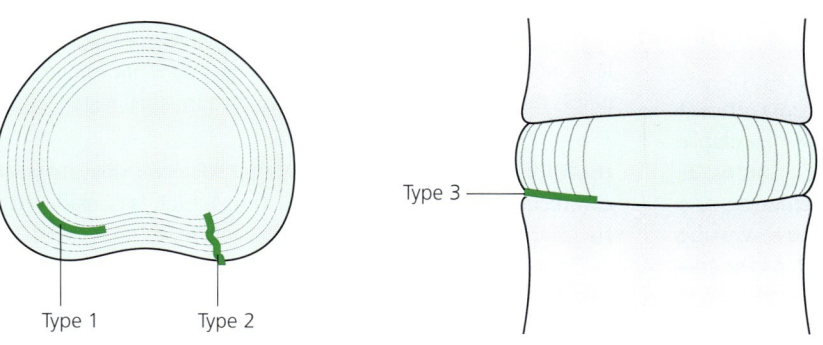

Figure 88.3 Three different types of annular tears.

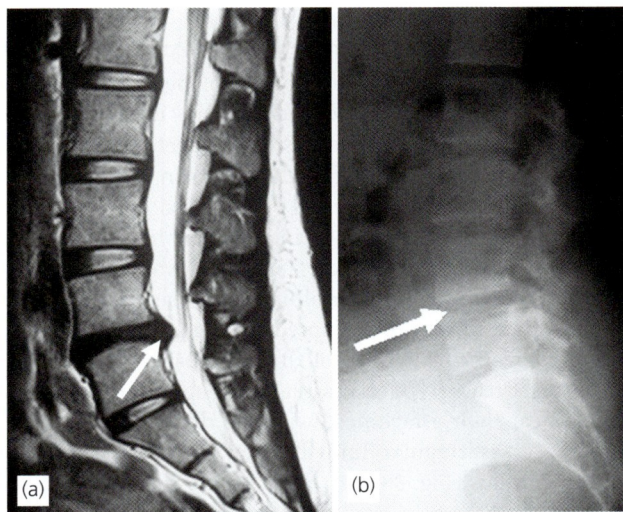

Figure 88.4 MRI demonstrating low signal intensity at the L4–L5 level with reduced intervertebral disc height shown in the lateral lumbosacral radiograph.

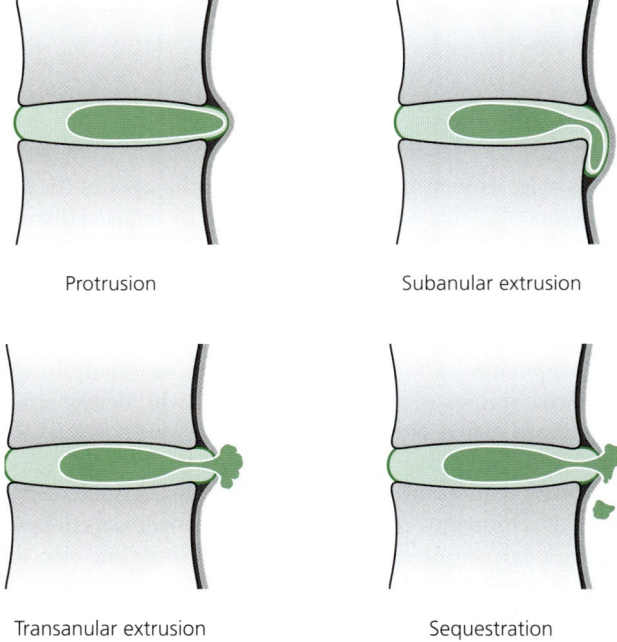

Figure 88.5 Four types of prolapsed disc (From McCulloch JA. Least invasive spine surgery at the L5–S1 level in adults. *Spine State of the Art Review* 1994;**11**:215–38).

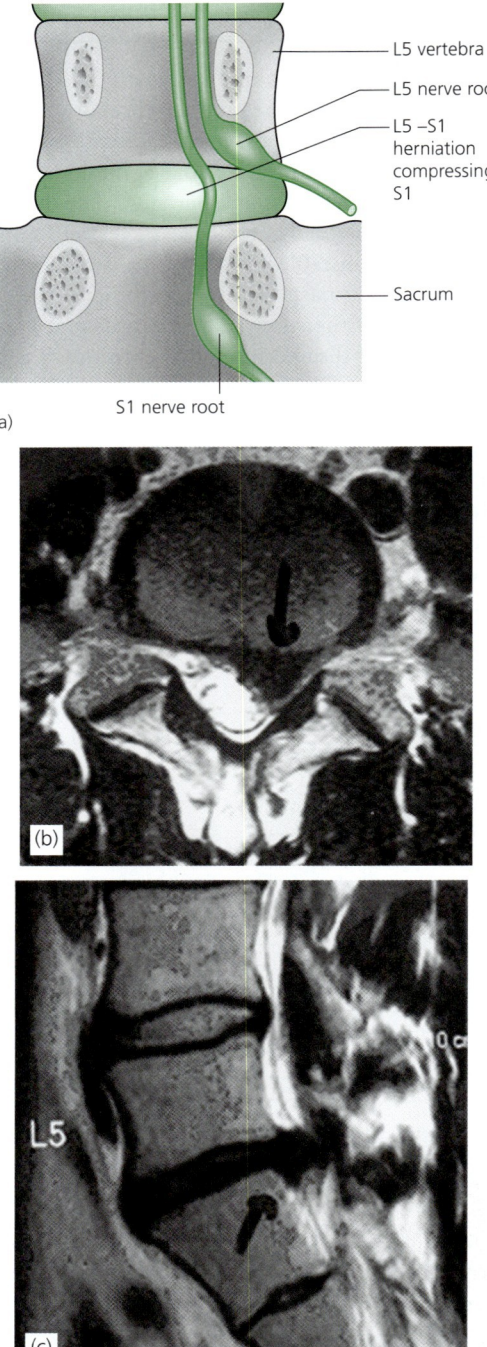

Figure 88.6 L5–S1 posterolateral prolapsed disc compressing the traversing nerve root S1, which is the nerve root exiting one level below the affected disc. The L5 nerve root is not compressed unless the prolapsed disc extends into the foraminal region.

In the lumbar spine, disc herniations occur most often at the lower lumbar levels at L4–L5 and L5–S1. Disc prolapse often occurs at the posterolateral aspect of the annulus, as this is the weakest portion of the annulus. Herniation of a disc at this site will result in compression of the traversing nerve root, which is located within the lateral recess just below the subarticular region. For example, a L5–S1 herniated disc usually impinges on the S1 traversing nerve root (Fig. 88.6). Occasionally, a large posterior disc prolapse can result in cauda equine syndrome, which is considered a surgical emergency.

The lumbar spinal canal is divided into the central canal and lateral canal. The lateral canal is further subdivided into (1) subarticular, (2) foraminal and

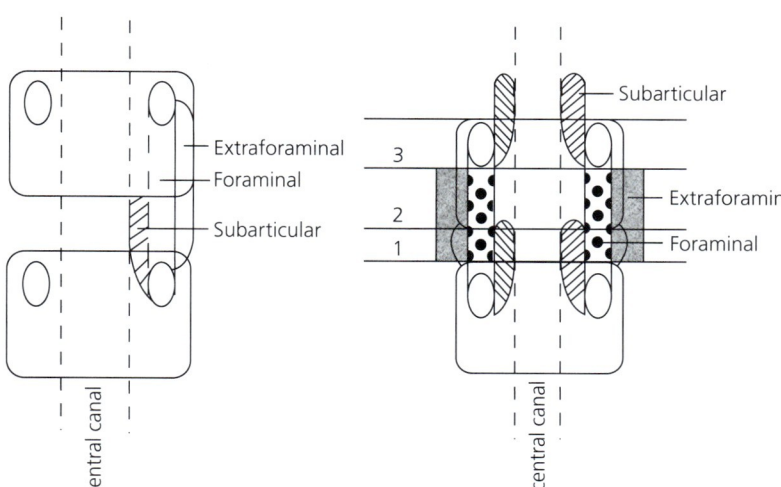

Figure 88.7 Diagram illustrates the central canal and lateral recess which further divides into the three zones: (1) subarticular, (2) foraminal and (3) extraforaminal. (From McCulloch JA. Microdiscetomy: The gold standard for minimally invasive disc surgery. *Spine State Art Rev* 1997;**11**:382)

(3) extraforaminal. The subarticular area can be narrowed by a posterolateral disc herniation anteriorly or by hypertrophy of the facet joint posteriorly. The foraminal space is further divided into two parts: the dorsal root ganglion occupies the upper region at the level of the vertebral body and the vascular pedicle occupies the intervertebral disc level (Figs 88.7–9).

A thoracic disc prolapse is uncommon, and represents approximately 1% of all symptomatic disc herniations. The low incidence rate is attributed to the stable rib cage support, small intervertebral disc and coronal orientation of the facet joints.

A cervical disc prolapse occurs most commonly at the C5–C6 and C6–C7 levels. The nerve affected is different from that seen with a lumbar disc prolapse. For example, a disc herniation at C6–C7 will result in compression of the C7 nerve root, which is the exiting nerve root of the respective level (Fig. 88.10). Significant compression may result in a neurological deficit involving the respective dermatome and myotome, whereas simple irritation will often result in only pain or discomfort which radiates into the shoulder, arm or hand. Occasionally, a central disc herniation can result in acute myelopathy due to cord compression (Fig. 88.11).

In the lumbar spine, as degeneration worsens, progressive disc resorption will occur where the disorganized

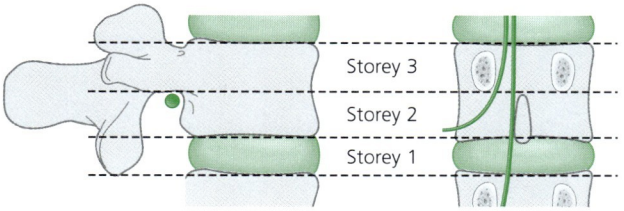

Figure 88.8 The spinal canal is also likened to a three-storey house. (From McCulloch JA. Microdiscetomy: The gold standard for minimally invasive disc surgery. *Spine State Art Rev* 1997;**11**:382)

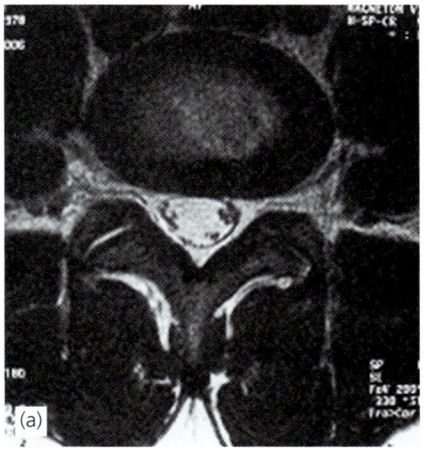
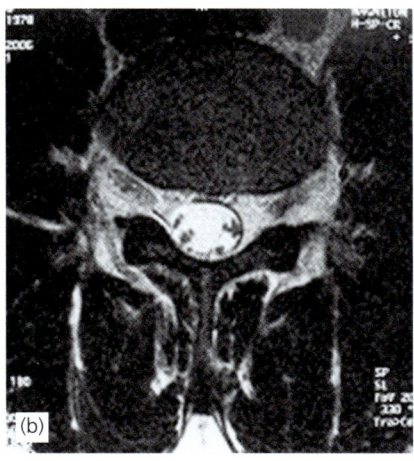
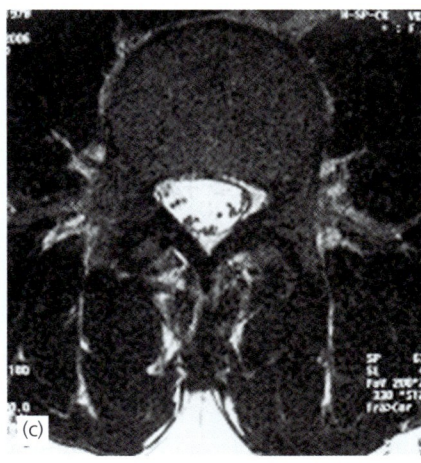

Figure 88.9 These transaxial MR images represent each of the storeys. Storey 1, disc space level, visualizing the traversing nerve root. Notice that there is no nerve located in the foramen on storey 1, as the nerve root is located in the extraforaminal region at this level. This level is useful to visualize an extraforaminal disc prolapse. Storey 2, dorsal root ganglion level, visualizing the dorsal root ganglion of the exiting nerve root which is located within the foraminal region. Storey 3, pedicle level.

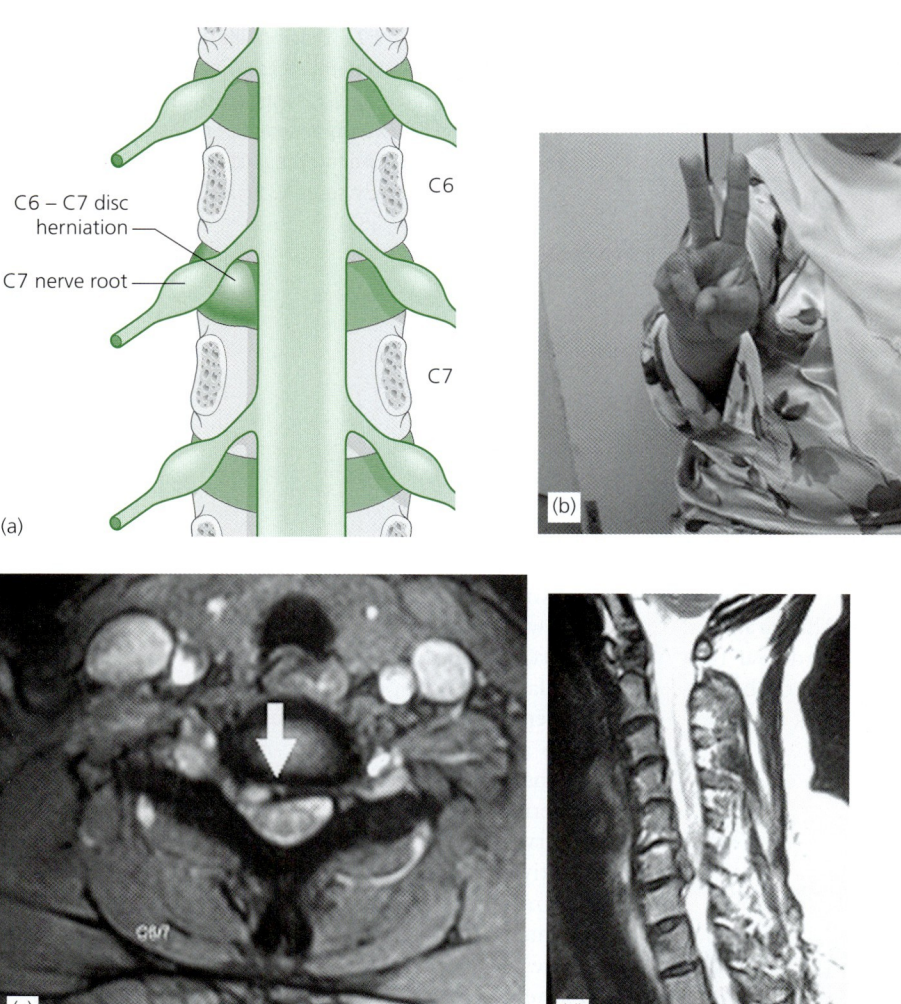

Figure 88.10 C6–C7 disc herniation will compress the C7 nerve root, which is exiting at the same level of the herniated disc. This patient complained of severe right-sided radicular pain associated with numbness of the right index and middle fingers and weakness of elbow extension.

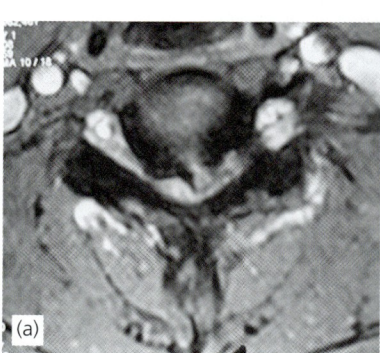
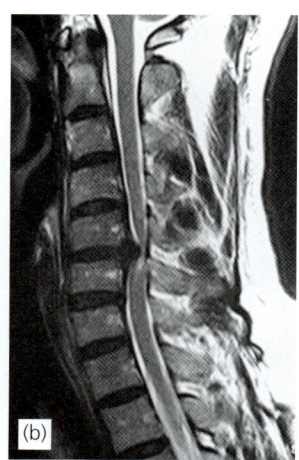

Figure 88.11 A large central prolapsed disc at C5–C6 causing severe central compression (left more than the right side) resulting in Brown–Sequard syndrome.

fibrous tissue replaces the normal structure of the nucleus pulposus, leaving no distinction between the nucleus and annulus. Tears that extend through the outer annulus will induce ingrowth of granulation tissue, which accelerates the degenerative process. The anterior intervertebral height reduces as a result of disc prolapse and/or progressive disc resorption. Formation of osteophytes along the anterior vertebral body will become more prominent, illustrated as spondylotic changes on plain radiography. At this stage, the posterior facet joints begin to bear more load, accelerating degeneration. Facet hypertrophy will compromise the lateral recess resulting in lateral canal stenosis (Fig. 88.12). The

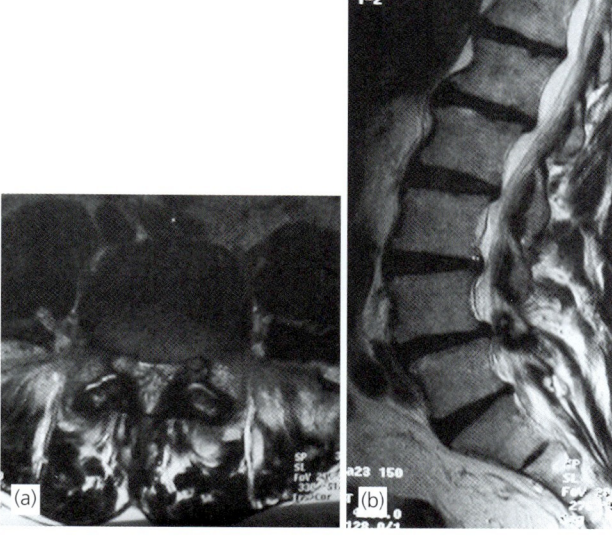

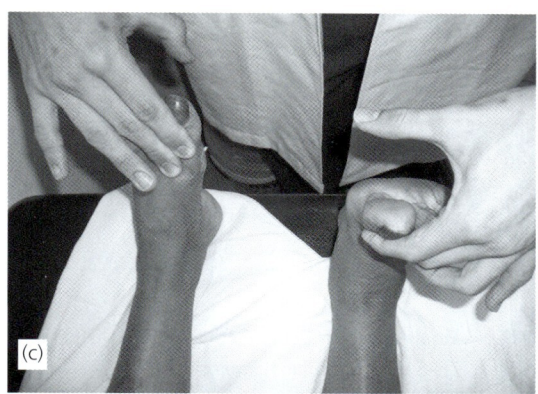

Figure 88.12 An axial magnetic resonance imaging scan demonstrating lumbar spinal stenosis, illustrated as a 'trefoil' shape to the spinal canal. The 'trefoil' shape is due to encroachment along the posterolateral aspects of the canal by hypertrophied facets. In this case, the L5 nerve root was compressed within the subarticular region resulting in weakness of left extensor hallucis longus with reduced sensation over the dorsum of the left foot.

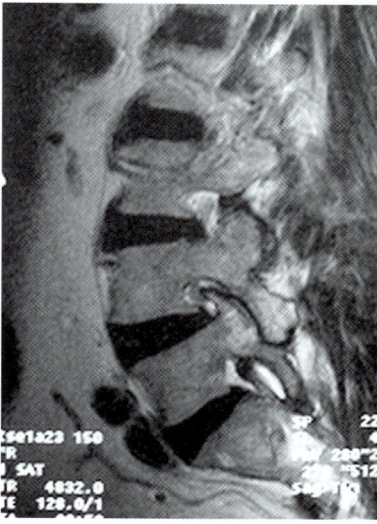

Figure 88.13 Facet hypertophy at L4–L5 will result in hyperthophy of the superior facet of L5 resulting in encroachment into the foraminal region which will potentially compress the exiting L4 nerve root. The lumbar neural foramen has the shape of an inverted teardrop, with the nerve root positioned in the superior aspect of the foramen. Small osteophytes project first into the inferior aspect of the foramen and are unlikely to compress the nerve root until they become quite large.

lateral recess area will become further compromised with the commencement of vertebral subluxation due to instability. Hypertrophy of the superior facet will cause encroachment into the foraminal region which may potentially compress the exiting nerve root (Fig. 88.13). The dorsal root ganglion within the foraminal region is quite resistant to compression compared with the nerve root traversing the subarticular region. Sometimes, a patient may remain asymptomatic despite severe compression occurring within the foraminal. As the posterior structures degenerate further, the ligamentum flavum begins to hypertrophy as well. The hypertrophied ligamentum flavum will gradually worsen central canal stenosis. Formation of posterior osteophytes along the vertebral body along with a bulging disc will further worsen central stenosis (Fig. 88.14).

When this condition becomes symptomatic, the patient will present with classical symptoms of spinal claudication.

In the cervical spine, the uncovertebral and facet joints are involved in the natural degenerative process. Osteophyte formation at these joints will cause compression within the foramen, resulting in impingement of the exiting nerve root. Similarly, the combination of flavum hypertrophy coupled with the presence of posterior osteophytes along with a bulging disc will result in central canal stenosis and possibly cervical myelopathy.

Degeneration of the intervertebral disc has indirect effects on the adjacent vertebral end plates and bone marrow, resulting in development of fissures over the cartilaginous end plates. Vascular granulation tissue grows into the fissures and induces an oedematous reaction and vascular congestion in the adjacent bone marrow.[25] Modic et al.[25] have classified the bone marrow changes according to the signal intensity on MR images (Table 88.1). Type 1 represents bone marrow oedema and vascular congestion, type 2 represents conversion of the bone marrow elements to a predominantly fatty marrow and type 3 represents chronic disc disease manifested as a dense sclerosis of the vertebral end plates and adjacent vertebral bodies. Kuisma et al.[26] reported that type I Modic changes at L5–S1 are more likely to be associated with low back pain than other types of Modic changes.

As the degenerative process continues, the facets may become unstable. Subluxation of the facet joints coupled

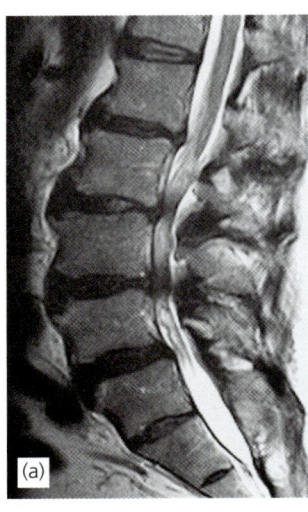 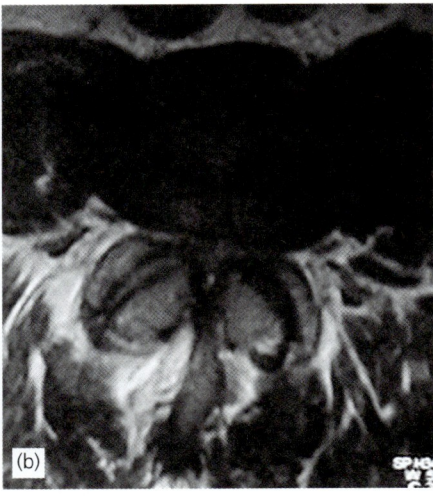

Figure 88.14 MRI scan showing severe central stenosis at L4–L5 due to the presence of posterior vertebral osteophytes, a disc bulge anteriorly, and hypertrophied facet joints and ligamentum flavum posteriorly.

Table 88.1 Modic classification of bone marrow changes according to signal intensity on MR images

	Type 1	Type 2	Type 3
T_1-weighted image	Hypointense	Hyperintense	Hypointense
T_2-weighted image	Hyperintense	Isointense or slightly hyperintense	Hypointense
Significance	Acute process with bone marrow oedema and vascular congestion	Chronic process with fatty degeneration of subchondral marrow	Chronic disc disease leads to dense sclerosis of the vertebral end plates

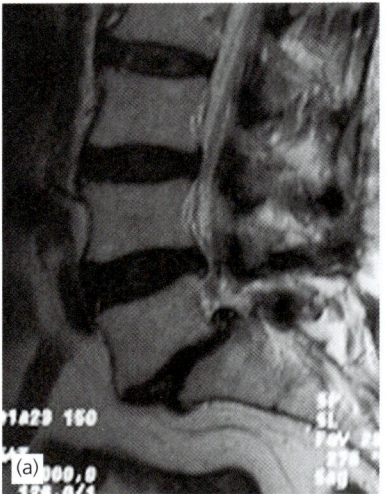 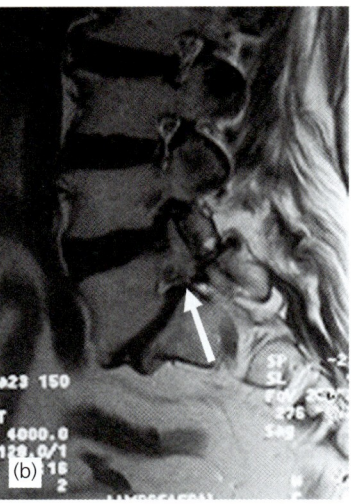

Figure 88.15 Degenerative spondylolisthesis of L5–S1 with foraminal stenosis.

with reduced intervertebral disc height will result in the cephalad vertebrae moving forward over the vertebrae below. This condition is called spondylolisthesis. Degenerative spondylolisthesis usually occurs at the level of L4–L5 and involves older patients (Fig. 88.15). Degenerative spondylolisthesis will result in central canal stenosis. More often this will be associated with bilateral foraminal stenosis affecting the bilateral exiting nerve root of the same level due to closure of the lower portion of the foramen as the vertebral body slips forward coupled with concomitant facet joints hypertrophy. Spondylolisthesis is graded according to the percentage of vertebral body slippage over the vertebrae below (see Figure 68.7, page xxx).

Stabilization phase

This stage is often seen in patients older than 60 years of age and is characterized by the development of hypertrophic bone over the disc and facet joints. Advanced degeneration leads to desiccation and destruction of the disc. Gas formation within the disc may occur, known as Knutsson's sign[27] or discal calcification (Fig. 88.16). Formation of hypertrophic osteophytes over the anterior body as well as the posterior facet joints will eventually fuse and lead to segmental ankylosis (Fig. 88.17).

The biomolecular changes that occur with the degenerative process occur both at the cellular and molecular level. Factors that may contribute to age-related changes in the intervertebral disc include declining nutrition, decreasing concentration of viable cells, cell senescence, post-synthetic modification of matrix proteins, accumulation of degraded matrix macromolecule and fatigue failure of the matrix.[28]

The intervertebral disc consists of cells that are sustained by diffusion of nutrients through the central part of the end plate.[29] Disc cell density is known to decrease with aging and the most critical factor that is responsible for these changes appears to be declining nutrition.[30] Gruber et al.[31] noted that cells within the degenerative disc will markedly alter their surrounding extracellular matrix; such extracellular matrix alterations, in turn, may affect disc cell function with a significant proportion of cells in the disc undergoing programmed cell death (apoptosis). A concomitant increase in cell senescence is also seen in the degenerating disc. The senescent disc cell population will accumulate over time within the disc. Since senescent cells cannot divide, senescence may reduce the disc's ability to generate new cells to replace existing ones lost to necrosis or apoptosis.[32]

The normal intervertebral disc consists of proteoglycans made up of chondroitin-6-sulphate, keratan sulphate, hyaluronic acid, and chondroitin-4-sulphate. As the disc degenerates, the proportion of the non-aggregated proteoglycans progressively increases. Proteoglycan content and the size of the individual molecules decrease dramatically.[33,34] There is an increase in the ratio of keratan sulphate to chondroitin sulphate. The end result is a decrease in the proteoglycan/collagen ratio. This will result in the disc losing its water-binding capacity with a concomitant decrease in its water content.[35] These changes are reflected by a 6% decrease in T_2-weighted MR signal intensity over a span of 80 years.[36]

Post-synthetic modification of the collagen proteins through increased collagen cross-linking also occurs with ageing. This will alter the mechanical properties of the intervertebral disc and is thought to increase the stiffness and decrease the disc's elasticity and resilience to mechanical loads.[37] Herniated lumbar disc's are noted to have increased amounts of matrix metalloproteinases, nitric oxide, prostaglandin E_2, and interleukin 6. These products may be involved in the biochemistry of disc degeneration and the pathophysiology of radiculopathy resulting in radicular pain.[38]

TREATMENT

Treatment of the degenerative spine is mainly directed toward patients' symptoms. However, the majority of the patients are asymptomatic; therefore, no treatment is

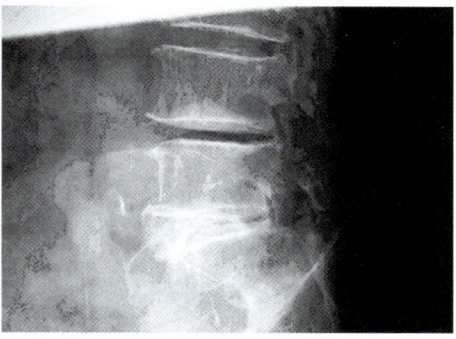

Figure 88.16 Knuttson's sign, also known as the vacuum sign, within the L4–L5 disc space seen on a lateral plain radiograph.

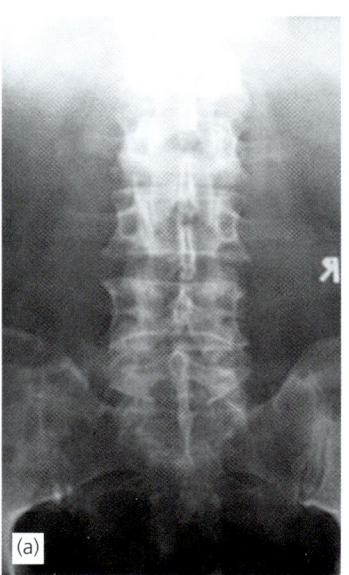
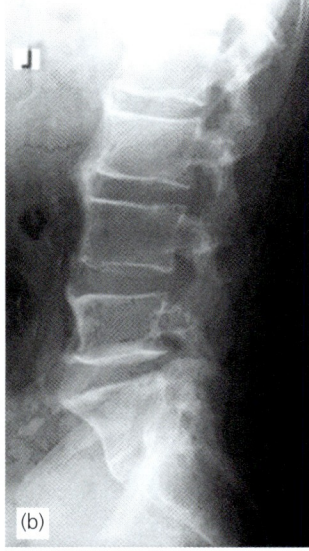

Figure 88.17 Segmental ankylosis noted over the L3–L4 disc level.

required. Only when symptoms emerge and are non-transient do patients seek medical advice and treatment.

Symptomatic degenerative disc disease

NECK AND BACK PAIN

The cause of neck and back pain can be very elusive and is often multifactorial in origin. See Table 88.2. Generally, pain may originate from the intervertebral disc, facet joints or musculo-ligament sources. Pain can be referred from other pathological conditions. Psychosocial factors have also been shown to play an important role as well. Generally, back pain is thought to arise from two main structures:

- Discogenic pain.
  - Pain is usually non-specific and aggravated by activities that increase the pressure within the intervertebral disc i.e. bending forward, prolonged sitting, coughing and sneezing.
- Facet joint pain.
  - Pain is usually more specific and noted over the facet joints region or localized only over the low back. This pain is aggravated by hyperextension, where facet joints capsular stretching occurs.

NEUROLOGICAL SYMPTOMS

- *Lateral canal stenosis* can occur within the cervical, thoracic or lumbar region resulting in radiculopathy. The patient may present with radicular pain (cervical or thoracic region) and sciatica (lumbar region). The radicular pain will be described as a shooting pain into the upper limb, trunk or posterior aspect of thighs, calves and feet. This pain can be associated with numbness, weakness, and reflex changes.
- *Central canal stenosis* will result in myelopathy (cervical and thoracic regions) or neurogenic claudication in the lumbar spine. Myelopathic symptoms range from incoordination of upper limb and lower limb movement, numbness, weakness, paraparesis and paraplegia. The symptoms of neurogenic claudication are described as bilateral lower extremity pain, aggravated by extension e.g. standing or walking upstairs and relieved by flexing of the lumbar spine e.g. sitting. Numbness and weakness are usually poorly localized but can be recreated by repeating the aggravating activities.

Back pain mainly occurs during the temporary dysfunctional stage. The initial treatment will be mainly conservative management. Pain can be relieved using anti-inflammatory drugs, rest with or without temporary immobilization, physiotherapy, spinal manipulation, etc. Exercise programmes to strengthen abdominal and spinal musculature will be initiated when the back pain improves. If the pain becomes intolerable or disturbs the patient's activities of daily living despite conservative management, diagnostic tests such as discogram[39] or facet joint injection/medial branch block[40] can be performed to assess the pain generator site. Occasionally, these procedures can be of therapeutic benefit as well.

Once the source of the pain generator is confirmed as originating from the disc, many treatment options exist. Some have attempted to use percutaneous modalities such as intradiscal electrothermal therapy (IDET), nucleoplasty, decompressor, radiofrequency annuloplasty, laser annuloplasty and transdiscal bipolar annuloplasty.[41–43] All these therapies have been shown to be effective in select groups of patients in low level evidence-based studies. Regarding presumed facet joint pain, medial branch block or radio frequency ablation can be performed to denervate the joint thus relieving potential facet pain. If back pain worsens and a single or two disc pain generator is identified the patient may become a candidate for surgical intervention.

Neurological symptoms usually require decompression surgery if objective compression is identified on advanced imaging studies. Discectomy surgery can be performed for a disc herniation if radicular pain does not improve

Table 88.2 Symptomatology of degenerative disease of the spine

	Symptoms	Anatomical site	Pathophysiology
Back pain	Discogenic pain	Intervertebral disc	Disc disruption mediated through the sinuvertebral nerve
	Facet pain	Facet joint	Facet synovitis or arthrosis mediated through the medial branch of the posterior rami
Neurological symptoms	Sciatica or radicular pain	Lateral recess stenosis (lumbar, thoracic and cervical spine)	Radiculopathy
	Intermittent or neurological claudication	Central canal stenosis (lumbar spine)	Lumbar spinal stenosis
	Upper motor neurone symptoms	Central canal stenosis (thoracic and cervical spine)	Myelopathy

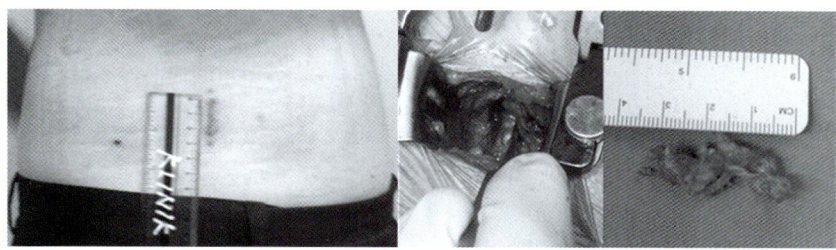

Figure 88.18 Microdiscectomy can be performed through a small incision. Intra-operative photo demonstrating the traversing nerve root which has been decompressed following removal of a large disc herniation.

despite conservative management for a duration of 6 to 12 weeks. Patients with symptomatic disc herniations often do not require surgery.[44] Research has shown that the larger the disc herniation, the more likely that the herniation will decrease in size. This is attributed to presence of greater vascularity or granulation tissue.[45] Indications for discectomy are failed conservative treatment, severe intolerable pain and the presence of a neurological deficit. Discectomy in the lumbar spine can be performed through conventional open or microdiscectomy techniques (Fig. 88.18). It can also be performed using percutaneous tools such as endoscopy. Based on the Cochrane review published in 2007 by Gibson and Waddell,[46] surgical discectomy for carefully selected patients with sciatica due to lumbar disc prolapse provides faster relief from an acute attack than conservative management. Microdiscectomy gives broadly comparable results to a standard open discectomy. The evidence for other minimally invasive techniques e.g. percutaneous endoscopic technique remains unclear.

Discectomy in the cervical spine is usually performed through a standard anterior open discectomy (Smith–Robinson approach) followed by fusion. Motion preserving instrumentation such as disc arthroplasty is gaining popularity in the cervical spine.[47] Cervical discectomy can also be performed using a percutaneous endoscopic method or through an open posterior neuro-foraminotomy approach.[48,49]

In the setting of a neurological deficit due to facet hypertrophy in the lumbar spine, a medial facetectomy can be performed safely to relieve compression of the traversing nerve root within the subarticular region. In the event of central canal stenosis, a central decompression can be performed through one of the following methods: laminotomy (partial removal of lamina without removal of spinous process or facet joints), laminoplasty (removal of the spinous process, bilateral osteotomy of lamin and dislocation dorsally, like a double door being swung open) or laminectomy (bilateral removal of lamina including spinous process with or without part of the facet joints, see Fig. 88.19). A complete central decompression will require a proper decompression (medial facetectomy) of the subarticular region to relieve compression of the traversing nerve at the respective level. Failure to do so will result in incomplete symptom relief after surgery. Central decompression of the cervical spine can be via an anterior approach by discectomy or copectomy followed by an instrumented fusion or via a posterior approach i.e. laminoplasty alone or laminectomy with lateral mass fusion (Fig. 88.20).

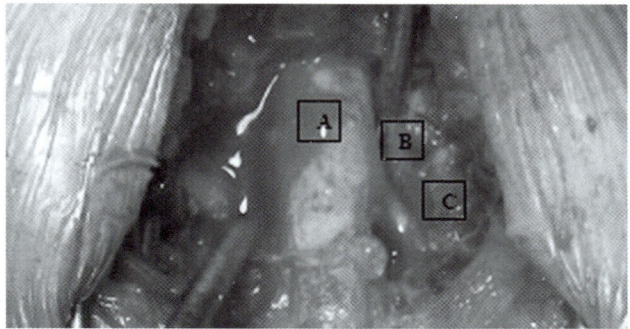

Figure 88.19 Intra-operative photo demonstrating a wide posterior laminectomy (A) decompressing the central stenosis along with a medial facetectomy (B) decompressing the traversing nerve root and foraminotomy (C) decompressing the foraminal stenosis exposing the proximal portion of the exiting nerve root.

A fusion is usually only required when there is the presence of symptomatic or impending spinal instability after a decompression surgery in the lumbar spine. Fusion can be achieved either by an instrumented or non-instrumented technique. Lumbar spine fusion can be performed through an anterior or posterior approach. Anterior approach lumbar discal fusion is also known as anterior lumbar interbody fusion (ALIF). A posterior approach lumbar fusion can be achieved through different techniques; posterior lumbar interbody fusion (PLIF), transforaminal lumbar interbody fusion (TLIF), posterolateral lumbar fusion (PLF) or 360° circumferential fusion (Fig. 88.21). Based on the Cochrane review in 2005 by Gibson and Waddell,[50] an instrumented fusion produces a higher fusion rate, but this does not translate into better clinical outcomes. No conclusions are possible about the relative effectiveness of anterior, posterior, or circumferential fusion. Recently, a new innovative technique of lumbosacral fusion through a percutaneous presacral approach has been introduced.[51,52]

FUTURE POTENTIAL THERAPY IN THE MANAGEMENT OF DEGENERATIVE DISEASE

Although degenerative disease of the spine is an inevitable phenomenon, identification of the various factors that may accelerate this process may help to decrease the progression. Methods to regenerate the disc are under research as this may not only help to decrease the severity

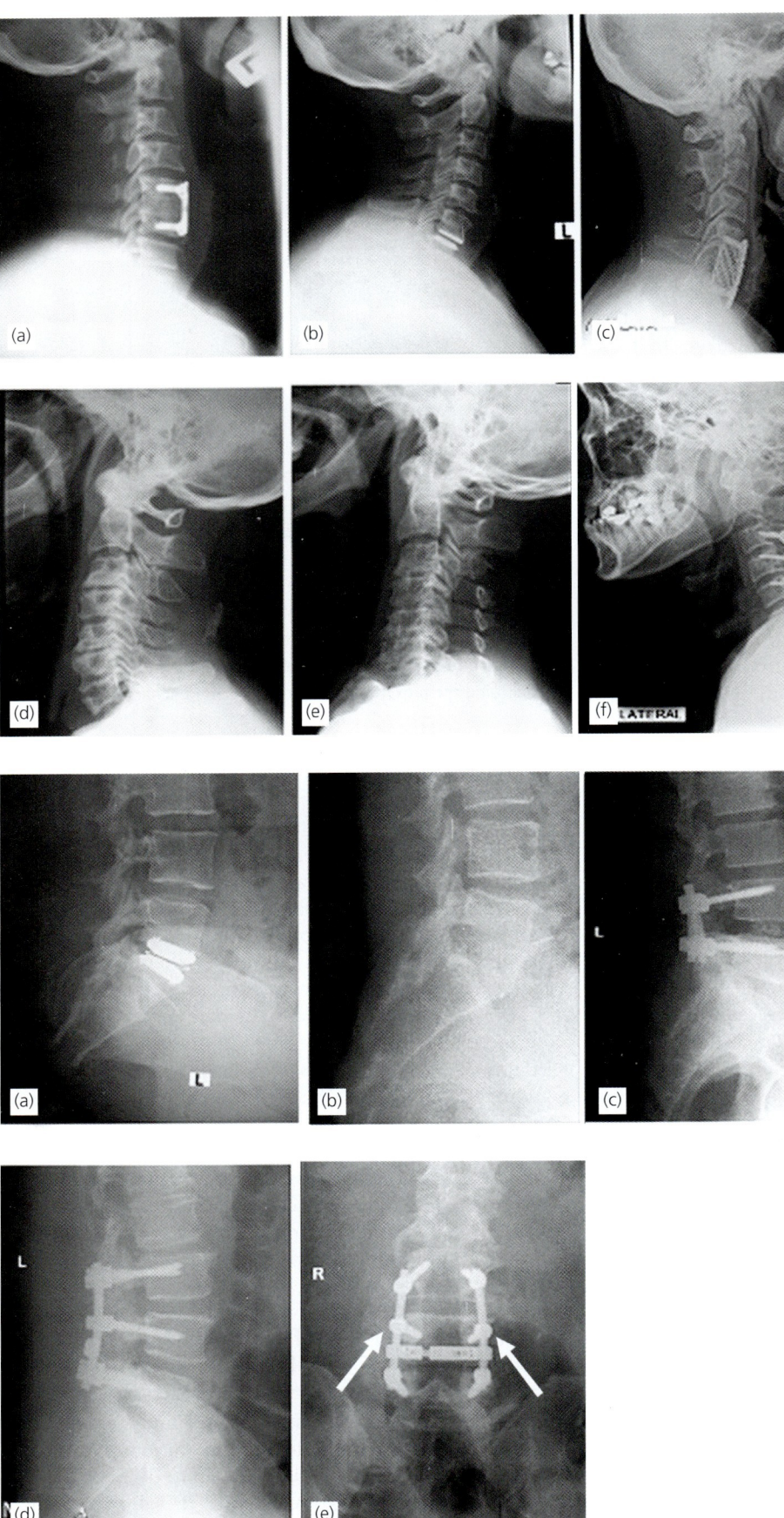

Figure 88.20 (a) Anterior cervical discectomy and fusion. (b) Anterior cervical total disc replacement. (c) Anterior cervical corpectomy and fusion. (d) Cervical spondylotic myelopathy (before laminoplasty). (e) Laminoplasty: notice that the lamina of the posterior cervical spine has been lifted up to decompress the central canal. (f) Posterior laminectomy with lateral mass fusion.

Figure 88.21 (a) Lumbar disc replacement L5–S1. (b) Anterior lumbar interbody fusion L5–S1. (c) Posterior interbody fusion – radiolucent polyethereneketone (PEEK) cage filled with bone graft was placed in between the vertebral bodies to achieve fusion. (d, e) Posterolateral lumbar instrumented fusion – a large amount of autogenous bone graft was laid over the posterolateral aspect of the posterior elements to achieve fusion.

of symptomatic degenerative disc disease but may also improve the natural history of the ageing process. Nucleus pulposus replacement has been introduced as a concept of motion-sparing which is intended to remove the pain generator without the associated morbidity of a surgical fusion.[53] Implantations of growth factors, and mesenchymal or chondrocytic cells are some of the possible options for future management of this condition. The intervertebral disc has been proven to be an appropriate environment for adenovirus-mediated transfer of exogenous genes which may lead to the production of therapeutic growth factors to help to regenerate the disc.[54]

REFERENCES

1. Hult L. The Munkfors investigation. *Acta Orthopaedica Scandinavica Supplementum* 1954;**16**:1.
2. Svensson HO, Andersson GBJ. Low back pain in 40- to 47-year-old men: work history and environment factors. *Spine* 1983;**8**:272.
3. Svensson HO, Andersson GBJ. The relationship of low-back pain, work history, work environment and stress: a retrospective cross-sectional study of 38- to 64-year-old women. *Spine* 1989;**14**:517.
4. Frymoyer JW, Cats-Baril WL. An overview of the incidences and costs of low back pain. *Orthopedic Clinics of North America* 1991;**22**:263–71.
5. Jensen MC, Brant-Zawadzki MN, Obuchowski N, et al. Magnetic resonance imaging of the lumbar spine in people without back pain. *New England Journal of Medicine* 1994;**331**:69–73.
6. Miller JA, Schmatz C, Schultz AB. Lumbar disc degeneration: correlation with age, sex, and spine level in 600 autopsy specimens. *Spine* 1988;**13**:173–8.
7. Deyo RA, Bass JE. Lifestyle and low-back pain: the influence of smoking and obesity. *Spine* 1989;**14**:501–6.
8. An HS, Silveri CP, Simeone FA, et al. Cigarette smoking as a risk factor for cervical and lumbar disc disease. *Journal of Spinal Disorders* 1994;**7**:369–73.
9. Frymoyer JW, Pope MT, Clements JH, et al. Risk factors in low-back pain: an epidemiological survey. *Journal of Bone and Joint Surgery* 1983;**65A**:213–18.
10. Magora A. Investigation of the relation between low back pain and occupation. *Industrial Medicine & Surgery* 1970;**39**:465–71.
11. Waddell G, Main CJ, Morris EW, et al. Chronic low-back pain, psychological distress, and illness behavior. *Spine* 1984;**9**:209–13.
12. Fahrni WH, Trueman GE. Comparative radiological study of the spines of a primitive population with North Americans and Northern Europeans. *Journal of Bone and Joint Surgery* 1965;**47B**:552–5.
13. Wilder DG, Woodworth BB, Frymoyer JW, Pope MH. Vibration and the human spine. *Spine* 1982;**7**:243–54.
14. Hall RA, Cassinelli EH, Kang JD. Degeneration, repair, and regeneration of the intervertebral disc. *Clinical Orthopaedics and Related Research* 2000;**11**:413–20.
15. Pedersen H, Blunck CFJ, Gardner E. The anatomy of lumbosacral posterior rami and meningeal branches of spinal nerves (sinu-vertebral nerves). *Journal of Bone and Joint Surgery* 1956;**38A**:2377–91.
16. Weishaupt D, Zanetti M, Hodler J, et al. Painful lumbar disk derangement: relevance of end plate abnormalities at MR imaging. *Radiology* 2001;**218**:420–7.
17. Botsford DJ, Esses SI, Ogilvie-Harris DJ. In vivo diurnal variation in intervertebral disc volume and morphology. *Spine* 1994;**19**:935–40.
18. Paajanen H, Lehto I, Alanen A, et al. Diurnal fluid changes of lumbar discs measured directly by magnetic resonance imaging. *Journal of Orthopedic Research* 1994;**12**:509–14.
19. Kirkaldy-Willis WH, Farfan HF. Instability of the lumbar spine. *Clinical Orthopaedics and Related Research* 1982;**165**:110–23.
20. Canale SC. (ed.) *Campbell's Operative Orthopaedics*. Philadelphia, PA: Mosby, 2003, 1960.
21. Yu SW, Sether LA, Ho PS, et al. Tears of the annulus fibrosus: correlation between MR and pathologic findings in cadavers. *American Journal of Neuroradiology* 1988;**9**:367–70.
22. Yu S, Haughton VM, Sether LA, Wagner M. Annulus fibrosus in bulging intervertebral disks. *Radiology* 1988;**169**:761–3.
23. Stadnik TW, Lee RR, Coen HL, et al. Annular tears and disk herniation: prevalence and contrast enhancement on MR images in the absence of low back pain or sciatica. *Radiology* 1998;**206**:49–55.
24. Ernst CW, Stadnik TW, Peeters E, et al. Prevalence of annular tears and disc herniations on MR images of the cervical spine in symptom free volunteers. *European Journal of Radiology* 2005;**55**:409–14.
25. Modic MT, Syeinberg PM, Ross JS, et al. Degenerative disk disease: assessment of changes in vertebral body marrow with MR imaging. *Radiology* 1988;**166**:193–9.
26. Kuisma M, Karppinen J, Niinimäki J, et al. Modic changes in endplates of lumbar vertebral bodies: prevalence and association with low back and sciatic pain among middle-aged male workers. *Spine* 2007;**32**:1116–22.
27. Knutsson F. The instability associated with disc herniation in the lumbar spine. *Acta Radiologica* 1944;**25**:593–609.
28. Buckwalter JA. Aging and degeneration of the human intervertebral disc. *Spine* 1995;**20**:1307–14.
29. Maroudas A, Stockwell RA, Nachemson A, Urban J. Factors involved in the nutrition of the human lumbar intervertebral disc: cellularity and diffusion of glucose in vitro. *Journal of Anatomy* 1975;**120**:113–30.
30. Buckwalter JA. Aging and degeneration of the human intervertebral disc. *Spine* 1995;**20**:1307–14.
31. Gruber HE, Hanley, Edward N Jr. Analysis of aging and degeneration of the human intervertebral disc: comparison of surgical specimens with normal controls. *Spine* 1998;**23**:751–7.

32. Gruber HE, Ingram JA, Norton HJ, Hanley EN. Senescence in cells of the aging and degenerating intervertebral disc: immunolocalization of senescence-associated [beta]-galactosidase in human and sand rat discs. *Spine* 2007;**32**:321-7.
33. Buckwalter JA. Aging and degeneration of the human intervertebral disc. *Spine* 1995;**20**:1307-14.
34. Gower WE, Pegrini V. Age-related variations in protein-polysaccharides from human nucleus pulposus, annulus fibrosus, and costal cartilage. *Journal of Bone and Joint Surgery* 1969;**51A**:1154-62.
35. Pearce RH, Grimmer BJ, Adams ME. Degeneration and the chemical composition of the human intervertebral disc. *Journal of Orthopedic Research* 1987;**5**:198-205.
36. Sether LA, Yu S, Haughton VM, Fiecher ME. Intervertebral disk: normal age-related changes in MR signal intensity. *Radiology* 1990;**177**:385-8.
37. Monnier VM, Sell DR, Pokharna H, Moskowitz R. Post-translational protein modification by the Maillard reaction: relevance to aging of the extracellular matrix molecules. In: Buckwalter JA, Goldberg VM, Woo SL-Y. (eds) *Musculoskeletal Soft Tissue Aging: Impact on Mobility*. Rosemont, IL: American Academy of Orthopaedic Surgeons, 1993:49-50.
38. Kang JD, Georgescu HI, McIntyre-Larkin L, *et al*. Herniated lumbar intervertebral discs spontaneously produce matrix metalloproteinases, nitric oxide, interleukin-6, and prostaglandin E2. *Spine* 1996;**21**:271-7.
39. Wolfer LR, Derby R, Lee JE, Lee SH. Systematic review of lumbar provocation discography in asymptomatic subjects with a meta-analysis of false-positive rates. *Pain Physician* 2008;**11**:513-38.
40. Sehgal N, Dunbar EE, Shah RV, Colson J. Systematic review of diagnostic utility of facet (zygapophysial) joint injections in chronic spinal pain: an update. *Pain Physician* 2007;**10**:213-28.
41. Maurer P, Block JE, Squillante D. Intradiscal electrothermal therapy (IDET) provides effective symptom relief in patients with discogenic low back pain. *Journal of Spinal Disorders & Techniques* 2008;**21**:55-62.
42. Boswell MV, Trescot AM, Datta S, *et al*. Interventional techniques: evidence-based practice guidelines in the management of chronic spinal pain. *Pain Physician* 2007;**10**:7-111.
43. Kapural L, Goyle A. Imaging for provocative discography and minimally invasive percutaneous procedures for treatment of discogenic lower back pain. *Techniques in Regional Anesthesia and Pain Management* 2007;**11**:73-80.
44. Weber H. Lumbar disc herniation. A controlled, prospective study with ten years of observation. *Spine* 1983;**8**:131-40.
45. Bozzao A, Gallucci M, Masciocchi C, *et al*. Lumbar disk herniation: MR imaging assessment of natural history in patients treated without surgery. *Radiology* 1992;**185**:135.
46. Gibson JN, Waddell G. Surgical interventions for lumbar disc prolapse: updated Cochrane Review. *Spine* 2007;**32**:1735-47.
47. Phillips FM, Garfin SR. Cervical disc replacement. *Spine* 2005;**30**(17 Suppl):S27-33.
48. Lee SH, Lee JH, Choi WC, *et al*. Anterior minimally invasive approaches for the cervical spine. *Orthopedic Clinics of North America* 2007;**38**:327-37.
49. Gala VC, O'Toole JE, Voyadzis JM, Fessler RG. Posterior minimally invasive approaches for the cervical spine. *Orthopedic Clinics of North America* 2007;**38**:339-49.
50. Gibson JN, Waddell G. Surgery for degenerative lumbar spondylosis: updated Cochrane Review. *Spine* 2005;**30**:2312-20.
51. Cragg A, Carl A, Casteneda F, *et al*. New percutaneous access method for minimally invasive anterior lumbosacral surgery. *Journal of Spinal Disorders & Techniques* 2004;**17**:21-8.
52. Ledet EH, Carl AL, Cragg A. Novel lumbosacral axial fixation techniques. *Expert Review of Medical Devices* 2006;**3**:327-34.
53. Goins ML, Wimberley DW, Yuan PS, *et al*. Nucleus pulposus replacement: an emerging technology. *Spine* 2005;**5**(6 Suppl):317S-24S. Review.
54. Nishida K, Kang JD, Gilbertson LG, *et al*. Volvo award winner in basic science studies. Modulation of the biologic activity of the rabbit intervertebral disc by gene therapy: an *in vivo* study of adenovirus-mediated transfer of the human transforming growth factor [beta]1 encoding gene. *Spine* 1999;**24**:2419-25. *In vivo* study demonstrating potential therapeutic benefits of gene therapy in the intervertebral disc.

89

Adult spinal deformity

WILLIAM C LAUERMAN, RYAN J CAUFIELD

| Introduction | 1007 | Adult kyphosis | 1014 |
| Adult scoliosis | 1007 | References | 1020 |

NATIONAL BOARD STANDARDS

- Knowledge of the natural history of scoliosis
- Know the indications for surgical treatment
- Understand the role of anterior, posterior and combined surgical approaches
- Understand the significance of kyphotic deformity, sagittal alignment and sagittal plane imbalance
- Be able to advise a patient with adult scoliosis
- Be able to advise a patient with adult kyphosis

INTRODUCTION

As our population lives longer and more active lives, adult spinal deformity continues to emerge as an important healthcare issue worldwide. Fortunately, recent research has led to increasing knowledge about the natural history of spinal deformity and a number of advances have been made in the evaluation and treatment of these disorders.

Management of spinal deformity in the adult patient, however, continues to present many challenges. Whereas the adolescent with spinal deformity typically reports minimal symptoms or disability, the adult patient often presents with significant pain and functional limitation. The deformity results from a wide variety of aetiologies with many associated symptoms, which include progressive deformity, degenerative osteoarthritis, spinal stenosis with radiculopathy, muscle fatigue from imbalance and cosmetic concerns.

Spinal deformity in the adult can arise from a variety of processes. The most common presentation is spinal deformity as a result of adolescent idiopathic scoliosis that was either untreated or failed non-surgical or even surgical treatment (Fig. 89.1). Spinal deformity may also develop in the adult patient *de novo* and is referred to as degenerative scoliosis (Fig. 89.2). *De novo* spinal deformity may be the result of progressive degenerative changes of the spinal column, iatrogenic instability after surgical procedures and fragility fractures from metabolic bone diseases such as osteoporosis. Although adult spinal deformity is often categorized as either scoliotic or kyphotic deformities, it is important to remember that those deformities are actually three-dimensional conditions that may present with combinations of coronal, sagittal and axial plane abnormalities.

The decision-making process regarding the method of treatment is complicated by the difficulty in accurately determining the individual's pain, the cosmetic effects of deformity and the impairment in quality of life. In regard to surgical treatment, the decision must not be taken lightly and the potential benefits must be weighed against the increased potential for complications in the adult patient.

The purpose of this chapter is to review the common forms of adult spinal deformity, discuss evaluation of the patient with spinal deformity, address the management options, and to provide insight into optimizing outcomes in this important problem.

ADULT SCOLIOSIS

Adult scoliosis refers primarily to a coronal plane curvature, occurring most commonly in the thoracic, thoracolumbar and lumbar spine, of a skeletally mature individual. Although the frontal curve is the most commonly recognized aspect

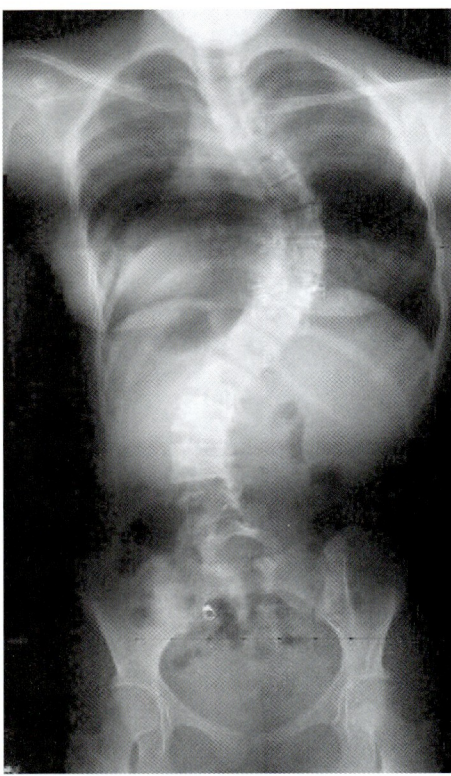

Figure 89.1 A 52-year-old woman with adult idiopathic scoliosis. She was originally diagnosed and followed as a teenager. Her curve was believed to be about 30° when she was last seen as a teenager, measured 50° at age 44 years, and has been followed and demonstrated to progress to 63° at this time.

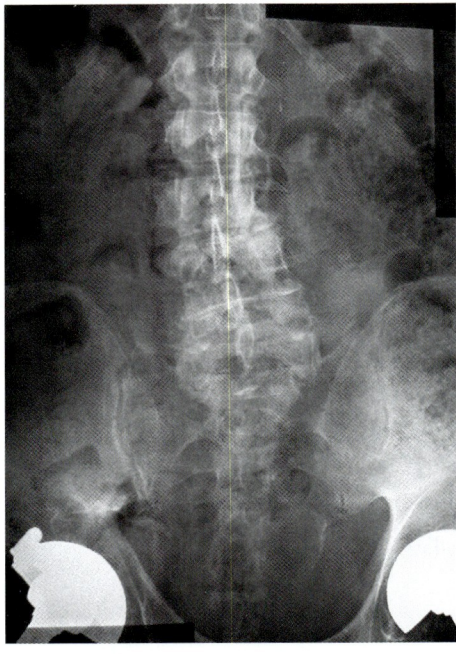

Figure 89.2 Plain anteroposterior radiograph of a 72-year-old man with degenerative scoliosis who has a longstanding history of low back pain and stiffness. Over the last 6 months he has developed more severe pain in his left buttock, posterior thigh and down the left leg. The radiograph demonstrates relatively mild scoliosis with degenerative changes at multiple levels. Significant degeneration and collapse is seen on the left at L4–L5 in the concavity of the lumbosacral fractional curve. This is a common site of nerve root entrapment in this setting and was responsible for this man's radicular symptoms.

of the deformity, scoliosis is a three-dimensional abnormality, with alterations in the sagittal and axial planes contributing significantly to the cosmetic deformity, as well as to the functional limitations and morbidity seen with this condition.

Adult scoliosis is a common condition across the skeletally mature population. Studies evaluating the overall prevalence of asymptomatic adult scoliosis have reported a range from 1.4% to 20% in the adult population.[1–3] However, when only the oldest segments of the population are considered, an even higher prevalence has been reported. Schwab et al.[4] evaluated an elderly population (older than 60 years) with no previous spinal surgery, no recent trauma and no prior diagnosis of spinal deformity. Using a 10 degree angulation in the coronal plane as the threshold for the definition of scoliosis, a 68% prevalence of scoliosis was identified.[4]

In the adult patient with scoliosis, the aetiology of the curve is frequently related to the age of the patient. Young and middle-aged adults frequently present with idiopathic scoliosis that may have been diagnosed in adolescence or may be newly identified. Older adults may have developed a scoliotic deformity secondary to degenerative changes of the spinal column without pre-existing scoliosis. In this situation, the deformity is referred to as degenerative scoliosis or *de novo* scoliosis. The older patient with new-onset scoliosis may also have a history of previous spinal surgery and/or osteoporosis.

The patients' presenting complaints will vary. Some patients will present for routine follow-up for a known curve whereas others may seek medical attention after a spinal curve is identified as an incidental finding (for example, following a chest radiograph). However, the most common presenting complaint in an adult with scoliosis is back pain. This is in contrast to the adolescent patients with scoliosis who are typically asymptomatic. Many orthopaedic surgeons feel that the older the patient, the more likely pain is to be the primary complaint.[5,6] In adult scoliosis, the aetiology of pain is multifactorial. The back pain may result from muscle fatigue on the convexity of the curvature, trunk imbalance, facet arthropathy in the concavity of the curve and degenerative disc disease. In the younger patient, the pain is often localized to their curvature secondary to asymmetric facet degeneration in the curve concavity. The older patient tends be more symptomatic in their lumbar curve as a result of disc degeneration.[1,7]

The evaluating physician must clearly identify the location of the pain and whether it is related to the curve or is the more typical low back pain. It is important to recognize that there is no clear-cut correlation between the presence of idiopathic scoliosis and back pain. A certain percentage of adults with scoliosis will develop persistent, at times worsening pain that is clearly related to their curve. These patients are good candidates for either non-surgical or surgical treatment of their curves. On the other hand, many patients with scoliosis present with non-specific low back pain. In this population, treatment directed at the scoliosis, particularly surgical treatment, is unlikely to be effective.

The overall prevalence of back pain in patients with adult scoliosis has been reported to range from 40% to 90%, and the overall prevalence of painful deformity ranges from 60% to 80%.[8] Historically, the contribution of scoliosis to back pain has been controversial. However, the natural history of adult scoliosis appears to be associated with more severe and more persistent back pain when compared with the non-scoliotic population. Although crippling pain is uncommon, the incidence of pain is felt to increase with age and degree of curvature.[9,10] Furthermore, those scoliosis patients with lumbar curves and those with thoracolumbar and lumbar curves exceeding 45° with apical rotation and coronal imbalance have a higher incidence of pain.[8]

The adult scoliosis patient may also present with complaints other than just isolated back pain. The patient may note a progressively worsening deformity. Curve progression is suggested by loss of height, particularly in young and middle-aged adults in whom height loss is uncommon, recognition that clothes fit differently or need special alteration, or sometimes by a spouse who will verify a change in appearance. This is often associated with diminished functional capacity in addition to cosmetic concerns. Adult scoliosis patients, particularly those with degenerative spinal disease, often experience symptoms consistent with spinal stenosis and radiculopathy. Additionally, although uncommon, patients may suffer from decreased pulmonary function or even respiratory failure. Those with more severe thoracic curves (>70–80°), especially when combined with thoracic lordosis, may have diminished vital capacity as a result of decreased volume of the chest cavity.[11] Although theoretically possible, there is no evidence to suggest that progression of deformity in an adult patient with previously normal pulmonary function will result in deterioration of pulmonary function unless there is underlying pulmonary disease or a history of smoking.[8,12]

It is important to be aware of the many psychosocial issues in patients with scoliosis. Although adults generally display fewer problems than adolescents, they still often experience significant psychosocial limitations.[13] The patients may suffer from poor body image, the burden of chronic pain and the perception of poor overall health. The Medical Outcomes Study 36-Item Short Form (SF-36) has been utilized to demonstrate that the presence of both minimal and significant scoliosis affects a patient's self-perception of health. Schwab et al.[14] found that adults with scoliosis averaged significantly lower SF-36 scores in seven of eight categories when compared with results from the general population of the United States. Thus, it is essential that treating physicians understand and appreciate the significant impact of scoliosis on a patient's perceived mental and physical functioning.

Evaluation

Evaluation of the patient with scoliosis should include a thorough history, careful physical examination and appropriate radiographs. The history should begin with a clear definition of why the patient is seeking treatment. A wide spectrum of non-specific problems is erroneously attributed, by patients and many physicians, to scoliosis. If pain is the presenting complaint, then a very detailed description of the exact location of the pain as well as sites of radiation should be sought. Pain localized near the curvature is often related to the deformity, whereas pain in the distal lower extremities is more likely secondary to spinal stenosis. The effects of the painful deformity on the patient's quality of life should be assessed (such as performance of activities of daily living, occupational activities, and recreational and social activities). Evidence of curve progression, such as loss of height or a notable change, over the last few years, in the fit of clothing, is important. Another essential aspect of the patient history is what, if any, treatments have been employed previously (both non-surgical and surgical) as well as their effectiveness. It is also important to ask about the patient's subjective sense of balance, particularly sagittal plane imbalance when previous surgery has been performed, suggestive of lumbar flat back syndrome. The patient interview should also include a past medical history regarding other comorbidities, as well as a social, family and occupational history. Patients with a history of smoking, substance abuse, depression, and workers' compensation injury have the potential for poorer outcomes following major spinal reconstructive surgery.

The physical examination must consist of evaluation of the spinal deformity, assessment of the musculoskeletal system, and documentation of the patient's neurological status. Examination should include careful evaluation of the patient's shoulders, trunk and waist. The presence of shoulder asymmetry, scapular prominence or a rotational rib or flank deformity should be noted. The magnitude and location of the spinal deformity must be assessed along with evaluation of gait, frontal and sagittal plane balance, and range of motion. It is often helpful, during the physical examination, to confirm the exact location of any pain complaints. The musculoskeletal examination evaluates the flexibility of the curve and the lower extremities. The hip and knee joints should be evaluated to assess the presence of any joint pathology. The range of motion of these joints and leg lengths should be evaluated as any associated pelvic obliquity or contracture may affect the patient's functional ability after correction of the deformity.

Neurological testing seeking both upper and lower motor neurone findings is carried out. This includes strength of both the upper and lower extremity muscles, elicitation of reflexes and sensory examination. Idiopathic scoliosis never results in spinal cord compression or dysfunction and the presence of upper motor neurone findings such as hyperreflexia, clonus or a positive Babinski sign should trigger a search for intraspinal pathology. If the history suggests any change in bowel or bladder function, a rectal examination, assessing sphincter tone and sensation, and bulbocavernosus reflex should be performed. For patients with symptoms suggestive of claudication, evaluation of the distal pulses by palpation and/or Doppler detection helps differentiate between neurogenic and vascular claudication.

Radiographic evaluation includes standing posteroanterior and lateral radiographs of the full spine. Preferably, long cassette 14 × 36 inch (35.6 × 91.4 cm) weight-bearing radiographs should be obtained to evaluate the extent of the primary curvature as well as any compensatory curves or imbalance. The patient must be positioned in a manner that the necessary vertebral segment and key landmarks are clearly visualized. Significant differences exist between positioning techniques, and it has been reported that a standing lateral radiograph with the subject's hands folded in the supraclavicular fossa provides significantly better overall visualization of critical vertebral landmarks.[15] As many patients may suffer from sagittal imbalance it is essential that the lateral view be performed with the knees and hips fully extended (Fig. 89.3). Dedicated supine views of the lumbar and lumbosacral spine may better define degenerative changes in this region. When surgery is being contemplated, bending films facilitate evaluation of spine flexibility and may aid in surgical planning. Additionally in patients with hyperkyphosis or sagittal imbalance, hyperextension lateral views may help in assessing flexibility and the potential need for an anterior release and fusion. Some authors have found that traction radiography performed under general anaesthesia demonstrates greater curve flexibility and prediction of correction with postoperative radiographs than the traditional supine bending radiography. This technique may permit avoidance of anterior release surgery without compromising postoperative correction.[16]

MRI should be obtained in cases of rapid curve progression, when any upper motor neurone findings are identified, when lumbar stenosis is suggested by history or physical examination, or with a left thoracic curve because of the increased risk of spinal cord pathology. MRI is also useful in evaluating the extent of degeneration in the lumbar discs and facet joints, aiding in the selection of distal fusion levels. In patients with previous spinal surgery, gadolinium enhancement helps differentiate postoperative scar from disc material. As metal artefact makes MRI of limited benefit in patients with prior spinal instrumentation, myelography followed by CT scan is the study of choice in these patients. In situations where a pseudarthrosis is suspected, CT with sagittal and coronal reconstructions is helpful. However, neither CT scanning, nor bone scan, nor oblique radiographs are highly predictable in diagnosing a pseudarthrosis.

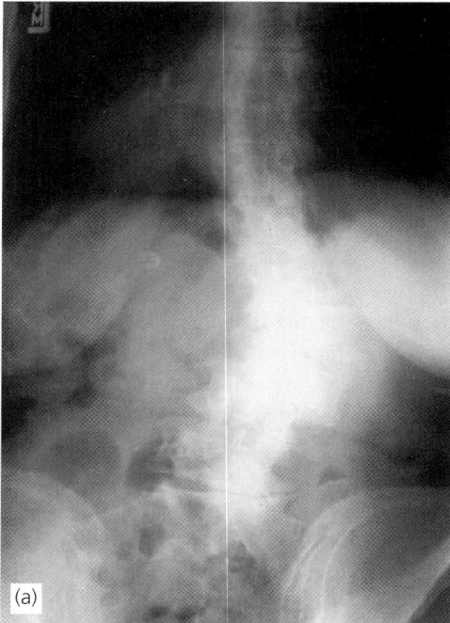

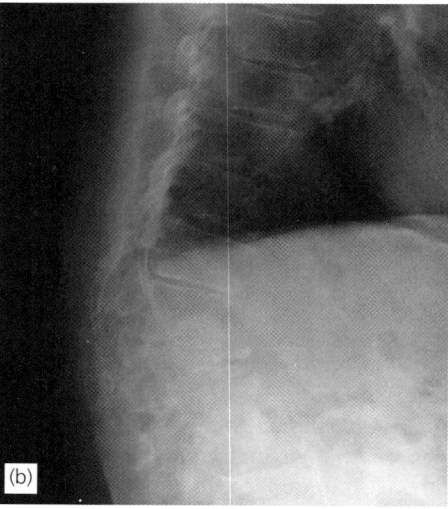

Figure 89.3 A 59-year-old woman with progressive, painful lumbar scoliosis. (a) The curve is seen to end proximally at about T12. The lateral view, however, (b) demonstrates significant kyphosis at the thoracolumbar junction, necessitating extension of the fusion to the mid-thoracic region to avoid the development of a junctional kyphosis.

Non-operative management

Many patients with scoliosis present for evaluation and treatment of their condition, but only rarely is surgical treatment necessary. Accurate identification of the patient's major source of concern will in many cases lead to observation as the appropriate form of management. When treatment is indicated, many patients either have low back pain, leading to non-operative management in most cases, or have mild to moderate curve-related pain, which will frequently respond to conservative treatment as well.

Non-steroidal anti-inflammatory medications, physical therapy and avoidance of pain-eliciting activities may help alleviate the back pain for many patients. Physical therapy should consist of trunk and back stretching and strengthening exercises.[17,18] When combined with aerobic exercise and a weight reduction programme, the benefits of physical therapy can be maximized in the adult scoliosis patient with pain. Localized injections such as epidural steroids or facet joint injections are also occasionally utilized. Other conservative treatment modalities that may improve symptoms include heat and ice, Pilates exercises, water aerobics and alternative medicine options, such as acupuncture, yoga, tai chi, among others.

Narcotic medications should be used judiciously and reserved only for acute pain episodes. Other medications such as muscle relaxants and neuropathic pain medications (such as Lyrica, Neurontin and Elavil) may also be beneficial as part of a pain management regimen.

There is no conservative treatment option that has been demonstrated to halt curve progression in the adult patient. Braces are not as useful in the adult as they are in the skeletally immature patient. They are often poorly tolerated and may even lead to brace dependence and loss of muscle tone. However, occasional clinical situations do exist when a custom-moulded brace may be beneficial to an individual who is a poor surgical candidate.[19]

Surgical treatment

Operative treatment is generally reserved for patients with documented curve progression, intractable pain clearly related to the curve itself that has failed non-operative management or a persistent pain pattern secondary to stenosis in a patient with degenerative scoliosis. Cosmesis is rarely identified as the primary indication for surgical treatment, although many patients will attest to its importance if questioned following the surgery. Surgery may also be occasionally offered to younger adults with significant clinical deformity and curves that are at significant risk for progression (i.e. thoracic curves greater than 50°, or lumbar curves greater than 40°).[8] Although very uncommon, patients with documented and ongoing decline in pulmonary function that is not attributable to underlying pulmonary disease may also benefit from surgical treatment.

It is essential that the patient's primary complaint be clarified. Whether the patient is primarily concerned about back pain, neurogenic claudication or deformity correction affects the surgical plan. The adult spinal deformity surgeon must have a careful discussion of the patient's goals of surgery. These goals may range from solely decompression of symptomatic stenosis to achievement of a solid fusion, stabilization of the curvature, and correction of sagittal and coronal imbalance. Furthermore, the risks and benefits of the procedure must be addressed followed by communication of a realistic assessment of the expected outcome.

The exact nature of the surgical procedure to be performed depends on many factors. The adult spinal deformity surgeon must consider the patient's coronal deformity, coronal balance, sagittal deformity, sagittal balance, rotational deformity, spinal stenosis, spondylolisthesis and lumbosacral degeneration. Furthermore, it is important to appreciate and consider the medical comorbidities that may be present in the ageing population with adult spinal deformity. Even the healthiest adult patient undergoing corrective spine deformity surgery can have significant medical complications after the procedure. Those with known comorbidities and older patients with more limited reserves are at even greater risk of experiencing medical complications.[20] Potential operative candidates should be evaluated for systemic disease, the appropriate medical consultations should be obtained, and the surgical plan carefully selected. Rarely are patients completely excluded from surgery due to medical problems, but many conditions, such as osteoporosis, obesity, deconditioning, coronary artery disease and diabetes, can be optimized prior to surgery, thereby lessening the risk of a poor outcome.

The surgical treatment of scoliosis consists of spinal fusion. Alternatives in surgical treatment include posterior fusion with posterior instrumentation, anterior fusion with anterior instrumentation, and combined anterior fusion with posterior fusion and instrumentation. Virtually all modern scoliosis surgery techniques include fusion and instrumentation. Segmental instrumentation utilizing pedicle screws, multiple hooks, sublaminar wires or combinations thereof is commonly used today. The entirety of the structural curve is typically included in the fusion, along with any levels that need decompression. When choosing the end vertebra, the fusion should end at a stable, neutral vertebra in both the coronal and sagittal planes. In adults, the compensatory curves often become structural, necessitating inclusion in the fusion to maintain truncal balance. It is essential to avoid ending the fusion in a region of kyphosis. As increased thoracic kyphosis is commonly seen in older patients as the result of osteoporosis with compression fractures, fusion up to the proximal thoracic spine may be required.

Posterior fusion with instrumentation is most often employed in isolated thoracic curves or when selective thoracic fusion is undertaken. Isolated posterior fusion with instrumentation is indicated for moderately severe curves and in particular curves that are more flexible (Fig. 89.4). Those patients with more rigid deformities may benefit from an additional anterior procedure that provides circumferential release. Thoracolumbar and lumbar curves may be treated with an isolated posterior approach when adequate correction of the curve and maintenance or restoration of coronal and sagittal balance can be achieved; this is more likely to be the case in younger and middle-aged adults.

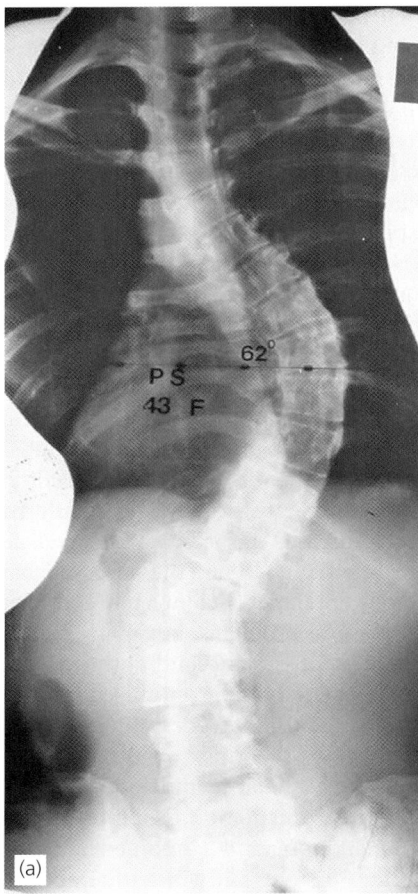 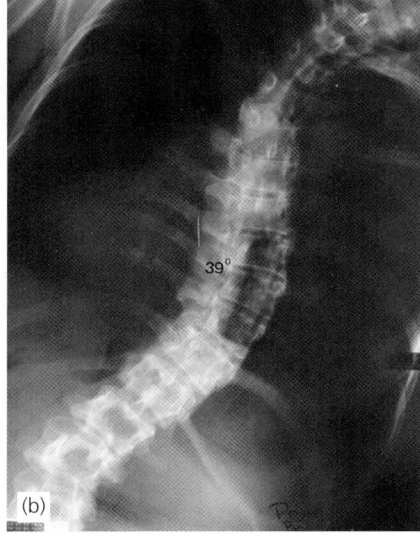 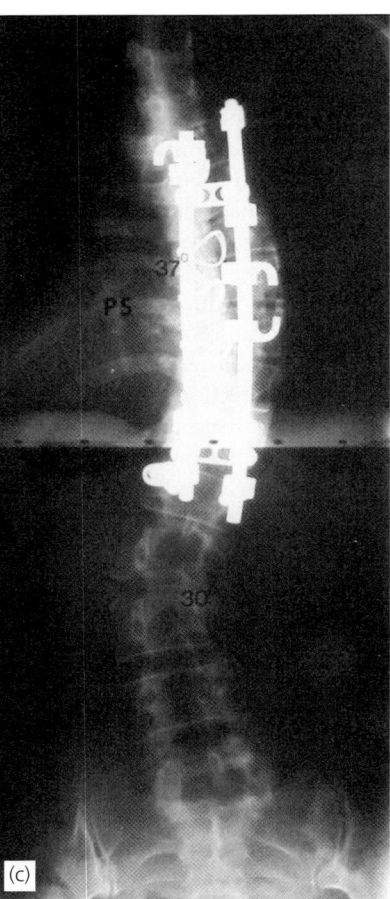

Figure 89.4 A 43-year-old woman who was essentially pain free but had documented progression of her thoracic curve (a) to 62°. The curve was moderately flexible (b) and a selective thoracic fusion (c) was performed, achieving the primary goal of arresting progression of the deformity.

Anterior fusion and anterior instrumentation, without posterior surgery, is commonly applied in adolescents with flexible thoracolumbar or lumbar curves in an attempt to save one or more distal fusion levels. Although it has been advocated for use in adults, factors such as the stiffness of the curve, the extent of degenerative changes and alterations in sagittal plane contour lower the threshold for utilizing a combined anterior and posterior approach for correctional surgery in most adults with spinal deformity.

Anterior release and fusion prior to posterior instrumentation offer three main advantages when compared with posterior surgery alone: an increase in flexibility of the curve, leading to an increase in correction of the deformity including imbalance; a decrease in the pseudarthrosis rate;[21] and a decrease in posterior instrumentation failure at the lumbosacral junction, in long fusions to the sacrum, when block structural support such as a femoral ring allograft or a cage is utilized at L4–5 and L5–S1. A combined anterior and posterior procedure is indicated, therefore, in several situations. When a curve exceeds 80–90°, is particularly rigid, extends into the thoracolumbar and certainly into the lumbar spine, causes sagittal imbalance, or the fusion crosses the lumbosacral junction, isolated posterior fusion with instrumentation frequently results in inadequate curve correction or an unacceptable risk of pseudarthrosis.[22] Patients at greatest risk of pseudarthrosis include those with inadequate or poor bone stock (i.e. after a wide laminectomy, prior radiation in the area or recent smoking history), previous infection, prior pseudarthrosis in the area, and those undergoing a long fusion to the sacrum. In these cases, a combined anterior approach employing bone graft or cages and generous removal of the discs down to the lowest anticipated level of fusion is employed as a first stage. Either during the same anaesthetic session or several days later, posterior fusion extending over the entire span of the deformity, utilizing segmental instrumentation, is performed. Postoperatively, if there is any question about the adequacy of fixation a custom-moulded thoracolumbosacral orthosis (TLSO) is utilized in most adults over the age of 30 years.

An even greater challenge is seen when a long scoliosis fusion needs to extend to the sacrum. There has been much debate regarding the caudal extent of long thoracolumbar fusions and whether the fusion should stop at L5 or cross the lumbosacral junction.[23] Fusion across the lumbosacral junction is indicated in patients in whom the L5–S1 level is felt to be the source of their pain, has been shown to have significant degenerative changes or has any tilt in the coronal plane. MRI, pain provocation discography, selective nerve root infiltration and differential facet blocks (Fig. 89.5) are all at times helpful in determining the status of the lower lumbar and lumbosacral motion segments and the extent to which each motion segment may be contributing to the patient's pain. Some surgeons prefer to terminate a fusion at L5 when the L5–S1 segment is free of pathology in order to preserve lumbar motion and avoid the higher risks and complications associated with fusion across the lumbosacral junction. Other surgeons, however, feel that any time a long fusion has to extend to L5, the results are less predictable and the risk of subjacent degenerative change at L5–S1, late lumbosacral pain, loss of sagittal balance and possible revision surgery is such that automatic extension to the sacrum should be undertaken.[24,25] In some series evaluating fusions across the lumbosacral junction the risks of implant loosening or failure, loss of lordosis, and nonunion have been shown to be excessive, leading to a number of potential solutions.[26–29] The most commonly employed alternative at this time is a combined anterior and posterior approach utilizing structural reconstruction, such as femoral ring allograft or titanium mesh, in the lowest disc spaces and segmental fixation with pedicle screws in the lumbar spine and sacral or iliac screws for distal fixation (Fig. 89.6). The advantages of this include better preservation of lordosis as well as a decrease in stress on the posterior implant.

Instrumentation

Over the past decade, as the indications for use have expanded and numerous spine surgeons have gained experience and familiarity with the technique, the use of pedicle screw fixation has become widespread and has changed the surgical management of spinal deformity. When compared to earlier fixation techniques, pedicle screw fixation has a number of potential benefits for both adolescent and adult patients. Lumbar spine fusion utilizing pedicle screw constructs has been reported to provide better control of correction and maintenance of correction in the coronal,

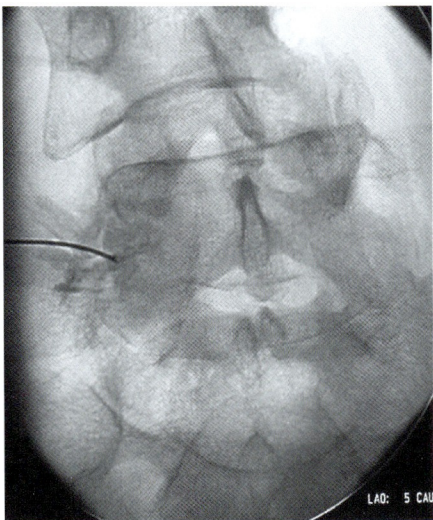

Figure 89.5 Procedure radiograph of a selective nerve root infiltration at L5–S1, blocking the L5 root to attempt to determine whether to extend the fusion in this patient to the L5 or the S1 level. Radiopacifier around nerve root and needle position medial to root can be seen. Because she manifested significant relief of her presenting left buttock pain it was elected to extend the fusion to the sacrum.

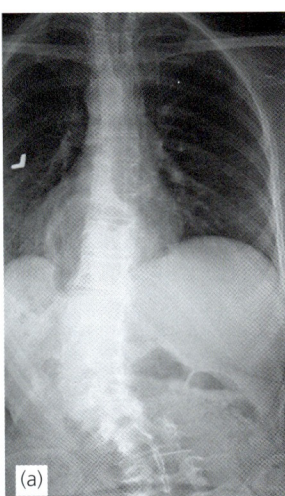
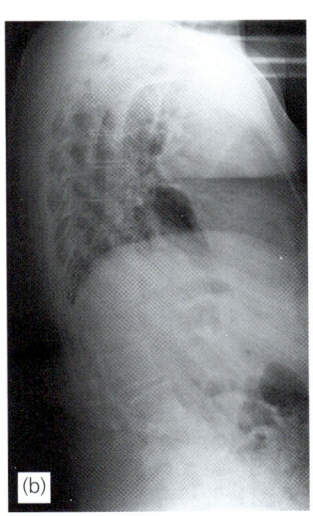
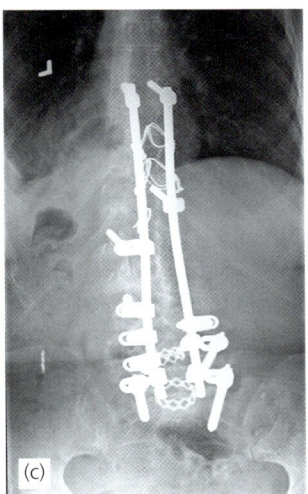
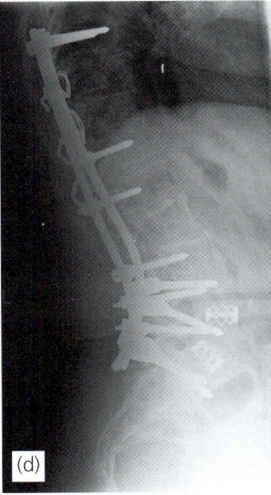

Figure 89.6 A 68-year-old woman with intractable left-sided thoracolumbar and lumbar pain. (a) Note the significant coronal plane imbalance as well as the lateral listhesis of L3 on L4 in the presence of a moderate curve. (b) Marked thoracolumbar kyphosis. (c, d) The results after a combined anterior and posterior fusion using cages for structural support at L4–5 and L5–S1 and posterior instrumentation.

sagittal and axial planes while shortening the length of fusion.[30–32] Additionally, some studies have demonstrated statistically higher fusion rates with pedicle screws and instrumentation.[33–35] This improved fixation and rate of fusion has led many surgeons to abandon the routine use of braces or casts postoperatively.[30]

Pedicle screws have been used routinely in the lumbar spine for a number of years, and evolution of pedicle screw technology and surgeon experience have permitted pedicle screw fixation in the thoracic spine to become a safe and effective procedure.[36,37] With strict adherence to the proper indications, meticulous technique and avoidance of the potential complications, pedicle screw fixation offers a great deal in the management of the adult with spinal deformity. Advocates of multilevel pedicle screw instrumentation report greater correction, lessening the need for combined anterior and posterior procedures.

Bone graft and bone graft alternatives

It is estimated that more than 200 000 spinal arthrodesis procedures are performed each year in the United States.[38] Although this is a commonly performed procedure, failure to obtain a solid bony union remains a relatively common complication even with modern segmental instrumentation techniques.[39] Successful spinal arthrodesis requires the incorporation of bone graft material into the fusion site. Traditionally, surgeons performing spinal fusion have utilized autograft obtained locally, from the excised rib after thoracoplasty, or from the iliac crest. Autogenous bone graft is considered the gold standard for inducing spinal fusion as it is readily available from most patients, there is no risk of rejection, and it contains osteoconductive matrix, osteoinductive factors and osteoprogenitor cells. However, autogenous bone grafting, particularly from the iliac crest, is not without its disadvantages. These include a limited quantity of available autogenous bone graft material, significant donor site morbidity (pain, infection, haematoma, pelvic instability and hernia formation) and excessive blood loss and increased operating room time.[40]

Cadaver allograft bone graft has been utilized as an alternative to autogenous bone graft. However, the processing and sterilization techniques (i.e. freezing, lyophilization, ethanol extraction and irradiation) alter the biological and mechanical properties of the bone affecting the potential of successful fusion. Furthermore, possible disease transmission remains a concern despite sterilization efforts.

Considerable research has been put into the quest for bone graft alternatives that promote union in spinal fusion while avoiding the limitations and disadvantages of traditional bone graft techniques. Bone morphogenic proteins (BMPs) and their osteoinductive properties have received particular attention in this regard. Recombinant human bone morphogenic protein-2 (rhBMP-2) with a collagen sponge carrier (INFUSE Bone Graft) has demonstrated the ability to achieve solid spinal fusions and has been approved by the Food and Drug Administration as a substitute for iliac crest bone graft for single-level anterior interbody fusion. Autogenous iliac crest bone graft remains the gold standard, but studies evaluating the efficacy of rhBMP-2 as a bone graft alternative in posterior spinal fusions and multilevel anterior interbody fusion appear to be promising.[41–43] One must keep in mind that at this time the use of BMPs is considered off-label in posterior spinal applications and multilevel anterior applications.

Outcomes

The results of surgery for scoliosis in the adult depend on a number of factors, including curve aetiology, severity, patient age and the patient's presenting complaint. Pain is the most common indication for surgery in adult scoliosis, but pain relief is frequently inadequate. Careful correlation of the patient's pain complaints with their spinal deformity, as well as establishing realistic goals for the surgery, offers the best hope for minimizing this problem. Curve correction certainly is less in adults than in adolescents, although this can be improved utilizing a combined anterior and posterior approach, in which case curve correction of 40–50% is routinely reported.[21,22] Implant-related complications and loss of correction are also seen; these problems are less common when segmental instrumentation is utilized. Pedicle screw fixation has been found to be quite effective in optimizing correction while minimizing implant loosening or dislodgement. Finally, cosmesis is a frequent secondary concern of the patient. Sponseller et al.[44] reported on the results of the surgical treatment of adults with scoliosis and noted, in addition to significant dissatisfaction in terms of pain relief, very high overall satisfaction with the extent of cosmetic improvement seen.

Various other studies have demonstrated the efficacy of surgical treatment of adult scoliosis. Dickson et al.[45] compared the outcomes of operative and non-operative care in symptomatic adults who were candidates for surgical management of scoliosis. When compared with those patients managed non-operatively, surgically treated patients were found to have a significantly greater improvement of pain, fatigue, self-image and functional ability.[45] Patient self-assessment instruments have also been utilized to evaluate the value of care as perceived by the recipient. Albert et al.[46] administered the SF-36 outcome measure to assess patients with spinal deformity managed by surgery. Significant improvement was demonstrated in regard to self-reported physical function, social function, bodily pain and perceived health change.[46]

ADULT KYPHOSIS

Historically, deformity in the coronal plane has garnered much of the attention in the study of spinal deformity. However, as adult spinal deformity has become better understood in recent years, deformity in the sagittal plane has gained increased attention. Kyphosis refers to the sagittal plane alignment of a segment of the spine with posterior convex angulation. Conversely, lordosis refers to the anterior convex sagittal alignment of a spinal segment. However, unlike coronal and axial plane alignment, where even minor deviations from neutral may be considered abnormal, some degree of kyphosis is normal in the thoracic and sacral spinal segments and some degree of lordosis is normal in the cervical and lumbar segments.

The amount of kyphosis varies considerably between individuals in both the normal state and pathological conditions. Typically, most kyphotic deformities seen in childhood are a result of congenital or developmental conditions. However, symptomatic kyphotic deformity is being increasingly seen in the adult population as the result of the general ageing of the population, collapse secondary to metabolic bone disease and the sequelae of older surgical techniques.

Before discussing abnormal sagittal plane alignment, the normal spinal sagittal contour must be addressed. Sagittal spinal balance is often defined by the C7 plumb line, which is considered to be the spine's weight-bearing axis. The C7 plumb line is drawn from the middle of the C7 vertebral body and extends vertically downwards. The horizontal distance between this line and the posterosuperior corner of the S1 vertebral body is then measured. When the C7 plumb line falls anterior or posterior to the S1 reference point, spinal balance is considered 'positive' or 'negative' respectively.[47] Normal sagittal balance is defined such that the head is centred over the pelvis in the sagittal plane.[48] From a purely radiographic point of view, neutral sagittal alignment follows a vertical axis from C2, in front of T7, behind L3 and across S2.[49]

As mentioned previously, kyphosis and lordosis are normal in certain segments of the spinal column. The thoracic and sacral segments exhibit kyphosis, whereas the cervical and lumbar segments demonstrate lordosis. Thoracic kyphosis typically ranges between 20 and 40° and is found to normally increase with ageing.[50] Normal lumbar lordosis ranges from 30 to 80° with increasing fractional lordosis in the caudad segments (between L4 and S1).[51] Decreases in normal lumbar lordosis of up to 20° have been recognized to result from ageing and degeneration.[52] Interestingly, despite this wide range of normal values, a proportional relationship seems to exist between thoracic kyphosis and lumbar lordosis in normal individuals. Although the total and segmental values may vary from person to person, the relative contribution of each segment to the total sagittal contour is relatively constant and the curves are fairly 'balanced'. The alternating lordotic and kyphotic curvature patterns between the cervical, thoracic, lumbar and sacral segments allow increased flexibility and force dampening than would be achievable by a straight vertebral column.[48] Sagittal balance is often compromised with ageing because, as thoracic kyphosis increases, lumbar lordosis is lost.

In the adult patient, certain aetiologies of kyphosis account for the majority of the deformities. The most common causes of adult sagittal plane deformity include Scheuermann's kyphosis, postural round back, osteoporotic deformity, flat back syndrome occurring as the result of prior spinal surgery, and post-traumatic kyphosis.

Scheuermann's kyphosis

Scheuermann first described the type of structural thoracic kyphosis that now bears his name in 1920. Over the years, there has been much debate regarding the aetiology of this deformity. In his initial description, Scheuermann observed an association between rigid juvenile kyphosis and the radiographic findings of epiphyseal irregularities and anterior wedging of the vertebral bodies. He hypothesized that avascular necrosis of the vertebral ring apophysis led to premature cessation of growth anteriorly with resultant wedging of the vertebral body. However, subsequent studies disproved this and a variety of other theories. Although an exact aetiology has yet to be elucidated, it appears an underlying genetic factor is likely.[53]

In 1964, Sorensen[54] reported on his experience with this deformity. Sorensen's criteria for the radiographic diagnosis of Scheuermann's kyphosis include greater than 5° of anterior wedging of at least three adjacent vertebral bodies, end plate irregularities and Schmorl's nodes (intervertebral disc herniation through the end plates of the vertebral bodies).[54] This definition is still widely used today to help differentiate Scheuermann's disease from other kyphotic deformities. Other radiographic findings that are often seen in association with anterior wedging include disc space narrowing, increased anteroposterior diameter of the vertebral bodies and, occasionally, mild scoliosis.[55]

Most series agree that the overall prevalence of Scheuermann's disease is between 0.4% and 8%, with males and females equally affected. The exact age of onset is difficult to establish as the radiographic findings used to diagnose Scheuermann's disease are not visible until the onset of puberty. Scheuermann's kyphosis may be diagnosed in the adult patient because, even though the deformity was present earlier as an adolescent, it was either ignored or considered to be the result of poor posture.[56]

Scheuermann's kyphosis is often asymptomatic or only mildly symptomatic. In the adolescent, the patient often presents with primarily cosmetic or postural complaints, although back pain and fatigue are also reported. In the adult patient, back pain is the most common complaint. Typically, the pain is located just distal to the apex of the deformity. However, degenerative disc disease and facet arthropathy may also be present and contribute to the overall pain pattern. Cord compression and cardiopulmonary complaints are rare findings in Scheuermann's disease, but their presence or absence should be included in the evaluation of the patient.[56]

When treating back pain in Scheuermann's kyphosis, conservative management consisting of exercise (postural and aerobic) and anti-inflammatory medications generally suffices. Brace treatment has little value in the skeletally mature patient. Surgery is reserved for patients with severe or progressive deformity, neurological compromise and/or recalcitrant pain.[55] In the adult patient, operative management usually requires combined anterior and posterior reconstruction and instrumented fusion. Correction of the deformity with compression instrumentation, rather than cantilever forces, is essential to avoid junctional kyphosis.

Postural kyphosis

Postural kyphosis is a sagittal plane deformity that is most commonly seen in adolescents. This condition, also known as postural round back, is related to poor posture and generally results in a mild to moderate increase in thoracic kyphosis with compensatory hyperlordosis of the lumbar spine. Postural round back is easily distinguished from Scheuermann's kyphosis by the flexibility of the curve, lack of acute apical angulation and the absence of the typical radiographic abnormalities. Surgical correction is rarely indicated. Postural education appears to be the most effective treatment, as bracing and exercise do little to alter the natural history of postural kyphosis.[48]

Osteoporotic kyphotic deformity

Osteoporosis is a common skeletal disorder characterized by compromised bone strength predisposing a person to an increased rate of fracture. As the population ages worldwide, the prevalence of osteoporosis will continue to increase and osteoporosis will remain a major public health problem facing post-menopausal women and elderly individuals of both sexes. The World Health Organization defines osteoporosis as a bone mineral density less than 2.5 SD below the average of young, healthy individuals. In the United States alone, it is estimated that anywhere from 10 to 24 million adults already suffer from osteoporosis with millions more having low bone mass.[57,58] These individuals are at increased risk of sustaining fragility fractures such as hip fractures, distal radius fractures, proximal humerus fractures and, most commonly, vertebral compression fractures. It has been estimated that more than 700 000 osteoporotic compression fractures occur annually in the United States, exceeding the combined total of hip (300 000 per year) and wrist (250 000 per year).[58] Osteoporosis and the associated vertebral compression fractures are the primary aetiologies of kyphotic spinal deformity in the ageing adult population.

Even in the absence of compression fractures, the ageing process is normally associated with an increase in thoracic kyphosis and loss of lumbar lordosis.[50,59] With increased age and decreased bone mineral density, elderly people are at risk for vertebral body compression fractures that may allow the kyphotic angulation to progress beyond the range of what is considered normal. Osteoporotic spinal deformity in the ageing adult can lead to a multitude of problems. The patient may suffer from pain, neurological deterioration, loss of height, sagittal imbalance, functional impairment, loss of appetite, compromise of pulmonary function and even development of hip osteoarthritis and flexion contracture. Furthermore, the presence of kyphotic deformity and vertebral compression fractures predisposes the patient to progression of deformity and occurrence of additional fractures at adjacent levels.[60] With collapse of a vertebral compression fracture, the kyphotic angulation places increased stress on the anterior cortex of the adjacent vertebral bodies and increases the risk of adjacent level fracture and collapse by fivefold.[61]

In the acute setting, the primary clinical finding in vertebral compression fractures is pain. However, neurological deficit resulting from compression of the anterior spinal cord or cauda equina, although rare, is also another possible finding that must be considered. Typically, the acute pain is described as intense, intermittent and aggravated by activity, usually lasting from 4 to 8 weeks. It has been reported that chronic disabling pain may develop in as many as 35% of patients.[62] Chronic pain following compression fracture may result from incomplete vertebral healing with progressive collapse, altered spine kinematics resulting from spinal deformity, or the development of a pseudarthrosis at the involved vertebra.[63] There are also many other potential long-term effects of compression fractures with associated loss of vertebral body height and subsequent kyphotic deformity. With decreased volume of the thoracic and abdominal cavities, patients may suffer from restrictive lung disease and early satiety.[64,65] These many consequences of vertebral compression fractures impact the affected individual's ability to successfully manage their activities of daily living, impair their quality of life and ultimately contribute to an increase in their relative risk of mortality.[64,66,67]

Treatment of patients with osteoporotic spinal pathology is mostly non-operative. In fact, an unknown number of vertebral compression fractures produce no or only mild symptoms and the individual never seeks acute medical attention. Symptomatic patients may benefit from analgesic medications, activity modification and administration of bisphosphonates. Bracing is often utilized, but there is much debate regarding its efficacy in pain control and in treating progression and correction of the deformity. Furthermore, compliance with bracing is often difficult given the limited independent functional ability of many patients.

Surgery for the treatment of osteoporotic spinal deformity is typically reserved for those with intractable pain, neurological signs or symptoms, and progressive disabling deformity. However, surgery in this patient population is complicated by a number of factors that require special consideration. In the setting of osteoporosis, the mechanical properties of the spine are altered, most notably by decreased bone stock. The risk of loss of fixation in osteoporotic bone calls for extra care in fusion technique.

The surgeon must be wary of overaggressive decompression that may result in iatrogenic instability. Anterior column insufficiency increases the risk of failure of a posterior-only decompression and fusion. An anterior approach may result in better correction of the deformity as it permits direct access to the vertebral body pathology and facilitates restoration of anterior column support. The addition of posterior instrumentation is often still required for adequate stabilization and correction of the deformity. In such combined anterior and posterior procedures, it is essential to select an appropriate anterior interbody graft as subsistence of graft materials is not uncommon in the osteoporotic spine. If the graft is small (i.e. fibular inlay) and does not distribute the load over a sufficiently large area of the adjacent end plate, it is at risk of telescoping into the adjacent levels. The use of larger implants (i.e. iliac crest, femoral or humeral grafts, or cages) lessens the risk of this problem.

Furthermore, the poor bone stock of the osteoporotic spine necessitates additional points of fixation to gain the necessary stability in instrumented fusions. This may be achieved with multiple pedicle screws alone or in combination with laminar hooks and/or sublaminar wires (Fig. 89.7). As the pedicles are often enlarged in the osteoporotic spine, the use of larger screws may improve purchase and increase pullout strength. It is under investigation if screws augmented with calcium hydroxyapatite resin or polymethylmethacrylate (PMMA) injection also increase the strength of the fixation construct.

An additional problem encountered is the overall decreased health status of the elderly patient, which often limits the degree of surgical intervention that can be safely performed. However, less invasive techniques that do not subject the elderly patient to inordinate risks or surgical trauma have been developed and are now options in the clinical management of vertebral compression fractures and kyphotic deformity in this patient population. Vertebroplasty and kyphoplasty are each minimally invasive procedures that offer promising results in the treatment of painful osteoporotic compression fractures and associated deformity.

Vertebroplasty consists of percutaneous augmentation of vertebral body volume and strength by injection of a hardening material in a liquid state. The initial uses of vertebroplasty were for treatment of painful haemangiomas of the vertebral body and as a supplementation to internal fixation during open procedures. After noting its successful analgesic effect, the indications for vertebroplasty were expanded to treat painful vertebral collapse in the setting of osteoporosis or tumour. The goals of vertebroplasty are to provide both analgesia and vertebral structural stabilization to prevent further vertebral collapse.[68]

Vertebroplasty may be performed under local or general anaesthesia in a radiology procedure room. With the patient prone on a radiolucent table, biplanar fluoroscopy is used to percutaneously insert a large gauge needle into the affected vertebral body via either a transpedicular or extrapedicular route. It must be verified that the needle is placed correctly within the vertebral body and not within a major venous outflow tract. Then, under fluoroscopic monitoring, a low-viscosity cement mixture (typically polymethylmethacrylate)

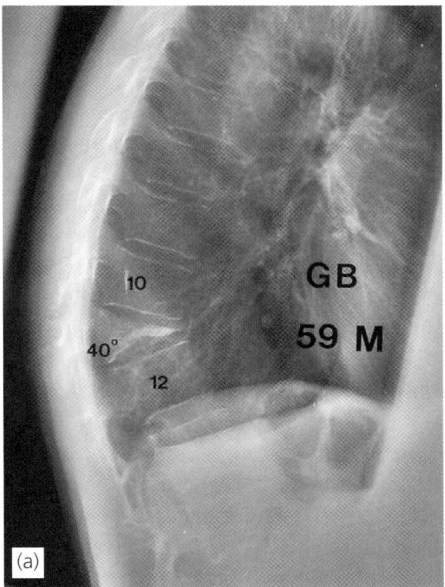
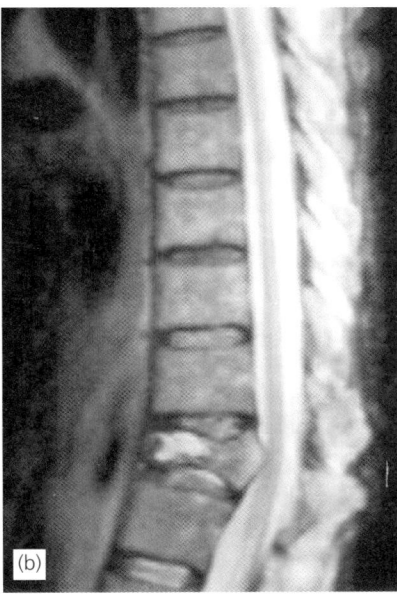
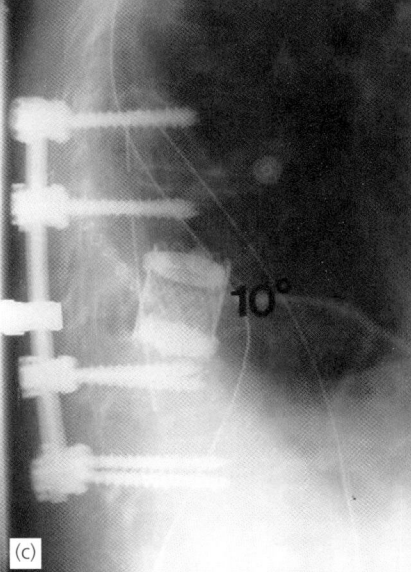

Figure 89.7 A 59-year-old man with a known diagnosis of osteoporosis who, 3 months prior to presentation, sustained a pathological fracture of T11. He presented with worsening and severe back pain, a worsening gibbus, and evidence of myelopathy including hyperreflexia and positive Babinski signs bilaterally. His plain lateral radiograph is seen in (a) and the sagittal MR image at the fracture site is seen in (b). Although only modest cord compression is seen on the supine MRI, the worsening kyphosis on the erect lateral radiograph (40°) explains the neurological signs. (c) The lateral radiograph following anterior vertebrectomy and decompression and combined anterior and posterior reconstruction.

with an opacifying agent and antibiotic is injected under pressure into the cancellous vertebral body. As the cement hardens, the fracture is stabilized.[68]

Kyphoplasty is a procedure similar to vertebroplasty that was first introduced in 1998. However, it not only provides increased vertebral stability, but also allows some correction of the kyphotic deformity resulting from compression fracture collapse. An inflatable balloon device (bone tamp) is inserted percutaneously and used to restore vertebral body height by elevating the end plates. The pre-created balloon cavity is subsequently filled with a low-pressure, high-viscosity injection of a hardening material (usually polymethylmethacrylate). After the polymethylmethacrylate has set, the vertebral compression fracture is stabilized along with restoration of vertebral body height and some correction of the kyphotic deformity.[63] It appears that the amount of correction obtained is related to the age and configuration of the fracture.[69]

The exact mechanism of the analgesic effect of vertebroplasty and kyphoplasty is not completely understood. The pain relief is thought to be the result of fracture stabilization and possibly the destruction of terminal nerve endings by the thermal effect of polymethylmethacrylate hardening. Reports on the outcomes of vertebroplasty demonstrate that the majority of patients experience complete or partial pain relief and improvement in function following the procedure. Early results suggest that kyphoplasty also provides excellent pain relief, but also can improve vertebral body height and reduce spinal kyphosis.[63,70–73]

Significant complications after vertebroplasty and kyphoplasty are fairly infrequent and both procedures are felt to be relatively safe. The reported complications include cement leakage, cerebrospinal fluid leak, cement embolization, cardiopulmonary collapse, infection and epidural haemorrhage.[68,74,75] Leakage of cement into the epidural or paravertebral areas is fairly common and has been reported to occur in 30–70% of vertebroplasties. Although the potential for serious neurological problems does exist, cement leakage is typically asymptomatic or results in only mild and transient neurological symptoms.[76]

Vertebroplasty and kyphoplasty are still relatively new techniques and additional outcome studies are needed, but early results are promising. With careful technique, proper patient selection, and thorough follow-up, these less invasive procedures are useful alternatives in the treatment of patients with symptomatic osteoporotic compression fractures and resultant kyphotic deformity.[77] See also Chapter 90.

Flat back syndrome

Flat back syndrome is another common sagittal plane deformity found in the adult patient. Surgical treatment of spinal conditions may result in loss of lumbar lordosis along with increased kyphosis more proximally. Flat back syndrome is a postural disorder of the spine that consists of a fixed loss of sagittal plane balance with associated pain symptoms. The original description of this symptomatic fixed sagittal imbalance was in scoliosis patients after the use of distraction instrumentation, such as Harrington rods, extending into the lumbar spine or sacrum for curve correction. Although distraction instrumentation into the lower lumbar spine or sacrum is the most common aetiology, iatrogenic loss of lumbar lordosis may also occur as a result of adjacent segment decompensation, anterior column collapse, posterior column incompetence, malaligned fusion and pseudarthrosis with progression of deformity or loss of correction. Other related instances of symptomatic sagittal imbalance resulting from lumbosacral fusions for kyphotic deformity correction or instrumentation of posttraumatic kyphosis have been termed 'kyphotic decompensation syndrome'. The term flat back syndrome is often utilized to include any aetiology of a symptomatic post-fusion condition attributable to severe loss of lumbar lordosis.[78]

Affected patients typically present with painful loss of lumbar lordosis and complain of a feeling of forward inclination with difficulty or inability to stand erect without hip and knee flexion. Often, there is a history of multiple spine surgeries. Low back pain, upper back pain, neck pain and thigh pain are often present along with the symptoms of imbalance. The muscle strain of attempting to maintain erect posture and horizontal gaze leads to pain and fatigue in these regions. Hip flexion contractures and abnormal pelvic tilt are commonly present. The fixed sagittal imbalance often results in an abnormal gait with decreased step and stride length along with diminished gait velocity.[79] Patients with flat back deformity particularly complain of difficulty ambulating on uneven ground, stumbling while walking, and catching feet on carpets.

Proper radiographic assessment is essential to define the problem in patients with flat back syndrome. Radiographic evaluation of a patient with suspected flat back syndrome should begin with a full-length standing lateral radiograph of the spine. The radiograph should be performed with the patient's hips and knees extended as failure to do so may result in artificial translation of the sagittal vertical axis. The sagittal vertical axis is best assessed with the C7 plumb line technique discussed earlier. The normal sagittal vertical axis falls within ±3 cm linear distance from the posterior-superior aspect of the S1 end plate.[78] Patients with flat back syndrome are found to have positive sagittal balance (plumb line falling anterior to the sacral promontory) along with flattening or even kyphosis of the lumbar segments.[80] Full-length standing anteroposterior radiographs help assess any associated coronal plane deformity, flexion and extension radiographs evaluate the remaining mobility and supine oblique radiographs and computed tomography may be useful in defining the presence and location of a pseudarthrosis.

Obviously, prevention is the preferred treatment for iatrogenic flat back syndrome. As revision spinal fusion is often associated with increased complication rates and residual deformity, appropriate pre-operative assessment and planning at the index procedure is essential. The patient must have adequate radiographs to assess his or her pre-operative sagittal, coronal and axial alignment. This way the operation can be planned so that the existing thoracic and lumbar curves and associated sagittal balance are either maintained or corrected. In situations involving lumbar degenerative disease, it is even often necessary to increase lumbar lordosis in anticipation of further degeneration and loss of curvature. Segmental instrumentation with pedicle screws, sublaminar wires or hooks should be utilized rather than distraction instrumentation (Harrington rods) and, when possible, the caudal extent of the fusion should be limited proximal to or at L3. Additionally, intra-operative positioning with the patient's hips extended helps preserve lumbar lordosis with lumbar fusion surgery.[78]

In those patients who do develop flat back syndrome, some may benefit from non-operative treatment consisting of hip extension, trunk stabilization and back extension exercises, hip flexor stretching, weight reduction and non-steroidal anti-inflammatory medications. However, these measures do not correct the deformity and often provide only temporary relief. Surgical correction is indicated after non-operative treatment has failed or the deformity has progressed.

The goals of surgery in the patient with flat back syndrome are to restore sagittal balance and to reduce pain. Prior to this undertaking, the problem must be properly defined. Where is the loss of lordosis? What is the degree of loss? Is a pseudarthrosis present? Is there associated distal degeneration or instability? Is there any proximal kyphosis? The site of the deformity and the presence and location of pseudarthrosis dictates the type and location of corrective osteotomies and the extent of fusion and instrumentation.

The two most common surgical techniques used to correct the fixed sagittal imbalance found with flat back syndrome include the extension (Smith–Petersen) osteotomy and the pedicle subtraction osteotomy. The Smith–Petersen osteotomy is performed by a posterior approach and entails resection of the posterior elements at the desired level of correction. To achieve lordosis, the posterior column is compressed and shortened while the anterior column is lengthened. It is important to note that complications have been associated with lengthening of the anterior column. Anterior column lengthening may predispose the patient to instrumentation failure, pseudarthrosis, spinal destabilization and even traction injury to the great vessels and viscera.[78] The Smith–Petersen (opening wedge) osteotomy is a technically less demanding procedure than other corrective procedures, but the associated potential for complications and loss of correction have led spine surgeons to seek a superior technique for treating fixed sagittal imbalance.

The pedicle subtraction osteotomy (also know as the transpedicular wedge resection procedure or transpediculer cortical decancellation procedure) is an alternative technique for treating fixed sagittal plane deformity. It is performed via a posterior approach and consists of a three-column posterior closing wedge osteotomy hingeing on the anterior cortex. All of the posterior elements, including the pedicles and the superior and inferior adjacent facet joints, are removed at the level of the correction. At this point, a posterior wedge of cancellous bone is removed from the vertebral body to permit the desired correction. The osteotomy is then closed with compression and fixation of instrumentation. Obtaining correction through all three columns prevents lengthening of the anterior column and avoids stretch on the soft tissue structures anterior to the spine, while the abundant cancellous bone contact maximizes the healing potential of the fusion. It has been reported that approximately 30° of curve correction is obtained through the osteotomy site.[81] Although the pedicle subtraction osteotomy is a technically demanding procedure that is not without its own complications (i.e. bleeding of the epidural venous plexus and cortical bone, thoracic pseudarthrosis cephalad to osteotomy site), it has many advantages and is a useful procedure for treating patients with fixed sagittal imbalance (Fig. 89.8).

Although the Smith–Petersen and pedicle subtraction osteotomies are posterior procedures, they are often combined with an anterior procedure such as discectomy, vertebrectomy and arthrodesis. A combined anterior procedure is generally indicated in the presence of multiple pseudarthroses, more extensive decompression and long fusions to the sacrum. Furthermore, as many patients suffering from flat back syndrome have had prior spine surgeries with instrumentation, staged procedures with initial removal of hardware and subsequent corrective surgery and reinstrumentation are often necessary.

Post-traumatic kyphosis

Kyphotic deformity also develops subsequent to traumatic injury to the spinal column. In compression fractures and burst fractures, the disruption of the anterior column with resultant shortening may lead to increased kyphosis of the thoracic spine or loss of lumbar lordosis. In the acute situation, a fracture is considered to be unstable and operative reconstruction and stabilization is recommended if there is greater than 50% collapse of anterior vertebral body height or more than 20° of sagittal angulation. In these situations, anterior column reconstruction procedures are often required to restore height and correct deformity, as well as to decompress the spinal canal when appropriate.

After healing of the fracture, late post-traumatic kyphotic deformity may occur as a result of untreated fractures or failed early reconstruction with an isolated posterior procedure. With lesser degrees of kyphosis (i.e. 30° or less), anterior column reconstruction alone (with autograft, allograft, cages, screws and plates) may be sufficient to address the deformity. In cases of greater degrees of kyphosis or more rigid deformity, combined anterior and posterior procedures may be necessary for adequate correction. Posterior column shortening with pedicle subtraction osteotomy and combined multilevel segmental instrumentation and fusion is another important option in the management of post-traumatic fixed sagittal plane deformity.

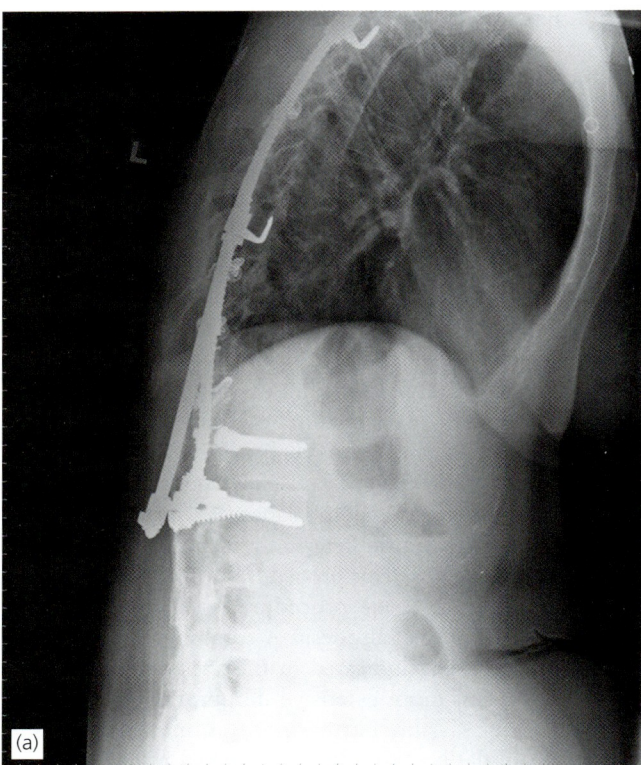 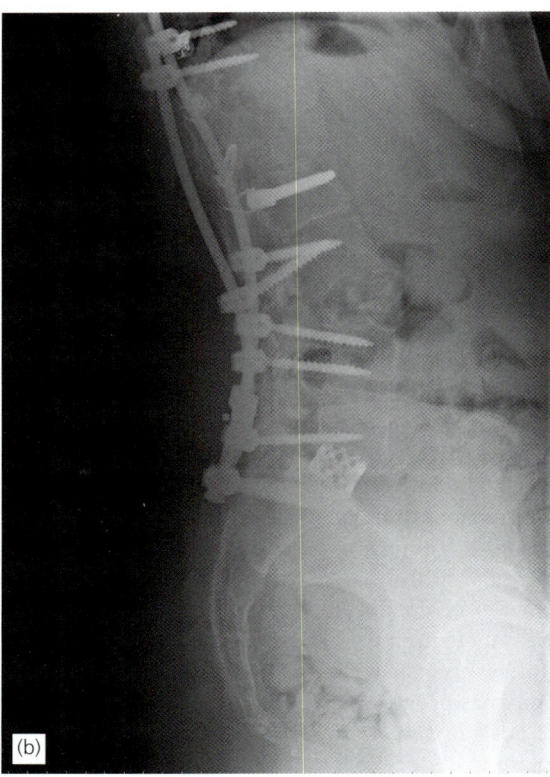

Figure 89.8 A 39-year-old woman who had scoliosis surgery from T4–L5 12 years ago followed 1 year later with removal of part of the instrumentation. She presents now with worsening postural imbalance and severe pain throughout her lower and upper back, at times extending into the neck. The pain is worse with extended standing. (a) A standing lateral radiograph demonstrating a marked sagittal plane imbalance as well as the complete loss of lumbar lordosis. (b) A lateral radiograph 2 months following anterior extension of the fusion to S1 with cage reconstruction supplemented with BMPs, pedicle subtraction osteotomy at L3 and revision posterior instrumentation. Her fatigue-type pain is completely resolved and she is now in normal sagittal balance.

KEY LEARNING POINTS

- Adult scoliosis has a mostly benign natural history but surgery is indicated in cases of intractable pain or documented curve progression.
- Scoliosis surgery in the adult requires careful attention to both coronal and sagittal curves; the fusion must end at a stable, neutral vertebra in both planes.
- Long fusions to the sacrum routinely require anterior column support.
- Surgery for osteoporotic deformity has a high complication rate which may be lessened by restoration of sagittal balance, multilevel fixation and, in some cases, anterior column support.
- Restoration of sagittal balance is essential in the operative treatment of flat back syndrome but other sources of pain and/or deformity such as pseudarthrosis, transition syndrome or thoracic deformity must be considered.

REFERENCES

1. Kostuik JP, Bentivoglio J. The incidence of low back pain in adult scoliosis. *Spine* 1981;**6**:268–73.
2. Biot B, Pendrix D. Frequence de la scoliose lombaire an l'age adult. *Annals of Medical Physics* 1982;**25**:251–4.
3. Perennou D, Marcelli C, Herisson C. Adult lumbar scoliosis. Epidemiologic aspects in a low back pain population. *Spine* 1994;**19**:123–8.
4. Schwab F, Dubey A, Gamez L, et al. Adult scoliosis: prevalence, SF-36, and nutritional parameters in an elderly volunteer population. *Spine* 2005;**30**:1082–5.
5. Deviren V, Berven S, Kleinstueck F, et al. Predictors of flexibility and pain patterns in thoracolumbar and lumbar idiopathic scoliosis. *Spine* 2002;**27**:2346–9.
6. Takahashi S, Delecrin S, Passuti N. Surgical treatment of idiopathic scoliosis: an age-related analysis of outcome. *Spine* 2002;**27**:1742–8.
7. Winter RB, Lonstein JE, Denis F. Pain patterns in adult scoliosis. *Orthopedic Clinics of North America* 1988;**19**:339–45.

8. Bradford DS, Tay BK, Hu SS. Adult scoliosis: surgical indications, operative management, complications, and outcomes. *Spine* 1999;**24**:2617–29.
9. Weinstein SL, Dolan LA, Spratt KF, *et al.* Health and function of patients with untreated idiopathic scoliosis – a 50 year natural history study. *Journal of the American Medical Association* 2003;**289**:559–67.
10. Jackson RP, Simmons EH, Stripinis D. Incidence and severity of back pain in adult idiopathic scoliosis. *Spine* 1983;**8**:749–56.
11. Upadhyay SS, Mullaji AB, Luk KD, *et al.* Relation of spinal and thoracic cage deformities and their flexibilities with altered pulmonary functions in adolescent scoliosis. *Spine* 1995;**20**:2415–20.
12. Pehrsson K, Bake B, Larsson S, *et al.* Lung function in adult idiopathic scoliosis: a 20 year follow up. *Thorax* 1991;**46**:474–8.
13. Tones M, Moss N, Polly DW. A review of quality of life and psychosocial issues in scoliosis. *Spine* 2006;**31**:3027–38.
14. Schwab FS, Dubey A, Pagala M, *et al.* Adult scoliosis: a health assessment analysis by SF-36. *Spine* 2003;**28**:602–6.
15. Horton WC, Brown CW, Bridwell KH, *et al.* Is there an optimal patient stance for obtaining a lateral 36" radiograph? A critical comparison of three techniques. *Spine* 2005;**30**:427–33.
16. Davis BJ, Gadgil A, Trivedi J, *et al.* Traction radiography performed under general anesthetic: a new technique for assessing idiopathic scoliosis curves. *Spine* 2004;**29**:2466–70.
17. van Dam BE. Nonoperative treatment of adult scoliosis. *Orthopedic Clinics of North America* 1988;**19**:347–51.
18. Ogilvie JW. Adult scoliosis: evaluation and nonsurgical treatment. *Instructional Course Lectures* 1992;**41**:251–5.
19. Weiss HR, Dallmayer R. Brace treatment of spinal claudication in an adult with lumbar scoliosis – a case report. *Research into Spinal Deformities* 2006;**5**:586–9.
20. Raffo CS, Lauerman WC. Predicting morbidity and mortality of lumbar spine arthrodesis in patients in their ninth decade. *Spine* 2006;**31**:99–103.
21. Byrd JA, Scoles PV, Winter RB, *et al.* Adult idiopathic scoliosis treated by anterior and posterior spinal fusion. *Journal of Bone and Joint Surgery (America)* 1987;**69**:843–50.
22. Bradford DS. Adult scoliosis: Current concepts of treatment. *Clinical Orthopaedics* 1988;**229**:70–87.
23. Polly DW Jr., Hamill CL, Bridwell KH. Debate: to fuse or not to fuse to the sacrum, the fate of the L5-S1 disc. *Spine* 2006;**31**:S179–S84.
24. Swamy G, Berven SH, Bradford DS. The selection of L5 versus S1 in long fusions for adult idiopathic scoliosis. *Neurosurgery Clinics of North America* 2007;**18**:281–8.
25. Eck KR, Bridwell KH, Ungacta FF, *et al.* Complications and results of long adult deformity corrections down to L4, L5, and the sacrum. *Spine* 2001;**26**:E182–E91.
26. Balderston MA, Winter RB, Moe JH, *et al.* Fusion to the sacrum for nonparalytic scoliosis in the adult. *Spine* 1986;**11**:824–9.
27. Boachie-Adjei O, Dendrinos GK, Ogilvie JW, *et al.* Management of adult spinal deformity with combined anterior-posterior arthrodesis and Luque-Galveston instrumentation. *Journal of Spinal Disorders* 1991;**4**:131–41.
28. Emami A, Deviren V, Berven S, *et al.* Outcome and complications of long fusions to the sacrum in adult spine deformity: Luque-Galveston, combined iliac and sacral screws, and sacral fixation. *Spine* 2002;**27**:776–86.
29. Islam NC, Wood KB, Transfeldt EE, *et al.* Extension of fusions to the pelvis in idiopathic scoliosis. *Spine* 2001;**26**:166–73.
30. Gaines, Jr. RW. Current concepts review: the use of pedicle-screw internal fixation for the operative treatment of spinal disorders. *Journal of Bone and Joint Surgery (America)* 2000;**82**:1458–76.
31. Barr SJ, Schuette AM, Emans JB. Lumbar pedicle screws versus hooks. Results in double major curves in adolescent idiopathic scoliosis. *Spine* 1997;**22**:1369–79.
32. Hamill CL, Lenke LG, Bridwell KH, *et al.* The use of pedicle screw fixation to improve correction in the lumbar spine of patients with idiopathic scoliosis. Is it warranted? *Spine* 1996;**21**:1241–9.
33. Zdeblick TA. A prospective, randomized study of lumbar fusion. Preliminary results. *Spine* 1993;**18**:983–91.
34. Yuan HA, Garfin SR, Dickman CA, *et al.* A historical cohort study of pedicle screw fixation in thoracic, lumbar, and sacral spinal fusions. *Spine* 1994;**20S**:2279S–96S.
35. Schwab FJ, Nazarian DG, Mahmud F, *et al.* Effects of spinal instrumentation on fusion of the lumbosacral spine. *Spine* 1995;**18**:2023–28.
36. Daubs MD, Kim YJ, Lenke LG. Pedicle screw fixation (T1, T2, T3). *Instructional Course Lecture* 2007;**56**:247–55.
37. Suk S, Kim W, Lee S, *et al.* Thoracic pedicle screw fixation in spinal deformities: are they really safe? *Spine* 2001;**18**:2049–57.
38. Boden SD. Overview of the biology of lumbar spine fusion and principles for selecting a bone graft substitute. *Spine* 2002;**27**:S26–S31.
39. Kim YJ, Bridwell KH, Lenke LG, *et al.* Pseudarthrosis in adult spinal deformity following multisegmental instrumentation and arthrodesis. *Journal of Bone and Joint Surgery (America)* 2006;**88**:721–8.
40. Ludwig SC, Boden SD. Osteoinductive bone graft substitutes for spinal fusion: a basic science summary. *Orthopedic Clinics of North America* 1999;**30**:635–45.
41. Luhman SJ, Bridwell KH, Cheng I, *et al.* Use of bone morphogenic protein-2 for adult spinal deformity. *Spine* 2005;**30**:S110–17.
42. Glassman SD, Carreon L, Djurasovic M, *et al.* Posterolateral lumbar spine fusion with INFUSE bone graft. *Spine Journal* 2007;**7**:44–9.

43. Dimar JR, Glassman SD, Burkus KJ, et al. Clinical outcomes and fusion techniques at 2 years of single-level instrumented posterolateral fusions with recombinant human bone morphogenic protein-2/compression resistant matrix versus iliac crest bone graft. *Spine* 2006;**31**:2534–9.
44. Sponseller PD, Cohen MS, Nachemson AL, et al. Results of surgical treatment of adults with idiopathic scoliosis. *Journal of Bone and Joint Surgery (America)* 1987; **69**:667–75.
45. Dickson JH, Mirkovic S, Noble PC, et al. Results of operative treatment of idiopathic scoliosis in adults. *Journal of Bone and Joint Surgery (America)* 1995;**77**:513–23.
46. Albert TJ, Purtill J, Mesa J, et al. Health outcome assessment before and after adult deformity surgery. *Spine* 1995;**20**:2002–5.
47. Jackson RP, McManus AC. Radiographic analysis of sagittal plane alignment and balance in standing volunteers and patients with low back pain matched for age, sex, and size. A prospective controlled clinical study. *Spine* 1994;**19**:1611–18.
48. Dykes DC, Ogilvie JW. Adult Kyphosis. In: Frymoyer JW, Wiesel SW, eds. *The Adult and Pediatric Spine*, 3rd edn. Philadelphia, PA: Lippincott Williams and Wilkins, 2003:479–90.
49. Berven SH, Deviren V, Smith J. Management of fixed sagittal plane deformity: Outcome of combined anterior and posterior surgery. *Spine* 2003;**28**:1710–16.
50. Fon GT, Pitt MJ, Thies AC Jr. Thoracic kyphosis: range in normal subjects. *AJR American Journal of Roentgenology* 1980;**134**:979–83.
51. Bernhardt M, Bridwell KH. Segmental analysis of the sagittal plane alignment of the normal thoracic and lumbar spines and thoracolumbar junction. *Spine* 1989;**14**:717–21.
52. Gelb DE, Lenke LG, Bridwell KH, et al. An analysis of sagittal spinal alignment in 100 asymptomatic middle and older aged volunteers. *Spine* 1995;**20**:1351–8.
53. Damborg F, Engell V, Andersen M, et al. Prevalence, concordance, and heritability of Scheuermann kyphosis based on a study of twins. *Journal of Bone and Joint Surgery (America)* 2006;**88**:2133–6.
54. Sorensen KH. *Scheuermann's Juvenile Kyphosis: Clinical Appearances, Radiography, Aetiology, and Prognosis*. Copenhagen: Munksgaard, 1964.
55. Lowe TG. Scheuermann Disease. *Journal of Bone and Joint Surgery (America)* 1990;**72**:940–5.
56. Tribus CB. Scheuermann's kyphosis in adolescents and adults: diagnosis and management. *Journal of the American Academy of Orthopedic Surgeons* 1998;**6**:36–43.
57. NIH Consensus Development Panel on Osteoporosis Prevention, Diagnosis, and Therapy. Osteoporosis prevention, diagnosis, and therapy. *Journal of the American Medical Association* 2001;**285**:785–95.
58. Riggs BL, Melton LJ 3rd. The worldwide problem of osteoporosis: insights afforded by epidemiology. *Bone* 1995;**17**(5 Supplement):505S–11S.
59. Korovessis PG, Stamatakis MV, Baikousis AG. Reciprocal angulation of vertebral bodies in the sagittal plane in an asymptomatic Greek population. *Spine* 1998;**23**:700–5.
60. Lindsay R, Silverman SL, Cooper C, et al. Risk of new vertebral fracture in the year following a fracture. *Journal of the American Medical Association* 2001;**285**:320–3.
61. Heaney RP. The natural history of vertebral osteoporosis. Is low bone mass an epiphenomenon? *Bone* 1992;**13**:S23–6.
62. Cooper C, Atkinson EJ, Jacobsen SJ, et al. Population-based study of survival after osteoporotic fractures. *American Journal of Epidemiology* 1993;**137**:1001–5.
63. Manson NA, Phillips FM. Minimally invasive techniques for the treatment of osteoporotic vertebral fractures. *Journal of Bone and Joint Surgery (America)* 2006;**88**:1862–72.
64. Schlaich C, Minne HW, Bruckner T, et al. Reduced pulmonary function in patients with spinal osteoporotic fractures. *Osteoporosis International* 1998;**8**:261–7.
65. Silverman SL. The clinical consequences of vertebral compression fracture. *Bone* 1992;**13**:S27–S31.
66. Melton LJ. Excess mortality following vertebral fracture. *Journal of the American Geriatric Society* 2000;**48**:338–9.
67. Johnell O, Kanis JA, Oden A, et al. Mortality after osteoporotic factures. *Osteoporosis International* 2004;**15**:8–42.
68. Spivak JM, Johnson MG. Percutaneous treatment of vertebral body pathology. *Journal of the American Academy of Orthopedic Surgeons* 2005;**13**:6–17.
69. Lieberman IH, Dudeney S, Reinhardt MK, et al. Initial outcome and efficacy of "kyphoplasty" in the treatment of painful osteoporotic vertebral compression fractures. *Spine* 2001;**26**:1631–8.
70. Prather H, Van Dillen L, Metzler JP, et al. Prospective measurement of function and pain in patients with non-neoplastic compression fractures with vertebroplasty. *Journal of Bone and Joint Surgery (America)* 2006;**88**:334–41.
71. Evan AJ, Jensen ME, Kip KE, et al. Vertebral compression fractures: pain reduction and improvement in functional mobility after percutaneous polymethylmethacrylate vertebroplasty – retrospective report of 245 cases. *Radiology* 2003;**226**:366–72.
72. Dudeny S, Lieberman IH, Reinhardt M, et al. Kyphoplasty in the treatment of osteolytic vertebral compression fractures as a result of multiple myeloma. *Journal of Clinical Oncology* 2002;**20**:2382–7.
73. Hiwatashi A, Moritani T, Numaguchi Y, et al. Increase in vertebral body height after vertebroplasty. *American Journal of Neuroradiology* 2003;**23**:185–9.
74. Birkenmaier C, Seitz S, Wegener B. Acute paraplegia after vertebroplasty caused by epidural hemorrhage: a case report. *Journal of Bone and Joint Surgery (America)* 2007;**89**:1827–31.
75. Harrington KD. Major neurological complications following percutaneous vertebroplasty with polymethylmethacrylate: a case report. *Journal of Bone and Joint Surgery (America)* 2001;**83**:1070–3.

76. Rao RD, Singrakhia MD. Painful osteoporotic vertebral fracture: pathogenesis, evaluation, and roles of vertebroplasty and kyphoplasty in its management. *Journal of Bone and Joint Surgery (America)* 2003;**85**:2010-22.
77. Hanley E, Green NE, Spengler DM. Orthopaedic forum: less invasive procedures in spine surgery. *Journal of Bone and Joint Surgery (America)* 2003;**85**:956-61.
78. Potter BK, Lenke LG, Kuklo TR. Prevention and management of iatrogenic flatback deformity. *Journal of Bone and Joint Surgery (America)* 2004;**86**:1793-808.
79. Sarwahi V, Boachie-Adjei O, Backus SI, Taira G. Characterization of gait function in patients with postsurgical sagittal (flatback) deformity: a prospective study of 21 patients. *Spine* 2002;**27**:2328-37.
80. Farcy JP, Schwab FJ. Management of flatback and related kyphotic decompensation syndromes. *Spine* 1997;**22**:2452-7.
81. Bridwell KH, Lewis SJ, Lenke LG, et al. Pedicle subtraction osteotomy for the treatment of fixed sagittal imbalance. *Journal of Bone and Joint Surgery (America)* 2003;**85**:454-63.

Surgical options in the osteoporotic spine

STEPHAN BECKER

Epidemiology and specific osteoporosis-related vertebral diseases and risks	1024	Minimally invasive treatment options in vertebral fractures	1032
Aetiology	1025	The use of injectable biomaterials in the osteoporotic spine	1039
Patient history	1026	Open surgery	1041
Clinical examination	1027	Postoperative management	1043
Differential diagnosis of osteoporosis	1029	References	1043

EPIDEMIOLOGY AND SPECIFIC OSTEOPOROSIS-RELATED VERTEBRAL DISEASES AND RISKS

The number of people affected by osteoporosis has become more significant worldwide over the last decade, and it is now regarded by the World Health Organization (WHO) as one of the 10 most serious global diseases. The ageing of society will probably present one of the most important changes in society throughout the next decades. In 2050 54% of the population in industrialized nations will be older than 65 years.[1,2]

The prevalence of osteoporosis, i.e. the number of people suffering from osteoporosis at a given time, will probably rise within the EU from 23.7 million in 2000 to 37.3 million in 2050, which means an increase of 57%.[3] Until 2020 men will present the larger fraction of pensioners, but until 2050 the ratio will change in favour of women. Accordingly the proportion of the high-risk population for osteoporosis, i.e. women of a pensionable age, will increase considerably, which explains the above-mentioned prevalence. The analysis of the progression of the prevalence of vertebral fractures within the first 10 years after starting vitamin D and calcium therapy shows a prevalence of 33% after 5 years and 55% after 10 years in women without previous fractures, i.e. half of the women treated without bisphosphonates suffer an osteoporotic fracture within the first 10 years of treatment. Eleven per cent of those women even suffer secondary or further vertebral fractures within the first 5 years and 29% within the first 10 years.[4]

The incidence of fractures as a consequence of osteoporosis increases exponentially with age.[5] The spine is the most common place for osteoporotic fractures.[6] Studies in the USA show indications of vertebral fractures in 25% of women older than 75 years and in more than 50% of women older than 80 years. The area affected most is the mid-thoracic spine and the transition area between the thoracic and lumbar spine.[7–9]

Every year 700 000 Americans and 490 000 EU citizens suffer an osteoporotic vertebral fracture.[1,10] The incidence in women over 50 years was 18 out of 1000 person-years in 1993,[11] and thus at that time already twice as high as the incidence of femoral neck fractures (6.2 of 1000 person-years). Furthermore it has to be taken into consideration that only every third osteoporotic fracture is diagnosed correctly, and only 10% of the diagnosed fractures need hospital treatment.[12] According to another study from the UK only every tenth fracture is diagnosed correctly.[13] Even if a fracture is seen on a radiograph, it is not always identified by the diagnosing radiologist, and thus does not show up in the patient's file.[14] Therefore, osteoporotic fracture as a sure sign of manifest osteoporosis is frequently missed, but unfortunately represents a major obstacle in spine surgery.

The main problem in this ageing population is on the one hand an osteoporotic fracture, on the other hand a degenerative scoliosis. Furthermore, degenerative scoliosis and osteoporotic fractures go hand in hand with scoliotic deformities being present in 36–48% of osteoporotic women. *De novo* scoliosis can rapidly emerge after an osteoporotic fracture and the clinical symptoms can deteriorate significantly. Lastly adult patients with scoliosis have a lower bone mass than the general population.[15,16]

Therefore, surgical strategies in treating osteoporotic spinal pathologies have been developed. They range from minimal-invasive stabilization like vertebroplasty (VP) and kyphoplasty (KP) to open fusion including screws/hooks and wire constructs.

Gender differences

It is without doubt that the danger of acquiring osteoporosis and thus the risk of osteoporotic fractures rises with increasing age. In general, women are regarded as the high-risk group, although exact figures that compare epidemiological data on the spine are missing; available data about men are poor and inconsistent.[17] Although the incidence in men is only 1.9 times lower than in women,[11] the EVOS study shows a higher prevalence of kyphotic deformity in men between 50 and 64 years than in women of the same age.[18] After reaching the age of 65 years, however, women show a higher prevalence of pathological kyphosis.[10] Thus it can be stated nowadays that osteoporosis is not only a problem affecting women.

AETIOLOGY

Natural course of the osteoporotic spine

During ageing, the bone decreases its capacity of remodelling. In a young adult there is a regular linked increase and decrease in the bone matrix that can be triggered with sports and exercise. It is important to know that until the age of 30 years, a dominant osteogenesis occurs and the bone mass reaches its peak. That is, at this crucial age, the individual reaches its life peak bone mass. After that age, there is a continuous loss of bone mass due to an irregular increase and decrease in the bone matrix, e.g. an irregular osteoblastic/osteoclastic activity.[19] This permanent loss of bone is in general a relatively linear bone loss of less than 2% per year. However, menopausal women may experience an accelerated bone loss up to 10% of cortical and 30% of trabecular bone over a period of 4–8 years.[20] This also means that every individual reaches a stage of osteoporosis sooner (e.g. with a primary low peak bone mass) or later in his/her life time.

Every moment, about 1 million basic multicellular units (BMUs) are active in the adult skeleton.[19] These units include the osteoclast-induced absorption of the bone, the osteoblast-formed new matrix and two phases of mineralization of the new matrix.[21] All of those stages may be affected during ageing. Those stages are furthermore controlled by hormones, mechanical stimulation and physical exercise or stress.[22] Therefore, a lack of any of those stimuli results in general or localized osteoporosis even in young adults (e.g. fracture of the wrist immobilized in a cast over 3 months results in local loss of bone). This mechanism is enhanced in patients with osteoporosis, where even relatively short bed rest after a trivial disease may exacerbate the bone loss.

Nowadays, we understand better the cellular mechanisms regulating the turnover of bone. Several known cytokines and regulatory proteins locally affect bone turnover.

Osteoblasts are secreting cells and can be differentiated from mature osteocytes by several members of the bone morphogenetic protein (BMP) family, which belongs to the transforming growth factor (TGF)-β superfamily. BMP-2, BMP-6, BMP-7 and TGF-β, insulin-like growth factor (IGF)-I, IGF-II and b-fibroblast growth factor (FGF), osteoblast specific factor (OSF)-1 and human osteosarcoma cell line SAOS-2 have been shown to have an osteogenetic effect on osteoblasts.[23] Currently, recombinant BMP-2 (Infuse, Medtronic, Minneapolis, MO) and BMP-7 (OP-1, Depuy, Warsaw, IA) are in topical clinical use for osteogenesis for spinal fusion.

Osteoclast activity is regulated by calcitonin, vitamin D3 and regulatory molecules produced by osteoblasts and stromal cells. Osteoblasts produce macrophage colony-stimulating factor (M-CSF), which leads to the expression of a specific receptor on the osteoclast progenitor cells, the receptor for activation of nuclear factor kappa B (RANK). This receptor allows osteoblasts and stromal cells to activate differentiation of precursor cells into mature osteoclasts by the RANK ligand (RANK-L). Furthermore, osteoclasts can deactivate this ligand, like a trigger, by secreting osteoprotegerin. Therefore, osteoblasts themselves secrete powerful proteins to modulate the osteoclastogenic process. This mechanism is currently used in clinical trials with a newly developed monoclonal antibody (Denosumab, AMG 162) which imitates the osteoprotegerin function by inhibiting RANK-L and therefore stops osteoclast differentiation.[23]

Histopathological changes in osteoporotic bone

Fractures can be considered as biomechanical failure of the bone; therefore, it is important to look at histological changes of bone architecture for fracture prediction.

Osteoporotic bone differs from healthy bone not only regarding decreased bone mineral density, but also in different bone architecture, tissue properties and a pathological accumulation of microscopic damage, e.g. microfractures.

Histological/micro-CT investigations assess the following parameters:

- bone volume/tissue volume (BV/TV): proportion or percentage of the volume of interest that is bone
- connectivity density (conn den): the number of connections normalized by the volume of interest
- structural model index (SMI): quantification of the prevalent type of trabecular elements
- Tb.N, Tb.Th, Tb.Sp (trabecular number, trabecular thickness and trabecular spacing)
- degree of anisotropy (DA): measure of preferential alignment of the trabeculae along a direction axis.

It has been shown in the spine that the BV/TV ratio not only decreases with age, but varies depending on the vertebral level.[24] The BV/TV was 5% lower over the whole spine if the individual was over 45 years of age than in those below the age of 45 years. Furthermore, the thoracic and lumbar spine showed 5% less bone than the cervical spine, independent of age. The BV/TV ratio was higher the more proximal the cervical level was, C1 having the highest BV/TV ratio of all vertebrae. Finally bone loss in L5 was found to be three times higher over the whole life span than loss in C4.

The parameters above change accordingly in osteoporosis:

- BV/TV decreases, which causes increased trabecular stress
- conn den decreases with a susceptibility to buckling of trabeculae
- SMI increases with more rod like elements and increased likelihood of bending and buckling
- Tb.N decreases, Tb.Th may increase or decrease and Tb.Sp increases
- DA decreases with a more isotropic trabecular orientation and a susceptibility to off axis loading.[24]

Therefore, in osteoporosis several crucial components of bone structure are weakened, which causes spontaneous failure of bone structure.

Furthermore, a study has shown that different vertebral levels are affected differently by osteoporosis, and there are also marked differences within the vertebra itself.[25] The posterior regions of the vertebrae have increased bone volume, more connections, reduced trabecular spacing and more plate-like isotropic structures, and are therefore more stable than the anterior regions of the vertebrae. In addition, the maximum failure load of the superior endplate varies from the inferior endplate, that is the superior endplate reaches only two-thirds of the stability of the inferior endplate.[26] This explains the pathological finding of osteoporotic vertebral fractures, which occur most often on the superior endplate and the anterior half of the vertebral body. Biomechanically this results in a pathological kyphosis that changes the alignment of the spine significantly and puts a much higher stress on adjacent structures, resulting in subsequent fractures rather than vertebra plana-like fractures.

The histological thickness of the superior endplate and the inferior endplate is different from the failure load, e.g. the superior endplate is thicker in four out of five segments (length of vertebra divided by five) than the inferior endplate, which makes it unnecessary to analyse the thickness of the endplate to predict vertebral failure.

It can be demonstrated[25,26] that the strength of a vertebra can be histologically best described by the BV/TV ratio, which is even more significant than BMD measurements. In order to predict vertebral failure, the most sensible part to analyse is the region next to the fracture site or the superior vertebral region.

Overall a histopathological assessment of a vertebra gives a much better idea about biomechanical failure, fracture prediction and osteoporosis than both BMD and osteoporotic serum/urine markers (see below).

Surgically it is important to analyse the specific anatomy of an osteoporotic spine. As mentioned above, differences regarding the level of the vertebra or differences within the vertebra exist. However, transpedicular screws in posterior fusion gain 80% caudocephalad stiffness and 60% pullout strength in the pedicle of a healthy spine. This can be enhanced by 20% if the screw is anchored 50% into the vertebral body and an additional 20% if it is anchored into the anterior cortex.[27,28] Therefore it makes sense to analyse not only the vertebral body but the pedicle in relation to osteoporosis. The trabecular portion, the strength of the subcortical portion and cortical parts of a pedicle vary in every spine, with the cortical bone being five times stronger than the trabecular bone.[27] In osteoporosis, this strength is reduced throughout the whole pedicle by 50%, which explains the high screw failure if the screw is only anchored within the pedicle[27] (for tips and tricks to enhance screw strength in the osteoporotic spine see below).

PATIENT HISTORY

The history of a spontaneous osteoporotic vertebral fracture is typical: it occurs without any particular event which the patient can remember. The patient very often just describes a sudden onset of localized pain; this can start on any movement/exertion. As we are dealing particularly with elderly patients who are used to sudden pain around or originating from the spine, patients may not think this pain is significantly different from other symptoms and therefore delay visiting a doctor. Overall, the lack of specific history leads to misdiagnosis by physicians (see above). Nevertheless, lack of early diagnosis may lead to kyphotic deformity or severe vertebral collapse. Therefore any patient presenting him/herself with sudden onset of vertebral pain and a history or suspicion of osteoporosis should be investigated thoroughly. However, 20% of fractures are incidental radiological findings, without the patient consciously experiencing pain.[12] In contrast, patients with advanced collapse of a vertebral body and a resulting deformity have a higher level of pain and thus are diagnosed sooner and treated earlier than patients with simpler fractures.[29]

The history reveals in general two types of patients. The first group show a distinctive vertebral collapse with immediate persisting pain that improves gradually in the following weeks and months with conservative therapy. The second group of patients presents only light fractures accompanied by mild, but lasting pain. However, either due to lack of follow-up or proper treatment this group is characterized by progressive collapse of one or several vertebrae[30] and by progressive loss of physiological posture.[31] A subgroup of this group includes patients with old, neglected osteoporotic vertebrae and a sudden onset of new fractures, which the patients describe as sudden worsening of the old persistent pain. This patient group may lead to misdiagnosis if they are only investigated with radiographs.

CLINICAL EXAMINATION

The clinically typical and persistent sign of an acute vertebral fracture is localized tenderness over the fracture site. Typically, no radicular pain is present; if this is the case, a more complex pathology (pathological fracture, burst fracture) has to be taken into consideration. The main point of tenderness may not always be the site of origin in thoraco-lumbar fractures, which may cause radiating pain over the lumbosacral ligaments and muscle groups towards the lumbosacral junction.[32] This group may be misdiagnosed, especially if they have some degenerative changes of the lumbosacral junction. Therefore, the thoracolumbar fracture should be always treated first and then treatment of the persisting pathology should be considered. However, it is possible in some patients that the fracture and misalignment may cause increased pain of the lumbosacral junction which will not be restored to the level prior to the fracture even after treatment; the patient is now much more aware of his/her secondary (lumbosacral) pathology and may also need surgical treatment of this pathology.

Pain persisting for more than 6 months should always be investigated for pseudarthrosis or osteonecrosis, which *per se* will not heal without surgical treatment (see below).

The clinical examination is completed in every case with a thorough neurological examination, although neurological deficit due to spontaneous osteoporotic fracture is extremely rare.

Additional investigations: markers of bone formation

Bone remodelling can be biochemically controlled by markers of the osteoblastic and osteoclastic pathway (Box 90.1). Those makers are widely used to monitor drug effectiveness in large studies.[19,33] However, it has not yet been proven that an increase in these markers towards normal levels has a positive impact on vertebral fractures.[34,35] The NIH consensus conference concluded in 2000 and 2003 that 'according to available data, marker levels do not predict bone mass or fracture risk and are only weakly associated with change in bone mass. Therefore, they are of limited utility in the clinical evaluation of individual patients.'[36] However, they may identify changes in bone remodelling within a relatively short time interval before changes in bone mineral density can be detected. These tests vary in sensitivity and specificity and overall cannot replace bone mineral density analysis. Densitometry measures the current bone status and the markers of the ongoing process of bone turnover. The current bone status is much more relevant in planning surgical treatment. Therefore, biochemical analysis plays only a minor role in management of osteoporotic fractures.

> **BOX 90.1: Biochemical markers of bone turnover**
>
> Osteoblast pathway (formation markers): serum alkaline phosphatase, serum osteocalcin (bone Gla-protein), serum procollagen I carboxy (PICP), serum N-terminal (PINP) extension peptides, bone sialoprotein
> Osteoclast pathway (resorption markers): urine hydroxyproline, urine pyridinium cross-links (total and free pyridinoline, total and free deoxypyridinoline), urine type I collagen telopeptide cross-links (C-telopeptide (CTX) and N-telopeptide (NTX)), serum tartrate-resistant acid phosphatase, serum carboxyterminal telopeptide of type I collagen (ITCP)

Additional upcoming analysis of bone turnover include measurements of homocystein, vitamins B6 and B12, and folate levels. It has been demonstrated in studies[37,38] that homocystein affects bone metabolism and can be used as a risk indicator for osteoporosis. However, more clinical studies are needed to clarify exactly the role of homocystein, vitamins B6 and B12, and folate in bone turnover.[38–40]

RADIOLOGICAL EVALUATION

Clinically it is important to diagnose a new osteoporotic vertebral fracture and to differentiate it from an old (healed) fracture. Plain standing up and lateral radiographs may document an acute fracture if we have older radiographs to compare, but it is often impossible to demonstrate the fracture age by radiographs alone.

However, for operative planning (multisegmental stabilization, etc.) normal radiographs remain important.

In order to evaluate the fracture age, it is necessary to perform MRI of the spine. MRI will show a decreased signal on T_1 and increased signal on T_2 in the case of a new fracture. A new fracture causes bleeding into the vertebra which can be easily picked up on MRI. If an older fracture is suspected, it is important to perform a suppressed T_2 technique (short tau inverted recovery (STIR)) that clearly shows an increased signal until the fracture is healed, which may take up to 12 months in the case of an osteoporotic fracture (Fig. 90.1).

Thus, the STIR image not only establishes the diagnosis of the osteoporotic fracture but it gives a good clinical picture about fracture healing. Injury of the posterior wall causing spinal stenosis is easily picked up on MRI, which is important in order to plan surgery. Furthermore, MRI is useful in difficult cases, such as young individuals with osteoporosis and traumatic accident, in order to exclude unstable fractures, e.g. injury of the posterior ligaments/bony structures.

Using these two methods, most spontaneous osteoporotic fractures can be diagnosed; however, in the case of a fall, or a traumatic fracture in older osteopathic patients, it is sometimes necessary to perform a CT scan.

The CT scan should reveal any split fractures (type A2 after Arbeitsgemeinschaft für Osteosynthesefragen AO[41] – Fig. 90.2.) or burst fractures (A3.3 after AO), which are a general contraindication to performing a stand-alone BKP or vertebroplasty (see next page). In general, CT has a lower sensitivity than MRI[42] and may in some cases confirm the diagnosis only in combination with bone scintigraphy. The latter, however, has a diagnostic window: the scintigraphy can be falsely negative in the acute phase following the fracture, and an already healed fracture can still show as a positive scan years after the event. The sensitivity of bone scintigraphy is also considerably lower than MRI.[43,44] Positron emission tomography examination is

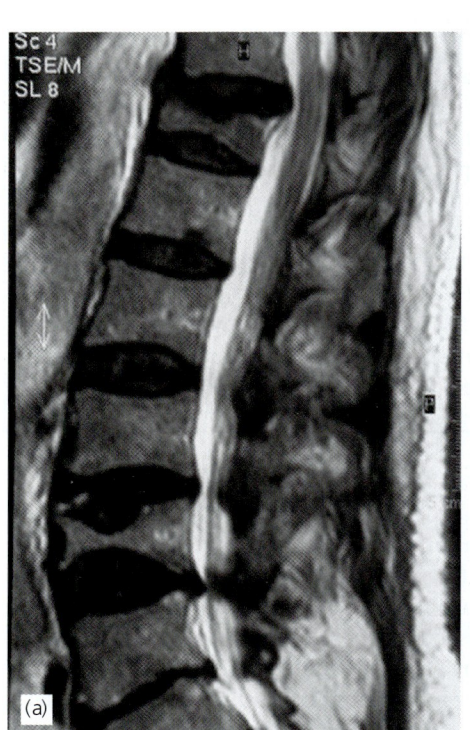

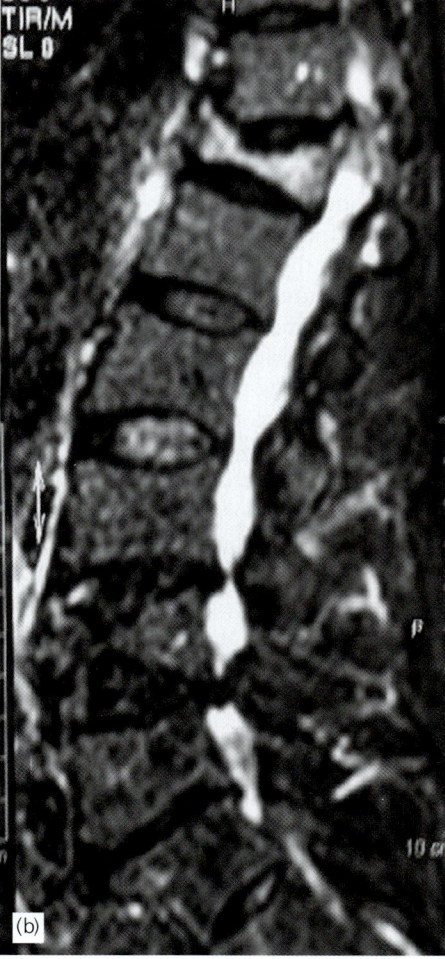

Figure 90.1 Female, 75 years with multiple fractures Th12 and L4 on MRI. (a) T_2 image without clear fracture signs. (b) Short tau inverted recovery image shows a hyperintense zone in Th12 as sign of a painful fracture.

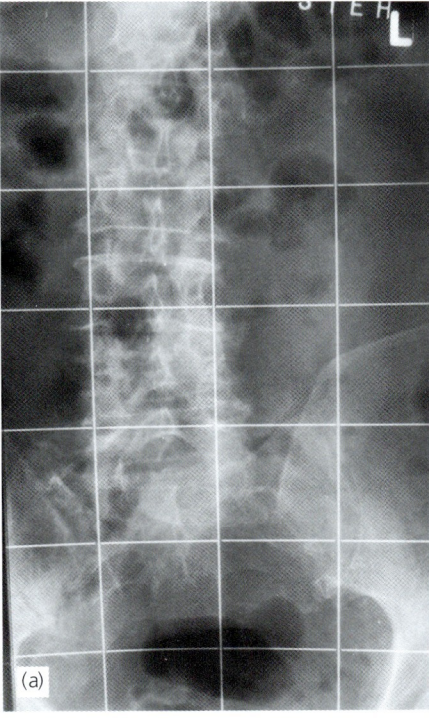
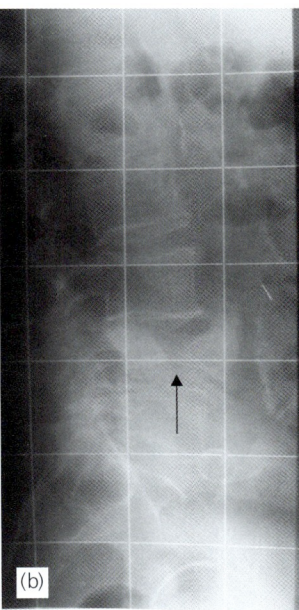

Figure 90.2 (a) Anteroposterior, (b) lateral image. Male 80 years, split fracture (type A2.3) L4, split clearly visible on radiograph (arrow) of lateral image.

not routinely applied in the diagnosis of osteoporotic vertebral fractures, but can also confirm diagnosis in specific cases.[45]

DIFFERENTIAL DIAGNOSIS OF OSTEOPOROSIS

We have to separate two main differential diagnosis groups: first the cause of the osteoporosis, and, second, different factors leading to an osteoporotic vertebral fracture.

The different conditions leading to secondary osteoporosis are manifold and are summarized in Table 90.1.

Besides those underlying conditions, the medications shown in Box 90.2 cause osteoporosis.

Glucocorticoids have by far the most potent impact on bone formation[46] and specifically affect the trabecular bone. The most rapid bone loss unfortunately occurs within the early stage of cortisone treatment and even a small dose (equivalent to 2.5–7.5 mg of prednisolone per day) is associated with an increased fracture risk.[13] Clinically cortisone-induced osteoporosis leads to multiple vertebral fractures, with a recurrent fracture risk in 50% of the cases, even after cementoplasty,[47] which leads to prophylactic multisegmental treatment in those patients.

It is obvious that any spontaneous event leading to a fracture is suspicious of underlying disease, e.g. metastatic lesions or osteonecrosis. Investigations such as MRI or CT and histology should reveal the diagnosis in most of the cases.

The treatment of benign and malign changes of the spine is dealt with in Chapter 69; the differential diagnosis of a spontaneous fracture outside those pathologies is vertebral osteonecrosis.

Osteonecrosis of the spine (Kümmel–Verneuil disease)

This pathology typically afflicts the osteoporotic spine. It has been named osteonecrosis, vascular necrosis, pseudarthrosis and Kümmel's spondylitis;[48–56] all these descriptions are simply different names for the same disease, a real vertebral osteonecrosis bearing the typical histological changes and is today mainly named after the first description in 1895, i.e. Kümmel–Verneuil disease.

The causes of this disease are manifold. In trauma, it has been postulated that a disruption of anterior perforating vessels results in pseudarthrosis, which is supported by the fact that these cases often show osteonecrosis of the anterior part of the vertebral body. Furthermore, malignancy, infection, radiation therapy, liver cirrhosis, alcoholism, steroid treatments, sarcoidosis haemoglobinopathies, such as sickle cell anaemia, Cushing syndrome, Gaucher syndrome and dysbarism after diving accidents can lead to osteonecrosis.[48,51,53,57–62] Nevertheless, osteoporosis is by far the main risk factor for developing osteonecrosis. This pathology shows typical changes on radiographs and MRI (Fig. 90.3). On radiographs or CT we typically find an intravertebral cleft, also described as the 'gas sign',

Table 90.1 Diseases that cause or contribute to secondary osteoporosis (after the US Department of Health and Human Services 2004)

Genetic disorders

Cystic fibrosis	Homocystinuria	Osteogenesis imperfecta
Ehlers–Danlos	Hypophosphatasia	Porphyria
Glycogen storage diseases	Idiopathic hypercalciuria	Riley–Day syndrome
Gaucher's disease	Marfan syndrome	
Haemochromatosis	Menkes steely hair syndrome	

Hypogonadal states

Androgen insensitivity	Hyperprolactinaemia	Turner and Klinefelter syndromes
Anorexia nervosa	Panhypopituitarism	
Athletic amenorrhoea	Premature ovarian failure	

Endocrine disorders

Acromegaly	Cushing syndrome	Hyperparathyroidism
Adrenal insufficiency	Diabetes mellitus (type I)	Thyrotoxicosis

Gastrointestinal diseases

Gastrectomy	Malabsorption	Primary biliary cirrhosis
Inflammatory bowel disease	Coeliac disease	

Haematological disorders

Haemophilia	Multiple myeloma	Systemic mastocytosis
Leukaemias and lymphomas	Sickle cell disease	Thalassaemia

Rheumatic and autoimmune diseases

Ankylosing spondylitis	Lupus	Rheumatoid arthritis

Miscellaneous

Alcoholism	Emphysema	Multiple sclerosis
Amyloidosis	End-stage renal disease	Muscular dystrophy
Chronic metabolic acidosis	Epilepsy	Post-transplant bone
Congestive heart failure	Idiopathic scoliosis	Disease
Depression	Immobilization	Sarcoidosis

BOX 90.2: Medication associated with secondary osteoporosis (after the US Department of Health and Human Services 2004)

Anticoagulants (heparin)
Anticonvulsants
Cyclosporine A and tacrolimus
Cancer chemotherapeutic drugs
Glucocorticoids (and ACTH)
Gonadotropin-releasing hormone agonists
Lithium
Methotrexate
Parenteral nutrition
Thyroxine

demonstrating fluid and gas in the intravertebral body.[63,64,65] On MRI we find fluid or gas in the vertebral body; this can be seen as a dark zone on T_1 and bright on T_2/STIR[49,53,64,65] (Fig. 90.4).

The clinically most dominant feature is the fact that this disease does not end in proper bone healing, but in instability of the vertebra on extension and flexion. The patient typically describes pain during sitting and walking with pain subsidence when lying.

This disease may be missed if only standing radiographs are performed; therefore a prone radiograph is indicated if there is any doubt, which will help in the diagnosis and treatment (Fig. 90.5, page 1035).

As in pseudarthrosis, severe collapse and kyphotic deformities are frequent and early surgical treatment with either KP or VP is indicated (Figs 90.3 and 90.4).

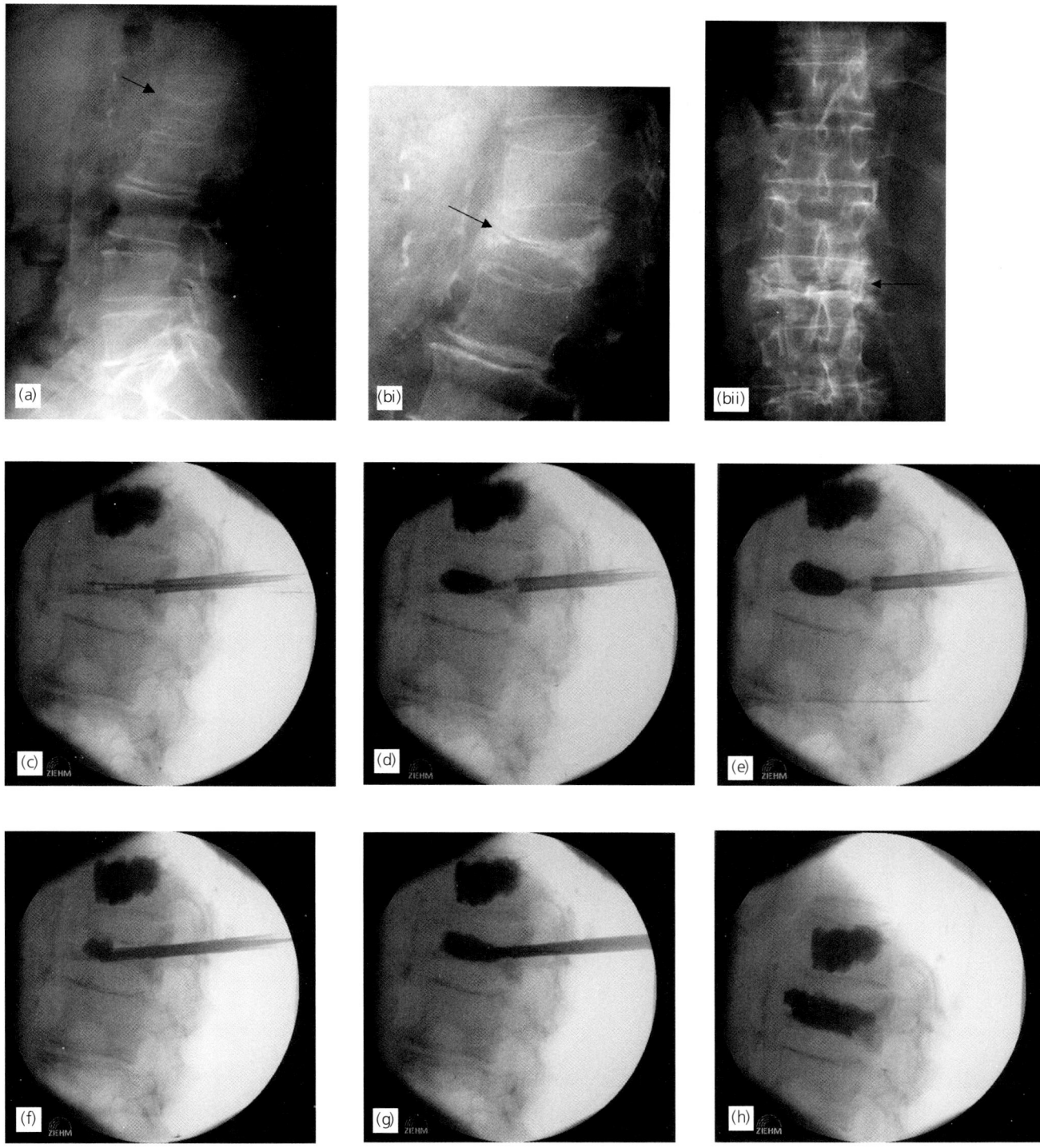

Figure 90.3 Female, 72 years, spontaneous fracture L1 (a), conservative treatment. Four months later, total collapse of L1 with osteonecrosis (b), balloon catheter in place (c) with enlarging of balloon (d, e), sequential filling (f, g) and result after balloon kyphoplasty (h). Note restoration of kyphotic deformity.

Osteonecrosis often involves the anterior wall, which leads to complete resorption of this part of the vertebral body with the risk of severe cement dislocation occurring (Fig. 90.6); therefore, stand-alone cementoplasties should be carefully considered, and very often a cement-augmented fusion is necessary to secure the cementoplasty. Kyphoplasty (KP) shows that cement dislocation and bone resorption also occurs, therefore new bone-preserving KP techniques are indicated (Fig. 90.7, page 11). This potential risk also exists in metastatic lesions with involvement of the anterior wall.

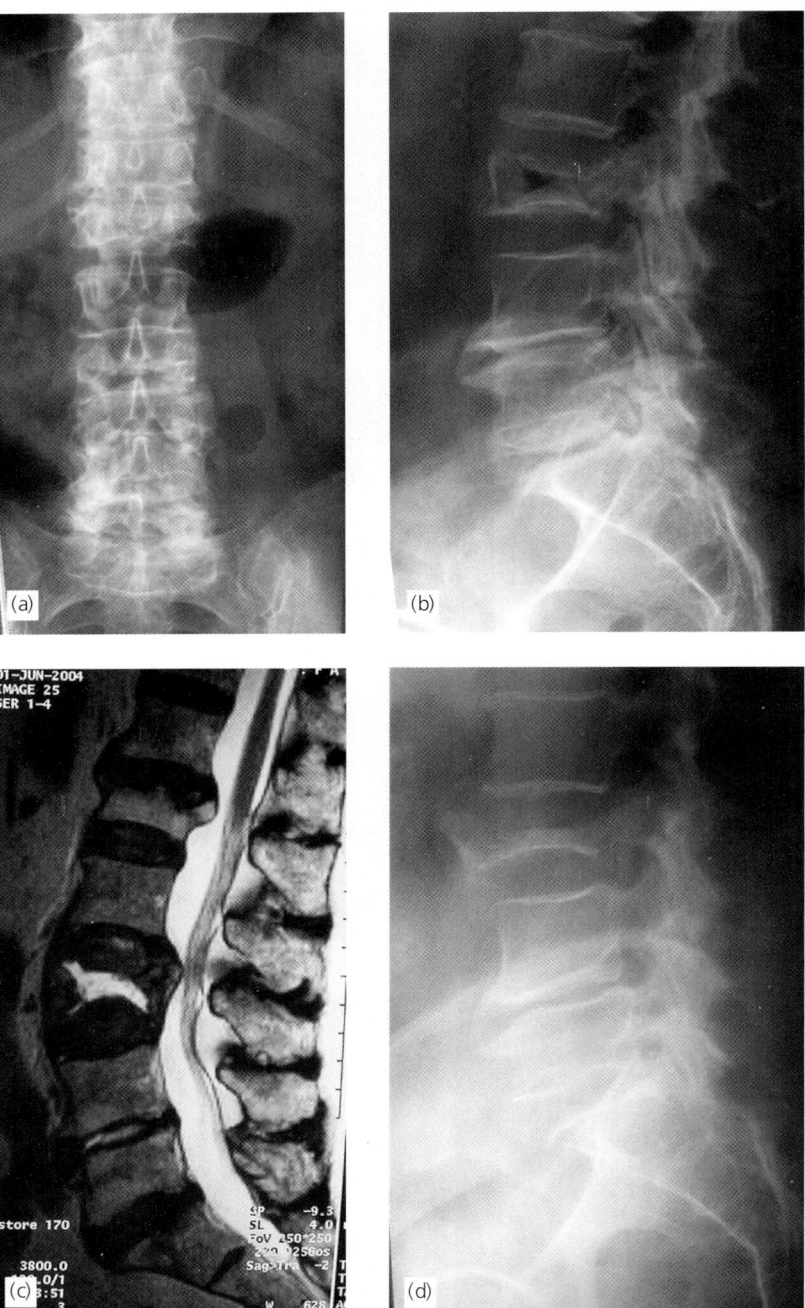

Figure 90.4 Female, 85 years, spontaneous fracture L3 with osteonecrosis, clearly visible on anteroposterior and lateral radiographs (a, b). MRI shows fluid within the vertebral body (c). Five months later after conservative treatment severe segmental collapse with chronic pain and immobility (d).

MINIMALLY INVASIVE TREATMENT OPTIONS IN VERTEBRAL FRACTURES

The general trend in spine surgery in recent years has clearly focused on minimally invasive techniques, leaving muscle, ligaments and joints intact. Several techniques have furthermore been developed to avoid fusion. A traumatic fracture of the vertebra with intact disc and intact posterior elements does not necessarily warrant fusion in order to achieve a pain-free situation. No other minimally invasive techniques in the spine realize those trends more than cementoplasties (VP and KP), especially in patients where other surgical treatment options are limited.

Vertebroplasty

One of the minimally invasive options to treat osteoporotic vertebral fractures is transpedicular injection of an artificial bone substitute (most often polymethylmethacrylate – PMMA, see below) into a vertebra, the VP (Fig. 90.8).

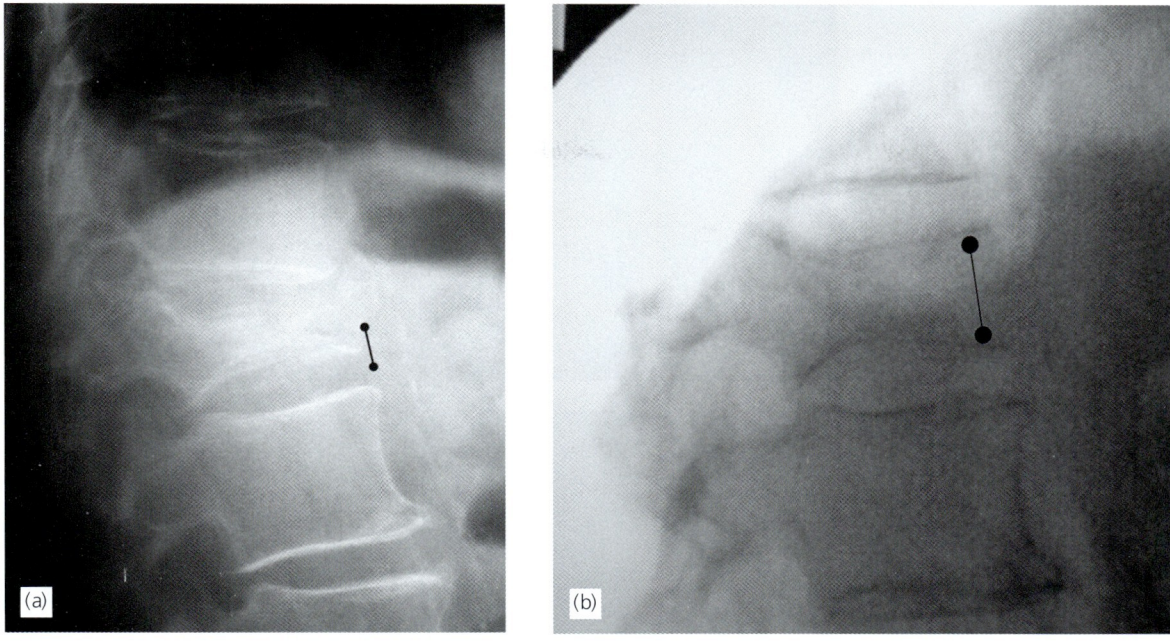

Figure 90.5 Male, 84 years, typical osteonecrotic instability L1. Although osteonecrosis is not clearly seen on radiographs (a), a total reduction of fracture occurs 4 weeks after onset of pain in prone position on OR table (b).

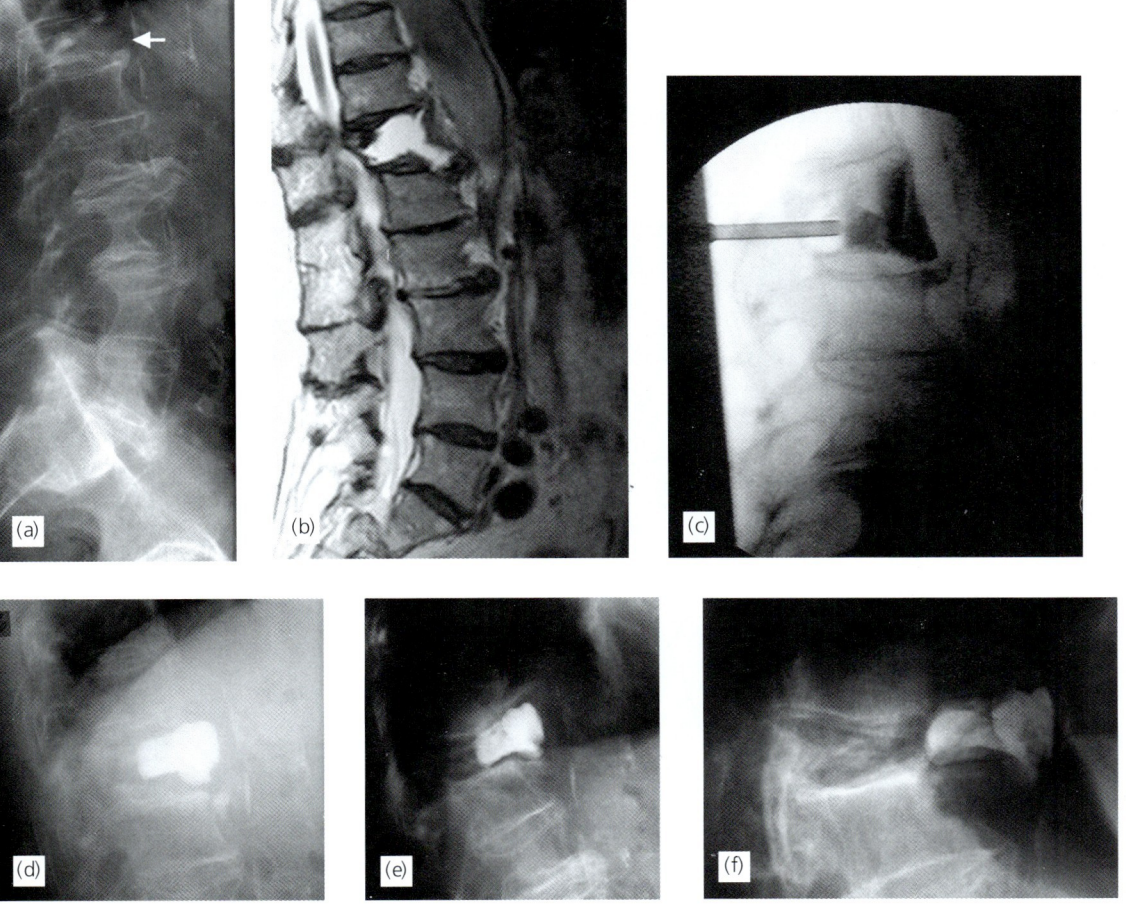

Figure 90.6 Female, 85 years, no tumour known, destruction of anterior wall of Th12 (a) and fluid in vertebra on MRI as in osteonecrosis (b). Vertebroplasty (c) and subsequent cement dislocation after 3 weeks (d), 9 and 24 months (e, f).

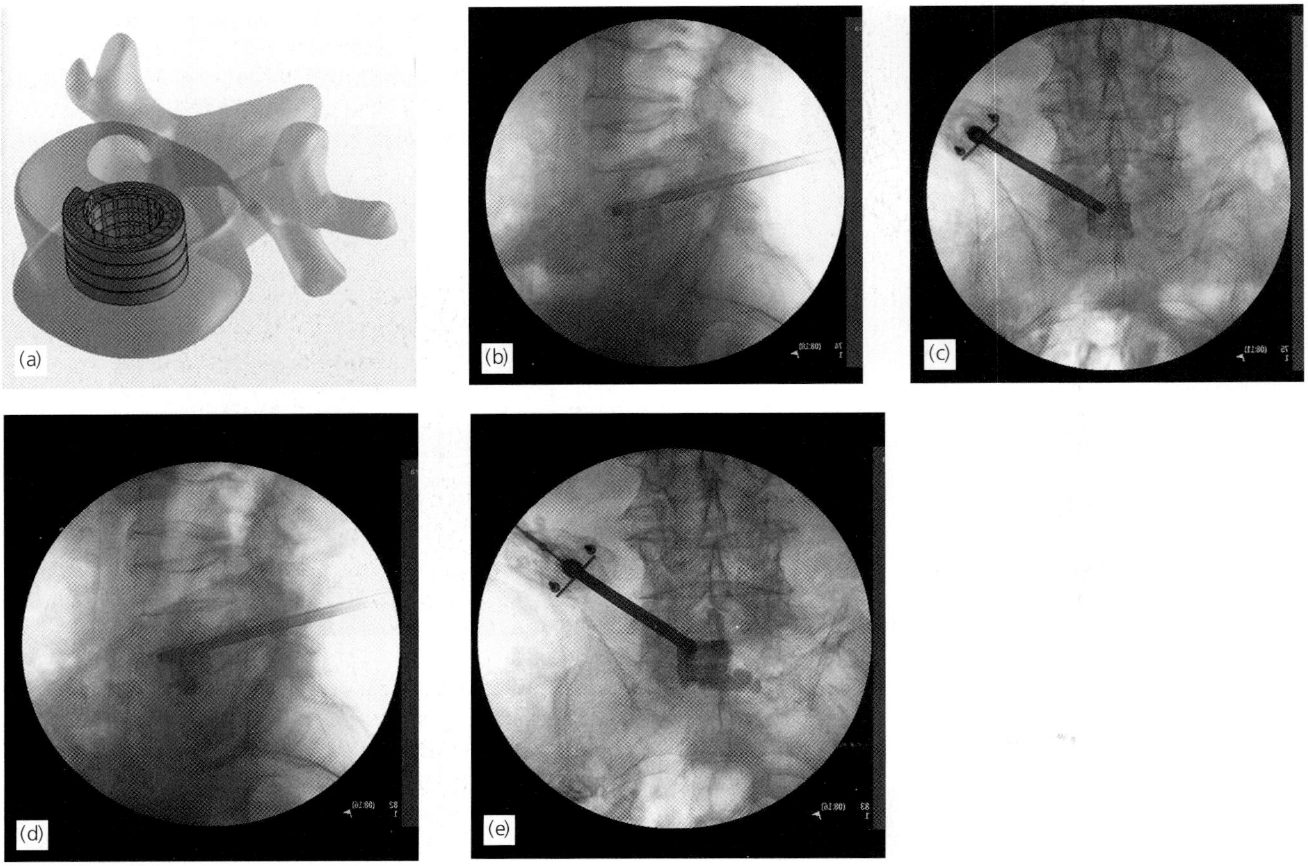

Figure 90.7 Bone-preserving kyphoplasty (KIVA, Benvenue Medical, Santa Clara, CA), schema of PEEK implant (a), intra-operative view of KIVA L5 without polymethylmethacrylate (PMMA) (b, c) and with 1.5 mL of PMMA cement (d, e).

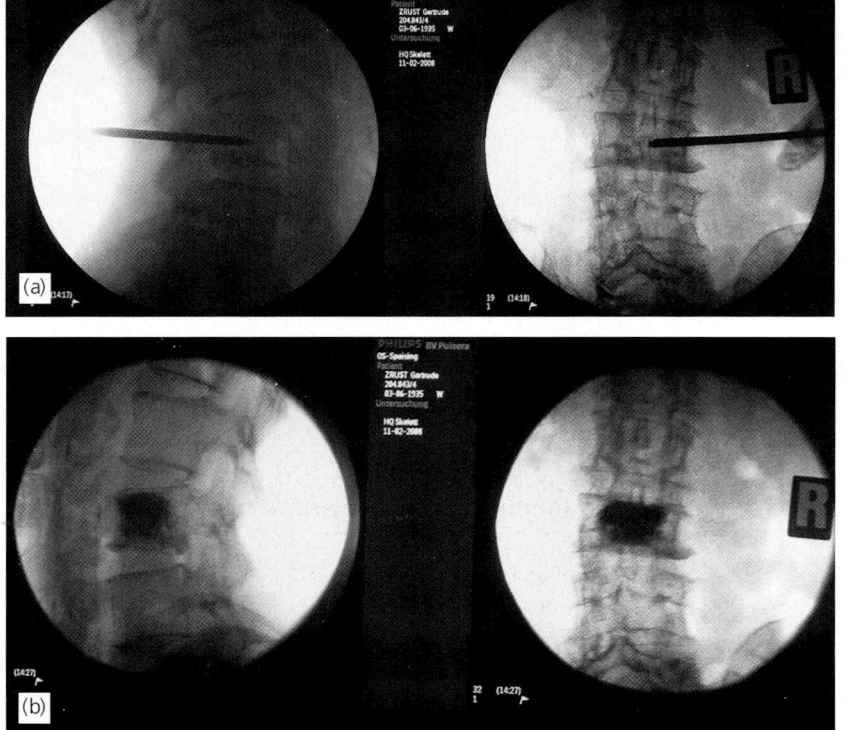

Figure 90.8 Unipedicular vertebroplasty of L3, note median position of injection needle (a) to allow median placement of cement (b). The cement reaches both endplates to provide good stabilization.

This technique was developed by Dr Galibert and Dr Deramond in France in 1984, primarily for the treatment of vertebral haemangioma.[66] It was only in the middle of the 1990s that it was used for treatment of metastases and increasingly for osteoporotic fractures of the spine.[67–69]

The goal of this method is the stabilization of macro- and microfractures, resulting in immediate pain reduction and allowing immediate full mobilization without a brace. Full weight bearing is possible after complete curing of the PMMA cement, which, depending on the product, is possible between 10 and 15 minutes after injection. In addition, it has the advantages of being applicable under local anaesthesia and the possibility to treat multiple levels. Long-term studies show a good cement tolerance without any dislocation (for specific advantages and disadvantages of injectable bone cements see below) as well as a persisting good vertebral stability. VP is generally used for treating fractured vertebra and for prophylactic treatment of vertebral fractures at risk (e.g. of the thoracolumbar junction).

In general, the AO classification[41] represents an efficient tool to assess spontaneous osteoporotic fractures. Indications for VP are all osteoporotic fractures with intact disc and fracture types A1 (all forms) and A3.1, according to the AO classification. Split fractures (type A2 fractures) are rare without trauma and are generally contraindicated as the cement may cause further dislocation of the fragments; furthermore, the cement tends to lie directly in the split, thus hindering bony remodelling (Fig. 90.9). In general, VP is indicated as long as an oedema is visible on MRI; once that sure sign of fracture has disappeared, the patient needs to be reassessed as the pain does not necessarily originate from the body itself but may have other causes, such as facet joints, ligaments, etc., which are clear contraindications to VP. Further indications include osteonecrotic fractures, cement augmentation for screw fixation (see below under open surgery) and tumours (see Chapter 92). For treatment schemes including conservative options see below.

Further contraindications for VP include infection, coagulation disorder, neurological deficit (if VP is performed as a stand-alone solution, see below) and inadequate visualization of the vertebra during surgery. Owing to osteoporosis, the vertebra itself may not be visible under an image intensifier; therefore, all additional aspects that can influence visualization (such as the quality of the image intensifier, etc.) need to be addressed. On this aspect, it is also important to get rid of bowel gas by administration of a laxative the day before surgery. Finally, possible PMMA allergies have to be considered.

TIPS AND TRICKS

VP can be performed transpedicularly (most often used) or extrapedicularly (in special cases on the lumbar spine or more often on the thoracic spine) under local anaesthesia.

It is recommended that the procedure is performed under slight sedoanalgesia. Regarding local infiltration, it is mandatory to anaesthetize the skin and the entry point into the pedicle, e.g. the facet joint. As VP is mainly carried out as a unilateral procedure, one-sided infiltration is enough. The insertion of the access needle into the vertebral body and the cement injection are usually not painful. It is recommended to limit VP under local anaesthesia to two to three levels for patients comfort.

Although the amount of cement needed for stabilization is still under debate, biomechanically it is important that the cement reaches the endplate, if possible both endplates, to avoid future fractures within the same vertebra. Furthermore, it is important in unilateral cases to use a filling which crosses the midline of the vertebra in order to avoid contralateral fractures. If this filling cannot be achieved, a bilateral approach may be considered. In multisegmental filling, it is advisable to alternate entry points in order to allow good handling of the injection needles (Fig. 90.10). A maximum of six vertebrae and a maximum of 25–30 ml of PMMA cement should not be exceeded in one session.[70,71]

In general, the risks of VP are not related to the approach, but to the cement. Resorbable and not resorbable cements may be used (see below). However it is important to use only cements that are designed for spinal applications. These cements are in general highly viscous and it has been demonstrated that the higher the cement viscosity the lower the complications, e.g. risk of leakage.[72]

The most common complication of VP, however, remains cement leakage; this can occur on any site, but posterior leakage is significant for neurological symptoms and anterior leakage for pulmonary emboli.

Leakage may occur in up to 70%,[73] but serious complications including pulmonary emboli or neurological deficit are rare and amount to 3%, mainly occurring during difficult cases such as tumours or severe destruction/ collapse of the vertebra.[74] However, these have to be considered and addressed when the patient gives consent. Recent developments focus on improving the cements, which now reach very fast high viscosity with long application times and new injection devices with lateral openings and remote controlled or tube controlled injection to limit radiation exposure of the hands.

The main disadvantage of VP has been described as a limited ability to reconstruct a kyphotic deformity, which can only be treated with VP in osteonecrosis or very early after the fracture by closed reduction on the operating table.

Clinical results and complication rates will be discussed together with BKP (see below).

Balloon kyphoplasty

Safety and kyphotic issues in VP led to the development of BKP in 1998.[75]

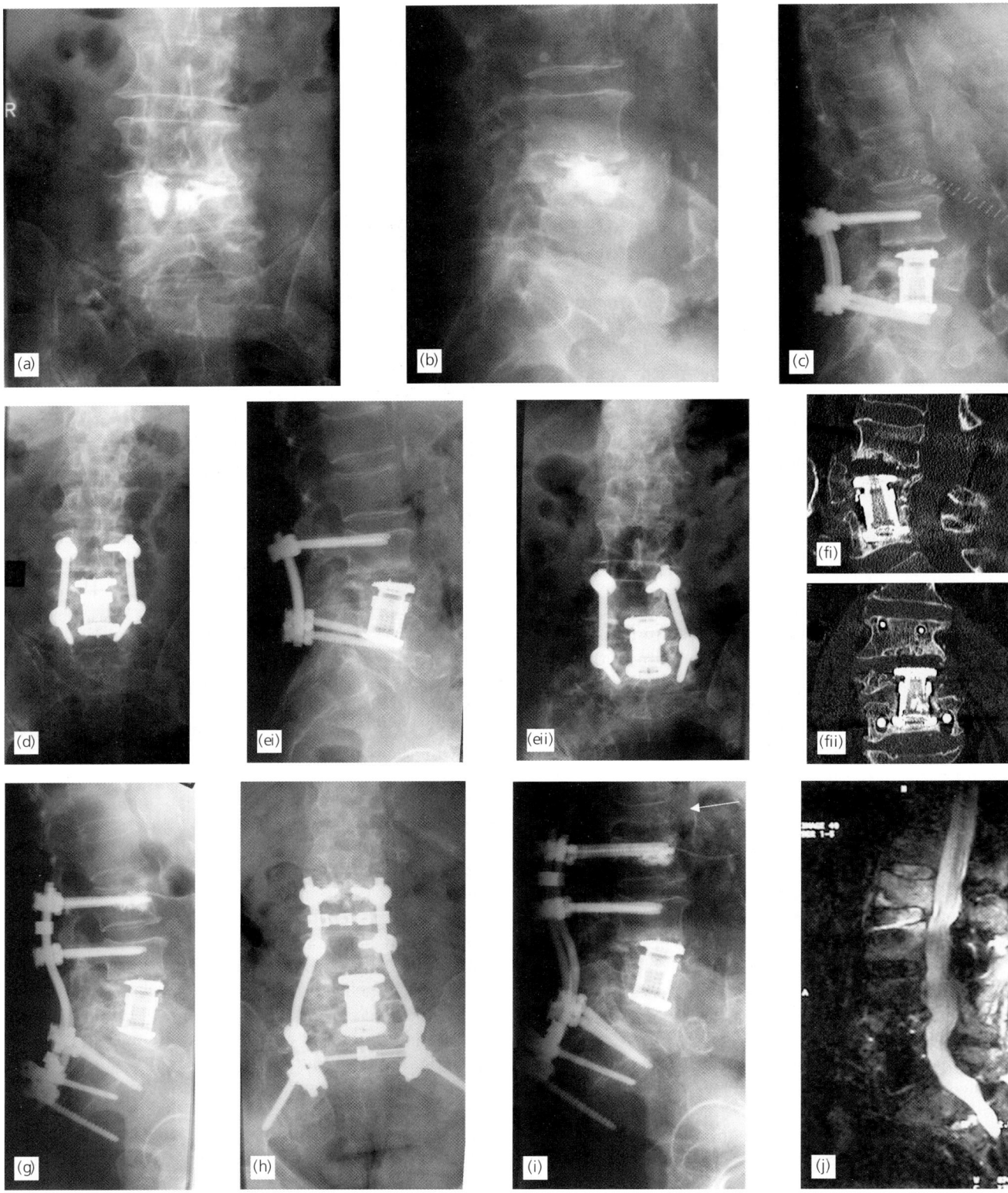

Figure 90.9 Same patient as Figure 90.2, 3 weeks after balloon kyphoplasty (a, b) with resorption and dislocation of the fracture segments. (c, d) One week after ventrodorsal stabilization with expandable cage (Synex, Synthes, Solothurn, Switzerland) and dorsal instrumentation L3–L5. Note cage subsidence. (e, f) Twenty-four months after ventrodorsal fusion; in the meantime the patient had a laminectomy L4 after increasing neurological symptoms and revision after local haematoma. Further subsidence of the cage into the osteoporotic bone, screw loosening and further dislocation of bony fragments. (g, h) Revision with dorsal fusion of L2–S1 and iliac screws. Cement augmentation of screws L2. (j) Three months after revision with adjacent fracture L1, confirmed by MRI (k).

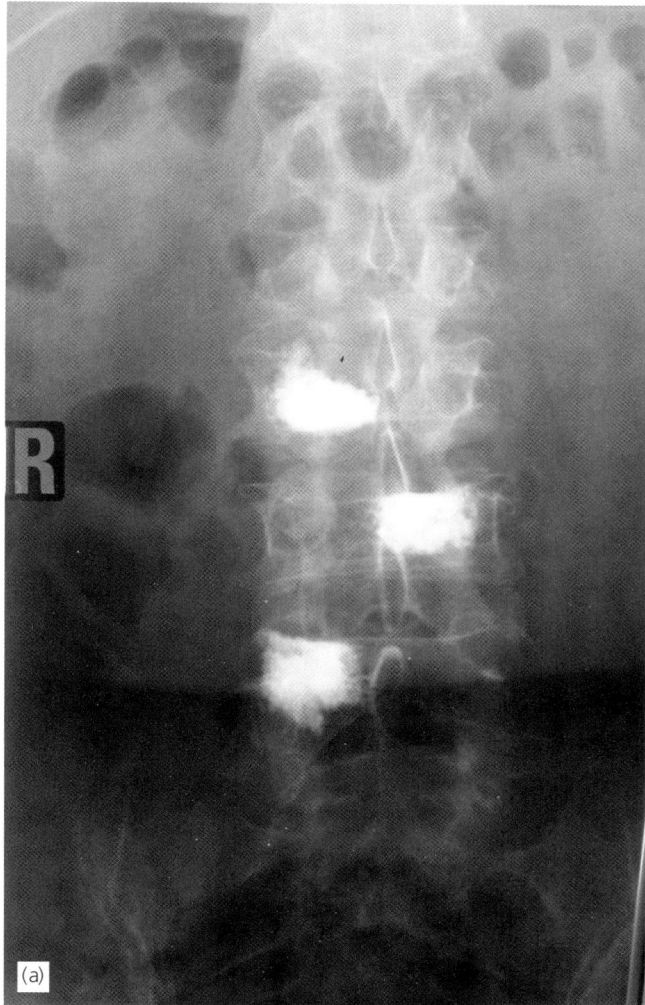 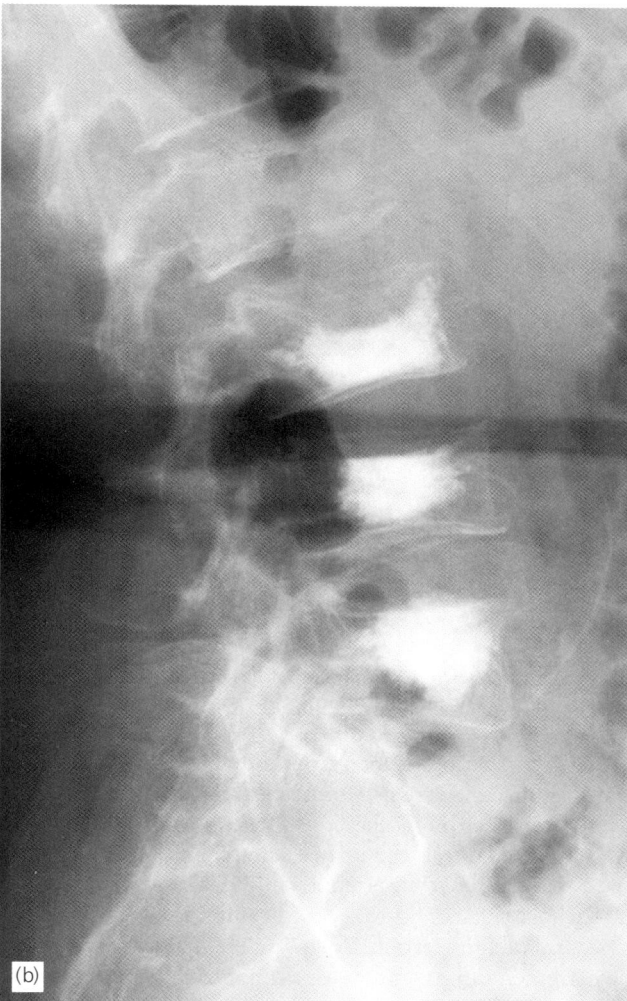

Figure 90.10 Triple level vertebroplasty with alternate unipedicular approach in order to avoid crowding of the injection needles.

This technique is based on the insertion of an expandable balloon into the vertebra, which after inflation may be able to restore vertebral height and correct the deformity (see Fig. 90.3). Further aspects include the formation of a void in the vertebra, which can be filled with prefilled bone fillers with lower risk of leakage. Specially designed balloons are available for all vertebra, and directable balloons, e.g. balloons opening only on one side, can be used in restoring the vertebral height. The balloons have been designed to withstand high pressures of up to 600 psi (41.4 bar) without disruption. In general, the more osteoporotic the vertebra and the more recent the fracture is, the lower the balloon pressure needs to be in order to restore vertebral height. The approach for BKP is the same as the approach for VP, but more care has to be taken to insert the balloons correctly in order to avoid breakage through the side of the vertebra. Furthermore, postoperative care remains the same as after VP, with early mobilization without a brace.

One particular aspect is (still) the need for the creation of a cavity in young patients. Currently, the primary load-bearing resorbable cements do not allow direct injection into the cancellous bone, and therefore the use of a BKP or other cavity creation device is necessary. However, recent research focuses on the development of new biomaterials omitting the use of BKP and allowing direct injection in a VP-like fashion (see below).

Since 1998, the use of BKP has helped the refinement and use of VP and both techniques now have their place in spine surgery.

Because of the potential kyphotic and vertebral height restoration effect of KP, several similar treatment methods focusing on minimally invasive restoration of the vertebral body height involving different implants such as nets or titanium implants are on the market or will appear in the near future. These techniques are based on balloons or mimic balloons, and do not differ much from BKP and have the same goal, so they have not been described separately in this chapter.

However BKP has been criticized as sacrificing bone in order to restore height and that there is no clinical evidence

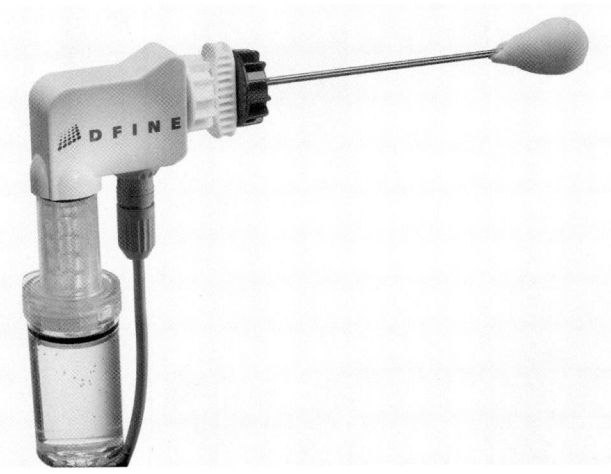

Figure 90.11 Radiofrequency-targeted vertebral augmentation (DFine, San Jose, CA). Radiofrequency is delivered to the cement during injection rendering it highly viscous and avoiding dripping. The cement will be injected in this state and has the potency to reduce mobile vertebral fractures whilst avoiding leakage.

in the literature that BKP changes kyphosis and the clinical outcome of height restoration.

The destruction of the vertebra by the balloon has had poor results in severe osteoporosis and osteonecrosis with cement dislocation.[76] Therefore, several improvements in KP have been developed by not using a balloon and avoiding destruction of the vertebra while restoring height, such as Kivaplasty (see Fig. 90.7) and radiofrequency-targeted vertebral augmentation (Fig. 90.11). These techniques have tremendous potential for the use of resorbable rather than primary load-bearing biomaterials. Furthermore, some of them have potential as a drug delivery platform.

The indications for KP and contraindications are the same as for VP (see above), with the exception of the potential use of VP in solid tumours after tumour debulking, which is currently contraindicated with KP.

KP can also be performed under local anaesthesia with sedoanalgesia; however, it is recommended to further limit the operation to a maximum of two levels, again for patient comfort. Difficult situations in general warrant general anaesthesia. In contrast to VP, it may be necessary to inject local anaesthetics into the fracture vertebra if height restoration is too painful; however, close monitoring of vital signs is then needed because of the cardiac depressive side-effects of local anaesthetics.

Clinical results and complication rates after VP and KP

The main differences between the techniques are the handling of the respective devices and surgical planning (which is more difficult with KP) and the price (KP being currently much more expensive). In recent years, there has been a lot of debate about which system is superior to the other, but now finally the consensus points towards the justified use of both techniques when indicated.

Both techniques have excellent clinical results with low complication rates.[77–79] No statistical differences between the techniques could be demonstrated regarding the clinical results and the adjacent fracture rates. The only statistical difference nowadays remains in the leakage rates. Leakage is strongly influenced by the experience of the user, indications (such as vertebral metastasis) and the cement properties. Owing to improvement both in handling and in cements, reduced complication rates can be expected in both techniques in the future. In particular, the development of high viscosity cements for VP has reduced leakage rates and improved safety tremendously over the last 3 years (Fig. 90.11). The current literature is still based on early VP techniques and results and does not yet include the development of instruments, techniques and cements.

Therefore the North American Neurosurgical and Orthopaedic Spine Societies (North American Spine Society, Society for the Advancement of Spine Surgery, American Association of Neurological Surgeons, Congress of Neurological Surgeons, Scoliosis Research Society) have declared in an open letter to the reimbursement authorities in the US that both techniques are indicated in the treatment of osteoporotic fractures and tumour, but that 'there is no value of KP over VP and … payment policy should be equivalent for both procedures'.[80] Actual numbers and trend therefore favour VP as the cheaper, easier and at least as safe procedure over KP, and it is probable that KP techniques in the future will be performed only for a small group of patients, whereas VP will be the first line of surgical treatment. Traditional BKP currently only plays a role in the treatment of traumatic fractures in young patients.

Treatment scheme

Not all patients will require operative intervention. Therefore, a clinical treatment scheme involving conservative treatment using both techniques is necessary; this scheme is shown in Fig. 90.12. The scheme is based on an early diagnosis of the fracture to be able to assess the feasibility of every treatment. One other important condition is the strict reassessment of patients treated conservatively to regroup them into the VP or bone-preserving KP arm if their condition meets VP/KP requirements. Therefore, strict clinical and radiological follow-ups have to be performed every 1–2 weeks to assess the pain condition and kyphotic state of the patient. In our clinical experience at least half of the patients can be treated conservatively without further risk using that scheme. Although the clinical restoration rates in KP have not yet been confirmed in prospective studies, in selected cases it is possible to restore the kyphosis better than with VP. Future results may prove the validity of new bone-preserving KP procedures in kyphosis and are therefore integrated into this treatment scheme avoiding the disadvantage of the more destructive BKP.

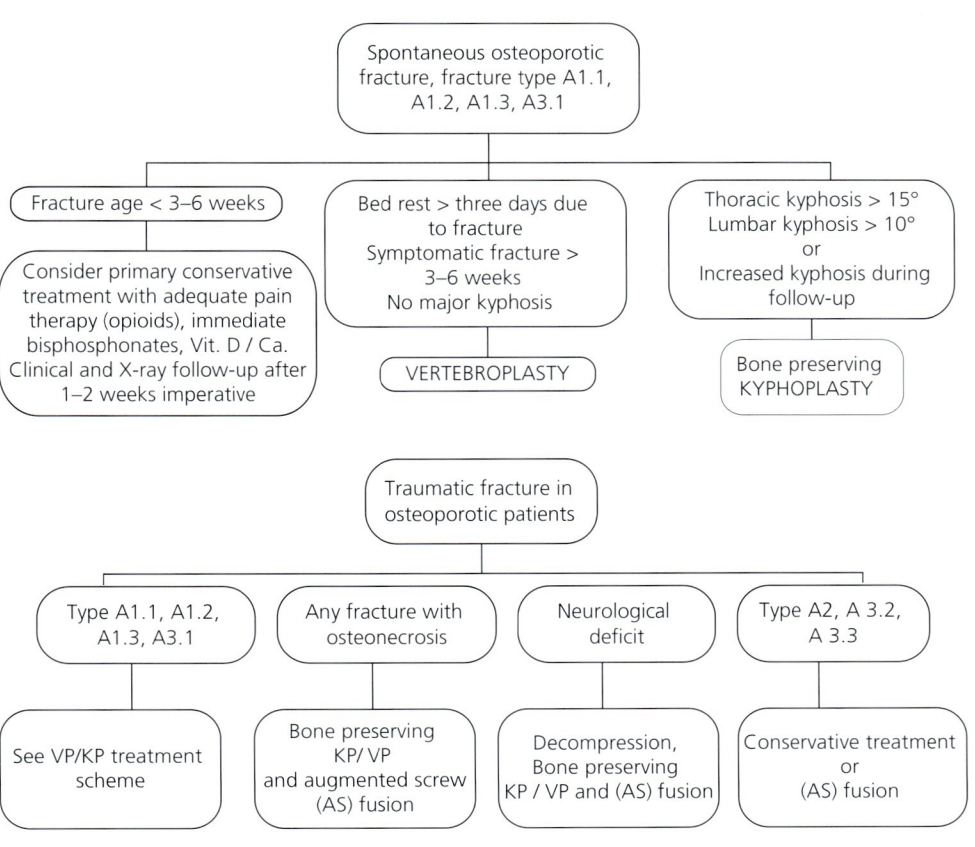

Figure 90.12 Treatment scheme after spontaneous osteoporotic vertebral fractures for fracture types A1.1, A1.2, A1.3, A3.1 (fracture classification after AO),[41] all other fracture types see Figure 90.13.

Figure 90.13 Treatment scheme in trauma (fracture classification after AO).[41]

Exceptions to this scheme are osteonecrotic fractures and cortisone-based fractures, which are generally not manageable with conservative treatment because of the high risk of recurrent fracture and collapse (see above). As already mentioned, VP and BKP techniques carry a risk in these patients and therefore a bone-preserving technique (VP, or new KP techniques) with a combination of a dorsal fixation is more often indicated.

Special considerations in trauma

In general, a spontaneous osteoporotic fracture has to be differentiated from a traumatic fracture in an osteoporotic patient, which may cause greater dislocation of the vertebra than spontaneous osteoporotic fractures. It may be difficult to assess the severity of the trauma looking at the patient's history alone, for 'easy' falls may cause severe vertebral fractures. Therefore, if there is any doubt of the severity of the trauma, the fracture type should be even more carefully assessed. Special trauma rules in osteoporosis should be applied in treating those patients with posterior instability (e.g. type B and C fractures, according the AO classification). It is clear that unstable fractures with posterior ligament disruption, disc disruption and severe dislocation of the vertebra cannot be treated with cementoplasties as stand-alone treatment. The indication for surgical treatment in trauma in osteoporosis is shown in Fig. 90.13 (please see also section below on screw augmentation).

In general, it has to be said that only the fracture types shown are amenable to stand-alone treatment, in all other cases or if there is any doubt open surgical stabilization with an augmented screw has to be performed to avoid complications such as cement dislocation (see Fig. 90.6) and subsidence of the fracture around the cement. Therefore, strict adherence to fracture classification is mandatory. As in trauma of other bones, the general approach is primarily to perform a radiograph and CT, but additional MRI may be necessary to safely rule out posterior structure injury before deciding on cementoplasty. Future techniques may combine percutaneous screws with VP augmentation in order to perform a purely percutaneous approach. Currently, the combination of new high viscosity cements in VP or new bone-preserving KP techniques for the fractured segment with dorsal fixation of adjacent segments play a bigger role in trauma in elderly people.

Again special attention has to be given to osteonecrosis in fractures. Because of a very high risk of cement dislocation an open solution should be generally preferred to stand-alone cemenoplasties.

THE USE OF INJECTABLE BIOMATERIALS IN THE OSTEOPOROTIC SPINE

For several years the idea of augmentation of an osteoporotic vertebral fracture or spinal implants has gained widespread acceptance. Early injectable substances have been refined over the years to meet specific requirements for spinal use.

In general, two substance groups are in use nowadays: non-resorbable polymers, mainly PMMA and, more recently, resorbable calcium phosphate cement (CPC).

PMMA cement

PMMA has been widely used for several years to enhance screw stability[71,81–84] or to perform VP and KP.[85] Spinal PMMA cements have been especially designed for spinal use, with superior capacity regarding radio-opacity, injection and thermal reaction during polymerization.[27, 86–89]

PMMA cements used for VP, KP or screw augmentation are polymers, with a ratio of liquid to powder phase of 2:3.[90] The changes necessary to make them applicable in spine surgery include optimization of injection properties, decreasing the powder to liquid ratio and the addition of substances for radio-opacity. The choice of radio-opaque substances is relatively easy because PMMA cements are not resorbable, so all radio-opaque non- or poorly soluble powders, such as metal salts ($BaSO_4$, ZrO_2, $SrCO_3$) or metal powders (Ti, Ta, W) can be used.[90] Those cements are now optimized for injection, but injection time varies greatly from manufacturer to manufacturer. Furthermore, the polymerization heat has been reduced from ~95°C in hip cements to ~50–70° in spine cements.[91] This reduction in the exothermic reaction is important in the preservation of neural tissues in the case of leakage.

INDICATIONS FOR PMMA, ADVANTAGES AND DISADVANTAGES

Clinical results of cementoplasties with PMMA support the use of vertebral cement in osteoporotic fractures. The reduction of up to 70% on the visual analogue scale, and significantly improved patient satisfaction, SF36 and ODI scores reflect the use of these cements in recent years.[71,74,75] However, failures also occur; the most common complication after PMMA injection into the vertebral body is not leakage or pulmonary emboli (this complication is fortunately rare) but subsequent fractures on adjacent bodies.[92–94] This has been mainly reported as being associated with the elasticity modulus of PMMA, but biomechanical and clinical results in this aspect are quite contradictory. As clinically too many factors influence the outcome (patient age, severity of deformity, DXA score, nutrition, mobilization, etc.), data are difficult to compare. However, what has been demonstrated is an average of 12–17% subsequent fractures after cementoplasties (VP or BKP). This number is still lower than the spontaneous refracture rate in conservatively treated osteoporotic vertebral fractures, which is as high as 58%.[95] Currently investigations are underway analysing the elastic modulus (E-mod) of PMMA cements and subsequent fracture rates. It has been demonstrated that E-mods from 0.5 MPa to 2 GPa show the best results regarding adjacent fracture rates.

Injectability is the main issue in VP and BKP. Methods differ for the respective techniques: in VP PMMA, being more viscous, is directly injected into the cancellous bone. In BKP, however, the balloon forms a void and the PMMA can be injected in a much less viscous state.

This fact is reflected by the cement extravasation rates, which range from 4% to 25% (average 8%) in BKP and 28–57% (average 43%) in VP (data without the new high-viscous cements).[74] Serious adverse events due to extravasations have been published, including fatal pulmonary emboli. Therefore, the ultimate goal to reduce leakage rates must be an optimized injection technique. The manufacturers of spinal PMMA prior to 2008 supplied general handling and application timelines that however varied largely depending on storage and environmental temperature. The guidelines in BKP can be more easily followed as less viscous cement can be injected, whereas VP surgeons tend to inject the cement prematurely.[90] BKP cement (KyphX HVR, Kyphon, Sunnyvale, USA) is ready for injection when it no longer sticks to surgical gloves or if it does not drip from the injection cannulla. VP cements have been further refined in 2007/2008, e.g. immediate optimal viscosity without time variation and the development of a direct syringe-based electroconductive measurement of cement viscosity (Skeltex, Boucherville, CA); the clinical impact of those developments has still to be shown.

However, even if the injection technique is optimized, some risks using PMMA cement remain. Owing to the exothermic reaction, they all create a more or less large necrotic zone around the cement, which is an issue in hip surgery, but which may not be so important in spine surgery. The remodelling of the surrounding bone is somewhat impaired by local toxicity of the polymers, and, furthermore, the persisting loss of liquid within the cement results in shrinkage of the cement.[90] This loss depends on the primary water content, which differs from cement to cement; therefore, shrinkage is difficult to assess individually.

Further disadvantages besides those mentioned above include monomer release with severe hypotension by action on vascular smooth muscles.[96,97] These disadvantages are also known from hip surgery, whether they also represent an important problem in spine surgery has not yet been observed.

One of the main advantages of PMMA is currently its low cost; PMMA is ~10 times cheaper than CPC. Further advantages are optimized handling properties and a primary rapid stability, which is generally reached within 20–30 minutes after injection.

Resorbable calcium phosphate cements

CPC cements are not as old as PMMA cements, which date back to the sixties; CPC cements were discovered two decades ago; the first *in vitro* trials in spine were performed a decade ago.[98,99]

Like PMMA, they generally consist of a powder and solution to be mixed together. The liquid to powder ratio has likewise been optimized over the years to improve injectability.[100] Most often the powder contains calcium phosphate compounds mixed with an aqueous solution to form crystals, which then typically form a porous structure. The final porosity is ~50% with pores ranging from 0.1 to 10 ∝m. CPCs are very resistant to compressive loads and less to shear forces (about 10 times higher compression properties). This is because the crystals are inadequately bonded.[100,101]

In general, two types of CPC are in clinical use: apatite (hydroxyapatite) and brushite (dicalcium phosphate dehydrate); most of the available CPCs are apatite CPC (e.g. Bone Source, Calcibon, Kyphos and Norian). The main difference between both CPC types is that brushite CPCs are resorbed much faster than apatite CPCs; this must be considered carefully in surgery.[101]

Radio-opacity in CPC is obtained by adding barium or strontium. A recently developed cement (Cerament), a hydroxyapatite and calcium sulphate mixture, allows injection into intact bone without the use of a KP procedure and, furthermore, contains iodine for radioopacity. This cement allows the use of a cheaper VP technique and, because of resorption of iodine within the first weeks, provides better follow-up regarding bone remodelling.

INDICATIONS FOR CPC, ADVANTAGES AND DISADVANTAGES

CPCs are currently in clinical trials in osteoporotic and traumatic fractures. Research focuses on use as stand-alone implants in traumatic vertebral fractures in young patients and the reduction of cement toxicity in older patients. As this chapter is discussing osteoporosis, only these indications are hereby discussed. It has been shown in elderly people that, although apatite CPC stays intact over 1-2 years, the remodelling of bone and bone ingrowth is minimal.[102] This may be different in young osteoporotic patients; however, clinical data are still lacking. The above-discussed disadvantage in CPC regarding shear forces must be taken into consideration in all cases. In elderly people, fractures are mainly primary stable fractures with reduced shear loads on the implants. However, in young patients, unstable or burst fractures are more common, which are clear contraindications for the use of CPC as a stand-alone treatment. The use of additional posterior fusion and CPC is still purely experimental; no prospective clinical data are available on this aspect.

Regarding screw augmentation, several experimental studies point out the benefit of CPC. The stability of the screw can be enhanced with CPC, currently up to 102%.[103] Nevertheless, there are some disadvantages which prevent CPC from widespread use in osteoporosis. The primary stability of the CPC depends on accurate injection technique. Poor injection technique and early mobilization prevent appropriate crystallization, which results in early resorption and subsequent loosening/implant failure. Five years ago, the surgeon had hardly time to inject cements, which hardened then within 30 seconds. Newer cements actually have longer handling and injection times. However, the time of definite crystallization and stability is long and, depending on the cement, may be as high as 24 hours, during which the patient has to remain in bed.

Generally the pores in CPCs are much too small for osteoblast ingrowth; therefore, CPCs are only resorbed from the outside, which explains the slower resorption rate than porous β-TCP (tri-calcium phosphate).[104] Finally, the type of CPC is important; cements with rapid resorption (brushite/trisulphate cements) run a risk of preliminary resorption and subsequent recurrence of the fracture.

This is not true for biphasic cements with a slow (e.g. HA) and fast resorption time (e.g. calcium sulphate), such as Cerament, which are injected in a VP fashion and remodelled more homogeneously. The slow resorption time maintains a certain stability over time. However, these cements are restricted for VP procedures, stable fractures or new KP procedures with implants such as PEEK (polyetheretherketone) (Fig. 90.7).

Although clinical progress in the treatment of primary vertebral fractures as stand-alone treatment with CPC has been made,[105] the indication in osteoporosis remains debatable and is probably not justified.

Resorption or even the question whether they resorb at all will probably never be predicted individually. The addition of radio-opaque substances like barium is necessary but also carries a risk; small particles are released over years and may represent a biohazard.[90] The impact of CPCs on the risk of adjacent fractures also has not been defined yet. Finally, CPCs are hydrophilic; they may therefore have a risk of thrombosis and blood clotting due to release of calcium phosphate particles.[106,107] This risk has also not been defined yet and depends largely on the formula of the different CPCs and their resorption rate.

Advantages of CPCs versus PMMA include the fact that, because of the slow crystallization, CPCs set isothermically without the risk of thermal damage to surrounding structures. Their greatest advantage surely lies in (more or less complete) remodelling into healthy bone, which avoids the long-term complications of PMMA.

OPEN SURGERY

Open decompression/fusion in osteoporotic spines is generally indicated in instabilities, multisegmental spinal stenosis, neurological deficits and degenerative scoliosis. It is generally accepted that transpedicular screws and anterior implants have a higher loosening and subsidence rate. Even long-segment fusions run a considerable risk in osteoporosis, the most common complication being progressive junctional cephalad kyphosis and screw loosening.[108]

Several studies have confirmed that osteoporotic patients have a significantly lower screw stability with more frequent screw movements within the vertebra than normal patients,[83,85,86,109,110] explaining the overall higher failure rates of up to 12%.[111]

Therefore, stand-alone transpedicular screws should not be used alone in an osteoporotic spine, they need to be somehow reinforced. This can be done with sublaminar hooks, wires, conical screws, iliac screws or expandable screws.[83,112] All of these additional techniques show higher stability than transpedicular screws alone in osteoporosis.[81,85,86]

As stated above, the operating technique for transpedicular screws is very important as the insertion depth of the screw plays a significant role. Screws that are implanted deeper than 50% into the vertebral body or bicortical screws perforating the anterior vertebral cortex and avoiding tapping enhance screw anchorage in the bone.[112–114]

Finally, the diameter of screws plays a role; in normal bone, screws with diameters of 7 mm and higher show better stability. However, in osteoporotic bone such screws may cause pedicle fractures in 24–40% of cases, which leads to premature screw failure.[89,112]

Nowadays, PMMA augmentation is regarded as the best method to enhance screw stability in osteoporotic bones. With injection of PMMA, screw stability can be enhanced up to 162%.[81,83] Furthermore, it has been demonstrated that anterior cages are better supported with augmented posterior screws as the failure of anterior implants is higher in osteoporosis than in normal bone[115] (see Fig. 90.8). Recent developments are now focusing on facilitating the injection technique using perforated screws. Those cementing techniques enhance the fixation of the screw within the vertebral body, transferring the biomechanical load anteriorly from the pedicle to the vertebra. However, clinical data using augmented screws are lacking because these operations are not performed very often and the individual range of diseases/fusion length/bone density is so large that prospective cohorts are difficult to recruit. Nevertheless, clinically screw augmentation with PMMA cement is indicated in cases where instability, neurological damage/multisegmental decompression or degenerative scoliosis are present and therefore instrumentation is necessary. The application of PMMA-augmented screws allows a shorter fusion segment than non-augmented screws.

Historically, cement augmentation was used before the insertion of the screw, which sometimes led to complications such as malpositioned screws and problems of insertion in cases where the cement rapidly hardened. Recently, perforated screws (either anterior or posterior) have gained popularity. These screws are cannulated and have several holes or slots where the cement can flow through. They are inserted in the normal way and positioning can be optimized if needed. Afterwards a spinal cement is injected via the screw into the vertebra, which facilitates the augmentation technique. In general, independent of the technique, it is enough to inject 1.5–2 mL of cement per screw. However, using conventional or perforated screws, it is important to observe the cementation rules mentioned above, because leakage is possible in both techniques, and to make sure that enough cement is located around the circumference of the screw (Fig. 90.14). Furthermore it has to be considered that screw augmentation requires more clinical experience and training as control of the cement injection is more difficult than in conventional VP. Newer resorbable or non-toxic and non-resorbable cements are being considered and tested

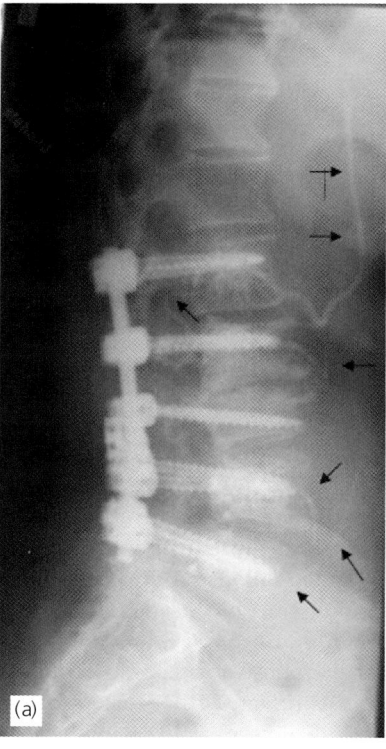 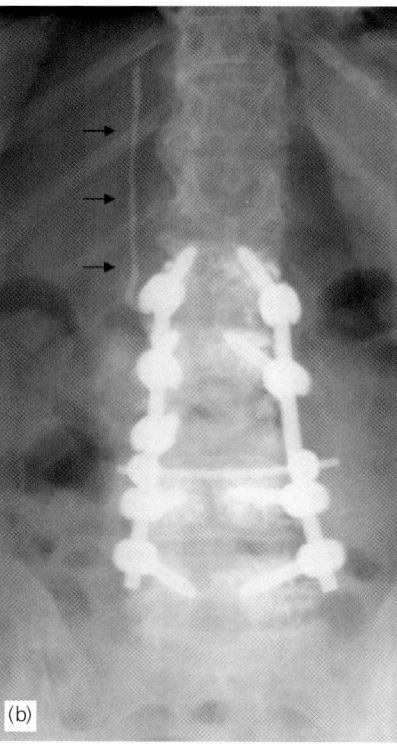

Figure 90.14 Multilevel stabilization and cement augmentation with perforated screws. Note cement extravasation on all aspects of the spine (arrows) and insufficient cement stabilization at least of the screw L5 right.

for use in open surgery and may play a more important role in this field in the future.

POSTOPERATIVE MANAGEMENT

Although surgery can achieve a proper reconstruction of a fracture, it cannot influence osteoporosis in the sense of healing, but is merely one element within an interdisciplinary treatment regimen.

Physiotherapy plays an important role in treatment after osteoporotic vertebral body fractures and in prevention of further fractures. The positive effect of physiotherapy in patients suffering from osteoporosis without VBF has been well documented scientifically.[116–118]

Furthermore, it has to be taken into account that after minimally invasive techniques such as VP or KP, we are dealing with healthy motion segments that make a major difference to the fused spine. Therefore special treatment regimens in osteoporotic patients particularly after VP and KP should be considered.

Please refer to specific literature on this topic where specialized treatment schemes are described.[119]

In summary, in all osteoporotic patients and even more so in those with persisting kyphosis, it is much more important to treat balance and gait disturbance than strength. Only balance training can reduce the most common complication in osteoporosis apart from vertebral fracture: falls resulting in femoral neck or radial fractures. It is easily understandable that patients with kyphosis have a general disturbance of equilibrium and that, although they are pain free postoperatively and even if we gain complete restoration of the kyphosis (which is not always the case), they have to gradually adapt postoperative changes: it is imperative that every osteoporotic patient is assessed individually and his/her fall risk is determined in order to start an individually adapted treatment scheme immediately. Only a strict scheme can avoid further complications. Current treatment schemes include balance training and training of the sensomotoric muscles as these involuntary muscle groups can reflectively control balance and posture.

It should therefore be the goal for all surgeons or interventional radiologists not only to enable a pain-free, but also a risk-free or less risky future life for their osteoporotic patients by offering optimal surgical and postoperative treatment options.

KEY LEARNING POINTS

- Osteoporosis is one of the most serious global diseases and will increase in significance due to increased live spans/aging.
- Osteoporosis is a problem in both genders.
- Most osteoporotic spontaneous fractures involve the spine and are overlooked.
- Patients with sudden backache should be sent for X-ray and MRI.
- Osteoporotic fractures are mainly painful as long as the intraosseus oedema persists.
- Minimal invasive cementoplasties (vertebroplasty or bone-preserving kyphoplasty) are indicated and show good results in osteoporotic vertebral fractures.
- Follow treatment schemes for osteoporotic or traumatic fractures in the elderly.
- Patients at risk for severe kyphosis and recurrent vertebral fractures are patients with osteonecrotic fractures and patients on cortisone; early stabilization (VP or KP) is advised in those groups.
- PMMA and resorbable bone cements can be used in VP and KP; biocements with a better bone adapted elastic modulus and less toxicity will play a larger role in the future.
- Prefer VP/KP with additional (augmented) screw fixation in severe bone destruction (osteonecrosis/metastasis).
- An individual postoperative adapted physical treatment scheme enhances bone quality and decreases the risk of falls, e.g. consecutive fractures of other bones.

REFERENCES

1. Riggs BL, Melton LJ 3rd. The worldwide problem of osteoporosis: insights afforded by epidemiology. *Bone* 1995;**17**(5 Suppl):505–11.
2. Crafts NFR. The human development index and changes in standards of living: some historical comparisons. *European Review of Economic History* 1997;**1**:299–322.
3. European Commission. Directorate-General for Employment, Industrial Relations and Social Affairs. Directorate V/F.2. *Report on Osteoporosis in the European Community*. Luxembourg: Office for Official Publications of the European Communities.
4. Lindsay R, Pack S, Li Z. Longitudinal progression of fracture prevalence through a population of postmenopausal women with osteoporosis. *Osteoporosis International* 2005;**16**:306–12.
5. Felsenberg D, Silman AJ, Lunt M, et al. For the European Prospective Osteoporosis Study (EPOS) Group. Incidence of vertebral fracture in Europe: results from the European Prospective Osteoporosis Study (EPOS). *Journal of Bone and Mineral Research* 2002;**17**:716–24.
6. Dennison E, Cooper C. Epidemiology of osteoporotic fractures. *Hormone Research* 2002;**54**(Suppl):58–63.
7. Melton LJ 3rd, Kan SH, Frye MA, et al. Epidemiology of vertebral fractures in women. *American Journal of Epidemiology* 1989;**129**:1000–11.

8. Kanis JA, Pitt FA. Epidemiology of osteoporosis. *Bone* 1992;**13**(Suppl 1):S7–15.
9. Lee YL, Yip KM. The osteoporotic spine. *Clinical Orthopaedics* 1996;**323**:91–7.
10. O'Neill TW, Felsenberg D, Varlow J, et al. The prevalence of vertebral deformity in European men and women: the European Vertebral Osteoporosis Study. *Journal of Bone and Mineral Research* 1996;**11**:1010–18.
11. Melton LJ 3rd, Lane AW, Cooper C, et al. Prevalence and incidence of vertebral deformities. *Osteoporosis International* 1993;**3**:113–19.
12. Cooper C, Atkinson EJ, O'Fallon WM, Melton LJ 3rd. Incidence of clinically diagnosed vertebral fractures: a population-based study in Rochester, Minnesota, 1985–1989. *Journal of Bone and Mineral Research* 1992;**7**:221–7.
13. van Staa TP, Dennison EM, Leufkens HG, Cooper C. Epidemiology of fractures in England and Wales. *Bone* 2001;**29**:517–22.
14. Gehlbach SH, Bigelow C, Heimisdottir M, May S, Walker M, Kirkwood JR. Recognition of vertebral fracture in a clinical setting. *Osteoporosis International* 2000;**11**:577–82.
15. Healey JH, Vigorita VJ, Lane JM. The coexistence and characteristics of osteoarthritis and osteoporosis. *Journal of Bone and Joint Surgery* 1985;**67**A:586–92.
16. DeWald CJ, Stanley T. Instrumentation-related complications of multilevel fusions for adult spinal deformity patients over age 65: surgical considerations and treatment options in patients with poor bone quality. *Spine* 2006;**31**(19 Suppl):144–51.
17. Harvey N, Cooper C. Epidemiology of vertebral fractures. *Advances in Osteoporotic Fracture Management* 2004;**3**:78–83.
18. EVOS. Europäische Studie zur vertebralen Osteoporose-Ergebnisse aus den deutschen Studienzentren. *Medizinische Klinik* 1998;**93**(Suppl II):3–66.
19. Resch H, Muschitz C. Drug therapy of osteoporosis. In: Becker S, Ogon M (eds) *Balloon Kyphoplasty*. New York, NY: Springer, 2008:5–15.
20. Faciszewski T, McKiernan F, Rao R. Management of osteoporotic vertebral compression fractures. In: Spivak JM, Connolly PJ (eds) *Orthopaedic Knowledge Update: Spine 3*. Rosemont, IL: American Academy of Orthopaedic Surgeons, 2006:377–86.
21. Parfitt AM. Quantum concept of bone remodelling and turnover: implications for the pathogenesis of osteoporosis. *Calcified Tissue International* 1979;**28**:1–5.
22. Bröll H, Dambacher MA (eds) *Osteoporosis: A Guide to Diagnosis and Treatment*. Basel, Switzerland: Krager, 1996.
23. Abraham Kierszenbaum. *Histology and Cell Biology*, 2nd edn. St. Louis, MO: Mosby, 2002.
24. Grote HJ, Amling M, Vogel M, et al. Intervertebral variation in trabecular microarchitecture throughout the normal spine in relation to age. *Bone* 1995;**16**:301–8.
25. Hulme PA, Boyd SK, Ferguson SJ. Regional variation in vertebral bone morphology and its contribution to vertebral fracture strength. *Bone* 2007;**41**:946–57.
26. Hulme PA, Ferguson SJ, Boyd SK. Determination of vertebral endplate deformation under load using micro-computed tomography. *Journal of Biomechanics* 2008;**41**:78–85.
27. Hirano T, Hasegawa K, Takahashi HE, et al. Structural characteristics of the pedicle and its role in screw stability. *Spine* 1997;**22**:2504–9.
28. Weinstein JN, Rydevik BL, Rauschning W. Anatomic and technical considerations of pedicle screw fixation. *Clinical Orthopaedics and Related Research* 1992;**284**:34–46.
29. Watts NB, Harris ST, Genant HK. Treatment of painful osteoporotic vertebral fractures with percutaneous vertebroplasty or kyphoplasty. *Osteoporosis International* 2001;**12**:429–37.
30. Lyritis GP, Mayasis B, Tsakalakos N, et al. The natural history of the osteoporotic vertebral fracture. *Clinical Rheumatology* 1989;**8**(Suppl 2):66–9.
31. Ryan PJ, Blake G, Herd R, Fogelman I. A clinical profile of back pain and disability in patients with spinal osteoporosis. *Bone* 1994;**15**:27–30.
32. Maigne R. Low-back pain of thoracolumbar origin. *Archives of Physical Medicine and Rehabilitation* 1980;**61**:389–95.
33. Miller PD, Barran DT, Bilezikian JT. Practical clinical applications of biochemical markers of bone turnover: consensus of an expert panel. *Journal of Clinical Densitometry* 1999;**2**:323–42.
34. Looker AC, Bauer DC, Chesnut III CH, et al. Clinical use of biochemical markers of bone remodeling: current status and future directions. *Osteoporosis International* 2000;**11**:467–80.
35. Marcus R, Holloway L, Wells B, et al. The relationship of biochemical markers of bone turnover to bone density changes in postmenopausal women: results from the Postmenopausal Estrogen/Progestin Interventions (PEPI) trial. *Journal of Bone and Mineral Research* 1999;**14**:1583–95.
36. NIH. Osteoporosis prevention, diagnosis, and therapy. *NIH Consensus Statement* 2000;**17**:1–45.
37. Morris MS, Jacques PF, Selhub J. Relation between homocysteine and B-vitamin status indicators and bone mineral density in older Americans. *Bone* 2005;**37**:234–42.
38. Gjesdal CG, Vollset SE, Ueland PM, et al. Plasma total homocysteine level and bone mineral density: The Hordaland Homocysteine Study. *Archives of Internal Medicine* 2006;**166**:88–94.
39. Herrmann M, Widmann T, Herrmann W. Homocysteine – a newly recognised risk factor for osteoporosis. *Clinical Chemistry and Laboratory Medicine* 2005;**43**:1111–17.
40. Selhub J. The many facets of hyperhomocysteinemia: Studies from the Framingham cohorts. *Journal of Nutrition* 2006;**136**(6 Suppl):1726–30.
41. Magerl F, Aebi M, Gertzbein SD, et al. A comprehensive classification of thoracic and lumbar injuries. *European Spine Journal* 1994;**3**:184–201.
42. Rhee PM, Bridgeman A, Acosta JA, et al. Lumbar fractures in adult blunt trauma: axial and single-slice helical abdominal and pelvic computed tomographic scans versus portable plain films. *Journal of Trauma* 2002;**53**:663–7.

43. Ryan PJ, Fogelman I. Osteoporotic vertebral fractures: diagnosis with radiography and bone scintigraphy. *Radiology* 1994;**190**:669–72.
44. Wiener SN, Neumann DR, Rzeszotarski MS. Comparison of magnetic resonance imaging and radionuclide bone imaging of vertebral fractures. *Clinical Nuclear Medicine* 1989;**14**:666–70.
45. Schmitz A, Risse JH, Textor J, et al. FDG-PET findings of vertebral compression fractures in osteoporosis: preliminary results. *Osteoporosis International* 2002;**13**:755–61.
46. Saag KG. Glucocorticoid use in rheumatoid arthritis. *Currunt Rheumatolology Reports* 2002;**4**(3):218–25.
47. Harrop JS, Prpa B, Reinhardt MK, Lieberman I. Primary and secondary osteoporosis: incidence of subsequent vertebral compression fractures after kyphoplasty. *Spine* 2004;**29**:2120–5.
48. Chou LH, Knight RQ. Idiopathic avascular necrosis of a vertebral body. Case report and literature review. *Spine* 1997;**16**:1928–32.
49. Hasegawa K, Homma T, Uchiyama S, Takahashi H. Vertebral pseudarthrosis in the osteoporotic spine. *Spine* 1998;**23**:2201–6.
50. Huy MD, Jensen ME, Marx WF, Kallmes DF. Percutaneous vertebroplasty in vertebral osteonecrosis (Kümmell's spondylitis). *Neurosurgery Focus* 1998;**1**, Article 2 (online journal).
51. Ito M, Motomiya M, Abumi K, et al. Vertebral osteonecrosis associated with sarcoidosis. Case report. *Journal of Neurosurgery Spine* 2005;**2**:222–5.
52. Jang JS, Kim DY, Lee SH. Efficacy of percutaneous vertebroplasty in the treatment of intravertebral pseudarthrosis associated with noninfected avascular necrosis of the vertebral body. *Spine* 2003;**28**:1588–92.
53. Maheshwari PR, Nagar AM, Prasad SS, et al. Avascular necrosis of spine: a rare appearance. *Spine* 2004;**29**:119–22.
54. Murakami H, Kawahara N, Gabata T, et al. Vertebral body osteonecrosis without vertebral collapse. *Spine* 2003;**28**:323–8.
55. Van Eenenaam DP, el-Khoury GY. Delayed post-traumatic vertebral collapse (Kummell's disease): case report with serial radiographs, computed tomographic scans, and bone scans. *Spine* 1993;**18**:1236–41.
56. Young WF, Brown D, Kendler A, Clements D. Delayed post-traumatic osteonecrosis of a vertebral body (Kummell's disease). *Acta Orthopaedica Belgica* 2002;**68**:13–19.
57. Allen BL Jr, Jinkins WJ 3rd. Vertebral osteonecrosis associated with pancreatitis in a child. A case report. *Journal of Bone and Joint Surgery (American)* 1987;**60**:985–7.
58. Brower AC, Downey EF Jr. Kummell disease: report of a case with serial radiographs. *Radiology* 1981;**141**:363–4.
59. Hutter CD. Dysbaric osteonecrosis: a reassessment and hypothesis. *Med Hypotheses* 2000;**54**(4):585–90.
60. Lieberman IH, Dudeney S, Reinhardt MK, Bell G. Initial outcome and efficacy of kyphoplasty in the treatment of painful osteoporotic vertebral compression fractures. *Spine* 2001;**26**:1631–8.
61. Maldague BE, Noel HM, Malghem JJ. The intravertebral vacuum cleft: a sign of ischemic vertebral collapse. *Radiology* 1978;**129**:23–9.
62. Van Bockel SR, Mindelzun RE. Gas in the psoas muscle secondary to an intravertebral vacuum cleft: CT characteristics. *Journal of Computer Assisted Tomography* 1987;**11**:913–15.
63. Bhalla S, Reinus WR. The linear intravertebral vacuum: a sign of benign vertebral collapse. *AJR American Journal of Roentgenology* 1998;**170**:1563–9.
64. McKiernan F, Faciszewski T. Intravertebral clefts in osteoporotic vertebral compression fractures. *Arthritis and Rheumatism* 2003;**48**:1414–19.
65. McKiernan F, Jensen R, Faciszewski T. The dynamic mobility of vertebral compression fractures. *Journal of Bone and Mineral Research* 2003;**18**:24–9.
66. Galibert P, Deramond H, Rosat P, Le Gars D. Preliminary note on the treatment of vertebral angioma by percutaneous acrylic vertebroplasty. *Neurochirurgie* 1987;**33**:166–8.
67. Cotten A, Dewatre F, Cortet B, et al. Percutaneous vertebroplasty for osteolytic metastases and myeloma: effect of the percentage of lesion filling and the leakage of methyl methacrylate at clinical follow-up. *Radiology* 1996;**200**:525–30.
68. Heini PF, Walchli B, Berlemann U. Percutaneous transpedicular vertebroplasty with PMMA: operative technique and early results. A prospective study for the treatment of osteoporotic compression fractures. *European Spine Journal* 2000;**9**:445–50.
69. Jensen ME, Evans AJ, Mathis JM, et al. Percutaneous polymethylmethacrylate vertebroplasty in the treatment of osteoporotic vertebral body compression fractures: technical aspects. *American Journal of Neuroradiology* 1997;**18**:1897–904.
70. Heini PF, Orler R. Vertebroplastik bei hochgradiger Osteoporose Technik und Erfahrung mit plurisegmentalen Injektionen. *Orthopäde* 2004;**33**:22–30.
71. Heini PF. The current treatment – a survey of osteoporotic fracture treatment. Osteoporotic spine fractures: the spine surgeon's perspective. *Osteoporosis International* 2005;**16**(Suppl 2):85–92.
72. Baroud G, Nemes J, Heini P, Steffen T. Load shift of the intervertebral disc after a vertebroplasty: a finite-element study. *European Spine Journal* 2003;**12**:421–6.
73. Bierschneider M, Boszczyk B, Jaksche H. Summary: the risks of kyphoplasty. In: Becker S, Ogon M (eds) *Balloon Kyphoplasty*. Vienna, Austria: Springer, 2008:79,83.
74. Taylor RS, Taylor RJ, Fritzell P. Balloon kyphoplasty and vertebroplasty for vertebral compression fractures: a comparative systematic review of efficacy and safety. *Spine* 2006;**31**:2747–55.
75. Becker S, Ogon M (eds). *Balloon Kyphoplasty*. Vienna, Austria: Springer, 2008.
76. Dabirrahmani D, Becker S, Hogg M, et al. Mechanical variables affecting balloon kyphoplasty outcome – a finite element study. *Computer Methods in Biomechanics and Biomedical Engineering* 2011 Apr 1:1 (Epub ahead of print).

77. Voormolen MH, Mali WP, Lohle PN, et al. Percutaneous vertebroplasty compared with optimal pain medication treatment: short-term clinical outcome of patients with subacute or chronic painful osteoporotic vertebral compression fractures: the VERTOS study. AJNR American Journal of Neuroradiology 2007;**28**:555–60.
78. Rousing R, Andersen MO, Jespersen SM, et al. Percutaneous vertebroplasty compared to conservative treatment in patients with painful acute or subacute osteoporotic vertebral fractures: three-months follow-up in a clinical randomized study. Spine 2009;**34**:1349–54.
79. Wardlaw D, Cummings SR, Van Meirhaeghe J, et al. Efficacy and safety of balloon kyphoplasty compared with non-surgical care for vertebral compression fracture (FREE): a randomised controlled trial. Lancet 2009;**373**:1016–24.
80. AANS, CNS, NASS, SRS, and SAS. Open letter. www.spine.org/Documents/final_NCD_response_092808.pdf (accessed 4 May 2011).
81. Sarzier JS, Evans AJ, Cahill DW. Increased pedicle screw pullout strength with vertebroplasty augmentation in osteoporotic spines. Neurosurgery 2002;**96**(3 Suppl):309–12.
82. Tan JS, Bailey CS, Dvorak MF, et al. Cement augmentation of vertebral screws enhances the interface strength between interbody device and vertebral body. Spine 2007;**32**:334–41.
83. Soshi S, Shiba R, Kondo H, Murota K. An experimental study on transpedicular screw fixation in relation to osteoporosis of the lumbar spine. Spine 1991;**16**:1335–41.
84. Becker S, Chavanne A, Spitaler R, et al. Assessment of different screw augmentation techniques and screw designs in osteoporotic spines. European Spine Journal 2008;**17**:1462–9.
85. Coe JD, Warden KE, Herzig MA, McAfee PC. Influence of bone mineral density on the fixation of thoracolumbar implants. A comparative study of transpedicular screws, laminar hooks, and spinous process wires. Spine 1990;**15**:902–7.
86. Halvorson TL, Kelley LA, Thomas KA, et al. Effects of bone mineral density on pedicle screw fixation. Spine 1994;**19**:2415–20.
87. Zdeblick TA, Kunz DN, Cooke ME, McCabe R. Pedicle screw pullout strength. Correlation with insertional torque. Spine 1993;**18**:1673–6.
88. Krag MH, Beynnon BD, Pope MH, et al. An internal fixator for posterior application to short segments of the thoracic, lumbar, or lumbosacral spine. Design and testing. Clinical Orthopaedics and Related Research 1986;**203**:75–98.
89. Brantley AG, Mayfield JK, Koeneman JB, Clark KR. The effects of pedicle screw fit. An in vitro study. Spine 1994;**19**:1752–8.
90. Bohner M. Injectable cements for vertebroplasty and kyphoplasty. In: Becker S, Ogon M (eds) Balloon Kyphoplasty. Vienna, Austria: Springer, 2008:143–8.
91. Belkoff SM, Molloy S. Temperature measurement during polymerization of polymethylmethacrylate cement used for vertebroplasty. Spine 2003;**28**:1555–9.
92. Berlemann U, Ferguson SJ, Nolte LP, Heini PF. Adjacent vertebral failure after vertebroplasty – A biomechanical investigation. Journal of Bone and Joint Surgery 2002;**84B**:748–52.
93. Polikeit A, Nolte LP, Ferguson SJ. The effect of cement augmentation on the load transfer in an osteoporotic functional spinal unit – Finite-element analysis. Spine 2003;**28**:991–6.
94. Baroud G, Nemes J, Heini P, Steffen T. Load shift of the intervertebral disc after a vertebroplasty: a finite-element study. European Spine Journal 2003;**12**:421–6.
95. Silverman SL, Minshall ME, Shen W, et al; Health-Related Quality of Life Subgroup of the Multiple Outcomes of Raloxifene Evaluation Study. The relationship of health-related quality of life to prevalent and incident vertebral fractures in postmenopausal women with osteoporosis: results from the Multiple Outcomes of Raloxifene Evaluation Study. Arthritis and Rheumatism 2001;**44**:2611–19.
96. Kim KC, Ritter MA. Hypotension associated with methyl methacrylate in total hip arthroplasties. Clinical Orthopaedics 1972;**88**:154–60.
97. Karlsson J, Wendling W, Chen D, et al. Methylmethacrylate monomer produces direct relaxation of vascular smooth muscle in vitro. Acta Anaesthesiologica Scandinavica 1995;**39**:685–9.
98. Bohner M, Lemaître J, Cordey J, et al. Potential use of biodegradable bone cement in bone surgery: holding strength of screws in reinforced osteoporotic bone. Orthopaedic Transactions 1992;**16**:401–2.
99. Schildhauer TA, Bennett AP, Tomin E, et al. Biomechanical evaluation of a new method for intra-vertebral body reconstruction with an injectable in situ setting carbonated apatite. Combined Orthopaedic Research Society Meeting, San Diego, California 1995:237.
100. Bohner M, Baroud G. Injectability of calcium phosphate pastes. Biomaterials 2005;**26**:1553–63.
101. Bohner M. Calcium orthophosphates in medicine: from ceramics to calcium phosphate cements. Injury 2000;**31**:37–47.
102. Libicher M, Hillmeier J, Liegibel U, et al. Osseous integration of calcium phosphate in osteoporotic vertebral fractures after kyphoplasty: initial results from a clinical and experimental pilot study. Osteoporosis International 2006;**17**:1208–15.
103. Moore DC, Maitra RS, Farjo LA, et al. Restoration of pedicle screw fixation with an in situ setting calcium phosphate cement. Spine 1997;**22**:1696–705.
104. Becker S, Maissen O, Ponomarev I, et al. Osteopromotion by a β-TCP/bone marrow hybrid implant for use in spine surgery. Spine 2006;**31**:11–17.
105 Maestretti G, Cremer C, Otten P, Jakob RP. Prospective study of standalone balloon kyphoplasty with calcium phosphate cement augmentation in traumatic fractures. European Spine Journal 2007;**16**:601–10.
106. Bernards CM, Chapman JR, Mirza SK. Lethality of embolized norian bone cement varies with the time between mixing and embolization. Proceedings of the 50th Annual Meeting of the Orthopaedic Research Society (ORS), San Francisco, 2004:254.

107. Axen N, Ahnfelt N-O, Persson T, Hermansson L, Sanchez J, Larsson R. Clotting behavior of orthopaedic cements in human blood. *Proceedings of the 9th annual meeting "Ceramics, cells and tissues"*, Faenza, 2004.
108. Pfeifer BA, Krag MH, Johnson C. Repair of failed transpedicle screw fixation. A biomechanical study comparing polymethylmethacrylate, milled bone, and matchstick bone reconstruction. *Spine* 1994;**19**:350–3.
109. Law M, Tencer AF, Anderson PA. Caudo-cephalad loading of pedicle screws: mechanisms of loosening and methods of augmentation. *Spine* 1993;**18**:2438–43.
110. Okuyama K, Abe E, Suzuki T, et al. Influence of bone mineral density on pedicle screw fixation: a study of pedicle screw fixation augmenting posterior lumbar interbody fusion in elderly patients. *Spine Journal* 2001;**1**:402–7.
111. Essens S, Sacs BL, Drezyin V. Complications associated with the technique of pedicle screw fixation: a selected survey of ABC members. *Spine* 1993;**18**:2231–9.
112. Zindrick MR, Wiltse LL, Widell EH, et al. A biomechanical study of intrapeduncular screw fixation in the lumbosacral spine. *Clinical Orthopaedics and Related Research* 1986;**203**:99–112.
113. Zdeblick TA, Kunz DN, Cooke ME, McCabe R. Pedicle screw pullout strength. Correlation with insertional torque. *Spine* 1993;**18**:1673–6.
114. Krag MH, Beynnon BD, Pope MH, et al. An internal fixator for posterior application to short segments of the thoracic, lumbar, or lumbosacral spine. Design and testing. *Clinical Orthopaedics and Related Research* 1986;**203**:75–98.
115. Tan JS, Bailey CS, Dvorak MF, et al. Cement augmentation of vertebral screws enhances the interface strength between interbody device and vertebral body. *Spine* 2007;**32**:334–41.
116. Bérard A, Bravo G, Gauthier P. Metaanalysis of the effectiveness of physical activity for the prevention of bone loss in postmenopausal women. *Osteoporosis International* 1997;**7**:331–7.
117. Sinaki M, Itoi E, Wahner HW, et al. Stronger back muscles reduce the incidence of vertebral fractures: a prospective 10 year follow-up of postmenopausal women. *Bone* 2002;**30**:836–41.
118. Wolff I, Croonenborg van JJ, Kemper HCG, et al. The effect of exercise training programs on bone mass: a metaanalysis of published controlled trials in pre- and postmenopausal women. *Osteoporosis International* 1999;**9**:1–12.
119. Becker S. Physiotherapeutic treatment after balloon kyphoplasty – aspects and concepts. In: Becker S, Ogon M (eds). *Balloon Kyphoplasty*. Vienna, Austria: Springer, 2008:148–60.

Spondylolysis and spondylolisthesis

ISTVÀN HOVORKA

Definitions	1048	Degenerative spondylolisthesis	1054
Spondylolisthesis by isthmic lysis	1048	References	1056

DEFINITIONS

Spondylolisthesis describes the condition when a vertebra shifts forward on the underlying vertebra. The shifting of vertebrae can be produced by specific and quite rare situations, such as tumours of the posterior arch or traumatic injuries as listed in the aetiological classification of Wiltse[1] (Table 91.1).

However it usually happens under two principal pathologies:

- by degenerative erosion of the articular surface leading to degenerative spondylolisthesis;
- by a fatigue fracture of the posterior arch occurring in the pars interarticularis. The pars fracture without displacement is named spondylolysis, and if the vertebra shifts, spondylolisthesis by isthmic lysis.

Table 91.1 Five-part Wiltse classification system of the aetiology of spondylolisthesis

Type I	Congenital (dysplastic)
Type II	Isthmic (defect in pars interarticularis)
	IIA spondylolytic (acquired stress fracture of pars region)
	IIB pars elongation (consolidated pars fracture)
	IIC acute traumatic fracture (exceptional)
Type III	Degenerative
Type IV	Post-traumatic (acute fractures of the posterior elements beside the pars region)
Type V	Pathological (destruction of the posterior elements from bone disease or iatrogenic)

SPONDYLOLISTHESIS BY ISTHMIC LYSIS

Epidemiology

Epidemiological studies note a 6% prevalence of isthmic spondylolisthesis[2,3] in the general population without any significant clinical differences in terms of symptomatology with the non-affected population.

Sports-related prevalence is much higher. Rossi[4] found isthmic abnormalities in 16.7% of a population of 1430 young athletes (15–27 years), with 15.7% of them with a confirmed isthmic lysis. Spondylolisthesis (mainly grade I) is associated with lysis in 32% of cases. The prevalence depends on the type of sport, i.e. 63% prevalence in divers, 36% prevalence in weight-lifting athletes, 33% prevalence in combat athletes and 22% prevalence in players of other sports. In addition, Jackson et al.[5] found a prevalence of 32.8% in gymnasts.

Aetiology

The congenital theory of the aetiopathology proposed initially is no longer accepted.

There is a *microtraumatic orig*in of an isthmic lysis.[6–8] Isthmic lysis occurs as a result of repeated stress applied on the antero-inferior cortical bone of the isthmus.

An acute traumatic origin of a spondylolisthesis – although claimed by some patients and thus creating medico-legal problems – is very rare since the pedicular and isthmic region represents the strongest area of the vertebrae.

There is a *hereditary predisposition* to the condition and a strong association with spina bifida occulta. Isthmic lysis occurs in 5–6% of the white adult population versus only 3% in the black adult population; it is four to five times greater in Eskimos, with a frequency up to 60% in some consanguine Inuit populations.[9] Wiltse et al.[8] found a family predisposition in 26% of the study population, Fredrikson et al.[2] report a family frequency of 17–34%. The hereditary transmission seems to be mulitfactorial.

Isthmic lysis never occurs in newborns, nor does it appear before walking age; moreover, it does not occur in apes who are able to stand up but lack lumbar lordosis. Age also has an effect on the prevalence and development of an isthmic lysis.[2] It occurs very rarely before 2 years of age,[10] but can reach 3% in the population between 2 and 6 years,[7] and 5–6% between 5 and 7 years, the same frequency as in the adult population.[11] The critical age for the appearance of an isthmic lysis appears to be between 5 and 7 years of age, when the child is *standing* and lumbar lordosis has already been acquired.

The high prevalence in cases of certain sporting activities can also be explained by hyperlordosis.

Pathomechanism

The isthmic defect happens as a result of compression caused by the lower articular process of the superior vertebra on the isthmic region in hyperlordosis (Fig. 91.1). This 'guillotine' mechanism is based on the anatomical constraints described by Louis.[12] The isthmus of L5 is more horizontal than on upper levels. During lumbar hyperextension movements, the L5 isthmus is caught between the L4 inferior and S1 superior articular processes. This results in a shear stress within the isthmus. A large inferior articular process of the upper vertebra represents an anatomical anomaly that results in a hyperextension stress force on the pars interarticularis.[12]

More recently, the relationship between pelvic parameters in regards to sagittal balance, including pelvic incidence and spondylolisthesis, has been reported.[13]

For Vidal and Marnay,[14] an isthmic lysis can be the consequence of an anteroposterior imbalance, and the secondary spondylolisthesis is a readjustment mechanism to adapt to a postural balance. In the standing position, the ideal balance line passes between the midline of the centres of the femoral heads in front of the L5 vertebral body. In some cases sagittal imbalance is observed with L4 and L5 in front of this line, with higher loads on the isthmus and a compensatory hyperlordosis. These subjects present with a higher risk of isthmic lysis due to a fatigue fracture.

Once a fracture occurs, the stability of the spine is compromised. The posterior articulations can no longer play their stabilizing role, and anterior listhesis of the cephalad vertebra becomes possible. This, along with the degree of sacral slope will have an impact on the stresses experienced at the level of the isthmic defect. Depending on the strength of the disc, which is the only regional stabilizer, vertebral slippage may commence.

If the shift is significant, it may disturb the sagittal balance; in addition, the displaced vertebra may result in localized kyphosis.

There are two compensation mechanisms.

- The first is progressive retroversion of the pelvis around the femoral heads by compensatory contraction of the iliocrural muscles. However, the more the pelvis is in retroversion, the greater the anterior force vector on the slipped vertebra, resulting in the potential for further slippage (Fig. 91.2).

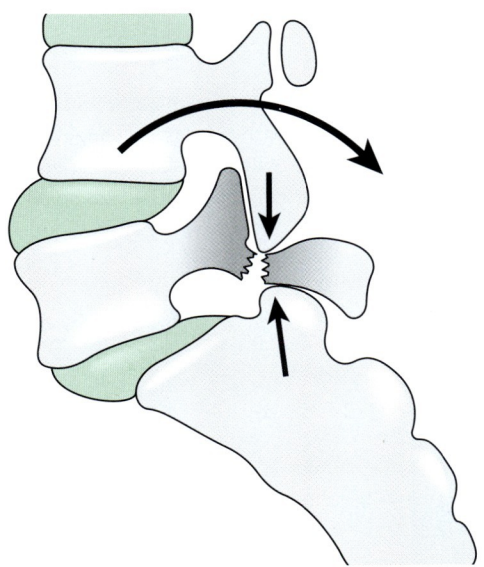

Figure 91.1   Mechanism causing isthmic lysis.

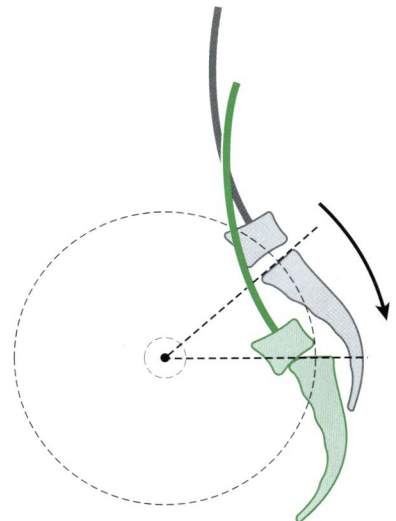

Figure 91.2   Pelvic retroversion caused by the vertebral shift.

- The second mechanism is a compensatory hyperlordosis to correct the kyphosis caused by the slipped vertebra. The stress of hyperlordosis generally focuses on the posterior articular processes with continued stress on the isthmic lysis that prevents any consolidation, and later promoting the development of articular pathology at this level. The hyperlordosis may adversely affect the superior disc, resulting in symptomatic degeneration. Hyperlordosis is sometimes associated with a compensatory retrolisthesis at the supradjacent level to compensate for sagittal imbalance.

Vertebral slippage usually occurs at an age when growth is not yet complete. The growth of the involved vertebrae will be affected by this process, with those vertebral elements exposed to excessive forces growing less than non-stressed vertebra. This explains the development of 'dysplastic forms', coupled with greater instability and difficulty in reducing a slippage surgically or with casting (Fig. 91.3).

The fact that the vertebral canal is enlarged with vertebral slippage mediates against the presence of any significant central canal stenosis. On the other hand, the foramens incur major distortion, which worsens with accelerated disc degeneration. Neurological symptomatology is often manifested via root compression involving the L5 nerve root (spondylolisthesis L5–S1), resulting in possible weakness of the foot extensors. This is often the result of a compression, not axial or anteroposterior load, and therefore may be countered via distraction of the contiguous vertebrae and not by simple decompression or anteroposterior translational reduction (Fig. 91.4).

There are cases where slipping is asymmetrical, resulting in secondary scoliosis representing a complex therapeutic challenge.

Diagnosis

Clinical examination may demonstrate on palpation a step-off between adjacent spinous processes, discomfort on palpation in the midline and paramedian location, neurological signs, and contractures of the quadriceps and ischiocrural muscles.

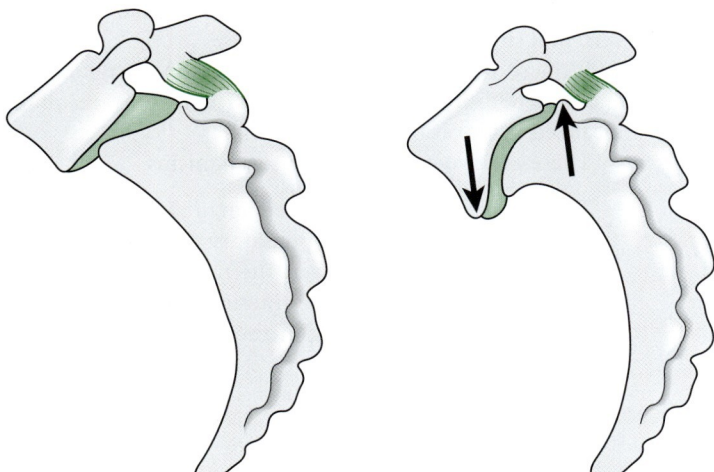

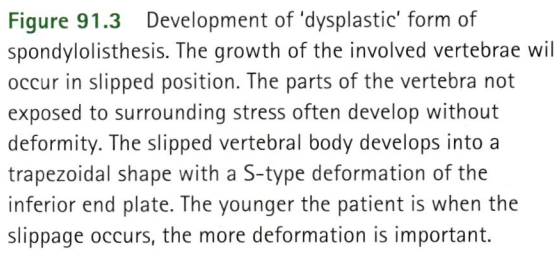

Figure 91.3 Development of 'dysplastic' form of spondylolisthesis. The growth of the involved vertebrae will occur in slipped position. The parts of the vertebra not exposed to surrounding stress often develop without deformity. The slipped vertebral body develops into a trapezoidal shape with a S-type deformation of the inferior end plate. The younger the patient is when the slippage occurs, the more deformation is important.

Figure 91.4 Foraminal stenosis due to listhesis with dysplastic changes. Posterior decompression may be ineffective, and intervertebral distraction can be necessary.

Imaging studies can demonstrate the degree of slippage and characteristic morphological changes to the involved vertebra such as a trapezoidal shape of the slipped vertebra.

A standing lateral long cassette plain radiograph demonstrates the patient's sagittal balance. CT with reconstruction can visualize the presence of isthmiclysis as well as the degree of foraminal stenosis (Fig. 91.5).

MRI is essential for surgical planning as it can demonstrate neurological compression with the foramen and the presence of disc degeneration. The transverse cuts may provide an image that gives the appearance of a herniated disc (Fig. 91.6). A disc herniation is rare in cases of isthmic spondylolisthesis, and a discectomy alone in this environment may worsen symptomatic instability.

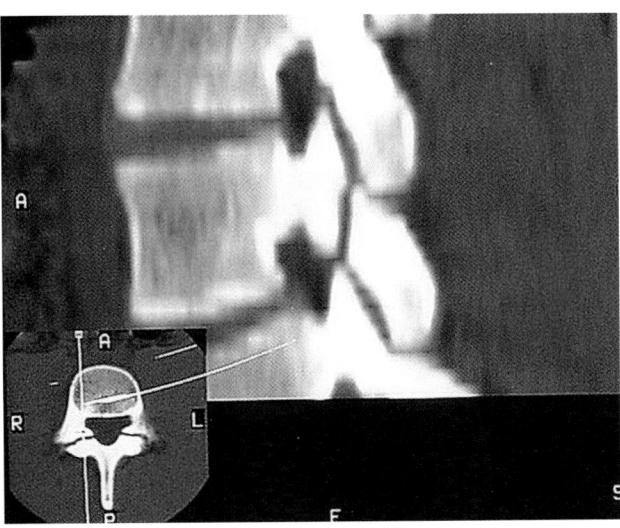

Figure 91.5 Paramedian CT scan reconstruction of a patient with spondylolisthesis showing the pars fracture.

In some cases, when seeking the source of pain, infiltration tests can be performed targeting the lysis level, or the supra-adjacent articulation.

Bone scintigraphy demonstrates increased activity if the pars fracture is recent.

Classification

The Meyerding classification[15] is the most popular (Fig. 91.7), describing vertebral shifting in relationship to the inferior end plate.

Natural history

Isthmic lysis is often discovered in young athletes. The characteristic symptom is low back pain that increases during training. Initial radiographs may be normal, but soon a perceived sclerosis of the isthmus develops. This is the first sign of isthmus fatigue. In the beginning, the isthmic lysis is unilateral but may progress to bilateral. The fracture is often not painful, and a history of trauma is rare. Healing may occur spontaneously following microfractures, resulting in lengthening of the isthmic region. Progression of a slip is unlikely after adolescence.

If pain develops and persists because of the pars fracture before disc degeneration occurs, surgical reconstruction may be a viable option. In the vast majority of cases the patient is not symptomatic or symptoms abate with activity restriction. As the disc is under considerable stress at the level of slippage, early degeneration may ensue. This may result in low back discomfort. Often symptomatic disc degeneration persists, potentially requiring surgical intervention, whereas in its absence patients can often live normally and have no difficulties

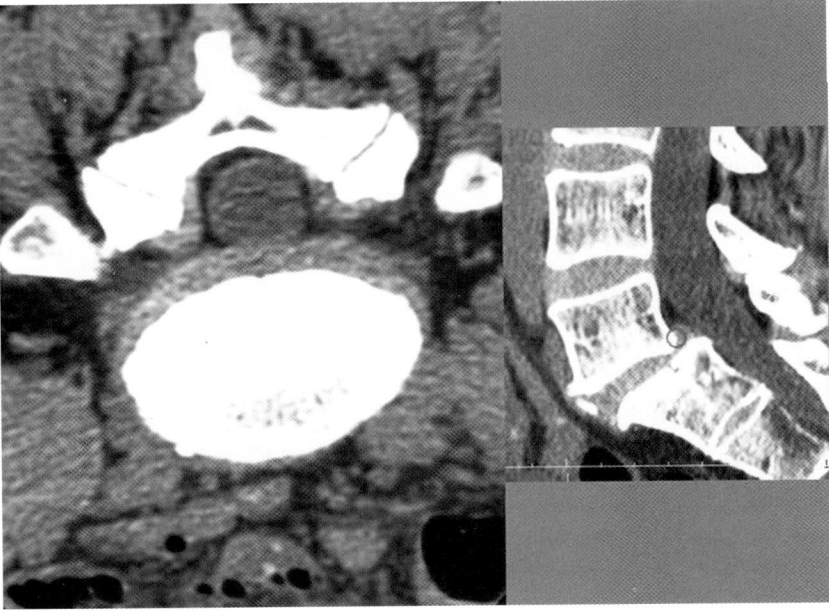

Figure 91.6 Scanner cut localized to the slipped level. The bulging disc is a result of the slippage, not of a real discal hernia.

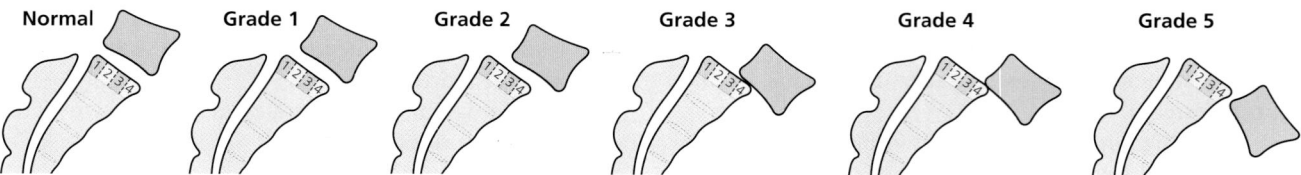

Figure 91.7 Meyerding classification of spondylolisthesis.

with their daily living activities. Radicular pain or neurological deficit related to foraminal stenosis may also require surgical intervention following failure of conservative treatment.

Conservative treatment

As disc degeneration is rarely painful, controversy often exists on the most effective management of symptomatic spondylolisthesis. The presence of slippage is by no means synonymous with the need for surgical treatment.

In children, success has been seen with the use of a custom-fit thoracolumbar orthosis or a 'hemi-bermouda' brace immobilizing the lumbosacral junction along with activity cessation for approximately 3 months followed by an organized physical therapy programme.[16] In children, this may allow for the healing of an isthmic lysis if the fracture is recent. This may be followed with bone scintigraphy. If there is increased activity, bracing is a viable option, but it is constraining, and its effectiveness remains modest. In the study of Fujii et al.[17] on 134 patients from 7 to 17 years of age, pars healing could be obtained in 62% at the early stages of a stress fracture, in 8.7% if the pars was actively fracturing, but in 0% of patients if a fracture was mature or at its terminal stage.

Symptomatic treatment with painkillers, anti-inflammatory drugs and injections will not heal the fracture but may limit pain.

Rehabilitation should involve stretching of the quadriceps, fighting against the effects of the constraints of hyperlordosis. Relaxation of the ischiocrural muscles can reduce the need for muscle contracture of the antagonistic muscles, the quadriceps.

If stopping or decreasing sport participation resolves symptoms, the existence of a spondylolisthesis does not justify a ban on all sporting activities. Sports that are recommended include swimming, or any activities that minimize loading of the intervertebral discs or movements in hyperlordosis.

Surgical treatment

Spondylolysis, if it is symptomatic and unresponsive to non-operative treatment in the absence of disc degeneration, may benefit from isthmic reconstruction.

This operation includes at least the resection of the lower part of the inferior articular process of the cephalad vertebra in order to remove the cartilaginous cap present in this region followed by the placement of grafting material to incite an osteosynthesis. To enhance healing, autologous graft in the form of corticocancellous chips can be applied over the contiguous spinous process to the tip of the transverse process to improve the grafting surface area.

Several surgical techniques are available:

- direct screw fixation as described by
- wire-based or wire screw fixation
- screwed hooks with compressive springs
- hooks associated with pedicular screws (Fig. 91.8a)
- pedicular screws with bent rod
- bicortical screw hooks with a transverse connection (Fig. 91.8b).

The results of isthmic reconstruction are usually very poor with up to a 40% incidence of pseudarthrosis and surgical failures. For example with a wire screw technique (modified Scott), Pai et al.[18] reported only a 50% fusion success. The fusion rate reported for the screw hook implants varies from 73% to 91%.[19,20] We have experienced improved fusion success with the bicortical screw hook technique combined with a transverse connector.

In cases of spondylolisthesis, the usual treatment is an instrumented arthrodesis. The objective of this operation is to restore stability and sagittal balance with a possible reduction of the slippage and correction of the kyphosis while ensuring foraminal decompression. Major difficulties exist: besides being a potentially unstable lesion, the surface area for fusion is often compromised (end plates are partly uncovered by each other, and the transverse processes of the slipped vertebrae are often very small and offer only small contact with bone graft). Decompression of the foramen often requires interbody distraction.

The posterior approach allows for foraminal decompression with decompression of the nerve root and resection of the isthmic hook (Gill's procedure), which may be followed with pedicular fixation for stabilization along with bone grafting.

A posterolateral fusion without anterior stabilization in an adult lumbar isthmic spondylolisthesis results in

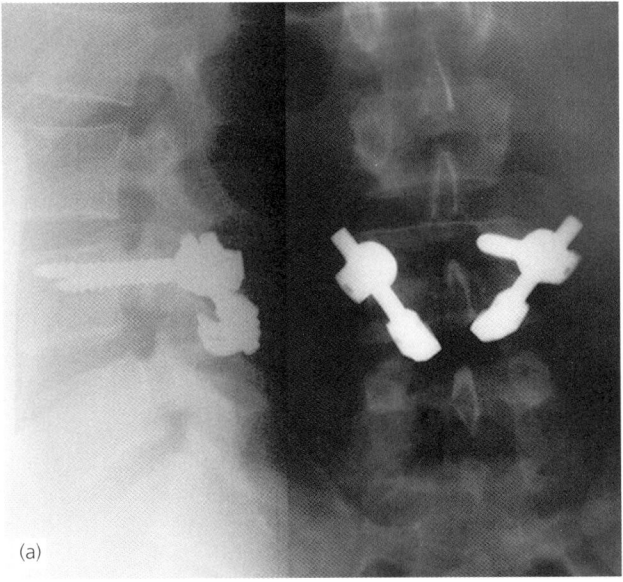

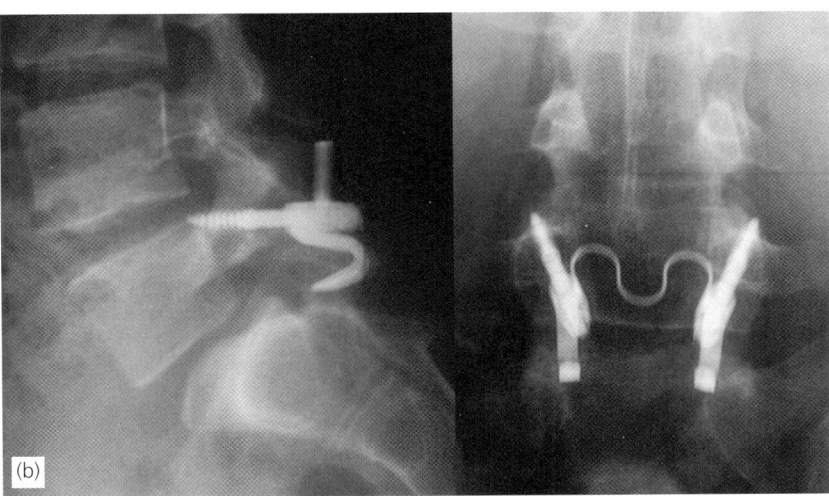

Figure 91.8 Examples of isthmic reconstruction methods. (a) Pedicular screws with hooks; (b) screw hook with transversal connection.

modest improvement over the long term compared with a 1 year exercise programme.[21]

An isolated posterior surgical approach has a reported high failure rate that justifies consideration for a combined anterior interbody fusion. This can be achieved via the introduction of an interbody graft or cages with a posterior lumbar interbody fusion (PLIF) or a transforaminal lumbar interbody fusion (TLIF) approach (Fig. 91.9). In some cases, fixation using a translumbosacral graft may be used. During vertebral reduction great care must be afforded not to compress the roots within the foramen. Also, care during attempted posterior compression to correct localized kyphosis should be taken to avoid nerve injury, especially if anterior distraction is not sufficient. Sometimes a partial sacral dome osteotomy is necessary for adequate correction.

The results are very good in case of a technically well-performed decompression and fusion. This can be explained by the fact that this is a mechanically unstable lesion that may be adequately stabilized with available technology. During the postoperative period, prolonged sitting should be avoided for 3 months so as not to exacerbate local muscular forces, and in the case of poor quality bone a brace is recommended.

The anterior approach is attractive for several reasons: the lordosis is more easily obtained partly by the positioning of the patient. Intervertebral distraction is easier and reduction is more efficient through tension on the non-resected annulus. Preservation of the posterior muscles is an advantage of the posterior approach. Osteosynthesis anteriorly in a stand alone procedure is essential; it is usually performed via application of a plate[22] or the use of transfixing screws.[23]

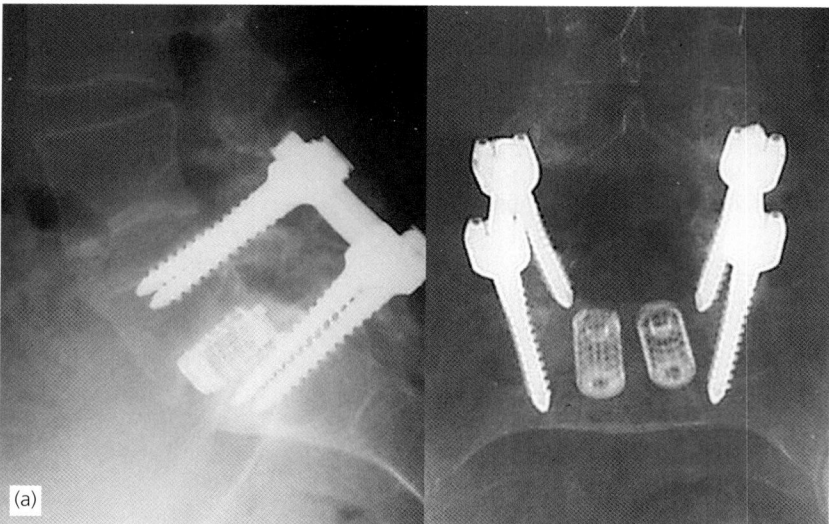
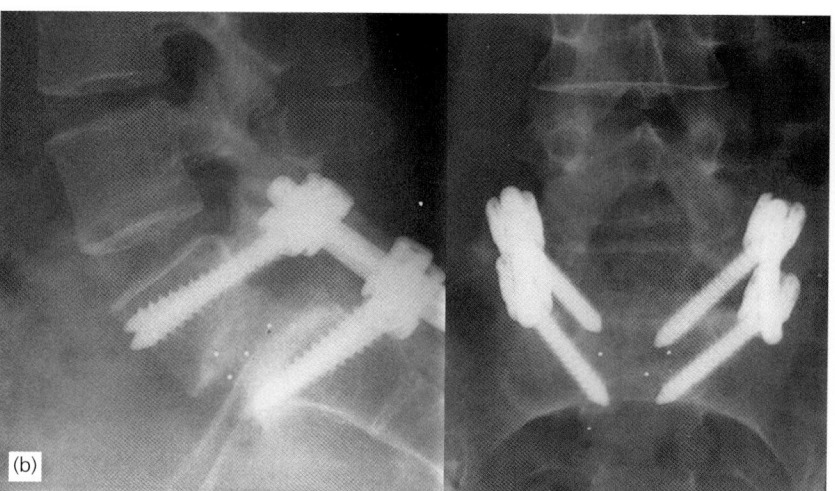
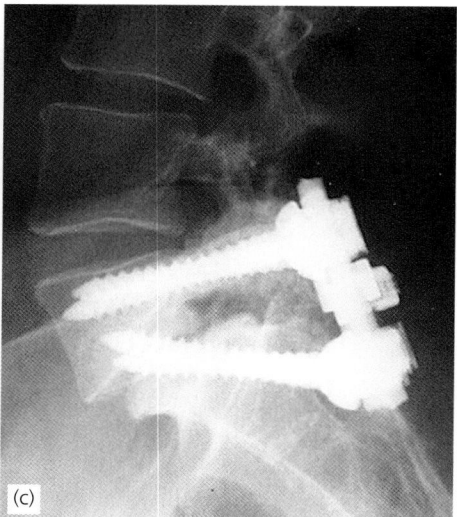

Figure 91.9 Posterior 360° arthrodesis method. (a) Posterior lumbar interbody fusion; (b) transforaminal lumbar interbody fusion; (c) trans-sacrolumbar screws.

The disadvantage of an anterior approach is the potential for retrograde ejaculation in men, and the fact that in some cases the inclination of the disc is so severe that its axis is below the pubic symphysis and access is difficult.

A combined approach may also be proposed to ensure optimum circumferential fixation with superior results to posterior fusion alone;[24] however, this is at the cost of longer and extended surgery. The failure of a posterior approach can be addressed with the addition of an anterior approach and vice versa.

More recently the possibility of circumferential reconstruction without fusion was proposed involving isthmus reconstruction via the posterior approach, followed by the application of a discal prosthesis by the anterior approach.

Simple decompression or discectomy must be avoided in the setting of spondylolisthesis because it may aggravate the presence of instability.

DEGENERATIVE SPONDYLOLISTHESIS

Epidemiology

Degenerative spondylolisthesis occurs with advanced age, more frequently among women.

Pathogenic mechanism

Degenerative slippage is usually the result of degenerative destruction of the posterior joints. Once this occurs the degenerative disc can no longer maintain vertebral relationships and the cephalad vertebra may move forward over the caudal vertebra. During this displacement, the inferior joints of the cephalad vertebrae contract and expand due to instability of the superior articular processes

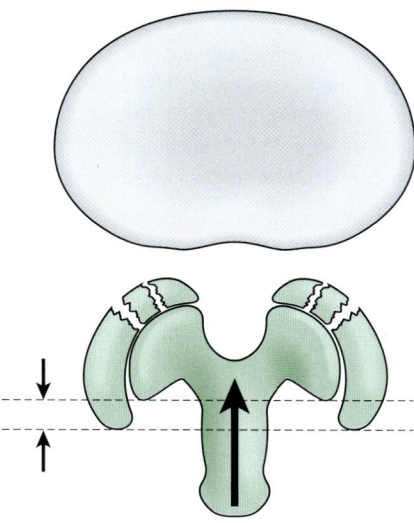

Figure 91.10 Aetiology of the origin of degenerative spondylolisthesis: articular destruction.

of the inferior vertebra, causing compensatory hypertrophy and canal stenosis (Fig. 91.10). This compression is not limited to the discal level, but as a result of remodelling of the posterior joints stenosis may extend into the subarticular and pedicular level. The amount of translation is limited by the length of the annular fibres, which can reach a maximum when disc height is completely lost.

As the shift occurs slowly, the neurological elements have time to adapt, and generally there is no neurological deficit at the time of consultation. Patients suffer from limited walking potential most of the time.

The sagittal orientation of the joints predisposes to this pathological process, which explains its rarity at L5–S1, and its frequency at the L3–L4 and L4–L5 levels.

Diagnosis

Clinical examination is directed by the patient's pain and neurological complaints. Spinal imaging in the standing position with dynamic views may demonstrate instability and displacement. Sagittal balance may be determined with long cassette views. A CT scan or MRI allows for visualization of the neural elements and the degree of neurological compression (Fig. 91.11).

Natural history and pathomechanism

Patients may experience progressive back pain due to loss of sagittal balance and instability. Muscle contractures and spasm due to sagittal imbalance can lead to pain and fatigue. This is especially evident in the gluteal muscles, with pain often localized at the insertion areas of the posterior iliac crest. The perimeter of walking is limited because of both pain and neurological compression. As truncal flexion increases canal diameter, patients often

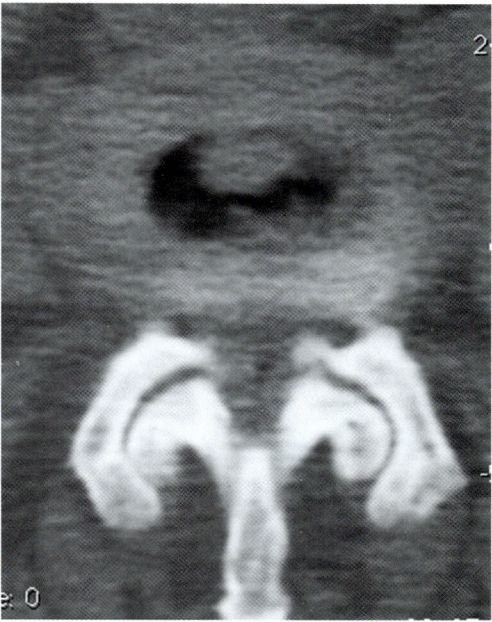

Figure 91.11 CT scanning showing spinal stenosis due to degenerative spondylolisthesis with facet hypertrophy.

bend more and more at the waist leading to imbalance and more localized vertebral kyphosis, with more pain and limited walking capacity. Radicular pain is caused initially by the central canal, but with further slippage foraminal compression may occur.

Spontaneous intervertebral fusion does not occur in this spinal disorder regardless of the advanced stage of degeneration.

In advanced stages of degeneration with stenosis, walking ability often becomes progressively compromised.

Conservative treatment

Medical treatment can reduce pain initially in the vast majority of patients. Epidural steroids are also a popular means of treatment for associated sciatica. Brace immobilization provides support and reduces muscle contractures; however, if it is well tolerated, patients quickly become complacent with its routine use. This treatment should be limited only to painful crises. Conservative treatment is often successful in the majority of patients. If unsuccessful, especially in the presence of a neurological deficit, intermittent claudication or vesicorectal disorder, surgical intervention is useful to address these issues.[25]

Surgical treatment

An isolated decompression should be avoided because it increases instability and makes a salvage secondary fusion more difficult and less likely to improve outcome.

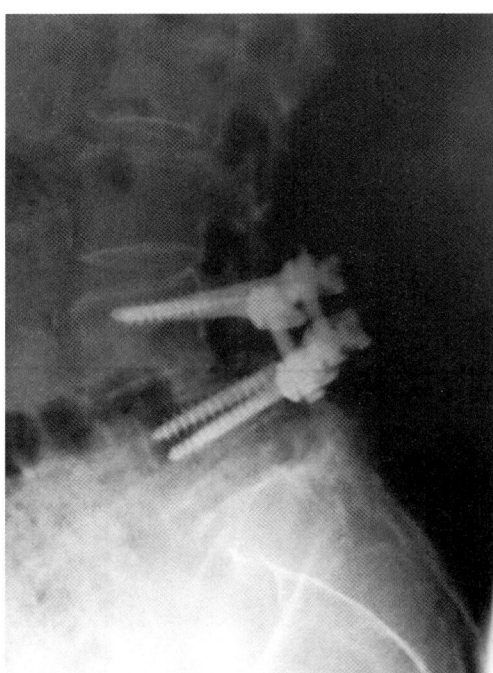

Figure 91.12 Surgical treatment by posterior approach and posterior stabilization.

An arthrodesis without instrumentation combined with a limited decompression is a viable option as the keystone of treatment is decompression associated with posterior arthrodesis. Decompression relieves radicular symptoms and neurogenic claudication, whereas fusion attempts to relieve back pain through the elimination of instability. The goals of instrumentation are to promote fusion and to correct deformity. Solid fusion produces better long-term outcomes than other procedures.[26]

The addition of an interbody arthrodesis improves stability, but makes the technical aspects of the operation more difficult, and is not always necessary since the area available for contact with the bone graft is greater in the absence of pars fracture (Fig. 91.12).

PLIF and TLIF techniques offer similarly excellent results, but TLIF is simpler to perform.[27]

Surgical results are often good as long as an adequate decompression is performed along with a stable fusion.

REFERENCES

1. Wiltse LLNP, MacNab I Classification of spondylolisthesis and spondylolysis. *Clinical Orthopaedics* 1976;**117**:17–22.
2. Fredrickson BE, Baker D, McHolick WJ, et al. The natural history of spondylolysis and spondylolisthesis. *Journal of Bone and Joint Surgery (America)* 1984;**66**:699–707.
3. Osterman K, Schlenzka D, Poussa M, et al. Isthmic spondylolisthesis in symptomatic and asymptomatic subjects, epidemiology, and natural history with special reference to disk abnormality and mode of treatment. *Clinical Orthopaedics and Related Research* 1993;65–70.
4. Rossi F. Spondylolysis, spondylolisthesis and sports. *Journal of Sports Medicine and Physical Fitness* 1978;**18**:317–40.
5. Jackson DW, Wiltse LL, Cirincoine RJ, Spondylolysis in the female gymnast. *Clinical Orthopaedics and Related Research* 1976:68–73.
6. Farfan HF, Osteria V, Lamy C. The mechanical etiology of spondylolysis and spondylolisthesis. *Clinical Orthopaedics and Related Research* 1976:40–55.
7. Pfeil E. [Experimental studies on the etiology of spondylolysis]. *Zeitschrift für Orthopädie und ihre Grenzgebiete* 1971;**109**:231–8.
8. Wiltse LL, Widell EH, Jr, Jackson DW. Fatigue fracture: the basic lesion is isthmic spondylolisthesis. *Journal of Bone and Joint Surgery (America)* 1975;**57**:17–22.
9. Semon RL, Spengler D. Significance of lumbar spondylolysis in college football players. *Spine* 1981;**6**:172–4.
10. Rowe GG, Roche MB. The etiology of separate neural arch. *Journal of Bone and Joint Surgery (America)* 1953;**35A**:102–10.
11. Porter RW, Hibbert CS. Symptoms associated with lysis of the pars interarticularis. *Spine* 1984;**9**:755–8.
12. Louis R. MC stabilisation chirurgicale avec réduction des spondylolyses et des spondylolisthésis. *International Orthopaedics* 1977;**1**:215–25.
13. Roussouly P, Gollogly S, Berthonnaud E, et al. Sagittal alignment of the spine and pelvis in the presence of L5-S1 isthmic lysis and low-grade spondylolisthesis. *Spine* 2006;**31**:2484–90.
14. Vidal J, Marnay T. [Morphology and anteroposterior body equilibrium in spondylolisthesis L5-S1]. *Revue de chirurgie orthopédique et réparatrice de l'appareil moteur* 1983;**69**:17–28.
15. Meyerding H. Spondylolisthesis. *Surgery, Gynecology & Obstetrics* 1932;**54**:371.
16. Kurd MF, Patel D, Norton R, et al. Nonoperative treatment of symptomatic spondylolysis. *Journal of Spinal Disorders & Techniques* 2007;**20**:560–4.
17. Fujii K, Katoh S, Sairyo K, et al. Union of defects in the pars interarticularis of the lumbar spine in children and adolescents. The radiological outcome after conservative treatment. *Journal of Bone and Joint Surgery (British)* 2004;**86**:225–31.
18. Pai VS, Hodgson B, Pai V. Repair of spondylolytic defect with a cable screw reconstruction. *International Orthopaedics* 2008;**32**:121–5.
19. Debusscher F, Troussel S. Direct repair of defects in lumbar spondylolysis with a new pedicle screw hook fixation: clinical, functional and CT-assessed study. *European Spine Journal* 2007;**16**:1650–8.
20. Hefti FSW, Morscher E. Repair of lumbar spondylolysis with a hook-screw. *International Orthopaedics* 1992;**16**:81–5.
21. Ekman P, Moller H, Hedlund R. The long-term effect of posterolateral fusion in adult isthmic spondylolisthesis: a randomized controlled study. *Spine Journal* 2005;**5**:36–44.

22. Aunoble S, Hoste D, Donkersloot P, et al. Video-assisted ALIF with cage and anterior plate fixation for L5-S1 spondylolisthesis. *Journal of Spinal Disorders & Techniques* 2006;**19**:471-6.
23. Wenger M, Vogt E, Markwalder TM. Double-segment Wilhelm Tell technique for anterior lumbar interbody fusion in unstable isthmic spondylolisthesis and adjacent segment discopathy. *Journal of Clinical Neuroscience* 2006;**13**:265-9.
24. Swan J, Hurwitz E, Malek F, et al. Surgical treatment for unstable low-grade isthmic spondylolisthesis in adults: a prospective controlled study of posterior instrumented fusion compared with combined anterior-posterior fusion. *Spine Journal* 2006;**6**:606-14.
25. Matsunaga S, Ijiri K, Hayashi K. Nonsurgically managed patients with degenerative spondylolisthesis: a 10- to 18-year follow-up study. *Journal of Neurosurgery* 2000;**93**:194-8.
26. Sengupta DK, Herkowitz HN. Degenerative spondylolisthesis: review of current trends and controversies. *Spine* 2005;**30**:S71-81.
27. Yan DL, Pei FX, Li J, et al. Comparative study of PILF and TLIF treatment in adult degenerative spondylolisthesis. *European Spine Journal* 2008;**17**:1311-6.

92

Tumours of the spine

STEPHAN BECKER, JASON BENG TECK LIM, VOLKER SCHIRRMACHER, HIMANSHU SHARMA

Introduction	1058	NEW TREATMENTS FOR SPINE METASTASES	1065
TUMOUR DIAGNOSIS	1058	Epidemiology	1065
Clinical presentation	1058	Location of spinal metastases	1065
Work-up	1059	Overall survival rates	1065
Tumour biopsy	1060	Surgical approaches	1066
Staging	1060	Modern additional cancer therapy	1068
Treatment principles	1061	Immuno-oncology	1068
TYPES OF SPINE TUMOURS	1061	References	1069
References	1064		

INTRODUCTION

Tumours of the spine can be either malignant or benign and can occur at all levels of the vertebral column. Early identification and appropriate management is crucial in order to improve the patient's quality of life and outcome. Malignant tumours of the spine are either primary tumours or secondary metastases. Metastases account for more than 95% of all spinal tumours, as the spine is one of the most frequent sites for metastasis.[1-3]

Metastatic spread to the spine from distant primary tumour sites takes place by three main mechanisms, which are (1) direct extension, (2) retrograde venous flow and (3) seeding of tumour emboli via the haematogenous route.[4] Both primary and metastatic tumours tend to originate in the vertebral body, involving either one or both pedicles. Other common sites affected by metastases include the pelvic bones and proximal ends of the femur and humerus, all of which contain haematogenous marrow receiving good blood supply.

Primary cancers that most commonly metastasize to the spine are mainly adenocarcinomas, arising from the breast (35%), lung (10%), kidney (5%), thyroid (2%) and prostate (30%). The first four are often seen as osteoclastic, lytic lesions on radiographs whereas prostate metastases are predominantly osteoblastic, sclerotic lesions.[5] Apart from these causes, it is important to note that any other tumour can also metastasize to the bone, such as colorectal carcinoma, which occurs in approximately 10% of metastases.[6] The relationship between the osteoclastic and osteoblastic remodelling processes determines whether a predominantly lytic, sclerotic or mixed pattern is seen on radiographs.[7,8]

TUMOUR DIAGNOSIS

CLINICAL PRESENTATION

Non-mechanical back pain and neurological deficits are the most common presenting features of spinal tumours. They usually arise from pathological fractures, nerve root or spinal cord compression, or invasion by the expanding vertebral cortex and surrounding tissues. But they can occur in patients with longstanding mechanical back pain. Spinal tumours often cause progressive and persistent non-mechanical back pain, night pain and well-localized pain on palpation and percussion over involved areas. If there is severe pain on walking, it indicates that bone destruction has progressed to the extent that a pathological fracture is imminent. In paediatric patients, the two most common reasons for presentations include pain and spinal deformities.[9,10]

Severe kyphosis can occur as a result of vertebral collapse. Scoliosis has been associated with benign tumours such as osteoid osteoma and osteoblastoma, which could also have other symptoms such as localized pain, muscle spasms and limited range of movement.[11–13] Early identification of spinal deformities allows conservative management, such as bracing, whereas a persistent and structural deformity may require surgical correction.

Neurological signs are very variable and they can range from slight weakness to complete paraplegia. There can be radicular signs from compression or invasion of nerve roots, or saddle anaesthesia/sphincter disturbance involving the cauda equina. The clinical signs to examine for are:[14]

- reduced range of spinal movement
- reduced straight leg raise
- neurological deficit (sensory, motor, reflex impairment), such as distribution of paraesthesias or sensory loss, reduced ankle and great toe dorsiflexion, knee and ankle reflexes.

Neoplastic disease can often be differentiated from other benign conditions such as herniated lumbar disc prolapse by a progressive and persistent pain that does not respond to rest. Also, a rapid progression of symptoms over months signifies a more aggressive, malignant tumour, whereas symptoms progressing over years are typical of a slow-growing and, often, benign tumour. Occasionally, a spinal tumour can present as a palpable lump.

Other presentations of bone metastases include hypercalcaemia, which manifests as bone pain, renal calculi and peptic ulcers. This is often due to lytic metastasis and also paraneoplastic syndrome that produces parathyroid hormone-related protein.[15]

WORK-UP

It is important to consider several differential diagnoses for the back pain and neurological symptoms. The investigations should be based upon relevant history-taking, physical examination of the breast, thyroid and rectum and stool guaiac to find the source of the primary tumour.[16,17]

The aims of investigations are:

- Identifying the tumour (benign or malignant):
  - history
  - radiology
  - biopsy.
- Staging of the tumour:
  - clinical
  - pathological.

Basic investigations for any spinal tumour include the following:

- Blood test:
  - full blood count
  - erythrocyte sedimentation rate and C-reactive protein to help distinguish between neoplastic and infectious processes
  - urea and electrolytes, noting particularly raised calcium levels, which can indicate neoplastic bone processes
  - serum and urine protein electrophoresis to evaluate the likelihood of multiple myeloma or plasmacytoma; if positive, bone survey and bone marrow aspirate.
- Plain radiography of the spine should be done as the most basic investigation to evaluate the trabecular architecture of the spine. Several radiological views, such as anteroposterior, lateral and oblique views of symptomatic spinal segments, can demonstrate abnormalities in up to 90% of patients with spinal neoplasm.
- Renal ultrasound.
- Chest with/without abdominal CT.
- Bone scan.
- MRI.
- Myelography.

The following points should be considered while interpreting the findings on any available imaging modalities:[18,19]

- Is the lesion lytic or sclerotic?
- What is the tumour doing to the bone?
- What is the bone doing to the tumour?
- Is the cortex intact, eroded or broken? Look for any pathological fractures or surrounding soft-tissue involvement.
- Is there Codman's triangle, suggesting periosteal lifting?
- Is there an onion skin appearance for fusiform tumours?
- Is there sun-ray calcification?

Radionuclide bone scan

Radionuclide imaging is useful in detecting:

- lesions before they become apparent
- the presence of any 'skip' lesions
- metastases
- recurrence of tumour after instituting treatment.

It has the advantage of being far more sensitive than plain radiographs in picking up early bone tumours, as evidence of bony destruction is not shown on plain radiographs until about 30–50% involvement of the trabecular bone.

Areas of increased uptake, or *hot spots*, denote areas of increased osteoblastic activity, particularly from prostate carcinoma. Bone metastases usually appear as multiple foci of increased activity, although they occasionally manifest as areas of decreased uptake.[20]

Although bone scan is a very sensitive test and often confers reassurance to patients when negative, it must be noted that false negatives do occur. This is particularly true in cases of *multiple myeloma*, in which lytic bone lesions may not be detected unless there is an associated pathological fracture.[21,22] Thus, it is necessary to gather further information from the patient's history or from other investigations such as a CT scan.[23]

Computed tomography scan

CT scan provides diagnostic information on small tumours that is early, before extensive bone destruction or intramedullary extension has occurred and before cortical erosion has occurred causing pathological fracture.

It provides unsurpassed imaging of bony architecture, and is also useful in the staging of the spine neoplasm by showing metastases to distant organs such as the lungs, liver and lymph nodes. It can be used for CT-guided needle biopsy of suspected metastases.

Magnetic resonance imaging

MRI is very sensitive for detecting soft-tissue tumour spread and any neurological involvement of the spinal cord, cauda equina or nerve roots without the need for intrathecal contrast.

With gadolinium enhancement, MRI can differentiate between osteoporotic and metastatic compression fractures of the vertebral body. The MRI features that are suggestive of malignancy include:

- convex posterior cortex
- epidural mass
- diffuse low-intensity T_1 signal within the vertebral body
- high or inhomogeneous signal intensity on T_2-weighted or after gadolinium injection.

Myelography

This was previously the gold standard for spinal imaging but it has largely been replaced by MRI. However, if MRI is contraindicated, myelography with post-myelogram CT may provide the same information as MRI.

TUMOUR BIOPSY

Despite all the imaging modalities available, biopsy is the definitive way to make a histological diagnosis of the tumour type to allow formulation of a treatment plan. However, there are some benign lesions with characteristic radiological features which may render biopsy unnecessary.

Several biopsy techniques may be used:

- fine-needle aspiration or trocar biopsy
- open, incisional biopsy
- open, excisional biopsy.

The choice of the technique depends on the location and extent of the tumour. Some important features in obtaining the biopsy include:

- The most direct route to the tumour should be taken as it has the least risk of tumour 'seeding' into adjacent compartments.
- The biopsy tract should also be in line with the future incision site for surgical resection of the tumour so that the biopsy tract can be excised with the specimen *en bloc*.
- Meticulous haemostasis must be obtained owing to the possibility of tumour spread and catastrophic haemorrhage particularly with renal cell metastases, which are highly vascular.
- A drain must be placed to prevent haematoma formation as this can pass tumour tissue through the soft tissues and seed into adjacent compartments.
- The drain should exit the skin in line with the incision, thus allowing excision together with the final specimen.

STAGING

Surgical staging is appropriate only after the diagnosis has been established and oncological staging has been determined. The main aims of surgical staging are to determine the surgical margins of resection and to facilitate future communication regarding treatment data and results.

Enneking system of staging

The Enneking system of surgical staging is described in Chapter 79.

Weinstein–Boriani–Biagini classification

A more practical approach for surgical staging of spinal tumours based on the principles of the Enneking system has been described by Weinstein, Boriani and Biagini.[19]

This system divides the transverse extension of a vertebral tumour into 12 radiating zones, numbered 1–12 in clockwise order, and into five layers (A–E; from the paravertebral extraosseous region to the dural involvement). The tumour location is defined further by the involvement of six areas:

A	Extraosseous soft tissue
B	Intraosseous (superficial)
C	Intraosseous (deep)
D	Extraosseous (extra-dural)
E	Extraosseous (intra-dural)
F	Metastasis

Tomita classification of spinal metastases

The Tomita classification built upon the Enneking system by incorporating a description of the affected anatomic site and the extent of metastasis. The tumour is categorized as involving one or more of the following:

1. the vertebral body
2. one or both pedicles
3. the lamina and spinous process
4. the epidural canal
5. the paravertebral area
6. adjacent vertebrae
7. skip lesions.

The lesions are then further subdivided into intra-compartmental (types 1–3) or extracompartmental (types 4–6). Multiple or skip lesions are designated as Tomita type 7. Resection of tumour can be attempted for types 1–3 if *en bloc* excision is possible. However, for types 4–6, intralesional debulking or total excision may be attempted using the posterior or combined approaches. For type 7, the only surgical option would be a posterior decompression and stabilization. This is the traditional teaching; more recent methods are covered later in this chapter.

Tokuhashi score

The Tokuhashi score was developed as an assessment tool to select the most suitable surgical procedure with respect to the predicted prognosis in order to help decision-making in the treatment of patients with spinal metastases. The score consists of six parameters that are used to measure the severity of the disorder:

1. general condition of the patient
2. number of extraspinal bone metastases
3. the number of spinal metastases
4. the number of metastases to major internal organs
5. the primary site of the cancer
6. spinal cord palsy.

Each parameter is rated from 0 to 2, with 0 signifying the worst state. Tokuhashi proposed a survival of ≤3 months for patients with a score of 0–4, a survival of 3–6 months for those with 5–8 points, and a survival of ≥12 months in patients with a total score of ≥9 points. Therefore, he recommended excisional surgery when the total score reached ≥9. Therefore, although all surgical procedures remain palliative by definition, it is important to know the prognosis before making a decision regarding the surgical procedure, which would be either a combined anterior and posterior approach or an isolated posterior instrumentation.

Cody Bunger incorporated the Tomita classification and a modification of the Tokuhashi score to create a more comprehensive algorithm to determine surgical strategy.

TREATMENT PRINCIPLES

The main foci in the treatment of spine tumours are:[26,27]

- *Pain management.* In addition to analgesia, radiotherapy is also effective in controlling pain and has the added benefit of preventing expansion of the lesion. Also anti-epileptic drugs or tricyclic antidepressants are sometimes used in addition to the traditional opioid analgesics and non-steroidal anti-inflammatory drugs (NSAIDs).
- *Symptomatic relief of hypercalcaemia* if present, particularly for lytic metastases. Initial treatment includes intravenous rehydration followed by bisphosphonates to inhibit osteoclastic function.
- *Controlling of local disease.* More information on the principles of surgical resection of tumours is found in Chapter 81.
- *Maintaining mechanical stability of the spine.* There are various methods of achieving mechanical stability, from the traditional posterior instrumentation, anterior and posterior instrumentation to newer techniques that include combined kyphoplasty and instrumentation, which are described below.

TYPES OF SPINE TUMOURS

Primary benign tumours of the spine

BENIGN CHONDROID-FORMING TUMOURS

Chondroid, cartilage-forming tumours have characteristic radiological features showing speckled calcification; they are slow growing with geographic lysis and central calcification.

Osteochondroma

- Constitutes up to 4% of all solitary spine tumours.
- Usually presents in patients aged 20–30 years.
- Frequently seen in the cervical spine.
- Arises in the posterior elements and is referred to as bony exostosis; may be associated with multiple hereditary exostoses.
- May present with neurological deficits and myelopathy.
- Treatment: complete surgical excision to prevent recurrence of the lesion and to rule out sarcomatous changes.

Osteoid osteoma

- Usually presents in children aged 10–20 years with male dominance.
- Common in the spine, most often in the lumbar region, followed by cervical, thoracic and sacral regions (in order of decreasing frequency).
- Predominantly arises in the posterior elements, in the facet joints, pedicles or laminae.

- Typically smaller than 2.0 cm in diameter.
- May present as painful scoliosis or radicular pain, which is often relieved by NSAIDs or aspirin.
- Treatment: conservatively by NSAIDs or aspirin to relieve back pain. Invasive treatments include open or percutaneous CT-guided surgical excision of the nidus. Alternatively, percutaneous radiofrequency ablation of the nidus.

Osteoblastoma

- Usually presents in adults aged 20–30 years with male dominance.
- Common in the spine and equal distribution in cervical, thoracic and lumbar regions.
- Often occurring in the posterior element and can extend to the vertebral body.
- Neurological complications occur in more than 50% of patients and often present with dull localized pain and paraesthesias. Paraparesis or even paralysis may occur.
- Typically larger than 2.0 cm in diameter.
- Treatment: wide local excision with posterior fusion is the treatment of choice if possible. This is because aggressive osteoblastomas have a high recurrence rate without good wide margins. They are not radiosensitive. When complete excision of the osteoblastoma is not feasible, curettage and bone grafting may provide an acceptable long-term result.

Note that scoliosis related to osteoid osteoma and osteoblastoma is often flexible and will usually improve or resolve after the lesion is removed. Instrumentation and fusion of the curve may be required if the scoliosis has been present for a long period and has become structural. Corrective surgery may be planned after the patient has recovered from the tumour surgery and has had a chance to improve spontaneously.

Haemangioma

- Benign vascular tumours of superficial cutaneous or deep intramuscular tissue or bone.
- Common, occurring in approximately 10% of all adults.
- Often asymptomatic and rarely cause deformities and pain.
- Treatment:
  - radiotherapy or vascular embolization are often beneficial
  - if vertebral collapse or neural compression occurs, surgical decompression and reconstruction through an anterior approach are indicated.

Eosinophilic granuloma

- Benign, self-limiting lesions commonly seen in children under the age of 10 years.
- Vertebral involvement occurs in approximately 15% of all cases.
- Treatment:
  - bracing and observation after establishing the diagnosis, usually by trocar biopsy
  - if neurological symptoms are present, either with or without vertebral collapse, the biopsy followed by irradiation and immobilization remains the most widely accepted treatment.

Giant cell tumour

- Benign giant cell tumours of the bone affect adults, usually in the third or fourth decade of life (more often women).
- Spine is the fourth most common site of occurrence; these tumours usually occur in the sacrum, followed by thoracic, cervical and lumbar regions (in order of decreasing frequency).
- Mostly benign, but malignant giant cell tumour can occur in about 5% of cases.
- They have a tendency to recur and there is a small chance of metastases to the lungs.
- Usually present as radicular back pain, but these tumours may be an incidental finding or discovered during a pathological fracture.
- Treatment:
  - CT scan/MRI are particularly important for planning of surgical treatment
  - complete excision with as wide a margin as possible is the key to eradicating these tumours and reducing recurrence
  - anterior/posterior vertebrectomy with an *en bloc* excision, followed by a combined reconstruction with bone cement
  - radiation is usually for surgically unresectable lesions
  - selective arterial embolization can be used for management.

Aneurysmal bone cyst

- These are characteristically multiloculated blood-filled spaces that are not lined by endothelium.
- Typically affect young patients, with 80% occurring in people younger than 20 years.
- Rarely involve the spinal column and usually involve posterior elements of the lumbar spine.
- These tumours demonstrate locally aggressive behaviour, which may extend into adjacent vertebrae, discs, ribs and paravertebral soft tissue.
- Treatment:
  - curettage or, if possible, complete excision, but there is a risk of damage to surrounding vascular or neurological structures
  - these tumours have a high recurrence rate of 20–30% but they can usually be treated by repeated curettage or excision
  - pre-operative embolization therapy and radiation may help to reduce the size of the tumour and decrease the amount of blood loss during surgical excision.

Primary malignant tumours of the spine

CHORDOMA

- One of the most common primary malignant tumours of the spine in adults; usually occurs in the age range 30–70 years.
- These occur almost exclusively in the axial skeleton, most often in the spine and in the sacrococcygeal area.
- They are typically slow-growing tumours, but there is relentless local extension of tumour and they can be very large at the time of presentation.
- Late and rare metastases (5%) but these tumours have an aggressive tendency to recur at the surgical site.
- Present with months or years of gradual onset of pain, numbness, motor weakness and constipation or incontinence.
- Treatment:
  - biopsy of a suspected chordoma through a posterior approach, after all other staging studies are done
  - surgical excision with a wide margin is the only curative procedure as they are generally unresponsive to radiotherapy and chemotherapy
  - a wide margin is crucial to local control and chemotherapy.

OSTEOSARCOMA

- Osteosarcomas of the spine is rare but has a poor prognosis, with median survival following diagnosis ranging from 6 to 18 months, irrespective of surgical approach.
- Typically present in patients in the fourth decade of life and predominantly in men.
- They can be found in all levels of the spine, but usually arise from the vertebral body and commonly occur in the lumbosacral region.
- They usually present as pain and a palpable mass with a varying degree of neurological symptoms (sensory deficits to paresis).
- There is an increased incidence in patients with Paget disease.
- Treatment:
  - combining current adjuvant chemotherapy and radiation therapy together with extensive anterior/posterior resections can improve local control and neurological function with some improved survival.

CHONDROSARCOMA

- One of the most common tumours affecting the spine (7–12% of all spinal tumours), and the thoracic spine is the most common site.
- Usually affect women.
- Slow growing, locally invasive and difficult to eradicate from the spinal column; these tumours have a poor prognosis with the mean survival for all patients with chondrosarcomas being 5.9 years.
- Treatment:
  - resistant to both radiotherapy and chemotherapy
  - complete resection with wide margins is most reliable for local control and cure but this is only possible for one-quarter of patients
  - intralesional resection is another surgical option.

EWING'S SARCOMA

- Most common non-lymphoproliferative primary malignant tumour of the spine in children aged between 10 and 20 years.
- May arise in the spine as a primary or metastatic tumour and more commonly as metastatic foci.
- Common sites include the sacrococcygeal region, lumbar and thoracic spine (in order of decreasing frequency) and rarely in the cervical spine.
- Occur in the centre of the vertebral body but may extend into the posterior elements.
- Treatment:
  - the mainstays of treatment are high-dose radiotherapy and multi-agent chemotherapy, which can achieve local control of the lesion in almost all patients and give a good long-term survival rate
  - surgical treatment is indicated to decompress neurological elements and stabilize the spinal column (thoracic and thoracolumbar laminectomies can be instrumented to prevent kyphosis).

SOLITARY PLASMACYTOMA AND MULTIPLE MYELOMA

- Represent two extremes for the continuum of malignant plasma B-cell lymphoproliferative diseases producing abnormal quantities of immunoglobulins.
- Multiple myeloma is the most common primary malignancy of bone and the spine. It is rapidly progressive and highly lethal, requiring little more than supportive care for spinal involvement.
- A solitary plasmacytoma (constituting only 3% of plasma cell neoplasms) may remain localized for years before eventually evolving to disseminated multiple myeloma with a rapidly lethal course.
- Treatment:
  - plasmacytoma and myeloma are generally sensitive to radiotherapy and chemotherapy
  - surgical treatment is indicated to stabilize the spine and reduce mechanical pain and to decompress neurological elements in patients with rapidly progressive symptoms
  - surgery is also indicated for those with recurrent disease or tumours resistant to radiotherapy
  - patients with plasmacytoma should be monitored for more than 20 years because of the risk of developing multiple myeloma
  - both tumours can be screened by MRI and serum protein electrophoresis to provide the earliest indication of recurrence or dissemination.

Metastatic bone disease of the spine

- The vertebral column is predisposed to metastatic disease because:
  - the vertebral trabecular bone is highly vascularized and its venous drainage is contiguous with that of the thoracic and abdominal viscera and retrograde venous flow allows a variety of tumours to spread to the vertebral body
  - the architectural structure of the red bone marrow of the vertebral body provides a physiologically favourable environment with little barrier to tumour cell expansion of the proximity to common sources of disease.
- Almost any neoplastic disease can have skeletal metastases, but the most common are primary breast, lung, prostate, renal and thyroid malignancy.
- Breast, prostate and renal carcinomas tend to establish spinal metastases early in the disease process, thus patients may need to have intervention to improve function and quality of life.
- Gastrointestinal carcinomas typically metastasize to the visceral organs such as liver and lungs before they produce spinal metastases.
- Patients with breast, prostate, renal, thyroid or gastrointestinal carcinoma may experience extended survivals with treatments that are currently available despite established metastases.
- Patients with multiple myeloma or pulmonary carcinoma typically deteriorate and die soon after metastasis.

REFERENCES

1. Perrin RG. Metastatic tumours of the axial spine. *Current Opinion in Oncology* 1992;**4**:525–32.
2. Weber K, Damron TA, Frassica FJ, Sim FH. Malignant bone tumours. *Instructional Course Lectures* 2008;**57**:673–88.
3. Sundaresan N, Rosen G, Boriani S. Primary malignant tumours of the spine. *Orthopedic Clinics of North America* 2009;**40**:21–36.
4. Peh W. *Imaging in Bone Metastases*. Available from: http://emedicine.medscape.com/article/387840-overview
5. Sama AA. *Spinal Tumors*. Available from: http://emedicine.medscape.com/article/1267223-overview
6. Katoh M, Unakami M, Hara M, Fukuchi S. Bone metastasis from colorectal cancer in autopsy cases. *Journal of Gastroenterology* 1995;**30**:615–18.
7. Imon JM, Kilpatrick SE. Pathology of skeletal metastases. *Orthopedic Clinics of North America* 2000;**31**:537–44, vii–viii.
8. Clines GA, Guise TA. Molecular mechanisms and treatment of bone metastasis. *Expert Reviews in Molecular Medicine* 2008;**10**:e7.
9. Mehlman CT, Crawford AH, McMath JA. Pediatric vertebral and spinal cord tumours: a retrospective study of musculoskeletal aspects of presentation, treatment, and complications. *Orthopedics* 1999;**22**:49–55; discussion 55–6.
10. Fraser RD, Paterson DC, Simpson DA. Orthopaedic aspects of spinal tumours in children. *Journal of Bone and Joint Surgery (British)* 1977;**59**:143–51.
11. Saifuddin A, White J, Sherazi Z, et al. Osteoid osteoma and osteoblastoma of the spine. Factors associated with the presence of scoliosis. *Spine* 1998;**3**:47–53.
12. Pettine KA, Klassen RA. Osteoid-osteoma and osteoblastoma of the spine. *Journal of Bone and Joint Surgery (American)* 1986;**68**(3):354–61.
13. Keim HA, Reina EG. Osteoid-osteoma as a cause of scoliosis. *Journal of Bone and Joint Surgery (American)* 1975;**57**:159.
14. Samanta J, Kendall J, Samanta A. 10-minute consultation: chronic low back pain. *British Medical Journal* 2003;**326**:535.
15. Fitch M, Maxwell C, Ryan C, et al. Bone metastases from advanced cancers: clinical implications and treatment options. *Clinical Journal of Oncology Nursing* 2009;**13**:701–10.
16. Hage WD, Aboulafia AJ, Aboulafia DM. Incidence, location, and diagnostic evaluation of metastatic bone disease. *Orthopedic Clinics of North America* 2000;**31**:515–28, vii.
17. Katagiri H, Takahashi M, Inagaki J, et al. Determining the site of the primary cancer in patients with skeletal metastasis of unknown origin: a retrospective study. *Cancer* 1999;**86**:533–7.
18. Greenspan A. *Orthopedic Imaging: a Practical Approach*, 4th edn. Philadelphia, PA: Lippincott Williams & Wilkins, 2004:529–70.
19. Rodallec MH, Feydy A, Larousserie F, et al. Diagnostic imaging of solitary tumours of the spine: what to do and say. *RadioGraphics* 2008;**28**:1019–41.
20. Love C, Din AS, Tomas MB, et al. Radionuclide bone imaging: an illustrative review. *RadioGraphics* 2003;**23**:341–58.
21. Valat JP, Eveleigh MC, Fouquet B, Born P. Bone scintigraphy in multiple myeloma. *Revue du Rhumatisme et des Maladies Ostéo-articulaires* 1985;**52**:707–11.
22. Leonard RC, Owen JP, Proctor SJ, Hamilton PJ. Multiple myeloma: radiology or bone scanning? *Clinical Radiology* 1981;**32**:291–5.
23. Lütje S, de Rooy JW, Croockewit S, et al. Role of radiography, MRI and FDG-PET/CT in diagnosing, staging and therapeutical evaluation of patients with multiple myeloma. *Annals of Hematology* 2009;**88**:1161–8.
24. Enneking WF, Spanier SS, Goodman MA. A system for the surgical staging of musculoskeletal sarcoma. *Clinical Orthopaedics and Related Research* 1980;**153**:106–20.
25. Boriani S, Weinstein JN, Biagini R. Primary bone tumours of the spine. Terminology and surgical staging. *Spine* 1997;**22**:1036–44.
26. Schmidt MH, Klimo Jr P, Vrionis FD. Metastatic spinal cord compression. *Journal of the National Comprehensive Cancer Network* 2005;**3**:711–19.

27. Yalamanchili M, Lesser GJ. Malignant spinal cord compression. *Current Treatment Options in Oncology* 2003;**4**:509–16.
28. Harrington KD. Orthopedic surgical management of skeletal complications of malignancy. *Cancer* 1997;**80** (Suppl. 8):1614–27.
29. Martin NS, Williamson J. The role of surgery in the treatment of malignant tumours of the spine. *Journal of Bone and Joint Surgery (British)* 1970;**52**:227–37.
30. Barr JD, Barr MS, Lemley TJ, et al. Percutaneous vertebroplasty for pain relief and spinal stabilization. *Spine* 2000;**25**:923–8.
31. Cortet B, Cotten A, Boutry N, et al. Percutaneous vertebroplasty in patients with osteolytic metastases or multiple myeloma. *Revue du Rhumatisme (English Ed.)* 1997;**64**:177–83.
32. Klimo Jr P, Schmidt MH. Surgical management of spinal metastases. *Oncologist* 2004;**9**:188–96.
33. Weigel B, Maghsudi M, Neumann C, et al. Surgical management of symptomatic spinal metastases. Postoperative outcome and quality of life. *Spine* 1999;**24**:2240–6.
34. Pointillart V, Vital JM, Salmi R, et al. Survival prognostic actors and clinical outcomes in patients with spinal metastases. *Journal of Cancer Research and Clinical Oncology* 2011;**137**:849–56.
35. Tokuhashi Y, Matsuzaki H, Toriyama S, et al. Scoring system for the preoperative evaluation of metastatic spine tumor prognosis. *Spine* 1990;**15**:1110–13.

NEW TREATMENTS FOR SPINE METASTASES

EPIDEMIOLOGY

Malignant tumours and metastases are more common in the spine than in any other bones. Around 60–70% of all tumour patients develop spinal metastases. Some of them are diagnosed coincidentally, e.g. 3% of osteoporotic spontaneous fractures are caused by undiagnosed primaries with spinal metastasis.[1] Furthermore ~10% of spinal metastasis are initially symptom free.

The overwhelming majority of spinal tumours are secondary metastasis. Primary malignant spinal tumours are mainly multiple myelomas[2] and rarely are other tumours, such as non-Hodgkin lymphoma.[3]

Multiply myeloma represents 50% of all primary spinal tumours. Of patients with multiple myelomas, 70–100% show skeletal involvement. Multiple myeloma causes bone resorption by stimulating the osteoclasts via the osteoclast activating factor.[4] This usually leads to a multilevel spinal disease with painful progressive vertebral compression fractures.[2] In the last few years the survival rates of multiple myeloma patients have increased significantly because of further development and improvement in chemotherapy.[5,6]

The prophylactic stabilization in multiple myeloma patients without a vertebral fracture is currently limited to individual cases where chemotherapy fails, but this remains an exeption.

The most common benign spinal tumour is a haemangioma, which can be extremely painful mimicking a fracture. They can be treated successfully either with minimally invasive cementoplasties or open instrumentation.[7–9]

LOCATION OF SPINAL METASTASES

The localization of spinal metastases is important as it directly dictates the surgical approach and treatment options. Ninety-eight per cent of metastases are located in the vertebral body, with a clear prevalence in the thoracic spine (70%, main vertebrae T4–T7). Lumbar (20%) and cervical (10%) metastases are less common. However, it is clinically important to screen for multiple metastases, as 50% of patients show multisegmental involvement.[10] Owing to the vascular supply of the vertebra, which favours the anterior part of the vertebral body, most of the metastases are localized in that area (60%), which results clinically in kyphotic deformity and may be overlooked as a normal osteoporotic fracture. The pedicle is involved in only 30% of patients. However, the missing pedicle 'eye' sign is important, as it might be readily seen on an anteroposterior radiographs (Fig. 92.1)

Primary cancers most frequently causing vertebral metastases are shown in Fig. 92.2. Originally it was important to distinguish osteolytic metastasis from osteoblastic metastases. Nowadays, minimally invasive options exist for all types, so that the difference between osteolytic and osteoblastic metastases remains relevant regarding their stability only.

OVERALL SURVIVAL RATES

The overall mean survival rate of all cancers with spinal metastases was only 10 months in 1995.[11] Even after development of more specific drugs, the mortality rates are still poor 10 years later.[12] They can be described in more detail for the different cancers: lung, osteosarcoma, stomach, bladder, oesophagus, pancreas, less than 6 months; liver, gallbladder, unidentified tumour, kidney, uterus, 6–12 months; and rectum, thyroid, breast, prostate, carcinoid tumour more than 12 months. The mean survival rate is especially poor after spinal metastasis with paraplegia (average survival rate 3 months).[11] Therefore, spine surgeons have to assess the risk of paraplegia under conservative treatment and adopt a more aggressive approach. It has to be taken into account that conservative measures such as chemotherapy and radiotherapy very often do not prolong survival. Therefore, the surgical goal must be to offer the patient a pain-free life with cancer and a stable spinal situation in order to improve life quality.

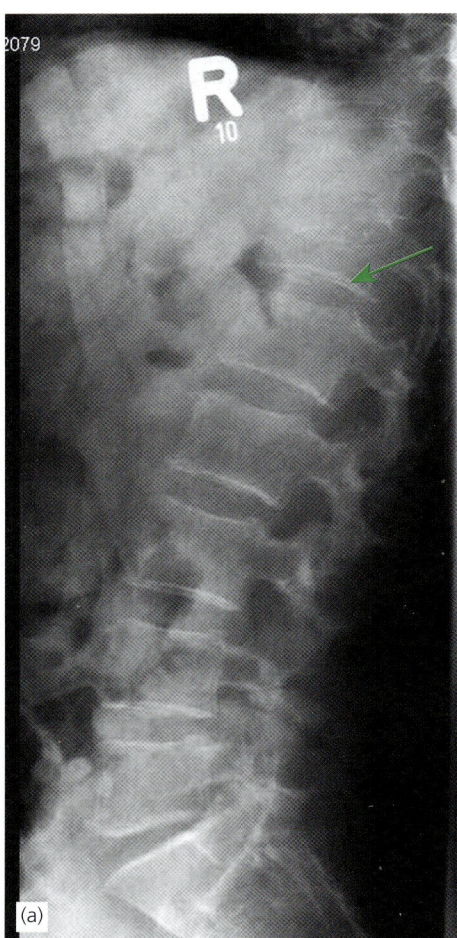
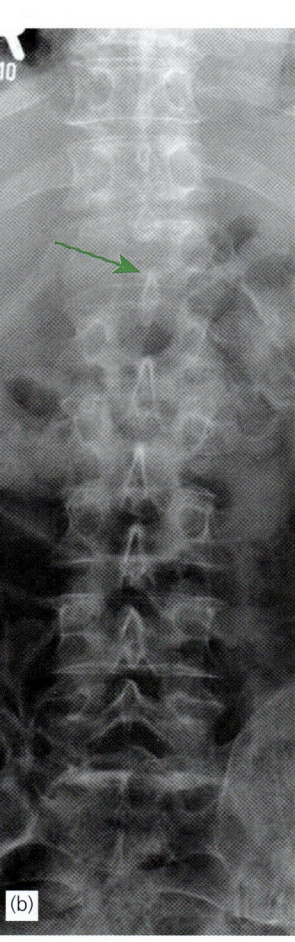

Figure 92.1 Sixty-year-old man: metastasis of a prostate carcinoma Th12 involving the right pedicle. Note pathological fracture Th12 (a) and destroyed right pedicle/missing eye sign (b).

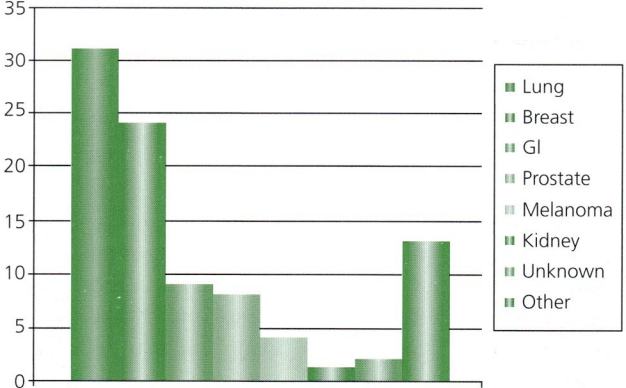

Figure 92.2 Cancer frequently causing vertebral metastasis (after Perrin RG. Metastatic tumors of the axial spine. *Current Opinion in Oncology* 1992;**4**(3):525–32).

SURGICAL APPROACHES

In order to achieve these goals, several surgical guidelines have been described[12,13] that all describe the surgical approach and treatment options depending on several prognostic factors, such as primary tumour, rapidity of growth and prevalence of visceral or bone metastases. The most widely known scores are the Tomita and revised Tokuhashi scores. They both propose conservative treatment, operative palliative surgery (decompression, limited tumour removal), in patients with a mean survival prognosis of ~6 months and large complete resection (vertebrectomy) with stabilization in patients with a mean survival rate of ~12 months. These scores do not take into account that the survival rate is not dependent on surgical treatment but on the effectiveness of the oncological and immuno-oncological treatment (see below). Furthermore, they do not take into account that surgical methods have been tremendously improved over the last years; mainly with the introduction of minimally invasive stabilization methods, such as vertebroplasty and kyphoplasty (see Chapter 67). These techniques have the advantages of significantly reducing surgical trauma, complication rates, intensive care unit and hospital stay and allow a fast return to normal ADL (activities of daily living). Good stabilization with excisional surgery and decompression yield a high morbidity rate and patients are often hospitalized over several weeks, which accounts for a significant part of their remaining life.

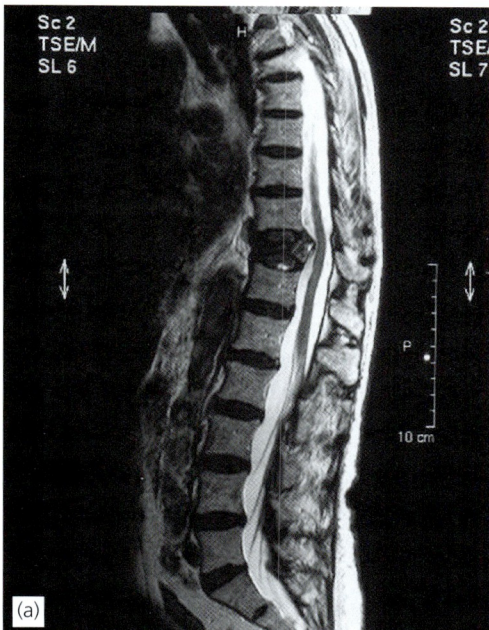
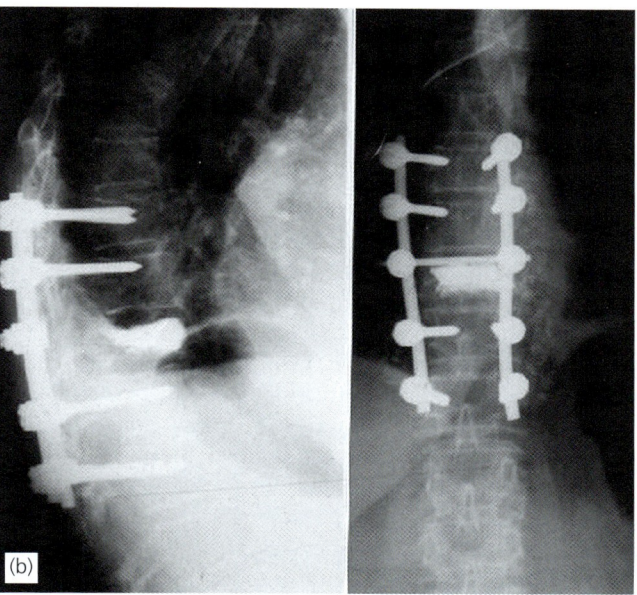

Figure 92.3 Eighty-year-old woman; metastasis Th12 (unknown primary) with fracture and incomplete paraplegia. (a) Postoperative improvement of neurological deficit after laminectomy, dorsal fusion Th9–L1 and kyphoplasty Th12 with polymethylmethacrylate bone substitute.

Minimally invasive cementoplasty techniques have been shown to result in stability and pain reduction in multiple myeloma[2,14] and metastases.[15,16] They also have the potential of reducing local tumour growth because of cement toxicity.[2,17,18] They can be performed easily on multiple levels and therefore play a dominant role in diseases involving multiple vertebrae (e.g. multiple myeloma, multiple metastases). These techniques can be combined with posterior fusion, resulting in a stable spine without using a more invasive anterior approach or complete resection of the vertebra (Fig. 92.3). Furthermore, it is easy to perform a biopsy during vertebra- or kyphoplasty that allows histology and immuno-oncological treatment (see below). Cementoplasties could only be used in the past in osteolytic tumours because of the possibility of dislocating tumour material during cement injection. Recently, good results have been achieved with minimally invasive tumour debulking methods (e.g. cryotherapy, coblation technology (Fig. 92.4)[19,20] or continuous aspiration/injection techniques),[21] which allow safer cement injection. Nowadays, osteoblastic tumours are no longer a contraindication for minimally invasive cementoplasty techniques. More and more, they are used as a first-line approach where possible and reduce the chance of longer inpatient treatment or a more invasive surgical procedure, while improving pain, stability and life quality.

Often there is agreement among surgical societies that there is a tendency to overtreatment following the Tomita and Tokuhashi scores. It has been shown that the combination of modern chemotherapy, radiation therapy

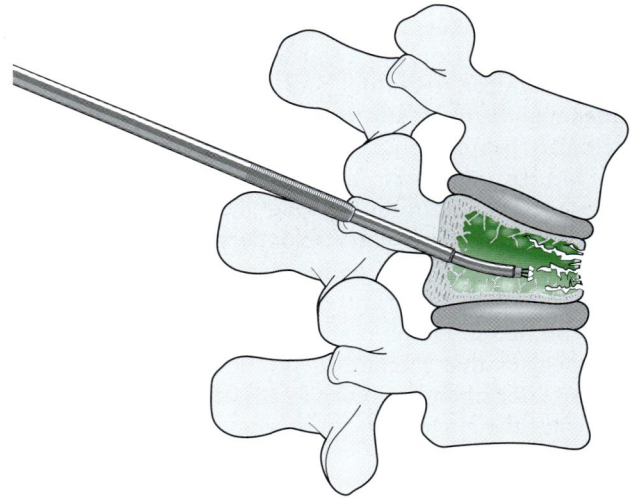

Figure 92.4 Schematic drawing of tumour ablation prior to vertebroplasty. Illustration copyright ArthroCare Corporation, Austin, TX, USA, redrawn with permission.

and bisphosphonates improved the quality of life in patients in whom the above-mentioned scores proposed wide excisional surgery.[22]

The following checklist may help better in deciding surgery than the above-mentioned scores: assessment of institution where treatment is performed (ICU, OR capacity, surgical experience); surgeon's opinion (pain management plus stability versus oncologist opinion); pain management plus tumour treatment, patient health and compliance and neurological deficit.[22]

MODERN ADDITIONAL CANCER THERAPY

An alternative for minimally invasive surgery is the CyberKnife stereotactic radiosurgery system (Accuracy, Sunnyvale, CA).[23] This improvement on gamma-knife technology allows the removal of tumours with selective ionization of tissue by means of high-energy beams of radiation. Unlike the gamma knife, the CyberKnife is applicable throughout the body. The downside of this technology is the cost, the need to implant surgically small metal markers (fiducials) in the treatment of soft-tissue cancer and the lack of long-term results.

However, long-term cancer survival is due to the ability to treat the underlying disease and not due to the surgical technique.

Recently, immunological treatment as an addition to surgery has become a strong focus of interest and offers new treatment options for cancer patients.

IMMUNO-ONCOLOGY

Basic knowledge

Lymphoid tissues are classified as generative organs, also called primary lymphatic organs, where lymphocytes first express antigen receptors and attain phenotypic and functional maturity, and as peripheral organs, also called secondary lymphoid organs, where lymphocyte responses to foreign antigens are initiated and develop. Lymphocytes mature in the bone marrow (B cells) and thymus (T cells) and enter secondary (peripheral) lymphoid organs as 'naïve' lymphocytes. Antigens are captured from their site of entry by dendritic cells (DCs) and concentrated in lymph nodes, where they activate naïve lymphocytes that migrate to the nodes through blood vessels. Effector and memory T cells develop in the nodes and enter the circulation, from where they may migrate to peripheral tissues.[24,25]

The bone marrow is unique among all lymphatic tissues because, according to recent findings,[26] it can perform primary organ as well as secondary organ immune functions.

Primary functions

Bone marrow is the site of generation of all circulating blood cells, including immature lymphocytes, in the adult and is the site of early events in B-cell maturation. All the blood cells originate from a common haematopoietic stem cell that becomes committed to differentiate along particular lineages (i.e. erythroid, megakaryocytic, granulocytic, monocytic and lymphocytic).

Secondary functions

In 2003 it was described for the first time that bone marrow can also function as a priming site for T-cell responses to blood-borne antigens.[26] Similar to spleen, bone marrow is vascularized by blood, but not by lymphatic vessels, and is part of the lymphocyte recirculation network. We and others have also observed an enrichment of antigen-specific memory T cells in bone marrow.[27] Tumour-specific memory T cells from bone marrow were involved in animal tumour studies in the control of tumour dormancy in the bone marrow,[28] and in studies with human cells xenotransplanted to mice, tumour-specific memory T cells from bone marrow were shown to exert therapeutic activity upon specific reactivation.[29] Antigen-specific naïve T cells were shown to home to bone marrow, where they can be primed. Antigen presentation to T cells in bone marrow is mediated via resident CD11c+ DCs. They are highly efficient in taking up exogenous blood-borne antigens (including circulating tumour cells) and processing them via major histocompatibility complex class I and class II pathways. T-cell activation correlated with DC T-cell clustering in bone marrow stroma. Primary CD4 and CD8+ T-cell responses could be generated in mice devoid of all secondary lymphoid organs autonomously in the bone marrow. The responses were not tolerogenic and resulted in the generation of cytotoxic T cells, protective anti-tumour immunity and immunological memory.[26]

These recent findings highlight the uniqueness of bone marrow as an organ important for haemato- and lymphopoiesis and for systemic T-cell-mediated immunity.

Thus it is of particular interest that the skeletal bones, a central organ, harbour and protect in their marrow perhaps the most important cell types for survival: haematopoietic stem cells and immunological memory cells. These are located in particular niches and share important properties, such as (1) a self-renewal capacity (response to homeostatic signals), (2) immortality and (3) pluripotentiality.[30] Bone surgeons should be aware of these hidden treasures!

Immunotherapy

Many current therapies for cancer rely on drugs that kill dividing cells or block cell division. Such treatments can have severe side-effects on normal proliferating cells, thereby increasing morbidity and mortality rates. In contrast, immune responses to tumours may be specific for tumour antigens and will not injure most normal cells. Therefore, immunotherapy has the potential of being the most tumour-specific treatment that can be devised. Tumour antigens recognized by cytotoxic T lymphocytes are the principal inducers of and targets for anti-tumour immunity. These antigens include mutants of oncogenes and other cellular proteins; normal proteins, whose expression is dysregulated or increased in tumours and products of oncogenic viruses.

Immunotherapy for tumours aims to augment the weak host immune response to tumours (active immunity) or to administer tumour-specific antibodies or T cells, a form of passive immunity. Cell-mediated immunity to tumours may be enhanced by expressing costimulators and cytokines in tumour cells (anti-tumour vaccination) and by treating tumour-bearing individuals with cytokines or non-specific immune stimulants that may affect natural killer cells, DCs and T cells. Oncolytic viruses have raised considerable interest as vectors for the treatment of human tumours in recent years.[31] One of these viruses, the avian paramyxovirus Newcastle disease virus (NDV), has been reported to have anti-neoplastic as well as immune stimulating properties.[32] The lentogenic NDV strain Ulster has been used to infect human tumour cells for preparation of the autologous virus-modified tumour vaccine ATV-NDV.[33] The rationale of this vaccine is to link multiple tumour antigens from individual patient-derived tumour cells with multiple immunological danger signals derived from virus infection. Danger signals, such as foreign viral RNA in the cytoplasm recognized by RIG-1 receptors, or viral HN protein recognized at the tumour cells' plasma membrane by receptors of NK cells, or type I interferons (IFN) induced by NDV in monocytes and plasmacytoid DCs, are recognized by cells of the innate immune system. IFN-α has a central role at the interface between the innate and the adaptive immune system. Postoperative vaccination of cancer patients with the vaccine ATV-NDV had beneficial effects on long-term survival. This was true even for very aggressive tumours refractory to standard treatments, such as glioblastoma[34] and head and neck squamous cell carcinoma. In a phase II study of primary operated breast cancer patients, the 5 year survival rate in vaccinated patients was more than 30% higher than in a similar control group.[35] The efficiency of adjuvant active-specific immunization with ATV-NDV was also reported for colon cancer patients following resection of liver metastases. The follow-up period was about 10 years. At this late time point 78.6% of patients from the control group had died whereas in the randomized vaccinated group only 30.8 % of the patients had died.[36]

We propose a unifying hypothesis that cancer patients contain pre-existing tumour-reactive memory T cells, which rest in particular reservoirs such as the bone marrow. These can be reactivated by anti-tumour vaccination with ATV-NDV and mobilized to circulate in the blood and to infiltrate tumour tissue, thereby causing anti-tumour effects.

NDV can also be used as a vector for gene therapy in cancer. Recently, reverse genetics technology has made it possible to clone the NDV genome and to introduce foreign genes, thus generating new recombinant viruses. The modular nature of gene transcription, the undetectable rate of recombination, and the lack of a DNA phase in the replication cycle make NDV a suitable candidate for the rational design of a safe and stable vaccine and gene therapy vector.[37]

Adaptive cellular therapy is another promising immunotherapy strategy. It involves the transfer of activated immune effectors, including tumour-specific T cells. The cells to be transferred are expanded from the lymphocytes of blood samples or from bone marrow aspirates[38] of patients with the tumour. In leukaemia patients, administration of alloreactive T cells together with haematopoietic stem cell transplants can contribute to eradication of the tumour (graft-versus-leukaemia effect).[39]

In this short overview we have given just a few examples of immunotherapeutic strategies and their application to cancer patients. From this it is apparent that surgeons and immunologists, upon proper cooperation, together can open the door for future better cancer treatments.

KEY LEARNING POINTS

- The most common malignant primary spine tumour is plasmocytoma.
- The spine is the most common organ for bone metastasis.
- Surgical approaches to spine metastasis should focus on spinal stability and life quality.
- Minimally invasive techniques such as vertebro- and kyphoplasty have a great impact on pain and stability whilst reducing peri-operative morbidity.
- Surgical treatment alone is not improving survival rates after cancer, additional focused treatments are necessary.
- Immunotherapy of bone metastases has the potential of being the most tumour-specific treatment that can be devised.
- Cancer patients often harbour in their bone marrow tumour-reactive memory T cells which can be re-activated by anti-tumour vaccination.

REFERENCES

1. Becker S, Ogon M (eds). *Balloon Kyphoplasty*. Vienna, Austria: Springer, 2008.
2. Dudeney S, Lieberman IH, Reinhardt MK, Hussein M. Kyphoplasty in the treatment of osteolytic vertebral compression fractures as a result of multiple myeloma. *Journal of Clinical Oncology* 2002;**20**:2382–7.
3. Becker S, Babisch J, Venbrocks R, *et al.* Primary non-Hodgkin lymphoma of the spine. *Archives of Orthopaedic and Trauma Surgery* 1998;**117**:399–401.

4. Callander NS, Roodman GD. Myeloma bone disease. *Seminars in Hematology* 2001;**38**:276–85.
5. Barlogie B, Jagannath S, Desikan KR, et al. Total therapy with tandem transplants of newly diagnosed multiple myeloma. *Blood* 1999;**1**:55–65.
6. Berenson JR, Yellin O. New drugs in multiple myeloma. *Current Opinion in Supportive and Palliative Care*. 2008;**2**:204–10.
7. Berlemann U, Müller CW, Krettek C. Perkutane Augmentierungtechniken der Wirbelsäule. *Orthopäde* 2004;**33**:6–12.
8. Castel E, Lazennec JY, Chiras J, et al. Acute spinal cord compression due to intraspinal bleeding from a vertebral hemangioma: two case-reports. *European Spine Journal* 1999;**8**:244–8.
9. Galibert P, Deramond H. Percutaneous acrylic vertebroplasty as a treatment of vertebral angioma as well as painful and debilitating diseases. *Chirurgie* 1990;**116**:326–34.
10. Heldmann U, Myschetzky PS, Thomsen HS. Frequency of unexpected multifocal metastasis in patients with acute spinal cord compression. Evaluation by low-field MR imaging in cancer patients. *Acta Radiologica* 1997;**38**:372–5.
11. Sioutos PJ, Arbit E, Meshulam CF, Galicich JH. Spinal metastases from solid tumors. Analysis of factors affecting survival. *Cancer* 1995;**76**:1453–9.
12. Tokuhashi M, Matsuzaki H, Oda H, et al. A revised scoring system for preoperative evaluation of metastatic spine tumor prognosis. *Spine* 2005;**30**:2186–91.
13. Tomita K, Kawahara N, Kobayashi T, et al. Surgical strategies for spinal metastases. *Spine* 2001;**26**:298–306.
14. Pflugmacher R, Schulz A, Schroeder RJ, et al. A prospective two-year follow-up of thoracic and lumbar osteolytic vertebral fractures caused by multiple myeloma treated with balloon kyphoplasty. *Zeitschrift für Orthopädie und ihre Grenzgebiete* 2007;**145**:39–47.
15. Fourney DR, Schomer DF, Nader R, et al. Percutaneous vertebroplasty and kyphoplasty for painful vertebral body fractures in cancer patients. *Journal of Neurosurgery Spine* 2003;**98**:21–30.
16. Pflugmacher R, Beth P, Schroeder RJ, et al. Balloon kyphoplasty for the treatment of pathological fractures in the thoracic and lumbar spine caused by metastasis: one-year follow-up. *Acta Radiologica* 2007;**48**:89–95.
17. Gough JE, Downes S. Osteoblast cell death on methacrylate polymers involves apoptosis. *Journal of Biomedical Materials Research* 2001;**57**:497–505.
18. Ciapetti G, Granchi D, Savarino L, et al. In vitro testing of the potential for orthopedic bone cements to cause apoptosis of osteoblast-like cells. *Biomaterials* 2002;**23**:617–27.
19. Gangi A, Tsoumakidou G, Buy X, Quoix E. Quality improvement guidelines for bone tumour management. *Cardiovascular and Interventional Radiology* 2010;**33**:706–13.
20. Georgy BA. Metastatic spinal lesions: state-of-the-art treatment options and future trends. *American Journal of Neuroradiology* 2008;**29**:1605–11.
21. Mohamed R, Silbermann C, Ahmari A, et al. Cement filling control and bone marrow removal in vertebral body augmentation by unipedicular aspiration technique: an experimental study using leakage model. *Spine* 2010;**35**:353–60.
22. Boriani S, Gasbarrini A. Point of view. *Spine* 2005;**30**:2227–9.
23. Koyfman SA, Tendulkar RD, Chao ST, et al. Stereotactic radiosurgery for single brainstem metastases: the Cleveland Clinic experience. *International Journal of Radiation Oncology, Biology, Physics* 2010;**78**:409–14.
24. Drayton DL, S Liao, RW Mcunzer, NH Ruddle. Lymphoid organ development: from ontogeny to neogenesis. *Nature Immunology* 2006;**7**:344–53.
25. Schluns KS, Lefrancois L. Cytokine control of memory T cell development and survival. *Nature Reviews Immunology* 2003;**3**:269–79.
26. Feuerer M, Beckhove P, Garbi N, et al. Bone marrow as a priming site for T cell responses to blood-borne antigen. *Nature Medicine* 2003;**9**:1151–7.
27. Feuerer M, Rocha M, Bai L, et al. Enrichment of memory T cells and other profound immunological changes in the bone marrow from untreated breast cancer patients. *International Journal of Cancer* 2001;**92**:96–105.
28. Khazaie K, Prifti S, Beckhove P, et al. Persistence of dormant tumor cells in the bone marrow of tumor cell vaccinated mice correlates with long-term immunological protection. *Proceedings of the National Academy of Sciences USA* 1994;**91**:7430–4.
29. Feuerer M, Beckhove P, Bai L, et al. Therapy of human tumors in NOD/SCID mice with patient-derived reactivated memory T cells from bone marrow. *Nature Medicine* 2001;**7**:452–8.
30. Rutishauser RL, Kaech SM. Generating diversity: transcriptional regulation of effector and memory CD8 T cell differentiation. *Immunological Reviews* 2010;**235**:219–33.
31. Harrington KJ, Vile RG, Pandha HS (eds). *Viral Therapy of Cancer*. Chichester, UK: John Wiley & Sons, Ltd, 2008.
32. Cassel WA, Garret RE. Newcastle disease virus as an antineoplastic agent. *Cancer* 1965;**7**:863–8.
33. Schirrmacher V, Ahlert T, Pröbstle T, et al. Immunization with virus-modified tumor cells. *Seminars in Oncology* 1998;**25**:677–96.
34. Steiner HH, Bonsanto MM, Beckhove P, et al. Anti-tumor vaccination of patients with glioblastoma multiforme in a case-control study: feasibility, safety and clinical benefit. *Journal of Clinical Oncology* 2004;**22**:4272–81.
35. Ahlert T, Sauerbrei W, Bastert G, et al. Tumor cell number and viability as quality and efficacy parameters of autologous virus modified cancer vaccines. *Journal of Clinical Oncology* 1997;**15**:1354.
36. Schulze T, Kemmner W, Weitz J, et al. Efficiency of adjuvant active specific immunization with Newcastle disease virus modified tumor cells in colorectal cancer patients following resection of liver metastases: results of a prospective

randomized trial. *Cancer Immunology, Immunotherapy* 2009;**58**:61–9.

37. Schirrmacher V, Fournier P. Newcastle disease virus: a promising vector for viral therapy, immune therapy, and gene therapy of cancer. In: Walther W, Stein US (eds) *Gene Therapy of Cancer.* Springer Protocols, Methods in Molecular Biology 542. Totowa, NJ: Humana Press, 2009:565–605.

38. Schuetz F, Ehlert K, Ge Y, *et al.* Treatment of advanced metastasized breast cancer with bone marrow-derived tumour-reactive memory T cells: a pilot clinical study. *Cancer Immunology, Immunotherapy* 2009;**58**:887–900.

39. Bleakley M, Riddel SR. Molecules and mechanisms of the graft-versus-leukemia effect. *Nature Review Cancer* 2004;**4**:371–80.

PART 9

ADULT RECONSTRUCTION SURGERY

EUGENE SHERRY

93	**Arthritis**	1077
	Sureshan Sivananthan, Ram Shah	
94	**History of the development of total hip arthroplasty**	1097
	Mukesh Hemmady	
95	**Biomechanics of the hip and total hip arthroplasty**	1105
	Asim Rajpura, Timothy N Board	
96	**Materials in hip arthroplasty**	1114
	Samuel S Rajaratnam, William L Walter	
97	**Perioperative considerations**	1123
	Daniel Kendoff, Thomas P Sculco, Friedrich Boettner	
98	**Primary total hip arthroplasty**	1135
	Ramankutty Sreekumar, Peter R Kay	
99	**Minimal incision surgery/mini-invasive total hip replacement**	1147
	Eugene Sherry, Declan O Sherry	
100	**Revision total hip arthroplasty**	1153
	Ardeshir Bonshahi, Timothy N Board, Martyn L Porter	
101	**Development of knee arthroplasty**	1171
	Shi-Lu Chia, Ser Kiat Tan	
102	**Total knee arthroplasty**	1176
	Shi-Lu Chia, Boon Keng Tay	
103	**Unicompartmental knee arthroplasty**	1186
	Seo-Kiat Goh, Seng Jin Yeo, Boon Keng Tay	
104	**Patellofemoral arthroplasty of the knee**	1193
	Erica D Taylor, Mark D Miller	
105	**Revision knee arthroplasty**	1198
	Shi-Lu Chia, Ngai-Nung Lo	
106	**Shoulder arthroplasty**	1207
	Gerald Williams	
107	**Ankle arthroplasty**	1241
	Norman Espinosa, Gerardo Juan Maquieira	
108	**Special considerations in young patients**	1253
	Minoo Patel	
109	**Osteotomies around the knee**	1260
	Andy Williams, Ali Narvani	
110	**Joint arthrodesis**	1268
	Nikolaos Giotakis, Rajiv Malhotra, Muhammed Arshad Nazar	

# SECTION 1

General considerations

93 **Arthritis** 1077
Sureshan Sivananthan, Ram Shah

93

Arthritis

SURESHAN SIVANANTHAN, RAM SHAH

Introduction	1077	Seronegative spondyloarthropathies	1089
Normal joint physiology	1077	Infectious arthropathies	1092
Degenerative arthropathies	1080	Haemophiliac arthropathy	1092
Inflammatory arthropathies	1084	References	1092

NATIONAL BOARD STANDARDS

- Understand normal joint physiology
- Be able to draw and explain the structural features and histology of normal cartilage
- Know the pathophysiology of osteoarthritis
- Understand non-surgical management options
- Know the common inflammatory arthritides
- Understand the role of cytokines and growth factors in osteoarthritis

INTRODUCTION

Advances in the diagnosis and treatment of arthritis include the identification of biochemical markers of normal and abnormal physiological states, the continued development of anatomical imaging studies and the evolution of function-associated treatment. The discussion of normal joint physiology has progressed from gross anatomy to cellular structure and function. Application of new findings in molecular biology to osseous and cartilaginous structures may lead to development of new treatments for arthritis. The widespread acceptance of MRI has increased knowledge of intra-articular anatomy in the various stages of arthritis, and advances in total joint replacement for all forms of end-stage arthritis have continued.

NORMAL JOINT PHYSIOLOGY

Synovial joints are composed of cartilage, bone and synovial tissue. Normal synovial tissue provides the necessary lubrication to assist in decreasing the friction of the moving joint surfaces. Subchondral bone provides the foundation of support for the articular surface. The articular surface is an avascular, aneural, hypocellular and alymphatic tissue composed of articular cartilage. The chondrocytes are encased by an extensive mass of extracellular matrix, which is a superhydrated material (approximately 75% water) composed predominantly of proteoglycans and type II collagen. The matrix provides articular cartilage with its material and structural properties and many of its characteristics. Although articular cartilage has little ability to repair itself, it functions well for an entire lifetime if the physical demands placed upon the joint are not excessive.

Cellular metabolism

CHONDROCYTES

Chondrocytes are metabolically very active cells that produce the collagenous and proteoglycan elements of the extracellular matrix as well as the enzymes necessary for the synthesis, maintenance and degradation of cartilage. Although the individual cells are physically isolated from each other, they are very responsive to various physical, pharmacological and hormonal perturbations.

ARTICULAR CARTILAGE

Articular cartilage is composed of four zones – superficial, transitional, deep (or radial) and calcified – characterized by morphological changes in chondrocytes as well as by a transition in chondrocyte metabolism. The superficial zone, the outermost and thinnest layer, contains densely packed chondrocytes oriented parallel to the joint surface. From the superficial zone through the top half of the calcified zone, the chondrocytes are more spheroidal and have increasing amounts of endoplasmic reticulum, Golgi apparatus, mitochondria, lysosomes and intracytoplasmic filaments, indicative of increased metabolic activity. Articular cartilage chondrocytes depend principally on diffusion of small (<100 kDa) molecules for nourishment and intercell communication. The small molecules are derived from a plasma transudate from the synovial vessels and, to a lesser extent, the subchondral bone plate. Because chondrocytes are physically isolated and totally dependent on diffusion mechanisms, their juxtacellular microenvironment is markedly different from those of most other cells. Chondrocytes are maintained in a higher level of carbon dioxide and a lower level of oxygen, allowing them to survive after extended periods of diminished or absent blood flow to a limb. When the pH is artificially increased or decreased from the normal value of 7.4, a variety of degradative processes are initiated. The chondrocyte differentiation pattern changes as a function of the chondrocyte age.

Chondrocytes respond to a number of growth factors, interleukins, pharmaceutical agents and mechanical perturbations. Growth hormone, insulin, calcitonin and androgens stimulate chondrocyte proliferation as well as the synthesis of type II collagen and proteoglycans. Dexamethasone decreases the cellular volume and the organelle content. Non-steroidal anti-inflammatory drugs (NSAIDs) reversibly decrease both proteoglycan synthesis and its secretion in cartilage explants and chondrocyte monolayer cultures. Cartilage-derived growth factor can increase hyaluronate synthesis while decreasing synthesis of sulphate glycosaminoglycans. Under dynamic, intermittent compression, the loss of macromolecules from cartilage is greater than that observed with a static compressive load. Further, chondrocyte synthesis of glycosaminoglycans under intermittent compression differs from that under static or no compression. Physiological hydrostatic pressures have been shown to stimulate matrix synthesis as a function of the pressure, time of application and the position of the joint. The dynamic compression of cartilage *in vitro* at physiological forces can accelerate the synthesis and release of matrix proteoglycans through physical phenomena, including tissue strain and fluid flow. Exposure to air reversibly decreases the glycosaminoglycan content of cartilage and leads to histological and ultrastructural changes.

In the past, the articular cartilage has been regarded as the target of, rather than an active contributor to, inflammation within a synovial joint. Recently, however, articular chondrocytes have been shown to be capable of producing a number of proinflammatory mediators, which result in leucocyte migration into the synovial joint. Thus, even chondrocytes have the potential to initiate and maintain an inflammatory process within the synovial joint.

Recent evidence suggests that nitric oxide is an important mediator of inflammation in both rheumatoid arthritis and osteoarthritis. Both synovial fibroblasts and macrophages appear to be the major sources of synovial nitric oxide, which may be produced as a non-specific synovial response to injury or inflammation. The tissue effects of nitric oxide are complex, and it appears to have both inflammatory and anti-inflammatory properties. Synovial cells have been shown to be activated by nitric oxide to produce tumour necrosis factor (TNF)-α, and possibly other proinflammatory cytokines. Nitric oxide also has been shown to regulate matrix metalloproteinase (MMP) production and may also inhibit matrix proteoglycan synthesis via interleukin (IL)-1β. Nitric oxide production within the chondrocyte is stimulated by the induction of nitric oxide synthase by IL-1 and TNF-α. Current evidence supports the association of nitric oxide with net catabolic activity in human articular cartilage.[1,2]

EXTRACELLULAR MATRIX

The extracellular matrix is composed of the chondrocyte products, type II collagen, proteoglycans, non-collagenous proteins, glycoproteins and water. Cartilage is a biphasic material composed of 80% water and 20% organic solid. The mechanical properties of articular cartilage are determined by individual mechanical and material properties of each of these macromolecules as well as by the highly ordered structure formed in the composite material. Water molecules are trapped within the collagen proteoglycan complex by hydrostatic forces. The concentration of water is greatest at the superficial zone, decreasing from 80% there to 65% in the calcified zone. The articular surface, the initial contact point for the resistance of tensile stresses, is stiffer than the deeper zones, reflecting a higher degree of collagen fibril orientation.

Collagen cross-linking determines the tensile strength of the extracellular matrix. These covalent cross-links, which are formed by the aldehydes produced by the reaction of lysine or hydroxylysine side chains with lysyl oxidase, increase the mechanical strength of the fibrils. In lathyrism this cross-linking mechanism is inhibited. The degradation of the cross-links produces an increase in urinary pyridinoline, a clinically useful indicator of bone turnover that is more sensitive than urinary hydroxyproline.

Proteoglycans, accounting for 5–10% of the wet weight of articular cartilage, are complex anionic glycoproteins that, in concert with the collagenous network, determine the load-bearing ability of the joint surface. Proteoglycans are made up of the glycosaminoglycans chondroitin-4-sulphate, chondroitin-6-sulphate and keratosulphate, which combine with a core protein to form the monomer, and are attached to a long hyaluronic acid chain by link protein. Proteoglycan aggregates typically stimulate the formation of type II collagen fibrils, and non-aggregating proteoglycans retard the formation of type II collagen fibrils except early in life when they strongly stimulate fibril formation in cartilage.

The distribution and structure of the proteoglycans in articular cartilage is heterogeneous and non-uniform. Variations in the amounts, chain length, degree of aggregation and distribution are observed in disease states and with ageing. Extracellular matrix homeostasis is controlled by the chondrocyte. Collagen turnover is relatively slow compared with that of the proteoglycans. In addition to synthesizing and secreting the synthetic elements of the matrix, chondrocytes synthesize and secrete the enzymes necessary for matrix degradation.

SUBCHONDRAL BONE

Although osteoarthritis is thought to be primarily a cartilage disease, there is mounting evidence that the supporting subchondral bone plate plays a vital, if not central, role in the maintenance of healthy articular cartilage.[3] The composite structure of the articular cartilage and supporting subchondral bone provides an ideal joint for locomotion and weight bearing. The subchondral bone, which is less resilient to pressure and friction than cartilage, is shielded from these forces by the articular surface. The thickness of articular cartilage is in direct proportion to the magnitude of the compressive forces in the subchondral plate. In most diarthrodial joints, there is a narrow range of normalized joint forces. The transmission of forces across the subchondral bone during normal daily activities is believed to be responsible for the maintenance of normal articular cartilage.

The architecture of the subchondral bone is influenced by those metabolic alterations that affect the supporting bone structures as well as by the calcified layer of articular cartilage. With damage originating in the underlying osseous structures, osteoclastic resorption proceeds, and there is an increase in vascularity and new bone formation. Normal ageing and immobilization lead to increased vascularity and eventual remodelling. Resorption of subchondral bone is the hallmark of osteonecrosis with eventual collapse of the supporting structure. An investigation of the short-term immobilization of rabbit hind limbs demonstrated that subchondral vascularization and metaphyseal resorption precede the articular surface changes. In osteoarthrosis, the subchondral bone is stiffer, with an increased trabecular volume and subchondral plate thickness and decreased mineralization, leading some authors to conclude that the primary defect resides in the bone and not in the cartilage See Fig. 93.1.

Damage to the articular surface alters the architecture of subchondral bone. At the site of cartilage damage, the underlying cancellous bone is replaced by vascularized dense bone. Transmission of excessive pressure to osseous structures causes cystic changes and growth of vascularized fibrous tissue in the bone. With normalization of the excessive joint forces, these cystic abnormalities are converted to bone. The anterior cruciate ligament resection model of osteoarthritis increases subchondral bone formation. Intra-articular injection of IL-1, as a model of inflammatory arthritis, produces erosion of subchondral bone and of articular surface. The subchondral bone is invaded by vascular channels that proceed from the marrow through the subchondral plate. Tetracycline labelling experiments demonstrate new bone formation in the trabecular network in the marrow and along the joint periphery as the bone attempts to return the joint forces to normal. Radiographically, these sclerotic changes are observed in the subchondral plate and in peri-articular osteophytes. New bone formation superficial to the subchondral plate, seen as replication of the calcified cartilage tidemark, occurs in osteoarthritis and can ultimately lead to articular cartilage detachment. The rate and magnitude of these changes can be altered by the mechanical environment.

SYNOVIUM AND SYNOVIAL FLUID

Synovium is a highly vascularized connective tissue that, although it lines the intra-articular cavity, does not have a basement membrane. Additionally, the synovial capillaries are fenestrated. The absence of any barrier between the synovial fluid and vasculature facilitates the diffusion of nutrients and waste materials. The synovial fluid is an ultrafiltrate of plasma with non-Newtonian characteristics, such that the shear rate and shear stress are not proportional. An increase in joint velocity is not accompanied by an increase in joint friction. A thin layer of fluid covers the articular surfaces under normal conditions; in diseased states, the volume of fluid increases. The diffusion rate to and from intravascular and intra-articular spaces is affected by many factors. Electrolyte and glucose concentration are typically identical to that of plasma, with glucose undergoing some form of facilitated diffusion. Large proteins are present in concentrations inversely proportional to their molecular size. Insulin-like growth factors are believed to be important regulators of synovial fluid proteoglycan synthesis.

The synovium is composed primarily of type A (phagocytic) and type B (secretory) cells with a smaller population of undifferentiated precursor cells. The cellular distribution increases from the capsular surface to the intra-articular surface and in those areas not subjected to mechanical stresses. The type A macrophage-like cells have prominent Golgi apparatuses and vacuoles, contain lysosomes and have abundant intracellular cytoskeletal filaments. These cells phagocytose debris that is present at the interface of the synovial fluid and the cell. The lymphatic system can also participate in the removal of particulates and large macromolecules. The type B fibroblast-like cells contain large rough endoplasmic reticulum complexes and have been shown to synthesize degradative enzymes and cytokines. The synovial cells also secrete macromolecules, such as glycoproteins, that are important for joint lubrication and nutrition.

PHYSIOLOGICAL SENESCENCE

With advancing age, the ability of cartilage to withstand compression decreases. Age-associated changes occur at the cellular as well as the structural level. The senescent chondrocyte is typically larger than younger cells and has an intracellular concentration of degradative enzymes that exceeds that required for normal remodelling. These older cells do not synthesize DNA and do not proceed through the mitotic stages of the cell cycle. The matrix components also exhibit age-related phenomena. The cellularity and absolute amounts of collagen or glycosaminoglycans do not change with age. Protein content increases while water content, proteoglycan half-life and subunit size, the ratio of chondroitin sulphate to keratan sulphate, and proteoglycan content all decrease with age. These age-related physiological changes in normal articular cartilage metabolism lessen the once advantageous mechanical and material properties of cartilage. These changes differ from those seen with cartilage damage, in which both cell replication and matrix synthesis increase. Load bearing and load history do not seem to be related to the onset of degenerative changes.

Structurally, with increasing age, the superficial layers of the cartilaginous surface become fibrillated. Fibrillation starts at the peripheral and superficial areas and proceeds centrally and to the deeper layers. The resultant surface irregularities can be observed arthroscopically as areas that lack the glossy finish of normal articular cartilage. Arthroscopic inspection with a probe reveals relatively softer areas of cartilage. The collagen concentration in these fibrillated areas does not vary; however, the concentration of glycosaminoglycans has been shown to be decreased, leading to a decrease in resilience and stiffness. Degenerated areas of cartilage may have a yellow discoloration that does not affect the material properties of the cartilage.

DEGENERATIVE ARTHROPATHIES

Osteoarthrosis

Osteoarthritis is commonly used to refer to a group of non-inflammatory arthritides. However, because the suffix, -itis, means inflammation, it should not be used when speaking of non-inflammatory conditions. While there is often an inflammatory component as part of the pathophysiology of this condition, it is generally agreed that the initiating events are mechanical, not inflammatory. The prevalence of osteoarthrosis generally increases with age. Osteoarthrosis is stratified into primary (idiopathic) disease and disease secondary to an associated factor. The most common of these associated factors is trauma, but there are many other associated factors, including congenital epiphyseal dysplasia, post-inflammatory arthritis, acromegaly, haemochromatosis, ochronosis and hyperparathyroidism.

AETIOLOGY

The aetiology of osteoarthrosis is multifactorial.[4] The theories can be stratified into two categories: excessive stresses on otherwise normal cartilage and the response of abnormal cartilage to normal forces. Ageing has been shown to decrease the fatigue strength of articular cartilage and increase susceptibility to osteoarthrosis. Moreover, genetic and constitutional factors are involved in both damage to and attempted repair of the cartilage matrix.

Under normal conditions, articular cartilage is loaded at roughly $20–25$ kg cm^{-2}. There is a narrow tolerance, because underloading reduces diffusion of cartilage nutrients and overloading enhances matrix breakdown. In a study of the effect of long-distance running on the development of osteoarthrosis, it was felt that, in the absence of other aetiological factors, recreational runners are not at risk for premature osteoarthrosis.

A canine model was used to examine osteoarthrotic changes after an acute transarticular load. In this study, an acute load (2170 N) was applied to the patellofemoral joint of a dog. Within 6 months, characteristic changes of osteoarthrosis had occurred, including surface fissures, loss of safranin-O staining, fibrillation and subchondral new bone formation. This study demonstrated the deleterious effects of a single transarticular load to the patellofemoral joint in a closed system, which may parallel the clinical syndrome of trauma-induced chondromalacia.

Pathophysiology of osteoarthritis

The standard teaching is that the earliest changes in osteoarthritis (cartilage swelling, increased hydration) can be attributed to a breakdown of the collagenous framework that allows further hydration of the matrix. Synthesis of proteoglycans (especially those richer in chondroitin sulphate) increases early in osteoarthrosis, presumably as an attempted repair mechanism. When mechanical overload persists, these repair mechanisms are overwhelmed, and overall proteoglycan degradation ensues. With further breakdown of the collagen framework and depletion of matrix proteins, structural changes, such as blistering, fibrillation and fissuring, appear. There are concomitant changes in the subchondral bone, and, eventually, the articular surface is denuded.

The role of cytokines and growth factors in the pathogenesis of osteoarthrosis and in attempts to counteract the cartilage damage was recently investigated. These cytokines and growth factors appear to be involved both in normal matrix homeostasis and in osteoarthrosis. For instance,

IL-1 and TNF-α stimulate chondrocytes and synovial fibroblasts to produce proteases, which can degrade matrix collagen and proteoglycans and suppress their synthesis. Moreover, growth factors such as transforming growth factor β (TGF-β) can counteract the effect of the cytokines.

A growing body of evidence suggests that osteoarthritis may be the indirect result of structural and biomechanical alterations in the subchondral bone, rather than simply the direct result of mechanical overloading of the articular cartilage itself. Eric Radin postulated this theory in 1976, and current evidence appears to support this 'bone first' theory. Microstructural and biomechanical changes within the subchondral bone have been demonstrated to precede the characteristic biochemical and histological changes typically associated with osteoarthritis. Alterations in the mechanical properties of the subchondral bone have significant effects on the mechanical stresses experienced by the overlying articular cartilage. Basically, the subchondral bone in the tibia is a spongy layer designed to take loading on the knee. In an overweight patient with poor bone quality, this subchondral bone begins to develop microfractures and fluid accumulates in the spaces. As time progresses this bone becomes hard, sclerotic and compacted and soon overlying cartilage damage begins to occur. In addition, the fluid that accumulates in the subchondral bone spaces is subject to *pressure effects*. Thus, when the atmospheric pressure is low (e.g. when it rains) the pressure in the subchondral bone fluid is high and the patient complains of increased pain. When the patient travels in an aeroplane where the cabin pressure is still lower, the pain may become excruciating, as the subchondral fluid pressure is comparatively very high. Therefore, one important clinical sign in the elderly patient with knee joint line pain with equivocal radiographic findings is the *joint line to subchondral bone pain ratio*. On palpation, the pain felt in the subchondral bone of the tibia will be far worse than the pain felt in the joint line. MRI of the knee will not show meniscal damage, but high signal changes in the subchondral bone. In addition, there may be varus or valgus laxity depending on whether the bone damage is on the medial or lateral side. Therefore, osteoarthritis should perhaps more appropriately be considered to be a disorder of disturbed balance between the degradation and repair of the articular cartilage and subchondral bone.

DIAGNOSIS

Osteoarthrosis is a long-term process with patients seeking medical care at variable stages of the disease. It is questionable whether early diagnosis and institution of therapy will modify the disease. Elevated levels of keratan sulphate were found in the serum of 125 patients with osteoarthrosis. Although there was a great variability in serum keratan sulphate levels in this study, serial measurements in individual patients may be helpful in following disease progression and monitoring response to treatment.

In another study, conventional radiography was compared with CT and MRI to assess the extent and severity of osteoarthrosis. MRI was found to be more sensitive in detecting changes in the least involved compartment, presence of early osteophytes and changes in the meniscal and ligamentous elements. Typical radiographic features are asymmetrical joint space reduction, subchondral sclerosis and marginal osteophyte formation.

TREATMENT

The non-surgical management of osteoarthrosis involves patient education, modification of function, weight reduction, physical therapy and analgesia.[5,6] Careful use of isometric and isokinetic exercises can strengthen periarticular soft tissues and decrease stresses across the damaged articular surface. The use of braces and other joint splints are frequently used for symptomatic pain relief.

The use of NSAIDs has not been shown to be chondroprotective in human osteoarthrosis.[7] A recent study compared the NSAID ibuprofen with the analgesic agent paracetamol (acetaminophen). Patients with osteoarthrosis who were treated for 4 weeks with ibuprofen in anti-inflammatory doses (2400 mg day^{-1}) or analgesic doses (1200 mg day^{-1}) were compared with a third group receiving paracetamol (4000 mg day^{-1}). There were no differences in pain, disability, walking distance or physician assessment during this brief study.

Surgical treatment of osteoarthrosis depends upon the extent and pattern of the disease as well as the patient's symptoms.[8–10] A recent review of the role of arthroscopy in osteoarthrosis pointed out the importance of deformity, loss of joint space and symptoms of internal derangement in the outcome of this procedure. Patients with little varus or valgus deformity and only slight radiographic changes do quite well. In these circumstances, removal of unstable meniscal and chondral flaps, lavage, excision of intercondylar osteophytes, and drilling of areas of exposed bone less than 1 cm in diameter may provide symptomatic relief for up to 5 years for 60–80% of patients.

Tibial osteotomy remains the treatment of choice for single-compartment osteoarthrosis of either the medial or lateral plateaus of the knee.[11] In general, medial osteoarthrosis is treated by high tibial osteotomy, and lateral osteoarthrosis is treated by supracondylar femoral osteotomy. A long-term follow-up study of high tibial osteotomy for medial osteoarthrosis of the knee indicated that, at 6 years, 50% of knees were good and over 75% were acceptable. At 11.9 years, 43% were good and 60% acceptable. The best results were obtained in patients with grade 1 (slight reduction in joint space) or grade 2 (obliteration of joint space) and if a mean angulation of 3–7° of mechanical valgus was obtained postoperatively.

Unicompartmental knee arthroplasty has been re-evaluated in terms of its role in the treatment of osteoarthrosis. Parallel survivorship curves comparing unicompartmental and total knee arthroplasty show that, at

10 years, survivorship is better in total knee arthroplasty. Analysis of the failures of unicompartmental knee arthroplasty show that most result from poor patient selection, errors in surgical technique and poor prosthetic design. Unicompartmental knee arthroplasty is contraindicated in patients with inflammatory arthritis, subluxation of the tibia on the femur, significant articular chondrocalcinosis, non-articular deformity and obesity. Total knee arthroplasty continues to provide excellent results in over 90% of patients at 10 years. Marked deformity, bone loss, flexion contracture and previous surgery present specific technical problems in performing total knee arthroplasty in patients with end-stage osteoarthrosis.

Molecular markers of arthritic disease

Articular cartilage and subchondral bone are dynamic tissues with continuous matrix turnover. Maintenance of health within the synovial joint requires maintenance of matrix homeostasis and structural integrity within both of these tissues. Pathological conditions, such as osteoarthritis, rheumatoid arthritis or trauma, disrupt the delicate balance between anabolic and catabolic processes within the matrix of these tissues, ultimately resulting in loss of articular cartilage. Structural macromolecules, or their fragments, are constantly released from the cartilage matrix by these metabolic processes. Quantification of these 'molecular markers' of joint disease is of considerable scientific and clinical interest, because they are potentially reflective of the relative state of matrix homeostasis within articular cartilage. Analysis of these markers of disease may help in elucidating the specific molecular events occurring in damaged or arthritic cartilage, and identify potential sites of therapeutic intervention.

As a result of the distinct zonal organization of articular cartilage, these molecular markers may allow for characterization of the anabolic and catabolic processes occurring in different zones (superficial, middle or deep), or different regions of proximity to the chondrocytes (pericellular, territorial or interterritorial). Because the recognized structural zones of articular cartilage each appear to be organized to serve a specific function, the consequences of damage in one zone may differ from that in another zone. Owing to the relative location with respect to chondrocyte proximity, matrix damage in the interterritorial region would not be expected to be as effectively repaired as damage in the pericellular region. Experimental evidence also suggests that, while loss of proteoglycan from the matrix may be reparable and potentially reversible, damage to matrix collagen may be considerably more difficult to repair. Identification of clinically relevant molecular markers of disease may thus be of diagnostic value, by establishing the presence of subclinical disease or the extent of disease within a joint. Molecular markers may also be useful in monitoring response to treatment or activity of disease.[12]

Several potentially relevant molecular markers have been identified in rheumatoid arthritis and osteoarthritis. A catabolic product of aggrecan degradation, hyaluronan binding region, has been shown to be associated with advanced, and probably irreversible, rheumatoid arthritis. Another cartilage matrix protein, cartilage oligomeric protein (COMP), appears to be a potentially useful serum marker for osteoarthritis and possibly rheumatoid arthritis.[13] COMP levels appear to increase with advancing osteoarthritis and remain constant in patients with non-progressive osteoarthritis. Bone sialoprotein is a bone-specific protein that appears to be increased in advanced, irreversible rheumatoid arthritis. Antibodies have also been generated that recognize epitopes of matrix macromolecules, including type II collagen and proteoglycans that are exposed during proteolytic cleavages associated with degradation. These epitopes are not recognized in normal cartilage, but can be detected in the serum or joint fluid, and thus show promise as additional markers for arthritis.

Therapeutic options for treatment of osteoarthritis

Activity modification, analgesics, NSAIDs and appropriate physical therapy have been the mainstay of treatment for osteoarthritis. Obesity is a potentially modifiable risk factor for development of osteoarthritis, and weight loss has been shown to slow progression of disease and to relieve symptoms in obese patients with osteoarthritis of the knee. Although low-impact exercise has not been shown to be a risk factor, several studies have documented the adverse effects of high-impact and high-intensity activity on the eventual development of osteoarthritis. Patients with abnormal joints as a result of previous ligament, meniscal or articular cartilage injuries will subject their joints to relatively increased mechanical loads, potentially accelerating the development of osteoarthritis. Secondary osteoarthritis developing as a result of a developmental or acquired skeletal deformity may potentially be reversed by a realignment osteotomy that normalizes the biomechanical loads on the involved joint. Unfortunately, these patients frequently present with degenerative changes that are too far advanced for an osteotomy to provide a reliable and satisfactory clinical result. Newer NSAIDs, with potentially reduced side-effects and increased efficacy, become available yearly. However, the potential side-effects of these medications are considerable in the older patient population typically afflicted with osteoarthritis. In general, the treatment of osteoarthritis in the past has been based primarily on alleviation of symptoms, rather than altering the normal progression of disease. Several recently available therapies and experimental therapies under development offer alternatives to previous treatment modalities, and may represent an opportunity to significantly alter the clinical course of osteoarthritis.

AUTOGENOUS CHONDROCYTE TRANSPLANTATION[14–17]

New therapeutic approaches incorporating cell-based technologies have been the subject of considerable interest in both the scientific and lay press. In general, these different techniques have been directed towards the repair of isolated, limited sized (2–7 cm^2) chondral defects of the knee. Although these lesions are probably pre-arthritic in nature, it is unknown whether these techniques will be applicable for the treatment of more extensive disorders of articular cartilage, such as established osteoarthritis.

The most popular of these procedures initially involves the arthroscopic harvesting of healthy autogenous articular chondrocytes from an uninvolved and non-load-bearing area of the knee. The isolated chondrocytes are then cultured for 2–3 weeks to increase the number of cells, and subsequently surgically reimplanted into the chondral defects to be treated. These autogenous transplants are held in place by a periosteal flap sutured over the defect. The early (2–3 years) reported clinical results with this technique are favourable, with 60–70% of patients experiencing a reduction in mechanical symptoms and improved function. Early clinical results with the treatment of chondral defects of the patella do not appear to be as favourable as the results of treatment of tibiofemoral defects.

Critics of this technique argue that it has not been subjected to the necessary scientific scrutiny obtainable only by a randomized clinical trial, or by comparing outcomes with untreated patients. It is not yet evident whether the same results may be obtainable with the use of a periosteal flap alone, considering the favourable reported results with the use of periosteal and perichondrial interpositional grafts for treatment of similar defects. In fact, results of a recent study using a canine model suggested no difference between periosteal flaps with and without transplanted autologous chondrocytes. The durability of the repair or regenerated tissue has not been established because of the short-term follow-up and the few clinical reports of this technique. Experimental evidence also suggests that cartilage regeneration following transplantation of mesenchymal stem cells may be superior to results obtained using autogenous chondrocytes. Autogenous chondrocyte transplantation (including the two associated surgical procedures) is expensive, and further documentation of the efficacy and cost-effectiveness of this procedure is warranted in this era of dwindling healthcare resources.

Focal chondral or osteochondral defects can also be managed by transplantation of osteochondral autografts. A technique, commonly referred to as 'mosaicplasty', of transplantation of multiple osteocartilagenous plugs or pegs from a non-weight-bearing or peripheral area of the joint into small defects has become more widely used. Autografts of up to 10 mm in diameter can be transferred into prepared defects in the femoral condyles. Reported clinical results with this technique are limited, however. The Steadman microfracture technique remains the gold standard for an isolated osteochondral defect with only one randomized controlled trial so far comparing it with autogenous chondrocyte implantation.

OTHER THERAPIES

Intra-articular administration of hyaluronic acid has become widely used for the treatment of osteoarthritis in Europe and Japan, and recently became available in the USA.[18] Although its mechanism of action is incompletely understood, exogenous synovial fluid hyaluronic acid acts as a lubricant in joints and has a pharmacological effect that results in stimulation of *de novo* synthesis of hyaluronic acid, inhibition of arachidonic acid release and inhibition of IL-1β-induced prostaglandin E2 (PGE2) synthesis by synoviocytes. Hyaluronic acid also influences leucocyte adherence, proliferation, migration and phagocytosis, and it protects against cellular damage caused by reactive oxygen species. Intra-articular injection of hyaluronic acid seems to be as effective as commonly used NSAIDs in relieving pain and improving function in patients with osteoarthritis of the knee, with a reduced incidence of side-effects. Intra-articular hyaluronic acid may be especially useful for the symptomatic treatment of osteoarthritis of the knee in elderly patients with a prior history of NSAID intolerance or unresponsiveness, or in patients with contraindications to the use of NSAIDs. Typically, a series of three to five hyaluronic acid injections, administered weekly, is recommended. Although the positive therapeutic effects of intra-articular hyaluronic acid have been documented to last for at least 6 months, long-term efficacy and the need for repeated series of injections are uncertain.

Glucosamine sulphate, administered orally, has been demonstrated to stimulate proteoglycan synthesis by chondrocytes and has mild anti-inflammatory properties. Several clinical trials in patients with osteoarthritis have demonstrated superior results with glucosamine sulphate compared with placebo. Efficacy of glucosamine sulphate appears to be comparable to that obtained with commonly used NSAIDs. Unlike NSAIDs, which exert their anti-inflammatory effects by inhibition of the cyclo-oxygenase system and prostaglandin synthesis, glucosamine sulphate appears to exert its therapeutic effects through a prostaglandin-independent mechanism. The reduced incidence of adverse events (principally gastrointestinal) with glucosamine sulphate, compared with NSAIDs, has been suggested to result from their differential effects on prostaglandin synthesis.

FUTURE DIRECTIONS

Although not yet clinically feasible, manipulation of the biological and environmental regulators of the chondrocyte would be logical targets of investigation into new therapies for the treatment of osteoarthritis and rheumatoid arthritis. The ability to stimulate the intrinsic self-reparative properties of damaged cartilage by growth factors, such as insulin-like growth factor I and

TGF-β, and to simultaneously inhibit the catabolic effects of cytokines, such as IL-1 and TNF, or MMPs, would probably have a profound effect on the treatment of these disorders. Further understanding of the specific events associated with the initiation and progression of cartilage degeneration and arthritis will probably result in the development of more effective therapies for these disorders.

INFLAMMATORY ARTHROPATHIES

Immunogenetic basis of inflammatory arthropathy

The pathology of most inflammatory arthritides results from the challenge of an immunogenetically susceptible host by a relevant antigen. The evidence for genetic susceptibility to most inherited diseases is seen in their widespread occurrence throughout affected families as well as by the presence of disease susceptibility markers on the major histocompatibility complexes (MHCs) of affected individuals.

Studies of families and of identical and fraternal twins suggest that there is a genetic influence on susceptibility to diseases such as rheumatoid arthritis, systemic lupus erythematosus (SLE), ankylosing spondylitis and Sjögren syndrome. These diseases are more likely to appear in first-degree relatives of affected patients than in the general population. Moreover, these diseases appear more frequently in monozygotic (identical) twins than in dizygotic (fraternal) twins, suggesting a stronger genetic than environmental association. Their lack of full penetrance in monozygotic twins demonstrates the environmental influence on the development of inflammatory arthropathies.

In humans, the MHC resides on the short arm of chromosome 6 and has three major loci. Class I loci consist of three related types of molecules, called HLA-A, HLA-B and HLA-C. Class I antigens are found on all cells except red blood cells and early embryonic tissue and are the primary factors in self-recognition and the development of tolerance. Class I antigens are responsible for graft rejection.

The class II (IA) loci encode for molecules termed HLA-DR, -DQ and DP. These molecules are involved in antigen presentation to helper/inducer T-lymphocytes (also called T cells) and are present on B-lymphocytes (also called B cells), macrophages and activated T cells. Class III loci are between the class I and class II loci in chromosome 6 and encode for soluble proteins that are involved primarily in the complement cascade.

Several rheumatic diseases have been associated with MHC class I and class II alleles. This association is defined by the relative risk, which is the increased chance that an individual with a disease-associated HLA antigen has of developing the disorder when compared with an individual lacking that antigen, and the absolute risk, which is the chance a patient with a disease-associated HLA antigen has of actually developing the disease. These associations vary when studied in different populations. The presence of an association between a known infectious arthritis such as Lyme disease and a class II HLA allele DR4 emphasizes the interaction of environmental and genetic factors in the development of rheumatic diseases.

The association of class II antigens with rheumatic disease is logical in that the receptors for these antigens on the presenting cells are the class II molecules. Processed antigen binds to these receptors and is then recognized by helper T-cell receptors complementary to the MHC–antigen complex. Most patients with rheumatoid arthritis carry DR1, DR4, or both. There is evidence that the presence of DR4 not only is involved in programming susceptibility to rheumatoid arthritis but also relates to disease severity.

The mechanism by which DR4 and DR1 can share responsibility for susceptibility to rheumatic arthritis is best understood by the concept of shared epitopes. Recombinant DNA technology has led to a better understanding of class II MHC molecular structure encoded on chromosome 6. Genes that code for the HLA-DR subregion include one alpha chain and several polymorphic beta chains. This allelic variability produces five subtypes of DR4 (Dw4, Dw10, Dw13, Dw14 and Dw15). The two subtypes (Dw4 and Dw14) of DR4 responsible for promoting susceptibility to rheumatoid arthritis share an epitope from amino acids 70 to 74 in the third hypervariable region of the beta chain. Subtypes of DR4 that do not have this specific amino acid sequence have no associated relative risk for the development of rheumatoid arthritis. Similar shared epitopes present on the DR1 subtypes may be responsible for conferring disease susceptibility. These new technologies should further elucidate the genetic control of disease susceptibility in rheumatic conditions.

Rheumatoid arthritis

The cause of rheumatoid arthritis is unknown.[19] Many putative agents have been associated with this disease and implicated in its aetiology. Epstein–Barr virus, human T-cell lymphotrophic virus type I, rubella virus, cytomegalovirus and herpesvirus have all been proposed as aetiological agents in rheumatoid arthritis. Although parvoviruses and other viral-related proteins have been identified in the synovium of patients with rheumatoid arthritis, no investigators have fulfilled Rivers' postulates, a series of requisites that must be met before a virus can be associated with disease aetiology.

The association of mycobacteria with rheumatoid arthritis has been postulated because these bacteria express heat shock proteins that are identical to the arthrogenic factors in a rat arthritis model. Moreover, elevated levels of antibodies to heat shock proteins from recombinant mycobacteria have been found in patients with rheumatoid arthritis.

Most investigators agree that altered immune reactivity or autoimmunity plays a major role in the progression of rheumatoid arthritis. There is less agreement as to whether autoimmunity has a role in causing it. Most theories of autoimmunity in rheumatoid arthritis implicate the development of autoantibodies towards collagen, proteoglycan and/or immunoglobulin (Ig) G.

The role of collagen autoimmunity in rheumatoid arthritis is demonstrated in a rat model in which intraperitoneal injection of denatured type II collagen produces a rheumatoid-like condition. Moreover, elevated titres of antibody to both native and denatured type II collagen have been reported in the serum of patients with rheumatoid arthritis. There is no evidence, however, that these antibodies precede the clinical onset of the disease, suggesting that the cartilage destruction exposes previously sequestered epitopes on degraded portions of collagen as an epiphenomenon of the disease. These collagen–antibody complexes precipitate within the superficial layers of cartilage and may serve as a chemoattractant for the invading pannus tissue.

Rheumatoid factor was first described in 1947. This class of antibodies is directed against antigenic determinants in the Fc region of IgG. Rheumatoid factors have been identified among IgM, IgA, IgG and IgE classes of immunoglobulin. The classic latex fixation test identifies the presence of IgM rheumatoid factor in the serum of patients. Approximately 80% of patients with rheumatoid arthritis have rheumatoid factor in their blood. The presence of this factor is associated with increased morbidity and nodule formation, and is considered an amplifier of the inflammatory response. The immune complexes produced by these factors can activate complement and serve as chemoattractants. In recent years, genes capable of encoding rheumatoid factors have been identified in humans. The presence of these genes has been associated with an increased risk (2.8 times) of the individual developing rheumatoid arthritis.

DIAGNOSIS

Rheumatoid arthritis is diagnosed on the basis of clinical criteria and not laboratory findings. These clinical criteria include: (1) morning joint stiffness lasting at least 1 hour; (2) peri-articular soft-tissue swelling around three or more joints; (3) swelling of the proximal interphalangeal, metacarpophalangeal or wrist joints; and (4) symmetric arthritis. These symptoms must be present for at least 6 weeks. The presence of subcutaneous nodules, a positive test for rheumatoid factor, and radiographic evidence of joint erosions and/or peri-articular osteopenia in the hands and wrists confirm the diagnosis. When these criteria are used, the diagnosis of rheumatoid arthritis can be confirmed with a 91–94% sensitivity and an 89% specificity. The diagnoses most likely to be confused with rheumatoid arthritis early in the course of the disease include SLE, psoriatic arthritis, ankylosing spondylitis, mixed connective tissue disease, Reiter syndrome, polymyalgia, Sjögren syndrome, crystal deposition disease and septic arthritis.

Laboratory tests alone cannot confirm the diagnosis of rheumatoid arthritis. Rheumatoid factors can be present (usually in low titres) in normal individuals and in association with other disease states. Common laboratory findings in rheumatoid arthritis include decreased haemoglobin, elevated acute phase reactants (sedimentation rate, C-reactive protein), elevated serum cryoglobulins and precipitating antibodies to soluble antigens.

DISEASE STAGE AND PATHOPHYSIOLOGY

Rheumatoid arthritis has been divided into five clinical stages based on pathology as well as symptoms, signs and radiographic findings. Stage I refers to the asymptomatic patient in whom a relevant antigen has been presented to an immunogenetically susceptible host. Stage II is characterized by B-cell and T-cell proliferation and synovial angiogenesis. Patients in stage II have symptoms of malaise and stiffness as well as early peri-articular swelling. There are no radiographic changes at this point.

Angiogenesis is essential for synovial proliferation, and it is controlled mainly by growth factors released from activated cells. Other factors, such as plasminogen activator, facilitate the invasion of newly formed vessels by activating the major metalloproteineases – collagenase and stromolysin.[20]

During neovascularization of the synovial membrane, circulating lymphocytes adhere to and migrate through the walls of the newly formed vessels. The presence of certain cytokines, interferon γ (IFN-γ), IL-1 and TNF-α, enhances lymphocyte adhesiveness. There are more T-lymphocytes than B-lymphocytes in the synovial membrane, and the helper/inducer T-lymphocytes adhere better than the cytotoxic/suppressor subset. The predominance of helper/inducer T cells intensifies the immune response. The activated T cells cause B-cell proliferation into antibody-secreting cells under the control of a variety of cytokines including IL-2. These combined B-cell and T-cell functions direct the humoral and cellular events leading to destruction of the rheumatoid joint.

Stage III is marked by a continuation of synovial cell proliferation and accumulation of neutrophils in the synovial fluid. Patients have increased constitutional symptoms as well as more soft-tissue swelling and evidence of synovitis. Radiographically, these patients demonstrate soft-tissue swelling.

In stage III disease, the complex interaction of cytokines becomes more evident. Different cytokines can stimulate proliferation of cells under some conditions and inhibit them in others. Cytokine interactions may be synergistic, additive or inhibitory. They may act at the level of cell–cell interaction or directly on gene expression. IL-2, -3 and -4 as well as IFN-γ are produced by T cells and act in the stimulation and amplification of cellular and humoral immune responses. IL-1 and -6, colony-stimulating factor 1 and TNF-α are synthesized primarily by macrophages and fibroblasts. Their major effects are on cell proliferation, prostaglandin production, matrix degradation and bone resorption.

Not all cytokines found in rheumatoid arthritis are destructive. TGF-β counteracts many of the effects of IL-1, IL-6 and TNF. It suppresses the production of collagenase by synovial cells and enhances the biosynthesis of matrix proteins. Moreover, identification of cytokine inhibitors in synovial tissue of patients with rheumatoid arthritis suggests that these effects could be downregulated.

Published reports on the role of cytokines in rheumatoid arthritis are confusing. This confusion is fostered by the cytokines' complex interactions as well as by the fact that they were usually named for their biological effect or the target organ. A cytokine might be called by more than one name, and cytokines that are active in synovium were frequently named for their non-synovial action(s). Reports of recent studies of cytokine messenger RNA (m-RNA) from patients with rheumatoid arthritis indicate that IL-6 was found in highest concentration in synovial tissue followed by IL-1βa, TNF-α, colony-stimulating factor, IFN-γ and IL-2.

The fact that neutrophils are found in high concentrations in synovial fluid of patients with rheumatoid arthritis, but rarely in the synovial membrane, suggests that the principal chemoattractants for neutrophils are in the joint space. These include an activated component of complement (C5a), leukotriene B4 and platelet-activating factor. The neutrophils are activated by phagocytosis of cellular debris and immune complexes. This activation results in the release of metalloproteinases, activation of arachidonic acid metabolism to produce prostaglandins and production of superoxide anions. These and other events in the joint fluid produce inflammation, amplify the response and induce matrix degradation. Other processes include the activation of the complement system, production of vasoactive kinins by kallikrein and activation of the clotting cascade.

Stage IV disease is marked by the initiation of the enzymatic degradation of cartilage. Patients become more symptomatic and MRI shows evidence of pannus formation and of peri-articular osteopenia. Stage V disease is marked by further erosion of subchondral bone as well as by radiographic evidence of joint destruction with narrowing of the joint space. Clinically, patients develop deformity because of cartilage loss and ligamentous laxity. There is limited range of motion, and flexion contractures develop.

TREATMENT

The multiple mechanisms and the complex interaction of events leading to cartilage destruction in rheumatoid arthritis explain why a single agent is incapable of blocking these events. Appropriate treatment requires the physician to classify the clinical stage of the disease as well as to develop objective criteria to evaluate disease activity.[21-24]

Self-management programmes are useful in the early stages of the disease. Patients should be educated as to the flares and remissions characteristic of rheumatoid arthritis as well as to means of protecting joints while sustaining muscle strength. A balance must be sought between activity, mobility and strengthening to maintain muscle tone and preserve range of motion versus overactivity with the resulting accelerated joint damage.

Drugs used for the treatment of rheumatoid arthritis have been classified into 'first-line' and 'second-line' drugs. The rationale for this classification was based primarily on the observed toxicity and risks of the various medications, rather their efficacy in halting the progress of the disease. In the past, use of second-line drugs was typically postponed until later in the course of the disease because of concerns about the potential side-effects of some of these medications. The adverse effects of these drugs are almost always reversible; however, articular damage due to inadequately controlled rheumatoid arthritis is virtually never reversible. The clinical course of rheumatoid arthritis is self-limited in fewer than 10% of patients, with the remainder of patients eventually progressing to chronic polyarticular rheumatoid arthritis. Recently, the necessity of early diagnosis and aggressive initial medical management in preventing irreversible articular damage in patients with rheumatoid arthritis has become more widely accepted. Unlike first-line drugs, several second-line drugs have been demonstrated to decrease the number of painful and swollen joints, suppress the acute-phase response, decrease the titre of rheumatoid factor, and retard the radiographic progression of rheumatoid arthritis. In view of the above, a more useful classification of drugs used to treat rheumatoid arthritis has been proposed, based on their effects and their ability to control the disease process. This classification categorizes therapeutic agents into symptom-modifying anti-rheumatic drugs (SMARDs) or disease-modifying anti-rheumatic drugs (DMARDs). NSAIDs traditionally are considered to be first-line drugs, and corticosteroids belong to the SMARD group.

Methotrexate and sulfasalazine are two of the most effective and widely used members of the DMARD group. Unlike many of the traditional second-line drugs, such as gold or hydroxychloroquine, which have a slow onset of action of 3–6 months, evidence of a positive clinical response may be seen after 3–6 weeks with methotrexate and sulfasalazine. Considering that irreversible joint destruction can occur rapidly after onset of rheumatoid synovitis, this is a significant advantage that allows for prompt modification of dosage or institution of other changes in the therapeutic regimen as necessary. Results of combined pharmacological therapy with both methotrexate and sulfasalazine may be superior to results obtained with either drug alone. Ciclosporin, a known inhibitor of T-lymphocyte function, in combination with methotrexate, has recently been shown to be effective in the treatment of severe rheumatoid arthritis.[25]

Serum markers of disease may be helpful in predicting severity of disease and response to treatment, and may be useful in monitoring disease activity during treatment. Experimental evidence suggests that COMP levels in the first year following diagnosis are elevated in patients who have rapid progression of disease. Genetic typing and analysis of HLA type in patients with rheumatoid arthritis show promise as potentially useful prognostic tools.

Corticosteroid administration is reserved for patients whose disease is refractory and those with severe non-articular manifestations of rheumatoid arthritis. While these agents block many of the pathological events in rheumatoid arthritis, harmful side-effects mitigate against their routine usage.

In patients with persistent synovitis without joint space narrowing, synovectomy may control symptoms in a specific joint. Surgical synovectomy can be performed either by open or by arthroscopic techniques. Radiation synovectomy has been used in multiple joints to control synovial proliferation. The efficacy of dysprosium (Dy165) ferric hydroxide macroaggregate in controlling symptoms and retarding disease progression in rheumatoid joints recently has been examined. These techniques do not work if there is significant cartilage destruction with the joint space narrowing. Early results suggest that the symptoms are controlled, but the long-term benefits in terms of disease progression are uncertain.

The role of total joint arthroplasty in the treatment of stage V disease is well established. Patients with rheumatoid arthritis require special consideration when total joint arthroplasty is contemplated. The presence of non-articular manifestations, such as vasculitis, neuropathy and pulmonary involvement, increase perioperative risk and may affect ultimate function. The polyarticular nature of rheumatoid arthritis often makes it difficult to assess which of the involved joints most affects patient function. Moreover, involvement of other extremities can influence postoperative physical rehabilitation. In general, multiply involved ipsilateral joints should be corrected from a proximal to distal direction; that is, total hip before total knee and total shoulder before total elbow. Fixation of implants is often difficult in rheumatoid patients and implants frequently must be cemented. In most cases, however, the prostheses function well and are protected by the physical limitations dictated by other manifestations of the disease. The reduced activity of most patients with stage V rheumatoid arthritis allows successful arthroplasties of the shoulder, elbow and ankle, which would have a higher failure rate in the more active individual with osteoarthritis.

Procedures such as hemiarthroplasty, osteotomy and unicondylar knee replacement are not indicated in patients with rheumatoid arthritis, because those procedures do not influence the destructive interaction between the synovium and the remaining cartilage.

Patients with rheumatoid arthritis require specific anaesthetic considerations. Micrognathia and cervical spine stiffness make these individuals difficult to intubate. Moreover, instability in cervical vertebra C1 and C2 increases the risk of spinal cord injury. Recent advances in epidural and other regional anaesthetics have reduced the risk in patients who often face multiple surgical procedures.

Biological agents for treatment of rheumatoid arthritis

Recent technological advancements have made it possible to identify cellular subtypes, cell surface markers and cell products important in the immunopathogenesis of rheumatoid arthritis. This evolving understanding of rheumatoid arthritis provides the opportunity for development of new therapies specifically targeted at many potential points along the disease pathway. Clinical use of these biological agents has been preliminary and, in general, limited to patients with refractory or longstanding disease. Some of these therapies, which may be relatively ineffective in the later stages of rheumatoid arthritis, may be effective in the early stages of the disease. In addition, successful treatment of rheumatoid arthritis may require combination therapy directed towards several targets involved in the disease process. Potential biological therapeutic agents for rheumatoid arthritis include monoclonal antibodies directed against cell surface markers (e.g. anti-CD4 antibodies, anti-cytokine antibodies), recombinant forms of natural inhibitor molecules (e.g. rIL-1Ra) or MMP inhibitors.[26]

T-CELL RECEPTOR RESPONSE

The central role of the T cell in the most widely accepted paradigm for the pathogenesis of rheumatoid arthritis has made it the target of many of these immunological therapies. Monoclonal antibodies directed at various T-cell surface markers (including CD4, CD7, CD5 and CD52) and at IL-2 receptors of activated T cells have been used in limited clinical trials. In general, the results of these attempts have been disappointing, prompting some to question the importance of the T cell in the perpetuation of rheumatoid arthritis.[27]

T-cell receptor (TCR) peptides and attenuated autologous T-lymphocytes have been used as vaccines in several controlled clinical trials in patients with rheumatoid arthritis. TCR vaccination may induce tolerance, depletion, suppression or inactivation of receptors on T cells that are specific for an inciting autoantigen. The lack of identification of a specific disease-inducing antigen in rheumatoid arthritis is the major potential limitation to this therapeutic approach.

Antigen-presenting cell (APC) activation of T cells can potentially be prevented by agents that block T-cell recognition by the APC. In rheumatoid arthritis, the obvious targets for this therapeutic approach are the class II MHC alleles associated with the disease (e.g. HLA-DR1 and HLA-DR4). Encouraging clinical responses have been noted in the few studies investigating the use of MHC antagonists.

CYTOKINE INHIBITION

The principal proinflammatory cytokines implicated in the pathogenesis of rheumatoid arthritis have been the target of many biological agents. Binding of IL-1 to its specific receptor (IL-1R) is the key event in the activation of target cells by this cytokine. Tenidap, a new antirheumatic drug, appears to reduce the number of IL-1 receptors and level of collagenase expression in human synovial fibroblasts in osteoarthritis and rheumatoid arthritis. Tenidap is also a potent inhibitor of cyclo-oxygenase, resulting in additional anti-inflammatory effects owing to suppression of prostaglandin synthesis.

Several naturally occurring inhibitors of the cytokines IL-1 and TNF-α have been isolated, including IL-1 receptor antagonist (IL-1Ra), soluble IL-1 receptors I and II (sIL-1R) and soluble TNF-α receptors I and II (sTNFR). Although levels of these inhibitors in serum and in the tissues (at sites of inflammation) are increased in rheumatoid arthritis, a relative excess of these cytokines in rheumatoid arthritis favours the proinflammatory effects of IL-1 and TNF-α.

IL-1Ra is a specific inhibitor of IL-1 activity that blocks the binding of IL-1 to cell surface receptors. The proinflammatory effects of IL-1 are overwhelmingly favoured because all IL-1 receptors on the cell surface must be blocked by IL-1Ra for complete inhibition of IL-1-induced functions. IL-1Ra concentrations over 100 times those of IL-1 are required to inhibit the activities of IL-1 *in vitro*. Clinical trials with recombinant human IL-1Ra have demonstrated promising short-term results in treatment of rheumatoid arthritis.

TNF INHIBITION

Another potentially useful therapeutic approach to the treatment of rheumatoid arthritis is inhibition of TNF. The biological effects of TNF-α and TNF-β are mediated through two cell surface receptors designated type I and type II. sTNFR are the shed extracellular portions of these two cell surface receptors. As is the case for IL-1Ra, there appears to be an excess of TNF compared with its natural inhibitor, sTNFR. To improve the pharmacokinetics of sTNFR, a recombinant sTNFR has been fused to the Fc portion of IgG1, forming a recombinant sTNFR fusion protein (rTNFR:Fc). sTNFRs, including rTNFR:Fc, function like antibodies by binding TNF and preventing its binding with the surface receptors on target cells and cell activation. Initial clinical trials with rTNFR:Fc have been encouraging.

IL-10 and IL-4 are regulatory cytokines that inhibit the release of and interfere with the activity of IL-1, TNF-α and other proinflammatory cytokines (IL-6 and IL-8), and increase synthesis of natural cytokine inhibitors including IL-1Ra and sTNFR. IL-10 and IL-4 also inhibit production of MMPs and thus may be clinically useful inhibitors of proinflammatory cytokines involved in rheumatoid arthritis.

Collagen degradation products have been suggested as potential antigenic stimuli for the initiation and/or perpetuation of synovitis in rheumatoid arthritis. Oral tolerance is a reduction in the systemic immune response to an antigen that occurs in response to feeding of the oral antigen. The exact mechanism underlying the development of oral tolerance is unknown. Several small studies of oral administration of type II collagen in rheumatoid arthritis have shown some decrease in disease activity.

Adhesion molecules expressed on the surface of endothelial cells and complementary sites on the surfaces of immune cells are important in recruitment and transvascular migration of a variety of cells (including neutrophils and macrophages) participating in the inflammatory synovitis of rheumatoid arthritis. Use of anti-adhesion molecules that block the above process may be a potential site of intervention into the pathogenesis of rheumatoid arthritis. Monoclonal antibodies to intracellular adhesion molecule 1 (ICAM-1) have been used in several clinical studies with promising results.

Therapeutic approaches directed towards modulation of MMPs are logical in the treatment of rheumatoid arthritis. Administration of exogenous TIMP, agents such as retinoids that can increase local production of TIMP, and synthetic inhibitors of MMPs have been used experimentally and may be clinically useful. Tetracycline and related antibiotics are inhibitors of MMPs and have been the subject of limited clinical trials in patients with rheumatoid arthritis.

The encouraging short-term clinical results with several of these biological therapies for rheumatoid arthritis require further investigation to establish whether these agents can truly modify the course of this disease and can be administered safely over long periods of time. Potential long-term toxicities of these biological agents include development of antibodies, opportunistic infections and lymphomas, which might potentially seriously limit their clinical usefulness.[28] Combinations of biological agents or the use of these agents in combination with traditional DMARDs may significantly enhance their clinical utility. As understanding of the pathogenesis of rheumatoid arthritis is refined by these investigations, more effective biological therapies that inhibit the critical events in the disease process will emerge.

Juvenile rheumatoid arthritis

Juvenile rheumatoid arthritis (JRA) affects 60 000–200 000 children in the USA. There are three specific subtypes of JRA: systemic onset (Still disease), polyarticular onset and pauciarticular onset. See chapter 63.

Approximately 20% of children with JRA have systemic onset. The ratio of boys to girls is equal. Clinical manifestations include fever, rash, lymphadenopathy, hepatosplenomegaly, and pericardial or pleural effusions. Leucocytosis and anaemia are common, but antinuclear antibodies and rheumatoid factor are generally absent. Chronic polyarthritis develops within weeks to months in many individuals. About 25% of patients develop a severe chronic arthritis.

Early-onset pauciarticular JRA is likely to be associated with characteristic HLA configurations and T-cell receptor genes. There is a recognized association between HLA phenotypes and the presence of antinuclear antibodies. Several studies have shown that the number of T cells of both CD4 and CD8 phenotypes is increased in polyarticular JRA patients. The number of T cells of CD4 phenotypes is increased in systemic JRA. Serum from patients with JRA contains immune complexes, rheumatoid factors (RFs) and other autoantibodies. These autoantibodies include several kinds of antinuclear antibodies in addition to RF. There is a particularly high frequency of the antibody against nucleoprotein in sera from patients with pauciarticular disease who have chronic uveitis.

Polyarticular JRA occurs in approximately 40% of patients. These children have constitutional symptoms: growth retardation, low-grade fever, mild organomegaly, adenopathy and anaemia. Cervical spine involvement, particularly at C2 and C3, is common in this form. Polyarticular JRA can occur at any age; girls are affected more often than boys by a ratio of 2:1. Latex fixation is positive in only 15% of children with polyarticular onset; in general, these children have a worse prognosis than those who are latex negative.

Pauciarticular-onset disease occurs in 40% of children with JRA. These patients often have serum antinuclear antibodies, but are rheumatoid factor negative. Inflammation of the anterior uveal tract (iridocyclitis) develops in 10–50% of children with pauciarticular disease; these patients require regular slit-lamp examinations by an ophthalmologist.

Although early diagnosis and appropriate therapy are important, the prognosis for most children with JRA is quite good. At least 75% of patients enter a long period of remission and have little or no residual disability.

The goals of therapy in JRA are relief of symptoms, maintenance of joint motion and preservation of function. Salicylates remain the basic anti-inflammatory medication in these patients. NSAIDs that have been approved for use in children are used for patients who cannot tolerate aspirin. Gold salts are as effective in the treatment of JRA as in the adult disease; antimalarials and penicillamine do not work as well in JRA. Corticosteroids are contraindicated in the treatment of JRA except in a crisis situation. Iridocyclitis can usually be managed with topical steroid preparations and dilating agents. Other second-line therapies remain experimental.

Synovectomy does not appear to benefit the course of the disease, but may be helpful in controlling symptoms. Total joint arthroplasty has proven to be beneficial in rheumatoid arthritis but requires special consideration in JRA. Total hip arthroplasty is often complicated by excessive coxa valga, anteversion and a narrow isthmus. Total knee arthroplasty may require posterior cruciate ligament substitution to decrease severe flexion contracture. This procedure requires careful pre-operative consideration, and frequently requires the use of modular or custom components.

SERONEGATIVE SPONDYLOARTHROPATHIES

These diseases include ankylosing spondylitis and juvenile ankylosing spondylitis, psoriatic arthritis, Reiter syndrome, arthritis of inflammatory bowel disease and undifferentiated spondyloarthropathies.[29,30] They often include inflammatory arthritis similar to rheumatoid arthritis, but they also frequently present as inflammation of the entheses (i.e. the cartilaginous site of attachment of a tendon or a ligament to bone). The peripheral arthritis is usually pauciarticular. The enthesopathy leads to localized pain, stiffness and often to local bone formation, causing spur formation or even ankylosis. The sacroiliac joint or the spine may be involved as well as other areas, such as the calcaneus where the Achilles tendon or the plantar fascia inserts.

Ankylosing spondylitis involves the sacroiliac joints, the spine and, to a lesser extent, the peripheral joints. Men are more commonly affected. Bilateral sacroiliitis with or without anterior uveitis in an HLA-B27 positive man is diagnostic. There is also an insidious onset of back pain with associated morning stiffness. Hip pain presents in the fourth decade with arthritis and protrusio. Although women have less progressive spinal disease, they are more likely to have peripheral joint manifestation.

A recent report reviewed 29 hip replacements performed in 19 patients with ankylosing spondylitis. While pain relief and functional improvement were significant at a mean 4 year follow-up, 23% of the hips developed Brooker class III or class IV heterotopic ossification. Another report of 53 total hip replacements in 31 patients with ankylosing spondylitis (mean follow-up 6.3 years) reported excellent durability with conventional cemented arthroplasty. Of these patients, 11% developed class III and class IV heterotopic ossification. Significant heterotopic ossification occurred only in those patients with previous hip surgery, postoperative infection or complete preoperative ankylosis. Prophylactic radiation was recommended for those patients who developed heterotopic ossification on the contralateral hip or were undergoing a reoperation.

Corrective spinal osteotomy was reported in 21 patients with ankylosing spondylitis treated over an 8 year period. The average correction for rigid thoracic kyphosis treated with a two-stage anterior and posterior procedure was 36°. Single-stage lumbar osteotomy with Harrington compression resulted in an average 30° correction. All but one patient in this series had improvement in pain and spinal alignment. There were no perioperative deaths and no permanent neurological abnormalities. Patients with ankylosing spondylitis are reported to have a higher incidence of spinal fracture with minimal trauma.[31] These fractures are associated with a higher risk of severe spinal cord injury and permanent neurological deficit.

Ankylosing spondylitis causes low back pain and can also involve larger peripheral joints. Ninety per cent of patients with this disease are HLA-B27 positive as compared with approximately 8% of the causcasian population generally. The disease is more commonly seen in men; however, it may more often be undiagnosed in women because of milder or uncharacteristic symptoms. In either sex, early onset of the disease and peripheral joint inflammation are indicative of a worse prognosis. Up to 25% of patients with ankylosing spondylitis develop iritis, but pulmonary and cardiovascular symptoms can also occur. Ankylosing spondylitis rarely develops after the age of 50 years.

The diagnosis of ankylosing spondylitis can sometimes be difficult, especially in the early stages. Decreased range of motion in the lower spine can usually be seen and thoracic expansion might be decreased. The sacroiliitis is often not apparent on radiographs; squaring of the vertebrae and vertical syndesmophytes may be seen. It develops on average 9 years after the onset of the disease. Bone scans may show an increased uptake earlier. In selective cases, HLA-B27 testing may be of diagnostic help.

It has recently been suggested that ankylosing spondylitis is a type of reactive arthritis to *Klebsiella* based on the more frequent findings of the bacterium in the faeces of patients with active ankylosing spondylitis compared with controls. However, additional investigations will be needed to confirm this association.

Reiter syndrome: reactive arthritis

This disease occurs shortly after an infection, but there is no evidence of a true infection of the joint itself. Up to 90% of patients are HLA-B27 positive. The disease occurs frequently after enteric infections caused by *Yersinia*, *Salmonella*, *Shigella* or *Campylobacter* species. It also occurs after venereal infections (e.g. infections caused by *Chlamydia*). There is inflammatory arthritis with effusion, particularly in the larger joints in the lower extremities. Some degree of back pain is common. Iritis, balanitis, stomatitis, skin rash and nail lesions can also occur. In Caucasian populations, the incidence of HLA-B27 positivity is high in Reiter syndrome, although in African Americans and Central Africans there is no apparent association. The course is variable, with recurrences, and, occasionally, the arthritis can persist for more than a year.

Enteropathic arthropathies

Patients with Crohn disease and ulcerative colitis frequently have arthritis. It is more common in Crohn disease. The arthritis often parallels the abdominal symptoms. Sacroiliitis is common, and about 50–70% of these patients are HLA-B27 positive.

Psoriatic arthritis

Two-thirds of patients with psoriasis have some degree of joint involvement. Nearly one-third have five or more involved joints. Although a symmetric oligoarthritis in the larger joints (e.g. the knees, hips, ankles or wrists) is the most common pattern of psoriatic arthritis, the distal interphalangeal joints sometimes are characteristically involved. The arthritis often accompanies pronounced psoriatic nail changes, but it may entirely precede the other manifestations. Spondylitis may occur in some of the patients with psoriasis and they are often HLA-B27 positive. RF or antinuclear antibodies are usually not found in psoriatic arthritis.

Treatment of spondyloarthropathies

NSAIDs, especially indomethacin, are usually effective. Education and physical therapy are equally important. In some patients with ankylosing spondylitis, sulfasalazine may provide significant relief from the peripheral symptoms. In chronic cases of Reiter syndrome, methotrexate or sulfasalazine can be considered. There is no proof of the value of antibiotics in the treatment of reactive arthritis.

Systemic lupus erythematosus

SLE is a chronic inflammatory disease resulting from abnormal immunoregulation. Its aetiology, like that of rheumatoid arthritis, is unknown, but both genetic and environmental factors are probably involved. SLE has a marked female predominance (greater than 9:1). It is more common among African Americans and certain Asian populations, with a prevalence reported to be from 2.9 to 400 per 100 000. The disease affects many organ systems, including bones, joints, tendons, skin, heart, kidney and the central nervous system. The diagnosis is made on the basis of clinical findings and a variety of laboratory tests. Patients are generally anaemic and have elevated acute-phase reactants. The fluorescent antinuclear antibody test is positive in most patients, with a homogeneous pattern indicating antibodies to nucleoprotein or a rim pattern indicating anti-DNA antibodies. Antibodies to double-stranded DNA or identification of extractable nuclear antigen may aid in the diagnosis. Treatment of the disease is related to its activity and the target organ. NSAIDs, corticosteroids, antimalarials and immunosuppressive agents all have a role in the treatment of SLE. Patients with SLE require careful monitoring by a rheumatologist.

The orthopaedic treatment of patients with SLE generally revolves around joint involvement and/or osteonecrosis. Patients undergoing total joint arthroplasty for SLE have increased perioperative risks, including infection. Ligamentous balance is more difficult because of soft-tissue involvement with SLE. Disease activity and corticosteroid therapy frequently produce osteopenia and predispose a patient to loosening and possible fracture.

A review of the use of bipolar hemiarthroplasty in patients with osteonecrosis secondary to SLE revealed a higher incidence of failure, leading to the recommendation for primary total hip arthroplasty in these patients. This higher incidence of failure presumably is caused by lupus synovitis.

Crystal arthritis

GOUT

The diagnosis of gouty arthritis is both overused and, at times, overlooked.[32] Gout cannot be diagnosed purely on the basis of clinical findings. Podagra, pain in the first metatarsophalangeal joint, is common in gout but not specific for that diagnosis. Moreover, gout may present in many joints, either as an acute event or as chronic arthritis. The diagnosis is confirmed by the identification of sodium urate crystals located within neutrophils in synovial fluid. These needle-like crystals are negatively birefringent when viewed with a polarized microscope and a first-order red compensator. Those crystals parallel with the compensator will appear bright yellow. This is in direct contrast to the short, rhomboidal calcium pyrophosphate crystals of chondrocalcinosis, which are weakly birefringent and appear blue when parallel to the compensator. Sodium urate crystals may also be identified in tophi. Early tophi may be detected on examination of the extensor surface of the elbow and particularly the pinna of the ear, aiding in the diagnosis of gout. Patients with an established diagnosis of gout should be monitored by a rheumatologist. The treatment of asymptomatic hyperuricaemia is controversial. This condition is more common in patients on thiazides or in association with alcohol consumption; moreover, it is seen with higher frequency in conditions such as psoriasis, a variety of haematological conditions, renal disease and hyperlipidaemia.

Patients with hyperuricaemia should undergo a 24 hour uric acid determination, because the risk of uric acid stones is closely related to urinary uric acid excretion. Of patients with urinary uric acid excretion over 1100 mg day^{-1}, 50% will ultimately develop renal stones and should receive chronic long-term treatment. A recent study suggests that patients with gout produce a urate crystal promoter, or perhaps lack an inhibitor of crystal formation. This may explain why some hyperuricaemic individuals develop gout and others remain asymptomatic.

Acute gout may be confused with other acute arthritides, including infection. Although major joints are frequently involved, the acute presentation can even be that of infectious tenosynovitis. If gout is suspected, a tissue specimen should be fixed in ethanol, because standard formalin fixation dissolves the sodium urate crystals.

Acute gouty attacks can be treated with NSAIDs, adrenocorticotropic hormone (ACTH), colchicine or allopurinol. Alternatively, colchicine can be given as two or three tablets followed by one tablet twice daily until side-effects occur. Colchicine should not be given intravenously because it is known to cause marrow depression, local venous irritation and potential cardiotoxicity. In a prospective comparison of 100 patients treated for 1 year with either a single intramuscular injection of ACTH (40 IU) or oral indometacin (40 mg, four times daily with meals) until the acute attack subsided, improvement in symptoms occurred much more rapidly with the ACTH (average 3 hours) than with indometacin (24 hours). None of the patients receiving ACTH developed side-effects, whereas more than 50% of those receiving indometacin developed gastrointestinal disturbance, headaches or other central nervous system symptoms.

Long-term treatment of patients with recurrent gouty episodes may prevent recurrent attacks. It is important to identify whether the patient is an underexcreter of uric acid (85–90% of primary gout) or an overproducer (10–15% of primary gout). These patients are generally managed with uricosuric agents (probenecid, sulphinpyrazone) or allopurinol, respectively. The frequency of side-effects of these agents is similar, but those to allopurinol are more severe. The allopurinol hypersensitivity syndrome is characterized by fever, eosinophilia, leucocytosis, impaired renal function, hepatocellular injury and rash. These reactions are severe and may be fatal. For this reason, allopurinol use should be carefully monitored, but still may be indicated in patients with tophi, renal insufficiency and a history of uric acid stones, and in those individuals with a 24 hour urinary uric acid over 1100 mg.

CHONDROCALCINOSIS

Chondrocalcinosis, or calcium pyrophosphate dihydrate deposition disease, has many clinical patterns, including asymptomatic calcium pyrophosphate dihydrate deposition disease, pseudogout, pseudorheumatoid arthritis and pseudo-osteoarthritis. The orthopaedic surgeon sees this disease most commonly either as an asymptomatic finding in association with arthritis or as an acute postoperative inflammatory arthritis. Calcium pyrophosphate dihydrate deposition disease is more common in patients with gout, rheumatoid arthritis, haemochromatosis, Wilson disease or hyperparathyroidism. The diagnosis is confirmed by identification of weakly positive, short, rhomboidal crystals of calcium pyrophosphate dihydrate seen in neutrophilic leucocytes.

The identification of calcium pyrophosphate crystals embedded in articular cartilage at the time of surgery is a relative contraindication of both osteotomy and unicondylar knee replacement. These crystals are believed to desiccate the articular cartilage and render it more susceptible to wear at normal loads. Moreover, significant chondrocalcinosis is often associated with a reactive synovitis that might persist after osteotomy or unicondylar replacement.

Pseudogout is often confused with infection and, in fact, a report indicated that 14 of 93 acute inflammatory pseudogout attacks were misdiagnosed as septic arthritis. Pseudogout tends to occur with greater frequency in the postoperative period. The diagnosis is confirmed by joint aspiration and crystal analysis. Aspiration of the involved joint and steroid injection, once the diagnosis of infection has been excluded, will usually control symptoms. Alternatively, NSAIDs may be used to control acute attacks.

INFECTIOUS ARTHROPATHIES

The advent of antibiotic therapy has decreased the destructive effects of acute septic arthritis.[33–35] In a *Staphylococcus aureus* infectious knee arthritis model in rabbits, prompt antibiotic therapy reduced but did not eliminate cartilage wear. In this model, untreated animals lost more than half of the glycosaminoglycan in articular cartilage by 3 weeks. Antibiotic administration 1 day after experimental infection reduced the overall loss of cartilage by 37%. This study highlighted the importance of prompt diagnosis and early treatment.

Arthroscopic lavage was used to treat 46 cases of septic arthritis of the knee. Fifteen of the cases were secondary to puncture and 20 resulted from postoperative infection. Positive cultures were obtained in only 63% of the cases. Treatment included arthroscopic lavage and prolonged antibiotic therapy (average 2 months). In this series, there were 36 cures (78.3%), five failures (10.9%) and five recurrences (10.9%) after apparent initial success. The role of arthroscopic lavage in the treatment of acute septic arthritis may be joint specific and related to the extent of synovitis. The knee seems most suitable for this form of treatment, because the surgery is easily performed and the results can be followed by physical examination; however, its role in the treatment of other major joint infections in adults is unclear.

A review of septic arthritis and osteomyelitis of the hand outlines both the surgical and medical management of these infections and the importance of prompt and adequate treatment to prevent osteomyelitis and other late complications. The need for proper diagnosis and therapy is emphasized in a review of acute septic arthritis in infancy and childhood that also covers the changing patterns of bacterial pathogens in this condition. A dosage schedule for commonly used antibiotics is included.

HAEMOPHILIAC ARTHROPATHY

Patients with severe haemophilia have a higher incidence of early arthritis of major joints. The most frequently involved joints, in order, are knees, ankles, elbows, shoulders and hips. The mechanism of arthritis in haemophiliacs is controversial, but most investigators agree that recurrent haemoarthrosis with subsequent free-radical formation predisposes the articular surface to injury. Patients with severe haemophilia can generally be maintained at home on factor VIII therapy. Factor VIII concentrates prepared from pooled donors are no longer used because of the high risk of HIV and non-A, non-B hepatitis. Preparations prepared by heat, detergent and solvent therapy carry a lower risk of viral transmission. Newer agents, such as monoclonal affinity column-purified factor VIII and pasteurized heat-treated factor VIII concentrate, are costly, but carry a low risk of viral transmission. Recombinant factor VIII is currently undergoing clinical trials.

Factor VIII levels of patients undergoing joint replacement surgery for haemophilic arthritis must be carefully monitored in the perioperative period. This monitoring should be done in consultation with the haematologist, but, generally, administration of 1 unit of factor VIII per kg of body weight will raise the level by 2%. It is generally recommended that factor VIII levels be maintained at 100–130% of normal for the first 2–3 days after surgery and at 50–60% of normal for the first 14 days. For 6 weeks the patients are maintained between 30% and 50% of normal, depending on their physical therapy and response to treatment. Patients known to have inhibitors to factor VIII should not undergo elective orthopaedic surgery.

Seventy per cent of haemophiliacs who have received pooled untreated factor VIII preparations are HIV positive, and as many as 90% of severe haemophiliacs are HIV positive. The T4 (helper/inducer T-cell subset) counts of these patients are carefully monitored, and zidovudine therapy is often begun when the T4 count falls below 500. The increased risk of infection in patients with low T4 counts makes elective total joint arthroplasty in this situation questionable.

Good to excellent results were reported for 13 of 19 total knee arthroplasties performed for haemophilic arthropathy, with an average follow-up of 9.5 years. Complications, including deep infection, superficial skin necrosis, nerve palsy and postoperative bleeding, occurred in 10 of the 19 knees. One hundred per cent factor VIII coverage was needed in the perioperative period.

REFERENCES

- ● = Key primary paper
- ◆ = Major review article

◆1. Abramson SB. Osteoarthritis and nitric oxide. *Osteoarthritis and Cartilage* 2008;**16** (Suppl. 2):S15–20.
2. van de Loo FA, Joosten LA, van Lent PL, et al. Role of interleukin-1, tumor necrosis factor alpha, and interleukin-6 in cartilage proteoglycan metabolism and destruction: effect of in situ blocking in murine antigen- and zymosan-induced arthritis. *Arthritis and Rheumatism* 1995;**38**:164–72.

- 3. Hulth A. Does osteoarthrosis depend on growth of the mineralized layer of cartilage? *Clinical Orthopaedics and Related Research* 1993;**287**:19-24.
- 4. Felson DT. The epidemiology of knee osteoarthritis: results from the Framingham Osteoarthritis Study. *Seminars in Arthritis and Rheumatism* 1990;**20** (Suppl. 1):42-50.
- 5. Hochberg MC, Altman RD, Brandt KD, et al. Guidelines for the medical management of osteoarthritis. Part I. Osteoarthritis of the hip: American College of Rheumatology. *Arthritis and Rheumatism* 1995;**38**:1535-40.
- 6. Hochberg MC, Altman RD, Brandt KD, et al. Guidelines for the medical management of osteoarthritis. Part II. Osteoarthritis of the knee: American College of Rheumatology. *Arthritis and Rheumatism* 1995;**38**:1541-6.
- 7. Brooks PM, Day RO. Nonsteroidal anti-inflammatory drugs: differences and similarities. *New England Journal of Medicine* 1991;**324**:1716-25.
- 8. Kirkley A, Birmingham TB, Litchfield RB, et al. A randomized trial of arthroscopic surgery for osteoarthritis of the knee. *New England Journal of Medicine* 2008;**359**:1169-70.
- 9. Ramsey DK, Briem K, Axe MJ, Snyder-Mackler L. A mechanical theory for the effectiveness of bracing for medial compartment osteoarthritis of the knee. *Journal of Bone and Joint Surgery (American)* 2007;**89**:2398-407.
- 10. Dandy DJ. Arthroscopic debridement of the knee for osteoarthritis. *Journal of Bone and Joint Surgery (British)* 1991;**73B**:877-8.
- 11. Ivarsson I, Myrnerts R, Gillquist J. High tibial osteotomy for medial osteoarthritis of the knee: a 5 to 7 and 11 year follow-up. *Journal of Bone and Joint Surgery (British)* 1990;**72B**:238-44.
- 12. Jimenez SA, Dharmavaram RM. Genetic aspects of familial osteoarthritis. *Annals of Rheumatic Diseases* 1994;**53**:789-97.
- 13. Lohmander LS, Saxne T, Heinegard DK: Release of cartilage oligomeric matrix protein (COMP) into joint fluid after knee injury and in osteoarthritis. *Annals of Rheumatic Diseases* 1994;**53**:8-13.
- 14. Brittberg M, Lindahl A, Nilsson A, et al. Treatment of deep cartilage defects in the knee with autologous chondrocyte transplantation. *New England Journal of Medicine* 1994;**331**:889-95.
- 15. Buckwalter JA, Mankin HJ. Articular cartilage. Part I. Tissue design and chondrocyte-matrix interactions. In: Cannon WD (ed.) *Instructional Course Lectures 47*. Rosemont, IL: American Academy of Orthopaedic Surgeons, 1998:477-86.
- 16. Buckwalter JA, Mankin HJ. Articular cartilage. Part II. Degeneration and osteoarthrosis, repair, regeneration, and transplantation. In: Cannon WD (ed.) *Instructional Course Lectures 47*. Rosemont, IL: American Academy of Orthopaedic Surgeons, 1998:487-504.
- 17. Messner K, Gillquist J. Cartilage repair: a critical review. *Acta Orthopaedica Scandinavica* 1996;**67**:523-9.
- 18. Muller-Fassbender H, Bach GL, Haase W, et al. Glucosamine sulfate compared to ibuprofen in osteoarthritis of the knee. *Osteoarthritis and Cartilage* 1994;**2**:61-9.
- 19. Isomaki H. Long-term outcome of rheumatoid arthritis. *Scandinavian Journal of Rheumatology* 1992;**95** (Suppl.):3-8.
- 20. Lohmander LS, Hoerrner LA, Dahlberg L, et al. Stromelysin, tissue inhibitor of metalloproteinases and proteoglycan fragments in human knee joint fluid after injury. *Journal of Rheumatology* 1993;**20**:1362-8.
- 21. American College of Rheumatology Ad Hoc Committee on Clinical Guidelines. Guidelines for the management of rheumatoid arthritis. *Arthritis and Rheumatism* 1996;**39**:713-22.
- 22. American College of Rheumatology Ad Hoc Committee on Clinical Guidelines: guidelines for monitoring drug therapy in rheumatoid arthritis. *Arthritis and Rheumatism* 1996;**39**:723-31.
- 23. Arend WP. The pathophysiology and treatment of rheumatoid arthritis. *Arthritis and Rheumatism* 1997;**40**:595-7.
- 24. Blackburn WD. Management of osteoarthritis and rheumatoid arthritis: prospects and possibilities. *American Journal of Medicine* 1996;**100**:24S-30S.
- 25. Kremer JM, Phelps CT. Long-term prospective study of the use of methotrexate in the treatment of rheumatoid arthritis: update after a mean of 90 months. *Arthritis and Rheumatism* 1992;**35**:138-45.
- 26. Horneff G, Burmester GR, Emmrich F, et al. Treatment of rheumatoid arthritis with an anti-CD4 monoclonal antibody. *Arthritis and Rheumatism* 1991;**34**:129-40.
- 27. Fox DA. The role of T cells in the immunopathogenesis of rheumatoid arthritis: new perspectives. *Arthritis and Rheumatism* 1997;**40**:598-609.
- 28. Fries JF, Williams CA, Morfeld D, et al. Reduction in long-term disability in patients with rheumatoid arthritis by disease-modifying antirheumatic drug-based treatment strategies. *Arthritis and Rheumatism* 1996;**39**:616-22.
- 29. Walker LG, Sledge CB. Total hip arthroplasty in ankylosing spondylitis. *Clinical Orthopaedics and Related Research* 1991;**262**:198-204.
- 30. Kilgus DJ, Namba RS, Goreck JE, et al. Total hip replacement for patients who have ankylosing spondylitis: the importance of the formation of heterotopic bone and of the durability of fixation of cemented components. *Journal of Bone and Joint Surgery (American)* 1990;**72A**:834-9.
- 31. Graham B, Van Peteghem PK. Fractures of the spine in ankylosing spondylitis. Diagnosis, treatment, and complications. *Spine* 1989;**14**:803-7.
- 32. McGill NW, Dieppe PA. Evidence for a promoter of urate crystal formation in gouty synovial fluid. *Annals of Rheumatic Diseases* 1991;**50**:558-61.
- 33. Shaw BA, Kasser JR. Acute septic arthritis in infancy and childhood. *Clinical Orthopaedics and Related Research* 1990;**257**:212-25.
- 34. Freeland AE, Senter BS. Septic arthritis and osteomyelitis. *Hand Clinics* 1989;**5**:533-52.
- 35. Thiery JA. Arthroscopic drainage in septic arthritis of the knee: a multicenter study. *Arthroscopy* 1989;**5**:65-9.

SECTION 2

The hip

TIM BOARD

94	History of the development of total hip arthroplasty *Mukesh Hemmady*	1097
95	Biomechanics of the hip and total hip arthroplasty *Asim Rajpura, Timothy N Board*	1105
96	Materials in hip arthroplasty *Samuel S Rajaratnam, William L Walter*	1114
97	Perioperative considerations *Daniel Kendoff, Thomas P Sculco, Friedrich Boettner*	1123
98	Primary total hip arthroplasty *Ramankutty Sreekumar, Peter R Kay*	1135
99	Minimal incision surgery/mini-invasive total hip replacement *Eugene Sherry, Declan O Sherry*	1147
100	Revision total hip arthroplasty *Ardeshir Bonshahi, Timothy N Board, Martyn L Porter*	1153

History of the development of total hip arthroplasty

MUKESH HEMMADY

Introduction	1097	More recent developments in total hip arthroplasty	1101
Developments in surgery of the hip	1097	References	1102

NATIONAL BOARD STANDARDS

- Know the importance of Sir John Charnley's contribution to low-friction arthroplasty
- Learn about the Exeter hip
- Understand how cementless implants developed
- Know about bearing surfaces

INTRODUCTION

Total hip replacement is a very successful operative procedure for improving quality of life in patients with severe arthritis of the hip. It was a pioneering operation which led the way for other joint replacements such as the knee, shoulder and elbow.

Although the first successful total hip replacement was performed at Wrightington Hospital, Wigan, UK, by the late Sir John Charnley in November 1962, there had been previous attempts, albeit unsuccessfully, by various surgeons.

Arthrodesis of the hip was a popular procedure before people realized that it had deleterious effects on the other joints of the body. The original aim of hip arthroplasty was to restore motion, but it was soon realized that, for an arthroplasty to be successful, it needs not only motion but also to provide stability. With this in mind various interposition arthroplasties were introduced.

DEVELOPMENTS IN SURGERY OF THE HIP

Osteotomy arthroplasty

In 1826, John Rhea Barton[1] of Lancaster, PA, performed an intertrochanteric osteotomy on an ankylosed hip with a view to creating a pseudarthrosis. He manipulated the 'joint' after 20 days postoperatively to maintain mobility.

In 1863, Sayre[2] reported an osteotomy for an ankylosed hip following resection of a bone fragment, which was essentially a modification of the above operation.

Interpositional arthroplasty

In Chicago, John Murphy[3] used a flap of fascia and fat between joint surfaces. William Baer,[4] the founder of the Orthopaedic Department at the Johns Hopkins Medical School, reported on the use of chromicized sheets of pig's bladder as interposing membrane. Autogenous fascia lata was also used by some surgeons. Colonna[5] used the capsule of the hip as an interposing membrane as well as a means to retain the hip in the acetabulum in the treatment of old, untreated congenital dislocation of the hip. Kallio,[6] in Helsinki, used the dermal layer of skin as an interposing membrane.

Reconstructive arthroplasty

Brackett[7] and Whitman[8] reconstructed the upper end of the femur to provide motion in the hip joint. Magnusen,[9] Luck[10] and Wilson[11] made their own modifications to the procedure to suit various indications. Sir Robert Jones[12] osteotomized the femoral neck to create a pseudarthrosis, and Girdlestone et al.[13] resected the head and neck to maintain motion. Charnley's[14] central dislocation–stabilization created a pain-free and stable hip in the pre-total hip era.

Replacement arthroplasty

In 1927, Groves,[15] in the UK, used ivory to replace the femoral head with limited success. Before this, Delbet,[16] in France, used a rubber prosthesis in 1919.

In 1940, Austin Moore and Harold Bohlman removed a tumour from the upper end of the femur and inserted the first metallic prosthesis. This was published as a case report in the *Reporter of the Columbia Medical Society* in South Carolina and in the *Journal of Bone and Joint Surgery*.[17] This was the first reported metallic hemiarthroplasty of the hip.[18]

In 1948, the Judet brothers[19] replaced the femoral head with a plastic (methylmethacrylate) prosthesis, which was widely used owing to the encouraging early results; however, breakage, loosening and osteolysis often required revision surgery and therefore the prosthesis fell into disrepute. The material of the prosthesis was subsequently changed to nylon and other synthetics available at the time. Their contribution is significant because it demonstrated that plastic materials could be used in arthroplasty of the hip with minimal soft-tissue reaction.[19]

Marius Nygaard Smith-Petersen of Boston began working on other materials to use for arthroplasties of the hip in 1923. He experienced failure with glass and Bakelite, an early plastic material. He achieved some success with the 'mold arthroplasty' 15 years later, in which he used cups made of Vitallium, the first non-reactive metal alloy to be used in orthopaedic surgery. The procedure was carried out through an anterior approach to the hip, which was described by him, and consisted of revision of both the head of the femur and the rim of the acetabulum using Vitallium cups of various diameters and depths. The results were impressive: 82% good or satisfactory results in 1000 cases.[20–22] This procedure became very popular, and John Schwartzman[23] showed this operation to be particularly useful in patients with rheumatoid arthritis.

Throughout the 1950s, more than 50 types of prosthesis were introduced that were essentially hemiarthroplasties of the hip. These were McBride's 'doorknob' and J.E.M. Thompson's 'light-bulb' prostheses.[24] The short-stem type was replaced by the long-stem type for stability, and the non-metallic type by metallic type for durability. Most of them bore resemblance to the prostheses developed by F.R. Thompson in 1950[25–27] and Austin Moore in 1952.[28] The acetabular replacement by a fixed cup was introduced by Urist[29] and others, but failure usually resulted from loosening of the devices.

Total hip arthroplasty

The hemiarthroplasty of the Judet brothers and the 'mold arthroplasty' of Smith-Petersen, although not entirely successful, stimulated surgeons all over the world to improve the technique and results. Themistocles Gluck, in Berlin, Germany, during the last decade of the nineteenth century, had designed total knee replacements of ivory that were fixed to bone with a mixture of resin and pumice or plaster of Paris. His experiments were initially on animals and later on human joints affected by tuberculosis. The important thing was that he had demonstrated that the human body could tolerate large foreign objects.[30,31] Philip Wiles[32] implanted matched pairs of stainless steel acetabular and femoral components in six patients with Still disease in 1938 in London, UK. The acetabulum was stabilized with screws and the femoral head with a stem, side plate and screws.[32] The Second World War intervened and the idea was not pursued any further.

With the rising popularity of the hemiarthroplasties of the hip, the operation was expanded to include the acetabulum. Metal-on-metal combinations were tried by Kenneth McKee[33] and John Watson Farrar[34] in London and Peter Ring[35] in Surrey, UK, and by Haboush, Urist and McBride in the USA.[36] Although this furthered the experience of total hip arthroplasty, as it was known then, the results were not satisfactory because of loosening of components and wear of the metallic bearing surfaces.

In 1956, Sir John Charnley observed a patient called Griffiths, who had a Judet Perspex replacement of the femoral head for hip arthritis. It emitted an audible squeak every time he moved. The patient sought Charnley's advice because his wife could not bear the sound – it went 'straight through her' – so much so that she could not even sit at the same table as him because, when he leaned forward to pick up the salt, his hip emitted a piercing squeak.[37] This led John Charnley to think that the basic fault with current joint replacements was deficient lubrication. Thereafter, he embarked on a study of the coefficient of friction of animal and human joints (Charnley 1959) in the basement of the physiology department of the University of Manchester, UK. He obtained an average value of 0.013 for the human knee joints, which is one-tenth of ice sliding on ice (0.03).[38,39] He directed his attention to polytetrafluoroethylene (PTFE) and used it as a 'synthetic cartilage' with concentric PTFE shells lining the acetabulum and covering the head of the femur (Fig. 94.1). Unfortunately, the technique had to be abandoned because of rapid wear and bone destruction. When he published his concept of the 'low-friction' arthroplasty as *Arthroplasty of the hip: a new operation*,[40] it would appear that the original concept of using interposition shells of PTFE was changing to the use of an Austin Moore and Thompson stem with a 1 and 5/8 inch (41.25 mm) head diameter articulating against PTFE shells, in the hope that a large femoral head would reduce the load per unit area. His engineering colleagues pointed out that reducing the

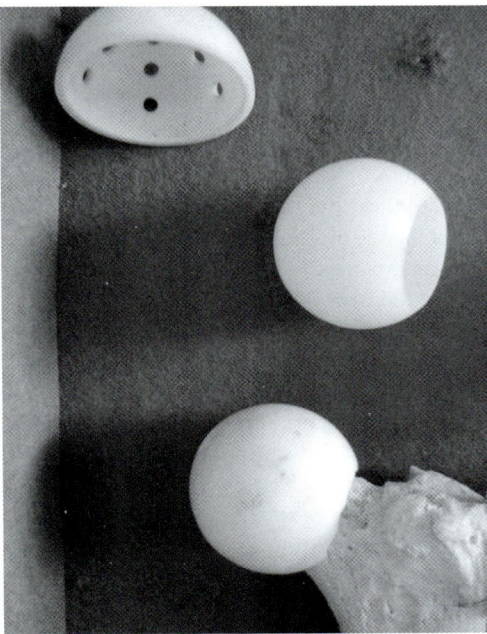

Figure 94.1 Charnley's original polytetrafluorethylene cups and femoral head.

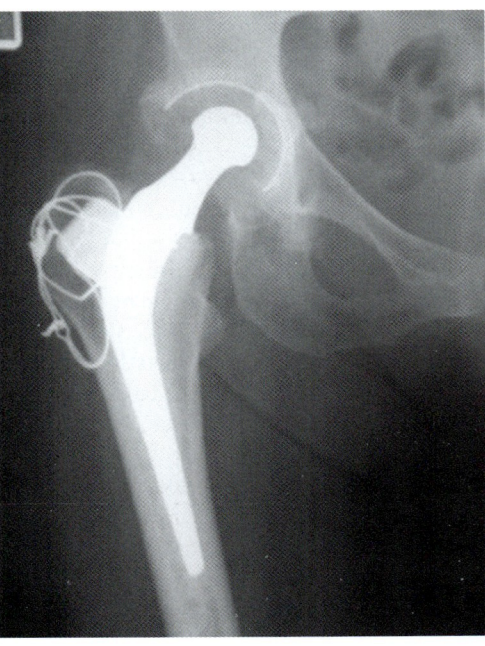

Figure 94.2 A Charnley flatback stem. Note the wires from the trochanteric osteotomy.

head diameter would reduce the frictional force between the head and the socket, and also that, if at the same time the radius of the exterior of the cup was made as large as possible, it would lessen the tendency of the cup to rotate against bone. Taking heed of this advice, Charnley reduced the diameter of the femoral head in stages from 1 and 5/8 inch to 7/8 inch (22.225 mm).[41] This fundamental change from low friction to 'low frictional torque' was the turning point in the evolution of low-frictional torque arthroplasty (LFA).

Charnley suspected that cup wear and loosening would be the most likely long-term problem and had used uncemented metal-backed cups, which he abandoned in favour of fixation with polymethylmethacrylate (PMMA). He did this after seeking the advice of Dr D.C. Smith of the Turner Dental School, University of Manchester, on fillings used in dentistry, and Smith advocated the use of PMMA, pink dental cement, to fix the stem. John Charnley was able to show that cement reduced the movement of the tip of the prosthesis by a factor of 200.[40]

In cooperation with Hugh Howarth, with his vast experience of air cleanliness in the brewing industry, the clean-air enclosure was designed, manufactured and put into use. By increasing the rate of air changes, eventually to 300 per hour, and introducing total-body exhaust suits, the deep infection rate was reduced from over 8% to about 1%.[42–45]

While the original Teflon-bearing surfaces were successful initially, after 12 months there was evidence of failure and mechanical loosening. At this stage, what was lacking was a suitable material for the cup. Introduction of ultra-high-molecular-weight polyethylene (UHMWPE) to arthroplasty was a fortuitous coincidence whereby the man-made fibre industry was looking for a replacement for buffalo hide used for washers in the spinning industry. Charnley's engineer, Harry Craven, saw the opportunity of testing the 'new' material for its wear properties. The results showed exceptionally low wear *in vitro*, which persuaded Charnley to use the material *in vivo*. As a result, the first LFA was performed by Sir John at Wrightington Hospital in November 1962 using the transtrochanteric approach (Fig. 94.2). The components were restricted to the residents trained by Charnley and senior surgeons who attended training courses. It was not until the second half of 1970, almost 8 years after the introduction of the operation into clinical practice, that the components became generally available, and even then under pressure from manufacturers because copies were appearing on the market. Charnley took no royalties, and £1 per set of components was the manufacturer's contribution to research. Charnley waited until 1972 to publish his results.[46] Surgeons from all over the world came to Wrightington Hospital to learn the operation from him.

The Charnley stem evolved from the original flatback to the Vaquasheen-finished stem with the cobra flanges. The flatback stem was changed to roundback in 1973 and the cobra flange was added in 1974. The neck diameter was reduced in 1982 to improve the head-to-neck ratio to reduce impingement and improve range of motion. In the same year, the material of the stem was changed to Ortron (high-nitrogen steel) to reduce stem fractures following the reduction of the neck diameter, and has remained unchanged since (Fig. 94.3). As regards the cups, the long posterior wall socket was introduced in 1972 and flanges in 1977 (PIJ cup). The Ogee cup was introduced in 1982, the angle bore in 1983 and the golf ball cup in 1997 (Fig. 94.4).

Charnley's work from 1954 to 1974 is best described in his own account of the evolution of LFA at Wrightington Hospital:[47,48]

1. Basic research into the lubrication of animal joints.
2. The use of PTFE or Teflon.
3. Low-friction arthroplasty as a principle.
4. Bonding of implant to living bone by quick-setting acrylic cement.
5. Introduction of high-density polyethylene.
6. Attempt to identify the cause of failures by introduction of clean-air enclosure to reduce infection.

Sir John Charnley's contribution to the understanding of total hip replacement is indeed a milestone in orthopaedic surgery. His work has had a world-wide influence on many surgeons and engineers, and it has been the mainspring of inspiration for development of other joint replacements.

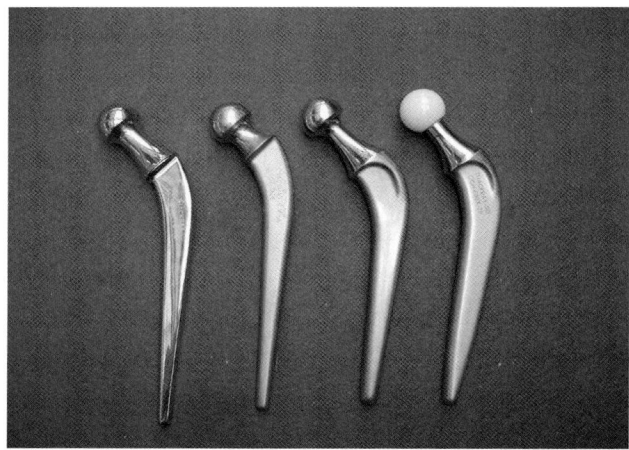

Figure 94.3 The evolution of the Charnley stem from the original flatback (far left) to the Vaquasheen finished roundback stem (1973), with the addition of the cobra flanges (1974).

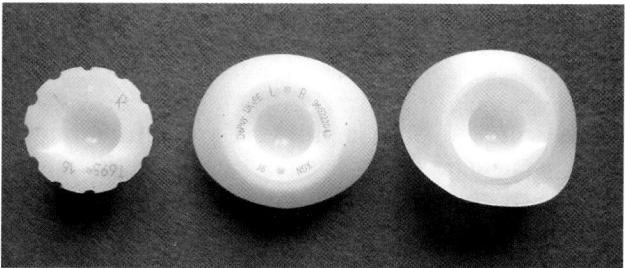

Figure 94.4 Evolution of the Charnley cemented socket. The long posterior wall (left), the flanged (middle) and Ogee (right).

Development of the Exeter stem

Robin Ling and his associates in Exeter, UK, were developing a stem to be inserted through the posterior approach. This was a smooth, double-taper stem made of the rather ductile stainless steel (EN58J) that was introduced into clinical practice in November 1970. Owing to the high incidence of stem and neck fractures, a new range of stems was introduced in 1976 that was slightly heavier in section, made from 316L stainless steel. Initially, the stem was polished, but a new matt version was introduced in 1976 as polishing the stem was expensive. Unfortunately, the matt stem fared rather badly; therefore, its use was discontinued in 1985, and Ling and associates returned to the original smooth finish, double-taper design, introducing the Exeter Universal series in 1988. The spigot at the head–neck junction was changed in 2001 to the V40 design to allow for seating of ceramic heads. The femoral head size evolved from the original 29.75 mm to 26 mm and then to 28 mm. In 1984, metal-backed cups were introduced and then abandoned in 1990 because of poor results.[49] Exeter stems have done well in terms of long-term revision for aseptic loosening. Indeed, surgeons at Exeter improved cementing techniques through pressure washing of the bone surface followed by subsequent plugging and retrograde filling of the femur with low-viscosity cement and 'closed cavity' pressurization to improve the micro-interlock and thereby improve the shear strength at the cement–bone interface.

Development of the uncemented hip

The US Food and Drug Administration approved the use of acrylic cement in the USA in 1968. Cemented hip replacements were the norm; however, some surgeons reported poor results in young patients, and also the term 'cement disease' was coined by Hungerford,[50] which later was found to be erroneous: it was the polyethylene debris and other factors which caused the osteolysis and not the cement. Chandler, from Boston, MA, and others,[51,52] reported early loosening of components in young patients with cemented hips. Total hip articular replacement by internal eccentric shell resurfacing was introduced in 1975 by Amstutz et al.,[53] with the primary goal of bone stock preservation and the hope of increased durability in the young patient.

In reaction to the perceived problems of methylmethacrylate, in both Europe and North America, efforts were made to promote a more 'biological fixation' by eliminating cement altogether and providing a surface to encourage bony ingrowth/ongrowth. Pillar and Galante,[54–56] Newsley and Osborn,[57] de Groot and Geesnik,[58,59] and other research groups[60–63] were pioneers in the study of this approach. The use of uncemented implants for both the stem and the cup started in the 1980s. Plasma spray technology provided the ability to coat orthopaedic metals with calcium salts, thus facilitating the emergence of 'bioactive' implants. In the UK, the first orthopaedic application seems to have been at St Thomas' Hospital, London, in 1981. The Furlong (JRI Ltd, London, UK) hydroxyapatite ceramic-coated hip replacement was introduced in 1985. Geesnik followed with the Omnifit hip (Stryker Howmedica Osteonics, Allendale, NJ) in 1986, and the ARTRO group began use of their Landos–Corail system in the same year. The ABG hip (Stryker Howmedica Osteonics) was first used in 1988.[64] There were some concerns regarding delamination of the hydroxyapatite coating and subsequent third-body wear of the bearing. Hybrid hip replacements (uncemented cup and cemented stem) became popular in the 1980s and 1990s, especially in young patients. However, metal-backed cups with conventional polyethylene have not done well in the long term; fixation was generally good but there has been a high rate of wear, osteolysis, aseptic loosening and dislocation.[65]

The evolution of *uncemented cups* can be mainly divided into devices designed to achieve mechanical fixation to the pelvis by virtue of their geometric shape, large pegs, threaded rings, etc., and designs intended to achieve biological fixation by bony ingrowth into a porous-coated surface. The results of cups using mechanical fixation devices were disappointing, perhaps because of the lack of initial stability and true micro-interlock between the cup and the acetabulum over the long term.[66] In an effort to improve long-term fixation, porous-coated cups were introduced to achieve biological fixation. Initially, supplemental fixation in the form of screws, spikes and pegs was used to provide initial stability for osseointegration. There were some concerns regarding excessive articular and back-side polyethylene wear with metal-backed cups and periacetabular osteolysis caused by wear debris travelling through screw holes in the metal shell.[67,68] Currently, the trend is to use a hemispheric porous/hydroxyapatite-coated implant without supplemental devices (press fit technique).

Earlier generations of *uncemented stems* had patchy coating proximally in the metaphyseal area and had problems of fixation, thigh pain, osteolysis and stress shielding.[69] Extensively coated stems have coating all along the length of the stem; stress shielding and difficulty in revision surgery are major problems.

Long-term results with some cementless stem and cup designs are encouraging, but this relates mainly to fixation of components and wear at the articular surface continues to be a problem.[70–72]

About 20 years after the first successful hip replacement at Wrightington Hospital in 1962, philosophical differences started emerging between North American and European orthopaedic surgeons; these occurred with the introduction of the term 'cement disease', which is when North American surgeons abandoned cemented implants. This paradigm shift led to a focus on product innovation in North America and an emphasis on procedural standardization and evidence-based practice in Europe. The latter led to the development of hip registries to assess the performance of various surgeons and implants, notably the Swedish and Norwegian arthroplasty registers.[73,74]

MORE RECENT DEVELOPMENTS IN TOTAL HIP ARTHROPLASTY

With the current trend towards the use of uncemented implants, attention has now moved to wear at the articular surface, which is perceived to be the main problem leading to failure of hip replacements, and the quest is on to find bearing surfaces with improved wear characteristics. Unsatisfactory results of polyethylene in metal-backed cups were attributed to the poor wear characteristics of conventional polyethylene and locking mechanisms. This saw the introduction of cross-linked and highly cross-linked polyethylene in North America. Cross-linkage was achieved by irradiation or chemical manipulation and has lately been improved by scavenging the free radicals with the use of vitamin E. Medium-term results suggest that, although there is a reduction of wear with highly cross-linked polyethylene, there have been concerns about reduced mechanical properties leading to fatigue failure and fracture. Some authors have attributed this to the reduced thickness of polyethylene consequent to the use of large-diameter femoral heads and also to malpositioning of components.[75] On the other hand, European surgeons have shown a preference for hard-on-hard bearings such as ceramic on ceramic and metal on metal with the use of large heads. In the UK, metal-on-metal resurfacing arthroplasty became extremely popular in the late 1990s.[76,77] The perceived advantages of hard-on-hard bearings are improved lubrication, less wear, improved stability and range of motion. However, they have had their share of problems as well: squeaking, fracture, chipping, stripe wear and reduced revision options with ceramic-on-ceramic articulations, and femoral neck fractures, neck thinning and aseptic lymphocytic, vasculitis and associated lesions or pseudotumours[78] with metal-on-metal bearings. In the hope of avoiding the deleterious effects of metal ions on soft tissues, ceramic-on-metal articulations are being tried to reduce the metal ion load on soft tissues.

Recently, there has been an increased demand from younger patients to maintain a very high level of activity, and therefore functionality has become an issue. Information available on the Internet and direct-to-consumer marketing by the companies has led to increased expectations from these joint replacements. This has led to the use of larger heads in conjunction with bearings that have shown low wear in the laboratory. For reduction of surgical trauma, minimally invasive surgery has been tried and computer-aided surgery was introduced to improve the accuracy of implant positioning; however, they have not met with universal acceptance. Although registry data from around the world and other reports suggest that, in the long term, with improved cementing techniques, revision rates remain very low with cemented hip replacements even in younger patients,[79–82] the tribe of cement users in total hip arthroplasty is dwindling rapidly, and it needs to be seen whether cementless hips with modern bearing surfaces and large femoral heads will stand the test of time; at the present time, there are no long-term studies to support a superior outcome. The functionality and the survival of hip replacements which have been subjected to excessive use by younger patients has yet to be determined.

> **KEY LEARNING POINTS**
>
> - Sir John Charnley's contribution to the evolution of low-friction arthroplasty; as the pioneer of arthroplasty, he addressed friction, fixation, wear, stability and infection. Gold standard in hip arthroplasty.
> - Development of the Exeter hip: this design evolved with time. Double polished taper stem is successful.
> - Evolution of cementless implants: hydroxyapatite-coated bone-conserving stems compared with fit and fill implants.
> - Advantages and disadvantages of newer bearings: no one clear winner at present.

REFERENCES

- ● = Key primary paper
- ◆ = Major review article

1. Barton JR. On the treatment of ankylosis by the formation of artificial joints. *North American Medical and Surgical Journal* 1827;**3**:279–92.
2. Sayre LA. A new operation for artificial hip joint in bony anchylosis. *Clinical Orthopaedics and Related Research* 1994;**298**:4–7.
3. Murphy JB. Arthroplasty. *Annals of Surgery* 1913;**57**:593–647.
4. Baer WS. Arthroplasty with the aid of animal membrane. *American Journal of Orthopedic Surgery* 1919;**16**:1–29;94–115;171–99.
5. Colonna PC. A new type of reconstruction operation for old ununited fracture of the neck of the femur. *Journal of Bone and Joint Surgery* 1935;**17**:110–22.
6. Kallio KE. Arthroplastia cutanea. Proceedings of Nordisk Ortopedisk Forenings Twenty-eighth Assembly in Helsinki, June, 1956. *Acta Orthopaedica Scandinavica* 1957;**26**:327.
7. Brackett EG. Fracture neck of the femur-operation of transplantation of the femoral head to trochanter. *Boston Medical and Surgical Journal* 1925;**192**:1118–20.
8. Whitman R. A new treatment for fracture of the neck of the femur. *Medical Record* 1904;**65**:441–7.
9. Magnuson PB. The repair of un-united fracture of the neck of the femur. *JAMA* 1932;**98**:1791–4.
10. Luck JV. A reconstruction operation for pseudarthrosis and resorption of the neck of the femur. *Iowa Medical Society* 1938;**28**:620–8.
11. Wilson PD. Trochanteric arthroplasty in the treatment of ununited fractures of the neck of the femur. *Journal of Bone and Joint Surgery* 1947;**29**:313–27.
12. Jones R (ed.). *Orthopaedic Surgery of Injuries.* London, UK: Frowde, 1921.
13. Girdlestone GR, Watson Jones R, Stamm T, Pridie KH. Discussion on the treatment of unilateral osteoarthritis of the hip. *Proceedings of the Royal Society of Medicine* 1945;**38**:363–8.
14. Charnley J. *Compression Arthrodesis, Including Central Dislocation as a Principle in Hip Surgery.* Edinburgh, UK: E&S Livingstone, 1953:242–55.
15. Groves EWH. Surgical treatment of osteoarthritis of the hip. *British Medical Journal* 1933;**1**:3–5.
16. Delbet P. Resultat eloigne d'un visage pour fracture transcervicale du femur. *Bulletin et Mémoires de la Société des Chirurgiens de Paris* 1919;**45**:434.
17. Moore AT, Bohlman HR. Metal hip joint-a case report. *Journal of Bone and Joint Surgery* 1943;**25**:688–92.
18. Moore AT. The self locking metal hip prosthesis. *Journal of Bone and Joint Surgery (American)* 1957;**39A**:811–27.
●19. Judet J, Judet R. The use of an artificial femoral head for arthroplasty of the hip joint. *Journal of Bone and Joint Surgery (British)* 1950;**32B**:166–73.
20. Smith-Petersen MN. Arthroplasty of the hip, a new method. *Journal of Bone and Joint Surgery* 1939;**21**:269–88.
●21. Smith-Petersen MN. Evolution of mould arthroplasty of the hip joint. *Journal of Bone and Joint Surgery (British)* 1948;**30B**:59–75.
22. Smith-Petersen MN. A new supra-articular subperiosteal approach to the hip joint. *American Journal of Orthopedic Surgery* 1917;**15**:592–5.
23. Schwartzmann JR. Arthroplasty of the hip in rheumatoid arthritis. *Journal of Bone and Joint Surgery (American)* 1959;**41A**:705–21.
24. Thompson JEM. A prosthesis for the femoral head: a preliminary report. *Journal of Bone and Joint Surgery* 1952;**34**:175–82.
25. Thompson FR. Vitallium intramedullary hip prosthesis-preliminary report. *New York State Journal of Medicine* 1952;**52**:3011–20.
26. Thompson FR. Two and a half years' experience with a Vitallium intramedullary hip prosthesis. *Journal of Bone and Joint Surgery (American)* 1954;**36A**:489–502.
27. Thompson FR. An essay on the development of arthroplasty of the hip. *Clinical Orthopaedics and Related Research* 1966;**44**:73–82.
28. Moore AT. Metal hip joint-new self locking Vitallium prosthesis. *South Medical Journal* 1952;**45**:1015–19.

29. Urist M. *Hip Arthroplasty*. Baltimore, MD: Williams and Wilkins, 1965.
30. Gluck T. Autoplastiktransplantation: implantation von Fremdkorpern. *Berliner Klinische Wochenschrift* 1890;**27**:421–7.
31. Gluck T. Referat uber die durch das modern chirurgische experiment gewonnenen positiven resultate, betreffend die naht und den Erastz von Defecten hoherer Gewebe, Sowie uber die Verwerthung resorbirbarer und lebendiger tampons in der Chirurgie. *Archiv für Klinische Chirurgie* 1891;**41**:187–239.
32. Wiles PW. The surgery of the osteoarthritic hip. *British Journal of Surgery* 1958;**45**:488–97.
33. McKee GK. Artificial hip joint. *Journal of Bone and Joint Surgery (British)* 1951;**33**:465.
●34. McKee GK, Watson-Farrar J. Replacement of arthritic hips by the McKee-Farrar prosthesis. *Journal of Bone and Joint Surgery (British)* 1966;**48**:245–9.
●35. Ring PA. Complete replacement arthroplasty of the hip by the Ring prosthesis. *Journal of Bone and Joint Surgery (British)* 1968;**50B**:720–31.
36. Haboush EJ. A new operation for arthroplasty of the hip based on biomechanics, photoelasticity, fast setting dental acrylic and other considerations. *Bulletin of the Hospital for Joint Diseases* 1953;**14**:242–7.
37. Hardinge K. The development of the Charnley low friction arthroplasty. In: Galasko CSB, Noble J (eds) *Current Trends in Orthopaedic Surgery*. Manchester, UK: Manchester University Press, 1988:242–5.
38. Charnley J. The lubrication of animal joints. *New Scientist* 1960;9 June:60–1.
39. Charnley J. The lubrication of animal joints in relation to surgical reconstruction by arthroplasty. *Annals of Rheumatic Diseases* 1960;**19**:10–18.
40. Charnley J. Arthroplasty of the hip: a new operation. *Lancet* 1961;**1**:1129–32.
41. Wroblewski BM. Charnley low-frictional torque arthroplasty of the hip. In: Faux JC (ed.) *After Charnley*. Chorley, UK: The John Charnley Trust, 2002:29–34.
42. Charnley J. A clean air operating enclosure. *British Journal of Surgery* 1964;**51**:202–5.
43. Charnley J, Efthekar N. Postoperative infection in total prosthetic replacement arthroplasty of the hip joint. With special reference to the bacterial content of the air of the operating room. *British Journal of Surgery* 1969;**56**:641–9.
●44. Lidwell O, Elson RA, Lowbury EJ, et al. Ultraclean air and antibiotics for the prevention of postoperative infection. A multi-centre study of 8052 joint replacement operations. *Acta Orthopaedica Scandinavica* 1987;**58**:4–13.
45. Lidgren L. Joint prosthetic infections: a success story. *Acta Orthopaedica Scandinavica* 2001;**72**:553–6.
●46. Charnley J. The long term results of low friction arthroplasty of the hip performed as a primary intervention. *Journal of Bone and Joint Surgery (British)* 1972;**54**:61–76.
47. Eftekar NS. A historical note on the development of hip arthroplasty. In: Eftekar NS (ed.) *Principles of Total Hip Arthroplasty*. St Louis, MO: CV Mosby, 1978:1–8.
48. Charnley J. Total hip replacement. *JAMA* 1974;**230**:1025–8.
●49. Gie GA, Lee ACJ, Ling RSM, Timperley AJ. The development of the Exeter hip. In: Faux JC (ed.) *After Charnley*. Chorley, UK: The John Charnley Trust, 2002:146–69.
50. Hungerford D. Cement disease. *Clinical Orthopaedics and Related Research* 1987;**225**:192–206.
51. Chandler HP, Reineck FT, Wixson RL, et al. Total hip replacement in patients younger than thirty years old: a five year follow-up study. *Journal of Bone and Joint Surgery (American)* 1981;**63A**:1426–34.
52. Collis DK. Cemented total hip replacement in patients who are less than fifty years old. *Journal of Bone and Joint Surgery (American)* 1984;**66A**:353–9.
53. Amstutz HC, Dorey F, O'Carroll PF. THARIES resurfacing arthroplasty: evolution and long term results. *Clinical Orthopaedics and Related Research* 1986;**213**:92–114.
●54. Bobyn JD, Pillar RM, Cameron HU, et al. Porous surfaced layered prosthetic devices. *Journal of Biomedical Engineering* 1975;**10**:126–31.
55. Bobyn JD, Pillar RM, Cameron HU, et al. The optimum pore size for fixation of porous surfaced metal implants by the ingrowth of bone. *Clinical Orthopaedics and Related Research* 1980;**150**:126–31.
56. Galante J. Symposium: total joint arthroplasty without cement. *Clinical Orthopaedics and Related Research* 1983;**176**:7–114.
57. Newsley H, Osborn JF. Structure and texture of calcium phosphate in ceramics. In: *Proceedings of the 3rd Conference on Materials for use in Medicine and Biology, Keele University, Manchester, 13–16 September 1978*. Manchester, UK: Manchester University Press.
58. De Groot K, Geesnik R, Klein CP. Plasma sprayed coatings of hydroxyapatite. *Journal of Biomedical Materials Research* 1987;**21**:375–81.
59. Geesnik R, de Groot K, Klein CPAT. Bonding of bone to apatite-coated implants. *Journal of Bone and Joint Surgery (British)* 1988,**70B**:17–22.
60. Cook SD, Thomas KA, Jarcho M. Hydroxyapatite-coated titanium for orthopaedic implant applications. *Clinical Orthopaedics and Related Research* 1988;**232**:225–43.
61. Soballe K, Hansen ES, Brockstedt-Rasmussen H, et al. Fixation of titanium hydroxyapatite coated implants in osteopenic bone. *Journal of Arthroplasty* 1991;**6**:307–16.
62. Jarcho M. Retrospective analysis of hydroxyapatite development for oral implant applications. *Dental Clinics of North America* 1992;**36**:19–26.
63. Geesnik RGT, Manley MT (eds) *Hydroxyapatite Coatings in Orthopaedic Surgery*. New York, NY: Raven Press, 1993.
64. Shepperd JAN, Apthorp H. A contemporary snapshot of the use of hydroxyapatite coating in orthopaedic surgery. *Journal of Bone and Joint Surgery (British)* 2004,**87B**;1046–9.

- 65. Hallan G, Dybvik E, Furnes O, Havelin LI. Metal-backed acetabular components with conventional polyethylene: a review of 9113 primary components with a follow-up of 20 years. *Journal of Bone and Joint Surgery (British)* 2010,**92B**:196–201.
66. Peters CL, Miller DM. The cementless acetabular component: In: Callaghan JJ, Rosenberg A, Rubash H (eds) *The Adult Hip*, vol. 2, 2nd edn. Philadelphia, PA: Lippincott Williams and Wilkins, 2007:946–68.
67. Barrack RL. Concerns with cementless modular acetabular components. *Orthopaedics* 1996;**19**:741–3.
68. Barrack RL, Folgueras A, Munn B, *et al*. Pelvic lysis and polyethylene wear at 5–8 years in an uncemented total hip. *Clinical Orthopaedics and Related Research* 1997;**335**;211–17.
69. Campbell AC, Rorabeck CH, Bourne RB, *et al*. Thigh pain after cementless arthroplasty hip. Annoyance or ill omen. *Journal of Bone and Joint Surgery (British)* 1992;**74**:63–6.
- 70. Hallan G, Lie SA, Furnes O, *et al*. Medium and long-term performance of 11516 uncemented primary femoral stems from the Norwegian Arthroplasty Register. *Journal of Bone and Joint Surgery (British)* 2007;**89B**:1574–80.
- 71. Havelin LI, Espehaug B, Engesaeter LB. The performance of two hydroxyapatite-coated acetabular cups compared with Charnley cups. From The Norwegian Arthroplasty Register. *Journal of Bone and Joint Surgery (British)* 2002;**84B**:839–45.
72. Della Valle CJ, Mesko NW, Quigley L, *et al*. Primary total hip arthroplasty with a porous-coated acetabular component. A concise follow-up, at a minimum of twenty years, of previous reports. *Journal of Bone and Joint Surgery (American)* 2009;**91**;773–82.
73. Garellick G, Malchau H, Herberts P. Survival of hip replacements. A comparison of a randomised trial and a registry. *Clinical Orthopaedics and Related Research* 2000;**375**:157–67.
74. Havelin LI. *Hip Arthroplasty in Norway 1987–1994*. The Norwegian Arthroplasty Register. Bergen, Norway: University of Bergen, 1995.
75. Tower SS, Currier JH, Currier BH, *et al*. Rim cracking of cross-linked Longevity polyethylene acetabular liner after total hip arthroplasty. *Journal of Bone and Joint Surgery (American)* 2007;**89A**:2212–17.
76. Daniel J, Pynsent PB, McMinn DJ. Metal-on-metal resurfacing of the hip in patients under the age of 55 years with osteoarthritis. *Journal of Bone and Joint Surgery (British)* 2004;**86**:177–84.
77. Treacy RBC, McBryde CW, Pynsent PB. Birmingham hip resurfacing arthroplasty: a minimum follow-up of five years. *Journal of Bone and Joint Surgery (British)* 2005;**87B**:167–70.
78. Pandit H, Glyn-Jones S, McLardy Smith P, *et al*. Pseudotumours associated with metal-on-metal hip resurfacings. *Journal of Bone and Joint Surgery (British)* 2008;**90**;847–51.
- 79. Callaghan JJ, Bracha P, Liu SS, *et al*. Survivorship of a Charnley total hip arthroplasty at a minimum of thirty five years, a concise follow-up of previous reports. *Journal of Bone and Joint Surgery (American)* 2009;**91**:2617–21.
- 80. Wroblewski BM, Siney PD, Fleming PA. Charnley low frictional torque arthroplasty; follow-up for 30–40 years. *Journal of Bone and Joint Surgery (British)* 2009;**91B**:447–50.
- 81. Wroblewski BM, Siney PD, Fleming PA. Charnley low-frictional torque arthroplasty in patients under the age of 51 years: follow-up to 33 years. *Journal of Bone and Joint Surgery (British)* 2002;**84**:540–3.
- 82. Ling RS, Charity J, Lee AJ, *et al*. The long term results of the original Exeter polished cemented femoral component: a follow-up report. *Journal of Arthroplasty* 2009;**24**:511–17.

# 95

Biomechanics of the hip and total hip arthroplasty

ASIM RAJPURA, TIMOTHY N BOARD

Introduction	1105	Optimizing fixation and the low frictional torque arthroplasty	1109
Relevant anatomy	1105	Reducing the joint reaction force in total hip arthroplasty	1110
Forces acting about the hip	1106		
Reducing the joint reaction force	1107		
Biomechanics of total hip arthroplasty	1108	Biomechanics of hip impingement	1110
Stability and range of motion	1108	References	1111

NATIONAL BOARD STANDARDS

- Understand the forces acting about the hip
- Know the biomechanics of total hip arthroplasty
- Understand the importance of low frictional torque arthroplasty
- Know the biomechanics of hip impingement

INTRODUCTION

A sound understanding of the biomechanics of the native hip joint allows one to appreciate the mechanics of pathologies about the hip and plan therapeutic interventions which may help reduce joint loading and subsequent symptomatology. Accurately restoring the original biomechanics of the diseased hip during hip arthroplasty may also help maximize function and longevity of the implants.

RELEVANT ANATOMY

The hip joint is a ball-and-socket joint formed by the acetabulum and femoral head. It has three degrees of freedom in rotation and zero degrees of freedom in translation. The three bones of the os coxae, the ilium, and pubis and ischium come together at the triradiate cartilage forming the acetabulum. Fusion occurs between the ages of 17 and 18 years.[1] The functional volume of the bony acetabulum is increased by the fibrocartilaginous labrum, which is attached along the acetabular rim and merges with the transverse acetabular ligament inferiorly. Normal values for acetabular orientation are estimated to be between 15° and 20° of anteversion with a mean lateral inclination angle of 51°.[2,3]

The femoral head is formed by two-thirds of a sphere. The femoral neck forms two angular relationships with the femoral shaft that are relevant to hip biomechanics. These are the neck–shaft angle and anteversion of the femoral neck, as shown in Fig. 95.1. Viewed in the coronal plane, the neck forms an oblique angle with the shaft that averages 135°.[4] This lateralizes the greater trochanter from the centre of rotation, giving the abductor muscles a mechanical advantage by increasing their lever arm. The implications of variations in the neck–shaft angle are discussed below. The anteversion of the femoral neck is the axial relationship of the long axis of the femoral neck and posterior condylar axis of the distal femur. This averages 8° in adults.[5] Anteversion of the neck allows a larger range of flexion before impingement occurs, and also helps to reduce horizontal turning moments.[6] The trabecular structure of the proximal femur follows the main lines of stress in the bone and is shown in Fig. 95.2.

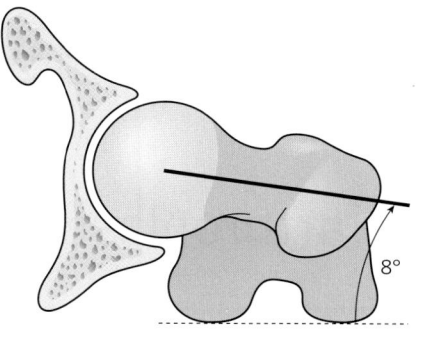
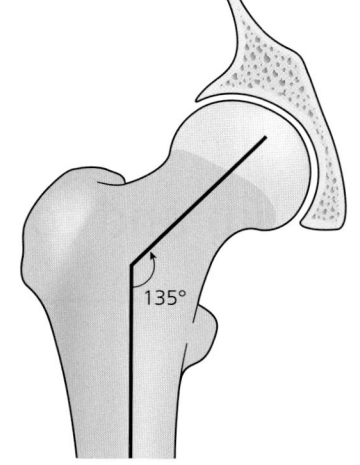

Figure 95.1 Femoral anteversion and the neck shaft angle of the proximal femur.

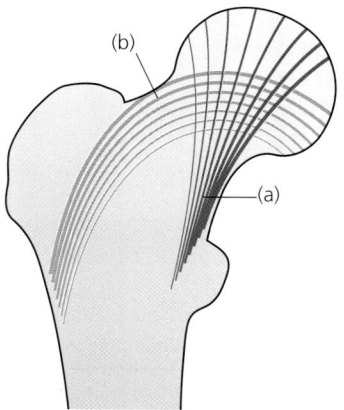

Figure 95.2 The trabecular structure of the femoral neck, demonstrating the primary compressive trabeculae (a) and the primary tensile trabeculae (b).

Stability of the joint is conferred mainly by the bony anatomy but also by the ligaments and musculature that cross the joint and the osseous arrangement as discussed above. The three main extracapsular ligaments of the hip are the iliofemoral, ischiofemoral and pubofemoral ligaments. The iliofemoral ligament is situated on the anterior aspect of the hip, resisting extension at the hip joint and therefore playing an important role in sagittal balance. The ischiofemoral ligament is located posteriorly and helps to control internal rotation. The pubofemoral ligament is located anteroinferiorly and resists external rotation.[7] With regards to muscles crossing the hip, the abductor muscle group is the most important in providing coronal plane stability. The gluteus medius is the primary abductor, accounting for 59% of the cross-sectional area of the abductor group.[8] Smaller contributions are provided by gluteus minimus, tensor fasciae latae, piriformis and the anterior fibres of gluteus maximus.

FORCES ACTING ABOUT THE HIP

Forces acting about the hip need to considered in both the sagittal and coronal planes, in both double- and single-leg stance.

Double-leg stance

In the *sagittal* plane the centre of gravity is located directly above the centre of the femoral heads. No turning moment is therefore generated about the hip; as a result, no muscular forces are required to maintain equilibrium. If the body leans backwards slightly and the centre of gravity moves posterior with respect to the centre of the femoral head, the anteriorly located iliofemoral ligament becomes taut and helps to maintain equilibrium.

In the *coronal* plane the load of the body weight minus the weight of the legs is distributed equally over the two hip joints, generating equal joint reaction forces (JRFs), as shown in Fig. 95.3.

Single-leg stance

When a single-leg stance is adopted, as occurs during walking, the hip joint acts as a fulcrum in a first-class lever system (Fig. 95.4). The hip therefore allows the body to pivot about its centre with respect to the stance leg. If a single leg is considered to be one-sixth of the body weight, then, with single-leg stance, the remaining five-sixths of the body weight generates a turning moment about the hip. In order to maintain balance, the hip abductors (HAs) contract, generating a counter-moment to maintain equilibrium. The length of the lever arm of the HAs is approximately half the length of the lever arm of the body weight. A HA force almost twice the body weight is therefore required to maintain balance. This

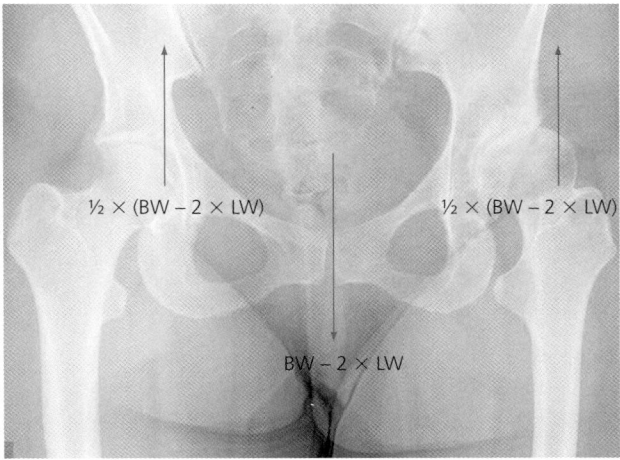

Figure 95.3 Forces acting at the hip joints with double-leg stance in the coronal plane. BW, body weight; LW, leg weight.

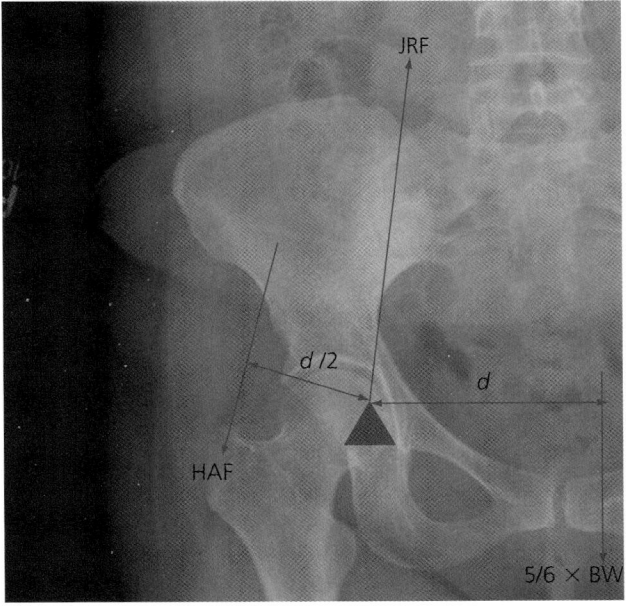

Figure 95.4 Free-body analysis of the hip joint during single-leg stance, and equation resolving moments about the hip joint. HAF, hip abductor force; BW, body weight; JRF, joint reaction force.
For equilibrium: HAF $\times$ ($d/2$) = $d \times$ (5/6 $\times$ BW)
$\therefore$ HAF = 2 $\times$ (5/6 $\times$ BW), if BW = 600N, then HAF = 1000N
JRF $\approx$ HAF + 5/6 $\times$ BW = 1500N

force, in combination with the body weight, generates a JRF of almost three times the body weight. The JRF is angled at approximately 14° towards the midline, exactly following the primary compressive trabeculae of the femoral head. JRFs can be approximately calculated by summing the HA force and five-sixths of the body weight. However, as the HA force is angled at approximately 20° with respect to body weight, accurate

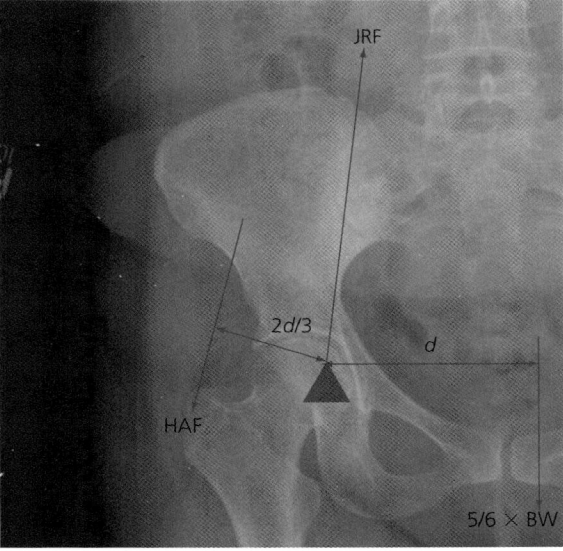

Figure 95.5 Free-body analysis of the hip joint during Trendelenburg gait, and equation resolving moments about the hip joint and showing the reduction in hip abductor force. HAF, hip abductor force; BW, body weight; JRF, joint reaction force.
For equilibrium: HAF $\times$ (2d/3) = $d \times$ (5/6 $\times$ BW)
$\therefore$ HAF = 3/2 $\times$ (5/6 $\times$ BW), if BW = 600N, then HAF = 750N
JRF $\approx$ HAF + 5/6 $\times$ BW = 1250N

calculation of the JRF requires resolution of the HA force into its horizontal and vertical vectors. The vertical component of the HA force is then combined with the body weight component as they act in the same direction. Pythagorean theorem can then be used to combine this summed vertical vector with the horizontal vector of the HA force to accurately calculate the JRF.

REDUCING THE JOINT REACTION FORCE

Strategies to reduce the JRF can help decrease pain in diseased hips, and in hip replacements it may reduce the load on the implants, potentially reducing loosening. As the JRF is a function of both body weight and HA force, the JRF can be reduced by either reducing the body weight-generated moment or reducing the required HA force. A reduction in the body weight-generated moment can be achieved by either reducing the body weight or reducing the body weight lever arm. This is the basis for the Trendelenburg gait. By swaying the upper body towards the diseased hip during single-leg stance, the body weight lever arm is reduced and therefore the moment generated is reduced. As a consequence, a lesser HA force is required to maintain equilibrium and therefore the JRF reduces, decreasing hip pain (Fig. 95.5).

The HA force can be reduced by increasing the HA lever arm or providing additional moments to help balance out the body weight moments. Altering the neck–shaft angle

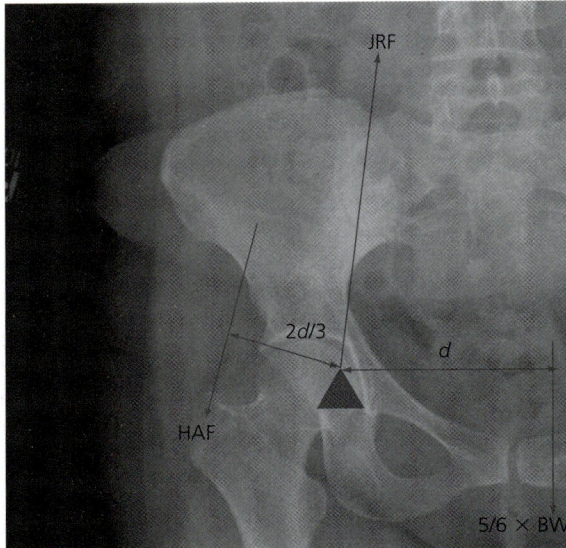

Figure 95.6 Free-body analysis of the hip joint during single-leg stance and a walking cane in the contralateral hand, and equation resolving moments about the hip joint and showing the reduction in hip abductor force and joint reaction force. HAF, hip abductor force; BW, body weight; JRF, joint reaction force; CF centre of femoral head.

For equilibrium: HAF $\times$ (d/2) + CF $\times$ 3d = d $\times$ (5/6 $\times$ BW)
$\therefore$ if BW = 600N, d = 0.1m and CF = 100N, then HAF = 400N
JRF $\approx$ HAF + 5/6 $\times$ BW = 900N

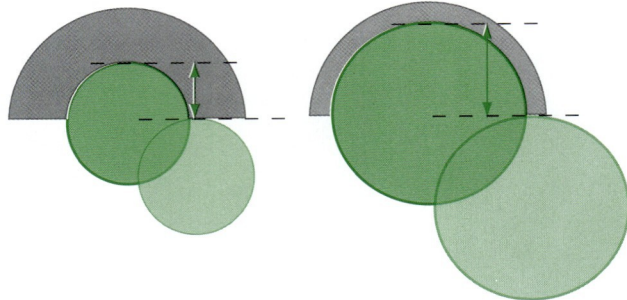

Figure 95.7 Jumping distance (indicated by the arrow) demonstrates the distance the head needs to travel before dislocation occurs. Increasing head size increases this distance.

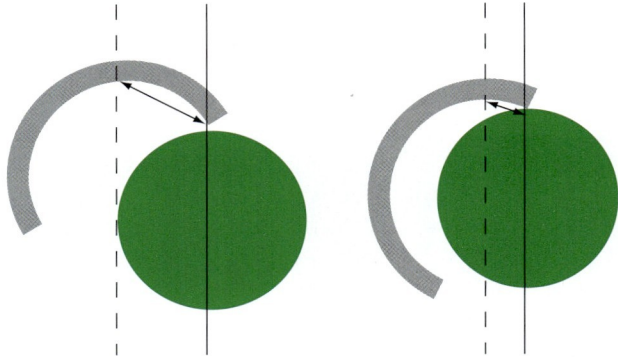

Figure 95.8 Jumping distance can also be influenced by component positioning; increasing the cup inclination reduces the jumping distance.

through varus osteotomy or varus placement of the femoral stem can help to increase the HA lever arm, reducing the required HA force needed to generate the appropriate counterbalancing moment. Increasing offset or medialization of the socket during total hip arthroplasty (THA) has the same effect. Additional moments to counterbalance the body weight moment can be generated through the use of a walking stick in the contralateral hand, as shown in Fig. 95.6. This again reduces the required HA force, consequently reducing the JRF. A similar effect can be seen with a load carried on the ipsilateral side. These effects have been demonstrated *in vivo* by using electromyographic (EMG) studies to measure HA activity during walking stick use and load carrying.[9–11] Using a stick on the contralateral side reduced HA EMG activity by 31%, and carrying a load equivalent to 10% of the body weight on the ipsilateral side reduced HA EMG activity by 17%.

BIOMECHANICS OF TOTAL HIP ARTHROPLASTY

The basic biomechanical concepts discussed above can be applied to THA to help achieve the aims of maximizing the range of motion (ROM) and stability of the implant while minimizing the risk of failure.

STABILITY AND RANGE OF MOTION

Implant-related factors that affect the stability and ROM of a THA include the head size, the head–neck ratio and implant design. Stability and ROM are inextricably linked and must be considered together.

Increasing the head diameter increases the *jumping distance* (i.e. the radius of the femoral head) required before dislocation occurs, as shown in Fig. 95.7. This has been clinically validated using data from both the Norwegian and Australian joint registries that have shown a reduction in rates of revision for dislocation with increasing head size.[12,13]

The jumping distance can also be influenced by component positioning, as increasing cup inclination effectively decreases the jumping distance in the coronal plane (Fig. 95.8).[14] For a hemispherical cup implanted with an inclination angle of 45°, the jumping distance is equal to 0.77 times the head radius.[14] Increasing the inclination to 65° decreases this distance to 0.43 times the head radius.

One of the major determinants of the impingement free ROM of a THA is the head–neck ratio. This is known as the *primary arc* of a joint and is depicted by the angle θ in Fig. 95.9. Increasing the head–neck ratio increases this arc, improving the ROM. A head diameter to neck diameter

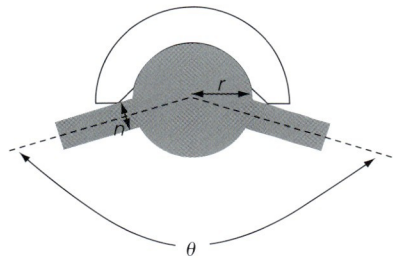 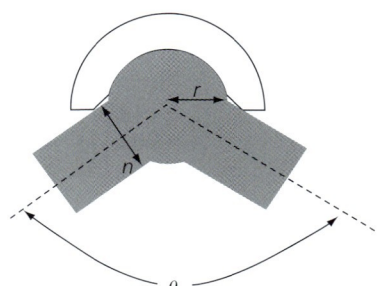

Figure 95.9 The primary arc (θ) of a total hip replacement. Note that the cup has bevelled edges and there is a large head–neck ratio allowing for larger range of motion. r, head radius; n, neck diameter.

ratio of less than 2:1 is said to greatly increase the risk of impingement.[15] The clinical consequences of impingement include fixation failure, limited function and dislocation. Neck geometry can also alter the head–neck ratio, as a trapezoidal or cut-away neck will reduce neck diameter compared with a standard neck, and this has been shown clinically to reduce dislocation rates.[16] Acetabular design features that can help increase the primary arc include the use of bevelled edges and cut-away portions of the socket. Lipped liners or semicaptive sockets that are greater than a hemisphere reduce the primary arc and may have a paradoxically adverse effect on stability. The original Charnley socket had a depth 2 mm greater than the radius of the head with unbevelled edges. This design had a small primary arc of only 90°. Many resurfacing monoblock sockets are subhemispherical in design, increasing primary arc but reducing jumping distance and predisposing to edge loading. The effect is magnified with decreasing size of socket in some designs, with the internal angle of the socket measuring as low as 144°.[17] This may be a factor in wear and soft-tissue reactions that have been recently described.[18–20]

Considerable debate exists regarding whether conventional THA or resurfacing provides a greater ROM. *In vitro* studies suggest that conventional THA has a greater ROM than resurfacing arthroplasty because of the more favourable head–neck ratio.[21–23] Clinical comparisons have been difficult owing to the differing patient cohorts that undergo conventional THA and resurfacing operations. Le Duff et al.[24] have, however, compared patients with bilateral hip arthroplasties, one side with a conventional THA and a contralateral resurfacing arthroplasty. They found no difference in ROM between the two designs and suggest that accurate component positioning to reduce impingement is a more critical factor.

OPTIMIZING FIXATION AND THE LOW FRICTIONAL TORQUE ARTHROPLASTY

Sir John Charnley, the father of THA, recognized at a very early stage that maintaining acetabular fixation was most likely to be the major long-term challenge.[25] His original designs were based on a low-friction concept in an attempt to replicate the low-friction environment of native joints. He used polytetrafluoroethylene (PTFE) press-fit acetabular

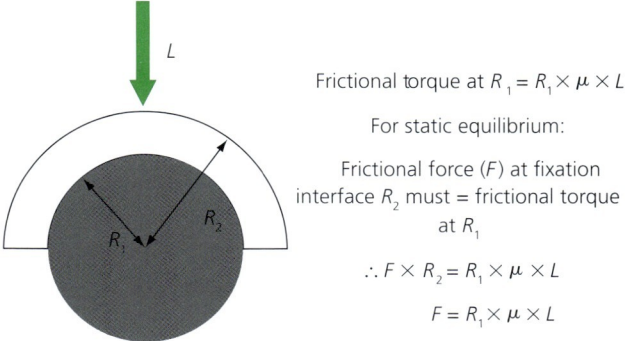

Figure 95.10 Diagram of a hip implant illustrating the basis of low frictional torque arthroplasty. R_1, radius of the femoral head; R_2, outer radius of the acetabular component; L, load; μ, frictional coefficient of the bearing couple. The equation demonstrates the relationship between the force (F) generated at the fixation interface and R_1 and R_2. As R_1 reduces compared with R_2, the frictional force at the fixation interface reduces.

liners with large metal heads. This design, however, had a high early failure rate because of high wear of the PTFE liner. Other early THA designs involving metal-on-metal bearings were equally unsuccessful.[26,27] This was thought to be due to the high incidence of equatorial bearing rather than polar bearing with these early designs. This generated high levels of frictional torque, leading to large torsional forces being transmitted to the fixation interface, which led to loosening. Charnley was therefore persuaded to move towards using smaller diameter heads while maximizing the outer diameter of the acetabular component.[28] This led to the concept of the low frictional torque arthroplasty.

As shown in Fig. 95.10, the frictional torque generated at the bearing surface is equal to the product of the coefficient of friction of the bearing surface, length of the lever arm, i.e. radius of the femoral head, and the load applied to the joint. This torque is transmitted to the cup, producing a turning force. In order to maintain static equilibrium, an equal but counter-directional frictional torque must be generated at the cup–cement or cement–bone interface. The forces generated at the fixation interface can therefore be minimized either by reducing the original frictional torque by reducing the size of the femoral head, or by maximizing the outer diameter of the cup, reducing the force needed at the fixation interface by increasing the lever arm. Reducing stresses at the fixation interface using these two strategies can therefore potentially reduce the risk of fixation failure. Charnley suggested that the ratio of the diameter of the cup to the head should be 2:1.[29] This is the basis behind the Charnley low frictional torque arthroplasty.

Sceptics of this approach state that the success of Charnley's THA was down to the low volumetric wear generated by the small 22.225 mm head and not its low frictional torque properties. Low wear minimizes the biological response induced, therefore reducing the incidence of aseptic loosening.[30] Wroblewski et al.[31] have compared the failure rate of a Charnley THA with 43 mm cups versus 40 mm cups, in which the volumetric wear was equal as judged by the depth of penetration of the 22.225 mm head. They showed a higher failure rate in the 40 mm group of a magnitude comparable to the increased relative level of stresses at the fixation interface owing to the reduction in outer cup diameter, as predicted by the equation in Fig. 95.5. This supports the concept of low frictional torque arthroplasty and suggests that low volumetric wear is not the key factor to the success of the Charnley THA.

Because of the additional stability afforded by larger head diameters there has been a recent move towards using larger heads. To offset the increase in frictional torque secondary to the increase in head diameter, the frictional coefficient can be reduced by the use of modern bearing materials such as ceramics. Metal-on-metal bearings are also becoming more prevalent again because even larger heads can be used as the thickness of acetabular component can be minimized. Earlier designs, such as the McKee–Farrar prosthesis, exhibited a high early failure rate, and therefore metal-on-metal bearings had become less popular.[26] The high early failure rate was thought to be due to a combination of impingement caused by a low head–neck ratio and an inadequate radial clearance, leading to equatorial bearing and resulting in high levels of frictional torque and subsequent loosening.[26,32] Charnley therefore abandoned the use of metal bearings as he thought hydrodynamic lubrication was not possible with metal bearings. There were, however, a proportion of McKee–Farrar prostheses that did function well and have survived for more than 20 years. These were thought to be correctly positioned prostheses with adequate radial clearance allowing polar bearing.[27] The manufacturing tolerances at the time were not good enough to allow reliable production of bearing couples with appropriate clearances and many couples had poor clearances leading to early failure.

The McKee–Farrar prostheses that did survive prompted the development of the second-generation metal bearings that are now widely and successfully used.[33,34] Radial clearance is now understood to be a critical factor in the success of these bearings, and manufacturing tolerances are much finer to allow reliable production of polar bearing implants. As discussed earlier, inadequate clearance results in equatorial bearing and high levels of friction. Metal bearings operate at their optimum with a mixed or ideally a fluid-film (hydrodynamic) lubrication regime. Clearances of the order of 100 μm are thought to be optimum in generating fluid films, which promote such lubrication regimes. Higher clearances have thinner films, increasing friction, whereas tighter clearances risk equatorial bearing if there is deformation of the acetabular component.[35]

REDUCING THE JOINT REACTION FORCE IN TOTAL HIP ARTHROPLASTY

Other key components of the Charnley THA included routine medialization of the socket and lateral displacement of the trochanter. Medialization of the socket helps to decrease the lever arm of the body weight, and lateral displacement of the trochanter helps increase the lever arm of the HAs. Both of these factors help to reduce the HA force required and therefore reduce the JRF and stress on the implants. These strategies are, however, now rarely practised as a move towards conservation of pelvic bone stock has led to anatomical placement of the socket, and, as trochanteric osteotomy is rarely practised, lateral trochanteric displacement is not usually on option.

'Modern day' equivalents of the above Charnley strategies include lateralizing the femoral component by increasing the horizontal femoral offset. This also helps to increase the HA lever arm, reducing the JRF as discussed previously. Inadequate restoration of offset results in HA insufficiency and soft-tissue laxity. This can predispose to dislocation and increased wear through increased JRF and microseperation during the gait cycle.[36–38] Excessive femoral offset can also predispose to failure by 'overtightening' the hip, increasing the stresses placed on the femoral fixation interface.[39] Offset can also be increased or decreased by varus or valgus alignment of the femoral stem, respectively. Intentional varus alignment is not advisable because of an increased risk of fixation failure secondary to thinning of cement mantle in zones 3 and 7.[40]

BIOMECHANICS OF HIP IMPINGEMENT

Impingement of the native hip joint has been increasingly purported as a possible cause for primary osteoarthritis of the hip.[41–43] Termed femoroacetabular impingement (FAI), this process involves abnormal contact between the proximal femur and the acetabular rim at the limits of the arc of motion. This is thought to result in abnormal articular contact stresses, leading to cartilage degeneration. This abutment can be a result either of bony abnormality in the proximal femur or acetabulum or of a supraphysiological ROM with normal bone architecture or very subtle bony abnormality.

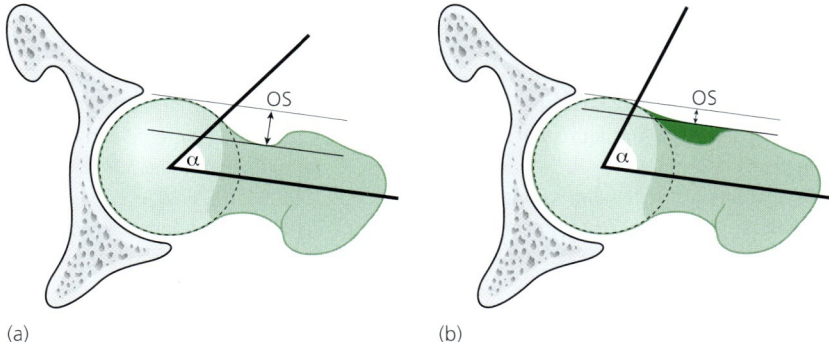

Figure 95.11 Radiographic abnormalities seen on axial imaging of the hip in cam-type femoroacetabular impingement. (a) Normal hip with α angle <55° and normal head–neck offset (OS). The α angle is the angle subtended between a line drawn from the centre of the femoral head along the long axis of the neck, and a line from the centre of the femoral head to the point where the neck protrudes anterior to a best fit circle drawn over the femoral head, i.e. the point where asphericity begins. OS is the difference between the anterior radius of the femoral head and the anterior radius of the femoral neck; less than 7 mm is abnormal. (b) Abnormal hip with an anterior neck bump demonstrating an increased α angle and reduced OS.

Two types of FAI exist: pincer and cam impingement. A mixed picture is, however, commonly seen.[44] Pincer impingement is due to effective overcoverage of the acetabulum. In contrast to hip dysplasia, the femoral head remains well centred within the acetabulum but the problem is primarily due to excessive coverage of the femoral head, resulting in impingement at the limits of the arc of motion. This excessive coverage can be global, as seen in protrusio acetabuli, or focal secondary to a malorientated acetabulum, as seen with acetabular retroversion leading to anterior impingement. Abutment between the abnormal acetabular rim and normal femoral neck leads to labral damage and secondary ossification. Chondral damage is initially limited to a narrow band at the acetabular rim.[44] Continued impingement levers the neck against the acetabular rim, leading to a 'contrecoup' lesion on the posteroinferior aspect of the femoral head.[44,45]

Cam impingement results from a deformity of the proximal femur. Bony prominence at the head–neck junction causes asphericity of the femoral head. Radiographically, this deformity results in a reduction in head–neck offset and increased α angle, as shown in Fig. 95.11. This 'neck bump', most commonly seen on the anterosuperior neck, jams into the acetabulum with hip flexion. This pushes the labrum away from the acetabular rim and compresses the cartilage, pushing it centrally. This can lead to cartilage delamination and subsequent joint degeneration. In contrast to pincer impingement, the damage is mainly seen anterosuperiorly.[44] Reduced femoral anteversion can also predispose to anterior impingement because of reduced clearance for flexion, especially in internal rotation. Ito et al.[43] noted a significant reduction in patients with femoral anteversion with FAI (15.7°) compared with a control group (9.7°).

> **KEY LEARNING POINTS**
>
> - The joint reaction force of the hip is a function of both the body weight and hip abductor-generated force.
> - Strategies to reduce the joint reaction force can help reduce the pain of a diseased hip and potentially reduce the stress on hip implants.
> - These strategies include increasing the hip abductor lever arm, reducing the lever arm of the body weight or providing additional counter-moments such as a walking stick.
> - Factors affecting the stability of a hip arthroplasty include the head size, head–neck ratio and internal socket profile.
> - Acetabular loosening remains one of the most frequent causes of hip arthroplasty failure, and frictional torque has been shown to play a key role in generating stresses at the fixation interface.
> - Hip impingement is a biomechanical cause of hip pathology that is related to proximal femoral and acetabular anatomy.

REFERENCES

● = Key primary paper
♦ = Major review article

● 1. Ponseti IV. Growth and development of the acetabulum in the normal child. Anatomical, histological, and roentgenographic studies. *Journal of Bone and Joint Surgery (American)* 1978;**60**:575–85.

2. Nagao Y, Aoki H, Ishii SJ, et al. Radiographic method to measure the inclination angle of the acetabulum. *Journal of Orthopaedic Science* 2008;**13**:62–71.
●3. Tonnis D, Heinecke A. Acetabular and femoral anteversion: relationship with osteoarthritis of the hip. *Journal of Bone and Joint Surgery (American)* 1999;**81**:1747–70.
●4. Hoaglund FT, Low WD. Anatomy of the femoral neck and head, with comparative data from Caucasians and Hong Kong Chinese. *Clinical Orthopaedics and Related Research* 1980;**152**:10–16.
●5. Kingsley PC, Olmsted KL. A study to determine the angle of anteversion of the neck of the femur. *Journal of Bone and Joint Surgery (American)* 1948;**30A**:745–51.
6. Tayton E. Femoral anteversion: a necessary angle or an evolutionary vestige? *Journal of Bone and Joint Surgery (British)* 2007;**89**:1283–8.
7. Martin HD, Savage A, Braly BA, et al. The function of the hip capsular ligaments: a quantitative report. *Arthroscopy* 2008;**24**:188–95.
8. Clark JM, Haynor DR. Anatomy of the abductor muscles of the hip as studied by computed tomography. *Journal of Bone and Joint Surgery (American)* 1987;**69**:1021–31.
●9. Neumann DA. Hip abductor muscle activity as subjects with hip prostheses walk with different methods of using a cane. *Physical Therapy* 1998;**78**:490–501.
10. Neumann DA, Cook TM. Effect of load and carrying position on the electromyographic activity of the gluteus medius muscle during walking. *Physical Therapy* 1985;**65**:305–11.
11. Neumann DA, Hase AD. An electromyographic analysis of the hip abductors during load carriage: implications for hip joint protection. *Journal of Orthopaedic and Sports Physical Therapy* 1994;**19**:296–304.
12. Conroy JL, Whitehouse SL, Graves SE, et al. Risk factors for revision for early dislocation in total hip arthroplasty. *Journal of Arthroplasty* 2008;**23**:867–72.
13. Bystrom S, Espehaug B, Furnes O, Havelin LI. Femoral head size is a risk factor for total hip luxation: a study of 42,987 primary hip arthroplasties from the Norwegian Arthroplasty Register. *Acta Orthopaedica Scandinavica* 2003;**74**:514–24.
14. Sariali E, Veysi V, Stewart T. (i) Biomechanics of the human hip: consequences for total hip replacement. *Current Orthopaedics* 2008;**22**:371–5.
15. Malik A, Maheshwari A, Dorr LD. Impingement with total hip replacement. *Journal of Bone and Joint Surgery (American)* 2007;**89**:1832–42.
16. Barrack RL, Butler RA, Laster DR, Andrews P. Stem design and dislocation after revision total hip arthroplasty: clinical results and computer modeling. *Journal of Arthroplasty* 2001;**16**(Suppl. 1):8–12.
17. Board TN, Walter W. When is 45 degrees not 45 degrees: an analysis of the subtended angle of resurfacing sockets. In: *Proceedings of the British Hip Society Annual Meeting, Manchester, UK, 11–13 March 2009.*
●18. Willert HG, Buchhorn GH, Fayyazi A, et al. Metal-on-metal bearings and hypersensitivity in patients with artificial hip joints. A clinical and histomorphological study. *Journal of Bone and Joint Surgery (American)* 2005;**87**:28–36.
19. Ollivere B, Darrah C, Barker T, et al. Early clinical failure of the Birmingham metal-on-metal hip resurfacing is associated with metallosis and soft-tissue necrosis. *Journal of Bone and Joint Surgery (British)* 2009;**91**:1025–30.
20. Pandit H, Glyn-Jones S, McLardy-Smith P, et al. Pseudotumours associated with metal-on-metal hip resurfacings. *Journal of Bone and Joint Surgery (British)* 2008;**90**:847–51.
21. Bengs BC, Sangiorgio SN, Ebramzadeh E. Less range of motion with resurfacing arthroplasty than with total hip arthroplasty: in vitro examination of 8 designs. *Acta Orthopaedica* 2008;**79**:755–62.
22. Kluess D, Zietz C, Lindner T, et al. Limited range of motion of hip resurfacing arthroplasty due to unfavorable ratio of prosthetic head size and femoral neck diameter. *Acta Orthopaedica* 2008;**79**:748–54.
23. Marker DR, Strimbu K, McGrath MS, et al. Resurfacing versus conventional total hip arthroplasty – review of comparative clinical and basic science studies. *Bulletin of the New York University Hospital for Joint Diseases* 2009;**67**:120–7.
24. Le Duff MJ, Wisk LE, Amstutz HC. Range of motion after stemmed total hip arthroplasty and hip resurfacing – a clinical study. *Bulletin of the New York University Hospital for Joint Diseases* 2009;**67**:177–81.
◆25. Wroblewski BM, Siney PD, Fleming PA. Charnley low frictional torque arthroplasty: clinical developments. *Orthopedic Clinics of North America* 2005;**36**:11–16.
◆26. Walker PS, Gold BL. The tribology (friction, lubrication and wear) of all-metal artificial hip joints. 1971. *Clinical Orthopaedics and Related Research* 1996;**329**(Suppl.):S4–10.
◆27. Amstutz HC, Grigoris P. Metal on metal bearings in hip arthroplasty. *Clinical Orthopaedics and Related Research* 1996;**329**(Suppl.):S11–34.
●28. Charnley J. Arthroplasty of the hip. A new operation. *Lancet* 1961;**1**:1129–32.
●29. Charnley J, Kamangar A, Longfield MD. The optimum size of prosthetic heads in relation to the wear of plastic sockets in total replacement of the hip. *Medical and Biological Engineering* 1969;**7**:31–9.
30. Mai MT, Schmalzried TP, Dorey FJ, et al. The contribution of frictional torque to loosening at the cement-bone interface in Tharies hip replacements. *Journal of Bone and Joint Surgery (American)* 1996;**78**:505–11.
●31. Wroblewski BM, Siney PD, Fleming PA. The principle of low frictional torque in the Charnley total hip replacement. *Journal of Bone and Joint Surgery (British)* 2009;**91**:855–8.
32. Dowson D, Jin ZM. Metal-on-metal hip joint tribology. *Proceedings of the Institution of Mechanical Engineers H* 2006;**220**:107–18.
33. Dorr LD, Long WT, Sirianni L, et al. The argument for the use of Metasul as an articulation surface in total hip

replacement. *Clinical Orthopaedics and Related Research* 2004;**429**:80–5.
34. Saito S, Ryu J, Watanabe M, *et al*. Midterm results of Metasul metal-on-metal total hip arthroplasty. *Journal of Arthroplasty* 2006;**21**:1105–10.
35. Brockett CL, Harper P, Williams S, *et al*. The influence of clearance on friction, lubrication and squeaking in large diameter metal-on-metal hip replacements. *Journal of Materials Science: Materials in Medicine* 2008;**19**:1575–9.
36. Fackler CD, Poss R. Dislocation in total hip arthroplasties. *Clinical Orthopaedics and Related Research* 1980;**151**:169–78.
37. Leslie IJ, Williams S, Isaac G, *et al*. High cup angle and microseparation increase the wear of hip surface replacements. *Clinical Orthopaedics and Related Research* 2009;**467**:2259–65.
38. Little NJ, Busch CA, Gallagher JA, *et al*. Acetabular polyethylene wear and acetabular inclination and femoral offset. *Clinical Orthopaedics and Related Research* 2009;**467**:2895–900.
39. Lecerf G, Fessy MH, Philippot R, *et al*. Femoral offset: anatomical concept, definition, assessment, implications for preoperative templating and hip arthroplasty. *Orthopaedics and Traumatology: Surgery and Research* 2009;**95**:210–19.
40. Devitt A, O'Sullivan T, Quinlan W. 16- to 25-year follow-up study of cemented arthroplasty of the hip in patients aged 50 years or younger. *Journal of Arthroplasty* 1997;**12**:479–89.
41. Ganz R, Parvizi J, Beck M, *et al*. Femoroacetabular impingement: a cause for osteoarthritis of the hip. *Clinical Orthopaedics and Related Research* 2003;**417**:112–20.
42. Wagner S, Hofstetter W, Chiquet M, *et al*. Early osteoarthritic changes of human femoral head cartilage subsequent to femoro-acetabular impingement. *Osteoarthritis and Cartilage* 2003;**11**:508–18.
43. Ito K, Minka 2nd MA, Leunig M, *et al*. Femoroacetabular impingement and the cam-effect. A MRI-based quantitative anatomical study of the femoral head-neck offset. *Journal of Bone and Joint Surgery (British)* 2001;**83**:171–6.
44. Beck M, Kalhor M, Leunig M, Ganz R. Hip morphology influences the pattern of damage to the acetabular cartilage: femoroacetabular impingement as a cause of early osteoarthritis of the hip. *Journal of Bone and Joint Surgery (British)* 2005;**87**:1012–18.
45. Pfirrmann CW, Mengiardi B, Dora C, *et al*. Cam and pincer femoroacetabular impingement: characteristic MR arthrographic findings in 50 patients. *Radiology* 2006;**240**:778–85.

Materials in hip arthroplasty

SAMUEL S RAJARATNAM, WILLIAM L WALTER

| Introduction | 1114 | Materials in implant design | 1120 |
| Bearing surfaces | 1116 | References | 1121 |

NATIONAL BOARD STANDARDS

- Understand the concepts of wear, lubrication and corrosion
- Know about bearing surfaces
- Appreciate the materials used in implant design

INTRODUCTION

The total hip replacement (THR) has been one of the most successful surgical interventions to date, and has resulted in reduced pain and improvement of function in many patients suffering from osteoarthritis of the hip. As the popularity of the procedure continues to increase, THRs are implanted in increasingly younger and more active patients. The long-term success of a THR depends on a number of factors, namely the surgical technique, the fixation of the implant to bone, bearing material wear, failure of implants, and bone and soft-tissue remodelling over the longer term.[1]

Tribology is the study of the interaction between two surfaces moving against each other. The consequence of this motion is wear, which over the long term can lead to failure of the joint replacement. Optimal lubrication of the articulating surfaces can reduce wear.

Wear

Wear is the removal of material from solid surfaces by mechanical action.[2] The hardness, microstructural surface profile and shape of the articulating surface influences the rate of wear in a joint replacement.

When the bonding forces between two moving surfaces are greater than that needed to fracture the surface of either material, *adhesive wear* occurs. A soft material scraping into a harder material results in abrasive wear. Both adhesive and abrasive wear are types of *interfacial wear*, in which two bearing surfaces articulate with each other. *Fatigue wear* occurs within a biomaterial as a result of cyclical loading and is distinct from the two types of interfacial wear described above.

In a prosthetic joint, four modes of wear have been described. *Mode 1 wear* describes material removed during movement between two articulating surfaces, e.g. between a cobalt chrome femoral head and a polyethylene liner. *Mode 2 wear* occurs between a primary articulating surface and a non-articulating surface, e.g. between a cobalt chrome head and the metal outer ring of a metal-backed cup, once the polyethylene liner has fractured (Fig. 96.1). *Mode 3 wear* occurs when debris gets between two primary articulating surfaces, e.g. cement debris between a metal and polyethylene articulation. Finally, *mode 4 wear* occurs between two non-articulating surfaces, e.g. impingement between a femoral neck and the metal backing of a cup. Mode 1 wear is intended by the design of an implant, whereas the other modes describe unintentional wear in an artificial joint. More than one of the above-described mechanisms of wear may be operating on the prosthesis at

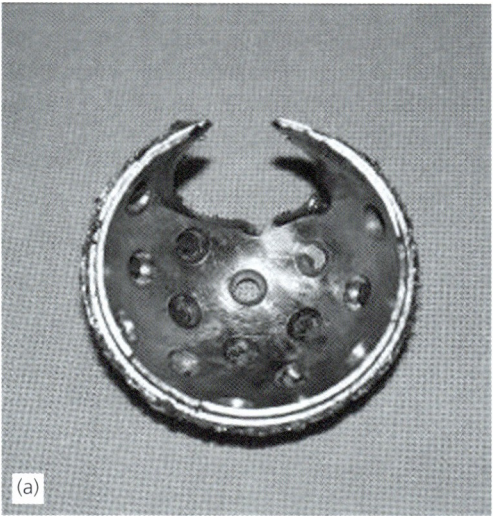

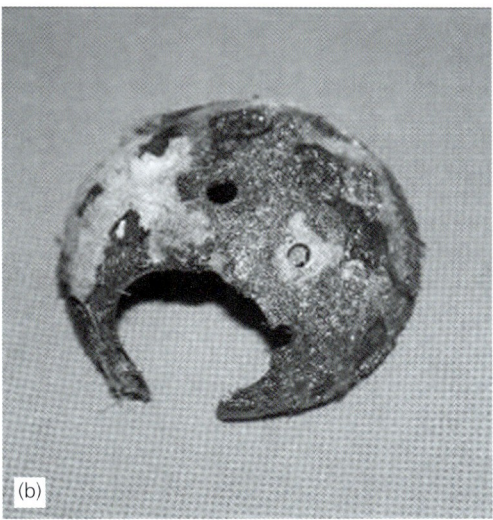

Figure 96.1 (a and b) A metal-backed cementless cup showing catastrophic wear of the metal shell due to articulation with the metal femoral head (mode 2).

any given time. Moreover, a THR may operate in a number of different wear modes over its life *in vivo*.

Lubrication

Lubrication between articulating surfaces dramatically reduces adhesive and abrasive wear. *Fluid-film lubrication* involves a film of fluid that completely separates two articulating surfaces. *Hydrodynamic lubrication* is the classic model of fluid-film lubrication that is seen to operate when hard-on-hard bearings articulate with each other. When two hard bearing surfaces move against each other, the relative motion draws fluid between the surfaces, dramatically reducing wear in the joint. The effectiveness of fluid-film lubrication depends on the thickness and viscosity of the fluid film, the microscopic surface asperities of the materials involved and their surface roughness, and the macroscopic design of the two surfaces in terms of clearance and size. Larger ceramic-on-ceramic (COC) or metal-on-metal (MOM) articulations with a polar bearing design with adequate clearance promote fluid-film lubrication of the bearing surfaces (Fig. 96.2).

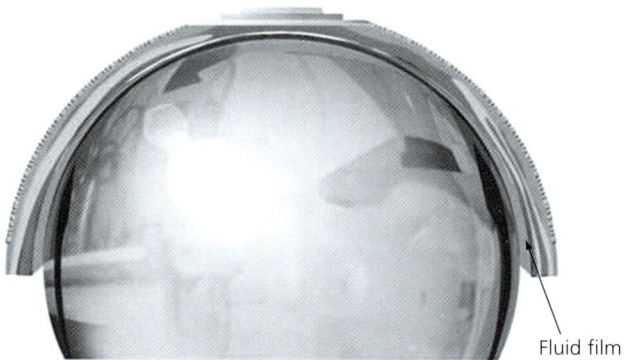

Figure 96.2 A metal-on-metal arthroplasty showing fluid-film lubrication.

Boundary lubrication occurs when a thin film of fluid is present on the surface of articulating bearings. This film of fluid is not sufficiently thick to prevent the surface asperities of the opposing surfaces from touching each other, but does prevent severe wear. In many instances, a joint operates under a combination of boundary and fluid-film lubrication, and this is known as *mixed lubrication*.

The ratio of the thickness of the fluid film separating two surfaces and the surface roughness of the two bearings is known as the lambda ratio (λ ratio). The greater the lambda ratio, the lower the expected wear in the joint.

Corrosion

Corrosion is a chemical reaction during which deterioration of a metal occurs.[3] Modern materials used in THR surgery are designed to prevent or minimize corrosion of all types. Nevertheless, it is important to consider the effects of corrosion when different metals and alloys are used in close proximity to each other in joint arthroplasty.

A number of different types of corrosion exist, including *galvanic corrosion*, *stress corrosion*, *fretting corrosion* and *pit corrosion*. Galvanic corrosion may occur when two reactive metals are used in close proximity to each other, e.g. a stainless steel femoral head and titanium femoral stem. Stress or crevice corrosion occurs at a crack on a metal and can cause propagation of the crack, leading to failure of the implant (Fig. 96.3). Fretting corrosion occurs when the surface layer of a metal is removed by movement between two surfaces leading to the removal of the protective 'passivating' oxide layer from the surface of the metal. Pit corrosion is a localized form of fretting corrosion.

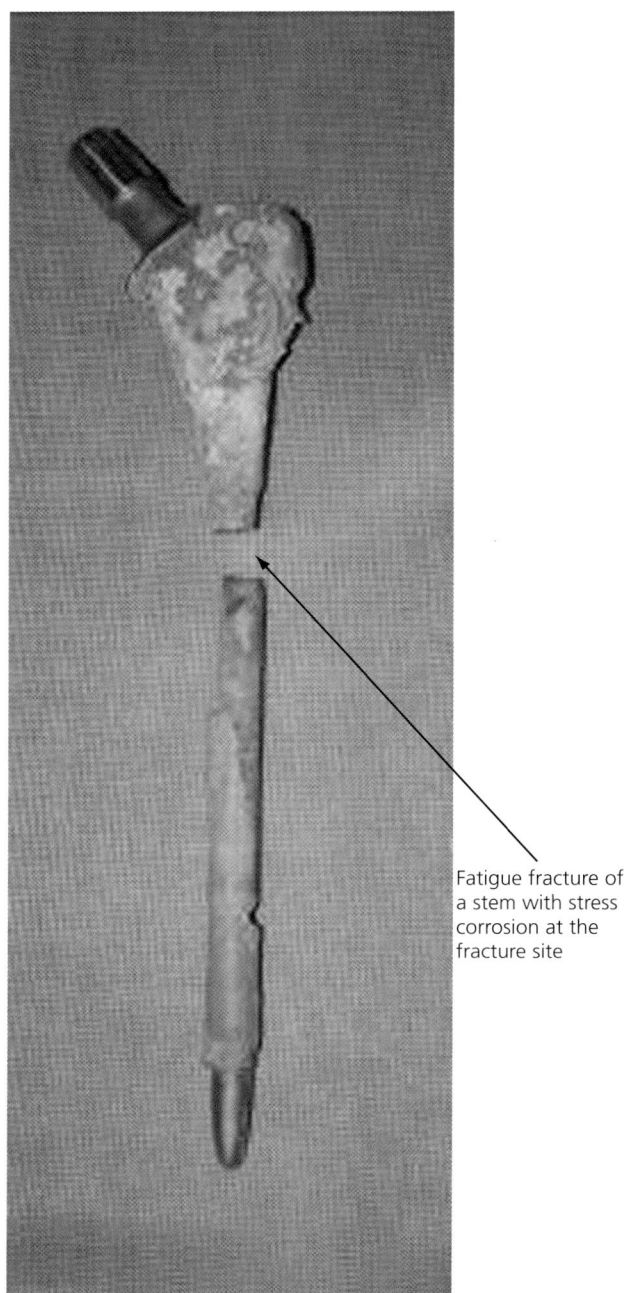

Figure 96.3 A fractured femoral stem.

The head–neck taper of a modular hip prosthesis is a potential site for fretting corrosion. This may be the result of a mismatch between the male and female components of the taper. Relative micromotion at the taper can result in the continued removal of the passivating oxide layer on the metal alloy. This can subsequently lead to corrosion and breakage of the implant. Galvanic corrosion can occur when two reactive metals are placed in contact with each other, e.g. a stainless steel femoral head and a titanium femoral stem.

Any of these processes can cause particulate debris in the effective joint space and local tissues and cause third-body wear in the articulating surface. More rarely, it can cause mechanical failure of the implant. A rise in systemic levels of measurable metal ions due to corrosion of metal implants has been reported, but the clinical significance of this phenomenon is currently unknown.

Osteolysis

It has been recognized for some time that particulate debris from an arthroplasty deposits in periprosthetic tissues, and can result in an inflammatory reaction and osteoclast-induced osteolysis around a THR. This is often associated with polyethylene wear and can lead to loosening of both cemented and uncemented implants. The osteolysis reduces the bone stock available at revision surgery, rendering fixation of revision implants more challenging. It is recognized that the extent and speed of progression of the osteolysis is determined by a number of factors, including type, size and number of particles within the 'effective joint space' of the arthroplasty. In recent years, much resource has been channelled to develop implants resistant to osteolysis through changes in manufacturing, material type and implant design.

BEARING SURFACES

The ideal bearing surface in a THR has to be wear resistant, biocompatible, resistant to gross failure and relatively easy to manufacture.[4] The quest for the ideal bearing surface has been ongoing for over a century. Early unsuccessful attempts at hip arthroplasty involved the use of interposing materials such as muscle, fat and even chromatized pig's bladder. The use of harder bearing surfaces such as glass (Smith-Peterson), acrylic (Judet) and various metals in mould arthroplasty still resulted in disappointing results, because of either loosening of the components or breakage of the implants. The introduction of polyethylene by Charnley in the late 1950s marked the dawn of the modern THR. Considerable advances have since been made in bearing material technology and manufacturing in the last three decades, but long-term follow-up data are required to show that the survival and wear of newer materials is better than those previously used.

Polyethylene

An acetabular component made of ultra-high-molecular-weight polyethylene (UHMWPE) has been used most commonly in THRs to date, often articulating with a metal or ceramic femoral head. Polyethylene is a long-chain polymer of the hydrocarbon monomer ethylene. UHMWPE used in total hip arthroplasty has a molecular weight of over 3–6 million g mol^{-1}.

Although there are many sources of particulate debris within the effective joint space, the greatest contribution

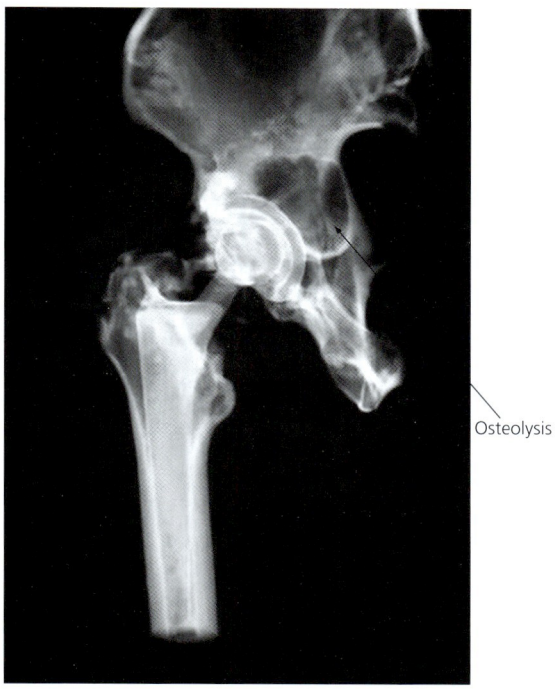

Figure 96.4 Digital subtraction CT showing polyethylene wear-related osteolysis around the acetabular component.

results from polyethylene particles generated under 'mode 1' wear conditions. The wear generated from the harder metal or ceramic head[5] is often negligible. The wear property of polyethylene is related to its molecular and structural properties, and to the manufacturing and sterilization of the components.

In vivo wear of a polyethylene acetabular component can be assessed radiographically and the sequential linear penetration can be measured (Figs 96.4 and 96.5). The two-dimensional linear penetration observed is often referred to as 'linear wear'. The use of a small femoral head (e.g. Charnley 22.225 mm head) is said to predispose to greater linear penetration, whereas there is greater volumetric wear seen in the acetabular component when large diameter femoral heads are employed (e.g. a 36 mm head). A 28 mm head diameter is thus considered by some to be the optimal size to minimize both linear and volumetric wear in metal-on-polyethylene articulation in THR surgery.

Oxidation of polyethylene can result in the shortening of the macromolecules and adversely affect the material properties of the implant, thus reducing its tensile strength and toughness. Until recently, many polyethylene components were sterilized with gamma irradiation in an air environment. The unstable free radicals created during irradiation then interacted with the oxygen in the environment, causing oxidation of the polyethylene. Subsurface oxidation sometimes leads to delamination of the polyethylene and cracking of the implant, and therefore to greater wear.

Modern manufacturing methods include vacuum gamma or electron beam irradiation of implants, thermal stabilization, and sterilization with gas plasma or ethylene oxide. These newer processes reduce oxidation of the polyethylene and increase intermolecular cross-linkage. Covalent cross-linkage of polyethylene can reduce intermolecular mobility and render implants more stable to deformation and wear. This can be achieved using chemicals (peroxides), electron beam irradiation or gamma irradiation of implants. The ensuing polyethylene product (often referred to as highly cross-linked polyethylene) has greatly improved in wear rates when compared with conventional UHMWPE in a joint simulator.

Conversely, the cross-linking between polyethylene molecules can undesirably alter the structural properties of the implant too and decrease its ultimate tensile strength. As highly cross-linked polyethylene has gained popularity over the last few years, reports of rim cracking of certain highly cross-linked polyethylene acetabular components have also emerged. Further studies on highly cross-linked polyethylene components are eagerly awaited in order to demonstrate its superiority to UHMWPE as a bearing surface.

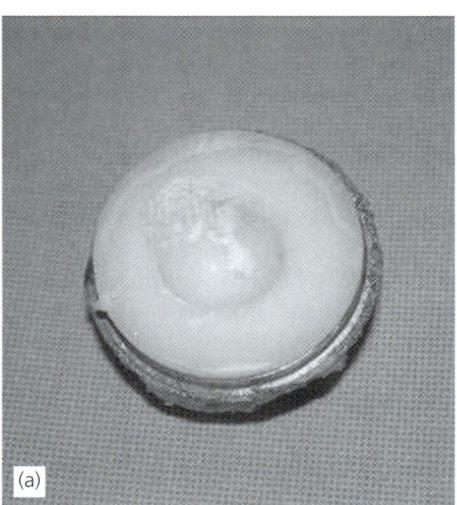
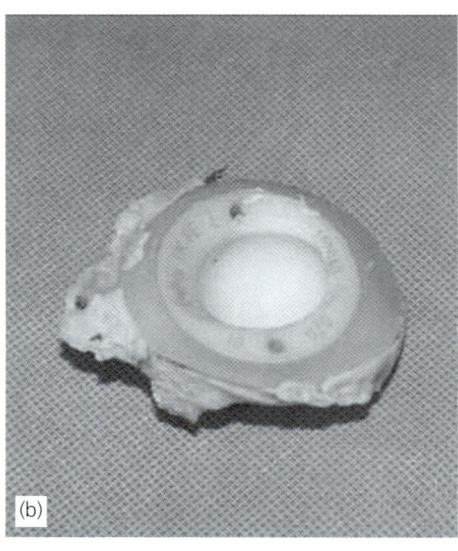

Figure 96.5 (a and b) Wear in a polyethylene liner (metal-backed cementless shell).

Polyethylene acetabular components have most often been implanted with either a metal or ceramic femoral head. Although the vast majority of wear in this type of 'soft-on-hard' articulation arises from polyethylene wear, important lessons regarding the counter-bearing surface have also been learned over the years. Titanium, which is a relatively soft metal, makes a poor bearing surface and can wear significantly, especially when the joint is operating under 'mode 3' conditions. Harder metal alloys such as cobalt chrome and stainless steel are commonly used materials for construction of femoral heads.

In recent years, there has been much interest in newer bearing surfaces such as oxidized zirconium (Oxinium; Smith & Nephew, Memphis, TN), which is a metal alloy with surface properties of a ceramic (Fig. 96.6). It is, therefore, thought to exhibit excellent fracture toughness like cobalt chrome alloy, but have the superior wear properties of a ceramic. Once again, long-term *in vivo* results are eagerly awaited.

Metal-on-metal bearing

The use of MOM articulation in hip arthroplasty predates the use of polyethylene as a bearing surface. Philip Wiles, a British surgeon, implanted total hip replacements with MOM bearing surfaces in 1938. Inadequate fixation of the femoral prosthesis led to early failures in Wiles' arthroplasty. Both Ring and McKee subsequently popularized their versions of MOM replacements in the 1950s and 1960s. The failure rates of these early MOM replacements, usually made of cast cobalt chrome alloy, were greater than Charnley's 'low-friction arthroplasty', mainly because of inadequate fixation of the implants, and they declined in popularity until the late 1980s.

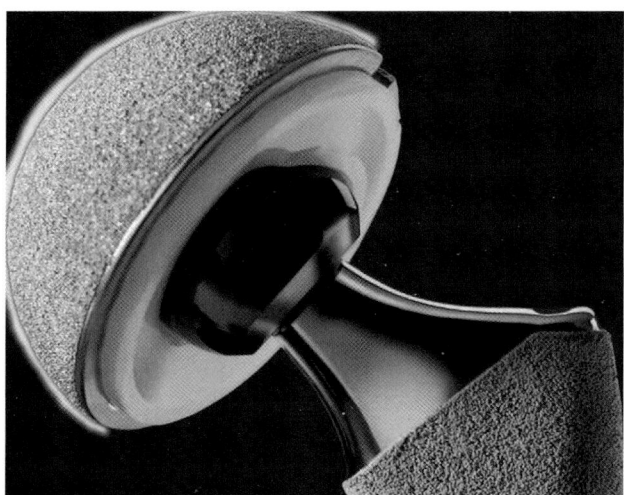

Figure 96.6 An Oxinium-on-polyethylene total hip replacement. Reproduced with permission from Smith & Nephew Orthopaedics Ltd.

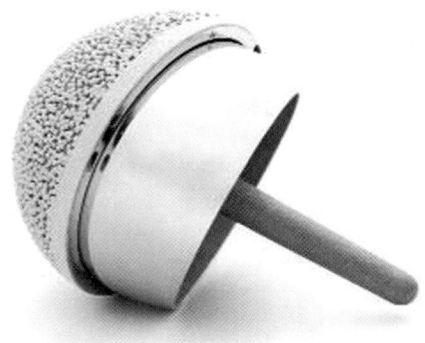

Figure 96.7 A metal-on-metal resurfacing hip replacement (Birmingham resurfacing). Reproduced with permission from Smith & Nephew, UK.

Polyethylene wear and osteolysis in conventional hip arthroplasty was recognized to be a problem over time, especially in young patients with a hard-on-soft bearing.[6] In the late 1980s modern MOM bearings regained popularity following McMinn's Birmingham hip-resurfacing procedure (Fig. 96.7), and Muller and Weber's Metasul bearing. Most large orthopaedic implant manufacturers now have their own MOM bearings made from cast cobalt chrome alloy for use as resurfacing and stemmed THRs.

Mechanical wear, surface corrosion or a combination of both these processes results in the production of metallic debris in MOM articulations. While the actual number of wear particles measured in MOM arthroplasty is often much greater than that of polyethylene in conventional hard-on-soft bearing THRs, the particle size is much smaller. This results in much less volumetric wear. It is thought that the linear wear measurable in MOM arthroplasty is approximately 25–35 μm per year in the initial 'run-in phase' and then decreases to approximately 5 μm per year thereafter.

Improved implant geometry and manufacturing has reduced the wear seen in MOM bearings. Wear in a MOM articulation is influenced by its surface roughness, clearance, sphericity and material hardness. Adequate clearance between the articulating surfaces can result in a polar bearing design, which can facilitate fluid-film lubrication of the two surfaces. Improved casting and polishing methods have resulted in smoother surface profiles of the implants. It is also suggested that increasing the carbon content in the cobalt chrome alloy reduces wear.

The recent interest in MOM bearing surfaces is partly related to the potential benefits of bone-conserving hip arthroplasty options. Metal resurfacing of the femur is bone conserving when compared with a standard femoral stem. If a revision arthroplasty is required at some point, femoral revision becomes easier as the femoral canal has not been altered by the primary resurfacing procedure.

Metallic wear debris from MOM arthroplasty has been known to deposit in the periprosthetic tissues over time. Although the number of metallic wear particles generated by MOM bearing surfaces is much greater than from equivalent metal-on-polyethylene arthroplasty, the local tissue reaction in periprosthetic tissues is much lower.

The metallic wear from a MOM arthroplasty can result in systemic dissemination of metal ions via the lymphatic and vascular systems. These measurable increases in metal ions can potentially affect every system in the body. Experimental studies using *in vivo* and *in vitro* models have shown the adverse effects of metal ion toxicity within the renal, respiratory, cardiovascular, nervous and immune systems. The principal ions known to affect these systems are Cr, Ni, Co and V.

A few studies showing a higher incidence of chromosomal abnormalities found in arthroplasty patients has raised concerns of a link between MOM arthroplasty and carcinogenesis. Metal ions can also traverse the placenta in pregnancy and potentially affect an unborn fetus. It must be stressed, however, that all the above concerns remain theoretical, and to date no proven link has been made between MOM arthroplasty and carcinogenesis or birth abnormalities.

A number of patients are known to suffer from topical metal allergies.[7] There have also been a few reports of MOM joint replacement failures owing to a unique localized hypersensitivity reaction in periprosthetic tissues. A dense perivascular lymphocytic infiltration is seen around the effective joint space of the affected patients, and this histological phenomenon is called aseptic lymphocytic vasculitis-associated lesions (ALVAL). Although it is recommended that a MOM arthroplasty should be avoided in a person with known metal allergy, the correlation between positive topical skin tests, known topical metal allergies and the development of ALVAL remains unclear.

Recent NJR data have shown increased failure rates in conventional large head MOM hip replacements. One explanation postulated is that the large number of metal ions generate result in trunion failure of these implants, along with an increased incidence of ALVAL.

Ceramics in orthopaedics[8]

Ceramics were introduced to orthopaedics by Pierre Boutin in 1971. They are a group of inorganic non-metallic materials that are typically crystalline in nature. Ceramics used in orthopaedics are either bioactive ceramics (e.g. hydroxyapatite coatings of implants) or bio-inert (e.g. alumina and zirconia used in bearing surfaces).[9]

Ceramic is a hard material and exhibits excellent wear characteristics. Its surface is also highly wettable, aiding lubrication between the bearing surfaces. The microstructural surface asperity profile of a ceramic bearing is different from a metallic bearing surface. Metal surfaces have microscopic 'peaks' and 'troughs' whereas ceramics generally exhibit 'troughs'. This may be one of the reasons for the superior wear characteristics seen in ceramics.

Ceramic components are brittle and can fracture. Moreover, they are expensive to manufacture. These two factors have limited their popularity in THR surgery over the last three decades. Early first-generation ceramic components occasionally fractured *in vivo*, necessitating immediate revision surgery. This problem has now been virtually eliminated with modern manufacturing methods and materials, and the current ceramic fracture rate is approximately 0.02% overall.

Modern third-generation alumina ceramic is manufactured by hot isostatic pressing of the base powder. This process reduces the grain size, reduces grain inclusions and impurities, increases burst strength and reduces wear.

CERAMIC-ON-POLYETHYLENE BEARINGS

Femoral heads made of ceramic have been shown to cause less polyethylene wear than comparable metal alloy heads *in vitro*. This is thought to be related to its highly polished nature, lower surface roughness and favourable asperity profile.

In the past, however, zirconia ceramic heads articulating with UHMWPE have been reported to undergo phase transformation after implantation.[10] This resulted in the surface roughness of the zirconia increasing dramatically after implantation because of grain pull-out (Fig. 96.8).[11] Increased surface roughness and third-body wear (due to the zirconia grains deposited between the bearing surfaces) contributed to vastly increased polyethylene wear in these particular articulations, and led to the abandonment of zirconia-on-polyethylene bearings.

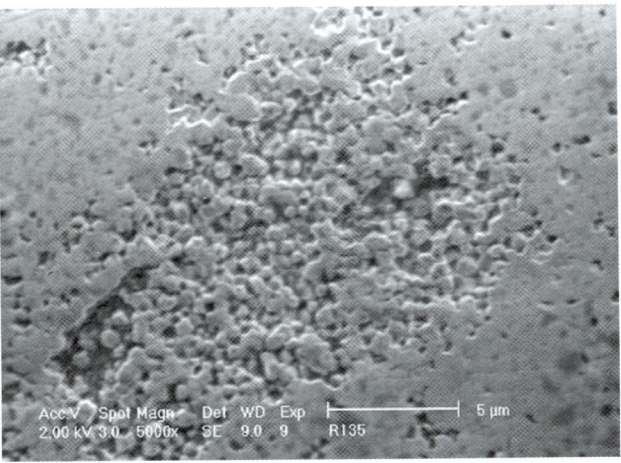

Figure 96.8 Scanning electron microscopic image of zirconia ceramic showing disintegration of the surface and grain pull-out resulting in a roughened surface. Bar, 5 μm.

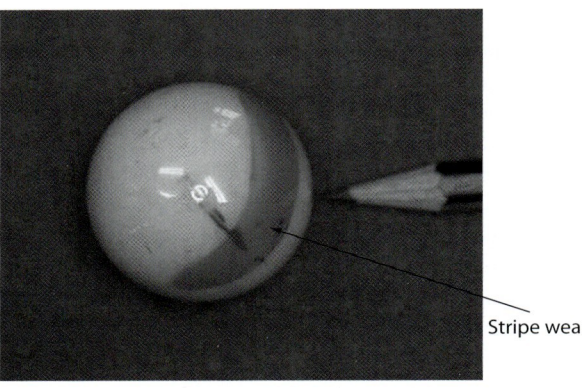

Figure 96.9 A ceramic-on-ceramic bearing showing 'stripe wear'.

CERAMIC-ON-CERAMIC BEARING SURFACES[12]

Retrieval analysis of alumina COC bearings used for over two decades shows extremely low wear rates compared with metal-on-polyethylene bearings. The pattern of wear commonly seen in COC articulation is often very different from that seen in metal-on-polyethylene bearings. The latter show surface-to-surface wear that is detectable radiologically as 'linear penetration' on serial radiographs. This type of surface-to-surface wear is radiographically undetectable in COC bearings. Ceramic femoral heads can, however, 'edge load' against the corresponding ceramic acetabular component at the extremes of movement of the artificial joint, leading to an area of localized 'stripe wear' on the femoral head (Fig. 96.9).[13] This unusual type of localized wear in ceramic bearings has been associated with steep acetabular cup orientation, suboptimal acetabular anteversion, revision surgery and young patients.[14]

Postoperative audible squeaking of a THR is a rare problem, and one that has been associated with a hard-on-hard bearing surface such as MOM or COC. Squeaking in COC bearings can occur in approximately 0.5% of cases and is of multifactorial aetiology. It is postulated that patient, implant and surgical factors may lead to squeaking THRs.[15]

MATERIALS IN IMPLANT DESIGN

The popularity of the THR has increased tremendously in the last four decades. During this period, two different rationales for the fixation of implants to bone have developed; namely, cemented and cementless fixation. Both methods aim for the implant to be able to adequately load the surrounding bone without prosthetic loosening or failure, throughout its working life.

Cemented hip arthroplasty

Polymethylmethacrylate (PMMA) bone cement was first introduced to orthopaedics in the 1950s and is a key component of cemented hip arthroplasty.[16] When set, it is a viscoelastic polymer that acts as a grout between the implant and bone. The modulus of elasticity of PMMA (approximately 2400 MPa) is lower than that of metals and bone, and is thus able to act as an elastic interlayer between two relatively stiff materials.

Prior to use, short chains of PMMA are mixed with liquid monomer and a catalyst, and this results in an exothermic polymerization reaction. The PMMA goes through a liquid phase, during which it is implanted, and, once set, acts as a solid material. It also exhibits time-dependent viscoelastic properties of creep and stress relaxation. The molecular weight, setting times and mechanical properties of PMMA vary between differing proprietary brands.

Various substances can be added to PMMA to affect its properties and functions. Barium sulphate is often added to make cement radio-opaque. Antibiotics are often added to reduce periprosthetic infection. Chlorophyll is also often used as a colouring agent in certain proprietary makes of PMMA.

Most cemented acetabular components involve the fixation of polyethylene cups to bone via macro-interlock of cement. As most cases of loosening of cemented acetabular components occur at the cement–bone interface, optimal cement interdigitation with bone is essential. This is often facilitated by creating lug-holes in bone, using pulsed lavage to prepare the bony bed and pressurizing cement during the polymerization process.

Cementless total hip replacement

Cementless hip arthroplasty involves the direct fixation of the implant to bone.[17] The initial fixation of the implant is achieved by an interference fit. Subsequently, bone ingrowth and ongrowth occurs and long-term implant stability can be achieved.

Sufficient surface roughness and porosity is required for stable cementless fixation to be achieved. Previous designs of components with beaded surfaces resulted in delamination of the metal beads over time. The ensuing metal debris occasionally entered the effective joint space, and resulted in third-body wear of the bearing surfaces. Modern cementless implants are often grit blasted or porous coated in order to achieve adequate surface roughness for bony ingrowth.

The addition of a hydroxyapatite coating to the surface of the cementless prosthesis often aids fixation.[18,19] Hydroxyapatite is one of the major mineral constituents of bone, and is a bioactive ceramic. It is usually plasma sprayed onto the surface of a cementless implant (Figs 96.10 and 96.11). The osteoinductive and osteoconductive hydroxyapatite layer is subjected to osteoclastic resorption *in vivo*, and is gradually replaced by direct bone ingrowth and ongrowth onto the prosthesis. Long-term results of hydroxyapatite-coated implants in THR surgery show implant survival rates that are at least as good as currently used cemented implants.

The optimal degree of porosity and surface roughness of a cementless implant continues to be debated. Recent variations include the tantalum trabecular metal implants (Zimmer, Warsaw, IN), which are said to have microstructural properties akin to cancellous bone. The trabecular microstructure of the implant is said to promote early bony interdigitation with the implant. Long-term studies will be required to validate the proposed benefits of this new prosthetic design.

Stress shielding of periprosthetic bone can occur during cementless and cemented hip arthroplasty and is related to the modulus of elasticity, design and fixation method of the implant. Cobalt chrome has a relatively high modulus of elasticity and has been known to stress shield periprosthetic bone. Titanium has a relatively low modulus of elasticity compared with cobalt chrome or stainless steel, and thus may causes less stress shielding. However, stress shielding of an implant is governed predominantly by implant geometry rather than its material property. Modern implants are designed to reduce stress shielding, and facilitate reliable load transfer to periprosthetic bone.

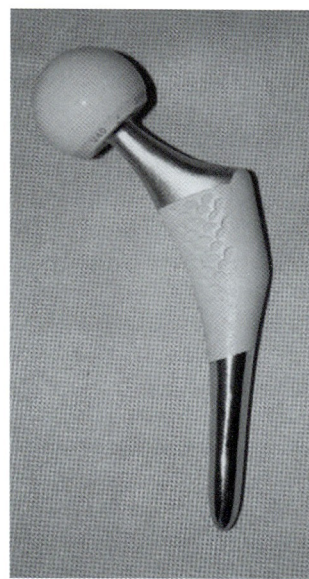

Figure 96.11 A proximally hydroxyapatite-coated stem (ABG; Stryker, USA).

REFERENCES

- ● = Key primary paper
- ◆ = Major review article

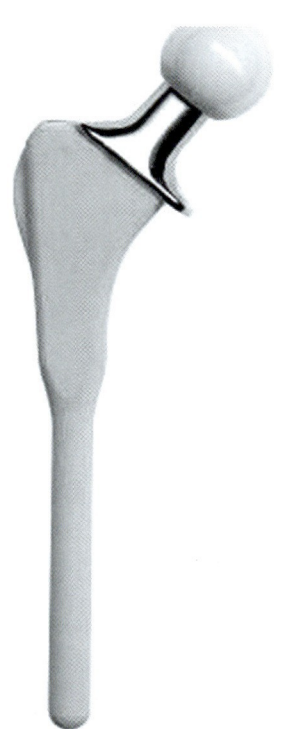

Figure 96.10 A fully hydroxyapatite-coated femoral stem (JRI; Furlong Ltd, UK).

◆1. Huo MH, Cook SM. What's new in hip arthroplasty. *Journal of Bone and Joint Surgery (American)* 2001;**83A**:1598–610.

◆2. Schmalzried TP, Callaghan JJ. Wear in total hip and knee replacements. *Journal of Bone and Joint Surgery (American)* 1999;**81**:115–36.

●3. Jacobs JJ, Gilbert JL, Urban RM. Corrosion of metal orthopaedic implants. *Journal of Bone and Joint Surgery (American)* 1998;**80**:268–82.

◆4. Heisel C, Silva M, Schmalzried TP. Bearing surface options for total hip replacement in young patients. *Instructional Course Lectures* 2004;**53**:49–65.

◆5. Amis AA. Is polyethylene still the best prosthetic bearing surface? *Journal of Bone and Joint Surgery (British)* 1996;**78**:345–8.

◆6. Parvizi J, Campfield A, Clohisy JC, *et al.* Management of arthritis of the hip in the young adult. *Journal of Bone and Joint Surgery (British)* 2006;**88**:1279–85.

◆7. Keegan GM, Learmonth ID, Case CP. Orthopaedic metals and their potential toxicity in the arthroplasty patient: a review of current knowledge and future strategies. *Journal of Bone and Joint Surgery (British)* 2007;**89**:567–73.

◆8. Hamadouche M, Sedel L. Ceramics in orthopaedics. *Journal of Bone and Joint Surgery (British)* 2000;**82**:1095–9.

●9. Dumbleton J, Manley MT. Hydroxyapatite-coated prostheses in total hip and knee arthroplasty. *Journal of Bone and Joint Surgery (American)* 2004;**86A**:2526–40.

- 10. Haraguchi K, Sugano N, Nishii T, et al. Phase transformation of a zirconia ceramic head after total hip arthroplasty. *Journal of Bone and Joint Surgery (British)* 2001;**83**:996–1000.
- 11. Gilbert JL, Buckley CA, Jacobs JJ, et al. Intergranular corrosion-fatigue failure of cobalt-alloy femoral stems. A failure analysis of two implants. *Journal of Bone and Joint Surgery (American)* 1994;**76**:110–15.
- 12. Lusty PJ, Tai CC, Sew-Hoy RP, et al. Third-generation alumina-on-alumina ceramic bearings in cementless total hip arthroplasty. *Journal of Bone and Joint Surgery (American)* 2007;**89**:2676–83.
- 13. Walter WL, Insley GM, Walter WK, Tuke MA. Edge loading in third generation alumina ceramic-on-ceramic bearings: stripe wear. *Journal of Arthroplasty* 2004;**19**:402–13.
- 14. Lusty PJ, Watson A, Tuke MA, et al. Orientation and wear of the acetabular component in third generation alumina-on-alumina ceramic bearings. An analysis of 33 retrievals. *Journal of Bone and Joint Surgery (British)* 2007;**89**:1158–64.
- 15. Walter WL, O'Toole GC, Walter WK, et al. Squeaking in ceramic-on-ceramic hips: the importance of acetabular component orientation. *Journal of Arthroplasty* 2007;**22**:496–503.
- 16. Webb JC, Spencer RF. The role of polymethylmethacrylate bone cement in modern orthopaedic surgery. *Journal of Bone and Joint Surgery (British)* 2007;**89**:851–7.
- 17. Scheerlinck T, Casteleyn PP. The design features of cemented femoral hip implants. *Journal of Bone and Joint Surgery (British)* 2006;**88**:1409–18.
- 18. Rajaratnam SS, Jack C, Tavakkolizadeh A, et al. Long-term results of a hydroxyapatite-coated femoral component in total hip replacement: a 15- to 21-year follow-up study. *Journal of Bone and Joint Surgery (British)* 2008;**90**:27–30.
- 19. Shepperd JA, Apthorp H. A contemporary snapshot of the use of hydroxyapatite coating in orthopaedic surgery. *Journal of Bone and Joint Surgery (British)* 2005;**87**:1046–9.

97

Perioperative considerations

DANIEL KENDOFF, THOMAS P SCULCO, FRIEDRICH BOETTNER

| Introduction | 1123 | Specific operative considerations | 1127 |
| General pre-operative considerations | 1123 | References | 1131 |

NATIONAL BOARD STANDARDS

- Understand the important perioperative problems of total hip arthroplasty
- Know the best choice of anaesthetic for total hip arthroplasty
- Learn the use of antibiotics and deep vein thrombosis prophylaxis
- Understand various surgical approaches and when to use them
- Learn the special considerations of patients with osteoarthritis, rheumatoid arthritis, ankylosing spondylitis and Paget disease

INTRODUCTION

A comprehensive pre-operative evaluation prior to total hip arthroplasty (THA) should focus on systematic conditions of relevance to pre-operative and intra-operative decision-making. It should focus on those factors that may have an impact on the approach and technical requirements or considerations. Thus, modern THA incorporates distinct protocols for antibiotic prophylaxis, thromboembolic prophylaxis, perioperative pain management and anaesthesia. This chapter describes some of the most relevant systematic conditions affecting patients undergoing THA so as to aid the surgeon to minimize perioperative complications and develop a patient-specific treatment plan.

GENERAL PRE-OPERATIVE CONSIDERATIONS

Neurological evaluation is a crucial part of the pre-operative work-up. This includes assessment of general neurological status with a subsequent focus on the affected lower extremity, ruling out pre-existing nerve deficits, nerve palsy, post-stroke sequelae or severe contractures of the pelvis or upper thigh muscles. An inability to mobilize and reliance on a walking frame or crutches makes the postoperative recovery less predictable. These patients rely on weight bearing, and this should be considered for implant selection and fixation technique.

Respiratory conditions, cardiac comorbidities and endocrine disorders may have an impact on the operative morbidity and mortality. Patients with diabetes mellitus require adequate pre-operative management of blood glucose levels. Patients with valvular heart disease may require a pre-operative assessment by their dentist. Renal disease has an impact on the perioperative fluid monitoring and administration. Anaemia may require a distinct work-up or necessitate pre-operative blood transfusion. A history of alcoholism or illicit drug use should be ruled out.

Anaesthesia

Regional anaesthesia is widely considered the method of choice for THA. Reduced blood loss and transfusion requirements, lower deep vein thrombosis (DVT) and pulmonary embolism rates have been reported, compared with general anaesthesia.[1–6]

Hypotensive anaesthesia has shown to significantly reduce intra-operative blood loss.[7] Studies have demonstrated a two- to fourfold reduction in intra-operative blood loss when the mean arterial pressure is reduced to 50 mmHg during surgery.[8,9] Reduced bleeding improves visualization of the surgical field and the dry osseous surface provides a superior bone–cement interface. An arterial line is recommended to monitor blood pressure continuously during hypotensive anaesthesia. However, a central venous line is rarely needed to manage intra-operative fluid even if a greater degree of blood loss is anticipated. Pulmonary artery lines should be reserved for one-stage bilateral hybrid THA, prolonged revision arthroplasty and patients with congestive heart failures, severe valvular heart disease or pulmonary hypertension. Low-dose intravenous adrenaline (epinephrine) infusions may be necessary to stabilize the circulation during hypotensive anaesthesia.

Spinal anaesthesia allows for rapid induction, but higher doses may also induce hypotension. In combination with adrenaline infusions, it has shown similar benefits to hypotensive epidural anaesthesia, including reduced blood loss and decreased DVT rates.[10–12] Continuous spinal anaesthesia is also used in some centres. It offers few advantages over continuous epidural techniques while conferring an increased risk of neurological complications.

Hypotensive epidural anaesthesia decreases arterial pressure while preserving an adequate heart rate, central venous pressure, stroke volume and cardiac output.[13,14] Additionally, patients can stay awake, allowing neurological monitoring. A significant reduction in mortality rate after THA was observed in the authors' institution after hypotensive anaesthesia was used routinely for THA.[15]

Hypotensive anaesthesia also resulted in a reduction in blood loss and transfusion requirements in our institution. The reduced incidence of DVT with hypotensive epidural anaesthesia may be attributed to the reduction in blood loss and the augmentation of lower extremity blood flow. Additionally, using hypotensive anaesthesia, several clinical studies at the current authors' institution have noted a reduction in the incidence of thromboembolism.[7,14–16]

Pain control

Intense pain after THA may impede mobilization and prolong hospitalization. Owing to the side-effects of parenteral opioid drugs, which can include nausea, vomiting, respiratory depression, reduced gastrointestinal motility and urinary retention, postoperative analgesia has been favoured on a local rather than systemic basis.

Recent multimodal pathways include peripheral nerve blocks, postoperative patient-controlled anaesthesia as well as oral pain medications. Peripheral nerve blocks include psoas compartment block of the lumbar plexus, sciatic nerve blocks and fascia iliaca blocks, which, however, will not reliably cover the complete lateral femoral side.[17,18] A large prospective survey demonstrated a significantly lower incidence of serious complications, such as cardiac arrest and neurological injuries, in patients with peripheral nerve blocks compared with patients who had undergone spinal or epidural anaesthesia.[19] Future directions include a comprehensive system that oversees the use of continuous peripheral nerve blocks outside the acute inpatient setting for several days postoperatively.

Recent techniques also include intra- and postoperative wound infiltration with multimodal narcotics that have been shown to reduce pain and the requirement for oral and intravenous narcotics after hip replacement, leading to faster postoperative recovery.[20] Furthermore inpatient applications include the use of intramuscular narcotics and patient-controlled intravenous analgesia (PCA). While the use of PCA has been somewhat controversial, a review of the literature supports its use over traditional intramuscular dosing. PCA has been shown to provide more effective analgesia than intramuscular dosing, and PCA administration is preferred over intramuscular dosing by both patients and nurses.[21,22]

Post-THA pain control also includes oral analgesics, which are usually selected for long-term usage in the rehabilitation time period. Regular oral analgesic regimens often combine the scheduled use of oral morphine and non-steroidal anti-inflammatory medications. The combination of a selective cyclo-oxygenase-2 inhibitor, paracetamol (acetaminophen) and oral morphine for at least 10 days postoperatively has demonstrated good results.[23]

Dental infections

Transient oral bacteraemia can be a source of deep implant infection following THA.[24–26] By penetrating the mucosal barrier, haematogenous spread with distant infections may occur. Bacteraemia can cause colonization of an artificial total joint implant and can lead to infection. The first 2 years postoperatively are the most critical period after joint placement and are the focus of prophylaxis.[27]

Routine dental procedures can produce transient bacteraemia of two to 10 colony-forming units per millilitre for up to 30 minutes.[28,29] More extensive oral procedures such as tooth extraction, periodontal scaling and endodontic surgery may increase bacterial load and potential risk for infection.[30] In general, patients at increased risk of implant infection include those with a pre-existing diagnosis of diabetes mellitus, rheumatoid arthritis, corticosteroid therapy use, immunosuppression, haemophilia or those undergoing revision surgery.[31,32] Patients who are being prepared for total joint arthroplasty should have good dental health prior to surgery, and should be encouraged to seek professional dental care if necessary. The risk of bacteraemia is far more substantial in a patient with ongoing dental issues. Any patient with a total joint prosthesis and coexisting acute orofacial infection should have aggressive treatment to eliminate the source of the infection. Antibiotic treatments are strongly recommended.

Although there is currently a paucity of substantial scientific evidence in the orthopaedic literature to support routine antibiotic prophylaxis prior to dental treatment in patients with total joint prostheses, guidelines are published by the National Institute for Health and Clinical Excellence (NICE) and the American Dental Association in combination with the American Academy of Orthopaedic Surgeons (AAOS).[27,33]

Dental procedures are divided into those with a low incidence or those with a high incidence of bacteraemia. The high-incidence group includes dental extractions, periodontal procedures, endodontal instrumentation, placement of dental implants, root canal surgery, initial placement of orthodontic bands, intraligamentary injections of local anaesthetic and prophylactic cleaning of teeth or implants when bleeding is anticipated. The recommended antibiotic prophylaxis regimen for patients who are not allergic to penicillin includes cephalexin, cephradine or amoxicillin, 1 hour before the dental procedure. Patients unable to take oral medications should receive cefazolin or ampicillin intramuscularly or intravenously 1 hour before the procedure. Patients allergic to penicillin should take clindamycin orally or intravenously 1 hour before dental procedures. No second doses are recommended for any of these dosing regimens.

Myocardial infarction

The emphasis on faster recovery times with reduced hospital stays for total hip replacement patients can also be problematic in patients with cardiovascular comorbidities. Perioperative cardiovascular complications are rare, yet they represent the most frequent serious complications after THA, with myocardial infarction being the most common adverse cardiovascular event.[34,35] The incidence of perioperative myocardial infarction has been reported in larger studies to be as high as 1.8% with an in-hospital mortality rate of between 0.2% and 0.3%.[36] Increased age, male sex and prior cardiovascular disease are the major risk factors. Perioperative myocardial infarction is more likely to occur in older patients (>70 years), when the rate may be as high as 0.4%, and can increase further to 1.6% for patients 80 years or older.[35] Delaying patient discharge until postoperative day 3 is likely to uncover 83% of cardiac events that could potentially occur in hospital and should be remembered amid the current trend of early discharge.[34]

Bladder catheterization

Although urinary tract infection (UTI) is a potential complication after THA, the use and timing of urethral catheterization remains controversial. Urinary retention can lead to UTI and subsequent implant infection through haematogenous spread; on the other hand, urethral catheterization also has been shown to cause THA infection.[37,38] An increased risk of UTI has been established with the use of an indwelling catheter for a period of greater than 48 hours.[39,40] A study investigating the routine use of a pre-operative bladder catheterization regimen versus a postoperative catheterization regime on a *pro re nata* (PRN) basis is warranted.

A recent study involving 719 patients demonstrated that universal routine pre-operative catheterization may not be warranted in patients who have THA. While the incidence of UTIs with general catheterization was comparable to that in a regimen of PRN catheterization, the overall costs were significantly increased.[41] Another recent study found that intermittent catheterization had a lower rate of UTI after THA than an indwelling catheter.[42] Therefore, it may be more cost-effective to observe patients for symptoms of urinary retention and insert a catheter if warranted. If subsequent catheterization is necessary, intermittent straight catheterization should be considered to avoid UTI, as recommended by some authors.

Diabetes mellitus

The prevalence of diabetes mellitus (DM) has more than tripled since 1970, and currently affects 6.2% of the US population and 4.26% in the UK. It is predicted that, by the year 2050, the prevalence will have increased by another 165%.[43]

DM affects almost every organ system. Of major relevance to THA is its effect on the vascular system. A thorough pre-operative cardiac and peripheral vascular evaluation should be carried out in every diabetic patient scheduled for THA. Documentation of the peripheral vascular status of the affected extremity is critical. General hyperglycaemia, secondary to diabetes, has an adverse effect on bone strength and fracture healing. Additionally, diabetic patients are more likely to develop osteopenia and postoperative infections than patients without DM.

Intra-operatively, particularly with regional anaesthesia, some medications may mask the symptoms of hypoglycaemia; therefore, the blood glucose level should be monitored at least every hour during surgery. Patients should be scheduled early to minimize prolonged fasting and hypoglycaemia. It should also be noted that diabetic nephropathy affects overall fluid management and use of nephrotoxic medications. Postoperatively, blood glucose levels should be closely monitored every 6 hours. An insulin sliding scale should be ordered to effectively allow treatment of increased glucose levels, which are frequently encountered during the early postoperative period. Because of their direct influence on blood glucose level, corticosteroids should be used with caution.

Antibiotics

Prophylactic antibiotics have been shown to reduce the incidence of infection in patients undergoing primary total joint arthroplasty.[44–46] Antimicrobial prophylaxis should be administered for as short a period as possible to prevent emergence of resistant organisms, reduce drug reactions, improve compliance and minimize costs. *Staphylococcus aureus* remains the most commonly encountered organism. Prophylactic antibiotics should be administered within 1 hour prior to skin incision.[47,48] If a proximal tourniquet is used, the antibiotic must be completely infused prior to the inflation of the tourniquet.

The current advisory statement of the AAOS recommends the following antibiotic prophylaxis regime.[49]

Cefazolin or cefuroxime are the preferred antibiotics for patients undergoing elective orthopaedic procedures.[50,51] Clindamycin or vancomycin may be used for patients with a confirmed β-lactam antibiotic allergy. Vancomycin may be used in patients with known colonization with meticillin-resistant *S. aureus* (MRSA) or in facilities with recent MRSA outbreaks.

Dosing should be in proportion to the patient's weight, with 1 g of cefazolin for patients <80 kg and 2 g for patients >80 kg.[52] Additional intra-operative doses of antibiotic are advised for procedures exceeding the half-life of the antibiotic or if significant blood loss is encountered during the procedure.[53] Vancomycin should be reserved for treatment of serious infection with β-lactam-resistant organisms or for treatment of infection in patients with a life-threatening allergy to β-lactam antimicrobials.[54]

The guidelines in terms of frequency of intra-operative administration are as follows: cefazolin every 2–5 hours; cefuroxime every 3–4 hours; clindamycin every 3–6 hours; vancomycin every 6–12 hours. Prophylactic antibiotics should be discontinued within 24 hours of surgery. The current literature does not support continuous use of antibiotics until all drains or catheters are removed and provides no evidence of benefit when they are continued past 24 hours.[55,56]

Thromboprophylaxis

Following THA, patients are at high risk for asymptomatic DVT, which has an incidence ranging from 40% to 60% and occurs at a median of 21 days postoperatively, and symptomatic venous thromboembolism, which has an incidence of 2–5% and occurs at a median of 34 days postoperatively.[57,58] Fatal pulmonary embolisms have been observed in one out of every 500 THA patients.

The first consensus on treatment recommendations for thromboprophylaxis in patients undergoing THA was published in 1986.[59] Although evidence-based guidelines derived from large randomized clinical studies have further refined these guidelines with collaboration between orthopaedic, haematological and thoracic societies, there still exists controversy as to optimal prophylaxis. Recently, in the USA, AAOS guidelines for the prevention of pulmonary embolism in patients undergoing total hip or knee arthroplasty have gained wider acceptance among orthopaedic surgeons. These guidelines have also facilitated more accurate identification of high- and low-risk patient cohorts.[60]

Multimodal thromboprophylaxis is commonly used in THA, including pharmaceutical and mechanical agents.[61]

The single use of mechanical prophylaxis has been less effective in preventing proximal DVTs than pharmacological anticoagulant strategies.[61] Recent anticoagulant-based prophylaxis strategies include the use of aspirin, vitamin K antagonists (such as warfarin), low-molecular-weight heparin (LMWH) and fondaparinux. Administration for 10–14 days postoperatively is recommended. While prolonged prophylaxis demonstrated reduced venous thromboembolism rates after 35 days of prophylaxis compared with 7–15 days, it remains unclear whether prophylaxis following THA should be extended beyond 10–14 days.[62]

As described above, the use of spinal or epidural regional anaesthesia has been associated with a significantly reduced incidence of DVT in THA patients. Evidence-based strategies at the authors' institution include the routine use of hypotensive epidural anaesthesia, anti-thromboembolic disease stockings or graduated elastic stockings, intra-operative heparin administration, automated pneumatic calf compression, early ambulation and mobilization and postoperative aspirin.[4,5,11,12,16] Administration of a single dose of unfractionated heparin (15 U kg^{-1}) at the time of cup insertion suppresses thrombogenesis during total hip replacement.[12,16,63] By combining intra-operative (hypotensive epidural anaesthesia and intra-operative heparin) and postoperative (pneumatic compression devices and aspirin) prophylaxis of deep venous thrombosis, the current authors were able to reduce the DVT rate to less than 10% and reduce the proximal deep venous thrombosis rate to 2%. In high-risk patients the authors would recommend warfarin over the use of aspirin.

However, the regimen described does not correlate with current guidelines recommended by the American College of Chest Physicians (ACCP) in North America or those recommended by NICE in the UK. Aspirin as a sole anticoagulant agent is not recommended in either set of guidelines.[59,61] The NICE guidelines for patients undergoing elective hip replacement without additional risk factors recommend mechanical prophylaxis and either LMWH or fondaparinux. Patients with one or more risk factors should have their LMWH or fondaparinux therapy continued for 4 weeks after surgery. Primary risk factors include age over 60 years, obesity (body mass index >30), immobility, active heart or respiratory disease, active cancer or cancer treatment, acute medical illness, central venous catheter *in situ*, inflammatory bowel disease or nephrotic syndrome. In Europe, the use of vitamin K antagonists has mostly been discontinued, owing to their delayed onset, variable response, need for frequent monitoring and the complexity of in-hospital and post-discharge supervision.

Recommendations from the ACCP are based on the following three anticoagulants: LMWH, fondaparinux or vitamin K antagonists (warfarin) with a minimum use of 10 days, without any emphasis placed on the use of one medication over the other. However, specific decisions should be individualized with attention to the specific patient, drug pricing and ability to safely monitor vitamin K antagonist use and duration of prophylaxis.

It is important to recognize that no prospective study has shown a reduction in fatal pulmonary embolism when comparing the use of aspirin, warfarin, LMWH or fondaparinux. However, a recent analysis involving evaluation of 20 studies with over 15 000 patients retrospectively concluded that all-cause mortality in patients after total hip or knee arthroplasty was higher in patients receiving LMWH than in patients receiving a combination of regional anaesthesia, aspirin and pneumatic compressions. The authors noted a higher proportion of clinical non-fatal pulmonary emboli.[5]

SPECIFIC OPERATIVE CONSIDERATIONS (FIGS 97.1–97.3)

Osteoarthritis

Primary osteoarthritis is the major indication for THA in Europe and North America. While around 600 000 THAs are performed in Europe yearly, the number of primary replacements is expected to increase consistently at least until the year 2030. An increase in the number of THAs being performed is mainly driven by a change in demographics, with a greater number of elderly people living longer and including more activity in their daily lives. Younger patients undergoing THA have higher expectations with regard to functional outcomes after surgery, including a swift return to work, sports and other activities. Therefore, current trends and discussion focus also on the young and middle-aged patient population.

The increasing number of young patients undergoing THA will result in an increase in revisions in the future. Therefore, maximizing implant survival is critical, including optimal positioning, reduced migration, reduced wear and improved osseointegration. With regard to implant selection in primary osteoarthritis, bone preservation remains one of the main surgical issues for young patients. The use of uncemented implants in the younger population has been well established over the past 20 years, and has shown excellent long-term results.

Modern trends in bone preservation techniques include the use of surface replacements and shorter hip stems, which are gaining more popularity. Although not every patient will meet the inclusion criteria, bone-preserving techniques should be kept in mind in order to save bone for a potential future revision.

Modern articulating options should also be considered, such as highly cross-linked polyethylene, metal-on-metal, ceramic-on-ceramic or ceramic-on-plastic solutions. In recent years, there has been a resurgence in prosthetic femoral heads with large diameters, with evidence of improved hip function and a reduced incidence of dislocation. Although

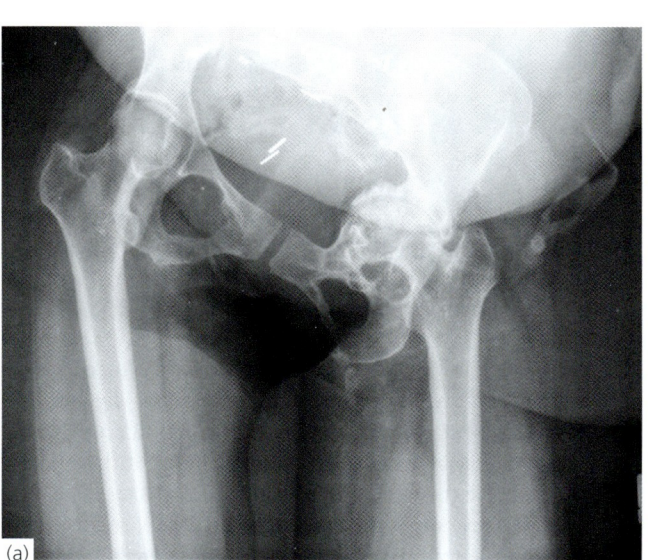
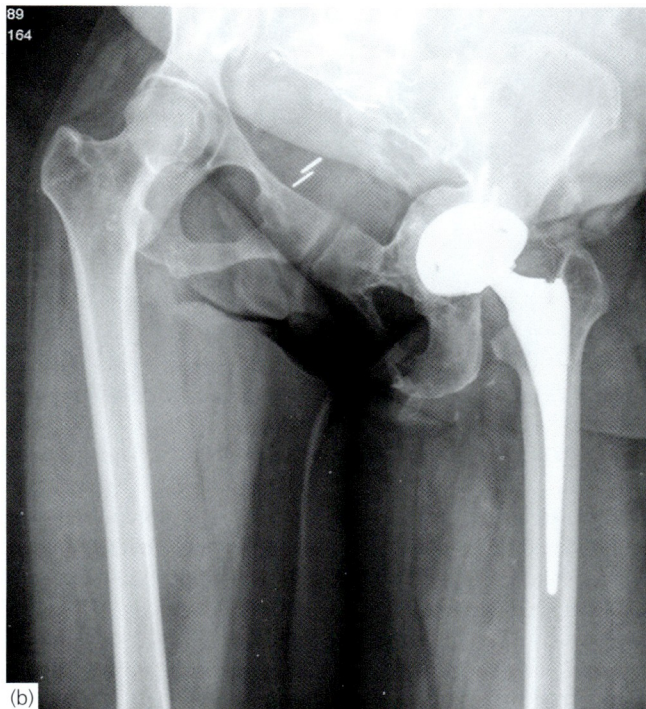

Figure 97.1 (a and b) Adjusting the cup position appropriately with respect to pelvic obliquity can be challenging.

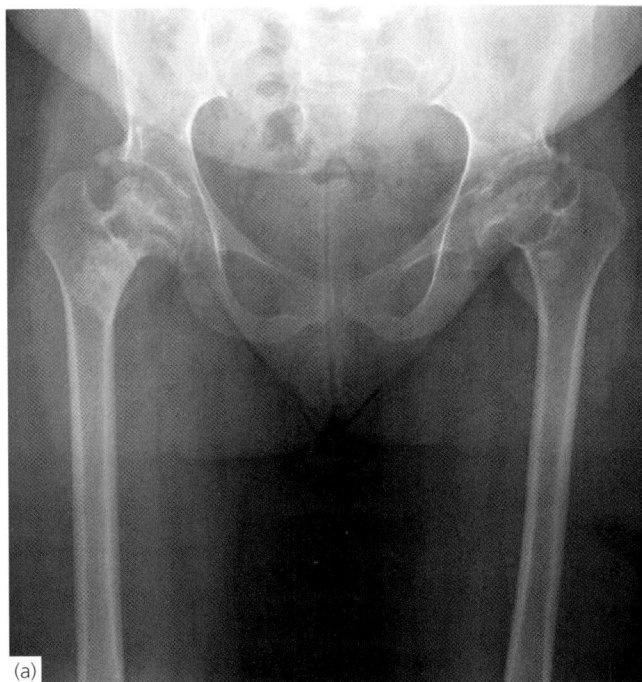 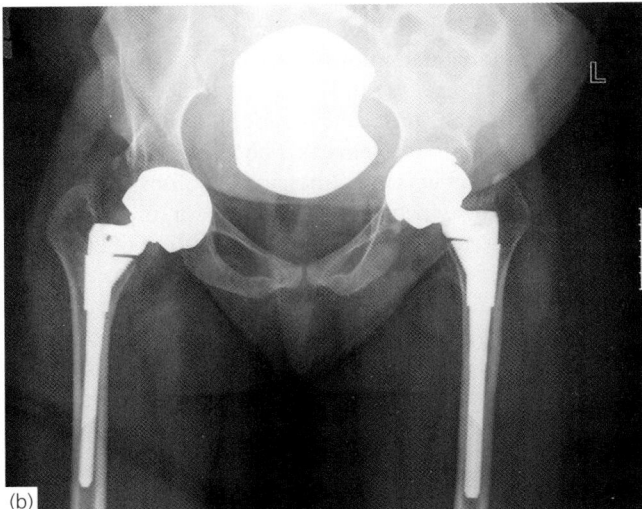

Figure 97.2 (a and b) Patients with achondroplasia require additional pre- and perioperative planning considerations so as to ensure correct implant size and placement.

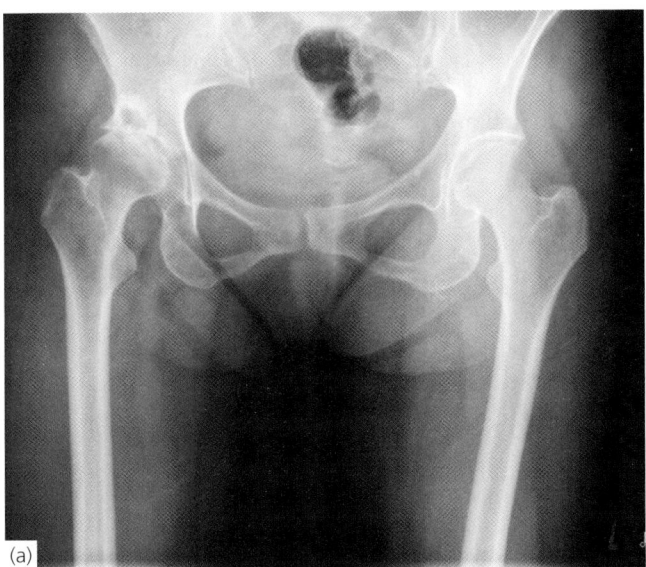 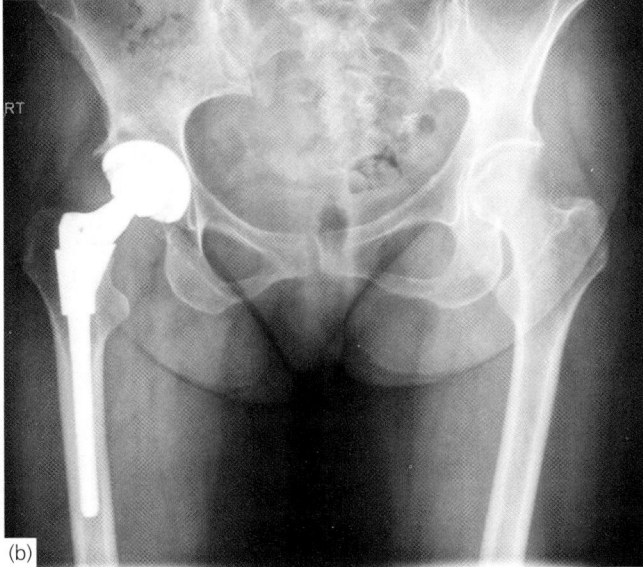

Figure 97.3 (a and b) Hip dysplasia will influence both perioperative management and implant choice.

current trends such as hip resurfacing, especially in young patients, exemplify the successful use of an alternative bone-preserving technique, there are no data supporting its long-term superiority.

Rheumatoid arthritis

The hip joint is involved in 15–30% of patients with rheumatoid arthritis.[64] However, the use of drugs which target certain inflammatory cytokines known to contribute to the development of rheumatoid arthritis, e.g. tumour necrosis factor α and other immunosuppressive agents, has resulted in a reduction in the overall number of rheumatoid arthritis patients requiring joint arthroplasty. THA in patients with rheumatoid arthritis presents a particular challenge. Rheumatoid patients are often younger than patients with osteoarthritis and bone quality is poor because of associated osteopenia and bone resorption. Rheumatoid patients are usually less active than other patients requiring THA owing to multiple joint involvements and associated systemic comorbidities. Rheumatoid patients may also have an increased incidence of delayed wound healing, sepsis and general complications due to their disease and the frequent use of oral steroids, anti-metabolic agents and non-steroidal anti-inflammatory drugs. A relatively high rate of wound-healing problems and infections in up to 19% of patients was observed in one clinical case series, and this was deemed to be most probably related to the systemic nature of rheumatoid arthritis.[65] Cemented THA in patients with rheumatoid arthritis has shown higher rates of infection than THA in patients with osteoarthritis.[66]

A distinct difference between the common problems associated with osteoarthritis and rheumatoid arthritis is the increased incidence of medial bone loss and protrusio acetabuli in patients with rheumatoid arthritis, which has been found to be present in up to 5% of all patients.[67] Traditionally, cemented THA has been preferred in patients with rheumatoid arthritis.[68] If THA for protrusio acetabuli is attempted, technical difficulties from an inadequate medial wall may be encountered, with the cement having insufficient support.

From a technical standpoint, direct dislocation of the hip in the severe protrusio can be difficult. Thus, resection of the femoral head *in situ* is sometimes necessary to reduce the force required for dislocation and reduce the risk of iatrogenic femoral fracture.

For cemented methods without bone grafting, bone cement mass filling, metal mesh and support rings have been introduced; however, loosening between the bone–cement interface can occur frequently in acetabular protrusions. A combination of bone graft using the resected femoral head and a support ring in rheumatoid arthritis patients has been shown to be effective,[69] but a high rate of loosening of both cemented acetabular and femoral components has been reported at medium-term follow-up compared with the rate in osteoarthritis patients. The loosening of cemented acetabular components is particularly progressive in patients with juvenile rheumatoid arthritis.[70] At the current authors' institution, good results have been demonstrated when a portion of the femoral head is removed and transferred as a bone graft to the acetabular cavity.

While cemented and uncemented techniques have demonstrated good results in the literature, a large Finnish arthroplasty registry study looking at more than 2500 patients reported that cemented all-polyethylene cups in combination with proximally uncemented, circumferentially porous-coated stems were the implants of choice for young patients with rheumatoid arthritis.[71–73] In contrast to the traditional techniques of cement fixation, uncemented press-fit acetabular component fixation with additional screws also has a high success rate in rheumatoid arthritis patients.[64] At the authors' institution, most surgeons prefer bone grafting with uncemented acetabular component fixation augmented with screws.

Rheumatoid arthritis has also been associated with longer rehabilitation times and lower functional outcome gain in patients with lower extremity arthroplasty. Such patients may require additional monitoring to ensure adequate rehabilitation.[74]

Ankylosing spondylitis

The incidence of hip joint involvement in patients with ankylosing spondylitis ranges from 30% to 50% of patients, with bilaterality in approximately 90% of these patients.[75,76] Ankylosing spondylitis of the hip joint generally results in severe disabling changes in function, posture and gait. Spinal deformities and their effect on posture should be considered for implant position and anaesthesia. For example, the presence of cervical spine fusion might necessitate fibre-optic-assisted intubation. Consequently, epidural or spinal anaesthetic may be preferred.

Ankylosing spondylitis of the hip usually results in flexion contractures and severe ankylosis; often, a disabling flexed position is present. Patients with ankylosing spondylitis typically undergo THA at a younger age than those patients requiring THA for osteoarthritis.[77] THA implant survival in ankylosing spondylitis patients is similar to that in other young patients with THA. Although it was previously thought that patients with ankylosing spondylitis were at a significantly greater risk of developing disabling heterotopic ossification, a careful review of the literature reveals that this may not be the case. Higher rates of heterotopic ossification in ankylosing spondylitis patients are not apparent when compared with similar groups of osteoarthritis patients.[78,79] High-risk patients with pre-operative ankylosis, previous hip surgery, previous infection or following a transtrochanteric approach should be considered for heterotopic ossification prophylaxis with indometacin or low-dose radiation.[80]

Correction of hip flexion contractures with THA should improve the sagittal balance and posture. Owing to the presence of a relative hyperextension of the hips after THA, patients are more prone to anterior dislocation when acetabular components are placed in their normal position relative to the pelvis.[81] When positioning the acetabular component in a patient with ankylosing spondylitis, the relationship of the pelvis to the lumbar spine should be considered in order to avoid anterior instability. Whether corrections of the spinal deformities should be performed before THA remains unclear.[80] Since an improvement in the range of motion of the hip and pain relief may obviate the need for spinal osteotomy in patients with severe hip flexion deformity,[82] determining an appropriate surgical sequence should be individualized. The long-term implant survival is comparable to that in patients with osteoarthritis.[73,83–85] According to recent clinical data, some authors support the use of uncemented acetabular and femoral components in all young, active patients, including those with ankylosing spondylitis.[83,86]

Paget disease

While most patients with Paget disease do not require surgical treatment, 10% of those who do need surgery undergo total hip replacement.[87] While uncemented and cemented techniques have both shown promising results, intra-operative technical difficulties arise mainly from the associated poor bone quality and anatomical abnormalities such as acetabular protrusion, coxa vara and extensive femoral bowing.[88–90]

The presence of sclerotic bone may also negatively affect reaming and acetabular component placement. Extreme cases may necessitate the use of a high-speed burr to aid bone preparation.[90,91] In addition, pagetoid bone may be hypervascular because of the increased metabolic activity, which can lead to increased bleeding especially in patients with active disease.

Restricted cemented fixation might result from extreme sclerosis and therefore uncemented implants may be preferred. Acetabular protrusion is often associated with severe medial wall bone defects and requires local bone grafting, oversized cups or even anti-protusion cages. Lateral offset acetabular liners can also compensate for a medial cup placement.[88]

With regard to the femur, coxa vara may be encountered, leading to severe varus malpositioning of the femoral component and difficulties in restoring the offset.[92] Trochanteric and realignment osteotomies are sometimes necessary to obtain adequate exposure and prevent varus malalignment. Of note, the use of custom-made prostheses has not demonstrated optimal outcomes, with reported early failures.[93]

Although it is not yet certain whether and how the bone in Paget disease influences ingrowth of uncemented implants, most reports in the literature show good midterm results up to 7 years.[91,94]

Postoperative heterotopic ossification is seen in 23–57% of cases.[90–92] Consequently, pre- and postoperative prophylaxis, such as local radiation and indometacin, are recommended. The perioperative blood loss is increased and perioperative cell savers should be considered.[89]

Osteopetrosis

Osteopetrosis is caused by defective osteoclast resorption, leading to hard and brittle bone.[95] While 40% of patients with autosomal dominant osteopetrosis are asymptomatic, degenerative osteoarthritis may develop secondary to coxa vara deformities.[96] Degenerative osteoarthritis is also a result of the increased density of the subchondral bone.

Pre-operative planning should consider the presence of scoliosis, spondylolisthesis and cervical spine fractures. Surgical difficulties often prolong the operative procedure and can result in increased blood loss.[97] In addition, the risk of deep infection is increased after THA in osteopetrotic bone.[98]

The hardness of osteopetrotic bone and obliteration of the medullary canal can cause iatrogenic fractures during implant placement. Thus, extreme caution is necessary during intramedullary reaming. High-speed burr or power drills can help to open the intramedullary canal. Breakage of drill bits and overheating has been reported.[99,100] The use of guidewires, increasing drill bit sizes and adequate cooling should also be implemented as necessary.

Although press fitting the femoral component may fracture the shaft, one study with a 10 year follow-up has shown promising results using a non-cemented stem.[101,102]

Use of a short and narrow stem simplifies placement. Some authors recommend a stem that is typically used for patients with congenital hip dislocation.[102] Recently, fluoroscopy-guided navigation has also been described to improve stem placement.[103]

Uncemented acetabular component placement is also recommended since sclerotic bone hinders the cement interdigitation. Resurfacing techniques are an appropriate choice when the intramedullary canal cannot be identified.

Despite the fact that osteopetronic bone can complicate THA, to date, there has not been a significant evaluation of potential complications among the few reports cited in the literature.[97,100]

> **KEY LEARNING POINTS**
>
> - A systematic review prior to hip arthroplasty is important.
> - Regional anaesthesia is widely considered the method of choice for total hip arthroplasty treatment.
> - Multimodal postoperative regimens are relevant after total hip arthroplasty.
> - Antibiotic prophylaxis prior to dental procedures is indicated.
> - Delayed hospital discharge after THA until day 3 will uncover 83% of cardiac events.
> - Urinary tract infections are a potential complication after total hip arthroplasty and a catheter should only be inserted if clinically indicated.
> - Prophylactic antibiotics reduce the incidence of infections after total hip arthroplasty.
> - Multimodal thromboprophylaxis is recommended after total hip arthroplasty.
> - Primary osteoarthritis is the major indication for total hip arthroplasty in Europe and the USA.
> - The hip is involved in 15–30% of patients with rheumatoid arthritis.
> - Patients with ankylosing spondylitis have hip (with flexion contractures) and spinal problems.
> - Ten per cent of Paget disease patients require total hip arthroplasty and there is the technical difficulty of coxa vara.

REFERENCES

● = Key primary paper
◆ = Major review article

●1. Keith I. Anaesthesia and blood loss in total hip replacement. *Anaesthesia* 1977;**32**:444–50.

●2. Modig J, Borg T, Karlstrom G, et al. Thromboembolism after total hip replacement: role of epidural and general anesthesia. *Anesthesia and Analgesia* 1983;**62**:174–80.

●3. Modig J, Karlstrom G. Intra- and post-operative blood loss and haemodynamics in total hip replacement when performed under lumbar epidural versus general anaesthesia. *European Journal of Anaesthesiology* 1987;**4**:345–55.

●4. Sharrock NE, Cazan MG, Hargett MJ, et al. Changes in mortality after total hip and knee arthroplasty over a ten-year period. *Anesthesia and Analgesia* 1995;**80**:242–8.

●5. Sharrock NE, Gonzalez Della Valle A, Go G, et al. Potent anticoagulants are associated with a higher all-cause mortality rate after hip and knee arthroplasty. *Clinical Orthopaedics and Related Research* 2008;**466**:714–21.

◆6. Sharrock NE, Salvati EA. Hypotensive epidural anesthesia for total hip arthroplasty: a review. *Acta Orthopaedica Scandinavica* 1996;**67**:91–107.

●7. Sharrock NE, Mineo R, Urquhart B, Salvati EA. The effect of two levels of hypotension on intraoperative blood loss during total hip arthroplasty performed under lumbar epidural anesthesia. *Anesthesia and Analgesia* 1993;**76**:580–4.

●8. Barbier-Bohm G, Desmonts JM, Couderc E, et al. Comparative effects of induced hypotension and normovolaemic haemodilution on blood loss in total hip arthroplasty. *British Journal of Anaesthesia* 1980;**52**:1039–43.

●9. Thompson GE, Miller RD, Stevens WC, Murray WR. Hypotensive anesthesia for total hip arthroplasty: a study of blood loss and organ function (brain, heart, liver, and kidney). *Anesthesiology* 1978;**48**:91–6.

●10. Thorburn J, Louden JR, Vallance R. Spinal and general anaesthesia in total hip replacement: frequency of deep vein thrombosis. *British Journal of Anaesthesia* 1980;**52**:1117–21.

11. Westrich GH, Farrell C, Bono JV, et al. The incidence of venous thromboembolism after total hip arthroplasty: a specific hypotensive epidural anesthesia protocol. *Journal of Arthroplasty* 1999;**14**:456–63.

●12. Westrich GH, Salvati EA, Sharrock N, et al. The effect of intraoperative heparin administered during total hip arthroplasty on the incidence of proximal deep vein thrombosis assessed by magnetic resonance venography. *Journal of Arthroplasty* 2005;**20**:42–50.

●13. Sharrock NE, Go G, Mineo R, Harpel PC. The hemodynamic and fibrinolytic response to low dose epinephrine and phenylephrine infusions during total hip replacement under epidural anesthesia. *Thrombosis and Haemostasis* 1992;**68**:436–41.

●14. Sharrock NE, Mineo R, Go G. The effect of cardiac output on intraoperative blood loss during total hip arthroplasty. *Regional Anesthesia* 1993;**18**:24–9.

●15. Lieberman JR, Huo MM, Hanway J, et al. The prevalence of deep venous thrombosis after total hip arthroplasty with hypotensive epidural anesthesia. *Journal of Bone and Joint Surgery (American)* 1994;**76**:341–8.

●16. Sharrock NE, Brien WW, Salvati EA, et al. The effect of intravenous fixed-dose heparin during total hip arthroplasty on the incidence of deep-vein thrombosis. A randomized, double-blind trial in patients operated on with epidural anesthesia and controlled hypotension. *Journal of Bone and Joint Surgery (American)* 1990;**72**:1456–61.

◆17. Indelli PF, Grant SA, Nielsen K, Vail TP. Regional anesthesia in hip surgery. *Clinical Orthopaedics and Related Research* 2005;**441**:50–5.

◆18. Pagnano MW, Hebl J, Horlocker T. Assuring a painless total hip arthroplasty: a multimodal approach emphasizing peripheral nerve blocks. *Journal of Arthroplasty* 2006;**21**(4 Suppl. 1):80–4.

◆19. Auroy Y, Narchi P, Messiah A, et al. Serious complications related to regional anesthesia: results of a prospective survey in France. *Anesthesiology* 1997;**87**:479–86.

●20. Andersen KV, Pfeiffer-Jensen M, Haraldsted V, Soballe K. Reduced hospital stay and narcotic consumption, and improved mobilization with local and intraarticular infiltration after hip arthroplasty: a randomized clinical trial of an intraarticular technique versus epidural infusion in 80 patients. *Acta Orthopaedica* 2007;**78**:180–6.

●21. Colwell Jr CW. The use of the pain pump and patient-controlled analgesia in joint reconstruction. *American Journal of Orthopedics* 2004;**33**(5 Suppl.):10–12.

22. Colwell Jr CW, Morris BA. Patient-controlled analgesia compared with intramuscular injection of analgesics for the management of pain after an orthopaedic procedure. *Journal of Bone and Joint Surgery (American)* 1995;**77**:726–33.

◆23. Skinner HB. Multimodal acute pain management. *American Journal of Orthopedics* 2004;**33**(5 Suppl.):5–9.

●24. Ahlberg A, Carlsson AS, Lindberg L. Hematogenous infection in total joint replacement. *Clinical Orthopaedics and Related Research* 1978;**137**:69–75.

●25. Bartzokas CA, Johnson R, Jane M, et al. Relation between mouth and haematogenous infection in total joint replacements. *British Journal of Medicine* 1994;**309**:506–8.

●26. Waldman BJ, Mont MA, Hungerford DS. Total knee arthroplasty infections associated with dental procedures. *Clinical Orthopaedics and Related Research* 1997;**343**:164–72.

◆27. American Academy of Orthopaedic Surgeons. *Antibiotic Prophylaxis for Dental Patients with Total Joint Replacements.* Rosemount, IL: AAOS, 2008.

◆28. American Heart Association. Prevention of bacterial endocarditis. *Journal of the American Dental Association* 1972;**85**:1377–9.

29. Robinson L, Kraus FW, Lazansky JP. Bacteremias of dental origin. II. A study of the factors influencing occurrence and detection. *Oral Surgery, Oral Medicine, Oral Pathology* 1950;**3**:923–36.
●30. Downes EM. Late infection after total hip replacement. *Journal of Bone and Joint Surgery (British)* 1977;**59**:42–4.
●31. Fitzgerald Jr RH, Nolan DR, Ilstrup DM, et al. Deep wound sepsis following total hip arthroplasty. *Journal of Bone and Joint Surgery (American)* 1977;**59**:847–55.
●32. Lachiewicz PF, Inglis AE, Insall JN, et al. Total knee arthroplasty in hemophilia. *Journal of Bone and Joint Surgery (American)* 1985;**67**:1361–6.
◆33. National Institute of Health and Clinical Excellence. *Prophylaxis Against Infective Endocarditis: Antimicrobial Prophylaxis Against Infective Endocarditis in Adults and Children Undergoing Interventional Procedures.* London, UK: NICE, 2008.
◆34. Gandhi R, Petruccelli D, Devereaux PJ, et al. Incidence and timing of myocardial infarction after total joint arthroplasty. *Journal of Arthroplasty* 2006;**21**:874–7.
◆35. Mantilla CB, Horlocker TT, Schroeder DR, et al. Frequency of myocardial infarction, pulmonary embolism, deep venous thrombosis, and death following primary hip or knee arthroplasty. *Anesthesiology* 2002;**96**:1140–6.
36. Marsch SC, Schaefer HG, Skarvan K, et al. Perioperative myocardial ischemia in patients undergoing elective hip arthroplasty during lumbar regional anesthesia. *Anesthesiology* 1992;**76**:518–27.
●37. Petersen MS, Collins DN, Selakovich WG, Finkbeiner AE. Postoperative urinary retention associated with total hip and total knee arthroplasties. *Clinical Orthopaedics and Related Research* 1991;**269**:102–8.
●38. Wroblewski BM, del Sel HJ. Urethral instrumentation and deep sepsis in total hip replacement. *Clinical Orthopaedics and Related Research* 1980;**146**:209–12.
39. Martinez OV, Civetta J, Merson K, et al. Bacteriuria in the catheterized surgical intensive care patient. *Critical Care Medicine* 1986;**14**:188–91.
40. Oishi CS, Williams VJ, Hanson PB, et al. Perioperative bladder management after primary total hip arthroplasty. *Journal of Arthroplasty* 1995;**10**:732–6.
●41. Iorio R, Whang W, Healy WL, et al. The utility of bladder catheterization in total hip arthroplasty. *Clinical Orthopaedics and Related Research* 2005;**432**:148–52.
●42. van den Brand IC, Castelein RM. Total joint arthroplasty and incidence of postoperative bacteriuria with an indwelling catheter or intermittent catheterization with one-dose antibiotic prophylaxis: a prospective randomized trial. *Journal of Arthroplasty* 2001;**16**:850–5.
●43. Meding JB, Reddleman K, Keating ME, et al. Total knee replacement in patients with diabetes mellitus. *Clinical Orthopaedics and Related Research* 2003;**416**:208–16.
●44. Doyon F, Evrard J, Mazas F, Hill C. Long-term results of prophylactic cefazolin versus placebo in total hip replacement. *Lancet* 1987;**1**(8537):860.
45. Hill C, Flamant R, Mazas F, Evrard J. Prophylactic cefazolin versus placebo in total hip replacement. Report of a multicentre double-blind randomised trial. *Lancet* 1981;**1**(8224):795–6.
46. Tang WM, Chiu KY, Ng TP, et al. Efficacy of a single dose of cefazolin as a prophylactic antibiotic in primary arthroplasty. *Journal of Arthroplasty* 2003;**18**:714–18.
◆47. Burke JP. Maximizing appropriate antibiotic prophylaxis for surgical patients: an update from LDS Hospital, Salt Lake City. *Clinics in Infectious Diseases* 2001;**33**(Suppl. 2):S78–83.
◆48. Classen DC, Evans RS, Pestotnik SL, et al. The timing of prophylactic administration of antibiotics and the risk of surgical-wound infection. *New England Journal of Medicine* 1992;**326**:281–6.
◆49. American Academy of Orthopaedic Surgeons. *Recommendations for the Use of Intravenous Antibiotic Prophylaxis in Primary Total Joint Arthroplasty.* Rosemount, IL: AAOS, 2008.
◆50. Dellinger EP, Gross PA, Barrett TL, et al. Quality standard for antimicrobial prophylaxis in surgical procedures. Infectious Diseases Society of America. *Clinics in Infectious Diseases* 1994;**18**:422–7.
◆51. Page CP, Bohnen JM, Fletcher JR, et al. Antimicrobial prophylaxis for surgical wounds. Guidelines for clinical care. *Archives in Surgery* 1993;**128**:79–88.
◆52. Hanssen AD, Osmon DR. The use of prophylactic antimicrobial agents during and after hip arthroplasty. *Clinical Orthopaedics and Related Research* 1999;**369**:124–38.
53. Bratzler DW, Houck PM. Antimicrobial prophylaxis for surgery: an advisory statement from the National Surgical Infection Prevention Project. *Clinics in Infectious Diseases* 2004;**38**:1706–15.
◆54. Haley RW, Culver DH, White JW, et al. The nationwide nosocomial infection rate. A new need for vital statistics. *American Journal of Epidemiology* 1985;**121**:159–67.
●55. Esler CN, Blakeway C, Fiddian NJ. The use of a closed-suction drain in total knee arthroplasty. A prospective, randomised study. *Journal of Bone and Joint Surgery (British)* 2003;**85**:215–17.
◆56. Oishi CS, Carrion WV, Hoaglund FT. Use of parenteral prophylactic antibiotics in clean orthopaedic surgery. A review of the literature. *Clinical Orthopaedics and Related Research* 1993;**296**:249–55.
57. Bjornara BT, Gudmundsen TE, Dahl OE. Frequency and timing of clinical venous thromboembolism after major joint surgery. *Journal of Bone and Joint Surgery (British)* 2006;**88**:386–91.
58. Heit JA, Silverstein MD, Mohr DN, et al. Risk factors for deep vein thrombosis and pulmonary embolism: a population-based case-control study. *Archives of Internal Medicine* 2000;**160**:809–15.
◆59. National Institute of Health and Clinical Excellence. *Venous Thromboembolism: Reducing the Risk of Venous Thromboembolism (Deep Vein Thrombosis and Pulmonary Embolism) in Inpatients Undergoing Surgery.* NICE Clinical Guideline 46. London, UK: NICE, 2007.

◆60. American Academy of Orthopaedic Surgeons. *Prevention of Symptomatic Pulmonary Embolism in Patients Undergoing Total Hip or Knee Arthroplasty. Summary of Recommendations*. Rosemount, IL: AAOS, 2007.

61. Geerts WH, Pineo GF, Heit JA, et al. Prevention of venous thromboembolism: the Seventh ACCP Conference on Antithrombotic and Thrombolytic Therapy. *Chest* 2004;**126**(3 Suppl.):338S-400S.

◆62. Friedman RJ. Optimal duration of prophylaxis for venous thromboembolism following total hip arthroplasty and total knee arthroplasty. *Journal of the American Academy of Orthopaedic Surgeons* 2007;**15**:148-55.

63. DiGiovanni CW, Restrepo A, Gonzalez Della Valle AG, et al. The safety and efficacy of intraoperative heparin in total hip arthroplasty. *Clinical Orthopaedics and Related Research* 2000;**379**:178-85.

●64. Thomason 3rd HC, Lachiewicz PF. The influence of technique on fixation of primary total hip arthroplasty in patients with rheumatoid arthritis. *Journal of Arthroplasty* 2001;**16**:628-34.

●65. Severt R, Wood R, Cracchiolo 3rd A, Amstutz HC. Long-term follow-up of cemented total hip arthroplasty in rheumatoid arthritis. *Clinical Orthopaedics and Related Research* 1991;**265**:137-45.

66. Poss R, Maloney JP, Ewald FC, et al. Six- to 11-year results of total hip arthroplasty in rheumatoid arthritis. *Clinical Orthopaedics and Related Research* 1984;**182**:109-16.

67. Hastings DE, Parker SM. Protrusio acetabuli in rheumatoid arthritis. *Clinical Orthopaedics and Related Research* 1975;**108**:76-83.

●68. Creighton MG, Callaghan JJ, Olejniczak JP, Johnston RC. Total hip arthroplasty with cement in patients who have rheumatoid arthritis. A minimum ten-year follow-up study. *Journal of Bone and Joint Surgery (American)* 1998;**80**:1439-46.

69. Mibe J, Imakiire A, Watanabe T, Fujie T. Results of total hip arthroplasty with bone graft and support ring for protrusio acetabuli in rheumatoid arthritis. *Journal of Orthopaedic Science* 2005;**10**:8-14.

70. Lachiewicz PF, McCaskill B, Inglis A, et al. Total hip arthroplasty in juvenile rheumatoid arthritis. Two to eleven-year results. *Journal of Bone and Joint Surgery (American)* 1986;**68**:502-8.

●71. Eskelinen A, Paavolainen P, Helenius I, et al. Total hip arthroplasty for rheumatoid arthritis in younger patients: 2,557 replacements in the Finnish Arthroplasty Register followed for 0-24 years. *Acta Orthopaedica* 2006;**77**:853-65.

72. Keisu KS, Orozco F, McCallum 3rd JD, et al. Cementless femoral fixation in the rheumatoid patient undergoing total hip arthroplasty: minimum 5-year results. *Journal of Arthroplasty* 2001;**16**:415-21.

73. Lyback CC, Lyback CO, Kyro A, et al. Survival of Bi-Metric femoral stems in 77 total hip arthroplasties for juvenile chronic arthritis. *International Orthopaedics* 2004;**28**:357-61.

74. Nguyen-Oghalai TU, Ottenbacher KJ, Caban M, et al. The impact of rheumatoid arthritis on rehabilitation outcomes after lower extremity arthroplasty. *Journal of Clinical Rheumatology* 2007;**13**:247-50.

75. Joshi AB, Markovic L, Hardinge K, Murphy JC. Total hip arthroplasty in ankylosing spondylitis: an analysis of 181 hips. *Journal of Arthroplasty* 2002;**17**:427-33.

76. Moll J. *Ankylosing Spondylitis*. Edinburgh, UK: Churchill Livingstone, 1980.

77. Sweeney S, Gupta R, Taylor G, Calin A. Total hip arthroplasty in ankylosing spondylitis: outcome in 340 patients. *Journal of Rheumatology* 2001;**28**:1862-6.

●78. Brinker MR, Rosenberg AG, Kull L, Cox DD. Primary noncemented total hip arthroplasty in patients with ankylosing spondylitis. Clinical and radiographic results at an average follow-up period of 6 years. *Journal of Arthroplasty* 1996;**11**:802-12.

◆79. Iorio R, Healy WL. Heterotopic ossification after hip and knee arthroplasty: risk factors, prevention, and treatment. *Journal of the American Academy of Orthopaedic Surgeons* 2002;**10**:409-16.

◆80. Kubiak EN, Moskovich R, Errico TJ, Di Cesare PE. Orthopaedic management of ankylosing spondylitis. *Journal of the American Academy of Orthopaedic Surgeons* 2005;**13**:267-78.

81. Tang WM, Chiu KY. Primary total hip arthroplasty in patients with ankylosing spondylitis. *Journal of Arthroplasty* 2000;**15**:52-8.

82. Lee ML. Orthopaedic problems in ankylosing spondylitis. *Rheumatism* 1963;**19**:79-82.

●83. Duffy GP, Berry DJ, Rowland C, Cabanela ME. Primary uncemented total hip arthroplasty in patients <40 years old: 10- to 14-year results using first-generation proximally porous-coated implants. *Journal of Arthroplasty* 2001;**16**(8 Suppl. 1):140-4.

●84. Joshi AB, Porter ML, Trail IA, et al. Long-term results of Charnley low-friction arthroplasty in young patients. *Journal of Bone and Joint Surgery (British)* 1993;**75**:616-23.

●85. Malchau H, Wang YX, Karrholm J, Herberts P. Scandinavian multicenter porous coated anatomic total hip arthroplasty study. Clinical and radiographic results with 7- to 10-year follow-up evaluation. *Journal of Arthroplasty* 1997;**12**:133-48.

●86. Crowther JD, Lachiewicz PF. Survival and polyethylene wear of porous-coated acetabular components in patients less than fifty years old: results at nine to fourteen years. *Journal of Bone and Joint Surgery (American)* 2002;**84**A:729-35.

●87. Graham J, Harris WH. Paget's disease involving the hip joint. *Journal of Bone and Joint Surgery (British)* 1971;**53**:650-9.

88. Lewallen DG. Hip arthroplasty in patients with Paget's disease. *Clinical Orthopaedics and Related Research* 1999;**369**:243-50.

89. McDonald DJ, Sim FH. Total hip arthroplasty in Paget's disease. A follow-up note. *Journal of Bone and Joint Surgery (American)* 1987;**69**:766–72.
●90. Parvizi J, Klein GR, Sim FH. Surgical management of Paget's disease of bone. *Journal of Bone and Mineral Research* 2006;**21**(Suppl. 2): P75–82.
91. Parvizi J, Schall DM, Lewallen DG, Sim FH. Outcome of uncemented hip arthroplasty components in patients with Paget's disease. *Clinical Orthopaedics and Related Research* 2002;**403**:127–34.
●92. Merkow RL, Pellicci PM, Hely DP, Salvati EA. Total hip replacement for Paget's disease of the hip. *Journal of Bone and Joint Surgery (American)* 1984;**66**:752–8.
93. Dunlop DJ, Donnachie NJ, Treacy RB. Failure after customized curved femoral stems in total hip arthroplasty for Paget's disease. *Journal of Arthroplasty* 2000;**15**:398–401.
94. Hozack WJ, Rushton SA, Carey C, et al. Uncemented total hip arthroplasty in Paget's disease of the hip: a report of 5 cases with 5-year follow-up. *Journal of Arthroplasty* 1999;**14**:872–6.
◆95. Tolar J, Teitelbaum SL, Orchard PJ. Osteopetrosis. *New England Journal of Medicine* 2004;**351**:2839–49.
96. Cameron HU, Dewar FP. Degenerative osteoarthritis associated with osteopetrosis. *Clinical Orthopaedics and Related Research* 1977;**127**:148–9.
97. Strickland JP, Berry DJ. Total joint arthroplasty in patients with osteopetrosis: a report of 5 cases and review of the literature. *Journal of Arthroplasty* 2005;**20**:815–20.
◆98. Shapiro F. Osteopetrosis. Current clinical considerations. *Clinical Orthopaedics and Related Research* 1993;**294**:34–44.
99. Casden AM, Jaffe FF, Kastenbaum DM, Bonar SF. Osteoarthritis associated with osteopetrosis treated by total knee arthroplasty. Report of a case. *Clinical Orthopaedics and Related Research* 1989;**247**:202–7.
◆100. Landa J, Margolis N, Di Cesare P. Orthopaedic management of the patient with osteopetrosis. *Journal of the American Academy of Orthopaedic Surgeons* 2007;**15**:654–62.
101. Gwynne Jones DP, Hodgson BF, Hung NA. Bilateral, uncemented total hip arthroplasty in osteopetrosis. *Journal of Bone and Joint Surgery (British)* 2004;**86**:276–8.
102. Matsuno T, Katayama N. Osteopetrosis and total hip arthroplasty. Report of two cases. *International Orthopaedics* 1997;**21**:409–11.
103. Egawa H, Nakano S, Hamada D, et al. Total hip arthroplasty in osteopetrosis using computer-assisted fluoroscopic navigation. *Journal of Arthroplasty* 2005;**20**:1074–7.

98

Primary total hip arthroplasty

RAMANKUTTY SREEKUMAR, PETER R KAY

Introduction	1135	Uncemented total hip replacement	1140
Indications	1135	Outcome	1142
Pre-operative assessment	1136	Trends in arthroplasty	1143
Surgical planning	1136	Functional outcome studies	1143
Surgical approaches	1136	References	1144
Cemented total hip replacement	1138		

NATIONAL BOARD STANDARDS

- Learn the indications, assessment and planning for total hip replacement
- Know the main surgical approaches
- Know that cemented total hip replacement is the gold standard
- Understand the importance of cementing techniques
- Know about osteolysis
- Learn about the National Joint Registry
- Know the NICE guidelines for THR

INTRODUCTION

Primary hip replacement is one of the most successful operations in orthopaedics. Although there were numerous previous attempts at carrying out hip replacements, it was the pioneering work of Sir John Charnley that laid the foundations for hip replacement surgery. There are numerous publications from Wroblewski and colleagues[1] outlining the technique and long-term results of the procedure. With increasing popularity and long-term survival of patients, attempts to improve on the work of the initial designs have led to a plethora of designs and techniques.

INDICATIONS

Total hip replacement (THR) is indicated in end-stage arthritis of the hip from any cause. Although initially offered for primary osteoarthritis, other conditions such as rheumatoid arthritis, secondary osteoarthritis due to trauma, avascular necrosis (AVN), developmental dysplasia (DDH) and slipped capital femoral epiphysis (SCFE) are now common indications for the procedure. In patients with idiopathic AVN, there are a multitude of surgical techniques which attempt to retain the femoral head, although the evidence for many of these is inconclusive.[2] Eventually, many of these patients progress to end-stage arthritis and require total hip arthroplasty. In DDH, the proximal femur and the acetabulum are often both abnormal and, therefore, the anatomy must be carefully considered.[3] Other indications include ankylosing spondylitis, fused hips, displaced intracapsular fracture of the neck of the femur and less common inflammatory arthropathies. The indications for THR have evolved over the years, from being offered only for pain relief in the later years of life to being offered for quality of life improvement in ever younger patients.

The technical aim of all hip replacement surgery should be to restore the hip biomechanics, including centre of rotation, to achieve good fixation of implants and to create a stable joint.

PRE-OPERATIVE ASSESSMENT

The key to achieving a successful outcome involves detailed pre-operative planning. This involves assessment of the patient's symptoms, confirmation of the diagnosis, and assessment of the ability of the patient to withstand a major operative procedure and comply with the postoperative regimen that is required. The standard investigations include an anteroposterior radiograph of the pelvis centred on the pubic symphysis. In cases of abnormal pathology of the femur, a cross-table lateral radiograph of the hip will be required.

Pain is the predominant symptom for which patients seek treatment. The pain is usually localized to the groin or upper thigh. Gluteal pain is often spinal in origin. Most patients with spinal pathology will describe the pain as radicular in nature. Pain from the hip is usually dull and aching but can be sharp. It is typically exacerbated by exercise. Care must be taken to rule out other causes of groin pain such as hernia or intrapelvic pathology. On occasions, patients with hip pathology will present with knee pain. Reproduction of pain with hip movements is helpful in clarifying the cause of pain. In addition, an intra-articular injection of local anaesthetic will often help to localize the site of pathology. Other causes of hip pain, including psoas tendinitis and trochanteric bursitis, must also be considered.

SURGICAL PLANNING

Standard radiographs are performed to confirm the diagnosis and evaluate the extent of the degeneration. The radiographs should be performed with the patient supine and the lower limbs internally rotated 15°. In cases of significant femoral deformity either long leg films of both lower limbs or a CT scanogram should be obtained. Templating is recommended in all hip arthroplasty and can be undertaken with traditional templating sheets or with digital templating software[4,5] (Fig. 98.1). It is important that the templating radiographs are taken with the hips in 15° of internal rotation in order to neutralize the femoral anteversion. Templating with malrotated limbs will cause inaccuracies in offset estimation. In cases of severe deformity, templating the contralateral hip can be helpful. In patients with previous acetabular fractures, Judet views may be helpful.

Consideration should be given to the internal shape of the femur. Dossick et al.[6] classified femurs based on the calcar canal ratio. The ratio of the outer diameter of the femur at the midportion of the lesser trochanter to the diameter at a point 10 cm distal is measured. If the ratio is less than 0.5, it is classified as type A; if it is over 0.75, it is classified as type C; those that fall between these figures are type B. Based on this, some authors advocate uncemented hips for type A femurs, cemented for type C femurs and either for type B.

Femoral bone stock can also be evaluated using the Dorr classification[7] of A, champagne flute shape; B, funnel shape; and C, cylindrical. A and B type femurs are often seen in younger patients and may best be treated by an uncemented stem, whereas cylindrical type C femurs are most often seen in the elderly and may be more appropriately treated with a cemented stem.

SURGICAL APPROACHES

A good surgical approach must provide sufficient exposure and facilitate orientation so that the procedure can be properly performed. McFarland and Osborne[8] classified approaches based on division or not of the tendon of the gluteus medius and the direction of approach: either anterior or posterior. When old scars exist around the hip, they should be incorporated as far as possible. However, adequate exposure is paramount and if an existing incision must be crossed then is it normally safe to do so.

Anterior approaches expose the hip through the sartorius–tensor fascia lata interval. These approaches provide limited exposure unless the gluteus medius is released or trochanteric osteotomy is performed.

Anterolateral approaches use the interval between the tensor fascia lata and gluteus medius. The anterior portion of the gluteus tendon is released to improve exposure.

Posterior approaches split the gluteus maximus in line with its fibres. The short external rotators are transected at their insertion and the capsule is divided along with them to expose the hip.

Anterior approach

This approach is truly internervous and is the most physiological approach. This approach gives good exposure of the acetabulum while retaining the abductor mechanism.[9]

The patient is positioned in a supine position with a sandbag under the sacrum. An incision is made from the anterior superior iliac spine (ASIS) to the tip of the greater

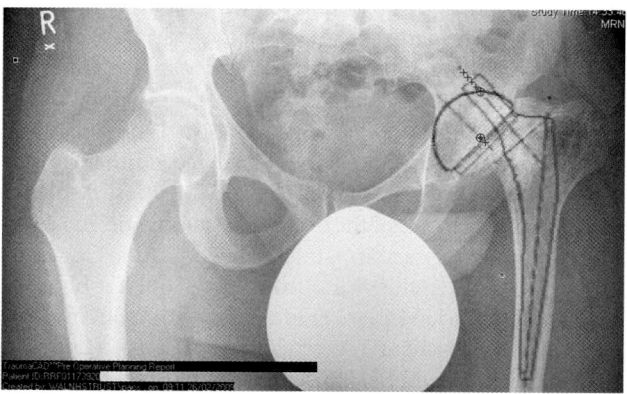

Figure 98.1 Anteroposterior pelvis radiograph showing digital templating with overlay of the planned implants.

trochanter. The tensor fascia lata is split longitudinally along the line of the fibres. The rectus femoris and sartorius are retracted anteriorly and the fascia lata is retracted posteriorly. The ascending branch of the lateral circumflex femoral artery is ligated. The anterior capsule is excised and the hip is exposed.

Anterolateral approach

This approach has been described by many authors but is usually described as the Watson Jones approach. This gives access to the anterior femoral neck and acetabulum. It is the approach of choice in patients who have scarring which prevents lateral or posterior approaches. It is useful in patients with spastic conditions such as Parkinson's disease, in which dislocation is a potential complication.[10]

Judging the position of the acetabulum is easier in this approach. It is also useful in the elderly as the patient is positioned supine. It may be difficult to perform in the obese and extension is difficult. The incision begins 2 cm posterior to the ASIS and curves distally to just posterior to the greater trochanter and then passes down the thigh parallel to the femur. The fascia lata is incised along the posterior border of the trochanter. After clearing the fatty tissue, the interval between the gluteus medius and the tensor fascia lata is developed. Small vessels are cauterized. The dissection should not be extended too proximally to avoid damaging the superior gluteal nerve. The gluteus minimus tendon is divided and the anterior part of the gluteus medius is released. The rectus femoris tendon is elevated and the capsule is exposed. A retractor is placed deep to the psoas tendon against the inferior acetabular margin. The capsule is then incised, exposing the femoral head. It is usually difficult to dislocate the hip in this approach and the neck is divided *in situ* and then delivered.

Posterior approach

This remains one of the most popular approaches for primary and revision hip surgery. Initially described by Von Langenback[11] and Kocher,[12] this was modified by many authors, including by Austin Moore[13] as the 'Southern approach'.

This approach involves dissection in internervous planes and preserves abductor musculature. It is extensile and can be used with extended trochanteric osteotomy for major revisions. One of the major concerns in this approach is the incidence of dislocation. With increasing numbers of surgeons carrying out repair of the soft tissues and capsule of the posterior aspect, the incidence of dislocation has reduced.[14,15]

The patient is positioned in the lateral decubitus position. The knee is kept flexed to reduce tension on the sciatic nerve. The incision is centred posterior to the prominence of the trochanter extending proximally in a curved fashion for about 8 cm. Distally it is extended for 8 cm. Increasingly, smaller incisions are utilized but the use of minimal incisions should not be at the expense of adequate visualization of the hip. The fascia lata is then incised along the length of the incision. Proximally, the gluteus maximus fibres are split along their length. The sciatic nerve is identified in the depth of the incision. The fat overlying the external rotators is cleared off by blunt dissection. Stay sutures are passed through the tendons of the piriformis, gemelli and obturator internus and they are divided close to their attachments to the trochanter. They are then retracted posteriorly, which further protects the sciatic nerve. Depending on the exposure needed, the quadratus femoris may be divided in part or in full. At the superior margin of the quadratus, branches of the medial circumflex femoral artery are seen and ligated. Rarely, the tendon of the gluteus maximus into the femur will need to be divided. The capsule is incised along the neck and the hip is dislocated by flexion, internal rotation and adduction. Closure will require careful reattachment of the stay sutures coupled with repair of the capsule.

Transtrochanteric

This approach, which was pioneered by Sir John Charnley, provides an excellent exposure of the hip joint (Fig. 98.2). It is useful in difficult primary hip replacements such as severe dysplasia and previous hip fusion. Trochanteric advancement when reattaching improves hip biomechanics and in the era of monoblock stems it provided an excellent

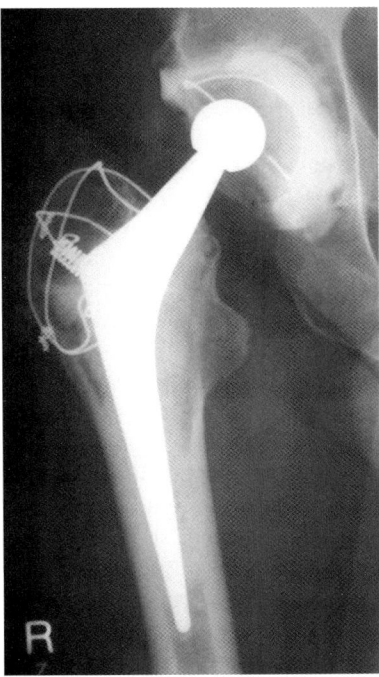

Figure 98.2 Postoperative anteroposterior pelvis radiograph showing total hip replacement performed through a trochanteric osteotomy.

method of restoring soft-tissue tension around the hip.[16] In spite of being the approach which perhaps provides the best exposure, non-union of the osteotomy has limited the use of this technique. The incidence varies between 3% and 20%. There are studies that indicate that it is the extent of the displacement of the trochanter rather than the non-union which causes a poorer outcome.

The patient is usually positioned supine, even though it can be done with the patient in the lateral position. The incision is a straight one centred on the greater trochanter and extending proximally for about 6 cm and distally for about 8 cm. The fascia lata is divided in line with the skin incision. The anterior capsule is exposed in the interval between the fascia lata and the gluteus medius. A curved forceps is passed from the anterior edge of the gluteus medius to its posterior edge and a Gigli saw is passed from back to front using the forceps. The origin of the vastus lateralis is reflected distally for a short distance. A pin is passed from the lateral aspect of the femur to the superior neck. This helps create a chevron shape when the Gigli saw is pulled distally when performing the osteotomy. The trochanter with the attached glutei is freed of capsular attachments and retracted proximally. The capsule is then opened in a T fashion and dislocation is carried out by flexion, adduction and external rotation. Reattaching the trochanter is with wires or cables.

Transgluteal (Hardinge)

This approach is a modification of an earlier approach described by McFarland and Osborne.[17] It provides a good exposure of the acetabulum and the proximal femur and still remains the most commonly used approach for primary hip replacement. The major problem with this approach appears to be a limp as a result of weak abductors. The dislocation rate is claimed to be much lower than in posterior approaches.

The patient can be positioned supine or lateral. A midlateral incision is made from the level of the ASIS to about 6 cm below the trochanter. The fascia lata is incised along the line of the incision. The gluteus medius insertion into the greater trochanter is identified and the fibres are split beginning in the middle of the trochanter. Distally this is carried down to the bone and carried slightly anteriorly and continued distally into the vastus lateralis for about 6 cm. The anterior fibres of the gluteus, the fascia of the vastus lateralis and the periosteum of the trochanter are elevated as a single layer using a sharp chisel and displaced forward. It is important not to go more than 3 cm above the upper border of the trochanter to avoid damage to the superior gluteal nerve. The tendon of the gluteus minimus is divided and the capsule of the hip is exposed and incised facilitating dislocation of the hip.

The National Joint Registry Report from England and Wales[18] shows that 46% of primary THRs carried out in the UK are still cemented, 30% are uncemented, 10% are resurfacings and 14% are hybrids. The trend over the past few years, however, indicates that more uncemented hips are being done. The report also shows that 88% of patients are operated in the lateral position. A total of 46% of patients have a posterior approach and 37% have a Hardinge approach; 16% of operations are anterolateral and only 3% of patients underwent a trochanteric osteotomy. Also, 69% of stems and 47% of cups are cemented, which are both less than in previous years.

CEMENTED TOTAL HIP REPLACEMENT

Design principles: stems

Cemented hip replacements remain the gold standard in hip arthroplasty. There are two major design philosophies[19] with regard to the stem. These are the composite beam and taper slip designs. The Charnley hip is an example of a composite beam (Fig. 98.3) and the Exeter and C-Stem (Fig. 98.4) designs are examples of the latter. Long-term follow-up of composite beam stems showed evidence of proximal femoral stress shielding, which was meant to be addressed by the taper slip designs.[20] In the taper slip designs, the stem is permitted to subside and becomes wedged in the cement mantle during loading, reducing proximal and distal pressures in the cement mantle. Radial compressive forces are transferred from the proximal cement mantle to the bone as hoop stresses. In the taper slip pattern, a void centralizer is used to allow for subsidence. The Wrightington School tend to use a bone block into which the stem of the implant is transfixed.[21] This is suggested to help in subsidence and also improve the long-term results. In the composite beam concept, the stem has to be rigidly held in the cement mantle. Subsidence will cause

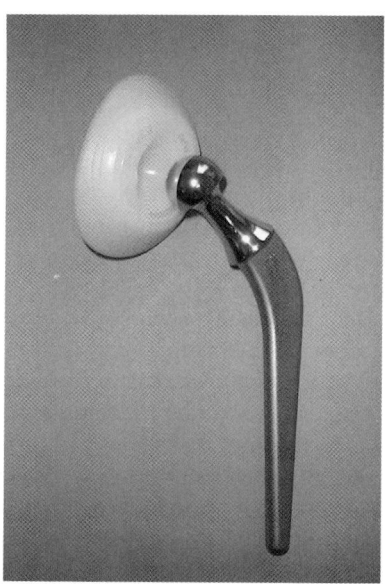

Figure 98.3 A Charnley stem with an all-polyethylene cemented socket. Note the roughened finish of the stem.

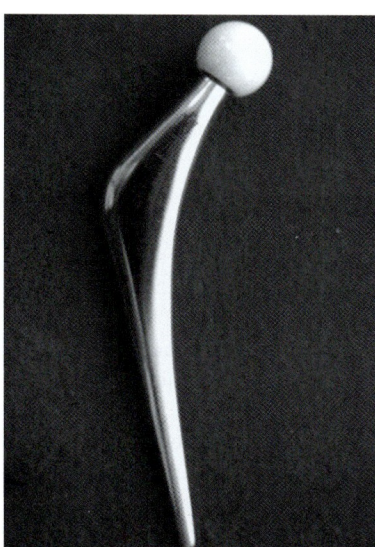

Figure 98.4 A C-stem femoral component. Note that the modular design allows use of a ceramic head, as pictured.

damage to the cement mantle with the generation of metal and cement debris. It is therefore important to avoid any voids distally while cementing. Taper slip designs tend to subside both axially and into retroversion in the first year, after which they tend to stabilize. Stems with the composite beam design tend to have greater stability initially.

A polished surface finish is the preferred choice in taper slip stems since this is less likely to generate metal debris with subsidence. A rough surface finish is desirable for composite beam stems to improve initial stability.

The use of a collar, which is a feature of a composite beam stem, is another controversial design issue.[22,23] Collars are claimed to reduce tensile stresses in the stem and transmit loads across the proximal femur. This is debatable as it is difficult to achieve an intimate fit between the collar and bone at the time of surgery. A collar could, however, prevent stem subsidence during loading, but does not appear to prevent micromotion. Resorption of bone at the calcar also decreases the intimate bone contact. Advocates of taper slip designs claim that the stem slips into a more stable design in the absence of a collar. A collar is only considered in situations in which a composite beam stem is undersized in relation to the broach. Studies, however, have not shown any advantage in survival with or without a collar. Crowninshield et al.,[24] in a detailed study of femoral stems, suggested that the ideal shape had a cross-sectional geometry that provides torsional stability within the cement mantle while avoiding sharp corners in areas that can cause cement fractures. Most of the current designs of cemented stems are made of cobalt chrome. Titanium is more biocompatible; however, it is soft and not scratch resistant, which increases wear. The finish of the stem also determines the long-term outcome. Rough surface stems debond less frequently than smooth finished ones, but, when they do, they cause marked osteolysis and clinical failure. Smooth surface stems debond more often but they cause less osteolysis and mechanical stability is maintained. Smooth taper slip stems are also said to cause increased hoop stresses in the proximal femur. Modular stems allow the use of multiple head sizes from 22 mm to 36 mm or even greater. Ceramic heads may provide improved wear characteristics over metal, although this has still not been proven.[25] Also, owing to the brittle nature of the material, they are prone to fractures. Modularity has the disadvantage of causing added wear debris.

Modifications of implants with a view to further improve the long-term results have not uniformly been successful.[26] An example is the Capital hip. This was marketed by 3M as similar to the Charnley-designed prosthesis. Unfortunately, following reports of very high failure rates, it was taken off the market. The surface roughness of the Capital hip was higher than that of the Charnley. Also, it incorporated four different designs. The hip was made of two different prosthetic geometries – round back and flanged – and they were designed to be made of steel or titanium. Of all the four designs, the stainless steel round-back stem, which was most similar to the Charnley, failed the least. Unfortunately, this was the stem that was distributed in least numbers.

Design principles: sockets

Cemented all-polyethylene sockets have been widely in use in primary hip arthroplasty with good long-term results (Fig. 98.3). In the USA, owing to loosening observed in cemented sockets at long-term follow-up, they are used only in elderly patients.[27] Failure patterns in cemented sockets can be decreased with increasing thickness of the sockets, increasing the cement mantle to the optimum of 3–5 mm. The greatest improvement in the long-term survival of cemented all-polyethylene sockets occurred as a result of cementation technique rather than design change. However, a change from first- to second-generation cementation techniques has resulted in far better results for the femoral component than for the socket.[28,29] Head size is not an important determinant as long as an 8 mm thickness of the polyethylene is realized at surgery. When cementing a cup in the acetabulum, it is important to retain the subchondral bone as it is better suited to handle stresses than cancellous bone. Oonishi[30] has indicated that, in addition to retaining the subchondral bone, the line of weight transmission should be directed posteriorly and superiorly. Metal-backed sockets were designed to reduce the stresses in polymethylmethacrylate (PMMA) and, although in theory they were effective, this advantage was not observed in clinical practice, with a few studies demonstrating disastrous results.[31,32] PMMA cement performs best under compressive loads and performs poorly under tension. All efforts to improve cement techniques have aimed at porosity reduction. Vacuum mixing and centrifugation[33] have both been shown to improve the consistency of cement. Of all the cement varieties commercially available, Simplex P outperforms others in fatigue

Table 98.1 Cementation of prosthesis: generation techniques

Generation	Mixing/porosity reduction	Canal preparation	Insertion	Centralization
First	Hand mix	Rasp only	Manual with finger packing	None
Second	Hand mix	Aggressive rasp, brushing, lavage	Cement gun, distal plug	Early distal centralizers
Third	Vacuum mix/centrifuge	Aggressive rasp, brushing, lavage	Cement gun with pressurization Distal plug	Proximal and distal centralizers

testing. Chilling of the monomer has a deleterious effect, which is overcome by porosity reduction. Miller and Stephenson[34] suggested the concept of a macro- and micro-interlock in cementing the prosthesis. Low-viscosity cement has better penetration than high-viscosity cement. PMMA penetration is a decreased function of the bone strength, with ultimate failure load capacity being a balance between bone porosity and strength of cancellous bone.

Technique

Bone preparation is vital in the performance of a cemented hip replacement (Table 98.1). Preparing a clean stable bony bed for cement integration is important in the longevity of the implant. This involves removing all loose cancellous bone but retaining the denser bone near the cortex to enhance interdigitation. Removing the calcar is an important part of the bony bed preparation, and studies by Wroblewski et al.[35] suggest less incidence of loosening in a medium-term study. Leaving only cortical bone would leave a smooth surface into which cement integration would be impossible. The aim is to achieve a 3–4 mm cement mantle around the implants.[36] This is usually achieved in the femur with specifically designed broaches. In the femur, distal plugging of the canal allows pressurization, which creates a uniform cement column. Lavaging the canal prior to pressurization removes all loose pieces of bone and fat.[37,38] Breusch has demonstrated improved cement impregnation following pulsed lavage. The bone bed should be dry, which can be facilitated by hypotensive anaesthesia, frequent cleaning and also hydrogen peroxide lavage.[39]

Centralizing the implant in the canal has been shown to increase the likelihood of long-term survival. There are commercially available centralizers that can help with the placement of the implant. There are many types of cement available, differing in viscosity, porosity and curing time. The ideal time for introduction of cement is when it is doughy and dull in appearance. Cement guns are valuable in introducing cement under pressurization, but will require the less viscous cements to be used.

On the acetabular side, the principles are largely the same in terms of preparation and cementation. The acetabulum is cleared of osteophytes and the labrum is excised in full. Circumferential reaming is done to expose bleeding cancellous bone in both the anterior and posterior column. Multiple fixation holes are made in the superior half of the acetabulum to permit cement interdigitation. Larger anchoring holes can also made in the pubis and the ischium. Any cysts should be cleared and the edges completely curetted out. Pulsed lavage can be used to clear the cavity prior to cementation. Cement is then introduced when in a doughy phase, pressurized and then the socket cemented in.

Assessment of the cement mantle is done radiographically both in the anteroposterior and lateral planes using Gruen zones[40] (Fig. 98.5). These zones are inspected to identify osteolysis, radiolucent lines and fractures of the cement mantle. On the acetabular side, similar assessment is done using the Charnley–De Lee zones (Fig. 98.6).

UNCEMENTED TOTAL HIP REPLACEMENT

Design principles: stem

To avoid the presumed complications of cement in the form of osteolysis affecting long-term results, uncemented hips, which aim to anchor the prosthesis to the parent bone and encourage host bone ingrowth, have been in use for some time now. Extensively porous-coated stems such as the anatomic medullary locking (AML) hip remain the most extensively used and studied cementless stems.[41,42] The initial stems were made of cobalt chrome with layers of sintered cobalt beads. Current designs are made of cobalt chromium, titanium or other composites. Many different surface finishes and treatments are also available (Figs 98.7 and 98.8). Subsequent uncemented designs have been proximal ingrowth stems that are either tapered stems or cylindrical stems. Bone ingrowth into porous-coated implant is dependent on the stability between implant and bone, contact area and pore size.[43] Gaps of over 2 mm between the implant and bone result in less bone ingrowth. Optimal fixation is achieved with gaps of less than 0.5 mm. Optimal pore sizes for fixation have been noted in several studies to be between 50 and 400 μm.[44]

Design principles: socket

Uncemented sockets have been advocated as being an easier alternative to cemented cups. In the presence of misshapen acetabula, there exists the option to orient modular liners

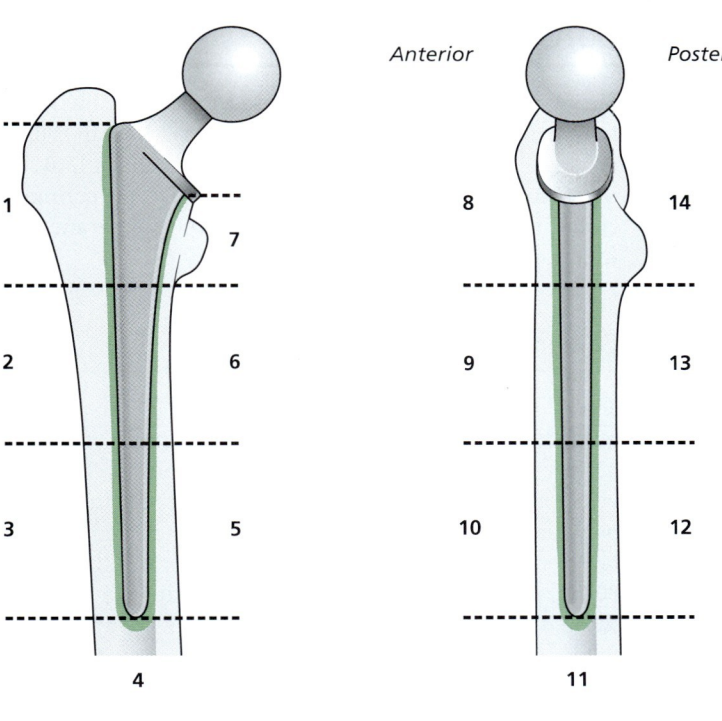

Figure 98.5 The Gruen zones around the femoral stem that are used to document radiolucent lines at the cement–bone interface.

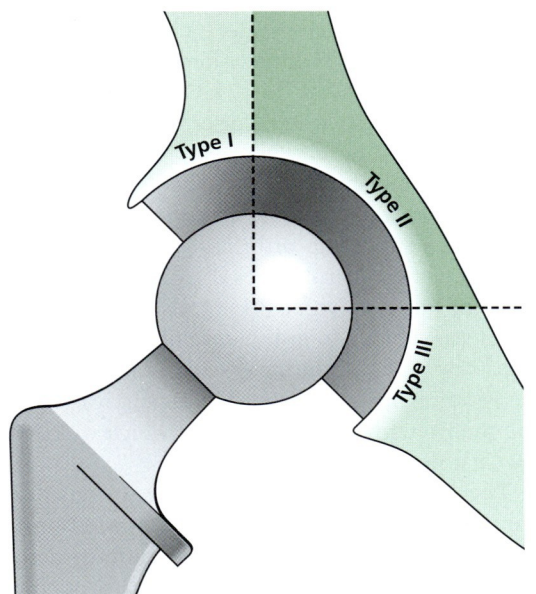

Figure 98.6 The Charnley–DeLee zone around the acetabular component which are used to document radiolucent lines at the cement–bone interface.

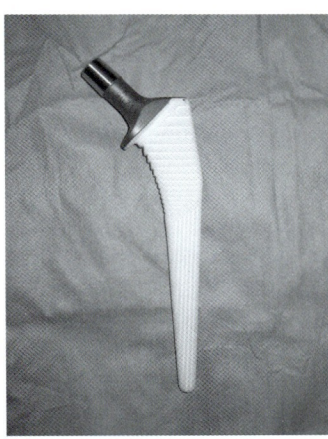

Figure 98.7 A Corail stem demonstrating the thick (150 μm) hydroxyapatite coating.

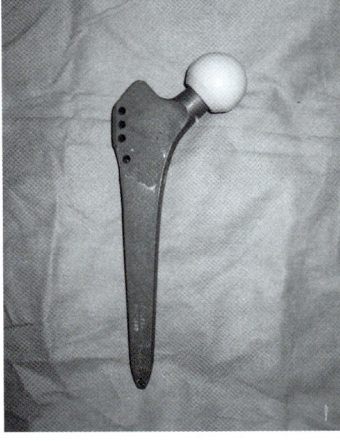

Figure 98.8 A 'Zweymuller'-type stem showing the rectangular cross-section and the roughened surface.

within the shells to introduce stability. There are a few basic designs for uncemented THR: threaded acetabular shell; hemispheric designs; transfixing screws; and a combination of the above. Hemispheric designs appear to be the most commonly used, with additional screws as required. More than three screws have not proved to be beneficial. Also there are concerns about cold flow and polyethylene-laden fluid pumping the pathway of the screws. This increases the effective joint space.[45,46] Most non-cemented implants currently in use are made of titanium, cobalt chromium or tantalum.

Technique

Femoral preparation involves femoral reaming to create a press-fit for the implant, achieving good initial stability. Reaming is done after creating an initial pilot hole in the piriform fossa and reaming straight distally as most porous-coated stems are straight stems. In younger patients, it is important to remove the hard bone at the lateral edge of the piriformis fossa as this could direct the reamers medially and cause fractures when an attempt is made to get the best fit in the canal. Regular washing is done to remove the reamed debris and also to cool the bone. Reaming should be carried out according to the prescribed size for the particular prosthesis. Usually, most commonly used systems advise under-reaming by about 0.5 mm. If required, depending on the implant shape, metaphyseal broaching may be required to accommodate a wider metaphyseal shape. Trial reduction is then done with the trial implants, and length, offset, soft-tissue tension and stability are checked before seating the definitive prosthesis. Care must be taken during impacting the stem to prevent any injury to the femoral shaft.

Prior to preparation of the acetabulum, all osteophytes and the labrum must be removed, as in the case of cemented acetabula. The true floor of the acetabulum is identified, removing any floor osteophytes if required, and then reaming of the socket is done with increasing diameter reamers. After subchondral bone is exposed and bleeding bone is seen, reaming is stopped and cysts, if any, are cleared. As in the case of the femur, under-reaming by about 1–2 mm provides good fixation. If this does not appear to be the case, additional screw fixation can be done. The liner is then oriented and any modifications can be done at this stage.

The advantages and disadvantages of cemented and uncemented arthroplasty are given in Table 98.2.

Table 98.2 The advantages and disadvantages of cemented and uncemented arthroplasty

Cemented	Uncemented
+Instant fixation	+Active fixation
+Good results with modern bearings	+Good results with modern bearings
+Control of implant position	+Choice of acetabular bearing
+Can use with antibiotics	+?Ease of use
+Use with bone grafting	+Quicker to perform
+Low fracture rate	+Low stress shielding femur
+?Easier to remove	−Fracture of femur
−?Technically demanding	−Difficult to control version of stem
−Cement wear	−Difficult to remove
−Difficult to train	−Stress shielding acetabulum

OUTCOME

Survivorship analysis is widely used to look at the long-term results of replacement arthroplasty. Kaplan–Meier analysis[47] is the most widely used method and it looks at the failure independent of time interval. The common endpoints used are revision, radiographic failure and low functional scores.

Cemented hips

Most long-term data of over 20 years of follow-up have been of the Charnley cemented stem. Berry et al.[48] in a 25 year follow-up of 2000 Charnley hips showed 82% survival for revision in patients below 40 years; 83% in patients between 40 and 49; 86% in patients between 50 and 59; 93% between 60 and 65; 97% between 70 and 75; and 100% over 80 years. Long-term results from Wrightington Hospital showed a clinical success rate of over 93.9% at a mean follow-up of 22 years. The authors also reported that the main long-term problem was the wear and loosening of the ultra-high-molecular-weight polyethylene socket. Reviewing their results in patients under 51 years, the same authors showed survivorship with revision as the endpoint as 93.7% at 10 years; 84.7% at 15; 74.3% at 20; and 55.3% at 27 years.[49,50] Sochart and Porter,[51] in a review of young patients with Charnley total hip arthroplasty, found a 25 year survivorship in 89% patients with hip dysplasia, 85% in those with rheumatoid arthritis, and 74% in those with degenerative hip arthritis.[51] Neumann et al.,[52] in a follow-up of 92 Charnley hips at 15–20 years, showed a 95% score for function with a 8.1% revision rate. They claimed that it was difficult to justify uncemented hip replacements with these results.[52] In the Swedish Arthroplasty Register, the Spectron hip had a better 10 year survival rate of 98.4%, and the Exeter had 94.1%, both of which were better than the Charnley and Stanmore at 92%.[53]

The results of all-polyethylene sockets have been impressive. There has been much confusion in the literature, but this is mainly due to variations in design, technique and definitions of failure. Wear rates of polyethylene sockets with metal heads have been shown to be 0.075 mm per year. Survivorship studies have also shown excellent long-term results. Wroblewski et al.[54] reported on the angle bore socket in association with a 22.225 mm head as showing a high level of success in preventing dislocations in revision hip replacements.

Uncemented hips

Reports have appeared in the literature showing 97% survival of the cementless AML stem at 12 years. However, 9% of these patients have pain-limiting activity.[55] The Porous-Coated Anatomic (PCA) hip was a cobalt chrome proximally coated stem with a good long-term survival.[56]

However, concerns with thigh pain led to many modifications of the designs. McLaughlin et al.[57] reported on 145 Taperloc prostheses with a 22 year follow-up showing a survivorship of 87%. The Corail stem, which has proved to be one of the most successful uncemented stems in terms of long-term follow-up, relies on a different technique of fixation. The stem is designed to preserve bone and achieves primary mechanical stability through compaction of cancellous bone rather than bone removal in 'fit and fill' type prostheses. It is fully coated with hydroxyapatite, which allows secondary biological integration. It has excellent survivorship, with the Norwegian register quoting over 95% at 15 years or more.[58,59] In a single-centre series, the stem has shown a 99.7% survivorship in 291 stems at a mean follow-up of 10 years.[60] In 2007, an independent analysis of the designing surgeons' results showed a 100% survival at minimum 10 years.[61] The implant now has good 25 year results reported.

Clohisy and Harris[62] reported on porous-coated acetabular components with screw fixation with an average 10 year follow-up and commented that the results were equal to or better than a cemented socket.[63] One hundred per cent survivorship has been documented with a press-fit porous-coated cup (Duraloc) in 100 patients at 10 years.[58]

Morshed et al.[64] carried out a meta-analysis comparing cemented and uncemented fixation in hip replacement. They found 20 studies (reporting 24 comparisons) that met their inclusion criteria. They found no significant benefit for either fixation method among subgroups defined by study setting (registry or multicenter vs single centre), study design (randomized vs non-randomized) or failure definition (type A (either component or both) vs type B (specific component failure)). The authors concluded that the published evidence suggests that cemented fixation still has superior survival among large subgroups studied and also that the results of uncemented fixation continue to improve. They also suggest that further research and improved methods of conducting the same are important to demonstrate relative benefits.

TRENDS IN ARTHROPLASTY

The Swedish Hip Registry shows that the Lubinus SP, Charnley and the Exeter are the three most common cemented hip replacements. The CLS, Allofit and Spotorno were the three most common uncemented. Generally, the universal trend towards uncemented hip replacements is mirrored in the register. Women outnumber men by 60% to 40%. The age at surgery also appears to be decreasing. The Norwegian Hip Registry[65] shows that there has been a slight fall in the cemented hip replacements, with a corresponding increase in hybrid replacements. There is no obvious increase in the use of uncemented hips, which have remained at about 8–10%. The Charnley, Exeter and the Titan remain the most common cemented hip replacements whereas the Corail remains the predominant uncemented stem.

FUNCTIONAL OUTCOME STUDIES

There are numerous scoring systems that look at the clinical results of total hip arthroplasty. Most of these do not look at the general function and the satisfaction of the patient. The scores from these are not comparable. The Charnley modification[66] of the Merle d'Aubigné score and the Harris hip score include assessment by both the surgeon and the patient. The Charnley modification scores pain, movements and walking on a scale of 0–6. The scores are not combined to create a total score. The Harris score[67] awards 0–44 points for pain, 0–47 for function, 0–5 for range of motion and 0–4 for absence of deformity, giving a total out of 100.

Patient-based assessment usually relates to:

1. Health-related quality of life analysis using the Short Form (SF)-36. The patients give their response to 36 questions about their physical functions, social functions and their mental health with no physician input. This has also been modified to a 12-item questionnaire (SF-12).[68]
2. Joint-specific assessment such at the Oxford Hip Score. The Oxford Hip Score[69] is a 12-item questionnaire for patients that was developed from patient interviews. It is validated, practical and useful in a clinical setting.
3. There are numerous studies looking at patient satisfaction after THR. These show that approximately 90% of patients are happy after a primary hip replacement.

KEY LEARNING POINTS

- Total hip replacement is indicated in end-stage arthritis of the hip and has been one of the most successful surgical interventions in orthopaedic surgery.
- Detailed pre-operative assessment and planning are mandatory for successful outcomes.
- Among the many approaches to the hip, the posterior and the anterolateral remain the most commonly used.
- Cemented hip replacements remain the gold standard in primary hip arthroplasty, with the Charnley, Exeter and Stanmore prostheses showing very good outcomes in long-term studies.
- Improvements in cementing techniques have further improved long-term outcomes.
- Osteolysis remains one of the problems affecting long-term outcome, but is also observed in uncemented hips.
- Among the many techniques to obtain uncemented fixation, recent results show good long-term outcomes with the hydroxyapatite-coated stems, i.e. Corail.
- Recent reports of the National Joint Registry continue to show better results for cemented hip arthroplasty over uncemented.

REFERENCES

● = Key primary paper
◆ = Major review article

●1. Wroblewski BM, Siney PD. Charnley low friction arthroplasty of the hip: long term results. *Clinical Orthopaedics and Related Research* 1993;**292**:191–201.
2. Urbaniak JR, Coogan PG, Gunneson EB, *et al.* Treatment of osteonecrosis of the femoral head with free vascularised fibular grafting: long term follow up study of one hundred and three hips. *Journal of Bone and Joint Surgery (American)* 1995;**77A**:681–94.
3. Trousdale RT, Ekkernkamp A, Ganz R, *et al.* Periacetabular and intertrochanteric osteotomy for the treatment of osteoarthrosis in dysplastic hips. *Journal of Bone and Joint Surgery (American)* 1995;**77A**:73–85.
◆4. D'Antonio JA. Preoperative templating and choosing implant for primary total hip arthroplasty in the young patient. *Instructional Course Lectures* 1994;**43**:339–46.
5. Whiddon DR, Bono JV. Digital templating in total hip arthroplasty. *Instructional Course Lectures* 2008;**57**:273–9.
6. Dossick PH, Dorr LD, Gruen T, Saberi MT. Techniques for preoperative planning and postoperative evaluation of non cemented hip arthroplasty. *Techniques in Orthopaedics* 1991;**6**(3):1–6.
●7. Dorr LD, Faugere MC, Mackel AM. Structural and cellular assessment of bone quality of proximal femur. *Bone* 1993;**3**:231–42.
8. McFarland B, Osborne G. Approach to the hip. A suggested improvement on Kocher's method. *Journal of Bone and Joint Surgery (British)* 1954;**36B**:364.
9. Light TR, Keggi KJ. Anterior approach to hip arthroplasty. *Clinical Orthopaedics and Related Research* 1980;**152**:55–60.
10. Watson Jones R. Fracture of the neck of the femur. *British Journal of Surgery* 1935;**23**:787.
11. Von Langenbeck B. Uber die Schussverletzungen des Huffgelenks. *Langenbecks Archiv für klinische Chirurgie* 1874;**16**:263.
12. Kocher T. *Textbook of Operative Surgery*, 3rd edn. London, UK: Adam & Charles Black, 1911.
13. Moore AT. The Moore self-locking vitallium prosthesis in fresh femoral neck fractures: a new low posterior approach (the Southern exposure). *Instructive Course Lectures* 1959;**16**:309.
●14. Pellicci PM, Bostrom M, Poss R. Posterior approach to total hip replacement using enhanced posterior soft tissue repair. *Clinical Orthopaedics and Related Research* 1998;**355**:224–8.
15. Kwon MS, Kuskowski M, Mulhall KJ, *et al.* Does surgical approach affect total hip arthroplasty dislocation rates? *Clinical Orthopaedics and Related Research* 2006;**447**:34–8.
●16. Charnley J. *Low Friction Arthroplasty*. Berlin, Germany: Springer, 1979.
●17. Hardinge K. The direct lateral approach to the hip. *Journal of Bone and Joint Surgery (British)* 1982;**64B**:17.
18. National Joint Registry for England and Wales. *Annual Report*. Hemel Hempstead, UK: National Joint Registry for England and Wales, 2007.
19. Scheerlink T, Casteleyn PP. The design features of cemented femoral hip implants. *Journal of Bone and Joint Surgery (British)* 2006;**88B**:1409–16.
●20. Wroblewski BM, Siney PD, Fleming PA. Triple taper polished cemented stem in total hip arthroplasty. *Journal of Arthroplasty* 2001;**16**(Suppl. 1):37–41.
●21. Wroblewski BM, Fleming PA, Hall RM, Siney PD. Stem fixation in the Charnley low-friction arthroplasty in young patients using an intramedullary bone block. *Journal of Bone and Joint Surgery (British)* 1998;**80B**:273–8.
22. Harris WH. Is it advantageous to strengthen the cement metal interface and use a collar for cemented femoral components of total hip replacements. *Clinical Orthopaedics and Related Research* 1992;**285**:67.
23. Ling RSM. The use of a collar and precoating on cemented femoral stems is unnecessary and detrimental. *Clinical Orthopaedics and Related Research* 1992;**285**:73.
24. Crowninshield RD, Brand RA, Johnston RC, Pederson DR. An analysis of collar function and the use of titanium in femoral prosthesis. *Clinical Orthopaedics and Related Research* 1981;**158**:220–7.
◆25. Schmalzried TP, Callaghan JJ. Current concepts review: wear in total hip and knee replacements. *Journal of Bone and Joint Surgery (American)* 1999;**81A**:115–36.
26. Massoud SN, Hunter JB, Holdsworth BJ, *et al.* Early femoral loosening in one design of cemented hip replacement. *Journal of Bone and Joint Surgery (British)* 1997;**79B**:603–8.
27. Ranawat CS, Deshmukh RG, Peters LE, Unlas ME. Prediction of the long term durability of all polythene cemented sockets. *Clinical Orthopaedics and Related Research* 1995;**317**:89–105.
◆28. Barrack RL, Mulroy Jr RD, Harris WH. Improved cementing techniques and femoral component loosening in young patients with hip arthroplasty: a 12 year radiographic review. *Journal of Bone and Joint Surgery (British)* 1992;**74B**:385–9.
29. Mulroy Jr RD, Harris WH. The effect of improved cementing techniques on component loosening in total hip replacement: an 11 year radiographic review. *Journal of Bone and Joint Surgery (British)* 1990;**72B**:757–60.
30. Oonishi H. Mechanical analysis of the human pelvis and its application to the artificial hip joint by means of the three dimensional finite element method. *Journal of Biomechanics* 1983;**16**:427.
31. Mattingley DA, Hopson CN, Kahn A, Gaennestras NJ. Aseptic loosening in metal backed acetabular components for total hip replacements. *Journal of Bone and Joint Surgery (American)* 1985;**67A**:387.
32. Ritter MA, Faris PM, Keating EM, Brugo G. Influential factors in cemented acetabular cup loosening. *Journal of Arthroplasty* 1992;**7**(Suppl.):365.

33. Davies JP, Jasty M, O'Connor DO, et al. The effect of centrifuging bone cement. *Journal of Bone and Joint Surgery (British)* 1989;**71B**:39–42.
34. Miller JE, Stephenson PK. Improved fixation in total hip arthroplasty using pressurised low viscosity cement: A radiological analysis. *Orthopaedic Transactions* 1987;**11**:489.
35. Wroblewski BM, Siney PD, Fleming PA, Bobak P. The calcar femorale in cemented stem fixation in total hip arthroplasty. *Journal of Bone and Joint Surgery (British)* 2000;**82B**:842–5.
36. Kwak BM, Lim OK, Kim YY, Rim K. An investigation of the effect of cement thickness on an implant by finite stress analysis. *International Orthopaedics* 1979;**2**:315–19.
37. Breusch S, Malchau H. *The Well Cemented Total Hip Arthroplasty: Theory and Practice*. Heidelberg, Germany: Springer, 2005.
●38. Majkowski RS, Miles AW, Bannister GC, et al. Bone surface preparation in cemented hip replacement. *Journal of Bone and Joint Surgery* 1993;**75**:459–63.
39. Breusch SJ, Namal T, Schneider U, et al. Lavage technique in total hip arthroplasty – jet lavage produces better cement penetration than syringe lavage in proximal femur. *Journal of Arthroplasty* 2000;**159**:21.
●40. Gruen TA, McNeice GM, Amstutz HC. Modes of failure of cemented stem-type femoral components. A radiographic analysis of loosening. *Clinical Orthopaedics and Related Research* 1979;**141**:17–27.
41. Engh CA. Recent advances in cementless hip arthroplasty using the AML prosthesis. *Techniques in Orthopaedics* 1991;**6**:59–72.
42. Engh Jr CA, Culpepper II WJ, Engh CA. Long term results of the anatomic medullary locking prosthesis in total hip arthroplasty. *Journal of Bone and Joint Surgery (American)* 1977;**79A**:177–84.
43. Engh CA, Bobyn JD, Glassman AH. Porous coated hip replacement, factors governing bone ingrowth, stress shielding and clinical results. *Journal of Bone and Joint Surgery (British)* 1987;**69B**:45–55.
44. Bobyn JD, Pilliar RM, Cameron HV, Weatherley GC. The optimum pore size for the fixation of porous surfaced metal implants by the ingrowth of bone. *Clinical Orthopaedics and Related Research* 1980;**150**:253.
45. Berman AT, Avolio A, Delgallo W. Acetabular osteolysis in total hip arthroplasty. Prevention and treatment. *Orthopaedics* 1994;**17**:963.
46. Cooper RA, McAllister CM, Borden LS, Bauer TW. Polyethylene debris induced osteolysis and loosening in uncemented total hip arthroplasty. A case of late failure. *Journal of Arthroplasty* 1992;**7**:285.
47. Kaplan El, Meier P. Nonparametric estimation from incomplete observations. *Journal of the American Statistical Association* 1958;**53**:457–81.
◆48. Berry DJ, Harmsen WS, Cabanela ME, Morrey BF. 25 year survivorship of 2000 consecutive primary Charnley total hip arthroplasties: factors governing acetabular and femoral component survivorship. *Journal of Bone and Joint Surgery (American)* 2002;**84A**:171.
49. Wroblewski BM, Siney PD, Fleming PA. Charnley low frictional torque arthroplasty in patients under the age of 51 years. *Journal of Bone and Joint Surgery (British)* 2002;**84B**:540–3.
◆50. Wroblewski BM, Fleming PA, Siney PD. Charnley low frictional torque arthroplasty of the hip. 20–30 year results. *Journal of Bone and Joint Surgery (British)* 1999;**81B**:427–30.
◆51. Sochart DH, Porter ML. The long term results of Charnley low-friction arthroplasty in young patients who have congenital dislocation, degenerative osteoarthritis or rheumatoid arthritis. *Journal of Bone and Joint Surgery (American)* 1997;**79**:1599–617.
52. Neumann L, Freund KG, Sorenson KH. Long term results of Charnley total hip replacement: review of 92 patients at 15 to 20 years. *Journal of Bone and Joint Surgery (British)* 1994;**76B**:245.
53. Swedish Hip Register 2005. http://www.shpr.se/en/default.aspx (accessed 6/7/2011).
54. Wroblewski BM, Siney PD, Fleming PA. The angle bore acetabular component and dislocation after revision of a failed total hip replacement. *Journal of Bone and Joint Surgery (British)* 2006;**88B**:184–7.
55. McAuley JP, Moore KD, Culpepper WJ, et al. Total hip arthroplasty with porous coated prostheses fixed without cement in patients who are 65 years of age or older. *Journal of Bone and Joint Surgery (American)* 1998;**80A**:1648–55.
56. Little BS, Wixson RL, Stulberg SD. Total hip arthroplasty with the porous-coated anatomic hip prosthesis: results at 11–18 years. *Journal of Arthroplasty* 2006;**21**:338–43.
57. McLaughlin JR, Lee KR, Total hip arthroplasty with uncemented tapered femoral component. *Journal of Bone and Joint Surgery (American)* 2008;**90**:1290–6.
58. American Academy of Orthopaedic Surgeons. *The Norwegian Arthroplasty Register 1987–2004. Prospective Studies of Hip and Knee Prostheses*. Rosemont, IL: AAOS, 2005.
◆59. Vidalain JP. Corail stem long term results based upon 15 years ARTRO group experience. In: Epinette JA, Manley MT (eds) *Fifteen Years Clinical Experience with Hydroxyapatite Coatings in Joint Arthroplasty*. Paris, France: Springer, 2004:217–24.
●60. Reikerås O, Gunderson RB. Excellent results of HA coating on a grit-blasted stem: 245 patients followed for 8–12 years. *Acta Orthopaedica Scandinavica* 2003;**74**:140–5.
●61. Froimson MI, Garino J, Machenaud A, Vidalain JP. Minimum 10-year results of a tapered, titanium, hydroxyapatite-coated hip stem: an independent review. *Journal of Arthroplasty* 2007;**22**:1–7.

62. Clohisy JC, Harris WH. The Harris Galante porous coated acetabular component with screw fixation: average 10 year follow up study. *Journal of Bone and Joint Surgery (American)* 1999;**81A**:66–73.
63. Grobler GP, Learmonth ID, Bernstein BP, Dower BJ. Ten-year results of a press-fit, porous-coated acetabular component. *Journal of Bone and Joint Surgery (British)* 2005;**87**:786–9.
◆64. Morshed S, Bozic KJ, Ries MD, *et al.* Comparison of cemented and uncemented fixation in total hip replacement. A meta-analysis. *Acta Orthopaedica* 2007;**78**:315–26.
65. The Norwegian Arthroplasty Register 2007. http://www.nrlweb.ihelse.net/eng/default.htm (accessed 6/7/2011).
66. Charnley J. Long term results of low friction arthroplasty of the hip performed as a primary intervention. *Journal of Bone and Joint Surgery (British)* 1972;**54**:61–76.
67. Harris WH. Traumatic arthritis of the hip after dislocation in acetabular fractures treatment by mold arthroplasty. *Journal of Bone and Joint Surgery (American)* 1969;**51**:737–55.
68. Ware JE, Kosinski M, Keller SD. A SF-12 an even shorter health survey. *Medical Outcomes Trust Bulletin* 1996;**4**:2.
69. Dawson J, Fitzpatrick R, Carr A, Murray D. Oxford Hip Score: questionnaire on the perceptions of patients about total hip replacement. *Journal of Bone and Joint Surgery* 1996;**78**:185–90.

99

Minimal incision surgery/mini-invasive total hip replacement

EUGENE SHERRY, DECLAN O SHERRY

Introduction	1147	Recommendations from national bodies	1149
The evidence to date for use of MIS hip replacement	1148	Recommendations	1149
How to perform MIS – surgical techniques described to date	1148	Conclusion	1150
		References	1150
Supplemental technology	1149		

NATIONAL BOARD STANDARDS

- Learn the definition of minimal incision surgery total hip replacement
- Understand the limitations and potential complications of this new technique

INTRODUCTION

Minimal incision surgery (MIS) hip replacement (also called minimally invasive total hip replacement, mini-incision or keyhole hip replacement) has been considered one of the big successes in orthopaedic surgery over the last 9 years but only now is there evidence that it actually represents a significant advance over the already successful conventional hip replacement. Its purported benefits over conventional incision (25–40 cm) are more rapid postoperative rehabilitation (as there is less pain and less swelling), less blood loss, less time in hospital and loss of time from work, with fewer soft-tissue and bony complications and a cosmetic scar. Such benefits have huge incentives for patients, health economics and employers (Table 99.1).

A summary of this is: make as small a skin incision (<12 cm) as possible that allows safe access to the hip joint with the least soft-tissue and bony disturbance.

Table 99.1 Parameters considered in defining minimal incision surgery (MIS) hip replacement

Parameter	Comment
Length of skin incision	Arbitrary
Extent of soft-tissue envelope disturbance	Sound principle. May play a role in the incidence of deep ven thrombosis (LOE III) and infection
Extent of bony resection	Sound principle. MIS femoral head resection (resurfacing) is old concept. Minimal acetabular resection is new
Size of the implant used	Sound principle to reduce the bulk of the implant

LOE, level of evidence.

THE EVIDENCE TO DATE FOR USE OF MIS HIP REPLACEMENT

Retrospective series

In 2003 Goldstein et al.[2] found no difference in postoperative parameters but continued with the smaller incision technique as patients expressed a preference for it.

The large amount of interest in the MIS hip technique in 2002/2003 prompted surgeons to report their experience with the use of small incision arthroplasty over the previous 20 years and found no real benefit for the technique.[1-7]

Case series (prospective series)

Similar experiences have been presented elsewhere.[8-12]

Comparative papers (prospective controlled studies)

In such series, outcomes improved with time and the experience of the surgeon.[13-17]

Randomized controlled trials

In 2005, Ogonda et al.[18] in a well-conducted randomized controlled trial of 209 operations could find no benefit, up to 6 weeks, from MIS (using a single incision posterior approach) over a conventional incision of 16 cm and nor did other surgeons[19-22] (Table 99.2).

HOW TO PERFORM MIS – SURGICAL TECHNIQUES DESCRIBED TO DATE

The surgical approaches described to date are summarized in Table 99.3.

In essence, the MIS incisions are based upon the well-described anterior, anterolateral, direct lateral and posterolateral incisions (Fig. 99.1) but only occupying a short segment of the longer incisions.

Two-incision approach

This technique uses two incisions; with the patient in the supine position, one incision is over the hip (the anterior surgical approach between sartorius/tensor fasciae and

Table 99.3 Surgical approaches described (see Fig. 99.1)

	One incision	Two incision
Anterior	Yes	Anterior with direct lateral (as per insertion of an intramedullary nail)
Anterolateral	Yes	
Direct lateral	Yes	
Posterolateral	Yes	

Table 99.2 Evidence for minimal incision surgery

Benefits (advantages)/disadvantages	Evidence for this	Level of evidence
Benefits (advantages)		
Less pain	The same[18,21,23]	I
Less swelling	The same[18]	I
More rapid rehabilitation	Yes but only for 6 weeks to 6 months[18,19,21-25]	I
Less blood loss	No[18,21,22,26,27]	I
(Better) cosmetic scar	No evidence[28-30]	II
Less time lost from work and recreation	No evidence	
Less time spent in hospital	Yes[16]	III
Less limp	Yes[21]	I
Less soft-tissue and bony complications	No or the same[2,18,21,26,29]	I
Disadvantages		
Higher complication rate	Mainly yes[18,21,24,25]	I
Dislocation rate higher	The same[18,21,31]	I
Fracture rate higher	The same[18,21,24,25]	I
Higher soft-tissue complications	The same[18,21,24,25]	I
Higher nerve injury	Yes[18,21,24,25]	I
(More) malposition of components	The same[18,21,26]	I
(More) skin problems	The same[18]	I
Steep learning curve (difficult technique)	Yes[24,25]	I

Level of evidence, LOE, as per *Journal of Bone and Joint Surgery* ref. 32.

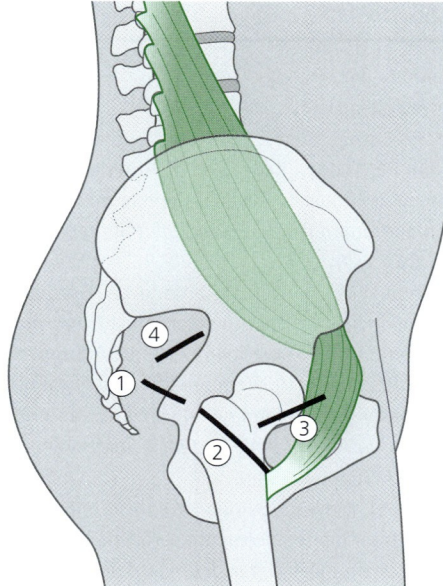

Figure 99.1 Minimal incision surgery incisions. 1, posterolateral; 2, anterolateral; 3 and 4, two-incision technique (anterior and lateral).

deeper between rectus femoris/tensor fasciae latae) and the second is over the lateral aspect of the greater trochanter (as per placing an intramedullary nail). Fluoroscopy is required. This has been called the 'two-incision' approach and was popularized by Berger.[33–36]

Two large groups do not recommend it.[36,37]

One-incision approach

POSTEROLATERAL (SOUTHERN)

In 2002 Sherry and co-workers[38,39,40] described a single-incision posterolateral approach using a 5–10 cm incision across the greater trochanter (curving posteriorly); at the same time, Berger described his two-incision technique.[33–35] Others followed.[9,4]

ANTERIOR (i.e. SMITH–PETERSEN)

In 2003 and 2004, Kennon et al.,[1,3] described the modified anterior MIS approach that they had been using for primary hip replacement and revision hip replacements. It is a single-incision technique which can be extended proximally (similar to the Smith–Petersen approach) or distally.

ANTEROLATERAL

This approach enters the hip through the fascia lata and takes down part (one-third) of gluteus medius (modification of the Hardinge approach).[42]

DIRECT LATERAL/TRANSGLUTEAL

O'Brien et al.[6] in 2005 reviewed their experience with the mini-incision technique via a direct lateral approach (similar to above).

SUPPLEMENTAL TECHNOLOGY

Use of specialized instrumentation

RETRACTORS

These include:

- a table-mounted self-retractor (called the Arthro-Tract; Omni-Tract Surgical, St Paul, MN)[1]
- the use of simple small self-retaining retractors (cerebellar retractors) throughout the case.[39,42]
- special illuminated retractors have been developed as well as curved retractors with increased handle length.[9]

SPECIALIZED INSTRUMENTS

These include:

- curved reamers (Chana reamer, Precimed SA, Orvin, Switzerland) and cup (dog-leg) inserters have been developed to aid access to the acetabulum
- other instruments include a device to osteotomize the femoral neck (avoid dislocation)
- drop-alignment gauge to insert and orientate the cup and a spacer system to balance the soft tissue (and avoid trial reductions).[39,42]

USE OF NAVIGATION

Many authors are now reporting the routine use of navigation especially with MIS surgery.[25,43,44]

RECOMMENDATIONS FROM NATIONAL BODIES

Such groups advise caution until more data are in and do not advise the two-incision technique.[37,45,46]

RECOMMENDATIONS

Surgeons wishing to use MIS techniques should work or seek training in centres where it is routinely used. It is important to practise on plastic bones and in cadaver laboratories.

An approach is outlined in Table 99.4.

Table 99.4 Considerations in decision-making for performing minimal incision surgery hip replacement

Patient's weight	Measure the body mass index
Length of incision	5–10 cm with option to extend. Limiting factor is the diameter of the cup to be used and size of acetabular reamer (the latter reduced with minimal resection of the acetabulum)
Surgical approach	Based on surgeon's experience. Two-incision technique is more demanding
Learning curve	Dependent upon institutional resources such as experienced colleagues, cadaver and animal laboratories, suitable models
Surgical aids	Use of navigation and/or specialized instruments
Anaesthetic techniques	To minimize blood loss, optimize visibility/access, for rapid rehabilitation, early mobilization and effective postoperative pain management

CONCLUSION

The scientific evidence to date does not definitively support the use of the popular MIS technique for hip replacement over a conventional incision.

This will require further significant technical improvements in visibility and the orientation of components with the use of navigation (already well-established in some centres for knee replacement and hip replacement), and improved equipment (reamers, retractors) and implant design.

In 2008, Huo et al.[47] in a full review of hip arthroplasty reported that the MIS technique offers no advantages after 12 months, has a higher rate of complications but is the stimulus to the development of better techniques, including MIS for resurfacing replacements.

More recently, MIS hip replacement has been reported as just as safe as conventional hip replacement, but shows no benefits after 3 months. Significantly, computer-assisted hip replacement showed better acetabular orientation than MIS techniques.[48]

KEY LEARNING POINTS

- Definition: as small a skin incision as possible (<12 cm) which allows safe access to the hip joint with the least soft-tissue and bony disturbance.
- Minimal incision surgery is a new technique which is sound in principle but still evolving and may well emerge as the new standard of care.
- No definitive evidence to support its use, although the trend is established.

REFERENCES

- ● = Key primary paper
- ◆ = Major review article

● 1. Kennon RE, Keggi J, Keggi J, et al. Anterior approach for total hip arthroplasty: beyond the minimally invasive technique. *Journal of Bone and Joint Surgery (American)* 2004;**86**:91–7.
● 2. Goldstein WM, Branson JJ, Berland KA, Gordon AC. Minimal-incision total hip arthroplasty. *Journal of Bone and Joint Surgery (American)* 2003;**85A**(Suppl.4): 33–8.
● 3. Kennon RE, Keggi JM, Wetmore RS, et al. Total hip arthroplasty through a minimally invasive anterior surgical approach. *Journal of Bone and Joint Surgery (American)* 2003;**85A**(Suppl.4):39–48.
● 4. Woolson ST, Mow CS, Syquia JF, et al. Comparison of primary total hip replacements performed with a standard incision or a mini-incision. *Journal of Bone and Joint Surgery (American)* 2004;**86A**:1353–8.
● 5. Matta JM, Shahrdar C, Ferguson T. Single-incision anterior approach for total hip arthroplasty on an orthopaedic table. *Clinical Orthopaedics and Related Research* 2005;**441**:115–24.
● 6. O'Brien DA, Rorabeck CH. The mini-incision direct lateral approach in primary total hip arthroplasty. *Clinical Orthopaedics and Related Research* 2005;**441**:99–103.
● 7. Teet JS, Skinner HB, Khoury L. The effect of the 'mini' incision in total hip arthroplasty on component position. *Journal of Arthroplasty*, 2006:**21**:503–7.
◆ 8. Berry DJ, Berger RA, Callaghan JJ, et al. Symposium: minimally invasive total hip arthroplasty. *Journal of Bone and Joint Surgery (American)* 2003;**85**:2235–46.
◆ 9. Berry DJ, Berger RA, Callaghan JJ, et al. Symposium: Minimally invasive total hip arthroplasty. *Journal of Bone and Joint Surgery (American)* 2003;**85**:2235–46.
◆ 10. Rachbauer F, Nogler M, Krismer M, Kessler O. Minimal invasive total hip arthroplasty via direct anterior single incision approach. Program and abstracts of the American Academy of Orthopaedic Surgeons 72nd Annual Meeting; February 23–27, 2005, Washington, DC. Course Number 141.
● 11. Swanson TV. Early results of 1000 consecutive, posterior, single-incision minimally invasive surgery total hip arthroplasties. *Journal of Arthroplasty* 2005;**20**(7 Suppl. 3):26–32.
● 12. Floren M, Lester DK. Durability of implant fixation after less-invasive total hip arthroplasty. *Journal of Arthroplasty* 2006;**21**:783–90.
● 13. Higuchi F, Gotoh M, Yamaguchi N, et al. Minimally invasive uncemented total hip arthroplasty through an anterolateral approach with a shorter skin incision. *Journal of Orthopaedic Science* 2003;**86**:812–17.
● 14. Inaba Y, Dorr LD, Wan Z, et al. Operative and patient care techniques for posterior mini-incision total hip arthroplasty. *Clinical Orthopaedics and Related Research* 2005;**441**:104–14.

15. Szendroi M, Sztrinkai G, Vass R, Kiss J. The impact of minimally invasive total hip arthroplasty on the standard procedure. *International Orthopaedics* 2006;**30**:167–71.
◆16. Howell JR, Masri BA, Duncan CP. Minimally invasive versus standard incision anterolateral hip replacement: a comparative study. *Orthopaedic Clinics of North America* 2004;**35**:153–62.
17. Nakata K, Nishikawa M, Yamamoto K, Hirota S. A clinical comparative study of direct anterior approach and mini-posterior approach in MIS-THA. AAOS Meeting. 15 February 2007, San Diego.
●18. Ogonda L, Wilson R, Archbold P, et al. A minimal incision technique in total hip arthroplasty does not improve early postoperative outcomes. A prospective, randomized, controlled trial. *Journal of Bone and Joint Surgery (American)* 2005;**87**:701–10.
●19. Lawlor M, Humphreys P, Morrow E, et al. Comparison of early postoperative functional levels following total hip replacement using minimally invasive versus standard incisions. A prospective randomized blinded trial. *Clinical Rehabilitation* 2005;**19**:465–74.
20. Wright J, Rosse D, Rosse S. A prospective randomized patient-blinded comparison of mini versus standard incision THA. Program and abstracts of the American Academy of Orthopaedic Surgeons 72nd Annual Meeting; 23–27 February 2005, Washington, DC. Course Number 139.
●21. Chimento GF, Pavone V, Sharrock N, et al. Minimally invasive total hip arthroplasty: a prospective randomized study. *Journal of Arthroplasty* 2005;**20**:139–44.
22. Dorr LD, Maheshwari AV, Long WT, et al. Early pain relief and function after posterior minimally invasive and conventional total hip arthroplasty. A prospective, randomized, blinded study. *Journal of Bone and Joint Surgery (American)* 2007;**89**:1153–60.
23. Ciminiello M, Parvizi J, Sharkey PF, et al. Total hip arthroplasty: is small incision better? *Journal of Arthroplasty* 2006;**21**:484–8.
24. DiGioia AM III, Plakseychuk AY, Levison TJ, Jaramaz B. Mini-incision technique for total hip arthroplasty with navigation. *Journal of Arthroplasty* 2003;**18**:123–8.
25. Bennett D, Ogonda L, Elliott D, et al. Comparison of gait kinematics in patients receiving minimally invasive and traditional hip replacement surgery: a prospective blinded study. *Gait and Posture* 2006;**23**:374–82.
26. Bal BS, Haltom D, Aleto T, Barrett M. Early complications of primary total hip replacement performed with a two-incision minimally invasive technique. *Journal of Bone and Joint Surgery (American)* 2005;**87**:2432–8.
27. Gunther KP. Potential benefit of MIS: comparison studies. Paper. Symposium 1. Mini-Invasive THR. EFFORT, 11 May 2007, Florence.
28. Mow CS, Woolson ST, Ngarmukos SG, et al. Comparison of scars from total hip replacements done with a standard or a mini-incision. *Clinical Orthopaedics and Related Research* 2005;**441**:80–5.
●29. McMinn DJW, Daniel J, Pysent PB, Pradhan C. Mini-incision resurfacing arthroplasty of hip through the posterior approach. *Clinical Orthopaedics and Related Research* 2005;**441**:91–8.
30. Peck CN, Foster A, McLauchlan GJ. Reducing incision length or intensifying rehabilitation: what makes the difference to length of stay in total hip replacement in a UK setting? *International Orthopaedics* 2006;**30**:395–8.
31. Sulco TP. 'Less invasive' hip replacement makes sense. AAOS Bulletin. August 2005. www2.aaos.org/aaos/archives/bulletin/aug05/fline12.asp.
32. Instructions to Authors. *Journal of Bone and Joint Surgery (British)* http://journals.jbjs.org.uk/tools/ifora.dtl.
33. Berger RA. Total hip arthroplasty using the minimally invasive two-incision approach. *Clinical Orthopaedics and Related Research* 2003;**417**:232–41.
34. Berger RA. Minimally invasive total hip arthroplasty with two incisions. *Operative Techniques in Orthopaedic* 2006;**16**:102–11.
●35. Berger RA Mini-incisions: two for the price of one! *Orthopedics* 2002;**25**:472–98.
36. Cigna HeathCare Coverage Position. CIGMA. minimally invasive total hip arthroplasty. Coverage Position 0217. revised date 11/15/2006. http://www.cigna.com/customer_care/healthcare_professional/coverage_positions/medical/mm_0217_coveragepositioncriteria_minimally_invasive_total_hip_arthroplasty.pdf.
37. NICE (National Institute for Health and Clinical Excellence). IPG 152 Single mini-incision hip replacement – guidance. http://www.nice.org.uk/guidance/index.jsp?action=download&r=true&to=31463.
●38. Sherry E, Egan M, Warnke PH, Henderson A. Minimally invasive techniques for total hip arthroplasty. *Journal of Bone and Joint Surgery (American)* 2002;**84A**:1481.
39. Sivananthan DKS, Sivananthan S, Egan, M, et al. Minimal invasive surgery for hip replacement using the NILNAV Hip System. Poster #512. Presented at the 70th Annual Meeting of the American Academy of Orthopaedic Surgeons, 5–9 Feb 2003, New Orleans.
●40. Sherry E, Egan M, Warnke PH, et al. Minimal invasive surgery for hip replacement: a new technique using the NILNAV Hip System. *Australia and New Zealand Journal of Surgery* 2003;**73**:157–61.
41. Blasser KE. Advances in total hip replacement: minimally invasive surgery. *Northeast Florida Medicine* 2006:**57**:21–3.
42. Howell JR, Garbuz DS, Duncan CP. Minimally invasive hip replacement: rationale, applied anatomy, and instrumentation. *Orthopaedic Clinics of North America* 2004;**35**:107–18.
●43. Wixson RL, MacDonald MA. Total hip arthroplasty through a minimal posterior approach using imageless computer-assisted hip navigation. *Journal of Arthroplasty* 2005,**20**:51–6.
44. Reininga IHF, Wagenmakers R, Van Den Akker-Scheek I, et al. Effectiveness of computer-navigated minimally invasive total hip surgery compared to conventional total hip arthroplasty: design of a randomized controlled trial. Study in progress. *BMC Musculoskeletal Disorders* 2007;**8**:4.

45. American Academy of Orthopaedic Surgeons (AAOS). Minimally invasive hip replacement. http://orthoinfo.aaos.org/fact/thr_report.cfm?Thread_ID=471.
46. American Association of Hip and Knee Surgeons (AAHKS). Minimally invasive and small incision joint replacement surgery: what surgeons should consider. http://www.goldsteinortho.com/MIS_patient_statement.pdf.
47. Huo MH, Parvizi J, Bal S, Mont MA. What's new in Total Hip Arthroplasty. *Journal of Bone and Joint Surgery (American)* 2008;**90**:2043-55.
●48. Reininga IHF, Zijlstra W, Wagenmakers R, *et al*. Minimally invasive and computer-navigated total hip arthroplasty: a qualitative and systematic review of the literature. *BMC Musculoskeletal Disorders* 2010;**11**:92.

100

Revision total hip arthroplasty

ARDESHIR BONSHAHI, TIMOTHY N BOARD, MARTYN L PORTER

Introduction	1153	Acetabular reconstruction	1158
Failure mechanisms of hip replacements	1153	Femoral reconstruction	1160
Bone loss	1156	One- or two-stage revision for infection	1161
Surgical approaches	1157	References	1162
Removal of implants	1157		

NATIONAL BOARD STANDARDS

- Learn the commonest indications for revision hip arthroplasty
- Know about the surgical approach
- Understand that the removal of implants is often the most difficult and time-consuming part
- Understand the techniques of reconstruction
- Realize that infection is a major consideration here

INTRODUCTION

The number of joint replacement procedures performed is growing faster than ever. In the USA alone, it has been estimated that nearly 600 000 hip replacements and 1.4 million knee replacements will be performed in the year 2015.[1] Similarly an increase in the number of revision total hip arthroplasties has been reported over the past 13 years. The revision burden – defined as the ratio of revision arthroplasties to the total number of arthroplasties – has remained relatively constant. This has led Kurtz et al.[2] to conclude that that a greater number of primary replacements will result in a greater number of revisions unless some limiting mechanism can be successfully implemented to reduce the future revision burden. Until this happens, revision hip replacement will remain an important issue and is the focus of this chapter.

FAILURE MECHANISMS OF HIP REPLACEMENTS

According to the National Institute for Health and Clinical Excellence guidelines,[3] for a hip prosthesis to be considered safe its mean survival rate should be at least 90% at 10 years. The failure rate is low but can vary greatly and is influenced by several factors, such as the type of prosthesis used, whether it is cemented or uncemented, patient characteristics, surgeon's experience and complications. Some of the common reasons for revision are discussed below.

Aseptic loosening: relation to polyethylene

Aseptic loosening accounts for more than 70% of the hip revisions in Sweden.[4] Osteolysis induced by particulate wear debris from implant materials results in aseptic loosening. Schmalzried et al.[5] hypothesized that wear particles from the polyethylene cup are dispersed into the effective joint space. The extent of access of wear particles within the effective joint space depends upon the contact between implant and bone, or between implant and cement, or between cement and bone. Macrophages activated by wear debris activate osteoclasts or become osteoclasts themselves and initiate bone resorption. This bone resorption results in an enlarged effective joint space, which eases the flow of joint fluid and the particles within it, eventually leading to loosening of the implant (Fig. 100.1). The polyethylene wear particles within

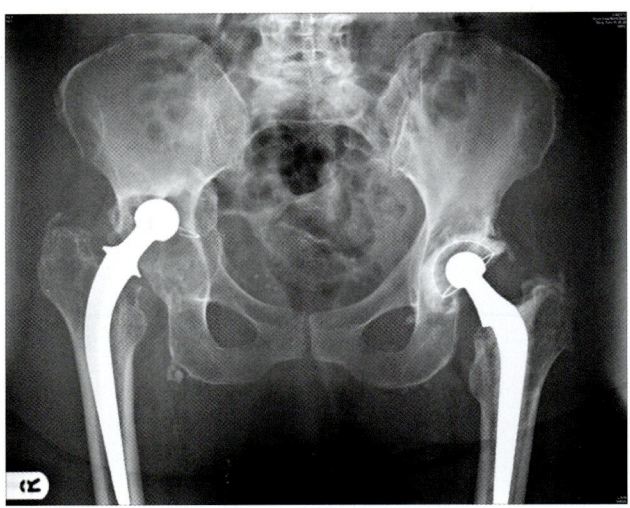

Figure 100.1 Aseptic loosening. Extensive osteolysis can be seen around the acetabular and femoral component.

an artificial joint vary in their size and shape, but it is proposed that the submicron-sized particles have the most effect on macrophages and bone remodelling.[6] The other factor that has a role in aseptic loosening is the high pressure of the joint fluid that moves the wear debris to the effective joint space, bringing it into greater contact with bone cells and the macrophages.[7]

Aseptic loosening: pressure effects of uncemented cups

The uncemented cup may have some areas without bone ingrowth, which results in access channels for joint fluid, and may result in expansile osteolysis. Also, screw holes in some acetabular cups act as a conduit for joint fluid. The presence of micromotion may result in a fibrous interface between prosthesis and bone. In an *in vivo* study in rabbits, fibrous membrane compression led to bone necrosis and cartilage formation, possibly because of fluid pressure or fluid flow, whereas the presence of high-density polyethylene particles led to the loss of bone with replacement of bone by fibrous tissue.[8] The cementless cup can be clinically asymptomatic even with severe osteolysis.

Aseptic loosening: relation to stem design

Among the most dramatic reports of early stem failures is that of the Capital Hip (3M Healthcare Ltd, Loughborough, UK). Definite loosening was present in 16% with an additional 8% possibly loose at follow-up of 26 months. Approximately 5000 stems were implanted throughout the UK with a failure rate at 5 years estimated at 20%.[9] A number of factors, including the stem design (modular flanged variety performing worse than the monoblock round back),

cement mantle thickness, type of cement and surgical technique, were implicated. A report on the performance of the 3M Capital Hip system published in 2001[10] concluded that it was not possible to identify one factor, or a combination of factors, that led to the poor performance of the flanged modular Capital Hip. This investigation, however, suggests that even a small modification in stem design may have the potential to lead to early failure. The Charnley Elite-Plus femoral component (De Puy International, Raynham, MA) highlights this issue. It was introduced in 1993, as an evolution of design of the Charnley stem, and included a modification of the shoulder flange, altered geometry of the stem and surface finish, improved material and new instrumentation.[11] Hauptfleisch *et al.*[12] reported a rate of survival of 83% at 10 years of the Elite-Plus femoral stem when revision was taken as the point of failure, and of 59% when radiological loosening of the stem was used. Their studies suggested that the Elite-Plus femoral stem was intrinsically rotationally unstable.

ZONES OF DEMARCATION

The acetabulum was divided into three zones by DeLee and Charnley.[13] The femur was divided into seven zones by Gruen *et al.*[14] The development of progressive radiolucent lines in these zones in either cemented or uncemented components suggests loosening. This should be differentiated from age-related radiolucent lines that do not have an area of adjacent sclerosis. Also non-progressive radiolucent lines, typically in zones 1 and 7 due to imperfect cement interlocking, were noted not to result in a disastrous outcome.[15]

Barrack *et al.*[16] graded the radiographic appearance of cementing on the immediate postoperative radiograph. Complete filling of the medullary cavity by cement, a so-called 'white-out' at the cement–bone interface was graded 'A'. Slight radiolucency of the cement–bone interface was defined as 'B'. Radiolucency involving 50–99% of the cement–bone interface or a defective or incomplete cement mantle was graded 'C'. Radiolucency at the cement–bone interface of 100% in any projection, or a failure to fill the canal with cement such that the tip of the stem was not covered, was classified 'D'.

A radiological assessment of Charnley total hip replacements (THRs) with aseptic loosening within 5 years of surgery found 69% of the failed stems had a Barrack C or D grading whereas only 19% of the failed stems belonging to Barrack grade A or B.[17]

Septic loosening

Deep infection following total joint arthroplasty is a challenging complication to both the patient and the surgeon. The risk of infection after joint arthroplasty is variable from 0.3%, reported by the British Medical Research Council,[18] to 2.2%, described in a large review of patients who underwent total hip arthroplasty.[19] Although the percentages are small, considering the increasing number of primary hip replacements, it relates to a large number of patients with periprosthetic infections who utilize a substantial amount of healthcare resources. The Swedish Hip Register reveals that 7.3% of total hip revisions are carried out for infection.[20]

Staphylococcus epidermidis is the most prevalent and persistent species found on most skin and mucous membranes, constituting 65–90% of all staphylococci. Of a confirmed 112 prosthetic joint infections, the most frequently isolated organisms were coagulase-negative staphylococci (47% patients) and meticillin-sensitive *Staphylococcus aureus* (44% patients); 8% grew meticillin-resistant *S. aureus* (MRSA) and 7% grew anaerobes.[21] Another study found that 43% of positive tissue cultures were coagulase-negative staphylococci, of which approximately 50% were meticillin resistant, suggesting therefore screening for meticillin-resistant *S. epidermidis* in addition to MRSA.[22]

Fitzgerald *et al.*[23] grouped prosthetic joint infections into stage I infections (acute fulminating infections), usually within 6 weeks; stage II infections (delayed sepsis), chronic indolent infection; and stage III infections (late haematogenous infections in a previously well-functioning hip replacement). Tsukayama *et al.*[24] proposed a fourth type in which a positive culture is found at the time of revision without previous evidence of infection.

Stem fracture

Early stem designs made of EN58J and 316L stainless steel had relatively high rates of failure that were due to the materials' low fatigue strength and metallurgical defects.[25–28] Fatigue fractures were produced by unfavourable biomechanics such as varus malposition or loss of proximal cement support, leading to exaggerated cantilever forces on the proximal stem relative to the well-fixed distal portion. In one study, scanning electron micrographs demonstrated a fatigue fracture that began through characters that had been etched on the implant with a laser.[26] Materials such as forged cobalt chrome, high-nitrogen stainless steel and titanium alloy used in modern stems have high strength and have made the incidence of this complication quite rare, with none reported in two long-term follow-up studies of matt and polished cemented stems.[29,30]

Ceramic bearing fractures

Fracture rates of ceramic bearings vary from 0% to 13%.[31] Higher fracture rates were seen in the older generation of alumina bearings and were related to the poor quality of the material and the difficulties in its fixation to the metallic stem. Introduction of the Morse taper after 1977 reduced the risk of fracture to less than 2%.[32] Third-generation ceramics are manufactured with hot isostatic pressing to reduce grain size and have greater burst strength and better wear properties.[33] These have had good clinical results.[34,35]

Under normal physiological conditions modern ceramic head fractures are rare. In contrast, ceramic liner fractures, though not well recognized, can occur as a result of multiple causes: dislocation, impingement, malpositioning and microseparation.[36] Overall, the choice of a high-quality alumina, a highly relevant design (avoid short neck) and, if possible, a thicker implant (especially for the cup) are of paramount importance to reduce the risk of fracture.

When a ceramic bearing fractures the ceramic fragments that have spread into the periarticular space are abrasive and can lead to early failure of the revision procedure.[37,38] Thorough debridement and synovectomy at the time of revision can reduce the incidence of this complication. The choice of bearing to use in the revision is controversial.

Dislocation

Dislocation is one of the most common complications of total hip arthroplasty. The reported incidence varies from 0.3% to 7% in primary THR and up to 25% in revision hip replacement. Early dislocation occurs within the first 3 months postoperatively and carries a better prognosis and a lower rate of recurrence with non-operative treatment.[39] In comparison, late dislocations have a multifactorial aetiology, including polyethylene wear and soft-tissue laxity, which leads to a higher recurrent dislocation rate.[40] Larger femoral heads have reduced the incidence of dislocation by increasing the head–neck ratio, thus improving the primary arc of motion, and by allowing a greater amount of translation before dislocation occurs.[41]

The treatment of late or recurrent dislocations depends on the cause. Some of the common causes are component malposition, polyethylene wear and abductor insufficiency. These are best treated with revision surgery. If the cause is unknown or multifactorial then the choice of surgery becomes less clear. The surgical options include augmentation of polyethylene socket with a posterior lip augmentation device, exchange of liner, revision of malpositioned components, constrained liner, bipolar or tripolar arthroplasty and soft-tissue reinforcement or greater trochanter advancement.

Periprosthetic fractures

Berry[42] reported an incidence of 0.3% in 20 859 primary cemented and 5.4% in 3121 uncemented total hip arthroplasties and an intra-operative fracture rate of 3.6% in cemented and 20.9% in uncemented revision total hip arthroplasties.

Treatment of periprosthetic fractures is difficult and depends upon the location of the fracture, stability of the implant, bone stock quality, the patient's comorbidities and age, and the surgeon's experience.[43] The Vancouver classification system aids this process and has three types based on fracture location: type A, involves the trochanteric region;

type B, a fracture around or just distal to the femoral stem; and type C, fractures that are so far below the stem that the treatment is independent of the hip replacement. Type B fractures are subdivided into B1 fractures, in which the femoral implant is well fixed; B2 fractures, in which the femoral implant is loose but the remaining bone stock is good; and B3 fractures, in which there is severe bone stock loss in the presence of a loose implant.[44]

If revision surgery is planned it is imperative to rule out infection by performing inflammatory markers and hip aspiration or biopsy. If positive, a two-stage procedure with an interim spacer is preferred to eradicate the infection while the fracture heals.[45] B1 fractures should be treated with open reduction and internal fixation with or without a cortical strut allograft. Augmentation with one anteriorly placed strut graft or just two strut grafts has a lower failure rate than fixation with cable plate alone.[46] We do feel that, in the case of a cemented stem of polished taper slip design, a B1 fracture through the cement mantle needs revision as the integrity of the cement mantle necessary to prevent excessive subsidence of these stems is lost and is difficult to restore through an open reduction. A longer femoral stem that bypasses a type B2 fracture by at least two canal diameters along with augmentation with strut grafts as biological plates is the treatment of choice, and has shown better outcomes.[47,48] Patients with B3 fractures are difficult to treat and often require the use of an allograft–prosthetic–composite revision, a tumour prosthesis or a custom implant. Patients with type C fractures are treated with standard open reduction and internal fixation techniques for the distal femur fracture.

FEMORAL NECK FRACTURE IN RESURFACING HIP ARTHROPLASTY

The incidence of femoral neck fractures reported from non-originator series ranges from 0.4% to 1.64%, most of which occur in the first year.[49–52] However, it is the commonest complication in resurfacing arthroplasty and accounts for 64% of the complications in one multicentre study[52] (Fig. 100.2). Conversion of a hip resurfacing with a femoral-side failure to a total hip arthroplasty appears to be comparable to primary total hip arthroplasty in terms of surgical effort, safety and early clinical outcomes.[53,54]

BONE LOSS

There are numerous classification systems for predicting bone loss in revision arthroplasty. The purpose of these systems is to plan the operation and ensure that the necessary prostheses, augmentation devices and bone graft are available at the time of surgery. The classification systems commonly used in revision hip surgery are the Endo-Klinik classification system for femoral bone loss[55] and the Paprosky classification system for acetabular[56] bone loss.

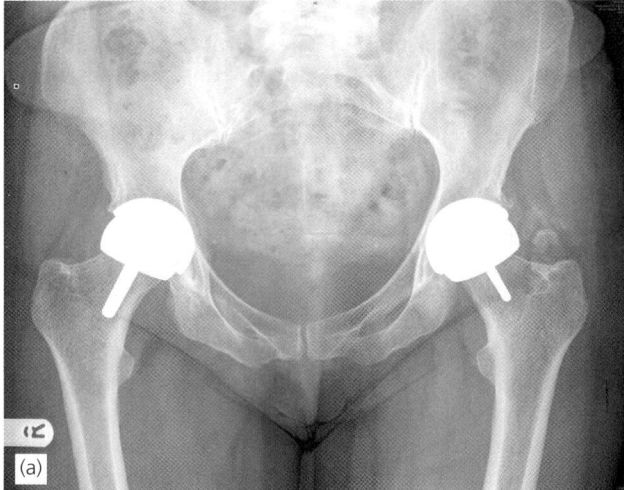
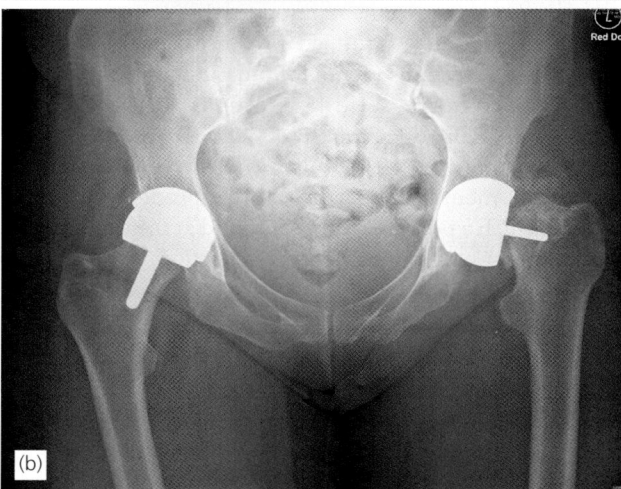

Figure 100.2 (a and b) Note neck thinning before the femoral neck fracture after left hip resurfacing.

In the Endo-Klinik classification system grade 1 represents a clinically loose prosthesis with radiolucent lines along the proximal half of the cement mantle. In grade 2, radiolucent lines are present circumferentially and there is endosteal erosion of the proximal femur. The bone loss is considered grade 3 when the proximal part of the femur is expanded with resultant widening of the medullary cavity with or without a cortical defect. Grade 4 bone loss is characterized by gross destruction of the proximal third of the femur that extends into the diaphysis.

The Paprosky classification system[56] is based upon the presence or absence of an intact acetabular rim and its ability to provide initial rigid support for an implanted acetabular component. Type 1 acetabular defects have an intact rim with contained lytic defects and no migration of the cup. In a type II defect, the acetabulum is distorted but there is adequate host bone to support a cementless acetabular component. There may be destruction of the dome and/or medial wall but the anterior and posterior columns remain intact. Type 3 defects represent major destruction of the acetabular rim and supporting structures that would not provide adequate initial trial component stability. The failed component has usually migrated more than 2 cm superiorly. Type 2 and 3 defects are further subdivided based upon the pattern of bone loss and resultant direction of component migration. Type 2A defects have superior bone lysis but the superior rim remains intact. Type 2B defects are similar to type 2A, but the dome is more distorted and the superior rim is absent. Type 3A defects show moderate lysis of the teardrop and ischium but, because the medial wall is still present, the component usually migrates superolaterally. Type 3B defects show complete obliteration of the teardrop and severe lysis of the ischium, usually resulting in superomedial component migration.

SURGICAL APPROACHES

The choice and extent of the surgical approach in revision arthroplasty depend upon the reason for revision, previous surgical approach, experience of the surgeon and presence of acetabular or femoral bone loss. An ideal approach should provide satisfactory exposure of both components, protect neurovascular structures, minimize bone and soft-tissue devitalization and allow for extension in case of complications.

The use of prior incisions is recommended when possible to avoid railroad-track scars and the potential risk of intervening skin necrosis. Laterally placed skin incisions can migrate with time and one could include the old scar in the new incision if skin laxity permits the correct fascial incision underneath.

There is no single surgical approach that it is most appropriate for all revision hip arthroplasties, but the surgeon needs to be familiar with the full gamut of surgical approaches to the hip joint so that the most appropriate one is used. In general, anterolateral approaches are not as extensile as the posterior or transtrochanteric approach.

Problems with the Hardinge approach[57] in revision surgery are a higher incidence of heterotopic bone formation and abductor weakness either through damage to the superior gluteal nerve[58] or failure of its reattachment, especially when limb lengthening is necessary. In addition, it is less extensile.[59]

The advantages of a posterior approach are good circumferential exposure of the acetabulum without disturbance of the abductor mechanism, posterior column visualization and a lower rate of heterotrophic ossification. The main disadvantage is a higher rate of posterior dislocation because of either loss of the posterior capsule and short external rotators or an inadequate acetabular component anteversion. A further advantage is the ease with which it can be extended distally by using the extended trochanteric osteotomy.

The extended trochanteric osteotomy[60] is an extremely useful technique when removing solidly fixed cemented and cementless stems. A posterior approach to the hip is extended distally along the posterolateral aspect of the femoral shaft. The vastus lateralis is elevated subperiosteally, leaving a small cuff at its insertion to the linea aspera to prevent retraction of perforators beyond the intermuscular septum. The perforating vessels are ligated or cauterized. A long osteotomy along the exposed posterior aspect of the femur, just anterolateral to the linea aspera, extending from the greater trochanter to a level on the femoral diaphysis determined by pre-operative templating, is performed with an oscillating saw blade or with multiple holes. Care should be taken not to strip the long trochanteric fragment of its muscle attachments, thereby depriving it of a blood supply. Once the unicortical distal and posterior cuts are made, a narrow osteotome is used to perforate the anterior femoral cortex through the vastus lateralis. Curved osteotomes are then inserted through the posterior osteotomy site to detach the bone fragment by fracturing the remaining bone along the anterior osteotomy line.

An *in vitro* cadaver study[61] demonstrated a reduction in torsional strength and energy required for fracture following an extended trochanteric osteotomy even after stem insertion and repair of the osteotomy. This finding suggests that postoperative rehabilitation protocols should be even more restrictive with regard to weight bearing.

REMOVAL OF IMPLANTS

The success of revision hip surgery to a great extent relies upon the quality of host bone remaining following implant removal. Depending upon the indication, the removal of implants during revision hip arthroplasty can be very technically demanding with potential for producing bone loss and fracture during the procedure. The goal is to minimize bone loss through careful pre-operative planning and to ensure that any specialized removal equipment that may be required is available.

The pre-operative plan for removal should include good anteroposterior and lateral radiographs, and, if necessary, Judet views of the acetabulum. It is necessary to know the implant manufacturer, size of implants, type of locking mechanism for the liner and type of screw heads, if used, from implant record labels in the case notes.

Removal of cemented cups

Cemented cups are removed following a good exposure of the periphery of the cup to delineate the polyethylene, cement and bone interfaces. Curved specialized osteotomes are used to develop the cup–cement interface to avoid damage to underlying bone stock. Once adequately mobilized all around the circumference the cup can be levered out of the cement mantle gently or a threaded extractor may be inserted into the polyethylene through a drill hole to allow disimpaction and removal of the cup. The cement is then carefully divided using a range of curved narrow osteotomes and removed piecemeal.

Removal of uncemented cups

The liner in an uncemented cup is removed first to allow access to any screws which may have been used. Many acetabular liners have locking mechanisms that may require specialized tools or techniques for removal. In other cases, it may be possible to use a small lever behind the rim to pry the liner out of place. If a polyethylene liner is used then a screw advanced through it will disengage the liner as the screw tip touches the metal shell.

Removal of an uncemented shell can be done using either the Explant system (Explant Acetabular Removal System; Zimmer, Warsaw, IN) or curved osteotomes as described above. The Explant system uses a curved blade specific to the diameter of the shell attached to a rotating handle device that is centred in the liner by a head component of appropriate size. First, a short blade is used to open up the interface between host bone and shell and then a full-length curved blade completely releases the implant from bone.

Removal of cemented stem

The principle in removing cemented stems is to remove the stem first followed by the cement. Following an adequate exposure the proximal and lateral aspect of the femur is cleared of cement and soft tissue using a combination of narrow gouges and osteotomes to allow extraction of the stem. In a curved stem it is essential to clear the cement beyond the shoulder before attempting stem removal, which reduces the risk of fracture. It is best to work from the cement–stem interface outwards in order to avoid unnecessary damage to adjacent bone. Once the implant has been extracted safely, any remaining cement must be removed by carefully splitting the cement and developing the interface between cement and bone. This is done using special long cement-splitting chisels and gouges. In the case of textured or precoated cement stems one could remove the stem either by loosening the stem from the cement using thin/flexible osteotomes from above or by an extended trochanteric osteotomy.

Apart from manual techniques the options include use of high-energy ultrasound delivered directly to the cement mantle; this heats and softens the polymethylmethacrylate, with little damage to cortical bone.[62,63] Our preferred technique involves using narrow gouges to remove the proximal cement followed by use of OSCAR (the Orthosonics System for Cemented Arthroplasty Revision) to breach the distal cement plug and then the use of reverse-cutting narrow long osteotomes to remove the remaining cement from below upwards.

Removal of uncemented stems

Removal of proximally coated cementless stems can be done using long thin flexible osteotomes from above. This can be difficult in some cases where the distal portion of the stem may have a rough surface with bone ongrowth. In such situations and in the case of fully coated stems an extended trochanteric osteotomy is preferred.

ACETABULAR RECONSTRUCTION

Impaction bone grafting

Impaction allografting of bone has been used successfully as a technique to reconstitute bone loss in both the femur and acetabulum in revision THR since the pioneering work of the groups in Nijmegen, the Netherlands,[64] and Exeter, UK.[65] The procedure involves progressive compaction of morsellized cancellous bone chips into the femoral canal or acetabular cavity. The prosthesis is then cemented in place, creating a three-layer composite of implant, cement and graft.

The raw material for impaction grafting is most commonly a whole femoral head received from a live donor at the time of primary THR. Bone is either fresh-frozen and stored at −80°C or freeze-dried and subsequently stored at room temperature. Freeze-dried bone is rarely used in impaction allografting. Most fresh-frozen femoral head allografts are not formally sterilized. Microbiological screening is performed, and stringent donor selection tests including hepatitis B, hepatitis C, HIV and syphilis are performed.

Initial stability of the impacted graft is obtained by interdigitation between different sized particles of graft created by a bone mill and some with a hand rongeur. Washing the graft has been shown to improve the shear strength of compacted allograft.[66] The mechanisms for this are twofold. First, the removal of fat and marrow fluid reduces the lubrication of particles, thereby increasing frictional resistance. Second, the removal of fat before compaction increases the compactability of the graft, allowing greater interdigitation between particles.

The original technique involves firm impaction of the graft particles into a contained acetabular defect with a hammer and impactors of different sizes. An alternative technique of reverse reaming of the graft slurry into a contained defect was tested *in vitro* and found to have suboptimal initial stability when compared with the original technique.[67]

The application of this technique is particularly attractive in young patients as one can reconstitute bone stock. In a series of 28 hips in patients younger than 50 years the 20 year survival rate was 80% with acetabular revision for any reason as the endpoint, and 91% with acetabular revision because of aseptic loosening as the endpoint.[68]

The prerequisite to success in impaction bone grafting is to provide a contained and stable acetabular cavity as movement or shear forces will produce graft resorption and loosening. Acetabular rim and medial wall mesh cages, as described by Slooff *et al.*,[69] are examples of containing

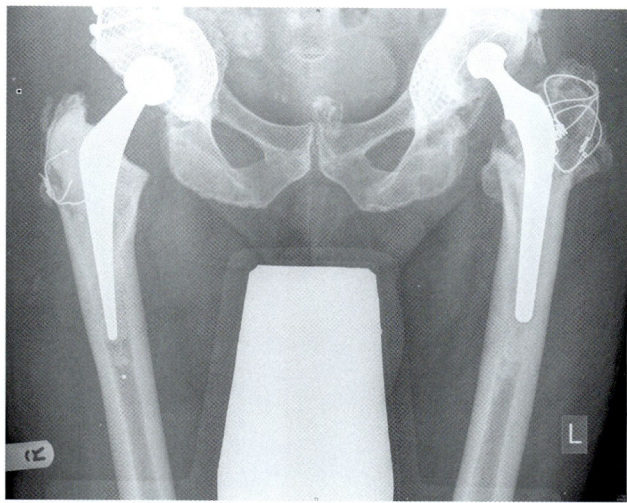

Figure 100.3 Peripheral and medial wall mesh used to contain the acetabular defect prior to impaction bone grafting.

devices that are designed to convert uncontained defects into contained defects (Fig. 100.3). The medial wall mesh is used to cover medial wall defects and prevents graft migration into the pelvic cavity. Peripheral segmental defects are converted into a contained defect by the application of a stainless steel mesh that needs to be securely fixed to the outer wall of the ilium with screws. The function of the mesh is to contain the graft and to produce a stable platform of particulate bone to support the cemented socket while revascularization and graft incorporation proceed.

With larger acetabular defects a metal reconstruction cage (e.g. Burch–Schneider cage) can be fixed to the pelvis with multiple screws to augment graft stability. The cage helps to contain the graft and prevents motion between the graft and acetabular component. An all-polyethylene acetabular component is usually cemented into the cage with favourable results up to 12 years.[70,71] However, some have reported a failure rate of 40% at 2–9 year follow-up.[72]

Uncemented acetabular revision

HEMISPHERICAL CUPS

In revising the acetabulum the remaining bone stock is often inadequate or sclerotic and may prevent optimal bone cement microinterlock. Reliable and durable fixation of cementless hemispherical acetabular components requires intimate contact between the implant and viable bone as well as mechanical stability (motion of less than 40–50 µm). The amount of host bone required to provide durable fixation is not known but most surgeons believe that 50–60% is necessary. The ability to supplement fixation of these implants with screws allows for their use in the presence of bone deficiency and has seen good results.[73] In select cases with severe bone loss the placement of the component at a high hip centre has not been found to be detrimental at a follow-up of minimum 15 years in one study.[74] The long-term results of uncemented porous-coated cups in revision surgery have shown good results in terms of re-revision rates.[75–78]

OBLONG/BILOBED CUPS

Bilobed or oblong-shaped cementless acetabular cups have been used in cases of extensive superior bone loss where standard or oversized hemispherical components would not achieve stability. The results are variable in the midterm for the bilobed cup with 0–24% failure rates.[79,80] In a series with an average follow-up of 9 years, the oblong cup remained *in situ* without further revision in 93% of the cases.[81]

TRABECULAR METAL

Acetabular components made from porous tantalum have been used to achieve primary stability in type III acetabular defects as an alternative to bone graft and cages. In cases of severe bone loss most of the support to a reconstruction cage is from the allograft rather than host bone. With remodelling and resorption of the allograft the cage is subject to high stresses, leading to fatigue failure. Trabecular metal augments act as a structural allograft, increasing the contact surface area with the host bone (Fig. 100.4). Acetabular deficiencies can be independently addressed and reconstructed, providing initial stability and, potentially, long-term biological fixation to host bone.[82] The early results with trabecular metal components suggest that these constructs are mechanically stable but longer follow-up is required.[83,84]

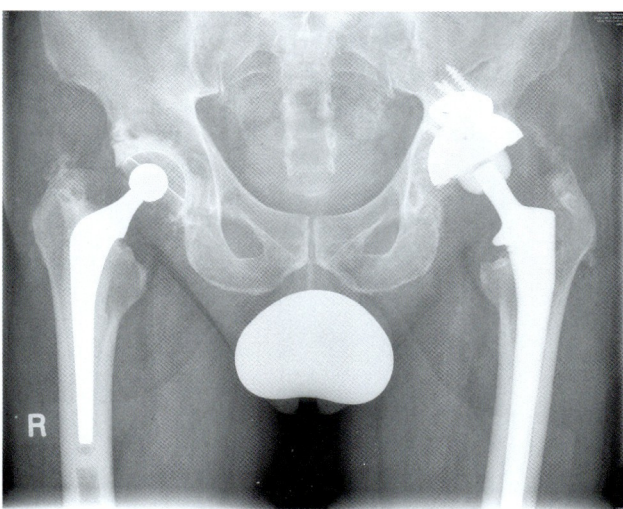

Figure 100.4 Large acetabular defect treated with a trabecular augment with a trabecular metal shell to restore the hip centre.

FEMORAL RECONSTRUCTION

Cemented revision

The advantages of using cemented femoral revision are immediate implant stability allowing for early weight bearing and the ability to add antibiotics to cement when dealing with infection. With modern cementing techniques the results are satisfactory with up to 10% re-revision at 11 years.[85–87] However, many early published series showed disappointing results,[88–91] with one reporting up to 53% stem loosening at 14 years.[92] The endosteal surface in revision is frequently smooth and sclerotic and does not allow for microinterlock and adequate cement bonding; hence, a strong fixation as in a primary THR cannot be achieved. Long cemented stems can be used to bypass the revised area or proximal bone deficiencies and overcome this problem by achieving distal fixation. However, with long stems there is difficulty of pressurizing cement and the risk of more bone loss if a long stem becomes loose. A 10 year survival rate of 91% using long tapered polished cemented stem revisions for aseptic loosening has been reported, with 70% survival using mechanical failure as an endpoint.[93] The mean age of patients in this series was 74 and this may have contributed to the good results. Occasionally, particularly in older patients or when a femoral component needs removal but the cement–bone interface is good, a cement-in-cement revision technique in which a new prosthesis is cemented into the existing cement mantle can be used (Figs 100.5 and 100.6).

Impaction bone grafting of femur

Impaction grafting in the femur was first described in cementless stem revision.[94] Gie *et al*.[65] adapted the technique described by Slooff *et al*.[64] for protrusio acetabuli and

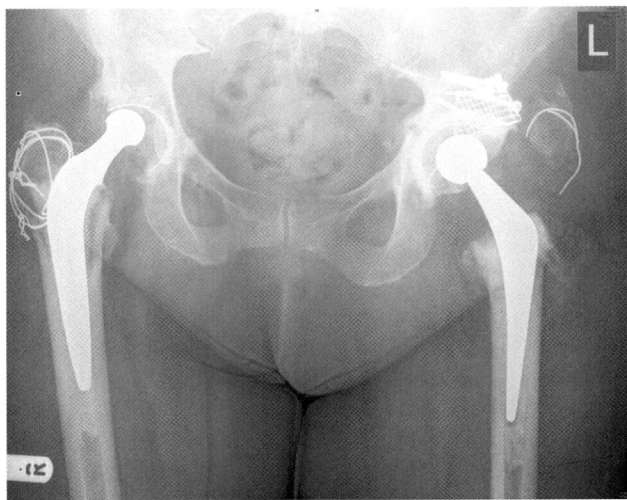

Figure 100.6 The same patient as in Fig. 100.5 treated with rim mesh and impaction bone grafting for the acetabulum and cement-in-cement revision of the femoral stem.

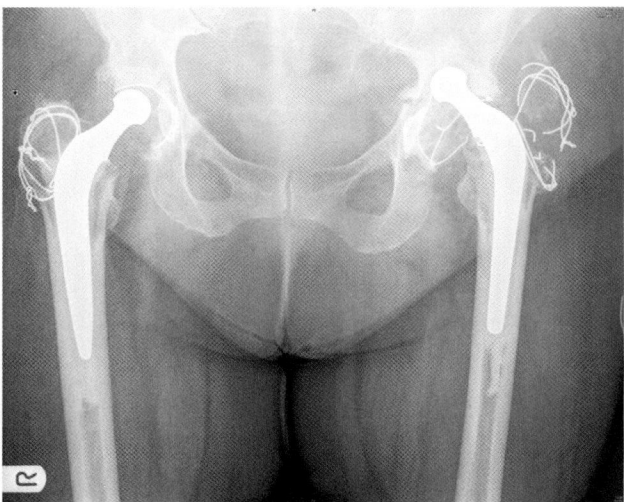

Figure 100.5 Acetabular failure with a well-fixed femoral component.

applied it to cemented stem revisions. The technique attempts to reconstitute a bone-deficient proximal femur by tightly packing morsellized cancellous bone graft within it. Insertion of the bone graft may be accomplished by hand or by using any number of commercially available instrument systems such as the X-Change system (Stryker, Mahwah, NJ). Most systems use cannulated tamps or impactors that pass over a threaded rod, which inserts into the distal canal-restricting plug or into the retained distal cement plug.[95,96] The graft impaction process needs to be vigorous such that the impactor is so tight that it is difficult to withdraw it without using the slap hammer, and it should be rotationally stable. This creates significant hoop stresses in the femur that can lead to intra-operative or postoperative fracture, which is the commonest complication of this procedure. To reduce this risk it is critical to locate cavitary and segmental defects in the femur, and areas of ectatic cortex that might require reinforcement with strut allografts or wire mesh.[65,97–99] *In vitro* studies have shown that the mechanical stability of impacted graft is related to the density, and hence compaction, of the graft.[100] It should be remembered, while undertaking the impaction, that the stiffness of the graft increases logarithmically up to approximately 30 impactions,[101] with little increase in stiffness after this. However, deciding when the construct has reached adequate stability remains largely a matter of experience. One study has suggested the use of a modified torque wrench to assess rotational stability of the femoral phantom.[102]

Excessive stem subsidence from additional packing of the graft during cyclic loading is another common complication. The original technique is described using a polished double-tapered stem where subsidence is considered to be beneficial and integral to the success of the technique. Subsidence inside the cement mantle might cause the mantle to expand radially, inducing radial stresses in the compacted bone graft that could stimulate graft remodelling. However a prospective, randomized study comparing the migration of Exeter and Charnley Elite stems with radiostereometric analysis[103] concluded that radial compression of the cement produced by a double-tapered design was not the essential stimulus for bone remodelling in impaction grafting. Stem subsidence has been associated with thigh pain, aseptic loosening and later dislocation.[98,104]

Cemented impaction grafting for the femur has revealed promising results and shows reconstitution in bone stock in a majority of cases.[65,96,105,106] In one large study, femoral reoperation because of symptomatic aseptic loosening as the endpoint was 1% at 10 years.[107]

Cementless femoral revision

Cementless femoral designs and revision surgical techniques vary and should not be amalgamated into one general category. There are numerous cementless stems with differing design philosophy and the results are not the same. There are those that depend on proximal fixation for stability and those that require distal osseous integration to achieve long-term stability and support.

Proximally porous-coated stems have had good results in the primary setting where good quality metaphyseal bone exists, but in revision arthroplasty the metaphysis is often deficient and sclerotic, making it difficult to achieve intimate bone contact and stability. Ideally, a proximal ingrowth design stem should transfer mechanical load to the top of the femur and increase proximal femoral bone stock through remodelling. The early designs of proximal ingrowth revision stems had unpredictable results with high subsidence rates.[108–111] Proximal ingrowth femoral components have evolved with new modular systems such as the S-ROM prosthesis (DePuy, Warsaw, IN), which relies on combined metaphyseal and diaphyseal support for stability with better results.[112–115] This design allows a porous-coated metaphyseal segment to be press-fitted proximally and mated with a slotted diaphyseal segment, which can provide initial stability through distal fixation. Modular systems allows for the construct to be assembled by the surgeon at the time of revision, enabling the establishment of the hip centre to restore joint stability and function.

Extensively porous-coated implants that achieve distal stability and bypass the compromised proximal femoral bone have had reliable results.[116–119] The rationale behind this technique is to obtain a scratch fit over a 5–7 cm segment of healthy distal femoral bone.[120] Poorer survivorship was seen among patients in whom the cortical bone damage extended more than 10 cm below the lesser trochanter.[121] The problems with extensively coated stems are stress shielding of the proximal femur and thigh pain.[118] Krishnamurthy et al.[117] report moderate to severe bone loss in 29% of femurs as a consequence of mechanically bypassing the proximal femur.

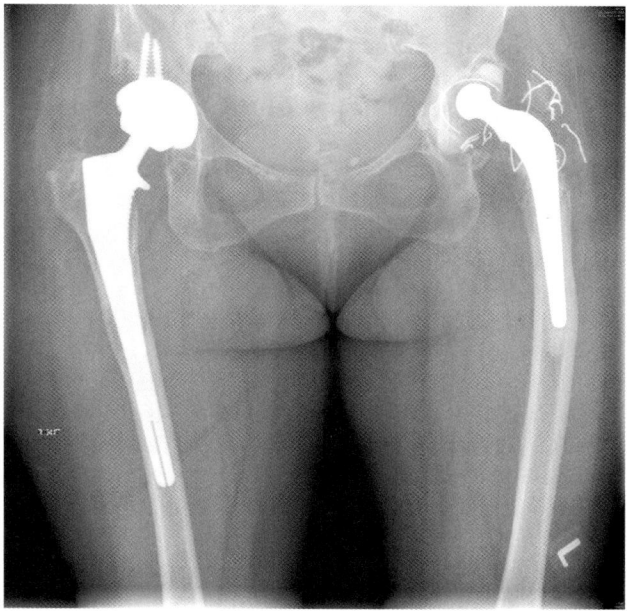

Figure 100.7 Revision of the right hip with a long fully hydroxyapatite-coated uncemented stem. Note that there is no distal hypertrophy and there was an absence of thigh pain in the patient. The left hip is awaiting revision.

A low degree of proximal bone loss and thigh pain is seen with hydroxyapatite-coated stems in revision surgery with good long-term results.[122,123] Also a low degree of distal bone hypertrophy was seen, suggesting a physiological weight distribution across both the proximal and distal portions of the stem to the femur[122] (Fig. 100.7).

ONE- OR TWO-STAGE REVISION FOR INFECTION

An infected arthroplasty is a major complication with a heavy economic burden and is often difficult to diagnose. A combination of clinical evaluation, blood investigations, imaging and microbiological assessment improves diagnostic ability. More importantly the combination of a negative erythrocyte sedimentation rate and C-reactive protein has a 95% specificity for ruling out the possibility of infection.[124] If either of these tests are positive and clinically one suspects infection, a hip aspiration has a high sensitivity and specificity and is recommended.[125–127] Nuclear imaging results vary in the literature from as low as 38% sensitivity[128] to 86% sensitivity[129] of a leucocyte-labelled scan.

Surgery in the form of a one- or two-stage component revision followed by antibiotics is the mainstay of treatment. In either case, eradication of infection can be difficult because of bacterial resistance to antibiotics, adhering to foreign bodies within biofilms,[130] poor penetration of antibiotics into infected bone,[131] presence of devascularized bone and occasionally inadequate debridement. Central to both one- and two-stage revision is local administration of high-dose antibiotics through a biocompatible medium such as polymethylmethacrylate cement. Addition of antibiotics to bone cement reduces its mechanical properties, but higher antibiotic levels can be achieved than with parenteral antibiotics.[132]

One-stage revision of an infected THR is attractive not only for the patient but has economic advantages and a reported success rate ranging from 77% to 100%.[133–135] In a literature review of one-stage revisions, 1299 cases were pooled from 12 studies; 83% were thought to be infection free at an average follow-up of 4.8 years. Antibiotic-impregnated bone cement was used in 99% of the cases, but there was a wide variability in the duration of parenteral antibiotic therapy, ranging from just 24 hours to 8 weeks. Factors associated with a successful direct result included: (1) absence of wound complications after the initial total hip replacement; (2) good general health of the patient; (3) meticillin-sensitive *S. epidermidis*, *S. aureus* and *Streptococcus* species; and (4) an organism that was sensitive to the antibiotic mixed into the bone cement. Factors associated with failure included (1) polymicrobial infection; (2) Gram-negative organisms, especially *Pseudomonas* species; and (3) certain Gram-positive organisms such as meticillin-resistant *S. epidermidis* and group D *Streptococcus*.[136]

Two-staged revision typically involves a thorough debridement and removal of the implant with placement of antibiotic cement in the form of beads, blocks or articulated spacers. An antibiotic-impregnated cement spacer can maintain soft-tissue tension and leg length and provide better function than a resection arthroplasty (Fig. 100.8). The total amount of antibiotics within the cement spacers varies considerably in the literature. In some series, as low as 2 g have been used, whereas other authors have placed close to 20 g of antibiotics per spacer without reported systemic side-effects. When comparing beads and spacers as antibiotic delivery systems, similar efficacy in eradication of infection was seen.[137] However, patient function in the interval between surgeries is though to be superior when spacers are used in comparison with beads. Most authors recognize 6 weeks of antibiotics as standard, and longer courses of antibiotics have not been beneficial.

A 94% success rate was obtained in two studies using antibiotic-impregnated spacers in two-stage revision for infection.[138,139] In one of the studies, the authors aspirated all the hip prior to reimplantation and intra-operative cultures were obtained at the time of reimplantation, which appeared to improve their overall success rate.[138] The main advantages of two-stage revision are a potentially lower reinfection rate, the ability to treat infections of unknown organism and the ability to use bone graft at the second stage.

KEY LEARNING POINTS

- The burden of revision surgery will inexorably rise in the future.
- The commonest indications for revision are aseptic loosening, infection, dislocation and periprosthetic fracture.
- The surgical approach must be guided by previous approaches, degree of bone loss and reason for revision.
- Removal of implants is often the most difficult and time-consuming part of revision surgery. Extreme care is needed to avoid further bone loss and intra-operative fractures. Many special techniques and devices are available.
- Reconstruction can be achieved with uncemented revision implants, cemented revision or by restoration of bone stock by impaction bone grafting (combined with cemented fixation).
- Revision for infection is a major problem, and debate remains over the merits of one- and two-stage revision.

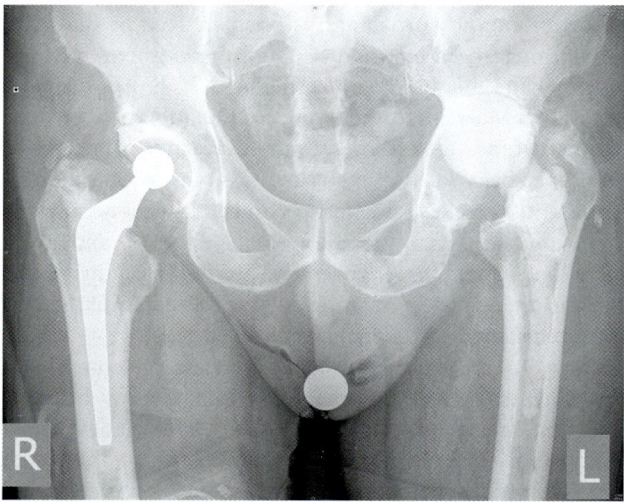

Figure 100.8 Articulating cement spacer made using commercially available prefabricated plastic cement moulds.

REFERENCES

- ● = Key primary paper
- ◆ = Major review article

1. Kim S. Changes in surgical loads and economic burden of hip and knee replacements in the US: 1997–2004. *Arthritis and Rheumatism* 2008;**59**:481–8.
◆2. Kurtz S, Mowat F, Ong K, et al. Prevalence of primary and revision total hip and knee arthroplasty in the United States from 1990 through 2002. *Journal of Bone and Joint Surgery (American)* 2005;**87**:1487–97.
3. National Institute for Health and Clinical Excellence. *Guidance on Selection of Prostheses for Primary Total Hip Replacement*. Technology Appraisal Guidance No. 2. London, UK: NICE, 2000.

4. Herberts, P, Malchau, H. Long-term registration has improved the quality of hip replacement: a review of the Swedish THR Register comparing 160,000 cases. *Acta Orthopaedica Scandinavica* 2000;**71**:111–21.
●5. Schmalzried TP, Jasty M, Harris WH. Periprosthetic bone loss in total hip arthroplasty. Polyethylene wear debris and the concept of the effective joint space. *Journal of Bone and Joint Surgery (American)* 1992;**74**:849–63.
●6. Green TR, Fisher J, Stone M, et al. Polyethylene particles of a 'critical size' are necessary for the induction of cytokines by macrophages in vitro. *Biomaterials* 1998;**19**:2297–302.
7. Aspenberg P, Van der Vis H. Fluid pressure may cause periprosthetic osteolysis Particles are not the only thing. *Acta Orthopaedica Scandinavica* 1998;**69**:1–4.
8. De Man FHR, Tigchelaar W, Marti RK, et al. Effects of mechanical compression of a fibrous tissue interface on bone with or without high-density polyethylene particles in a rabbit model of prosthetic loosening. *Journal of Bone and Joint Surgery (American)* 2005;**87**:1522–33.
9. Muirhead-Allwood SK. Lessons of a hip failure: if we want improved prostheses we must regulate their use. *British Medical Journal* 1998;**16**:644.
10. The Royal College of Surgeons of England. *An Investigation of the Performance of the 3M Capital Hip System*. London, UK: RCS, 2001. Available at: http://www.rcseng.ac.uk/publications/docs/investigation_3m_capital_hip.html
11. DePuy. *Elite Plus Total Hip Replacement System. Product Rationale*. Leeds, UK: DePuy International Ltd, 1993.
12. Hauptfleisch J, Glyn-Jones S, Beard DJ, et al. The premature failure of the Charnley Elite-Plus stem: a confirmation of RSA prediction. *Journal of Bone and Joint Surgery (British)* 2006;**88B**:179–83.
●13. DeLee JG, Charnley J. Radiological demarcation of cemented sockets in total hip replacement. *Clinical Orthopaedics and Related Research* 1976;**121**:20–32.
●14. Gruen TA, McNeice GM, Amstutz HC. 'Modes of failure' of cemented stem-type femoral components: a radiographic analysis of loosening. *Clinical Orthopaedics and Related Research* 1979;**141**:17–27.
15. Iwak H, Scott G, Freeman MA. The natural history and significance of radiolucent lines at a cemented femoral interface. *Journal of Bone and Joint Surgery (British)* 2002;**84**:550–5.
●16. Barrack RL, Mulroy Jr RD, Harris WH. Improved cementing techniques and femoral component loosening in young patients with hip arthroplasties: a 12-year radiographic review. *Journal of Bone and Joint Surgery (British)* 1992;**74B**:385–9.
17. Chambers IR, Fender D, McCaskie AW, et al. Radiological features predictive of aseptic loosening in cemented Charnley femoral stems. *Journal of Bone and Joint Surgery (British)*. 2001;**83**:838–42.
◆18. Lidwell OM. Clean air at operation and subsequent sepsis in the joint. *Clinical Orthopaedics and Related Research* 1986;**211**:91–102.
19. Sculco TP. The economic impact of infected total joint arthroplasty. *Instructional Course Lectures* 1993;**42**:349–51.
20. Swedish National Arthroplasty Register. *Annual Report 2006*. Available from: http://www.jru.orthop.gu.se/
21. Moran E, Masters S, Berendt AR, et al. Guiding empirical antibiotic therapy in orthopaedics: the microbiology of prosthetic joint infection managed by debridement, irrigation and prosthesis retention. *Journal of Infection* 2007;**55**:1–7.
22. Mohanty SS, Kay PR. Infection in total joint replacements. Why we screen MRSA when MRSE is the problem? *Journal of Bone and Joint Surgery (British)* 2004;**86**:266–8.
23. Fitzgerald Jr RH, Nolan DR, Ilstrup DM, et al. Deep wound sepsis following total hip arthroplasty. *Journal of Bone and Joint Surgery (American)* 1977;**59A**:847–55.
24. Tsukayama DT, Estrada R, Gustilo RB. Infection after total hip arthroplasty: a study of the treatment of one hundred and six infections. *Journal of Bone and Joint Surgery (American)* 1996;**78A**:512–23.
25. Wroblewski BM. The mechanism of fracture of the femoral prosthesis in total hip replacement. *International Orthopaedics* 1979;**3**:137–9.
26. Woolson ST, Milbauer JP, Bobyn JD, et al., Fatigue fracture of a forged cobalt-chromium-molybdenum femoral component inserted with cement. A report of ten cases. *Journal of Bone and Joint Surgery (American)* 1997;**79**:1842–8.
27. Miller A, Shastri R, Shih C. Fracture failure of a forged vitallium prosthesis. *Journal of Bone and Joint Surgery (American)* 1982;**64**:1359–63.
28. Marmor L, Gruen T. Stem fractures of extra-heavy cobra femoral hip prostheses. *Clinical Orthopaedics and Related Research* 1984;**190**:148.
29. Williams H, Browne G, Gie G, et al., The Exeter universal cemented femoral component at 8 to 12 years. A study of the first 325 hips. *Journal of Bone and Joint Surgery (British)* 2002;**84**:45.
30. Berli B, Schafer D, Morscher E. Ten-year survival of the MS-30 matt-surfaced cemented stem. *Journal of Bone and Joint Surgery (British)* 2005;**87B**:928.
31. Toni A, Sudanese A, Busanelli L, et al: Cementless arthroplasty using alumina ceramics as a coating and bearing material. In: Sedel L, Cabanela M (eds) *Hip Surgery Materials and Developments*. London, UK: Martin Dunitz, 1998:267–76.
32. Bizot P, Nizard R, Hamadouche M, et al. Prevention of wear and osteolysis: alumina-on-alumina bearing. *Clinical Orthopaedics and Related Research* 2001;**393**:85–93.
33. Willmann G. Ceramic femoral head retrieval data. *Clinical Orthopaedics and Related Research* 2000;**379**:22–8.
34. D'Antonio J, Capello W, Manley M, et al. Alumina ceramic bearings for total hip arthroplasty: five-year results of a prospective randomized study. *Clinical Orthopaedics and Related Research* 2005;**436**:164–71.
35. Bizot P, Hannouche D, Nizard R, et al. Hybrid alumina total hip arthroplasty using a press-fit metal-backed socket in patients younger than 55 years. A six- to 11-year evaluation. *Journal of Bone and Joint Surgery (British)* 2004;**86**:190–4.

36. D'Antonio J, Capello W, Manley M, Bierbaum B. New experience with alumina-on-alumina ceramic bearings for total hip arthroplasty. *Journal of Arthroplasty* 2002;**17**:390-7.
37. Kempf I, Semlitsch M. Massive wear of a steel ball head by ceramic fragments in the polyethylene acetabular cup after revision of a total hip prosthesis with fractured ceramic ball. *Archives of Orthopaedic and Trauma Surgery* 1990;**109**:284-7.
38. Allain J, Goutallier D, Voisin MC, Lemouel S. Failure of a stainless-steel femoral head of a revision total hip arthroplasty performed after a fracture of a ceramic femoral head: A case report. *Journal of Bone and Joint Surgery (American)* 1998;**80A**:1355-60.
39. Woo RY, Morrey BF. Dislocations after total hip arthroplasty. *Journal of Bone and Joint Surgery (American)* 1982;**64**:1295.
40. von Knoch M, Berry DJ, Harmsen WS, et al. Late dislocation after total hip arthroplasty. *Journal of Bone and Joint Surgery (American)* 2002;**84A**:1949.
41. Berry DJ, von Knoch M, Schleck CD, Harmsen WS. Effect of femoral head diameter and operative approach on risk of dislocation after primary total hip arthroplasty. *Journal of Bone and Joint Surgery (American)* 2005;**87**:2456-63.
42. Berry DJ. Epidemiology of periprosthetic fractures after major joint replacement: hip and knee. *Orthopedic Clinics of North America* 1999;**30**:183-90.
43. Beals RK, Tower SS. Periprosthetic fractures of the femur: an analysis of 93 fractures. *Clinical Orthopaedics and Related Research* 1996;**327**:238-46.
♦44. Duncan CP, Masri BA. Fractures of the femur after hip replacement. *Instructional Course Lectures* 1995;**45**:293-304.
45. Masri BA, Meek RM, Duncan CP. Periprosthetic fractures evaluation and treatment. *Clinical Orthopaedics and Related Research* 2004;**420**:80-95.
46. Haddad FS, Duncan CP, Berry DJ, et al. Periprosthetic femoral fractures around well-fixed implants: Use of cortical onlay allografts with or without a plate. *Journal of Bone and Joint Surgery (American)* 2002;**84A**:945-50.
47. Tsiridis E, Haddad FS, Gie GA. Dall-Miles plates for periprosthetic femoral fractures: a critical review of 16 cases. *Injury* 2003;**34**:107-10.
48. Sledge III JB, Abiri A. An algorithm for the treatment of Vancouver type B2 periprosthetic proximal femoral fractures. *Journal of Arthroplasty* 2002;**17**:887-92.
49. Marker DR, Seyler TM, Jinnah RH, et al. Femoral neck fractures after metal-on-metal total hip resurfacing: a prospective cohort study. *Journal of Arthroplasty* 2007;**22**(Suppl. 3):66-71.
50. Mont MA, Seyler TM, Ulrich SD, et al. Effect of changing indications and techniques on total hip resurfacing, *Clinical Orthopaedics and Related Research* 2007;**465**:63-70.
51. Shimmin AJ, Back D. Femoral neck fractures following Birmingham hip resurfacing. *Journal of Bone and Joint Surgery (British)* 2005;**87**:463-4.
52. Khan M, Kuiper JH, Edwards D, et al. Birmingham hip arthroplasty five to eight years of prospective multicenter results. *Journal of Arthroplasty* 2009;**24**:1044-50.
53. Ball ST, Le Duff MJ, Amstutz HC. Early results of conversion of a failed femoral component in hip resurfacing arthroplasty. *Journal of Bone and Joint Surgery (American)* 2007;**89**:735-41.
54. McGrath MS, Marker DR, Seyler TM, et al. Surface replacement is comparable to primary total hip arthroplasty. *Clinical Orthopaedics and Related Research* 2009;**467**:94-100.
55. Engelbrecht E, Heinert K. *Klassifikation und Behandlungsrichtlinien von Knochensubstanzverlusten bei Revisionsoperationen am Huftgelenkmittelfristige Ergebnisse. Primare und Revisionsalloarthroplastik Hrsg: Endo-Klinik.* Berlin, Germany: Springer-Verlag, 1987.
●56. Paprosky WG, Perona PG, Lawrence JM. Acetabular defect classification and surgical reconstruction in revision arthroplasty: a 6-year follow-up evaluation. *Journal of Arthroplasty* 1994;**9**:33-44.
57. Hardinge K. The direct lateral approach to the hip. *Journal of Bone and Joint Surgery (British)* 1982;**64**:17-19.
58. Ramesh M, O'Byrne JM, McCarthy N, et al. Damage to the superior gluteal nerve after the Hardinge approach to the hip. *Journal of Bone and Joint Surgery (British)* 1996;**78**:903-6.
59. Horwitz BR, Rockowitz NL, Goll SR, et al. A prospective randomized comparison of two surgical approaches to total hip arthroplasty. *Clinical Orthopaedics and Related Research* 1993;**291**:154-63.
●60. Younger TI, Bradford MS, Magnus RE, Paprosky WG. Extended proximal femoral osteotomy: a new technique for femoral revision arthroplasty. *Journal of Arthroplasty* 1995;**10**:329-38.
61. Noble AR, Branham DB, Willis MC, et al. Mechanical effects of the extended trochanteric osteotomy. *Journal of Bone and Joint Surgery (American)* 2005;**87**:521-9.
62. Brooks AT, Nelson CL, Stewart CL, et al. Effect of an ultrasonic device on temperatures generated in bone and on bone-cement structure. *Journal of Arthroplasty* 1993;**8**:413-18.
63. Callaghan JJ, Elder SH, Stranne SK, et al. Revision arthroplasty facilitated by ultrasonic tool cement removal: an evaluation of whole bone strength in a canine model. *Journal of Arthroplasty* 1992;**7**:495-500.
64. Slooff TJ, Huiskes R, van Horn J, Lemmens AJ. Bone grafting in total hip replacement for acetabular protrusion. *Acta Orthopaedica Scandinavica* 1984;**55**:593-6.
65. Gie GA, Linder L, Ling RSM, et al. Impacted cancellous allografts and cement for revision total hip arthroplasty. *Journal of Bone and Joint Surgery (British)* 1993;**75B**:14-21.
66. Dunlop DG, Brewster NT, Madabhushi SP, et al. Techniques to improve the shear strength of impacted bone graft: the effect of particle size and washing of the graft. *Journal of Bone and Joint Surgery (American)* 2003;**85A**:639-46.

67. Bolder SB, Verdonschot N, Schreurs BW. Technical factors affecting cup stability in bone impaction grafting. *Proceedings of the Institution of Mechanical Engineers Part H* 2007;**221**:81–6.
◆68. Schreurs BW, Busch VJ, Welten ML, *et al*. Acetabular reconstruction with impaction bone-grafting and a cemented cup in patients younger than fifty years old. *Journal of Bone and Joint Surgery (American)* 2004;**86A**:2385–92.
69. Slooff TJ, Schimmel JW, Buma P. Cemented fixation with bone grafts. *Orthopedic Clinics of North America* 1993;**24**:667–77.
70. Wachtl SW, Jung M, Jakob RP, *et al*. The Burch-Schneider antiprotrusio cage in acetabular revision surgery: a mean follow-up of 12 years. *Journal of Arthroplasty* 2000;**15**:959.
71. Perka C, Ludwig R. Reconstruction of segmental defects during revision procedures of the acetabulum with the Burch-Schneider anti-protrusio cage. *Journal of Arthroplasty* 2001;**16**:568.
72. Sporer SM, O'Rourke M, Paprosky WG. The treatment of pelvic discontinuity during acetabular revision. *Journal of Arthroplasty* 2005;**20**(Suppl. 2):79.
73. Weeden SH, Paprosky WG. Porous-ingrowth revision acetabular implants secured with peripheral screws. A minimum twelve-year follow-up. *Journal of Bone and Joint Surgery (American)* 2006;**88**:1266–71.
74. Hendricks KJ, Harris WH. High placement of noncemented acetabular components in revision total hip arthroplasty. A concise follow-up, at a minimum of fifteen years, of a previous report. *Journal of Bone and Joint Surgery (American)* 2006;**88**:2231–6.
75. Lachiewicz PF, Poon ED. Revision of a total hip arthroplasty with a Harris-Galante porous coated acetabular component inserted without cement. A follow-up note on the results at five to twelve years. *Journal of Bone and Joint Surgery (American)* 1998;**80A**:980.
76. Chareancholvanich K, Tanchuling A, Seki T, *et al*. Cementless acetabular revision for aseptic failure of cemented hip arthroplasty. *Clinical Orthopaedics and Related Research* 1999;**361**:140.
77. Garcia-Cimbrelo E. Porous coated cementless acetabular cups in revision surgery: a 6–11 year follow-up study. *Journal of Arthroplasty* 1999;**14**:397.
78. Jones CP, Lachiewicz PF. Factors influencing the longer-term survival of uncemented acetabular components used in total hip revisions. *Journal of Bone and Joint Surgery (American)* 2004;**86**:342–7.
79. Berry DJ, Sutherland CJ, Trousdale RT, *et al*. Bilobed oblong porous coated acetabular components in revision total hip arthroplasty. *Clinical Orthopaedics and Related Research* 2000;**371**:154.
80. Chen WM, Engh Jr CA, Hopper RH, *et al.*, Acetabular revision with use of a bilobed component inserted without cement in patients who have acetabular bone-stock deficiency. *Journal of Bone and Joint Surgery (American)* 2000;**82A**:197.
81. Köster G, Rading S. Revision of failed acetabular components utilizing a cementless oblong cup: an average 9-year follow-up study. *Archives of Orthopaedic and Trauma Surgery* 2009;**129**:603–8.
82. Paprosky WG, Sporer SS, Murphy BP. Addressing severe bone deficiency: what a cage will not do. *Journal of Arthroplasty* 2007;**22**(4 Suppl. 1):111–15.
83. Siegmeth A, Duncan CP, Masri BA, *et al*. Modular tantalum augments for acetabular defects in revision hip arthroplasty. *Clinical Orthopaedics and Related Research* 2009;**467**:199–205.
84. Flecher X, Sporer S, Paprosky W. Management of severe bone loss in acetabular revision using a trabecular metal shell. *Journal of Arthroplasty* 2008;**23**:949–55.
85. Estok DM, Harris WH. Long term results of cemented femoral revision using second generation techniques. An average 11 year follow-up evaluation. *Clinical Orthopaedics and Related Research* 1994;**299**:190–202.
86. Katz RP, Callaghan JJ, Sullivan PM, *et al*. Results of cemented femoral revision total hip arthroplasty using improved cementing techniques. *Clinical Orthopaedics and Related Research* 1995;**319**:178–83.
87. Pierson JL, Harris WH. Effect of improved cementing techniques in the longevity of fixation in revision cemented femoral arthroplasties. Average 8.8-year follow-up period. *Journal of Arthroplasty* 1995;**105**:581–91.
88. Amstutz HC, Steven ME, Ma SM, *et al*. Revision of aseptic loose total hip arthroplasties. *Clinical Orthopaedics and Related Research* 1982;**170**:21–33.
89. Englebrecht DJ, Weber FA, Sweet MBE, *et al*. Long term results of revision hip arthroplasty. *Journal of Bone and Joint Surgery (British)* 1990;**72B**:41–5.
90. Marti RK, Schuller HM, Besselaar PP, *et al*. Results of revision of hip arthroplasty with cement: a five to fourteen year follow-up study. *Journal of Bone and Joint Surgery (American)* 1990;**72A**:346–54.
91. Pellicci PM, Wilson Jr PD, Sledge CB, *et al*. Long term results of revision total hip replacement: a follow up report. *Journal of Bone and Joint Surgery (American)* 1985;**67A**:513–16.
92. Morrey BF, Kavanagh BF. Complications with revision of the femoral component of total hip arthroplasty. Comparison between cemented and uncemented techniques. *Journal of Arthroplasty* 1992;**7**:71–9.
93. Howie DW, Wimhurst JA, McGee MA, *et al*. Revision total hip replacement using cemented collarless double-taper femoral components. *Journal of Bone and Joint Surgery (British)* 2007;**89**:879–86.
94. Nelson IW, Bulstrode CJ, Mowat AG. Femoral allografts in revision of hip replacement. *Journal of Bone and Joint Surgery (British)* 1990;**72B**:151–2.
95. Capello WN. Impaction grafting plus cement for femoral component fixation in revision hip arthroplasty. *Orthopedics* 1994;**17**:878–9.

96. Leopold SS, Berger RA, Rosenberg AG, et al. Impaction allografting with cement for revision of the femoral component: a minimum four-year follow-up study with use of a precoated femoral stem. *Journal of Bone and Joint Surgery (American)* 1999;**81A**:1080–92.
97. Knight JL, Helming C. Collarless polished tapered impaction grafting of the femur during revision total hip arthroplasty: pitfalls of the surgical technique and follow-up in 31 cases. *Journal of Arthroplasty* 2000;**15**:159–65.
98. Masterson EL, Masri BA, Duncan CP. The cement mantle in the Exeter impaction allografting technique. A cause for concern. *Journal of Arthroplasty* 1997;**12**:759–64.
99. Pekkarinen J, Alho A, Lepisto J, et al. Impaction bone grafting in revision hip surgery: a high incidence of complications. *Journal of Bone and Joint Surgery (British)* 2000;**82B**:103–7.
100. Kuiper JH, Soliman A, Cheah K, Richardson JB. Stability of impaction-grafted hip and knee prostheses: surgical technique, implant design and graft compaction. In: Delloye C, Bannister G (eds) *Impaction Bone Grafting in Revision Arthroplasty*. New York, NY: Marcel Dekker, 2004:75–94.
101. Bavadekar A, Cornu O, Godts B, et al. Stiffness and compactness of morselized grafts during impaction: an in vitro study with human femoral heads. *Acta Orthopaedica Scandinavica* 2001;**72**:470–6.
102. Hostner J, Hultmark P, Karrholm J, et al. Impaction technique and graft treatment in revisions of the femoral component. *Journal of Arthroplasty* 2001;**16**:76–82.
103. van Doorn WJ, ten Have BL, van Biezen FC, et al. Migration of the femoral stem after impaction bone grafting. First results of an ongoing, randomised study of the Exeter and Elite Plus femoral stems using radiostereometric analysis. *Journal of Bone and Joint Surgery (British)* 2002;**84**:825–31.
104. Eldridge JD, Smith EJ, Hubble MJ, et al. Massive early subsidence following femoral impaction grafting. *Journal of Arthroplasty* 1997;**12**:535–40.
105. Meding JB, Ritter MA, Keating EM, Faris PM. Impaction bone-grafting before insertion of a femoral stem with cement in revision total hip arthroplasty. A minimum two-year follow-up study. *Journal of Bone and Joint Surgery (American)* 1997;**79A**:1834–41.
106. Wraighte PJ, Howard PW. Femoral impaction bone allografting with an Exeter cemented collarless, polished, tapered stem in revision hip replacement: a mean follow-up of 10.5 years. *Journal of Bone and Joint Surgery (British)* 2008;**90**:1000–4.
107. Halliday BR, English HW, Timperley AJ, et al. Femoral impaction grafting with cement in revision total hip replacement. Evolution of the technique and results. *Journal of Bone and Joint Surgery (British)* 2003;**85**:809–17.
108. Malkani AL, Lewallen DG, Cabanela ME, et al. Femoral component revision using an uncemented, proximally coated, long-stem prosthesis. *Journal of Arthroplasty* 1996;**11**:411–18.
109. Woolson ST, Delaney TJ. Failure of a proximally porous-coated femoral prosthesis in revision total hip arthroplasty. *Journal of Arthroplasty* 1995;**10**(Suppl.):22–8.
110. Hussamy O, Lachiewicz PF. Revision total hip arthroplasty with the BIAS (Biologic Ingrowth Anatomic System) femoral component: three to six-year results. *Journal of Bone and Joint Surgery (American)* 1994;**76A**:1137–48.
111. Berry DJ, Harmsen WS, Ilstrup D, et al. Survivorship of uncemented proximally porous-coated femoral components. *Clinical Orthopaedics and Related Research*. 1995;**319**:168–77.
112. McCarthy JC, Lee JA. Complex revision total hip arthroplasty with modular stems at a mean of 14 years. *Clinical Orthopaedics and Related Research* 2007;**465**:166–9.
113. Cameron HV. The long-term success of modular proximal fixation stems in revision total hip. *Journal of Arthroplasty* 2002;**17**(Suppl.):138–41.
114. Christie MJ, DeBoer DK, Tingstad EM, et al. Clinical experience with a modular noncemented femoral component in revision total hip arthroplasty: 4- to 7-year results. *Journal of Arthroplasty* 2000;**15**:840–8.
115. Walter WL, Walter WK, Zicat B. Clinical and radiographic assessment of a modular cementless ingrowth femoral stem system for revision hip arthroplasty. *Journal of Arthroplasty* 2006;**21**:172–8.
116. Hamilton WG, Cashen DV, Ho H, et al. Extensively porous-coated stems for femoral revision: a choice for all seasons. *Journal of Arthroplasty* 2007;**22**(4 Suppl. 1):106–10.
117. Krishnamurthy AB, MacDonald SJ, Paprosky WG. 5-13-year follow study on cementless femoral components in revision surgery. *Journal of Arthroplasty* 1997;**12**:839–47.
118. Engh CA, Culpepper WJ, Kassapidis E. Revision of loose cementless femoral prostheses to larger porous coated components. *Clinical Orthopaedics and Related Research*. 1998;**347**:168–78.
119. Kim YH. Long-term results of the cementless porous-coated anatomic total hip prosthesis. *Journal of Bone and Joint Surgery (British)* 2005;**87**:623–7.
120. McAuley JP, Engh Jr CA. Femoral fixation in the face of considerable bone loss: cylindrical and extensively coated femoral components, *Clinical Orthopaedics and Related Research* 2004;**429**:215
121. Engh Jr CA, Hopper Jr RH, Engh CA. Distal ingrowth components. *Clinical Orthopaedics and Related Research* 2004;**420**:135–41.
122. Reikerås O, Gunderson RB. Excellent results with femoral revision surgery using an extensively hydroxyapatite-coated stem: 59 patients followed for 10–16 years. *Acta Orthopaedica* 2006;**77**:98–103.
123. Crawford CH, Malkani AL, Incavo SJ, et al. Femoral component revision using an extensively hydroxyapatite-coated stem. *Journal of Arthroplasty* 2004;**19**:8–13.
124. Spangehl MJ, Masri BA, O'Connell JX, Duncan CP. Prospective analysis of preoperative and intraoperative investigations for the diagnosis of infection at the sites of two hundred and two revision total hip arthroplasties. *Journal of Bone and Joint Surgery (American)* 1999;**81**:672–82.

125. Lachiewicz PF, Rogers GD, Thomason HC. Aspiration of the hip joint before revision total hip arthroplasty. Clinical and laboratory factors influencing attainment of a positive culture. *Journal of Bone and Joint Surgery (American)* 1996;**78**:749-54.
126. Spangehl MJ, Younger ASE, Masri BA, Duncan CP. Diagnosis of infection following total hip arthroplasty. *Journal of Bone and Joint Surgery (American)* 1997;**79**:1578-88.
127. Ali F, Wilkinson JM, Cooper JR, et al. Accuracy of joint aspiration for the preoperative diagnosis of infection in total hip arthroplasty. *Journal of Arthroplasty* 2006;**21**:221-6.
128. Kraemer WJ, Saplys R, Waddell JP, Morton J. Bone scan, gallium scan, and hip aspiration in the diagnosis of infected total hip arthroplasty. *Journal of Arthroplasty* 1993;**8**:611-15.
129. Palestro CJ, Kim CK, Swyer AJ, et al. Total-hip arthroplasty: periprosthetic indium-111-labeled leukocyte activity and complementary technetium-99m-sulfur colloid imaging in suspected infection. *Journal of Nuclear Medicine* 1955;**31**:1950-5.
130. Costerton JW. Biofilm theory can guide the treatment of device-related orthopaedic infections. *Clinical Orthopaedics and Related Research* 2005;**437**:7-11.
131. Wilson KJ, Mader JT. Concentrations of vancomycin in bone and serum of normal rabbits and those with osteomyelitis. *Antimicrobial Agents and Chemotherapy* 1984;**25**:140-1.
132. Wahlig H, Dingeldein E, Bergmann R, Reuss K. The release of gentamicin from polymethylmethacrylate beads: an experimental and pharmacokinetic study. *Journal of Bone and Joint Surgery (British)* 1978;**60B**:270-5.
133. Buchholz HW, Elson RA, Engelbrect E, et al. Management of deep infection of total hip replacement. *Journal of Bone and Joint Surgery (British)* 1981;**63**:342-52.
134. Ure KJ, Amstutz HC, Nasser S, Schmalzried TP. Direct-exchange arthroplasty for the treatment of infection after total hip arthroplasty. An average ten-year follow-up. *Journal of Bone and Joint Surgery (American)* 1998;**80**:961-8.
135. Callaghan JJ, Katz RP, Johnston RC. One-stage revision surgery of the infected hip. A minimum 10-year followup study. *Clinical Orthopaedics and Related Research* 1999;**369**:139-43.
136. Jackson WO, Schmalzried TP. Limited role of direct exchange arthroplasty in the treatment of infected total hip replacements. *Clinical Orthopaedics and Related Research* 2000;**381**:101-5.
137. Hsieh P, Shin C, Chang Y, et al. Two stage revision hip arthroplasty fro infection. *Journal of Bone and Joint Surgery (American)* 2004;**86**:1989-97.
138. Younger AS, Duncan CP, Masri BA, McGraw RW. The outcome of two-stage arthroplasty using a custom-made interval spacer to treat the infected hip. *Journal of Arthroplasty* 1997;**12**:615-23.
139. Hofmann AA, Goldberg TD, Tanner AM, Cook TM. Ten-year experience using an articulating antibiotic cement hip spacer for the treatment of chronically infected total hip. *Journal of Arthroplasty* 2005;**20**:874-9.

SECTION 3

The knee

SHI-LU CHIA, MARK G FREEMAN

101	**Development of knee arthroplasty** *Shi-Lu Chia, Ser Kiat Tan*	1171
102	**Total knee arthroplasty** *Shi-Lu Chia, Boon Keng Tay*	1176
103	**Unicompartmental knee arthroplasty** *Seo-Kiat Goh, Seng Jin Yeo, Boon Keng Tay*	1186
104	**Patellofemoral arthroplasty of the knee** *Erica D Taylor, Mark D Miller*	1193
105	**Revision knee arthroplasty** *Shi-Lu Chia, Ngai-Nung Lo*	1198

101

Development of knee arthroplasty

SHI-LU CHIA, SER KIAT TAN

Early developments	1171	Emerging trends in knee arthroplasty	1174
The modern era	1172	References	1175

NATIONAL BOARD STANDARD

- To understand the development of knee arthroplasty and the objectives/principles of implant design

EARLY DEVELOPMENTS

The first account of knee arthroplasty is often attributed to Verneuil, who in 1860 described the formation of a 'false articulation' within the arthritic knee by using soft-tissue interposition. Later in the nineteenth century, Dr Theophilus Gluck designed a knee prosthesis made of ivory, which he implanted in patients using a combination of plaster of Paris and colophony (a type of resin) (Fig. 101.1). As might be expected, these early attempts met with little success and often had disastrous results because of infection and loss of fixation.

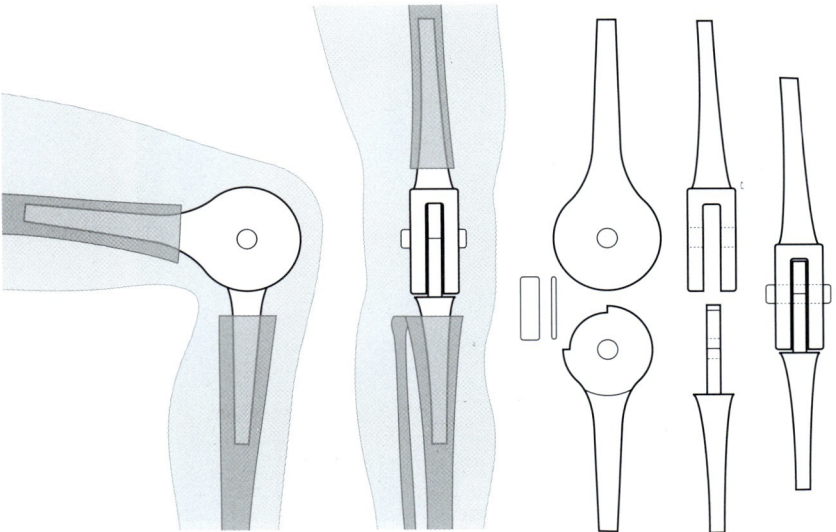

Figure 101.1 The Gluck knee prosthesis, made of ivory and bonded to the bone using a type of resin and plaster of Paris.

THE MODERN ERA

The development of prosthetic knee arthroplasty in the modern era was inspired by the positive results obtained with hip arthroplasty. Encouraging results from early mould hip arthroplasty stimulated Campbell to develop femoral mould interposition arthroplasty in 1940, and also spurred the development of the Massachusetts General Hospital mould femoral hemiarthroplasty during the same period. This prosthesis acted like a spacer and was not attached to the underlying femur; therefore, although it brought some symptomatic relief, the outcomes were neither predictable nor durable.

In the 1950s, MacIntosh developed a knee hemiarthroplasty comprising an acrylic tibial prosthesis, and McKeever developed a similar prosthesis at the Brigham and Women's Hospital in Boston, MA. These devices would today be more accurately described as unicompartmental spacer prostheses. The McKeever prosthesis is still in limited use today for patients who are too young and active for unicompartmental knee replacement and are not candidates for osteotomy (Fig. 101.2).[1]

Modern total knee arthroplasty arguably began in 1968 with Frank Gunston's design. Gunston was a Canadian orthopaedic surgeon who was working at the Charnley Hip Centre at Wrightington Hospital, Wigan, UK. His design incorporated metallic runners in the distal femur that articulated with polyethylene troughs that were embedded in the proximal tibia. These components were affixed to the bone with acrylic cement, the forerunner of today's polymethylmethacrylate bone cement. Hence, all the components recognizable in a modern knee replacement were present: a metallic femoral component that articulates with a plastic tibial component, both of which were securely attached to the underlying bone with a fixative (cement) (Fig. 101.3). This was a predecessor of unicompartmental designs.

Freeman and co-workers[2] developed this concept even further into the design known as the Freeman–Swanson prosthesis (Fig. 101.4). The ICLH (Imperial College London Hospital) prothesis was a modification of the Freeman-Swanson Prosthesis. Freeman et al.[2] considered the following to be important objectives in the design of a knee prosthesis:

- A *salvage* procedure should be available. It was suggested then that there should remain enough bone stock for arthrodesis.
- The tendency for implant *loosening* should be minimized by:
  - avoidance of complete constraint between the femoral and tibial components
  - low friction
  - limitation of hyperextension, which should be via a gradual mechanism
  - the load that is transmitted across the components should be spread over as large an area as possible.
- The rate of production of *wear debris* should be minimized.
- The probability of *infection* should be minimized.
- The *consequences of infection*, should it occur, should be minimized by avoiding long intramedullary extension of the implants.
- *Insertion* of the prosthesis should be standardized and repeatable.
- The prosthesis should allow *movement* from 5° hyperextension to at least 90° of flexion.
- *Stability* of the prosthetic joint should be afforded by the soft tissues, and in particular the collateral ligaments.

Not everyone agreed with Freeman's opinion regarding constraint, and, from the 1950s onwards, a series of fully constrained hinged prostheses were developed. One of the earliest examples was the Walldius prosthesis, and this was followed by other hinged implants that were all unce-

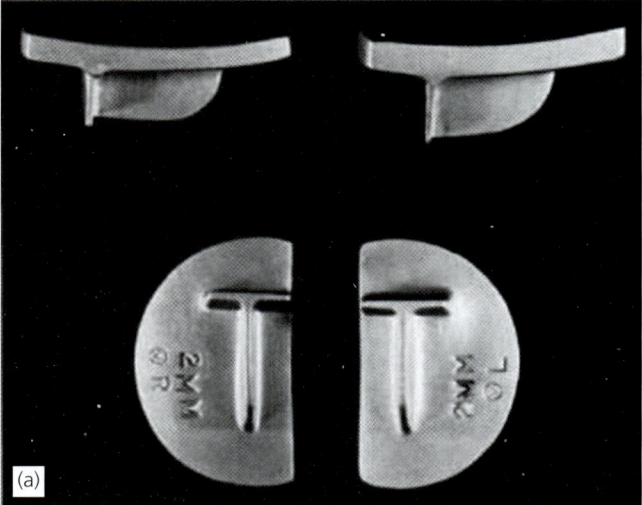
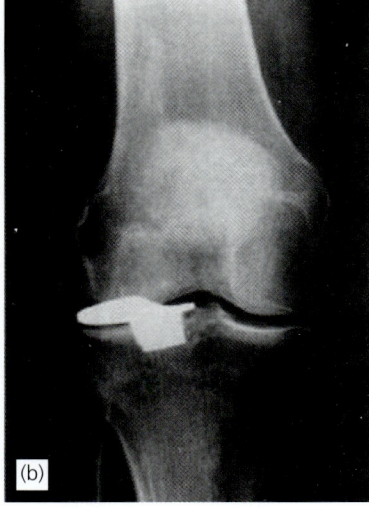

Figure 101.2 McKeever hemiarthroplasty. (a) McKeever knee hemiarthoplasty prostheses. (b) Plain radiograph of McKeever prosthetic arthroplasty in a patient with lateral compartment osteoarthritis. Reproduced with permission from Scott et al.[5]

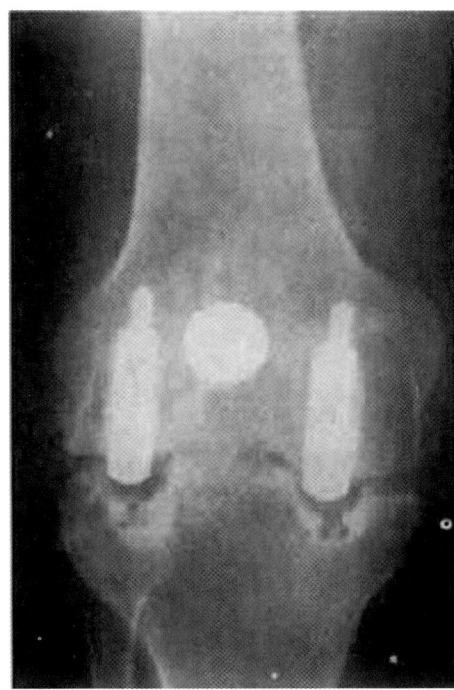
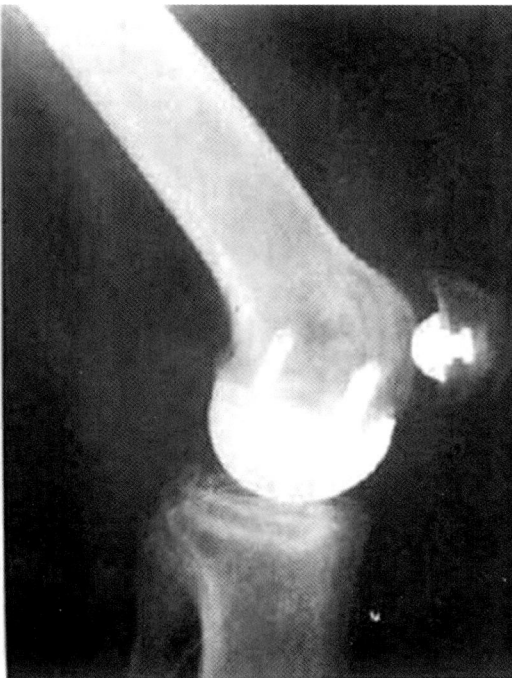

Figure 101.3 Gunston knee prosthesis. Gunston knee arthroplasty incorporating metallic femoral runners that articulate with polyethylene tibial troughs. Note also the metallic patellar button prosthesis. Reproduced with permission from Gunston FH et al. *Clinical Orthopaedics and Related Research* 1976;**120**:11–17.

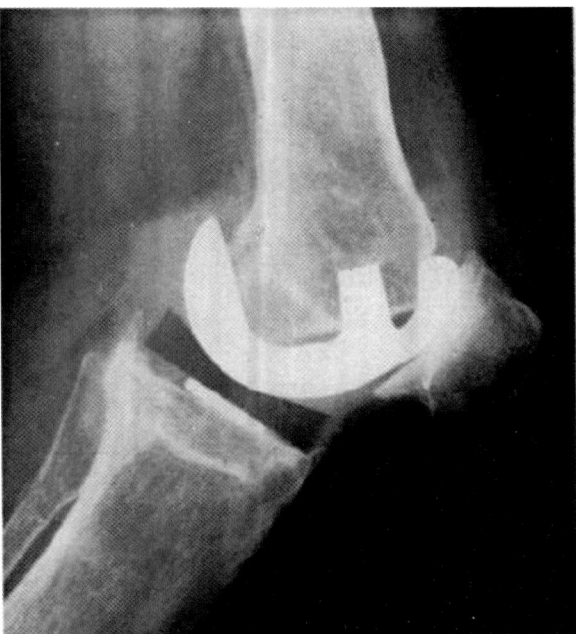
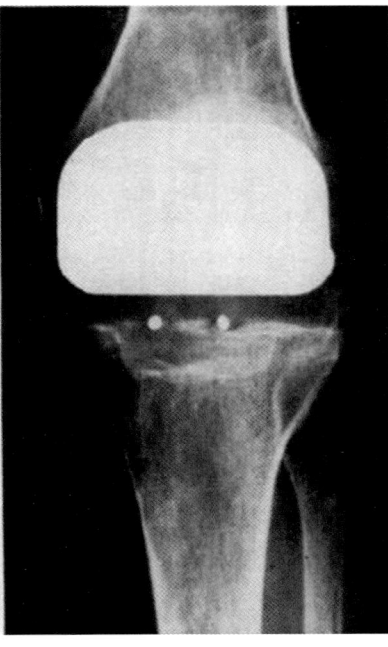

Figure 101.4 Freeman–Swanson knee arthroplasty. Reproduced with permission from Gibbs AN et al. *Journal of Bone and Joint Surgery (British)* 1979;**61**:358–61.

mented. The attractions of using hinged prostheses included the ease of alignment of the limb, and the ability to disregard, to some extent, the condition of the periarticular soft tissues as the hinge meant that such implants were intrinsically stable.[3] However, as predicted by Freeman et al.,[2] the main problem with these implants was their tendency towards loosening because of increased stresses at the implant–bone interface.

In the USA, the Marmor prosthesis succeeded the McKeever prosthesis. The Marmor could be used as a unicompartmental or bicompartmental prosthesis. The Marmor worked well for unicompartmental disease, and an evolved version is in current use as a successful unicompartmental replacement, but the bicompartmental version suffered issues with coronal subluxation.[4] Thus, in the early 1970s, the duocondylar prosthesis replaced the Marmor prosthesis for the treatment of bicompartmental knee osteoarthritis. However, the duocondylar prosthesis did not address the patellofemoral compartment, and hence many patients suffered residual patellofemoral symptoms.[5]

Also in the 1970s, Peter Walker, Chitranjan Ranawat and John Insall developed the total condylar and duopatellar prostheses. The total condylar prosthesis sacrificed both cruciate ligaments, and is the immediate forerunner of modern cruciate-sacrificing/cruciate-substituting knee arthroplasty (Fig. 101.5). In stark contrast, the duopatellar

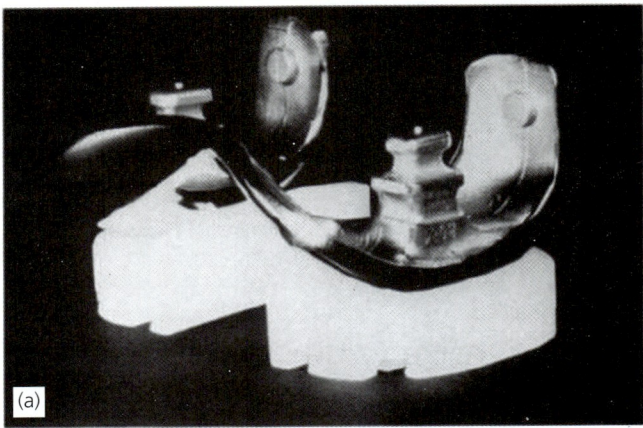
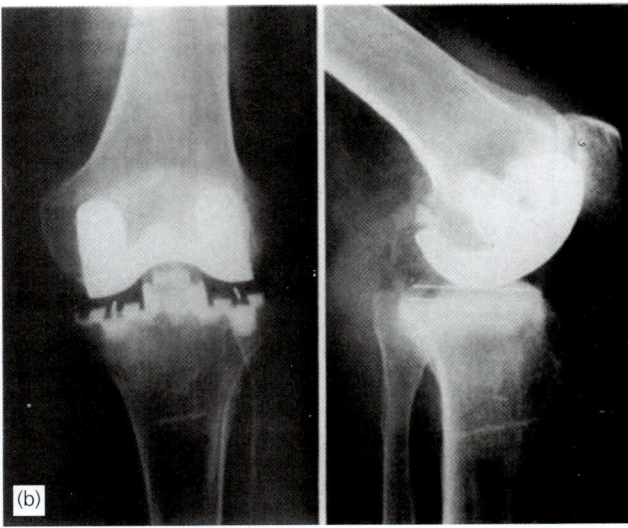

Figure 101.5 Total condylar knee prosthesis. (a) Instrumentation for tibial and femoral cuts for the total condylar knee replacement. (b) Plain radiographs of total condylar knee replacement. Reproduced with permission from Insall et al.[6]

design, much like the duocondylar design, preserved both ligaments, and the tibial component comprised two separate tibial trays divided by the tibial spines. However, because of the small contact areas of the individual trays, the tibial component was prone to loosening. Thus, the design was changed to a one-piece all-polyethylene component, which was similar in many ways to that of the total condylar prosthesis. The duopatellar knee prosthesis was thus one of the key forerunners of today's cruciate-retaining designs.

The total condylar design had higher conformity and contact area, thus giving it better stability but with the disadvantage of a reduced range of motion that was typically limited to 90°.[6] The duopatellar design was less conforming and allowed more rollback and better motion, but required a more meticulous surgical technique for alignment and soft-tissue balance.[7] The further significance of these implants was twofold: (1) they incorporated specific cemented components for the femur, tibia and patella, allowing for total condylar replacement, and (2) they were designed together with specific instrumentation for their implantation.

EMERGING TRENDS IN KNEE ARTHROPLASTY

With improvements in materials, implant design and surgical technique, the survivorship of modern knee replacement is excellent. The challenge seems to lie in developing implants that better reproduce normal knee kinematics. Many feel that the path to this end lies in implants that conserve more bone and soft tissue. This would also help to reduce surgical trauma and improve the recovery experience.

As with many cases of technology evolution, the development of knee arthroplasty seems to have come full circle. Hence, we are looking again at compartment-specific knee replacement, and at implants which are truly surface replacing. There is also great interest in custom implants, which are manufactured based on detailed anatomical images of the patient's knee. As always, advances in materials science are improving the longevity of artificial joints, and hopefully together with improved manufacturing this will help reduce costs as well.

KEY LEARNING POINTS

- A salvage procedure should be available (arthrodesis).
- Implant loosening should be minimized by avoidance of complete constraint; low friction; limitation of hyperextension; and the load transmitted should be spread over as large an area as possible.
- The rate of production of wear debris should be minimized.
- Infection should be minimized.
- The consequences of infection should be minimized by avoiding long intramedullary extension of the implants.
- Insertion of the prosthesis should be standardized and repeatable.
- The prosthesis should allow movement from 5° hyperextension to at least 90° of flexion.
- The stability of the prosthetic joint should be afforded by the soft tissues, and in particular the collateral ligaments.
- The challenge is to develop implants which better reproduce normal knee kinematics.

In the future, we may also be able to manufacture implants which are biological–prosthetic composites with self-renewal capabilities, or perhaps even fully biological knee replacements that will finally fulfil the early promises of tissue engineering.

REFERENCES

1. Springer BD, Scott RD, Sah AP, Carrington R. McKeever hemiarthroplasty of the knee in patients less than sixty years old. *Journal of Bone and Joint Surgery (American)* 2006;**88**:366–71.
2. Freeman MA, Swanson SA, Todd RC. Total replacement of the knee using the Freeman-Swanson knee prosthesis. *Clinical Orthopaedics and Related Research* 1973;**94**:153–70.
3. Insall J, Clarke HD. Historic development, classification and characteristics of knee prostheses. In: Insall J, Scott WN (eds) *Surgery of the Knee*. Philadelphia, PA: Churchill Livingstone, 2001:1516–52.
4. Scott RD. *Total Knee Arthroplasty*. Philadelphia, PA: Elsevier, 2006:1–7.
5. Scott RD, Joyce MJ, Ewald FC, Thomas WH. McKeever metallic hemiarthroplasty of the knee in unicompartmental degenerative arthritis. Long-term clinical follow-up and current indications. *Journal of Bone and Joint Surgery (American)* 1985;**67**:203–7.
6. Insall J, Ranawat CS, Scott WN, Walker P. Total condylar knee replacement: preliminary report. *Clinical Orthopaedics and Related Research* 1976;**120**:149–54.
7. Ranawat CS, Insall J, Shine J. Duo-condylar knee arthroplasty: hospital for special surgery design. *Clinical Orthopaedics and Related Research* 1976;**120**:76–82.

Total knee arthroplasty

SHI-LU CHIA, BOON KENG TAY

Introduction	1176	Implant choices and configurations	1178
Indications for total knee arthroplasty	1176	Surgical considerations	1181
Surgical goals in total knee arthroplasty	1177	Results of total knee arthroplasty	1184
Pre-operative assessment and planning	1177	References	1184

NATIONAL BOARD STANDARD

- To understand the principles of total knee arthroplasty including indications, goals, planning, implant choices, surgical technique and the results.

INTRODUCTION

Despite advances in our understanding of cartilage biology and osteoarthrosis (see Chapter 6), and the promise of chondrocyte implantation techniques for chondral defects, the most reliable option for symptomatic control and functional restoration in the end-stage osteoarthritic knee is prosthetic replacement.

Arthroplasty, or joint replacement, can be most simply defined as the functional substitution of the articulating surfaces of the joint. This definition draws together the many variants of arthroplasty that exist:

- *conventional* prosthetic arthroplasty in which the diseased cartilage and adjoining bone are resected and replaced with metal and/or plastic
- *resurfacing* arthroplasty in which only the diseased portion is removed and the contour reconstituted, typically with a biological graft such as cells or an allograft
- *interpositional* arthroplasty in which the diseased surfaces are left *in situ* and a biological or prosthetic graft is placed between these surfaces to restore smooth articulation.

This chapter concerns conventional total prosthetic arthroplasty of the knee, in which the articulating surfaces of the femur and tibia are replaced in their entirety by an artificial joint. In these cases, the native patella may or may not be resurfaced with a prosthetic patella.

INDICATIONS FOR TOTAL KNEE ARTHROPLASTY

It is important to recognize that the indication for total knee arthroplasty (TKA) in the arthritic patient is relative and the decision to proceed with TKA is primarily based on the patient's symptom severity and his or her functional requirements. Indications include:

- Severe osteoarthritis, whether primary or secondary, affecting one or more compartments of the knee, which cannot be satisfactorily managed by conservative or other surgical means. Although unicompartmental arthroplasty is possible for patients with disease restricted to one knee compartment, some patients may still choose to proceed with TKA after being counselled on the merits/demerits of compartmental arthroplasty versus TKA. In general, TKA is offered to elderly patients (typically >70 years old), whereas in younger patients other techniques are preferred to control symptoms until they reach an age where prosthetic arthroplasty becomes definitive treatment. The primary consideration here is the longevity of the implant, and the likelihood that the patient would require revision surgery in his or her lifetime. However, in some cases when the osteoarthritis is severe and no other effective option is available, TKA may be offered to younger

patients, e.g. patients who are unsuitable for tibial or femoral realignment osteotomy, young patients with severe haemophiliac arthropathy.
- Joint reconstruction using special megaprostheses as an alternative to allografts in limb-preserving surgery for tumours involving the knee.
- Joint reconstruction following severe trauma resulting in non-reconstructible loss of the articular surfaces, as an alternative to allografts.

The only absolute contraindication to TKA is ongoing sepsis, whether localized to the knee or systemic.

SURGICAL GOALS IN TOTAL KNEE ARTHROPLASTY

The success of TKA is critically dependent on proper implant positioning and limb alignment. Surgical aims include:

- preservation of the joint line
- restoration of a normal mechanical axis, i.e. 0°
- balanced flexion and extension bone gaps
- balanced soft-tissue restraints, maintaining adequate medial/lateral (coronal) and anteroposterior (sagittal) joint stability
- good patellar tracking (maintaining or restoring a normal Q angle).

If the above goals are met, then the knee will be stable and have a good range of motion, and forces should be optimally distributed across the articulating surfaces, promoting implant longevity.

PRE-OPERATIVE ASSESSMENT AND PLANNING

Clinical

Look out for (conditions indicated in parentheses are considered as complex cases which may require specialized techniques/equipment/prostheses):

- extent of varus and valgus deformity (varus deformity >15° and valgus deformity >20°)
- range of motion of the knee (range of motion <90° is considered a stiff knee)
- amount of fixed flexion deformity (FFD; >20°)
- degree of hyperextension of the knee if present (hyperextension >15°)
- competency of the collateral ligaments
- competency of the posterior cruciate ligament (PCL), if a cruciate-retaining prosthesis is planned
- vascular status of the limb should be assessed; the absence of palpable distal pulses should prompt a vascular work-up
- neurological status of the limb, particularly the lateral peroneal nerve in a valgus knee
- status of the skin, and presence of previous incisions which may affect the vascularity of the planned incision
- presence of ipsilateral hip disease.

Radiological

The standard set of films for the primary TKA patient is as follows (Fig. 102.1):

- anteroposterior weight bearing
- lateral weight bearing, with the knee in 30–45° flexion
- axial view of the patella, e.g. Merchant's view.

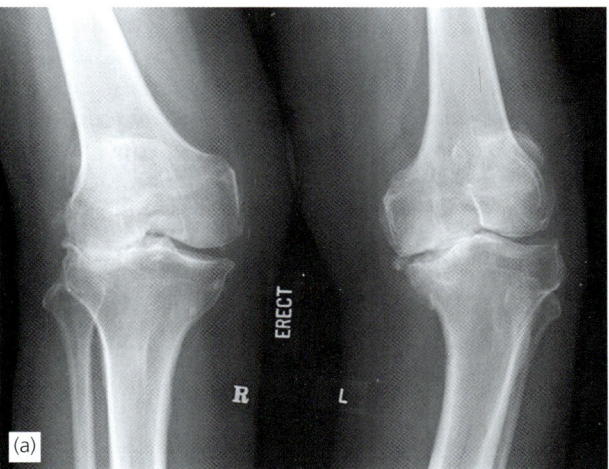
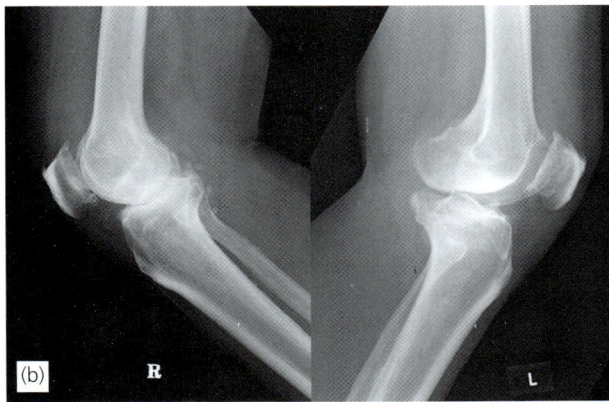
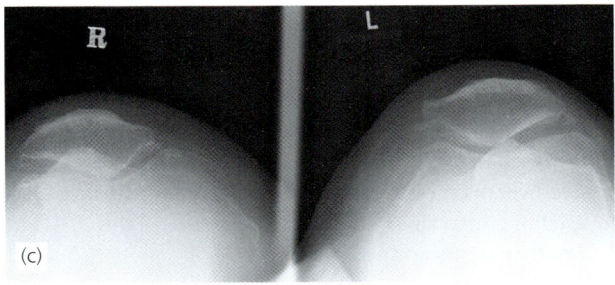

Figure 102.1 Standard set of plain radiographs of the knee for pre-operative evaluation of the patient under consideration for knee arthroplasty. (a) Anteroposterior; (b) lateral weight bearing; (c) skyline views of the patellae.

Typically, both knees are imaged, and long-leg films from the hip to the feet are preferred for evaluation of the mechanical axis.

The radiographs are examined for:

- confirmation of joint disease
- degree of coronal deformity
- amount of bone loss at the femoral and tibial articular surfaces
- presence of bony abnormalities that may affect judgement of component alignment intra-operatively, e.g. malunited tibial or femoral fractures
- planning of distal femoral and proximal tibial cuts (see below)
- sizing of the implants; the anteroposterior film is used for sizing of the tibial component as the medial–lateral dimension is important for good plateau coverage, whereas the lateral film is typically used for sizing of the femoral component since the anteroposterior dimension of the femoral component is more critical, e.g. to avoid notching of the anterior femoral shaft
- patellofemoral disease.

IMPLANT CHOICES AND CONFIGURATIONS

The parts of a typical total knee prosthesis comprise the (Fig. 102.2):

- femoral component
- tibial component
- tibial articular surface (component)
- patellar component.

The femoral and tibial components are typically made of metals such as cobalt chrome or titanium, whereas the articular and patellar components are typically made of ultra-high-molecular-weight polyethylene (UHMWPE). The tibial component may also be of a 'monoblock' configuration and be completely fabricated from UHMWPE ('all-polyethylene tibial component').

Under certain circumstances, such as in the presence of significant bony defects, metallic blocks/wedges (augments) may be fixed to the femoral and/or tibial components. To better distribute the transfer of stresses, metallic stems may also be attached to the femoral and/or tibial components (see below).

The main decisions regarding implant type and configuration are:

- PCL-retaining versus substituting
- fixed versus mobile bearing tibial articular surface
- level of constraint
- whether stems are necessary
- whether to resurface the patella or not.

The components are usually all cemented into position, although some designs feature a porous-coated cementless femoral component (a hybrid design consists of a cemented tibial component with a cementless femoral component).

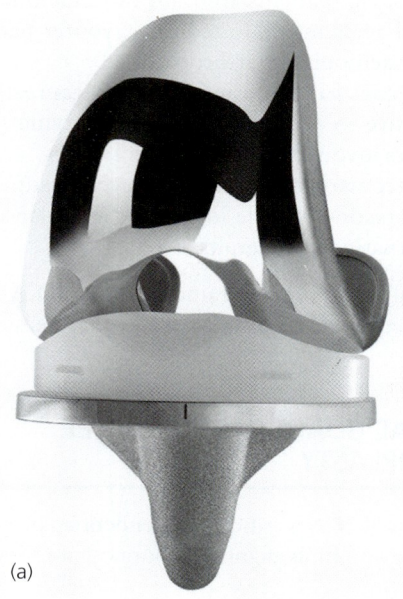

(a)

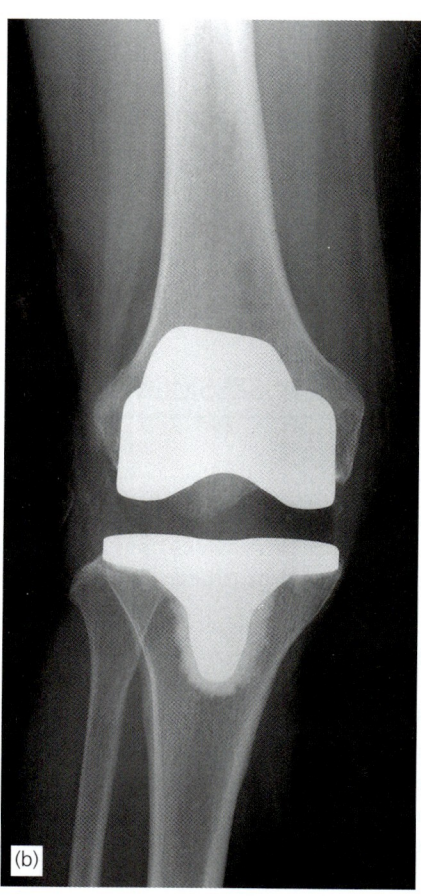

(b)

Figure 102.2 (a) A modern knee replacement prosthesis with cobalt chrome femoral and tibial components, and modular polyethylene articular insert. This is a cruciate-retaining, mobile bearing design. (b) Radiograph of a knee replacement with the prosthesis seen in (a).

In general, arguments can be made and evidence can be found for choosing almost every TKA configuration mentioned above; obviously, designs with poor results would already have been eliminated from the market.

PCL-retaining versus substituting total knee arthroplasty

The advantages/disadvantages of either are generally theoretical except in certain special circumstances (Table 102.1), as the reported clinical results of both designs are comparable, in terms of both implant survival and performance.

The most cited advantage of retaining the PCL is preservation of femoral 'roll-back'. Femoral roll-back refers to the shift of the femoral condyle posteriorly on the tibial plateau as the knee flexes, i.e. the femoral–tibial contact point in the sagittal plane 'rolls' to the 'back' as the knee moves into flexion. This roll-back facilitates high degrees of knee flexion by preventing the posterior femur from impinging on the posterior tibia. Roll-back only occurs if the PCL is intact; otherwise, the femur will tend to sublux anteriorly off the tibia. Roll-back in a knee replacement can also only occur if the tibial articular surface is relatively flat, but the penalty for this is increased contact stresses on the polyethylene. Finally, it should be noted that 'normal' roll-back has not been consistently demonstrated in cruciate-retaining knees using videofluoroscopic techniques. This should not be entirely surprising since physiological roll-back requires an intact anterior cruciate ligament as well as an intact PCL.

Fixed versus mobile bearing total knee arthroplasty

In a fixed bearing design, the polyethylene articular surface is firmly affixed to the tibial component via a locking mechanism. The all-polyethylene tibial component is naturally also considered a fixed bearing design.

In a mobile bearing design, the polyethylene insert is not fixed to the tibial component, but is free to move or rotate (hence the synonymous term 'rotating platform') on the underlying tibial tray as the knee moves. The theoretical advantage of a mobile bearing design is lower polyethylene wear, owing to better stress distribution across an additional interface during repeated flexion–extension cycles. Another purported advantage is the more forgiving nature of such a design in instances of small degrees of tibiofemoral malalignment, and this may help to reduce tibiofemoral contact stresses and also improve patellar tracking.

However, given the already excellent survivorship of modern knee replacements, coupled with ever-improving polyethylene technology, the purported advantages of mobile bearing knee replacement over conventional fixed bearing design have yet to be proven.[1,2]

Constraint

The stability of a knee replacement is related both to the soft tissues (primarily the collateral ligaments) and the prosthesis itself. The level of constraint in a prosthesis design refers to the degree to which the eventual stability of the knee is due to the prosthesis. Theoretically, the greater the level of constraint, the greater the level of stress

Table 102.1 Comparison of cruciate-retaing and cruciate-substituting designs

	Cruciate-retaining design	Cruciate-substituting design
Advantages	Better kinematics by facilitating joint line preservation, may translate into less mid-flexion instability Facilitates physiological 'roll-back' of the femur on the tibia during high knee flexion, thus increasing knee flexion Femoral component is more bone-conserving owing to lack of the 'box'-cut needed to accommodate the tibial post in cruciate-substituting designs Preservation of proprioception associated with the PCL	Technically easier, procedure more easily reproducible More conforming articular surface reduces contact stresses and wear
Disadvantages	Soft-tissue balancing more difficult Subsequent loss of PCL competency may render the knee unstable Tibial articular surface is flatter to allow roll-back and hence less conforming; this increases stresses on the polyethylene and may increase wear	More conforming articular surface will, however, transfer more stresses to the implant–bone interface, increasing the risk of loosening Absence of roll-back may reduce flexion Greater disruption of knee kinematics and proprioception

PCL, posterior cruciate ligament.

transfer to the implant–bone interface, and hence a higher risk of implant loosening.

- *Unconstrained prosthesis.* Few modern total knee replacement designs are truly unconstrained. This would typically refer to a design in which the femoral compartment articulates on a flat tibial insert, such as in some cruciate-retaining designs. The stability of such a knee replacement would be mainly dependent on the integrity and balance of the periarticular soft tissues.
- *Semiconstrained prosthesis* (Fig. 102.3). Most designs would fall into this category. The degree of constraint is usually related to the degree of conformity between the femoral component and the tibial insert, which is curved.
- A further level of constraint, typically *varus–valgus constraint* (VVC), which offers resistance to coronal instability, is often used in instances where the competency of the medial and/or lateral collateral ligaments is questionable, e.g. severe varus or valgus deformity. VVC is often afforded by the provision of a tall central peg arising from the tibial polyethylene insert into an open 'box' in the middle of the femoral component, which resists varus–valgus deforming forces at the joint line. Some degree of resistance to tibiofemoral rotation is also given by such designs. It should be noted that in many posterior-stabilized designs, the central tibial peg (or 'post' in the post–cam mechanism) also gives some degree of VVC.
- *Fully constrained prosthesis.* This conventionally refers to a hinged prosthesis, in which the femoral and tibial components are linked. Such a design does not depend on the integrity of the surrounding soft tissues, and is useful in cases of substantial disruption of the soft tissues (multiligamentous knee injury, bone loss due to trauma or tumour resection). One critical characteristic of a hinged prosthesis is that it gives stability not only in the coronal plane but also in the sagittal plane. Only a hinged prosthesis can provide adequate sagittal stability in cases where it is absent, e.g. in marked knee recurvatum.

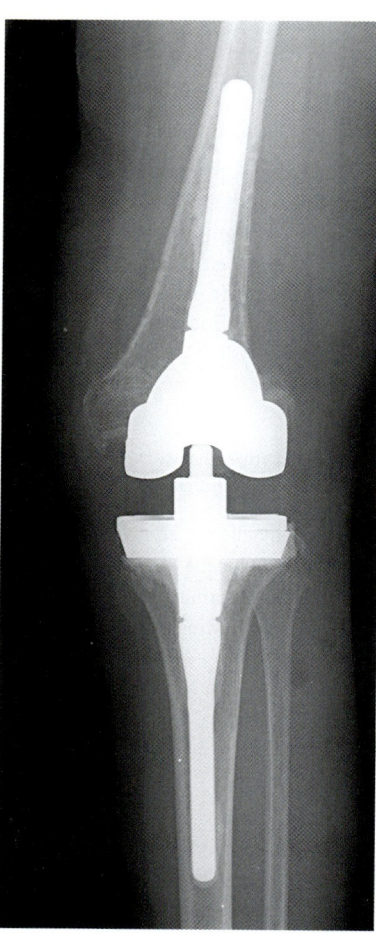

Figure 102.3 An example of a varus–valgus constrained knee replacement. Note the prominent and tall central, reinforced post extending from the tibial component into the femoral notch, affording greater coronal stability.

Role of stems

Stems are rods that can be attached to the femoral or tibial components, and placed intramedullarly.

They perform a few functions:

- Transfer stresses away from the implant–bone interface, and improve implant stability on the cut bone surfaces. Thus, stems are often used in instances when the host bone is poor and/or deficient, whether bone grafts, augments or cement are used to address such deficiencies. Also, with implants with higher levels of constraint, stems help to reduce the stresses at the principal component–bone interface. One useful way of thinking about stems is the analogy to building construction: if the surface on which the building is being constructed is suspect, one would do well to use deeper foundations.
- Bypass cortical defects. Stems are intramedullary devices, and can be used to bypass cortical deficiencies, e.g. after osteotomies or when dealing with periprosthetic fractures.

Patellar resurfacing

This is a controversial issue. In general, the evidence in the literature does not support any definite advantage of replacing over not replacing the patella, and vice versa. Some investigators have reported less anterior knee pain and better stair-climbing in patients with resurfaced patellae,[3,4] but many others have reported equivalent results in long-term studies.[5–8] Complications associated with patellar resurfacing include prosthesis loosening and patellar fracture.

SURGICAL CONSIDERATIONS

Surgical goals have been discussed above, but the desired outcome is that of a stable, pain-free knee with an acceptable range of motion and good power.

Exposure

A midline skin incision is preferred for its versatility and safety. When previous incisions are present, the general rule is to use the most lateral incision as the cutaneous blood supply is predominantly medially based.

The most common approach is medial to the patella. Variations to this approach exist, and differ in terms of how much of the extensor mechanism is violated. The common medial parapatellar approach incises into or adjacent to the quadriceps tendon, whereas the midvastus approach incises along the oblique fibres of the vastus medialis. The subvastus approach spares the vastus fibres completely, and develops the fascial plane below the vastus medialis. The more medial the approach, the greater the 'sparing' of the quadriceps mechanism, which conceptually should reduce postoperative pain and improve recovery, although this has not always been borne out in clinical practice. The downside of the quadriceps-sparing approaches is more difficult knee access, including difficulty with patellar eversion and/or retraction. The subvastus approach is not recommended in large patients with very bulky quadriceps, as the subsequent exposure will be limited (Fig. 102.4).

In cases of difficult exposure, often the result of a contracted extensor mechanism such as patella baja due to a shortened patellar tendon, the extensor mechanism may have to be released to facilitate exposure. Many techniques have been described, but in general fall into two broad categories:

- *soft-tissue releases* such as quadriceps snip, quadriceps turn-down and V–Y quadricepsplasty
- *bony procedures*, typically a tibial tubercle osteotomy with subsequent repair/reconstruction.

The lateral parapatellar approach has been advocated by some for knee replacement in patients with valgus deformity, since it necessarily incorporates a lateral release (commonly needed in these patients) and provides direct exposure to the more involved compartment of the knee. Some also feel that the lateral approach better protects the patellar tendon from avulsion. However, exposure and access to the knee can be difficult with this exposure, and medial approaches have been used with equal efficacy, safety and ease in patients with valgus knees.

Surgical technique

Naturally, there are many ways of performing a knee replacement, but certain principles and key concepts hold true, and are summarized below.

AXIS RESTORATION AND PRINCIPAL BONE CUTS

The goal is to restore the coronal mechanical axis to 0°, or between 5° and 7° of tibiofemoral valgus (Fig. 102.5).

To achieve this, the proximal tibia is cut such that it will be parallel to the plane of the ground when the patient is upright, i.e. perpendicular to the long axis of the tibia. This means that the mechanical coronal alignment of the tibial component will be 0°. As the proximal

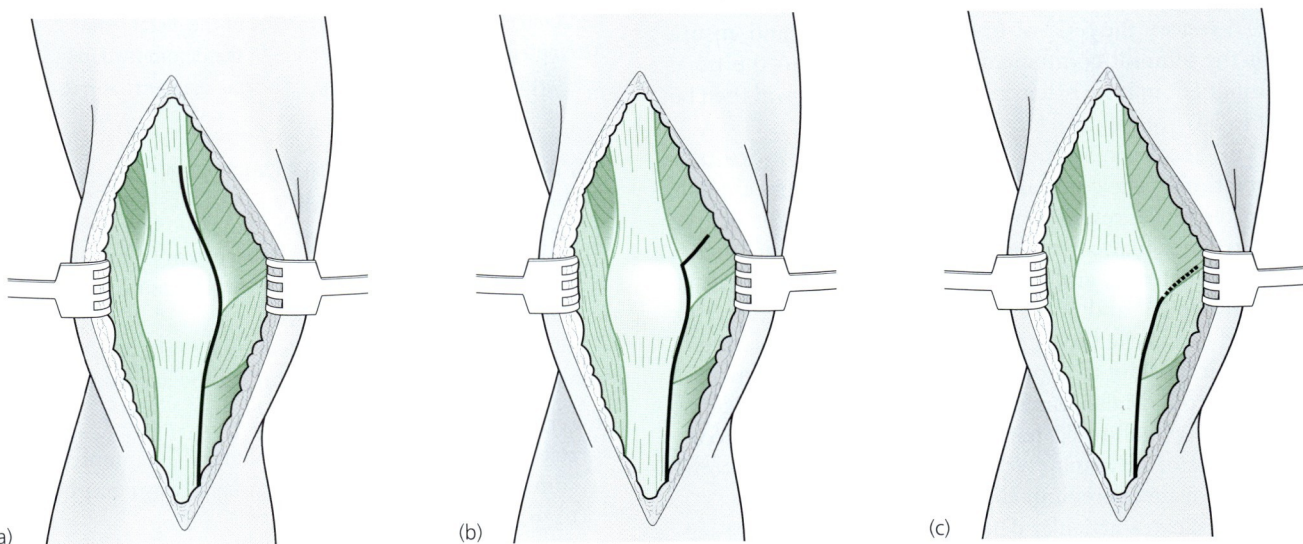

Figure 102.4 Some examples of surgical exposures for total knee replacement. The black lines denote the incision. (a) Medial parapatellar; (b) medial midvastus; (c) medial subvastus. Both (b) and (c) are known as 'quad-sparing' as they do not violate the quadriceps tendon, but exposure and patellar eversion are more difficult with these exposures.

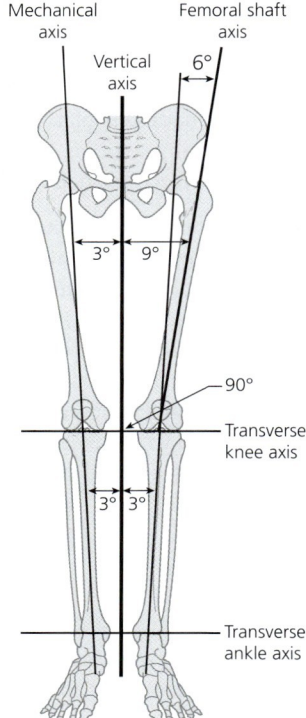

Figure 102.5 Coronal mechanical and anatomical axes of the knee. Note that the mechanical axis passes between the centre of the femoral head and the middle of the talus (this is 3–5 mm medial to the midpoint of the intermalleolar line), whereas anatomical axes are generally referenced to the shafts of the femur and tibia. The anatomical femorotibial axis is between 5° and 7°.

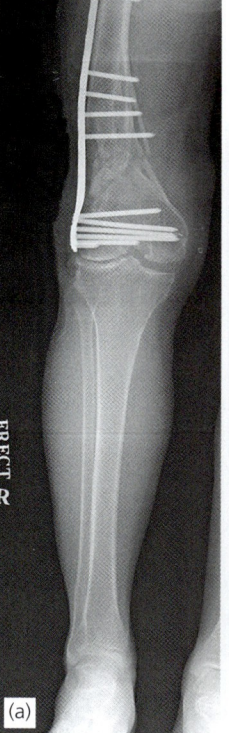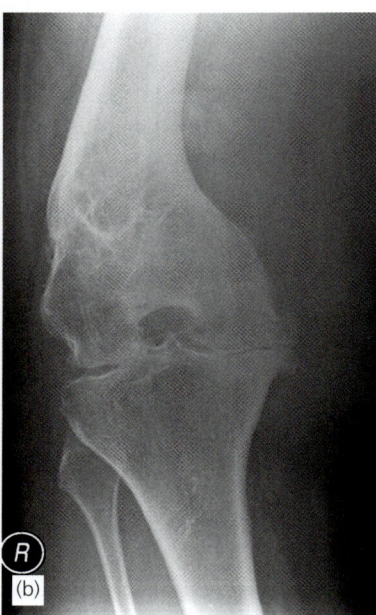

Figure 102.6 Extra-articular deformity. (a) Previous fixation of a supracondylar fracture with femoral shaft malalignment and bone loss also precludes use of intramedullary femoral guides. (b) Complex, severe triplanar deformity of the distal femur. Attempted intra-articular correction of the deformity during knee arthroplasty may place the collateral ligaments at risk.

tibial surface is normally in 3° of varus relative to the tibial shaft, we normally cut the tibia in 3° of valgus to achieve this.

To restore the 5–7° of tibiofemoral valgus and ensure that the femoral component will be parallel to the tibial component in knee extension, the distal femur will then be cut in 5–7° of valgus relative to the shaft.

The above bone cuts bring about an *intra-articular* correction of the coronal deformity. More severe angular deformities represent a significant challenge. The degree of intra-articular correction is limited by the attachments of the collaterals, and commonly this limit has been put at between 25° and 30° of varus and valgus; however, this should be checked by careful pre-operative templating.

It is important to appreciate where the malalignment is arising from. Malalignment that is mainly extra-articular, e.g. from a malunited femoral or tibial fracture or congenital deformity, may require a realignment osteotomy to achieve adequate limb alignment (Fig. 102.6).

Even if extra-articular deformities do not require a separate corrective osteotomy, they may preclude the use of intramedullary alignment jigs. In such situations, extramedullary jigs, gap balancing or computer navigation techniques will be useful.

SOFT-TISSUE RELEASES FOR CORRECTION OF VARUS/VALGUS DEFORMITY

The aim of tissue releases and subsequent bone cuts are to *create equal and rectangular flexion and extension gaps*. This ensures good knee kinematics.

In *varus* knees, the medial tissues are relatively tight and medial releases are required. This can be accomplished by:

- removal of medial osteophytes
- release of the deep medial collateral ligament (MCL); some of the superficial MCL must always be preserved to maintain medial stability
- release of the pes anserinus tendons
- release of semimembranosus.

In *valgus* knees, lateral releases are required. It is important to remember not to be too aggressive in releasing the

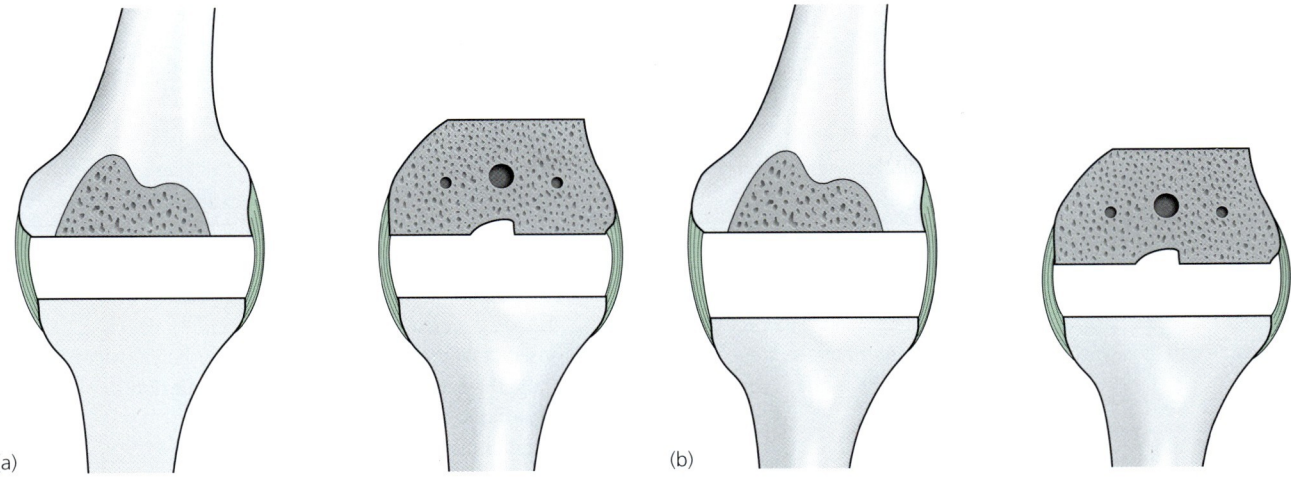

Figure 102.7 Flexion and extension gaps following femoral and tibial bone cuts should be equal and rectangular, as in (a). In (b), the gaps are unequal, so, for a given polyethylene insert, the knee will be either too loose in extension or too tight in extension.

lateral soft-tissue restraints, as the medial structures are already very lax in these cases and a very loose and unstable knee with very large gaps can result. In general, the following order of release has been recommended (O! CLIP LIPS!):

- Osteophytes removal
- Capsule attachments to the lateral tibia
- Lateral patellofemoral ligament
- Iliotibial band released from Gerdy's tubercle
- Popliteus
- Lateral collateral ligament from the femur
- Intermuscular septum (from the vastus lateralis)
- Posterior cruciate ligament
- BicepS tendon off fibula head (usually the last to be released).

Varus cut should be avoided. If at the end of these releases the knee becomes too loose in extension, usually in the presence of a severely attenuated MCL, then a varus–valgus constrained prosthesis will have to be used.

FLEXION DEFORMITY

Most types of FFD, typically up to 15°, may be managed by a combination of:

- osteophyte removal
- appropriate soft-tissue releases (particularly posterior capsule release)
- relevant bone cuts, typically further resection of the distal femur.

FFD above 15° may necessitate extra distal femoral bone cuts to achieve full extension. Under some circumstances, it may be impossible to achieve full extension at the time of surgery because of residual soft-tissue contractures, and there is some evidence in the literature that, with proper physiotherapy, the FFD will improve over time.

Very severe FFD, e.g. over 40–45°, may benefit from serial casting pre-operatively to reduce the FFD to a more manageable level (30° and below) at the time of surgery.

BONE CUTS FOR BALANCING FLEXION AND EXTENSION GAPS

When the bone cuts and soft-tissue releases have been completed, trial components or spacer blocks can be used to assess the stability and range of motion. Typically, the knee is tested in full extension (extension gap) and at 90° of flexion (flexion gap) (Fig. 102.7). It is important to remember that what is done to the proximal tibia affects both flexion and extension gaps equally, but what is done to the distal femur may either affect the extension gap or flexion gap separately, but not both.

Hence:

- The level of tibial resection affects *both* the flexion and extension gaps.
- The level of *distal* femoral resection affects the *extension* gap, but not the flexion gap.
- The level of *posterior* femoral resection affects the *flexion* gap, but not the extension gap.

The algorithm shown in Table 102.2 is often recommended for dealing with problems at this stage.

MANAGEMENT OF BONY DEFECTS

Bone loss on either the femoral or tibial side may generally be managed in the following ways:

- Small defects <10 mm: if contained (i.e. with bone all around), fill with cement; if uncontained, can still use cement but with screw augmentation ('rebar technique').
- Larger defects: bone graft or metallic augments.

Table 102.2 Flexion gap considerations

	Flexion gap tight	**Flexion gap normal**	**Flexion gap loose**
Extension gap tight	• Resect more proximal tibia • Use a thinner polyethylene insert	• Resect more distal tibia • Posterior capsular release	• Resect more distal femur and use a thicker insert • Posterior capsular release
Extension gap normal	• Downsize the femur • Create more posterior slope • Release the PCL	• Success!	• Upsize the femur
Extension gap loose	• Downsize the femur and use a thicker polyethylene insert	• Use a thicker insert to address the extension gap, then, as the flexion gap is now tight, act as for 'extension gap normal, flexion gap tight' • Augment the distal femur, or cement the femur proud	• Use a thicker polyethylene insert • Tibial augmentation

PCL, posterior cruciate ligament.

RESULTS OF TOTAL KNEE ARTHROPLASTY

The results of primary modern TKA are generally excellent. For adequately prepared patients, both morbidity and mortality are very low. Overall 30 day morbidity from all causes in specialist centres is frequently reported to be below 10%,[9] and 30 day mortality less than 0.3%.[10]

After TKA, patients experience statistically and clinically significant improvements in both general health scores, such as the Short Form 36, and disease-specific scores, such as the Oxford Knee Score and Knee Society Rating System. These results have been reported from both centre-specific studies and registry studies.[11]

Implant survival, for cementless and particularly for cemented prostheses, is also excellent, with 10 year implant survival generally in excess of 90%, and in some cases above 95%.[12,13] Negative factors for implant survival include male sex, young age (<60 years) and post-traumatic osteoarthritis as the primary diagnostic indication for TKA.

KEY LEARNING POINTS

- The indications for total knee arthroplasty are: severe osteoarthritis in patients (typically >60 years old), while in younger patients other techniques are preferred; joint reconstruction in limb-preserving surgery for tumours; joint reconstruction after severe trauma.
- The only absolute contraindication to total knee arthroplasty is ongoing sepsis.
- The success of total knee arthroplasty is critically dependent on proper implant positioning and limb alignment.
- Pre-operative assessment and planning is critical and includes clinical and radiological assessment.
- Implant choice is based upon consideration of posterior cruciate ligament-retaining versus substituting; fixed versus mobile bearing tibial articular surface; level of constraint; use of stems; whether to resurface the patella or not.
- Surgical considerations include: the exposure (usually midline incision and medial to the patella); surgical technique (axis restoration, soft-tissue releases and bone gaps); and the management of bone defects.
- A useful algorithm for bone gaps is to look at the extension gap (too tight, normal or too loose).

REFERENCES

1. Oh KJ, Pandher DS, Lee SH, et al. Meta-analysis comparing outcomes of fixed-bearing and mobile-bearing prostheses in total knee arthroplasty. *Journal of Arthroplasty* 2009;**24**:873–84.
2. Smith TO, Ejtehadi F, Nichols R, et al. Clinical and radiological outcomes of fixed-versus mobile-bearing total knee replacement: a meta-analysis. *Knee Surgery, Sports Traumatology, Arthroscopy* 2010;**18**:325–40.
3. Bourne RB, Burnett RS. The consequences of not resurfacing the patella. *Clinical Orthopaedics and Related Research* 2004;**428**:166–9.
4. Pakos EE, Ntzani EE, Trikalinos TA. Patellar resurfacing in total knee arthroplasty. A meta-analysis. *Journal of Bone and Joint Surgery (American)* 2005;**87**:1438–45.

5. Ikejiani CE, Leighton R, Petrie DP. Comparison of patellar resurfacing versus nonresurfacing in total knee arthroplasty. *Canadian Journal of Surgery* 2000;**43**:35–8.
6. Barrack RL, Bertot AJ, Wolfe MW, *et al*. Patellar resurfacing in total knee arthroplasty. A prospective, randomized, double-blind study with five to seven years of follow-up. *Journal of Bone and Joint Surgery (American)* 2001;**83A**:1376–81.
7. Peng CW, Tay BK, Lee BP. Prospective trial of resurfaced patella versus non-resurfaced patella in simultaneous bilateral total knee replacement. *Singapore Medical Journal* 2003;**44**:347–51.
8. Burnett RS, Haydon CM, Rorabeck CH, Bourne RB. Patella resurfacing versus nonresurfacing in total knee arthroplasty: results of a randomized controlled clinical trial at a minimum of 10 years' followup. *Clinical Orthopaedics and Related Research* 2004;**428**:12–25.
9. Memtsoudis SG, Gonzalez Della Valle A, Besculides MC, *et al*. In-hospital complications and mortality of unilateral, bilateral, and revision TKA: based on an estimate of 4,159,661 discharges. *Clinical Orthopaedics and Related Research* 2008;**466**:2617–27.
10. Memtsoudis SG, Della Valle AG, Besculides MC, *et al*. Trends in demographics, comorbidity profiles, in-hospital complications and mortality associated with primary knee arthroplasty. *Journal of Arthroplasty* 2009;**24**:518–27.
11. Kane RL, Saleh KJ, Wilt TJ, Bershadsky B. The functional outcomes of total knee arthroplasty. *Journal of Bone and Joint Surgery (American)* 2005;**87**:1719–24.
12. Furnes O, Espehaug B, Lie SA, *et al*. Early failures among 7,174 primary total knee replacements: a follow-up study from the Norwegian Arthroplasty Register 1994–2000. *Acta Orthopaedica Scandinavica* 2002;**73**:117–29.
13. Gioe TJ, Killeen KK, Grimm K, *et al*. Why are total knee replacements revised? Analysis of early revision in a community knee implant registry. *Clinical Orthopaedics and Related Research* 2004;**428**:100–6.

Unicompartmental knee arthroplasty

SEO-KIAT GOH, SENG JIN YEO, BOON KENG TAY

Introduction	1186	Indications for unicompartmental arthroplasty	1190
Surgical solutions	1186	Choice of prosthesis	1190
Early development of unicompartmental knee arthroplasty	1187	Surgical technique	1190
		Future directions	1190
Re-emergence of unicompartmental knee arthroplasty	1188	References	1191
Unicompartmental knee arthroplasty survivorship today	1189		

NATIONAL BOARD STANDARDS

- Know the indications for unicompartmental knee arthroplasty
- Learn the indications and exclusion criteria for unicompartmental knee arthroplasty
- Know the surgical approach for unicompartmental knee arthroplasty

INTRODUCTION

Unicompartmental osteoarthritis of the knee refers to the condition whereby there are degenerate changes in the articular cartilage that are mainly confined to either the medial or lateral aspect of the tibiofemoral joint. Although it may be idiopathic in primary osteoarthritis, it may be, in cases of secondary arthritis, associated with tibiofemoral mechanical malalignment, meniscal tear or ligamentous instability. When this condition occurs in younger, more active patients, the natural history is believed to be progressive.[1] An early subtype of medial compartmental osteoarthritis, known as anteromedial osteoarthritis (Fig. 103.1), has been described in Oxford, UK. It is believed that early treatment of this subtype of lesion can delay, or even prevent, subsequent development of advanced osteoarthritis.[2]

SURGICAL SOLUTIONS

Surgical treatment options for unicompartmental osteoarthritis include arthroscopic debridement, proximal

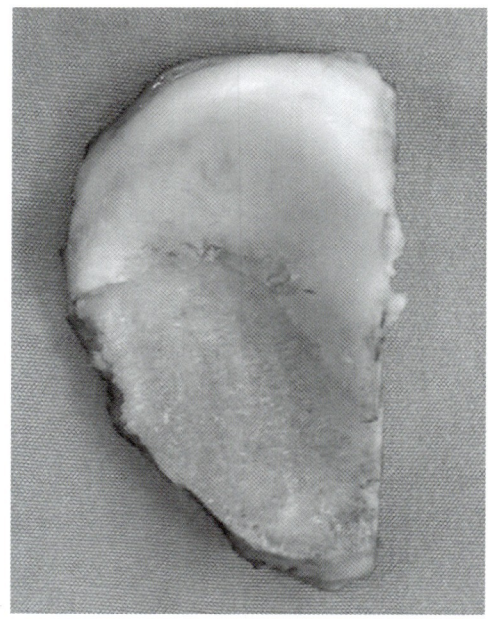

Figure 103.1 Anteromedial osteoarthritis of the knee.

tibial osteotomy, unicompartmental and total knee arthroplasty.

Although arthroscopy is a useful tool in the diagnostic work-up of patients with symptomatic unicompartmental osteoarthritis, its therapeutic value has been controversial at best. Arthroscopic debridement does not improve the knee alignment and, thus, in patients with malalignment of the knee, arthroscopy does not alter the natural history of the disease.[3] It has also been suggested that there may be a significant component of placebo effect in patients who do respond, albeit temporarily, to arthroscopic debridement of knee osteoarthritis.[4]

Proximal tibial osteotomy generally requires a long postoperative rehabilitation to enable bone healing. Also, it does not provide effective long-term relief of pain. In a group of patients (92 knees) who had undergone high tibial osteotomy for gonoarthritis, Insall et al.[5] reported that only 61% of this patient cohort had maintained good or excellent function at 8.9 years.

The total knee replacement, on the other hand, has been a remarkable success story in the modern history of orthopaedic surgery.[6] Relief of pain can be reliably achieved in the most degenerate tricompartmental osteoarthritic knees, and total knee replacement has enjoyed long survival rates of more than 15 years in some series. However, despite its longevity, a total knee arthroplasty does have a definite life span. There is also evidence to show that total knee arthroplasties in younger, physically more active, patients do not last as long as those in older, more sedentary, patients. Some series have reported that the survivorship of total knee replacements in patients younger than 60 years can be as low as 76% at 10 years. Revision total knee arthroplasty is, and is likely to remain, technically demanding surgery with significant operative morbidity.

Unicompartmental knee arthroplasty (UKA) in this select group can provide excellent pain relief and good long-term results.

EARLY DEVELOPMENT OF UNICOMPARTMENTAL KNEE ARTHROPLASTY

The idea of resurfacing a single knee articular compartment was introduced in the 1950s by MacIntosh (and modified by McKeever), who inserted a prosthetic disc (Howmedica Inc., Rutherford, NJ) into the diseased tibial plateau; the disc functioned effectively as a joint spacer (Fig. 103.2).[7] Marmor[8] subsequently designed the first unicompartmental knee prosthesis, which is the forerunner of present-day designs.

However, early results from these prostheses were poor because of the high incidence of prosthetic loosening (Fig. 103.3) and deterioration of osteoarthritis in the contralateral compartment (Fig. 103.4). Revision rates then were as high as 22% at 2 years of follow-up.[9] In

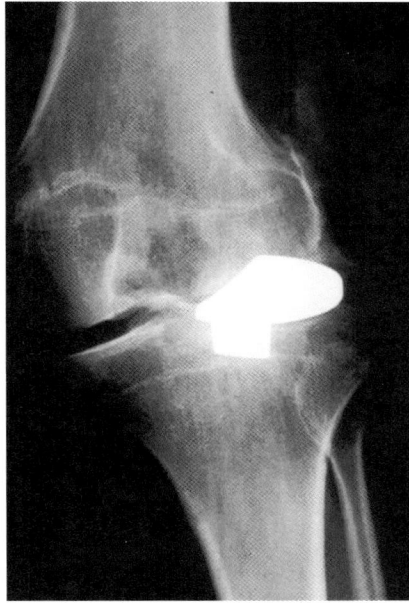

Figure 103.2 An early version of unicompartmental knee arthroplasty; a prosthetic disc placed in the medial plateau with poor results.

another series, Insall and Walker[10] reported that only 43% of 24 cases of UKA had a good outcome at 2–4 years of follow-up.

The reasons for early failure were multifactorial, and can be categorized as follows.

Implant design and instrumentation

The early designs had relatively thinner polyethylene tibial inserts to accommodate the metal tibial trays. Early flat-on-flat designs led to edge loading with malpositioning. Finally, early surgical instrumentations were crude and often led to suboptimal alignment of the implanted early prostheses.

Surgical technique

Overcorrection of the deformity led to accelerated osteoarthritic wear of the opposite compartment. Severe undercorrection of the knee alignment also led to increased stresses on the prostheses, and hence increased polyethylene wear (Fig. 103.5). The present trend is to achieve a slight undercorrection of the alignment.[11]

Poor patient selection

Patient selection was not as stringent in the older series and included patients who would not be suitable candidates today, such as those with inflammatory arthritis.

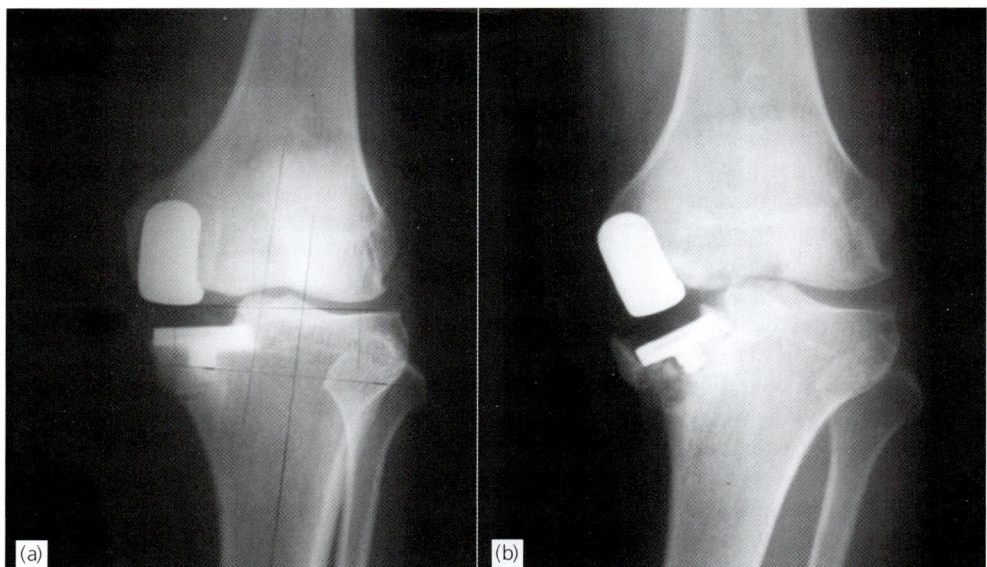

Figure 103.3 (a) Marmor unicompartmental knee arthroplasty. (b) Prosthetic failure from loosening.

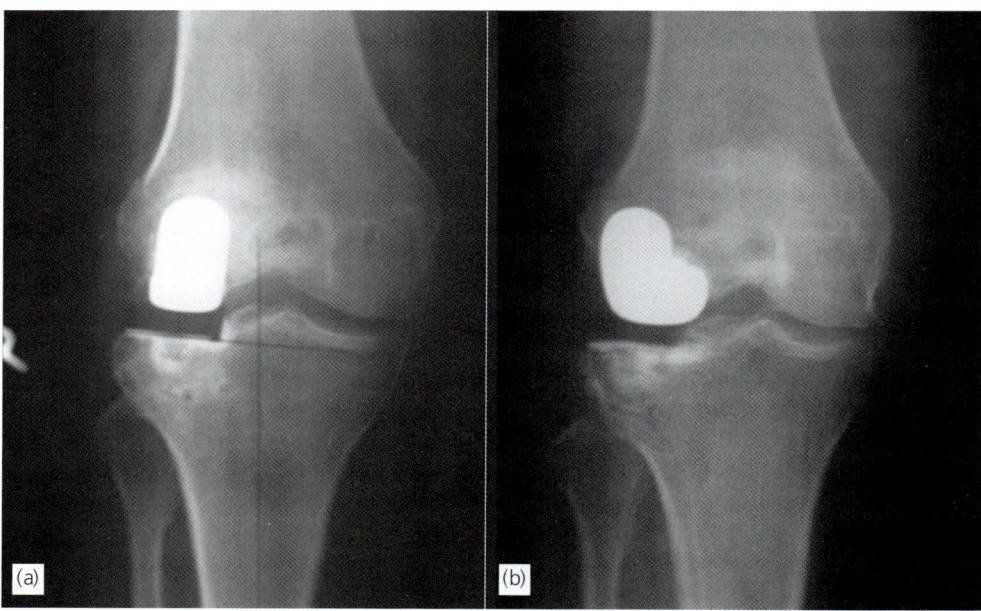

Figure 103.4 (a) Unicompartmental knee arthroplasty functioning well, but (b) result compromised by development of arthritis in lateral compartment.

RE-EMERGENCE OF UNICOMPARTMENTAL KNEE ARTHROPLASTY

Despite the early dismal results, the theoretical advantages and subsequent design improvements to UKA continued to make this an alluring option for the management of unicompartmental osteoarthritis by means of:

- *Conservative surgery*: the ability to adequately treat unicompartmental osteoarthritis disease with conservation of the normal contralateral compartment provides an option for later conversion to total knee arthroplasty, should it become necessary. Revision of a unicompartmental arthroplasty to total knee arthroplasty is thought to be easier than a revision total knee arthroplasty.[12]
- *Better knee kinematics* as a result of retention of the cruciate mechanisms. This enables the UKA knee to function with the four-bar linkage system, which is more physiological.[13]
- *Less invasive surgical techniques and newer instrumentation* have been developed. These minimally invasive techniques have made UKA increasingly more popular as a treatment modality. UKA can now be carried out with less disruption to the quadriceps mechanism, better cosmesis (Fig. 103.5 103.6), faster postoperative rehabilitation and less surgical pain.[14]

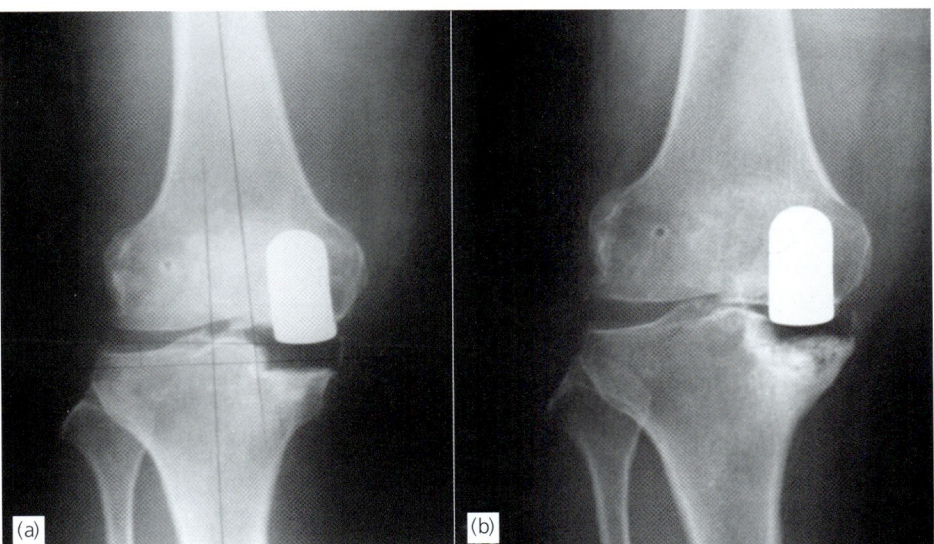

Figure 103.5 (a) Under-correction of knee alignment; (b) result is increased polyethylene wear.

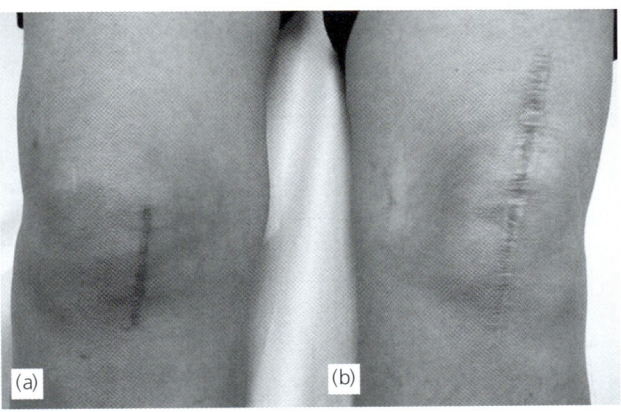

Figure 103.6 (a) Smaller scar can mean less disruption of quadriceps mechanism, better cosmesis, faster rehabilitation and less pain. (b) In contradistinction to the traditional long surgical scar of total knee replacement.

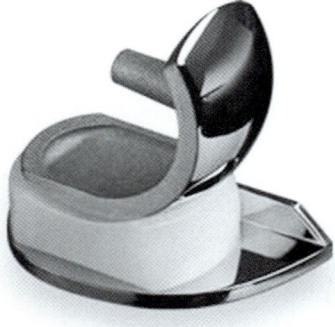

Figure 103.7 Oxford mobile bearing unicompartmental knee arthroplasty.

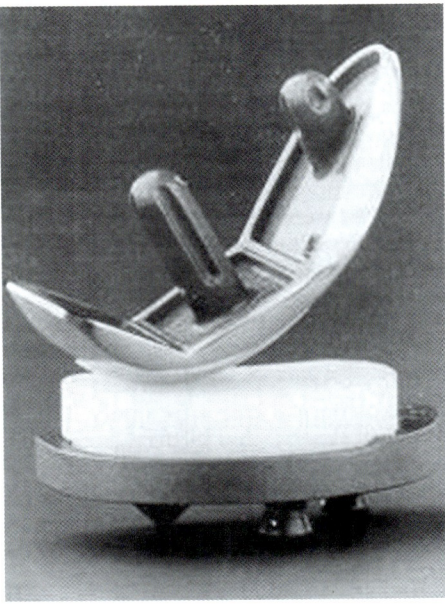

Figure 103.8 Fixed bearing design unicompartmental knee arthroplasty.

UNICOMPARTMENTAL KNEE ARTHROPLASTY SURVIVORSHIP TODAY

There have been several encouraging results from a few centres on the long-term surivivorship of UKA.

Both fixed bearing and mobile bearing designs have equivalent good long-term results. Berger et al.[15] from Chicago, IL, reported a 98% survivorship of the Miller–Galante fixed bearing unicompartmental knee system (Zimmer, Warsaw, IN; Fig. 103.6) in elderly patients (mean age 68) at 10 years. In Oxford, UK, Murray et al.[16] also reported similar results with the Oxford mobile bearing unicompartmental arthroplasty system (Fig. 103.7). Using a fixed bearing design in our own institution, we have demonstrated medium-term results of 8 year survivorship of 95% (Yeo SJ, unpublished data; Fig. 103.8).

Interestingly, the Oxford group has shown that UKA may protect the knee from further deterioration of the joint when compared with a control population.[2]

In a series of young, active patients (aged 35–60) who had received UKA, Pennington et al.[17] reported that the survivorship was 92% at 11 years of follow-up. This challenges the traditional view that UKA should be reserved for only elderly patients.

On the other hand, unicompartmental arthroplasty appears to have a poorer result when done to the lateral compartment. The Bristol Knee Group has reported a 10 year survival rate of 83%.[18]

INDICATIONS FOR UNICOMPARTMENTAL ARTHROPLASTY

We believe that careful patient selection is crucial for a successful outcome following UKA. The following is the list of criteria by which patients are selected for UKA in our institution:

- *Age of patients*. UKA is generally reserved for men older than 60 or women older than 50.
- *Presence of unicompartmental disease only*. History and examination should indicate that the pain originates from either the medial or lateral compartment only. Pain should be present on walking on flat surfaces and climbing down stairs. A history of pain when climbing up stairs or getting up from a chair may indicate patellofemoral osteoarthritis. Such patients with patellofemoral pain syndrome are unlikely to benefit from this surgery.
- *Both cruciate ligaments should ideally be intact*. The unicompartmental knee implant is unrestrained in the anteroposterior plane and is thus heavily reliant on the cruciate mechanisms for a stable knee. However, mild to moderate anterior cruciate ligament (ACL) laxity may be acceptable for some surgeons when a fixed bearing implant is used for the medial part of the knee.
- *Degree of knee malalignment*. The valgus–varus deformity should be mild and can be passively correctable to at least neutral alignment. The usual degree of deformity in this plane is taken as 15°. There should be no more than 15° flexion contracture and the patient should be able to flex to more than 90°.
- *Radiographic investigations* (anteroposterior, lateral and Merchant views) of the knee should confirm that the degenerative process is largely confined to one compartment. Other views that have been suggested include a valgus stress view to look at the integrity of the cartilage in the opposite compartment and a standing lateral view to assess competency of the ACL.
- Exclusion criteria:
  - *Gross ligamentous instability*. The unicompartmental prosthesis is not a constrained device and requires a stable knee to function optimally.
  - *Inflammatory arthritis*, such as crystal arthropathy and rheumatoid arthritis, affects all three knee compartments.
  - *Anterior knee pain syndrome*. This could be a problem of patellar maltracking or patellofemoral osteoarthritis. Again, the unicompartmental arthroplasty does not correct these issues at all.

CHOICE OF PROSTHESIS

Most modern fixed bearing designs (Fig. 103.8) allow for the minimum of constraint to accommodate for the natural kinematics of the knee. This consists of an anatomical femoral component with a flat tibial component of at least 6 mm of polyethylene. Mobile bearing designs (Fig. 103.7) have an unconstrained mobile tibial insert and therefore are more technically demanding during surgery. The latter are not recommended for lateral compartment disease.

SURGICAL TECHNIQUE

The unicompartmental arthroplasty is performed through a medial or lateral arthrotomy without violation of the quadriceps mechanism.

However, with this technique, the operating surgeon would have less access to the anatomical landmarks that will be essential for accurate placement of the prosthesis.

A few salient points should be highlighted:

- It is vital that the limb alignment is restored to neutral, or at least to slight undercorrection. Gross undercorrection will lead to accelerated implant wear. Overzealous correction will aggravate osteoarthritis in the opposite compartment. It has been shown that the quality of cartilage in the 'non-diseased' compartment is generally inferior to that in normal individuals. Therefore, minimal soft-tissue release should be performed and alignment is achieved by the natural ligament balance of the knee with the resurfacing procedure of the UKA.
- The proximal tibia cut should be made as shallow as possible to allow preservation of bone stock and restoration of the joint after implantation of the tibial component. This will facilitate future conversion to total knee arthroplasty.
- Ligament balancing and gap balancing are crucial and must be done correctly in both flexion and extension.

FUTURE DIRECTIONS

The increasing demand for minimally invasive surgery and the necessity for accurate anatomical implantation of the UKA prosthesis pose two diametric challenges to the knee arthroplasty surgeon: small incisions limit visualization, leading to less accurate surgery. There are reports of this new approach adversely affecting the outcome of an already technically demanding operation (Kasodekar et al., unpublished results).

The unifying solution to both challenges lies in computer-assisted surgery. A few studies have already demonstrated that minimally invasive unicompartmental arthroplasty achieves better alignment with the aid of computer navigation.

> **KEY LEARNING POINTS**
>
> - Unicompartmental osteoarthritis of the knee is a condition of degenerate changes in the articular cartilage of mainly the medial or lateral aspect of the tibiofemoral joint.
> - Surgical treatment options for this include: arthroscopic debridement, proximal tibial osteotomy, and unicompartmental and total knee arthroplasty.
> - The advantages of unicompartmental knee arthroplasty include conservation of the normal contralateral compartment (with an option for later conversion to total knee arthroplasty); better knee kinematics (from retention of the cruciate mechanisms); and a less invasive surgical technique and newer instrumentation.
> - Both fixed bearing and mobile bearing designs have equivalent good long-term results (with the exception of lateral compartment unicompartmental knee arthroplasty).
> - The indications for unicompartmental knee arthroplasty are age (men older than 60; women older than 50); unicompartment disease only; both cruciate ligaments intact; the valgus–varus deformity should be mild (<15°) and passively correctable to at least neutral alignment with <15° flexion contracture and flexion >90°; and radiographs confirm that the degenerative process is largely confined to one compartment (mild to moderate changes in the opposite and patellofemoral compartments can be ignored, if asymptomatic).
> - Exclusion criteria are: gross ligamentous instability; inflammatory arthritis; and anterior knee pain syndrome (from patellar maltracking or patellofemoral osteoarthritis).
> - Most modern fixed bearing designs allow for the minimum of constraint (an anatomical femoral component with a flat tibial component of at least 6 mm of polyethylene).
> - Surgical technique: unicompartmental knee arthroplasty is performed through a medial or lateral arthrotomy without violation of the quadriceps mechanism.
> - Minimally invasive unicompartmental arthroplasty may give better alignment with the aid of computer navigation.

REFERENCES

1. Iorio R, Healy WL. Unicompartmental arthritis of the knee. *Journal of Bone and Joint Surgery (American)* 2003;**85A**:1351–64.
2. Weale AE, Murray DW, Crawford R, et al. Does arthritis progress in the retained compartments after 'Oxford' medial unicompartmental arthroplasty? A clinical and radiological study with a minimum ten-year follow-up. *Journal of Bone and Joint Surgery (British)* 1999;**81**:783–9.
3. Salisbury RB, Nottage WM, Gardner V. The effect of alignment on results in arthroscopic debridement of the degenerative knee. *Clinical Orthopaedics and Related Research* 1985;**198**:268–72.
4. Moseley JB, O'Malley K, Petersen NJ, et al. A controlled trial of arthroscopic surgery for osteoarthritis of the knee. *New England Journal of Medicine* 2002;**347**:81–8.
5. Insall JN, Joseph DM, Msika C. High tibial osteotomy for varus gonarthrosis. A long-term follow-up study. *Journal of Bone and Joint Surgery (American)* 1984;**66**:1040–8.
6. Rand JA, Trousdale RT, Ilstrup DM, Harmsen WS. Factors affecting the durability of primary total knee prostheses. *Journal of Bone and Joint Surgery (American)* 2003;**85A**:259–65.
7. MacIntosh DL. Hemi-arthroplasty of the knee using a space occupying prosthesis for painful varus and valgus deformities. Proceedings of the Joint Meeting of the Orthopaedic Associations of the English Speaking World. *Journal of Bone and Joint Surgery (American)* 1958;**40A**:1431.
8. Marmor L. The Marmor knee replacement. *Orthopedic Clinics of North America* 1982;**13**:55–64.
9. Laskin RS. Unicompartmental tibiofemoral resurfacing arthroplasty. *Journal of Bone and Joint Surgery (American)* 1978;**60**:182–5.
10. Insall JN, Walker P. Unicondylar knee replacement. *Clinical Orthopaedics and Related Research* 1976;**120**:83–5.
11. Kennedy WR, White RP. Unicompartmental arthroplasty of the knee. Postoperative alignment and its influence on overall results. *Clinical Orthopaedics and Related Research* 1987;**221**:278–85.
12. Chesnut WJ. Preoperative diagnostic protocol to predict candidates for unicompartmental arthroplasty. *Clinical Orthopaedics and Related Research* 1991;**273**:146–50.
13. Patil S, Colwell Jr CW, Ezzet KA, D'Lima DD. Can normal knee kinematics be restored with unicompartmental knee replacement? *Journal of Bone and Joint Surgery (American)* 2005;**87**:332–8.
14. Price AJ, Webb J, Topf H, et al. Oxford Hip and Knee Group. Rapid recovery after oxford unicompartmental arthroplasty through a short incision. *Journal of Arthroplasty* 2001;**16**:970–6.
15. Berger R, Nedeff D, Barden R, et al. Unicompartmental knee arthroplasty: clinical experience at 6-10 year follow up. *Clinical Orthopaedics and Related Research* 1999;**367**:50.

16. Murray DW, Goodfellow JW, O'Connor JJ. The Oxford medial unicompartmental arthroplasty: a ten year survival study. *Journal of Bone and Joint Surgery (British)* 1998;**80**:983-9.
17. Pennington DW, Swienckowski JJ, Lutes WB, Drake GN. Unicompartmental knee arthroplasty in patients sixty years of age or younger. *Journal of Bone and Joint Surgery (American)* 2003;**85A**:1968-73.
18. Ashraf T, Newman JH, Evans RL, Ackroyd CE. Lateral unicompartmental knee replacement survivorship and clinical experience over 21 years. *Journal of Bone and Joint Surgery (British)* 2002;**84**:1126-30.

104

Patellofemoral arthroplasty of the knee

ERICA D TAYLOR, MARK D MILLER

Introduction	1193	Clinical outcomes	1196
Patellofemoral arthritis	1193	The future of patellofemoral arthroplasty	1196
Treatment modalities	1194	References	1197
Patellofemoral arthroplasty implant development	1195		

NATIONAL BOARD STANDARDS

- Understand the signs and symptoms of isolated patellofemoral osteoarthritis
- Know the investigations needed to diagnose patellofemoral osteoarthritis

INTRODUCTION

A variety of treatment options for isolated patellofemoral arthritis of the knee have gained increasing attention in orthopaedic practice over the past few decades. When conservative measures fail in the absence of patellar malalignment, patellofemoral arthroplasty is a viable option. The design of implants for anterior knee resurfacing evolved to evade the previous pitfalls that formerly led to failure, such as progressive tibiofemoral cartilage degeneration and patellofemoral maltracking. The long-term clinical outcomes data after patellofemoral joint replacement are sparse and variable, although a few available studies suggest that the success and satisfaction ratings of the newer implants are acceptable. The objective of this chapter is to provide an overview of patellofemoral arthritis, non-arthroplasty treatment options, and the current literature on outcomes following patellofemoral replacement.

PATELLOFEMORAL ARTHRITIS

Isolated patellofemoral arthritis of the knee is an interesting concept that has gained increasing attention in orthopaedic practice. Despite the complex interplay of forces that control loading mechanics across the tricompartmental knee joint, patients can indeed be predisposed to degeneration of cartilage isolated just to the patellofemoral articulation. Termed patellofemoral arthritis, this condition has been associated with potentially disabling anterior knee pain which, historically, was relatively refractory to conservative treatment modalities.

The classic definition of patellofemoral arthritis refers to loss of articular cartilage on the surfaces of the patella or the trochlear groove of the femur, in isolation or in combination, with the greatest prevalence of chondral wear found on the lateral patellar facet.[1] Several factors have been attributed to the accelerated development of this single-compartment degeneration, including patella alta, trochlear dysplasia, increased quadriceps angle, weakened vastus medialis oblique muscle, contracted lateral retinaculum, and weakened or absent medial patellofemoral ligament.[2] Extrinsic factors linked to patellofemoral joint degeneration include excess weight, accumulated microtrauma with intense activity level, and traumatic injury. Patients may present with anterior knee pain exacerbated by stair climbing and descent, prolonged seated position (the so-called 'movie theatre sign'), squatting and rising from a seated position. The constellation of these anterior joint symptoms is also referred to as *patellofemoral pain*. In addition to obtaining a clear history and physical examination, it is recommended that the evaluation of these patients includes a true lower extremity alignment assessment. From an imaging standpoint, standing anteroposterior, flexion posteroanterior, lateral and sunrise radiographic views of the knee should be obtained. In cases of suspected maltracking or anatomical dysplasia, CT scans may be helpful.

In 2002, Davies et al.[3] reported the results of a radiological study that demonstrated the prevalence of isolated patellofemoral arthritis in 9.2% of their patients over the age of 40. Another epidemiological study found isolated patellofemoral arthritis in 11% of men and 24% of women aged 55 years or older who presented with symptomatic osteoarthritis of the knee.[4] Furthermore, women constitute up to 75% of patellofemoral arthroplasty patients in most reported series, postulated to be the result of the increased frequency of joint malalignment and dysplasia in the female population.[5]

TREATMENT MODALITIES (Table 104.1)

Non-operative treatment

Conservative modalities exist as the initial treatment for isolated patellofemoral pathology, and the majority of patients experience improvement of their symptoms without surgical intervention. The non-operative approach may include activity modification, weight loss and physiotherapy. A comparison study by Quilty et al.[6] compared the short-term outcomes of a commonly used therapy programme (patellar taping, quadriceps strengthening, postural education and functional exercises) with a non-treatment group. The treatment group experienced a reduction in pain and increases in quadriceps strength at 10 weeks after treatment; however, after 12 months, no differences in patient outcome measures were noted between the two groups. Intra-articular injections and viscosupplementation have also been assessed in non-randomized trials, but the quality of evidence supporting their effective use in patellofemoral joint arthritic conditions is low.

Operative treatment

It is important to recognize the spectrum of operative techniques that have been implemented in the surgical treatment of isolated patellofemoral arthritis. Once conservative measures have failed to provide relief for the patient, the underlying aetiology of the patellofemoral pathology dictates the appropriate surgical intervention. Arthroscopic debridement, chondroplasty, extensor mechanism realignment (with or without lateral release) and arthroplasty are the commonly used techniques to address isolated patellofemoral disease.

There are only a few studies that describe the effectiveness of arthroscropic debridement of articular cartilage for the specific patient population with isolated single-compartment disease. However, a systemic literature review found two high-quality studies that described no differences in outcomes when arthroscopic debridement was compared with placebo arthroscopy and arthroscopic debridement plus physiotherapy in the treatment of generalized osteoarthritis of the knee.[7] Chondroplasty procedures have also been studied in a retrospective fashion and are found to be only somewhat beneficial in the younger patient population with

Table 104.1 Current treatment options for isolated patellofemoral arthritis of the knee

Non-operative treatment options	
Physiotherapy	May include quadriceps strengthening, isometrics, activity modification education, and patellar taping
Anti-inflammatory medications	Side-effects are self-limiting
Intra-articular injections of corticosteroids or viscous supplementation	Low evidence to support efficacy of treatment
Patellar unloader bracing	No significant evidence to support their efficacy
Operative treatment options	
Arthroscopic debridement	Little difference in outcome when compared with non-operative treatment
Isolated lateral retinacular release	May have some utility in the setting of radiographic tilt without instability
Chondroplasty	Includes advanced techniques such as autologous chondrocyte implantation, chondral shaving or removal of a degenerated lateral facet
Tibia tubercle osteotomies	Current techniques include anteromedial transfer of the tubercle. Carries surgical complications, but also corrects underlying biomechanical pathology
Patellectomy	Eliminates a pain generator, but leads to chronic weakness and extensor lag
Total knee arthroplasty	Produces satisfactory results short term, but can lead to persistent anterior knee pain and be technically challenging when instability is present
Patellofemoral arthroplasty	Has potential advantages of preserving natural knee kinematics, but implant durability has not yet been fully elucidated or maximized

cartilage defects.[8] Extensor mechanism realignment procedures, such as the anterior or anteromedial displacement osteotomies, are not without their own set of surgical complications, but do address underlying biomechanical abnormalities that could potentiate the development of patellofemoral arthritis. Whether or not the risks outweigh the potential long-term benefits is yet to be determined.

Before the development of reliable patellofemoral replacement implants, osteoarthritis of the patellofemoral joint was most often treated similarly to tricompartmental osteoarthritis – with total knee arthroplasty. The 5–7 year results demonstrated this to be a satisfactory treatment option for this patient population in multiple studies.[7] However, most early total knee replacement designs did not include resurfacing of the patellofemoral joint, leading to progression of patellofemoral arthritis and anterior knee pain (up to 20% of patients per report).[9] It was not until the late 1970s that total knee implants with a patellofemoral articulation and patellar component become the standard for total knee replacement. Nevertheless, it is still unclear whether patellar resurfacing results in better outcomes in isolated patellofemoral arthritis.[10] Furthermore, because of the concomitant patellar instability that can accompany patellofemoral disease, total knee replacement in patients with isolated patellofemoral arthritis can be technically demanding. There is little evidence to support total knee arthroplasty as a recommended treatment for this disease process, although Mont et al.[11] suggested total knee arthroplasty as a preferred treatment option for patients aged >55 years with primarily patellofemoral arthritis.

Finally, patellofemoral arthroplasty, when compared with a total knee arthroplasty, has the potential advantages of retaining the menisci and cruciate ligaments and can be considered in the presence of true end-stage single-compartment arthrosis. In theory, the natural kinematics of the knee joint are retained by the maintenance of the native ligaments and menisci. However, the most feared pitfall of this treatment option has been identified as the durability of the arthroplasty, with the main reasons for failure being malalignment, polyethylene wear, soft-tissue impingement and disease progression in adjacent compartments.[4] Therefore, patellofemoral arthroplasty should be performed only after a careful clinical evaluation has proved the patellofemoral joint to be the definite cause of symptoms.

PATELLOFEMORAL ARTHROPLASTY IMPLANT DEVELOPMENT

In general, patellofemoral arthroplasty is appropriate for patients with isolated patellofemoral arthritis in the absence of lower extremity malalignment. The ideal patient age range has yet to be determined, but it is postulated that is it best restricted to patients younger than 60 years who have not developed arthrosis in the adjacent compartments. The current indications and contraindications for patellofemoral arthroplasty are highlighted in

Table 104.2 Indications and contraindications for patellofemoral arthroplasty

Indications	Contraindications
Patellofemoral pain secondary to isolated patellofemoral arthrosis	Large quadriceps angle (>20° in women; >15° in men) or excessive maltracking
Patellofemoral dysplasia in the absence of limb malalignment	Tibiofemoral chondromalacia or arthrosis
Patient age >40	Chondromalacia/superficial cartilage injury of the patellofemoral joint
	Inflammatory arthritis

Table 104.2. These patient factors have been evaluated since the inception of patellofemoral replacement and were identified from the pitfalls of previous designs.

Patellofemoral-specific devices were initially designed to selectively resurface only the patella, using a metallic implant.[5] However, because of pre-existing or progressive trochlear chondromalacia, persistent anterior knee pain was common. In an effort to improve results, first-generation patellofemoral devices were developed to consist of a polyethylene patellar component and a metallic trochlear component. In 1955, McKeever and associates published the first account of patellar resurfacing as a better pain-relieving alternative to patellectomy and patellar shaving for the treatment of patellofemoral arthritis. This conclusion was reinforced by subsequent studies, and long-term success was outlined by Pickett and Stoll,[12] who documented satisfactory results in 39 of 45 patients with McKeever prostheses at 22 years of follow-up.

Nevertheless, the original descriptions of patellofemoral arthroplasty did not address the strict criteria for patient selection, the potential technical pitfalls or the possible need for realignment of the extensor mechanism prior to arthroplasty.[2] As a result, reports of these earlier designs were overall disappointing when evaluated by independent authors and surgeons. For some surgeons, this led to renovation of the implant design, while other groups proceeded with general abandonment of the procedure itself.[13] However, recent newer device designs that address the above-mentioned pitfalls and attempt to more accurately replicate patellofemoral joint motion and function have been introduced. For example, the Avon Patellofemoral Arthroplasty (Stryker Howmedica Osteonic, Allendale, NJ) was introduced in the early twenty-first century and, by 2007, studies had reported survivorship of up to 95.8% at 5 years with significant improvement in pain and function.[14] This implant design was based on the patellofemoral compartment of a related total knee arthroplasty implant. The femoral flange and patellar components were both designed to avoid impingement in deep flexion as well as to aid in consistent and appropriate patellar tracking. An independent study of this implant suggested 100% survival rates of the Avon implant with good functional outcome at 5 years.[15] Similar approaches have been initiated among various industry companies to help regenerate popular opinion in favour of patellofemoral arthroplasty. In addition, use of components based on a total knee design allows for easier conversion to total knee arthroplasty should the patellofemoral replacement not be successful. An example of a conventional patellofemoral arthroplasty is shown in Fig. 104.1.

In the past few years, the idea of customized implants has been introduced to recreate the patient's unique native trochlear anatomy, similar to previous customized implants designed for hip acetabular revision. Three-dimensional CT scan imaging software is used to reconstruct a custom implant modelled on the patient's femoral groove characteristics. In a 2006 study by Sisto and Sarin,[16] results of 25 custom implants were reviewed, demonstrating good to excellent results after 6 years.

CLINICAL OUTCOMES

The clinical success of patellofemoral arthroplasty has varied, depending on the chosen indications for surgery and implant design features, as outlined in the previous section. In 2010, van Jonbergen et al.[17] published an important study on the long-term results of patellofemoral replacement in relation to primary diagnosis, age, sex and body mass index. The authors studied 161 patients who had undergone replacement for isolated patellofemoral arthritis with the Richards type II prosthesis and found implant survival rates of 84% at 10 years and 69% at 20 years. Primary diagnosis, sex and age did not significantly affect the rate of revision, whereas excess weight did have a significant correlation.

A significant proportion of technical failures of patellofemoral arthroplasty relates to patellar instability arising from uncorrected patellar malalignment, soft-tissue imbalance or component malposition.[7] Problems related to these issues generally become clinically evident within months of surgery. As emphasized before, it is important to recognize pre-operative extremity malalignment or patellar maltracking and instability so that these compounding factors can be addressed prior to implant of a prosthesis, decreasing the need for revision arthroplasty in the future. Interestingly, there have been case reports of medial patellofemoral ligament reconstruction for treatment of subluxating patellofemoral arthroplasty, although the level of evidence to support the success of this technique is low.[18] Strain shielding of the distal femur after patellofemoral replacement as a cause of implant-related bone loss has also been studied biomechanically, with higher rates of this overload phenomenon occurring with regular deep knee bending activity.[19]

Progression of femorotibial osteoarthritis has been highlighted in patients who have undergone patellofemoral replacement and is considered one of the most important reasons for conversion to total knee arthroplasty. Conversion rates of 20% have been reported after an average of 7–16 years.[7] It remains unclear which patients are at risk of developing progressive patellofemoral arthritis. Recently, the results of revision to total knee arthroplasty were described, demonstrating improved Knee Society scores after conversion.[5] Finally, according to current literature, patellofemoral arthroplasty does not appear to have a negative effect on the outcome of later total knee arthroplasty.[20]

THE FUTURE OF PATELLOFEMORAL ARTHROPLASTY

Patellofemoral arthroplasty is an increasingly common procedure that has been shown to provide alleviation of symptoms caused by patellofemoral osteoarthritis in both

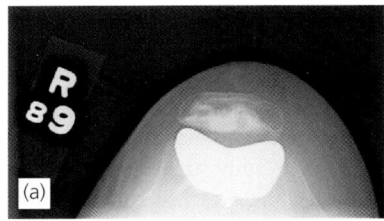
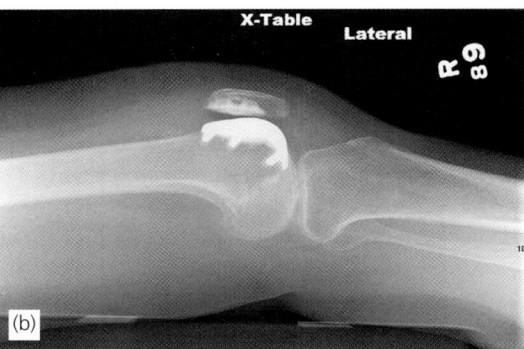
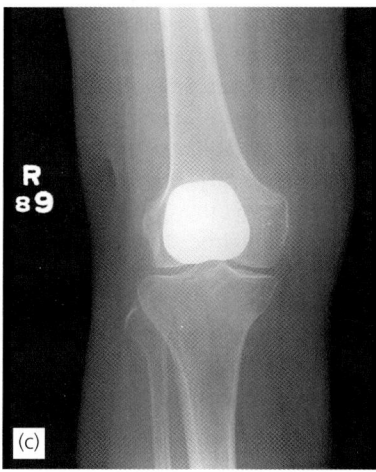

Figure 104.1 Sunrise (a), laterak (b) and anteroposterior (c) radiographs of a 58 year old woman with isolated patellofemoral arthrosis after arthroplasty. Note the absence of tibiofemoral joint degeneration and the central position of the patellar component in the trochlea, both of which are key considerations in patient selection and technique.

short-term and intermediate-term studies. Nevertheless, high-quality clinical evidence to support the long-term durability of this treatment modality is still sparse. Further investigations will be necessary to determine how patients progress in the long term after patellofemoral replacement with regard to achievable functional activity levels and the longevity of the prosthesis. Proper patient selection cannot be emphasized enough, as it is a key factor in the determination of outcomes and also in the prevention of the previously described modes of implant failure. With the advent of custom prostheses for the patellofemoral joint and newer implant designs that address the appropriate intrinsic biomechanics of this compartment, it is possible that the rates of revision will continue to decline, as they have over the past few years.

KEY LEARNING POINTS

- The spectrum of treatment for isolated patellofemoral arthritis ranges from conservative physical therapy measures to surgical intervention options.
- Patellofemoral arthroplasty is an increasingly common procedure that has been shown to provide reliable alleviation of symptoms in short-term and immediate-term studies.
- Advancements in implant design that recreate natural knee biomechanics have improved the success rate in long-term studies of patellofemoral replacement.
- Persistent patellofemoral symptoms after replacement may be caused by component malposition, limb malalignment, prosthetic design, improper patellar preparation or soft-tissue imbalance.
- The rate of revision arthroplasty has been linked to patient factors such as obesity, with conversion to total knee arthroplasty demonstrating satisfactory results.

REFERENCES

1. Saleh KJ, Arendt EA, Eldridge K, et al. Symposium. Operative treatment of patellofemoral arthritis. *Journal of Bone and Joint Surgery (American)* 2005;**87**:659–71.
2. Minkowitz RB, Bosco JA. Patellofemoral arthritis. *Bulletin of the New York University Hospital for Joint Diseases* 2009;**67**:30–8.
3. Davies AP, Vince AS, Shepstone L, et al. The radiologic prevalence of patellofemoral osteoarthritis. *Clinical Orthopaedics and Related Research* 2002;**402**:206–12.
4. McAlindon TE, Snow S, Cooper C, Dieppe PA. Radiographic patterns of osteoarthritis of the knee joint in the community: the importance of the patellofemoral joint. *Annals of Rheumatic Diseases* 1992;**51**:844–9.
5. Lonner JH. Patellofemoral arthroplasty. *Journal of the American Academy of Orthopaedic Surgeons* 2007;**15**:495–506.
6. Quilty B, Thucker M, Campbell R, Dieppe P. Physiotherapy, including quadriceps exercises and patellar taping, for knee osteoarthritis with predominant patello-femoral joint involvement: randomized controlled trial. *Journal of Rheumatology* 2003;**30**:1311–17.
7. van Jonbergen HPW, Poolman RW, van Kampen A. Isolated patellofemoral osteoarthritis: A systematic review of treatment options using the GRADE approach. *Acta Orthopaedica* 2010;**81**:199–205.
8. Spak RT, Teitge RA. Fresh osteochondral allografts for patellofemoral arthritis: long-term follow-up. *Clinical Orthopaedics and Related Research* 2006;**444**:193–200.
9. Barrack RL, Wolfe MW. Patellar resurfacing in total knee arthroplasty. *Journal of the American Academy of Orthopaedic Surgeons* 2000;**8**:75–82.
10. Thompson NW, Ruiz AL, Breslin E, Beverland DE. Total knee arthroplasty without patellar resurfacing in isolated patellofemoral osteoarthritis. *Journal of Arthroplasty* 2001;**16**:607–12.
11. Mont MA, Haas S, Mullick T, Hungerford DS. Total knee arthroplasty for patellofemoral arthritis. *Journal of Bone and Joint Surgery (American)* 2002;**84**:1977–81.
12. Pickett JC, Stoll DA. Patellaplasty or patellectomy. *Clinical Orthopaedics and Related Research* 1979;**144**:103–6.
13. Grelsamer RP. Patellofemoral arthritis. *Journal of Bone and Joint Surgery (American)* 2006;**88**:1849–60.
14. Ackroyd CE, Newman JH, Evans R, et al. The Avon patellofemoral arthroplasty: five-year survivorship and femoral results. *Journal of Bone and Joint Surgery (British)* 2007;**89B**:310–15.
15. Odumenya M, Costa ML, Parsons N, et al. The Avon patellofemoral joint replacement: five-year results from an independent centre. *Journal of Bone and Joint Surgery (British)* 2010;**92B**:56–60.
16. Sisto DJ, Sarin VK. Custom patellofemoral arthroplasty of the knee. *Journal of Bone and Joint Surgery (American)* 2006;**88**:1475–80.
17. Van Jonbergen HPW, Werman DM, Barnaart LF, van Kampen A. Long-term outcomes of patellofemoral arthroplasty. *Journal of Arthroplasty* 2010;**25**:1066–71.
18. Carmont MR, Crane T, Thompson P, Spalding T. Medial patellofemoral ligament reconstruction for subluxating patellofemoral arthroplasty. *Knee* 2011;**18**:130–2.
19. Meireles S, Completo A, Simoes JA, Flores Paulo. Strain shielding in distal femur after patellofemoral arthroplasty under different activity conditions. *Journal of Biomechanics* 2010;**43**:477–84.
20. van Jonbergen HPW, Werkman DM, van Kampen A. Conversion of patellofemoral arthroplasty to total knee arthroplasty. A matched case-control study of 13 patients. *Acta Orthopaedica* 2009;**80**:62–6.

Revision knee arthroplasty

SHI-LU CHIA, NGAI-NUNG LO

Introduction	1198	Principles of revision knee arthroplasty	1200
Causes of total knee arthroplasty failure	1198	Results of revision knee arthroplasty	1202
Clinical evaluation	1199	References	1203

NATIONAL BOARD STANDARDS

- Understand the causes of and options after total knee arthroplasty failure
- Know the clinical, radiological and laboratory evaluation of failed total knee arthroplasty
- Understand the planning for revision of a total knee arthroplasty
- Surgical approaches and techniques/considerations for this surgery
- Learn the results of this surgery

INTRODUCTION

Modern knee arthroplasty is a very successful procedure with low morbidity and high patient satisfaction. However, despite improvements in implant design and exacting surgical technique, some knee replacements fail. In this unfortunate situation, the orthopaedic surgeon has several options:

- revision of part of, or the entire, knee replacement to new implants; this procedure may be staged
- arthrodesis
- excision arthroplasty
- amputation.

This chapter deals with the first of these options, whereby components that have failed are removed and replaced by new ones, restoring knee function.

Note that the alternatives can be remembered as the three As: Arthrodesis, excision arthroplasty forming a pseudo-Arthrosis and Amputation.

CAUSES OF TOTAL KNEE ARTHROPLASTY FAILURE

The most common reason for failure of total knee arthroplasty (TKA) today is infection.[1,2] If the infection cannot be eradicated without removing the original implants, revision to new implants will be necessary following adequate resolution of the infection.

Thus, failure modes for TKA are often categorized into *septic* and *aseptic* causes. Aseptic causes include:

- loosening, including periprosthetic fracture (Fig. 105.1)
- instability, which can be in either flexion or extension, or both
- malalignment, which is a common cause contributing to component failure and increased polyethylene wear[3]
- extensor mechanism failure, such as patellar instability, causing anterior knee pain or patellar subluxation, and patellar fracture.

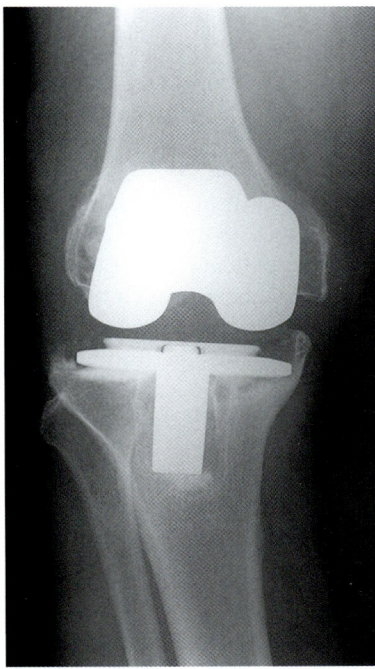

Figure 105.1 Knee radiograph showing a loose tibial implant with component movement and breakage of the cement mantle.

CLINICAL EVALUATION

The clinical problem is that of a patient who is unhappy with his/her knee replacement. The presentation may occur within a few days of or many years after the index surgery.

The key to successful revision surgery is obtaining an accurate cause for the TKA failure. Hence, meticulous history-taking and physical examination, together with appropriate radiological and laboratory investigations, are mandatory.[4]

If the cause for persistent knee pain cannot be found, then revision TKA will have only limited success. In their series, Mont and co-workers[5] reported that only 41% of such patients had excellent/good results after TKA, and, if patients had a good range of motion pre-operatively and complained only of pain, excellent/good results were obtained in only a dismal 17% of such patients.

The first thing to ask is what is troubling the patient. Is it:

- Pain?
- Instability?
- Stiffness?
- Swelling? Deformity?
- Non-resolution of pre-operative symptoms?

Non-resolution of pre-operative symptoms should alert one to an incorrect indication for the index knee replacement procedure. For instance, pain in the knee may be referred from hip or spine pathology, and it is important to exclude these if the patient experiences no change in symptoms following knee replacement.

Pain is probably the most common presenting complaint for the patient with a failing knee replacement. It is important to differentiate between mechanical and non-mechanical pain. Non-mechanical symptoms, such as persistent pain, night pain, systemic symptoms, should alert one to the possibility of infection, fracture or, less commonly, a flare-up of an inflammatory arthritis such as gout. Mechanical symptoms could indicate any of the other causes for aseptic failure (loosening, instability, malalignment, extensor problems), and in themselves may not be terribly helpful. However, the location of the pain may help in localizing the problem. Pain on initiation of movement after a period of inactivity ('start-up pain') is commonly associated with implant loosening.

Physical examination should focus on identifying any evidence of infection such as effusion, erythema or sinuses. One should also look for periarticular bursitis, and assess the knee's range of motion and stability. Stability testing should evaluate both coronal (varus–valgus) as well as sagittal (?recurvatum) stability. Moreover, midflexion instability should be specifically looked for, i.e. varus–valgus instability at differing degrees of knee flexion.

The condition of the soft tissues should be noted. Is there any evidence of vascular problem or neurological deficits? Is there any possibility of a chronic regional pain syndrome, or perhaps a traumatic neuralgia associated with the wound? One should also exclude deep vein thrombosis or phlebitis.

The *stiff knee* is a common presentation, and has its particular aetiological considerations:

- effusion from any cause
- infection
- arthrofibrosis
- contracted soft tissues
- extensor mechanism weakness/failure
- anterior tilt of the tibial component (reverse tilt)
- posteriorly tilted/extended femoral component
- overstuffing of joint, gaps balanced too tightly
- component loosening and dislodgement
- mechanical block owing to loose bodies, e.g. retained cement.

Imaging investigations

Imaging investigations include:

- *Plain radiographs*. Look for loosening, fractures, loose bodies and alignment. One should also consider imaging the hips and lumbar spine.
- *Bone scans*. Standard bone scans may be of limited specificity, but may indicate loosening or infection.[6] The value of more specialized scans such as gallium and white-cell indium-labelled scans remains unclear.

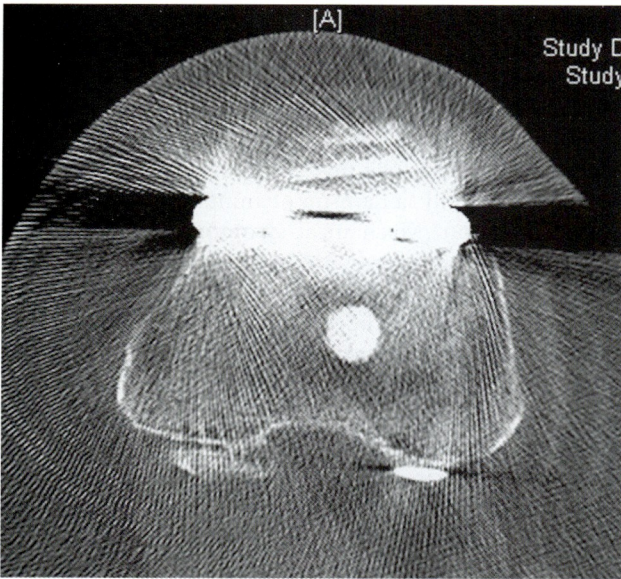

Figure 105.2 CT scan of a patient with a malrotated femoral component with patellofemoral instability.

- *CT scans.* These may be useful in assessing component alignment, particularly with respect to those parameters that cannot be accurately assessed on plain radiographs, e.g. rotation of the femoral and tibial components (Fig. 105.2).
- *MRI.* The use of MRI for investigation of the failed TKA is still evolving. With metallic artefact reduction algorithms, MRI scanning may yet prove useful for the evaluation of loosening and infection, particularly when osteomyelitis is present.[7]

Laboratory investigations

Blood investigations are mainly carried out to assess the probability of infection. The total leucocyte count, erythrocyte sedimentation rate (ESR) and C-reactive protein (CRP) levels, when interpreted together, are reasonably predictive for infection, or its lack thereof.[8]

Aspiration of the knee is also useful, particularly when the ESR and CRP values suggest underlying sepsis. Different studies report differing diagnostic thresholds, but generally a white cell count of less than 1000 μL^{-1} and a polymorphonuclear cell fraction of less than 60% has an excellent negative predictive value for infection.[9] Naturally, positive cultures would be diagnostic, but a negative culture does not preclude infection.

At the time of revision surgery, if the available histopathological expertise is available, the presence of 10 or more polymorphonuclear leucocytes per high-power field of a frozen section of tissue obtained intra-operatively, is considered presumptive evidence of infection.

Other tests

The following are other procedures that we have found to be useful in the evaluation of these patients:

- *Intra-articular injection of local anaesthetic.* The injection of 10–15 mL of a local anaesthetic into the knee can sometimes be useful in ascertaining whether the source of the patient's complaints arises from the knee. In most instances in which the primary problem comes from the knee, the patient will experience significant relief while performing weight-bearing activities after the injection has been administered. Such patients would be more likely to benefit from revision surgery.
- *Bracing.* When instability is suspected to be the cause of the patient's complaints, a trial of bracing may be useful to confirm the diagnosis. The type of bracing, whether constraining coronal or sagittal mobility, can also be useful in confirming the direction of instability.
- *Physiotherapy and pain management.* When no cause can be identified, expert physiotherapy and pain management consultation may bring about a satisfactory resolution of the patient's complaints. We have witnessed many cases whereby non-compliance with prescribed physiotherapy, or simply slow muscular recovery on a background of poor physical conditioning, has resulted in a poor functional outcome. Such patients would respond well to persistent, sensitively administered physiotherapy.

PRINCIPLES OF REVISION KNEE ARTHROPLASTY

Revision knee arthroplasty is complex and should not be undertaken lightly. If the surgeon is relatively inexperienced, expert assistance should be enlisted until such a time that the surgeon's expertise has developed.

Meticulous preparation with adequate contingency planning is necessary for a smooth and successful procedure. All necessary implants and instruments must be available during the surgery; therefore, the surgeon should notify theatre staff and the implant vendors before surgery if specialist implants and instruments are required.

As the surgery is typically more prolonged and more invasive than primary arthroplasty, patients undergoing revision knee surgery have a higher risk for morbidity and mortality; hence, the level of perioperative care needs to be heightened (see chapter 73).

Hence,

- prepare the patient
- prepare the staff
- prepare instruments and implants
- prepare yourself
- prepare a plan for the surgery, with contingency plans as well.

Goals of revision knee arthroplasty

- Eradicate infection, if present.
- Restore knee stability, and kinematics as far as possible. Stability should be considered before kinematic restoration as a surgical goal.
- Preserve soft-tissue integrity and function.

Exposure

The knee will have had at least one previous operation, and there may be more than one previous incision. Use the original incision if possible; otherwise, follow the usual axiom concerning use of the most lateral incision if possible.

Exposure will be difficult owing to:

- altered anatomy
- soft-tissue contractures, including quadriceps and patellar tendon contractures, making patellar mobility difficult and increasing the risk of patellar avulsion
- arthrofibrosis
- synovitis with friable tissues.

The revision surgeon should be well versed in the various methods of improving exposure: quadriceps snip, V–Y quadricepsplasty, tibial tubercle osteotomy, etc.

Adequate arthrolysis and synovectomy should be performed, and the appropriate tissue and fluid cultures taken at this time.

Implant removal

Typically, the polyethylene insert is removed first. If the dedicated insert remover is available then this can be used; otherwise, the polyethylene insert of a modular implant can usually be knocked out using osteotomes. For an all-polyethylene tibial component, the tray can be separated from the intramedullary peg by using a saw at the component–cement interface. The tray portion can then be knocked out. The same principle is applied for the removal of the insert of a mobile bearing tibial component: the insert is separated from the tray beneath, after which the insert can be easily removed.

The femoral or tibial implant can then be removed in turn, depending on which is more accessible. The implants are usually removed with a combination of saws and osteotomes. The Gigli saw can be used on the femoral flange, and stacked osteotomes can also be useful. Specialized instruments for component removal are also available and can be useful for to hard-to-reach areas, e.g. the femoral notch, posterior femoral condyles and posterior tibia. These instruments are directed at the implant–cement interface, and the goal is to remove the implant while preserving as much bone stock as possible (Fig. 105.3).

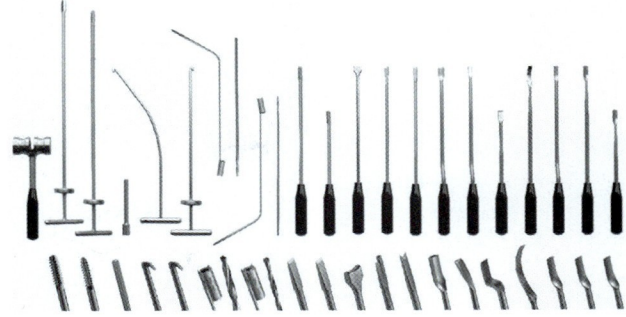

Figure 105.3 Revision knee arthroplasty instruments for implant removal.

All remaining cement is then removed, and special instruments (cement splitters, gouges, reverse hooks and curettes) may be necessary for this. A high-speed burr is also useful in this situation.

Tibial and femoral reconstruction

The proximal tibia is recut so that the surface is perpendicular to the mechanical axis of the lower limb. The femoral cuts are then made, typically using a combination of measured resection and gap-balancing techniques to produce rectangular flexion and extension gaps. Normally the only remaining landmark for judging femoral rotation is the epicondylar axis. Computer navigation is an emerging technique for guiding axis restoration and bone cuts during revision knee arthroplasty.

Depending on the integrity of the collateral ligaments, a varus–valgus constrained prosthesis may be needed. In extreme cases with severe bone and soft-tissue disruption, a hinged prosthesis may be necessary to achieve adequate stability.

Consideration is made regarding how to address bone loss. An assessment has to be made regarding its location(s), size and containment. A commonly used classification system is that of the Anderson Orthopaedic Research Institute. This system is based on the radiographic determination of the metaphyseal bone of the distal femur and proximal tibia. Femoral and tibial defects are preceded by F and T respectively, then further subdivided into three types: I, II and III. Type I defects have *intact, structurally stable metaphyseal bone* with no evidence of component subsidence, i.e. the component is stable. Type II defects have *damaged metaphyseal bone* with implant subsidence and/or joint line alteration, i.e. the implant is unstable (Fig. 105.4). Femoral type II defects are further subdivided into A (single condyle involved) and B (both condyles involved). Type III defects are more severe than type II defects with *deficiency* of the metaphysis that affects a major portion of the distal femur or tibial plateau. In the femur, this commonly refers to defects that

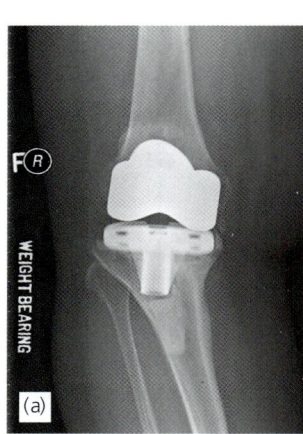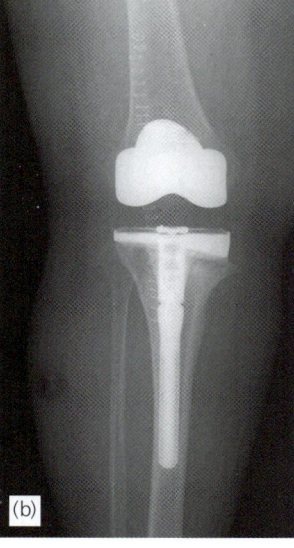

Figure 105.4 (a) Anderson Orthopaedic Research Institute type II bony defect. (b) Postoperative radiograph of the same patient following revision knee arthroplasty, with a stemmed tibial component and a metallic wedge augment to address the medial tibial bone loss.

extend to the level of the epicondyles, whereas in the tibia the defect typically extends to and below the fibula head.

Options for dealing with bone defects include:

- *Bone cement*.
- *Bone graft*. This may be an autograft, e.g. from distal femoral resection, or an allograft. Bone grafts may be used in morcellized or structural form.
- *Component augmentation*. This involves the use of wedges, stems and metaphyseal sleeves.
- *Allograft–prosthetic composite*.
- Distal femoral/proximal tibial replacement (megaprostheses).

For FI/TI defects, bone cement or morcellized graft is sufficient, whereas metal augments are typically needed for type II and III defects, and stemmed components will be necessary.

Stem extensions may be needed for the femoral and tibial components, to provide additional stability to the components and to transfer stresses away from the component–bone interface at the level of the joint line. Stem extensions may be necessary as a result of:

- poor bone stock
- use of augments/bone graft/cement for filling of bony deficiencies
- increasing prosthesis constraint, i.e. varus valgus constrained and hinged prostheses
- any requirement to bypass cortical defects in the metaphysis and diaphysis.

Another consideration relates to restoration of the native joint line. The native joint line may be estimated as:

- 1 cm below the distal pole of the patella
- 1 cm above the fibula head
- 2.5 cm and 1 cm below the medial and lateral femoral epicondyles, respectively. This distance can be more accurately judged using measurements from the contralateral knee, if it is not diseased.

When trying to balance flexion and extension gaps, an effort should be made to return to the normal joint line. For instance, if the extension gap is smaller than the flexion gap, cutting more distal femur will balance the gaps but lead to joint line elevation. A better solution might be to upsize the femoral component or use posterior augments to reduce the flexion gap. It is advisable not to raise the joint line by more than 8 mm.

Patellar reconstruction

If the patella has not previously been resurfaced, then it may be either left alone or resurfaced.

If the patella has previously been resurfaced, then it may be left alone if minimally worn and well fixed, or revised. Metal-backed patellar prostheses should be removed.[10] If the bone stock is poor, the patella may be reconstructed using bone graft, e.g. pouch technique,[11] or using an augment, e.g. trabecular metal, into which the prosthesis can be cemented.[12]

Patellectomy should be avoided as it significantly reduces the quadriceps function.

RESULTS OF REVISION KNEE ARTHROPLASTY

Current outcomes for revision knee arthroplasty are good, but fall short of the excellent outcomes seen following primary knee replacement.[13] Excellent and good results following revision probably average 80–85%. Actual outcomes depend on the mode of failure of the index procedure, with revision for sepsis having poorer outcomes.[14] As stated earlier, revision surgery for unexplained pain in an otherwise well-functioning knee has very poor results.[15]

Revision knee replacement is associated with higher morbidity and mortality[16] than primary knee replacement. Complications may occur in as many as 30% of patients, with wound and soft-tissue problems being particularly common. It also has reduced survivorship compared with primary arthroplasty, with failure rates estimated to range from 1% to 2% per year.[17]

KEY LEARNING POINTS

- When a total knee arthroplasty fails a surgeon has these options: revision; arthrodesis; excision arthroplasty or amputation.
- Causes of total knee arthroplasty failure are septic and aseptic. Aseptic causes include: loosening and periprosthetic fracture; instability; malalignment; and extensor failure (such as patellar instability, patellar subluxation, patellar fracture).
- Clinical evaluation should look at: pain; instability; stiffness, swelling; deformity; non-resolution of pre-operative symptoms and any evidence of infection.
- Causes of stiffness include: effusion; infection; arthrofibrosis; contracture; extensor mechanism weakness/failure; anterior or posterior tilt of components; overstuffing of the joint; loosening and loose bodies.
- Imaging includes: radiographs; bone scans; CT scans; and MRI.
- Blood tests to exclude infection include: leucocyte count, erythrocyte sedimentation rate, and C-reactive protein.
- Aspiration is useful to exclude infection.
- Frozen section of tissue with >10 polymorphonuclear cells per high-power field indicates infection.
- Other measures include: intra-articular injection of local anaesthetics; bracing; and physiotherapy and pain management.
- In general, for revision total knee arthroplasty, prepare the patient/staff/instruments and implants/yourself/and a plan for surgery.
- Goals of revision total knee arthroplasty are: eradicate infection; restore knee stability and kinematics; and preserve the soft tissues.
- Exposure can be difficult because of altered anatomy and scarring.
- The previous implant is removed stepwise.
- Tibial and femoral reconstruction are guided by the mechanical axis.
- Bone defects need consideration of use of: cement; bone graft; component augmentation; allograft; or megaprostheses.
- Stems may be needed: when there is poor bone stock; when augments/bone graft/cement have been used; when the prosthesis is constrained; and to bypass metaphysical or cortical defects.
- Restore the native joint line.
- The patella may need to be left alone, resurfaced or revised. But avoid patellectomy.
- Revision total knee arthroplasty is 85% successful.

REFERENCES

- ● = Key primary paper
- ◆ = Major review article

◆1. Mulhall KJ, Ghomrawi HM, Scully S, et al. Current etiologies and modes of failure in total knee arthroplasty revision. *Clinical Orthopaedics and Related Research* 2006;**446**:45–50.

●2. Vessely MB, Whaley AL, Harmsen WS, et al. The Chitranjan Ranawat Award: Long-term survivorship and failure modes of 1000 cemented condylar total knee arthroplasties. *Clinical Orthopaedics and Related Research* 2006;**452**:28–34.

●3. Werner FW, Ayers DC, Maletsky LP, Rullkoetter PJ. The effect of valgus/varus malalignment on load distribution in total knee replacements. *Journal of Biomechanics* 2005;**38**:349–55.

◆4. Brown 3rd EC, Clarke HD, Scuderi GR. The painful total knee arthroplasty: diagnosis and management. *Orthopedics* 2006;**29**:129–36; quiz 137–8.

●5. Mont MA, Serna FK, Krackow KA, Hungerford DS. Exploration of radiographically normal total knee replacements for unexplained pain. *Clinical Orthopaedics and Related Research* 1996;**331**:216–20.

●6. Klett R, Steiner D, Laurich S, et al. Evaluation of aseptic loosening of knee prostheses by quantitative bone scintigraphy. *Nuklearmedizin* 2008;**47**:163–6.

●7. Vessely MB, Frick MA, Oakes D, et al. Magnetic resonance imaging with metal suppression for evaluation of periprosthetic osteolysis after total knee arthroplasty. *Journal of Arthroplasty* 2006;**21**:826–31.

●8. Greidanus NV, Masri BA, Garbuz DS, et al. Use of erythrocyte sedimentation rate and C-reactive protein level to diagnose infection before revision total knee arthroplasty. A prospective evaluation. *Journal of Bone and Joint Surgery (American)* 2007;**89**:1409–16.

●9. Ghanem E, Parvizi J, Burnett RS, et al. Cell count and differential of aspirated fluid in the diagnosis of infection at the site of total knee arthroplasty. *Journal of Bone and Joint Surgery (American)* 2008;**90**:637–43.

◆10. Rorabeck CH, Mehin R, Barrack RL. Patellar options in revision total knee arthroplasty. *Clinical Orthopaedics and Related Research* 2003;**416**:84–92.

11. Hanssen AD. Bone-grafting for severe patellar bone loss during revision knee arthroplasty. *Journal of Bone and Joint Surgery (American)* 2001;**83A**:171–6.

●12. Nelson CL, Lonner JH, Lahiji A, et al. Use of a trabecular metal patella for marked patella bone loss during revision total knee arthroplasty. *Journal of Arthroplasty* 2003;**18**(7 Suppl. 1):37–41.

●13. Hossain F, Patel S, Haddad FS. Midterm assessment of causes and results of revision total knee arthroplasty. *Clinical Orthopaedics and Related Research* 2010;**468**:1221–8.

- 14. Deehan DJ, Murray JD, Birdsall PD, Pinder IM. Quality of life after knee revision arthroplasty. *Acta Orthopaedica* 2006;**77**:761-6.
- 15. Piedade SR, Pinaroli A, Servien E, Neyret P. Revision after early aseptic failures in primary total knee arthroplasty. *Knee Surgery, Sports Traumatology, Arthroscopy* 2009;**17**:248-53.
- 16. Memtsoudis SG, Gonzalez Della Valle A, Besculides MC, et al. In-hospital complications and mortality of unilateral, bilateral, and revision TKA: based on an estimate of 4,159,661 discharges. *Clinical Orthopaedics and Related Research* 2008;**466**:2617-27.
- 17. Sheng PY, Konttinen L, Lehto M, et al. Revision total knee arthroplasty: 1990 through 2002. A review of the Finnish arthroplasty registry. *Journal of Bone and Joint Surgery (American)* 2006;**88**:1425-30.

SECTION 4

The shoulder

106 **Shoulder arthroplasty**   1207
     Gerald Williams

106

Shoulder arthroplasty

GERALD WILLIAMS

Introduction	1207	Glenohumeral arthritis	1223
Rotator cuff tears	1207	Summary	1233
Glenohumeral instability	1214	References	1233

NATIONAL BOARD STANDARDS

- Learn about rotator cuff pathology and its surgical care
- Understand glenohumeral instability and the surgical treatment
- Know glenohumeral arthritis and the surgical options

INTRODUCTION

The field of adult shoulder reconstruction has enjoyed explosive growth over the last two decades. As recently as the early 1990s, most American orthopaedic residency programmes did not include attending orthopaedic surgeons with specialty training in shoulder surgery. Most graduating residents saw a reasonable number of open rotator cuff repairs but experienced only an occasional open Bankart procedure and few if any shoulder arthroplasties. As a result of the burgeoning interest in adult shoulder reconstruction, important clinical and basic science advances have improved the training received by our residents and the care received by our patients.

One of the biggest advances in the field of adult shoulder reconstruction has been the advent of arthroscopic techniques to manage many clinical problems. In fact, in many contemporary shoulder centres, including ours, arthroscopic management of most rotator cuff tears and glenohumeral instability problems is the norm. However, open procedures still have a substantial role in the treatment of many adult shoulder disorders. Moreover, arthroscopic management of adult shoulder problems is discussed elsewhere in this text.

Therefore, the purpose of this chapter is to discuss the role of open techniques in adult shoulder reconstruction. Discussion of all open procedures used in adult shoulder reconstruction is not possible within the confines of a single chapter. The focus, then, of this section will be the open surgical management of rotator cuff tears, glenohumeral instability and glenohumeral arthritis.

ROTATOR CUFF TEARS

Historical background

Rotator cuff tears were recognized in some of the earliest medical writings.[1] Although rotator cuff repair in the context of treatment of glenohumeral instability was described as early as 1889, it was not until the early 1900s that rotator cuff repair for isolated rotator cuff tears was reported.[2,3] Codman[2] is credited with one of the first reports of a supraspinatus tendon repair in 1911. Codman's technique evolved over time and eventually included an incision in Langer's lines, a deltoid-splitting approach, avoidance of an acromial osteotomy, rotation of the arm to improve visualization of different portions of the cuff and repair of the retracted tendon edge to bone.[4] Codman's privately published book, *Rupture of the Supraspinatus Tendon and Other Lesions In or About the Subacromial Bursa*,[5] outlines many of Codman's observations and techniques and is still one of the true classics in orthopaedic literature.

Controversy regarding the aetiology of rotator cuff tears has always existed. Traumatic tears of otherwise normal tendons are uncommon and probably represent no more than 5–10% of all rotator cuff tears.[6] Neer[6] emphasized subacromial impingement as an important aetiological factor in rotator cuff tears. Intrinsic tendon degeneration is also, undoubtedly, a substantial contributing factor to most rotator cuff defects.[7,8] Although debate continuously occurs regarding the relative contributions of these three aetiological factors, it is likely that almost all rotator cuff tears are the result of some combination of age-related degeneration, trauma and subacromial impingement.

Radical acromionectomy was a popular surgical treatment for subacromial impingement and rotator cuff lesions prior to 1972. Neer[6] was the first to recognize that subacromial impingement lesions occurred on the undersurface of the anterolateral aspect of the acromion and not on the lateral acromion. In addition, he recognized the potentially devastating complications associated with radical acromionectomy.[9] Therefore, in 1972, Neer[6] published his classic article on anterior acromioplasty in the management of rotator cuff lesions. Anterior acromioplasty became one of the most common shoulder procedures performed in the USA over the ensuing three decades. More recently, some have questioned the role of acromioplasty in the surgical management of rotator cuff tears.[10–13] However, most surgeons continue to perform acromioplasty or some form of subacromial smoothing when repairing chronic rotator cuff tears.

Pertinent anatomy

The rotator cuff comprises four musculotendinous units and their corresponding neurovascular bundles. The two largest muscles are the infraspinatus posteriorly and the subscapularis anteriorly. The supraspinatus muscle occupies the supraspinatus fossa superiorly and its tendon is most commonly involved in rotator cuff tears. The teres minor is the smallest rotator cuff muscle and its tendon is the most inferior of the posterior rotator cuff tendons. The supra- and infraspinatus are both supplied by the suprascapular nerve, which can be affected by retraction associated with posterosuperior rotator cuff tears.[14–16] The teres minor is supplied by the axillary nerve, following its exit from the quadrilateral space posteriorly. The subscapularis is supplied by the upper and lower subscapular nerves.

The deltoid muscle is the power elevator of the arm and acts in concert with the rotator cuff and other shoulder girdle muscles. It arises from the anterior clavicle, acromion and scapular spine. The raphe between its middle and anterior thirds is commonly used to gain entrance into the subacromial space.[6] The deltoid is supplied by the axillary nerve, which innervates the muscle from posterior to anterior as it courses along the deltoid undersurface approximately 5 cm distal to the lateral acromial margin.[17,18]

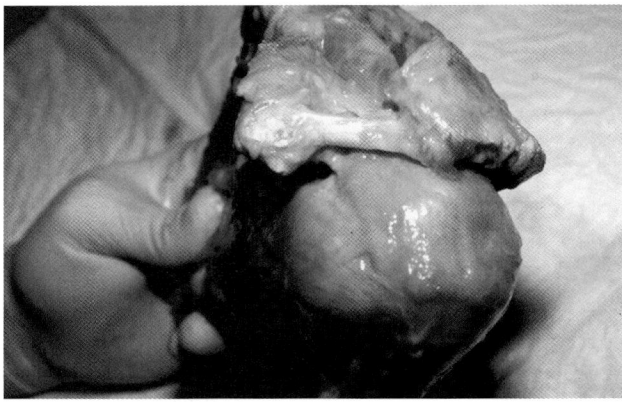

Figure 106.1 The coracoacromial arch is a bone–ligament structure consisting of the coracoid process, the coracoacromial ligament and the acromion. The supraspinatus travels under this arch during arm elevation.

The coracoacromial arch is a bone–ligament complex consisting of the anterior acromion, coracoacromial ligament and coracoid process (Fig. 106.1). It acts as a restraint to anterosuperior subluxation, especially in the presence of a large rotator cuff tear.[19–21] Loss of the coracoacromial arch can cause disabling anterosuperior instability in large rotator cuff tears.[21,22] In addition to the undersurface of the acromioclavicular joint, the coracoacromial arch forms a tunnel through which the supraspinatus tendon passes during elevation of the arm. The coracoacromial arch and acromioclavicular joint have been implicated in the development of impingement syndrome and rotator cuff tears.[23]

Clinical evaluation

HISTORY AND PHYSICAL EXAMINATION

In the absence of severe trauma or repetitive overuse injuries, rotator cuff tears most commonly occur after the fourth decade of life. In addition, many patients with rotator cuff tears will report past episodes of transient shoulder pain that may have been diagnosed as tendonitis or bursitis. Therefore, in patients over the age of 40 years who complain of anterior shoulder pain, the rotator cuff should at least be considered as the cause of pain. A recent history of trauma, particularly if it were associated with weakness or loss of elevation, is important to elicit and suggests an acute or an acute-on-chronic full-thickness rotator cuff tear.

Neer[6] described the impingement sign, which is elicited by passively pushing the arm into maximal elevation (Fig. 106.2a). This presumably causes pain by compressing the inflamed subacromial bursa and rotator cuff against a

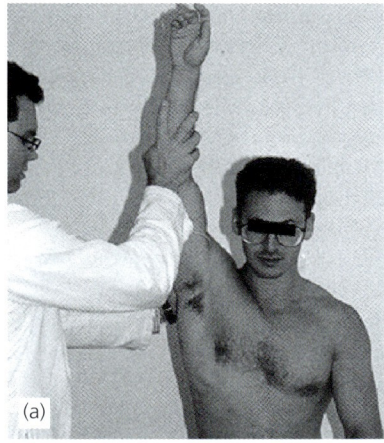

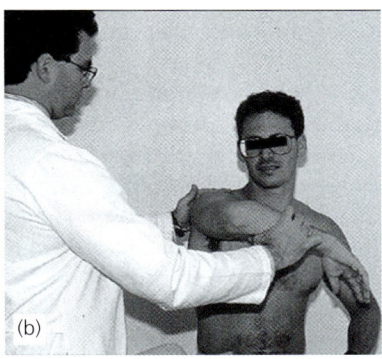

Figure 106.2 The Neer impingement sign (a), and the Hawkins impingement reinforcement sign (b) are positive in patients with subacromial impingement syndrome. Reprinted from Arroyo JS, Flatow EL. Management of rotator cuff disease: intact and reparable cuff. In Iannotti JP, Williams GR (eds) *Disorders of the Shoulder: Diagnosis and Management*. Philadelphia, PA: Lippincott, Williams, and Wilkins, 1999:35.

prominent anterior acromion. If the pain associated with the impingement sign is relieved following subacromial injection of a local anaesthetic, the diagnosis of impingement syndrome is confirmed.[6] The impingement reinforcement sign or Hawkins sign is performed with the arm in 90° of elevation in the scapular plane (Fig. 106.2b).[24] The humerus is internally rotated so that the greater tuberosity passes under the coracoacromial arch. This causes pain in patients with impingement syndrome, and the pain is more pronounced as the arm is brought anterior to the scapular plane. Subacromial injection of a local anaesthetic, just as with the classic Neer impingement sign, usually relieves the pain.

Inability to raise the arm is a sign of stiffness, pain or weakness. Symmetrical loss of both active and passive range of motion is a sign of stiffness. If pain is severe enough to interfere with range of motion assessment, it can be mitigated by injection of a local anaesthetic followed by repeat examination. Lack of active motion in the absence of stiffness or pain severe enough to prevent motion testing is a sign of weakness. If it is new in onset following a traumatic event, a large, acute or acute-on-chronic rotator cuff tear should be suspected. Alternatively or concomitantly, a nerve injury (i.e. axillary nerve) may be present. However, in patients over 40 years, a large rotator cuff defect should be excluded when shoulder weakness following trauma is identified.

Specific strength tests can be used to identify weakness in each of the rotator cuff muscles. Although it is difficult, if not impossible, to completely isolate the function of individual rotator cuff muscles, testing in certain planes of motion can indicate strength of portions of the rotator cuff. In general, three types of tests are performed to gauge strength. First, the patient is asked to actively perform a motion. Second, the force with which they can perform the requested motion is measured or estimated. Third, the examiner passively places the arm in a position of maximum excursion in a given plane and the patient's ability to maintain that position is evaluated. This last manoeuvre is termed a lag sign.[25] Obviously, full or near full passive range of motion is a prerequisite for accurate strength testing.

Active external rotation is tested with the arm at the side as well as with the arm at 90° of elevation in the scapular plane. In the former position, external rotation strength is likely to be a function of the supraspinatus and upper portion of the infraspinatus. In the latter position, external rotation strength is determined by the teres minor and lower portion of the infraspinatus. Likewise, external rotation lag signs are performed in both arm positions and are indicative of weakness of the same muscles (Fig. 106.3). A severe external rotation lag sign at 90° of elevation is also known as a 'horn blower's sign'.

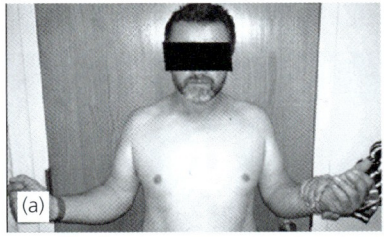

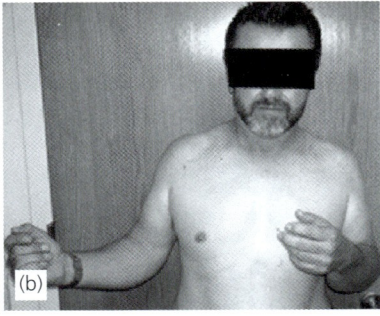

Figure 106.3 The external rotation lag sign is positive on this patient's left arm. The test is performed by passively externally rotating the arm (a) and determining that he cannot hold it there actively (b). Reprinted from Arroyo JS, Flatow EL. Management of rotator cuff disease: intact and reparable cuff. In Iannotti JP, Williams GR (eds) *Disorders of the Shoulder: Diagnosis and Management*. Philadelphia, PA: Lippincott, Williams, and Wilkins, 1999:33.

Supraspinatus strength can also be evaluated using abduction in the scapular plane. The patient is asked to hold the arm at 90° of elevation in the scapular plane against resistance and the strength is estimated. Alternatively, an abduction lag sign is tested when the examiner passively positions the arm into maximum scapular plane abduction and the patient's ability to maintain that position is assessed.

Subscapularis strength can be evaluated by testing internal rotation. The patient is asked to place the back of their hand against their sacrum or lower back. They are then asked to lift their hand away from their body by internally rotating their humerus. Inability to do so, in the absence of loss of passive internal rotation, is indicative of subscapularis weakness. This has been termed the 'lift-off' test by Gerber and colleagues.[25,26] The abdominal compression test may be easier to perform and also implies subscapularis weakness.[27] The internal rotation lag sign can be performed in either of these positions and also indicates subscapularis weakness (Fig. 106.4).[25]

IMAGING

Potential imaging modalities in patients with suspected rotator cuff tears include routine radiography, arthrography, ultrasound, CT arthrography, MRI and MRI arthrography. Plain radiographs should be obtained in most cases. In large, chronic rotator cuff tears, proximal humeral migration and a diminished acromiohumeral interval may be identified. In addition, specialized views, such as the supraspinatus outlet view and the 30° caudal tilt view, can aid in assessing acromial shape (Fig. 106.5).[28–30]

Sonography is a cost-effective and accurate method of identifying rotator cuff tears.[31,32] Rotator cuff tear size and chronicity as well as biceps tendon abnormalities can be assessed with ultrasound. In addition, it may be the best modality for evaluation of the postoperative rotator cuff.[33] However, the technique is operator dependent and information regarding other intra-articular abnormalities is limited.

MRI is probably the most commonly used method of rotator cuff imaging in the USA. It has the advantages of excellent accuracy,[34] accessibility and versatility, in that it potentially provides information about many other soft-tissue and osseous structures about the shoulder. Atrophy and fatty degeneration of the rotator cuff muscles can also be identified (Fig. 106.6).[35] It is, however, expensive and scan quality can vary widely depending on the scanning equipment.

Arthrography was very commonly used to identify full-thickness rotator cuff tears in the 1970s and 1980s.[36,37] Although it can reliably distinguish between full-thickness rotator cuff tears and intact and partially torn rotator cuff tendons, information regarding the size and location of the tear and the presence of atrophy is limited. CT arthrography has been used more recently and provides more information on tear size and location than plain radiography. In addition, fatty degeneration of the rotator cuff muscles can also be identified.[38] MRI arthrography can be particularly helpful in the postoperative setting.

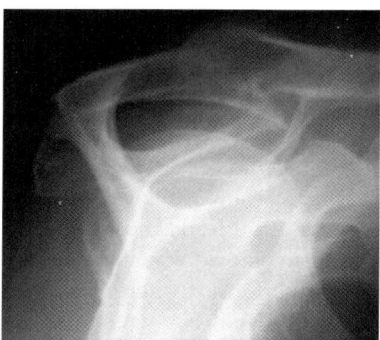

Figure 106.5 The outlet view demonstrates anteroinferior spur formation in patients with subacromial impingement syndrome.

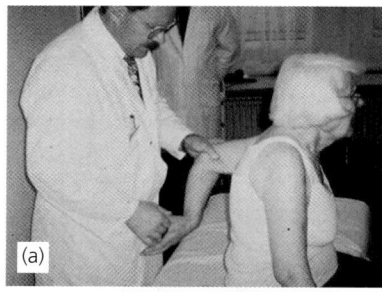
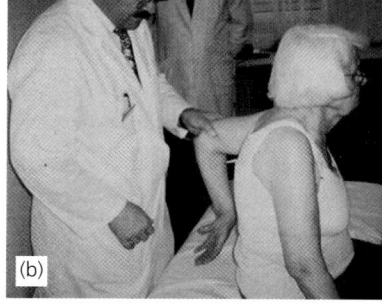

Figure 106.4 The internal rotation lag sign is indicative of subscapularis weakness and is performed by passively internally rotating the arm (a) and asking the patient to hold it there. The test is positive when the arm recoils back to the sacrum (b). Images courtesy of Christian Gerber, MD.

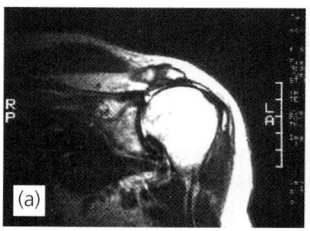
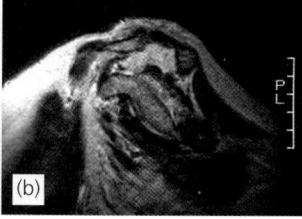

Figure 106.6 MRI scanning reveals a retracted tear of the supra- and infraspinatus (a) with severe atrophy and fatty infiltration of both muscles (b).

The timing of rotator cuff imaging is dependent on patient age, functional demand, injury history and physical findings. The cuff should be imaged early (within days to weeks) after an injury in a young patient with new onset of weakness and loss of overhead function. In an older, sedentary patient with good overhead elevation, and no history of recent injury, imaging can be delayed until non-operative management has failed (3 months). Many patients will fall somewhere between these two extremes. The timing of rotator cuff imaging in these patients should be individualized. In general, imaging is indicated earlier in the treatment process for younger, more active patients.

Treatment

NON-OPERATIVE

Most patients with chronic rotator cuff tears and acute rotator cuff tears without substantial retraction are candidates for non-operative management. The mainstays of non-surgical treatment of rotator cuff tears are pain control, activity modification and physiotherapy. Pain management includes analgesics, non-steroidal anti-inflammatory medications and occasional corticosteroid injections. Narcotic analgesics are rarely needed. The frequency of corticosteroid injections is controversial and few data exist to solve the controversy. A frequency of three injections per year is used as a guideline by many surgeons.

The goals of therapeutic exercises are to restore or maintain passive motion, strengthen the remaining rotator cuff and deltoid muscles, and improve coordination between the scapular rotators and the remaining rotator cuff. Stiffness may accompany rotator cuff tears and can have a negative influence on the outcome of surgical repair. Therefore, when stiffness is present, passive range of motion and stretching exercises are performed. The posterior capsule is often contracted and should be especially targeted. Once passive range of motion has been restored, strengthening exercises for the remaining rotator cuff, deltoid and scapular rotators are instituted. Many exercise protocols exist and an in-depth discussion of all of them is beyond the scope of this chapter. However, in general, rotator cuff and deltoid exercises include external rotation with the arm at the side, scapular plane abduction, flexion, extension and internal rotation. Scapular strengthening exercises comprise shoulder shrugs, upright rowing and wall push-ups. When non-operative management is indicated, a trial of 3–6 months is appropriate.

OPEN ROTATOR CUFF REPAIR

Rotator cuff repair is indicated in most patients with an acute tear with retraction, an acute-on-chronic tear with new onset of weakness and poor function, and a chronic tear that has not responded to non-operative management for a minimum of 3 months. The decision to repair the rotator cuff open, as opposed to arthroscopically, should be individualized and is based on surgeon and patient preference, cuff tear size and chronicity, and patient age and activity level. When an open rotator cuff repair has been chosen, certain technical steps are important. These steps include anaesthesia and patient positioning, skin incision, deltoid and coracoacromial ligament detachment, acromioplasty, cuff mobilization and repair, and deltoid and coracoacromial ligament reattachment. In addition, symptomatic acromioclavicular joint arthropathy and biceps tendonitis, subluxation or partial tearing may require treatment. Appropriate postoperative rehabilitation is also an important element of success.

ANAESTHESIA AND PATIENT POSITIONING

Anaesthetic choices for open rotator cuff repair include general, regional (i.e. interscalene block) or a combination of general and regional. Each method has associated risks and benefits. The patient should choose the anaesthetic method after a discussion with the anaesthetist. Many patients elect either regional or combined general and regional anaesthesia because of the added benefit of prolonged postoperative analgesia.

The most commonly used position for open rotator cuff repair is the 'beach chair' position. The back of the table may be elevated 70–80° to allow complete access to the superior aspect of the shoulder. The hips and knees should be flexed to avoid excessive tension on the sciatic nerve. The head and neck should be stabilized in a neutral position to prevent injury to the brachial plexus, cervical nerve roots and other neurovascular structures. All bony and neurological prominences should be padded to minimize pressure. Surgical drapes should be placed to allow access to the anterior, superior and posterior aspects of the shoulder as well as the acromioclavicular joint and the entire upper extremity.

SKIN INCISION

The rotator cuff tear is approached through an 8–10 cm incision in Langer's skin lines, approximately parallel to the lateral margin of the acromion (Fig. 106.7). The incision begins at the mid-portion of the lateral acromial margin and extends anteriorly. If acromioclavicular excision is also

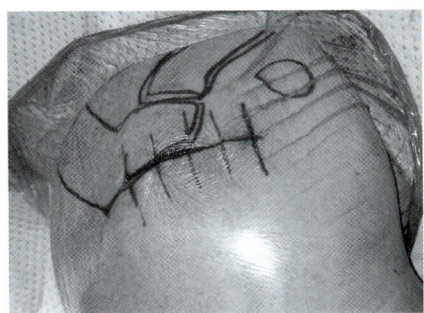

Figure 106.7 The skin incision for open rotator cuff repair is made in Langer's skin lines, paralleling the lateral margin of the acromion.

planned, the incision should be more medial, midway between the lateral acromial margin and the acromioclavicular joint. The incision is carried to the level of the deltoid fascia and full-thickness subcutaneous flaps are developed medially and laterally. This allows visualization of the proximal portion of the deltoid, the anterior half of the acromion and the acromioclavicular joint.

DELTOID AND CORACOACROMIAL LIGAMENT DETACHMENT

The deltoid is split in line with its fibres, starting at the anterolateral corner of the acromion and extending distally for approximately 4 cm. The split should lie within the raphe between the anterior and middle portions of the deltoid. This split is developed through the deltoid to the level of the roof of the subacromial bursa, which is likewise split from the anterolateral acromial corner distally for approximately 4 cm. The incision between the anterior and middle thirds of the deltoid is then extended onto the dorsal surface of the acromion from its anterolateral corner and is extended medially to a point 1 cm medial to the acromioclavicular joint. The incision should be made parallel to the long axis of the distal clavicle approximately 0.5–1.0 cm posterior to the anterior acromial margin. The anterior deltoid, roof of the subacromial bursa, anterior acromioclavicular joint capsule and acromial attachment of the coracoacromial ligament are then detached from the anterior acromion in a single layer. This method of detachment creates a thick, fibrous edge for secure reattachment at the completion of the procedure.

ACROMIOPLASTY

With the deltoid retracted, the undersurface of the acromion can be palpated. If it is prominent, an anterior acromioplasty is performed. The goal is to create a smooth, relatively flat subacromial surface. The anterior extent of the residual acromion should be even with the anterior cortical border of the distal clavicle. This typically requires removal of a wedge of bone that includes the anterior acromion, from the anterolateral corner to the acromioclavicular joint, and the undersurface of its anterior third (Fig. 106.8). This wedge should be thickest anteriorly and taper posteriorly. The acromioplasty can be performed with an osteotome or micro-sagittal saw, with final smoothing of the acromial undersurface with a rasp or burr. In addition, the bone can be removed in two steps (anterior acromionectomy and inferior bevelling), as described by Rockwood and Lyons,[30] or in one step, as described by Neer.[6] Care should be taken to avoid excessive anteroposterior (AP) shortening or thinning of the acromion. The subacromial area should be copiously irrigated and cleared of all visible bone debris to minimize the development of postoperative heterotopic ossification.

CUFF MOBILIZATION AND REPAIR

Successful rotator cuff repair requires firm reattachment of the torn tendon to bone without excessive tension. In

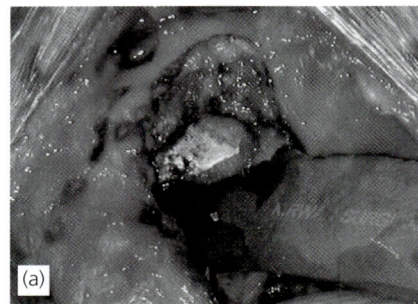

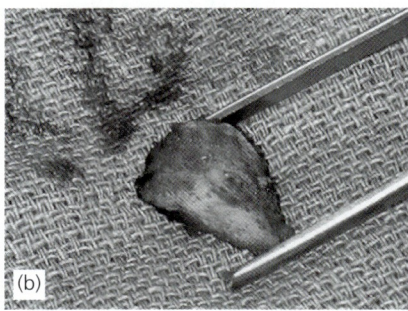

Figure 106.8 In patients with a prominent anterior acromial spur (a), an acromioplasty is performed that removes a small wedge of bone that is widest anteriorly and tapers posteriorly (b).

some cases, the rotator cuff tear is small and minimally retracted. Under these circumstances, the cuff can be repaired to bone without substantial mobilization. In larger tears, however, the torn tendon is retracted. In chronic and most acute-on-chronic cases, the tendon cannot be advanced to the greater tuberosity or anatomic neck without soft-tissue releases and lateral mobilization. Even after extensive mobilization techniques have been performed, some rotator cuff tears cannot be repaired with the arm at the side under minimal tension.

Mobilization of retracted rotator cuff tears comprises three basic steps: (1) release of adhesions on the superficial surface, (2) release of the capsule on the deep surface and (3) longitudinal release of the anterior and/or posterior leading edges of the retracted tendon. Mobilization is facilitated by placing multiple traction sutures in the edge of the retracted tendon and displacing the humeral head inferiorly. Superficial adhesions are released using scissors and blunt dissection. The capsule deep to the retracted tendon is released sharply at the glenoid margin. Dissection medial to the superior or posterior glenoid rim should be limited to 1–2 cm to avoid injury to the suprascapular nerve.[39] The need for anterior and posterior interval releases is dictated by tear configuration. If the anterior edge of the tear is retracted and the posterior edge is not, the tear is L-shaped and an anterior interval release is required.[40] If the posterior edge is retracted and the anterior edge is not, the tear is reverse L-shaped and a posterior interval release is required.[41] If both edges are retracted, the tear is U-shaped and both anterior and posterior interval releases may be required. Obviously, complicated tear configurations beyond these three basic types are common and the need for longitudinal releases should be individualized accordingly.

The rotator cuff can be repaired to bone using multiple sutures passed through bone and tied over the lateral cortex of the humerus. These tendon-to-bone sutures are supplemented with side-to-side sutures in any longitudinal interval releases that were created to mobilize the tendon (Fig. 106.9). The number of sutures depends on the tear size. In general, tendon-to-bone sutures should be 1.0–1.5 cm apart. Initial pull-out strength can be maximized by passing the sutures through the tendon in a Mason–Allen configuration.[42] The tendon footprint can be maximized by passing the deep suture through the anatomic neck and the superficial suture more laterally, through the tip of the greater tuberosity. Addition of a soft-tissue button or plate at the lateral cortex minimizes suture pull-through.[42]

DELTOID AND CORACOACROMIAL LIGAMENT REPAIR

The anterior deltoid and roof of the subacromial bursa are reattached in a single layer. In addition, since loss of the coracoacromial ligament may result in anterosuperior escape of the humeral head should the cuff repair fail, it is also repaired with the deltoid and the roof of the bursa.[43] Non-absorbable sutures are passed through the entire thickness of the detached tissue, including the acromial periosteum and anterior deltoid fascia, the posterior deltoid fascia, the roof of the subacromial bursa and the coracoacromial ligament. The suture is then passed through the anterior

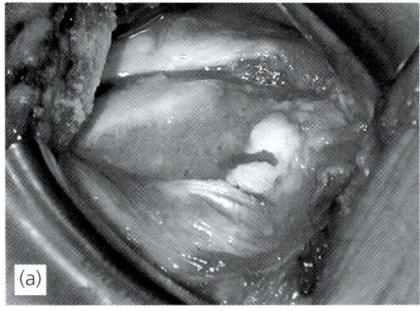
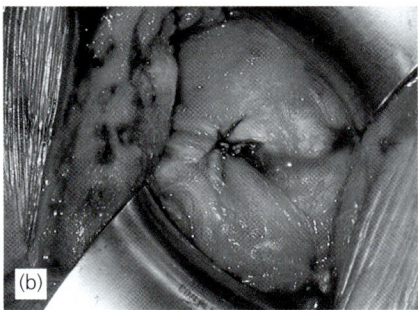

Figure 106.9 This rotator cuff tear involves the right shoulder and is a reverse-L configured tear, with an avulsion of the supraspinatus and a longitudinal tear between the retracted supraspinatus and the infraspinatus (a). It was repaired with three tendon-to-bone sutures and one side-to-side suture in the posterior longitudinal split (b).

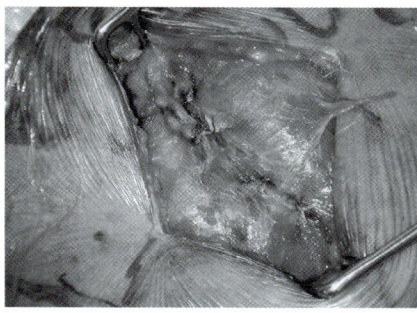

Figure 106.10 The deltoid is repaired to the bone of the acromion as well as to the deltoid fascia and acromioclavicular joint capsule.

acromion and the dorsal fascia (Fig. 106.10). Soft-tissue repair is performed medially, using the acromioclavicular joint capsule, and laterally, using the middle deltoid fascia. The anterolateral deltoid split is repaired using interrupted sutures. The skin incision is closed with interrupted absorbable sutures in the subcutaneous layer and a running, subcuticular stitch using a non-absorbable monofilament suture in the skin.

ACROMIOCLAVICULAR ARTHROPATHY

Symptomatic acromioclavicular joint arthropathy may be present in conjunction with a rotator cuff tear and is managed with acromioclavicular joint excision. The distal clavicular periosteum and superior acromioclavicular joint capsule are elevated from the distal clavicle. A micro-sagittal saw is used to resect 0.5–1.0 cm of the distal clavicle, taking care to preserve the posterior capsule. The superior capsule and periosteum are repaired to the residual distal clavicle through drill holes and the anterior deltoid is repaired as described above.

BICEPS TENDON LESIONS

Failure to address associated biceps pathology in patients undergoing rotator cuff repair may result in persistent pain postoperatively. The biceps tendon should be inspected for partial tearing and subluxation in all patients at the time of rotator cuff repair.[44] If partial tearing of greater than 25% of the tendon substance or subluxation is identified, the tendon is tenodesed into the proximal humerus. A grasping suture is placed in the long head of the biceps at the level of the superior extent of the bicipital groove. The tendon is excised proximal to the suture and a burr hole large enough to accept the residual end of the biceps tendon is made in the bicipital groove. One suture end is passed posteriorly through the burr hole and out the greater tuberosity. The other suture end is passed anteriorly through the burr hole and out the lesser tuberosity. The suture ends are then pulled tightly to bring the tendon end into the burr hole and are tied over the bicipital groove.

POSTOPERATIVE REHABILITATION

A polysling with a small abduction pillow is used after most rotator cuff repairs. Following repair of large, chronic, two-tendon tears, a larger abduction pillow may be used. Keeping the arm slightly abducted and in neutral rotation presumably minimizes the tension on the repair and may improve tendon healing. Active and active-assisted range of motion are avoided for 6–8 weeks postoperatively. For the first 2 weeks postoperatively, even passive range of motion may be avoided in order to allow early adherence of the tendon to the bone of the humerus. If, however, any pre-operative stiffness were present, passive range of motion is instituted immediately postoperatively. Passive range of motion is maintained for 6–8 weeks postoperatively, at which time active range of motion, rotator cuff and deltoid strengthening, and scapular stabilizing exercises are instituted. Strengthening is performed using elastic straps until 3 months postoperatively, when hand weights may be added.

Complete recovery requires approximately 1 year. Guidelines for return to activity include no active use of the shoulder for 6 weeks, active use of the arm with no lifting from 6–12 weeks, lifting of up to 10 pounds (4.5 kg) with both arms from 12–24 weeks, lifting of up to 20 pounds (9 kg) with both arms from 24–36 weeks and activity as tolerated at 36 weeks.

Results

The clinical results of rotator cuff repair are good or excellent in approximately 90% of cases.[6,45–47] In general, results correlate with tear size and chronicity as evidenced by rotator cuff muscle atrophy and fatty degeneration.[38] These results are typically maintained in a high percentage of cases with long-term follow-up.[48] In addition, despite good clinical results, re-rupture of the rotator cuff happens frequently and at a rate that is related to the size of the tear, the age of the patient, and the chronicity of the tear.[49] However, even though most patients are satisfied following rotator cuff repair, regardless of repair integrity, the patients with an intact repair at follow-up are the most satisfied and exhibit the highest functional scores. Therefore, the goal of rotator cuff repair remains a permanently healed tendon to bone.

Complications

Complications of rotator cuff repair, except for recurrence of the tear, are relatively uncommon.[50] Reported complications include infection, deltoid detachment, frozen shoulder, heterotopic ossification, recurrent rotator cuff tear, axillary nerve injury, anterosuperior instability, reflex sympathetic dystrophy, deep vein thrombosis and death. Most complications can be avoided or minimized through good surgical technique. Prophylactic antibiotics are used to minimize the rate of infection. The deltoid should be detached and reattached carefully. Avoid detaching the deltoid distal to its tendon of origin so that good tissue is available for repair. Irrigate frequently and excise or remove all visible bone debris. Avoid splitting the deltoid more than 4 cm distal to the lateral edge of the acromion. Repair the coracoacromial ligament along with the deltoid and avoid excessive acromial bone removal.

A high index of suspicion is necessary to recognize complications early. Any patient with a subcutaneous haematoma within the first two postoperative weeks has a deltoid detachment until proven otherwise. If a deltoid detachment is recognized, it should be repaired as soon as possible, since the results of deltoid repair correlate closely with time from surgery.[51] Postoperative infection following rotator cuff surgery must be treated aggressively with debridement and long-term antibiotics and more than one debridement may be necessary.[52–54] Infection is often accompanied by deltoid detachment and failure of the cuff repair. The deltoid should be repaired at the time of the initial debridement. Consideration is given to early re-repair of the rotator cuff. The use of a monofilament, absorbable suture for early deltoid or rotator cuff repair may decrease the incidence of recurrence of the infection.

GLENOHUMERAL INSTABILITY

Historical background

For as long as humans have been physically active, glenohumeral dislocations are likely to have occurred. It is not surprising that the earliest human writings contain descriptions of shoulder dislocations and their treatment.[1] Hippocrates, the father of modern medicine, provided much information about glenohumeral instability, including normal and pathological anatomy, classification of dislocations and treatment – both surgical and non-surgical.[55]

In the mid-1800s, study of autopsy and museum specimens revealed the anterior glenoid rim defects, posterolateral humeral head impression fractures, capsular avulsions and occasional rotator cuff ruptures associated with traumatic and recurrent dislocations.[56,57] With the advent of radiographs in 1895, the association of osseous defects of both the humerus and glenoid with glenohumeral instability became even more recognized. Hill and Sachs,[58] in 1940, produced an exhaustive review of the published information on the posterolateral humeral head defect; this defect subsequently has borne their names.

Although Bankart[59] was not the first to recognize the anterior capsulolabral avulsion lesion in recurrent anterior dislocations, he believed it was the 'essential lesion' in most recurrent dislocations and recommended its repair to prevent further dislocations. Many subsequent surgeons have reported the results of surgical repair of recurrent anterior dislocations using some modification of Bankart's original technique. One of the most often quoted series is that of Rowe et al.,[60] who reported 97% good or excellent results in 161 patients who underwent open Bankart repair. The presence of a glenoid rim defect of up to 25% of the articular surface had no effect on outcome and a 'moderate to severe' Hill–Sachs defect increased the risk of recurrence 'only slightly'. More recently, the importance of glenoid and humeral bone defects has become more recognized.[61–63]

Posterior instability is less common than its anterior counterpart and, traditionally, has not responded as well to surgical treatment. This is most likely at least partially because of the overlap of generalized ligament laxity and scapular dyskinesis that seems more common in patients with posterior instability. In this difficult patient population, non-operative management in the form of physiotherapy deserves greater emphasis. The most commonly performed surgical techniques are capsular procedures – either repair or plication.

The 'essential lesion' in most patients with multi-directional instability is increased capsular volume.[64,65] Neer and Foster[65] described the inferior capsular shift as a means of decreasing capsular volume in patients with multidirectional instability. They recommended performing the operation from both anterior as well as posterior approaches, depending on the most prominent direction of the symptoms. Although rotator interval closure was a component of Neer and Foster's original technique for anteroinferior capsular shift, its importance was emphasized more strongly by subsequent authors.[66]

Pertinent anatomy

In general, stability of the glenohumeral joint is maintained through the combined efforts of the static and dynamic stabilizers. The static restraints include the humerus, glenoid, labrum and capsular ligaments; the dynamic stabilizers include the rotator cuff, long head of the biceps, deltoid and scapular rotators. Stability throughout mid-ranges of motion is primarily the result of the concavity-compression mechanism created by the combination of bony/labral constraint and axial compression of the rotator cuff.[67,68] Osseous constraint of the glenohumeral joint is relatively poor compared with other ball-and-socket joints. The depth of the glenoid socket, when the articular cartilage and labrum are included, is only 5–9 mm.[69] The addition of a compressive force improves stability substantially.[68] Loss of the glenoid rim causes a significant decrease in the force required for dislocation.[67]

The glenohumeral ligaments are thickenings of various regions of the joint capsule and act primarily as restraints to excessive rotation and translation at the extremes of motion (Fig. 106.11). The superior glenohumeral and coracohumeral ligaments are part of the rotator interval

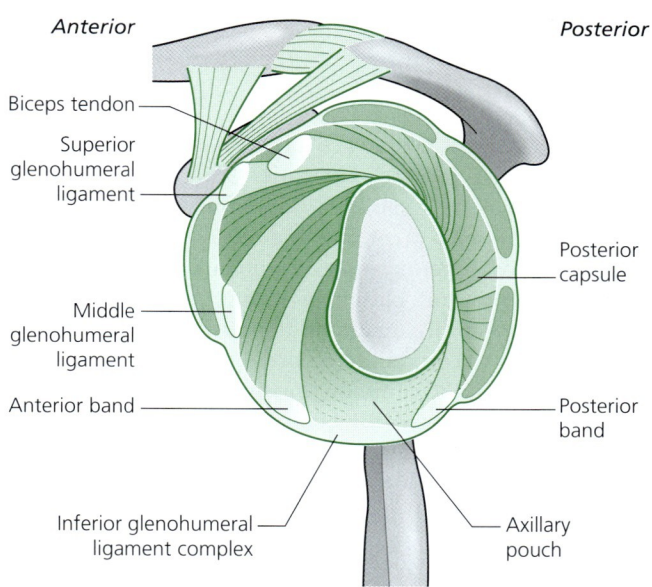

Figure 106.11 The glenohumeral ligaments are thickenings in the joint capsule and provide stability at the extremes of motion.

capsule and limit external rotation and inferior translation with the arm at the side. The inferior glenohumeral ligament consists of an anterior band, posterior band and intervening axillary pouch.[70] Overall, the inferior glenohumeral ligament limits passive abduction and inferior translation with the arm at 90° of elevation in the scapular plane. The anterior band limits external rotation and anterior translation, whereas the posterior band limits internal rotation and posterior translation of the elevated arm.[71]

Surgical approaches to the glenohumeral joint during instability operations require knowledge of important neurological structures. The axillary nerve arises from the posterior cord of the brachial plexus and traverses the anterior surface of the subscapularis muscle to reach the inferior aspect of the glenohumeral joint. It enters the quadrilateral space bounded medially by the long head of the triceps, laterally by the humeral neck, inferiorly by the teres major, and superiorly by the subscapularis. Upon exiting the quadrilateral space, the axillary nerve supplies the teres minor and the deltoid as well as sensation to the lateral portion of the shoulder. The musculocutaneous nerve is a terminal branch of the lateral cord of the brachial plexus and enters the posterior surface of the conjoined tendon of the coracobrachialis and short head of the biceps a variable distance from the tip of the coracoid. The suprascapular nerve is a terminal branch of the superior trunk of the brachial plexus and supplies the supra- and infraspinatus muscles. The interval between the infraspinatus and teres minor is an internervous plane commonly exploited during posterior approaches to the shoulder.

Clinical evaluation

CLASSIFICATION

Glenohumeral instability is a spectrum of disease that cannot be divided into tidy categories easily. Nevertheless, it helps to think of instability in certain patterns. Instability has been classified according to direction (anterior, posterior, inferior, superior, multidirectional), degree (subluxation or dislocation), chronicity (acute, chronic, recurrent) and mechanism (traumatic, atraumatic, congenital, microtraumatic). Classification according to mechanism has been the basis of common treatment algorithms which have been developed for certain types of glenohumeral instability.[72–74] Patients with a documented traumatic history are most likely to have a discrete anatomic lesion (i.e. Bankart lesion) which will respond favourably to surgical intervention. Conversely, patients with atraumatic recurrent instability often demonstrate bilateral, multidirectional laxity which is best managed with a rehabilitative exercise programme. Surgical stabilization is reserved for those few patients with disabling instability despite compliance with rehabilitation and consists of decreasing capsular volume through an inferior capsular shift and, often, a rotator interval plication.[64,65,75–77]

HISTORY AND PHYSICAL EXAMINATION

History taking should be aimed at eliciting information that may influence surgical prognosis. Patients with a traumatic history of a dislocation that required a reduction by a health professional and was accompanied by a period of substantial disability are likely to have an anatomic cause for their instability that is correctable. Patients with a seizure history are likely to have bone defects. Moreover, their seizures should be well controlled before proceeding with surgery. A history of multiple dislocations is likely to signal a component of capsular stretching that requires more than just labral reattachment. Participation in contact sports such as wrestling and football may suggest a greater likelihood of recurrence after surgery.

Physical findings in patients with recurrent glenohumeral instability are also important. It is critical to remember that instability and laxity are different. Instability requires symptoms and laxity may be normal for a given patient. Comparison with the asymptomatic side will help discern laxity from instability. In addition, other joints such as the knee, elbow and metacarpophalangeal joints should be tested for excessive motion as generalized ligamentous laxity may suggest an underlying collagen–vascular disorder, a poor surgical prognosis, or, at the very least, a tendency to stretch out after repair (Fig. 106.12).

An in-depth discussion of all physical examination tests that have been described in the diagnosis of glenohumeral instability is beyond the scope of this chapter. However, several points deserve emphasis. First, apprehension in

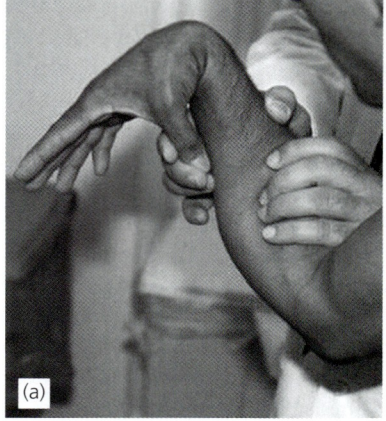
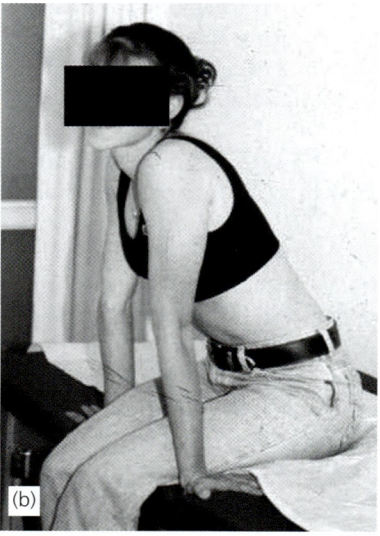

Figure 106.12 Laxity of other joints such as the metacarpophalangeal joint of the thumb (a) or the elbows (b) indicates generalized ligamentous laxity that may be a poor prognostic sign for surgery.

abduction and external rotation is a reliable sign of anterior instability, especially when it is relieved with a posteriorly directed force on the humerus.[78] Second, decreased external rotation of the abducted arm indicates relative shortening of the anterior band of the inferior glenohumeral ligament and suggests the presence of a medially healed Bankart lesion.[79] Third, translation of the humerus on the glenoid is normal, especially in a neutral position. When the translation is associated with pain or a sense of instability when compared with the normal side, it may be a sign of instability. Fourth, rotator cuff tears and neurological injuries can accompany instability. Strength testing of the rotator cuff and neurological testing should be done in all patients with glenohumeral instability. Finally, especially in patients with posterior and multidirectional instability, scapular dyskinesis and true scapular winging can be present. This should be recognized and corrected in addition to any instability problem.

Glenohumeral instability

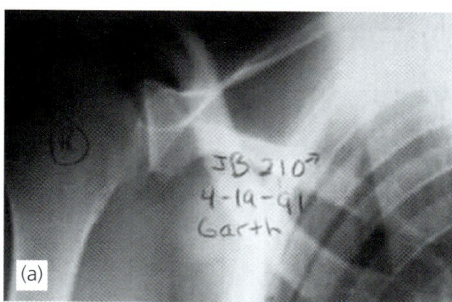

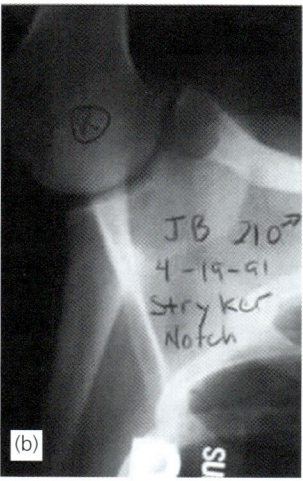

Figure 106.13 Anterior glenoid rim calcification or fractures (a) and Hill–Sachs defects (b) can be appreciated on the apical oblique (Garth) and Stryker notch views.

IMAGING

Radiographic views which may be used in the evaluation of glenohumeral instability include an AP view in the scapular plane, an axillary view, an apical oblique or Garth view,[80] a Stryker notch view[81] and a West Point view.[82] The last three views will demonstrate Hill–Sachs defects and calcification or fracture of the anterior glenoid rim in patients who have sustained traumatic anterior subluxations or dislocations (Fig. 106.13). The axillary view may suggest abnormal glenoid retroversion or localized posterior glenoid hypoplasia.

CT and MRI are often indicated in the evaluation of glenohumeral instability. Abnormalities of glenoid version or subtle glenoid dysplasia or hypoplasia suspected on routine axillary view may be verified and quantified with CT scan (Fig. 106.14). Labral detachment as well as abnormalities of the articular surface in cases of suspected hypoplasia or dysplasia may be visualized using intra-articular contrast in combination with either CT or MRI.[4,83–85]

Examination under anaesthesia

Examination under anaesthesia (EUA) is a useful supplement to office evaluation in the assessment of the degree and

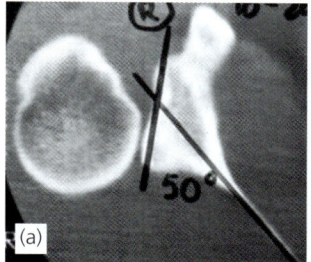 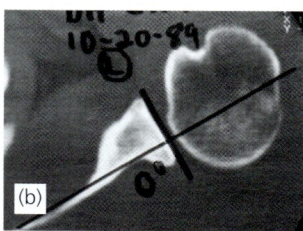

Figure 106.14 CT scanning of the involved (a) and normal (b) shoulders of this patient with recurrent posterior instability reveals 50° of retroversion.

direction of capsular laxity.[65,86,87] However, it may be very difficult to perceive movement of the humeral head on the glenoid in muscular patients with large shoulders. Since the patient is anaesthetized and muscular forces are minimized, assessment of the magnitude of humeral translation on the glenoid is probably more accurate with EUA than in the awake patient. As in the awake patient, glenohumeral translations demonstrate significant individual variation and the amount of translation documented in the pathological shoulder should be compared with the normal shoulder. Information obtained during EUA should be interpreted in the context of all previous clinical information obtained. Although quantification of humeral translation may be more accurate during EUA than during office evaluation in the awake patient, examination of the awake patient allows for interpretation of symptoms associated with humeral translation. Caution should be exercised when the findings of EUA differ substantially from the overall clinical picture established through synthesis of information obtained from history, physical examination and diagnostic testing. When significant disagreement between the overall clinical picture and the findings of EUA exists, further clarification of the instability pattern may be accomplished with diagnostic arthroscopy.

Treatment

NON-OPERATIVE

Non-operative management of glenohumeral instability consists of a combination of bracing, activity modification and physiotherapy. Strengthening exercises are aimed at the rotator cuff, deltoid and scapular rotators. The programme is very similar to what has been described for rotator cuff problems above. Exercises are more likely to be successful in patients with atraumatic instability than in those with traumatic instability.[72] In the subset of patients with atraumatic multidirectional instability, rehabilitation should be pursued for 9–12 months prior to consideration for surgical stabilization.[88]

In patients with traumatic anterior instability, the likelihood of recurrence following the first dislocation is directly related to age and is highest in patients under the age of 20 years.[89,90] Young, active patients may be candidates for stabilization after the first dislocation.[91] However, some patients may want to complete the athletic season before stabilization. Therefore, in certain circumstances, the use of a brace that restricts abduction and external rotation may allow the completion of a season without further dislocations. In addition, recent data suggest that immobilization in external rotation following the first dislocation may prevent recurrence more efficiently than immobilization in a sling in internal rotation.[92,93] Consequently, a trial of therapeutic exercises following a period of immobilization in external rotation may be indicated in most patients with a first time dislocation.

Open Bankart repair

ANAESTHESIA AND PATIENT POSITIONING

As with open rotator cuff repair, open Bankart repair can be performed under general, regional (i.e. interscalene block) or combined general and regional anaesthesia. The patient is positioned supine, at the edge of the operating table, so that the scapula, shoulder and arm are unsupported and fall slightly posteriorly. A padded roll may be placed under the patient, medial to the scapula, in order to elevate the ipsilateral hemithorax and allow the shoulder girdle to fall further posteriorly. Given the scapula's normal inclination on the thorax, this technique facilitates exposure of the anterior aspect of the scapula and glenohumeral joint. The table is placed in the semirecumbent (i.e. beach chair) position with the back of the table elevated approximately 30–40° from the horizontal (i.e. floor).

SKIN INCISION AND SUPERFICIAL DISSECTION

A 6–8 cm anterior axillary incision is made from the tip of the coracoid process to the anterior axillary fold (Fig. 106.15). Full-thickness skin flaps are developed superomedially and inferolaterally to expose the cephalic vein and deltopectoral interval. The deltopectoral interval is developed and the cephalic vein and deltoid are retracted laterally while the pectoralis major is retracted medially to expose the underlying clavipectoral fascia and conjoined tendon of the coracobrachialis and short head of the biceps.

DEEP DISSECTION

The clavipectoral fascia is incised at the lateral margin of the conjoined tendon starting at the upper border of the pectoralis major and extending to the coracoacromial ligament. Division of the coracoacromial ligament is not necessary for adequate exposure. The plane between the conjoined tendon and the subscapularis is developed and the conjoined tendon is retracted medially. Digital palpation is used to verify the position of the axillary nerve,

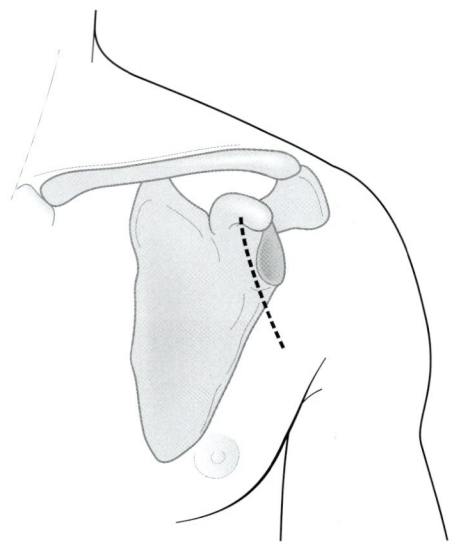

Figure 106.15 An anterior axillary incision is used for open Bankart repairs and anterior capsular shifts.

which is protected throughout the procedure. The undersurface of the conjoined tendon is also palpated to determine the proximity of the musculocutaneous nerve to the tip of the coracoid. If the nerve enters the posterior surface of the conjoined tendon close to the coracoid tip (1.5–2.0 cm), extreme care should be exercised when retracting the conjoined tendon medially.

The subscapularis tendon is incised approximately 1.5–2.0 cm medial to its attachment site on the lesser tuberosity (Fig. 106.16). The incision should begin at the most superior extent of the subscapularis tendon at the rotator interval and extend distally to include the superior two-thirds of the tendon. At the junction of the superior two-thirds and inferior one-third of the subscapularis, the incision is carried medially, in line with the subscapularis fibres. The anterior capsule is then exposed by reflecting the detached superior two-thirds of the subscapularis musculotendinous unit medially. If the entire thickness of the subscapularis tendon has been incised and reflected, there will always be a defect in the superior capsule. This is the same capsular defect through which the intra-articular portion of the subscapularis tendon is visualized during routine glenohumeral arthroscopy. In many patients with multidirectional instability and some patients with anteroinferior instability, this capsular defect will be enlarged.

The humeral attachment site of the anterior capsule is exposed by carefully reflecting the lateral stump of the subscapularis tendon laterally. The anterior capsule is then incised approximately 1–1.5 cm medial to its attachment site on the humerus. This incision begins superiorly at the defect in the rotator interval capsule and extends inferiorly to the axillary recess. A humeral head retractor is placed

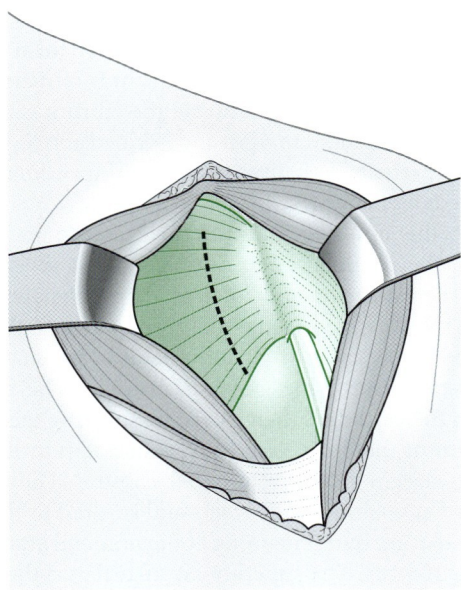

Figure 106.16 The subscapularis is incised 1–2 cm medial to its insertion on the lesser tuberosity. With a routine Bankart repair, the incision involves only the upper two-thirds of the tendon; with a formal anteroinferior capsular shift, the entire tendon may be incised.

within the glenohumeral joint and the humerus is retracted posteriorly to expose the glenoid.

LABRAL REATTACHMENT

A probe is used to identify the Bankart lesion. An elevator is placed between the labrum and the anterior glenoid rim and the labrum and attached periosteum are stripped from the anterior glenoid. This creates a mobile capsulolabral complex. A Bankart retractor is then placed along the anterior scapular neck and the labrum and capsule are retracted medially to expose the glenoid rim. A burr is used to expose a bleeding bone surface on the anterior glenoid rim. However, a minimum amount of bone should be removed. The Bankart retractor is then placed on the scapular neck in an extra-articular position, between the capsule and the subscapularis. The labrum can then be reattached using suture anchors or bone tunnels (Fig. 106.17). Whichever method is chosen, the labrum should be shifted superiorly and laterally so that its reattachment site is on the glenoid rim and not medially on the scapular neck. This ensures that the socket-deepening effect of the labrum has been recreated.

CAPSULE AND SUBSCAPULARIS REPAIR

The medial capsular flap is repaired to the lateral capsular stump with non-absorbable suture. If the patient has had fewer than three dislocations and does not have underlying

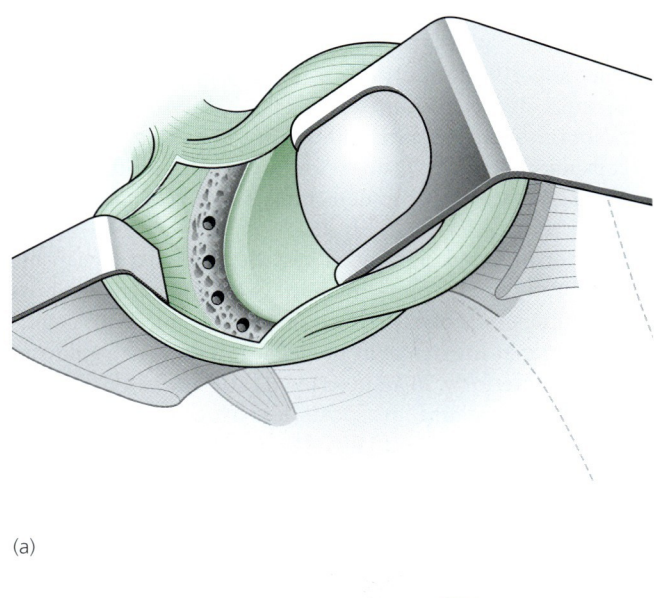

(a)

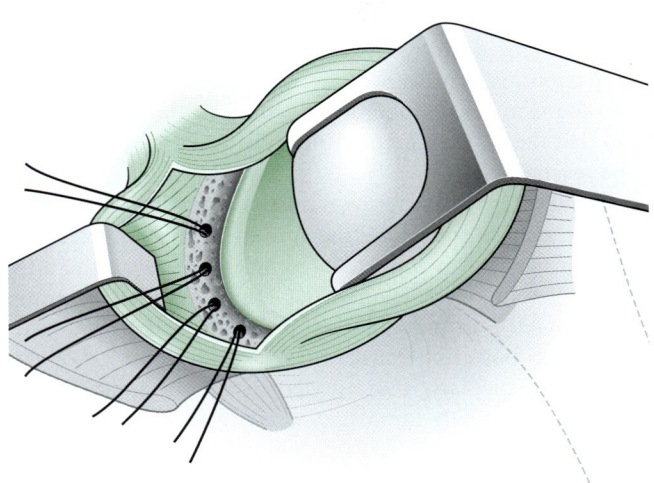

(b)

Figure 106.17 When a Bankart lesion is present, the anterior glenoid rim is abraided and a drill hole may be placed for suture anchor placement (a). The anchors are placed along the glenoid rim and the sutures are used to repair the labrum (b).

multidirectional laxity, the capsule is repaired anatomically. Otherwise, the capsule is shifted superiorly and laterally and the rotator interval is closed. The subscapularis is repaired anatomically with heavy, non-absorbable sutures.

CLOSURE

Digital palpation is used to verify the integrity of the axillary nerve. The wound is then closed with interrupted, absorbable sutures in the subcutaneous layer and a running, subcuticular suture using a non-absorbable, monofilament suture.

Open anteroinferior capsular shift

The superficial approach for an open anteroinferior capsular shift is the same as for a Bankart repair. From that point on, there are some differences. The extent of inferior capsular release is greater for a capsular shift and the release is facilitated by detachment and reflection of the entire subscapularis. This may require sacrifice of the anterior humeral circumflex vessels. The anterior capsule is then incised approximately 1–1.5 cm medial to its attachment site on the humerus. This incision begins superiorly at the defect in the rotator interval capsule and extends inferiorly, in an inverted 'L' configuration,[94] to the axillary recess and the posterior band of the inferior glenohumeral ligament (PIGHL). Exposure of the inferior humeral capsular attachment is facilitated by simultaneous external rotation and slight abduction in the scapular plane. It is also helpful to avoid extension of the shoulder during inferior capsular release by maintaining the arm in or anterior to the scapular plane. Sequential placement of sutures along the free edge of the anterior capsule as the capsulotomy proceeds inferomedially provides a mechanism for maintaining traction on the capsular flap so that the most posteroinferior portion of the capsule can be reached.

The extent of posterior release is a function of the size of the axillary pouch and the amount of posterior translation with the arm abducted. Complete release of the inferior glenohumeral ligament (IGHL) complex (including the PIGHL) is particularly important in patients with increased posterior translation with the arm at 90° of elevation, particularly those patients with atraumatic instability. It is equally important to avoid excessive posterior release and anterior shift in patients with traumatic and microtraumatic multidirectional instability, as this will result in significant loss of rotation in abduction.

A humeral head retractor is placed within the glenohumeral joint, which is inspected for the presence of labral abnormalities. In cases of traumatic and, rarely, microtraumatic multidirectional instability, a Bankart lesion may be identified. The detached labrum is retracted anteriorly, the glenoid is prepared, and the labrum is repaired to the anterior glenoid margin as described above. Bankart lesions in patients with atraumatic multidirectional instability are not encountered.

Once the anterior and inferior capsule have been released, the resultant large capsular flap is divided into two smaller superior and inferior flaps (Fig. 106.18) by incising the anterior capsule slightly superior to the anterior band of the inferior glenohumeral ligament from its free, lateral edge to the glenoid labrum.[65] The superior defect in the capsule is then closed by suturing the superior margin of the most superior capsular flap to the most anterior margin of the reinforced capsule. The inferior capsular flap is shifted superiorly and sutured to the anterior capsular margin remaining at the humeral attachment site (Fig. 106.18). The superior capsular flap is then shifted inferiorly, over the previously shifted inferior capsular flap, and sutured to the lateral capsular margin (Fig. 106.18).

Based upon the reciprocal relationship between various regions of the capsule, selective tensioning of the capsular flaps has been recommended.[94] The exact recommended arm positions for capsular tensioning are somewhat arbitrary and are probably less important than the overall concept. The inferior capsular flap is shifted superiorly and sutured into the remaining lateral capsular attachment site with the humerus in approximately 40–45° of abduction in the scapular plane and 30–35° of external rotation. The superior capsular flap is then shifted inferiorly, over the previously shifted inferior capsular flap, and sutured into the remaining lateral capsular attachment site with the humerus in approximately 20–25° of abduction in the scapular plane and 25–30° of external rotation.

The subscapularis is repaired anatomically and the remainder of the closure is the same as Bankart repair.

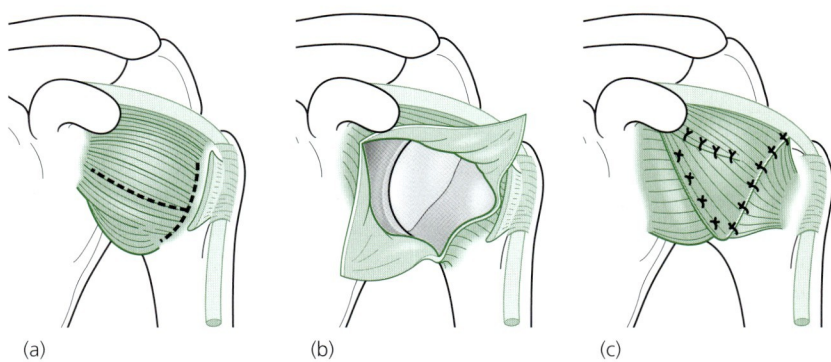

Figure 106.18 In a laterally based anteroinferior capsular shift (Neer), the anterior capsule is released near its lateral attachment and is split medial-to-lateral at the superior border of the inferior glenohumeral ligament (a and b). The superior capsular flap is shifted inferiorly over the superiorly shifted inferior capsular flap (c).

Posterior reconstruction

Posterior reconstruction usually involves posterior capsular shift, with or without labral repair. The patient is placed in the lateral decubitus position with the assistance of either a hip positioner or 'bean bag'. General anaesthesia is preferred over regional (i.e. interscalene block) anaesthesia as interscalene block provides poor coverage of the posteroinferior shoulder.

The glenohumeral joint is approached through a posterior axillary, deltoid splitting incision.[95] The skin incision begins at the posterior axillary fold and extends superiorly towards the scapular spine to a point slightly inferior and medial to the posterolateral corner of the acromion. The posterior deltoid is split in line with its fibres, beginning at the scapular spine and extending inferiorly for a distance of approximately 4–5 cm.[95] Exposure of the infraspinatus and teres minor may be improved by releasing a small portion of the deltoid origin on the scapular spine, especially lateral to the deltoid split.

The posterior capsule can be approached by splitting the posterior cuff muscles (either by splitting the infraspinatus[96] or by developing the interval between infraspinatus and teres minor) or by incising the infraspinatus tendon and reflecting it medially. In patients without severe redundancy of the axillary pouch, the infraspinatus splitting approach is preferred. Patients with atraumatic multidirectional instability, with a very patulous axillary pouch, require an inferior capsular incision which extends anteriorly towards the anterior band of the inferior glenohumeral ligament (AIGHL). Although this may be accomplished through a rotator cuff splitting incision, exposure is facilitated by reflecting the infraspinatus. When this approach is utilized, the infraspinatus is incised 1.5–2.0 cm from its attachment site on the greater tuberosity. Caution is exercised during medial retraction of the musculotendinous unit to avoid injury to the suprascapular nerve.

The posterior capsule is incised in a mediolateral direction from the lateral humeral capsular attachment site to the glenoid labrum.[65] The capsulotomy should be made approximately 1.5–2.0 cm inferior to the posterior border of the supraspinatus and parallel to it (Fig. 106.19). The capsule is then incised in the superoinferior direction approximately 1.5–2.0 cm medial to the lateral humeral capsular attachment site. The capsular incision begins at the previously placed mediolateral capsulotomy and extends inferomedially to include the axillary recess and the AIGHL. The capsule superior to the mediolateral capsulotomy is also incised in the superoinferior direction approximately 1.5–2.0 cm medial to the lateral humeral capsular attachment site. This creates a superior capsular flap to shift inferiorly over the inferior capsular flap.

The use of a humeral head retractor allows the glenohumeral joint to be inspected for evidence of articular or labral injury. This occurs in patients with traumatic and microtraumatic instability. In patients with a large axillary recess (i.e. atraumatic instability) the humeral head may be displaced significantly anteriorly with the humeral head retractor to allow visualization of the entire anterior glenoid. If detachment of the posterior labrum (i.e. posterior Bankart lesion) is identified, the posterior glenoid rim is prepared and the labrum and capsule are reattached to the glenoid margin (Fig. 106.20). The presence of a posterior Bankart lesion in patients with multidirectional instability is even more uncommon than an anterior Bankart lesion. However, when one is encountered, it is repaired prior to commencing with the inferior capsular shift.

The concept of reciprocal tightening of the superior and inferior regions of the capsule as a function of arm position, as applied to the anterior capsule, is probably also relevant to posterior capsular tensioning. Therefore, in patients with traumatic and microtraumatic instability, the inferior capsular flap is shifted superiorly and sutured to the lateral capsular remnant with the humerus abducted 40–45° in the scapular plane and internally rotated 10–15°. The superior capsular flap is shifted inferiorly, over the previously shifted inferior capsular flap, and sutured to the lateral capsular remnant with the humerus abducted 20–25° in the scapular plane and internally rotated 0–5° (Fig. 106.21). Fixation in external rotation and shortening of the infraspinatus in these patients (i.e. traumatic and microtraumatic instability) are avoided in order to prevent loss of motion. In patients with atraumatic instability and a large axillary recess, the shift is performed in less abduction (i.e. 10–20°) and internal rotation (0–5°).

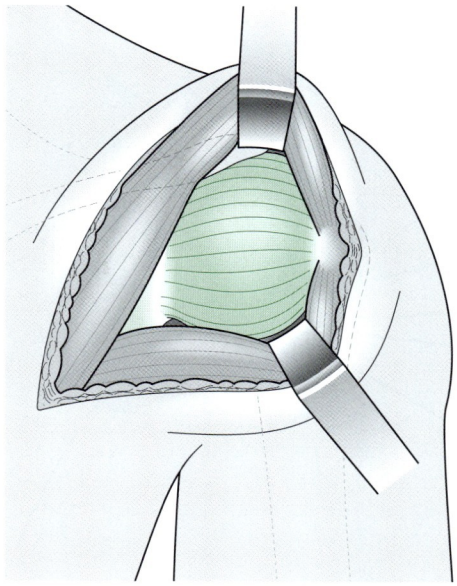

Figure 106.19 The posterior capsule is incised in a medial-to-lateral direction.

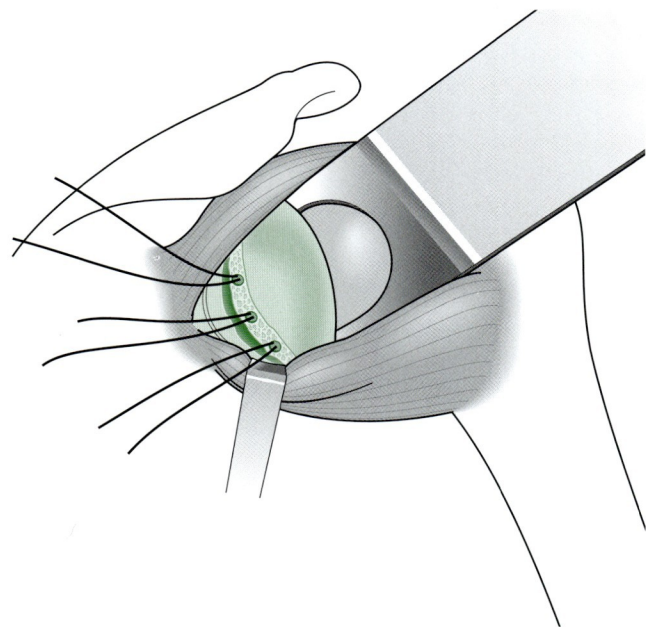

Figure 106.20 When a posterior Bankart lesion is present, the posterior glenoid rim is prepared and sutures are placed for reattachment of the posterior labrum.

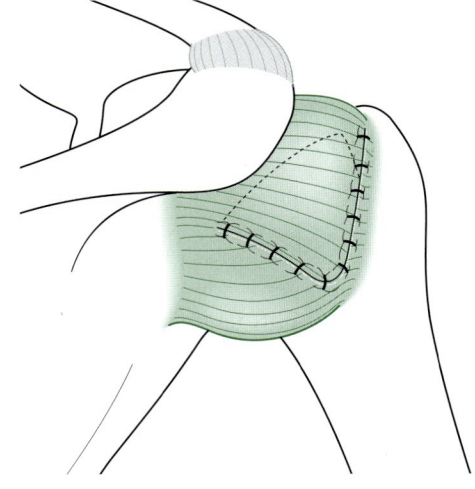

Figure 106.21 A posterior capsular shift is performed by shifting the superior capsular flap inferiorly over the superiorly shifted inferior capsular flap.

The infraspinatus is repaired with non-absorbable suture utilizing a 'tendon grasping' configuration (i.e. modified Kessler). In patients with atraumatic instability, the infraspinatus can be repaired anatomically or it can be imbricated or overlapped to provide additional support to the posterior capsular repair. However, shortening of the infraspinatus in traumatic and microtraumatic instability may result in significant loss of motion. Therefore, it is repaired anatomically in these subgroups of patients.

Postoperative rehabilitation

The type and length of postoperative protection as well as the timing of rehabilitation varies depending on the procedure performed. Following open anterior Bankart repair, the patient is placed in a sling for 7–10 days. Pendulum exercises, passive external rotation to 30° and passive elevation to 130° are then instituted and continued for the next 3–4 weeks. At 6 weeks postoperatively, manual stretching and strengthening exercises are begun. Strengthening is aimed at the rotator cuff, deltoid, and scapular rotators and begins with elastic bands. At 3 months postoperatively, strengthening advances to weights and sports-specific training. Return to non-contact sports is allowed 4–6 months postoperatively. Contact sports are avoided until 9–12 months postoperatively.

Patients undergoing formal anteroinferior capsular shift are maintained in a sling and pillow or brace that maintains neutral rotation and mild abduction for 4–6 weeks postoperatively. Pendulum exercises, passive external rotation to 30° and passive elevation to 130° are then instituted. At 6–8 weeks postoperatively, manual stretching and strengthening exercises are begun and the rehabilitation proceeds as with a Bankart repair thereafter.

A brace is used following open posterior reconstruction. This brace maintains the arm in slight abduction and 10–20° of external rotation. The brace is maintained for 4–6 weeks. Rehabilitation then follows the same protocol as described above for anteroinferior capsular shift.

Results

The results following shoulder instability procedures are based not only on postoperative function and pain but also on the presence or absence of recurrent instability. In general, the results are best in patients undergoing anterior Bankart repair for unidirectional instability, followed by posterior and multidirectional instability. Reported results of anterior Bankart repair range from 85% to 97% satisfactory results with 3–13% recurrence of instability.[60,97–99]

The management of posterior instability has undergone substantial change over the years. The percentage of good and excellent results has ranged from 50% to 97% with recurrence rates ranging from 3% to 50%.[76,100–105] More recent series have reported consistently better results with current capsular repair and plication techniques.[102,103,105] However, the results are still not as predictable as anterior instability.

Reported results of surgical management of multidirectional instability are difficult to interpret primarily because of differences in inclusion criteria. The percentage of patients with a Bankart lesion and primarily anteroinferior instability, which presumably carry a better prognosis, varies significantly among reported series. In addition, surgical technique has also varied. The reported results are mid-term (i.e. less than 10 years) and reveal that 85–90% of patients are satisfied, the recurrence of symptomatic instability is in the 10–15% range, and patients without symptomatic recurrent instability frequently (20–25%) have feelings of apprehension when the shoulder is stressed.[65,106–109] In comparison, long-term follow-up of patients with multidirectional instability who were initially treated non-operatively reveals that less than half have satisfactory outcomes.[110]

Complications

Potential complications following open glenohumeral instability include recurrent instability, stiffness, post-traumatic arthritis, nerve injury, rotator cuff repair failure (i.e. subscapularis and infraspinatus), capsular insufficiency and infection. The rates of recurrent instability have been discussed above in the Results section. However, it should be emphasized that failure to recognize multidirectional instability in patients undergoing Bankart repair and posterior instability repairs is a common cause of failure.[111–113] In addition, when instability is associated with soft-tissue and bone deficiency, it can be very difficult to manage.

The incidence of post-traumatic arthritis following open instability surgery is difficult to determine because separating the effect of the instability itself from the effect of the surgery is often impossible. Several conclusions can be made on the basis of review of current literature. First, similar glenohumeral arthritic changes can occur following glenohumeral instability with or without surgical repair.[114–116] Second, the incidence of arthritis increases with age and time from initial injury.[114–116] Third, the development of arthritis seems to be accelerated in patients who have developed stiffness, particularly in external rotation, following surgery.[117] Finally, prominent hardware also results in particularly severe and progressive degenerative changes.[118–120]

GLENOHUMERAL ARTHRITIS

Historical background

Glenohumeral arthritis is a spectrum of disease processes with varying involvement of the articular cartilage, bony supporting structures (i.e. glenoid and humerus), and the periarticular soft tissues (i.e. capsule and rotator cuff). On one end of the spectrum is avascular necrosis, which spares the rotator cuff and has focal changes in the humeral bone. The glenoid is spared until the final stages of the disease. On the other end of the spectrum is cuff tear arthropathy, which is characterized by irreparable rotator cuff deficiency, scant osteophyte formation and bone destruction.[121] Osteoarthritis is the most common type of glenohumeral arthritis and is manifested by relative sparing of the rotator cuff, large humeral osteophyte formation and asymmetrical posterior wear of the glenoid.[122] Rheumatoid arthritis produces progressive destruction of the articular cartilage, bone and rotator cuff. In the later stages, it can resemble cuff tear arthropathy.

Prosthetic replacement for glenohumeral arthritis was first performed by Pean[123] in 1893 in a patient with tuberculosis of the shoulder. The device was constrained and failed 2 years after implantation because of recurrent infection. However, the modern era of shoulder replacement with unconstrained, anatomically designed implants began in the mid- to late 1950s.[124–126] The first reported results following shoulder replacement for glenohumeral arthritis in a large series of patients was by Neer in 1974.[122] Although two of the 48 patients in this series received a glenoid component, more routine use of a glenoid component was added by Neer in approximately 1977.[127] Unconstrained shoulder arthroplasty based on normal anatomy has become the standard and, although some controversy still exists, total shoulder arthroplasty provides more reliable pain relief than hemiarthroplasty in patients with an intact or reparable rotator cuff.[128–131] In patients with irreparable cuff insufficiency and proximal humeral migration, the potential for early glenoid component loosening favours hemiarthroplasty over anatomic total shoulder arthroplasty.[132] Pain relief is usually good but functional return is variable and dependent on preoperative function.[133]

Pain relief and restoration of overhead function can be restored in patients with glenohumeral arthritis, irreparable cuff insufficiency and poor elevation with reverse total shoulder arthroplasty as introduced by Grammont in the late 1980s.[134,135] This prosthetic design differs from other reverse prostheses in that the glenosphere is large with no neck so that the centre of rotation is medialized. In addition, the neck shaft angle of the humeral component is more valgus (155°) than the anatomic humerus. These features are likely to contribute to its success.

Pertinent anatomy

The goal of shoulder arthroplasty in patients with an intact or reparable cuff is to recreate normal anatomy with the prosthetic reconstruction. Consequently, knowledge of certain normal anatomic dimensions is required. The central 80% of the humeral head is spherical and the peripheral 20% is elliptical.[136] However, if one assumes that the entire articular surface is spherical, the humeral head radius of curvature, humeral head thickness, retrotorsion with respect to the humeral shaft and neck–shaft angle are extremely variable.[136–139] Both humeral head radius and thickness correlate strongly with humeral shaft length and patient height.[136] However, the ratio of humeral head thickness to humeral head radius of curvature is remarkably constant at approximately 0.7–0.9, regardless of patient height or humeral shaft size.[136,139,140] The surface arc of the humerus available for contact with the glenoid is directly proportional to the ratio of humeral head thickness to humeral head radius and is, therefore, also relatively constant.[140]

The humeral head centre and the centre of the intramedullary canal of the humerus do not coincide in all cases. The distance between the centre of the humeral head and the central axis of the intramedullary canal is defined as the humeral head offset.[83,137,140] Humeral head offset is approximately 7–9 mm medial and 2–4 mm posterior to the central axis of the intramedullary canal.[83,137,140]

The angle between the plane of the humeral head and the epicondylar axis of the humerus is known as the humeral retroversion. Humeral retrotorsion averages 20–30°, with a wide range of approximately 20–55°.[83,137,139,140] The vertical distance between the highest point of the humeral articular surface and the highest point of the greater tuberosity (i.e. head to greater tuberosity height) is approximately 8 mm and shows a relatively small range of interspecimen variability.[136,140] The neck–shaft angle is defined as the angle subtended by the central intramedullary axis of the humeral shaft and the base of the articular segment. The average neck–shaft angle is 40–45°.[83,136,140] However, more importantly, the humeral neck–shaft angle demonstrates significant individual variation with a range of 30–55°. Normal glenoid version also exhibits significant individual variation.[141–143] Direct measurement of glenoid retroversion in cadaver specimens indicates that the glenoid is retroverted 1.23° and is slightly more retroverted in Caucasian males (2.63°) than in African American males (0.20°).[141]

Clinical evaluation

HISTORY AND PHYSICAL EXAMINATION

Patients with glenohumeral arthritis typically present with an insidious onset of pain, which has been slowly progressive over past years. Progressive stiffness is often associated with the discomfort. As is the case in other arthritic joints, the pain is often activity related. Patient complaints will often relate to functional limitations such as difficulty internally rotating to reach their back pocket or fastening a brassiere. Questioning the patient as to how their symptoms have interfered with their daily routines will provide insight into the degree of pain and disability. Understanding the patient's occupation, hobbies and activity levels also helps gauge the impact of their disease. Documentation of treatments that have been or are being used also gives information about disease course and severity.

Arthritic conditions of the glenohumeral joint cause progressive global loss of motion, with particular loss of external rotation in osteoarthritis. Any internal rotation contracture must be noted and documented as it dictates whether subscapularis releases are required at the time of surgery. Active and passive motion should be compared and the rotator cuff strength noted. This can sometimes be difficult to determine on physical examination alone, as there is often pain-related weakness. Painful crepitus is common. Tenderness to palpation over the acromioclavicular joint can indicate arthritis, which potentially can contribute to the symptom complex. This is an important finding to identify as it can also be addressed at the time of surgery if needed.

Imaging

Plain radiographs are the single most important investigation required in the diagnosis of osteoarthritis and arthroplasty planning. A standard radiograph series (AP, transcapular lateral and axillary lateral) is typically performed and each provides different information required for pre-operative preparation. The AP radiograph, which often is performed in internal and external rotation, allows assessment of bone quality, identification of inferior osteophytes and measurement of the diameter of the humeral canal. Although not universally reliable because of slight variations in the angle of beam projection, evaluation of the acromiohumeral distance can suggest the presence of significant rotator cuff deficiency if the distance measures <7 mm. The axillary radiograph is useful in identifying glenoid version as well as the posterior glenoid wear and resultant posterior subluxation that is often associated with osteoarthritis (Fig. 106.22).

CT scan provides a more definitive assessment of glenoid bone stock and version. It also allows accurate determination of whether glenoid replacement is feasible and whether bone grafting may be necessary (Fig. 106.23). Since posterior glenoid erosion and posterior subluxation are common with severe internal rotation contracture, CT scanning is ordered in all patients with external rotation of 30° or less or in any patient whose axillary view is insufficient to determine glenoid morphology.

MRI may be useful in cases of suspected rotator cuff tear. In general, full-thickness rotator cuff tears are uncommon in patients with osteoarthritis or osteonecrosis (5%). However, in patients who have had prior rotator cuff surgery or who demonstrate a decreased acromiohumeral distance on plain radiography, rotator cuff tears may be more common. In addition, rheumatoid arthritis is associated with a higher rate of rotator cuff insufficiency than osteoarthritis or avascular necrosis. Under these circumstances, MRI scanning can reveal glenoid erosion, abnormal glenoid version, as well as full-thickness rotator cuff tears (Fig. 106.24).

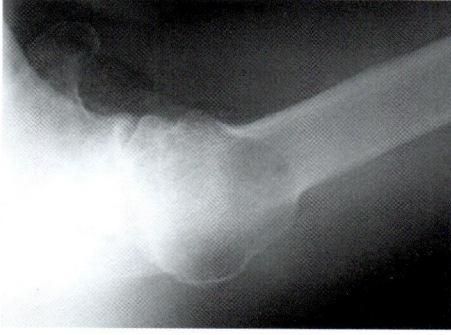

Figure 106.22 In patients with osteoarthritis, an axillary radiograph may demonstrate posterior glenoid wear and posterior humeral subluxation.

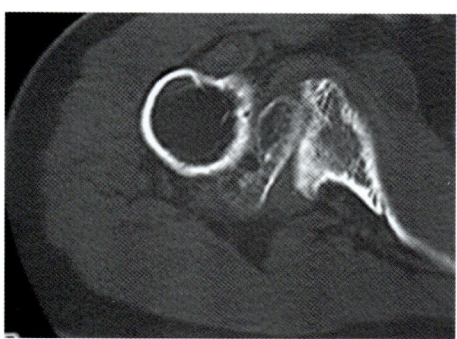

Figure 106.23 Posterior glenoid wear and posterior humeral subluxation can be confirmed and quantified using CT scanning.

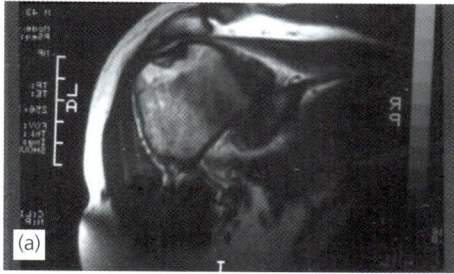

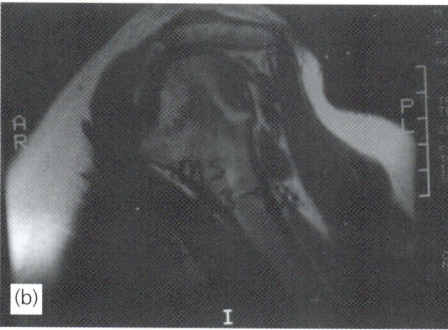

Figure 106.24 MRI reveals supraspinatus thinning (a) and severe humeral erosions (b) in this patient with rheumatoid arthritis.

Treatment

Shoulder replacement is indicated when patients have symptomatic glenohumeral arthritis that has not responded to non-operative management. Anatomic arthroplasty, hemiarthroplasty or total shoulder arthroplasty are indicated in patients with an intact or reparable rotator cuff. Hemiarthroplasty is preferred in patients with pre-operative elevation of 120° or more and who are young and active (i.e. under the age of 65 or 70 years).

Total shoulder arthroplasty results in better pain relief and is preferred in patients over the age of 50 years who do not participate in heavy weight lifting or other activities that put excessive stress across the shoulder. Patients with arthritis and irreparable rotator cuff deficiency require a reverse shoulder arthroplasty.

NON-OPERATIVE

All patients with glenohumeral arthritis should exhaust non-operative management before considering surgical replacement. Non-operative treatment modalities include activity modification, non-steroidal anti-inflammatory medications, intra-articular corticosteroid injections and limited physiotherapy. In patients with rheumatoid arthritis, consultation with a rheumatologist for the possible use of newer remittive agents is indicated. Although passive stretching exercises to maximize range of motion may decrease pain, excessive physiotherapy may increase pain. Therefore, progress should be carefully monitored and exercises should be modified or terminated if progressive pain occurs.

Operative: anatomic total shoulder replacement

ANAESTHESIA AND PATIENT POSITIONING

Anaesthetic options for shoulder arthroplasty, like the other procedures described in this chapter, include general anaesthesia, regional anaesthesia (i.e. interscalene block) or a combination of general anaesthesia and an interscalene block. Using a combination of general anaesthesia and an interscalene block combines the advantages of both methods. Namely, excluding interactions with the patient during surgery and prolonged postoperative pain control. For these reasons, a combination of anaesthetic methods is often used.

Following induction of anaesthesia, the patient is placed in the beach chair position, with the torso at approximately 30–45° to the horizontal. The head and body should be well stabilized and all pressure points padded appropriately. The affected arm should be free enough to be placed into a fully extended and adducted position (in order to allow dislocation of the humeral

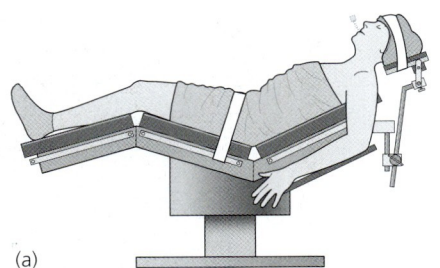 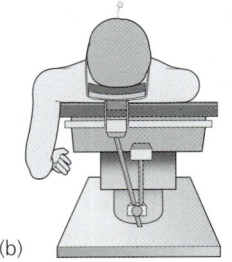

Figure 106.25 The patient is positioned beach chair (a) with the shoulder unsupported off the edge of the table and a special headrest (b) to allow full extension and adduction of the arm.

head) without restriction by the bed or positioning devices (Fig. 106.25).

INCISION AND SUPERFICIAL EXPOSURE

The deltopectoral approach is the standard access for shoulder arthroplasty. The skin incision is approximately 10 cm long, beginning just superior and medial to the tip of the coracoid and extending distally towards the deltoid insertion, along the estimated location of the deltopectoral groove (Fig. 106.26). Subcutaneous fat is split in line with the incision and the cephalic vein is identified, serving as a landmark for the deltopectoral groove. The cephalic vein is then taken laterally with the deltoid while the pectoralis major is taken medially. With the deltoid and pectoralis major retracted, the deep exposure can be carried out.

DEEP EXPOSURE

The clavipectoral fascia is incised at the most lateral extent of the conjoined tendon and associated muscles. This incision is carried distally to the level of the inferior most extent of the subscapularis and proximally to the coracoacromial ligament. Digital palpation is used to identify the axillary nerve as it courses along the superficial surface of the subscapularis to reach the quadrilateral space at the inferior aspect of the glenohumeral joint. The musculocutaneous nerve enters the deep aspect of the conjoined tendon a variable distance from the tip of the coracoid.[144] Therefore, it cannot always be palpated within the surgical field. One should attempt to palpate it, however, because it can enter the conjoined tendon within 1.5–2.0 cm from the tip of the coracoid. In this position, the nerve could be injured while retracting the conjoined tendon.

The incision in the clavipectoral fascia stops superiorly at the anterior border of the coracoacromial ligament. This ligament is an important restraint to anterosuperior subluxation, especially in patients with large or massive rotator cuff tears.[19,21,145,146] The coracoacromial ligament may be incised, excised or partially excised in order to improve visualization of the superior glenoid. However,

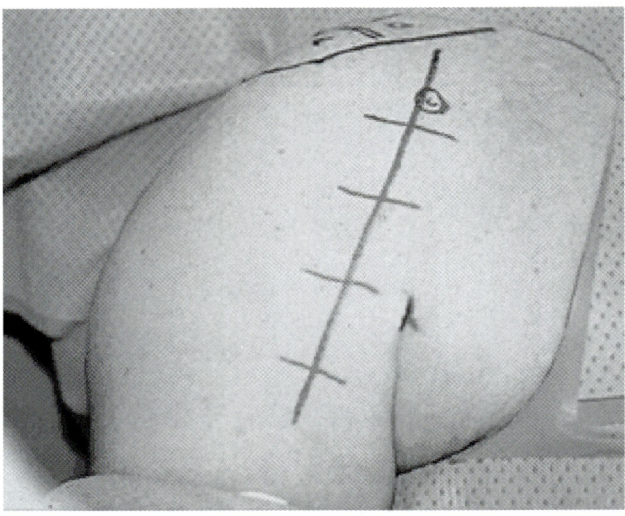

Figure 106.26 Shoulder arthroplasty is performed through an anterior, deltopectoral incision. Reprinted from Schenk T, Iannotti JP. Prosthetic arthroplasty for glenohumeral arthritis with an intact or reparable rotator cuff: indications, techniques, and results.

exposure is almost always adequate without coracoacromial ligament sacrifice. Moreover, rotator cuff tears can develop after shoulder arthroplasty. Therefore, the coracoacromial ligament can be completely preserved during shoulder arthroplasty, even if the rotator cuff is intact.

With the conjoined tendon retracted medially and the deltoid retracted laterally, the humerus is externally rotated approximately 30° and the anterior humeral circumflex vessels are clamped, cut and tied-off or coagulated. The long head of the biceps is routinely tenodesed to soft tissue at the level of the pectoralis major tendon and the biceps is then excised proximal to the tenodesis site all the way to the supraglenoid tubercle. This requires that the rotator interval be incised from the bicipital groove to the glenoid.

SUBSCAPULARIS REFLECTION AND CAPSULAR RELEASE

Subscapularis management is predicated on the amount of internal rotation contracture present. The goal is to restore optimal subscapularis length with the assumption that optimal function will follow. In many cases of primary osteoarthritis, significant loss of external rotation exists. When the internal rotation contracture is mild (passive external rotation is greater than 0° with the arm at the side, under anaesthesia), the subscapularis can be reflected with a lesser tuberosity osteotomy[147] or an intratendinous incision and repaired anatomically. With moderate degrees of internal rotation contracture (passive external rotation of 0° but not less than minus 30°), the subscapularis is removed from the lesser tuberosity with maximum length and is advanced medially and repaired to the cut surface of the humeral osteotomy. In the most severe cases of internal rotation contracture (passive external rotation of less than minus 30°), a coronal z-plasty of the subscapularis and capsule is performed.

Lesser tuberosity osteotomy as a means of reflecting the subscapularis in total shoulder arthroplasty yields a high rate of normal subscapularis function postoperatively.[148] Therefore, when passive external rotation exceeds 0°, an osteotomy is performed using a large curved osteotome. The interval between the capsule and subscapularis is developed inferiorly and the lesser tuberosity and attached subscapularis are released from the underlying capsule, working inferior to superior. Once the release has been carried into the rotator interval, the subscapularis and lesser tuberosity are retracted medially (Fig. 106.27). The anterior capsule is then released from the anatomic neck. In cases of moderate internal rotation contracture, subscapularis advancement is indicated. The subscapularis is incised at its most lateral extent and is elevated along with the humeral capsule. Inferiorly, the subscapularis and capsule are released in a single layer.

With either of the two above-mentioned methods of subscapularis and capsular release, the inferior capsule must be released to or past the 6 o'clock position. At the anteroinferior aspect of the humeral head, electrocautery is used to raise a periosteal/capsular flap that includes the upper 1 cm of the latissimus dorsi, the inferior periosteum, and the anteroinferior capsule to at least the 6 o'clock position. This can be performed safely by progressively externally rotating the humerus and using a blunt Homan retractor between the inferior most portion of the humeral head and the overlying capsule. As the incision gets close to the 6 o'clock position, the electrocautery is switched to a surgical knife to avoid inadvertent electrical injury to the axillary nerve by conduction through the metallic retractor. This inferior soft-tissue release is a critical manoeuvre to allow not only adequate delivery of the humerus into the wound but also adequate glenoid exposure.

Rarely is subscapularis z-lengthening required. When z-lengthening is indicated, the subscapularis must be elevated separately from the anterior capsule. The subscapularis is released from its attachment as far laterally as possible. As the tendon is being reflected medially, the interval between the capsule and subscapularis can be deter-

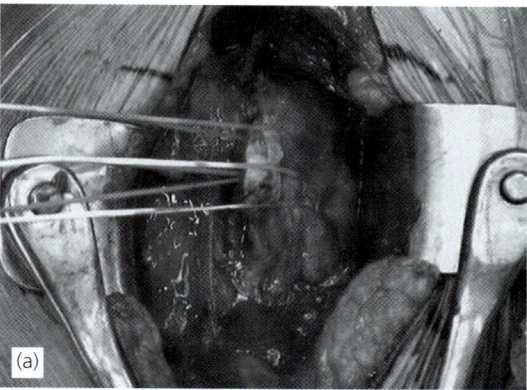
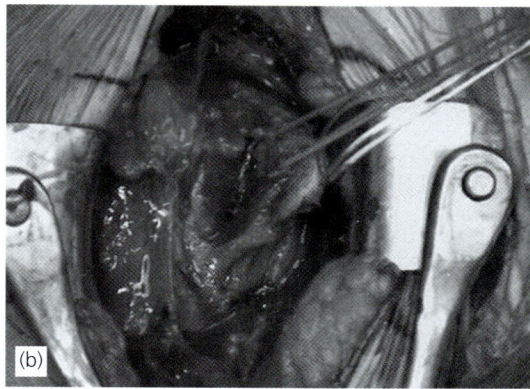

Figure 106.27 In patients with mild to moderate internal rotation contractures, the subscapularis is detached using a lesser tuberosity osteotomy (a). The lesser tuberosity and subscapularis are then reflected medially (b).

mined distally, where the inferior third of the subscapularis attachment is muscular rather than tendinous. This interval is bluntly dissected to provide the appropriate interval for dissection. The subscapularis tendon is then completely detached and reflected medially. A small portion of the tendon and muscle can be left behind on the anterior capsule for reinforcement. With the subscapularis released and retracted medially, the capsule is released from its glenoid attachment, starting superiorly and extending to the 6 o'clock position on the glenoid. With the axillary nerve retracted, the capsule is then incised in a mediolateral direction from the inferior glenoid margin to the humerus. This then creates a laterally based capsular flap that can be used to lengthen the subscapularis during closure. The remainder of the inferior capsule is released from the inferior humerus along with a small portion of latissimus dorsi and inferior humeral periosteum as described above.

HUMERAL EXPOSURE AND OSTEOTOMY

The humerus is delivered into the wound using simultaneous adduction, external rotation and extension. All humeral osteophytes are removed. The humeral head is then removed using an oscillating saw. The osteotomy begins anteriorly along the anatomic neck and proceeds posteriorly so that it exits 5 mm medial to the infraspinatus insertion. Superiorly, the osteotomy will exit 2–3 mm medial to the supraspinatus. In this way, native retroversion has been recreated (Fig. 106.28). The osteotomy can be made free-hand, with an extramedullary guide or with an intramedullary guide. The use of a prosthesis with a variable neck–shaft angle allows some flexibility in osteotomy placement.

The humeral head size is estimated by placing various humeral head trial implants on the osteotomy surface and selecting the one that most closely covers the osteotomy surface. The humerus is then retracted posteriorly to expose the glenoid. In some systems, a metallic humeral head cover can be used to protect the humeral metaphysis during glenoid preparation.

GLENOID EXPOSURE, PREPARATION AND COMPONENT PLACEMENT

Obtaining adequate glenoid exposure may be the most difficult part of total shoulder arthroplasty. Even if the glenoid is not going to be resurfaced, virtually every soft-tissue release required for glenoid exposure should still be carried out in order to maximize postoperative range of motion following hemiarthroplasty. Therefore, the integral manoeuvres for total shoulder arthroplasty[149] and hemiarthroplasty are the same.

There are four basic requirements for adequate glenoid exposure, all of which are within the control of the surgeon or surgical team: adequate humeral bone resection, proper arm positioning, appropriate soft-tissue contracture releases and proper glenoid retractors. Glenoid exposure is easiest in thin, small patients in whom there is little tissue between the skin and the glenoid. In more massive patients, particularly muscular males, glenoid exposure can be extremely challenging and all of the above-mentioned 'requirements' take on added importance.

Failure to resect enough humeral bone may lead to difficulties in glenoid exposure. As mentioned above, there should be very little bone (2–3 mm) between the osteotomy and the supraspinatus insertion. There will be slightly more bone between the osteotomy and the infraspinatus insertion. The persistence of humeral osteophytes is another source of inadequate bone resection in cases of osteoarthritis. The inferior humeral osteophyte is the largest and most obvious of the humeral osteophytes. It should be removed entirely before attempted glenoid exposure and, preferably, before humeral resection. However, osteophyte formation on the humeral head occurs circumferentially. Any bony structure that makes the humerus wider than normal will make posterior displacement of enough humerus to adequately expose the glenoid difficult. Therefore, humeral osteophytes should be excised circumferentially before attempted glenoid exposure.

During glenoid exposure, the arm should be positioned such that the intact soft tissues will allow maximum posterior humeral displacement. Assuming that the anterior and inferior capsules have been adequately released or excised and that there are no other remaining soft-tissue tethers, only the posterior and superior capsules remain. These two capsular regions are made slack by a combination of abduction, extension and external rotation. Therefore, this is the preferred position for the arm during glenoid exposure. However, in some cases, a more neutral position may allow better exposure. The optimal position should be selected and the arm can be held there using an assistant, a padded Mayo stand, or a mechanical arm-holding device.

Soft-tissue releases are the most important steps in glenoid exposure. The anterior and inferior capsular regions have been released from the humeral side as far posteriorly as the 6 o'clock position during humeral exposure and preparation. With the humerus retracted posteriorly with a humeral head retractor, the anteroinferior capsule is separated from the subscapularis. If the capsule is thickened, it is excised, starting slightly posterior to the 6 o'clock position and extending to the base of the coracoid. Otherwise, the capsule can be released from the labrum from the inferior aspect of the glenoid to the base of the coracoid. The last step in soft-tissue release is labral excision. The labrum is excised circumferentially.

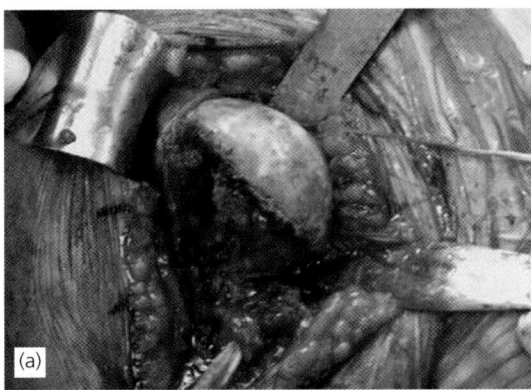
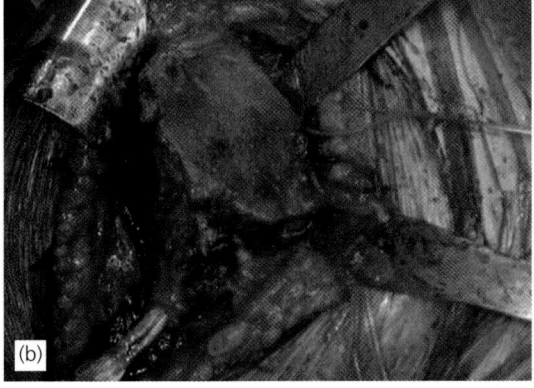

Figure 106.28 After removing the humeral osteophytes, the anatomic neck is marked (a) and the humeral head is removed. The osteotomy surface should be slightly medial to the rotator cuff attachment site (b).

Care is taken to preserve the posterior capsule attachment in cases of posterior glenoid wear and posterior subluxation of 25% or greater.

The choice of retractors and their placement are key elements in attaining good glenoid exposure. The basic retractors include a humeral head retractor (i.e. a Fukuda ring), a large Darrach retractor and a single pronged Bankart retractor or reverse Homan retractor. The Fukuda ring retractor is placed between the humerus and glenoid, with the ring cupping the posterior glenoid rim and the T-handle of the instrument retracting the humerus posteriorly. The large Darrach retractor is placed through the anterior capsulotomy along the anterior glenoid neck, deep to the subscapularis. It is used to retract the anterior soft tissues anteriorly. When the Fukuda is being levered posteriorly and the Darrach is being levered anteriorly, there is potential for axillary nerve traction. Therefore, when using either one of these retractors vigorously, the other should be reciprocally relaxed. The final basic retractor is the single pronged Bankart retractor, which is placed posterosuperiorly, along the posterosuperior glenoid rim. These three retractors (the Darrach anteriorly, the Fukuda ring posteriorly and the single pronged Bankart posterosuperiorly) are usually adequate for excellent glenoid exposure (Fig. 106.29). Occasionally, it is useful to place a fourth retractor (i.e. a reverse or blunt Homan) inferiorly. However, this is not routinely necessary. Having a variety of humeral head retractors, of different types and sizes, may also be helpful.

With the glenoid exposed, the surface is prepared and the component is placed (Fig. 106.30). Preparation of the glenoid requires concentric reaming so that the posterior surface of the component matches the surface of the glenoid.[150] In many cases of osteoarthritis, posterior glenoid bone loss is present. Management of these defects is beyond the scope of this chapter. However, most often they are managed through asymmetrical reaming of the high, anterior side. Bone grafting is not commonly performed but may be necessary in some cases. Once the glenoid surface has been adequately reamed, anchoring points for the glenoid component are made. The types and numbers of these anchoring holes depend on the system. Central slots are made for keels and drill holes are made for pegs. Most often, cemented all polyethylene components are used.

HUMERAL PREPARATION AND COMPONENT PLACEMENT

After the glenoid component has been placed, the humerus is redelivered into the wound with simultaneous adduction, extension and external rotation. Preparation of the humerus is dependent on the replacement system being used. In general, the humeral canal is reamed with sequentially larger cylindrical reamers until distal purchase can be felt against the intramedullary canal. The canal should not be over-reamed as endosteal notching can cause intra-operative fracture.

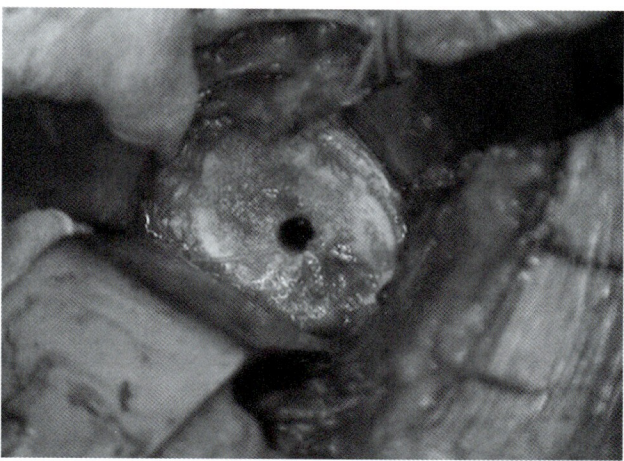

Figure 106.29 Glenoid exposure is obtained using a Fukuda ring retractor posteriorly, a single prong Bankart retractor superiorly, and a large Darrach retractor anteriorly.

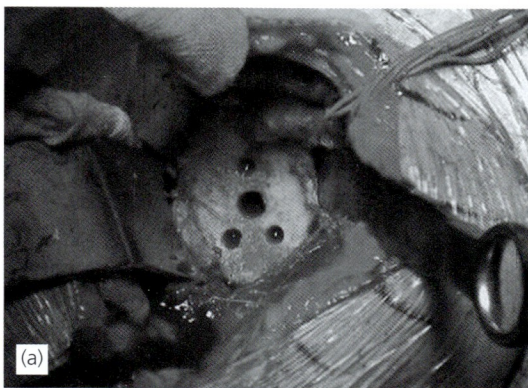

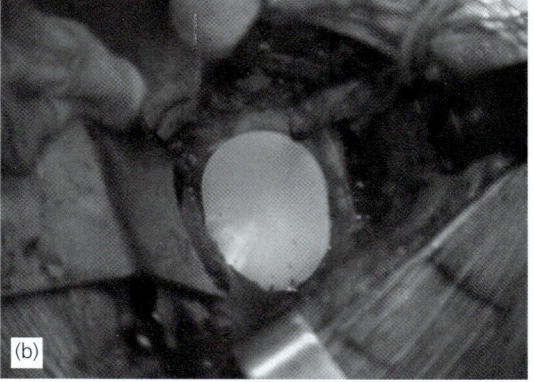

Figure 106.30 After glenoid reaming, the anchoring holes for a pegged glenoid component are drilled (a) and the component is placed (b).

After reaming, the appropriately sized broach is placed. With the broach in place, a trial humeral head is selected. In most systems, a choice will have to be made with regard to humeral head diameter, thickness (i.e. neck length) and offset. In many systems, the neck–shaft angle can also be selected. The goal is to select the humeral head size that precisely covers the osteotomy surface in a position that recreates the appropriate greater tuberosity head height and lateral offset of the normal shoulder. With the trial head in place, the humerus is reduced and tested for stability and adequate subscapularis length (Fig. 106.31). With the humerus reduced and the arm in neutral position, posterior translation should be 50–75% and the subscapularis should easily reach the insertion site with the arm in 30° of external rotation. The humerus is then redislocated, the trial is removed and the real implant is placed. Cancellous graft can be used from the resected head to impact into the proximal before final seating of the implant to create a good press fit. If there is any question of implant fixation, it is cemented.

CLOSURE

The most important component of wound closure is a secure subscapularis repair. If a lesser tuberosity has been performed, it is secured with three groups of sutures: (1) a soft-tissue to soft-tissue repair at the rotator interval, (2) interfragmentary sutures passed around the tuberosity and through the osteotomy surface and (3) a suture from the implant (placed before seating it) to the bone–tendon junction of the lesser tuberosity (Fig. 106.32). If the subscapularis was incised intratendinously, it is repaired anatomically, tendon-to-tendon. If the subscapularis was released from its insertion at the lesser tuberosity because of the need for tendon lengthening, it is repaired to the anterior edge of the humeral osteotomy through drill holes.

The subscapularis repair is performed with a z-lengthening in cases of severe internal rotation contracture. There are two flaps of anterior soft tissue that are used to perform this repair: the medially based subscapularis tendon and the laterally based capsular flap that may contain some remaining subscapularis tendon and muscle fibres. The laterally based flap is brought deep to the medial flap and horizontally

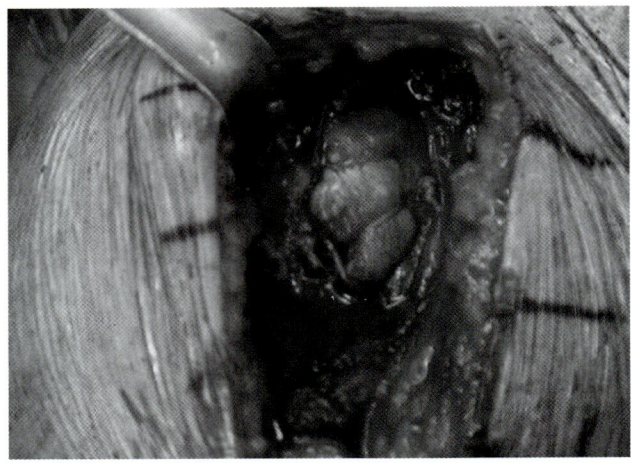

Figure 106.32 The lesser tuberosity, with its attached subscapularis, has been reduced and stabilized with sutures.

based mattress sutures are passed through the two superimposed flaps from deep to superficial. The sutures are passed so that external rotation of 45° with the arm at the side is permitted without untoward tension on the sutures. The lateral most extent of the medially based subscapularis tendon is then sutured to the underlying lateral capsular flap, more lateral than the previously placed sutures. The rotator interval is then closed laterally.

The deltopectoral interval is sutured closed over a closed suction drainage system using absorbable suture. The subcutaneous tissue and skin are closed routinely with interrupted absorbable and running subcuticular monofilament suture (Fig. 106.33).

Operative: reverse shoulder arthroplasty

Reverse total shoulder arthroplasty can be performed through either a standard deltopectoral approach or a superior, deltoid-splitting approach. There are advantages and disadvantages to both. Most surgeons in the USA use a standard deltopectoral approach. The surgical technique is similar to what has been described above for anatomic total shoulder arthroplasty with a few important exceptions.

SUBSCAPULARIS REFLECTION AND CAPSULAR RELEASE

The subscapularis is routinely released from the lesser tuberosity with maximum length. Both the capsule and subscapularis are released posterior to the 6 o'clock position. The axillary nerve is identified and protected throughout the procedure.

HUMERAL OSTEOTOMY AND DISTAL REAMING

With the humerus delivered into the wound, a saw is used to remove a small sliver of the humeral head at its highest

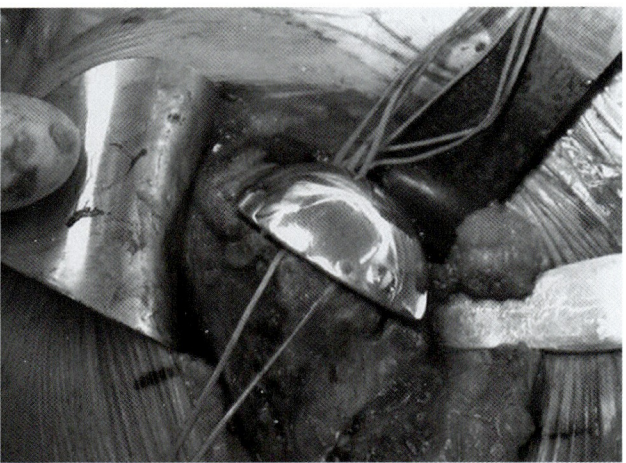

Figure 106.31 The final humeral component is placed. The sutures for reattachment of the lesser tuberosity can be visualized.

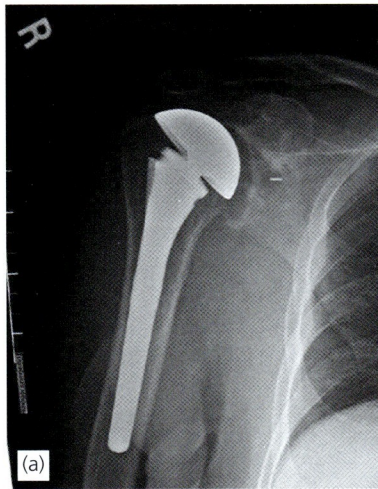

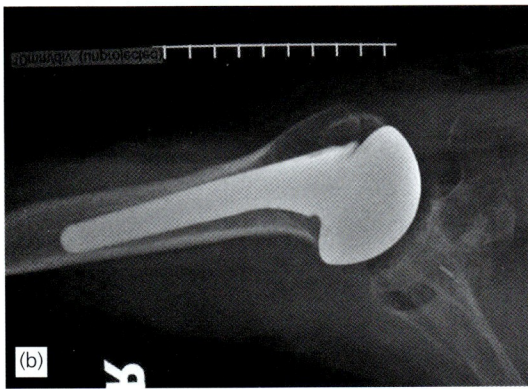

Figure 106.33 Postoperative anteroposterior (a) and axillary (b) radiographs reveal anatomic placement of the implants.

point. This will allow easy entry of the humeral reamers into the intramedullary canal. The humeral shaft is reamed until the reamers begin to purchase the endosteal surface of the canal. An appropriately sized intramedullary cutting guide handle is placed into the humeral canal and the cutting guide is placed on the handle in 0° of retroversion compared with the epicondylar axis of the humerus. The humeral osteotomy is then made at a neck–shaft angle of 155° and the humeral head is removed. A humeral metaphysis protector is placed in the humerus and the humerus is retracted posteriorly, similar to the technique described above.

GLENOID EXPOSURE, PREPARATION, AND TRIAL COMPONENT PLACEMENT

The joint capsule is released from the glenoid at the glenoid–labral junction circumferentially. This is particularly important inferiorly. The entire inferior glenoid rim must be visualized so that the proximal extent of the lateral angle of the scapula is palpable. This is an important landmark for placement of the inferior screw in the glenoid baseplate.

The central guide pin is placed in the glenoid using the hand-held guide to ensure proper placement and orientation. It should be placed so that the inferior margin of the glenoid baseplate aligns with the most inferior margin of the glenoid rim and the pin should be oriented in a neutral plane in both the superoinferior and AP directions. The glenoid is then reamed over the guide pin. Both the inferior glenoid and the superior glenoid should be reamed to accept the glenoid baseplate and glenoid sphere, respectively. The central drill hole is then made over the guide pin, the guide pin is removed and the glenoid baseplate is placed. The orientation of the baseplate should be slightly clockwise (right shoulder) from the superoinferior axis of the glenoid to ensure that the superior screw is in the base of the coracoid and the inferior screw is in the lateral angle of the scapula. The four screws are then placed with the superior and inferior screws being placed first. At a minimum, the superior and inferior screws should lock to the baseplate. The trial glenoid sphere is then placed. If possible, a 42 mm sphere is used.

HUMERAL EPIPHYSIS PREPARATION AND TRIAL COMPONENT PLACEMENT

The humerus is redelivered into the wound and the metaphyseal protector is removed. The proximal reaming guide is placed into the humeral canal in 0° of retroversion. The humeral epiphysis is reamed using either a size 1 or 2 reamer, depending on the size of the humerus. The reamer guide is removed and a trial humeral component is placed in 0° of retroversion. A trial liner is placed and the joint is reduced. Joint stability and motion as well as tension in the conjoined tendon are evaluated. With the arm at the side, traction should cause 1–2 mm of component gapping. When the arm is externally rotated at the side, the anterior aspect of the joint should gap open only slightly at the end range.

FINAL COMPONENT PLACEMENT

The joint is redislocated and the trial implants are removed. The final glenoid sphere is impacted into position and secured with the central screw (Fig. 106.34). The final humeral component is placed in 0° of retroversion. The humerus is most often cemented using antibiotic impregnated cement. However, with good bone quality, a cementless stem may be used. The appropriate final liner is placed and the joint is reduced (Fig. 106.35).

CLOSURE

If the subscapularis can be reattached to the bone of the humerus without compromising motion, this will presumably decrease the likelihood of postoperative dislocation. The remainder of the closure is as described above for anatomic replacement.

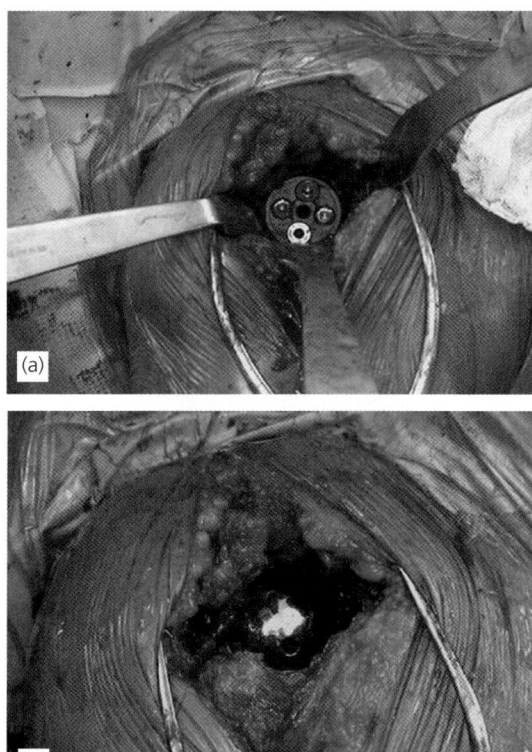

Figure 106.34 The glenoid baseplate should be fixed with four screws, at least two of which should be locking (a). The glenoid sphere is then seated onto the baseplate (b).

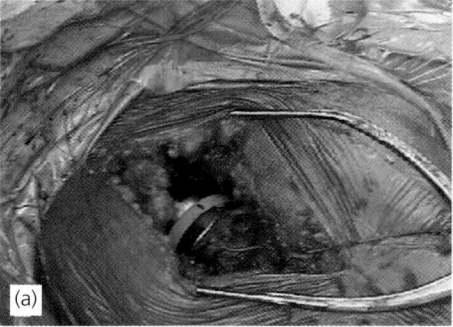
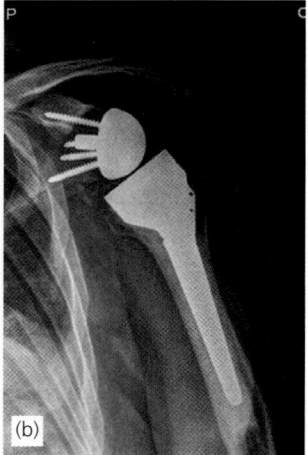

Figure 106.35 After the humeral component is placed, it is reduced onto the glenoid sphere (a). A postoperative anteroposterior radiograph reveals a reduced joint with the inferior margin of the glenoid sphere aligned with the inferior glenoid rim (b).

Postoperative rehabilitation

Postoperative management differs depending on whether the replacement is anatomic or reverse. At the time of anatomic replacement, the safe zone of passive motion is identified by moving the arm through a range of motion after closure of the subscapularis. Passive range of motion within those limits along with pendulum exercises are begun on postoperative day 1. This is continued for the first 6 weeks. Then formal stretching, active range of motion and strengthening exercises are instituted. Full recovery of range of motion and strength will require 12–15 months. However, formal exercises are required for 2–3 months.

Physiotherapy is not required after reverse shoulder arthroplasty. The shoulder is kept in a sling for protection for 10–14 days. The patient is then asked to use the arm for daily activities within their limits of pain. Maximum recovery will again require 12–15 months.

Results

The results of anatomic arthroplasty are disease dependent. In properly selected patients, shoulder arthroplasty provides dramatic relief of pain, improvement in function and patient satisfaction. Approximately 90% of patients report complete or near complete pain relief.[151–156] Return of function is more variable and is dependent on the status of the rotator cuff. Total shoulder arthroplasty provides more reliable pain relief than hemiarthroplasty but adds the possibility of component wear and loosening. Survivorship of total shoulder arthroplasty is 85–87% at 15 years.

Patients with glenohumeral arthritis and irreparable rotator cuff insufficiency are a heterogeneous population. Hemiarthroplasty provides reliable pain relief in most patients. However, postoperative function is variable and most dependent on pre-operative active motion.[157] Reverse[158] arthroplasty also provides excellent pain relief. However, it also offers the possibility of overhead function in patients who did not have it pre-operatively.[159,160] Polyethylene wear is a significant potential problem with reverse arthroplasty and 10–15 year survivorship data are not available.

Complications

The complication rate for anatomic shoulder arthroplasty has dropped substantially as experience has increased.[161]

When all potential complications are considered, including minor ones, the overall rate of complications with current shoulder arthroplasty techniques is approximately 10%. Potential complications include infection, instability, neurological injury, complex regional pain syndrome (reflex sympathetic dystrophy), rotator cuff tear, stiffness, component dissociation and aseptic loosening. The rate of postoperative glenoid lucent lines is 30–90% and their significance is not known. However, it is likely that a substantial percentage of them, particularly those that are progressive, represent loosening or impending loosening.

The complication rate associated with reverse arthroplasty is higher than with anatomic arthroplasty and ranges from 20% to 50%.[158,160] It is highest in patients undergoing reverse arthroplasty for revision of a failed prosthesis and lowest in patients with primary cuff tear arthropathy. Potential complications include dislocation, infection, acromial stress fracture, glenoid fracture, nerve injury, component dissociation, periprosthetic humeral fracture, haematoma, deltoid detachment (anterosuperior approach only) and scapular notching. Scapular notching is common (40%) when designs are used that have minimal lateral offset. Notching can probably be minimized by placing the glenoid component as low on the glenoid as possible. The effect on outcome of scapular notching is not yet known and catastrophic failure is rare.

SUMMARY

Adult shoulder reconstruction is an enormous field that encompasses a variety of diagnoses and treatments. Even if the discussion is limited to open reconstructive procedures, the amount of information is impossible to put in one chapter. This chapter includes only the most common open reconstructive procedures performed, and, even then, in broad terms. Important topics that could not be discussed include proximal humeral fractures, glenoid fractures, clavicle fractures, glenohumeral instability with bone loss, revision arthroplasty, and many others. The interested reader is encouraged to further his or her education by reading the many books now available on shoulder reconstruction. There are more resources from which to learn about the management of shoulder problems than ever before. It is hoped that this chapter serves as an adequate platform from which to expand one's knowledge.

KEY LEARNING POINTS

- Most patients with chronic rotator cuff tears and acute rotator cuff tears without substantial retraction are candidates for non-operative management.
- Rotator cuff repair is indicated in most patients with an acute tear with retraction, an acute-on-chronic tear with new onset of weakness and poor function, and a chronic tear that has not responded to non-operative management for a minimum of 3 months.
- The 'essential lesion' in most patients with multidirectional instability is increased capsular volume.
- Non-operative management of glenohumeral instability consists of a combination of bracing, activity modification and physiotherapy.
- Surgical options include open Bankart repair, capsular shift and posterior reconstruction.
- Shoulder replacement is indicated when patients have symptomatic glenohumeral arthritis that has not responded to non-operative management. Anatomic arthroplasty, hemiarthroplasty or total shoulder arthroplasty are indicated in patients with an intact or reparable rotator cuff. Total shoulder arthroplasty results in better pain relief and is preferred in patients over the age of 50 years who do not participate in heavy weight lifting or other activities that put excessive stress across the shoulder. In patients with arthritis and irreparable rotator cuff deficiency, hemiarthroplasty is preferred in patients with pre-operative elevation of 120° or more and who are young and active (i.e. under the age of 65 or 70 years).

REFERENCES

- ● = Key primary paper
- ◆ = Major review article

1. Smith E. *Edwin Smith's Surgical Papyrus*. Chicago, IL: University of Chicago Press, 1930.
●2. Codman E. Complete rupture of the supraspinatus tendon: operative treatment with report of two successful cases. *Boston Medical and Surgical Journal* 1911;**164**:708–10.
3. Perthes G. Uber operationen bei habitueller schulterluxation. *Deutsche Zeitschrift für Chirurgie* 1906;**85**:199–227.
●4. Codman EA. Rupture of the supraspinatus. *American Journal of Surgery* 1938;**42**:603–6.
5. Codman EA. *Rupture of the Supraspinatus Tendon and Other Lesions In or About the Subacromial Bursa*. Boston, MA: Thomas Todd, 1934.
●6. Neer CS 2nd. Anterior acromioplasty for the chronic impingement syndrome in the shoulder: a preliminary report. *Journal of Bone and Joint Surgery (American)* 1972;**54**:41–50.
7. Keyes EL. Anatomical observations on senile changes in the shoulder. *Journal of Bone and Joint Surgery* 1935;**17A**:953–60.
●8. Keyes EL. Observations on rupture of supraspinatus tendon based upon a study of 73 cadavers. *Annals of Surgery* 1933;**97**:849–56.

9. Neer CS 2nd, Marberry TA. On the disadvantages of radical acromionectomy. *Journal of Bone and Joint Surgery (American)* 1981;**63**:416–19.
●10. Budoff JE, Nirschl RP, Guidi EJ. Debridement of partial-thickness tears of the rotator cuff without acromioplasty. Long-term follow-up and review of the literature. *Journal of Bone and Joint Surgery (American)* 1998;**80**:733–48.
●11. Gartsman GM, O'Connor DP. Arthroscopic rotator cuff repair with and without arthroscopic subacromial decompression: a prospective, randomized study of one-year outcomes. *Journal of Shoulder and Elbow Surgery* 2004;**13**:424–6.
●12. Goldberg BA, Lippitt SB, Matsen FA 3rd. Improvement in comfort and function after cuff repair without acromioplasty. *Clinical Orthopaedics and Related Research* 2001;**Sep**:142–50.
13. McCallister WV, Parsons IM, Titelman RM, Matsen FA 3rd. Open rotator cuff repair without acromioplasty. *Journal of Bone and Joint Surgery (American)* 2005;**87**:1278–83.
14. Albritton MJ, Graham RD, Richards RS 2nd, Basamania CJ. An anatomic study of the effects on the suprascapular nerve due to retraction of the supraspinatus muscle after a rotator cuff tear. *Journal of Shoulder and Elbow Surgery* 2003;**12**:497–500.
15. Costouros JG, Porramatikul M, Lie DT, Warner JJ. Reversal of suprascapular neuropathy following arthroscopic repair of massive supraspinatus and infraspinatus rotator cuff tears. *Arthroscopy* 2007;**23**:1152–61.
16. Mallon WJ, Wilson RJ, Basamania CJ. The association of suprascapular neuropathy with massive rotator cuff tears: a preliminary report. *Journal of Shoulder and Elbow Surgery* 2006;**15**:395–8.
17. Burkhead W, Scheinberg R, Box G. Surgical anatomy of the axillary nerve. *Journal of Shoulder and Elbow Surgery* 1992;**1**:31–6.
18. Kulkarni RR, Nandedkar AN, Mysorekar VR. Position of the axillary nerve in the deltoid muscle. *Anatomical Record* 1992;**232**:316–17.
19. Flatow EL, Wang VM, Kelkar R, et al. The coracoacromial ligament passively restrains anterosuperior humeral subluxation in the rotator cuff deficient shoulder. *Transactions of the Orthopaedic Research Society* 1996;**21**:229.
20. Soslowsky LJ, An CH, DeBano CM, Carpenter JE. Coracoacromial ligament: in situ load and viscoelastic properties in rotator cuff disease. *Clinical Orthopaedics and Related Research* 1996;**Sep**:40–4.
21. Wiley AM. Superior humeral dislocation. A complication following decompression and debridement for rotator cuff tears. *Clinical Orthopaedics and Related Research* 1991;**263**:135–41.
22. Flatow E, Connor P, Levine W, et al. Coracoacromial arch reconstruction for anterosuperior subluxation after failed rotator cuff surgery. *Journal of Shoulder and Elbow Surgery* 1997;**6**:228.
●23. Neer CS 2nd. Impingement lesions. *Clinical Orthopaedics and Related Research* 1983;**173**:70–7.
●24. Hawkins RJ, Hobeika P. Physical examination of the shoulder. *Orthopedics* 1983;**6**:1270–8.
25. Hertel R, Ballmer FT, Lombert SM, Gerber C. Lag signs in the diagnosis of rotator cuff rupture. *Journal of Shoulder and Elbow Surgery* 1996;**5**:307–13.
26. Gerber C, Krushell RJ. Isolated rupture of the tendon of the subscapularis muscle. Clinical features in 16 cases. *Journal of Bone and Joint Surgery (British)* 1991;**73**:389–94.
●27. Tokish JM, Decker MJ, Ellis HB, et al. The belly-press test for the physical examination of the subscapularis muscle: electromyographic validation and comparison to the lift-off test. *Journal of Shoulder and Elbow Surgery* 2003;**12**:427–30.
28. Kitay GS, Iannotti JP, Williams GR, et al. Roentgenographic assessment of acromial morphologic condition in rotator cuff impingement syndrome. *Journal of Shoulder and Elbow Surgery* 1995;**4**:441–8.
29. Neer CS II, Poppen NK. Supraspinatus outlet. *Orthopedic Transactions* 1987;**11**:234.
●30. Rockwood CA, Lyons FR. Shoulder impingement syndrome: diagnosis, radiographic evaluation, and treatment with a modified Neer acromioplasty [see comments]. *Journal of Bone and Joint Surgery (American)* 1993;**75**:409–24.
31. Mack LA, Matsen FA 3rd, Kilcoyne RF, et al. Ultrasound evaluation of the rotator cuff. *Radiology* 1985;**157**:205–9.
●32. Yamaguchi K, Tetro AM, Blam O, et al. Natural history of asymptomatic rotator cuff tears: a longitudinal analysis of asymptomatic tears detected sonographically. *Journal of Shoulder and Elbow Surgery* 2001;**10**:199–203.
33. Mack LA, Nyberg DA, Matsen FR 3rd, et al. Sonography of the postoperative shoulder. *AJR American Journal of Roentgenology* 1988;**150**:1089–93.
34. Zlatkin MB, Iannotti JP, Roberts MC, et al. Rotator cuff tears: diagnostic performance of MR imaging. *Radiology* 1989;**172**:223–9.
35. Fuchs B, Weishaupt D, Zanetti M, et al. Fatty degeneration of the muscles of the rotator cuff: assessment by computed tomography versus magnetic resonance imaging. *Journal of Shoulder and Elbow Surgery* 1999;**8**:599–605.
36. Hattrup SJ, Cofield RH, Berquist TH, et al. Shoulder arthrography for determination of size of rotator cuff tears. *Journal of Shoulder and Elbow Surgery* 1992;**1**:98–105.
37. Mink JH, Harris E, Rappaport M. Rotator cuff tears: Evaluation using double-contrast shoulder arthrography. *Radiology* 1985;**153**:621–3.
38. Goutallier D, Postel JM, Bernageau J, et al. Fatty muscle degeneration in cuff ruptures. Pre- and postoperative evaluation by CT scan. *Clinical Orthopaedics and Related Research* 1994;**Jul**:78–83.
39. Warner J, Krushell R, Masquelet A, Gerber C. Anatomy and relationships of the suprascapular nerve: anatomical constraints to mobilization of the supraspinatus and infraspinatus muscles in the management of massive rotator cuff tears. *Journal of Bone and Joint Surgery (American)* 1992;**74A**:36–45.

◆40. Cordasco FA, Bigliani LU. The rotator cuff. Large and massive tears. Technique of open repair. *Orthopedic Clinics of North America* 1997;**28**:179–93.
41. Miller SL, Gladstone JN, Cleeman E, et al. Anatomy of the posterior rotator interval: implications for cuff mobilization. *Clinical Orthopaedics and Related Research* 2003;**408**:152–6.
42. Gerber C, Schneeberger AG, Beck M, Schlegel U. Mechanical strength of repairs of the rotator cuff. *Journal of Bone and Joint Surgery (British)* 1994;**76**:371–80.
43. Flatow E, Weinstein D, Duralde X, et al. Coracoacromial ligament preservation in rotator cuff surgery. *Journal of Shoulder and Elbow Surgery* 1994;**3**:S73.
●44. Walch G, Nove-Josserand L, Boileau P, Levigne C. Subluxations and dislocations of the tendon of the long head of the biceps. *Journal of Shoulder and Elbow Surgery* 1998;**7**:100–8.
45. Iannotti J, Bernot M, Kuhlman J et al. Prospective evaluation of rotator cuff repair. *Journal of Shoulder and Elbow Surgery* 1993;**2**:S9.
46. Romeo AA, Hang DW, Bach BR Jr, Shott S. Repair of full thickness rotator cuff tears. Gender, age, and other factors affecting outcome. *Clinical Orthopaedics and Related Research* 1999;**Oct**:243–55.
●47. Watson EM, Sonnabend DH. Outcome of rotator cuff repair. *Journal of Shoulder and Elbow Surgery* 2002;**11**:201–11.
●48. Galatz LM, Griggs, S, Cameron BD, Iannotti JP. Prospective longitudinal analysis of postoperative shoulder function: a ten-year follow-up study of full-thickness rotator cuff tears. *Journal of Bone and Joint Surgery (American)* 2001;**83A**:1052–6.
49. Harryman DT, Mack LA, Wang KY, et al. Repairs of the rotator cuff. Correlation of functional results with integrity of the cuff. *Journal of Bone and Joint Surgery (American)* 1991;**73**:982–9.
◆50. Mansat P, Cofield RH, Kersten TE, Rowland CM. Complications of rotator cuff repair. *Orthopedic Clinics of North America* 1997;**28**:205–13.
51. Sher JS, Iannotti JP, Warner JJ, et al. Surgical treatment of postoperative deltoid origin disruption. *Clinical Orthopaedics and Related Research* 1997;**Oct**:93–8.
52. Athwal GS, Sperling JW, Rispoli DM, Cofield RH. Deep infection after rotator cuff repair. *Journal of Shoulder and Elbow Surgery* 2007;**16**:306–11.
53. Mirzayan R, Itamura JM, Vangsness CT Jr, et al. Management of chronic deep infection following rotator cuff repair. *Journal of Bone and Joint Surgery (American)* 2000;**82A**:1115–21.
54. Settecerri JJ, Pitner MA, Rock MG, et al. Infection after rotator cuff repair. *Journal of Shoulder and Elbow Surgery* 1999;**8**:1–5.
55. Adams F. *The Genuine Works of Hippocrates.* New York, NY: William Woods, 1886.
56. Flower W. On pathologic changes produced in the shoulder joint by traumatic dislocation. *Transactions of the Pathological Society of London* 1861;**12**:179–200.
57. Joessel D. Ueber die recidine der humerus-luxationen. *Deutsche Zeitschrift für Chirurgie* 1880;**13**:167–84.
58. Hill HA, Sachs MD. The grooved defect of the humeral head: a frequently unrecognized complication of dislocations of the shoulder joint *Radiology* 1940;**35**:690–700.
59. Bankart ASB. The pathology and treatment of recurrent dislocation of the shoulder joint. *British Journal of Surgery* 1939;**26**:23–9.
60. Rowe CR, Patel D, Southmayd WW. The Bankart procedure: a long-term end-result study. *Journal of Bone and Joint Surgery (American)* 1978;**60**:1–16.
61. Burkhart SS, De Beer JF. Traumatic glenohumeral bone defects and their relationship to failure of arthroscopic Bankart repairs: significance of the inverted-pear glenoid and the humeral engaging Hill-Sachs lesion. *Arthroscopy* 2000;**16**:677–94.
62. Lo IK, Parten PM, Burkhart SS. The inverted pear glenoid: an indicator of significant glenoid bone loss. *Arthroscopy* 2004;**20**:169–74.
63. Weishaupt D, Zanetti M, Nyffeler RW, et al. Posterior glenoid rim deficiency in recurrent (atraumatic) posterior shoulder instability. *Skeletal Radiology* 2000;**29**:204–10.
●64. Cooper RA, Brems JJ. The inferior capsular shift procedure for multidirectional instability of the shoulder. *Journal of Bone and Joint Surgery* 1992;**74A**:1516–29.
65. Neer CS 2nd, Foster CR. Inferior capsular shift for involuntary inferior and multidirectional instability of the shoulder. A preliminary report. *Journal of Bone and Joint Surgery (American)* 1980;**62**:897–908.
66. Harryman DT, Sidles JA, Harris SL, Matsen FA. The role of the rotator interval capsule in passive motion and stability of the shoulder. *Journal of Bone and Joint Surgery (American)* 1992;**74**:53–66.
67. Lazarus MD, Sidles JA, Harryman DT 2nd, Matsen FA 3rd. Effect of a chondral-labral defect on glenoid concavity and glenohumeral stability. A cadaveric model. *Journal of Bone and Joint Surgery (American)* 1996;**78**:94–102.
68. Lippitt SB, Vanderhooft JE, Harris SL, et al. Glenohumeral stability from concavity-compression: a quantitative analysis. *Journal of Shoulder and Elbow Surgery* 1993;**2**:27–35.
69. Howell SM, Galinat BJ. The glenoid-labral socket: a constrained articular surface. *Clinical Orthopaedics and Related Research* 1989;**243**:122–5.
70. O'Brien SJ, Neves MC, Arnoczky SP, et al. The anatomy and histology of the inferior glenohumeral ligament complex of the shoulder. *American Journal of Sports Medicine* 1990;**18**:449–56.
71. O'Brien SJ, Schwartz RS, Warren RF, Torzilli PA. Capsular restraints to anterior-posterior motion of the abducted shoulder: a biomechanical study. *Journal of Shoulder and Elbow Surgery* 1995;**4**:298–308.
72. Burkhead W, Rockwood CA Jr. Treatment of instability of the shoulder with an exercise program. *Journal of Bone and Joint Surgery* 1992;**74A**:890–6.
●73. Matsen FA, Harryman DT, Sidles JA. Mechanics of glenohumeral instability. *Clinics in Sports Medicine* 1991;**10**:783–8.

74. Rowe CR. Prognosis in dislocations of the shoulder. *Journal of Bone and Joint Surgery* 1956;**38A**:957-77.
75. Bigliani LU, Kurzweil PR, Schwartzbach CC, et al. Inferior capsular shift procedure for anterior-inferior shoulder instability in athletes. *American Journal of Sports Medicine* 1994;**22**:578-84.
76. Bigliani LU, Pollock RG, McIlveen SJ, et al. Shift of the posteroinferior aspect of the capsule for recurrent posterior glenohumeral instability. *Journal of Bone and Joint Surgery (American)* 1995;**77**:1011-20.
●77. Lebar RD, Alexander AH. Multidirectional shoulder instability. Clinical results of inferior capsular shift in an active-duty population. *American Journal of Sports Medicine* 1992;**20**:193-8.
78. Speer KP, Hannafin JA, Altchek DW, Warren RF. An evaluation of the shoulder relocation test. *American Journal of Sports Medicine* 1994;**22**:177-83.
79. Deutsch A, Ramsey ML, Williams GR. Loss of passive external rotation at 90 degrees abduction is predictive of a medially healed Bankart lesion. *Arthroscopy* 2006;**22**:710-15.
80. Garth WP, Slappey CE, Ochs CW. Roentgenographic Demonstration of instability of the shoulder: the apical oblique projection. *Journal of Bone and Joint Surgery (American)* 1984;**66A**:1450-3.
81. Hall RH, Isaac F, Booth CR. Dislocations of the shoulder with special reference to accompanying small fractures. *Journal of Bone and Joint Surgery (American)* 1959;**41A**:489-94.
82. Rokous JR, Feagin JA, Abbott HG. Modified axillary roentgenogram. A useful adjunct in the diagnosis of recurrent instability of the shoulder. *Clinical Orthopaedics and Related Research* 1972;**82**:84-6.
83. Boileau P, Walch G. The three-dimensional geometry of the proximal humerus. Implications for surgical technique and prosthetic design. *Journal of Bone and Joint Surgery (British)* 1997;**79**:857-65.
84. Flannigan B, Kursunoglu-Brahme S, Snyder S, et al. MR arthrography of the shoulder: comparison with conventional MR imaging. *AJR American Journal of Roentgenology* 1990;**155**:829-32.
85. Jahnke AH Jr, Petersen SA, Neumann C, et al. Prospective comparison of computerized arthrotomography and magnetic resonance imaging of the glenohumeral joint. *American Journal of Sports Medicine* 1992;**20**:695-700; discussion 700-1.
86. Cofield RH, Irving JF. Evaluation and classification of shoulder instability. With special reference to examination under anesthesia. *Clinical Orthopaedics and Related Research* 1987;**223**:32-43.
●87. Cofield RH, Nessler JP, Weinstabl R. Diagnosis of shoulder instability by examination under anesthesia. *Clinical Orthopaedics and Related Research* 1993;**291**:45-53.
88. Burkhead WZ, Schiffern SC, Krishnan SG. Use of GraftJacket as an augmentation for massive rotator cuff tears. *Seminars in Arthroplasty* 2007;**18**:11-18.
89. Hovelius L, Eriksson K, Fridin H, et al. Recurrences after initial dislocation of the shoulder. *Journal of Bone and Joint Surgery (American)* 1983;**65A**:343-9.
●90. Hovelius L, Lind B, Thorling J. Primary dislocation of the shoulder. Factors affecting the two-year prognosis. *Clinical Orthopaedics and Related Research* 1983;**Jun**:181-5,.
91. DeBerardino TM, Arciero RA, Taylor DC, Uhorchak JM. Prospective evaluation of arthroscopic stabilization of acute, initial anterior shoulder dislocations in young athletes. Two- to five-year follow-up. *American Journal of Sports Medicine* 2001;**29**:586-92.
92. Itoi E, Hatakeyama Y, Sato T, et al. Immobilization in external rotation after shoulder dislocation reduces the risk of recurrence. A randomized controlled trial. *Journal of Bone and Joint Surgery (American)* 2007;**89**:2124-31.
93. Yamamoto N, Itoi E, Abe H, et al. Contact between the glenoid and the humeral head in abduction, external rotation, and horizontal extension: a new concept of glenoid track. *Journal of Shoulder and Elbow Surgery* 2007;**16**:649-56.
94. Warner JJ, Johnson D, Miller M, Caborn DN. Technique for selecting capsular tightness in repair of anterior-inferior shoulder instability. *Journal of Shoulder and Elbow Surgery* 1995;**4**:352-64.
95. Wirth MA, Butters KP, Rockwood CA Jr. The posterior deltoid-splitting approach to the shoulder. *Clinical Orthopaedics and Related Research* 1993;**296**:92-8.
96. Shaffer BS, Conway J, Jobe FW, et al. Infraspinatus muscle-splitting incision in posterior shoulder surgery. An anatomic and electromyographic study. *American Journal of Sports Medicine* 1994;**22**:113-20.
97. Protzman RR. Anterior instability of the shoulder. *Journal of Bone and Joint Surgery (American)* 1980;**62**:909-18.
98. Levine WN, Richmond JC, Donaldson WR. Use of the suture anchor in open Bankart reconstruction. A follow-up report. *American Journal of Sports Medicine* 1994;**22**:723-6.
99. Loomer R, Fraser J. A modified Bankart procedure for recurrent anterior/inferior shoulder instability. A preliminary report. *American Journal of Sports Medicine* 1989;**17**:374-9,.
100. Fuchs B, Jost B, Gerber C. Posterior-inferior capsular shift for the treatment of recurrent, voluntary posterior subluxation of the shoulder. *Journal of Bone and Joint Surgery (American)* 2000;**82**:16-25.
●101. Hawkins RJ, Koppert, G, Johnston G. Recurrent posterior instability (subluxation) of the shoulder. *Journal of Bone and Joint Surgery (American)* 1984;**66**:169-74.
102. Rhee YG, Lee DH, Lim CT. Posterior capsulolabral reconstruction in posterior shoulder instability: deltoid saving. *Journal of Shoulder and Elbow Surgery* 2005;**14**:355-60.
●103. Shin RD, Polatsch DB, Rokito AS, Zuckerman JD. Posterior capsulorrhaphy for treatment of recurrent posterior glenohumeral instability. *Hospital for Joint Diseases* 2005;**63**:9-12.
104. Tibone J, Ting A. Capsulorrhaphy with a staple for recurrent posterior subluxation of the shoulder [see comments]. *Journal of Bone and Joint Surgery (American)* 1990;**72**:999-1002.

105. Wolf BR, Strickland S, Williams RJ, et al. Open posterior stabilization for recurrent posterior glenohumeral instability. *Journal of Shoulder and Elbow Surgery* 2005;**14**:157–64.
106. Altchek DW, Warren RF, Skyhar MJ, Ortiz G. T-plasty modification of the Bankart procedure for multidirectional instability of the anterior and inferior types. *Journal of Bone and Joint Surgery (American)* 1991;**73**:105–12.
107. Choi CH, Ogilvie-Harris DJ. Inferior capsular shift operation for multidirectional instability of the shoulder in players of contact sports. *British Journal of Sports Medicine* 2002;**36**:290–4.
●108. Cooper RA, Brems JJ. The inferior capsular-shift procedure for multidirectional instability of the shoulder. *Journal of Bone and Joint Surgery (American)* 1992;**74**:1516–21.
109. van Tankeren E, de Waal Malefijt MC, van Loon CJ. Open capsular shift for multi directional shoulder instability. *Archives of Orthopaedic and Trauma Surgery* 2002;**122**:447–50.
110. Misamore GW, Sallay PI, Didelot WA. Longitudinal study of patients with multidirectional instability of the shoulder with seven- to ten-year follow-up. *Journal of Shoulder and Elbow Surgery* 2005;**14**:466–70.
●111. Flatow EL, Miniaci A, Evans PJ, et al. Instability of the shoulder: complex problems and failed repairs: Part II. Failed repairs. *Instructional Course Lectures* 1998;**47**:113–25.
●112. Flatow EL, Warner JI. Instability of the shoulder: complex problems and failed repairs: Part I. Relevant biomechanics, multidirectional instability, and severe glenoid loss. *Instructional Course Lectures* 1998;**47**:97–112.
113. Hawkins RH, Hawkins RJ. Failed anterior reconstruction for shoulder instability. *Journal of Bone and Joint Surgery (British)* 1985;**67**:709–14.
114. Cameron ML, Kocher MS, Briggs KK, et al. The prevalence of glenohumeral osteoarthrosis in unstable shoulders. *American Journal of Sports Medicine* 2003;**31**:53–5.
115. Matsoukis J, Tabib W, Guiffault P, et al. Shoulder arthroplasty in patients with a prior anterior shoulder dislocation. Results of a multicenter study. *Journal of Bone and Joint Surgery (American)* 2003;**l85A**:1417–24.
116. Samilson RL, Prieto V. Dislocation arthropathy of the shoulder. *Journal of Bone and Joint Surgery (American)* 1983;**65**:456–60.
117. Hawkins RJ, Angelo RL. Glenohumeral osteoarthrosis. A late complication of the Putti-Platt repair. *Journal of Bone and Joint Surgery (American)* 1990;**72A**:1193–7.
118. Athwal GS, Shridharani SM, O'Driscoll SW. Osteolysis and arthropathy of the shoulder after use of bioabsorbable knotless suture anchors. A report of four cases. *Journal of Bone and Joint Surgery (American)* 2006;**88**:1840–5.
119. Kaar TK, Schenck RC Jr, Wirth MA, Rockwood CA Jr. Complications of metallic suture anchors in shoulder surgery: A report of 8 cases. *Arthroscopy* 2001;**17**:31–7.
120. Zuckerman JD, Matsen FA 3rd. Complications about the glenohumeral joint related to the use of screws and staples. *Journal of Bone and Joint Surgery (American)* 1984;**66**:175–80.
121. Neer CS, Craig EV, Fukuda H. Cuff-tear arthropathy. *Journal of Bone and Joint Surgery (American)* 1983;**65**:1232–44.
122. Neer CS. Replacement arthroplasty for glenohumeral osteoarthritis. *Journal of Bone and Joint Surgery (American)* 1974;**56**:1–13.
123. Pean JE. The classic: on prosthetic methods intended to repair bone fragments. *Clinical Orthopaedics and Related Research* 1973;**94**:4–7.
124. Krueger FJ. A vitallium replica arthroplasty on the shoulder. *Surgery* 1951;**30**:1005–11.
125. Neer C. Articular replacement for the humeral head. *Journal of Bone and Joint Surgery (American)* 1955;**37A**:215–28.
126. Neer CS. Indications for replacement of the proximal humeral articulation. *American Journal of Surgery* 1955;**89**:901–7.
127. Neer CS II. Total shoulder replacement. a preliminary report. *Orthopedic Transactions* 1977;**1**:244–5.
●128. Edwards TB, Kadakia NR, Boulahia A, et al. A comparison of hemiarthroplasty and total shoulder arthroplasty in the treatment of primary glenohumeral osteoarthritis: results of a multicenter study. *Journal of Shoulder and Elbow Surgery* 2003;**12**:207–13.
129. Gartsman GM, Roddey TS, Hammerman SM. Shoulder arthroplasty with or without resurfacing of the glenoid in patients who have osteoarthritis. *Journal of Bone and Joint Surgery (American)* 2000;**82**:26–34.
130. Jain NB, Hocker S, Pietrobon R, et al. Total arthroplasty versus hemiarthroplasty for glenohumeral osteoarthritis: role of provider volume. *Journal of Shoulder and Elbow Surgery* 2005;**14**:361–7.
131. Orfaly RM, Rockwood CA, Esenyel CZ, Wirth MA. Shoulder arthroplasty in cases with avascular necrosis of the humeral head. *Journal of Shoulder and Elbow Surgery*, 2007;**16**(3 Suppl.):527–32.
132. Franklin JL, Barrett WP, Jackins SE, Matsen FA 3rd. Glenoid loosening in total shoulder arthroplasty. Association with rotator cuff deficiency. *Journal of Arthroplasty* 1988;**3**:39–46.
133. Williams GR Jr, Rockwood CA Jr. Hemiarthroplasty in rotator cuff-deficient shoulders. *Journal of Shoulder and Elbow Surgery* 1996;**5**:362–7.
●134. Boileau P, Watkinson DJ, Hatzidakis AM, Balg F. Grammont reverse prosthesis: design, rationale, and biomechanics. *Journal of Shoulder and Elbow Surgery* 2005;**14**(1 Suppl S):147S–61S.
135. Grammont PM, Baulot E. Delta shoulder prosthesis for rotator cuff rupture. *Orthopedics* 1993;**16**:65–8.
136. Iannotti JP, Gabriel JP, Schneck SL, et al. The normal glenohumeral relationships. An anatomical study of one hundred and forty shoulders. *Journal of Bone and Joint Surgery (American)* 1992;**74**:491–500.
137. Ballmer FT, Sidles JA, Romeo AA, Matsen FA III. Humeral head prosthetic arthroplasty: surgically relevant geometric considerations. *Journal of Shoulder and Elbow Surgery* 1993;**2**:296–304.
138. Hertel R, Knothe U, Ballmer FT. Geometry of the proximal humerus and implications for prosthetic design. *Journal of Shoulder and Elbow Surgery* 2002;**11**:331–8.

139. Pearl ML, Volk AG. Retroversion of the proximal humerus in relationship to prosthetic replacement arthroplasty. *Journal of Shoulder and Elbow Surgery* 1995;**4**:286–9.
140. Pearl ML, Volk AG. Coronal plane geometry of the proximal humerus relevant to prosthetic arthroplasty. *Journal of Shoulder and Elbow Surgery* 1996;**5**:320–6.
141. Churchill RS, Brems JJ, Kotschi H. Glenoid size, inclination, and version: an anatomic study. *Journal of Shoulder and Elbow Surgery* 2001;**10**:327–32.
142. Couteau B, Mansat P, Darmana R, et al. Morphological and mechanical analysis of the glenoid by 3D geometric reconstruction using computed tomography. *Clinical Biomechanics (Bristol, Avon)* 2000;**15**(Suppl 1):S8–12.
143. Friedman RJ, Hawthorne KB, Genez BM. The use of computerized tomography in the measurement of glenoid version. *Journal of Bone and Joint Surgery (American)* 1992;**74**:1032–7.
144. Flatow EL, Bigliani LU, April EW. An anatomic study of the musculocutaneous nerve and its relationship to the coracoid process. *Clinical Orthopaedics and Related Research* 1989;**244**:166–71.
145. Lazarus M, Yung S, Sidles J, Harryman D. Anterosuperior humeral displacement: limitation by the coracoacromial arch. In: *American Shoulder and Elbow Surgeons Eleventh Open Meeting*, Orlando, FL. 1995:28.
146. Soslowsky LJ, An CH, Johnston SP, Carpenter JE. Geometric and mechanical properties of the coracoacromial ligament and their relationship to rotator cuff disease. *Transactions of the Orthopaedic Research Society* 1993;**18**:139.
147. Gerber C, Pennington SD, Yian EH, et al. Lesser tuberosity osteotomy for total shoulder arthroplasty. Surgical technique. *Journal of Bone and Joint Surgery (American)* 2006;**88**(Suppl 1 Pt 2):170–7.
148. Gerber C, Yian EH, Pfirrmann CA, et al. Subscapularis muscle function and structure after total shoulder replacement with lesser tuberosity osteotomy and repair. *Journal of Bone and Joint Surgery (American)* 2005;**87**:1739–45.
149. Cofield RH. Integral surgical maneuvers in prosthetic shoulder arthroplasty. *Seminars in Arthroplasty* 1990;**1**:112–23.
150. Collins D, Tencer A, Sidles J, Matsen F III. Edge displacement and deformation of glenoid components in response to eccentric loading: the effect of preparation of the glenoid bone. *Journal of Bone and Joint Surgery (American)* 1992;**74A**:501–7.
151. Cofield RH. Total shoulder arthroplasty with the Neer prosthesis. *Journal of Bone and Joint Surgery (American)* 1984;**66**:899–906.
152. Iannotti JP, Norris TR. Influence of preoperative factors on outcome of shoulder arthroplasty for glenohumeral osteoarthritis. *Journal of Bone and Joint Surgery (American)* 2003;**85A**:251–8.
153. Matsen FA 3rd. Early effectiveness of shoulder arthroplasty for patients who have primary glenohumeral degenerative joint disease. *Journal of Bone and Joint Surgery (American)* 1996;**78**:260–4.
154. Matsen FA 3rd, Antoniou J, Rozencwai R, et al. Correlates with comfort and function after total shoulder arthroplasty for degenerative joint disease. *Journal of Shoulder and Elbow Surgery* 2000;**9**:465–9.
●155. Neer CS 2nd, Watson KC, Stanton FJ. Recent experience in total shoulder replacement. *Journal of Bone and Joint Surgery (American)* 1982;**64**:319–37.
156. Torchia ME, Cofield RH, Settergren CR. Total shoulder arthroplasty with the Neer prosthesis: long-term results. *Journal of Shoulder and Elbow Surgery* 1997;**6**:495–505.
157. Williams G, Rockwood C. Massive rotator cuff defects and glenohumeral arthritis. In: Frieman RJ (ed.) *Arthroplasty of the Shoulder.* New York, NY: Thieme Medical Publishers, Inc., 1994:204–14.
158. Boileau P, Watkinson D, Hatzidakis AM, Hovorka I. Neer Award **2005**: the Grammont reverse shoulder prosthesis: results in cuff tear arthritis, fracture sequelae, and revision arthroplasty. *Journal of Shoulder and Elbow Surgery* 2006;**15**:527–40.
159. Matsen FA 3rd, Boileau P, Walch G, et al. The reverse total shoulder arthroplasty. *Journal of Bone and Joint Surgery (American)* 2007;**89**:660–7.
160. Werner CM, Steinmann PA, Gilbart M, Gerber C. Treatment of painful pseudoparesis due to irreparable rotator cuff dysfunction with the Delta III reverse-ball-and-socket total shoulder prosthesis. *Journal of Bone and Joint Surgery (American)* 2005;**87**:1476–86.
161. Chin PY, Sperling JW, Cofield RH, Schleck C. Complications of total shoulder arthroplasty: Are they fewer or different? *Journal of Shoulder and Elbow Surgery* 2006;**15**:19–22.

SECTION 5

The ankle

107 **Ankle arthroplasty** 1241
Norman Espinosa, Gerardo Juan Maquieira

107

Ankle arthroplasty

NORMAN ESPINOSA, GERARDO JUAN MAQUIEIRA

Introduction	1241	Theoretic aspects	1245
Aetiology	1241	Patient evaluation	1245
Pathophysiology	1241	Surgical technique	1245
Basic science	1242	Results	1246
Types of osteoarthritis	1242	Complications	1246
Presentation and diagnosis	1242	ALLOGRAFT TOTAL ANKLE REPLACEMENT	1246
Management	1242	Background	1246
Radiography	1243	Basic science	1246
TOTAL ANKLE REPLACEMENT	1243	Problems associated with allograft transplant	1247
Anatomy and biomechanics of the ankle joint and total ankle replacement	1243	Indications	1247
		Results	1247
Surgery	1244	Outlook	1247
Results	1244	Summary	1248
Complications	1245	References	1248
DISTRACTION ARTHROPLASTY	1245		
Introduction	1245		

NATIONAL BOARD STANDARDS

- Understand the aetiology, pathophysiology, types and management of osteoarthritis of the ankle
- Know the indications for surgery

- Understand total ankle replacement, distraction arthroplasty and allograft total ankle replacement

INTRODUCTION

Proper understanding of the various forms of osteoarthritis in the ankle is essential. The anatomy and the biomechanics of the ankle joint and total ankle replacement differ significantly when compared with that of total hip and knee arthroplasty. This chapter provides a review of the basic knowledge concerning surgical treatment of ankle arthrosis.

AETIOLOGY

The most frequent cause of ankle osteoarthritis is trauma (70%), which is then followed by rheumatoid arthritis (12%). Primary osteoarthritis occurs in approximately 7–9% of trauma cases. Other causes are quite rare, for example neuropathy, septic conditions, gout, haemophilia and osteonecrosis. Among all sequelae from trauma, rotational ankle fractures and chronic ankle instability predominantly account for the establishment of osteoarthrosis.[1,2]

PATHOPHYSIOLOGY

The rarity of primary osteoarthritis of the ankle might be the result of the congruency, stability and restrained motion of the ankle joint, tensile properties and metabolic characteristics of ankle articular cartilage, or a combination of these factors. The thin ankle articular cartilage and the small contact area result in high peak contact stresses, making the cartilage more susceptible to post-traumatic osteoarthritis. In particular, the thinner, stiffer articular cartilage of the ankle may be less able to adapt to articular surface incongruity and increased contact stresses than the thicker articular cartilage of the hip and knee, and contact stresses may be higher in the ankle.[3-5]

Any damage to the articular cartilage and subchondral bone creates articular surface incongruences and decreases joint stability. Post-traumatic ankle osteoarthritis seems to be the result of elevated contact stress that exceeds the capacity of the joint to repair itself or adapt. In secondary osteoarthritis, like neuropathies or necrosis of the talus, an incongruity of the articular surface is caused. This can occur because the loss of positional sense leads to undetected ligamentous or articular surface injuries that create localized regions of increased contact stress. This then leads to joint degeneration.

In contrast, there are patients who develop progressive joint degeneration without apparent articular surface damage, alteration of joint anatomy or instability. Other patients with articular surface incongruity or joint instability do not develop progressive joint degeneration. Thus, the pathogenesis of ankle osteoarthritis is more complex than it appears, and more studies are needed.

BASIC SCIENCE

The biology of osteoarthritic cartilage continues to be a focus of ongoing research. We know that there are changes in the biochemical and biomechanical nature of the osteoarthritic articular cartilage. At the beginning there is continuous deterioration of the articular cartilage secondary to progressive destruction of the collagen network and loss of cartilage molecules including proteoglycans. Finally, the molecular structure of the cartilage is altered, including its mechanical properties. In an attempt to repair the damage to the cartilaginous surface, chondrocytes dedifferentiate and begin to produce inappropriate matrix molecules such as catabolic cytokines and matrix proteases, which lead to further degradation of the cartilage.[6] Additionally, the subchondral bone is altered and becomes dense. Radiographically, subchondral sclerosis suggests increased bone density. It remains unclear whether these subchondral changes are the result of alterations in the articular cartilage itself or whether they are the catalyst for such changes.[7-9]

TYPES OF OSTEOARTHRITIS[10,11]

Idiopathic osteoarthritis of the ankle

The main characteristics of primary or idiopathic osteoarthritis are loss of cartilage tissue and hypertrophy of the bone. The exact mechanisms that lead to cartilage degeneration are still unclear. On conventional radiography, narrowing of the joint space, subchondral sclerosis, subchondral cysts and osteophytes can be observed. Normally, there is no juxta-articular osteoporosis.

Post-traumatic osteoarthritis of the ankle

Injuries to the ankle joint may result in lesions of the bony and cartilaginous structures as well and end in post-traumatic osteoarthritis. Most often it is secondary as a result of fracture (malleolar, pilon fracture, talar body fractures, etc.). However, chronic ankle instability due to ligamentous incompetency and dislocation of the ankle may also result in arthrosis. In contrast to idiopathic forms of ankle arthrosis, post-traumatic osteoarthritis involves the soft tissues as well. The latter may be scarred and as such have inelasticity that poses significant risk for further treatment. Besides the radiographic signs as seen for idiopathic osteoarthritis, patients with post-traumatic osteoarthritis of the ankle also present with incongruence of the ankle joint or misalignment and/or dislocation.

Systemic arthritis

This comprises rheumatoid arthritis, inflammatory systemic diseases (primarily involving the soft tissues) and synovial diseases of unknown origin. Usually, there is symmetric narrowing of the joint space and erosions (but no osteophytes) found on conventional radiography. Normally, patients with arthritic degeneration of the ankle joint also present with osteopenia.

PRESENTATION AND DIAGNOSIS

A thorough history and proper clinical examination provide enough information to establish the correct diagnosis and to define an adequate treatment plan. It is necessary to identify activities that could cause ankle pain or limit function. Think about further diagnoses such as anterior or posterior impingement, subtalar or talonavicular joint disease, misalignment or soft-tissue disorders.

MANAGEMENT

Once diagnosis of symptomatic ankle arthritis is confirmed, there are various possibilities for medical and surgical treatment.

Non-operative treatment

Non-operative treatment includes non-steroidal anti-inflammatory drugs, intra-articular injections (steroids), mechanical unloading and application of ankle-foot orthoses or adapted footwear.

Evaluation of surgical treatment

Surgical options for the treatment of ankle arthritis include fusion, total ankle replacement, distraction arthroplasty and replacement of the joint by allograft tissue. Additionally, there are various osteotomies for correction of deformities, which could be used alone or in conjunction with the former treatments.

RADIOGRAPHY[12–14]

Standard weight-bearing anteroposterior and lateral views of the ankle provide sufficient information about the type of ankle arthritis and ankle deformities. Occasionally, CT scans, with or without three-dimensional reconstructions, might be used to understand and evaluate complex deformity. If any supramalleolar deformity is suspected on clinical and radiographic examination or in case of limb length discrepancy, standing full-length lower extremity anteroposterior and lateral radiographs from the hip to the ankle should be obtained. If one considers distraction ankle arthroplasty, then it is important to exclude any advanced deformity in the coronal plane.

TOTAL ANKLE REPLACEMENT

ANATOMY AND BIOMECHANICS OF THE ANKLE JOINT AND TOTAL ANKLE REPLACEMENT

The ankle joint is a highly constrained articulation, which comprises three important bones (tibia, talus, fibula) that provide stability together with the tendons, ligaments and syndesmosis. Tendons and ligaments contribute to some dynamic stabilization of the joint.

The talus articulates with the tibial plafond superiorly, the tibia medially and the fibula laterally. The greatest contact between tibiotalar and tibiofibular is achieved during mid-stance phase and averages 7 cm². The articulations act as a combined osseous and soft-tissue (ligaments, capsule, retinacula) support complex, which provides proprioception, stabilization and control over the movement of the talus and calcaneus around their axes of motion. The tibiotalar angulation averages 93°, which is important to know when considering reconstructive interventions at the ankle joint. The strongest part of the tibial plafond is found posteromedially. Resection of the subchondral layer reduces the compressive resistance of the bone by 30–50%. When resecting 1 cm of the distal tibia, compressive resistance is reduced 70–90%.[1,10,11,15–19]

Under weight-bearing conditions the congruency of bones provides 100% of stability for eversion and inversion but only 30% of rotational stability. The ligamentous complexes predominantly control rotatory stability and anteroposterior tibiotalar shifting. The lateral ligamentous complex includes three important structures: the anterior talofibular ligament (ATFL), calcaneofibular ligament (CFL) and the posterior talofibular ligament (PTFL). Among these, the CFL uniquely spans both the tibiotalar and talocalcaneal joints. The cervical ligament is located within the sinus tarsi and runs in an oblique fashion from the neck of the talus to the superior surface of the calcaneus. A stable ankle results from a perfect interplay of static (bones, ligaments, retinaculum) and dynamic (muscles, tendons) anatomical structures. The role of bony and ligamentous stabilizers of the ankle and subtalar joints depends on the load and position of the foot and ankle in space. They provide proprioception, stabilization and limitation of non-physiological motion about the lateral ankle. The sural nerve courses behind and inferior to the lateral malleolus and the average distance from the tip has been found to be 13 mm.

Although studies have found the articular surfaces contribute to stability in rotation and inversion, these results must be interpreted with caution. Motion at the ankle is multiplanar and also linked to the tibia. The complex and dynamic configuration of the rotational axis of the ankle joint might be responsible for some implant failures at the ankle. Several studies using different types of methodology tried to identify the direction of axis of all of them, confirming a shift of the instant centre of rotation from posterior inferior to anterior superior. It is important to realize that the ankle joint is not a simple hinge joint, and this fact should influence current and future implant designs. The course of movement within the ankle joint is predominantly from plantarflexion (range 23–56°) to dorsiflexion (range 13–33°), but contains mild degrees of internal (1.9 ± 4.12°) and external rotation (7.2 ± 3.8°). For normal gait an average dorsiflexion of 10° and plantarflexion of 15° is needed. In contrast to the ankle joint, the subtalar joint follows more complex kinematics. The calcaneus rotates around the interosseous ligament, resulting in a screw-like motion associated with translation and rotation. According to Inman,[20,21] motion at the subtalar joint is triplanar, comprising inversion (calcaneus turns inward) and eversion (calcaneus turns outward). The subtalar joint due to its unique axis has been compared to a 'torque convertor' as it converts foot rotation to leg rotation.

As noted, ankle motion is highly dependent on the supporting ligamentous lateral structures. In plantarflexion the ATFL becomes taut and the calcaneofibular ligament remains loose. The ATFL primarily restricts internal rotation of the talus in the mortise. Biomechanical studies revealed that the ATFL has the highest degree of deformation, i.e. greatest strain, but the lowest load to failure when compared with the CFL. The relative strength of the CFL is approximately three times greater than that of the ATFL. The CFL stabilizes the subtalar joint and inhibits adduction and exerts its greatest effect in the neutral and dorsiflexed position. In dorsiflexion, the CFL approaches a vertical position with respect to the subtalar joint and acts as a true collateral ligament, preventing talar tilting.

Cass and Settles and colleagues[22,23] concluded that there was a tandem function of the ATFL and CFL in preventing talar tilt. They also showed that external rotation of the leg occurred with inversion averaging 11° in the intact specimen. Interestingly, this external rotation increased with further sectioning of the ATFL and CFL. Other authors have demonstrated that the anterolateral joint capsule adds mechanical stability to the ankle. The deltoid ligament and its deep fibres are extremely important to stabilize the talus against lateral and anterior translation.[15,24] As stated by Hintermann and colleagues,[25,26] inversion is accompanied by a mandatory external rotation of the leg. In the intact hind foot this rotation takes place at the subtalar joint whereas in the injured ankle joint without stabilizing ligaments this rotation is happening at the tibiotalar joint.

During normal gait the ankle joint is loaded with a force approximately six times bodyweight. In a degenerated ankle joint this force is reduced down to three times bodyweight. However, it is assumed that when total ankle replacement is considered the strength of bone should be at least three times higher than that under normal conditions to compensate for the forces exerted under higher performance activities in order to avoid any subsidence of the components. Thus, proper fixation techniques are needed. Fixation of ankle prostheses has seen significant changes. Contemporary designs use biological integration of the components. The surfaces are covered with calcium hydroxyapatite sometimes combined with porous coating of the component. The advantages of biological cementless fixation include less extensive resections of the tibia and talus; smaller sizes of implants; reduction in body wear; and avoidance of heat destruction of the soft tissues and bones. Full integration is achieved within 4–12 weeks after implantation, but remodelling of the implant–bone interface is completed up to 24 months postoperatively.

Polyethylene wear depends on geometry, strength (ultrastructure) and alignment of the components. There is no information about the adequate thickness of polyethylene that should be used in total ankle replacement. The optimal polyethylene should be thin and strong without the risk of impairing bony strength at the bone–implant interface. An adequate prosthesis should be shaped as anatomically correct as possible and mimic the kinetics and kinematics of a normal joint.[27–30]

SURGERY

Indications

Indications for total ankle replacement include primary osteoarthritis, secondary osteoarthritis (due to rheumatoid arthritis; haemochromatosis; haemophilia; scleroderma and lupus erythematosus; synovial diseases; psoriasis) and post-traumatic osteoarthrosis. Adequate bone quality, ligamentous stability, proper vascular status and immunological conditions as well as a well-aligned hindfoot with sufficient pre-operative range of motion at the ankle are prerequisites for an acceptable outcome.

Relative contraindications

Relative contraindications encompass status after major trauma (open ankle fractures, fracture–dislocations of the talus, segmental bony defects), infection, avascular necrosis of the talus (25–50% involvement), severe osteopenia or osteoporosis, longstanding steroid treatment (either systemic or local); diabetes mellitus; and moderate physical demands (tennis, skiing, jogging).

Absolute contraindications

Absolute contraindications include neuropathic feet, active joint infections, avascular necrosis of the talus (>50% involvement), severe hypermobility of the joints and hyperlaxity, periarticular compromise of the soft tissues, and high physical demands.

RESULTS

Table 107.1 provides a synopsis of widely used total ankle replacements and their outcomes.

Table 107.1 The table lists a group of (TAR) designs that are frequently used in the USA, Europe and Asia total ankle replacement

Authors	TAR	N	PTA (%)	PRA (%)	SA (%)	Follow-up	Satisfaction (%)	Loosening (%)	Revision (%)
Hintermann et al.[48]	HINTEGRA	122	75	13	12	28	84	2	7
Valderrabano et al.[49]	S.T.A.R.	68	71	13	16	44	97	13	34
Knecht et al.[33]	AGILITY	132	46	29	25	108	90	76	35
Tanaka and Takakura[50]	TNK 3^d G	70	39	0	31	63	71	24	4
Bonnin et al.[51]	SALTO	98	69	0	29	35	n.a.	2	6
Büchel et al.[52]	Buechel-Pappas	75	73	5	12	60	88	11	6

PRA, post-rheumatoid arthritis; PTA, post-traumatic arthritis; SA, post-septic arthritis.
Modified after Hintermann.[11]

COMPLICATIONS

The current literature reveals a high complication rate associated with total ankle replacement. Some of those complications could be prevented by proper indication. A frequently found complication is the fracture of one or both malleoli depending on the approach and technique used, which may occur in up to 22% of cases. The medial malleolus is the most affected one. Neurovascular structures are in close proximity. When using the anterior approach visualization of the posterior capsule may be difficult and could result in laceration of the posteromedial tendons from saw cuts (posterior tibial; flexor hallucis longus and flexor digitorum longus tendon). Excessive traction on the wound margins bears the potential for local damage to the anterior tibial tendon. In addition, the peroneus longus and brevis tendons can also be injured. Wound-healing problems are not unusual and in very severe cases they may need a transfer of a flap. Superficial infections or delayed wound healing both may happen in 2–24% of all cases. The management comprises local and/or systemic antibiotics. Severe wound-healing problems were reported to occur in up to 7% of all patients. In such cases revision surgery, conversion into arthrodesis or amputation must be taken into consideration. Swelling may persist up to 18 months after initial surgery. Aseptic loosening of the total ankle is another possible complication. However, if there is any doubt a CT or a single-photon-emission tomography CT scan could help to identify any weakness at the bone–implant interface.[30–36]

DISTRACTION ARTHROPLASTY

INTRODUCTION

The treatment aim of ankle osteoarthritis is to reduce pain, limit disability, preserve foot function and slow progression. Conservative treatment options are medications and injections, physical therapies, modification of activities, orthotic devices and footwear modifications. When these measures fail and the patient continues to be impaired and experiencing significant pain, surgical intervention may be warranted.

Among all surgical options to treat osteoarthrosis of the ankle, ankle distraction arthroplasty represents a relatively new treatment option, which intends to preserve ankle joint mobility. Judet and Judet[37] were among the first to describe distraction arthroplasty for the ankle joint.

THEORETICAL ASPECTS

The hypothesis that osteoarthritic cartilage has the potential to repair itself, once mechanical stresses are reduced or diminished at the articular surface, serves as the primary background for joint distraction arthroplasty.[38] However, the mechanism by which this reparative process occurs is unclear. One of the most popular theories is that generation of intermittent fluid pressure while prohibiting mechanical loading has an effect on the healing capacity of the chondrocytes.[39] One hypothesis is that subchondral bone alterations play a significant role in articular cartilage repair. The subchondral bone appears to have decreased density on radiographs after treatment with distraction arthroplasty. However, we do not know whether the decreased density leads to healing of the articular cartilage or whether the healthier cartilage, acted on by another mechanism, leads to stress shielding of the subchondral bone and, therefore, decreases density.

Other mechanisms such as action-like positive effects on nerve endings, decreased synovial inflammation, stretching of the joint capsule, decreased joint reaction forces or the formation of intra-articular fibrous tissue have also been discussed.[39]

PATIENT EVALUATION

To evaluate an appropriate indication for surgery such as distraction arthroplasty the following approach is suggested.

Evaluate the indications for and acceptance of distraction arthroplasty with the patient. The patient has to be informed about treatment and results. Physically demanding occupations might not allow for optimal clinical results with ankle distraction arthroplasty. After ankle distraction, swimming and bicycling are the preferred advised recreational activities.

Exclude contraindications such as active infection, joint ankylosis, and significant loss of bone stock and advanced coronal plane deformity.

The ideal candidate for distraction arthroplasty is suggested to be a young patient whose symptoms are refractory to conservative measures, and who is unwilling to undergo arthrodesis or joint replacement.

SURGICAL TECHNIQUE

Both ankle arthroscopy and open ankle debridement remain optional before applying the distraction device. An arthroscopy may be helpful to remove loose bodies or areas of unstable cartilage, tibiotalar osteophytes or inflamed synovial tissue. Additionally, microfracturing or subchondral drilling can be performed to increase local blood flow and provide an environment for healing. Joint debridement can improve pain and dorsiflexion, which is imperative to the function of distraction arthroplasty. Other surgical procedures to improve function are Achilles tendon lengthening or gastrocnemius recession. Ankle joint malalignment caused by deformities may be the cause of ankle joint degeneration. In such cases an adjunctive reorientation procedure such as supramalleolar osteotomy must be considered.

The external fixator consists of a two-ring leg construct connected by threaded rods to a foot ring or foot plate. First, a two-ring tibial base frame is applied orthogonal to the tibia by using wires and half pins. Fluoroscopic imaging is helpful for correct positioning of the wires and frame and for joint alignment. After the tibial base frame is applied, a temporary centre of rotation reference guidewire is placed from the tip of the lateral malleolus to the tip of the medial malleolus. Thus alignment of the joint and frame is assessed. The leg rings are secured and the foot plate or foot ring stabilized. The foot ring is usually fixed to the foot by means of three to five wires. The foot ring has to be positioned at the mid-portion of the calcaneus and superior to the sole of the foot so as not to inhibit weight bearing.

Next, medial and lateral threaded rods are attached from the tibial ring to the foot ring. Optional hinges are secured to threaded rods, which are attached to the distal tibial ring, and the hinges are aligned relative to the guidewire. After the hinge is properly positioned, the temporary axis guidewire is removed. With the apparatus in place the ankle joint is acutely distracted 3–5 mm from the pre-operative position using the threaded rods attached to the hinges.[8,9] This distraction is usually performed on the tibial ring attachment sites. Fluoroscopic evaluation is carried out with the ankle in the neutral position, and lateral radiographs are made to assess satisfactory ankle range of motion and confirm the absence of ankle subluxation with motion. Wounds are dressed in routine fashion with dressings and elastic bandages.

RESULTS

There are several published articles investigating the effect of joint distraction on ankle arthritis.[35,38,39] All series report a clinical success rate ranging from 70% to 80%. Most patients report improved pain and function. The average follow-up among the studies ranged from 1 to 10 years. Between 10% and 50% of patients presented a radiographic increase in joint space or decrease in subchondral sclerosis. A more recent prospective study of 57 patients showed a progressive improvement after an average follow-up of 2.8 years. Patients who received joint distraction arthroplasty had significantly better results than those with ankle joint debridement alone.[38] Comparable results have been achieved when ankle distraction was used for arthritis in conjunction with osteotomy for deformity correction. However, the most recent reports of Paley and colleagues[39,40] questioned the benefit of hinged distraction treatment. The group confirmed a decrease in outcome after 5 years, and radiographically the joint distraction space of the ankle could not be maintained. The failure rate (i.e. conversion into ankle fusion or total ankle replacement) of distraction arthroplasty in these series was 11% and 28%.

COMPLICATIONS

The most common complications of ankle distraction arthroplasty include pin tract inflammation or infection and hardware failure, which was found to be between 28% and 14%, respectively in one of these series.[38] Forefoot wires or half pins seem to loosen quite often and then have to be retensioned or changed.

Other potential risks are direct neurovascular injury resulting from pin placement, or a distraction injury of the posterior tibial nerve and tarsal tunnel syndrome.

ALLOGRAFT TOTAL ANKLE REPLACEMENT

BACKGROUND

The treatment of ankle arthritis in a young patient can be difficult. Although ankle fusion remains an option, the negative long-term effects on adjacent joints cannot be ignored. It is highly probable that total ankle arthroplasty will not withstand the loads exerted by the daily activities of a young individual unless there are only low demands expected. In such cases either extended fusions or revision total ankle replacement should be considered. In an attempt to overcome these limitations, transplantation of total allograft ankle replacement has become an option, which more recently has found recognition among foot and ankle surgeons.

BASIC SCIENCE

Based on the experience of using allogenic tissue to reconstruct larger focal defects in the knee joint, a similar approach has been tried to reconstruct the ankle joint. As reported, the allogenic chondrocytes seem to survive the cold storage period. Williams and colleagues[41] presented a study that confirmed 82% chondrocyte viability in failed allografts at an average of 42 months after retrieval. Addition of fetal bovine serum to the medium increases chondrocyte viability and cell density compared with serum-free medium alone. Usually, the underlying allograft bone that supports the cartilage heals to the host by creeping substitution. However, one very important aspect is when to implant the allograft transplant. Recent studies revealed that fresh allografts that were stored *in vitro* for more than 28 days showed significant decline in chondrocyte viability and density. The loss of viable chondrocytes has been found in the critically important superficial zone of the cartilage. Allograft tissue that is stored for 14 days or less is of better quality.

PROBLEMS ASSOCIATED WITH ALLOGRAFT TRANSPLANT

Analysis of allograft total ankle replacement determined that the risk factors for failure of an ankle transplant were (1) size mismatch of the allograft to the host and (2) tibial or talar allografts that were cut too thin. Although no statistically significant difference in the average graft thickness between the failure and success groups was found, technical errors in cutting the graft too thin was considered a risk factor. In the study by Jeng et al.[42] two tibial allografts and one talar allograft measured less than 0.7 cm in thickness and failed. Each of these subsequently fractured in the early postoperative period. The same group identified factors that were found to be significantly different between the success and failure groups. All of them were host related. They included (1) the patient's body mass index, (2) the patient's age and (3) the amount of pre-operative varus or valgus ankle malalignment on radiographs. Transplant surgeries performed in hosts with a lower body mass index, older age and less pre-operative deformity were more likely to survive. However, it may be difficult to interpret the actual clinical importance of these findings in light of the subtle differences in the numbers and the overall high failure rate in this series. The factors that were not found to be statistically different between the success and failure groups were the donor's age, the time from death of the donor to implantation, the thickness of the tibial and talar allografts and the postoperative radiographic ankle alignment.

The mechanisms of ankle failure included tibial graft fracture, talar graft fracture, tibial graft collapse, loss of joint space and infection. We found multiple factors, including a combination of mechanical, technical and immunological reasons.

INDICATIONS

Indications (according to Jeng et al.[42]) include patients who

- are too young for ankle replacement
- have a low body mass index
- refuse ankle arthrodesis.

RESULTS

Gross et al.[43] reported the earliest results of fresh osteochondral allograft tissue use in the ankle. They evaluated the outcome of unipolar transplants to the talus. Most of those allografts were used to treat osteochondritis dissecans lesions. Six out of nine allografts survived after 11 years. All three failures were revised to ankle arthrodesis.

Later Brage and colleagues[44] were first to present the results of bipolar ankle transplantation. They reported an 87% allograft survival rate, with only three ankles (from 16 in total) requiring revision to an arthrodesis.

The failures were due to graft fragmentation, graft subluxation and non-union. Kim and colleagues[45] published the results of seven ankle transplants followed for 148 months. They showed a 42% long-term failure rate. Allografts failed due to graft fragmentation, malunion and non-union. When compared with pre-operative values the patients' Short Form-12 general health survey scores at final follow-up were not significantly improved. Tontz and colleagues[46] reviewed the results of 12 patients followed for 21 months using a newer technique to prepare the allograft. Nine patients had a bipolar tibiotalar allograft, two patients had a unipolar talar allograft and one patient had a unipolar tibial allograft. Only one allograft (a partial unipolar allograft of the lateral talar dome) had to be revised due to graft collapse. The remaining 11 allografts were still *in situ* at the final follow-up. Meehan et al.[47] used similar techniques. They followed 11 ankle transplants using the agility cutting jig for an average of 33 months. Six of the 11 allografts survived. Of the five failures, three underwent repeat allografting, one had a prosthetic total ankle replacement, and one was a radiographic failure but had not yet been revised. Interestingly, the patients in those series were tested for serum cytotoxic HLA antibodies. At 6 months postoperatively, 91% of the patients were positive for antibodies. The investigators speculated that the immune response of the host may play a more important role in fresh osteochondral allograft survival than previously believed. Recently, Jeng et al.[42] reported their results of the largest study group ever investigated for allograft total ankle replacement. Twenty-nine patients underwent bipolar osteochondral allograft for the ankle joint. Removal of allograft was defined as the endpoint. At an average follow-up of 2 years, the survival rate was found to be 52%. Among all 29 patients in the study there were 15 successful transplants and 14 failures. However, six patients were not yet revised but had clear evidence of radiographic failure. If those six patients had been added to the 14 failures the overall survival rate had been reduced down to 31% at 2 years. The average AOFAS ankle–hindfoot score was 84 (range 71–96) at final follow-up. The average for the pain component of the AOFAS score was 31 out of a possible 40. The average for the function component of the AOFAS score was 44 out of a possible 50. No pre-operative scores were available for comparison. When the nine successful allograft patients were asked whether they would undergo the procedure again, 67% responded yes, 11% responded no, and 22% were unsure.

OUTLOOK

As stated by Jeng the continued use of ankle transplantation as an alternative to ankle arthrodesis for the treatment of end-stage ankle arthritis should be viewed with some scepticism. The high failure rate and salvage of failed allografts has proved to be extremely challenging and unsatisfying for patients. Future prospective studies should be performed in order to evaluate the true effectiveness of allograft total ankle replacement. However, the current results published in the literature do not speak in favour of this technique for a large number of patients. Correct indication as usual determines the outcome after such intervention.

SUMMARY

Total ankle replacement became increasingly important throughout recent decades and has become a valuable alternative treatment modality to ankle fusion. Biomechanically sound designs of total ankle replacement, improved materials and adequate selection of patients provide good to excellent outcomes. For some patients ankle distraction arthroplasty might be an option to salvage the ankle joint. However, based on the sparse information in the literature it can only be used in a selected patient population suffering from ankle arthrosis. Fresh osteochondral total ankle transplant is an alternative to ankle arthrodesis and artificial ankle replacement for the treatment of end-stage ankle arthritis. However, with its prohibitively high failure rate, it should be considered only under very rare circumstances. Among all surgical options to treat ankle arthrosis, ankle fusion and total ankle replacement remain the gold standards.

KEY LEARNING POINTS

- The most frequent cause of ankle osteoarthritis is trauma (70%), followed by rheumatoid arthritis (12%). Primary osteoarthritis occurs in about 9–12% cases of trauma.
- The main characteristics of primary or idiopathic osteoarthritis are loss of cartilage tissue and hypertrophy of the bone.
- Non-operative treatment of ankle arthritis includes non-steroidal anti-inflammatory drugs, intra-articular injections (steroids), mechanical unloading and application of ankle–foot orthoses or adapted footwear.
- Surgical options for the treatment of ankle arthritis include arthroscopy, fusion, total ankle replacement, distraction arthroplasty and replacement of the joint by allograft tissue.
- Total ankle replacement has become a valuable alternative treatment modality to ankle fusion. Biomechanically sound designs of total ankle replacement, improved materials and adequate selection of patients provide good to excellent outcomes.
- For some patients ankle distraction arthroplasty might be an option to salvage the ankle joint. However, based on the sparse information in the literature it can only be used in a selected patient population suffering from ankle arthrosis.
- Fresh osteochondral total ankle transplant is an alternative to ankle arthrodesis and artificial ankle replacement for the treatment of end-stage ankle arthritis. However, with its prohibitively high failure rate, it should be considered only under very rare circumstances.
- Among all surgical options to treat ankle arthrosis, ankle fusion and total ankle replacement remain the gold standards.

REFERENCES

- ● = Key primary paper
- ◆ = Major review article

◆1. Hintermann B, Valderrabano V. [Total ankle joint replacement]. *Zeitschrift für ärztliche Fortbildung und Qualitätssicherung* 2001;**95**:187–94.

◆2. Brown TD, Johnston RC, Saltzman CL, et al. Posttraumatic osteoarthritis: a first estimate of incidence, prevalence, and burden of disease. *Journal of Orthopaedic Trauma* 2006;**20**:739–44.

◆3. Seiler H. [The upper ankle joint. Biomechanics and functional anatomy]. *Orthopade* 1999;**28**:460–8.

◆4. Seiler H. [Biomechanics of the upper ankle joint]. *Orthopade* 1986;**15**:415–22.

◆5. Tochigi Y, Rudert MJ, Brown TD, et al. The effect of accuracy of implantation on range of movement of the Scandinavian Total Ankle Replacement. *Journal of Bone and Joint Surgery (British)* 2005;**87**:736–40.

◆6. Buckwalter JA, Saltzman CL. Ankle osteoarthritis: distinctive characteristics. *Instructional Course Lectures* 1999;**48**:233–41.

●7. Li B, Aspden RM. Mechanical and material properties of the subchondral bone plate from the femoral head of patients with osteoarthritis or osteoporosis. *Annals of the Rheumatic Diseases* 1997;**56**:247–54.

●8. Li B, Aspden RM. Composition and mechanical properties of cancellous bone from the femoral head of patients with osteoporosis or osteoarthritis. *Journal of Bone and Mineral Research* 1997;**12**:641–51.

●9. Li B, Aspden RM. Material properties of bone from the femoral neck and calcar femorale of patients with osteoporosis or osteoarthritis. *Osteoporosis International* 1997;**7**:450–6.

◆10. Hintermann B, Valderrabano V. Total ankle replacement. *Foot and Ankle Clinics* 2003;**8**:375–405.

◆11. Hintermann B. *Total Ankle Arthroplasty. Historical Overview, Current Concepts and Future Perspectives.* New York, NY: Springer-Verlag, 2005.
●12. Hayes A, Tochigi Y, Saltzman CL. Ankle morphometry on 3D-CT images. *Iowa Orthopedic Journal* 2006;**26**:1–4.
●13. Tochigi Y, Suh JS, Amendola A, et al. Ankle alignment on lateral radiographs. Part 1: sensitivity of measures to perturbations of ankle positioning. *Foot and Ankle International* 2006;**27**:82–7.
●14. Tochigi Y, Suh JS, Amendola A, Saltzman, CL. Ankle alignment on lateral radiographs. Part 2: reliability and validity of measures. *Foot and Ankle International* 2006;**27**:88–92.
◆15. Espinosa N, Smerek J, Kadakia AR, Myerson MS. Operative management of ankle instability: reconstruction with open and percutaneous methods. *Foot and Ankle Clinics* 2006;**11**:547–65.
16. Valderrabano V, Hintermann B, Nigg BM, et al. Kinematic changes after fusion and total replacement of the ankle. Part 2: movement transfer. *Foot and Ankle International* 2003;**24**:888–96.
17. Valderrabano V, Hintermann B, Nigg, BM, et al. Kinematic changes after fusion and total replacement of the ankle. Part 1: range of motion. *Foot and Ankle International* 2003;**24**:881–7.
18. Valderrabano V, Hintermann B, von Tscharner V, et al. [Muscle biomechanics in total ankle replacement]. *Orthopade* 2006;**35**:513–20.
19. Valderrabano V, Nigg BM, von Tscharner V, et al. Leonard Goldner Award 2006. Total ankle replacement in ankle osteoarthritis: an analysis of muscle rehabilitation. *Foot and Ankle International* 2007;**28**:281–91.
20. Inman VT. The human foot. *Manitoba Medical Review* 1966;**46**:513–15.
21. Inman VT. The influence of the foot-ankle complex on the proximal skeletal structures. *Artificial Limbs* 1969;**13**:59–65.
●22. Cass JR, Morrey BF, Chao EY. Three-dimensional kinematics of ankle instability following serial sectioning of lateral collateral ligaments. *Foot and Ankle* 1984;**5**:142–9.
23. Cass JR, Settles H. Ankle instability: in vitro kinematics in response to axial load. *Foot and Ankle International* 1994;**15**:134–40.
◆24. Espinosa N, Smerek JP, Myerson MS. Acute and chronic syndesmosis injuries: pathomechanisms, diagnosis and management. *Foot and Ankle Clinics* 2006;**11**:639–57.
25. Hintermann B, Nigg BM. [Movement transfer between foot and calf in vitro]. *Sportverletz Sportschaden* 1994;**8**:60–6.
26. Hintermann B, Sommer C, Nigg B. The influence of ligament transection on tibial and calcaneal rotation with loading and dorsi-plantarflexion. *Foot and Ankle International* 1995;**16**:567–71.
27. Nicholson JJ, Parks BG, Stroud CC, Myerson MS. Joint contact characteristics in agility total ankle arthroplasty. *Clinical Orthopaedics and Related Research* 2004;**424**:125–9.
28. Bell CJ, Fisher J. Simulation of polyethylene wear in ankle joint prostheses. *Journal of Biomedical Materials Research Part B Applied Biomaterials* 2007;**81**:162–7.
29. Collier MB, Engh CA Jr, McAuley JP, Engh GA. Factors associated with the loss of thickness of polyethylene tibial bearings after knee arthroplasty. *Journal of Bone and Joint Surgery (American)* 2007;**89**:1306–14.
30. Hoffmann AH, Fink B. [Modern three-piece total ankle replacement: Frequency and causes of luxation and premature wear of the polyethylene bearing.]. *Orthopade* 2007;**36**:908–16.
◆31. Conti SF, Wong YS. Complications of total ankle replacement. *Foot and Ankle Clinics* 2002;**7**:791–807, vii.
◆32. Stamatis ED, Myerson MS. How to avoid specific complications of total ankle replacement. *Foot and Ankle Clinics* 2002;**7**:765–89.
●33. Knecht SI, Estin M, Callaghan JJ, et al. The Agility total ankle arthroplasty. Seven to sixteen-year follow-up. *Journal of Bone and Joint Surgery (American)* 2004;**86A**:1161–71.
34. Raikin SM, Myerson MS. Avoiding and managing complications of the Agility Total Ankle Replacement system. *Orthopedics* 2006;**29**:930–8.
◆35. Deorio JK, Easley ME. Total ankle arthroplasty. *Instructional Course Lectures* 2008;**57**:383–413.
36. Liao X, Gao Z, Huang S, Yang, S. [Prevention and treatment of perioperative period complication of total ankle replacement]. *Zhongguo Xiu Fu Chong Jian Wai Ke Za Zhi* 2008;**22**:40–3.
●37. Judet R, Judet T. [The use of a hinge distraction apparatus after arthrolysis and arthroplasty (author's transl)]. *Revue de Chirurgie Orthopédique et Réparatrice de l'Appareil Moteur* 1978;**64**:353–65.
38. Marijnissen AC, Van Roermund PM, Van Melkebeek J, et al. Clinical benefit of joint distraction in the treatment of severe osteoarthritis of the ankle: proof of concept in an open prospective study and in a randomized controlled study. *Arthritis and Rheumatism* 2002;**46**:2893–902.
●39. Paley D, Lamm BM, Purohit RM, Specht, SC. Distraction arthroplasty of the ankle: how far can you stretch the indications? *Foot and Ankle Clinics* 2008;**13**:471–84.
40. Paley D, Lamm BM. Ankle joint distraction. *Foot and Ankle Clinics* 2005;**10**:685–98.
41. Williams SK, Amiel D, Bull S, et al. Prolonged storage effects on the articular cartilage of fresh human osteochondral allografts. *Journal of Bone and Joint Surgery (American)* 2003;**85**:2111–20.
●42. Jeng CL, Kadakia A, White KL, Myerson MS. Fresh osteochondral total ankle allograft transplantation for the treatment of ankle arthritis. *Foot and Ankle International* 2008;**29**:554–60.
●43. Gross AE, Agnidis Z, Hutchison CR. Osteochondral defects of the talus treated with fresh osteochondral allograft transplantation. *Foot and Ankle International* 2001;**22**:385–91.

44. Meehan R, McFarlin S, Bugbee W, Brage M. Fresh ankle osteochondral allograft transplantation for tibiotalar joint arthritis. *Foot and Ankle International* 2005;**26**:793–802.
45. Kim CW, Jamali A, Tontz WL, *et al*. Treatment of posttraumatic ankle arthrosis with bipolar tibiotalar osteochondral shell allografts. *Foot and Ankle International* 2002;**23**:1091–102.
●46. Tontz WL Jr, Bugbee WD, Brage ME. Use of allografts in the management of ankle arthritis. *Foot and Ankle Clinics* 2003;**8**:361–73, xi.
47. Meehan R, McFarlin S, Bugbee W, Brage M. Fresh ankle osteochondral allograft transplantation for tibiotalar joint arthritis. *Foot and Ankle International* 2005;**26**:793–802.
●48. Hintermann B, Valderrabano V, Dereymaeker G, Dick W. The HINTEGRA ankle: rationale and short-term results of 122 consecutive ankles. *Clinical Orthopaedics and Related Research* 2004;**424**:57–68.
●49. Valderrabano V, Hintermann B, Dick W. Scandinavian total ankle replacement: a 3.7-year average followup of 65 patients. *Clinical Orthopaedics and Related Research* 2004;**424**:47–56.
50. Tanaka Y, Takakura Y. [The TNK ankle: short- and mid-term results]. *Orthopade* 2006;**35**:546–51.
●51. Bonnin M, Judet T, Colombier JA, *et al*. Midterm results of the Salto Total Ankle Prosthesis. *Clinical Orthopaedics and Related Research* 2004;**424**:6–18.
●52. Buechel FF Sr, Buechel FF Jr, Pappas MJ. Ten-year evaluation of cementless Buechel-Pappas meniscal bearing total ankle replacement. *Foot and Ankle International* 2003;**24**:462–72.

SECTION 6

Arthritis in the younger adult

108	**Special considerations in the younger adult** *Minoo Patel*	1253
109	**Osteotomies around the knee** *Andy Williams, Ali Narvani*	1260
110	**Arthrodeses** *Nikolaos Giotakis, Rajiv Malhotra and Muhammed Arshad Nazar*	1268

108

Special considerations in the younger adult

MINOO PATEL

Introduction	1255	Ankle arthroplasty	1257
Aetiology	1255	Shoulder arthroplasty	1257
Hip arthroplasty	1255	Elbow arthroplasty	1258
Knee arthroplasty	1256	References	1259

NATIONAL BOARD STANDARDS

- Know the place of joint arthroplasty for younger patients (under 50–55 years)
- Learn the indications and potential problems
- Understand the different treatment options available
- Know the principles of non-surgical management

INTRODUCTION

Joint arthroplasty in younger patients (defined as those under 50–55 years) presents with a different set of issues from those in the usual 55–75 years age group. These relate not only to the obvious issue of longevity or survival of the implant, but also to the likelihood of future revision surgery and its implications for bone stock. Younger patients tend to be high demand.

AETIOLOGY

Aetiology includes a higher proportion of inflammatory arthritis at one end of the spectrum and post-traumatic arthritis at the other. There are sequelae of childhood joint infections, and other paediatric conditions such as developmental dysplasia of the hip (DDH), Perthes' disease and slipped upper femoral epiphysis (SUFE). There are other joint-specific aetiologies such as instability arthritis of the shoulder.

HIP ARTHROPLASTY

Common indications

Common indications for hip arthroplasty in the young are inflammatory arthritis including ankylosing spondylitis, avascular necrosis (AVN) of the femoral head (primary or secondary to steroid therapy for inflammatory arthritis or organ transplant), post-traumatic hip arthritis or destruction. An important subgroup is hips with sequelae of paediatric conditions such as DDH, Perthes' disease, SUFE, septic hip and juvenile rheumatoid arthritis.

Technical considerations

In a lot of these cases the acetabulum either is absents, as happens in the case of a septic hip in early childhood, or is deformed by a high articulating hip or even replaced by a pseudo-acetabulum, higher than the original acetabulum in cases of DDH. Special oblong acetabular components may have to be used to allow better bone coverage.

The acetabulum can be seated at the site of the original acetabulum, although it may be difficult to bring the femoral 'head' down to this anatomical level. The 'station' of the femoral head can be improved by preoperative limb traction or skeletal traction with external fixation as described Lopes et al.,[1] although this may lead to excessive stretching of the abductors and subsequent weakness. An additional problem is a difficult 'tight' intra-operative reduction, which may also lead to increased wear.

Conversion of an ankylosed or fused hip can also be challenging.

A proximal femoral osteotomy with femoral shortening can prevent excessive abductor stretch and ease intra-operative reduction. Osteotomy fixation is achieved with a long-stem uncemented femoral stem and may be augmented with a unicortical locking plate.

In many cases the femoral canal can be narrow and may need customized implants.

Abductor weakness due to disuse or stretching may also affect gait and predispose to a tendency to dislocate. There is also an increased risk of heterotopic ossification, especially in ankylosing spondylitis.

Renal and other organ transplant patients and patients with inflammatory arthritis may be on immune suppression medical treatment, including corticosteroids, disease-modifying antirheumatic drugs and ciclosporins, which may increase infection risk. Corticosteroid treatment can also result in osteoporosis.

The relatively high mid- to long-term mortality rates in various series reflects the range of medical comorbidity in this group of patients.[2–12]

Longevity and survival

Uncemented acetabulum and uncemented femoral stems appear to be the implants of choice,[2,4,7–9,11] although Joshi et al.[13] reported a 20 year survivorship of 86% for femoral stems and 84% for acetabular components in 218 hips in 141 patients under the age 40 years using Charnley cemented arthroplasty. Similarly others have shown very favourable long-term results with the Charnley hip, which remains the gold standard.[3,5,10,14] Mont et al.[15] demonstrated that long-term results in young patients with osteonecrosis (AVN) with uncemented implants were similar to those with osteoarthritis. Wroblewski et al.[16] reported a 74% survival using revision as an endpoint in a cohort of 292 hips in 195 cases with rheumatoid arthritis.

Polyethylene wear with or without osteolysis remains a concern.[7] The wear resistance of polyethylene has been improved by cross-linking. Ceramic femoral heads have been associated with up to 50% lower *in vivo* polyethylene wear rates than with metallic heads.[17] Although ceramic-on-ceramic bearings have the lowest wear rates, they are associated with a risk of *in vivo* fracture especially in the younger high-demand patient.[17] Ceramic-on-ceramic and metal-on-metal bearings are also more sensitive to implant position with the possibility of higher dislocation rates.[17] There also remain ongoing concerns with long-term exposure to metal particles and ions in younger patients, especially those on immune suppression treatments.[17]

Hip resurfacing

Hip resurfacing has gained in popularity, especially in young patients.[18–21] Although the potential of a bone-sparing femoral implant is attractive, the implants are position sensitive. There is also the added risk of a proximal femur pathological fracture. A dual energy X-ray absorptiometry scan should be considered in patients having hip resurfacing arthroplasty. Although short- to mid-term results are promising, the long-term benefits of hip resurfacing are yet to be determined.

Hip resurfacing also has issues relating to the metal-on-metal articulation and the associated risks of pseudo-tumours and elevated serum cobalt and chromium levels.[22–25]

The thrust plate[26] is an attractive alternative to hip resurfacing, although the numbers reported are still small.

Alternatives

Varus and valgus femoral osteotomies remain alternatives to hip arthroplasty, as does triple innominate osteotomy (TIO). Conversion from TIO to a total hip replacement can be technically more demanding.[27] Peters et al.[27] also report poorer pain relief and increased intra-operative blood loss.

Hip arthrodesis is an option attractive in the very young, especially those unsuited for arthroplasty.

Pelvic support osteotomy (Ilizarov hip reconstruction) is an attractive option in septic hips,[28] DDH,[29–32] excision hip arthroplasty[33] and with caution in unstable hips.[34]

KNEE ARTHROPLASTY

Common indications

Common indications include haemophilic arthropathy, post-traumatic osteoarthritis, inflammatory arthritis, including rheumatoid arthritis and seronegative arthritis, instability-related arthritis, primary osteoarthritis, arthritis secondary to osteochondritis dissecans and arthritis associated with metabolic diseases such as rickets and bone deformity such as genu varum or valgum, tibia vara (Blount's), femoral and/or tibial bowing.

Technical considerations

Total knee arthroplasty (TKA) for post-traumatic arthritis can be technically challenging. TKA following tibial plateau fractures can be associated with high peri-operative complication rates.[35]

Longevity and survival

Rand et al.[36] in a study based on Mayo clinic data from over 11 000 cases showed a 10 year survivorship of 83% those in patients under 55 years of age, 89% in those aged 56–70 years and 94% in those aged over 70 years. Excluding age, the other significant factors affecting survivorship were the type of implant, gender of the patient, diagnosis, type of fixation and design of the patellar component.[36] In the ideal situation, when treating a woman over the age of 70 years who has inflammatory arthritis with a non-modular, metal-backed tibial component, cement fixation, an all-polyethylene patellar component and retention of the posterior cruciate ligament, the 10 year survivorship of the prosthesis was estimated to be 98%.[36]

Gioe et al.[37] reported from a community joint registry that cemented TKAs performed best, with a cumulative revision rate of 15.5%, compared with 34.1% in cementless designs. Men had a higher cumulative revision rate than women, 31.9% compared with 20.6%.[37] Cemented knee arthroplasty remains the gold standard, although there have been a few studies showing good mid- to long-term results with cementless TKR.[38,39]

There is no evidence to show lower aseptic loosening in either posterior cruciate-retaining (CR) implants or cruciate-substituting (CS) implants at 10 years. CS designs may be beneficial in post-traumatic arthritis and in joints with previous heterotopic ossification, allowing for better joint balancing and giving more predictable range of motion. Prior patellectomy on the other hand is an indication for CR knees for better anteroposterior stability.

The use of mobile bearings may reduce wear, but the data are far from conclusive. Mono-bloc tibial components may have the theoretical advantage of decreased wear. With studies showing an almost 16% linear exchange rate at 10 years,[39] modularity of implants would be an advantage.

Unicompartmental knee replacement

Although unicompartmental knee replacement (UCKR) remains an attractive option as a bone-sparing and minimally invasive alternative, it is technically demanding and is associated with higher early and late failure rates, especially in the younger patient population, than TKR. Gioe et al.[37] reported a 32.3% cumulative revision rate in unicompartmental knee arthroplasty compared with 15.5% for cemented TKR, although this was less than the revision rate of 34.1% in cementless designs. Pennington et al.[40] and Swienckowski and Pennington[41] showed over 92% survivorship for UCKR at 10 years in patients under 60 years.

Patellofemoral replacement

Similarly primary patellofemoral (patellotrochlear) replacements have a higher revision rate for patients under 55 years. The Australian National Joint Replacement registry reports 3.6 vs 1.8 revisions per 100 observed component years for patients under 55 years and over 75 years respectively (http://www.dmac.adelaide.edu.au/aoanjrr/publications.jsp?section=reports2008).

Alternatives

Knee fusion (arthrodesis) remains an option especially for infection, bone loss or in paralytic limbs.

ANKLE ARTHROPLASTY

Ankle fusion remains the preferred option for younger patients, unless there is bilateral disease or associated subtalar and foot arthritis.[42]

Fresh osteochondral total ankle allograft transplantation is a promising alternative with survival rates between 50% and 92% at 1–12 years' follow-up.[43,44]

SHOULDER ARTHROPLASTY

Common indications

Apart from inflammatory arthritis, post-instability (recurrent dislocation) arthritis[45] forms the bulk of shoulder arthritis cases requiring arthroplasty in the younger population. Other indications include haemophilic arthropathy, post-traumatic arthritis, AVN and post-arthroscopy chondrolysis.[46] Cuff tear arthropathy and pseudo-paralysis are also seen in inflammatory arthritis and occasionally in neglected cuff tears.

Patients with post-traumatic arthritis, AVN and haemophilic arthropathy do well with hemi-arthropathy. Patients with rheumatoid arthritis do better with a total shoulder arthroplasty.[47] Burroughs et al.[47] did not report any deterioration of shoulder function at 5.5 years.

Glenoid wear remains a concern with shoulder hemi-arthroplasty.[48] Mean constant scores of 71% were associated with a joint space of greater than 1 mm, whereas a joint space less than 1 mm was associated with a significantly lower score of 50%.[48] Eccentric glenoid wear (usually anterior or anterosuperior) can lead to joint subluxation and/or cuff dysfunction.

Sperling et al.[49] reported estimated survival of the hemi-arthroplasty prostheses of 92% at 5 years, 83% at 10 years, and 73% at 15 years compared with an estimated survival of the total shoulder prostheses of 97% (92–100%) at 5 years, 97% at 10 years, and 84% at 15 years, in patients under 50 years.

Hemi-arthroplasty may be combined with concentric glenoid reaming,[50] although biological resurfacing may be a better option.[51,52] Various biological materials have been used from autografts such as joint capsule, to allografts such as Achilles tendon and lateral meniscus, and acellular xenografts such as the porcine dermis (Graftjacket membrane). True cartilage metaplasia may be seen with capsule interposition. Allografts used for resurfacing usually disintegrate over the short to mid-term, and may force conversion to a total shoulder.

Humeral resurfacing implants not only preserve bone stock, but also recreate the host anatomy, replicating the humeral neck–shaft angle, version and articular posterior offset. The implants however can over-stuff the shoulder, especially if the glenoid is also resurfaced. These implants are usually uncemented.

Cuff-deficient shoulders

Total shoulder arthroplasty has high failure and revision rates when performed in cuff-deficient shoulders.[49] If the cuff is irreparable a CTA head implant should be considered.

On current evidence, reverse total shoulder arthroplasty should be reserved for patients over 65 years. Newer modular interchangeable humeral and glenoid systems, such as the SMR (Lima LTO, Italy), allow easy conversion between reverse total shoulder replacement and anatomic total shoulder replacement components, both for humeral stems as well as for the glenoid.

ELBOW ARTHROPLASTY

Common indications

Rheumatoid arthritis and inflammatory arthritis together are the single largest cause of elbow arthritis requiring total elbow arthroplasty in the young. Other reasons include post-traumatic arthritis and haemophilic arthropathy.

Technical considerations

Semi-constrained implants with a sloppy hinge such as the Conrad–Morrey design are preferable to unconstrained joints because of ligamentous instability in inflammatory arthritis. Elbow implants tend to be cemented and most implant designs incorporate the anterior flange. Newer designs such as the Latitude and Acclaim allow initial insertion of a non-constrained implant with theoretical advantages of less implant loosening in the young. This can be converted to a semi-constrained design without having to remove the original implant. The Latitude implant also allows for lateral compartment or radial head arthroplasty, thereby decreasing the valgus medial load.

Longevity and survival

Connor and Morrey[53] reported an improvement in the average Mayo elbow performance score from 31 points pre-operatively to 90 points at an average of 7.4 years after the operation in 24 elbow replacements for rheumatoid arthritis. Early complications included a fracture of the olecranon, subluxation of the prosthesis, stiffness of the elbow and problems with wound healing not affecting eventual outcome. Late complications of aseptic loosening, instability and worn bushings led to three poor results. Importantly, none of the 18 semi-constrained prostheses had radiographic evidence of loosening at their most recent evaluation.

Wright and Hastings.[54] reported on mid- to late-term failures relating to bushing wear in the Coonrad–Morrey arthroplasty in young patients. Common associated factors were post-traumatic arthritis, supracondylar non-union, male sex, young age, and high activity level.

In a study involving elbow arthroplasty for gunshot injuries in very young patients with a mean age of 23 years, Demiralp et al.[55] reported good initial results but poor long-term results in five out of seven cases at a minimum 8 years' follow-up with loosening of ulnar and humeral components. Two cases had infections and three had aseptic loosening. All required revision.

Alternatives

Biological resurfacing interposition arthroplasty using fascia lata or dermis autograft, Achilles tendon allograft or Graftjacket xenograft, as described by Cheng and Morrey,[56] can be a useful alternative and may be used as a stopgap measure to delay eventual prosthetic arthroplasty. Interposition arthroplasty may however damage bone stock and make future total joint arthroplasty technically challenging.

Elbow resurfacing and hemi-arthroplasty are newer less invasive alternatives available especially for localized osteochondritis dissecans, lateral compartment arthritis or post-traumatic articular damage. Local capitellum resurfacing with radial head replacement can be used for localized lateral compartment disease and may be a better long-term option than radial head excision.

Elbow hemi-arthroplasty, replacing the distal humerus, has been used for severe intra-articular fractures in older patients, but may be used as a bone-preserving option for younger patients.

KEY LEARNING POINTS

- Joint arthroplasty in younger patients (defined as those under 50–55 years) presents with issues of longevity or survival of the implant, future revision surgery and worries relating to bone stock.
- Aetiology is inflammatory arthritis and post-traumatic arthritis.
- For total hip replacement (THR), the aetiology is inflammatory arthritis, ankylosing spondylitis, avascular necrosis, post-traumatic hip arthritis or destruction and sequelae of developmental dysplasia of the hip, Perthes' disease, slipped upper femoral epiphysis, septic hip and juvenile rheumatoid arthritis.
- The acetabulum maybe absent or deformed.
- Conversion of an ankylosed or fused hip is difficult.
- Uncemented acetabulum and uncemented femoral stems appear to be the implants of choice.
- Hip resurfacing is popular.
- Alternatives to THR are: varus and valgus femoral osteotomies and triple innominate osteotomy, hip arthrodesis and pelvic support osteotomies or Ilizarov hip reconstruction.
- Total knee replacement (TKR): common indications include haemophilic arthropathy, post-traumatic osteoarthritis, inflammatory arthritis, instability-related arthritis, primary osteoarthritis, arthritis secondary to osteochondritis dissecans and metabolic diseases (rickets) and bone deformity (genu varum or valgum, tibia vara (Blount's), femoral and or tibial bowing).
- TKR for post-traumatic arthritis is difficult.
- Unicompartmental knee replacement and primary patellofemoral (patellotrochlear) replacements are technically demanding and have higher early and late failure rates.
- Knee fusion (arthrodesis) is an option especially for infection, bone loss or in paralytic limbs.
- Total shoulder replacement: most common indications are inflammatory arthritis and post-instability (recurrent dislocation).
- Total elbow replacement: common indications are rheumatoid arthritis and inflammatory arthritis.
- Semi-constrained implants with a sloppy hinge such as the Conrad–Morrey design are preferred.
- Alternative is: biological resurfacing interposition arthroplasty.

REFERENCES

- ● = Key primary paper
- ◆ = Major review article

1. Lopes NC, Jacinto J, Escada C, et al. Treatment of late neglected adult congenital dislocation of the hip with hybrid Ilizarov or monolateral distractor and total hip replacement. A new methodology. In Proceedings of the International Congress On External Fixation & Bone Reconstruction, Barcelona, Spain, 20–22 October 2010. Available from: http://www.scribd.com/doc/56598091/Treatment-of-late-neglected-adult-congenital-dislocation-of-the-hip-with-hybrid-Ilizarov-monolateral-distractor-and-total-hip-replacement-A-new-method.
●2. Hartofilakidis G, Karachalios T, Zacharakis N. Charnley low friction arthroplasty in young patients with osteoarthritis. A 12- to 24-year clinical and radiographic followup study of 84 cases. *Clinical Orthopaedics and Related Research* 1997;**Aug**:51–4.
●3. Sochart DH, Porter ML. The long-term results of Charnley low-friction arthroplasty in young patients who have congenital dislocation, degenerative osteoarthrosis, or rheumatoid arthritis. *Journal of Bone and Joint Surgery (American)* 1997;**79**:1599–617.
●4. Kumar MN, Swann M. Uncemented total hip arthroplasty in young patients with juvenile chronic arthritis. *Annals of the Royal College of Surgeons of England* 1998;**80**:203–9.
●5. Wroblewski BM, Fleming PA, Hall RM, Siney PD. Stem fixation in the Charnley low-friction arthroplasty in young patients using an intramedullary bone block. *Journal of Bone and Joint Surgery (British)* 1998;**80**:273–8.
●6. McLaughlin JR, Lee KR. Total hip arthroplasty in young patients. 8- to 13-year results using an uncemented stem. *Clinical Orthopaedics and Related Research* 2000;**Apr**:153–63.
7. Chiu KY, Tang WM, Ng TP, et al. Cementless total hip arthroplasty in young Chinese patients: a comparison of 2 different prostheses. *Journal of Arthroplasty* 2001;**16**:863–70.
8. Nercessian OA, Wu WH, Sarkissian H. Clinical and radiographic results of cementless AML total hip arthroplasty in young patients. *Journal of Arthroplasty* 2001;**16**:312–16.
●9. Ince A, Lermann J, Göbel S, et al. No increased stem subsidence after arthroplasty in young patients with femoral head osteonecrosis: 41 patients followed for 1–9 years. *Acta Orthopaedica* 2006;**77**:866–70.
●10. Wroblewski BM, Siney PD, Fleming PA. Charnley low-frictional torque arthroplasty in young rheumatoid and juvenile rheumatoid arthritis: 292 hips followed for an average of 15 years. *Acta Orthopaedica* 2007;**78**:206–10.
●11. Raj D, Jaiswal PK, Sharma BL, Fergusson CM. Long term results of the Corin C-Fit uncemented total hip arthroplasty in young patients. *Archives of Orthopaedic and Trauma Surgery* 2008;**128**:1391–5.

- 12. Burgess DL, McGrath MS, Bonutti PM, et al. Shoulder resurfacing. *Journal of Bone and Joint Surgery (American)* 2009;**91**:1228–38.
- 13. Joshi AB, Porter ML, Trail IA, et al. Long-term results of Charnley low-friction arthroplasty in young patients. *Journal of Bone and Joint Surgery (British)* 1993;**75**:616–23.
♦ 14. White SH. The fate of cemented total hip arthroplasty in young patients. *Clinical Orthopaedics and Related Research* 1988;**Jun**:29–34.
  15. Mont MA, Yoon TR, Krackow KA, Hungerford DS. Clinical experience with a proximally porous-coated second-generation cementless total hip prosthesis: Minimum 5-year follow-up. *The Journal of Arthroplasty* 1999;**14**(8):930–939.
  16. Wroblewski BM, Siney PD, Fleming PA. Charnley low-frictional torque arthroplasty in young rheumatoid and juvenile rheumatoid arthritis: 292 hips followed for an average of 15 years. *Acta Orthop.* 2007;**78**(2):206–10.
♦ 17. Heisel C, Silva M, Schmalzried TP. Bearing surface options for total hip replacement in young patients. *Instructional Course Lectures* 2004;**53**:49–65.
  18. Amstutz HC, Ebramzadeh E, Sarkany A, et al. Preservation of bone mineral density of the proximal femur following hemisurface arthroplasty. *Orthopedics* 2004;**27**:1266–71.
- 19. Boyd HS, Ulrich SD, Seyler TM, et al. Resurfacing for Perthes disease: an alternative to standard hip arthroplasty. *Clinical Orthopaedics and Related Research* 2007;**465**:80–5.
- 20. Little JP, Taddei F, Viceconti M, et al. Changes in femur stress after hip resurfacing arthroplasty: response to physiological loads. *Clinical Biomechanics* 2007;**22**:440–8.
  21. Akbar M, Mont MA, Heisel C, et al. [Resurfacing for osteonecrosis of the femoral head]. *Orthopade* 2008;**37**:672–8.
  22. Amstutz HC, Le Duff MJ, Campbell PA, et al. Complications after metal-on-metal hip resurfacing arthroplasty. *Orthopedic Clinics of North America* 2011;**42**:207–30.
  23. De Smet KA, Van Der Straeten C, Van Orsouw M, et al. Revisions of metal-on-metal hip resurfacing: lessons learned and improved outcome. *Orthopedic Clinics of North America* 2011;**42**:259–69.
  24. Canadian Hip Resurfacing Study Group. A survey on the prevalence of pseudotumors with metal-on-metal hip resurfacing in Canadian academic centers. *Journal of Bone and Joint Surgery (American)* 2011;**93** (Suppl. 2):118–21.
  25. Kim PR, Beaule PE, Dunbar M, et al. Cobalt and chromium levels in blood and urine following hip resurfacing arthroplasty with the Conserve Plus implant. *Journal of Bone and Joint Surgery (American)* 2011;**93** (Suppl. 2):107–17.
- 26. Zelle BA, Gerich TG, Bastian L, et al. Total hip arthroplasty in young patients using the thrust plate prosthesis: clinical and radiological results. [see comment]. *Archives of Orthopaedic and Trauma Surgery* 2004;**124**:310–16.
- 27. Peters CL, Beck M, Dunn HK. Total hip arthroplasty in young adults after failed triple innominate osteotomy. [see comment]. *Journal of Arthroplasty* 2001;**16**:188–95.
- 28. Rozbruch SR, Paley D, Bhave A, Herzenberg JE. Ilizarov hip reconstruction for the late sequelae of infantile hip infection. *Journal of Bone and Joint Surgery (American)* 2005;**87**:1007–18.
  29. Edelson JG, Taitz C. Pelvic support osteotomy in an unusual congenital dislocation of the hip. A 52-year follow-up study. *Clinical Orthopaedics and Related Research* 1991;**Mar**:228–31.
- 30. Aksoy MC, Musdal Y. Subtrochanteric valgus-extension osteotomy for neglected congenital dislocation of the hip in young adults. *Acta Orthopaedica Belgica* 2000;**66**:181–6.
- 31. Kocaoglu M, Eralp L, Sen C, Dinçyürek H. The Ilizarov hip reconstruction osteotomy for hip dislocation: outcome after 4–7 years in 14 young patients. *Acta Orthopaedica Scandinavica* 2002;**73**:432–8.
  32. Inan M, Alkan A, Harma A, Ertem K. Evaluation of the gluteus medius muscle after a pelvic support osteotomy to treat congenital dislocation of the hip. *Journal of Bone and Joint Surgery (American)* 2005;**87**:2246–52.
- 33. Emara KM, Emara KM. Pelvic support osteotomy in the treatment of patients with excision arthroplasty. *Clinical Orthopaedics and Related Research* 2008;**466**:708–13.
  34. El-Mowafi H, El-Mowafi H. Outcome of pelvic support osteotomy with the Ilizarov method in the treatment of the unstable hip joint. *Acta Orthopaedica Belgica* 2005;**71**:686–91.
  35. Weiss NG, Parvizi J, Trousdale RT, et al. Total knee arthroplasty in patients with a prior fracture of the tibial plateau. *Journal of Bone and Joint Surgery (American)* 2003;**85A**:218–21.
♦ 36. Rand JA, Trousdale RT, Ilstrup DM, Harmsen WS. Factors affecting the durability of primary total knee prostheses [see comment]. *Journal of Bone and Joint Surgery (American)* 2003;**85A**:259–65.
- 37. Gioe TJ, Novak C, Sinner P, et al. Knee arthroplasty in the young patient: survival in a community registry. *Clinical Orthopaedics and Related Research* 2007;**464**:83–7.
  38. Otte KS, Larsen H, Jensen TT, et al. Cementless AGC revision of unicompartmental knee arthroplasty. *Journal of Arthroplasty* 1997;**12**:55–9.
- 39. Hofmann AA, Heithoff SM, Camargo M. Cementless total knee arthroplasty in patients 50 years or younger. *Clinical Orthopaedics and Related Research* 2002;**Nov**:102–7.
- 40. Pennington DW, Swienckowski JJ, Lutes WB, Drake GN. Unicompartmental knee arthroplasty in patients sixty years of age or younger. *Journal of Bone and Joint Surgery (American)* 2003;**85A**:1968–73.
  41. Swienckowski JJ, Pennington DW. Unicompartmental knee arthroplasty in patients sixty years of age or younger. *Journal of Bone and Joint Surgery (American)* 2004;**86A**(Suppl 1, Pt 2):131–42.
- 42. McGuire MR, Kyle RF, Gustilo RB, Premer RF. Comparative analysis of ankle arthroplasty versus ankle arthrodesis. *Clinical Orthopaedics and Related Research* 1988;**Jan**:174–81.

- 43. Tontz WL Jr, Bugbee WD, Brage ME. Use of allografts in the management of ankle arthritis. *Foot and Ankle Clinics* 2003;**8**:361-73.
44. Jeng CL, Kadakia A, White KL, Myerson MS. Fresh osteochondral total ankle allograft transplantation for the treatment of ankle arthritis. *Foot and Ankle International* 2008;**29**:554-60.
- 45. Brems JJ. Arthritis of dislocation. *Orthopedic Clinics of North America* 1998;**29**:453-66.
46. Levy JC, Virani NA, Frankle MA, *et al.* Young patients with shoulder chondrolysis following arthroscopic shoulder surgery treated with total shoulder arthroplasty. *Journal of Shoulder and Elbow Surgery* 2008;**17**:380-8.
- 47. Burroughs PL, Gearen PF, Petty WR, Wright TW. Shoulder arthroplasty in the young patient. *Journal of Arthroplasty* 2003;**18**:792-8.
48. Parsons IM 4th, Millett PJ, Warner JJ. Glenoid wear after shoulder hemiarthroplasty: quantitative radiographic analysis. *Clinical Orthopaedics and Related Research* 2004;**Apr**:120-5.
- 49. Sperling JW, Cofield RH, Rowland CM. Neer hemiarthroplasty and Neer total shoulder arthroplasty in patients fifty years old or less. Long-term results. [see comment]. *Journal of Bone and Joint Surgery (American)* 1998;**80**:464-73.
50. Lynch JR, Franta AK, Montgomery WH Jr, *et al.* Self-assessed outcome at two to four years after shoulder hemiarthroplasty with concentric glenoid reaming. *Journal of Bone and Joint Surgery (American)* 2007;**89**:1284-92.
51. Nicholson GP, Goldstein JL, Romeo AA, *et al.* Lateral meniscus allograft biologic glenoid arthroplasty in total shoulder arthroplasty for young shoulders with degenerative joint disease. *Journal of Shoulder and Elbow Surgery* 2007;**16**(5 Suppl):S261-6.
- 52. Elhassan B, Ozbaydar M, Diller D, *et al.* Soft-tissue resurfacing of the glenoid in the treatment of glenohumeral arthritis in active patients less than fifty years old. *Journal of Bone and Joint Surgery (American)* 2009;**91**:419-24.
- 53. Connor PM, Morrey BF. Total elbow arthroplasty in patients who have juvenile rheumatoid arthritis. *Journal of Bone and Joint Surgery (American)* 1998;**80**:678-88.
54. Wright TW, Hastings H. Total elbow arthroplasty failure due to overuse, C-ring failure, and/or bushing wear. *Journal of Shoulder and Elbow Surgery* 2005;**14**:65-72.
- 55. Demiralp B, Komurcu M, Ozturk C, *et al.* Total elbow arthroplasty in patients who have elbow fractures caused by gunshot injuries: 8- to 12-year follow-up study. *Archives of Orthopaedic and Trauma Surgery* 2008;**128**:17-24.
- 56. Cheng SL, Morrey BF. Treatment of the mobile, painful arthritic elbow by distraction interposition arthroplasty. *Journal of Bone and Joint Surgery (British)* 2000;**82**:233-8.

109

Osteotomies around the knee

ANDY WILLIAMS, ALI NARVANI

Introduction	1260	Techniques	1263
Osteotomies for osteoarthritis	1260	Complications of osteotomies	1266
Osteotomies for patients with ligamentous dysfunction	1262	Conclusion	1266
Calculation of correction required	1263	References	1266

NATIONAL BOARD STANDARDS

- Understand the role of osteotomy in managing osteoarthritis
- Know the planning of an osteotomy

INTRODUCTION

In recent years osteotomies around the knee have regained popularity in management of osteoarthritis (OA), deformities and ligament instability. In OA, the aim of the procedure is deliberately to realign the mechanical axis to shift knee loading to the compartment with the healthy articular surface.[1] In patients with damaged ligaments, especially those with varus alignment and lateral ligament complex insufficiency, osteotomies may be employed to 'fine-tune' alignment in favour of stability.

To appreciate the principles involved in osteotomies, it is important to consider the normal alignment of the lower limb. In the coronal plane, although the weight-bearing line is assumed to pass through the centres of the hip, knee and ankle, it usually passes through the medial compartment of the knee. The angle of intersection between the shaft of the femur and tibia is, approximately, between 5° and 7°. The tibial surface is in 3° of varus to the long axis of the tibia, which also means that in bipedal stance, with a horizontal tibial joint line, the mechanical and vertical axis intersect at 3° (Fig. 109.1).[2] The radiographic assessment of lower limb alignment is problematic. Long-leg (hips to ankles) weight-bearing radiographs represent, still, the best method available. However, since it is a two-dimensional representation of three-dimensional reality the lower limb rotation at the time of X-ray exposure can have a big impact on apparent coronal alignment. For example, because of the femoral bow, external rotation increases apparent varus alignment of the limb. CT scanning lacks the important aspect of weight-bearing.

In the sagittal plane, it is widely accepted that the tibia has a posterior slope. It is, however, important to note that this posterior slope really only applies to the medial tibia where there is a slope from anterior to posterior in the anterior half (the posterior half of the medial tibia is flat). In the lateral tibia, there is a central flat surface from which the anterior and posterior surfaces slope downwards. In the sagittal plane the weight-bearing line passes anterior to the midpoint of the knee resulting in a slight tendency to hyperextension in stance. This is useful in minimizing the muscular effort required for standing. This hyperextension tendency is countered by tension within the strong posterior capsule and fine-tuning contraction of the lower limb muscle groups. No major effort is required, unless, of course, the knee is unable to 'lock out' straight because of fixed flexion. Fixed flexion deformities require active quadriceps contraction to maintain stance, and this is hard to sustain for long periods.

OSTEOTOMIES FOR OSTEOARTHRITIS

Osteotomies may have a role in management of those patients with symptomatic OA in whom:

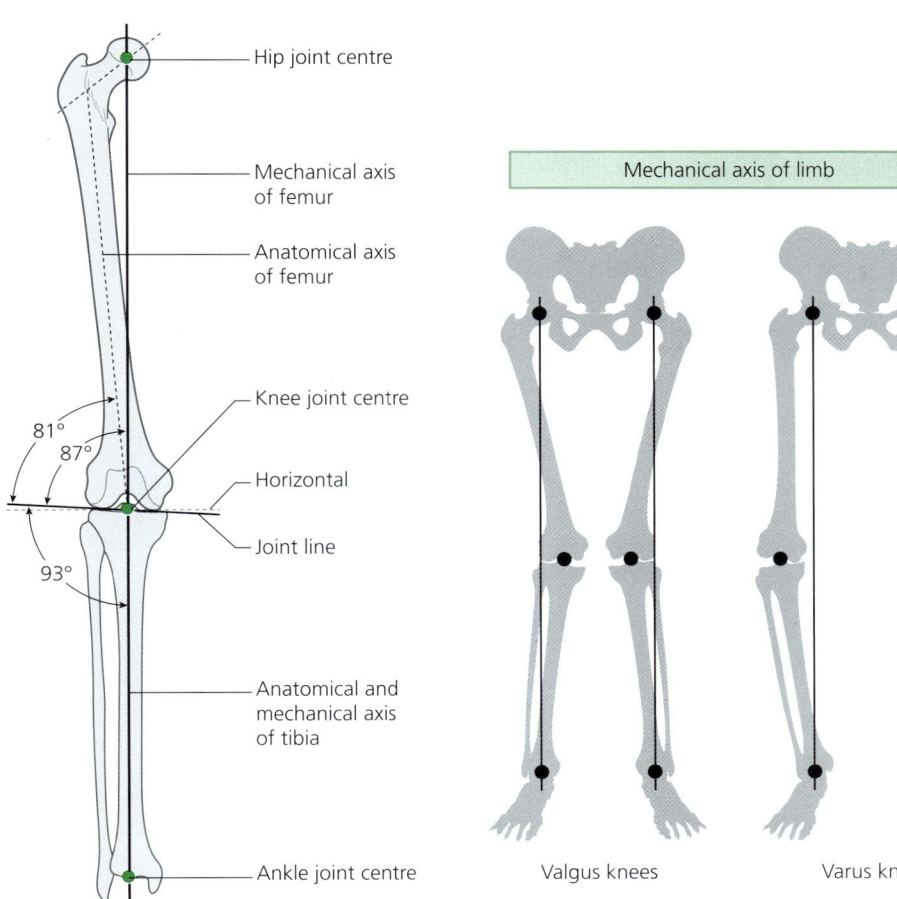

Figure 109.1 Normal alignment of the lower limb. The mechanical axis is medial and lateral to the centre of the knee in varus and valgus knees respectively.

1. degenerative change is restricted to either the medial or lateral compartment
2. coronal plane deformity is not more than 15–20°
3. fixed flexion deformity is not more than 15°
4. flexion is at least 100°.[3]

Of course these factors are relevant to patients having knee replacement. There is surprising confusion among orthopaedic surgeons regarding the decision between joint replacement and osteotomy. An illogical and completely unnecessary debate has been created about whether high tibial osteotomy (HTO) or unicompartmental knee replacement (UKR) is best for treating patients with medial OA. Perhaps this is fuelled by the promotion of the concept that UKR is somehow a lesser joint replacement than total knee replacement (TKR). As a result of undoubted improvements in design and implantation techniques, UKR is more popular than it was. It has been forgotten that it is still a step that commits a patient to arthroplasty for the rest of their life. It can wear and loosen, and it may need revision that is often not straightforward, and no less major than revision of many TKR cases. It is increasingly being promoted as an operation for the young and active. Paradoxically perhaps, the perfect patient in many ways is actually the elderly and frail patient in whom UKR is better tolerated than TKR. The argument of whether UKR or HTO is better is completely pointless because they are appropriate for different groups of patients who happen to have the same pattern of disease. If a patient wishes to run, jump, twist and jar their knee or load it in deep flexion, or play sport, or is young enough to mean revision arthroplasty could be problematic, osteotomy should be seriously considered. The decision in patients with OA is whether they are candidates for osteotomy or arthroplasty (they are different patient groups) and if best suited by arthroplasty then the decision is between TKR and UKR. The majority of patients clearly fall into one or other group; only a few do not. In this minority a decision should then be based on prognostic factors: the older, obese, smokers, poorly motivated, poorly compliant, those lacking proximal tibial varum (see below) are usually better off with arthroplasty.

The aim of osteotomy in OA is to intentionally shift the weight-bearing line to load the unaffected/healthier compartment. The malalignment due to osteoarthritis loads the diseased compartment of the joint, so exacerbating symptoms and disease progression (Fig. 109.2a,b). The degree of correction is of vital importance as overcorrection leads to instability, excessive overloading and failure of the healthier compartment and poor cosmetic appearance. Similarly, undercorrection can result in unsatisfactory outcome. The degree of correction can be determined from the position of the desired weight-bearing line. For medial OA, suggested

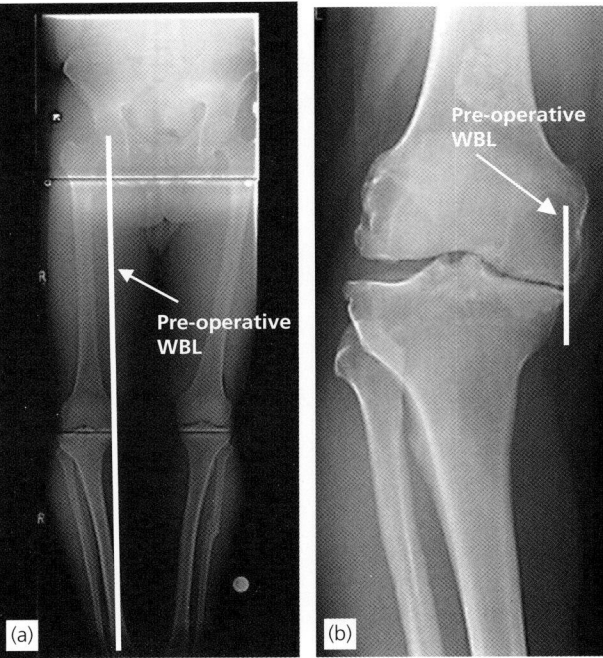

Figure 109.2 (a, b) Medial shift of weight-bearing line in varus knee. WBL, weight-bearing line.

guides for placement of the weight-bearing line should intersect a point 62% of the way along a horizontal line joining the lateral edge of the tibia to the medial edge of the tibial plateau. This approximates to its intersection with the lateral edge of the base of the lateral tibial spine in most cases (Fig. 109.3).[4]

There are some prognostic factors worth considering. Complications are more likely, and results worse, in the obese and in smokers, where there is evidence of significant bone loss, and when patient age is over 50 years. Another important prognostic factor is patient morphology. Varus deformity is either due to metaphyseal tibial varus or acquired OA resulting in medial compartment wear. The former group have always been bow-legged in their lives and osteotomy is therefore a corrective procedure and usually has a better outcome. In those who have varus secondary to osteoarthritic change alone, the results are less satisfactory and the osteotomy is effectively 'palliative'. It simply creates deformity to offload a problem.[5]

OSTEOTOMIES FOR PATIENTS WITH LIGAMENTOUS DYSFUNCTION

Ligament injuries result in not only structural damage but also proprioceptive deficit. Proprioceptive feedback is crucial in maintaining dynamic stability during limb loading. In the congenitally varus-aligned limb, which is a common occurrence, the mechanical axis is situated medially and this leads to medial joint compartment compression and relative tension across the lateral compartment.

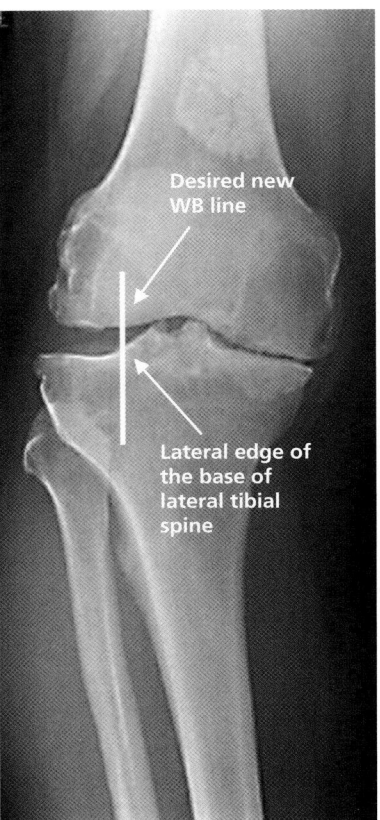

Figure 109.3 Placement of weight-bearing (WB) line.

Proprioceptive-mediated dynamic neuromuscular control counters this. Under loading conditions the lateral compartment of the knee is held compressed by the action of muscles such as biceps femoris and lateral gastrocnemius. Without this control, lateral compartment opening leads to excess tension in the lateral collateral ligament (LCL), leading to attritional stretching of that ligament. In fact, this can occur in a varus knee with chronic proprioceptive deficit from an initial isolated anterior cruciate ligament (ACL) deficiency. Also if, for example, an ACL reconstruction is performed in a knee with varus alignment, since it can never provide normal proprioception, there is a risk of the graft stretching out when subject to uncontrolled dynamic varus. In such situations an osteotomy may be required to 'fine tune the alignment in favour of stability'.[6] The most common situation for an osteotomy in ligament insufficiency is with LCL laxity in a varus-aligned limb. In this situation a valgizing HTO is employed. Of course the osteotomy can counter LCL laxity directly by compression of the lateral joint compartment, but not directly the posterolateral rotatory laxity often occurring in injuries to the posterolateral ligament complex. However, if the osteotomy causes an increase in tibial slope (common when medial opening wedge upper tibial osteotomy is undertaken) there is a tendency for tibial internal rotation, which counters the excess external rotation seen in posterolateral

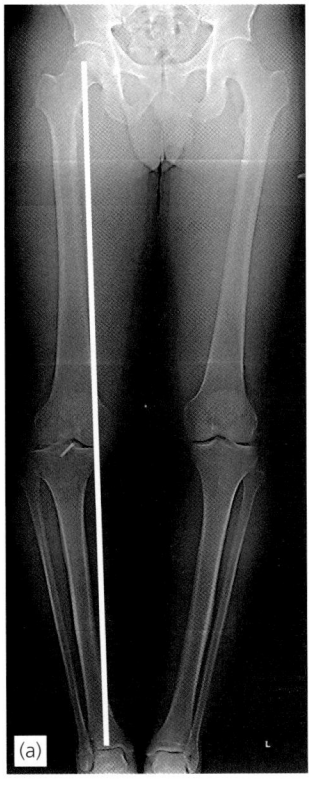 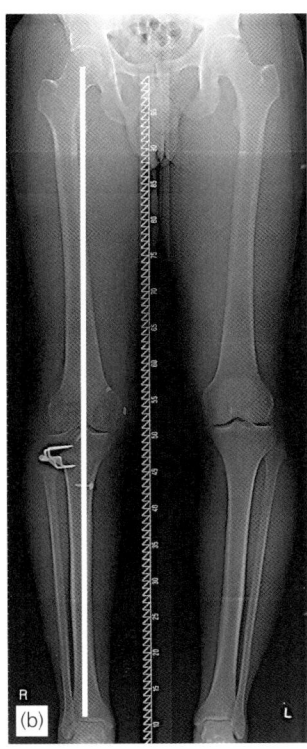

Figure 109.4 Valgizing high tibial osteotomy for optimal alignment in a case of posterior and lateral cruciate ligament laxity. Note that no 'overcorrection' is produced. (a) Pre-operative; (b) postoperative.

rotatory laxity. Rarely is varizing distal femoral osteotomy required for uncontrolled MCL laxity.

The osteotomy for situations of instability aims simply to place the mechanical axis through the centre of the knee. When this is achieved varus/valgus thrust is eliminated. Therefore, unlike osteotomy for OA minor 'fine-tuning' corrections are required when osteotomy is used to treat ligament deficiencies (Fig. 109.4).

Sagittal alignment is also of great importance regarding knee stability. The tibial slope has a potent effect on tibial translation in the anteroposterior direction. An excessive slope produces anterior tibial translation when the knee is loaded, and reduced or reversed slope produces posterior tibial translation.

During an osteotomy procedure a surgeon can deliberately alter the slope to favour stability. Increased slope will favour posterior cruciate ligament deficiency whereas a reduction favours anterior cruciate ligament deficiency.

CALCULATION OF CORRECTION REQUIRED

Having chosen the desired point of the intersection of the weight-bearing line with the joint line, a simple way to calculate the required correction is by measuring the angle subtended by two lines passing from this point to the centre of the femoral head and another to the centre of the ankle (Fig. 109.5). During the operation it is important to know the length of the base of the wedge created or removed during osteotomy. This should be calculated from pre-operative weight-bearing radiographs which have been calibrated for magnification. Many surgeons however employ a rough guide that every degree of correction requires a wedge width of 1 mm.

It is important to note that the varus witnessed on standing radiographs of patients requiring HTO could be a combination of

- proximal tibial varus
- medial joint line loss
- lateral ligament joint laxity.

Any degree of the varus which is secondary to LCL laxity must be excluded from the calculation of the correction. Failure to do this results in overcorrection because, as soon as the mechanical axis crosses the midline of the knee, lateral joint compression occurs so eliminating the contribution to original varus from the LCL laxity. This lateral ligament laxity can be detected pre-operatively by assessing the degree of excess lateral joint line opening on the plain radiograph. As a rough guide, each millimetre of excess lateral joint opening compared with the normal knee, in standing views, results in an extra 1° of varus. This amount should be subtracted from the correction angle calculated.

TECHNIQUES

There are a number of techniques which could be utilized. In medial OA the pathology involves the tibia. In lateral

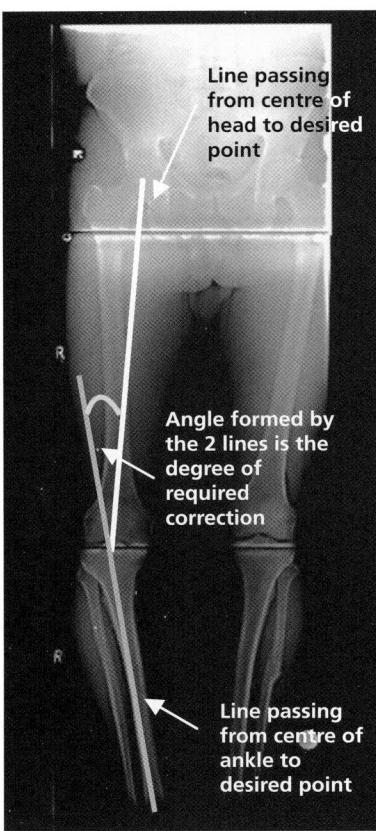

Figure 109.5 Calculation of the required correction angle.

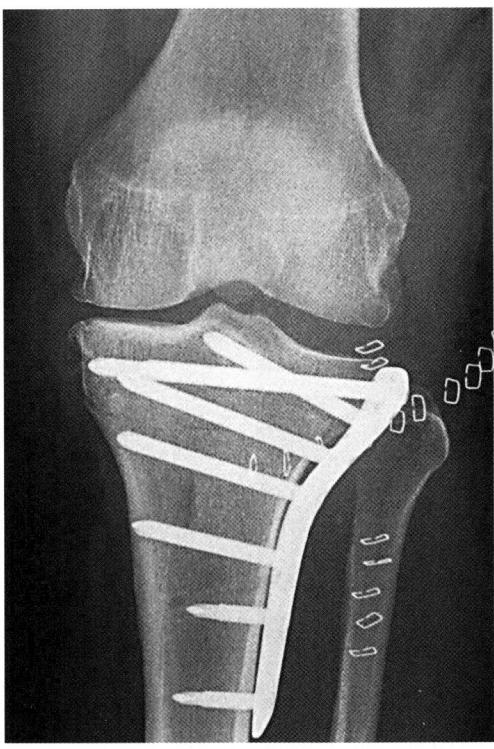

Figure 109.6 Anteroposterior radiograph demonstrating closing wedge high tibial osteotomy.

OA the disease commonly affects the femur. To maintain a horizontal joint line it is best to place the osteotomy as close to the deformity as possible: hence usually HTO for medial OA and distal femoral osteotomy (DFO) for lateral OA.

With both HTO and DFO to maximize the chance of bony union the osteotomy should pass through the metaphyseal cancellous bone. For HTO this means that the patellar tendon poses an obstruction and is at risk of damage as the osteotomy line should be above the tibial tubercle. However, good technique means this is rarely an issue. Furthermore, osteotomies distal to a tibial tuberosity have a significant non-union rate.

The most common scenario is HTO for medial OA. Classically closing wedge high tibial osteotomy (CWHTO) (Fig. 109.6) was employed but recently there has been a great surge in popularity of the opening wedge high tibial osteotomy (OWHTO) (Fig. 109.7a–c). This is largely due to the development of strong fixation devices. There are advantages and disadvantages with each technique. As there is direct bone-to-bone contact, the union rates with CWHTO are very good; however, this is at the expense of greater risk of damage to the common peroneal nerve, the need to divide the fibula or the proximal tibiofibular joint to allow unimpeded closure of the osteotomy, loss of height and, by producing inevitable tibial deformity, potentially more challenging future arthroplasty as the tibial shaft would be medial to the centre of the metaphyseal bone. With OWHTO, the risk of injury to the peroneal nerve is less and the integrity of the fibula/superior tibiofibular ligament is maintained. However, OWHTO has a higher non-union rate (hence the need for possible bone grafting), lowers the patella with respect to the joint surface (unless the anterior osteotomy is taken obliquely below the tibial tubercle in a biplanar technique and prominent subcutaneous metalware).

With both CWHTO and OWHTO one important factor to take into consideration is the influence of the osteotomy on the tibial slope, which in turn has a significant effect on anterior/posterior stability. With OWHTO, there is a high likelihood of increasing the tibial slope. With a CWHTO there is a tendency to decrease the tibial slope. This is mainly because the osteotomy alters the alignment of a bone of triangular cross-section, and with the OWHTO that the approach is actually usually anteromedial rather than truly medial. These effects on the tibial slope are useful in choosing the best technique in cases of associated cruciate ligament deficiency.[7]

DFO is much less commonly required since lateral OA is only 5% of the total cases of OA (Fig. 109.8a,b). Although opening wedge techniques are attractive since they involve a much simpler surgical lateral approach, the fixation device failure is higher than for closing wedge techniques.

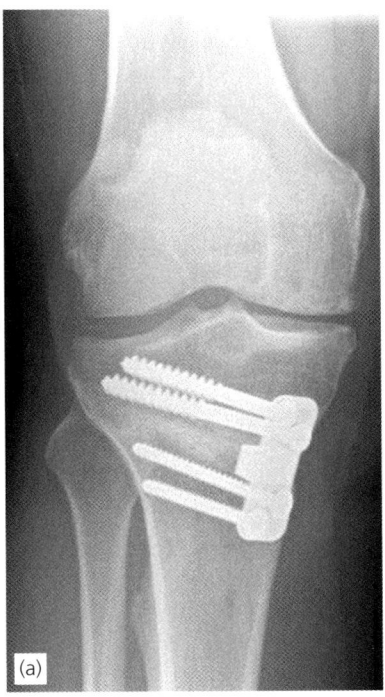 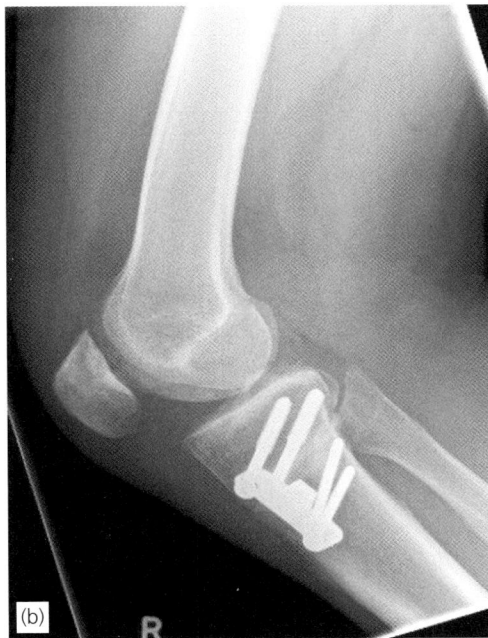 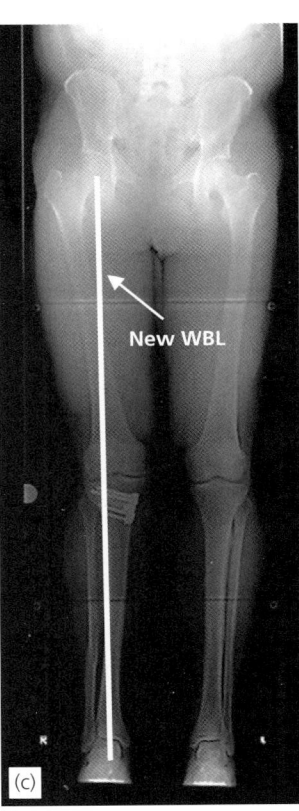

Figure 109.7 (a) Anteroposterior plain radiograph following opening wedge high tibial osteotomy. (b) Lateral postoperative view of opening wedge high tibial osteotomy. (c) Postoperative long leg view illustrating the new weight-bearing line (WBL).

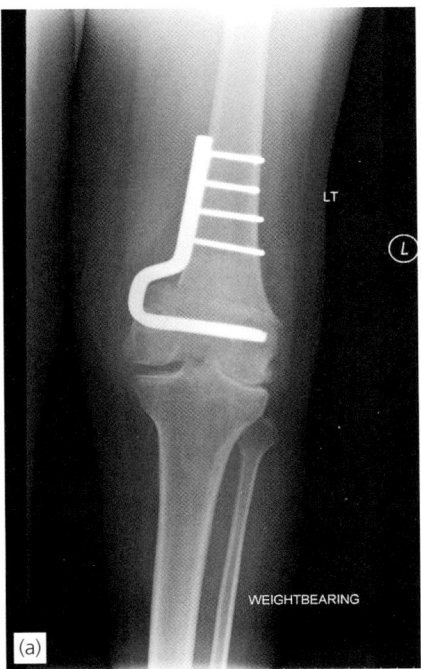 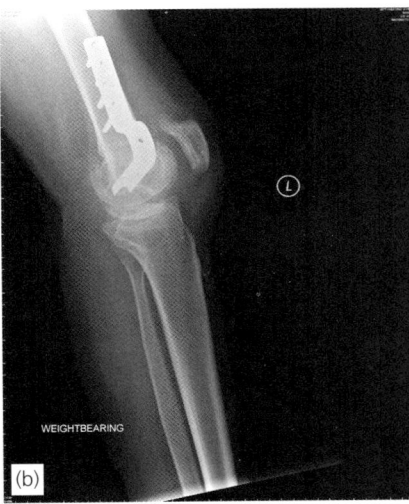

Figure 109.8 (a) Anteroposterior view of distal femoral osteotomy. (b) Lateral view of distal femoral osteotomy.

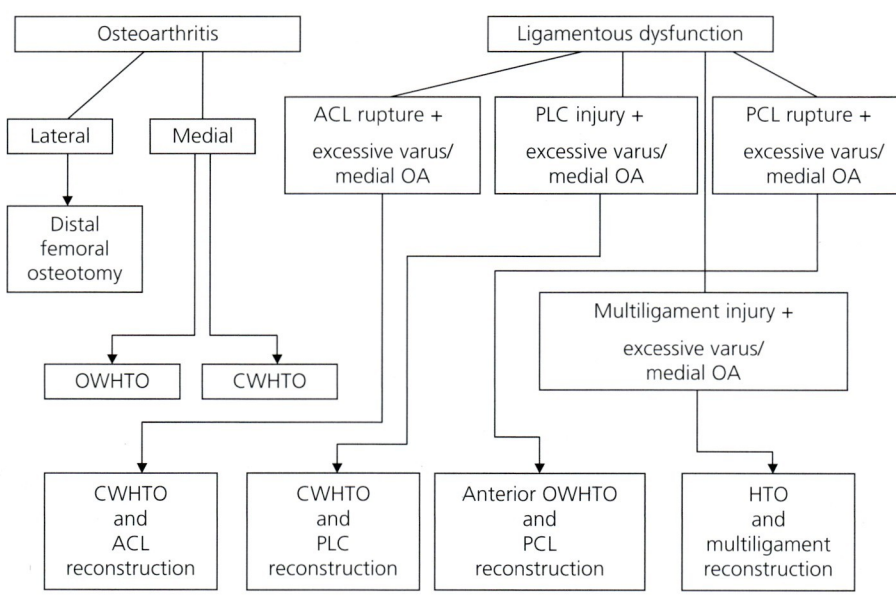

Figure 109.9 Algorithm for management of different situations. CWHTO, closing wedge high tibial osteotomy; OWHTO, opening wedge high tibial osteotomy; OA, osteoarthritis; HTO, high tibial osteotomy; PCL, posterior cruciate ligament; ACL, anterior cruciate ligament; PCL, posterolateral corner.

One of the key advances allowing 'modern' osteotomy to become reliable and successful is the development of fixation devices which allow early limb mobilization. One of the main reasons for the poor reputation of 'old' osteotomy was the need for cast immobilization with high rates of fat pad contracture causing patellar baja.

COMPLICATIONS OF OSTEOTOMIES

Osteotomies are major operations and complications occur. These risks can be reduced by careful patient selection, accurate pre-operative planning, selection of the correct technique, good surgical skills and an appropriate rehabilitation programme. The risks include

- peroneal nerve injury or dysfunction
- vascular injury
- compartment syndrome
- deep vein thrombosis/pulmonary emboli
- tibia plateau fracture
- delayed/non-union
- patella baja
- undercorrection
- overcorrection (see above).

CONCLUSION

The role of osteotomies in the management of OA and ligamentous problems is important. When performed, pre-operative planning is crucial. Although surgeons must select and perform techniques of osteotomies that they are comfortable with, it is important to appreciate that one technique does not fit all patients. Each type of osteotomy has its own particular advantages and disadvantages. Good outcome is dependent on careful selection of the patient and technique, precise pre-operative planning, sound surgical skills and an appropriate rehabilitation programme. A suggested algorithm for management of different situations has been provided in Fig. 109.9.

KEY LEARNING POINTS

- Osteotomies have an important role in management of osteoarthritis.
- Equally, their role in 'fine-tuning' alignment of some ligament instability cases must not be disregarded.
- Careful patient selection is crucial.
- Complications do occur and can be reduced by careful planning.
- One technique does not fit all patients.

REFERENCES

- ● = Key primary paper
- ◆ = Major review article

◆1. Williams A, Devic N. Osteotomy in the management of knee osteoarthritis and ligamentous instability. *Current Orthopaedics* 2006;**20**:112–20.
◆2. Hart A, Carrington R, Allen P. Biomechanics and joint replacement of the knee. In: Ramachandran M (ed.) *Basic Orthopaedic Sciences, the Stanmore Guide*. London, UK: Holder Arnold, 2007:170–9.
◆3. Puddu G, Franco V, Cipolla M, *et al*. Opening wedge osteotomy – proximal tibia and distal femur. In: Jackson DW (ed.) *Reconstructive Knee Surgery*. Philadelphia, PA: Wolters Kluwer/Lippincott Williams & Wilkins, 2008:433–50.

- ◆4. Dugdale TW, Noyes FR, Styer D. Preoperative planning for high tibial osteotomy. *Clinical Orthopaedics and Related Research* 1992;**274**:248–64.
- ●5. Bonnin M, Chambat P. Current status of valgus angle, tibial head closing wedge osteotomy in medial gonarthrosis. *Orthopäde* 2004;**33**:135–45.
- ●6. Noyes FR, Barber-Westin SD. High tibial osteotomy in knees with associated chronic ligament deficiencies. In: Jackson DW (ed.) *Reconstructive Knee Surgery*. Philadelphia, PA: Wolters Kluwer/Lippincott Williams & Wilkins, 2008:315–59.
- ◆7. Amendola A. The role of osteotomy in the multiple ligament injured knee. Instructional course. *Arthroscopy: Journal of Arthroscopic Related Surgery* 2003;**19**(Suppl 1).

110

Joint arthrodesis

NIKOLAOS GIOTAKIS, RAJIV MALHOTRA, MUHAMMED ARSHAD NAZAR

Introduction	1270	Specific joints	1271
Work-up	1271	References	1275

NATIONAL BOARD STANDARDS

- Understand when fusion is indicated
- Know the common sites and positions for fusion
- Be able to request appropriate tests for planning
- Know the surgical approaches
- Learn the surgical steps for major joints
- Know the main complications

INTRODUCTION

Fusion is a treatment option following advanced destruction of the joint when arthroplasty is not possible or has failed. It is commonly performed in the spine, foot and ankle. Other sites are the wrist, knee, elbow, shoulder and hip. It should usually follow failure of conservative treatment. Radiographs are usually diagnostic of advanced joint disease but do not always correlate with symptoms. They also highlight the presence of associated deformities. CT is commonly employed for better surgical planning whereas MRI and white cell scans are used in cases of suspected infection. Exposure, preparation, coaptation of surfaces and stable fixation are the key stages of the surgical technique. Bone grafting is required in the presence of defects. The presence of infection usually requires a two-stage approach, particularly when bone grafting is anticipated.

Patients need to have very clear expectations on outcomes and complications. These are generally high, with malpositioning and non-union being the most common.

Successful fusion in a good position has high satisfaction rates.

In the cervical spine, rheumatoid arthritis (RA) is a common condition requiring fusion. Common candidates are patients with atlanto-axial subluxation, subaxial subluxation or both, requiring C1–2 or occipitocervical fusions.

In the lumbar spine, which is the commonest site of the spine requiring fusion, posterior, anterior or combined approaches are used preferably with instrumentation.

Arthrodesis is surgical fusion of a joint as opposed to ankylosis, which occurs spontaneously via a pathological process.

Arthroplasty has for some time been the treatment of choice for osteoarthritis of the hip and knee and more recently for the shoulder and elbow. In joints where stiffness allows satisfactory function, arthrodesis can be the optimal treatment. This is often the case in the foot and ankle, and the spine.

Table 110.1 illustrates the sites that will be discussed in this chapter and the recommended joint position for fusion.

Table 110.1 The table illustrates the sites of joint arthrodesis discussed in this chapter and the recommended position of fusion

Common sites	Positions for fusion
Shoulder	30° abduction, 30° forward flexion, 40° int. rotation
Elbow	70–90° flexion
Wrist	10–20° extension
Hip	30° flexion, 0–5° adduction, 0–15° ext. rotation
Knee	0–15° flexion, 5–8° valgus, 10° int. rotation
Ankle	Neutral plantarflexion with 5° valgus, 10° of ext. rotation
Hallux	Average 15° dorsiflexion (10–30°)
Proximal interphalangeal joint	Neutral

All causes must have as a common denominator a process leading to deterioration and destruction of the joint cartilage, producing a chronically painful joint unresponsive to conservative methods of treatment (Box 110.1).

> **BOX 110.1: This most common causes leading to the possible need for arthrodesis**
>
> - Primary osteoarthritis
> - After traumatic joint degeneration
> - Inflammatory joint disease, i.e. rheumatoid arthritis
> - After septic arthritis
> - After failed arthroplasty
> - After resection of tumours
> - Spinal trauma, deformities, tumour

The diagnosis of the underlying cause of the symptoms will play an important role in the treatment strategy.

Joint pain is usually associated with loss of movement and advanced arthritic radiographic changes.

WORK-UP

Surgical planning in most instances will be based on imaging studies.

- Plain radiographs are usually sufficient to demonstrate the degree of deterioration of the joint. They can offer clues on the presence of associated deformities. The indication to fuse is mainly based on symptoms. Radiographic signs of osteoarthritis do not necessarily coincide with the severity of symptoms.
- CT will give valuable information about the joint and subchondral bone.
- Inflammatory markers, white cell scan and MRI can be deployed in cases when infection may be a possible cause. In the presence of infection a two-stage approach is preferred, particularly when bone-grafting procedures are required.

In patients where risk factors to healing are present (such as smoking, metabolic disease, bone-suppressive medication) these should be addressed when possible. It is very important to give a realistic picture of the outcomes, and, if possible, to introduce other patients who have already had such surgery.

Surgical stages

EXPOSURE

This must be obtained via one or more anatomic approaches which will allow full visualization of the joint. Recently, arthroscopy has also been introduced in ankle fusion.

PREPARATION

This will involve removal of cartilage and non-viable bone.

COAPTATION

It is essential to optimize bone-to-bone contact. The direction of bone cuts has to be very precise in order to obtain contact in the appropriate alignment. In the presence of defects, the use of autologous corticocancellous bone graft and BMPs may be indicated.

STABLE FIXATION

This aims to minimize movement at the arthrodesis site. Internal fixation is the most commonly employed. External fixation is often the choice in the presence of previous infection, in cases of bone loss or when combined techniques of length restoration are necessary.

SPECIFIC JOINTS

Ankle and foot

Arthrodesis is the most common procedure in advanced foot and ankle arthritis.

The aim is to achieve a plantigrade, stable and pain-free foot.

Limiting fusion to the symptomatic joint will offer better function.

Some joints are more mobile and their preservation if unaffected will offer a better outcome. These are the ankle, subtalar, naviculocuneiform and fourth–fifth tarsometatarsal joints.

Long-term studies indicate that hindfoot or ankle fusion can lead to gradual deterioration of adjacent joints. In one of these,[1,2] subtalar joint fusion was associated with radiographic changes in all ankle joints, and some midfoot joints in long-term evaluation. However, long-term patient satisfaction remained high (95%).[2]

IMAGING

- Weight-bearing foot and ankle radiographs are always obtained.
- The axial view of the calcaneus (Cobey view) shows alignment of the heel.
- CT can provide more information on the condition of the hindfoot joints, bone defects and avascular bone.
- A bone scan can help diagnose concomitant osteoarthritis in other foot joints.

CLINICAL ASSESSMENT

Joint motion, pain and response to non-surgical treatment are the most important assessment tools. Examination of all foot joints is crucial.

Prior to considering fusion in less severe degenerative disease, use of cushion heels and rocker bottom sole and the temporary use of a walking cast can be helpful. Intra-articular injections can have both diagnostic and therapeutic value.

SCENARIOS

- *Early stages of ankle arthritis:* ankle debridement via arthrotomy or arthroscopy can offer temporary relief. The use of arthrodiastasis with external fixators has also been described at the early stage of disease particularly after trauma.
- *Flexible deformities of the hindfoot:* imbalance can be treated with tendon transfers and or corrective osteotomies. Some can be simply due to muscle imbalance.
- *Degenerated joints with no deformity:* fusion *in situ* is indicated.
- *Rigid deformity* requires realignment and then arthrodesis to hold the correction. Arthrodesis may relieve symptoms, but poor alignment will eventually cause problems in other parts of the limb. For example if a valgus hindfoot (flat foot) is fused *in situ*, valgus forces will continue to be transmitted across the ankle, resulting in degeneration.

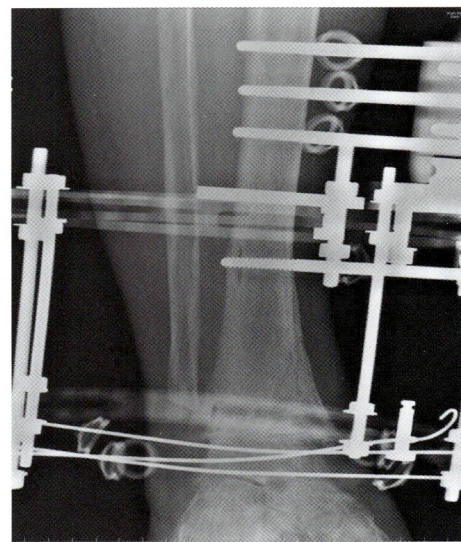

Figure 110.1 This is a case of ankle fusion with the use of a circular frame following septic ankle arthritis.

ANKLE FUSION

Approaches

Arthroscopic or minimally invasive fusion is indicated in the presence of no or minimal deformity. Winson and Robertson[3] reported a 92.4% success rate in 116 cases. In the presence of significant deformity open surgery is chosen.

The most common approaches are dual lateral transfibular, and medial. When possible the medial malleolus is preserved. An alternative is the posterior approach for the use of blade plates (Fig. 110.1).

The lateral transfibular approach allows excellent visualization of the tibiotalar joint.

Preparation of the surfaces is done by curettage of cartilage and any sclerotic bone or via resection to create two flat parallel surfaces. On average the latter will result in 1 cm shortening.

A large contact area will optimize the chances of union. In cases where defects are present the use of autologous corticocancellous bone graft is recommended. The use of BMPs may also be considered.

The desired foot position is plantigrade with 5° valgus and 10° of external rotation.

Fixation

This is achieved by the use of large cannulated screws with washers or posterior neutralization plates.

In the presence of infection, the use of circular frames is indicated (Fig. 110.1).

More complex is the treatment of non-unions, failed arthrodesis or arthroplasty, in osteonecrosis of the talus and Charcot arthropathy. These require radical debridement and bone grafting. Non-union, infection and malunion are common complications.

TIBIOCALCANEAL FUSION

This is necessary when both the ankle and the subtalar joints are affected. It is inappropriate to fuse the subtalar joint if this is normal.

A transfibular approach can be used to expose all joints. Compression screws, neutralization plates, retrograde nails and circular frames are used. If a posterior blade plate is used then a posterior and medial approach can be combined. Intramedullary nails of modern design allow multiple distal locking screw positions, which may overcome the relatively poor purchase on cancellous bone. Structures at risk with nails are the lateral plantar artery and nerve.

TRIPLE ARTHRODESIS

This involves fusion of the talocalcaneal, calcaneocuboid and talonavicular joints. Persistent pain with or without deformity is the classic presentation. Anaesthetic blocks are very useful for identifying the joints from which the pain originates (Fig. 110.2).

The combined lateral and medial approaches allow optimal exposure of all joints.

Osteoarthritis of adjacent joints is common. Nonunion of the talonavicular joint is another frequent problem (5–10%) particularly when the lateral approach alone has been used.

PANTALAR FUSION

This is necessary when the ankle and hindfoot joints are symptomatic.

It results in pain relief but with less good function owing to the overall stiffness. As a result, there will be a noticeable limp. The use of a rocker bottom sole can be helpful.

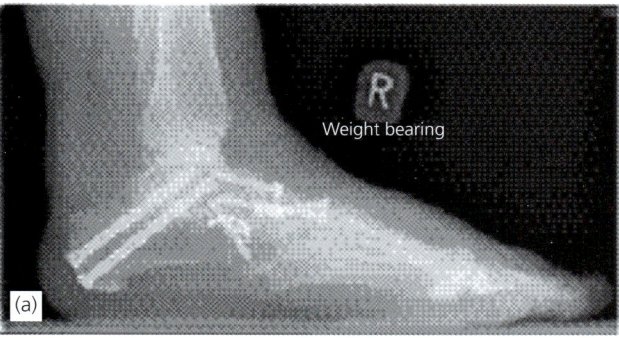
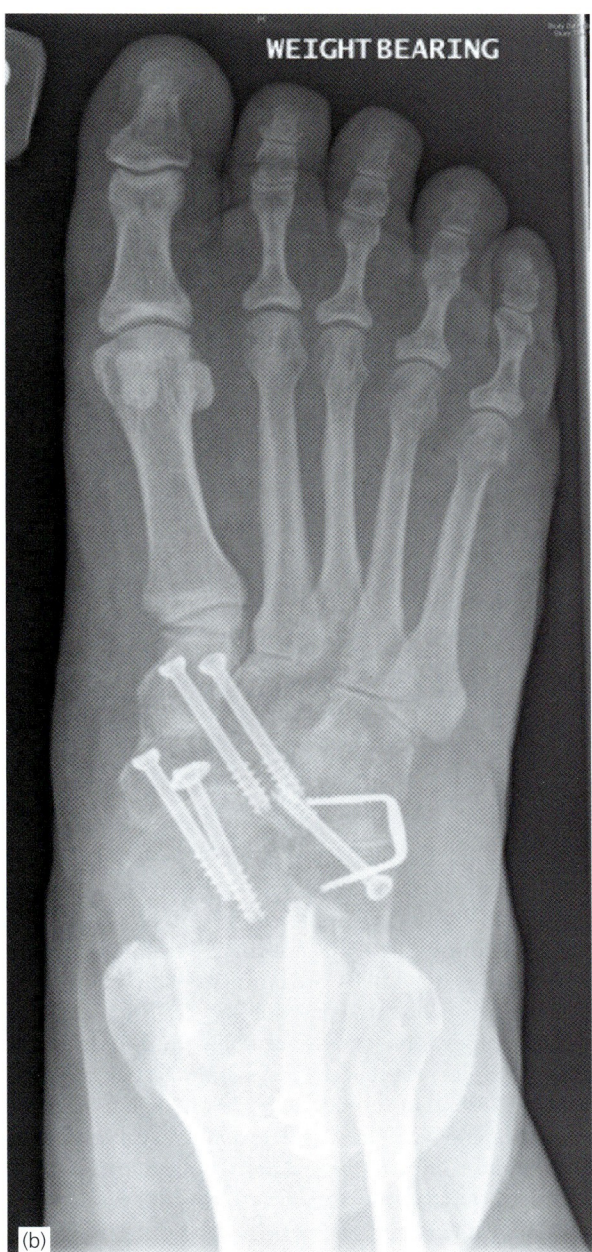

Figure 110.2 (a) Triple arthrodesis with the use of cannulated lag screws and staple (lateral view). (b) Triple arthrodesis with the use of cannulated lag screws and staple (anteroposterior view).

Fusion of the talonavicular joint requires a medial and lateral approach to visualize the joints entirely and to allow surface preparation.

The use of internal screws and staple can be used at the calceneocuboid joint.

LISFRANC JOINT

Untreated Lisfranc injuries or symptomatic internally fixed injuries represent common indications for fusion. Most frequently, the symptoms are related to the medial three joints (usually the most stiff).

The approach is the same as that used for fixation of acute injuries. Fixation can be achieved with the use of small fragment screws across each joint.

Rigid fixation with bone grafting in complex cases can address associated deformity.

In the presence of varus or valgus deformity, medial or lateral column lengthening with bone grafting may need to be undertaken.

Fusion of the lateral column (more mobile) is more disabling as it is associated with significantly increased stiffness. Recent small studies with alternative methods of treatment, such as tendon interposition arthroplasty and ceramic interposition arthroplasty, have reported good outcomes.

HALLUX METATARSOPHALANGEAL JOINT

This is indicated in grade 3 and 4 hallux rigidus when pain is not responsive to conservative treatment.

APPROACHES: MEDIAL, DORSOMEDIAL

The recommended position is 15–30° dorsiflexion, depending on the hallux declination angle, to clear the ground and prevent adjacent osteoarthritis in the proximal interphalangeal (PIP) joint.

There are high fusion rates (90–100%) with different techniques (suturing, wires, plates).

LESSER TOES PROXIMAL INTERPHALANGEAL JOINT

Fusion is the treatment of choice for painful toe deformities unresponsive to splintage (i.e. fixed hammertoe). It is more common in women in association with hallux valgus or when the second toe is longer. Pain needs to be differentiated from interdigital neuroma.

The ideal position of fusion is neutral. Peg and socket method is used and the commonest complication is malposition.

Knee

The commonest indication is failure of knee arthroplasty. Others are pain/instability post infection, trauma, in paralysis and after tumour resection.

APPROACHES

Careful preservation of the blood supply to the skin is necessary to avoid wound-healing problems. Longitudinal or transverse incisions can be used. In the presence of multiple previous incisions, the most biological approach is the longitudinal lateral parapatellar.[4] Good bone contact, adequate blood supply and stable fixation are key for success. The removal of avascular bone, prosthetic components, menisci, cruciate ligaments and cement is essential.

FIXATION

Intramedullary nails

These have been often employed in cases with extensive bone loss such as post-infected arthroplasty. Such bone loss would generally require the addition of large bone grafts or allograft. In post-infected cases, a two-stage approach with use of spacers and systemic antibiotics has been suggested with a fusion rate of 85–95%. These are, however, associated with long surgical times, blood loss and frequent complications.

Special arthrodesis nails are available or can be custom made. They can be locked for added stability and rotational control. The disadvantages are mainly lack of compression and risk of intramedullary osteomyelitis in cases of recurrence of infection.[4]

External fixators

The use of circular frames has advantages in terms of weight bearing and the ability to maintain and apply gradual compression. These can be utilized successfully in the presence of little bone loss and with good bone-to-bone contact. Charnley and Lowe[5] have reported excellent results in terms of union (98.9%) with the use of external fixation in primary arthrodesis. Most of the cases were for osteoarthritis, tuberculosis and RA. None was post total knee arthroplasty.

The success rates tends to drop significantly (38–65%) in cases associated with large defects such as those created by failed arthroplasty.

Pin site infections are common; patient compliance may also be difficult. The use of dual-compression plates and the combination of intramedullary nails with plates have been reported. Successful fusion will offer satisfactory relief of knee pain and will allow weight bearing. The main disadvantages are the presence of a very obvious limp, difficulty on using transportation and space requirements when sitting.

Hip

Fusion is rarely performed because of the debilitating effect of complete loss of movement of the hip.

The position in flexion is always an impossible compromise between walking and sitting, and backache and knee problems are very common. Multiple revisions and grafting if needed now seem to be the norm, trying to preserve as much function as possible, with excision arthroplasty (Girdlestone's procedure) as a last resort.

Requirements are the presence of a normal contralateral hip and ipsilateral knee. Fixation is performed via plating with a Cobra plate or a sliding screw. Supra-acetabular or subtrochanteric osteotomy has been reported to improve positioning. Complications are malpositioning, non-union, knee and lower back pain, and limb length inequality.

Wrist

Although arthrodesis of the wrist is less common than in the past, there are instances where it still represents the most viable solution. Indications are post-traumatic painful joints, infection, tumour resection and RA. Stabilization of the wrist in the presence of paralysis, failed arthroplasty or complex instability can also be treated by fusion.

The preferred position for most tasks and hand grip is 10–20° dorsiflexion while maintaining the third metacarpal in line with the radius. This can allow preservation of full pronation–supination. Mild ulnar deviation (radius in line with the second metacarpal) can maximize hand grip.

APPROACHES

The most commonly used is dorsal. Alternatively, a radial or ulnar approach can be used. Removal of cartilage from the third carpometacarpal, capitolunate, radioscaphoid and radiolunate joints is required. This can be extended to other symptomatic carpal joints.

FIXATION

The use of low-profile DCP type plates with autologous bone grafting has a successful rate of fusion of around 90%, as reported by several authors.[6] AO pre-contoured type plates are commonly used. Alternative techniques involve the use of intramedullary rods or external fixation.

Although union rates, particularly with use of plates, are high,[6] complications are common: wound dehiscence, removal of plate for tendon and skin irritation range from 50% to 75%. Distal radio-ulnar joint pain/instability, carpal tunnel syndrome, metacarpophalangeal (MCP) joint stiffness and complex regional pain syndrome can occur.

Patient satisfaction rates are high with regard to pain relief and correction of deformities. Grip strength and digital range of motion do not change drastically from pre-operative levels. Perianal care, pronation–supination under resistance, and use of the hand in tight spaces are the most commonly limiting tasks following wrist arthrodesis.

Shoulder

The widespread use of arthroplasty and the elimination of tuberculosis and polio in many parts of the world have limited the indications for arthrodesis to the shoulder.

It is still a useful procedure in cases of persistent infection and in the presence of paralytic disorders, particularly when both the deltoid and the rotator cuffs are involved. Post failed arthroplasty is also an indication if revision is not appropriate, as well as the ultimate treatment of multidirectional instability, tumour resections and recurrent dislocations.

Common approaches used are anterosuperior and posterior.

Internal or external fixation techniques can be used, with the latter preferred in infected cases. Bone grafts are required in cases of associated bone loss. When the acromion is included the contact between the humeral head and the glenoid fossa is improved. Single plates or double plates are sometimes used, as well as a combination of rush pin with tension band and muscle pedicle flaps.[4]

Contact with compression and stable fixation are essential. Complications are infection, non-union, malunion, painful hardware and humeral stress fractures.

Elbow

Indications for fusion are conditions causing a painful arthritic elbow, where arthroplasty is not preferable (i.e. post-infective arthritis, failed fixation or arthroplasty).

A position of 90° is ideal for personal hygiene whereas fusion at 70° is better for other activities.

The standard approach is posterior. Both internal and external fixation techniques are employed. The presence of bone loss increases the risk of failure. Resection of the radial head allows pronation–supination.

Non-union, malunion and hardware-related problems are common complications.

For arthrodesis in the spine, see chapter 89.

> **KEY LEARNING POINTS**
>
> - Fusion is more tolerated in less mobile joints.
> - Considered only after failure of conservative treatment.
> - Do not fuse healthy joints (no pain, no deformity).
> - Bone grafts in defects.
> - Internal fixation when no infection.
> - Frames for infected and some cases with large defects.
> - Two-stage surgery, particularly when bone grafting after infection.
> - Non-union and malpositioning are the commonest complications.
> - Hip fusion is very disabling.
> - Cord injury is the commonest complication in spinal fusion.
> - The approaches to the spine are anterior and posterior, or a combination.
> - Grafting with bone graft or BMPs increases fusion rates.

ACKNOWLEDGEMENTS

Thanks to David Neal Smith for his help in editing the chapter and Robin Pilay, Marcus De Matas, Siva Sirikonda and Badri Narayan for kindly providing clinical pictures.

REFERENCES

● = Key primary paper
◆ = Major review article

● 1. Coester LM, Saltzman CL, Leupold J, Pontarelli W. Long-term results following ankle arthrodesis for posttraumatic arthritis. *Journal of Bone and Joint Surgery (American)* 2001;**83**:219–28.

● 2. Saltzman CL, Fehrle MJ, Cooper RR, *et al*. Triple arthrodesis: twenty-five and forty-four-year average follow-up of the same patients. *Journal of Bone and Joint Surgery (American)* 1999;**81**:1391–402.

● 3. Winson IG, Robertson E. Arthroscopic ankle arthrodesis. *Journal of Bone and Joint Surgery (British)* 2005;**87B**:343–7.

◆ 4. Canale ST. *Campbell's Operative Orthopaedics*, vol. 1, 10th edn. St Louis, MN: Mosby, 2003:155–219.

● 5. Charnley J, Lowe HB. A study of the end results of compression arthrodesis of the knee. *Journal of Bone and Joint Surgery (British)* 1958;**40B**:633.

● 6. Hastings H II, Weiss APC, Quenzer D, *et al*. Arthrodesis of the wrist for post-traumatic disorders. *Journal of Bone and Joint Surgery (American)* 1996;**78**:897–902.

PART 10

HAND AND UPPER LIMB

TED MAH

111	**Finger injuries**	**1277**
	A Bobby Chhabra, Jesse Seamon	
112	**Tendon injuries**	**1292**
	S Raja Sabapathy, Praveen Bhardwaj	
113	**Nerve injuries**	**1302**
	Rolfe Birch	
114	**Hand infections**	**1309**
	Tunku Kamarul Zaman	
115	**Replantation and microsurgery**	**1315**
	Tunku Kamarul Zaman	
116	**Dupuytren's contracture**	**1324**
	William YC Loh, Wee-Leon Lam	
117	**Arthritis of the hand**	**1333**
	Ashish Sharma, Edward T Mah	
118	**Carpal instability**	**1351**
	Ng Eng Seng, Edward T Mah	
119	**The distal radial ulnar joint**	**1365**
	Edward T Mah, Ng Eng Seng	
120	**Hand tumours**	**1373**
	Graham Cheung, Gillian L Cribb	
121	**The elbow**	**1382**
	Ashish K Sharma, Kamarul Khalid, Edward T Mah	

111

Finger injuries

A BOBBY CHHABRA, JESSE SEAMON

Injuries to the flexor tendons	1277	Fingertip and nail bed injuries	1287
Injuries to the extensor tendons	1280	References	1290

NATIONAL BOARD STANDARDS

- Understand finger tip injuries
- Know trigger finger, mallet finger, boutonnière and swan neck deformities

- Learn how to manage proximal interphalangeal joint dislocations, phalangeal fractures and traumatic finger tip amputations

INJURIES TO THE FLEXOR TENDONS

Trigger finger/thumb

Trigger finger, also called stenosing tenosynovitis, can affect any of the digits but most commonly affects the thumb, ring and middle fingers.[1] The incidence is greatest in women, with the average age being between 52 and 62 years.[2] The great majority of cases involve obstruction of the flexor tendon at the A1 pulley. Trigger finger has been associated with a number of systemic conditions, including amyloidosis, mucopolysaccharidosis and rheumatoid arthritis.[3]

The mechanism of injury is repetitive friction occurring between the flexor tendon and its associated tendinous sheath within the annular pulley system.[4] The majority of reactive inflammatory change occurs within the inner layer of the A1 pulley, and is associated with concurrent thickening of the pulley system, sometimes to three times the original size.[3] Histologically, chondroblast and synovial proliferation are observed within the inner layer of the A1 pulley; usually no changes are noted in the tenosynovium of the flexor tendon.[3,5] These changes create a mismatch between the volume of the flexor tendon and the available space through the A1 pulley and lead to catching or locking of the tendon with attempted joint flexion.[4]

Patients present with pain over the volar metacarpal head that continues along the flexor tendon sheath. Initially, a complaint can usually be elicited of a locking or popping sensation with flexion of the affected digit, progressing to a more painful condition with inability to smoothly flex or extend the digit. Eventually, the finger may become locked, usually in flexion. Although this injury is typically seen in older individuals due to degenerative change, it may be seen in younger individuals, including young athletes, secondary to pressure from holding tennis racquets or baseball bats.[2–4]

Initial treatment is conservative, with corticosteroid injections, activity modification, non-steroidal anti-inflammatory drugs (NSAIDs) and splinting. Splinting should be reserved for less severe cases when only one finger is involved, and triggering of the affected digit is relatively mild. In these cases NSAIDs can be a useful adjuvant to treatment.[3] Corticosteroid injections into the flexor tendon sheath are the cornerstone of conservative management. This treatment is effective for most individuals, with reported cure rates ranging from 57% to 84%.[2,4] Betamethasone is the steroid of choice, although effective results have been obtained with methylprednisolone and triamcinolone.[3] If conservative treatment fails, or there is complete locking of the affected digit, surgical intervention with release of the A1 pulley is indicated.[4] In general, the entire A1 pulley should be released, leading to approximately 10% increased effort with flexion. This is usually not apparent clinically, and almost all patients have resolution of symptoms with open A1 pulley release.[3] Complications of surgery include bowstringing of the tendon from inadvertent damage to the A2 pulley and digital nerve injury.[3,4]

Finger and palm lacerations

Lacerations of the palm and fingers are extremely common. These lacerations must be taken seriously because of the anatomic proximity of vital tendons, nerves and arteries to the subcutaneous tissue. All lacerations of the palm and fingers require a thorough physical examination to rule out injury to tendinous and neurovascular structures. A history should be elicited including the time and mechanism of injury and the potential for contamination with foreign and infectious materials. The patient's occupation, hobbies and handedness should be elicited.[6,7]

The wound should not be explored in the Accident and Emergency Department as it only causes more bleeding and considerable discomfort to the patient. Bleeding vessels should not be clamped, as a nerve could be inadvertently damaged in the process. The wound should be covered with sterile gauze, bandaged and elevated until bleeding has been controlled. Vascular integrity is assessed by checking for appropriate colour, warmth and capillary refill of the fingers. Neurological integrity is assessed by checking for the presence or absence of sensation to light touch, along with the use of two-point discrimination testing with a paper clip or callipers. The flexor digitorum profundus (FDP) is assessed by asking the patient to flex the distal interphalangeal (DIP) joint while the examiner holds the proximal interphalangeal (PIP) joint in extension. The flexor digitorum superficialis (FDS) is tested by asking the patient to flex the finger at the PIP joint while all other fingers are held in full extension. It is important to test resisted flexion at these joints as pain and weakness may be a sign of a partial tendon disruption.[6,7]

Initial management of the laceration is saline irrigation and debridement followed by saline-soaked gauze over the wound and wound bandaging. Surgical intervention involves primary repair of the tendon or free tendon grafting if primary repair is not possible for flexor tendon lacerations. Primary repair or delayed primary repair (within 10 days) has similar outcomes. The indications for primary repair are complete tendon ruptures and lacerations of greater than 50% of the tendon diameter. Contraindications to immediate and primary repair include contaminated wounds, severe crush injuries, significant volar skin loss and extensive soft-tissue injury.[8]

The tendon is repaired using core suture techniques to rejoin the tendon stumps followed by circumferential epitendinous sutures to smooth out the repair site and add tensile strength. Care must be taken to conserve the A2 and A4 pulleys intra-operatively to prevent bowstringing of the flexor tendons. Repair of the flexor sheath should be initiated for disruption of the A2 and A4 annular pulleys with reconstruction accomplished using free tendon grafts or retinacular grafts. Repair of the membranous portions of the tendon sheath does not appear to be beneficial.[8]

Lacerations of the volar portion of the hand are anatomically localized using a modification of Verdan's zones of the hand, which divides the hand into five distinct zones[9] (Fig. 111.1). Similarly eight zones are used to define the dorsal (extensor) portion of the hand and wrist[10] (Fig. 111.2).

ZONE I INJURIES – JERSEY FINGER

Zone I injuries occur in the region of the finger at or distal to the FDS insertion. The forceful disruption of the FDP insertion at the base of the volar distal phalanx is

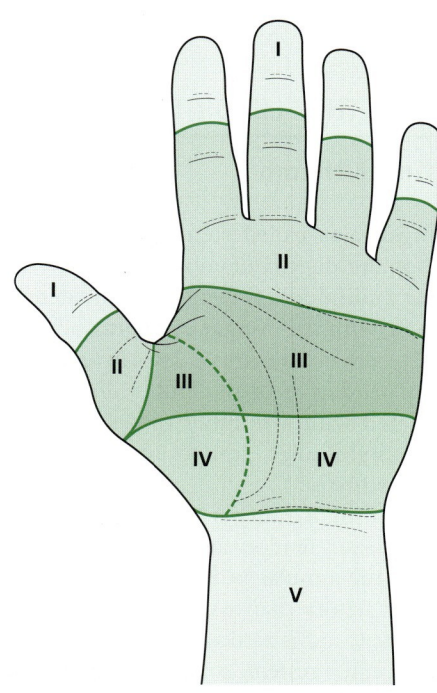

Figure 111.1 Flexor tendon zones. Redrawn with permission from Green D, Hotchkiss R, Pederson W (eds). *Green's Operative Hand Surgery*, vol. 1, 5th edn. Philadelphia, PA: Elsevier Churchill Livingstone, 2005:221.

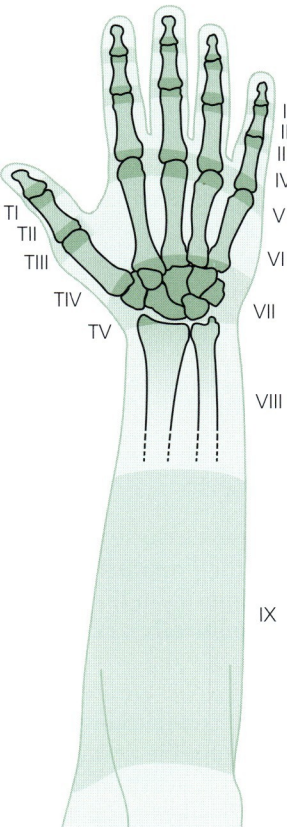

Figure 111.2 Extensor tendon zones. Redrawn with permission from Green D, Hotchkiss R, Pederson W (eds). *Green's Operative Hand Surgery*, vol. 1, 5th edn. Philadelphia, PA: Elsevier Churchill Livingstone, 2005:190.

called a jersey finger injury.[11] Most commonly, this injury is seen in football players following a tackle in which the actively flexed DIP joint is forced into hyperextension. The bony insertion of the FDP tendon is the site of rupture the vast majority of the time, although mid-substance ruptures may be seen in patients with rheumatoid arthritis, tenosynovitis, lacerations or fractures of the hook of the hamate.[11–13] The ring finger is involved in over three-quarters of cases.[11,14] Cadaver studies have shown a relative weakness of the FDP insertion on the ring finger compared with the middle finger, perhaps due to the tethering of the FDP tendon by the lumbricals in the distal palm.[11] Other factors related to the increased incidence may include the prominence of the ring finger during grip and the fact that the ring finger has the least independent motion of all the fingers.[12]

Jersey finger occurs because of blunt trauma or a forceful hyperextension across the DIP joint. The injury is most common among football and rugby players.[13] On clinical examination, the patient will display an inability to flex the DIP joint when asked to make a fist. Alternatively, FDP integrity can be tested by stabilizing the PIP joint in extension and asking the patient to flex the fingertip. In either case, inability to flex the finger at the DIP joint indicates loss of FDP function.[11,15] On palpation along the length of the flexor tendon there is often a point of maximal tenderness, which represents the proximally retracted tendon stump. If the diagnosis is suspected but clinical examination is equivocal, ultrasound and/or MRI are useful for determining the location of the tendon stump.[12] Pain, swelling and ecchymosis are not reliably present with jersey finger injuries.[13]

Leddy and Packer[14] have classified jersey finger injuries into three categories depending on the degree of tendon retraction. In a type I injury the tendon retracts into the palm with subsequent loss of vinicular blood supply. Accordingly, the tendon must be reinserted within 7–10 days to prevent muscle contracture. Surgical intervention involves the identification of the avulsed tendon, followed by introduction of a flexible catheter passed distal to proximal to the level of the A1 pulley. At the A1 pulley the tendon is sutured to the catheter and pulled through the synovial sheath to its insertion on the base of the volar distal phalanx. Reattachment to the distal phalanx is with a pull-out wire and button technique using synthetic monofilament suture in a criss-cross fashion or steel wire to secure the tendon to the bone. Suture anchors can also be used. Care must be taken not to damage the volar plate of the DIP joint or to extend the tendon more then 1 cm past the original insertion as this can cause flexion contractures or result in quadrigria.[10,11,15] Boyer et al.[8] emphasize that the A4 pulley should not be partially released during repair; rather, a paediatric urethral dilator should be used to sequentially dilate the pulley until the FDP tendon can pass through.

In type II injuries the FDP tendon retracts to the level of the PIP joint, thus maintaining blood supply from the long viniculum. On clinical examination a lack of active flexion at the DIP joint is characteristically present and flexion at the PIP joint is typically disrupted as well.[11,15] A small piece of bone may avulse with the FDP tendon, allowing it to get caught in the chiasm formed by the FDS tendon, accounting for its position at the level of the PIP joint.[12] The window for reinsertion is 6–12 weeks for these injuries because nutritional supply to the tendon is maintained by the long viniculum.[11,12,15] Nevertheless, surgical repair is still recommended in the acute phase of these injuries.[12,13]

In a type III injury there is avulsion of the FDP with an associated large bony fragment that is often caught in the A4 pulley[13] (Fig. 111.3). Repair should be attempted in the acute setting with open reduction and internal fixation (ORIF) of the avulsed fragment.[12,13] Rarely, the FDP may rupture separately from the fracture fragment; the so-called type IIIb (also called type IV) injuries. These injuries are treated in a two-stage manner. First the avulsion

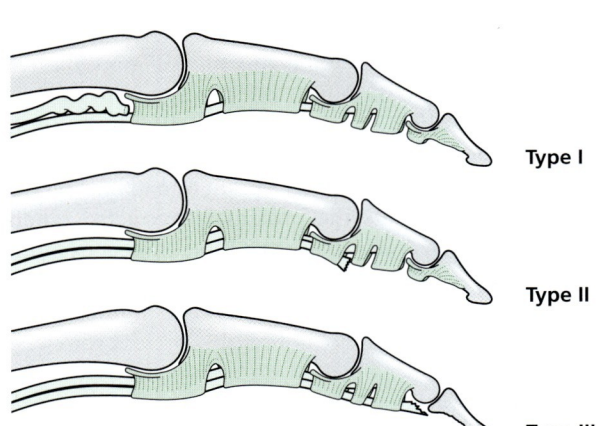

Figure 111.3 Flexor digitorum profundus rupture, types I–III. Redrawn with permission from Green D, Hotchkiss R, Pederson W (eds). *Green's Operative Hand Surgery*, vol. 1, 5th edn. Philadelphia, PA: Elsevier Churchill Livingstone, 2005:226.

fracture is corrected with ORIF using K-wires or mini-fragment screws; second the flexor tendon is repaired in the same fashion as a type I injury.[11–13,15]

For patients who present with chronic jersey finger injuries, treatment options are varied and include FDS flexor tendon grafts, arthrodesis of the DIP joint and observation without surgical intervention.[11,15] Leddy and colleagues[11,13] have suggested that asymptomatic patients with FDP injuries of the ring finger should receive no treatment because most patients have full motion of the PIP joint 6 months after injury and maintain good enough function of the ring finger for athletic performance. Repair with flexor tendon graft is indicated for musicians or technicians who require use of the DIP joint of the ring finger, and DIP fusion is recommended for most patients with continued DIP instability.[11] Tendon stump excision is undertaken when the retracted tendon causes a painful lump in the palm.[12,13]

ZONE II INJURIES

Zone II injuries occur in the region defined by the area just proximal to the FDS insertion on the middle phalanx and extend distally to the distal volar crease. Also known as 'no man's land', zone II injuries are notoriously difficult to treat because of the high incidence of postoperative adhesions.[8]

Both the FDP and the FDS tendons are involved, in contrast to zone I where only the FDP tendon is involved. Intra-operative repair with combined core and epitendinous suturing techniques are used for primary repair.[8] Both the FDP and FDS tendons should be repaired, with the FDS tendon being repaired before the FDP tendon.[8] In general, partial lacerations that constitute more than 50–60% of the tendon should be repaired primarily with a core and epitendinous suture technique.[8,9]

Aggressive postoperative hand therapy is aimed at movement across the DIP and PIP joints to prevent adhesions without disrupting the primary repair.[8,10] Passive motion is initiated soon after surgery, with active motion delayed until 4 weeks postoperatively when the tendon repair is of adequate strength. Passive 'place and hold' technique encourages differential gliding of the tendons to reduce tendon adhesion. Many different postoperative regimens have been used in various parts of the world and depend primarily on the strength of repair. Compliance with an appropriate hand therapy regimen is essential for the best outcome. Subsequent tenolysis may be required if adhesions persist limiting functional motion 3 months after surgery despite therapy.[8,10]

ZONE III AND IV INJURIES

Zone III injuries involve the region proximal to the distal volar crease at the proximal A1 pulley and distal to the carpal tunnel. Injuries in this region can damage the flexor tendons, lumbricals and digital neurovascular structures.[10]

Zone IV injuries involve the area of the wrist contained within the transverse carpal ligament (TCL) or carpal tunnel. Injuries may involve the flexor tendons, as well as the ulnar or median nerve. Results of repair can be compromised by difficulty in identifying tendinous structures.[10] Injuries to tendons in zone IV are relatively rare because of the protection provided by the TCL and adjacent carpal bones. Repair should preserve or reconstruct the TCL as it prevents prolapse of flexor tendons during postoperative wrist flexion.[16] As in zone II, postoperative adhesion is a concern in zone IV.[9]

ZONE V INJURIES

Zone V injuries occur in the distal forearm proximal to the carpal tunnel. Primary repair with appropriate postoperative therapy is indicated. Adhesions are less problematic in this region. Results are poorer in this region because of damage of the underlying neurovascular structures including the median and ulnar nerves and the radial and ulnar arteries.[10,16]

INJURIES TO THE EXTENSOR TENDONS

Zone I injuries – mallet finger

The disruption of the terminal tendon of the extensor mechanism insertion at the base of the dorsal distal phalanx is known as a mallet finger injury. It is the most common closed tendon injury among athletes and is seen among baseball players, American football wide receivers and basketball players.[11,15] It is also commonly seen in middle-aged people as a result of simple tasks such as making up beds.

The mechanism of injury is an acute force causing hyperflexion of the extended distal phalanx at the DIP joint, such as a blow to the fingertip while attempting to catch a ball.[11,15] In some cases, the injury is caused by severe hyperextension leading to a fracture at the base of the dorsal distal phalanx with concomitant loss of the extensor mechanism at the fracture site when the distal phalanx impacts into the middle phalanx. A twisting-type injury to the DIP joint can cause a tear in one of the merging lateral bands, leading to a mallet finger injury.[12]

On physical examination the affected DIP joint is flexed because of the unopposed action of the FDP muscle. This extensor lag can vary from 15° to greater than 60°, and pain may or may not be present.[17] The patient will be unable to actively extend the fingers. Surprisingly, only a minority of patients report difficulty with activities of daily living, although athletes typically will have greater levels of disability with regards to their specific sport. Care should be taken in ruling out mallet finger because of a negative physical examination as the deformity may take several days to develop. Radiographs are also recommended to rule out an associated fracture or joint subluxation[5,17] (Fig. 111.4).

Mallet finger may be classified on the basis of several systems that take into account both the mechanism and degree of injury. Doyle[18] has classified mallet finger into four types depending on the mechanism of injury. A type I mallet finger is caused by forced flexion of an extended finger and involves disruption of the extensor digitorum communis (EDC) tendon just proximal to the insertion point and is sometimes associated with an avulsion fracture. Type II injuries are lacerations that extend through the EDC tendon at or just proximal to the insertion of the tendon at the distal phalanx. Type III injuries are deep abrasions that involve the EDC tendon around its insertion at the dorsal distal phalanx. Type IV injuries are produced by three types of fractures: a transepiphyseal plate injury in children, a hyperflexion injury involving 20–50% of the articular surface and hyperextension injuries leading to fracture of greater than 50% of the articular surface with associated volar subluxation of the distal phalanx.[5,12,18] McCue and Wooten[19] have proposed a five-tier classification system as follows: type I is tendon attenuation, type II is tendon rupture, type III is rupture with an avulsion fracture, type IV is fracture, and type V is physeal fracture.[15]

Treatment of closed acute mallet finger injuries is usually undertaken by splinting the DIP joint continuously 24/7 in extension for 8–12 weeks while leaving the PIP joint free to move normally. Following 8–12 weeks of splinting in this fashion, the splint may be worn at night for an additional 4 weeks and during athletic activities for 2 months.[11,15,20] Even patients presenting a late as 1–3 months may be treated with splinting successfully.[11,12,15,17]

Tuttle et al.[12] recommend that surgical intervention be considered based on the degree of subluxation of the distal phalanx on lateral radiographs with the DIP joint splinted in extension. They advocate operative intervention when there is lack of collinearity of the affected distal and middle phalanx secondary to volar subluxation of the distal phalanx.

Mallet finger injuries that involve greater than one-third of the articular surface with volar dislocation, or injuries associated with avulsion of large bony fragments may be treated with surgical intervention.[11,20] This is achieved via ORIF of the avulsed fragment and reduction of the dislocated DIP joint (Fig. 111.5). Longitudinal K-wire placement across the DIP joint is usually adequate to maintain reduction of the injured joint.[11] Another method for reducing the mallet fracture is to place a K-wire at a 45° angle through the terminal extensor tendon just proximal to the fracture fragment followed by extension of the DIP joint to reduce the fragment. As described above, a K-wire should be placed longitudinally through the DIP joint to

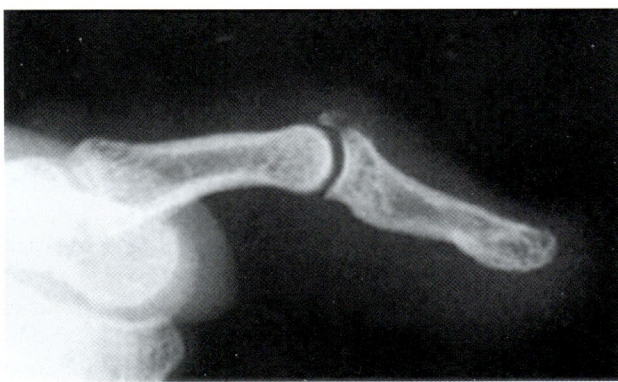

Figure 111.4 Mallet finger.

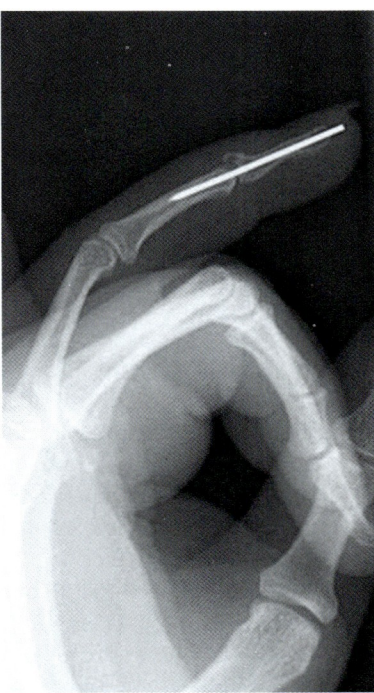

Figure 111.5 Open reduction and internal fixation of mallet finger.

hold the reduction following this procedure. In some cases a third K-wire may be passed through the fracture fragment to further stabilize the reduction.[12] Following surgery, the DIP joint should be splinted for 6 weeks before rehabilitation is begun.[11]

Ephipyseal plate fractures in children, which mimic mallet finger deformity, are treated with closed reduction. ORIF is reserved for unstable reductions. Open mallet fingers should be irrigated and debrided followed by primary repair of the extensor tendon. The splinting regimen is the same as for a closed mallet finger injury following surgery.[11]

Mallet deformities of the thumb are rare injuries accounting for approximately 3% of mallet finger injuries. Current treatment recommendations are to splint the interphalangeal joint of the thumb in extension for 6–8 weeks.[15]

Chronic mallet finger deformities (defined as greater than 4 weeks) are often treated successfully with additional splinting for up to 10–18 weeks followed by 2–4 weeks of night splinting.[12,21] Treatment can be initiated up to 12 weeks after injury with good success. Some untreated mallet fingers will progress to swan neck deformities where there is flexion posturing of the DIP joint and hyperextension of the PIP joint.[17] The mechanism whereby this occurs and the surgical treatment options for this condition are discussed in the section on swan neck deformities.

Zone II injuries

Zone II injuries involve the middle phalanx proximal to the DIP and distal to the PIP. Injuries in this zone are typically incomplete lacerations secondary to the width and curvature of the extensor mechanism.[1] Lacerations involving greater than 50% of the tendon should be repaired primarily, while smaller lacerations are treated with protected splinting.[20,22] Appropriate postoperative therapy is required to protect tendon repairs with gradual progression of motion.[22]

Zone III injuries – boutonnière deformity

Boutonnière deformity is caused by the disruption of the central slip of the extensor mechanism at the base of the dorsal middle phalanx. Three main mechanisms are responsible for the boutonnière deformity. They are acute forceful hyperflexion of the PIP joint, volar and lateral dislocation of the PIP joint, and deep contusion along the proximal middle phalanx.[20] Volar lateral dislocations of the PIP joint are believed to be the most common mechanism of injury.[11]

The boutonnière deformity develops as a result of central slip rupture. When the central slip ruptures, the lateral bands gradually migrate volar to the PIP joint axis, stretching the triangular ligament and concentration of the lateral bands' extension force at the DIP joint. This, in combination with central slip rupture, causes the classic

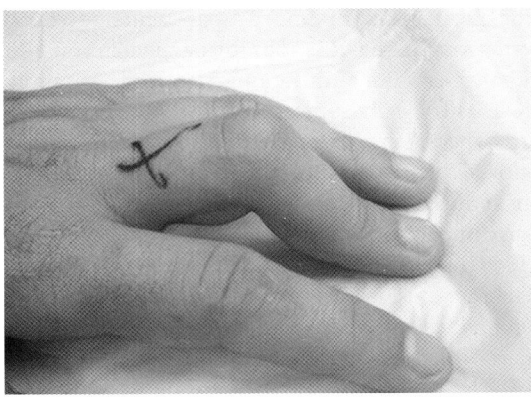

Figure 111.6   Boutonnière deformity.

posturing of the finger in flexion at the PIP joint and extension at the DIP joint. This classic type boutonnière deformity typically develops over a period of 7–14 days[11,15,20,22] (Fig. 111.6). In the acute setting a central slip injury may manifest as swelling, erythema and tenderness at the base of the dorsal middle phalanx, although these findings are not reliably present. Diagnosis in the acute phase depends on a careful history and a high index of suspicion. One method for making the diagnosis is to test active extension at the PIP joint following a digital block to provide pain relief. Weakness suggests a central slip injury. Alternatively, the metacarpophalangeal (MCP) and wrist joints can be held in full flexion while asking the patient to actively extend the PIP joint. An extensor lag of greater than 20° is indicative of a central slip injury.[21]

Treatment for acute closed boutonnière deformities is with immobilization of the PIP joint in extension allowing for free motion of the DIP joint for 6–8 weeks. This treatment regimen assumes that there is full passive extension of the PIP joint.[11,15] Free motion of the DIP joints prevents stiffness and reduces the chance of contracture of the lateral bands and oblique retinacular ligament. Night splinting should be continued for an additional 2–3 weeks following continuous splinting.[22]

The window for treatment of acute closed central slip ruptures in this fashion is 3 weeks. After 3 weeks, signs of fixed deformity may already be present, and splinting should be attempted for at least 3 months as long as the joint is supple and passively correctable.[22] Typically, splinting is required for at least 8 weeks in these cases and is achieved in the same fashion as for acute injuries. If the PIP joint is not passively correctable, a dynamic splint is used until the PIP joint deformity has resolved followed by a dorsal extension splint for at least 8 weeks.[21]

Injuries presenting later than 3 weeks that are associated with marked joint stiffness are referred to as chronic boutonnière deformities.[22] A trial of splinting for these injuries is not unreasonable as most surgical options are complicated procedures requiring up to a year of rehabilitation and therapy along with strong patient commitment for optimum results.[21] Surgical intervention includes repair and shortening of the central slip, anatomic relocation of the lateral bands, free tendon grafting and release of associated adhesions.[11,21] K-wires are used to hold the PIP joint in extension for 3 weeks postoperatively followed by 6 weeks of splinting after removal of the K-wire. It is important to note that splinting and hand therapy should be utilized pre-operatively to attain full passive motion of the PIP joint prior to surgery.[11]

A two-stage reconstruction procedure is required for the stiffened PIP joint deformity that does not respond to dynamic splinting. First, the volar plate and lateral bands are released until the PIP joint can be placed in the neutral position. Following 6–8 weeks of dynamic splinting the central slip can be reconstructed.[21] Surgical treatment for the acute boutonnière deformity is advocated for volar dislocations of the PIP joint with soft-tissue interposition and for large avulsion fractures.[11,15,21]

Zone IV–VIII injuries

Zone IV injuries are lacerations of the proximal phalanx distal to the MCP joint and proximal to the PIP joint. Complete lacerations are rare, and partial lacerations may undergo primary repair using 4-0 or 5-0 non-absorbable suture if they are greater than 50% of the total tendon width.[20,22] Splinting of the PIP joint in neutral with the MCP joint in 30° of flexion and the wrist joint in 30° of extension can help prevent flexion posturing of the PIP joint postoperatively due to volar migration of the lateral bands. Appropriate therapy protocols are critical to preventing adhesions at the MCP and PIP joints.[20] Primary repair is indicated for greater than 50% rupture of the EDC tendon.[22]

Zone V injuries involve the area of the MCP joint and are a common location for abrasions and lacerations of the hand, with the long and ring fingers being most frequently involved. Care must be taken to inspect, clean and irrigate all wounds in the zone V region as the thin joint capsule can easily be disrupted in this region. The presence of a puncture wound should be considered to be a human bite until proven otherwise. These wounds should be treated with surgical debridement followed by antibiotics. Primary repair of the extensor tendons and sagittal bands should be delayed until the infection clears.[20] Primary repair is indicated for greater than 50% rupture of the EDC tendon.[22] Less than 50% of lacerations with extension against resistance is an indication for protective splinting and supervised mobilization.

Zone VI injuries involve the area of the metacarpals proximal to the DIP joint and distal to the carpometacarpal joint. The thin subcutaneous tissue in this region makes injury to the underlying EDC common, even with relatively benign lacerations. Injury to the dorsal ulnar and superficial radial nerves can occur. Dynamic splinting with the wrist in 30° of extension and the MCP joint in neutral along with early protected range of motion (ROM) exercises is utilized postoperatively to minimize the risk of adhesions.[20] Primary repair is indicated for greater than 50% rupture of the extensor tendon. Less than 50% lacerations with extension against resistance is an indication for protective splinting and supervised mobilization.[22]

Injuries to zone VII involve the wrist and injuries to zone VIII involve the distal forearm. Zone VII injuries are complex because they involve the extensor retinaculum.[20] Primary repair for tendons with a greater than 50% laceration is recommended but care must be taken to avoid adhesions and to preserve the extensor retinaculum to prevent bow stringing of extensor tendons.[20,22] Repair can be difficult secondary to retracted proximal tendons in the forearm. Postoperatively the wrist is maintained in 20° of extension with the MCP joints in the neutral or partially flexed position.[22]

Swan neck deformity

A swan neck deformity refers to hyperextension of the PIP joint with flexion of the DIP joint.[23] In athletes this deformity is seen in chronic untreated mallet finger or untreated volar plate injury.[11] The deformity is most commonly seen in patients with rheumatoid arthritis, but may be present in individuals with spasticity or fracture malunion with associated ligamentous laxity[11,23] (Fig. 111.7).

Depending on the initial injury, the incompetence of the volar plate or the disruption of the distal extensor mechanism can lead to concentration of the extensor mechanism at the PIP joint as the terminal tendon insertion slides proximally.[21] The lateral bands then migrate dorsally leading to relative lengthening of the extensor mechanism.[5,11] Thus, the intrinsic muscles increase deformity at the PIP joint, whereas increased relative pull of the FDP increases the deformity at the DIP joint. Both exercise and splinting

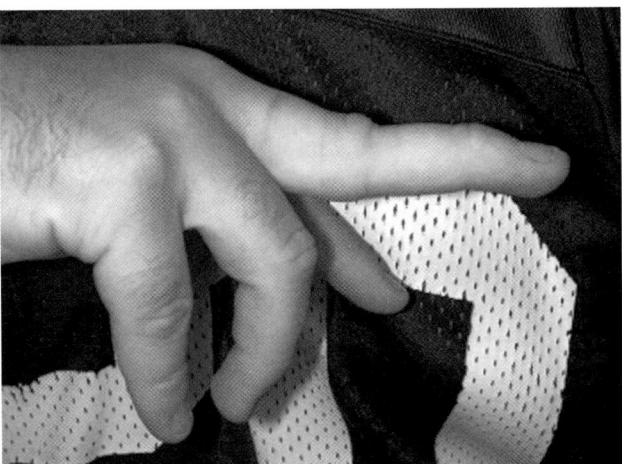

Figure 111.7 Swan neck deformity. Reproduced from Green D, Hotchkiss R, Pederson W (eds). *Green's Operative Hand Surgery*, vol. 1, 5th edn. Philadelphia, PA: Elsevier Churchill Livingstone, 2005:193.

may be attempted to relieve intrinsic muscle tightness and fixed contractures.[5,11] However, definitive treatment of a swan neck deformity is surgical intervention.[12,21]

Two surgical methods are commonly employed for correction of a swan neck deformity and include the Fowler procedure and oblique retinacular ligament reconstruction.[12,21] The Fowler method involves a central slip tenotomy and can often be performed under local anaesthesia.[12] The removal of the central slip extension force at the PIP joint allows the FDS to be opposed only by the dorsally migrated lateral bands and often restores balance at the joint. If adequate scar is present at the disrupted terminal extensor tendon (after mallet finger injury) then the DIP joint often resets into neutral.[21] Oblique retinacular ligament reconstruction, which was originally described by Thompson,[24] involves the use of a free tendon graft that is first fixed to the dorsal base of the distal phalanx and then passed around the digit at the level of the PIP joint in such a way as to pass dorsal to the neurovascular bundle but volar to the flexor pulleys before being attached to the middle phalanx radially.[12,21,24] The tendon graft is secured in a volar position that allows for full extension of the DIP joint with the PIP joint in 15–25° of flexion.[5,11] Tuttle et al.[12] recommend the use of the Fowler procedure because of its technical simplicity, proven record of success and decreased risk of overcorrection, which can occur with oblique retinacular ligament reconstruction. In patients with severe damage to the PIP joint, an arthrodesis or arthroplasty should be considered rather than primary correction of the swan neck deformity.[5,11,12]

PIP joint injuries

Injuries occurring at the PIP joint include dislocations, fracture–dislocations and collateral ligament injuries. Dislocation of the PIP joint is common in ball-handling sports and is often reduced in the field by 'pulling the finger' of the affected athlete. Unfortunately, because PIP joint dislocations can involve ligamentous damage and in some cases are fracture–dislocations, it is critical to not dismiss these injuries as they can result in long-term disability. Dislocations of the PIP joint are usually dorsal, with lateral and volar dislocations also occurring but not as frequently. The most common mechanism of injury is an axial force causing hyperextension of the joint.[22]

In a dorsal dislocation of the PIP joint the middle phalanx is displaced dorsally to the proximal phalanx.[25] Dorsal dislocations result in rupture of the volar plate with longitudinal disruption of the collateral ligaments.[22,25,26] Typically, these injuries are reducible and stable.[25] Reduction is accomplished by applying axial traction to the finger with PIP flexion to reduce the joint. Following reduction, injury to the collateral ligaments should be ruled out in both extension and slight flexion of the PIP joint.[22] In certain situations when a dorsal dislocation occurs in combination with a twisting-type force the head of the proximal phalanx may displace and buttonhole between the volar plate and flexor tendon, making closed reduction difficult or impossible. Additionally, the volar plate, lateral band or profundus tend may be interposed within the PIP joint preventing closed reduction. In these situations surgical intervention is usually necessary to obtain adequate reduction.[25]

Dorsal dislocations can be classified into three categories. In type I dislocations there is avulsion of the volar plate from the middle phalanx and a small longitudinal tear in the collateral ligaments, but the articular surfaces remain in contact. Treatment for a type I dislocation is acute reduction and buddy taping to adjacent fingers with early ROM until resolution of symptoms. Type II injuries are defined by avulsions of the volar plate from the middle phalanx with large longitudinal splits in the collateral ligaments and dorsal dislocation of the middle phalanx so that it rests on the dorsal condyle of the proximal phalanx. These dislocations are reduced as described above and treated with buddy taping for 3 weeks, allowing for early ROM. Lastly, a type III injury involves a fracture dislocation. Treatment of fracture dislocation of the PIP joint is discussed separately below.[26]

Lateral dislocations occur due to avulsion (partial or complete) of the volar plate from the middle phalanx and rupture of one collateral ligament.[25] Treatment is controversial for lateral dislocations. McCue et al.[19] advocate surgical repair of ruptured collateral ligaments and associated volar plate injuries for lateral dislocations in athletes.[22] Freiberg et al.[25] advocate treatment with simple buddy taping to the adjacent fingers for 3 weeks.

Volar dislocation of the PIP joint is a rare injury and can be classified as straight volar, lateral volar or rotatory.[15] The most common mechanism of injury is a longitudinally directed compressing force with concurrent rotation of the semi-flexed middle phalanx along the PIP joint.[26] This leads to rupture of one collateral ligament, followed by volar dislocation of the middle phalanx and disruption of the central slip. Partial disruption of the transverse retinacular ligaments and volar plate can also occur.[22] Straight volar and volar lateral dislocations occur from varus or valgus forces in concert with a volar blow to the middle phalanx.[15] Initial treatment is closed reduction followed by splinting of the PIP joint in extension to prevent the formation of a boutonnière deformity. PIP splinting should be continued for 6 weeks.[15] McCue et al.[19] recommend surgical repair for these injuries with repair of the central slip and collateral ligaments along with transarticular pinning of the PIP joint in full extension for 3 weeks.[22] In most rotatory-type volar dislocations, closed reduction is not possible because the dorsal condyle of the proximal phalanx is buttonholed between the central slip and lateral band.[26] Open reduction is the preferred treatment in these cases with open repair of the central slip and transarticular pinning of the PIP joint for 3 weeks.[15] Failure to appropriately recognize and treat a volar dislocation of the PIP joint can result in chronic boutonnière deformity.[22]

Most collateral ligament injuries of the PIP joint involve the radial collateral ligament (RCL). They are usually secondary to axially directed forces causing 'jamming of the finger', and may be treated with splinting, buddy taping, and early ROM. The index finger is most commonly involved. Minimal laxity may only require splinting for 7–10 days whereas moderate laxity may require splinting for 2–3 weeks. Complete tears of the RCL are a rare occurrence and should be repaired surgically if the index finger is involved, soft-tissue interposition is present, or there is dynamic instability manifested by subluxation of the PIP joint with active ROM.[15] McCue recommends repair of all complete collateral ligament ruptures in athletes.[22]

Fracture dislocation of the PIP joint occurs by the same mechanism as simple dislocation of the PIP joint and is classified as a type III dislocation injury.[15,22] Fracture dislocations may be either volar or dorsal, although dorsal fracture dislocations are much more common.[27] Dorsal fracture dislocations occur as the base of the middle phalanx is driven proximally and dorsally into the proximal phalanx resulting in a volar base fracture of the middle phalanx and a dorsal dislocation of the PIP joint.[27] Because this area of the middle phalanx serves as an attachment for collateral ligaments and the volar plate, instability can become severe with relatively small avulsion fractures of the volar articular surface.[15,26]

Type III dislocation injuries are classified as stable or unstable based on the degree of bony involvement.[26,27] A stable type III dislocation involves less than 30% of the articular surface, allowing a portion of the collateral ligament to remain intact on the middle phalanx. In an unstable type III dislocation injury greater than 40% of the articular surface is involved, leading to complete separation of the volar plate and collateral ligaments from the middle phalanx.[26,27] Unsupported lateral radiographs are critical to making the diagnosis, and examination with fluoroscopy may be utilized if lateral radiographs fail to provide a clear picture of the extent of bony involvement.[15] Reduction of these injuries is undertaken by applying longitudinal traction to the PIP joint followed by flexion of the PIP joint.[27,28] If a concentric reduction is achieved with flexion of the PIP joint for injuries involving less than 30–40% (type II stable) of the articular surface, Glickel and Barron[27] recommend splinting these injuries in a dorsal extension block splint, which maintains the level of flexion necessary for the initial reduction (Fig. 111.8). The patient is then followed up weekly to confirm by radiographs that the PIP joint is well aligned. The extension block is decreased by 15° each week, with radiographic confirmation that the joint is still stable after increasing the amount of extension allowed at the joint. Patients usually gain full extension in 3–8 weeks, and are then splinted for an additional 2 weeks, usually with buddy taping to the adjacent digit.[27] The most common complication following the conservative treatment of these injuries is a stiff PIP joint that often takes months to regain acceptable ROM.[28]

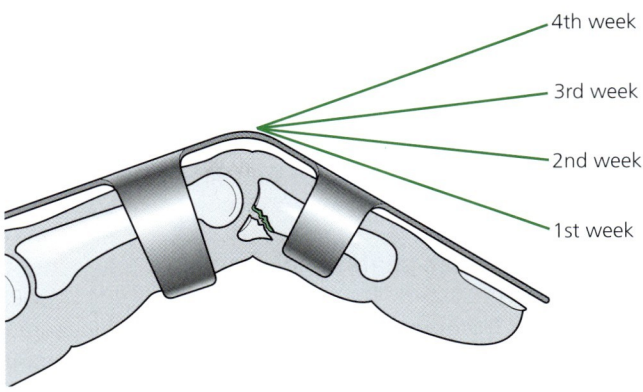

Figure 111.8 Dorsal blocking splint.

For injuries involving greater than 30–40% of the articular surface treatment recommendations vary. Fracture dislocations with minimally comminuted fragments can be treated by ORIF of the large bony fragment, closed reduction with percutaneous pinning and a dorsal extension blocking splint, and the use of a dorsal extension blocking splint alone if the PIP joint is stable in flexion.[15,26,27] For comminuted and chronic fracture dislocations volar plate arthroplasty as described by Eaton and Malerich[29] may be necessary.[15]

PIP joint intra-articular fractures

Intra-articular fractures of the PIP joint may be simple, involving only one or two bony fragments, or may be extensively comminuted to the point of total joint destruction.[25] PIP joint intra-articular fractures typically involve the condyles of the proximal phalanx or the articular surface of the middle phalanx. Fractures may involve one or both condyles and are usually oblique in nature.[22] Fractures without displacement may be treated with splinting of the involved PIP joint in slight flexion along with the MCP joint and the adjacent finger. Care must be taken to obtain weekly radiographs following splinting, as both unicondylar and especially bicondylar fractures can be associated with late malunion causing rotary displacement secondary to the pull of the collateral ligaments.[22] Fractures that involve one or two large bony fragments are considered unstable and often require surgical intervention.[25] For those fractures with greater than 1–2 mm of displacement, marked obliquity, rotational deformity and large intra-articular fragments, ORIF with K-wires or mini-screw fixation is advisable.[15,22,25] Freiberg et al.[25] recommend internal fixation or percutaneous pinning for the fracture patterns just described as it allows for early active motion postoperatively with the use of an extension blocking splint. Return to sports should be delayed 3–6 weeks to allow for complete healing of the fracture site.[15,22] Severely comminuted pylon-type fractures are best managed by dynamic traction and early ROM (Fig. 111.9a–c). The extent of soft-tissue damage should be considered when determining treatment options.

Extra-articular phalangeal fractures

Phalangeal fractures are a common injury in athletes and should be taken seriously, as derangement in phalangeal function can affect the function of the entire hand. Fractures along the phalangeal shaft are classified as comminuted, transverse, oblique or spiral in nature.[30] Direct blows to the phalanges are likely to cause transverse or comminuted fractures, whereas twisting forces often result in spiral or oblique fracture patterns. In many cases phalangeal fractures display angular deformity and displacement, which is secondary to the pull of the intrinsic hand musculature on the associated fracture fragments and the initial mechanism of injury.[31]

The initial evaluation of phalangeal fractures includes a clinical examination to elicit the mechanism of injury and rule out associated soft-tissue damage to tendons, ligaments and neurovascular structures.[32] The alignment of the digit should be determined in both full flexion and extension with careful comparison with the contralateral hand to rule out clinically obvious deformity, malrotation or misalignment. Local anaesthesia may be necessary to appropriately assess alignment of the phalanges as the patient may be too uncomfortable initially to fully flex or extend the digit. Radiographic examination consists of oblique, posteroanterior and lateral films of the injured finger. Placing the wrist and hand in 10–15° of supination provides a better lateral view of the fourth and fifth metacarpals; the same degree of pronation provides a better lateral view of the second and third metacarpals.[31]

Phalangeal fractures which are non-displaced as indicated by no rotational deformity and less than 10° of angulation can be treated conservatively with buddy taping and splinting with protected ROM initiated at 3 weeks.[30] Following reduction, any phalangeal fracture with greater than 5 mm of shortening, greater than 15° of angular deformity or any rotational deformity should be treated surgically.[31] Percutaneous pinning may be possible with K-wires, although in some cases interposed soft-tissue (ligaments of Cleland and Grayson) may make this difficult and ORIF becomes necessary.[28,31]

Fractures of the proximal phalanx (P1) tend to displace with dorsal angulation secondary to the pull of the interossei on the proximal fragment of the phalanx.[32] The dorsal angulation is increased by the transmitted extension force through the PIP joint from the central slip of the extensor mechanism.[31] In athletes fracture most frequently occurs distally in the neck of the proximal phalanx, although fractures can occur in the diaphysis and base of P1 as well.[32]

Fractures at the base of P1 are typically transverse and may be treated with immobilization alone if stable after reduction or percutaneous pinning if stability is not achieved as outlined by the criteria above. Stable fractures are immobilized with the MCP joint in flexion and should allow for free motion of the PIP joint. Unstable fractures following reduction are treated with percutaneous pinning.[32] Following pinning, these fractures are immobilized as described for stable fractures. K-wires should be removed at 3 weeks and protected ROM initiated.[32]

Diaphyseal fractures of the proximal phalanx tend to be stable secondary to the fibrous tissue surrounding the involved phalange. They occur from direct blows to the proximal phalanx. Non-displaced fractures are treated with buddy taping to the adjacent finger and early ROM.[15,32] Unstable fractures may be treated with closed reduction by applying traction with PIP joint flexion followed by percutaneous pinning to stabilize the reduction.

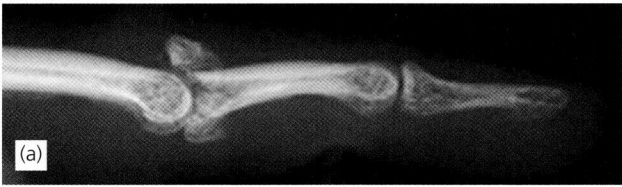

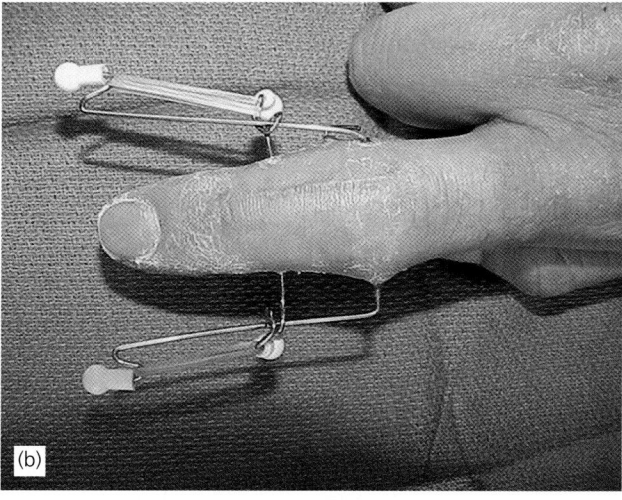

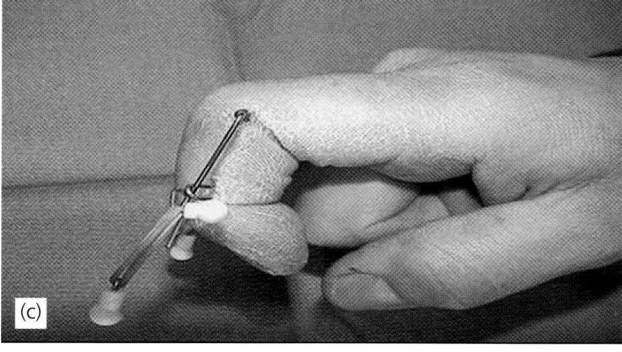

Figure 111.9 (a) Pilon fracture. (b) Dynamic traction splint. (c) Dynamic traction splint allows finger range of motion.

Following reduction, the digit should be splinted to the adjacent finger(s).[32]

For spiral and oblique fractures, rotational misalignment becomes a concern. Accordingly, either ORIF or percutaneous pinning is the appropriate treatment, with care to keep K-wires and screws perpendicular to the fracture line.[31] Fractures of the distal neck of P1 frequently undergo rotational deformity. Treatment usually requires closed reduction and percutaneous pinning. This is accomplished by placing crossed K-wires through the condyles of P1.[32] In certain cases (athletes) lag screw fixation is the preferred treatment method to allow early rehabilitation.

Fractures of the middle phalanx (P2) are relatively uncommon compared with the distal and proximal phalanx because of the load-absorbing properties of the surrounding PIP and DIP joints along with the inherent characteristics of its hard cortical bone. Fractures are usually transverse or oblique in nature and occur from direct blows to P2.[32] Fractures distal to the FDS insertion in the distal half of the bone display apex volar angulation whereas more proximal fractures may display dorsal angulation secondary to the pull of the central slip of the extensor mechanism.[31] Regardless of fracture site, both the FDS and central slip exert deforming forces on the bone, and fractures in the middle two-thirds of the bone may not display angulation in the sagittal plane.[32] In some cases, an extensor lag or flexion contracture may be observed.[31]

Proximal fractures which are non-displaced may be treated with buddy taping and splinting with ROM initiated as soon as tolerated. Displaced and unstable fractures should be treated with closed reduction and percutaneous pinning or rigid screw fixation to maintain appropriate alignment. If dorsal angulation is severe, it may be necessary for the splint to include the wrist to stabilize the deforming forces of the FDS. Fractures of the distal portion of P2 can be associated with severe volar angulation secondary to the strong pull of the FDS on the proximal fragment. If adequate reduction cannot be obtained by closed means, percutaneous pinning or ORIF may be necessary. Fractures in this region may be slow to heal, and improper treatment or malunion can result in a swan neck deformity or an extensor lag of the DIP joint secondary to extensor tendon adhesions.[32]

Fractures of the distal phalanx (P3) constitute over half of all hand fractures, with the middle finger being most commonly affected.[32] Fracture tends to occur at the tuft of the distal phalanx from a crushing force or at the base from an axially directed force.[31] Avulsion fractures of the dorsal and volar lip can occur secondary to mallet and jersey finger-type injuries respectively.[11] Associated nail bed injuries must be managed appropriately along with fractures to the tuft of the distal phalanx, and the pain with these fractures may be severe due to rapid haematoma formation from the rich blood supply of the fingertip and nail bed.[33]

Fractures at the base of P3 occur in sports such as baseball, football and karate where axially directed forces across the DIP joint are common.[31] Non-displaced proximal fractures of P3 can be managed with a DIP splint extending past the fingertip that allows for free motion of the PIP joint and is worn for 3 weeks. Displaced and angulated fractures may require percutaneous pinning with K-wires across the DIP joint kept in place for 3 weeks.[32]

Associated injuries to the nail bed such as lacerations or nail plate avulsion may occur. In some cases an avulsed nail plate may interpose between the fracture fragments, necessitating irrigation of the wound and nail bed repair with or without K-wire fixation of the associated fracture.[31]

Distal tuft fractures of P3 are typically comminuted, but the fragments are often held in place by the fibroseptae volarly and the nail plate dorsally.[31,32] In some of these patients a subungual haematoma will be present. If the haematoma takes up more than 50% of the nail bed then evacuation of the haematoma with nail bed exploration is traditionally indicated.[5] Some recent studies have suggested that, in an uncomplicated injury, even large subungual haematomas may not have to be drained.[34–36] Recommended treatment is placement of a splint across the DIP joint for 3 weeks, with return to regular activities or athletics typically possible in approximately 7–14 days.[31,32] Unfortunately, up to 70% of patients have continued pain in the fingertip 6 months after injury, with up to one-third having malunion of the fracture site. A hand therapist can play an important role in the rehabilitation of these patients.[32]

FINGERTIP AND NAIL BED INJURIES

Anatomy review

The nail and its surrounding structures are known as the perionychium, which consists of the nail plate, nail bed and hyponychium[37] (Fig. 111.10). The nail plate is the tough keratinized covering of the dorsal distal finger, often referred to as the fingernail. The nail bed lies deep to the nail plate and consists of a germinal and sterile matrix. The germinal matrix, which is responsible for the majority of nail growth, begins at the origin of the nail bed and inserts distal to the extensor tendon insertion at the lunula. The lunula is

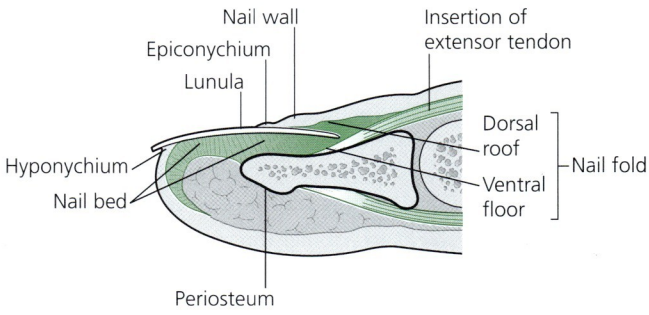

Figure 111.10 Nail anatomy. Redrawn with permission from Green D, Hotchkiss R, Pederson W (eds). *Green's Operative Hand Surgery*, vol. 1, 5th edn. Philadelphia, PA: Elsevier Churchill Livingstone, 2005:390.

the proximal white semicircular portion of the nail.[38] The sterile matrix begins at the lunula and ends at the hyponychium. The hyponychium is the intersection of the skin of the fingertip with the sterile matrix. The eponychium refers to the soft tissue on the proximal portion of the nail, which is an extension of the skin on the dorsal finger. The nail fold consists of the eponychium, the dorsal nail plate and the nail wall. The paronychium refers to the folds on each side of the nail plate where the nail meets the skin of the finger.[37,38]

Fingertip lacerations

Lacerations of the fingertip are common and are typically treated by the Accident and Emergency physician.[39] The management of these injuries must take into account the degree of tissue loss, damage to the nail bed and associated distal phalanx fractures.[40] It is important to obtain radiographs to rule out fracture and check for the possibility of foreign bodies.[39]

Simple volar lacerations of the fingertip that do not extend to the bone or involve visible ligament or tendon injury can be repaired primarily.[40] Treatment involves copious irrigation and debridement of the laceration followed by closure with non-absorbable monofilament sutures that may be removed in 1 week's time. Wounds that are obviously contaminated should be left open following thorough irrigation and debridement.[39]

Dorsal lacerations often involve the underlying nail bed, and thus treatment for these injuries involves primary repair of the injured nail bed. To treat these injuries the nail plate must be removed with a small curved elevator or curved iris scissors. In either case, care is taken to avoid further damage to the underlying nail bed when removing the nail plate.[37] Lacerations of the nail bed can be repaired under loupe magnification with 6-0 or 7-0 chromic suture (Fig. 111.11). The nail plate is then cleaned, trimmed at the corners and positioned back in to the nail fold and may be sutured back into place at the hyponychium with nylon suture. Alternatively, the nail plate may be reattached proximally at the nail fold. This provides a protective biological cover for the nail bed.[37,41] If the nail is not available to be reattached, an artificial nail can be used as a substitute.[41] Brown[37] recommends the use of 0.05 cm (0.020 inch) silicone because it is malleable enough to fit under the nail fold, and strong enough to provide adequate protection. Alternative materials include the aluminium foil from suture packaging (e.g. 1 nylon). Following repair, the wound can be wrapped in gauze dressing, which is removed at 5–10 days.[41] A cap splint can then be worn for an additional 2 weeks to protect the repair.[37]

More complex stellate lacerations of the nail bed can still be repaired primarily by reapproximating the various fragments of nail bed. It is important to carefully inspect the underside of the nail bed for portions of matrix, as they can be reapplied to the nail bed directly as a graft.[37,41] If portions of the sterile matrix are lost, a split-thickness graft

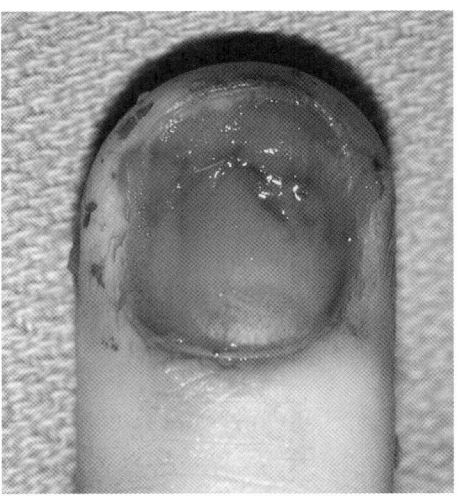

Figure 111.11 Nail bed repair.

is necessary for proper repair of the nail bed. The split-thickness sterile matrix graft can often be taken from the adjacent finger, and is sutured in place with 7-0 chromic suture.[37,41] The graft can be harvested with a 15 blade scalpel, and a template is taken from the matrix defect to ensure that the proper size graft is harvested.[37] Large defects in the sterile matrix that represent greater than 50% of the total area should be replaced with split-thickness grafts from the great toe.[41] The graft should be less than 0.03 cm (0.011 inches) thick to prevent deformity at the donor site.[42] Shepard[43] reports that, in a series of 84 patients treated with sterile matrix grafts, 75 obtained good results postoperatively. Moreover, in the nine patients who had suboptimal results, the defect in the nail occurred at the site of original injury, not at the donor site.[43]

Avulsions that result in the loss of the germinal matrix are more difficult to treat than sterile matrix injuries. The first option for replacement of the germinal matrix is the presence of the original tissue on the underside of the damaged nail plate.[37] If this is not available, a graft of germinal matrix can often be taken from one of the toes, usually the great toe. The graft must be full thickness, and will leave a nail defect in the donor digit.[41] If a large graft is necessary (greater than 33–50%), the entire nail bed of the donor digit should be ablated to prevent the formation of nail spikes. The germinal matrix graft can be sutured to the injured matrix with 7-0 chromic suture.[37] Nail deformity is common.

Subungual haematoma

A direct blow or crushing injury to the fingernail can cause bleeding from the fingernail's rich vascular bed. Subungual haematomas can be so small that they are missed clinically or so large they create enough pressure to cause separation of nail from the underlying finger. Small haematomas require no treatment as the blood will gradually be reabsorbed on its own.[33] Traditionally, a haematoma that involved

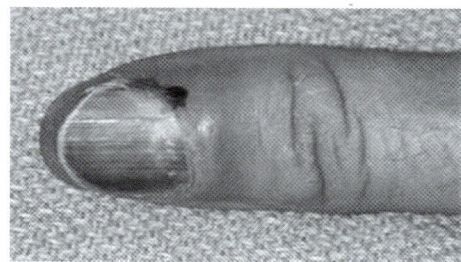

Figure 111.12 Subungual haematoma.

greater than 50% of the nail bed is an indication for nail plate removal and exploration[32,33,37,41,42] (Fig. 111.12). More recent studies have suggested that all nail bed haematomas can be treated with trephining alone.[34–37,40] Trephinization can be accomplished by making a hole in the fingernail with a hot microcautery unit followed by soaking in sterile water or betadine.[33] If the nail plate is dislodged from the nail bed or side walls then removal of the nail with exploration of the nail bed is indicated.[37] Care should be taken when draining a large haematoma, as many of these may be associated with open distal phalanx fractures, thus converting a closed to an open fracture.

Radiographs are mandatory as approximately half of nail bed injuries are associated with distal phalanx fractures.[37] Antibiotics following irrigation and debridement should be considered if an open fracture is present.[32,33,37] Comminuted fractures of the distal tuft can often be treated with nail bed repair and splinting alone. More proximal fractures often require pinning with K-wires to prevent rotation of the fracture fragment following reduction. Fractures that are more proximal with minimal displacement can be stabilized with the nail plate alone. This is accomplished by reattaching the nail plate with a dorsal figure-of-eight suture just distal to the hyponychium and just proximal to the nail fold that is tied back on itself.[37]

Traumatic amputations of the fingertips

Amputation of the fingertip can lead to loss of superficial skin, subcutaneous tissue, sensory nerve structures, and in severe cases loss of a portion of the tuft of the distal phalanx.[39] Associated loss of all or a portion of the nail bed can make the treatment of these injuries difficult. A decision must often be made in regards to ablating the nail bed and appropriate coverage of the remaining fingertip.[37]

The degree of tissue loss can be used to help differentiate among treatment options.[33] For wounds smaller than 1 cm², healing by secondary intention is appropriate treatment.[33,42] The advantage of this treatment is its simplicity, high patient satisfaction and relatively few complications.[42] Complete healing can be expected in 3–5 weeks, and daily soaks in a warm solution of water and peroxide should begin at 7–10 days after injury and continue until the wound has healed. Bandaging is accomplished with non-adherent dressing and a fingertip protector.[33,42]

Larger wounds should be managed surgically with the application of a skin graft. If the fingertip is being covered with a graft, it should be full thickness to provide for maximum sensation and durability with decreased contraction and tenderness postoperatively. The hypothenar area is the preferred donor site because of the durability of the skin and its relative similarity to the skin of the fingertip. Skin grafts as large as 2 cm can be taken and still allow for primary closure of the donor site. For transverse or dorsal oblique amputations a V–Y flap is often appropriate (Fig. 111.13). Regional flaps such as a cross-finger flap (Fig. 111.14) or a thenar flap are often necessary for volar oblique amputations or for replacing large losses of fingertip pulp tissue.[42]

In cases of soft-tissue loss that result in exposure of bone, primary closure is usually not possible.[42] In certain situations, a rongeur can be used to trim back the exposed bone, and then healing by secondary intention can be attempted but is often associated with nail plate deformities.[40,42] If there is loss of bony support, it is generally best to shorten the nail bed back to the level of the remaining distal phalanx.[37] Coverage of the defect is then attempted with primary closure or the use of local or regional flaps.[42] In either case, care should be taken to avoid tension in the primary repair or grafted skin as this can lead to curvature of the distal nail plate causing a painful hook-nail deformity.[37]

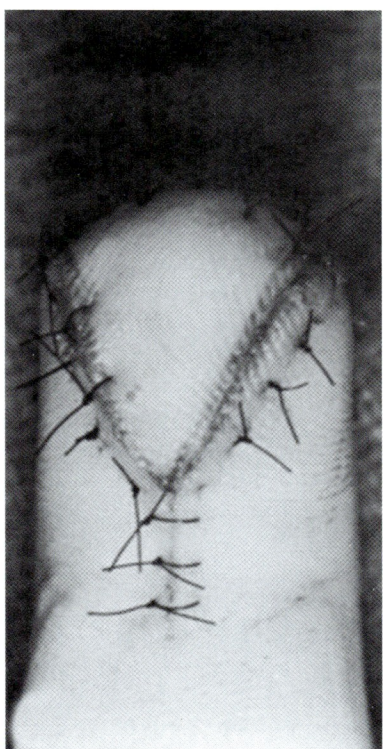

Figure 111.13 V–Y advancement flap. Reproduced from Green D, Hotchkiss R, Pederson W (eds). *Green's Operative Hand Surgery*, vol. 1, 5th edn. Philadelphia, PA: Elsevier Churchill Livingstone, 2005:1668.

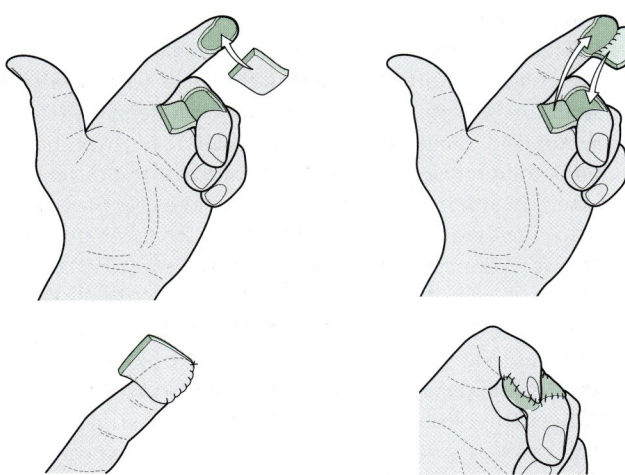

Figure 111.14 Cross-finger flap. Redrawn with permission from Green D, Hotchkiss R, Pederson W (eds). *Green's Operative Hand Surgery*, vol. 1, 5th edn. Philadelphia, PA: Elsevier Churchill Livingstone, 2005:1670.

KEY LEARNING POINTS

- Trigger finger, also called stenosing tenosynovitis, most commonly affects the thumb, ring and middle fingers.
- Finger lacerations must be taken seriously and not explored in the Accident and Emergency Department.
- Volar lacerations are localized using a modification of Verdan's zones of the hand (five distinct zones) and eight zones dorsally.
- Mallet finger, disruption of the terminal tendon of the extensor mechanism insertion at the base of the dorsal distal phalanx, is the most common closed tendon injury. Either splint or operate when it involves more than one-third of the articular surface with volar dislocation.
- The boutonnière deformity is from central slip rupture.
- A swan neck deformity is hyperextension of the proximal interphalangeal (PIP) joint with flexion of the distal interphalangeal joint.
- PIP joint dislocations can result in long-term disability.
- Phalangeal fractures should be taken seriously, as malfunction here can affect the function of the entire hand.
- For traumatic amputations of the fingertips with exposure of bone, primary closure may not be possible; it is better to shorten the nail bed back to the level of the remaining distal phalanx and then carry out primary closure.

REFERENCES

● = Key primary paper
◆ = Major review article

1. Bonnici AV. Survey of trigger finger in adults. *Journal of Hand Surgery* 1988;**13**:202–3.
2. Fleish SB, Spindler KP, Lee DH. Corticosteroid injections in the treatment of trigger finger: a level I and II systematic review. *Journal of the American Academy of Orthopedic Surgeons* 2007;**15**:166–71.
◆3. Ryzewicz M, Wolf JM. Trigger digits: principles, management, and complications. *Journal of Hand Surgery* 2006;**31A**:135–46.
◆4. Rettig AC. Wrist and hand overuse syndromes. *Clinical Sports Medicine* 2001;**20**:591–611.
5. Craig EV. *Clinical Orthopaedics*. Philadelphia, PA: Lippincot Williams and Wilkins, 1999.
6. Overton DT, Uehara DT. Evaluation of the injured Hand. *Emergency Medicine Clinics of North America* 1993;**11**:585–600.
◆7. American Society for Surgery of the Hand. *The Hand: Examination and Diagnosis*, 3rd edn. Rosemont, IL: ASSH, 1990.
◆8. Boyer MI, Strickland JW, Engles DR, et al. Flexor tendon repair and rehabilitation: state of the art in 2002. *Journal of Bone and Joint Surgery (American)* 2002;**84**:1684–706.
9. Steinberg DR. Flexor tendon lacerations in the hand. *University of Pennsylvania Orthopaedic Journal* 1997;**10**:5–11.
10. Steinberg DR. Acute flexor tendon injuries. *Orthopedic Clinics of North America*. 1992;**23**:125–40.
◆11. Aronowitz ER, Leddy JP. Closed tendon injuries of the hand and wrist in athletes. *Clinical Sports Medicine* 1998;**17**:449–67.
12. Tuttle HG, Olvey SP, Stern PJ. Tendon avulsion injuries of the distal phalanx. *Clinical Orthopaedics and Related Research* 2006;**445**:157–68.
13. Stamos BD, Leddy JP. Closed flexor tendon disruption in athletes. *Hand Clinics* 2000;**16**:359–65.
●14. Leddy JP, Packer JW. Avulsion of the profundus tendon insertion in athletes. *Journal of Hand Surgery* 1977;**2**:66.
◆15. Rettig AC. Athletic injuries of the wrist and hand. Part II. Overuse injuries of the wrist and traumatic injuries to the hand. *American Journal of Sports Medicine* 2004;**32**:262–73.
16. Meals RA. Flexor tendon injuries. *Journal of Bone and Joint Surgery (American)* 1985;**67**:817–21.
17. Patel MR, Shekhar SD, Bassini-Lipson L. Conservative management of chronic mallet finger. *Journal of Hand Surgery* 1986;**11**:570–3.
●18. Doyle JR. Extensor tendons-acute injuries. In: *Green's Operative Hand Surgery*. New York, NY: Churchill Livingstone 1992:1925–54.
●19. McCue FC III, Wooten, SL. Closed tendon injuries of the hand in athletics. *Clinical Sports Medicine* 1970;**5**:741–56.

20. Blair WF, Steyers CM. Extensor tendon injuries. *Orthopedic Clinics of North America* 1992;**23**:141–8.
21. Scott SC. Closed injuries to the extensor mechanism of the digits. *Hand Clinics* 2000;**16**:367–73.
22. Brunton LM, Chhabra AB. Hand, upper extremity, and microvascular surgery. In: Miller MD (ed.) *Review of Orthopaedics*, 5th edn. Philadelphia, PA: W.B. Saunders, 2008:505–70.
23. Nalebuff EA. The rheumatoid swan-neck deformity. *Hand Clinics* 1989;**5**:203–14.
◆24. Thompson RV. An evaluation of flexor tendon grafting. *British Journal of Plastic Surgery* 1967;**2**:21–44.
25. Freiberg A, Pollard BA, Macdonald MR, Duncan MJ. Management of proximal interphalangeal joint injuries. *Hand Clinics* 2006:**22**;235–42.
◆26. Palmer RE. Joint injuries of the hand in athletes. *Clinics in Sports Medicine* 1998;**17**:513–31.
27. Glickel SZ, Barron OA. Proximal interphalangeal joint fracture dislocations. *Hand Clinics* 2000:**16**:333–44.
28. Culver JE, Anderson TE. Fractures of the hand and wrist in athletes. *Clinics in Sports Medicine* 1992;**11**:101–28.
◆29. Eaton RG, Malerich MM. Volar plate arthroplasty of the proximal interphalangeal joint: a review of ten years of experience. *Journal of Hand Surgery* 1980;**5**:250–68.
30. Peterson JJ, Bancroft LW. Injuries of the fingers and thumbs in athletes. *Clinics in Sports Medicine* 2006;**25**:527–42.
◆31. Lee SG, Jupiter JB. Phalangeal and metacarpal fractures of the Hand. *Hand Clinics* 2000:**16**:323–32.
◆32. Capo JT, Hastings H. Metacarpal and phalangeal fractures in athletes. *Clinics in Sports Medicine* 1998;**17**:491–511.
33. Hart RG, Kleinert HE. Fingertip and nail bed injuries. *Emergency Medicine Clinics of North America* 1993;**11**:755–65.
34. Roser SE, Gellman H. Comparison of nail bed repair versus nail trephination for subungual hematomas in children. *Journal of Hand Surgery* 1999;**24**:1166–70.
35. Seaberg DC, Angelos WJ, Pairs PM. Treatment of subungual hematomas with nail trephination: a prospective study. *American Journal of Emergency Medicine* 1991;**9**:209–10.
36. Batrick N, Hashemi K, Freij R. Treatment of uncomplicated subungual hematoma. *Emergency Medicine Journal* 2003;**20**:65.
◆37. Brown RE. Acute nail bed injuries. *Hand Clinics* 2002;**18**:561–75.
38. Zook EG. Anatomy and physiology of the perionychium. *Hand Clinics* 2002;**18**:553–9.
39. Stevenson TR. Fingertip and nailbed injuries. *Orthopedic Clinics of North America* 1992;**23**:149–59.
40. Brown DJ, Jaffe JE, Henson JK. Advanced laceration management. *Emergency Medicine Clinics of North America* 2007;**25**:83–99.
41. Van Beek AL, Kassan MA, Adson MH, Dale V. Management of acute fingernail injuries. *Hand Clinics* 1990;**6**:23–35.
42. Fassler PR. Fingertip injuries: evaluation and treatment. *Journal of the American Academy of Orthopedic Surgeons* 1996;**4**:84–92.
43. Shepard GH. Management of acute nail bed avulsions. *Hand Clinics* 1990;**6**:39–56.

Tendon injuries

S RAJA SABAPATHY, PRAVEEN BHARDWAJ

Introduction	1292	Acknowledgement	1301
Flexor tendon injuries in the hand	1292	References	1301
Extensor tendon injuries in the hand	1298		

NATIONAL BOARD STANDARDS

- Review of the knowledge of flexor tendon anatomy
- Biology of tendon healing
- Clinical examination
- Indications and techniques of primary repair
- Postoperative therapy protocols
- Complications
- Secondary repair and flexor tendon grafting
- Extensor tendon anatomy
- Techniques of repair
- Specific deformities following extensor tendon injury
- Mallet deformity, boutonnière deformity

INTRODUCTION

Tendons convey the power of the muscles to their insertions at the bones and cause joint movement. To increase mechanical efficacy, they are structurally well adapted. Flexor tendon injury has attracted more attention than extensor, but management of the latter is neither simple nor complication free. Primary repair of tendons in all zones is recommended, provided expertise and adequate infrastructure is available.

The goal of tendon repair is to provide adequate tensile strength at the repair site to allow application of early mobilization protocols to reduce adhesions and promote healing. It is difficult to obtain good functional outcome in zone II flexor tendon repair because of the repair site being within the confines of the pulley system. Good results are now possible by the use of multistrand suturing techniques and early controlled motion protocols in the previously termed 'no man's land'. Ruptures of repair and adhesion formation are two important complications.

While managing extensor tendon injuries one has to remember that loss of finger flexion due to a tightly repaired extensor is more disabling than extensor lag due to weak extensor action. Delay in the diagnosis and treatment in the specific zones may result in mallet or boutonnière deformities. Over the dorsum of the hand and wrist, extensor tendons have a synovial sheath similar to flexor tendons and hence they are likely to develop adhesions after repair. To prevent this, early mobilization is advisable. Zone-specific therapy protocols are followed at other levels.

FLEXOR TENDON INJURIES IN THE HAND

Introduction

Tendons are like cables transmitting the power of the muscles to their insertion in the bones to produce movement in the joints. The large forearm muscles can generate high tensile loads, up to as much as 120 N in the index finger profundus tendon with strong pinch grip.[1] Newmeyer[2] reported that, in the two decades from 1974 to 1994, the maximum number of scientific papers published in the *Journal of Hand Surgery* for any specific condition was on flexor tendon repair. Even in 2009, hand surgeons remain interested in refining the techniques of tendon repair and rehabilitation. Research continues to aim at modifying the healing process in order to improve outcome. Extensor tendon injuries have not commanded such a position in the literature, but obtaining good outcomes in the event of their injury is as demandinas, if not more than, flexor tendon repairs.

Anatomy of flexor tendons

Each finger has two long flexors, flexor digitorum superficialis (FDS) and flexor digitorum profundus (FDP), inserting into the bases of the middle and terminal phalanx respectively. The profundus takes origin from the proximal medial and anterior surfaces of the ulna and the ulnar half of the interosseous membrane, and as it passes distally all the tendons lie in the same plane up to the carpal tunnel. There is one musculotendinous unit for the middle, ring and little fingers and a separate musculotendinous unit for the index finger, which can act independently. The superficial flexor takes origin from the medial epicondyle of the humerus and the volar surface of the ulna and radius. As it passes distally, the tendons of the index and little fingers lie dorsal to the tendons of the middle and ring fingers, which become the most superficial finger flexors at the wrist level. The FDS of the little finger is thin and may sometimes be absent. At the wrist level the median nerve is more superficial than the finger flexors and its injury must always be excluded in lacerations at this level. The FDS tendon splits into two slips in the palm, allowing the profundus to pass between them with the slips passing around the FDP tendon to be inserted in the base of the middle phalanx. The lumbricals take origin from the FDP tendon as it courses along the metacarpal shaft, remain volar to the metacarpophalangeal (MCP) joint and are inserted into the lateral band of the extensor mechanism on the radial side. The thumb has only one long flexor tendon, the flexor pollicis longus (FPL), taking origin from the anterior surface of the middle third of the radius and inserting into the base of the terminal phalanx of the thumb.

THE PULLEY SYSTEM

A series of pulley systems keep the flexor tendons close to the bones (Fig. 112.1). By maintaining a short moment arm they allow conversion of limited excursion of flexor tendons to produce large joint motions needed for functional hand and finger motion. This system allows a 3 cm flexor tendon excursion to result in an arc of motion of 260°. Absence of pulleys would lead to bowstringing of tendons:

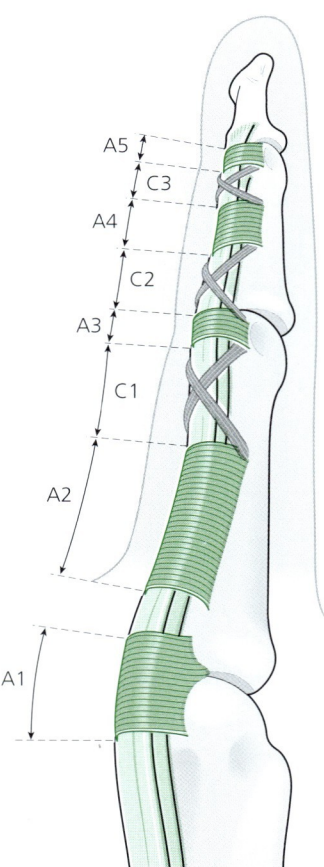

Figure 112.1 Flexor tendon pulleys in the finger. A1–A5 are the annular pulleys. C1–C3 are the cruciate pulleys.

the range of motion of a joint would be markedly decreased and the ability to straighten the fingers would be limited, leading to joint contractures.[3]

Flexor tendons enter a synovium-lined fibro-osseous tunnel at the base of the finger. Doyle and Blythe[4] in 1975 described four annular pulleys and three cruciate pulleys and later another annular pulley, A5, was described distal to the A4 pulley. The A1, A3 and A5 pulleys originate from the palmar plates of the metacarpophalangeal, proximal interphalangeal and distal interphalangeal joints respectively. The A2 and A4 pulleys are continuous with the periosteum of the proximal and the middle phalanx respectively. There are three thin cruciate pulleys and they are located between A2 and A3 (C1), between A3 and A4 (C2) and between A4 and A5 (C3). The A2 and A4 pulleys are considered to be functionally more important. The thumb has two annular pulleys and an oblique pulley with no cruciate pulleys. The oblique pulley is considered the most important (Fig. 112.2).

One centimetre proximal to the A1 pulley, the transverse fascicular fibres and paratendinous bands of the palmar aponeurosis form a 'pulley' called the palmar aponeurosis pulley (PA pulley).[5] This along with the flexor retinaculum completes the pulley system of the flexor tendons.

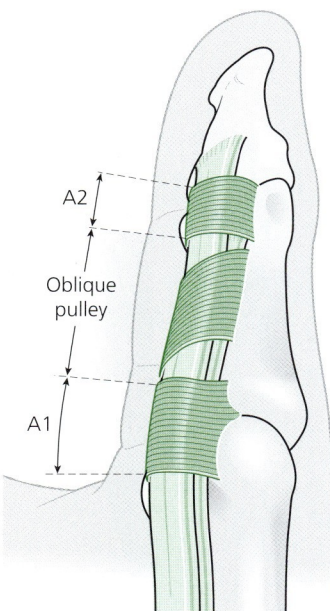

Figure 112.2 Flexor tendon pulleys in the thumb. A1 and A2 are the annular pulleys.

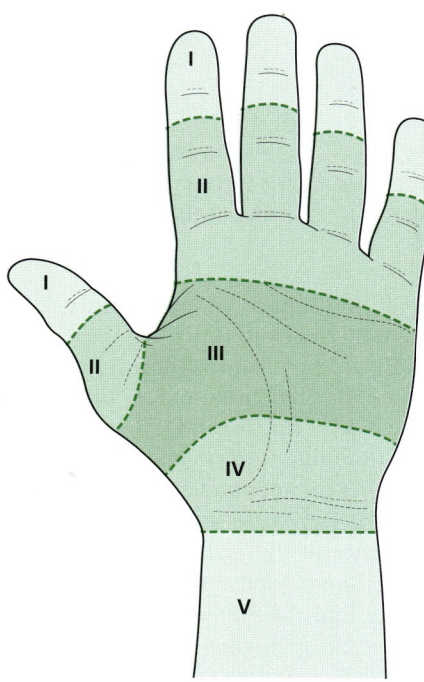

Figure 112.3 Flexor tendon zones (I–V).

ZONES OF THE FLEXOR TENDONS

The flexor tendons in the hand are divided into five zones (Fig. 112.3).

- Zone I extends from the insertion of FDP at the distal phalanx to the distal edge of the insertion of the FDS tendon into the middle phalanx. This zone contains only one tendon (FDP).
- Zone II extends from the distal edge of the FDS insertion to the proximal edge of the A1 pulley. This is the critical area where both the tendons pass through the pulleys and was referred by to as 'no man's land' by Bunnell.
- Zone III extends from the proximal edge of the A1 pulley to the distal edge of the carpal tunnel.
- Zone IV includes the flexor tendons within the carpal tunnel.
- Zone V is the zone proximal to the carpal tunnel.

In the thumb, zone I is at the region of the interphalangeal joint and the insertion of the FPL, zone II extends from the interphalangeal joint to the proximal edge of the A1 pulley and zone III is the area of the thenar eminence. Zones IV and V are the same as for the long fingers.

Tendon nutrition and biology of tendon healing

Flexor tendons get their nutrition from the local vascular networks and in addition the synovial fluid contributes to nutrition of the intrasynovial part of the tendon. Tendons heal by a combination of extrinsic and intrinsic mechanisms and the proportion of each differs in various situations. Extrinsic healing causes adhesions to the surrounding structures.

Tendon healing can be divided into three stages.

- Stage I is the inflammatory phase and lasts for about 72 hours.
- Stage II is the fibroblastic collagen production phase and it extends from 3 days to 28 days.
- Stage III is the remodelling phase, which extends from 28 days to 3 months.

Collagen fibre maturation has been found to increase with the application of early passive movement, thereby leading to more rapid recovery of tensile strength, and thus this has been applied in rehabilitation protocols, commonly called the 'place and hold' technique.[6] Controlled motion reduces adhesions, improves excursion and increases tendon nutrition, as it encourages intrinsic healing and reduces extrinsic healing and scar formation. Sutures need to be strong enough to prevent gap formation since during the inflammatory phase the strength reduces by 10–60%. Between 5 and 21 days the repair strength is essentially due to the suture. Active motion should be started before day 5, as starting after this point increases the risk of rupture.[7]

Clinical examination

In the acute situation the posture of the finger reveals the diagnosis. Partially divided tendons cannot be diagnosed by posture alone and so all lacerations along the

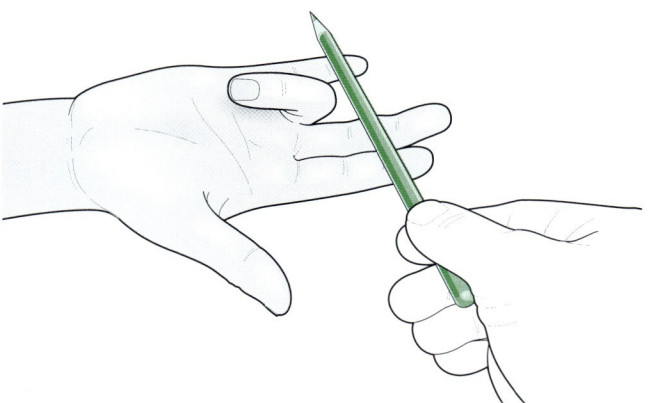

Figure 112.4 Test for flexor digitorum superficialis (FDS) of middle, ring and little fingers. Blocking the other fingers in extension prevents flexor digitorum profundus function, providing isolated FDS action.

course of the flexor tendons must be explored under tourniquet. Squeezing the volar aspect of the forearm at the level of the musculotendinous junction makes the fingers flex in a cascade. If there is a lag in the finger, the flexor is probably injured. This test is particularly useful in children. At all times sensation distal to the injury must also be tested since there is a high likelihood of combined injuries.

In elective situations, FDP is tested by the ability to flex the distal interphalangeal (DIP) joint when the middle phalanx is supported. FDS is tested by the ability to flex the proximal interphalangeal joint (PIP) joint with the other fingers held in extension (Fig. 112.4). The interconnection of the FDP tendons of the ulnar three fingers makes this test reliable for testing of the FDS of the little, ring and middle fingers. The index FDS is tested by asking the patient to perform the index–thumb pinch with the DIP joint of the index extended. In the absence of FDS, pinch is possible only with DIP flexion (Fig. 112.5).

Management of flexor tendon injuries

SURGICAL TREATMENT

Primary repair of the injured flexor tendons is recommended in all zones. Previously tendon grafting was preferred for zone II injuries. Kleinert and colleagues[8–10] showed that with meticulous surgical technique and institution of regimented postoperative therapy protocols it was safe to repair tendons in all zones and excellent results could be achieved. Tendon repairs done within 2–3 days have given equally good results, as repairs done immediately and hence primary repairs have to be carried out under ideal conditions. A good regional block anaesthesia, tourniquet, loupe magnification and experienced surgeon are essential requirements. Repair performed within 24 hours is called primary repair; between 24 hours and 10 days, delayed primary repair; 10 days to 4 weeks the

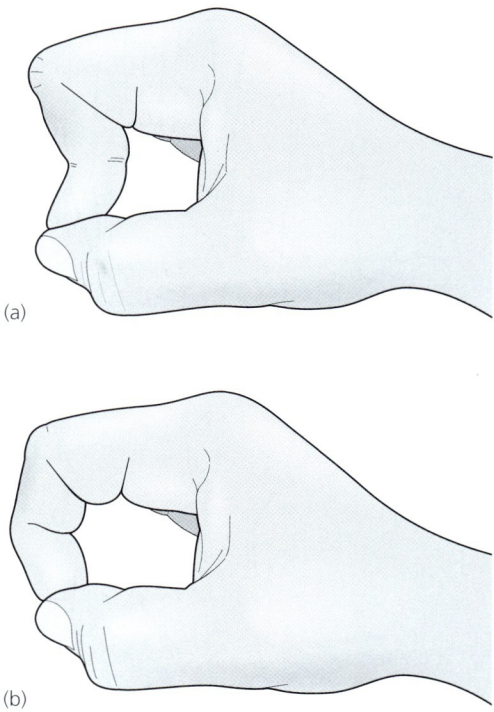

Figure 112.5 Test for flexor digitorum superficialis (FDS) of the index. Forceful tip pinch with the distal interphalangeal (DIP) joint in hyperextension (a) can only be achieved by an intact FDS tendon. If the DIP joint flexes while applying force (b), it means that FDS is either absent or non-functional.

repair is called secondary; and after 4 weeks, late secondary repair.[11]

The wound is extended by oblique Bruner's incisions, midlateral incisions (Fig. 112.6) or a combination of both. The location of the cut flexor tendon ends depends upon the posture of the fingers at the time of injury. If injury happens with flexed fingers the distal end will be very distal when the finger is extended. If the injury happens with the fingers in extension, the tendon ends will be nearer to the wound. If the distal end is easily seen when flexing the finger, the wound is extended proximally; otherwise, the wound is extended distally. Special techniques may be needed to deliver the proximal cut ends.[12]

The aim of surgery is to have a strong enough repair that allows early active mobilization and prevents tendon gapping. Early mobilization encourages intrinsic healing and reduces adhesions. Suture techniques involve a core suture and a circumferential epitendinous suture. The strength of repair increases with the number of strands in the core suture and the thickness of the suture.[13,14] A four-strand single knot core suture with 3-0 polypropylene suture and a running suture with 6-0 polypropylene has been found sufficient for the commonly followed therapy protocols (Fig. 112.7). A circumfentrial epitendinous suture is used to smoothen the tendon repair, improve gliding, reduce gapping and increase strength by 10–59%.[7] Locking epitendinous sutures give greater strength.

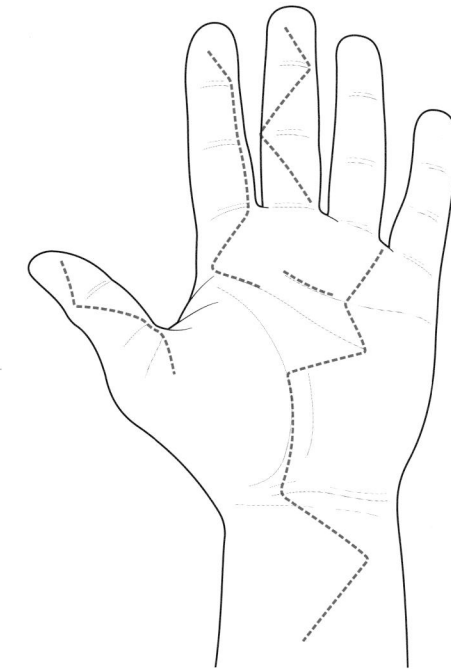

Figure 112.6 Exposure for flexor tendon repair. Either midlateral or Bruner-type incisions can be used. Straight incisions should never be placed over the flexor side of the joints.

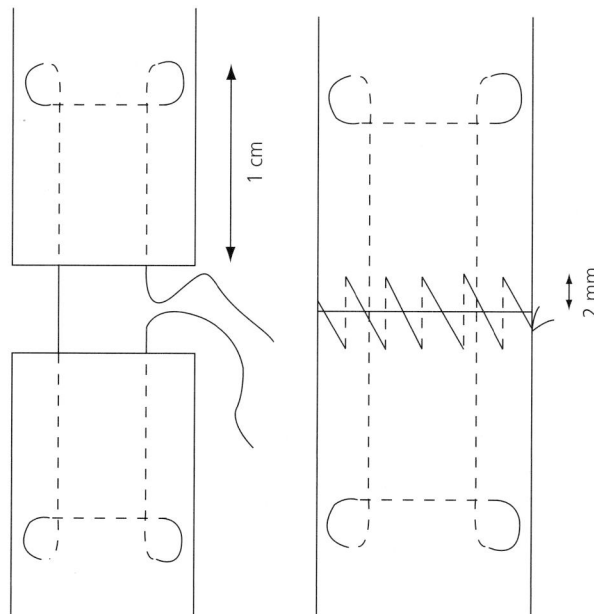

Figure 112.7 Flexor tendon suturing techniques. (a) The modified two-strand Kessler repair with the knot between the cut ends. A four-strand repair is created either by using a double suture (looped suture) or by placing a second Kessler suture next to the first one. (b) Epitendinous running suture.

ZONE I INJURY

The FDP tendon alone is injured in this zone, either by avulsion or by laceration. Avulsion occurs when forced hyperextension of the DIP joint occurs against a maximally contracting force (jersey finger). Depending upon the location of the avulsed end, Leddy and Packer[15] classified the injury into three types.

- Type I: the avulsed end has retracted to the palm.
- Type II: the avulsed end retracts to the level of FDS decussation at the level of the PIP joint.
- Type III: avulsion occurs with a large piece of bone and it is held up at the level of the A4 pulley.

Type I injuries need to be repaired immediately. Since both vinculae are injured the tendon suffers from ischaemia, the muscle undergoes adaptive shortening and the other FDP tendons suffer from the quadriga effect. The long vincula remains intact in type II injury, and hence this injury can be addressed up to 3 months with good results as long as the tendon has not further retracted. Type III injuries are managed according to the size of the bone fragment. If large, a screw can be inserted, or if small the tendon is reinserted into the base of the distal phalanx either by pull through suture or bone anchor sutures.

ZONE II INJURIES

Primary repair of both FDS and FDP tendons is recommended in zone II injuries. The advantages are that it allows independent movement of both the PIP and the DIP joints; repaired FDS provides a gliding surface for the FDP tendon and acts as a dynamic pulley. Special concern in tendon repair in this zone is that repair of the two tendons must not make it bulky to pass through the pulleys and to restore the anatomical orientation of the profundus between the slips of FDS. If the superficialis tendon is injured at the middle of zone II, the two ends may rotate 90° but in opposite directions, and the ends would, deceivingly, look to be matching. If the correct orientation is not restored, it will block the excursion of FDP.

Part of the pulley system may need to be sacrificed to gain access, but at least some part of A2 and A4 pulleys must be maintained or repaired. If the bulky repair site is tethered at the free edge of the pulley, the pulley may be vented by incising along the attachment.[16] Up to one-third of the pulley can be divided either proximally or distally without compromising the outcome. Sheath closure is not considered essential.

Primary repair of the isolated injury of superficialis or the profundus can be easily achieved. In neglected situations isolated FDP injury may need a tendon graft. Flexor tendon grafting in the presence of intact FDS needs careful consideration, as it is fraught with the danger of joint stiffness. Simpler options are tenodesis, arthrodesis of the DIP joint or no treatment at all.

ZONE III, IV AND V

The technique of repair is essentially the same as in zone II. Because the tendons are less confined at these levels than in the finger, the prognosis is better. In zone III, tendon injuries are usually associated with injury to the common digital neurovascular bundles. When exploring cut tendons in zone IV (the region of carpal tunnel) it is better to retain a part of the transverse carpal ligament to prevent bowstringing. If complete release is required for adequate exposure, the ligament can be divided in z-lengthening configuration and later repaired. If the transverse carpal ligament is completely divided and cannot be reconstructed, even partly, it is advisable to immobilize the wrist in at least neutral position instead of flexion. Tension on the repaired tendon can be reduced by increasing the flexion at the fingers. Zone V injuries often involve multiple lacerated wrist and finger flexor tendons, associated median and ulnar nerve injuries and arterial injury. For this reason a zone V injury is also referred to as 'the spaghetti wrist'. Matching the correct tendon ends is essential and is aided by testing their action on the fingers and size matching.

POSTOPERATIVE REHABILITATION PROTOCOL

Immobilization was historically used after flexor tendon repair to prevent rupture. It is now well accepted that immobilization results in marked adhesions and leads to severe stiffness and poor outcome. Presently it is used only in children and adults who do not comply with the mobilization protocol. Most hand units use any one of the following three mobilization protocols with some modification to suit their system and patients.

The modified Kleinert method

This method involves passive flexion and active extension of the finger during the healing phase of the tendon. The patient is given a dorsal protective splint to hold the wrist in 30–40° of palmar flexion, metacarpophalangeal joints in 60–70° of flexion and full extension at the proximal and distal interphalangeal joints. An elastic band is attached distally to the injured fingertip by means of a string passed through the nail or a hook glued to the nail and proximally tied to a band at the forearm. In the commonly used modification a palmar bar is added at the level of the palm as a pulley for the rubber bands to obtain a greater degree of interphalangeal joint flexion.[17] The elastic band is detached at night and the fingers are strapped to the splint in extension to prevent flexion contracture. Mobilization is started on the first day. Patients are taught to perform active extension and allow the finger to flex with the tension of the rubber band. They are taught not to perform passive extension or active flexion. At 3 weeks the dorsal splint can be removed and a wristband with hooks for the rubber band is applied and mobilization is continued in the same manner. At 6 weeks a dynamic extension splint is given to prevent flexion contracture. Strengthening exercise is started at about 8 weeks and the patient is encouraged in normal use of the hand at 12 weeks.

Duran–Houser method

This method described by Duran and Houser[18] involves controlled passive finger flexion. The patient is put on a dorsal splint with the wrist in 20° of flexion, the MCP joint in 50° of flexion and the interphalangeal joints in full extension. Mobilization is started under supervision initially and patients can later be taught to perform the exercises for themselves. The protocol involves 10 passive DIP joint extensions with PIP and MCP joint flexions, and 10 passive PIP joint extensions with MCP and DIP joint flexions hourly within the splint for 4–5 weeks. The main advantage of this method over the methods using rubber band traction is decreased incidence of flexion contracture of the PIP joint.

Belfast regimen

In the last couple of decades, an early active motion protocol is being used by more and more surgeons.[19] Belfast surgeons reported their results of this method of mobilization for repaired flexor tendons in zone II; hence it is referred to as the 'Belfast method'. Early active mobilization is made possible by the improvement of the suturing techniques. The repair has to be strong to allow early active motion lest the disastrous complication of tendon rupture will occur. The patient is put on a posterior above elbow splint with the wrist in mid-flexion, the MCP joint slightly less than 90° of flexion and the interphalangeal joints straight. Mobilization is started on the second postoperative day. Under supervision of hand therapists, the exercises consist of two passive movements followed by two active movements and are performed at 2 hour intervals. During the first week, the PIP joint is actively flexed through about 30° and the DIP joint through 5–10°. In subsequent weeks, the range of active motion is gradually increased. The splint is removed by the sixth week and blocking exercises of the interphalangeal joints are started.

Outcome measurement

The total active range of motion and the grip strength determine the final outcome of flexor tendon repair. Outcome should be determined no sooner than 3 months after surgery, when postoperative therapy is complete and before most patients would return to work.

Complications

- *Rupture.* This occurs in 4–17% of zone II repairs and 3–17% with FPL in various series. If rupture occurs, immediate surgical repair is advocated. After 3 weeks the chances of successful secondary repair are low and such cases would require tendon grafting.
- *Adhesion formation.* Dense adhesions restricting movement of the tendon occur as a result of excessive extrinsic healing. This may be prevented by proper hand therapy. Chemicals enhancing tensile strength of the repaired tendons and preventing adhesions are not

useful in regular clinical practice. Tenolysis may be performed to release adhesion if the passive range of movement exceeds the active range of movement at that joint. The conditions to be fulfilled before tenolysis are (1) minimal 3 months post-primary repair; (2) associated fractures must be well healed; (3) skin over the repair site must be soft and supple; (4) the repaired tendon must be in continuity; and (5) the patient must be compliant and motivated to undergo therapy.

- *Joint stiffness.* Unresolved adhesions will result in joint stiffness. Joint stiffness must be corrected before tenolysis.
- *Quadriga effect.* If a tendon, particularly the FDP, is shortened by more than 1 cm, the finger will reach the palm before the remaining fingers when the patient attempts to flex his fingers. This will reduce the ability to flex the uninjured fingers. The best way to prevent this is by resorting to tendon grafting if there is excessive tension at the time of tendon repair.

Flexor tendon grafting

When primary repair of injured tendons in zone I and zone II has not been done, tendon grafting has to be carried out. If the skin and the pulley systems are not badly damaged, one-stage flexor tendon grafting can be performed. Delayed treatment or multiple failed efforts to restore continuity in the flexor tendon can result in severe scarring of the digit. In this case a staged reconstruction using the initial placement of a silicon implant in the tendon bed, followed later by the replacement of that implant with a tendon graft, can offer realistic salvage possibilities.[20] An interval of 3 months is usually given between the placement of the silicone rod and the replacement of the tendon graft. Palmaris longus, plantaris and long toe extensors of the middle three toes are the sources of tendon grafts.

EXTENSOR TENDON INJURIES IN THE HAND

Introduction

Extensor tendon injuries are more common than those of the flexors because of their superficial location on the dorsum of the hand. They can be complicated by loss of overlying skin. Two important points need to be remembered when dealing with extensor tendon injuries. One, the loss of finger flexion due to tightly sutured extensors is more disabling than extensor lag.[21] The other is that neglected extensor tendon injuries can cause deformities that are difficult to correct.

Anatomy of extensor tendons

The main extensor of the digits, the extensor digitorum communis (EDC), takes origin from the lateral epicondyle of the humerus. The slip to the ring finger may be double

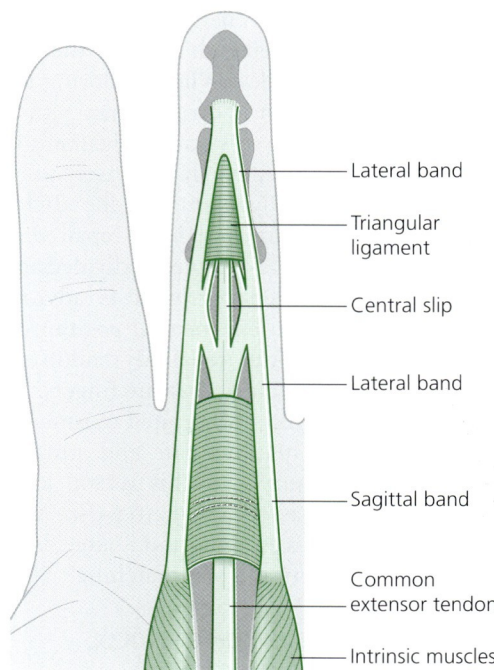

Figure 112.8 Anatomy of the extensor tendon at the finger. There is an intricate balance between the central slip arising from the common extensor digitorum and the lateral bands arising from the intrinsic muscles.

and that to the little may be absent.[22] The index and the little fingers have another separate extensor, the extensor indicis proprius and extensor digiti quinti, which lie ulnar to the communis tendon. The slips on the dorsum are interconnected by juncturae tendinum. At the dorsum of the MCP joint the extensor tendons are joined by the lumbricals on the radial side and the interossei. Together they form a triangular fibro-aponeurotic sheet called the extensor expansion. Fig. 112.8 shows the formation of the extensor expansion. The long extensors are the main extensors of the metacarpophalangeal joint. Interphalangeal extension is by the intricate balance between the long extensors and the intrinsic muscles. The thumb has two extensors, the extensor pollicis longus and brevis. The former is responsible for extension of the interphalangeal joint and the latter for the extension of the MCP joint.

Extensor tendons have been divided into nine zones (Fig. 112.9). Zones with odd numbers overly the joints and even numbered zones overly the intervening bones.[23]

Management of extensor tendon injuries

Injuries occurring over the expansion (zones I–V) are usually partial. The extensor expansion over the digits is very flat and it is not possible to apply a core suture. In these zones the preferred technique of repair is by horizontal mattress or by figure-of-eight sutures (Fig. 112.10). In zones VI, VII and VIII the extensor tendons are more oval and

Extensor tendon injuries in the hand 1299

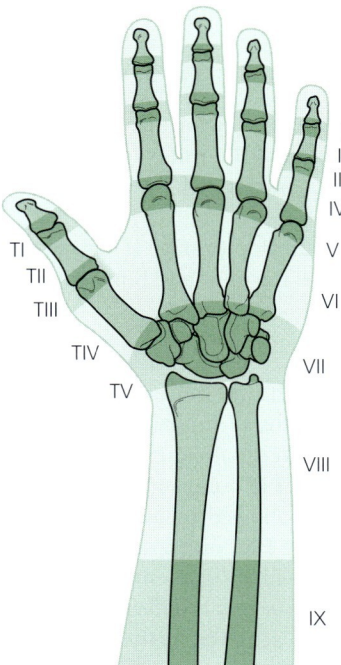

Figure 112.9 Extensor tendon zones of injury. The odd numbers overly the joints. Zone 9 is the extensor muscle.

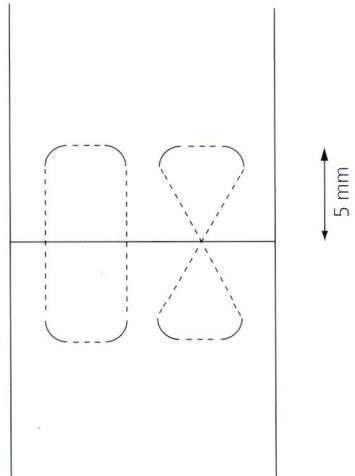

Figure 112.10 Repair of a flat extensor tendon with horizontal mattress sutures.

permit inserting a core suture with epitendinous sutures. The extensor tendons in zones VI and VII have a synovial sheath and hence the healing process is similar to flexor tendons in their synovial sheaths and adhesions after repair are common. Thus repaired tendons are likely to get stuck in their canals as they heal. To prevent this, it has been advised to partly excise the extensor retinaculum. Recently, there has been strong argument for retaining the extensor retinaculum and following an early controlled mobilization protocol to prevent adhesions.[24,25] In zone IX, since the muscle does not hold the suture well, one should identify the fibrous muscular septae and use these to hold the sutures. In zone IX and sometimes in zone VIII exact matching of the tendons may be difficult. Priority should be given to restoration of independent wrist and thumb extension. In zones I, II and III, the repair has to be protected for about 6 weeks. If patient compliance is of concern it may be necessary to fix the corresponding interphalangeal joint in extension with a transarticular K-wire. When core sutures are applied, early controlled mobilization is presently preferred.[24]

Two specific deformities due to extensor injury are discussed in detail.

MALLET FINGER

Injury to the extensor tendon in zone I results in flexion deformity of the distal interphalangeal joint. The typical deformity seen after the injury is called 'mallet finger' (Fig. 112.11b). Injury to the extensor tendon in this zone can be due to division of the tendon or more commonly avulsion of the extensor insertion. It is usually caused by forced flexion of the distal interphalangeal joint but can also occur in forced hyperextension with fracture of the

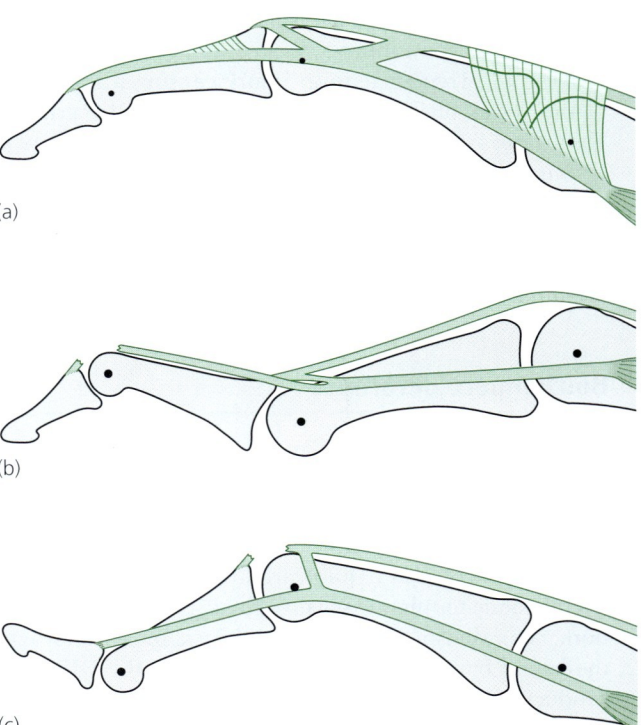

Figure 112.11 Biomechanics of mallet and boutonnière deformity. (a) Lateral view of the normal extensor tendon anatomy. (b) Mallet deformity. The extensor tendon insertion at the distal phalanx is ruptured. Compensatory hyperextension in the proximal interphalangeal joint can lead to swan neck deformity. (c) Boutonnière deformity. Rupture or attenuation of the central slip eventually leads to migration of the lateral bands volar to the axis of the proximal interphalangeal (PIP) joint. This increases the flexion deformity in the PIP joint and leads to hyperextension in the distal interphalangeal joint.

terminal phalanx and dorsal displacement. Mallet deformity can be of four types.[11]

- *Type 1.* Closed injury with or without an avulsion fracture. These are best managed with a rigid splint for the DIP in neutral alignment or hyperextension for 8–10 weeks followed by 2 weeks of night splinting. If patient compliance is a concern, it is best to fix the DIP in extension with a transarticular K-wire. The degree of displacement of the bone fragment does not influence the outcome.[26]
- *Type 2.* Open laceration of the tendon at the DIP can be repaired with a figure-of-eight non-absorbable suture or a mattress suture and splinted as above, or with a temporary K-wire across the DIP joint.
- *Type 3.* Deep abrasion with loss of tendon and overlying tissues requires thorough debridement and soft-tissue cover. Delayed reconstruction of the tendon or DIP arthrodesis may be required.
- *Type 4A.* Transphyseal fracture in a child. This is also known as a Seymour fracture. These can be managed by closed reduction and splinting for 3–4 weeks.
- *Type 4B.* Hyperflexion injury with a fracture involving 20–50% of the articular surface. The management is similar to type 1 injury.
- *Type 4C.* Hyperextension injury causing a fracture of the distal phalanx (involving >50% of the articular surface) with dorsal displacement. The management of this is controversial. Some authors feel that it can be best managed by open reduction and fixation with an interosseous wire loop. This is a tricky procedure and there is an argument for treating these injuries by simple splinting.[26]

Boutonnière deformity

Loss of continuity of the central slip leads to inability to extend the PIP joint and persistent flexion at the PIP joint. If left untreated, the transverse retinacular and triangular ligaments, which normally maintain the lateral bands dorsal to the axis of the PIP joint, are stretched. This allows the lateral bands to migrate volar to the PIP joint axis of rotation. The extensor forces of the intrinsic muscles through the lateral band are then concentrated on the DIP joint, producing hyperextension of the joint.[27] If left untreated, the lateral bands will remain in this abnormal volar position by the contracture of the volar portion of the transverse retinacular ligament, with subsequent lateral band shortening (Fig. 112.11c). In chronic cases there is shortening of the oblique retinacular ligament and contracture of the PIP joint collateral ligaments, capsule and volar plate and intra-articular fibrosis. Eventually bony changes set in. The combination of flexion at the PIP joint and extension at the DIP joint is called boutonnière deformity, the French word for buttonhole, as the head of the proximal phalanx buttonholes through the dorsal defect, allowing the lateral bands to migrate volar to the PIP joint axis of rotation.

Boutonnière deformity can be divided into three stages.[28]

- Stage I is a dynamic deformity with passively correctable deformity of the PIP joint.
- Stage II is characterized by a fixed PIP joint flexion contracture.
- Stage III in addition to stage II has secondary soft-tissue contracture at the joint and bony changes in longstanding cases.

Surgical correction of the boutonnière deformity is technically difficult and not always successful. In stage I, even after 6 months of injury, the preferred treatment is splinting and exercises. The exercise programme consists of active assisted PIP joint extension to stretch the tight volar structures followed by active assisted flexion of the DIP joint with the PIP joint in extension. This will stretch the oblique retinacular ligament and lateral bands.

In stage II the surgery is deferred until full range of passive movement is achieved at the PIP joint. In a few cases end-to-end repair of cut ends may be possible. The PIP joint should be able to passively flex fully without rupturing the repair. In most of cases the gap in the central slip will require reconstruction.

In stage III arthrodesis of the PIP joint is the preferred option

KEY LEARNING POINTS

Flexor tendon
- Specific tests can aid in diagnosing flexor digitorum superficialis and flexor digitorum profundus injuries.
- Associated nerve or arterial injury is common and should always be looked for.
- Flexor tendon repair requires a meticulous technique to allow smooth gliding with adequate tensile strength for early controlled motion.
- The A2 and the A4 pulleys are essential and need to be at least partially preserved in zone II.
- Early controlled motion prevents adhesion formation and promotes tendon healing.
- Delay or a failed repair in zone II requires a staged repair with grafting of the tendon.

Extensor tendon
- Extension of the fingers depends on the intricate balance of common extensors and intrinsic muscles.
- In zones I–V the tendon is flat and cannot hold a core suture. The repair consists mainly of mattress or figure-of-eight sutures.
- In zones VI, VII and VIII the tendon is round and can hold a core suture and an epitendinous suture.

- Mallet deformity results from a zone I extensor tendon injury and consists of a flexed distal interphalangeal joint (DIP) joint with inability to extend.
- Boutonnière deformity results from a central slip injury in zone III and consists of a flexion deformity of the proximal interphalangeal joint joint with compensatory hyperextension at the DIP joint.
- Closed zone I and III injuries have equally good results with splinting as with surgical treatment.

ACKNOWLEDGEMENT

The authors would like to thank Dr Katleen Libberecht for creating the illustrations and for editorial help.

REFERENCES

- ● = Key primary paper
- ◆ = Major review article

◆1. Strickland JW. The scientific basis for advances in flexor tendon surgery. *Journal of Hand Therapy* 2005;**18**:94–110; quiz 1.

◆2. Newmeyer WL 3rd. History of the journal of hand surgery: 1976–1999. *Journal of Hand Surgery (American)* 2000;**25**:5–13.

◆3. Goodman HJ, Choueka J. Biomechanics of the flexor tendons. *Hand Clinics* 2005;**21**:129–49.

◆4. Doyle JR, Blythe W. The finger flexor tendon sheath and pulleys: anatomy and reconstruction. In: Hunter JM, Schneider LH (eds) *AAOS Symposium on Tendon Surgery in the Hand*. St. Louis, MO: Mosby, 1975:81–7.

●5. Manske PR, Lesker PA. Palmar aponeurosis pulley. *Journal of Hand Surgery (American)* 1983;**8**:259–63.

●6. Gelberman RH, Woo SL, Lothringer K, et al. Effects of early intermittent passive mobilization on healing canine flexor tendons. *Journal of Hand Surgery (American)* 1982;**7**:170–5.

◆7. Rust PA, Eckersley R. Twenty questions on tendon injuries in the hand. *Current Orthopaedics* 2008;**22**:17–24.

●8. Kleinert HE, Kutz JE, Ashbell TS, Martinez E. Primary repair of lacerated flexor tendons in 'no man's land'. *Journal of Bone Joint Surgery (American)* 1967;**49A**:577.

●9. Kleinert HE, Kutz JE, Atasoy E, Stormo A. Primary repair of flexor tendons. *Orthopedic Clinics of North America* 1973;**4**:865–76.

●10. Lister GD, Kleinert HE, Kutz JE, Atasoy E. Primary flexor tendon repair followed by immediate controlled mobilization. *Journal of Hand Surgery (American)* 1977;**2**:441–51.

◆11. Wright II PE. Flexor and extensor tendon injuries. In: Canale ST (ed.) *Campbell Operative Orthopaedics*, 9th edn. St. Louis, MO: Mosby, 2004:3318–76.

●12. Sourmelis SG, McGrouther DA. Retrieval of the retracted flexor tendon. *Journal of Hand Surgery (British)* 1987;**12**:109–11.

●13. Thurman RT, Trumble TE, Hanel DP, et al. Two-, four-, and six-strand zone II flexor tendon repairs: an in situ biomechanical comparison using a cadaver model. *Journal of Hand Surgery (American)* 1998;**23**:261–5.

●14. Winters SC, Gelberman RH, Woo SL, et al. The effects of multiple-strand suture methods on the strength and excursion of repaired intrasynovial flexor tendons: a biomechanical study in dogs. *Journal of Hand Surgery (American)* 1998;**23**:97–104.

●15. Leddy JP, Packer JW. Avulsion of the profundus tendon insertion in athletes. *Journal of Hand Surgery (American)* 1977;**2**:66–9.

◆16. Elliot D. Primary flexor tendon repair – operative repair, pulley management and rehabilitation. *Journal of Hand Surgery (British)* 2002;**27**:507–13.

●17. Cooney WP, Lin GT, An KN. Improved tendon excursion following flexor tendon repair. *Journal of Hand Therapy* 1989;**2**:102–13.

◆18. Duran RE, Houser RG. Controlled passive motion following flexor tendon repair in zones two and three. In: *The American Academy of Orthopaedic Surgeons: Symposium on Tendon Surgery in the Hand*. St. Louis, MO: Mosby, 1975:105–14.

●19. Savage R, Risitano G. Flexor tendon repair using a 'six strand' method of repair and early active mobilisation. *Journal of Hand Surgery (British)* 1989;**14**:396–9.

◆20. Strickland JW. Delayed treatment of flexor tendon injuries including grafting. *Hand Clinics* 2005;**21**:219–43.

●21. Newport ML, Blair WF, Steyers CM, Jr. Long-term results of extensor tendon repair. *Journal of Hand Surgery (American)* 1990;**15**:961–6.

●22. von Schroeder HP, Botte MJ. Anatomy of the extensor tendons of the fingers: variations and multiplicity. *Journal of Hand Surgery (American)* 1995;**20**:27–34.

◆23. Kleinert HE, Verdan C. Report of the Committee on Tendon Injuries (International Federation of Societies for Surgery of the Hand). *Journal of Hand Surgery (American)* 1983;**8**(Pt 2):794–8.

●24. Chow JA, Dovelle S, Thomes LJ, et al. A comparison of results of extensor tendon repair followed by early controlled mobilisation versus static immobilisation. *Journal of Hand Surgery (British)* 1989;**14**:18–20.

●25. Evans RB, Burkhalter WE. A study of the dynamic anatomy of extensor tendons and implications for treatment. *Journal of Hand Surgery (American)* 1986;**11**:774–9.

◆26. Watts AC, Hooper G. Extensor tendon injuries in the hand. *Current Orthopaedics* 2004;**18**:477–83.

◆27. Mah ET, Ng YO. Repair and reconstruction of extensor tendons. In: Venkataswami R (ed.) *Surgery of the Injured Hand: Towards Functional Restoration*: Maidenhead, UK: McGraw Hill, 2010:260.

◆28. Burton RI, Melchior JA. Extensor tendons-late reconstruction. In: Green DP (ed.) *Operative Hand Surgery*, 4th edn. New York, NY: Churchill Livingstone, 1999:1988–2021.

113

Nerve injuries

ROLFE BIRCH

Peripheral nerve injuries	1302	Acknowledgement	1307
Nerve injuries in fractures and dislocations	1306	References	1307
When should the injured nerve be explored?	1306	Further reading	1308

NATIONAL BOARD STANDARDS

- Know the structure, function and classification of peripheral nerves
- Understand the importance of the level of injury, depth of injury and factors in the prognosis
- Learn some common nerve injuries and when to explore them

PERIPHERAL NERVE INJURIES

The consequences of nerve injury are severe. The immediate effects of laceration of a main nerve include (1) paralysis, (2) loss of sensation and (3) sometimes severe neuropathic pain. The later consequences include (1) atrophy of the skin and soft tissues, (2) unnoted injury, (3) progressive deformity from muscle imbalance and (4) growth disturbance in children.

The concentration of so much functional and relay capacity concentrated in so small a volume of tissue is unique to the nervous system. The peripheral nerves contain motor fibres to end plates in skeletal muscle, sensory fibres from organs and endings in skin, muscle, tendon, periosteum and bone and joint, efferent autonomic fibres to smooth muscle and blood vessels, sweat glands and hair follicles and visceral afferent fibres. Nerve fibres are classified as A, B or C based upon whether they are myelinated, their diameter and their conduction velocity (Table 113.1).

The essential component of the system is the neurone, the nerve cell body with its dendrites and its prolongation, the axon (Fig. 113.1). The nerve fibre is defined as the axon, its axolemma and the enveloping Schwann cells. The Schwann cell is far more than a supporting element, for

Table 113.1 Nerve type classification

Axon type	Myelination	Diameter (μm)	Speed (m s^{-1})	Function
Aα	Yes	20	80	Efferent to skeletal muscle; afferent from muscle spindles and tendon
Aβ	Yes	10	50	Afferent: Merkel, Meissner, Pacinian, Ruffini, hair follicle
Aγ	Yes	5	20	Efferent to muscle spindles
Aδ	Yes	5	20	Fast pain, cold sensation (e.g. a knife)
B	Yes	3	10	Preganglionic autonomic
C	No	1	2	Post-ganglionic autonomic – slow pain and thermoreceptors

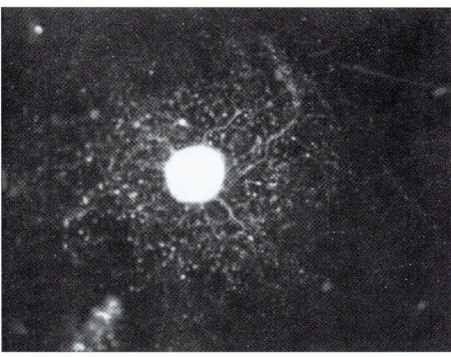

Figure 113.1 Cultured human dorsal root ganglion neurone immunostained for Gap 43 (growth-associated protein) showing the cell body and neurites arising from the cell body (×40). Courtesy of Dr Uma Anand.

without it the development, maturation, survival and regeneration of the neurone cannot occur. Nerve fibres possess two special properties, both of which are ATP driven; both are blocked by anoxia.

- *Axoplasmic transport* is the mechanism by which the cell body communicates with the periphery, and receives signals and sustenance from it. The fast systems convey neurotransmitters to the periphery and neurotrophins from the periphery to the cell body. The slow system delivers structural proteins and membrane components to the periphery. Loss of centrifugal transport blocks conduction and axon growth while loss of the centripetal process leads to degeneration and to death of the cell body.
- *Nerve conduction.* The action potential is a brief, self-propagating reversal of membrane polarity and it depends on an initial influx of sodium ions which causes a reversal of polarity to about 40 mV followed by a rapid return towards the resting potential as potassium ions flow out. In the unmyelinated fibre, the wave of depolarization spreads continuously along the axon, limiting the velocity of conduction to about 1 m s^{-1}. In the myelinated fibre the myelin sheath acts as a capacitor and limits radial resistance at the internodes, so that most of the current flows axially along the fibre; conduction velocity may be up to 80 m s^{-1}. The calibre of unmyelinated axons varies from 0.4 to 1.25 μm, that of myelinated fibres from 2 to 22 μm. The largest, fasting conducting fibres are concerned with somatic afferent and efferent activity; the smallest and slowest conducting fibres subserve autonomic activity and delayed pain sensitivity. The influx and efflux of ions across the axon membranes occurs through voltage-gated ion channels which are uniformly distributed along the axon membrane of non-myelinated fibres. In myelinated nerve fibres the excitatory sodium ion channels are densely concentrated at the nodes of Ranvier whereas the inhibitory potassium channels are concentrated in the axon membrane at the juxtaparanode.

Nerve fibres lie in the endoneurium, chiefly composed of collagen fibres and fibroblasts. They are organized into bundles (fascicles) by a strong cellular envelope, the perineurium. Bundles are aggregated into a nerve trunk by the epineurium, which is a well-defined translucent envelope. Translucent arcades of connective tissue, the paraneurium, pass to the nerve trunk, which provides a pathway for the extrinsic blood supply and enables gliding of the nerve trunk. The extrinsic blood supply interconnects with the intrinsic network of blood vessels within the epi-, peri- and endoneurium.

Although the blood supply to peripheral nerves is generally abundant there are important variations. At the knee the supply to the common peroneal nerve is much weaker than it is to the tibial nerve.[1] The blood supply to the ventral and dorsal roots of the spinal nerves is much less than it is to the nerve itself. However, radicular vessels, passing with roots through the intervertebral foramina, provide vital contributions to the longitudinal systems nourishing the spinal cord, especially to the anterior spinal artery. Their occlusion, by interscalene or other forms of nerve block, may lead to infarction of the cord. Main nerves and vessels are often enclosed within sleeves of fascia, predisposing the nerve to ischaemia and compression from bleeding (Fig. 113.2).

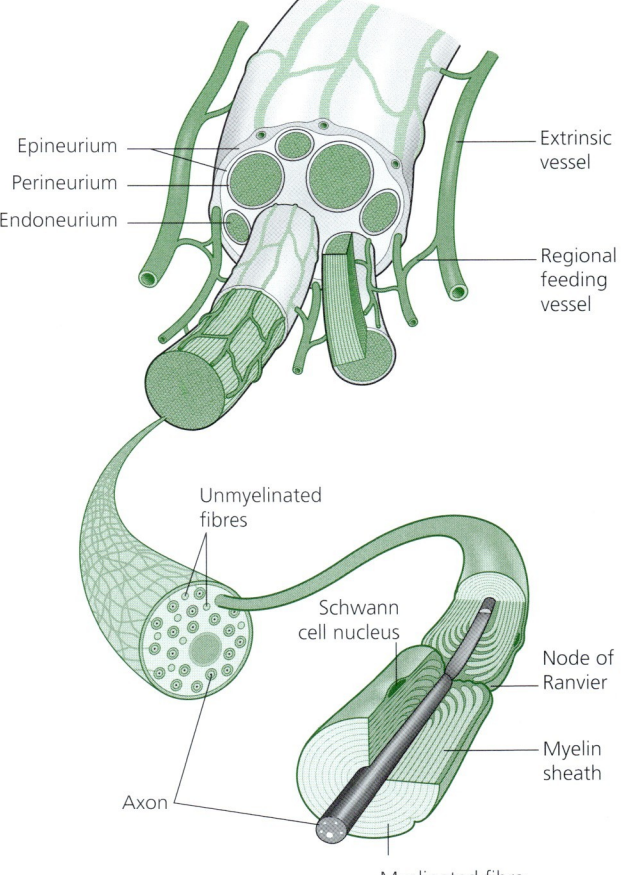

Figure 113.2 Fascicular arrangement of nerve fibres and their supporting structures, the vascular systems of the peripheral nerve.

Some peripheral nerves are particularly vulnerable in skeletal injuries. The sacral nerve is particularly at risk in fractures involving the sacral foramina. The great mobility of the shoulder girdle puts the brachial plexus at risk from traction. The proximity to bone of the main nerves at the elbow render all three vulnerable to skeletal injury. The radial nerve is relatively fixed in the tunnel through the intermuscular septum, the sciatic trunk at the sciatic notch and the common peroneal nerve at the neck of the fibula.

Clinical examination usually shows where the nerve is injured and whether that injury is complete or incomplete. It is more difficult to distinguish between the lesion of conduction block (neurapraxia) from the deeper lesions of Wallerian degeneration (axonotmesis, neurotmesis).

The level of the injury to the nerve

Accurate diagnosis of the level of the lesion requires a sound knowledge of the course and distribution of the main nerves in the limbs and of the site of their main branches.[2] Lesions of the sciatic nerve are often, incorrectly, placed at the knee, to the common peroneal nerve. Such errors are prevented by examining gluteus medius (superior gluteal nerve), gluteus maximus (inferior gluteal nerve) and biceps femoris (common peroneal division). The level of injury to the posterior cord or radial nerve can be determined by examining the teres major (inferior scapular nerve), latissimus dorsi (thoracodorsal nerve) and deltoid (circumflex nerve). The nerves to the long head of the triceps leave the main trunk within the axilla; those to the medial head leave at the entrance to the spiral groove. Branches to the lateral head leave the main nerve more distally. The nerve to the brachioradialis consistently passes away from the radial nerve about three fingers' breadth of the lateral epicondyle; the nerve to extensor carpi radialis longus comes off about one finger's breadth more distal.

Depth of injury

Neurotmesis occurs when a main nerve is severed by a fragment of bone or ruptured by violent traction. All modalities of function are lost. Wallerian degeneration ensues. The distal segment of the axon disintegrates. Conduction diminishes and, after several days, disappears altogether. Wallerian degeneration affects the whole neurone and the central changes are intensified by the violence of the injury and by proximity to the cell body. They may culminate in the death of the neurone. A nerve which has been transected or ruptured cannot recover until it is repaired and the sooner that is done the better.[3]

In *axonotmesis* the axons are divided, the columns of Schwann cells and the basal lamina remain intact. There is Wallerian degeneration, but spontaneous regeneration can occur. Neurotmesis and axonotmesis can be distinguished only by exploration of the nerve or by awaiting events.

Conduction block (neurapraxia) is a non-degenerative lesion: the axon is intact.

The mildest form is produced by the transient ischaemia of a tourniquet and it affects principally the large myelinated fibres. There is little interference with sudomotor and vasomotor (sympathetic) function. It is caused by anoxia of the voltage-gated ion channels. Recovery occurs within minutes of release of the cuff and it is accompanied by painful, spontaneous sensory symptoms (dysaesthesia). Displaced fractures or missile wounds cause conduction block by displacement, or stretching, of the nerve trunk. Paralysis exceeds loss of sensation, proprioceptive fibres are more deeply affected than those light touch fibres and sympathetic function is least affected. Distortion of the myelin sheath caused by a bone fragment or haematoma, or external pressure leads to prolonged conduction block (Fig. 113.3).

It should never be forgotten that the continuing action of the responsible agent will transform the lesion of the nerve from a conduction block to a much less favourable one[4] (Fig. 113.4).

The depth of the lesion often varies between groups of nerve fibres. The sciatic trunk injured by posterior dislocation of the hip is usually a mixture of neurapraxia, axonotmesis and neurotmesis. A diagnosis of neurapraxia of the whole nerve is extremely unlikely in the following circumstances:

1. High-energy transfer injury. If there is a wound over the line of the nerve, and if there is any suggestion of loss of sensibility or impairment of motor function in the distribution of that nerve, then *it must be regarded as having been cut until and unless it is proved otherwise.*

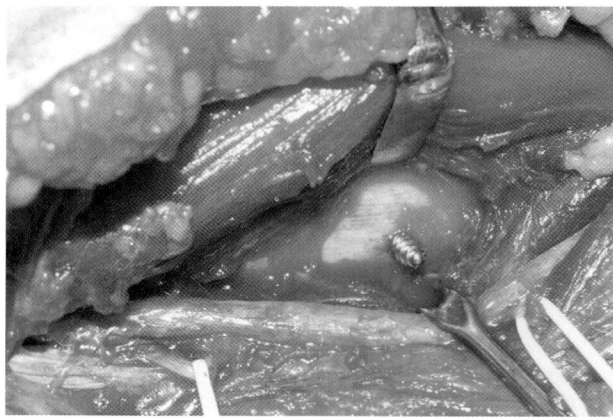

Figure 113.3 Conduction block. The radial nerve shown tented over the tip of the screw 10 days after operation for fracture. There was a painful deep radial palsy. Conduction in the distal segment was preserved but there was no conduction across the lesion. Conduction in the nerve to brachioradialis (left-hand sling) was preserved. Stimulation of the radial nerve above the level of lesion did not evoke response through the nerve to extensor carpi radialis longus (right-hand sling). The screw was shortened. Recovery was complete by 24 hours.

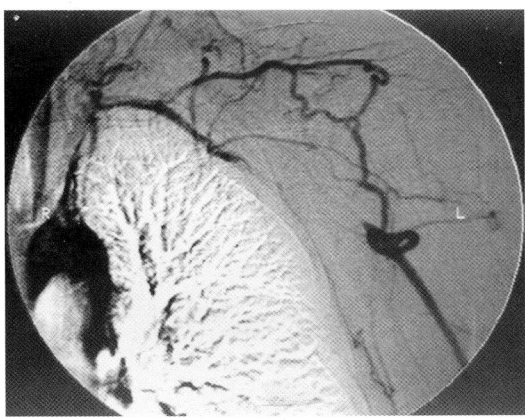

Figure 113.4 Rupture of the axillary artery from fracture of the proximal humerus in a 68-year-old woman. The robust collateral circulation contributed to delay in diagnosis. A large haematoma in the axilla caused pain and deepening of the nerve lesion.

2. Sympathetic paralysis. One almost infallible sign is always present in the first 48 hours after degenerative (axonotmesis, neurotmesis) injury of a nerve with a cutaneous sensory component: the skin in the distribution of the affected nerve is warm and dry.
3. Persisting neuropathic pain indicates that the responsible agent remains active. Neuropathic pain is recognized by its distribution: the pain from a lesion of the tibial nerve in the thigh is felt in the sole of the foot, that from a lesion of the median nerve in the axilla is felt in the hand. Some characteristic qualities include: shooting, burning or crushing, often associated with sensory symptoms such as intense pins and needles (dysaesthesiae). *Allodynia*, in which a stimulus that is normally not painful is perceived as a painful one, suggests a severe, incomplete injury. Neuropathic pain may signify impending critical ischaemia.[5]
4. Tinel's sign indicates that axons have been ruptured and it is detectable on the day of injury in a conscious patient with a closed lesion. The examiner's finger percusses along the line of the affected nerve from distal to proximal. The patient is asked to indicate when that percussion induces a wave of pins and needles into the distribution of the nerve. The level of the sign is measured from a fixed bony point, and that interval is measured at subsequent examinations. A static Tinel's sign indicates that regenerating axons are blocked; a strong advancing sign indicates that they are advancing. The sign is most valuable in lesions of the radial, the median, the ulnar and the tibial nerves. It is less reliable in the common peroneal nerve because of the common association with ischaemia. It cannot be elicited in most cases of circumflex palsy.
5. A firm diagnosis of neurapraxia should never be made unless 1 week after the injury stimulation of the nerve below the level of the lesion produces a motor response proving that the distal axons had not undergone Wallerian degeneration.

The demonstration of conduction *across* the lesion on the day of injury or at any time after indicates that some nerve fibres are intact and working.

Factors in prognosis

The most important is the continuity of the Schwann cell column and the basal lamina. Recovery is good in conduction block and axonotmesis *if the cause is removed*. The prognosis for recovery after repair is governed by

1. the violence of the injury
2. the extent of destruction of the nerve, the skin and, above all, the blood vessels
3. by the proximity of the injury to the cell body
4. by the urgency of the repair (Fig. 113.5).

Delay before repair is especially harmful because of (1) atrophy and death of the cell body, (2) atrophy and fibrosis of the distal stump and the target organs, (3) the decreasing inability of the Schwann cells to support regenerating axons, (4) increasing technical difficulty, (5) the increasing requirement for grafting in place of suture and (6) unnecessary uncertainty and prolongation of disability for the patient.

Factors of lesser importance include

- *Level*. Repair of a ruptured radial nerve in the axilla only rarely restores extension of the digits.[6]

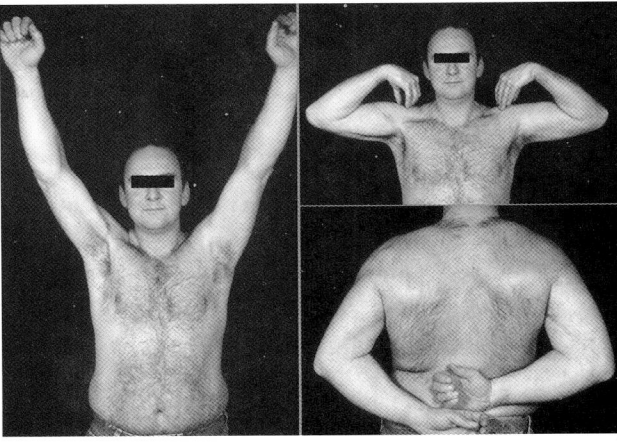

Figure 113.5 Rupture of the axillary artery and of the musculocutaneous and circumflex nerves during dislocation of the right shoulder. The function at 26 months after urgent repair.

- *Age.* The assumption that children always do better is incorrect. Sensory recovery is often good but motor recovery much less so.[7] Atrophy, limb shortening and deformity may be severe. There is no justification for neglecting the older patient.

NERVE INJURIES IN FRACTURES AND DISLOCATIONS

Recovery can be anticipated in nerves injured by closed fractures of the long bones in the upper limb if two conditions are met: 'the first is reasonable apposition of the bony fragments and the other *complete certainty that there is no threat of ischaemia of the forearm muscles*'.[8] The prognosis for nerves injured by skeletal injury is worse in dislocation or fracture/dislocation, in the lower limb, and after vascular injury (Table 113.2).

1. Recovery can be expected in about 80% of circumflex palsies caused by simple closed dislocations in younger patients. The outlook is worsened by associated fracture, rupture of the rotator cuff and increasing age. Inability to abduct at the glenohumeral joint signifies injury to the suprascapular nerve, the supraspinatus muscle and its insertion. Abduction is little short of normal in most cases of isolated paralysis of the deltoid (Fig. 113.6).
2. The incidence of radial palsy in low-energy transfer fractures of the shaft of the humerus is 8%.[9] Spontaneous recovery occurs in 80% or more. The Tinel sign is particularly helpful and it should be possible to distinguish between axonotmesis and neurotmesis by no later than 6 weeks after injury.
3. The outlook for injuries to the sciatic trunk and the tibial and common peroneal nerves is poor. Less than one-half of degenerative lesions recovered spontaneously.

Table 113.2 Circumflex, radial and common peroneal nerves injured by fracture/dislocation. Operated and non-operated cases 1965–2007

Nerve	Number of nerves	Arterial injury/ compartment syndrome	Nerves showing good spontaneous recovery
Circumflex	464	55	231
Radial	1015	125	404
Common peroneal	518	148	201
Total	1997	328	836

Most cases were referred because of the severity of the injury. The proportion of nerves injured during operation for internal fixation has increased, and accounted for nearly 25% in the years 2000–7. There has been a corresponding increase in the number of neglected cases of ischaemia.[11]

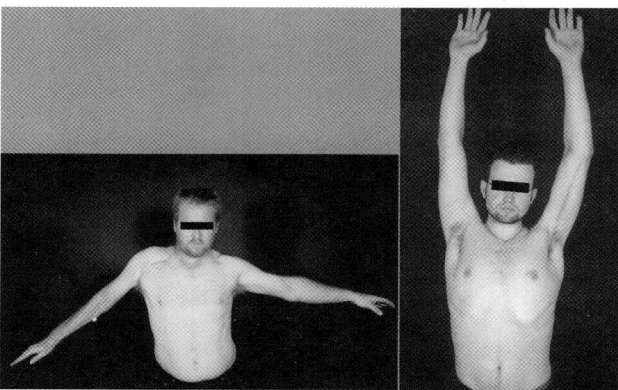

Figure 113.6 Combined injuries to the suprascapular and circumflex nerves. (Left) The range of elevation in a patient with irreparable injury to the right suprascapular nerve but with a good result after repair of the circumflex nerve. (Right) The elevation in another patient in whom repair of the left suprascapular nerve was successful but whose circumflex nerve injury was irreparable.

WHEN SHOULD THE INJURED NERVE BE EXPLORED?

The indications include when:

1. the fracture needs internal fixation
2. there is associated vascular injury
3. wound exploration of an open fracture is necessary
4. a fracture or dislocation is irreducible
5. the lesion deepens while it is under observation
6. the lesion occurred during operation for internal fixation
7. there are incomplete lesions of the main nerves in the lower limb.

If a surgeon elects to convert a closed fracture to an open one by whatever technique, then the lesion of the nerve should be exposed. The nerve, indeed the nerve with the adjacent artery, may be in the fracture or in the joint. Both will certainly be displaced from their normal position.[10] The surgeon must be on the alert for impending compartment syndrome after intramedullary nailing of the long bones of the lower limb (Fig. 113.7).

The return of function in an injured limb is determined by recovery of injured nerves and by ischaemia. The first intervention is no more than the first step in the process of rehabilitation, which must remain the responsibility of the fracture surgeon from start to finish. That process may include further operations such as musculotendinous transfers, the provision of orthoses which must always be carefully monitored by the fracture surgeon and the recognition and treatment of continuing pain. Rehabilitation ends when the patient is able to return to independent living, to work, to retraining or to study.

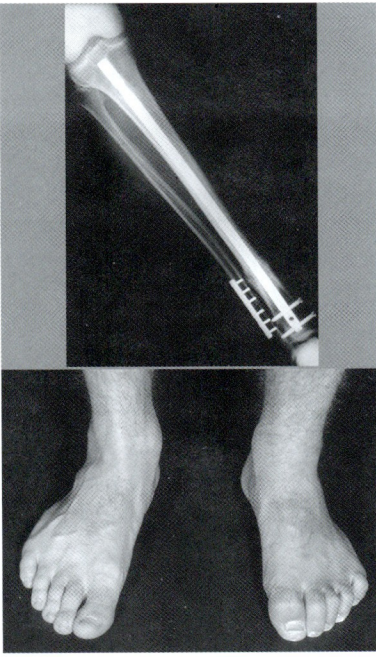

Figure 113.7 'Closed' intramedullary nailing of fracture of long bone. The tibial nerve and the posterior tibial artery were in the fracture. The muscles of the deep flexor compartment were fibrosed, causing severe clawing of the toes.

> - Deepening of the nerve lesion while the patient is under observation, in association with persisting neuropathic pain, signifies critical ischaemia of the nerve and perhaps of the limb unless and until proven otherwise.
> - A nerve which stops working after an operation in the vicinity of that nerve, in the presence of sympathetic paralysis, has been cut unless or until proven otherwise.
> - Most patients with isolated circumflex (axillary) palsy are able to abduct at the shoulder to 150° or more. A patient with paralysis of the deltoid who is unable to abduct the shoulder has associated injury to the rotator cuff and/or the suprascapular nerve until proven otherwise.

ACKNOWLEDGEMENT

The figures in this chapter have previously appeared in *Surgical Disorders of the Peripheral Nerves* and are reproduced by kind permission of Springer UK.

REFERENCES

- ● = Key primary paper
- ◆ = Major review article

> **KEY LEARNING POINTS**
>
> - Divided peripheral nerves will not recover unless and until they have been repaired.
> - Divided peripheral nerves should be repaired as soon as is reasonably possible. Where the wounding of the nerve is associated with wounding of an adjacent main artery, emergency repair of both is preferable.
> - A diagnosis of conduction block (neurapraxia) should not be made when there is sympathetic paralysis or when there is persisting neuropathic pain, and is unwise if there is any wound over the course of the nerve.
> - Neuropathic pain is recognized by the onset of painful, spontaneous, sensory symptoms (dysaesthesiae) and by intolerance of examination of the part (allodynia). Neuropathic pain is expressed in the distribution of the nerve often remote from the site of injury so that a lesion of the sciatic nerve at the hip evokes pain in the foot, whereas a lesion of the medial cord in the axilla evokes pain in the hand.
> - Neuropathic pain signifies that the noxious agent responsible for the lesion is still active.

●1. Kadiyala RK, Ramirez A, Taylor AE, *et al.* The blood supply of the common peroneal nerve in the popliteal fossa. *Journal of Bone and Joint Surgery (British)* 2005;**87B**:337–42.

◆2. O'Brian M (ed.). *Aids to the Examination of the Peripheral Nervous System*, 4th edn. London, UK: Elsevier, 2000.

●3. Birch R, Raji ARM. Repair of median and ulnar nerves. *Journal of Bone and Joint Surgery (British)* 1991;**73B**:154–7.

●4. Stenning M, Drew S, Birch R. Low energy arterial injury at the shoulder with progressive or delayed nerve palsy *Journal of Bone and Joint Surgery (British)* 2005;**87B**:1102–6.

●5. Blakey CM, Biant LC, Birch R. Ischaemia and the pink, pulseless hand complicating supracondylar fractures of the humerus in children. *Journal of Bone and Joint Surgery (British)* 2009;**91B**:1487–98.

6. Shergill G, Birch R, Bonney G, Munshi P. The radial and posterior interosseous nerves: results of 2560 repairs. *Journal of Bone and Joint Surgery (British)* 2000;**83**:646–9.

●7. Anand P, Birch R. Restoration of sensory function and lack of long-term chronic pain syndromes after brachial plexus injury in human neonates. *Brain* 2002;**125**:113–22.

♦8. Seddon HJ. Common causes of nerve injury. In: *Surgical Disorders of Peripheral Nerves*, 2nd edn. Edinburgh, UK: Churchill Livingstone, 1975:67–88.

♦9. Ekholm R, Adami J, Tidermark J, *et al*. Fractures of the shaft of the humerus. *Journal of Bone and Joint Surgery (British)* 2006;**88B**:1469–73.

10. Bottomley N, Williams A, Birch R, *et al*. Displacement of the common peroneal nerve in postero-lateral corner injuries of the knee. *Journal of Bone and Joint Surgery (British)* 2005;**87B**:1225–6.

●11. Birch R. Iatrogenous lesions of nerves and arteries in the leg and foot. *Foot and Ankle Surgery* 2008;**14**:130–7.

FURTHER READING

Birch R. *Surgical Disorders of the Peripheral Nerves*, 2nd edn. London, UK: Springer, 2011.

114

Hand infections

TUNKU KAMARUL ZAMAN

Introduction	1309	Other infections of the hand	1313
Common organisms	1310	Surgical approach for treating hand infections	1313
Treatment	1310	References	1314
Common hand infections	1310		

NATIONAL BOARD STANDARDS

- Understand hand infections according to anatomical planes
- Learn how to diagnose and treat hand infections
- Be able to suggest the best treatment option for all types of hand infections
- Understand the pathophysiology of hand infections and the common causative organisms
- Know the different surgical (and medical) approaches to managing hand infections
- Know Kanavel's four cardinal signs

INTRODUCTION

Very few body parts are as complex as the human hand, mainly because of its highly sophisticated anatomy designed to perform unique functions. The hand consists of multiple compartments and planes, and thus the knowledge of normal hand anatomy is crucial for the basic understanding of the pathophysiology, diagnosis and treatment of hand infections. So important is this knowledge that, in most literature, hand infections are described according to the involved anatomical planes.[1-7]

Although the overall incidence of hand infections is lower than those of lower extremities, a number of local or systemic factors can influence the outcomes of hand infections (Tables 114.1 and 114.2). The causative organism in any hand infection is usually directly related to how the organism was first introduced (e.g. infection following trauma is usually due to *Staphylococcus aureus* as this organism is found commonly on the skin). Bacterial infections account for 65% of all hand infections, with *S. aureus* being responsible for over 50% of these cases.[1]

However, other causative organisms may also cause hand infections, and they vary according to the type and location of the injury. The patient's health status (e.g. reduced immunity against infection) may also be a contributing factor. The causative organisms in paediatric patients occur in different frequencies from adult patients (Table 114.2).

Table 114.1 A summary of local and systemic factors that can influence the occurrence or progression of hand infections

Factors influencing hand infections	
Local factors	**Systemic factors**
Pathogen virulence	Systemic diseases (e.g. diabetes, HIV, immunocompromised etc.)
Tissue disruption	Drug treatment (chemotherapy)
Foreign material	
Previous injury	
Blood supply	

COMMON ORGANISMS

Good history taking can suggest the possible causative organisms (and even possible underlying diseases) in hand infection (Fig. 114.1 and Table 114.1). Presentations may differ from one patient to another but, in general, infections of the hand appear as cellulitis, swellings or abscesses. It is very rare that hand infections present with septic arthritis or osteomyelitis (Fig. 114.1). These presentations usually result in pain with or without loss of finger function.[1]

Table 114.2 Common organisms causing infection in the adult and paediatric population

Paediatrics	Adult
Aerobic	*Aerobic*
Staphylococcus aureus (37%)	*Staphylococcus aureus* (50–80%)
Streptococcus pyogenes (20%)	*Streptococcus pyogenes* (10%)
Aerobic Gram (−) rods (13%)	Aerobic Gram (−) rods
Aerobic Gram (+) cocci (20%)	Aerobic Gram (+) cocci
Anaerobic	*Anaerobic* (<5%)
Gram (+) cocci (20%)	Gram (+) cocci
Gram (−) rods (13%)	Gram (−) rods
Gram (+) rods (3%)	Gram (+) rods
Fungal (3%)	Fungal (1–2%)
Eikenella corrodens (6%)	*Eikenella corrodens* (20%)

Note that the total numbers do not add up to 100% as in 22% of cases more than one causative organism is found.

Blood investigations and radiographs are generally not helpful as diagnostic tools, except in cases where prolonged osteomyelitis is present. However, related investigations to determine underlying causes (e.g. tuberculosis) are generally useful and in most instances necessary. The use of ultrasound may be useful as a diagnostic tool, but very frequently hand infections can be easily recognized using clinical judgement alone.

TREATMENT

In general, treatment for hand infections involves the use of antibiotics. The choice of antibiotics depends on the causative organism, although in cases where the causative organism is unknown empirical therapy may be used. A guideline of the recommended antibiotics is described in Table 114.3. However, please note that the antibiotics recommended here are merely a guide and that it is wise to follow local hospital antibiotic policies and the advice of microbiology services. In cases where abscess is present, surgery must be performed early.

COMMON HAND INFECTIONS

Relatively common types of infections seen in the hand are

- paronychia (acute or chronic)
- eponychia (acute or chronic)
- subungal abscess.

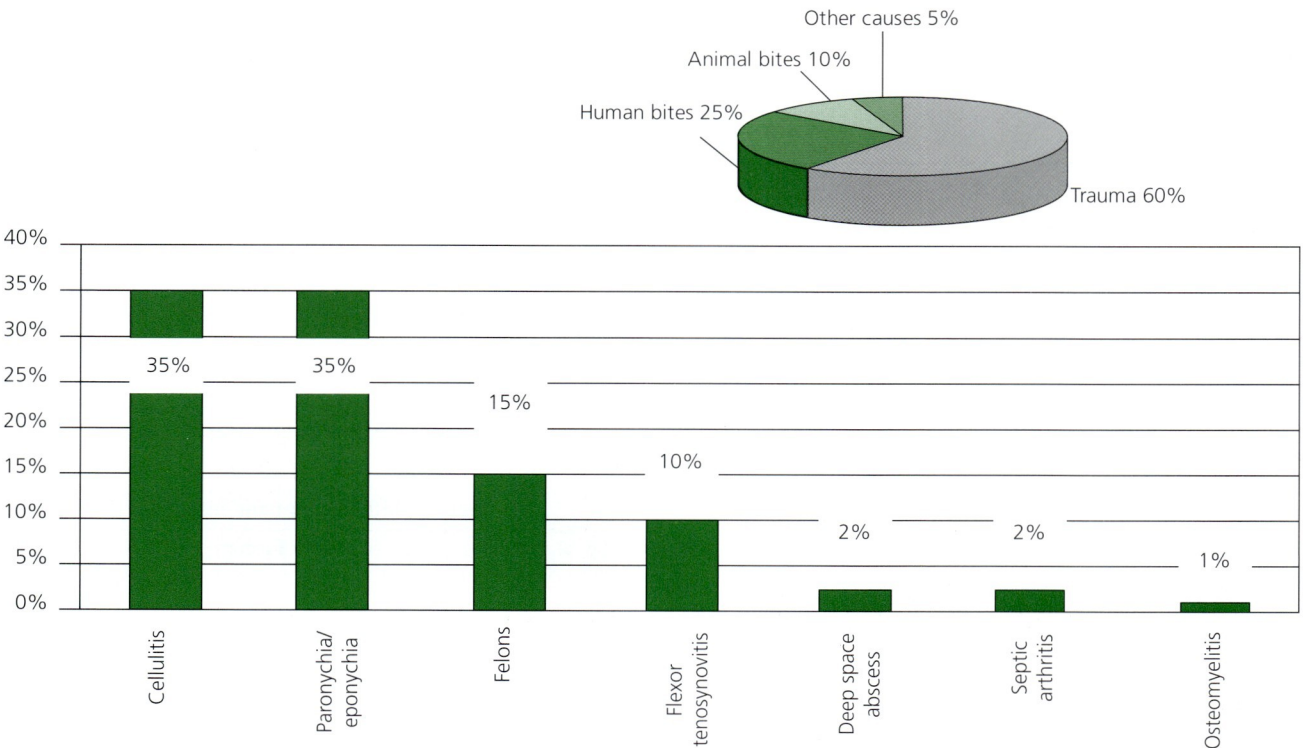

Figure 114.1 Causes of hand infections and the clinical presentations that are commonly seen.

Table 114.3 Guideline for the use of antimicrobials for different presentations of hand infections

Type of infection	Causative organisms	Empirical antibiotic treatment	
		First-line drug	Second-line drug
Simple laceration without any contamination		None required but requires immediate surgical intervention	
Wound infections	S. aureus	Flucloxacillin + penicillin	Cephalosporin (first generation)
Cellulitis	Streptococci		
Septic arthritis	S. aureus	Cephalosporin (first generation)	Vancomycin + gentamicin
Acute osteomyelitis	Streptococci		
Light to moderate contaminated wound			
Severely infected wound	S. aureus	Cephalosporin (second generation) + gentamicin + metronidazole	Vancomycin + gentamicin + metronidazole
Immunocompromised patients	Streptococci		
Bite wounds	Gram (−) bacilli Anaerobes		
Suspected infection with resistant organism	Meticillin-resistant S. aureus	Cephalosporin (second generation) + gentamicin + metronidazole	

Acute paronychia is infection of an area on the lateral nail fold (paronychium) and is typically due to superficial trauma ranging from self-inflicted nail biting to work-related accidental trauma (Table 114.1).[3] In most instances paronychia begins with cellulitis, progressing slowly to form abscess(es). In some instances, infections can spread to the proximal nail edge, developing to what is known as *eponychia*. Occasionally, infection can spread under the nail plate itself, resulting in a *subungual abscess*. Although not as common as acute infections, *chronic paronychia* does sometimes occur. Treatment of this condition is much more difficult as it commonly occurs in people whose hands are exposed to water or other irritants. This condition can also be present in patients who are immunocompromised, suffering from metastatic cancer, subungual melanoma and squamous cell cancer.[4]

Treatment of acute paronychia depends on whether or not an abscess is present. If an abscess is not present, treatment should include frequent hot soaks and a short course of antibiotics (e.g. flucloxacillin for 5 days).[3] In cases where abscesses are present, urgent surgical drainage is required in most instances. A single incision on the side of the nail where the abscess is located is the preferred surgical approach. The incision made must avoid the nail bed to prevent future nail deformity. Once the abscess is completely drained, the empty spaces are packed with dressings. In conditions where the abscess extends around both sides of the nail, larger incisions may be needed and sometimes involve removing part of the nail. In chronic paronychia, prevention or avoidance of the underlying cause(s) (e.g. repeated exposure to irritants) must be maintained in addition to receiving antimicrobial therapy.[5]

Felon – subcutaneous abscess of the pulp

Because the pulp on the ends of fingers possesses a relatively large subcutaneous space, this area forms a potential area for infection to occur. The pulp can be divided into tiny compartments by strong fibrous septa traversing from skin to bone. There is also a fibrous curtain present at the distal finger crease which is in continuity to these septa. Owing to these anatomical arrangements, any swelling occurring in this area causes immediate pain. Abscesses forming in this area may also extend into the periosteum of the distal phalanx, around the nail bed or proximally, through the fibrous curtain or through the skin. Therefore, it is important that felon is treated early and aggressively. Surgeons must also be aware that felons can present with other concomitant conditions (e.g. osteomyelitis) or underlying predisposing factors (e.g. diabetes).[5]

Treatment must include surgical drainage, as in most instances abscesses are usually present. A single incision giving access to the infected space(s) is preferred. It is worth noting that attempts must be made to avoid incision to the tip of the finger just before the distal nail tip. Fish mouth incisions and direct cuts breaching the periosteum must also be avoided.[5,6]

Deep fascial space (and web space) infection

The deep fascial spaces of the hand are potential spaces for infection to occur which consist of (Fig. 114.2).

1. dorsal subaponeurotic space (dorsal to the extensor tendons)

2. subfascial web space (demarcated by the palmar interosseous muscles dorsally and the flexor tendons of the third, fourth and fifth digits ventrally)
3. midpalmar space (continuous with the dorsal subcutaneous space)
4. thenar space (area between the adductor pollicis muscle dorsally and the flexor tendon of the second digit ventrally passing mainly through the thenar eminence).

Infections in these areas may be due to (1) direct penetrating injury, (2) spread from neighbouring compartments or from (3) haematogenous spread. Patients may present with a swelling, tenderness along the described anatomical planes and pain on moving the affected fingers; because venous and lymphatic drainage occurs mainly at the dorsum of the hand, infection originating from the palmar side can be seen to affect the dorsum of the hand. Treatment with antibiotics is usually adequate unless the abscess has formed within these spaces, in which case surgical drainage is necessary.

Infection of bursas (radial and ulnar)

Because of the close anatomical location of the ulnar and radial bursas being extensions of the flexor sheaths for flexor pollicis longus and flexor digitorum profundus of the thumb and little finger respectively (Fig. 114.2), penetrating injury along the flexor tendons of the thumb or little fingers can result in infection of these structures. These infections can spread along the tendon sheath proximally to the forearm. As is often the case where these bursas may be in communication (via Parona's space), infection in one bursa may affect the other. This condition is known as a 'horseshoe abscess', where pus moves freely from one bursa to the other. Treatment of these conditions involves the incision and drainage of the abscess followed by the use of intravenous (i.v.) antibiotics. In certain cases, continuous or multiple lavages maybe be required.[1]

Suppurative flexor tenosynovitis

This condition occurs in the flexor tendon sheath and, like infection of the bursas, can spread along the flexor sheath towards the forearm as well as to the neighbouring tendons via the shared bursas or anatomical spaces (Fig. 114.2). Failure to treat suppurative flexor tenosynovitis (SFT) early can result in tendon adhesions or tendon ruptures.

First described by Kanavel,[7,8] SFT can be diagnosed using simple examination techniques. Upon careful examination, the point of entry for infections can sometimes be identified (e.g. puncture wound at the tip of finger). A detailed history also helps to identify the point at which infection started and/or the causative organism.[4-6] However, in most cases the causative organism is usually due to a surface bacterium such as *S. aureus*.

Kanavel's four cardinal signs are

1. finger held in a flexed position
2. sausage digit (symmetrical swelling)
3. severe percussion tenderness along the tendon sheath
4. intense pain on passive extension of the finger.

Treatment of SFT usually involves surgical drainage as patients usually present late for medical care. In cases where infections are detected early (i.e. less than 48 hours), i.v. antibiotics (i.e. flucloxacillin plus penicillin) alone may be sufficient.[4,5] However, where i.v. antibiotics do not elicit response within 24 hours, urgent surgical intervention is required.[5,6] Incision using a Brunner approach is the preferred method as this helps to prevent future wound contractures. Incisions of the A2 and A4 pulleys must be avoided as cutting these structures and leaving them unrepaired will result in a 'bowstringing effect' of the involved

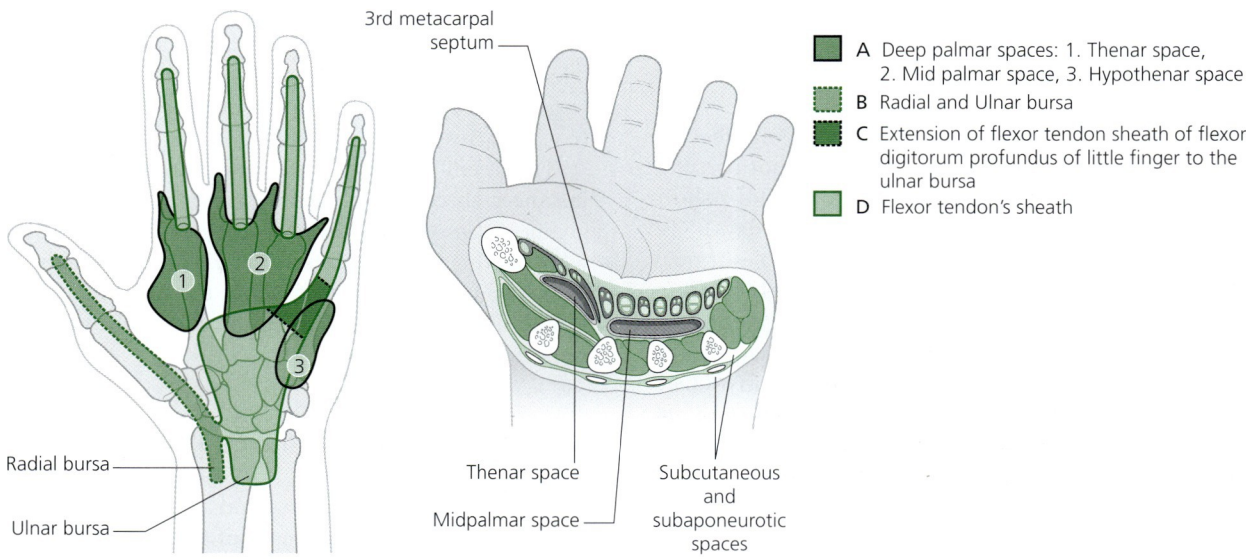

Figure 114.2 The anatomical locations of the deep fascial spaces and their relation to the ulna/radial bursas.

fingers. A less invasive method is to use a flexible catheter to to drain the abscess by flushing it from an entry site proximal to the infection and exiting the wash at the end away from the infection site (Fig. 114.2). Irrigation is continued until all pus is absent and the fluid is clear. Known as flexor tendon sheath irrigation, this technique is used to great effect in cases where the infection is confined within the flexor sheath and is not extensive.

OTHER INFECTIONS OF THE HAND

- *Osteomyelitis.* Treatment principles are similar to other cases of osteomyelitis. It is rare that infection of the hand requires amputation but, if necessary, the surgeon may need to consider amputation proximal to the joint of the affected bone. Erosion of the distal phalanx as the result of pulp infections heals well by removing the abscess followed by a course of antibiotic therapy.
- *Fight bite injury.* In one published report, it has been noted that 82% of cases heal well with adequate treatment but the remaining 18% of cases required some form of amputation. In men, this form of injury is usually due to 'knuckles to teeth' contact resulting in injury to the third and fourth metacarpal regions (42% of male cases). However, this form of injury usually does not occur in women as they tend to have 'true bite' injuries to the hands. Treatment must be early, correct and comprehensive. Aggressive and immediate surgical intervention with antibiotic administration (broad spectrum, covering both aerobic and anaerobic organisms) is mandatory.
- *Animal bite injury.* Treatment should be just as aggressive as for human bite injuries. The use of anti-tetanus toxoid has been advocated in some centres but does not appear to be part of the standard recommended treatment protocol. Treatment also depends on the species of animal that bit the patient (e.g. the organism involved after a dog bite is usually (>50%) *Pasteurella multocida,* which is resistant to flucloxacillin and erythromycin). Some animals have venom (e.g. snakes, certain spiders, scorpions) and may require anti-venoms as part of their treatment.
- *Mycobacterial infections.* Identified organisms that cause hand infections include *Mycobacterium marinum* (found in stagnant clear water, e.g. swimming pools, fish tanks, etc.), *Mycobacterium tuberculosis,* which may be as a result of infection from a primary site (i.e. lung), *Mycobacterium avium-intracellulare* (found in infected poultry) and *Mycobacterium kansasii.* In some cases, especially if tuberculosis is suspected, other investigations must be performed (e.g. chest radiograph). Surgical debridement is usually not required as the infection heals well with a prolonged but appropriate antimicrobial therapy regimen.
- *Herpetic whitlow.* Caused by herpes simplex type I virus (and rarely type II). It may be related to certain occupations (e.g. dental nurses may contract the virus from a patient's cold sores). This condition is usually self-limiting, but supportive care may be needed (e.g. splinting and antiviral drugs such as acyclovir may be helpful to relieve pain).

SURGICAL APPROACH FOR TREATING HAND INFECTIONS

In managing infection of the hand, surgery is preferable in cases where abscess is present.[1] Certain principles must be observed when performing surgery.

1. A direct incision always leads to the abscess site. Adequate exposure is needed to ensure that all the pus can be drained completely.
2. Avoid incision across the finger and palm creases and if possible a 'zig-zag' incision is preferable to a straight incision.
3. Avoid cutting into the nail bed as this can lead to nail deformity.
4. Be vigilant when incising over important structures (e.g. digital artery, tendon) as repairing the damage caused to these structures can be daunting.
5. Use copious amounts of wash to ensure you are rid of the infection.
6. Do not suture incised wounds as this creates potential space for further infection. It is better to allow healing by secondary intention.
7. Surgery alone is not sufficient for treating infections. This has to be supplemented with the use of antibiotic/antimicrobials.

Suggested incisions for drainage of abscesses are summarized in Fig. 114.3.

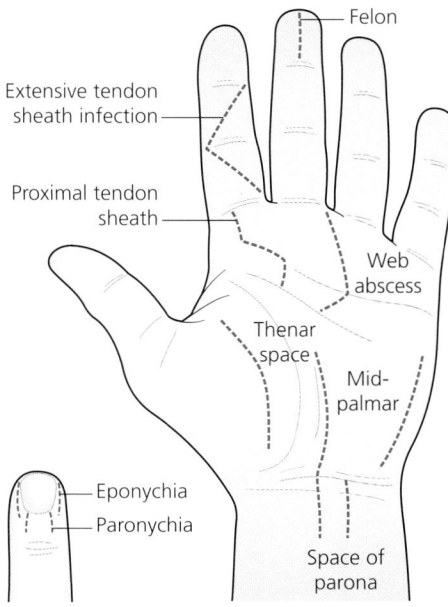

Figure 114.3 Examples of surgical incision to approach various types of infection of the hand and fingers.

KEY LEARNING POINTS

- Hand infections are divided according to anatomical planes and can present as an acute or chronic condition.
- Investigations are rarely needed as good clinical examination is usually adequate to make an accurate diagnosis.
- Hand infections can present (in the order of commonest first) as cellulitis, abscess, septic arthritis and rarely osteomyelitis.
- Antibiotics are required as treatment when abscesses have not developed.
- Knowledge of causative organisms is important in order to deliver the most effective antimicrobial therapy. However, when this information is not available, in most cases empirical therapy may be adequate as a treatment.
- Note that 50–80% of infections in adults are caused by *S. aureus*.
- Surgery is needed in cases where abscesses are present, but it is important that the surgeon has an extensive knowledge of hand anatomy to ensure that the best result is achieved without causing further complications.

REFERENCES

● = Key primary paper
♦ = Major review article

♦1. Neviaser RJ. Acute infections. In: Green DP, Hotchkiss RN, Pederson WC (eds) *Green's Operative Hand Surgery*, 4th edn. Edinburgh, UK: Churchill Livingstone, 1999:1033–47.

●2. Harness N, Blazaar PE. Causative microorganisms in surgically treated pediatric hand infections. *Journal of Hand Surgery* 2005;**30**:1294–7.

♦3. Abrams RA, Botte MJ. Hand infections: treatment recommendations for specific types. *Journal of the American Academy of Orthopaedic Surgeons* 1996;**4**:219–30.

♦4. Haussman MR, Lisser SP. Hand infections. *Orthopedic Clinics of North America* 1992;**23A**:171–85.

♦5. Spiegel JD, Szabo RM. A protocol for the treatment of severe infections of the hand. *Journal of Hand Surgery* 1988;**13A**:254–9.

♦6. Siegel DB, Gelberman RH. Infection of the hand. *Orthopedic Clinics of North America* 1988;**19**:779–89.

●7. Kanavel AB. An anatomical, experimental, and clinical study of acute phlegmons of the hand. *Surgery, Gynecology and Obstetrics* 1905;**1**:221–59.

♦8. Kanavel AB. *Infections of the Hand: A Guide to the Surgical Treatment of Acute and Chronic Suppurative Processes in the Fingers, Hand, and Forearm*, 6th edn. Philadelphia, PA: Lea & Febiger, 1933.

115

Replantation and microsurgery

TUNKU KAMARUL ZAMAN

Introduction	1315	Microsurgical technique	1318
Early management	1316	Repairing other structures (non-microsurgery)	1319
Ischaemia time	1317	Postoperative care	1320
Decision (indications) for replantation	1317	Outcome of surgery	1320
Contraindications	1317	Ring avulsion injuries	1321
Surgical technique	1318	References	1323

NATIONAL BOARD STANDARDS

- Classify upper limb amputations according to various clinical presentations
- Predict clinical outcome based on the initial presentation, and make a decision on when surgery is required
- Understand the principles of managing amputations
- Recognize the various surgical techniques implemented in the replantation procedure and its related microsurgical skills

INTRODUCTION

Replantation and microsurgery is a highly skilled and demanding surgical technique which yields good to excellent outcomes in the hands of experienced and well-equipped surgical teams. Because the procedure is labour intensive and ultimately consumes a large amount of resources, careful selection of cases is needed in order to maximize good outcomes for the benefit of patients. Presentations of amputations have been described in detail to determine the levels and severity (including ring avulsion injuries) of an amputation. These have been done to not only assist in making the right decision of replanting an amputated part, but also to predict future clinical outcomes. A series of protocols and techniques in managing the potential replant patient have been established over the years, detailing the procedure required as soon as an amputation has occurred up to the time of rehabilitation. These methods have been widely accepted and practised in many centres. Detailed preparation and understanding of this information are important to ensure favourable outcomes. Despite the acclaimed success of replantation procedures, a replanted appendage is expected to have certain long-term limitations and complications, especially cold intolerance of the replanted part, which can make the decision to replant difficult.

The exact incidence of traumatic amputation involving the upper limb in the UK is currently unknown, but the extrapolated prevalence of all types of amputations in the UK is approximately 0.2–0.7% in the current population. Of these, 63% of the amputation cases are the result of trauma.[1,2] Amputation is best categorized according to

1. The anatomical site of the amputation (e.g. through a joint, though the metacarpals)
2. The level of amputation (e.g. finger tip amputations, wrist amputations)
3. The mechanisms resulting in the amputation (i.e. guillotine, crush or avulsion)
4. The duration from the occurrence of amputation and the manner in which the amputated part had been transported (i.e. cold or warm ischaemic time).

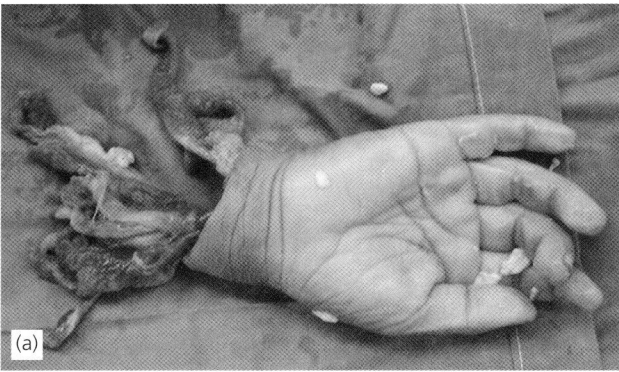

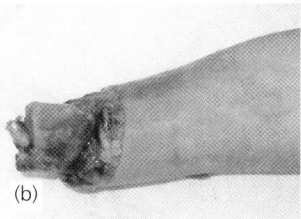

Figure 115.1 Pictures of amputation in a 4-year-old boy whose hand got caught in a cake mixer. Note that, although the skin appears to be a clean 'guillotine' amputation, this injury is classified as an avulsion-type injury which can be noted from the muscle bulk on the amputated part. A complete history taking would have suggested this mechanism in the first instance. In this case, the decision to continue the replantation was based on the patient's age and that the hand appeared to have initially survived. However, it was later found that the hand did not appear to be functional as there were complete losses of forearm muscles.

The categories listed above are important considerations in determining the decision for replantation and the associated surgical outcome (Fig. 115.1). Certain definitions have also been described, including the degree of amputation as well as the appropriate surgical management (Box 115.1). Upper extremity replantation has been the topic of interest in the past 25–30 years.[2] In this chapter, we will discuss the evidence-based approach to the management of upper limb amputation based on the current published data.

EARLY MANAGEMENT

Management of the amputated part starts from the time of amputation. Care of the amputated part is of the utmost importance, with gentle handling of the remaining tissues to be applied at all times. It is highly advisable that the amputated part be preserved for replantation as soon as possible to slow the process of tissue degradation. Depending on the mechanisms of injury, the amputated part can rapidly be transported to a medical centre where replantation procedures can take place, provided that the amputation is 'clean' (i.e. guillotine type) and adequate preparation/preservation of the amputated part is performed prior to transportation. However, if the amputation conditions appear 'dirty' or other than the guillotine type (i.e. crushed, avulsed, etc.), washing with adequate amounts of Hartman's solution (or at least normal saline) is required to reduce contamination and bio-burden. In instances where proper irrigation solutions are not readily available on site, irrigation using clean water is acceptable, but must be performed gently to avoid any tissue damage. With or without irrigation, the amputated part is then wrapped with wet gauze and placed in a plastic bag, which is then immersed in ice water to maintain low temperature (4°C) during transportation. Take care not to freeze the amputated part. Direct immersion of the amputated part into ice-cooled normal or Hartman's saline has also been described in the literature, despite some concerns of its effect in causing the remaining tissue to become oedematous or macerated. In either case, the exact manner in which the amputated part is preserved should be clearly communicated to the clinical staff at the referral centre.[2–6]

Care of the amputated stump must also be carried out as quickly as possible. Haemostasis must be maintained by proper bandaging without the use of vessel clips or tourniquet. Equal and constant pressure of the amputated stump must be maintained and bandages should be left in place until the time of surgery. Prevention of further blood loss is necessary, especially in forearm amputations, as uncontrolled blood loss can result in haemorrhagic shock.[6]

Overall patient care must be maintained before and after the surgery. More importantly, the management of the patient's major injuries apart from the amputated part take precedence to the management of the amputation. The patient's condition needs to be stabilized. Adequate fluid replacement following blood loss due to the injury must be performed as soon as possible. The patient must be reassured at all times, as an extreme amount of stress may result in an inappropriate sympathetic response causing profound vasoconstriction. This will impede reperfusion of the amputated part and may result in poor surgical outcomes.[2,4,6]

BOX 115.1: A list of common definitions used to describe the degree of amputation and the various interventions that can be performed

- Complete amputations: a body part that has been completely severed without any attachments
- Incomplete amputations: a body part that has been partially severed
- Subtotal replantation: a procedure necessary to restore viability of the partial amputation
- Revascularization: reconstruction of the blood vessels that are damaged to prevent the ischaemic part becoming non-viable

Table 115.1 A general comparison of the ischaemic times allowed for the different levels of amputations and the environment of which the amputated part had been transported

	Warm ischaemia time	Cool ischaemia time (4°C)
Digit	12 hours	24 hours
Significant amount of muscle	6 hours	12 hours

ISCHAEMIA TIME

Ischaemia time is defined as the duration of complete absence of perfusion in the amputated part.[2,6] It is important to note that the duration of ischaemia serves as a guide for operating surgeons to reattach the amputated part to establish adequate reperfusion. Failure to do so before this time would result in irreversible tissue damage. The Louisville group found that survival was inversely proportional to ischaemia time, warm or cold.[7] Proximal amputation is less likely to tolerate longer ischaemia time because of the larger amount of muscle involved in the amputation (Table 115.1). As muscle does not tolerate hypoxia well, in the event that reperfusion is not established early, muscle necrosis will ensue, leaving the patient with a non-functioning limb. This would not only create a ground for microbial contamination, but also release harmful tissue toxins (as a result of myonecrosis) into the systemic circulation. Successful transplant also depends upon the duration of which perfusion of the amputated part has been re-established, and the environment in which the part had been preserved before being replanted. An appendage which is stored in a cool environment (i.e. packed in ice water at 4°C) has twice the estimated survival time without reperfusion as one stored at room temperature (e.g. at 25°C). A summary of ischaemic time that may be used as a guideline for replantation is listed in Table 115.1. In the digits, late replantation (i.e. more than 24 hours) is associated with only minimal risk of replantation failure due to involvement of a relatively smaller amount of muscle tissue. Successful replantation of cooled digits has been reported at 30 hours or longer following amputation.[1–3,5–7]

DECISION (INDICATIONS) FOR REPLANTATION

The decision whether or not to replant an amputated appendage during its initial presentation is of paramount importance.[1–8] It is worth noting that, in most cases, replantation surgery may consume a large amount of time, manpower and financial resources. Furthermore, the amount of stress imposed on the patient during the procedure and rehabilitation process is an additional factor to consider if the surgical outcome would only achieve poorer function than a complete amputation with early rehabilitation using a prosthesis. It is therefore important that surgeons select cases prudently to ensure that patients will benefit from the replantation surgery (Fig. 115.1).

In general, the accepted indications for replantation are as follows:

1. thumb amputation
2. multiple digit amputations
3. metacarpal amputation
4. almost any body part in a child
5. wrist or forearm amputation
6. individual digit distal to flexor digitorum superficialis (FDS) insertion; replantation at the level distal to the insertion of FDS often results in satisfactory function
7. partial hand amputations (through the palm)
8. elbow and above elbow where the amputation has been sharp or moderately sharp.

These indications are merely guidelines to ensure that successful outcome is achieved. The success rate of any replantation is also dependent upon the experience and skill of the operating surgeon. Relative indications have also been described (see below), with the final decision to perform surgery determined by the surgeon's assessment of the individual cases:

1. duration of warm and cold ischaemia time based on the level of the amputation (especially when considering warm ischemia time and in more proximal amputations)
2. age of the patient: older patients with lesser demand for upper limb function may be better with an amputation as they generally have poorer tissue regenerative ability and tend to tolerate prolonged stress poorly
3. segmental injuries to the amputated part
4. patient's general condition, including other major injuries or diseases
5. rehabilitation potential of patient (occupation and intelligence)
6. economic factors.

To ensure a successful replantation, certain contraindications to this procedure must also be identified. These not only assist in predicting those patients who may do well after an operation, but also exclude patients from undergoing an unnecessary replantation procedure when there is a high prediction of failure.

CONTRAINDICATIONS

1. Local
   a. severely crushed or mangled parts
   b. amputations at multiple levels of the same limb
   c. distal amputations; amputations distal to the distal interphalangeal joint are difficult to replant since the digital artery begins to branch and dorsal veins are hard to find.

2. General
   a. amputations in patients with other serious injuries or diseases
   b. arteriosclerotic vessels
   c. mentally unstable patients
   d. patients with pre-existing disease that may affect peripheral blood circulation
   e. severe chronic or uncompensated medical illnesses such as coronary artery disease, myocardial infarction, peptic ulcer disease, malignant neoplasms and chronic renal or pulmonary disease may increase the anaesthetic risk enough to preclude replantation.

SURGICAL TECHNIQUE

The Louisville group presented one of the first large series (86 replants in 71 patients) and established some of the basic technical steps in the sequence.[3]

1. Bilateral (or more) midline incision to expose bone and other structures. This technique allows the identification of the important structures that need to be reattached/reanastomosed (i.e. blood vessels, nerves, etc.).
2. Bone shortening and fixing.
3. Repairing the extensor followed by the flexor tendons.
4. Repairing the nerves.
5. Repairing the artery followed by the veins before releasing the tourniquet.
6. Skin and/or soft-tissue coverage.
7. The use of local heparin and lidocaine liberally.
8. A bolus of 3000 U of heparin after completion of the anastomoses.
9. After surgery, patients receive heparin and low molecular weight dextran for 3–7 days.

In later years, a number of experienced surgeons described improvements to these basic steps in an effort to further improve surgical outcomes.[3–9] Some of these measures include flushing the vessels in the amputated part of the body with heparinized saline to ensure removal of intravascular clotting prior to revascularization. According to Tamai et al.,[8] following careful experimental and clinical trials, blood should be milked at the amputated part and flushed out with heparinized saline. The authors also stated that the need for perfusion depended on the degree of injury; if there is extensive crushing, the probability of intervascular clotting is much higher and washing out the part is indicated, particularly in the case of double crush levels.[2] These recommendations have been further described in the report of the Subcommittee on Replantation, presented at the Third Meeting of the International Society for Surgery of the Hand.[6] Other methods have also been described, including vessel transport, tissue transplant, etc.; however, these techniques are best discussed and performed by experienced surgeons as they require high levels of skill and expertise.[9–14]

Fasciotomy and decompression (and even carpal tunnel release) must be performed in cases where amputation involves the more proximal part of the upper limb (i.e. major limb replantation) as pressure and oedema that occur as a result of trauma or prolonged surgery may result in compression of the restored vessel. These areas can be managed later by either skin grafts or flaps.[6,7]

MICROSURGICAL TECHNIQUE

The success of a replantation procedure is heavily dependent on the outcome of the microsurgery technique adopted during the procedure, specifically during the microvascular anastomoses.[2] It is therefore important that, in order for any replantations to be successful, the operating surgeon must be experienced, well trained and competent to perform microsurgery. The operating theatre is not a setting for practise (Fig. 115.2).

It is important to note that, in order to accomplish successful microsurgery, two main areas need to be fulfilled: (1) surgeon and (2) equipment/facility requirements.

Considerations from the perspective of the surgeon include

1. the experience of the surgical team and its ability to work together
2. the surgeon's knowledge of the physiology of microcirculation
3. the training received followed by the amount of laboratory and clinical practice.

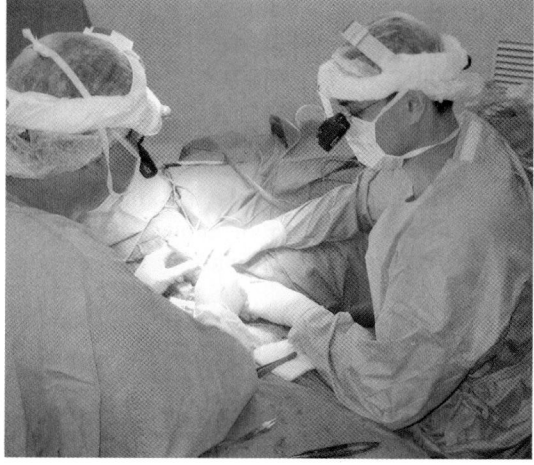

Figure 115.2 Example of a replantation in progress showing two microsurgeons working using 5× magnification loupes. As hours of microsurgery are required to perform this procedure, it is advisable that there are more than two teams on standby to ensure that the whole surgery can be performed without putting too much strain on the surgeons.

Table 115.2 The microsurgical equipment and accessories required to perform a replantation in optimal conditions

Microsurgical equipment	
Magnification	Microscopes
	Operating loupes
Instruments	Forceps
	Scissors
	Vascular clamps
	Dilators
	Fogarty catheters
	Irrigation tips
	Suture material (sizes 4-0, 6-0 for tendons and 8-0, 9-0, 10-0 for vessel repair)
	Needle drivers
Other equipment	Warm heparinzed Ringer's lactate
	Bipolar electrocautery

Adequate and appropriate instruments, equipment and facilities are also major factors to be considered when performing microsurgery. A summary of the required materials is listed in Table 115.2.

Details on the methods of use of these instruments and techniques of performing microsurgery are beyond this chapter; however, the principles of repair will be briefly described. This is because microsurgical techniques and skills are highly specialized, and attempts to discuss this topic in general terms may be inadequate for the inexperienced trainee. Please refer to specialized text books detailing precise microsurgical techniques for further information.

Blood vessel repair

There are four major principles to adhere to when attempting to anastomose a damaged vessel.

1. Vessel ends are dissected sharply on either side until normal tissue is seen. Damaged vessel walls will lead to intravascular thrombosis once blood flow is established and thus must be avoided.
2. Both ends of the vessels are trimmed with straight, sharp scissors under high-power microscopy. Note that the intima has to be normal in appearance with any overhanging adventitia removed. Dilatation of the proximal part of the artery may be needed if flow is impaired. Locally acting dilating agents (e.g. lidocaine and papaverine) may be used concomitantly.
3. No anastomosis should be under tension and therefore bone shortening has to be performed prior to this procedure. In the event that this effort is not adequate, a vein graft can be used to bridge the gap.
4. Meticulous technique must be maintained during any vessel repair. Adequate length must be maintained at the end of the anastomosis, but not too long as this will result in kinking of the vessels and impeding blood flow.

Other points to note when performing vessel repair.

1. Arteries have larger diameters and thicker walls making them relatively easier to anastomose, whereas veins have smaller luminal diameters and thinner walls, which are relatively more difficult to repair.
2. As a rule, for every artery anastomosed, two veins need to be patent and reanastomosed to ensure return blood circulation is maintained and not pooled into the replanted part.
3. When handling the vessels, every attempt should be made to not damage the intima layer as this would lead to possible thrombus formation.
4. Sutures used for these vessels are non-absorbable monofilament types to ensure adequate strength is achieved while allowing the vessel to undergo tissue repair.

REPAIRING OTHER STRUCTURES (NON-MICROSURGERY)

Bone fixation

Although there have been some debates regarding the use of external fixators (including K-wires) versus internal fixators (e.g. plates) for the fixation of bone, one thing is for certain, fixation of the bone can only be carried out after shortening is performed to ensure that the other repaired structures are not stretched or in tension. Fixation is done so that the bone being fixed is stable and will not cause further damage to the surrounding structures. Problems commonly noted after bone fixation include poor bone alignment following the fixation, and, in the case of finger replantation, rotational malalignment. It is therefore important that fixation is done well at the first instance, as readjustment after completing repair can be extremely difficult and daunting to the operating surgeon.

Tendon repair

Tendon repair usually follows bone fixation, and extensor tendons are repaired before the flexor tendons. When repairing tendons there are a number of rules that need to be observed. See chapter 112 for more details.

1. Repair sutures should be the strong monofilament non-resorbable type; large calibre sizes are preferred for the larger tendons (generally size 3-0 or 4-0).
2. As much as possible, sutures must remain within the core of the tendon as any structures protruding on the external smooth surfaces of the tendon can result in poor tendon gliding and thus poor tendon function.

3. Four-strand repair is preferred to two-strand repair, as the larger the numbers of opposing sutures, the better the repair quality and also allows earlier rehabilitation. However, studies have shown that six-strand repairs offer no further advantage than four-strand repairs. It is also worth noting that the more sutures introduced within a tendon, the more likely 'strangulation' of the tendon will occur, thus preventing good tendon healing.
4. Ensure that the appropriate tendons are repaired to the proximal tendon ends. Poor results can be expected if an antagonist muscle is now pulling an opposing tendon function (e.g. tendon from a flexor muscle is attached to a tendon which extends a finger).

Nerve repair

Nerve repair is relatively easy, as once all other structures have been repaired, tension at the suture line is no longer a problem. Their return of function depends mainly on the physiological repair process taking place. It is therefore wise that any attempts to repair damaged nerves should be made in the direction of the pre-injury anatomical arrangements. In larger motor nerve trunks, repair of the epineurium is preferred. The use of fascicular repair has been suggested; however, this technique places a strain on the operating surgeon as it is more tedious, and the results of this technique have not been shown to improve the final outcome. It is important to note that, during the epineurium repair, opposing the fascicles of the possible original order may be helpful for better return of nerve function. The use of 'tissue/fibrin glue' has been suggested as a useful method to not only reduce the time of surgery but also to produce better outcomes. However, this method is not standard practice or advocated widely by many established microsurgeons.

Skin coverage and dressing

The skin has to be loosely approximated and not impede or place pressure on the underlying structures. In the event that the skin cannot completely cover the wound, secondary reconstruction at a later date can be performed by using either skin flaps or skin grafts. Loose bulky dressing should be used to cover the wands with minimal compression applied. Circumferential constriction must be avoided at all times. The replanted limb needs to be immobilized and elevated/ lowered to ensure circulation is maintained during the healing process.

POSTOPERATIVE CARE

Postoperative care remains one of the most important aspects of the replantation procedure.[2-9] The distal area of the reattached part must be reviewed half-hourly or

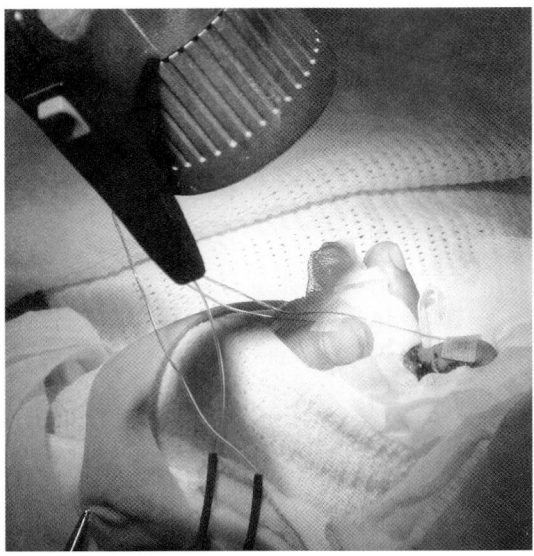

Figure 115.3 Example of the use of a warming light and temperature probe to ensure that the vessels repaired during the replantation do not undergo vasospasm.

hourly, as vascular insufficiency can develop over a short period of time. Continuous i.v. infusion of fluids including antithrombolytic/anticoagulant (e.g. heparin or dextran) is recommended to ensure maintenance of perfusion. In many instances, the use of heating lights and a temperature probe for maintenance and monitoring of skin temperature (>30°C) have been found useful to maintain perfusion and/or indicate inadequate perfusion to the replanted part (Fig. 115.3). In the event that vascular insufficiency has occurred, early detection and repair can help to avoid complete failure of the replantation. Foreknowledge of early complications is helpful for medically trained staff to monitor replanted body parts to prevent poor outcomes (Box 115.2).

Wound dressings are usually not opened until after 2 weeks to prevent unwanted vasospasm, and therefore reduce blood flow to the replanted part (Fig. 115.4). This is especially true in replantation of the digits.

Despite the initial success of the replantation procedure, certain complications may develop over time and are only seen during follow-up in clinics. These include functional difficulties, cold intolerance and poor return of sensation (Box 115.3).[14-20]

OUTCOME OF SURGERY

In the Louisville report, the results of initial survival rates of replantation were reported to be low (69–70%),[3,14] but subsequently increased to 90% in later years. These investigators stressed the importance of experience and a careful operative technique. These results were further confirmed by Tamai in his Founder's Lecture to the Hand Society in 1980, where he reviewed 20 years' experience of

> **BOX 115.2: Early complications: detecting these changes early can help to restore viability of the replantation by early intervention**
>
> - Arterial insufficiency
> When this occurs first inspect for constrictions and loosen dressing. Change of hand position may help blood flow/circulation. The use of regional blocks (e.g. brachial or stiletto block) may improve poor blood flow due to vasoconstriction. Bolus injection of i.v. heparin (3000–5000 units) may help thrombolysis but can be dangerous as it may create a systemic embolus. In the event that no improvement is seen within 4–6 hours, return to theatre for redo anastomosis, which can bring about 50–60% success rate in re-establishing perfusion
> - Venous insufficiency
> Elevation of the limb can help to reduce venous congestion. When no venous repair is possible, venous drainage can be accomplished by removing the nail and placing a concentrated heparin sponge on the exposed nail bed. The French popularized the use of leeches, which can be placed on the exposed nail bed (or the replanted site) to treat venous congestion. However the use of antibiotics is needed to cover against aeromonas hydrophilia
> - Infections
> In the series reported by the Subcommittee on Replantation presented at the Third Meeting of the International Society for Surgery of the Hand, almost no infection was found. However, it is noted that infection is more common in upper extremity replantations which develop as the result of myonecrosis

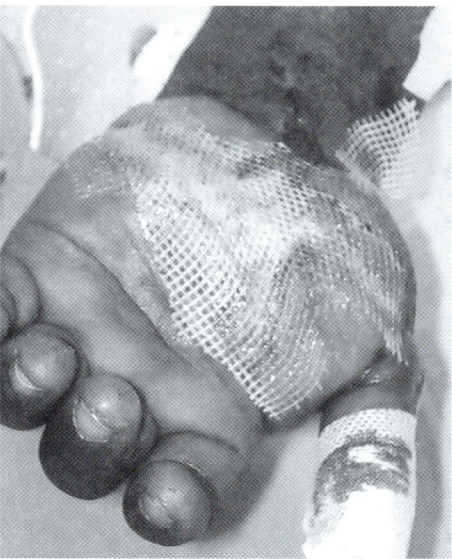

Figure 115.4 An example of a 2-week-old wound following a replantation of a mid-palmar amputation that occurred during a fight.

> **BOX 115.3: Long-term complications are expected in replantation cases and are worth noting in patient follow-up**
>
> - Functional difficulties
> As tissues tend to scar onto the underlying tendons or wounds adhering to one another onto tendons, differential gliding as well as adhesions prevent adequate motion occurring. Scarring itself restricts joint motions even when the tendons are not involved
> - Cold intolerance
> Although this problem is said to improve after a period extending up to 2 years, a recent long-term study has shown otherwise. In a number of case series, almost all patients undergoing replantation will experience cold intolerance of the replanted part
> - Poor return of sensation
> From several reports, a large number of patients who have undergone replantation have a return of sensation of 10 mm or better although the recovery may occur over a long period, as nerve regeneration occurs at a rate of approximately 1 mm day^{-1}. However, it is noted that fine tactile discrimination very rarely recovers

replants of the upper extremities. He analysed 293 cases that had an overall survival rate of 88%.[5,6]

An accepted overall functional recovery has not been established universally due to the multifaceted nature of the injury and variation in the assessment methods. However, continuous monitoring and assessment of a patient's recovery over a long period of time must be performed to ensure achievement of optimal recovery. Assessment of the overall outcome should include tests involving active range of motion, cold intolerance, nerve recovery and cosmetic appearance. Although the aim of replantation is to restore normal function of the amputated part to its state prior to the injury, this rarely occurs because of some inherent limitations. An example of functional evaluation following replantation is shown in Table 115.3. Although published and described in the text book, very few authors have ever reported the use of these scores in the literature (Table 115.3).[15,16]

RING AVULSION INJURIES

Ring avulsions have received special attention over the years. There has been much debate whether or not replantation should be attempted at the first instance because of

Table 115.3 Chen criteria for the evaluation of function after extremity replantation. Although published here, very rarely has this been reported in practising centres

Grade	Function
I	Able to resume original work. Range of motion (ROM) is between 60% and 100% of normal ROM. Complete or nearly complete recovery of sensibility. Muscle power grades 4 and 5
II	Able to resume suitable work; ROM exceeds 40% of normal. Nearly complete sensibility. Muscle power grades 3 and 4
III	Able to carry out activities of daily life. ROM exceeds 30% of normal. Partial recovery of sensibility. Muscle power grade 3
IV	Almost no usable function of survived limb

From Chen et al.[16]

Table 115.4 Urbaniak classification for the description of degloving injury of the fingers/hand

Class I	Disruption of the soft tissues with intact circulation. This requires standard bone and soft-tissue treatment
Class II	Disruption of the soft tissues down to the underlying fibrocartilage structures and bone with disruption of the neurovascular structures. The circulation is deemed inadequate and therefore requires vessel repair
Class III	Complete degloving injury or complete amputation

the severe nature of the injury. Urbaniak et al.[20] reported one of the early series of ring avulsions in which nine of the 24 cases reviewed were replanted. Based on the findings, the investigators have classified ring avulsions into three different groups (Table 115.4). The complete ring avulsion usually includes the distal phalanx and the long flexor with the nerves avulsed with the amputated part. Replantation almost always requires long vein and nerve grafts (Fig. 115.5). With careful attention to these details, success rates have been high. The success of replantation has been reported to be between 45% and 71%.[14,15,20] A major complication noted in all cases was cold intolerance. With no specific treatment for this complication, attempts to replant these injuries remain questionable, especially in areas of constant cold climate, such as in Scandinavian countries.[1,21,22]

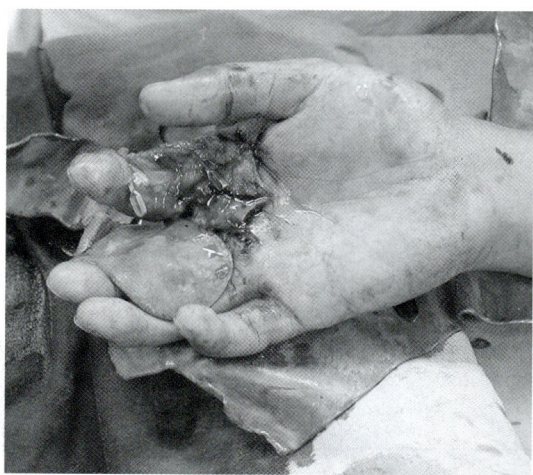

Figure 115.5 Example of an extensive (degloving) amputation of the index finger. Note that, because of the high amount of soft-tissue damage in these injuries, the radial side of the digital artery is insufficient for repair as part of the artery has been lost. A vein graft was then used to re-establish perfusion on the ulnar side.

KEY LEARNING POINTS

- Amputations of the upper limb, although uncommon, require vigilant and immediate medical care.
- Although care of the amputation is important, immediate and general care of the patient takes precedence (i.e. fluid/blood resuscitation and prevention of further blood loss).
- Amputation can be classified according the mode of injury (e.g. guillotine, crush) or level of amputation (e.g. mid-palmar, wrist) or duration of when the amputation occurred (i.e. cold or warm ischaemia time).
- It is important to ensure maintenance of tissue viability prior to the surgery. Early preservation of the amputated part in cold but properly managed conditions must be done to ensure that the amputated part can be preserved as long as possible.
- The decision for replantation must be made based on strict criteria, as the process of surgery, recovery and rehabilitation is long and expensive. Failure to do so results in poor survival rates and surgical outcomes.

- The overall success rates for replantations are approximately 80%; however, this can only be achieved in well-equipped centres manned by experienced surgical teams.
- The techniques used in replantation must be performed by an experienced and well-trained surgeon as they require high levels of microsurgical skill.
- In early complications of replantation, immediate management can assist in long-term survival of the replanted part. In contrast, late complications can be managed conservatively or by planned surgery.
- Ring avulsion injuries are of special interest as repair of these cases requires even higher levels of expertise.

REFERENCES

- ● = Key primary paper
- ◆ = Major review article

● 1. Nylander G, Vilki S, Östrup L. The need for replantation surgery after traumatic amputations of the upper extremity – an estimate based upon the epidemiology of Sweden. *Journal of Hand Surgery (European)* 1984;**9**:257.

◆ 2. Buncke HJ. 25th Anniversary Presentation. Microvascular hand surgery – transplants and replants – over the past 25 years. *Journal of Hand Surgery* 2000;**25A**:415–28.

● 3. Weiland AJ, Villarreal-Rios A, Kleinert HE, et al. Replantation of digits and hands: analysis of surgical techniques and functional results in 71 patients with 86 replantations. *Journal of Hand Surgery* 1977;**2**:1–12.

◆ 4. Urbaniak JR. Digital replantation. *Journal of Hand Surgery* 1977;**2**:82 (letter).

◆ 5. Tamai S. Twenty years' experience of limb replantation – review of 293 upper extremity replants. *Journal of Hand Surgery* 1982;**7**:549–56.

● 6. Tamai S, Michon J, Tupper J, Fleming J. Report of the Subcommittee on Replantation. *Journal of Hand Surgery* 1983;**8**:730–2.

● 7. Arakaki A, Tsai TM. Thumb replantation: survival factors and re-exploration in 122 cases. *Journal of Hand Surgery* 1993;**18B**:152–6.

● 8. Tamai S, Tatsumi Y, Shimizu T, et al. Traumatic amputation of digits: the fate of remaining blood. An experimental and clinical study. *Journal of Hand Surgery* 1977;**2**:13–21.

● 9. May JW Jr, Toth BA, Gardner M. Digital replantation distal to the proximal interphalangeal joint. *Journal of Hand Surgery* 1982;**7**:161–6.

● 10. Goldner RD, Stevanovic MV, Nunley JA, Urbaniak JR. Digital replantation at the level of the distal interphalangeal joint and the distal phalanx. *Journal of Hand Surgery* 1989;**14A**:214–20.

● 11. Slattery P. Distal digital replantation using a solitary digital artery for arterial inflow and venous drainage. *Journal of Hand Surgery* 1994;**19A**:565–6.

● 12. Gordon L, Leitner DW, Buncke HJ, Alpert BS. Partial nail plate removal after digital replantation as an alternative method of venous drainage. *Journal of Hand Surgery* 1985;**10A**:360–4.

● 13. Moiemen NS, Elliot D. Composite graft replacement of digital tips. 2. A study in children. *Journal of Hand Surgery* 1997;**22B**:346–52.

● 14. Arakaki A, Tsai TM. Thumb replantation: survival factors and re-exploration in 122 cases. *Journal of Hand Surgery* 1993;**18B**:152–6.

◆ 15. Ch'en CW, Meyer VE, Kleinert HE, Beasley RW. Present indications and contraindications for replantation as reflected by long-term functional results. *Orthopedic Clinics of North America* 1981;**12**:849.

● 16. Chen CW, Qian YQ, Yu ZJ. Extremity replantation. *World Journal of Surgery* 1978;**2**:513.

● 17. Nylander G, Nylander E, Lassvik C. Cold sensitivity after replantation in relation to arterial circulation and vasoregulation. *Journal of Hand Surgery* 1987;**12B**:78–81.

● 18. Backman C, Nystrom A, Backman C. Cold-induced arterial spasm after digital amputation. *Journal of Hand Surgery* 1991;**16B**:378–81.

● 19. Koman LA, Nunley JA. Thermoregulatory control after upper extremity replantation. *Journal of Hand Surgery* 1986;**11A**:548–52.

● 20. Urbaniak JR, Evans JP, Bright DS. Microvascular management of ring avulsion injuries. *Journal of Hand Surgery* 1981;**6**:25–30.

● 21. Povlsen B, Nylander G, Nylander E. Cold-induced vasospasm after digital replantation does not improve with time. A 12-year prospective study. *Journal of Hand Surgery* 1995;**20B**:237–9.

● 22. Kay S. Venous occlusion plethysmography in patients with cold related symptoms after digital salvage procedures. *Journal of Hand Surgery* 1985;**10B**:151–4.

Dupuytren's contracture

WILLIAM YC LOH, WEE-LEON LAM

Introduction	1324	Surgical treatment	1327
Epidemiology	1324	Release of proximal interphalangeal joint flexion contracture	1329
Anatomy	1324		
Pathogenesis	1325	Complications after surgery	1330
Clinical presentation	1325	Postoperative management and rehabilitation	1330
Treatment	1326	References	1331

NATIONAL BOARD STANDARDS

- Understand the incidence, risk factors, pathology and clinical features of Dupuytren's contracture
- Common sites for the disease
- Surgical approaches especially for the metacarpophalangeal and proximal interphalangeal joint contractures
- Learn the main complications of surgery

INTRODUCTION

Dupuytren's contracture is a condition of unknown aetiology that affects the palmar fascia of the hand, leading to a progressive worsening contracture of the fingers and potentially loss of hand function. Since its initial description in 1777 by Henry Cline, and a later description of its treatment by Guillaume Dupuytren in 1831 (resulting in his name becoming synonymous with the condition), Dupuytren's contracture continues to generate widespread interest with regards to its aetiology, pathogenesis and treatment.

EPIDEMIOLOGY

Worldwide, Dupuytren's contracture remains largely a disease of Caucasians over the age of 40 years, with exceptions in the Japanese.[1] There is a particular strong link between people of northern European descent and men, with the male to female ratio up to 10:1.[2] Besides a familial tendency,[3] there are other well-known risk factors, including alcoholism, diabetes, chronic liver disease and epilepsy, although the proportion of patients in these groups who require surgical treatment is probably small. Hueston[4] was the first to suggest the concept of 'Dupuytren diathesis', a condition characterized by a particularly aggressive disease presentation. McFarlane[5] further strengthened the concept of a 'Dupuytren's diathesis' by describing five factors that are found to influence the course of disease: involvement of more than the hand; early onset; bilateral disease; family history; and more than two rays involved. The first two factors listed above are thought to be particularly important.

ANATOMY

Anatomically, the condition of Dupuytren's contracture can be described in three regions: palmar, palmodigital and digital. In the palm, the fascia is arranged in three layers: longitudinal, transverse and vertical.[6] Dupuytren's contracture mainly affects the longitudinal fibres, believed

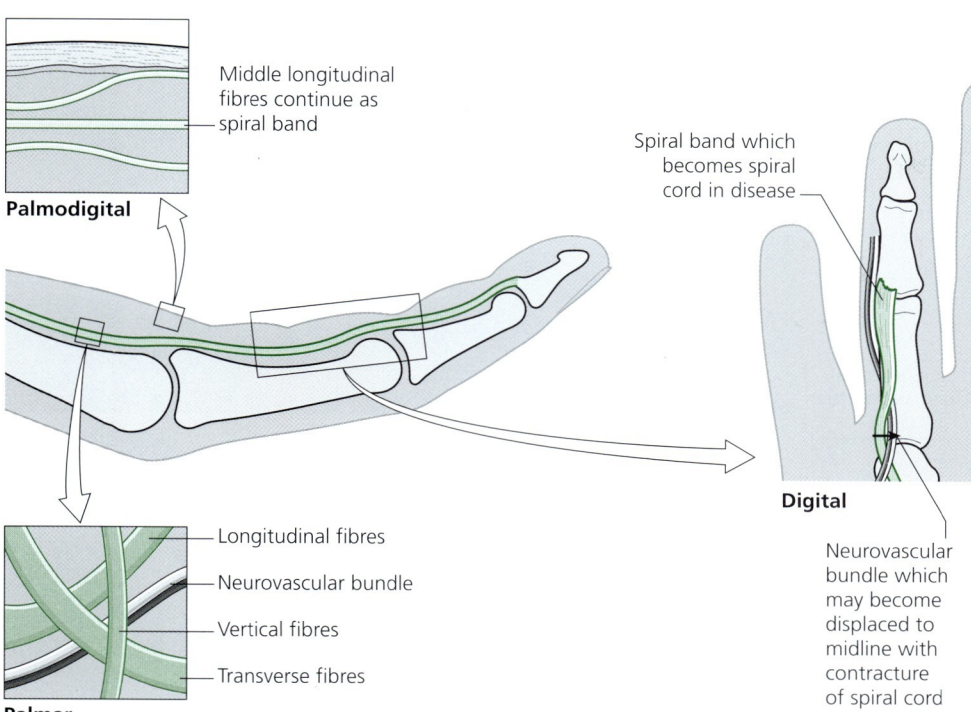

Figure 116.1 Anatomy of palmodigital fascias (bands) and corresponding diseased fascias (cords).

to be a result of a tension hypothesis.[7] The affected fibres become shortened cords that progressively contract and flex the metacarpophalangeal (MCP) joint. As the longitudinal fibres continue into the palmodigital area, they further split into three layers, with the middle layer continuing into the digit. When disease affects this middle layer, it forms a potential spiral cord comprising the spiral band, natatory ligament, lateral digital sheet and Grayson's ligament. Subsequent shortening of the cord can result in displacement of the neurovascular bundle to a more central and superficial position, rendering it susceptible to damage during surgical dissection (Fig. 116.1).

PATHOGENESIS

Pathologically, Dupuytren's contracture is believed to be a fibroproliferative disease. Luck[8] classified the disease into three stages: proliferative, involutional and residual. In the proliferative stage, the disease is characterized by proliferative whorls of cells that macroscopically are thought to correspond to the nodules seen in the condition. The final residual stage is thought to represent the 'burnt out' stage, where only diseased, shortened cords are left that progressively shorten resulting in a worsening of the contracture.

The central cell responsible for the disease pathogenesis is thought to be the myofibroblast.[9] These cells possess the properties not only of fibroblasts in laying down collagen and secreting key growth factors for cell proliferation, but also of smooth muscle cells in their ability to contract and produce macroscopic contracture through their interaction with the surrounding extracellular matrix.[10] This hypothesis is supported by the observation that the ratio of type III to type I collagen decreases with disease progression,[11] a condition seen in wound healing, and that myofibroblasts are thought to be the key cells responsible for wound healing. Another important factor seems to be tension, which seems in some ways to perpetuate the differentiation of fibroblasts into myofibroblasts under the influence of transforming growth factor (TGF) $\beta1$.[12] A simplified flow diagram of events in disease pathogenesis is shown in Fig. 116.2a.

CLINICAL PRESENTATION

The appearance of pitting and thickening of the palmar skin is an early manifestation. More commonly a non-tender nodule is found in the palm. In some patients, the appearance of a palmar nodule is associated with discomfort and leads to medical consultation. The palmar nodules classically progress to form a cord which, over time, contracts and may result in the fixed flexion deformities of digital MCP and proximal interphalangeal (PIP) joints. The progressive deformity of the PIP joint causes a permanent joint contracture. In severe cases where the distal interphalangeal joint is affected by the Dupuytren's contracture, a 'pseudo-boutonnière' deformity of the digit appears (Fig. 116.3a–c).

Finger contracture is a common presenting complaint. Common daily activities, such as hand shake, wearing gloves, washing, dressing, etc., become difficult and troublesome. The ring and little fingers are most commonly affected. There is usually a bilateral hand involvement. In

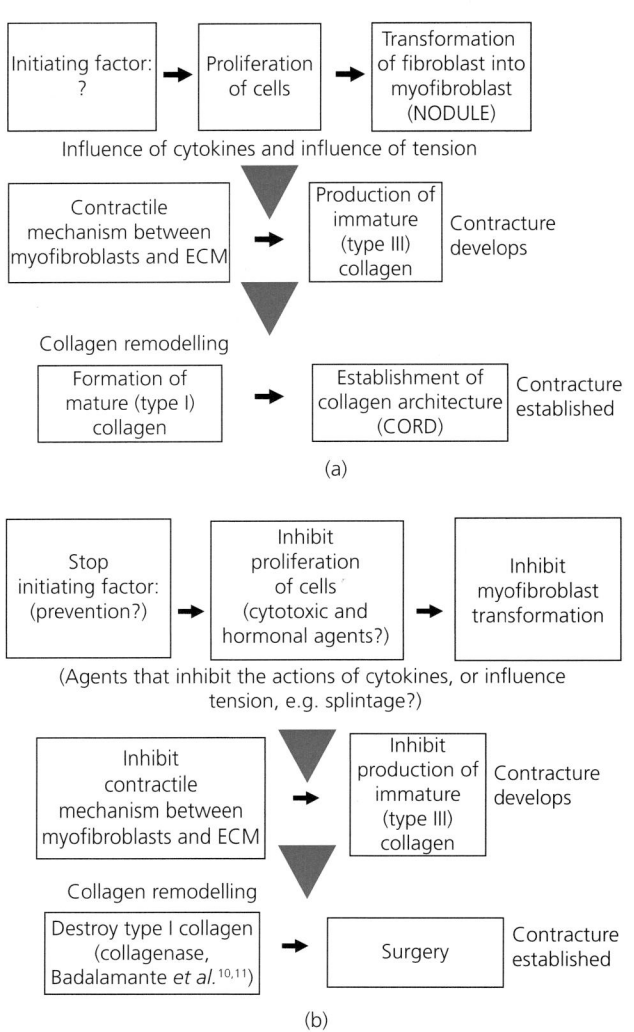

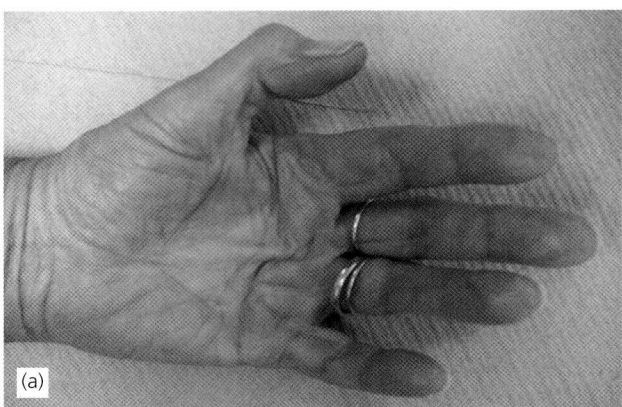

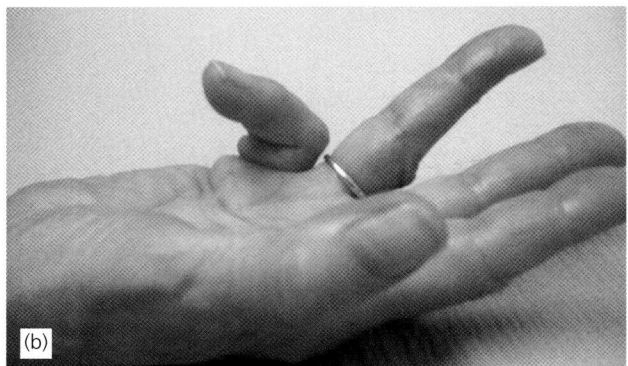

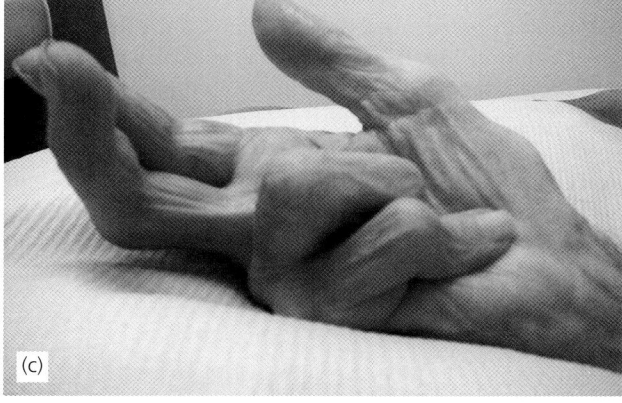

Figure 116.2 (a) Sequence of events in the pathogenesis of Dupuytren's disease. Reproduced with permission from Lam et al.[11] (b) A corresponding flowchart of potential pharmacological targets that may be available. ECM, extracellular matrix.

patients with a strong familial history of Dupuytren's disease, the radial side of the palm and radial digits tend to be more affected. If the disease is more severe or aggressive, it carries a more serious prognosis. Dupuytren's diathesis is recognized in many young Caucasian men with a strong family history, bilateral involvement, severe disease and manifestations outside the hand. Garrod's knuckle pads over the dorsal aspects of the digital PIP joints, plantar fibromatosis (Ledderhose disease) and penile fibromatosis (Peyronie disease) are seen in the other areas of the body in more severe cases.

TREATMENT

Currently, the mainstay of treatment for Dupuytren's contracture remains surgical, but ongoing developments in our understanding of disease pathogenesis have increased

Figure 116.3 (a) Dupuytren's contracture involving the metacarpophalangeal joint. (b) Dupuytren's contracture affecting both metacarpophalangeal and proximal interphalangeal joints. (c) Pseudo-boutonnière deformity of little finger.

the possibility of treating the condition with non-surgical modalities. An effective non-surgical treatment would obviously be an attractive option as it obviates the need for surgery and possibly prevents recurrences. Pharmacological modalities that have been suggested include steroids, tamoxifen, androgen therapy and even interferon. Fig. 116.2b shows a corresponding flowchart of potential pharmacological targets that may be available. One of the most encouraging results has come from the use of injection of clostridial collagenase,[13,14] which has recently been approved for clinical use in both the USA and Europe.

This therapy theoretically bypasses all the other disease processes prior to the formation and maturity of type I collagen and may be considered as a form of fasciotomy. Isolated clostridial collagenase injected into cords has been shown to result in a reduction in contracture almost back to the normal joint range of motion in about 90% of patients.[15] The future of Dupuytren's contracture treatment is likely to be a combination of specific surgical and pharmacological regimens designed for various stages of the disease.

SURGICAL TREATMENT

The majority of patients with Dupuytren's disease do not require any treatment. However when an intervention is deemed necessary, there are a number of treatment options. There are both subjective (patient's perspective) and objective (surgeon's perspective) indications for treatments.

The subjective indications include the painful palmar nodule, deteriorated daily hand function and cosmetic appearance of the affected hand. The objective indications for surgical treatments are the severe palmar skin involvement, joint contracture, positive table-top test and web space contracture (Table 116.1).

The *palmar nodule* is usually associated with discomfort when the hand grasps an object. Patients usually complain of pain before noticing the appearance of the palmar nodule. These patients are sometimes helped by a local steroid injection to the area. It is not advisable to excise the nodule as the process of fibromatosis is still actively taking place, otherwise it may result in a poor surgical outcome and early recurrence.

The pre-tendinous bands of the palmar aponeurosis become the cords as the Dupuytren's disease process progresses. These bands, which normally insert into the palmar skin distal to the distal crease of the palm, thicken and distort the skin. This disease process may diffusely involve the whole palmar aponeurosis. Skin puckering, skin pitting and painful skin induration without any finger joint contracture are the early presenting signs. Painful and matured palmar skin thickening may need excision in the absence of joint contracture.

Table 116.1 Indications for treatments of Dupuytren's disease

Subjective indications	Objective indications
Painful palmar nodule	Palmar skin involvement
Impaired hand function	Positive table-top test
Cosmetic effect	Joint contracture
	Web space contracture

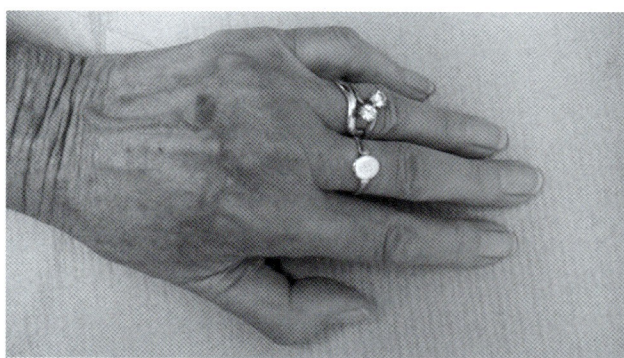

Figure 116.4 Positive table-top test.

Finger joint contracture is a common indication for surgery. A positive table-top test (Fig. 116.4) signifying increased severity of joint contracture and deterioration of hand function warrants surgical intervention. The MCP joint is the most frequently contracted but is most readily corrected because only the pre-tendinous band of the Dupuytren's diseased palmar aponeurosis (i.e. the central cord) is involved. A flexion contracture of the MCP joint of 30° or more is a good indication for surgical intervention.[16] There is no urgency for surgical correction because the MCP joint contracture could usually be readily corrected regardless of the duration of contracture.

The PIP joint flexion contracture is more difficult to correct. This is because of the involvement of multiple fascial bands by Dupuytren's disease. This includes the central, spiral, lateral and retrovascular cords either in isolation or in combination. A flexion contracture of the PIP joint of 15° or beyond is an indication for surgery. The longer standing the contracture and the greater the degree of flexion contracture of the PIP joint, the more difficult it is to fully correct the deformity. Prolonged PIP joint contracture also affects the joint capsule, volar plate, accessory lateral collateral ligament and lateral collateral ligament proper, flexor sheaths, flexor tendons and extensor expansion adhesion and contracture. Hence, early surgical intervention is advisable in order to obtain a good surgical correction. The patient should be warned that a PIP joint contracture could be improved but may not be fully corrected.

The involvement of the distal interphalangeal (DIP) joint by Dupuytren's contracture is uncommon. The hyperextension deformity at the DIP joint seen in the 'pseudo-boutonnière' deformity (Fig. 116.5) is difficult to correct. This is not due to Dupuytren's fascial tissue contracture but is due to secondary prolonged postural deformity as in other boutonnière deformity aetiology. The dolphin procedure involving tenotomy of the conjoint lateral bands of the extensor expansion only and taking care to preserve the oblique retinacular ligament and its insertion

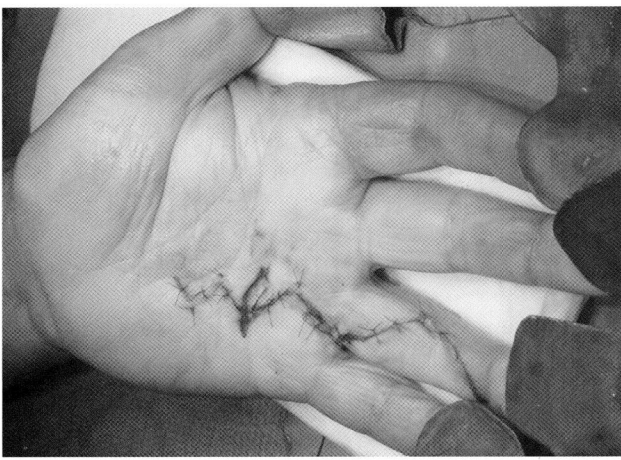

Figure 116.5 McCash and Bruner incisions.

Table 116.2 Types of operations

Fasciotomy	Needle fasciotomy
	Stab fasciotomy
	Segmental aponeurectomy
Fasciectomy	Partial/subtotal fasciectomy with or without PIP joint contracture release
	Dermofasciectomy + full skin thickness graft ± PIP joint contracture release
Others (usually for severe contracture)	Digital amputation
	Dolphin's conjoint lateral band tenotomy
	Arthrodesis of PIP joint
	Arthroplasty of PIP joint

PIP, proximal interphalangeal.

to the terminal tendon may improve DIP joint flexion.[17] However, the appearance of pseudo-boutonnière deformity in a Dupuytren's diseased finger carries a poorer prognosis. The deformity indicates both the severity and the chronicity of Dupuytren's contracture of the finger. This usually results in finger amputation to optimize the remaining hand function. The DIP joint flexion deformity is also difficult to treat because the involved fascial strands are intermingled in between the terminal branches of the digital neurovascular bundles.

Web space contracture is due to the disease affecting the natatory ligament of the palm. It is troublesome and causes a decrease in the hand span. The contracture prevents the separation of the fingers and makes hand hygiene difficult. The most commonly affected web space involves the first web of the thumb. This contracture is a result of the combination of central cord thickening of the terminal transverse fibres of the palmar aponeurosis and the natatory ligament. In severe cases, the thumb is not able to extend or abduct.

The aim of surgery is to restore function and correct deformity with minimal complications. The purpose of surgery, the risks to the neurovascular structure and what may be achieved must be explained to patients. The patients must also be counselled about the possible recurrence of the Dupuytren's contracture. The timescale of recurrence is unpredictable. The types of operations available for Dupuytren's contracture are summarized in Table 116.2.

In general, fasciotomy means that the Dupuytren's cord is simply divided, whereas fasciectomy implies that the diseased fascia is excised. Fasciotomy can be performed under local anaesthesia in the outpatient department. It is usually performed for elderly people who may be medically unfit for more extensive surgery. Early recurrence and neurovascular injuries are the common complications.

Needle fasciotomy

Needle fasciotomy carried out under local anaesthetic is an effective way of correcting the MCP joint flexion contracture. The diseased fascia (central cord) is divided by the bevelled part of a hypodermic needle after the skin area has been anaesthetized. In this procedure, the surrounding neurovascular bundles and flexor tendons are at risk. However, it is a good procedure for elderly and unfit patients in whom Dupuytren's disease is quiescent and recurrence is less likely. Needle fasciotomy is unable to correct the PIP or DIP joint flexion contracture.

Segmental aponeurectomy and stab incision fasciotomy

Segmental aponeurectomy and stab incision fasciotomy are also useful techniques during open surgery of Dupuytren's contracture. An approximately 1 cm segment of the diseased cord is excised to correct the finger and palmar deformities particularly when local excision is deemed too risky for the surrounding neurovascular structures or when the patient is unable to tolerate prolonged general anaesthesia. However, like needle fasciotomy, disease recurrence is high because most diseased tissue is left behind.

Partial or subtotal fasciectomy

Partial or subtotal fasciectomy is usually carried out under regional anaesthesia or general anaesthesia as a day surgery procedure. Since only the macroscopically diseased fascia is excised, this form of surgery is most suitably performed on the palm. In contrast, in the finger, the result of partial fasciectomy is less satisfactory because it is difficult to differentiate diseased from local normal tissue, especially when dealing with recurrent disease.

The surgical skin incisions can vary and are carried out according to the preference and training of the surgeon. Dupuytren's contracture surgery is performed with an inflated tourniquet applied to the affected upper limb. Under a bloodless field and using loupe magnification, the diseased fascia is identified and removed. In general, a longitudinal incision provides good exposure of the cord and the neurovascular structures and z-plasty may be used to overcome the longitudinal skin tension during wound closure. The longitudinal incision with z-plasty can be utilized in the palm and finger. Other incisions such as a transverse palmar incision with a Bruner digital incision are also popular. They provide not only good exposure of the diseased fascia but also good wound closure with little tension in the palm and finger. The open palm technique is a useful alternative and a versatile technique in some patients undergoing partial fasciectomy.[18] The transverse palmar wound is left open at the end of fasciectomy. The open palm method prevents haematoma formation and relaxes the wound tension. This reduces swelling of the hand and may reduce finger stiffness. It has also been claimed by some authors that postoperative pain is reduced and early mobilization is possible. The McCash palmar incision is usually accompanied by digital and palmar Bruner incisions to adequately remove the diseased palmar fascia (Fig. 116.5). The transverse palmar wound is left to heal by secondary intention. The combination of marginal epithelialization and contracture of the wound edges contributes to the gradual healing of the open wound.[19] The McCash open wound principle can also be applied to the finger when the PIP joint contracture is released during fasciectomy. Alternatively, the open digital wound may be covered with a partial thickness skin graft.

In the palm, ideally under loupe magnification (between 3.5 and 4.5 times), the central cord, adjacent neurovascular bundles, lumbrical muscles and flexor tendons are identified. Having retracted and protected the aforementioned important structures, the central cord is excised by a sharp dissection. At the palm level, only the longitudinal layer (but sometimes the vertical layer) of the palmar aponeurosis is diseased and contracted. The diseased fascia can be safely excised superficial to the transverse layer of the palmar aponeurosis, thereby avoiding injury to the important neurovascular structures underneath.[20]

At the palmodigital area, a very careful dissection is needed. There are numerous diseased fascial structures such as the central cord, spiral cord, lateral cord and retrovascular cord distorting the normal local anatomy and particularly displacing the neurovascular bundle superficially. This superficial displacement of the neurovascular bundle renders iatrogenic injury during dissection possible. The mechanism of distortion of the neurovascular bundle by the diseased cords is usually predictable, particularly in the finger. The spiral cord displaces the neurovascular bundle both medially and superficially. The central cord conceals a part of the medially displaced neurovascular bundle from the surgeon. The neurovascular bundle may pierce through the central cord tissue at the level of the middle phalanx.

The tourniquet is released at the completion of dissection, and bleeding is controlled with bipolar cautery. The longitudinal and Bruner wounds are closed with non-absorbable sutures. At the conclusion of a McCash open palm technique, the wound is covered with a non-adherent gauze dressing such as Mepitel (Molnlycke Health Care AB). A bulky fluff dressing is placed in the palm and between the fingers. A crepe bandage is applied to the hand, which is placed in the 'Edinburgh' functional position. The hand is elevated in a Cory sling (Cory Brothers Ltd). Postoperative wound care is important. The Mepitel dressing is changed weekly until the open wound has healed. This dressing is so light and simple that early and normal finger mobilization is not affected. The time taken for the wound to close is proportional to the size of wound defect and it usually varies from 1 to 4 weeks.

Dermofasciectomy and full skin thickness graft

Hueston[21] introduced the excision of the overlying skin and diseased fascia during fasciectomy. The defect is then covered with a full-thickness skin graft. He believed that recurrence is very unlikely to develop deep to a skin graft. The indications for this extensive procedure are recurrent Dupuytren's joint contracture and young patients with strong Dupuytren's diathesis. Possible donor sites for the full-thickness skin graft include the supraclavicular area, volar distal forearm, volar elbow crease area, post-auricular area and groin area.

Although the open palm technique can be employed to aid the fasciectomy in Dupuytren's disease with severe PIP joint contracture, it has been shown that wound closure with a full-thickness skin graft yields a far better outcome.[22]

RELEASE OF PROXIMAL INTERPHALANGEAL JOINT FLEXION CONTRACTURE

As the PIP joint flexion deformity progresses into chronicity, both internal and external joint structures become tightened and contracted. If only the diseased fascias (e.g. spiral cord, central cord, lateral cord and retrovascular cord) are excised, the PIP joint contracture usually persists. These internal and external structures restricting the PIP joint extension must be carefully assessed and systematically released. The structures to be considered include the flexor tendon sheath, flexor tendons, volar plate, transverse retinacular ligaments, accessory collateral ligaments, collateral ligaments and intra-articular fibrosis/adhesion.[23] In order to expose the volar plate of the PIP joint, the A3 pulley is excised and flexor tendons are atraumatically retracted. Flexor tendolysis is performed if necessary. The checkrein ligaments are incised proximally and transversely. The volar plate is then released from the proximal to distal direction to relieve the contracture. If the PIP joint fails to extend passively, both sides of the accessory collateral ligaments may need to be sequentially released. If necessary, a portion of proper collateral ligaments is released to aid the extension of the PIP joint without compromising the PIP joint stability.

COMPLICATIONS AFTER SURGERY

In general, complications are rare and are more likely to occur with severe disease and after extensive surgery for recurrence. The majority of complications are generally minor – wound infection, haematoma, skin necrosis/loss during the first 4 weeks postoperatively (Table 116.3). Intra-operative complications are rare (1–2%) and include digital nerve or vessel injury and buttonholing of skin flap.[24] The neurovascular bundle injury may cause a delay in postoperative recovery. The patient complains of cold intolerance and has been shown to develop postoperative joint stiffness.

Complex regional pain syndrome (CRPS II) and finger gangrene are the more serious major complications. CRPS II may develop in 5% of patients after extensive surgery. It is more common in female patients and usually results in permanent disability.

Recurrence is common after surgery (up to 60%), especially in patients with aggressive disease.[25] Patients should be counselled carefully prior to surgery that surgery does not cure the disease and, over time, recurrence and extension of the disease is possible. Patients with diathesis carry the worst prognosis and their hand function is likely to be impaired.

Table 116.3 Complications after surgery

Early	Late
Haematoma	Finger gangrene
Wound infection	Complex regional pain syndrome II
Skin necrosis/loss	Recurrence

POSTOPERATIVE MANAGEMENT AND REHABILITATION

The treatment goals after surgery are as follows.

1. Promote wound healing especially in the open palm technique.
2. Control of postoperative oedema.
3. Maintain range of movement of uninvolved joints and fingers.
4. Maintain and improve the active and passive range of movement of operated digits in both flexion and extension.
5. Minimize postoperative scarring and guide scar formation.
6. Restore strength to the hand.

Hand therapy is started immediately after surgery to promote the aforementioned goals. During the first week, the bulky dressing and bandage are replaced with a non-adhesive dressing (e.g. Mepitel) and a volar removable thermoplastic extension splint is applied. The splint is worn continuously except for exercise and hygiene. In severe cases, the extension splint is worn at night for 3 months throughout the period of scar maturation. The splint may need to be adjusted during the rehabilitation stage to achieve full finger extension and flexion.

A whirlpool with the upper limb placed horizontally is used early in treatment with an open palm wound. Appropriate wound care is instituted until the wound heals completely. The non-adhesive dressing (e.g. Mepitel) is changed to an Opsite dressing (from Smith & Nephew) as the wound is healing.

Hand elevation and active exercise, Coban retrograde massage and occasionally pressure gloves are employed to control postoperative oedema. Persistent oedema may compromise the surgical outcome by causing peri-articular fibrosis and permanent joint contracture.

Regular active, active and passive assisted exercises to the finger joints are initiated as soon as possible following surgery. Delay or special care in these exercises is considered when the skin grafting procedure has been undertaken. These exercises are carried out to maintain the gains obtained from the surgery. Both flexion and extension exercises are practised several times a day.

Moulded materials like silastic elastomer may be used to mould thickened scar during the scar maturation phase. Local massage and use of vitamin E cream may also help to soften the scar.

Finally, light activities of daily living and light strengthening exercises are introduced as soon as the wounds have healed, oedema is well controlled and the scar is 'desensitized'.

KEY LEARNING POINTS

- A condition of unknown aetiology that affects the palmar fascia of the hand, leading to a progressive worsening contracture of the fingers and potentially loss of hand function.
- A disease of Caucasians over the age of 40 years, with exceptions in the Japanese, with a particular strong link to men of northern European descent, with a male to female ratio of up to 1:10.
- Well-known risk factors include alcoholism, diabetes, chronic liver disease and epilepsy (although the proportion of patients in these groups who require surgical treatment are probably small).
- The 'Dupuytren diathesis' is a condition characterized by a particularly aggressive disease presentation, and has five factors: involvement of more than the hand; early onset; bilateral disease; family history; and more than two rays involved.
- There are three regions: palmar (arranged in three layers; longitudinal, transverse and vertical; mainly affecting the longitudinal fibres) palmodigital and digital. Note the tension hypothesis. The affected fibres become shortened cords which contract and flex the metacarpophalangeal (MCP) joint. The spiral cord may render damage possible during surgical dissection of the neurovascular bundle.
- A fibroproliferative disease with three stages: proliferate, involutional and residual.
- The central cell responsible for disease pathogenesis is the myofibroblast.
- Clinically there is pitting and thickening of the palmar skin and a non-tender nodule. This palmar nodule may progress to form a cord which contracts to cause fixed flexion deformities of the MCP and proximal interphalangeal (PIP) joints, resulting in permanent joint contracture. (With the distal interphalangeal joint affected, a pseudo-boutonnière deformity appears.)
- Finger contracture is a common presenting complaint. Also note Garrod's knuckle pads over the dorsal aspects of the digital PIP joints, plantar fibromatosis (Ledderhose disease) and penile fibromatosis (Peyronie disease).
- Treatment is surgical but non-surgical options include steroids, tamoxifen, androgens, interferon and injected collagenase.
- Indications for treatment include the painful palmar nodule, impaired hand function, cosmesis, palmar skin involvement, joint contracture, positive table-top test and web space contracture.
- A flexion contracture of the MCP joint is readily correctable and when >30° should be corrected; the PIP flexion contracture is more difficult to correct and so when >15° should be corrected; web space contracture of the thumb when it impairs hand hygiene may require correction.
- Needle fasciotomy (division of the cord) under local anaesthesia, to correct the MCP joint, is a good procedure for elderly and unfit patients. Segmental aponeurectomy and stab incision fasciotomy are also useful but also carry high recurrence.
- Partial or subtotal fasciectomy is the definitive surgical procedure.
- Dermofasciectomy and full-thickness skin graft may be required for recurrence or severe disease in young patients.
- More extensive surgery may be required for PIP joint flexion deformity.
- Complications after surgery are rare and include wound infection, haematoma, skin necrosis/loss, digital nerve or vessel injury, buttonholing of skin flap, cold intolerance and joint stiffness, complex regional pain syndrome (CRPS II), finger gangrene. Recurrence is common (up to 60%). Patients with diathesis carry the worst prognosis.
- Goals after surgery are to promote wound healing; control postoperative oedema; maintain range of movement of uninvolved joints and fingers; maintain and improve the active and passive range of movement of operated digits in both flexion and extension; minimize postoperative scarring and guide scar formation and restore strength to the hand.
- This is achieved with immediate postoperative hand therapy.

REFERENCES

- ● = Key primary paper
- ◆ = Major review article

●1. Egawa T, Senrui H, Horikia A, Egama M. Epidemiology of the oriental patient. In: McFarlane R, McGrouther D, Flint M (eds) *Dupuytren's Disease*. Edinburgh, UK: Churchill Livingstone, 1990:239–45.

●2. Brouet JP. Etude de 1000 dossiers de maladie de Dupuytren. In: Tubiana R, Hueston JT (eds) *La Maladie Dupuytren*. Paris, France: Expansion Scientifique, 1986:98–105.

●3. Ling RSH. The genetic factor in Dupuytren's disease. *Journal of Bone and Joint Surgery (British)* 1963:**45B**;709.

●4. Hueston JT. Recurrent Dupuytren's contracture. *Plastic and Reconstructive Surgery* 1963;**31**:66–9.

●5. McFarlane RM. Some observations on the epidemiology of DD. In: Hueston JT, Tubiana R (eds) *Dupuytren's Disease*. Edinburgh, UK: Churchill Livingstone, 1990:250–2.

- 6. McGrouther DA. The microanatomy of Dupuytren's contracture. *Hand* 1982;**14**:215–36.
- 7. Tarlton JF, Meagher P, Brown RA, *et al*. Mechanical stress in vitro induces increased expression of MMPs 2 and 9 in excised Dupuytren's disease tissue. *Journal of Hand Surgery (British)* 1998;**23**:297–302.
- 8. Luck J. A new concept of the pathogenesis correlated with surgical management. *Journal of Bone and Joint Surgery (American)* 1959;**41A**:635–64.
- 9. Gabbiani G, Majno G. Dupuytren's contracture: fibroblast contraction? An ultrastructural study. *American Journal of Pathology* 1972;**66**:131–46.
- 10. Tomasek JJ, Haaksma CJ. Fibronectin filaments and actin microfilaments are organised into a fibronexus in Dupuytren's diseased tissue. *Anatomical Record* 1991;**230**:175–82.
- 11. Lam WL, Rawlins JM, Karoo RO, *et al*. Re-visiting Luck's classification: a histological analysis of Dupuytren's disease. *Journal of Hand Surgery, European Volume* 2010;**35**:312–17.
- 12. Badalamente MA, Sampson SP, Hurst LC, *et al*. The role of transforming growth factor beta in Dupuytren's disease. *Journal of Hand Surgery (American)* 1996;**21**:210–15.
- 13. Badalamente MA, Hurst LC. Enzyme injection as nonsurgical treatment of Dupuytren's disease. *Journal of Hand Surgery (American)* 2000;**25**:629–36.
- 14. Badalamente MA, Hurst LC, Hentz VR. Collagen as a clinical target: nonoperative treatment of Dupuytren's disease. *Journal of Hand Surgery (American)* 2002;**27**:788–98.
- 15. Hurst LC, Badalamente MA, Hentz VR, *et al*. Injectable collagenase clostridium histolyticum for Dupuytren's contracture. *New England Journal of Medicine* 2009;**361**:968–79.
- 16. Smith AC. Diagnosis and indications for surgical treatment. *Hand Clinics* 1991;**7**:635–43; Discussion 643.
- 17. Dolphin JA. Extensor tenotomy for chronic boutonniere deformity of the finger. *Journal of Bone and Joint Surgery (American)* 1965;**47A**:161–4.
- 18. McCash CR. The open palm technique in Dupuytren's contracture. *British Journal of Plastic Surgery* 1964;**17**:271.
- 19. Kleinman WB. Dupuytren's contracture: treatment by the open palm technique. In Strickland JW, Streichen JB (eds) *Difficult Problems in Hand Surgery*. St. Louis, MO: C V Mosby, 1982.
- 20. Skoog T. The transverse elements of the palmar aponeurosis in Dupuytren's contracture. *Scandinavian Journal of Plastic Surgery* 1967;**1**:15–63.
- 21. Hueston JT. Dermofasciectomy for Dupuytren's disease. *Bulletin of the Hospital for Joint Diseases Orthopaedic Institute* 1984;**44**:224.
- 22. Ketchum LD, Hixson FP. Dermatofasciectomy and full thickness grafts in the treatment of Dupuytren's contracture. *Journal of Hand Surgery (American)* 1987;**12A**:659–63.
- 23. Curtis RM. Capsulectomy of the interphalangeal joints of the fingers. *Journal of Bone and Joint Surgery (American)* 1954;**36A**:1219–32.
- 24. Bulstrode NW, Jemec B, Smith PJ. The complications of Dupuytren's contracture surgery. *Journal of Hand Surgery (American)* 2005;**30**:1021–5.
- 25. Rodrigo J, Niebauer JJ, Brown RL, Doyle JR. Treatment of Dupuytren's contracture: long term results after fasciotomy and fascial excision. *Journal of Bone and Joint Surgery (American)* 1976;**58**:380–7.

117

Arthritis of the hand

ASHISH SHARMA, EDWARD T MAH

Introduction	1333	Metacarpophalangeal joint osteoarthritis	1343
Osteoarthritis	1333	Proximal interphalangeal joint osteoarthritis	1344
Trapeziometacarpal joint osteoarthritis	1334	Distal interphalangeal joint osteoarthritis	1346
Finger CMC joint osteoarthritis	1342	References	1348

NATIONAL BOARD STANDARDS

- Know the sites and causes of arthritis in the hand
- Learn surgical options including joint arthroplasty, interposition arthroplasty, resectional arthroplasty or arthrodesis according to the site
- Understand when fusion is indicated
- Know how to manage mucous cyst

INTRODUCTION

Pain and loss of function of the small joints in the hand may result from primary osteoarthritis (OA), post-traumatic osteoarthritis or inflammatory arthritis. The common types of inflammatory arthritides of the hand are rheumatoid arthritis, systemic lupus erythematosus, psoriatic arthritis, scleroderma, gout and post-infective arthritis. Osteoarthritis is the most common form of hand arthritis; the next common is rheumatoid arthritis.

OSTEOARTHRITIS

Basic science

OA is characterized by degeneration of the articular cartilage of the joint affected. Hand joints most commonly involved in primary OA are the thumb carpometacarpal (CMC) joint, distal interphalangeal (DIP) joints of the fingers and the proximal interphalangeal (PIP) joints of the fingers. Metacarpophalangeal (MCP) joints are rarely involved in primary OA. Osteoarthritic changes in a joint are manifested by pain, swelling, stiffness, contracture, angular deformity and joint enlargement with osteophyte formation, with or without joint subluxation. OA of the hand joints may have a genetic predisposition and may be associated with OA of other joints of the body. Post-traumatic arthritis of the first CMC joint is often a sequel to incongruous healing of fractures or fracture dislocations of the CMC joint, most commonly the base of first metacarpal fractures and fracture dislocations. Primary OA is more common in elderly women than men in the corresponding age range. More than 90% of women and 85% of men older than 80 years suffer from primary OA of the trapeziometacarpal (TM) joint.[1] It has been found to be so common in radiological reviews that TM joint arthritis had been considered a part of the normal ageing process.[1] However, the prevalence of a severe grade of arthritis of the TM joint (totally destroyed joint) in those older than 80 years is 66% in women and 23% in men.[1] A patient's clinical presentation and the radiological appearance of joint destruction may show a great discrepancy. Patients may present with severe pain and disability with little evidence of arthrosis in radiographs. On the contrary, patients may have few, if any, symptoms in a radiologically advanced stage of joint destruction. Often the arthritis is discovered incidentally in radiographs carried out for a different purpose (e.g. for fracture of the distal radius). Psychosocial aspects are increasingly recognized as factors explaining such varied clinical presentation.[2]

TRAPEZIOMETACARPAL JOINT OSTEOARTHRITIS

The TM or first CMC joint is the second most common joint of the hand (after the distal interphalangeal joints) to be affected by OA. The first CMC joint is however considered the most important; arguably contributing to man's evolution by having a vital role in the hand's grip, pinch and dexterity. It thus helped in the evolution of man's ability to use tools. The first CMC joint or the TM joint is a saddle joint and motion occurs over the reciprocal concave articular surfaces of the base of the first metacarpal and the convex distal articular surface of the trapezium. Large amounts of loads, both axial and cantilever bending loads, are transmitted to the trapezium and TM joint during pinch and grip. The shape of the joint gives it a large freedom of movement, but makes it inherently unstable. Thus, the stability of the joint is largely dependent upon ligamentous supports. As many as 16 ligaments have been shown to contribute to the stability of the TM joint and trapezium, 14 of which insert into the trapezium, and two independently attach to the base of the first metacarpal.[3]

The ligaments attaching to the trapezium are:

- superficial anterior oblique (SAOL)
- deep anterior oblique ('beak' ligament/dAOL)
- dorsoradial (DRL)
- posterior oblique (POL)
- ulnar collateral
- dorsal trapezio-trapezoid
- volar trapezio-trapezoid
- dorsal trapezio-second metacarpal (DTSML)
- volar trapezio-second metacarpal (VTSML)
- volar trapezio-third metacarpal (VTTML)
- volar scapho-trapezial
- radial scapho-trapezial
- transverse carpal
- trapezio-capitate ligament (TCL).

The two ligaments attached to the base of the first metacarpal are:

- proper intermetacarpal ligament
- dorsal intermetacarpal ligament.

The ligaments mainly responsible for the stability of the TM joint are listed below.

1. The deep anterior oblique ligament (dAOL or 'beak' ligament)[4] tightens in thumb pronation, as in forceful lateral pinch, when it is the primary stabilizer against dorsal translation of the first metacarpal on the trapezium. Its attrition or loss shifts the metacarpal pivot point distally, causing dorsal translation of the metacarpal on the trapezium and thereby inducing subluxation and the degenerative process.
2. The DRL[3,5] is the primary restraint to dorsal and dorsoradial translation of the first metacarpal at the TM joint. The dAOL and DRL ligaments are vital stabilizers of the TM joint during lateral pinch. Attenuation or incompetence of one or either of them causes dorsal translation of the metacarpal base, resulting in pain.
3. The DTSML, the VTSML and VTTML are the chief tensile restraints to the cantilever forces acting across the CMC joint.[3]
4. The dorsal expansion of the abductor pollicis longus (APL) is the chief stabilizer of the TM joint in supination, but is not as important as the beak ligament because pinch is rarely performed in supination.

Pathophysiology of first CMC joint osteoarthritis

The early stage of joint synovitis is initiated by ligament laxity. Next, the disease progresses to the stage of arthritis, when chondromalacia is followed by degeneration of joint surfaces and formation of osteophytes. Late stages often involve dorsoradial subluxation of the thumb metacarpal on the trapezium and adduction contracture of the thumb due to adductor pollicis muscle and APL muscle overactivity. The scapho-trapezial (ST) joint may also be involved in advanced stages of first CMC joint OA. Since primarily the first CMC and ST joints are in the compression line of the thumb axis, 'pan-trapezial arthritis' typically involves these two joints.

Eaton and Glickel staging[6] for basal joint arthritis is the most widely used as a rationale for treatment of TM joint OA. It is based upon true lateral radiographs of the thumb and defines CMC and ST joint involvement in the arthritic process.

- Stage 1 (*pre-arthritic*): normal articular contours; occasional joint widening due to effusion or ligament laxity.
- Stage 2 (*early arthritis*): mild joint space narrowing; minimal or absent subchondral sclerosis; joint debris or osteophytes measuring 2 mm or less in diameter.
- Stage 3 (*advanced arthritis*): joint space is further narrowed; subchondral sclerosis present; osteophytes

and loose bodies greater than 2 mm; no abnormalities in ST joint.
- Stage 4 (*pan-arthritis*): degeneration involving CMC and ST joints.

However, since there is poor correlation between radiographic and clinical disease, the treatment should be based on clinical assessment and not on radiological appearance.

Management

HISTORY

Thumb basal joint arthritis most commonly affects postmenopausal women. Patients may complain of progressive weakness and pain over the radial aspect of the hand and wrist. They often have difficulty in performing activities involving pinch and grip. The dexterity in hand movements is affected. Activities involving pinching, grasping and torsional motions aggravate the pain, whereas rest and non-steroidal anti-inflammatory drugs (NSAIDs) often bring about relief.

Examination – signs and symptoms

Clinical presentation varies in severity according to the stage of the disease. The thumb may look normal in the early stages of the disease. Patients in later stages of the disease may present with increasing pain, tenderness and joint enlargement due to inflammation and osteophyte formation. Adduction contracture (restriction of TM joint abduction and extension) (Fig. 117.1a,b) and dorsal subluxation of the first metacarpal base may be seen in the late stages. Stress loading of the metacarpal base may elicit joint stiffness, crepitus and pain. Nearly a quarter of the patients needing surgery may also have associated carpal tunnel syndrome.[7] However, a lax and unstable TM joint may be part of a generalized joint laxity, which may also be elicited in the uninvolved opposite TM joint. This may be important to confirm, as it may change the management decisions. But, it is also important to remember that TM joint arthritis is often bilateral.

Investigations

Thumb CMC joint radiographs in the posteroanterior (PA), oblique and lateral views will show the severity of CMC joint arthritis (Fig. 117.2) and the palmar beak. A 30° stress PA view of both thumbs (with the patient pressing both thumbs firmly) may reveal the degree of radial subluxation. A stress lateral view taken while performing lateral pinch shows dorsal subluxation.[8] True PA and lateral views are used to stage the disease according to the Eaton and Glickel staging system.[6]

Differential diagnosis

The most common condition mistaken for TM joint OA is de Quervain's tenosynovitis of the first dorsal compartment, which is often confirmed with a positive

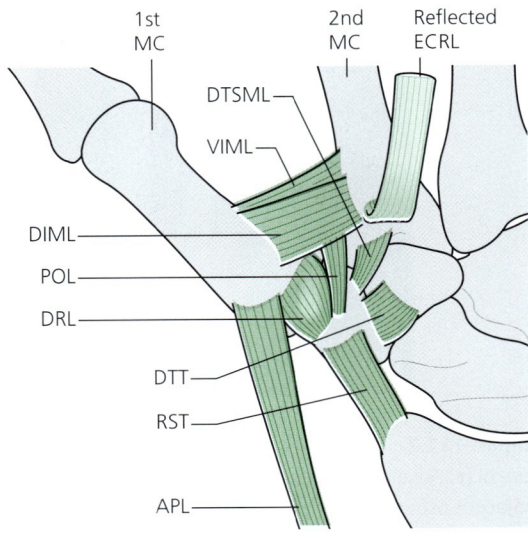

Figure 117.1 (a) Deep volar ligaments of the carpometacarpal joint. (b) Dorsal ligaments of the carpometacarpal joint. APL, abductor pollicis longus; DIML, dorsal intermetacarpal ligament; DRL, dorsoradial ligament; DTSML, dorsal trapezio-second metacarpal; DTT, dorsal trapezio-trapezoidal ligament; ECRL, extensor carpi radialis longus; FCR, flexor carpi radialis; ICL, intercarpal ligament; POL, posterior oblique ligament; RST, radial scapho-trapezial ligament; dAOL, deep anterior oblique ligament (beak ligament); VIML, volar intermetacarpal ligament; VST, volar scapho-trapezial ligament; VTSML, volar trapezio-second metacarpal; VTTML, volar trapezio-third metacarpal; VTT, volar trapeziotrapezoidal ligament.

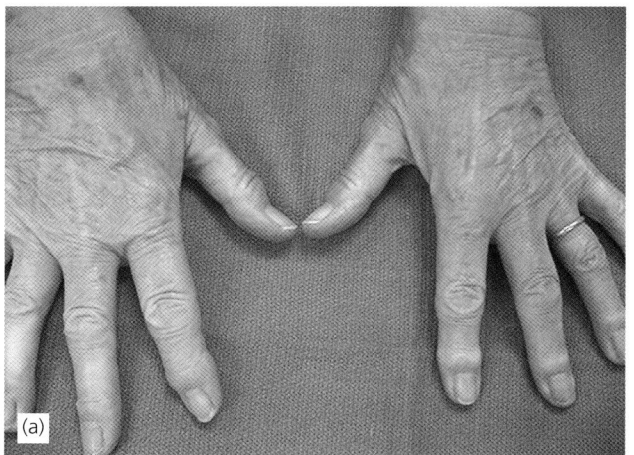
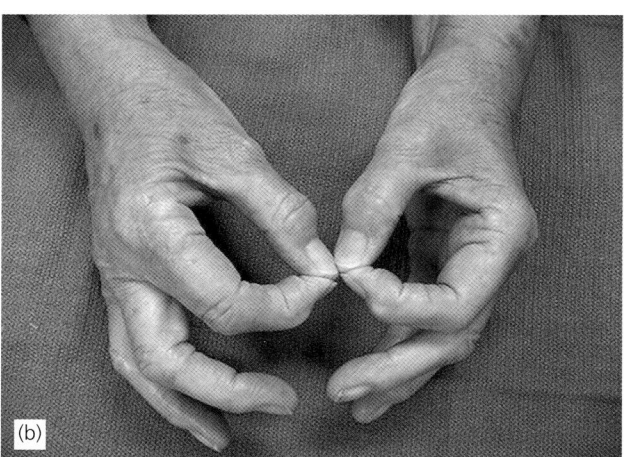
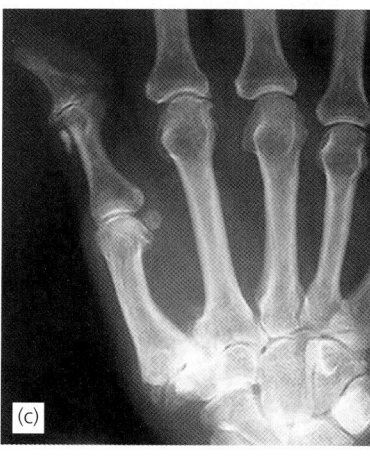

Figure 117.2 Loss of first web span: (a) in extension and (b) on pinch. (c) Advanced degeneration of carpometacarpal joint with adjacent osteophytes.

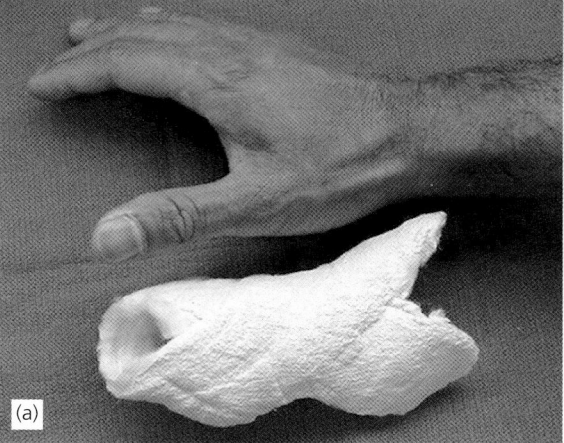
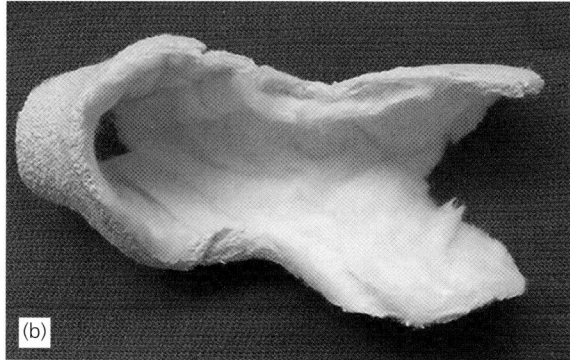
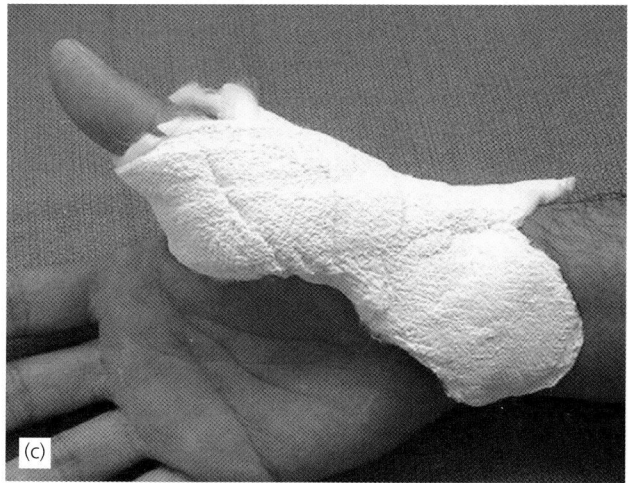

Figure 117.3 (a–c) A plaster of Paris splint over the thumb for temporary relief.

Finkelstein's test. Other conditions to differentiate are neuritis of the dorsal cutaneous branch of the radial nerve, second dorsal compartment tenosynovitis, OA of the scapho-trapezio-trapezoid (STT) joint, metacarpophalangeal (MP) joint arthritis and radiocarpal joint arthritis.

Non-operative treatment

Every patient in any stage of the disease should be given a trial of conservative treatment,[9] although symptomatic relief is more common in the early stages than late stages of the disease.[10] NSAIDs, thumb splinting for 3–4 weeks and modification of activities should be tried initially (Fig. 117.3). Patients refractory to these may be injected with cortisone injection into the CMC joint. Nearly all patients get some relief, often temporary, from these measures. But if symptoms return, then surgery should be offered to the patient.

Operative treatment

The most common surgical procedure for advanced stages of the disease (Eaton IV) is *resectional arthroplasty* (Figs 117.4 and 117.5). A variety of techniques of resection arthroplasty have been described in the literature, with good results in different studies. Other procedures described for advanced disease include *arthrodesis, interposition arthroplasty* and *joint replacement* (Fig. 117.6). Most procedures provide some degree of pain relief, but the functional outcome varies according to the type of the procedure. For example, excision with or without ligament reconstruction provides good mobility but results in slight weakness. Arthrodesis provides better grip and pinch strength but has the disadvantage of limiting the range of motion. Interposition arthroplasty and joint replacement provide good mobility and strength but have the risk of implant failure and so are not good options in young, active and high-demand patients.

TM joint arthroscopy is indicated for early stages (Eaton I, II and III) for evaluation, and arthroscopic staging (Badia Arthroscopic Classification for TM arthritis)[11] for a more logical decision-making about the management. Depending upon the arthroscopic findings, Badia[11] has proposed three stages of TM joint OA:

- Stage I: intact cartilage; disrupted DRL, diffuse synovial hypertrophy, inconsistent attenuation of AOL.
- Stage II: cartilage eburnated on the ulnar third of the first MC base and central third of the trapezium; disrupted DRL, more intense synovial hypertrophy; constant attenuation of the AOL.
- Stage III: widespread, full-thickness cartilage loss with or without a peripheral rim on both articular surfaces. Less severe synovitis. Frayed volar ligaments with laxity.

Depending on the arthroscopic staging, Badia[11] has advised the following treatments:

- Badia stage 1 (stable): synovectomy and debridement.
- Badia stage 1 (dorsal subluxation): thermal capsulorraphy and casting for 4 weeks.
- Badia stage 2: debridement, thermal capsulorraphy and extension/abduction osteotomy of the first metacarpal base.
- Badia stage 3: interposition arthroplasty – arthroscopic (with capsular shrinkage if clinically unstable) or open.
- Eaton stage 4 (with severe STT changes) and for recurrent pain: open trapeziectomy and LRTI (ligament reconstruction and tendon interposition).

There is a paucity of evidence regarding the role of capsular shrinkage in stabilizing the TM joint. Although some recent studies[11] have claimed good results with capsular shrinkage for TM joint subluxation, these have not been

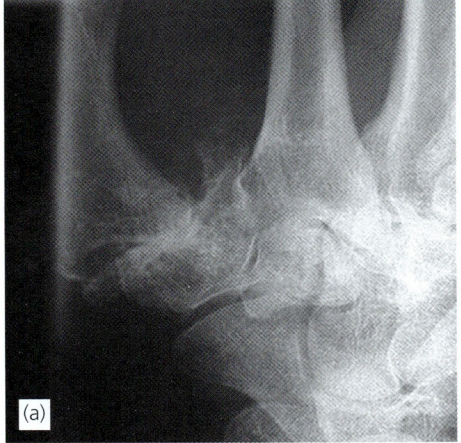

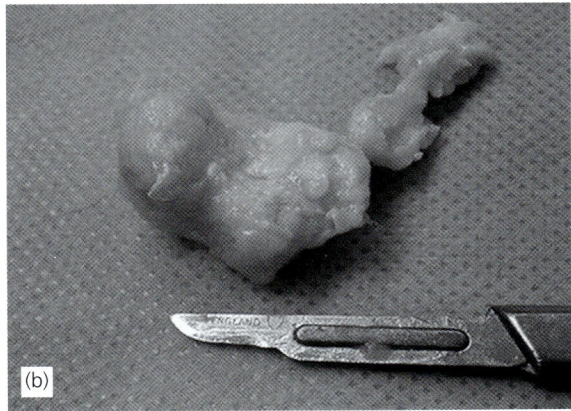

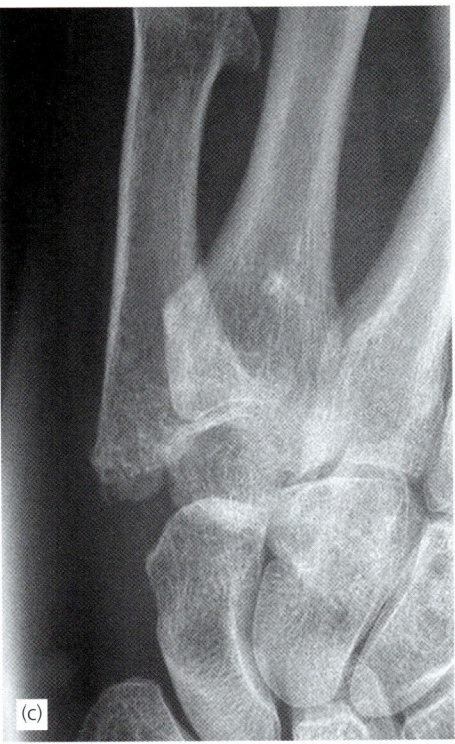

Figure 117.4 (a) Carpometacarpal osteoarthritis, (b) resected trapezium and (c) postoperative radiograph.

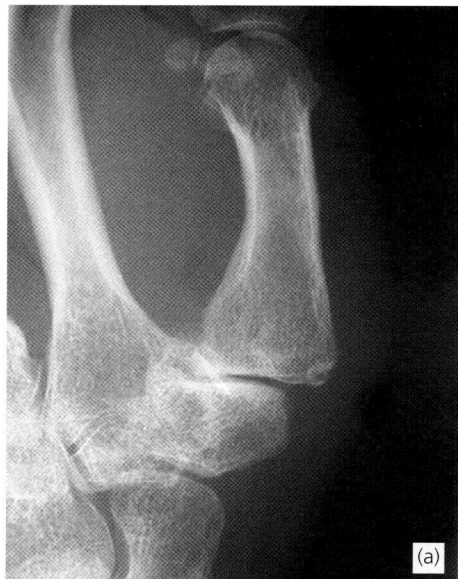
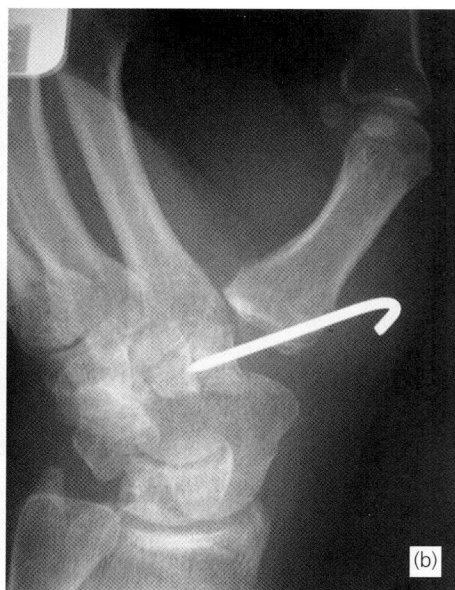

Figure 117.5 (a and b) Pre-operative and K-wire used to span the space following trapezium excision.

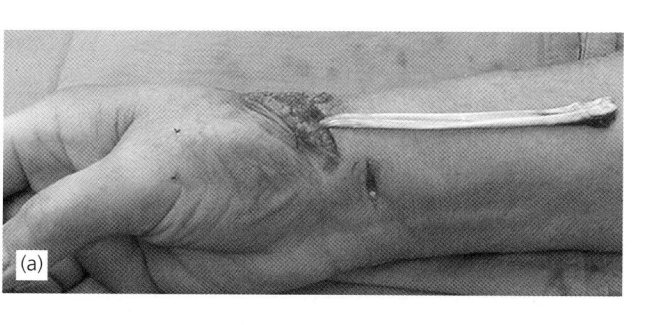
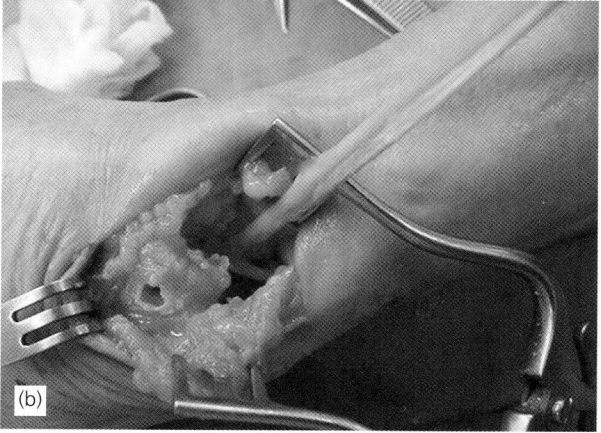
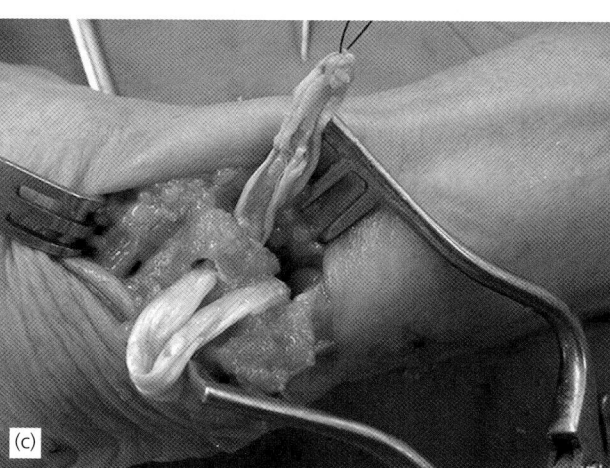
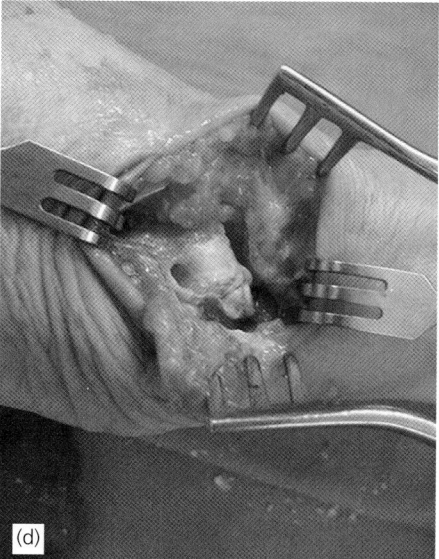

Figure 117.6 (a) Harvested half flexor carpi radialis (FCR) tendon; (b) drill hole is made in the base of the metacarpal for passage of the tendon; (c) half the FRC tendon is looped to suspend the base of the metacarpal and tensioned with the remaining FCR in slight wrist flexion; (d) completion of suspension arthroplasty.

reproduced by other author. Others[12] have recommended metacarpal extension osteotomy for stage 1 of the disease instead of capsular shrinkage.

Palmar ligament reconstruction[13] is recommended for Eaton stage 1, where one-half of the flexor carpi radialis (FCR) tendon is placed into a drill hole made in the base of the first metacarpal, looping it back under the attached part of the FCR and suturing it under tension to the dorsal periosteum of the metatarsal. The metacarpal needs to be pronated, abducted and reduced palmarly over the trapezium during tensioning. Following surgery, the hand is immobilized in a thumb spica cast in abduction and pronation for 4 weeks. Mobilization is begun for the interphalangeal and MCP joints at 4 weeks and the CMC joint at 2 months. Pinch and grip strengthening is begun at 3 months.

Metacarpal extension osteotomy for stage 1 has been advised by some[4,12] who are not satisfied by the long recovery period and fairly stiff TM joint after ligament reconstruction. They advocate 30° extension osteotomy of the metacarpal base, 1 cm distal to the TM joint and removing a dorsally based wedge. A thumb spica cast is applied for 6 weeks, leaving the interphalangeal joint free, followed by gentle TM joint mobilization in a forearm-based thumb spica splint. Grip and pinch strength exercises are started 2 months after surgery.

Trapeziectomy alone, first described by Gervis[14] in 1949, can be used in low-demand elderly patients and after failed infected implant arthroplasty. This has been unpopular because of the chief complication of proximal migration of the thumb, leading to weakness and instability. There are some reports of similar pain relief to other popular procedures.[15]

Distraction arthroplasty after trapeziectomy[16] is another modification of trapeziectomy alone, where the gap is kept distracted for 6 weeks by a 1.6 mm K-wire with the thumb in wide palmar abduction, slight opposition and distraction. The aim is to let a dense haematoma convert into fibroblastic tissue and ultimately a dense fibrous scar. Varley et al.[15] have claimed the results of distraction arthroplasty to be equal to or superior to the LRTI procedures.

LRTI was first described by Burton and Pellegrini[17] in 1986, using half the FCR tendon to reconstruct the beak ligament by passing through a drill hole in the base of the thumb metacarpal. Usually trapeziectomy is performed to simplify the procedure in all stages and the remaining FCR is rolled into an 'anchovy', placed into the trapeziectomy gap and sewn to the FCR tendon. It improves grip and pinch strength.

Suspensionplasty was reported by Thompson[18] in 1986 using the APL tendon. The procedure involved trapeziectomy followed by detaching the APL tendon proximally and passing it into a drill hole from the dorsal cortex of the first metacarpal to its articular surface and then through a drill hole in the index metacarpal and then weaving it into the ECRL tendon. Thompson[18] reported results similar to LRTI and relies on this procedure for all stages beyond stage 1.

Modifications of suspensionplasty have been reported by Weilby.[19] After trapeziectomy, one-half of the FCR tendon is harvested and looped around the APL tendon and the remaining tendon of the FCR.

We advocate a more reliable technique of suspension arthroplasty using half the FCR tendon. The trapezium is completely excised and half of the FCR tendon is harvested with the tendon graft freed proximally and looped through the base of the metcarpal through a drill hole. It is then looped multiple times onto the remaining FCR tendon like a spindle, so as to 'tension' the tendon graft with every loop while the wrist is kept in slight flexion. The joint capsule is then closed and a plaster slab is applied to immobilize the thumb in the abducted position for 2 weeks before changing to a forearm-based thumb splint. Active mobilization of the thumb is commenced after 2 weeks of immobilization.

The world literature has uniformly reported favourable outcomes of suspensionplasties in terms of excellent pain relief, significant improvement in pinch and grip strength and marked improvement in hand functions. However, in a Cochrane Library database search for studies on TM joint arthritis surgeries, Wajon et al.[20] did not find superiority of any procedure over the other. The procedures included trapeziectomy alone, trapeziectomy with soft-tissue interposition, trapeziectomy with ligament reconstruction, trapeziectomy with interposition and reconstruction and joint replacement.

New techniques in interposition arthroplasty have been reported.[21–27] A variety of materials, besides tendon, have been used for interposition arthroplasty, including fascia late allograft,[26] costochondral graft,[23] porous expanded polytetrafluoroethylene (ePTFE) vascular grafts (Gore-Tex) and gelfoam.[22] Reports of silicon synovitis and implant dislocation have put silicon interposition arthroplasty out of favour.[25] Gore-Tex implants have shown problems with particulate debris, synovitis and osteolysis, similar to silicon.[27] Polypropylene (Marlex) as interpositional material was found to be a valuable alternative to tendon for interpositional arthroplasty.[22] Adams et al.[21] have described *arthroscopic debridement, hemitrapeziectomy* and *interposition arthroplasty* with an acellular dermal matrix allograft (Graft-Jacket) for Eaton stages II and III symptomatic OA of the first CMC joint, with results similar to other series. However, cadaver grafts are used reluctantly due to the possibility of transmission of viral disease. Therefore, alternative materials have been introduced, such as the pyrolytic carbon spacer (PyroDisc) for interpositional arthroplasty, but long follow-up studies are needed as there is some concern regarding the chances of disc dislocation.

Artelon Spacer CMC (SBi) is a biocompatible, degradable, woven, textile device made of polycaprolactone-based polyurethaneurea (PUUR) for implantation into the first CMC joint as an interpositional spacer between the trapezium and the first metacarpal bone. This implant design offers a less invasive surgical alternative to minimally invasive arthroscopic implantation, requiring only 1–2 mm resection of the distal end of the trapezium.

This is conceived to work on the principle of *resorbable interposition arthroplasty*, whereby it acts as a temporary spacer until the host scar tissue proliferates into the space to create stability. The material slowly resorbs, eventually transferring load-bearing function entirely to the scar tissue. This again lacks long-term studies at present (Fig. 117.7).

Arthrodesis of the TM joint is an option for stages II, III and early stage IV of the disease. Complications include delayed union (12%), non-union (9%), reduced adduction/abduction (72%) and reduced flexion/extension (61%).[28] Successful fusion provides good grip and pinch power but residual stiffness and inability to place the palm flat onto a flat surface has to be accepted. Luckily it usually does not affect function in most patients and is a good option in young manual labourers with post-traumatic arthritis who require a strong grip for their occupation (Figs 117.8–117.11).

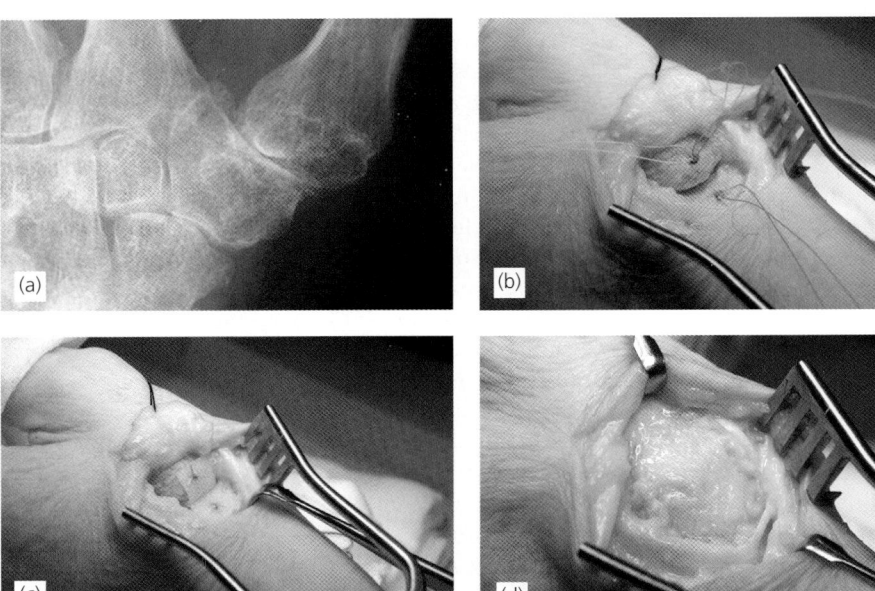

Figure 117.7 (a) Pre-operative patient selection – not more than 25% subluxation of carpometacarpal joint is suitable; (b) insertion of small bone anchors to hold the implant *in situ*; (c) suturing the implant onto the decorticated trapezium and base of metacarpal; (d) complete capsular closure for stability is essential.

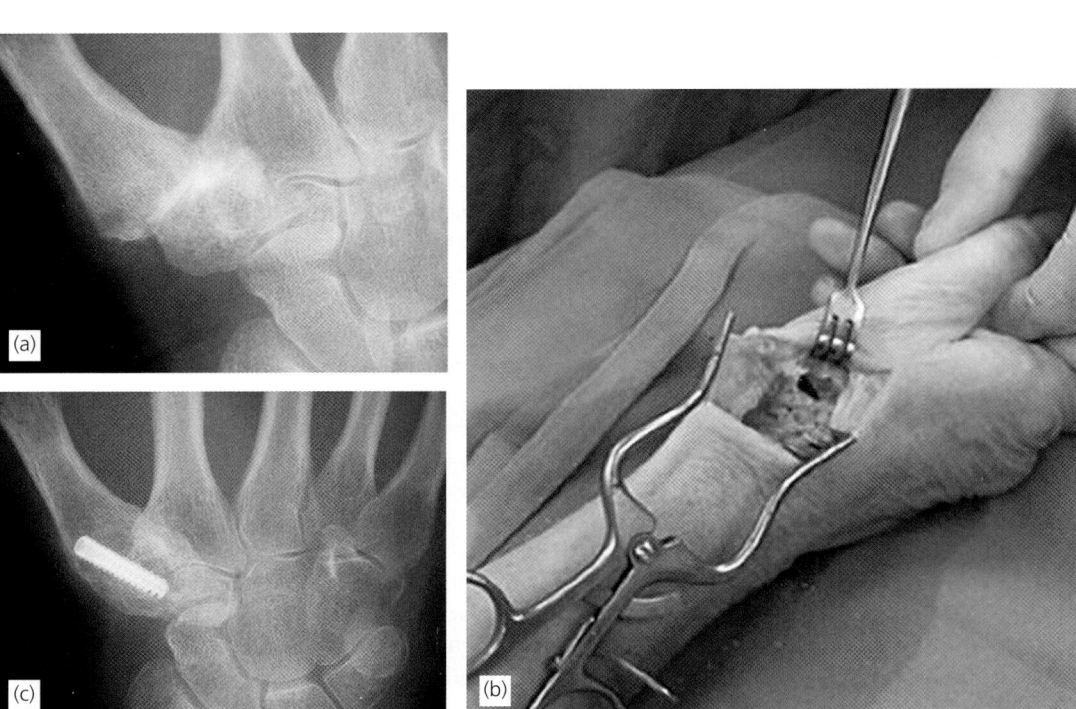

Figure 117.8 (a) Pre-operative radiograph; (b) decorticate the carpometacarpal joint before packing with bone graft from the distal radius; (c) radiograph following insertion of a mini Acutrack screw.

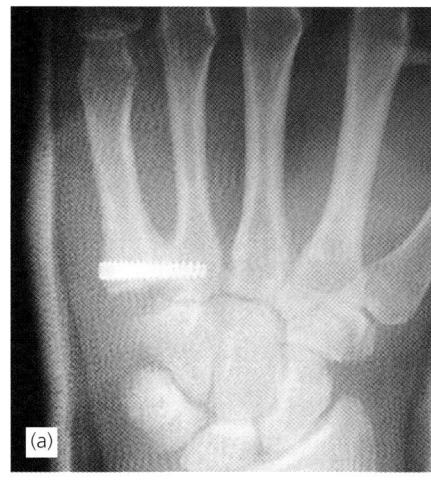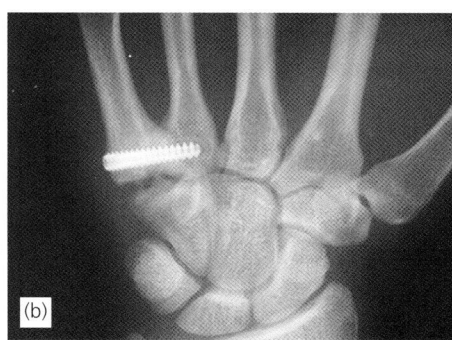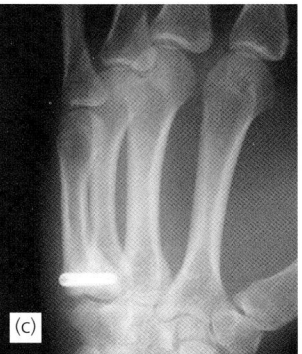

Figure 117.9 (a) Resection of base of the fifth metacarpal and fusion of fourth and fifth metacarpals; (b, c) solid fusion.

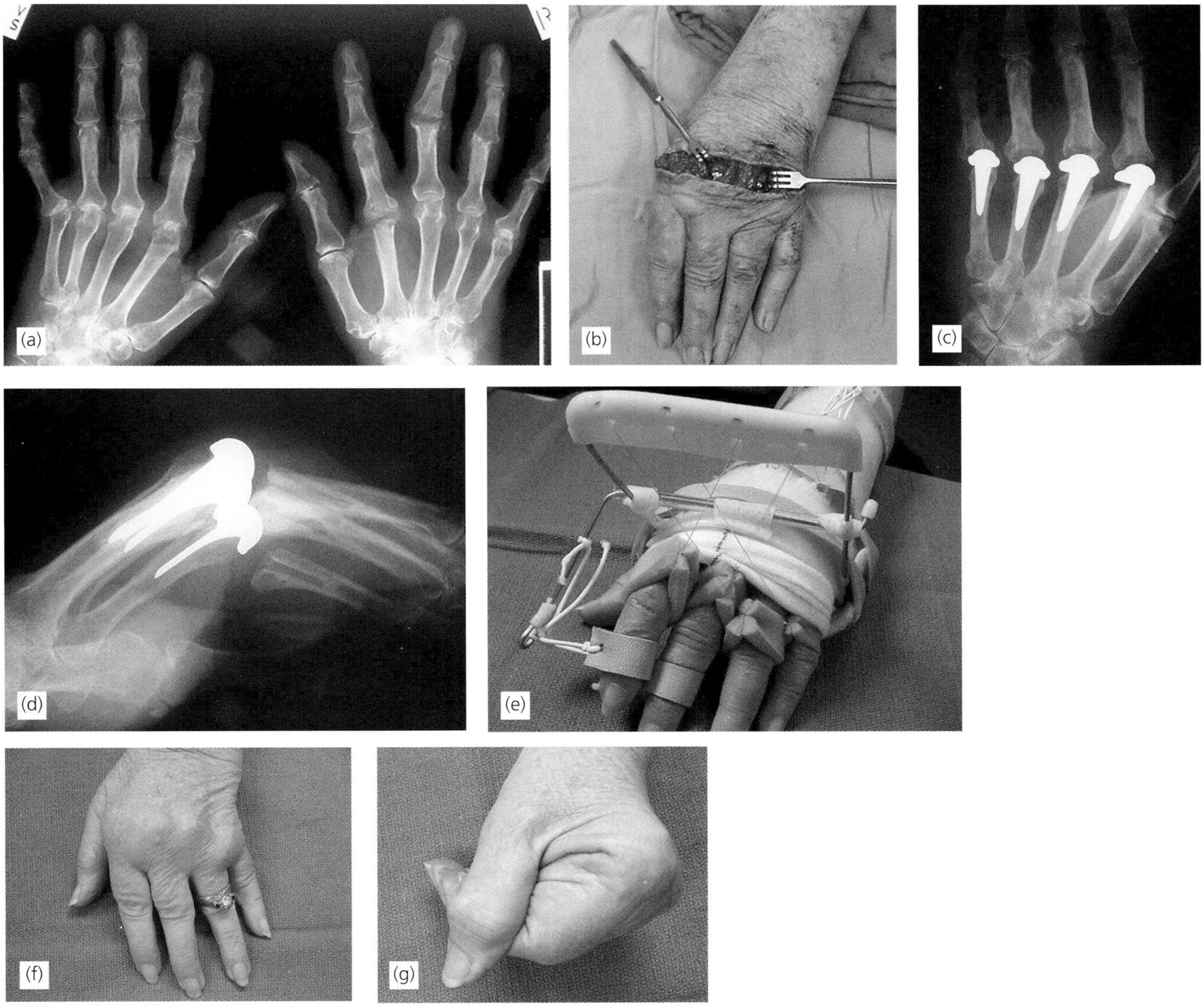

Figure 117.10 (a) Pre-operative radiograph; (b) intra-operative trial implant to check sizing and stability; (c, d) postoperative radiographs showing implant position; (e) postoperative splint, maintaining radial deviation; (f, g) hand function following the surgery.

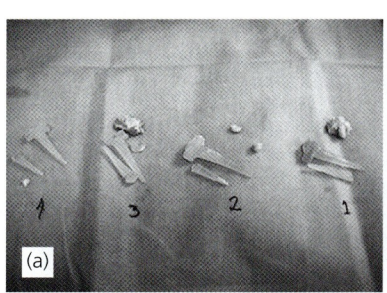
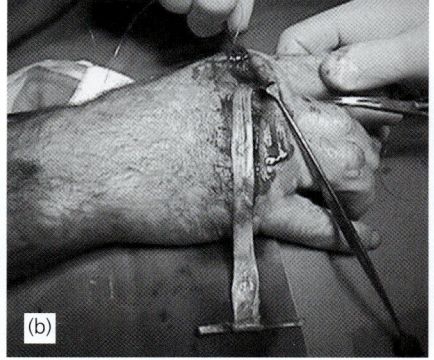
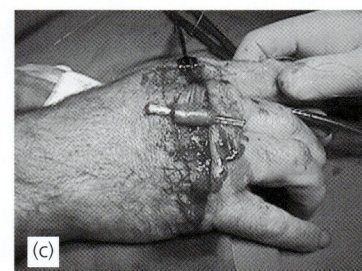
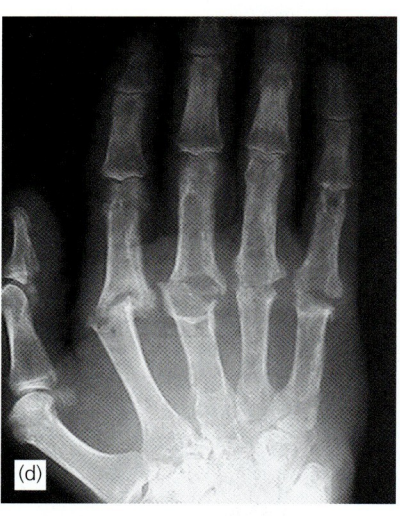
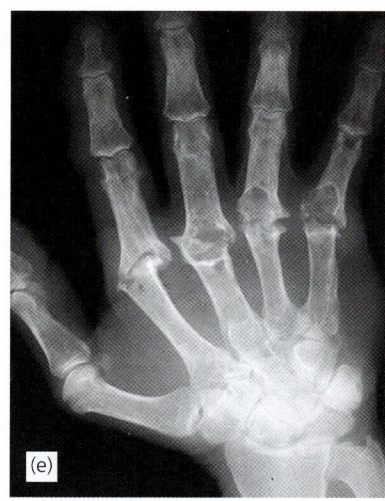
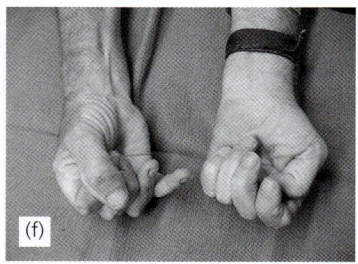

Figure 117.11 (a) broken silicon implants with resected synovitis; (b, c) fascia lata used to wrap around a vicryl pin as a temporary stabilizer; (d) radiograph at 6 weeks after operation; (e, f) 2 year follow-up, showing reasonably good hand function and radiograph.

FINGER CMC JOINT OSTEOARTHRITIS

Introduction and basic science

CMC joint OA of the index and middle fingers is relatively rare because of the inherent stability of their CMC joints compared with the ring and little fingers, whose CMC joints are more mobile in flexion and extension (range of movement 20–30°), and also allow some degree of rotation. The CMC joints of the fingers are classified as plane joints with one degree of freedom. However, the fifth CMC joint is the most mobile of the four finger joints and is often classified as a semi-saddle joint with conjunctional rotation[29] (first CMC joint being a true saddle joint).

Management

HISTORY AND CLINICAL EXAMINATION

Fifth CMC joint OA is commonly post-traumatic, secondary to fractures and dislocations. Onset is usually insidious, with a history of fracture or dislocation many years earlier. The most common aetiology is intra-articular malunion due to a reverse Bennett's fracture and ligament instability due to CMC joint dislocation. Patients present with a tender swelling over the dorsum of the hand (carpal boss). Arthritic joints may be associated with ganglion in 30% patients.[30]

NON-OPERATIVE TREATMENT

This includes rest, NSAIDs, splints for immobilization and adaptive devices to assist hand function. Corticosteroid injections may be tried in refractory cases for symptomatic relief.

OPERATIVE TREATMENT

This is indicated in patients not responding to conservative treatment or those with recurrence of symptoms. Chronically dislocated CMC joints can be open reduced with satisfactory results.[31–33] Debridement and synovectomy may be an option in select cases with painful synovial hypertrophy.

Reconstruction options include arthrodesis,[34] resection and interposition arthroplasty using a silastic prosthesis,[35] tendon[36] or other material, e.g. Artelon spacer. Silastic arthroplasty is not recommended because of reports of instability, breakage and silicon synovitis.[37] Generally, arthrodesis of the CMC joint is recommended for index to ring finger CMC joint OA. For fifth CMC joint OA, resection of the base of the fifth metacarpal with fusion of the fifth to fourth metacarpal and bone grafting is recommended.[38,39] It has shown good results with relief of pain and improvement in grip strength and is the recommended operation for this problem.

METACARPOPHALANGEAL JOINT OSTEOARTHRITIS

Introduction

MCP joint OA is usually secondary to joint incongruity in malunited intra-articular fractures, joint instability due to ligamentous injury or chondral damage from a previous joint sepsis, which is very common to this joint. The degenerative disease process of the joint involves synovitis and effusion in the early stages, with the later stages showing joint destruction and deformity. Sometimes, the collateral ligaments (usually radial) catch on the marginal osteophyte causing locking of the MCP joint.[40]

Management

HISTORY AND CLINICAL EXAMINATION

The patient may give a history of previous trauma to the joint involved. Mild to moderate pain may be the only symptom in the early stages. More advanced disease may present with swelling, stiffness, difficulty in making a tight grip, occasional popping digits and rarely an ulnar drift of the arthritic joint.

INVESTIGATIONS

Radiographs will show joint space narrowing, subchondral bone sclerosis, osteophyte formation and evidence of old malunited intra-articular fracture or angular deformity. Osteophytes may be more evident in oblique views.[41]

DIFFERENTIAL DIAGNOSIS

Differential diagnosis of MCP joint OA should include rheumatoid arthritis, which is the most common arthritis affecting the MCP joints. It often involves multiple MCP joints and is often bilaterally symmetrical. Other conditions in the differential diagnosis include one or multiple trigger finger(s) and extensor tendon subluxation. Differential diagnosis of a mono-articular arthopathic MCP joint must include psoriatic arthropathy. Differential diagnosis of a locked MCP joint must include locked trigger finger at the level of the A1 pulley, with a painful volar nodule between the mid-palm and the PIP joint. Rarely, the extensor tendon may be subluxed over the metacarpal head, which may present with pain centred over the MCP joint.

NON-OPERATIVE TREATMENT

This should be tried initially with rest, NSAIDs, hand-based splints and customized hand devices to assist hand function. Local intra-articular corticosteroid injections are indicated for patients not responding to conservative treatment and are often most gratifying in symptomatic relief. However, steroids must be used judiciously, since excessive use may lead to further chondral damage or tendon rupture. It is not recommended to have more than three cortisone injections per region per year.

OPERATIVE TREATMENT

This is indicated when an appropriate period of conservative treatment is unsuccessful or if patients have a locked MCP joint.

MCP joint reconstruction may be carried out by implant arthroplasty or soft-tissue interpositional arthroplasty. Arthrodesis is generally not recommended because of the resultant stiffness and dysfunction.

Implant arthroplasty remains the procedure of choice for reconstruction of the arthritic MCP joint. MCP reconstruction implant designs include hinged (constrained),[42] semi-constrained and unconstrained types. Silicone implants have been shown to provide relief from pain and improve cosmesis.[43] However, they have a high complication rate because of inherent design limitations, such as silicon synovitis, progressive bone destruction, implant fracture and an inability to achieve a normal range of movements. Eight-two per cent of silicone implants have been reported to fracture after 5 years.[44–46] Notwithstanding these factors, silicone-based arthroplasty remains the gold standard for prosthetic replacement of the MCP joint. NeuFlex (DePuy) is a new modification of the Swanson MCP joint design, made from Anasil silicone elastomer material with an improved range of motion, but it still has the problem of radiological loosening.[47] A silicone–elastomer constrained implant remains the most common type used today.

Metal-on-polyethylene semi-constrained implants may be a better choice when soft-tissue constraints are intact in primary and post-traumatic OA. Soft-tissue repair and balance is an essential part of implant arthroplasty.

Recently, unconstrained total joint implant designs of pyrolytic carbon have become available for MCP joint replacement. Pyrolytic carbon has excellent wear properties and long-term biological compatibility. It has an elastic modulus similar to that of cortical bone and thus theoretically lowers implant–bone interface loosening.

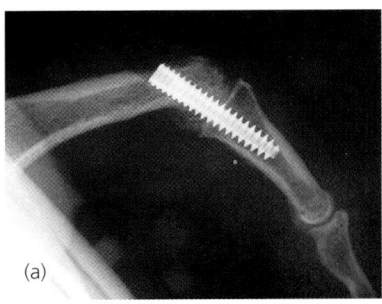 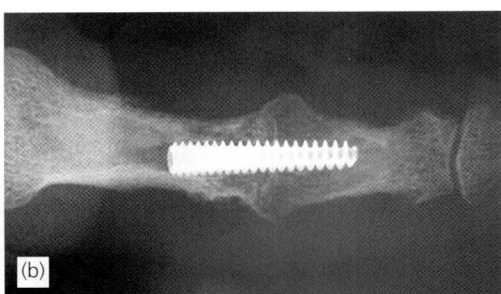

Figure 117.12 (a and b) Mini Acutrack screw to fuse a proximal interphalangeal joint.

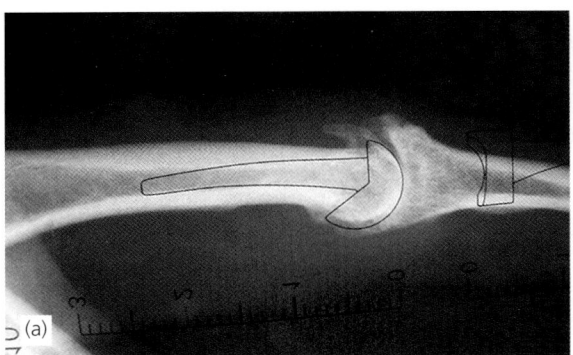 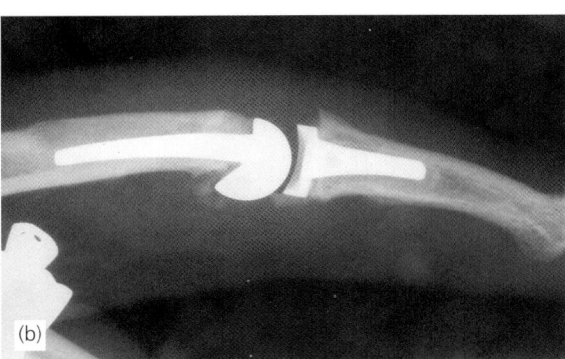

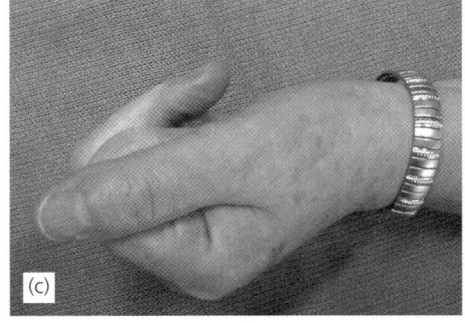 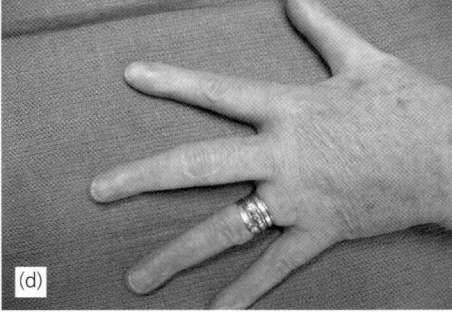

Figure 117.13 (a) Templating the proximal interphalangeal joint before surgery; (b) radiograph after surgery; (c, d) hand function after surgery.

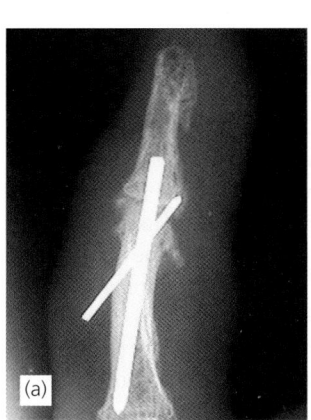 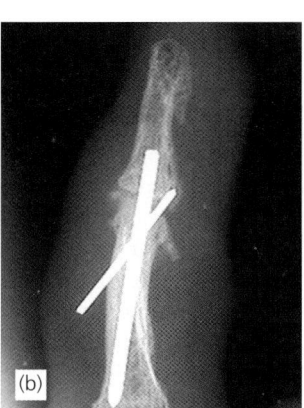 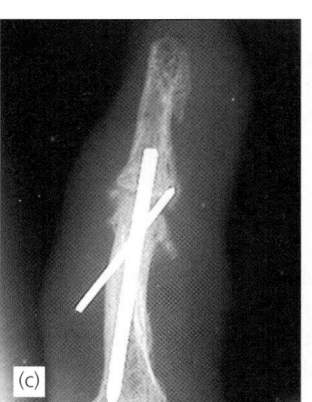 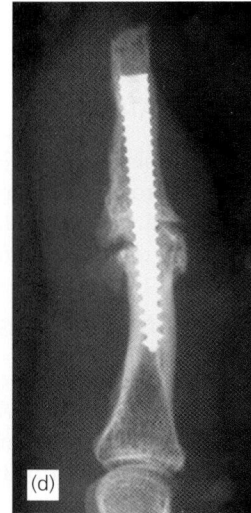

Figure 117.14 (a–c) Arthrodesis using intramedullary and cross K-wire; (d) arthrodesis using a mini Acutrack screw.

But unconstrained implants require more careful sizing, intact collateral ligaments and optimal soft-tissue balancing to maintain joint stability and joint biomechanics. Hilker et al.[47] in a prospective study with a mean follow-up of 4 years evaluated pyrocarbon prostheses for the MCP joint and have reported radiolucent lines in 46%, loosening in 25% and revision to a silicone implant in 15%, and have abandoned the use of this implant.

Resection arthroplasty may have a role in failed implant arthroplasty, post-infectious arthrosis and following trauma, with loss of soft-tissue restraints or excessive bone loss. The principles of resection arthroplasty include resection of an adequate amount of bone to correct the deformity and permit motion, and tissue interposition between the resected surfaces to prevent painful impingement or fusion. Various techniques have been described for resection arthroplasty using extensor retinaculum,[48] volar plate[49] extensor tendon,[50] fascia lata[51] and rib periosteum.[52]

Arthrodesis is rarely indicated but may be considered in deficient ligamentous supports leading to compromised intrinsic function, especially in manual labourers. Arthrodesis in 20–30° of flexion is generally recommended, since it allows prehensile function to some extent.[53]

Revision arthroplasty of failed primary MCP joint implant arthroplasty using fascia lata is considered a salvage procedure. It is more commonly carried out in failed silicon MCP joint arthroplasty. The procedure involves removal of failed implants, synovectomy and harvesting autologous fascia lata to be used as strips to wrap around a vicryl rod for temporary stability. Soft-tissue repair and balance is an integral part of the procedure, followed by intensive hand therapy and splintage.

PROXIMAL INTERPHALANGEAL JOINT OSTEOARTHRITIS

Introduction

PIP joint OA is more commonly secondary to malunited intra-articular fractures and fracture dislocations of the PIP joint. Primary OA of the PIP joint is less common, unlike rheumatoid arthritis, which commonly involves PIP joints and MP joints.

Basic science

The PIP joint is a simple diarthroidal (hinge) joint with movements in one plane. The strong radial and ulnar collateral ligaments give lateral stability. The biconvex shape of the head of the proximal phalanx with a central intercondylar groove articulating with the biconcave shape of the base of the middle phalanx with the central articular ridge gives secondary stability to the joint. The range of movement of the PIP joint is 0–105°.

Management

HISTORY AND PHYSICAL EXAMINATION

Insidious onset of pain and stiffness of the affected PIP joint are the main symptoms. Varying degrees of angular deformity, swelling and Bouchard's nodes may be present. The affected joint may be tender. Pinch and grip strength is usually weak because of pain.

INVESTIGATIONS

Radiographs may show varying grades of joint space narrowing, subchondral bone sclerosis, marginal osteophytes and subchondral cyst formation. Laboratory tests such as complete blood counts, erythrocyte sedimentation rate, rheumatoid factor and uric acid must be obtained to rule out other inflammatory diseases.

DIFFERENTIAL DIAGNOSIS

This most commonly must include rheumatoid arthritis, which often involves multiple joints of both hands and feet, and often causes considerable destruction and deformity in advanced stages. Other types of inflammatory arthritis such as psoriatic arthritis, gout and Reiter disease must also be differentiated.

NON-OPERATIVE TREATMENT

Non-operative treatment of PIP joint OA is aimed at pain relief and includes modifying activities which cause pain, use of adaptive devices, gentle mobilization for increasing range of movements and strengthening exercises for increasing the pinch and grip strength. Short-term immobilization with wrist-based splints and NSAIDs may be needed during periods of acute flare-up of pain and swelling of the osteoarthritic joint. Intra-articular steroids may be administered carefully and judiciously for temporary symptomatic relief in very painful acute flare-ups. Repeated steroid injections may cause further chondral damage or may lead to boutonnière deformity if the resulting attenuated central slip of the extensor tendon ruptures.[54]

OPERATIVE TREATMENT

This is indicated when non-operative treatments have failed to provide pain relief and to improve function. Surgical options include *arthrodesis* and *joint arthroplasty*. The surgical option is determined by the patient's age, occupational and recreational demands, lifestyle, bone stock and status of collateral ligaments of the arthritic PIP joint. Priority may also be given for lateral stability of the radial digits for key pinch strength and providing a pain-free flexion arc in the ulnar digits for grip strength.

Arthrodesis is indicated in young, active patients, index finger PIP joint arthritis with loss of bone stock, collateral ligament deficiency, stiff joint (flexion arc less than 30°) and failed previous implant arthroplasty (Figs 117.13 and 117.14). There is no ideal position for arthrodesis of the PIP joint. However, generally, the index finger is usually arthrodesed in 30–40° of flexion, 40–45° of flexion for the middle finger, 50° of flexion for the ring finger and 55° of flexion for the little finger. Common techniques for arthrodesis include crossed K-wires,[55] intra-osseous wiring, tension band wiring,[56–60] compression screw fixation,[61–63] external fixators[64,65] and moulded mini-plate fixation.[66,67]

Arthroplasty is commonly indicated for older individuals with post-traumatic PIP joint OA of the middle, ring and little fingers, adequate bone stock, intact collateral ligaments and preserved functional arc of motion. It is generally not recommended for joints with current or past infection. Various techniques of non-prosthetic and prosthetic arthroplasty have been described in the literature. Non-prosthetic arthroplasty is usually recommended for patients younger than 40 years[68] and in arthritic fingers of previous healed pyoarthrosis.

Techniques of non-prosthetic PIP joint arthroplasty include resection arthroplasty and volar plate interposition (with or without flexor digitorum superficialis (FDS) tenodesis and perichondral grafting).

Prosthetic PIP joint arthroplasty has evolved significantly since Burman reported using a vitallium cap for PIP joint arthroplasty in 1940.[69] The first generation of implants were hinge type, which had a high failure rate because of non-anatomic centres of rotation, a high coefficient of friction of the hinge mechanism, metallic debris reaction and eventual implant breakage.[70,71]

Classically, silicone implants have been used since 1966 when Swanson developed his silicon rubber flexible implant and started using it. This is a joint spacer strictly speaking, but has predictable pain relief. It has remained the most popular implant arthroplasty for more than four decades and is still considered by many to be the gold standard for PIP joint arthroplasty with 81% survivorship at 9 years.[72] Chief complications of silicone PIP joint implants include implant fracture, lateral instability, particulate synovitis and implant dislocation. Moreover, the collateral ligaments have to be sacrificed, which makes silicone implants undesirable in the index and middle finger PIP joints.

The second generation of implants were ball and socket designs, attempting to add adduction and abduction motion to the flexion and extension. However, these had a high failure rate because of a high incidence of instability, poor mobility, hypertrophic new bone formation and proximal phalangeal component failure.

The current generation of implants for the PIP joint fall into the category of surface replacement prostheses as they closely resemble the anatomic configuration of the head of the proximal phalanx and the base of the middle phalanx. Thus, these need intact collaterals and less deformity or destruction of the joint.

Almost all short-term studies have reported satisfactory arc of motion and that loosening is not an early problem.[73] There are only a few long-term follow-up studies, but most have reported good to fair results in the majority of the patients.[74]

The pyrolytic carbon PIP joint is the newly introduced US Food and Drug Administration-approved prosthesis made of graphite substrate coated with pyrocarbon gas. Its surface is extremely hard and less vulnerable to wear than previous materials. Short-term results show that pyrolytic carbon implants are promising for the treatment of PIP joint arthritis, but the available data in a recent study did not show a conclusive superiority over silicone PIP joint implants.[75]

A mean 5 year follow-up study of cemented versus uncemented surface replacement arthroplasty of the PIP joint showed no difference in postoperative pain scores or the arc of motion, but the uncemented group showed significantly more radiological subsidence, loosening and revision rate than the cemented group.[76] Other studies also have recommended cementing of the surface replacement arthroplasty implant.[77]

DISTAL INTERPHALANGEAL JOINT OSTEOARTHRITIS

Introduction

Distal interphalangeal joint OA can be primary or post-traumatic. Primary OA of the DIP joint is fairly common in elderly people. It is considered a multifactorial disease, being predisposed by genetic factors, age and systemic causes. The DIP joint is the joint most commonly affected by OA in the hand.

Basic science

The DIP joint too is a simple diarthroidal joint like the PIP joint, allowing motion only in one plane. Primary stabilizing factors of the joint are the strong collateral ligaments, with secondary constraints being the bony architecture of the opposing articular surfaces of the phalanges. The DIP joint allows 0–85° range of motion.

Natural history of the disease

Chondral damage and fibrillation is initiated and perpetuated by abnormal mechanical stresses leading to bony eburnation, osteophyte formation, a decrease in joint space, subchondral sclerosis and frequent angular deformity due to asymmetric joint damage. This may further lead to joint instability, deformity and pericapsular contracture with painful and restricted range of movements.

Management

HISTORY AND PHYSICAL EXAMINATION

Patients usually complain of insidious onset of pain and stiffness of the finger joint, causing weakness of grip and pinch strength. A variable degree of angular deformity, more commonly ulnar deviation of the joint, may be seen. Heberden's nodes are often present on the dorsum of the joint. Mucous cysts of variable size may be present adjacent to the involved joint. These mucous cysts may occasionally press on the germinal matrix of the nail, which may cause grooving of the nail plate.

INVESTIGATIONS

Radiographs in true posteroanterior, lateral and oblique views are all that is required. Radiographs will show asymmetric joint space narrowing in the early stage. Subchondral sclerosis and marginal osteophytes appear in the later stages. Radiographs of the advanced arthritic joint may show subchondral cysts, a broadened base of phalanx and gross joint malalignment.

DIFFERENTIAL DIAGNOSIS

This includes other inflammatory arthritic conditions such as rheumatoid arthritis, gout, psoriatic arthritis and rarely Reiter syndrome. These usually show symmetric joint space narrowing and gross joint destruction. Laboratory tests such as the erythrocyte sedimentation rate, C-reactive protein, rheumatoid factor, serum uric acid and complete blood count are needed to further evaluate the arthritic process.

NON-OPERATIVE TREATMENT

This is mainly symptomatic and should be the first line of management. Hand therapy strategies to control pain, swelling and stiffness include modifying or eliminating activities that put pressure on the arthritic joint during pulp-to-pulp pinch or key pinch. Use of adaptive devices, gentle mobilization and strengthening exercises may help reduce symptoms. Acute flare-up of the disease may need splinting of the joint and judicious use of NSAIDs. Intra-articular steroids may be administered carefully and judiciously in refractory cases for symptomatic relief. Repeated steroid injections may lead to subcutaneous fat atrophy and depigmentation.

OPERATIVE TREATMENT

This is indicated when pain is refractory to non-operative treatment or gross deformity is interfering with pinch or grip function. The main surgical procedures include mucous cyst excision, arthrodesis and arthroplasty.

Mucous cyst excision is indicated in large cysts and cysts causing longitudinal grooving on the nail plate. Cysts may rupture through the skin and create a channel from skin to the joint, leading to septic arthritis. Therefore, simple incision and drainage of the mucous cyst may not cure the mucous cyst, but may rather cause septic arthritis. Mucous cyst excision must be combined with osteophyte excision and joint debridement to minimize recurrence.[78,79] However, patients need to be counselled that this procedure will not cure them of the OA disease process.

Arthrodesis is the most common and reliable surgical procedure for DIP joint OA. It provides a pain-free, stable and normally aligned finger with improved grip and pinch strength, and improved function of the hand. Various techniques have been used in fixation of DIP joint arthrodesis in slight flexion (10–15°), and include single K-wire,[80] crossed K-wires,[81] multiple longitudinal K-wires, interosseous wire loop,[82] tension band wiring and compression screw.[83–85]

Although the K-wire fixation and screw fixation techniques have a similar union time and non-union rate,[86] screw fixation allows better compression and immediate stability than K-wire(s). It also provides higher torsional rigidity than tension-band wire fusion techniques.[87] Headless full threaded compressive screw (mini Acutrak and micro Acutrak Acumed) has proven successful in DIP joint arthrodesis.[88]

Arthroplasty of the PIP joint is rarely indicated. It may be indicated in patients who need fine finger movements in their occupations and need some painless range of motion of the DIP joint affected by OA. A relative indication is multiple digit involvement of the same hand. The essential prerequisite is adequate bone stock, intact collateral ligaments, and functioning flexor and extensor tendons. However, the patient needs to be counselled regarding the higher incidence of complications and survivorship issues of arthroplasty surgery. The chief complications of arthroplasty are infection, instability, skin erosion, implant breakage and loosening.

KEY LEARNING POINTS

- The hand joints most commonly involved in primary osteoarthritis (OA) are thumb carpometacarpal (CMC) joint, distal interphalangeal (DIP) joints of fingers and proximal interphalangeal (PIP) joints of fingers.
- The trapeziometacarpal (TM) or first CMC joint is the second most common joint of the hand (after the distal interphalangeal joints) affected.
- The most common condition mistaken for TM joint OA is de Quervain's tenosynovitis of the first dorsal compartment.
- The most common surgical procedure for advanced stages of the disease (Eaton IV) is *resectional arthroplasty*. Other procedures are *arthrodesis*, *interposition arthroplasty* and *joint replacement*.

- CMC joint OA of the index and middle fingers is rare.
- Metacarpophalangeal (MCP) joint OA is usually secondary to joint incongruity in malunited intra-articular fractures, joint instability due to ligamentous injury or chondral damage from previous joint sepsis (common). MCP joint reconstruction may be done by implant arthroplasty or soft-tissue interpositional arthroplasty.
- PIP joint OA is more commonly secondary to malunited intra-articular fractures and fracture dislocations of the PIP joint. Surgical options include *arthrodesis* and *joint arthroplasty*.
- DIP joint OA can be primary or post-traumatic. The main surgical procedures include mucous cyst excision, arthrodesis and arthroplasty.

REFERENCES

- ● = Key primary paper
- ◆ = Major review article

●1. Sodha S, Ring D, Zurakowsk ID, JupiterJB. Prevalence of osteoarthrosis of the trapeziometacarpal joint. *Journal of Bone and Joint Surgery (American)* 2005;**87**:2614-18.

●2. Keefe FJ, Rumble ME, Scipio CD, *et al*. Psychosocial aspects of persistent pain: current state of the science. *Journal of Pain* 2004;**5**:195-211.

●3. Bettinger PC, Linscheid RL, Berger RA, *et al*. An anatomic study of the stabilizing ligaments of the trapezium and trapeziometacarpal joint. *Journal of Hand Surgery (American)* 1999;**24**:786-98.

4. Pellegrini VD Jr, Olcott CW, Hollenberg G. Contact patterns in the trapeziometacarpal joint: the role of the palmar beak ligament. *Journal of Hand Surgery (American)* 1993;**18**:238-44.

●5. Strauch RJ, Behrman MJ, Rosenwasser MP. Acute dislocation of the carpometacarpal joint of the thumb: an anatomic and cadaver study. *Journal of Hand Surgery (American)* 1994;**19**:93-8.

●6. Eaton RG, Glickel SZ. Trapeziometacarpal osteoarthritis: staging as a rationale for treatment. *Hand Clinics* 1987;**3**:455-71.

●7. Florack T, Miller R, Pellegrini VD Jr, *et al*. The prevalence of carpal tunnel syndrome in patients with basal joint arthritis of the thumb. *Journal of Hand Surgery (American)* 1992;**17**:624-30.

●8. Eaton RG, Littler JW. Ligament reconstruction for the painful thumb carpometacarpal joint. *Journal of Bone and Joint Surgery (American)* 1973;**55A**:1655-66.

◆9. Wolock BS, Moore JR, Weiland AJ. Arthritis of the basal joint of the thumb: a critical analysis of treatment options. *Journal of Arthroplasty* 1989;**4**:65-78.

10. Swigart CR, Eaton RG, Glickel SZ, *et al*. Splinting in the treatment of arthritis of the first carpometacarpal joint. *Journal of Hand Surgery (American)* 1999;**24**:86-91.

◆11. Badia A. Trapeziometacarpal arthroscopy: a classification and treatment algorithm. *Hand Clinics* 2006;**22**:153-63.

12. Tomaino MM. Thumb by metacarpal extension osteotomy: rationale and efficacy for Eaton stage I disease. *Hand Clinics* 2006;**22**:137-41.

●13. Eaton RG, Littler JW. Ligament reconstruction for the painful thumb carpometacarpal joint. *Journal of Bone and Joint Surgery (American)* 1973;**55A**:1655-66.

●14. Gervis WH. Excision of the trapezium for osteoarthritis of the trapeziometacarpal joint. *Journal of Bone and Joint Surgery (British)* 1949;**31B**:537-39.

15. Varley GW, Calvey J, Hunter JB, *et al*. Excision of the trapezium for osteoarthritis at the base of the thumb. *Journal of Bone and Joint Surgery (American)* 1959;**41**:609-25.

◆16. Mahoney JD, Meals RA. Trapeziectomy *Hand Clinics* 2006;**22**:165-9.

◆17. Burton RI, Pellegrini VD Jr. Surgical management of basal joint arthritis of the thumb. Part II. Ligament reconstruction with tendon interposition arthroplasty. *Journal of Hand Surgery (American)* 1986;**11**:324-32.

◆18. Thompson J. Surgical management of trapeziometacarpal arthrosis. *Advances in Orthopaedic Surgery* 1986;**10**:105.

●19. Weilby A. Tendon interposition arthroplasty of the first carpo-metacarpal joint. *Journal of Hand Surgery (British)* 1988;**13**:421-5.

20. Wajon A, Ada L, Edmunds I. Surgery for thumb (trapeziometacarpal joint) osteoarthritis. *Cochrane Database of Systematic Reviews* 2005;**4**:CD004631.

21. Adams JE, Merten SM, Steinmann SP. Arthroscopic interposition arthroplasty of the first carpometacarpal joint. *Journal of Hand Surgery (European)* 2007;**32**:268-74.

●22. Nusem I, Goodwin DR. Excision of the trapezium and interposition arthroplasty with gelfoam for the treatment of trapeziometacarpal osteoarthritis. *Journal of Hand Surgery (British)* 2003;**28B**:242-5.

23. Trumble TE, Rafijah G, Gilbert M, *et al*. Thumb trapeziometacarpal joint arthritis: partial trapeziectomy with ligament reconstruction and interposition costo-chondral allograft. *Journal of Hand Surgery (American)* 2000;**25A**:61-76.

◆24. Pellegrini VD Jr, Burton RI. Surgical management of basal joint arthritis of the thumb. Part I. Long-term results of silicone implant arthroplasty. *Journal of Hand Surgery (American)* 1986;**11A**:309-24.

25. Henk GJ, van Cappelle RD, van Horn J. Use of the Swanson silicone trapezium implant for treatment of primary osteoarthritis: long-term results. *Journal of Bone and Joint Surgery (American)* 2001;**83**:999-1004.

●26. Taghinia AH, Al-Sheikh AA, Upton J. Suture anchor suspension and fascia lata interposition arthroplasty for basal joint arthritis of the thumb. *Plastic and Reconstructive Surgery* 2008;**122**:497-504.

27. Muermans S, Coenen L. Interpositional arthroplasty with Gore-Tex, Marlex or tendon for osteoarthritis of the trapeziometacarpal joint. A retrospective comparative study. *Journal of Hand Surgery (British)* 1998;**23**:64–8.
28. Bamberger HB, Stern P, Keifhaber TR, et al. Trapeziometacarpal joint arthrodesis: a functional evaluation. *Journal of Hand Surgery (American)* 1992;**17**:605–11.
◆29. Moran CA. Anatomy of the hand. *Physical Therapy* 1989;**69**:1007–13.
◆30. Cuono CB, Watson HK. The carpal boss: surgical treatment and etiological considerations. *Plastic and Reconstructive Surgery* 1979;**63**:88–93.
31. Hagstrom P. Fracture dislocation in the ulnar carpometacarpal joints. *Scandinavian Journal of Plastic and Reconstructive Surgery* 1975;**9**:249–51.
◆32. Waugh RL, Yancey AG. Carpometacarpal dislocations. *Journal of Bone and Joint Surgery (American)* 1948;**30A**:397–404.
◆33. Bora FW Jr, Didizian NH. The treatment of injuries to the carpometacarpal joint of the little finger. *Journal of Bone and Joint Surgery (American)* 1974;**56A**:1459–63.
34. Green D, O'Brien E. Fractures of the thumb metacarpal. In: Hotchkiss RN, Pederson WC, Kozin SH, Green DP (eds) *Green's Operative Hand Surgery*. New York, NY: Churchill Livingstone, 1999:809–64.
35. Green WL, Kilgore ES Jr. Treatment of the fifth digit carpometacarpal arthritis with Silastic prosthesis. *Journal of Hand Surgery (American)* 1981;**5A**:510–14.
36. Gainor BJ, Stark HH, Vender MD. Tendon arthroplasty of the fifth carpometacarpal joint for treatment of post traumatic arthritis. *Journal of Hand Surgery (American)* 1991;**16A**:520–4.
37. Swanson AB. Silicone rubber implants for replacement of arthritic or destroyed joints in the hand. *Surgical Clinics of North America* 1968;**48**:1003–13.
38. Dubert T. [Stabilized arthroplasty of the 5th metacarpal bone. A therapeutic proposal for the treatment of old fracture-luxations of the 5th metacarpal bone]. *Annales de Chirurgie de la Main et du Membre Superieur* 1994;**13**:363–5.
39. Bain GI, Unni PMR, Mehta JA, Eames MHA. Arthrodesis of ring finger and little finger metacarpal bases for little finger carpometacarpal joint arthritis. *Journal of Hand Surgery (British)* 2004;**29B**:449–52.
40. Rankin EA, Uwagie-Ero S. Locking of the metacarpophalangeal joint. *Journal of Hand Surgery (American)* 1986;**11A**:868–71.
41. Posner MA, Langa V, Green SM. The locked metacarpophalangeal joint: diagnosis and treatment. *Journal of Hand Surgery (American)* 1986;**11A**:249–53.
42. Blair WF, Shurr DG, Buckwalter JA. Metacarpophalangeal joint arthroplasty with a metallic hinged prosthesis. *Clinical Orthopaedics and Related Research* 1984;**184**:156–63.
43. Rettig LA, Luca L, Murphy MS. Silicone implant arthroplasty in patients with idiopathic osteoarthritis of the metacarpophalangeal joint. *Journal of Hand Surgery* 2005;**30**:667–72.
44. Beckenbaugh RD, Dobyns JH, Linscheid RL, et al. Review and analysis of silicone-rubber metacarpophalangeal implants. *Journal of Bone and Joint Surgery* 1976;**58**:483–7.
45. Kay AG, Jeffs JV, Scott JT. Experience with silastic prosthesis in the rheumatoid hand. A 5-year followup. *Annals of Rheumatic Disease* 1978;**37**:255–8.
46. Kirschembaum D, Schneider LH, Adams DC, et al. Arthroplasty of the metacarpophalangeal joints with use of silicone-rubber implants in patients who have rheumatoid arthritis. Long-term results. *Journal of Bone and Joint Surgery* 1993;**75**:3–12.
47. Hilker A, Miehlke RK, Schmidt K. [Prosthetics of metacarpophalangeal joints]. *Zeitschrift Rheumatologie* 2007;**66**:366–75.
48. Netscher D, Eladoumikdachi F, Gao YH. Resurfacing arthroplasty for metacarpophalangeal joint osteoarthritis: a good option using either perichondrium or extensor retinaculum. *Plastic and Reconstructive Surgery* 2000;**106**:1430–3.
49. Tupper JW. The metacarpophalangeal volar plate arthroplasty. *Journal of Hand Surgery (American)* 1989;**14**:371–5.
50. Vainio K. Vainio arthroplasty of the metacarpophalangeal joints in rheumatoid arthritis. *Journal of Hand Surgery (American)* 1989;**14**:367–8.
51. Fowler SB. Arthroplasty of the metacarpophalangeal joint in rheumatoid arthritis. *Journal of Bone and Joint Surgery* 1962;**44**:1037.
52. Seradge H, Kutz JA, Kleinert HE, et al. Perichondria resurfacing arthroplasty in the hand. *Journal of Hand Surgery (American)* 1984;**9**:880–6.
53. Moberg E. Arthrodesis of finger joints. *Surgical Clinics of North America* 1960;**40**:465–70.
●54. Stern PJ, Ho S. Osteoarthritis of the proximal interphalangeal joint. *Hand Clinics* 1987;**3**:405–12.
55. Das GA, Belskey MR. Arthrodesis of the proximal interphalangeal joint with K-wire technique. In: Blair WF (ed.) *Hand Surgery Techniques*. Baltimore, MD: Williams & Wilkins, 1996:816–23.
56. Allende BT, Engelem JC. Tension-band arthrodesis in the finger joints. *Journal of Hand Surgery* 1980;**5**:269–71.
57. Khuri MS. Tension band arthrodesis in the hand. *Journal of Hand Surgery* 1986;**11**:41–5.
58. Uhl RL, Schneider LH. Tension band arthrodesis of the finger joints: a retrospective review of 76 consecutive cases. *Journal of Hand Surgery* 1992;**17**:518–22.
59. Stern PJ, Gates NT, Jones TB. Tension band arthrodesis of small joints in the hand. *Journal of Hand Surgery* 1993;**18**:194–7.
60. Ijsselstein CB, van Egmond, DB, Kovius SE, et al. Results of small-joint arthrodesis: comparison of Kirschner wire fixation with tension band wire technique. *Journal of Hand Surgery* 1992;**17**:952–6.
61. Ayres JR, Goldstrohm GL, Miller GJ, et al. Proximal interphalangeal joint arthrodesis with the Herbert screw. *Journal of Hand Surgery* 1988;**13**:600–3.

62. Katzman SS, Gibeault JD, Dickson K, et al. Use of a Herbert screw for interphalangeal arthrodesis. *Clinical Orthopaedics* 1993;**296**:127–32.
63. Leibovic SJ, Strickland JW. Arthrodesis of the proximal interphalangeal joint of the finger: comparison of the use of the Herbert screw with other fixation methods. *Journal of Hand Surgery* 1994;**19**:181–8.
64. Kleinert JM, Gateley D. Proximal interphalangeal joint fusion: special situations. *Atlas of Hand Clinics* 998;**3**:31–39.
65. Bishop AT. Small joint arthrodesis. *Hand Clinics* 1993;**9**:683–9.
66. Leibovic SJ, Strickland JW. Arthrodesis of the proximal interphalangeal joint of the finger: comparison of the use of the Herbert screw with other fixation methods. *Journal of Hand Surgery* 1994;**19**:181–8.
67. Wright CS, McMurtry RY. AO arthrodesis in the hand. *Journal of Hand Surgery* 1983;**9**:932–5.
68. Seradge H, Kutz JA, Kleinert HA. Perichondral resurfacing arthroplasty in the hand. *Journal of Hand Surgery* 1984;**9**:880–6.
69. Burman MS. Vitallium cap arthroplasty of metacarpophalangeal and interphalangeal joints of fingers. *Bulletin of the NYU Hospital for Joints Diseases* 1940;**1**:79–89.
70. Linscheid RL. Implant arthroplasty of the hand: retrospective and prospective considerations. *Journal of Hand Surgery (American)* 2000;**25**:796–816.
♦71. Beevers DJ, Seedhom BB. Metacarpophalangeal joint prostheses: a review of past and current designs. *Proceedings of the Institute of Mechanical Engineers* 1993;**207**:195–206.
72. Iselin F, Conti E. Long-term results of proximal interphalangeal joint resection arthroplasties with a silicone implant. *Journal of Hand Surgery* 1995;**20**:S95–7.
73. Murray PM. New-generation implant arthroplasties of the finger joints *Journal of the American Academy of Orthopaedic Surgeons* 2003;**11**:295–301.
74. Sauerbier M, Cooney WP, Berger RA, Linscheid RL [Complete superficial replacement of the middle finger joint – long-term outcome and surgical technique]. *Handchirurgie, Mikrochirurgie, Plastische Chirurgie* 2000;**32**:411–18.
75. Branam BR, Tuttle HG, Stern PJ, Levin L. Resurfacing arthroplasty versus silicone arthroplasty for proximal interphalangeal joint osteoarthritis. *Journal of Hand Surgery (American)* 2007;**32**:775–88.
76. Johnstone BR, Fitzgerald M, Smith KR, Currie LJ. Cemented versus uncemented surface replacement arthroplasty of the proximal interphalangeal joint with a mean 5-year follow-up. *Journal of Hand Surgery (American)* 2008;**33**:1565–72.
77. Jennings CD, Livingstone DP. Surface replacement arthroplasty of the proximal interphalangeal joint using the PIP-SRA implant: results, complications, and revisions. *Journal of Hand Surgery* 2008;**33**:1565.e1–1565.
78. Eaton RG, Dobranski AI, Littler JW. Marginal osteophyte excision in treatment of mucous cysts. *Journal of Bone and Joint Surgery (American)* 1973:**55A**:570–4.
79. Kleinert HE, Kutz JE, Fishman JH, et al. Etiology of the so-called mucous cyst of the finger. *Journal of Bone and Joint Surgery* 1972;**54**:1455–8.
80. Nemethi CE. Phalangeal fractures treated by open reduction and Kirschner wire fixation. *Industrial Medicine* 1954;**23**:148.
81. Bunnell S. Joints. In: Boyes J (ed.) *Surgery of the Hand*, 4th edn. Philadelphia, PA: J.B. Lippincott Co, 1948:320–4.
82. Lister G. Intraosseous wiring of the digital skeleton. *Journal of Hand Surgery* 1978;**3**:427–35.
●83. Faithfull DK, Herbert TJ. Small joint fusions of the hand using the Herbert bone screw. *Journal of Hand Surgery* 1984;**9**:167–8.
84. Bednar MS. Distal interphalangeal joint fusion. *Atlas of Hand Clinics* 1988;**3**:1–16.
85. Teoh LC, Yeo SJ, Singh I. Interphalangeal joint arthrodesis with oblique placement of an AO lag screw. *Journal of Hand Surgery* 1994;**19**:208–11.
86. Engel J, Tsur H, Farin I. A comparison between K-wire and compression screw fixation after arthrodesis of the distal interphalangeal joint. *Plastic and Reconstructive Surgery* 1977;**60**:611–14.
87. Wyrsch B, Dawson J, Aufranc S, et al. Distal interphalangeal joint arthrodesis comparing tension band wire and Herbert screw: a biomechanical and dimensional analysis. *Journal of Hand Surgery* 1996;**21**:438–43.
88. Brutus JP, Palmer AK, Mosher JF, et al. Use of a headless compressive screw for distal interphalangeal joint arthrodesis in digits: clinical outcome and review of complications. *Journal of Hand Surgery (American)* 2006;**31**:85–9.

118

Carpal instability

NG ENG SENG, EDWARD T MAH

Introduction	1351	Physical examination	1353
Functional anatomy	1351	Investigation	1353
Carpal biomechanics	1352	Classification	1354
Pathomechanics	1352	Scapholunate injury	1355
Diagnosis	1353	References	1362
History	1353		

NATIONAL BOARD STANDARDS

- Understand the functional anatomy of the wrist
- Know common types of carpal injuries, including the Larsen classification
- Know how to diagnose and assess these carpal injuries
- Understand the SLAC (scapholunate advanced collapse) wrist
- Learn how to treat these common carpal injuries

INTRODUCTION

Carpal instability was not given much attention until the classic papers written by Linscheid et al.[1] and Dobyns et al.[2] Currently enormous experimental and clinical research has been carried out worldwide on wrist ligamentous injuries and the information has enabled better understanding of the biomechanical properties of the wrist, and diagnosing and treating this condition. Unfortunately, many cases are still missed or neglected and lead to chronic wrist dysfunction. It is then a great challenge for the hand surgeon to restore hand function. In this chapter, we attempt to give an overall description of wrist ligamentous injuries and highlight common injuries.

FUNCTIONAL ANATOMY

The wrist has complex bony and ligamentous structures. It forms a link between the forearm and the hand. Bony structures include distal radius and ulna, proximal carpal row (scaphoid, lunate, triquetrum and pisiform), distal carpal row (trapezium, trapezoid, capitate and hamate) and the bases of the metacarpal bones. The bony components contribute little to wrist stability. The main stabilizer for the wrist is the complex ligamentous structure. In general, the palmar ligaments are stronger and more complex than the dorsal ligaments. They are classified into extrinsic (those from the forearm to the carpal bone) and intrinsic (those with origin and insertion within the carpal bones) (Fig. 118.1). The two most important intrinsic ligaments are the scapholunate (SL) ligament and the lunotriquetral (LT) ligament. Both have dorsal, proximal fibrocartilagenous membrane and palmar components. The strongest component of the SL ligament is located dorsally whereas that of the LT ligament is located palmarly.[3–6] The three strong palmar extrinsic ligaments are the radioscaphocapitate (RSC), and the long and short radiolunate ligaments. The space between the former two ligaments is called the space of Poirier. This is the capsular weak point at which lunate dislocation occurs.[7] At the ulnar side, there are ulnolunate and ulnotriquetral ligaments that are considered part

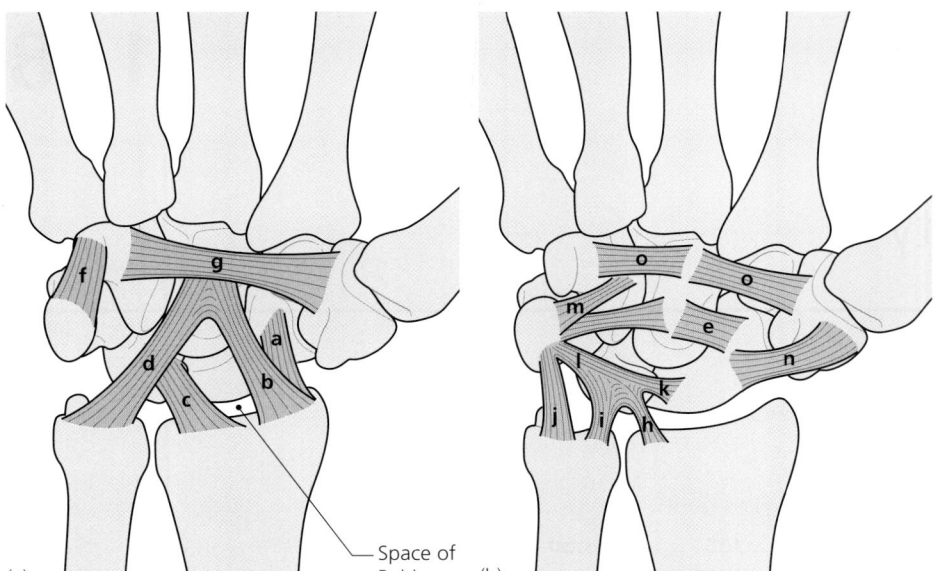

Figure 118.1 Schematic representation of the ligaments of the wrist. (a) Palmar superficial ligaments. (b) Palmar deep ligaments. a, Radioscaphoid; b, radiocapitate; c, long radiolunate; d, ulnocapitate; e, scaphocapitate; f, pisohamate; g, flexor retinaculum; h, short radiolunate; i, ulnolunate; j, ulnotriquetral; k, palmar scapholunate; l, palmar lunotriquetral; m, triquetral-hamate-capitate; n, scaphotrapezial; o, palmar transverse interosseous ligament. Arrow, the space of Poirier.

of the triangular fibrocartilagenous complex (TFCC). The dorsal wrist ligaments (dorsal radiocarpal and dorsal intercarpal ligaments) are structured in a V configuration centred at the triquetrum.

CARPAL BIOMECHANICS

There is extensive information on both wrist kinematics (wrist motion) and carpal kinetics (load transmission across the wrist) in the literature. The main role of the wrist is to provide a mobile and yet stable joint for the hand to function. This is achieved by the interaction between the bony articular surfaces, carpal ligaments and the dynamic tendon contraction across the wrist.

In the normal wrist, there is minimal movement between the carpal bones of the distal row.[8] In contrast, the carpal bones of the proximal row are less tightly bounded and they move in variable amounts on wrist movement.[8,9] There are no direct tendinous attachments on the carpal bones of the proximal row, and muscle contraction will move the distal row first until the midcarpal ligament reaches a certain tension before moving the proximal row secondarily.[8,10] In flexion–extension of the wrist, both rows synchronously move into flexion and extension in variable magnitude. As the wrist moves from radial to ulnar deviation, the proximal row moves from flexion to extension.[8,11] Many theories have been described on the mechanism of wrist movement, including column theories[12–15] and ring theories.[16]

The wrist is subjected to a vast amount of load that could reach 10 times the load exerted from finger pinching.[17] Hence it must be able to sustain these loads without yielding. In a normal wrist position, most of the load is transmitted through the scapho-lunate-capitate column. In the radiocarpal joint, about 50% of the load is transmitted through the radioscaphoid, 35% through the radiolunate and 15% through the ulnolunate joint.[18] More loads are transmitted through the ulnar side if the wrist is held in ulnar deviation. Many theories have postulated how the wrist is capable of sustaining the load without yielding.[1,14,15,19–21] The scaphoid is the key of the carpal, it lies obliquely across both the carpal rows; hence, it provides stability to both the carpal rows as a slider crank (so-called three-bar linkage mechanism) preventing the wrist from collapsing.[1]

PATHOMECHANICS

Carpal ligaments can be injured by direct or indirect forces. A large direct force may dislocate the wrist joint as the load is exerted directly on the carpal bone. Most carpal injuries result from an indirect force when the subject falls on an extended outstretched hand with variable amounts of radial or ulnar deviation and midcarpal supination or pronation. Mayfield et al.[22] described a pathomechanic event around the radial side of the wrist joint that leads to four stages of carpal instability around the lunate bone (perilunate instability). In stage I of perilunate instability, as the wrist is placed in extension, the distal carpal row is held in extension and the palmar midcarpal ligament to the scaphoid becomes taut and the force is transmitted to the lunate bone through the SL ligament. This tears the SL ligament as the lunate is strongly held by the radiolunate ligaments. In some cases, instead of a ligament tear the scaphoid may fracture. In stage II, as wrist extension increases, the RSC ligament will rupture and the capitate dislocate dorsally in relation to the lunate through the space of Poirier. As the extension load progresses, the triquetral capitate (TqC) ligament becomes taut and the force is transmitted to the triquetrum bone leading to TqC ligament rupture; sometimes the triquetrum bone is fractured (stage III). Finally in stage IV, all the perilunate ligaments are ruptured except the palmar radiolunate ligament; the dorsally displaced capitate may exert a palmar force that pushes the lunate palmarly leading to lunate dislocation.

DIAGNOSIS

Early diagnosis and appropriate treatment of carpal ligament injury is essential to provide a good outcome. However, diagnosis is often delayed or missed, especially when the injury occurs in isolation with minimal symptoms or is masked by other more serious injuries.[23,24] Carpal ligament injuries are commonly associated with distal radial fracture[25] and scaphoid fracture.[26] Diagnosis of these injuries is based on detailed history taking, physical examination and appropriate investigations.

HISTORY

Carpal ligament injury should be suspected in patients who complain of wrist pain after a fall on an outstretched hand with the wrist in dorsiflexion. A detailed history of the mechanism of injuries is essential. Symptoms may be mild if the ligament injury is incomplete or isolated. Patients may accept the injury as wrist sprain until chronic wrist dysfunction occurs. In more severe cases, such as carpal dislocation, the initial symptoms are usually greater. Carpal ligament injuries can be missed if associated with other injuries such as scaphoid or distal radius fractures. Other factors such as age, hand dominance, job and expectation should be considered as these may influence treatment options.

PHYSICAL EXAMINATION

The patient must be in a comfortable position and the normal hand should be examined as well for comparison. The patient should point out the maximum point of tenderness as this usually indicates the underlying pathology. For example, tenderness at the dorsum of the wrist distal to Lister's tubercle indicates SL injuries. Hence, a clear understanding of the anatomical structure and the surface anatomy of the wrist is important to complement wrist examination.

In acute injuries, tenderness and swelling may be minimal in isolated injuries. Swelling may be more diffuse with underlying haematoma. Diffuse swelling may also be associated with underlying dislocation or fracture. The range of movement and grip strength is limited by pain.

In chronic injuries, swelling may have settled and local tenderness may be more obvious. There is wrist dysfunction with reduced grip, pinch strength and movement.

Various special and provocative tests have been described to diagnose various carpal ligament injuries and this will be discussed under specific topics.

Examination is completed with a thorough vascular and neurological examination of the hand.

INVESTIGATION

Investigation of carpal injuries are essential. Various modalities of investigation are available but a good-quality, standardized test is required. Reading and interpreting an investigation of carpal ligament injuries requires a high index of suspicion and experience.

A plain radiograph is essential not only for diagnosis of ligament injuries but also for various measurements to assess the severity of the malalignment. Owing to vast normal variations, it is best to compare with the contralateral radiographs. Routine plain radiograph in a suspected wrist injury should include wrist posteroanterior (PA), lateral, PA in ulnar deviation and 45° semi-prone views.[27,28] A true PA view of the wrist is performed with the shoulder in 90° abduction, elbow in 90° flexion and the wrist in neutral rotation. The true lateral view is performed with the wrist in neutral rotation and the elbow adducted to the side of the body. In a normal neutral PA view, three smooth curved lines (Gilula arcs) connect the proximal and distal cortical surface of the proximal row and the proximal cortical surface of the distal carpal row (Fig. 118.2). A break in this line or step-off indicates carpal derangement.[29] The distance between the carpal bones is usually uniform and constant, any widening between the carpal bones indicates dissociation of the ligament between these carpal bones. The classic sign is the 'Terry Thomas' sign, which indicates SL ligament injury with widening of the SL interval.[30] In the lateral view of the wrist, various angles can be drawn to demonstrate malalignment based on several lines.

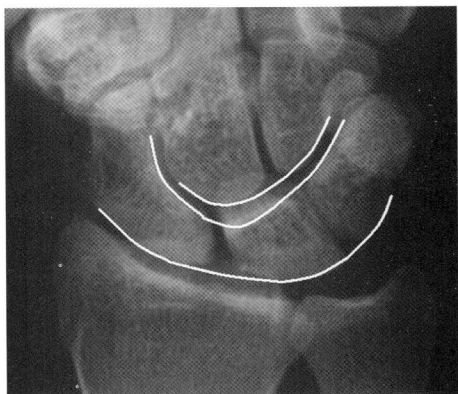

Figure 118.2 A normal neutral posteroanterior view of the wrist. Three smooth lines (Gilula's line) can be drawn connecting the proximal and distal cortical surface of the proximal row and the proximal cortical surface of the distal carpal row. Any break in this line or step-off indicates carpal derangement.

A scaphoid line is drawn along the most ventral points of the proximal and distal poles of the scaphoid. The lunate line runs through the midpoints of the convex proximal and concave distal surfaces of the lunate. The capitate line joins the mid-portion of the proximal convex and the distal surface of capitate and the radial line is along the longitudinal axis of the radius. The common angles that are used are the SL, capitolunate (CL) and radiolunate (RL). The capitolunate angle is formed between the capitate and the lunate lines. The normal value is 0°±15°.[31,32] Abnormality in the CL angle indicates midcarpal malalignment. The SL angle is the angle formed between the scaphoid and lunate lines. The normal value is 30–60°.[1] Angles more than 80° and less than 30° indicate a dorsal intercalated segment instability (DISI) and volar intercalated segment instability (VISI) pattern of malalignment respectively.[29] The radiolunate angle is the angle that is formed between the radial and lunate lines. Angles with more than 15° of dorsal tilt of lunate suggest a DISI deformity.[1] Various special views are described to confirm the specific malalignment. The commonly performed view is the clenched fist view or stress view.[2] The malalignment will be exaggerated if the wrist is loaded (Fig. 118.3).

Tomography has been replaced by CT. CT is useful in assessing malunion of the scaphoid with wrist pain and assessing carpal fusion; three-dimensional reconstruction is very helpful in pre-operative planning for treating complex carpal bone fractures and carpal fracture dislocations.

Wrist arthrography is useful in assessing intracarpal ligament injuries. Any leakage of dye from the radiocarpal joint into the midcarpal joint indicates either SL or LT ligament rupture. However, many studies have shown high positive arthrography in normal wrists, especially in older patients where asymptomatic degenerative ligament perforation is not uncommon.[33,34] Similarly, a small leak between the lunate and triquetrum is common and often regarded as a normal variant.

MRI allows carpal ligament injuries to be viewed, especially with dedicated wrist coils or combined with intra-articular contrast (gadolinium) injection.

Wrist arthroscopy has developed rapidly recently and currently it is the gold standard in diagnosing carpal ligament injuries. It is also useful in assessing a patient with chronic wrist pain. It allows direct visualization of the intra-articular pathology; various therapeutic procedures can be carried out arthroscopically. Wrist arthroscopy allows good visualization of the radiocarpal, midcarpal and distal radioulnar joints. The SL and LT ligaments can be seen on the radial side, and the triangular fibrocartilagenous complex can be seen on the ulnar side. It also can be used in assisting reduction and fixation in distal radius or a scaphoid fractures.

CLASSIFICATION

The main purposes of the classification of carpal injury are to provide an aid for the surgeon in managing the patient. The most comprehensive and practical classification is the one from Larsen and colleagues.[35,36] This classification divides carpal ligament injuries into six categories (chronicity, constancy, aetiology, location, direction and pattern). In general, the repair and healing potential of a ruptured ligament is best in the acute setting immediately after injury. Injury for more than 6 weeks is considered chronic, where the damaged ends are fibrosed and retracted making repair difficult. In between 1 and 6 weeks is considered subacute, when the ruptured ligament is probably still reparable but with poorer healing potential. In the category of constancy, a predynamic injury is where the ligament is partially torn with no malalignment under stress. Dynamic instability is where the ligament is completely torn and exhibits only under certain loading condition. Static instability is where there is complete rupture with permanent malalignment. The displacement is reducible initially but may become irreducible if left untreated as fibrosis occurs. Carpal instability is commonly caused by trauma and other causes such as inflammatory or congenital/developmental may lead to instability. In the location category, an instability occurs between the

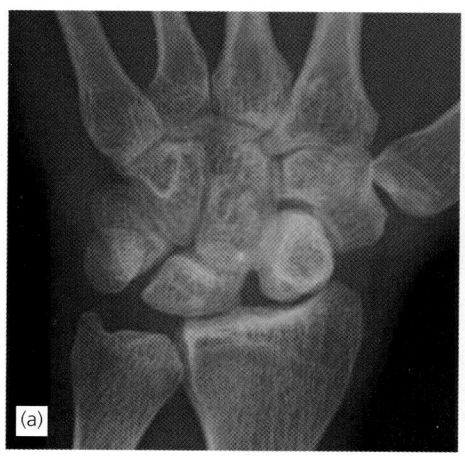
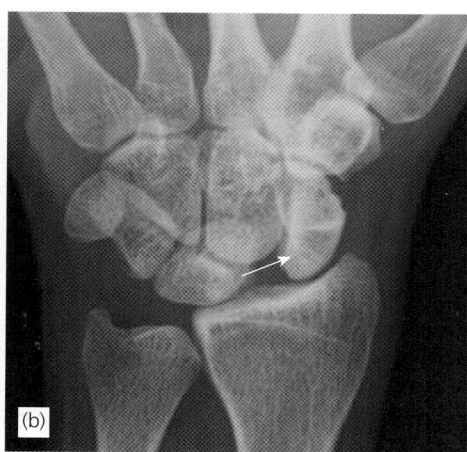

Figure 118.3 In dynamic scapholunate instability, the radiological feature of malalignment is exaggerated on clenched fist stress view. (a) Slight widening in the scapholunate interval (Terry Thomas's sign) that becomes more prominent after the wrist is loaded. (b) The scaphoid is held in abnormal flexion and will have a foreshortened appearance and 'cortical ring sign' as the scaphoid tubercle overlaps with the distal pole of the scaphoid (arrow).

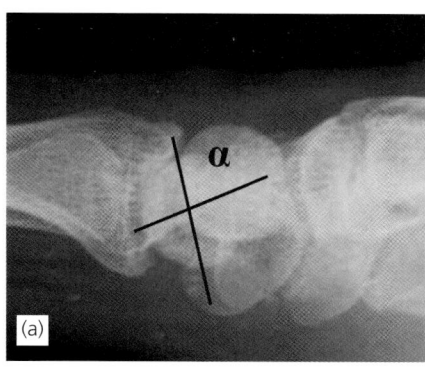
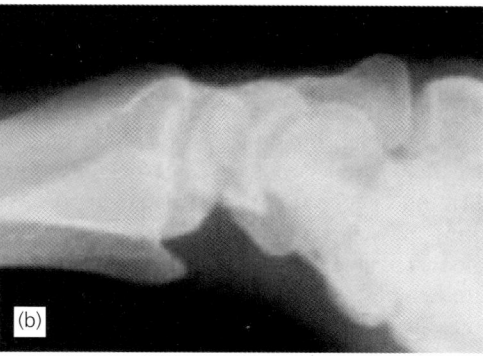

Figure 118.4 (a) Dorsal intercalated segment instability; scapholunate angle α is more than 80°. (b) Volar intercalated segment instability; lunate bone faces volarly.

Table 118.1 Pattern of carpal instability

Carpal instability dissociative (CID)	Scapholunate dissociation
	Lunotriquetral dissociation
	Scaphoid malunion or non-union
	Kienbock disease
Carpal instability non-dissociative (CIND)	Radiocarpal CIND
	Ulnar translocation
	Radial translocation
	Radiocarpal dislocation
	Midcarpal CIND
	Dorsal midcarpal
	Palmar midcarpal
Carpal instability complex (CIC)	Dorsal perilunate dislocation (lesser arcs)
	Dorsal perilunate fracture dislocation (greater arcs)
	Palmar perilunate dislocation
	Axial dislocation
	Isolated carpal dislocation
Carpal instability adaptive (CIA)	Malunited distal radius fracture

radiocarpal, midcarpal, carpometacarpal or intercarpal joints. Several types of carpal malalignment have been described. The commonest are DISI and VISI (Fig. 118.4), and ulnar and radial translocations.[1] The pattern of carpal instability is classified into four groups.[37,38] *Carpal instability dissociative* (CID) is where the injury occurs between the bones in the same row of carpal bones. In *carpal instability non-dissociative* (CIND), there is dissociation between the distal radius, ulna and the proximal, and distal carpal row with a normal relationship between the carpal bones in similar rows. *Carpal instability complex* (CIC) is a group of carpal derangement when it involves bones not only in the same carpal row (CID) but also between the carpal rows (CIND). Lastly, *carpal instability adaptive* (CIA) is carpal instability secondary to pathology outside the wrist joint. The instability in these different patterns is shown in Table 118.1.

SCAPHOLUNATE INJURY

Anatomy

The SL ligament is an important intrinsic ligament connecting the scaphoid and the lunate. It consists of three components: the dorsal ligament, the palmar ligament and the proximal fibrocartilagenous membrane.[3] The dorsal ligament is the major component and maintains the stability of the joint.[4] It is composed of transversely oriented collagen fibres. The palmar component has oblique orientated collagen fibres and plays a relatively minor role in stability.[3] The fibrocartilagenous membrane forms a membrane between the two bones from the dorsal to the volar and it prevents communication between the radiocarpal and the intercarpal joint.[39]

A SL ligament injury is produced by a combination of hyperextension, ulnar deviation and midcarpal supination of the wrist.[22] In hyperextension, the palmar midcarpal ligaments that connect to the scaphoid become taut and the force is transmitted to the lunate via the SL ligament. Hence there is progressive tearing of the SL ligament from the volar to the dorsal and eventually leads to complete SL ligament dissociation. In complete SL disruption, the scaphoid is unconstrained. The wrist will progress into DISI deformity, where the lunate and triquetrum rotate into abnormal extension while the scaphoid becomes abnormally flexed.[23] Furthermore, the force is abnormally transmitted across the wrist joint with excessive load on the radioscaphoid joint leading to radioscaphoid degenerative changes.[40,41]

Diagnosis

A SL ligament injury should be suspected in patients who fall on an outstretched hand with the wrist in dorsiflexion. Diagnosis is often delayed or missed, especially when the injury is partial or occurred in isolation with minimal symptoms or is overshadowed by other more serious injuries.[23,24] These injuries may occur with distal radial fracture[25] or scaphoid fracture.[26] The signs and symptoms depend on the severity and duration or whether it is an isolated injury.

In acute injury, there is usually pain and swelling of the wrist. In chronic injury, the swelling may be minimal but there is wrist dysfunction with pain, stiffness and weakness that usually leads to a poor outcome.

In an acute SL ligament injury, there is localized pain and maximal point tenderness at the site of the ligament that is located one finger breadth distal to Lister's tubercle on the dorsum of the wrist. Swelling may be minimal, and diffuse swelling usually indicates more serious injury with associated fractures. Movement of the wrist will usually aggravate the pain. Classically, a positive scaphoid shift test (Watson's test) is suggestive of SL dissociation.[42] This is performed with the examiner placing four fingers over Lister's tubercle dorsally and the thumb over the scaphoid tubercle palmarly. The wrist is moved from the ulnar to the radial position. The scaphoid extends in the ulnar position and flexes in the radial deviation. The thumb will prevent the scaphoid from flexing in the radial position; in the presence of a SL injury, the scaphoid will subluxate dorsally, inducing pain. Release of the fingers will allow reduction of the scaphoid and typical snapping or clunking may be felt. This test should be compared with the normal wrist. Another useful test is the finger extension test (FET), where patient is asked to extend the index and middle finger against resistance with the wrist held in 90° flexion. Pain is usually elicited at the ligament in the presence of acute dissociation.

In SL injuries, on the wrist PA view, the gap between the SL joint is wider (Terry Thomas sign) (Fig. 118.3) than normal, and a gap more than 5 mm is said to be diagnostic of SL dissociation.[30] The scaphoid will have a foreshortened appearance as it collapses into flexion and a 'cortical ring sign' as the scaphoid tubercle overlaps with the distal pole of the scaphoid (Fig. 118.3). In the lateral view, there will be DISI deformity with the SL angle more than 60°. In the normal wrist, a wide C line can be drawn by connecting the palmar margin of the scaphoid and the radius; when the scaphoid is abnormally flexed, the scaphoid and the radius intersect in an acute angle producing a V pattern (Figs 118.4 and 118.5). In dynamic instability, a special projection with a clenched fist is required to show the abnormality.

Wrist arthrography is commonly used in the diagnosis of a SL ligament tear. In the normal wrist, there is usually no communication between the radiocarpal and the intercarpal joint. Any abnormal flow of contrast from one articular space to another is interpreted as pathogenic.

Currently, wrist arthroscopy is the gold standard for diagnosing a carpal ligament injury.[38,43] It allows direct visualization of the injury and also diagnosis of other associated injuries of the wrist, for example TFCC injury or an osteochondral fracture. A radiocarpal and midcarpal arthroscopy is required. Geissler et al.[25] divided the intercarpal interosseous ligament into four grades. In grade I injury, there is attenuation and haemorrhage of the ligament with normal SL congruency of alignment in the midcarpal space. In grade II injury there is step-off and a slight gap (less than the width of a probe) between the SL intervals. In grade III injury, there is step-off and gapping that allow the probe to pass through. In grade IV injury, the gap is huge and a scope can pass through and sometimes the capitate bone can be seen from the interval.

Treatment

Treatment of SL ligament injuries depends on several factors. These include whether the ligament injury is partial or complete, the timing of presentation, the condition of the ruptured ligament stump, whether it is dynamic or static, whether it is reducible and the presence of degenerative changes. Patient expectation and the surgeon's capability must also be taken into consideration. Injury to the SL ligament can be partial and usually involves the volar component, which is not essential in maintaining joint stability. However, the natural history of this injury is still unknown. The timing of presentation is essential. If they present late, the ruptured stumps are fibrosed and retracted, and repair with good healing is impossible. Fibrosis may also have occurred around the joint and makes reduction impossible. The

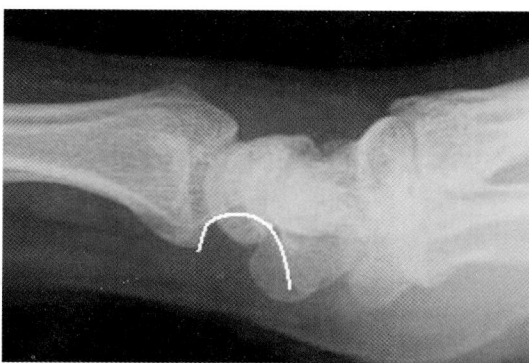 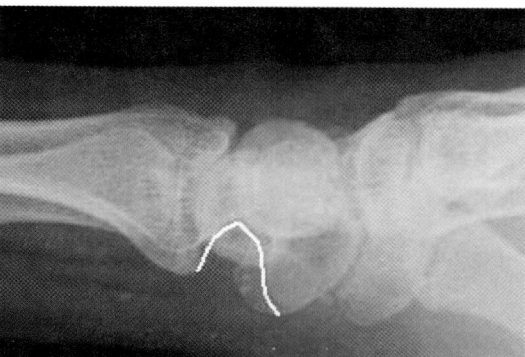

Figure 118.5 In a normal wrist, a wide C line can be drawn by connecting the palmar margin of the scaphoid and the radius; when the scaphoid is abnormally flexed, the scaphoid and the radius intersect in an acute angle producing a V pattern.

scaphoid is usually held in its normal position by various other ligaments (secondary stabilizers). Rupture of the SL ligament with intact secondary stabilizers will produce dynamic instability. If both the ligaments are ruptured, this will produce static instability.

ACUTE SCAPHOLUNATE DISSOCIATION

An acute injury is when the patient presents within 3 weeks of injury. The principle of treating acute SL dissociation is to reduce and maintain the reduction of the SL joint and allow healing of the ligament. The healing potential of the ligament is better[35,36] in the acute setting when the ligament stumps have not retracted and there is good blood perfusion. Primary ligament repair is recommended up to 6 weeks after the injury.[44]

Many approaches have been used ranging from closed reduction to surgery. SL disruption is reduced by dorsiflexion of the wrist followed by cast immobilization. However, it is difficult to maintain the reduction throughout the period of cast immobilization as the load of the capitate on the SL joint is significant. One technique is to maintain the reduction by percutaneous K-wire fixation. K-wires are inserted to transfix the scaphoid to the lunate and another to transfix from the scaphoid to capitate. An optional third wire may be used to transfix the distal radius to the lunate. Reduction is ensured by an image intensifier or wrist arthroscopy. An above-elbow cast is applied for 6–8 weeks. This technique is not reliable as the ruptured ligaments are not visualized and repaired.

The best approach to treat acute SL disruption is by open reduction, ligament repair and internal fixation. This allows direct visualization, reduction, direct repair of the torn ligaments and stabilization of the dissociation.[45] The dorsal approach is commonly used as it is more important to restore the dorsal ligament than the volar ligament. The joint is approached between the third and fourth compartment. Dissection through the wrist joint capsule will expose the scaphoid and lunate. Cartilaginous damage of the scaphoid and lunate is not uncommon (Fig. 118.6) and any attached or free cartilaginous fragments are removed. After direct reduction of the SL dissociation, it is stabilized with two or three K-wires as described above. Direct repair of the dorsal SL interosseous ligament is performed where possible, and if this is not possible then small bone anchor sutures (one in each of scaphoid and lunate) are a good alternative (Fig. 118.7). Reinforcement of the ligament repair using a strip of the dorsal capsule, as described by Blatt,[46] may be used. Typically, two cross K-wires are inserted intra-operatively in the manner described above to hold the carpus for a period of 6 weeks before removal. Postoperatively, the wrist is immobilized in a below-elbow cast with neutral wrist position. The cast and K-wires are removed after 6–8 weeks and active range-of-motion exercises commenced before strengthening exercises in a progressive manner.

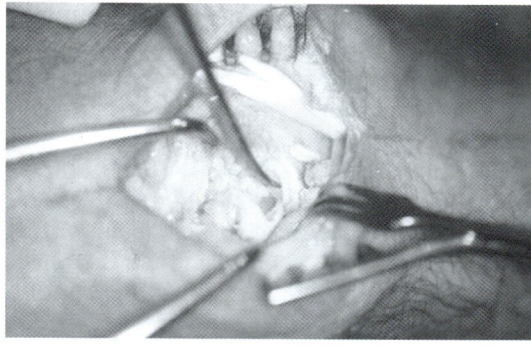

Figure 118.6 Catilaginous damage of the carpal bone (scaphoid) after scapholunate injury. Loose fragments should be removed.

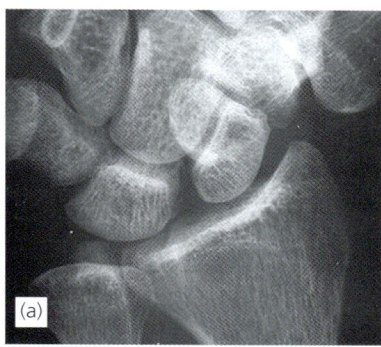

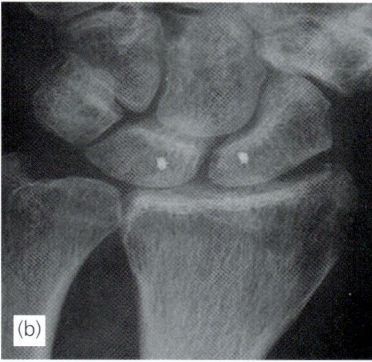

Figure 118.7 Acute scapholunate ligament injury. (a) Widening of the scapholunate interval suggestive of scapholunate tear. (b) The wrist is explored acutely through a dorsal approach and the scapholunate ligament is repaired using bone anchor sutures.

SUBACUTE SCAPHOLUNATE DISSOCIATION

The injury is regarded as subacute if it is 3–6 weeks after injury. The SL joint is reducible but the ligament stumps have started to retract and fibrose, precluding a direct repair. There is no general rule on the duration, and it all depends on the condition of the stumps intra-operatively and whether a delayed repair can be carried out.

The rationale of treating a subacute injury is the same as an acute injury. The SL joint may be reducible and the ligament is repaired with similar methods to those described above. If primary repair is not possible, ligament reconstruction is performed using the remnants of the ligaments augmented by capsulodesis. Capsulodesis was popularised by Blatt[46] with the use of a proximal flap of wrist capsule to stabilize the unstable scaphoid bone. The requirement for a capsulodesis is that the SL joint is able to reduce anatomically. Capsulodesis reduces some mobility of the wrist, especially volar flexion. A standard dorsal approach is used. A 1 cm wide flap is created from the dorsal wrist capsule; the proximal origin on the dorsum of the distal radius will be left attached. The abnormal scaphoid flexion and the SL dissociation are reduced. The scaphoid is stabilized with K-wires transfixing the scaphoid to the capitate and lunate. The flap is attached to the dorsum of the distal pole of the scaphoid distal to the mid-axis of rotation of the scaphoid with either a pull-through technique or using bone anchor sutures. Apply a below-elbow cast for 6–8 weeks. The K-wires are removed at the time of removal of the plaster, and progressive active and passive assisted range-of-motion exercises commence. Various modifications of capsulodesis have been described. Herbert et al.[47] used a reversed capsular flap with the base attached to the scaphoid; the proximal end is sutured into Lister's tubercle. Linschied and Dobbyns[48] used the distal half of the dorsal intercarpal ligament and released its insertion from the triquetrum. This flap is inverted to the dorsum of the radius and sutured to Lister's tubercle.

CHRONIC SCAPHOLUNATE DISSOCIATION

An injury is termed chronic if the injury is over 6 weeks old. In this situation the ruptured SL ligament is irreparable. The key point at this stage is to determine whether the dissociation is reducible. The SL gap can be filled with fibrous tissue and the wrist ligaments can be either retracted or stretched out. A joint is considered reducible only if the dissociation can be reduced by vertical traction and radial deviation of the wrist. This may be attempted under anaesthesia and image intensification or during reconstructive surgery. Treatment of this group of patients is difficult. Many studies have shown that untreated SL ligament injuries may eventually lead to carpal degeneration and carpal dysfunction.[40,49]

Several surgical options may be considered in these groups of patients. A wrist arthroscopy debridement may improve the patient's wrist pain for a certain period of time until salvage surgery is carried out. If the SL joint is reducible, a bone–tendon–bone graft or a free tendon graft (e.g. palmaris longus) using bone anchor sutures as described previously may be considered. Ligament reconstruction is technically demanding and the outcome is unpredictable. A bone–tendon–bone graft such as using either the autologous or the allographic hemiphalangeal joint is technically demanding and clinical experience of this technique is very limited. Most patients can expect to have some loss of wrist motion and grip strength after tendon reconstruction. Various local grafts or free grafts have been used. Almquist et al.[50] use the extensor carpi radialis brevis (ECRB) tendon to recreate the transverse portion of the dorsal SL ligament through drill holes at the scaphoid, lunate, capitate and radius. The drawback of this method is that it does not stabilize the distal scaphoid and the drill holes are placed close to the vascularly compromised SL joints. Brunelli and Brunelli[51] use the flexor carpi radialis (FCR) tendon graft to stabilize the SL joint by passing the tendon near the scaphoid tubercle and suturing with the SL remnant and finally anchoring to the distal radius. Linschied and Dobbyns[48] use the ECRB tendon passed through the drill hole at the distal scaphoid and swept around the SL joint and finally passed under the LT ligament, looped around and sutured to itself. The last two modifications stabilize both the proximal and distal scaphoid and do not devascularize the scaphoid and lunate bones. All these methods produced only moderate mid-term results[48,50,51] and the long-term outcome is unknown.

If the SL joint is irreducible, a limited wrist fusion is performed. This preserves some wrist movement. Various limited wrist fusions have been described to treat various wrist problems. The commonest method in treating this injury is scaphoid–trapezium–trapezoid (STT) fusion, also known as triscaphoid fusion. The goal of this fusion is to try to realign the proximal scaphoid pole with the scaphoid fossa of the radius so the radioscaphoid congruency is restored and reduces the risk of developing radioscaphoid arthritis. It is also essential to gain correct alignment of the scaphoid, and Ambrose et al.[52] and Watson have suggested that the scaphoid is placed about 50° to the long axis of the forearm in lateral view. The overall non-union rate is about 14% and these are always associated with reduced wrist strength and movement. Other methods of limited fusion are SC (scaphoid–capitate) fusion and SLC (scaphoid–lunate–capitate) fusion. Direct SL (scaphoid–lunate) fusion is the most anatomically logical approach in treating this injury but clinical experience showed that this fusion is difficult to achieve and hence it gives poor results in treating SL dissociation.[53–55]

DEGENERATIVE CHANGES

Longstanding untreated SL injury will lead to cartilage degeneration of the radial carpal joint. Watson and Ballet[41] described arthrosis after SL dissociation as SLAC (scapholunate advanced collapse) wrist. In stage IA, arthritis occurs around the radial styloid with narrowing of the radioscaphoid articulation. This may progress to involve the entire radioscaphoid joint in stage IB. In stage II SLAC wrist, the arthritis involves the capitolunate joint, and, in stage III, there is involvement of the entire wrist joint.

In stage I SLAC wrist, a radial styloidectomy will usually produce a favourable outcome. Stage II wrist can be treated by proximal row carpectomy or four-corner fusion (excision of the scaphoid with fusion of the lunate, capitate, triquetrum and hamate). The prerequisite for proximal row carpectomy is a normal articular surface of the capitate and the lunate facet of the radius so the proximal end of the capitate can articulate with the lunate fossa of the radius. In our experience, both procedures reduced some movement of the wrist joint but four-corner fusion produces better wrist grip strength. Proximal row carpectomy is done through a dorsal approach, and the scaphoid, lunate and triquetrum bones are removed leaving the pisiform bone. The capitate is then seated onto the lunate fossa of the radius with some capsulodesis to provide some initial stability. The patient is put on a plaster backslab for 3 weeks and active mobilization is allowed gradually. Four-corner fusion (Fig. 118.8) is carried out by a dorsal approach and the proximal pole of the scaphoid is excised. The fusion surface between the lunate, triquetrum, capitate and hamate is debrided. An iliac bone graft is used and the bones are stabilized using K-wires (triquetrum to lunate, capitate to lunate, hamate to lunate and triquetrum to capitate), staples or various newer four-corner fusion devices. Postoperatively plaster is needed until the bones fuse. In stage III SLAC wrist, four-corner fusion is preferable to preserve some wrist movement, while in advanced stage IV disease, total wrist fusion is the best option to provide the patient with a painless and functional wrist.

Lunotriquetral instability

LT joint instability is not uncommon. However, there is poor awareness and understanding of this condition compared with the SL instability. This condition is often missed or ignored, and is confused with TFCC injury or midcarpal instability.

As in the SL ligament, the LT ligament consists of dorsal and palmar components and proximal fibrocartilagenous membrane with the stronger volar component. LT joint instability may be caused by a traumatic event or degenerative process. In traumatic causes, it commonly occurs in lunate or perilunate dislocation together with a SL ligament tear and lunocapitate joint dislocation (Mayfield stage III). It also can be caused by isolated injury with a fall on an outstretched hand with the wrist in radial deviation and pronation.[56] LT instability can also occur in ulnar impaction syndrome or as a chronic TFCC injury.

LT ligament injury may be considered as predynamic if the ligament is only partially torn. In dynamic injury, only the LT ligament is ruptured, whereas the secondary ligaments around the triquetrum are still intact. If all the ligaments are ruptured, this will produce a static instability. After LT ligament rupture, the carpal bones will classically go into a VISI deformity.

DIAGNOSIS

Signs and symptoms after LT ligament tears depend on the severity and the duration of the injury. In predynamic injury, the signs and symptoms may be minimal or absent. However, in a classical complete LT ligament tear, the pain and point tenderness are located over the dorsal aspect of the joint[6] and aggravated by ulnar deviation and supination.[57] In advanced cases with VISI collapse, the wrist will have a slight forklike deformity with prominent distal ulna.[5,58] A ballottement test described by Reagan et al.[6] may be positive in LT instability. It is performed by ballotting the LT joint with the thumb and index finger stabilizing the lunate while the other hand holds the triquetrum and pisiform bones. A positive test will demonstrate pain, crepitus and ballottable LT joint.

A plain radiograph is often unremarkable in LT instability. In the PA view, there may be narrowing of the LT joint. In complete LT tear, there may be disruption of the Gilula line with step-off over the lunate and triquetrum bone.[6] This finding can sometimes be produced under stress in dynamic instability. In static instability, the lunate has a moonlike appearance and the SL distance may slightly increase with a positive ring sign of the scaphoid. In the lateral view, there may be typically VISI deformity. Wrist arthrography may show a communication of dye between the radiocarpal and midcarpal joint.[59.] It must be borne in mind that developmental and degenerative perforation of the LT ligament is common in those with ulnar positive variance[60] and elderly people respectively. Wrist arthroscopy is currently the gold standard in diagnosis and assessment of LT injury and also ulnar wrist pain.

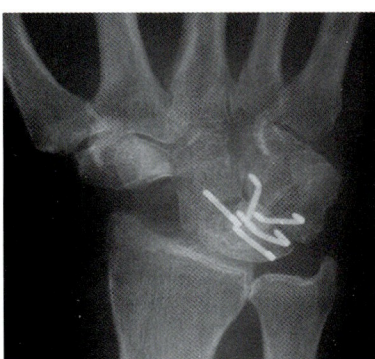
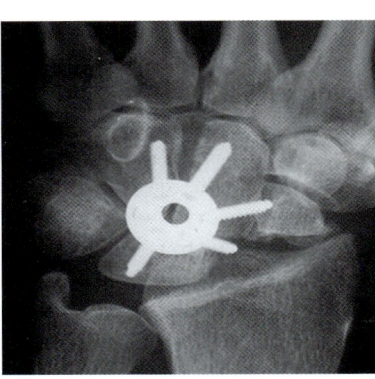

Figure 118.8 Four-corner fusions. The lunate, capitate, hamate and triquetral bones are fused using staples and spider rings.

TREATMENT

Treatment depends on the time of presentation. With the routine use of arthroscopy as a diagnostic tool in assessing patients with ulnar wrist pain, more cases of early acute LT ligament injury are being detected. Early rupture has a good prognosis of healing after repair. Another factor to consider in treating these patients is whether the lesion is dynamic or static. In dynamic lesions, the secondary constraints (extrinsic ligaments) are intact and competent.

In an acute dynamic rupture of LT ligament injury, it can be treated conservatively with a well-padded above-elbow cast in the neutral position to limit supination and pronation for 6 weeks. A below-elbow cast may lead to failure of the ligament to heal with secondary attenuation of the extrinsic ligament and VISI collapse. Another option is to perform a percutaneous K-wiring from the triquetrum to the lunate under fluoroscopy or arthroscopy. The wrist is then placed in a short arm cast for 6 weeks. This approach produces excellent results.[5] In chronic cases where there is poor healing of the ligament, arthroscopic debridement may decrease pain or even result in complete resolution.[61] In general, the result of arthroscopic debridement in this condition is better than SL ligament tear as less load is exerted on the ulnar side of the wrist. Ligament reconstruction using a distally based extensor carpi ulnaris tendon to restore the linkage of the LT joint by passing the tendon through drill holes at the lunate and triquetrum.[6] Alternatively, bone anchor sutures may be used for the reconstruction. In patients with static instability, most ligament reconstruction is not reliable and the best option is a combined LT fusion and a radiolunate fusion.[62]

RADIOCARPAL INSTABILITY

The radiocarpal joint is constrained by the palmar and ulnar inclined distal radius, and the proximal row is held to the distal radius by strong radioscaphoid, RSC long and short radiolunate and ulnolunate ligaments. Hence disruption of these anatomical constraints may lead to radiocarpal instability. This is usually caused by inflammatory arthritis and less commonly by trauma.

The proximal carpal row can be displaced radially or ulnarly. In ulnar translocation, the whole carpal is displaced ulnarly and palmarly.[63] The space between the radial styloid and the scaphoid is widened. On plain radiographs, the amount of translocation can be measured by measuring the perpendicular distance between the centre of the capitate and the radial styloid.[64] Treatment of this injury is difficult. The resulting ligament repair is unsatisfactory and fusion of the radiolunate joint is probably the best option in providing a stable wrist.[64] Radial translocation of the radiocarpal joint is rare and may occur after a malunited distal radius fracture that is radially inclined with the ulnar side ligament injury (short radiolunate and ulnolunate) rupture. Treatment mainly involves correction of the malunited radius. A pure traumatic radiocarpal dislocation is extremely rare compared with radiocarpal dislocation with a radial styloid fracture. Treatment is by radial styloid fixation.

MIDCARPAL INSTABILITY

Midcarpal instability (MCI) involves dissociation between the proximal and distal carpal row and sometimes involves the radiocarpal joint as well.[65] The midcarpal is stabilized by the midcarpal crossing ligaments, particularly the palmar triquetral–hamate–capitate (TqHC), dorsal STT and scaphocapitate ligaments.[66–68] These ligaments ensure a smooth transition of the proximal row from flexion to extension as the wrist deviates ulnarly. Hence, damage or attenuation of these ligaments allows the wrist to fall into VISI deformity and lose smooth transition and produce a sudden clunk on ulnar deviation.

Midcarpal injury is commonly associated with generalized ligament laxity and is rarely due to trauma. Common MCI is called palmar MCI,[69] where the proximal row is held in flexion producing VISI instability. Classically there is sagging of the midcarpal palmarly. There is a painful clunk when the wrist is ulnarly deviated and pronated; the sag is corrected in ulnar deviation.[68,70] There is also generalized ligament laxity. On plain radiographs, the condition appears as classical VISI deformity on the lateral view and in the AP view the scaphoid is held in a flexed position with a moon-shaped lunate bone. A stress view may exaggerate the abnormality by a palmarly applied load on the capitate.[71,72] The condition is best demonstrated by fluoroscopy to show the snapping as the wrist is ulnarly deviated in pronation. These patients are usually treated conservatively initially with anti-inflammatory drugs, splinting and activity modification. A strengthening programme includes flexor carpi ulnaris strengthening that acts as a dynamic stabilizer to prevent clunking. If this treatment fails and the patient remains symptomatic, then surgery is indicated, which involves triquetral hamate joint fusion or tendon reconstruction using the ECRB tendon to reconstruct the palmar TqC.[73]

Dorsal perilunate dislocation/lunate dislocation

These injuries occur when there is a fall on an outstretched hand with the wrist in dorsiflexion. Both dorsal perilunate and lunate dislocation represent different stages of the same pathomechanic process described by Mayfield as stage IV perilunate instability.[22] A lunate or perilunate dislocation is an unstable condition, for almost all the carpal ligaments attaching to the lunate are disrupted except the strong palmar radiolunate ligaments. The patient usually presents with an acute painful swollen wrist joint with severe pain and reduced wrist movement. The lunate bone that has displaced palmarly may compress on the median nerve causing carpal tunnel syndrome. Unfortunately, this condition is still commonly missed either through ignorance of the patient or by the physician in the emergency room. A high index of suspicion is required when interpreting the radiograph. In the normal PA radiograph, any disruption of the Gilula arc[29] or overlapping of the carpal bones suggest a carpal derangement. A lateral view radiograph reveals either a dorsal perilunate or a lunate dislocation. Associated fractures of the carpal or distal radius should be identified, particularly the radial styloid, scaphoid or the capitate, and triquetrum bones (Fig. 118.9).

TREATMENT

Dislocation must be reduced as soon as possible to restore the anatomy and to reduce compression of the median nerve. It is more difficult to reduce if the dislocation has been in place for some time. In chronic cases, fibrosis occurs and reduction is impossible. Good analgesia and complete muscle relaxation is essential for closed reduction. With continuous traction for about 10 minutes, and with traction maintained, the wrist is brought into hyperextension, while the thumb stabilizes the lunate at the palmar side. The wrist is brought from extension to flexion and will usually allow the capitate to snap back into the lunate fossa.[74,75] After reduction, a radiograph confirms the reduction, and visualizes any fracture. A SL angle of >80° and SL gap more than 3 mm is associated with a poor prognosis.[76]

Owing to inherent instability of this injury, reduction is difficult to maintain throughout the course of conservative treatment. Unless the patient is contraindicated for surgery, the authors advocate treating this condition surgically. If this is treated conservatively, a below-elbow thumb spica is applied with the wrist in neutral or slight flexion for 6–12 weeks. Reduction must be checked weekly for three consecutive weeks to ensure the reduction is maintained.

An alternative to surgery is percutaneous pinning to allow the ligament to heal. This is carried out using an image intensifier or arthroscopically. The lunate is first aligned to the distal radius and a K-wire is inserted from the distal radius radially to the lunate and through the LT joint once the joint is reduced. The SL joint is reduced and another K-wire is inserted from the scaphoid to the lunate thorough the snuffbox. Finally the capitolunate joint is reduced and a K-wire is inserted from the scaphoid to the capitate and the lunate to the capitate. A plaster cast is applied as mentioned for 6 weeks before mobilization.

The authors advocate open surgery for this injury. Surgery is needed to ensure good reduction, removal of loose osteocartilagenous fragments, ligament repair and median nerve decompression. We commonly use a dorsal approach through the three or four compartments and reduction is easy in the early stage; if this fails an additional volar approach is added. The dislocation is reduced through the dorsal wound, and the ligament is repaired either by direct repair or using bone anchor sutures. The volar side is approached only when carpal tunnel release is required. K-wires are inserted as previously described with similar postoperative regimens (Fig. 118.9). In most cases it is possible to return to pre-injury activities after 6 months.[77,78]

Dorsal perilunate fracture dislocation

As mentioned under Pathomechanics, ligament injury will depend on the load and position of the wrist during injury. Various perilunate bones can be fractured. Many perilunate fracture dislocations have been described: trans-scaphoid perilunate dislocation,[77–80] trans-scaphoid trans-capitate perilunate dislocation, trans-triquetral perilunate dislocation,[81,82] trans-scaphoid trans-triquetral perilunate dislocation or a trans-radial styloid transscaphoid dislocation. In general, fracture dislocations have a better prognosis than pure ligamentous dislocations, because fractures can be reduced anatomically and secure fixation can be achieved to ensure union. A similar approach is used, and the fracture is fixed by various methods (K-wire, headless screw) and ligaments are repaired.

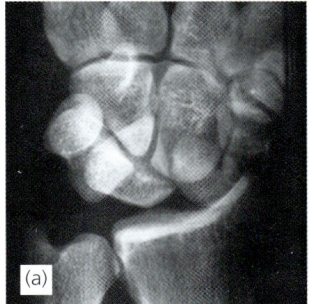
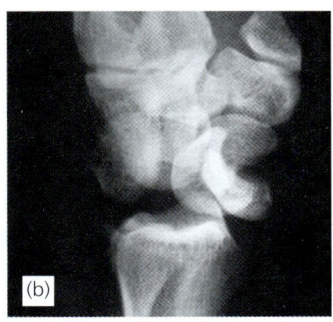
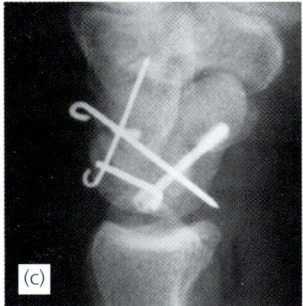
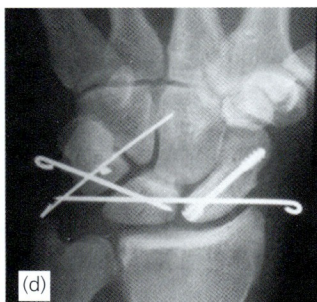

Figure 118.9 Trans-scaphoid dorsal perilunate dislocation. (a) In the posteroanterior view of the wrist, there is break in Gilula's line and overlapping of the carpal bones. (b) In the lateral view, the lunate is displaced volarly by the capitate bone. (c and d) The dislocation is reduced through a dorsal approach and the scaphoid fracture is stabilized with a headless screw and the lunotriquetral and midcarpal joints are stabilized with K-wires.

Carpal instability adaptive

This is carpal instability secondary to pathology outside the wrist joint. The most common recognized cause is a malunited distal radius fracture.[2] In a dorsally displaced malunited fracture, the lunate is dorsiflexed in relation to the capitate. In due course this will lead to progressive pain at the midcarpal joint with an occasional midcarpal click. In the Taleisnik and Watson series,[83] corrective osteotomy of the distal radius provides resolution of pain and midcarpal instability.

KEY LEARNING POINTS

- The wrist forms a link between the forearm and the hand; its role is to provide a mobile and yet a stable joint for the hand to function.
- The wrist is subjected to loads up to 10 times the load from finger pinching.
- Most carpal injuries result from an indirect force after a fall onto an extended outstretched hand with variable amounts of radial or ulnar deviation and midcarpal supination or pronation.
- Radiographs to image carpal injuries are a true posteroanterior view of the wrist with the shoulder in 90° abduction, elbow in 90° flexion and the wrist in neutral rotation.
- The classic radiograph sign of scapholunate ligament injury with widening of the scapholunate interval is called the Terry Thomas sign.
- The most comprehensive and practical classification is Larsen's.
- A positive scaphoid shift test (Watson's test) is suggestive of scapholunate dissociation.
- Wrist arthroscopy is the gold standard in diagnosing a carpal ligament injury.
- Treat acute scapholunate disruption with open reduction, ligament repair and internal fixation.
- Arthrosis after scapholunate dissociation is SLAC (scapholunate advanced collapse) wrist.
- The lunotriquetral joint instability is not uncommon but is poorly known.
- A lunate or perilunate dislocation is an unstable condition (with damage to the median nerve), often missed but can be easily seen on lateral radiographs

REFERENCES

- ● = Key primary paper
- ◆ = Major review article

◆1. Linscheid RL, Dobyns JH, Beabout JW, Bryan RS. Traumatic instability of the wrist. Diagnosis, classification and pathomechanics. *Journal of Bone and Joint Surgery (American)* 1972;**54A**:1612-32.

◆2. Dobyns JH, Linscheid RL, Chao EYS, et al. Traumatic instability of the wrist. *Instructional Course Lectures.* 1975;**24**:182-99.

●3. Berger RA. The gross and histologic anatomy of the scapholunate interosseous ligament. *Journal of Hand Surgery (American)* 1996;**21A**:170-8.

●4. Kobayashi M, Berger RA. Kinametic analysis of the scapholunate interosseous ligament repair. *Orthopaedic Transactions* 1995;**19**:129.

●5. Osterman AL, Seidman GD. The role of arthroscopy in the treatment of lunatotriquetral ligament injuries. *Hand Clinics* 1995;**11**:41-50.

●6. Reagan DS, Linscheid RL, Dobyns JH. Lunotriquetral sprains. *Journal of Hand Surgery (American)* 1984;**9**:502-14.

●7. Mayfield JK. Patterns of injury to carpal ligaments: a spectrum. *Clinical Orthopaedics* 1984;**187**:36-42.

●8. Ruby LK, Cooney WP III, An KN, et al. Relative motion of selected carpal bones: A kinematic analysis of the normal wrist. *Journal of Hand Surgery (American)* 1988;**13**:1-10.

●9. Seradge H, Sterbank PT, Seradge E, Owens W. Segmental motion of the proximal carpal row: Their global effect on the wrist motion. *Journal of Hand Surgery (American)* 1990;**15**:236-9.

●10. Youm Y, McMurtry RY, Flatt AE, Gillespie TE. Kinematics of the wrist: I. An experimental study of radial-ulnar deviation and flexion-extension. *Journal of Bone and Joint Surgery (American)* 1978;**60**:423-31.

●11. Craigen MAC, Stanley JK. Wrist kinematics: Row, column or both? *Journal of Hand Surgery (British)* 1995;**20**:165-70.

◆12. Navarro A. Anatomy and physiology of the carpus. *Anales del Instituto de Clinica Quirurgica y Cirugia Experimental*, Montevideo, Uruguay, 1935;166-89.

◆13. Taleisnik J. Wrist: anatomy, function and injury. *Instructional Course Lectures* 1978;**27**:61-87.

◆14. Weber ER. Biomechanical implications of scaphoid wrist fractures. *Clinical Orthopaedics and Related Research* 1980;**149**:83-90.

◆15. Weber ER. Concepts governing the rotational shift of the intercalated segment of the carpus. *Orthopedic Clinics of North America* 1984;**15**:193-207.

●16. Lichtman DM, Schneider JR, Swafford AR, Mack GR. Ulnar midcarpal instability-clinical and laboratory analysis. *Journal of Hand Surgery (American)* 1981;**6**:515-23.

●17. An KN, Chao EY, Cooney WP, Linscheid RL. Forces in the normal and abnormal hand. *Journal of Orthopaedic Research* 1985;**3**:202-11.

●18. Hara T, Horii E, An KN, et al. Force distribution across the wrist joint: Application of pressure-sensitive conductive rubber. *Journal of Hand Surgery (American)* 1992;**17**:339-47.

●19. Gilford WW, Bolton RH, Lambrinudi C. The mechanism of the wrist joint with special reference to fractures of the scaphoid. *Guy's Hospital Reports* 1943;**92**:52-9.

●20. Landseer JMF. Studies in the anatomy of articulation: I. The equilibrium of the 'intercalated' bone. *Acta Morphologica Neerlando-Scandinavica* 1961;**3**:287-303.

- 21. Fisk GR. Carpal instability and the fractured scaphoid. *Annals of the Royal College of Surgeons of England* 1970;**46**:63–76.
- 22. Mayfield JK, Johnson RP, Kilcoyne RF. The ligaments of the human wrist and their functional significance. *Anatomical Record* 1976;**186**:417–28.
- 23. Taleisnik J. Carpal instability. *Journal of Bone and Joint Surgery (American)* 1988;**70A**:1262–7.
- 24. Jones WA. Beware of the sprained wrist: The incidence and diagnosis of scapholunate instability. *Journal of Bone and Joint Surgery (British)* 1988;**70B**:293–7.
- 25. Geissler WB, Freeland AE, Savoy FH, et al. Intracarpal soft tissue lesions associated with an intraarticular fracture of the distal end of radius. *Journal of Bone and Joint Surgery (American)* 1996;**78A**:357–65.
- 26. Palmer AK, Levinsohn EM, Kuzma GR. Arthrography of the wrist. *Journal of Hand Surgery* 1983;**8**:15–23.
- 27. Peh WC, Gilula LA. Imaging of the wrist: a customized approach. *Current Orthopaedics* 1994;**8**:23–31.
- 28. Gilula LA, Destitute JM, Weeks PM, et al. Roentgenographic diagnosis of the painful wrist. *Clinical Orthopaedics and Related Research* 1984;**187**:52–64.
- 29. Gilula LA, Weeks PM. Post-traumatic ligamentous instabilities of the wrist. *Radiology* 1978;**129**:641–51.
- 30. Frankel VH. The Terry-Thomas sign (letter). *Clinical Orthopaedics* 1977;**129**:321–2.
- 31. Nakamura R, Hori M, Imamura T, et al. Method for measurement and evaluation of carpal bone angles. *Journal of Hand Surgery (American)* 1989;**14**:412–16.
- 32. Sarrafian SK, Melamed JL, Goshgarian GM. Study of wrist motion in flexion and extension. *Clinical Orthopaedics and Related Research* 1977;**126**:153–9.
- 33. Viejas SF, Patterson RM, Hokanson JA, Davis J. Wrist anatomy: Incidence, distribution, and correlation of anatomic variations, tears, and arthrosis. *Journal of Hand Surgery (American)* 1993;**18**:463–75.
- 34. Herbert TJ, Faithfull RG, McCann DJ, Ireland J. Bilateral arthrography of the wrist. *Journal of Hand Surgery (British)* 1990;**15**:233–5.
- 35. Hodge JC, Gilula LA, Larsen CF, Amado PC. Analysis of carpal instability: II. Clinical applications. *Journal of Hand Surgery (American)* 1995;**20**:765–76.
- 36. Larsen CF, Amado PC, Gilula LA, Hodge JC. Analysis of carpal instability: I. Description of the scheme. *Journal of Hand Surgery (American)* 1995;**20**:757–64.
- 37. Amado PC. Carpal kinematics and instability: a clinical and anatomic primer. *Clinical Anatomy* 1991;**4**:1–12.
- 38. Cooney WP, Dobbins JH, Linscheid RL. Arthroscopy of the wrist: anatomy and classification of carpal instability. *Arthroscopy* 1990;**6**:133–40.
- 39. Palmer AK, Levinsohn EM, Kuzma GR. Arthrography of the wrist. *Journal of Hand Surgery* 1983;**8**:15–23.
- 40. Watson HK, Ryun J. Evolution of arthritis of the wrist. *Clinical Orthopaedics and Related Research* 1986;**202**:57–67.
- 41. Watson HK, Ballet FL. The SLAC wrist: Scapholunate advanced collapse pattern of degenerative arthritis. *Journal of Hand Surgery* 1984;**9A**:358–65.
- 42. Watson HK, Ashamed D IV, Makhlouf MV. Examination of the scaphoid. *Journal of Hand Surgery* 1988;**13A**:657–60.
- 43. Weiss APC, Akelman E, Lambiase R. Comparison of the findings of triple injection cinearthrography of the wrist with those of arthroscopy. *Journal of Bone and Joint Surgery (American)* 1996;**78A**:348–56.
- 44. Cooney WP III, Linschied RL, Dobbins JH. Fracture and dislocation of the wrist. In; Rockwood CA Jr, Green DP, Bocholt RW (eds) *Fracture in Adults*, 3rd edn. Philadelphia, PA: J.B. Lippincott, 1991:354–9.
- 45. Louis DS, Hankins FM, Greene TL, et al. Central carpal instability-capitolunate instability pattern. Diagnosis by dynamic displacement. *Orthopedic* 1984;**7**:1693–6.
- 46. Blatt G. Capsulodesis in reconstructive hand surgery: Dorsal capsulodesis for the unstable scaphoid and volar capsulodesis following the excision of the distal ulna. *Hand Clinics* 1987;**3**:81–102.
- 47. Herbert TJ, Hargreaves IC, Clarke AM. A new surgical technique for treating rotatory instability of the scaphoid. *Hand Surgery* 1996;**1**:75–7.
- 48. Linschied RL, Dobbyns JH. Treatment of scapholunate dissociation. *Hand Clinics* 1992;**8**:645–52.
- 49. Sebald JR, Dobbins JH, Linschield RL. The natural history of collapse deformities of the wrist. *Clinical Orthopaedics and Related Research* 1974;**104**:140–8.
- 50. Almquist EE, Bach AW, Sack JT, et al. Four bone ligament reconstruction for treatment of chronic complete scapholunate separation. *Journal of Hand Surgery* 1991;**16A**:322–7.
- 51. Brunelli GA, Brunelli GR. A new surgical technique for carpal instability with scapholunate dislocation: eleven cases. *Annales de Chirurgie de la Main et du Membre Supérieur* 1995;**14**:207–13.
- 52. Ambrose L, Posner MA, Green SM, Stuchin S. The effect of scaphoid intercarpal stabilization on wrist mechanics: An experimental study. *Journal of Hand Surgery (American)* 1992;**17A**:429–37.
- 53. Siegel JM, Ruby Elk. A critical look at intercarpal arthrodesis. Review of literatures. *Journal of Hand Surgery (American)* 1996;**21A**:717–23.
- 54. Frykman EB, Ekenstam FA, Wading K. Triscaphoid arthrodesis and its complication. *Journal of Hand Surgery (American)* 1988;**13A**:844–8.
- 55. Hom S, Ruby Elk. Attempted scapholunate arthrodesis for chronic scapholunate dissociation. *Journal of Hand Surgery (American)* 1991;**16A**:334–9.
- 56. Brown IW. Volar intercalary carpal instability following a seemingly innocent wrist fracture. *Journal of Hand Surgery (British)* 1987;**12**:54–6.
- 57. Christodoulou L, Bainbridge LC. Clinical diagnosis of triquetrolunate ligament injuries. *Journal of Hand Surgery (British)* 1999;**24**:598–600.
- 58. Viejas SF, Patterson RM, Peterson PD, et al. Ulnar-sided perilunate instability: An anatomic and biomechanics study. *Journal of Hand Surgery (American)* 1990;**15**:268–78.
- 59. Alexander CE, Lichtman DM. Ulnar carpal instabilities. *Orthopedic Clinics of North America* 1984;**15**:307–20.

◆60. Chun S, Palmer AK. The ulnar impaction syndrome: follow-up of ulnar shortening osteotomy. *Journal of Hand Surgery (American)* 1993;**18**:46–53.

●61. Weiss APC, Sachar K, Glowacki KA. Arthroscopic debridement alone for intercarpal ligament tears. *Journal of Hand Surgery (American)* 1997;**22**:344–9.

●62. Taleisnik J. Radiolunate arthrodesis. In: Blair WF (ed.) *Techniques in Hand Surgery*. Baltimore, MD: Williams & Wilkins, 1996:879–86.

●63. Rayhack JM, Linscheid RL, Dobbins JH, Smith JH. Posttraumatic ulnar translation of the carpus. *Journal of Hand Surgery (American)* 1987;**12**:180–9.

●64. Camay A, Della Santa D, Vilaseca A. Radiolunate arthrodesis factor of stability for the rheumatoid wrist. *Annales de Chirurgie de la Main* 1983;**2**:5–17.

●65. Wright TW, Dobbins JH, Linscheid RL, et al. Carpal instability non-dissociative. *Journal of Hand Surgery (British)* 1994;**19**:763–73.

●66. Bell MJ, McMurtry RY. Volar intercalated segment instability as a result of spontaneous rupture of the supporting ligaments of the wrist due to long-term systemic steroid medication. *Journal of Hand Surgery (British)* 1985;**10**:395–8.

●67. Garcia-Elias M. Kinetic analysis of carpal stability during grip. *Hand Clinics* 1997;**13**:151–8.

●68. Lichtman DM, Schneider JR, Swafford AR, Mack GR. Ulnar midcarpal instability-clinical and laboratory analysis. *Journal of Hand Surgery (American)* 1981;**6**:515–23.

◆69. Lichtman DM, Bruckner JD, Culp RW, Alexander CE. Palmar midcarpal instability: Results of surgical reconstruction. *Journal of Hand Surgery (American)* 1993;**18**:307–15.

●70. Feinstein WK, Lichtman DM, Noble PC, et al. Quantitative assessment of the midcarpal shift test. *Journal of Hand Surgery (American)* 1999;**24**:977–83.

●71. Johnson RP, Carrera GF. Chronic capitolunate instability. *Journal of Bone and Joint Surgery (American)* 1986;**68**:1164–76.

●72. Ono H, Gilula LA, Evanoff BA, Grand D. Midcarpal instability: is capitolunate instability pattern a clinical condition? *Journal of Hand Surgery (British)* 1996;**21**:197–201.

◆73. Gracia-Elias M, Grislier WB. Carpal instability. In: Green DP, Hotchkiss RN, Pederson WC, Wolfe SW (eds) *Green's Operative Hand Surgery*, 5th edn. Edinburgh, UK: Churchill Livingstone, 2005.

74. Watson-Jones R. Carpal semilunar dislocations and other wrist dislocations with associated nerve lesions. *Proceedings of the Royal Society of Medicine* 1929;**22**:1071–86.

75. Watson-Jones R. *Fractures and Joint Injuries*, 3rd edn. Edinburgh, UK: E & S Livingstone, 1943:568–77.

◆76. Rawlings ID. The management of dislocations of the carpal lunate. *Injury* 1981;**12**:319–30.

●77. Herzberg G, Comet JJ, Linscheid RL, et al. Perilunate dislocations and fracture-dislocations: a multicenter study. *Journal of Hand Surgery (American)* 1993;**18**:768–79.

●78. Sotereanos DG, Misiones GJ, Giannakopoulos PN, et al. Perilunate dislocation and fracture-dislocation: A critical analysis of the volar-dorsal approach. *Journal of Hand Surgery (American)* 1997;**22**:49–56.

●79. Garcia-Elias M, Irisarri C, Henriquez A, et al. Perilunar dislocation of the carpus: A diagnosis still often missed. *Annales de Chirurgie de la Main* 1986;**5**:281–7.

●80. Lacour C, de Peretti F, Barraud O, et al. Perilunar dislocations of the carpus: Value of surgical treatment. *Revue de Chirurgie Orthopédique et Réparatrice de l'Appareil Moteur* 1993;**79**:114–23.

●81. Stevanovic M, Schnall SB, Filler BC. Trans-scaphoid, trans-triquetral, volar lunate fracture-dislocation of the wrist. *Journal of Bone and Joint Surgery* 1996;**78**:1907–10.

●82. Labia JL, Vachaud M, Rouge D, Ficat P. Trans-scapho-perilunar dislocations with internal instability of the carpal bones. *Revue de Chirurgie Orthopédique et Réparatrice de l'Appareil Moteur* 1986;**72**:53–62.

83. Taleisnik J, Watson HK. Midcarpal instability caused by malunited fractures of the distal radius. *Journal of Hand Surgery (American)* 1984;**9**:350–7.

119

The distal radial ulnar joint

EDWARD T MAH, NG ENG SENG

Introduction	1365	Management	1368
Anatomy	1365	Chronic DRUJ injury without osteoarthritis	1369
Classification	1366	Chronic DRUJ injury with osteoarthritis	1371
Diagnosis	1366	References	1371

NATIONAL BOARD STANDARDS

- Understand the distal radial ulnar joint (DRUJ)
- Know DRUJ and triangular fibrocartilaginous complex instability
- Learn how to manage acute and chronic DRUJ instability

INTRODUCTION

The distal radial ulnar joint (DRUJ) is one of the least understood joints in the body. Disorder of DRUJ is an important cause of ulnar sided wrist pain and yet is often underdiagnosed or misdiagnosed. Palmer[1] termed DRUJ problems as 'low back pain of the wrist'. Over the last 20 years, there has been a surge in research regarding the anatomy, function, biomechanics and treatment of DRUJ. Despite the volume of information currently available, there is still no consensus in treating DRUJ pathology. Recent advances in arthroscopic surgery have opened a new horizon in diagnosis and treatment of DRUJ problems. In this chapter, we review the clinical anatomy, diagnosis, classification and management of DRUJ problems.

ANATOMY

DRUJ is a diarthrodial, trochoid joint that forms between the concave sigmoid notch of the distal radius and the ulnar head (Fig. 119.1). Together with the radiocapitellar joint, proximal radial ulnar joint, radius and ulna bone and the interosseous membrane (IOM), it acts as a pivot for forearm supination–pronation. The axis of forearm rotation extends from the radial head proximally to the ulnar head distally.[2]

The bony structures of DRUJ provide little inherent stability for the joint. A cadaveric study by Tolat et al.[3] showed that 42% of the DRUJs had flat sigmoid notches that make the joint inherently unstable and 80% of the specimens had a palmar osteocartilaginous lip that prevents palmar displacement. The soft tissues are the prime stabilizers for DRUJs. They can be divided into 'static' and 'dynamic' stabilizers. The static stabilizers are the triangular fibrocartilaginous complex (TFCC) and the IOM; the dynamic stabilizers include the pronator quadratus and the extensor carpi ulnaris (ECU) tendon[4]

The TFCC was first described by Palmer and Werner.[5] It consists of the triangular fibrocartilage (TFC), dorsal and palmar radioulnar ligaments, extensor carpi ulnaris (ECU) sheath and ulnocarpal ligaments (ulnolunate and ulnotriquetral ligaments) (Fig. 119.1). The TFC or articular disc is attached to the dorsal and volar edges of the sigmoid notch to blend peripherally with the dorsal and palmar radioulnar ligaments. These ligaments merge at the apex of the TFC and have dual insertion onto the midportion and fovea of the ulnar styloid. It also inserts indirectly onto the lunate and triquetrum bone as the ulnolunate and

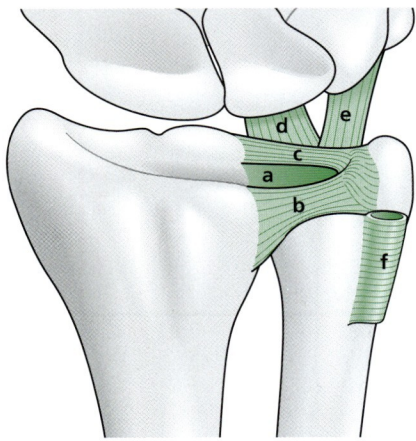

Figure 119.1 Structures of distal radius ulnar joint (DRUJ) and triangular fibrocartilagenous complex (TFCC). a, triangular fibrocartilage; b, dorsal radiocarpal ligament; c, palmar radioulnar ligament; d, ulnolunate ligament; e, ulnotriquetral ligament; f, extensor carpi ulnaris tendon sheath.

Table 119.1 Classification of triangular fibrocartilaginous complex instability

Causes	Chronicity	Degree	Direction	Types
Trauma	Acute	Mild	Dorsal	Dynamic
Inflammatory	Chronic	Moderate	Palmar	Static
Developmental	Acute on chronic	Severe	Multidirectional	
Others				

ulnotriquetral ligament. Hence the carpus is suspended not only from the radius, but also from the distal ulna at the ulnar styloid and the structures that inserted to it.[6] Fracture of the base of the styloid process could affect DRUJ stability. The dorsal and palmar radioulnar ligaments are the important structures that maintain DRUJ stability and provide stability in full supination and pronation respectively.[7] The ulnocarpal ligament resists dorsal displacement of the distal ulna relative to the radiocarpal unit. The IOM plays a role in force transmission through the forearm and is taut during supination and tethers the radius and ulna bone.[2] The ECU sheath strengthens the dorsal capsule and together with the dynamic ECU tendon resists dorsal dislocation in pronation and palmar dislocation in supination.[4] The pronator quadratus coapts the ulnar head in the sigmoid notch during pronation.

The TFCC receives its blood supply from the dorsal and palmar radiocarpal branches of the ulnar artery and anterior interosseous artery.[8] The pattern of blood supply determines the healing potential of the TFCC. The triangular cartilage receives blood only at its outer 15%, leaving the central portion avascular.[9] There are rich blood supplies at the fovea attachment and the dorsal and palmar ligaments, indicating good healing potential of the periphery after injury. No vessels cross the radial attachment to enter the TFCC.[10]

CLASSIFICATION

DRUJ instability can be classified according to causation, chronicity, degree, direction, and types of instability (Table 119.1).

DRUJ instability may be caused by trauma, inflammatory processes in the surrounding soft tissue or developmental ligament laxity. Traumatic DRUJ instability is the commonest and can result from direct or indirect injuries. In direct injury, the DRUJ will dislocate dorsally after a fall with the wrist in extension and forearm in hyperpronation; this will lead to palmar dislocation. In more severe injuries the DRUJ may be unstable both dorsally and palmarly, resulting in 'multidirectional' instability. The commonest causes of indirect injuries to the DRUJ are distal radius fracture, Galeazzi's or radial head fractures. The DRUJ is affected in 60% of forearm fractures.[11] Inflammatory processes such as rheumatoid arthritis cause synovitis of the DRUJ and erosion of the ulnar styloid. This will damage the structures attached to the styloid and lead to instability. Furthermore, the ECU tendon can be ruptured by osteoarthritic DRUJ caused by the inflammatory process.

TFCC injury is best treated acutely where reduction of the DRUJ joint is easy and the healing potential of the damaged structure is good. In chronic injury, the injured ligament will fibrose and retract, making ligament repair difficult and healing poor. Reduction may be difficult due to fibrosis. There is no consensus on the duration of chronicity, but in general an injury more than 6 weeks old is considered chronic.

DRUJ instability may be dynamic or static. In dynamic instability, static radiography will not show any abnormality and instability is only shown on the dynamic view as the joint is loaded (Fig. 119.2). In static instability the ulna is subluxed or dislocated either dorsally or volarly, and the deformity can be easily demonstrated with static radiography.

As a guide for treatment, a simple dislocation is where the subluxation or dislocation can be reduced spontaneously or easily with closed reduction or after fixation of associated fractures (distal radius, Galeazzi's or radial head fractures). Complex dislocation is where the subluxation or dislocation is irreducible or requires forceful reduction. These are usually due to high-energy injuries with significant styloid fracture, severe TFCC rupture or interposed soft tissue. The ECU tendon may be detached from the distal ulna together with the TFCC and slipped volarly into the DRUJ.

DIAGNOSIS

Diagnosis of DRUJ disorder and injury to specific structures of the TFCC are a great challenge for clinician.

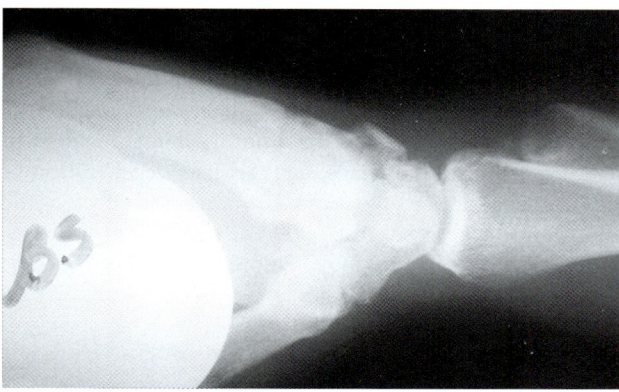

Figure 119.2 Dorsal subluxation of the distal ulna on dynamic view. The ulnar head is subluxed dorsally on loading.

Other causes of the ulnar side wrist pain must be ruled out and this requires an understanding of the various underlying anatomical structures. A thorough history, physical examination and investigation are always important.

History includes age, hand dominance, occupation, detailed mechanism of injury, with the position of the wrist during injury and the characteristic details of the symptoms. Pain is usually located at the ulnar side of the wrist. In acute injury, there may be associated swelling with painful forearm rotation. Chronic DRUJ dysfunction is not uncommon and is commonly seen in malunited distal radius fractures. Isolated DRUJ injury is less common. Patients usually present months after injury with a history of so-called wrist sprain that has been ignored or neglected. Besides the pain on the ulnar side, there may be associated clicking. Patients may have difficulties with daily activity involving rotation, such as turning doorknobs or opening lids of jars.

Physical examination of the wrist should always include a comparison with the normal side. There may be obvious dorsal displacement of the distal ulna, especially on pronation. Tenderness over the TFCC is best palpated at the soft spot between the flexor carpi ulnaris (FCU), ECU, ulnar styloid and pisiform bone. ECU tendonitis is located at the groove over the dorsum of the ulna radial to the styloid. Localized ulnar styloid tenderness indicates a styloid fracture or non-union, and tenderness over the DRUJ dorsally suggests underlying DRUJ osteoarthritis. DRUJ instability is demonstrated by the ballottement test. The clinician will ballot the ulnar head with the wrist in pronation. A positive 'piano key sign' is when there is very little resistance on the ballottement test. We prefer to perform this with a 90° flexed elbow on the table using one hand to stabilize the patient's wrist and the other hand holding the distal ulna and to try to displace it both dorsally and palmarly (Fig. 119.3). The test is performed with the wrist in the neutral position and full supination and full pronation. Wrist motion and pronation–supination are usually reduced secondary to pain or altered biomechanics.

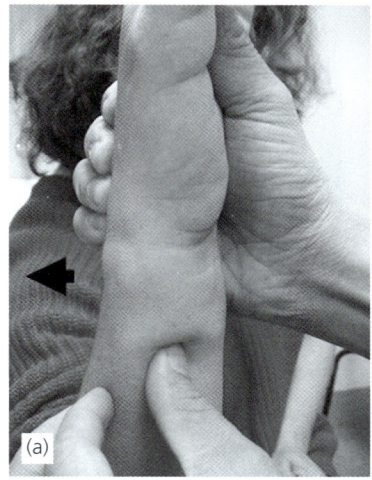

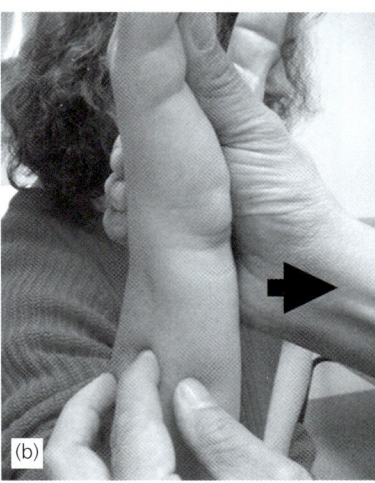

Figure 119.3 (a, b) Test for distal radius ulnar joint instability. The patient's elbow is flexed 90° on the table. The physician uses one hand to stabilize the patient's wrist and the other hand to hold the distal ulnar and to try to displace dorsally (a) and palmarly (b).

Imaging techniques for assessment of DRUJ include plain radiograph, CT, MRI, arthrography and wrist arthroscopy. Diagnosis from plain radiographs is difficult as rotation of the wrist can yield a false negative result in regard to DRUJ instability. It is important to obtain a true lateral and posteroanterior (PA) radiographs. These plain films must be compared with the contralateral side for radioulnar widening, ulnar displacement, ulnar variant and DRUJ osteoarthritis. In dorsal displacement, the ulna is displaced dorsally in the lateral view with DRUJ widening on the PA view. In contrast, in volar displacement, the ulna is displaced volarly on the lateral view with overlapping of the distal radius and ulna on the PA view (Fig. 119.4). CT of both wrists may enable one to assess chronic DRUJ instability.[12] Besides, CT is a valuable tool in assessing fracture, developmental deformities of the sigmoid notch and osteoarthritis. Arthrography was once an important tool in assessing TFCC injury but has now been replaced by other modalities. Its

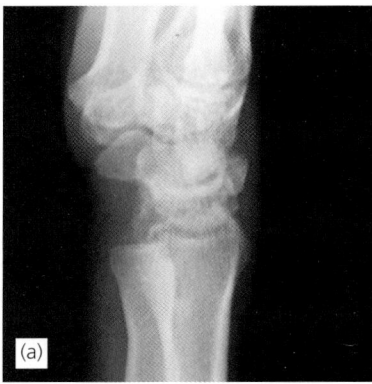
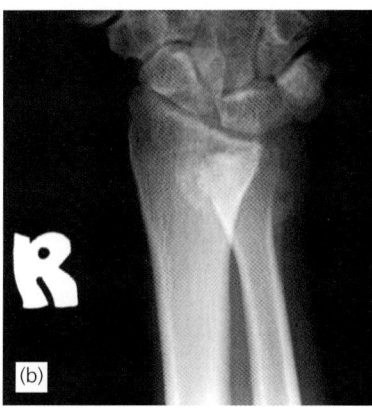

Figure 119.4 Volar distal radius ulnar joint (DRUJ) subluxation. In the posteroanterior view (a), there is overlapping of the DRUJ, and in the lateral view (b) the ulna is displaced volarly.

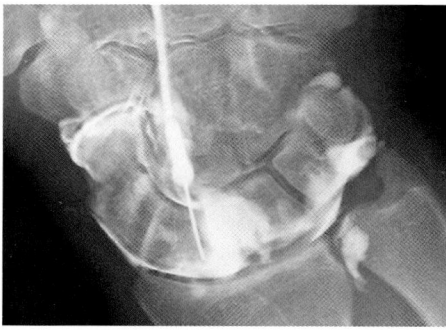

Figure 119.5 Wrist arthrography in triangular fibrocartilagenous complex (TFCC) injury. Dye is injected into the radiocarpal joint; leakage of dye to the distal radius ulnar joint indicates a possible TFCC tear.

findings showed poor clinical correlation[13] with a high incidence of perforation detected in an asymptomatic wrist, especially in elderly people[14,15] (Fig. 119.5).

The utility of high-resolution MRI, particularly with a dedicated surface coil, allows diagnosing and localizing a TFCC tear. Potter et al.[16] found MRI to have a sensitivity of 100%, specificity of 90% and accuracy of 97% in TFCC injuries.

Wrist arthroscopy is currently the gold standard for evaluation and treatment of DRUJ instability. The arthroscope is inserted into the 3/4 portal while the probe is in the 6U/6R portal. It allows us to visualize and localize the TFCC tear, the integrity of the ulnocarpal ligament and to assess the chondral damage, e.g. cartilage degeneration of the articular surface. A loss of the 'trampoline effect' of the TFCC on probing suggests a TFCC tear.[17] Many studies have shown that arthroscopy is more sensitive and specific than other imaging modalities.[18]

MANAGEMENT

Acute DRUJ injury

Acute isolated dorsal dislocation is generally more common than volar dislocation. In most cases, this may be reduced easily with a closed method. In dorsal dislocation, it is reduced by supinating the forearm with direct volar pressure. On the other hand, in volar dislocation, the ulna is reduced ulnarward and dorsally in a pronated forearm. Sometimes, there may be difficulty in reduction because of the deforming force of the pronator quadratus. The reduction is checked for congruent reduction with radiographs, and the forearm is tested for stability in supination and pronation. If the stability can only be maintained in extreme rotation, it is advised to pin the DRUJ in the reduced position with one or two K-wire(s) proximal to the DRUJ and parallel to the radiocarpal joint under radiological guidance. If the reduction is congruent and stable, an above-elbow cast is applied with the wrist in supination for dorsal dislocation and pronation for volar dislocation for 6 weeks. Range of movement exercises are started after removal of wire(s) and/or plaster.

The commonest cause for traumatic DRUJ instability is following a distal radius fracture. Instability after an accurate fracture reduction and union is uncommon. The prognostic factors for persistent DRUJ instability after a distal radius fracture are DRUJ widening and radial height shortening, as the radioulnar ligaments can tolerate no more than 5–7 mm of shortening before the ligaments fail;[19] this ligament is commonly torn at the ulnar attachment.[20]

Surgery is indicated if reduction is unstable or irreducible. In unstable reduction, it will redislocate easily, or reduction is maintained only by extreme rotation. If the dislocation is irreducible or could only maintained by undue force, there may be interposed soft tissue causing the problem. Incongruity of DRUJ on radiographs may also suggest soft-tissue interposition. In these circumstances, forceful reduction with K-wiring fixation is contraindicated. This is usually associated with a significant ulnar styloid fracture or ECU tendon detachment from the distal ulna with the TFCC and slipped volarly into the DRUJ. Exploration of the DRUJ using a dorsal approach is recommended. A longitudinal incision is made radial to the ECU tendon. The digiti minimi is released and retracted radially. The interposed structure is removed or relocated and any DRUJ intra-articular cartilaginous or bony fragments are removed. The ulnar styloid is stabilized or the TFCC is repaired with the anchor suture or pull-through techniques at the base of the ulnar styloid. The DRUJ may need to be K-wired if it remains unstable. Various options of arthroscopic repairs have been described for TFCC injury. An outside repair can be performed using mulberry knots[21] or an inside repair using a meniscus fastener.[22]

Dislocation after 6 weeks is difficult to reduce, especially a volar dislocation where reduction is prevented by the contracted pronator quadratus muscle. The distal pronator quadratus must be released for reduction and every attempt must be made to repair the TFCC or fix the styloid fracture.

The ulnar styloid is fractured in about 61% of distal radius fractures.[23] Owing to the attachment of the TFCC on the styloid shaft and base, fractures at its tip will not compromise DRUJ stability. A displaced basal fracture will usually require fixation to restore DRUJ stability. It can be stabilized with screws, tension band wiring or ulnar plates. In painful chronic non-union, the styloid may be excised subperiosteally if the DRUJ is stable. In unstable DRUJ, every attempt should be made to stabilize the ulnar styloid fracture and to repair the TFCC to the base.[24]

CHRONIC DRUJ INJURY WITHOUT OSTEOARTHRITIS

Managing chronic DRUJ instability is a great challenge. The TFCC and surrounding structures are retracted and fibrosed. Repair of these structures is difficult and healing may be poor. Many of these patients are asymptomatic and have fairly good function. It is unclear if there is a natural progression from chronic DRUJ instability to osteoarthritis. Hence, surgical intervention is indicated only if it is symptomatic or disturbing daily activities. Restoration of full painless supination and pronation with stable joints is the goal of treatment for chronic DRUJ instability. Treatment of chronic instability depends on the severity, the direction of instability and the patient's symptoms. Mild instability can be treated with a short-term splint, to restrict rotation, and anti-inflammatories followed by a range of movement and strengthening exercises. Pain in DRUJ instability is usually due to ulnar impaction, ECU tendonitis or osteoarthritis of the DRUJ or ulnocarpal joint. These must be identified and treated accordingly.

In chronic instability without DRUJ osteoarthritis, a diagnostic wrist arthroscopic and debridement of the TFCC is performed. Positive ulnar variance must be treated with various methods of shortening, and malunion or non-union of the distal radius is corrected. Ulnar shortening may tighten the TFCC and stabilize the DRUJ joint. Many soft-tissue reconstructions have been described that involved creating a direct distal radioulnar joint link extrinsic to the joint,[25] indirect radioulnar links via an ulnocarpal sling[26,27] or direct reconstruction of the distal radioulnar ligaments.[28–30] Direct reconstruction is the most anatomic approach and can restore DRUJ stability without substantial loss of movement and strength. In radioulnar ligament reconstruction, a free graft (palmaris longus or plantaris) is used to reconstruct dorsal and palmar radioulnar ligaments by threading the graft around the sigmoid notch of the distal radius towards the ulna and suturing to itself (Fig. 119.6a–c). The outcome is good with pain relief, restoration of range of movement (ROM) and improvement in grip strength.[28–30] We prefer to stabilize the dorsal dislocation with half of the ulna-based extensor retinaculum. The retinaculum is passed

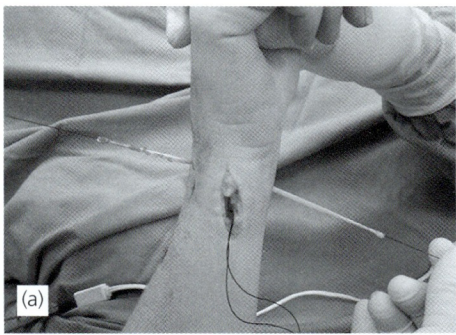

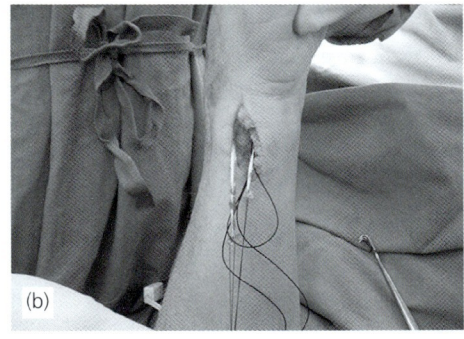

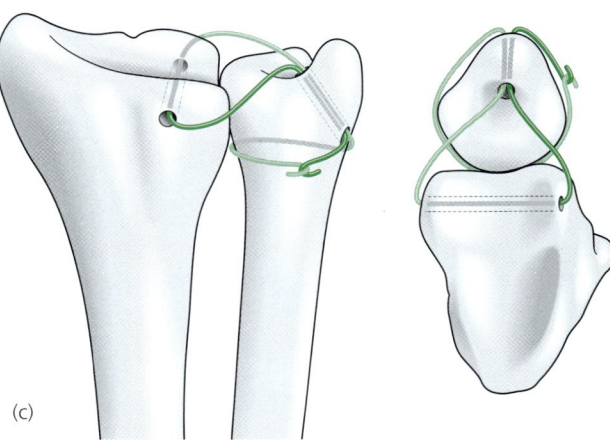

Figure 119.6 (a) Reconstruction of the distal radioulnar joint using a free palmaris longus graft. (b) The free palmaris longus graft is threaded around the sigmoid notch of the distal radius toward the ulna and sutured to itself. (c) Schematic diagram of the procedure.

below the ECU tendon and is tethered to the distal radius with anchor sutures (Fig. 119.7a–c). This method has shown excellent results in 93% of patients after a mean follow-up of 38 months.[31] Alternatively, stabilization using half of either the flexor (for volar instability) or the extensor (for dorsal instability) carpi ulnaris tendons to zig-zag through the ulnar may be considered for more severe DRUJ instability (Fig. 119.8a–c). Most of these reconstructions have been performed on small series of patients and require long-term review.

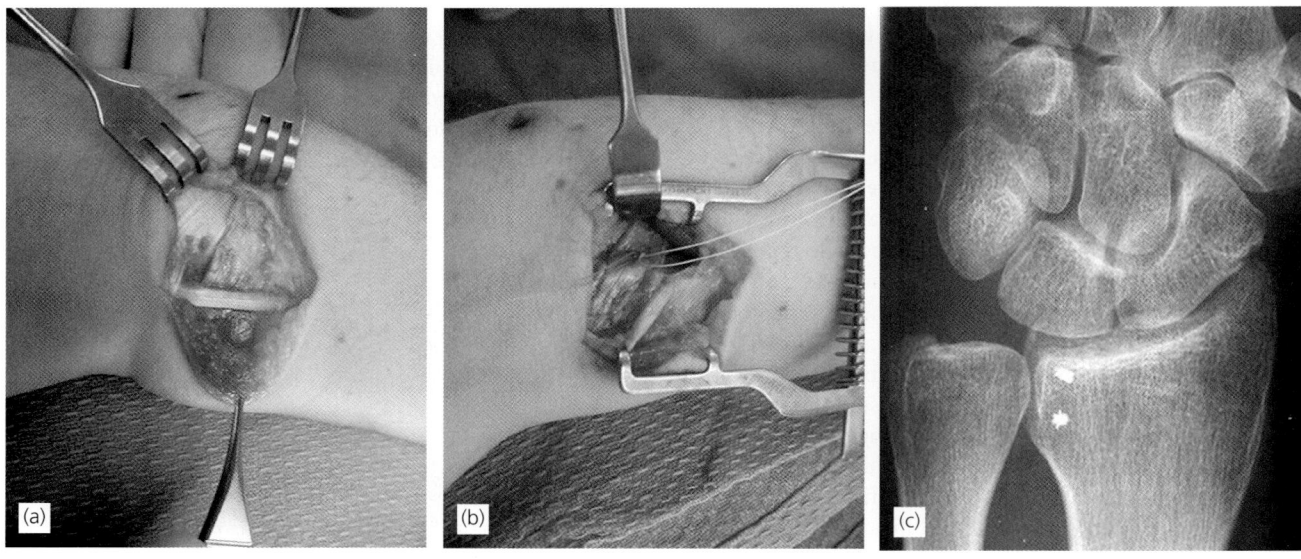

Figure 119.7 (a, b) Distal radius ulnar joint stabilization using extensor retinaculum. Half of the ulna-based extensor retinaculum is harvested. The extensor retinaculum is passed below the extensor carpi ulnaris tendon and is tethered to the distal radius with suture anchors. (c) Postoperative radiograph.

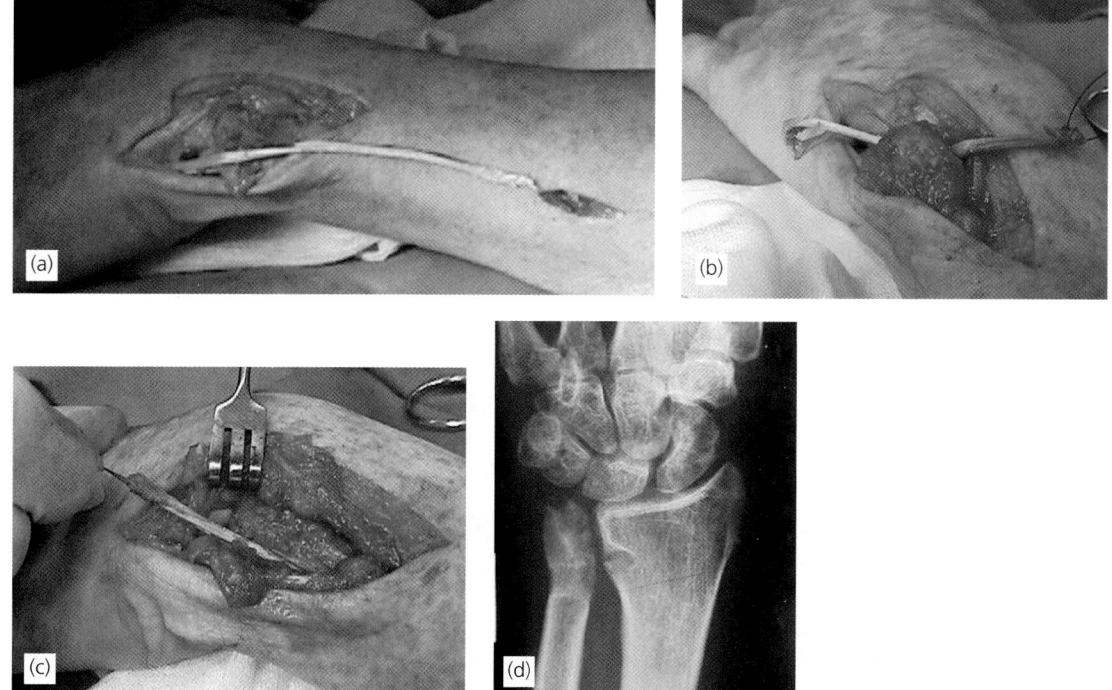

Figure 119.8 Use of extensor carpi ulnaris tendon graft to treat severe dorsal distal radioulnar instability. (a) Harvest half of the extensor carpi ulnaris tendon graft; (b) loop through the base of the ulnar sigmoid notch; (c) zig-zag through the radius and ulna; (d) postoperative radiograph.

CHRONIC DRUJ INJURY WITH OSTEOARTHRITIS

DRUJ reconstruction is contraindicated in the presence of DRUJ osteoarthritis. Various procedures have been used to treat DRUJ osteoarthritis. The classical Darrach procedure involves excision of the distal ulna with preservation of the periosteal sleeve and the ulnar styloid. Bowers[32] introduced the hemiresection interpositional technique (HIT), which involves hemiresection of the ulna at the sigmoid notch followed by soft-tissue interposition using a tendon graft (Fig. 119.8a). This preserves the ulnar attachments of the TFCC ligaments compared with the Darrach procedure.[32] Sauve and Kapandji[33] in 1936 introduced fusion of the distal radius and ulna, creating an ulnar pseudoarthrosis proximal to the fusion. The fusion is maintained by screws and the ulnar gap is interposed with the pronator quadratus, preventing regrowth or fusion of the pseudoarthrosis (Fig. 119.9b,c). Implant arthroplasty of the distal ulna combined with adequate soft-tissue repair has been performed to improve pain and strength of the wrist. However, this method is still unpopular and may need greater clinical assessment to determine long-term success.[34]

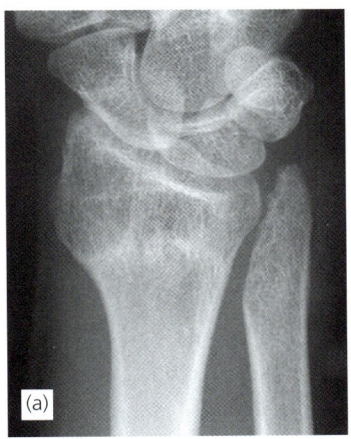
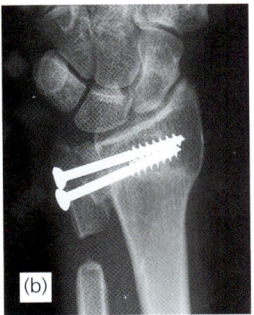
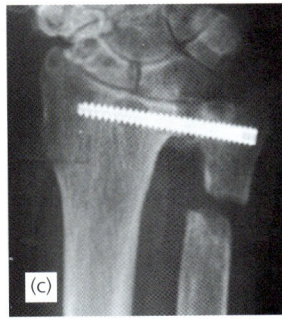

Figure 119.9 Various methods of treating distal radioulnar osteoarthritis. (a) Bowers hemiresection of the ulnar head; (b) Sauve-Kapandji procedure (using AO screws); (c) Sauve-Kapandji procedure (using mini Acutrack screw).

KEY LEARNING POINTS

- The bony structures of the distal radial ulnar joint (DRUJ) provide little inherent stability for the joint.
- DRUJ instability may be from trauma, inflammatory causes or developmental lax ligaments.
- Triangular fibrocartilaginous complex (TFCC) injury is best treated acutely when reduction of the DRUJ joint is easy.
- DRUJ instability may be dynamic or static.
- TFCC instability is classed as either trauma, inflammatory or developmental.
- Diagnosis of a DRUJ disorder and injury to specific structures of the TFCC is difficult.
- Chronic DRUJ dysfunction is commonly seen in malunited distal radius fractures.
- Wrist arthroscopy is the gold standard in evaluation and treatment of DRUJ instability.
- Late dislocation (after 6 weeks) is difficult to reduce.
- Managing chronic DRUJ instability is difficult and involves some sort of reconstruction.
- DRUJ reconstruction is contraindicated in the presence of osteoarthritis.
- The Darrach procedure involves excision of the distal ulna with preservation of the periosteal sleeve.

REFERENCES

- ● = Key primary paper
- ◆ = Major review article

◆1. Palmer AK. The distal radioulnar joint. *Orthopedic Clinics of North America* 1984;**15**:321–35.
◆2. GrahamTJ, Fischer TJ, Hotchkiss RN, Kleinman WB. Disorders of the forearm axis. *Hand Clinics* 1998;**14**:305–6.
●3. Tolat AR, Stanley JK, Trail IA. A cadaveric study of the anatomy and stability of the distal radioulnar joint in the coronal and transverse planes. *Journal of Hand Surgery (British)* 1996;**21**:587–94.
◆4. Garcis-Elias M. Soft tissue anatomy and relationships about the distal ulna. *Hand Clinics* 1998;**14**:165–76.
●5. Palmer AK, Werner FW. The triangular fibrocartilage complex of the wrist-anatomy and function. *Journal of Hand Surgery (American)* 1981;**6**:153–62.
●6. Wiesner L, Rumelhart C, Pham E, Comtet JJ. Experimentally induced ulno-carpal instability. A study on 13 cadaver wrists. *Journal of Hand Surgery (British)* 1996;**21**:24–9.
◆7. af Ekenstam F, Hagert CG. Anatomical studies on the geometry and stability of the distal radio-ulnar joint. *Scandinavian Journal of Plastic Reconstructive Surgery* 1985;**19**:17–25.

8. Thiru RG, Ferlic DC, Clayton ML, McClure DC. Arterial anatomy of the triangular fibrocartilage of the wrist and its surgical significance. *Journal of Hand Surgery (American)* 1986;**11**:258-63.
9. Chidgey LK, Dell PC, Bittar ES, Spanier SS. Histologic anatomy of the triangular fibrocartilage. *Journal of Hand Surgery (American)* 1991;**16**:1084-100.
10. Bednar MS, Arnoczky SP, Weiland AJ. The microvasculature of the triangular fibrocartilage complex: Its clinical significance. *Journal of Hand Surgery (American)* 1991;**16**:1101-5.
11. Goldber HD, Young JW, Reiner BI, et al. Double injuries of the forearm: a common occurrence. *Radiology* 1992;**185**:223-7.
◆12. Mino DE, Palmer AK, Levinsohn EM. Radiography and computerized tomography in the diagnosis of incongruity of the distal radio-ulnar joint: A prospective study. *Journal of Bone and Joint Surgery (American)* 1985;**67**:247-52.
13. Metz VM, Mann FA, Gilula LA. Three-compartment wrist arthrography: correlation of pain site with location of the uni- and bidirectional communications. *AJR American Journal of Roentgenology* 1993;**160**:819-22.
●14. Herbert TJ, Faithfull RG, McCann DJ, Ireland J. Bilateral arthrography of the wrist. *Journal of Hand Surgery (British)* 1990;**15**:233-5.
●15. Kirschenbaum D, Sieler S, Solonick D, et al. Arthrography of the wrist: assessment of the integrity of the ligaments in young asymptomatic adults. *Journal of Bone and Joint Surgery (American)* 1995;**77**:1207-9.
●16. Potter HG, Asnis Ernberg L, Weiland AJ, et al. The utility of high-resolution magnetic resonance imaging in the evaluation of the triangular fibrocartilage complex of the wrist. *Journal of Bone and Joint Surgery (American)* 1997;**79**:1675-84.
17. Hermansdorfer JD, Kleinman WB. Management of chronic peripheral tears of the triangular fibrocartilage complex. *Journal of Hand Surgery (American)* 1991;**16**:340-6.
●18. Cooney WP. Evaluation of chronic wrist pain by arthrography, arthroscopy, and arthrotomy. *Journal of Hand Surgery (American)* 1993;**18**:815-22.
19. Adams BD. Effects of radial deformity on distal radioulnar joint mechanics. *Journal of Hand Surgery (American)* 1993;**18**:492-8.
●20. Melone CP Jr, Nathan R. Traumatic disruption of the triangular fibrocartilage complex: pathoanatomy. *Clinical Orthopaedics and Related Research* 1992;**275**:65-73.
●21. Zachee B, De Smet L, Gabry G. Arthroscopic suturing of TFCC lesions. *Arthroscopy* 1993;**9**:242-3.
●22. Bohringer G, Schadel-Hopfner M, Petersson J. A method of all inside arthroscopic repair of palmer IB triangular fibrocartilage tears. *Arthroscopy* 2002;**18**:211-13.
23. Friedman SL, Palmer AK. The ulnar impaction syndrome. *Hand Clinics* 1991;**7**:295-310.
●24. Hauck RM, Skahen J 3rd, Palmer AK. Classification and treatment of ulnar styloid nonunion. *Journal of Hand Surgery (American)* 1996;**21**:418-22.
25. Lichtman DM, Alexander AH. *The Wrist and Its Disorder*. Philadelphia, PA: Saunders, 1997.
●26. Hui FC, Linscheid RL. Ulnotriquetral augmentation tenodesis: a reconstructive procedure for dorsal subluxation of the distal radioulnar joint. *Journal of Hand Surgery (American)* 1982;**7**:230-6.
◆27. Boyes JH. Surgical repair of joints. In: Bunnell S (ed.) *Bunnell's Surgery of the Hand*. Philadelphia, PA: Lippincott, 1970:294-313.
●28. Adams BD, Berger RA. An anatomic reconstruction of the distal radioulnar ligaments for posttraumatic distal radioulnar joint instability. *Journal of Hand Surgery (American)* 2002;**27**:243-51.
●29. Johnston Jones K, Sanders WE. Posttraumatic radioulnar instability: treatment by anatomic reconstruction of the volar and radioulnar ligaments. *Orthopedic Transactions* 1995-1996;**19**:832.
30. Scheker LR, Belliappa PP, Acosta R, German DS. Reconstruction of the dorsal ligament of the triangular fibrocartilage complex. *Journal of Hand Surgery (British)* 1994;**19**:3108.
●31. Gupta RK, Singh H, Sandhu VP. Stabilisation of the distal radioulnar joint with a double-breasted slip of extensor retinaculum. *Journal of Bone and Joint Surgery (British)* 2008;**90**:200-2.
●32. Bowers WH. Distal radioulnar joint arthroplasty: the hemiresection-interposition technique. *Journal of Hand Surgery (American)* 1985;**10**:169-78.
33. Sauve L, Kapandji M. Nouvelle technique de traitement chirurgical des luxations recidivantes isolées de l'extremité inferièure du cubitus. *Journal de Chirurgie* 1936;**47**:589.
●34. Willis AA, Berger RA, Cooney WP. Arthroplasty of the distal radioulnar joint using a new ulnar head endoprosthesis: preliminary report. *Journal of Hand Surgery (American)* 2007;**32**:177-89.

120

Hand tumours

GRAHAM CHEUNG, GILLIAN L CRIBB

| Introduction | 1373 | Bone lesions | 1377 |
| Soft-tissue lesions | 1374 | References | 1380 |

NATIONAL BOARD STANDARDS

- Know the commonest hand tumours and how to manage them
- Be able to formulate a sound differential diagnosis when presented with a mass in the hand
- Know the presentation and management of enchondrome

INTRODUCTION

A broad spectrum of benign and malignant tumours and tumour-like features can arise from the hand. Thankfully, the majority of these will be benign,[1] of which ganglions, epidermoid cysts, giant cell tumours of tendon sheath and the nodules of Dupuytren will constitute the majority.[2,3] As in other parts of the musculoskeletal system, the principles of diagnosis and treatment remain the same, that is timely assessment by a multidisciplinary team, with a musculoskeletal radiologist and a pathologist (Fig. 120.1). Before definitive treatment, the surgeon should be confident of the diagnosis. In certain cases, it may be appropriate to rely on the combination of clinical picture and radiological findings, if the imaging has been reviewed by an experienced musculoskeletal radiologist. If a tissue diagnosis is required, a Trucut needle biopsy or open biopsy may be performed (rather than fine needle aspiration for cytology). In some cases, such as in the distal finger, where amputation is the only option if a malignancy is diagnosed, an excision biopsy may be appropriate. The biopsy should be performed by the surgeon performing the definitive surgery, along sound oncological principles, which are covered in chapter 79.

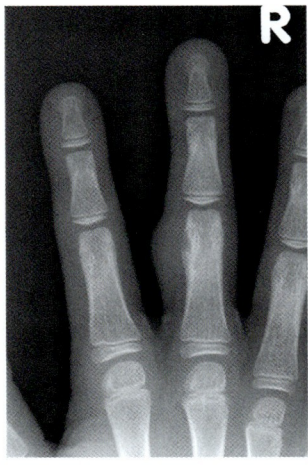

Figure 120.1 Staphylococcal osteomyelitis needs to be differentiated from tumour.

SOFT-TISSUE LESIONS

Benign

GANGLION

Ganglia are the most common soft-tissue mass occurring in the hand and wrist. Although the exact aetiology is unknown, they are thought to arise due to mucoid degeneration of collagen. They are not true cysts as they lack an epithelial lining, but instead have a few fibroblasts and mesenchymal cells in the collagen fibres. They contain a clear jelly-like fluid of glucosamine, globulin and hyaluronic acid.[4] They are commoner in women than in men. Dorsal wrist ganglions account for 70% of all ganglions, and usually arise from the scapholunate joint; whereas volar ganglions account for approximately 20% and tend to arise either from the radioscaphoid or scaphotrapezial joint. They typically present as a smooth, firm mass, which is occasionally painful. Once sufficiently large, they will transilluminate. Occasionally volar ganglia can cause compression of the median or ulnar nerve depending on their location.

Most patients merely require reassurance that the lesion is benign. Other treatments include injections with and without steroids or hyaluronidase, with success rates quoted between 15% and 89%. Varley et al.[5] found no difference with the addition of steroid compared with aspiration alone, with a success rate of 33%. Paul and Sochart[6] found the addition of hyaluronidase to steroid aspiration improved results from 57% to 89%. Such techniques should be avoided in the case of volar radiocarpal ganglia, because of the risk of injury to the radial artery. Most surgeons advocate leaving the capsule open after resection of the origin of the ganglion.

A mucoid cyst is usually associated with degeneration of a joint, most commonly the distal interphalangeal (DIP) joint, although the presence of an osteophyte may not always be appreciable on plain radiographs. Usually these can be treated conservatively (Fig. 120.2). Steroid injection should be avoided as this will result in thinning of the overlying skin. Should excision be undertaken, any osteophytes should be removed. Care should be taken to avoid injury to the germinal matrix of the nail or the extensor tendon. Often local flaps or full-thickness skin graft are required for coverage. Should significant degenerate changes be present an arthrodesis will reduce further the risk of recurrence (see chapter 117).

EPIDERMAL INCLUSION CYST

Epidermal inclusion cysts result from deposition of keratin-producing cells into the soft tissues from penetrating trauma. They tend to be slow growing, firm, painless masses on tactile surfaces of the digit. They can occasionally extend to the bone, mimicking a neoplastic infective lesion of the bone. Treatment can be merely symptomatic or by marginal excision, or with curettage and grafting of lesions affecting the bone. Recurrence is uncommon.[7]

FIBROMATOSIS

Dupuytren's disease is a superficial palmar fibromatosis affecting the palmar fascia of the hand. See chapter 116 for more details. The diagnosis may not be evident on initial presentation with a nodule. The presence of persistent, especially night-time, pain particularly should alert surgeons to the rare fibrosarcoma.[8]

GOUT AND PSEUDOGOUT

Gout is caused by the deposition of monosodium urate crystals in the synovial and tenosynovial tissues. Pseudogout is characterized by calcium pyrophosphate deposition.

ANEURYSMAL LESIONS

True aneurysms of the palmar arch or digital vessels are caused by weakening of the vessel wall from blunt trauma. This most commonly occurs in manual labourers who use their hypothenar pad as a hammer, causing injury to the ulnar artery.[9] False aneurysms develop as a consequence of penetrating injury. A haematoma forms at the site of the injury, which organizes and recanalizes and forms an outer wall for the vessel. Both types usually present as a painless, but not always, pulsatile mass. Local symptoms from its expanding mass effect may also occur.

Treatment is the same for true and false aneurysms. Because the natural history is to progressively increase in size, with possible thrombosis and emboli, resection is recommended. The decision on whether to ligate, repair or reconstruct the artery with vein graft depends on the adequacy of the collateral circulation and the size of the resultant defect.[10]

GIANT CELL TUMOUR OF THE TENDON SHEATH

A giant cell tumour of the tendon sheath (fibrous xanthoma of synovium or localized pigmented villonodular synovitis) is the second most common tumour of the hand.[11] They present as a firm, slow-growing, non-tender mass over the flexor surface of the digit. They do not always arise from

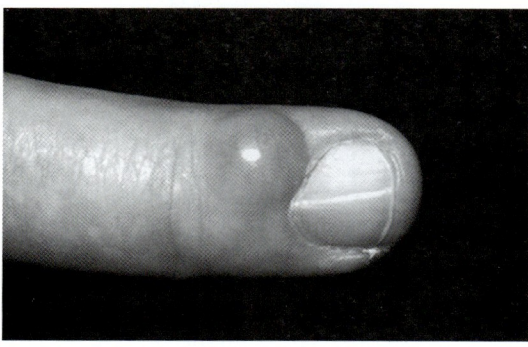

Figure 120.2 Mucous cyst with ridging of the nail.

the tendon sheath, but may also arise from the synovium. Microscopically the lesion contains multinucleated giant cells, polygonal mononuclear cells and histiocytes (which may contain abundant haemosiderin or lipid). Pigmented villonodular synovitis can also occur as a diffuse form and a localized form, but the diffuse form is much less common in the hand and has a higher rate of recurrence. With time, they can erode cortical bone and cause tendon damage. Treatment is by careful, meticulous excision. Although a benign condition, there is a high recurrence rate of up to 48% quoted.[12] This has led to some authors advocating the use of radiotherapy in the presence of a high risk of recurrence, in those who had either mitotic figures or possible incomplete excision.[13] Radiotherapy in the hand can lead to poor function and is therefore difficult to recommend in a benign condition.

LIPOMA

Lipomas are well-circumscribed, mobile masses of mature fat cells, which can grow to a large size and still remain asymptomatic.[10] On MRI they are well-circumscribed, homogeneous lesions, with a signal similar to the surrounding fat. When lesions of greater than 5 cm are present, they should be considered malignant until proven otherwise.[14] Marginal excision is the procedure of choice for both lipomas and well-differentiated lipoma-like liposarcomas. However, if imaging or biopsy shows a more aggressive lesion, a more radical approach should be undertaken (Fig. 120.3).[15]

HAEMANGIOMA

A haemangioma consists of a proliferating group of blood vessels which tends to appear within the first few years of life. They are true neoplasms and separated from vascular malformations.[16] They are commoner in female patients and on the volar aspect of the hand.[17] Typically, the tumour has a rapidly growing proliferative phase that may last up to a year, followed by an involutional phase, during which the tumour gradually fades and regresses. Approximately 50% will involute by 5 years and 70% by 7 years.[10] Those that occur within the first decade of life and are present for less than 1 year may be observed. Should they become symptomatic, they should be excised. Certain lesions may be suitable for embolization as the results of excision can be disappointing and unpredictable.

GLOMUS TUMOUR

A glomus body is an apparatus for regulating normal blood flow and temperature in the dermal reticular layer of the skin. Although glomus bodies are situated throughout the body, they are most common in the subungual areas, the lateral aspects of the digits and the palm. A glomus tumour is a benign tumour of modified perivascular smooth muscle cells. Clinically, the blue-red subungual

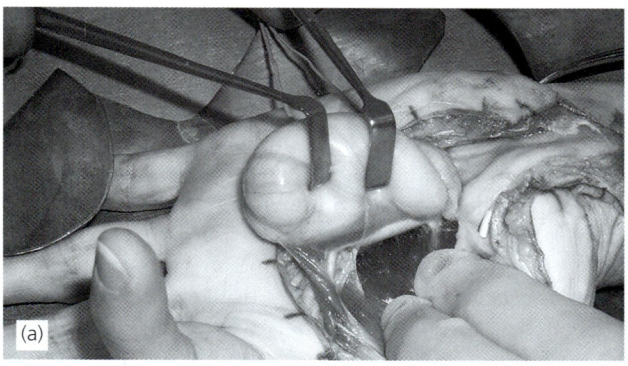

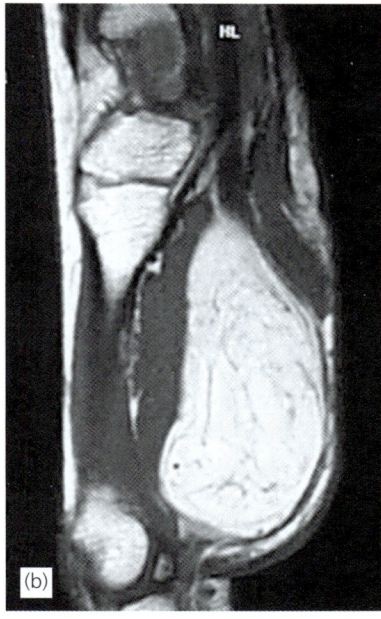

Figure 120.3 (a) Atypical lipoma. (b) MRI of atypical lipoma.

lesions cause pain, tenderness and cold intolerance out of proportion to the size of the lesion. Surgical excision is usually curative.

NEURILEMOMA AND NEUROFIBROMA

Neurilemoma and neurofibroma (and malignant peripheral nerve sheath tumours) originate from Schwann cells. Benign tumours tend to grow slowly with few symptoms, and neural dysfunction is not typically a feature. Nerve tumours make up only 5% of upper extremity tumours in adults and 2% in chidren. Inappropriate surgery can result in irreversible loss of function.[18]

The neurilemoma or schwannoma is a benign peripheral nerve sheath tumour and is the most common solitary tumour of the peripheral nerve. The tumour typically presents in the middle decades of life. Patients with neurofibromatosis type 1 (NF-1) may suffer from multiple schwannomas involving large peripheral nerve trunks. Patients with neurofibromatosis type 2 (NF-2) suffer from bilateral acoustic schwannomas.

Schwannomas are typically painless, slow-growing, isolated, firm, round soft-tissue masses less than 2.5 cm in diameter. In the upper limb, they are more common on the flexor owing to the presence of the larger nerves in the palm and volar forearm. The tumours may be found tethered in the longitudinal axis of the forearm and in the line of the peripheral nerve, although sometimes there is no nerve association.

At surgery, the tumour is found to arise eccentrically from the nerve sheath, often with a pedicle or a well-lobulated shape. The tumour is well encapsulated, preventing nerve fascicle, whereas tumours of small nerves may expand the entire nerve. Operative treatment may be indicated for symptomatic tumours, or to reach a diagnosis where there is a concern for potential malignancy. Surgery involves an excisional biopsy, with intraneural dissection enucleating the tumour and leaving the fascicular groups intact. Incisional biopsy should be performed if the tumour is not well encapsulated or adherent to the soft tissues.

Neurofibroma is another benign lesion of Schwann cell origin. Neurofibromas can be localized, dermal or plexiform. Clinical symptoms and signs are indistinguishable from schwannomas, although pathological features and surgical techniques differ.

NF-1 should be suspected in the presence of family history, axillary freckling, Lisch nodules, café-au-lait spots, optic gliomas, orthopaedic manifestations and neurofibroma (FALCON mnemonic). Dermal neurofibromas originate from small nerves in the skin and infiltrate the dermis and subcutaneous plaque-like swellings. Plexiform neurofibromas form palpable masses of thickened tortuous tissue along the course of small and large nerves.

Surgical exploration of the localized or plexiform neurofibroma reveals a characteristic incorporation of fascicles within the lesion. Unlike the eccentric schwannomas, neurofibromas are central, less well encapsulated, but not adherent to the soft tissues.

Malignant change of neurofibromas is rare in the absence of NF-1, where it may be as high as 15%.[10] Again where malignancy is suspected, a diagnostic incisional biopsy should be performed. Complete excision of neurofibromas requires excision of the affected part of the nerve and either direct approximation or cable grafting.[18]

SYNOVIAL CHONDROMATOSIS

Synovial chondromatosis infrequently occurs in the tendon sheaths and small joints of the hand. The tumour arises from cartilaginous metaplasia of synovial tissue, giving rise to mature, lobulated masses of hyaline cartilage. Clinically patients present with pain, swelling and reduced range of motion. Radiologically, lesions may have calcification. MRI may also be useful, as the hyaline cartilage with its high water content will be very bright on T_2 sequences. Treatment involves excision, which can be arthroscopic when within the joint and open when extra-articular.

Malignant

SKIN CANCERS

Suspicious skin lesions should be under the care of a multidisciplinary team headed by a dermatologist.

MALIGNANT MELANOMA

Melanomas are malignant lesions of the skin associated with sun exposure, which occur commonly in the upper limb. When faced with a pigmented lesion, one should remember the ABCDE of malignant melanoma:

- Asymmetry – is there asymmetry?
- Border – does it have an uneven border?
- Colour – is the colour uneven?
- Diameter – is it greater than 6 mm across?
- Evolution – has it changed in size, shape, pigmentation, symptoms?

Acral lentiginous melanoma is the least common subtype of malignant melanoma, accounting for 2–8% in the white population, but up to 72% in dark-skinned individuals, in whom the diagnosis may be delayed. Acral lentiginous melanoma occurs on the palms, on the soles or beneath the nail. A low index of suspicion should be maintained even in the presence of a history of trauma.

Suspicious pigmented lesions should be assessed by way of full-thickness biopsy to allow assessment of the Breslow thickness. As melanomas typically spread via the lymphatics, upper limb lesions should be accompanied by examination of the epitrochlear, axillary and supraclavicular lymph nodes.

For lesions greater than 2 mm an excisional margin of greater than 3 cm is recommended.[19] In the hand, adequate excision may require ray amputation to obtain clearance.

SQUAMOUS CELL CARCINOMA

Squamous cell carcinoma is the commonest malignant skin lesion of the hand, making up 74% of all malignant or potentially malignant skin lesions.[20] They most commonly affect the skin on the dorsum of the hand, in pale-skinned, blue-eyed men with significant sun exposure. Chronic infection, ulcers, sinuses and the presence of premalignant conditions such as actinic keratosis also predispose to squamous cell carcinomas. The macroscopic appearance can range from dry, scaly erythematous lesions to large fungating masses.

The mainstay of treatment is surgical excision. Brodland and Zitelli[21] recommend a 6 mm margin for high-risk lesions. High risk was defined as size of 2 cm or larger, histological grade 2 or higher, invasion of the subcutaneous tissue and location in high-risk areas (which included the hand). The use of radiation is important in the medically unfit, with cure rates in the region of 90%.[22] Radiation therapy as a primary treatment lacks margin control, has a prolonged course of treatment and increases the risk of future squamous cell carcinomas within the radiation field. It may be useful though as adjuvant therapy or for the treatment of regional lymph nodes.[23] Topical treatments, such as 5-fluorouracil, are indicated in the treatment of premalignant lesions only.

SOFT-TISSUE SARCOMAS

Soft-tissue sarcomas are rare, and are typically misdiagnosed so that treatment is delayed. Lesions that are deep to the fascia, greater than 5 cm, rapidly enlarging and are painful should arouse suspicion. The most common soft-tissue sarcomas of the upper extremity are epithelioid sarcoma, clear cell sarcoma, synovial cell sarcoma and malignant fibrous histiocytoma (MFH).[24,25]

Epithelioid sarcoma

The most common presentation for this tumour is a slow-growing firm nodule, typically affecting the digits, the palm of the hand or the volar forearm in the young patient between 14 and 50 years old (mean 31 years).[26] Lesions may ultimately ulcerate and drain, leading to the misdiagnosis of infection, or be mistaken for palmar fibromas or Dupuytren's disease. MRI may reveal that the tumour involvement is much greater than would otherwise have been expected.[25]

Clear cell sarcoma

Clear cell sarcoma is often referred to as malignant melanoma of soft parts. Clear cell sarcoma should be considered when suspicious masses are found close to tendons or aponeurotic junctions. Typically they are slow growing with high rates of local and lymph node recurrence following treatment. They are so called as histologically the tumour has round cells with clear cytoplasm.

Synovial cell sarcoma

Synovial cell sarcoma presents as slow-growing painless masses, arising in close proximity to bursas and joints, in patients aged 15–40 years old. (See chapter 82 for the histology)

Malignant fibrous histiocytoma

Although regarded by some investigators as the most common sarcoma of the upper limb, MFH is rarely reported in the hand. These tumours are often painless, only being noticed after trauma. Most patients will be in their sixth to eighth decade. The histology is classically of spindle-shaped fibroblasts in a storiform pattern.[25] Unlike epithelioid and synovial sarcoma, lymphatic spread is uncommon.

LIPOSARCOMA

Should be treated depending on their grade; see chapter 82.

TREATMENT

Soft-tissue sarcomas of the hand should be treated by wide local excision. An inadequate margin of excision results in a 12 times greater risk of local recurrence than those in whom a wide margin of excision has been achieved. To achieve a wide local excision, either plastic surgical reconstruction or amputation may be required. There is no role for radiotherapy in decreasing the risk of local recurrence when there was an inadequate margin of excision. Patients with an inadequate margin of excision have a much higher risk of both local recurrence and metastasis than those with wide margins.[24]

MALIGNANT PERIPHERAL NERVE SHEATH TUMOUR

Malignant peripheral nerve sheath tumours (MPNSTs) arise either *de novo* or from a malignant degeneration of a benign tumour, usually a plexiform neurofibroma. In general, MPNSTs arise in the fourth and fifth decades, except in NF-1 when they tend to arise a decade earlier. MPNSTs usually arise from large deep nerves, although a nerve is not always apparent. Superficial nerves, including digital nerves, may also be involved. Approximately 20% of all MPNSTs occur in the upper extremities.[25] In the upper limb, 3% of all malignant tumours are MPNSTs, of which half are associated with neurofibromatosis.[27]

BONE LESIONS

Benign

INTRA-OSSEOUS GANGLIA

Intra-osseous ganglia are the most common cystic bony lesions of the hand and wrist. They most commonly occur in the lunate. Histologically they are identical to the soft-tissue ganglia of the wrist. There may be a link between dorsal wrist ganglia and intra-osseous ganglia; with one MRI study showing that 47% of patients with a dorsal wrist ganglion also had an intra-osseous ganglion.[28] Many lesions will be asymptomatic incidental radiographic findings after trauma, whereas others will cause an aching discomfort. Radiographs may be normal, or reveal a sclerotic well-marginated lesion. In the absence of such changes, bone scanning and MRI may provide further clues to their presence.[29] The treatment of symptomatic lesions is by curettage and bone grafting.

ANEURYSMAL BONE CYSTS

Aneurysmal bone cysts (ABCs) can arise primarily or secondary to lesions such as a giant cell tumour or chondroblastoma. They are uncommon in the hand and represent approximately 5% of ABCs.[30] They present most commonly in the second decade of life as either a painful or painless expanding mass. Occasionally they present as a pathological fracture. Radiographs show a central, expansile, metaphyseal lesion that can extend into the epiphysis, and thins the cortex. Lesions in the hand may be purely lytic and lack the sclerotic margin, appearing more destructive, much like a giant cell tumour.[31] MRI is often useful in providing a definitive diagnosis if there are fluid–fluid levels. The treatment principles are the same as elsewhere for extended curettage. There are technical difficulties when using a high-speed burr or liquid nitrogen in the small bones of the hand. Amputation may be required in large destructive lesions, especially in the distal phalanx.

Cartilage lesions

Most cartilage lesions of bone are benign, of which enchondromas are the most common.

ENCHONDROMA

Enchondroma is the most common primary bone tumour of the hand (Fig. 120.4). It affects most commonly the proximal phalanx, the metacarpal and the middle phalanx in that order. Patients are often diagnosed in the second or third decade of life, either through an incidental finding in the asymptomatic patient after trauma, when radiographs are taken, or due to pain from expansion of the lesion, or fracture. The radiographs characteristically have well-defined margins with a central cloudy cartilage matrix with punctuate calcification and endosteal scalloping. Malignant potential for isolated enchondromas is low, but is elevated to 25% if the patient has Ollier's disease (Fig. 120.5) or to approaching 100% if the patient has Maffuci's syndrome.[32] Enchondromas form part of a spectrum, from atypical enchondromas to frank chondrosarcomas. Treatment of enchondromas can be via observation of asymptomatic lesions. Treatment of symptomatic lesions is usually with curettage with or without bone grafting, with samples from the lesion bone interface sent for histology to look for malignancy. Chondroid lesions are often downgraded by surgeons, as metastases are extremely rare. In those patients with a pathological fracture, it is usually best to treat the fracture conservatively and contain the lesion, thus avoiding internal fixation and curettage and spreading lesional cells. Once the fracture has united, curettage can be considered to try to prevent further pathological fracture.

Although recurrence is uncommon, it may indicate malignancy. Should there be frank malignancy, the treatment is with wide local excision, which in the hand usually requires amputation. See chapter 81 for more detail.

OSTEOCHONDROMA

Osteochondroma (Fig. 120.6) is a benign bony prominence with a cartilage cap. Most are diagnosed in the second decade of life and are associated with similar lesions elsewhere in the body. If they are solitary, they are most likely to occur on the proximal phalanx. Symptoms are from either local soft-tissue impingement or fracture at the base of the stalk. Growth disturbances may also occur. The key radiographic feature is continuity between the lesion with the medulla of the underlying parent bone.[33] Treatment is with either reassurance and observation or excision. Osteochondromas can be differentiated from subungal exostoses, the latter being a posttraumatic event. The two conditions can be distinguished

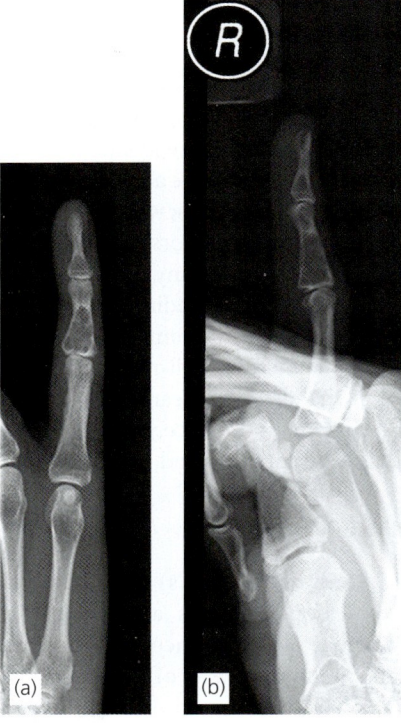

Figure 120.4 Enchondroma.

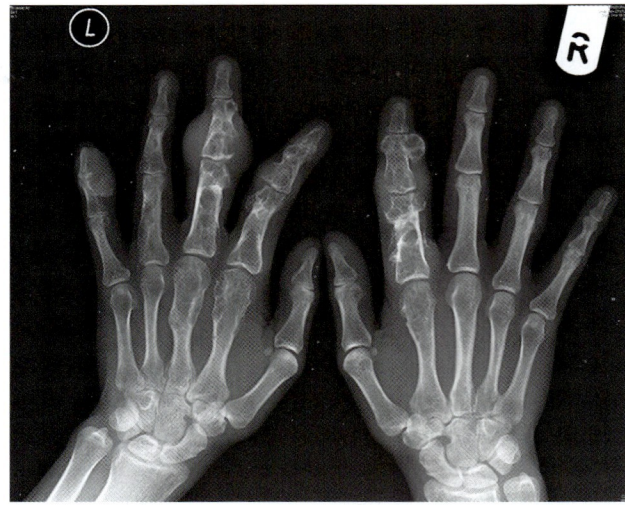

Figure 120.5 Ollier's disease.

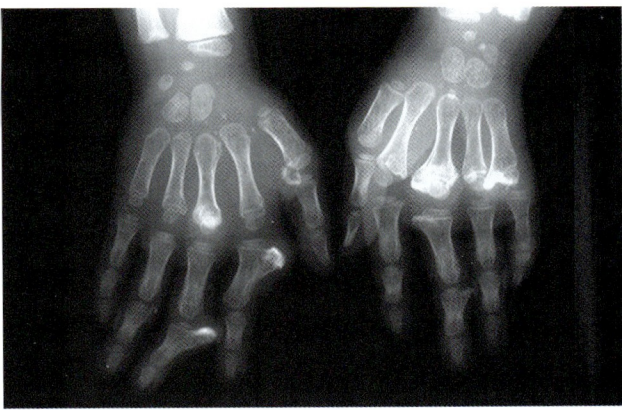

Figure 120.6 Osteochondromata in diaphyseal aclasia.

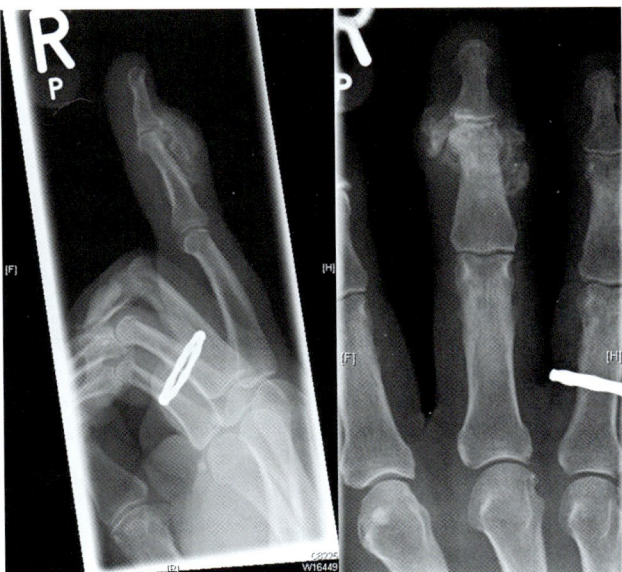

Figure 120.7 Exostosis.

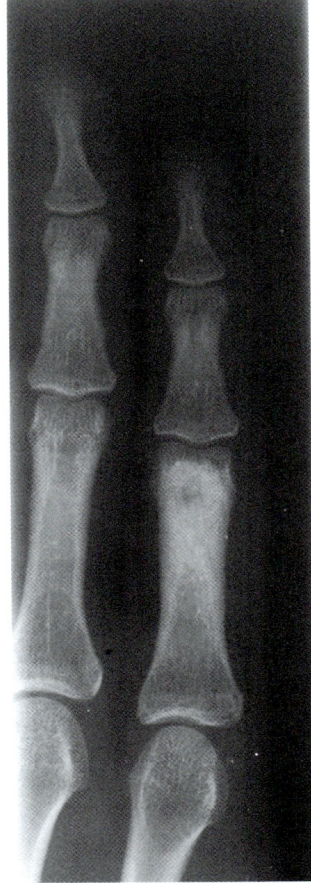

Figure 120.8 Proximal phalanx osteoid osteoma.

radiologically: the stalk of a true osteochondroma must be in continuity with the intramedullary cavity and a post-traumatic exostosis does not have such a connection (Fig. 120.7).

BONE-FORMING LESIONS

Osteoid osteoma

Osteoid osteoma (Fig. 120.8) is a relatively uncommon benign osteoblastic tumour. The hand and wrist are relatively infrequent sites to be affected, with 10% of all osteoid osteomas affecting the hand: 6% in the phalanges, 2% in the metacarpals and 2% in the carpal bones.[34] Patients are usually in their second to third decades and complain of gradually increasing pain that is worse at night and may be relieved by aspirin or non-steroidal anti-inflammatory drugs. Physical findings include swelling, point tenderness, heat and redness of the overlying skin and joint restriction, depending on the location of the lesion.[35] As with elsewhere in the body, radiofrequency ablation or curettage may be utilized. Radiofrequency ablation can be difficult, because of the lack of surrounding soft tissue to stabilize the needle, in which case curettage may be preferred.

Osteoblastomas

Osteoblastomas are similar in presentation and histologically to osteoid osteomas, but tend to be greater than 2 cm in diameter. Treatment is dependent on the location of the lesion, but recurrence is lowest with en bloc excision. Simple curettage is associated with less morbidity but a higher rate of recurrence.[36]

Malignant

OSTEOSARCOMA

Osteosarcoma is a primary malignant tumour of mesenchymal origin in which the proliferating cellular stroma directly produces an immature neoplastic osteoid. Osteosarcoma is very rare in the hand. Metacarpals and phalanges are more commonly involved than the carpus. The hand is the primary site in approximately 0.18% of cases. Patients tend to present with pain, swelling and pathological fractures.[36] The clinical and radiological features and treatment principles are the same as for other places within the body.

EWING'S SARCOMA

Ewing's sarcoma may occur in virtually any bone in the body, but is most common in the long bones and the pelvis. It occurs in the shoulder girdle in 5–10% of cases and only rarely in the hand. Case reports would suggest that the metacarpal is the most common location in the hand.[36] These neoplasms occur primarily in the second decade of life, with a male preponderance. The treatment of Ewing's sarcoma is difficult to define, as they occur so rarely in the hand. Based on current evidence, wide local resection and chemotherapy are the mainstay of treatment.

METASTATIC DISEASE

Metastatic tumours of the hand and wrist are rare, representing 0.1% of all skeletal metastases. Most hand metastases involve bone, although there are reports of soft-tissue involvement. The most common primary sites for metastases to the hand are lung (40%), kidney (13%), breast (10%), colon (5%) and oesophagus (3%). All of the bones of the hand and wrist can be involved in metastatic disease. The distal phalanges are most commonly affected, followed by the proximal and middle phalanges, metacarpals and the carpus. That the hand is at the distal-most portion of the upper extremity and the bones of the carpus and hand do not contain a significant amount of red marrow accounts for the low frequency of metastatic disease compared with the axial skeleton. The biomechanical mediators of the metastatic process (chemokines, chemotactic factors and parathyroid hormone-related protein) are found predominantly in bone and synovial tissue (not cartilage), and may account for the high frequency of bone involvement and sparing of soft tissues.[37]

The presence of metastases in the hand is a poor prognostic indicator with a median survival of approximately 5 months.[38] Although renal cell carcinoma with solitary metastasis and nephrectomy can have excellent survival,[39] for most lesions the aim of treatment is symptomatic pain relief and preservation of function. This should include close liaison with medical oncologists for an understanding of the possible prognosis. Treatment options include conservative measures, chemotherapy, radiotherapy and surgery. Radiotherapy is not widely used as post-radiation scarring may result in scarring and fibrosis, which can lead to scarring of the hand.[37] Surgery can be in the form of amputation or curettage with cementation. Conservative measures of splintage and analgesia should be considered in those with milder symptoms, or those with a very short expected survival.

KEY LEARNING POINTS

- A broad spectrum of benign and malignant tumours and tumour-like features can arise from the hand.
- Ganglia are the most common soft-tissue mass occurring in the hand and wrist.
- True aneurysms of the palmar arch or digital vessels are caused by weakening of the vessel wall from blunt trauma.
- Giant cell tumour of the tendon sheath is the second most common tumour of the hand.
- Glomus tumour presents as a blue-red subungual lesion and causes pain, tenderness and cold intolerance out of proportion to the size of the lesion.
- Melanomas are malignant lesions of the skin associated with sun exposure, which occur commonly in the upper limb.
- Synovial chondromatosis infrequently occurs in the tendon sheaths and small joints of the hand.
- Squamous cell carcinoma is the commonest malignant skin lesion of the hand.
- Soft-tissue sarcomas are rare.
- Intra-osseous ganglia are the most common cystic bony lesions of the hand and wrist.
- Enchondroma is the most common cartilage primary bone tumour of the hand.
- Ewing's sarcoma may occur in virtually any bone in the body, but is most common in the long bones and the pelvis.
- Metastatic tumours of the hand and wrist are rare, representing 0.1% of all skeletal metastases.

REFERENCES

1. Enneking WF. *Musculoskeletal Tumour Surgery*. New York, NY: Churchill Livingstone, 1983:469–82.
2. Murray PM. Soft tissue neoplasms: benign and malignant. In: Trumble T (ed.) *Hand Surgery*, update 3. Rosemont, IL: American Society for Surgery of the Hand, 2003:569–81.
3. Enneking WF, Spanier SS, Goodman MA. A system for the surgical staging of musculoskeletal sarcoma. *Clinical Orthopaedics and Related Research* 2003;**415**:4–18.
4. Soren A. Pathogenesis and treatment of ganglion. *Clinical Orthopaedics and Related Research* 1966;**48**:173–9.
5. Varley GW, Needoff M, Davis TR, Clay NR. Conservative management of wrist ganglia. Aspiration versus steroid infiltration. *Journal of Hand Surgery (British)* 1997;**22**:636–7.
6. Paul AS, Sochart DH. Improving the results of ganglion aspiration by the use of hyaluronidase. *Journal of Hand Surgery (British)* 1997;**22**:219–21.

7. Athanasian EA. Bone and soft tissue tumours. In: Wolfe SW, Hotchkiss RN, Pederson WC, Kozin SH (eds) *Green's Operative Hand Surgery*, 6th edn. Philadelphia, PA: Elsevier, 2011:2141-95.
8. Wilbrand S, Ekbom A, Gerdin B. Dupuytren's contracture and sarcoma. *Journal of Hand Surgery (British)* 2002;**27**:50-2.
9. Conn J Jr, Bergan JJ, Bell JL. Hypothenar hammer syndrome: posttraumatic digital ischemia. *Surgery* 1970;**68**:1122-8.
10. Plate A, Lee SJ, Steiner G, Posner M. Tumorlike lesions and benign tumors of the hand and wrist. *Journal of the American Academy of Orthopedic Surgeons* 2003;**11**:129-41.
11. Jones FE, Soule EH, Coventry MB. Fibrous xanthoma of synovium (giant-cell tumor of tendon sheath, pigmented nodular synovitis). A study of one hundred and eighteen cases. *Journal of Bone and Joint Surgery (American)* 1969;**51**:76-86.
12. Granowitz SP, D'Antonio J, Mankin HL. The pathogenesis and long-term end results of pigmented villonodular synovitis. *Clinical Orthopaedics and Related Research* 1976;**114**:335-51.
13. Kotwal PP, Gupta V, Malhotra R. Giant-cell tumour of the tendon sheath. Is radiotherapy indicated to prevent recurrence after surgery? *Journal of Bone and Joint Surgery (British)* 2000;**82**:571-3.
14. Johnson CJ, Pynsent PB, Grimer RJ. Clinical features of soft tissue sarcomas. *Annals of the Royal College of Surgeons of England* 2001;**83**:203-5.
15. Cribb GL, Cool WP, Ford DJ, Mangham DC. Giant lipomatous tumours of the hand and forearm. *Journal of Hand Surgery (British)* 2005;**30**:509-12.
16. Mulliken JB, Glowacki J. Hemangiomas and vascular malformations in infants and children: a classification based on endothelial characteristics. *Plastic and Reconstructive Surgery* 1982;**69**:412-22.
17. Palmieri TJ. Subcutaneous hemangiomas of the hand. *Journal of Hand Surgery (American)* 1983;**8**:201-4.
18. Forthman CL, Balazr PE. Nerve tumours of the hand and upper extremity. *Hand Clinics* 2004;**20**:233-42.
19. Thomas JM, Newton-Bishop J, A'Hern R, et al; United Kingdom Melanoma Study Group; British Association of Plastic Surgeons; Scottish Cancer Therapy Network. Excision margins in high-risk malignant melanoma. *New England Journal of Medicine* 2004;19;**35**:757-66.
20. Chakrabarti I, Watson JD, Dorrance H. Skin tumours of the hand. A 10-year review. *Journal of Hand Surgery (British)* 1993;**18**:484-6.
21. Brodland DG, Zitelli JA. Surgical margins for excision of primary cutaneous squamous cell carcinoma. *Journal of the American Academy of Dermatology* 1992;**27**(2 Pt 1):241-8.
22. Rowe DE, Carroll RJ, Day CL Jr. Prognostic factors for local recurrence, metastasis, and survival rates in squamous cell carcinoma of the skin, ear, and lip. Implications for treatment modality selection. *Journal of the American Academy of Dermatologists* 1992;**26**:976-90.
23. Hepper DM, Hepper CT, Anadkat M. Treatment options for squamous cell carcinoma of the dorsal hand including Mohs micrographic surgery. *Journal of Hand Surgery (American)* 2009;**34**:1337-9.
24. Pradhan A, Cheung YC, Grimer RJ, et al. Soft-tissue sarcomas of the hand: oncological outcome and prognostic factors. *Journal of Bone and Joint Surgery (British)* 2008;**90**:209-14.
25. Murray PM. Soft tissue sarcoma of the upper extremity. *Hand Clinics* 2004;**20**:325-33.
26. Herr MJ, Harmsen WS, Amadio PC, Scully SP. Epithelioid sarcoma of the hand. *Clinical Orthopaedics and Related Research* 2005;**431**:193-200.
27. Wehbé MA, Mickelson MR. Malignant schwannoma in neurofibromatous elephantiasis of the upper extremity. *Clinical Orthopaedics and Related Research* 1982;**167**:164-7.
28. Van den Dungen S, Marchesi S, Ezzedine R, et al. Relationship between dorsal ganglion cysts of the wrist and intraosseous ganglion cysts of the carpal bones. *Acta Orthopaedica Belgica* 2005;**71**:535-9.
29. Magee TH, Rowedder AM, Degnan GG. Intraosseous ganglia of the wrist. *Radiology* 1995;**195**:517-20.
30. Frassica FJ, Amadio PC, Wold LE, Beabout JW. Aneurysmal bone cyst: clinicopathologic features and treatment of ten cases involving the hand. *Journal of Hand Surgery (American)* 1988;**13**:676-83.
31. Athanasian EA. Aneurysmal bone cyst and giant cell tumor of bone of the hand and distal radius. *Hand Clinics* 2004;**20**:269-81.
32. Schwartz HS, Zimmerman NB, Simon MA, et al. The malignant potential of enchondromatosis. *Journal of Bone and Joint Surgery (American)* 1987;**69**:269-74.
33. O'Connor ML, Bancroft LW. Benign and malignant cartilage tumours of the hand. *Hand Clinics* 2004;**20**:317-23.
34. Jackson RP, Reckling FW, Mants FA. Osteoid osteoma and osteoblastoma. Similar histologic lesions with different natural histories. *Clinical Orthopaedics and Related Research* 1977;**128**:303-13.
35. Marcuzzi A, Acciaro AL, Landi A. Osteoid osteoma of the hand and wrist. *Journal of Hand Surgery (British)* 2002;**27**:440-3.
36. Sfrzo CR, Scarborough MT, Wright TW. Bone-forming tumors of the upper extremity and Ewing's sarcoma. *Hand Clinics* 2004;**20**:303-15.
37. Hayden RJ, Sullivan LG, Jebson PJL. The hand in metastatic disease and acral manifestations of paraneoplastic syndromes. *Hand Clinics* 2004;**20**:335-43.
38. Amadio PC, Lombardi RM. Metastatic tumors of the hand. *Journal of Hand Surgery (American)* 1987;**12**:311-16.
39. Brodsky G, Garnick MG. Renal tumours in the adult patient. In: Tisher CC, Brenner BM (eds) *Renal Pathology with Clinical and Functional Correlations*. Philadelphia, PA: Lippincott, 1989:1540-67.

The elbow

ASHISH K SHARMA, KAMARUL KHALID, EDWARD T MAH

Introduction	1382	Olecranon bursitis	1388
Static stabilizing factors	1382	Lateral and medial epicondylitis	1389
Dynamic stabilizing factors	1383	Cubital tunnel syndrome	1397
Nerves around the elbow	1384	References	1409
Biomechanics of the elbow	1386		

NATIONAL BOARD STANDARDS

- Understand the anatomy and biomechanics of the elbow joint
- Learn common disorders of the elbow: including nerve compressions, olecranon bursitis, epicondylitis and cubital tunnel syndrome

INTRODUCTION

The elbow joint has a key role in the functions of the upper limb, such as feeding, washing and toilet care. Its hinge action and strong static collateral stability, combined with dexterity and versatility of the shoulder, hand and forearm, enable the hand to be put in almost any position on the body. The elbow is inherently a stable joint. Both static as well as dynamic factors contribute to its stability. Numerous biomechanical studies have contributed to our understanding of the elbow stabilizing factors and elbow dynamics.

STATIC STABILIZING FACTORS

The *static* stabilizing factors for the elbow joint are a combination of joint (bony) congruity and capsulo-ligamentous (soft-tissue) constraints.

Osteoarticular anatomy

The trochlear notch of the proximal ulna and its central ridge grips and articulates with the spool-shaped trochlea and its central groove for nearly 180°, giving the elbow joint a stable medial column. The radial head and the capitellum, as well as the proximal radioulnar joint contribute to the lateral column support for the elbow joint. During flexion of the elbow joint, the osseous stability is augmented when the coronoid process of the proximal ulna locks in the coronoid fossa of the distal humerus and the radial head lodges into the radial fossa of the distal humerus. During extension, the osseous stability is augmented when the tip of the olecranon lodges into the olecranon fossa of the distal humerus.

Capsulo-ligamentous units

The capsulo-ligamentous units around the elbow contribute to the soft-tissue stability of the elbow joint. The anterior and posterior joint capsule and the medial and lateral collateral ligament complexes are the static soft-tissue stabilizers of the elbow joint.

The *anterior capsule* is attached proximally to the articular margin of the distal humerus above the coronoid and radial fossae. Distally, it is attached to the margins of the coronoid process, extending laterally to attach to the annular ligament. The *posterior capsule* is attached proximally to the margins of the olecranon fossa, and distally to the margins of the greater sigmoid notch, extending laterally to attach to the annular ligament. The anterior capsule is the chief stabilizer of the elbow in extension, becoming taut to prevent hyperextension. The posterior capsule also becomes taut in flexion.

The collateral ligaments are thickenings of the joint capsule.

The *medial collateral ligament (MCL) complex* consists of three parts – the anterior bundle, the posterior bundle and the transverse ligament.[1] The anterior and posterior bundles of the MCL complex originate from the anteroinferior surface of the medial epicondyle. The anterior bundle inserts on the anteromedial aspect of the coronoid process and is the chief soft-tissue stabilizer to valgus stress. It has three bands – the anterior band, which is taut in extremes of joint positions, the intermediate band, which is taut in intermediate joint positions, and the posterior (isotonic) band, which is taut in full arc of joint movement. The posterior bundle of the MCL complex is a less discrete structure and inserts on the medial olecranon. It is taut in flexion of the elbow and contributes to valgus stability of the elbow in pronation. The transverse ligament consists of horizontally placed fibres from coronoid to the tip of the olecranon. It is often an ill-defined structure and does not contribute to joint stability as it is limited only to the ulna (Fig. 121.1).[2]

The *lateral collateral ligament (LCL) complex* consists of four components – the radial collateral ligament, the lateral ulnar collateral ligament (UCL), the annular ligament and the accessory collateral ligament. The annular ligament is attached to the anterior and posterior margins of the lesser sigmoid (radial) notch of the proximal ulna, the ligament itself encircling and supporting part of the head and neck of the radius. The accessory collateral ligament is attached to the annular ligament and the supinator crest of the ulna. The radial collateral ligament is attached to the lateral epicondyle proximally, and merges distally with annular ligament, contributing to stability of the radial head. The lateral UCL originates from the lateral epicondyle proximally, and inserts on the supinator crest of the proximal ulna, posterior to the attachment of the annular ligament.

The lateral UCL is one of the primary lateral stabilizers of the elbow and its insufficiency is the 'essential lesion' in posterolateral rotatory instability of the elbow,[3,4] although some studies suggest that both the lateral UCL and the radial collateral ligament have a key role in prevention of posterolateral rotatory instability of the elbow (Fig. 121.2).[5]

Some studies have stressed that the primary restraints to rotatory instability are the lateral UCL and the annular ligament, whereas the secondary restraints of the lateral aspect of the elbow are the extensor muscles with their fascial bands and the intermuscular septa.[6]

DYNAMIC STABILIZING FACTORS

The musculotendinous units which cross the elbow joint provide dynamic stability to the joint when they contract. The four groups of muscle which cross the elbow joint are the elbow flexors, elbow extensors, common forearm flexor–pronators and common forearm extensors. Muscle groups contract during strenuous activities and augment the static stability of the joint when failure strength of the collateral ligaments is less than the deforming forces. Biomechanical studies have shown that the flexor–pronator mass dynamically stabilizes the elbow against valgus torque. The flexor carpi ulnaris (FCU) is the primary stabilizer, and the flexor digitorum superficialis (FDS) is the secondary stabilizer. The pronator teres contributes least to dynamic stability against valgus torque.[7]

Thus, when considering injury prevention and rehabilitation in throwing athletes, emphasis should be given to optimizing the function of the FCU and FDS. Similarly, during surgery, the importance of reducing morbidity of the FCU and FDS has been emphasized, e.g. muscle splitting approach for MCL reconstruction.[8–10]

In summary, the primary static constraints for the elbow joint are the ulnohumeral articulation, the anterior

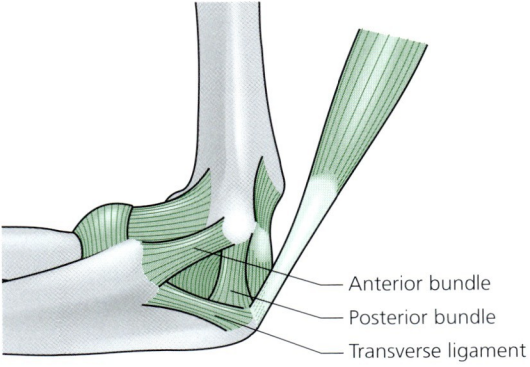

Figure 121.1 The medial collateral ligament.

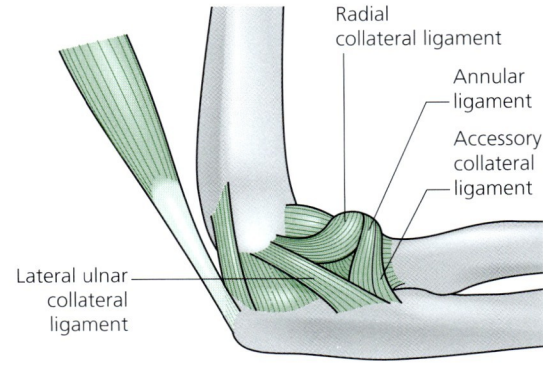

Figure 121.2 The lateral collateral ligament.

bundle of the MCL and the LCL complex. Secondary static constraints are the radiocapitellar articulation, common flexor tendon, common extensor tendon and the joint capsule. The dynamic stabilizers are the muscles that cross the elbow joint.[11]

NERVES AROUND THE ELBOW

Ulnar nerve (C7–8, T1)

This passes posteriorly through the medial intermuscular septum, 8 cm proximal to the medial epicondyle, and continues distally along the medial aspect of triceps. It enters the cubital tunnel posterior to the medial epicondyle. Upon exiting the tunnel, the ulnar nerve enters the forearm deep to the *arcade of Osborne*, a fibrous band between the two heads of the FCU.[12]

Ulnar nerve entrapment may be at variable levels in the elbow (Fig. 121.3).[13]

1. Proximal to the cubital tunnel, the ulnar nerve may be compressed under the so-called *arcade of Struthers*.[14–16] It is actually a 5.7 cm fibrous canal that begins 9.6 cm proximal to the medial epicondyle, through which the ulnar nerve travels from the anterior compartment to the posterior compartment in the arm. Its V-shaped proximal opening is formed by the medial intermuscular septum and the internal brachial ligament.[17] This is an important structure to be considered during anterior transposition of the ulnar nerve as it may kink the transposed nerve if not adequately released.[18] To date only three cases of high ulnar nerve entrapment proven by electrodiagnostic examination to be 7–10 cm proximal to the medial epicondyle have been reported.[19]
2. In the cubital tunnel. This is formed by the ulnar groove of the medial epicondyle and MCL (floor), and the cubital retinaculum (roof).[20] A shallow ulnar groove of the medial epicondyle, hypoplastic humeral trochlea or cubital retinaculum insufficiency may lead to recurrent ulnar nerve subluxation or dislocation during flexion in one-sixth of elbows.[20,21] Entrapment neuropathy of the ulnar nerve in the cubital tunnel with no known trauma is known as *cubital tunnel syndrome*.[22]
3. Distal to the cubital tunnel, where the ulnar nerve enters the forearm, deep to the arcade of Osborne, which is present in three out of four individuals. The arcade tightens in elbow flexion and can compress the nerve.

A more detailed description regarding ulnar nerve entrapment will be discussed later in this chapter.

Radial nerve (C6–8, T1)

This passes from the posterior compartment to the anterior compartment of the arm through the lateral intermuscular septum about 10 cm proximal to the lateral epicondyle. While coursing between the brachioradialis and the lateral half of brachialis in the anterior compartment, it supplies motor fibres to both. It enters the radial tunnel at the level of the radiohumeral joint. The *radial tunnel* extends from the radiohumeral joint to the proximal edge of the superficial head of the supinator. The floor of the radial tunnel is formed by the joint capsule proximally and the deep head of the supinator distally. The roof and lateral wall of the radial tunnel are formed by the brachioradialis, the extensor carpi radialis longus (ECRL) and extensor carpi radialis brevis (ECRB). The radial nerve divides into the superficial cutaneous branch exiting the tunnel proximally and the posterior interosseous nerve, passing posterolaterally beneath the proximal border of superficial head of the supinator muscle, the *arcade of Frohse* (Fig. 121.4).

The arcade of Frohse is the fibrous semicircular proximal edge of the superficial head of supinator. It is attached to the tip of the lateral epicondyle, arching down for 1 cm, and attaching to the meeting point of the capitellum and the lateral epicondyle. The arcade of Frohse may compress the posterior interosseous nerve in pronation (Fig. 121.5).

The radial nerve may be predisposed to compression at different levels around the elbow:

1. in the arm, by the fibrous arch of the lateral head of triceps
2. proximal to the supinator by the flat, rigid medial edge of the ECRB
3. at the level of the neck radius, by a fan of vessels, including the *recurrent branch of the radial artery*, and the muscular branches to the mobile wad crossing the posterior interosseous nerve *(leash of Henry)*
4. the *arcade of Frohse*, where the posterior interosseous nerve enters between the two heads of supinator
5. occasionally, at the exit of the posterior interosseous nerve over the distal border of supinator.

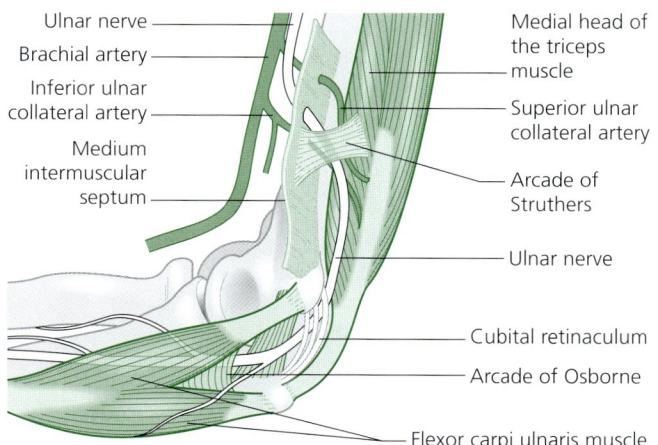

Figure 121.3 The course of the ulnar nerve at the elbow.

Nerves around the elbow

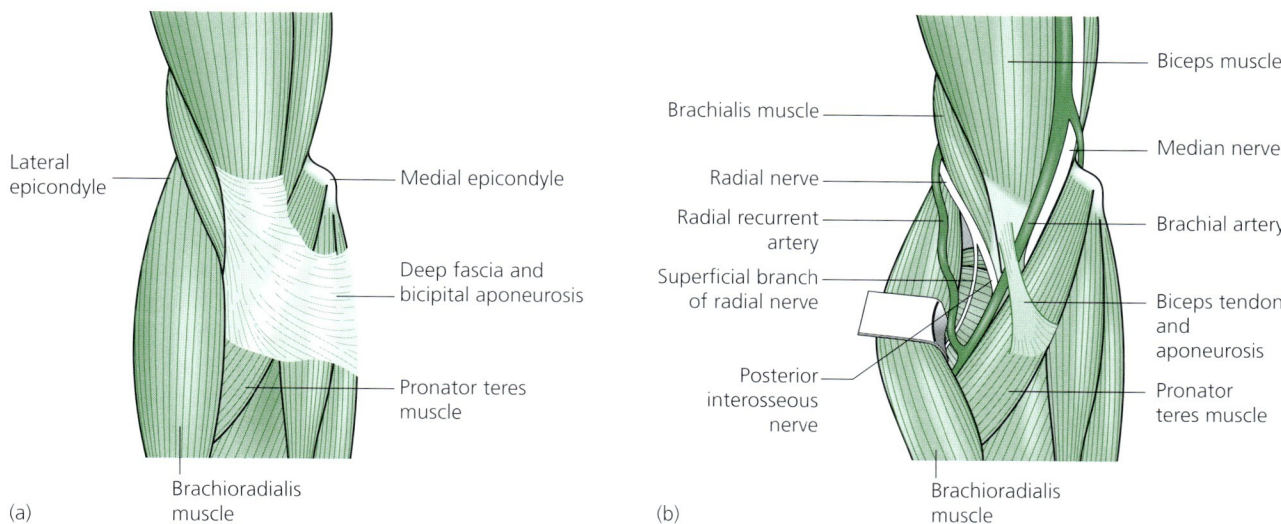

Figure 121.4 The superficial anatomy of the course of the radial nerve.

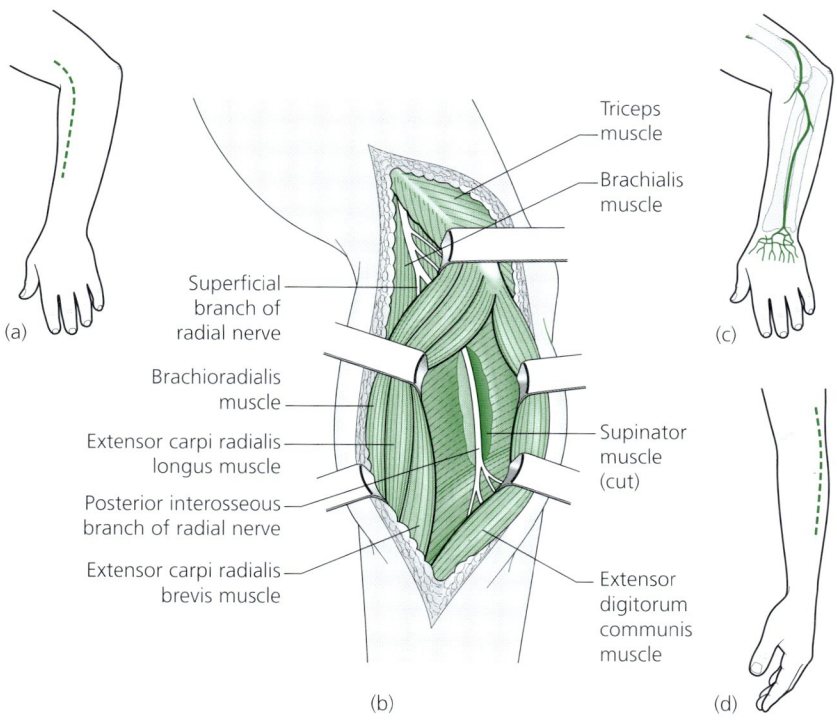

Figure 121.5 Exposure of the posterior interosseous branch of the radial nerve for repair or decompression in radial tunnel syndrome. (a) Line of incision, forearm prone, elbow flexed. (b) Nerve exposed. (c) The course of the nerve with the arm in position (a). (d) Line of incision, elbow extended. Modified from Mayer JH Jr, Mayfield FH. *Surgery, Gynecology and Obstetrics* 1947;**84**:979.

Compression of the radial nerve at the elbow can present as either motor palsy (*posterior interosseous nerve syndrome*) or lateral elbow and forearm pain (*radial tunnel syndrome*). Although the location of compression is the same, the factors that cause posterior interosseous nerve palsy in some and radial tunnel syndrome in others are still not clear.

1. *Posterior interosseous nerve syndrome* presents as progressive weakness of the digital extensors and extensor carpi ulnaris (ECU), sparing the muscles of the mobile wad which are innervated by muscular branches arising more proximally. The aetiology for compression may be ganglia, rheumatoid nodules, radiocapitellar synovitis, unstable radial head or idiopathic. Differential diagnosis includes extensor tendon rupture, sagittal band rupture or inflammatory arthritis of the MP joints causing palmar–ulnar subluxation of the digits.

2. *Radial tunnel syndrome* mainly causes pain in the dorsal aspect of proximal forearm, with actual motor involvement being quite rare. Night pains or pain aggravated by activities like forearm rotation and extremes of wrist flexion/extension. Symptoms of the more common lateral epicondylitis (tennis elbow) often overlap those of radial tunnel syndrome. Nearly half the patients with radial tunnel syndrome also have tennis elbow,[23] whereas one in 20 patients with tennis elbow also has radial tunnel syndrome.[24] Patients with radial tunnel syndrome are tender over the mobile wad, as opposed to patients with tennis elbow, who are tender over the lateral epicondyle. Differential lidocaine injections may help differentiate lateral epicondylitis from radial tunnel syndrome. Electrodiagnostic studies may be normal in radial tunnel syndrome and lateral epicondylitis, but show motor palsy of digital extensors and ECU in posterior interosseous nerve syndrome.

The median nerve (C6–8, T1)

This lies parallel and anterior to the intermuscular septum in the lower arm, just medial to the brachial artery. It passes under the lacertous fibrosus (bicipital aponeurosis) in front of the brachialis, medial to the brachial artery and bicipital tendon to enter the cubital fossa. The median nerve enters the forearm between the two heads of pronator teres, and then passes into the forearm under the proximal arch of flexor digitorum superficialis, the tendinous bridge that connects the humero-ulnar head and the radial head of FDS, where it lies on flexor digitorum profundus (FDP). The anterior interosseous nerve is given off from the median nerve as it passes between the two heads of pronator teres, just after the origin of branches to the superficial flexor forearm muscles. In the forearm, it lies between the flexor digitorum and flexor pollicis muscles anterior to the interosseous membrane, accompanied by the anterior interosseous artery.

The median nerve can be compressed at the elbow and can present as anterior interosseous nerve syndrome and pronator syndrome. These can be atraumatic, but more commonly post-traumatic or iatrogenic due to damage to the nerve during surgery.

1. *Anterior interosseous nerve syndrome* is caused by compression of the anterior interosseous nerve at the fibrous arch of flexor digitorum superficialis or below the pronator teres. It presents mainly as motor palsy, with patients complaining of weakness of pinch (weak FPL and FDP) and an inability to write normally. Patients if asked to make an 'OK sign' pinch would compensate by making a key pinch (an ulnar nerve action). These manifestations of motor weakness may be preceded by episodes of spontaneous forearm pain. Repetitive elbow flexion and forearm pronation may be a cause of dynamic compression of the nerve in the proximal forearm. Differential diagnosis includes post-viral or post-immunization brachial neuritis, of which a large majority involve the anterior interosseous nerve.
2. *Pronator syndrome* may mimic carpal tunnel syndrome, with symptoms of pain and paraesthesias of the radial three and one-half digits. Tinel's sign is usually elicited at the site of maximum compression at the elbow or forearm. Night pains waking up the patient are more common in carpal tunnel syndrome. Patients with pronator syndrome will have a negative Phalen's test and may have thenar eminence hypoaesthesia (innervated by the palmar cutaneous branch of the median nerve, which off-shoots proximal to the flexor retinaculum and pierces the deep fascia, or at the proximal edge of the flexor retinaculum, to innervate the thenar eminence). Resisted forearm pronation or resisted flexion–supination of the elbow may reproduce the pain of nerve compression below pronator teres or lacertous fibrosus, respectively.

Electrodiagnostic studies are useful in differentiating the three conditions, i.e. anterior interosseous nerve palsy in anterior interosseous nerve syndrome, compromised nerve conduction in carpal tunnel syndrome and normal study in pronator teres syndrome.

BIOMECHANICS OF THE ELBOW

Unlike the shoulder joint, the elbow joint is a more constrained joint, with limited range of movements. Elbow biomechanics plays a very important role in daily functions and sports.

Flexion–extension

The normal range of elbow flexion–extension is 0–140°, with the elbow functioning as a loose hinge. The axis of flexion–extension was described in earlier studies as a stationary axis passing through the centre of the trochlea.[25–27] Recent studies, using electromagnetic tracking techniques, have indicated that the axis is not fixed, but changes in position and orientation throughout the arc of movement.[28,29]

A recent *in vivo* study analysed the axis of movement in the normal elbow during flexion using radiostereoisometric analysis (RSA) and found an intra-individual variation in the inclination of the axis ranging from 2.1° to 14.3° in the frontal plane and from 1.6° to 9.8° in the horizontal plane during flexion–extension.[30]

The inclination of the mean axis of rotation varied within a range of 12.7° in the frontal plane and 4.6° in the horizontal plane, and was closely located in both planes to a line joining the centres of the trochlea and capitellum. There also was an intra- and interindividual variation of the axis of flexion of the elbow. This variation in the flexion axis throughout the range of flexion–extension is often described in terms of the *screw displacement axis* (SDA). The SDA shows the instantaneous rotation and position of the axis throughout the range of flexion–extension. Duck et al.[31] have shown that the variability and repeatability of the flexion axis (and SDA) is attributable to the forearm *position* (pronation–supination) or the *mode* of loading (active/passive) employed to bring about elbow flexion.

These concepts are important in designing of endoprosthesis and dynamic external fixators for ligament reconstructions. To properly mimic normal joint motion, an elbow endoprosthesis should be modelled similar to a 'loose' hinge with slight freedom of variability of flexion axis rather than a 'pure' hinge joint.

Pronation–supination

The normal range of forearm pronation is 80–90°, and supination is approximately 90°.[32]

Of the nearly 180° range of forearm rotation, about 100° range (50° each of pronation and supination) is required for most activities of daily living. The shoulder can compensate for loss of pronation to a certain extent, but compensation for loss of supination is usually poorly compensated. At the level of the elbow, the movements of pronation–supination occur at the radiocapitellar and proximal radioulnar joints. The normal axis of forearm pronation–supination runs from the centre of the radial head to the centre of the distal ulna. Recently, Moore et al.[33] have shown that the axis of rotation shifts slightly ulnar and volar during supination, and slightly radial and dorsal during pronation.

Some recent research has shown that forearm rotation plays an important role in stabilizing the elbow in some ligamentous deficiencies like those of MCL, LCL or the anterior band of the medial collateral ligament (AMCL) (anterior band of medial collateral ligament) and fractures of the coronoid (Table 121.1).

Table 121.1 Effects of elbow flexion and forearm rotation on valgus laxity of the elbow

Elbow destabilizing factors	Position of forearm rotation for maximum stability
MCL deficiency, passive flexion	MCL deficiency, passive flexion[34]
LCL deficiency, passive flexion	Pronation[35]
Fractures of more than 50% coronoid	Supination[36]
AMCL deficiency, valgus stress	Pronation[37]

AMCL, anterior band of medial collateral ligament; LCL, lateral collateral ligament; MCL, medial collateral ligament.

Coronoid

Coronoid fractures are pathognomonic for an episode of elbow instability.[38]

The 'terrible triad' is classically defined as elbow dislocation associated with fractures of the radial head and coronoid. Fractures involving more than 50% of the coronoid cause increased varus–valgus laxity, even after repair of the collateral ligaments. This is because the anterior band of the MCL attaches near the base of the coronoid process; thus large fractures of the coronoid process may result in incompetence of this ligament.[36,39,40]

Olecranon

Excision of more than 50% of the olecranon increases joint pressure, which may lead to early arthritic changes.[41] Resection of only a quarter of the olecranon process decreases the resistance of the elbow to valgus force by 50%.

Radial head

The radial head is an important secondary stabilizer of the elbow joint, contributing to nearly 30% of its valgus stability.[42–44]

Radial head excision has been classically performed for displaced fractures of the radial head in adults. However, new studies have shown that radial head excision increases varus–valgus laxity. There are also increased chances of posterolateral rotatory instability of the elbow joint, possibly caused by decreased tension of the lateral UCL after radial head excision.[40,45] Proximal migration of the radius leading to distal radial ulnar joint (DRUJ) problems could occur some months or years later.

Medial collateral ligament

The MCL is the chief soft-tissue restraint to valgus stress. The anterior band of the MCL complex is tauter during valgus stress in extension, whereas the posterior band of the MCL complex is tauter during valgus stress in flexion.[46]

Therefore, valgus stress in extension may cause damage to the anterior band, whereas valgus stress in flexion may cause damage to the whole MCL. The posterior bundle has a limited role in valgus instability, but it has an important role in posteromedial rotatory instability of the elbow joint. The 'moving valgus stress test'[47] has been described as a highly sensitive and specific test for diagnosing valgus instability of the elbow due to MCL insufficiency. A constant moderate valgus stress is applied to a fully flexed elbow and the elbow is quickly extended. The test is positive if medial elbow pain is reproduced at the MCL, and it is maximum between the 120° and 70° arc.

Lateral collateral ligament

The LCL complex is the chief constraint to external rotation and varus stress to the elbow joint. The radial collateral ligament and the lateral UCL are attached to the inferior surface of the lateral epicondyle. The flexion–extension axis passes through the origin of the LCL attachment at the lateral epicondyle. Although the SDA varies by approximately 3–6° in orientation and 1.4–2.0 mm in translation,[29] there is uniform tension in the LCL throughout the arc of flexion.[2]

In the sequence of injuries in elbow dislocation, the LCL is often the first to be disrupted.[48]

Muscles

The musculotendinous units which cross the elbow joint provide dynamic stability to the joint when they contract. For example, during throwing motion, the valgus torque puts strain on the UCL that exceeds its failure strength. But the flexor–pronator muscle mass contracts against valgus torque to provide dynamic stability.[7]

The FCU is the primary dynamic stabilizer and flexor digitorum superficialis and flexor carpi radialis are secondary dynamic stabilizers, whereas pronator teres is the weakest stabilizer of the flexor–pronator group.[7]

Joint forces

Even though the elbow joint is a non-weight-bearing joint, the joint forces can be significant under some conditions, such as falls on outstretched hand, performing push-ups, and contact sports like boxing. Fall on an outstretched hand is the most common cause of dislocation of the elbow joint. The axial joint compression force at the elbow due to fall on an outstretched hand with the elbow extended from a height of only 6 cm has been estimated to be about 50% of the body weight.[49]

Increasing the fall height significantly increases the axial loading force at the elbow joint. Joint reaction forces vary with elbow position. The peak forces and the peak torque exerted onto the elbow joint vary with the hand positions; these are significantly different for 'normal' hand position, for 'hands apart' position and 'hands together' position.[50]

Ulnohumeral and radiocapitellar joints share 43% and 57% of the load transmitted, respectively, across the joint.[51] Across the radiocapitellar joint, greatest force is transmitted between 0° and 30° of flexion, and continues to decrease with increased flexion. Also, pronation of the forearm caused more force transmission than supination across the radiocapitellar joint (Fig. 121.6).[52]

Across the ulnohumeral joint, more forces are transmitted to the coronoid process in extension and to the olecranon in flexion.[53]

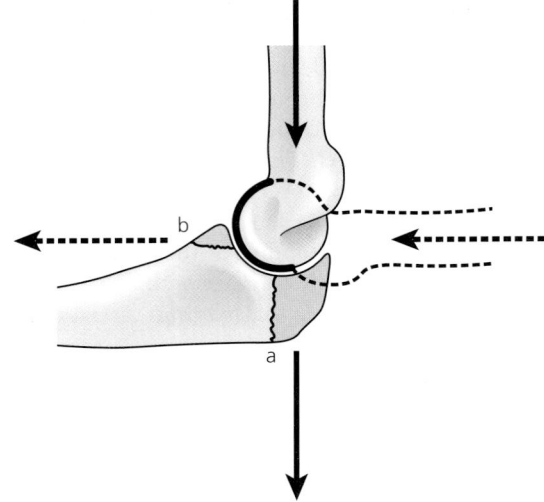

Figure 121.6 Concentration of the force at the ulnohumeral joint varies with flexion and extension of the elbow. When the elbow is flexed at 90°, force (solid line) is concentrated at the olecranon. When the elbow is extended the force (dashed line) is concentrated at the coronoid. The resulting olecranon fracture (a) and coronoid fracture (b) are shown. Adapted from Wake H, Hashizume H, Nishida K, et al. Biomechanical analysis of the mechanism of elbow fracture-dislocations by compression force. *Journal of Orthopedic Science* 2004;**9**:49; with permission.

OLECRANON BURSITIS

Introduction

Olecranon bursitis is an inflammation of the bursa overlying the olecranon process between the bone and skin. Other synonyms for olecranon bursitis are student's elbow, miner's elbow and draftsman's elbow.

Aetiology

The common causes of olecranon bursitis are

1. *Post-traumatic* – acute haemorrhagic bursitis due to direct trauma.
2. *Chronic* – repetitive rubbing on hard surfaces.
3. *Inflammatory* – gout, pseudo-gout, uraemia, rheumatoid arthritis, pigmented villonodular synovitis.
4. *Infection* – pyogenic, tuberculosis.

Basic science and history

Olecranon bursitis is relatively common in adults but less so in children. Normally, the bursa prevents soft-tissue tears by providing a mechanism for skin to glide freely over the olecranon process.

Direct trauma to the area in sports or from injury leads to acute swelling as the bursa fills up with blood and effusion. There may be associated fractures of the olecranon spurs. It is important to rule out underlying fractures and ligament injuries in the differential diagnosis.

Chronic aseptic bursal swelling is the most common form of olecranon bursitis.[54–56] It occurs most commonly from repetitive rubbing of the olecranon on hard surfaces and is often asymptomatic. Patients often consult to explore the cause and allay their fears.

Inflamed and infected olecranon bursitis is the most difficult to treat. It is often difficult to differentiate septic from aseptic inflammatory arthritis and often needs microbiological confirmation.

EXAMINATION

Acute post-traumatic bursitis may present as a tender, fluctuant, fluid-filled swelling with aspiration yielding haemorrhagic fluid.

Patients with chronic, aseptic bursitis present with painless swelling overlying the olecranon process and often give a history of repetitive rubbing of the elbows on hard surfaces.

Patients with systemic conditions like rheumatoid arthritis, gout, uraemia and other medical conditions may present with painful swelling of the olecranon bursa(e).[54,56–58]

Septic olecranon bursitis may be primary (haematogenous spread) or secondary to local cortisone injections. Patients may have local signs of inflammation with or without discharging sinus, with some patients presenting with systemic signs of infection.

DIFFERENTIAL DIAGNOSIS

The differential diagnosis of acute bursitis includes underlying fractures and ligamentous injuries. Rarely, a synovial cyst may mimic bursitis of the elbow.

LABORATORY STUDIES

For suspicion of infection or inflammation, a complete blood count (CBC), differential count of white blood cells (DLC), erythrocyte sedimentation rate (ESR), C-reactive protein (CRP), serum uric acid and rheumatoid factor should be assessed. Aspirate of the bursa fluid should be sent for Gram stain, bacterial culture and crystal analysis (monosodium urate crystals in gout, calcium pyrophosphate crystals in pseudo-gout, and hydroxyapatite crystals).

IMAGING

Radiographs are mandatory for post-traumatic onset bursitis to rule out fracture. Ultrasound studies may reveal an underlying abscess or fluid collection.[59]

MRI may reveal underlying abscess or osteomyelitis not apparent in the radiographs.[60]

Treatment

Acute post-traumatic bursitis can be treated conservatively initially with rest, ice, a compression dressing, elevation and non-steroidal anti-inflammatory drugs (NSAIDs) to decrease swelling and pain. Excessive swelling may need to be aspirated, sometimes repeatedly, if the swelling is too much or in case of urgency to return back to sports. However, in patients not responding to conservative treatment for a long time, surgical bursectomy may be indicated.

Patients with chronic, aseptic bursitis of idiopathic aetiology or from repeated rubbing of the elbow can be given protective pads for elbows, ice, instructions regarding avoiding repetitive trauma, NSAIDs and reassurance. Cortisone injections may be indicated in refractory cases, but only after ascertaining that there is no infection. Aspiration and corticosteroid injection have been shown to result in more rapid recovery at 6 months than only NSAID treatment.[61]

Surgical bursectomy is indicated for recalcitrant cases who fail to respond to long period of conservative treatment.

Septic bursitis should be treated with aspiration, intravenous or oral antibiotics, rest, ice, compression, elevation and occasional splinting. Incision and drainage may be needed if aspiration alone fails to control symptoms.

Inflammatory, non-pyogenic bursitis may be better controlled by treating the underlying systemic illness, e.g. disease-modifying antirheumatic drugs (DMARDs) for control of rheumatoid arthritis, colchicine and allopurinol to control gout, etc.

LATERAL AND MEDIAL EPICONDYLITIS

Introduction

Epicondylitis is the most common condition to occur in the elbow. The term 'lawn tennis arm' was first coined by Morris in 1882 for a condition that he was inflicted with, but the first documented description of ulnar neuropathy at the elbow (post-traumatic tardy ulnar nerve palsy) was actually by Runge in 1873.[62] In 1883 Major described it as a painful condition of the lateral aspect of the elbow among tennis players but Morris gave further details of his affliction in the same year as being on the inner side of the humerus. From the beginning the similarity between lateral and medial epicondylitis has been obvious.

Lateral epicondylitis has become synonymous with the term 'tennis elbow' ever since the beginning. It has also been known by a plethora of terms like lateral epicondylalgia, tendinosis and tendinopathy. However, the most appropriate term in clinical practice seems to be *lateral elbow tendinopathy*.[63] This is because inflammation of a low degree is present only in the very early stages of the disease and the condition has been shown to be a degenerative tendinopathy of the ECRB tendon.[64] Tennis elbow is extremely common in today's active lifestyle. It has been reported to occur in 10–50% of regular tennis players at some point of their careers,[65] but it actually occurs more commonly in non-tennis players and the general public, affecting 1–3% of adults each year.[66]

The incidence is equal among men and women in the general population, but, among tennis players, it affects males more than females. The age group most commonly affected is 35–55 years and the typical patient is a recreational player (tennis, squash, fencing, badminton, cricket) or someone having a rigorous active lifestyle (plumbers, bricklayers, weavers, painters, musicians, drummers, butchers), more commonly affecting the dominant arm. Overexertion of the extremity with repetitive wrist extension and forearm pronation–supination has been postulated to be the precipitating factor in the majority of patients.[67]

Current or prior tobacco users have an increased risk of developing lateral epicondylitis.[68]

Medial epicondylitis is much less common than lateral epicondylitis. However, there are very disparate figures in the literature regarding just how much less common it can be. Medial epicondylitis has been cited to occur anywhere from between five to nine times[69] and 7–20 times[70] less commonly than lateral epicondylitis in the population.

A Finnish population study in 2006 showed a prevalence of 0.4% for medial epicondylitis as opposed to 1.3% for lateral epicondylitis.[68] It is most commonly found in the fourth and fifth decades although it has been reported in patients as young as 12 years and as old as 80 years. It seems to be equally prevalent in both men and women with 75% having it in the dominant arm.[71] Smoking, obesity, repetitive movements and forceful activities are independently associated with having medial epicondylitis.[68]

Although the term 'golfer's elbow' has historically been coined for this condition, lateral epicondylitis is the more common problem among golfers.[72] In amateur golfers medial elbow injury is found to be almost five times less common than lateral elbow injury.[73,74] Other athletes that have been reported to have this complaint are javelin throwers, bowlers, racquetball players, footballers, archers, weightlifters, golfers and even tennis players. It can also be commonly found in those with occupations involving repetitive elbow, hand and wrist motions that impart large valgus stresses across the elbow, such as carpentry (hammering and using the screwdriver), plumbing, bricklaying, typing, textile production and meat cutting.[70,71]

Basic science

Lateral epicondylitis has been described as a degenerative tendinopathy of the ECRB muscle. Currently, the most popular theory for pathogenesis of tennis elbow is that of 'repetitive microtrauma to ECRB muscle from overuse', resulting in tendinosis of ECRB, with or without involvement of extensor digitorum communis (EDC) muscle. This is primarily thought to be due to internal stress from tension forces on the ECRB tendon. In a cinematographic and electromyography study of tennis players with lateral epicondylitis, increased activity of ECRB and altered swing mechanics was demonstrated.[75] Tennis players who have a two-handed backhand rarely develop tennis elbow, as the non-dominant hand absorbs most of the energy. Electromyogram (EMG) studies have shown reduced amplitude in the extensor muscles in two-handed stroke players.[76]

Tennis elbow has been linked to a player's technique and not the grip size of the tennis racquet. Recently published research[77] did not find any significant differences in forearm muscle firing pattern between small, recommended, or big grips of tennis racquets (as per Nirschl's hand measurement technique to determine a player's 'recommended' grip size[64]).

The 'anatomic vulnerability of ECRB origin to attrition' theory mentions that the ECRB origin on the humerus lies slightly medial and superior to the outer edge of the capitellum. During extension, the undersurface of ECRB rubs against the lateral edge of the capitellum, together with the ECRL compressing the ECRB against the underlying bone. This might cause abrasion of the tissues leading to ECRB tendinosis.[78]

The pathological findings are of degenerative tendinopathy of the origin of ECRB. Goldie[67] first described granulation tissue in ECRB of tennis elbow patients. Nirschl[65] noted grey, friable tissue associated with varying degrees of tears of ECRB, with histopathological findings of disorganized immature collagen formation, and immature fibroblastic and vascular elements, which he called 'angiofibroblastic hyperplasia' (now called 'angiofibroblastic tendinosis'). Regan et al.[79] reported microscopic histopathology findings of degeneration rather than inflammation in recalcitrant lateral epicondylitis. However, despite the absence of inflammatory cells, it is quite painful and tender. Some recent studies have suggested neurogenic inflammation after showing the presence of neuropeptides (substance P and calcitonin gene-related peptide) in a subgroup of small vessels in the origin of ECRB.[80,81]

Medial epicondylitis has been closely associated with the pitching mechanism in baseball players and the biomechanics involved at the medial elbow and the flexor–pronator muscles.[82] During the acceleration phase of the throwing motion, the elbow is being rapidly extended and it places a large valgus tensile stress across the elbow, specifically on the flexor–pronator mass.[83] Pronation of the forearm with the elbow in extension further stresses the flexor–pronator origin. The peak angular velocity and valgus forces during this phase exceed the tensile strength of the medial musculotendinous and ligamentous structures. These forces are initially transmitted to the flexor–pronator mass at its origin on the medial epicondyle and subsequently to the MCL and the ulnar nerve deep to it. The high overhand serve and late forehand strokes in tennis have similar biomechanics,[84] accounting for medial elbow pain being more common in the experienced and aggressive player.[85,86] In golf, improper technique of throwing the club from the apex of the backward swing downward to hit the ball also generates excessive valgus forces on the dominant elbow, causing tension overload of the flexor–pronator mass.[87]

In medial epicondylitis, pathological changes occur mostly within the flexor–pronator mass, especially pronator teres and flexor carpi radialis, close to their attachment to the medial epicondyle. Occasionally it can also be seen in the FCU. Very rarely, flexor sublimis degeneration and rupture into the elbow joint medially with secondary pseudo-bursal formation is also seen.[88] In the majority of cases the changes are macro- and microscopically similar to what is observed for lateral epicondylitis.[69] Sufficient repetitive stress leads to muscle fatigue, weakness and microtears within musculotendinous junctions near their origins. This repetitive microtrauma is followed by fibroblastic tendinosis with proliferation of vascular granulation tissue (angiofibroblastic tendinosis). With a failed healing response, the process becomes chronic and the histology of the tendon becomes abnormal. It can ultimately lead to frank avulsion of the flexor–pronator origin.

Nirschl[64] has categorized the stages of repetitive microtrauma for epicondylar tendinosis. Stage 1 injury is purely inflammatory and is not associated with pathological changes. It is very likely to resolve with non-surgical treatment. Stage 2 injury is associated with the aforementioned angiofibroblastic tendinosis and degenerative changes. Pathological tissue appears grey and friable on gross examination. In stage 3 injury there is rupture of the tissue along with the pathological changes. Stage 4 injury has the features of stage 2 or stage 3 injury but is also associated with other changes such as fibrosis, soft matrix calcification and hard osseous calcification. Stage 4 injury changes can also be related to the use of local cortisone injections.[64] Both lateral and medial epicondylitis undergo the same stages of injury.

Transmission of the damaging forces to the ulnar nerve may also occur, hence the common association of ulnar nerve neuritis with medial epicondylitis in baseball pitchers with medial elbow pain. When stretched, the ulnar nerve can sustain direct injury with an inflammatory response leading to neuritis, compression and entrapment symptoms.[71]

Medial elbow instability is another condition associated with medial epicondylitis. Poor biomechanics, improper conditioning, lack of flexibility or fatigue when doing strenuous activities may cause muscle strain, which can lead to increased transmission of forces to the MCL. Subsequent repeated excessive stress to the MCL can lead to microdamage, and eventually to ligamentous insufficiency and elbow instability.[71]

Management of lateral epicondylitis

HISTORY

Typically, a patient between the ages of 35 and 55 years will complain of insidious-onset pain over the lateral aspect of the elbow, which exacerbates with activities involving active wrist extension or passive wrist flexion with the elbow in extension. Patients will often describe aggravating activities such as backhand stroke in tennis, bowling action in cricket, overuse of a screwdriver, wringing clothes, painting a wall, teachers attempting to write on a blackboard, holding a cup of coffee, etc. Pain may radiate to the back of the forearm, but the most common site to which the patients point is 1.5 cm distal to the origin of the ECRB.

PHYSICAL EXAMINATION

Examination of a patient presenting with lateral elbow pain should start with examination of the cervical spine, and then to include the entire upper limb, including the shoulder, wrist and hand.

Patient reports maximum tenderness about 1–2 cm distal to the origin of ECRB and EDC muscles, which is slightly anterior and distal to the lateral epicondyle (Fig. 121.7). There is often weakness of grip because of the pain. Resisted wrist dorsiflexion with the elbow in full extension reproduces the pain of tennis elbow.

Maximal passive wrist flexion with the elbow in extension stretches the ECRB and also reproduces the pain (Fig. 121.8).

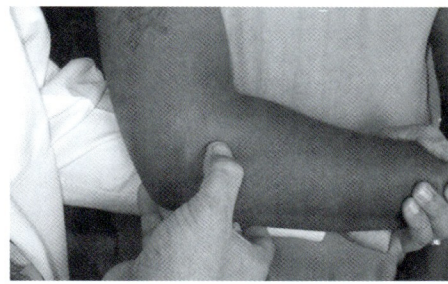

Figure 121.7 Patient reports maximum tenderness about 1–2 cm distal to the origin of the extensor carpi radialis brevis and extensor digitorum communis muscles, which is slightly anterior and distal to the lateral epicondyle.

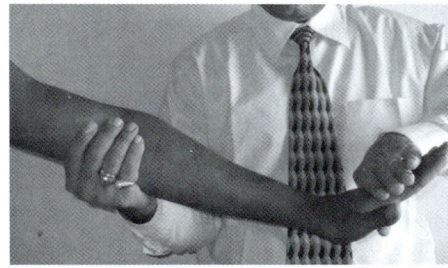

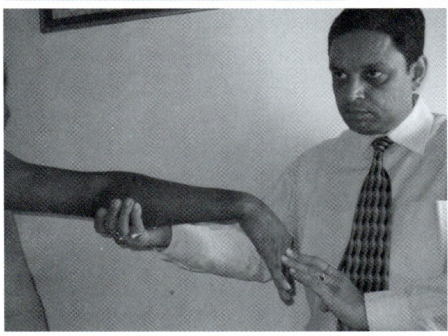

Figure 121.8 There is often weakness of grip because of the pain. Resisted wrist dorsiflexion with the elbow in full extension reproduces the pain of tennis elbow.

DIFFERENTIAL DIAGNOSIS

Radial nerve compressive neuropathy at the elbow can present either as *radial tunnel syndrome* (lateral elbow and forearm pain) or *posterior interosseous nerve syndrome* (progressive motor weakness of the digital extensors and the ECU, but sparing the muscles of the mobile wad, which are innervated by the muscular branches more proximally). Nearly half the patients with radial tunnel syndrome also have tennis elbow,[23] whereas one in 20 patients with tennis elbow also has radial tunnel syndrome. Maximal tenderness in radial tunnel syndrome is typically over the mobile wad, 3–4 cm distal and anterior to the lateral epicondyle. Unlike lateral epicondylitis, resisted thumb and index finger extension may be painful in radial tunnel syndrome, but not resisted wrist extension. Also, resisted forearm supination may be painful in radial tunnel syndrome because of compressive neuropathy of the posterior interosseous nerve within the supinator muscle. Differential lidocaine injections may help to differentiate lateral epicondylitis from radial tunnel syndrome. Electrodiagnostic studies may be normal in radial tunnel syndrome and lateral epicondylitis, but may show motor palsy of the digital extensors and ECU in posterior interosseous nerve syndrome.

Radiocapitellar osteoarthritis may mimic lateral epicondylitis, and radiographs may confirm the diagnosis.

Posterolateral plica as a cause of refractory lateral elbow pain has been recently reported by Ruch et al.[89] It can be diagnosed by palpating for painful clicks over the radiocapitellar joint upon pronation/supination of a flexed elbow.

Posterolateral rotatory instability of the elbow may remain undiagnosed and can mimic lateral epicondylitis.

Other differential diagnoses to be considered are cervical radiculopathy, elbow and forearm overuse injuries, little league elbow syndrome, osteochondritis dissecans of the capitellum and loose body in the joint.

INVESTIGATIONS

Often, lateral epicondylitis is a clinical diagnosis and no investigations are needed. Radiographs of recalcitrant lateral epicondylitis may occasionally show calcifications within the extensor muscle mass. These are associated with persistent disease and do not affect the treatment.[90] Laboratory studies are usually not useful in investigating tennis elbow. Ultrasound is useful to demonstrate local inflammation and ligament erosion or tears. MRI may be considered to rule out osteochondritis dissecans and stress fractures of the distal humerus.

Management of medial epicondylitis

HISTORY

Patients typically give a history of chronic medial elbow pain that occurs during activities involving forearm pronation and wrist flexion. A progressive history with insidious onset is common. A detailed history is required to distinguish it from other possible causes of medial elbow pain, especially UCL instability or ulnar neuritis. Radiation of pain to the forearm and a weak grasp is more suggestive of UCL sprain or partial tear.[91]

PHYSICAL EXAMINATION

Patients will have tenderness at the medial epicondyle and origin of the flexor–pronator mass, usually over the pronator teres and flexor carpi radialis muscles. Maximum tenderness is approximately 5–10 mm distal and anterior to the midpoint of the medial epicondyle.[71] Wrist flexion and pronation against resistance will elicit the pain.

There may be local swelling and increase in temperature.[92] Normal strength and sensation of the limb is typically noted with medial epicondylitis alone.

During initial disease the elbow range of motion is usually full but with time it may become limited and lead to flexion contracture, which is commonly noted in the throwing athlete with chronic symptoms.[91]

There is higher than normal prevalence for patients with recalcitrant medial epicondylitis to have other musculotendinous dysfunction such as cubital tunnel syndrome, lateral epicondylitis, carpal tunnel syndrome or rotator cuff problems. Gabel and Morrey[93] reported a 62% (16 out of 26 patients) prevalence in their study. Therefore, it is important to examine the entire upper limb when managing this type of patient.

DIFFERENTIAL DIAGNOSIS

Many other conditions give rise to pain at the medial elbow and can make the diagnosis of medial epicondylitis difficult. Among them are osteoarthritis of the ulnohumeral joint, anterior interosseous nerve (AIN) entrapment, cervical radiculopathy, cubital tunnel syndrome, loose bodies in the elbow joint, arthrofibrosis, medial epicondyle avulsion injury, synovitis, tardy ulnar nerve palsy, valgus extension overload, UCL instability and the presence of osteophytes. A complete history, physical examination and additional investigations should be used to make the correct diagnosis/diagnoses.

The two most important conditions to consider when examining patients with medial elbow pain are primary ulnar nerve neuritis and primary UCL instability. These conditions may coexist with medial epicondylitis, especially in the overhead athlete. Apart from examination of the elbow, a thorough examination of the cervical spine, shoulder and wrist, as well as a complete neurological examination of the affected limb, should be performed.

Ulnar neuropathy, when present, gives rise to a positive Tinel's sign. This is indicated by local pain and numbness with distal radiation of tingling when compression is applied to the ulnar nerve at the elbow. If it is positive proximal to the cubital tunnel it may indicate ulnar nerve compression at the level of the *arcade of Struthers*. If at the medial epicondyle, it may be due to compression by osteophytes, loose bodies or synovitis. A positive Tinel's sign distal to the medial epicondyle implies ulnar nerve compression as it passes between the two heads of the FCU. A provocative test for ulnar nerve neuritis at the elbow is the *elbow flexion test*, which is performed by fully flexing the elbow in pronation with the wrist extended for about 1–3 minutes. The presence of ulnar neuropathy will cause the patient to experience medial elbow pain, with numbness and tingling of the ring and little fingers. The ulnar nerve may sublux on elbow flexion and extension. This can be demonstrated by palpating the ulnar nerve and feel it flop over the medical epicondyle.

UCL instability is indicated when there is focal pain along the UCL on applying valgus stress to the elbow at 30° of flexion. Pain when pulling on the thumb with the elbow flexed and forearm supinated, the *milking test*, is also indicative of instability. For the elite overhead athlete it is very important to distinguish medial epicondylitis from a UCL injury, but diagnosis may be difficult as medial epicondylitis can be secondary to an initial UCL injury.[71,91]

INVESTIGATIONS

Just as in lateral epicondylitis, diagnosis for medial epicondylitis is mainly clinical. However, additional investigations may be important to exclude conditions listed in the differential diagnosis.

Radiological examination should include not only the anteroposterior and lateral views of the elbow, but also an axial view. About 25% of patients have soft-tissue calcifications adjacent to the medial epicondyle.[94] A traction spur off the medial epicondyle or calcification of the MCL, especially in throwing athletes, may indicate a chronic UCL tear.[95]

Bone scans may be helpful if the patient has uncharacteristic pain but normal radiographs. The presence of osteoid osteomas or osteoblastomas usually will not show up in radiographs but will show an increased uptake on a technetium-99 bone scan.

MRI or dynamic ultrasonography is a useful adjunct if the patient has confounding medial elbow symptoms. It is able to more accurately define underlying pathological changes within the musculotendinous and adjacent structures. However, when contemplating an MRI study, the use of coils and imaging protocols specifically for the elbow is required. In cases of recalcitrant medial epicondylitis, it is useful in evaluating the integrity of the structures around the elbow. The presence of full-thickness tears may indicate a requirement for earlier and more aggressive surgical treatment, especially in athletes.

Patients with abnormal neurological findings on examination will require electrodiagnositc studies for further evaluation. Previous authors have reported that 23–53% of patients undergoing surgical treatment for medial epicondylitis also have concomitant ulnar nerve involvement.[93,96] Treatment should be directed towards both the neuropathy and the epicondylitis to maximize functional outcome.

Treatment

There is very little consensus in the literature regarding the treatment protocol. Even though there are many published clinical studies on the treatment of lateral epicondylitis, a recent review of 54 prospective randomized therapeutic trials reported in the literature from 1950 to 2005 found that most of them are actually of low level of evidence.[97] Two independent reviewers found that the vast majority of the studies (>90%) are only level II according to the Oxford Levels of Evidence, or unsatisfactory according to the Coleman Methodology Score (almost 90% of reports) and CONSORT score (about 63% of reports).

The aim of any treatment is to reduce pain, increase strength and improve the quality of life as fast as possible, with minimum possible side-effects of treatment. Various treatment modalities have been proposed in the literature that are suitable for both lateral and medial epicondylitis.

Nirschl and Ashman[88] have proposed treatment concepts for elbow tendinosis designed to parallel the biological healing response. These treatment concepts are in the form of:

1. pain relief with control of exudation or haemorrhage
2. promotion of specific tissue healing
3. promotion of general fitness
4. control of force loads
5. surgical removal of pain-producing pathological tissue if non-operative measures fail.

NON-OPERATIVE TREATMENT

The same basic principles of non-surgical treatment for lateral epicondylitis apply to medial epicondylitis. In the overhead-throwing athlete the initial treatment goal is to diminish pain and inflammation with non-operative measures while maintaining the elbow's flexibility. Previous authors have reported success rates of 82–96% for the treatment of lateral and medial epicondylitis using non-operative measures.[98–101]

Non-operative treatment can be divided into three phases.[71] The initial phase of treatment consists of rest from the causal/aggravating activity to provide early relief of inflammation and pain. Complete immobilization or inactivity is not recommended. Use of ice, NSAIDs, night splinting, local corticosteroid injection,[102] ultrasound and high-voltage galvanic stimulation in this phase may provide adjuvant benefit. Counterforce bracing is helpful in athletes with symptoms during activities of daily living and also when they attempt to return to sport.

The second phase of treatment should be initiated once the acute pain and inflammation has improved with treatment during the first phase. A guided rehabilitation programme is started with establishment of a full and painless wrist and elbow range of motion as its first goal. The ultimate goal is to achieve similar or greater than pre-injury strength. If the patient can satisfactorily complete a sports or occupational simulation they can be gradually reinitiated back into the sport or occupation with increasing exposure and intensity.

The third phase is more for athletes who have returned to sport. The athlete, coaches and trainers need to identify equipment and training inadequacies that may contribute to a recurrence of the symptoms and take proper preventive measures to address them. This includes technique correction or enhancement, equipment modification and continued conditioning of the entire body along with the affected extremity. Conditioning is best performed with a slow, structured interval programme monitored by the coach, trainer and team physician.

Available non-operative treatment modalities include the following.

Rest and NSAIDs reduce inflammation in acute lateral epicondylitis, thus relieving tendon strain, so that the tendon gets time to heal. There is no conclusive evidence for the effectiveness of topical NSAIDs.[103] However, NSAIDs do not show long-term efficacy of treatment.[104] Rest should involve avoidance of abuse but not abstinence from activity, e.g. grasping or lifting with the elbow in slight flexion; and the forearm supinated and not pronated.[88]

A *physical therapy* protocol as described by Nirschl,[64] and also found to be effective in the majority of patients by the authors, focuses on increasing forearm strength, flexibility and endurance. Patients are taught stretching of the extensor origin by flexing the wrist with the elbow extended and forearm pronated. Isometric and concentric strengthening exercises are also added to the physical therapy regimen. Recently, electrical muscle stimulation has been found to cause muscle hypertrophy, thereby augmenting its tensile strength and decreasing the strain from the tendon. However, it has not proved to have significant advantages over stretching with or without concentric strengthening.[105,106]

Initially, rehabilitation for medial epicondylitis is with wrist flexor and forearm pronator stretching and progressive isometric exercises. Eccentric and concentric resistive exercises are added later when there is improvement of flexibility, strength and endurance.[95]

Ergonomic measures/biomechanical correction: correcting faulty technique while at work, work station or play may prevent pain or improve pain scores. Each sport or activity in an individual suffering from the disease must be analysed and aberrant biomechanics corrected.

In sports, player biomechanics, player characteristics and correct equipment may help in preventing lateral epicondylitis. For example, tennis players with lateral epicondylitis have been found to have a significantly greater activity of wrist extensors during ball impact and early follow through. This is possibly by an aberrant technique of 'leading elbow', wrist extension and ball contact occurring with an open face racquet or ball hitting the lower half of the strings. This not only scales down performance, but also predisposes the wrist extensors to injury. Tennis players should be advised to hit the ball in front of the body with an extended wrist and elbow in a forehand stroke. This minimizes stress on the wrist extensors, with the upper body and torso providing the majority of the power for the stroke. Similarly, a two-handed backstroke should be encouraged, as the force is shared between the two extremities.

Equipment-related factors which diminish load transmission to the elbow include tennis racquets with mid-sized frames of a low-vibration, medium-flex material such as graphite and epoxies, racquets with low string tension or a high string count per unit area, and playing on slow surfaces like 'clay courts'.[107]

Steroid injections have shown better results during early follow-up (5 days to 6 weeks) than NSAIDs, physical therapy or placebo.[108–110] However, long-term results of corticosteroids have shown a high recurrence rate and significantly poorer outcome at 52 weeks compared with physical therapy.[108,109] Steroids could weaken the tendon directly by decreasing collagen production and tenocyte replication,[111] or indirectly because of patients adding more stress after early relief from pain.[109]

Other complications of local steroids are local skin depigmentation, fat necrosis and rarely common extensor tendon rupture.[112]

Similarly, in the treatment of medial epicondylitis, local injection with a mixture of methylprednisolone and lidocaine is shown to provide short-term pain relief only.[113]

Injection of botulinum toxin A, an anticholinergic agent which acts by blocking the presynaptic release of acetylcholine, into the forearm extensor muscles has been found to be effective in treating chronic lateral epicondylitis.[114] Local muscle paralysis relaxes the tendon, allowing it to heal better. However, there is increased incidence of side-effects such as weakness of finger and wrist extension.[115] However, there is still a lack of consensus regarding the dose of injection.[114] Moreover, there is no long-term evidence regarding the efficacy of botulinum.

Extracorporeal shock wave therapy provides little or no benefit in terms of pain and functions in patients with lateral epicondylitis and should not be recommended.[116,117]

Orthotic devices, which include proximal forearm bands (Fig. 121.9) and wrist cock-up splints, are commonly prescribed for the treatment of lateral epicondylitis.

Forearm bands work as counterforce devices, diffusing overuse forces over a broader area while maintaining muscle balance, thus offloading the elbow tendons. EMG analysis of tennis players has shown reduced muscle activity while wearing braces during play. Braces should be applied firmly about 10 cm distal to the lateral epicondyle. However, care must be taken as compression of the anterior interosseous nerve[118] and posterior interosseous nerve entrapment[119] have been reported with use.

Cock-up splints restrict wrist extension, thus relaxing the extensor tendons. However, these are not as popular among practitioners as forearm bands, and there is not much evidence to prove which is more effective between the two.[120,121]

Other treatment modalities

Local ultrasound therapy has a modest pain reduction effect.[117,122]

Autologous blood injection locally is promising and has shown good early results, but more evidence is needed for clinical recommendation.[123]

Buffered platelet-rich plasma injection has shown promising results in a study, but more evidence is needed.[124]

Laser light therapy has been reported to not be beneficial in the treatment of lateral epicondylitis.[125,126] However, a recent systematic review of the literature found that low-level laser therapy with optimal doses of 904 nm and 632 nm wavelengths applied directly to the lateral elbow tendon insertions seem to offer short-term relief with less disability.[127]

Acupuncture has proved effective for short-term pain relief to some extent.[128,129]

Topical nitrates have proved effective in the treatment of lateral epicondylitis, but more evidence is needed.[130]

SURGICAL TREATMENT

Surgical treatment is usually indicated if, after 6–12 months, non-operative treatment has failed to relieve the patient's pain and functional disability.

In high-performance athletes, surgical treatment is recommended if they fail to respond to a disciplined 3–6 month programme of non-operative treatment,[102] provided all other possible pathological causes for the elbow pain have been excluded. If examination and imaging studies indicate a musculotendinous disruption, operative treatment can be even sooner, as non-operative treatment alone will be insufficient for the high-level athlete to return to peak performance.

Historically, a number of techniques have been described in the literature for the surgical treatment of resistant tennis elbow. A chronological list of these procedures is in Table 121.2. Most of these techniques have a high incidence of complications, such as weakening of extensors, persistent pain and injury to the LCL complex (sometimes leading to posterolateral rotatory instability). Therefore, none is worth recommendation.

Currently recommended techniques for lateral epicondylitis include debridement of grey, friable, angiofibrotic tissue, lengthening of the involved tendons and decortication of the lateral epicondyle. This can be performed by open, mini-open or arthroscopic techniques.

Although reports on the surgical treatment of medial epicondylitis are few, available results using similar surgical techniques for lateral epicondylitis described above are encouraging. Vangsness and Jobe[96] reported that 88% of patients have either excellent (69%) or good (19%) results

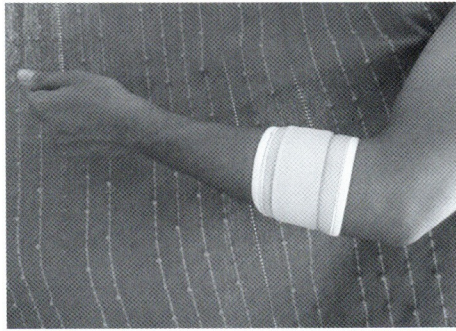

Figure 121.9 Braces should be applied firmly about 10 cm distal to the lateral epicondyle.

Table 121.2 Techniques for the surgical treatment of resistant tennis elbow

Procedure	Author	Year
Epicondylar osteotomy	Franke[131]	1910
Excision of subcutaneous tissue	Fischer[132]	1923
Incision of the extensor carpi radialis brevis belly	Hohmann[133]	1927
Partial regional (lateral) denervation	Tavernier[134]	1946
Partial resection of the orbicular (annular) ligament	Bosworth[135]	1955
Partial ventral degeneration	Kaplan[136]	1959
Lengthening of the extensor carpi radialis brevis distally	Garden[137]	1961
Complete denervation	Wilhelm and Gieseler[138]	1962
Excision of subtendinous pathological tissue	Goldie[67]	1964
Decompression of the posterior interosseous nerve	Capener[139]	1966
Radial tunnel decompression	Roles and Maudsley[140]	1972
Epicondylectomy with partial (distal part) excision of annular ligament	Boyd and McLeod[98]	1973
Decompression of the radial nerve	Wilhelm[141]	1977
Proximal lengthening of extensor carpi radialis brevis	Narakas[142]	1987

in their series of 35 patients who were treated surgically. Time to full recovery is from 3 to 24 months, with all patients having some improvement and 86% no limitations to their daily living or sport activities. Gabel and Morrey[93] reported an 87% rate of excellent or good results in their series of 30 elbows that underwent open surgery for medial epicondylitis. In their series less than half of the patients with concomitant moderate or severe ulnar neuropathy did well, in contrast to 24 out of 25 patients with no or mild concurrent ulnar nerve symptoms.

Open surgical technique – lateral epicondylitis

Skin incision is made on the lateral aspect of the elbow, from 1 cm proximal to the lateral epicondyle, extending to just distal of the radiocapitellar joint. The interval between the ECRL and the extensor aponeurosis is split (Fig. 121.10). The ECRB lies deep and posterior to the ECRL. With a soft-tissue elevator, the ECRL is peeled off the ECRB. This will expose the ECRB tendon, which may look healthy superficially, but, once it is incised, the pathological granulation tissue (grey, friable) may be seen. If present, this needs to be curetted out. Similarly, the EDC tendon may also be debrided if found to be pathological in some patients. A lateral epicondyle decortication with or without radial nerve exploration may be carried out, but drilling holes into the lateral epicondyle has been found to have high chances of residual pain, stiffness and wound bleeding (Fig. 121.10).[143]

Depending on the extent of debridement, either the remaining tendon is reattached to the lateral epicondyle or the fascia is closed over the extensor muscles. A 2.8 mm bone anchor suture may be used to supplement the repair of the avulsed extensor tendon. Postoperatively, a sling for support is given for 10 days, followed by range of motion exercises, with strengthening exercises to commence after 6 weeks.

Open surgical technique – medial epicondylitis

A 5–10 cm oblique incision is made just anterior to the medial epicondyle in the affected limb with the patient lying supine and under tourniquet control. Care is taken to identify and protect the branches of the medial antebrachial cutaneous nerve within the subcutaneous tissue. The incision can be extended proximally if concurrent anterior transposition of the ulnar nerve is required.

The common flexor–pronator origin and the ulnar nerve are then identified. A longitudinal incision of the pronator teres–flexor carpi radialis interval is developed to enable visualization and removal of abnormal tissue. In most instances this is easily done by simply scraping off the abnormal tissue with a scalpel blade held perpendicular to the tendon, the 'scratch test' as described by Nirschl and Ashman.[88] Budoff et al.[144] demonstrated the effectiveness of this technique to differentiate between normal tendon and diseased tissue (angiofibroblastic tendinosis).

Less commonly, when the pathology is diffuse, a transverse incision is required to enable it to be completely excised. Dellon et al.[145] had suggested that denervation of the medial epicondyle may be considered in patients who failed to respond to conservative treatment.

The UCL, deep to the flexor–pronator mass, should be evaluated together for possible concurrent pathology. Surgical management of concurrent ulnar nerve and UCL pathology is performed as appropriate.

The medial epicondyle needs to be prepared to provide a sufficiently vascular bed prior to reattachment of the common flexor–pronator origin; 2.8 mm or 3.5 mm bone anchors are used for reattaching the tendon to bone.

The deep fascia is closed with a smooth, resorbable monofilament suture. Closure of the subcutaneous tissue and skin is best carried out using a shorter acting resorbable monofilament suture to minimize inflammation and scar formation. An above-elbow plaster splint may be applied with the elbow in 90° flexion and the forearm in the neutral position.

Postoperatively the elbow is kept immobilized with a Duke of Edinburgh sling for support. A gradual rehabilitation programme is initiated at 2 weeks and will continue to until at least 6 weeks after surgery. For athletes, isometric exercises can be initiated at 2–4 weeks and progressive resistance training initiated at 6–8 weeks. However, if substantial detachment of the flexor–pronator origin was performed, aggressive progressive resistance training may need to be delayed to 8 or 10 weeks after surgery.[146]

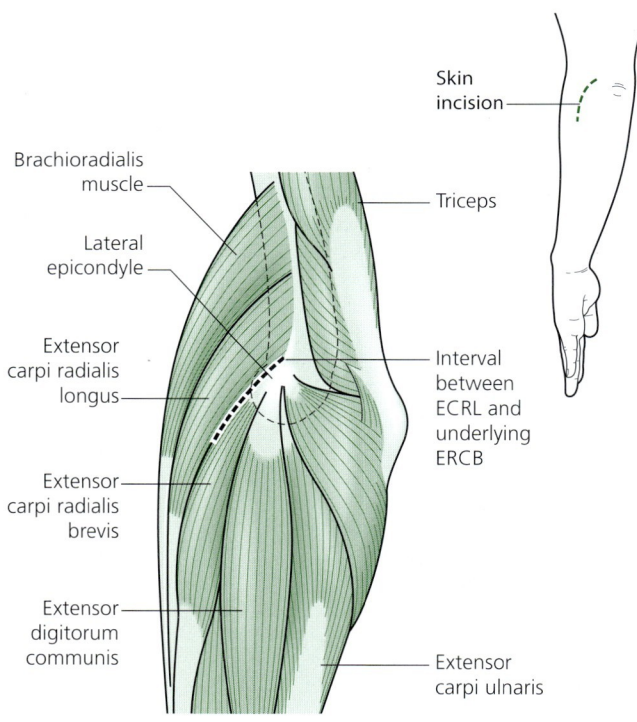

Figure 121.10 Surgical exposure. ECRB, extensor carpi radialis brevis; ECRL, extensor carpi radialis longus.

In summary, surgical treatment of medial epicondylitis consists of the following steps:[71]

1. excise portion of affected tendon that has undergone pathological changes
2. enhance local vascularity to stimulate healing response
3. reattach any avulsed tendon origin back to the epicondyle
4. repair of any resultant defects
5. management of concomitant ulnar nerve or UCL disorders.

Arthroscopic debridement

Recent reports regarding long-term follow-up of arthroscopic lateral release for recalcitrant lateral epicondylitis has proved it to be a reliable treatment option.[147] However, the close proximity of both the ulnar nerve and the UCL contraindicates its use for the treatment of medial epicondylitis.

Arguments have been made against arthroscopic management, citing lateral epicondylitis to be an extra-articular pathology, and, therefore, the need to manage it by an open approach. Yet, recent reports comparing open and arthroscopic lateral release for lateral epicondylitis have found no significant differences in outcomes. Rather, arthroscopic cases did better in the short term with regards to earlier return to work and less postoperative therapy.[148]

Advantages of arthroscopy include the opportunity to examine the joint for occult pathology. Any infolded tissue that may impinge within the radiocapitellar joint is debrided. The degenerative lateral joint capsule and the undersurface of the ECRB are released from the lateral epicondyle, restricting resection away from the muscular ECRL insertion and the LCL complex. Keeping debridement parallel to the anterior half of the radial head protects injury to the LCL complex.[149] The bony surface of the lateral epicondyle can be decorticated using a high-speed burr. Postoperatively, sling support is needed for few days and range-of-motion exercises are commenced a few days postoperatively. Strengthening exercises can begin as soon as pain and swelling resolves.

CUBITAL TUNNEL SYNDROME

Introduction

The term cubital tunnel syndrome was originally coined in 1958 by Feindel and Stratford.[22] Many proscribed the first description on ulnar nerve compression at the elbow to Panas in 1878. Prior to that, however, Earle reported in 1816 on the surgical sectioning of the ulnar nerve in a 14-year-old girl with symptoms characteristic of ulnar nerve compression that did not respond to 3 years of conservative treatment.[150]

Compression of the ulnar nerve is a common condition. It can occur anywhere along the course of the nerve as a result of focal trauma or disease but most commonly occurs at the elbow. Apart from compression within the cubital tunnel itself, the ulnar nerve can less commonly be compressed at the proximal end of the so-called arcade of Struthers[14–17] by the medial intermuscular septum proximally or the arcade of Osborne (also known as the deep flexor pronator aponeurosis[151] or Osborne's fascia)[152] distally.[153]

Cubital tunnel syndrome is the second most common nerve compression syndrome after carpal tunnel syndrome and is often idiopathic.[154] Cubital tunnel syndrome can be classified as follows.[155]

1. *Physiological.* This is due to an exaggeration of the normal physiology where the reduction in the cubital tunnel volume during elbow flexion is enough to cause symptoms. This probably accounts for the 'sleep palsy' described by Gowers in 1892.
2. *Acute.* Compression to the ulnar nerve occurs with a single episode of trauma, which may be severe. It is seen in substance abusers who lie in a position that puts pressure on the ulnar nerve for prolonged periods of time.
3. *Subacute.* Compression is due to the medial elbow being in contact with a surface over a period of minutes or hours. It is seen in individuals who continually rest on their elbows or those confined to bed or wheelchair.
4. *Chronic* compression of the ulnar nerve is caused by any space-occupying lesion within the cubital tunnel. It can also be due to a lateral shift of the proximal ulna with a subsequent decrease in the cubital tunnel volume following injury to the capitellum epiphysis in childhood. In chronic cubital tunnel syndrome there is usually flattening of the ulnar nerve at the level of the compression with a fusiform swelling proximal to it.

Various non-operative and surgical treatment options have been described. Choice of treatment mainly depends on the severity of the symptoms and signs.

Basic science

Feindel and Stratford[156] named the fibro-osseous tunnel that the ulnar nerve passes through at the elbow as the cubital tunnel because of the similarity between ulnar nerve compression at the elbow and median nerve compression in the carpal tunnel. The role of occupation in nerve compression disorders remains controversial.[157,158] Cubital tunnel syndrome occurs more frequently in men than in women and is probably due to the smaller coronoid body and more abundant subcutaneous fat found in women.[159,160]

The large arc of motion that the elbow typically goes through to place the hand in positions of function during the day produces an associated decrease in the cubital tunnel volume[155,161] as the FCU aponeurosis[162] and cubital tunnel retinaculum[163] become stretched. With the elbow in extension it is almost round in shape but with flexion becomes flatter and narrower with a decrease in height of 2.5 mm[164] and resultant decrease of about 55% in volume.[161] This brings about a resultant increase in the pressure within the cubital tunnel.[165] With elbow flexion maximum extraneural pressure in the cubital tunnel has been recorded intra-operatively by Iba et al.[166] at 1 cm distal to the proximal edge of the cubital tunnel retinaculum. It is 105 ± 47 mmHg compared with only 9 ± 14 mmHg with full elbow extension. The measured extraneural pressure decreases the more distal along the cubital tunnel.

A clinical study by Werner et al.[167] on 10 patients with clinically proven elbow ulnar neuropathy showed that the mean extraneural cubital tunnel pressure increased from 9 mmHg in full extension to 63 mmHg when the elbow is flexed at 120°. However, with maximal contraction of the FCU the mean pressure increased to 92 mmHg and 209 mmHg respectively.

Gelberman et al.[168] agreed with this but also showed that during flexion of the elbow greater than 90° there is a much more significant increase in the intraneural pressure. It can go up to 45% higher than the extraneural pressure. They also found that the ulnar nerve cross-sectional area decreases up to 50% when the elbow is flexed beyond 90° without evidence of direct extrinsic compression. They believe that the significant decrease in area and parallel increase in intraneural pressure is caused by traction-related deformity of the ulnar nerve itself. Another study reported a more than three times increase in the intraneural pressure from resting level when the elbow is flexed and the wrist is extended.[169] Further elbow flexion and wrist extension combined with shoulder abduction during the throwing motion increased the intraneural pressure by up to six times the resting level. Chronic changes associated with elbow valgus overload, such as scar tissue formation, UCL calcification, traction spurs and degenerative changes within the ulnar groove, which tethers down the ulnar nerve, can cause further increases in the intraneural pressure. This can impair the intraneural microcirculation.[170]

Stretching and longitudinal excursion of the ulnar nerve occurs with elbow flexion as its course is posterior to the axis of rotation. Apfelberg and Larson[161] reported that the ulnar nerve is stretched approximately 4.7 mm during elbow flexion, while Schuind et al.[163] reported that the ulnar nerve underwent an average of 18% elongation proximal to the elbow (between the arcade of Struthers and the cubital tunnel) on full elbow flexion. However, they also reported no significant change in the ulnar nerve between the ulnar and humeral heads of the FCU. Stretching of the nerve is known to cause increased permeability of the perineurium and also interferes with the nerve microcirculation.[171] Sensory conduction is affected first before motor conduction when the nerve is stretched.

Management

HISTORY

A detailed history, including assessment of work or leisure time activities that aggravate the condition, is essential. Pain is not a typical symptom in most cases of early cubital tunnel syndrome[162] and patients, therefore, often present with late disease. Athletes tend to present with early disease as their performance is affected early on in the disease even before motor changes occur.

Typically, patients commonly present with numbness, paraesthesias and weakness in the distribution of the ulnar nerve that is gradual in onset. In early disease patients may simply state that their hands fatigue quickly with repetitive activities. When present, weakness of grip is usually with activities that require application of torque. Patients with recurrent ulnar nerve subluxation or dislocation may complain of painful popping or snapping sensations at the elbow.

Symptoms can vary and may include severe pain on the medial aspect of the elbow and paraesthesia radiating distally to the hand and sometimes proximally to the shoulder and neck. Depending on the severity, the paraesthesias might be intermittent or constant. Sensory involvement on the ulnar dorsal aspect of the hand also suggests cubital tunnel syndrome as the dorsal cutaneous branch is given off proximal to Guyon's canal.[172]

Past or present history of systemic conditions that predispose to a lower threshold for nerve irritation, such as diabetes mellitus, renal disease, multiple myeloma, amyloidosis, chronic alcohol abuse, malnutrition and leprosy should be always kept in mind.

PHYSICAL EXAMINATION

Physical examination should always start at the neck and along the course of the brachial plexus for possible peripheral nerve compression more proximally.

The elbow is then inspected for deformity followed by measurements of the normal carrying angle and active range of motion. The ulnar nerve is palpated for any enlargement or associated mass and is also clinically evaluated during elbow flexion for subluxation or dislocation.[173] Local tenderness along its course may aid in identifying the site of compression.

Tinel's sign is positive when percussion of the ulnar nerve at the medial epicondyle reproduces paraesthesias in the ring and little fingers, although it can be positive in up to 24% of asymptomatic people.[174]

Neurological examination shows initial loss of vibratory and light touch (monofilament) sensation at the autonomous zone for ulnar nerve sensation, which is the pulp of the little finger, with early disease. Disease progression will gradually lead to a two-point discrimination deficit.

A provocative test, the elbow flexion test, is performed with the elbow flexed, the forearm supinated and the wrist in extension for up to 3 minutes[175,176] and is positive when the ulnar nerve symptoms are reproduced. Similar to Phalen's test, the elbow flexion test is more sensitive than specific, and false positive results have been reported in 10% of normal individuals when it is performed with the wrist and shoulder in the neutral position.[174] The number of false positives increased when the test was performed with the shoulder abducted and the wrist extended.

Tinel's sign, the elbow flexion test (30 seconds), the pressure provocation test (30 seconds), and the combined pressure provocation with elbow flexion test is found to be 70%, 32%, 55%, and 91% sensitive, respectively.[177] Specificity is very high for all four tests at 95–99%. The sensitivity of the elbow flexion test and pressure provocation test increased to 75% and 89%, respectively, when the duration is greater (60 seconds) with very little decease in specificity. With a duration of 60 seconds, combining the elbow flexion and pressure provocation tests gives a sensitivity and specificity of 98% and 95%, respectively, with a positive predictive value of 91% and negative predictive value of 99%. Novak et al.[177] reported that 43 of the 60 participants with cubital tunnel syndrome had positive results while only two of 66 normal control subjects experienced ulnar nerve symptoms when doing the pressure provocation and elbow flexion tests in combination.

Motor deficits and muscle wasting occurs later in the disease, with intrinsic muscles of the hand being affected first as their motor fibres lie more superficial within the ulnar nerve in the cubital tunnel.[155,162] Involvement of the forearm muscles (FDP and FCU) is usually associated with more severe and advanced disease as their motor fibres lie deeper within the nerve and are better protected. In severe cases, patients will have intrinsic muscle atrophy and ulnar paradox clawing of the hand.

With disease progression the patient can develop a positive Jeanne sign (loss of key pinch due to weakness of adductor pollicis), Froment sign (flexion of the thumb interphalangeal joint with FPL during key pinch to compensate for adductor pollicis dysfunction), Duchenne sign (clawing of the ring and little fingers) and Wartenberg sign (spontaneous abduction of the little finger on extension of the fingers due to unopposed extensor digiti minimi action).[178]

DIFFERENTIAL DIAGNOSIS

As previously mentioned, there are many conditions affecting the ulnar nerve or its origins that can mimic ulnar nerve compression symptoms.

Cervical disc disease or arthritis causing cervical nerve root compression may be indicated by limitation of neck movement that is accompanied with pain, especially when there is radicular pain on axial compression of the spine (positive Spurling test). Progression to *cervical spondylitic myelopathy* leads to development of upper motor neurone signs.[179]

Brachial plexus compression will have tenderness or a positive Tinel's sign at the supraclavicular and infraclavicular areas.[175]

Thoracic outlet syndrome most commonly involves the lower trunk of the brachial plexus and can reproduce symptoms similar to cubital tunnel syndrome. Provocative tests for thoracic outlet syndrome, such as Adson's manoeuvre, Wright's manoeuvre, Roos's test and the costoclavicular manoeuvre, are frequently positive in normal individuals and are therefore non-specific in patients with mainly neurogenic complains. For any of these tests to be relevant when positive it should reproduce the patient's symptoms also. Also, look for weakness of periscapular and proximal arm muscles and multiple nerve involvements.

An apical tumour of the lung can also compress or invade the inferior brachial plexus causing ulnar nerve symptoms.

Pancoast tumour should be considered whenever a history of smoking with ulnar nerve symptom and shoulder pain is reported. Presence of a Horner's syndrome distinguishes it from ulnar neuropathy.[179] A chest radiograph will be necessary to rule it out.

Syringomelia, a cavitary lesion of the spinal cord, usually affects C8 motor and pain/temperature sensory functions while sparing large-fibre sensation. Biceps reflex is also affected. There is multiple nerve involvement with patchy sensory loss.

Amyotrophic lateral sclerosis affects multiple nerves but sensory function is intact. There are muscle fasciculations present.

Systemic and metabolic disorders such as diabetes mellitus, hypothyroidism, alcoholism, malignancies and vitamin deficiencies should also be included in the differential diagnosis. Presence of any of these conditions does not exclude the possibility of a concomitant ulnar nerve compressive neuropathy.

Other conditions that might present with similar symptoms are amyotrophic lateral sclerosis, Guillain–Barré syndrome, Charcot–Marie–Tooth disease and hereditary neuropathy with liability to pressure palsies and should be considered in likely patients during the history and physical examination.

INVESTIGATIONS

The diagnosis of cubital tunnel syndrome is primarily clinical. Electrodiagnostic testing can confirm the site of ulnar nerve compression and quantify its severity. However, it is not sensitive enough to be used as a screening tool. It is important to remember that the results of electrodiagnostic testing are very dependent on the skills of the technician performing it and, to a certain extent, on the level of cooperation by the patient.[173] Exchange of information between the clinician and the electromyographer would greatly help in understanding of the problem being evaluated and the proper electrodiagnostic studies required to help with the diagnosis.[180]

Guidelines have been formulated on the use of nerve conduction studies as a diagnostic aid, such as the American Association of Electrodiagnostic Medicine criteria,[181] where positive diagnosis of ulnar neuropathy includes one of the following:

1. absolute slowing of nerve conduction at the elbow
2. decreased conduction velocity of more than 10 m s^{-1} across the elbow
3. decreased amplitude of more than 20%
4. absence of sensory responses
5. evidence of muscle atrophy.

Conduction velocities are measured across the elbow with the intrinsic musculature used for motor velocity and the small finger for sensory velocity. Parameters for accurate testing include flexing the elbow between 70° and 90° when measuring conduction at the elbow,[182] although others have advocated flexing at 135°.[180] The recommended length to obtain the most accurate measurement of conduction across the elbow is 100 mm,[183] although previous studies have supported lengths of 50–80 mm.[184] An absolute measurement for motor conduction velocity of less than 50 m s^{-1} across the elbow or a difference of more than 10 m s^{-1} between measurements across the elbow and below the elbow is indicative of compression.[185] Other electrodiagnostic abnormalities that may indicate cubital tunnel syndrome are distal motor latency of more than 8.7 ms with stimulation from above the elbow to the abductor digiti minimi,[186] motor latency of 3.5 ms or more from the wrist to the hypothenar muscles and a sensory latency of 3 ms and greater from the little finger to the wrist,[22] and a surface short segment incremental stimulation latency change of greater than 0.4 ms over a 1 cm segment.[187] Abnormal electrodiagnostic findings of the asymptomatic contralateral limb may be found in up to 36.7% of patients, although it is only found bilaterally in 8–19% of patients.[188]

Electromyography will reveal whether axonal degeneration has occurred, which is usually in advanced disease. The first dorsal interosseous muscle is most commonly affected. The abductor pollicis brevis should be examined to exclude a C8/T1 nerve root or inferior brachial plexus lesion.

Interestingly, a recent study found that the prognosis of patients with focal demyelination of the ulnar nerve (presenting with a motor conduction block of ⩾50% on electrodiagnostic examination) is more favourable than those without (motor conduction block ⩽20%).[189] However, the sample size in the study is relatively small and a prospective randomized study is required to evaluate this hypothesis further.

Radiographic examination of the elbow is useful in a small percentage of patients, i.e. those with arthritis, history of trauma or abnormal elbow motion or carrying angle as revealed by physical examination. Associated bony pathological changes may be seen on plain radiographs, especially with the cubital tunnel view.[155] When comparing the findings with this view between patients with cubital tunnel syndrome and normal control subjects, St John and Palmaz[190] found medial trochlear lip osteophytes in 20% of the patients with none in the controls. They also found that 29% of patients have a greater than 5 mm difference in the projection of the trochlea and the olecranon versus 6% only in control subjects.

Ultrasonography can also be used to aid in the diagnosis. Although it is operator dependent, has a long learning curve, produces images that can be difficult to interpret and provides a limited range of information, it is a dynamic examination modality with none of the contraindications for MRI and is largely preferred by patients.[191] Subluxation and dislocation of the ulnar nerve on elbow flexion are easily identifiable with ultrasound examination. Presence of a bony spur, ganglion, thickened retinaculum or an anomalous anconeus epitrochlearis muscle compressing the ulnar nerve in the cubital tunnel can be also be demonstrated.

Staging and grading

A number of classification systems have been developed since the mid-twentieth century to attempt to stage the severity of the disease. As with any staging classification, the main purpose of having one is twofold: to standardize the reporting of patients with cubital tunnel syndrome, and as a tool for the prognosis and planning of treatment options. With a common standard made available the results after an intervention, both non-operative and surgical, could be critically evaluated. A review of the staging or grading classifications found in the literature is presented below.

The first staging classification was introduced by McGowan in 1950.[192] It is based mainly on the severity of the ulnar nerve motor dysfunction at the time of surgery. There are three grades of severity and in his series of 46 patients six were grade I, 27 grade II and 13 grade III. He defined grade I as *minimal lesions with no detectable motor weakness of the hand*. However, in the text of his paper, the associated symptoms in the patients with grade I disease were paraesthesia in the ulnar area and a feeling of clumsiness in the affected hand. Examination reveals no wasting or weakness of the ulnar intrinsic muscles but mild paraesthesia is present. The sweating test may reveal a slight but definite hyperhidrosis of the ulnar area.

Grade II was defined as *intermediate lesions*, in which there is obvious intrinsic muscle wasting but some voluntary power is usually retained. In assessing the motor function the interossei were frequently more severely affected than the hypothenar or proximal muscles. Sensory disturbance can vary from paraesthesia (tingling sensation) to anaesthesia and analgesia. Sweating was always preserved with hyperhidrosis present in some patients.

The definition for grade III was *severe lesions with paralysis of one or more of the ulnar intrinsic muscles*. The interossei were found to be paralysed in all patients with marked weakness of the hand. However, weak voluntary power may be retained in the first dorsal interosseous and hypothenar muscles in some patients, with preservation of the forearm muscles in most. There is marked hypoaesthesia to complete anaesthesia and analgesia. Sweating is preserved with hyperhidrosis in most.

As evidenced above, McGowan's staging can be very subjective and may be difficult to be exactly reproduced by another examiner or in another set of patients. Furthermore, it may not be accurate in staging the disease because, as we now know, sensory dysfunction occurs earlier than motor dysfunction in nerve compression neuropathy.

Wilson and Krout[193] described a postoperative grading system to help them analyse the results of 16 patients who had *in situ* decompression performed. Excellent is defined as having an essentially normal elbow with minimal motor or sensory changes and no tenderness over the site of surgery. Good is when there is general resolution of symptoms with occasional ache/tenderness at the site of surgery and mild residual decreased sensibility but no motor loss along the ulnar nerve distribution. Fair is improved symptoms but with persistent moderate sensory changes, residual motor weakness, discomfort at the surgical site and positive elbow flexion test. Poor shows no improvement or a worse outcome postoperatively.

A more objective rating system that can be useful in reporting clinical data was described in 1986.[194] A score of between 0 (worse) and 3 (normal) is given for pain and dysfunction of the ulnar sensory and motor components in the hand (Table 121.3). A lower score denotes more severe symptoms.

Using this rating system Gabel and Amadio[195] were better able to classify the results on their series of patients who underwent reoperation for a failed ulnar nerve decompression. Results are deemed excellent if the score is 9 points; good if the score is ≥2 points for each category with a total score increase of ≥1 point, or total score increase of ≥4 points; fair if the score is <2 points in any category but the total score increase is 1–3 points; and poor if there is no change in scores or a decrease in the total score, when comparing the pre-operative and postoperative scores.

In the same year another classification system that incorporates both nerve conduction study findings and clinical symptoms in grading ulnar neuropathy was also described. It is divided into five stages as shown in Table 121.4. Okamoto and colleagues used the Akahori grading system to correlate severity of the ulnar neuropathy and their ultrasonography findings. Currently, this method of classifying ulnar neuropathy in cubital tunnel syndrome is probably the most objective available as it utilizes the findings of an investigation modality commonly used to aid the diagnosis of this condition, instead of just physical examination signs alone. Further investigation is warranted to validate its use in reporting clinical study results.

A staging classification that incorporates not only the sensory and motor findings but also specific tests performed during physical examination was later developed by Dellon[196] (Table 121.5). It is based on the pathophysiological concepts of chronic nerve compression available at that time. Using this staging system he attempted to reinterpret the results of 50 published reports on more than 2000 patients who were treated for ulnar nerve compression at the elbow between 1898 and 1988.

The 12-point Bishop rating system was used by Kleinman and Bishop[197] to objectively and subjectively grade the surgical results on their series of 45 anterior intramuscular transpositions. It is a point demerit system that assesses the patient satisfaction, strength, sensation, residual symptoms, improvement, work status and leisure activity (Table 121.6). Black *et al.*[198] also used this rating

Table 121.3 Rating scale for ulnar neuropathy at the elbow as first described by Amadio in 1986

Score	Description
Category: pain	
0	Need regular narcotics
1	Constant pain but intermittent medication
2	Intermittent pain
3	No pain
Category: sensory findings	
0	2-PD >10 mm with anaesthesia
1	2-PD >6 mm with constant numbness
2	2-PD normal with intermittent paraesthesia
3	No numbness
Category: motor findings	
0	Intrinsic muscle paralysis with ulnar clawing, muscle power grade 0 or 1
1	Obvious intrinsic muscle atrophy, muscle power grade 2 or 3
2	Weaker than unaffected side, muscle power grade 4
3	Muscle power grade 5 (McGowan grade 1)

2-PD, 2-point discrimination.
Adapted from Gabel GT, Amadio PC. Reoperation for failed decompression of the ulnar nerve in the region of the elbow. *Journal of Bone and Joint Surgery (American)* 1990;**72**:213–19.

Table 121.4 Classification system for ulnar neuropathy as first described by Akahori in 1986

Stage	Conduction velocity			Clinical symptoms		
	Motor nerve	Sensory nerve	Sensory	Muscle atrophy	Muscle weakness	Ulnar clawing
I	Normal	Normal	Normal or mild paraesthesia	Mild	Mild	Absent
II	Normal	Slowed	Hypoaesthesia+	Present	Mild	Mild
III	Normal or slowed	Slowed or unmeasurable	Hypoaesthesia+	Present	Present	Mild or present
IV	Slowed	Unmeasurable	Hypoaesthesia++	Severe	Severe	Severe
V	Slowed or unmeasurable	Unmeasurable	Hypoaesthesia++ or analgesia	Severe	Severe	Severe

Adapted from Okamoto M, Abe M, Shirai H, Ueda N. Diagnostic ultrasonography of the ulnar nerve in cubital tunnel syndrome. *Journal of Hand Surgery (British)* 2000;**25**:499–502.

Table 121.5 Staging of ulnar nerve compression at the elbow

Stage	Description	Sensory	Motor	Tests
0	Normal	No pain or numbness	No weakness	No positive findings
1	Mild	Intermittent paraesthesia, increase vibration perception	Subjective weakness, clumsiness or loss of coordination	Elbow flexion test and/or Tinel's sign may be positive
2	Moderate	Intermittent paraesthesia, normal or decreased vibration perception	Measureable weakness for pinch and/or grip strength	Positive elbow flexion test and/or Tinel's sign, finger crossing may be abnormal
3	Severe	Persistent paraesthesia, decreased vibration perception, abnormal 2-PD (static ⩾6 mm, moving ⩾4 mm)	Measurable weakness in pinch and grip with muscle atrophy present	Positive elbow flexion test and/or Tinel's sign, finger crossing usually abnormal

Adapted from Dellon AL. Review of treatment results for ulnar nerve entrapment at the elbow. *Journal of Hand Surgery (American)* 1989;**14**:688–700.

system to grade the long-term outcome of their series of 51 anterior subcutaneous transpositions. A score of 10–12 points is deemed excellent, 7–9 points good, 4–6 points fair and 0–3 points as poor.

A scoring system that evaluated the amount of numbness, sensation, muscle strength and muscle atrophy was developed in 1997[199] (Table 121.7). It is based on the work done by Stuffer et al.[200] Grading of the patient depends on the total score achieved, with a score of 0–3 as poor, 4–6 as fair, 7–9 as good and 10–12 as excellent.

In 2001, Dellon[201] put forward a grading system that assigns a numerical value for actual measurements of the sensory and motor functions of the ulnar nerve (Table 121.8), which he has actually been using since 1991. A higher value indicates a more severe degree of impairment. The sensory, motor and overall values can be mathematically analysed using parametric statistical methods. Application of this numerical grading system is rather exhaustive and is probably useful only when applied in a prospective clinical study.

With the myriad systems available to stage or grade cubital tunnel syndrome pre- and postoperatively, it is no wonder there is much difficulty comparing the results of the numerous clinical data published to date relating to the various treatments. It is interesting to note that most of these systems were developed within a short space of time in the mid-1980s to late 1990s. It is very possible that a standard staging and grading system will need to be devised in consensus by an authoritative body before a well-designed proper multicentre prospective randomized study can be undertaken to firmly decide on the best course of treatment for cubital tunnel syndrome.

Treatment

In many patients symptoms of ulnar nerve compression are often transient and are related to the resting position of the limb. Most individuals do not seek treatment and learn to avoid positions that bring on the symptoms. It is important to note that approximately half of patients with untreated cubital tunnel syndrome have been reported to improve spontaneously.[202]

Although there have been many papers published in the literature with regards to ulnar nerve compression at the elbow and its treatment, no specific or standard guidelines are available yet. In general, non-operative treatment modalities for cubital tunnel syndrome are indicated in mild to moderate disease.[203] Patients with intermittent symptoms, no muscle wasting and mild electrodiagnostic findings are the ones who usually respond well non-operatively. Surgical treatment is indicated in failure of non-operative treatment and in those with severe or end-stage ulnar nerve dysfunction.

NON-OPERATIVE TREATMENT MODALITIES

Conservative treatment for patients presenting with ulnar nerve compression at the elbow has only been suggested in the literature from 1970.[196,204] This seems to be related to an increase in the number of reports on patients with ulnar nerve compression at the elbow who have no history of trauma. Prior to that reports on ulnar neuropathy are usually associated with a history of elbow fracture and dislocation or direct soft-tissue injury to the elbow.

Non-operative treatment is indicated for cases without objective neurological deficit.[153] The goals for non-operative treatment are

1. to decrease the frequency of symptoms or eliminate them altogether
2. to prevent further progression of the condition.

A review of the literature by Dellon[196] found that approximately half of patients with mild compression symptoms recover with non-operative treatment. Another study by him demonstrated that 89% of patients without electrodiagnostic findings do not require surgery, as opposed to 67% of those with threshold changes in the sensorimotor system and 38% with decreased innervation density in the sensorimotor system.[204] In other words, the resolution of symptoms with non-operative treatment has an inverse relationship to the severity of the condition at the start of treatment, whereas the likelihood of having surgery is directly proportional.

In their series of patients, Beekman et al. found that, in 46 elbows undergoing non-operative treatment, 11% had complete remission, 24% improved, 39% did not change and 26% progressed after an average follow-up period of 16.3 months. This is compared with 25% remission, 36% improvement, 39% stable and 14% progression

Table 121.6 The 12-point Bishop rating system for grading final postoperative outcomes for cubital tunnel syndrome

Criteria	Points
Satisfaction	
Satisfied	2
Satisfied with reservation	1
Dissatisfied	0
Improvement	
Better	2
Unchanged	1
Worse	0
Severity of residual symptoms (pain, paraesthesia, dysaesthesia, weakness, clumsiness)	
Asymptomatic	3
Mild/occasional	2
Moderate	1
Severe	0
Work status	
Working or able to work at previous job	1
Not working due to symptoms	0
Leisure activity	
Unlimited	1
Limited	0
Strength	
Grasp and pinch ≥80% of unaffected side	2
Either one only is <80%	1
Both grasp and pinch <80%	0
Sensibility (static 2-PD)	
Normal (≤5 mm)	1
Abnormal (>5 mm)	0
Maximum total points	12

Adapted from Kleinman WB, Bishop AT. Anterior intramuscular transposition of the ulnar nerve. *Journal of Hand Surgery (American)* 1989;**14**:972–9.

Table 121.7 The scoring table for the modified method of Stuffer *et al.* scoring system

Criteria	0	1	2	3
Numbness	Severe, ADL disturbed	Moderate as a complaint	Slight not complained	None
Sensation	Lacking, below 5/10	Diminished (+) 6/10 to 7/10	Diminished (±) 8/10 to 9/10 abnormal 2-PD	Normal, 10/10
Muscle strength	Paralysis	Weakness (+)	Weakness (±)	Normal
Manual muscle testing	Below poor, claw finger	Fair	Good, Froment sign (+)	
Muscle atrophy	Severe, FDIO + other muscles	Moderate FDIO (+)	Slight FDIO (±)	None

ADL, activities of daily living; FDIO, first dorsal interosseus muscle.
Adapted from Tada H, Hirayama T, Katsuki M, Habaguchi T. Long term results using a modified King's method for cubital tunnel syndrome. *Clinical Orthopaedics and Related Research* 1997;**336**:107–10.

Table 121.8 Numerical grading of ulnar nerve compression at the elbow. S2-PD, static two-point discrimination; m2-PD, moving two-point discrimination

Numerical score Sensory	Motor	Description of impairment
0	0	None
1		Intermittent paraesthesia
	2	Mild weakness of pinch/grip ♀10–14/26–39 lbs (4.5–6.4/12–18 kg) ♂13–19/31–59 lbs (6–9/14–27 kg)
3		Abnormal threshold SW monofilament 3.22–3.61 Biothesiometer 3–10 Pressure-specified sensory device <45 years old, ≤3 mm at 1.0–20.0 g mm^{-2} ≥45 years old, ≤4 mm at 1.9–20.0 g mm^{-2}
	4	Weakness of pinch/grip ♀6–9/15–25 lbs (3–4/9–11 kg) ♂6–12/15–30 lbs (3–5.5/9–13.5 kg)
5		Persistent paraesthesia
6		Abnormal 2-PD little finger: s2-PD 7–10 mm, m2-PD 4–6 mm Pressure-specified sensory device <45 years old, ≥4 mm <8 mm at any g mm^{-2} ≥45 years old, ≤5 mm <9 mm at any gm mm^{-2}
	7	Muscle wasting (1–2/4)
8		Abnormal 2-PD little finger: s2-PD ≥11 mm, m2-PD ≥7 mm Pressure-specified sensory device <45 years old, ≥8 mm at any g mm^{-2} ≥45 years old, ≥9 mm at any g mm^{-2}
9		Anaesthesia
	10	Muscle wasting (3–4/4)

Adapted from Dellon AL. Clinical grading of peripheral nerve problems. *Neurosurgery Clinics of North America* 2001;**12**:229–40.

in 28 elbows that were treated surgically with an average follow-up period of 13.8 months.

Seradge and Owen[205] reported that, out of 336 patients from their cohort of 347 patients with cubital tunnel syndrome, 176 (52.3%) responded to non-operative treatment of between 2 and 57 months (mean period of 8 months). They also found that the length of non-operative management did not adversely affect the eventual surgical outcome. Therefore, based on the above studies, a period of at least 3–6 months of supervised non-operative treatment for all patients presenting with this condition is advocated.

Non-surgical treatment modalities for cubital tunnel syndrome consist of the following.

1. *Patient education.* Many patients are unaware of the cause of their discomfort and pain. Understanding their anatomy can be very informative for patients and enables them to modify their daily activities to protect the ulnar nerve at the elbow.

2. *Activity modification/ergonomic measures.* Avoidance of tasks with repetitive elbow flexion and extension can be difficult as few hand tools are available that can substitute this motion. Limiting the arc of motion to a more extended range and decreasing repetition is helpful; however, some sort of job modification may be required. Among steps that can be taken are: replacing hand tools with pneumatic ones, adjusting chair height and distance from the keyboard, removing chair arms, the padding of desk edges, moving the car seat further away from the steering wheel, using a telephone headset or shoulder cradle, avoiding the crossing of forearms and resting the forearms in supination on the thighs.[204,206] All these measures can decrease stress across the cubital tunnel and also limit the need for elbow-flexed positions. An elbow pad can also be used during work to help prevent direct pressure on the ulnar nerve. It can also help to remind the patient to avoid flexing the elbow.[206]

3. *NSAIDs.* There are no studies available that specifically look at the efficacy of these medications in cubital tunnel syndrome. Their use as part of the non-operative treatment regimen should be individualized to the patient's specific needs and problems.

4. *Splinting.* An effective method for treating cubital tunnel syndrome and has played a successful role when used together with activity modification. The type and durability of the splint used and the patient's compliance are important considerations to ensure effectiveness of the treatment protocol. A patient's compliance with treatment depends on the comfort, practicality and cosmetic appearance of the splint being used.[207,208]

Splints that prevent elbow flexion beyond 90° help to reduce the strain and increase in pressure on the ulnar nerve. An overall improvement of 86.3% had been reported with the use of long-term (average 8.7 months) long-arm splinting that not only limits elbow flexion to between 45° and 70° but also supports the wrist to decrease tension on the FCU.[208]

Night splinting has also been shown to be beneficial.[209] It is suggested that the elbow is kept from going beyond 60° of flexion with the forearm in neutral rotation during sleep. Protecting the ulnar nerve may be done by having a pillow between the upper limb and the trunk. Wrapping a towel around the elbow at night or using an elbow pad in reverse over the antecubital fossa effectively limits elbow flexion.[185,204,206] Better immobilization can be achieved by using a thermoplastic long-arm splint over the volar aspect of the arm. However, it is important to ensure that none of the straps used to secure it cross over the ulnar nerve at the cubital tunnel.

There is no widely accepted consensus available on the duration of treatment, type of splinting and degree of splinting. When there is constant pain and paraesthesia a rigid thermoplastic splint keeping the elbow at less than 45° flexion can be applied, usually on the volar side. Initially, it should be worn all the time but can be worn at night only when symptoms subside.[206] The splint should also be worn while at work, although this may relegate the patient to being one-handed.[185,210] Necessary adjustments specific to the individual patient will have to be made by the resident therapist and surgeon during clinical visits.

5. *Physical therapy.* Exercises are mainly for athletes who want to maintain their strength while preventing further irritation to the ulnar nerve. Isometric and isotonic strengthening of elbow flexors and extensors within a 0–45° arc minimize stretch to the nerve. Ulnar nerve gliding exercises that mobilize the entire course of the nerve require a skilled therapist to implement. General stretching and strengthening exercises to the chest, shoulder, back and neck can help to modify posture.

6. *Steroid injections.* Response of patients with cubital tunnel syndrome to steroid injections is questionable. There are limited studies available that either recommend perineural steroid injections[211] or find it not beneficial.[212] Some authors advise against its use[213,214] in cubital tunnel syndrome or caution against its use[173] because of concerns regarding potential complications, such as skin depigmentation, possible intraneural injection and subcutaneous fat atrophy.

In throwing athletes a trial of conservative treatment is usually initiated with rest, ice and NSAIDs.[183] A period of elbow immobilization for 2–3 weeks may be necessary, especially if the ulnar nerve is clinically subluxating or dislocating. The athlete's throwing mechanics should also be reviewed to make sure that it is not contributing to the occurrence of the condition.[102] Local injections of steroids are not recommended. For many athletes a recurrence of symptoms can occur on resumption of throwing activities, especially if they have associated valgus instability of the elbow, and ultimately will require surgical intervention of some sort.[95]

SURGICAL TREATMENT

There are a number of methods that have been well described in the literature for the surgical treatment of cubital tunnel syndrome, namely

1. *in situ* decompression
2. medial epicondylectomy
3. anterior transposition, which can be
   a. subcutaneous
   b. intramuscular
   c. submuscular.

Other less well-known surgical techniques that have been recently described in the literature are anterior subfascial transposition[215,216] and cubital tunnel reconstruction.[217] However, the number of patients in these studies is far too small to draw any conclusions despite the good outcomes reported.

Previous reviews of the literature, including the use of meta-analysis and systematic review methods,[154,196,218,219] failed to find a mutual consensus on the best surgical treatment that can be applied on all patients with cubital tunnel syndrome.[220] Medical practitioners treating this condition will have to keep abreast of the latest developments as more information regarding the pathophysiology and disease spectrum for cubital tunnel syndrome becomes available. Hopefully this will lead to the formation of a treatment algorithm using a standardized staging classification for the treatment of cubital tunnel syndrome in the near future. Careful selection of patients and, if required, choosing the most suitable surgical treatment option will have to be tailored on a case-by-case basis by the attending surgeon.[221,222] Knowledge and experience of the different surgical methods may be necessary to enable a fallback procedure should intra-operative findings necessitate a change in the type of surgery required. Sometimes the pathology is identified to be at a specific location other than the cubital tunnel and may necessitate either an additional procedure or another procedure on its own.[151]

In situ decompression

In situ decompression of the cubital tunnel was probably first reported by Fèvre in 1878 as liberation and elongation of the ulnar nerve,[150] although other authors[210,223] attribute the first description to Buzzard in 1922.[224] The presence of what is now known as the arcade of Osborne was first described during the British Orthopaedic Association Autumn Meeting in 1957 by Geoffrey Osborne.[12] He considered that tardy ulnar neuritis is due to compression by this fibrous band and reported a good outcome, similar to anterior transposition, with simple division of this band in 13 patients. However, it was in the following year that the surgical technique of *in situ* decompression of the ulnar nerve was first described in detail by Feindel and Stratford.[156]

Since then there have been a number of papers that reported good results with the use of this method.[193,225–237] Most are on a small number of patients. Nathan et al.[238] reported excellent outcomes in their series of 102 elbows on intermediate and long-term follow-up of up to 12.4 years. They also recommended an early start to rehabilitation on the day after surgery as it is associated with an early return to work (within 3 weeks postoperatively) and activities of daily living.[232] After reviewing the records of 100 patients, Macnicol[239] recommended *in situ* decompression in cases with a short history of ulnar nerve compression and no obvious ulnar nerve dislocations or adhesions in the region. As to be expected, patients with more severe electrodiagnostic findings (absent sensory nerve conduction) have less improvement of sensory symptoms after surgery, be it *in situ* decompression or anterior subcutaneous decompression.[240]

Prospective studies that compared *in situ* decompression with anterior subcutaneous transposition,[241–243] anterior submuscular transposition[244,245] or both anterior subcutaneous and submuscular transposition[221] showed no real difference in the postoperative outcomes, even in patients with severe (Dellon stage 3) disease.[245] In their prospective randomized controlled study, Bartels et al.[241] reported a lower complication rate (9.6%) with *in situ* decompression than with anterior subcutaneous transposition (31.1%). This is also demonstrated by Biggs and Curtis[244] with three out of 21 patients in the anterior submuscular transposition group experiencing deep infection compared with none in the *in situ* decompression group. Bartels et al.[246] also reported a median cost that is 2.5 times lower with *in situ* decompression than with anterior subcutaneous transposition. Gervasio et al.[245] demonstrated that patients returned to work earlier after having *in situ* decompression by an average of 9 days than after anterior submuscular transposition. Foster and Edshage[247] found better relief of paraesthesia and return of intrinsic muscle function with anterior subcutaneous transposition than *in situ* decompression in their series of 48 patients, although relief from pain and dysaesthesia is equal.

When the literature was reviewed by Dellon in 1989[196] and Mowlavi et al.[218] in 2000 postoperative outcomes were similar in patients with mild compression for all surgical treatment methods. In their meta-analysis of four randomized controlled trials comparing *in situ* decompression with anterior transposition (two subcutaneous and two submuscular), Zlowodzki et al.[219] found no significant difference in the postoperative clinical outcomes or motor nerve conduction velocities and suggested that *in situ* decompression is a reasonable alternative to anterior transposition for the surgical management of cubital tunnel syndrome.

Because of these studies, *in situ* decompression is only recommended for selected patients, those with a short history and mild disease conditions, because it has fewer complications and is also less invasive.[223] However, this surgical technique has fallen out of favour among the orthopaedic surgeons and orthopaedic hand surgeons[223] in recent years, probably due to the evidence suggesting, as discussed in more detail earlier in this chapter, that traction injury of the ulnar nerve contributes more towards the development of cubital tunnel syndrome. Current opinion in the orthopaedic literature suggests that *in situ* decompression is contraindicated in severe compressive neuropathy, especially when there is perineural and nerve bed scarring, a space-occupying lesion in the ulnar groove, or habitual ulnar nerve subluxation/dislocation.[210] It is also not recommended in patients with abnormal two-point discrimination testing or evidence of progressive motor loss and when the elbow flexion test is positive.[223] Recent neurosurgical literature is advocating the use of *in situ* decompression over anterior transposition as the initial procedure in first-time patients.[248]

Medial epicondylectomy

This is another form of ulnar nerve decompression that allows the nerve to lie anterior to the axis of rotation of the elbow. However, instead of transposing the nerve itself, the floor of the cubital tunnel is removed to enable anterior displacement of the nerve.

Medial epicondylectomy was first described by King in 1950.[249] Morgan contributed an appendix to King's report that briefly described the surgical technique in which >40% of the medial epicondyle was removed. Their follow-up paper in 1959[250] reported no more pain in 19 of 20 patients with complete sensory recovery in 11 and complete motor recovery in eight out of 16 patients with motor loss. Over the next 20 years few reports on this technique were found in the literature.[251,252]

From 1979 onwards, there have been many papers published[199,205,253–260] that report relatively good results with the use of this surgical method in treating cubital tunnel syndrome. Good or excellent results ranged from 65% to 98%. Unfortunately, the staging classifications and grading criteria used are not uniform and most series are small, ranging from 19 to 46 patients. Follow-up periods were also wide-ranging. Although most are prospective studies others[205,256] are retrospective analyses of case notes.

Seradge and Owen[205] performed medial epicondylectomy on 160 out of 347 patients, the biggest series to date, with 93% having McGowan grade II or III cubital tunnel syndrome preoperatively. Using Wilson and Krout's[193] postoperative grading system, described earlier, they reported 87% (139 patients) with excellent or good results, 12% (19 patients) with fair and 1% (two patients) with poor outcomes. However, this is a retrospective study, rather than a prospective one.

From 43 patients in their report, Heithoff et al.[257] were able to look at the postoperative radiographs of 34 patients and found that only 16 patients (47%) had a complete osteotomy of the medial epicondyle; of the remaining 18 patients, 12 and six patients had partial or minimal osteotomies, respectively. They also noted a 5–10% loss in grip and pinch strength measurements in their patients with excellent or good results, but believed that this was not due to the medial epicondylectomy procedure itself.

In their prospective randomized study, Geutjens et al.[261] reported that patients were more satisfied after having medial epicondylectomy than after anterior transposition. However, objective outcomes that were measured are similar.

One of the most mentioned complications for medial epicondylectomy is potential medial instability of the elbow joint due to injury to the AMCL. O'Driscoll et al.[262] demonstrated that the AMCL arises from the anteroinferior surface of the medial epicondyle and is preserved if only 20% or less (1–4 mm) of the medial epicondyle is removed in the coronal plane. More bone can be removed if the plane for the osteotomy is made obliquely between the sagittal and coronal planes. When more than 40% of the medial epicondyle is removed valgus instability of the elbow was significantly greater.[263]

Anterior transposition

This has been in use since the late nineteenth century for the treatment of ulnar neuropathy at the elbow, well before *in situ* decompression became popular. It relieves the biomechanical factors believed to contribute towards the nerve injury by placing the ulnar nerve anterior to the axis of movement in the elbow.[264]

Watchmaker *et al.*[265] defined the intraneural topography of the first motor branch to the ulnar nerve and found that it could be traced back between 6.0 cm and 7.5 cm within the main ulnar nerve trunk before interfascicular mingling occurred. They concluded that proximal separation of this branch of up to 6 cm within the main trunk may be performed to facilitate anterior transposition.

The most voiced concerns for anterior transposition of the ulnar nerve are relative ischaemia due to the disruption of its blood supply and adhesions due to increased perineural scarring. The mesoneurium not only provides the framework for the segmental supply to the nerve, it also facilitates the excursion of the nerve without disrupting its blood supply.[266] Damaging the mesoneurium during dissection could potentiate tethering of the nerve, via adhesions, to the surrounding tissues, resulting in increased traction forces to the nerve. In 1985 Ogata *et al.*[267] reported their study on the effects of *in situ* decompression, medial epicondylectomy and anterior subcutaneous transposition on the regional blood flow to the ulnar nerve in non-human primates. They demonstrated a significant decrease in the blood flow after anterior subcutaneous transposition, not seen with *in situ* decompression or medial epicondylectomy, which lasted for at least 3 days postoperatively. However, this relative ischaemia is transient and adequate longitudinal intraneural collateral circulation is restored by the fourth to seventh postoperative day. To address this issue, some authors[268] advocated performing anterior transposition of the ulnar nerve together with its vascular bundle and have reported good results. In this instance the ulnar nerve was transposed either submuscularly or intramuscularly. Another study in baboons found no significant adherence of the ulnar nerve to the flexor–pronator muscles 3 months after either intramuscular or submuscular anterior transposition.[269]

There is also the potential risk of creating new areas of compression when rerouting the nerve. Therefore it is important to ensure that all potential sites of compression are released during anterior transposition and the ability of the transposed ulnar nerve to glide unimpeded in its new bed is diligently checked time and again before closure.

Anterior subcutaneous transposition was first described in 1898 by Curtis.[270] He reported performing the procedure on a patient with ulnar neuritis following trauma to the elbow. With this technique the ulnar nerve is dissected out and rerouted subcutaneously anterior to the axis of rotation of the elbow. It is reported to be the most commonly used technique as it is the least difficult technically and has a high success rate.[271] Richmond and Southmayd[272] reported the results on their series of 18 anterior subcutaneous transpositions with epineurial neurolysis performed on 16 patients as being 83% good to excellent, 5% satisfactory and 12% unsatisfactory. The transposed ulnar nerve was sutured to the underlying deep fascia to keep it in place.

In 1980 Eaton *et al.*[273] described a modification of this technique where a 'fasciodermal sling' is created to prevent the nerve from slipping back posteriorly and also to provide additional soft-tissue cover. Recent publications[274,275] and clinical papers[198,242,276,277] on anterior subcutaneous transposition describe Eaton's modification. Another modification using the medial intermuscular septum as a fascial sling was described in 1998 by Pribyl and Robinson.[278] In both methods early elbow rehabilitation was recommended. Black *et al.*[198] reported a much earlier return to work if immediate range of motion is initiated postoperatively (10 days on average) than in patients who were immobilized with a cast for the first 2 weeks (30 days on average).

Although subcutaneous transposition is technically easier to perform, many authors caution its use in the thin patient who does not have enough subcutaneous fat to adequately protect the transposed ulnar nerve, and also in athletes as they run the risk of reinjuring the relatively unprotected nerve. Interestingly, in Eaton's paper,[273] seven out of the 16 patients that he reported on were baseball pitchers of varying levels who experienced transient but severe ulnar nerve paraesthesias when throwing. All returned to pitching postoperatively without further symptoms. In the management of athletes with cubital tunnel syndrome, anterior subcutaneous transposition has gained popularity over the traditional submuscular technique because of the more aggressive rehabilitation that can be done following surgery.[146] Typically, range of motion exercises can begin within the first 10 days, flexor–pronator strengthening exercises can commence as early as the third to fourth week, with a return to competition between 12 and 16 weeks. In contrast, elbow range of motion is only started by the second week after anterior submuscular transposition, with aggressive flexor–pronator strengthening only commencing at 8 weeks postoperatively and a typical return to sports at 5–6 months.

Anterior intramuscular transposition was described as a technique used after repair of a transacted nerve by Klauser in 1917.[150] Maintenance of the anteriorly transposed ulnar nerve by intramuscular stabilization was proposed by Adson[279] in 1918. With this technique the transposed ulnar nerve is placed within a 5 mm trough created in the flexor–pronator muscle mass and closed over with the repaired flexor–pronator fascia. Platt[280] reported on its use for treating ulnar nerve palsy in 1926 and by the mid-twentieth century it had become the treatment of choice for post-traumatic tardy ulnar nerve paralysis.[281]

Comparatively, there are fewer reports available in the literature on the outcomes of performing anterior intramuscular transposition. Gay and Love[281] used the technique described by Adson, but without the fascial sleeve, in 95 of the 100 cases that they reported on. Although they mentioned 70% of the patients as having satisfactory results, they did not quantify their results sufficiently to enable it to be compared with other methods of anterior transposition. Fifty-four of the patients also had neurolysis performed at the same time and only four patients had anterior subcutaneous transposition done.

Kleinman and Bishop[197] reported on 43 cases that had anterior intermuscular transposition with a mean follow-up period of 28 months: 87% were graded as excellent or good using the Bishop rating system. No patients required reoperation in their series.

Leone and colleagues[282] reported on 34 patients with Dellon stage 3 (severe) cubital tunnel syndrome who had 39 anterior intramuscular transposition procedures done. Initial results showed clinical improvement in 77% of patients at an average of 3.34 months follow-up, which later decreased to 62% at a mean follow-up period of 30.9 months. Younger patients (<50 years old), patients who have it as a second procedure, and those who had concurrent external neurolysis have less satisfactory results.

A modified anterior intramuscular transposition technique that incorporates features of the classical intramuscular method with the submuscular method was described by Henry[283] in 2006. However, no clinical studies using this modification are available to date.

In 1942, 44 years after Curtis, the *anterior submuscular transposition* technique was described in detail by Learmonth.[284] In his description, the ulnar nerve is transposed deep to the flexor–pronator muscles alongside the median nerve. The main advantages of this technique are release of all potential sites of compression, and better protection of the transposed nerve. However, the disadvantages include longer postoperative immobilization, possible weakness of the flexor–pronator muscles, and a technically demanding procedure.[178,285]

A variation of the anterior submuscular transposition, the musculofascial lengthening technique by Dellon,[286] has been reported and described in great detail in the literature.[287–291] The major difference between this technique and Learmonth's is that the flexor–pronator muscle mass is lengthened with a step-cut (Z-lengthening) technique. In a study on 50 cadavers, Dellon et al.[292] determined that musculofascial lengthening was the only surgical technique that reduced intraneural ulnar nerve pressure for all degrees of flexion (0°, 30°, 60° and 90°) at all three sites (proximal, within and distal to the cubital tunnel) measured, when compared with *in situ* decompression, medial epicondylectomy, anterior subcutaneous transposition and Learmonth's anterior submuscular transposition techniques.

The above are the three techniques for anterior transposition currently most commonly in use. A subfascial anterior transposition technique has recently been described by Chuang and Treciak.[215] A small retrospective study[216] on eight patients with severe (Dellon[196] stage 3) disease gave excellent results after an average follow-up of 2 years and 9 months.

There are many reports and studies published in the literature comparing the usefulness of anterior transposition in its various forms.[221] Anterior transposition as a whole has been reported to be just as successful as *in situ* decompression or medial epicondylectomy. Reports for the three techniques are also comparable to each other. Hagstrom[293] suggested anterior transposition, whether subcutaneous or submuscular, as the treatment of choice. However, Stuffer et al.[200] concluded from a series of 51 patients that the results after anterior subcutaneous transposition are clinically and electrically better than after anterior submuscular transposition. Unfortunately, as discussed before, there is still no well-designed prospective randomized study available to conclusively state which technique is better.

Endoscopic release

Use of the endoscope to assist with the surgical decompression of the ulnar nerve is a relatively new procedure. Tsai et al.[294] published a series of 76 patients (85 elbows) that showed 87% excellent and good results after an average follow-up period of 32 months, following use of an endoscope and custom-made glass rods. Using a 2–3 cm incision, the authors were able to release the ulnar nerve up to 10 cm proximal and 10 cm distal to the medial epicondyle.

Bain and Bajhau[295] reported on the use of the Agee endoscopic system (3M, Orthopedic Products, St. Paul, MN) for ulnar nerve decompression at the elbow in a cadaveric model. They concluded that it is both safe and effective for this purpose.

In 2007 Ahcan and Zoman[296] reported on 36 patients who underwent endoscope-assisted ulnar nerve decompression via a 3.5 cm incision: 20 cm of the ulnar nerve was able to be released, with 33 patients (91.7%) having excellent or good results after an average of 14 months' follow-up. Minimal complications were reported and all patients had electrophysiological improvement with return to full activities within 3 weeks after having the procedure.

Further clinical studies and prospective randomized studies are needed before this technique can be widely accepted.

Failed surgical treatment

Failure rates of approximately 25% for surgical treatment of cubital tunnel syndrome have been quoted.[297] Causes of failed surgery for cubital tunnel syndrome can be divided into pre-operative, intra-operative and postoperative factors.[298] Pre-operative factors include making an incorrect diagnosis for the symptoms, additional pathology that was unrecognized and unrealistic expectations by the patient. Intra-operatively, failure of the procedure can be due to inadequate decompression, creation of new compressive sites,[299] unrecognized ulnar nerve instability and iatrogenic injury to branches of the medial antebrachial cutaneous nerve, MCL of ulnar nerve motor fascicles. Postoperative causes include perineural fibrosis, elbow instability, recurrent ulnar nerve subluxation, heterotopic bone formation and elbow contracture.

For many authors anterior submuscular transposition is the fallback procedure for revision surgery of a failed primary cubital tunnel surgery.[195,300,301] However, others advocate the proper use of anterior intramuscular transposition,[297] especially when the primary procedure is submuscular,[302] anterior subcutaneous transposition[303] and even *in situ* decompression.[304,305] Treatment of these cases can be challenging and very complex. A thorough knowledge of the ulnar nerve and elbow anatomy, with the various treatment options, is required to successfully treat them.

For recalcitrant and chronic nerve pain after a failed decompression direct nerve stimulation[306] or neurolysis with vein wrapping of the nerve using the autogenous saphenous vein[307,308] (autologous vein insulator) has been reported to be useful. However, these are largely experimental solutions that require further research to determine their usefulness in the long term.

KEY LEARNING POINTS

- The elbow joint has a hinge action with strong static collateral stability.
- The trochlear notch, its central ridge, the spool-shaped trochlea and its central groove give the elbow a stable medial column.
- The anterior bundle of the medial collateral ligament (MCL) is the chief soft-tissue stabilizer to valgus stress.
- Ulnar nerve entrapment may occur at variable levels in the elbow: the arcade of Struthers, in the cubital tunnel and distal to the cubital tunnel.
- Compression of the radial nerve at the elbow can be either a motor palsy (*posterior interosseous nerve syndrome*) or lateral elbow and forearm pain (*radial tunnel syndrome*).
- The median nerve, compressed at the elbow, can present as the anterior interosseous nerve syndrome or the pronator syndrome; differentiated by electrodiagnostic studies.
- Coronoid fractures are pathognomonic for an episode of elbow instability; the 'terrible triad' is elbow dislocation with fractures of radial head and coronoid.
- Excision of more than 50% of the olecranon increases joint pressure, which may lead to early arthritic changes.
- Radial head is an important secondary stabilizer of the elbow joint, contributing to nearly 30% of its valgus stability.
- The MCL is the chief soft-tissue restraint to valgus stress.
- The lateral collateral ligament complex is the chief constraint to external rotation and varus stress to the elbow joint.
- The common causes of olecranon bursitis are post-traumatic, chronic and infection.
- Epicondylitis is the most common condition to occur in the elbow.
- Compression of the ulnar nerve is common, especially cubital tunnel, the diagnosis of which is clinical; it may need to be treated surgically with anterior transposition.

REFERENCES

- ● = Key primary paper
- ◆ = Major review article

1. Fuss FK. The ulnar collateral ligament of the human elbow joint. Anatomy, function and biomechanics. *Journal of Anatomy* 1991;**175**:203–12.
◆2. Morrey BF, An KN. Functional anatomy of the ligaments of the elbow. *Clinical Orthopaedics and Related Research* 1985;**201**:84–90.
●3. O'Driscoll SW, Morrey BF, Korinek SL, An KN. The pathoanatomy and kinematics of posterolateral rotatory instability (pivot-shift) of the elbow. *Transactions of the Orthopaedic Research Society* 1990;**15**:6.
4. Osborne G, Cotterill P. Recurrent dislocation of the elbow. *Journal of Bone and Joint Surgery (British)* 1966;**48**:340–6.
◆5. Dunning CE, Zarzour ZD, Patterson SD, et al. Ligamentous stabilizers against posterolateral rotatory instability of the elbow. *Journal of Bone and Joint Surgery (American)* 2001;**83A**:1823–8.
◆6. Cohen MS, Hastings H 2nd. Rotatory instability of the elbow. The anatomy and role of the lateral stabilizers. *Journal of Bone and Joint Surgery (American)* 1997;**79**:225–33.
7. Park MC, Ahmad CS, Park MC, Ahmad CS. Dynamic contributions of the flexor-pronator mass to elbow valgus stability. *Journal of Bone and Joint Surgery (American)* 2004;**86A**:2268–74.
●8. Ahmad CS, Lee TQ, ElAttrache NS, et al. Biomechanical evaluation of a new ulnar collateral ligament reconstruction technique with interference screw fixation. *American Journal of Sports Medicine* 2003;**31**:332–7.
9. Smith GR, Altchek DW, Pagnani MJ, Keeley JR. A muscle-splitting approach to the ulnar collateral ligament of the

elbow. Neuroanatomy and operative technique. *American Journal of Sports Medicine* 1996;**24**:575–80.
10. Thompson WH, Jobe FW, Yocum LA, Pink MM. Ulnar collateral ligament reconstruction in athletes: muscle-splitting approach without transposition of the ulnar nerve. *Journal of Shoulder and Elbow Surgery* 2001;**10**:152–7.
◆11. Bryce CD, Armstrong AD. Anatomy and biomechanics of the elbow. *Orthopedic Clinics of North America* 2008;**39**:141–54.
12. Osborne GV. The surgical treatment of tardy ulnar neuropathy. (Proceedings and reports of universities, colleges, councils and association. Great Britain. British Orthopaedic Association Autumn Meeting 1957). *Journal of Bone and Joint Surgery (British)* 1957;**39**:782.
◆13. Osterman AL, Kltay GS. Compression neuropathies: Ulnar. In: Peimer CA (ed.) *Surgery of the Hand and Upper Extremity*. New York, NY: McGraw-Hill, 1995;1339–62.
14. Bartels RHMA, Grotenhuis JA, Kauer JMG. The arcade of Struthers: an anatomical study. *Acta Neurochirurgica (Wien)* 2003;**145**:295–300.
15. Bartels RH, Bartels RHMA. Redefining the 'arcade of Struthers'.[comment]. *Journal of Hand Surgery (American)* 2004;**29**:335; author reply.
16. De Jesus R, Dellon AL. Historic origin of the 'arcade of Struthers'. *Journal of Hand Surgery (American)* 2003;**28**:528–31.
17. von Schroeder HP, Scheker LR. Redefining the 'arcade of Struthers'. *Journal of Hand Surgery (American)* 2003;**28**:1018–21.
◆18. Campbell WW, Landau ME. Controversial entrapment neuropathies. *Neurosurgery Clinics of North America* 2008;**19**:597–608.
19. Ochiai N, Honmo J, Tsujino A, Nisiura Y. Electrodiagnosis in entrapment neuropathy by the arcade of Struthers. *Clinical Orthopaedics and Related Research* 2000;**378**:129–35.
◆20. O'Driscoll SW, Horii E, Carmichael SW, Morrey BF. The cubital tunnel and ulnar neuropathy. *Journal of Bone and Joint Surgery (British)* 1991;**73**:613–17.
21. Childress HM. Recurrent ulnar-nerve dislocation at the elbow. *Clinical Orthopaedics and Related Research* 1975;**108**:168–73.
22. Feindel W, Stratford J. The role of the cubital tunnel in tardy ulnar nerve palsy. *Canadian Journal of Surgery* 1958;**1**:287–300.
23. Werner CO. Lateral elbow pain and posterior interosseous nerve entrapment. *Acta Orthopaedica Scandinavica Supplementum* 1979;**174**:1–62.
24. Klab K, Gruber P, Landsleitner B. (Compression syndrome of the radial nerve in the area of the supinator groove. Experiences with 110 patients). *Handchirurgie Mikrochirurgie Plastiche Chirurgie* 1999;**31**:303–10.
25. Morrey BF, Chao EY. Passive motion of the elbow joint. *Journal of Bone and Joint Surgery (American)* 1976;**58**:501–8.
◆26. Youm Y, Dryer RF, Thambyrajah K, *et al.* Biomechanical analyses of forearm pronation-supination and elbow flexion-extension. *Journal of Biomechanics* 1979;**12**:245–55.
27. London JT. Kinematics of the elbow. *Journal of Bone and Joint Surgery (American)* 1981;**63**:529–35.
28. Stokdijk M, Meskers CG, Veeger HE, *et al.* Determination of the optimal elbow axis for evaluation of placement of prostheses. *Clinical Biomechanics* 1999;**14**:177–84.
29. Bottlang M, Madey SM, Steyers CM, *et al.* Assessment of elbow joint kinematics in passive motion by electromagnetic motion tracking. *Journal of Orthopaedic Research* 2000;**18**:195–202.
30. Ericson A, Arndt A, Stark A, *et al.* Variation in the position and orientation of the elbow flexion axis. *Journal of Bone and Joint Surgery (British)* 2003;**85**:538–44.
31. Duck TR, Dunning CE, King GJ, *et al.* Variability and repeatability of the flexion axis at the ulnohumeral joint. *Journal of Orthopaedic Research* 2003;**21**:399–404.
32. Boone DC, Azen SP. Normal range of motion of joints in male subjects. *Journal of Bone and Joint Surgery (American)* 1979;**61**:756–9.
33. Moore DC, Hogan KA, Crisco JJ 3rd, *et al.* Three-dimensional in vivo kinematics of the distal radioulnar joint in malunited distal radius fractures. *Journal of Hand Surgery (American)* 2002;**27**:233–42.
◆34. Dunning CE, Zarzour ZD, Patterson SD, *et al.* Muscle forces and pronation stabilize the lateral ligament deficient elbow. *Clinical Orthopaedics and Related Research* 2001;**388**:118–24.
35. Dunning CE, Duck TR, King GJ, Johnson JA. Simulated active control produces repeatable motion pathways of the elbow in an in vitro testing system. *Journal of Biomechanics* 2001;**34**:1039–48.
36. Beingessner DM, Dunning CE, Stacpoole RA, *et al.* The effect of coronoid fractures on elbow kinematics and stability. *Clinical Biomechanics* 2007;**22**:183–90.
37. Safran MR, McGarry MH, Shin S, *et al.* Effects of elbow flexion and forearm rotation on valgus laxity of the elbow. *Journal of Bone and Joint Surgery (American)* 2005;**87**:2065–74.
◆38. McKee MD, Jupiter JB. Trauma of the adult elbow and fractures of the distal humerus. In: Browner BD, Jupiter JB, Levine AM, *et al.* (eds) *Skeletal Trauma: Basic Science, Management, and Reconstruction*, 3rd edn. Philadelphia, PA: Saunders, 2003:1404–80.
39. Hull JR, Owen JR, Fern SE, *et al.* Role of the coronoid process in varus osteoarticular stability of the elbow. *Journal of Shoulder and Elbow Surgery* 2005;**14**:441–6.
◆40. Schneeberger AG, Sadowski MM, Jacob HAC. Coronoid process and radial head as posterolateral rotatory stabilizers of the elbow. *Journal of Bone and Joint Surgery (American)* 2004;**86A**:975–82.
41. Moed BR, Ede DE, Brown TD, *et al.* Fractures of the olecranon: an in vitro study of elbow joint stresses after tension-band wire fixation versus proximal fracture fragment excision. *Journal of Trauma* 2002;**53**:1088–93.
42. Morrey BF, An KN. Articular and ligamentous contributions to the stability of the elbow joint. *American Journal of Sports Medicine* 1983;**11**:315–19.

43. Hotchkiss RN, Weiland AJ. Valgus stability of the elbow. *Journal of Orthopaedic Research* 1987;**5**:372–7.
◆44. Morrey BF, Tanaka S, An KN. Valgus stability of the elbow. A definition of primary and secondary constraints. *Clinical Orthopaedics and Related Research* 1991;**265**:187–95.
45. Charalambous CP, Stanley JK. Posterolateral rotatory instability of the elbow. *Journal of Bone and Joint Surgery (British)* 2008;**90**:272–9.
●46. Callaway GH, Field LD, Deng XH, et al. Biomechanical evaluation of the medial collateral ligament of the elbow. *Journal of Bone and Joint Surgery (American)* 1997;**79**:1223–31.
●47. O'Driscoll SW, Lawton RL, Smith AM, et al. The 'moving valgus stress test' for medial collateral ligament tears of the elbow. *American Journal of Sports Medicine* 2005;**33**:231–9.
48. O'Driscoll SW, Jupiter JB, King GJ, et al. The unstable elbow. *Instructional Course Lectures* 2001;**50**:89–102.
49. Chou PH, Chou YL, Lin CJ, et al. Effect of elbow flexion on upper extremity impact forces during a fall. *Clinical Biomechanics* 2001;**16**:888–94.
50. Donkers MJ, An KN, Chao EY, Morrey BF. Hand position affects elbow joint load during push-up exercise. *Journal of Biomechanics* 1993;**26**:625–32.
51. Halls AA, Travill A. Transmission of pressures across the elbow joint. *Anatomical Record* 1964;**150**:243–7.
52. Morrey BF, An KN, Stormont TJ. Force transmission through the radial head. *Journal of Bone and Joint Surgery (American)* 1988;**70**:250–6.
53. Wake H, Hashizume H, Nishida K, et al. Biomechanical analysis of the mechanism of elbow fracture-dislocations by compression force. *Journal of Orthopaedic Science* 2004;**9**:44–50.
54. McFarland EG. Olecranon and prepatellar bursitis. *Physician and Sports Medicine* 2000;**28**:40–52.
55. Singer KM, Butters KP. Olecranon bursitis. In: DeLee JC, Drez D (eds) *Orthopaedic Sports Medicine*, 2nd edn. Philadelphia, PA: WB Saunders, 1994:890–5.
56. McAfee JH, Smith DL. Olecranon and prepatellar bursitis. Diagnosis and treatment. *Western Journal of Medicine* 1988;**149**:607–10.
57. Morrey BF. Bursitis. In: Morrey BF (ed.) *The Elbow and its Disorders*. Philadelphia, PA: W.B. Saunders, 2000:901–8.
◆58. Stell IM. Septic and non-septic olecranon bursitis in the accident and emergency department—an approach to management. *Journal of Accident & Emergency Medicine* 1996;**13**:351–3.
59. Tran N, Chow K, Tran N, Chow K. Ultrasonography of the elbow. *Seminars in Musculoskeletal Radiology* 2007;**11**:105–16.
60. Floemer F, Morrison WB, Bongartz G, et al. MRI characteristics of olecranon bursitis. *AJR American Journal of Roentgenology* 2004;**183**:29–34.
●61. Smith DL, McAfee JH, Lucas LM, et al. Treatment of nonseptic olecranon bursitis. A controlled, blinded prospective trial. *Archives of Internal Medicine* 1989;**149**:2527–30.
62. Thurston AJ. The early history of tennis elbow: 1873 to the 1950s. *Australian and New Zealand Journal of Surgery* 1998;**68**:219–24.
63. Stasinopoulos D, Johnson MI. 'Lateral elbow tendinopathy' is the most appropriate diagnostic term for the condition commonly referred to as lateral epicondylitis. *Medical Hypotheses* 2006;**67**:1400–2.
◆64. Kraushaar BS, Nirschl RP. Tendinosis of the elbow (tennis elbow). Clinical features and findings of histological, immunohistochemical, and electron microscopy studies. *Journal of Bone and Joint Surgery (American)* 1999;**81**:259–78.
65. Nirschl RP. Elbow tendinosis/tennis elbow. *Clinics in Sports Medicine* 1992;**11**:851–70.
◆66. Calfee RP, Patel A, DaSilva MF, Akelman E. Management of lateral epicondylitis: current concepts. *Journal of the American Academy of Orthopaedic Surgeons* 2008;**16**:19–29.
67. Goldie I. Epicondylitis lateralis humeri (epicondylalgia or tennis elbow). A pathogenetical study. *Acta Chirurgica Scandinavica Supplementum* 1964;**57**(339):1.
68. Shiri R, Viikari-Juntura E, Varonen H, Heliovaara M. Prevalence and determinants of lateral and medial epicondylitis: a population study. *American Journal of Epidemiology* 2006;**164**:1065–74.
69. Maffulli N, Wong J, Almekinders LC. Types and epidemiology of tendinopathy. *Clinics in Sports Medicine* 2003;**22**:675–92.
70. Jobe F, Ciccotti M. Lateral and medial epicondylitis of the elbow. *Journal of the American Academy of Orthopaedic Surgeons* 1994;**2**:1–8.
71. Ciccotti MC, Schwartz MA, Ciccotti MG. Diagnosis and treatment of medial epicondylitis of the elbow. *Clinics in Sports Medicine* 2004;**23**:693–705.
72. Stockard AR. Elbow injuries in golf.[see comment]. *Journal of the American Osteopath Association* 2001;**101**:509–16.
73. McCarroll JR, Rettig AC, Shelbourne KD. Injuries in the amateur golfer. *Physician and Sports Medicine* 1990;**18**:122–6.
74. McCarroll JR. Overuse injuries of the upper extremity in golf. *Clinics in Sports Medicine* 2001;**20**:469–79.
75. Kelley JD, Lombardo SJ, Pink M, et al. Electromyographic and cinematographic analysis of elbow function in tennis players with lateral epicondylitis. *American Journal of Sports Medicine* 1994;**22**:359–63.
●76. Giangarra CE, Conroy B, Jobe FW, et al. Electromyographic and cinematographic analysis of elbow function in tennis players using single- and double-handed backhand strokes. *American Journal of Sports Medicine* 1993;**21**:394–9.
77. Hatch GF 3rd, Pink MM, Mohr KJ, et al. The effect of tennis racket grip size on forearm muscle firing patterns. *American Journal of Sports Medicine* 2006;**34**:1977–83.
78. Bunata RE, Brown DS, Capelo R, et al. Anatomic factors related to the cause of tennis elbow. *Journal of Bone and Joint Surgery (American)* 2007;**89**:1955–63.
79. Regan W, Wold LE, Coonrad R, Morrey BF. Microscopic histopathology of chronic refractory lateral epicondylitis. *American Journal of Sports Medicine* 1992;**20**:746–9.

- 80. Ljung BO, Forsgren S, Friden J. Substance P and calcitonin gene-related peptide expression at the extensor carpi radialis brevis muscle origin: implications for the etiology of tennis elbow. *Journal of Orthopaedic Research* 1999;**17**:554-9.
- 81. Zeisig E, Ohberg L, Alfredson H, et al. Extensor origin vascularity related to pain in patients with Tennis elbow. *Knee Surgery, Sports Traumatology, Arthroscopy* 2006;**14**:659-63.
82. Sisto DJ, Jobe FW, Moynes DR, Antonelli DJ. An electromyographic analysis of the elbow in pitching. *American Journal of Sports Medicine* 1987;**15**:260-3.
83. Rizio L, Uribe JW. Overuse injuries of the upper extremity in baseball. *Clinics in Sports Medicine* 2001;**20**:453-68.
◆ 84. Marx RG, Sperling JW, Cordasco FA. Overuse injuries of the upper extremity in tennis players. *Clinics in Sports Medicine* 2001;**20**:439-51.
85. Ben Kibler W, Sciascia A. Kinetic chain contributions to elbow function and dysfunction in sports. *Clinics in Sports Medicine* 2004;**23**:545-52.
◆ 86. Hotchkiss RN. Common disorders of the elbow in athletes and musicians. *Hand Clinics* 1990;**6**:507-15.
87. Ciccotti MG, Charlton WP. Epicondylitis in the athlete. *Clinics in Sports Medicine* 2001;**20**:77-93.
◆ 88. Nirschl RP, Ashman ES. Elbow tendinopathy: tennis elbow. *Clinics in Sports Medicine* 2003;**22**:813-36.
89. Ruch DS, Papadonikolakis A, Campolattaro RM. The posterolateral plica: a cause of refractory lateral elbow pain. *Journal of Shoulder and Elbow Surgery* 2006;**15**:367-70.
90. Pomerance J, Pomerance J. Radiographic analysis of lateral epicondylitis. *Journal of Shoulder and Elbow Surgery* 2002;**11**:156-7.
91. Dlabach JA, Baker CL Jr. Lateral and medial epicondylitis in the overhead athlete. *Operative Techniques in Orthopaedics*. 2001;**11**:46-54.
92. Bennett JB. Lateral and medial epicondylitis. *Hand Clinics* 1994;**10**:157-63.
93. Gabel GT, Morrey BF. Operative treatment of medical epicondylitis. Influence of concomitant ulnar neuropathy at the elbow. *Journal of Bone and Joint Surgery (American)* 1995;**77**:1065-9.
◆ 94. Ciccotti MG. Epicondylitis in the athlete. *Instructional Course Lectures* 1999;**48**:375-81.
95. Chen FS, Rokito AS, Jobe FW. Medial elbow problems in the overhead-throwing athlete. *Journal of the American Academy of Orthopaedic Surgeons* 2001;**9**:99-113.
96. Vangsness CT Jr, Jobe FW. Surgical treatment of medial epicondylitis. Results in 35 elbows. *Journal of Bone and Joint Surgery (British)* 1991;**73**:409-11.
◆ 97. Cowan J, Lozano-Calderon S, Ring D, et al. Quality of prospective controlled randomized trials. Analysis of trials of treatment for lateral epicondylitis as an example. *Journal of Bone and Joint Surgery (American)* 2007;**89**:1693-9.
98. Boyd HB, McLeod AC Jr. Tennis elbow. *Journal of Bone and Joint Surgery (American)* 1973;**55**:1183-7.
99. Coonrad RW, Hooper WR. Tennis elbow: its course, natural history, conservative and surgical management. *Journal of Bone and Joint Surgery (American)* 1973;**55**:1177-82.
100. Nirschl RP, Pettrone FA. Tennis elbow. The surgical treatment of lateral epicondylitis. *Journal of Bone and Joint Surgery (American)* 1979;**61**:832-9.
101. Leach RE, Miller JK. Lateral and medial epicondylitis of the elbow. *Clinics in Sports Medicine* 1987;**6**:259-72.
102. Grana W. Medial epicondylitis and cubital tunnel syndrome in the throwing athlete. *Clinics in Sports Medicine* 2001;**20**:541-8.
103. Burton AK. A comparative trial of forearm strap and topical anti-inflammatory as adjuncts to manual therapy in tennis elbow. *Manual Medicine* 1988;**3**:141-3.
104. Labelle H, Guibert R. Efficacy of diclofenac in lateral epicondylitis of the elbow also treated with immobilization. The University of Montreal Orthopaedic Research Group. *Archives of Family Medicine* 1997;**6**:257-62.
- 105. Martinez-Silvestrini JA, Newcomer KL, Gay RE, et al. Chronic lateral epicondylitis: comparative effectiveness of a home exercise program including stretching alone versus stretching supplemented with eccentric or concentric strengthening. *Journal of Hand Therapy* 2005;**18**:411-19.
106. Svernlov B, Adolfsson L. Non-operative treatment regime including eccentric training for lateral humeral epicondylalgia. *Scandinavian Journal of Medicine & Science in Sports* 2001;**11**:328-34.
107. Hennig EM, Rosenbaum D, Milani TL. Transfer of tennis racket vibrations onto the human forearm. *Medicine and Science in Sports and Exercise* 1992;**24**:1134-40.
108. Bisset L, Beller E, Jull G, et al. Mobilisation with movement and exercise, corticosteroid injection, or wait and see for tennis elbow: randomised trial. *British Medical Journal* 2006;**333**:939.
- 109. Smidt N, van der Windt DAWM, Assendelft WJJ, et al. Corticosteroid injections, physiotherapy, or a wait-and-see policy for lateral epicondylitis: a randomised controlled trial.[summary for patients in *Australian Journal of Physiotherapy* 2002;**48**:239; PMID: 12369566]. *Lancet* 2002;**359**:657-62.
110. Hay EM, Paterson SM, Lewis M, et al. Pragmatic randomised controlled trial of local corticosteroid injection and naproxen for treatment of lateral epicondylitis of elbow in primary care. *British Medical Journal* 1999;**319**:964-8.
111. Wong MW, Tang YY, Lee SK, et al. Effect of dexamethasone on cultured human tenocytes and its reversibility by platelet-derived growth factor. *Journal of Bone and Joint Surgery (American)* 2003;**85A**:1914-20.
112. Smith AG, Kosygan K, Williams H, Newman RJ. Common extensor tendon rupture following corticosteroid injection for lateral tendinosis of the elbow. *British Journal of Sports Medicine* 1999;**33**:423-4; discussion 4-5.
113. Stahl S, Kaufman T. The efficacy of an injection of steroids for medial epicondylitis. A prospective study of

sixty elbows. *Journal of Bone and Joint Surgery (American)* 1997;**79**:1648-52.
- ●114. Placzek R, Drescher W, Deuretzbacher G, et al. Treatment of chronic radial epicondylitis with botulinum toxin A. A double-blind, placebo-controlled, randomized multicenter study. *Journal of Bone and Joint Surgery (American)* 2007;**89**:255-60.
115. Wong SM, Hui AC, Tong PY, et al. Treatment of lateral epicondylitis with botulinum toxin: a randomized, double-blind, placebo-controlled trial.[summary for patients in *Annals of Internal Medicine* 2005;**143**:I48; PMID: 16330786]. *Annals of Internal Medicine* 2005;**143**:793-7.
116. Buchbinder R, Green SE, Youd JM, et al. Systematic review of the efficacy and safety of shock wave therapy for lateral elbow pain. *Journal of Rheumatology* 2006;**33**:1351-63.
117. Bisset L, Paungmali A, Vicenzino B, Beller E. A systematic review and meta-analysis of clinical trials on physical interventions for lateral epicondylalgia. *British Journal of Sports Medicine* 2005;**39**:411-22; discussion, 22.
118. Enzenauer RJ, Nordstrom DM. Anterior interosseous nerve syndrome associated with forearm band treatment of lateral epicondylitis. *Orthopedics* 1991;**14**:788-90.
119. Field LD, Savoie FH. Common elbow injuries in sport. *Sports Medicine* 1998;**26**:193-205.
120. Van De Streek MD, Van Der Schans CP, De Greef MH, et al. The effect of a forearm/hand splint compared with an elbow band as a treatment for lateral epicondylitis. *Prosthetics and Orthotics International* 2004;**28**:183-9.
121. Struijs PA, Smidt N, Arola H, et al. Orthotic devices for the treatment of tennis elbow.[update of *Cochrane Database Systematic Review* 2001;CD001821; PMID: 11406011]. *Cochrane Database Systematic Review* 2002:CD001821.
122. D'Vaz AP, Ostor AJ, Speed CA, et al. Pulsed low-intensity ultrasound therapy for chronic lateral epicondylitis: a randomized controlled trial. *Rheumatology (Oxford)* 2006;**45**:566-70.
123. Edwards SG, Calandruccio JH, Edwards SG, Calandruccio JH. Autologous blood injections for refractory lateral epicondylitis. *Journal of Hand Surgery (American)* 2003;**28**:272-8.
124. Mishra A, Pavelko T, Mishra A, Pavelko T. Treatment of chronic elbow tendinosis with buffered platelet-rich plasma. *American Journal of Sports Medicine* 2006;**34**:1774-8.
125. Smidt N, Assendelft WJ, Arola H, et al. Effectiveness of physiotherapy for lateral epicondylitis: a systematic review. *Annals of Medicine* 2003;**35**:51-62.
126. Basford JR, Sheffield CG, Cieslak KR. Laser therapy: a randomized, controlled trial of the effects of low intensity Nd:YAG laser irradiation on lateral epicondylitis. *Archives of Physical Medicine and Rehabilitation* 2000;**81**:1504-10.
127. Bjordal JM, Lopes-Martins RA, Joensen J, et al. A systematic review with procedural assessments and meta-analysis of low level laser therapy in lateral elbow tendinopathy (tennis elbow). *BMC Musculoskeletal Disorders* 2008;**9**:75.
128. Assendelft W, Green S, Buchbinder R, et al. Tennis elbow.[update of *Clinical Evidence* 2002;1290-300; PMID: 12603940]. *Clinical Evidence* 2004;1633-44.
129. Ramsay DJ, Bowman MA, Greenman PE, et al. Acupuncture - NIH Consensus Development Panel on Acupuncture. *Journal of the American Medical Association* 1998;**280**:1518-24.
130. Paoloni JA, Appleyard RC, Nelson J, et al. Topical nitric oxide application in the treatment of chronic extensor tendinosis at the elbow: a randomized, double-blinded, placebo-controlled clinical trial. *American Journal of Sports Medicine* 2003;**31**:915-20.
131. Franke F. Uber epicondylitis humeri [Lateral humeral epicondylitis]. *Deutsche Medizinische Wochenschrift* 1910;**36**:13-16.
132. Fischer AN. Uber die epicondylus und styloideusneuralgie, ihre pathogenese und zweckmbgige therapic [Epicondylitis and styloid neuralgia: its pathogenesia and treatment]. *Langenbecks Archiv für klinische Chirurgie vereinigt mit Deutsche Zeitschrift für Chirurgie* 1923;**125**:749-75.
133. Hohmann G. Ober den tennisellbogen [Tennis elbow]. *Verhandlungen der Deutschen Orthopadischen Gesellschaft* 1927;**21**:349-54.
134. Tavernier L. Epicondylite tenace guerie par enervation sensitive regionale [Chronic epicondylitis treated by regional denervation]. *Revue d'Orthopedie* 1946;**32**:61-2.
135. Bosworth DM. The role of the orbicular ligament in tennis elbow. *Journal of Bone and Joint Surgery (American)* 1955;**37**:527-33.
136. Kaplan EB. Treatment of tennis elbow (epicondylitis) by denervation. *Journal of Bone and Joint Surgery (American)* 1959;**41**:147-51.
137. Garden RS. Tennis elbow. *Journal of Bone and Joint Surgery (British)* 1961;**43**:100-6.
138. Wilhelm A, Gieseler H. Die behandlung der epicondylitis humeri radialis durch denervation [Treatment of epicondylitis humeri radialia by denervation]. *Chirurgie* 1962;**33**:118-22.
139. Capener N. The vulnerability of the posterior interosseous nerve of the forearm. A case report and an anatomical study. *Journal of Bone and Joint Surgery (British)* 1966;**48**:770-3.
140. Roles NC, Maudsley RH. Radial tunnel syndrome: resistant tennis elbow as a nerve entrapment. *Journal of Bone and Joint Surgery (British)* 1972;**54**:499-508.
141. Wilhelm A. [Management of epicondylitis humeri radialis through the decompression of the radial nerve]. *Handchirurgie* 1977;**9**:185-7.
142. Narakas AO. Allongement proximal du 2eme radial et neurolyse du nerf radial dans les epicondylalgies rebelles [Proximal lengthening of the ECRB tendon and neuralgia of the radial nerve in the chronic epicondylitis]. *Schweizerische medizinische Wochenschrift* 1987;**9**:50-2.
- ●143. Khashaba A. Nirschl tennis elbow release with or without drilling. *British Journal of Sports Medicine* 2001;**35**:200-1.
144. Budoff JE, Hicks JM, Ayala G, Kraushaar BS. The reliability of the 'scratch test'. *Journal of Hand Surgery (European)* 2008;**33**:166-9.

145. Dellon AL, Ducic I, Dejesus RA. The innervation of the medial humeral epicondyle: implications for medial epicondylar pain. *Journal of Hand Surgery (British)* 2006;**31**:331–3.
146. Curl LA. Return to sport following elbow surgery. *Clinics in Sports Medicine* 2004;**23**:353–66.
147. Baker CL Jr, Baker CL 3rd. Long-term follow-up of arthroscopic treatment of lateral epicondylitis. *American Journal of Sports Medicine* 2008;**36**:254–60.
148. Peart RE, Strickler SS, Schweitzer KM Jr, et al. Lateral epicondylitis: a comparative study of open and arthroscopic lateral release. *American Journal of Orthopedics (Chatham, NJ)* 2004;**33**:565–7.
149. Smith AM, Castle JA, Ruch DS, et al. Arthroscopic resection of the common extensor origin: anatomic considerations. *Journal of Shoulder and Elbow Surgery* 2003;**12**:375–9.
150. Bartels RH. History of the surgical treatment of ulnar nerve compression at the elbow. *Neurosurgery.* 2001;**49**:391–400.
151. Amadio PC, Beckenbaugh RD. Entrapment of the ulnar nerve by the deep flexor-pronator aponeurosis. *Journal of Hand Surgery (American)* 1986;**11**:83–7.
152. Polatsch DB, Melone CP Jr, Beldner S, Incorvaia A. Ulnar nerve anatomy. *Hand Clinics* 2007;**23**:283–9.
153. Collier A, Burge P. Management of mechanical neuropathy of the ulnar nerve at the elbow. *Current Orthopaedics* 2001;**15**:256–63.
154. Bartels RH, Menovsky T, Van Overbeeke JJ, Verhagen WI. Surgical management of ulnar nerve compression at the elbow: an analysis of the literature. *Journal of Neurosurgery* 1998;**89**:722–7.
◆155. Wadsworth TG. The external compression syndrome of the ulnar nerve at the cubital tunnel. *Clinical Orthopaedics and Related Research* 1977;**124**:189–204.
156. Feindel W, Stratford J. Cubital tunnel compression in tardy ulnar palsy. *Canadian Medical Association Journal* 1958;**78**:351–3.
157. Mackinnon SE, Novak CB. Repetitive strain in the workplace. *Journal of Hand Surgery (American)* 1997;**22**:2–18.
158. Hadler NM. Repetitive upper-extremity motions in the workplace are not hazardous. *Journal of Hand Surgery (American)* 1997;**22**:19–29.
159. Contreras MG, Warner MA, Charboneau WJ, Cahill DR. Anatomy of the ulnar nerve at the elbow: potential relationship of acute ulnar neuropathy to gender differences. *Clinical Anatomy* 1998;**11**:372–8.
160. Richardson JK, Green DF, Jamieson SC, Valentin FC. Gender, body mass and age as risk factors for ulnar mononeuropathy at the elbow. *Muscle and Nerve* 2001;**24**:551–4.
161. Apfelberg DB, Larson SJ. Dynamic anatomy of the ulnar nerve at the elbow. *Plastic Reconstructive Surgery* 1973;**51**:79–81.
◆162. Vanderpool DW, Chalmers J, Lamb DW, Whiston TB. Peripheral compression lesions of the ulnar nerve. *Journal of Bone and Joint Surgery (British)* 1968;**50**:792–803.
163. Schuind FA, Goldschmidt D, Bastin C, Burny F. A biomechanical study of the ulnar nerve at the elbow. *Journal of Hand Surgery (British)* 1995;**20**:623–7.
164. Patel W, Heidenreich FP Jr, Bindra RR, et al. Morphologic changes in the ulnar nerve at the elbow with flexion and extension: a magnetic resonance imaging study with 3-dimensional reconstruction. *Journal of Shoulder and Elbow Surgery* 1998;**7**:368–74.
165. Macnicol MF. Extraneural pressures affecting the ulnar nerve at the elbow. *Hand* 1982;**14**:5–11.
166. Iba K, Wada T, Aoki M, et al. Intraoperative measurement of pressure adjacent to the ulnar nerve in patients with cubital tunnel syndrome. *Journal of Hand Surgery (American)* 2006;**31**:553–8.
●167. Werner CO, Ohlin P, Elmqvist D. Pressures recorded in ulnar neuropathy. *Acta Orthopaedica Scandinavica* 1985;**56**:404–6.
168. Gelberman RH, Yamaguchi K, Hollstien SB, et al. Changes in interstitial pressure and cross-sectional area of the cubital tunnel and of the ulnar nerve with flexion of the elbow. An experimental study in human cadavera. *Journal of Bone and Joint Surgery (American)* 1998;**80**:492–501.
169. Pechan J, Julis I. The pressure measurement in the ulnar nerve. A contribution to the pathophysiology of the cubital tunnel syndrome. *Journal of Biomechanics* 1975;**8**:75–9.
170. Lundborg G, Dahlin LB. Anatomy, function, and pathophysiology of peripheral nerves and nerve compression. *Hand Clinics* 1996;**12**:185–93.
171. Grewal R, Xu J, Sotereanos DG, Woo SL. Biomechanical properties of peripheral nerves. *Hand Clinics* 1996;**12**:195–204.
172. Szabo RM, Kwak C, Szabo RM, Kwak C. Natural history and conservative management of cubital tunnel syndrome. *Hand Clinics* 2007;**23**:311–18.
173. McPherson SA, Meals RA. Cubital tunnel syndrome. *Orthopedic Clinics of North America* 1992;**23**:111–23.
174. Rayan GM, Jensen C, Duke J. Elbow flexion test in the normal population. *Journal of Hand Surgery (American)* 1992;**17**:86–9.
175. Posner MA. Compressive ulnar neuropathies at the elbow: I. Etiology and diagnosis. *Journal of the American Academy of Orthopaedic Surgeons* 1998;**6**:282–8.
176. Buehler MJ, Thayer DT. The elbow flexion test. A clinical test for the cubital tunnel syndrome. *Clinical Orthopaedics and Related Research* 1988;**233**:213–16.
177. Novak CB, Lee GW, Mackinnon SE, Lay L. Provocative testing for cubital tunnel syndrome. *Journal of Hand Surgery (American)* 1994;**19**:817–20.
178. Elhassan B, Steinmann SP. Entrapment neuropathy of the ulnar nerve. *Journal of the American Academy of Orthopaedic Surgeons* 2007;**15**:672–81.
179. Anto C, Aradhya P. Clinical diagnosis of peripheral nerve compression in the upper extremity. *Orthopedic Clinics of North America* 1996;**27**:227–36.
180. Hilburn JW. General principles and use of electrodiagnostic studies in carpal and cubital tunnel

syndromes. With special attention to pitfalls and interpretation. *Hand Clinics* 1996;**12**:205–21.

181. American Association of Electrodiagnostic Medicine, American Academy of Neurology, American Academy of Physical Medicine and Rehabilitation. Practice parameter for electrodiagnostic studies in ulnar neuropathy at the elbow: summary statement. *Muscle and Nerve* 1999;**22**:408–11.

182. Britz GW, Haynor DR, Kuntz C, et al. Ulnar nerve entrapment at the elbow: correlation of magnetic resonance imaging, clinical, electrodiagnostic, and intraoperative findings. *Neurosurgery.* 1996;**38**:458–65; discussion 65.

183. de Araujo MP. Electrodiagnosis in compression neuropathies of the upper extremities. *Orthopedic Clinics of North America* 1996;**27**:237–44.

184. Kern RZ, Kern RZ. The electrodiagnosis of ulnar nerve entrapment at the elbow. *Canadian Journal of Neurological Sciences* 2003;**30**:314–19.

185. Idler RS. General principles of patient evaluation and nonoperative management of cubital syndrome. *Hand Clinics* 1996;**12**:397–403.

186. Eisen A, Danon J. The mild cubital tunnel syndrome. Its natural history and indications for surgical intervention. *Neurology* 1974;**24**:608–13.

187. Campbell WW, Pridgeon RM, Sahni KS. Short segment incremental studies in the evaluation of ulnar neuropathy at the elbow. *Muscle and Nerve* 1992;**15**:1050–4.

188. Harmon RL. Bilaterality of ulnar neuropathy at the elbow. *Electromyography and Clinical Neurophysiology* 1991;**31**:195–8.

189. Dunselman HH, Visser LH, Dunselman HHAM. The clinical, electrophysiological and prognostic heterogeneity of ulnar neuropathy at the elbow. *Journal of Neurology, Neurosurgery, and Psychiatry* 2008;**79**:1364–7.

190. St John JN, Palmaz JC. The cubital tunnel in ulnar entrapment neuropathy. *Radiology* 1986;**158**:119–23.

191. Beggs I. Ultrasound of the shoulder and elbow. *Orthopedic Clinics of North America* 2006;**37**:277–85.

192. McGowan AJ. The results of transposition of the ulnar nerve for traumatic ulnar neuritis. *Journal of Bone and Joint Surgery (British)* 1950;**32B**:293–301.

193. Wilson DH, Krout R. Surgery of ulnar neuropathy at the elbow: 16 cases treated by decompression without transposition. Technical note. *Journal of Neurosurgery* 1973;**38**:780–5.

194. Amadio PC. Anatomical basis for a technique of ulnar nerve transposition. *Surgical and Radiologic Anatomy* 1986;**8**:155–61.

195. Gabel GT, Amadio PC. Reoperation for failed decompression of the ulnar nerve in the region of the elbow. *Journal of Bone and Joint Surgery (American)* 1990;**72**:213–19.

196. Dellon AL. Review of treatment results for ulnar nerve entrapment at the elbow.[see comment]. *Journal of Hand Surgery (American)* 1989;**14**:688–700.

197. Kleinman WB, Bishop AT. Anterior intramuscular transposition of the ulnar nerve. *Journal of Hand Surgery (American)* 1989;**14**:972–9.

198. Black BT, Barron OA, Townsend PF, et al. Stabilized subcutaneous ulnar nerve transposition with immediate range of motion. Long-term follow-up. *Journal of Bone and Joint Surgery (American)* 2000;**82A**:1544–51.

199. Tada H, Hirayama T, Katsuki M, Habaguchi T. Long term results using a modified King's method for cubital tunnel syndrome. *Clinical Orthopaedics and Related Research* 1997;**336**:107–10.

200. Stuffer M, Jungwirth W, Hussl H, Schmutzhardt E. Subcutaneous or submuscular anterior transposition of the ulnar nerve? *Journal of Hand Surgery (British)* 1992;**17**:248–50.

●201. Dellon AL. Clinical grading of peripheral nerve problems. *Neurosurgery Clinics of North America* 2001;**12**:229–40.

202. Padua L, Aprile I, Caliandro P, et al. Natural history of ulnar entrapment at elbow. *Clinical Neurophysiology* 2002;**113**:1980–4.

203. Spinner M. Management of nerve compression lesions of the upper extremity. In: Omer G, Spinner M (eds) *Management of Peripheral Nerve Problems.* Philadelphia, PA: W.B. Saunders, 1980:569–605.

204. Dellon AL, Hament W, Gittelshon A. Nonoperative management of cubital tunnel syndrome: an 8-year prospective study.[see comment]. *Neurology* 1993;**43**:1673–7.

205. Seradge H, Owen W. Cubital tunnel release with medial epicondylectomy factors influencing the outcome. *Journal of Hand Surgery (American)* 1998;**23**:483–91.

206. Sailer SM. The role of splinting and rehabilitation in the treatment of carpal and cubital tunnel syndromes. *Hand Clinics* 1996;**12**:223–41.

207. Apfel E, Sigafoos GT. Comparison of range-of-motion constraints provided by splints used in the treatment of cubital tunnel syndrome—a pilot study. *Journal of Hand Therapy* 2006;**19**:384–91; quiz 92.

208. Dimond M, Lister G. Cubital tunnel syndrome treated by long-term splintage. Proceedings of the 1985 American Society for Surgery of the Hand Annual Meeting. *Journal of Hand Surgery (American)* 1985;**10**:430.

209. Seror P. Treatment of ulnar nerve palsy at the elbow with a night splint. *Journal of Bone and Joint Surgery (British)* 1993;**75**:322–7.

210. Posner MA. Compressive ulnar neuropathies at the elbow: II. Treatment. *Journal of the American Academy of Orthopaedic Surgeons* 1998;**6**:289–97.

211. Pechan J, Kredba J. Treatment of cubital tunnel syndrome by means of local administration of corticosteroids. I. Short-term follow-up. *Acta Universitatis Carolinae - Medica* 1980;**26**(3–4):125–33.

212. Hong CZ, Long HA, Kanakamedala RV, et al. Splinting and local steroid injection for the treatment of ulnar

213. Brady RL, Catalano LW, Barron OA. Ulnar nerve entrapment and cubital tunnel syndrome: do's and don'ts. *Current Opinion in Orthopedics* 2003;**14**:296-301.
214. Salama A, Stanley D. Nerve compression syndromes around the elbow. *Current Orthopaedics and Related Research* 2008;**22**:75-9.
215. Chuang DC, Treciak MA. Subfascial anterior transposition: a modified method for the treatment of cubital tunnel syndrome (CuTS). *Techniques in Hand & Upper Extremity Surgery* 1998;**2**:178-83.
216. Teoh LC, Yong FC, Tan SH, Andrew Chin YH. Anterior subfascial transposition of the ulnar nerve. *Journal of Hand Surgery (British)* 2003;**28**:73-6.
217. Tsujino A, Itoh Y, Hayashi K, Uzawa M. Cubital tunnel reconstruction for ulnar neuropathy in osteoarthritic elbows. *Journal of Bone and Joint Surgery (British)* 1997;**79**:390-3.
218. Mowlavi A, Andrews K, Lille S, et al. The management of cubital tunnel syndrome: a meta-analysis of clinical studies. *Plastic Reconstructive Surgery* 2000;**106**:327-34.
219. Zlowodzki M, Chan S, Bhandari M, et al. Anterior transposition compared with simple decompression for treatment of cubital tunnel syndrome. A meta-analysis of randomized, controlled trials. *Journal of Bone and Joint Surgery (American)* 2007;**89**:2591-8.
220. Chung KC. Treatment of ulnar nerve compression at the elbow. *Journal of Hand Surgery (American)* 2008;**33**:1625-7.
221. Adelaar RS, Foster WC, McDowell C. The treatment of the cubital tunnel syndrome. *Journal of Hand Surgery (American)* 1984;**9A**:90-5.
222. Lundborg G. Surgical treatment for ulnar nerve entrapment at the elbow. *Journal of Hand Surgery (British)* 1992;**17**:245-7.
223. Waugh RP, Zlotolow DA. In situ decompression of the ulnar nerve at the cubital tunnel. *Hand Clinics* 2007;**23**:319-27.
224. Buzzard EF. Some varieties of traumatic and toxic ulnar neuritis. *Lancet* 1922;**1**:317-19.
225. Miller RG, Hummel EE. The cubital tunnel syndrome: treatment with simple decompression. *Annals of Neurology* 1980;**7**:567-9.
226. Clark CB. Cubital tunnel syndrome. *Journal of the American Medical Association* 1979;**241**:801-2.
227. Fannin TF. Local decompression in the treatment of ulnar nerve entrapment at the elbow. *Journal of the Royal College of Surgeons of Edinburgh* 1978;**23**:362-6.
228. Lavyne MH, Bell WO. Simple decompression and occasional microsurgical epineurolysis under local anesthesia as treatment for ulnar neuropathy at the elbow. *Neurosurgery* 1982;**11**(Pt 1):6-11.
229. Osborne G. Compression neuritis of the ulnar nerve at the elbow. *Hand* 1970;**2**:10-13.
230. Thomsen PB. Compression neuritis of the ulnar nerve treated with simple decompression. *Acta Orthopaedica Scandinavica* 1977;**48**:164-7.
231. Filippi R, Farag S, Reisch R, et al. Cubital tunnel syndrome. Treatment by decompression without transposition of ulnar nerve. *Minimally Invasive Neurosurgery* 2002;**45**:164-8.
232. Nathan PA, Keniston RC, Meadows KD. Outcome study of ulnar nerve compression at the elbow treated with simple decompression and an early programme of physical therapy.[see comment]. *Journal of Hand Surgery (British)* 1995;**20**:628-37.
233. Nathan PA, Myers LD, Keniston RC, Meadows KD. Simple decompression of the ulnar nerve: an alternative to anterior transposition.[see comment]. *Journal of Hand Surgery (British)* 1992;**17**:251-4.
234. Cho Y-J, Cho S-M, Sheen S-H, et al. Simple decompression of the ulnar nerve for cubital tunnel syndrome. *Journal of the Korean Neurosurgical Society* 2007;**42**:382-7.
235. Manske PR, Johnston R, Pruitt DL, Strecker WB. Ulnar nerve decompression at the cubital tunnel. *Clinical Orthopaedics and Related Research* 1992;**274**:231-7.
236. LeRoux PD, Ensign TD, Burchiel KJ. Surgical decompression without transposition for ulnar neuropathy: factors determining outcome. *Neurosurgery* 1990;**27**:709-14.
237. Lankester BJ, Giddins GE. Ulnar nerve decompression in the cubital canal using local anaesthesia. *Journal of Hand Surgery (British)* 2001;**26**:65-6.
238. Nathan PA, Istvan JA, Meadows KD. Intermediate and long-term outcomes following simple decompression of the ulnar nerve at the elbow. *Chirurgie de la Main* 2005;**24**:29-34.
239. Macnicol MF. The results of operation for ulnar neuritis. *Journal of Bone and Joint Surgery (British)* 1979;**61B**:159-64.
240. Taha A, Galarza M, Zuccarello M, Taha J. Outcomes of cubital tunnel surgery among patients with absent sensory nerve conduction. *Neurosurgery* 2004;**54**:891-6.
241. Bartels RHMA, Verhagen WIM, van der Wilt GJ, et al. Prospective randomized controlled study comparing simple decompression versus anterior subcutaneous transposition for idiopathic neuropathy of the ulnar nerve at the elbow: Part 1. *Neurosurgery* 2005;**56**:522-30.
242. Nabhan A, Ahlhelm F, Kelm J, et al. Simple decompression or subcutaneous anterior transposition of the ulnar nerve for cubital tunnel syndrome.[see comment]. *Journal of Hand Surgery (British)* 2005;**30**:521-4.
243. Nabhan A, Kelm J, Steudel WI, et al. [Cubital tunnel syndrome—simple nerve decompression or decompression with subcutaneous anterior transposition?].[see comment]. *Fortschritte der Neurologie-Psychiatrie* 2007;**75**:168-71.

244. Biggs M, Curtis JA. Randomized, prospective study comparing ulnar neurolysis in situ with submuscular transposition. *Neurosurgery* 2006;**58**:296–304.
245. Gervasio O, Gambardella G, Zaccone C, Branca D. Simple decompression versus anterior submuscular transposition of the ulnar nerve in severe cubital tunnel syndrome: a prospective randomized study.[erratum appears in *Neurosurgery* 2005;**56**:409]. *Neurosurgery* 2005;**56**:108–17.
246. Bartels RHMA, Termeer EH, van der Wilt GJ, et al. Simple decompression or anterior subcutaneous transposition for ulnar neuropathy at the elbow: a cost-minimization analysis – Part 2. *Neurosurgery* 2005;**56**:531–6.
247. Foster RJ, Edshage S. Factors related to the outcome of surgically managed compressive ulnar neuropathy at the elbow level. *Journal of Hand Surgery (American)* 1981;**6**:181–92.
248. Toussaint CP, Zager EL. What's new in common upper extremity entrapment neuropathies. *Neurosurgery Clinics of North America* 2008;**19**:573–81.
249. King T. The treatment of traumatic ulnar neuritis; mobilization of the ulnar nerve at the elbow by removal of the medial epicondyle and adjacent bone. *Australian and New Zealand Journal of Surgery* 1950;**20**:33–42.
250. King T, Morgan FP. Late results of removing the medial humeral epicondyle for traumatic ulnar neuritis. *Journal of Bone and Joint Surgery (British)* 1959;**41B**:51–5.
251. Gore D, Larson S. Medial epicondylectomy for subluxing ulnar nerve. *American Journal of Surgery* 1966;**111**:851–3.
252. Neblett C, Ehni G. Medial epicondylectomy for ulnar palsy. *Journal of Neurosurgery* 1970;**32**:55–62.
253. Jones RE, Gauntt C. Medial epicondylectomy for ulnar nerve compression syndrome at the elbow. *Clinical Orthopaedics and Related Research* 1979;**139**:174–8.
254. Froimson AI, Zahrawi F. Treatment of compression neuropathy of the ulnar nerve at the elbow by epicondylectomy and neurolysis. *Journal of Hand Surgery (American)* 1980;**5**:391–5.
255. Craven PR Jr, Green DP. Cubital tunnel syndrome. Treatment by medial epicondylectomy. *Journal of Bone and Joint Surgery (American)* 1980;**62**:986–9.
256. Goldberg BJ, Light TR, Blair SJ. Ulnar neuropathy at the elbow: results of medial epicondylectomy. *Journal of Hand Surgery (American)* 1989;**14**(2 Pt 1):182–8.
257. Heithoff SJ, Millender LH, Nalebuff EA, Petruska AJ Jr. Medial epicondylectomy for the treatment of ulnar nerve compression at the elbow. *Journal of Hand Surgery (American)* 1990;**15**:22–9.
258. Froimson AI, Anouchi YS, Seitz WH Jr, Winsberg DD. Ulnar nerve decompression with medial epicondylectomy for neuropathy at the elbow. *Clinical Orthopaedics and Related Research* 1991;**265**:200–6.
259. Robinson D, Aghasi MK, Halperin N. Medial epicondylectomy in cubital tunnel syndrome: an electrodiagnostic study. *Journal of Hand Surgery (British)* 1992;**17**:255–6.
260. Tomaino MM, Brach PJ, Vansickle DP. The rationale for and efficacy of surgical intervention for electrodiagnostic-negative cubital tunnel syndrome. *Journal of Hand Surgery (American)* 2001;**26**:1077–81.
261. Geutjens GG, Langstaff RJ, Smith NJ, et al. Medial epicondylectomy or ulnar-nerve transposition for ulnar neuropathy at the elbow? *Journal of Bone and Joint Surgery (British)* 1996;**78**:777–9.
262. O'Driscoll SW, Jaloszynski R, Morrey BF, An KN. Origin of the medial ulnar collateral ligament. *Journal of Hand Surgery (American)* 1992;**17**:164–8.
263. Amako M, Nemoto K, Kawaguchi M, et al. Comparison between partial and minimal medial epicondylectomy combined with decompression for the treatment of cubital tunnel syndrome. *Journal of Hand Surgery (American)* 2000;**25**:1043–50.
264. Kleinman WB. Cubital tunnel syndrome: anterior transposition as a logical approach to complete nerve decompression. *Journal of Hand Surgery (American)* 1999;**24**:886–97.
●265. Watchmaker GP, Lee G, Mackinnon SE. Intraneural topography of the ulnar nerve in the cubital tunnel facilitates anterior transposition. *Journal of Hand Surgery (American)* 1994;**19**:915–22.
266. George V, Smith AG. Anatomic considerations of the peripheral nerve in compressive neuropathies of the upper extremity. *Orthopedic Clinics of North America* 1996;**27**:211–18.
267. Ogata K, Manske PR, Lesker PA. The effect of surgical dissection on regional blood flow to the ulnar nerve in the cubital tunnel. *Clinical Orthopaedics and Related Research* 1985;**193**:195–8.
268. Messina A, Messina JC. Transposition of the ulnar nerve and its vascular bundle for the entrapment syndrome at the elbow. *Journal of Hand Surgery (British)* 1995;**20**:638–48.
269. Dellon AL, MacKinnon SE, Hudson AR, Hunter DA. Effect of submuscular versus intramuscular placement of ulnar nerve: experimental model in the primate. *Journal of Hand Surgery (British)* 1986;**11**:117–19.
270. Curtis BF. Traumatic ulnar neuritis: Transplantation of the nerve. *Journal of Nervous and Mental Disease* 1898;**25**:480–4.
271. Farzan M, Mortazavi SMJ, Asadollahi S. Cubital tunnel syndrome: review of 14 anterior subcutaneous transpositions of the vascularized ulnar nerve. *Acta Medica Iranica* 2005;**43**:197–203.
272. Richmond JC, Southmayd WW. Superficial anterior transposition of the ulnar nerve at the elbow for ulnar neuritis. *Clinical Orthopaedics and Related Research* 1982;**164**:42–4.
●273. Eaton RG, Crowe JF, Parkes JC 3rd. Anterior transposition of the ulnar nerve using a non-compressing fasciodermal sling. *Journal of Bone and Joint Surgery (American)* 1980;**62**:820–5.

274. Catalano LW 3rd, Barron OA. Anterior subcutaneous transposition of the ulnar nerve. *Hand Clinics* 2007;**23**:339–44.
275. Gelberman RH, Eaton R, Urbaniak JR. Peripheral nerve compression. *Journal of Bone and Joint Surgery (American)* 1993;**75**:1854–78.
276. Hashiguchi H, Ito H, Sawaizumi T, et al. Stabilized subcutaneous transposition of the ulnar nerve. *International Orthopaedics* 2003;**27**:232–4.
277. Lascar T, Laulan J. Cubital tunnel syndrome: a retrospective review of 53 anterior subcutaneous transpositions. *Journal of Hand Surgery (British)* 2000;**25**:453–6.
278. Pribyl CR, Robinson B. Use of the medial intermuscular septum as a fascial sling during anterior transposition of the ulnar nerve. *Journal of Hand Surgery (American)* 1998;**23**:500–4.
279. Adson AW. The surgical treatment of progressive ulnar paralysis. *Minnesota Medicine* 1918;**1**:455–60.
280. Platt H. The pathogenesis and treatment of traumatic neuritis of the ulnar nerve in the post-condylar groove. *British Journal of Surgery* 1926;**13**:409–31.
281. Gay JR, Love JG. Diagnosis and treatment of tardy paralysis of the ulnar nerve: based on a study of 100 cases. *Journal of Bone and Joint Surgery (American)* 1947;**29**:1087–97.
282. Leone J, Bhandari M, Thoma A. Anterior intramuscular transposition with ulnar nerve decompression at the elbow. *Clinical Orthopaedics and Related Research* 2001;**387**:132–9.
283. Henry M. Modified intramuscular transposition of the ulnar nerve. *Journal of Hand Surgery (American)* 2006;**31**:1535–42.
284. Learmonth JR. Technique for transplantation of the ulnar nerve. *Surgery, Gynecology and Obstetrics* 1942;**75**:792–3.
285. Siegel DB. Submuscular transposition of the ulnar nerve. *Hand Clinics* 1996;**12**:445–8.
286. Dellon AL. Operative technique for submuscular transposition of the ulnar nerve. *Contemporary Orthopaedics* 1988;**16**:17–24.
287. Dellon AL, Coert JH. Results of the musculofascial lengthening technique for submuscular transposition of the ulnar nerve at the elbow. *Journal of Bone and Joint Surgery (American)* 2003;**85A**:1314–20.
288. Dellon AL, Coert JH. Results of the musculofascial lengthening technique for submuscular transposition of the ulnar nerve at the elbow. *Journal of Bone and Joint Surgery (American)* 2004;**86A** (Suppl 1, Pt 2):169–79.
289. Pasque CB, Rayan GM. Anterior submuscular transposition of the ulnar nerve for cubital tunnel syndrome. *Journal of Hand Surgery (British)* 1995;**20**:447–53.
290. Nouhan R, Kleinert JM. Ulnar nerve decompression by transposing the nerve and Z-lengthening the flexor-pronator mass: clinical outcome. *Journal of Hand Surgery (American)* 1997;**22**:127–31.
291. Williams EH, Dellon AL. Anterior submuscular transposition. *Hand Clinics* 2007;**23**:345–58.
292. Dellon AL, Chang E, Coert JH, Campbell KR. Intraneural ulnar nerve pressure changes related to operative techniques for cubital tunnel decompression. [see comment]. *Journal of Hand Surgery (American)* 1994;**19**:923–30.
293. Hagstrom P. Ulnar nerve compression at the elbow. Results of surgery in 85 cases. *Scandinavian Journal of Plastic Reconstructive Surgery* 1977;**11**:59–62.
294. Tsai TM, Chen IC, Majd ME, Lim BH. Cubital tunnel release with endoscopic assistance: results of a new technique. [see comment]. *Journal of Hand Surgery (American)* 1999;**24**:21–9.
295. Bain GI, Bajhau A. Endoscopic release of the ulnar nerve at the elbow using the Agee device: a cadaveric study. *Arthroscopy* 2005;**21**:691–5.
296. Ahcan U, Zorman P. Endoscopic decompression of the ulnar nerve at the elbow. *Journal of Hand Surgery (American)* 2007;**32**:1171–6.
●297. Lowe JBI, Mackinnon SE. Management of secondary cubital tunnel syndrome. *Plastic Reconstructive Surgery* 2004;**113**:e1–e16.
298. Ruchelsman DE, Lee SK, Posner MA. Failed surgery for ulnar nerve compression at the elbow. *Hand Clinics* 2007;**23**:359–71.
299. Jackson LC, Hotchkiss RN. Cubital tunnel surgery. Complications and treatment of failures. *Hand Clinics* 1996;**12**:449–56.
300. Rogers MR, Bergfield TG, Aulicino PL. The failed ulnar nerve transposition. Etiology and treatment. *Clinical Orthopaedics and Related Research* 1991;**269**:193–200.
301. Bartels RH, Grotenhuis JA, Bartels RHMA. Anterior submuscular transposition of the ulnar nerve. For post-operative focal neuropathy at the elbow. *Journal of Bone and Joint Surgery (British)* 2004;**86**:998–1001.
302. Kleinman WB. Revision ulnar neuroplasty. *Hand Clinics* 1994;**10**:461–77.
303. Caputo AE, Watson HK. Subcutaneous anterior transposition of the ulnar nerve for failed decompression of cubital tunnel syndrome. *Journal of Hand Surgery (American)* 2000;**25**:544–51.
304. Dagregorio G, Saint-Cast Y. Simple neurolysis for failed anterior submuscular transposition of the ulnar nerve at the elbow. *International Orthopaedics* 2004;**28**:342–6.
305. Antoniadis G, Richter HP. Pain after surgery for ulnar neuropathy at the elbow: a continuing challenge. *Neurosurgery* 1997;**41**:585–91.
306. Strege DW, Cooney WP, Wood MB, et al. Chronic peripheral nerve pain treated with direct electrical nerve stimulation. *Journal of Hand Surgery (American)* 1994;**19**:931–9.
307. Varitimidis SE, Vardakas DG, Goebel F, Sotereanos DG. Treatment of recurrent compressive neuropathy of peripheral nerves in the upper extremity with an autologous vein insulator. *Journal of Hand Surgery (American)* 2001;**26**:296–302.
308. Vardakas DG, Varitimidis SE, Sotereanos DG. Findings of exploration of a vein-wrapped ulnar nerve: report of a case. *Journal of Hand Surgery (American)* 2001;**26**:60–3.

PART 11

FOOT AND ANKLE

ANISH KADAKIA

122	**Tendon pathologies** *Clifford L Jeng*	1421
123	**Hallux valgus** *Shamal Das De, Krishna Lingaraj*	1434
124	**Disorders of the hallucal sesamoids and related great toe pathologies** *Andrew Moore, Anish Raj Kadakia*	1442
125	**Lesser toe deformities** *Andrew P Molloy, Moez S Ballal*	1449
126	**Pes cavus and pes planus** *Anthony Perera, Mark S Myerson*	1460
127	**The diabetic foot** *Aziz Nather, Fu Cai Han*	1466
128	**Neurological disorders** *Norman Espinosa*	1472
129	**Inflammatory and osteoarthritis of the foot and ankle** *Andrew P Molloy, Edward V Wood*	1484
130	**Nerve compression syndromes of the foot and ankle** *Giselle Tan, Norman Espinosa, Anish Raj Kadakia*	1500

122

Tendon pathologies

CLIFFORD L JENG

Posterior tibial tendon dysfunction	1421	Anterior tibial tendon rupture	1429
Achilles tendon rupture	1424	Flexor hallucis longus tenosynovitis	1430
Achilles tendinosis	1426	References	1431
Peroneal tendons	1428		

NATIONAL BOARD STANDARDS

- Understand the pathoanatomy and pathophysiology of tendon pathology of the foot and ankle
- Know the rationale for choosing conservative treatments
- Understand the indications for surgical intervention and the appropriate techniques for tendon disorders
- Be able to appropriately evaluate and treat an acute Achilles tendon rupture

POSTERIOR TIBIAL TENDON DYSFUNCTION

Aetiology

The tibialis posterior is the second strongest muscle in the leg. Its main function is to invert the subtalar joint and to adduct the transverse tarsal joints, opposing the actions of its antagonist the peroneal tendons. Its proper functioning is critical to maintaining arch height and neutral heel alignment.

Posterior tibial tendon dysfunction (PTTD) is the most common cause of an acquired flat foot in the adult (Table 122.1). The average age at presentation is between 50 and 60 years. PTTD is more common in women than in men. It has also been associated with obesity, previous surgery or trauma, diabetes, steroid exposure and hypertension.[1]

The aetiology is believed to be an overuse phenomenon, with repetitive stresses causing an inflammatory response around the tendon. Anatomically, the tendon takes a sharp turn beneath the medial malleolus, which can cause

Table 122.1 Johnson classification for posterior tibial tendon dysfunction (PTTD) (with Myerson modification)

Stage	Description
I	Posterior tibial tendininitis with no deformity
II	Posterior tibial tendinosis with heel valgus, collapsed arch, forefoot abduction, still flexible
III	Progressive deformity, fixed forefoot varus, stiffness
IV	Stage III PTTD with valgus angulation of talus within ankle mortise

mechanical degeneration of the posterior tibial tendon with age. In addition, there is a hypovascular zone within the tendon (4 cm from the medial navicular tuberosity and extends proximally 14 mm) that increases its sensitivity to stresses.[2] Rupture of the tendon usually occurs between the tip of the medial malleolus and the insertion of the tendon.

Once the posterior tibial tendon fails, the spring ligament, which is a static stabilizer of the arch, attenuates because of repeated overload. Multiple structural changes then occur. The talar head plantarflexes, the transverse tarsal joint abducts and the calcaneus moves into a valgus position. When the heel goes into valgus, the Achilles tendon changes from a relative invertor to an evertor of the subtalar joint as its insertion moves laterally. Longstanding valgus results in contracture of the Achilles tendon as well. The above changes, in combination with the relative overpull of the now unopposed peroneus brevis muscle, result in the characteristic deformity of a collapsed longitudinal arch, heel valgus and forefoot abduction.

Clinical presentation

Patients with posterior tibial tendon dysfunction typically present with either pain or deformity of the foot and ankle. The pain is typically located over the postero-medial ankle along the course of the tendon with variable amounts of swelling. Later in the course of the disease with worsening valgus malalignment, the pain may shift from the medial to the lateral aspect of the ankle due to impingement of the lateral wall of the calcaneus under the fibula.

On standing examination, particularly in unilateral disease, the malalignment of the heel can be striking (Fig. 122.1). The 'too many toes' sign describes the finding where the fourth and fifth toes can be seen deviating beyond the lateral border of the foot when viewing the patient from behind.[3] This is a result of severe forefoot abduction. The single leg heel rise test is performed with the patient standing only on the affected leg a few inches away from a wall and attempting to elevate the heel completely off the floor.[3] This requires a functioning posterior tibial tendon to invert the heel, which locks the transverse tarsal joints, providing a stable lever arm for the Achilles tendon to pull upon.

On physical examination in patients with PTTD, the range of motion of the ankle, subtalar, and transverse tarsal joints should be carefully assessed and compared with the contralateral limb. Tenderness to palpation is elicited medially over the course of the tendon both proximally and distally. There may also be lateral hindfoot tenderness due to subfibular impingement.

Standing radiographs of the foot may reveal collapse of the longitudinal arch. Meary's angle (lateral talus–first metatarsal angle) is often negative (Fig. 122.2). The anteroposterior foot radiograph shows abduction through the transverse tarsal joints with uncovering of the talar head by the navicular. Degenerative arthritis may be present in the hindfoot joints. In stage IV disease, the ankle may be arthritic as well, showing valgus tilting of the talus within the mortise due to deltoid ligament disruption (Fig. 122.3).

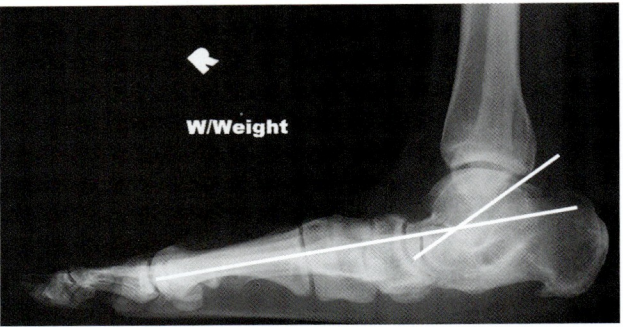

Figure 122.2 Lateral weight-bearing radiograph of a patient with posterior tibial tendon dysfunction. Meary's angle (lateral talus–first metatarsal angle) is demonstrated. Note the plantarflexed talus.

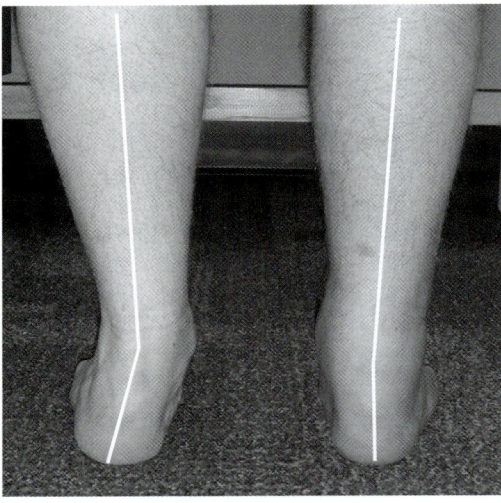

Figure 122.1 Evaluation of the alignment of the hindfoot demonstrating increased valgus on the left leg compared with the right.

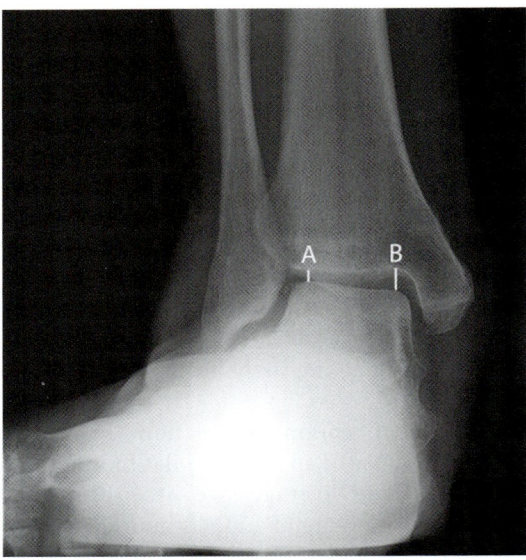

Figure 122.3 Anteroposterior ankle weight-bearing radiograph of a patient with stage IV posterior tibial tendon dysfunction. Note the valgus angulation at the tibiotalar joint. Note the increased superior clear space medially (B) compared with laterally (A).

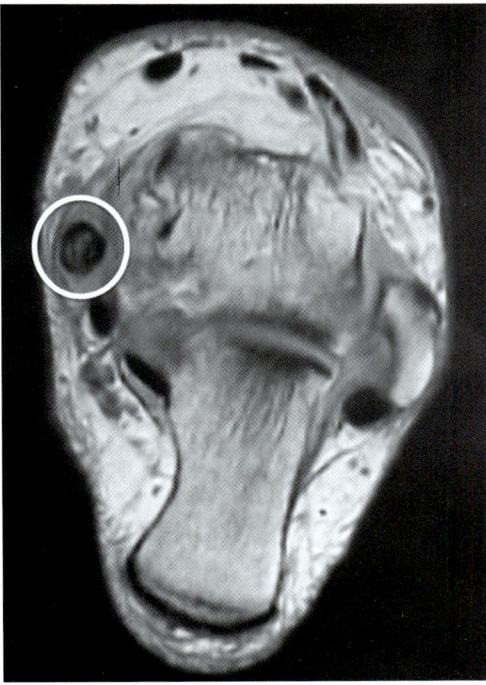

Figure 122.4 Axial T_1 MRI of a patient with posterior tibial tendon dysfunction. Note the enlargement of the tendon with intrasubstance degeneration noted by the signal changes within the tendon.

MRIs, which are typically not required to make the diagnosis of PTTD, show variable amounts of fluid signal surrounding the tendon on T_2-weighted images. T_1 images show enlargement of the tendon with intrasubstance degeneration (Fig. 122.4).

Management

Conservative management of PTTD includes cryotherapy, non-steroidal anti-inflammatory medications, immobilization or correction of the hindfoot deformity with orthoses and physical therapy. If the deformity is flexible, medially posted orthotics and custom or off-the-shelf ankle braces can correct the heel valgus malalignment to a more neutral position. This decreases the strain on the diseased tendon and relieves pain. In rigid stage III PTTD, where the deformity is not correctable, the aim of bracing is to immobilize the painful joints *in situ*. Physical therapy in conjunction with an orthosis has been shown to be effective in managing stage I and stage II PTTD.[4] Cortisone injections in or around the tendon are typically not recommended because of concerns that the degenerated tendon may further weaken, leading to greater deformity. In refractory patients, a short period of immobilization in a cast or cam boot can be beneficial.

For stage I disease that has failed conservative management, operative tenosynovectomy and debridement of the

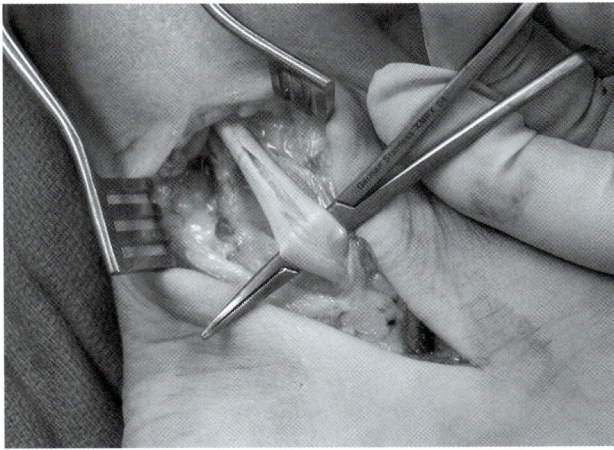

Figure 122.5 Intra-operative photograph demonstrating a longitudinal tear of the posterior tibial tendon in a patient with stage I disease.

tendon allows for return of function and improvement of subjective symptoms in 84% of patients (Fig. 122.5).[5]

In stage II PTTD with flexible flat foot deformity, surgical treatment must address both the foot deformity as well as the lack of a functioning invertor. Realignment of the deformity is typically managed with a medial displacement calcaneal osteotomy (MDCO), which corrects the hindfoot valgus.[6] The MDCO also repositions the Achilles tendon insertion medially to correct its pathological eversion effect. An alternative bony procedure is an Evan's lateral column lengthening. A transverse osteotomy is made 1.5 cm proximal to the calcaneocuboid joint. The calcaneal osteotomy is then distracted and held open with a structural bone graft to correct the abduction deformity through the transverse tarsal joints. Calcaneocuboid joint distraction arthrodesis with an intercalary structural bone graft is an alternative technique for lengthening of the lateral column. However, there is a 10–20% non-union rate associated with this procedure.[7,8] In longstanding stage II disease with significant heel valgus, there may be a compensatory forefoot varus with rigid elevation of the first metatarsal. When the hindfoot is corrected by a calcaneal osteotomy, it may be necessary in these cases to perform a dorsal opening wedge osteotomy of the medial cuneiform (Cotton osteotomy) to depress the first metatarsal and restore a plantigrade foot.[9]

SURGICAL TECHNIQUE FOR MEDIAL SLIDE CALCANEAL OSTEOTOMY

1. The patient is positioned with a large bump under the operative hip to bring the lateral hindfoot into better view for the osteotomy. The bump is removed in the middle of the procedure.
2. A thigh tourniquet is used for haemostasis during the procedure.

3. An oblique skin incision is made starting from the posterior/distal border of the fibula and continuing down to the border of the glabrous skin parallel to the course of the peroneal tendons.
4. Careful Metzenbaum dissection is performed to find and protect the sural nerve, which typically runs obliquely across the proximal third of the incision.
5. Once the nerve has been dissected out and retracted proximally, full-thickness dissection down to bone along the lateral wall of the calcaneus can be performed safely.
6. An elevator is used to lift the periosteum of the lateral wall of the calcaneus proximally and distally off the site of the planned osteotomy cut. The dorsal and plantar aspects of the tuberosity are also defined with a blunt elevator and retractors are placed dorsal and plantar to the tuberosity to protect the saw blade.
7. A large sagittal saw blade is used to make a transverse calcaneal osteotomy. Great care is taken to not overpenetrate the medial wall and risk damaging the medial neurovascular bundle.
8. Once the osteotomy is completed, a smooth lamina spreader is inserted across the osteotomy and spread open to relax the soft tissues. An elevator can be used to gently release the medial periosteum through the osteotomy.
9. The calcaneal tuberosity is translated 1 cm medially and fixed with a partially threaded 6.5 mm or 7.0 mm cannulated screw through the centre of the heel into the anterior process of the calcaneus.
10. The lateral wound is closed with subcuticular stiches and staples for the skin. Remember to staple the incision in the heel as well.

The lack of a functioning posterior tibial tendon must also be corrected during PTTD reconstruction. This is most often addressed with a flexor digitorum longus tendon transfer to the plantar aspect of the navicular through a separate medial foot incision. This restores inversion and adduction strength to oppose the antagonistic peroneus brevis and prevents recurrence of the deformity.[10,11] The soft-tissue component of the PTTD reconstruction may also include a repair or imbrication of the disrupted spring ligament to help support the longitudinal arch.[12]

SURGICAL TECHNIQUE FOR FLEXOR DIGITORUM LONGUS TRANSFER TO NAVICULAR

1. A long longitudinal incision is made starting from the tip of the medial malleolus and extending to the midshaft of the first metatarsal. Numerous veins, which are typically present just below the skin, are cauterized. Deep dissection involves reflecting the abductor hallucis muscle belly plantarly off the first metatarsal to expose the origin of the flexor hallucis brevis, where it attaches to the plantar midfoot. A self-retaining retractor is placed between the first metatarsal and the plantar soft tissues to put the flexor hallucis brevis on maximal tension, and then the origin is divided transversely, being careful not to injure the flexor hallucis longus (FHL), which lies just deep to this.
2. Blunt dissection with the index finger is carried out to identify the FHL and flexor digitorum longus deep to the released flexor hallucis brevis origin. The flexor digitorum longus runs plantar and medial to the FHL. To confirm that the correct tendon has been identified, retract on the tendons and note which toes move. The intertendinous attachments between the flexor digitorum longus and FHL are released and the two tendons are tenodesed as far distally as possible. The flexor digitorum longus is then transected just proximal to the tenodesis site and is then tagged with 2-0 Ethibond sutures.
3. Dissect dorsally over the navicular and identify the tibialis anterior tendon inserting into the medial cuneiform. With fluoroscopic assistance, a guide pin for a 4.5 mm cannulated drill bit is advanced into the medial aspect of the navicular from dorsal to plantar. Be careful not to position the drill hole too far medially, which may risk fracturing the hole during tensioning of the graft.
4. The flexor digitorum longus tendon is then passed through the drill hole in the navicular from plantar to dorsal using a suture passer. While the heel is held in maximal inversion and the tendon is maximally tensioned, the flexor digitorum longus transfer is sutured down onto the medial periosteum overlying the navicular and cuneiforms using no. 1 Ethibond sutures. An additional stitch is placed plantarly at the entry site of the tendon into the navicular for additional fixation of the graft.
5. The wound is irrigated and the abductor hallucis muscle belly is reattached to the dorsal soft tissues with absorbable sutures. This layer of closure is important to cover the Ethibond suture knots, which may later cause irritation of the overlying skin. The subcuticular layer is closed and the skin is reapproximated with staples.

In stage III PTTD, the hindfoot deformity is rigid and the joints are arthritic and painful. The only treatment option is a triple arthrodesis (fusion of the subtalar, talonavicular and calcaneocuboid joints) with realignment of the foot.

ACHILLES TENDON RUPTURE

Aetiology

The Achilles tendon is the most commonly ruptured tendon in the lower extremity. The frequency of Achilles ruptures has increased significantly with increasing emphasis on fitness in middle-aged adults. The peak incidence of Achilles tendon ruptures is in the third to fifth decade of life. Only 10% of patients will experience prodromal symptoms in the Achilles prior to rupture.

There are two primary mechanisms of injury: direct and indirect. Direct injury typically involves a blow to the posterior ankle, a crushing injury or a laceration of the tendon. Indirect injuries differ in that they are non-contact injuries. They occur because of a sudden forceful overload of the Achilles tendon. This can be seen during unexpected or violent dorsiflexion of the ankle, for example stepping into a pothole. A common indirect mechanism during sports is forcefully pushing off with the affected leg while the knee is fully extended. Multiple predisposing risk factors for Achilles tendon ruptures have been described. These include intratendinous degeneration, the use of fluoroquinolone antibiotics, intratendinous corticosteroid injections and inflammatory arthritis.

The most vulnerable region for Achilles tendon injury is the area between 2 and 6 cm proximal to the calcaneal insertion. This is the watershed zone for bloodflow to the tendon. Proximally the tendon is supplied by the gastrocnemius–soleus muscle belly. Distally it is fed by the osseous blood supply from the Achilles insertion. The central watershed zone is supplied only by the mesotenon on the tendon's ventral surface. Microscopic evaluation has documented a decrease in the number and size of blood vessels in this region.[13] This peritendinous circulation may also be compromised in patients who have chronic tendinitis.

Clinical presentation

On physical examination, a palpable or visible gap over the posterior ankle is diagnostic of Achilles tendon rupture (Fig. 122.6). Motor strength testing will usually reveal weakness with resisted plantarflexion; however, this can be disguised in patients who can adequately recruit the long toe flexors to plantar flex the ankle. The Thompson test is the most common examination described for Achilles tendon rupture. Squeezing the calf muscle causes passive plantarflexion of the ankle in patients with an intact gastroc–soleus–Achilles tendon unit. With rupture of the Achilles tendon, no plantarflexion occurs.[14] The initial diagnosis of Achilles tendon rupture may be missed in up to 20% of cases.

Management

Management of acute Achilles tendon ruptures should be by direct end-to-end repair. In two level I prospective randomized controlled trials comparing operative repair with non-operative management, surgical patients had earlier return to sports, less calf atrophy, greater ankle range of motion and fewer complaints.[15,16] According to two meta-analyses of level I studies, there was a significantly lower rerupture rate in acute Achilles ruptures repaired surgically (3–4% with surgery versus 13% with non-operative management).[17,18] In rare circumstances when medical comorbidities prohibit surgery, non-operative treatment with an equinus cast or boot gradually dorsiflexing the ankle to neutral over 8 weeks is appropriate. Weight-bearing is permitted between 8 and 12 weeks with a dorsiflexion block orthosis or boot.[19]

SURGICAL TECHNIQUE FOR ACHILLES TENDON RUPTURE REPAIR

1. Surgery is delayed until soft-tissue swelling has resolved to avoid wound-healing problems. The surgery may be carried out either in prone position or with a bump beneath the contralateral hip.
2. The location of the proximal stump of the Achilles tendon is carefully localized and a 5 cm incision is made at this level. The distal stump can be delivered into the incision for suturing by plantarflexing the ankle.
3. The incision is made 1 cm medial to the Achilles tendon and is carried down full thickness into the peritenon sheath to avoid undermining the skin.
4. The haematoma is evacuated and the 'mop-ends' debrided sharply to healthy tendon.
5. A heavy, non-absorbable suture is used in a Krackow stitch fashion to secure the proximal and distal stumps of the Achilles tendon.
6. The tendon ends are reapproximated with the ankle plantarflexed and the suture ends tied together (Fig. 122.7). The repair is tightened to match the resting equinus angle of the contralateral limb.
7. An additional running epitenon suture can be added to provide additional strength to the repair.
8. Meticulous closure of the peritenon is performed, followed by careful subcuticular and skin closure. The ankle is splinted in 20° of equinus to maximize blood flow to the skin flaps.

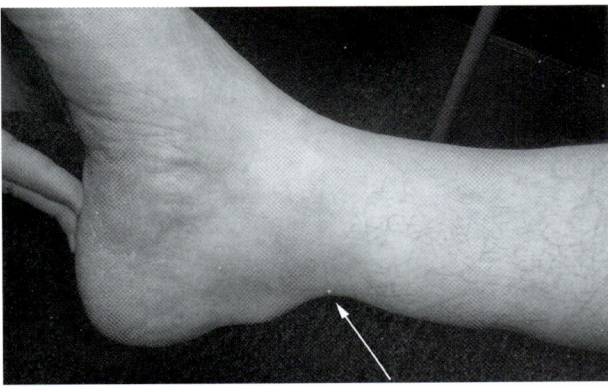

Figure 122.6 Clinical photograph of a patient with an Achilles rupture. Note the defect in the posterior aspect of the leg (arrow) that corresponds to the site of the rupture.

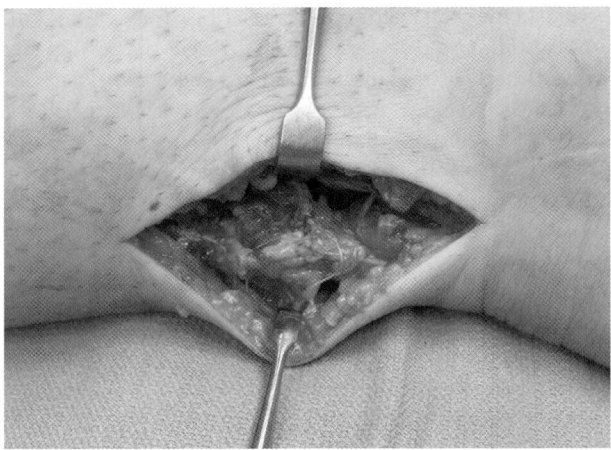

Figure 122.7 Intra-operative photograph demonstrating the apposition of the proximal and distal stumps in an Achilles tendon rupture. An epitenon suture can be added at this stage to increase the strength of the repair.

Multiple level I prospective randomized controlled studies have shown that early functional bracing following Achilles tendon rupture repair has multiple advantages over cast immobilization. Patients who are allowed early protected mobilization of the ankle have improved range of motion, earlier return to work and sports, fewer adhesions and greater satisfaction with their surgery. There was no difference in tendon lengthening, rerupture or infection with early rehabilitation protocols.[20,21]

Percutaneous repair of Achilles tendon ruptures has gained popularity since its first description by Ma and Griffith.[22] A minimally invasive approach is desirable because of the significant risk of wound-healing complications following surgery due to the thin soft-tissue envelope in the posterior aspect of the ankle. However, blindly passing sutures percutaneously may potentially place the nearby sural nerve at risk for injury. In a level I study comparing percutaneous with open repair techniques, the percutaneous group had significantly fewer wound complications (0% versus 21%) and no difference in rerupture rate or nerve injury. In a second level I study, the isokinetic strength of Achilles tendons repaired percutaneously or open was equivalent at 1.5 years postoperatively.[23,24]

Management of missed or neglected Achilles tendon ruptures more than 4–6 weeks old can be technically challenging. The algorithm for treatment is based on the size of the resulting defect in the tendon. Patients with less than a 1 cm defect can be successfully treated with direct end-to-end repair. In patients with a 1–2 cm defect, longitudinal traction on the proximal limb of the ruptured Achilles can usually restore adequate length for repair. With defects between 2 and 5 cm, a V–Y lengthening of the proximal gastrocnemius fascia may be necessary to reapproximate the ends of the tendon. Finally, with larger gaps of greater than 5 cm, a FHL tendon transfer to the calcaneal tuberosity is indicated.[25]

ACHILLES TENDINOSIS

Aetiology

Achilles tendinosis describes a degenerative tendinopathy of the Achilles tendon. With increasing age, there is a significant decrease in the diameter and overall production of collagen fibres within the Achilles tendon, and a relative increase in matrix proteoglycans. This may be due to an imbalance between proteolytic enzymes, matrix metalloproteases (MMPs) and their antagonists, tissue inhibitors of MMPs (TIMP).

These changes lead to weakening of the ageing tendon. In addition, the Achilles tendon sees forces of up to 10 times body weight during strenuous training or activity. The combination of these two factors results in micro-tears within the tendon that progress over time to macroscopic tears. These tears manifest themselves clinically with thickening and nodularity of the Achilles tendon.

The histology of Achilles tendinosis reveals mucoid degeneration and necrosis similar to lateral epicondylitis in the elbow, without any significant inflammatory infiltrate present. The pain from this condition is thought to arise from increased levels of glutamate or substance P within the tendon.[26]

Clinical factors that are believed to be associated with the development of Achilles tendinosis include overuse, errors in training, inflammatory arthritis and postural deformities. Valgus hindfoot malalignment during midstance may cause excessive tension and vascular 'blanching' of the Achilles. Heel varus may similarly place the tendon at risk.

The classification of Achilles tendinosis is based on the location of symptoms. Achilles tendinopathy can be located either in the mid-substance of the tendon (non-insertional) or near its insertion into the heel (insertional). Insertional Achilles tendinosis is often associated with either a Haglund's deformity or intratendinous calcifications.

Achilles tendinosis is also classified by the pathology present within the tendon: peritendinitis (stage I); peritendinitis with tendinosis (stage II); and tendinosis (stage III).[27] Physical examination in patients with pure peritendinitis (stage I) has been described by swelling and tenderness that remains in the same location regardless of ankle dorsiflexion and plantarflexion due to global inflammation along the entire length of the peritenon. In pure tendinosis (stage III), the location of tenderness and swelling moves proximally and distally with ankle dorsiplantarflexion due to the focal degeneration within one area of the tendon (Fig. 122.8).

There are various bony problems that may be associated with insertional Achilles tendinosis. A Haglund's deformity is a prominence of the posterosuperior calcaneal tuberosity that can cause underlying mechanical irritation to the Achilles tendon and to the retrocalcaneal bursa. The Haglund's deformity results in posterior heel pain, especially with footwear. It is classically measured on the lateral radiograph by parallel pitch lines. A line is drawn

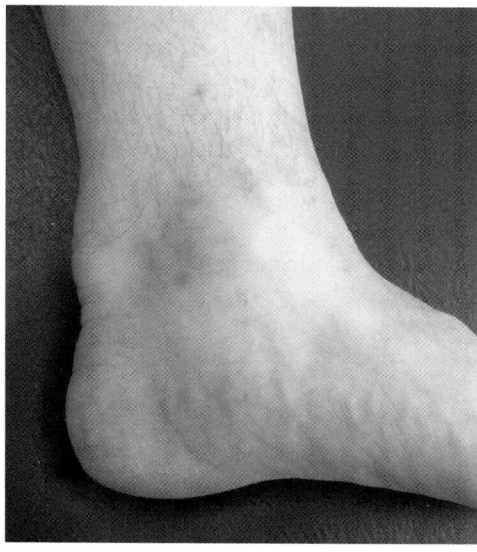

Figure 122.8 Clinical photograph of a patient with Achilles tendinosis. Note the thickened Achilles with the typical posterior prominence.

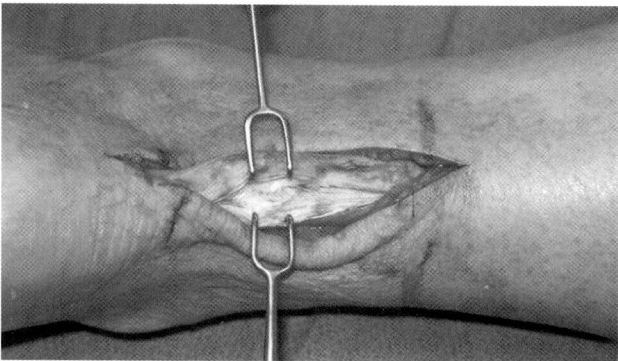

Figure 122.9 Intra-operative photograph demonstrating disorganized collagen in the centre of the Achilles tendon with no visible longitudinal fibre orientation consistent with Achilles tendinosis.

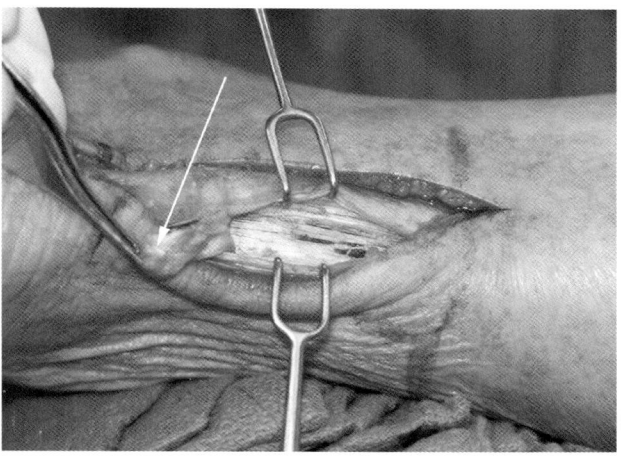

Figure 122.10 Intra-operative photograph demonstrating excision of the non-viable tendinotic tissue of the Achilles (arrow) revealing viable healthy tendon anteriorly.

from the antero-inferior to the postero-inferior aspect of the calcaneus. A second parallel line is then drawn starting from the superior most aspect of the posterior facet of the subtalar joint and extending posteriorly. If the postero-superior calcaneal tuberosity extends above the second line, then a Haglund's deformity is present.[28] A recent clinical study, however, showed no significant difference in the parallel pitch line measurements between patients with symptoms of insertional tendinopthy and asymptomatic control subjects.[29]

Intratendinous calcifications may occur within the Achilles tendon near its insertion onto the calcaneus. Repetitive mechanical stress and overuse lead to microtears within the distal tendon. These tears lead to collagen degeneration, fibrosis and eventual calcific metaplasia of the tendon.[30] Surgical findings show that the Achilles tendon does not attach to this posterior spur.[31] These calcifications can be an additional source of bony impingement in the posterior heel and ankle.

Management

Conservative management of Achilles tendinosis includes rest, heel lifts and immobilization in a cam boot to relieve mechanical stress upon the tendon. Non-steroidal anti-inflammatories, cryotherapy and orthotics, which correct excessive pronation, can be useful adjuncts to treatment.

In a prospective controlled study, physical therapy focusing on eccentric stretching exercises of the Achilles tendon was effective in reducing pain and restoring strength and normal activity.[32] Topical glyceryl trinitrate applied to chronic non-insertional Achilles tendinopathy has also shown early promise in relieving symptoms associated with tendinosis.[33] Finally, extracorporeal shock wave therapy for non-insertional Achilles tendinopathy has been shown to be significantly more effective than other non-operative therapies in treating patients with chronic symptoms.[34]

Surgery for non-insertional Achilles tendinosis should be considered only after 6 months of failed conservative treatment. In general, most surgical procedures for non-insertional Achilles tendinosis involve debridement of the diseased portion of the tendon, which is considered to be the primary source of pain. A longitudinal incision into the Achilles at the site of greatest thickening of the tendon is made. This reveals disorganized collagen in the centre of the nodular thickening with no visible longitudinal fibre orientation (Fig. 122.9). This damaged tissue is excised sharply until healthy tendon fibres are visible (Fig. 122.10). Once the split in the tendon is repaired, the weakened tendon should be reinforced. This can be done using local tissues such as the plantaris tendon or turndown repair, or by using an allograft tendon (Fig. 122.11).[35] In patients with more severe disease, the FHL tendon can be transferred into the calcaneus to provide additional plantarflexion strength to

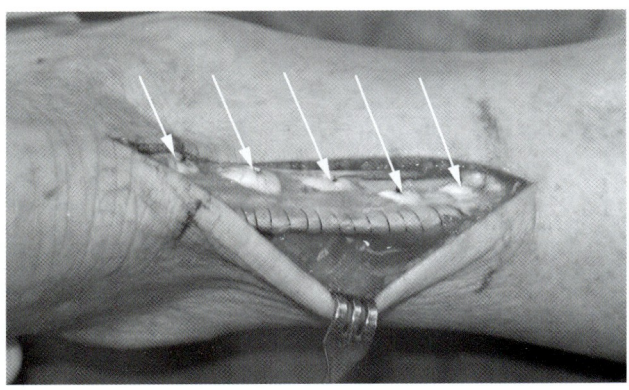

Figure 122.11 Intra-operative photograph demonstrating closure of the Achilles defect after removal of the diseased tissue and augmentation with an allograft weave (arrows).

an Achilles that has been significantly weakened from the debridement. Published results of Achilles debridement and FHL tendon transfer show high rates of patient satisfaction but a significant loss of overall plantarflexion strength.[36–38]

Surgical management of insertional Achilles tendinosis can be done through either a medial J-shaped incision, a lateral incision or a central tendon-splitting approach. The Haglund's deformity, if present, is removed with an osteotome. Then the diseased tendon and retrocalcaneal bursa is excised near the insertion of the tendon. If greater than 50% of the tendon attachment is released during exposure of the Haglund's deformity, a suture anchor should be used to secure the tendon to the exposed cancellous surface of the calcaneus to avoid complete rupture.[39] Good to excellent results in 82–97% have been reported in the literature following this treatment.[40,41] Completely arthroscopic debridement of Haglund's deformities and retrocalcaneal bursitis have been described with low rates of complications and rapid return to function.[42,43]

PERONEAL TENDONS

Aetiology

The peroneus brevis tendon inserts onto the base of the fifth metatarsal and functions as the primary evertor of the hindfoot. It is compressed between the peroneus longus and the posterior aspect of the distal fibula, which makes it susceptible to attritional tears. The sharp angle that the peroneus brevis makes beneath the tip of the fibula further adds to the stress to which the tendon is exposed.

The peroneus brevis and peroneus longus pass superior and inferior to the peroneal tubercle, respectively. The two tendons then enter their individual tendon sheaths. The peroneus longus passes beneath the cuboid, where either a fibrocartilagenous sesamoid or an os peroneum is present within the tendon. The peroneus longus passes beneath the foot to insert under the base of the first metatarsal and the medial cuneiform. It functions to plantar flex the first metatarsal, support the arch and weakly evert the subtalar joint.

The blood supply of the peroneal tendons reveals two hypovascular zones. Both the peroneus brevis and longus show decreased blood flow at the tip of the fibula. In addition, the peroneus longus has a second hypovascular zone at the cuboid tunnel, where it turns sharply to enter the plantar aspect of the foot. These sites correspond to the most common areas where tendinopathy occurs.[44]

One risk factor for peroneal tendon injury is recurrent ankle instability. Frequent inversion injuries lead to increased traction on the tendons, which are secondary restraints to ankle sprain.[45] Another risk factor for peroneal injury is the presence of an accessory peroneus quartus muscle, which can occur in 13–22% of the population. A peroneus quartus or a low-lying muscle belly of the peroneus brevis can cause increased pressure within the peroneal tunnel. This results in further compression to the already vulnerable tendons. Hypertrophy of the peroneal tubercle has also been reported as a source of friction for both tendons, which can lead to tears.[46]

Clinically, patients with a peroneal tendon injury will complain of posterolateral ankle pain and swelling. In many cases there is a history of either an ankle sprain or an overuse injury, and recurrent ankle instability may be present. On examination, ankle clicking or popping may be present. There may be significant laxity of the lateral ankle ligaments with inversion stress testing. It is also critical to evaluate for peroneal subluxation (Fig. 122.12), ankle instability and heel varus malalignment. In general, peroneus brevis tears occur above the tip of the fibula with tenderness in the retromalleolar area. In contrast, peroneus longus tears occur most frequently distal to the tip of the fibula, and therefore are most tender to palpation in the region near the peroneal tubercle or os peroneum.

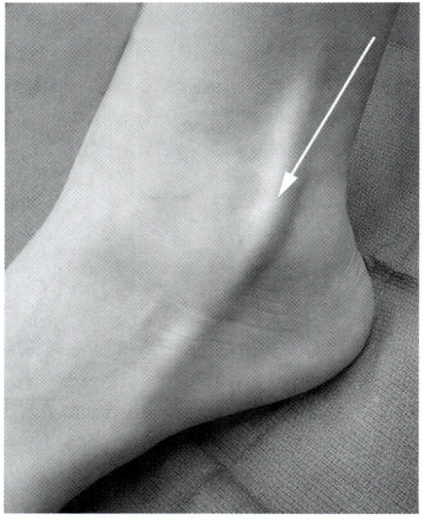

Figure 122.12 Clinical photograph of a patient with dislocation of the peroneal tendons. Note the prominence of the tendons underneath the skin (arrow).

Management

Conservative management of peroneal tendon injuries includes rest, cryotherapy and non-steroidal anti-inflammatories. An ankle brace or cam walker boot can immobilize the tendons to help alleviate symptoms. Similarly, a laterally posted foot orthosis can place the heel into valgus and offload the injured peroneals. Physical therapy may be helpful to rehabilitate weakened eversion strength. Some authors have recommended brisement or injection of local anaesthetic into the peroneal tendon sheaths to free adhesions to the tendon. Lidocaine injection may also be helpful in the diagnosis of peroneal pathology. MRI allows visualization of the peroneal tendons to aid in pre-operative planning with respect to the extent of the tears and the fibular groove (Fig. 122.13). Conservative treatment of peroneal tendon pathology has a success rate of approximately 20%, with the remaining patients requiring surgery.[46,47]

Surgical management of the peroneal tendons depends upon the pathology present. In patients with pure tenosynovitis, a simple debridement of the inflammatory tissues with meticulous repair of the peroneal retinaculum is often successful. If there is a tear in either tendon, treatment is dictated by the size of the tear. In grade I tears, where there is a large percentage of the tendon intact and only a small sliver of tendon torn, the smaller portion of tendon can be excised and the remainder tubularized with a running suture. In grade II tears, where greater than 50% of the tendon is torn, the diseased segment should be debrided and a tenodesis performed to the intact peroneal tendon. If both tendons are irreparable, a flexor digitorum longus tendon transfer to the peroneus brevis can be performed to restore eversion power.[47,48]

Associated pathology must also be addressed in the initial surgery to prevent early recurrence of the injury. This includes surgical procedures that correct superior peroneal retinaculum laxity, chronic ankle instability, prominent osteophytes, hindfoot varus and the presence of a peroneus quartus. Results of peroneal tendon surgery show a majority of patients achieving good to excellent results, although return to maximum function may be prolonged.[47]

Peroneal tendon dislocation is the condition where the peroneal tendons either subluxate or dislocate out of the retrofibular groove (Fig. 122.12). This occurs from a dorsiflexion inversion type injury associated with a sudden contraction of the peroneals, which disrupts the superior peroneal retinaculum (SPR). The SPR is the primary restraint to tendon dislocation. Also important to the stability of the tendons is the fibrocartilagenous cap on the posterolateral ridge of the fibula, as well as the shape of the posterior aspect of the distal fibula. Eighty-two per cent of patients have a concave groove, which is the most stable situation. Eleven per cent have a flat fibula, and 7% have a convex fibula.[49]

On examination, resisted dorsiflexion and eversion can elicit palpable or visible dislocation of the tendons. Patients may have significant apprehension with this manoeuvre, which is relieved by the examiner manually holding the tendons in place. Some patients are able to voluntarily dislocate their peroneal tendons.

Delay in diagnosis and treatment of peroneal pathology has been shown to lead to poorer clinical results and greater recurrence.[50] Conservative treatment involves casting the ankle in plantarflexion and inversion for 6 weeks in order to contain the peroneals behind the fibula while the SPR heals. Failure rates of this treatment have been reported between 43% and 86%. Surgery is indicated for chronic peroneal subluxation and may be considered as primary treatment in young, athletic patients.

There are several surgical procedures that have been described for the stabilization of the peroneal tendons. The most popular of these are direct repair with imbrication of the superior peroneal retinaculum, and groove deepening of the fibular groove. Direct repair can either be performed by dividing the retinaculum and repairing it in a pants over vest fashion, or by directly suturing the posterior portion of the retinaculum to the malleolar ridge through drill holes. Success rates have been reported in the literature between 85% and 100%.[51,52] Groove deepening is performed by elevating an osteoperiosteal flap on the posterior aspect of the distal fibula with a saw, burring out the cancellous bone from beneath the flap, and then impacting the flap into the deepened groove to create a concave fibula. Groove deepening has been reported to have 100% good to excellent results in one case series.[53]

ANTERIOR TIBIAL TENDON RUPTURE

Aetiology

The tibialis anterior muscle is the primary dorsiflexor of the ankle, providing 80% of dorsiflexion power. It is primarily

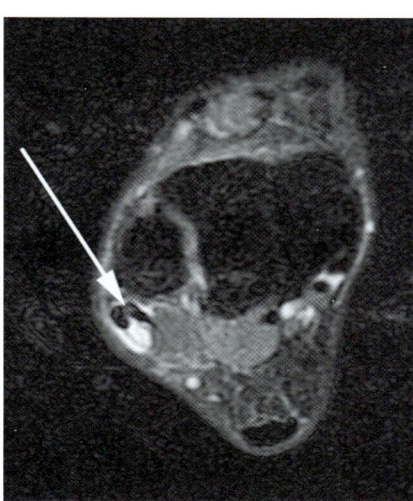

Figure 122.13 Axial T_2-weighted MRI demonstrating fluid within the peroneal sheath and a tear of the peroneus brevis (arrow).

active during the swing phase of gait to allow the foot to clear the floor, and during heel strike to prevent a foot slap gait. An avascular zone of the anterior tibial tendon has been identified in the anterior half of the tendon where it passes beneath the extensor retinaculum.[54] This is a common site of rupture of the anterior tibial tendon. Another frequent site of rupture is 2–3 cm proximal to its insertion, especially when underlying osteophytes are present in the midfoot.

Anterior tibial tendon ruptures have a bimodal age distribution. Young patients with ruptures typically present early after their injury with acute pain and swelling. The mechanism is by an eccentric load on the tendon, most commonly following forced or excessive plantarflexion against a contracted tibialis anterior. In contrast, the classic presentation in the older age group is a 50–70 year old man who has a painless foot drop. There is often no history of trauma or only minimal injury. The average delay in diagnosis is 10 weeks in this older group of patients.

On clinical examination, there is a visible and palpable lump over the anterior ankle at the site of rupture. Excessive swelling may disguise the lump, however. Patients will have weakness with dorsiflexion and will recruit their extensor hallucis longus and extensor digitorum longus to compensate for their deficit. Patients will be unable to heel walk.

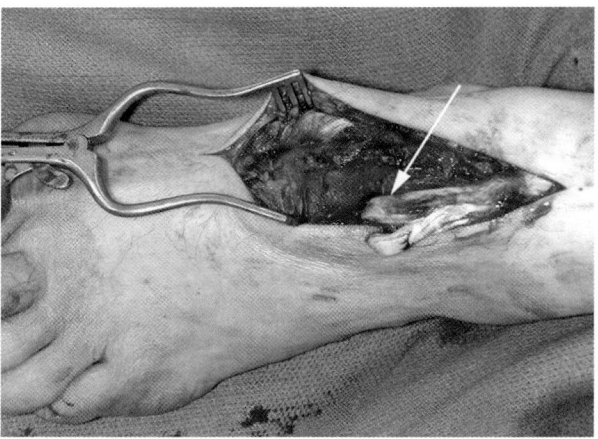

Figure 122.14 Intra-operative photograph demonstrating an insertional tear of the anterior tibial tendon (arrow).

Management

In young patients, anterior tibial tendon ruptures should be repaired primarily to maximize function and strength. However, in older patients, particularly if the rupture is greater than 4 weeks old, non-operative treatment can be considered. In two studies there was no significant clinical difference found between operative and non-operative treatment of anterior tibial tendon ruptures in elderly patients. There was minimal disability found at final follow-up with non-operative treatment.[55,56]

Surgery for acute anterior tibial tendon ruptures is by direct end-to-end repair. In cases where the tendon has avulsed from its insertion and there is inadequate length to reach the medial cuneiform, the ruptured tendon can be reinserted into the navicular (Fig. 122.14). For neglected ruptures, the surgical options are either a sliding anterior tibial tendon graft or an extensor hallucis longus or extensor digitorum longus tendon transfer.

FLEXOR HALLUCIS LONGUS TENOSYNOVITIS

Aetiology

The FHL runs behind the ankle joint and then passes into a fibro-osseous tunnel to enter the midfoot. Stenosis of this tendon can occur at three different sites: (1) in the posterior ankle, (2) in the midfoot at the knot of Henry and (3) distally where the FHL runs between the hallucal sesamoids. FHL pathology typically occurs because of overuse syndromes, postural abnormalities, trauma and inflammatory arthropathies. Ballet dancers are particularly prone to FHL tenosynovitis due to the en pointe position, which places excessive pressure upon the tendon.

Clinically, patients present with posteromedial ankle pain. Fifty per cent of them will report having crepitus behind the ankle, and if significant nodularity of the tendon develops there may be actual triggering, known as hallux saltans. On physical examination, there is tenderness with deep palpation over the FHL tendon behind the ankle, and there is weakness and pain with resisted hallux interphalangeal joint flexion.

Management

Conservative treatment of FHL tenosynovitis includes resting the tendon with a cam walker boot, non-steroidal anti-inflammatories and physical therapy with stretching of the muscle–tendon unit. Non-operative care can be successful in up to 64% of patients.[57]

Surgery is indicated in recalcitrant cases that have failed at least 6 months of conservative care. Through a posteromedial approach with the patient in the prone position, the tendon sheath is released as far distally as the fibro-osseous tunnel. Once the tendon is exposed, surgical findings may include tendon hypertrophy, synovial adhesions or synovitis, a low-lying FHL muscle belly, longitudinal tendon tears or nodular thickening of the tendon. Any nodular areas are resected and tendon tears are repaired. Operative treatment is successful in up to 81% of patients.[58]

> **KEY LEARNING POINTS**
>
> - The tibialis posterior is the second strongest muscle in the leg.
> - Posterior tibial tendon dysfunction (PTTD) is the most common cause of acquired flat foot in adults.
> - The Johnson classification for PTTD (with Myerson modification) is the standard.
> - Conservative care consists of cryotherapy, non-steroidal anti-inflammatory drugs (NSAIDs), orthoses, physical therapy.
> - The medial slide calcaneal osteotomy is useful for stage II PTTD along with a flexor digitorum longus transfer to navicular.
> - Stage III PTTD requires a triple arthrodesis.
> - Rupture of the Achilles tendon is the most common ruptured tendon in the leg.
> - The Thompson test is diagnostic.
> - Treatment of Achilles tendon rupture is a direct end-to-end repair.
> - A pecutaneous repair technique may be prone to sural nerve injury.
> - Missed or neglected Achilles tendon ruptures will require repair with possible V–Y lengthening or flexor hallucis longus tendon transfer.
> - Achilles tendinosis is a degenerative tendinopathy of the Achilles tendon with mucoid degeneration and necrosis (similar to tennis elbow). There maybe a Haglund's deformity.
> - Conservative management is rest, heel lifts, a cam boot, NSAIDs, cryotherapy and orthotics. Surgery may be necessary after 6 months of treatment.
> - Peroneal tendon injury is typically treated with tenosynovectomy and tendon repair. Associated conditions must also be addressed, such as ankle instability, heel varus or dislocating peroneal tendons.
> - Anterior tibial tendon rupture should be repaired (unless an old rupture in an older patient).
> - Flexor hallucis longus tenosynovitis should be treated by open tenosynovectomy from a posteromedial approach after 6 months of failed conservative care.

REFERENCES

- ● = Key primary paper
- ◆ = Major review article

●1. Holmes GB, Jr, Mann RA. Possible epidemiological factors associated with rupture of the posterior tibial tendon. *Foot and Ankle* 1992;**13**:70–9.

●2. Frey C, Shereff M, Greenidge N. Vascularity of the posterior tibial tendon. *Journal of Bone and Joint Surgery (American)* 1990;**72**:884–8.

●3. Johnson KA. Tibialis posterior tendon rupture. *Clinical Orthopaedics and Related Research* 1983;**Jul–Aug**:140–7.

●4. Alvarez RG, Marini A, Schmitt C, Saltzman CL. Stage I and II posterior tibial tendon dysfunction treated by a structured nonoperative management protocol: an orthosis and exercise program. *Foot and Ankle International* 2006;**27**:2–8.

●5. Teasdall RD, Johnson KA. Surgical treatment of stage I posterior tibial tendon dysfunction. *Foot and Ankle International* 1994;**15**:646–8.

●6. Koutsogiannis E. Treatment of mobile flat foot by displacement osteotomy of the calcaneus. *Journal of Bone and Joint Surgery (British)* 1971;**53**:96–100.

●7. Toolan BC, Sangeorzan BJ, Hansen ST Jr. Complex reconstruction for the treatment of dorsolateral peritalar subluxation of the foot. Early results after distraction arthrodesis of the calcaneocuboid joint in conjunction with stabilization of, and transfer of the flexor digitorum longus tendon to, the midfoot to treat acquired pes planovalgus in adults. *Journal of Bone and Joint Surgery (American)* 1999;**81**:1545–60.

●8. van der Krans A, Louwerens JW, Anderson P. Adult acquired flexible flatfoot, treated by calcaneocuboid distraction arthrodesis, posterior tibial tendon augmentation, and percutaneous Achilles tendon lengthening: a prospective outcome study of 20 patients. *Acta Orthopaedica* 2006;**77**:156–63.

●9. Tankson CJ, The Cotton osteotomy: indications and techniques. *Foot and Ankle Clinics* 2007;**12**:309–15, vii.

●10. Mann RA, Thompson FM, Rupture of the posterior tibial tendon causing flat foot. Surgical treatment. *Journal of Bone and Joint Surgery (American)* 1985;**67**:556–61.

●11. Myerson MS, Badekas A, Schon LC. Treatment of stage II posterior tibial tendon deficiency with flexor digitorum longus tendon transfer and calcaneal osteotomy. *Foot and Ankle International* 2004;**25**:445–50.

●12. Gazdag AR, Cracchiolo A, 3rd. Rupture of the posterior tibial tendon. Evaluation of injury of the spring ligament and clinical assessment of tendon transfer and ligament repair. *Journal of Bone and Joint Surgery (American)* 1997;**79**:675–81.

●13. Carr AJ, Norris SH. The blood supply of the calcaneal tendon. *Journal of Bone and Joint Surgery (British)* 1989;**71**:100–1.

●14. Thompson TC, Doherty JH. Spontaneous rupture of tendon of Achilles: a new clinical diagnostic test. *Journal of Trauma* 1962;**2**:126–9.

●15. Cetti R, Henriksen LO, Jacobsen KS. Operative versus nonoperative treatment of Achilles tendon rupture. A prospective randomized study and review of the literature. *American Journal of Sports Medicine* 1993;**21**:791–9.

●16. Moller M, Movin T, Granhed H, et al. Acute rupture of tendon Achillis. A prospective randomised study of comparison between surgical and non-surgical treatment. *Journal of Bone and Joint Surgery (British)* 2001;**83**:843–8.

- 17. Bhandari M, Guyatt GH, Siddiqui F, et al. Treatment of acute Achilles tendon ruptures: a systematic overview and metaanalysis. *Clinical Orthopaedics and Related Research* 2002;**Jul**:190-200.
- 18. Khan RJ, Fick D, Keogh A, et al. Treatment of acute achilles tendon ruptures. A meta-analysis of randomized, controlled trials. *Journal of Bone and Joint Surgery (American)* 2005;**87**:2202-10.
- 19. McComis GP, Nawoczenski DA, DeHaven KE. Functional bracing for rupture of the Achilles tendon. Clinical results and analysis of ground-reaction forces and temporal data. *Journal of Bone and Joint Surgery (American)* 1997;**79**:1799-808.
- 20. Cetti R, Henriksen LO, Jacobsen KS. A new treatment of ruptured Achilles tendons. A prospective randomized study. *Clinical Orthopaedics and Related Research* 1994;**Nov**:155-65.
- 21. Mortensen HM, Skov O, Jensen PE. Early motion of the ankle after operative treatment of a rupture of the Achilles tendon. A prospective, randomized clinical and radiographic study. *Journal of Bone and Joint Surgery (American)* 1999;**81**:983-90.
- 22. Ma GW, Griffith TG. Percutaneous repair of acute closed ruptured achilles tendon: a new technique. *Clinical Orthopaedics and Related Research* 1977;**Oct**:247-55.
- 23. Lim J, Dalal R, Waseem M. Percutaneous vs. open repair of the ruptured Achilles tendon – a prospective randomized controlled study. *Foot and Ankle International* 2001;**22**:559-68.
- 24. Goren D, Ayalon M, Nyska M. Isokinetic strength and endurance after percutaneous and open surgical repair of Achilles tendon ruptures. *Foot and Ankle International* 2005;**26**:286-90.
- 25. Myerson MS. Achilles tendon ruptures. *Instructional Course Lectures* 1999; **48**:219-30.
- 26. Andersson G, Danielson P, Alfredson H, Forsgren S. Presence of substance P and the neurokinin-1 receptor in tenocytes of the human Achilles tendon. *Regulatory Peptides* 2008;**150**:81-7.
- 27. Puddu G, Ippolito E, Postacchini F. A classification of Achilles tendon disease. *American Journal of Sports Medicine* 1976;**4**:145-50.
- 28. Pavlov H, et al. The Haglund syndrome: initial and differential diagnosis. *Radiology* 1982;**144**:83-8.
- 29. Lu CC, Cheng YM, Fu YC, et al. Angle analysis of Haglund syndrome and its relationship with osseous variations and Achilles tendon calcification. *Foot and Ankle International* 2007;**28**:181-5.
- 30. Johnson KW, Zalavras C, Thordarson DB. Surgical management of insertional calcific achilles tendinosis with a central tendon splitting approach. *Foot and Ankle International* 2006;**27**:245-50.
- 31. Myerson MS, McGarvey W. Disorders of the Achilles tendon insertion and Achilles tendinitis. *Instructional Course Lectures* 1999;**48**:211-18.
- 32. Alfredson H, Lorentzon R. Chronic Achilles tendinosis: recommendations for treatment and prevention. *Sports Medicine* 2000;**29**:135-46.
- 33. Paoloni JA, Appleyard R, Nelson J, Murrell G. Topical glyceryl trinitrate treatment of chronic noninsertional achilles tendinopathy. A randomized, double-blind, placebo-controlled trial. *Journal of Bone and Joint Surgery (American)* 2004;**86A**:916-22.
- 34. Furia JP. High-energy extracorporeal shock wave therapy as a treatment for chronic noninsertional Achilles tendinopathy. *American Journal of Sports Medicine* 2008;**36**:502-8.
- 35. Nelen G, Martens M, Burssens A. Surgical treatment of chronic Achilles tendinitis. *American Journal of Sports Medicine* 1989;**17**:754-9.
- 36. Martin RL, Manning CM, Carcia CR, Conti SF. An outcome study of chronic Achilles tendinosis after excision of the Achilles tendon and flexor hallucis longus tendon transfer. *Foot and Ankle International* 2005;**26**:691-7.
- 37. Wilcox DK, Bohay DR, Anderson JG. Treatment of chronic achilles tendon disorders with flexor hallucis longus tendon transfer/augmentation. *Foot and Ankle International* 2000;**21**:1004-10.
- 38. Monroe MT, Dixon DJ, Beals TC, et al. Plantarflexion torque following reconstruction of Achilles tendinosis or rupture with flexor hallucis longus augmentation. *Foot and Ankle International* 2000;**21**:324-9.
- 39. Kolodziej P, Glisson RR, Nunley JA. Risk of avulsion of the Achilles tendon after partial excision for treatment of insertional tendonitis and Haglund's deformity: a biomechanical study. *Foot and Ankle International* 1999;**20**:433-7.
- 40. Sammarco GJ, Taylor AL. Operative management of Haglund's deformity in the nonathlete: a retrospective study. *Foot and Ankle International* 1998;**19**:724-9.
- 41. McGarvey WC, Palumbo RC, Baxter DE, Leibman BD. Insertional Achilles tendinosis: surgical treatment through a central tendon splitting approach. *Foot and Ankle International* 2002;**23**:19-25.
- 42. van Dijk CN, van Dyk GE, Scholten PE, Kort NP. Endoscopic calcaneoplasty. *American Journal of Sports Medicine* 2001;**29**:185-9.
- 43. Ortmann FW, McBryde AM. Endoscopic bony and soft-tissue decompression of the retrocalcaneal space for the treatment of Haglund deformity and retrocalcaneal bursitis. *Foot and Ankle International* 2007;**28**:149-53.
- 44. Petersen W, Bobka T, Stein V, Tillmann B. Blood supply of the peroneal tendons: injection and immunohistochemical studies of cadaver tendons. *Acta Orthopaedica Scandinavica* 2000;**71**:168-74.
- 45. Sammarco GJ, DiRaimondo CV. Chronic peroneus brevis tendon lesions. *Foot and Ankle* 1989;**9**:163-70.
- 46. Sobel M, Pavlov H, Geppert MJ, et al. Painful os peroneum syndrome: a spectrum of conditions responsible for plantar lateral foot pain. *Foot and Ankle International* 1994;**15**:112-24.

- 47. Krause JO, Brodsky JW. Peroneus brevis tendon tears: pathophysiology, surgical reconstruction, and clinical results. *Foot and Ankle International* 1998;**19**:271-9.
- 48. Redfern D, Myerson M, The management of concomitant tears of the peroneus longus and brevis tendons. *Foot and Ankle International* 2004;**25**:695-707.
- 49. Edwards ME. The relations of the peroneal tendons to the fibula, calcaneus, and cuboideum. *The American Journal of Anatomy* 1928;**42**:213-253.
- 50. Escalas F, Figueras JM, Merino JA. Dislocation of the peroneal tendons. Long-term results of surgical treatment. *Journal of Bone and Joint Surgery (American)* 1980;**62**:451-3.
- 51. Eckert WR, Davis EA Jr. Acute rupture of the peroneal retinaculum. *Journal of Bone and Joint Surgery (American)* 1976;**58**:670-2.
- 52. Hui JH, Das De S, Balasubramaniam P. The Singapore operation for recurrent dislocation of peroneal tendons: long-term results. *Journal of Bone and Joint Surgery (British)* 1998;**80**:325-7.
- 53. Zoellner G, Clancy W Jr. Recurrent dislocation of the peroneal tendon. *Journal of Bone and Joint Surgery (American)* 1979;**61**:292-4.
- 54. Petersen W, Stein V, Tillmann B. Blood supply of the tibialis anterior tendon. *Archives of Orthopaedic and Trauma Surgery* 1999;**119**(7-8):371-5.
- 55. Markarian GG, Kelikian AS, Brage M, *et al*. Anterior tibialis tendon ruptures: an outcome analysis of operative versus nonoperative treatment. *Foot and Ankle International* 1998;**19**:792-802.
- 56. Ouzounian TJ, Anderson R. Anterior tibial tendon rupture. *Foot and Ankle International* 1995;**16**:406-10.
- 57. Michelson J, Dunn L. Tenosynovitis of the flexor hallucis longus: a clinical study of the spectrum of presentation and treatment. *Foot and Ankle International* 2005;**26**:291-303.
- 58. Hamilton WG, Geppert MJ, Thompson FM. Pain in the posterior aspect of the ankle in dancers. Differential diagnosis and operative treatment. *Journal of Bone and Joint Surgery (American)* 1996;**78**:1491-500.

123

Hallux valgus

SHAMAL DAS DE, KRISHNA LINGARAJ

Introduction	1434	Radiographic evaluation	1436
Pathoanatomy	1434	Treatment	1437
Aetiology	1435	References	1440
Clinical features	1436		

NATIONAL BOARD STANDARDS

- To know the definition and causes of hallux valgus
- Common sites and positions for fusion
- To request the correct radiographs for planning
- The essential surgical procedures based on deformity approaches
- Learn what are the main complications of surgery

INTRODUCTION

Hallux valgus can be defined as a complex progressive deformity affecting the forefoot, in which the lateral deviation of the great toe is the most obvious feature.[1] The complex may also involve rotation of the hallux, metatarsus primus varus, overriding of the second toe over the hallux, overriding of the lateral toes, and hammer and claw deformities of the lateral toes. The term bunion refers to the swelling that occurs because of the medial eminence of the metatarsal head, overlying bursitis and, on occasion, skin callosity. Hallux valgus is a common disorder that may cause pain, difficulty with footwear and restriction of function. It affects both adolescents and adults, and the underlying pathophysiology in each group varies.

PATHOANATOMY

Excessive lateral deviation of the first metatarsophalangeal (MTP) joint of more than 35° leads to pronation of the big toe. As a result of this, the normal static and dynamic stabilizers of the first MTP joint become destabilizers (Fig. 123.1). The abductor hallucis, which normally prevents lateral deviation of the toe, moves further plantarward from its normal position, and leaves the medial capsular ligament as the only medial restraining structure. The adductor hallucis, which is now unopposed by the abductor hallucis, increases the lateral deformity and causes attenuation of the medial capsular structures. This allows the metatarsal head to shift medially.[2]

The tibial sesamoid then exerts pressure on the sesamoid ridge or crista on the plantar surface of the first metatarsal head causing it to flatten. This allows the fibular sesamoid to displace into the first intermetatarsal space and leads to increased weight transfer to the lesser metatarsal heads. In addition, the flexor hallucis brevis and the flexor hallucis longus increase the valgus moment at the first MTP joint, thereby deforming the first ray. Eventually there may be chronic shortening and contracture of the adductor hallucis, flexor hallucis brevis and lateral capsuloligamentous structures.

The valgus deformity of the first MTP joint may be either congruent or incongruent. In a congruent deformity, there is inherent soft-tissue and articular stability, which prevents

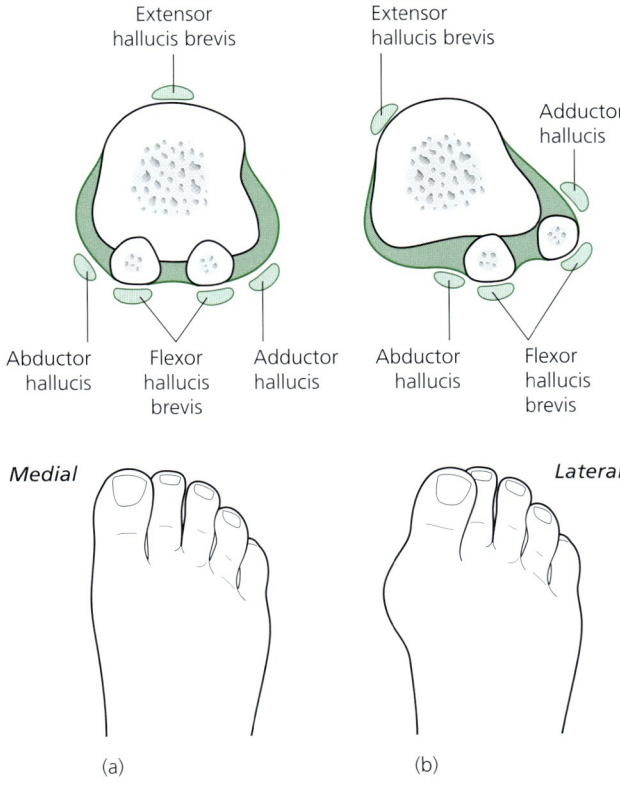

Figure 123.1 Pronation of the hallux is a key factor in the development of the hallux valgus deformity. (a) Normal; (b) pronation results in plantar shift of the abductor hallucis and lateral shift of the sesamoids and their associated intrinsic muscles.

may also cause a hammer toe-like deformity and overriding of the second toe, as well as splaying of the forefoot.

AETIOLOGY

Many factors are believed to contribute to the development of the hallux valgus deformity. The role of inappropriate footwear in the aetiology of this deformity is suggested by the increased incidence in shoe-wearing populations, particularly those wearing fashion shoes in which there is insufficient space for the forefoot. In Hong Kong, hallux valgus has been found to be 17 times as common among shoe-wearers as in the unshod population.[4] Pre-existing metatarsus primus varus, or medial deviation of the first metatarsal, may also contribute to increased laterally directed pressure on the hallux. This may be an isolated feature or secondary to instability or hypermobility of the first metatarsal–cuneiform joint. Generalized ligamentous laxity may also be a contributory factor, and could be the most common cause in males with hallux valgus. These patients have planovalgus feet with pronation of the great toe.

Another anatomical variant that may be contributory is the presence of an increased distal metatarsal articular angle (DMAA), which refers to the valgus tilt of the distal articular surface of the first metatarsal. Increased valgus tilt of the proximal phalangeal articular surface, termed hallux valgus interphalangeus (HVI), contributes to the hallux valgus deformity. Other anatomic variants associated with, though not proven to be causally related to, hallux valgus include pes planus, a rounded metatarsal head and a relatively long first metatarsal. Causes of secondary hallux valgus include inflammatory arthropathies, such as rheumatoid arthritis, spastic disorders, such as cerebral palsy, and trauma, in which there is disruption of the soft-tissue envelope of the first MTP joint. Amputation of the second toe can lead to iatrogenic hallux valgus, but the presence of an os intermetatarsum can also lead to the development of this deformity.

subluxation of the joint. In an incongruent deformity, lateral subluxation of the joint occurs as a result of musculotendinous imbalance, and this deformity often increases with time. Piggot[3] has proposed a classification system for the degree of congruence in the first MTP joint (Fig. 123.2). In severe cases, valgus subluxation of the first MTP joint can lead to osteoarthritis. The valgus deformity of the big toe

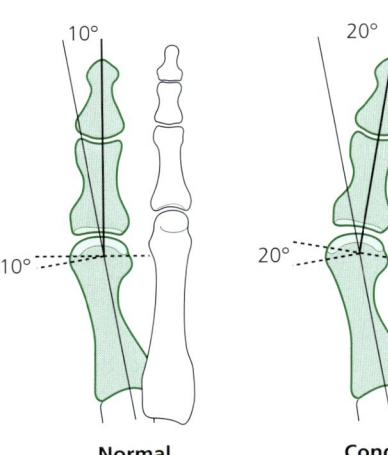
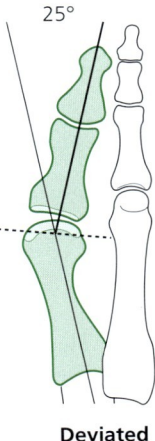
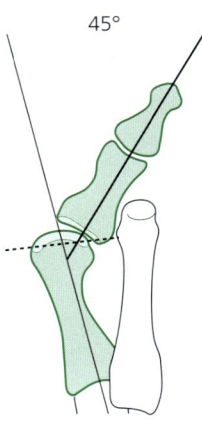

Normal Congruous Deviated Subluxated

Figure 123.2 Classification of the congruence of the first metatarsophalangeal joint in the hallux valgus, as defined by Piggot.

In adolescent patients, footwear is less of a contributory factor. Underlying metatarsus primus varus, increased DMAA, HVI, pes planus, ligamentous laxity and hypermobility of the first metatarsal–cuneiform joint are considered to be the more likely causative factors.

CLINICAL FEATURES

Hallux valgus is often asymptomatic. In symptomatic patients, pain is often the primary complaint, and the site of pain is of diagnostic importance. Pain on the medial aspect of the first MTP joint is associated with bursitis, whereas that on the dorsal aspect is associated with osteoarthritis. Plantar pain may signal involvement of the sesamoids. Similarly, pain in the metatarsal heads of the lesser toes suggests transfer metatarsalgia. Pain resulting from the hallux valgus deformity may affect the patient's daily work and recreational activities. Cosmesis is often a concern, especially among adolescents, although this should not be a primary consideration for treatment.

Clinical examination will reveal lateral deviation and often pronation of the big toe (Fig. 123.3). The range of motion of the first MTP joint after passive correction of the deformity will indicate the expected post-surgical range of motion. Soft-tissue swelling, callosity and sometimes ulceration may be observed over the medial eminence of the metatarsal head. As alluded to earlier, the site of tenderness is of diagnostic importance. The second toe may exhibit a hammer-toe deformity or be overriding. Plantar callosities beneath the metatarsal heads of the lesser toes would indicate excessive weight transfer from the first ray to the lesser toes. The first metatarsal–cuneiform joint may also demonstrate hypermobility.

Other findings that may be present include pes planus deformity, heel valgus, Achilles tendon contracture and generalized ligamentous laxity. The vascularity and sensation of the foot should be assessed in all patients, particularly those afflicted with diabetes and peripheral vascular disease.

RADIOGRAPHIC EVALUATION

Radiographic evaluation requires weight-bearing anteroposterior (AP), lateral and oblique views of the foot. The AP view of the foot is used to assess the extent of the deformity. To this end, several angular measurements are made. These include the hallux valgus angle (HVA), which is marked by the intersection of a line bisecting the diaphysis of the first metatarsal and a line bisecting the proximal phalangeal shaft. A normal hallux valgus angle is 15° or less (Fig. 123.4a). The first–second intermetatarsal angle (IMA_{1-2}) is defined by lines bisecting the first and second metatarsal shafts. This should normally measure less than 9° (Fig. 123.4b).

The lateral tilt of the distal articular surface of the first metatarsal is measured by the DMAA. This is measured between the longitudinal axis of the first metatarsal and a line connecting the medial and lateral margins of the chondral surface. A measurement of more than 10° is considered abnormal (Fig. 123.4c). The proximal phalangeal articular angle (PPAA) is defined by a line bisecting the proximal phalanx and a line perpendicular to the base of the proximal phalanx. This should normally be less than 10° (Fig. 123.4d). An increase in this angle is a predisposing factor for the development of hallux valgus. It is also useful in identifying hallux valgus interphalangeus.[5]

Other radiographic findings to note include congruency of the joint (implied by an increased DMAA or HVI), the presence of subluxation, arthritic changes, pes planus, dorsal subluxation of the first metatarsocuneiform joint and the relative lengths of the first and second metatarsals.

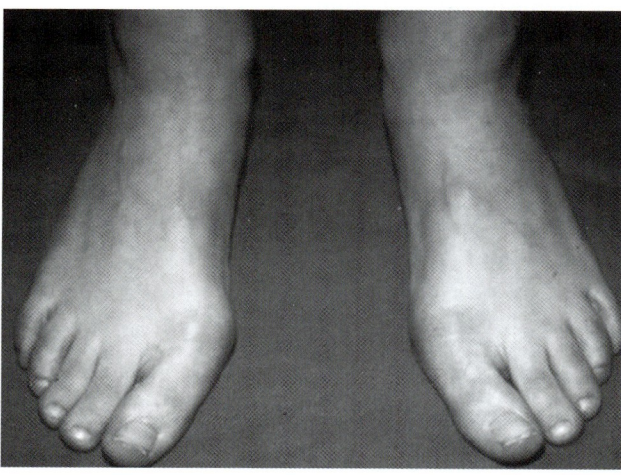

Figure 123.3 Typical patient with bilateral hallux valgus deformity.

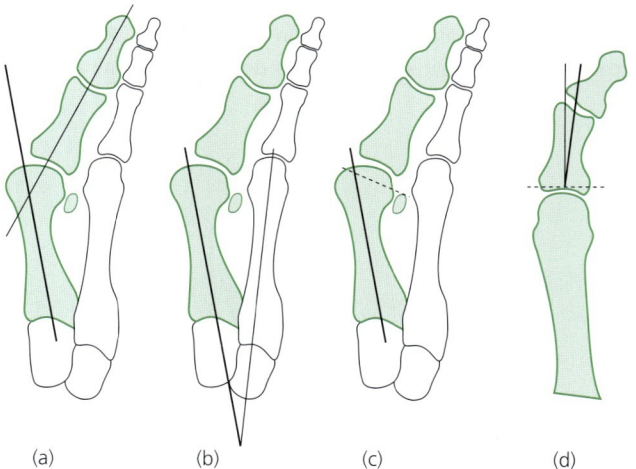

Figure 123.4 The various angular measurements of the hallux valgus deformity. (a) Hallux valgus angle; (b) first–second intermetatarsal angle; (c) distal metatarsal articular angle; (d) proximal phalangeal articular angle.

An axial sesamoid view is sometimes used to assess sesamoid translation and the presence of metatarsal–sesamoid arthrosis.

TREATMENT

Non-operative

Modification of footwear is often helpful. The patient should be advised to wear shoes with a wide toe box. Shoes with extra depth may be helpful when there are associated hammer toe or crossover deformities. Stretching of the leather over the bunion may be helpful, as would the application of padding devices or cushions. Splinting or strapping is sometimes used to reduce the deformity. Orthoses such as longitudinal arch supports and toe spacers may be prescribed.

Operative

The indications for operative treatment include failure of non-operative measures, persistent pain that interferes with daily, work or recreational activities, and severe deformity and pain that are unlikely to respond to non-operative treatment.

Specific considerations that influence the choice of operative treatment include age, functional demand, comorbid medical conditions, severity of the deformity, varus deviation of the first metatarsal, pronation of the toe, increased distal metatarsal articular angle, congruency of the joint, arthrosis of the joint, hypermobility of the first metatarsal–cuneiform joint, hallux valgus interphalangeus, and the intrinsic and extrinsic musculotendinous balance. We propose a simple treatment algorithm, which is based on some of these considerations and is adapted from Mann[6] (Fig. 123.5).

There are more than 130 procedures described for the surgical treatment of hallux valgus. As such, the scope of this chapter allows for the description of only the more commonly performed of these (Fig. 123.6).

DISTAL SOFT-TISSUE PROCEDURE

Also known as the modified McBride's procedure, it involves release of contracted lateral structures, specifically the adductor hallucis, transverse metatarsal ligament and lateral capsule, as well as resection of the medial eminence and medial capsulorrhaphy. The modification from the original McBride's procedure is the retention of the lateral sesamoid, which helps to prevent hallux varus.

It is seldom used in isolation and only in cases of mild deformity (HVA >25°; IMA_{1-2} ≤13°).[2] It is used more often as an adjunct to other bony techniques such as a proximal metatarsal osteotomy in patients with incongruent deformities to allow reduction of the subluxed MTP joint. Complications of this procedure include recurrence and hallux varus.

DISTAL METATARSAL OSTEOTOMY

The *chevron osteotomy* is an intracapsular distal metatarsal osteotomy that is useful in younger patients with a hallux valgus angle of less than 25° and an intermetatarsal angle of less than 13°.[2,6] It consists of medial eminence removal, V-shaped intracapsular osteotomy through the first metatarsal head (an angle of 60–70° between the limbs of the osteotomy maximizes the metaphyseal cancellous bone contact while maintaining stability of the osteotomy once it is displaced), lateral displacement of the capital fragment (this should be about 5 mm and not exceed

Hallux valgus <25°	
Congruent joint	Chevron or Mitchell osteotomy
Incongruent joint	Chevron or Mitchell osteotomy
Hallux valgus 25–40°	
Congruent joint	Mitchell osteotomy
Incongruent joint	Mitchell osteotomy or Distal soft-tissue procedure with proximal osteotomy
Severe hallux valgus 25–40°	
Congruent joint	Double osteotomy (Mitchell with proximal osteotomy or Akin with chevron)
Incongruent joint	Distal soft-tissue procedure with proximal osteotomy
Hypermobile first metatarsocuneiform joint	Distal soft-tissue procedure with fusion of first metatarsocuneiform joint

Figure 123.5 Proposed treatment algorithm for hallux valgus.

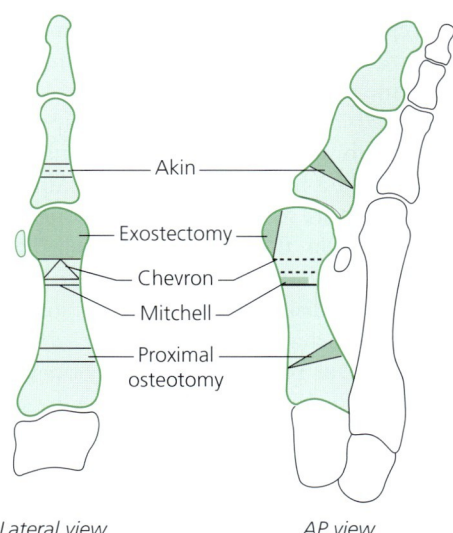

Figure 123.6 Pictorial representation of some common procedures performed for hallux valgus.

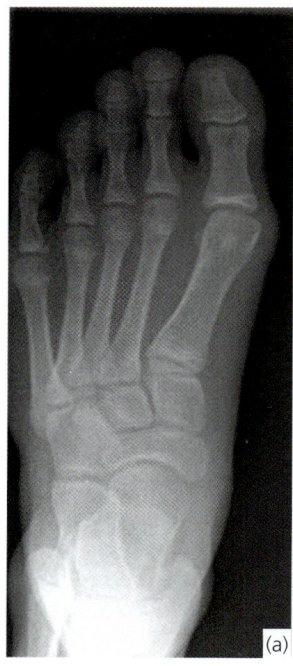
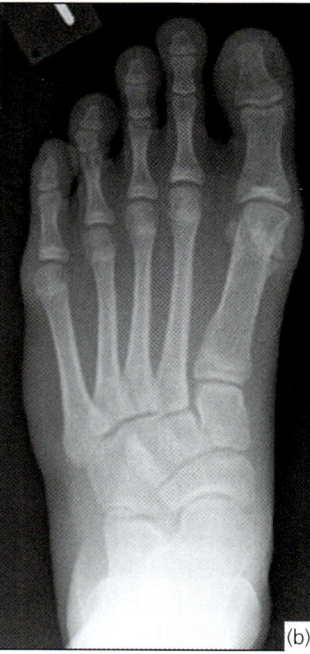

Figure 123.7 Pre-operative and postoperative radiographs of a 13-year-old girl who has undergone a chevron osteotomy of the distal first metatarsal. HV, hallux valgus angle; IM, intermetatarsal angle.

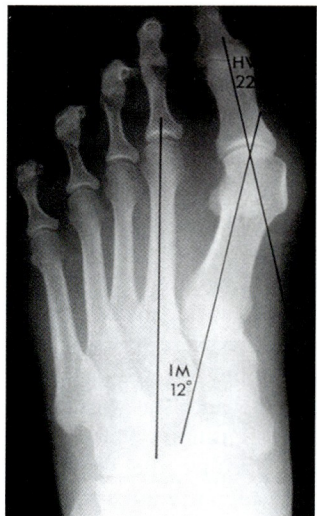
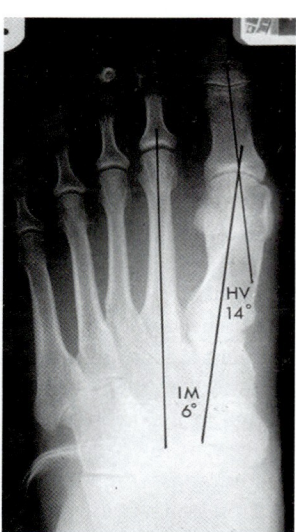

Figure 123.8 Pre-operative and postoperative radiographs of a patient who has undergone a Mitchell osteotomy of the distal first metatarsal. HV, hallux valgus angle; IM, intermetatarsal angle.

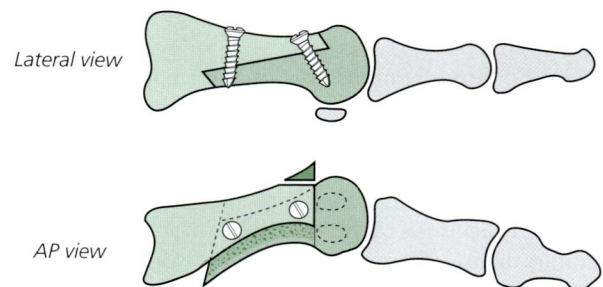

Figure 123.9 Pictorial representation of Scarf osteotomy, showing lateral displacement and fixation of distal fragment.

40–50% of the width of the metatarsal), removal of the resulting first metatarsal projection and medial capsulorrhaphy (Fig. 123.7). Fixation of the osteotomy may be supplemented with one or two Kirschner wires, a cortical screw or a biodegradable pin.[2] A concomitant lateral capsular release may be performed to improve correction, although this should be done as distally as possible to avoid devascularizing the metatarsal head.

A specific complication associated with this procedure is osteonecrosis of the metatarsal head, with rates of up to 20% being reported in some series. Other complications of this procedure include osteotomy malunion, MTP joint stiffness and metatarsalgia.[7]

The *Mitchell osteotomy* is an extracapsular distal metatarsal osteotomy. It is used in cases of mild to moderate deformity with a hallux valgus angle of up to 40°. Its ability to correct more severe deformities is due to its more proximal location in the distal metatarsal. This is the procedure of choice of the senior author. It involves excision of the medial eminence, step-cut osteotomy at the metaphyseal–diaphyseal junction and medial capsulorrhaphy. Our preference is to use a percutaneous K-wire rather than drill holes and sutures to secure the osteotomy. Splintage is then maintained in a cast for 5 weeks, after which the K-wire is removed.

We have previously reported good results with the Mitchell osteotomy in separate series of adolescent and middle-aged patients[8,9] (Fig. 123.8). Complications of this procedure include metatarsalgia, attributable to dorsiflexion malunion of the distal fragment and excessive shortening of the metatarsal,[2] as well as late recurrence of the hallux valgus deformity. Fokter et al.[10] found that their good to excellent results deteriorated from 97%, at follow-up ranging from 2 to 11 years, to 64%, at follow-up ranging from 15 to 24 years, primarily because of the recurrence of deformity with medial eminence pain.

METATARSAL SHAFT OSTEOTOMY

The *Scarf osteotomy* is used in moderate to severe deformities, where the hallux valgus angle is more than 25° and the intermetatarsal angle is more than 13°. It has gained popularity because of its inherent stability, minimal shortening of the first metatarsal and ease of internal fixation.[11] The procedure is preceded by a lateral soft-tissue release and involves a Z-step cut osteotomy of the first metatarsal (Fig. 123.9). This is followed by lateral translation of the plantar fragment, screw fixation, excision of the medial eminence and overhanging edge of bone and medial capsulorrhaphy. It is often combined with an Akin closing wedge osteotomy of the proximal phalanx. Reported complications include infection, transfer metatarsalgia, osteonecrosis of the first metatarsal head, fracture of the first metatarsal and prominent screws.[11] A potential complication unique to the Scarf osteotomy is 'troughing', which refers to an impaction of the two osteotomy fragments, resulting in loss of metatarsal height.[12]

PROXIMAL METATARSAL OSTEOTOMY

A proximal first metatarsal osteotomy is indicated in severe deformities, where the HVA is more than 35°, the IMA is more than 13° and when varus of the first metatarsal contributes to the hallux valgus complex[2] (Fig. 123.10). Advantages of proximal osteotomies include the ability to correct large angles between the first and second metatarsals with small changes in osteotomy position, minimal shortening of the first metatarsal and narrowing of the forefoot, which improves footwear choice.

The *crescentic osteotomy* is an example of a proximal osteotomy. The osteotomy is placed convex distally and performed 1 cm distal to the metatarsal–cuneiform articulation. This is followed by lateral translation of the distal fragment. A screw may be used to internally fix the osteotomy. A 93% success rate has been reported with this procedure.[13] Such osteotomies are carried out in association with a distal lateral soft-tissue release and medial eminence excision. The major complications of the crescentic osteotomy are hallux varus, dorsiflexion malunion of the osteotomy site with transfer metatarsalgia and stiffness of the MTP joint.[2,13]

PROXIMAL PHALANGEAL OSTEOTOMY

The medial closing wedge osteotomy of the proximal phalanx or Akin osteotomy is used in combination with

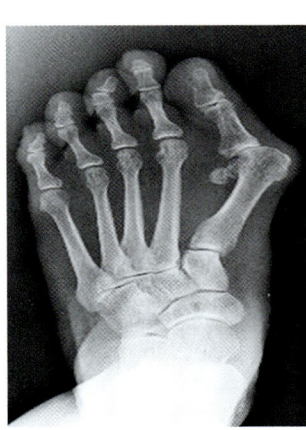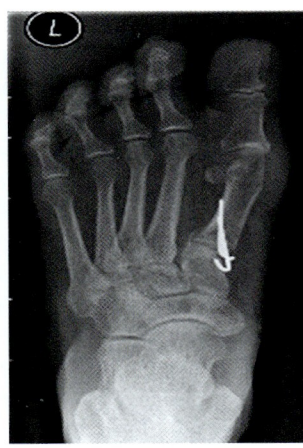

Figure 123.10 Pre-operative and postoperative radiographs of a patient who has undergone a proximal metatarsal osteotomy and distal soft-tissue release for severe hallux valgus deformity.

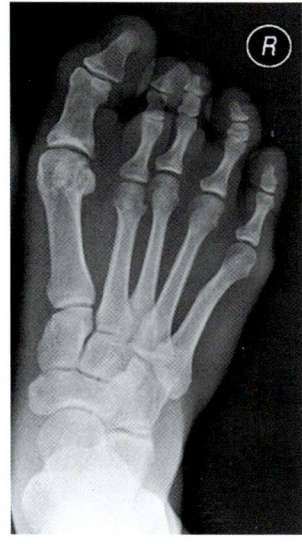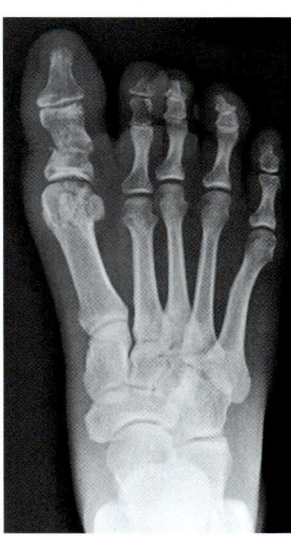

Figure 123.11 Pre-operative and postoperative radiographs of hallux valgus interphalangeus treated with an Akin osteotomy.

osteotomies of the distal or proximal metatarsal, particularly in cases where there is concomitant hallux valgus interphalangeus[14] (Fig. 123.11). Complications of this procedure include recurrence and delayed or non-union.

ARTHRODESIS OF THE FIRST METATARSAL–CUNEIFORM JOINT

Arthrodesis of the first metatarsal–cuneiform joint or the modified Lapidus procedure is indicated in cases where there is moderate to severe deformity resulting from metatarsus primus varus and hypermobility of the first ray. It is usually combined with a distal soft-tissue release. However, first ray hypermobility remains a controversial finding and a diagnostic challenge, particularly on physical examination. Radiographic features that have been suggested to indirectly determine hypermobility of the first ray include second metatarsal diaphyseal hypertrophy, a medially oriented first tarsometatarsal (TMT) joint, and first TMT joint obliquity.[15] Early reports identified non-union rates of 10–12%, while more recent series have reported much lower rates of between 0% and 4%.[12] Other complications include malunion and transfer metatarsalgia.

RESECTION ARTHROPLASTY

Resection arthroplasty of the first metatarsophalangeal joint or Keller's procedure involves excision of the base of the proximal phalanx, stabilization of the hallux with a K-wire and medial capsulorrhaphy[16] (Fig. 123.12). Many authors have reported poor results with this procedure, with complications such as recurrence of the deformity and transfer metatarsalgia.[12] As such, its indication is limited

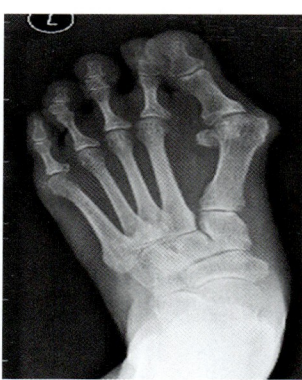
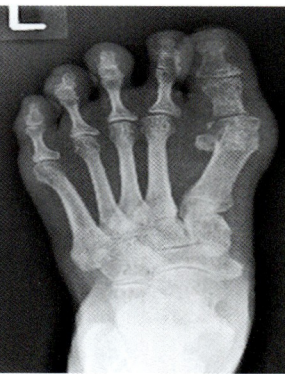

Figure 123.12 Pre-operative and postoperative radiographs of an elderly patient who has undergone a Keller excision arthroplasty.

to elderly patients with reduced functional demand where there is severe degeneration of the joint.

ARTHRODESIS OF THE MTP JOINT

Arthrodesis of the first MTP joint is reserved for patients with severe hallux valgus deformity, hallux valgus associated with arthrosis of the joint, failed prior surgical correction, a neuromuscular disorder, such as cerebral palsy, or rheumatoid arthritis. Various fixation methods have been used, including screws, plates and K-wires.[2] Complications of this procedure include non-union and degenerative arthritis of the interphalangeal joint of the hallux. The non-union rate has been reported in one series to be 5%.[17]

> **KEY LEARNING POINTS**
>
> - Hallux valgus (HV) is a complex progressive deformity of the forefoot with rotation of the hallux, metatarsus primus varus, overriding of the second toe over the hallux, overriding of the lateral toes, and hammer and claw deformities of the lateral toes. The lateral deviation of the great toe is the most obvious feature.
> - Bunion refers to the swelling from the medial eminence of the metatarsal head, with overlying bursitis, and skin callosity.
> - Excessive lateral deviation of the first metatarsophalangeal (MTP) joint of more than 35° leads to pronation of the big toe.
> - HV is caused by inappropriate footwear and increased distal metatarsal articular angle.
> - Often asymptomatic; pain is otherwise the main complaint.
> - Required radiographs are weight-bearing AP, lateral and oblique views of the foot.

> - Treatment is modification of footwear (a wide toe box), distal soft-tissue procedure (McBride's operation) for mild deformity, distal metatarsal ostetomy (the chevron osteotomy is intracapsular; the Mitchell osteotomy is extracapsular) for moderate deformity, metatarsal shaft osteotomy (Scarf osteotomy) for moderate to severe deformity, proximal metatarsal osteotomy for severe deformity, proximal phalangeal osteotomy combined with the above, arthrodesis of the first metatarsal–cuneiform joint for moderate to severe deformity, resection arthroplasty (not recommended) and arthrodesis of the MTP joint for failed previous surgery, where osteoarthritis of the MTP joint, or where neuromuscular disorders.

REFERENCES

- ♦ = Major review article
- • = Key primary paper

- •1. Stamm TT. Surgical treatment of hallux valgus. *Guy's Hospital Reports* 1963;**112**:21–6.
- ♦2. Richardson EG, Donley BG. Disorders of hallux. In: Canale ST (ed.) *Campbell's Operative Orthopaedics*. St Louis, MO: Mosby, 2002:3915–4015.
- •3. Piggot H. Natural history of hallux valgus in adolescence and early adult life. *Journal of Bone and Joint Surgery (British)* 1960;**42**:749–60.
- •4. Sim-Fook L, Hodgson AR. A comparison of foot forms among the non-shoe and shoe-wearing Chinese population. *Journal of Bone and Joint Surgery (American)* 1958;**40**:1058–62.
- ♦5. Campbell JT. Hallux valgus: adult and juvenile. In: Richardson EG (ed.) *Orthopaedic Knowledge Update: Foot and Ankle 3*. Rosemont, IL: American Academy of Orthopaedic Surgeons 2003:3–16.
- ♦6. Mann RA. Decision-making in bunion surgery. *Instructional Course Lectures* 1990;**39**:3–13.
- ♦7. Mann RA. Complications associated with the Chevron osteotomy. *Foot and Ankle* 1982;**3**:125–9.
- •8. Das De S. Distal metatarsal osteotomy for adolescent hallux valgus. *Journal of Pediatric Orthopaedics* 1984;**4**:32–8.
- •9. Das De S, Hamblen DL. Distal metatarsal osteotomy for hallux valgus in the middle-aged patient. *Clinical Orthopaedics and Related Research* 1987;**218**:239–46.
- •10. Fokter SK, Podobnik J, Venqust V. Late results of modified Mitchell procedure for the treatment of hallux valgus. *Foot and Ankle International* 1999;**20**:296–300.
- •11. Jones S, Al Hussainy HA, Ali F, *et al*. Scarf osteotomy for hallux valgus: A prospective clinical and pedobarographic study. *Journal of Bone and Joint Surgery (British)* 2004;**86**:830–6.

- ◆12. Easley ME, Trnka HJ. Current concepts review: hallux valgus part II: Operative treatment. *Foot and Ankle International* 2007;**28**:748–58.
- ●13. Mann RA, Rudicel S, Graves SC. Repair of hallux valgus with a distal soft-tissue procedure and proximal metatarsal osteotomy. *Journal of Bone and Joint Surgery (American)* 1992;**74**:124–9.
- ●14. Frey C, Jahss M, Kummer FJ. The Akin procedure: An analysis of results. *Foot and Ankle* 1991;**12**:1–6.
- ◆15. Easley ME, Trnka HJ. Current concepts review: hallux valgus part I: Pathomechanics, clinical assessment and non-operative management. *Foot and Ankle International* 2007;**28**:654–9.
- 16. Richardson EG. Keller resection arthroplasty. *Orthopaedics* 1990;**13**:1049–53.
- ●17. Mann RA, Oates JC. Arthrodesis of the first metatarsophalangeal joint. *Foot and Ankle* 1980;**1**:159–66.

124

Disorders of the hallucal sesamoids and related great toe pathologies

ANDREW MOORE, ANISH RAJ KADAKIA

Introduction	1442	Arthritis	1446
Anatomy	1442	Sesamoiditis	1446
TRAUMATIC DISORDERS	1443	RELATED DISORDERS	1447
Turf-toe injuries	1443	Hallux varus	1447
Sesamoid fractures	1445	Hallux valgus	1448
NON-TRAUMATIC DISORDERS	1446	References	1448
Osteochondritis	1446		

NATIONAL BOARD STANDARDS

- Understand the pathoanatomy and pathophysiology sesamoid disorders
- Know the rationale for choosing conservative treatments
- Be able to advise patients with traumatic sesamoid/hallux disorders
- Be able to advise patients with non-traumatic afflictions of the sesamoids

INTRODUCTION

The tibial and fibular sesamoids of the great toe metatarsophalangeal (MTP) joint function to stabilize the first ray, increase the mechanical advantage of the flexor hallucis brevis (FHB) as a toe plantarflexor, and assist in weight bearing. Because greater than 50% of body weight is transmitted through the first MTP joint, it is not surprising that the sesamoids are involved in the pathogenesis of traumatic disorders affecting the first ray, including turf toe and sesamoid fractures. Furthermore, several non-traumatic disorders, which indeed may result from repetitive stress at the first MTP joint, include osteochondritis, arthritis and sesamoiditis. Discussion of the role of the sesamoids in hallux valgus deformity of the first ray is found elsewhere in this text.

ANATOMY

The medial (tibial) and lateral (fibular) sesamoids of the great toe are contained within the tendons of the FHB, corresponding to its medial and lateral heads.[1] They articulate with corresponding facets on the plantar surface of the first metatarsal head, separated by an osteocartilaginous crista, and form part of the plantar plate complex, which also comprises the plantar portions of the abductor and adductor hallucis tendons, the intersesamoidal ligament, the joint capsule and the collateral ligaments. The plantar plate complex inserts onto the base of the proximal phalanx; the flexor hallucis longus tendon runs between and plantar to the sesamoids and inserts onto the distal phalanx (Figs 124.1 and 124.2)

TURF-TOE INJURIES

Turf toe injuries involve traumatic capsuloligamentous disruption of the first MTP joint of variable severity.[5] These result in a range of clinical manifestations, from short-lived pain with push-off in sports activities to chronic pain and weakness, post-traumatic hallux rigidus, hallux valgus or hallucal cock-up deformity.

Pathophysiology

Hyperextension at the first MTP joint during an axial load with a foot fixed in equinus is the most commonly reported mechanism of injury.[2] This can produce dorsal translation or dislocation of the hallux, resulting in avulsion of the plan-tar structures from the metatarsal neck, joint capsule disruption and possibly plantar plate avulsion from the sesamoids permitting proximal retraction of the sesamoids (Fig. 124.3).[3] Diastasis of bipartite sesamoids, sesamoid fractures, disruption of FHB tendon insertions, and intra-articular osteochondral injuries are occasionally seen. Postulated predisposing factors include flexible shoes, hardness of playing surface, and patient factors such as weight, MTP joint morphology and adjacent joint flexibility.[2,4,5]

Clinical presentation

Patients typically present following an athletic injury with complaints of pain with weight bearing, especially at toe-off, as well as swelling and ecchymosis at the first MTP joint. Clinical evaluation should include the following:

- alignment of the hallux, including clinical MTP joint reduction, or the presence of an intrinsic-minus posture (MTP extension, interphalangeal flexion), suggesting disruption of FHB tendon insertion

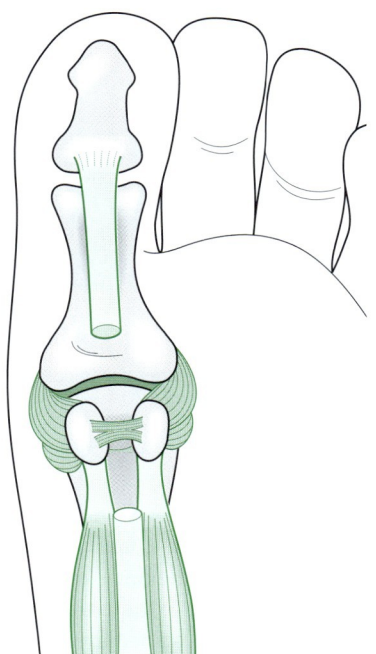

Figure 124.1 Diagram of the sesamoid complex viewed from the plantar aspect. Note the attachment of the flexor hallucis brevis to the sesamoids and their location just proximal to the first metatarsophalangeal joint.

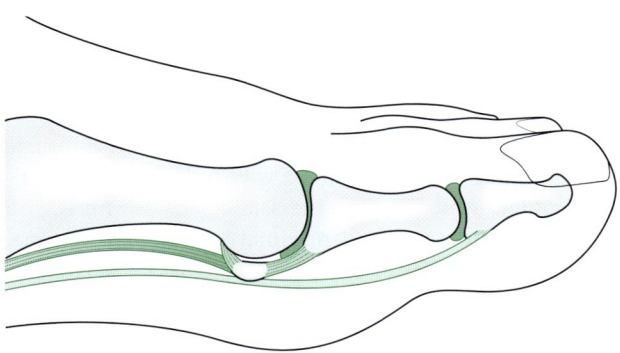

Figure 124.2 Diagram of the sesamoids complex viewed from the medial aspect. Note again the location of the sesamoids and their location just proximal the first metatarsophalangeal joint. The capsuloligamentous attachment to the proximal phalanx is critical in maintaining their position and function.

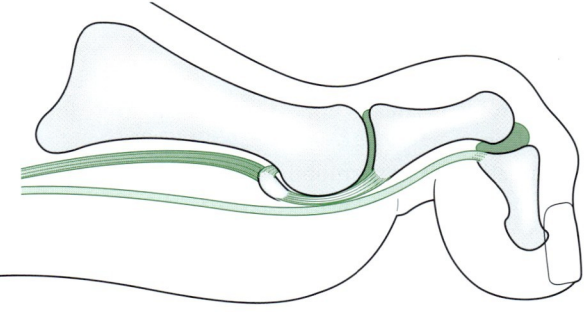

Figure 124.3 Diagram of the sesamoids following a severe turf-toe injury with avulsion of the plantar structures from the metatarsal neck, joint capsule disruption and plantar plate avulsion from the sesamoids permitting proximal retraction of the sesamoids. Note the claw hallux deformity.

TRAUMATIC DISORDERS

Turf-toe injuries and sesamoid fractures share similar mechanisms of injury, but have many distinct clinical features, and are considered separately here.

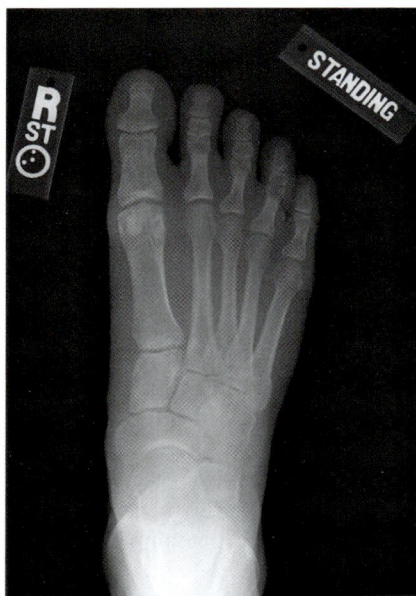

Figure 124.4 Anteroposterior weight-bearing radiograph of the foot demonstrating a fracture of the fibular (lateral) sesamoid.

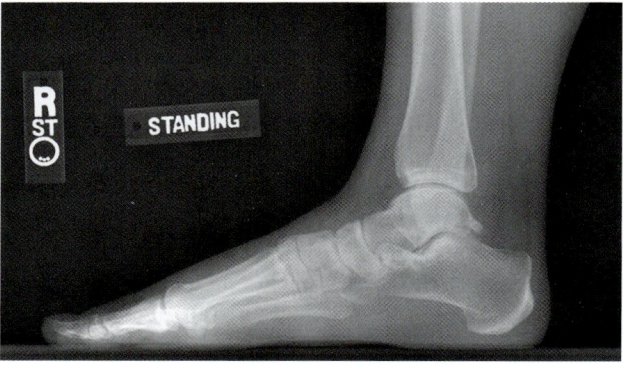

Figure 124.5 Lateral weight-bearing radiograph of the foot in a patient with a fractured fibular (lateral) sesamoid.

- careful palpation of plantar (including individual sesamoids), lateral and dorsal structures for focal tenderness
- evaluation of hypermobility or a mechanical block at the MTP compared with the contralateral side.

Radiographic evaluation

Plain radiographs are the mainstay of radiographic evaluation. Weight-bearing anteroposterior (AP) and lateral views (Figs 124.4 and 124.5) as well as a non-weight-bearing medial oblique view and an axial sesamoid view (Fig. 124.6) are recommended to assess for joint reduction, impaction fractures, sesamoid bipartition or fractures, and proximal

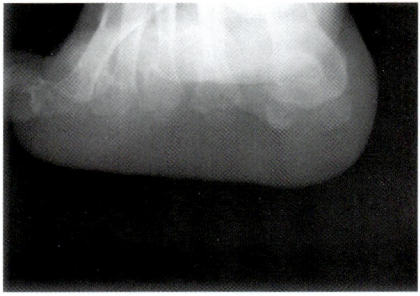

Figure 124.6 Axial sesamoid view of a patient with a fractured tibial (medial) sesamoid. Note the irregularity compared with the fibular (lateral) sesamoid.

migration of the sesamoids, suggesting a complete plantar plate disruption. The last two conditions can be further assessed with a forced dorsiflexion lateral under a local anaesthetic. Comparison with the contralateral side frequently can be helpful; the distance from the distal pole of the sesamoid to the MTP joint line should be within 3.0 mm of the contralateral side for the tibial sesamoid and 2.7 mm for the fibular sesamoid.[6] Likewise, dorsoplantar drawer and varus/valgus stress radiographs may detect injuries to the plantar plate complex and collateral ligaments, respectively.

Natural history

The natural history is based on the severity of injury, which is graded by the extent of capsular or capsuloligamentous injury.[3,7] Grade 1 disease involves an incomplete tear of the capsule, is associated with mild swelling, localized plantar or medial tenderness, and generally heals with rapid return to sport and minimal loss of playing time. Grade 2 injury involves a more extensive capsular tear, moderate swelling, ecchymosis, more diffuse tenderness and some initial loss of range of motion. Typically, athletes with grade 2 injury are unable to play for 3–14 days and recover fully with symptomatic management. Grade 3 disease involves a complete capsuloligamentous disruption, attended by marked swelling, ecchymosis, inability to bear weight and patients may require 4–6 weeks for return to play. In severe, repetitive or untreated cases, persistent instability may lead to chronic synovitis and pain, or progression to degenerative arthrosis/hallux rigidus.

Non-surgical treatment

Grade 1 and 2 injuries typically respond to an initial programme of rest, ice and elevation coupled with anti-inflammatories and analgesics to control symptoms. Return to play may benefit from taping to prevent dorsiflexion or the use of a carbon fibre plate in the forefoot region of the shoe, or a custom insert with a Morton's extension. Grade 3 injuries may require a period of 4–6 weeks of immobilization with a walker boot or short leg cast with a toe extension. As a rule, in these cases, 50–60° of painless dorsiflexion at the MTP joint is advocated prior to return to competitive sport.

Surgical treatment

Surgical indications include intra-articular loose bodies and chondral flaps, displaced sesamoid fractures, bipartite sesamoids with diastasis, proximal retraction of the sesamoids and traumatic hallux valgus.[3] Surgical intervention is based on the specific pathology. In the case in which turf-toe-type injury has produced a disruption of the plantar plate complex and proximal migration of both the tibial and fibular sesamoids has been observed, operative repair is indicated to prevent chronic instability of the MTP joint as well as development of an intrinsic-minus (due to disruption of FHB tendon insertion) or cock-up toe deformity. This is described below.

With the patient positioned prone, and under tourniquet control, a curvilinear or C-shaped plantar medial incision is carried out at the level of the MTP joint, with proximal and distal limbs of the incision more medial and the apex just lateral to the lateral sesamoid. Longitudinal blunt dissection is carried down with care to protect the plantar digital nerves. The long flexor tendon lies just plantar to the tibial and fibular sesamoids, which are inspected, and if avulsed from the plantar plate a suture repair is carried with drill holes or suture anchors in the sesamoid bones. This repair is generally protected from dorsiflexion moments by means of a cast with toe extension for 8 weeks followed by another 4–6 weeks in a hard-soled shoe.

SESAMOID FRACTURES

Sesamoid fractures include fractures of non-bipartite sesamoids, diastasis of bipartite sesamoids, and stress fractures.

Pathophysiology

Greater than 50% of body weight is transmitted through the first MTP joint. The sesamoids therefore are susceptible to acute and repetitive injuries both from dorsiflexion injuries of the great toe and from direct trauma. It is thought that a bipartite sesamoid may be more susceptible to acute injury resulting in diastasis. The larger tibial sesamoid is more frequently injured; it is also four times more frequently bipartite (Fig. 124.7). In all, the tibial sesamoid is bipartite in 10% of the population, and in 25% of these cases the condition is bilateral.[8] Multipartite tibial sesamoid, with three or four parts, has also been reported.

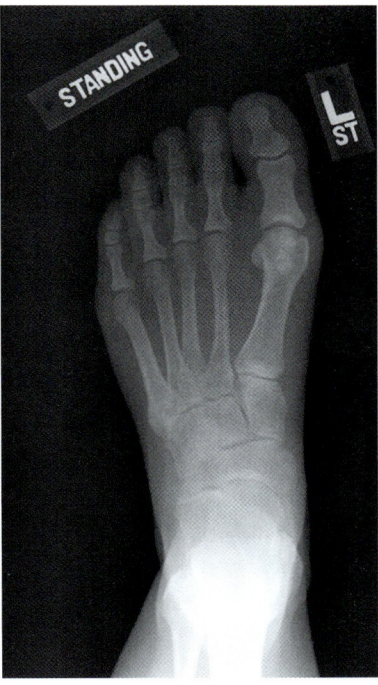

Figure 124.7 Anteroposterior weight-bearing radiograph of the foot demonstrating an asymptomatic bipartite tibial sesamoid.

Clinical presentation

Patients complain of pain at the plantar aspect of the hallux, often with a gradual or insidious onset. There may be mild swelling or a history of discrete trauma in the case of an acute sesamoid fracture. Pain is worsened with athletic activities, stair climbing and walking barefoot. Patients may report walking on the outside of their foot to avoid pain with toe-off. Occasionally, numbness is reported, signalling compression of a digital nerve. On examination, careful attention should be given to the following:

- the specific location of tenderness and swelling, if present
- foot deformity and callosities, as discussed in the next section, which may also be associated with non-traumatic disorders of the sesamoids
- MTP range of motion compared with the other side, which may relate to a joint effusion or underlying arthrosis
- a positive Tinel's sign in the presence of nerve compression.

Radiographic evaluation

Standard radiographic assessment for a suspected sesamoid fracture is the same as that for the evaluation of a turf-toe injury, including weight-bearing AP and lateral, oblique and axial sesamoid views. Contralateral films are often helpful. If these are normal, bone scan may have clinical utility in the setting of suspected fracture, particularly in distinguishing a fracture from a bipartite sesamoid. Specific projections must be used during the bone scan so that intra-articular pathology of the first MTP joint can be distinguished from sesamoid disorders.[9] CT scan can also be useful in evaluation of traumatic sesamoid disorders and for distinguishing between a fracture and bipartite sesamoid. Comparison of the contralateral side is readily made by including both feet in the gantry.

Non-surgical treatment

Non-surgical treatment is indicated for the initial management of non- or minimally displaced fractures. Most authors recommend immobilization in a short leg walking cast with a toe extension for 6 weeks, followed by a removable boot, or a moulded orthosis with a well and a metatarsal pad if tenderness has subsided after 6 weeks of casting. This regimen may also be used for the initial management of stress fractures.

SURGICAL TREATMENT

Surgical management is indicated for displaced sesamoid fractures and those that fail to heal despite 6 months of non-operative treatment. Techniques include partial or complete sesamoidectomy with soft-tissue repair (described in the next section). In general, excision of both the tibial and fibular sesamoids is not advocated because of loss of FHB tendon function and cock-up deformity of the hallux.

Open reduction and internal fixation (ORIF) of acute displaced sesamoid fractures has been advocated as an alternative to sesamoidectomy. For treatment of the more commonly fractured tibial sesamoid, a longitudinal plantar medial incision is made over the first MTP joint and carried down plantar to the abductor hallucis tendon, affording an extra-articular exposure of the sesamoid. The fracture is reduced, clamped and fixed with a small headless screw, with subsequent suture repair of the adjacent soft-tissue disruption.

Successful healing after bone grafting of symptomatic sesamoid fracture non-union has been reported in 19 of 21 patients by Anderson and McBryde.[10] A similar approach as for ORIF is performed, followed by curettage of the non-union site and packing with bone graft harvested locally through a cortical window in the medial eminence of the first metatarsal head.

NON-TRAUMATIC DISORDERS

Common non-traumatic causes of hallucal sesamoid pain include osteochondritis, arthritis and sesamoiditis. Although these are distinct clinical entities, they share many similar features; this section will therefore review collectively their clinical and radiographic evaluation, as well as their non-surgical and surgical management.

OSTEOCHONDRITIS

Osteochondritis of the hallucal sesamoids involves a process of osteonecrosis and subsequent regeneration, often with excessive calcification. The disease may progress from an initial phase of pain and minimal radiographic abnormality to later fragmentation, collapse and subsequent repair, with symptoms gradually resolving even without treatment over 6–12 months. The aetiology is unknown, but may be due to repetitive trauma, and is most frequently seen in young adult females, but may be seen in any age or gender.

ARTHRITIS

Arthritis may be present at the metatarsal–sesamoid articulation as a result of trauma, osteochondritis, chronic subluxation or dislocation (as in hallux valgus deformity, covered elsewhere in this text), or in association with degenerative or inflammatory arthritis of the first MTP joint.

SESAMOIDITIS

Sesamoiditis is a non-specific term referring to pain localized to the sesamoids that is not clearly attributable to other causes, such as sesamoid fracture, arthritis or osteochondritis. This condition more often affects the tibial sesamoid due to its larger size and prominence, and is found most frequently in teenagers and young adults. There may or may not be an association with repetitive trauma. This term is often associated with other conditions, such as intractable plantar keratosis, digital nerve compression and tendinitis.

Clinical presentation

Patients with non-traumatic disorders of the sesamoids may or may not report a history of trauma. The pain generally localizes to the plantar aspect of the base of the hallux, and is typically worse at toe-off in terminal stance phase. Athletes may consider these disorders disabling. Particular attention should be directed to the following.

- Cavus foot deformity with a stiff, plantarflexed first ray, which may cause elevated pressure under the first metatarsal head and increased axial loading of particularly the tibial sesamoid.

- Hallux valgus deformity, in which the tibial sesamoid may become dislocated laterally from its sulcus with respect to the medially translated metatarsal head, resulting in painful impingement against the crista.
- Pain with resisted hallucal interphalangeal joint plantarflexion, suggesting tenosynovitis of the flexor hallucis longus tendon.
- Radiating pain and/or a positive Tinel's sign heralding the presence of digital nerve compression.
- Range of motion at the first MTP joint compared with the other side, which may be decreased in the presence of a joint effusion or associated hallux rigidus

Radiographic evaluation

Standard AP, medial oblique, lateral oblique and axial sesamoid views are most useful in the initial radiological evaluation of suspected sesamoid pathology. In the non-traumatic setting, lateral views may be less helpful. If radiographs are normal, bone scan may reveal evidence of sesamoid pathology, but may require specific projections (and thus clear communication with the nuclear medicine physician) to distinguish sesamoid from first MTP joint disease. CT may elucidate post-traumatic osseous changes. In this setting, MRI is most useful in the setting of suspected osteomyelitis.

Non-surgical treatment

Most non-traumatic disorders of the hallucal sesamoids respond to non-surgical treatment. Mild to moderate pain can be controlled with anti-inflammatory medication, a stiff-soled or rocker-bottom shoe, and a metatarsal pad. In simple cases, taping to prevent dorsiflexion of the hallux during athletics and modification of footwear to include avoidance of high-heeled shoes and use of a shoe with a widened toe box may be all that are needed. Occasionally, a period of restricted weight bearing and cast immobilization may be required to lessen symptoms. In this case, making diagnosis of osteochondritis can be helpful, as this process often requires a period of lengthy immobilization for symptomatic management, but has a favourable prognosis without surgery.

Surgical treatment

Cases that have failed non-operative treatment, generally for a minimum of 6 months, are candidates for surgical treatment. Surgical treatment includes tibial or fibular sesamoidectomy, as well as sesamoid shaving. Removal of both tibial and fibular sesamoids is rarely indicated, as it predictably results in the development of a cock-up and intrinsic-minus deformity of the hallux.

Tibial sesamoidectomy is carried out through a plantar medial longitudinal incision at the level of the first MTP joint, with care taken to protect the medial plantar digital nerve.[11] The hallux is flexed, relaxing the flexor hallucis longus tendon, which is retracted. The intersesamoidal ligament is then incised, and the tibial sesamoid is pulled medially, releasing its attachment to the surrounding FHB tendon and plantar fibres of the abductor hallucis tendon. The capsule and skin are closed, taking care to close the defect from the excision of the sesamoid with no. 0 suture.

Fibular sesamoidectomy is less frequently required, and can be accomplished through either a dorsal or a plantar incision. The technique for dorsal excision is described here.[12]

A 7 cm longitudinal incision is made in the first intermetatarsal space, ending several centimetres proximal to the web space, and is carried down between the adductor hallucis and the joint capsule, taking care to protect the branches of the deep peroneal nerve. The capsule is opened, and the adductor hallucis tendon and the lateral capsulosesamoid ligament are incised from the fibular sesamoid. The sesamoid is grasped with either forceps or a threaded K-wire, and pulled laterally; the intersesamoidal ligament is incised, taking care not to cut the tendon of the flexor hallucis longus. The attachments of the FHB tendon are then released proximally and distally, and the sesamoid is removed from the wound.

Tibial shaving may be indicated for an intractable plantar keratosis as an alternative to sesamoidectomy.[13] If there is an associated cavovarus foot deformity with a rigidly plantarflexed first ray, a dorsiflexion osteotomy of the first ray is preferred to isolated sesamoid shaving due to the likelihood of recurrence in the presence of this deformity.

A longitudinal plantar medial incision is made as for tibial sesamoidectomy, with careful protection of the medial plantar nerve. The MTP joint is flexed, the plantar fat pad and flexor hallucis longus tendon are protected, and the plantar half of the tibial sesamoid is removed with a sagittal saw. Edges are smoothed with a rongeur, followed by routine closure and protection in a rigid-soled shoe or cast for 2–3 weeks postoperatively.

RELATED DISORDERS

HALLUX VARUS

This term refers to medial deviation of the great toe. The most common aetiology is iatrogenic, as a consequence of surgical correction for hallux valgus (e.g. McBride procedure, as discussed elsewhere in this text). Other causes are congenital, idiopathic, rheumatic and post-traumatic.

Though uncommon, the precise incidence is unknown for these non-iatrogenic forms. Congenital hallux valgus may be due to overpull of the abductor hallucis tendon, or secondary to other congenital anomalies, such as metatarsus adductus, longitudinal epiphyseal bracket syndrome or delta phalanx. Idiopathic hallux valgus deformity arises without a clear aetiological factor, is usually passively correctable and tends to improve with shoe wear. Inflammatory causes include psoriatic and rheumatoid arthritis, and involve destruction of articular surfaces, distension of the joint capsule and collateral ligament attenuation by pannus, and intrinsic muscle contracture producing the deformity. Traumatic hallux varus has been reported, and is thought to result from rupture of the lateral collateral ligament and conjoined tendon.

Surgical treatment is reserved for patients who fail non-operative measures such as shoe wear modification. Supple deformities can be treated with a transfer of the extensor hallucis brevis or split transfer of the extensor hallucis longus to the proximal phalanx.[14] Fixed deformities or joints with concomitant degenerative changes should be treated with arthrodesis.

HALLUX VALGUS

This complex deformity of the first ray involves lateral deviation of the great toe and is discussed elsewhere in this text.

KEY LEARNING POINTS

- Hallucal sesamoid disorders can be disabling, particularly in athletes, but most respond to non-surgical treatment.
- The standard radiographic evaluation of a patient with suspected sesamoid pathology includes AP, lateral, oblique and axial sesamoid views. Other modalities useful in specific circumstances include bone scan, stress views and, less frequently, CT and MRI.
- There are clear surgical indications in the management of traumatic disorders of the sesamoids and related structures, which include plantar plate avulsion and some displaced fractures, which can produce deformity and instability of the hallux.

REFERENCES

1. Richardson EG. Hallucal sesamoid pain: causes and surgical treatment. *Journal of the American Academy of Orthopaedic Surgeons* 1999;**7**:270-8.
2. Bowers Jr KD, Martin RB. Turf-toe: a shoe-surface related football injury. *Medicine and Science in Sports* 1976;**8**:81-3.
3. Anderson RB. Turf toe injuries of the hallux metatarsophalangeal joint. *Techniques in Foot and Ankle Surgery* 2002;**1**:102-11.
4. Coker TP, Arnold JA, Weber DL. Traumatic lesions of the metatarsophalangeal joint of the great toe in athletes. *American Journal of Sports Medicine* 1978;**6**:326-34.
5. Rodeo SA, O'Brien S, Warren RF, et al. Turf-toe: an analysis of metatarsophalangeal joint sprains in professional football players. *American Journal of Sports Medicine* 1990;**18**:280-.
6. Rodeo SA, Warren RF, O'Brien SJ, et al. Diastasis of bipartite sesamoids of the first metatarsophalangeal joint. *Foot and Ankle* 1993;**14**:425-34.
7. Clanton TO, Butler JE, Eggert A. Injuries to the metatarsophalangeal joints in athletes. *Foot and Ankle* 1986;**7**:162-76.
8. Leventen, EO: Sesamoid disorders and their treatment. *Clinical Orthopaedics and Related Research* 1991;**269**:236-40.
9. Chisin R, Peyser A, Milgrom C. Bone scintography in the assessment of hallucal sesamoids. *Foot and Ankle International* 1995;**16**:291-4.
10. Anderson RB, McBryde Jr AM. Autogenous bone grafting of hallux sesamoid nonunions. *Foot and Ankle International* 1997;**18**:293-6.
11. Lee S, James WC, Cohen BE, et al. Evaluation of hallux alignment and functional outcome after isolated tibial sesamoidectomy. *Foot and Ankle International* 2005;**26**:803-9.
12. Dedmond BT, Cory JW, McBryde Jr A. The hallucal sesamoid complex. *Journal of the American Academy of Orthopaedic Surgeons* 2006;**14**:745-53.
13. Mann RA, Wapner K. Tibial sesamoid shaving for treatment of intractable plantar keratosis. *Foot and Ankle* 1992;**13**:196-8.
14. Myerson MS, Komenda GA. Results of hallux varus correction using an extensor hallucis brevis tenodesis. *Foot and Ankle International* 1996;**17**:21-7.

125

Lesser toe deformities

ANDREW P MOLLOY, MOEZ S BALLAL

Introduction	1449	Congenital overlapping of the fifth toe	1456
Anatomic considerations	1449	Congenital underlapping of the fifth toe	1457
Initial assessment	1450	Congenital short fourth toe (brachymetatarsia)	1457
Hammer toe	1451	Curly toes	1457
Claw toe	1452	Mucous cysts of the toes	1458
Mallet toe	1454	Hard corns	1458
Bunionette deformity	1454	Soft corns	1458
Crossover second toe	1455	References	1459

NATIONAL BOARD STANDARDS

- Review anatomy of lesser toes.
- Understand the development and symptoms of lesser toe pathologies.
- Understand the conservative treatment of deformities.
- Understand the surgical treatment of deformities and how the modality of surgical treatment alters with the severity of the deformity.

INTRODUCTION

Normal alignment of the lesser toes relies upon static and dynamic stabilizers maintaining the bony relationships. Any disruption of the normal balance between these factors can manifest in a lesser toe deformity. The symptoms from these deformities vary and can range from being asymptomatic to disabling.

The aetiology of these deformities can be multifactorial, including neuromuscular, rheumatological, mechanical, congenital and traumatic factors. The underlying causes of such deformities are frequently attributed to high-fashion footwear because of the high incidence of these problems in women.[1] These deformities can involve one or multiple toes. The second toe is the most common affected toe as it typically has the longest metatarsal of the lesser toes. The common problems encountered in the forefoot include mallet toes, hammer toes, claw toes, interdigital corns, lateral corns on the fifth toe and crossover fifth toes.

ANATOMIC CONSIDERATIONS

Bony stability arises from the congruency of the metatarsophalangeal and interphalangeal joints.

Soft-tissue stabilization is maintained by the joint capsule, plantar aponeurosis and the collateral ligaments. The plantar plate is a confluence of the last two structures and supports the metatarsal heads and resists hyperextension of the metatarsophalangeal joint (MTPJ).

Dynamic stabilization is formed by the intrinsic and extrinsic foot muscles.

Extrinsic muscles

- *Extensor digitorum longus (EDL)*. The tendon runs through the extensor sling dorsally and distally divides into three slips. The central slip attaches at the middle phalanges and the remaining two attach at the sides of the

distal phalanges. The tendon is a strong dorsiflexor of the MTPJ. When the MTPJ is in a neutral or flexed position, the EDL can dorsiflex the proximal interphalangeal joint (PIPJ) and distal interphalangeal joint (DIPJ).
- *Flexor digitorum longus (FDL).* The tendon runs under the metatarsal heads and inserts at the plantar aspect in the base of distal phalanges. The FDL is a very strong DIPJ plantarflexor and weak MTPJ plantarflexor.

Intrinsic muscles

- *Extensor digitorum brevis (EDB).* Inserts at the lateral aspect of the EDL tendon of only the second, third and fourth toes. The primary function of the EDB is to extend the PIPJ.
- *Flexor digitorum brevis (FDB).* The tendon splits into two branches at the level of the MTPJ running at the sides of the FDL and finally joining and inserting the middle phalanges of the second to fifth toes. Its main action is as a flexor of the PIPJ. It is also a weak MTPJ flexor.
- *The lumbricals.* They arise from the FDL tendon and insert on the tibial side of the plantar plate and the extensor sling at the level of the MTPJ. When the MTPJ is in neutral position, the lumbricals are strong plantarflexors at this level. They lose the function if the MTPJ is dorsiflexed.
- *The interossei.* There are four dorsal and three plantar. These insert on the medial side of the proximal phalanges of the second to the fifth toes. They flex the proximal phalanges on the metatarsals and extend the middle and distal phalanges of the second to fifth toes (Box 125.1).

> **BOX 125.1: Pathophysiology of flexion deformities**
>
> The lumbricals and the interossei are the main plantarflexors of the MTPJ. Their mechanical axis as they insert at the base of the proximal phalanx is plantar to the rotational axis MTPJ. If there is dorsal subluxation at the MTPJ together with flexion at the PIPJ their axis moves dorsal to the centre of rotation of the MTPJ so that they now become MTPJ extensors. This will obviously accelerate the aforementioned deformities. This applies to the second to fifth toes. This concept is crucial to understanding the development of these deformities.

INITIAL ASSESSMENT

History

A thorough history is essential to identify the symptoms, functional deficit and progression of any lesser toe deformity. It is also essential to identify if there is any underlying deformity.

Specific points from the history should include areas of any tenderness or rubbing on footwear and the ability to purchase appropriately fitting footwear. Any history of ulceration or infection is crucial to potential lines of treatment. The speed of progression of deformity as well as any family history of deformity will help delineate prognosis. One should closely enquire about any hindfoot or ankle problems as well as any history of trauma to the foot or lower limb.

A thorough neurovascular history, including any central nervous system problems, should be elicited. If the onset of deformities has been during childhood or adolescence, then a birth and developmental history should be taken. One should also enquire about any history of an inflammatory arthropathy and potential associated conditions (e.g. nail lesions, skin lesions and rheumatoid nodules).

General examination tips

Full exposure of the lower limb should be obtained so that the anatomical alignment of the lower limb may be assessed. The lower limb should be inspected from all sides with particular reference to surgical scars, muscle wasting and trophic changes (skin quality, hair distribution, nail changes and hallmarks of venous or arterial disease). There should be careful inspection for any ulceration (including between the toes) and callosities (Fig. 125.1). The position of the fat pads with regards to the metatarsal heads should be assessed. All four limbs should be inspected for any evidence of an inflammatory arthropathy.

Forefoot, midfoot, hindfoot and ankle alignment should be determined, both non-weight bearing and weight bearing, together with observation throughout the gait cycle. The effect of these on lesser toe deformities should be determined. Particular reference should be paid to the position of the MTPJ on weight bearing.

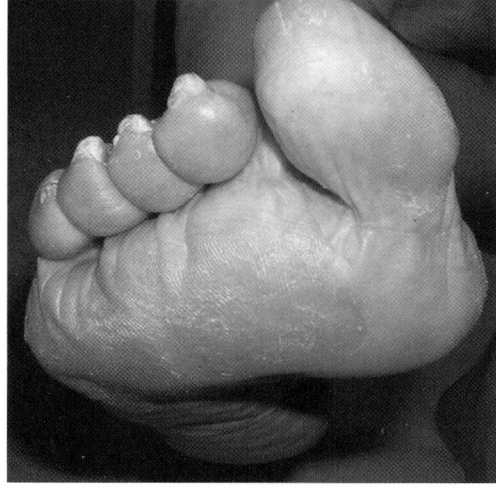

Figure 125.1 Callosities at the plantar surface of the foot over the metatarsal heads.

The range of movement of all joints of foot and ankle should be assessed. The most crucial determinant is whether the lesser toe deformities are flexible or fixed. Active power of all stabilizing muscles of the foot and ankle should be graded (particularly tibialis posterior and peroneus brevis).

A thorough neurovascular examination of the lower limb should be undertaken. This should include examination of the spine, Semmes Weinstein monofilament testing and Doppler ultrasound examination as necessary.

Investigations

PLAIN RADIOGRAPHS

Weight-bearing anteroposterior (AP) and lateral views of the foot as well as an oblique view should be taken. Standard weight-bearing views of the ankle should be taken if there is any evidence of ankle disease. Coby's view (posteroanterior view of the ankle in flexion which includes the distal half of the tibia, the ankle joint and the calcaneum) is useful in accurately determining hindfoot alignment.

MAGNETIC RESONANCE IMAGING

This modality is useful is determining synovitis, tendinopathies and any articular erosive changes.

NUCLEAR MEDICINE

This is only normally indicated in determining whether there is chronic osteomyelitis (e.g. in diabetes mellitus). This would normally involve a bone scan and white cell-labelled scan.

HAMMER TOE

Definition

A hammer toe is defined as flexion deformity at the PIPJ. This can be associated with an extended MTPJ and DIPJ. This most commonly affects the second toe, although all toes may be affected.

The deformity is most commonly seen in association with hallux valgus or hallux interphalangeus (Fig. 125.2). Again, it most commonly affects the second toe only in this clinical scenario. There is also a predisposition with an overly long second toe (so-called Greek foot morphology). When the condition affects the fifth toe and it is severe where the proximal phalanx articulates at a nearly 90° angle to the fifth metatarsal, the deformity is called a cock-up toe deformity.

The causes of toe hammering are multifactorial. In cases without a primary systemic disease it is believed that footwear, and its shape and fitting, is causative. There is a far higher incidence of hammer toes in populations where shoe-wearing is endemic. There is also a far higher

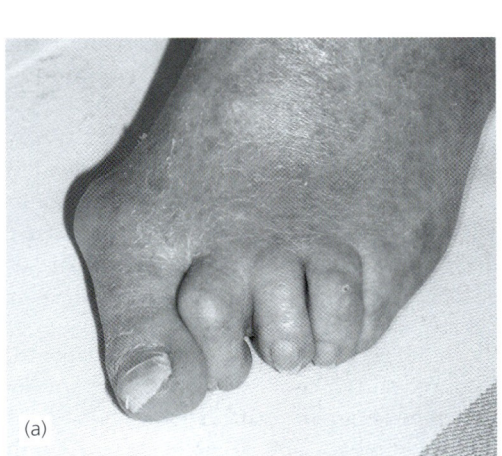
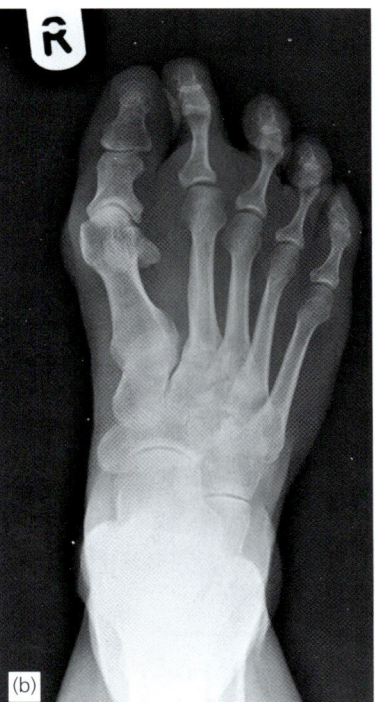
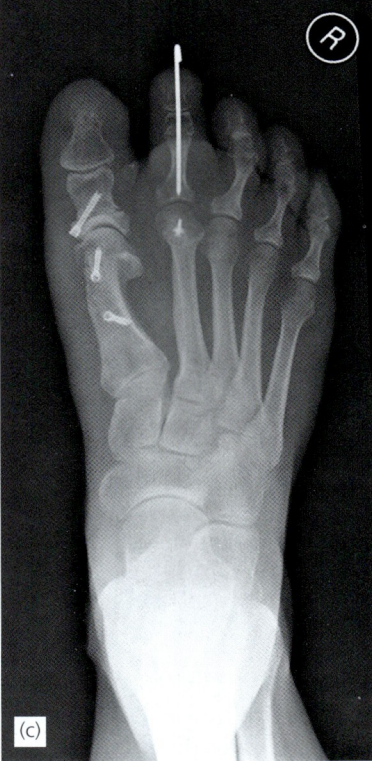

Figure 125.2 (a) Hammer toe deformity associated with hallux valgus, (b) radiographic images and (c) postoperative images.

incidence of the toe deformity in females. There are also associations with arthritides (e.g. rheumatoid, psoriatic), diabetes mellitus (especially with concomitant neuropathy) and neuromuscular diseases (e.g. Charcot–Marie–Tooth, myelodysplasia).

Pathophysiology

Attenuation of the collateral ligaments and the plantar plate as a result of MTPJ synovitis due to any underlying cause such as repeated trauma to the toe because of a long second metatarsal that leads to extension of the MTPJ.[2] When the longitudinal axis of the intrinsic flexors and the interossei displaces dorsal to the rotation axis of the MTPJ, the entire extensor function is expended at the MTPJ and offers no resistance to the flexors at the interphalangeal joint. The PIPJ becomes angulated as a result of the lumbricals. With disease progression, the EDL and the FDL lose their function. Displacement of the plantar plate distally and dorsally depresses the metatarsal head plantarwards.

Examination

The most crucial determinant of surgical treatment is the flexibility of the deformity. This relates to the position of the MTPJ upon standing. Any hyperextension deformity of the DIPJ is of limited importance. However, if the FDL is thought to be tight it may be tenotomized at the time of surgery.

A flexible deformity is defined as a lack of a fixed contracture at the MTPJ or PIPJ. Deformity increases on weight bearing. Semiflexible deformities can either have fixed or partially fixed contracture at the PIPJ. The MTPJ is fully correctable. A fixed deformity occurs when there is fixed flexion contracture at the PIPJ with fixed extension contracture of the MTPJ or subluxation/dislocation of the base of the proximal phalanx on the metatarsal head.

For operative treatment of a fixed or flexible deformity to be successful, there needs to be sufficient room for the toes to rest in their natural position. Therefore, any hallux valgus or interphalangeus must also be addressed. Surgical treatment of these deformities, even if they are asymptomatic, is indicated as part of the surgical treatment of a symptomatic hammer toe.

It must not be assumed that hammer toe is simply an idiopathic deformity. Signs of any of the aforementioned deformities should be sought and any secondary investigations carried out.

Treatment

Conservative treatment of a mild flexible deformity may simply be correctly fitting shoes. A simple tip during the consultation is to get the patient to stand barefoot on a piece of paper, trace round it and compare with their own footwear. With more severe deformities, padding and accommodative shoes with a wide and deep toe box may be indicated. A metatarsal bar or in-shoe orthosis may relieve local pressure symptoms under the metatarsal heads.

Operative treatment of a fully flexible hammer toe is usually with a flexor to extensor tendon transfer. However, if there is a secondary plane to the deformity then a bony procedure should be considered.

Operative treatment of a fixed deformity can be performed by either a proximal phalanx condylectomy[3] or a PIPJ arthrodesis. The latter is normally reserved for severe deformities or revision cases. If there is any residual dorsiflexion deformity at the MTPJ after the PIPJ has been addressed then a MTPJ release is carried out. This involves a dorsal capsular release plus release of the medial and lateral capsule if necessary. In more severe cases, typically in longstanding cases, extensor tendon lengthening may be necessary. With these more severe deformities a K-wire used to transfix the interphalangeal joints can be driven across the MTPJ to provide temporary stabilization. In the case of a relatively long metatarsal, usually the second and occasionally the third, then a metatarsal-shortening osteotomy may be considered.

CLAW TOE

Definition

There is hyperextension of the MTPJ combined with flexion of the distal and proximal interphalangeal joint. The key element in differentiating this deformity from a hammer toe is the presence of hyperextension at the MTPJ (Fig. 125.3). As the deformity progresses the MTPJ subluxes or can dislocate. With the increasing deformity the plantar surface of the metatarsal head becomes progressively uncovered. This is due to the attachment of the fat pad to the proximal phalanx; as the proximal phalanx dorsiflexes, the fat pad is drawn anteriorly and the metatarsal can 'dislocate' through the thinner posterior attachments of the fat pad.

Symptoms are usually related to local pressure effects. Callosities may develop over the interphalangeal joints, the tip of the toes and over the uncovered metatarsal heads. This last group of callosities is exaggerated if there is dysfunction of the first ray secondary to hallux valgus. It may also be difficult to obtain footwear that the forefoot will fit into. Ulceration may develop over any of the bony prominences, especially if there is a primary systemic disease causing trophic changes of local soft tissues (e.g. diabetes, rheumatoid arthritis).

There are many conditions associated with clawing of the lesser toes and even the hallux: rheumatoid arthritis, diabetes mellitus, advanced age, compartment syndrome involving the deep posterior compartment, pes cavus (and its primary neurological causes), Charcot–Marie–Tooth disease, poliomyelitis. Constrictive footwear is also felt to be a contributory factor.

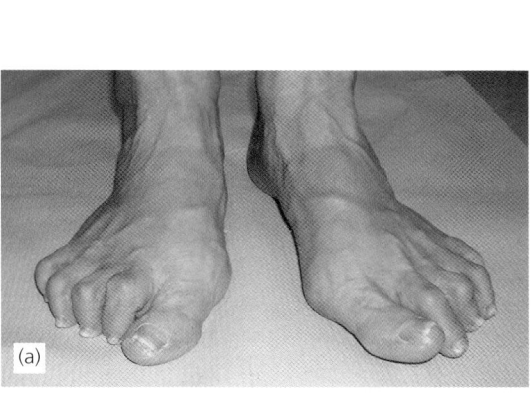
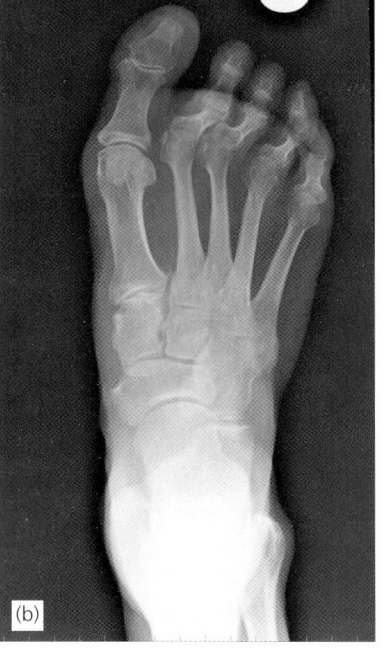

Figure 125.3 (a) Claw toe deformity of the second to fifth toes, and (b) the weight-bearing radiographs.

Pathophysiology

There is weakness of the plantar plate and the collateral ligaments leading to dorsiflexion at the MTPJ. This will lead to transferring of the axis of the interossei dorsal to the rotational axis of the MTPJ. The interossei as a result will become weak extensors or even functionless. The PIPJ and DIPJ subsequently flex. The deformity at this stage is still flexible. With a longstanding deformity, the collateral ligaments along the sides of the PIPJ and DIPJ become contracted and lose their flexibility and the deformity becomes fixed. When the deformity is a result of an underlying neuromuscular disease, there is imbalance between the extrinsic extensor tendons and the intrinsic muscles.

Examination

The assessment of flexibility of the claw toe is crucial to choosing the correct modality of treatment. The simplest method of this is whether there is any clawing with the ankle at neutral (i.e. clawing only develops with ankle dorsiflexion). Assessment of the extent of flexion deformity at the interphalangeal joints is most accurately seen if the MTPJs can be reduced.

The remainder of the foot should be assessed for any signs of pes cavus as this will tend to depress the metatarsal heads. Treatment of the midfoot and hindfoot deformities will be necessary to fully correct the forefoot deformity.

It is critical to examine for any of the hallmarks of any of the systemic diseases. The symmetrical polyarthropathy of rheumatoid arthritis (including the common progressive pes planovalgus and upper limb involvement) should be fully assessed. Inspection of the lower limb should reveal any trophic changes to the lower limb, although one needs to be thorough in checking for typically punched-out arterial ulcers. A thorough assessment of the vascular status of the foot should be undertaken including both manual and Doppler assessment. A consultation from a vascular surgeon should be sought if necessary. Semmes Weinstein filament testing may be a necessary part of neurological evaluation. If there is any suspicion of Charcot–Marie–Tooth then nerve conduction and electromyographic studies should be undertaken together with a consultation from a neurologist. If there are any upper motor neuron signs then brain and spine MRI should be undertaken.

Treatment

Conservative measures include padding of bony prominences and accommodative shoe wear with a wide and deep toe box. A metatarsal bar or in-shoe orthosis may relieve local pressure symptoms under the metatarsal heads.

If the claw toe is flexible then treatment is possible with a flexor to extensor tendon transfer. This is performed at the proximal flexor crease. It may be necessary to release the MTPJ if complete correction is not achieved. If the primary condition is an old posterior compartment syndrome then it may be possible to carry out lengthening more proximally of the posterior compartment muscles.

If the clawing is fixed, in addition to dorsal MTPJ release (including the collaterals) and extensor tendon lengthening, the interphalangeal joints will need to be addressed.

Normally the PIPJ is addressed first with either a Du Vries arthroplasty or arthrodesis. An osteoclasis of the DIPJ will then usually suffice. If the MTPJ is still not fully reducible then a metatarsal shortening osteotomy is performed. Our preference is for a Weil's oblique distal metatarsal osteotomy as it is easily reproducible and the approach has already been made when performing the MTPJ release.

Longstanding fixed deformity may also produce contracture of the neurovascular bundle. Care must be taken to resect enough bone so that reduction is relatively atraumatic. If a tourniquet is used then it should always be deflated during skin closure so that vascular compromise maybe dealt with (immediate removal of the K-wire and further resection if necessary). This is critical if there is any prior history of vascular compromise.

MALLET TOE

Definition

A mallet toe is defined as a plantarflexion deformity at the level of the DIPJ. This may occur alone or with other lesser toe deformities (Fig. 125.4). Aetiology may be traumatic or atraumatic. Traumatic mallet toes are less common and are due to an axially loaded hyperflexion injury.

Pathophysiology

They represent a tear of the extensor tendon. One theory states that repeated trauma to toes or impingement from tight shoes leads to weakness or even rupture of the EDL tendon at the level of the DIPJ. As a result, there will be no opposition of the flexion force of the FDL tendon at the DIPJ level thus resulting in the deformity.

Mallet toes may be associated with diabetes or an inflammatory arthropathy. However, they are far more commonly idiopathic. Footwear is thought to be a major factor. They have equal incidence in the second, third and fourth toes. The affected toe or toes tend to be overly long.

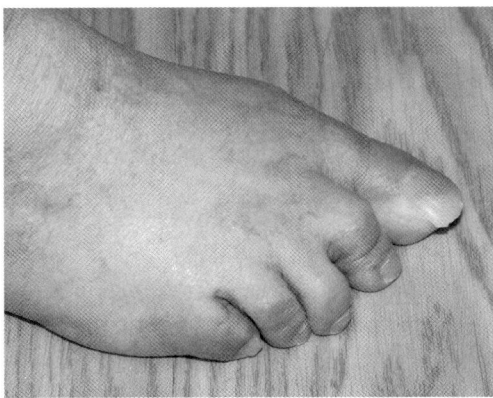

Figure 125.4 Mallet toe deformity at the third toe.

Symptoms are usually due to the development of a painful callosity at the tip of the toe. These may become infected in diabetic patients. The majority of these deformities are fixed. Fully flexible deformities have usually developed in childhood/adolescence. These deformities may be associated with a delta phalanx.

Treatment

Conservative treatment involves footwear with a sufficient toe box that allows for the height of the flexed distal phalanx. Padding of toes and soft toe cap over the tip of the toe may also be beneficial.

If the mallet toe is fully flexible then a FDL tenotomy at the distal flexion crease may be sufficient. If there is an underlying delta phalanx then an excision arthroplasty will be necessary.

In the more typical fixed deformities a phalangeal condylectomy and flexor tenotomy with K-wire fixation is undertaken. In chronic deformities with gross skin changes, usually in the old and infirm, patients may sometimes opt for a tip amputation. This operation, although cosmetically unacceptable for most, has a low morbidity.

BUNIONETTE DEFORMITY

Definition

This is defined as a painful osseous prominence on the lateral aspect of the fifth metatarsal head. This may include an inflamed overlying bursa and callosity, and a varus deformity of the fifth toe (Fig. 125.5). Its original terminology was a tailor's bunion; it was commonly seen in tailors who used to position themselves cross-legged and barefoot on the floor to cut cloth thereby putting constant pressure on the lateral border of the foot.[4]

Aetiology

Commonly it is an idiopathic condition. It is associated with various morphologies of the fifth metatarsal and surrounding structures: wide head of the fifth metatarsal, lateral bowing of the fifth metatarsal, short or dumbbell-shaped fifth metatarsal, an increase in the fourth–fifth intermetatarsal angle (>10°), supernumerary ossicles attached to the lateral side of the fourth metatarsal pushing the fifth metatarsal laterally. It may also be associated with rheumatoid arthritis, and may have a potentially worse outcome in the presence of peripheral neuropathy of any cause.

Bunionettes may also be associated with hallux valgus, splaying of the forefoot (laxity of the intermetatarsal ligaments), pes planovalgus and may be aggravated by a cavus foot position.

Patients will normally complain of localized pain over the fifth metatarsal head as well as soft-tissue swelling and

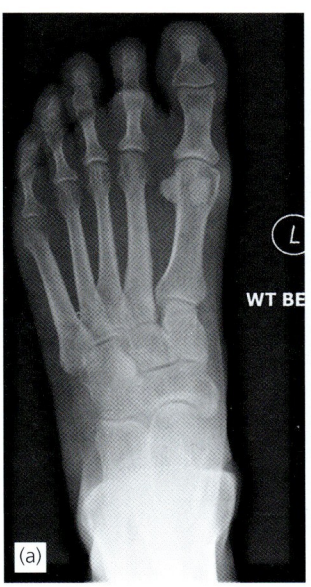
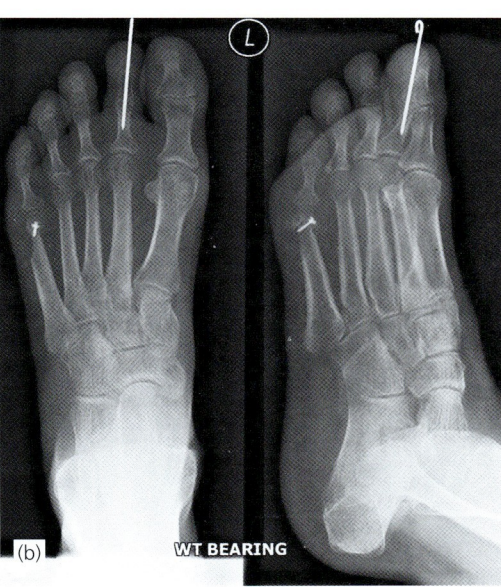

Figure 125.5 (a) Radiographic image of a bunnionette, and (b) the postoperative images.

Table 125.1 Classification of bunionette

Type	Description	Associations	Incidence (%)
Type 1	Enlargement of the lateral aspect of the fifth metatarsal head	Lateral exostosis hypertrophy of the lateral condyle dumb-bell metatarsal	27
Type 2	Lateral bowing of the distal diaphysis of the fifth metatarsal		23
Type 3	Widened fourth to fifth intermetatarsal angle	Splayed foot; hallux valgus	50
Type 4	Combination of at least two of the above types	Systemic pathologies such as rheumatoid arthritis	

callosities. These may be exacerbated by ill-fitting footwear and increase in sporting activities (particularly long-distance running and skiing). If there is splaying of the forefoot and hallux valgus, it may be difficult to purchase appropriate footwear. Ulceration over bony prominences may occur in rheumatoid and neuropathic patients.

Classification

Originally Coughlin[5] described three types of bunionette, now a fourth type is recognized (Table 125.1).

Karasick[6] described radiological parameters that can be used to assess bunionette on the AP weight-bearing view.

- *Fourth–fifth intermetatarsal angle.* This should normally measure less than 8°. It usually averages more than 10° in symptomatic patients.
- *Fifth metatarsophalangeal angle.* This should normally measure less than 10°. It usually averages more than 16° in symptomatic individuals.
- *Lateral bowing of the fifth metatarsal.* This normally measures less than 3°. It averages 8° in symptomatic patients.

Treatment

Conservative treatment includes appropriate footwear with a wide toe box, padding and chiropody. In-shoe orthoses may be appropriate if there is a predisposing hindfoot deformity.

Operative treatment is dependent upon the type of bunionette. A type 1 bunionette may be treated with an exostectomy. The other types are usually treated with a combination of exostectomy and metatarsal osteotomy. The authors' preferred osteotomy is a chevron osteotomy with internal fixation. Patients may immediately weight bear in a stiff-soled postoperative shoe.

CROSSOVER SECOND TOE

Definition

There is dorsomedial deviation of the second toe in relation to the hallux and the third toe leading to overlapping of the second toe on the hallux. It is a progressive deformity which starts usually with pain in the early stages at the plantar plate and second MTPJ, with a slight increase in the interval

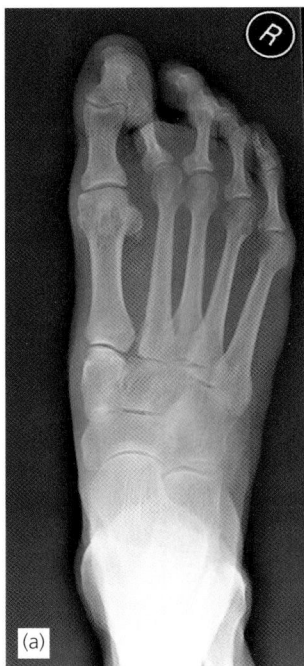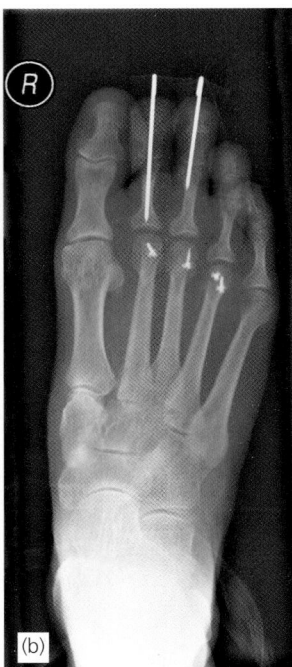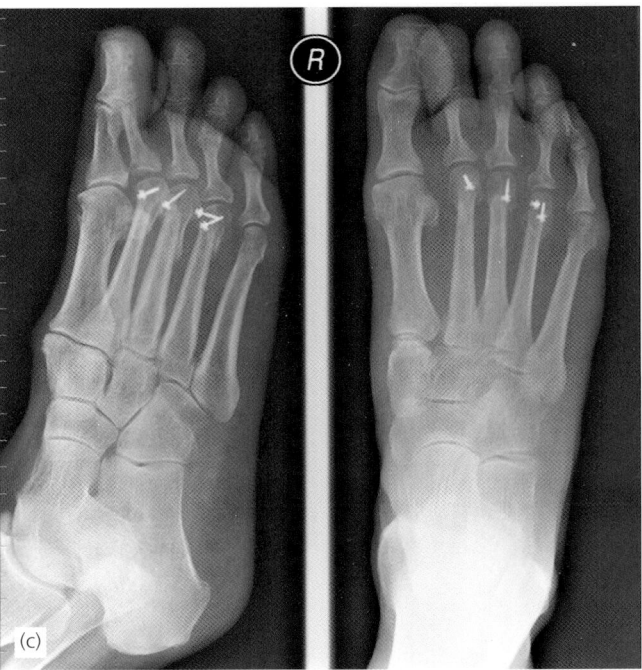

Figure 125.6 Crossover second toe (a), postoperative radiographic images (b) and the follow-up images (c).

between the second and third toes due to medial deviation of the second toe. If left untreated, this can progress into the late stage, which involves hyperextension of the second MTPJ with subluxation, overriding of the second toe on the hallux and dislocation of the MTPJ (Fig. 125.6).

Pathophysiology

The condition is characterized by second MTPJ instability. This is probably due to attenuation of the lateral collateral ligament complex alone or in combination with the plantar plate, which leads to joint instability, pain and subsequent MTPJ deformity. The medial collateral ligament can be contracted. The presence of a positive Lachman sign usually indicates MTPJ instability.

Extrinsic factors such as trauma, high-fashion footwear, pressure on the second toe from a hallux valgus deformity, impingement from the neighbouring third toe and gastrosoleus contracture leading to forefoot overloading are thought to contribute to this deformity.

Hyperextension of the second toe proximal phalanx due to an anomalous muscle slip or muscular imbalance between the intrinsic and extrinsic musculature of the toes have also been postulated to be a cause of second MTPJ instability. Other factors such as long second metatarsal and first ray hypermobility leading to overloading the second metatarsal can lead to subsequent second MTPJ deformity.

The classical clinical sign is the presence of gap between the second and the third toe. In the early stages, diagnosis can be difficult as the pain can be misdiagnosed as a Morton's neuroma. The drawer sign is the first objective sign of MTPJ instability. Pressing on the MTPJ and checking for stability and radiographic pictures can aid in establishing diagnosis.[7]

Treatment

Conservative treatment is effective in the early stages of the disease before deviation and subluxation of the second toe MTPJ. This includes splinting of the toe and strapping, non-steroidal anti-inflammatory drugs, custom shoe insoles, and rest and immobilization.

Surgical treatment involves release of the dorsal and medial MTPJ capsule, medial collateral ligament and EDL tendon. Some authors recommended amputation of the second toe in people over 70 years of age. Flexor to extensor tendon transfer has also been described. Weil's osteotomy can also be performed if a long second metatarsal bone is the underlying cause.

CONGENITAL OVERLAPPING OF THE FIFTH TOE

Definition

The fifth toe in this deformity overlaps the fourth toe and is held in this varus (adduction) position due to dorsal and medial contracture of the capsule. It is often a bilateral deformity. Other components in this condition include external rotation of the fifth toe, contracture of the extensor tendon and dislocation at the fifth MTPJ. The condition is not rare and often surgical advice is sought, either for the cosmetic appearance or for the relief of disturbances which occur from the friction of the footwear on the misplaced little toe.

Pathophysiology

The condition exists at birth. Prolonged malposition of the fifth toe during intra-uterine life appears to be the cause. It affects both sexes equally and it can be unilateral or bilateral. The tendon of the EDL of the fifth toe is displaced medially and shortened, and the skin, fascia, and the capsule at its mediodorsal surface are contracted. A dorsal callus is commonly seen.

Treatment

Treatment is often sought due to either cosmetic reasons or difficulties with footwear. Conservative treatment by passive starching or strapping of the toe can have some effect in very young children with flexible deformity.

Operative treatment is often sought because conservative measures are often unsuccessful. Surgical correction usually involves release of the dorsal medial tight structures with or without lengthening or release of EDL tendon. V–Y skin advancement to the contracted dorsomedial skin or Z-plasty to dorsomedial skin have also been described in correction.[8] Toes are kept in the over-corrected position by taping or use of a K-wire for 3–6 weeks, depending on the type of correction.

Procedures such as syndactylization of the fifth toe to the fourth toe or the Ruiz–Mora procedure have been described as salvage options.

CONGENITAL UNDERLAPPING OF THE FIFTH TOE

Definition

This is also termed congenital curly fifth toe. The fifth toe is externally rotated into a varus position, and lies under the fourth toe with plantarflexion at the MTPJ. It is often a bilateral deformity.

Pathophysiology

There is weakness of the dorsal MTPJ capsule and EDL. This is associated with contracture of the FDL tendon and the plantar medial MTPJ capsule. In the young children group, it is commonly a flexible deformity.

Treatment

In the flexible type, soft-tissue surgery alone often gives good results. This includes tenotomy of both the FDL and the FDB tendons and splinting of the toe postoperatively.

In adults, the deformity is usually of the fixed type. The Thompson[9] technique has been described for the correction of this deformity with good results. This procedure includes skin Z incision and plasty, resection of the head of the proximal phalange of the fifth toe, flexor to extensor tendon transfer and derotation soft tissue procedure. The correction is held in position by strapping or use of a K-wire for 3–6 weeks postoperatively.

CONGENITAL SHORT FOURTH TOE (BRACHYMETATARSIA)

Definition

This is a congenital shortening of a metatarsal with the fourth being the most affected. The diagnosis is confirmed when the metatarsal ends 5 mm or more proximal to the parabolic arc.[10] It is most commonly seen in Far Eastern countries in females and is most commonly a bilateral disease.

Aetiology

Its exact aetiology is unknown but is thought to represent premature closure of the distal metatarsal epiphysis. It may also be present following poliomyelitis, when it is a unilateral disease. Other causes may include post-traumatic, post-surgical or linked to specific disease processes such as Down syndrome, sickle-cell anaemia and diastrophic dwarfism.

Patients may present with metatarsalgia. However, it is commonly asymptomatic. It represents a cosmetic deformity that can have social stigmata in cultures where shoe and sock wear are socially unacceptable indoors.

Treatment

Surgical treatment involves lengthening of the affected metatarsal. This may be achieved acutely with one-stage lengthening and interpositional autograft and internal fixation or by gradual lengthening through distraction osteogenesis.

CURLY TOES

Definition

These are a common childhood disorder describing flexion at the interphalangeal joints. This is usually due to tight flexor tendons, although it may also be associated with a delta phalanx. There is normally neither subluxation nor dislocation at the MTPJ.

Curly toes are often associated with a rotational deformity as well as adduction. In severe cases this can become an overlapping or underlapping toe.

Treatment

The majority of curly toes are asymptomatic and respond to conservative treatment as well as reassurance for the parents. This can be a self-resolving condition.

If surgical treatment is required then the majority of cases respond to a flexor tenotomy at the level of the proximal flexor crease. If however there is severe malrotation plus adduction, a more widespread release (such as a Butler's procedure) is necessary. This would involve release of all deforming structures at the MTPJ. This may be approached through a tennis racket incision based dorsally at the MTPJ so that an advancement V–Y-plasty of skin contractures may be simultaneously performed.

MUCOUS CYSTS OF THE TOES

Definition

This is a cystic lesion located eccentrically on the dorsum of the distal phalanx of a finger or lesser toe. It represents a herniation of synovial tissue from the interphalangeal joint similar to other joint ganglia. The majority of patients are between the ages of 40 and 70 years.[11]

Presentation

They commonly present as a firm cystic lesion located eccentrically on the dorsum of the distal phalanx of a lesser toe and less commonly they present over the interphalangeal joint of the thumb or great toe. The skin overlying the cyst is usually thin and occasionally ulcerated, especially when caused by the trauma of tight-fitting shoes. They can cause significant disability due to pain and difficulty in fitting appropriate footwear. Spontaneous resolution of the cyst may occur, but the timeframe for this is unpredictable and recurrent discharge with subsequent infection may be troublesome.

Treatment

Methods such as needle aspiration and puncture, electrical and chemical cautery, cryotherapy, injection of steroids or sclerosing agents, and irradiation all have a high recurrence rates.

Aggressive surgical excision with skin grafts or advancement of local flaps has been employed with reported recurrence rates of 0–5%.

HARD CORNS

These are due to chronic abrasion of bony prominences against footwear, causing hypertrophy of the skin. These are commonly seen over the dorsal or the dorsal lateral side of the PIPJ due to hammering or clawing and at the tips of the toes or over the dorsum of the DIPJ with clawing or mallet toe deformity. They result from pressure from the bony prominence and external pressure over the exposed fifth toe. They are usually associated with an underlying toe deformity such as a hammer toe or a rotational deformity.

Treatment

Conservative treatment includes shaving the corn followed be removal of the central part of the corn. Modifying and wearing wider shoes to decrease pressure placed on the toe can also be helpful. Protective padding can be useful to decrease shoe friction.

Surgical correction is reserved for conditions where conservative measures fail. This includes decompression of bony prominences by treatment of the underlying deformity as outlined in the relevant previous sections.

SOFT CORNS

These develop as a result of abrasion between two adjacent toes due to deformity. The softness of the corn is due to sweat that is unable to evaporate. These lesions are most common over the lateral fourth PIPJ, medial fifth PIPJ or DIPJ, or deep in the web space. The skin overlying the affected toe is friable, macerated and associated with thick callus.

Treatment

Conservative treatment includes accommodative shoe wear as well as absorptive paddings and toe spacers to ease pressure on corns.

Surgical treatment includes excision of the bony prominences as well as the skin lesion if this is involved in the approach to the deformity. The resection should address the underlying deformities of both toes as outlined in previous sections.

KEY LEARNING POINTS

- The causes of lesser toe deformities are multifactorial (neuromuscular, rheumatological, mechanical, congenital and traumatic factors) but mainly from women's high-fashion footwear.
- Mallet toes, hammer toes, claw toes, interdigital corns, lateral corns on the fifth toe, and crossover fifth toes.
- Dynamic stabilization is formed by the intrinsic (extensor digitorum brevis, flexor digitorum brevis, lumbricals and interossei) and extrinsic foot muscles (extensor digitorum longus, flexor digitorum longus).

- For flexion deformities, dorsal subluxation at the metatarsophalangeal joint (MTPJ), the lubricals and interossei shift from being flexors to being extensors.
- Check for pain, footwear friction and fitting problems, ulceration and infection and do a neurovascular examination.
- Weight-bearing anteroposterior, lateral and oblique radiographs.
- Hammer toe is a flexion deformity at the proximal interphalangeal joint (PIPJ) with an extended MTPJ and distal interphalangeal joint (DIPJ), often of the second toe. Seen with hallux valgus or hallux interphalangeus. Access flexibility. Hallux valgus or interphalangeus will also have to be corrected.
- Treatment of hammer toe is flexor-to-extensor tendon transfer, proximal phalanx condylectomy or PIPJ arthrodesis.
- Claw toe is hyperextension of the MTPJ combined with flexion of the distal and proximal interphalangeal joint. Check for flexibility. Exclude systemic diseases. A fixed deformity may require a Weil's oblique distal metatarsal osteotomy.
- Mallet toe is a plantarflexion deformity at the DIPJ. Usually idiopathic. Often there is a painful callosity at the tip.
- Bunionette is a painful osseous prominence over lateral aspect of fifth metatarsal head often associated with hallux valgus. Treatment is a chevron osteotomy with internal fixation.
- Congenital overlapping of the fifth toe over the fourth is due to capsular contracture. Surgical correction is difficult. Underlapping of the same toe is called curly fifth toe.

REFERENCES

- ◆ = Major review article
- ● = Key primary paper

●1. Thompson FM, Coughlin MJ. The high price of high-fashion footwear. *Journal of Bone and Joint Surgery* 1994;**76A**:1586-93. An article describing relation between ill-fitting shoes and forefoot deformity. They concluded that shoe-wearing patterns in the USA have a distinct and unequivocal influence on the development of forefoot problems in women. Changing societal footwear habits requires an awareness of the dangers of and damage done by ill-fitting, tight shoes. Proper shoe fit is critical for good foot health.

●2. Bhatia D, Myerson MS, Curtis MJ, *et al.* Anatomical restraints to dislocation of the second metatarsophalangeal joint and assessment of a repair technique. *Journal of Bone and Joint Surgery* 1994;**76A**:1371-5. A study on cadaveric feet examining the forces required to dislocate the MTPJ following division of the collateral ligaments and the joint capsule. Stability was then observed following repair by flexor tendon transfer.

◆3. Coughlin MJ. Lesser-toe abnormalities. *Journal of Bone and Joint Surgery* 2002;**84A**:1446-69. This is from selected instructional course lectures on lesser toe deformities. Common lesser toe deformities have been reviewed along with physical examinations tips and treatment options.

◆4. Koti M, Maffulli N. Bunionette. *Journal of Bone and Joint Surgery* 2001;**83A**:1076-82. This is a current concepts review on bunionettes. They have discussed aetiology, clinical presentations, imaging studies, classifications, management options, and scoring system.

●5. Coughlin MJ. Treatment of bunionette deformity with longitudinal diaphyseal osteotomy with distal soft tissue repair. *Foot and Ankle* 1991;**11**:195-203. Twenty patients with symptomatic bunionettes refractory to conservative care underwent longitudinal diaphyseal osteotomy, lateral condylectomy and distal metatarsophalangeal realignment. At an average of 31 months follow-up, 93% noted good or excellent results.

●6. Karasick D. Preoperative assessment of symptomatic bunionette deformity: radiologic findings. *AJR American Journal of Roentgenology* 1995;**164**:147-9. The author illustrated the radiographic abnormalities of bunionettes and described angular measurements related to the preoperative evaluation.

●7. Kaz AJ, Coughlin MJ. Crossover second toe: demographics, etiology, and radiographic assessment. *Foot and Ankle International* 2007;**28**:1223-37. This is a retrospective study of 326 patients diagnosed with cross over second toe that had surgical treatment between 2001 and 2006. The demographics, aetiology and radiographic findings associated with a crossover second toe deformity were discussed.

●8. Goodwin FC, Swisher FM. The treatment of congenital hyperextension of the fifth toe. *Journal of Bone and Joint Surgery* 1943;**25A**:193-6. Surgical correction of varus fifth toe through a dorsal Y-shaped incision over the fifth MTPJ is described and the outcome in 20 patients is reported.

9. Thompson FM, Deland JT. Flexor tendon transfer for metacarpophalangeal instability of the second toe. *Foot and Ankle* 1993;**14**:385-8.

●10. Bartolomei FJ. Surgical correction of brachymetatarsia. *Journal of the American Podiatric Medical Association* 1990;**80**:76-82. The author proposes specific criteria for the objective diagnosis of brachymetatarsia and discusses one such surgical technique.

●11. Calder JDF, Buch B, Hennessy MS, Saxby TS. Treatment of mucous cysts of the toes. *Foot and Ankle International* 2003;**24**:490-3. This study reports on the treatment of mucous cysts of the toes by simple excision and joint debridement in 15 patients with a 2 years follow up. One cyst recurred at 9 months. A review of literature is also included.

Pes cavus and pes planus

ANTHONY PERERA, MARK S MYERSON

| Introduction | 1460 | Pes planus | 1462 |
| Pes cavus | 1460 | References | 1465 |

NATIONAL BOARD STANDARDS

- Revise the biomechanics of the foot
- Understand the pathophysiology of pes cavus and planus
- Thorough knowledge of the evaluation of pes cavus and planus
- Be able to make a management plan for pes cavus and planus
- Revise your knowledge of hereditary sensory motor neuropathy

INTRODUCTION

The high-arched cavus foot and the flat planus foot have some important features in common. First, they are not diagnoses but phenotypes, representing the summation of various biomechanical changes in the complex kinematic coupling of the foot. Failure to recognize all of these alterations will affect the success of surgery. Second, many abnormalities may be present, so it is important to recognize those that are symptomatic, those that may be become symptomatic and also occasionally those that are asymptomatic but require correction nonetheless. Many severely deformed feet will remain totally trouble-free and require no treatment. Finally, both have a number of different causes that are quite disparate in their nature and natural history; therefore, there is no 'one-rule-for-all'.

PES CAVUS

The cavus foot is a high-arched foot that fails to flatten on weight bearing. If the foot is thought of as a tripod, then the points (first and fifth metatarsal heads and the heel) describe a triangle that shortens and, in the cavovarus foot, topples to the lateral side. Claw toes are commonly seen; these may be due to the primary pathology or a knock-on effect of the changes.

Aetiology

It is essential to appreciate that there are serious and treatable causes (Box 126.1). Spinal pathology is particularly important; failure to look for this can be disastrous.

Twenty per cent of cases will be idiopathic and are non-progressive, unlike neurological cases.

Pathophysiology

A number of biomechanical abnormalities can cause these changes.

- The intrinsic muscles can fail, e.g. crush injury or compartment syndrome.
- The forefoot may be in plantaris (weak extensors) or pronated (overpull of peroneus longus), e.g. hereditary sensory motor neuropathy (HSMN).
- The heel may be in calcaneus (weak Achilles with normal tibialis anterior), e.g. polio.

> **BOX 126.1: Causes of pes cavus**
>
> - Congenital
> - Idiopathic
> - Congenital talipes equinovarus
> - Acquired
> - Spinal: dysraphism, tethered cord, tumours
> - Neuromuscular: polio
> - Central: cerebral palsy, Friedrich's ataxia
> - Peripheral: hereditary sensory motor neuropathy
> - Traumatic
> - Crush injury
> - Compartment syndrome
> - Burns
> - Iatrogenic
> - Overlengthening of the Achilles

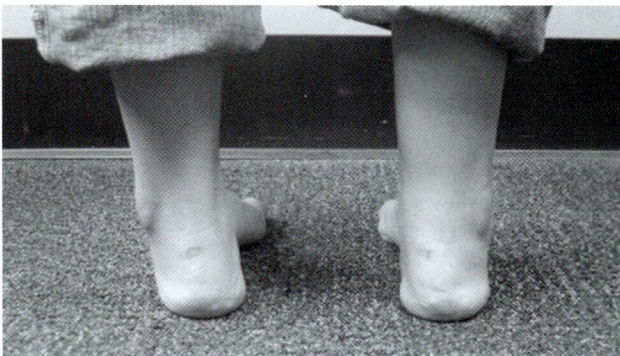

Figure 126.1 Cavovarus feet (left unoperated).

- Congenital field change, e.g. the tight plantar fascia and deformed osteology residual to congenital talipes equinovarus (CTEV).

CLINICAL FEATURES

These mechanical changes can cause various problems, e.g.

- muscle imbalance: toe clawing, weak dorsiflexion, varus instability
- plantarflexion of the metatarsals: metatarsalgia, plantar keratosis, clawing, metatarsophalangeal subluxation
- varus foot: stiffness, lateral soft-tissue problems (collateral ligament and peroneals), lateral loading
- abnormal loading: foot fatigue, stress fractures, degeneration (Fig. 126.1).

EVALUATION

- *Aetiology.* Family history is found in both the idiopathic type and the HSMN type. Beware the unilateral and increasing deformity, a treatable cord lesion such as tethering or tumour should not be missed. Any neurological abnormalities mandate full investigation.
- *Assessment of symptoms.* Many deformities may be present, but often the patient may complain of just one. Sometimes even the most severe clawing can be asymptomatic. Spend some time on the history and examination to elucidate what is troublesome and what is not. Be aware of any evidence of joint degeneration.
- *Biomechanical assessment.* Finding out what is driving the deformity is an important part of the examination.

EXAMINATION

First look at the gait for muscle balance (especially tibialis anterior) and instability. Describe the appearance of the foot, including the plantar aspect (Fig. 126.2). Palpate for bony and soft-tissue pain. Look for joint degeneration such as stiffness, pain, crepitation. Determine whether the deformities (e.g. claw toes) are fixed or mobile. If heel varus is present is it correctable and is it is driven by a plantar flexed first ray (using the Coleman block test) or is there a pronation of the whole forefoot? Test sensation and power and look for muscle imbalance. In Charcot–Marie–Tooth disease the tibialis anterior and peroneus brevis are relatively weak whereas the tibialis posterior and peroneus longus are relatively strong (Table 126.1). Some patients may have peroneal or lateral ligament pathology.

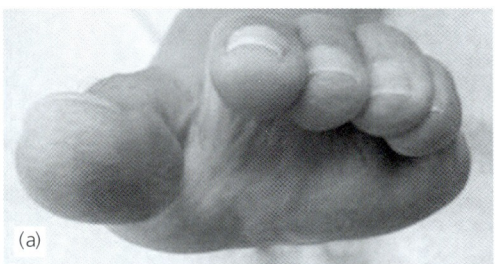
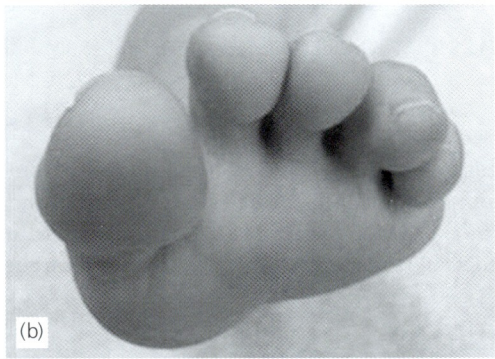

Figure 126.2 Plantar flexed first ray (a) pre- and (b) postoperatively.

Investigations should include plain radiographs (cavus = calcaneal pitch >30° (Fig. 126.3); if forefoot plantaris is present Meary's angle is increased). Degenerative changes

Table 126.1 Deformity in hereditary sensory motor neuropathy[1]

Deformity	Weak	Intact
Equinus	Tibialis anterior	Gastrosoleus
Adduction and hindfoot varus	Peroneus brevis	Tibialis posterior
Plantar flexed first ray	Tibialis anterior	Peroneus longus
Lesser toe clawing (and also metatarsal head depression)	Intrinsics	Long flexors
Clawed hallux	Intrinsics	Flexor hallucis longus, extensor hallucis longus (especially if tibialis anterior poor)

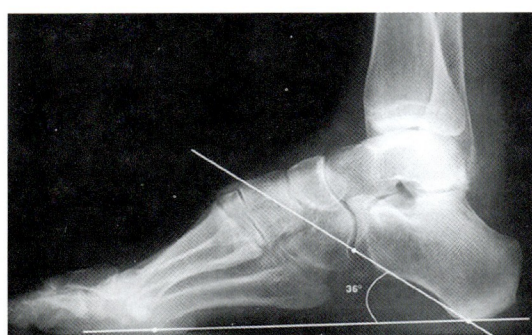

Figure 126.3 Cavus foot calcaneal pitch angle >30°.

and joint laxity may be present in more severe cases. Electromyogram (EMG) and nerve conduction studies can rule out HSMN, and MRI for spinal pathology. Nonetheless, neurological referral may be required.

CLASSIFICATION

There is no widely used system; instead, management is 'à la carte'. That is, each patient has to be treated individually with procedure selection based on the symptomatic deformities present.

CONSERVATIVE MANAGEMENT

Orthotics with metatarsal padding, arch support and lateral heel pads accommodate and cushion the deformity. For patients with marked clawing shoes with a high toe-box are advised. Ankle braces have a role to play in patients with lateral instability. Some patients may benefit from physical therapy and treatment of callosities.

SURGICAL MANAGEMENT

The aim of surgery is a pain-free, plantigrade, stable foot (Table 126.2). Knowledge of the aetiology, the problematic issues and underlying biomechanical abnormalities is essential to creating an individualized treatment plan that may involve multiple separate procedures. In general, the possible options can be divided into soft-tissue and bony procedures.

Clearly, when the foot is totally paralysed, stiff or degenerate then arthrodesis is necessary. However, the best outcome is a mobile, flexible foot and so releases, tendon transfers and osteotomies should be considered whenever possible.

PES PLANUS

Flat feet are very common affecting 20–30% of the population, although most will remain asymptomatic. This chapter refers to acquired or progressive symptomatic pes planus (or planovalgus if the heel is also everted). Although some will go on to develop a stiff foot if it is longstanding or degenerate, it does not include the rigid flat foot of talocalcaneal coalition or even congenital vertical talus, both of which occasionally present in adults.

Aetiology

Posterior tibial tendon dysfunction (PTTD) is the most common cause of acquired adult flat foot deformity, but there are other causes. Consideration should be given to congenital conditions, arthritides (rheumatoid, seronegative and osteoarthritis), bony trauma (to the medial arch or midfoot), soft-tissue trauma (to the spring ligament) and neuropathic (Charcot) collapse.

Pathophysiology

The medial longitudinal arch is maintained by a balance between its static and dynamic restraints. The most frequent disruption is an injury to the posterior tibial tendon. It is the most powerful invertor of the foot and if it fails the loss of this movement prevents the foot from locking at the transverse tarsal joint and becoming a rigid lever for push-off. It is postulated that the loss of this dynamic support places greater stress on static stabilizers. Thus, the

Table 126.2 Problem-based surgical approach

Problem	Procedure
Cavus	Steindler plantar fascia release
Varus (that does not correct on Coleman block test)	Lateral closing wedge calcaneal osteotomy
Metatarsalgia	Closing wedge metatarsal osteotomy
Peroneal imbalance leading to lateral weakness and first metatarsal pronation	Peroneus longus to peroneus brevis transfer
Weak ankle dorsiflexion	Tibialis posterior transfer if tibialis anterior poor
	Long extensor transfer (also reduces their contribution to clawing)
Hallucal clawing	Interphalangeal fusion +
	Jones transfer: extensor hallucis longus transfer to first metatarsophalangeal neck (also reduces its contribution to clawing and improves ankle dorsiflexion) or
	Flexor hallucis longus transfer to proximal phalanx
Lesser toe clawing	IP fusion +
	Flexor to extensor transfer
	Flexor tenotomy and extensor recession
Stiffness or arthritis	Triple fusion

spring and talocalcaneal ligaments can fail leading to increased arch collapse and ankle deformity in severe cases if the deltoid also fails.

PTTD is more common in older women, especially if obese, and 60% of patients will have diabetes, hypertension, previous corticosteroids, trauma or surgery to the midfoot.[2] Because acute dysfunction can occur in a long-standing flat foot, a degenerative mechanism is likely. An area of hypovascularity is seen in the tendon at malleolar level, where ruptures are most common. A subset of younger patients has also been identified who have features of spondyloarthropathy and enthesopathies at multiple sites.[3]

CLINICAL FEATURES

Typically this starts with pain and swelling on the medial side of the ankle with a gradual medial arch collapse causing increased wear on the inner border of the shoe. As this deteriorates, the heel goes into valgus, and the midfoot can abduct, giving the 'too-many-toes' sign. As the valgus deteriorates the patient may complain of lateral ankle pain from a sinus tarsi syndrome or lateral impingement and the medial pain may even settle completely.

With dysfunction of the posterior tibial tendon, heel inversion deteriorates as does the ability to perform single heel raise. Eventually the ability to invert the heel on even passive motion is lost.

Frequently the longstanding heel valgus results in a tight gastrocnemius. Often, the tendon is stretched out rather than ruptured, but this has little practical difference. In severe longstanding cases the foot can become stiff and eventually the joints including the ankle can become degenerate.

EVALUATION

Diagnosis is made on clinical grounds and the classification system used relies on the examination findings. As with pes cavus, it is important to assess the relationship between the forefoot and hindfoot (Fig. 126.4); if the forefoot is still fixed in supination on correction of the heel, then hindfoot surgery alone will be inadequate. A tight gastrocnemius must be identified as this too can predispose to failure.

Radiographs are used for surgical planning, for instance looking for joint degeneration and assessing ankle instability. There are some measures of severity (talo–first metatarsal angle, talonavucular coverage, medial cuneiform to floor distance and calcaneal pitch) but they are of little diagnostic use. An MRI scan can be used but it is of poor reliability and little value in planning. Screening for rheumatoid and seronegative arthritis should be considered.

CLASSIFICATION

The Johnson and Strom[4] system has been modified by Myerson[5] and is useful in guiding management.

Stage 1 Peritendinitis: swelling and inflammation along the tendon but it remains functional.
Stage 2 Tendon dysfunction: loss of single heel raise but the foot remains flexible.
Stage 3 Rigid flatfoot: the foot becomes stiff due to longstanding PTTD and deformity.
Stage 4 Ankle valgus and degeneration: after failure of the deltoid ligament.

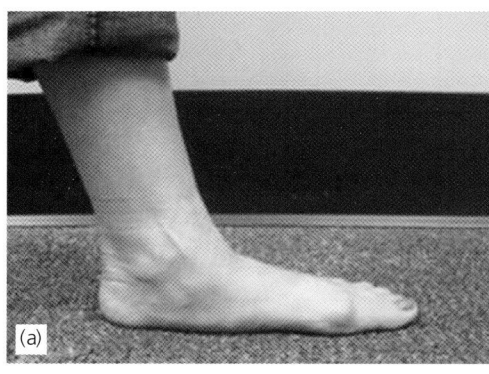

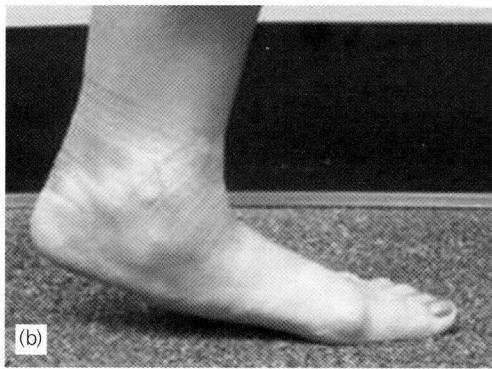

Figure 126.4 Pes planus with midfoot break.

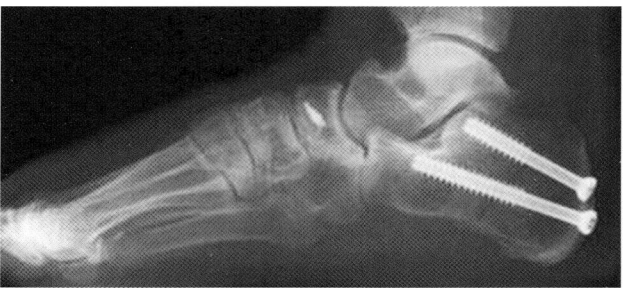

Figure 126.5 Pes planus after surgery.

This system is used to guide management but it does have some weaknesses. The stages are not well demarcated and thus there is an observer variation. Furthermore, the majority of patients fall into the second stage with a huge difference in severity within this group. This system has been updated by Bluman et al.[6] to take into account the deformities that occur throughout the whole foot secondary to the planus. This is useful for planning the additional procedures that may be required and makes the management decisions much more specific. For instance, if the forefoot is in fixed supination once the heel is corrected then hindfoot surgery alone will be inadequate.

MANAGEMENT

There is a bewildering array of footwear and devices designed to manage pes planus and its sequelae. There is good evidence that conservative measures are of benefit in early flexible flat feet. In stage I disease semirigid arch supports or tibialis posterior tendon bracing can settle the acute synovitis, occasionally a period of immobilization in a boot or cast and anti-inflammatory medication is required prior to this. Steroid injections are contraindicated, as they risk further weakening to the tendon (although they can be useful in a sinus tarsi syndrome). In stage II disease, a UCBL (University of California Biomechanics Laboratory) orthosis in addition to a more rigid brace can improve heel control. Studies have shown that a significant number of patients will settle with conservative measures.

But this is intensive and requires long-term bracing and significant lifestyle changes. Subsequently patient compliance can be poor.

The only role for conservative measures in stage III and IV disease is in accommodating the deformity in patients inappropriate for surgery.

When conservative measures are pursued, it is important to keep close follow-up; if there is deterioration or lack of improvement, surgery should be considered. Once the foot becomes rigid and degenerate, the surgical options are less satisfactory.

Surgical management

There is a limited role for debridement and tenosynovectomy in stage I disease. The majority of patients present in stage II, but there is a wide range of deformity in this group. The classic treatment is a reconstruction using the flexor digitorum longus tendon. If this is harvested proximal to the knot of Henry control of toe flexion is still possible via the flexor hallucis longus tendon. Experience has shown that this transfer needs to be protected with a medial slide calcaneal osteotomy; this corrects the heel and shifts the moment arm of the Achilles so that it becomes a medial force rather than a deforming force. Subtalar arthrosis in adults can be associated with lateral pain or extrusion and is mainly reserved for children (Fig. 126.5). Gastrocnemius and peroneus brevis tendon tightness are common and may require lengthening.

In more severe disease midfoot deformity may be present, either abduction of the midfoot or elevation of the first ray due to fixed supination of the forefoot. Lateral column lengthening through a calcaneal (Evans) osteotomy or via a calcaneocuboid fusion can correct the abduction and talonavicular uncovering. Elevation of the first ray may similarly be treated by either a plantarflexion cuneiform (Cotton) osteotomy or a medial fusion procedure. A lapidus procedure can be useful for symptomatic hallux valgus.

In stage III disease, the fixed nature of the deformity necessitates bony surgery. Moreover, it generally signifies advanced degeneration throughout the hindfoot, and therefore a triple fusion is recommended. This can be approached in a number of ways, but in the longstanding severely deformed foot there can be issues with skin closure and healing of a lateral wound and therefore a familiarity with an 'all medial approach' is important.

The talonavicular joint has 10% risk of non-union, although not all of these patients will require further surgery. In patients with longstanding triple arthrodeses, arthrosis of adjacent joints is commonly seen; again not all will be symptomatic.

Stage IV disease involves additional ankle degeneration. The treatment for this is a pantalar fusion or a tibiotalocalcaneal fusion.

KEY LEARNING POINTS

- Many severely deformed feet will remain totally trouble-free and require no treatment.
- The cavus foot is a high-arched foot that fails to flatten on weight bearing.
- Spinal pathology is particularly important for pes cavus; failure to look for this may be disastrous.
- Causes of pes cavus can be idiopathic, spinal, neuromuscular, central nervous system, peripheral nervous system, trauma, iatrogenic or congenital talipes equinovarus.
- Surgical management of pes cavus is directed at the cavus, varus, metatarsalgia, weakness of dorsiflexion, clawing of toes and arthritis.
- The aim of surgery is a pain-free, plantigrade, stable foot.
- Pes planus is common.
- Posterior tibial tendon dysfunction is the most common cause of acquired pes planus.
- The Johnson and Strom system, modified by Myerson, is useful in guiding management.
- Conservative management is good for flexible flat feet.
- The classic treatment of stage II is a reconstruction using the flexor digitorum longus tendon, midfoot deformity may require a lateral column lengthening, stage III disease requires bony surgery, and stage IV will require a fusion.

REFERENCES

- ● = Key primary paper
- ◆ = Major review article

●1. Mann RA, Hsu JD. Triple arthrodesis in the treatment of fixed cavovarus deformity in adolescent patients with Charcot-Marie-Tooth. *Foot and Ankle* 1992;**13**:1–6.

◆2. Holmes GB, Jr, Mann R. Possible epidemiological factors associated with rupture of the posterior tibial tendon. *Foot and Ankle* 1992;**13**:70–9.

●3. Myerson M, Solomon G, Shereff M. Posterior tibial tendon dysfunction: its association with seronegative inflammatory disease. *Foot and Ankle* 1989;**9**:219–25.

◆4. Johnson KA, Strom D. Tibialis posterior tendon dysfunction. *Clinical Orthopaedics and Related Research* 1989;**239**:196–206.

◆5. Myerson M. Adult acquired flatfoot deformity: treatment of dysfunction of the posterior tibial tendon. *Instructional Course Lectures* 1997;**46**:393–405.

●6. Bluman EM, Title CI, Myerson MS. Posterior tibial tendon rupture: a refined classification system. *Foot and Ankle Clinics* 2007;**12**:233–49.

The diabetic foot

AZIZ NATHER, FU CAI HAN

Introduction	1466	Surgical treatment	1469
Pathogenesis	1466	Predictive factors for limb salvage	1470
Classifications for diabetic foot	1467	Strategy for managing diabetic foot	1470
Assessment of a diabetic foot	1467	Acknowledgement	1470
Conservative treatment	1469	References	1471

NATIONAL BOARD STANDARDS

- Know about diabetic foot problems and the main complications
- Understand King's Classification
- Learn surgical treatment and the indications for distal or major amputation
- Learn about the team approach and effective clinical pathways
- Know the role of annual foot screening

INTRODUCTION

Diabetes mellitus is a very common disorder, and diabetic foot complications account for about 10% of all emergency admissions in orthopaedics, National University Hospital.[1] There is a need to develop a subspecialty for the diabetic foot. This is a neglected area, confounded by the fact that patients mainly belong to the lower socioeconomic group.

Need for a multidisciplinary team

The diabetic foot is best managed by a multidisciplinary team, involving an orthopaedic surgeon, endocrinologist, infectious disease consultant, podiatrist, and nurses specializing in wound care and foot care.[2] Nather[2] showed that, with a team approach, the average length of stay was reduced from 20.4 to 14 days, the average hospitalization cost per patient was reduced from US$5900 to US$5100, and the hospital readmission rate decreased from 13% to 7%.[2] Most importantly, the major amputation rate was reduced significantly from 31% to 20%. In addition to a team approach, an effective clinical pathway also needs to be implemented.

PATHOGENESIS

This consists of the diabetic triad that includes neuropathy, vasculopathy and immunopathy. The incidence of sensory neuropathy is 42.1% and the incidence of vasculopathy (based on an ankle brachial index <0.8, indicating ischaemia) is 54.2% in our series.[1]

Microbiology

Common bacteria include mainly Gram-positive cocci, e.g. *Staphylococcus aureus*, group B *Streptococcus pyogenes*, group A *Streptococcus agalactiae* and meticillin-resistant *Staphylococcus aureus*. Other infections include Gram-negative rods: *Proteus vulgaris*, *Escherichia coli* and *Pseudomonas aeruginosa*. Anaerobes are commonly present: *Bacteroides fragilis* and *Peptostreptococcus*.

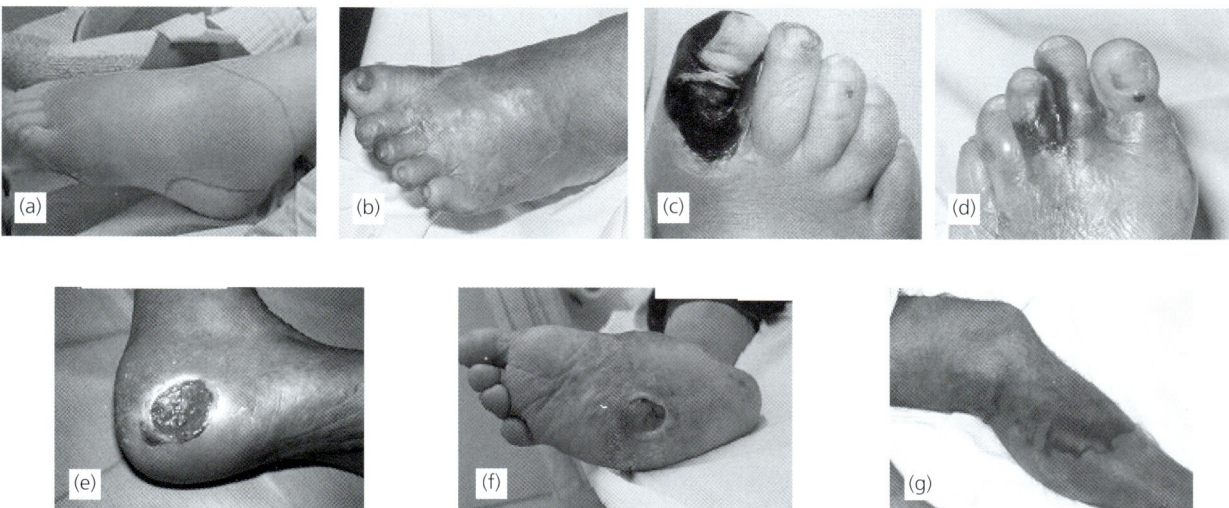

Figure 127.1 (a) Cellulitis; (b) abscess; (c) dry gangrene; (d) wet gangrene; (e) ulcer; (f) Charcot joint disease; (g) necrotizing fasciitis with classical haemorrhagic blisters.

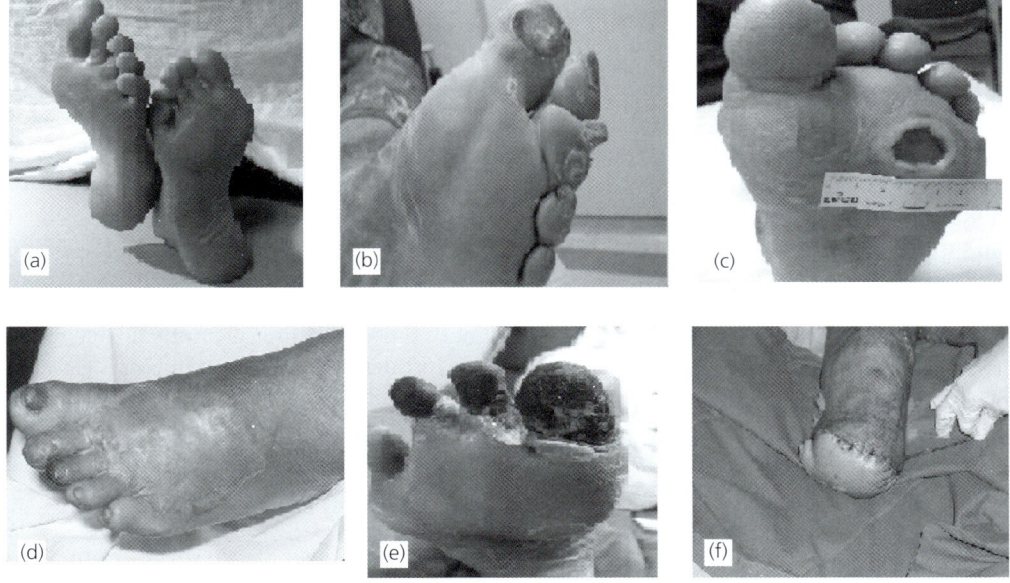

Figure 127.2 (a) The normal foot; (b) the high-risk foot; (c) the ulcerated foot; (d) the cellulitic foot; (e) the necrotic foot; (f) major amputation.

Modes of clinical presentation

Diabetic foot presents as cellulitis, abscess, osteomyelitis, septic arthritis, dry gangrene, wet gangrene, ulcers, Charcot joint disease and necrotizing fasciitis (Fig. 127.1).

CLASSIFICATIONS FOR DIABETIC FOOT

The King's College Foot Classification (Fig. 127.2) is the international classification now used.[3] It has superseded Wagner's Classification and the University of Texas Classification.

ASSESSMENT OF A DIABETIC FOOT

Patient profile

Patients are commonly in the fifth and sixth decades of life, mean age being 60. Males are equally affected as females.

Presenting complaint(s)

- *Pain.* Including the presence of rest pain and vascular claudication.

- *Ulcer.* Describe site, size, edge, floor and contents of the ulcer; a painful ulcer is usually due to infection or ischaemia, a non-painful ulcer is typically due to a neuropathic foot (Charcot joint disease).
- *Swelling.* Unilateral swelling indicates infection or Charcot joint disease. With an abscess, the swelling is fluctuant. In the case of septic arthritis, severe pain occurs with joint motion. Fever, chills and rigours may be present with abscess, osteomyelitis or septic arthritis. Such a systemic response is often absent in diabetic patients.
- *Joint deformity.* Clawing of the toes may be present due to motor neuropathy. Patients also have loss of the longitudinal arch and, in advanced cases, rocker bottom foot occurs in Charcot joint disease.
- *Gangrene.* Dry (not infected) or wet gangrene (with superimposed infection) may be present.
- *Neuropathy.* Motor neuropathy (weakness), sensory neuropathy (paraesthesia, glove and stocking distribution) and autonomic neuropathy may be present.

RELATED HISTORY

- Self-inflicted trauma, e.g. digging of nails.
- Foreign body penetration.
- Self-medication or use of traditional medication.
- Use of footwear: Nather[4] found that 70% of diabetics wear slippers or no footwear most of the time. Diabetic patients should be counselled to wear appropriate footwear at all times.
- Diabetes history: duration, type of diabetes, diabetic medications used and patients' compliance with medications. Diabetic patients should be monitoring their capillary blood glucose level regularly.
- Complications of diabetes: peripheral vascular disease, retinopathy, cataracts, nephropathy and neuropathy.
- Comorbidities: ischaemic heart disease, cerebrovascular accidents, hypertension and renal failure.
- Risk factors, e.g. smoking, hyperlipidaemia and hypertension.
- Family history, especially the patient's caregiver.

Physical examination

The authors recommend a systematic approach in examining the diabetic foot instead of the traditional look, feel and move approach for the examination of an orthopaedic problem. In examining a diabetic foot, inspection should be followed by examination for sensory neuropathy, examination for vasculopathy and examination for immunopathy. A general examination must be performed first, including vital signs and examination of heart, lungs and abdomen. The local examination is then performed wearing gloves.

Inspection

EXAMINATION FOR SENSORY NEUROPATHY

This is carried out using the pinprick test, Semmes Weinstein 5.07 gauge monofilament test[5] (Fig. 127.3), tendon reflex (ankle jerk), vibration sense (using a 128 Hz tuning fork placed over bony prominences – malleoli, tibial crest, tips of toes and using a biothesiometer), and position sense of toes (test proprioception).

EXAMINATION FOR VASCULOPATHY

This is then performed, including colour of skin, temperature of skin, capillary refill and palpation of pulses, including femoral, popliteal, dorsalis pedis and posterior tibial pulse (Fig. 127.4).

One could also perform the Buerger's test, when one or both pulses are clinically not palpable.

In Buerger's test, when the leg is elevated, at about 30°, the sole of the foot turns pale due to ischaemia in patients where one or both foot pulses are clinically not palpable.

EXAMINATION FOR IMMUNOPATHY

Palpate for deep tenderness in the foot to exclude osteomyelitis of the underlying bones, ray by ray from toes

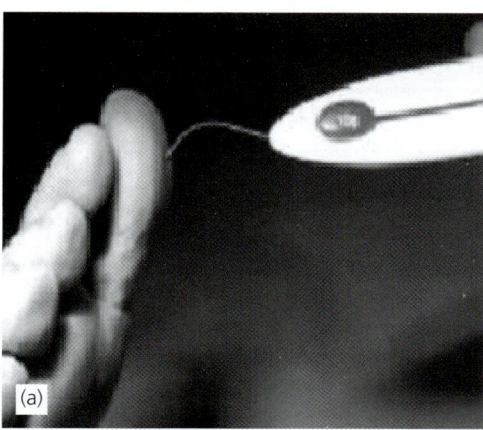
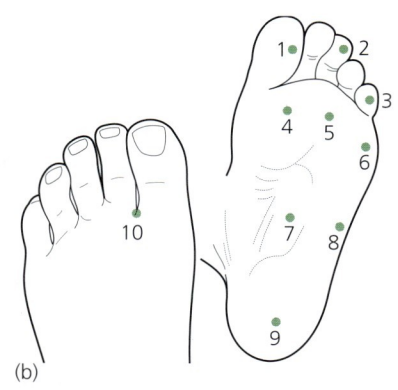

Figure 127.3 (a) Ten gram force applied until filament bends. (b) Ten sites for Semmes Weinstein Monofilament testing. Sensation present in seven or fewer sites equals loss of protective sensation.

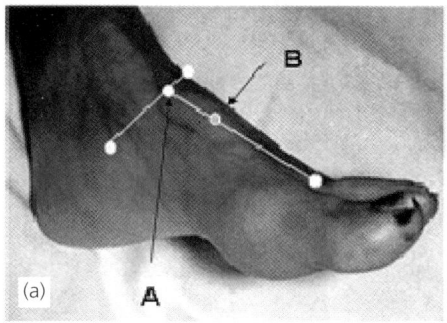 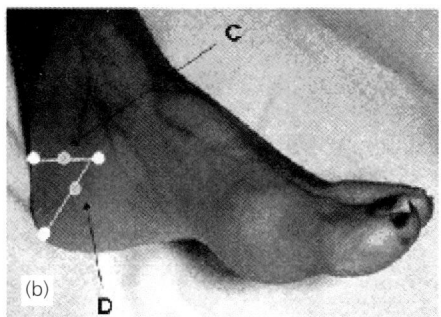

Figure 127.4 (a) A, mid-point of the line between the malleoli and, B, one-third down the line from A to the first interdigital cleft. (b) C, one-third posteriorly along the line between the medial malleolus and tendo-Achilles and, D, one-third down the line between the medial malleolus and the point of the heel.

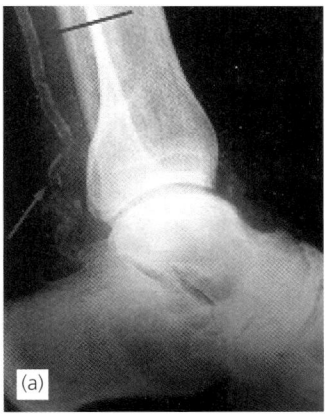 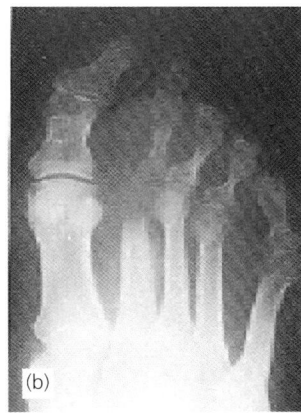 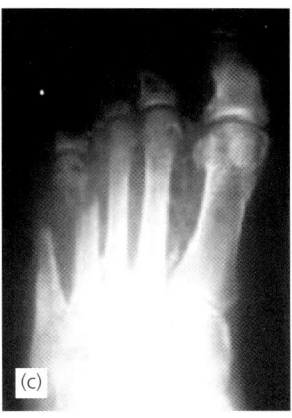

Figure 127.5 (a) Calcification of arteries; (b) septic arthritis of the second metatarsophalangeal joint; (c) gas in between the third and fourth rays and pathological fracture of the fourth metatarsal bone due to osteomyelitis.

to ankle, first in the dorsum and second in the sole of the foot. Move the interphalangeal joint and metatarsophalangeal joints to look for septic arthritis.

Investigations

Investigations performed include full blood count and markers of infection, erythrocyte sedimentation rate (ESR) and C-reactive protein (CRP). Other blood tests include urea and electrolytes; glycosylated haemoglobin (HbA1C); the capillary blood glucose test is performed four times daily, for marking on the diabetes chart. Wound swab culture and blood cultures (for aerobic and anaerobic culture) should be carried out in all cases, even in the absence of a spike of fever, as there is often no response in elderly or immunocompromised people. Broad-spectrum antibiotics are the treatment of choice for diabetic wound infections, as typically they are polymicrobial. Cultures should be taken before antibiotics are started as this will help detect resistant organisms and guide treatment.

Other investigations include electrocardiogram, chest radiographs, and radiographs of the foot or ankle. Findings include loss of soft-tissue planes; the presence of gas is an ominous sign that could indicate serious life-threatening infection (necrotizing fasciitis), osteomyelitis, septic arthritis, neuropathic changes of Charcot joint disease, and calcification of dorsalis pedis or posterior tibial arteries (Fig. 127.5).

CONSERVATIVE TREATMENT

Infection is treated with antibiotics once culture has been taken and ulcers are managed with daily dressings. Technology has advanced a great deal in the management of wounds. In addition to the use of simple gauze and tulle gras dressing, one can now use low-adherent, transparent film, hydrocolloid, hydrogel, alginate, foam, hydrofibre, antimicrobial and de-odourizer dressings.[6]

New-generation dressings[7] can be used for the treatment of diabetic wounding, e.g. Biatain Ag, SeaSorb Ag, Aquacel Ag, Hydrofibre, Carboflex odour control, Kaltostat, COPA, Ultra-soft foam and Safetec soft silicon E adhesive technology Vacuum-assisted closure therapy can be used for the management of large wounds.[8]

SURGICAL TREATMENT

Abscesses must be drained adequately as soon as possible. Wound debridement must be radically performed in order to save the foot from unnecessary amputation. Ultrasonic debridement can be used for selective cases.

Distal amputations can only be performed if foot pulses are palpable. The presence of both foot pulses indicates a good chance of success. One palpable pulse gives only a fair chance of success. Distal amputation (ray amputation) should not be performed when both pulses are not palpable. Non-invasive vascular examinations should be performed to aid in predicting healing potential. These include ankle brachial index (>0.5), absolute toe pressure (>45 mmHg) and transcutaneous partial pressure of oxygen ($TcPO_2$ >30 mmHg). Distal amputation should be avoided if non-invasive studies demonstrate poor vascularity. The patient's general nutritional status should also be evaluated as both an albumin level of at least 3 g dL^{-1} and a total lymphocyte count of greater than 1500 μL^{-1} have been associated with increased healing potential.

Distal amputations include ray amputation, transmetatarsal amputation and Syme's amputation. No prosthesis is required. Special shoes can be fitted.

Major amputations include below-knee amputation (BKA), through-knee amputation and above-knee amputation (AKA).

Indications include infection extending up to the ankle; severe, ischaemic/gangrene involving the whole foot; ankle brachial index <0.5; the presence of rest pain in the foot; and gangrene involving the heel.

Prosthesis is required for BKA and AKA. A special rehabilitation programme must be provided.

Amputations at the transmetatarsal level and distal level provide for the lowest energy expenditure. The next lowest level of energy expenditure is a Syme's amputation. Energy expenditure for a BKA fitted with a prosthesis is at least 1.5 times the normal energy used for walking.

PREDICTIVE FACTORS FOR LIMB SALVAGE

The most dreaded complication of diabetic foot is major amputation of the lower limb. This has serious emotional and psychological problems, and significant morbidity and mortality. The risk of mortality is about 10% intra-operatively and increases to 30% within 1 year, 50% within 3 years and 70% within 5 years.[9]

Nather et al.[1] found predictive factors for limb salvage to be age above 60 years, stroke and ischaemic heart disease, nephropathy, peripheral vascular diseases, sensory neuropathy, HbA1C level >7%, ankle brachial index <0.8 and the presence of gangrene.

STRATEGY FOR MANAGING DIABETIC FOOT

The strategy is prevention and early intervention with prevent the development of complications.[10] Early detection of risk factors – the triad of neuropathy, vasculopathy and immunopathy – is a key component in the overall management of diabetic foot disorders and amputation prevention programmes.[10]

All diabetic subjects are advised to comply with certain guidelines, which include dietary restriction, an exercise regimen, quarterly measurement of HbA1c levels, regular capillary blood glucose monitoring, yearly measurement of creatinine level and yearly foot, renal and eye screening (Singapore's Ministry of Health Guidelines).[11]

Annual foot screening detects the foot at 'high risk' early, so that appropriate measures can be taken to prevent development of diabetic foot complications. Several co-workers have shown annual foot screening to have reduced the amputation rate.[12]

Care of a diabetic foot must be directed at the community level by public education programmes and foot-screening programmes. The use of proper footwear is potentially important.[4]

In Singapore, annual foot screening is performed by nurses trained in podiatric screening. The National University Hospital runs annual training courses.[12] This programme has been found to be successful and has attracted participation from nurses in neighbouring countries, including Indonesia, Malaysia and Hong Kong. Three courses have been run annually and 60 nurses have been trained.

> ### KEY LEARNING POINTS
>
> - Diabetic foot complications are due to a triad of neuropathy, vasculopathy and immunopathy.
> - King's Classification is used.
> - Careful assessment is required, including inspection, assessment for neuropathy, vasculopathy and immunopathy.
> - Aggressive drainage or wound debridement is needed to save the limb.
> - Distal amputation can be performed if one or both foot pulses are palpable, when the ankle brachial index/toe brachial index is more than 0.5.
> - Major amputation is needed if both pulses are not palpable, when the ankle brachial index/toe brachial index is less than 0.5.
> - Team approach and effective clinical pathway reduces major amputation rate.
> - Annual foot screening prevents foot complications, thereby reducing limb loss.

ACKNOWLEDGEMENT

The authors would like to thank the NUH Multi-Disciplinary Team for Diabetic Foot Problems for all the support in the management of patients with diabetic foot.

REFERENCES

◆ = Major review article
● = Key primary paper

◆1. Nather A, Chionh SB, Chan YH, et al. Epidemiology of diabetic foot problems and predictive factors for limb loss. *Journal of Diabetes Complications* 2008;**22**:77-82.
●2. Nather A. Team approach for diabetic foot problems – The Singapore experience. In: Nather A (ed.) *Diabetic Foot Problems*. Singapore: World Scientific, 2008:29-40.
◆3. Edmonds ME, Foster AVM. *Managing the Diabetic Foot*, 2nd edn. London, UK: Blackwell, 2005.
◆4. Nather A, Singh E. Diabetic footwear: Current status and future directions. In: Nather A (ed.) *Diabetic Foot Problems*. Singapore: World Scientific, 2008:527-39.
●5. Sosenko JM, Kato M, Sato R, Bild DE. Comparison of quantitative survey threshold measures for their associates with foot ulceration in diabetic patients. *Diabetes Care* 1990;**13**:1057-61.
●6. Tsao T, Nather A. Types of dressings for diabetic foot ulcers. In: Nather A (ed.) *Diabetic Foot Problems*. Singapore: World Scientific, 2008:403-15.
7. Nather A, Tsao T. New generation dressings for diabetic wounds. In: Nather A (ed.) *Diabetic Foot Problems*. Singapore: World Scientific, 2008:417-44.
◆8. Peng YP. Vacuum assisted closure in the treatment of diabetic foot ulcers. In: Nather A (ed.) *Diabetic Foot Problems*. Singapore: World Scientific, 2008:485-501.
◆9. Bakker K, Foster A, Van Houtum W, Riley P. *Diabetes and Foot Care: Time to Act*. Brussels, Belgium: Internal Diabetes Federation, 2005:34.
◆10. Frykberg RG. Diabetic foot ulcer: current concepts. *Journal of Foot and Ankle Surgery* 1998;**37**:440-6.
◆11. Singapore Ministry of Health. *Clinical Practice Guidelines for Managing Diabetes Mellitus*. Singapore: Ministry of Health, 2006.
●12. Nather A, Cheng JCC, Devi GP et al. Foot screening for diabetics. In: Nather A (ed.) *Diabetic Foot Problems*. Singapore: World Scientific, 2008:169-77.

Neurological disorders

NORMAN ESPINOSA

CONGENITAL NEUROLOGICAL DISORDERS	1472	Stroke (cerebrovascular accident)	1477
Introduction	1472	Traumatic brain injury	1478
Charcot–Marie–Tooth disease	1472	Spinal cord injury	1479
Myelomeningocele (spina bifida)	1474	Peripheral nerve injury	1479
Cerebral palsy	1475	Postpoliomyelitis syndrome	1480
Duchenne's muscular dystrophy	1477	Parkinson's disease	1481
ACQUIRED NEUROLOGICAL DISORDERS	1477	Summary	1481
Introduction	1477	References	1482

NATIONAL BOARD STANDARDS

- Be aware of the complex presentation of neurological and nerve disorders
- Learn a thorough anatomical and pathophysiological knowledge as the basis for the correct diagnosis and treatment
- Know that clinical examination surpasses the power of conventional radiography
- Understand that non-operative treatment is acceptable prior to surgery
- The surgeon needs to know that surgical results are not as good as other orthopaedic interventions
- Understand to provide proper information and education to the patients

CONGENITAL NEUROLOGICAL DISORDERS

INTRODUCTION

The current chapter reviews the different forms of congenital and acquired neurological disorders and nerve disorders respectively. It is fundamental to understand the mechanisms of lesions in order to apply any type of treatment. Selection of treatment is based on clinical findings and additive diagnostic examinations and should improve function.

CHARCOT–MARIE–TOOTH DISEASE

Introduction

Charcot–Marie–Tooth (CMT) disease is an inherited progressive peripheral neuropathy. CMT is referred to as hereditary motor–sensory neuropathies (HMSNs).[1]

Pathogenesis

Type I HMSN is the most common presentation of CMT disease (75%). Although not definitively clear it is thought to result from myelination abnormalities. It is autosomal dominantly inherited and occurs as a familial disorder. The nerve conduction velocities are dramatically slow. Specific genetic sequences are associated with a subset of type I patients. The majority of type I presentations are linked to chromosome 17 and designated CMT-1A.[2] CMT disease affects the longest nerves to the smallest muscles first. Thus the symptomatic presentation of feet before hands. Type II HMSN (axonal form) has a similar presentation but is less pronounced and appears later in life. Nerve conduction velocities are rarely slow and, if so, only mildly.

Presentation and diagnosis

Patients suffering from CMT usually start to present the typical clinical signs in their second decade of life. Although

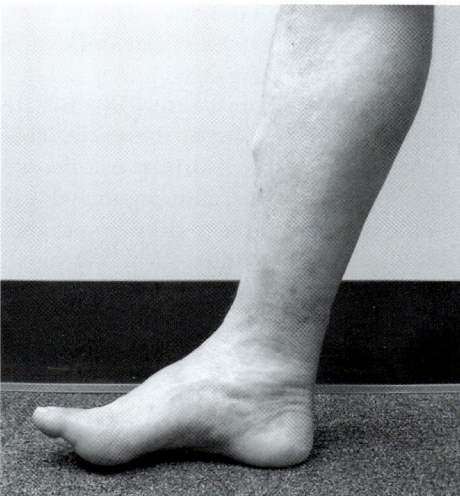

Figure 128.1 Clinical photograph of a patient with longstanding Charcot–Marie–Tooth disease with the characteristic cavus foot. Note the plantarflexed first ray and high arch.

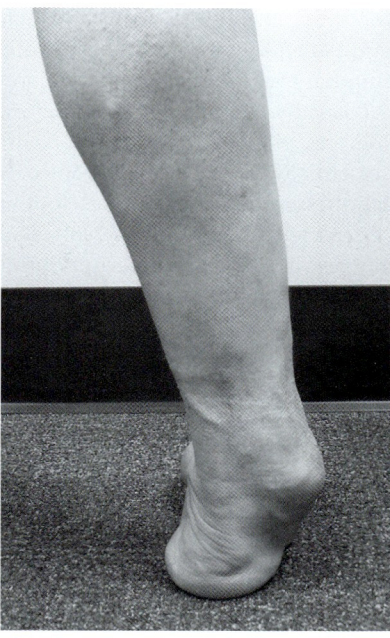

Figure 128.2 Clinical photograph demonstrating severe hindfoot varus in a patient with long-standing Charcot–Marie–Tooth. In such severe cases careful attention must be paid to the lateral collateral ligaments which will require reconstruction in addition to correction of the bony deformity.

it is a familial inherited disorder, it shows a great disparity in the amount of disability and presentation among family members. Involvement progresses from distal to proximal.[2]

Motor abnormalities include[3] cavus feet (Fig. 128.1), often bilateral (up to two-thirds of patients); weakness of the anterior tibial and peroneus brevis muscles (most common early presentation); the first ray is plantarflexed due to peroneus longus hyperactivity, creating a relative forefoot valgus; hindfoot varus results to compensate for the forefoot valgus; unopposed pull of the posterior tibial muscle against the weakened peroneus brevis aggravates hindfoot varus (Fig. 128.2); intrinsic minus deformity at the metatarsophalangeal (MTP) and interphalangeal (IP) joints; the clinician sees the clinical presentation of hindfoot varus, midfoot cavus to forefoot valgus, to clawing of the toes (increased by the pull of the extensor hallucis longus muscle and extensor digitorum muscle); progressive weakness in the upper extremities (delayed onset compared with the foot findings); metatarsalgia, claw toes, tarsal prominence and recurrent ankle sprains. Besides these findings, dysplastic hips (5%) and scoliosis (10%) also are found.

Sensory alterations include[1] primarily loss of proprioceptive and vibratory sense. However, sensory presentations vary.

A thorough neurological evaluation is mandatory to establish diagnosis and to plan surgery.[4] The examination first encompasses testing the weakness of the anterior tibial and peroneus brevis muscles and then examining all extrinsic motor muscles around the foot and ankle. The sensory impairment appears later and is usually not as severe; however, up to 25% of patients do have significant sensory impairment. Vibration, two-point discrimination and proprioception are affected first and should be evaluated. When the patient ambulates, careful observation reveals a combination of dorsiflexion weakness, fixed equinus and difficulties with proprioception. These findings give the characteristic steppage gait. The examiner should focus on relative hindfoot varus and atrophy of the medial longitudinal arch, as well as tarsal bossing and some degree of toe clawing. CMT causes significant muscle atrophy below the knee. The primary deformity of the forefoot is a depressed first ray, but over time the second and third rays may be similarly depressed in relation to the lateral border of the foot. In longstanding deformity, limited dorsiflexion is present because of an abutment of the talar neck against the anterior tibia. The classic test described by Coleman and Chestnut is useful to identify the flexibility of the hindfoot.[5]

A series of weight-bearing radiographs should be taken of both feet and the ankles. Finally, because CMT is a sensory neuropathy, these images are useful in the evaluation of possible Charcot's changes in the foot and ankle. CT scans can be helpful to evaluate the extent of deformities and in order to plan surgical correction.

Management

CONSERVATIVE TREATMENT

In the early phase of disease (in children), observation at regular intervals might be enough. Physical therapy plays a minor role, but occasionally in a young child range of motion can be improved. Orthotic management and shoe modifications are important. The main goals are proper positioning of the hind- and forefoot, and to compensate for a degree of footdrop. Orthotics require total agreement of the parents and patients as well. However, those measures are only of temporary value because of the progressive character of the neuropathy and corresponding deformity.[6–8]

Orthotic devices play an important role in the adult patient who essentially has a paralysed foot or significant footdrop. Orthotics protect the insensate foot and reduce some of the energy expenditure of the so-called steppage gait. They may prevent or delay deformity but cannot be used to correct the deformity.[9]

SURGICAL TREATMENT

Decision-making for surgical treatment in these patients can be complex. The patient's goals, expectations and demands should be taken into consideration. A foot may become so deformed (severe hindfoot varus or midfoot equinus) that the rationale for surgery comes down to correcting the deformity so that orthotics can be used.

Motor status around the foot and ankle, reducibility of the deformity and degree of sensory impairment dictate the type surgery. When surgical treatment is warranted then the following procedures can be carried out: plantar fascia release (seldom performed alone); calcaneal slide osteotomy (to correct varus deformity); dorsiflexion metatarsal osteotomy (to compensate for fixed plantarflexed first metatarsal); transfer of the peroneus longus to the brevis (to oppose adduction by the posterior tibial tendon or to aid in dorsiflexion of the foot and to reduce overactivity of the peroneus longus muscle); modified Jones procedure (correction of clawing of the great toe with transfer of the extensor hallucis longus (EHL) tendon); posterior tibial tendon transfer; midfoot osteotomies (in addition to the above-mentioned measures) (Fig. 128.3). Triple arthrodesis should be used only as a salvage procedure for a completely rigid deformity that shows signs of degenerative joint disease of the transverse tarsal joints and the rest of the hindfoot. The surgeon must ensure that no lateral ligamentous instability is present at the ankle. The key to successful correction of the deformity is a derotation of the calcaneus under the talus, allowing the talus to plantar flex and the hindfoot varus to drop into slight valgus. Ankle instability must be addressed by means of a peroneus longus to brevis transfer or, if possible, by anatomic reconstruction.[8,10–12]

MYELOMENINGOCELE (SPINA BIFIDA)

Introduction

Myelomeningocele is defined as a congenital malformation of the central nervous system (CNS) resulting in dysplasia of the vertebral elements as well as the spinal cord. The defect is present at birth but may not be detected until later. Males and females are equally affected.[13]

Incidence

Spina bifida occulta occurs in 2–3% of the population. In the USA the overall incidence of neural tube defects is about 1 per 1000.

Classification

Classification follows the level of involvement: thoracic, upper lumbar, lower lumbar and sacral. By definition the thoracic and upper lumbar patients are paralysed below the knee but might have involuntary motors affecting foot position. The pattern of sensory and motor loss is rarely symmetric.

Pathogenesis

As a disorder of the CNS, involvement of both lower motor neurons (flaccid paralysis and lack of sensation) and upper motor neurons (spasticity) must be considered. Growth can also change the basic neurological picture because of tethering of the cord from soft-tissue scars or bony anomalies within the vertebral column.[14]

Presentation

There is a wide range of deformities, beginning with congenital presentations to modelling changes in the growing foot and fixed conditions in the skeletally mature patient.

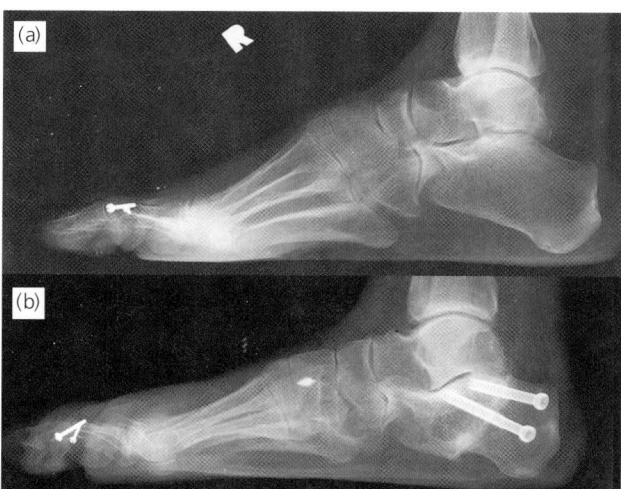

Figure 128.3 Lateral pre-operative (a) and postoperative (b) weight-bearing radiographs of a patient who underwent a reconstruction of a cavus foot with a lateral closing wedge calcaneal osteotomy and posterior tibial tendon transfer to the midfoot. Note the improvement in the lateral talometatarsal angle.

Management

The primary goal in treatment of these foot deformities focuses on a plantigrade foot. Because of the wide variations of paralytic and sensory deficit and variable functional capacity, treatment becomes complex. An important long-term prognostic factor is foot sensibility. Most of the children have an insensate foot and loss of proprioception unless they are suffering from the lowest lumbar or sacral level involvement. Deformity might result in increased focal pressures and lead to ulcerations. Patient and parent education is essential. Orthotics as a protective measure for the insensate foot and a preventive measure against the deforming forces (to balance the foot) should be applied. It is recommended that these children avoid walking barefoot and they must have some form of protective footwear. Generally, it is not recommended to fuse the joints in these patients, because rigidity of the foot and ankle reduces the ability of the foot to accommodate irregularities of the ground and increases the risk for ulcerations. Additionally, it poses a risk for Charcot's neuroarthropathy. Triple arthrodesis is an excellent procedure for patients with remaining sensation. In the older or non-ambulatory patient who has problems with fitting shoes or braces, however, it is a good compromise to obtain a plantigrade foot even if it is insensate. In the case of a non-healing ulcer or for protection of soft tissues after surgical correction total-contact casting can be considered. However, the cast must be checked at weekly intervals to prevent skin break down. Casts to correct deformity are prohibited. Surgery must be performed in a latex-free environment.

Up to one-half of children with myelomeningocele have some type of significant foot deformity. The most common congenital foot deformities associated with myelomeningocele are talipes equinovarus (clubfoot); vertical talus; calcaneus and equinus of the hindfoot with components of valgus or varus. In case of surgical correction, each of these deformities must be addressed.[14–16]

CEREBRAL PALSY

Introduction

Cerebral palsy is defined as a static encephalopathy that most frequently results from a cerebral injury in the perinatal period. It presents with a wide range of functional disabilities, starting with the totally involved, non-ambulatory patients to the less involved, spastic diplegic and hemiplegic patients. Spasticity is the primary problem in these patients, and acts as the main deforming force. Patients present with poor balance that impairs normal ambulation. In general, if these children have not begun ambulating by age 6, they will not develop the ability later in life.[17]

Incidence

This disorder affects 1–2% of all children.[18]

Aetiology

Known causes for cerebral palsy include a prenatal brain dysplasia, a maternal infection, fetal hypoxia (especially perinatal), a vascular event, encephalitis, trauma and kernicterus.[5,19]

Classification

Classification is based on both anatomic (hemiplegic: ipsilateral arm and leg; diplegic: both legs; totally involved) and physiological types (spastic, athetoid, mixed and dystonic).[20]

Management

GENERAL CONSIDERATIONS

It is important to evaluate the entire child when planning the appropriate treatment. All surgical procedures have to be carried out during childhood before skeletal maturity is reached. Thus, the highest functional ability is achieved with minimal external bracing. Contractures should be prevented, which could lead to abnormal modelling of the foot and ankle. A plantigrade foot provides a broad base of pressure and contact with the footrest of the wheelchair and footwear. The surgeon should make sure that the functional goals and needs of the patient are met.

Physical therapy might maintain or prolong range of motion. Gait training may be necessary. Two basic types of foot and ankle deformities are seen in the cerebral palsy population. The varus or equinovarus deformity is noted most often in the hemiplegic patient, whereas the equinovalgus deformity is seen more often in the spastic diplegic patient.

TREATMENT OF EQUINUS DEFORMITY

General aspects

The examiner must differentiate between increased tone and fixed contracture. Additionally, distinction between the components of the triceps surae musculature is mandatory. The gastrocnemius heads originate proximal to the knee joint while the soleus originates on the proximal posterior tibia. Silferskjöld's test is performed to differentiate between gastrocnemius-only and gastrocnemius–soleus contracture.[21]

Conservative treatment

Physical therapy is a very important treatment and is more effective in the case of a supple foot. In the younger child with a very mild equinus, it may be managed with continuous therapy, a night-time dorsiflexion splint, and a submalleolar orthosis or an ankle–foot orthosis (AFO). In a child with minimal fixed contracture, physical therapy, night-time splinting and a daytime orthosis can be applied. With older age and increased fixed contractures those measures are not effective enough. Serial casting must be taken into consideration (usually less than 6 weeks). However, recurrence must be expected. The older child who has developed significant pronation is very difficult to treat by serial casting alone.[22–24]

During recent years, botulinum type A toxin has gained increasing popularity in the treatment of spasticity. Botulinum type A toxin blocks transmission at the neuromuscular junction. It is useful particularly in the hamstring musculature combined with physical therapy (including stretching of the contracted muscles and strengthening of the antagonists). The peak effect is usually seen 2 weeks after injection, and it may last 3–6 months.[25]

Surgical treatment

The major issue in surgical decision-making for the patient with cerebral palsy is to perform all the procedures aimed at functional goals at the same time. Surgery includes recession of the gastrocnemius aponeurosis or percutaneous Achilles tendon lengthening (in case of soleus contracture).[23,26–29]

TREATMENT OF EQUINOVARUS DEFORMITY

General considerations

The most common deforming force in a hemiplegic patient with a spastic equinovarus deformity is the posterior tibial muscle. The flexibility of the entire foot must be assessed to choose adequate treatment. Ideally, any fixed deformity must be corrected before the transfer, although these can be all carried out at the same time.

Surgical treatment

For a younger child with a flexible deformity (i.e. the foot reaches neutral position or pronates slightly), a split transfer of the posterior tibial tendon may be indicated. Results with the complete transfer of the tendon have been inconsistent, and therefore this is not advised. In the patient whose foot cannot be brought out of supination, the surgeon must consider a medial release, often with lengthening of the posterior tibial tendon at the navicular and transfer of the split portion to the peroneus brevis tendon. In general, the equinus position must be corrected first, followed by addressing the rest of the deformities. Calcaneal slide osteotomies help to correct a fixed varus deformity. Closing wedge osteotomies of the cuboid and opening wedge osteotomy of the medial cuneiform can be used to correct an adductus deformity. In the rare case of an adult patient suffering from extremely severe deformity and a rigid hindfoot, a subtalar joint or triple arthrodesis may be considered.

TREATMENT OF EQUINOVALGUS DEFORMITY

General aspects

This kind of deformity is mainly seen in patients with spastic diplegia. There is a combination of spasticity of the triceps surae and the peroneal muscles, which results in an altered growth and remodelling of the foot into a spastic flat foot. The proximal, angular and rotational alignment at the hips and knees must be examined.

Conservative treatment

In the presence of mild tightness of the Achilles tendon and the peroneals (as seen in the early stage), physical therapy with stretching exercises and orthotics and night-time splints might be enough to control deformity. In the older child who is beginning to have difficulty maintaining the position and to develop irritation from the orthosis, serial casting or botulinum A toxin injections may be used.

Surgical treatment

Once a cerebral palsy patient is not able to wear the orthotics surgery becomes necessary. The common stabilizing procedure for the hindfoot valgus is subtalar fusion. If a graft is required, a good source of cancellous bone (e.g. iliac crest, calcaneal tuberosity) should be used. An important aspect during surgery is to rotate the calcaneus medially underneath the talus to obtain a more physiological hindfoot position. In the presence of severe deformity with arthritic changes in both the subtalar and the transverse tarsal articulations, triple arthrodesis may be indicated in the ambulatory patient.

Although not intended for use in patients with neurological disease the Evans procedure has proved its efficacy in treating the spastic flat foot. Depending on the stage of flexibility, it might be enough to combine the Evans procedure with tendon lengthening procedures alone. With advanced skeletal maturity, permanent collapse of the longitudinal arch combined with forefoot varus often results in subluxation, dorsal angulation and instability of the naviculocuneiform joint. Thus additional stabilizing procedures (e.g. Miller procedure) must be performed, again followed by Achilles tendon lengthening and possibly peroneus brevis lengthening.

These lateral and medial column procedures require a structural bone graft. The literature has established the efficacy of allograft for the Evans procedure. Personally, I think that the autologous iliac crest graft surpasses the quality of allograft bone and should almost always be chosen, although it may have a higher morbidity. Besides the Evans procedure, calcaneocuboid distraction arthrodesis, the Miller procedure (plantarflexion arthrodesis of navicular–medial cuneiform articulation), can be carried out.

DUCHENNE'S MUSCULAR DYSTROPHY

Introduction

Duchenne's muscular dystrophy is a sex-linked disorder transmitted as a recessive trait. The disease is non-inflammatory and has its clinical onset usually between the third and sixth years of life. The life expectancy of these patients is limited because of pulmonary complications, and most of them die between 20 and 30 years of age.[9,30–33]

Incidence

Duchenne's muscular dystrophy occurs in 1 in 3500 live male births.

Presentation

Although the skeletal musculature is affected, the child might have slight developmental delay. Additionally, the child might be a toe walker, or might have difficulty running and jumping. Pseudohypertrophy of the calf muscles is a pathognomonic finding.

Management

CONSERVATIVE TREATMENT

Primary treatment consists of physical therapy: aggressive range of motion exercises to try to prevent contractures, and strength training through resistance exercises are carried out. Serial casting is performed in order to correct possible equinus deformity at the ankle or flexion deformity at the knee. A night-time orthosis should follow casting to prevent recurrence. A below-knee AFO should be used as soon as the child's ambulation becomes increasingly unstable. As weakness and instability progress, use of a knee–ankle–foot orthosis (KAFO) and usually a walker must be instituted. However, with progression of the disease, patients usually become wheelchair-bound by 10–13 years. The anterior tibial and peroneus brevis muscles are weakened early in the course of the disease, and because of unopposed posterior tibial muscle function, equinus contractures occur at the ankle first, followed by equinovarus contractures. As non-ambulatory wheelchair-bound patients still require plantigrade feet, tenotomies or transfers to correct the equinus and the equinovarus deformities may be needed. However, orthotics maintain foot position after surgery.

SURGICAL TREATMENT

The timing of surgery is crucial. It should be performed before the child becomes non-ambulatory. In general, all lower extremity deformities should be corrected at the same time to allow effective orthotic management postoperatively, followed by immediate weight bearing and ambulation. Surgery includes tendon lengthening and transfers as well as corrective osteotomies and fusions.

ACQUIRED NEUROLOGICAL DISORDERS

INTRODUCTION

Acquired neurological disorders primarily involve the CNS. Cerebrovascular accident (stroke), traumatic brain injury and spinal cord injury are the main causes for this condition. In general, patients present with spasticity, which should be treated properly. These three aetiologies are treated similarly and differ primarily in age of occurrence and variable neurological recovery time. The main goal in treating these patients lies in establishing as much function as possible.

STROKE (CEREBROVASCULAR ACCIDENT)

Incidence

Stroke is the primary cause of adult hemiplegia. It is the third leading cause of death in the USA. The average life expectancy after the initial event is expected to last longer than 5 years. Among patients who have sustained a stroke, many have significant foot and ankle deformity that requires orthopaedic intervention.

Pathophysiology

Injury of the CNS leads to disruption of the upper motor neuron inhibitory pathways. By so doing muscle spasticity is the result, which is characterized by a pathological increase in muscle tone and hyperactive reflexes. The range of motion of the joints is reduced, followed by fixed positioning of the limbs. Contracture may be avoided with appropriate management of the spasticity in the post-injury period. Of course, patterns of spasticity are specifically related to the anatomic region affected. Stroke most often involves the middle cerebral artery. This results in a hemiplegic picture with greater spasticity in the upper extremities and face. When affecting an anterior cerebral artery, lower extremity involvement is more likely. The initial spasticity can improve over time and is characteristic of the cause of the upper motor neuron lesion. In the stroke patient, this improvement can occur over a 6 month period.

Presentation and diagnosis

The initial and acute flaccid paralysis of the extremities gradually changes into increased muscle tone over the first 48 hours, which then ends in spasticity, typically involving the hip adductors, knee extensors and ankle plantarflexors. Another concern considers the ability to move the limb voluntarily and coordinate synergistic patterns of motion properly. Sensory deficiencies are important symptoms in this patient population.

Examination includes thorough motor assessment (strength, phase activity of motor groups, presence or absence of clonus and normal reflexes). Stability during the stance phase, balance reactions and voluntary hip flexion are important prerequisites for ambulation. Spasticity leading to contracture can involve all soft tissues from the joint capsule, including tendons, ligaments, neurovascular structures and even the skin. Longstanding immobilization results in degeneration of the cartilage and arthrofibrosis. Conventional radiography might reveal degeneration of the joints and MRI could be helpful in assessing fatty infiltration of the musculature (as this may preclude any possibility of ambulation).

Management

CONSERVATIVE TREATMENT

Non-operative measures are almost always the first step in treating patients suffering from stroke. The treatment modalities used include intensive physical therapy; serial casting and splinting are recommended.

In addition to physical therapy, casting and splinting, other treatment strategies have become important. Lidocaine and phenol blocks have been widely used to block the tibial nerve for varying periods of relief. As seen for cerebral palsy patients botulinum type A toxin injections have recently been used to provide temporary relief from spasticity.

Equinovarus is a frequently found deformity in patients with spastic diplegia and manifests as a spastic varus deformity of the hindfoot and forefoot. Besides this, equinus deformity at the ankle and midfoot might be present and toe flexion as well. The deforming force is the anterior tibial muscle while the posterior tibial muscle remains silent. The varus of the mid- and hindfoot is the result of exaggerated supination. In conjunction with contracture of the triceps musculature, equinus posture of the foot is the result. Spasticity in the flexor hallucis longus, flexor digitorum longus and intrinsic musculature of the foot can be found, causing toe flexion deformities and contributing further to the equinus posture of the foot and the ankle. If only mild deformity and spasticity are found AFOs could be helpful in redressing the foot and ankle. Strong inversion secondary to dynamic overpull or contracture of the anterior tibial muscle is often not braceable. Thus surgery must be considered to make the foot and ankle braceable. To correct equinus and varus a split anterior tibial tendon transfer is recommended.

In the presence of a triceps surae contraction, percutaneous Achilles tendon lengthening can be performed. However, in cases of scarring from a previous procedure or when severe contracture is present, an open Z-plasty with complete posterior release is the better approach to this problem.

Procedures to correct claw toes include lengthening of the extrinsic toe flexors behind the medial malleolus at the midfoot and combined intrinsic and extrinsic procedures at the level of the toes. The latter seems to be easier and efficacious for preventing late recurrence. Flexor tenotomy and resection arthroplasties of the proximal interphalangeal joints should be considered.

Although not as frequent as other deformities, spastic flat foot can occur. Patients often are predisposed to pes planus, and contracture of the triceps surae and peroneal muscles enhance the deformity. Mild to moderate deformities usually respond very well to Achilles tendon and peroneus brevis tendon (only seldom peroneus longus) lengthening. Posterior tibial tendon insufficiency needs to be addressed by performance, either lateral column lengthenings, subtalar arthrodesis or triple arthrodesis, depending on the extent of deformity and degree of arthrosis.

TRAUMATIC BRAIN INJURY

Incidence

Traumatic brain injury typically affects a younger segment of the adult population. Most of them sustain a motor vehicle accident. In general, patients often have significant foot and ankle deformities that need to be treated.

Aetiology

Motor vehicle accidents are the main reason for traumatic brain injury. Gunshot wounds and suicide attempts can also be identified.

Pathophysiology

Direct brain lesion or ischaemia result in injury of the neural structure of the brain (macro- and microscopically). Depending on the extent of ischaemia the brain damage may be relatively focal or global. The patient who sustains a neurological injury to the lateral cortex appears much the same as the patient with hemiplegia secondary to a stroke. The issues of cognitive impairment, motor function and sensibility require the same thorough evaluation. The recovery period usually lasts longer than that for stroke or spinal cord injury patients. Improvements may be noted 2–4 years after the initial event.

Management

The longer recovery period prolongs the phase of mobilization and prevention of contractures and usually requires an evolution of orthotic management.

The longer recovery period requires surgery to be delayed longer than in the stroke patient. As reported for stroke patients phenol nerve blocks and botulinum type A toxin muscle injections can be useful. The equinovarus foot deformities are treated similar to those in stroke patients.

SPINAL CORD INJURY

Incidence

Men between 30 and 40 years of age are the most affected individuals. Approximately 30% of all patients with polytrauma are diagnosed to have a spinal cord injury.

Aetiology

As for traumatic brain injuries, motor vehicle accidents are the main reason. A high incidence of polytrauma occurs among these patients. As the whole body may be injured, rehabilitation and reconstruction are complicated and delayed. Frequently traumatic brain injury and spinal cord injury often occur together. Early and aggressive medical and surgical treatment of both the spinal cord injury and the concomitant musculoskeletal injuries significantly improves the potential rehabilitation for many of these patients.

Management and its aspects

The factors that differentiate spinal cord injury from other upper motor neuron lesions are age, concomitant musculoskeletal injuries and a lower motor neuron component. Cognitive impairment is found in the presence of traumatic brain injury. Patients with spinal cord injuries who receive methylprednisolone within 3 hours and are maintained for 24 hours have significant improvement of motor function. In addition, those who are given methylprednisolone within 3–8 hours and continued for 48 hours show similar findings.

The degree of cognitive skills and residual motor function are the most important factors that determine outcome. The recovery of spasticity in the incomplete lesion may require a year. The patient might still be left with complete motor and sensory loss in a pattern characteristic of spinal cord injury.

PERIPHERAL NERVE INJURY

General

Regarding the foot and ankle, injuries of the sciatic, peroneal and posterior tibial nerves have the greatest relevance.

Aetiology

The common peroneal nerve and its branches are most at risk for injury in the lower extremity. At the level of the fibular head, the nerve is very superficial to the skin. The mechanism is either a direct blow (resulting in fracture) or a laceration, whereas injury to the deep peroneal nerve usually results from a penetrating injury. Compression injuries, the most common type of injury, usually resolve spontaneously. Injuries to the common peroneal nerve at the level of the fibular head and to the deep peroneal nerve both cause a drop foot during swing phase because of loss of anterior tibial function. Tibial fractures represent the most common injury to the tibial nerve in the leg.

Besides other high-impact accidents, sciatic nerve injuries are usually the result of gunshot wounds to the upper thigh (especially in the USA). Other reasons for sciatic nerve lesions are posterior dislocation of the hip, an intramuscular injection or an iatrogenic injury during a reconstructive surgical procedure.

Pathology

Neurotmesis (complete disruption of the nerve) has no potential for regeneration unless the endoneurium and axon are reapproximated. Injuries to the nerve where the endoneurial structure remains intact (neuropraxia) or without continuity of the axon (axonotmesis) have a much better prognosis for axonal regeneration and recovery of function. Among the last two forms the former has a significantly better prognosis than the latter one.

Management

Most of the injuries to peripheral nerves are treated surgically. However, there are differences of functional outcome regarding the surgical repair of peripheral nerve lacerations. In general, repair of peripheral nerve lacerations in the lower extremity usually provide less satisfactory functional outcome than those in the upper extremity. Recent studies show that an early anatomic repair of some disrupted lower extremity peripheral nerves leads to improved results.

PERONEAL NERVE LESIONS

Early repair of a simple transection of the peroneal nerve appears to be much more favourable and up to two-thirds of patients have a satisfactory functional outcome, including proper dorsiflexion and control of the foot during swing phase. However, sensation usually does not return but this is of no real functional consequence. The deformity resulting from an injury to the common peroneal nerve can easily be understood. The drop foot results from loss of the dorsiflexor (tibialis anterior muscle) and loss of the evertor (peroneus brevis and longus muscles) functions of the foot. The unopposed pull of the posterior tibial muscle leads to supination of the mid- and forefoot area. In cases of isolated injury to the deep peroneal nerve, the drop foot occurs only during swing phase because the peroneus brevis and longus functions remain preserved. Surgical treatment includes restoration of dorsiflexion and eversion. This is best achieved by means of a posterior tibial tendon transfer through the interosseous membrane to the dorsum of the foot (out of phase transfer) (Fig. 128.4). Some authors advocate transferring the flexor digitorum longus to the navicular at the same time to oppose the active pull of the peroneus brevis muscle. Alternatively, a simple AFO, with or without a plantarflexion stop hinge, can be used to treat drop foot following peroneal nerve injury.

SCIATIC NERVE LESIONS

The results of anatomic repair of the sciatic nerve following transection are less favourable, but, interestingly, the hamstrings and calf muscles have a better chance of recovery following repair than distally innervated muscles. Sensory recovery appears limited to only protective sensation at best.

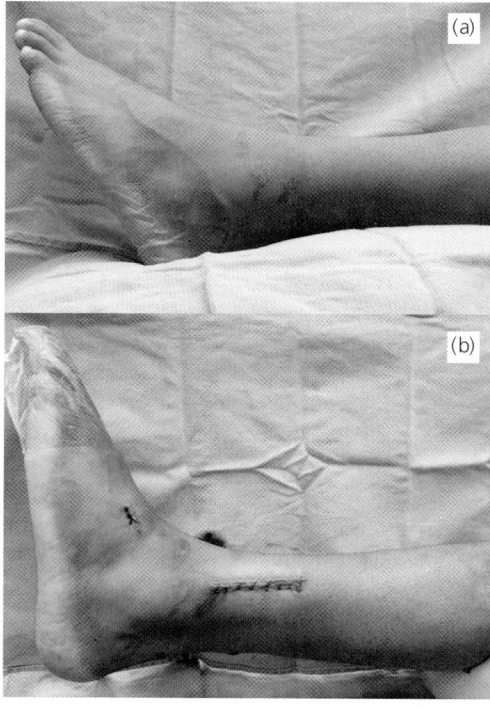

Figure 128.4 Pre-operative (a) and immediate postoperative (b) photographs of a patient with a foot drop after a posterior tibial tendon transfer through the interosseous membrane. Note the resting position of the foot after the tendon transfer. A concomitant Achilles lengthening was performed to allow 10° of dorsiflexion.

Traumatic dislocation of the hip primarily involves only the peroneal portion of the nerve. A tendon transfer may be considered. As the tibial portion of the sciatic nerve provides sensation to the majority of the sole and dorsum of the foot, except for an area along the medial arch, this finding is very important. In contrast, involvement of the entire sciatic nerve (common peroneal and tibial nerves) results in an insensate and inoperable foot. A rigid AFO can help in such cases but the patient must be advised and educated to care for the insensate foot. If some motor function and sensation return, a tendon transfer can be taken into consideration.

A tibial nerve injury in the popliteal fossa results in an insensate foot and partial or complete paralysis of the triceps surae. A calcaneal gait is the result. Tendon transfers are inadequate in the adult but may have some efficacy in the child younger than 10 years. A well-moulded anterior-shell, rear-entry AFO can provide stability from midstance to toe-off during gait. The concern again is loss of sensation on the plantar aspect of the foot. A surgeon should consider whether the chance of primary repair of the nerve and its sequels outweigh primary amputation in the grade IIIC open tibia fracture.

POSTPOLIOMYELITIS SYNDROME

Definition

Recent studies show that an early anatomic repair of some disrupted lower extremity peripheral nerves leads to improved results.

The onset of fatigue, weakness and joint pain occurs approximately 30–40 years after recovery from the initial infection.

Incidence

The syndrome occurs in approximately 25% of all former polio patients. Poliomyelitis continues to be a relatively common infectious paralytic disease in developing countries.

Aetiology of postpoliomyelitis syndrome

The true aetiology remains debated. There are several theories to explain late recurrence, but the most accepted explanation is overuse. There seems to be a relation to overuse of unaffected muscles working in concert to compensate for paralysed or partially paralysed muscles. Some studies reveal that patient age at the time of initial acute infection and response to the severity of the acute infection might predispose individuals to postpoliomyelitis syndrome. The symptomatic lower extremity is often the limb that is less involved acutely.

Pathophysiology of poliomyelitis

The acute infection destroys the anterior spinal neuron cells. Normally, the acute infection encompasses asymmetric motor weakness with no sensory component. In the recovery phase, strength may return as a result of adaptation at the neuromuscular junction or of muscle hypertrophy.

Presentation of postpoliomyelitis syndrome

The most common feature is easy fatigability. The triceps surae musculature remains an important site of weakness below the knee. Push-off is lost, and apparently a calcaneal gait can be found. No stability exists as the weight progresses from hindfoot to midfoot. The most common presenting foot deformity of postpoliomyelitis patients is a valgus hindfoot with midfoot collapse.

Management

The goal of treatment is to achieve a functional and plantigrade foot.

CONSERVATIVE TREATMENT

Ideally, if the patient is willing, limited resistive and aerobic exercises performed well below the patient's level of maximal muscle capacity can help to increase endurance and reduce this fatigability. In contrast, strenuous exercise can exacerbate symptoms and should be avoided. Lifestyle modification is the most important aspect of treatment in order to conserve energy. Bracing or use of orthotics is the main orthopaedic management of postpoliomyelitis patients. In the patient with a plantigrade foot and preserved ankle motion, a hinged AFO (with a 5–10° dorsiflexion stop and free plantarflexion) provides support to the foot and ankle. When calcaneal gait is controlled it decreases quadriceps overuse during the early portion of the gait cycle as a compensatory mechanism. In patients with severe weakness or contracture at the knee, bracing that crosses the knee (hinged above-knee orthosis) must be considered. The primary function is to provide stability during the stance phase. Patients who have adequate upper extremity strength but severe lower extremity weakness and fatigability are particularly good candidates for the use of walking aids. If the patient has substantial upper extremity weakness, however, a wheelchair may be the only option for community ambulation.

SURGICAL TREATMENT

The use in patients suffering from postpoliomyelitis syndrome is limited. Surgery is required to make orthotic management possible. As a general rule, the true benefit to the patient after surgery must be evaluated. Soft-tissue procedures and tendon transfers may improve strength or at least produce a tenodesis effect, allowing stability and adequate load transmission through the lower leg and ankle. Additionally, they provide a basis for proper orthotic management.

Arthrodesis of the joints at the ankle, hindfoot and midfoot should be considered when orthotic management has failed either to relieve symptoms in arthritic joints or to provide stability. There are many reports in the literature that show the successful and functional outcome after fusions.

PARKINSON'S DISEASE

Introduction

An abnormality within the basal ganglion is thought to be the cause.

Presentation

It appears clinically as a motor disturbance with rigidity and tremor. Balance impairment appears to be related to abnormal postural reflexes and inability to modify these reflexes. Up to one-third of patients have foot and ankle findings. Foot dystonia is the most common clinical finding in Parkinson's disease. The classic dystonia-induced contracture of the foot in untreated Parkinson patients involves plantarflexion of the ankle, supination at the subtalar joint with plantarflexion of the lesser toes, and extension of the hallux.

Management

Primary treatment of Parkinson's disease is carried out by levodopa (L-dopa) therapy. The medication improves all the symptoms except for the dystonic foot spasms. The latter bear the potential of increasing severity. Foot symptoms appear in up to 40% of Parkinson patients on sustained L-dopa therapy. Because of treatment, however, this foot dystonia seldom manifests as a fixed contracture. The primary orthopaedic concern is then prevention of fixed deformity and enhancement of balance.

SUMMARY

The foot and ankle specialist must be aware of the complex presentation of neurological and nerve disorders. A thorough anatomical and pathophysiological knowledge is the basis to establish the correct diagnosis and to choose adequate treatment. Clinical examination most often surpasses the power of conventional radiography. Despite rates of reduced compliance, non-operative treatment offers an acceptable approach for both the patient and the physician and might increase a patient's tolerance for possible subsequent surgery if it does fail. For neurological disorders of the foot and ankle, surgery is less effective than for many other orthopaedic conditions.

KEY LEARNING POINTS

- Charcot–Marie–Tooth (CMT) disease is an inherited progressive peripheral neuropathy, referred to as hereditary motor–sensory neuropathies (HMSNs); type I HMSN is the most common presentation of CMT disease (75%).
- Patients with CMT disease present in their second decade.
- Clinically there is hindfoot varus, midfoot cavus to forefoot valgus, clawing of the toes, progressive weakness in the upper extremities (after the foot findings); metatarsalgia, claw toes, tarsal prominence, recurrent ankle sprains; dysplastic hips (5%); and scoliosis (10%).
- Sensory alterations include loss of proprioceptive and vibratory sense.
- Motor status of the foot and ankle, reducibility of the deformity and degree of sensory impairment dictate the type of surgery required.
- Myelomeningocele is a congenital malformation of the CNS resulting in dysplasia of the vertebral elements and the spinal cord.
- Classification follows the level of involvement.
- Being a disorder of the CNS, involvement of both lower motor neurons (flaccid paralysis and lack of sensation) and upper motor neurons (spasticity) must be considered.
- The primary goal of treatment is to produce a plantigrade foot and so a prognostic factor is foot sensibility. Half of these patients have a foot deformity.
- Cerebral palsy (CP) is a static encephalopathy that most frequently results from a cerebral injury in the perinatal period.
- Classification is based on both anatomic (hemiplegic: ipsilateral arm and leg; diplegic: both legs; totally involved) and physiological types (spastic, athetoid, mixed and dystonic).
- All surgical procedures have to be carried out during childhood before skeletal maturity is reached.
- Botulinum type A toxin has gained increasing popularity in the treatment of spasticity.
- In CP, perform all the procedures aimed at functional goals at the same time.
- The most common deforming force in a hemiplegic patient with a spastic equinovarus deformity is the posterior tibial muscle.
- Equinovarus deformity: a younger child with a flexible deformity (i.e. the foot reaches neutral position or pronates slightly), a split transfer of the posterior tibial tendon may be indicated.
- Equinovalgus deformity: this kind of deformity is mainly seen in patients with spastic diplegia.
- Duchenne's muscular dystrophy is a sex-linked disorder transmitted as a recessive trait; the child might be a toe walker, or might have difficulty running and jumping. Pseudohypertrophy of the calf muscles is a pathognomonic finding.
- Surgery should be performed before the child becomes non-ambulatory.
- Stroke is the primary cause of adult hemiplegia.
- Motor vehicle accidents are the main reason for traumatic brain injury and spinal cord injury.
- Patients with spinal cord injuries who receive methylprednisolone within 3 hours and are maintained for 24 hours have significant improvement of motor function.
- Peripheral nerve injury: sciatic nerve injuries are usually the result of gunshot wounds to the upper thigh (especially in the USA); early anatomic repair of some disrupted lower extremity peripheral nerves leads to improved results.
- Parkinson's disease is a motor disturbance with rigidity, tremor and balance impairment; primary treatment is L-dopa therapy.

REFERENCES

- ● = Key primary paper
- ◆ = Major review article

●1. Holmes JR, Hansen ST, Jr. Foot and ankle manifestations of Charcot-Marie-Tooth disease. *Foot and Ankle* 1993;**14**:476–86.
●2. Guyton GP, Mann, RA. The pathogenesis and surgical management of foot deformity in Charcot-Marie-Tooth disease. *Foot and Ankle Clinics* 2000;**5**:317–26.
●3. Newman CJ, Walsh M, O'Sullivan R, *et al.* The characteristics of gait in Charcot-Marie-Tooth disease types I and II. *Gait and Posture* 2007;**26**:120–7.
14. Jahss MH. Evaluation of the cavus foot for orthopedic treatment. *Clinical Orthopaedics and Related Research* 1983;**181**:52–63.

- ●5. Younger AS, Hansen ST, Jr. Adult cavovarus foot. *Journal of the American Academy of Orthopaedic Surgeons* 2005; **13**:302–15.
- ●6. Vinci P, Gargiulo P. Poor compliance with ankle-foot-orthoses in Charcot-Marie-Tooth disease. *European Journal of Physical and Rehabilitation Medicine* 2008;**44**:27–31.
- ●7. Refshauge KM, Raymond J, Nicholson G, van den Dolder PA. Night splinting does not increase ankle range of motion in people with Charcot-Marie-Tooth disease: a randomised, cross-over trial. *Australian Journal of Physiotherapy* 2006;**52**:193–9.
- ●8. Olney B. Treatment of the cavus foot. Deformity in the pediatric patient with Charcot-Marie-Tooth. *Foot and Ankle Clinics* 2000;**5**:305–15.
- 9. Sackley C, Disler PB, Turner-Stokes L, Wade DT. Rehabilitation interventions for foot drop in neuromuscular disease. *Cochrane Database Systematic Review* 2007:CD003908.
- ●10. Oganesyan OV, Istomina IS, Kuzmin VI. Treatment of equinocavovarus deformity in adults with the use of a hinged distraction++ apparatus. *Journal of Bone and Joint Surgery (American)* 1996;**78**:546–56.
- ●11. Mann DC, Hsu JD. Triple arthrodesis in the treatment of fixed cavovarus deformity in adolescent patients with Charcot-Marie-Tooth disease. *Foot and Ankle* 1992;**13**:1–6.
- ●12. Wetmore RS, Drennan JC. Long-term results of triple arthrodesis in Charcot-Marie-Tooth disease. *Journal of Bone and Joint Surgery (American)* 1989;**71**:417–22.
- ●13. Yalcin S, Kocaoglu B, Berker N, Erol B. [Talectomy for the treatment of neglected pes equinovarus deformity in patients with neuromuscular involvement]. *Acta Orthopaedica et Traumatoogica Turcica* 2005;**39**:316–21.
- 14. Westcott MA, Dynes MC, Remer EM, et al. Congenital and acquired orthopedic abnormalities in patients with myelomeningocele. *Radiographics* 1992;**12**:1155–73.
- ●15. Segal LS, Mann DC, Feiwell E, Hoffer MM. Equinovarus deformity in arthrogryposis and myelomeningocele: evaluation of primary talectomy. *Foot and Ankle* 1989;**10**:12–16.
- ●16. Sharrard WJ, Grosfield I. The management of deformity and paralysis of the foot in myelomeningocele. *Journal of Bone and Joint Surgery (British)* 1968; **50**:456–65.
- ◆17. Samilson RL. Current concepts of surgical management of deformities of the lower extremities in cerebral palsy. *Clinical Orthopaedics and Related Research* 1981:99–107.
- ●18. Graham HK, Baker R, Dobson F, Morris ME. Multilevel orthopaedic surgery in group IV spastic hemiplegia. *Journal of Bone and Joint Surgery (British)* 2005;**87**:548–55.
- ●19. Greene WB. Cerebral palsy. Evaluation and management of equinus and equinovarus deformities. *Foot and Ankle Clinics* 2000;**5**:265–80.
- ●20. Kyzer SP, Stark SL. Congenital idiopathic clubfoot deformities. *AORN Journal* 1995;**61**:492–506; quiz 508–12.
- ●21. Strayer LM, Jr. Recession of the gastrocnemius; an operation to relieve spastic contracture of the calf muscles. *Journal of Bone and Joint Surgery (American)*. 1950;**32A**:671–6.
- ●22. Phillips JP, Sullivan, KJ, Burtner PA, et al. Ankle dorsiflexion fMRI in children with cerebral palsy undergoing intensive body-weight-supported treadmill training: a pilot study. *Developmental Medicine and Child Neurology* 2007;**49**:39–44.
- ●23. Rodda JM, Graham HK, Nattrass GR, Galea, MP, et al. Correction of severe crouch gait in patients with spastic diplegia with use of multilevel orthopaedic surgery. *Journal of Bone and Joint Surgery (American)* 2006;**88**:2653–64.
- ◆24. Carlson WE, Vaughan CL, Damiano DL, Abel MF. Orthotic management of gait in spastic diplegia. *American Journal of Physical Medicine & Rehabilitation* 1997;**76**:219–25.
- ●25. Dimitrijevic L, Stankovic I, Zivkovic V, et al. [Botulinum toxin type A for the treatment of spasticity in children with cerebral palsy]. *Vojnosanitetski Pregleg* 2007;**64**:513–18.
- ●26. Schwering L. Surgical correction of the true vertical talus deformity. *Operative Orthopadie und Traumatologie* 2005;**17**:211–31.
- ●27. Karol LA. Surgical management of the lower extremity in ambulatory children with cerebral palsy. *Journal of the American Academy of Orthopaedic Surgeons* 2004;**12**:196–203.
- ◆28. Gough M, Eve LC, Robinson RO, Shortland AP. Short-term outcome of multilevel surgical intervention in spastic diplegic cerebral palsy compared with the natural history. *Developmental Medicine and Child Neurology* 2004;**46**:91–7.
- ●29. Doderlein L. [The surgical management of spastic foot deformities]. *Orthopade* 2004;**33**:1152–62.
- ●30. Roposch A, Scher DM, Mubarak S, Kotz R. [Treatment of foot deformities in patients with Duchenne muscular dystrophy]. *Zeitschrift fur Orthopadie und Ihre Grenzgebiete* 2003;**141**:54–8.
- ●31. Letts M, Davidson D. The role of bilateral talectomy in the management of bilateral rigid clubfeet. *American Journal of Orthopedics* 1999;**28**:106–10.
- ◆32. Roberts, A, Evans, GA. Orthopedic aspects of neuromuscular disorders in children. *Current Opinion in Pediatrics* 1993;**5**:379–83.
- ●33. Law PK, Goodwin TG, Fang Q, et al. Cell transplantation as an experimental treatment for Duchenne muscular dystrophy. *Cell Transplantation* 1993;**2**:485–505.

129

Inflammatory and osteoarthritis of the foot and ankle

ANDREW P MOLLOY, EDWARD V WOOD

Introduction	1484	Midfoot	1489
Initial assessment	1484	First metatarsophalangeal joint	1490
Examination	1485	Lesser MTP joint OA/Freiberg disease	1492
OSTEOARTHRITIS	1486	Charcot neuroarthropathy	1492
Pathophysiology	1486	INFLAMMATORY ARTHRITIS	1493
Principles of treatment	1486	Rheumatoid arthritis	1494
Ankle osteoarthritis	1486	Gout	1496
Ankle impingement	1488	Psoriatic arthropathy	1496
Hindfoot – subtalar	1488	Ankylosing spondylitis	1497
Hindfoot – triple arthrodesis	1489	Reiter syndrome/reactive arthritis	1497
Adult-acquired flat foot and tibialis posterior tendonopathy	1489	Systemic lupus erythematosis	1497
		References	1498

NATIONAL BOARD STANDARDS

- Principles of clinical assessment of the foot and ankle
- Revise the pathology of degenerative joint disease
- Revise the pathology of rheumatoid foot and ankle disease
- Principles of treatment of foot and ankle disorders
- Appreciate the indications for and limitations of different modes of treatment

INTRODUCTION

This chapter aims to cover both osteo- and inflammatory arthritis of the foot and ankle.

Although patients with these conditions present with different problems, the clinical assessment of a patient with foot and ankle arthritis follows the same principles regardless of the underlying cause. We will initially consider osteoarthritis (OA) and its involvement in the different areas of the foot and ankle, before considering inflammatory arthritis.

INITIAL ASSESSMENT

History

A thorough history is essential and should enable the clinician to determine the site, extent and underlying cause of the condition and should also identify any associated conditions or significant comorbidities. Specific critical points are listed below.

- *Pain.* Understanding the functional limitation secondary to pain and how many areas are affected is critical. Progressive instability and/or deformity may affect treatment modality.
- *Comorbidities.* Diabetes mellitus, peripheral vascular disease, neurological disorders, any diagnoses (or undiagnosed signs or symptoms) of an inflammatory arthropathy.
- *Treatment.* Previous (including any preceding trauma) and current treatment should be documented, including medication, orthotics and surgical procedures.
- *Social history.* Occupation (and requirements for continuing to work), domestic circumstances, potential ability to non-weight bear (e.g. rheumatoid upper limb disease).

- *Smoking.* An important risk factor to identify as it has been shown to lead to a 16-fold increase in the non-union rate following arthrodesis.[1]

EXAMINATION

The patient must be adequately exposed to allow assessment of the overall lower limb alignment and facilitate thorough examination of the foot and ankle. Specific detailed points are listed below.

- *Deformity.* It is imperative to assess the level and plane of deformity (e.g. tibial malunion with ankle OA). The flexibility of any deformity also needs to be ascertained.
- *Gait.* Usually the diagnosis can be facilitated from observing patients walking and the effect the condition has on the three rockers of gait and foot position.
- *Ankle.* Range of motion may determine potential treatment as total ankle replacement does not significantly improve the functional arc. Tightness of the tendo-Achilles causes reduced dorsiflexion, and if present Silfverskiöld's test will determine the degree of gastroc-nemius involvement: if the contracture is in the gastroc-nemius alone dorsiflexion of the ankle will increase on knee flexion; if the contracture is in the soleus as well, there will be no change. It is also imperative to ascertain any instability.
- *Hindfoot and midfoot.* Alignment should be assessed, with particular attention paid to deviation from the normal 5° of hindfoot valgus, the medial longitudinal arch and the relation of the forefoot to the midfoot in terms of abduction/adduction and pronation/supination. Tiptoe standing is used to assess hindfoot flexibility and the function of the tibialis posterior tendon. If varus is present, Coleman's block test should be used to determine hindfoot flexibility and whether the cavus is hindfoot or forefoot driven. This is performed with a block under the lateral border of the foot, which neutralizes the effect of a plantarflexed first ray. If a midfoot break or medial column insufficiency is present a reverse Coleman's block test can be undertaken. This involves placing blocks under the first metatarsal head until the hindfoot valgus is corrected; this gives an indication of the site and degree of medial column insufficiency and can be confirmed radiographically.
- *Inflammatory arthritis.* Careful inspection and examination should be undertaken for any polyarthropathy as well as any of the extra-skeletal manifestations of the inflammatory arthritides (e.g. nail and skin lesions).

To complete the examination it is essential to check the neurovascular status of the feet. Pedal pulses should be palpated and if there is any doubt a formal ankle brachial pressure index (ABPI) should be taken. If abnormal, a formal vascular surgical opinion may be sought. Sensation should also be assessed and, in a diabetic patient, formal examination with Semmes Weinstein monofilaments should be undertaken, looking for reduced protective sensation (5.07 monofilament). The condition of the skin should be observed particularly for scars in those with a history of previous trauma. Nail and skin changes associated with inflammatory arthritis should also be looked for. Footwear should be inspected for signs of abnormal wear, and any orthotics and walking aids noted. Rheumatoid patients require clinical and radiological assessment of the cervical spine prior to planned general anaesthesia, to exclude cervical instability.

Blood tests

If an inflammatory arthritis is suspected, blood should be taken for full blood count, erythrocyte sedimentation rate, C-reactive protein, auto-antibodies and rheumatoid factor as an initial screen.

Radiographs

Specific radiographs will be detailed in the following sections. An important principle is to use weight-bearing films, as non-weight-bearing films can mask an underlying deformity and loss of joint space. Standard orthogonal anteroposterior (AP) and lateral views are not sufficient for assessment of the foot. Additional oblique views are required and form part of the standard series. Cobey views are weight-bearing posteroanterior (PA) films that allow assessment of hindfoot alignment at the ankle and subtalar joints in the coronal plane. Long-leg standing films should be obtained if there is a coexistent coronal plane deformity elsewhere in the lower limb. Characteristic changes of OA are loss of joint space, subchondral sclerosis, subchondral cyst formation and osteophyte formation. Characteristic changes in inflammatory arthritis are soft-tissue swelling, peri-articular osteoporosis, marginal cortical erosions, central joint destruction, subluxation or dislocation of the lesser toes. These vary according to the condition.

Special tests

DIAGNOSTIC INJECTION UNDER FLUOROSCOPY

In the foot it can be difficult to isolate the symptomatic joint with examination and plain radiographs alone. Sequential injection of the joints with local anaesthetic under fluoroscopic control followed by immediate weight bearing is an effective technique in this situation.

MAGNETIC RESONANCE IMAGING

This allows assessment of the soft tissues and the presence of inflammation, marrow oedema, avascular necrosis, osteochondral defects (OCDs) and the condition of the joint surfaces.

COMPUTED TOMOGRAPHY

This allows assessment of anatomy and bone quality in post-traumatic OA. It is also useful in demonstrating a tarsal coalition.

NUCLEAR MEDICINE

Nuclear medicine is most often used to exclude the presence of osteomyelitis in diabetic neuroarthropathy or aggressive inflammatory arthritis. Combining a standard technetium bone scan with a leukoscan improves the accuracy in this context.

OSTEOARTHRITIS

PATHOPHYSIOLOGY

OA is a non-inflammatory, degenerative, synovial joint disease, characterized by progressive loss of articular cartilage with associated new bone formation and capsular fibrosis. It is commonly classified into primary (idiopathic) or secondary (due to trauma, congenital deformity, infection or metabolic disorder).

The aetiological factors are

- failure of chondrocytes to repair damaged cartilage
- a disparity between wear and repair
- genetic predisposition.

Articular cartilage is subject to enormous loads, between 10 and 20 MPa during normal activity.[2] Loads greater than this lead to chondrocyte damage and formation of fissures. This can result from a single traumatic event or from repeated lower energy injury. Joint instability reduces joint congruence and surface area of contact. This leads to an increase in the number and intensity of impact loadings and an increase in shear and compression forces across the joint. Loss of sensory innervation accelerates this degeneration, as seen in Charcot joints, otherwise referred to as a neuroarthropathy. In the foot and ankle, in the Western world, this is commonly the result of diabetes.

PRINCIPLES OF TREATMENT

Initial management is usually non-operative: activity modification, analgesia, non-steroidal anti-inflammatory drugs, load reduction and support of painful or unstable joints. Shoe modification and orthoses play an important role. Intra-articular injection of corticosteroid or viscosupplementation may be indicated in certain cases to provide short-term pain relief. Surgical treatment is usually arthroplasty or arthrodesis, with the aim of providing a pain-free, plantigrade, shoeable foot. There is however a role for corrective osteotomy in certain cases of OA associated with an underlying deformity.

ANKLE OSTEOARTHRITIS

Primary OA of the ankle is infrequent. It is most commonly the result of trauma, for example following an ankle or pilon fracture. It may also be associated with other conditions, including chronic lateral ligamentous instability, arthrodesis of adjacent joints, congenital deformity and avascular necrosis of the talus.

Presentation

Pain with exacerbation on activity or prolonged standing is common, as is stiffness, particularly on start-up. Loose bodies may cause locking, and symptoms of instability may be due to deformity or ligamentous instability. Examination may reveal tenderness localized to the anterior or posterior joint line or it may be generalized. Range of motion is often reduced, and it is important to isolate the ankle when assessing this, as movement in the midfoot can mask loss of motion here (normal: 20° dorsiflexion to 40° plantarflexion). The condition of the surrounding joints should be determined along with any deformity or instability.

Investigation

The standard radiographic series consists of weight-bearing ankle AP, mortise (AP with ankle internally rotated 15–20°) and lateral films (Fig. 129.1). A radiological scoring system is described (Table 129.1). Coronal plane malalignment can be assessed with Cobey views. Long limb alignment radiographs are suggested if there is evidence of more proximal malalignment.

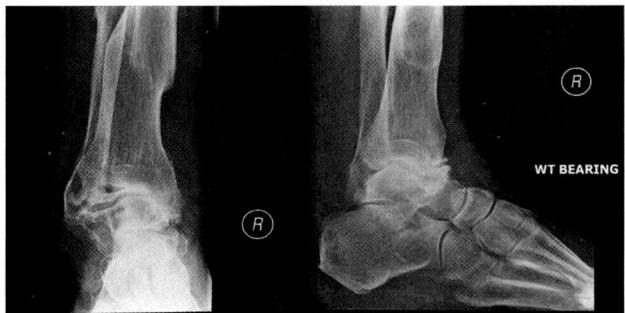

Figure 129.1 Anteroposterior and lateral radiographs showing varus ankle osteoarthritis.

Table 129.1 Pell radiological score for ankle arthritis[3]

0	No narrowing, no osteophytes
1	>3 mm joint space, minimum narrowing of joint space compared with contralateral side, osteophytes
2	1–3 mm joint space, moderate narrowing compared with contralateral side, marked formation of osteophytes, bone sclerosis
3	Obliteration of joint space

Conservative treatment

Along with the usual conservative measures, orthoses may be beneficial. Heel lifts reduce the amount of dorsiflexion, others may benefit from an ankle–foot orthosis with rocker sole shoe or lace-up leather gauntlet ankle braces.

Debridement of joint

Open or arthroscopic debridement of the joint may be indicated in those with symptomatic tibiotalar osteophytes, or with loose bodies associated with OA but with otherwise well-preserved joint space.

Lateral ligament reconstruction

Chronic lateral ligament instability can predispose to early ankle OA. Lateral ligament reconstruction has been shown to halt the progression of early to moderate OA and restore ankle stability.[4]

Arthrodiatasis

Temporary joint distraction using the Ilizarov system has been shown to improve symptoms for 2 years in patients with ankle OA.[5]

Arthrodesis

Arthrodesis is the historical gold standard treatment for end-stage OA of the ankle. Gait analysis studies have shown the best position to be plantigrade, 5° of hindfoot valgus, 5–10° of external rotation and posterior translation of the talus to reduce the lever arm. With a well-positioned arthrodesis, gait efficiency achieves 90% of normal and requires only 3% greater energy expenditure over a normal counterpart at a similar pace of walking. The mild valgus positioning of the hindfoot allows pronation of the foot that 'unlocks' the mid-tarsal joints, which are used as a compensatory mechanism, allowing more natural motion of the hindfoot. Loss of 60–70% of sagittal plane motion does however occur leading to a foreshortened stride, which in turn reduces gait velocity by 16%. A wide variety of techniques have been described to achieve an arthrodesis, but most contemporary methods use compressive internal fixation following decortication of the joint surfaces and correction of deformity (Fig. 129.2). This can be done either open or arthroscopically, with the latter reserved for those with minimal deformity. Union rates are in the region of 90–95% using modern techniques. Arthrodesis increases the risk of developing OA in adjacent joints. The reported rates of subtalar degeneration following ankle arthrodesis ranges from 2.8% to 33%.

Total ankle replacement

Early generations of total ankle prostheses produced poor results, but modern designs are more reliable, leading to a resurgence in total ankle arthroplasty (Fig. 129.3). The benefits of total ankle replacement (TAR) are partial preservation of ankle motion, which produces an improved, but not normalized, gait and reduces the load on adjacent joints, thus reducing the rate of secondary OA.[6,7] The long-term results reported by the inventors of the prostheses are excellent, with 92% survival at 12 years with the Buechel–Pappas,

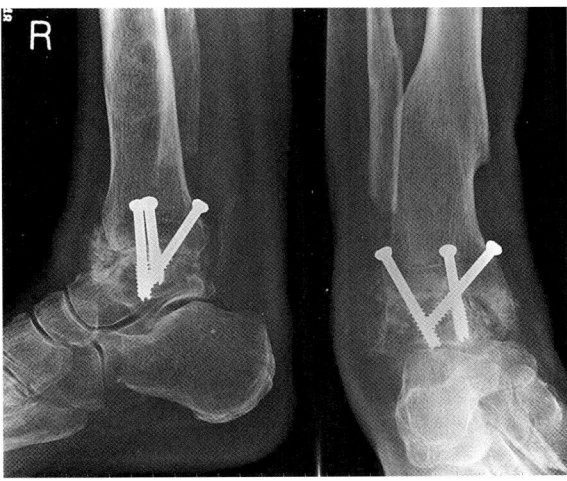

Figure 129.2 Postoperative films showing ankle arthrodesis of the patient in Figure 129.1.

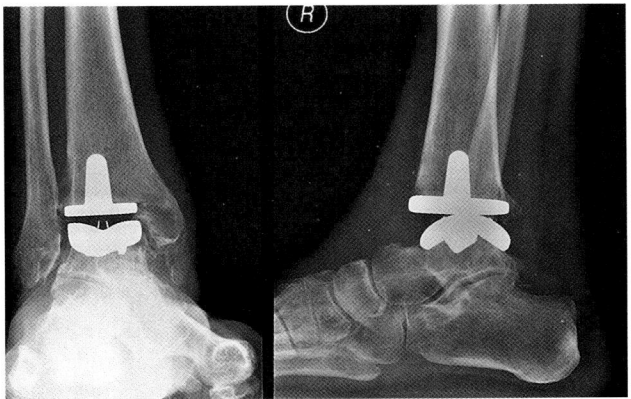

Figure 129.3 Radiographs of a total ankle replacement.

95% 12 year survival for the STAR and 85% survival at 10 years for the Agility. Results for the three prostheses from the National Joint Registries are however less favourable, with 5 year survival of 85% and 89% in the New Zealand and Norwegian registers respectively.[8,9]

Supramalleolar osteotomies

Ankle arthritis associated with a coronal plane deformity can be successfully treated with a corrective osteotomy if the degenerative changes are isolated to either the medial or lateral half of the plafond. Normalizing or slight overcorrection allows unloading of the arthritic area of the joint and loads the more normal cartilage. Although there is limited experience with this technique and the indications have yet to be well defined, it appears to be an effective, if underutilized, method.[10]

Tibiotalocalcaneal arthrodesis

Conditions that produce arthritis in both the ankle and subtalar joints are amenable to this procedure. It can also be indicated in salvage of a failed TAR, neuroarthropathy and ankle fractures in elderly people. A number of methods can be used, including compressive internal fixation with screws, a blade plate, locking plate or intramedullary nail fixation. Techniques using external fixation have also been described. Fusion of both the ankle and subtalar joints significantly limits hindfoot motion and is associated with an increased incidence of subsequent OA in adjacent joints; for this reason it is used mainly as a salvage procedure.

ANKLE IMPINGEMENT

Although impingement is not an arthritic process, it is included here as it may mimic OA on presentation. Impingement can be anterior or posterior and is characterized by pain on dorsiflexion or plantarflexion respectively. The exact cause is unknown but it is thought that soft tissue becomes caught between the tibia and the talus in these positions. The soft tissue may be abnormal, with hypertrophy following trauma or meniscoid lesions from ligamentous damage. The bone is also often abnormal, with the presence of bony spurs from the tibia and talus. Posterior impingement may also be due to an os trigonum or fracture of the posterior process of the talus.

Presentation

Patients present with pain, often on the lateral side of the ankle, and often mechanical symptoms of locking or giving way. Examination may show joint line tenderness, with a small reduction in dorsiflexion. Pressure on the joint line with dorsiflexion will increase the symptoms (Molloy's impingement test).[11]

Investigation

Lateral radiographs will often show a bony spur from the tibial joint line and a spur or boss on the talar neck. The standard weight-bearing lateral film will show anterolateral osteophytes, but is less reliable at demonstrating anteromedial ones, which can be shown with the oblique anteromedial impingement view (leg in 30° external rotation and X-ray beam tilted 45° craniocaudally). These can be supplemented by lateral films in plantar- and dorsiflexion. MRI will identify synovitis, and is useful in excluding other intra-articular pathology such as an osteochondral lesion of the talus (OCLT).

Treatment

Instability and synovitis should initially be addressed with a combination of physiotherapy and intra-articular injection. If conservative treatment is unsuccessful, an open or arthroscopic debridement may be undertaken. This involves an anterior synovectomy and resection of the bony spurs. The rest of the joint should be inspected, particularly for a tibiofibular impingement lesion or OCLT, which should again be debrided. Posterior debridement can also be undertaken arthroscopically or open, with resection of the os trigonum and inspection of the joint surface.

HINDFOOT – SUBTALAR

Subtalar (talocalcaneal) OA is often idiopathic or secondary to tibialis posterior tendon insufficiency, but can also be due to a previous calcaneal or talar fracture or associated with a talocalcaneal tarsal coalition. It is also associated with neuromuscular disorders, such as hereditary motor sensory neuropathy and polio. Coronal plane deformity in the ankle or knee, or previous ankle arthrodesis, will also be compensated for by the subtalar joint, which may lead to early degenerative changes.

Presentation

Patients present with activity-related pain experienced around the hindfoot, which is worse on uneven ground. They may also complain of locking or giving way. On examination, there is often tenderness in the sinus tarsi. The range of motion is reduced in the subtalar joint.

Investigation

Investigation includes standard foot series and a Cobey view if malalignment present. MRI or CT can be used for investigation of a suspected coalition. Diagnostic injections under fluoroscopy can also be useful.

Treatment

Conservative management includes the use of talar-neutral orthoses, such as the Arizona orthosis (Arizona AFO, Mesa, AZ). Surgical treatment usually involves arthrodesis when the joint is degenerate, although some authors describe success with arthroscopic debridement in early disease. In an arthrodesis the subtalar joint is usually approached through a lateral or Ollier incision. Following preparation of the joint surfaces the heel should be placed in 5° valgus for the reasons outlined above. Fixation is achieved with one or two compression screws. Union rates are in the region of 90–95%. Approximately 5% of patients following a calcaneal fracture will go on to require a subtalar arthrodesis.[12] This can be performed using a standard technique; however, if there is a loss of calcaneal height a bone-block, distraction, subtalar arthrodesis can performed. This procedure may need to be combined with peroneal tendon relocation, lateral wall decompression and correction of heel varus – all sequelae of calcaneal fractures.

HINDFOOT – TRIPLE ARTHRODESIS

Triple arthrodesis involves fusion of the talonavicular, calcaneocuboid and subtalar joints. Arthritis of these joints may be post traumatic, but is often due to rheumatoid disease, diabetic neuroarthropathy or stage 3 tibialis posterior tendon deficiency with a non-correctable deformity. The position of fusion is critical; again the heel needs to be in 5° valgus, and the transverse tarsal joints in 5–10° of abduction. Compressive internal fixation is the method of choice (Fig. 129.4).

ADULT-ACQUIRED FLAT FOOT AND TIBIALIS POSTERIOR TENDONOPATHY

Adult-acquired flat foot (AAFF) may be due to arthritic changes or posterior tibial tendon dysfunction (PTTD). With AAFF failure and arthritis of the medial column or first metatarsomedial cuneiform joint occurs. PTTD describes a spectrum of disorders: from isolated tendonopathy to a stiff planovalgus foot. Stages 1 and 2 tendonopathy may be treated with tendon reconstruction or transfer and a

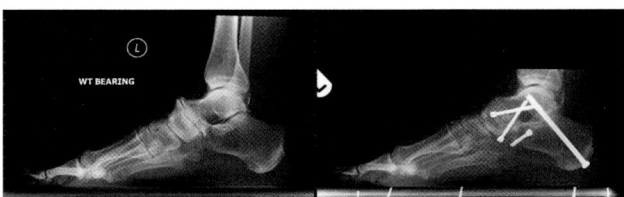

Figure 129.4 Lateral radiograph showing hindfoot arthritis, pre- and postoperative films.

calcaneal osteotomy. As the deformities become fixed arthrodeses are necessary. These range from additional isolated medial column arthrodesis to a triple or even pantalar arthrodesis.

MIDFOOT

The metatarsocuneiform (MTC) joints are also known as the Lisfranc joints. They are key to maintenance of the longitudinal arches of the foot. The second and third MTC joints allow the least movement and are the most frequent sources of symptomatic OA in the midfoot. Failure of the first MTC joint can lead to appearances similar to tibialis posterior tendon dysfunction with midfoot collapse and should be differentiated from this. Lisfranc fracture dislocations are notorious for producing secondary arthritis in these joints.

Presentation

Patients present with ill-defined pain in the midfoot, worse on activity. Dorsal osteophytes produce a boss, which may put pressure on the deep and superficial peroneal nerves, particularly in tight footwear, producing additional symptoms. OA of these joints may be associated with instability and failure of the medial column. This is appreciated by loss of the medial longitudinal arch and the stability of these joints should be assessed, as described previously.

Investigation

The radiological findings may be unremarkable in early disease and one should have a low threshold for undertaking diagnostic injections under fluoroscopy. When present radiological abnormalities include dorsal joint space reduction associated with dorsal osteophytes. These are best viewed on a weight-bearing lateral radiograph of the foot.

Treatment

Non-surgical treatment includes orthoses to support the medial longitudinal arch and hindfoot, and full-length stiff insoles combined with rocker-soled footwear. If the deformity is marked, with midfoot collapse, forefoot supination and abduction, a custom moulded insole and accommodative footwear can be used. Surgical treatment is arthrodesis for disease involving the medial three rays. This can be achieved using a variety of techniques, but commonly involves resection of the joint surfaces and fixation with either screws or plates or both. Where bone destruction is present bone graft may be required. During arthrodesis it is important to achieve the correct sagittal and coronal plane position to avoid offloading or overloading the metatarsal head and producing transfer metatarsalgia. Arthrodesis is not suitable for the fourth and fifth MTC joints however. These joints need to retain their flexibility to allow the foot to accommodate to the ground during gait. OA here has been successfully treated with resection arthroplasty and more recently by interposition arthroplasty, with reasonable results.[13,14]

FIRST METATARSOPHALANGEAL JOINT

OA affecting the first metatarsophalangeal joint (MTPJ) is called hallux rigidus (HR). It is twice as common in females and is often associated with a history of trauma, although it can be due to gout, infection or other inflammatory arthropathy. Its course is usually benign and slowly progressive.

Presentation

HR often presents with dorsal pain and limited dorsiflexion associated with dorsal osteophyte formation. Pressure from footwear may cause a painful callus or bursa. Progression brings increasing stiffness of the first MTPJ and compensatory hyperextension of the interphalangeal joint, which may itself become symptomatic. Examination often reveals clearly palpable dorsal osteophytes with a reduction in the range of motion (normal: 80° dorsiflexion, 40° plantarflexion). Pain may be elicited only at the extremes of movement in early disease, but will affect the midrange of motion as it progresses. This can be confirmed using the grind test, with axial loading of the toe and rotation in the coronal plane.

Investigation

Standard weight-bearing AP and lateral radiographs of the foot (Fig. 129.5). A radiographic and clinical score is described by Coughlin et al.[15] (Table 129.2).

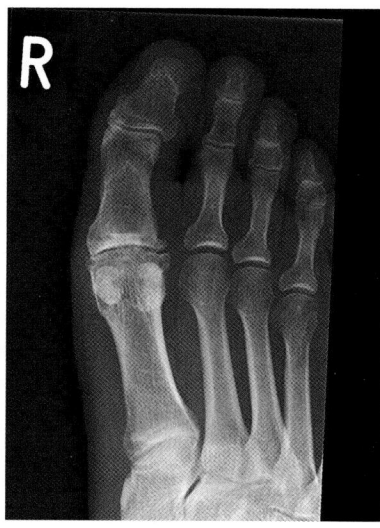

Figure 129.5 First metatarsophalangeal joint osteoarthritis.

Treatment

A large proportion of patients can be managed non-operatively with accommodative footwear, a stiff-soled shoe, stiff full-length orthotic and simple analgesics. Some authors have reported good results with first MTPJ corticosteroid and hyaluronic acid injections. The main surgical treatments are cheilectomy and arthrodesis, but other options are available, as outlined below.

Cheilectomy

Via a dorsomedial approach the dorsal osteophyte and a variable amount of the joint surface is removed (0–30%). Good results are reported with early to moderate disease (stage 1 or 2), but patients with mid-range pain or more advanced disease do not respond as well.

Dorsiflexion phalangeal osteotomy

A dorsal closing wedge osteotomy of the proximal phalanx increases the dorsiflexion and has been combined with a limited cheilectomy, with good results in a limited number of small series.

Metatarsal osteotomies

A number of procedures have been described which aim to decompress the joint by shortening the first metatarsal, realigning the joint surface and correcting the metatarsus primus elevatus. It is difficult to draw conclusions from the literature due to the wide variety of techniques and outcome measures used.

First metatarsophalangeal joint arthrodesis

Arthrodesis is indicated in more advanced disease (stage 3). The position of fusion is important: neutral or plantarflexion will prevent roll through of the foot, increasing forces through the interphalangeal joint, which may become symptomatic. Excessive dorsiflexion will cause shoe fitting problems. Dorsiflexion of 20–30° in relation to the metatarsal is suggested, with neutral rotation and 5° of valgus or more in the rheumatoid foot or for revision bunion surgery. Although a number of techniques are described, biomechanically the most stable method is a compression screw combined with a dorsal compression plate (Fig. 129.6).[16] Union rates are between 90% and 100%. Compared with Keller's procedure and hemiarthroplasty, arthrodesis produces equivalent or superior results with fewer complications and remains the gold standard for treatment of stage 3 OA.[17]

Table 129.2 Coughlin's classification of first metatarsophalangeal joint arthritis

Grade	Dorsiflexion	Radiographic findings	Clinical findings
0	40–60° and/or 10–20% loss compared with normal side	Normal	No pain; only stiffness and loss of motion on examination
1	30–40° and/or 20–50% loss compared with normal side	Dorsal osteophyte is main finding, minimal joint space narrowing, minimal peri-articular sclerosis, minimal flattening of the metatarsal head	Mild or occasional pain and stiffness, pain at extremes of dorsiflexion and/or plantarflexion on examination
2	10–30° and/or 50–75% loss compared with normal side	Dorsal, lateral, and possibly medial osteophytes giving flattened appearance to metatarsal head, no more than one-quarter of dorsal joint space involved on lateral radiograph, mild-to-moderate joint-space narrowing and sclerosis, sesamoids not usually involved	Moderate-to-severe pain and stiffness that may be constant; pain occurs just before maximum dorsiflexion and maximum plantarflexion on examination
3	≤10° and/or 75–100% loss compared with normal side. There is notable loss of metatarsophalangeal plantarflexion as well (often ≤10° of plantarflexion)	Same as in grade 2 but with substantial narrowing, possibly peri-articular cystic changes, more than one-quarter of dorsal joint space involved on lateral radiograph, sesamoids enlarged and/or cystic and/or irregular	Nearly constant pain and substantial stiffness at extremes of range of motion but not at mid-range
4	Same as in grade 3	Same as in grade 3	Same criteria as grade 3 *but* there is definite pain at mid-range of passive motion

Interpositional arthroplasty

A small number of authors have reported good results with various types of interpositional arthroplasty, using extensor hallucis brevis, plantaris tendon and gracillis tendon, although others have used a temporary metal spacer.

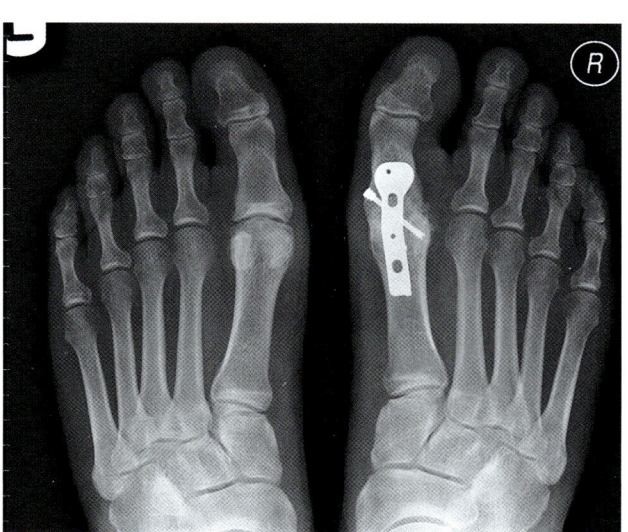

Figure 129.6 First metatarsophalangeal joint arthrodesis.

As yet, there is insufficient evidence to recommend one technique over the others.

Silastic arthroplasty

Results with single-stemmed implants have been poor with a 30% failure rate and granuloma formation in 70%.[18] Results with double-stemmed, metal-cuffed implants are more promising but are still best reserved for the elderly low-demand patient.

Hemi-arthroplasty

Hemi-arthroplasty usually involves resurfacing of the proximal phalanx, although metatarsal head surface replacement has also been described. There is little high-quality evidence to support its use, with most series reporting high failure and revision rates.

Total joint arthroplasty

Total joint arthroplasty can be performed using metallic or ceramic components. There is a paucity of level 1 or 2 evidence regarding total joint arthroplasty of the first

MTPJ. Several studies have shown promising early results, but the medium- to long-term results have shown problems with radiological loosening and subsidence in up to 30% of patients, regardless of the method of fixation.

Resection arthroplasty

The Keller procedure has fallen out of favour in recent years. It is an excision arthroplasty with removal of the proximal part of the proximal phalanx and soft-tissue reconstruction. Although it decompresses the joint and improves the range of motion, it weakens the hallux, leads to a cock-up deformity and metatarsalgia. If used, it is best reserved for elderly and low-demand patients.

LESSER MTP JOINT OA/FREIBERG DISEASE

Freiberg disease is an osteochondrosis of a lesser metatarsal head that causes degeneration of the MTPJ. It most often affects teenage or young adult females and usually involves the second metatarsal head, although it can be seen in the third and fourth. The exact aetiology is unknown but osteonecrosis and subchondral collapse may be due to trauma, increased coaguability, raised intraosseous pressure, overload, from a long metatarsal, and iatrogenic, from forefoot surgery.

Presentation

Patients presenting early in the course of the disease will have pain isolated to the affected joint, which is worse on weight bearing. Examination will reveal an irritable joint with a limited range of motion.

Investigation

There will be little to see on initial radiographs. As revascularization occurs the metatarsal head can collapse making the joint incongruent, which predisposes to osteophyte formation and subsequent degenerative changes (Fig. 129.7).

Treatment

In the acute phase, conservative measures should be used: analgesics and anti-inflammatories, metatarsal pads or dome insoles to offload the metatarsal head, toe strapping and steroid injection. If these are not successful, a rocker-soled shoe can be prescribed. Early in the disease, synovectomy and core decompression may be effective. For later disease a multitude of different surgical techniques have

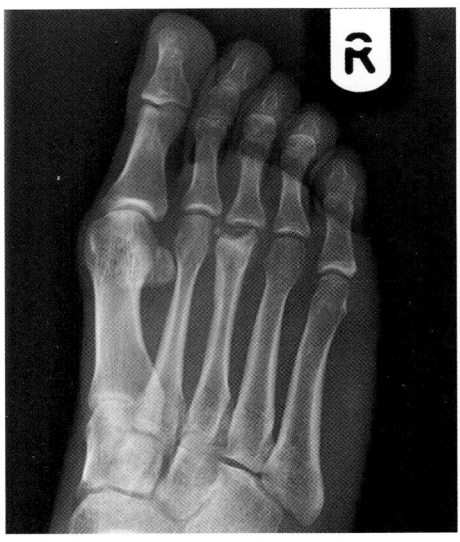

Figure 129.7 Freiberg disease of the third metatarsal.

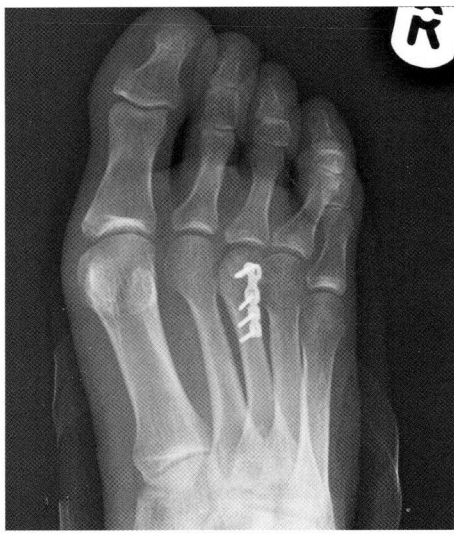

Figure 129.8 Freiberg disease treated with a dorsal closing wedge osteotomy.

been described, including arthrotomy with removal of loose bodies and debridement, drilling, dorsal closing wedge osteotomy (Fig. 129.8), interpositional tendon arthroplasty, proximal phalangeal resection, metatarsal head resection, metatarsal shortening and joint replacement. The degree of joint destruction will obviously guide the technique used. The evidence base regarding the type of treatment remains limited to small case series.

CHARCOT NEUROARTHROPATHY

Charcot or neuroarthropathy was originally described in tertiary syphilis, but now most commonly occurs secondary to diabetes, affecting approximately 0.3% of diabetic

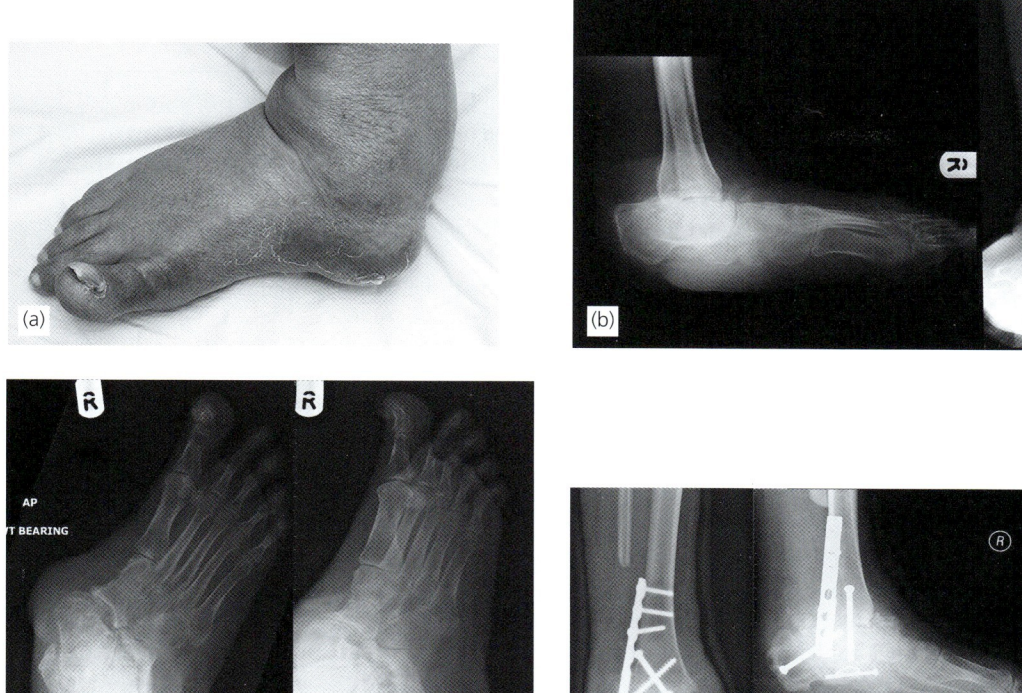

Figure 129.9 (a) Clinical photograph of a Charcot foot deformity. (b) Anteroposterior (AP) and lateral ankle radiographs of the same patient. (c) AP and oblique foot radiographs of the same patient. (d) Postoperative radiographs following tibiotalocalcaneal arthrodesis with a blade plate.

patients. It is a severe, non-infectious, destructive arthropathy associated with dislocation and peri-articular fracture in any patient with loss of protective sensation. Charcot arthropathy probably begins with trauma, either as a single event or from repeated microtrauma. Peripheral neuropathy reduces protective behaviour and increases the risk of injury through reduced proprioception. Abnormal vasomotor control leads to hyperaemia, increased osteoclast activity and subsequent bone demineralization. These combine to produce a rapidly destructive arthropathy associated with deformity and skin pressure and ulceration (Fig. 129.9).

The stages of the disease are described by the Eichenholtz classification:

Stage 1   Destruction: hyperaemia, fragmentation, dislocation
Stage 2   Coalescence: reduced warmth and oedema, new bone formation
Stage 3   Consolidation: healing, often with residual deformity.

Brodsky classified the region of the foot involved as follows:

Type 1   involves the midfoot
Type 2   involves the hindfoot
Type 3A   involves the ankle
Type 3B   fractures of the calcaneus.

The tarsometatarsal joints being the most commonly affected.

Treatment

It is important to establish tight control of the diabetes and prevent deformity and ulceration. The latter is achieved by support of the foot in either a total contact cast or diabetic walker boot. Surgery is indicated in severe instability and persistent or recurrent ulceration. Corrective surgery should be avoided in stage 1 as the bone is of poor quality and markedly osteopenic.

INFLAMMATORY ARTHRITIS

Inflammatory arthritis covers a broad spectrum of conditions including synovial joint disorders, crystal deposition and connective tissue disorders. Synovial joint disease can be divided into seropositive (rheumatoid arthritis) and seronegative (Reiter's, psoriasis, ankylosing spondylitis). Crystal deposition disorders include gout and pseudogout and the connective tissue disorders include systemic lupus erythematosis (SLE), Crohn disease and ulcerative colitis, among others.

RHEUMATOID ARTHRITIS

Rheumatoid arthritis is a systemic disease causing a symmetrical polyarthropathy affecting both small and large joints. It affects up to 1% of the population, more commonly women than men. The feet and hands are the most commonly affected primary areas. The prevalence of rheumatoid foot disease is up to 90%.

Pathophysiology

The pathological abnormalities seen in rheumatoid arthritis are caused by the immune-mediated formation of pannus. Initially this is confined to the peri-articular recesses of the joints but as the disease progresses it invades more centrally. Joint and soft-tissue destruction are caused by immune-mediated enzymatic degradation. Joint capsule, ligament and tendon destruction lead to progressive deformity. This is most commonly seen in the lesser toes as well as pes plano valgus and associated tibialis posterior problems. Altered mechanics of the joint lead to abnormal pressure loading above the mechanical yield point of the already damaged articular surface. This accelerates the destruction of the joint and can lead to secondary OA. This may be compounded by peripheral neuropathy where decreased nocioception and proprioception reduces protective behaviour. Loss of bone stock, osteoporosis (secondary to relative hyperaemia) and immunological destruction weaken the subchondral bone so that once the subchondral plate is breached progression of deformities may be rapid.

Diagnosis

Box 129.1 shows the criteria for diagnosis of rheumatoid arthritis set out by the American Rheumatological Association. The course of rheumatoid disease can be split into three clinical patterns: polycyclic, monocyclic and progressive. Polycyclic disease (70%) follows a remitting and relapsing course where multiple episodes of synovitis cause erosive joint changes. Monocyclic disease (20%) involves a single, often prolonged, exacerbation of synovitis and tends to have minor erosive changes. Progressive disease (10%) describes a constant and rapidly progressive disease with no remitting episodes. As rheumatoid arthritis is a systemic autoimmune disease there are multiple extra-articular manifestations. Rheumatoid nodules present as discrete firm lesions that may be fixed to the tissues. These are normally on the extensor surfaces of the body. Peripheral neuropathy may occur either systemically or due to local nerve compression. Tendonopathies are common, particularly of the extensor tendons to the lesser toes and tibialis posterior in the foot. Renal, cardiac and pulmonary disease is also prevalent and should be taken into consideration during any pre-operative work-up. Arterial insufficiency must be thoroughly investigated before any surgical procedures are considered.

> **BOX 129.1: The American Rheumatism Association 1987 revised criteria for the classification of rheumatoid arthritis**
>
> 1. Morning stiffness in and around joints lasting at least 1 hour before maximal improvement
> 2. Soft-tissue swelling (arthritis) of three or more joint areas observed by a physician
> 3. Swelling (arthritis) of the proximal interphalangeal, metacarpophalangeal, or wrist joints
> 4. Symmetric swelling (arthritis)
> 5. Rheumatoid nodules
> 6. The presence of rheumatoid factor
> 7. Radiographic erosions and/or peri-articular osteopenia in hand and/or wrist joints.
>
> Criteria 1–4 must have been present for at least 6 weeks. Four out of seven of the criteria are necessary for a diagnosis of rheumatoid arthritis

Rheumatoid – ankle

The ankle joint is less commonly affected than other joints of the foot. The prevalence is determined by the duration of the disease. It is relatively uncommon to see gross primary deformities of the ankle. If present, these are normally secondary to hindfoot deformities. Therefore, if surgical treatment is to be undertaken then both the ankle and hindfoot deformities will need to be addressed.

TREATMENT

Conservative treatments include pharmacological agents and bracing. The bracing may range from a simple stirrup brace to a more substantial orthotic to prevent ankle motion. Arthrodesis of the ankle is historically seen as the gold standard for treatment of ankle rheumatoid arthritis. Complications of surgery include wound breakdown, infection, neurovascular damage and non-union. One must be mindful of the chance of progression of rheumatoid arthritis throughout the hindfoot and the future need for a pantalar fusion. TAR is being used more frequently now, and the largest series of rheumatoid patients reported by Wood et al.[19] showed an overall 8 year survivorship of 88%. However, in patients with normal alignment the survivorship increased to 97%.

Rheumatoid – hindfoot

The prevalence of hindfoot involvement in rheumatoid patients is related to the duration of disease. This is due to ligamentous, tendinous and articular damage accumulated by the mechanical stresses of weight bearing over time. The talonavicular joint is the most commonly affected followed by the calcaneocuboid, then the subtalar joint. This is also the sequence in which they become involved. Ligamentous and articular destruction of the talonavicular joint followed by the other hindfoot and medial column joints leads to a progressive pes plano valgus deformity. Associated tibialis posterior dysfunction will also contribute to this deformity. Pes plano valgus deformity places additional stresses across the ankle and can cause a secondary deformity due to deltoid ligament insufficiency, bony erosion or stress fractures. Examination should determine if the deformity is fixed or flexible, which joints are involved and if there is medial column involvement.

TREATMENT

Non-operative treatment of the hindfoot includes rest and mobilization and pharmacological agents. Orthotics may help with symptomatic relief but are not proven to affect the overall progression of the disease. In the earlier stages, an in-shoe orthosis with neutral heel clasp, medial posting and medial longitudinal arch support can provide enough stabilization for symptomatic improvement. As deformities progress, custom-made shoes and even a calliper with an inside iron and outside strap may be necessary. The latter is rarely acceptable to patients and is usually reserved for patients unwilling to undergo surgery or who are unfit. Patients should be counselled thoroughly about the progressive nature of the disease, including the potential to develop ankle deformities, soft-tissue problems upon correction of pes plano valgus deformity, and regarding the functional result of an eventual tibiotalocalcaneal fusion.

Rheumatoid – talonavicular disease

Previously an isolated talonavicular fusion was seldom performed due to frequent involvement of the other hindfoot joints. The advent of immune system-modifying drugs brings the potential to halt disease progression. Talonavicular arthrodesis may therefore become more common. Historically the non-union rate ranged from 3% to 37%. More modern techniques, using internal fixation, push fusion rates towards the more successful end of this range. Patients should be counselled regarding the risk of developing calcaneocuboid and subtalar joint disease that may require further surgery.

Rheumatoid – triple arthrodesis

The most commonly performed operation is a triple arthrodesis, usually undertaken through a standard lateral and dorsomedial approach. If, however, there are long-standing severe deformities with contracture of the soft tissues on the lateral side, an isolated medial approach may be used. This is technically more difficult, but can prevent the complication of wound breakdown on the lateral side secondary to undue tension from correction of the deformities. The ideal position for fusion is with the heel in 5° of valgus with a neutral forefoot (abduction is fully corrected with no pronation or supination).

Rheumatoid – midfoot

Approximately two-thirds of patients with rheumatoid arthritis will develop midfoot disease. Deformities associated with midfoot disease can be accelerated by hindfoot-driven pes plano valgus deformity. It is common for an ankylosis to develop in midfoot joints. This is due to the inherent stability and limited range of movement in the midfoot, where there is a high level of bony congruency. Consequently, rheumatoid disease of this area is rarely the primary complaint.

TREATMENT

Conservative treatment is usually adequate, but there are two scenarios where operative treatment is indicated. First, in cases of severe pes plano valgus where the hindfoot has driven the midfoot into extremes of abduction and flattening. The second is hypermobility of the first metatarsal cuneiform joint. Surgery involves an extended medial column fusion with the more lateral joints being addressed as necessary.

Rheumatoid – forefoot

Rheumatoid forefoot deformities are typically hallux valgus, dorsal subluxation or dislocation of the lesser MTPJs, and flexible or fixed deformities of the interphalangeal joints of the lesser toes (Fig. 129.10). However, any

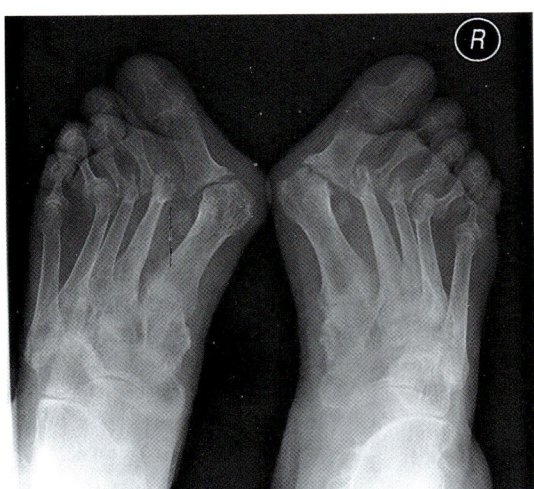

Figure 129.10 Anteroposterior radiograph showing severe rheumatoid forefoot deformity.

conceivable deformity of the toes may be present, depending on how many of the stabilizing structures of the joints have been destroyed. As the lesser toes sublux or dislocate dorsally, the plantar fat pad subluxes anteriorly because of its attachment of the proximal phalanx. This uncovers the metatarsal heads.

TREATMENT

Conservative treatment includes chiropody, padding over prominent bony surfaces and accommodative shoe wear with a wide, deep toe box with a cushioned orthotic sole. Standard surgical treatment is first MTPJ fusion with lesser metatarsal head resection and proximal interphalangeal joint (PIPJ) fusion.[20] An alternative to metatarsal head resection is resection of a portion of the proximal part of the proximal phalanges as described by Stainsby.[21] In both these scenarios, extensor tendon tenotomy is carried out. With the advent of immune system-modifying drugs, interest has concentrated on joint-sparing surgery. This includes hallux valgus correction with lesser metatarsal shortening (e.g. Weil osteotomy) plus closed osteoclasis or PIPJ fusion with Kirschner wiring.

GOUT

Gout is a monosodium urate crystal arthropathy secondary to hyperuricaemia. Primary gout is due to an inborn error of metabolism, whereas secondary gout is an acquired disorder or a side-effect of certain medications. The predilection for crystal formation in the foot is due to factors that decrease the solubility of urate crystals, lower ambient pH and lower temperature.

Presentation

Gout usually starts as a mono-arthropathy but can develop into an asymmetric polyarthropathy. Involvement of the first MTPJ is the most common presenting feature. Clinical features are of rapid onset of severe pain, swelling and erythema. With chronicity gouty tophi develop. These may precipitate ulceration and secondary infection.

Investigation

Laboratory tests should include serum urate level, liver function tests, and urea and electrolytes along with the standard inflammatory series. Early in the disease, radiographs may appear normal. As it progresses the characteristic radiographic findings are punched out peri-articular lesions, sclerotic joint surfaces and overhanging joint margins. In severe cases, massive destruction of the first metatarsal and proximal phalanx may occur, and in these cases one must be mindful of secondary osteomyelitis. The key laboratory test is joint fluid analysis for Gram stain, cell count and differential, culture and sensitivity and microscopy for crystals. The finding of needle-shaped, negatively birefringent crystals is diagnostic for gout and the other tests are important to exclude septic arthritis in the acute presentation. Synovial biopsy may be required if an aspirate is not possible.

Treatment

The mainstay of treatment is pharmacological. In the acute attack, non-steroidal anti-inflammatory drugs (NSAIDs) provide symptomatic relief. When NSAIDs are insufficient, colchicine or steroids may be added. To prevent further attacks the serum urate level needs to be reduced. This is through a combination of lifestyle and diet changes and urate-lowering drugs, such as allopurinol and probenicid. Gouty arthritis of the first MTPJ is usually treated with an arthrodesis. In cases of unresolving tophaceous ulceration, it may be necessary to excise the ulcer and gouty tophi. This does however have a high complication rate: 53% delayed wound healing and 7% digit amputation.[22]

PSORIATIC ARTHROPATHY

Psoriasis affects up to 4% of the population with an almost 1:1 male to female ratio. Approximately 10% of these patients will develop an asymmetric polyarthropathy of both small and large joints. Patients are normally rheumatoid factor negative.

Presentation

Psoriasis is characterized by its dermatological lesions: plaqueing, white scaly lesions and vesicles (particularly long and medial longitudinal arch of the foot). One should be aware that these lesions are not always obvious to the patient (e.g. on the scalp). Nail pitting and oncholysis are also common. The distal interphalangeal joint (DIPJ) of the lesser toes are most commonly affected. Erythema and fusiform swelling give rise to 'sausage' toes. Enthesopathies are common, as are tendonopathies. Heel pain is therefore one of the commonly presenting features.

Investigation

Psoriatic arthropathy is characterized radiographically by marginal joint erosions without peri-articular osteoporosis. At the DIPJ 'pencil-in-cup' deformities are virtually pathognomonic. Periostitis and proliferated bone formation may be present particularly on the plantar surface of the calcaneum.

Treatment

Foot deformities are often similar to rheumatoid arthritis. The conservative and surgical management of the two conditions is similar. Deformities in psoriatic arthropathy tend to be much stiffer than the rheumatoid feet and care should be taken not to compromise the vascular supply.

ANKYLOSING SPONDYLITIS

This is a human leucocyte antigen (HLA) B27-associated, seronegative spondyloarthropathy characterized by sacroiliitis, acute anterior uveitis and spinal disease. Any tendon or ligament insertion may be affected. Common presentations in the foot and ankle include insertional Achilles tendonopathy and heel pain. Although the prevalence of foot disease in ankylosing spondylitis may be up to 60%, it is usually the axial skeleton manifestations that are more symptomatic.

The majority of treatment in the foot and ankle is non-operative, with physiotherapy to maintain flexibility of joints and eccentric loading exercises for Achilles tendonopathy, NSAIDs and orthotics.

REITER SYNDROME/REACTIVE ARTHRITIS

Presentation

The classical presentation of Reiter syndrome is arthritis, urethritis and conjunctivitis, with painless oral ulcers and keratoderma blennorrhagica (pustules on the soles and palms). Up to 80% of patients are HLA B27 positive. There is also thought to be an association with gastrointestinal and genitourinary infection. Acute arthritic episodes may resemble septic arthritis or gout. Patients may present with asingle 'sausage' digit. Enthesopathies, particularly at the calcaneus, are common and may be associated with periostitis and proliferative new bone formation. Recurrent arthritic exacerbations are common and may lead to erosion of the metatarsal heads.

Treatment

Treatment is usually only necessary for the acute phase and is similar to that of ankylosing spondylitis. Surgical treatment of foot deformities follows the same principles as rheumatoid disease.

SYSTEMIC LUPUS ERYTHEMATOSIS

SLE mainly affects young women. It is an autoimmune condition characterized by a butterfly malar rash, photosensitivity, oral ulcers and arthritis. Vasculitis, photosensitivity, pericarditis, pancytopenia and peripheral neuropathy are the commonest extra-osseous manifestations. Up to 80% of patients are anti-nuclear antibody positive and around a third rheumatoid factor positive.

Presentation

The presentation of its polyarthropathy is similar to rheumatoid disease, although it tends to be less deforming.

Investigation

Radiographically SLE is not as erosive as rheumatoid disease.

Treatment

Treatment of SLE is also similar to that of rheumatoid disease. One must always be mindful of the prevalence of vasculitis and other comorbidities in the pre-operative work-up.

> **KEY LEARNING POINTS**
>
> - The clinical assessment of a patient with foot and ankle arthritis follows the same principles regardless of the underlying cause.
> - Use weight-bearing films (non-weight-bearing films can mask an underlying deformity and loss of joint space).
> - Articular cartilage is subject to enormous loads, between 10 and 20 MPa during normal activity.
> - Surgical treatment is broadly arthroplasty or arthrodesis, with the aim of providing a pain-free, plantigrade, shoeable foot.
> - Primary osteoarthritis (OA) of the ankle is infrequent.
> - Open or arthroscopic debridement of the joint may be indicated in those with symptomatic tibiotalar osteophytes, or with loose bodies associated with OA, but with otherwise well-preserved joint space.
> - Chronic lateral ligament instability can predispose to early ankle OA.
> - Arthrodesis is the historical gold standard treatment for end-stage OA of the ankle.
> - Total ankle replacement (TAR): the long-term results reported by the inventors of the prostheses are excellent with 92% survival at 12 years with the Buechel–Pappas, 95% 12 year survival for the Star and 85% survival at 10 years for the Agility.
> - Tibiotalocalcaneal arthrodesis for conditions that produce arthritis in both the ankle and the subtalar joints; it can also be indicated in salvage of a failed TAR, neuroarthropathy and ankle fractures in elderly people.

- Ankle impingement is not an arthritic process, but may mimic OA.
- Subtalar (talocalcaneal) osteoarthritis is often idiopathic or secondary to tibialis posterior tendon insufficiency.
- Triple arthrodesis (fusion of the talonavicular, calcaneocuboid and subtalar joints) may be required for arthritis of these joints. May be post-traumatic, but is often due to rheumatoid disease, diabetic neuroarthropathy, or stage3 tibialis posterior tendon deficiency with a non-correctable deformity.
- In adult-acquired flat foot and tibialis posterior tendinopathy, arthrodesis is required when the deformities become fixed.
- OA affecting the first metatarsophalangeal joint (MTPJ) is called hallux rigidus; treatment is cheilectomy and arthrodesis; silastic replacements have a 30% failure rate.
- Freiberg disease is an osteochondrosis of a lesser metatarsal head, which causes degeneration of the MTPJ (usually the second MT head) and occurs in teens or young female adults.
- Rheumatoid arthritis is a systemic disease causing a symmetrical polyarthropathy affecting both small and large joints; it can be polycyclic, monocyclic or progressive.
- Rheumatoid foot: the talonavicular joint is the most commonly involved, requiring talonavicular arthrodesis but triple arthrodesis is the most common operation.
- Rheumatoid forefoot problems are hallux valgus, subluxed/dislocated MTPJs and involved interphalangeal joints.
- Gout is a monosodium urate crystal arthropathy secondary to hyperuricaemia; the mainstay of treatment is pharmacological.
- Psoriatic arthropathy is characterized radiographically by marginal joint erosions without peri-articular osteoporosis.
- The classical presentation of Reiter syndrome is arthritis, urethritis and conjunctivitis.
- Systemic lupus erythematosus is an autoimmune condition characterized by a butterfly malar rash, photosensitivity, oral ulcers and arthritis.

REFERENCES

- ● = Key primary paper
- ◆ = Major review article

●1. Cobb TK, Gabrielsen TA, Campbell DC, et al. Cigarette smoking and nonunion after ankle arthrodesis. *Foot and Ankle International/American Orthopaedic Foot and Ankle Society [and] Swiss Foot and Ankle Society* 1994;**15**:64–7.

2. Urban JP. The chondrocyte: a cell under pressure. *British Journal of Rheumatology* 1994;**33**:901–8.

3. Pell IV RF, Myerson MS, Schon LC. Clinical outcome after primary triple arthrodesis. *Journal of Bone and Joint Surgery (American)* 2008;**82**:45–57.

4. Harrington KD. Degenerative arthritis of the ankle secondary to long-standing lateral ligament instability. *Journal of Bone and Joint Surgery (American)* 1979;**61**:354–61.

5. van Valburg AA, van Roermund PM, Lammens J, et al. Can Ilizarov joint distraction delay the need for an arthrodesis of the ankle? A preliminary report. *Journal of Bone and Joint Surgery (British)* 1995;**77**:720–5.

◆6. SooHoo NF, Zingmond DS, Ko CY. Comparison of reoperation rates following ankle arthrodesis and total ankle arthroplasty. *Journal of Bone and Joint Surgery (American)* 2007;**89**:2143–9.

7. Kofoed H, Sturup J. Comparison of ankle arthroplasty and arthrodesis. A prospective series with long-term follow-up. *Foot* 1994;**4**:6–9.

◆8. Hosman AH, Mason RB, Hobbs T, Rothwell AG. A New Zealand national joint registry review of 202 total ankle replacements followed for up to 6 years. *Acta Orthopaedica* 2007;**78**:584–91.

◆9. Fevang BS, Lie SA, Havelin LI, et al. 257 ankle arthroplasties performed in Norway between 1994 and 2005. *Acta Orthopaedica* 2007;**78**:575–83.

10. Tanaka Y, Takakura Y, Hayashi K, et al. Low tibial osteotomy for varus-type osteoarthritis of the ankle. *Journal of Bone and Joint Surgery (British)* 2006;**88**:909–13.

●11. Molloy S, Solan MC, Bendall SP. Synovial impingement in the ankle. A new physical sign. *Journal of Bone and Joint Surgery (British)* 2003;**85**:330–3.

◆12. Zwipp H, Rammelt S, Barthel S. Calcaneal fractures—open reduction and internal fixation (ORIF). *Injury* 2004;**35**(Suppl. 2):SB46–54.

13. Berlet GC, Hodges Davis W, Anderson RB. Tendon arthroplasty for basal fourth and fifth metatarsal arthritis. *Foot and Ankle International/American Orthopaedic Foot and Ankle Society [and] Swiss Foot and Ankle Society* 2002;**23**:440–6.

14. Shawen SB, Anderson RB, Cohen BE, et al. Spherical ceramic interpositional arthroplasty for basal fourth and fifth metatarsal arthritis. *Foot and Ankle International/American Orthopaedic Foot and Ankle Society [and] Swiss Foot and Ankle Society* 2007;**28**:896–901.

◆15. Coughlin MJ, Shurnas PS. Hallux rigidus. Grading and long-term results of operative treatment. *Journal of Bone and Joint Surgery (American)* 2003;**85A**:2072–88.

16. Politi J, John H, Njus G, et al. First metatarsal-phalangeal joint arthrodesis: a biomechanical assessment of stability. *Foot and Ankle International/American Orthopaedic Foot and Ankle Society [and] Swiss Foot and Ankle Society* 2003;**24**:332–7.

17. Raikin SM, Ahmad J, Pour AE, Abidi N. Comparison of arthrodesis and metallic hemiarthroplasty of the hallux metatarsophalangeal joint. *Journal of Bone and Joint Surgery (American)* 2007;**89**:1979–85.

- 18. Rahman H, Fagg PS. Silicone granulomatous reactions after first metatarsophalangeal hemiarthroplasty. *Journal of Bone and Joint Surgery (British)* 1993;**75**:637–9.
- 19. Wood PLR, Crawford LA, Suneja R, Kenyon A. Total ankle replacement for rheumatoid ankle arthritis. *Foot and Ankle Clinics* 2007;**12**:497–508, vii.
- 20. Coughlin MJ. Rheumatoid forefoot reconstruction. A long-term follow-up study. *Journal of Bone and Joint Surgery (American)* 2000;**82**:322–41.
- 21. Stainsby GD. Pathological anatomy and dynamic effect of the displaced plantar plate and the importance of the integrity of the plantar plate-deep transverse metatarsal ligament tie-bar. *Annals of the Royal College of Surgeons of England* 1997;**79**:58–68.
- 22. Kumar S, Gow P. A survey of indications, results and complications of surgery for tophaceous gout. *New Zealand Medical Journal* 2002;**115**:U109.

130

Nerve compression syndromes of the foot and ankle

GISELLE TAN, NORMAN ESPINOSA, ANISH RAJ KADAKIA

Introduction	1500	Anterior tarsal tunnel syndrome	1505
Anatomy	1500	Entrapment of the superficial peroneal nerve	1506
Interdigital plantar neuroma (Morton's neuroma)	1500	Summary	1506
Tarsal tunnel syndrome	1502	References	1507
Lateral plantar nerve entrapment	1504		

NATIONAL BOARD STANDARDS

- Understand the pathoanatomy and pathophysiology of nerve compression disorders
- Understand the critical history and physical examination points in diagnosing nerve compression disorders
- Know the rationale for choosing conservative treatments and the appropriate indications for surgical intervention

INTRODUCTION

Nerve entrapment pathology of the foot and ankle constitutes an important yet frequently unrecognized aetiology of foot pain. The more common entities include interdigital neuroma (Morton's neuroma), tarsal tunnel syndrome, compression of the lateral plantar nerve, anterior tarsal tunnel syndrome (compression of deep peroneal nerve) and compression of the superficial peroneal nerve. It is important to understand the neuroanatomy of the foot and ankle to diagnose and treat these entrapment neuropathies. Treatment modalities range from conservative management with footwear modification designed to decrease pressure on the pathological nerve to surgical decompression or excision.

ANATOMY

There are five major nerves that enter the foot. The tibial nerve lies posteromedially and divides into the calcaneal branches and the medial and lateral plantar nerve. Note that the lateral plantar nerve courses deep to the abductor hallucis muscle and the first branch supplies the nerve to the abductor digiti quinti. The saphenous nerve courses with the saphenous vein over the medial aspect of the ankle. The deep peroneal nerve travels with the anterior tibial artery between the extensor hallucis longus (EHL) and extensor digitorum longus (EDL) and courses deep to the extensor retinaculum to supply sensation to the first web space. The superficial peroneal nerve exits the deep fascia anterolaterally, which can vary between 8 and 12 cm above the tip of the lateral malleolus, to supply the dorsum of the foot. The sural nerve runs lateral to the Achilles tendon adjacent to the short saphenous vein innervating the lateral aspect of the foot.

INTERDIGITAL PLANTAR NEUROMA (MORTON'S NEUROMA)

Aetiology

Plantar interdigital neuroma, also commonly referred to as Morton's neuroma, is a benign perineural and endoneural fibrosis of the common plantar digital nerve.[1]

This was described in the English language first by Durlacher[2] in 1845 and then by Morton[3] in 1876. It occurs in women nearly 10 times more frequently than in men, possibly secondary to fashion footwear. The nerve changes appear distal to the deep transverse metatarsal ligament[4] and is most common in the third web space followed by the second web space. This condition is thought to be mechanically induced and not a true neuroma but rather an entrapment neuropathy. It is hypothesized that constant traction of the nerve against the ligament when the toes are brought into a dorsiflexed position causes degeneration of the nerve fibres. Excessive motion between the third and fourth metatarsal heads as well as traumatic factors have also been cited as possible causes. There are many conditions that can mimic symptoms seen in patients with interdigital neuroma that makes adequate treatment difficult and even more complex in the presence of recurrent interdigital neuroma.

Anatomic factors

It has been hypothesized that in some individuals communicating branches between the lateral plantar nerve (LPN) and medial plantar nerve (MPN) within the third webspace attribute to a thicker common digital nerve. However, the frequency of such communicating branches has only been found to be about 28%.

Symptoms

Patients usually present with localized pain, burning or aching in the plantar aspect of the metatarsal head region. Many patients describe radiation of the pain into the toes (62%). Some also report the feeling of having a pebble in the metatarsal head region. Pain is typically exacerbated by walking (92%), wearing tight-fitting or high-heeled shoes and relieved by rest (89%) and shoe removal (70%). Numbness is less frequently reported (40%).

Physical examination

Focal tenderness may be reproduced by squeezing the metatarsal heads together. This Morton's test is performed by grasping the heads of the first and fifth metatarsals and compressing them together. Mulder's click sign consists of milking the small mass of nerve and bursal tissue between the involved metatarsal heads with alternating thumb and forefinger pressure while simultaneously compressing these same metatarsal heads. A palpable click and pain are considered positive findings when this test is performed and are thought to be caused by a large neuroma being forced plantarly by the compressed metatarsal heads.[5] Pain between the interspaces should be distinguished from pain in the metatarsophalangeal joint. The 'mini-Lachmann' test (dorsal and plantar stress testing of the metatarsophalangeal (MTP) joint) is performed to evaluate the MTP joints for possible instability.

Imaging studies

Although radiographs will not show a Morton's neuroma, plain radiographs should be obtained for each foot to determine possible pathology of the MTP joint as the cause of symptoms. There are multiple reports suggesting use of advanced imaging such as MRI and ultrasound. These studies may aid in localization of pathology as well as evaluation of the size of a neuroma prior to surgical intervention,[6] but it is highly operator dependent and, at least in the case of MRI, a prevalence of 30% of presumed Morton's neuroma has been seen in asymptomatic volunteers.[7]

Treatment

CONSERVATIVE MANAGEMENT

Conservative management begins with footwear modification. This includes wearing shoes with a wide toe box and low heels. The use of a metatarsal pad to offload the area of the neuroma and spread apart the metatarsal heads can minimize compression of the nerve. More than 60% of patients in a recent study had complete resolution of symptoms after 1 year follow-up with conservative treatment.[8] Steroid injection into the web space can also diminish a symptomatic Morton's neuroma. The mechanism for this effect is that the steroid induces atrophy of the web space tissue, which decreases the compression and inflammation of the nerve. Reports of 50–80%[9] pain relief have been reported but the concern of local fat atrophy, hypopigmentation and local skin thinning may make this option less desirable, especially in patients requiring multiple injection treatments. Additionally, it is not recommended to perform surgery within 4 weeks after local injection of steroids. Radiofrequency ablation and alcohol nerve injections have been reported to be less traumatic. A recent study presented more than 90% of patients having a partial or total symptomatic relief after ultrasound-guided injections with alcohol (70% carbocaine–adrenaline (noradrenaline) and 30% ethylic alcohol).

Surgical intervention

In patients who have failed conservative management, surgical excision of the nerve can be performed. There are multiple surgical incisions described in the literature. The two most common incisions involve a longitudinal dorsal or plantar approach. A retrospective analysis showed no difference in clinical outcome or patient satisfaction with either approach. However, proponents of the dorsal approach claim that there are fewer problems observed with scar formation. If a keloid develops from any plantar incision the symptoms can become very difficult to treat.

Surgical technique

TECHNIQUE FOR DORSAL APPROACH

An incision is made in the dorsal aspect of the foot, starting in the web space over the affected common interdigital nerve. The length of the incision varies but usually measures 3 cm. Take care not to cut one of the dorsal digital nerves. The incision is deepened through the subcutaneous tissue. The innominate fascia is explored and incised. Afterwards a laminar spreader is placed between the metatarsal heads. After spreading the transverse metatarsal ligament becomes taut. This can now be split. The spreader is placed a little bit deeper. The nerve is explored and the proximal part of it identified. Ensure that you can follow the proximal part of the common digital nerve until it passes underneath the intrinsic musculature. Proximally, the common digital nerve is cut proximal to the metatarsal heads. The nerve is then dissected out distally past the bifurcation and excised. Make sure to remove any accessory branch to either the common or the interdigital nerves. The nerve specimen is sent for histological examination (Fig. 130.1).

TECHNIQUE FOR PLANTAR APPROACH

The incision must be strictly kept between the metatarsals. An improper incision is unforgiving. The incision is carried out through the subcutaneous tissue. The common digital nerve is exposed and traced down to the bifurcation. The nerve branches are cut and the specimen sent to pathology.

The success rate of surgical intervention is in the 70–80% range with an approximately 7–24% failure rate.[10] This failure rate may be secondary to incorrect diagnosis prior to surgical intervention versus the development of a recurrent neuroma. This recurrent neuroma can be a true neuroma following transaction of the common digital nerve. This can occur if the transaction is not made proximal enough or the nerve has become trapped or scarred beneath the metatarsal head. A Tinel's sign is often positive in these cases. If the pain is well localized, re-exploration can be performed and the nerve transected to a more proximal level or transposed into muscle.[11] However, results of revision neuroma surgery are poor.

TARSAL TUNNEL SYNDROME

Aetiology

Tarsal tunnel syndrome is a compression neuropathy of the tibial nerve or one of its branches. It was described independently by Keck[12] and Lam[13] in 1962 when they released the fibro-osseous tunnel created by the flexor retinaculum over the distal tibia, talus and calcaneous. This condition affects men and women equally and in long-standing cases can progress to development of sensory and motor paralysis.[14] Space-occupying lesions, such as engorged varicose veins, neurilemoma (benign nerve sheath tumour), pigmented villonodular synovitis, lipomas, synovial cysts, intraneural degenerative cysts and ganglion cysts (flexor hallucis longus tendon sheaths), can result in tibial nerve entrapment. Trauma may be the most common cause of tarsal tunnel syndrome as displaced fractures of the talus, calcaneus, distal tibia or recurrent sprains of the deltoid ligament lead to decreased area in the tarsal tunnel leading to tibial nerve entrapment.[15] A varus or valgus hindfoot along with a pronated forefoot has an increased susceptibility to tarsal tunnel syndrome.[16] An accessory soleus and the flexor digitorum accessorius longus have also been implicated as causes of this syndrome.[17,18]

Tarsal tunnel syndrome can be divided into proximal and distal syndromes. The proximal tunnel syndrome affects the entire tibial nerve whereas the distal syndrome affects one of its terminal branches. The distal end of the tunnel is a connective tissue partition between the medial and lateral plantar nerves that originates from the medial calcaneus and is attached to the fascia of the abductor hallucis.

The lateral plantar nerve is the most vulnerable to entrapment in the tarsal tunnel. It usually travels in its own separate and more proximal slip of the tarsal tunnel and it changes from an inferior to lateral direction beneath the abductor hallucis. The first branch of the lateral plantar nerve supplies the abductor digiti quiti.

'Jogger's foot' described by Rask[19] is the local entrapment of the medial plantar nerve at the fibromuscular tunnel outlined by the abductor hallucis and its border with the navicular. There is a strong association with a valgus foot and long-distance running. This is usually characterized by exercise-induced pain in the medial plantar nerve distribution with radiation to the medial arch and toes.

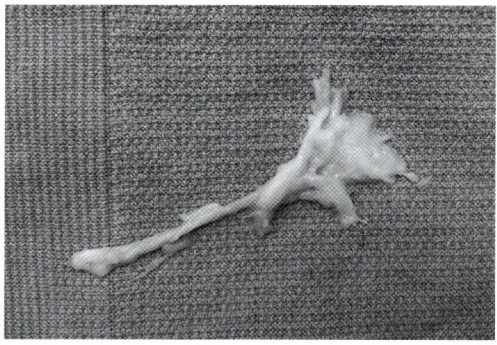

Figure 130.1 Pathological specimen of an interdigital neuroma.

Anatomy

The tarsal tunnel is formed by the fibro-osseous tunnel of the flexor retinaculum as it wraps around the posterior aspect of the medial malleolus encasing all the medial structures of the ankle. The floor is formed by the medial talar surface, the sustentaculum tali and the medial calcaneal wall. The flexor retinaculum, which is renamed the lacinate ligament, forms the roof of the tarsal tunnel. The lacinate ligament encases the posterior tibial, flexor digitorum longus and flexor hallucis longus tendons as well as the posterior tibial artery and tibial nerve in its own compartment. The base of the flexor retinaculum is the superior edge of the abductor hallucis.

The volume in the tunnel is greatest when the foot is in the neutral position, decreasing in inversion and eversion. A specific test for tarsal tunnel syndrome has been described.[20] In this test, the ankle is passively and maximally dorsiflexed and everted while all metatarsophalangeal joints are maximally dorsiflexed. This position is held for 5–10 seconds. A positive result occurs if the patient reports recreation of their pain and numbness.

Symptoms

Patients report a poorly localized tingling or a burning or aching sensation over the plantar aspect of the foot along with pain in this distribution when the foot is inverted or everted or when direct pressure applied along the nerve. Tinel's sign can be elicited in the distribution of the tibial nerve or its branches. Sensory loss in this distribution is manifested by a decrease in two-point discrimination over the plantar aspect of the foot. Pain may also radiate proximally to the calf, which is known as the Valliex phenomenon. This phenomenon may also be present in a more proximal nerve entrapment creating a so-called 'double crush' nerve disorder. Discomfort is worse after activity and at the end of the working day. Some patients report night pain that wakes them from sleep. Symptoms are relieved with rest, elevation and wearing of loose shoes. This syndrome may present with similar symptoms to plantar fasciitis, in which pain is over the origin of the plantar fascia on the medial calcaneal tuberosity.

Imaging studies

Plain weight-bearing radiographs of the foot and ankle should be obtained to rule out bony pathology that may cause pain, such as fractures, accessory ossicles and spurs in the area of the tarsal tunnel. If no bony abnormality is seen, an MRI can assess for the contents of the tarsal tunnel.[21] This is particularly useful if a mass is suspected in the tunnel and makes surgical planning more facile.

Electromyography can also help with diagnosis of tarsal tunnel syndrome. Many groups have likened tarsal tunnel syndrome to carpal tunnel syndrome in the hand. A retrospective review of electromyogram (EMG) studies of tarsal tunnel syndrome reported an 82% abnormal sensory conduction velocity and a 74% distal motor latency abnormality in either the abductor hallucis or abductor digiti quinti.[22] Given that some patients with tarsal tunnel syndrome have a normal EMG study, it is recommended that the diagnosis be made only if the patient has all of the following symptoms: pain and paraesthesias in the foot, positive Tinel's sign and a positive EMG.[23]

Treatment

CONSERVATIVE MANAGEMENT

In the absence of any lesion that could lead to nerve entrapment, non-operative measures are recommended. This can consist of administration of non-steroidal anti-inflammatory drugs (NSAIDs) to reduce the inflammatory response, oral vitamin B6 and tricyclic antidepressants (imipramine, nortryptiline, desipramine, amitriptyline). Besides those medications, there are also selective serotonin reuptake inhibitors (sertraline, paroxetine, duloxetine) or antiseizure drugs (gabapentin, topiramate, pregabalin, carbamazepine) that can be used. Currently there are no clear guidelines in the literature to help guide treatment.

Initial treatment should also be geared towards correcting any foot deformity that may decrease the volume of the tarsal tunnel. For flexible hindfoot deformities, orthotics can be used: lateral heel wedges for a varus hindfoot, medial arch supports for a valgus heel and splinting in a neutral position work well as initial treatment. Physical therapy to strengthen the intrinsic and extrinsic muscles of the foot to restore the medial longitudinal arch is a modality that should be suggested to all patients. Local corticosteroid injections can be used to decrease the inflammatory response of the nerve.

SURGICAL INTERVENTION

A symptomatic space-occupying lesion in the tarsal tunnel is one of the few clear indications for surgical decompression. Surgical exploration of the tarsal tunnel is a good option for patients with documented focal compression of the tibial nerve. Patients should be warned that pain symptoms may not be completely relieved.

SURGICAL TECHNIQUE

The patient is positioned supine, and under tourniquet control a curved incision is made parallel to the flexor tendons just posterior to the posterior tibial artery above and below the medial malleolus. The dissection is carried down to the flexor retinaculum (Fig. 130.2) The tibial nerve is identified proximally and protected as the lacinate

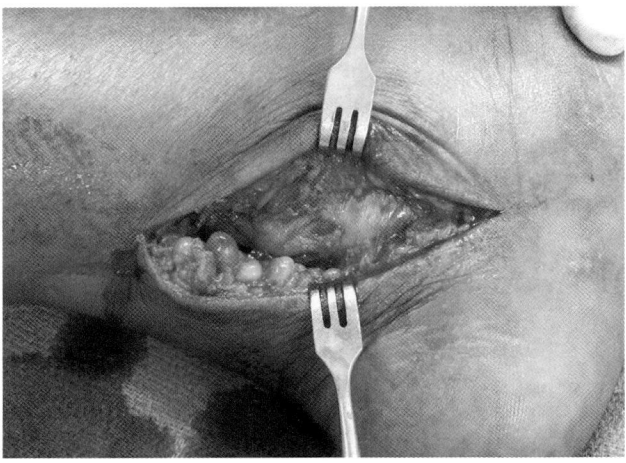

Figure 130.2 Intra-operative photograph demonstrating an intact flexor retinaculum that must be incised to release the tarsal tunnel.

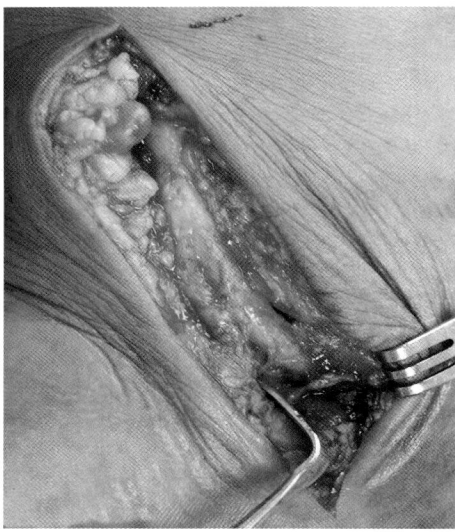

Figure 130.3 Intra-operative photograph demonstrating a full release of the tarsal tunnel. Note the bifurcation distally and the length of the incision required to perform the release.

ligament is incised. The calcaneal, medial plantar and lateral plantar nerve branches are identified and exposed along their course to the plantar foot, releasing the septa between these nerves from the lacinate ligament. The fascia of the abductor hallucis is incised to the level of the plantar fascia. The main trunk of the posterior tibial nerve is inspected, and any constricting bands of tissue are released (Fig. 130.3). The wound is irrigated and the tourniquet released. Meticulous haemostasis should be maintained. The incision is closed in layers, leaving the flexor retinaculum open. The leg is placed in a well-padded posterior splint with the ankle in neutral.

Patients should be instructed to be non-weight-bearing for 10–14 days and the extremity should be elevated for the first few days. Sutures are removed in 2 weeks and weight bearing can be advanced as tolerated. No further splinting is necessary and physical therapy is not necessary.[24]

There are many reports on outcomes after surgical decompression of the tarsal tunnel. Patient satisfaction is usually linked to pain relief, functional activities, appearance and motion. Patients with longstanding symptoms greater than 1 year have less satisfaction with their outcomes than patients with symptoms less than 1 year. Patients with space-occupying lesions had better outcomes than patients with idiopathic, post-traumatic or anomalous muscle causes of tarsal tunnel syndrome. Generally patients report from 44% to 95% satisfaction after surgical exploration.[25–28]

LATERAL PLANTAR NERVE ENTRAPMENT

Aetiology

Among all patients suffering from chronic heel pain up to 20% are thought to have an entrapment of the first branch of the lateral plantar nerve. Entrapment of the first branch of the lateral plantar nerve occurs mainly between the fascia of the abductor hallucis muscle and the medial caudal margin of the quadratus plantae.

Anatomy

The first branch of the lateral plantar nerve runs between the abductor hallucis muscle and the quadratus plantae in an oblique direction. The first branch then divides into three branches that innervate the periosteum of the medial process of the calcaneal tuberosity, the flexor digitorum brevis, the plantar ligament and the abductor digiti minimi muscle.

Symptoms

The diagnosis is made based on clinical findings. More proximal and distal nerve entrapments must be excluded. Patients often report chronic heel pain. The symptoms might be worse during higher activity levels, for example running. The pain radiates from the medial inferior aspect of the heel more proximally into the medial area of the ankle or laterally and plantar into the foot. Tenderness (reproducible symptoms and radiation of pain proximally and distally of the spot) over the first branch of the lateral plantar nerve deep to the abductor hallucis muscle is a pathognomonic finding.

Treatment

The problem of lateral plantar nerve entrapment is that it often goes mis- or undiagnosed. Many patients are treated for plantar fasciitis instead of the nerve disease. Thus, the delay until proper treatment can be started has been found to average 22 months since initial presentation of symptoms.

CONSERVATIVE MANAGEMENT

Non-operative measures include rest, NSAIDs, contrast baths, ice massage, physical therapy and steroid injections (in athletes). A shock-absorbing heel pad could help to diminish inflammation and pressure. Excessive pronation can be decreased by means of orthotic devices.

SURGICAL TREATMENT

When conservative treatment fails release of the first branch of the lateral plantar nerve is recommended.

ANTERIOR TARSAL TUNNEL SYNDROME

Aetiology

This syndrome was first described by Kopell and Thompson[29] in 1960, when they identified compression of the deep peroneal nerve under the inferior extensor retinaculum on the dorsum of the foot. The compression resulted in paraesthesias that radiated into the hallux and second toe. Osteophyte formation at the talonavicular or metatarsocuneiform joint may also compress the nerve as it courses along the dorsal surface of the foot. This was termed 'anterior tarsal tunnel syndrome' by Marinacci[30] in 1968. The most common cause of this relatively rare entrapment syndrome is local trauma such as a sprain of the ankle or midfoot. Space-occupying lesions such as ganglions or tight footwear have also been implicated in producing nerve irritation.

Anatomy

The anterior tarsal tunnel is a fibro-osseous tunnel between the inferior extensor retinaculum and the fascia overlying the talus and navicular. The superficial branch of the deep peroneal nerve and the anterior tibial artery pass longitudinally through this tunnel and between the EHL and EDL tendons. Proximal to the ankle the nerve has motor and sensory components and at about 1.5 cm proximal to the head of the talus it divides into the medial and lateral branches, which supply sensation to the first web space and motor innervation to the extensor digitorum brevis.

Symptoms

Patients often complain of continuous paraesthesias with aching and numbness radiating from the dorsum of the foot to the hallux and second toe. Patients also complain of weakness in hallux extension and fatigue when walking. Dorsiflexion of the foot improves symptoms whereas plantarflexion and wearing high-heels and tight shoe laces exacerbate them. Pain and paraesthesias can also awaken patients at night as the foot falls into plantarflexion.

A careful history can delineate the patient's course of paraesthesias. On examination there is weakness of the hallux extension with sensation impaired in the skin of the first web space. Percussion of the nerve as it courses over the anterior tarsal tunnel just lateral to the EHL tendon often produces a positive Tinel's sign. Wasting of the extensor hallucis brevis and extensor digitorum brevis may also be seen.

The differential diagnosis includes L5 radiculopathy. Occasionally referred pain in the distribution of the superficial branch of the deep peroneal nerve may be secondary to anterior exertional compartment syndrome.

Imaging studies

Plain radiographs of the foot and ankle should be obtained to evaluate for possible osteophytes that may compress the nerve along its course in the midfoot. Electromyograms may also be performed to evaluate for involvement of the extensor digitorum brevis. Normal distal latency of the extensor digitorum brevis is 4.53 ms.[31] If this is increased, it suggests a lesion proximal to the inferior extensor retinaculum.

Treatment

CONSERVATIVE MANAGEMENT

Initial management should attempt to keep pressure off the area of entrapment either by padding the tongue of the shoe or creating a pad that keeps pressure off the nerve. An injection of corticosteroid with local anaesthetic into the area of entrapment is also useful in diagnosis and treatment of this syndrome.

SURGICAL INTERVENTION

When conservative management fails, the nerve may be decompressed by releasing the anterior tarsal tunnel.

Surgical technique

A 6 cm longitudinal incision is made along the lateral border of the EHL tendon below the ankle. Care must be used to protect the lateral subcutaneous branch of the superficial peroneal nerve. The inferior extensor retinaculum is incised and the deep peroneal nerve and anterior tibial artery are identified. The nerve should not be excessively manipulated and unnecessary dissection of the loose areolar tissue around the nerve should be avoided. Remove any prominent osteophytes or obstructing ganglions. The extensor retinaculum is not repaired and the skin is closed. A soft dressing is applied and gradual resumption of activity is allowed over the next 4–6 weeks.

ENTRAPMENT OF THE SUPERFICIAL PERONEAL NERVE

Aetiology

Entrapment of the superficial peroneal nerve as it emerges from the subfascial to the subcutaneous tissue in the peroneal tunnel was initially described by Henry in 1945.[32] The age of affection averages 28 years for athletic individuals and 36 years for the non-athletic population. The most common presenting symptom is pain across the ankle joint and dorsum of the foot. Chronic ankle sprains can lead to stretching of the superficial peroneal nerve and induce a focal lesion. Other causes include previous anterior compartment fasciotomy, direct trauma, ganglion, fibular fracture, exertional compartment syndrome, muscle herniation, syndesmotic sprains, lower extremity oedema and neoplasia.

Anatomy

The superficial peroneal nerve exits the deep fascia of the lateral compartment approximately 8–12 cm above the tip of the fibula. Here the nerve typically exits in a fibrous tunnel. The nerve can be compressed at several sites as it exits this fibrous tunnel. Several authors have also found that the superficial peroneal nerve may have an anomalous course into the anterior compartment. The anomalous course does not imply increased likelihood of developing entrapment of the nerve but it does increase the awareness that decompression of the nerve in the lateral compartment may not be sufficient.[33]

Symptoms

Patients often have pain and numbness over the lateral aspect of the ankle extending into the foot. Styf and Morberg[34] report three provocative tests: first, pressure is applied where the nerve emerges from the deep fascia while the patient actively dorsiflexes and everts against resistance; second, the foot is passively plantarflexed and inverted without local pressure over the nerve; and, finally, while maintaining passive stretch gentle percussion over the course of the nerve is applied. Symptoms with any of these tests suggest entrapment of the superficial peroneal nerve. Nerve pain must be distinguished from joint pain in these tests as ankle instability may also mimic nerve pain in this distribution.[35]

Imaging studies

Plain radiographs of the foot, ankle and leg should be taken to rule out possible stress fracture of other bony pathology. EMGs can be obtained to evaluate anterior tibial and peroneal muscle conduction velocities. A conduction velocity below 44 ms was considered abnormal. It should be noted that a normal study does not exclude this diagnosis.

Treatment

Conservative management includes adding lateral wedges to shoes and physical therapy to increase the stability of the ankle. A trial injection of corticosteroids along with local anaesthetic can be diagnostic and therapeutic and help delineate the location of entrapment. In most cases patients have had symptoms for quite some time with the mean duration of symptoms in a large study documented to be nearly 5 years. In longstanding cases surgical release of the superficial peroneal nerve is warranted. Approximately 80% of patients report good to excellent results after surgical decompression.[34] Should the symptoms persist after release, then re-exploration and transection and burial into muscle as well is considered.

SUMMARY

Nerve entrapment syndromes of the foot and ankle are difficult to diagnose and treat. The operative treatments available will invariably lead to a poor result if the diagnosis is not correct. A careful physical examination with a detailed focus on the location and type of pain is critical in obtaining the correct diagnosis. Adjuvant studies, which have become prevalent in orthopaedics, do not supersede in importance a thorough history and physical examination for nerve entrapment disorders.

> **KEY LEARNING POINTS**
>
> - Nerve entrapment about the foot and ankle is a common cause of foot pain.
> - The diagnosis is difficult, a careful clinical examination is paramount (especially Tinel's test).
> - Common entities include interdigital neuroma (Morton's neuroma), tarsal tunnel syndrome, compression of the lateral plantar nerve, anterior tarsal tunnel syndrome (compression of the deep peroneal nerve) and compression of the superficial peroneal nerve.
> - Plantar interdigital neuroma (Morton's neuroma) is a benign perineural and endoneural fibrosis of the common plantar digital nerve.
> - Focal tenderness may be reproduced by squeezing the metatarsal heads together (Morton's test).
> - When footwear modification fails, surgical excision of the nerve may be required (dorsal or plantar approaches).

- Tarsal tunnel syndrome is a compression neuropathy of the tibial nerve or one of its branches (akin to carpal tunnel syndrome); the lateral plantar nerve is the most vulnerable to entrapment. A symptomatic space-occupying lesion in the tunnel is one of the few clear indications for surgical decompression.
- Lateral plantar nerve entrapment is often missed.
- Anterior tarsal tunnel syndrome is where there is paraesthesias, aching and numbness from the dorsum of the foot to the first and second toes. The nerve may need to be decompressed.
- Entrapment of the superficial peroneal nerve presents with pain and numbness over the lateral ankle to the foot. Exclude a stress fracture. Surgical decompression release may be required in longstanding cases.

REFERENCES

- ● = Key primary paper
- ◆ = Major review article

●1. Giannini S, Bacchini P, Ceccarelli F, Vannini F. Interdigital neuroma: clinical examination and histopathologic results in 63 cases treated with Excision. *Foot and Ankle International* 2004;**25**:79-84.

◆2. Durlacher L. *Treastise on Corns, Bunions, the Disease of the Nails and the General Management of Feet.* London, UK: Simpkin and Marshal, 1845:52.

●3. Morton TG. A peculiar and painful affection of the fourth metatarsophalangeal articulation. *American Journal of Medical Science* 1876;**71**:37.

●4. Kim J, Choi JH, Park J, et al. An anatomical study of Morton's Interdigital neuroma: the relationship between the occurring site and deep transverse metatarsal ligament. *Foot and Ankle International* 2007;**28**:1007-10.

◆5. Reider B. The orthopaedic physical examination, 2nd edn. Elsevier Saunders, 2005:292-4.

●6. Biasca N, Zanetti M, Zollinger H. Outcomes after partial neurectomy of Morton's neuroma related to preoperative case histories, clinical findings, and findings on magnetic resonance imaging scans. *Foot and Ankle International* 1999;**20**:568-75.

7. Zanetti M, Strehle J, Zollinger H, Hodler J. Morton's neuroma and fluid in the intermetatarsal bursae on MR images of 70 asymptomatic volunteers. *Radiology* 1997;**203**:516-20.

●8. Saygi B, Yildirim Y, Saygi EK, et al. Morton neuroma: comparative results of two conservative methods. *Foot and Ankle International* 2005;**26**:556-9.

●9. Markovic M, Crichton K, Read JW, et al. Effectiveness of ultrasound-guided corticosteroid injection in the treatment of Morton's neuroma. *Foot and Ankle International* 2008;**29**:483-7.

●10. Akermark C, Crone H, Saartok T, Zuber Z. Plantar versus dorsal incision in the treatment of primary intermetatarsal Morton's neuroma. *Foot and Ankle International* 2008;**29**:136-41.

●11. Stamatis ED, Myerson MS. Treatment of recurrence of symptoms after excision of an interdigital neuroma. *Journal of Bone and Joint Surgery (British)* 2004;**86**:48-53.

●12. Keck C. The tarsal tunnel syndrome. *Journal of Bone and Joint Surgery* 1962;**44**:180-2.

●13. Lam SJS. A tarsal tunnel syndrome. *Lancet* 1962;**2**:1354-5.

●14. Lam SJS. Tarsal tunnel syndrome. *Journal of Bone and Joint Surgery (British)* 1967;**49B**:87-92.

◆15. Lau JTC, Daniels TR. Tarsal tunnel syndrome: a review of the literature. *Foot and Ankle International* 1999;**20**:202-9.

◆16. Radin EL. Tarsal tunnel syndrome. *Clinical Orthopaedics and Related Research* 1982;**181**:167-70.

17. Sammarco GJ, Stephens MM. Tarsal tunnel syndrome caused by the flexor digitorum accessorius longus. *Journal of Bone and Joint Surgery* 1990;**72A**:453-4.

18. Kinoshita M, Okuda R, Morikawa J, Abe M. Tarsal tunnel syndrome associated with an accessory muscle. *Foot and Ankle International* 2003;**24**:132-6.

19. Rask MR. Medial plantar neuropraxia (Jogger's foot): report of 3 cases. *Clinical Orthopaedics* 1978;**134**:193-5.

●20. Kinoshita M, Okuda T, Morikawa J, et al. The dorsiflexion-eversion test for diagnosis of tarsal tunnel syndrome. *Journal of Bone and Joint Surgery* 2001;**83A**:1835-9.

●21. Frey C, Kerr R. Magnetic resonance imaging and the evaluation of tarsal tunnel syndrome. *Foot and Ankle* 1993;**14**:159-64.

22. Mondelli M, Morana P, Padua L. An electrophysiological severity scale in tarsal tunnel syndrome. *Acta Neurologica Scandinavica* 2004;**109**:284-9.

●23. Galardi G, Amadio S, Maderna L, et al. Electrophysiologic studies in tarsal tunnel syndrome: a diagnostic reliability of motor distal latency, mixed nerve and sensory nerve conduction studies. *American Journal of Physical Medicine and Rehabilitation* 1994;**73**:193-8.

24. Bailie DS, Kelikian AS. Tarsal tunnel syndrome: diagnosis, surgical technique and functional outcome. *Foot and Ankle International* 1998;**19**:65-72.

25. Turan I, Rivero-Melian C, Guntner P, Rolf C. Tarsal tunnel syndrome: outcome of surgery in long standing cases. *Clinical Orthopaedics and Related Research* 1997;**343**:151-6.

26. Takakura Y, Kitada C, Sugimoto K, et al. Tarsal tunnel syndrome: causes and results of operative treatment. *Journal of Bone and Joint Surgery (British)* 1991;**73B**:125-8.

27. Urguden M, Bilbasar H, Ozdemir H, et al. Tarsal tunnel syndrome: the effect of the associated features on outcome of surgery. *International Orthopaedics* 2002;**26**:253-6.

28. Sammarco GJ, Chang L. Outcome of surgical treatment of tarsal tunnel syndrome. *Foot and Ankle International* 2003;**24**:125–31.
29. Kopell HP, Thompson WAL. Peripheral entrapment neuropathies of the lower extremity. *New England Journal of Medicine* 1960;**262**:56–60.
●30. Marinacci AA. Neurological syndromes of the tarsal tunnels. *Bulletin of the Los Angeles Neurological Society* 1968;**33**:90–100.
31. Zongzhao L, Jiansheng Z, Li Z. Anterior tarsal tunnel syndrome. *Journal of Bone and Joint Surgery (British)* 1991;**73B**:470–3.
32. Rosson GD, Dellon AL. Superficial peroneal nerve anatomic variability changes surgical technique. *Clinical Orthopaedics and Related Research* 2005;**438**:248–52.
33. Henry AK. *Extensive Exposure*. Edinburgh, UK: E. & S. Livingstone, 1945:163.
●34. Styf J, Morberg P. The superficial peroneal tunnel syndrome: results of treatment by decompression. *Journal of Bone and Joint Surgery (British)* 1997;**79B**:801–3.
◆35. Beskin JL. Nerve entrapment syndromes of the foot and ankle. *Journal of the American Academy of Orthopaedic Surgeons* 1997;**5**:261–9.

PART **12**

NEW TECHNOLOGIES AND BEST CLINICAL PRACTICE

PATRICK WARNKE AND SURESHAN SIVANANTHAN

131	**Computer-assisted navigation in orthopaedic surgery** *Kamal Deep*	1511
132	**Orthopaedic tissue engineering** *Patrick H Warnke*	1524
133	**Medical ethics** *Rachel G Geddes, Suresh Sivananthan*	1531
134	**Outcomes, databanks (joint registries), medical coding** *Eugene Sherry, Sureshan Sivananthan, Raquel Gehr*	1536
135	**Informed consent** *Eugene Sherry, Raquel Gehr*	1539
136	**Work-related injuries and assessment for compensation** *Eugene Sherry, Raquel Gehr*	1542
137	**Evidence-based medicine and orthopaedic surgeons** *Patrick H Warnke, Eugene Sherry, Conor sherry*	1545
138	**Risk management through burnout prevention in orthopaedic surgeons** *Sue Besomo*	1549

131

Computer-assisted navigation in orthopaedic surgery

KAMAL DEEP

Introduction	1511	Surgical control	1515
Registration	1511	Use of computer-assisted navigation	1515
Communication	1513	Future of computer assistance in orthopaedic surgery	1522
Computation and presentation	1514	References	1523

NATIONAL BOARD STANDARDS

- Knowledge of the basic process of computer navigation and various surgeries were it may be used
- Knowledge of various registration methods and their advantages and disadvantages
- Understanding of the biomechanics of knee and hip joint replacements and the potential advantages of CAOS on TKR and THR
- Knowledge of the advantages and disadvantages of using computer navigation

INTRODUCTION

Computer-assisted navigation has been one of the most striking developments in orthopaedic surgery in recent times. While joint replacement arthroplasty became popular and developed through the 1960s to 1990s, the most effective change so far in the twenty-first century seems to be the use of computer assistance in orthopaedic surgery.

Although limited to spine, knee and hip joint arthroplasty in the beginning, the scope of computer assisted orthopaedic surgery (CAOS) is expanding to other fields. It has been used in anterior cruciate ligament (ACL) reconstruction, trauma, osteotomies and oncology, and the list keeps on growing.

Historically, the use of CAOS in orthopaedics began in the spine, following on from neurosurgical navigation. Its use in joint arthroplasty came about in the early 1990s, when robotic joint replacements were attempted. Then came computer-assisted navigation. Although both use computers, the difference between robotic surgery and computer navigation is that bone cuts in the former are performed by robots and in the latter by surgeons. More recently, there have been attempts to combine the two and exploit the advantages of both.

The basic process of computer navigation involves five steps: registration, communication, computation, presentation and surgical control.

REGISTRATION

This is the process by which the patient-specific anatomy is fed into the computer so that a virtual three-dimensional (3D) model of the required anatomical elements can be formed. There are different ways of doing this, including CT scan, fluoroscopy, ultrasound and imageless methods. Each has its advantages and disadvantages.

CT scan

A CT scan is done pre-operatively; digital format is required to process the information. Next, a 3D reconstruction of the

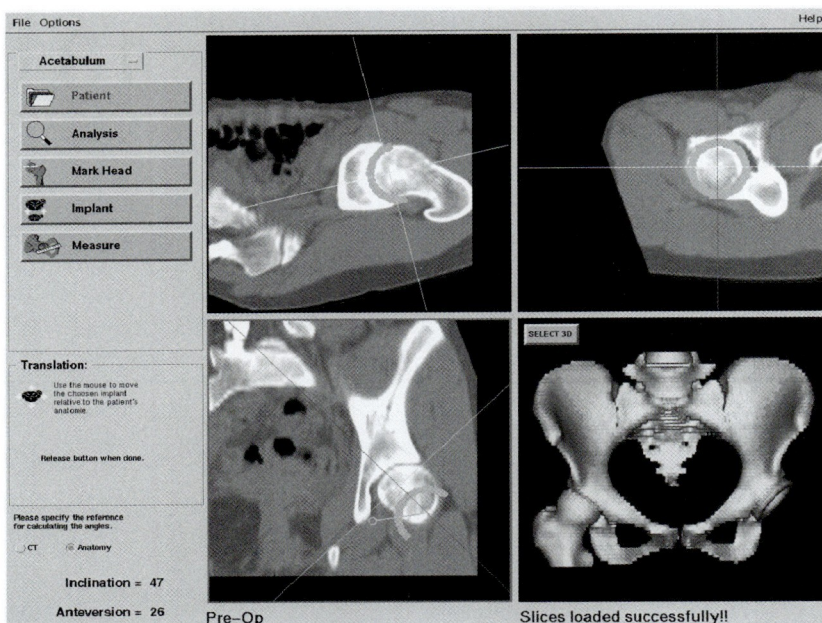

Figure 131.1 CT scan-based registration of anatomy.

acquired CT images is produced. To do this, some specific reference points on the CT scan are marked (Fig. 131.1). These reference points denote specific important bony landmarks that can be used to make a virtual model of bones and joints for that patient. These points are then cross-referenced during the surgical procedure. With the advent of intra-operative CT facilities in some centres, the possibility of intra-operative CT registration is now being investigated.

ADVANTAGES

- Accuracy.
- The data from the CT scan can be cross-checked pre-operatively and post-operatively.
- Proponents claim it is time saving during the procedure.

DISADVANTAGES

- Exposes the patient to more radiation.
- Time consuming, as the surgeon has to spend a lot of time planning on the CT images before the operation.
- Involves more manpower and space.
- It has financial implications.
- The surgeon has to be specifically trained to interpret the CT pictures and plan the surgery.

Fluoroscopy

Fluoroscopy can be used intra-operatively to delineate patient anatomy by means of computer software. Two-dimensional images are used to portray the virtual anatomy. Specific calibration is required to maintain accuracy. A calibrated grid with markers that have known size and spatial relationship is combined with the image. Images are taken with the dynamic reference base (DRB) in place to obtain a virtual model that allows the fluoroscopic image to be navigated. More advanced versions are now available and these are more useful in spinal surgery.

ADVANTAGES

- Intra-operative registration.
- Accuracy.
- Less time consuming than CT scan registration.
- More economical than CT scan registration.

DISADVANTAGES

- Cumbersome to use during surgery.
- Exposes the patient and the surgical team to radiation.

Ultrasound

The use of ultrasound for registration is still under development. It is used mainly for total hip replacement arthroplasty. It requires the surgeon to focus the ultrasound beam on specific points such as the anterior superior iliac spines to register the pelvic plane.

ADVANTAGES

- It has the potential advantage of registering deep bony points, especially in obese patients.

DISADVANTAGES

- The surgeon needs to be trained in ultrasonography.
- The ultrasound gel is a potential source of infection.
- The accuracy of the process needs to be validated and is operator dependent.

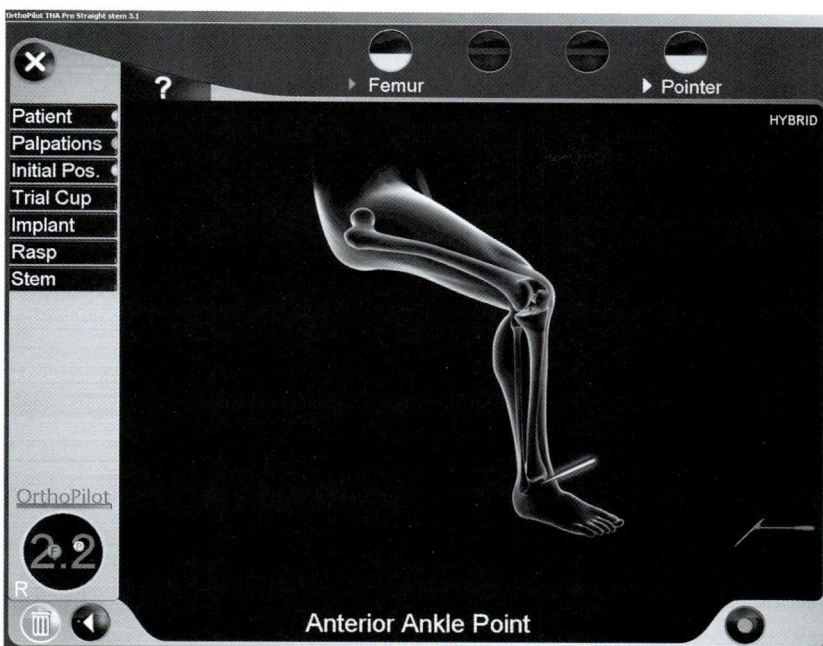

Figure 131.2 Point-based registration of anatomy. Screenshot from OrthoPilot® Navigation System. Image reproduced with permission from B. Braun Meslungen AG.

Imageless registration

This is the most frequently used form of registration for knee and hip arthroplasty. The surgeon has a pointed probe that he/she places on different bony landmarks of importance to produce a virtual model of the patient's bones using a program such as OrthoPilot® (Fig. 131.2). It can be used by a point-touching method, in which only specific points are touched, or by a surface-painting method, in which the probe is moved over the surfaces of the bones and the computer program registers all the points and selects the relevant ones.

ADVANTAGES

- It is simple to use, quicker and more economical than other methods.
- It does not expose the patient or the surgeon to radiation.
- It does not need any pre-operative processing of information.

DISADVANTAGES

- It is surgeon dependent.
- It can be difficult to use in obese patients, especially for total hip replacement.

COMMUNICATION

This is the process by which the computer program can track the patient's bones and instrumentation in 3D space. Fiducial markers (also called trackers or markers) are attached to the bones and instruments of interest. They consist of at least three non-collinear points on a fixed body at different distances and spatial orientation from each other, so that the camera can detect the separate markers and recognize them individually. These form a DRB. Thus, any movement of these fixed trackers can be detected by the camera in 3D space. As these are attached rigidly (or at least intended to be fixed rigidly) to the bone and instruments, the computer translates the tracker movements into the movements of bones and instruments. The communication process involves optical or electromagnetic methods.

Optical communication

Optical methods use infrared waves or visible light rays. Most commonly used are the infrared waves, which are produced by a source near the camera in passive tracking methods or by active light-emitting diodes on the trackers in the active tracking method (Fig. 131.3). In the passive tracking method, the waves are reflected back by round reflective rigid balls that form the DRB (Fig. 131.3); these are then picked up by the camera system by two or more charge-coupled devices. In the active tracking method, the waves come directly from the DRB. The sensor camera system thus configures the different DRBs in space in different orientations and feeds the information into the computing system. It is the different and specific orientations of the DRBs that enable the computer to recognize what it is tracking.

The DRB trackers need to be fixed rigidly to the bone. The tracker can encounter different forces produced accidentally during the procedure by surgeon or assistants.

We studied the strength of fixation in a laboratory setting using different diameter pins and constructs.[1] We found that, in the single pin fixations, bicortical fixations

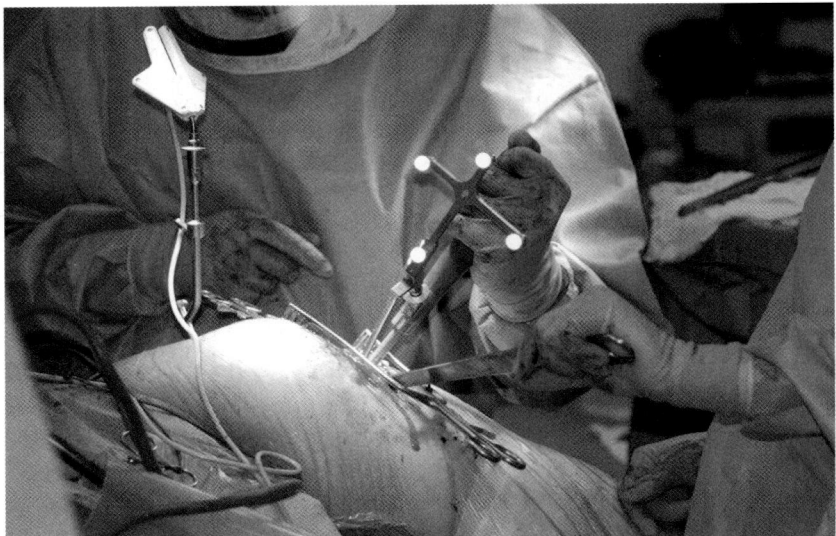

Figure 131.3 The active tracker can be seen in the top left corner attached to the wire, and the passive tracker can be seen with reflective balls as the dynamic reference base in the left hand of the surgeon during a total hip replacement.

were better than unicortical and the greater the diameter, the better the hold. Bicortical pins of 4 mm diameter or more give translatory resistance equivalent to the force required for displacement. Different forces that usually can be accidentally produced during an operation were also measured as 153–208 N, which was at the safety limit for the translatory forces on single bicortical pins (of ⩾4 mm diameter) but exceeded the rotatory resistance (15–30 N) of the single pins. Three-pin fixation of the tracker to the bone gave the best rotational and translatory stability to the construct.

ADVANTAGES

- Easy, accurate and user friendly.
- There are usually no wires involved except in some active trackers produced by specific companies.

POTENTIAL DISADVANTAGES

- Requires a direct line of sight; if there is more than one surgical assistant, he or she may need to move during the operation so that the camera can be aimed directly at the trackers.
- The configuration of the passive reflector balls has to be perfectly round in order to reflect the waves properly.
- The passive balls need to be kept clean during the operation as any blood stains can interfere with their function. This does not seem to be a problem with active trackers.
- The trackers are usually large, although the size has decreased dramatically over the years and these are now much smaller and lighter.
- The other method in optical communication is the use of visible light rays. This method utilizes stickers and discs with a certain orientation of black and white geometric combinations which a camera can pick up. Thus, the computer recognizes various black and white corners of combinations at the point. This method is not as accurate as the infrared waves and operating theatre lights can interfere with recognition. It is not as user friendly as infrared waves.

Electromagnetic communication

This method involves communicating with trackers that can be followed by an electromagnetic field-producing device which is held close to the operating site. This method could be very useful because of its advantages, but, unfortunately, it still has limited use because of metal interference.

ADVANTAGES

- Uses small size trackers, equivalent to the size of a coin; thus, it is more suitable for use in minimally invasive procedures (Fig. 131.4).
- Fixation and stability during the procedure are not a major problem as the trackers sit directly on the bone and are usually away from the surgeon's working area.
- No direct line of sight is required.

DISADVANTAGES

- The major disadvantage is signal interference by metal from instruments and implants.
- The electromagnetic field-producing device needs to be close to the operating field and can be heavy to hold.
- Wires are attached to the trackers; these can interfere in the surgical field.

COMPUTATION AND PRESENTATION

The data from the cameras are fed into the computer, which has complex algorithms to handle all the information in real time. The algorithms are used to produce the virtual model of the patient's anatomy and to track the bones and instruments in space and present all the information to the

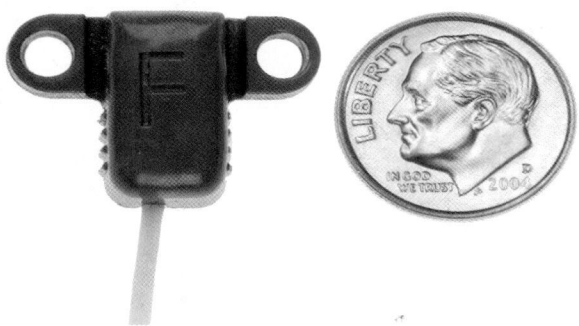

Figure 131.4 The electromagnetic tracker is very small, comparable in size to a coin.

surgeon in a concise and user-friendly way. Although the data presented to the surgeon are limited, a huge number of software calculations are required to produce the data that the surgeon is interested in. The form in which the data are presented to the surgeon can be different for each company producing the navigation system. The software handling the data may also be different for each. But the common thing is that all of these aim to produce the 3D model of patient-specific anatomy and present to the surgeon the orientation of bones and instruments with all six degrees of freedom in space. Some systems try to show very detailed information, but other manufacturers believe that too much information is not desirable or necessary for actually carrying out the steps in the operative process.

SURGICAL CONTROL

The navigation systems allow the surgeon to be in full control of the surgical procedure; this is in contrast to robotic surgery, in which the surgeon sets the steps but cannot control them fully in many prevalent robotic systems. In navigation, the surgeon may, under certain circumstances, overrule the computer if there are doubts about the accuracy of registration or fixity of the markers. Most navigation systems have a method by which the surgeon can navigate the different computer screens and look at the desired data. Some use a foot-controlled switch for this, whereas others use a touch-screen technique with a sterile transparent cover over the screen. In some active systems, the tracker device has triggers that can act as a mouse, and the surgeon can control the computer from the operative field itself. At first, most surgeons need an assistant to control the computer part for them; this is usually a company representative.

USE OF COMPUTER-ASSISTED NAVIGATION

CAOS is undergoing rapid development and is becoming simpler and more user friendly. There are different fields of orthopaedics and trauma in which CAOS techniques are already commonly used, including total knee replacement, total hip replacement, resurfacing hip replacement and spinal procedures. There are also certain areas that are undergoing development; the originators are working in these areas, but they are not as popular in other centres. The developmental areas include ACL reconstructions, unicompartmental knee replacement and osteotomies for tibia, femur and radius. In trauma surgery the uses include intramedullary nailing and pelvic reconstruction surgery. There are other procedures for which CAOS is being developed, including orthopaedic deformity correction surgery, oncology surgery, shoulder arthroplasty and ankle arthroplasty.

The most commonly used single application is for knee arthroplasty, followed by hip arthroplasty.

The uses of CAOS are no longer limited to surgical procedures. It is also being used for research and training, in which it has huge potential.

Further information on total knee arthroplasty and total hip arthroplasty is given in the following sections.

Total knee arthroplasty

The biomechanics of the knee joint are complex and are still not properly understood. The aim of the surgical procedure in total knee arthroplasty is to achieve a stable, well-balanced, well-aligned knee with good function. This requires accurate placement of the components and a good soft-tissue balance. It is desirable to achieve a biomechanical axis, which is an imaginary line passing through the centre of the head of the femur, the knee and the ankle. The biomechanical axis differs in every patient and is not a constant entity. When considering the operative procedure for total knee arthroplasty, one has to analyse each component of it, including the femoral mechanical axis, the tibial mechanical axis and the soft tissues holding these together. The femoral mechanical axis extends from the centre of the femoral head to the centre of the knee. It is conventionally taken as a 6° angle to the anatomical axis that passes through the midline of the femoral shaft. This is not true for every patient. A study carried out at our hospital by Sarungi and associates on 158 patients, including 174 primary total knee replacements, revealed that the angle can range from 2° to 9°, and in 23.6% of cases was either less than 5° or more than 7°[2]. The study used long leg radiographs to calculate both the anatomical and biomechanical axis and to compare them. A standard distal femoral 5° or 7° valgus cut to the anatomical axis, used in the conventional technique of knee replacement surgery, may not produce the desired cut of 90° to the biomechanical axis.

Also, the position of the intramedullary rod used in conventional surgery for referencing the distal femoral cut can vary considerably because the medullary canal is much wider than the diameter of the guiding rod on which the jig sits.

Similarly, for the femoral rotational cut, many surgeons use a 3° external rotation to the dorsal condylar line as their standard conventional measurement for deciding the rotation of the femoral component. It has been suggested that the transepicondylar axis represents the axis around which the knee movements take place. We conducted a study in our hospital on 48 knees. The relationship between the dorsal condylar line and the transepicondylar line was measured. The difference in the two rotational planes ranged from 10° internal rotation to 7° external rotation with a mean of −0.75° and a standard deviation of 3.7°; 52% of the knees had a difference of more than 3°.[3] These studies indicate that the desired biomechanical and rotational axis may not even be known in conventional surgery. Using computer navigation, one can actually see on the computer screen exactly where the cut is being made or the implant is being placed. In addition to the exact bone cuts, it is very important that the correct soft-tissue balance is also achieved for a well-functioning knee. Computer navigation can be very helpful in achieving this. A major advantage of computer-assisted navigation is that one can see the exact results while operating and can correct any errors during the procedure. It does not restrict the surgeon to a specific instruction but shows exactly what the surgeon is doing, thus helping to achieve the best outcome.

CAOS has also challenged the traditional concept of varus or valgus deformity of the knee. In conventional surgery, the soft-tissue releases are done on the basis of the initial deformity in full extension. For a varus deformity in knee extension, soft-tissue release of various structures on the medial side is done in succession until the surgeon judges subjectively that the deformity has been corrected. The same holds true for valgus deformity of the knee, in which the lateral structures are released. It is very difficult to predict what effect these releases will have on the final biomechanics of the knee. The use of computer navigation has shown that the kinematics of an arthritic knee are different in various degrees of flexion. Thus a dynamic mechanical axis may be completely different from what a static mechanical axis represents in an extended knee.

As a result, we conducted a study on the kinematics of arthritic knees.[4] This was done on 283 knees and it was observed that the patterns were not constant varus or valgus but behaved in different ways. We classified these knees into four different types, with further subtypes (Box 131.1).

The neutral type denotes a neutral axis and the varus/valgus types denote varus or valgus as the starting point in

BOX 131.1: Classification of coronal deformity of arthritic/replaced knee[3] (extension to 90° flexion)

- Neutral
- Varus/valgus (starting position in extension) when the knee flexes
- Group 1
  A Deformity remains the same
  B Increasing deformity
- Group 2
  A Decreasing deformity but does not reach neutral
  B Decreasing deformity reaches neutral
- Group 3
  Decreasing deformity and crosses to opposite (varus becomes valgus and valgus becomes varus as the knee flexes) deformity
- Group 4
  A Deformity first increases and then decreases but does not reach neutral
  B Deformity first increases and then decreases to neutral
  C Deformity first increases and then decreases to cross over to opposite deformity

(Tables 131.1 and 131.2 show the frequencies of each type)

Table 131.1 Coronal deformity navigation classification: different types with numbers and percentages in pre-implant arthritic knees

Group	Neutral (n)	Neutral (%)	Varus (n)	Varus (%)	Valgus (n)	Valgus (%)
Neutral	1	0.4				
1A			16	5.7	3	1.1
1B			14	4.9	5	1.8
2A			52	18.4	4	1.4
2B			21	7.4	4	1.4
3			43	15.2	17	6.0
4A			36	12.7	25	8.8
4B			11	3.9	7	2.5
4C			9	3.2	13	4.6

Table 131.2 Coronal deformity navigation classification: different types with numbers and percentages in postimplant replaced knees

Group	Neutral (n)	Neutral (%)	Varus (n)	Varus (%)	Valgus (n)	Valgus (%)
Neutral	144	50.8				
1A			12	4.2	25	8.8
1B			6	2.1	9	3.2
2A			3	1.1	2	0.7
2B			13	4.6	4	1.4
3			30	10.6	14	4.9
4A			1	0.4	9	3.2
4B			2	0.7	5	1.8
4C			1	0.4	3	1.1

extension, and then the group types denote how the deformity behaves when the knee flexes. Only 6.8% of knees behave in a true varus or valgus (group 1a) fashion. The majority (93.2%) of the knees do not behave in this way.[3]

It has also been observed that the knees may not behave in a constant fashion beyond 90° of flexion. This has also been divided into similar groups. One can easily see from Table 131.1 and Fig. 131.5 that a group 3 or group 4C knee is one deformity in extension and the opposite deformity in flexion; therefore, the surgeon needs to be very careful in

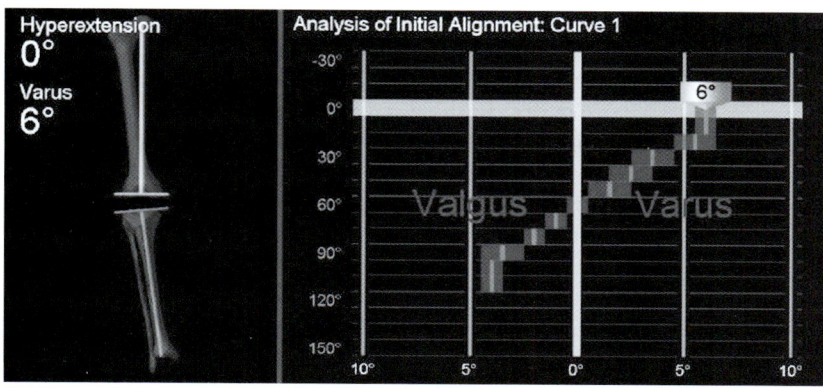

Figure 131.5 Analysis of varus–valgus. Knee kinematics (varus group 3) in the coronal plane as the knee flexes from the extended position. Screenshot from OrthoPilot® Navigation System. Image reproduced with permission from B. Braun Meslungen AG.

doing any ligamentous release for these deformities. Thus, a global medial or lateral release for a group 3 or group 4C knee may be completely unnecessary or even counterproductive leading to flexion instability.

RATIONALE OF USING CAOS IN TOTAL KNEE ARTHROPLASTY

- CAOS provides the surgeon with a replica of the individual patient's specific anatomy, based on which the surgeon can formulate the plan for making bone cuts and balancing the ligaments.
- A patient-specific biomechanical axis is created and the most appropriate cuts are suggested to achieve the best results.
- It helps with the ligamentous balancing. Thus, with stress testing, the surgeon is able to balance the knee not only in extension but also throughout the range of flexion.
- It has been proved in various studies that CAOS increases the accuracy of anatomical placement compared with conventional means.[4] This has been shown by a meta-analysis that included 29 studies and that concluded that the incidence of malalignment of the biomechanical axis by more than 3° happened in 9% of knee joint arthroplasties with computer navigation compared with 31% with conventional techniques.[5] However, there was one study that did not find this benefit.[6]
- It has also been proved in various studies that malaligned knees do not function well and fail earlier than well-aligned knees. In a study carried out in 1991, it was shown that the rate of loosening at a median of 8 years was 3% in knees that had a biomechanical axis within the 3° range compared with 24% for those that fell outside this range.[7] It is thus hoped that CAOS can prevent early failures and potentially lead to better function and increased survival of the implants. As the CAOS techniques are in their infancy, it is too early to state whether these statements will hold true.
- The use of CAOS has also been shown to reduce blood loss in some studies,[8] but not in others. This could be explained by the use of intramedullary jigs in conventional surgery, which violate on the medullary canal and lead to increased bleeding.
- CAOS has also been shown to reduce the incidence of cranial emboli compared with conventional methods.[9] This may be significant in patients with pulmonary compromise and when simultaneous bilateral knee arthroplasty is done. It has also been shown to produce a gait pattern more like a natural knee than arthroplasty carried out with conventional surgery.[10] Finally, it has been shown to be helpful in training young surgeons and can give consistent results in trainees' hands that compare well with those of experienced surgeons.[11]

DISADVANTAGES

- The weakest link in the chain is the surgeon. If the surgeon does not register the exact anatomy the results will not be as good. The computer can only tell the surgeon what to do; it is the surgeon's job to achieve the best results.
- During the learning period, which is very short, there is an increase in the operating time. But, as the surgeon becomes more experienced, the operating time equates to that of conventional surgery.
- There is a potential for tracker attachment site morbidity as the surgeon needs to make a hole in the bone to attach the trackers.

OPERATIVE TECHNIQUE

We describe here the procedures used in the imageless registration method, which is the most commonly used technique. We shall only describe the steps that are important from a navigation point of view. The surgeon should know how to perform a conventional knee replacement arthroplasty. CAOS involves various stages, as does conventional surgery.

System set-up

Patient and part preparation is carried out as in conventional surgery. The limb is prepared from the upper thigh to the foot and left in clear view. It is important that one can access the ankle and foot for proper registration of the anatomy. The knee joint is exposed as usual.

Patient data and side are fed into the system. The trackers and instruments are registered and calibrated if needed by the system. The trackers are attached to the tibia and femur by various means, depending on the computer system being used (Fig. 131.6). The camera is adjusted so that it can both detect the trackers and is at an appropriate distance to be out of the surgical field but still give accurate readings. Normally, the computer will indicate whether the camera cannot detect any of the trackers properly. The registration process may seem lengthy while reading, but, in practice, takes only 3–5 minutes.

Registration of biomechanical axis

The hip centre is then calculated by taking the leg through multiple circular movements that pivot on the centre of motion of the hip joint. Some systems use other methods, such as only one circle of 10–15° of arc that not only calculates the hip centre but also gives the plane for the distal femoral cut (Fig. 131.7). Once the hip centre has been calculated, the distal femoral centre is marked by a pointer. The knee centre calculation can differ according to which system is being used; automatic kinematic calculation of the centre can be done by the computer, as with the hip centre. The knee is put through external and internal rotation and flexion–extension, which helps the computer algorithm to calculate the centre of the knee. The centre of the tibia is then registered with a pointer. The ankle centre is calculated by registration of the medial and lateral malleolus, and the centre is marked on the anterior part with a pointer in line with the second metatarsal. In some systems, it can also be calculated kinematically by attaching a tracker with a rubber strap to the foot and taking the ankle through the motions of dorsiflexion and plantarflexion. This completes the information for the computer to calculate the biomechanical axis for that patient.

Distal femoral anatomy registration

Registration of the distal femoral anatomy is then done by one of various methods used in different systems, with either single point registration or surface painting. The distal femoral condyles are marked. Some systems also use the posterior femoral condyle registration to calculate the size of the component required. The anterior femoral cortex is then marked. One should be careful to include the most anterior part of the femoral cortex, especially on the lateral aspect, to avoid notching. The femoral rotation is registered using the anteroposterior axis (Whiteside's line) and/or the transepicondylar axis. The importance of accurate registration of this point cannot be overemphasized as the femoral component rotation depends on this. We explored a method of palpating the epicondyles in 50 consecutive patients undergoing total knee replacement. It was not possible to feel the clear prominence of the medial and lateral epicondyles by routine palpation through normal exposure in 32 cases. However, by using scissors with closed tips and pushing it through the synovium in the medial and lateral gutters at the level of epicondyles, and opening the limbs of the scissors and withdrawing with the limbs open, this creates a space in the synovium through which the surgeon's finger and pointer can go posterior to the synovial fold. By this means, one can feel the epicondyles very easily in over 90% of cases accurately registered.

Proximal tibial anatomy registration

Next, the anatomy of the proximal tibia is registered. The deepest points of the tibial plateaus are registered by either a single point method or surface painting. The anteroposterior axis of the tibia is also registered in some systems, keeping the registration pointer in line with the junction of the medial third of the tibial tuberosity, although the validity of this method is disputed, as in conventional surgery.

Femoral cuts

The surgeon is now ready to make the bone cuts. The distal femoral cut is normally guided by the computer at 90° to the biomechanical axis independent of where the anatomical

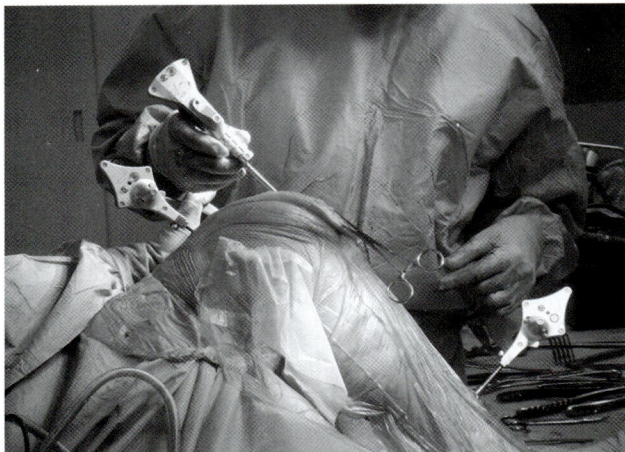

Figure 131.6 The trackers are attached to the femur and the tibia in a total knee replacement procedure.

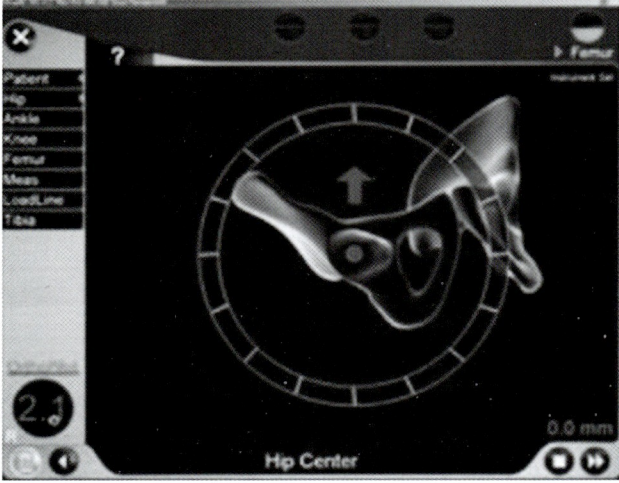

Figure 131.7 Hip centre detection for registration. Screenshot from OrthoPilot® Navigation System. Image reproduced with permission from B. Braun Meslungen AG.

axis is, as is the case with conventional surgery. It also shows the thickness/depth of the cut being made in comparison with the registered medial and lateral femoral condyles. Any deviation from the mechanical axis in the coronal plane is shown on the screen (Fig. 131.8). The jig that has the tracker attached is fixed in the correct orientation to the femur and the cut is made.

The frontal femoral cut is oriented according to the surgeon's preference. Some surgeons use the transepicondylar line as their reference for femoral rotation whereas others use Whiteside's line as the reference. We use the transepicondylar axis as our reference for femoral rotation (Fig. 131.9). In some software versions it may be determined by soft-tissue tension used for balancing.

The size of the femoral component can now be indicated by the computer with most systems, but the final decision lies with the surgeon, who must make sure of the correct size before making any cuts as adjustments can be done at this stage. One should ensure that there is no potential for notching of the anterior cortex. It is suggested that beginners use the angel wing or similar tool to identify any notching before making the cut. This is also useful if registration of the anatomy is doubtful. The potential for any notching is also shown by the computer. In addition, the orientation in the sagittal plane can be seen. The cutting jig with the tracker attached is fixed to the femur in the appropriate orientation and the remaining cuts to the femur are made.

The osteophytes are excised and posterior condylar clearance is carried out. If the surgeon is using posterior cruciate sacrificing or stabilization of the implant, the appropriate cut is made using the jigs.

Tibial cut

The tibial jig with the tracker attached is fixed to the tibia in the correct orientation. The computer shows the orientation of the sagittal and coronal planes. Although it can also show the orientation of the axial plane, this is currently ignored as the desired standard landmark of the rotational alignment of the tibia is not known. The computer also shows the depth of the tibial cut in relation to the registered medial and lateral tibial plateau. Once the desired position is achieved the tibial cut is made. Osteophytes are excised.

Component implantation

Once the cuts are made, the trial femoral and tibial components are put on the prepared ends of the bone and an appropriate thickness tibial insert is used. The knee is flexed, and range of movement, any deformities in the coronal plane, patellar tracking, stability and ligamentous balance are noted. If ligamentous release is required to correct the varus or valgus deformity, it is done at this stage. In our experience it is only rarely necessary to do any additional ligamentous release apart from the release needed to expose the joint sufficiently to make the femoral and tibial cuts. This is possibly because, with computer navigation, the appropriate biomechanics can be produced. One can clearly see on the computer screen any deviations from the expected results in different planes at any point of flexion, and the range of movement. The surgeon can also assess the stability by using varus and valgus stress and assessing the deformity produced in the coronal plane. Thus, the surgeon is able to balance the knee not only in extension but also throughout the range of flexion. When the desired result has been achieved, the tibial rotation is marked on the trial component and femoral drilling is done for the lug holes, if they are required by the design of the prosthesis.

The upper end of the tibia is then prepared for the tibial component to be inserted. The routine used in conventional surgery is then followed. For uncemented components, the prosthesis is inserted. For cemented components the bone ends are washed and cleared of any debris and the prosthesis

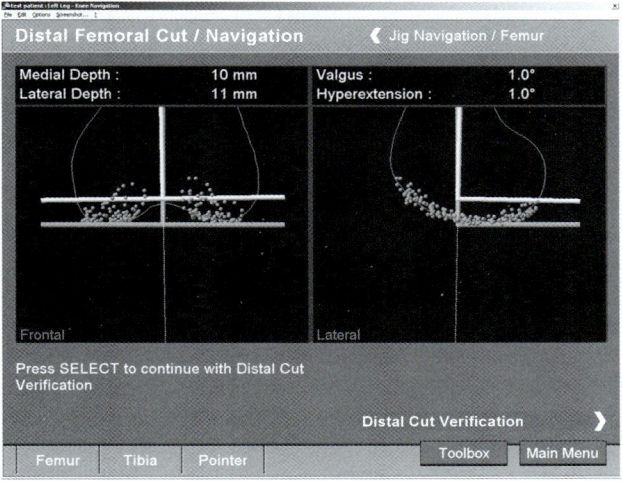

Figure 131.8 The computer screen showing the orientation of sagittal and coronal planes and the depth of medial and lateral cuts of femoral condyles.

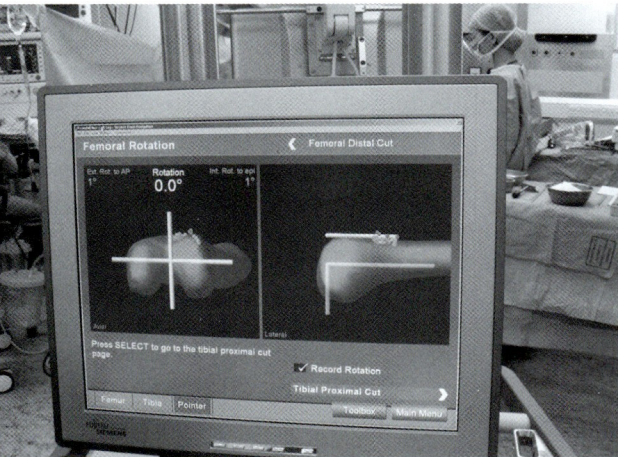

Figure 131.9 Rotation of the femoral component guided by computer navigation; also shows the impingement on the registered anterior cortex of the femur.

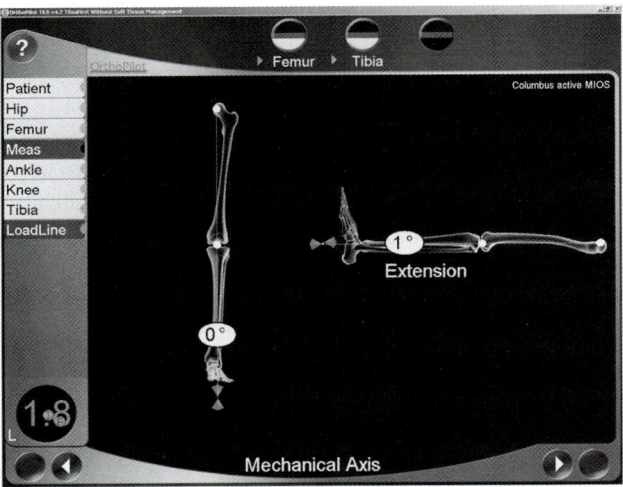

Figure 131.10 Biomechanical axis assessment in different ranges of flexion can be carried out once the prosthesis is implanted. Screenshot from OrthoPilot® Navigation System. Image reproduced with permission from B. Braun Meslungen AG.

is cemented in place. The final result is then noted and recorded by the computer (Fig. 131.10). The final kinematics are recorded and assessment is made again of range of movement, coronal deformity, stability and patellar tracking.

Thus, CAOS helps at every stage of the surgical procedure, including pre-operative kinematic analysis, intra-operative guidance at every step and postoperative kinematic analysis. The surgeon is immediately able to objectively document the result of the procedure.

Total hip replacement

The use of CAOS in total hip replacement is a recent development, and it is not yet as popular in total hip replacement as it is in total knee arthroplasty. The main reason for this is that the majority of misplaced total hip implants do not cause as many visible problems as do misplaced total knee replacements. However, surgeons are now realizing its potential advantages in total hip replacement in achieving good biomechanical results. The problems related to implant malposition with conventional surgery include dislocation, impingement, leg length discrepancy and early failure.[12–14] Impingement has been shown recently to be a significant problem, especially with use of ceramics.[14,15] Also, with metal-on-metal bearings, the metal ion concentration is much higher with malplaced implants.[16]

There is no consensus on the standard position of the acetabular cup, although some safe zones have been described.[17] The functional plane may be different for every individual, and there can be contractures of various degrees in the arthritic hip. This also holds true for conventional surgery.

Most of the computer navigation systems presently use the anterior pelvic plane as the reference plane for registering the pelvis. While this plane gives consistent fixed bony points, it may not represent a true reference for every individual functional position. Alternatives have been explored but have not been proved to be better than the anterior pelvic plane. These include the posterosuperior iliac spines and the transverse acetabular ligament. The most common difficulty with the anterior pelvic plane is registration in imageless navigation, especially if the surgeon uses the lateral position for the surgery. Acetabular central axis (ACA) software has recently been developed which uses local acetabular anatomy rather than anterior pelvic plane.

POTENTIAL ADVANTAGES

- CAOS provides individual patient-specific anatomy, based on which the surgeon can formulate a plan to prepare the bone and produce the optimum result. For the acetabular cup, it can show, in real time, the orientation in which the surgeon is placing the cup in six degrees of freedom. It can give inclination, anteversion, flexion, any anteroposterior, mediolateral and superoinferior shifts that the surgeon produces, and can correct them at the time of surgery. Similarly, for the femoral stem, it can show flexion, varus, anteversion, offset and leg length changes. Most of the systems available should be able to show the above parameters.
- It has been proved in various studies that CAOS increases the accuracy of anatomical placement compared with conventional means, even in experienced hands.[12]
- It has also been shown to correct leg length discrepancy better than conventional techniques.[14,18] Thus, the problems with conventional surgery that are related to implant malposition such as dislocation, impingement and leg length discrepancy can be addressed.
- The pelvis can move during the procedure without the knowledge or control of the surgeon, leading to possible misplacement of the cup. With navigation, any movement of the pelvis will be detected by the computer and the likelihood of misplacement is minimal.
- It is hoped that CAOS can prevent early failures and potentially lead to better function and increased survival of the implants. As CAOS techniques are in their infancy, it is too early to say whether this will hold true.
- CAOS has been shown to be helpful in training young surgeons and can give consistent results in trainees' hands that compare well with the results of experienced surgeons.[19] It is also helpful if minimally invasive approaches are being used in which the field of view is limited.[20] It guides the surgeon through various stages of the procedure and shows in real time what he/she is doing.

POTENTIAL DISADVANTAGES

- There is potential for tracker attachment site morbidity as a hole has to be made in the bone to attach the trackers.

- The trackers have the potential to move as the pelvis can be porotic, especially in older patients, in whom total hip replacement is generally performed.
- Registration can be difficult, especially in obese patients, when the surgeon operates in lateral position.
- The procedure may take longer than the conventional technique. For beginners, this can be up to 30 minutes longer, which decreases to about 10 minutes as the surgeon's experience increases and the operating staff become accustomed to the system.

OPERATIVE TECHNIQUE

We describe here the technique used in the imageless registration method, which is the most commonly used technique. We shall only describe the steps that are important from the navigation point of view. The surgeon must know how to perform a conventional hip replacement arthroplasty. CAOS involves various stages, as does conventional surgery. The method described here is the one we use, but there may be variations with the different commercial systems available.

System set-up

Patient and part preparation is done as for conventional surgery. The position of the patient can be supine or lateral. The limb is prepared from the lower chest to the foot and left in clear view. It is important that the surgeon can access the knee, iliac crest and pelvis for proper registration of the anatomy and for attaching the trackers to the bone. In obese individuals, if the surgeon is using the lateral position with the posterior approach, it may be easier to leave the patient first in a sloppy lateral position until registration of the pelvis is done and then tighten the posterior supports. Cardiac leads may also be used to guide the opposite anterosuperior iliac spine and pubic symphysis under the drapes for registration of the pelvis.

Patient data and side are fed into the system. The trackers and instruments are registered and calibrated, if required by the system. The trackers are attached to the pelvis and femur by various means, depending on the system being used (Fig. 131.11). The camera is adjusted so that it can both detect trackers and is at an appropriate distance to be out of the surgical field but still give accurate readings. Normally, the computer screen will indicate whether the camera cannot detect any of the trackers properly.

Registration of pelvis and acetabulum

This can be image based or imageless. In the image-based method, pre-operative CT scan or fluoroscopy may be used. We use the imageless method of registration. The pelvis is registered by the frontal plane, by means of the two anterosuperior iliac spines and the pubic tubercles or pubic symphysis. Some systems also register a functional plane, which consists of the mid-axillary point and the greater trochanter with the leg in neutral position. This can be difficult to reproduce as neither of these

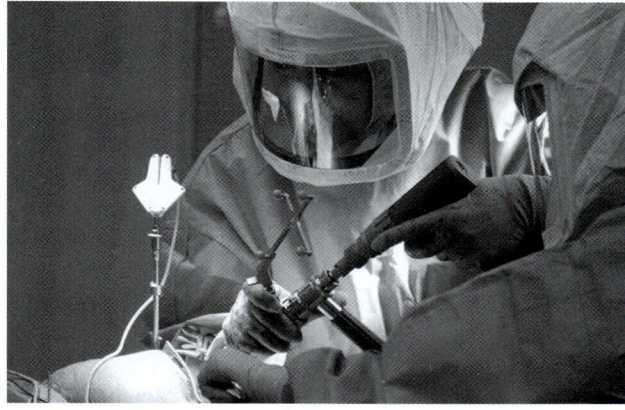

Figure 131.11 The active tracker is attached to the pelvis and the passive tracker with reflective balls is attached to the reamer handle.

points is a single discrete bony point; thus, this is open to errors. This process can be difficult in obese patients, especially when using the lateral position. The hip joint is then exposed as in conventional surgery, the neck osteotomy is performed and the head part extracted. The acetabular registration is done by denoting the true medial wall, the acetabular surface and the circumference of the margin. This will give an approximate diameter of the acetabulum and a native anatomy. A reamer of the same diameter can be used to insert in the acetabulum and the centre of the hip is thus registered by the computer as the centre of that reamer. This centre acts as a reference for further calculations.

Femoral registration

The trochanteric fossa is registered first, followed by popliteal fossa, which can be registered either as a single point or as two femoral epicondyles. Then, the knee is bent to 90° to avoid any effect of leg rotation and the midpoint of the Achilles tendon is registered. The centre of the ankle may also be registered. This forms a virtual femoral plane by combining all these points to act as a reference for the femoral components.

Acetabular cup

Acetabular reamers are then used to prepare the cup bed after good exposure is achieved. A tracker is attached to the reamer handle that communicates with the computer to give the orientation and position of the reamer in all six degrees of freedom, including inclination, version, flexion and the superoinferior, anteroposterior and mediolateral positions (Fig. 131.12). Similar information is given when the cup is inserted, as a tracker is attached to the cup insertion handle. For uncemented cups it is important to be very careful when using the reamers that they are in the correct orientation. For cemented cups, the position of the cup within the cement mantle can be changed to some extent before the cement sets.

Femoral stem

The femur is prepared in the normal fashion, taking care to achieve the correct orientation, which is shown by the computer as a tracker is attached to the femoral broach handle. It shows the position in all six degrees of freedom, including flexion, varus, version, offset and lengthening (Fig. 131.13). Similar readings are given when inserting the stem component. Again, in uncemented stems, it is important to be careful at the time of preparation of the bed, and, in cemented stems, one can alter the position to some extent in the cement mantle.

Final steps

A virtual reduction can be done and the effect of various lengths of femoral neck can be seen even without the actual hip trial reduction (Fig. 131.13). A trial reduction is then done with selected components and the new hip centre seen. A change of leg length and offset can be seen, which can be changed to an extent even at this stage by varying the neck length. The final range of movements and points of impingement are recorded by the computer and the procedure is finished as in the conventional technique.

Considerable development in CAOS technology that is specific to total hip replacement needs to take place before CAOS is accepted as a conventional technique by all. The present methods need to be modified; the instrumentation needs to be modified for use with CAOS; and a whole new range of implants need to be developed to properly reproduce the optimal biomechanics. The registration process needs to be simplified and the reference plane needs to be standardized.

Patient specific jigs

Recently there has been renewed interest in patient specific jigs. This technology utilises pre-operative imaging in the form of MR scans, CT scans or long leg radiographs. Different commercial companies use different imaging techniques. This is an extended use of pre-operative planning process. The surgeon/engineers plan the optimal position of the cuts to be made during the surgery based on the images. For these cuts to be reproduced during the surgery, specific jigs are made for individual patients. These jigs fit to the femur and tibia of the patients and planned cuts can thus be achieved perioperatively. Long term results of these jigs are yet not available but they seem to give promising results in majority of patients in short term.

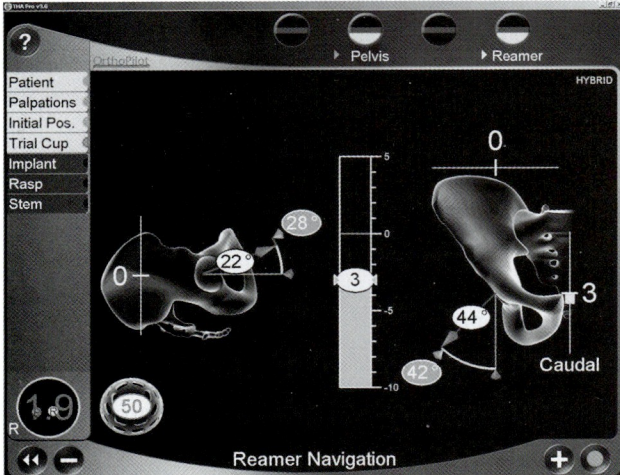

Figure 131.12 The acetabular reaming screen showing the reamer size and the anteroposterior, mediolateral and craniocaudal positions. It also shows the inclination, anteversion and distance to the true floor. Screenshot from OrthoPilot® Navigation System. Image reproduced with permission from B. Braun Meslungen AG.

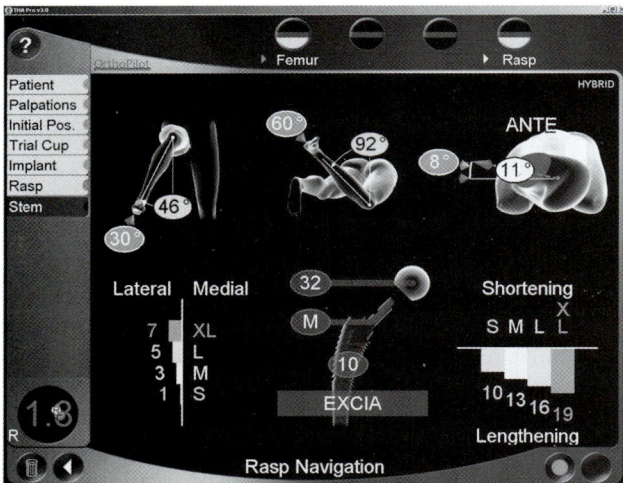

Figure 131.13 Femoral rasping showing the internal and external rotations that will be achieved by anteversion of the rasp position shown. The lower part of the screen shows the virtual trial, including the offset, the size of the head, neck and stem and the changes that would be made to the leg length. Screenshot from OrthoPilot® Navigation System. Image reproduced with permission from B. Braun Meslungen AG.

FUTURE OF COMPUTER ASSISTANCE IN ORTHOPAEDIC SURGERY

It is the author's opinion that the technology will be much simpler and more user friendly in the future. It will be used for all joint arthroplasties and for most other orthopaedic surgery, including deformity correction and spinal, trauma and tumour surgery. It will even be used for pre-operative and postoperative evaluation of kinematics and implants, and will track their progress with time, recognizing early failures before they happen. CAOS is also going to be helpful in training surgeons, and can act as an evaluating tool for examination purposes. Its potential for research and understanding of biomechanics of humans is huge, and will no doubt assist us to give better outcomes for our patients.

REFERENCES

1. Deep K, Donnelly W, Morar Y, et al. Biomechanical force displacement analysis of strength of fixation of tracker holding devices to bone in computer aided joint replacements. *Journal of Bone and Joint Surgery (British)* 2006;**88B** (Suppl. 3):439.
2. Sarungi M, Basanagoudar P, Nunang P, Deakin AH. The femoral mechanical angle and the preoperative varus–vulgus limb alignment: x-ray analysis of 174 hip-knee-ankle films. *Journal of Bone and Joint Surgery (British)* 2011;**93B**(Suppl. 3):385.
3. Deep K, Smith B, Nunag P, Wilcox N. A comparison of posterior condylar axis with transepicondylar axis as the reference for rotational orientation of femoral component in total knee replacement: conventional vs. computer navigation. In: Davies BL, Joskowicz L, Murphy SB (ed). *Proceedings of CAOS International 2009, Boston, MA, 17–20 June 2009.* California: Wingspan Publishing.
4. Deep K, Picard F, Baines J, et al. An analysis of knee kinematics with computer navigation: a classification of kinematics and nomenclature for arthritis of knee. *Journal of Bone and Joint Surgery (British)* 2011;**93B**:391.
5. Mason JB, Fehring TK, Estok R, et al. Meta-analysis of alignment outcomes in computer-assisted total knee arthroplasty surgery. *Journal of Arthroplasty* 2007;**22**:1097–106.
6. Kim YH, Kim JS, Choi Y, Kwon OR. Computer-assisted surgical navigation does not improve the alignment and orientation of the components in total knee arthroplasty. *Journal of Bone and Joint Surgery (American)* 2009;**91**:14–19.
7. Jeffery R, Morris, Rehman R. Coronal alignment after total knee arthroplasty. *Journal of Bone and Joint Surgery (British)* 1991;**73**:709–14.
8. Kalairajah Y, Simpson D, Cossey AJ, et al. Blood loss after total knee replacement: effects of computer-assisted surgery. *Journal of Bone and Joint Surgery (British)* 2005;**87**:1480–2.
9. Kalairajah Y, Cossey AJ, Verrall GM, et al. Are systemic emboli reduced in computer-assisted knee surgery? A prospective, randomised, clinical trial. *Journal of Bone and Joint Surgery (British)* 2006;**88**:198–202.
10. Dillon JM, Clarke JV, Kinninmonth A, et al. Dynamic functional outcome assessment in navigated TKR using gait analysis. *Journal of Bone and Joint Surgery (British)* 2008;**90B**:567.
11. Stulberg SD. Computer navigation as a teaching instrument in knee reconstruction surgery. *Journal of Knee Surgery* 2007;**20**:165–72.
12. Wixson RL. Computer-assisted total hip navigation. *Instructional Course Lectures* 2008;**57**:707–20.
13. Ecker TM, Murphy SB. Application of surgical navigation to total hip arthroplasty. *Proceedings of the Institute of Mechanical Engineers [H]* 2007;**221**:699–712.
14. Sugano N, Nishii T, Miki H, et al. Mid-term results of cementless total hip replacement using a ceramic-on-ceramic bearing with and without computer navigation. *Journal of Bone and Joint Surgery (British)* 2007;**89**:455–60.
15. Murali R, Bonar SF, Kirsh G, et al. Osteolysis in third-generation alumina ceramic-on-ceramic hip bearings with severe impingement and titanium metallosis. *Journal of Arthroplasty* 2008;**23**:1240.e13–19.
16. Onda K, Nagoya S, Kaya M, Yamashita T. Cup-neck impingement due to the malposition of the implant as a possible mechanism for metallosis in metal-on-metal total hip arthroplasty. *Orthopedics* 2008;**31**:396.
17. Lewinnek GE, Lewis JL, Tarr R, et al. Dislocations after total hip-replacement arthroplasties. *Journal of Bone and Joint Surgery (American)* 1978;**60**:217–20.
18. Confalonieri N, Manzotti A, Montironi F, Pullen C. Leg length discrepancy, dislocation rate, and offset in total hip replacement using a short modular stem: navigation vs conventional freehand. *Orthopedics* 2008;**31**(10 Suppl. 1):ii.
19. Gofton W, Dubrowski A, Tabloie F, Backstein D. The effect of computer navigation on trainee learning of surgical skills. *Journal of Bone and Joint Surgery (American)* 2007;**89**:2819–27.
20. Judet H. Five years of experience in hip navigation using a mini-invasive anterior approach. *Orthopedics* 2007;**30**(10 Suppl):S141–3.

Orthopaedic tissue engineering

PATRICK H WARNKE

Introduction	1524	Bioreactors	1527
The basic principles	1525	Examples of clinical applications of tissue engineering	
Scaffold materials and shape	1525	in skeletal reconstruction	1527
Cells	1526	References	1529
Signals	1527		

NATIONAL BOARD STANDARDS

- Be able to summarize the technological challenges and influencing factors in tissue engineering for orthopaedic surgery
- Be able to characterize the different potentials and associated concerns in various cell types to grow tissue anew
- Be aware of first case studies and clinical trials applying stem cells and regenerative technologies
- Be confident to enter the discussion on 'modern stem cell technologies' with patients who bring this up

INTRODUCTION

Tissue engineering is an emerging field in orthopaedic surgery. The translation of fundamental new discoveries in laboratory science into concrete advancements in patient care may lead to essential changes in clinical treatment options. The term *tissue engineering* was originally coined to denote the construction in the laboratory of a device containing viable cells and biological mediators such as growth factors in a synthetic or biological matrix that could be implanted into patients to facilitate regeneration of particular tissues.[1]

The popular media often incorrectly use terms such as *tissue engineering, regenerative medicine, bionics, biomimetic materials* and *stem cell therapy* as synonyms.[2,3] Thus, increasing numbers of patients come to orthopaedic clinics requesting miracle-like 'stem cell therapies' to cure their diseases, which may not meet current therapy standards.

Regenerative medicine is the general term for all techniques that focus on regeneration of damaged or missing tissue in the human body. 'Regeneration' means the repair of damaged tissue by growing it anew. Some organisms such as *Hydra* or amphibians (e.g. *Ambystoma mexicanum*) are able to regenerate missing body parts *de novo* even in the adult stage. Much can be learned from these species as they provide the basic guide to how tissue can form. The focus of *regenerative medicine* is to mimic these or embryological growth patterns by means of tissue engineering techniques.[4] Thus, most orthopaedic operations, such as artificial joint implantation or bone graft transplantation, are mainly a repair of skeletal structures but are never a kind of regeneration.

Bionics is the combination of artificial electronic mechanisms and living tissue to work together as one unit. Bionic implants differ from simple prostheses by mimicking the original function very closely, or even surpassing it. While the technologies that make bionic implants possible are still in a very early stage, a few bionic items already exist, the best known being the cochlear implant – an electronic ear device for deaf people.[5] Significant further progress is expected with the advent of nanotechnologies and superior computer chip development.

Biomimetic materials mimic living tissue surfaces. The biomimicry of artificial ceramic bone substitutes such as hydroxyapatite can be enhanced by the incorporation of collagen type I, which is the main organic component of bone[6] and which supports the adhesion and proliferation of osteoblasts.[7,8] With the aim of exploiting the benefits of both materials simultaneously, several groups have produced hydroxyapatite/collagen composite scaffolds.[9–11]

Even though the field of life sciences is moving forward at a rapid pace, the repair of bony defects from congenital malformations, trauma, infection or tumour resection remains a challenge in modern orthopaedic or maxillofacial surgical practice.[12] The reconstruction of long bones, spine and the skull must meet high mechanical and aesthetic demands.

Major discontinuity defects of more than 5 cm are repaired with an autologous vascularized fibula, scapula, iliac crest or rib transplant. However, a major disadvantage of these techniques is that harvesting the required bone grafts creates another skeletal defect that is associated with significant morbidity.[13]

This chapter highlights recent advances in the promising field of regenerative medicine that may offer new solutions for reconstructive and orthopaedic surgeons to handle critical size bone and cartilage defects. The crucial essentials of tissue engineering techniques are put into plain words to shed light on this new discipline in orthopaedic surgery.

THE BASIC PRINCIPLES

Tissue engineering generally involves the use of artificial or inert scaffold materials and living cells with the goal of growing a desired tissue with its characteristic biological function. To manipulate the cells in the required way mediators or signals are utilized. Thus, *tissue engineering* has been represented as a static triangle consisting of scaffolds, cells and signals (Fig. 132.1).[1]

However, a fourth factor, the choice of the bioreactor to provide an environment for cell growth on scaffolds, is also of fundamental importance. Although *in vitro* tissue engineering techniques using artificial bioreactors have been a focus of many research groups, more recently interest has begun to shift to tissue engineering techniques *in vivo*.

The missing vascular supply of engineered tissue in artificial bioreactors limits the size of the constructs. Cultivation of substantial bone-like tissue of volume greater than 1 mL is currently an almost unachievable challenge *in vitro*. In contrast, *tissue engineering in vivo* allows for vascular supply and blood perfusion of the cultivated tissue. Thus, considerable amounts of bone can already be engineered *in vivo*.[14] Vascular supply is therefore the fifth factor influencing tissue engineering.

Calcified tissues such as bone and cartilage require special mechanical environments during cultivation. Functional loading or mechanical stimulation is crucial for a proper remodelling at certain phases of tissue growth. Thus, *functional stimulation* of the engineered tissue is the essential sixth factor to achieve the desired biological performance. These further biological aspects have just been introduced into modern *tissue engineering* (Fig. 132.1). Many more may come in the future. We may now need to consider good manufacturing practice (GMP) as a seventh factor. GMP processing protocols, GMP certified staff and GMP cleanroom facilities are important to be able to apply tissue engineering in clinical practice. For example, many preclinical studies based on DNA alteration with viral vector transfection cannot be translated into humans without significant protocol changes.

SCAFFOLD MATERIALS AND SHAPE

Scaffolds or matrices should allow cell adhesion, if necessary display growth factors on their surfaces and direct growth. For bone tissue engineering resorbable and non-resorbable scaffolds have been used, in some cases extensively as bone

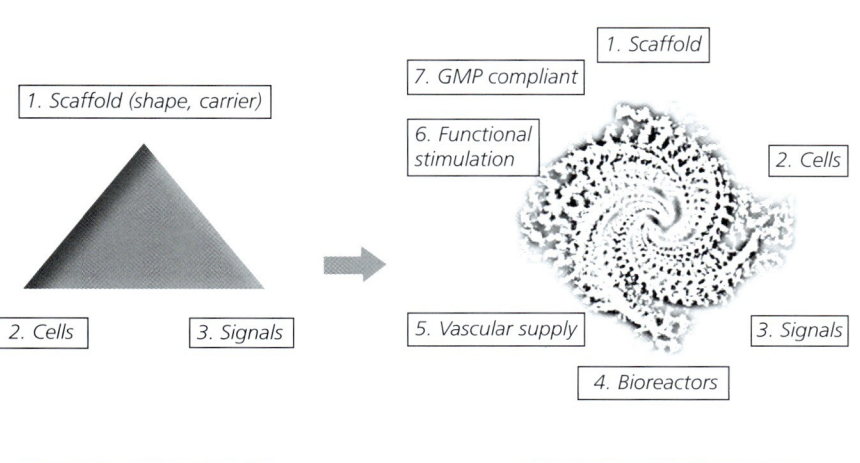

Figure 132.1 Today, the classic triangle of three factors influencing tissue engineering has changed into a vivid spiral of seven crucial factors. Many more factors may be identified in the future.

replacement materials in implantology. Resorbable materials degrade at the site of implantation and, optimally, are replaced by bone. The degradation progress can lead to undesirable changes in the local environment and mechanical and contour instability. Non-resorbable materials retain their basic stability but may interfere with remodelling processes in bone.[15] One important issue is that scaffolds provide shape to the cultivated tissue. *Rapid prototyping* techniques such as selective laser melting (SLM) computer-aided design (CAD) can be used to produce three-dimensional (3D) scaffolds.[16] Often, these scaffolds are designed on the basis of virtual imaging data from a patient's CT scans.[14] CAD provides a practical and precise method of customizing replacement scaffolds to produce a perfect fit for each individual defect. CAD techniques have already been used to construct titanium alloy scaffolds[16] by SLM and ceramic[17] scaffolds by 3D printing with subsequent sintering. In contrast to materials previously used for bone contact and bone replacement, these scaffolds have precisely defined external geometry and internal dimensions such as pore size.

Some scaffolds may also serve as carriers for cells and cytokines.

> **BOX 132.1: Potency of stem cells**
>
> - *Totipotent* stem cells have the ability to form an entire organism. The fertilized oozyte and the cells after the first cleavage divisions are considered *totipotent*.
> - *Pluripotent* stem cells are able to form all three germ layers including germ cells, but not the placenta and umbilical cord. Cells of the inner cell mass of the blastocyst are *pluripotent*. When these cells are brought into culture, they are called *embryonic stem cells*.
> - *Multipotency* means the ability to form multiple cell types. Adult mesenchymal stem cells are multipotent and can differentiate into cells that form bone, cartilage and fat for example.
> - *Oligopotent* stem cells can differentiate into two or more lineages, e.g. neural stem cells that can form a subset of neurones in the brain.
> - *Unipotency* is the ability to form cells from a single lineage, e.g. spermatogonial stem cells.
>
> From Jukes et al.[19]

CELLS

Regarding the choice of cells, two main approaches have been followed. In general *differentiated cells*, such as osteoblasts, can be cultivated on scaffolds which are then inserted into defects. *Differentiated cells*, however, generally proliferate poorly and, therefore, a large amount of tissue must be harvested to obtain a sufficient cell number. Furthermore, in contrast to such tissue constructs, native tissues always contain more than one cell type.

The alternative is the use of pluripotent or multipotent *stem cells*, which usually self-replicate more quickly than differentiated cells and which can be transformed into the targetted cell type by the application of the correct growth or differentiation factor. Stem cells can be harvested at different sites and may potentially provide an unlimited supply of cells that can form any of the hundreds of specialized cells with limitations according to their potency (Box 132.1). Human embryonic stem cells have been reported to proliferate for years and go through hundreds of population doublings.[18,19] However, the identity of stem cells must be established by testing their ability to differentiate into the desired cell types. Adult stem cells are rare in the human body, and their identification requires technical support and experienced laboratory staff. Often, in practice, the cells do not possess the level of multipotence expected.

In general stem cells can be divided into two main groups: *embryonic* and *adult or somatic* stem cells. *Embryonic stem cells* are responsible for embryonic and fetal development and growth. In the human body, *adult stem cells* are responsible for growth, tissue maintenance and regeneration of compromised tissue.[19] However, recently engineered induced pluripotent stem cells (IPSC) make up a novel third group and may play a pivotal role for tissue engineering in the future. IPSCs are a sort of pluripotent stem cells derived from a non-pluriotent cell, typically an adult specialized somatic cell, by inducing a 'forced' expression of genes. In other words, you pick an adult differentiated cell such as a skin fibroblast and reprogram it backwards, so that it becomes a stem cell again. IPSC have a similar high pluripotency as embryonic stem cells, but are derived from adult cells. Transfection or reprogramming is typically achieved through viral vectors and integration of transcription factors and some are unfortunately oncogenes, which carry the risk of mutations and malignancies. However, researchers are now working to develop protocols without viral transfection or oncogene integration for translation of this cell type into clinical practice. It has yet to be proven if this stem cell type will be feasible for the clinical environment.

The most advantageous and defining property of a stem cell is its ability to differentiate into a more specialized cell. The number of cell types that a stem cell can differentiate into is determined by its potency (Box 132.1).[19]

Embryonic stem cells would be most advantageous for regeneration of compromised bone or cartilage in orthopaedic surgery because of their pluripotency. But this raises ethical concerns as this entails harvesting cells from an embryo. Therefore, human embryonic stem cells are not freely available today. Thus, *adult stem cells* are the sole multipotent cell available for orthopaedic tissue engineering currently.

Adult stem cells have been derived from many human tissues, such as bone marrow, peripheral blood, brain, spinal cord, dental pulp, blood vessels, skeletal muscle, heart, epidermis, mucosa, cornea, liver and pancreas.[20]

Today, adult *haematopoietic stem cells* that can be harvested from bone marrow have found wide clinical acceptance and play an important role in the treatment of leukaemias to reconstitute the haematolymphoid system.

For orthopaedic surgery a second population of multipotent adult stem cells existing in the bone marrow is important as these can be easily harvested by orthopaedic surgeons; these are *mesenchymal stem cells*.

Adult *mesenchymal stem cells* can be used to generate differentiated cells of mesenchymal origin, such as osteoblasts or chondrocytes. Therefore, many scientific groups use mesenchymal stem cells to improve regenerative therapies for bone and cartilage defects.

SIGNALS

Signals or mediators used in *tissue engineering* are usually growth factors or cytokines, which exert a mitogenic (cell division activating) and/or a morphogenic (cell differentiating) effect. Different tissue components require different cocktails of signals applied in appropriate form. Particularly relevant for bone tissue cultivation are the growth factors platelet-derived growth factor, fibroblast growth factor, insulin-like growth factor, vascular endothelial growth factor and the isoforms of transforming growth factor and bone morphogenetic protein (BMP). BMPs are especially important as they induce the differentiation of mesenchymal precursor cells to osteoblasts and have been successfully applied in humans.[14,21]

BIOREACTORS

Once the desired scaffold system and the targeted tissue cell line have been developed, they have to be put together in order to direct the scaffold–cell combination into a living tissue via mediators. Bioreactors, which provide an environment for growth of engineered tissue, can be divided into three classes, namely *in vitro*, *in vivo* and *in silico*.

In vitro bioreactors attempt to condition tissue engineering constructs before subsequent implantation in the recipient, often by attempting to simulate conditions *in vivo*. Advantages include better control over culture and ease of checking the quality of the engineered tissue. Disadvantages are the risks of infection and rejection and the limitations in the size of the tissue which can be engineered, e.g. by the need for a vascular system capable of sustaining the engineered tissue. Vascularization of large engineered tissues is not yet possible *in vitro* and remains a major challenge.[22]

Currently, *in vivo* endocultivation techniques offer greater potential.[4,14] In 'endocultivation', the patient serves as his or her own *in vivo* bioreactor, whereby the required tissue is cultivated inside the patient's own body on an individualized matrix, making *in vitro* bioreactors unnecessary.[14,23,24] The use of *in vivo* bioreactors minimizes the risk of immunological rejection by using the patient's own cells and enables the development of a vascular system. CAD of scaffolds allows the endocultivation of customized replacements. However, the growth of the engineered tissue in the recipient is harder to control.

In the newest class of bioreactor, the *in silico* variety, tissue growth processes are simulated using computers as virtual bioreactors.[12,25] Computer models could allow optimization of the positioning of cells within an engineered tissue as well as the timing and manner of their stimulation (e.g. with growth factors). The usefulness of this approach is still awaiting final evaluation.

EXAMPLES OF CLINICAL APPLICATIONS OF TISSUE ENGINEERING IN SKELETAL RECONSTRUCTION

Endocultivation: tissue engineering of customized vascularized bone replacements *in vivo*

Endocultivation is a pioneering technique used to grow individually shaped bone replacements within the latissimus dorsi muscle of patients with severe skeletal defects. The goal is to use the patient as a living bioreactor to avoid the common problems associated with engineering tissue *in vitro* in the laboratory. The replacement scaffolds are individually designed prior to surgery using CAD to enable a perfect fit. The two major advantages of the endocultivation technique are the production of an optimal 3D aesthetic outcome and the prevention of the creation of a secondary skeletal defect. In addition, good vascularization can be achieved using endocultivation, which remains a major challenge in the engineering of thick tissues *in vitro*.[22]

The choice of a prepared muscle pouch inside the latissimus dorsi has proven to be a highly successful site as a bioreactor in animal and early clinical studies with substantial evidence of heterotopic bone growth and remodelling within the graft.[23,26,27] The muscular bioreactor allows for neovascularization of the bone replacement by means of the thoracodorsal artery and vein, thereby allowing subsequent free-flap transfer into the desired recipient region. This independent vascular supply makes it possible to grow constructs of the size of a mandible or, in the future, possibly of a joint or even a complex organ.

In 2004 we started using endocultivation techniques to grow customized computer-designed vascularized jaw replacements in the latissimus dorsi muscles of patients for subsequent transplantation to reconstruct their previously resected jaws (Fig. 132.2).[14,23] These types of jaw replacements allowed for immediate masticatory function after transplantation into the recipient region (Fig. 132.3). Besides this, patients are provided with a significantly superior quality of life given their improved aesthetic appearance and enhanced ability to speak.

Experience in humans with this computer-assisted endocultivation technique is currently very limited.[16,23,28,29]

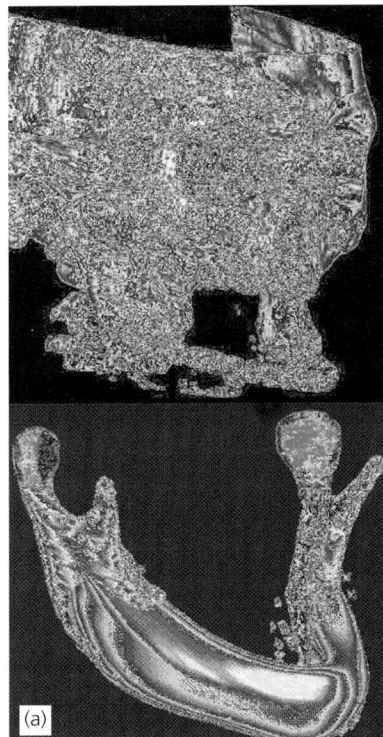
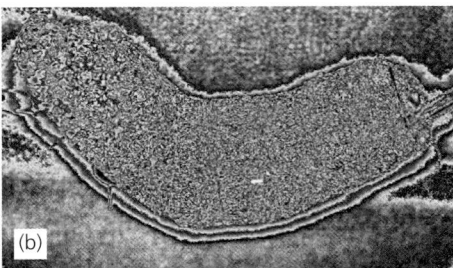
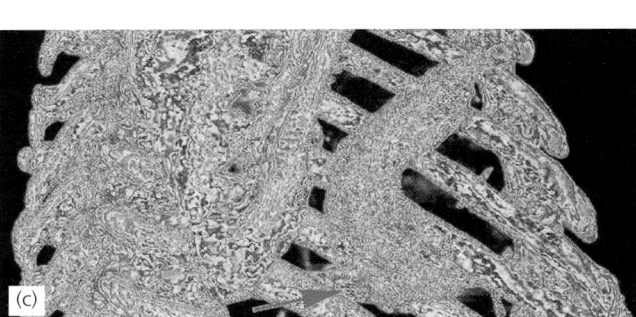
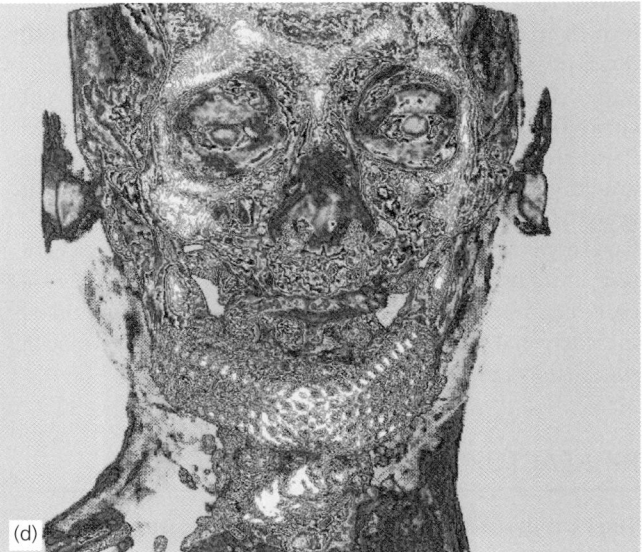

Figure 132.2 Endocultivation allows tissue engineering of computer-designed customized vascularized bone replacements *in vivo*. In this patient with a severe mandibular defect, a virtual mandible replacement was designed using computer-aided design (a). The computer data were used to create a titanium scaffold that was loaded with hydroxyapatite, bone morphogenetic protein and bone marrow cells (b). The scaffold was implanted into the latissimus dorsi muscle for neovascularization and bone growth for 7 weeks (c). After transplantation the perfect fit replacement received mechanical loading as immediate masticatory function was possible (d).[14,23]

It should be emphasized that as the endocultivation technique is still very new such prefabricated flaps are currently indicated only for patients who have poor skeletal donor sites and no other choice of reconstruction.

Autologous stem cell injection: regeneration of cartilage defects *in vivo*

Autologous chondrocyte implantation (ACI) is the most widely used cell-based surgical procedure for the treatment of symptomatic chondral and osteochondral defects of the knee. Challenges to successful ACI outcomes include limitation in defect size and geometry as well as inefficient cell retention. ACI has undergone considerable development since its inception in 1994.[30]

The original ACI technique involved the injection of a suspension of cultured chondrocytes into a debrided chondral defect beneath a periosteal cover.[31]

Second-generation ACI procedures have thus focused on developing 3D constructs using native and synthetic biomaterials. Clinically significant and satisfactory results from applying autologous chondrocytes seeded in fibrin within a biodegradable polymeric material were recently reported. In the future, third-generation cell-based articular cartilage regeneration will focus on the use of chondroprogenitor cells and biofunctionalized biomaterials for more extensive and permanent repair.[32]

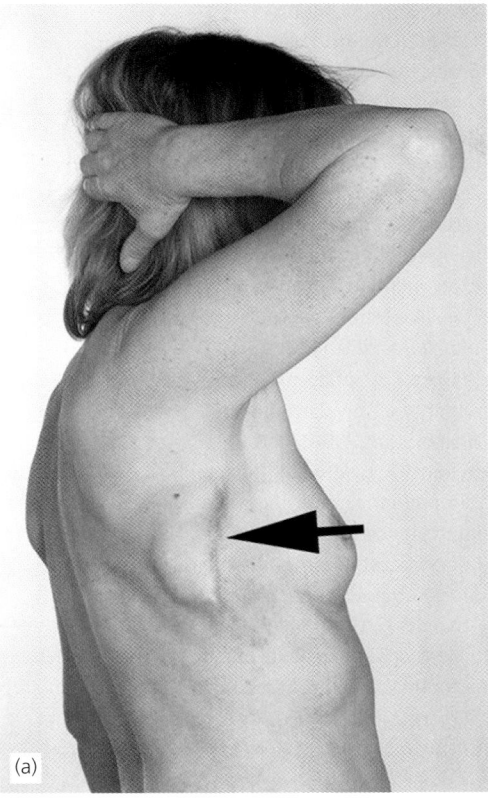
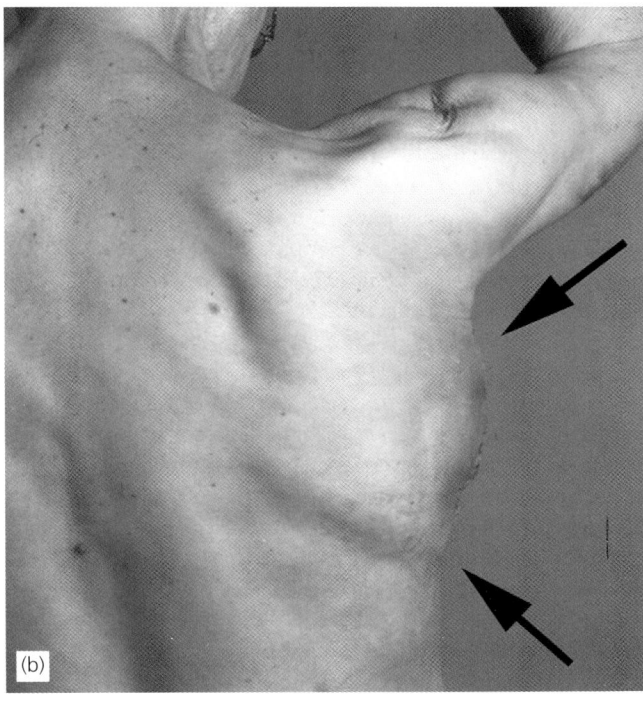

Figure 132.3 (a, b) Endocultivation bioreactor: patients growing new jawbones in their back muscles.

Another highlighted improvement with second-generation ACI is the application of mesenchymal stem cells (MSCs), instead of articular chondrocytes, in order to minimize additional donor site morbidity caused by cartilage harvesting.[32] Targeted gene therapy might further enhance the activities of MSCs. Delivery of MSCs might be attained by direct intra-articular injection or by graft of engineered constructs derived from cell-seeded scaffolds.[33] To accomplish this, the scaffold used could also serve the purpose of delivering chondroinductive factors and signals.[32] However, many of these novel approaches to cartilage regeneration are still at the animal model level.

REFERENCES

1. Lynch SE, Genco RJ, Marx RE (eds). *Tissue Engineering: Applications in Maxillofacial Surgery and Periodontics*. Chicago, IL: Quintessence Publishing, 1999.
2. Jayasuriya AC, Shah C, Ebraheim NA, Jayatissa AH. Acceleration of biomimetic mineralization to apply in bone regeneration. *Biomedical Materials* 2008;**3**:15003.
3. Crevier MC, Richard M, Rittenhouse DM, et al. Artificial exomuscle investigations for applications: metal hydride. *Biomedical Materials* 2007;**2**:S1–6.
4. Spector M. Basic principles of tissue engineering. In: Lynch SE, Genco RJ, Marx RE (eds) *Tissue Engineering: Applications in Maxillofacial Surgery and Periodontics*. Chicago, IL: Quintessence Publishing, 1999.
5. Fallon JB, Irvine DR, Shepherd RK. Cochlear implants and brain plasticity. *Hearing Research* 2008;**238**:110–17.
6. Weiner S, Wagner HD. The material bone: structure-mechanical function relations. *Annual Review Materials Science* 1998;**28**:271–98.
7. Park BS, Heo SJ, Kim CS, et al. Effects of adhesion molecules on the behavior of osteoblast-like cells and normal human fibroblasts on different titanium surfaces. *Journal of Biomedical Materials Research A* 2005;**74**:640–51.
8. Roehlecke C, Witt M, Kasper M, et al. Synergistic effect of titanium alloy and collagen type I on cell adhesion, proliferation and differentiation of osteoblast-like cells. *Cells Tissues Organs* 2001;**168**:178–87.
9. Dawson JI, Wahl DA, Lanham SA, et al. Development of specific collagen scaffolds to support the osteogenic and chondrogenic differentiation of human bone marrow stromal cells. *Biomaterials* 2008;**29**:3105–16.
10. Rodrigues CVM, Serricella P, Linhares ABR, et al. Characterization of a bovine collagen-hydroxyapatite composite scaffold for bone tissue engineering. *Biomaterials* 2003;**24**:4987–97.
11. Brodie JC, Goldie E, Connel G, et al. Osteoblast interactions with calcium phosphate ceramics modified by coating with type I collagen. *Journal of Biomedical Materials Research A* 2005;**73A**:409–21.

12. MacArthur BD, Oreffo ROC. Bridging the gap. *Nature* 2005;**433**:19.
13. Takushima A, Harii K, Asato H, *et al.* Mandibular reconstruction using microvascular free flaps: a statistical analysis of 178 cases. *Plastic and Reconstructive Surgery* 2001;**108**:1555–63.
14. Warnke PH, Springer IN, Wiltfang J, *et al.* Growth and transplantation of a custom vascularised bone graft in a man. *Lancet* 2004;**364**:766–70.
15. Vogelin E, Jones NF, Huang JI, *et al.* Healing of a critical-sized defect in the rat femur with use of a vascularized periosteal flap, a biodegradable matrix, and bone morphogenetic protein. *Journal of Bone and Joint Surgery (American)* 2005;**87**:1323–31.
16. Wehmöller M, Warnke PH, Zilian C, Eufinger H. Implant design and production: a new approach by selective laser melting. *International Congress Series* 2005;**1281**:690–5.
17. Seitz H, Rieder W, Irsen S, *et al.* Three-dimensional printing of porous ceramic scaffolds for bone tissue engineering. *Journal of Biomedical Materials Research B Applied Biomaterials* 2005;**74B**:782–8.
18. Hoffmann LM, Carpenter MK. Human embryonic stem cell stability. *Stem Cell Reviews* 2005;**1(2)**:139–44.
19. Jukes J, Both S, Post J, *et al.* Stem cells. In: Van Blitterswijk C, Williams DF, Lindahl A (eds) *Tissue Engineering*. Academic Press Series in Biomedical Engineering. London, UK: Elsevier, 2008:1–27.
20. Bianco P, Gehron Robey P, Pennesi G, Cancedda R. Cell source. In: Van Blitterswijk C, Williams DF, Lindahl A (eds) *Tissue Engineering*. Academic Press Series in Biomedical Engineering. London, UK: Elsevier, 2008:279–306.
21. Warnke PH, Coren AJ. First experiences with recombinant human bone morphogenetic protein 7 (osteogenic protein 1) in a human case in maxillofacial surgery. *Plastic and Reconstructive Surgery* 2003;**111**:2471–2.
22. Ko HCH, Milthorpe BK, McFarland CD. Engineering thick tissues: the vascularisation problem. *European Cells and Materials* 2007;**14**:1–19.
23. Warnke PH, Wiltfang J, Springer IN, *et al.* Man as living bioreactor: fate of an exogenously-prepared customized tissue-engineered mandible. *Biomaterials* 2006;**27**:3163–7.
24. Warnke PH: Repair of a human face by allotransplantation. *Lancet* 2006;**368**:181–3.
25. García-Aznar JM, Kuiper JH, Gómez-Benito MJ, *et al.* Computational simulation of fracture healing: influence of interfragmentary movement on the callus growth. *Journal of Biomechanics* 2007;**40**:1467–76.
26. Terheyden H, Warnke P, Dunsche A, *et al.* Mandibular reconstruction with prefabricated vascularized bone grafts using recombinant human osteogenic protein-1: an experimental study in miniature pigs. Part 2. Transplantation. *International Journal of Oral and Maxillofacial Surgery* 2001;**30**:469–78.
27. Warnke PH, Springer IN, Acil Y, *et al.* The mechanical integrity of in vivo engineered heterotopic bone. *Biomaterials* 2006;**27**:1081–7.
28. Heliotis M, Lavery KM, Ripamonti U, *et al.* Transformation of a prefabricated hydroxyapatite/osteogenic protein-1 implant into a vascularised pedicled bone flap in the human chest. *International Journal of Oral and Maxillofacial Surgery* 2006;**35**:265–9.
29. Arnander C, Westermark A, Veltheim R, *et al.* Three-dimensional technology and bone morphogenetic protein in frontal bone reconstruction. *Journal of Craniofacial Surgery* 2006;**17**:275–9.
30. Brittberg M, Lindahl A, Nilsson A, *et al.* Treatment of deep cartilage defects in the knee with autologous chondrocyte transplantation. *New England Journal of Medicine* 1994;**331**:889–95.
31. Bartlett W, Skinner JA, Gooding CR, *et al.* Autologous chondrocyte implantation versus matrix-induced autologous chondrocyte implantation for osteochondral defects of the knee: a prospective, randomised study. *Journal of Bone and Joint Surgery (British)* 2005;**87**:640–5.
32. Tuan RS. A second-generation autologous chondrocyte implantation approach to the treatment of focal articular cartilage defects. *Arthritis Research and Therapy* 2007;**9**:109.
33. Nöth U, Steinert AF, Tuan RS. Technology insight: adult mesenchymal stem cells for osteoarthritis therapy. *Nature Clinical Practice Rheumatology* 2008;**4**:371–80.

Medical ethics

RACHEL G GEDDES, SURESHAN SIVANANTHAN

Introduction	1531	Best interests and informed consent	1533
Applied principlism	1531	References	1535
Applying ethics	1532		

INTRODUCTION

Ethics are based on philosophical theories and can often seem abstract and removed from real-life situations. Also, those who tend to choose medicine or surgery as their profession intuitively want to treat their patients in a way that will be most beneficial to the patient's quality of life. For these reasons, many clinicians see medical ethics either as impractical to apply in daily practice or as common sense. It is, we believe, more useful to use medical ethics as a set of tools. If we have a good understanding of ethical concepts, these tools can be used in situations we encounter every day – not just in life or death situations, but also during ward rounds, in outpatient clinics, in theatre or in the emergency department. This chapter has two objectives. First, to give the reader a clear and concise explanation of applied principlism as a revision tool or 'recap'. Second, to expand on these concepts to give a deeper understanding of how applied principlism can be used in modern medical and surgical practice.

APPLIED PRINCIPLISM

Applied principlism is also known as the 'four ethical principals'. It was developed by Beauchamp and Childress in the 1970s specifically to make ethics more relevant to everyday clinical practice, and to give the clinician the 'tools' to make ethical decisions. Applied principlism recognizes the fact that ethical dilemmas in medicine are never black and white – there are always complexities and each patient and each doctor has a different way of looking at the world. Even though every human body is different, we still use anatomical landmarks to know where to make an incision. Similarly, in applied principlism, we can still use the four principles in any medical dilemma to orientate ourselves and approach the decision-making process within an ethical framework. Next, we will define the four principles that make up applied principlism (Box 133.1).

> **BOX 133.1: Definitions of the four principles that make up applied principlism**
>
> - Autonomy: deliberated self rule[1]
> - Beneficence: doing good
> - Non-maleficence: to do no harm
> - Justice: to treat equals equally

Autonomy

As medical professionals, we are expected to have respect for patient autonomy. The patient makes decisions relating to his or her life after deliberating the pros and cons of the intervention. This means that a patient has the right to decide whether to undergo a medical intervention, even if refusal to undergo the intervention may result in harm or perhaps death.[2] The best definition of autonomy is therefore 'deliberated self-rule'.[3] Patient confidentiality can be described as respecting autonomy because it builds trusting relationships between doctors and patients.[4]

Beneficence

This literally means 'doing good'.[5] The idea of beneficence is often the driving force behind people's desire to become doctors. In practical terms, beneficence may involve working with and supporting families, communities or medical charities, and providing the highest standard of care possible through using an evidence-based approach to treatment. Examples of beneficence can be seen in the UK General Medical Council's *Good Medical Practice: Duties of a Doctor*,[6] and best practice recommendations. Of course, sometimes the treatment may cause some harm (such as gastrointestinal disturbances in antibiotic use), but prescribing the antibiotics in the first place is still a beneficent act as the aim of the treatment is to remove infection.

Non-maleficence

The literal meaning of non-maleficence is 'to do no harm'. This is related to the concept of beneficence, and ideally we weigh up the two principles against each other. Non-maleficence is not the opposite of beneficence; for example, the same treatment may be ideal in one situation and harmful in another. This means the decision to administer the treatment requires us to weigh up risk and benefit to act in a non-maleficent way. We also need to consider our (modern) understanding of 'harm'. Common medications such as pain relief can have side-effects such as gastric ulcers or liver damage, and organ and tissue transplants require powerful immunosuppressants that leave the patient susceptible to a multitude of pathogenic complications. The disease itself and the treatment both have the potential to cause 'harm'.[7] In cases 2 and 3 described below, we will consider the fine line between 'doing good' and 'doing no harm'.

Justice

This principle dictates that we should 'treat equals equally'.[8] Justice is a difficult concept to grasp, and many different forms of justice exist. In medicine, our main rationale for treatment should be based on clinical need.[8] Broadly speaking, this means that two patients with the same diagnosis and prognosis should be offered the same treatment, regardless of lifestyle, culture, beliefs, ethnicity or sexuality. Justice-based areas in medicine include human rights, financial allocation and funding for certain medical procedures, and access to healthcare.

APPLYING ETHICS

Autonomy, agency and decision-making

The concept of autonomy has been interpreted in different ways by various authors. For example, Beauchamp and Childress, the forefathers of applied principlism, believe that a truly autonomous patient is one who acts with understanding, intention of an outcome, and without interference from other agents.[1] This definition is valid and accepted, but still makes assumptions. First, it assumes that patients will always act rationally and with reason. If we examine this definition more closely, the first thing we notice is the assumption that the patient acts with *understanding*. In terms of medical ethics, this means that the patient has received all of the information necessary to make his or her decision, and has the ability to make sense of the information. This, of course, is linked with the concept of informed consent and capacity, which we will discuss later. The next assumption is that the patient will act with *intent*. This means not only that the patient understands the consequences of his or her decision but also that he or she actively wishes the outcome of that decision to be met; therefore, the decision is compliant with the treatment plan. Third, the patient is acting without *interference* from other agents. Put simply, an agent is an individual who is not a passive bystander to the social world around them, but one who can shape and make decisions within this social world. If we understand this concept, it becomes difficult to imagine how a patient can make a decision about treatment without being influenced by someone else. When patients are consented for surgery, for example, we can give them the facts and figures on the likelihood of postoperative bleeding, infection or the need for further surgery, but we can never do this in a completely objective way. We are all agents and have emotions, beliefs and moral standards; therefore, even the way in which we present the information will, to some extent, influence the decision made. Similarly, when patients go through the process of making a decision about a surgical procedure, they will (hopefully) seek advice and opinion from family, friends and those involved in their care. On the one hand, a patient who has done this is more informed. On the other hand, another agent will have influenced the decision in some way. This is another key point, as, once we understand this, we can accept that the most important factor in autonomy is *critical reflection*[1] by patients. That is, they have weighed up the relevant information, gathered from the sources *they have selected* and have made their decision. Patient autonomy should therefore be seen as a process, and, as surgeons, our role is effective communication with patients, their families and the multidisciplinary team to ensure optimum care.[8] This is discussed further in case 3 (see below).

When autonomy does not apply: capacity and children

Autonomous patients are those who can weigh up the information given to them, and make a decision based on that information. Clearly, not all patients are autonomous! For example, neonates are not able to make autonomous decisions, and those with severe mental illness may be unable to make autonomous decisions. In both these cases, we can probably expect this type of individual to become autonomous or capable of making decisions about their care at some point in time, e.g. when the child grows up or the mentally ill person is in remission. In other cases, such as in individuals who are mentally impaired owing to progressive neurodegenerative conditions, we may not expect them to make autonomous decisions in the future. This should not affect immediate decisions regarding treatment, unless an advance directive is in place. The ability to make autonomous decisions is *capacity*. In paediatric cases, which we will use as the example in this section, we would normally expect a child to gain capacity and be able to make decisions for themselves at some point in time. Of course, this point will be at different ages for some children, and as clinicians we must not make assumptions about a child's capacity (or lack of it).

Adolescents may be deemed competent to participate in decision-making, and their competence to determine their treatment is measured by their capacity to understand the issue in question, which involves cognitive ability, rationality, self-identity and the ability to reason.[9] Even if a child does not have the capacity to make a decision for him- or herself, if the child is undergoing a surgical procedure, he or she should still have the procedure explained in a way that he or she can understand. In explaining a procedure to a child, it is useful to remember that, even though the child may not have the capacity to decide whether or not to have surgery, the child may have the capacity to decide which clothes, books or games to bring to the ward. It may, therefore, be possible to offer the child some choices regarding treatment (e.g. to offer a liquid or tablet form of antibiotic). Perhaps the most important aspect to consider is how best to work in the patient's best interests. An individual should rarely make decisions regarding care for a patient with reduced capacity. In paediatric cases, the ability to consent is passed to the birth mother,[8] and the consent-holder's wishes should be upheld unless the doctor in charge believes those wishes are against the best interests of the patient (see Best interests and informed consent, and case 2). Similarly, in a trauma case involving a child, if no one can be contacted who could consent to, say, emergency surgery, the doctor is expected to act in the child's best interests.

BEST INTERESTS AND INFORMED CONSENT

In simple terms, the best interests of a patient involve the doctor weighing up the risks and benefits of an intervention against not having that intervention. Table 133.1 gives the example of the potential risks and benefits of a total knee joint replacement. Looking at the risks and benefits, it is likely that, in most cases, the benefits would outweigh the risks; therefore, the procedure would be in the patient's best interests. This is a straightforward example to illustrate the point, and we acknowledge that real-life situations are often more complex! Case 3 (see below) considers the best interests of a trauma patient, introducing the idea of temporarily diminished capacity discussed in the previous section.

Along with establishing best interests for a patient, we also need to consider how to effectively consent the patient for the procedure. This is to ensure that we have gained appropriately *informed* consent. This not only is for legal protection, but also it is a professional requirement.[6,10] Informed consent should be seen as a process, and not as a means to complete our mental checklist in an outpatient clinic. It requires that we explain procedures to patients using terms they understand, and in a way that allows the patients to ask us questions. It is also a key aspect of respecting patients' autonomy and allowing them to begin the process of critical reflection. A good example of effective informed consent can be seen when patients are offered the opportunity to take part in randomized controlled trials (RCTs). On the one hand, researchers need to maximize recruitment and make results as representative for the sample group as possible, thus acting in a beneficent way to 'the greater good'. On the other hand, disclosing a greater amount of information about what is potentially at stake for the patient has been shown to reduce recruitment for trials.[11] Thus, a delicate balancing act is required of the researcher, as individual autonomy must be respected, even though it may be in the social 'best interests' for an individual to take part in the trial. Of course, it is down to the individual to make the decision after a period of critical reflection, and, as researchers and clinicians, we should give the patient the option of current and proven treatment options outside the RCT to establish whether the patient has preferences for treatment. If the researcher is in doubt about treatment preferences, or if the patient is not in the best position to make that choice, the researcher should avoid putting the patient forward for an RCT.[11]

Table 133.1 Risks and benefits to establish whether a knee joint replacement is in the best interests of a patient

	Risks	Benefits
Surgical intervention	Adverse drug reactions, risk of anaesthetic, postsurgical complications, e.g. pulmonary embolism, deep vein thrombosis	Patient free from pathology; patient has an enhanced quality of life
No surgical intervention	Chronic pain, disability, deformity; decreased quality of life	Patient may not want surgery; avoids risks related to surgery

In the following sections, we will consider three hypothetical cases using the most recent evidence available. These cases have been designed to highlight the concepts and dimensions we have discussed so far.

Case 1

You are a consultant surgeon, and you have been called by your junior colleague on the surgical assessment ward. A 65-year-old Jehovah's Witness has been admitted with haemorrhagic shock from a perforated duodenal ulcer. The patient has capacity, and has already had the treatment plan explained to him in a comprehensive manner by the ward surgeon, according to the patient's best interests. This involves an urgent blood transfusion to restore circulating volume, and surgical intervention to arrest the bleed. After considering the treatment plan and speaking to his wife, the patient decides a blood transfusion is morally wrong according to his beliefs, and he would like you to proceed with the surgery using available non-blood products. The patient accepts the increased risks involved, but stands firm in his decision. His wife supports his decision.

DISCUSSION

Legally, you cannot give the patient a blood transfusion if the patient is aware of the risks and has made the decision to refuse the treatment. The key points in this case are, first, that the patient has capacity and, second, that the patient has been informed of the risks and benefits of the procedure, including the outcome of refusing the blood transfusion.[12] The patient believes the harm of a blood transfusion outweighs the benefits. This is a difficult situation to accept, as a surgeon wants to act in the best interests of the patient. However, you can still act with beneficence, as you can still offer the patient the best alternative treatment (i.e. surgery without a blood transfusion). Non-maleficence is present as the alternative treatment will not harm the patient, even though it may not be as effective as if blood products were given. Justice is upheld as the best available treatment has been offered to the patient. The autonomy of the patient has clearly been respected, even if you believe that the patient's decision is not in his best interests. On balance for this case, the principle of autonomy has swayed the treatment of the patient.

Case 2

This case involves a similar presentation (haemorrhagic shock), but the patient is a 12-year-old trauma patient with an internal bleed. You are the surgeon, and the patient's mother is insisting that you operate but do not give a blood transfusion, or she will take legal action against you and the hospital.

DISCUSSION

You could potentially give the blood transfusion in this case. As the patient lacks capacity, you must act in the best interests of the patient, and clearly this would involve a blood transfusion. Even if the patient's mother was present and refused the transfusion, you could still administer the optimum treatment available as the principle of autonomy does not apply here. You would still be acting in a beneficent, non-maleficent way, while upholding justice. You would be 'doing good' by using the best treatment available according to the current evidence base in the short term. You would also be acting with non-maleficence in terms of the treatment and outcome, but it could be argued that, culturally, the patient will be 'harmed' because of being given allogeneic blood. In addition, you may harm the doctor–patient (and doctor–family) relationship, which should be based foremost on trust. In the long term, the family may not bring the children to hospital again for fear that they may be treated against the family's wishes, and this could lead to a tragic outcome. This would also conflict with the principle of beneficence. In summary, you may take the views of the parent into account, but you would be professionally obliged to act in the patient's best interests.[8,12] At the same time, however, you should seek legal counsel and the opinions of other suitably qualified staff.

Case 3

A 68-year-old woman is brought into the emergency department with a fractured neck of femur. You perform a surgical repair, and you meet her the next day on the ward. Before the surgery, you quickly explained the procedure and she signed a consent form. However, postoperatively, she seems confused and is not sure why she needed to go to theatre. You suspect that she did not fully understand the procedure she had, and may have been suffering from a delirium. Her family wants to know why you did not explain the surgery to her, and are now worried about the risk of postsurgical complications.

DISCUSSION

In this case, you acted in the patient's best interests. In a trauma case, this is legally all that is required of a surgeon, i.e. consent is not necessarily required (e.g. if the patient lacks capacity).[8] However, most people would agree that it is good practice to attempt to obtain some form of consent! Consenting trauma patients is challenging. There is often insufficient time to question the patient's understanding of surgical procedures, and patients may be confused as they have suddenly been brought into hospital, and may be in pain. Even though this type of presentation does not allow for the ideal period of critical reflection by the patient, it is still vitally important to respect the patient's autonomy. This may be achieved by giving patients the salient points regarding the surgery and complications, and may be enhanced by giving them some information in written form (such as a leaflet).[13] Respect for autonomy involves building a trusting relationship with the patient. Open communication is crucial and the patient should always be given an opportunity to ask questions. It may be worth referring to the patient's notes and explaining to the patient how capacity was measured before consent was obtained. In addition, studies have shown that trauma patients would like to have verbal information repeated several times,[13] which may be difficult on a busy ward, but would be wise and could prevent problems down the line. In terms of beneficence, you were clearly acting in the best interests of the patient, and the risks and benefits of undergoing surgery versus withholding surgery should be explained to the patient (and family). Non-maleficence was carried out at the time of the operation; however, in this case, it would be worth spending time with the patient, exploring her concerns and explaining possible postsurgical complications to avoid harm in the future. Justice has also been taken into account, as the patient was offered the best treatment based on her clinical need.

KEY LEARNING POINTS

- Autonomy is a process by which clinicians should promote and facilitate critical reflection.
- When capacity is diminished, the clinician should work in the best interests of the patient and seek the views of the consent-holder, or the patient's family.
- In randomized controlled trials, the researcher should offer the participant all the alternative treatments.
- In trauma cases, the process of obtaining consent should be well documented in the notes.

REFERENCES

1. Stiggelbout AM, Molewijk AC, Otten W, et al. Ideals of patient autonomy in clinical decision-making: a study on the development of a scale to assess patients' and physicians' views. *Journal of Medical Ethics* 2004;**30**:268–74.
2. General Medical Council. Seeking patient consent: the ethical considerations. London, UK: GMC, 1998. Available from: http://www.gmc-uk.org/Seeking_patients_consent_The_ethical_considerations.pdf_25417085.pdf.
3. Dworkin G. *The Theory and Practice of Autonomy.* New York, NY: Cambridge University Press, 1988.
4. Gillon R. Medical ethics: four principles plus scope. *British Medical Journal* 1994;**309**:184.
5. Boyd K (ed.) *The New Dictionary of Medical Ethics.* London, UK: BMJ Publishing Group, 1997.
6. General Medical Council. Good medical practice: duties of a doctor. London, UK: GMC, 2010. Available from: http://www.gmc-uk.org/guidance/good_medical_practice/duties_of_a_doctor.asp.
7. Wolpe PR. The triumph of autonomy in American bioethics: a sociological view. In: DeVries R, Subedi J (eds) *Bioethics and Society: Constructing the Ethical Enterprise.* Upper Saddle River, NJ: Prentice Hall, 1998.
8. Sokol D, Bergson G. *Medical Ethics and Law. Surviving on the Wards and Passing Exams.* London, UK: Trauma Publishing, 2005.
9. Larcher V. ABC of adolescence. Consent, competence, and confidentiality. *British Medical Journal* 2005;**330**:353–6.
10. Pitts D, Rowley DI, Marx C, et al. A competency based curriculum specialist training in trauma and orthopaedics. London, UK: British Orthopaedic Association, 2007. Available from: https://www.iscp.ac.uk/orthocurriculum/Content/15350_Whole_Doc_19.pdf.
11. Lilford R. Ethics of clinical trials from a Bayesian and decision analytic perspective: whose equipoise is it anyway? *British Medical Journal* 2003;**326**:980.
12. Gillon R. Four scenarios. *Journal of Medical Ethics* 2003;**29**:267–8.
13. Bhangu A, Hood E, Datta A. Is informed consent effective in trauma patients? *Journal of Medical Ethics* 2008;**34**:780–2.

Outcomes, databanks (joint registries), medical coding

EUGENE SHERRY, SURESHAN SIVANANTHAN, RAQUEL GEHR

Outcomes	1536	Medical coding	1537
Databanks	1536	References	1538
Stakeholders of healthcare	1537		

NATIONAL BOARD STANDARDS

- Learn what audit is in modern surgical practice
- Learn the role of databanks
- To understand what medical coding is

OUTCOMES

Continuing professional development is all about your work as a surgeon without the consideration of fees.

It includes documentation of self-directed learning (reading journals, internet education, workshops, group activity); clinical and consulting activities (hospital meetings, grand rounds, journal clubs, visits to other units, peer involvement, supervision of trainees, voluntary work, medico-legal work); teaching and related activities (with students, residents, registrars, college and academy activities, examination involvement, mentoring); scientific and research activities (papers, scientific presentations, basic and clinical research); credentialing (by the hospital where you work); and audit (morbidity, mortality meetings, adverse events, caseload summaries, peer review).

Clinical outcomes are important for the review of our clinical practice and to improve patient care. This is done by an audit. Most professional bodies take this matter seriously and require all their members to participate in regular audits of their surgical care (including their medico-legal work).

The Royal Australasian College of Surgeons (RACS) defines surgical audit as 'the regular documented critical analysis of the outcomes of the surgical care'. It is to be reviewed by peers and then used to improve surgical practice. Audit is said to answer the question 'Are we doing what we think we are doing?' The next step is to use this as parts of 'peer review', where you and colleagues use such information to modify and improve practice, education, best-practice models and protocols.

Guidelines and online and paper booklets are provided for surgeons to meet these requirements of the RACS.[1] Similar requirements exist in the UK, Europe and Asia.[2–4]

DATABANKS

Surgeons have always reviewed their work: getting together in formal meetings to discuss difficult cases and to seek the advice of colleagues about how to proceed. But now it has become a requirement of their own professional bodies, medical licensing boards and even government. Governments are keen to make it law, but most professional associations prefer to keep it 'in house' as a requirement of membership of their body.

Such self-regulation appears to be an orderly and mature way of running such activities rather than giving it over to government, where regulations are 'imposed' on the profession that may become irrational or onerous.

Also, it is important to not allow insurance companies and government to 'hijack' such information and use something collected voluntarily to be then used against the members contributing such information freely.

National joint registries

The only well-organized databanks in orthopaedics are joint registries to collect information on joint replacements. Such registries define the epidemiology of joint replacement and so identify trends regarding failure. They exist in Sweden (the first), Finland, Norway, Denmark, Hungary, Canada, New Zealand, Australia and the UK.

The information derived from the Swedish databank has shown for total hip replacement that surgical technique and implant type are the main determinants for a good outcome (non-cemented acetabular component with a cemented femoral implant).[5]

Obviously, insurance companies and government are interested in this information as total hip replacement, although expensive, is repeatedly documented as the best elective operation performed across all surgical disciplines with a seen increasing demand for it.

Background databanks

COCHRANE

The Cochrane Library is a collection of databases in healthcare set up by the Cochrane Collaboration and other organizations. The Cochrane Reviews, a database of systematic reviews and meta-analyses, summarizes and interprets the results of high-quality medical research. It is supported by epidemiologists with the belief that so-called evidence-based medicine is only a recent phenomenon in medicine and that all clinical decisions are based on published papers. It does not recognize that busy clinicians seldom publish and so a huge resource of experience is ignored with this approach.

CORPORATE DATABANKS: MICROSOFT AND GOOGLE HEALTH DATABASES

Microsoft has announced the formation of Health Vault, an online personal health information database. Google has set up Google Health. It is likely that these databases are the biggest and most profitable social databases ever.

Electronic health records are being established in many countries, including Australia.

It seems everyone wants to own and collect clinical data. The motives are clear, profit, even though improving clinical outcomes are talked about. But surgeons need to realize that they are the originators of these clinical data and should not readily lose ownership as there are examples of government databanks breaching patient confidentiality.

STAKEHOLDERS OF HEALTHCARE

Numerous groups act as 'stakeholders of healthcare': the profession (as above), and patient advocate or consumer groups, both recent (e.g. the Leapfrog Group) and long term (the RAND Corporation, MedWatch from the US Food and Drug Administration).[6]

Insurance companies (recently Medibank Private of Australia) and goverments (in Australia, the Health Insurance Corporation; in the USA, the Centres for Medicare and Medicaid Services) have criticized the use of more expensive modern hip implants rather than cheaper cemented implants (based on data from national joint registries).

The USA appears to have the most formalized and structured approach to these organizations, but that has not stopped healthcare in the USA spiralling to 16% of GDP (2.5 times the Organization for Economic Cooperation and Development average) and threatening to bankrupt the economy with an average life expectancy of 78 years (the global average is 69 years, Australia 81 years, Switzerland 82 years, China 69 years, Sudan 58 years).[7]

These various groups' interests are summarized in Table 134.1.

The profession's response to this pressure has been to provide clinical practice guidelines (an initiative of the American Academy of Orthopaedic Surgeons) for the management of common conditions (e.g. carpal tunnel syndrome) that focus on best outcomes and the reasonable costs to achieve this. It seems prudent to keep doctors and surgeons in the forefront of developing such guidelines to prevent other stakeholders or third parties introducing absurdities into clinical practice (e.g. the current practice of Worker's Compensation case managers in Australia, with modest medical training, overruling the surgeon's clinical decision of whether a knee arthroscopy is required by insisting upon expensive MRI technology and numerous second opinions that increase the cost of the procedure by >100%).

MEDICAL CODING

Medical classification, or *medical coding*, is defined by Wikipedia as the process of transforming descriptions of

Table 134.1 Stakeholders in healthcare

Group or stakeholder	Goal	Measure
Financial or the payer	Value for money	Benefit–cost analysis
Healthcare regulator	Efficiency of services	Outcome–cost analysis
Government	Successful management	Total cost of healthcare as % of gross domestic product

Table 134.2 Requirement for designing a coding system

Designers	Involvement of the clinicians who generate the data
Data	Easily collected
Data	Transferable so can be used for planning of clinical services, research and clinical treatment

medical diagnoses and procedures/operations into universal medical code numbers. Sources include medical records, laboratory results, radiograph/imaging results, and other sources. Such diagnostic codes can be used to track diseases. Users of such data include government health programmes, private health insurance companies, workers' compensation insurers, and others.

Other applications include statistical analysis of diseases and therapy, reimbursement (based on diagnostic related groups), knowledge-based and decision support systems and direct surveillance of epidemic or pandemic outbreaks

This is a system whereby clinical data (including operations) from a hospital are collected, assigned a numeric code, collated and then compiled to document this clinical activity. The information is held by government health departments. The requirement for such a coding system is clear (Table 134.2).

However, many coding systems have been devised with minimal involvement of surgical professional bodies and are seldom if ever used in textbooks, research papers or online (in surgical sites such as Wheeless Textbook of Orthopaedics). It is as if the system has developed separately in parallel with medical knowledge. The information is collected without the involvement of the treating doctors or surgeons so it is not unusual for the coders to have great difficulty assigning a code to a particular operation, thereby casting doubt over the accuracy of the data. Further, the data are not used by surgeons for research or clinical work. In fact, there is evidence of misuse of such data by hospital administrators in New South Wales, Australia, using such data to run vendettas and to discredit doctors working at the same hospital.

KEY LEARNING POINTS

- Audit, a measure of clinical outcomes, is an important and essential part of surgical practice.
- The best-known databanks in orthopaedic surgery are national joint registries.
- Medical coding collects medical information by translating it into universal medical code numbers. It has limited clinical value.

REFERENCES

- ● = Key primary paper
- ♦ = Major review article

● 1. Guide by the RACS-Surgical Audit and peer review, 2002. Available from: http://www.surgeons.org/Content/NavigationMenu/FellowshipandStandards/CPDRecertification/default.htm
● 2. Royal College of Surgeons. *Continuing Professional Development of the Royal College of Surgeons.* Available from: www.rcseng.ac.uk/standards
● 3. European Federation of National Associations of Orthopaedics and Traumatology (EFFORT). Available from: http://www.efort.org/
● 4. Asia Pacific Orthopaedic Association (APOA). Available from: http://www.apoa-home.org/index.html
5. Swedish Joint Register. Available from: http://www.jru.orthop.gu.se/
6. The Leapfrog Group. Available from: www.leapfrog.org
7. The Costs of US HealthCare. Available from: http://www.cfr.org/publication/13325/%20

135

Informed consent

EUGENE SHERRY, RAQUEL GEHR

Background	1539	Competency	1540
Specifics of informed consent	1539	Informed consent and the right to refuse treatment	1540
Decision-making capacity (competency)	1540	Children and consent	1540
Disclosure	1540	Clinical trials and research	1541
Documentation of consent	1540	References	1541

NATIONAL BOARD STANDARDS

- To understand the implications of informed consent for treatment and clinical trials

BACKGROUND

Contemporary doctors and surgeons are well aware of the need to obtain informed consent prior to treatment or surgery, but this was not always the case. For example, the Nuremberg Code was enacted in the 1940s after Nazi human experimentation, and the Declaration of Helsinki was enacted in 1964 to create a code of research ethics. In addition, Institutional Review Boards were set up as a result of the outrage caused by the Tuskegee Study, in which Black men with syphilis were left untreated from 1932 to 1972 despite penicillin becoming available in the 1940s.[1,2]

It is important for doctors to know about consent issues, even though many organizations, including governments, want to take ownership of this basic medical entity, because, in the final analysis, it is the treating doctor who bears all or most of the responsibility. Also, lawyers seek to exploit any deficiencies or errors in the system.

This is further complicated by the fact that, at times, various healthcare advocates can place 'impossible' demands upon doctors by patients refusing reasonable treatment but shifting responsibility back to the doctor.

Informed consent is said to be about professional negligence, and is about a 'breach of care owed to the patient and causation in English Law'. It concerns disclosing the risks of surgery in the UK, Singapore and Malaysia, but, in the USA, Australia and Canada, it is said to be a 'more patient-centered approach' in which the significant risks of such surgery, as 'well as the risks which would be of particular importance to that patient' are explained.

General medical consent is to do with assault or battery. The patient must understand the nature and purpose of the procedure.

SPECIFICS OF INFORMED CONSENT

As part of informed consent, before surgery or a procedure, the doctor must explain (in layperson's terms) the risks and benefits of the treatment. There is an exchange of information between the surgeon and the patient (verbal, written and even audiovisual) that should be easily understood by the patient. It must be freely given. It is not required for many 'minor' or routine procedures, such as physical examination or inserting an intravenous line (putting out your arm implies consent). Here, informed consent is assumed. However, for invasive tests or tests or treatments with significant risks or alternatives, informed consent is required.

If not obtained, the surgeon may face allegations of assault, battery or trespass against the patient.[3] Exceptions to this include an emergency or incompetence (young, very old, mentally incompetent), when the patient is not able to give permission.

The four components of informed consent are: (1) the patient's capacity (or ability) to make the decision; (2) the requirement that the doctor must disclose the expected benefits and risks; (3) the likelihood of each of the benefits and risks occurring; and (4) the patient must understand the likelihood of the risks and benefits and that the procedure is voluntary.

DECISION-MAKING CAPACITY (COMPETENCY)

This is a very important part of informed consent. It includes: the patient being able to understand the options; the patient being able to understand the consequences of choosing each of the options; the patient's ability to evaluate the personal cost and benefit of each of the consequences; and the patient being able to relate these to his or her own set of values and priorities.

If the patient does not understand, then family members, court-appointed guardians or others (as determined by state law) may act as 'surrogate decision-makers' and make these decisions on the patient's behalf.

DISCLOSURE

The doctor or healthcare provider must supply information so that a reasonable person can make an intelligent decision. This information includes the risks, and the likelihood (or probability) of each of the risks, and the benefits, and the likelihood (or probability) of each of the benefits. Questions should be encouraged.

In the USA, two standards are applied: professional or reasonable doctor standard (customary practice of your region) and the patient's viewpoint standard (what a reasonable person would expect to know).

DOCUMENTATION OF CONSENT

For routine blood tests, radiographs, and splints or casts, consent is implied. No written consent process is required. For many invasive tests or surgery a written consent form and a verbal explanation are required. The components of this are: an explanation of the medical problem that requires the test, procedure or treatment; an explanation of the purpose and benefits of the test, procedure or treatment; an explanation or description, including possible complications or adverse events, of the test, procedure or treatment; alternative treatments, procedures or tests; and the consequences of not accepting the test, procedure or treatment.

A long form (with all the specific details of the discussion), a short form (in which it states that the risk/benefits have been discussed) or a detailed note in the patient's chart (often combined with the short or long form to make the so-called double consent) may be used.

The consent form should be signed and dated by the doctor and the patient. An adult signs for a child.

COMPETENCY

Competency indicates that a patient has the ability to make, and be held accountable for, decisions. A patient can be declared 'incompetent' only by a court of law.

INFORMED CONSENT AND THE RIGHT TO REFUSE TREATMENT

Apart from legally authorized involuntary treatment, patients who are legally competent to make medical decisions, and who can be considered to have decision-making capacity, have the legal and moral right to refuse any or all treatment. This is true even if the patient chooses to make a 'bad decision' that may result in serious disability or even death (although great care needs to be exercised when a patient makes such a decision, i.e. the doctor should seek another medical opinion or even refuse to be involved). Such patients are requested to sign an Against Medical Advice form.

However, a doctor may decide that, because of intoxication, injury, illness, emotional stress or any other reason, a patient does not have decision-making capacity and so the patient may not be able to refuse treatment. The law presumes that the average reasonable person would consent to treatment in most emergencies to prevent permanent disability or death.

Advance directives and living wills are filled out by patients to determine care in the face of an emergency. These legal documents direct doctors and other healthcare providers about specific treatments. Extreme caution has to be exercised in these cases.

CHILDREN AND CONSENT

Minors usually do not have legal empowerment to give informed consent. Therefore, the parents or authorized decision-makers may give informed consent on the child's behalf. Parents are assumed to act in the best interests of their children. But, when the parents and the doctor disagree (e.g. parents refusing blood transfusions for their child), authority comes from state laws to empower the doctor to give the considered appropriate treatment. Thus, disagreements may result in court orders that specify what treatment should occur (e.g. blood transfusions) or in the court-ordered appointment of a guardian to make medical decisions for the child. Be aware that many US states have laws that designate certain minors as emancipated and entitled to the full rights of adults (self-supporting and/or not living at home, married, pregnant or a parent, in the military, declared emancipated by a court). Similarly, decision-making authority is given to otherwise unemancipated minors with decision-making capacity (mature minors) who require care for certain medical conditions (drug or alcohol abuse, pregnancy or sexually transmitted diseases).

CLINICAL TRIALS AND RESEARCH

Patients may want to take part in clinical studies or trials for various reasons, such as receiving a new drug or treatment before it is generally available or receiving drugs for which no payment is made. Informed consent is required setting out why the research is being done and what is involved.

Clinical studies are the backbone of modern orthopaedic practice, as there are constant improvements in surgical technique and implant design. In the USA the Food and Drug Administration (with the Institutional Review Board) and in Australia the Therapeutic Goods Administration regulate clinical trials to evaluate new techniques or implants, unless the new entity involves a variation of a previous surgical technique (e.g. mini-incision surgery) or a minor modification of an existing implant.

> **KEY LEARNING POINTS**
>
> - Written informed consent is required for most procedures apart from minor ones (e.g. putting in an intravenous line).
> - Informed consent requires explanation of the risks of surgery to avoid an allegation of negligence.
> - Clinical research needs to be done under guidelines (Institutional Review Board or Therapeutic Goods Administration).

REFERENCES

● = Key primary paper
◆ = Major review article

● 1. Clarkfield AM. Nazi medicine and the Nuremberg trials: from medical war crimes to informed consent. *New England Journal of Medicine* 2006;**295**:2668–9.
2. Baker SM, Brawley OW, Marks LS. Effects of untreated syphilis in the Negro male, 1932–1972: a closure comes to the Tuskegee study, 2004. *Urology* 2005;**65**:1259–62.
3. National Cancer Institute. A guide to informed consent. Available from: http://www.cancer.gov/clinicaltrials/conducting/informed-consent-guide

136

Work-related injuries and assessment for compensation

EUGENE SHERRY, RAQUEL GEHR

Background	1542
Return to work: too soon or too late	1543
Third-party involvement	1543
The assessment of permanent disability: guidelines and the 'battery hen' industry	1543
Specifics of work-related injuries: injury rate, occupation, types of injury, cause of injury	1543
Summary	1544
References	1544

NATIONAL BOARD STANDARDS

- To understand the role of orthopaedic surgeons in work-related injuries and worker's compensation, and the obligations of orthopaedic surgeons
- Learn the types of workers' compensation injuries

BACKGROUND

Most industrial societies have some kind of statutory insurance scheme for patients injured at work to pay the costs for medical care and lost wages on a no-fault basis.[1] It is like any other health insurance policy but with important differences: it is paid for by a third party – the employer, who is legally obliged to carry such insurance for employees. Therefore, the employer and insurance provider have a vested interest in the injury being resolved as soon as possible (i.e. rapid treatment and rehabilitation) with the return of the employee to work.

The features of workers' compensation are summarized in Table 136.1, with further detail below.

Table 136.1 Advantages and disadvantages of workers' compensation

	Advantages	Disadvantages
The injured worker	Prompt treatment in private system	Delay in treatment may result in second gains or further problems such as psychiatric
	Works well for self-limited injuries	Excluded from national insurance cover (e.g. Medicare in Australia) for long-term treatment of serious injuries
The workers' compensation insurance company/carrier	Legal fees contained	Premium rise pressure (from exaggerated or fraudulent claims)
The treating doctor/surgeon	Allows prompt treatment	A lot of paperwork/documentation (sometimes onerous but required by legislation)
		Third party (the case worker and various treatment therapists) placed in the doctor–patient relationship

RETURN TO WORK: TOO SOON OR TOO LATE

Employers' perspective

In industrial sectors of the economy, having employees off work with injury can result in penalties in the tendering process for future project/work contracts. Therefore, there is little interest in delaying treatment by second-guessing the treating doctor's diagnosis and treatment advice (as seen in the 'battery hen' second opinion industry; see below).

In contrast, in more corporate areas the 'battery hen' industry allows insurance companies to delay treatment (and therefore costs), resulting in an injured worker being out of work for a long time with secondary medical (including psychiatric) problems.

Employees' perspective

Employees may not see things in the same way as the employer. They may feel that they are being pressured to return to work too soon, and may wish to optimize the time away from work and the extent of residual disability to maximize a financial settlement (permanent disability) on the injury, given that litigation (tort) is limited.

This can provide an incentive to 'stay unwell', and workers' compensation surgical cases are often referred to in a separate category in the surgical literature when poor results are expected.[1]

Low back pain is prone to 'slow recovery', and so systems such as Waddell's non-organic physical signs exist to determine whether the injury is organic/physical.

Orthopaedic surgeons should keep to the principles they learnt in their training, with objective documentation of symptoms and signs and making a diagnosis and recommendation of treatment based upon sound science.

The area of repetitive strain injuries/trauma may not 'fit' here, and a second opinion or psychiatric referral may be required.

Disputes

The above can result in a dispute between the injured employee and the employer/insurance company. In the past, this has led to the involvement of lawyers on behalf of the injured. Such a situation in Australia and the USA resulted in an explosion of the costs of such insurance in the 1960s to 1990s, with the subsequent introduction of legislation for the resolution of such cases to minimize the involvement of lawyers in dispute resolution. Settlement amounts are now largely fixed, although they may be understated for a serious injury when a worker is permanently disabled and is not able to return to the work force.

Independent review panels now exist in many countries to decide such matters.

THIRD-PARTY INVOLVEMENT

Workers' compensation insurance introduces *case workers* to oversee the treatment and rehabilitation process (this is done by few other health insurance carriers; in addition, therapists not chosen by the treating doctor or patient are involved). Specialists in rehabilitation and occupational medicine are also involved.

This results in a case worker, well intentioned but in a *de facto* way, orchestrating and reviewing the treatment, i.e. a third party is introduced between the treating doctor and the patient. This often results in the unnecessary ordering of MRI examinations, as if such examinations can replace clinical judgement of whether surgery is required and of when treatment is completed.

THE ASSESSMENT OF PERMANENT DISABILITY: GUIDELINES AND THE 'BATTERY HEN' INDUSTRY

The assessment of permanent disability after injury translates into a financial settlement for the injured worker. The determination of this percentage disability or impairment is usually carried out using the American Medical Association *Guides to the Evaluation of Permanent Impairment*. This is a book of tables, figures and charts that quantify impairment; however, most surgeons do not realize that they are arbitrary and non-scientific.

Also, lucrative allied businesses (so-called 'battery hen' orthopaedic assessments) have been established around this assessment process, employing (usually) retired orthopaedic surgeons (attracted as the risks of operating are eliminated and the stress of clinical care is absent) even though it can be a repetitive process with little resemblance to the vigours of clinical orthopaedic practice (resulting in the reduction of the orthopaedic workforce for clinical and surgical care). The task here is to offer a second/'independent' opinion regarding the need for treatment, whether the injury is work related and to assess progress and whether the condition has reached the maximum possible improvement, in order to avoid the bias that would be expected from the treating doctor (who is required to act in the patient's interests). How necessary and independent they are is open to question.

SPECIFICS OF WORK-RELATED INJURIES: INJURY RATE, OCCUPATION, TYPES OF INJURY, CAUSE OF INJURY

There are a lot of data about work-related injuries. Injuries of the musculoskeletal system account for >33% of all such injuries.

In Australia, a 12 month review of injuries from 2005 to 2006 showed that, in the workforce of 10.8 million, 6.4%

were injured.[2] Most (86%) continued in the same job; 7.5% changed jobs; and 6.8% became unemployed. Two-thirds (63%) were men (54% of the workforce is male). The 15–19 year age group was more likely to be injured (78 per 1000 people), with the >55 years age group having the lowest rate (50 per 1000 people).

The industries with the highest work-related injury or illness rates were agriculture, forestry and fishing (109 per 1000 employed people), manufacturing (87 per 1000 employed people) and construction and mining (each 86 per 1000 employed people). The industries with the lowest rates were finance/insurance (19 per 1000 employed people), property/business services (36 per 1000 employed people) and communications (37 per 1000 employed people).

With regard to types of injury, the most common were sprains or strains (30%), followed by cuts or open wounds (19%) and chronic joint or muscle conditions (19%).

The mechanism of injury was from lifting, pushing or pulling an object (32%), hitting, being hit or cut by an object, falls on the same level and repetitive movements.

Of note, salaries were paid to >50% by workers' compensation and >50% had some time off work.

A similar picture exists in Canada, and also showed that the rate of injury increased in the 1980s, with a decline from 48.9 per 1000 in 1987 to 18.8 per 1000 in 2007.[3]

Death from injury at work is rare. In the UK, there were 180 deaths from injury at work in 2008/9 (a rate of fatal injury of 0.6 per 100 000 workers), having decreased from the average rate for the previous 5 years.[4]

Areas of controversy include whether carpal tunnel syndrome is related to computer use (probably not) and whether ergonomic intervention in the workplace makes any difference (a lot less than might be expected).[5]

SUMMARY

Statutory workers' compensation is a compromise, guaranteeing workers medical care and continued payment but on a no-fault basis. But there is a cost, with an interruption of the doctor–patient relationship and a huge paper trail burden placed upon all participants. Workers' compensation is also a major cost to business.

KEY LEARNING POINTS

- Workers' compensation is, in principle, a good system of health insurance to provide the speedy and effective care of injured workers that limits litigation and so directly minimizes the costs to the economy. However, it does introduce interference in the doctor–patient relationship (seldom highlighted in the literature).
- Workers' compensation entails a lot more documentation, letters and reports by treating surgeons and doctors, with the questionable growth and value of the allied workers' compensation-related health industry.
- Workers' compensation works well for self-limited injuries with a small permanent impairment, but the associated exclusion of a worker with significant impairment from national health schemes is a major disadvantage.
- One-third of such injuries are musculoskeletal injuries in young men working in physical industries, and the overall work injury rate is declining.

REFERENCES

◆ = Major review article

1. Harris I, Mulford J, Solomon M, *et al*. Association between compensation status and outcome after surgery: a meta-analyses. *Journal of the American Medical Association* 2005;**293**:1644–52.
2. Australian Bureau of Statistics, *6324.0*, 2005–6. Available from: http://www.actu.org.au/Images/Dynamic/attachments/6514/factsheet_death_at_work_0409.pdf Work-Related Injuries, Australia
3. Human Resources and Skills Development Canada. Work-related injuries in Canada. Available from: http://www4.hrsdc.gc.ca/.3ndic.1t.4r@-eng.jsp?iid=20.
4. Health and Safety Executive UK. Fatal injury statistics. Available from: http://www.hse.gov.uk/statistics/fatals.htm.
◆5. American Academy of Orthopaedic Surgeons. *Orthopaedic Knowledge Update*, 9th edn. Rosemount, IL: AAOS, 2008:158–9.

137

Evidence-based medicine and orthopaedic surgeons

PATRICK H WARNKE, EUGENE SHERRY, CONOR SHERRY

| Introduction | 1545 | What is evidence-based medicine? | 1547 |
| Background | 1545 | References | 1548 |

NATIONAL BOARD STANDARDS

- Understand the role of evidence-based medicine in modern orthopaedic practice
- Know that evidence-based medicine has limitations in the process of surgical break throughs

INTRODUCTION

Evidence-based medicine (EBM), or the reliance on current scientific evidence to reach medical decisions, has been embraced as a new paradigm to standardize clinical care in many disciplines in medicine. A situation of uncertainty for clinical decision-making is unfamiliar to the experienced orthopaedic surgeon. Therefore, EBM has its limitations in surgery and is often neglected by orthopaedic surgeons. This chapter describes the elements of EBM required to understand the process of EBM-originated decision-making.

BACKGROUND

The term 'Evidence-Based Medicine' has flooded the clinically relevant literature in the past two decades. Together with this new topic in medicine, leaders and institutes in that field have come to influence 'clinical decision-making' and to evaluate the quality of a doctor's patient management. The reliance on current scientific evidence to reach medical decisions has even been embraced as a new paradigm to standardize clinical care .[1]

> It has been said that EBM is the last refuge of doctors escaping from patient care.

These statements predict that there is a lot of controversy about EBM and the doctors involved. This chapter may help one to understand current criticism on EBM and the dilemma it may face in orthopaedic surgery. So, what is important to know about EBM and its methods for 'clinical decision-making'?

One of the major textbooks on EBM for today's medical students starts with this paragraph:

> Clinical practice is about making choices. Shall I order a test? Should I treat the patient? What should I treat them with? The decision depends on the doctors' knowledge, skills and attitudes, and on what resources and tests are available. The patient's concerns, expectations and values also need to be taken into account...[2]

This may sound very unfamiliar to the orthopaedic consultant and experienced surgeon, because it resembles a clinical scenario full of doubt and uncertainty. You would rarely start an operation if you are in doubt about how to proceed after the incision. Orthopaedic surgery would not have its high standards today, or even exist, if this scenario was to be true for surgeons in an operating theatre. During his/her training the surgeon has learnt and acquired certain surgical skills to use in the theatre. One of the most important is confidence. Thus, a scenario of confidence and certainty is more realistic with orthopaedic surgeons in particular, as it is said that there are a lot of alpha males/females in this discipline.

Also, surgery is, unlike the prescribing of tablets, not a cookery book, where you can apply the same 'recipe' to every patient, which would easily allow for designing and performing reliable multicentre randomized controlled studies.

No operation is exactly the same: every surgeon does it a little bit different from his/her colleagues. Therefore, it is hard to compare one operation to another. The surgeon can quickly see the outcome for the particular operation and so evaluate it for him/herself. This way, the surgeon can identify problems and improve the technique. Each operation needs to be adapted to the patient and the constantly changing situations while operating. Also, each operation must address the individual patient expectations and values. It is as if every operation is an ongoing clinical experiment. This is a concept alien to many non-surgeons in medicine.

Another important factor for the clinical decision-making of surgeons is the situation in which the patient is presented. It makes a difference whether a patient presents for emergency or for elective surgery. In emergency situations you may not have all the relevant information you want. You may have to operate at 3 am in an emergency theatre without an EBM facility and without the convenient environment of a private hospital. These factors may influence the outcome of an operation and are not adequately recognized in EBM. It is thought or expected that a surgeon is performing each operation under circumstances that can be measured by EBM and quality assessment methods. There is also the problem of litigation, which influences clinical decision-making to follow non-scientific pathways.

Surgical training is also a steep learning curve. If you want to acquire these skills and perfect your surgical technique, you have to operate on many cases. This gives you confidence in clinical decision making, in and out of the theatre.

It comes down to this:

> The surgeon who rarely performs a certain operation has a high complication rate. The surgeon who frequently performs a certain operation has a low complication rate. Only those surgeons who never operate have no complications.
>
> Franz Härle, Kiel, Germany

The experience of a surgeon is very important and hard to measure. It is from this that a surgeon learns and has to make decisions as an individual under pressure, most often in the theatre, without the comfort of complicated statistical proof (Fig. 137.1).

However, review studies are possible in certain topics in orthopaedic surgery, for example to compare different surgical approaches to the hip – such as the posterior versus the anterior approach to hip arthroplasty. There are groups such as the 'The Swedish National Hip Arthroplasty Registry' (www.jru.orthop.gu.se) reviewing and reporting

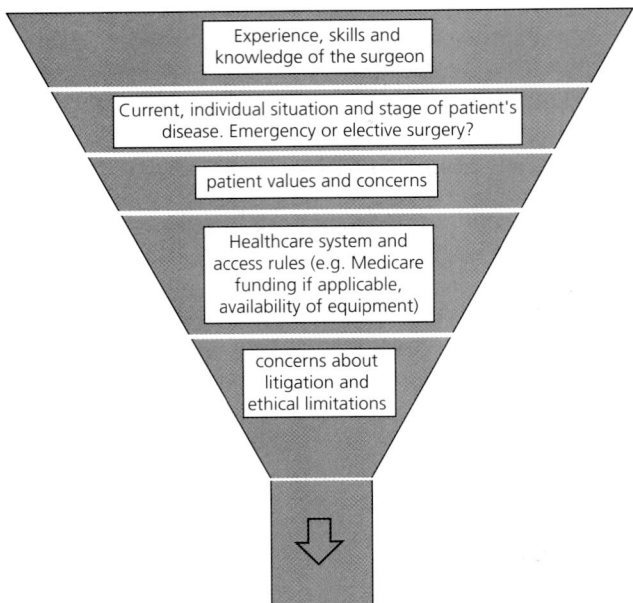

Figure 137.1 Clinical decision-making in orthopaedic surgery. The experience and skills of a surgeon play a pivotal role in this scenario. Some factors are critical for decision-making and standardized methods in EBM fail reliability when applied here or when evaluating the clinical outcome.

on the success rates of Swedish hip replacement surgery. But how do you reliably compare the outcome if different surgeons with different teams and instrumentation are performing the operations? Statistics rely on standardized methods that are difficult to apply here.

Pioneering surgical methods are not amenable to statistical testing, which may come later, when the new technique is in widespread use.

But such pioneering surgical approaches are essential. Surgical breakthroughs occur by first showing that a new (or first) type of operation is technically feasible, and then by repetition and follow-up to show that this new operation has long-term success. For example, surgical pioneer and Nobel laureate (in 1990) Dr Joe Murray has privately said that he knew that his new operation was a success when he saw the flow of urine within minutes of the first kidney transplant in 1954. In his Nobel Prize acceptance speech he said 'All the elements for a sound renal transplant program were in order: experienced knowledge in renal disease, availability of dialysis, and skilled imaginative surgeons'.[3]

The Nobel prizes awarded in medicine in the twentieth century were not EBM but often brain models developed in the minds of the scientists first. For example, the description of the DNA molecule in 1953 was not EBM or peer reviewed. Even the original publication itself was not a full study article, but a simple plain letter in Nature with one sketch of the suggested DNA structure.[4] It would have one of the lowest levels of evidence in EBM today, but this letter benefited medical science and patient care more than EBM ever will. The list goes on: Charnley's development of modern hip arthroplasty[5] or the first heart transplant in 1967;[6] the first tissue-engineered individualized body replacement in 2004;[7] and the first face transplant in 2005.[8] These would never have occurred if EBM had ruled the hands and minds of those pioneering surgeons. This doesn't mean that surgeons 'have more guts' and are braver than others, but in other areas of medicine such single-case breakthroughs are rare.

'Gut feeling' in surgery is something that every surgeon has experienced. It is hard to explain to non-surgeons and it is impossible to represent in EBM. But a surgeon's 'gut feeling' might be of higher importance for the patient than we ever thought. In 2005 Markus et al.[9] determined the predictive accuracy of the surgeon's 'gut feeling' in estimating the postoperative outcomes of patients undergoing major hepatobiliary or gastrointestinal surgery. Immediately after completion of surgery the surgeons were asked to predict the possible development of postoperative complications on a scale from 0 to 100. These predictions were compared with the actual outcome and with statistical predictions made using the Physiological and Operative Severity Score for the enumeration of Mortality and Morbidity (POSSUM). Surprisingly, the surgeon's gut feeling was more accurate in the prediction of morbidity than the relevant clinicopathological score-based evaluation.

In conclusion, we do not say that that EBM has no place in surgery, but it may have severe limitations when being applied in surgery. Therefore, we believe that the paradigm shift towards standardized clinical care can only be performed when the individual surgeon can be integrated into decision-making recommendations and when his/her quality and skills can be evaluated in an appropriate manner.

In the following paragraphs we summarize the nature of EBM and its goals.

WHAT IS EVIDENCE-BASED MEDICINE?

In the early 1990s David Sackett and his colleagues implemented the term Evidence-Based-Medicine at McMaster University in Ontario, Canada.[2] Sackett defined 'Levels of Evidence' for effectiveness of treatment and brought those in relation to clinical recommendations being set up for patient management.[10]

On the one hand, EBM is about trying to improve the quality of the information on which decisions in clinical practice are based. The goal is to integrate the best available research evidence – from the scientific method to decision-making – together with clinical expertise and patient values in order to achieve the best possible patient management.[2] On the other hand, its associated Cochrane Collaboration and the EBM recommendations help the practitioner to identify the risks and benefits of a clinical treatment and to avoid non-useful 'information overload' for finding the best clinical decision.[2]

The hallmark of this approach is said to be the Cochrane Collaboration. The Cochrane Collaboration was founded in response to Professor Archie Cochrane's call for systematic up-to-date reviews of all relevant randomized trials of healthcare in his influential postulations made in 1972.[11] He criticized the great collective unawareness at that time of the effects and benefits of healthcare to the patient.[2] He was concerned that doctors did not have ready access to reliable reviews of available evidence.[2] He requested a collection of systematic reviews, for which contributing authors are asked to provide detailed and repeatable literature reviews of a topic. Once this is done the treatment is said to be categorized as 'likely to be beneficial', 'likely to be harmful' or 'evidence did not support either benefit or harm'. In the early 1990s, funds were provided by the UK National Health Service to establish a Cochrane Centre in Oxford.[2] Today, the international Cochrane Collaboration publishes systematic reviews electronically in the Cochrane Library of Systematic reviews. The database can be accessed online at http://www.cochrane.org.

When performing systematic reviews inside the EBM frame you have to follow a certain pattern. However, at first 'you must admit that you don't know'.[2] Then you follow five steps that are listed in Box 137.1.

BOX 137.1: Steps in evidence-based medicine (FIRES)[2]

Step 1 Formulate an answerable question of interest for patient management

Step 2 Identify the best evidence of outcomes available

Step 3 Review and critically judge the evidence (How good is it?)

Step 4 Employ evidence (integrate results with clinical expertise and patient values)

Step 5 Summarize effectiveness and efficiency of the process (to improve next time)

Following those steps a practitioner will be able to gather valuable information to assist in optimal decision-making.

In conclusion, EBM is a very complex topic that you may simplify as follows:

1. EBM is about decision-making and clinical outcomes. The goal is to treat patients in the best and most scientifically valid way.
2. EBM is about systematically reviewing the medical literature and data to identify the best studies with the highest levels of evidence on the topic of interest.
3. EBM is about informing colleagues of findings and giving recommendations for patient management assisting in decision-making.

Levels of evidence

For clinical decision-making the information provided in the scientific medical literature plays a pivotal role. EBM categorizes different types of clinical evidence, as not every article or study has the same quality and relevance as another. For example, the strongest evidence for therapeutic interventions is provided by systematic reviews of randomized, double-blind and placebo-controlled trials involving a homogeneous patient population and medical condition. In contrast, least scientific value is given to patient testimonials, case reports and expert opinions or personal communications. In addition articles in non-peer-reviewed journals have a weak level of evidence.

There have been several attempts, such as by the US Preventive Services Task Force, the UK National Health Service or the Australian National Health and Medical Research Council (NHMRC),[12] at ranking the evidence about the effectiveness of treatments or screenings in levels of evidence (LOE) so that the assessed studies can be categorized (Box 137.2). A complex and detailed definition of LOE is published online by the Oxford Centre for Evidence-based Medicine (http://www.cebm.net/). However, defining LOE and improved systems to stratify evidence by quality are under constant development. For example, a more recent system has been developed by 'the GRADE Working Group' which takes into account more dimensions than just the quality of medical evidence with the use of 'Extrapolations'.[13] Extrapolation is used in a situation where potentially clinically important differences from the original study situation need to be considered. Thus, both the 'clinical directness of the data' and the quality of the research can be applied to decision-making.

However, the appropriate integration or extrapolation of the crucial influential factor – 'The Surgeon' – to evaluate the LOE of studies is a milestone in EBM yet to be achieved.

BOX 137.2: Levels of evidence defined by the Australian NHMRC

Level I	Evidence obtained from a systematic review of all relevant randomized controlled trials (RCTs).
Level II	Evidence obtained from at least one properly designed RCT.
Level III-1	Evidence obtained from well-designed pseudo-RCTs (alternate allocation or some other method).
Level III-2	Evidence obtained from comparative studies with concurrent controls and allocation not randomized (cohort studies), case–control studies or interrupted time series with a control group.
Level III-3	Evidence obtained from comparative studies with historical control, two or more single-arm studies or interrupted time series without a parallel control group.
Level IV	Evidence obtained from case series, either post-test or pre-test and post-test expert opinions (http://www.nhmrc.gov.au/PUBLICATIONS/synopses/cp30syn.htm).

KEY LEARNING POINTS

- Understand the basics of EBM and components of clinical decision-making.
- Identify the 'levels of evidence' in clinical studies.
- Describe the steps in EBM and types of clinical studies to find an answer to a question.

REFERENCES

- ● = Key primary paper
- ◆ = Major review article

◆1. Timmermans S, Angell A. Evidence-based medicine, clinical uncertainty, and learning to doctor. *Journal of Health and Social Behavior* 2001;**42**:342–59.

◆2. Glasziou P, Del Mar C. *Evidence-based Medicine Workbook. Finding and Applying The Best Evidence to Improve Patient Care.* London, UK: BMJ Books, 2003.

●3. Murray, JE. The first successful organ transplants in man. See http://nobelprize.org/nobel_prizes/medicine/laureates/1990/murray-lecture.html.

●4. Watson JD, Crick FH. Molecular structure of nucleic acids; a structure for deoxyribose nucleic acid. *Nature* 1953;**171**:737–8.

●5. Wroblewski BM. Professor Sir John Charnley (1911–1982). *Rheumatology (Oxford)* 2002;**41**:824–5.

●6. Barnard CN. The operation. A human cardiac transplant: an interim report of a successful operation performed at 'Groote Schuur Hospital', Cape Town. *South African Medical Journal* 1967;**41**:1271–4.

●7. Warnke PH, Springer IN, Wiltfang J, et al. Growth and transplantation of a custom vascularised bone graft in a man. *Lancet* 2004;**364**:766–70.

●8. Devauchelle B, Badet L, Lengelé B, et al. First human face allograft: early report. *Lancet* 2006;**368**:203–9.

●9. Markus PM, Martell J, Leister I, Horstmann O, et al. Predicting postoperative morbidity by clinical assessment. *British Journal of Surgery* 2005;**92**:101–6.

10. Sackett DL. Rules of evidence and clinical recommendations on the use of antithrombotic agents. *Chest* 1989;**95**:2S–4S.

◆11. Cochrane AL. Archie Cochrane in his own words. Selections arranged from his 1972 introduction to 'Effectiveness and Efficiency: Random Reflections on the Health Services' 1972. *Control Clinical Trials* 1989;**10**:428–33.

◆12. The Australian Government. National Health and Medical Research Council (NHMRC): A guide to the development, evaluation and implementation of clinical practice guidelines. See http://www.nhmrc.gov.au/PUBLICATIONS/synopses/cp30syn.htm.

◆13. The 'GRADE working group'. http://www.gradeworkinggroup.org/.

Risk management through burnout prevention in orthopaedic surgeons

SUE BESOMO

Introduction	1549	Signs and symptoms of burnout	1551
What is burnout?	1549	Risk management through burnout prevention	1551
Stressors in orthopaedic surgery	1550	References	1552

NATIONAL BOARD STANDARDS

- Identify stressors that place orthopaedic surgeons at risk for burnout
- Describe the signs and symptoms of burnout
- Manage professional risk using evidence-based burnout prevention strategies

INTRODUCTION

Practising as an orthopaedic surgeon puts you at risk for burnout. Working as a doctor in any specialty attracts more than the average amount of work-related stress, and orthopaedic surgeons have a specific group of pressures that can be added to these. This chapter will describe the pressures inherent in orthopaedic surgical practice and the signs and symptoms of burnout. Evidence-based strategies for burnout prevention will follow.

WHAT IS BURNOUT?

The word burnout was first coined in 1974 by Herbert Freudenberger. This German psychologist noticed that certain clients he was treating were suffering from feelings of meaninglessness and disillusionment as well as physical exhaustion. He named this syndrome 'burnout' and concluded that it is a state of depletion and exhaustion caused by overcommitment to work or to other areas of a person's life.[1]

A clearer picture of burnout emerged in the early 1980s when behavioural researchers Veninga and Spradley[2] studied burnt out workers from more than 100 occupations. They found burnout to be a state of psychological debilitation caused by unrelieved work stress resulting in fatigue, lowered resistance to illness, dissatisfaction, pessimism and inefficiency at work.[2] Psychologists Pines and Aronsen[3] further defined burnout after completing 10 years of formal research on more than 5000 participants from many occupations. They concluded that burnout is 'a state of physical, mental and emotional exhaustion caused by long term involvement in situations that are emotionally demanding'.[3]

Landmark research by Maslach[4] in the 1980s identified three clear dimensions of burnout as being emotional exhaustion, depersonalization and a sense of low personal accomplishment. Subsequent application and analysis of Maslach's Burnout Inventory over the past 20 years has confirmed the veracity of these dimensions.[5] In 1993, Powell's work[6] drew attention to personality constructs that may contribute to burnout. These include perfectionism, idealism and vigorous conscientiousness – attributes that are often consistent with a career in medicine.

STRESSORS IN ORTHOPAEDIC SURGERY

Burnout is the end result of a sustained unrelieved experience of stress. Stressors that have an impact on medical practice in general include the emotional demands of serving a sick and often difficult client population, long hours, uncertain success, failure to live up to one's own expectations, unrewarded altruism, competitive practice, geographical or professional isolation, the threat of lawsuits, healthcare reform, managed care, new regulations for quality control, increased cost of public health, decreased resources and the constant requirement to update knowledge and skills.

Certain pressures that fall into the domain of orthopaedic surgeons intensify the risk of burnout even further.[7] Such pressures include a growing workload with the ageing population; long waiting lists; increased scope for litigation; budgetary concerns; night and weekend emergency work;[8] and disputes with hospital administrators regarding access to facilities.[9] Professional jealousy may become more likely as the orthopaedic surgeon develops a high professional profile, adding a further stressor to the list. When many of these are combined with a conscientious and committed personality, such as that of most professional doctors, the stage is set for burnout.[10]

Several orthopaedic surgeons have recently written personal accounts of the stress they experienced in their professional lives. In *Hot Lights, Cold Steel*, Michael J. Collins gives an account of his struggle to reconcile his high ideals as an orthopaedic surgeon with what is possible as a human being.[11] His account of the professional and personal pressures he experienced spans his development from a junior surgeon to Chief Resident in Orthopaedic Surgery at the Mayo Clinic. He recounts the scientific hazards of the act of orthopaedic surgery in replacing a hip:

> But there were pitfalls everywhere. Damage the sciatic nerve, and the patient could be partially paralysed. Mal-orient the components and the hip could dislocate. Cut the femoral artery and the patient could bleed to death. Over-ream the acetabulum and you could break through the wall of the pelvis. Impact the stem too vigorously and you could fracture the femur. Kink the femoral vein and the patient could die of a pulmonary embolus. Repair the abductors improperly and the patient could limp for the rest of his life. Rush the cementing and the prosthesis could loosen prematurely. Take too long with the cementing and the patient could go hypotensive and die on the table. Break your sterile technique and the patient could get an infection. Fail to evaluate the medical condition and the patient could die of a heart attack. And all the time you are doing this [operating] you are living with the realization that a mistake could ruin your career.

These and other pressures left Collins wondering who he was and whose life he was living. He saw his salvation from burnout in the strong family life that was there for him with his wife and children.

Laurent Sedel,[12] a high-profile French orthopaedic surgeon, wrote a book entitled *Surgeon Close to Burnout*, stating that he wrote it so the layperson could understand it.

> I explained how the fear of judges progressively replaces the fear of malpractice. In each chapter I concentrated on a subject that contributes to our stress such as quality control systems, cost containment programs, debates regarding nosocomial infection, and increasing litigation, and for each of these subjects I explained how they are beneficial for insurance companies, lawyers, for-profit companies that own hospitals, and manufacturers of supplies, but in no way are beneficial to quality control, cost containment or surgeon efficacy.

Sedel found that the writing of this book was an effective method of stress reduction for him, and suggests that it may help other surgeons under pressure.

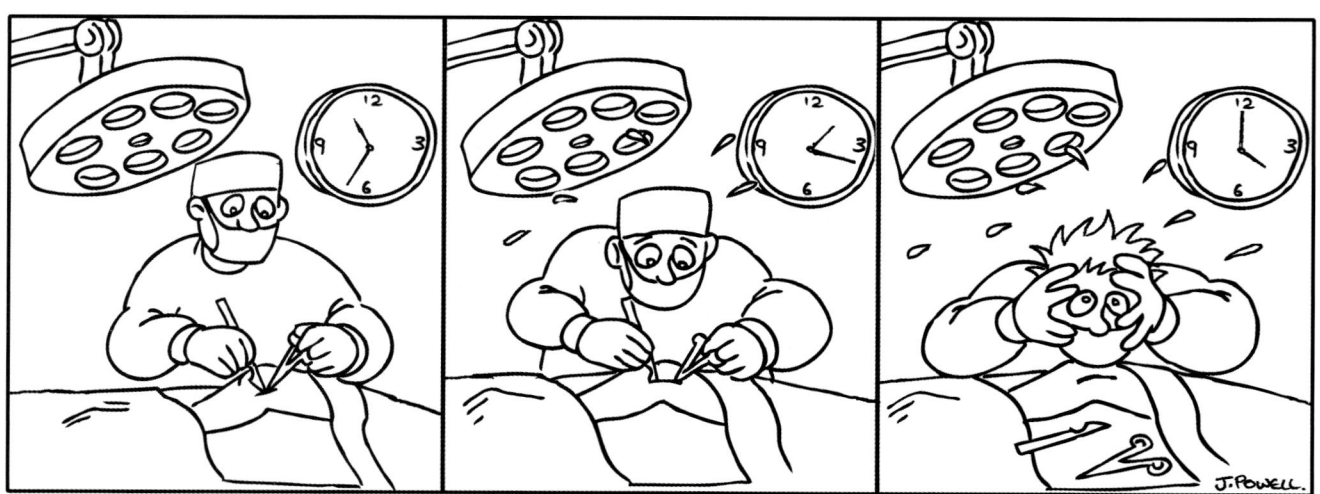

SIGNS AND SYMPTOMS OF BURNOUT

Burnout has been reported as multidimensional exhaustion resulting from unrelieved emotionally taxing work demands.[3] The onset of specific signs and symptoms that indicate burnout can be swift or gradual, depending upon the person and his or her circumstances. Quite often, others will notice early signs in sufferers before they do themselves, particularly with the onset of emotional exhaustion as this is a significant component of burnout. Manifestations of burnout can be considered under the headings of emotional, mental and physical exhaustion,

Emotional exhaustion includes depersonalization, meaninglessness and a sense of low personal accomplishment or fulfilment.[5] Depersonalization is a very strong indicator of burnout and most often manifests as a loss of concern and feeling for others. The emotional capacity of the burnt out person is so reduced that they do not relate to others with their customary warmth or with some degree of humanness. Research conducted in Belgrade showed that orthopaedic surgeons suffer higher depersonalization levels than general practitioners.[7] Feelings of entrapment and anger may also characterize emotional exhaustion.

Mental exhaustion can manifest in any combination of the following: forgetfulness; inability to concentrate; inefficiency; negative attitudes toward self and others; inflexibility; indifference; and generalized dissatisfaction. Some of the signs of mental exhaustion are due to a condition identified as 'brain fog', which is characterized by a lack of clarity and concentration in performing everyday mental tasks.[13] Some of the negative attitudes that also signal mental exhaustion can be detected in the comments and attitudes of the person who is burning out. Such a person can often be heard to say 'Everything gets on my nerves', or they may even demonstrate sustained indifference to events and other people around them. Mental exhaustion can, by its very nature, limit the sufferer's ability to see that they are burning out.

Physical exhaustion experienced in burnout is usually characterized by fatigue and stress-related illnesses, indicating reduced immune system function. Diminished immune system function has been linked to chronic patterns of resentment, disillusionment and helplessness,[14] providing a possible link between emotionally demanding work and the development of burnout.[15] The mechanism that accounts for the link between chronic negative thought patterns and the development of burnout may involve the emotion-mediating neuropeptide receptors that are located not only in the brain but also on immune system cells.[16,17] Whatever the explanation for it, the struggling immune system that is evident in burnt out individuals seems to claim the available energy reserves, leaving the person feeling fatigued and unwell.

RISK MANAGEMENT THROUGH BURNOUT PREVENTION

The clinical implications of burnout relate to the ability of the orthopaedic practitioner to deliver high-quality specialized care. Apart from the health and wellbeing of the surgeon, the success of the orthopaedic intervention and the safety of the patient are at risk in the burnt out practitioner owing to a compromised ability to function optimally in his or her professional practice. Burnout prevention is an essential component of risk management in professional practice.[18]

It is entirely possible to prevent yourself from burning out.

Certain personality traits will increase an individual's resistance to burnout, and these have been collectively termed the *hardy personality*.[19] There are three identified facets to the hardy personality, the first being a sense of commitment (as opposed to alienation) to oneself and the various areas in one's life, including work. This commitment reflects the hardy person's curiosity and consequent sense of meaning about life. The second hardiness facet is a belief that an individual has the power to influence the course of events in their own life, as opposed to a feeling of helplessness and subordination to the direction of others. The third characteristic of the hardy personality is the ability to see a stressor as a challenge rather than a threat, epitomizing the expectation that it is normal for life to change and for development to be stimulated. Hardiness is associated with fewer mental and physical symptoms of stress[10] and can be developed or strengthened through the specific strategies outlined below.

The first strategy is for the practitioner to identify the personal meaning that is inherent in the various areas of their life and, in particular, their practice of medicine. A clear identification of the personal reasons, whatever they may be, for practising in the field of orthopaedic surgery will strengthen commitment to it. Feelings of alienation are more likely to occur in the absence of a personal connection to the work that is done. Dr Hunter (Patch) Adams, although not an orthopaedic surgeon, is a medical doctor who provides an extraordinary example of the impact of personal connection of the practitioner to his medical practice. When asked why he does not burn out given his hectic worldwide speaking schedule as a professional doctor and clown, his building of and practice in a free hospital in West Virginia, and his propensity to sleep little and eat haphazardly, he responded with 'I never do anything that goes against my personal truth' (H. Adams 1999, personal communication). This is an extreme example of one aspect of a hardy personality, but serves to exemplify the power of commitment and connection to a life work.

The next strategy is the need to acknowledge stressors. Denial that stress exists in a person's life builds up exhausting internal tension, whereas acknowledging the truth can release built-up energy. In his book about the experience of serving in the Australian Army in Vietnam, Barry Heard[20] acknowledges for the first time the stressful experiences he had to deny in order to survive those years in combat situations. He describes the damage that denial had on his own mental health and that of Vietnam veterans who were unable to acknowledge what was truly happening.[20] The practice of medicine can induce a type of battle fatigue that is not unlike that experienced by wartime soldiers, and includes the chronic build-up of tension. The insistent need to release such tension may be destructively expressed in substance abuse or other types of addiction when stressors remain unacknowledged. Once acknowledged, a stressor can be seen as a challenge rather than a threat. This approach builds hardiness and creates the opportunity to use problem-solving skills – a practice that offers desensitization to chronic stress.

Further burnout resistance can be derived from the consistency of the match between what a person wants to achieve and what is humanly possible. Medicine lends itself to high ideals and expectations as well as the engagement of emotions – a combination that favours burnout. Holding realistic expectations of self and others will minimize the build-up of tense expectant energy and diminish the potential for disillusionment.

It is almost impossible for a person to burn out if they lead a fairly balanced life. Extremes of anything will alter the natural rhythms and patterns that balance energy. Attention to physiological patterns such as breathing deeply, promoting balanced rhythmic eating habits, and finding a balance between sensory and intellectual input can minimize build-up of body tension. Whether your work makes emotional, physical or mental demands of you, taking short breaks that enable a contrast in activity can restore some balance. For example, an orthopaedic surgeon may need solitude after working intensively with people; or a few moments of fresh air and sunlight after hours in the air-conditioned clinic or operating theatre. If the practice of orthopaedic surgery lacks artistic expression, occasional engagement with the arts offers a way to restore balance.

Social support is widely documented as a powerful defence against stress and burnout. Emotional intensity is an inevitable part of dealing with individuals who need health intervention – as well as dealing with their significant others – and yet medicine traditionally values emotional restraint.[21] Ensuring an effective social support system such as family, friends or a peer support group that fosters meaning and purpose in professional practice will protect against compassion fatigue and burnout.[21]

Ultimately, the efficient and effective practice of orthopaedic surgery is dependent upon the health and well-being of the surgeon. Professional risk management must include burnout prevention. The burnout-resistant personality is characterized by optimism and confidence in meeting challenges; a strong commitment to internally held values; and feelings of connectedness to others and the environment. Further burnout resistance can be achieved by holding realistic professional expectations of self, striving for balance in areas of living, and shoring up an effective social support system. Consciously engaging

Table 138.1 Burnout prevention summary

Strategy	Rationale
Approach stressors as challenges	Builds hardiness
Take action to influence your own life	Builds hardiness
Find meaning in your work	Builds hardiness
Hold realistic expectations	Eases performance pressure
Engage social support	Protects against compassion fatigue
Create balance	Increases vitality

these strategies will go a long way towards preventing professional burnout in the orthopaedic surgeon. Table 138.1 summarizes burnout prevention strategies.

> ### KEY LEARNING POINTS
>
> - Burnout is the end result of sustained, unrelieved stress associated with emotionally demanding work.
> - Orthopaedic surgeons are exposed to specific stressors as well as those generally associated with medical practice.
> - Signs of burnout include depersonalization, emotional exhaustion and dissatisfaction with personal accomplishment.
> - The hardy personality will resist burnout. Hardiness includes a sense of commitment, an internal locus of control, and ability to see stressors as challenges.

REFERENCES

1. Freudenberger JH. *Burnout: The High Cost of Success – and How to Cope with It.* New York, NY: Doubleday, 1980.
2. Veninga RL, Spradley JP. *The Work Stress Connection: How to Cope with Job Burnout.* Boston, MA: Little Brown, 1981.
3. Pines A, Aronson E. *Career Burnout: Causes and Cures.* New York, NY: Free Press, 1988:9.
4. Maslach C, Jackson SE. The measurement of experienced burnout. *Journal of Occupational Behaviour* 1981;**2**:99–113.
5. Maslach C, Jackson SE, Leiter MP. *Maslach Burnout Inventory Manual*, 3rd edn. Palo Alto, CA: Consulting Psychologists Press, 1996.
6. Powell K. *Burnout: What Happens When Stress Gets Out of Control and How to Regain Your Sanity.* London, UK: Thorsons, 1993.
7. Lesi AR, Stefanovic NP, Peronicic I, et al. Burnout in Belgrade orthopaedic surgeons and general practitioners: a preliminary report. *Acta Chirurgica Iugoslavica* 2009;**56**:53–9.

8. LeBlanc C, Heyworth J. Emergency physicians: burned out or fired up. *Canadian Journal of Emergency Medical Care* 2007;**9**:121–3.
9. Saleh KJ, Quick JC, Sime WE, Einhorn TA. Recognising and preventing burnout among orthopaedic leaders. *Clinical Orthopaedics and Related Research* 2009;**467**:558–65.
10. Kobasa S, Maddi S, Courington S. Personality and constitution as mediators in the stress-illness relationship. *Journal of Health & Social Behaviour* 1981;**22**:368–78.
11. Collins MJ. *Hot Lights, Cold Steel*. New York, NY: St Martins Press, 2005.
12. Sedel L. Letter to the Editor: Recognising and preventing burnout among orthopaedic leaders. *Clinical Orthopaedics and Related Research* 2009;**467**:1111.
13. Rothstein B. *Brain Fog: Solve the Mysteries of Decreased Mental Capacity and Keep your Brain Fit and Functional Throughout Your Life*. Lincoln, NE: iUniverse, 2005.
14. Pert CB. The wisdom of the receptors: neuropeptides, the emotions, and bodymind. *Advances in Mind–Body Medicine* 2002;**18**:30–5.
15. Everly GS, Jun Smith KJ, Welzant V. Cognitive-affective resilience indicia as predictors of burnout and job-related outcome. *International Journal of Emergency Mental Health* 2008;**10**:185–9.
16. Pert C, Ruff MR, Weber RJ, Herkenham M. Neuropeptides and their receptors: a psychosomatic network. *Journal of Immunology* 1985;**135**(Suppl. 2):820s–6s.
17. Pert C. *Molecules of Emotion*. New York, NY: Simon & Schuster, 1997.
18. Wallace JE, Lemaire JE, Ghali WA. Physician wellness: a missing quality indicator. *Lancet* 2009; **374**(9702):1653.
19. Kobasa S. The hardy personality. In: Sanders G, Suls J (eds) *Social Psychology of Health and Illness*. Hillsdale, NJ: Lawrence Erlbaum Associates, 1989.
20. Heard B. *Well Done, Those Men*. Carlton North, Australia: Scribe Publications, 2007.
21. Benson J, Magraith K. Compassion fatigue and burnout: the role of Balint groups. *Australian Family Physician* 2005;**34**:497–8.

Subject Index

Note: *vs* denotes differential diagnosis or comparisons

Abbreviations:
    ACL - anterior cruciate ligament
    ATLS - advanced trauma life support
    CAOS - computer-assisted orthopaedic surgery
    DDH - development dysplasia of hip
    DIP - distal interphalangeal joint
    DRUJ - distal radial ulnar joint
    DVT - deep vein thrombosis
    MTP - metatarsophalangeal
    PCL - posterior cruciate ligament
    PET - positron emission tomography
    PIP - proximal interphalangeal joint
    SCFE - slipped capital femoral epiphysis
    TFCC - triangular fibrocartilage complex
    TKA - total knee arthroplasty

A1 pulley
  jersey finger 1279, 1296
  trigger finger 1277, 1278
A-band, muscle 108, 699
abatacept therapy, juvenile idiopathic arthritis 595
abbreviated injury scale (AIS) 233
ABCDE management 234, 235–7
  acute compartment syndrome 280
  concussion 721
  pelvic injuries 239
  spinal cord injury 440, 442
  unconscious patients with head injury 467
  see also Advanced Trauma Life Support (ATLS)
abdominal compression test 1210
abdominal examination, developmental disorders of bone 550
abdominal injuries, children 499–500
abduction lag sign 1210
abductor digiti minimi (ADM), testing 16
abductor hallucis
  atrophy 848
  in hallux valgus 1434, 1435
abductor pollicis brevis (APB), power 16
abductor pollicis longus (APL) 1334
above-knee amputation (AKA) 962
  diabetic foot 1470
abscess
  Brodie's 224, 586
  cold (tuberculosis) 225, 987, 988, 990
  epidural, of spine 983
  'horseshoe' (hand) 1312
  psoas, in tuberculosis 987
  subcutaneous, of pulp of fingers 1311
  subperiosteal 225
  subungual 1311
absolute stability, fixation 269–70
acceleration 204
  angular 206
  definition 175
  linear *see* linear acceleration
accessory collateral ligament (elbow) 1383
accessory peroneus quartus muscle 1428

acetabular anteversion angle 419, 1105
acetabular component 189–90
  Charnley–DeLee zone 1141
  history 1098, 1109
  materials for 190
  mechanical testing 198, 199
  one-/two-piece designs 190
  osteopetrosis 1130
  polyethylene 1118
  wear 1117
  PTFE shells 1098–9
  young patients 1253–4
  see also acetabular cups
acetabular cups
  cemented 1139–40
    bone preparation techniques 1140
    Charnley, evolution 1100, 1109
    design 1139–40
    removal 1157
  Charnley cemented, evolution 1100, 1109
  computer-assisted navigation, THA 1521
  design
    cemented arthroplasty 1139–40
    stability 1109
    uncemented arthroplasty 1101, 1140–1
  development 1098, 1099–100
  hemispherical, revision surgery 1159
  jumping distance and 1108
  loosening 1139
  materials used 190, 1098
  mechanical fixation 1101
  oblong/bilobed, revision surgery 1159
  pelvic obliquity and 1127
  trabecular metal, revision surgery 1159
  uncemented 1140–2
    design 1101, 1140–1
    development 1101
    outcome 1143
    pressure effect, aseptic loosening 1154
    removal 1158
    revision 1159
  uncemented press-fit 1101
    rheumatoid arthritis 1129
  Vitallium 1098
  see also acetabular component
acetabular fossa 772
acetabular fractures 419–24, 1563–4
  associated fracture patterns 422
  classification 421–2
  clinical presentation 420
  CT role 422
  dislocation with 420
  indications for surgery 422–3
  injuries associated (incidence) 420
  patterns 421–2
  radiology 420–1
  roof arch angle 422, 423
  superior roof 422, 423
  treatment
    non-operative 423
    operative/approaches 423
    results 423–4
acetabular index, DDH assessment 647

acetabular labrum
  anatomy 772
  assessment 21
  tears 778
acetabular ligament 772
acetabular liners 1109, 1117
acetabular screw placement, zones 71
acetabulum
  abduction angle 772
  anatomy 69–70, 419, 772, 773, 1105–6
    radiology and Judet lines 420–1
  anterior column 419, 420, 421
  anterior orientation 419
  defects
    impaction bone grafting for 1158–9
    tantalum trabecular metal implants 1159
  development/growth 645
  fractures *see* acetabular fractures
  inferior orientation 419
  Letournel's column concept 419, 420
  pincer impingement 1111
  posterior column 419, 420, 421
  preparation for hip arthroplasty 1140, 1142
  reconstruction, revision hip arthroplasty 1158–9
  registration, computer-assisted surgery 1521
  roof arch angle 422, 423
  surgical approaches 73
  transverse angle 419
  zone of demarcation 1154
acetaminophen (paracetamol) 128–9
  osteoarthritis treatment 1081
  side-effects 129
acetyl Co-A 703
acetylcholine 109, 700
  receptors, antibodies to 700–1
acetylcholinesterase 109, 700
N-acetylcysteine 129
acetylsalicylic acid (aspirin) 128
  in hip arthroplasty 1126
  pre-operative considerations 128
Achilles tendon 78
  age-related changes 1426
  anatomy 829
  blood supply 1425
  collagen types 831
  degenerated 829, 1426
  direct injury 1425
  indirect injury 1425
  intratendinous calcifications 1427
  lengthened and failure 829
  lengthening, in amputations 961
  paratendonitis 833–4
  paratenon 829
  peritendinitis 832, 1426
  repetitive stress/overuse 1427
  rupture/tears 113, 393, 829–31, 1424–6
    aetiology 393, 829, 1424–5
    clinical presentation 1425
    complete 830, 832
    complete, treatment 831, 1425–6
    delayed/missed diagnosis 830, 1426
    end-to-end repair 1425–6

    examination/imaging 830
    gap distance 829
    incidence 1424–5
    mechanisms of injury 1425
    partial 830, 832
    partial, treatment 830
    pathophysiology 393, 829
    percutaneous repair 1426
    treatment 393, 830–1, 1425–6
  tendinosis/tendinitis 831, 832, 833–4, 1426–8
    aetiology 1426–7
    classification 832, 1426
    clinical features 832, 1426, 1427
    insertional 831, 832, 1426
    investigations 832
    management 1427–8
    non-insertional 831, 1427, 1428
    non-operative treatment 833, 1427
    pathology 1426–7
    surgery 833, 1427–8
    surgical results 1428
  tendonopathy 831–4
    aetiology and pathology 831
    classification 831–2
    degenerative 1426
    evaluation and imaging 832–3
    non-operative treatment 833
    operative treatment 833–4
  vulnerable region 1425
  zone of hypovascularity 112, 1425
Achilles tenotomy, congenital clubfoot 690
achondrogenesis, prevalence 542
achondroplasia 570, 572
  clinical features 556, 572
  hip arthroplasty 1128
  management 556–8
acid–base, monitoring in trauma 236
acquired brain injury, management after 969–70
acquired neurological disorders 1477–82
acquired patellar dislocation 666–7
acral lentiginous melanoma 1376
acromial spur, anterior 1212
acromioclavicular (AC) joint 9
  anatomy 53, 285
  arthropathy, rotator cuff repair and 1213
  examination 10, 285
  excision, rotator cuff tears 1211–12
  fractures 1556
  injuries 285–7
    classification 286
    clinical evaluation 285
    complications 286
    mechanism 285
    non-operative treatment 286
    operative treatment 286
    radiography 285–6
acromioclavicular (AC) ligament 285
  injuries 286
acromion 52
  anterior 1208
acromionectomy, radical 1208
acromioplasty, anterior 1208, 1212
acrylic cement 1100
ACTH injection, in gout 1091
actin 108

actin–myosin cross-bridge 108, 109, 699, 701
  age-related changes 122
action potential
  motor unit 213, 700
  nerve 109, 1303
  skeletal muscle 109
activated partial thromboplastin time (APTT) 130
active damping 185
activities of daily living, spinal cord injury determining 970
acupuncture, lateral epicondylitis 1395
acute compartment syndrome *see* compartment syndrome
acute haematogenous osteomyelitis (AHO) 221, 582–6
  aetiology and pathogenesis 582–3
  clinical features 583
  clinical investigations 584
  differential diagnosis 583
  management 582, 584–6
acute inflammatory response *see* inflammation/inflammatory response
acute lengthening procedures, leg length discrepancy 683
acute osteomyelitis *see* osteomyelitis, acute
acute phase proteins 145, 147
  see also C-reactive protein (CRP)
acute shortening procedures, leg length discrepancy 681–2
Acutrack screw 1344
adalimumab therapy, juvenile idiopathic arthritis 594
Adam's forward bend test 540
adaptive immune system *see* immune system, adaptive
adductor hallucis, in hallux valgus 1434, 1435
adductor lengthening, cerebral palsy 602–3
adductor longus
  origin, palpation 19
  strains 774
adductor magnus, transection 962
adductor strain injuries 774
adenosine triphosphate (ATP) 140, 702
  cleavage, energy release 702
  muscle contraction 109, 699, 701, 702
  sources, metabolic pathways 702–3
adhesion molecules, in rheumatoid arthritis 1088
adipocytic tumours 916, 917
adjuvant chemotherapy, definition 878
adolescent(s)
  ACL injury and reconstruction 810
  ankle fractures (transitional) 498
  avulsion injuries, pelvis 493, 777
  decision-making capacity 1533
  foot examination 539
  hallux valgus 1436
    surgical treatment 1438
  hip examination 539–40
  pelvic fractures 426
  postural kyphosis 1016
  Scheuermann's kyphosis 1015
  see also children
adolescent idiopathic scoliosis 636–8, 639, 1007
  adult scoliosis *vs* 1007, 1008
adolescent postural kyphosis 638, 640
adrenal hormones 704
adrenaline *see* epinephrine
adrenocorticotropic hormone (ACTH), injection, in gout 1091
Adson's test 33
adult kyphosis *see* kyphosis
adult respiratory distress syndrome (ARDS) 240
adult scoliosis *see* scoliosis (adult)
adult stem cells, tissue engineering 1526–7
adult-acquired flat foot (AAFF) 1489
adult-acquired spasticity 969, 970
advance directives 1533, 1540
advanced life support 233–43
Advanced Trauma Life Support (ATLS) 234
  definition of patient condition after 237–8

'golden hour' 234, 440
  initial assessment, trauma room 235, 440
  open injuries of limbs 248–9
  pelvic fractures 239, 426, 430
    children 493
  protocol 234
  specific orthopaedic situations 238–9
  spinal cord injury 235, 238–9, 440, 444–5
  steps/process 234–7
  unconscious patients with head injury 467
  see also ABCDE management; trauma/injury, management
aerobic metabolism 702, 703
agarose gel electrophoresis 141–2
ageing/age-related changes 120–3
  articular cartilage 102, 103, 1080
  degenerative disc disease 993, 994, 995
  intervertebral disc 106–7
  kyphosis and lordosis changes 1016
  nerve repair and prognosis 1306
  physiology 120–3
  skeletal muscle 121
  tendons 120–1
agency 1532
aggrecan 83, 101, 548
  functions 101
airway, management in trauma 234–5
Aitken classification, proximal focal femoral deficiency 650
Akahori grading, cubital tunnel syndrome 1401, 1402
Akin osteotomy 1439
Albee, Fred Houdlett 5
Albright syndrome 93
albumin 83
aldosterone 704
alendronic acid 132
alkaline phosphatase 83, 93, 543
  elevated, bone tumours 866, 900
  metastases 930, 931
  tissue non-specific 86
'all hazards approach', mass casualty 244
alleles 140, 150
Allen–Ferguson classification 1556
allodynia 1305
allograft/allograft transplantation
  ACL reconstruction 810
  adult scoliosis treatment 1014
  advantages/disadvantages 944
  ankle replacement *see* ankle arthroplasty (total)
  bone 148–9
  chondrocyte survival 1246
  complications 944–5
  definition 148
  fractures, healing 520, 944
  harvesting/storage 944
  intercalary structural reconstruction 944
  limb reconstruction 944–5
  massive 944
  meniscus 105
  osteochondral *see* osteochondral autograft/allograft transfer
  shoulder hemiarthroplasty 1256
  survival rates 944
allograft–prosthetic composites, limb reconstruction 946
allopurinol 1091
alpha errors (type I) 42
α-fetoprotein 608
ALPSA lesion 730
alteplase 132
alternative hypothesis (hypothesis-testing) 40
alumina ceramic 189, 1119
AMBRI shoulder dislocation 300
AMC Mobile Knee System 191, 192
amenorrhoea, female athletes 708, 822
American Academy of Orthopedic Surgeons (AAOS) 1125, 1126
American College of Chest Physicians (ACCP) 1126, 1127
American Joint Committee on Cancer (AJCC), tumour staging 871, 914
American Spinal Injury Association (ASIA) 441
  spinal cord injury terminology 442

aminoglycosides
  open fractures 254
  open injuries of limbs 253
amplification refractory mutation system (ARMS) 141
amputations 957–63
  amputated part, early management 1316
  biological level 959
  cognitive ability requirement 959
  complete 1316
  end bearing, load transfer 957, 958
  energy expenditure 957
  general principles 960
  incomplete 1316
  indications/conditions requiring 957, 959
    diabetic foot 1470
    fracture non-union 521, 524
    infections 959
    metastatic bone lesions 936
    open injuries 252–3
    soft-tissue sarcoma 915
    tumours 915, 959
    vascular disease 959
  'internal' forequarter 296
  limb salvage *vs*, in open injuries 252–3
  limb-sparing surgery *vs* 942
  lower limb, levels 960–2
    above-knee *see* above-knee amputation (AKA)
    ankle 961
    below-knee *see* below-knee amputation (BKA)
    foot 960–2
    metatarsal bones 961
    through-knee 962
  major, diabetic foot 1470
  paediatric 958–9
  soft-tissue envelope 957, 960
  transfemoral *see* transfemoral amputation
  transhumeral 963
  transtibial *see* transtibial amputation
  traumatic 959
    categorization 1315
    'clean' (guillotine type) 1316
    early management 1316
    fingertips 1289
    ischaemia time 1317
    replantation *see* replantation (upper limb)
    upper limb 1315
  upper limb
    levels 961, 963
    traumatic *see* amputations, traumatic
  see also individual amputations
amyotrophic lateral sclerosis, cubital tunnel syndrome *vs* 1399
anaerobic metabolism 702, 703
anaesthesia
  anatomic total shoulder replacement 1225–6
  for arthroscopy 713
  epidural, in hip arthroplasty 1124, 1126
  for hip arthroplasty 1123–4
  history 4
  hypotensive, for hip arthroplasty 1124
  for open Bankart's repair 1218
  regional, for hip arthroplasty 1123–4, 1126
  in rheumatoid arthritis 1087
  for rotator cuff tear repair 1211
anaesthetics, local *see* local anaesthetics
anakinra therapy, juvenile idiopathic arthritis 595
anal wink 441
analgesics 126–9
  forearm fracture reduction 263
  hip arthroplasty 1124
  NSAIDs *see* non-steroidal anti-inflammatory drugs (NSAIDs)
  opioid 126–8, 1124
  rotator cuff tear management 1211
  see also opioid analgesics; pain control
analysis of variance (ANOVA) 44
anatomy (surgical) 52–81
  see also individual bones and joints
Andersen classification, congenital pseudarthrosis of tibia 675

Anderson and D'Alonzo classification 1556
  odontoid fractures 450
Anderson and Montesano classification 1555
  occipital condyle fractures 446–7
Anderson Orthopaedic Research Institute 1201, 1202
Anderson–Green–Messner growth-remaining charts 679–80
androgens, use by athletes 707
androstenedione, use by athletes 707
Andry, Nicholas 3
anencephaly 608
aneuploidy 152
aneurysmal bone cyst (ABC) 868, 869, 888–9
  hand 1377–8
  secondary 888, 892
  spine 1062
aneurysmal lesions, hand 1374
aneurysmal phenomenon, vertebral bodies 988
angiofibroblastic hyperplasia 750, 1390
angiofibroblastic tendinosis 1390, 1396
angiogenesis
  metastases 927
  synovial proliferation, rheumatoid arthritis 1085
angiography
  pelvic 430
  renal/thyroid metastases, surgery 935
angiolipoma 917
angiosarcoma
  chemotherapy 880
  of soft tissue 919
angle of pennation 121
angle of Wiberg 419
angular acceleration 206
angular displacement 174–5, 206
  of knee during gait 206–7
angular motion 174–5
angular movement 204
  assessment of control 207
angular speed 174
angular velocity 206
  of knee during gait 206–7
animal bite injury 1313
anisotropy, degree of (DA) 1026
ankle
  anatomy 27, 77–80, 386, 838
    arthrology 78, 386, 387, 1243
    blood supply 79–80
    ligaments 392, 840, 1243
    neuromuscular 78–9
    osteology 77–8, 392
  in ankylosing spondylitis 1497
  anterior soft-tissue impingement 838–9
    examination/evaluation 838–9
    treatment 839
  anterior synovial fold 838
  arthritis 1484–97
    arthrodesis 1269, 1270, 1478, 1488
    clinical assessment 1484–6
    inflammatory arthritis 1485, 1493–7
    osteoarthritis *see* osteoarthritis
    rheumatoid arthritis 1241, 1494
    see also specific types
  arthrodesis 1255, 1268, 1269–72
    approaches and fixation 1270
    arthritis 1269, 1270, 1487, 1488
    imaging and assessment 1269–70
    osteoarthritis 1487, 1488
    pantalar fusion 1270–1
    tibial plafond fractures 384–5
    triple 1270, 1271
    see also tibiocalcaneal fusion
  arthroplasty *see* ankle, distraction arthroplasty; ankle arthroplasty (total)
  arthroscopy *see* arthroscopy
  articular cartilage 1241
    damage 1242
  biomechanics 186, 1243–4
  braces 1423, 1429
  clinical examination 26–31
    in arthritis 1485
    inspection 27–8
    movement 27, 29–30
    palpation 28–9
    resisted movements 29
    special tests 30–1

deformities
  arthritis, examination 1485
  in children with cerebral palsy,
    management 604–5
  in children with myelomeningocele
    610
  valgus 1464
  see also specific disorders
degeneration 1242
  forces 1244
disarticulation/amputation 961
dislocation 386
  treatment 388
distraction arthroplasty 1245–6
  complications 1246
  external fixator 1246
  patient evaluation 1245
  principles/theory 1245
  results 1246
  technique 1245–6
dynamic equinus 969
force through, during gait 186, 1244
fractures 386–93, 1567
  chondral injuries with 388
  classification 387–8
  closed treatment 266
  complications 391
  low risk of DVT 261
  mechanism of injury 386, 387, 388
  open 386
  open, treatment 391
  paediatric 498
  pronation–abduction (PA) force
    387, 388
  pronation–external rotation (PER)
    force 387, 388
  supination–adduction (SA) force
    387, 388
  supination–external rotation (SER)
    387, 388, 498
  transitional, paediatric 498
  treatment 388–91
  see also malleolar fractures
in gait 955, 956, 1243, 1244
gait analysis, in children 566, 567
'giving way' 840, 841
'high ankle sprains' 391
history-taking 26–7, 1484–5
impingement 1488
  see also ankle, posterior
    impingement
injuries 386–93
  clinical evaluation 386
  inversion 391, 834, 838, 841
  mechanisms 386, 387, 388
  radiographic evaluation 387
  sports-related see under sports
    injuries
instability
  lateral 840–2
  osteoarthritis after 1242
  peroneal tendon injuries 1428
internal/external rotation 1243
lateral ligament complex 840
lateral ligament reconstruction in
  arthritis 1487
lateral ligamentous instability 840–2
  aetiology and pathology 840–1
  evaluation/examination 841
  treatment 841–2
loose bodies 716, 1245, 1486
malalignment 1245–6
movements 79
  clinical examination 27, 29–30
  in gait 955, 956, 1243, 1244
  normal range 29, 186, 1243, 1244
nerve compression syndromes 1500–6
  interdigital plantar (Morton's)
    neuroma 1500–2
  lateral plantar nerve 1504–5
  superficial peroneal nerve 1506
  tarsal tunnel syndrome see tarsal
    tunnel syndrome
  see also Morton's neuroma
neurological disorders affecting
  1472–82
  see also specific disorders
observational gait analysis, in
  children 566, 567
osteoarthritis see osteoarthritis
pain 26, 839
plantarflexion and dorsiflexion 29,
  391, 840, 1243
  Achilles tendon rupture and 1425

plantarflexion/knee extension couple
  566, 567
posterior impingement 839–40
  examination 840
  treatment 840
pronation 387, 388
proprioception 1243
radiography 1243
  normal 387
range of motion 29, 186, 1243, 1244
reconstruction 948
replacement see ankle arthroplasty
  (total)
rheumatoid arthritis 26–7, 1241,
  1494
sprains 391, 843
  evaluation and treatment 391
  external rotation stress test 392–3
  syndesmotic see syndesmotic
    sprains, ankle
stability 27, 1243
subchondral bone 1242, 1245
supination 387, 388
surgical approaches 80
synovial fold, anterior 838
tendons 78
  resisted movements 29
twisting 391
valgus deformity 1464
  myelomeningocele 610
weight supported by 27
see also medial malleolus; talus; tibia,
  distal
ankle arthroplasty (total) 1243–50,
  1487–8, 1494
  allograft 1246–8
    failure 1247
    indications 1247
    principles 1246
    problems associated 1247
    results 1247
  ankle anatomy and 1243
  biomechanics and 1243–4
  bipolar, results 1247
  cementless 1244
  complications 1245
  contraindications (relative/absolute)
    1244
  fixation methods 1244
  future prospects 1247–8
  indications 1244
  materials used for 192, 1244
  prostheses, design 1244
  results 1244
  young patients 1255
  see also ankle, distraction arthroplasty
ankle–foot orthosis (AFO) 968, 969
  cerebral palsy 605
  Charcot–Marie–Tooth disease 614
  Duchenne muscular dystrophy 1477
  postpoliomyelitis syndrome 1481
  stroke patients 1478
ankylosing spondylitis 1089–90, 1497
  examination 33
  foot/ankle presentations 1497
  of hip 1089, 1129
  hip arthroplasty 1129
  spinal deformities 1129
  surgical treatment 1089–90
ankylosis 1268
  degenerative disc disease leading to
    1001
  segmental 1001
annular ligament (elbow) 1383
annulus fibrosus 66
  defects 107
  disc degeneration 106–7, 978
  outer and inner segments 106, 107,
    994
  posterolateral deficiency 994
  structure 106, 994
  tears 993–4
    concentric 995
    granulation tissue growth 998,
      999
    radial 995
    transverse 995
    types 995
  Young's modulus 188
  see also intervertebral disc
ANOVA 44
antalgic gait 31, 567
antegrade femoral nail 349
anterior acromioplasty 1208

anterior cervical corpectomy and fusion
  1003, 1004
anterior cord syndrome 443
anterior cruciate ligament (ACL) 25
  anatomy 807
  bracing 211
  bundles
    (anteromedial/posterolateral)
    807
    double-bundle reconstruction 811
  deficient knee 808, 1262
  management 211
  diagnosis/testing 25
    anterior drawer test 211, 807
    pivot shift test 807– 808
  healing 113
  imaging 808–9
  injury
    children/adolescents 810
    female athletes 810
    in multiligamentous injury of knee
      814, 815
    non-operative management 809
    operative treatment 809–10
    quadriceps role 211
    treatment 809–10
  insertion, site 375, 807
  intercondylar eminence avulsions
    497
  medial collateral ligament injury with
    806, 807
  physical examination 807–8
  reconstruction 211, 809–10, 1262
    double-bundle 811
    female athletes 810
    graft selection 810
    in knee dislocation 815
    postoperative rehabilitation 810
    resection model (osteoarthritis) 1079
    skeletally immature patient 810
  rupture/tears 23, 24, 807–11
    adolescents 497
    in knee dislocation 365
    in unicompartmental knee
      arthroplasty 1190
anterior drawer test
  foot/ankle 30, 841
  knee 24, 25, 211, 807
  shoulder 11
anterior epiphysiodesis, cerebral palsy
  604
anterior impingement test, hip 21
anterior inferior iliac spine 69
anterior interosseous nerve 1386
  testing 16, 17
anterior interosseous nerve syndrome
  1386
anterior knee pain syndrome 1190
anterior longitudinal ligament (ALL)
  65, 976
anterior lumbar interbody fusion
  (ALIF) 1003, 1004
  degenerative disc disease 1003, 1004
anterior superior iliac spine (ASIS) 19,
  69
  in hip inspection 18
  palpation 19
anterior talofibular ligament (ATFL)
  78, 840, 1243
  in ankle motion 1243, 1244
  palpation 28
  repair 842
  testing 30
anterior tarsal tunnel syndrome 1505–6
anterior tibial artery 77
anterior tibial tendon
  avascular zone 1430
  rupture 1429–30
    management 1430
anthropometric measurements, bone
  developmental disorders 550
anti-adhesion molecules 1088
antibiotics
  acute haematogenous osteomyelitis in
    children 584, 585–6
  acute paronychia 1311
  in bone cement 1120, 1161
  choice
    in open injuries of limbs 253
    for specific infections 220
  diabetic foot 1469
  hand infections 1310, 1311
  hip arthroplasty 1125, 1126
    cement impregnated 1161

mechanisms of action 221
open fractures 253, 254
open injuries of limbs 253
prophylaxis
  hip arthroplasty 1125, 1126
  rotator cuff tear repair 1214
pyogenic spinal infections 985
septic arthritis 1092
  in children 581
antibodies 148
  anti-DNA 1090
  antinuclear, juvenile idiopathic
    arthritis 589–90, 591, 593
  specificity 148
  see also specific immunoglobulins
antibody-mediated immunity 147–8
  see also B lymphocytes (B cells)
anticoagulants 130–2
  classification 130–1
  clinical use 131, 132
  direct-acting 131
  drug interactions 131–2
  in hip arthroplasty 1126
  indirect-acting 130–1
  pre-operative considerations 131
  retrobulbar haematoma risk
    reduction 476
  side-effects 131
  see also heparin; warfarin
anti-DNA antibodies 1090
antifibrinolytic agents, in trauma 237
antigen(s), antibody specificity 148
antigen presentation, to T cells 1068,
  1084
antigen-presenting cells 145, 149, 1084
  inhibition, rheumatoid arthritis
    therapy 1087
anti-inflammatory drugs 126–9
  non-steroidal see non-steroidal anti-
    inflammatory drugs (NSAIDs)
antinuclear antibodies (ANAs), juvenile
  idiopathic arthritis 589, 591, 593
anti-osteoporotic drugs 132–4
  classification 132–3
anti-rheumatic drugs 1086
antisense oligonucleotides, Duchenne
  muscular dystrophy 612
antisepsis
  history 4
  see also antibiotics
antitubercular chemotherapy 225,
  989
Antoni A and B tissue 920
AO Child Survey 499
AO classification 6, 258, 269
  ankle fractures 387–8, 389
  fractures in children 499
  osteoporotic fractures 1034
  proximal femoral fractures in
    children 493
  thoracolumbar spine fractures
    462–3
  tibial shaft fractures 378
apical ectodermal ridge (AER) 542
aponeurectomy, segmental,
  Dupuytren's contracture 1328
apophyseal joints see facet (apophyseal)
  joints
apophysitis, iliac crest, athletes 777
apoptosis 542
  disc cells 1001
applied principlism 1531–2
apprehension tests
  hip 21
  multidirectional shoulder instability
    738
  shoulder stability 11
    anterior instability 731
    posterior instability 735
Arbeitsgemeinschaft für
  Osteosynthesefragen see AO
  classification
arcade of Frohse 1384
arcade of Osborne 1384
arcade of Struthers 1384, 1393
arm
  anatomy 56–61
    arthrology 57
    blood supply 58
    muscles 57
    nerves 57–8
    neuromuscular 57–8
    osteology 56–7
  inability to raise 1209

1558 Subject Index

arm – continued
    surgical approaches 57–61
        to elbow 60–1
        to humerus 58–9
        internervous planes 58–9, 60
    see also upper limb; *specific anatomical structures*
Arnold–Chiari malformation 608
aromatase inhibitors 929
Artelon Spacer CMC 1339
arterial injuries
    acute compartment syndrome due to 279, 504
    compartment syndrome *vs* 510
arterial injury theory, compartment syndrome 504
arterial insufficiency, replantation (upper limb) complication 1321
arterial spasm 504, 505
arteries, microsurgical repair 1319
arteriography, compartment syndrome 510
arteriovenous gradient theory, compartment syndrome 507
arteriovenous pressure gradient (AV) 507
artery of Adamkiewicz 68
arthritis 1077–94
    crystal 1091–2
    foot/ankle *see* ankle; foot
    gonococcal 226
    hallucal sesamoids 1446
    hand *see* osteoarthritis
    inflammatory *see* inflammatory arthritis
    juvenile idiopathic *see* juvenile idiopathic arthritis (JIA)
    osteo- *see* osteoarthritis
    post-traumatic *see* post-traumatic arthritis
    psoriatic *see* psoriatic arthritis
    reactive *see* reactive arthritis
    rheumatoid *see* rheumatoid arthritis
    septic *see* septic arthritis
    systemic, ankle osteoarthritis in 1242
    tuberculous 226
arthrodesis 1268–73
    ankle osteoarthritis *see* ankle, arthrodesis
    causes leading to 1269
    distraction, calcaneocuboid joint 1423
    first metatarsal–cuneiform joint 1439
    first MTP joint 1440
    fixation methods *see* fixation
    hallux rigidus 1490
    hindfoot *see* hindfoot
    hip *see* hip
    imaging before 1268, 1269
    knee *see* knee, arthrodesis
    midfoot *see* midfoot
    positions for, by joint 1268
    shoulder 618, 1268, 1273
    spinal *see* spinal arthrodesis; spinal fusion
    subtalar *see* subtalar joint, arthrodesis
    surgical stages 1269
    talonavicular joint 1495
    work-up 1269
    wrist 1268, 1272, 1358
    see also specific joints
arthrodesis nails 1272
arthrodiastasis, ankle osteoarthritis 1487
arthrography
    MR *see* magnetic resonance arthrography
    rotator cuff muscles 1210
    wrist 1354, 1356, 1367–8
arthrology *see specific joints*
arthropathy
    Charcot 1492–3
    degenerative 1080–4
        see also osteoarthritis
    enteropathic 1090
    haemophiliac 1092
    infectious 1092
    inflammatory 1084–9
        immunogenetic basis 1084
        see also rheumatoid arthritis
    psoriatic 1496
    see also arthropathies

arthroplasty
    ankle *see* ankle arthroplasty
    definition 1176
    elbow *see* elbow, arthroplasty
    hallux rigidus 1491–2
    hip *see* hip arthroplasty
    interpositional *see* interpositional arthroplasty
    knee *see* knee arthroplasty
    resection
        hallux rigidus 1491–2
        hallux valgus 1439–40
    resurfacing 1176
    shoulder *see* shoulder arthroplasty (total)
    in trapeziometacarpal osteoarthritis 1337
    wrist *see* wrist, joint replacement
    see also joint replacement; *specific types*
arthroscope 712, 713
arthroscopic surgeon 713
arthroscopy 712–19
    anaesthesia for 713
    ankle 716
        in distraction arthroplasty 1245
        indications and positioning 716
        portal placement and anatomy 716
    capsulolabral repair 731–4
    complications 718
    concepts 713
    debridement, lateral epicondylitis 1397
    diagnostic 713
        ankle 716
        elbow 717
        hip 716
        knee 714
        shoulder 715
        wrist 718
    elbow 716–17
        indications 716
        portal placement and anatomy 717
        positioning 716–17
    equipment/instrumentation 712–13
    hip 715–16
        indications 715
        portal placement and anatomy 716
        positioning 715–16
        sports injuries 779
    irrigation fluid for 713
    knee 713–14
        ACL injuries 809
        indications 713–14
        medial plica syndrome 783
        osteoarthritis 1081
        pigmented villonodular synovitis 784–5
        portal placement and anatomy 714
        positioning 714
        synovial chondromatosis 784
        unicompartmental osteoarthritis 1187
    knot tying 713
    lavage, septic arthritis 1092
    osteoarthritis 1081
    shoulder 714–15, 1207
        anterior instability, capsulolabral repair 731–4
        glenohumeral arthritis 732
        glenohumeral ligaments 715
        indications 714
        multidirectional instability 738–9
        portal placement and anatomy 714–15, 732, 733, 736, 742–3
        positioning 714, 742
        posterior instability 736
        rotator cuff tear repair 742–3
        SLAP lesions 740–1
    trapeziometacarpal (TM) joint osteoarthritis 1337
    triangulation 713
    wrist 717–18, 1354, 1356, 1358, 1368
        indications and positioning 717
        portal placement and anatomy 717–18
arthrotomy, septic arthritis management 581
articular cartilage 101–3, 1077, 1078
    age-related changes 102, 103, 1080
    calcified zone 101, 1078
    chondrocytes 101, 1078
        see also chondrocytes

composition 101, 1077, 1078
    collagen 101, 102
    extracellular matrix 101, 1077, 1078–9
    proteoglycans 101, 1078–9
    as contributor to inflammation 1078
damage, subchondral bone damage 1079
excessive stress on, osteoarthritis 1080
fibrillation 1080
functions 101, 102, 1077
glycoproteins 101–2
growth factors 1078
injury and healing 102–3
    injury types 103
    MRI scan 171
layers 102
matrix metalloproteinases 102, 1088
mechanical properties 102
microstructure 102
MRI appearance 161, 168
normal loading 1080
in osteoarthritis 102, 103, 1242
superficial zone 1078
thickness 1079
tidemark zone 102, 103
Young's modulus 188
    see also Young's modulus (E)
zones 1078
    anabolic/catabolic processes, markers 1082
arylsulphatase E 549
ascending tracts, spinal cord 66, 67
ascorbic acid, Charcot–Marie–Tooth disease treatment 615
aseptic loosening
    endoprosthetic reconstruction complication 943
    femoral stem (implants) 1154
    hip implants *see* hip arthroplasty (total)
    knee arthroplasty 1198, 1199
aseptic lymphocytic vasculitis-associated lesions (ALVAL) 1119
aseptic surgery, history 4
aspirin *see* acetylsalicylic acid (aspirin)
ataxia 568
athletes
    injuries *see* sports injuries
    nutrition *see* nutrition, sports and
athletic pubalgia 776
atlantoaxial joint 64–5
    anatomy 65–6, 449
    fusion 450
    instability, traumatic 448–9
    rotary subluxation/dislocation 449–50
    transverse ligament 449
atlantodens interval 446, 448
atlanto-occipital joint
    anatomy 65
    dislocation, sports injuries 725
atlas
    anatomy 64–5
    fractures 447–8, 725
        classification 448
    sporting injuries 725
    see also atlantoaxial joint
ATLS *see* Advanced Trauma Life Support (ATLS)
ATP–phosphocreatine system 702, 703
ATV-NDV tumour vaccine 1069
atypical lipomatous tumour 917
Australian National Health and Medical Research Council (NHMRC) 1548
autogenous chondrocyte transplantation *see* autologous chondrocyte implantation (ACI)
autogenous zones 16
autografts
    ACL reconstruction 810
    adult scoliosis treatment 1014
    extracorporeal irradiation/reimplantation 946
    fixation 945
    harvesting, arthroscopy 713
    limb reconstruction 945–6
    osteochondral *see* osteochondral autograft/allograft transfer
autoimmunity, rheumatoid arthritis and 1085
autologous blood injection 1395

autologous chondrocyte implantation (ACI) 1528–9
    criticisms 1083
    knee cartilage injuries 790–1
    osteoarthritis 1083
    procedure 790, 1083
autonomic dysreflexia, spinal cord injury determining 970
autonomy 1531, 1532
autosomal dominant disorders 152
autosomal dominant inheritance 150–1
autosomal recessive disorders 152
autosomal recessive inheritance 151
Avanta finger replacement 193
avascular necrosis (AVN) *see* osteonecrosis (avascular necrosis)
average speed 174
average velocity 174, 204
'aviator's astragalus' 394
Avon Patellofemoral Arthroplasty 1195–6
avulsion fracture
    athletes 777
    fifth metatarsal 846
    greater tuberosity of humerus 304
    intercondylar eminence of tibia 497
    olecranon 318
    pelvis, hip and thigh 777
    tibial plateau, lateral 366
    tibial spine 808
    tibial tuberosity 497
avulsion injuries, ring 1321–2
axillary artery 54
    branches 54, 55
axillary nerve 1208, 1215
    injury, proximal humerus fractures 303
    rupture 1305
    in total shoulder replacement 1226
axillary pouch 1215
axis (C2)
    anatomy 64–5
    blood supply 450
    development 64–5
    hangman's fracture 445, 451, 452, 1556
    sports injuries 725–6
    traumatic spondylolisthesis 451, 452
    see also atlantoaxial joint; odontoid process
axonotmesis 1304
axons
    injuries 1304
    presynaptic 700
axoplasmic transport 1303
axotomy 720
azathioprine 149

B lymphocytes (B cells) 147–8, 1068, 1084
    B-cell lymphoma 907–8
    rheumatoid arthritis pathophysiology 1085
Babinski reflex 33
Babinski sign 1010
'baby Bennett's fracture' 768
back muscles 66
back pain
    adult scoliosis 1008, 1009
    costs 993
    degenerative disc disease 993, 1002
    idiopathic scoliosis 633
    non-mechanical, spinal tumours 1058
    postoperative pyogenic infections 985
    Scheuermann's kyphosis 1016
    spinal infections 983
    spinal tuberculosis 987
    vertebral body compression fractures, osteoporotic 1016
    see also low back pain (LBP)
baclofen therapy, cerebral palsy 602
bacteraemia, oral 1124
Badia's staging, trapeziometacarpal osteoarthritis 1337
Bado's classification, Monteggia fracture 324
'bag of bones' technique 312
Bag1 gene 547
BAK Vista (Zimmer) cage 197
Baker's cyst, MRI 162, 163
balance training, osteoporotic spinal surgery 1043

balloon kyphoplasty (BKP) 1036–8
    criticisms 1038–9
    PMMA cement 1040
    technique 1038
ballottement test, distal radioulnar joint 759, 1367
Bankart retractor 1219, 1229
Bankart tear 730
Bankart's lesion 297, 731, 1214
    bony 298
    capsular 298
    medially healed, glenohumeral instability 1216
    posterior 1221, 1222
    see also glenoid labrum, tear
Bankart's repair, open 1218–19
    anaesthesia and positioning 1218
    capsule/scapularis repair 1219
    closure 1219
    deep dissection 1218–19
    history 1214–15
    incision and superficial dissection 1218
    labral reattachment 1219
    results 1215
Barlow test 539, 643, 646
Barrack grading, hip prosthesis loosening 1154
Barton fracture 329, 1560
    treatment 330
Barton-type fractures 327
baseball, medial epicondylitis pathogenesis 1390
basic multicellular units (BMUs) 1025
basilar fractures 478
basivertebral nerve 976
Bateson's paravertebral plexus 927
Batson's venous plexus 983, 987
Baumann angle 487
Baxter's nerve 79
Bayly–Walker shoulder 948
B-cell lymphoma 907–8
beach chair positioning 1211, 1226
    open anterior capsulorrhaphy 732, 1218
    rotator cuff tear repair 742, 1211
    shoulder arthroscopy 714, 731, 732
beam, definition 180
Becker muscular dystrophy 610
Belfast regimen 1297
belly press tests, Napoleon/La Fosse 10, 11
below-knee amputation (BKA) 961–2
    diabetic foot 1470
Bence–Jones protein 906
bench presses 701
bending 181
beneficence 1532
Bennett's fracture 763
best interests, patient 1533–5
beta defensins 471, 472
beta errors (type II) 42
β-blockers, use by athletes 707
β-oxidation 702–3
betamethasone dipropionate 129
    trigger finger 1277–8
bias 39
    selection 40
    types 39
biceps (biceps brachii)
    anatomy 322
    examination/tests 11
biceps curl 701
biceps tendon
    dynamic stabilizer of shoulder 730
    lacertous fibrous fascia 505
    lesions, rotator cuff repair and 1213
    long head, in total shoulder replacement 1226
    tearing/subluxation 1213
bicipital aponeurosis 505
bifid uvula 552
Bigelow manoeuvre 336
    reverse manoeuvre 339
biglycan 83, 101
bimalleolar fractures 386
    treatment 389–91
Bi-Metric stem 190
biocompatible materials 188
biofeedback 214
biofilm
    acute osteomyelitis pathogenesis 222
    chronic osteomyelitis pathogenesis 223

biological materials see biomaterials
biological plate fixation 272–4
    tibial shaft fracture 379
biological reconstruction 944–6
    allograft–prosthetic composites 946
    allografts 944–5
    autografts 945–6
    long-term complications 951
    see also allograft/allograft transplantation; autografts
biological therapy, rheumatoid arthritis 1087–8
biomaterials 188–9
    biocompatible 188
    injectable, osteoporotic spine 1039–40
        PMMA 1040
        resorbable calcium phosphate cement 1040–1
    natural tissues 188
    synthetic 188–9
        for ankle implants 192
        fixation of implants 194
        for fracture fixation devices 195
        for hand/wrist replacement 192–4
        for hip implants 188, 189, 190
        for knee implants 191–2
        mechanics 183
        preclinical testing 197–9
        for shoulder and elbow implants 192
        for spinal implants 196, 197
        tibial shaft fracture fixation 379
    tough 183
    see also material(s)
biomechanics 173–201
    bones 82–3, 88
    boutonnière deformity 1299
    carpal bones 1352
    cubital tunnel syndrome 1398
    dynamics vs statics 184–5
    fracture/bone healing 270–1, 518–20
    joints (normal) 186–8
        ankle 186, 1243–4
        control and stability 207–11
        elbow see elbow
        in fingers 187
        hip 186, 1105–13
        knee 186–7
        shoulder 187
        wrist 187
    knee 186–7, 665–6
    ligaments 112
    mallet finger 1299–300
    medial collateral ligament 805
    multidirectional instability of shoulder 737
    muscle see muscle (skeletal)
    natural tissues 188
    osteoarthritis 102, 1242, 1333–4
    osteoporosis 1026
    patella 665–6
    posterior shoulder instability 735
    principles 173–8
    radial head 1387
    spine 187–8
    tendons 112
    total hip arthroplasty see hip arthroplasty (total)
    see also loading
biomimetic materials 1524–5
bionics 1524
biopsy
    muscle, muscular dystrophy 611
    pyogenic spinal infections 985, 986
    sarcoma 941
    soft-tissue sarcoma 915
    spinal tuberculosis 988–9
    spinal tumours 1060
    tumours 870, 886–7, 915, 941
        metastatic 931
bioreactors, tissue engineering 1527
Birbeck granules 890, 891
birth injuries see obstetric brachial plexus birth palsy (OBPP)
Bishop rating system, cubital tunnel syndrome 1401–2, 1403
bisphosphonates 132, 133
    bone metastases and 933
    mechanism of action 133
    side-effects 133
bite injuries, to hand 1313
black eye 468, 469, 475
bladder

catheterization
    hip arthroplasty 1125
    spinal injuries 445
disruptions, pelvic fractures with 427
bleeding
    anticoagulant side-effect 131
        management 131
    ATLS management 236, 239, 445
    finger/palm lacerations 1278
    from nose or ear 468
    open injuries of limbs 248
    see also blood loss; haemorrhage
Blickenstaff and Morris classification 1565
blinding, in trials 40
blindness 469, 475
blood cultures
    acute haematogenous osteomyelitis 584
    spinal infections 984
blood flow
    arteriovenous pressure gradient and 507
    raised compartmental pressure reducing 507
blood loss
    hip/femur fractures 239
    hypovolaemic shock 236
    intra-operative, reduction in hip arthroplasty 1124
    pelvic fractures 239
    see also bleeding
blood pressure, hypovolaemic shock 236
blood supply
    Achilles tendon 1425
    arm 58
    bones 271
        fracture healing 520
    elbow 58
    femoral epiphysis 653
    femoral head see femoral head
    foot and ankle 79–80
    forearm 62, 505
    hip and pelvis 71–2
    humerus 57
    leg 77, 377
    ligaments 111
    meniscus 103–4, 105
    to peripheral nerves 1303
    peroneal tendon 1428
    shoulder 54, 55, 56
    skeletal muscle 108
    spine 68
    tendons 111–12
    thigh 75
    tibia and fibula 377
    triangular fibrocartilage complex (TFCC) 1366
    ulnar nerve 1407
blood tests
    acute haematogenous osteomyelitis 584
    foot/ankle arthritis 1485
    septic arthritis in children 579–80
blood transfusion
    pelvic injuries 239
    primary survey after trauma 236, 237
blood vessels
    in amputations 960
    injury in fractures, effect on healing 517–18
    ligation, bleeding after trauma 239
    repair, microsurgical 1319
    transmural pressure (TM) 506
Blount disease 670–1
blow-out fracture 469, 472
    maxillofacial 472
Blumensaat line 370
BMP-2, recombinant human 1014
BMP-7 545
body-image awareness 969, 970
body's line of gravity 955
Böhler, Lorenz 5
Böhler's tuber joint angle 399
bone(s) 82–97
    age-related changes 122–3
    allograft transplantation 148–9
    in amputations 960
    aspiration, acute haematogenous osteomyelitis 584
    atrophy, maxillofacial fractures 472
    biomechanical properties 82–3
        adaptation to environment 88
    biopsy 886

blood supply
    fracture healing 517–18, 520
    fractures 271
blood supply loss 96
    see also osteonecrosis
brittle 1130
bruise see bone bruising
cancellous 85–6, 88, 885
    formation 89
    remodelling 88
    screws for fracture fixation 195
    turnover rate 88
    Young's modulus 188
chemotherapy effects on 929
chronic stress injury, MRI scan 169
compact see bone(s), cortical (compact)
components 82–3
    extracellular matrix proteins 82, 83
    inorganic 82, 86
    organic matrix 82, 83
compressive strength 82
contusion, MRI 163
cortical (compact) 84–5, 88, 885
    MRI appearance 161, 167
    remodelling 88
    sclerotic rim 867, 885
    screws for fracture fixation 195
    turnover rate 88
    Young's modulus 188
cysts 867
    aneurysmal see aneurysmal bone cyst (ABC)
    simple/unicameral 887–8
densitometry, spinal osteoporosis 1027
density
    assessment in chemotherapy 929
    decreased, diseases with 94
    increased, diseases with 96
destruction
    mechanisms, in metastases 928
    osteolytic metastases 927
    patterns, in tumours 867
development and growth 86, 88–91
    children 482–3
    enchondral growth 52
    see also ossification
embryology 52
enchondral growth 52
erosion, juvenile idiopathic arthritis 590
formation 86, 543, 544, 885
    markers of, in osteoporosis 1027
    periosteal, patterns 867
    in tumours 867, 885
    see also ossification
graft see bone grafts/grafting
healing 517–20
    biological treatment 520–1
    direct (primary) 519
    indirect (secondary) 519–20
    shear stress effect 519
    see also fracture(s), healing
immature (woven) 84
infarcts 867
infection see osteomyelitis
intramedullary cyst 887–8
lamellae 85, 885
    circumferential 85
lamellar (cancellous and compact types) 84–6, 885
ligament attachment 111
loss 98
    age-related 122, 1025
    cancer treatment-induced (CTIBL) 929, 933
    in fracture non-union, management 524
    osteoporosis 183
    postmenopausal 122–3, 1025
    radius non-union 527
    revision hip arthroplasty 1156–7
    revision knee arthroplasty 1201–2
    spinal cord injury 95
    see also bone(s), resorption
mass, peak 98, 1025
matrix 885
    composition 82, 83
medullary 885
metabolism
    metastases 927, 928, 929
    normal 92, 97
    regulation 92, 98

bone(s) – continued
    metastases see metastases (skeletal)
    mineralization 82, 84, 86, 91, 885
        failure 93
        process 86
        see also calcification
    number in skeleton 52
    nutrient supply 85–6
    pagetoid 1130
    permeative/non-permeative growth of tumours 885
    raised intracompartmental pressure effect 508
    remodelling 84, 87, 88
        after fracture healing 145, 519
        age-related changes 122, 1025
        control 88, 1027
        induction by osteocytes 87
        process 88
    replacements, endocultivation 1527–8
    resection
        fracture non-union, infected 521
        subchondral bone 1079
    resorption 885
        in hip prosthesis loosening 1153–4
        mechanism 87
        metastases 928, 929, 1065
        osteoclast role 87
        TGF-β and PTHrP role 928
    resorption cavity 87
    sclerotic rim 867, 885
    stress fractures see stress fractures
    structure 82–3, 86, 885
    tendon attachment 111
    trabecular 885
        MRI appearance 161, 167
    trauma, MRI application 169
    tumours see bone tumours
    turnover
        rate 88
        regulation 1025
    turnover markers 928, 931, 1025
        in osteoporosis 1027
    viability, conditions affecting 96
    viable, feature of (punctate bleeding) 222
    woven 84, 885
        metastases 929
bone bruising 103
    in ACL injuries 808
bone cells 86–7
    osteoprogenitor 86, 88
    see also osteoblast(s); osteoclast(s); osteocyte(s)
bone cement see cement
bone collar, formation 543
bone densitometry, spinal osteoporosis 1027
'bone first' theory, osteoarthritis 1081
bone grafts/grafting
    adult scoliosis 1014
    alternatives, adult scoliosis 1014
    arthroplasty in rheumatoid arthritis 1129
    donor site 520
    fracture healing 520
    impaction see impaction bone grafting
    in revision knee arthroplasty 1202
bone in-growth techniques 194
bone marrow 89, 1068
    age-related changes 122
    formation 543
    functions 1068
    MRI appearance 161, 167
    red 161, 167
    tumours, MRI 171, 869
        see also myeloma
    yellow 161, 167
bone morphogenetic proteins (BMPs) 1025
    BMP-7 gene 545
    fracture healing 520
    recombinant human BMP-2 (rhBMP-2) 1014
    spinal fusions and 1014
    tissue engineering role 1527
bone multicellular units (BMUs) 88
bone pain
    syphilis 224
    tumours 884
    see also pain

bone sarcoma see osteosarcoma; sarcoma; other specific sarcomas
bone scans 156–8
    acute haematogenous osteomyelitis 584
    clinical uses 157, 171
    metastases 930
    method 156–7
    for revision knee arthroplasty 1199
    spinal tuberculosis 988
    spinal tumours 1059–60
    strengths/weaknesses 157
    tumours 157, 158, 867–8
    see also radionuclide imaging
bone sialoprotein 83
bone substitute, in vertebroplasty 1032, 1035
bone tamp 1018
bone tissue
    structure 82–3
    types 83–6
bone tumours 882–912
    benign
        aneurysmal bone cyst see aneurysmal bone cyst (ABC)
        eosinophilic granuloma 890–1, 1062
        epidemiology 884
        fibrous dysplasia 891, 892
        giant cell see giant cell tumour of bone
        of hand 1377–8
        simple/unicameral bone cysts 887–8
    benign osteoblastic
        osteoblastoma see osteoblastoma
        osteoid osteoma see osteoid osteoma
    biopsy 870, 886–7
    bone formation in 867, 1379
    clinical presentation 884–5
    diagnosis 885
    diaphyseal 886
    epidemiology 883–4
    epiphyseal 886
    genetics 886
    history-taking 866
    incidence 884
    intramedullary 885
    limb-sparing surgery 941, 942
    lymphoma 907–8
    malignant
        chondrosarcoma see chondrosarcoma
        epidemiology 883–4
        Ewing's sarcoma see Ewing's sarcoma
        malignant fibrous histiocytoma 904, 919, 1377
        osteosarcoma see osteosarcoma
    metaphyseal 886
    metastatic see metastases (skeletal); spinal metastases
    MRI scans 171
    non-permeative growth 885
    occult, MRI scan 171
    pathology 887
    permeative growth 885, 897, 901
    radiography 866–7
    radiological diagnosis 885–7
        information provided by 886
    radionuclide imaging 157, 158, 867–8, 886
    risk factors 884
    sarcoma see osteosarcoma; sarcoma; other specific sarcomas
    sclerotic rim 867, 885
    staging, Enneking system 870
    WHO classification 883, 887
bone volume/tissue volume (BV/TV) 1026
bone-healing organ (BHO) 517–20
bone-lining cells 88
bone–tendon–bone graft, chronic scapholunate ligament injury 1358
bony Bankart's lesion 297
bony erosion, juvenile idiopathic arthritis 590
'bony pincers' theory 977
borderline patients, after trauma 238, 241
botulinum toxin A (BTX-A) therapy
    cerebral palsy 602, 1476
    lateral epicondylitis 1394
    stroke patients 1478

boundary lubrication 184, 1115
boutonnière deformity 1282–3, 1300, 1562
    biomechanics 1299
    mechanisms of injury 765, 1282
    pseudo- 766, 1325, 1326, 1327
    sports injuries 765–6
    stages 1300
    testing 17, 1282
    treatment 765–6, 1282–3, 1300
    two-stage reconstruction 1283
Bouvier's test 17
Bowers and Martin classification, first MTP joint injuries 414, 415
bowstring test 35
bowstringing effect, tendons 1293, 1312
Box Total Ankle Replacement 192
Boyd amputation 961
Boyd and Griffin classification, intertrochanteric fractures 347
Boyd classification, congenital pseudarthrosis of tibia 675
Boye's test 17
braces/bracing
    adult scoliosis 1011
    ankle 1423, 1429
    anterior cruciate ligament 211
    functional see functional bracing
    genu valgum/varum 669
    glenohumeral instability 1218, 1222
    knee see knee, braces/bracing
    lateral epicondylitis 1394, 1395
    osteoporotic vertical compression fractures 1016
    for patellofemoral pain 210–11
    spinal see spinal bracing
brachial artery 58
    anatomy 505
    compartment syndrome
        aetiopathogenesis 505
    injury, humeral shaft fractures 309
brachial plexus
    anatomy 53–4
    compression
        cubital tunnel syndrome vs 1399
        see also obstetric brachial plexus birth palsy (OBPP)
    injuries 1304
        sports 722
    lateral cord 58
    medial cord 58
    palsy 54
    posterior cord 58
    pre/post-ganglionic lesions 54
brachioradialis, nerve to 1304
brachydactyly type A 546
brachymetatarsia 1457
brachytherapy 875
    soft-tissue sarcoma 876
bracing see braces/bracing
Bradford, Edward 5
bradycardia, neurogenic shock in spinal cord injury 443
brain
    herniation 721
    in skull fractures 478
    trauma see traumatic brain injury (TBI)
breast cancer 926, 927, 929, 933
    bisphosphonates in 933
    Li–Fraumeni syndrome 930
    pathological fracture 934
breathing, in trauma management 235
bridge plates, for fractures 273–4
brittle bones 1130
brittle fracture (of material) 182, 183
Brodie's abscess 224, 586
Brown–Séquard syndrome 443, 998
Brucella spondylitis 986
Bruner's incisions 1295, 1296, 1328, 1329
Brunner approach 1312
brushite (dicalcium phosphate dehydrate) 1041
Bryan and Morrey classification 1558
Bryant's triangle 18
buckle fracture, children 483, 493, 495
buckle handle fractures, non-accidental injuries 501
buddy taping, PIP joint dislocations 1284
buffered platelet-rich plasma injection 1395
Buford complex 715

bulbocavernosus reflex 67, 441
'bulge' test, knee 23–4
bunionette deformity 1454–5
    aetiology 1454–5
    classification 1455
    treatment 1455
Bunnel–Littler test 17
bupivacaine 129
burnout 1549–52
    definition 1549
    resistance 1551, 1552
    risk management through prevention 1551–2
    signs and symptoms 1551
    stressors in orthopaedic surgery 1550
bursae, infections 1312
bursectomy, olecranon 1389
bursitis
    around hip 775
    iliopsoas 775
    ischial 775
    olecranon see olecranon bursitis
    pelvis, hip and thigh, sports injuries 775
    precalcaneal 832
    retrocalcaneal 832
    trochanteric 775
burst fractures
    osteoporotic 1028
    post-traumatic kyphosis after 1019
    subaxial cervical spine 454–5, 456
    thoracolumbar spine see thoracolumbar spine injuries

C3 and C3b 145
C3a and C5a 145
C7 plumb line 1015, 1018
Caffey disease (infantile cortical hyperostosis) 96, 547
cage(s) 1012
    acetabular defects, impaction bone grafting 1158, 1159
    isthmic spondylolisthesis 1053
calcaneal exostosis 832
calcaneal fractures 398–402
    anterior process 399, 401
    body fractures 401
    classification 399–400
        Essex–Lopresti 399–400
        Sanders (CT-based) 400
    clinical evaluation 398
    complications 401
    displaced, treatment 400
    extra-articular features 399
        treatment 400
    frequency 398
    intra-articular features 399–400
        treatment 400–1
    lateral process 401
    mechanism of injury 398
    medial process 399, 401
    posterior tuberosity 399, 401
    primary fracture line 399
    radiographic evaluation 398–9
    secondary fracture 399
    sustentacular 399
    treatment 400–1
        guidelines 401
calcaneal osteotomy
    cerebral palsy 605, 1476
    medial slide 1423–4
calcaneal pitch 1461, 1462
calcaneocuboid joint 403
    distraction arthrodesis 1423
calcaneofibular ligament (CFL) 78, 840, 842, 1243
    in ankle motion 1243, 1244
    palpation 28
    repair 842
calcaneovalgus, congenital 691
calcaneus 398
    anatomy 77
    deformity, myelomeningocele 610
    exostosis 832
    fractures see calcaneal fractures
    osteotomy see calcaneal osteotomy
    posterior superior tuberosity 832
    see also heel
calcific tendonitis, Achilles tendon 832
calcification
    'arc and ring' 867
    'chicken wire' 895
    glenoid rim 1217
    intervertebral disc 1001

tumours 867
zone, growth plate 544
zone of provisional 93
see also bone(s), mineralization
calcitonin 87
as anti-osteoporotic drug 133
bone metabolism control 98
calcium and phosphate metabolism 98
clinical uses 133
interaction with osteoclasts 87
calcium
absorption/reabsorption 97
bone metabolism regulation 98
daily requirements 97
deficiency 94
child athletes 708
function in bone 97
influx
action potential 109
muscle injury 110, 704
metabolism 97
regulation 98
plasma levels 97
release, muscle contraction 109, 701
calcium phosphate cement, resorbable 1040–1
advantages/disadvantages 1041
indications 1041
types 1041
calcium pyrophosphate dihydrate deposition disease 1091–2
calcium/calmodulin-dependent kinase II (CaMKII) 547
calf muscle abnormalities
in cerebral palsy 604
pseudohypertrophy 611
calf squeeze test 830
callosities
over interphalangeal joints, claw toe 1452
over metatarsal heads 1450
plantar 1436
callotasis 683–4
callus 145
foot 27, 28
fracture healing by 270, 275, 517, 519–20
children, diaphyseal greenstick fracture 483
hypertrophic non-union 516
fracture healing without 270
callus distraction 684
caloric intake, athletes 706
child athletes 708
female athletes 708
caloric restriction 706
female athletes 708
cameras, in CAOS 1513, 1514, 1518, 1521
CaMKII (calcium/calmodulin-dependent kinase II) 547
campomelic syndrome, prevalence 542
Canale and Kelley classification, talar neck fractures 395
Canale view, radiography, talar neck fractures 395
canaliculi 86
cancer treatment-induced bone loss (CTIBL) 929, 933
cancers see tumours (musculoskeletal); specific cancers
capacity, decision-making 1532, 1533, 1540
Capanna scoring 936
capillary occlusion, compartment syndrome pathogenesis 507
Capital Hip 1139, 1154
capitate
in four-corner fusions 1359
in scapholunate degenerative changes 1359
capitellum
fracture 313–14, 1558
osteochondritis dissecans 753–4
capitolunate (CL) angle 1354
capitolunate (CL) joint, reduction, in dislocations 1361
capsular plication, multidirectional instability of shoulder 739
capsulolabral repair, arthroscopic
anterior instability 731–3
posterior instability 736

capsulorrhaphy, anterior
arthroscopic 731–3
open, technique 734–5
capsulotomy, shoulder 734
caput membranaceum 552
carbohydrate sulphotransferase 3 549
carbohydrates, intake and metabolism 706
child athletes 708
female athletes 708
Carbon Copy II/III foot 964
carbon fibre dynamic-response foot 964
carbon monoxide 704
carbonic acid, bone resorption 87
carbonic anhydrase 87
γ-carboxy glutamic acid-containing proteins 83
carcinogens 149
cardiac output 703
hypovolaemic shock 236
cardiac tamponade 235
cardiogenic shock 235
cardiopulmonary system, in exercise 703–4
cardiovascular examination, developmental disorders of bone 550
carotid (Chassaingnac's) tubercle 65
carpal bones
anatomy 64, 1351
biomechanics 1352
distal row 1351
fractures 330, 1361
in athletes 755–6
hook of hamate fractures 756–7
see also scaphoid fractures
injuries 1352, 1354
proximal row 1351
carpectomy 1359
dissociation with distal row 1360
instability 1360
see also wrist
carpal instability 1351–64
adaptive 1362
causes/mechanism 1352–3, 1354–5
classification 1354–5
diagnosis 1353
dorsal intercalated segment instability (DISI) 1354, 1355, 1356
dorsal perilunate dislocation 1360–1
dorsal perilunate fracture dislocation 1361
history and examination 1354
investigations/imaging 1353–4
lunotriquetral see lunotriquetral instability
midcarpal 1360
patterns 1355
radiocarpal 1360
scapholunate injury see scapholunate ligament (SLL), injury
volar intercalated segment instability (VISI) 1354, 1355, 1359, 1360
see also carpal ligaments, injuries
carpal instability adaptive (CIA) 1355
carpal instability complex (CIC) 1355
carpal instability dissociative (CID) 1355
carpal instability non-dissociative (CIND) 1355
carpal ligaments 1351
anatomy 1351, 1352
injuries 1352
chronic 1353, 1354
classification 1354–5
clinical features 1353
diagnosis 1353
grades 1356
history and examination 1353
imaging 1353–4
investigation 1353–4
see also scapholunate ligament (SLL)
carpal tunnel, zone IV flexor tendon injuries 1280
carpal tunnel syndrome 848, 1361
examination/testing 15
pronator syndrome vs 1386
see also median nerve, compression
carpectomy, proximal row 1359
carpometacarpal (CMC) joint
anatomy 1333, 1335
dislocations 768

fifth
osteoarthritis 1342–3
resection/fusion 1341
first, osteoarthritis see trapeziometacarpal (TM) joint
ligaments 1335
osteoarthritis 1333, 1334–41, 1342–3
see also carpal bones; metacarpals
carrying angle 57, 311, 1400
Carter's strain theories 518–19
cartilage
acute necrosis (chondrolysis) 660
articular see articular cartilage
calcified zone 101, 1078
cap, osteochondroma 895
defects, regeneration in vivo 1528–9
see also autologous chondrocyte implantation (ACI)
growth plate see growth plate
hyaline see articular cartilage
injury, knee 788–91
matrix, calcification, in tumours 886
cartilage degeneration zone, growth plate 544
cartilage model, ossification 89
cartilage oligomeric matrix protein (COMP) 101–2
osteoarthritis marker 1082
rheumatoid arthritis marker 1087
cartilage tumours 883, 897
benign 894–5
enchondroma 896–8
hand 1378–9
osteochondroma 895–6
spine 1061–2
see also enchondroma; osteochondroma
malignant 896–8
see also chondrosarcoma
case series 42
case workers, workers' compensation 1543
case–control study 41–2, 45
cast wedging, paediatric fractures 485
casts/cast immobilization
above-elbow 263
congenital clubfoot 690
fractures 260
ankle 266, 389
in children 485
complications 261
distal humerus 313
distal radius 261
forearm 263
humeral shaft 264, 308
tibial shaft 265–6
method 260
three-point rule 260, 261
synthetic materials for 260
cataract, congenital 552
categorical data 43
cathepsin K 549
catheterization
hip arthroplasty 1125
spinal injuries 445
Catterall classification 654
cauda equina syndrome 443, 978
history-taking and symptoms 32
lumbar disc herniation 996
spinal infections and 983
caudal reflex arcs 441
cavus foot see pes cavus
CBFA1 (core binding factor α1) gene 545
cdk2 protein 149
cefazolin
hip arthroplasty 1126
open fractures 254
cefuroxime, hip arthroplasty 1126
cell(s), tissue engineering 1526–7
cell biology 139–45
cell-mediated immunity 147, 148, 1069
adoptive, in tumour therapy 1069
tumours 1068, 1069
see also T lymphocytes (T cells)
cellulitis 219, 220, 1310
antibiotic treatment 220
diabetic foot 1467
organisms causing 219
cement (bone)
acrylic 1100
antibiotic impregnated 1161
calcium phosphate see calcium phosphate cement, resorbable

for hip arthroplasty 1140
introduction methods, in arthroplasty 1140
for joint implant fixation 194
PMMA see polymethylmethacrylate (PMMA)
spinal 1040
vertebroplasty 1032, 1036
cement disease 1100, 1101
cement spacer, cement impregnated 1161
cementation technique, proximal femur reconstruction 947
cementoplasty 1067
osteonecrosis of spine 1031
with PMMA, osteoporotic fractures 1040
spinal metastases 1067
see also kyphoplasty; vertebroplasty
central cord syndrome 443
central venous line, hip arthroplasty 1124
central venous pressure, in trauma 236
centre of gravity 954, 955, 1106
centre of rotation of angulation (CORA) 528
cephalic vein 1226
Ceracup 190
Cerament 1041
ceramic
description 1119
fractures 1119, 1155
for implants 189, 1119–20
ceramic-on-ceramic bearings
hip 1120
lubrication 1115
ceramic-on-polyethylene bearings 1119
cerebral autoregulation, loss 721
cerebral palsy 598–608, 1475–6
aetiology 598–9, 1475
classification 599–600, 1475
clinical evaluation 600–1
definition 598
epidemiology 598, 1475
gait abnormalities 568, 601
hip instability 606–7
knee kinematics during walking
angular displacement 206–7
angular velocity 207
pathophysiology of muscular abnormalities 599
spinal deformities 607
static physical examination 600–1
unilateral, gait 601
upper extremity disorders 607
cerebral palsy management 601–7, 1475–6
equinovalgus deformity 605, 1476
equinovarus deformity 604–5, 1476
equinus deformity 604, 1475–6
general considerations 1475
hip instability 606–7
medical therapy 602, 1476
non-ambulatory patients 605–6
postoperative rehabilitation after multilevel surgery 605
priorities and goals 600
spinal deformities 607
surgical procedures
at calf, ankle and foot 604–5, 1476
at hip 602–3, 606–7
at knee 603–4
at spine 607
upper extremity problems 607
cerebrospinal fluid (CSF) 478
leakage (rhinorrhoea) 468
cerebrovascular accident 1477–8
surgery for 969–71
cervical collar 238
in trauma 235, 238, 440, 442
cervical cord injury 440, 445
neurogenic shock 443
cervical disc disease
after stingers 724
cubital tunnel syndrome vs 1399
herniation/prolapse 455, 997, 999
C5–C6 998
C6–C7 997, 998
cervical ligament (ankle) 1243
cervical myelopathy
gait and 31
testing for 33
see also cervical spondylotic myelopathy

cervical nerve pinch syndrome 720, 722
cervical neuropraxia ('stinger') 720, 722, 724
　initial management 724
　mechanism of injury 722, 724
　return to play 724, 725
　signs/symptoms 722, 724
cervical radiculopathy
　history-taking and symptoms 32
　tests for 33
cervical spine
　anatomy 64–5
　anterior column 453
　anterior corpectomy and fusion 1003, 1004
　apophyseal joints 66
　arthritis, cubital tunnel syndrome vs 1399
　C1 see atlas
　C2 see axis (C2)
　C3–C7 see cervical spine, subaxial
　C5–C6 disc prolapse 998
　C6–C7 disc prolapse 997, 998
　canal diameter 65
　columns (three) 65, 453
　decompression, degenerative disc disease 1003
　degeneration 999
　disc herniation 455, 999
　　see also cervical disc disease
　discectomy 1003, 1004
　dislocations 445
　examination 32–3
　fractures see under cervical spine injuries
　fusion
　　C2–3 452
　　rheumatoid arthritis 1268
　imaging, after sporting injury 725
　immobilization, after trauma 234, 235, 725
　injury see cervical spine injuries
　instability 448–9
　　checklist for diagnosis 454
　metal artefacts, CT scan 159
　middle column 453
　movements 32–3
　orthoses 969
　polyarticular juvenile rheumatoid arthritis 1089
　posterior column 453
　protection in trauma 235, 238
　space for cord 445, 447
　special tests 33
　subaxial (C3–7) 453–8
　　columns 65, 453
　　injuries see under cervical spine injuries
　　ligamentous complexes 453
　　radiographs, assessment 454
　surgical approaches
　　anterior 68–9
　　posterior 68, 69
cervical spine injuries 445–59
　atlantoaxial rotary subluxation/dislocation 449–50
　atlanto-occipital dislocation 725
　C1-2 sports injuries, management 725
　causes/mechanisms 445
　fractures 1555–6
　　burst, CT scan 158, 456
　　C1 447–8, 725, 1555
　　C1–2 rotary 1555
　　C2 445, 451, 452, 725–6, 1556
　　C3 454, 1556
　　C4–C7 1556
　　immobilization 445
　　sports injuries 725–6
　gunshot 459
　history and examination 724–5
　imaging 724–5
　　CT scan 158
　immobilization for 235, 238, 440, 442, 445
　mortality 446
　occipitocervical dislocation 447
　occiput–C1–C2 complex 446–52, 725–6
　　occipital condyle fractures 446–7, 725
　　odontoid process fractures 450–1
　　protection from 235, 238
　　pure transverse ligament 448–9

radiographic evaluation 445–6
sports injuries 724–6
　lower spine, 726
　upper spine 725–6
sprains/strains, sports injuries 726
subaxial (C3–7) 453–8
　bifacetal dislocations 456, 457
　burst fractures 454–5, 456
　C6–7 bifacetal dislocation 456
　classification 453–8
　compression–extension (CE) injuries 457, 458, 726
　compression–flexion (CF) injuries 453–4, 455, 726
　distraction–extension (DE) injuries 457–8, 459, 726
　distraction–flexion (DF) injuries 455, 456, 457, 726
　facet dislocations 456, 457
　lateral flexion (LF) injuries 458, 459
　mechanisms 453
　sports injuries 726
　vertical compression (VC) fractures 454–5, 456
transient quadriplegia 726
traumatic C1–C2 instability 448–9
traumatic spondylolisthesis of C2 445, 451, 452
cervical spondylotic myelopathy 1004
　cubital tunnel syndrome vs 1399
　symptoms 32
cervical sympathetic ganglia 68
'chair test', lateral epicondylitis 750
Chance fracture 460, 461–2
Chaput osteotomy 837
Charcot joint disease, diabetic foot 1467, 1468
Charcot neuroarthropathy 1492–3
Charcot–Marie–Tooth disease 613–15, 1472–4
　causative genes 613, 614
　clinical features 613–15, 1472–3
　　claw toe and 1453
　　pes cavus 1461
　diagnosis 1473
　pathogenesis 1472
　treatment 615, 1473–4
　　conservative 1473–4
　　surgical 1474
Charité device 197
Charnley, Sir John 5, 259, 1097, 1098, 1099, 1109, 1135
　contribution to hip arthroplasty 1098–100, 1109–10, 1116
　PTFE prostheses and 1098, 1099
　transtrochanteric approach to hip 1137–8
　use of PMMA 1099
Charnley acetabular component 190
Charnley Elite-Plus femoral component 1154, 1161
Charnley femoral head/stem 190
Charnley hip 1098–9, 1100, 1109–10, 1138
　aseptic loosening 1154
　modular hip 189, 190
　outcome 1142
Chassaingnac's (carotid) tubercle 65
chauffeur's fracture 329, 1560
cheilectomy 1490
chemotherapy 874, 878–81
　adjuvant 878
　adverse effects on bone 929
　combination vs single agents 879–80
　drug resistance 879
　general principles 878–9
　isolated limb perfusion 880
　limitations 878
　for metastases 881
　neoadjuvant 879
　palliative 879
　rationale for 878
　for sarcomas 880, 951
　side-effects 879
　targeted therapy 878
Chen criteria, function evaluation after replantation 1322
chevron osteotomy 1437–8
'chicken wire calcification' 895
child abuse 500–1
children
　ACL reconstruction 810
　amputations 958–9

athletic, nutrition 708
bone and joint infections 578–88
clinical assessment 535–40
dislocations
　diagnosis 484–5
　frequency 484
　reduction 486
foot disorders see foot deformities
fractures 481–502
　causes 482
　characteristics 483–4
　classifications 499
　clinical examination 484
　diagnosis 484–5
　epidemiology 481–2
　non-accidental 500
　osteochondral 484
　radiography/imaging 485
　radius and ulna shaft, non-operative treatment 262
　treatment 485–6, 500
　see also individual bones
gait see gait
Glasgow Coma Scale (GCS) 499, 500
gymnast's wrist 761
hip disorders see hip disorders
informed consent and 1532–3, 1540–1
isthmic spondylolisthesis 1052
knee disorders see knee, disorders in children
leg disorders see leg, disorders in children
ligament injuries 484
limb reconstruction 950–1
multiply injured 499–500
　treatment 500
neuromuscular disorders see neurological/neuromuscular disorders
non-accidental injury 500–1
orthoses for 969
patellar tendon rupture 791
radiography 485
skeletal development 482–3
skeletal injury characteristics 483–4
spinal disorders see spinal deformities
spinal infections 983
spinal tuberculosis 990, 991
see also entries beginning infantile, juvenile; specific disorders
Childress duck waddle test 26
chloride, release, bone resorption 87
chlorophyll, in bone cement 1120
chondral injuries, pelvis, hip and thigh 779
chondroblastic tumours, radiography 886
chondroblastoma 894–5
chondrocalcinosis 1091–2
chondrocyte maturation defects 547
chondrocytes 1077–8
　age-related changes 1080
　allogenic, survival 1246
　in articular cartilage 101, 1078
　autologous transplant see autologous chondrocyte implantation (ACI)
defects
　hypertrophic 547
　maturation 547
　proliferative 545–6
endochondral ossification 89, 91
function 1077
growth factors affecting 1078
harvesting and culture for transplantation 790, 1083
hypertrophic 89, 547
in intervertebral disc 106
in osteoarthritis 102
chondrodiastasis 683–4
chondrodysplasia 541
　see also developmental disorders of bone
chondrogenesis, in vivo, after chondrocyte transplantation 143
chondroid-forming tumours, spine 1061–2
chondroitin sulphate 102
　supplements 134
chondroitin-6-sulphotransferase 549
chondrolysis, slipped capital femoral epiphysis 660

chondroplasty, patellofemoral arthritis 1194–5
chondrosarcoma 896–8
　chemotherapy 880
　dedifferentiated 898, 899
　'grade half' 897
　metastatic spread 898
　multiple enchondromatosis 575
　multiple hereditary exostosis 575
　pathology/histology 897–8, 899
　pelvic reconstruction after resection 947
　radiography 886, 897, 899
　spine 1063
　synovial chondromatosis vs 784
Chopart amputation 961
Chopart joint see midtarsal joint
Chopart joint line 403
chordoma 904–6
　clinical features 904–5
　radiology 905
　spine 1063
chromosomal non-disjunction 152
chromosomal translocation 152
　in Ewing's sarcoma 904
chromosomes 140
　aberrant number 152
　chromosome 17, aneurysmal bone cyst and 888
　number (human) 140
　osteosarcoma and 901
chronic exertional compartment syndrome (CECS) 824, 825–6
　aetiology 825
　evaluation/imaging 825–6
　pathology 825–6
　treatment 826
chronic inflammation 145
chronic osteomyelitis see osteomyelitis, chronic
chronic recurrent multifocal osteomyelitis 586
ciclosporin, rheumatoid arthritis 1086
Cierny–Mader classification 222, 223
Cierny's infected host types 223
circulation, assessment/maintenance, in trauma 235–6, 239
circumflex nerve
　injury by fracture/dislocation 1306
　palsy 1306
　rupture 1305
Clarke's sign 26
claudication
　lumbar spine stenosis pain vs 977
　spinal (lumbar canal stenosis) 32
clavicle 52, 288
　anatomy 52, 288
　fractures 288–91, 1556
　　classification 289
　　clinical evaluation 288
　　complications 289–90
　　malunion 289
　　neurovascular injury 290
　　non-operative treatment 289
　　non-union 289–90
　　open, operative treatment 289
　　operative treatment 289
　　radiography 288–9
clavipectoral fascia 1226
claw toe 1452–4, 1460
　pathophysiology, examination 1453
　treatment 1453–4
clear cell sarcoma, hand 1377
cleidocranial dysplasia (CCD) 545
clexane 132
clindamycin, hip arthroplasty 1126
clinical assessment, paediatric patients 535–40
clinical decision-making 1546
clinical examination 8–35
　lower limb 17–35
　　gait, foot and ankle 26–31
　　hip 17–22
　　knee 22–6
　　spine 31–5
　upper limb 9–17
　　elbow 11–13
　　hand 15–17
　　shoulder 9–11
　　wrist 13–15
　see also individual anatomical structures/conditions; specific disorders

Subject Index 1563

clinical trials
  informed consent 1541
  see also randomized controlled trials (RCT)
clodronate 933
cloning, human 143
  types 143
closed kinetic chain (CKC) 203–4
  exercises, functionality 204
  open kinetic chain *vs* 203–4
closed reduction, developmental dysplasia of hip 648
closing cone 88
closing wedge high tibial osteotomy (CWHTO) 1264
clostridial collagenase 1326–7
clotting *see* coagulation
clover leaf skull 552
club foot *see* talipes equinovarus
CLUMP tumour 897
coagulation 130
  pathways 130
  trauma patient, evaluation/management 241
coagulopathy, after trauma 236
cobalt chrome alloy
  hip prostheses 1118, 1121, 1139
  knee prostheses 1177
cobalt–chrome–molybdenum alloy 188
  femoral components 189, 190
Cobb angles 631, 632
  adolescent idiopathic scoliosis 635, 636
  infantile idiopathic scoliosis 634
  juvenile idiopathic scoliosis 635
coccygeus muscle 429
coccyx, anatomy 65
Cochrane Collaboration 1537, 1547
Cochrane Library 1537, 1547
Cochrane Reviews 1537, 1547
'cock robin' position, head 449
codeine (methylmorphine) 127
coding, medical 1537–8
Codivilla, Alessandro 5
Codivilla technique 370
Codman's technique 1207–8
Codman's triangle 867, 886, 900
codons 140, 151
coefficient of friction 184
cohort study 41, 45
'coin test' 983
COL1A1 gene mutations 547, 570
COL1A2 gene mutations 547, 570
COL2A1 gene mutations 547–8, 570, 573
COL9 gene mutations 548, 572
COL10A1 gene mutations 548
colchicine 1091
cold abscess 225, 987, 988, 990
cold intolerance, replantation (upper limb) complication 1321
Coleman block test 30, 841
collagen 100–1
  age-related changes 120, 121, 1001
  in articular cartilage 101, 102
    osteoarthritis 102
  autoantibodies 1085
  in bone 82, 83
    lamellar bone 84
    woven bone 84
  cross-linking
    ageing and 121, 1001
    extracellular matrix strength 1078
  defects 547–8, 571
    see also specific disorders
  in intervertebral discs 106, 994
  in meniscus 103
  post-synthetic modification, ageing and 1001
  properties 100
  structure 100
  synthesis 100
  in tendons 111
    Achilles tendon 831
  type I 100, 101, 547
    in annulus fibrosus 106
    in bone 82–3
    Dupuytren's contracture pathogenesis 1325
    in tendons 111
  type II
    antibodies to epitopes 1082
    in articular cartilage 101, 1078
    autoantibodies 1085

in inner annulus fibrosus 106
oral tolerance induction 1088
type XI copolymerized with 101
type IX 101, 548
type X 548
type XI 101
  types 100
  in musculoskeletal system 101
collagen degradation products, rheumatoid arthritis 1088
collagenase, clostridial 1326–7
collar *see* cervical collar
collateral ligaments
  elbow *see* lateral collateral ligament (LCL) complex (elbow); medial collateral ligament (MCL) complex (elbow)
  knee *see* lateral collateral ligament (LCL) (knee); medial collateral ligament (MCL) (knee)
collateral vessels, flexor compartment of forearm 505–6
Colles fracture 327, 328, 1560
  non-operative treatment 261–2
  reverse (Smith fracture) 328–9
Collins, Michael J., *Hot Lights, Cold Steel* 1550
colloid administration, polytrauma 237
common iliac arteries 71
common iliac vessels 71
common peroneal nerve 76, 79
  entrapment 826–7
    aetiology 826
    evaluation/examination 827
    pathology 826–7
    treatment 827
  injury by fracture/dislocation 1306
communication, in CAOS 1513–14, 1515
COMP gene mutations 92
compartment(s) (osteofascial) 940
  forearm 278, 511
  hand 511
  leg 278, 279, 511
compartment syndrome, acute 278–81, 503–14
  anatomic considerations 505–6
  causes 278–80, 504, 505, 506
    injury types 506
  clinical examination 508–9
  clinical features 280, 378, 509
    six P's 509
  definition 278, 503
  diagnosis 508
    delay 510
  differential diagnosis 510
  forearm 323, 505
  fractures causing 279
    femoral shaft fractures 356
    forearm fractures 323, 505
    talar neck fractures 394–5
    tibial shaft fractures 378, 380, 506
  history 503–5
  impending, treatment 510
  investigations 280
  management 280–1, 508–10
  open injuries and 248
  pathogenesis 278, 504, 505, 506–8, 825
    arteriovenous gradient theory 507
    critical closing pressure theory 506
    effect on bone 508
    effect on muscle 507–8
    effect on nerve 508
    Matsen's unified concept 507
    microvascular occlusion theory 507
  pathophysiology 278, 506–8
    Hargen's and Akenson's 508
  prevention
    forearm fractures 263, 323
    traction for fractures 259
  sites 278, 378, 503, 504, 505
    characteristics of 505
  thigh 774
  treatment
    fasciotomy 280, 504, 511
    general principles 510–12
    in leg 511
    non-operative 510–11
  see also Volkmann ischaemic contracture
compartment syndrome, exertional *see* chronic exertional compartment syndrome (CECS)

compartmental pressure *see* intracompartmental pressure (ICP)
compensation, workers *see* workers' compensation
competency (decision-making) 1532, 1533, 1540
complement system 145
  activation pathways 145, 146
  in acute inflammation 147
complex regional pain syndrome (CRPS II) 1330
compliant material 179
component implantation, computer-assisted navigation, TKA 1519–20
Comprehensive Classification of Fractures (Müller) 342
compression fractures
  proximal tibia 498
  vertebral *see* vertebral body, compression fractures
compression plates, fracture fixation 272
compressive force 175
computation, in CAOS 1514–15
computed tomography (CT) 158–9
  arthrodesis 1268, 1269
  arthrography, rotator cuff muscles 1210
  in CAOS 1511–12
  clinical uses 158–9
  guided biopsy, pyogenic spinal infections 985, 986
  helical 158
  history 155–6
  injuries assessment 239
  needle biopsy of tumours 868
  New Orleans Criteria (head injury) 471
  pelvic 430
  Sanders classification of calcaneal fractures 400
  specific conditions/injuries
    acetabular fractures 422
    adult scoliosis 1010
    ankle/foot arthritis 1486
    cervical spine injuries 446, 450
    compartment syndrome 510
    congenital vertebral anomalies 631
    developmental disorders of bone 554
    fracture non-union 516, 517
    glenohumeral arthritis 1224
    glenohumeral instability 1217
    head and face trauma 471
    hip dislocation 336
    isthmic spondylolisthesis 1051
    juvenile idiopathic arthritis 594
    leg length discrepancy 679
    metastatic tumours 931
    odontoid fractures 450
    osteoporotic fractures 1028, 1029
    patellar dislocation 667
    revision knee arthroplasty 1200
    Scheuermann's kyphosis 640
    septic arthritis in children 580, 583
    soft-tissue sarcoma 913
    spinal cord injuries 444
    spinal tuberculosis 988
    spinal tumours 1060
    thoracolumbar spine injuries 460
    tibial torsion 674
    tumours 868
    wrist injuries 1354
  strengths/weaknesses 158
computer-aided design (CAD), tissue engineering scaffolds 1526
computer-assisted continuous infusion, morphine 127
computer-assisted orthopaedic surgery (CAOS) 1511–22
  applications 1511, 1515–22
    total hip replacement *see* hip arthroplasty (total)
    total knee arthroplasty *see* knee arthroplasty
  communication 1513–14
  computation and presentation 1514–15
  future aspects 1522
  patient-specific jigs 1522
  pelvic fractures 436
  registration of anatomy 1511–13
    total hip replacement 1521
    total knee arthroplasty 1518
  surgical control 1515

concentric contraction 701, 955
concurrent shift 204
concussion, in sport 718, 720–2
  definition 720
  grading scales 722, 723
  history and examination 721
  long-term deficits 720, 722
  management 723
    initial 721, 723
  pathophysiology 720
  return to play 721–2
  signs/symptoms 721, 722
conduction velocities, nerves at elbow 1400
condylar blade plate 359
condylar buttress plates, distal femoral fractures 360
confidence intervals 46
congenital calcaneovalgus 691
congenital cataract 552
congenital club foot *see* talipes equinovarus
congenital convex pes valgus *see* congenital vertical talus
congenital dislocation of knee (CDK) 664–5
congenital hyperextension of knee 665
congenital muscular dystrophy 613
congenital patellar dislocation 666
congenital posteromedial bowing of tibia 674–5
congenital pseudarthrosis of tibia (CPT) 675–7
congenital subluxation of knee 664
congenital talipes equinovarus (CTEV) *see* talipes equinovarus
congenital vertebral anomalies 628–30
  myelomeningocele 609
  patient evaluation 630–1
  treatment 631–2
  see also spinal deformities
congenital vertical talus 691–2
  in myelomeningocele 610
connective tissue
  age-related changes 121
  skeletal muscle structure 698
connective tissue syndromes 92
connectivity density (conn den) 1026
consent
  general medical 1539
  informed *see* informed consent
constitutional disorders of bone *see* developmental disorders of bone
content validity 39
continuing professional development, clinical outcomes and 1536
continuous data 43
contractures
  Dupuytren's *see* Dupuytren's contracture
  fingers 1325–6
  flexion *see* flexion contractures
  hand
    testing 17
    web space 1328
  ischaemic, history 504
  myelomeningocele 610
  obstetric brachial plexus palsy 617
  paediatric assessment 538
  paralytic, history 504
  shoulder, internal rotation 1227
  Volkmann's ischaemic *see* Volkmann ischaemic contracture
  see also specific types
contrecoup injury 478, 720
control group
  case–control study 41–2
  randomized trials 40
contusions
  bone, MRI 163
  pelvis, hip and thigh region 773, 774
conus medullaris 66, 67
conus medullaris syndrome 443
cool ischaemia time 1317
Copeland test 830
coracoacromial arch 1208
coracoacromial ligament 52, 1208
  detachment, rotator cuff tear repair 1212
  injuries 286
  repair 1213
  in total shoulder replacement 1226
coracoclavicular (CC) ligament 285, 288

coracohumeral ligament 1215
coracoid 52
coracoid process 1208
Cormet hip resurfacing 191
corner fractures, non-accidental injuries 501
corns
  hard 1458
  soft 1458
  treatment 1458
coronary ligament sprain 26
coronoid fractures 1559
corporate databanks 1537
correlations 44, 45
corrosion, implants 1115–16
  types 1115–16
'cortical ring sign' 1354, 1356
corticospinal tracts 66–7
corticosteroid(s)
  anterior tarsal tunnel syndrome 1505
  bone metabolism control 98
  cubital tunnel syndrome 1405
  Duchenne muscular dystrophy 612
  entrapment of superficial peroneal nerve 1506
  interdigital plantar (Morton's) neuroma 1501
  juvenile idiopathic arthritis 594
  lateral epicondylitis 1394
  olecranon bursitis 1389
  rheumatoid arthritis 1087
  rotator cuff tears 1211
  trigger finger 1277
  see also glucocorticoid(s); specific corticosteroids
cortisol 704
cortisone, osteoporosis associated 1029, 1030
Cotton fractures 391
Cotton osteotomy 1423, 1465
Coughlin's classification 1490, 1491
coup injury 478, 720
COX-1 128
COX-2 128
COX-3 128
coxa anteverta 419
coxa retroverta 419
coxa vara 651–2
  developmental 651–2
  Paget disease 1130
Craig's test 21
cranial fossa
  fractures 478
  middle, fractures 478
cranial nerve palsies, occipital condyle fractures 446
craniocervical junction 446
craniofacial disjunctions (Le Fort III fractures) 474
craniosynostosis 553
craniovertebral dissociations (occipitocervical dislocation) 447
crank-shaft phenomenon 635
Craven, Harry 1099
Crawford classification, congenital pseudarthrosis of tibia 675
C-reactive protein (CRP) 147
  acute haematogenous osteomyelitis in children 584, 585
  acute osteomyelitis 221–2
  juvenile idiopathic arthritis 593
  pyogenic spinal infections 984
  before revision hip arthroplasty 1161
  before revision knee arthroplasty 1200
  septic arthritis in children 579, 580, 581
creatine
  impact on muscle and exercise performance 706–7
  muscle levels 707
creatine kinase 699, 702, 706
creatine phosphate (CP) 702, 706
creep, definition 181
crescent fractures, pelvis 432
  treatment 432
crescentic osteotomy 1439
criterion validity 39
critical closing pressure theory 506
critical damping 185
critical reflection, autonomous patient 1532
cross-finger flap, traumatic fingertip amputations 1290

'crossing sign' 794
crossover second toe 1455–6
'crossover' sign 35
cross-sectional surveys 42
crouch gait 567
cruciate anastomosis 71
cruciate ligaments see anterior cruciate ligament (ACL); posterior cruciate ligament (PCL)
crush injuries, tibial/fibular shaft fractures 377
crush syndrome 278
  pathophysiology 508
crystal arthritis 1091–2
crystalloids administration, polytrauma 237
C-spine see cervical spine
C-Stem 1138, 1139
CT see computed tomography (CT)
cubital tunnel 1384
  anatomy 1384, 1397
  decompression (in situ) 1405–6, 1407
  pressure 1398
  volume changes in flexion/extension 1398
cubital tunnel retinaculum 1398
cubital tunnel syndrome 1384, 1397–409
  acute 1397
  basic science/anatomy 1397–8
  biomechanics and 1398
  chronic 1397
  classification 1397
  differential diagnosis 1399
  historical aspects 1397
  history-taking 1398
  intermediate lesions 1401
  investigations 1399–400
  management 1398–400
  non-operative treatment 1403–5
    goals 1403
  pathogenesis 1398
  physical examination 1398–9
  physical therapy 1405
  physiological 1397
  provocation tests 1399
  scoring for symptoms 1402, 1403
  staging and grading 1400–2, 1404
  subacute 1397
  surgical treatment 1405–8
    anterior intramuscular transposition 1407–8
    anterior subcutaneous transposition 1407
    anterior submuscular transposition 1408, 1409
    anterior transposition 1407–8
    endoscopic release 1408
    failed/failure rates 1408–9
    fallback procedure after failures 1409
    in situ decompression 1405–6, 1407
    medial epicondylectomy 1406–7
  treatment 1402–9
cubitus valgus 489
cubitus varus 489
cuboid 77, 403
  fractures 405
  nutcracker fracture 404, 405
culture (organisms), chronic osteomyelitis diagnosis 223
cumulative incidence 37
cuneiform bones 77, 78, 403
  first metatarsal bone joint, arthrodesis 1439
  fractures 405
  injuries 843
curare 700
curly toes 1457–8
customized vascular bone replacements, endocultivation 1527–8, 1529
cutaneous nerves
  of arm 62
  of forearm 62, 1384
  of leg 77
  see also lateral femoral cutaneous nerve
cutting cone 88, 519
CyberKnife stereotactic surgery 1068
cyclo-oxygenase (COX) 128
cyclosporine, graft rejection reduction (animals) 149
cyst(s)

aneurysmal bone see aneurysmal bone cyst (ABC)
Baker's 22, 162
epidermal inclusion 1374
ganglion see ganglion/ganglion cysts
intraspinal, low back pain 979
lumbar spine 979
meniscus 786
mucous see mucous cysts
occult dorsal ganglion 762
perimeniscal 786
popliteal 22, 162
simple bone 887–8
cystogram 430
cytochrome P450 oxidoreductase 545
cytokines 147, 1086
  anti-inflammatory 1088
  inhibition, rheumatoid arthritis therapy 1088
  juvenile idiopathic arthritis pathogenesis 590
  osteoarthritis pathophysiology 1080–1
  produced by T cells 1085–6
  proinflammatory
    inhibition, rheumatoid arthritis therapy 1088
    rheumatoid arthritis 1085–6, 1088, 1128
  in synovial joints 1078
  rheumatoid arthritis pathophysiology 1085–6, 1128
cytotoxic drugs 878

dabigatran 131, 132
dactylitis, syphilitic 224
damage control orthopaedic (DCO) concept 239, 240
'damage control resuscitation' 237, 238
Dameron and Rockwood classification 1556
damping, critical 185
'dancer's fracture' 846, 847
Danis, Robert 6
Danis–Weber classification, ankle fractures 387–8, 389
Darrach procedure 1372
Darrach retractor 1229
data, types 43
databanks 1536–7
Davy, Sir Humphry 4
de Quervain's tenosynovitis
  clinical features 760
  sports injuries causing 760
  trapeziometacarpal joint osteoarthritis vs 1335–6
  treatment 760
'dead arm syndrome' 730
deafness 478
debridement
  acute osteomyelitis 222
  ankle arthritis 1487
  chronic osteomyelitis 222, 223
  open injuries of limbs 253–5, 256
  principles 253–5
decision-making, clinical 1546
decision-making capacity 1532, 1533, 1540
decompression surgery
  achondroplasia 557
  cubital tunnel syndrome 1405–6, 1407
  degenerative disc disease 1002
  degenerative spondylolisthesis 1056
  isthmic spondylolisthesis 1052
  osteoporotic spines 1041
  upper limb amputations (traumatic) 1318
decorin 83, 101
deep anterior oblique ligament (dAOL) 1334
deep femoral artery 75
deep peroneal nerve 76, 79, 1500
  compression 1505–6
deep tendon reflexes, upper limb 9
deep vein thrombosis (DVT)
  arthroscopy complication 718
  management, thrombolysis 132
  pelvic fracture patients 435
  prophylaxis see thromboprophylaxis
  reduction, regional anaesthesia for hip arthroplasty 1123–4, 1126
  risk, cast immobilization of fractures 261

β-defensins 471, 472
deflazacort therapy, Duchenne muscular dystrophy 612
deformity
  bone tumour presenting with 884
  fracture malunion 527
  see also specific deformities/joints
degenerative disc disease 993–1006
  advanced 1000–1
  aetiology 994
  anatomy 994
  cervical 997, 999
  definition 993–4
  future potential therapy 1003, 1005
  lumbar 996–7, 997–8
  neck/back pain 1002
  neurological symptoms 1002–3
  pathophysiology 995
  repetitive injury 994
  spondylolisthesis and 1050, 1051, 1052
  stabilization phase 1000–1
  symptomatic, treatment 1002–3
  temporary dysfunction stage 995, 1002
  thoracic 997
  treatment 1001–3
  unstable phase 995–1000
  see also intervertebral disc
degenerative spine disease 993
  degenerative spondylolisthesis 1054–6
  disc disease see degenerative disc disease
  symptoms and treatment 1002–3
degloving injuries, pelvic fractures with 426
degree of anisotropy (DA) 1026
dehydroepiandrosterone (DHEA), use by athletes 707
Dejerine–Sottas syndrome 615
delamination 87
delayed onset of muscle soreness (DOMS) 701, 704
Delpech, Jacques-Malthieu 4
delteparin 131
deltoid atrophy 731
deltoid ligament (ankle)
  disruption, malleolar fractures 387, 390
  sprains 843
deltoid muscle 1208
  atrophy 731
  detachment, rotator cuff repair complication 1214
  repair, in rotator cuff repair 1213, 1214
  splitting 1207, 1212, 1214
  reverse shoulder arthroplasty 1230
deltopectoral approach 1226
deltopectoral interval 1230, 1231
denaturing high-performance liquid chromatography (DHPLC) 142
dendritic cells 1068
Denis classification
  sacral fractures 463, 464
  thoracolumbar spine injuries 460, 1556
Denis spine columns 65, 453, 460
Denosumab 1025
dental infections, hip arthroplasty and 1124–5
dental occlusion
  malocclusion, in mandibular fractures 470
  reduction/fixation of midfacial/mandibular fractures 476
depolarization
  motor neurone 109, 213, 700
  myofibres 109
  unmyelinated vs myelinated fibres 1303
dermatomes
  hand 16
  L3 773
  lower limb 773
dermofasciectomy, Dupuytren's contracture 1329
Desault bandage 486
descending geniculate artery 77
descending tracts, spinal cord 66, 67
descriptive statistics 43–4
desmoid-type fibromatoses 918

development
  embryological see embryological development
  post-natal
    hip 645
    spinal column 627–8
developmental coxa vara 651–2
developmental disorders of bone 541–58
  classification 549, 570, 571
  diagnostic considerations 549–56
  embryological see embryological development
  epidemiology 541–2
  management 556–8
  molecular pathogenesis 544–9
  physical examination 550–1, 552–3
  see also skeletal dysplasia; specific disorders
developmental dysplasia of hip (DDH) 642–50
  epidemiology 646
  hip arthroplasty and 1135, 1253
  incidence 642
  natural history 647
  neglected DDH in older childhood 649–50
  pathoanatomy 646
  physical examination 643, 646
  risk factors 643, 646
  screening/diagnosis 539, 642–5, 646–7
    clinical screening 643
    radiography 645
    ultrasound 643–4
  treatment 647–9
    newborn 647–8
    up to 6 months of age 648
    patients aged 6-18 months 648–9
    patients older than 18 months 649
    postoperative immobilization 649
dexamethasone 129, 1078
dextropropoxyphene 127
diabetes mellitus
  amputations 959
  Charcot neuroarthropathy 1492–3
  hip arthroplasty and 1125
  prevalence 1125
diabetic foot 1466–70
  assessment 1467–8
  classifications 1467
  clinical presentation 1467
  conservative treatment 1469
  joint deformity 1468
  management strategy 1470
  pathogenesis 1466
  physical examination 1468–9
  predictive factors for limb salvage 1470
  surgical treatment 1469–70
diabetic nephropathy 1125
diagnostic tests 38
  'gold standard' 38
dial test 24, 813
diamorphine (heroin) 127
diaphyseal aclasia 895, 1379
diaphysis
  bone tumours located in 886
  endochondral ossification in 89
  fractures 483
  pathological fractures, operative treatment 935, 936
  see also individual bone shafts
Dias–Tachdjian classification, ankle fractures 498
diastrophic dysplasia (DTD) 549
dichotomous data 43
diet
  carbohydrate intake 706
  high-fat 706
  vegetarian 706, 707–8
diffuse-type giant cell tumour (DTGCT) see pigmented villonodular synovitis (PVNS)
1,25-dihydroxyvitamin D 98
dinner fork-type deformity, wrist 261, 328
diplopia 469
disability 202, 203
  assessment in trauma 236
disc see intervertebral disc
discectomy
  cervical spine 1003, 1004
  degenerative disc disease 1002
  lumbar spine 1003

discitis
  lumbar 978
  postoperative 985
disclosure, informed consent 1540
discogenic pain 978, 1002
disease-modifying anti-rheumatic drugs (DMARDs) 1086, 1088
disimpaction forceps 477
dislocated hip see hip dislocations
dislocations
  in children see children
  nerve injuries in 1306
  see also specific joints
displacement
  angular see angular displacement
  linear see linear displacement
disputes, return to work following work-related injuries 1543
distal amputations, diabetic foot 1470
distal femoral anatomy registration, in CAOS 1518
distal femoral osteotomy (DFO) 1264, 1265
  extension osteotomy, cerebral palsy 604
distal femur see femur, distal
distal interphalangeal (DIP) joint
  anatomy 1346
  arthrodesis 1347
  arthroplasty 1347
  boutonnière deformity 1282
  carpometacarpal joint 1333
  Dupuytren's contracture 1327
  extensor tendon injuries 1281
  jersey finger 1279
  lesser toes 1450
    claw toe 1453
    hammer toe 1451
    plantarflexion deformity (mallet toe) 1454
  mallet finger 1281
  mucous cyst excision 1347
  osteoarthritis 1346–7
  psoriatic arthropathy 1496
  zone II injuries 1280
distal metatarsal articular angle (DMAA) 1435, 1436
distal metatarsal osteotomy 1437–8
distal radial ulnar joint (DRUJ) 1365–72
  anatomy 1365–6
  bony structures 1365
  chronic dysfunction 1367
  dislocation 1366
    children 493
  Galeazzi fracture see Galeazzi fracture
  imaging 1367–8
  injuries
    acute, management 1368–9
    causes/types 1366
    chronic with osteoarthritis 1371
    diagnosis 1366–8
    management 1368–71
  instability 1387
    chronic, management 1369–70
    chronic without osteoarthritis 1369–70
    classification 1366
    diagnosis 1366–8
    multidirectional 1366
    testing 14, 759, 1367
    traumatic 1366, 1368
  interosseous membrane (IOM) 1365, 1366
  osteoarthritis 1367, 1371
  reconstruction 1369–70
  'static'/'dynamic' stabilizers 1365
  testing 759, 1367
  volar, subluxation 1367, 1368
  see also triangular fibrocartilage complex (TFCC)
distal tarsal tunnel syndrome 1502
distal tibial (supramalleolar) derotational osteotomy, cerebral palsy 605
distal tibiofibular syndesmosis, testing 30
distraction arthrodesis, calcaneocuboid joint 1423
distraction arthroplasty
  after trapeziectomy 1339
  ankle see under ankle
distraction instrumentation, lumbar spine, flat back syndrome and 1018, 1019

distraction osteogenesis
  congenital pseudarthrosis of tibia 676–7
  infected fracture non-union 524
  limb reconstruction 946
DNA (deoxyribonucleic acid) 139–40
  heteroduplex 141
  ligation 141
  probes 143
  replication 139, 140
  structure 139, 140
DNA testing kits, developmental disorders of bone 554, 556
'docking technique', ulnar collateral ligament repair 753
documentation, informed consent 1540
'doping', in sports 707
Doppler flowmetry, compartment syndrome 510
Doppler pressure, amputations and 958
Doppler ultrasonography, amputation outcome 958
Dorr classification 1136
dorsal impingement syndrome, wrist 762
dorsal intercalated segment instability (DISI) 1354, 1355, 1356
dorsal perilunate dislocation 1360–1
dorsal perilunate fracture dislocation 1361
dorsal root ganglion 997, 999
  neuron, cultured 1303
dorsalis pedis artery 79–80
dorsiflexion phalangeal osteotomy, hallux rigidus 1490
dorsoradial ligament (DRL) 1334
double blinded trials 40
'double crush' nerve disorder, tarsal tunnel syndrome 1503
Down syndrome 152
draftsman's elbow see olecranon bursitis
drainage
  acute haematogenous osteomyelitis 586
  septic arthritis 581
dressings
  diabetic foot wounds 1469
  Dupuytren's contracture surgery 1329, 1330
  replantation of/in upper limb 1320
drop-foot gait 567
drug(s)
  acetylcholinesterase inhibitors 700
  fracture healing affected by 518
  illegal use in sports 707
  interactions, anticoagulants 131–2
  resistance, of tumours to chemotherapy 879
  secondary osteoporosis due to 1029, 1030
  see also individual drugs/drug groups
drug addiction, opioids, pain in 128
dry gangrene, diabetic foot 1467, 1468
dual-action bone agent (DABA) 134
Duchenne muscular dystrophy (DMD) 610–12, 1477
  clinical picture 611, 1477
  incidence 1477
  management 612, 1477
Duchenne sign 1399
ductile fracture (of material) 183
Duke of Edinburgh sling 1396
Duncan Ely test (rectus femoris) 20, 600
duopatellar knee prosthesis 1173–4
Dupuytren's contracture 1324–32, 1374
  anatomy 1324–5
  clinical presentation 1325–6
  epidemiology 1324
  palmar, palmodigital and digital regions 1324–5
  pathogenesis 1325, 1326
  postoperative management/rehabilitation 1330
  recurrence 1330
  surgical treatment 1327–9
    complications 1330
    dermofasciectomy and skin graft 1329
    fasciectomy 1328–9
    fasciotomy 1328
    indications 1327

PIP joint flexion contracture release 1329–30
  segmental aponeurectomy 1328
  treatment 1326–7
Dupuytren's diathesis 1324, 1326
Dupuytren's disease 918, 1374
  see also Dupuytren's contracture
dural stretch test (slump test) 34
Duran–Houser method 1297
dynamic compression plate (DCP) 273
dynamic condylar screw (DCS), distal femoral fractures 360
dynamic hip screw 344, 348
dynamic parameters
  angular motion 177
  translational motion 176
dynamic reference base (DRB), in CAOS 1512, 1513
dynamic traction splint, phalangeal fractures 1286
dynamics 184–5
  control 185
  definition 176
dynamometers
  hand-held, muscle strength testing 212, 213
  isokinetic, muscle strength testing 212, 213
dysaesthesia 1304
dysostoses 541, 571
  see also developmental disorders of bone
dysostosis multiplex 549
dyspareunia, pelvic fracture complication 435
dysprosium (Dy165) 1087
dystonia 568
dystrophinopathies 610–12

E (energy) 179
E (Young's modulus) see Young's modulus (E)
early total care (ETC) approach 239–40, 240–1
East Baltimore lift 337
eating disorders, female athletes 708
Eaton and Glickel staging, trapeziometacarpal joint osteoarthritis 1334–5, 1337
eccentric contraction 109, 701, 955
Echinococcus granulosus 986
ectoderm 51
effect size 42
Effendi and Francis classification 452, 1556
Ehlers–Danlos syndrome 92
Eichenholz classification 1493
eicosanoids, biosynthetic pathway 128
  inhibition by glucocorticoids 129
  inhibition by NSAIDs 128
'8' plates, leg length discrepancy 681
elastic fibres, age-related changes 121
elastic material 179
elastic stable intramedullary nailing (ESIN)
  femoral shaft fractures 494
  paediatric fractures 486
elasticity 178–80
  modulus of, PMMA 1120
elbow 1382–418
  anatomy 57, 316, 1382–6
    blood supply 58
    capsulo-ligamentous units 1382–3
    dynamic stabilizing factors 1383–4, 1388
    muscles 57–8, 1383–4
    nerves 57–8, 1384–6
    osteoarticular 1382
    secondary stabilizer 1387
    static stabilizing factors 1382–3
  angular relationships 316
  anterior capsule 1382–3
  anterior structures, examination 12
  arthrodesis 1268, 1273
  arthroplasty
    biological resurfacing interposition 1256
    endoprosthesis design 1387
    indications 1256
    longevity and survival 1256
    young patients 1256–7
  arthroscopy see arthroscopy
  axis of rotation 57

elbow – continued
  biomechanics 1383, 1386–8
    coronoid fractures 1387
    joint forces 1388
    lateral collateral ligament 1388
    medial collateral ligament 1387
    muscles 1388
    olecranon 1387
    pronation–supination 1387
    radial head 1387
  carrying angle 57, 311, 1400
  clinical examination 11–13, 1398–9
    inspection 11
    movement 12
    palpation 11–12
    special tests 13
  disarticulation 963
  dislocation 316–18
    children 490
    clinical examination 317
    mechanism of injury 317, 1388
    posterior 317
    posterior rotatory instability after 754
    radiography 317
    treatment 317
  extension 12, 1386–7
    cubital tunnel volume 1398
  extraneural pressure 1398
  flexion 12, 173, 174, 1386–7
    axis, variation 1387
    cubital tunnel volume 1398
    effect on valgus laxity 1387
    intraneural pressure increase 1398
  flexion test 1393, 1399
  flexion–extension 1386–7, 1388
    normal range 1386
  fracture dislocations 317–18
    complications 318
  fractures around 1558
    condylar fractures 1559
    coronoid fractures 1387
    intercondylar fractures 1558
    paediatric 487–8, 488–90
    supracondylar fractures 1558
    see also humerus, distal; radial head, fractures
  fractures at, olecranon 318–19, 1559
    see also olecranon, fractures
  functions 1382
  golfer's see medial epicondylitis
  hemiarthroplasty 1256
  hyperextension 738
  instability
    children 490
    coronoid fractures 1387
    medial epicondylitis 1391
    posterolateral see elbow, posterolateral rotatory instability
    testing 13
  intercondylar fractures 1558
  intraneural pressure 1398
  lateral aspects, examination 11
  ligaments 57, 1383
  locking 11
  loose bodies 11, 317, 716, 752, 753, 754, 1392
  medial aspects, examination 12
  nerves around 1384–6
  nursemaid's 491
  olecranon bursitis see olecranon bursitis
  orthoses 968
  ossification centres around 487, 488
  pain
    cubital tunnel syndrome 1398
    lateral epicondylitis 750, 1391
    medial epicondylitis 751, 1392
    osteochondritis dissecans 753–4
    posterolateral plica 1391
  posterior capsule 1383
  posterior structures, examination 12
  posterolateral rotatory instability (PLRI) 754–5, 1392
    clinical features 754–5
    lateral pivot-shift test 13, 755
    lateral UCL insufficiency 1383
    mechanism of injury and stages 754
    treatment 755
  pressure provocation test 1399
  pronation–supination 1387
    test 13

provocation tests 12–13
pulled 491
range of movement 1386–7
  cubital tunnel volume and 1398
replacement (total) 313
  materials used for 192
resurfacing 1256
screw displacement axis (SDA) 1387, 1388
sports injuries see sports injuries; specific injuries
stiffness, distal humerus fractures in children 489
supracondylar fractures 1558
surgical approaches 60–1
  anterolateral (Henry's) 60, 61
  medial 60
  posterior 60
  posterolateral (Kocher's) 60–1
tennis see lateral epicondylitis
'terrible triad' 317, 1387
valgus extension overload syndrome 751
valgus laxity, effect of flexion/pronation on 1387
valgus stress 751, 1387
valgus testing 13
varus testing 13
elderly patients
  femoral neck fractures 340, 342
  pelvic fractures 426
electrodiagnostic testing, cubital tunnel syndrome 1399–400
electrolyte balance, athletes 706
electromagnetic communication 1514, 1515
electromyography (EMG) 213–14
  anterior tarsal tunnel syndrome 1505
  clinical and biofeedback 214
  cubital tunnel syndrome 1400
  entrapment of superficial peroneal nerve 1506
  onset and offset 214
  tarsal tunnel syndrome 1503, 1505
electrons, radiotherapy 875
Ellis buttress plate 330
Ellis–van Creveld syndrome 550
Elson's test 17
Ely's test 20
embryo cloning 143, 144
embryological development 51–2
  myelomeningocele development 608
  skeletal system 542–4
    hip 645
    vertebral column 628–9
embryonic stem cells, tissue engineering 1526
emergency surgery, warfarin use and 131
Emery–Dreifuss muscular dystrophy 612
emotional exhaustion, as burnout manifestation 1551
employees' perspective, return to work 1543
employers' perspective, return to work 1543
'empty can' test 10
enchondroma 896–8
  atypical 897
  biopsy 897
  clinical features 897
  hand 1378
  pathology/histology 897–8, 899
  radiography 886, 897, 898, 899
enchondromatosis 896
  Maffucci's syndrome 546, 575, 896, 1378
  multiple 575, 896
endochondral ossification 89–91, 101, 543, 544
  in diaphysis and epiphysis 89
  in growth plate 89–91
endocrine abnormalities, SCFE association 657
endocultivation 1527–8, 1529
Endo-Klinik classification, revision hip surgery 1156
endomysium 698, 699
endoneurium 1303
endoprostheses
  aseptic loosening 943
  design 943

failure/fracture 943
fixation 943
long-term complications 951
pathological fractures treatment 933–4
endoprosthetic reconstruction 942–3
  in children 950, 951
  distal femur 948
  hip, complications 943
  pelvis 947
endoscopic release, ulnar nerve, in cubital tunnel syndrome 1408
endosteal scalloping 867, 897
endosteum 85, 87–8
  formation, during remodelling 88
endotenon 111, 112
endothelin 928
endurance exercise 704
  energetics 703
endurance training 698, 703
  vegetarian diets and 707
energy 176, 178
  balance in athletes, nutrition and 705
  demands/requirements
    by age/sex 709
    athletes 706
  for high-intensity exercise 703
  intake by female athletes 708
  metabolism 702–3
    hormones affecting 704
  sources 702–3, 706
  transmitted by injury mechanism 248
engineering strain 178
engineering stress 178
Enneking and Dunham classification, pelvic resection 946
Enneking system 940
  benign bone tumours 870
  malignant bone tumours 870
  spinal tumours 1060
enoxaparin 131, 132
enteropathic arthropathies 1090
enthesis-related arthritis (ERA) 590, 593
enthesopathy 1089
entrapment neuropathies see nerve compression syndromes
environment control, primary survey in trauma 236–7
enzyme(s)
  defects, skeletal dysplasias 549, 574
  extracellular matrix (ECM) 102
  see also individual enzymes
enzyme-linked immunosorbent assay (ELISA), spinal tuberculosis 988
eosinophilic granuloma (EG) 890–1, 1062
eosinophils 145
epicondylitis 1389
  lateral see lateral epicondylitis
  medial see medial epicondylitis
epidemiology 36–48
  definition 36, 37
  importance 36
  terminology 37–9
epidermal inclusion cyst 1374
epidural abscess, spine 983
epidural anaesthesia, in hip arthroplasty 1124, 1126
epimysium 698
epinephrine 704, 713
  infusion in hip arthroplasty 1124
epiphyseal axis angle 496
epiphyseal collapse, Perthes disease 654, 655
epiphyseal distraction, limb reconstruction 950
epiphyseal dysplasia, multiple (MED) 572–3, 653
epiphyseal extrusion, Perthes disease 654, 655
epiphyseal stapling, leg length discrepancy 681
epiphyses 88
  bone tumours located in 886
  endochondral ossification in 89
  femoral see femoral epiphysis
  fractures 483–5
    distal femur 495, 496
    proximal tibia 496
  loosening, Salt-Harris I fracture 483
  separation of distal femur 495

epiphysiodesis
  Blount disease 671
  genu varum/valgum 670
  leg length discrepancy 681
epitenon 111, 112
epithelioid sarcoma, hand 1377
epitopes
  proteoglycans/collagen, antibodies to 1082
  shared 1084
eponychia 1288, 1310, 1311
Epstein classification, anterior hip dislocations 338, 339
equilibrium (mechanics) 177–8, 184
equinovalgus deformity, in cerebral palsy, management 605, 1476
equinovarus deformity see talipes equinovarus
equinus deformity see talipes equinus
Erb palsy 617
Erb–Duchenne palsy 54, 615, 616
erectile dysfunction, pelvic fracture complication 435
ergogenic aids 706–7
ergonomic measures
  cubital tunnel syndrome 1404
  lateral/medial epicondylitis 1394
error, in experimental studies 42
  type I (alpha) 42
  type II (beta) 42
erysipelas 220
  antibiotic treatment 220
erythrocyte sedimentation rate (ESR)
  juvenile idiopathic arthritis 591, 593
  pyogenic spinal infections 983–4
  before revision hip arthroplasty 1161
  before revision knee arthroplasty 1200
  septic arthritis in children 579, 580, 581
  spinal tuberculosis 988
erythropoietin, recombinant, use by athletes 707
Essex-Lopresti classification, calcaneal fractures 399–400
Essex-Lopresti lesion 319, 320
Essex-Lopresti technique, calcaneal fracture treatment 401
ET-1 928
etanercept therapy, juvenile idiopathic arthritis 594
ethics see medical ethics
Evans classification, intertrochanteric fractures 347, 1565
Evan's lateral column lengthening 1423, 1465
Evans procedure, equinovalgus deformity treatment 1476
evidence, levels 46–7
evidence-based medicine (EBM) 46–7, 1545–8
  definition 46, 1547–8
  evidence levels 46–7
  levels of evidence 1547–8
  origin of 36–7
  steps 1547
Ewing's sarcoma 883, 902–4
  bone scintigraphy 868
  chemotherapy 880
  epidemiology 884, 902
  genetic translocations 904
  hand 1380
  histology 903–4
  pathology/macroscopic appearance 903
  PNET variant 902, 903
  prognosis 904
  radiography 867, 886, 903
  radiotherapy 941
  sites/location 902
  spine 1063
  tumours mimicking 903
EWS gene 904
examination techniques see clinical examination
examination under anaesthesia (EUA), glenohumeral instability 1217
exercise performance 703–5
  cardiopulmonary system 703–4
  hormones and effects on muscle 704
  muscle damage/disuse 704–5
exercise physiology 697–705
  energy metabolism 702–3
  skeletal muscle 697–702

exercise programmes
　adult scoliosis 1011
　degenerative disc disease 1002
　rotator cuff tear management 1211
exercise training 703
Exeter femoral head 190
Exeter stem 190, 1138, 1143, 1161
　development 1100
exhaustion, as burnout manifestation 1551
exostosis 895
　calcaneal 832
　hand 1379
　multiple hereditary 574–5
experimental study 40
experimental study designs 40–2
　observational 40, 41–2
　RCTs as gold standard 40–1
exposure, primary survey in trauma 236–7
EXT1 gene mutations 574, 575
extended oligoarticular juvenile idiopathic arthritis 590, 591
extensor carpi radialis brevis (ECRB)
　anatomy 1384
　chronic scapholunate dissection treatment 1358
　degenerative tendinopathy 1390
　extension, epicondylitis pathogenesis 1390, 1391
　intersection syndrome 761
　in lateral epicondylitis 1390, 1391
　　open surgical technique 1396
　tenderness 11
　vulnerability to attrition, theory 1390
extensor carpi radialis longus (ECRL)
　anatomy 1384
　intersection syndrome 761
　in lateral epicondylitis surgery 1396
extensor carpi ulnaris (ECU) 60, 1365
　acute DRUJ injury management 1368
　anatomy 1365, 1366
　subluxation 761
　tendinitis 761, 1367
　tendon graft, in chronic DRUJ injury 1370
extensor digitorum avulsion 1562
extensor digitorum brevis (EDB) 78, 1450
extensor digitorum communis (EDC)
　anatomy 1298
　in lateral epicondylitis 1390, 1391
　mallet finger 1281
　testing 16
extensor digitorum longus (EDL) 1449–50
extensor hallucis longus (EHL) 79, 80
extensor lurch 31
extensor mechanism (knee) see under knee
extensor pollicis longus (EPL), testing 16
extensor retinaculum, DRUJ stabilization 1369, 1370
extensor tendons, fingers see finger(s)
external fixation
　congenital pseudarthrosis of tibia 676–7
　fractures see fracture fixation, external
　see also fixation
external fixators
　ankle distraction arthroplasty 1246
　for fractures 196, 255
　knee arthrodesis 1272
　in open injuries 255
　ring, for fractures 196
external iliac artery 75
external iliac vessels 428
external rotation lag test 10, 1209
external rotation stress test, syndesmotic ankle sprains 392–3
external rotation/recurvatum test, knee 24, 26
external validity 39
EXT genes 895
extracellular matrix (ECM) 82
　articular cartilage 101, 1077, 1078–9
　　age-related changes 1080
　bone 82, 83
　　bone resorption 87
　　formation/mineralization 86, 88–9, 543
　　secretion by osteoblasts 84, 86

composition 82, 83, 100, 1078
enzymes 102
intervertebral disc 106
ligaments and tendons 111, 113
　age-related changes 120–1
meniscus 103
nucleus pulposus 106
protein defects 548
extracompartmental sites 940
extracorporeal irradiation and reimplantation, autografts 946
extracorporeal shock wave therapy, lateral epicondylitis 1394
extrapolation, evidence-based medicine 1548
eyeball movement, examination in head injury 469
eyes
　examination in head injury 468
　screening for uveitis, juvenile idiopathic arthritis 591, 592

Fab domains, immunoglobulins 148
FABER position, septic arthritis of hip 225
FABER test 20–1
face trauma see head and face trauma
facet (apophyseal) joints
　anatomy 66
　capsule, low back pain generation 976
　hypertrophy 998, 999, 1003
　lumbar 975
　　low back pain 977
　orientation by spinal region 66
　pain 977, 1002
　separations/injuries, children 484
　subluxation 999–1000
facetectomy, medial 1003
facioscapulohumeral muscular dystrophy 612–13
factor VIII 1092
'fallen leaf' sign 887
falls
　distal femoral fractures 358
　distal humeral fractures 313
　distal radial ulnar joint injuries 1366
　distal radius fractures 327
　elbow dislocation 317, 1388
　femoral neck fractures 340
　femoral shaft fractures 353
　proximal humeral fractures 303
　radial and ulnar shaft fractures 324
　radial head fractures 319
　radial neck fractures, children 490
　tibial plafond fractures 382
　tibial plateau fractures 372
　wrist injuries 1355, 1360
false aneurysms, hand 1374
false negatives 38
false positives 38
familial syndromes, hypercalcaemia 93
fascia lata 773
fascicles 697, 1303
fasciectomy, Dupuytren's contracture 1328–9
fasciocutaneous flaps, open injuries of limbs 257
fasciodermal sling 1407
fasciotomy
　acute compartment syndrome 280, 504, 511
　chronic exertional compartment syndrome 826
　Dupuytren's contracture 1328
　intracompartmental pressure level indicating 280, 511
　leg 511
　needle, Dupuytren's contracture 1328
　stab incision, Dupuytren's contracture 1328
　upper limb amputations (traumatic) 1318
fat
　intramuscular, age-related changes 121
　MRI appearance 161, 166, 167
fat (dietary)
　intake and metabolism, female athletes 708
　metabolism 702–3, 706
　sources and intake 706
fat embolism, femoral shaft fractures 356

fat pad sign 487
'fat saturation', MRI 162–3
fatigue (materials) 183
　hip implants 1116
fatigue (muscle) 705
fatigue fracture
　femoral stem 1116, 1155
　pars interarticularis see pars interarticularis
　see also stress fractures
fatty acids 706
fee weights and springs, muscle strength testing 212, 213
feet see foot
Feiss line 30
felons 1310, 1311
felypressin 129
female athletes see women
femoral anteversion, assessment 537
　tibial torsion 674
femoral artery 71, 75
femoral component (hip replacement) 189–90
　Charnley Elite-Plus 1154, 1161
　failure, reconstruction after 1160
　materials for 189, 190
　modular 189
　osteopetrosis 1130
　see also femoral head (implants); femoral stem (implants)
femoral component (knee replacement) 1177
　computer-assisted navigation 1519
　removal in revision surgery 1201
　stem extensions 1202
　stems 1180
femoral cuts, computer-assisted navigation 1518–19
femoral deficiency, proximal focal 650–1
femoral epiphysis
　blood supply 653
　in Perthes disease 652, 653, 654, 655, 656
　see also slipped capital femoral epiphysis (SCFE)
femoral fractures
　blood loss 239
　diaphyseal 353
　　in children 494
　　see also femoral shaft fractures
　distal 358–62, 1566
　　in children 495
　　classification 358, 359
　　clinical/radiological evaluation 358
　　complications 361
　　epiphyseal separation 495
　　external fixation 361
　　implant choice 359–61
　　intra-articular 359
　　non-operative treatment 359
　　operative treatment 359–60
　　postoperative management 361
　　supracondylar 358
　　treatment 359–61
　　unicondylar fractures 361
　　vascular injury 358, 361
　extracapsular 346
　femoral head see femoral head, fractures
　femoral neck see femoral neck fractures
　greater trochanteric 349
　intertrochanteric (peritrochanteric) see intertrochanteric fractures
　intracondylar 359, 361
　leg shortening by 528
　lesser trochanteric 349
　malunion 527
　metaphyseal, non-union 523
　non-union, management 521, 523
　proximal
　　children 493
　　pathological, treatment 933–4
　　sports injuries 776
　　see also femoral neck fractures
　salvage 523
　shaft see femoral shaft fractures
　spiral, non-accidental injuries 501
　subtrochanteric see subtrochanteric fracture
　supracondylar 359, 361
femoral head
　anatomy 772, 1105–6

arthroplasty in younger patients 1254
blood supply 70, 75, 493
　age-dependent changes 70
　containment, Perthes disease treatment 655–6
　deformity, Perthes disease 652, 653, 654
　fractures 1564
　　type V posterior fracture dislocation with 337–8
　　injuries, with anterior hip dislocation 339
　osteonecrosis 97
　preparation for hip arthroplasty 1140, 1142
　prosthetic replacement see femoral head (implants)
　subluxation, in acetabular fractures 423
　tip (implant)–apex distance 348
femoral head (implants) 189
　ceramic 1119, 1120
　Charnley's prostheses 1098, 1099
　diameter and designs 190
　history 1098
　materials used for 189, 190
　mechanical testing 198, 199
　metastatic tumours 935
　size 190, 1100, 1109, 1117
　　historical aspects 1100
　　jumping distance and 1108
　　larger heads, development/use 1101, 1110, 1117, 1127
　stripe wear 1120
　wear 1120
　see also femoral component (hip replacement); femoral stem (implants)
femoral head coverage (FHC) 644
femoral head–neck offset 1111
femoral head–neck ratio, hip arthroplasty 1108–9
femoral neck
　anatomy 1105
　anteversion 74, 1105, 1106
　Craig's test 21
　shaft angle 74, 1105, 1106
　trabecular structure 1106
femoral neck fractures 340–5, 1564
　avascular necrosis see osteonecrosis
　basicervical 341
　classification 341–2
　clinical evaluation 340–1
　complications 342, 344–5
　displaced, treatment 342
　elderly patients 340, 342
　fatigue/stress 345
　impacted/non-displaced, treatment 342
　insufficiency, bone scan 157
　internal fixation failure 345
　mechanisms of injury 340
　non-union 344
　pathological 342, 934, 935
　with posterior hip dislocation 338
　prevalence and age groups 340
　radiography 341
　in resurfacing hip arthroplasty 1156
　shaft fractures with 355–6
　stress fractures 345, 777, 1565
　subcapital 341, 342
　transcervical 341
　treatment 342–4
　　closed/open reduction 342
　　fixation 343
　　in situ screw fixation 342
　　operative treatment principles 342–3
　　prosthetic replacement 343
　　results/outcome 344
　young patients 340, 342
femoral neck–shaft angle 74, 1105, 1106
femoral nerve 71, 79, 429
　anatomy 74
　palsy, pelvic fractures and 435
femoral neurovascular structures 773
femoral ossification centre, DDH assessment 647
femoral osteotomy
　proximal 652, 1254
　　slipped capital femoral epiphysis 659
　varus derotational see femoral varus derotational osteotomy

femoral registration, in CAOS
    total hip replacement 1521
    total knee replacement 1518
'femoral roll-back' 187, 1179
femoral shaft fractures 353–7, 1105,
        1566
    in children 494
        incidence 482
    classification 353–4
    clinical/radiological evaluation 353
    complications 356
    femoral neck fractures with 355–6
    floating knee with 356
    non-union 356
    open 356
    in polytrauma 355
    stress fractures 777
    treatment 354–5, 494
        bridge plating 273
        children 494
        external fixation 274, 355
        implant choice 354–5
        intramedullary nailing 275,
            354–5
        non-operative 354
        operative, principles 354
        plate fixation 355
femoral stem (implants) 189–90,
        1138–9
    aseptic loosening and 1154
    bone preparation techniques 1140
    cemented arthroplasty 1138–9
        removal, in revision 1158
        revision, femoral reconstruction
            1160
    Charnley flatback 1099, 1138
    collars 1139
    composite beam 1138–9
    computer-assisted navigation 1522
    Corail 1141, 1143
    C-Stem 1138, 1139
    Exeter 1100, 1138, 1143, 1161
    extensions, revision arthroplasty
        1202
    failures, Capital Hip 1139, 1154
    fatigue fracture 1116, 1155
    fractures 1155
    Gruen zones 1140, 1141, 1154
    history 1099–100
    hydroxyapatite-coated 1121
    in knee replacement 1180
        revision arthroplasty 1202
    materials for 189, 190, 1155
    matt 1100
    mechanical testing 198, 199
    modifications 1139
    Morse 1155
    polished finish vs rough 1139
    porous-coated, revision 1161
    reaming for 1142
    roundback 1099, 1139
    taper 1099, 1100, 1116
    taper slip design 1138–9
    uncemented 1101, 1140
        outcomes 1143
        removal, in revision 1158
        revision 1161
    Vaquasheen 1099, 1100
    Wrightington School 1099, 1138
    Zweymuller-type 1141
    see also femoral component (hip
        replacement); femoral head
        (implants)
femoral stretch test 35
femoral triangle 773
    anatomy 71
femoral trochlear dysplasia 795 796
femoral varus derotational osteotomy
    cerebral palsy 603, 606
    Perthes disease 655
femoroacetabular impingement
        1110–11
    athletes 778
    cam 778, 1110, 1111
    pincer 778, 1111
femorotibial osteoarthritis 1196
femur
    adductor magnus attachment 962
    amputation 962
    anatomical and mechanical axes
        1261
    anatomy 73–4
    arthrodesis, pelvic reconstruction
        947

bone defects
    classification 1201
    impacting grafting, revision hip
        arthroplasty 1160
    management 1202
    revision knee arthroplasty 1201–2
deficiency, proximal focal 650–1
distal
    endoprosthetic reconstruction 943
    fractures see femoral fractures,
        distal
    reconstruction 947–8
    rotationplasty after resection 950
greater trochanter, fractures 349
head see femoral head
impaction bone grafting 1160–1
lengthening, after fractures 528
lesser trochanter, fractures 349
neck see femoral neck
in Paget disease 97
proximal
    anatomy 70
    cam impingement 1111
    focal deficiency 650–1
    fractures see femoral fractures,
        proximal
    metastases 925, 926
    osteolytic metastases 928
    reconstruction 947
reaming, uncemented arthroplasty
        1142
reconstruction 948
    cementless 1161
    revision hip arthroplasty 1160–1
    revision knee arthroplasty 1201–2
resurfacing 1118
rotation, assessment, paediatric 537
rotational deformity 527
shaft
    autograft, reconstruction 945
    fractures see femoral shaft
        fractures
shape, hip arthroplasty planning
        1136
shortening 18, 19
surgical approaches 75
tibial articular conformity, meniscus
        and 104
'true' shortening 18
fenbufen 129
fentanyl patches 127
Fernandez mechanism-based
    classification 329
fetal bone 89, 90
fever, spinal infections 983
FGF-2 (fibroblast growth factor 2) 143
FGF23 gene 546
FGFR3 (fibroblast growth factor
    receptor 3 gene) 546
    mutations 546, 554, 570
fibrillation, articular cartilage 1080
fibrillin 1 and 2 83
fibrin clot 103, 105, 113
    meniscal repairs 786
fibroblast(s)
    in annulus fibrosus 106
    in ligaments and tendons 111
fibroblast growth factor 2 (FGF-2) 143
fibroblast growth factor receptor 3 gene
    see FGFR3 (fibroblast growth factor
        receptor 3 gene)
fibroblast growth factors 546
fibroblastic tumours 916, 918
fibrocartilage 103
    MRI appearance 161, 168
    tears, MRI scan 171
fibrochondrocyte 103
fibrogenic tumours 883
fibrohistiocytic tumours 883, 916,
        918–19
fibromatoses 1326, 1327
    desmoid-type 918
    hand 918, 1374
    see also Dupuytren's contracture
    superficial 918
fibromodulin 101
fibronectin 83
fibroproliferative disease, Dupuytren's
    contracture 1325
fibrosis, after muscle injury 110
fibrous dysplasia 891
    monostotic/polyostotic 891
    pathology/histology 891, 892
    radiography 867, 891, 892

fibula
    anatomy 76, 377
    blood supply 377
    fractures
        in bimalleolar fractures 390
        comminuted, compartment
            syndrome and 279
        compartment syndrome 279
        Danis–Weber classification 387–8
        shaft see fibular shaft fractures
    lateral malleolus see lateral malleolus
    surgical approach to, lateral 80
    transection, for amputation 961
    vascularized grafts see vascularized
        fibular grafts
fibula osteotomy 521
fibular sesamoid 1442
    anatomy 1442, 1443
    fracture 1444
    in hallux valgus 1434
    see also sesamoid bones (foot)
fibular sesamoidectomy 1447
fibular shaft fractures 377–81
    classification 378
    complications 380
    isolated 380
    mechanism of injury 377
    radiography 378
    treatment 378–80
fibular tunnel, in common peroneal
    nerve entrapment 826–7
Fick equation 703
fiducial markers, in CAOS 1513–14,
        1515
Fielding and Hawkins classification
        1555
    atlantoaxial rotatory displacement
        449–50
Fielding classification, subtrochanteric
    fracture 350–1
fight bite injury 1313
fine needle aspiration cytology (FNAC)
        931
fine needle biopsy, tumours 887
finger(s)
    biomechanics 187
    contractures 1325–6
        Dupuytren's see Dupuytren's
            contracture
    degloving injury 1322
    epiphyseal plate fractures 1282
    extensor tendons
        anatomy 1298
        central slip rupture 1282
        hyperextension 1300
        injuries 1298–300
        injuries, management 1298–300
        normal 1299
        swan neck deformity 1283–4
        zone I injuries 1280–2, 1299–300
        zone II injuries 1282
        zones 1298, 1299
        see also boutonnière deformity
    flexor tendons 1292–8
        A1 pulley 1293, 1294
        A1 pulley, jersey finger repair
            1279, 1296
        A1 pulley, trigger finger 1277, 1278
        A2 pulley 1293, 1294, 1296
        A3, A4, A5 pulleys 1293, 1294,
            1296
        adhesion formation 1297–8
        anatomy 1293–4
        annular (A1-A5) pulleys 1293
        clinical examination 1294–5
        complications of injuries 1297–8
        cruciate (C1-C3) pulleys 1293
        healing 1294
        injuries 1277–80
        postoperative rehabilitation 1297
        pulley system 1293–4
        rupture after repair 1297
        surgical management of injuries
            1295–7
        suturing technique 1295–6
        zone I injuries (jersey) 762,
            1278–80, 1296
        zone II injuries 1280, 1295, 1297
        zones 1278, 1294
    fractures 766–7, 1561
        epiphyseal plate 1282
    infections 1310–13
        surgical incisions for 1313
        see also hand, infections

injuries 1277–91, 1294–300
    extensor tendons 1280–7,
        1298–300
    flexor tendons 1277–80, 1294–8
    jersey see jersey finger
    joint replacement 192–4
    joint stiffness 1298
    lacerations 1278–80
    mallet see mallet finger
    phalangeal fractures see phalangeal
        fractures
    proximal interphalangeal (PIP) joint
        injuries 1284–5
    replantation see replantation (upper
        limb)
    ring avulsion injuries 1321–2
    swan neck deformity 1283–4
    tendons, ultrasound assessment 159
    traumatic amputations, early
        management 1316
    see also fingertip; hand; thumb
'finger escape' sign 33
finger extension test (FET) 1356
'finger fatigue' test 33
fingertip
    anatomy 1287–8
    injuries 1287–90
        lacerations 1288
    pulp, subcutaneous abscess 1311
    traumatic amputation 1289
finite-element modelling 198
Finkelstein's test 14, 760
'first hit phenomenon' 240
First World War, orthopaedic surgery in
        4
fixation
    allografts 944
    arthrodesis
        ankle 1270
        knee 1272
        shoulder 1273
        wrist 1272
    autografts 945
    bones, in replantation of upper limb
        1319
    devices see fracture fixation devices
    external see external fixation
    fractures see fracture fixation
    of joint replacement implants 194
    in rheumatoid arthritis 1087
    open reduction and internal fixation,
        mallet finger 1281–2
    plate, allografts 944
    three-point principle 260, 261
fixators
    external see external fixators
    external ring, for fractures 196
flaps
    fasciocutaneous, open injuries of
        limbs 257
    medial myocutaneous 962
    open injuries of limbs 256–7
    osteochondral, femoral head
        osteonecrosis 97
    skin, in amputations 960
    traumatic fingertip amputations
        1289
    V-Y advancement, traumatic
        fingertip amputations 1289
flat back syndrome 1018–19
    after surgery 1018
    prevention 1018
flat foot 692–3, 1270
    adult-acquired (AAFF) 1489
    assessment 538, 539
    flexible 692–3
    infantile 691
    posterior tibial tendon dysfunction
        1421, 1422, 1423, 1462–3
    rigid 693
    see also pes planus
fleck sign 408
Flex Foot 964
flexibility, lower extremity, paediatric
    assessment 538
flexible flat foot 692–3
Flexicore device 197
flexion contractures
    forearm 17
    hip see hip, flexion contractures
    knee 610
    myelomeningocele 610
    proximal interphalangeal (PIP) joint
        1327, 1329–30

flexion–adduction test, hip 21
flexor carp radialis (FCR)
  in chronic scapholunate dissection treatment 1358
  in trapeziometacarpal osteoarthritis surgery 1337, 1338, 1339
flexor carpi ulnaris (FCU) 1383
  dynamic stabilizer, elbow 1388
flexor digitorum brevis (FDB) 1450
flexor digitorum longus (FDL) 1450
  transfer to navicular 1424
flexor digitorum profundus (FDP)
  anatomy 1293
  assessment, in lacerations 1278
  avulsion 762, 1279, 1562
  disruption/ruptures
    types I-III jersey finger 1279–80, 1296
    ultrasound scan 159
    zone II injuries 1280, 1296
  median nerve anatomy 1386
  testing 16, 1295
flexor digitorum superficialis (FDS) 505
  anatomy 1293, 1383
  assessment, in lacerations 1278
  middle phalanx fractures and 1287
  testing 16, 1295
  zone II injuries 1280, 1296
flexor hallucis brevis (FHB) 1442
  hallux valgus 1434, 1435
  sesamoid bone attachment 1442, 1443
flexor hallucis longus (FHL) muscle 839
flexor hallucis longus (FHL) tendon 839
  hallux valgus 1434, 1435
  stenosis 839–40
  tenosynovitis 1430
flexor pollicis longus (FPL) 1293
flexor retinaculum 1293
flexor tendons
  fingers see finger(s)
  grafting 1295, 1296, 1298
  hand see hand
flexor tenosynovitis, suppurative 1310, 1312–13
floating shoulder 289, 295
flow (mechanics) 180–1
  resistance (viscosity) 180
fluid
  administration
    crystalloids vs colloids, in trauma 237
    hypovolaemic shock 236
    in polytrauma 237
    pre-hospital care in trauma 234–5
    warmed, in hypothermia 236
  flow (mechanics) 180
  intake, child athletes 708
  irrigation, for arthroscopy 713
  MRI appearance 161, 167
  Newtonian and non-Newtonian 181
  see also water intake
fluid warmers 236
fluid-film lubrication 184, 1115
18F-fluorodeoxyglucose (18F-FDG) 157–8, 869
fluoroscopy
  in CAOS 1512
  diagnostic injection under, foot arthritis 1485
  intra-operative, pelvic fractures 434
folate 1027
folic acid supplementation
  juvenile idiopathic arthritis 594
  myelomeningocele prevention 608
fondaparinux, in hip arthroplasty 1126, 1127
foot
  amputations 960–2
  anatomy 27, 77–80
    blood supply 79–80
    nerves 78–9, 1500
    neuromuscular 78–9
    osteology 77–8, 403
  in ankylosing spondylitis 1497
  arch 1463
  arthritis 1484–97
    arthrodesis 1269, 1270, 1478, 1488
    clinical assessment 1484–6
    inflammatory arthritis 1485, 1493–7
    osteoarthritis 1486–93
    rheumatoid arthritis 1241, 1494

arthrodesis 1269–72
bone number in 77
cavovarus 1461
cavus see pes cavus
clinical examination 26–31
  arthritis 1485
  children 538–9
  inspection 27–8
  movement 27, 29–30
  palpation 28–9
  resisted movements 29
  special tests 30–1
club see talipes equinovarus
deformity see foot deformities
diabetic see diabetic foot
elastic keel 965
flat (valgus hindfoot) see flat foot; pes planus
fractures 1567
in gait 955
high-arched see pes cavus
hindfoot see hindfoot
history-taking 26–7, 1484–5
lateral wedging, in knee osteoarthritis 210
medial longitudinal arch 1463
midfoot see midfoot
movements, examination 29
nerve compression syndromes 1500–6
  interdigital plantar (Morton's) neuroma 1500–2
  lateral plantar nerve entrapment 1504–5
  superficial peroneal nerve entrapment 1506
  tarsal tunnel syndrome see tarsal tunnel syndrome
neurological disorders affecting 1472–82
  see also specific disorders
normal, pedobarographs 1460
normal weight-bearing 27
observational gait analysis, in children 566, 567
orthoses see foot orthoses
prosthetic 964–5
  dynamic response 964
  gait abnormalities 967
reconstruction 948
rheumatoid arthritis 26–7
SACH (solid ankle, cushioned heel) 965, 968
SAFE (stationary ankle flexible endoskeletal) 965
screening, diabetic foot 1470
single-axis (prosthetic) 965
supination and pronation 29
surgery see foot surgery
surgical approaches 80
tendon pathologies 1421–33
  see also individual tendons
types 27
see also toes
foot deformities
  arthrodesis 1270
  in children 688–93
    cerebral palsy, management 605, 1475–6
    Charcot–Marie–Tooth disease 613–14, 1473
    clubfoot see talipes equinovarus
    congenital vertical talus see congenital vertical talus
    metatarsus adductus 692
    with myelomeningocele 610, 1475
    pes planus see flat foot; pes planus
    self-limiting 691
    skewfoot 692
  see also specific deformities
foot orthoses 968
  Charcot–Marie–Tooth disease 1473–4
  flat foot 693
  hindfoot osteoarthritis 1489
  hindfoot rheumatoid arthritis 1495
  leg length discrepancy 680
  midfoot osteoarthritis 1489
  myelomeningocele 1475
foot progression angle 30
foot surgery
  anterior tarsal tunnel syndrome 1505–6
  Charcot–Marie–Tooth disease 1474

in children
  cerebral palsy 605, 1476
  congenital clubfoot 690–1
  flat foot 693
entrapment of superficial peroneal nerve 1506
forefoot rheumatoid arthritis 1496
Freiberg disease 1492
hallux rigidus 1490–2
hallux valgus see hallux valgus
hindfoot osteoarthritis 1489
hindfoot rheumatoid arthritis 1495
interdigital plantar (Morton's) neuroma 1501–2
midfoot osteoarthritis 1489–90
stroke patients 1478
tarsal tunnel syndrome 1503–4
see also specific conditions/procedures
foot–thigh angle 30
footwear see shoes
4Titude Ligament Knee Brace 212
force 175–6
  acting on specific joints 186, 187
  component of 176
  definition 176
  to initiate movement 185
  muscle strength testing and 211
forearm
  anatomy 61–4, 322
  arthrology 61
  blood supply 62, 505
  muscles 61–2, 322, 505
  nerves 62, 505
  neuromuscular 61–2
  osteology 61, 322
  compartments 278, 511
  distal, fractures, cast wedging in children 485
  flexor compartment
    acute compartment syndrome 505
    anatomy 505
  flexor contracture 17
  fractures 262, 322
    angular correction 491
    children 491–3
    children, incidence 482
    closed treatment 262–3
    greenstick 491
    indication for surgery 491
    non-union, management 523, 527
    oblique 263
    open 322
    see also under radius; ulna
  injuries 322
  pronation 13, 14, 1387
    effect on valgus laxity of elbow 1387
    medial epicondylitis pathogenesis 1390
  proximal
    fracture-dislocations 490
    fractures, children 490–1
  supination 14
  surgical approaches 62–4
    anterior (Henry's) 62–3
    posterior (Thompson) 63, 64
    of radius 62–3, 64
    of ulna 63–4
forearm bands, in lateral epicondylitis 1394
forearm muscles 61–2, 322, 505
  in cubital tunnel syndrome 1399
forefoot
  fractures 411–13
  MTP joints 415
  pain 843–9
  pes cavus 1461
  pes planus 1463
  phalangeal 415–16
  rheumatoid arthritis 1495–6
  stress fractures 411
  see also metatarsal bones; metatarsophalangeal (MTP) joints
foreign bodies, ultrasound detection 160
forward bend test, Adam's 540
4Titude Ligament Knee Brace 212
four-corner fusions, wrist 1359
four-point force system, translational stability of knee 211, 212
fovea capitis 772
Fowler procedure 1284

fracture(s) 183, 1555–68
  of allografts 944
  callus formation 270, 275
  in children see children
  classifications
    paediatric 499
    see also individual classifications/bones
  closed treatment 258–68
    ankle fractures 266
    casts 260
    clavicle fractures 289
    complications 260–1
    distal femoral fracture 359
    distal radius fractures 261–2, 329
    femoral neck fractures 342–3
    forearm fractures 262–3, 323, 324
    functional braces 260
    humeral shaft fractures 263–4, 308
    paediatric fractures 485–6
    principles 259
    proximal humeral fractures 263, 304
    splints 260
    three-point rule 260, 261
    tibial plafond fractures 383
    tibial plateau fractures 373
    tibial shaft fractures 264–6, 378–9, 380
    traction 259
    types of fractures 259
    see also other individual bones
  clot around bone ends 517
  comminuted, relative instability of fixation 271
  common, closed treatment 258–68
  compartment syndrome due to see compartment syndrome, acute
  complications 515–31
    psychosocial aspects 528
  compound 247
  contamination 248
  definition 269, 1025–6
  delayed union 515
  external fixation see fracture fixation, external
  fatigue see stress fractures
  fixation see fracture fixation
  healing 145, 270
    augmenting 520–1
    biological environment and 271
    biomechanics 270–1, 518–20
    blood supply importance 271, 517–18, 520
    callus formation 270, 275
    in children 482–3
    direct (primary) 519
    direct process 270
    drugs affecting 518
    indirect (secondary) 519–20
    indirect process 270
    infections 518
    mechanical environment and 270–1
    mechanobiology 518–20
    physical treatments for 521
    remodelling after 145
    slow, delayed union 515
    smoking affecting 518, 524
  iatrogenic, hip arthroplasty in osteopetrosis 1130
  indirect reduction 273
  infected 223, 518, 520, 521
    active vs quiescent 521
  intra-articular, open reduction internal fixation 258–9
  malunion 527–8
    clavicle fractures 289
    deformities 527
    distal femoral fractures 361
    femoral 527
    femoral shaft fractures 356
    Ilizarov technique for 528
    tibial 527
    tibial pilon 527
  metaphyseal, pathological, treatment 935
  metaphyseal fragments, assessment, wound debridement 254
  morphology, non-union and fixation 521–2
  nerve injuries in 1306
  non-operative management see fracture(s), closed treatment

fracture(s) – continued
  non-union 515–27
    aetiology (biological/mechanical) 517
    atrophic (rat's tail) 516
    biological factors affecting 517–18, 520
    classification 517
    clavicle fractures 289–90
    definition 515
    diagnosis 515–16
    femoral neck fractures 344
    femoral shaft fractures 356
    hypertrophic (elephant's foot) 516
    infected 223, 518, 520, 521, 524
    lower limb, fixation 521
    mechanobiology 518–20
    oblique 522
    odontoid fractures 451
    pathological fractures 934
    'peg and socket', CT scans 516, 517
    pelvic fractures 435
    psychosocial aspects 528
    scaphoid fractures 756
    shear causing 518–19, 525
    spiral 522
    subtrochanteric fracture 352
    tibial plafond fractures 385
    tibial shaft fractures 380
    transverse 522
    upper limb, fixation 521
    Weber-Cech classification 516–17
  non-union, management 520–7
    amputation 521, 524
    biological treatment 520–1
    bone grafts 520
    femur 523
    fixation methods 521–2
    forearm 523
    humerus 523
    infected 223, 520, 521
    mechanical environment optimization 521
    tibia 523
  open 247–57
    antibiotics for 253, 254
    assessment 248
    blood loss and management 239
    bone stabilization 255–6
    debridement 253–5
    definition 247
    femoral shaft fractures 356
    fixation see fracture fixation devices
    Gustilo–Anderson classification 249, 250
    infection rate and infections 253
    maxillofacial 471
    pathophysiology 248
    see also open injuries, of limbs
  operative fixation see fracture fixation
  pathological see pathological fractures
  radiographically occult 156, 170
  reduction see fracture(s), closed treatment
  simple patterns, stable fixation 271, 272
  stress see stress fractures
  tables 1555–68
  treatment
    non-operative see fracture(s), closed treatment
    operative see fracture fixation
  union
    assessment by CT 159
    Perkins' rules 515
  see also individual bones/fractures
fracture (of materials, in mechanics) 182–3
fracture braces 969
fracture clinics, history 4
fracture fixation 258, 269–77
  absolute stability 269–70
    interfragmental compression 271, 272
    lag screw use 271, 272
    methods for 271–2
  acute osteomyelitis, management 222
  aim 270
  biological environment for 271
  in children 486

closed treatment and see fracture(s), closed treatment
complications 258
compression plating, humeral non-union 525
decision-making over type 259
devices for see fracture fixation devices
elastic stable intramedullary nailing (ESIN) 486
external 274
  complications and infections 274
  distal radius fractures 330
  femoral shaft fractures 355
  fracture non-union treatment 522
  hybrid, tibial plafond fractures 383
  indications 274
  tibial plafond fractures 383–4
  tibial shaft fractures 380
failure, pathological fractures 934
goals 269
humeral shaft fractures 308, 309
internal
  contraindications 522
  femoral neck fractures 342–3
  in fracture non-union 522
  pathological fractures 933–4
mechanical environment for 270–1, 272
non-union management 521–2
open fractures 255–6
open reduction internal fixation (ORIF) 258–9
  ankle fractures 389
  Bennett's fracture 763
  calcaneal fractures 400
  distal radius fractures 330
  hook of hamate fractures 756–7
  humeral shaft fractures 308
  patellar fractures 369
  phalangeal fractures (hand) 766
  scaphoid fractures 756
  sesamoid fractures 1446
  talar neck fractures 395
  tibial plateau fractures 374
pathological fractures 933–4
percutaneous pinning, distal radius fractures 329–30
plating 271–2
  see also fracture fixation devices, plates
prophylactic, pathological fractures 932
relative stability 270, 272
  biological plate fixation 272–4
  external fixation 274
  indirect reduction 273
  intramedullary nailing 274–5
  methods for 272–5
retrograde nailing, femoral shaft fractures 355
screw osteosynthesis 486
stable, concept 269–70, 271
surgical strategies 239–40
tension band wiring, patellar fractures 369
see also individual fractures/bones
fracture fixation devices 195–6
  external devices see external fixators
  external ring fixators 196, 255
  interlocking nails 255, 275
    femoral shaft fractures 355
    humeral shaft fractures 308
    subtrochanteric fracture 351, 352
  intramedullary nails 195–6, 274
    distal femoral fractures 360–1
    elastic stable, in children 486
    femoral shaft fractures 354–5
    fracture non-union treatment 522
    for humeral non-union 526
    humeral shaft fractures 308
    open fractures 255
    pathological shaft fractures 935
    pubis ramus fractures 431
    reaming, pathological fractures 935
    subtrochanteric fracture 351
    tibial nerve injury 1307
    tibial shaft fracture 379, 380
    tibial stress fractures 823
    unreamed 355
  intramedullary pins 289
  intramedullary screws, hip 349

K-wire osteosynthesis 486
  see also Kirschner (K) wire
lag screw 271, 272
  distal humeral fractures 312, 313, 314
  talar neck fractures 395
locking plates 255–6
  distal femoral fractures 360
  for humeral non-union 526
  tibial shaft fractures 255, 379
nails
  antegrade femoral 349
  Gamma 349
  reamed vs unreamed, tibial shaft fractures 379
plates 195, 255, 271–2
  biological, tibial shaft fracture 379
  bridge plates 273
  compression and tension band 272
  condylar blade (95°) 359
  condylar buttress 360
  distal femoral fractures 359–60
  distal humeral fractures 313
  dynamic compression (DCP) 273
  femoral shaft fractures 355
  fracture non-union treatment 522
  limited contact (LCP) 273
  locking see above
  micro- and miniplates, midfacial fractures 476, 477
  neutralization and buttress 271, 272
reamed nails 255, 379
screws 195, 255
  compression hip 351
  distal femoral fractures 359
  dynamic condylar 360
  dynamic hip 344, 348
  iliosacral 433
  interfragmentary lag 359
  intramedullary hip 349
  lag see fracture fixation devices, lag screw
  sliding hip 348
unreamed nails 255, 379
fracture gap 270, 519
  non-union 521–2
  strain and 519
'fracture of necessity' (Galeazzi fracture) 325
'fracture personality' 259
frame acopia 527
free body diagram 177
  hip 186, 1106, 1107, 1108
  spine 187
free vascularized fibular grafting see vascularized fibular grafts
Freeman–Swanson prosthesis 1172, 1173
Freiberg's disease 28–9, 1492
fretting corrosion 1115, 1116
friction 178, 183–4
friction force 183
Froment sign 1399
Froment' test 16
Frykman classification, distal radius fractures 328, 1560
Fukuda ring retractor 1229
functional bracing
  anterior cruciate ligament injuries 809
  for fractures 260
  humeral shaft fractures 264, 265, 308
functional stimulation, engineered tissue 1525
functioning, international classification 202, 203
fungal infections, spinal 986
fused ribs 631
fusion, joints see arthrodesis

G protein, α-subunit, gene encoding 891
gadolinium (Gd) 160, 163–6
  adverse effect 163
  intra-articular 166
  intravenous 163–5
  see also under magnetic resonance imaging (MRI)
gait 563, 954–7
  antalgic 31, 956
  assessment 31, 32
  see also gait analysis

asymmetry, tibial stress fractures due to 822
ataxic 31
attributes 563
broad-based 31
in children 563–8
  analysis see gait analysis
  normal 563, 564
  pathological 566–8, 601
circumducting 31
crouch 208, 567
cycle 564, 565
  distance and time 955, 956
determinants (motion patterns) 563, 955
double-limb support 954, 957
  forces acting at hip 1106
dynamics 954
extensor lurch 31
gluteus maximus 31
high-stepping 31
in hip inspection 18
in-toeing 30
in knee inspection 23
knee kinematics during see under knee
knee stability and 208
leg length discrepancy 31, 567
line of progression 565
metabolic cost 957
muscle action 955–6
normal 27, 31
  ankle movements 1243
  in children 563, 564
osteoporotic spinal surgery 1043
pathological 27, 955–6, 957
  cerebral palsy 601
  in children 566–8, 601
  see also Trendelenburg gait
pes cavus 1461
pistoning during 957, 967
prosthetic foot abnormalities 967, 968
quadriceps avoidance 957
sagittal plane moments, control 208
single-limb support 954
  forces acting at hip 1106–7
stance and swing phases 31, 954, 955, 956
steppage 31
stiff-legged 977
Trendelenburg see Trendelenburg gait
vaulting 31
gait analysis 31, 32
  instrumented three-dimensional 563, 564
  cerebral palsy 601
  observational see observational gait analysis
  paediatric patients 564–6
    with cerebral palsy 601
  physical setting force
Galeazzi fracture 324–5
  children 493
  distal radial ulnar joint injury 1366
  reverse 325
Galeazzi sign 539, 646, 678
Galeazzi's test 19
gallium, pyogenic spinal infections 984
galvanic corrosion 1115, 1116
gamekeeper's thumb 763–4
Gamma nail 349
Ganga Hospital Open Injury Severity Score 249–52, 253
  covering tissues (skin/fascia) 250, 251
  functional tissues (muscles/tendons/nerves) 250
  skeletal tissues (bones/joints) 250, 251
ganglion/ganglion cysts
  dorsal 1374
  hand/wrist 1374
  intra-osseous 1377
  occult dorsal 762
  see also mucous cysts
gangrene 958
  diabetic foot 1467, 1468
  gas see gas gangrene
gap junctions 86, 700
Garden classification, femoral neck fractures 341, 342, 1564
'garden spade' deformity, wrist 328

Gardner–Wells tong traction 445
Garrod's knuckle pads 1326
Garrod's pads 918
Gartland classification, supracondylar fracture of humerus 488
gas gangrene 220
  antibiotic treatment 220
'gas sign' 1029
gastritis, haemorrhagic 445
gastrocnemius
  action and function 956
  lengthening, cerebral palsy management 604, 1476
  weakness, gait 957
Gaussian distribution 43
gender differences, osteoporosis 1024, 1025
gene(s) 140–5, 150
  mutations, cancer aetiology 149
gene chip technology 143
gene therapy 143–5
  adverse effects/toxicity of vectors 145
  Duchenne muscular dystrophy 612
  ex vivo and in vivo delivery 143
  prerequisites 144
  somatic 143
  vectors 144, 145, 1069
    classification 144
gene transfer 143
general medical consent 1539
generalizability (external validity) 39
genetic disorders
  inheritance mechanisms 151–2
  orthopaedic 152
  techniques for studying 141–3
genetic fingerprinting 141
genetic techniques 141–3
genetics 150–2
  bone tumours 882
  susceptibility, inflammatory arthropathies 1084
geniculate arteries, meniscus blood supply 104
genitofemoral nerve 71
genitourinary complications, pelvic fractures 435
genome, sequence 140
genomic imprinting 151
genomic screening 141
genu valgum 667–70
  aetiology 668
  see also knee, valgus deformity
genu varum 667–70
  aetiology 668
  Blount disease vs. 670
  see also knee, varus deformity
Gerber's lift-off test 10, 1210
Gerdy's tubercle 75
giant cell tumour, diffuse-type see pigmented villonodular synovitis (PVNS)
giant cell tumour of bone 883, 885, 889–90
  age range and sex ratio 889
  malignant transformation 890
  pathology/histology 889
  spine 1062
  treatment 890, 1062
giant cell tumour of tendon sheath 918
  hand 1374–5
Gigli saw 1201
Gilbert and Tassin's method 616
Gilchrist bandage 486
Gill's procedure 1052
Gilula arcs/line 1353, 1361
Girdlestone, Gathorne Robert 5
Girdlestone's procedure 1272
Glasgow Coma Scale (GCS) 236, 467–8
  details 468
  paediatric 499, 500
  skull fractures 478
glenohumeral joint
  anatomy 52, 57, 1215
  anterior capsule
    exposure 1218, 1220
    humeral attachment 1218
    posterior vs 735
    release 1220
  anterior instability 730–5, 1214
    arthroscopic capsulolabral repair 731–4
    athletes 730–5
    clinical features 730–1
    imaging 731

open anterior capsulorrhaphy 734–5, 1218–19
open anteroinferior capsular shift 1220
open Bankart repair 1218–19
physical examination 731, 1216
recurrence 1217
surgical indications 731
surgical techniques 731–5, 1218–21
traumatic 1217
see also Bankart's repair
anterosuperior instability 1208
arthritis 1223–33
  history and examination 1224
  imaging 1224
  non-operative treatment 1225
  operative treatment 1225–30
  post-traumatic 1223
  treatment 1225
  see also shoulder arthroplasty
arthroscopy 732
capsule
  anterior see glenohumeral joint, anterior capsule
  'circle' concept 737
  inferior release 1220
  inferior shift 1215
  in open Bankart's repair 1218, 1219
  plication, multidirectional instability 739
  posterior see glenohumeral joint, posterior capsule
  posterior release 1220
  release, anatomic total shoulder replacement 1226–7
  release, reverse shoulder arthroplasty 1231
  static stabilizer 730
  thickenings 1215
  volume increase 1215
capsulolabral repair
  arthroscopic 731–3, 736–7
  open 1218–21
dislocations 297–302, 1214
  anterior 298–300, 1214
  classification/types 297, 298
  clinical evaluation 298, 300
  complications 299–300, 301
  history 1214
  inferior (luxatio erecta) 301
  mechanism 298, 300
  posterior 300–1
  radiographic evaluation 298–9, 300
  recurrent 298, 299, 300, 301, 1214
  superior 301
  treatment 299, 301
immobilization, external rotation 1218
instability 729–39, 1214–23
  after acute dislocation 300, 301
  anterior see glenohumeral joint, anterior instability
  anteroinferior 1220, 1223
  anterosuperior 1208
  arthritis after 1223
  causes 730
  classification 1216
  clinical evaluation 1215–17
  complications of repair 1223
  dynamic inferior 737
  dynamic stabilizers 730, 735, 1215
  'essential lesion' 1215
  examination 1216
  examination under anaesthesia 1217
  exercises for 1217, 1222
  history of repair 1207
  history-taking 1216
  imaging 1217
  laxity vs 1216
  multidirectional see glenohumeral joint, multidirectional instability
  non-operative treatment 1217–18
  open anteroinferior capsular shift 1220
  open Bankart repair 1218–19
    see also Bankart's repair
  open posterior capsular shift 1221–2
  posterior see glenohumeral joint, posterior instability

posterior reconstruction 1221–2
postoperative rehabilitation 1222
recurrent 300, 1216, 1223
results of surgery 1222–3
sports injuries 729–39, 1216
static stabilizers 729–30, 737
testing 11
traumatic vs atraumatic 1216
TUBS 300
voluntary 730
multidirectional instability 731, 737–9
  biomechanics 737
  clinical features 737–8
  non-operative management 1217
  physical examination 738
  radiography 738
  surgical decision-making 738
  surgical results 1222–3
  surgical techniques 738–9
negative pressure gradient 730
posterior capsular shift 1221–2
posterior capsule
  anterior vs 735
  release 1220
  surgical approach 1221
posterior instability 729–30, 735–7, 1215
  biomechanics 735
  clinical features 735
  physical examination 735
  postoperative care 737
  radiography 735
  reconstruction 1221–3
  surgical decision-making 736
  surgical results 1223
  surgical technique 736–7, 1221–2
post-traumatic arthritis 1223
rheumatoid arthritis 1223
safe zone of passive motion 1232
surgical approaches 1215, 1218, 1220, 1221
translations, examination 1217
unstable
  linear acceleration of hand during reaching task 205–6
  linear displacement of hand during reaching task 205
  linear velocity of hand during reaching task 205
  see also glenohumeral joint, instability
  see also shoulder
glenohumeral ligaments 298
  anatomy 730
  arthroscopy 715
  humeral avulsion of (HAGL) lesion see HAGL lesion
glenohumeral stabilizers 52, 297, 298
glenoid
  baseplate, reverse shoulder arthroplasty 1231, 1232
  bone loss 732
  defects, glenohumeral instability 1214
  exposure/preparation
    anatomic total shoulder arthroplasty 1228–9
    reverse shoulder arthroplasty 1231
  soft-tissue releases 1228, 1229
  fractures 295, 1557
  lucent lines 1233
  normal version 1224
  posterior bone loss 1229
  posterior wear 1224, 1225
  reaming 1229
  retroversion 1224
  rim 739
    anterior calcification/fractures 1217
    open Bankart's repair 1219
  socket depth 1215
  wear, arthroplasty in young patients 1255
glenoid component, placement
  anatomic total shoulder arthroplasty 1228–9
  reverse shoulder arthroplasty 1231
glenoid fossa 297
glenoid labrum 297, 730
  avulsion 297
  detachment 1217, 1220
  posterior instability, repair 736

reattachment, open Bankart's repair 1219
static stabilizer of shoulder 729, 730
superior labrum tears see SLAP tears/lesions
tear
  arthroscopic capsulolabral repair 731–4
  open repair 734, 1218
  see also Bankart's lesion
glenoid ligament see glenoid labrum
glide test 26
global stabilizing muscles, spine 979
glomus body 919, 1375
glomus tumour 919
  hand 1375
glucagon 704
Gluck knee prosthesis 1171
glucocorticoid(s) 129–30
  classification based on potency 129–30
  clinical uses 130
  osteoporosis associated 1029, 1030
  pharmacokinetics 130
  receptors 129
  side-effects 130
  see also corticosteroid(s)
glucocorticoid response elements (GREs) 129
gluconeogenesis 703
glucosamine hydrochloride, supplements 134
glucosamine sulphate, osteoarthritis treatment 1083
glucose, metabolism 702, 706
gluteal pain 1136
gluteus maximus 773
  gait 31, 956
  weakness, gait 957
gluteus medius 773
  gait 956
  weakness, gait 957
glycaemic index (GI) foods 706
glycocalyx, definition 221
glycogen 702
  resynthesis 706
glycoproteins
  in articular cartilage 101–2
  in bone 83
glycosaminoglycans 101, 104, 1078, 1079
  mucopolysaccharidoses 573–4
gold salts
  juvenile rheumatoid arthritis 1089
  rheumatoid arthritis 1086
'gold standard', diagnostic test 38
golf players, medial epicondylitis pathogenesis 1390–1
golfer's elbow see medial epicondylitis
Golgi tendon organ-like mechanoreceptors 215
Golgi tendon organs 212, 215
gonococcal arthritis 226
good manufacturing practice (GMP), tissue engineering 1525
Google Health 1537
Gore-Tex 1339
gout 1091, 1496
  acute 1091
  chronic 1091
  hand 1374
  radiography 156
Gower manoeuvre 611
gradient echo (GRE) sequence 161
granulation tissue 145
  degenerative disc disease 998, 999, 1003
  fracture gap 270
granulomas 219
  eosinophilic 890–1, 1062
  infections characterized by 219
granulomatous infection 219
greater sciatic nerve 71
greater sciatic notch 69
greater trochanteric fractures 349
Greenspan view, radial head fractures 319
greenstick fractures
  children 483, 491, 493
  forearm 491, 493
  maxillofacial 471–2
Greulich–Pyle atlas 680
Gross Motor Functional Classification System (GMFCS) 599–600

growth
  post-natal, spinal column 627–8
  stimulation, short limbs 683
growth disturbances
  juvenile idiopathic arthritis 590
  septic arthritis complication 582
growth factors
  bone metabolism control 98
  implantations, degenerative disc disease 1005
  osteoarthritis pathophysiology 1080–1
  release, muscle injury 110
growth hormone (GH) 546
  bone metabolism control 98
  effect on muscle, in exercise 704
  growth plate control 91
  use by athletes 707
growth plate 89
  endochondral ossification 89–91
  formation 543
  histology 544
  hormones affecting 91
  hypertrophic and calcification zone 544
  zones 89, 90, 91
Gruen zones 1140, 1141, 1154
'guillotine' mechanism 1049
gunshot injuries
  cervical spine 459
  thoracolumbar spine 463
gunstock deformity 489
Gunston knee prosthesis 1172, 1173
Gustilo–Anderson classification 249, 250
gymnast's wrist 761–2

H band 108
habitual patellar dislocation 666
haemangioma
  hand 1375
  spine 1062, 1065
haemarthrosis, in tibial plateau fractures 372
haematoma
  floor of mouth 470
  hand 1374
  monocle (orbit) 468, 469, 475
  retrobulbar see retrobulbar haematoma
  in soft-tissue healing 105
  subcutaneous, rotator cuff tear repair 1214
  subungual 1288–9
haematopoietic stem cells 1068, 1527
haematopoietic tumours 883
haematosinus 475, 476
haematuria
  micro-, in tumours 866
  pelvic fractures and 427
haemodynamic stabilization, trauma 444–5
haemoglobin 958
haemophiliac arthropathy 1092
Haemophilus influenzae infection
  acute haematogenous osteomyelitis 582, 585
  septic arthritis in children 580, 581
haemorrhage
  life-/major organ-threatening 131
  pelvic fractures 239, 425–6, 427, 437
  see also bleeding
haemorrhagic gastritis 445
haemosiderin 918
Hagie pin 289
HAGL lesion 297, 730
  arthroscopic capsulolabral repair 732
Haglund's deformity 832, 1426–7
  surgery 1428
Hahn-Steinthal fragment 313
hallux
  amputations 960
  arthrodesis 1268
  examination 28, 29
  interphalangeal joint dislocation 416
  lateral deviation 1435, 1436
  medial deviation 1447–8
  MTP joint, arthrodesis 1271
  MTP joint injuries 414–15
  pronation 1434, 1435
hallux interphalangeus 1451
hallux rigidus 1490–2
  arthrodesis for 1271

hallux valgus 28, 29, 1434–41
  aetiology 1435–6
  classification 1435
  clinical features 1436
  definition 1434
  hammer toe with 1451
  non-operative treatment 1436
  operative treatment 1436–40
    complications 1438
    distal metatarsal osteotomy 1437–8
    distal soft-tissue procedure 1437
    first metatarsal–cuneiform joint arthrodesis 1439
    first MTP joint arthrodesis 1440
    metatarsal shaft osteotomy 1438–9
    proximal metatarsal osteotomy 1439
    proximal phalangeal osteotomy 1439
    resection arthroplasty 1439–40
  pathoanatomy 1434–5
  radiographic evaluation 1436–7
  secondary 1435
  in sesamoiditis 1447
  treatment algorithm 1437
hallux valgus angle (HVA) 1436, 1439
hallux valgus interphalangeus (HVI) 1435
hallux varus 1447–8
'halo' sign, CSF leakage 468
halo traction, atlas fractures 448
hamate
  in four-corner fusions 1359
  fractures 1561
  hook of, fractures 756–7
Hamilton Russell, Robert 4
hammer toe 1451–2
  pathophysiology, examination 1452
  treatment 1452
hamstring muscles
  action and function 774, 956
  autograft tissue, ACL reconstruction 810
  length, examination/testing 21
  lengthening, cerebral palsy 603–4
  quadriceps balance 211, 213
  strain 774
  translational stability of knee 211
hamstring/quadriceps (HQ) ratio 213
hand
  amputation, early management 1316
  anatomy 64
  aneurysmal bone cyst (ABC) 1377–8
  aneurysmal lesions 1374
  arthritis 1333–50
    see also osteoarthritis
  avulsion-type injury 1316
  cartilage lesions 1378–9
  clear cell sarcoma 1377
  clinical examination 15–17
    inspection and palpation 15
    motor/movement 16
    special tests 16–17
  compartments 511
  contractures, testing 17
  deep fascial spaces
    anatomy 1312
    infections 1311–12
  degloving injury 1322
  dermatomes 16
  displacement 173–4
  enchondroma 1378
  epithelioid sarcoma 1377
  Ewing's sarcoma 1380
  exostosis 1379
  extensor tendon(s)
    anatomy 1298
    suturing 1298, 1299
    zones 1278, 1279, 1298, 1299
  extensor tendon injuries 1280–7, 1298–300
    repair 1292, 1298–300
    zone I (mallet finger) 1280–2, 1299–300
    zone II 1282
    zone III (boutonnière) 1282–3, 1300
    zone IV-VIII 1283
  false aneurysms 1374
  flexor tendon(s)
    anatomy 1293–4
    bowstringing 1293, 1312
    pulleys 1293–4

suturing technique 1295–6
  zones 1278, 1294
  see also finger(s), flexor tendons
flexor tendon injuries 1278–80, 1292–8
  adhesions 1297–8
  clinical examination 1294–5
  complications 1297–8
  outcome measurement 1297
  postoperative rehabilitation 1297
  rupture/lacerations 1278, 1297
  surgical management 1278, 1280, 1295–7
  zone I (jersey finger) 1278–80, 1296
  zone II 1280, 1296
  zone III and IV 1280, 1296–7
  zone V 1280, 1297
  fractures 766–8, 1561
    phalangeal see phalangeal fractures
    PIP joint intra-articular 1285–6
  giant cell tumour of tendon sheath 1374–5
  glomus tumour 1375
  gout 1374
  haemangioma 1375
  incisions 1313
  infections 1309–14
    causative organisms 1309, 1310
    common types 1310–13
    incisions for 1313
    prognostic factors 1309
    surgical approach 1313
    treatment 1310
  injuries 762–8
  intra-osseous ganglia 1377
  'intrinsic plus' 17
  intrinsic tightness 17
  joint replacement 192–4
    implant materials 189
  lacerations to palm 1278–80
  linear displacement during reaching task 205
  linear velocity during reaching task 205
  lipoma 1375
  liposarcoma 1377
  malignant fibrous histiocytoma 1377
  malignant peripheral nerve sheath tumour 1377
  metastatic disease 1380
  nerve injuries 1302–8
  neurilemoma 1375
  neurofibroma 1375, 1376
  orthoses 969
  osteoblastoma 1379
  osteochondroma 1378–9
  osteoid osteoma 1379
  osteology 64
  osteomyelitis 1092
  osteosarcoma 1379–80
  pseudogout 1374
  reconstruction 950
  rehabilitation, after Dupuytren's contracture 1330
  replantation see replantation (upper limb)
  sensation, testing 16–17
  septic arthritis 1092, 1310
  skin cancers 1376–7
  soft-tissue sarcoma 1377
  sports injuries see sports injuries; specific injuries
  squamous cell carcinoma 1376–7
  staphylococcal osteomyelitis 1373
  surgical approach 1313
  synovial cell sarcoma 1377
  synovial chondromatosis 1376
  tumours 1373–81
    benign bone 1377–8
    benign cartilage 1378–9
    benign soft-tissue 1374–6
    bone 1377–80
    diagnosis/assessment 1373
    malignant bone 1379–80
    malignant soft-tissue 1376–7
    soft-tissue 1374–7
  Verdan's zones 1278, 1294
  web space
    contracture 1328
    infections 1311–12
  see also finger(s); thumb; wrist
handlebar palsy 760
'hanging drop' sign 476

hangman's fracture (C2 vertebra) 445, 451, 452, 1556
  sports injuries 725–6
Hardinge approach, to hip 72–3, 1138, 1149
hardy personality, burnout resistance 1551
Harrington compression, ankylosing spondylitis 1089
Harrington rods 1018, 1019
Harris basion–axial interval (BAI)/basion–dental interval (BDI) method 447
Harris score, modified 18
Hartman's saline 1316
Haversian canal 85
Haversian systems (osteons) 85
Hawkin test 10
Hawkins classification, talar neck injuries 395
Hawkins impingement reinforcement sign 1209
Hawkins sign 395
Hawkins–Kennedy sign 742
head and face trauma 466–80
  children 499
  clinical diagnosis 467–71
    extraoral examination 468–9
    intraoral examination 469–70
    neurological examination 467–8
    radiological examination 471
  closed injury, surgery for 969–71
  evaluation in concussion 721
  fractures
    examination for 468, 469
    mandible see mandibular fractures
    maxillofacial see maxillofacial fractures
    midfacial see Le Fort fractures; midfacial fractures
    reduction and fixation 476
    skull see skull fractures
  general considerations 466
  incidence 466
  indications for consultation 467
  long-term sequelae 468
  minor, sequelae 468
  scale of head injuries 468
  in sport 718–28
    concussion see concussion
  tenderness, palpation 469
  types/causes of injuries 466
healing
  amputation wounds 958
  articular cartilage 102–3
  fractures see fracture(s), healing
  intervertebral disc 107
  ligaments 113
  meniscus 104, 105
  phases 113
  skeletal muscle 110
  soft tissues 100
  stages/sequence 105
  tendons see tendon(s)
health status, joint assessment principles 202–3
Health Vault 1537
heart rate, maximum 704
heat shock proteins
  HSP90 129
  rheumatoid arthritis aetiology 1084
heel
  malalignment 1422
  normal appearance 27
  pain 847
  see also calcaneus
heel bisector 30
heel raise stance 28
height, peak see peak height velocity (PHV)
hemiarthroplasty
  bipolar (hip)
    femoral neck fractures 342, 343, 344
    in SLE 1091
  calcar replacement, intertrochanteric fractures 349
  elbow 1256
  in femoral neck fractures 342, 343, 344
  hallux rigidus 1491
  history 1098
  knee 1172
  McKeever 1172

reconstruction after tumour resection 947
shoulder 1223, 1232
  young patients 1256
unipolar, in femoral neck fractures 343
hemiplegia
  gait 957
  stroke patients 1477
hemiresection interpositional technique (HIT) 1372
Henneman principle 700
Henry approach
  to elbow 60, 61
  to forearm (radius) 62–3
  to shoulder 55, 56
heparin 131–2
  antagonism 132
  clinical use and side-effects 132
  in hip arthroplasty 1126
  mechanism of action 131–2
hepatic microsomal enzymes 131–2
hereditary motor–sensory neuropathies (HMSNs) 613–15, 1462
  see also Charcot–Marie–Tooth disease; specific disorders
hereditary multiple exostosis 574–5
hereditary neuropathies 613–15
hereditary osteochondromatosis 895
hernias, pelvic fracture complication 434
heroin (diamorphine) 127
herpetic whitlow 1313
Herring classification 654
heteroduplex analysis 141
Hickman, Henry 4
high tibial osteotomy (HTO) 1261
  closing wedge 1264
  indications 1262, 1263
  opening wedge 1264, 1265
  osteoarthritis (knee) 1081
    medial compartment 209–10
  technique 1264
  valgizing 1262, 1263
  see also osteotomy, around knee
high-altitude training 704
high-energy injuries
  nerves 1304–5
  open injuries of limbs 247
  skull fractures 478
high-energy phosphates 702
high-velocity injuries 248
Hilgenreiner epiphyseal (HE) angle, coxa vara 651, 652
Hilgenreiner line, DDH assessment 646, 647
Hill–Sachs lesion 298, 731, 732, 1214, 1215
  radiography 1217
  reverse 300, 735
Hilton's law 56
hindfoot
  arthrodesis 1269, 1424
    osteoarthritis 1489
    rheumatoid arthritis 1495
  examination, arthritis 1485
  flexion deformities, arthrodesis 1270
  osteoarthritis 1422, 1488–9
  rheumatoid arthritis 1494–5
  triple arthrodesis 1489
  valgus (flat foot) see flat foot
  varus, Charcot–Marie–Tooth disease 1473
hip
  abduction 70
    examination 19–20
    see also hip abductors
  abduction contractures, myelomeningocele 610
  adduction 70
    adductor action and function 956
    examination 20
  anatomy 69–73, 772–3
    arthrology 70, 419, 772–3, 1105–6
    blood vessels 71–2
    ligaments 70, 772–3, 1106
    muscles 70–1, 773, 1106
    nerves 70–1, 773
    osteology 69–70
    see also acetabulum; femoral head
  ankylosing spondylitis of 1089, 1129
  arthrodesis 1097, 1268, 1272
    young patients 1254
  arthroplasty see hip arthroplasty

arthroscopy see arthroscopy
biomechanics 186, 1105–13
blood supply 70
bursitis 775
capsular restriction, pattern 17
capsule 772–3
centre of joint 1261
chondral injuries 779
clinical examination 18–22
  inspection (look) 18–19
  movement 19–20
  paediatric 539–40
  palpation (feel) 19
  schedule 22
  special tests 20–1
contusions 773–4
coronal plane 1106
development 645, 1105
developmental dysplasia see developmental dysplasia of hip (DDH)
disarticulation 962, 963
dislocations see hip dislocations
disorders, childhood see hip disorders, in children
dysplasia
  in Charcot–Marie–Tooth disease 614
  implant choice 1128
  see also developmental dysplasia of hip (DDH)
embryology and development 645
extension, examination 19
extensors 70
external rotation 70
  assessment 20
flexion
  examination 19
  paediatric assessment 538
flexion contractures
  ankylosing spondylitis 1129
  myelomeningocele 609
flexion–adduction test 21
flexors 70
forces acting on 186, 1106–7
  double-leg stance 1106
  single-leg stance 1106–7
fracture dislocations
  type V, with femoral head fracture 337–8
fractures 1564
  athletes 776, 777
  blood loss 239
  children 776
  intertrochanteric see intertrochanteric fractures
  stress fractures 345, 777, 1565
  see also femoral neck fractures
free body diagram 186
as fulcrum, during walking 1106
history of surgery 1097–101
history-taking 17–18
hyperextension, in ankylosing spondylitis 1129
impingement 1110–11
  biomechanics 1110–11
  tests 21
  see also femoroacetabular impingement
instability, cerebral palsy 606–7
internal rotation 70
  assessment 20, 21
intra-articular disorders, sports-related 778–9
irritable 660
joint reaction forces (JRFs) 1106, 1107
  reducing 1107–8
  total hip arthroplasty 1108, 1110
joint replacement see hip arthroplasty
jumping distance, biomechanics 1108
ligaments 70, 772–3, 1106
loose bodies 778, 779
movements 773
  degrees of freedom 1105
muscle strains 774–5
nerve entrapment around 775
observational gait analysis 566
pain 17, 21
  ankylosing spondylitis 1089, 1129
  decrease, reduction of joint reaction force 1107–8

labral tears 778
night 17
pre-arthroplasty assessment 1136
range of motion 186, 1108–9
reconstruction 947
referred pain 71
replacement see hip arthroplasty
resurfacing see hip resurfacing
revision arthroplasty see revision hip arthroplasty
sagittal plane 1106
scars 1136
scissoring 955
septic, arthroplasty in young patients 1253
sports injuries 772–81
  see also sports injuries; specific injuries
stability 772, 1106, 1108–9
stiffness 17
subluxation
  athletes 776–7
  traumatic, in children 493
  see also hip dislocations
surgery in children
  cerebral palsy 602–3, 606–7
  developmental coxa vara 652
  developmental dysplasia of hip 648–9
  Perthes disease 655
  proximal focal femoral deficiency 651
  slipped capital femoral epiphysis 658–9
surgical approaches 72–4
  anterior (Smith–Peterson) 72, 1136–7, 1149
  anterolateral (Watson-Jones) 72, 73, 1136, 1137, 1149
  lateral (Hardinge) 72–3, 1138, 1149
  for minimal incision hip arthroplasty 1149
  posterior (Moore; Southern) 73, 74, 1136, 1137, 1149, 1157
  for revision hip arthroplasty 1157
  for total hip replacement 1136–8
  transgluteal (Hardinge) 1138, 1149
  transtrochanteric 1137–8
symptoms involving 17
telescoping (pistoning) 21
tumours 778
windswept deformity, cerebral palsy 606
hip abductors 1105
  action and function 956, 1106
  force 1106–7
    joint reaction force reduction 1107–8
    lever arm, action 1106–7, 1108, 1110
  reconstruction 947
hip adductors, action and function 956
hip arthroplasty 189–91
  history 1097–101, 1109
  interpositional 1097
  intertrochanteric fractures 349
  'mold' (Smith-Petersen) 1098
  osteotomy 1097
  reconstructive 1097–8
  resurfacing see hip resurfacing
  revision see revision hip arthroplasty
hip arthroplasty (total) 1097, 1098–100, 1135–46
  achondroplasia 1128
  aim 1135
  anaesthesia 1123–4
  ankylosing spondylitis 1129
  antibiotic prophylaxis 1125, 1126
  aseptic loosening 1153–4
    polyethylene associated 1099, 1117, 1139, 1153–4
    stem design and 1154
    uncemented cup pressure effects 1154
    zones of demarcation 1154
  bearing surfaces 1116–20
    see also specific bearings below
  biological fixation 1100–1
  biomechanics 1105–13
    range of motion maximization 1108
  bone preservation techniques, in osteoarthritis 1127
  cardiovascular complications 1125

cemented 1099, 1138–40
  bone preparation 1140
  generation techniques 1140
  outcome 1142
  sockets for 1139–40
  stems for 1139
  uncemented arthroplasty vs 1142
cementless see hip arthroplasty (total), uncemented
ceramic-on-ceramic bearings 1120, 1254
  fractures 1155
  lubrication 1115
ceramic-on-polyethylene bearings 1119
computer-assisted navigation 1520–2
  operative technique 1521–2
  patient-specific jigs 1522
  potential advantages 1520
  potential disadvantages 1520–1
corrosion 1115–16
dental infections 1124–5
failure mechanisms 1153–6
  aseptic loosening see hip arthroplasty (total), aseptic loosening
  ceramic bearing fracture 1155
  dislocation 1155
  infections 1161
  periprosthetic fractures 1155–6
  septic loosening 1154–5
  stem fracture 1155
  in femoral neck fractures 343
femur shape in planning 1136
fixation optimization 1109–10, 1120, 1140
functional outcome 1143
guidelines 1153
  antibiotic prophylaxis 1125, 1126
  thromboprophylaxis 1126–7
'hard-on-soft' 1118
head–neck ratio 1099, 1108–9
head–neck taper, fretting corrosion 1115, 1116
history of development 1097–104
indications 1127, 1135, 1253
infections after 1124–5
  assessment 1161
  loosening due to 1154–5
  rate 1099
  revision for 1156, 1161–2
  in rheumatoid arthritis 1129
  urinary tract 1125
joint reaction force reduction 1108, 1110
loosening 1099, 1100, 1120
  aseptic see aseptic loosening (above)
  cemented sockets 1139, 1153–4
  rheumatoid arthritis 1129
  septic 1154–5
low-friction (Charnley) 1098–9, 1100, 1109–10
low-frictional torque (LFA) 1098–9, 1100, 1109–10
lubrication 184, 1110, 1115
  biomechanics 1109–10
  historical issues 1098
materials used for 188, 189, 190, 1098, 1099, 1100, 1139
  ceramics 1119–20
  highly cross-linked polyethylene 1101, 1116, 1117
  metal alloys 1118
  oxidized zirconium 1118
  Oxinium-on-polyethylene 1118
  PMMA 1099, 1120, 1139
  polyethylene see polyethylene
  PTFE 1098, 1099, 1109
  range of combinations used 190
  Teflon 1099
  UHMWPE 190, 1099, 1119
  see also individual materials
medialization of socket 1108, 1110
metal-on-metal (MOM) 1098, 1101, 1109, 1110, 1118–19, 1254
  history 1098
  lubrication 1110, 1115
  problems 1101, 1118, 1119
  wear 1118, 1119
minimal incision surgery/mini-invasive 1147–52
  decision-making 1150
  evidence supporting use 1148
  one-incision approach 1149

hip arthroplasty (total) – *continued*
  minimal incision surgery/
    mini-invasive – *continued*
      parameters for defining 1147
      randomized trials 1148
      recommendations 1149–50
      supplemental technology 1149
      techniques 1148–9
      two-incision approach 1148–9
  number per annum 1127, 1153
  osteoarthritis 1127–8, 1129
  osteolysis 1116, 1117, 1118, 1153, 1154
  osteopetrosis 1130
  outcome 1114, 1142–3
    functional 1143
  Paget disease 1130
  pain control 1124
  perioperative aspects 1123–34
    general considerations 1123–7
    in specific conditions 1127–30
  periprosthetic fractures 1155–6
  pre-operative assessment 1136
  primary 1135–46
  prostheses
    ABG 1101, 1121
    anatomic medullary locking 1140
    bone scan 157
    design 1108, 1120–1
    development, history 1098–101
    Furlong 1101, 1121
    history 1098
    hybrid 1101
    Judet Perspex 1098, 1116
    Landos–Corail system 1101
    McKee–Farrar 1110
    Omnifit 1101
    Porous-Coated Anatomic (PCA) 1142–3
    removal, in revision surgery 1157–8
    Smith-Peterson 1116
    sockets 1139–40
    stems 1138–9
    see also acetabular component; acetabular cups; femoral component (hip replacement); femoral stem (implants)
  range of motion 1108–9
    hip resurfacing *vs* 1109
  recent developments 1101–2, 1110
  resurfacing *see* hip resurfacing
  revision *see* revision hip arthroplasty
  rheumatoid arthritis 1128–9
  'soft-on-hard' 1118
  squeaking 1098, 1120
  stability and 1108–9
  success, factors affecting 1114
  surgical approaches 1136–8
    anterior 1136–7, 1149
    anterolateral 1136, 1137, 1149
    posterior 1136, 1137, 1149
    transgluteal (Hardinge) 1138, 1149
    transtrochanteric 1099, 1137–8
  surgical planning 1136
  templating 1136
  thromboprophylaxis 1126–7
  trends 1143
  types 1114–15
  uncemented 1101, 1102, 1120–1, 1138–40, 1140–2
    aseptic loosening 1154
    cemented arthroplasty *vs* 1142
    design principles 1140–2
    development 1100–1
    osteopetrosis 1130
    outcome 1142–3
    Paget disease 1130
    porosity/roughness for 1121
    rheumatoid arthritis 1129
    sockets 1140–1
    stems 1140
    technique 1142
    see also acetabular cups; femoral stem (implants)
  USA *vs* Europe 1101
  wear 1101, 1114–15, 1117, 1118
    Charnley's low-frictional torque (LFA) 1110
    debris 1153
    low, benefits 1110
    osteolysis associated 1116, 1117, 1118, 1153, 1154

    polyethylene particles 1099, 1117, 1139, 1153–4
    stripe, on femoral head 1120
    types 1114–15
    see also wear, joint replacement/implants
  younger patients 1101–2, 1127, 1128, 1253–4
    longevity and survival 1254
  see also acetabular component; femoral component (hip replacement); hemiarthroplasty
hip centre registration, in CAOS 1518
hip dislocations 335–9
  anterior 338–9
    classification 338, 339
    clinical features and treatment 339
  arthroplasty in rheumatoid arthritis 1129
  athletes 776–7
  endoprosthetic reconstruction complication 943
  hip arthroplasty complication 1155
  in myelomeningocele 609–10
  paediatric assessment 539
  posterior 335–8
    classification 336, 337
    clinical evaluation 335
    complications 338
    with femoral head fracture 337–8
    with femoral neck fracture 338
    management guidelines 338
    mechanism of injury 335
    prognosis 338
    radiography 335–6
    treatment 336–8
    type I, treatment 336–7
    type II, III, and IV, treatment 337
    type V, treatment 337–8
  sciatic trunk injury 1304
hip disorders, in children 18, 642–62
  DDH *see* developmental dysplasia of hip (DDH)
  developmental coxa vara 651–2
  with myelomeningocele 609–10
  Perthes disease *see* Perthes disease
  proximal focal femoral deficiency 650–1
  slipped capital femoral epiphysis 656–9, 661–2
  transient synovitis *see* transient synovitis
  see also specific disorders
'hip pointer' 774
hip prostheses *see* hip arthroplasty (total), prostheses
hip resurfacing 190–1
  femoral neck fractures 1156
  implants for 190–1
  range of motion 1109
  young patients 1254
hip screws
  compression 351
  dynamic 347, 348
  intramedullary 349
  sliding 348
hip spica cast, developmental dysplasia of hip (DDH) treatment 648, 649
hip–knee–ankle–foot orthoses 968
Hippocrates 3, 1214
  shoulder dislocation reduction 299
histamine 145
histocompatibility antigens 147
  see also entries beginning HLA
history (orthopaedics) 3–7
  acute compartment syndrome 503–5
  anaesthesia 4
  antisepsis 4
  arthroscopy 712
  developments (1810-1950) 4–5
  early pioneers and founding fathers 3–4
  glenohumeral instability 1214–15
  hip arthroplasty 1097–104
    see also hip arthroplasty
  knee arthroplasty 1171–3
    unicompartmental 1187
  limb reconstruction 940
  modern orthopaedics 5
  rotator cuff tears 1207–8
  shoulder arthroplasty 1223
  technique development 5–6
  X-rays and imaging 155–6

history-taking 8–35
  elbow 11
  foot and ankle 26–7, 1484–5
  hip 17–18
  knee 22–3
  method 8–9
  shoulder 9, 1216
  spine 32
  see also specific conditions
hitchhiker thumb 552
HIV infection, haemophilia and 1092
HLA antigens (human leucocyte antigens) 147
HLA DR1 1084
HLA DR4 1084
  subtypes 1084
HLA-B27 1089, 1090
  juvenile idiopathic arthritis 590, 593
Hoffman's sign 33
Holland, Charles Thurstan 155
Holstein–Lewis pattern 263–4
Holstein–Lewis syndrome 308–9
homeobox (*HOX*) genes 545
Homer–Wright rosettes 903
homocysteine 1027
homocystinuria 92
hook of hamate fractures 756–7
Hooke's law 179
hormones
  abnormalities, SCFE association 657
  skeletal muscle and 704
'horn blower's sign' 10, 1209
Horner syndrome 617
'horseshoe abscess' 1312
Hospital Incident Command System (HICS) 244
hospital transfer, in trauma/polytrauma 234
host defence system 145
Hot Lights, Cold Steel (Collins) 1550
Hotchkiss injury 317
Howarth, Hugh 1099
Howship's lacunae 88
HQ (hamstring/quadriceps) ratio 213
α_2-HS glycoprotein 83
HSP90 129
Huckstep, Ronald L 6
Hughston's plica test 26
human cloning 143
human embryonic stem cells (HESC), cell lines 144
human genome, sequence 140
Human Genome Project 140, 141
humeral avulsion of glenohumeral ligaments lesion *see* HAGL lesion
humeral component
  anatomic total shoulder replacement 1230
  reverse shoulder arthroplasty 1231
humeral head 57, 303
  centre and intramedullary canal centre 1224
  offset 1224
  osteophytes 1228
  preparation, anatomic total shoulder replacement 1229–30
  radius and thickness 1223–4
  radius of curvature 1223–4
  removal, anatomic total shoulder arthroplasty 1227–8
  resurfacing 1256
  size, anatomic total shoulder arthroplasty 1228, 1229–30
  see also humerus, proximal
humeral head component, total shoulder replacement 1229–30
humeral head retractor 1220, 1221, 1229
humeral retrotorsion 1224
humeral retroversion 1224
humeral shaft *see* humerus, shaft
humeroradial articulation 57
humeroulnar articulation 57
humerus
  amputations 963
  anatomical neck, fractures 303, 304
  anatomy 56–7, 505, 1224
    blood supply 57
  capitellum
    fracture 313–14, 1558
    osteochondritis dissecans 753–4
  defects, glenohumeral instability 1214

  diaphyseal, fractures
    in children 486–7
    see also humerus, shaft fractures
  distal
    anatomy 311
    lateral approach to 60
    reconstruction 949
  distal, fractures 311–15
    bicolumnar 311, 312
    capitellum 313–14
    in children 487, 488–90
    in children, incidence 482
    classification 311
    clinical evaluation 312
    comminuted 312
    complications 313
    epicondylar 314, 490
    intercondylar 312
    lateral condyle, children 489
    mechanism of injury 312
    medial condyle, children 490
    radiography 312
    supracondylar *see* supracondylar fracture of humerus (SCH)
    transcondylar 313
    treatment 312–13
    trochlear 314
    Y-type 490
  epiphysis, preparation, reverse shoulder arthroplasty 1231
  Ewing's sarcoma 867
  fracture non-union, management 523, 525, 526
  greater tuberosity 53, 57, 303
    avulsion fracture 304
    fractures 304
    see also humerus, proximal
  lesser tuberosity 53, 57, 303
    in anatomic total shoulder replacement 1230
    fractures 304
    osteotomy 1227
    see also humerus, proximal
  neck–shaft angle 1224
  osteophytes 1228
  proximal 303
    fracture dislocation 304, 305
    metastases 926
    reconstruction 948–9
    tumour resection 948
  proximal, fractures 303–6, 1558
    classification 304, 1558
    clinical evaluation 303
    closed reduction 263
    complications 305
    four-part, treatment 305
    mechanism of injury 303
    minimally displaced 304
    paediatric 486, 487
    pathological 935
    radiography 304
    sites 303
    subcapital 486
    three-part, treatment 305
    treatment 304–5
    two-part, treatment 304
    valgus impacted 305
  shaft 57, 303
    anatomy 307
  shaft fractures 307–10, 1558
    birth trauma 488
    in children 486–7
    in children, incidence 482
    classification 308
    clinical evaluation 307
    closed reduction 263–4, 308
    complications 308–9
    mechanism of injury 307
    operative treatment 308, 309
    radiography 307
    treatment 308
  subluxation, posterior 1225
  supracondylar fracture *see* supracondylar fracture of humerus (SCH)
  surgical approaches
    anterior 58–9
    lateral 60
    posterior 58, 59
  surgical neck, fractures 303, 304
humoral immunity 147–8
Hunter, John 3–4
Hunter syndrome 574
Hurler syndrome 574

Hurricane Katrina, mass casualty management 245
Hutchinson fracture 329
hyaline cartilage *see* articular cartilage
hyaluronan (HA) 83, 545
hyaluronan binding region 1082
hyaluronic acid
　functions 1083
　intra-articular administration, osteoarthritis 1083
hydrocephalus 608
hydrochloric acid, bone resorption 87
hydrocortisone 129
hydrodynamic lubrication 1115
hydroxyapatite/hydroxyapatite coating 1041
　endoprostheses 943
　hip prostheses 1101, 1120–1
hydroxychloroquine, rheumatoid arthritis 1086
hypercalcaemia
　causes 93
　conditions with 93
　metastatic tumours 929, 932–3, 1059
　management 1061
hypercapnia 467
hyperlordosis 1049, 1050
　compensatory, in isthmic lysis 1050
hyperparathyroidism
　brown tumours 889
　primary 93
hypersensitivity 149–50
hypertonia 568
　cerebral palsy 599
hypertrophic and calcification zone, growth plate 544
hypertrophic chondrocyte defects 89, 547
hypertrophic zone 89
hyperuricaemia 1091
hypocalcaemia
　causes 93–4
　conditions with 93–4, 133
hypoglycaemia, in hip arthroplasty 1125
hyponychium 1287
hypoparathyroidism, primary/secondary 93
hypophosphataemic rickets, molecular pathogenesis 546
hypophosphatasia 94
hypotension
　hypovolaemic shock 236
　neurogenic shock in spinal cord injury 443
　'permissive' in polytrauma 237
hypothenar hammer syndrome 760
hypothermia, primary survey in trauma 236
hypothesis generation 40
hypothesis testing 39–40
hypothyroidism, SCFE association 657
hypotonia 568
hypovolaemic shock 236
　management 236
　neurogenic *vs* 443
　stages 236
hypoxia 467
hypoxia inducible factor-1 929
hysteresis 181, 182

I-band 108, 699
ibuprofen 129, 1081
Ideberg's classification 1557
idiopathic juvenile osteoporosis 95
idiopathic scoliosis 632–8
　adolescent *see* adolescent idiopathic scoliosis
　adult 1008, 1009, 1010
　infantile 633–5
　juvenile 635–6
　morbidity 633
IGF-1 (insulin-like growth factor 1) 546
IHH (Indian hedgehog gene) mutations 546
IHH (Indian hedgehog) proteins 545
iliac blood vessels 428
iliac crest
　apophysitis, athletes 777
　bone graft 1014
　contusion 774
iliac wing fractures 431–2
iliacus haematoma, spontaneous 71

iliofemoral approach, extended, acetabular fracture fixation 423, 424
iliofemoral ligament 69, 70, 772–3, 1106
iliohypogastric nerves 429
ilioinguinal approach, acetabular fracture fixation 423, 424
ilioinguinal nerve 429
iliolumbar ligament, anatomy 66
iliopsoas bursitis 775
iliopsoas muscle
　action and function 956
　anatomy 69
　power, assessment 19
　strains 775
iliopsoas tendon, snapping 775–6
iliosacral screws 433
iliotibial band, snapping 776
iliotibial band syndrome, Noble compression test for 21
ilium 69, 1105
　anatomy 773
Ilizarov, Gavriil Abramovich 5–6
Ilizarov frame 196
　construction 528
Ilizarov's method 528
　for deformity after fracture malunion 528
imageless registration, computer-assisted surgery 1513
imaging 155–72
　see also individual disorders; individual modalities/techniques
immobilization
　postoperative, in DDH 649
　see also casts/cast immobilization
immune deficiency 958
immune system
　adaptive 145, 147–8
　　hypersensitivity 149–50
　　oncology and 1068
　　see also cell-mediated immunity
　innate 145–7
immunoglobulin(s), classes/structure 148
immunoglobulin A (IgA) 148
immunoglobulin D (IgD) 148
immunoglobulin E (IgE) 145, 148
immunoglobulin G (IgG) 148
immunoglobulin M (IgM) 148
　rheumatoid factor 1085
immunology 145–50
immuno-oncology 1068–9
immunopathy, diabetic foot 1466
　examination 1468–9
immunosuppression, in transplants/bone grafts 149
immunotherapy, tumours 1068–9
impaction bone grafting 1158
　acetabular reconstruction, revision arthroplasty 1158–9
　femur 1160–1
　　cemented 1161
　raw material source 1158
　reverse reaming method 1158
impingement sign (Neer's) 10, 742, 1208, 1209
impingement test
　ankle 838
　subtalar soft-tissue impingement 839
implants
　fixation 194
　hip *see* hip arthroplasty (total)
　infected
　　acute/chronic osteomyelitis 222
　　management algorithm 222
　knee *see* knee arthroplasty
　materials for *see* biomaterials, synthetic; metals (for implants)
　mechanical testing 198–9
　metallic, pyogenic spinal infections and 985
　spinal *see* spinal implants
　wear and wear debris 194
　see also joint replacement; prostheses; *specific implants/joints*
imprinting 151
in extremis patients, after trauma 238, 240, 241
in situ fusion, congenital spine deformities 631, 632
incidence 37–8
　cumulative 37
　prevalence comparison 37–8

incidence rate, and calculation 37
Incident Command System (ICS) 244
index–thumb pinch 1295
Indian hedgehog gene (*IHH*) mutations 546
Indian hedgehog (IHH) proteins 545
Indian hedgehog/PTH-related peptide pathway 91
indometacin 1091
induced growth arrest, leg length discrepancy treatment 681
induced pluripotent stem cells (IPSCs) 1526
inertia 176
　moment of 177
　rotational 177
infantile cortical hyperostosis (Caffey disease) 96, 547
infantile flat foot 691
infantile idiopathic scoliosis 633–5
infantile-onset tibia vara 670, 671
infants
　hip examination 539
　proximal femur injuries 493
　see also children; neonates
infections (musculoskeletal) 219–27
　amputations for 959
　antibiotic choice for 220
　bone *see* osteomyelitis
　diabetic foot 1466
　endoprosthetic reconstruction complication 943
　fracture healing affected by 518
　　active infections 521
　　management 223, 520, 521
　　quiescent infections 521
　　treatment 520
　hand *see* hand, infections
　joint *see* septic arthritis
　juvenile idiopathic arthritis triggers 590
　MRI scans 164, 171
　olecranon bursitis 1389
　open injuries of limbs 253
　risk factors 253
　rotator cuff repair complication 1214
　soft-tissue *see* soft-tissue infections
　spine *see* spinal infections
　tibial plafond fractures 385
　total hip arthroplasty *see* hip arthroplasty (total)
　total knee arthroplasty 1172, 1198
　see also specific infections
infectious arthropathies 1092
inferential statistics 43–4
inferior drawer test 11
inferior geniculate artery 77
inferior glenohumeral ligament (IGHL) complex 730, 735, 1215
　anterior band (AIGHL) 1215, 1221
　in open anteroinferior capsular shift 1220
　posterior band (PIGHL) 1215, 1220
inferior gluteal artery 79, 773
inferior gluteal nerve 79
inferior sulcus test 738
inferior tibiofibular joint 78
inflammation/inflammatory response
　Achilles tendon 831
　acute 147, 219
　after trauma 240
　cardinal signs 147, 219
　cartilage as contributor 1078
　chronic 145
　surgical strategy after trauma and 240
inflammatory arthritis
　foot/ankle 1485, 1493–7
　gadolinium contrast MRI 165
　young patients 1253
　see also rheumatoid arthritis; *specific types*
inflammatory cells, skeletal muscle injury 110
inflammatory mediators 1078
　release, muscle injury after exercise 704
　in synovial joints 1078
infliximab therapy, juvenile idiopathic arthritis 594
informed consent 1533, 1539–41
　children and 1532–3, 1540–1
　clinical trials and research 1541
　decision-making capacity 1532, 1533, 1540

disclosure 1540
documentation 1540
right to refuse treatment and 1540
specifics 1539–40
INFUSE Bone Graft 1014
inguinal hernia, pelvic fracture complication 434
inheritance
　mechanisms 150–1
　non-Mendelian 151–2
injury *see* trauma/injury
injury severity score (ISS) 233
　paediatric 500
innate immune system 145–7
innominate bones 69, 428
inorganic behaviour, Waddell's five signs of 35
Insall–Salvati index 667
inspection
　cervical spine 32
　elbow 11
　foot and ankle 27–8
　hand 15
　head, face and scalp 468–9
　hip 18–19
　knee 23
　lumbar spine 34
　shoulder 9–10
　thoracic spine 33
　wrist 13
instrumentation
　arthroscopy 712–13
　microsurgery 1319
　revision knee arthroplasty 1201
　spinal fusion with *see* spinal fusion
　see also specific procedures/instruments
instrumented 3D gait analysis *see* gait analysis
insulin 704
　actions 704
　resistance, muscle mass loss 121
　use by athletes 707
insulin sliding scale 1125
insulin-like growth factor 1 (IGF-1) 546
insulin-like growth factors (IGFs)
　growth plate control 91
　osteoarthritis treatment 1083–4
intent 1532
interbody fusion cage 196
intercalary structural allograft reconstruction 944
intercarpal interosseous ligament, injury grades 1356
intercondylar eminence avulsions 497
interdigital plantar neuroma 1500–2
interference fit and screws 194
interferons 147
　type I (IFN-α/β) 147
　　role in tumour immunotherapy 1069
　type II (IFN-γ) 147
interfragmentary strain theory 270, 518
interleukin-1 (IL-1) 1078, 1085–6
　inhibitors, rheumatoid arthritis therapy 1088
　osteoarthritis pathophysiology 1081
　subchondral bone erosion 1079
interleukin-1 (IL-1) receptor (IL-1R) 1088
　IL-1Ra 1088
interleukin-2 (IL-2), receptors, rheumatoid arthritis treatment 1087
interleukin-4 (IL-4) 1088
interleukin-6 (IL-6), rheumatoid arthritis pathophysiology 1086
interleukin-10 (IL-10) 1088
interlocking nails, fracture fixation *see* fracture fixation devices
interlocking screws 275
intermetatarsal angle, first–second 1436, 1437
internal iliac vessels 428
　somatic segmental branches 428, 429
internal rotation lag sign 1210
International Classification of Functioning, Disability and Health (ICF) 202, 203
international normalized ratio (INR) 130

International Nosology and Classification of Constitutional Diseases of Bone 549, 570, 571
interobserver reliability 39
interossei, lesser toes 1450
interosseous membrane (IOM), dorsal radial ulnar joint 1365, 1366
interphalangeal joint
 distal see distal interphalangeal (DIP) joint
 hallux, dislocation 416
 lesser toes, injuries 416
 proximal see proximal interphalangeal (PIP) joint
interpositional arthroplasty 1176
 hallux rigidus 1491
 hip 1097
 new techniques 1339
 resorbable 1340
 trapeziometacarpal osteoarthritis 1337, 1339, 1340
interpubic disc 428
intersection syndrome 761
interspinous ligaments 65, 976
intertrochanteric fractures (femur) 346–9, 1565
 classification 347
 clinical/radiological evaluation 346
 complications 349
 mechanism of injury 346
 mortality rates 346, 347
 reverse obliquity 347
 stable 347, 348
 treatment 347–9
  fixation failures 348
  implant choice/positioning 348
  reduction 348
intervertebral disc 105–7
 age-related changes 106–7, 993, 994, 995
 anatomy 66, 994
 calcification 1001
 cell density 1001
 cervical, disease see cervical disc disease
 degeneration 106–7, 995, 999
  biochemistry 1001
  lumbar 976, 977, 978
 degenerative disease see degenerative disc disease
 extracellular matrix 106
 functions 105, 106
 growth factor implantations 1005
 height reduction 995, 996, 998
 injury and healing 107
 low back pain 976
 lumbar 975
  degeneration 976, 977, 978
  herniation 107, 978, 996
  injuries, low back pain 978
  replacement 1003, 1004
 prolapse (herniation) 107, 993–4
  cervical see cervical disc disease
  decrease in size 1003
  isthmic spondylolisthesis 1050, 1051
  L4–L5 and L5–S1 996
  lumbar spine 107, 978, 996
  posterolateral direction 994
  prevention 107
  protrusion 996
  recurrent, rates 107
  sequestration 996
  thoracic 997
  types 996
 replacement devices 197
 resorption, in degeneration 997–8
 rupture 65
 size 105
 structure 105–6, 994, 1001
  see also annulus fibrosus; nucleus pulposus
 volume 994
intervertebral disc space
 inflammation 978
 lateral, foraminal 997
intracellular adhesion molecule 1 (ICAM-1) 1088
intracompartmental pressure (ICP) 278, 503
 continuous monitoring 511
 history 505

measurement 280, 505, 509–10
 distance from fracture 511
 methods 509–10, 511
 normal 505, 507
 raised 507–8
  chronic exertional compartment syndrome 825
  compartment syndrome 278, 503, 505, 507
  duration 507, 508
  effect on bone 508
  effect on muscle 507–8
  effect on nerves 508
  level indicating fasciotomy 280, 511
  magnitude 508
  threshold, variations 280, 508
  tibial shaft fractures 378
  variations in tolerance 511
 reducing, measures 281
 see also compartment syndrome, acute
intramedullary fixation/grafting, congenital pseudoarthrosis of tibia 676, 677
intramedullary hip screw 349
intramedullary nails/nailing 180
 elastic stable 486, 494
 for fracture fixation see fracture fixation devices
 knee arthrodesis 1272
intramedullary pins, fracture fixation 289
intramembranous ossification 543
intramuscular myxoma 920
intramuscular pressure
 compartment syndrome 507
 normal 507
intraoral examination 469–70
intra-osseous ganglia, hand 1377
intraspinal cysts, lumbar 979
involucrum 587
 definition 221
ionophoretic drug administration, morphine 127
iontophoresis 127
iridocyclitis, juvenile rheumatoid arthritis 1089
iron deficiency
 child athletes 708
 female athletes 708
irritable hip 660
ischaemia
 pathogenesis, in compartment syndrome 507
 see also muscle (skeletal)
 types 504–5
ischaemia time 1317
 cool 1317
 warm 1317
ischaemia–oedema cycle 504
 ischaemia types 504–5
ischaemic index 958
ischiofemoral ligament 772–3, 1106
ischium 69, 1105
 anatomy 773
isocentric contraction 955
isoinertial contraction 109
isokinetic contraction 109, 701
isokinetic testing, muscle strength 212, 213
isolated limb perfusion, chemotherapy 880
isometric contraction 701
isometric testing, muscle strength 213
isotonic contraction 109, 701
isthmic lysis 1048, 1049
 development, age effect 1049
 natural history 1051–2
 pathomechanism 1049–50
 spondylolisthesis see spondylolisthesis
 see also vertebral isthmus

J sign 26
Jahss classification, first MTP joint injuries 415
Jamshidi needle 886–7
jaw, wiring 476
jawbone
 replacement, endocultivation 1527–8, 1529
 see also mandible
Jeanne sign 1399

jerk test, knee 25
jersey finger (zone I injuries) 762, 1278–80, 1296
 chronic 762, 1280
 classification (type I-III) 1279, 1280, 1295
Jobe's test 10, 11
'jogger's foot' 1502
Johnson and Strom system, pes planus classification 1464
joint(s)
 arthrodesis see arthrodesis
 assessment, principles 202–3
 biomechanics see biomechanics
 control 207–11
  'six degrees of freedom' 207
  see also joint(s), stability
 deformity see specific joints
 disarticulation see specific joints
 formation 543–4
 infection see septic arthritis
 lubrication 101
  meniscus role 104
 movement see joint movement
 normal physiology 1077–80
 stability 207–11
  alignment correction (surgical) 209–10
  orthotic management 210
  rotational in coronal plane 208–10
  rotational in sagittal plane 208
  translational 211, 212
  transverse plane (knee) 210–11
 see also specific joints
joint depression type, calcaneal injury 399
joint disease, molecular markers 1082
joint movement 109, 204–7
 angular 204
 importance of assessment of control 207
 knee kinematics during gait 206–7
 linear 204
 importance of assessment of control 207
 during reaching task with hand 205–6
joint position sense (JPS) 214
joint reaction forces (JRFs), hip 1106, 1107
joint registries 1537
joint replacement 189–94
 fixation of implants 194
 in hand and wrist 192–4
 hip see hip arthroplasty
 implants see implants
 knee see knee arthroplasty
 metastatic tumours/pathological fractures 934, 935
 preclinical testing 197–9
 in rheumatoid arthritis 1087
 spinal 197
 synthetic biomaterials used in 188–9
 thromboprophylaxis, newer anticoagulants 132
 tribology of implants 194
 wrist see wrist, joint replacement
 young patients 1253–9
 see also arthroplasty
Jones, Robert 4, 155
Jones fracture, fifth metatarsal 846, 847
Judet Perspex prosthesis 1098
Judet's hemiarthroplasty 1098
Judet's lines, acetabular anatomy 420–1
jumper's knee 791
jumping distance, THA biomechanics and 1108
justice 1532
juvenile idiopathic arthritis (JIA) 589–95
 aetiology 589–90
 classification 589, 590
 clinical manifestations 591–3
 definition 589
 epidemiology 589
 laboratory findings 593–4
 pathophysiology 590
 prognosis and outcomes 595
 radiography 594
 treatment 594–5
juvenile idiopathic scoliosis 635–6
juvenile rheumatoid arthritis (JRA) 1088–9
 early-onset pauciarticular 1089

polyarticular 1089
 subtypes 1088
 therapy 1089

Kanaval's four cardinal signs 1312
Kapandji 'intrafocal' pinning 330
Keller's procedure 1439–40
keratan sulphate
 chondroitin sulphate ratio 1001
 elevated, osteoarthritis 1081
ketoacids 703
Kim lesion 735, 736
Kim test 735
Kim's biceps load test 740
kinaesthesia 214
kinematics 175
 measurement 175
 parameters for angular motion 175
 parameters for translational motion 175
 of a reaching task 205–6
 tibiofemoral joint 187
kinesiology 202–18
 joint movement see joint movement
 joint stability/control see joint(s), stability
 muscle 109–10
 muscle strength 211–13
 principles, open/closed kinetic chains 203–4
 proprioception 214–15
kinetic energy 176, 178
 open injuries of limbs and 247
Kingella kingae infection
 acute haematogenous osteomyelitis 582, 585
 septic arthritis 580
King's College Foot Classification 1467
Kirk Watson's scaphoid shift test 14, 15
Kirschner (K) wire 259
 acute scapholunate dissociation repair 1357
 DIP joint fixation 1347
 distal femoral fractures 495
 distal radius fractures fixation 329–30, 491, 492, 493
 DRUJ injury repair 1368
 lateral condyle fractures (distal humerus) 489
 mallet finger treatment 1281–2
 olecranon fracture fixation 319
 paediatric fractures 486
 subacute scapholunate dissociation repair 1358
 supracondylar fractures of humerus 489
KIVAplasty 1034, 1038
Klebsiella, reactive arthritis to, ankylosing spondylitis 1090
Kleiger's test 30
Kleinert method, modified 1297
Kleinman shear test (shuck test) 15
Klein's line, slipped capital femoral epiphysis 657–8
Klumpke palsy 54, 615, 616
knee 807–8
 adduction moment 209
 alignment 667, 668, 1260, 1261
  correction (surgical) 209–10
 amputations
  above-knee 962, 1470
  below knee 961–2
  through-knee 962
 anatomy 75–7, 665–6
  lateral side, anatomic layers 812–13
  ligaments 665, 805–6, 807, 812–13
  neuromuscular 76–7
  osteology 75–6, 666
 arthrodesis 1255, 1268, 1271–2
  approaches and fixation 1272
 arthroscopy see arthroscopy
 biomechanics 186–7, 665–6
 braces/bracing 212
  trial before revision arthroplasty 1200
  valgus 210
 cartilage injury 788–91
  autologous chondrocyte implantation 790–1
  microfracture technique 789
  osteochondral autograft/allograft 790

cartilage loss, microfracture
    technique for 789
in children
    normal alignment 667, 668
    observational gait analysis 566
clinical examination 22–6
    inspection and palpation 23
    movement 23
compressive load through, meniscus
    role 104
constant friction (prosthesis) 965
coronal mechanical/anatomic axes
    1181, 1182
defects, management in TKA 1183
disarticulation 962
dislocations 365–7, 813–15
    arterial injury 365
    classification 366, 814
    clinical evaluation 365–6, 815
    complications 367
    congenital 664–5
    mechanism of injury 365, 366
    neurological injury 814
    posterolateral 366, 814
    posterolateral corner injuries
        812
    radiography 366, 814
    rotatory 366, 814
    sports-related 813–15
    treatment 366–7, 665, 815
    vascular injury 365, 366, 814
    see also patellar dislocation
disorders in children 664–71
    Blount disease 670–1
    with cerebral palsy, management
        603–4
    congenital dislocation of knee
        664–5
    genu valgum 667–70
    genu varum see genu varum
    with myelomeningocele 610
    patellar dislocations 665–7
    see also specific disorders
effusion 23
    examination 23–4
extension contractures,
    myelomeningocele 610
extension gap 1183
extensor mechanism
    anatomy 370
    injuries 370, 791–6
flexion 104
flexion contractures,
    myelomeningocele 610
flexion deformity, in TKA 1183
flexion gap 1183, 1184
floating, femoral shaft fractures and
    356
fluid-control (prosthesis) 965
forces across, in gait 957
fractures around 1566
    in children 495
    see also specific bones
in gait 955
'giving way' 23
hemiarthroplasty 1172
history-taking 22–3
hyperextension 1260
    congenital 665
infectious arthritis, model 1092
injury 23
    intra-articular bleeding 102–3
instability 24
    anterolateral 24
    children 496
    intercondylar eminence avulsions
        497
    one-plane 24
    posterolateral rotatory 24
    revision arthroplasty for 1199
    rotatory 24
    symptoms 23
    testing 24
    TKA failure 1198
    unicompartmental knee
        arthroplasty exclusion 1190
    see also patellar instability
intra-articular injection of anaesthetic
    1200
joint line to subchondral bone pain
    ratio 1081
jumper's 791
kinematic analysis with computer
    navigation 1516–17

kinematics during gait
    angular displacement 206–7
    angular velocity 207
    unicompartmental arthroplasty
        1188
lateral compartment, loading 208,
    209
ligament injury
    in knee dislocation 365, 366
    sports-related 805–20
    see also specific ligaments
locking 23
loose bodies 783, 784
malalignment
    correction (surgical) 209–10
    osteoarthritis 1261
    TKA failure 1198
    unicompartmental knee
        arthroplasty 1190
manual locking (prosthesis) 965
medial compartment
    excessive loading prevention 209
    loading 208, 209
    osteoarthritis 208–9
medial plica syndrome 783
meniscus see meniscus
Morel–Lavallée lesion (MLL) 426,
    795–6
movement, normal 23
multiligamentous injury see knee,
    dislocations
non-ligamentous injuries 782–804
    cartilage injury 788–91
    extensor mechanism 370, 791–6
    meniscus injury 785–8
    pigmented villonodular synovitis
        784–5
    plicae 783
    sports-related 782–804
    synovial chondromatosis 783–4
    synovial disease 782–3
open/closed kinetic chain exercises
    204
osseous metaphyseal ligament
    ruptures 496
osteoarthritis see osteoarthritis
osteochondritis dissecans see
    osteochondritis dissecans (OCD)
osteotomy around see osteotomy
pain 22, 783
    anterior 22, 1193
    in hip pathology 1136
    persistent 1199
    physiotherapy 1200
pigmented villonodular synovitis
    784–5
    recurrence 785
plicae 783
polycentric (four-bar linkage) 965
'pop', extensor mechanism 370
posterior horn medial meniscus root
    tear 787–8
postoperative, MR arthrography 166
prosthetic 965–6
    characteristics 966
    see also knee arthroplasty
range of motion 186–7
reconstruction
    after trauma 1177
    for tumours 1177
    see also knee arthroplasty
recurvature 497
replacement see knee arthroplasty
septic arthritis 1092
single compartment degeneration
    1193
'six degrees of freedom' modelling
    207–8
stability 104, 208
    ACL deficiency, management 211
    alignment correction (surgical)
        209–10, 1262
    coronal plane during walking in
        OA 208–9
    orthotic management 210
    sagittal plane moments during
        walking 208
    screw home mechanism 208
    translational 211, 212
    transverse plane 210–11
stance-phase control (prosthesis) 965
stiffness
    after tibial plateau fractures 375
    revision arthroplasty for 1199

subluxation, congenital 664
surgery in children
    Blount disease 671
    congenital dislocation of knee 665
    genu varum/valgum 669–70
    patellar dislocation 667
    see also specific procedures
surgical approaches
    medial midvastus 1181
    medial parapatellar 1181
    medial subvastus 1181
swelling 22–3
symptoms 22
synovectomy 784–5
synovial disease 782, 784
synovial osteochondromatosis 783–4
synovium 782, 783
    plicae 783
in tibial plateau fractures 372
valgus deformity 498, 667–70, 1261
    measurement 207–8
    measurement errors due to internal
        rotation 207–8
    soft-tissue releases 1182–3
    see also genu valgum
valgus stress 805
valgus stress test 25, 806
variable friction (prosthesis) 965
varus deformity 667–70, 1261, 1262
    after distal femoral fractures 361
    osteotomy 1262
    realignment 209
    soft-tissue releases 1182
    tibial malunion 527
    see also genu varum
varus stress test 25
knee arthroplasty 191–2, 1515
    computer-assisted navigation
        1515–20
        disadvantages 1517
        operative technique 1517–20
        rationale for use 1517
    design of implants 191, 1172
        objectives for 1172
    development (history) 1171–5
        early 1171
        modern era 1172–4
        emerging trends 1174
    fixed bearing designs 191, 1179
        unicompartmental 1189
    implant choices 1177–80
    indications 1254
    infections 1172, 1198
    loosening 1172
        aseptic 1198, 1199
    materials used for implants 191–2
    megaprostheses 1202
    mobile bearing designs 191–2, 1179
        unicompartmental 1189
        young patients 1255
    movement after 1172
    pain persistence 1199
    patellofemoral see patellofemoral
        arthroplasty of knee
    prostheses 1177–80
        components 1177
        constraint 1179–80
        duopatellar design 1173–4
        Freeman–Swanson 1172, 1173
        fully constrained 1180
        Gluck 1171
        Gunston's design 1172, 1173
        Marmor 1173
        McKeever 1172
        semiconstrained 1180
        stems 1180
        tibial component see tibial
            component (knee
            replacement)
        total condylar 1173–4
        unconstrained 1180
        for unicompartmental arthroplasty
            1190
        varus–valgus constraint (VVC)
            1180
        Walldius 1172–3
    quad-sparing approaches for 1181
    radiography 1177–8
    revision see revision knee arthroplasty
    stability 1172, 1179–80
    total (TKA) 1176–85, 1515
        bony defects management 1183
        cemented vs cementless, young
            patients 1255

computer-assisted navigation
    1519–20
constraint 1179–80
contraindication 1177
effect on varus angle and adduction
    moments 209
extra-articular deformities and
    1182
failures, causes 1198
failures, management 1198
fixed vs mobile bearing 1179
flexion deformity 1183
flexion/extension gaps 1183, 1184
indications 1176–7
infections 1198
longevity/survival, young patients
    1255
malalignment 1182
for osteoarthritis 1176–7
for patellofemoral arthritis 1195
patellofemoral arthroplasty vs
    1195
PCL-retaining vs substituting 1178
for post-traumatic arthritis in
    young patients 1255
pre-operative assessment 1177–8
results 1184, 1187
scar 1189
surgical exposure/incisions 1181
surgical goals 1177, 1181
surgical planning 1177–8
surgical technique 1181–3
survivorship 1187
varus/valgus deformity 1182–3
younger patients 1187, 1254–5
unicompartmental (unicondylar)
    (UKA) 192, 1176, 1186–92
    contraindications 1082
    early development 1187
    early failures, reasons 1187
    fixed bearing design 1189
    future directions 1190–1
    implant designs 1187
    indications 1190
    Marmor 1187, 1188
    mobile bearing designs 1189
    in osteoarthritis 1081–2, 1186,
        1261
    prosthesis choice 1190
    re-emergence, reasons 1188
    results 1189–90
    scar 1189
    surgical technique 1187, 1190
    survivorship 1189–90
    trends 1261
    under-correction of alignment
        1188, 1189
    young patients 1255, 1261
    younger patients 1187, 1254–5, 1261
knee–ankle–foot orthosis 968
    Blount disease 671
    Duchenne muscular dystrophy 611,
        1477
    genu varum 669
knot tying, arthroscopic 713
Knutsson's sign 1001
Kocher–Langenbeck approach 423, 424
Kocher–Lorenz fragment 313
Kocher's approach
    to elbow 60–1
    shoulder dislocation reduction 299
Kreb cycle 702, 703
Kümmel–Verneuil disease see
    osteonecrosis (avascular necrosis),
    spine
Küntscher, Gerhard 5, 6
Küntscher nail 274–5
Kyle and Gustilo classification,
    intertrochanteric fractures 347
kyphoplasty 1017, 1018
    analgesic action 1018
    bone-preserving 1031, 1034, 1038
    complications 1018, 1038
    indications/contraindications 1038
    osteonecrosis of spine 1031, 1034,
        1039
    osteoporotic kyphosis 1017
    results 1038
    in spinal metastases 1066, 1067
    see also balloon kyphoplasty (BKP)
kyphosis 630
    adolescent postural 638, 640
    adult 1014–20
    definition 1014–15

Subject Index

kyphosis – continued
    examination for 33
    flat back syndrome 1018–19
    in isthmic lysis 1049
    myelomeningocele 609
    normal 1015
    osteoporotic deformity 1016–18, 1043
        kyphoplasty 1017, 1018
        pain in 1016
        surgical treatment 1016–18
        vertebroplasty 1017–18, 1035
    post-traumatic 1019–20
    post-tubercular 991
    postural 1016
    Scheuermann's see Scheuermann's kyphosis
    spinal tumours 1059
    thoracic 1015
        adult scoliosis 1011
        age-related increase 1016
        ankylosing spondylitis 1089
    thoracolumbar 1013
    tuberculosis 987, 988, 990, 991
    see also congenital vertebral anomalies; spinal deformities
kyphotic decompensation syndrome 1018

labrum see acetabular labrum; glenoid labrum
lacerations
    finger and palm 1278–80, 1283
    fingertip 1288
    nail bed 1288
    nerve 1302
lacertous fibrosus, compartment syndrome and 505
lacertous fibrous fascia, biceps tendon 505
Lachman's test 25, 807, 808
lactate threshold 704
lactic acid
    accumulation 702
    tumour cells producing 929
lactic acidosis 703
lacuna 86
lag screws see fracture fixation devices
lag sign 1209
lag test 10, 1209
lambda ratio (λ ratio) 1115
Lambotte, Albin 5
lamellae
    annulus fibrosus 994
    bone 85, 885
laminectomy
    degenerative disc disease 1003
    pyogenic spinal infections and 985
    in spinal metastases 1067
laminoplasty 1003, 1004
laminotomy 1003
Lane, William Arbuthnot 4
Langenskiold classification, Blount disease 670–1
Langerhan's histocytic cells 890, 891
Langer's lines 1207, 1211
Laplace's law 506
Lasègue's sign 21, 35
Lasègue's test, reverse 35
laser light therapy, lateral epicondylitis 1395
late-onset tibia vara 670
lateral collateral ligament (LCL) (knee) 25, 813
    diagnosis 813
    examination 25
        palpation 23
    functions 1262
    laxity, osteotomy for 1262, 1263
    in meniscal repairs 786
    treatment 813
lateral collateral ligament (LCL) complex (elbow) 57, 1383
    anatomy 1383
    biomechanics 1388
lateral corticospinal tract 66–7
lateral elbow tendinopathy 1389
    see also lateral epicondylitis (tennis elbow)
lateral epicondylitis (tennis elbow) 750–1, 1389–97
    basic science 1390
    causes 750, 1390
    differential diagnosis 1392
        PIN syndrome vs 13, 1392

epidemiology/incidence 750, 1389–90
examination 11, 750, 1391–2
history-taking 1391
investigations/imaging 1392
management 750–1, 1391–2
pain 750, 1391
pathogenesis 1390
provocation tests 12–13, 750, 1391–2
repetitive microtrauma 1391
resistant/treatment failure
    arthroscopic treatment 1397
    surgery for 1395
return to sport 1394
stages 1391
terminology 1389
treatment 1393–7
    aims/treatment concepts 1393
    arthroscopic debridement 1397
    guided rehabilitation programme 1393–4
    non-operative 1393–5
    open surgical technique 1396
    physical therapy protocol 1394
    surgery indications 1395
    surgical 1395–7
lateral femoral cutaneous nerve 71, 74, 429, 773
    entrapment 775
    injuries, in pelvic fractures 435
lateral ligament reconstruction, ankle arthritis 1487
lateral ligamentous instability see under ankle
lateral malleolus 76, 1500, 1518
    examination 28
    fractures, treatment 389
    'snapping' over 27
    total ankle replacement 1243, 1246
lateral pivot-shift test 13, 755
lateral plantar nerve 79, 1500, 1504
    entrapment 847–8, 1504–5
        aetiology/pathology 847–8
        evaluation/treatment 848
lateral process fractures 396
lateral spinothalamic tract 66
lateral talus–first metatarsal angle (Meary's) 1422, 1461
lateral ulnar collateral ligament (LUCL) 57, 1383
    injury 754
    insufficiency, as 'essential lesion' 1383
lateral wedging, of foot, in knee osteoarthritis 210
lathyrism 1078
Lauge-Hansen classification, ankle fractures 387, 388, 1567
lavage, open injury wounds 254
'lawn tennis arm' 1389
laxity see ligamentous laxity
laxity tests, shoulder 11
Le Fort classification 473
Le Fort fractures 470, 471, 473
    clinical signs 473
    Le Fort I fractures 474, 476
        treatment 476, 477
    Le Fort II fractures 474
        treatment 477
    Le Fort III fractures 474
        treatment 477
'leading elbow' technique 1394
lean body mass, age-related decline 121
leash of Henry 13, 1384
Ledderhose disease 918, 1326
Leddy and Packer classification 1562
LeForte–Wagstaffe fracture 388
leg
    anatomy 75–7
        blood supply 77
        nerves 76–7
        neuromuscular 76–7
        osteology 75–6
    compartment releases 76
    compartments 278, 279, 511
    disorders in children 673–85
        congenital pseudarthrosis of tibia 675–7
        limb length inequality see leg length discrepancy (LLD)
        torsional/bowing deformities of tibia 673–5
    exercise-induced pain 821–9
    'heavy' 978

lengthening after fractures 528
muscles 76–7
sports injuries see sports injuries
tendon problems in athletes 829–36
see also lower limb
leg holder, arthroscopy, cautions 713, 714
leg length
    examination/assessment 18–19, 536–7
    fractures affecting 528
    inequality see leg length discrepancy (LLD)
    'true', measurement 18, 19
leg length discrepancy (LLD) 18–19, 528, 677–84, 950
    aetiology 678
    assessment/imaging 678–9
    gait alterations 31, 567
    prediction 679–80
    treatment 680–4
        leg-shortening procedures 681–2
        limb-lengthening procedures see leg-lengthening procedures
        orthoses 680
Legg–Calvé–Perthes disease 776
leg-lengthening procedures
    achondroplasia 556–7
    acute lengthening 683
    congenital posteromedial bowing of tibia 675
    gradual lengthening 683–4
    leg length discrepancy 682–4
    proximal focal femoral deficiency 651
    stimulation of natural growth 683
leg-shortening procedures 681–2
leiomyosarcoma 880, 919
lesser metatarsophalangeal joint, osteoarthritis 1492
lesser sciatic foramen 70
lesser toes
    anatomy 1449–50
    crossover second toe 1455–6
    deformities 1450–60
        bunionette 1454–5
        examination 1450–1
        history-taking 1450
        initial assessment 1450–1
        investigations 1451
        mallet 1454
        see also claw toe; hammer toe
    dynamic stabilization 1449–50
    extrinsic muscles 1449–50
    fifth
        congenital overlapping 1456–7
        congenital underlapping 1457
    flexion deformities 1450
    fourth, congenital short 1457
    interphalangeal joint injuries 416
    intrinsic muscles 1450
    MTP joint injuries 415
    PIP joint, arthrodesis 1271
    range of movement 1451
lesser trochanteric fractures 349
lesser tuberosity see humerus, lesser tuberosity
Letournel's column concept 419, 420
leucocytosis, pyogenic spinal infections 983–4
leukaemia 95, 583
levator ani muscle 429
levels of evidence (LOE) 1545–8
Levine and Edwards' modification 452, 1555
levodopa therapy 1481
Lhermitte's sign 33
lidocaine 129
Li-Fraumeni syndrome 149, 901, 913
    breast cancer 930
    osteosarcoma 901, 913, 930
lift-off test (Gerber's) 10, 1210
ligament(s) 110–14
    attachment to bone 111
    blood supply 111
    function 110–11
    healing 113
    injuries 112–13
        children 484
        MRI scan use 169, 171
        see also specific ligaments
    MRI appearance 161, 168
    structure 111
    tears 183
    weakest zones 113

Young's modulus 179
see also specific ligaments
ligamentotaxis 327
ligamentous laxity
    generalized 738, 1215, 1216
        hallux valgus aetiology 1435
    joint instability vs 1216
    medial collateral ligament (knee) 807
    shoulder ligaments 730, 738
ligamentum flavum 65, 976
    hypertrophy 65, 999
ligamentum nuchae 65
ligamentum teres 772
    ruptured 779
limb
    lengthening see leg-lengthening procedures
    morphogenesis 542
    open injuries see open injuries, of limbs
    prolonged compression, compartment syndrome 279–80
    vascular injury, signs 248
    see also lower limb; upper limb
limb girdle muscular dystrophy 612
limb reconstruction 940–53
    after sarcoma resection 942–6
    assessment of limb function after 941
    biological 944–6, 951
    children 950–1
    see also allograft/allograft transplantation; autografts
    bone sarcomas 941, 942–6
    in children/adolescents 950–1
    distraction osteogenesis 946
    endoprosthetic reconstruction 942–3, 950, 951, 953
    see also endoprosthetic reconstruction
    historical perspective 940
    multidisciplinary team 941
    options 940–1
    regional 946–50
        distal femur 947–8
        distal humerus 949
        distal radius 949–50
        distal talus 948
        foot and ankle 948
        hand and wrist 950
        hip and proximal femur 947
        pelvis 946–7
        proximal humerus 948–9
        proximal tibia 948
        total femur 948
    soft tissue sarcomas 941, 951
limb replantation see replantation (upper limb)
limb salvage
    amputation vs, in open injuries 252–3
    predictive factors, diabetic foot 1470
    upper limb 964
limb-patterning defects 544–5
limb-sparing surgery
    amputation vs 942
    contraindications 942
    reconstruction after see limb reconstruction
    for sarcoma 941, 942
    stages 942
    surgical margins 942
limp, transient synovitis 660
line of progression, gait 565
Lineage acetabular component 190
linear acceleration 204
    of hand during reaching task 205–6
linear displacement 204
    of hand during reaching task 205
linear movement 204
    assessment of control 207
linear regression 44
linear velocity 204
    of hand during reaching task 205
liners
    hip prostheses 1109, 1117
        removal, in revision 1158
    lower limb prostheses 966, 967
lipogenic tumours 883
lipoma 912, 917
    atypical, hand 1375
    hand 1375
lipomatous tumours 917
    atypical 917
    limb-sparing surgery 942

liposarcoma 917
  chemotherapy 880
  hand 1377
  myxoid/round cell 917
  types 917
Lisfranc joint complex 407
  arthrodesis 1271
  homolateral type dislocation 409
  injuries 407
    indirect 844
  osteoarthritis 1489–90
  sprains 843–5
  see also tarsometatarsal (TMT) joint
Lisfranc joint line 403
Lisfranc ligament 78, 843
  injuries 843
  rupture 845
  sprain 844, 865
Lisfranc tarsal–metatarsal amputations 961
Lister, Joseph 4
Lister's tubercle 61, 1356, 1358
Little, William John 4
living wills 1540
load and shift manoeuvre
  anterior instability of shoulder 731
  posterior instability of shoulder 735
loading
  end bearing amputations 957, 958
  knee 208, 209
  normal, articular cartilage 1080
  skeletal muscle lengthening 109
  tendons 1292–3
    excessive 112
  see also biomechanics
local anaesthetics 129
  intra-articular, revision knee arthroplasty 1200
  mechanism of action 129
  side-effects 129
local stabilizing muscles, spine 979
locking plates, for fractures see fracture fixation devices
log-rolling 442, 445
long bone fractures
  ATLS management 239
  children
    frequency 482
    non-accidental injuries 500–1
  longitudinal growth of physes, children 482
  see also specific bones
long thoracic nerve, injury 54
longitudinal septa 89
loose bodies
  ankle 716, 1245, 1486
  elbow 11, 317, 716, 752, 753, 754, 1392
  hip 778, 779
  knee 783, 784
  shoulder 714
  wrist 1335
loosening, implants see aseptic loosening; specific arthroplasties
lordosis 1015
  age-related loss 1016
  normal 1015, 1018
  see also lumbar lordosis
loss modulus (E″) 182
low back pain (LBP) 975–81
  ankylosing spondylitis 1089, 1090
  degenerative disc disease and 993
  history-taking and symptoms 32
  lumbar spine injuries 976
    acute soft-tissue injuries 978–9
    bone 977–8
    intervertebral disc 978
    intraspinal cysts 979
    muscle strain/sprains 978
    nerve 978
    paravertebral musculature 978–9
  non-specific 976
  pain generators 976, 1002
  prevalence/incidence 975, 993
  'red flag' symptoms 32
  see also back pain
low-energy injuries, skull fractures 478
lower extremity screen, paediatric patients 536–8
  with cerebral palsy 600–1
lower limb
  after acquired brain injury, management 969
  alignment, angles 1260, 1261

amputation levels 960–2
  see also amputations
anatomy 773
clinical examination see clinical examination
dermatomes 773
flexibility, paediatric assessment 538
fractures 1563–8
  non-union, fixation 521
injuries in children 499
innervation 79
ligamentous dysfunction 1262–3
myotomes 18
normal alignment 667, 668
open/closed kinetic chain 204
prostheses see prostheses
reconstruction see limb reconstruction
temporary arrest of growth, genu varum/valgum 669
weight-bearing line 1261, 1262, 1263
see also leg; specific anatomical structures
low-molecular-weight heparins (LMWHs) 131
  clinical use and side-effects 132
  in hip arthroplasty 1126, 1127
  in major joint replacements 132
  safety and use 131–2
  thromboprophylaxis 132
low-volume resuscitation, in polytrauma 237
Lubinus acetabular component 190
Lubinus SP II 190
lubrication 184, 1115
  hip arthroplasty (total) 1115
lumbar lordosis 65
  age-related loss 1016
  exaggerated, normal 34
  loss, flat back syndrome 1018–19
  normal 1015, 1018
lumbar nerve roots
  compression, tests for 34–5
  L4, injuries, pelvic ring injuries with 427
lumbar plexus 70–1, 429
  anatomy 429
lumbar spinal canal 996–7
  central 996, 997
    stenosis 999, 1000, 1002
    disc herniations and 997
  lateral 996–7, 998
    extraforaminal zone 997
    foraminal space 997
    stenosis 998, 1002
    subarticular zone 997
  stenosis 977–8, 998–9, 1000, 1002
    history-taking and symptoms 32
lumbar spine
  anatomy 65, 975–6
  cysts 979
  degenerative changes 976, 997–8
  discectomy 1003
  discs see degenerative disc disease; intervertebral disc
  distraction instrumentation, flat back syndrome 1018
  dynamic stability 976
  examination 34–5
  fusion 1013–14, 1268
    adult scoliosis 1013–14
    degenerative disc disease 1003
    see also spinal fusion
  gadolinium contrast MRI 165
  hyperextension 1049
  infections see spinal infections
  injuries
    bone injuries, pain 977–8
    disc 978
    low back pain 976, 978
    nerve 978
    paravertebral musculature 978–9
    sports injuries 977
    see also thoracolumbar spine injuries
  isthmic spondylolisthesis 1050, 1051, 1052
  L4–L5, collapse 1008
  L5, sports injury 977
  ligaments 976
    injuries 978–9
  lordosis see lumbar lordosis
  movements 34
  muscular pain 976

pain generators 976, 1002
  see also low back pain (LBP)
repetitive hyperextension 977
scars vs disc detection, gadolinium contrast MRI 165
scoliosis 1010
special tests 34–5
spinal cord 976
spinal cord injury 440
sports injuries 977
static stability 976
stenosis see lumbar spinal canal, stenosis
stiffness 17
structure/function 975–6
surgical approaches
  anterior (transperitoneal) 68, 69
  anterolateral (retroperitoneal) 69
  posterior 69
vertebral body infections 983
see also thoracolumbar spine
lumbosacral plexus 70, 429
  sports-related nerve entrapment 775
lumbosacral spine, fusion 1003, 1012–13
lumbricals 1450
lumican 101
lunate
  damage, scapholunate ligament dissociation 1357
  dislocation 1351, 1360–1
  in four-corner fusions 1359
  instability around 1352
lung, apical tumour 1399
lung carcinoma 927, 930, 934
lunotriquetral ballottement test (Reagan test) 15, 1359
lunotriquetral instability 1359–60
  causes, and diagnosis 1359
  testing 15, 1359
  treatment 1360
lunotriquetral (LT) ligament 1351
  injury 1359, 1360
  reconstruction 1360
  tears 1359, 1360
lunula (nail) 1287–8
luxatio erecta 301
Lyme disease 1084
lymphoid organs 145, 1068
lymphoma 907–8
  high-grade B-cell 907–8
  T-cell 908
lysosomal storage disorders 549, 574

M line 108
Macewen, Sir William 4
Mc/Mac names see entries beginning Mc
macrophage 145
macrophage activation syndrome (MAS) 593
macrophage colony-stimulating factor (M-CSF) 1025
Maffucci's syndrome 546, 575, 896, 1378
magnetic resonance arthrography (MRA) 166, 735–6
magnetic resonance imaging (MRI) 160–71
  artefacts 161–2, 168
    bloom artefact 868
    susceptibility 161, 162
  fat saturation 161
  gadolinium contrast agents 163–6
    arthrography 166
    intravenous 163–5
    tumours 868
  gradient echo (GRE) sequence 161
  hardware for 160
  'high field strength' machines 160
  history 156
  image analysis 166
  imaging planes 160
  musculoskeletal tissue appearance 161, 166–9
  principles 160–1
  pulse sequences 161
  short tau inverted recovery (STIR), osteoporotic fractures 1027, 1028
  specific conditions/injuries
    Achilles tendonopathy 832–3
    ACL injuries 808, 809
    acute haematogenous osteomyelitis 584
    adult scoliosis 1010

ankle soft-tissue impingement 838
ankle/foot arthritis 1485
cervical spine hyperextension 446
congenital vertebral anomalies 631
developmental disorders of bone 554
glenohumeral arthritis 1224–5
glenohumeral instability 1217
infantile idiopathic scoliosis 635
isthmic spondylolisthesis 1051
juvenile idiopathic arthritis 594
juvenile idiopathic scoliosis 636
lesser toes 1451
medial epicondylitis 1393
medial tibial stress syndrome 824
musculoskeletal applications 169, 171
osteoarthritis 1081
osteochondral lesions of talus 837
osteoporotic fractures 1028
patellar dislocation 667
patellar tendon rupture 791
PCL injury 812
pigmented villonodular synovitis 162, 784, 918
posterior instability of shoulder 735–6
pyogenic spinal infections 984, 986
revision knee arthroplasty 1200
rotator cuff tears 1210
scaphoid fractures 755
septic arthritis in children 580, 583
soft-tissue sarcoma 913
spinal cord injuries 444
spinal tuberculosis 988
spinal tumours 1060
synovial chondromatosis (knee) 784
thoracolumbar spine injuries 460
tibial stress fractures 822–3
tumours 868–9, 1060
ulnar collateral ligament rupture 752
wrist injuries 1354
surface coil 160
T_1 and T_2 161
T_1-weighted sequence 161, 162, 163, 166, 167
  tumours 868, 869
T_2-weighted sequence 161, 162–3, 166, 167
  tumours 868
tissue characterization 161, 166–9
Maisonneuve fracture 387
major histocompatibility complex (MHC) 1084
  class I loci 1084
  class II loci 1084, 1087
  class III loci 1084
  inflammatory arthropathies and 1084
  see also entries beginning HLA
Malgaigne fracture 1563
malignant fibrous histiocytoma (MFH) 904
  hand 1377
  pleomorphic 919
malignant melanoma see melanoma, malignant
malignant peripheral nerve sheath tumour (MPNST) 913, 920–1
  hand 1377
malleolar fractures 386
  bimalleolar 389–91
  classification and mechanism 387
  isolated lateral/medial, treatment 389
  trimalleolar (Cotton) 391
malleolus see lateral malleolus; medial malleolus
mallet finger 762–3, 1280–2, 1299–300, 1562
  biomechanics 1299–300
  causes and mechanism 1280–1
  chronic 1282
  classification/types 1281, 1300
  treatment 1281
mallet toe 1454
malnutrition, muscle wasting, age-related 122
malocclusion, mandibular fractures 470
mandible
  exposure, for fracture fixation 477
  replacement, endocultivation 1527–8, 1529

mandibular fractures 469, 472–3
  clinical signs 472
  condylar neck 470, 477
  condylar process 473
  in children 477
  direct/indirect 473
  malocclusion in 470
  reduction and fixation 476
  sites 472, 473
  treatment 476–7
Mangled Extremity Severity Score (MESS) 252, 253
manipulative therapy, congenital clubfoot 690
Mann–Whitney U-test 44
marble bone disease (osteopetrosis) 96
Marfan syndrome 92
marine injuries, antibiotic treatment 220
Marmor prosthesis 1173
  unicompartmental 1187, 1188
Maroteaux–Lamy syndrome 574
Mason's classification, radial head fracture 319, 320, 1559
mass, definition 175–6
mass casualty, definition 244
mass casualty management 244–6
  checklist/elements in 245
  command personnel/systems 244–5
  critical mortality rate reduction 245
  planning, importance 245
mast cells 145
  degranulation 145, 147
material(s)
  biocompatible 188
  cyclical deformity 182
  damage due to stress 182
  elastic 178–80
  fatigue 183
  fracture 182–3
  friction 183–4
  mechanical properties see mechanical properties
  strong, or tough 183
  viscoelastic 179, 181–2
  wear 184
  see also biomaterials
Matles' test 830
matrilin-3 548
matrix see extracellular matrix (ECM)
matrix extracellular phosphoglycoprotein (MEPE) 83
matrix Gla protein 83
matrix metalloproteinases (MMPs) 102, 1078, 1088
  Achilles tendinosis 1426
  inhibitors 102, 1088, 1426
  tendon healing 113
Matsen's unified concept, compartment syndrome 507
mattress sutures 1298, 1299
maturation zone, growth plate 544
maxilla, examination 470
maxillary sinus, zygoma fractures 474
maxillofacial bones 466
  osteomyelitis 471
maxillofacial fractures 471–2
  blow-out 472
  in bone atrophy 472
  closed/open 471
  complicated 471
  defects/missing bone fragments 472
  direct/indirect 472
  impacted 472
  modes 471–2
  pathological 472
  relation to overlying tissues 471
  see also Le Fort fractures
maxillofacial trauma 466
  clinical diagnosis 467–71
  incidence 466
maxillo-mandibular fixation 476, 477
Mazabraud syndrome 891
McAfee's classification, thoracolumbar spine injuries 460–3
McBride's procedure 1437
McCash incision 1328, 1329
McCash open palm technique 1329
McCune–Albright syndrome 891
McGowan's staging, cubital tunnel syndrome 1400–1
McKee–Farrar prosthesis 1110
McKee's classification, capitellum fractures 1559

McKeever prosthesis 1172
McMurray's test 26
MCP joint see metacarpophalangeal (MCP) joint
mean (statistics) 43
Meary's angle 1422, 1461
mechanical energy 178
mechanical factors, pathological gait 567
mechanical hysteresis 181
mechanical principles 173–8
mechanical properties, of materials 178–84
  bending and twisting 180
  elasticity 178–80
  flow 180–1
  viscoelasticity 181–2
mechanical testing, implant materials/devices 198–9
mechanobiology, fracture/bone healing 518–20
mechanoreceptors 214
  meniscus 104
  in proprioception 214, 215
  tendons 112
medial clear space, ankle 387
medial collateral ligament (MCL) (knee) 25
  ACL injury with 806, 807
  anatomy 805–6
  biomechanics 805
  chronic laxity 807
  healing 113
  imaging 806
  injury 24
    grades I, II and III 25, 806–7
    sports-related 805–7
  in meniscal repairs 786
  physical examination 12, 25, 806
  posterior oblique (POL) 805
  sprain 805
  superficial 805
  treatment 806–7
medial collateral ligament (MCL) complex (elbow) 57, 316, 1383
  anatomy 1383
  anterior bundle 1383
  biomechanics 1387, 1391
  microdamage, medial epicondylitis 1391
  posterior bundle 1383
  transverse ligament 1383
medial coronary ligament sprain 26
medial deltoid ligament, testing 30
medial displacement calcaneal osteotomy (MDCO) 1423
medial epicondylectomy, cubital tunnel syndrome treatment 1406–7
medial epicondylitis (golfer's elbow) 751, 1389–97
  basic science 1390–1
  causes 1390
  differential diagnosis 1392–3
  epidemiology 1390
  examination 12, 751, 1392
  history-taking 1392
  investigations/imaging 1393
  management 1392–3
  pathogenesis 751, 1390–1
  pathology 1391
  provocation tests 13, 751, 1392
  repetitive microtrauma 1391
  return to sport 1394
  stages 1391
  treatment 751, 1393–7
    aims/treatment concepts 1393
    guided rehabilitation programme 1393–4
    non-operative 1393–5
    open surgical technique 1396–7
    physical therapy protocol 1394
    surgical 1395–7
medial femoral circumflex artery 71, 75
medial gap, DDH assessment 647
medial malleolus 1518
  evaluation, posterior tibial tendon pathology 835
  fractures, treatment 389
  surgical approach to 80
  in total ankle replacement 1245, 1246
medial myocutaneous flap 962
medial patellofemoral ligament (MPFL) 667, 793, 795
  reconstruction 795

medial plantar nerve 79
  entrapment 847–8
  tenderness 848
medial plica syndrome 783
medial slide calcaneal osteotomy 1423–4
medial tibial stress syndrome (MTSS) 824–5
median, definition 43
median nerve
  anatomy 58, 62, 505
    at elbow 1386
    branches 1386
  compression
    at elbow 1386
    in forearm 505
    see also carpal tunnel syndrome
  examination at elbow 12
  injuries, distal radius fractures 330
  neuropathy after distal radius fracture treatment 262
  testing 16
mediators
  inflammatory see inflammatory mediators
  tissue engineering 1527
medical coding 1537–8
medical ethics 1531–5
  applied principlism 1531–2
  applying 1532–3
  best interests 1533–5
  informed consent see informed consent
mediopatella plica test 26
Medoff bi-axial compression plate 348
Mehne and Matta classification, distal humeral fractures 311, 312
Meissner's corpuscles 215
melanoma, malignant
  ABCDE of 1376
  hand 1376
membrane attack complex (MAC)(complement) 145
Mendel, Gregor 150
Mendelian inheritance 150–1
Menelaus method 680
meniscectomy
  joint contact stress after 104
  partial, arthroscopic 713
meniscofemoral ligaments 811
meniscus 103–5
  allograft transplantation 105
  anatomy 103–4
  blood supply 103–4, 105
  nerve supply 104
  composition 103
  cysts 786
  examination/testing 26
  functions 103, 104
  healing 104, 105
    improving/developments 105
  injuries 785–8
    sports-related 785–8
  lateral 104, 785
    tears, repair 786
  mechanoreceptors 104
  medial 104, 785
    tears, repair 786
  medial posterior root injury 787–8
  pathology, arthroscopy for 713
  'red zone' 104, 105, 785
  'red–white zone' 104, 105, 785
  tears 104, 785, 786
    chronic 23
    healing 105
    inside-out repair technique 786
    MRI scan 171
    outside-in repair technique 786–7
    patterns 785
    repair 785–6
    repair techniques 786–7
    in 'white–white' zone 105
  ultrastructure 103
  'white zone' 104, 105, 785
  zones of vascularity 104, 105
mental exhaustion, as burnout manifestation 1551
MEPE (matrix extracellular phosphoglycoprotein) 83
Mepitel dressing 1329, 1330
meralgia paraesthetica 775
Merkel's discs 215
mesenchymal cells
  bone formation 88

chondral ossification 89
intramembranous ossification 88
mesenchymal stem cells, tissue engineering 1527, 1529
mesenchymal tumours 912
mesoderm 51
mesotenon 112
messenger RNA (mRNA) 140, 149
meta-analysis 40, 42
metabolic bone diseases 92–9
metabolic disorders
  cubital tunnel syndrome vs 1399
  developmental disorders 549
  see also specific disorders
metabolic syndrome 121
metacarpals
  anatomy 64
  base
    fractures 768
    resection 1341
  extension osteotomy 1339
  fifth, fracture 1561
  first, Bennett's fracture 763, 1561
  fractures 767
    comminuted 768
    metacarpal neck 767
    metacarpal shaft 767
    oblique and spiral 767–8
  ligaments attaching 1334
metacarpophalangeal (MCP) joint
  arthrodesis 1345
  arthroplasty 1343
    resection 1345
    revision 1345
  biomechanics 187
  Dupuytren's contracture 1325, 1327
  extensor tendon injuries 1283
  flexor tendons
    anatomy 1293
    rehabilitation 1297
  osteoarthritis 1333, 1343–5
  reconstruction 1343
  replacement, implants 193
  sports injuries 764
  testing 16, 17
Métaizeau technique, leg length discrepancy treatment 681
metal allergies 1119
metal alloys, implants 1118
metal artefact, CT scan 159
metal ions, hip arthroplasty 1119
metal-on-metal arthroplasty
  hip see hip arthroplasty (total)
  lubrication for 1110, 1115
metals (for implants) 188–9
  Young's modulus 188
metaphyseal arteries, blockage, pyogenic spinal infections 983
metaphyseal chondroplasia, Schmid type (MCDS) 548
metaphysis/metaphyseal
  bone tumours located in 886
  defects, revision knee arthroplasty 1201–2
  fractures 483
    distal femur 495
    distal tibial 156, 498
    femoral, non-union 523
    pathological, treatment 935
    proximal tibial 498
metastases
  definition, and biology 927
  lymph node, soft-tissue sarcoma 915
metastases (skeletal) 925–39
  assessment 930–1
  biology 927
  biopsy 931
  bone structure in 929
  chemotherapy 881
    adverse effects on bone 929
  classes 932, 933
  cortical 927
  fractures see pathological fractures
  haematogenous spread of tumours 927
  in hand/wrist 1380
  imaging
    MRI scan 171
    PET scans 869, 870
    radionuclide scans 157, 868
  management 926, 929–30
    ET-1 antagonist action 928
  medullary 927
  osteoblastic 927, 928–9

pathways/mechanisms 928–9
osteolytic 927–8, 930
patient groups/categorization 932, 933
primary tumours causing 926, 930, 1058, 1064, 1380
prognosis 925, 926, 931, 932
  effect on operative treatment 933, 934
  prediction of life expectancy 931
sites 926
  operative treatment and 935
soft-tissue sarcoma 915
solitary, operative treatment 935
spinal *see* spinal metastases
treatment 925, 932–6
  amputation 936
  non-operative 932–3
  operative 933–6
  tumour–bone interaction 927
of unknown origin 930
see also pathological fractures
metatarsal bones 78
amputations 961
base fractures 411, 412
fifth metatarsal, lateral bowing 1455
fifth metatarsal fractures 412–13, 846–7
  aetiology/pathology 846
  avulsion fracture 846
  evaluation 846–7
  spiral 413
  stress fractures 846, 847
  treatment 412–13, 847
  types/locations 846
  zone I 412
  zone II and zone III 412, 413
first metatarsal
  distal osteotomy 1437–8
  medial deviation 1435, 1447–8
  proximal osteotomy 1439
  shaft osteotomy 1438–9
  valgus tilt of distal articular surface 1435
first to fourth metatarsal fractures 411–12
  base, neck or shaft 412
  clinical/radiographic evaluation 411
  complications 412
  treatment 411–12
first–cuneiform joint, arthrodesis 1439
neck fractures 412
osteonecrosis 1438
osteotomy, hallux rigidus 1490
shaft fractures 412
stress fractures 411
see also hallux
metatarsalgia 27
metatarsocuneiform (MTC) joints, osteoarthritis 1489–90
metatarsophalangeal (MTP) angle, fifth 1455
metatarsophalangeal (MTP) joints
anatomy 414
examination 29
first joint/toe
  arthrodesis 1440
  capsuloligamentous disruption 1443–4
  congruence, classification 1435
  dislocations 415
  hyperextension 1443
  injuries 414–15
  lateral deviation 1434
  normal 1435
  osteoarthritis 1490–2
  resection arthroplasty 1439–40
  sesamoids *see* sesamoid bones (foot)
  static/dynamic stabilizers 1434
  stress fracture 848–9
  valgus deformity 1434–5
  see also hallux rigidus; hallux valgus
in gout 156
injuries 414–16
lesser toes 1449, 1450
  dislocations and fractures 415
  in hammer toe 1452
  hyperextension, claw toe 1452, 1453
  injuries 415
  osteoarthritis 1492

second toe
  crossover deformity 1455–6
  instability 1456
  stabilization 1449–50
metatarsus adductus 27, 30, 692
metatarsus primus varus 1435, 1436
methotrexate
  juvenile idiopathic arthritis 594
  rheumatoid arthritis 1086
methylprednisolone 129, 130
  spinal cord injury 445, 1479
meticillin-resistant *Staphylococcus aureus* (MRSA) 1126
  acute haematogenous osteomyelitis 582
  hip arthroplasty infections 1155
Meyerding classification, spondylolisthesis 1051
Meyers and McKeever classification 497, 1566
MGP gene 547
microbiology
  diabetic foot 1466
  hand infections 1309, 1310
microdiscectomy 1003
microfracture technique 789, 1083
  osteochondral lesions of talus 837
micro-RNA genes 149
Microsoft Health Vault 1537
microsurgery 1318–19
  blood vessel repair 1319
  hand/finger replantation 1318–19
  obstetric brachial plexus birth palsy 617
microsurgical equipment 1319
microvascular disease, fracture healing affected by 518
microvascular occlusion theory, compartment syndrome 507
midcarpal instability 1360
middle geniculate artery 77
middle glenohumeral ligament (MGHL) 730
midface, instability, Le Fort fractures, examination for 470
midfacial fractures 468–9, 473–8
  Le Fort classification 473
  in polytrauma 476
  reduction and fixation 476
  see also Le Fort fractures
midfoot
  anatomy 403, 404
  arthrodesis 409, 1489–90
  examination, arthritis 1485
  fractures 403–6
    classification 404
    clinical/radiographic evaluation 404
    complications 405
    tarsal navicular 405
    treatment 404–5
    see also Lisfranc joint complex injuries 404
  lateral/medial stress injury 404
  ligaments 403, 404
  longitudinal stress injury 404
  navicular dislocation 405
  osteoarthritis 1485, 1489–90
  pain 843–9
  plantar stress injury 404
  rheumatoid arthritis 1495
  sprains 404
  see also cuboid; cuneiform bones; metatarsal bones; navicular bone
midpalmar space, infections 1312
midtarsal joint (Chopart joint)
  amputation at 961
  anatomy 403
  movements 29
  see also calcaneocuboid joint; talonavicular joint
Milch technique, shoulder dislocation reduction 299
military
  mass casualty management 244
  medial tibial stress syndrome 824
  tibial stress fractures 821, 823
milking manoeuvre 752
milking test 1393
mineralization of bone *see under* bone(s)
miner's elbow *see* olecranon bursitis
'mini-Lachmann' test 1501

minimal invasive plate osteosynthesis (MIPO) 258
minimally invasive percutaneous plate osteosynthesis (MIPPO) 274
minimally invasive techniques
  chronic exertional compartment syndrome 826
  hip replacement *see* hip arthroplasty (total)
  kyphoplasty *see* kyphoplasty
  in spinal metastases 1067
  tumour debulking 1067
  vertebroplasty *see* vertebroplasty
miR-15a and miR-16-1 149
Mirel score 931–2
Mitchell osteotomy 1438
mitochondria, dysfunction, age-related 122
mitochondrial DNA 139
M-line 699
mnemonics
  ABCDE (trauma management) 234, 430
  AMPLE (secondary survey after trauma) 238
  CRITOL (ossification centres around elbow) 487, 488
  FALCON (neurofibroma) 1376
  PACES (gait assessment) 31
  SALTR (physeal fractures) 483, 484
  SNOW DROP (Southern/Northern blotting) 142
  TAN (elbow examination) 12
  TUBS and AMBRI shoulder instability 300
mobility, spinal cord injury determining 970
mode (statistics) 43
modern orthopaedic developments 6
Modic changes/signs 976
  bone marrow changes 999, 1000
  degenerative disc disease 999
molecular analyses, developmental disorders of bone 554, 556
molecular biology 139–45
Molloy's impingement test 1488
moment of inertia 177
moments (mechanics) 188
momentum 176
monocyte colony-stimulating factor (M-CSF) 87
monosodium urate crystals 1091, 1374
Montegia fracture 323–4, 325, 490
  Bado's classification 324
  children 490, 491
  treatment 324
Moore, Austin Talley 5
Moore approach, to hip 73, 74, 1137
Morel–Lavallee lesion (MLL), knee 426, 795–6
morphine 127
morphine analogues 127
morphogenesis
  limb 542
  skeletal 543–4
Morquio syndrome 574
mortality
  cervical spine injuries 446
  intertrochanteric fractures (femur) 346, 347
  pyogenic spinal infections 985
  trauma and polytrauma *see* trauma/injury
Morton, W.T.G. 4
Morton's neuroma 29, 78, 1500–2
  testing 30
Morton's test 1501
mosaicplasty 790, 1083
Moseley straight-line graph 680
motor end plate 700
motor neurone 108
  action potential 109, 1303
  degeneration, age-related 121–2
motor point 108
motor unit 108, 699–700
  action potential 213, 700
  depolarization 109, 213, 700
  loss, age-related 121–2
  size 699, 700
movement, kinesiology principles *see* joint movement; kinesiology
'movie theatre sign' 1193
'moving valgus stress test' 1387

MRSA *see* meticillin-resistant *Staphylococcus aureus* (MRSA)
mucopolysaccharidoses (MPS) 549, 573–4
mucosa-associated lymphoid tissue 145
mucous cysts
  hand/wrist/fingers 1374
  excision 1347
  toes 1458
  see also ganglion/ganglion cysts
Mulder's click sign 1501
Mulder's sign 29, 30
Müller, Maurice E 6
Müller classification
  distal femoral fractures 358, 359
  femoral neck fractures 342
Muller hip 190
multidisciplinary care/team
  achondroplasia 557–8
  diabetic foot 1466
  limb reconstruction 941
  oncology 874
multiple enchondromatosis 575, 896
multiple epiphyseal dysplasia (MED) 572–3, 653
multiple hereditary exostosis 574–5
multiple myeloma *see* myeloma
multiple organ dysfunction syndrome (MODS) 240
multiplier method 680
multipotent stem cells 1526
multivariate analysis 44
Munster socket 964
muscle (skeletal) 107–10
  action/electrical activity 213–14
  adaptation/training 703
  age-related changes 121, 122
  agonist 109, 122, 955
  in amputations 960
  antagonist 109, 955
    age-related changes 122
    balance between, HQ ratio and 213
    control of motion of body 185
  atrophy, age-related 122
  balance/imbalance
    hamstring and quadriceps 211, 213
    testing 213
  biomechanics 109–10
    age-related changes 121
  biopsy, muscular dystrophy 611
  blood supply 108
  central fatigue 705
  composition 107, 697–8
  contractile proteins 108, 699
  contraction 107, 109, 699–700, 701–2
    concentric 701, 955
    eccentric 109, 701, 955
    isocentric 955
    isoinertial 109
    isokinetic 109, 701
    isometric 701
    isotonic 109, 701
    mechanism 109, 700, 701–2
    nerve signal for 700
    open/closed kinetic chain exercises 204
    sequence of events 109
  cross-bridges *see* actin–myosin cross-bridge
  damage and disuse 704
  electromyogram 213–14
  endurance training *see* endurance training
  energetics 702–3
  fatigue 705
  fatty atrophy, MRI scan 171
  fibres *see* muscle fibres
  force, transmission 701–2
  force and length 109, 698
  force and motor units recruited 700
  in gait 955–6
  hormones and 704
  immobilization, effects 704
  infarction 278
  injuries 110
    from exercise 704
    healing 110
    injury types 110
    MRI scan 169, 171
    scar tissue formation 110
  intracompartmental pressure rise effects 507–8

muscle (skeletal) – continued
　ischaemia 503, 504
　　duration 507
　　pathogenesis 507–8
　　raised compartmental pressure
　　　effect 507–8
　　see also compartment syndrome,
　　　acute
　kinesiology 109–10
　lengthening in response to load 109
　mass, decline with age 121
　MRI appearance 161, 168
　necrotic, after compartment
　　syndrome 281
　normal pressure 507
　passive stretching, pain,
　　compartment syndrome 509
　peripheral fatigue 705
　physiology 697–702
　power, loss, age-related 122
　rupture, pelvic fracture complication
　　434
　soreness after exercise 704
　strains 705
　strength, age-related loss 122
　strength testing 211–13
　　advantages/disadvantages of
　　　methods 212
　　general considerations 211
　　objective assessment methods
　　　212–13
　strength training 703
　strengthening 109
　strenuous activity effects 704–5
　structure 107–8, 697–8, 698–9
　　macrostructure 698
　　microstructure 108, 699
　tears 705
　tumours 919
　ultrastructure 108, 699
　wasting, age-related 122
　weakness
　　Charcot–Marie–Tooth disease
　　　613
　　compartment syndrome 509
　　gait problems 955, 957
　　pathological gait 567
muscle fibres 107, 697–8
　arrangements 697–8
　mature 107
　sizes 107
　　age-related changes 121
　structure 697–8
　type I (red/slow-twitch)(aerobic)
　　109–10, 698, 699
　　ischaemia effect 507
　type II (white/fast-twitch) 110, 121,
　　507, 699
　　ischaemia effect 507
　type IIA (intermediate aerobic)
　　110, 698, 699
　type IIB (anaerobic) 110, 698, 699
　types 109–10, 698, 699
　　characteristics 699
　see also myofibre
muscle spindle 215
muscle-splitting approach, ulnar
　collateral ligament repair 752–3
muscular dystrophy 610–13
　Becker 610
　congenital 613
　Duchenne see Duchenne muscular
　　dystrophy (DMD)
　Emery–Dreifuss 612
　facioscapulohumeral 612–13
　limb girdle 612
musculocutaneous nerve 57, 1215
　anatomy 58, 1215
　rupture 1305
　in total shoulder replacement 1226
musculoskeletal imaging 155–72
　see also specific modalities
Musculoskeletal Tumour Society Score
　(MSTS) 941
myasthenia gravis 700–1
mycobacteria
　hand infections 1313
　rheumatoid arthritis and 1084
Mycobacterium avium-intracellulare
　1313
Mycobacterium kansasii 1313
Mycobacterium marinum 1313
Mycobacterium tuberculosis 224, 587,
　987, 1313

myelin sheath 1303
　distortion, injuries 1304
myelodysplasia see myelomeningocele
myelography, spinal tumours 1060
myeloma 95, 906–7
　clinical features 906
　differential diagnosis 906
　epidemiology 906
　imaging 906
　　bone scan insensitivity 157,
　　　1059–60
　　MRI 161, 869
　osteolytic metastases 927
　spinal lesions 1059–60, 1063
　spinal metastases 1065
　　stabilization 1065
　treatment 1063
myelomeningocele 608–10, 1474–5
　aetiology 608
　classification 1474
　general considerations 608–9
　incidence 608, 1474
　orthopaedic management 609, 1475
　regional assessment 609–10
　pathogenesis 1474
　presentation 1474
myelopathy 1002
Myerson classification, tarsometatarsal
　injuries 408, 409
myocardial infarction, hip arthroplasty
　and 1125
myodesis 960, 962
myoelectric prostheses 964
myofascial pain syndrome 979
myofibre 107
　autodigestion, injury 110
　depolarization 109
　in motor units 109
　regeneration after injury 110
　see also muscle fibres
myofibrils 108, 699
　injury from exercise 704
　light/dark bands 699
myofibroblastic tumours 916, 918
myofibroblasts, Dupuytren's
　contracture pathogenesis 1325
myogram see electromyography (EMG)
myoplasty 960
myosin 108, 699
　cross-bridges see actin–myosin cross-
　　bridge
myosteatosis 121
myotendinous junction (MTJ) 111, 112
　force transmitted across 701–2
myotomes
　lower limb 18
　upper limb 9
myxofibrosarcoma 918
myxoma, intramuscular 920

nail
　anatomy 1287–8
　germinal matrix 1287
　　loss/injuries 1288
　infections 1311
　ridging, mucous cyst 1374
nail bed 1287
　haematoma 1288–9
　injuries 1287
　lacerations 1288
　repair/grafts 1288
nail fold, infections 1311
nail plate 1287–8
nail–patella syndrome (NPS) 551
naloxone hydrochloride 127
Napoleon/La Fosse belly-press test 10
naproxen 129
narcotic drugs
　adult scoliosis 1011
　see also opioid analgesics
National Acute Spinal Cord Injury
　Study (NASCIS) 130, 445
National Cancer Institute (NCI) 883,
　884, 915
National Collegiate Athletic Association
　(NCAA) (US) 705, 707
National Institute (for health) and
　Clinical Excellence (NICE)
　antibiotic prophylaxis 1125
　anticoagulant guidelines 132
　hip prosthesis guidelines 1153
　thromboprophylaxis 1126
national joint registries 1537
natural killer (NK) cells 145, 147

navicular bone 77, 403, 404
　dislocation 405
　flexor digitorum longus transfer 1424
　fractures 405
　stress fractures 845–6
NCAA Injury Surveillance System 705
near-infrared spectroscopy(NIRS) 510
　intracompartmental pressure
　　measurement 510
neck
　anterior region 66
　muscles 66
　neuromuscular anatomy 66
　osteology 64–5
　pain
　　degenerative disc disease 993, 1002
　　spinal injuries 444
　posterior region 66
　rotation 65
'neck bump' (femoroacetabular
　impingement) 1111
neck of femur (NOF), fractures see
　femoral neck fractures
necrosis
　caseous 219
　non-caseous 219
necrosis bridge 496
necrotizing fasciitis 220
　antibiotic treatment 220
　diabetic foot 1467
needle test, Achilles tendon 830
Neer, CS, subacromial impingement
　lesion 1208
Neer's classification
　clavicular fractures 289, 1556
　distal femoral fractures 1566
　proximal humerus fractures 304,
　　1558
Neer's laterally based anteroinferior
　capsular shift 1220
Neer's sign 10, 742, 1208, 1209
nefopam (Acupan) 128
negative predictive value (NPV) 38, 39
Nelaton's line 19
neoadjuvant, definition 879
neonates
　developmental dysplasia of hip
　　screening 642–5
　treatment 647–8
　see also children; infants
neoplasia (musculoskeletal) see
　tumours (musculoskeletal)
nerve(s)
　in amputations 960
　anatomy see specific
　　nerves/anatomical regions
　conduction 1303
　　block (neurapraxia) 1304–5
　conduction velocities, at elbow 1400
　diameters/functions of types 1302
　injuries see nerve injuries
　raised intracompartmental pressure
　　effect 508
　repair, in replantation of/in upper
　　limb 1320
　signal, flow 700
　synapses 108, 700
　transection, in amputation 960
　types 1302
　see also specific nerves
nerve blocks 969
nerve compression syndromes
　ankle see ankle, nerve compression
　　syndromes
　deep peroneal nerve 1505–6
　median nerve see median nerve
　posterior interosseous nerve (PIN)
　　13
　radial nerve, around elbow 1384–6,
　　1392
　superficial peroneal nerve 1506
　tibial nerve see tarsal tunnel
　　syndrome
　ulnar nerve see cubital tunnel
　　syndrome; ulnar nerve
nerve fibre 1302
　anatomy 1303
　bundles 1303
　myelinated 1302, 1303
nerve injuries 1304
　compartment syndrome vs 510
　delay before repair 1305
　depth 1304–5
　exploration, indications 1306

fracture non-union, management
　524
in fractures and dislocations 1306
hand/upper limb 1302–8
high-energy transfer 1304–5
laceration 1302
level 1304
prognostic factors 1305–6
recovery 1305
types/causes 1304–5
Wallerian degeneration 1304
see also specific nerves
nerve roots see spinal nerve roots
neural tumours 883, 920–1
neurapraxia 1304–5
neurilemoma 920
　hand 1375
neurofibroma 920
　gadolinium contrast MRI 164
　hand 1375, 1376
　soft-tissue sarcoma 913
neurofibromatosis
　congenital pseudarthrosis of tibia
　　675
　type 1 (NF-1) 1375
　type 2 (NF-2) 1375
neurogenic claudication 1002
neurogenic shock 235, 443
　hypovolaemic shock vs 443
neurological examination
　Charcot–Marie–Tooth disease 1473
　head trauma 467–8
　juvenile idiopathic scoliosis 636
　paediatric spine screen 540
neurological signs, spinal tumours
　1059
neurological testing, adult scoliosis
　1010
neurological/neuromuscular disorders
　acquired 1477–82
　as cause of pathological gait 568
　congenital/in children 598–625,
　　1472–7
　brachial plexus birth palsy see
　　obstetric brachial plexus birth
　　palsy (OBPP)
　cerebral palsy see cerebral palsy
　hereditary motor–sensory
　　neuropathies 613–15
　　see also Charcot–Marie–Tooth
　　　disease
　muscular dystrophy see muscular
　　dystrophy
　myelomeningocele see
　　myelomeningocele
　foot/ankle abnormalities 1472–82
　see also specific disorders
neuroma, interdigital plantar
　(Morton's) see Morton's neuroma
neuromuscular junction 108–9
　age-related changes 122
　nerve signal 700
　substances affecting 700
neurone 1302
neuropathic pain 1305
neuropathy(ies)
　diabetic foot 1466, 1468
　　examination 1468
　hereditary motor–sensory 613–15
　see also Charcot–Marie–Tooth
　　disease
neurotmesis 1304
neurotransmitters 700
neurotrophin 3, Charcot–Marie–Tooth
　disease treatment 615
neurovascular injury
　clavicle fractures 290
　Dupuytren's contracture surgery
　　1330
　shoulder dislocation 297
　supracondylar fracture of humerus
　　489
neutraceuticals, as anti-osteoporotic
　agents 134
neutralization plate 272
neutrophils 145
　rheumatoid arthritis pathophysiology
　　1085, 1086
New Orleans Criteria, for CT in head
　injury 471
newborns see neonates
Newcastle disease virus (NDV) 1069
Newtonian fluids 181
nicoumalone 130

night splints
  Achilles tendonopathy 833
  cubital tunnel syndrome 1404
nightstick fractures 262, 322, 323
  clinical/radiographic features 324
  treatment 324
nitrates, topical, lateral epicondylitis 1395
nitric oxide 1078
  synthesis 1078
'no man's land', zone II injuries 1280, 1292
Noble compression test 21
nodes of Ranvier 1303
non-accidental injury (NAI), children 500–1
non-Hodgkin's lymphoma
  high-grade B-cell 907–8
  T-cell 908
non-maleficence 1532
non-Newtonian fluids 181
non-ossifying fibroma 866–7
non-parametric statistics 44
non-steroidal anti-inflammatory drugs (NSAIDs) 128–9
  adult scoliosis 1011
  adverse effects 128
  classification 128
  cubital tunnel syndrome 1404
  effect on articular cartilage 1078
  fracture healing and non-union 518
  gout 1496
  juvenile idiopathic arthritis 594
  juvenile rheumatoid arthritis 1089
  lateral epicondylitis 1394
  lumbar spine muscle injuries 979
  mechanism of action 128
  medial epicondylitis 1394
  olecranon bursitis 1389
  osteoarthritis treatment 1081, 1082, 1083
  tarsal tunnel syndrome 1503
  trigger finger 1277
norepinephrine 704
normal distribution 43, 44
Notch signalling pathway, disturbance 629–30
notochordal tumour 883
  see also chordoma
no-touch technique, introduction/history 4
N-telopeptide 928, 931
nuclear medicine, ankle/foot arthritis 1486
nuclear medicine scans see radionuclide imaging
nucleosomes 140
nucleotides 139, 140
nucleus pulposus 66
  dehydration 978, 995
  disc degeneration 106–7, 978
  functions 106
  replacement 1005
  replacement devices 197
  structure/composition 106, 994
  Young's modulus 188, 197
null hypothesis 40
'nutcracker' mechanism 977
nutrition, sports and 705–9
  carbohydrate/protein/fat sources/intake 705–6
  child athletes 708
  ergogenic aids 706–7
  older adults 708–9
  specific groups 707–9
  vegetarians 706, 707–8
  women athletes 708
nutrition, tendons 1294

Ober's test 20
obesity
  osteoarthritis risk factor 1082
  sarcopenic 121
oblique retinacular ligament reconstruction 1284
O'Brien's active compression test 739
observational gait analysis 564–5
  foot/ankle osteoarthritis 1485
  paediatric patients 536, 563, 564–6, 567
    with cerebral palsy 600
    with tibial torsion 674
observational study 40, 41–2

obstetric brachial plexus birth palsy (OBPP) 615–18
  classification 616
  clinical features 617
  diagnosis 617
  incidence 615
  natural history 616
  prognostic indicators 616
  risk factors 615
  theories of causation 615
  treatment 617–18
obturator nerve 74, 79, 429
  entrapment 775
occipital condyle fractures 446–7, 1555
  classification/management 446–7, 725
  sports injuries 725
occipitocervical dislocation 447
  anterior 447
  distraction separation 447
  posterior 447
occipitocervical spine, radiography 445, 446
occupational therapy, juvenile idiopathic arthritis 595
odds ratio 45–6
  calculation 46
odontoid process
  anatomy 450
  fractures 450–1, 1556
    classification 725
    non-union 451
    sporting injuries 725
    types I–III 450, 451
  radiography 446
oedema, compartment syndrome and 505
oesophageal carcinoma 927
oestrogen
  bone metabolism control 98
  female athletes 708
  growth plate activity and 91
  postmenopausal levels, bone loss and 122–3
  receptors, on osteoblasts 122
Ogee cup 1099–100
'OK sign' 16, 17, 1386
older adults
  nutrition for athletes 708–9
  see also elderly patients
olecranon
  anatomy 318
  avulsion fractures 318
  excision 1387
  fractures 318–19, 1559
    children 490
    classification 318
    clinical evaluation 318
    complications 319
    radiography 318
    treatment 318–19
olecranon bursitis 1388–9
  aetiology and science 1388–9
  chronic 1389
  examination/imaging 1389
  septic 1389
  treatment 1389
oligoarticular juvenile idiopathic arthritis 590, 591, 592, 594
oligonucleotide ligation assay 141
oligopotent stem cells 1526
Ollier's disease 575, 896, 1378
onapristone, Charcot–Marie–Tooth disease 615
oncogenes 149
  17p 888
oncology (musculoskeletal) 149, 865–972
  see also tumours (musculoskeletal)
oncolytic viruses 1069
'onion skin' pattern, bone tumours 867, 886, 903
onset of condition 8
open injuries, of limbs 247–57
  classification 249–53
    Ganga Hospital Open Injury Severity Score 249–52, 253
    Gustilo–Anderson 249
    Mangled Extremity Severity Score 252, 253
  infections 253
    factors increasing risk 253
  initial evaluation/management 248–9
  limb salvage vs amputation 252–3

pathophysiology 247–8
treatment 253–7
  antibiotics 253
  bone stabilization 255–6
  debridement 253–5, 256
  soft-tissue reconstruction 255, 256–7
  see also fracture fixation devices
vascular injury, signs 248
see also fracture(s), open
open kinetic chain 203–4
  exercises, functionality 204
open palm technique 1329
opening wedge high tibial osteotomy (OWHTO) 1264, 1265
opiates 126
opioid addicts, pain in 128
opioid analgesics 126–8
  adverse effects 1124
  classification 127
  mechanism of action 126
opsonization 147
optical communication, in CAOS 1513–14
Optimom large diameter metal-on-metal Total Hip Replacement system 191
orbital floor, fracture 468–9, 475
orbital haematoma 468
orbital trauma 468, 469
ordinal data 43
Orthopaedic Infirmary (London) 4
orthopaedic surgeons, burnout see burnout
orthopaedic tissue engineering see tissue engineering
Orthopaedic Trauma Association (OTA) classification, tibial plafond fractures 384
orthopaedics
  demand for 6
  history see history (orthopaedics)
  modern 6
OrthoPilot® 1513
orthoroentgenograph, leg length discrepancy 679
orthoses/orthotic management 967–71
  ankle–foot orthosis see ankle–foot orthosis (AFO)
  direct 210
  elbow 968
  foot see foot orthoses
  function 967–8
  hand 969
  hip–knee–ankle–foot 968
  indirect 210
  knee–ankle–foot orthosis see knee–ankle–foot orthosis
  paediatric 969
  specific conditions
    Achilles tendonopathy 833
    ankle osteoarthritis 1487
    ankle rheumatoid arthritis 1494
    knee stability management 210
    lateral ankle instability 841
    lateral epicondylitis 1394
    leg length discrepancy 680
    postpoliomyelitis syndrome 1481
  spine 969, 1052
    see also spinal bracing
  wedged insoles 210
  wrist 969
  see also braces/bracing; splints/splinting
Ortolani test 539, 643, 646
Ortron 1099
os coxae 1105
os tibiale externum 404
OSCAR (Orthosonics System for Cemented Arthroplasty Revision) 1158
OSF2 (osteoblast-specific transcription factor) 545
Osgood–Schlatter disease 497
osseous metaphyseal ligament ruptures 496
ossification 52, 88, 543, 544
  centres
    around elbow 487, 488
    primary 88
    secondary 88, 90
  chondral 88, 89–91
  endochondral see endochondral ossification

foot 78
heterotopic
  ankylosing spondylitis 1129
  postoperative, Paget disease 1130
intramembranous 88–9, 543
secondary 52
see also bone(s), development and growth; bone(s), formation
osteitis pubis, athletes 777–8
osteoarthritis 1080–4
  ACL resection model 1079
  aetiology 1080
    femoroacetabular impingement 1110
  ankle 1241–3, 1486–8, 1486–93
    aetiology 1241
    arthrodesis 1269, 1270
    distraction arthroplasty 1245–6
    idiopathic 1242
    imaging 1243
    management 1242–3
    pathophysiology 1241–2
    post-traumatic 1242
    presentation and diagnosis 1242
    secondary 1242
    in systemic arthritis 1242
    types 1242
    young patient, treatment 1246
    see also ankle arthroplasty (total)
  articular cartilage changes 102, 103, 1242
  biochemistry/biomechanics 102, 1242, 1333–4
  clinical features 1333
  diagnosis 1081
  distal radial ulnar joint (DRUJ) 1367, 1371
  femorotibial 1196
  glenohumeral joint 1223, 1227
    see also glenohumeral joint, arthritis
  hand 1333–50
    distal interphalangeal (DIP) joint 1346–7
    finger carpometacarpal joint 1342–3
    joints involved 1333
    metacarpophalangeal (MCP) joint 1343–5
    post-traumatic 1333
    proximal interphalangeal (PIP) joint 1345–6
    trapeziometacarpal (TM) joint see trapeziometacarpal (TM) joint
  hindfoot 1422, 1488–9
  hip arthroplasty for 1127–8, 1129
  knee 23
    adduction moment 209
    anteromedial 1186
    coronal plane knee stability during gait 208–9
    lateral, distal femoral osteotomy 1264
    lateral wedging of foot 210
    malalignment 1261
    medial, osteotomy 1261–2, 1263
    medial, surgical management 209–10
    medial compartment 208
    meniscal injuries 104, 105
    osteotomy for 1260–2
    pathophysiology 1081
    post-traumatic 361, 375
    surgical management 1186–7
    total arthroplasty for 1176–7
    unicompartmental 1186
    valgus bracing 210
  metacarpophalangeal (MCP) joint 1343–5
  metatarsophalangeal (MTP) joint
    first 1490–2
    lesser (Freiberg disease) 1492
  midfoot 1489–90
  molecular markers 1082
  obesity as risk factor 1082
  patellofemoral see patellofemoral joint, arthritis
  pathophysiology 1080–1, 1486
    'bone first' theory 1081
  prevalence 1080
  progression, glucosamine salts/chondroitin sulphate effect 134

osteoarthritis – continued
  radiocapitellar joint 1392
  secondary 1082
  shoulder see glenohumeral joint, arthritis
  therapeutic options 1082–4
  trapeziometacarpal (TM) joint see trapeziometacarpal (TM) joint
  treatment 1081–2
    autologous chondrocyte transplantation 1083
    future directions 1083–4
    non-surgical 1081, 1083
    principles, foot/ankle 1486
    surgical 1081–2
osteoarthrosis 1080
  see also osteoarthritis
osteoblast(s) 86, 543, 544, 1025
  age-related changes 122
  bone formation 86, 885
    markers 1027
  in bone remodelling 88
  endochondral ossification 91
  factors secreted 1025
  formation 86, 88, 145
  function 84, 86
  intramembranous ossification 88–9
  monolayer 892
  oestrogen receptors 122
  osteoclast interaction 87, 927, 929
  regulation 1025
  structure 86
osteoblastic tumours
  metastases 927, 928–9
  radiography 886
osteoblastoma (OBL) 891–4
  age range and sex ratio 892
  hand 1379
  radiology 892–3
  size 891
  spine 1062
  treatment 892, 1062
osteocalcin 83
osteocartilaginous exostoses 895
osteochondral, knee, autografts 790
osteochondral autograft/allograft transfer
  advantages 790
  ideal lesions for 790
  knee cartilage injuries 790
  osteoarthritis 1083
  thickness and donor sites 790
osteochondral flap, femoral head osteonecrosis 97
osteochondral fractures
  children 484
  classification 370
osteochondral lesion of talus (OCLT) 1488
osteochondral lesions (OCLs) 836
  MR arthrography 166
  talus see talus, osteochondral lesions
osteochondritis, hallucal sesamoids 1446
osteochondritis dissecans (OCD)
  humeral capitellum 753–4
    treatment 754
  knee 788–9
    incidence/epidemiology 788
    non-operative treatment 789
    operative treatment 789
    unstable lesions 789
osteochondrodysplasia 541
  see also developmental disorders of bone
osteochondroma 895–6
  hand 1378–9
  spine 1061
osteochondromatosis, multiple hereditary 574–5
osteochondrosis 96
  severe, Achilles tendon 832
osteoclast(s) 87, 543, 885, 1025
  age-related changes 122
  bone resorption 87, 88
    markers 1027
  control 87, 1025
  formation 87
  function 87
  osteoblast interaction 87, 927, 929
  osteolytic metastases 927
osteocyte(s) 86–7
  function 87
  in lamellar bone 85

osteofascial compartments see compartment(s)
osteogenesis, distraction see distraction osteogenesis
osteogenesis imperfecta 95, 547
  prevalence 542
osteogenic tumours 883
osteogenic zone, growth plate 544
osteoid 86, 89, 885
  production in osteosarcoma 898, 901
osteoid osteoma (OO) 891–4
  age range and sex ratio 892
  clinical features 892
  hand 1379
  radiology 867, 892
  size 891
  spine 1061–2
  treatment 892, 1062
osteoinductive factors, fracture healing 520
osteology 52
  see also specific bones
osteolysis 928
  periprosthetic tissues 1116, 1117, 1118, 1153
osteomalacia 93
osteomyelitis 221–5, 226
  acute 221–2
    causes 221–2
    deep infection 222
    management 222
    poorly treated 222, 224
  acute haematogenous see acute haematogenous osteomyelitis (AHO)
  causative agents 221
    unusual 224
  chronic 222–3
    causes 222
    Cierny's infected host types 223
    diagnosis 223
    management 223
    type I (medullary) 222, 223
    type II (superficial) 222, 223
    type III (localized) 222, 223
    type IV (diffuse) 222–3
  chronic, in children 586–8
    primary types 586–7
    secondary type 587–8
  chronic multifocal 224
  chronic recurrent multifocal 586
  chronic sclerosing 224
  classification 221–3
  definition 221
  epiphyseal 224
  hand 1092, 1313, 1373
  maxillofacial 471
  method of spread 224
  MRI scans 171
  post-traumatic 223
  pyogenic vertebral 982
  radionuclide imaging 157, 171
  sclerosing 586
  septic arthritis vs. 580
  staphylococcal, of hand 1373
  subacute 224
  in syphilis 224
  tuberculous 224–5, 586–7
osteonecrosis (avascular necrosis) 96
  after proximal humerus fractures 305
  DDH treatment and 648, 649
  femoral head 97
    athletes 777
    hip arthroplasty in younger patients 1254
  femoral neck fractures and 342, 344
  hip subluxation and 777
  idiopathic 96
  metatarsal bones 1438
  Perthes disease 652, 653, 656
  slipped capital femoral epiphysis 658, 659–60
  spine
    kyphoplasty 1031, 1034
    osteoporosis as risk factor 1029
    osteoporosis vs 1029–31
    radiographs 1030, 1031, 1032, 1033
    vertebroplasty 1031, 1033
  talus 528, 529
osteonectin 83
osteons 85, 88

osteopenia 94
  of rickets 95
  subchondral bone 984
osteopetrosis 96
  hip arthroplasty 1130
  radiograph 97
osteophytes
  humeral 1228
  lumbar disc degenerative disease 998, 999, 1001
  trapeziometacarpal joint osteoarthritis 1336
osteopoikilosis (spotted bone disease) 96
osteopontin 83
osteoporosis 94, 1016, 1024–47
  age-related 122, 1025
  bone loss 183, 1025
  definition 94, 1016
  differential diagnosis 1029–31
  female athletes 708
  fractures
    age-related 122
    vertebral see under osteoporosis, spinal
  idiopathic juvenile 95
  idiopathic transient 95
  prevention 133
  secondary 1029, 1030
  types 95
osteoporosis, spinal 1024–47
  aetiology 1025–6
  biomaterials (injectable) use 1039–40
  biomechanics 1026
  bone turnover markers 1027
  clinical examination 1024–9
  conservative treatment 1038
  differential diagnosis 1029–31
  epidemiology 1024
  gender differences 1024, 1025
  histopathological changes in bone 1025–6
  history-taking 1026–7
  minimally invasive treatment 1032–9
    kyphoplasty see kyphoplasty
    vertebroplasty see vertebroplasty
  natural course 1025
  open surgery 1041–3
  postoperative management 1043
  radiography/radiology 1028–9
  spinal deformity 1016, 1025
    anterior column insufficiency 1017
    kyphosis in see kyphosis
    surgical treatment 1016–18
    surgical treatment problems 1017
  transpedicular screws, strength/failure 1026
  vertebral collapse 1027
  vertebral fractures 1016, 1024, 1025–6
    age evaluation 1028
    AO classification 1034
    burst 1028
    compression 1016
    incidence 1024
    kyphoplasty see kyphoplasty
    minimally invasive treatment 1032–9
    old/neglected 1027, 1028
    open surgery 1041–3
    pathological 1017
    split 1028, 1029
    thoracolumbar 1027
    in trauma 1039
    treatment scheme 1038–9
    vertebroplasty see vertebroplasty
  vertebral levels affected 1026
  vertebral pain 1027
osteoprogenitor cells 86, 88, 89
osteoprotegerin (OPG) 87, 927, 929, 1025
osteosarcoma 898–901
  age range and sex ratio 900
  bone surface 899, 901
  chemotherapy 880
  clinical features 900
  epidemiology 884
  hand 1379–80
  high-grade primary intramedullary 899–900
  histology 892, 900, 901
  intra-cortical 899
  Li–Fraumeni syndrome 901, 913, 930

  limb-sparing surgery 941
  medullary 899
  'normalization' 901
  osteoblast monolayer 892
  osteoblastic 900, 901
  parosteal 899, 901–2
    age range and sex ratio 901
    pathology/histology 902
  pathology 900, 901
  periosteal 899
  primary 899
  radiography 867, 900
  secondary 899
  spine 1063
  subtypes 899
osteosynthesis
  Kirschner (K) wire, paediatric fractures 486
  midfacial/mandibular fractures 476
  screw, paediatric fractures 486
osteotendinous junction (OTJ) 111, 112
osteotomy
  acute lengthening procedure 683
  acute shortening procedure 681, 682
  Akin 1439
  around knee 1260–7
    aims 1260, 1261
    algorithm for management 1266
    calculation of required correction 1263
    complications 1266
    ligamentous dysfunction 1262–3
    osteoarthritis 1260–2
    techniques 1263–6
    see also high tibial osteotomy (HTO)
  Blount disease 671
  calcaneal see calcaneal osteotomy
  cerebral palsy 603, 604, 605, 606, 1476
  Charcot–Marie–Tooth disease 615
  chevron 1437–8
  closing wedge 528
  congenital posteromedial bowing of tibia 675
  Cotton 1423, 1465
  coxa vara 652
  crescentic 1439
  distal femoral 1264, 1265
  distal metatarsal 1437–8
  femoral realignment 344
  fibula 521
  genu varum/valgum 670
  hallux rigidus 1490
  high tibial see high tibial osteotomy (HTO)
  humeral 1230–1
  intertrochanteric, history 1097
  lesser tuberosity 1227
  medial closing wedge, of proximal phalanx 1439
  medial displacement calcaneal (MDCO) 1423
  medial slide calcaneal, technique 1423–4
  metacarpal extension 1339
  metatarsal shaft 1438–9
  Mitchell osteotomy 1438
  multiple epiphyseal dysplasia 573
  pedicle subtraction 1019
  pelvic support 1227
  Perthes disease 655
  in posterior tibial tendon dysfunction 1423
  proximal femoral 652, 659, 1254
  proximal metatarsal 1439
  proximal phalangeal 1439
  proximal tibial 1187
  in revision hip arthroplasty 1157, 1158
  Scarf 1438–9
  Smith–Petersen 1019
  spinal, ankylosing spondylitis 1089
  supracondylar femoral, osteoarthritis 1081
  tibial, in osteoarthritis 1081
  tibial torsion 674
  trochanteric, hip replacement 1137
    extended, in revision arthroplasty 1157
  varus/valgus femoral 1254
  see also specific indications, types
osteotomy arthroplasty, hip 1097

otorrhoea 468, 478
outcome measures 39
outcomes 1536
outpatient review, acute haematogenous osteomyelitis 586
overdamping 185
overtriage 245
overuse injuries 112
  Achilles tendon injuries 1427
  degenerative disc disease 994
  lateral epicondylitis (tennis elbow) 1391
  medial epicondylitis (golfer's elbow) 1391
  posterior tibial tendon 1421
  sesamoid bones (foot) 1445
Oxford hip score 18
Oxford scale, muscle strength testing 212
Oxford shoulder replacement 193
β-oxidation 702–3
Oxinium 190, 191
Oxinium-on-polyethylene hip replacement 1118
oxygen
  consumption
    amputations and 957
    during exercise 703–4
  hyperbaric, in acute compartment syndrome 510–11
  transcutaneous partial pressure 958

p21 protein 149
p53 gene 149
  mutations 913
PACES acronym, gait assessment 31
Pacinian corpuscle 215
paediatric patients *see* children
Paediatric Trauma Score (PTS) 500
Paget disease 96
  hip arthroplasty 1130
  radiograph 97
pain
  acute compartment syndrome 280
  back, idiopathic scoliosis 633
  bone tumour presenting with 884
    osteosarcoma 900
  compartment syndrome 509
  diabetic foot 1467
  foot/ankle arthritis, assessment 1484
  hip *see* hip
  knee *see* knee
  metastases 932
  spine 32
  tumours causing 866
pain control
  head and face trauma, cautions 469
  hip arthroplasty 1124
  postoperative, pelvic fractures 434
  spinal tumours 1061
  see also analgesics
paired *t*-test 44
Paley multiplier method 680
palliative surgery, spinal metastases 1066
palliative therapy 932
  chemotherapy 879
  radiotherapy 874
palm, lacerations 1278–80
palmar aponeurosis 1293
  re-tendinous bands 1327
palmar ligament 1351
  reconstruction 1339
palmar midcarpal injury (MCI) 1360
palmar nodules 1325, 1327
palmaris longus, free graft 1369–70
Palmer's classification, TFCC tears 758–9
palmodigital fascia, anatomy 1325
palpation
  cervical spine 32
  elbow 11–12
  foot and ankle 28–9
  hand 15
  head and face 469
  hip 19
  knee 23
  lumbar spine 34
  shoulder 10
  thoracic spine 33
  wrist 13
pamidronate 933
Pancoast tumour 1399
pannus formation 1086

pantalar fusion 1270–1
Panton–Valentine leucocidin (PVL) 582–3
Papineau technique 520
paprika sign 222
Paprosky classification, revision hip surgery 1156–7
paracetamol *see* acetaminophen (paracetamol)
paraesthesia, compartment syndrome 509
paralysis 1304
  sympathetic 1305
paramedics 234
parametric statistics 44
paraneoplastic syndrome 1059
paraplegia, spinal metastases with 1065
parasitic infections, spinal 986
paraspinal muscles
  injuries 978–9
  poor strength/endurance 979
parasymphyseal fractures, treatment 431
paratenon 111, 112
  Achilles tendon 829
parathyroid hormone (PTH)
  as anti-osteoporotic agent 133
  bone metabolism control 98
  calcium and phosphate metabolism 98
  osteoclast control, bone resorption 87
  recombinant (teriparatide) 133
parathyroid hormone-related peptide (PTHrP) 545, 928
  prostate-specific antigen action 928–9
  PTHrP gene mutations 545–6
paravertebral plexus 927
Parkinson's disease 1481
paronychia 1310
  acute 1311
pars interarticularis
  bilateral fractures (hangman's fracture) 445, 451, 452, 725–6, 1556
  fatigue fracture 977, 1048, 1051
  see also spondylolisthesis; spondylolysis
partial fusion, congenital spine deformities 631, 632
passive damping 185
patella 665–6
  accessory 75
  anatomy 75, 665–6
  biomechanics 665–6
  bipartite 75, 368–9
  dislocation *see* patellar dislocation
  facets 793
  fractures *see* patellar fractures
  instability *see* patellar instability
  lateral deviation 26
  mobility, testing 26
  reconstruction, revision knee arthroplasty 1202
  resurfacing 1180
patella alta 26, 370
patella baja 26, 370, 1181
patella partita 497
patellar apprehension test 26
patellar 'bulge' test 23–4
patellar component 1177
patellar compression test 26
patellar dislocation 363–4, 665–7
  acquired, in children 666–7
  classification 666
  complications 364
  congenital 666
  evaluations 363–4, 667, 794
  habitual 666
  intra-articular 363
  lateral 363, 364, 666, 793, 795
  mechanism and classification 363, 793
  medial 363, 794
  non-operative treatment 795
  osteochondral fractures 370
  recurrent 364, 795
    in children 667
  superior 363
  traumatic, in children 666–7
  treatment 364, 667, 794–5
patellar fractures 368–71
  children 497–8

classification 369
clinical features 368
comminuted 369
complications 369
mechanism/causes of injury 368
osteochondral fractures 370
radiography 368–9
transverse 368, 369
treatment 369, 497–8
patellar instability 793–5
  causes/pathophysiology 793
  non-operative treatment 795
  patellofemoral arthroplasty failure 1196
  surgical treatment 793–5
patellar 'sleeve fracture' 791
patellar tap 23
patellar tendinopathy 22
patellar tendon 26, 665
  autograft tissue, ACL reconstruction 810
  partial tears 370
  prostheses 967
  rupture 370, 791–2
    Achilles tendon 829
    children 791
    chronic 791
    mechanism/causes 791
    repair 791
    sports injury 791–2
  shortening/advancement, in cerebral palsy 604
patellar tendon-bearing cast 266
patellar tilt test 26
patellectomy 369
patellofemoral arthroplasty of knee 1193–7
  Avon implant 1195–6
  early failures/problems 1195
  future prospects 1196–7
  implant development 1195–6
  indications/contraindications 1195
  results/outcomes 1195, 1196
  young patients 1255
patellofemoral joint
  arthritis 1193–4
    non-operative treatment 1194
    operative treatment 1194–5
    treatment options 1193–4
  degeneration, causes 1193
  forces acting on 187
  instability 793, 1200
  resurfacing 1195
  testing 26
  transverse plane knee stability 210–11
patellofemoral pain 1193
  taping and bracing for 210–11
patellofemoral pain syndrome (PEPS) 214
pathological fractures 925
  assessment 930–1
    phase I 930
    phase II 930–1
    phase III 931
  bone tumour presenting with 884
  causes 925–6
  defect size, assessment 932
  definition 925
  femoral neck 342
  femoral shaft 353
  history-taking 866
  major tumours causing 926
  management 926, 929–30
  maxillofacial 472
  metabolic causes 925–6
  myeloma 906, 907
  neoplastic 926
    primary *vs* metastatic tumours 929–30
    see also metastases (skeletal)
  operative treatment 933–6
    amputation 936
    fixation methods 934, 935
    primary tumour influence 934–5
    principles 933–4
    prosthetic replacement 934, 935
  osteonecrosis of spine 1031
  osteoporosis 1017
  prediction of life expectancy 931
  prophylactic fixation 932
  risk, prediction 931–2
  risk factors 931–2
  simple bone cysts and 887
  treatment 932–6

  see also metastases (skeletal)
pathological gait *see under* gait
patient categories (condition)
  after trauma/polytrauma 237–8
    borderline 238, 241
    in extremis 238, 241
    stable 237, 241
    unstable 238, 241
  mass casualty 245
patient-controlled analgesia (PCA)
  hip arthroplasty 1124
  morphine 127
patient's condition after trauma *see* patient categories (condition)
patient-specific jigs, in CAOS 1522
Patrick test 20–1
patterning defects, limbs 544–5
Patte's test 10
Pauwels' classification, femoral neck fractures 341
Pavlik harness
  congenital dislocation of knee 665
  developmental dysplasia of hip 647–8
  septic arthritis management 582
Pax gene family 545
peak height velocity (PHV) 628
  adolescent idiopathic scoliosis 637
  juvenile idiopathic scoliosis 636
Pearson correlation test 44
pedicle screws 1013–14
  fixation
    adult scoliosis 1013–14
    osteoporotic kyphosis 1016, 1017
    isthmic spondylolisthesis 1052, 1053
    osteoporosis 1026
  see also transpedicular screws
pedicle subtraction osteotomy 1019
PEEK cages 197
Pell radiological score, ankle arthritis 1487
'pelvic deltoid' 773
pelvic floor muscles 429
pelvic fractures 425–38, 1563
  aetiology 426
  anatomy relevant to 428–9
    neurological structures 429
    vascular structures 428–9
  children 493, 499
  classification 427–8
  clinical evaluation 427
  complications 434–5
  degloving injuries with 426
  elderly 426
  frequency (incidence) 426
  future issues and controversies 436
  haemorrhage 239, 425–6, 427, 437
  high-energy 425, 426
  low-energy 426
  management 427–8
    ATLS management 239, 426, 430
    goal 427
  nerve injuries/palsy with 433, 435
  outcome and prognosis 435–6
  presentation 426–7
  radiography 429–30
  postoperative 435
  sacral fractures with 463
  soft-tissue injuries 426
    Morel–Lavallee lesion 426
  surgical treatment 425, 431–3
    crescent fractures 432
    follow-up 435
    iliac wing fractures 431–2
    intra-operative management 434
    postoperative care 434
    pre-operative templating of plates 434
    pubic ramus fractures 431
    sacral fractures 433
    sacroiliac joint disruption 432–3
    symphysis pubis disruptions 431
  treatment 430–3
    medical 430
    non-operative 425
    operative *see* pelvic fractures, surgical treatment
    pre-operative care 433–4
  unstable 425–6
  vertical shear 428
  work-up 429–30
pelvic girdle 69
pelvic ligaments, anatomy 428
pelvic obliquity, acetabular cup position 1127

pelvic osteotomy, cerebral palsy 603
pelvic resection, tumours 946
pelvic ring, anatomy 428
pelvic ring injuries/disruptions
  children 499
  clinical evaluation 427
  controversies and future prospects 436
  deformities from 426
  operative management 425
  outcome and prognosis 435–6
  sacral fractures with 433
  vascular/neurological injuries 427
  see also pelvic fractures
pelvic rotation 955
pelvic stability, definition 436
pelvic support osteotomy 1254
pelvis
  anatomy 69–73, 772–3
    blood vessels 71–2, 428–9
    muscle groups around 429
    neurological structures 429
    osteology 69–70, 428
  as conduit for neurovascular structure 428–9
  false 428
  fractures see pelvic fractures
  injuries
    ATLS management 239, 426, 430
    avulsion, children/adolescents 493, 777
    see also pelvic ring injuries/disruptions
  MRI scan 161
  muscle strains 774–5
  neurological structures 429
  reconstruction 946–7
  registration, in CAOS 1521
  retroversion, in isthmic lysis spondylolisthesis 1049
  sports injuries 772–81
    see also sports injuries; specific injuries
  stress fractures 777
  surgical approaches 72–4
  true 428
  tumours 778
    metastases 928
    resection 946
  see also entries beginning pelvic
penicillin
  open fractures 254
  open injuries of limbs 253
percutaneous internal fixation, SFCE treatment 658, 662
periacetabular pelvic osteotomy, cerebral palsy 603
perichondrium 89
pericytic tumours 916, 919
perilunate dislocation 1560
  dorsal 1360–1
perilunate fracture dislocation 1361
perilunate instability 1352
perimeniscal cyst 786
perimeniscal plexus 104
perimysium 698
perionychium 1287
periosteal circulation, in fracture fixation 271, 272
periosteum 84, 87–8
  formation 543
  structure 87
  tibial, traction injury 824
  in tumours 867, 886
peripheral analgesia, morphine 127
peripheral nerve(s)
  anatomy 1303
  blood supply to 1303
peripheral nerve injuries
  foot/ankle 1479–80
  hand/upper limb 1302–6
  see also nerve injuries
peripheral neuropathy, affecting foot 26
periprosthetic fractures, hip arthroplasty 1155–6
peritalar dislocation 397
peritendinitis 1464
  Achilles tendon 831, 832, 1426
peritrochanteric fractures see intertrochanteric fractures
perivascular (pericytic) tumours 916, 919
Perkins line, DDH assessment 646–7
Perkins' rules 515

perlecan 548
permanent disability, assessment, work-related injuries 1543
permanent epiphysiodesis
  genu varum/valgum 670
  see also epiphysiodesis
peroneal nerve 1500
  deep see deep peroneal nerve
  idiopathic palsy 827
  injuries/lesions 1479–80
    in knee dislocation 365
  superficial see superficial peroneal nerve
  see also common peroneal nerve
peroneal tendon 1428–9
  blood supply 1428
  disorders 834–5
    complete rupture 834, 1429
    dislocation 834, 1428, 1429
    evaluation/examination 834, 1429
    treatment 834–5, 1429
  injuries 1428–9
    management 1429
    stabilization/repair 1429
    tears 834, 1429
peroneal tenosynovitis 1429
peroneus brevis 30, 846
peroneus brevis tendon 1428
peroneus longus 29, 1428
Perren's interfragmentary strain theory 270, 518
persistent oligoarticular juvenile idiopathic arthritis 590, 591
persistent patellar dislocation 666
Perthes disease 652–6
  aetiology 652
  classification 654
  clinical features 652–3
  differential diagnosis 653, 660
    multiple epiphyseal dysplasia vs. 572–3, 653
  epidemiology 652
  natural history 652–3
  pathology 652
  prognostic factors 653–4
  treatment 654–6
    indications/contraindications 656
pes cavus 1460–2
  aetiology 1461
  Charcot–Marie–Tooth disease 613–14, 1473
  classification 1462
  clinical features 1461
  definition 1460
  evaluation/examination 1461
  management 1462
  pathophysiology 1461
  in sesamoiditis 1446
  surgical management 1462, 1463
pes planus 27, 1460, 1462–5
  aetiology 1462–3
  classification 1464
  clinical features 1463
  evaluation 1463–4
  management 1464
  pathophysiology 1463
  posterior tibial tendon dysfunction 1421, 1422, 1423, 1462–3
  rigid 1464
  surgical management 1464–5
  see also flat foot; posterior tibial tendon dysfunction (PTTD)
pes valgus, congenital convex see congenital vertical talus
PET scans see positron emission tomography (PET)
Peyronie disease 918, 1326
phagocytic cells 145, 147, 148
phagocytosis, in rheumatoid arthritis 1086
phalangeal fractures 766–7
  forefoot 415–16
  hand/fingers 766–7, 1286–7, 1562
    diaphyseal 1286–7
    distal 767, 1287
    distal tuft of P3 1287
    middle 766, 1287
    non-displaced, treatment 1286, 1287
    oblique/spiral 1287
    proximal 766, 1286
phalanges, anatomy
  foot 78
  hand 64

Phalen's test 15
pharmacology (orthopaedic) 126–35
phase difference 182
phenindione 130
Phillip and Fowler angle 832
phosphagens 702, 703
phosphate
  in bone 97
    daily requirement and plasma levels 97
  deficiency 94
  metabolism regulation 98
phosphofructase 825
phrenic nerve, palsy 617
physaliphorous cells 905
physeal bar excision, genu varum/valgum 669
physeal damage, septic arthritis 582
physeal surgery, genu varum/valgum 669–70
physical examination see clinical examination; specific conditions
physical exhaustion, as burnout manifestation 1551
physical therapy
  Charcot–Marie–Tooth disease 1473
  cubital tunnel syndrome 1405
  Duchenne muscular dystrophy 612, 1477
  juvenile idiopathic arthritis 595
  lateral epicondylitis 1394
  medial epicondylitis 1394
  obstetric brachial plexus birth palsy 617
Physician Rating Scale 564
physiological state, after trauma, patient types 240, 241
physiotherapy
  osteoporotic spinal surgery 1043
  before revision knee arthroplasty 1200
physis
  development and growth (%) 482–3
  fractures 483–4
    around knee 495, 496–8
    Salter and Harris classification 483–4
'piano key' sign/test 14, 759, 1367
Piggot's classification, MTP joint congruence 1435
pigmented villonodular synovitis (PVNS) 784, 918–19
  clinical features 784, 918
  incidence and pathophysiology 784
  localized 918
    hand 1374–5
    knee 784–5
  MRI 162, 784, 918
  sites 918
  treatment 784–5, 918–19
pilon fracture
  phalangeal 1286
  tibial see tibial plafond fractures
pinning
  prophylactic, SCFE 659
  see also fracture fixation
Pipkin classification 337, 1564
Pirani classification 689
piriformis muscle 70, 71, 74, 429
piriformis syndrome 775
  features and treatment 776
piriformis test 21
Pirogoff amputation 961
'pistoning' of bone 957, 967
pit corrosion 1115
pivot shift tests
  knee 24, 25, 807–8
  lateral, of elbow 13
  reverse, PCL 26
'place and hold' technique 1280, 1294
plafond fractures, tibial see tibial plafond fractures
plagiocephaly, infantile idiopathic scoliosis 635
plantar fasciitis 27
plantar nerve 1500
  entrapment 847–8
  interdigital plantar neuroma 1500–2
  lateral see lateral plantar nerve
  medial see medial plantar nerve
plasma cell neoplasms 906
  multifocal see myeloma
  solitary see plasmacytoma
plasma spray technology 1100–1, 1120

plasmacytoma 906–7
  spine 1063
  treatment 1063
plasmid vectors 142
plaster of Paris, casts 260
plastic deformation 182
plate osteosynthesis, open fractures 255
plates see fracture fixation devices, plates
plating
  fractures 271–2
  leg length discrepancy treatment 681
pleomorphic malignant fibrous histiocytoma 919
pleomorphic sarcoma, undifferentiated high-grade 919
plicae 783
  medial 26
pluripotent stem cells 1526
PMMA see polymethylmethacrylate (PMMA)
pneumatic antishock garments
  contraindications 427
  pelvic fractures 427
pneumothorax 235
podagra 1091
point prevalence 37
point-based registration, in CAOS 1513
Poirier, space of 1351, 1352
Poisson's ratio 180
poliomyelitis 971, 1481
  post-polio syndrome 971, 1480–1
polyarticular juvenile idiopathic arthritis 590, 591–2, 594
  RF negative 591–2
  RF positive 592
polydactyly 552
polydioxanone (PDS), Le Fort fracture treatment 477
polyetherenekeone (PEEK) 1004, 1034, 1041
polyethylene 1116–17
  ankle prostheses 1244
  ceramic-on, hip prosthesis 1119
  cross-linking 1117
    tensile strength reduction 1117
  highly cross-linked 189
    acetabular component 190, 1101
  hip prostheses 1101, 1116–18, 1139
    loosening 1099, 1117, 1139, 1153–4
  knee prostheses
    fixed vs mobile bearing design 1179
    modular inserts 1177
    removal, in revision surgery 1201
  oxidation 1117
  reduction 1117
  structure 1116–17
  wear
    ankle prostheses 1244
    hip arthroplasty in younger patients 1254
    rates 1142
    wear-related osteolysis 1117, 1118, 1142
polymerase chain reaction (PCR) 141
  spinal tuberculosis 988
polymethylmethacrylate (PMMA) 194, 1040
  advantages/disadvantages 1040
  augmentation, with transpedicular screws 1042
  for bone defects with pathological fractures 934
  calcium phosphate cement vs 1041
  composition 1040
  hip arthroplasty 1120, 1139
    history 1099
    substances added to 1120
  indications 1040
  modulus of elasticity 1120
  problems with 1100–1
  vertebroplasty 1032, 1035, 1040
    in osteoporotic kyphosis 1017–18
polypropylene 1295, 1339
polytetrafluoroethylene (PTFE) 1098
  Charnley's prostheses 1098, 1099, 1109
polytrauma 233–43
  children 499–500
  definition 233
  head and face trauma 466
    midfacial fractures 476

injury severity score 233
management 234
resuscitation 237
spinal cord injury and 442–3
see also trauma/injury
polyurethaneurea (PUUR) 1339
Ponseti method 689, 690
Popeye sign 11
popliteal artery 77
injury, in knee dislocation 814
trifurcation, in tibial plateau fractures 372
popliteal cysts 22
popliteus muscle 24
population of patients 38
poroelasticity 182
position vector 174
positive predictive value (PPV) 38, 39
positron emission tomography (PET) 157–8
clinical uses 157–8
history 156
metastatic tumours 931
osteoporotic fractures 1028–9
pyogenic spinal infections 984
soft-tissue sarcoma 913
tumours 869–70
post-concussion syndrome 720, 722
posterior cord syndrome 443
posterior cruciate ligament (PCL) 25–6
anatomy 811
bundles (anterolateral/posteromedial) 811
clinical evaluation 811
deficient knees 811, 812
imaging 811–12
injury 24, 811–12
in multiligamentous injury of knee 814, 815
sports-related 811–12
reconstruction, in knee dislocation 815
rehabilitation 812
retaining *vs* substituting in TKA 1178
rupture, in knee dislocation 365
testing 25–6, 811
treatment 812
non-operative 812
operative 812
posterior cuff, examination/tests 10
posterior drawer test
knee 25, 211, 811
shoulder 11
posterior horn medial meniscus root tear (PHMMRT) 787–8
repairs 788
posterior ilium, crescent fractures 432
posterior impingement test, hip 21
posterior interosseous artery 505
posterior interosseous nerve (PIN)
anatomy 1384, 1385
compression, lateral epicondylitis *vs* 13
testing 16
posterior interosseous nerve (PIN) syndrome 14, 1385, 1392
posterior longitudinal ligament (PLL) 65, 976
posterior lumbar interbody fusion (PLIF) 1003, 1004
degenerative disc disease 1003, 1004
degenerative spondylolisthesis 1056
isthmic spondylolisthesis 1053
posterior oblique ligament (POL) (knee) 805
posterior osseoligamentous complex (POLC) 459
posterior process fractures 396
posterior sag test, PCL injury 811
posterior talofibular ligament (PTFL) 78, 840, 1243
palpation 28
posterior tibial artery 77, 80
intramedullary nailing of fracture 1307
posterior tibial nerve 104
posterior tibial tendon 30, 78, 835
anatomy 1421
failure 1422
overuse 1421
split tendon transfer/lengthening 604–5

tears/ruptures 835–6, 1423
partial 836
tendinosis 835, 836
tenosynovitis 835–6
posterior tibial tendon dysfunction (PTTD) 1421–4, 1489
aetiology 1421–2, 1463
clinical features 1422–3
epidemiology 1463
flat foot 1421, 1422, 1423, 1462–3
investigation/imaging 1422–3
Johnson classification 1421, 1464
management 1423–4, 1464
non-operative treatment 1423
surgical treatment 1423–4
see also pes planus
posterior tibialis muscle 835
posterior/posteromedial releases, congenital clubfoot 690–1
posterolateral corner (PLC) complex
anatomy 812–13
injuries 812–13
treatment 813
posterolateral plica 1392
posterolateral rotatory instability (PLRI), of elbow *see under* elbow
posterolateral rotatory instability (PLRI), of knee 24
post-natal growth and development, spinal column 627–8
postoperative care *see specific conditions/procedures*
postoperative immobilization, developmental dysplasia of hip 649
postoperative infections, spinal (pyogenic) 985–6
postoperative rehabilitation *see* rehabilitation (post-operative)
post-polio syndrome 971, 1480–1
post-traumatic arthritis
ankle fractures 391
calcaneal fractures 401
distal humeral fractures 313
knee 361, 375
talar neck fractures 396
see also osteoarthritis
post-traumatic kyphosis 1019–20
post-tubercular kyphosis 991
postural kyphosis 638, 640, 1016
postural round back 1016
potential energy 176, 178, 179
Pott, Percivall 3
power 176, 178
peak 213
power (statistical), in experimental studies 42
power grip test 16
Powers ratio 446, 447
precalcaneal bursitis 832
precision pinch tests 16
preclinical testing, joint replacement devices 197–9
predictive values 38, 39
calculation 39
prednisolone, Duchenne muscular dystrophy 612
prednisone
Duchenne muscular dystrophy 612
juvenile idiopathic arthritis 594
pre-hospital care 234–5
spinal cord injury 235, 440
pre-hospital trauma life support (PHTLS) 234
prematurity, as cerebral palsy risk factor 599
prenatal diagnosis
congenital clubfoot 689
skeletal dysplasia 554
presenting complaint 8
press fit, joint implant fixation 194
prevalence 37–8
calculation 37
primary bone marrow cavities 89
primary hip arthroplasty *see* hip arthroplasty (total)
primary spongiosa 89, 91
primary survey, trauma 235–7, 239
open injuries of limbs 248
spinal injuries 440, 442, 444–5
primitive neuroectodermal tumours (PNET) 902, 903
primordial skeleton 89
probability 42

pro-collagen 100–1
ProDisc C 197
profunda femoris 71
proliferation zone, growth plate 544
proliferative chondrocyte defects 545–6
proliferative zone 89
pronator syndrome 12, 1386
carpal tunnel syndrome *vs* 1386
medial epicondylitis *vs* 13
pronator teres, anatomy 322, 505, 1383
prophylactic pinning, slipped capital femoral epiphysis 659
proprioception 214–15
components 214
deficits
assessment 215
conditions with 214–15
factors leading to 215
definition 214–15
functional relevance 215
mechanoreceptors involved 214, 215
testing 215
prospective cohort study 41
prostaglandin E2 (PGE2), synthesis inhibition 1083
prostaglandin synthesis
inhibition by hyaluronic acid 1083
inhibition by NSAIDs 128
prostate cancer 926, 927
chemotherapy effect on bone 929
metastases 926, 927, 928, 1066
management 933
osteoblastic 928
radiographs 928, 929
prostate-specific antigen (PSA) 866, 928–9, 930
prostheses 963–7
body-powered 964
bone scan 157
gait abnormalities 967, 968
hip *see under* hip arthroplasty (total)
knee *see under* knee arthroplasty
lower limb 964–7
ankle 1244
common problems 967
feet 964–5
knees 965–6
shanks 965
sockets 966, 967
suspension systems 966–7
myoelectric 964
upper limb 963–4
elbow 1387
shoulder 1253
see also implants
prosthetic arthroplasty 1176
see also joint replacement; *individual joints*
protection plate (neutralization plate) 272
protein (dietary), sources/intake 706
child athletes 708
protein S 83
protein truncation test 141
proteoglycans
aggregates 1079
antibodies to epitopes 1082
in articular cartilage 101, 1078–9
distribution/structure 1079
degradation, in osteoarthritis 1080
increased synthesis in early osteoarthritis 1080
in intervertebral disc 106, 994, 1001
in tendons 111
protons
in MRI 161, 167
radiotherapy 875
proto-oncogenes 149
protrusio acetabuli 1129
provocation tests
elbow 12–13
cubital tunnel syndrome 1399
lateral epicondylitis 12–13, 750, 1391–2
medial epicondylitis 13, 751, 1392
pronator syndrome 12
sacroiliac 21
proximal femoral osteotomy 659, 1254
proximal femur *see* femur, proximal
proximal focal femoral deficiency 650–1
proximal humerus *see* humerus, proximal

proximal interphalangeal (PIP) joint (hand)
anatomy 1345
arthrodesis 1268, 1344, 1345, 1346
failure 1346
arthroplasty 1345, 1346
implants 1346
assessment, in lacerations 1278
boutonnière deformity 1282
collateral ligament injuries 1285
dislocation 1284
dorsal 1284
dorsal, classification 765, 1284
lateral 765, 1284
sports injuries 764–5, 1284
stable/unstable 1285
treatment 1284–5
types I and II 1284
types III 1285
volar 765, 1284
Dupuytren's contracture 1325, 1326, 1327
flexion contracture 1327
release 1329–30
fracture dislocation 765, 1285
dorsal 1285
fractures 1562
intra-articular 1285–6
hyperextension (swan neck deformity) 1283–4
injuries 1284–5
osteoarthritis 1333, 1345–6
templating before surgery 1344
testing 17
volar plate avulsion 1284
zone II injuries 1280
proximal interphalangeal (PIP) joint (lesser toes) 1450
arthrodesis 1271
in claw toe 1453
flexion deformity 1451–2
proximal metatarsal osteotomy 1439
proximal phalangeal articular angle (PPAA) 1436
proximal phalangeal osteotomy 1439
proximal tarsal tunnel syndrome 1502
proximal tibial anatomy registration 1518
proximal tibial fractures *see* tibia, proximal
pseudarthrosis
congenital, of tibia 675–7
definition 675
partial, diaphyseal greenstick fracture 483
risk in spinal fusion for scoliosis 1012
synovial 517
pseudoachondroplasia 550–1
pseudoboutonnière deformity 766, 1325, 1326, 1327
pseudogout 1092
hand 1374
pseudohypoparathyroidism 93
pseudoisometric muscle contraction 204
Pseudomonas, open fracture infections 253
Pseudomonas aeruginosa, cellulitis 219
psoas abscess, in tuberculosis 987
psoas lengthening, cerebral palsy 602
psoas muscle 429
psoriatic arthritis 1090, 1496–7
juvenile 590, 593
psychosocial factors
adult scoliosis 1009
degenerative disc disease 1002
spinal cord injury management 970
PTHrP *see* parathyroid hormone-related peptide (PTHrP)
PTHrP gene mutations 545–6
pubalgia, athletic 776
puberty, precocious 91
pubic ramus fractures 464
neurological injury 435
treatment 431
pubis 69, 1105
anatomy 773
pubofemoral ligament 773, 1106
pudendal nerve, entrapment 775
pulled elbow syndrome 491
pulley system, flexor tendons (fingers) 1293–4
pulmonary artery line, hip arthroplasty 1124

pulmonary embolism
　hip arthroplasty and 1127
　management, thrombolysis 132
　pelvic fracture patients 435
pulmonary function
　adult scoliosis 1009
　idiopathic scoliosis 633, 634
pulmonary implants, chondroblastoma 895
pulse
　absent, open injuries of limbs 248
　acute compartment syndrome 509
　knee dislocation and 815
　open injuries of limbs 248
pulsed-field gel electrophoresis (PFGE) 142
pulvinar 772
'pump bump' 832, 833
purines 139
Putti, Vittorio 5
P-value 42, 44
pyogenic spinal infections *see* spinal infections
pyrimidines 139
pyrolytic carbon 1339, 1343, 1346

Q angle 26, 665–6
quadrangular (quadrilateral) space 57, 58
quadriceps angle (Q angle) 26, 665–6
quadriceps muscle
　ACL injury and 211
　action and function 956
　in avulsions of tibial tuberosity 497
　contractions, hamstring action 204
　contusions 774
　hamstring muscle balance 211, 213
　translational stability of knee 211
　weakness, gait 957
　weakness, muscular dystrophy 611
quadriceps tendon
　incomplete tear 370
　mid-substance tears 370
　rupture 370, 792–3
　　causes/mechanism 792–3
　　clinical features 793
　　incomplete/partial 793
　　treatment 793
quadriceps-sparing approaches, TKA 1181
quadriga phenomenon 16, 1298
quadriplegia 442
　transient, sports injuries 726
quality of life, adult scoliosis 1009
quasistatic behaviour 188
Quenu and Kuss classification, tarsometatarsal injuries 408

'r' value 44
racoon sign 468, 469
radial artery
　anatomy 62, 505
　recurrent branch 1384
radial bow, non-operative treatment of fractures 262
radial bursa
　infections 1312
　location 1312
radial collateral ligament (RCL) 1383
　injuries 1285
radial head 1382
　anatomy 319
　biomechanics 1387
　dislocation
　　children 490, 491
　　Monteggia fracture 324, 325, 490, 491
　　excision 320, 1387
　fractures 319–20, 1559
　　children 490
　　classification 319, 320
　　clinical evaluation 319
　　complication 320
　　in fracture dislocation of elbow 317
　　mechanism of injury 319
　　radiography 319
　　treatment 320
　subluxation 490, 491
radial neck fractures 320
　children 490
radial nerve 57
　anatomy 58, 62, 307, 1385
　at elbow 1384–5

compression around elbow 1384–6
　lateral epicondylitis *vs* 1392
conduction block 1304
injury, humeral shaft fractures 307, 308–9
injury by fracture/dislocation 1306
palsy 1306
　humeral shaft fractures, treatment 264
posterior interosseous branch *see* posterior interosseous nerve (PIN)
superficial cutaneous branch 1384
testing 16
radial styloid process, fracture (avulsion) 329
radial tunnel 1384
radial tunnel syndrome 1385, 1392
　clinical features 1386
　lateral epicondylitis *vs* 1392
radians 174
radiation dose, CT 159
radiation synovectomy 1087
radicular pain 1002
radiocapitellar joint 1365
　forces 1388
　osteoarthritis 1392
radiocapitellar joint line 11
radiocapitellar overload syndrome 752
radiocarpal joint
　anatomy 61
　instability 1360
radiofrequency (RF), in MRI 160, 161
'radiographically occult fracture' 156, 170
radiography 156
　Canale view 395
　cervical spine series 444, 445
　　after sports injury 725
　　subaxial, assessment criteria 454
　clinical uses 156
　'four-view', for fracture non-union 515, 516
　history 155
　pelvic, inlet and outlet 430
　pelvis (AP), 'six lines' 430
　specific indications/conditions
　　achondroplasia 572
　　acute haematogenous osteomyelitis 584
　　adolescent idiopathic scoliosis 637–8, 639
　　adult scoliosis 1010
　　ankle impingement 1488
　　ankle osteoarthritis 1486–7
　　anterior tarsal tunnel syndrome 1505
　　arthrodesis 1268, 1269
　　Blount disease 670
　　bone tumours 866–7, 886
　　bone/joint tuberculosis 225
　　Charcot–Marie–Tooth disease 1473
　　chronic osteomyelitis 587
　　compartment syndrome 510
　　congenital posteromedial bowing of tibia 674
　　congenital pseudarthrosis of tibia 675
　　congenital vertebral anomalies 631
　　cubital tunnel syndrome 1400
　　DDH 645, 646–7
　　developmental coxa vara 651, 652
　　foot/ankle arthritis 1485, 1486–7
　　fracture non-union 515–16
　　Freiberg disease 1492
　　glenohumeral arthritis 1224
　　hallux rigidus 1490
　　head and face trauma 471
　　infantile idiopathic scoliosis 635
　　juvenile idiopathic arthritis 594
　　knee arthroplasty planning 1177
　　leg length discrepancy 679
　　midfoot osteoarthritis 1489
　　multiple epiphyseal dysplasia 572–3
　　multiple hereditary exostosis 575
　　paediatric fractures/dislocations 485
　　patellar dislocation 667
　　pyogenic spinal infections 984
　　rotator cuff tears 1210
　　Scheuermann's kyphosis 640

septic arthritis 580
simple bone cyst 887
skeletal dysplasias 554, 555, 572–3, 575
skull fractures *vs* sutures 479
slipped capital femoral epiphysis 657
spinal cord injuries 444
spondyloepiphyseal dysplasia 573
superficial peroneal nerve entrapment 1506
tarsal tunnel syndrome 1503
thoracolumbar spine 459–60
tibial torsion 674
traction, adult scoliosis 1010
tuberculous osteomyelitis 587
wrist injuries 1353–4
see also other specific conditions
strengths and weaknesses 156
swimmer's view, cervical spine 445
radiohumeral joint 316
see also elbow
radiology
　bone tumours *see* bone tumours
　head and face trauma 471
　history 155–6
　'spine at risk' 990, 991
　see also specific modalities
radiolunate (RL) angle 1354
radionuclide imaging 156
　history 156
　hot spots, spinal tumours 1059
　lesser toes 1451
　pyogenic spinal infections 984
　spinal tuberculosis 988
　tumours 157, 158, 867–8, 886
　　metastatic 930
see also bone scans
radioscaphocapitate (RSC) ligament 1351
　ruptures 1352
radioscaphoid joint, arthritis/degenerative changes 1358–9
radiostereoisometric analysis (RSA) 175
　elbow movement 1386–7
radiotherapy 874–8, 941
　adjuvant 874
　in benign disease 878
　general principles 874–5
　kilovoltage 875
　megavoltage 875
　neo-adjuvant 875
　palliative 874
　pre-operative 877, 941
　radiation types, characteristics 875
　radical 874
　for sarcomas 876–8, 941, 951
　　see also soft-tissue sarcoma
　side-effects 875
radioulnar joint
　distal *see* distal radial ulnar joint (DRUJ)
　Galeazzi fracture 324–5
　proximal 316
　see also elbow
radioulnar ligaments 1366
radioulnar synostosis, post-traumatic 323
radius
　amputations 963
　anatomy 61, 322, 327
　distal
　　anatomy 327
　　normal radiographic measurements 328
　　in normal wrist (C line) 1356
　　reconstruction 949–50
　　V pattern with scaphoid 1356
　distal, fractures 327–31, 1369
　　cast wedging in children 485
　　children 482, 491–3
　　classification 318, 328, 329
　　clinical evaluation 327
　　complications 329–30
　　mechanism of injury 327
　　non-operative treatment 261–2
　　radiography 328
　　treatment 329–30
　fractures
　　non-operative treatment 262–3
　　non-union, cancellous graft 527
　head *see* radial head
　neck, fractures 320, 490

shaft, fractures 262, 322–6, 324–5
　children 491–3
　clinical evaluation 322, 325
　complications 323, 325
　radiography 322–3, 325
　treatment 323, 325
　with ulna shaft fractures 322–3
surgical approaches
　anterior (Henry's) 62–3
　posterior (Thompson) 63, 64
raloxifene 132, 133
randomization 40
randomized controlled trials (RCT) 40–1
　minimal incision surgery, hip arthroplasty 1148
　outcome evaluation 40
range of motion (ROM)
　ankle 29, 186, 1243, 1244
　in cerebral palsy 600–1
　hip 186, 1108–9
　　adolescents 539–40
　knee 186–7
　shoulder 187, 297
　spine 187–8
　wrist 187
RANK 1025
　RANK-L binding 87, 927
RANK-L 927, 1025
　osteoblast/osteoclast interaction 87, 927, 929
　osteoclast control 87
Ranvier, nodes of 1303
rapid prototyping techniques, tissue engineering scaffolds 1526
rapport-building, with children 535–6
ray amputation, diabetic foot 1470
Raymedica prosthetic disc nucleus (PDN) 197
RB1 gene 149
reaching task, kinematics 205–6
reactive arthritis 1497
　Reiter syndrome 1090
reactive zone, around tumour 940, 942
Reagan test (lunotriquetral ballottement test) 15, 1359
reaming
　femoral
　　method 1142
　　shaft fracture fixation 355
　　uncemented hip arthroplasty 1142
　glenoid 1229
　humerus, reverse shoulder arthroplasty 1231
　intramedullary nails, reamed *vs* unreamed 255, 379
　pathological fracture fixation 935
　reverse, in impaction bone grafting 1158
　tibial shaft fractures fixation 379
receptor activator of nuclear factor kappa B ligand *see* RANK-L
recoil 179
reconstruction, limb *see* limb reconstruction
rectus abdominis muscle
　metastasis in, PET scan 869
　rupture, pelvic fracture complication 434
rectus femoris
　strains 774
　test 20
　transfer, in cerebral palsy 604
'red flag' symptoms, lower back pain 32
reduction, closed, of fractures *see* fracture(s), closed treatment
reflexes
　sacral, in spinal cord injury 441
　upper limb 9
refusal of treatment 1540
Regan and Morrey classification, coronoid fractures 1559
regenerative medicine 1524
　see also tissue engineering
'regiment badge area' 303
registration, in CAOS *see under* computer-assisted orthopaedic surgery (CAOS)
regression 44
regression analyses 44–5
rehabilitation (post-operative)
　ACT reconstruction 810
　Duchenne muscular dystrophy 612
　Dupuytren's contracture 1330

finger flexor tendons injuries 1297
glenohumeral joint instability 1222
lateral epicondylitis 1393–4
medial epicondylitis 1393–4
multilevel surgery, cerebral palsy 605
rotator cuff tears 1214
shoulder arthroplasty 1232
Reiter syndrome 1090, 1497
rejection of grafts 148–9
  timing, animal studies 149
relative risk 45–6
  calculation 45
reliability 39
relocation test of Jobe 11, 731
renal carcinoma 928, 930, 934, 935, 1380
  hypervascularity 935
renal failure, myelomeningocele 609
renal osteodystrophy 93
repetition maximum (RM), concept 213
repetitive injuries *see* overuse injuries
replantation (upper limb) 1315–23
  bone fixation 1319
  contraindications 1317–18
  early complications 1321
  early management before 1316
  indications 1317
  long-term complications 1321
  microsurgical technique *see* microsurgery
  nerve repair 1320
  outcome 1320–1, 1322
  postoperative care 1320
  skin coverage and dressing 1320
  subtotal 1315
  surgical technique 1318
  tendon repair 1319–20
reproductive cloning 143
research, informed consent 1541
research methods 36–48
  applicability of results to practice 47
  hypothesis testing 39–40
  statistics 43–6
  study design *see* experimental study designs
resection arthroplasty
  hallux rigidus 1492
  hallux valgus 1439–40
reserve cartilage zone 544
reserve zone 89
resistance training 698
  older adults 709
resorption, bone *see* bone(s), resorption
resorption cavity, bone 87
respiration, in trauma management 235
respiratory rate, in exercise 704
responsiveness 39
resting zone 89
restriction enzymes 141
resurfacing arthroplasty 1176
  hip *see* hip resurfacing
resuscitation
  damage control, in polytrauma 237, 238
  endpoints 237
  low-volume, in polytrauma 237
  polytrauma 237
  spinal cord injury and 442–3
  see also Advanced Trauma Life Support (ATLS)
resuscitation systems, 'smart' 237
retractors
  humeral head 1220, 1221, 1229
  minimal incision hip arthroplasty 1149
retrobulbar haematoma 469, 475
  risk reduction 476
retrocalcaneal bursitis 832
retropulsion sign 990
retrospective cohort study 41
return to work, following work-related injuries 1543
revascularization 1316
reversal zone 88
reverse pivot-shift test, knee 26
reverse shoulder arthroplasty *see* shoulder arthroplasty (total), reverse
revision arthroplasty, metacarpophalangeal (MCP) joint 1345
revision hip arthroplasty 1118, 1153–67
  acetabular reconstruction 1158–9

impaction bone grafting 1158–9
  uncemented revision 1159
  assessment before 1156
  bone loss 1156–7
  burden/number of procedures 1153
  femoral reconstruction 1160–1
    cemented 1160–1
    cementless 1161
    impaction bone grafting 1160–1
  imaging 1199–200
  implant removal 1157–8
  for infections 1161–2
  one-stage 1161–2
  for periprosthetic fractures 1156
  rates 1102
  reasons for primary arthroplasty failures 1153–6
    see also hip arthroplasty (total)
  surgical approaches 1157
  two-stage 1156, 1161–2
  see also hip arthroplasty (total)
revision knee arthroplasty 1198–204
  clinical evaluation before 1199–200
  femoral reconstruction 1201–2
  goals 1201
  implant removal 1201
  indications 1198
  instruments for 1201
  laboratory investigations/tests 1200
  patellar reconstruction 1202
  principles 1200–2
  results 1202
  surgical approach 1201
  tibial reconstruction 1201–2
RGD-containing glycoproteins 83
rhabdomyosarcoma 919
  embryonal 912, 919
rheumatic fever, septic arthritis *vs.* 580
rheumatoid arthritis 1084–9, 1494–6
  ankle 1241, 1494
  atlantoaxial joint 65
  autoantibodies 1085
  cause 1084
  cervical spine, fusion 1268
  cytokines role 1086, 1128
  diagnosis 1085, 1494
  finger/hand deformities 1283–4
  foot and ankle 26–7, 1453
    forefoot 1495–6
    hindfoot 1494–5
    midfoot 1495
  genetic susceptibility 1084
  glenohumeral joint 1223, 1225
    see also glenohumeral joint, arthritis
  hip 1128
  HLA DR4 subtypes 1084
  juvenile *see* juvenile rheumatoid arthritis (JRA)
  MHC allele association 1084
  molecular markers 1082, 1087
  pathophysiology 1085–6, 1087, 1088, 1128, 1494
  polyarticular 1087
  self-management 1086
  stages 1085–6, 1087
  talonavicular disease 1495
  treatment 1086–7
    biological agents 1087–8
    drugs 1086
    total joint replacement 1087
  triple arthrodesis 1495
rheumatoid factor 1085
rhinorrhoea 468
rhisomelic chondrodysplasia punctata, prevalence 542
rib fusions 631
rib vertebral angle difference (RVAD) 634–5
rickets 93
  hereditary types 94
  hypophosphataemic 94, 546
  osteopenia of 95
  vitamin D-dependent 94
  vitamin D-resistant 94
rigid flat foot 693
rigidity 180
ring avulsion injuries 1321–2
'ring' sign, CSF leakage 468
Riseborough and Radin classification 1558
risk, estimation, incidence as 37
risk management, through burnout prevention 1551–2

Rivaroxaban 131, 132
road traffic accidents, children 499
Rockwood pin 289
roentgen stereophotometric analysis *see* radiostereoisometric analysis (RSA)
Rolando fracture 763, 1561
roll-back, knee arthroplasty 187, 1179
Romberg's sign 33
Röntgen, Wilhelm Conrad 155
roof arch angle, acetabular fractures 422, 423
Roos' test 33
Rotaglide 191, 192
rotation flaps, open injuries of limbs 257
rotational inertia 177
rotational profile assessment, children 537–8
rotationplasty 950
  proximal focal femoral deficiency 651
rotator cuff muscles 53, 297, 1208
  anatomy 1208
  atrophy and fat degeneration 1210
  dynamic stabilizer of shoulder 730
  in humeral shaft fractures 264
  imaging 1210–11
  innervation 53
  testing/evaluation 1208–10, 1216
rotator cuff tears 741–4, 1207–14
  aetiology 1208
  anteroinferior, examination 10
  clinical evaluation 743, 1208–11
  examination and special tests 10, 742, 1208–10
  in glenohumeral arthritis 1223
  glenohumeral instability and 1216
  history (repair) 1207–8
  history-taking 1208–9
  imaging 1210–11
  timing 1211
  non-operative treatment 1211
  presentation 741
  radiography 742
  recurrence 1214
  retracted, mobilization 1212–13
  sporting injuries 741–4
  strength tests 1209
  surgical management 742–4, 1211–14
    acromioclavicular arthropathy 1213
    acromioplasty 1212
    anaesthesia and positioning 1211
    arthroscopic repair 742–3
    biceps tendon repair 1213
    complications 1214
    coracoacromial ligament detachment 1212
    coracoacromial ligament repair 1213
    deltoid repair 1213
    deltoid splitting 1212
    guidelines for return to activity 1214
    incision 1211–12
    indications 1211
    L-shaped and reverse L-shaped tears 1212–13
    mobilization and repair 1212–13
    postoperative rehabilitation 1214
    repair 743–4
    results 744, 1214
    tendon reattachment to bone 1212
rotator cuff-deficient shoulder, arthroplasty 1256
rotator interval
  anatomy 730, 737
  capsule 1215
  closure 737, 1215
Royal Australasian College of Surgeons (RACS), surgical audit 1536
Rüedi and Allgöwer classification, tibial plafond fractures 383, 384, 1567
Ruffini ending 215
running 954
Russell–Taylor classification, subtrochanteric fracture 351, 352, 1565

SACH (solid ankle, cushioned heel) foot 965, 968
sacral fractures 433, 463–4, 1556
  classification (Denis) 463, 464

neurological injury 435
pelvic fractures with 427, 463
surgical management 464
treatment 433
sacral nerve, injury 1304
sacral plexus 429
sacral promontory 65
sacral reflexes, in spinal cord injury 441
sacral sparing, spinal fractures 440
sacroiliac joint 975
  anatomy 70
  crescent fracture treatment 432
  disruption 432–3
    treatment 432–3
  examination 34
  low back pain generation 976
  testing 21
sacroiliac ligaments 428
sacroiliac provocation test 21
sacrospinous ligament 70, 428
sacrotuberous ligament 70, 428
sacrum
  anatomy 65
  chordoma 905, 906
  fractures *see* sacral fractures
  palpation 34
saddle anaesthesia 978
saddle prosthesis 947
SAFE (stationary ankle flexible endoskeletal) foot 965
sagittal plane deformity 638
SAID principle 703
saline retention test 368
saline solutions, hypertonic–hyperoncotic, in trauma 237
Salmonella
  acute haematogenous osteomyelitis 221, 585
  septic arthritis in children 580, 581
Salter and Harris classification, fractures of physis 483–4, 496, 498
Salter osteotomy, developmental dysplasia of hip 649
sample of population 38
  size 42
sample size 42
Sanders classification, calcaneal fractures 400
Sanfilippo syndrome 574
saphenous nerve 71, 74, 77, 1500
sarcolemma 107, 699
sarcoma
  biopsy 941
  chemotherapy 880
  clear cell, hand 1377
  epithelioid, hand 1377
  Ewing's *see* Ewing's sarcoma
  limb reconstruction *see* limb reconstruction
  limb-sparing surgery 941, 942
  osteosarcoma *see* osteosarcoma
  radiotherapy 876, 941
  small round cell *see* Ewing's sarcoma
  soft-tissue *see* soft-tissue sarcoma
  spindle cell 902
  synovial *see* synovial sarcoma
sarcomeres 108, 699
  age-related changes 121
sarcopenia 121
  causes 121–2
  definition/calculation 121
  functional consequences 121, 122
sarcopenic obesity 121
sarcoplasm 107, 699
sarcoplasmic reticulum 107, 109
Sarmiento functional bracing 264, 266
satellite cells 107, 110
Sauvé–Kapanji procedure 1372
SC joint *see* sternoclavicular joint
scaffolds, tissue engineering 1525–6
scalar 173
scalp, inspection, after head injury 468
scanogram, leg length discrepancy 679
scaphoid bone 1352
  C line with radius (normal) 1356
  in scapholunate instability 1354
  in scapholunate ligament dissociation 1357
  in scapholunate ligament injury 1356
  stabilization, scapholunate dissociation repair 1357, 1358
  V pattern with radius 1356

scaphoid fractures 1561
  in athletes 755–6
    clinical features/examination 755
    treatment 755–6
scaphoid impaction syndrome 761
scaphoid shift test 1356
scaphoid–trapezium–trapezoid (STT)
  fusion 1358
scapholunate advanced collapse (SLAC)
  wrist 1358–9
scapholunate angle 757, 758, 1354,
  1355
scapholunate ballottement 14
scapholunate interosseous ligament
  (SLIL), injury 757
scapholunate interval
  widening, in acute dissociation 1357
  widening, in chronic dissociation
    1358
scapholunate joint
  degenerative changes 1358–9
  dissociation 1356
    acute, treatment 1357
    chronic, treatment 1358
    subacute, treatment 1357–8
  fusion 1358
  hyperextension 1355
  malalignment 1354
  reduction 1357, 1358
scapholunate ligament (SLL) 1351
  anatomy 1355
  complete disruption 1355, 1356
  degenerative changes 1358–9
  dorsal, palmar and fibrocartilagenous
    membrane 1355
  injury 14, 1355–62
    acute 1356, 1357
    chronic 1358
    clinical features 1356
    diagnosis 1355–6
    mechanism 1355
    partial 1356
    sign 1353
    subacute 1357–8
    treatment 1356–9
  instability 1354
    dynamic 757–8, 1354
    mechanism of injury 757
    radiography 757
    severity and features 757
    sports injury 757–8
    testing 14
    treatment 757–8
  reconstruction 1358
  tears 1352, 1355
scapho-trapezial joint, osteoarthritis
  1334
scaphotrapeziotrapezoidal (STT) joint,
  arthritis, test 14
scapula 296
  anatomy 52, 294
  fractures 294–6, 1557
    classification 295
    clinical evaluation 294
    complications 295
    mechanism 294
    radiography 294–5
    treatment 295
  neck, fractures 295
scapular dyskinesis 1215, 1216
scapular notching 1233
scapular spine 52
scapular strengthening exercises 1211
scapulectomy, partial/total 949
scapulohumeral arthrodesis 948
scapulohumeral rhythm 10
scapulothoracic amputation 963
scapulothoracic dissociation 295–6
scapulothoracic joint, anatomy 53
scapulothoracic stabilizers 730
scar tissue, after muscle injury 110
Scarf osteotomy 1438–9
Scarf test 9, 10
Schanz pins 330
Schatzker, J 259
Schatzker's classification
  distal radius fractures 318
  proximal tibial fractures 1566
  tibial plateau fractures 373, 374
Scheibel's test 10
Scheie syndrome 574
Scheuermann's kyphosis 640, 1015–16
  adolescents 1015
Schmorl's nodes 1015

Schober's test, modified 34
Schwann cells 920, 1302
schwannoma 920, 1375–6
  hand 1376
Schwartz–Jampel syndrome (SJS) 548
SCI see spinal cord injury
sciatic list (gait) 31
sciatic nerve 79
  anatomy 74
  compression, by piriformis 776
  entrapment 775
  injuries 1304, 1479, 1480
    posterior hip dislocation 335, 338
  palsy
    fracture non-union, management
      524
    pelvic fractures 433
sciatic notch 773
sciatic stretch test 35
sciatic trunk, injuries 1304, 1306
sciatica 1002
  examination/testing 21, 35
scintigraphy see radionuclide imaging
SCIWORA syndrome (spinal cord
  injury without radiographic
  abnormalities) 499
sclerosing osteomyelitis 586
scoliosis 630
  adolescent idiopathic see adolescent
    idiopathic scoliosis
  examination for 33
  idiopathic see idiopathic scoliosis
  paediatric patients
    clinical assessment 540
    with myelomeningocele 609
    see also congenital vertebral
      anomalies
  see also spinal deformities
scoliosis (adult) 1007–14
  adolescent idiopathic scoliosis vs
    1007, 1008
  aetiology 1008
  back pain 1008, 1009
  clinical presentation 1008
  de novo 1007, 1025
  definition 1007–8
  degenerative 1007, 1008, 1025
  evaluation 1009–10
  idiopathic 1008, 1009, 1010
  imaging 1010
  lumbar 1010
  neurological testing 1010
  non-operative management 1010–11
  osteoid osteoma and osteoblastoma
    1062
  physical examination 1009
  prevalence 1008
  surgical treatment 1011–13
    bone grafts/graft alternatives 1014
    indications 1011
    instrumentation and grafts
      1013–14
    outcomes 1014
    pedicle screws 1013–14
    pre-operative evaluation 1011
    spinal fusion 1011–13
'scratch test' 1396
screening tests 38
screw displacement axis (SDA) 1387
screw fixation
  fractures see fracture fixation devices
  joint implants 194
screw home mechanism, knee stability
  208
screw hook technique, isthmic
  spondylolisthesis 1052, 1053
screw osteosynthesis, paediatric
  fractures 486
scurvy 95
seat belt-type fractures, thoracolumbar
  spine 460, 461–2
Seattle foot 964
'second hit phenomenon' 240
second impact syndrome 720, 722
secondary spongiosa 89
secondary survey, after trauma 238,
  239
Sedel, Laurent, Surgeon Close to Burnout
  1550
sedlin 549
Segond fracture 808
Segond sign 366
Seinsheimer classification,
  subtrochanteric fracture 350–1

seizures, glenohumeral instability and
  1216
selective dorsal rhizotomy (SDR),
  cerebral palsy 602
selective laser melting (SLM) 1526
selective oestrogen receptor modulators
  132, 133
Semmes Weinstein filament testing
  1453
Semmes Weinstein monofilament test
  1468
sensation
  changes, compartment syndrome
    509
  hand, testing 16–17
  proprioception 214–15
sensitivity 38
  calculation 38, 39
sensory neuropathy
  diabetic foot 1466, 1468
    examination 1468
  see also neuropathy(ies)
septic arthritis 225–6, 226–7
  in children 578–82
    complications and sequelae 582
    differential diagnosis 580, 660,
      661, 662
    history 578
    investigations 579–80
    pathogenesis/pathology 578–9
    physical examination 578
    predicted probability 661
    treatment 580–2
  diagnosis 225
  differential diagnosis 225–6
  emergency management 225
  hand 1092, 1310
  knee 1092
  syphilitic 226
  treatment 226
sequestrum 587
  definition 221
seronegative spondyloarthropathies
  1089–92
  treatment 1090
sesamoid bones (foot) 415, 1442
  anatomy 1442, 1443
  fractures 415, 1445–6
    clinical features/imaging 1445–6
    non-surgical treatment 1446
    pathophysiology 1445
    surgical treatment 1446
  injuries 1443–6
    turf-toe injuries 1443–5
  lateral see fibular sesamoid
  medial see tibial sesamoid
  non-traumatic disorders 1446–7
  pain 1446, 1447
  repetitive injuries 1445
  stress fractures 848–9
  see also fibular sesamoid; tibial
    sesamoid
sesamoiditis 1446–7
SF-36, adult scoliosis 1009, 1014
shaft (support in torsion) 180
shanks, prosthetic 965
shared epitopes 1084
Sharpey's fibres 87, 994
  rupture 995
shear
  bone healing affected by 518–19, 521
  fracture non-union 518–19, 525
  simple, bending and rotational types
    519
shear force 175
shear modulus (G) 180
shear stress 180
  effect on bone healing 519
shear thickening 181
shear thinning 181
Shenton's line 335
  DDH assessment 647
shepherd's crook deformity 892
'shin splints' 821
shock
  cardiogenic 235
  evaluation and management 241
  hypovolaemic see hypovolaemic
    shock
  neurogenic 235, 443
  trauma patient 235, 241
shock absorption 185, 955
  meniscus role 104

shoe inserts
  flat foot 693
  see also foot orthoses
shoe lifts, leg length discrepancy 680
shoes 968
  hallux valgus management 1437
  inappropriate, hallux valgus 1435
short stature 570
  surgical interventions,
    achondroplasia 556–7
short stature homeobox gene (SHOX)
  545
shoulder 9
  anatomy 52–6, 297, 298
    arthrology 52–3, 297, 298, 729,
      1215, 1223–4
    blood supply 54, 55, 56
    dynamic stabilizers 297, 298, 730,
      735, 1215
    ligaments 297, 298, 729, 1215
    muscles 53, 297, 1208, 1215
    nerves 53–4
    osteology 52
    static stabilizers 297, 298, 729–30,
      735, 1215
    see also glenohumeral joint;
      glenohumeral ligaments;
      rotator cuff muscles
  anterior capsular tear 297, 298
  arthritis see glenohumeral joint,
    arthritis
  arthrodesis 618, 1268, 1273
  arthroscopy see arthroscopy
  biomechanics 187
  capsule see glenohumeral joint
  clinical examination 9–11
    inspection 9–10
    movement 10
    palpation 10
    special tests 10–11
  deformities
    brachial plexus birth palsy 616,
      617–18
    see also specific types
  disarticulation 963
  dislocation 297
    anterior 297, 298–300
    clinical evaluation 298, 300
    complications 299–300, 301
    frequency 297
    historical aspects 1214
    immediate reduction 299
    inferior glenohumeral dislocation
      301
    pathoanatomy 297–8
    posterior 300–1
    post-reduction treatment 299
    radiographic evaluation 298–9,
      300–1
    recurrent 298, 299, 301, 1214
    superior glenohumeral dislocation
      301
    treatment 299, 301
    types 298
    see also glenohumeral joint,
      dislocations
  double-jointed, adolescent 300
  downward sagging 285
  external rotation
    loss 1224, 1227
    test 1209
  hemiarthroplasty 1223, 1232
    young patients 1256
  history-taking 9
  impingement, rotator cuff tears 741
  instability see glenohumeral joint
  internal rotation contracture 1227
  labrum see glenoid labrum
  laxity 730, 738
  ligaments 298
  loose bodies 714
  pain
    anterior 1208
    impingement syndrome 1209
    posterior instability 735
    rotator cuff tears 741
  'popping' 739
  prostheses 963–4
  range of motion 187, 297
  reconstruction 1207
  replacement see shoulder
    arthroplasty (total)
  sporting injuries see sports injuries;
    specific injuries

stability
  concavity-compression mechanism 297, 1215
  static/dynamic stabilizers 297, 298, 729–30, 1215
  see also glenohumeral joint
stiffness 1209
  after proximal humerus fractures 305
  rotator cuff tears and 1211, 1214
subluxation, posterior instability 735
surgical approaches 54–6, 1207, 1215
  anterior (Henry) 55, 56
  deltopectoral incision 1226
  lateral and anterolateral 55–6
  posterior 56
tenderness, diffuse 10
unstable see glenohumeral joint, instability
winging 54
see also acromioclavicular (AC) joint; glenohumeral joint
shoulder abduction (relief) test 33
shoulder arthroplasty (total) 193, 1225–33
  anatomic 1225–30
    anaesthesia and positioning 1225–6
    closure 1230
    deep exposure 1226
    glenoid component placement 1228–9
    glenoid exposure, preparation 1228–9
    humeral component placement 1229–30, 1231
    humeral exposure, osteotomy 1227–8
    humeral preparation 1229–30
    incision and superficial exposure 1226
    results 1232, 1233
    subscapularis reflection, capsular release 1226–7
  complications 1232–3
  goal 1223
  history 1223
  indications 1255
  materials used for 192
  postoperative rehabilitation 1232
  prostheses 963–4
  prosthetic designs 1223
  results 1232–3
  reverse 1230–2
    closure 1231
    complications 1233
    final components placement 1231
    glenoid component trial placement 1231
    glenoid exposure and preparation 1231
    humeral component trial placement 1231
    humeral osteotomy and reaming 1230–1
    results 1232
    subscapularis reflection, capsular release 1230
  rotator cuff-deficient shoulder 1256
  unconstrained 1223
  young patients 1255–6
shoulder spaces 57, 58
SHOX (short stature homeobox gene) 545
shuck test (Kleinman shear test) 15
sialoprotein, rheumatoid arthritis marker 1082
SIBLING proteins 83
sickle cell anaemia
  osteomyelitis 585
  septic arthritis 580, 581
side swipe injuries 312
sigmoid notch 318
signals, tissue engineering 1527
silastic arthroplasty, hallux rigidus 1491
Silfverskiold test 29, 31, 601
silicone, for implants 189
  fingers 193, 1339, 1343, 1346
Simmond's test 31
Simond's calf squeeze test 830
simple bone cyst (SBC) 887–8
Simplex P 1139–40
single leg heel rise test 1422

single-photon emission CT (SPECT) 157
single-stranded conformation polymorphism analysis (SSCP) 141
sinus tarsi 28
sinus tarsi syndrome 1464
sinuvertebral nerve 995
'six degrees of freedom' 207
  knee 207–8
skaters' heel 832
skeletal development
  children 482–3
  see also embryological development
skeletal dysmorphology syndrome see developmental disorders of bone
skeletal dysplasia 541, 570–5
  classification 570–5
  histopathological examination 554, 556
  pathophysiology 570, 571
  radiography see under radiography
  see also developmental disorders of bone; specific disorders
skeletal morphogenesis 543–4
skeletal muscle see muscle (skeletal)
skeletal survey, children, non-accidental injuries 501
skeletal system, development see embryological development
skewed distribution 43
skewfoot 692
skier's thumb 763–4
skiing accidents 382
skin, in amputations 960
skin cancer, hand 1376–7
skin flaps, in amputations 960
skin graft, full thickness, Dupuytren's contracture 1329
'skip' lesions
  bone tumours 886, 900, 948
  spinal infections 984
  spinal tuberculosis 987
  spinal tumours 1059, 1061
skull 478
  sutures, vs fractures (radiography) 479
skull fractures
  base of skull 478
  children 478
  classification 478–9
  depressed 478–9
  linear 478
  open 479
  surgical treatment 479
  temporal bone 478
SLAC wrist 1358–9
SLAP tears/lesions 739–41, 1557
  classification 739
  clinical features 739
  imaging 740
  management 740
  outcome after repair 741
  physical examination 739–40
  surgical technique 740–1
sleep palsy 1397
sliding filament theory 109
sliding hip screws 348
SLIL (scapholunate interosseous ligament) tears 757, 758
slipped capital femoral epiphysis (SCFE) 656–9, 661–2, 770
  classification and natural history 657
  clinical features and imaging 657–8
  complications management 659–60
  physical examination 657
  stable 657, 659
  treatment 658–9
  unstable 657, 658–9
slump test 34
Smith fracture (reverse Colles fracture) 328–9, 1560
Smith-Petersen, Marius Nygaard 1098
Smith-Petersen osteotomy 1019
Smith–Peterson approach to hip 72, 1136–7, 1149
  DDH treatment 649
smoking
  degenerative disc disease 994
  fracture healing affected by 518, 524
smooth muscle tumours 883, 916, 919
snapping iliopsoas tendon 775–6
snapping iliotibial band 776
snowboarder fractures 396

socioeconomic burden, spinal cord injury 440
sockets, lower limb prostheses 966
sodium urate crystals 1091, 1374
soft tissue(s) 100–19
  amputations and 957, 960
  fracture non-union management 522
  healing 100
soft-tissue haemangioma, MRI 869
soft-tissue infections 219–21
  gadolinium contrast MRI 164
  management 220, 221
soft-tissue injuries
  acute compartment syndrome due to 279
  lumbar spine, low back pain 978–9
  Morel–Lavallee lesion 426
  pelvic fractures and 426
  trauma, evaluation/management 241
soft-tissue mass, gadolinium contrast MRI 163, 171
soft-tissue reconstruction, open injuries of limbs 255, 256–7
soft-tissue sarcoma 912–24
  aetiology 912–13
  age and location 912
  amputation 915
  biopsy 915
  chemotherapy 880, 951
  clinical features 913
  epidemiology 912
  grade and size 915
  hand 1377
  imaging 878, 913
  metastases 915
  radiotherapy 876–8, 941, 951
    algorithm, with surgery 877
    clinical target volume 877
    gross target volume 877
    planning, principles 877–8
    postoperative 877
    pre-operative 877, 941
    randomized trials
      excision with radiotherapy 876
      surgery only 876
  staging 914–15
  surgical treatment
    limb-sparing surgery 941, 942
    margin width for excision 915, 942
    planes of dissection 915
    principles 915–16
    reconstruction after resection 951
  treatment
    brachytherapy 876
    radiotherapy with surgery 877
    surgery 876
soft-tissue tumours
  benign 912, 913, 914, 916, 920
  hand 1374–6
  classification 913–14, 916
  clinical features 913
  history-taking 866
  imaging 866, 921
  intermediate (locally aggressive) 914, 916
  intermediate (rarely metastasizing) 914, 916
  malignant 914, 916
    hand 1376–7
    see also liposarcoma; soft-tissue sarcoma
  pathology 916–21
  recurrence 921
  surgical treatment, principles 915–16
  surveillance strategies 921
  of uncertain differentiation 920
soleus muscle
  action and function 956
  lengthening in cerebral palsy 604
  weakness, gait 957
somatic cell nuclear transfer 143
somites 542, 629
Sorensen's criteria, Scheuermann's kyphosis 1015
Southern approach to hip 73, 74, 1137, 1149
Southern blotting 142
SOX9 545
space of Poirier 1351, 1352
spasticity 568
  adult-acquired 969, 970
  cerebral palsy examination 600–1
  stroke patients 1477–8

Spearman rank order 44
specific adaptations to imposed demands (SAID) principle 703
specificity 38
  calculation 38, 39
speed 174
  angular 174
  average 174
Speed's test 11, 739
sphenoid bone 474
spica cast, DDH treatment 648, 649
spicules 89
spina bifida see myelomeningocele
spina bifida occulta 608
spinal accessory nerve, injuries 54
spinal anaesthesia, in hip arthroplasty 1124, 1126
spinal arthrodesis 1014, 1052
  in spondylolisthesis 1052, 1056
  see also spinal fusion
spinal bracing
  achondroplasia 557
  adolescent idiopathic scoliosis 638
  cerebral palsy 607
  congenital spine deformities 632
  infantile idiopathic scoliosis 635
  juvenile idiopathic scoliosis 636
  myelomeningocele 609
  Scheuermann's kyphosis 640
spinal canal
  lumbar see lumbar spinal canal
  stenosis
    central 999, 1000, 1002
    degenerative spondylolisthesis 1055
    lateral 998, 1002
    lumbar 32, 998–9, 1000, 1050
  zones 996–7
spinal claudication (lumbar canal stenosis) 32
spinal cord 439
  anatomy 66–7
    arterial supply 68
    ascending/descending tracts 66–7
    compression, tuberculosis 990
    lumbar 976
    space for 446, 447
spinal cord injury 1479
  associated injuries 442–3
  bone loss from 95
  cervical 440, 445
    neurogenic shock 443
    see also cervical cord injury
  children 499
  classification 441–2
  complete 440, 441
  epidemiology 439–40
  'golden hour' 234, 440
  incomplete 440, 441–2
  patterns 443
  lumbar 440
  management
    evaluation in emergency department 442–3
    pharmacological 445
    pre-hospital care 440
    primary survey and ABCDE 235, 238–9, 440, 442, 444–5
  neurological classification (ASIA) 441, 725
  pathophysiology 440
  patterns 67, 443
  primary injury 440
  radiographic evaluation 444
  secondary injury 440
  'shutdown' after injury 441
  socioeconomic burden 440
  terminology 442
  thoracic 32, 443
  treatment by functional level 970–1
  without radiographic abnormalities (SCIWORA) 499
  see also spinal injuries
spinal decompression see decompression surgery
spinal deformities 630
  adult 1007–23
    causes 1007
    kyphosis see kyphosis
    management 1007
    in sagittal plane 1015
    see also kyphosis
    scoliosis see scoliosis (adult)
    spinal tumours 1059

spinal deformities – *continued*
  in children 627–40
    adolescent postural kyphosis 638, 640
    with cerebral palsy 607
    with Charcot–Marie–Tooth disease 614
    congenital *see* congenital vertebral anomalies
    idiopathic scoliosis *see* idiopathic scoliosis
    with myelomeningocele 609
    sagittal plane deformity 638
    Scheuermann's kyphosis 640
  see also kyphosis; scoliosis
spinal dysraphism 608
spinal fractures 238–9, 439–65, 1555–6
  ankylosing spondylitis 1089–90
  neural injury 440–2
  osteoporotic *see* osteoporosis, spinal
  principles of treatment 444–5
  see also vertebral body, compression fractures
spinal fusion 196, 1014, 1052
  in adult scoliosis treatment 1011–13
    extent 1011, 1012
    to sacrum 1012–13, 1020
  anterior, with instrumentation
    adult scoliosis 1011, 1012
    osteoporotic kyphosis 1017
  combined anterior/posterior and instrumentation
    adult scoliosis 1011, 1012, 1013
    osteoporotic kyphosis 1017
    post-traumatic kyphosis 1019
  congenital spine deformities 631, 632
  degenerative disc disease 1003
  devices for 196–7
  interbody techniques *see* posterior lumbar interbody fusion (PLIF); transforaminal lumbar interbody fusion (TLIF)
  juvenile idiopathic scoliosis 636
  lumbar 1013–14
  lumbosacral 1003, 1012–13
  muscular dystrophy 611
  number of procedures performed 1014
  in osteoporosis 1041
  posterior, with instrumentation
    adult scoliosis 1011
    anterior release/fusion before 1011, 1012
    osteoporotic kyphosis 1017
    spondylolisthesis 1052, 1053
  posterior 360° method 1053, 1054
  posterolateral, in spondylolisthesis 1052–3
  revision, complications 1018–19
  segmental instrumentation with 1013–14
    adult scoliosis 1011, 1012
    flat back syndrome and 1018, 1019
  in spinal cord injury 970
  in spondylolisthesis 1052, 1056
  thoracic 1012
spinal immobilization 445
  after injury 235, 238, 440, 442, 445
spinal implants 196–7
  disc replacement devices 197
  fusion devices 196–7
  nucleus replacement devices 197
spinal infections 982–92
  Brucella spondylitis 986
  in children 983
  fungal 986
  parasitic 986
  prognosis 982, 985
  pyogenic 982–5
    aetiology 983
    clinical presentation 983
    conservative treatment 985
    diagnostic imaging 984
    differential diagnosis 985
    histopathology 985
    incidence/epidemiology 982
    investigations 983–5
    mortality 985
    pathophysiology/infection route 983
    postoperative 985–6
    risk factors 983
    surgical treatment 985

surgical treatment 982
tuberculosis *see* tuberculosis
spinal injuries 439–65
  cervical *see* cervical spine injuries
  children 499
    non-accidental 501
  cord injuries *see* spinal cord injury
  CT scans 158
  epidemiology 439–40
  fractures *see* spinal fractures
  immobilization and realignment 235, 238, 440, 442, 445
  lumbar *see* lumbar spine, injuries
  resuscitation 440, 442, 444–5
  in sport 718–28
  thoracolumbar *see* thoracolumbar spine injuries
  see also spinal cord injury
spinal ligaments 65–6
spinal metastases 926, 1058, 1064, 1065–9
  CyberKnife stereotactic surgery 1068
  epidemiology 1065
  hypercalcaemia 1059
  immuno-oncology 1068–9
  location 1065
  palliative surgery 1066
  paraplegia with 1065
  primary tumours causing 1064, 1065, 1066
  stabilization 1065
  surgical approaches 1066–8
    overtreatment 1067
  survival rates 1065
  Tokuhashi score 1061, 1066
  Tomita classification 1060–1, 1066
spinal nerve roots 67–8
  chemical irritation 976
  compression 976
  injury 443
spinal nerves 67–8
spinal shock 440, 441
  resolution, testing 441
spinal stenosis *see* spinal canal, stenosis
spinal tumours 1058–71
  biopsy 1060
  clinical presentation 1058–9
  diagnosis 1058–65
  immunotherapy 1068–9
  metastatic *see* spinal metastases
  radionuclide bone scan 1059–60
  staging 1060–1
  treatment principles 1061
  types 1061–4, 1065
    primary benign 1061–2, 1065
    primary malignant 1063
    secondary *see* spinal metastases
  work-up 1059–60
spindle cell sarcoma 902
spine 973–1071
  alignment 439
    realignment after injury 445
  anatomy 64–9, 975–6
    columns (Denis) 65, 453, 460
    muscles 66
    nerves 66–7
    neuromuscular 66–8
    osteology 64–6
    vascular supply 68
  anterior column insufficiency, in osteoporosis 1017
  biomechanics 187–8
  cleared 444
  clinical examination 31–5
    cervical 32–3
    lumbar 34–5
    thoracic 33–4
  deformities *see* spinal deformities
  degenerative disease 993
    see also degenerative disc disease; degenerative spine disease
  epidural abscess 983
  examination, in children 540
    with cerebral palsy 601
  fractures *see* spinal fractures
  free body diagram 187
  gadolinium contrast MRI 165
  global stabilizing muscles 979
  growth and development 627–8
  history-taking 32
  ideal balance line 1049
  infections *see* spinal infections
  instability, in osteoporotic kyphosis 1017

local stabilizing muscles 979
metastases *see* spinal metastases
motion segment 105
orthoses 969
  see also spinal bracing
osteonecrosis *see* osteonecrosis (avascular necrosis), spine
osteoporosis *see* osteoporosis, spinal
osteotomy, ankylosing spondylitis 1089
pain 32, 1136
posterior elements 975
range of motion 187–8
sagittal balance 1015, 1018, 1049
  ideal balance line 1049
  imbalance 1018, 1049
sagittal plane
  deformity 1015
  normal 1015, 1018
stability 65
  management in spinal tumours 1061
surgery in children
  achondroplasia 557
  cerebral palsy 607
  congenital spine deformities 631, 632
  infantile idiopathic scoliosis 635
  see also specific types of spinal surgery
surgical approaches 68–9
  anterior (to cervical spine) 68–9
  anterior (to lumbar spine) 68, 69
  anterolateral (retroperitoneal) 69
  posterior (to cervical spine) 68, 69
  posterior (to lumbar spine) 69
  to thoracic spine 69
tumours *see* spinal tumours
vertebrae number 64
  see also cervical spine; lumbar spine; thoracic spine; vertebrae
'spine at risk' 991
  in tuberculosis 990
spine board 445
spinoglenoid notch 52
spinothalamic tracts 66, 67
splints/splinting
  boutonnière deformity 1282
  coaptation, humeral shaft fractures 308
  cock-up, in epicondylitis 1395
  cubital tunnel syndrome 1404–5
  dynamic traction, phalangeal fractures 1286
  flexor tendon injuries 1297
  for fractures 260
  history 4
  PIP joint dislocations 1285
  sugar tong
    distal radius fractures 261
    forearm fractures 263
    humeral shaft fractures 264
  trigger finger 1277
split thickness skin graft, open injuries of limbs 256
spondylitis
  in brucellosis 986
  Kümmel's *see* osteonecrosis (avascular necrosis), spine
spondyloarthropathies, treatment 1090
spondylodiscitis 984
  postoperative 986
spondyloepiphyseal dysplasia (SED) 570, 573
spondyloepiphyseal dysplasia congenita 573
spondyloepiphyseal dysplasia tarda (SEDT) 547, 548, 549, 573
spondylolisthesis 1048–57
  C2 1556
  classification 1048, 1051
  definition 1000, 1048
  degenerative 1000, 1048, 1054–6
    conservative treatment 1055
    diagnosis 1055
    natural history 1055
    pathogenic mechanism 1054–5
    surgical treatment 1055–6
  dysplastic form 1050
  by isthmic lysis 1048–54
    aetiology 1048–9
    classification 1051
    conservative treatment 1052
    diagnosis 1050–1

    disc degeneration 1050, 1051, 1052
    epidemiology 1048
    imaging 1051
    natural history 1051–2
    pathomechanism 1049–50
    surgical treatment 1052–4
  low back pain 977
  traumatic 1048
    C2 vertebrae 451, 452
    classification 451
spondylolysis 65, 977
  surgical treatment 1052
spondyloperipheral dysplasia 547–8
sports injuries
  ankle 836–43
    anterior/subtalar joint impingement 838–9
    deltoid ligament sprains 843
    flexor hallucis longus stenosis 839–40
    lateral ligamentous instability 840–2
    osteochondral lesions of talus 836–7
    posterior impingement 839–40
    syndesmotic sprains 842–3
  elbow 750–5
    cubital tunnel syndrome 1405
    lateral epicondylitis 750–1, 1390, 1394
    medial epicondylitis 751, 1390, 1394
    osteochondritis dissecans 753–4
    posterolateral rotatory instability 754–5
    ulnar collateral ligament rupture 751–3
    valgus extension overload syndrome 753
  epidemiology 705
  hand 762–8
    Bennett's fracture 763
    boutonnière deformity 765–6, 1282–3
    extra-articular phalangeal fractures 1286–7
    fractures 766–8
    jersey finger 762, 1279, 1296
    mallet finger 762–3, 1280–2
    PIP joint dislocations 764–5, 1284–5
    pseudoboutonnière deformity 766
    Rolando fracture 763
    skier's and gamekeeper's thumb 763–4
  knee, ligamentous 805–20
    anterior cruciate ligament 807–11
    medial collateral ligament 805–7
    multiligamentous 813–15
    posterior cruciate ligament 811–12
    posterolateral corner 812–13
    see also specific ligaments
  knee, non-ligamentous 782–804
    meniscal 785–8
    see also knee, non-ligamentous injuries
  leg 821–36
    common peroneal nerve entrapment 826–8
    exercise-induced pain 821–9
    exertional compartment syndrome 825–6
    medial tibial stress syndrome 824–5
    peroneal tendon problems 834–5
    posterior tibial tendon problems 835–6
    superficial peroneal nerve entrapment 827–9
    tendon problems 829–36
    tibial stress fractures 821–3
    see also Achilles tendon
  lumbar spine 977
  midfoot/forefoot pain 843–9
    fifth metatarsal fractures 846–7
    first MTP joint stress fractures 848–9
    lateral/medial plantar nerve entrapment 847–8
    Lisfranc sprains 843–5
    navicular stress fractures 845–6
    turf-toe injuries 1443
  MRI scan use 169
  nutrition *see* nutrition

pelvis, hip and thigh 772–81
    bone disorders 776–8
    bursitis 775
    contusions 773, 774
    intra-articular disorders 778–9
    muscle strains 774–5
    nerve entrapment 775
    syndromes 775–6
premature osteoarthritis and 1080
prevention 705
shoulder
    instability 729–39, 1216
    rotator cuff tears 741–4
    SLAP lesions 739–41
spine, isthmic spondylolisthesis 1048, 1051, 1052
types 705
wrist 755–62
    de Quervain's tenosynovitis 760
    dorsal wrist syndromes 761–2
    extensor carpi ulnaris tendinitis/subluxation 761
    gymnast's wrist 761–2
    handlebar palsy 760
    hook of hamate fractures 756–7
    hypothenar hammer syndrome 760
    intersection syndrome 761
    scaphoid fractures 755–6
    scapholunate instability 757–8
    triangular fibrocartilage complex (TFCC) 758
    see also individual anatomical structures/injuries
sports medicine 697–862
spotted bone disease (osteopoikilosis) 96
Spry1 gene 547
Spurling's compression test 33
squamous cell carcinoma (SCC), hand 1376–7
squeaking, hip replacement 1098, 1120
squeeze and turn test 14
squeeze test
    ankle injuries 386, 1425
    syndesmotic sprains 392
    foot 28
    Simond's, calf 830
    syndesmotic sprains, ankle 843
stability, of fixation 269–70
stabilization, skeletal 255
stable patients, after trauma 237, 241
stable slipped capital femoral epiphysis 657, 659
stainless steel 188
stair climbing, prosthetic problem 967
stakeholders of healthcare 1537
STALIF TT 197
standard deviation 43
Stanmore implant 942
Stanmore Juvenile Tumour System 950
Staphylococcus aureus
    acute haematogenous osteomyelitis 221, 582, 585
    cellulitis 219
    hand infections 1309
    hip arthroplasty infections 1126
    knee arthritis model 1092
    meticillin-resistant see meticillin-resistant *Staphylococcus aureus* (MRSA)
    open fracture infections 253
    septic arthritis in children 580, 581
    spinal infections 983, 985
Staphylococcus epidermidis
    cellulitis 219
    hip arthroplasty infections 1155
statics 178
statistical analyses 44–6
statistics 43–6
    descriptive vs inferential 43–4
    parametric and non-parametric 44
statutory workers' compensation see workers' compensation
Steadman microfracture technique 1083
Steinmann, Fritz 5
Steinmann pin 259
stem cells
    haematopoietic 1068, 1527
    human embryonic (HESC) cell lines 144
    induced pluripotent (IPSCs) 1526

mesenchymal 1527, 1529
    potency 1526
    tissue engineering 1526–7
        autologous chondrocyte implantation 1528–9
stems, in hip replacement see femoral stem (implants)
Stener's lesion 764
stenosing tenosynovitis see trigger finger/thumb
step-off sign 25
sternoclavicular joint
    anatomy 52, 291
    dislocations 292
        anterior 291, 292
        complications 292
        posterior 291–2
    injuries 291–6
        clinical evaluation 291–2
        complications 292
        mechanism 291
        radiography 292
        treatment 292
sternocleidomastoid muscle 66
steroids 129
    fracture non-union 518
    see also corticosteroid(s); glucocorticoid(s)
Stewart–Treves syndrome 919
Stickler syndrome 573
stiffness, tensile, definition 178
Stimson prone reduction technique 299
stimulants, use by athletes 707
'stinger' see cervical neuropraxia ('stinger')
storage modulus (E') 181–2
Stout–Obwegeser ligatures 477
straight leg raise (SLR) test 21, 35
    for prolapse disc 34–5
strain, fractures 270, 271
    healing affected by 518
strain theory, fracture healing 270
strap muscles, of neck 66
strength testing, muscles see under muscle (skeletal)
strength training 703
streptococcal infections
    acute haematogenous osteomyelitis in children 585
    septic arthritis in children 580, 581
Streptococcus pyogenes, cellulitis 219
streptokinase 132
stress (mechanical) 178–9
    definition 178
    engineering 178
    repetitive, to viscoelastic material 182
    true 178
stress corrosion 1115, 1116
stress fractures
    aetiology, by tissue 821–2
    athletes 777
    compression-sided, femoral neck 345
    femoral neck 345, 777, 1565
    femoral shaft 777
    fifth metatarsal 846, 847
    first MTP joint 848–9
    forefoot 411
    MRI scan 169, 171
    navicular bone 845–6
    pars interarticularis 977
    pelvis 777
    sesamoid bones 848–9
    tension-sided, femoral neck 345
    tibia see tibia, stress fractures
stress injuries, midfoot 404
stress relaxation 181
'stress shielders' 211
stressors, in orthopaedic surgery 1550
    see also burnout
stress–strain curve 179
    Hooke's law and 179
    hysteresis 181, 182
    non-Hookean curve 179
    tendons 112
    ultimate tensile strength 182
    yield point 182
stretching
    Achilles tendonopathy 833
    adult scoliosis 1011
stride 954, 955
stroke 1477–8
    surgery for 969–71
stroke volume 704
Stromeyer, Louis 4

strontium (Protelos) 133–4
strontium ranelate 134
    structure 133
structural model index (SMI) 1026
structural protein defects 547–8
    see also specific disorders
strut grafts, periprosthetic fracture management 1156
Stryker manometer 509
'stubbing' injuries 415, 416
student's elbow see olecranon bursitis
Student's t-test 44
study designs 40–2
'stutter' test 26
styloidectomy 1358–9
subacromial impingement 1208
    radiography 1210
    tests 10
subchondral bone 1077, 1079
    ankle 1242, 1245
    architecture, factors affecting 1079
    damage 1079
    functions 1079
    in hip arthroplasty 1139
    joint line to pain ratio 1081
    osteopenia 984
    resorption 1079
    structural/mechanical changes, osteoarthritis 1081, 1242
    tibia, osteoarthritis 1081
    type III cartilage injuries 103
subchondral bone spaces, pressure effect, osteoarthritis 1081
subclavian artery 54
subdental synchondrosis 64–5
subscapularis muscle 1208
    anatomic shoulder replacement 1226–7
    as dynamic stabilizer 735
    examination/tests 10, 1210
    reflection, reverse shoulder arthroplasty 1230–1
    repair
        anatomic total shoulder arthroplasty 1230
        open Bankart's repair 1219
    z-lengthening 1227, 1230
subscapularis tendon
    detachment, in total shoulder replacement 1226–7
    incision, open Bankart's repair 1218, 1219
subtalar joint 27, 78
    arthrodesis
        cerebral palsy 605, 1476
        hindfoot osteoarthritis 1489
    dislocation 397
    inversion and eversion 29
    movements 29, 1243
    osteoarthritis 1488–9
    soft-tissue impingement 838–9
        examination/evaluation 838–9
        treatment 839
subtalar joint ligaments, tears 838
subtrochanteric fracture 97, 350–2, 1565
    classification 350–1
    clinical/radiological evaluation 350
    complications 352
    mechanism of injury 350
    pathological, treatment 934
    treatment 351
        implant choice 351–2
subungual abscess 1311
subungual haematoma 1288–9
succinylcholine 700
'suction sign' 30
sulcus sign, positive 731
sulfasalazine, rheumatoid arthritis 1086
sulphate transport defects 549
'sun ray' appearance 900
superficial femoral artery 71, 75
superficial peroneal nerve 76, 79, 1500, 1506
    entrapment 827–9, 1506
        aetiology 827–8
        evaluation/examination 828
        pathology 828
        treatment 828–9
superior glenohumeral ligament (SGHL) 730, 1215
superior gluteal nerve 71, 79
superior labrum anterior to posterior (SLAP) tears see SLAP tears/lesions
superior lateral geniculate artery 77

superior peroneal retinaculum (SPR) 1429
    avulsion 834
superior shoulder suspensory complex (SSC), disruptions 295
supination–external rotation (SER), ankle fractures 387, 388, 498
support phases, gait cycle 564
suppurative flexor tenosynovitis (SFT) 1310, 1312–13
supracondylar femoral osteotomy 1081
supracondylar fracture of humerus (SCH)
    children 488–9
    classification 488–9
    compartment syndrome pathogenesis 505
    nerve injuries 489
    non-union, treatment 527
supracondylar suspension (lower limb prosthesis) 966
supramalleolar derotational osteotomy, cerebral palsy 605
supramalleolar osteotomy, ankle osteoarthritis 1488
suprapatellar plica syndrome 783
suprascapular nerve 1208, 1215
    injuries 1306
suprascapular notch 52
supraspinatus muscle
    avulsion 1213
    examination/tests 10
    strength testing 1209, 1210
    tears, examination/imaging 10, 1210
    thinning, in arthritis 1225
supraspinous ligament 65, 976
sural nerve 77, 1500
Surgeon Close to Burnout (Sedel) 1550
surgery
    strategy in polytrauma 239–41
    see also individual procedures/indications
surgical audit 1536
surgical control, in CAOS 1515
surgical margins
    limb-sparing surgery 942
    sarcomas 915, 942
surgical wound infections 220
    antibiotic treatment 220
    pelvic fractures 435
Surveillance Epidemiology and End Result (SEER) programme 883, 884
suspension systems, prostheses 966–7
suspensionplasty, trapeziometacarpal osteoarthritis 1337, 1339
Sutter implant 193
suturing
    extensor tendons 1298, 1299
    flexor tendons 1295–6
    microsurgical repair of blood vessels 1319
swan neck deformity 1283–4
Swanson finger implant 192, 193, 1343, 1346
Swanson wrist implants 193, 194
Syme's amputation 958, 961
sympathetic chain, cervical 68
symphysis pubis 428
    anatomy 70, 428
    disruptions, treatment 431
    external fixation 431
    injuries, in athletes 777–8
symptom-modifying anti-rheumatic drugs (SMARDs) 1086
symptoms of condition 8–9
synapses 108, 700
    description 700
synaptic cleft 700
syndesmosis 842
syndesmotic sprains, ankle 391–3, 842–3
    aetiology/pathology 842
    evaluation 842–3
    external rotation stress test 391–3
    treatment 843
syndesmotic stabilization, fibular fractures above plafond 390
synovectomy
    juvenile rheumatoid arthritis 1089
    pigmented villonodular synovitis 784–5
    radiation 1087
    rheumatoid arthritis 1087

synovial A cells 782, 1079
synovial abrasion, meniscal tear surgery 105
synovial B cells 782, 1079–80
synovial chondromatosis 783–4
   hand 1376
synovial disease, knee 782
synovial fluid 1079–80
   analysis
      juvenile idiopathic arthritis 594
      septic arthritis 580
   juvenile idiopathic arthritis 590
   rheumatoid arthritis 1086
synovial fluid fistula 718
synovial joints 1077–80
   age-related changes 1080
   cellular metabolism 1077–80
   nitric oxide and inflammation 1078
   replacement 189–94
   see also individual joints
synovial membrane see synovium
synovial osteochondromatosis 783–4
synovial plica syndrome 22
synovial pseudarthrosis 517
synovial sarcoma 920
   chemotherapy 880
   epidemiology 912
   hand 1377
synovial tendon sheaths
   inflammation see tenosynovitis
   structure 111
synoviocytes 782
synovitis
   persistent, rheumatoid arthritis 1087
   transient see transient synovitis
   trapeziometacarpal (TM) joint osteoarthritis 1334
synovium 782, 1079–80
   appearance in disease 782
   MRI appearance 169
   neovascularization, rheumatoid arthritis 1085
   proliferation 783
      rheumatoid arthritis 1085
   structure 1079–80
   type A (phagocytic) cells 782, 1079
   type B (macrophage-like) cells 782, 1079–80
Synthes (end caps) 494
synthetic biomaterials see biomaterials, synthetic
syphilis
   joint infection 226
   osteomyelitis in 224
syringomyelia, cubital tunnel syndrome vs 1399
systematic reviews 42
systemic lupus erythematosus (SLE) 1090–1, 1497
systemic-onset juvenile idiopathic arthritis 590, 591, 592–3, 594

T cell receptor (TCR), vaccination, in rheumatoid arthritis 1087
T lymphocytes (T cells) 147, 1068
   antigen presentation 1068, 1084
      prevention, rheumatoid arthritis therapy 1087–8
   CD8 type (cytotoxic) 1068
   cytokines formed 1085
   helper (CD4) 1068, 1084
      HIV-positive haemophiliacs 1092
   increased, juvenile rheumatoid arthritis 1089
   memory cells 1068, 1069
      reactivation by tumour vaccination 1069
   monoclonal antibodies to 1087
   rheumatoid arthritis pathophysiology 1085
      biological therapy 1087–8
   transplant rejection 148
   tumour-specific, transfer 1069
T4 ligase 141
table-top test 1327
tachycardia
   hypovolaemic shock 236
   polytrauma in children 500
talar body fractures 397
talar dome, mapping 836–7
talar head fractures 396
talar neck fractures 394–6
   classification 395
   clinical evaluation 394–5
   complications 396
   mechanism of injury 394
   radiology 395
   treatment 395–6
talar shift, ankle fractures 266
talar tilt test 30, 841
talipes equinovarus 552, 688–91
   aetiology 688–9
   anatomy 689
   in cerebral palsy, management 604–5, 1476
   classification 689
   congenital 688–91
   epidemiology 688
   examination 689
   in myelomeningocele 610
   prenatal diagnosis 689
   stroke patients 1478
   treatment 689–91
talipes equinus
   in cerebral palsy 601
      management 604, 1475–6
   in myelomeningocele 610
   stroke patients 1478
talocalcaneal joint
   dislocation at 397
   osteoarthritis 1488–9
talocrural angle 387
talonavicular joint 403
   arthrodesis 1495
   dislocation at 397
   in pes planus 1465
   rheumatoid disease 1495
talus 77
   anatomy 394, 1243
   avascular necrosis 528, 529
   dislocation 397
   excision 528
   fractures 394–6
      head 396
      lateral process 396
      neck see talar neck fractures
      posterior process 396
      talus body 397
   osteochondral lesions 836–7
      aetiology 836–7
      evaluation 837
      lateral and medial lesions 837
      non-operative treatment 837
      operative treatment 837
Tanner staging, juvenile idiopathic scoliosis 636
tantalum trabecular metal implants 1121, 1159
taper 1140
'target' sign 920
targeted therapy 878
tarsal coalition, rigid flat foot 693
tarsal navicular see navicular bone
tarsal tunnel 28
   anatomy 1503
tarsal tunnel syndrome 28, 1502–4
   anterior 1505–6
   distal 1502
tarsometatarsal (TMT) joint 78
   anatomy 407
   examination 28, 29
   fracture dislocations 409
   injuries 407–10
      classification 408, 409
      clinical/radiographic evaluation 407–8
      treatment 408–9
   movements 29
   radiography 407, 408
   see also Lisfranc joint complex
tarsus 77
   ossification 78
Taylor spatial frame fixator 528
T-cast wedging 485
technetium-99m diphosphonate 156, 930
teeth
   loose 470
   in maxillomandibular fixation 477
teleroentgenograph, leg length discrepancy 679
temperature (body), trauma patient 241
templating
   hip arthroplasty 1136
   pelvic fractures 434
   PIP joint 1344
temporal bone, fractures 478
temporary arrest of growth, genu varum/valgum treatment 669
temporomandibular joint (TMJ), factures 469
tendinitis
   Achilles tendon see Achilles tendon
   tenosynovitis vs, foot 28
tendinopathy
   Achilles tendon see Achilles tendon
   aetiology 113
tendon(s) 110–14
   acute rupture 113
   age-related changes 120
   attachment to bone 111
   biomechanics 112
   blood supply 111–12
   bowstringing effect 1293, 1312
   degeneration 120
   dry mass 111
   excessive loading 112
   function 111, 1292
   grafts, flexor tendons of hand 1295, 1296, 1298
   healing 113, 1294
      extrinsic/intrinsic 113
      factors affecting 114
   injuries 112–13
      MRI scan use 169
   loads 1292–3
   low metabolic rate 113
   mechanoreceptors 112
   microtrauma 113
   MRI scans 162
      normal appearance 161, 168
   nerve supply 112
   nutrition 1294
   pain perception 112
   repair
      flexor tendons 1295–7
      goal 1292
      replantation of upper limb 1319–20
      suturing 1295–6
   repetitive overload 112
   strength, age-related decrease 121
   structure 111
   tears 183
   transfer see specific tendons
   ultrasound assessment 159
   ultrastructure 111
   see also specific tendons
tendon cells, age-related changes 120
tendon sheath
   giant cell tumour 918
   inflammation see tenosynovitis
   structure 111
tendon-to-bone sutures, rotator cuff tear repair 1213
tenidap 1088
tennis elbow see lateral epicondylitis
tennis players
   lateral epicondylitis pathogenesis 1390
   lateral epicondylitis treatment 1394
tenosynovitis 1429
   de Quervain's see de Quervain's tenosynovitis
   flexor hallucis longus 1430
   flexor suppurative 1310, 1312–13
   posterior tibial tendon 835–6
   stenosing see trigger finger/thumb
   tendinitis vs, foot 28
tenotomy, Achilles, congenital clubfoot 690
tensile force 175
tensile stiffness 178
tensile strength, ultimate 182, 183
   metals used in implants 189
tension band plates, fracture fixation 272
teratocarcinoma 149
teres minor 1208, 1215
teriparatide 133
'terrible triad injury' 317, 1387
Terry Thomas sign 757, 1353, 1354, 1356
testosterone esters, use by athletes 707
test–retest reliability 39
tetanus prophylaxis 469
tetracycline, subchondral bone and 1079
THA see hip arthroplasty (total)
thanatophoric dysplasia, prevalence 542
thenar eminence hypoaesthesia 1386
thenar space, infections 1312

therapeutic cloning 143
thigh
   anatomy 73–5, 773
      blood supply 75
      neuromuscular 74–5
      osteology 73–4
   muscle anatomy 774
   muscle strains 774
   sports injuries 772–81
      see also sports injuries; specific injuries
   surgical approaches 75
thixotropy (shear thinning) 181
Thomas, Hugh Owen 4
Thomas' test 20
   modified 20
Thompson, Frederick Roeck 5
Thompson and Epstein classification, posterior hip dislocation 336
Thompson's approach, to radius (posterior) 63, 64
Thompson's test 31, 393, 1425
thoracic cord injury 443
   compression 32
thoracic outlet syndrome (TOS) 1399
   cubital tunnel syndrome vs 1399
   history-taking and symptoms 32
   tests for 33, 1399
thoracic spine
   anatomy 65
   examination 33–4
   injuries, children 500
   metastases 1065
   movements 33–4
   special tests 34
   see also thoracolumbar spine
thoracobrachial immobilization, humeral shaft fractures 308
Thoracolumbar Injury Classification and Severity Score (TLICS) 463
thoracolumbar junction, injuries/fractures at 459
thoracolumbar spine
   injury/fractures see thoracolumbar spine injuries
   kyphosis 1013
   orthoses 969, 1052
   three-column concept 460
   tuberculosis 990
   see also lumbar spine; thoracic spine
thoracolumbar spine injuries 459–64
   burst fractures 460, 461, 977
      load sharing classification 461
      stable 461
      unstable 461
   Chance fracture 460, 461–2
   children 499
   classification 460–3
      AO system 462–3
      Denis 460
      McAfee's 460–3
   compression fractures 460–1
   distraction–flexion 460, 461–2
   fractures 1556
      causes/mechanisms 459
      osteoporotic 1027
   gunshot 463
   minor 462–3
   radiographic evaluation 459–60
   severity, scores/system 463
   translational (fracture dislocations) 460, 462
   see also lumbar spine, injuries
Thoracolumbar Spine Severity Score (TLISS) 463
thoracolumbosacral orthosis (TLSO) 1012
thread shape factor 195
three rockers pattern, ankle 566, 567
three-dimensional gait analysis 563, 564
   cerebral palsy 601
three-point rule, casts/cast immobilization 260, 261
thrombin
   direct inhibitors 131
   indirect inhibitor (heparin) 131–2, 1126
thrombolysis 132
thrombolytics 132
   clinical use 132
thromboprophylaxis 132
   hip arthroplasty 1126–7
   intra-operative with postoperative, hip arthroplasty 1126

metastatic carcinoma 932
pelvic fracture management 433, 434
thrombospondin (TSP) 83, 548
thrombospondin-5 (TSP5) 548
thrombus (thrombi), anticoagulant uses 132
thumb
　anatomy 1335
　base, Rolando fracture 763
　in Dupuytren's contracture 1327, 1328
　flexor tendon, anatomy 1293
　fractures 1561
　gamekeeper's 763–4
　ligaments 1335
　mallet deformities 763, 1282
　osteoarthritis see trapeziometacarpal (TM) joint
　in scapholunate ligament injury 1356
　skier's 763–4
　splint, trapeziometacarpal joint osteoarthritis 1336
　trigger 1277–8
thumb carpometacarpal (CMC) joint arthritis test 14
thyroid cancer 926, 928, 935
thyroid hormones
　bone metabolism control 98
　deficiency, SCFE and 657
tibia
　amputations 957, 961–2, 967
　anatomical and mechanical axis 1261
　anatomy 75, 377
　posterior slope 1260
　anterior translation, Lachman test 807
　blood supply 377
　bone defects
　　classification 1201
　　in revision knee arthroplasty 1201–2
　congenital posteromedial bowing 674–5
　congenital pseudarthrosis (CPT) 675–7
　diaphysis, fractures 498
　　stress fractures 822
　　see also tibial shaft fractures
　distal, fractures
　　in children 482, 484
　　explosion fracture see tibial plafond fractures
　　intra-articular see tibial plafond fractures
　　malunion 527
　　metaphyseal 156, 498
　　transition 484
　　tri-plane 484
　　two-plane 484
　　see also tibial plafond fractures
　distal, reconstruction 948
　femoral articular conformity, meniscus and 104
　fractures 264
　　comminuted 279
　　compartment syndrome 279
　　condylar 373
　　distal see tibia, distal, fractures
　　infection non-union 223
　　ipsilateral, with femoral shaft fractures 356
　　leg shortening by 528
　　malunion 527
　　malunion, two-box/four-ring frame 528, 529
　　non-union, management 521, 523, 524, 525
　　plateau see tibial plateau fractures
　　proximal see tibia, proximal, fractures
　　shaft see tibial shaft fractures
　　stress see tibia, stress fractures
　　see also tibial plafond fractures
　intercondylar eminence, avulsions 497
　lengthening, after fractures 528
　medial malleolus see medial malleolus
　medial stress syndrome 824–5
　open injuries/fracture fixation 255, 256
　　flap for 257

periosteum, traction injury 824
posterior sag 25
post-traumatic osteomyelitis 223
proximal, fractures 380, 1566
　children 496, 497
　compression fractures 498
　metaphysis, children 498
　stress fracture 823
proximal, reconstruction 948
pseudarthrosis, congenital 675–7
reconstruction, in revision knee arthroplasty 1201–2
rotation assessment, children 537–8
shortening 18, 19
stress fractures 380, 821–4
　aetiology 821–2
　children 498
　evaluation 822
　imaging 822–3
　pathology 822
　physical examination 822
　site 822
　treatment 823
subchondral bone, osteoarthritis 1081
torsional and bowing deformities 673–5
transection, for amputation 961
'true' shortening 18, 19
tuberosity, fractures 497
tibia vara (Blount disease) 670–1
tibial arteries, anterior/posterior 77
tibial articular surface (component), knee prosthesis 1177
tibial collateral ligament (TCL), injuries 373
tibial component (knee replacement) 1177
　computer-assisted navigation 1519–20
　fixed bearing design 1179
　mobile bearing design 1179
　removal in revision surgery 1201
　rotating platform 1179
　stem extensions 1202
　stems 1180
tibial condylar fractures 373
tibial cut, computer-assisted navigation 1519
tibial eminence fractures 375–6
tibial nerve 74, 76, 79, 1500
　compression neuropathy see tarsal tunnel syndrome
　intramedullary nailing of fracture 1307
　neuropathic pain 1305
tibial plafond, anatomy 1243
tibial plafond fractures 382–5, 1567
　classification 383, 384
　clinical evaluation 382
　complications 385
　displaced 383
　malunion 527
　mechanism of injury 382
　radiography 382–3
　treatment 383–5
　　external fixation 384
　　non-operative 383
　see also tibia, distal, fractures
tibial plateau, lateral, avulsion fracture 366
tibial plateau fractures 372–6, 814
　bicondylar 372
　classification 373, 374
　clinical evaluation 372–3
　complications 375
　high-energy 372, 373
　mechanism of injury 372, 373
　neurovascular injuries 372
　radiography 373
　treatment 373–5
　　guidelines 374–5
　　non-surgical 373
　　peri-articular, 'raft' 375
　　surgical 373–5
tibial sesamoid 1442
　anatomy 1442, 1443
　bipartite 1445
　fracture 1444
　in hallux valgus 1434
　multipartite 1445
　sesamoiditis 1446
　see also sesamoid bones (foot)
tibial sesamoidectomy 1447

tibial shaft fractures 377–81, 498
　children 482, 498
　classification 378
　closed treatment 264–6, 485
　compartment syndrome see compartment syndrome, acute
　complications 380
　diaphyseal, plating of 380
　evaluation 378
　fixation 270
　mechanism of injury 377
　pathological, treatment 934
　prevalence 377
　radiography 378
　special situations 380
　stress fractures 380, 822
　treatment 378–80
　　external fixation 380
　　non-operative 378–9, 380
　　operative 379–80
　treatment, 'closed' intramedullary nailing 1307
tibial shaving 1447
tibial spine fractures 375–6, 1566
　avulsion fracture 808
tibial torsion 673–4
　assessment 30, 674
tibial tuberosity, avulsions 497
tibialis anterior (TA) 29
　action and function 956
　anatomy 1429–30
　palpation 28
　weakness, gait 957
tibialis anterior tendon transfer (TATT)
　cerebral palsy management 605
　congenital clubfoot 690
tibialis posterior 30, 1421
　split tendon transfer/lengthening 604–5
　see also posterior tibial tendon
tibiocalcaneal fusion 528, 529
　method 1270
tibiofemoral joint
　alignment, paediatric patients 536
　forces acting on 187
　kinematics 187
　transverse plane knee stability 210–11
tibiofemoral load transmission, meniscus role 104
tibiofibular articulation 1243
tibiofibular clear space 387
tibiofibular overlap 387
tibiofibular syndesmotic ligamentous injuries 391–3
tibiotalar articulation 1243
　angulation 1243
　valgus angulation 1422
tibiotalocalcaneal arthrodesis, ankle osteoarthritis 1488
tidemark zone 102
　cartilage injuries 103
Tile classification, pelvic fractures 427–8
Tillaux fracture 484, 498
Tillaux-Chaput fracture 388
tiludronic acid 132
Tinel's sign 30, 1305, 1306
　axon rupture 1305
　cubital tunnel syndrome 1398
　handlebar palsy 760
　medial epicondylitis 751
　static 1305
　ulnar neuropathy 1392–3
Tinel's test 12
　carpal tunnel syndrome 15
　tarsal tunnel syndrome 28
tinzaparin 131, 132
tissue engineering 1524–9
　basic principles 1525
　bioreactors 1527
　cells 1526–7
　clinical applications in skeletal reconstruction 1527–9
　　autologous chondrocyte implantation 1528–9
　　endocultivation 1527–8, 1529
　in silico 1527
　in vitro 1525, 1527
　in vivo 1525, 1527
　scaffold materials and shapes 1525–6
　signals 1527
tissue inhibitors of metalloproteinases (TIMPs) 102, 1088, 1426

tissue pressure, compartment syndrome see intracompartmental pressure (ICP)
tissues, biomechanics 188
titanium alloy 188
　hip implants 1121, 1139
titanium grommets 193, 194
titanium implants, pyogenic spinal infections and 985
TKA see knee arthroplasty, total
tocilizumab therapy, juvenile idiopathic arthritis 595
'toddler's fracture' 498
toeing-in 419
toeing-out 419
toes
　amputations 960–1
　claw see claw toe
　curly 1457–8
　hammer see hammer toe
　lateral deviation 1434
　length, foot type 27
　lesser, deformities/conditions see lesser toes
　mallet 1454
　mucous cysts 1458
　pain 1436
　see also hallux; hallux valgus; lesser toes
Tokuhashi score 1061
　spinal metastases 1061, 1066
Tom Smith arthritis 578
　see also septic arthritis
Tomita classification, spinal metastases 1060–1, 1066
tomogram, history 155–6
'too many toes' sign 27, 1422, 1463
Toronto Extremity Salvage Score 941
torque 176–7, 180
　peak 213
torsion 673
　tibial see tibial torsion
total ankle replacement (TAR) see ankle arthroplasty (total)
total hip replacement see hip arthroplasty (total)
total joint replacement see joint replacement
total knee replacement see knee arthroplasty, total (TKA)
total lean body mass, age-related decline 121
total plexus palsy 616, 617
total shoulder replacement see shoulder arthroplasty (total)
total-elastic suspension (TES) belt 966, 967
totipotent stem cells 1526
tourniquets 713
　complications 718
　hip arthroplasty 1126
　neurapraxia due to 1304
toxic shock syndrome 220
　antibiotic treatment 220
trabeculae
　formation 89
　immature 89
　primary 89
　secondary 89
trabecular bone 885
　MRI appearance 161, 167
trabecular number (Tb.N) 1026
trabecular spacing (Tb.Sp) 1026
trabecular thickness (Tb.Th) 1026
trackers, in CAOS 1513–14, 1515
traction
　cervical spine injury 445
　continuous, complications 259
　forearm fracture reduction 263
　halo, atlas fractures 448
　method 259
　paediatric fractures 486
　pre-operative, pelvic fractures 433
　reduction of fractures 259
　shoulder dislocation reduction 299
　skeletal, force 259
　skin, force 259
tramadol 127
tranexamic acid, in trauma 237
transcription 140
transcription factor defects 545
transdermal medications, morphine 127
transfemoral amputation 962
　prosthetic problem 967

transfemoral sockets (prostheses) 966–7
transfemoral suspension (prostheses) 966
transforaminal lumbar interbody fusion (TLIF)
  degenerative disc disease 1003, 1004
  degenerative spondylolisthesis 1056
  isthmic spondylolisthesis 1052, 1053
transformation (using plasmids) 142
transforming growth factor β (TGF-β) 928, 1025
  Dupuytren's contracture pathogenesis 1325
  osteoarthritis pathophysiology 1081, 1084
  rheumatoid arthritis pathophysiology 1086
transgenic animals 142
transhumeral amputation 963
transient synovitis 660–1
  differential diagnosis 653, 660, 662
translation 140
translational motion
  dynamic parameters 176
  kinematic parameters 175
translational stability, joints (knee) 211, 212
transmetatarsal amputation 961
transmural pressure (TM), vessels, compartment syndrome 506
transpedicular cortical decancellation procedure 1019
transpedicular injection, bone substitute 1032, 1035, 1036
transpedicular screws
  diameter 1042
  loosening 1041
  osteoporosis 1026, 1041–3
  perforated 1042
  technique for use 1042
  see also pedicle screws
transpedicular wedge resection procedure 1019
transphyseal screws, leg length discrepancy 681
transplantation see allograft/allograft transplantation
transradial amputation 963
trans-scaphoid perilunate dislocation 1361
transtibial amputation 957, 961–2, 967
  prosthetic problem 967
transtibial sockets (prostheses) 967
transverse acetabular ligament 772
transverse carpal ligament (TCL), zone IV injuries 1280
transverse ligament, atlantoaxial joint 449
transverse metatarsal ligament 78
transverse septa 89
trapeziectomy 1339
trapeziometacarpal (TM) joint
  anatomy and stability 1334, 1335
  arthrodesis 1340
  arthroplasty 1337, 1339, 1340
  movement and function 1334
  osteoarthritis 1333, 1334–41
    arthroscopy 1337
    differential diagnosis 1335–6
    history and examination 1335
    interpositional arthroplasty 1337, 1339, 1340
    investigations/imaging 1335, 1336
    ligament reconstruction, tendon interposition 1337, 1339
    non-operative treatment 1336–7
    operative treatment 1337–8
    pan-arthritis 1335
    pathophysiology 1334–5
    stages 1334–5, 1337
trapezium
  fractures 1561
  ligaments attaching 1334
  resection 1337, 1338
trauma team 234, 235
trauma/injury
  advanced life support 233–43
    see also Advanced Trauma Life Support (ATLS)
  amputations see amputations, traumatic
  asymptomatic, cleared spine 444
  clearing spine 444

energy transmitted by injury mechanism 248
'golden hour', death reduction 234, 440
as leading cause of death 233
management 234
  definition of patient's condition 237–8
  initial, goal 235
  initial assessment (trauma room) 234, 235
  operating room, strategy 239–41
  pelvic injuries 239
  pre-hospital care 234–5, 440
  primary survey 235–7, 239, 248, 444–5
  secondary survey 238, 239
  spinal injuries 238–9, 440, 442–3, 444–5
  see also Advanced Trauma Life Support (ATLS)
mass casualty management 244–6
mortality 233–4
  reduction 234
  timing/distribution 232–4
open, of limbs see fracture(s), open; open injuries
osteoporotic fracture treatment 1039
paediatric 481–2
patient's condition after see patient categories (condition)
preceding, in history 9
specific orthopaedic situations 238–9
trimodal distribution of deaths (timing) 233–4
work-related see work-related injuries
see also polytrauma; specific injuries
traumatic brain injury (TBI) 1478–9
  children 499, 500
Traynelis classification, occipitocervical dislocation 447
treatment, refusal of 1540
'trefoil' shape, lumbar spinal stenosis 999
Trendelenburg gait 31, 567
  developmental coxa vara 651
  developmental dysplasia of hip 646
  fee-body analysis of hip 1107
  Perthes disease 653
Trendelenburg test 18, 31
trephinization, subungual haematoma 1289
Treponema pallidum 224, 226
triage system
  errors, mass casualty 245
  mass casualty management 245
triamcinolone 129
triangular fibrocartilage (TFC) 1365
triangular fibrocartilage complex (TFCC)
  anatomy 61, 327, 758, 1351–2, 1365–6
  arthrography 1367–8
  blood supply 1366
  in chronic DRUJ injury treatment 1369–70
  complications in distal radius fractures 330
  injuries 1366
    classification 758–9
    diagnosis 1366–8
    treatment 1366
  instability, classification 1366
  sports injuries 758–60
    causes/mechanisms 758
    clinical features 759
    repair of tears 759–60
    testing 14, 759
triangular interval 57, 58
triangular space 57, 58
triangulation, arthroscopy 713
triceps muscle 57
  nerve supply 1304
trigeminal nerve 469
trigger finger/thumb 1277–8
  mechanism of injury 1277
  treatment 1277–8
trigger points, myofascial 979
triglycerides 706
trigonal process 839
trimalleolar fractures 391
trinucleotide repeat disorder 151

tri-plane fracture 484
triple arthrodesis
  hindfoot osteoarthritis 1489
  hindfoot rheumatoid arthritis 1495
'tripod' fracture (zygoma fracture) 469, 475
triquetral bone, in four-corner fusions 1359
triquetral capitate (TqC) ligament 1352–3
triscaphoid fusion 1358
trisomy 152
trisomy 21 (Down syndrome) 152
trochanteric bursitis 775
tropocollagen fibrils 101, 111
tropomyosin 701
troponin(s) 109, 701
'trough' sign 300
true strain 178
true stress 178
trunk, centre of gravity 954–5
trust-building, with paediatric patients 535–6
TSP (thrombospondin) 83, 548
TSP5 (thrombospondin-5) 548
t-tests 44
T-tubules 108
tuberculosis
  antitubercular chemotherapy 225, 989
  arthritis 226
  bone/joint 224–5
    diagnosis and imaging 225
    natural history 225
    treatment 225
  cold abscess 225, 987, 988, 990
  osteomyelitis 224–5, 586–7
  paraplegia, stages 988
  spinal 987–91
    abscess 225, 987, 988, 990
    children 990, 991
    clinical features 987
    deformity prevention 990
    differential diagnosis 987–8
    'middle path regimen' 989
    neurological complications 987, 988
    prognosis 990
    surgical treatment 989–90
    treatment 989–90
    workup 988–9
tuberculum intercondylare mediale 375
TUBS shoulder instability 300
tumour antigens, cytotoxic T cell recognition 1068
tumour cells
  haematogenous spread 927
  metastases development, biology 927
tumour necrosis factor α (TNF-α) 1085–6
  inhibition/inhibitors 1088
    juvenile idiopathic arthritis therapy 594–5
    rheumatoid arthritis therapy 1088
  osteoarthritis pathophysiology 1081
  receptor 1088
  synovial joints, inflammation 1078
tumour necrosis factor β (TNF-β) 1088
tumour suppressor genes 149
tumour vaccine 1069
tumours (musculoskeletal)
  aetiology 149
  amputations for 959
  benign 865, 870
    radiotherapy principles 878
  biopsy 870, 886–7, 915, 941
  clinical evaluation 865–6
  clinical features, pain 866
  diagnosis, 'red flags' 866
  hand see hand, tumours
  history-taking 865–6
  imaging 866–70
    CT scans 868
    MRI 868–9
    PET 869–70
    radiography see below
    scintigraphy see radionuclide imaging
  immuno-oncology 1068–9
  immunotherapy 1068–9
  laboratory studies 866
  limb reconstruction see limb reconstruction
  malignant, spread 927

malignant transformation, bone scan signs 867–8
management, multidisciplinary team for 874, 941
missed diagnoses 865
multiple, genetic conditions predisposing 930
physical examination 866
radiographic features 866–7, 886
  bone destruction patterns 867
radiology 885–7
reactive zone around 940, 942
resection, gadolinium contrast MRI after 164
spinal see spinal tumours
staging 870–1
  AJCC system 871, 915
  Enneking 870
  by MRI 868
  soft-tissue sarcoma 914–15
treatment
  chemotherapy see chemotherapy
  radiotherapy see radiotherapy
see also specific tumours
turf-toe injuries 1443–5
  natural history 1444
  non-operative management 1444–5
  radiography 1444
twisting, mechanics 180
2 X 2 table 38, 42
two-plane fracture 484

UKA see knee arthroplasty, unicompartmental
ulcers, diabetic foot 1467, 1468, 1469
ulna 262
  anatomy 61, 318, 322
  coronoid process, fractures 1559
  exposure/surgical approach 63–4
  fractures 262, 1559
    non-operative treatment 262–3
  medial epicondyle
    groove of 1384
    surgery for medial epicondylitis 1396
  medial epicondylectomy, cubital tunnel syndrome 1406–7
  proximal, fractures, children 490
  shaft, fractures 262, 322–6, 323–4
    clinical evaluation 322
    complications 323
    radiography 322–3
    with radius shaft fractures 322–3
    treatment 323
ulna impingement test 14
ulnar artery
  anatomy 62, 505
  subluxation/dislocation, elbow flexion 1400
ulnar bursa
  infections 1312
  location 1312
ulnar collateral ligament (UCL) 764
  disruption/rupture 751–3
    mechanism of injury 751
    skier's thumb 763
    sporting injury 751–3
    surgical treatment 752–3
  instability 1393
  lateral see lateral ulnar collateral ligament (LUCL)
  in medial epicondylitis 751, 1393
  open surgical technique 1396
  partial injuries 752
  thumb, chronic laxity 763
ulnar nerve
  anatomy 58, 62, 1407
    at elbow 1384, 1397–8
  anterior transposition 1407–8
    intramuscular 1407–8
    subcutaneous 1407
    submuscular 1408, 1409
  blood supply 1407
  compression
    at elbow 12, 1384, 1392–3, 1397
    at elbow, grading 1404
    at elbow, staging 1400–2
    handlebar palsy 760
    see also cubital tunnel syndrome
  conduction velocities 1400
  decompression
    endoscopic release 1408
    in situ 1405–6, 1407
    medial epicondylectomy 1406–7

entrapment, elbow 1384
examination at elbow 12
injury, medial epicondylitis 1391
intraneural/extraneural pressure, elbow flexion 1398
neuritis, medial epicondylitis vs 1392
palsy 489
testing, hand 16
ulnar neuropathy 1392–3
  medial epicondylitis vs 1392
ulnar paradox 16
ulnar styloid, fracture 1369
ulnohumeral joint 316
  forces 1388
  see also elbow
ultimate tensile strength 182, 183
  metals used in implants 189
ultra-high-molecular-weight polyethylene (UHMWPE) 189, 1116, 1117
  disc replacement devices 197
  hip implants 190, 1119
    history 1099
  knee implants 191, 1177
  wear debris 194
ultrasound 159–60
  Achilles tendonopathy 832
  in CAOS 1512
  clinical uses 159–60
  compartment syndrome 510
  cubital tunnel syndrome 1400
  developmental disorders of bone 551, 554
  developmental dysplasia of hip 643–5, 646
    reliability 644–5
    technique 644
  high-intensity, fracture healing 521
  lateral epicondylitis therapy 1395
  rotator cuff tears 1210
  septic arthritis 580
  soft-tissue sarcoma 913
  strengths/weaknesses 159
  transient synovitis 660
unconscious patients
  cervical spinal cord injury 724
  head injury, management 467
underdamping 185
'under-powered' study 42
understanding, autonomous patient 1532
unicameral bone cyst 887–8
unicompartmental knee arthroplasty see knee arthroplasty, unicompartmental (unicondylar) (UKA)
uniparental disomy 152
unipotent stem cells 1526
units, size, prefixes 175
unstable patients, after trauma 238, 241
unstable slipped capital femoral epiphysis 657, 658–9
upper limb
  after acquired brain injury, management 969–70
  amputation levels 961, 963
  clinical examination see clinical examination
  congenital deficiency 958–9
  deep tendon reflexes 9
  disorders
    cerebral palsy 607
    see also specific disorders
  examination, cerebral palsy 601
  fractures 1556–62
    non-union, fixation 521
  limb salvage 964
  myotomes 9
  nerve injuries 1302–8
  prosthetics 963–4
  reconstruction see limb reconstruction
  traumatic amputations 1315
    early management 1316
    replantation see replantation (upper limb)
  see also arm
Urbaniak classification 1322
urethral disruption, pelvic fractures with 427
urethrogram, retrograde 430
uric acid, gout 1091

uricosuric agents 1091
urinary tract infections, hip arthroplasty 1125
urine, output, hypovolaemic shock assessment 236
U-slab 264
uveitis, juvenile idiopathic arthritis 589, 590, 591, 593, 594

'vacant glenoid' sign 300
vacuum sign 1001
valgus alignment, paediatric patients 536
valgus bracing, knee osteoarthritis 210
valgus deformity
  ankle 610, 1464
  knee see knee
  MTP joints 1434–5
valgus extension overload syndrome 753
  elbow 751
  mechanism of injury 753
  treatment 753
valgus stress test
  medial collateral ligament (elbow) 1387
  ulnar collateral ligament rupture 752
valgus testing, elbow 13
validity 39
Valleix phenomenon 1503
vancomycin, hip arthroplasty 1126
Vancouver classification, periprosthetic fractures 1155–6
variables 39–40
  independent and dependent 39–40
variance 42
varus derotational osteotomy, femoral see femoral varus derotational osteotomy
varus testing, elbow 13
vascular bone replacements, endocultivation 1527–8, 1529
vascular endothelial growth factor (VEGF) 89, 91
vascular spasm 504, 505
vascular tumours 883, 916, 919
vascularized fibular grafts 945
  children 950
  complications 945–6
  congenital pseudarthrosis of tibia 676
  surgical technique 945
vasculopathy, diabetic foot 1466
  examination 1468, 1469
vastus medialis obliquus (VMO), bulk, assessment 26
vectors
  gene therapy 144, 145, 1069
  plasmid 142
vectors (mechanical) 173–4
  definition 173
vegetarians, nutrition for 706, 707–8
velocity 174, 204
  angular see angular velocity
  average 174, 204
  linear 204, 205
Velpeau dressing, humeral shaft fractures 308
venous cutdown, primary survey after trauma 236
venous insufficiency, replantation (upper limb) complication 1321
venous pressure, in acute compartment syndrome 505
venous thromboembolism
  prophylaxis 132
  treatment 132
  see also deep vein thrombosis (DVT); thromboprophylaxis
ventral corticospinal tract 67
ventral spinothalamic tract 67
Verdan's zones of hand 1278, 1294
versican 83
vertebrae
  anatomy 64–6, 975
  blood supply, metastases and 1065
  collapse, spinal tumours 1059
  congenital anomalies see congenital vertebral anomalies
  displacement, low back pain 977
  fractures see osteoporosis, spinal; vertebral body, compression fractures

growth, spondylolisthesis development 1050
injury evaluation in emergency department 442–3
levels, osteoporosis 1026
lumbar 64
metastases see spinal metastases
number 64
range of motion and 187–8
shifting see spondylolisthesis
structure 65
see also spine
vertebral artery 68, 450
vertebral augmentation, radiofrequency-targeted 1038
vertebral body
  aneurysmal phenomenon 988
  compression fractures 460–1
    traumatic 1019
  compression fractures, osteoporotic 1016
    incidence 1024
    pain 1016
  fractures, low back pain 977
  intervertebral disc between 105
  lumbar 975
  pyogenic spinal infections 983
  spinal metastases 1065
vertebral canal, in pyogenic infections 983
vertebral end plates
  disc degeneration effect 999
  superior, in osteoporosis 1026
vertebral infections see spinal infections
vertebral isthmus
  fatigue/microfractures 1051
  reconstruction 1052–3
    circumferential 1054
  see also isthmic lysis
vertebroplasty 1017–18
  analgesic action 1018
  calcium phosphate cement, resorbable 1041
  cement 1036
  cement leakage 1036, 1038
  complications 1018, 1036, 1038
  contraindications 1034
  indications 1034, 1036
  osteonecrosis of spine 1031, 1033, 1039
  osteoporotic kyphosis 1017–18, 1035
  osteoporotic vertebral fractures 1032, 1033, 1035
  results 1038
  spinal metastases and tumour ablation 1067
  transpedicular 1032, 1036
  triple level 1038
  unipedicular 1034
vertical expanding prosthetic titanium rib (VEPTR) 631, 632
vertical talus, congenital see congenital vertical talus
vesicles 700
vibration, degenerative disc disease 994
viruses
  gene therapy vector 144, 145, 1069
  hand infections 1313
  oncogenic 1069
viscoelasticity 179, 181–2
  materials 181–2
  natural tissues 188
viscosity 180
  fluids 180
Vitallium cups 1098
vitamin(s), deficiencies, vegetarian diets and 707–8
vitamin B6 1027
vitamin B12 1027
vitamin D
  bone metabolism control 98
  deficiency 94
  metabolism 99
vitamin D derivatives, as anti-osteoporotic drug 133
vitamin K
  antagonists, in hip arthroplasty 1126–7
  warfarin inhibition of carboxylation 131
vitronectin 83
volar intercalated segment instability (VISI) 1354, 1355, 1359, 1360

Volkmann, Richard von 503–4
Volkmann ischaemic contracture 279, 503
  aetiopathogenesis 504, 505
  anatomic considerations 505–6
  history 503–4
  muscles involved 505
  supracondylar fracture of humerus in children 489
  testing for 17
  treatment 504
  see also compartment syndrome, acute
Volkmann's canals 85
Volkmann's vessels 85
von Mises strain 183
von Mises stress 198
V-Y advancement flap 1289

Wackenheim line 446
Waddell's five signs of inorganic behaviour 35
walking see gait
walking aids 957
walking stick, hip abductor activity 1108
Wallerian degeneration 1304
warfarin 130
  dextropropoxyphene interaction 127
  dosage 131
  mechanism of action 131
  pre-operative considerations 131
  side-effects 131
warm ischaemia time 1317
Wartenberg sign 760, 1399
Wartenberg's neuritis 16
Wartenberg's sign 16
Wartenberg's test 14
water intake (athletes) 706
  child athletes 708
Watson, Kirk 14, 15
Watson-Jones, Sir Reginald 5
Watson-Jones anterolateral approach 72, 73, 947
  femoral neck fracture reduction 342
  hip arthroplasty 1136, 1137
Watson-Jones classification
  extensor digitorum avulsion 1562
  tibial tuberosity fractures 497
Watson's manoeuvre 757
Watson's test (scaphoid shift test) 1356
wear, joint replacement/implants 194, 1114–15
  adhesive 1114
  definition 184, 1114
  fatigue 1114
  hip prostheses see hip arthroplasty (total)
  interfacial 1114
  mechanical testing 198–9
  mode 1 1114, 1117
  mode 2 1114
  mode 3 1114, 1116, 1119
  mode 4 1114–15
web space
  contracture 1328
  infections 1311–12
Weber–Cech non-union classification 516–17
weight, of objects 176
weight bearing, fracture non-union and 521
weight loss, female athletes 708
weights and springs, muscle strength testing 212, 213
Weinstein–Boriani–Biagini classification, spinal tumours 1060
Wells, Horace 4
wet gangrene, diabetic foot 1467, 1468
wheelchairs 971
white blood cell (WBC) count
  acute haematogenous osteomyelitis 584
  septic arthritis in children 579–80
Whitesides straight needle manometer method 509, 511
whitlow, herpetic 1313
Wiberg, angle of 419
Wilcoxon rank-sum test 44
Wilcoxon signed rank 44
Wiles, Philip 1098, 1118

Wiltse classification, spondylolisthesis 1048
Windlass mechanism 28
wink sign, atlantoaxial rotary subluxation 449
Winquist and Hansen classification, femoral shaft fractures 354, 1566
Wnt proteins 545
Wolff's law 88
WOMAC Osteoarthritis Index 18
women athletes
    ACL injury and reconstruction 810
    nutrition for 708
    tibial stress fractures 822
work (mechanical) 176, 178
workers' compensation 1542
    assessment of permanent disability 1543
    third-party involvement 1543
work-related injuries 1542–4
    assessment of permanent disability 1543
    return to work issues 1543
    specifics 1543–4
World Health Organization (WHO)
    bone tumour classification 883, 887
    osteoporosis definition 1016
    soft-tissue tumour classification 913–14, 916
wormian bones, multiple 553
wound(s)
    amputations 958
    healing problems, in total ankle replacement 1245
    infections 219
        open injuries of limbs 253
        pelvic fractures 435
        surgical *see* surgical wound infections
    infiltration with narcotics, hip arthroplasty 1124
    lavage 254

    management
        debridement in diabetic foot 1469–70
        debridement in open injuries 253–5
        diabetic foot 1469
        open injuries of limbs 248
    primary closure
        delayed, open injuries 256
        open injuries and 256
wrist
    anatomy 64, 1351–2
        bony components 1351
        ligaments 1351–2
    arthrodesis 1268, 1272, 1358
    arthrography 1354, 1356, 1367–8
    arthroscopy *see* arthroscopy
    biomechanics 187
    C line from scaphoid to radius 1356
    clinical examination 13–15
        inspection and palpation 13
        movement 13–14
        special tests 14–15
    dinner fork-type deformity 261
    disarticulation 963
    dorsal, ganglions 762, 1374
    dorsal syndromes 761–2
    dorsiflexion (extension) 13
    extensor tendon injuries 1283
    flexion (palmar) 13, 14
    flexor tendon injuries 1280
    foreign body, ultrasound for 160
    four-corner fusions 1359
    fractures around 1560
        see also Colles fracture; radius, distal; scaphoid fractures
    ganglion 1374
    gymnast's 761–2
    hyperextension 1355
    injuries 1355, 1360
        dorsal perilunate dislocation 1360–1

        radiography 1353–4
        see also scapholunate ligament (SLL), injury
    instability 1351–64
        see also carpal instability; carpal ligaments, injuries
    joint replacement 192–4
        biaxial implant 194
        implant materials 189
    kinematics 1352
    loads, transmission 1352
    loose bodies 1335
    normal movements 13, 1352
    occult dorsal ganglion cysts 762
    orthoses 969
    pain 1356, 1379
        differential diagnosis 15
        gymnast's wrist 761
    pathomechanics 1352–3
    range of motion 187
    reconstruction 950
    scapholunate advanced collapse (SLAC) 1358–9
    sports injuries *see* sports injuries; *specific injuries*
    sprain 1367
    stability 1352
    stabilizers 1351–2
    swelling 1356
    tendinitis 760, 761
        see also de Quervain's tenosynovitis
    ulnar deviation 1356, 1360
    V pattern of scaphoid and radius 1356
    see also carpal bones

X chromosome, inactivation 151
xenografting 148
X-linked dominant disorder 152
X-linked dominant inheritance 151
X-linked recessive chondrodysplasia punctata (CDPX1) 549

X-linked recessive disorders 152
X-linked recessive inheritance 151
X-rays 155, 156
    see also radiography

Y ligament of Bigelow 69, 70
Yergason's test 11, 739
yield point 182
Young and Burgess classification, pelvic fractures 428, 1563
Young's modulus (E) 179, 180
    metals used in implants 188, 189
    for natural tissues 188, 197
    plates for fracture fixation and 195

Z line 108
Zasloff test 10
Zdrakovich and Damholt classification 1557
Ziehl–Neelsen staining 225
zirconia implants 189
    femoral head 1119
    oxidized 1118
z-lengthening, subscapularis muscle 1227, 1230
Z-line 699
zoledronic acid 132
zone of degeneration 91
zone of provisional calcification 93
zone of resorption 91
z-plasty, fasciectomy in Dupuytren's contracture 1329
zygapophyseal joints *see* facet (apophyseal) joints
zygoma 474
    anatomy 474, 475
    fracture 469, 470, 474–5
        clinical signs 475
        CT scans 475
        treatment 477–8
zygomatic arch 475
zygomatic process 475